220.00
W9-CEH-532

Fundamental Immunology

Fundamental Immunology

Sixth Edition

EDITOR

WILLIAM E. PAUL, MD

Wolters Kluwer | Lippincott Williams & Wilkins
Health
Philadelphia • Baltimore • New York • London
Buenos Aires • Hong Kong • Sydney • Tokyo

Acquisitions Editor: Frances DeStefano
Managing Editor: Julia Seto
Project Manager: Alicia Jackson
Senior Manufacturing Manager: Benjamin Rivera
Marketing Manager: Kimberly Schonberger
Designer: Risa Clow
Cover Designer: Melissa Walter
Production Service: Aptara, Inc.

530 Walnut Street
Philadelphia, PA 19106 USA
LWW.com

Printed in the USA

Library of Congress Cataloging-in-Publication Data

Fundamental immunology / [edited by] William E. Paul. —6th ed.
p. ; cm.
Includes bibliographical references and index.
ISBN–13: 978-0-7817-6519-0 (alk. paper)
ISBN–10: 0-7817-6519-6 (alk. paper)
1. Immunology. I. Paul, William E.
[DNLM: 1. Immunity. QW 540 F981 2008]
QR181.F84 2008
616.07′9—dc22

2008011406

To purchase additional copies of this book, call our customer service department at (800) 638-3030 or fax orders to (301) 223-2320. International customers should call (301) 223-2300.

Visit Lippincott Williams & Wilkins on the Internet: at LWW.com. Lippincott Williams & Wilkins customer service representatives are available from 8:30 am to 6 pm, EST.

10 9 8 7 6 5 4 3 2 1

For Julien Stehlik Paul Mezey
In Loving Memory

Nature's first green is gold,
Her hardest hue to hold.
Her early leaf's a flower;
But only so an hour.
Then leaf subsides to leaf.
So Eden sank to grief,
So dawn goes down to day.
Nothing gold can stay.

Robert Frost, 1923

CONTRIBUTORS

Eitan M. Akirav, PhD
Postdoctoral Associate
Immunobiology Section
Department of Human Translational Immunology
Yale University School of Medicine
New Haven, Connecticut

Albert Bendelac, MD, PhD
Professor
Department of Pathology
University of Chicago
Howard Hughes Medical Institute
Chicago, Illinois

Ira J. Berkower, MD, PhD
Chief, Lab of Immunoregulation
Division of Viral Products
Office of Vaccines
Center for Biologies, FDA
Bethesda, Maryland

Jay A. Berzofsky, MD, PhD
Chief, Vaccine Branch
Center for Cancer Research
National Cancer Institute
Bethesda, Maryland

Nicolas Bidère, PhD
Postdoctoral Fellow
Laboratory of Immunology
National Institute of Allergy and Infectious Diseases
National Institutes of Health
Bethesda, Maryland

R. Chris Bleackley, PhD
Professor
Department of Biochemistry
University of Alberta
Edmonton, Alberta, Canada

Rebecca H. Buckley, MD
J. Buren Sidbury Professor of Pediatrics and Professor of Immunology
Departments of Pediatrics and Immunology
Duke University School of Medicine
Durham, North Carolina

Yueh-Hsiu Chien, PhD
Professor
Departments of Microbiology and Immunology
Stanford University School of Medicine
Stanford, California

Shane Crotty, PhD
Assistant Professor
Division of Vaccine Discovery
La Jolla Institute for Allergy and Immunology
La Jolla, California

Mark M. Davis, PhD
Professor
Departments of Microbiology and Immunology
Stanford University School of Medicine
Stanford, California

Anthony L. DeFranco, PhD
Professor and Chair
Microbiology and Immunology
University of California, San Francisco
San Francisco, California

Lélia Delamarre, PhD
Department of Cell Biology
Yale School of Medicine
New Haven, Connecticut

Betty Diamond, MD
Investigator/Head
Center for Autoimmune and Musculoskeletal Disease
The Feinstein Institute for Medical Research
Manhasset, New York

Manfred P. Dierich, MD
Professor
Department of Hygiene, Microbiology and Social Medicine
Innsbruck Medical University
Innsbruck, Austria

Charles A. Dinarello, MD
Professor of Medicine
University of Colorado Health Sciences Center
Denver, Colorado

Louis Du Pasquier, PhD
Professor
Institute of Zoology and Evolutionary Biology
University of Basel
Basel, Switzerland

Suzanne L. Epstein, PhD
Associate Director for Research
Office of Cellular, Tissue and Gene Therapies
Center for Biologics Evaluation and Research
Food and Drug Administration
Rockville, Maryland

Hildegund Ertl, MD
Professor and Immunology Program Leader
The Wistar Institute
Philadelphia, Pennsylvania

Martin F. Flajnik, PhD
Professor
Departments of Microbiology and Immunology
University of Maryland at Baltimore
Baltimore, Maryland

Siamon Gordon, MD
Glaxo Wellcome Professor of Cellular Pathology
Sir William Dunn School of Pathology
University of Oxford
Oxford, United Kingdom

Neil S. Greenspan, MD, PhD
Professor
Department of Pathology
Case Western Reserve University
Director, Histocompatibility and Immunogenetics Laboratory
Department of Pathology
University Hospitals Case Medical Center
Cleveland, Ohio

Richard R. Hardy, PhD
Senior Member
Division of Basic Science
Fox Chase Cancer Center
Philadelphia, Pennsylvania

Dirk Homann, MD
Assistant Professor
Departments of Pediatrics, Immunology and Microbiology
University of Colorado Health Sciences Center, Fitzsimmons
Aurora, Colorado

Hiroshi Kiyono, DDs, PhD
Professor
Division of Mucosal Immunology
The University of Tokyo Institute of Medical Science
Tokyo, Japan

Gary A. Koretzky, MD, PhD
Leonard Jarett Professor of Pathology and Laboratory Medicine
Vice Chair for Research and Chief Scientific Officer
Investigator & Director, Signal Transduction Program, Abramson Family Cancer Research Institute
Department of Medicine
University of Pennsylvania School of Medicine
Philadelphia, Pennsylvania

Jun Kunisawa, PhD
Division of Mucosal Immunology
The University of Tokyo Institute of Medical Science
Tokyo, Japan

Michael J. Lenardo, MD
Chief, Molecular Development Section
Laboratory of Immunology
National Institute of Allergy and Infectious Diseases
National Institutes of Health
Bethesda, Maryland

Warren J. Leonard, MD
Chief, Laboratory of Molecular Immunology
Director, Immunology Center
National Heart, Lung, and Blood Institute
National Institutes of Health
Bethesda, Maryland

Norman L. Letvin, MD
Professor
Department of Medicine
Harvard Medical School
Chief, Division of Viral Pathogenesis
Department of Medicine
Beth Israel Deaconess
Boston, Massachusetts

Shan Liao, PhD
Postdoctoral Fellow
Department of Radiation Oncology
Massachusetts General Hospital
Boston, Massachusetts

David H. Margulies, MD, PhD
Chief, Molecular Biology Section
Laboratory of Immunology
National Institute of Allergy and Infectious Diseases/National Institutes of Health
Bethesda, Maryland

Jeanette I. Webster Marketon, PhD
Assistant Professor
Department of Internal Medicine
The Ohio State University
Columbus, Ohio

Edward E. Max, MD, PhD
Associate Director for Research
Office of Biotechnology Products
Food and Drug Administration
Bethesda, Maryland

James McCluskey, BMedSci, MBBS, MD
Professor and Head
Departments of Microbiology and Immunology
The University of Melbourne
Parkville, Victoria, Australia

Jerry R. McGhee, PhD
Microbiology
The University of Alabama at Birmingham
Birmingham, Alabama

Michael McHeyzer-Williams, PhD
Associate Professor
Department of Immunology
The Scripps Research Institute
La Jolla, California

Ruslan Medzhitov, PhD
Investigator, Howard Hughes Medical Institute
David W. Wallace Professor of Immunobiology
Yale University
New Haven, Connecticut

Ira Mellman, PhD
Professor
Cell Biology and Immunology
Yale Medical School
New Haven, Connecticut

Jiri Mestecky, MD, PhD
Professor
Department of Microbiology
University of Alabama, Birmingham
Birmingham, Alabama

Muriel Moser, PhD
Research Director
Department of Molecular Biology
Université Libre de Bruxelles
Gosselies, Belgium

Philip M. Murphy, MD
Chief
Laboratory of Molecular Immunology
National Institute of Allergy and Infectious Diseases
National Institutes of Health
Bethesda, Maryland

Moon H. Nahm, MD
Professor
Departments of Pathology and Microbiology
University of Alabama, Birmingham
Birmingham, Alabama

Kannan Natarajan, PhD
Staff Scientist
Laboratory of Immunology, NIAID
National Institutes of Health
Bethesda, Maryland

Falk Nimmerjahn, PhD
Associate Professor
Medical Department
University of Erlangen
Erlangen, Germany

G.J.V. Nossal, MD, PhD
Professor Emeritus
Department of Pathology
The University of Melbourne
Parkville, Victoria, Australia

Eric Pamer, MD
Immunology Program
Sloan-Kettering Institute
Attending Physician
Infectious Disease Service, Department of Medicine
Memorial Sloan Kettering Cancer Center
New York, New York

Wolfgang M. Prodinger, MD
Associate Professor
Department of Hygiene, Microbiology and Social Medicine
Innsbruck Medical University
Innsbruck, Austria

Jeffrey V. Ravetch, MD, PhD
Theresa and Eugene M. Lang Professor
Head, Laboratory of Molecular Genetic and Immunology
The Rockefeller University
New York, New York

Steven L. Reiner, MD
Professor
Department of Medicine
University of Pennsylvania
Philadelphia, Pennsylvania

Nicholas P. Restifo, MD
Senior Investigator
Surgery Branch
National Cancer Institute
National Institutes of Health
Bethesda, Maryland

Eleanor M. Riley, PhD
Professor of Immunology
London School of Hygiene & Tropical Medicine
London, United Kingdom

Paul F. Robbins, PhD
Staff Scientist
Surgery Branch
National Cancer Institute
National Institutes of Health
Bethesda, Maryland

Steven A. Rosenberg, MD, PhD
Chief of Surgery
Surgery Branch
National Cancer Institute
National Institutes of Health
Bethesda, Maryland

Jamie Rossjohn, MD
Australian Research Council Federation Fellow
Departments of Biochemistry and Molecular Biology
Monash University
Clayton, Victoria, Australia

Ellen V. Rothenberg, PhD
Albert Billings Ruddock Professor of Biology
Division of Biology
California Institute of Technology
Pasadena, California

Nancy H. Ruddle, PhD
John Rodman Paul Professor
Department of Epidemiology and Public Health
Yale University School of Medicine
New Haven, Connecticut

David H. Sachs, MD
Paul S. Russel/Warner-Lambert Professor of Surgery
Department of Surgery
Harvard Medical School
Director, Transplantation Biology Research
Massachusetts General Hospital
Boston, Massachusetts

David L. Sacks, PhD
Section Chief
Laboratory of Parasitic Diseases
National Institute of Allergy and Infectious Diseases
National Institutes of Health
Bethesda, Maryland

Stephen P. Schoenberger, PhD
Member
Laboratory of Cellular Immunology
La Jolla Institute for Allergy and Immunology
La Jolla, California

Harry W. Schroeder, Jr., MD, PhD
Professor
Departments of Medicine, Microbiology, and Genetics
The University of Alabama at Birmingham
Birmingham, Alabama

Ronald H. Schwartz, MD, PhD
Chief
Laboratory of Cellular and Molecular Immunology
National Institutes of Health
Bethesda, Maryland

Alan Sher, PhD
Laboratory Chief
Laboratory of Parasitic Diseases
National Institutes of Health
Bethesda, Maryland

Ethan M. Shevach, MD
Chief, Cellular Immunology Section
Laboratory of Immunology
National Institute of Allergy and Infectious Diseases
National Institute of Health
Bethesda, Maryland

Cornelia Speth, MD
Associate Professor
Department of Hygiene, Microbiology and Social Medicine
Innsbruck Medical University
Innsbruck, Austria

Esther M. Sternberg, MD
Director, Integrative Neural Immune Program
Chief, Section on Neuroendocrine Immunology and Behavior
National Institute of Mental Health
National Institutes of Health
Bethesda, Maryland

Heribert Stoiber, MD
Associate Professor
Department of Hygiene, Microbiology and Social Medicine
Innsbruck Medical University
Innsbruck, Austria

Helen C. Su, MD, PhD
Clinical Investigator
Chief, Human Immunological Diseases Unit
Laboratory of Host Defenses
National Institute of Allergy and Infectious Diseases
National Institutes of Health
Bethesda, Maryland

Megan Sykes, MD
Professor of Surgery and Medicine
Departments of Surgery and Medicine
Harvard Medical School
Immunologist
Massachusetts General Hospital
Boston, Massachusetts

Matthias G. von Herrath, MD
Professor
Department of Immunology
La Jolla Institute for Allergy and Immunology
La Jolla, California

David Wald, MD, PhD
Resident Department of Pathology
University Hospitals Case Medical Center
Cleveland, Ohio

Carl F. Ware, PhD
Head
Division of Molecular Immunology
La Jolla Institute for Allergy & Immunology
La Jolla, California

Jeffrey N. Weiser, MD
Associate Professor
Department of Microbiology
University of Pennsylvania School of Medicine
Philadelphia, Pennsylvania

Marsha Wills-Karp, PhD
Professor
Department of Immunobiology
Cincinnati Children's Hospital Medical Center
Cincinnati, Ohio

Kathryn Wood, MD
Professor
Nuffield Department of Surgery
University of Oxford
Oxford, United Kingdom

Reinhard Würzner, MD
Associate Professor
Department of Hygiene, Microbiology and Social Medicine
Innsbruck Medical University
Innsbruck, Austria

Thomas A. Wynn, PhD
Section Chief
Laboratory of Parasitic Diseases
National Institute of Health
Bethesda, Maryland

Wayne M. Yokoyama, MD
Investigator
Howard Hughes Medical Institute
Sam J. & Audrey Loew Levine Chair for Research on Arthritis
Professor of Medicine and of Pathology and Immunology
Rheumatology Division
Washington University School of Medicine
St. Louis, Missouri

Mary A. Yui, PhD
Senior Research Fellow
Department of Biology
California Institute of Technology
Pasadena, California

PREFACE

Immunology is the quintessential medical science. Indeed, no branch of the medical sciences has improved the health of people more than the application of immunologic principles to prevention of disease. Smallpox has been eliminated from the planet as a natural infection, as has poliomyelitis from the Western Hemisphere. Hepatitis B vaccine has prevented more cancers than any intervention other than smoking cessation. The newly introduced human papilloma virus vaccine promises to cut strikingly the toll of cervical cancer.

The continued need for progress in immunology is clear. The HIV epidemic roars on. Disappointing results from vaccine trials require a redoubled effort to understand how to build the new generations of vaccines that can attack the really hard problems, including HIV, tuberculosis, and malaria, among infectious diseases. Highly effective therapeutic vaccines for cancers still elude us, but progress in understanding the innate immune system and regulatory T cells places new tools in our hands to continue the attack on this major problem.

Understanding the basis of inflammation and the cytokine world has given us effective drugs to treat rheumatoid arthritis and other autoinflammatory/autoimmune diseases. The value of the interventions based on this knowledge, such as the use of tumor necrosis factor (TNF), interleukin-6 (IL-6), and IL-1 blockers, is now established. The application of anti-CD20 in the treatment of autoimmune disorders shows great promise.

Fundamental Immunology has the goal of aiding in the education of a new generation of immunologists who can both probe more deeply into the organizing principles of the immune system and can translate this new information into effective treatments and preventatives that can extend and enlarge on the record of immunologic science in bettering the lot of humankind.

Were I beginning the task of preparing a comprehensive text of immunology today, I might have titled it *Immunology, Endless Fascination*. Certainly that describes my own view of this science over the more than 25 years that I have been working on the six editions of *Fundamental Immunology*. I had believed that scientific progress was marked by periods of intense creativity, during which new concepts were established, followed by longer periods of consolidation, when work that made important but anticipated advances would dominate. Perhaps that will prove to be true of modern immunology as well when it is looked at by a disinterested observer, but for one in the midst, the pace of discovery seems to speed up with each passing year. *Endless fascination* certainly describes my experience of immunology.

During the interval since the previous edition, there have been major advances in every field of immunology. Indeed, in one of the most striking pieces of work, an entirely new adaptive immune system has been discovered. Pancer, Cooper, and their colleagues have shown that jawless vertebrates, rather than using an adaptive immune system based on the immunoglobulin superfamily T-cell and B-cell receptors, evolved an entirely distinct adaptive system based on the use of leucine-rich repeat molecules as the recognition elements. The understanding of innate immunity continues to grow with the deepening understanding of the range of microbial sensors and of how they link to the adaptive immune system. The 2007 Lasker Prize for Basic Medical Sciences went to Ralph Steinman for his discovery of dendritic cells, which interpret the messages of the innate system to the adaptive system. The importance of regulatory T cells continues to grow, as does our insight into the mechanisms of their action. The cytokine biology field expands and broadens in its importance. The number of interleukins is now into the mid-30s, and some of the more recently discovered molecules have the most important functions. The application of imaging technologies that allow the visualization of the in vivo behavior of the cells and tissues of the immune system has provided spectacular insights into the structure and dynamics of the system and promises still more amazing results in the future. The field of systems immunology, still in its infancy, has given notice that it will be a major approach to our science in the next decades.

I hope that this sixth edition will convey this dynamism and provide the reader with both a solid grounding in our field and with much of the very latest that has been achieved. As with each of the previous editions, most of the chapters are entirely new and not simple reworkings of the chapter in the previous edition. In order to contain the sixth edition within one volume, a decision was made to limit the number of references that will be printed in the text. For those chapters in which there are substantially in excess of 200 references cited in the text, the authors have selected 200 to be included in the print version of the book. All are included in the electronic version. The electronic version can be accessed at www.fundamentalimmunology.com.

As before, this edition begins with an introductory chapter, "The Immune System," aimed at giving an overview of modern immunology and providing those new to the field with the basis to go on to the subsequent chapters. This is followed by an "expanded introduction" provided by the sections, "Organization and Evolution of the Immune System," "Immunoglobulins and B Lymphocytes," and "T lymphocytes." I have introduced a new and extended section, "The Intersection of Innate and Adaptive Immunity," which is followed by the section, "Regulation and Effector Functions of the Immune Response." The book concludes with sections devoted to the immune system's role in protection against pathogenic microorganisms, "Immunity to Infectious Agents," and on how the immune system is involved in a variety of human disorders, "Immunologic Mechanisms in Disease."

I repeat a word of caution that has been in the Preface to each edition. Immunology is moving very fast. Each of the chapters is written by an expert in the field, but in some areas there may be differences of opinion expressed by equally accomplished authors. I ask the reader to take note of the differences and to follow developments in the field.

William E. Paul
Washington, DC

ACKNOWLEDGMENTS

The preparation of the sixth edition required the efforts of many individuals. I particularly wish to thank each of the authors. Their contributions, prepared in the midst of extremely busy schedules, are responsible for the value of this book. Julia Seto of Lippincott Williams & Wilkins saw that the process of receiving, editing, and assembling the chapters went as smoothly as possible, as she did for the fifth edition. Without her efforts, the completion of this edition would have been immeasurably more difficult. Frances DeStefano's counsel was of utmost importance in planning this edition and in making key decisions about its organization. I wish to gratefully acknowledge the efforts of each of the members of the editorial and production staffs of Lippincott Williams & Wilkins who participated in the preparation of this edition.

CONTENTS

SECTION VI: REGULATION AND EFFECTOR FUNCTIONS OF THE IMMUNE RESPONSE *631*

SECTION VII: IMMUNITY TO INFECTIOUS AGENTS *1097*

SECTION VIII: IMMUNOLOGIC MECHANISMS IN DISEASE *1291*

Everything should be made as simple as possible, but not simpler.

ALBERT EINSTEIN

From my teachers I have learned much, from my colleagues still more, but from my students most of all.

The Talmud

Discovery consists of seeing what everybody has seen and thinking what nobody has thought.

ALBERT SZENT-GYORGYI

. . . the clonal selection hypothesis . . . assumes that . . . there exist clones of mesenchymal cells, each carrying immunologically reactive sites . . . complementary . . . to one (or possibly a small number) of potential antigenic determinants.

FRANK MACFARLANE BURNET

In the fields of observation, chance favors the prepared mind.

LOUIS PASTEUR

In all things of nature there is something of the marvelous.

ARISTOTLE

Fundamental Immunology

SECTION I

Introduction

Chapter 1

The Immune System

William E. Paul

The immune system is a remarkable defense mechanism. It makes rapid, specific, and protective responses against the myriad potentially pathogenic microorganisms that inhabit the world in which we live. The tragic examples of acquired immunodeficiency syndrome (AIDS) and the inherited severe combined immunodeficiencies (SCID) graphically illustrate the consequences of a nonfunctional adaptive immune system. AIDS patients and children with SCID often fall victim to infections that are of little or no consequence to those with normally functioning immune systems. The immune system also has a role in the rejection of tumors and, when dysregulated, may give rise to a series of autoimmune diseases, including insulin-dependent diabetes mellitus, multiple sclerosis, rheumatoid arthritis, systemic lupus erythematosus, and inflammatory bowel diseases, among others.

Fundamental Immunology has as its goal the authoritative presentation of the basic elements of the immune system, of the means through which the mechanisms of immunity act in a wide range of clinical conditions, including recovery from infectious diseases, rejection of tumors, transplantation of tissue and organs, autoimmunity and other immunopathologic conditions, and allergy, and how the mechanisms of immunity can be marshaled by vaccination to provide protection against microbial pathogens.

The purpose of this opening chapter is to provide readers with a general introduction to our current understanding of the immune system. It should be of particular importance for those with a limited background in immunology, providing them with the preparation needed for subsequent chapters of the book. Rather than providing extensive references in this chapter, each of the subject headings will indicate the chapters that deal in detail with the topic under discussion. Those chapters will not only provide an extended treatment of the topic, but will also furnish the reader with a comprehensive reference list.

KEY CHARACTERISTICS OF THE IMMUNE SYSTEM

Innate Immunity (Chapters 14, 15, and 18)

Powerful nonspecific defenses prevent or limit infections by most potentially pathogenic microorganisms. The epithelium provides both a physical barrier to the entry of microbes and produces a variety of antimicrobial factors. Agents that penetrate the epithelium are met with macrophages and related cells possessing "microbial sensors" that recognize key molecules characteristic of many microbial agents. These "pattern recognition receptors" include several families of molecules, of which the most intensively studied are the Toll-like receptors (TLRs). Each TLR recognizes a distinct substance (or set of substances) associated with microbial agents: TLR4 recognizes lipopolysaccharides; TLR3, double-stranded RNA; and TLR9, unmethylated CpG-containing DNA. Since the recognized substances are generally indispensable to the infectious agent, microbial sensors provide a highly efficient means to recognize potential pathogens.

The interaction of a TLR with its ligand induces a series of intracellular signaling events of which activation of the NF-κB system is particularly important. Macrophage activation with enhancement of the cell's phagocytic activity and the induction of antimicrobial systems aid in the destruction of the pathogen. The induction of an inflammatory response as a result of the activation of the innate immune system recruits other cell types, including neutrophils, to the site.

The innate immune system also acts to recruit antigen-specific immune responses, not only by attracting cells of the immune system to the site of the infection, but also through the uptake of antigen by dendritic cells (DC) and its transport by these cells to lymphoid tissues where primary immune responses are initiated. Activated DCs express cell surface costimulatory molecules and produce cytokines that can regulate the quality of the immune response so that it is most appropriate to combating the infectious agent.

Primary Responses (Chapters 9 and 13)

Primary immune responses are initiated when a foreign antigenic substance interacts with antigen-specific lymphocytes under appropriate circumstances. The response generally consists of the production of antibody molecules specific for the antigenic determinants of the immunogen and of the expansion and differentiation of antigen-specific helper and effector T lymphocytes. The latter include cytokine-producing cells and killer T cells, capable of lysing infected cells. Generally, the combination of the innate immune response and the primary adaptive response are sufficient to eradicate or to control the microbe. Indeed, the most effective function of the immune system is to mount a response that eliminates the infectious agent from the body—so-called *sterilizing immunity*.

Secondary Responses and Immunologic Memory (Chapters 9, 13, and 28)

As a consequence of initial encounter with antigen, the immunized individual develops a state of immunologic *memory*. If the same (or a closely related) microorganism is encountered again, a secondary response is made. This generally consists of an antibody response that is more rapid, greater in magnitude, and composed of antibodies that bind to the antigen with greater affinity and are more effective in clearing the microbe from the body. A more rapid and more effective T cell response also ensues. Thus, an initial infection with a microorganism often initiates a state of immunity in which the individual is protected against a second infection. In the majority of situations, protection is provided by high-affinity antibody molecules that rapidly clear the reintroduced microbe. This is the basis of most licensed vaccines; the great power of vaccines is illustrated by the elimination of smallpox from the world and by the complete control of polio in the western hemisphere.

The Immune Response Is Highly Specific and the Antigenic Universe Is Vast

The immune response is highly specific. Primary immunization with a given microorganism evokes antibodies and T cells that are specific for the antigenic determinants found on that microorganism but that generally fail to recognize (or recognize only poorly) antigenic determinants expressed by unrelated microbes. Indeed, the range of antigenic specificities that can be discriminated by the immune system is enormous.

The Immune System Is Tolerant of Self-antigens (Chapters 29 and 30)

One of the most important features of the immune system is its ability to discriminate between antigenic determinants expressed on foreign substances, such as pathogenic microbes, and potential antigenic determinants expressed by the tissues of the host. The failure of the system to make full-blown immune responses to self-antigens is referred to as *immunologic tolerance*. Tolerance is a complex process that actually involves several distinct mechanisms. One element, perhaps the most important, is an active process involving the elimination or inactivation of cells that can recognize self-antigens. In addition, there are mechanisms through which cells that encounter antigens (e.g., self-antigens) in the absence of cues from the innate immune system may fail to make a response, may make a minimal response or may be inactivated through a process referred to as *anergy*. Finally, a specialized set of T cells exist, designated regulatory cells that actively *suppress* responses against self-antigens. Indeed, individuals who have mutations in the key transcription factor Foxp3 expressed by the regulatory cells develop severe multiorgan autoimmunity (polyendocrinopathy, enteropathy X-linked [IPEX] syndrome). The critical necessity to control self-reactivity is clearly shown by this multilayered system that involves elimination, inactivation, and suppression.

Immune Responses Against Self-antigens Can Result in Autoimmune Diseases (Chapters 41 and 42)

Failure in establishing immunologic tolerance or unusual presentations of self-antigens can give rise to tissue-damaging immune responses directed against antigenic determinants on host molecules. These can result in autoimmune diseases. As has already been mentioned, a group of extremely important diseases are caused by autoimmune responses or have major autoimmune components, including systemic lupus erythematosus, rheumatoid arthritis, insulin-dependent diabetes mellitus, multiple sclerosis, myasthenia gravis, and regional enteritis. Efforts to treat these diseases by modulating the autoimmune response are a major theme of contemporary medicine.

AIDS Is an Example of a Disease Caused by a Virus That the Immune System Generally Fails to Eliminate (Chapter 39)

Immune responses against infectious agents do not always lead to elimination of the pathogen. In some instances, a chronic infection ensues in which the immune system adopts a variety of strategies to limit damage caused by the organism or by the immune response. Indeed, herpes viruses, such as human cytomegalovirus (CMV), frequently are not eliminated by immune responses and establish chronicity in which the virus is controlled by immune responses. One of the most notable infectious diseases in which the immune response generally fails to eliminate the organism is AIDS, caused by the human immunodeficiency virus (HIV). In this instance, the principal infected cells are those of the immune system itself, leading to an eventual state in which the individual can no longer mount protective immune responses against other microbial pathogens. Indeed, under the assault of HIV, control of viruses such as CMV is lost and they may cause major tissue damage.

Major Principles of Immunity

The major principles of the immune response are:

Elimination of many microbial agents through the nonspecific protective mechanisms of the innate immune system.

Cues from the innate immune system inform the cells of the adaptive immune system as to whether it is appropriate to make a response and what type of response to make.

Cells of the adaptive immune system display exquisitely specific recognition of foreign antigens and mobilize potent mechanisms for elimination of microbes bearing such antigens.

The immune system displays memory of its previous responses.

Tolerance of self-antigens.

The remainder of this introductory chapter will describe briefly the molecular and cellular basis of the system and how these central characteristics of the immune response may be explained.

CELLS OF THE IMMUNE SYSTEM AND THEIR SPECIFIC RECEPTORS AND PRODUCTS

The immune system consists of several distinct cell types, each with important roles. The lymphocytes occupy central stage because they are the cells that determine the specificity of immunity. It is their response that orchestrates the effector limbs of the immune system. Cells that interact with lymphocytes play critical parts both in the presentation of antigen and in the mediation of immunologic functions. These cells include DCs and the closely related Langerhans cells, monocyte/macrophages, natural killer (NK) cells, neutrophils, mast cells, basophils, and eosinophils. In addition, a series of specialized epithelial and stromal cells provide the anatomic environment in which immunity occurs, often by secreting critical factors that regulate migration, growth and homeostasis, and gene activation in cells of the immune system. Such cells also play direct roles in the induction and effector phases of the response.

The cells of the immune system are found in peripheral organized tissues, such as the spleen, lymph nodes, Peyer's patches of the intestine, and tonsils, where primary immune responses generally occur (see Chapter 2). Many of the lymphocytes comprise a recirculating pool of cells found in the blood and lymph, as well as in the lymph nodes and spleen, providing the means to deliver immunocompetent cells to sites where they are needed and to allow immunity that is initiated locally to become generalized. Activated lymphocytes acquire the capacity to enter nonlymphoid tissues, where they can express effector functions and eradicate local infections. Some memory lymphocytes are "on patrol" in the tissues, scanning for reintroduction of their specific antigens. Lymphocytes are also found in the central lymphoid organs, the thymus, and bone marrow, where they undergo the developmental steps that equip them to mediate the responses of the mature immune system.

Individual lymphocytes are specialized in that they are committed to respond to a limited set of structurally related antigens. This commitment exists before the first contact of the immune system with a given antigen. It is expressed by the presence on the lymphocyte's surface of receptors specific for determinants (epitopes) of the antigen. Each lymphocyte possesses a population of receptors, all of which have identical combining sites (this is a slight oversimplification, as occasionally T cells and less frequently B cells may express two populations of receptors). One set, or clone, of lymphocytes differs from another clone in the structure of the combining region of its receptors and thus in the epitopes that it can recognize. The ability of an organism to respond to virtually any non–self-antigen is achieved by the existence of a very large number of different lymphocytes, each bearing receptors specific for a distinct epitope. As a consequence, lymphocytes are an enormously heterogeneous group of cells. Based on reasonable assumptions as to the range of diversity that can be created in the genes encoding antigen-specific receptors, it seems virtually certain that the number of distinct combining sites on lymphocyte receptors of an adult human can be measured in the millions.

Lymphocytes differ from each other not only in the specificity of their receptors but also in their functions. There are two broad classes of lymphocytes: the B lymphocytes, which are precursors of antibody-secreting cells, and the T (thymus-derived) lymphocytes. T lymphocytes express important helper functions, such as the ability to aid in the development of specific types of immune responses, including the production of antibody by B cells and the increase in the microbicidal activity of macrophages. Other T lymphocytes are involved in direct effector functions, such as the lysis of virus-infected cells or certain neoplastic cells. Regulatory T lymphocytes have the capacity to suppress immune responses.

B LYMPHOCYTES AND ANTIBODY

B Lymphocyte Development (Chapter 7)

B lymphocytes derive from lymphoid progenitor cells, which in turn are derived from hematopoietic stem cells (Figure 1.1). A detailed picture has been obtained of the molecular mechanisms through which committed early members of the B lineage develop into mature B

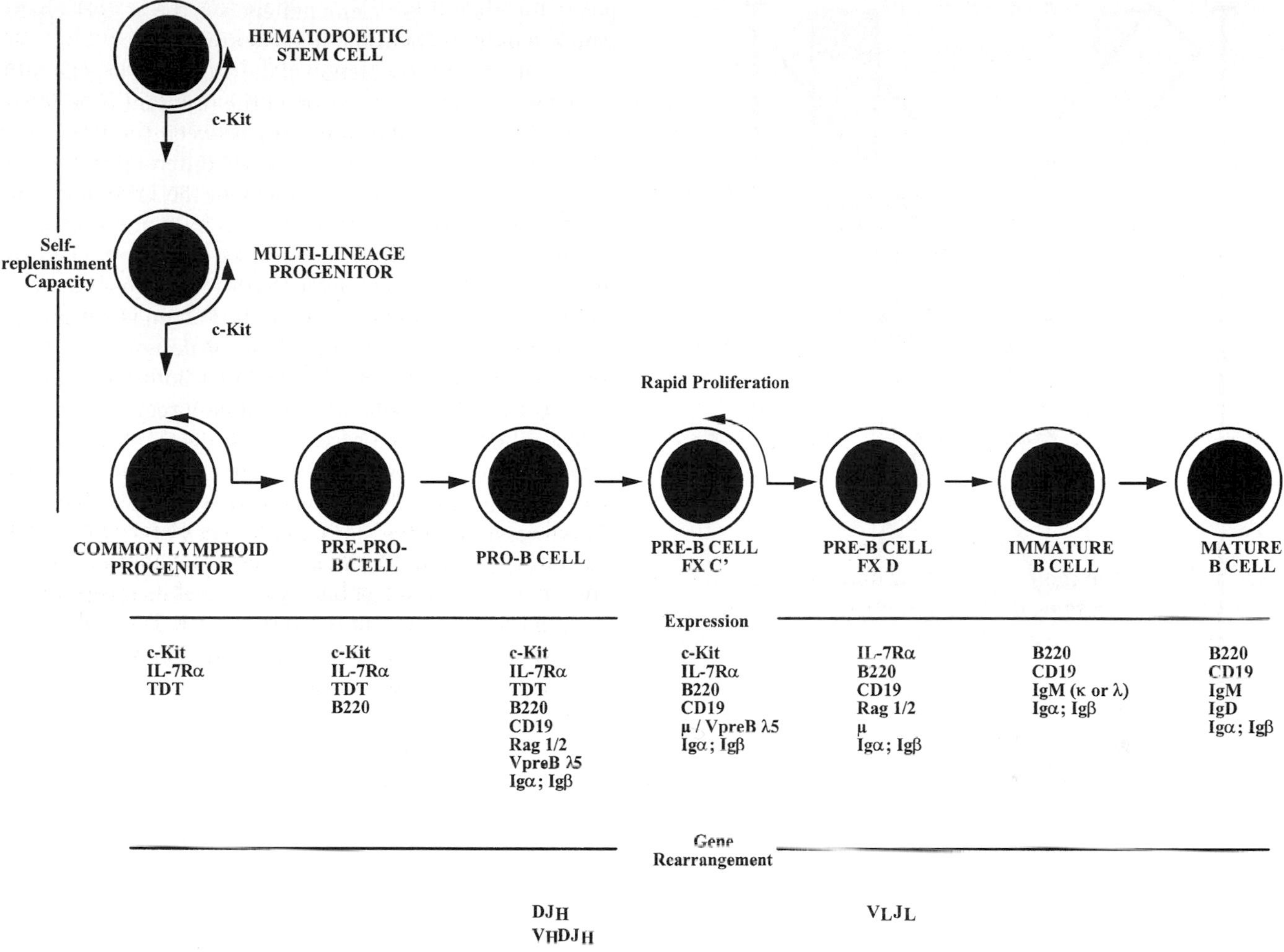

FIGURE 1.1 The patterns of gene expression, timing of gene rearrangement events, and capacity for self-replenishment and for rapid proliferation of developing B lymphocytes are indicated. (Adapted from Richard R. Hardy and Kyoko Hayakawa, B cell development pathways, *Annual Review of Immunology*. 2001;19:595–621.)

lymphocytes. These events occur in the fetal liver and, in adult life, in the bone marrow. Interaction with specialized stromal cells and their products, including cytokines such as interleukin (IL)-7 and B cell activating factor of the TNF family (BAFF) are critical to the normal regulation of this process.

The key events in B cell development involve commitment to the B lineage and repression of the capacity to differentiate to cells of other lineages. In pro-B cells and pre-B cells, the genetic elements that encode the antigen-specific receptors are assembled. These receptors are immunoglobulin (Ig) molecules specialized for expression on the cell surface. Igs are heterodimeric molecules consisting of heavy (H) and light (L) chains, both of which have variable (V) regions, which contribute to the binding of antigen and that differ in sequence from one Ig molecule to another (see Chapters 4 and 6), (Figure 1.2), and constant (C) regions.

The genetic elements encoding the variable portions of Ig H and L chains are not contiguous in germline DNA or in the DNA of nonlymphoid cells (see Chapter 6) and (Figure 1.3). In pro- and pre-B cells, these genetic elements are translocated to construct an expressible V region gene. This process involves a choice among a large set of potentially usable variable (V), diversity (D), and joining (J) elements in a combinatorial manner and depends upon the RAG proteins, RAG1 and RAG2, that are essential for the recombination process. Such combinatorial translocation, together with the addition of diversity in the course of the joining process, results in the generation of a very large number of distinct H and L chains. The pairing of H and L chains in a quasi-random manner further expands the number of distinct Ig molecules that can be formed.

The H chain variable region is initially expressed in association with the product of the μ constant (C) region

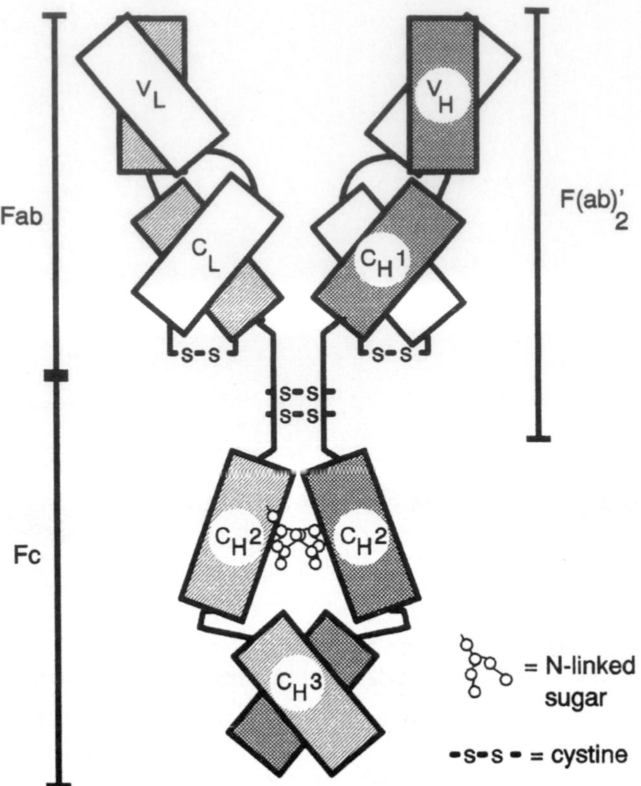

FIGURE 1.2 A schematic representation of an Ig molecule indicating the means through the V regions and the CH1 and CL regions of H and L chains pair with one another and how the CH2 and CH3 regions of the H chains pair.

gene. Together these elements encode the μ IgH chain, which is used in Igs of the IgM class.

The successful completion of the process of Ig gene rearrangement and the expression of the resultant IgM on the cell surface marks the transition between the pre-B and B cell states (Figure 1.1). The newly differentiated B cell initially expresses surface Ig solely of the IgM class. The cell completes its maturation process by expressing on its surface a second class of Ig composed of the same L chain and the same H chain variable (VDJ) region but of a different H chain C region; this second IgH chain is designated δ, and the Ig to which it contributes is designated IgD, so that the mature naïve B cells expresses both IgM and IgD surface molecules that share the same V region.

The differentiation process is controlled at several steps by a system of checks that determines whether prior steps have been successfully completed. These checks depend on the expression on the surface of the cell of appropriately constructed Ig or Ig-like molecules. For example, in the period after a μ chain has been successfully assembled but before an L chain has been assembled, the μ chain is expressed on the cell surface in association with a surrogate light chain, consisting of VpreB and $\lambda5$. Pre-B cells that fail to express this μ–VpreB $\lambda5$ complex do not move forward to future differentiation states or do so very inefficiently.

B Lymphocyte Activation (Chapter 8)

A mature B cell can be activated by an encounter with antigen expressing epitopes that are recognized by its cell surface Ig (Figure 1.4). The activation process may be a

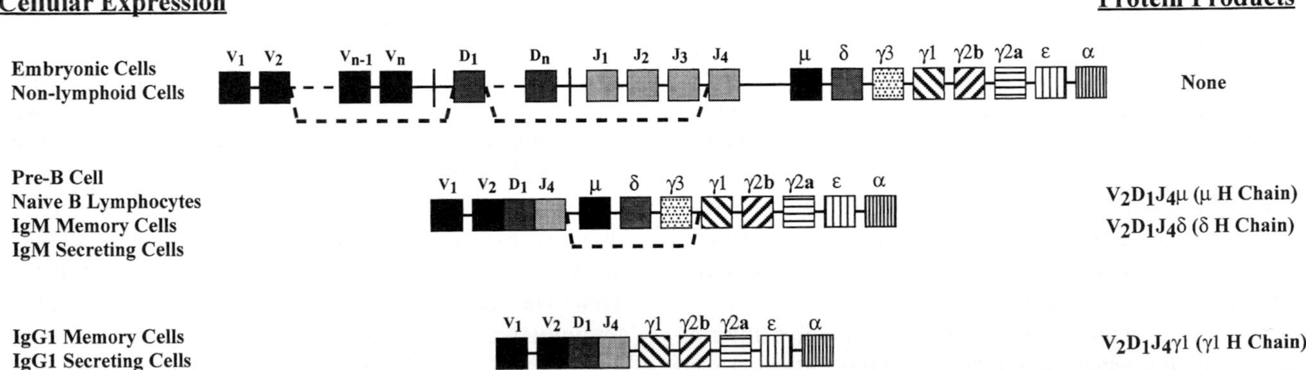

FIGURE 1.3 Organization and translocation of mouse IgH genes. IgH chains are encoded by four distinct genetic elements: Igh-V (V), Igh-D (D), Igh-J (J), and Igh-C. The V, D, and J genetic elements together specify the variable region of the H chain. The Igh-C element specifies the C region. The same V region can be expressed in association with each of the C regions (μ, δ, $\gamma3$, $\gamma1$, $\gamma2b$, $\gamma2a$, ε and α). In the germline, the V, D, and J genes are far apart, and there are multiple forms of each of these genes. In the course of lymphocyte development, a VDJ gene complex is formed by translocation of individual V and D genes so that they lie next to one of the J genes, with excision of the intervening genes. This VDJ complex is initially expressed with μ and δ C genes but may be subsequently translocated so that it lies near one of the other C genes (e.g., $\gamma1$) and in that case leads to the expression of a VDJ $\gamma1$ chain.

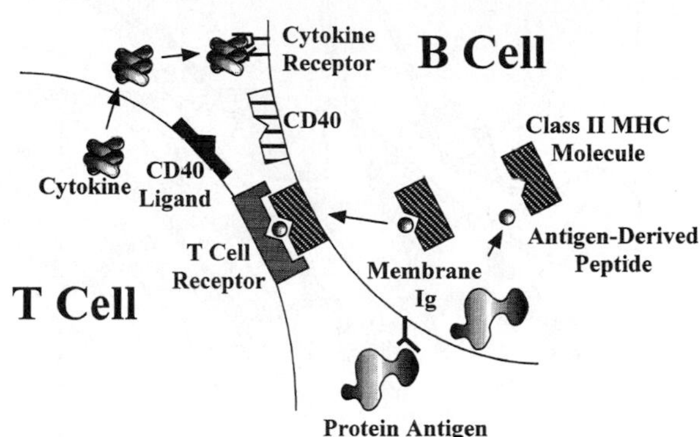

A

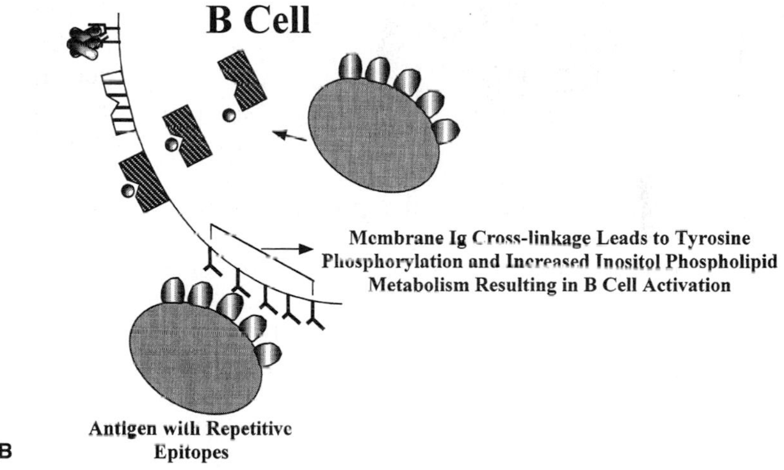

B

FIGURE 1.4 Two forms of B cell activation. **A:** Cognate T cell/B cell help. Resting B cells can bind antigens that bear epitopes complementary to their cell surface Ig. Even if the antigen cannot cross-link the receptor, it will be endocytosed and enter late endosomes and lysosomes where it will be degraded to peptides. Some of these peptides will be loaded into class II MHC molecules and brought to the cell surface, where they can be recognized by $CD4^+$ T cells that bear receptors specific for that peptide–class II complex. This interaction allows an activation ligand on the T cells (CD40 ligand) to bind to its receptor on B cells (CD40) and to signal B cell activation. In addition, the T cells secrete several cytokines that regulate the growth and differentiation of the stimulated B cell. **B:** Cross-linkage-dependent B cell activation. When B cells encounter antigens that bear multiple copies of an epitope that can bind to their surface Ig, the resultant cross-linkage stimulates biochemical signals within the cell leading to B cell activation, growth, and differentiation. In many instances, B cell activation events may result from both pathways of stimulation.

direct one, dependent on cross-linkage of membrane Ig molecules by the antigen (*cross linkage–dependent B cell activation*), or an indirect one, occurring most efficiently in the context of an intimate interaction with a helper T cell, in a process often referred to as *cognate help*.

Because each B cell bears membrane Ig molecules with identical variable regions, cross-linkage of the cell surface receptors requires that the antigen express more than one copy of an epitope complementary to the binding site of the receptor. This requirement is fulfilled by antigens with repetitive epitopes. Among these antigens are the capsular polysaccharides of many medically important microorganisms such as pneumococci, streptococci, and meningococci. Similar expression of multiple identical epitopes on a single immunogenic particle is a property of many viruses because they express multiple copies of envelope proteins on their surface. Cross linkage–dependent B cell activation is a major protective immune response mounted against these microbes. The binding of complement components (see Chapter 33) to antigen or antigen–antibody complexes can increase the magnitude of the cross linkage–dependent B cell activation due to the action of a receptor for complement, which, together with other molecules, increases the magnitude of a B-cell response to limiting amounts of antigen.

Cognate help allows B cells to mount responses against antigens that cannot cross-link receptors and, at the same time, provides costimulatory signals that rescue B cells from inactivation when they are stimulated by weak cross-linkage events. Cognate help is dependent on the binding of antigen by the B cell's membrane Ig, the endocytosis of the antigen, and its fragmentation into peptides within the endosomal/lysosomal compartment of the cell. Some of the resultant peptides are loaded into a groove in a specialized set of cell surface proteins, the class II major histocompatibility complex (MHC) molecules (Figure 1.5). The resultant class II–peptide complexes are expressed on the cell surface. As will be discussed, these complexes are the ligands for the antigen-specific receptors of a set of T cells designated CD4 T cells. CD4 T cells that have

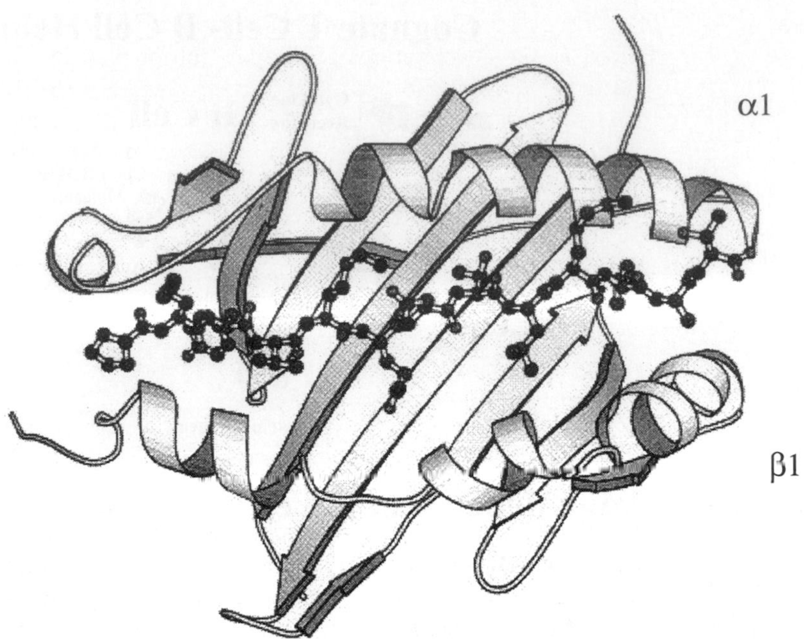

FIGURE 1.5 Illustration of the structure of the peptide binding domain (α1 and β1) of a class II MHC molecule (HLA-DR; protein data bank designation 1DLH) bound to an antigenic peptide from influenza hemagglutinin. (Adapted by D. H. Margulies from Stern, L. J., et al. Crystal structure of the human class II MHC protein HLA-DR1 complexed with an influenza virus peptide. *Nature,* 1994;368(6468):215–221.)

receptors specific for the class II–peptide complex expressed on the B cell surface recognize and interact with that B cell. That interaction results in the activation of the B cell through the agency of cell surface molecules expressed by the T cells (e.g., the CD40 ligand [CD154]) and cytokines produced by the T cell (Figure 1.4). The role of the B cell receptor for antigen is to create the T cell ligand on the surface of antigen-specific B cells; activation of the B cell derives largely from the action of the T cell. However, in many physiologic situations, receptor cross-linkage stimuli and cognate help synergize to yield more vigorous B cell responses. Recently, it has been shown that the association of ligands for TLRs with antigen will strikingly enhance B cell responses.

B Lymphocyte Differentiation (Chapters 7 and 9)

Activation of B cells prepares them to divide and to differentiate either into antibody-secreting cells or into memory cells, so that there are more cells specific for the antigen used for immunization. Those cells that differentiate into antibody-secreting cells account for primary antibody responses. Some of these antibody-secreting cells migrate to the bone marrow where they may continue to produce antibody for an extended period of time and may have lifetimes in excess of one year.

Memory B cells give rise to antibody-secreting cells upon re-challenge of the individual. The hallmark of the antibody response to rechallenge (a secondary response) is that it is of greater magnitude, occurs more promptly, is composed of antibodies with higher affinity for the antigen, and is dominated by Igs expressing γ, α, or ε C regions (IgG, IgA, or IgE) rather than by IgM, which is the dominant Ig of the primary response.

Division and differentiation of cells into antibody-secreting cells is largely controlled by the interaction of the activated B cells with T cells expressing CD154 and by their stimulation by T cell–derived cytokines.

The differentiation of activated B cells into memory cells occurs in a specialized microenvironmental structure in the spleen and lymph nodes, the germinal center (GC). The increase in antibody affinity occurs also takes place within the GC. This process, designated *affinity maturation,* is dependent on somatic hypermutation. The survival of B cells within the GC depends on their capacity to bind antigen so that as the amount of antigen diminishes, B cells that have higher affinity receptors, either naturally or as a result of the hypermutation process, have a selective survival and growth advantage. Thus, such cells come to dominate the population.

The process through which a single H chain V region can become expressed with genes encoding C regions other than μ or δ is referred to as *Ig class switching*. It is dependent on a gene translocation event through which the C region genes between the genetic elements encoding the V region and the newly expressed C gene are excised, resulting in the switched C gene being located in the position that the Cμ gene formerly occupied (Figure 1.3). This process also occurs mainly in GCs. Both somatic hypermutation and Ig class switching depend upon the action of activation-induced cytidine deamidase (AID) that plays an important role in the breakage and repair of DNA, which is essential for recombination events.

B1 and Marginal Zone B Lymphocytes (Chapters 7 and 9)

B lymphocytes consist of at least three distinct populations: conventional B cells, B1 B cells, and marginal zone (MZ) B cells. B1 B cells were initially recognized because some express a cell-surface protein, CD5, not generally found on other B cells. In the adult mouse, B1 B cells are found in relatively high frequency in the peritoneal cavity but are present at low frequency in the spleen and lymph nodes. B1 B cells are quite numerous in fetal and perinatal life. B1 B cells appear to be self-renewing, in contrast to conventional B cells, in which division and memory are antigen driven.

MZ B cells are localized in a distinct anatomical region of the spleen (the marginal zone) that represents the major antigen-filtering and scavenging area. Like B1 B cells, MZ B cells express a repertoire biased toward bacterial cell wall constituents and senescent self-components. MZ and B1 B cells respond very rapidly to antigenic challenge, likely independently of T cells. Uniquely, among all populations of B cells, MZ B cells are dependent on Notch-2 signaling for their development.

B1 B cells and MZ B cells are responsible for the secretion of the serum IgM that exists in nonimmunized mice, often referred to as *natural IgM*. Among the antibodies found in such natural IgM are molecules that can combine with phosphatidyl choline (a component of pneumococcal cell walls) and with lipopolysaccharide and influenza virus. B1 B cells also produce autoantibodies, although they are generally of low affinity and in most cases not pathogenic. There is evidence that B1 B cells are important in resistance to several pathogens and may have a significant role in mucosal immunity.

B Lymphocyte Tolerance (Chapter 29)

One of the central problems facing the immune system is that of being able to mount highly effective immune responses to the antigens of foreign, potentially pathogenic, agents while ignoring antigens associated with the host's own tissues. The mechanisms ensuring this failure to respond to self-antigens are complex and involve a series of strategies. Chief among them is elimination of cells capable of self-reactivity or the inactivation of such cells. The encounter of immature, naïve B cells with antigens with repetitive epitopes capable of cross-linking membrane Ig can lead to elimination of the B cells, particularly if no T cell help is provided at the time of the encounter. This elimination of potentially self-reactive cells is often referred to as *clonal elimination*. Many self-reactive cells, rather than dying upon encounter with self-antigens, undergo a further round of Ig gene rearrangement. This *receptor editing* process allows a self-reactive cell to substitute a new receptor and therefore to avoid elimination.

There are many self-antigens that are not encountered by the developing B cell population or that do not have the capacity to cross-link B cell receptors (BCR) to a sufficient degree to elicit the receptor editing/clonal elimination process. Such cells, even when mature, may nonetheless be inactivated through a process that involves cross-linkage of receptors without the receipt of critical costimulatory signals. These inactivated cells may be retained in the body but are unresponsive to antigen and are referred to as *anergic*. When removed from the presence of the anergy-inducing stimulus, anergic cells may regain responsiveness.

Immunoglobulins

Structure (Chapter 4)

Igs are the antigen-specific membrane receptors and secreted products of B cells. They are members of a large family of proteins designated *the Ig supergene family*. Members of the Ig supergene family have sequence homology, a common gene organization, and similarities in three-dimensional structure. The latter is characterized by a structural element referred to as the *Ig fold*, generally consisting of a set of seven β-pleated sheets organized into two apposing layers (Figure 1.6). Many of the cell surface proteins that participate in immunologic recognition processes, including the T cell receptor (TCR), the CD3 complex, and signaling molecules associated with the BCR (Ig-α and Ig-β), are members of the Ig supergene family.

The Igs themselves are constructed of a unit that consists of two H chains and two L chains (Figure 1.2). The H and L chains are composed of a series of domains, each consisting of approximately 110 amino acids.

The L chains, of which there are two types (κ and λ), consist of two domains. The carboxy-terminal domain is essentially identical among L chains of a given type and is referred to as the *constant (C) region*. As already discussed, the amino-terminal domain varies from L chain to L chain and contributes to the binding site of antibody. Because of its variability, it is referred to as the *variable (V) region*. The variability of this region is largely concentrated in three segments, designated the *hypervariable* or *complementarity-determining regions* (CDR). The CDRs contain the amino acids that are the L chain's contribution to the lining of the antibody's combining site. The three CDRs are interspersed among four regions of much lower degree of variability, designated framework regions (FR).

The H chains of Ig molecules are of several classes determined by their constant regions (μ, δ, γ [of which there are several subclasses], α and ε). An assembled Ig molecule, consisting of one or more units of two identical H and L chains, derives its name from the C region of the H chain that it possesses. Thus, there are IgM, IgD, IgG, IgA, and IgE antibodies. The H chains each consist of a single amino-terminal V region and three or four C regions.

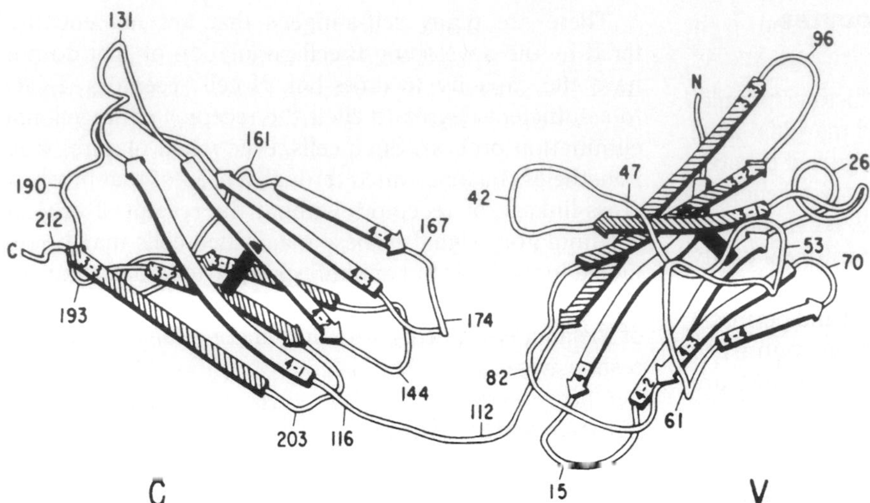

FIGURE 1.6 Schematic drawing of the V and C domains of an Ig L chain illustrating the "Ig fold." The β strands participating in the antiparallel β-pleated sheets of each domain are represented as arrows. The β strands of the three-stranded sheets are shaded, whereas those in the four-stranded sheets are white. The intra-domain disulfide bonds are represented as black bars. Selected amino acids are numbered with position 1 as the N terminus. (Reprinted with permission from Edmundson AB, Ely KR, Abola EE, et al. Rotational allomerism and divergent evolution of domains in immunoglobulin light chains. *Biochemistry* 1975;14:3953–3961.)

In many H chains, a hinge region separates the first and second C regions and conveys flexibility to the molecule, allowing the two combining sites of a single unit to move in relation to one another so as to promote the binding of a single antibody molecule to an antigen that has more than one copy of the same epitope. Such divalent binding to a single antigenic structure results in a great gain in energy of interaction (see Chapter 5). The H chain V region, like that of the L chain, contains three CDRs lining the combining site of the antibody and four FRs.

The C region of each H-chain class conveys unique functional attributes to the antibodies that possess it. Among the distinct biologic functions of each class of antibody are the following:

IgM antibodies are potent activators of the complement system (Chapter 33).

IgA antibodies are secreted into a variety of bodily fluids and are principally responsible for immunity at mucosal surfaces (Chapter 31).

IgE antibodies are bound by specific receptors (FcεRI) on basophils and mast cells. When cross-linked by antigen, these IgE–FcεRI complexes cause the cells to release a set of mediators responsible for allergic inflammatory responses (Chapter 43).

IgD antibodies act virtually exclusively as membrane receptors for antigen.

IgG antibodies, made up of four subclasses in both humans and mice, mediate a wide range of functions including transplacental passage and opsonization of antigens through binding of antigen–antibody complexes to specialized Fc receptors on macrophages and other cell types (Chapters 18 and 22).

IgD, IgG, and IgE antibodies consist of a single unit of two H and L chains. IgM antibodies are constructed of five or six such units, although they consist of a single unit when they act as membrane receptors. IgA antibodies may consist of one or more units. The antibodies that are made up of more than a single unit generally contain an additional polypeptide chain, the J chain, that appears to play a role in the polymerization process. In addition, secreted IgA expresses a chain, secretory piece, that is derived from the receptor for polymeric IgA, which plays a role in the transport of IgA across the cells lining the lumen of the gut.

Each of the distinct Igs can exist as secreted antibodies and as membrane molecules. Antibodies and cell surface receptors of the same class made by a specific cell have identical structures except for differences in their carboxy-terminal regions. Membrane Igs possess a hydrophobic region, spanning the membrane, and a short intracytoplasmic tail, both of which are lacking in the secretory form.

Immunoglobulin Genetics (Chapter 6)

The components of the Ig H chain gene have already been alluded to. To reiterate, the IgH chain gene of a mature lymphocyte is derived from a set of genetic elements that are separated from one another in the germline. The V region is composed of three types of genetic elements: V_H, D, and J_H. More than 100 V_H elements exist; there are more than 10 D elements and a small number of J_H elements (four in the mouse). An H chain $V_H D J_H$ gene is created by the translocation of one of the D elements on a given chromosome to one of the J_H elements on that chromosome, generally with the excision of the intervening DNA. This is followed by a second translocation event in which one of the V_H elements is brought into apposition with the assembled DJ_H element to create the $V_H D J_H$ (V region) gene (Figure 1.3). Although it is likely that the choice of the V_H, D, and J_H elements that are assembled is not entirely random, the combinatorial process allows the creation of a very large number of distinct H chain V region genes.

Additional diversity is created by the imprecision of the joining events and by the deletion of nucleotides and addition of new, untemplated nucleotides between D and J_H and between V_H and D, forming N regions in these areas. This further increases the diversity of distinct IgH chains that can be generated from the relatively modest amount of genetic information present in the germline.

The assembly of L chain genes follows generally similar rules. However, L chains are assembled from V_L and J_L elements only. Although there is junctional diversity, no N regions exist for L chains. Addition diversity is provided by the existence of two classes of L chains, κ, and λ.

An Ig molecule is assembled by the pairing of an IgH chain polypeptide with an IgL chain polypeptide. Although this process is almost certainly not completely random, it allows the formation of an exceedingly large number of distinct Ig molecules, the majority of which will have individual specificities.

The rearrangement events that result in the assembly of expressible IgH and IgL chains occur in the course of B cell development in pro-B cells and pre-B cells, respectively (Figure 1.1). This process is regulated by the Ig products of the rearrangement events. The formation of a μ chain signals the termination of rearrangement of H chain gene elements and the onset of rearrangement of L chain gene elements, with κ rearrangements generally preceding λ rearrangements. One important consequence of this is that only a single expressible μ chain will be produced in a given cell, since the first expressible μ chain shuts off the possibility of producing an expressible μ chain on the alternative chromosome. Comparable mechanisms exist to ensure that only one L chain gene is produced, leading to the phenomenon known as *allelic exclusion*. Thus, the product of only one of the two alternative allelic regions at both the H and L chain loci are expressed. The closely related phenomenon of L chain isotype exclusion ensures the production of either κ or λ chains in an individual cell, but not both. An obvious but critical consequence of allelic exclusion is that in most cases an individual B cell makes antibodies, all of which have identical H and L chain V regions, a central prediction of the clonal selection theory of the immune response. During the process of receptor editing, secondary rearrangements may occur, and, in some instances, the receptor editing process is associated with the expression of both κ and λ L chain genes by an individual B cells

Class Switching (Chapter 6)

An individual B cell continues to express the same IgH chain V region as it matures but it can switch the IgH chain C region it uses (Figure 1.3). Thus, a cell that expresses receptors of the IgM and IgD classes may differentiate into a cell that expresses IgG, IgA, or IgE receptors and then into a cell-secreting antibody of the same class as it expressed on the cell surface. This process allows the production of antibodies capable of mediating distinct biologic functions but that retain the same antigen-combining specificity. When linked with the process of affinity maturation of antibodies, Ig class switching provides antibodies of extremely high efficacy in preventing reinfection with microbial pathogens or in rapidly eliminating such pathogens. The associated phenomena of class switching and affinity maturation account for the high degree of effectiveness of antibodies produced in secondary immune responses.

The process of class switching is known to involve a recombination event between specialized switch (S) regions, containing repetitive sequences, that are located upstream of each C region (with the exception of the δ C region). Thus, the S region upstream of the μ C_H region gene (Sμ) recombines with an S region upstream of a more 3′ isotype, such as Sγ1, to create a chimeric Sμ/Sγ1 region and in the deletion of the intervening DNA (Figure 1.7). The genes encoding the C regions of the various γ chains (in the human γ1, γ2, γ3, and γ4; in the mouse γ1, γ2a, γ2b, and γ3), of the α chain, and of the ε chain are located 3′ of the Cμ and Cδ genes.

The induction of the switching process is dependent on the action of a specialized set of B cell stimulants. Of these, the most widely studied are CD154, expressed on the surface of activated T cells, and the TLR ligands such as bacterial lipopolysaccharide (LPS). The targeting of the C region that will be expressed as a result of switching is largely determined by cytokines. Thus, IL-4 determines that switch events in the human and mouse will be to the ε C region and to the γ4 (human) or γ1 (mouse) C regions. In the

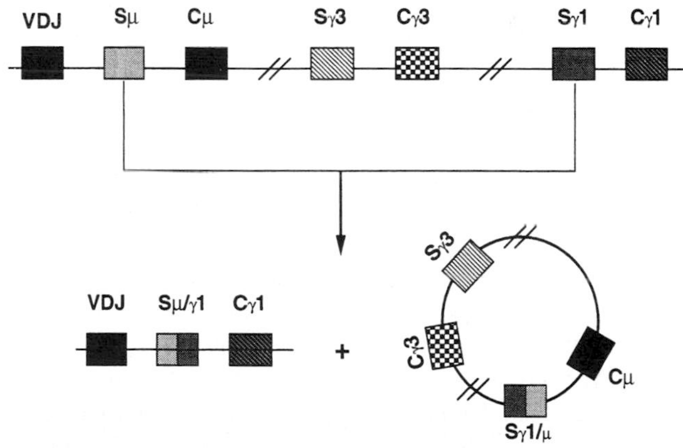

FIGURE 1.7 Ig class switching. The process through which a given VDJ gene in a stimulated B cell may switch the C region gene with which it is associated from μ to another, such as γ1, is illustrated. A recombination event occurs in which DNA between a cleavage point in Sμ and one in Sγ1 forms a circular episome. This results in Cγ1 being located immediately downstream of the chimeric Sμ/γ1 region, in a position such that transcription initiating upstream of VDJ results in the formation of VDJCγ1 mRNA and γ1 H-chain protein.

mouse, interferon-gamma (IFN-γ) determines switching to γ2a and transforming growth factor-beta (TGF-β) determines switching to α. A major goal is to understand the physiologic determination of the specificity of the switching process. Because cytokines are often the key controllers of which Ig classes will represent the switched isotype, this logically translates into asking what regulates the relative amounts of particular cytokines that are produced by different modes of immunization.

As already noted, both the switching process and somatic hypermutation depend upon the AID. Mice and humans that lack AID fail to undergo both Ig class switching and somatic hypermutation.

Affinity Maturation and Somatic Hypermutation (Chapters 6 and 9)

The process of generation of diversity embodied in the construction of the H and L chain V region genes and of the pairing of H and L chains creates a large number of distinct antibody molecules, each expressed in an individual B cell. This primary repertoire is sufficiently large so that most epitopes on foreign antigens will encounter B cells with complementary receptors. Thus, if adequate T cell help can be generated, antibody responses can be made to a wide array of foreign substances. Nonetheless, the antibody that is initially produced usually has a relatively low affinity for the antigen. This is partially compensated for by the fact that IgM, the antibody initially made, is a pentamer. Through multivalent binding, high avidities can be achieved even if individual combining sites have only modest affinity (see Chapter 5). In the course of T cell–dependent B cell stimulation, particularly within the GC, a process of somatic hypermutation is initiated that leads to a large number of mutational events, largely confined to the H chain and L chain V region genes and their immediately surrounding introns.

During the process of somatic hypermutation, mutational rates of 1 per 1,000 base pairs per generation may be achieved. This implies that, with each cell division, close to one mutation will occur in either the H or L chain V region of an individual cell. This creates an enormous increase in antibody diversity. Although most of these mutations will either not affect the affinity with which the antibody binds its ligand or will lower that affinity, some will increase it. Thus, some B cells emerge that can bind antigen more avidly than the initial population of responding cells. Because there is an active process of apoptosis in the GC from which B cells can be rescued by the binding of antigen to their membrane receptors, cells with the most avid receptors should have an advantage over other antigen-specific B cells and should come to dominate the population of responding cells. Thus, upon rechallenge, the affinity of antibody produced will be greater than that in the initial response. As time after immunization elapses, the affinity of antibody produced will increase. This process leads to the presence in immunized individuals of high-affinity antibodies that are much more effective, on a weight basis, in protecting against microbial agents and other antigen-bearing pathogens than was the antibody initially produced. Together with antibody class switching, affinity maturation results in the increased effectiveness of antibody in preventing reinfection with agents with which the individual has had a prior encounter.

T LYMPHOCYTES

T lymphocytes constitute the second major class of lymphocytes. They derive from precursors in hematopoietic tissue, undergo differentiation in the thymus (hence the name *thymus-derived [T] lymphocytes*) and are then seeded to the peripheral lymphoid tissue and to the recirculating pool of lymphocytes (see Chapter 12). T cells are subdivided into two distinct classes based on the cell surface receptors they express. The majority of T cells express antigen-binding receptors (TCRs) consisting of α and β chains. A second group of T cells express receptors made up of γ and δ chains. Among the α/β T cells are two important sublineages: those that express the coreceptor molecule CD4 (CD4 T cells) and those that express CD8 (CD8 T cells). These cells differ in how they recognize antigen and mediate different types of regulatory and effector functions.

CD4 T cells are the major *helper* cells of the immune system. Their helper function depends both on cell surface molecules such as CD154, induced upon these cells when they are activated, and on the wide array of cytokines they secrete when activated. CD4 T cells tend to differentiate, as a consequence of priming, into cells that principally secrete the cytokines IL-4, IL-13, IL-5, IL-6, and IL-10 (T_{H2} cells), into cells that mainly produce IFN-γ and lymphotoxin (T_{H1} cells) or into cells that produce IL-17 and related cytokines (T_{H17} cells). T_{H2} cells are very effective in helping B cells develop into antibody-producing cells, T_{H1} cells are effective inducers of cellular immune responses, involving enhancement in the microbicidal activity of monocytes and macrophages and consequent increased efficiency in lysing microorganisms in intracellular vesicular compartments, while T_{H17} cells are efficient recruiters of granulocytes and other cells of the inflammatory system and play a major role in responses to extracellular bacterial pathogens. Naïve CD4 T cells can also be stimulated to differentiate into induced regulatory T cells (iT_{regs}). However, most T_{regs} develop as a independent lineage of CD4 T cells. T_{regs} express the forkhead transcription factor Foxp3 and many express large amounts of the α chain of the IL-2 receptor (CD25).

T cells mediate important effector functions. Some of these are determined by the patterns of cytokines they

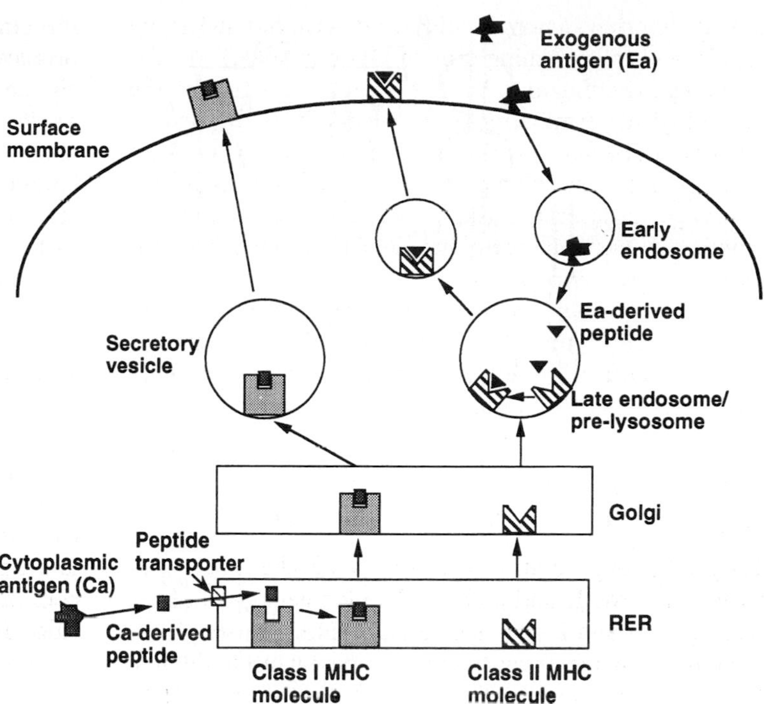

FIGURE 1.8 Pathways of antigen processing. Exogenous antigen (Ea) enters the cell via endocytosis and is transported from early endosomes into late endosome or prelysosomes, where it is fragmented and where resulting peptides (Ea derived peptides) may be loaded into class II MHC molecules. The latter have been transported from the RER through the Golgi apparatus to the peptide-containing vesicles. Class II MHC molecules–Ea-derived peptide complexes are then transported to the cell surface, where they may be recognized by TCR expressed on CD4+ T cells. Cytoplasmic antigens (Ca) are degraded in the cytoplasm and then enter the RER through a peptide transporter. In the RER, Ca-derived peptides are loaded into class I MHC molecules that move through the Golgi apparatus into secretory vesicles and are then expressed on the cell surface where they may be recognized by $CD8^+$ T cells (Reprinted with permission from Paul WE, in Gallin JI, Goldstein, I, Snyderman, R, eds. *Inflammation*. New York: Raven, 1992:776.)

secrete. These powerful molecules can be directly toxic to target cells and can mobilize potent inflammatory mechanisms. In addition, T cells, particularly CD8 T cells, can develop into cytotoxic T lymphocytes (CTLs) capable of efficiently lysing target cells that express antigens recognized by the CTLs.

T Lymphocyte Antigen Recognition (Chapters 10, 20, and 21)

T cells differ from B cells in their mechanism of antigen recognition. Ig, the BCR's receptor, binds to individual antigenic epitopes on soluble molecules or on particulate surfaces. BCRs recognize epitopes expressed on the surface of native molecules. Antibody and BCRs evolved to bind to and to protect against microorganisms in extracellular fluids.

By contrast, T cells invariably recognize cell-associated molecules and mediate their functions by interacting with and altering the behavior of such *antigen-presenting cells* (APCs). Indeed, the TCR does not recognize antigenic determinants on intact, undenatured molecules. Rather, it recognizes a complex consisting of a peptide, derived by proteolysis of the antigen, bound into a specialized groove of a class II or class I MHC protein. Indeed, what differentiates a CD4 T cell from a CD8 T cell is that the CD4 T cells recognize peptide–class II complexes, whereas the CD8 T cells recognize peptide–class I complexes.

The TCR's ligand (i.e., the peptide–MHC protein complex) is created within the APC. In general, class II MHC molecules bind peptides derived from proteins that have been taken up by the APC through an endocytic process (Figure 1.8). These endocytosed proteins are fragmented by proteolytic enzymes within the endosomal/lysosomal compartment, and the resulting peptides are loaded into class II MHC that traffic through this compartment. Peptide-loaded class II molecules are then expressed on the surface of the APC where they are available to be bound by CD4 T cells that have TCRs capable of recognizing the expressed cell surface peptide–MHC protein complex. Thus, CD4 T cells are specialized to largely react with antigens derived from extracellular sources.

In contrast, class I MHC molecules are mainly loaded with peptides derived from internally synthesized proteins, such as viral gene products. These peptides are produced from cytosolic proteins by proteolysis within the proteasome and are translocated into the rough endoplasmic reticulum. Such peptides, generally nine amino acids in length, are bound by class I MHC molecules. The complex is brought to the cell surface, where it can be recognized by CD8 T cells expressing appropriate receptors. This property gives the T cell system, particularly CD8 T cells, the ability to detect cells expressing proteins that are different from, or produced in much larger amounts than, those of cells of the remainder of the organism (e.g., viral antigens [whether internal, envelope, or cell surface] or mutant antigens [e.g., active oncogene products]), even if these proteins, in their intact form, are neither expressed on the cell surface nor secreted.

Although this division of class I–binding peptides being derived from internally synthesized proteins and class II–binding peptides from imported proteins is generally

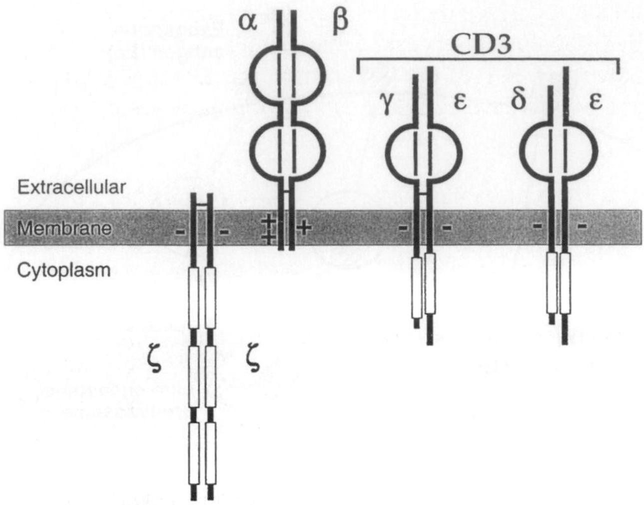

FIGURE 1.9 The T cell antigen receptor. Illustrated schematically is the antigen binding subunit comprised of an $\alpha\beta$ heterodimer, and the associated invariant CD3 and ζ chains. Acidic (–) and basic (+) residues located within the plasma membrane are indicated. The open rectangular boxes indicate motifs within the cytoplasmic domains that interact with protein tyrosine kinases.

correct, there are important exceptions to this rule that are central for the function of the immune system. The most effective priming of naïve CD8 T cells occurs in response to peptide–MHC-I complexes expressed by DCs, and yet many viruses do not infect these cells but rather target other cell types. It is now recognized that viral antigens produced by infected cells can be taken up by DCs and loaded into class I molecules in a process referred to as cross-presentation.

T Lymphocyte Receptors (Chapter 10)

The TCR is a disulfide-linked heterodimer (Figure 1.9). Its constituent chains (α and β, or γ and δ) are Ig supergene family members. The TCR is associated with a set of transmembrane proteins, collectively designated the CD3 complex, that play a critical role in signal transduction. The CD3 complex consists of γ, δ (note that the CD3 γ and δ chains and the TCR γ and δ chains are distinct polypeptides that, unfortunately, have similar designations), and ε chains and is associated with a homodimer of two ζ chains or a heterodimer of ζ and η chains. CD3 γ, δ, and ε consist of extracellular domains that are Ig supergene family members. The cytosolic domains of CD3 γ, δ, and ε and of ζ and η contain one or more copies of the immunoreceptor tyrosine-based activation motif (ITAM) (D/ExxYxxLxxxxxxxYxxL/I) that is found in a variety of chains associated with immune recognition receptors. This motif appears to be very important in the signal transduction process and provides a site through which protein tyrosine kinases can interact with these chains to propagate signaling events.

The TCR chains are organized much like Ig chains. Their N-terminal portions are variable and their C-terminal portions are constant. Furthermore, similar recombination mechanisms are used to assemble the V-region genes of the TCR chains. Thus, the V region of the TCR β chain is encoded by a gene constructed from three distinct genetic elements ($V\beta$, D, and $J\beta$) that are separated in the germline. Although the relative numbers of $V\beta$, D, and $J\beta$ genes differ from that for the comparable IgH variable region elements, the strategies for creation of a very large number of distinct genes by combinatorial assembly are the same. Both junctional diversity and N region addition further diversify the genes, and their encoded products. TCR β has fewer V genes than IgH but much more diversity centered on the D/J region, which encodes the equivalent of the third CDR of Igs. The α chain follows similar principles, except that it does not use a D gene.

The genes for TCR γ and δ chains are assembled in a similar manner except that they have many fewer V genes from which to choose. Indeed, γ/δ T cells in certain environments, such as the skin and specific mucosal surfaces, are exceptionally homogeneous. It has been suggested that the TCRs encoded by these essentially invariant γ and δ chains may be specific for some antigen that signals microbial invasion and that activation of γ/δ T cells through this mechanism constitutes an initial response that aids the development of the more sophisticated response of α/β T cells.

T Lymphocyte Activation (Chapter 11)

T cell activation is dependent on the interaction of the TCR–CD3 complex with its cognate ligand, a peptide bound in the groove of a class I or class II MHC molecule, on the surface of a competent APC. Through the use of chimeric cell surface molecules that possess cytosolic domains largely limited to the ITAM signaling motif alluded to earlier, it is clear that cross-linkage of molecules containing such domains can generate some of the signals that result from TCR engagement. Nonetheless, the molecular events set in motion by receptor engagement are complex ones. Among the earliest steps are the activation of tyrosine kinases leading to the tyrosine phosphorylation of a set of substrates that control several signaling pathways. Current evidence indicates that early events in this process involve the src family tyrosine kinases $p56^{lck}$, associated with the cytosolic domains of the CD4 and CD8 coreceptors, and $p59^{fyn}$, and ZAP-70, a Syk family tyrosine kinase that binds to the phosphorylated ITAMs of the ζ chain. The protein tyrosine phosphatase CD45, found on the surface of all T cells, also plays a critical role in T cell activation.

A series of important substrates are tyrosine phosphorylated as a result of the action of the kinases associated with the TCR complex. These include a (i) set of adapter proteins that link the TCR to the ras pathway; (ii) phospholipase Cγ1, the tyrosine phosphorylation of which increases its catalytic activity and engages the inositol phospholipid metabolic pathway, leading to elevation of intracellular free calcium concentration and activation of protein kinase C; and (iii) a series of other important enzymes that control cellular growth and differentiation. Particularly important is the phosphorylation of LAT, a molecule that acts as an organizing scaffold to which a series of signaling intermediates bind and upon which they become activated and control downstream signaling.

The recognition and early activation events result in the reorganization of cell surface and cytosolic molecules on the T cell, and correspondingly, on the APC to produce a structure, the *immunological synapse*. The apposition of key interacting molecules involving a small segment of the membranes of the two cells concentrates these interacting molecules in a manner that both strengthens the interaction between the cells and intensifies the signaling events. It also creates a limited space into which cytokines may be secreted to influence the behavior of the interacting cells. The formation of the immunological synapse is one mechanism through which the recognition of relatively small numbers of ligands by TCRs on a specific T cell can be converted into a vigorous stimulatory process.

In general, normal T cells and cloned T cell lines that are stimulated only by TCR cross-linkage fail to give complete responses. TCR engagement by itself may often lead to a response in which the key T cell–derived growth factor, IL-2, is not produced and in which the cells enter a state of anergy such that they are unresponsive or poorly responsive to a subsequent competent stimulus (see Chapter 29). Full responsiveness of a T cell requires, in addition to receptor engagement, an accessory cell–delivered costimulatory activity. The engagement of CD28 on the T cell by CD80 or CD86 on the APC (or the engagement of comparable ligand/receptor pairs on the two cells) provides a potent costimulatory activity. Inhibitors of this interaction markedly diminish antigen-specific T cell activation *in vivo* and *in vitro*, indicating that the CD80/86–CD28 interaction is physiologically very important in T cell activation (see Chapters 13 and 15).

The interaction of CD80/86 with CD28 increases cytokine production by the responding T cells. For the production of IL-2, this increase appears to be mediated both by enhancing the transcription of the IL-2 gene and by stabilizing IL-2 mRNA. These dual consequences of the CD80/86–CD28 interaction cause a striking increase in the production of IL-2 by antigen-stimulated T cells.

CD80/86 has a second receptor on the T cell, CTLA-4, that is expressed later in the course of T cell activation. The bulk of evidence indicates that the engagement of CTLA-4 by CD80/86 leads to a set of biochemical signals that terminate the T cell response. Mice that are deficient in CTLA-4 expression develop fulminant autoimmune responses.

T Lymphocyte Development (Chapter 12)

Upon entry into the thymus, T cell precursors do not express TCR chains, the CD3 complex, or the CD4 or CD8 molecules (Figure 1.10). Because these cells lack both CD4 and CD8, they are often referred to as *double-negative (DN) cells*. Thymocytes develop from this DN pool into cells that are both CD4$^+$ and CD8$^+$ (double-positive cells) and express low levels of TCR and CD3 on their surface. In turn, double-positive cells further differentiate into relatively mature thymocytes that express either CD4 or CD8 (single-positive cells) and high levels of the TCR–CD3 complex.

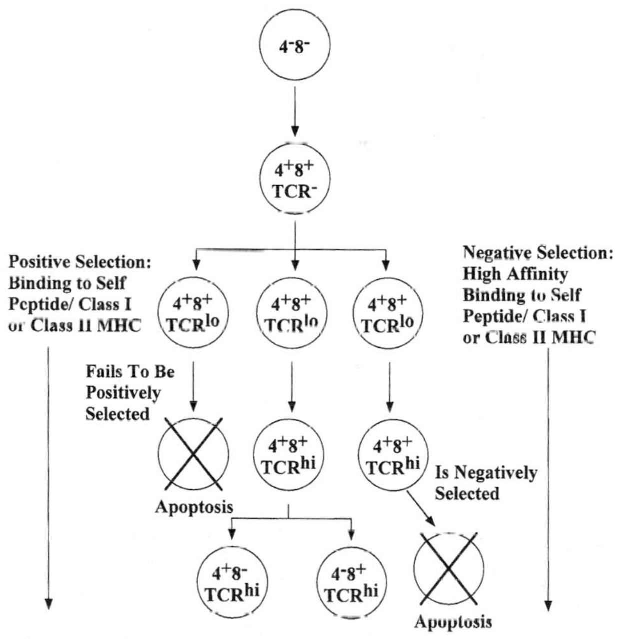

FIGURE 1.10 Development of α/β T cells in the thymus. Double-negative T cells (4^-8^-) acquire CD4 and CD8 (4^+8^+) and then express α/β TCRs, initially at low levels. Thereafter, the degree of expression of TCRs increases and the cells differentiate into CD4 or CD8 cells and are then exported to the periphery. Once the T cells have expressed receptors, their survival depends upon the recognition of peptide/MHC class I or class II molecules with an affinity above some given threshold. Cells that fail to do so undergo apoptosis. These cells have failed to be *positively selected*. Positive selection is associated with the differentiation of 4^+8^+ cells into CD4 or CD8 cells. Positive selection involving peptide/class I MHC molecules leads to the development of CD8 cells whereas positive selection involving peptide/class II MHC molecules leads to the development of CD4 cells. If a T cell recognizes a peptide/MHC complex with high affinity, it is also eliminated via apoptosis (it is *negatively selected*).

The expression of the TCR depends on complex rearrangement processes that generate TCR α and β (or γ and δ) chains. Once TCR chains are expressed, these cells undergo two important selection processes within the thymus. One, termed *negative selection,* is the deletion of cells that express receptors that bind with high affinity to complexes of self-peptides with self-MHC molecules. This is a major mechanism through which the T cell compartment develops immunologic unresponsiveness to self-antigens (see Chapters 12 and 29). In addition, a second major selection process is *positive selection,* in which T cells with receptors with "intermediate affinity" for self-peptides bound to self-MHC molecules are selected, thus forming the basis of the T cell repertoire for foreign peptides associated with self-MHC molecules. It appears that T cells that are not positively selected are eliminated in the thymic cortex by apoptosis. Similarly, T cells that are negatively selected as a result of high-affinity binding to self-peptide–self-MHC complexes are also deleted through apoptotic death. These two selection processes result in the development of a population of T cells that are biased toward the recognition of peptides in association with self-MHC molecules from which those cells that are potentially autoreactive (capable of high-affinity binding of self-peptide–self-MHC complexes) have been purged.

One important event in the development of T cells is their differentiation from double-positive cells into $CD4^+$ or $CD8^+$ single-positive cells. This process involves the interaction of double-positive thymocytes with peptide bound to class II or class I MHC molecules on accessory cells. Indeed, CD4 binds to monomorphic sites on class II molecules, whereas CD8 binds to comparable sites on class I molecules. The capacity of the TCR and CD4 (or of the TCR and CD8) to bind to a class II MHC (or a class I MHC) molecule on an accessory cell leads either to the differentiation of double-positive thymocytes into $CD4^+$ (or $CD8^+$) single-positive T cells or to the selection of cells that have "stochastically" differentiated down the CD4 (or CD8) pathway.

Less is understood about the differentiation of thymocytes that express TCRs composed of γ/δ chains. These cells fail to express either CD4 or CD8. However, γ/δ cells are relatively numerous early in fetal life; this, together with their limited degree of heterogeneity, suggests that they may comprise a relatively primitive T cell compartment.

T Lymphocyte Functions (Chapter 13)

T cells mediate a wide range of immunologic functions. These include the capacity to help B cells develop into antibody-producing cells, the capacity to increase the microbicidal action of monocyte/macrophages, the inhibition of certain types of immune responses, direct killing of target cells, and mobilization of the inflammatory response. In general, these effects depend on their expression of specific cell-surface molecules and the secretion of cytokines.

T Cells That Help Antibody Responses (Chapter 13)

Helper T cells can stimulate B cells to make antibody responses to proteins and other T cell–dependent antigens. T cell–dependent antigens are immunogens in which individual epitopes appear only once or only a limited number of times so that they are unable to cross-link the membrane Ig of B cells or do so inefficiently. B cells bind the antigen through their membrane Ig, and the complex undergoes endocytosis. Within the endosomal and lysosomal compartments, the antigen is fragmented into peptides by proteolytic enzymes and one or more of the generated peptides are loaded into class II MHC molecules, which traffic through this vesicular compartment. The resulting complex of class II MHC molecule and bound peptide is exported to the B cell surface membrane. T cells with receptors specific for the peptide/class II molecular complex recognize that complex on the B cell.

B cell activation depends not only on the binding of peptide–class II MHC complexes on the B cell surface by the TCR but also on the interaction of T cell CD154 with CD40 on the B cell. T cells do not constitutively express CD154; rather, it is induced as a result of an interaction with an activated APC that expresses a cognate antigen recognized by the TCR of the T cell. Further, CD80/86 are generally expressed by activated but not resting B cells so that interactions involving resting B cells and naïve T cells generally do not lead to efficient antibody production. By contrast, a T cell already activated and expressing CD154 can interact with a resting B cell, leading to its upregulation of CD80/86 and to a more productive T cell/B cell interaction with the delivery of cognate help and the development of the B cell into an antibody-producing cell. Similarly, activated B cells expressing large amounts of class II molecules and CD80/86 can act as effective APC and can participate with T cells in efficient cognate help interactions. Cross-linkage of membrane Ig on the B cell, even if inefficient, may synergize with the CD154/CD40 interaction to yield vigorous B cell activation.

The subsequent events in the B cell response program, including proliferation, Ig secretion, and class switching either depend on or are enhanced by the actions of T cell–derived cytokines. Thus, B cell proliferation and Ig secretion are enhanced by the actions of several type I cytokines, including IL-2 and IL-4. Ig class switching is dependent both on the initiation of competence for switching, which can be induced by the CD154/CD40 interaction, and on the targeting of particular C regions for switching, which is determined, in many instances, by cytokines. The best studied example of this is the role of IL-4 in determining switching to IgG1 and IgE in the mouse and to IgG4 and IgE in the human. Indeed, the central role of IL-4 in the production of IgE is demonstrated by the fact that mice that lack the IL-4 gene or the gene for the IL-4 receptor α chain, as a result of homologous recombination-mediated gene knockouts, have a marked defect in IgE production.

Although $CD4^+$ T cells with the phenotype of T_{H2} cells (i.e., IL-4, IL-13, IL-5, IL-6, and IL-10 producers) are efficient helper cells, T_{H1} and T_{H17} cells also have the capacity to act as helpers. Because T_{H1} cells produce IFN-γ, which acts as a switch factor for IgG2a in the mouse, T_{H1}-mediated help often is dominated by the production of IgG2a antibodies.

Induction of Cellular Immunity (Chapters 13 and 18)

T cells also may act to enhance the capacity of monocytes and macrophages to destroy intracellular microorganisms. In particular, IFN-γ enhances several mechanisms through which mononuclear phagocytes destroy intracellular bacteria and parasites, including the generation of nitric oxide and induction of tumor necrosis factor (TNF). T_{H1} cells are particularly effective in enhancing microbicidal action because they produce IFN-γ. By contrast, three of the major cytokines produced by T_{H2} cells, IL-4, IL-13 and IL-10, block these activities; IL-4 and IL-13 induce an alternative gene activation program in macrophages resulting in *alternatively activated macrophages*, characterized (in the mouse) by the expression of arginase 1 and chitinase. Thus, T_{H2} cells often oppose the action of T_{H1} cells in inducing cellular immunity and in certain infections with microorganisms that are intracellular pathogens of macrophages, a T_{H2}-dominated response may be associated with failure to control the infection.

Regulatory T Cells (Chapter 30)

There has been a longstanding interest in the capacity of T cells to diminish as well as to help immune responses. Cells that mediate such effects are referred to as T_{regs}. T_{regs} may be identified by their expression of Foxp3 and of CD25, the IL-2 receptor alpha chain. These cells inhibit the capacity of both CD4 and CD8 T cells to respond to their cognate antigens. The mechanisms through which their suppressor function is mediated are still somewhat controversial. In some instances, it appears that cell–cell contact is essential for suppression, whereas in other circumstances, production of cytokines by T_{regs} has been implicated in their ability to inhibit responses. Evidence has been presented for both IL-10 and TGFβ as mediators of inhibition.

T_{regs} have been particularly studied in the context of various autoimmune conditions. In the absence of T_{regs}, conventional T cells cause several types of autoimmune responses, including autoimmune gastritis and inflammatory bowel disease. T_{regs} express cell surface receptors, allowing them to recognize autoantigens and their responses to such recognition results in the suppression of responses by conventional T cells. Whether the receptor repertoire of T_{regs} and the conventional T cells are the same has not been fully determined, although there is increasing evidence that T_{regs} derive from a thymic CD4 T cell population with relativley high affinity for self-antigen. As noted earlier, iT_{regs} can be derived in the periphery from naïve CD4 T cell populations. This is seen when naive cells are stimulated by their cognate ligands in the presence of TGFβ.

Cytotoxic T Cells (Chapter 34)

One of the most striking actions of T cells is the lysis of cells expressing specific antigens. Most cells with such cytotoxic activity are CD8 T cells that recognize peptides derived from proteins produced within the target cell, bound to class I MHC molecules expressed on the surface of the target cell. However, CD4 T cells can express CTL activity, although in such cases the antigen recognized is a peptide associated with a class II MHC molecule; often such peptides derive from exogenous antigens.

There are two major mechanisms of cytotoxicity. One involves the production by the CTL of perforin, a molecule that can insert into the membrane of target cells and promote the lysis of that cell. Perforin-mediated lysis is enhanced by a series of enzymes produced by activated CTLs, referred to as *granzymes*. Many active CTLs also express large amounts of fas ligand on their surface. The interaction of fas ligand on the surface of the CTL with fas on the surface of the target cell initiates apoptosis in the target cell.

CTL-mediated lysis is a major mechanism for the destruction of virus-infected cells. If activated during the period in which the virus is in its eclipse phase, CTLs may be capable of eliminating virus and curing the host with relatively limited cell destruction. However, vigorous CTL activity after a virus has been widely disseminated may lead to substantial tissue injury because of the large number of cells that are killed by the action of the CTLs. Thus, in many infections, the disease is caused by the destruction of tissue by CTLs rather than by the virus itself. One example is hepatitis B, in which much of the liver damage represents the attack of HBV-specific CTLs on infected liver cells.

It is usually observed that CTLs that have been induced as a result of a viral infection or intentional immunization must be reactivated *in vitro* through the recognition of antigen on the target cell. This is particularly true if some interval has elapsed between the time of infection or immunization and the time of test. This has led to some question being raised as to the importance of CTL immunity in protection against reinfection and how important

CTL generation is in the long-term immunity induced by protective vaccines. However, in active infections, such as seen in HIV$^+$ individuals, CTL that can kill their targets cells immediately are often seen. There is much evidence to suggest that these cells play an active role in controlling the number of HIV$^+$ T cells.

CYTOKINES (Chapters 23, 24, 25, and 26)

Many of the functions of cells of the immune system are mediated through the production of a set of small proteins referred to as cytokines. These proteins can now be divided into several families. They include the type I cytokines or hematopoeitins that encompass many of the interleukins (i.e., IL-2, IL-3, IL-4, IL-5, IL-6, IL-7, IL-9, IL-11, IL-12, IL-13, IL-15, IL-21, IL-23, and IL-27), as well as several hematopoietic growth factors; the type II cytokines, including the interferons and IL-10; the TNF-related molecules, including TNF, lymphotoxin, and Fas ligand; Ig superfamily members, including IL-1, IL-18, and IL-33; and the chemokines, a growing family of molecules playing critical roles in a wide variety of immune and inflammatory functions. IL-17 and its congeners, including IL-25, constitute a structurally unique set of cytokines.

Many of the cytokines are T cell products; their production represents one of the means through which the wide variety of functions of T cells are mediated. Most cytokines are not constitutive products of the T cell. Rather, they are produced in response to T cell activation, usually resulting from presentation of antigen to T cells by APCs in concert with the action of a costimulatory molecule, such as the interaction of CD80/86 with CD28. Although cytokines are produced in small quantities, they are very potent, binding to their receptors with equilibrium constants of $\sim 10^{10}$ M^{-1}. In some instances, cytokines are directionally secreted into the immunological synapse formed between a T cell and an APC. In such cases, the cytokine acts in a paracrine manner. Indeed, many cytokines have limited action at a distance from the cell that produced them. This appears to be particularly true of many of the type I cytokines. However, other cytokines act by diffusion through extracellular fluids and blood to target cells that are distant from the producers. Among these are cytokines that have proinflammatory effects, such as IL-1, IL-6, and TNF, and the chemokines, that play important roles in regulating the migration of lymphocytes and other cell types.

Chemokines (Chapter 26)

A large family of small proteins that are *chemotactic cytokines* (chemokines) have been described. While members of this family have a variety of functions, perhaps the most dramatic is their capacity to regulate leukocyte migration and thus to act as critical dynamic organizers of cell distribution in the immune and inflammatory responses. The receptors for chemokines are seven transmembrane-spanning, G protein–coupled receptors.

The chemokines are subdivided based on the number and positioning of their highly conserved cysteines. Among chemokines with four conserved cysteines, the cysteines are adjacent in one large group (the CC chemokines) while in a second large group they are separated by one amino acid (CXC chemokines). There are also rare chemokines in which the cysteines are separated by three amino acids (CX3C) or in which there are only two conserved cysteines (C chemokines).

Individual chemokines may signal through more than one chemokine receptor and individual receptors may interact with more than one chemokine, producing a very complex set of chemokine/chemokine receptor pairs and providing opportunities for exceedingly fine regulation of cellular functions.

THE MAJOR HISTOCOMPATIBILITY COMPLEX AND ANTIGEN PRESENTATION (see Chapters 19 and 20)

The MHC has already been introduced in this chapter in the discussion of T cell recognition of antigen-derived peptides bound to specialized grooves in class I and class II MHC proteins. Indeed, the class I and class II MHC molecules are essential to the process of T cell recognition and response. Nonetheless, they were first recognized not for this reason but because of the dominant role that MHC class I and class II proteins play in transplantation immunity (see Chapter 44).

When the genetic basis of transplantation rejection between mice of distinct inbred strains was sought, it was recognized that although multiple genetic regions contributed to the rejection process, one region played a dominant role. Differences at this region alone would cause prompt graft rejection, whereas any other individual difference usually resulted in a slow rejection of foreign tissue. For this reason, the genetic region responsible for prompt graft rejection was termed the *major histocompatibility complex*.

In all higher vertebrates that have been thoroughly studied, a comparable MHC exists. The defining features of the MHC are the transplantation antigens that it encodes. These are the class I and class II MHC molecules. The genes encoding these molecules show an unprecedented degree of polymorphism. This, together with their critical role in antigen presentation, explains their central role as the target of the immune responses leading to the rejection of organ and tissue allografts.

The MHC also includes other genes, particularly genes for certain complement components. In addition, genes for the cytokines TNF-α and lymphotoxin (also designated TNF-β) are found in the MHC.

Class I MHC Molecules (Chapter 19)

Class I MHC molecules are membrane glycoproteins expressed on most cells. They consist of an α chain of approximately 45,000 daltons noncovalently associated with $\beta 2$-microglobulin, a 12,000-dalton molecule (Figure 1.11). The gene for the α chain is encoded in the MHC, whereas that for $\beta 2$-microglobulin is not. Both the α chain and $\beta 2$-microglobulin are Ig supergene family members. The α chain is highly polymorphic, with the polymorphisms found mainly in the regions that constitute the binding sites for antigen-derived peptides and that are contact sites for the TCR.

The class I α chain consists of three extracellular regions or domains, each of similar length, designated $\alpha 1$, $\alpha 2$, and $\alpha 3$. In addition, α chains have a membrane-spanning domain and a short carboxy-terminal cytoplasmic tail. The crystal structure of class I molecules indicates that the $\alpha 1$ and $\alpha 2$ domains form a site for the binding of peptides derived from antigens. This site is defined by a floor consisting of β sheets and bounded by α-helical walls. The polymorphisms of the class I molecule are mainly in these areas.

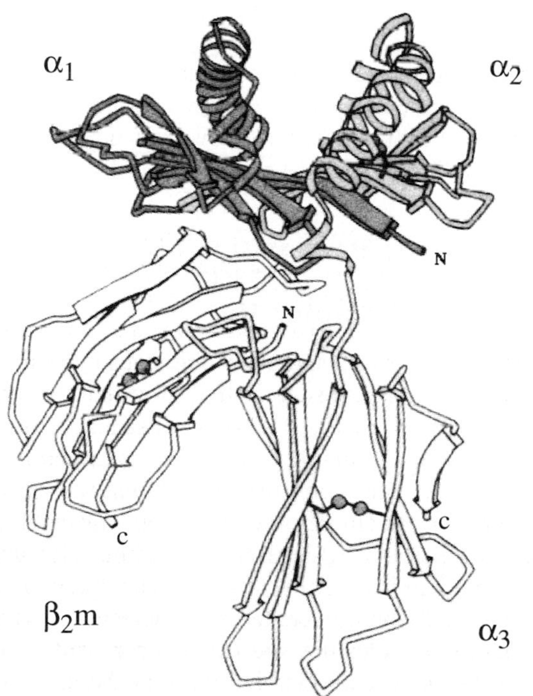

FIGURE 1.11 Model of the class I HLA-A2 molecule. A schematic representation of the structure of the HLA-A2 class I MHC molecule. The polymorphic $\alpha 1$ and $\alpha 2$ domains are at the top. They form a groove into which antigen-derived peptides fit to form the peptide–MHC class I complex that is recognized by TCRs of $CD8^+$ T cells. (Reprinted from Bjorkman PJ, et al. *Nature.* 1987;329:506–512).

In the human, three loci encoding classical class I molecules have been defined; these are designated HLA-A, HLA-B, and HLA-C. All display high degrees of polymorphism. A similar situation exists in the mouse. In addition, there are a series of genes that encode class I–like molecules (class Ib molecules). Some of these have been shown to have antigen-presenting activity for formulated peptides, suggesting that they may be specialized to present certain prokaryotic antigens. The class Ib molecule CD1 has been shown to have antigen-presenting function for mycobacterial lipids, providing a mechanism through which T cells specific for such molecules can be generated. CD1d, presenting certain endogenous or exogenous phospholipids, is recognized by a novel class of T cells (NK T cells) that produce large amounts of cytokines upon immediate stimulation.

Class II MHC Molecules (see Chapter 19)

Class II MHC molecules are heterodimeric membrane glycoproteins. Their constituent chains are designated α and β; both chains are Ig supergene family members, and both are encoded within the MHC. Each chain consists of two extracellular domains ($\alpha 1$ and $\alpha 2$; $\beta 1$ and $\beta 2$, respectively), a hydrophobic domain, and a short cytoplasmic segment. The overall conformation of class II MHC molecules appears to be quite similar to that of class I molecules. The peptide-binding site of the class II molecules is contributed to by the $\alpha 1$ and $\beta 1$ domains (Figure 1.5); it is within these domains that the majority of the polymorphic residues of class II molecules are found.

A comparison of the three-dimensional structures of class I and class II molecules indicates certain distinctive features that explain differences in the length of peptides that the two types of MHC molecules can bind. Class I molecules generally bind peptides with a mean length of nine amino acids, whereas class II molecules can bind substantially larger peptides.

In the mouse, class II MHC molecules are encoded by genes within the I region of the MHC. These molecules are often referred to as I region–associated (Ia) antigens. Two sets of class II molecules exist, designated I-A and I-E, respectively. The α and β chains of the I-A molecules (Aα and Aβ) pair with one another, as do the α and β chains of I-E (Eα and Eβ). In heterozygous mice, α and β chains encoded on alternative chromosomes (i.e., $A\alpha^b$ and $A\beta^k$) may cross-pair so that heterozygous mice can express both parental and hybrid class II molecules. However, the degree of cross-pairing is allele specific; not all hybrid pairs are formed with equal efficiency.

In the human, there are three major sets of class II molecules, encoded in the DR, DQ, and DP regions of the HLA complex.

Class II molecules have a more restricted tissue distribution than do class I molecules. Class II molecules are found on B cells, DCs, epidermal Langerhans cells, macrophages, thymic epithelial cells, and, in the human, activated T cells. Levels of class II molecule expression are regulated in many cell types by interferons and in B cells by IL-4. Indeed, interferons can cause expression of class II molecules on many cell types that normally lack these cell surface molecules. Interferons also can cause striking upregulation in the expression of class I MHC molecules. Thus, immunologically mediated inflammation may result in aberrant expression of class II MHC molecules and heightened expression of class I molecules. Such altered expression of MHC molecules can allow cells that do not normally function as APCs for $CD4^+$ T cells to do so and enhances the sensitivity of such cells to CD8 T cells. This has important consequences for immunopathologic responses and for autoimmunity.

Antigen Presentation (Chapter 20)

As already discussed, the function of class I and class II MHC molecules is to bind and present antigen-derived peptides to T cells whose receptors can recognize the peptide–MHC complex that is generated. There are two major types of antigen-processing pathways, specialized to deal with distinct classes of pathogens that the T cell system must confront (Figure 1.8).

Extracellular bacteria and extracellular proteins may enter APCs by endocytosis or phagocytosis. Their antigens and the antigens of bacteria that live within endosomes or lysosomes are fragmented in these organelles and peptides derived from the antigen are loaded into class II MHC molecules as these proteins traverse the vesicular compartments in which the peptides are found. The loading of peptide is important in stabilizing the structure of the class II MHC molecule. The acidic pH of the compartments in which loading occurs facilitates the loading process. However, once the peptide-loaded class II molecules reach neutral pH, such as at the cell surface, the peptide–MHC complex is very stable. Peptide dissociation from such class II molecules is very slow, with a half-time measured in hours. The peptide–class II complex is recognized by T cells of the CD4 class with complementary receptors. As already pointed out, the specialization of CD4 T cells to recognize peptide–class II complexes is partly due to the affinity of the CD4 molecule for monomorphic determinants on class II molecules. Obviously, this form of antigen processing can only apply to cells that express class II MHC molecules. Indeed, APCs for CD4 T cells principally include cells that normally express class II MHC molecules, including DCs, B cells, and macrophages.

T cells also can recognize proteins that are produced within the cell that presents the antigen. The major pathogens recognized by this means are viruses and other obligate intracellular (non–endosomal/lysosomal) microbes that have infected cells. In addition, proteins that are unique to tumors, such as mutant oncogenes, or are overexpressed in tumors also can be recognized by T cells. Endogenously produced proteins are fragmented in the cytosol by the proteases in the proteasome. The resultant peptides are transported into the rough endoplasmic reticulum through the action of a specialized transport system. These peptides are then available for loading into class I molecules. In contrast to the loading of class II molecules, which is facilitated by the acid pH of the loading environment, the loading of class I molecules is controlled by interaction of the class I α chain with $\beta 2$-microglobulin. Thus, the bond between peptide and class I molecule is generally weak in the absence of $\beta 2$-microglobulin, and the binding of $\beta 2$-microglobulin strikingly stabilizes the complex. (Similarly, the binding of $\beta 2$-microglobulin to the α chain is markedly enhanced by the presence of peptide in the α chain groove.) The peptide-loaded class I molecule is then brought to the cell surface. In contrast to peptide-loaded class II molecules that are recognized by CD4 T cells, peptide-loaded class I molecules are recognized by CD8 T cells. This form of antigen processing and presentation can be performed by virtually all cells because, with a few exceptions, class I MHC molecules are universally expressed.

Although the specialization of class I molecules to bind and present endogenously produced peptides and of class II molecules to bind and present peptides derived from exogenous antigens is generally correct, there are exceptions, many of which have physiologic importance. Particularly important is the representation by class II^+ cells of antigens derived from class II^- cells.

T Lymphocyte Recognition of Peptide–MHC Complexes Results in MHC-Restricted Recognition (Chapter 10)

Befor the biochemical nature of the interaction between antigen-derived peptides and MHC molecules was recognized, it was observed that T cell responses displayed *MHC-restricted antigen recognition*. Thus, if individual animals were primed to a given antigen, their T cells would be able to recognize and respond to that antigen only if the APCs that presented the antigen shared MHC molecules with the animal that had been immunized. The antigen would not be recognized when presented by APCs of an allogeneic MHC type. This can now be explained by the fact that the TCR recognizes peptide bound to an MHC molecule. MHC molecules display high degrees of polymorphism, and this polymorphism is concentrated in the regions of the class I and class II molecules that interact with the peptide and that can bind to the TCR. Differences in structure of the MHC molecules derived from different individuals (or different inbred strains of mice) profoundly affect the recognition process. Two obvious explanations exist to account for this. First, the structure of the grooves in different class I or class II MHC molecules may determine that a different range of peptides are bound or, even if the same peptide is bound, may change the conformation of the surface of the peptide presented to the TCR. Second, polymorphic sites on the walls of the α-helices that are exposed to the TCR can either enhance or diminish binding of the whole complex, depending on their structure. Thus, priming an individual with a given antigen on APCs that are syngeneic to the individual will elicit a response by T cells whose TCRs are specific for a complex consisting of a peptide derived from the antigen and the exposed polymorphic residues of the MHC molecule. When the same antigen is used with APCs of different MHC type, it is unlikely that the same peptide/MHC surface can be formed, and thus the primed T cells are not likely to bind and respond to such stimulation.

Indeed, this process also occurs within the thymus in the generation of the T cell repertoire, as already discussed. T cells developing within the thymus undergo a positive selection event in which those T cells capable of recognizing MHC molecules displayed within the thymus are selected (and the remainder undergo programmed cell death). This leads to the skewing of the population of T cells that emerges from the thymus so that the cells are specialized to respond to peptides on self-MHC molecules. One of the unsolved enigmas of positive selection within the thymus is how the vast array of T cells with receptors capable of reacting with a very large set of foreign peptides associated with self-MHC molecules are chosen by self-MHC molecules that can only display self peptides. It is believed that a high degree of cross-reactivity may exist so that T cells selected to bind a given class I (or class II) molecule plus a particular self-peptide can also bind a set of other (foreign) peptides bound to the same MHC molecule. Further, the affinity of an interaction required for positive selection in the thymus appears to be considerably lower than that required for full activation of peripheral T cells. Thus, thymocytes selected by a given self-peptide–self-MHC complex will generally not mount a full response when they encounter the same peptide–MHC complex in the periphery, although they will respond to a set of foreign peptide–MHC complexes to which they bind with higher affinity. Recognition of the self-peptide–self-MHC complex in the periphery may nonetheless have important consequences such as sustaining the viability of resting lymphocytes.

Our modern understanding of T cell recognition also aids in explaining the phenomenon of immune response (Ir) gene control of specific responses. In many situations, the capacity to recognize simple antigens can be found in only some members of a species. In most such cases, the genes that determine the capacity to make these responses have been mapped to the MHC. We would now explain Ir gene control of immune responses based on the capacity of different class II MHC molecules (or class I MHC molecules) to bind different sets of peptides. Thus, for simple molecules, it is likely that peptides can be generated that are only capable of binding to some of the polymorphic MHC molecules of the species. Only individuals who possess those allelic forms of the MHC will be able to respond to those antigens. Based on this, some individuals are nonresponders because of the failure to generate a peptide–MHC molecule complex that can be recognized by the T cell system.

This mechanism also may explain the linkage of MHC type with susceptibility to various diseases. Many diseases show a greater incidence in individuals of a given MHC type. These include reactive arthritides, gluten-sensitive enteropathy, insulin-dependent diabetes mellitus, and rheumatoid arthritis (see Chapters 41 and 42). One explanation is that the MHC type that is associated with increased incidence may convey altered responsiveness to antigens of agents that cause or exacerbate the disease. Indeed, it appears that many of these diseases are due to enhanced or inappropriate immune responses.

Antigen-presenting Cells (Chapter 15)

T cells recognize peptide–MHC complexes on the surface of other cells. Such cells are often referred to as *antigen-presenting cells*, or *APC*. Although effector cells can mediate their functions by recognizing such complexes on virtually any cell type, naïve cells are most efficiently activated by a set of specialized APC, the DCs. DCs are a multimember family including the plasmacytoid DCs which are the principal source of type I interferons in viral infections.

In general, in their immature form, DCs are resident in the tissues where they are efficient at capturing and endocytosing antigen. Their antigen capture activity is dependent upon expression of several surface receptors including Fc receptors, receptors for heat shock proteins, and C-type lectins. If they receive signals, such as various inflammatory stimuli, often mediated by TLRs, they down-regulate the expression of these molecules but increase their expression of surface MHC molecules and various costimulatory molecules such as CD80/86. In addition, such stimulation induces expression of chemokine receptors, such as CCR2 and CCR7. The latter allow stimulated DCs to follow signals from the chemokines CCL19 and CCL21 and to migrate into the T cell zone of lymph nodes. As part of the maturation process, they may also acquire the capacity to produce cytokines and express surface molecules that can aid in determining the polarization of T cell priming. This includes the production of IL-12 , IL-23, IL-6 and the expression of inducible costimulator (ICOS) ligand and of Notch ligands. Interaction of naïve

T cells with immature DCs may induce a state of peripheral tolerance.

One important function of DCs is the ability to acquire antigen from virally infected cells and to *cross present* it through the class I pathway. This allows DCs to aid in the priming of precursors of cytotoxic T cells specific for viruses that do not infect the DCs themselves.

EFFECTOR MECHANISMS OF IMMUNITY

The ultimate purpose of the immune system is to mount responses that protect the individual against infections with pathogenic microorganisms by eliminating these microbes or, where it is not possible to eliminate infection, to control its spread and virulence. In addition, the immune system may play an important role in the control of the development and spread of some malignant tumors. The responses that actually cause the destruction of the agents that initiate these pathogenic states (e.g., bacteria, viruses, parasites, tumor cells) are collectively the effector mechanisms of the immune system. Several have already been alluded to. Among them are the cytotoxic action of CTLs, which leads to the destruction of cells harboring viruses and, in some circumstances, expressing tumor antigens. In some cases, antibody can be directly protective by neutralizing determinants essential to a critical step through which the pathogen establishes or spreads an infectious process. However, in most cases, the immune system mobilizes powerful nonspecific mechanisms to mediate its effector function.

Effector Cells of the Immune Response

Among the cells that mediate important functions in the immune system are cells of the monocyte/macrophage lineage, NK cells, mast cells, basophils, eosinophils, and neutrophils. It is beyond the scope of this introductory chapter to present an extended discussion of each of these important cell types. However, a brief mention of some of their actions will help in understanding their critical functions in the immune response.

Monocytes and Macrophages (Chapter 18)

Cells of the monocyte/macrophage lineage play a central role in immunity. One of the key goals of cellular immunity is to aid the macrophages in eliminating organisms that have established intracellular infections. In general, nonactivated macrophages are inefficient in destroying intracellular microbes. However, the production of IFN-γ and other mediators by T cells can enhance the capacity of macrophages to eliminate such microorganisms. Several mechanisms exist for this purpose, including the development of reactive forms of oxygen, the development of nitric oxide, and the induction of a series of proteolytic enzymes, as well as the induction of cytokine production. Macrophages can act as APCs and thus can enlist the "help" of activated, cytokine-producing CD4$^+$ T cells in regulating their function.

Although macrophages function as APCs for attracting activated T cells, they do not appear to be particularly effective in the activation of naïve CD4 T cells. In instances in which they are the site of infection or have phagocytosed infectious agents or their proteins, antigens from these agents may be transferred to DCs. In such cases the DCs would be the principal APCs that activate naive or possibly resting memory CD4 T cells. This process is often described as cross-presentation. Such activated T cells would then be available to help infected macrophages.

Natural Killer Cells (Chapter 16)

Natural killer, or *NK*, cells play an important role in the immune system. Indeed, in mice that lack mature T and B cells due to the *scid* mutation, the NK system appears to be highly active and to provide these animals a substantial measure of protection against infection. NK cells are closely related to T cells. They lack conventional TCR (or Ig) but express two classes of receptors. They have a set of activating receptors that allow them to recognize features associated with virally infected cells or tumor cells. They also express receptors for MHC molecules that shut off their lytic activity. Thus, virally infected cells or tumor cells that escape the surveillance of cytotoxic T cells by down-regulating or shutting off expression of MHC molecules then become targets for efficient killing by NK cells because the cytotoxic activity of the latter cells is no longer shut off by the recognition of particular alleles of MHC class I molecules.

In addition, NK express a receptor for the Fc portion of IgG (FcγRIII). Antibody-coated cells can be recognized by NK cells, and such cells can then be lysed. This process is referred to as antibody-dependent cellular cytotoxicity (ADCC).

NK cells are efficient producers of IFN-γ. A variety of stimuli, including recognition of virally infected cells and tumor cells, cross-linkage of FcγRIII and stimulation by the cytokines IL-12 and IL-18, cause striking induction of IFN-γ production by NK cells.

Mast Cells and Basophils (Chapter 43)

Mast cells and basophils play important roles in the induction of allergic inflammatory responses. They express cell surface receptors for the Fc portions of IgE (FcεRI) and for certain classes of IgG (FcγR). This enables them to bind antibody to their surfaces, and when antigens capable of reacting with that antibody are introduced, the resultant cross-linkage of FcεRI or FcγR results in the prompt release of a series of potent mediators such as histamine, serotonin, and a variety of enzymes that play critical roles in initiating allergic and anaphylactic-type responses. In addition, such stimulation also causes these cells to produce a set of cytokines, including IL-3, IL-4, IL-13, IL-5, IL-6, granulocyte-macrophage colony-stimulating factor (GM-CSF), and TNFα, that have important late consequences in allergic inflammatory responses.

Granulocytes

Granulocytes have critical roles to play in a wide range of inflammatory situations. Rather than attempting an extended discussion of these potent cells, it may be sufficient to say that in their absence it is exceedingly difficult to clear infections with extracellular bacteria and that the immune response plays an important role in orchestrating the growth, differentiation, and mobilization of these crucial cells. Recent work indicates that T_{H17} cells are particularly important because of their role in recruiting granulocytes to sites of immune responses.

Eosinophils (Chapter 43)

Eosinophils are bone marrow–derived myeloid cells that complete their late differentiation under the influence of IL-5. They migrate to tissue sites in response to the chemokine eotaxin and as a result of their adhesion receptors. Since T_{H2} cells can produce IL-5 and stimulate the production of eotaxin, eosinophil accumulation is often associated with T_{H2}-mediated inflammation. Eosinophils store a series of proteins in their secondary granules including major basic protein, eosinophil cationic protein and eosinophil peroxidase. When released, these proteins are responsible for much of the damage that eosinophils mediate both to helminthic parasites and to the epithelium. Eosinophils have been implicated as important in protective responses to helminths and in the tissue damage seen in allergic inflammation in conditions such as asthma.

The Complement System (Chapter 33)

The complement system is a complex system of proteolytic enzymes, regulatory and inflammatory proteins and peptides, cell surface receptors, and proteins capable of causing the lysis of cells. The system can be thought of as consisting of three arrays of proteins. Two of these sets of

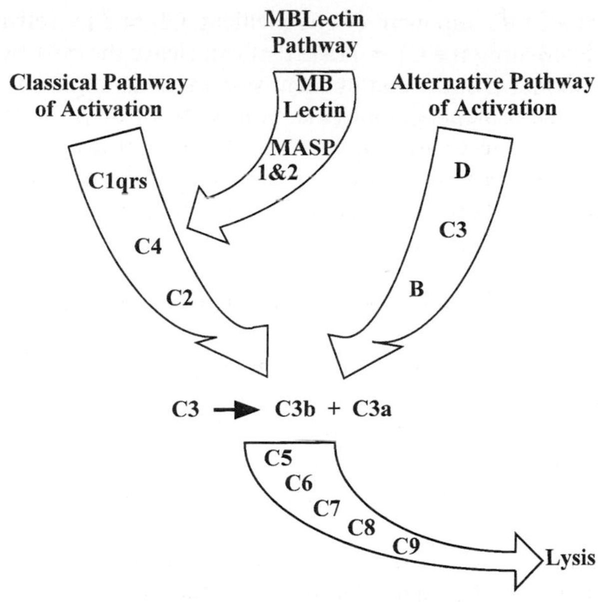

FIGURE 1.12 The complement system. The classical pathway of complement activation, usually initiated by the aggregation of C1 by binding to antigen–antibody complexes, resulting in the formation of an enzyme, a C3 convertase, that cleaves C3 into two fragments, C3b and C3a. The classical pathway can also be initiated by the aggregation of MBL as a result of binding sugars expressed in the capsules of many pathogenic microbes. The components of the MBL pathway appear to mimic the function of C1qrs. The alternative pathway of complement activation provides a potent means of activating complement without requiring antibody recognition of antigen. It results in the formation of a distinct C3 convertase. The fragments formed by cleaving C3 have important biologic activities. In addition, C3b, together with elements of the classical pathway (C4b, C2a) or the alternative pathway (Bb, properdin), form enzymes (C5 convertases) that cleave C5, the initial member of the terminal family of proteins. Cleavage of C5 leads to the formation of the membrane attack complex that can result in the osmotic lysis of cells.

proteins, when engaged, lead to the activation of the third component of complement (C3) (Figure 1.12). The activation of C3 releases proteins that are critical for opsonization (preparation for phagocytosis) of bacteria and other particles and engages the third set of proteins that insert into biologic membranes and produce cell death through osmotic lysis. In addition, fragments generated from some of the complement components (e.g., C3a and C5a) have potent inflammatory activities.

The Classical Pathway of Complement Activation

The two activation systems for C3 are referred to as the *classical pathway* and the *alternative pathway*. The classical pathway is initiated by the formation of complexes of antigen with IgM or IgG antibody. This leads to the binding of the first component of complement, C1, and its activation, creating the C1 esterase that can cleave the next two components of the complement system, C4 and C2.

C4 is a trimeric molecule, consisting of α, β, and γ chains. C1 esterase cleaves the α chain, releasing C4b, which binds to surfaces in the immediate vicinity of the antigen–antibody–C1 esterase complex. A single C1 esterase molecule will cause the deposition of multiple C4b molecules.

C2 is a single polypeptide chain that binds to C4b and is then proteolytically cleaved by C1 esterase, releasing C2b. The resulting complex of the residual portion of C2 (C2a) with C4b (C4b2a) is a serine protease whose substrate is C3. Cleavage of C3 by C4b2a (also referred to as *the classical pathway C3 convertase*) results in the release of C3a and C3b. A single antigen–antibody complex and its associated C1 esterase can lead to the production of a large number of C3 convertases (i.e., C4b2a complexes) and thus to cleavage of a large number of C3 molecules.

The components of the classical pathway can be activated by a distinct, non–antibody-dependent mechanism. The mannose-binding lectin (MBL) is activated by binding to (and being cross-linked by) repetitive sugar residues such as N-acetylglucosamine or mannose. The activation of MBL recruits the MBL-associated serine proteases MASP-1 and MASP-2, which cleave C4 and C2 and lead to the formation of the classical pathway C3 convertase. Because the capsules of several pathogenic microbes can be bound by MBL, this mechanism provides an antibody-independent pathway through which the complement system can be activated by foreign microorganisms.

The Alternative Pathway of Complement Activation

Although discovered more recently, the alternative pathway is the evolutionarily more ancient system of complement activation. Indeed, it, and the MBL activation of the classical pathway, can be regarded as important components of the innate immune system. The alternative pathway can be activated by a variety of agents such as insoluble yeast cell wall preparations and bacterial lipopolysaccharide. Antigen–antibody complexes also can activate the alternative pathway. The C3 convertase of the alternative pathway consists of a complex of C3b (itself a product of cleavage of C3) bound to the b fragment of the molecule factor B. C3bBb is produced by the action of the hydrolytic enzyme, factor D, that cleaves factor B; this cleavage only occurs when factor B has been bound by C3b.

Apart from the importance of the alternative pathway in activating the complement system in response to nonspecific stimulants, it also can act to amplify the activity of the classical pathway, because the C3 convertase of the classical system (C4b2a) provides a source of C3b that can strikingly enhance formation of the alternative pathway convertase (C3bBb) in the presence of factor D.

The Terminal Components of the Complement System

C3b, formed from C3 by the action of the C3 convertases, possesses an internal thioester bond that can be cleaved to form a free sulfhydryl group. The latter can form a covalent bond with a variety of surface structures. C3b is recognized by receptors on various types of cells, including macrophages and B cells. The binding of C3b to antibody-coated bacteria is often an essential step for the phagocytosis of these microbes by macrophages.

C3b is also essential to the engagement of the terminal components of the complement system (C5 through C9) to form the membrane attack complex that causes cellular lysis. This process is initiated by the cleavage of C5, a 200,000-dalton two-chain molecule. The C5 convertases that catalyze this reaction are C4b2a3b (the classical pathway C5 convertase) or a complex of C3bBb with a protein designated properdin (the alternative pathway C5 convertase). Cleaved C5, C5b, forms a complex with C6 and then with C7, C8, and C9. This C5b/C9 complex behaves as an integral membrane protein that is responsible for the formation of complement-induced lesions in cell membranes. Such lesions have a donutlike appearance, with C9 molecules forming the ring of the donut.

In addition to the role of the complement system in opsonization and in cell lysis, several of the fragments of complement components formed during activation are potent mediators of inflammation. C3a, the 9,000-dalton fragment released by the action of the C3 convertases, binds to receptors on mast cells and basophils, resulting in the release of histamine and other mediators of anaphylaxis. C3a is thus termed an *anaphylotoxin,* as is C5a, the 11,000-dalton fragment released as a result of the action of the C5 convertases. C5a is also a chemoattractant for neutrophils and monocytes.

Finally, it is important to note that the process of activation of the complement cascade is highly regulated. Several regulatory proteins (e.g., C1 esterase inhibitor, decay accelerator factor, membrane cofactor protein) exist that function to prevent uncontrolled complement activation. Abnormalities in these regulatory proteins are often associated with clinical disorders such as hereditary angioedema and paroxysmal nocturnal hemoglobinuria.

CONCLUSION

This introductory chapter should provide the reader with an appreciation of the overall organization of the immune system and of the properties of its key cellular and molecular components. It should be obvious that the immune system is highly complex, that it is capable of a wide range of effector functions, and that its activities are subject to potent, but only partially understood, regulatory processes. As the most versatile and powerful defense of higher organisms, the immune system may provide the key to the development of effective means to treat and prevent a broad range of diseases. Indeed, the last two sections of this book deal with immunity to infectious agents and immunologic mechanisms in disease. The introductory material provided here should be of aid the uninitiated reader in understanding the immunologic mechanisms brought into play in a wide range of clinical conditions in which immune processes play a major role either in pathogenesis or in recovery.

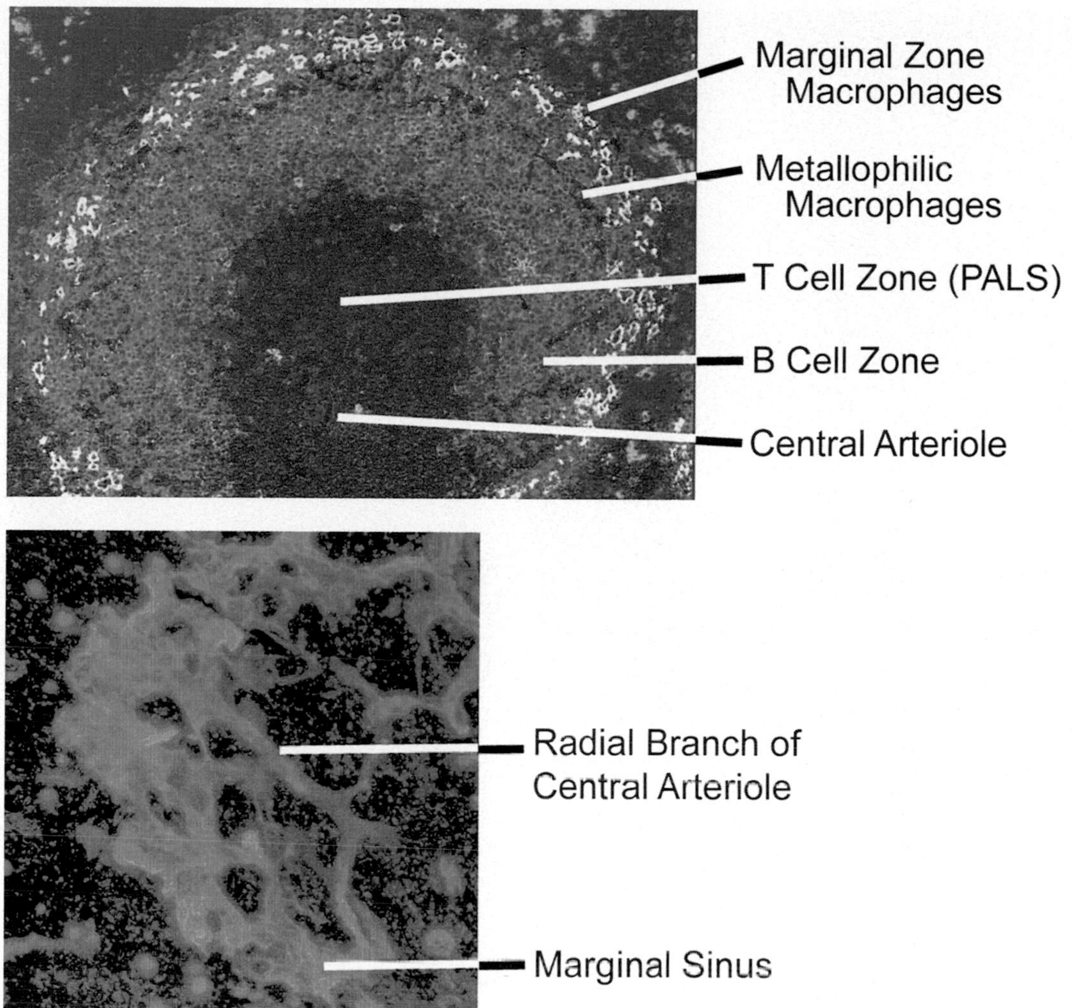

FIGURE 2.4 Organization of the spleen white pulp. **Top panel:** Immunofluorescent staining of a white pulp unit in the mouse spleen. T cells (anti-CD4$^+$anti-CD8$^+$, red) are localized around the central arteriole. B cells (anti-IgM, green) are localized in follicles around the T cell area, surrounded by a layer of metalophillic macrophages (labeled with monoclonal antibody-MOMA-1) and a more peripheral layer of marginal zone macrophages (labeled with monoclonal antibody ERTR9, orange). The marginal zone (MZ) is located between the metalophillic macrophage and the MZ macrophage layers (not shown) (307). **Bottom panel:** Structure of the marginal sinus in a thick (100 micrometer) frozen section of mouse spleen with targeted insertion of the *LacZ* gene into the ephrin B2 locus. Eprhrin B2 is expressed at high levels in the central arteriole, in radial branches of the central arteriole, and in the marginal sinus. LacZ is visualized by staining with FITC-labeled anti-LacZ antibody. Note the transition from discrete arteriolar vessels to a network of flattened vessels at the transition to the marginal sinus plexus (C. Zindl, University of Alabama at Birmingham, Birmingham, AL). From Chaplin (308), with permission.

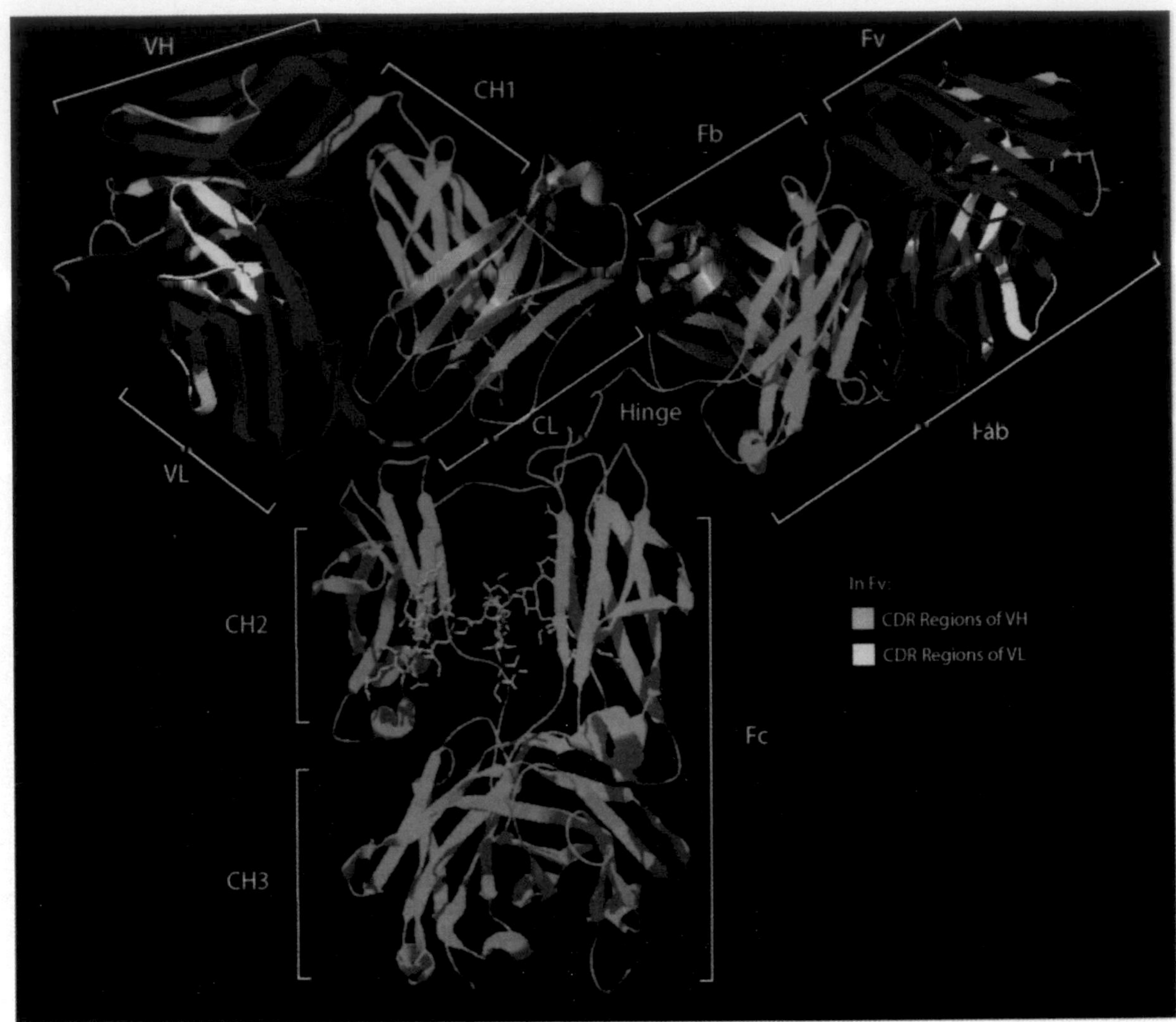

FIGURE 4.2 Ribbon diagram of a complete IgG1 crystal (1 hzh in PDB from data of Harris et al [190]). The major regions of the immunoglobulin are illustrated. The heavy-chain constant regions (green) also include the hinge (yellow) between the first two domains. CH2 is glycosylated (also seen in yellow). The heavy- and light-chain variable regions (red and dark blue, respectively) are N terminal to the heavy-(green) and light-chain (light blue) constant regions. CDR loops in the heavy- and light-chain variable regions (yellow and white) are illustrated as well.

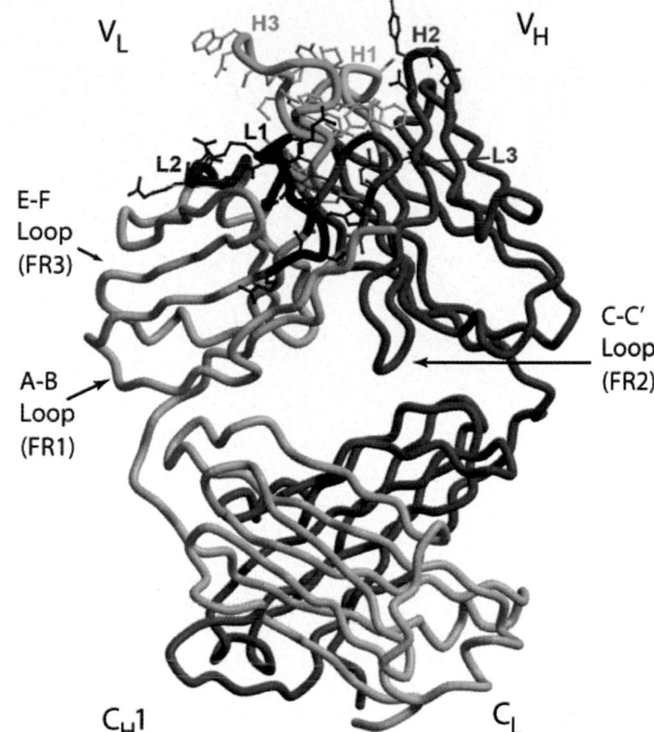

FIGURE 4.6 The structure of an Fab. The antigen binding site is formed by the H and L chain B-C, C′-C″, and F-G loops. Each loop encodes a separate complementarity determining region, or CDR. The location of CDRs H1, H2, H3, L1 L2, and L3 are shown. The opposing H and L chain C-C′ strands and loop help stabilize the interaction between VH and VL. This C-C′ structure is encoded by the second V framework region, FR2. The inclusion of this structure permits the V domains to interact in a head-to-head fashion. The E-F strands and loop are encoded by the FR3 region and lie directly below the antigen binding site. The A-B strands and loop encode FR1 and lie between the C_H1 and CL domains and the rest of the Vs. The beta sheet strands of the C_H1 and CL domains rest crosswise to each other. The illustration is modified from (191).

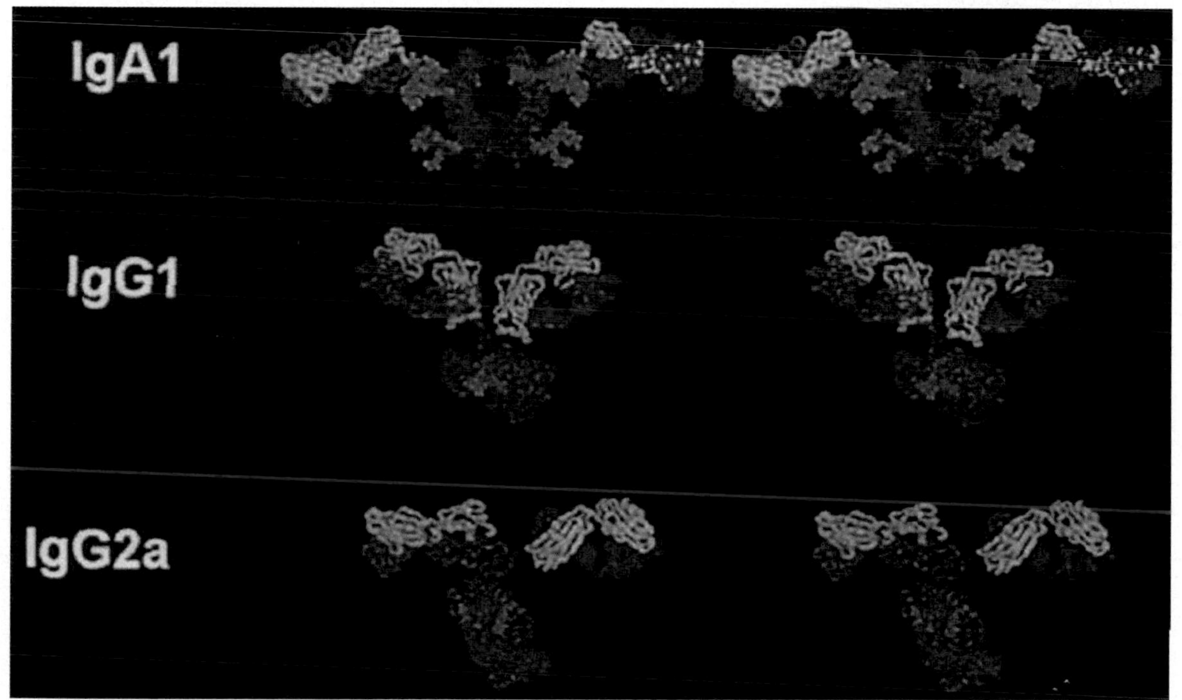

FIGURE 4.12 A comparison of an x-ray and neutron-solution-scattering theoretical model (human IgA1) and x-ray crystal (murine IgG1 and IgG2a) structures. Light chains (yellow), heavy chains (red and dark blue), and glycosylation (light blue) are illustrated. The extended length of IgA1 over that of IgG can be seen along with extensive glycosylation that characterizes this isotype. (From Boehm et al. [192], with permission.)

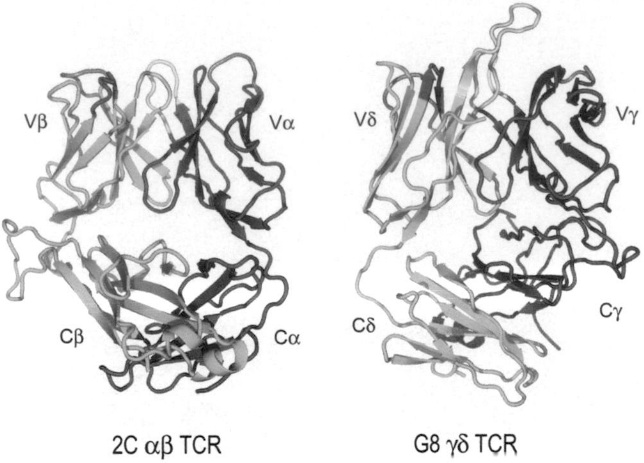

FIGURE 10.6 Ribbon diagrams of the T cell receptor (TCR) structures. This shows the structures of the 2C$\alpha\beta$TCR (150) versus the G8$\gamma\delta$ TCR (153). The TCRβ and the TCRγ chains are in cyan, and the TCRα and γ chains are in vermillion. The CDRs of both are in yellow. The very long TCRδCDR3 in G8, which binds the T10/T22 ligands, is very apparent here but are shorter in most other $\gamma\delta$ TCRs. Note the different C region interactions with these TCRs and the deviations from the classic "β barrel" structure in both Cα and Cδ. The prominent Cβ loop to the left is also unusual and may mediate interactions with CD3 or other molecules on the T cell surface. (Figure courtesy of Dr. K. C. Garcia.)

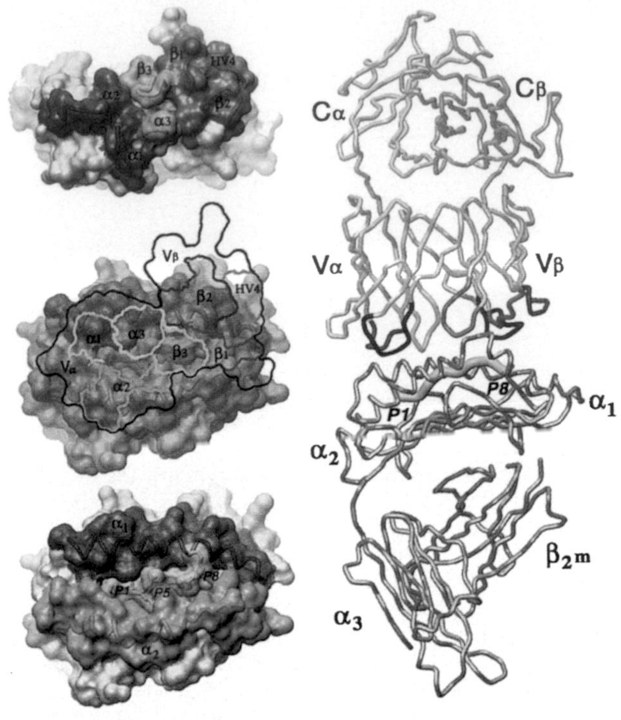

FIGURE 10.9 T cell receptor (TCR)-peptide/major histocompatibility complex (MHC) crystal structure of a TCR-peptide/MHC complex. Peptide and complementary-determining regions are portrayed in different colors (150).

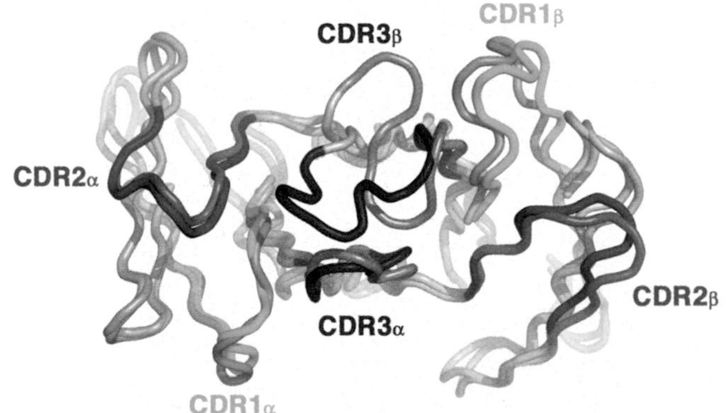

FIGURE 10.10 CDR3 movement in $\alpha\beta$ T cell receptor (TCR) binding. In most cases where there is a structure for an $\alpha\beta$ TCR as well as for one (or more) for that TCR in complex with a peptide-MHC, there is a marked movement of one or the other of the Vα or Vβ CDR3s. This example from Mallissen et al. (209) shows a particularly large (14 Å) movement of CDR3β with binding. This meshes well with thermodynamic data showing an "induced fit" binding mechanism for most TCRs (173,211).

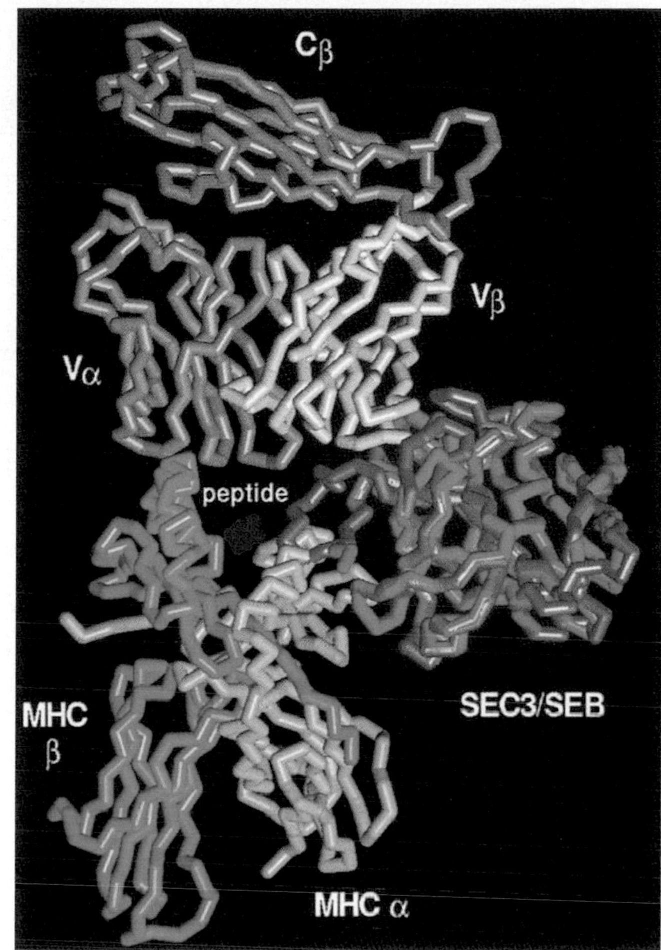

FIGURE 10.12 Crystal structure of a T cell receptor (TCR) β/superantigen (SAg) complex. Fields et al. (253) crystallized TCR-SAg complexes and from the structure of the same superantigens with a class II major histocompatibility complex (MHC) molecule and were able to deduce the relative spatial arrangement of the three molecules. This model suggests that TCR does not contact the MHC very strongly, which is consistent with the relative peptide insensitivity of SAg activation.

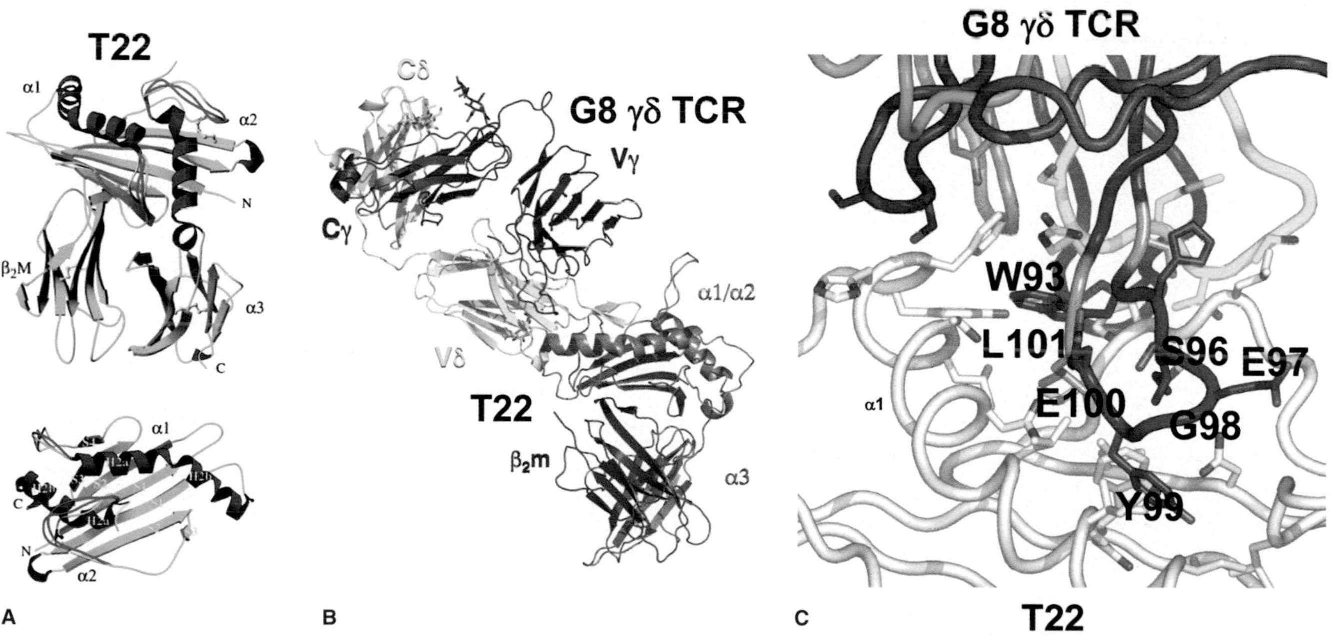

FIGURE 10.14 The T22 structure and the interaction with the G8 γδ TCR. **A:** The structure of a T22 molecule, a nonclassical class I MHC that is missing half of an alpha helix and does not bind peptides (270). **B, C:** The intersection with the G8 TCR, where the long TCR δ CDR3 accounts for almost all of the contact residues (153).

	Vδ	P/N	Dδ1 (GTGGCATATCA)	P/N	Dδ2 (ATCGGAGGGATACGAG)	P/N	Jδ1 (CTACCGACAAACTC)
G8	TGT GCT GCT GA C A A D	C AC T	G TGG CAT AT W H I		A TCG GAG GGA TAC GAG S E G Y E	CTC GG L G	T ACC GAC AAA CTC T D K L
KN6	TGT GCC TCG GGG C A S G		TAT Y	TG W	G GAG GGA TAC GAG E G Y E	CTG L	ACC GAC AAA CTC T D K L
Vδ6	TGT GCT CTC TGG GAG CTG C A L W E L	GAG E			TCG GAG GGA TAC GAG S E G Y E	CTC G L A	CC GAC AAA CTC D K L
	TGT GCT CTC TGG GAG CTG C A L W E L	GTT A V M	TG GC A		A TCG GAG GGA TAC GAG S E G Y E	CTA L	ACC GAC AAA CTC T D K L
	TGT GCT CTC TGG GAG CTG C A L W E L		AT I		A TCG GAG GGA TAC GAG S E G Y E	CTA L	ACC GAC AAA CTC T D K L
Vδ4	TGT GCT CTC ATG GAG C A L M E	GGT ATA G I	TGG CAT AT W H I		A TCG GAG GGA TAC GAG S E G Y E	CTT G L A	CT ACC GAC AAA CTC T D K L
	TGT GCT CTC ATG GAG CG C A L M E R	A	AT I		A TCG GAG GGA TAC GAG S E G Y E	CTG GA L D	C GAC AAA CTC D K L
Vδ5	TGT GCC TCG GGG T C A S G S	CC CCC P	CAT AT H I	A TGG CTC GG W L G	A TCG GAG GGA TAC GAG S E G Y E	CTC CTC G L L A	CT ACC GAC AAA CTC T D K L
	TGT GCC TCG GGG TAT C A S G Y	AT M	G TGG W	AGC AT S I	A TCG GAG GGA TAC GAG S E G Y E	CTT G L A	CT ACC GAC AAA CTC T D K L

A

Vγ1	Vδ6	$t_{1/2}$ (min)	K_D (nM)
CAVWI LS GTSWVKIF	CALWEL E SEGYEL A DKL	64 ± 7	12.0 ± 0.5
CAVWI P GTSWVKIF	CALWEL VMA SEGYEL T DKL	86 ± 22	17.2 ± 2.8
CAVWI T GTSWVKIF	CALWEL I SEGYEL T DKL	109 ± 19	13.8 ± 2.8

B

FIGURE 10.15 Conserved TCRδCDR3 sequences correlate with T10/T22 specificity in $\gamma\delta$ T cells. Sequence data from Shin et al. (290) showing that both established cell lines (G8 and KNG) and $\gamma\delta$ T cells from clonal cultures that are specific for the T10/T22 share highly conserved TCRδCDR3 sequences. These are largely derived from the Dδ2 gene segment and from the structural data (Adams et al., color plate 4, 153). These conserved sequences constitute the main interaction between these $\gamma\delta$ T cell receptors and their ligand.

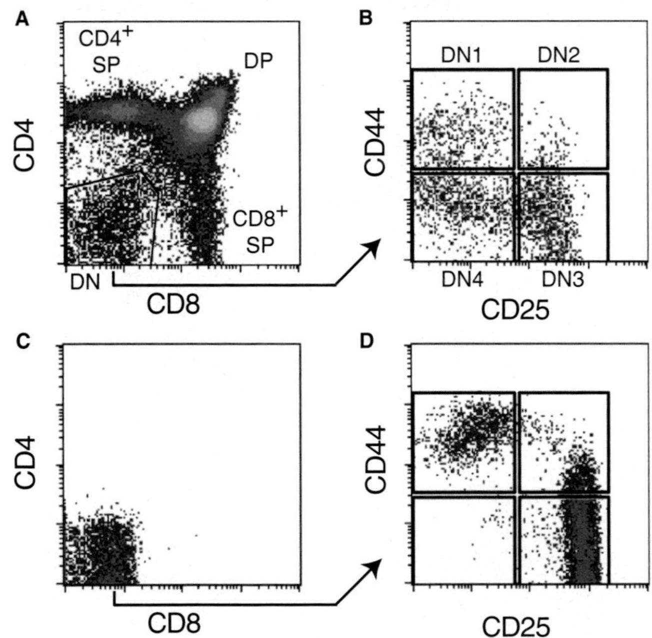

FIGURE 12.1 Subsets of T cell precursors: normal development versus development without TCR gene rearrangement. The major subsets of cells discussed in this chapter are shown in a typical flow cytometric analysis. Top panels (**A** and **B**) show normal thymocytes, and bottom panels (**C** and **D**) show thymocytes from RAG-deficient mice, which cannot rearrange any TCR genes. Cells are stained with fluorescent antibodies against CD4 and CD8 (**A** and **C**), and the DN cells (boxed in **A**) are further analyzed with fluorescent antibodies against CD44 and CD25 (**B** and **D**). The axes show increasing levels of these surface molecules on a 4-decade logarithmic scale (10^4-fold range) of staining intensity. The main populations discussed in Figure 12.2 are indicated (DN, DP, CD4 SP, CD8 SP) (**A**), and the DN cells are subdivided into DN1, DN2, DN3, and DN4 (**B**). The recombinase-deficient thymocytes are developmentally arrested in the DN stages (**C;** cf. **A**), and these DN cells accumulate in the DN3 state and are blocked from progressing forward to the DN4 state (**D;** cf. **B**). RAG-deficient thymocytes also accumulate to only about 1/100 as many cells per thymus as wild-type (~4 × 10^6 versus ~3 × 10^8).

FIGURE 16.4 Crystal structures of NK cell receptors in complex with their ligands. **A:** Mouse Ly49A bound to H2D^d at site 1 (PDB ID = 1QO3) (170). Site 2 interaction is not shown. **B:** Mouse Ly49C bound to H2K^b at site 2 (PDB ID = 1P1Z) (193). Ly49A interaction with site 1 of H2D^d is very similar (170). **C:** Human LILRB1 (LIR1, ILT2) bound to HLA-A2 (PDB ID = 1P7Q) (266). Figures were produced using the UCSF Chimera package from the Resource for Biocomputing, Visualization, and Informatics at the University of California, San Francisco (www.cgl.ucsf.edu/chimera) *(776)*. The structures are viewed from the side with the NK cell positioned at the top of the figure and the target cell surface at the bottom. The MHC molecules are oriented similarly.

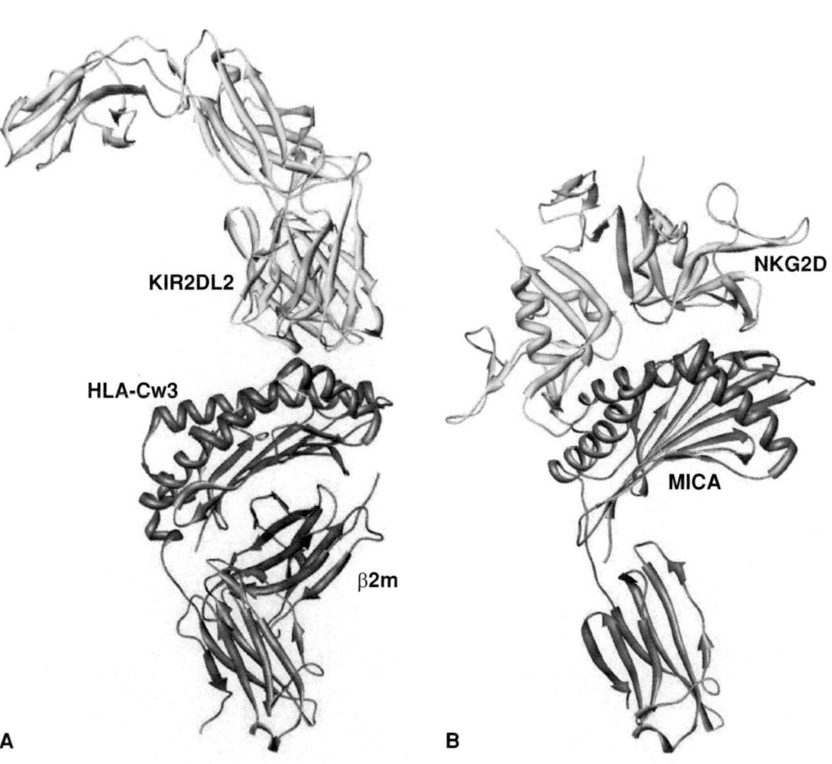

FIGURE 16.5 Additional structures of NK cell receptors in complex with their ligands. **A:** Human KIR2DL2 with HLA-Cw3 (PDB ID = 1EFX) (236). Two KIR molecules are apparent in the crystal structure with only one molecule (KIR A) contacting the HLA molecule. In this view, the D2 domain of the KIR A obscures the D1 domain behind it. **B:** Human NKG2D with MICA (PDB ID = 1HYR) (412). The figures were produced and oriented as described in Figure 16.4.

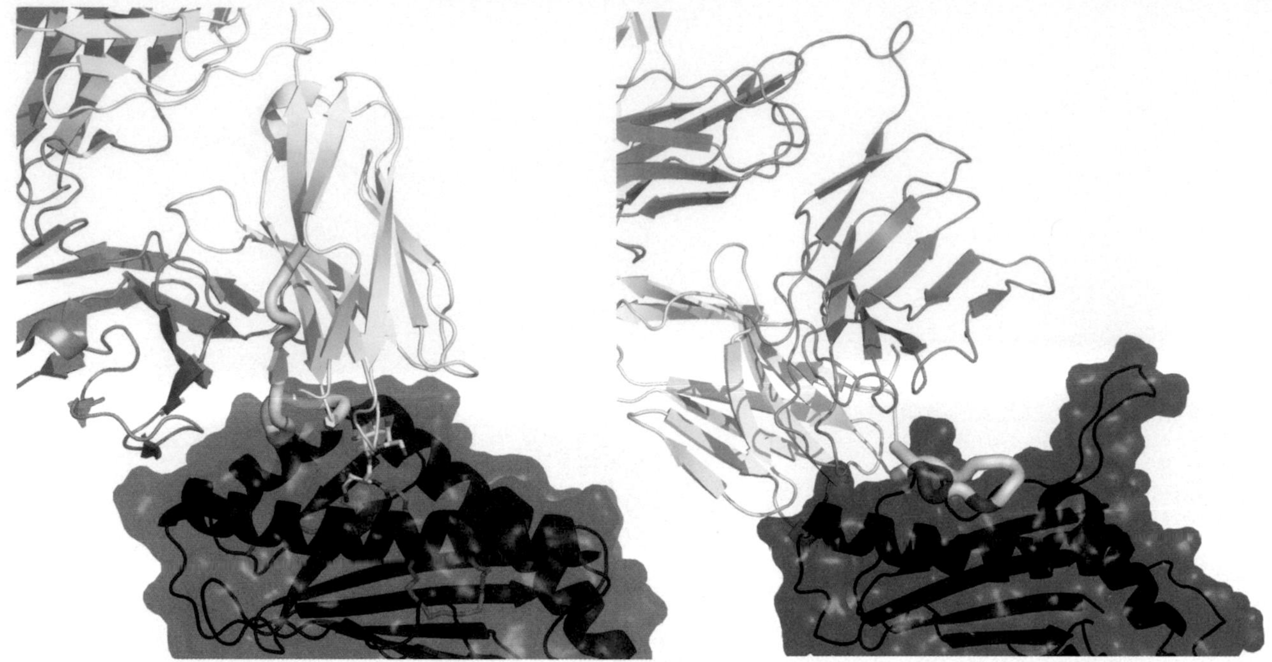

FIGURE 17.5 Structural determinants of ligand recognition. Left: The rearranged TCR α chain of NKT cells exclusively use Jα18, shown as a thick tube in the structure of the human Vα24-Jα18/Vβ11 TCR. The CDR3α of the NKT TCRs are nearly identical in amino acid sequence between mouse and human and provide most of the contact points with CD1d complexed with an α-galactosylceramide ligand (99a). Right: $\gamma\delta$ T cells specific for the H-2T22 MHC class I molecule use a conserved amino acid motif (W.EGYEL) in their CDR3δ loop, shown as a thick tube in the structure of the G8 $\gamma\delta$ TCR in complex with H-2T22. These amino acids, which are encoded by the germline V region and D segments, contribute most of the contact points with H-2T22 (7). (Courtesy of Erin Adams, University of Chicago, Chicago, IL, USA.)

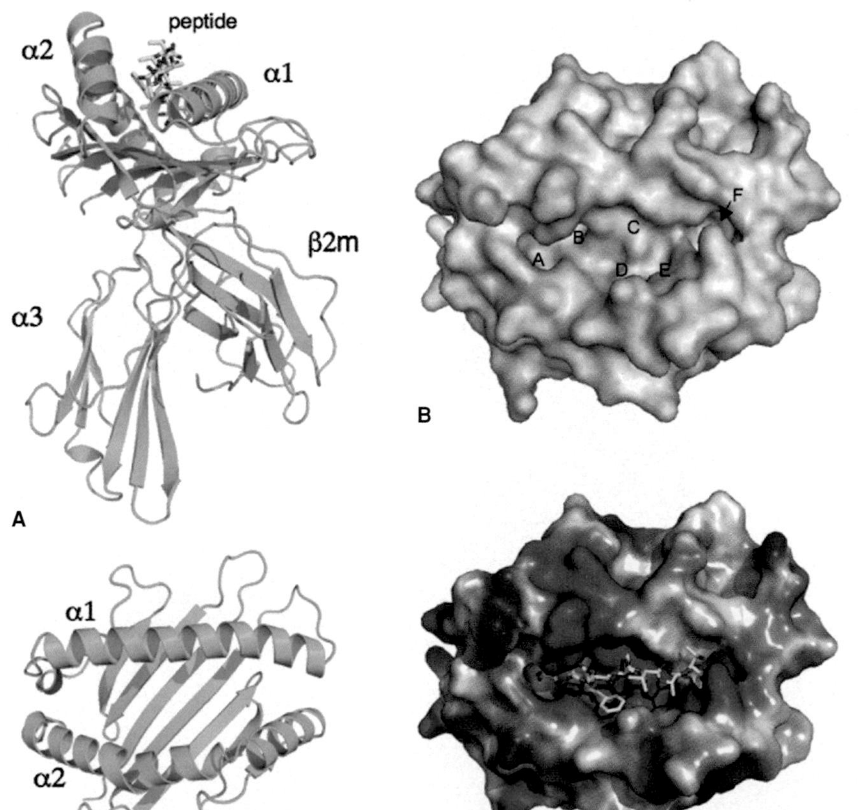

FIGURE 19.6 Structure of HLA-A*0201. **A:** Ribbon representation of HLA-A2 heavy chain (green), β2m light chain (cyan), and bound peptide (yellow). **B:** Ribbon representation of the peptide-binding groove. **C:** Surface representation of the binding groove, with pockets labeled. **D:** Surface representation of binding groove with peptide shown in stick illustration. Figure generated from protein data bank (*508*) structure 2BSV using PyMol (*509*).

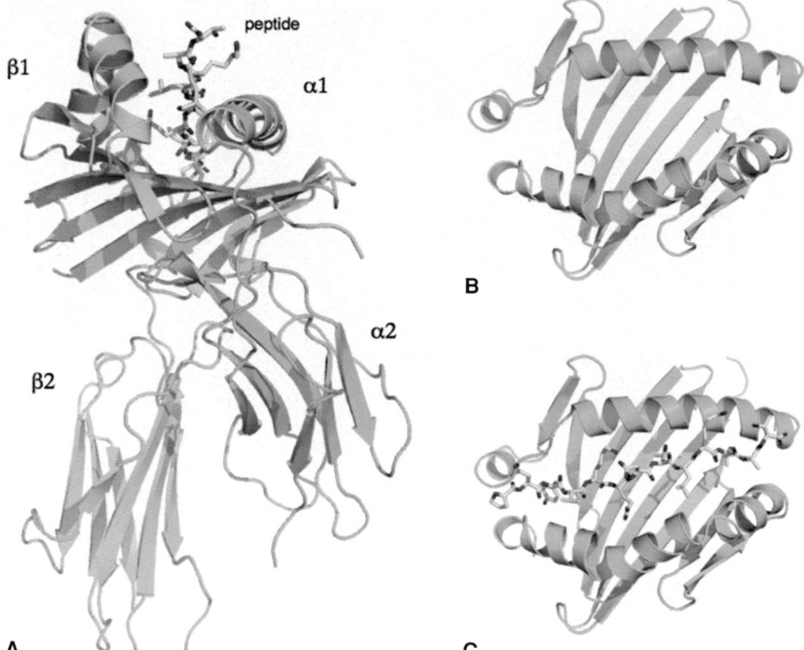

FIGURE 19.7 Color ribbon representation of HLA-DR1. **A:** Side view; α chain is in green, β chain is in blue, peptide in stick representation is in yellow. **B:** Top view. **C:** Top view with bound peptide (PKYVKQNTLKLAT) visualized. The illustration was made with PyMol (*509*) based on the protein data bank (*508*) coordinates of 1DLH.

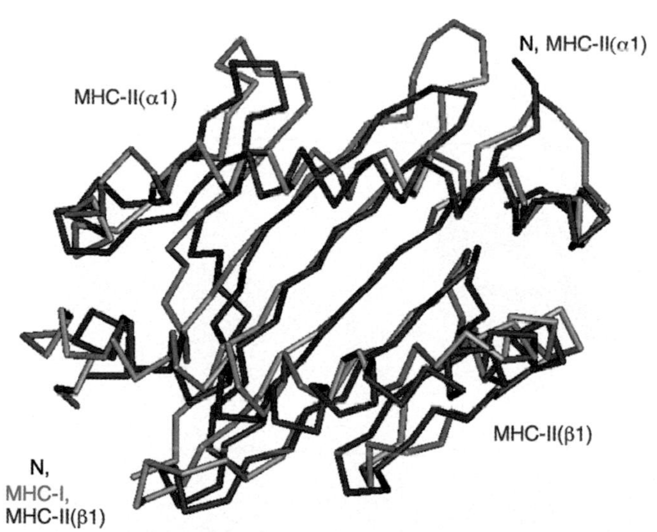

FIGURE 19.8 Superposition of the α-carbon backbones of an MHC-I [PDB (*508*)], 3HLA (*363*), and an MHC-II [1DLH (383)] molecule. The backbone tracings were displayed and superposed with QUANTA 97 (Molecular Simulations, Inc). MHC-I is shown in blue, MHC-II in red. Amino termini are labeled N.

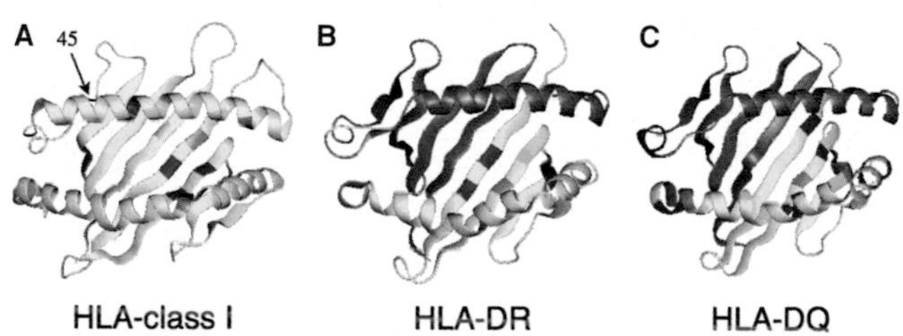

FIGURE 19.9 Location of polymorphic amino acid residues in MHC-I and MHC-II molecules. Variability plots were calculated according to the method of Kabat and Wu (*382*) and the level of variability illustrated on ribbon diagrams. Generated in QUANTA 2000 (Accelrys) of 3HLA (*363*) (HLA-class I), 1DLH (383) (HLA-DR), and 1JK8 (*510*) (HLA-DQ), where greatest variability is red, intermediate is green, and least is blue.

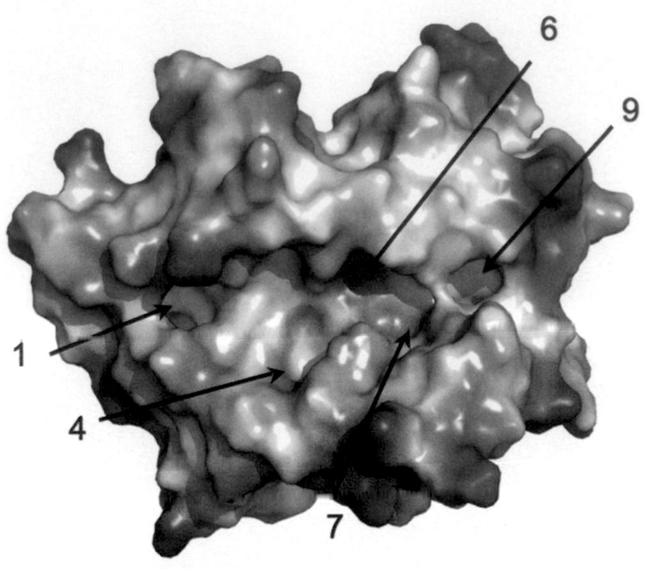

FIGURE 19.10 Location of pockets in HLA-DR1 based on the cocrystal of HLA-DR1 with a peptide derived from the influenza hemagglutinin. The surface representation of the molecule, looking into the cleft, is shown colored based on electrostatics—red, acidic; blue, basic. Numbering of the major binding pockets of HLA-DR1 is according to (383).

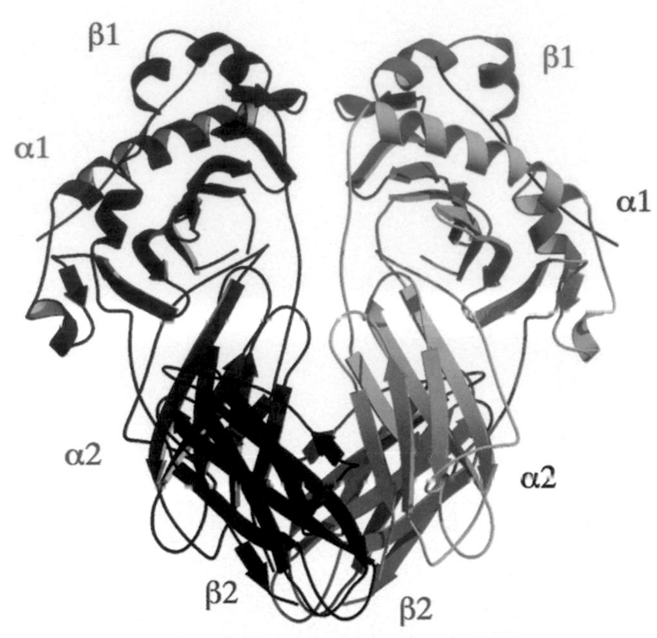

FIGURE 19.11 Ribbon diagram of the structure of HLA-DR1 showing the dimer of dimers and the individual domains of the protein. α chains are in blue and I, β chains are in red and green. Peptide is in red. The illustration was generated from 1DLH (383) in MOLSCRIPT (*511*) and rendered in RASTER3D (*512*).

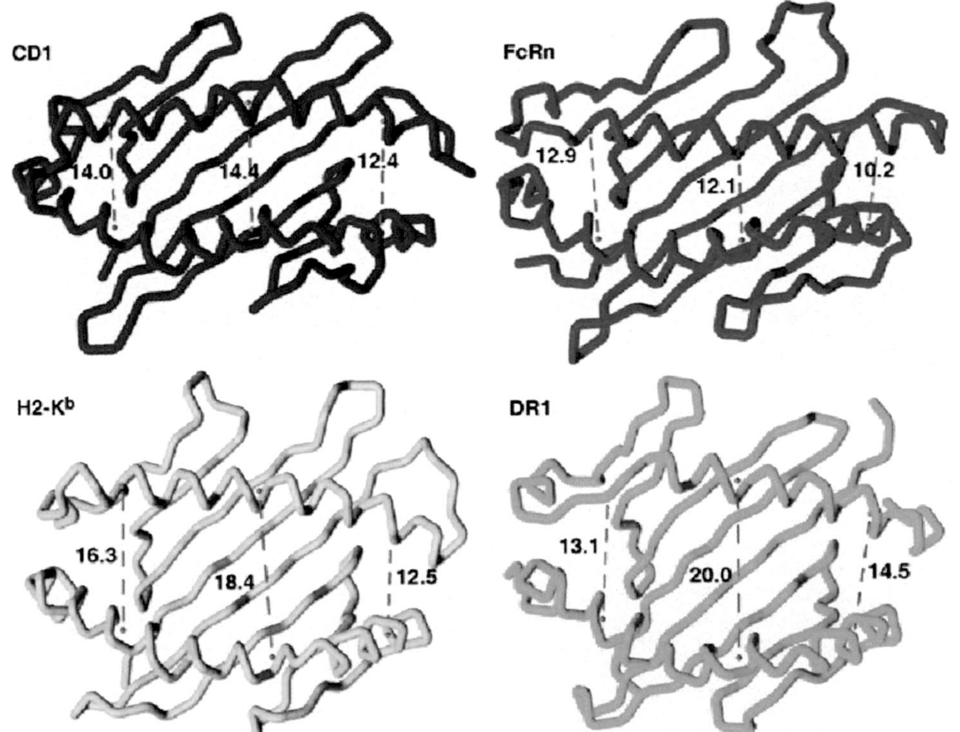

FIGURE 19.12 Comparison of the α-carbon backbone tracings and size of the potential peptide-bindng cleft of MHC-I molecule H2-K^b, MHC-II HLA-DR1, and MHC-Ib molecules CD1d, and FcRn. (From (*397*), with permission.)

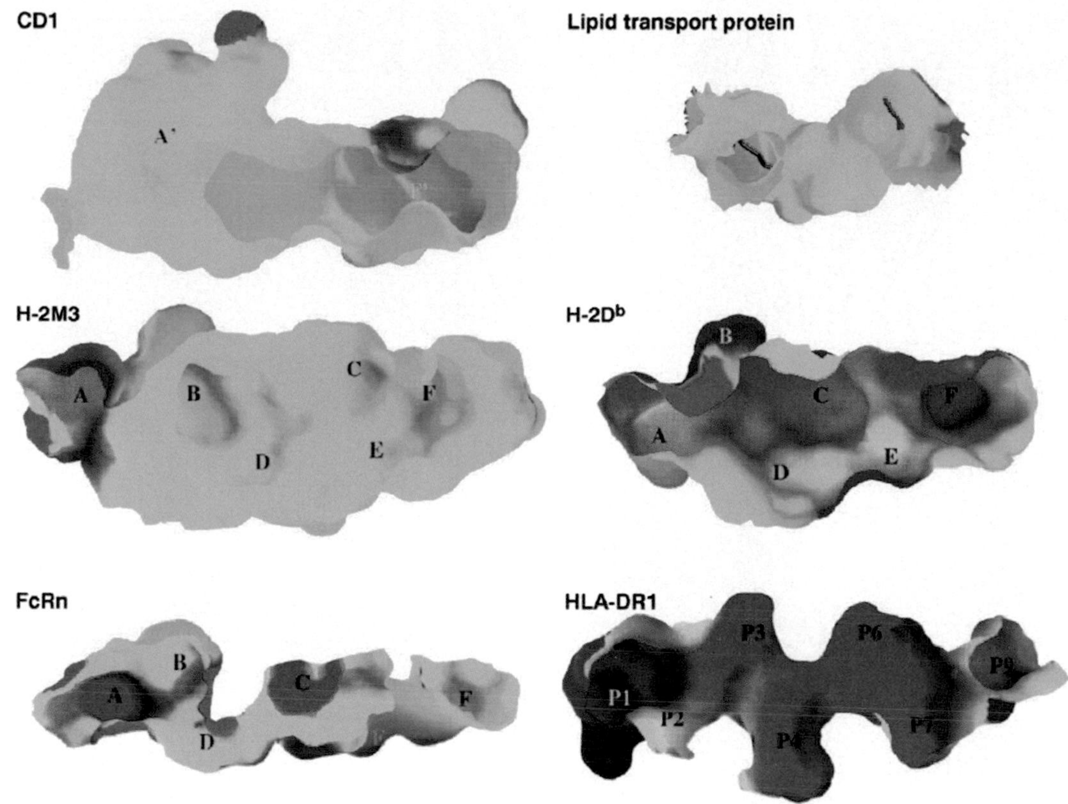

FIGURE 19.13 Shape, size, and charge of the binding groove of CD1d compared with those of several other MHC molecules and with a lipid-transport protein. Surface representation of the ligand-bindng cleft is displayed with acidic regions in red, basic regions in blue, and hydrophobic regions in green. (From (*397*), with permission.)

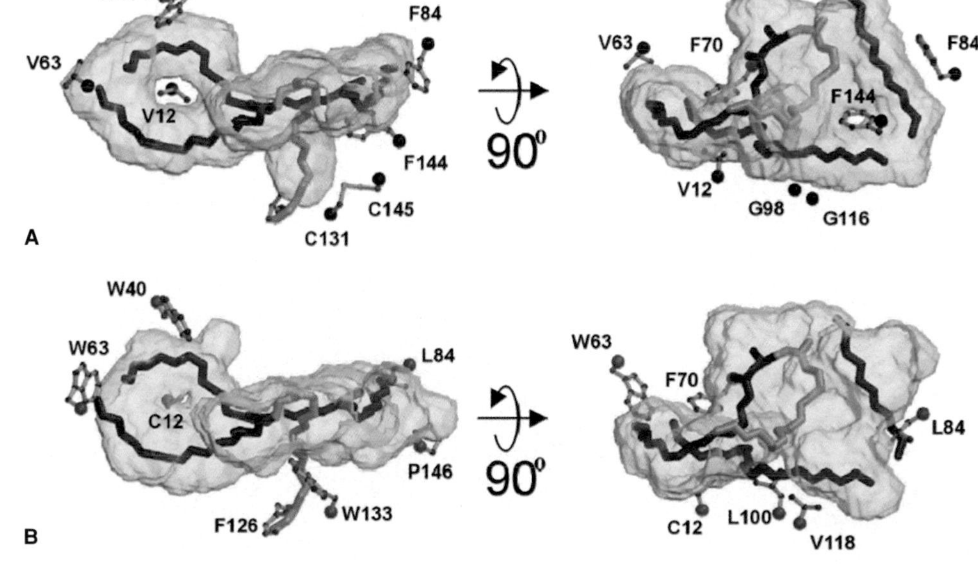

FIGURE 19.14 Structural differences between the binding grooves of CD1b and CD1d. **A:** Orthogonal views for CD1b. **B:** Orthogonal views for CD1d. The hydrophobic groove and key side chains for CD1b and CD1d are in blue and green, respectively. Position of alkyl chains and detergent visualized in CD1b are colored with respect to the binding channels they occupy: A′ (red), C′ (yellow), F′ (pink), and T′ (violet). (From (*398*), with permission.)

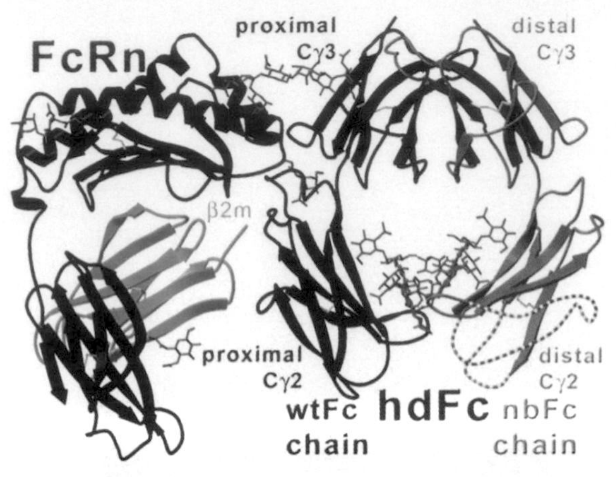

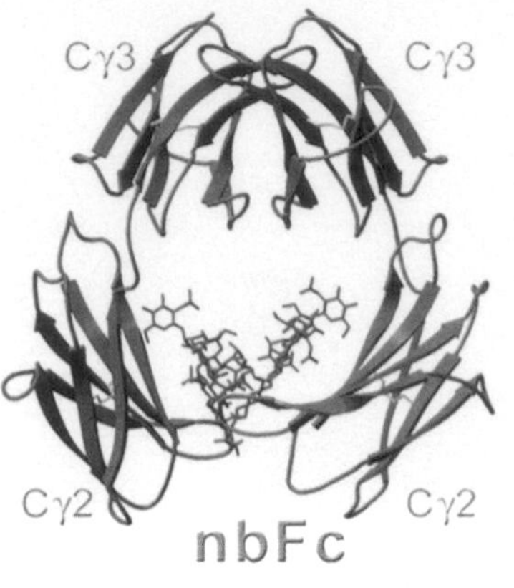

FIGURE 19.15 Structure of the FcRn complexed with Fc. Ribbon diagram of the FcRn (purple), β2m (green) interacting with the Fc (magenta and brown) heterodimer consisting of the wild-type (wt) and nonbinding (nb) engineered chain. For comparison, the homodimer of the nbFc is shown on the right. These are PDB (*508*) files, 1I1A and 1I1C (*513*), respectively. (From (*513*), with permission.)

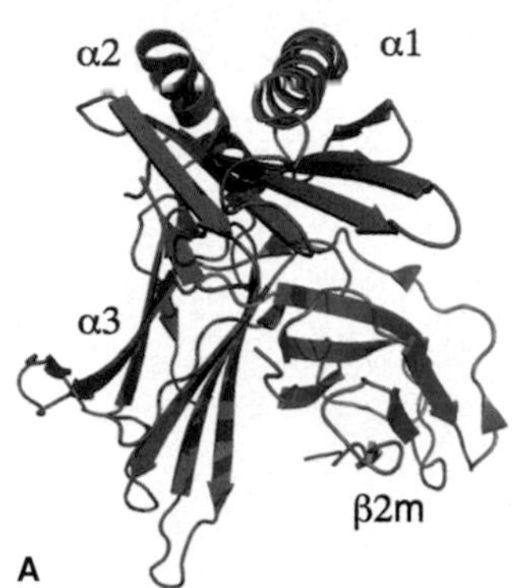

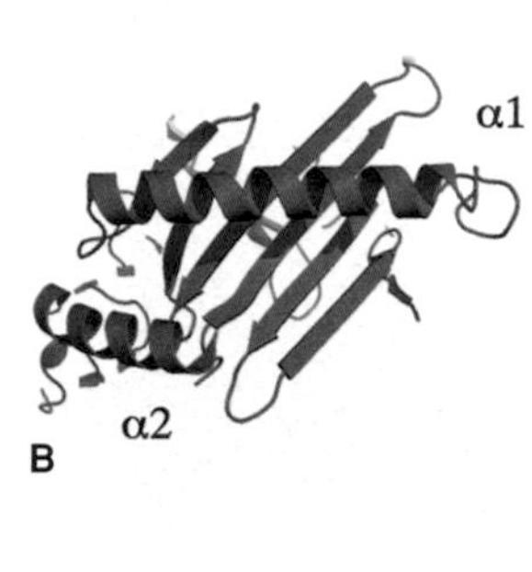

FIGURE 19.16 Structure of the MHC-Iv molecule, m144 (27), is shown. Heavy chain is in magenta, β2m light chain is in blue.

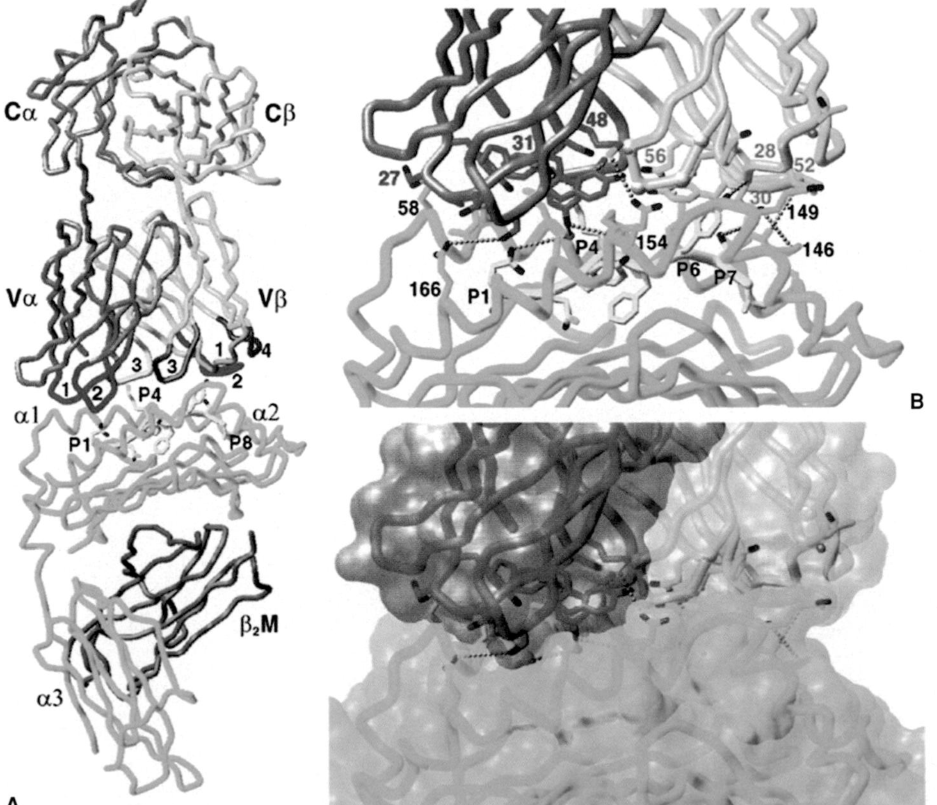

FIGURE 19.17 Structure of an MHC-I/peptide/TCR complex. H2-K^b bound to the peptide dEV8 (EQYKFYSV) in complex with the 2C TCR is shown. The TCR α and β chains (magenta and light blue) as well as H2-K^b (green) and peptide (yellow) are shown. Complementarity-determining regions (CDRs) of the TCR, colored in contrasting colors, and labeled 1, 2, and 3, are also indicated. (From (429), with permission.)

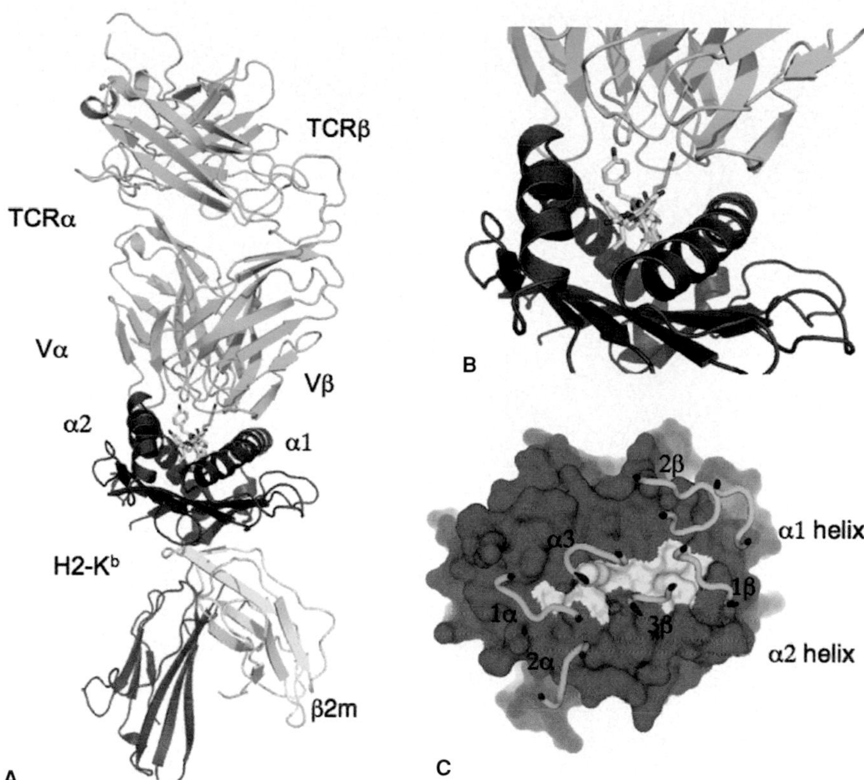

FIGURE 19.18 Footprint of CDRs. The structure of the H2-K^b/dEV8/2CTCR complex (2TCR) was displayed in PyMol (*509*). **(A)** shows the full complex, **(B)** a close-up of the TCR/MHC/peptide interface, and **(C)** shows the surface of the MHC (magenta)/peptide (yellow) complex with the CDR loops of the TCR Vα (green) and Vβ (blue) shown and labeled.

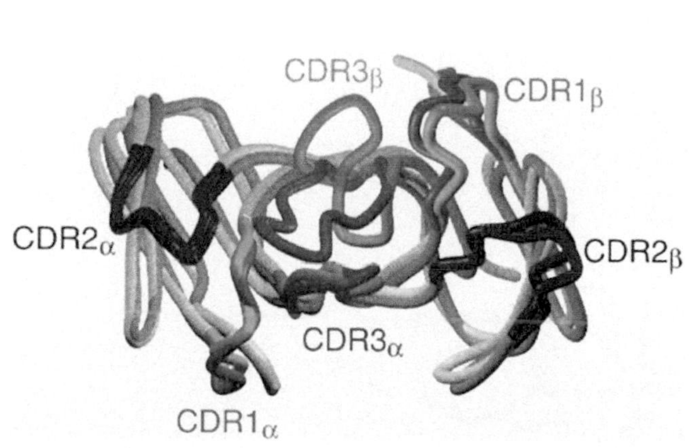

FIGURE 19.19 CDR3 plasticity. Backbone tracings of the KB5-C20 TCR CDR loops free or bound to the MHC/peptide complex are superposed. The unliganded forms are in lighter colors. (From (*430*), with permission.)

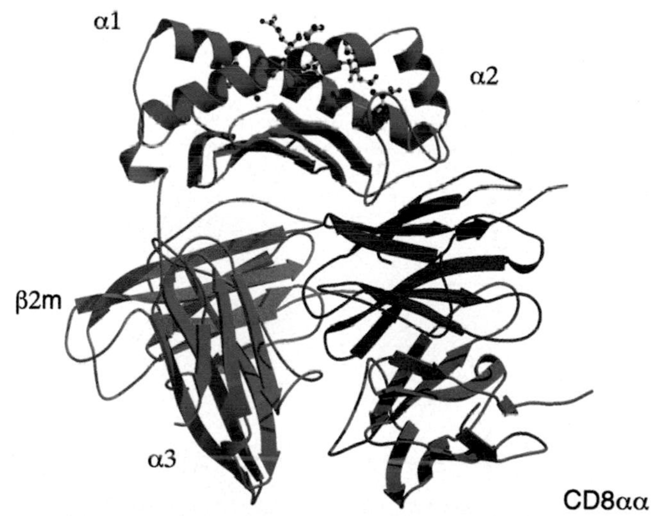

FIGURE 19.20 MHC-I–binding site for CD8$\alpha\alpha$ homodimer lies beneath the peptide-binding groove. HLA-A2 heavy chain, red, β2m, orange, and peptide (ball-and-stick) are shown in complex with the CD8$\alpha\alpha$ homodimer (red and blue). MOLSCRIPT (*511*) illustration based on the PDB (*508*) file 1AKJ (82).

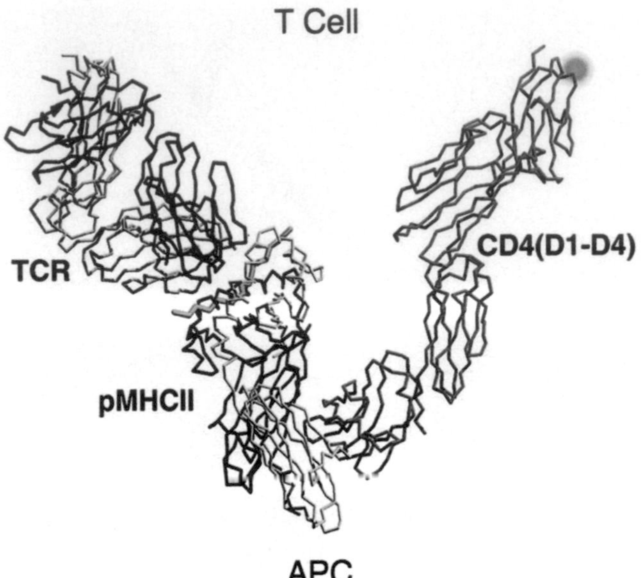

FIGURE 19.21 Model of TCR/MHC-II/peptide complex interacting with CD4. Superposition of MHC-II/CD4 D1D2 structure with that of a complete D1-D4 CD4 structure results in this model suggesting how MHC-II may contribute to multimerization of a TCR/CD4 complex. (From (78), with permission.)

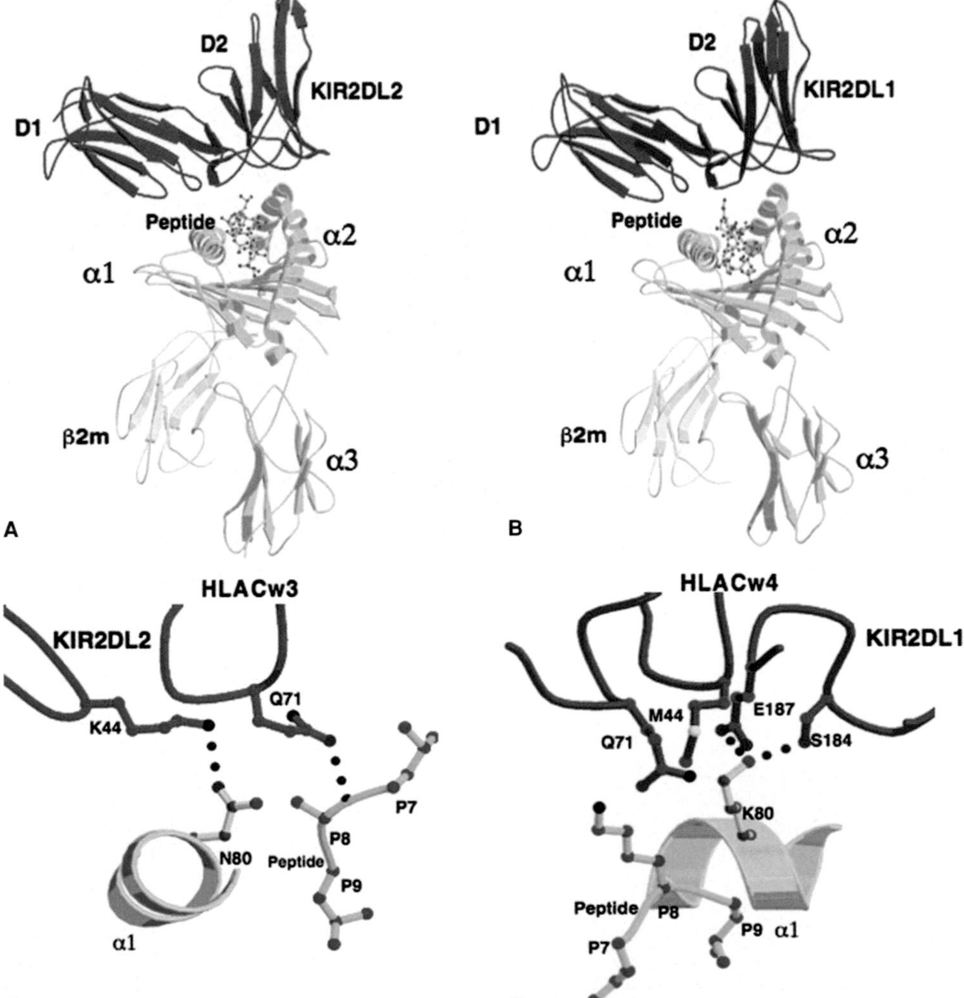

FIGURE 19.22 Interactions of KIR2D molecules with their HLA-Cw ligands. KIR2DL2 **(A, C)** and KIR2DL1 **(B, D)** are shown (magenta) in complex with their respective HLA-Cw3 and HLA-Cw4 ligands. (From (13), with permission.)

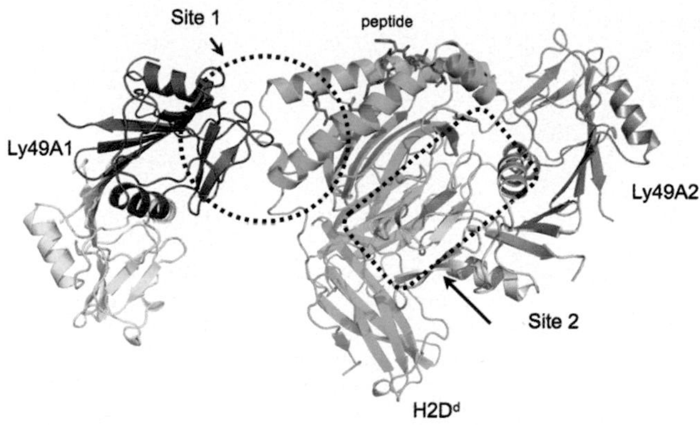

FIGURE 19.23 H2-D^{d} interactions with the C-type lectinlike receptor, Ly49A. The crystallographic determination of two distinct sites of H2-D^{d} interacting with the Ly49A homodimer is shown. Extensive mutagenesis and binding studies suggest that the functional site of interaction is site 2. (From (13), with permission.)

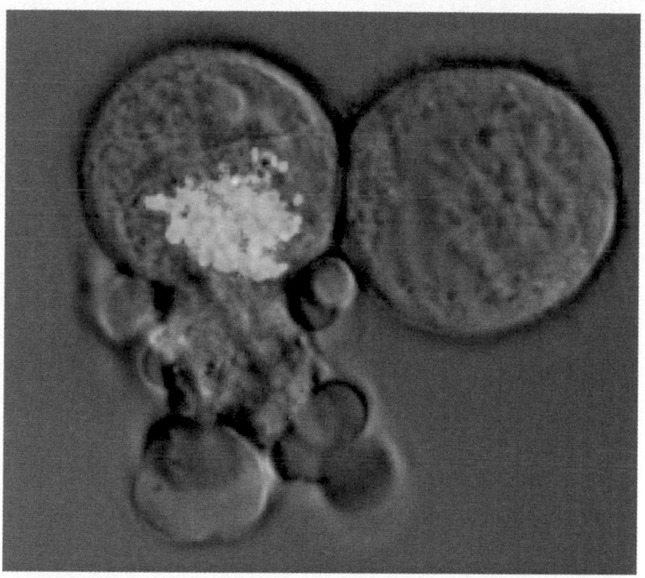

FIGURE 34.3 Killing in action. This cytotoxic cell appears to contact two targets (red); however, the granules (green) are polarized to the left-hand target. The cell exhibits the characteristic blebbing of apoptosis. The other target seems unaffected. Figure provided by Dr. I.S. Goping, University of Alberta.

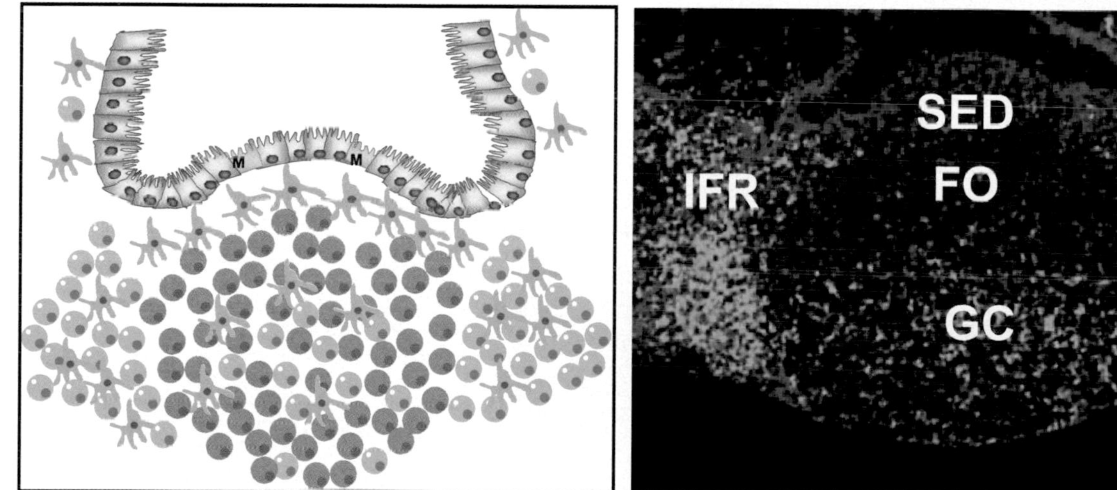

FIGURE 31.5 Segregated cell distribution in the PPs. CD4^{+} T cells (green) are mainly present in the intrafollicular regions (IFRs) and B cells (red) are located in the subepithelial dome (SED) and follicle (FO) regions. DCs (blue) are distributed in the SED and IFRs. GCs are enriched in B cells with small numbers of T cells and DCs for the creation of a cellular environment for the efficient generation of IgA-committed B cells.

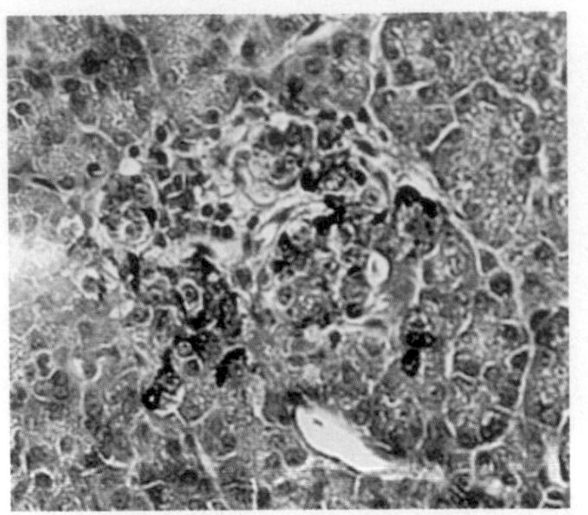

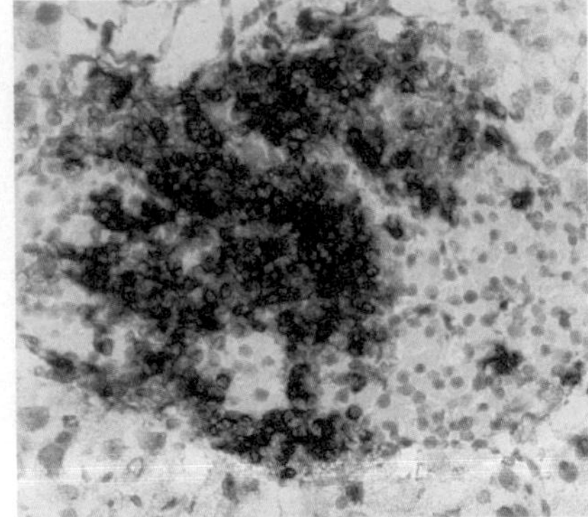

FIGURE 42.6 Human and mouse insulitic lesions. Comparison of human insulitis **(left)** and insulitis from a rat insulin promoter-lymphocytic choriomeningitis virus (LCMV) mouse 14 days postinfection with LCMV **(right)**. (Left panel courtesy of Francesco Dotta, University La Sapienzia, Rome, Italy; right panel courtesy of von Herrath laboratory, La Jolla Institute for Allergy and Immunology, La Jolla, California.)

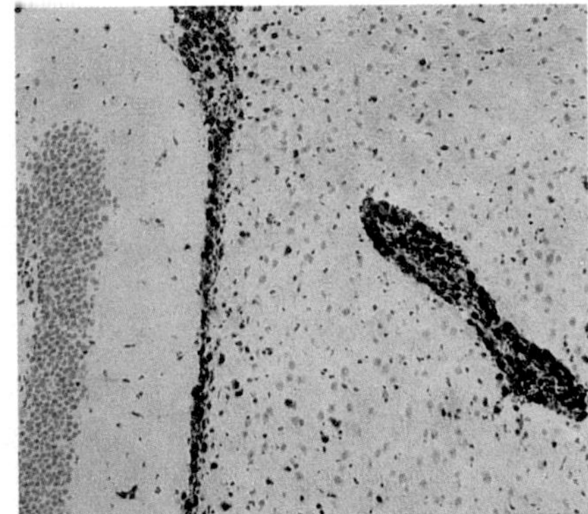

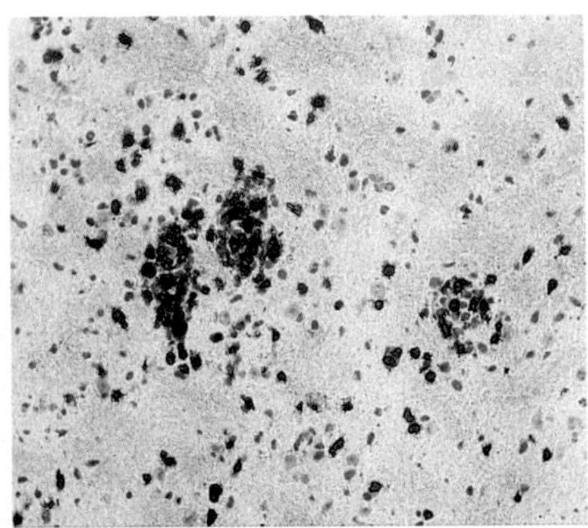

FIGURE 42.8 Induction of experimental allergic encephalitis in SJL mice with proteolipoprotein peptide amino acids 139 to 151 and adjuvant. (Courtesy of Andreas Holz, Max Planck Institute for Neurobiology, Munich, Germany.)

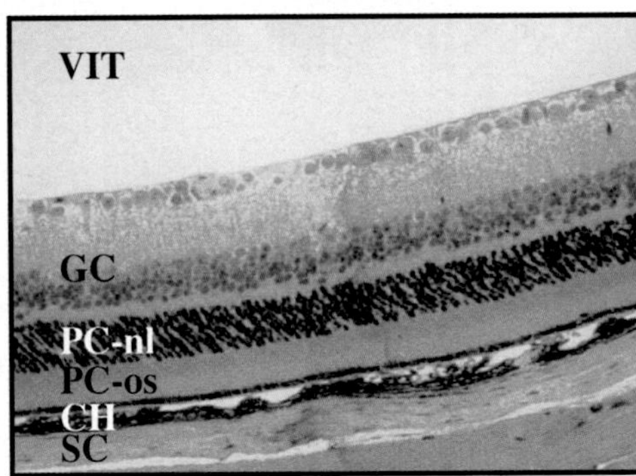

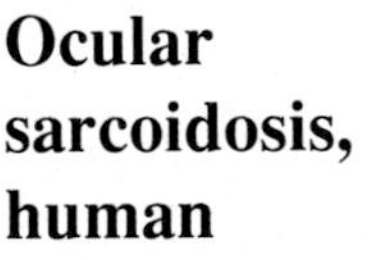

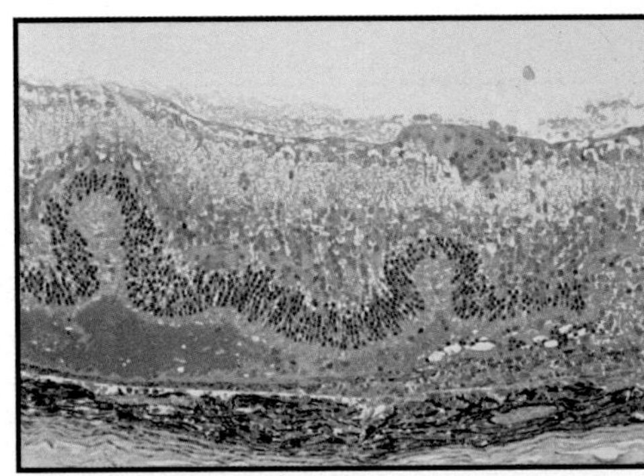

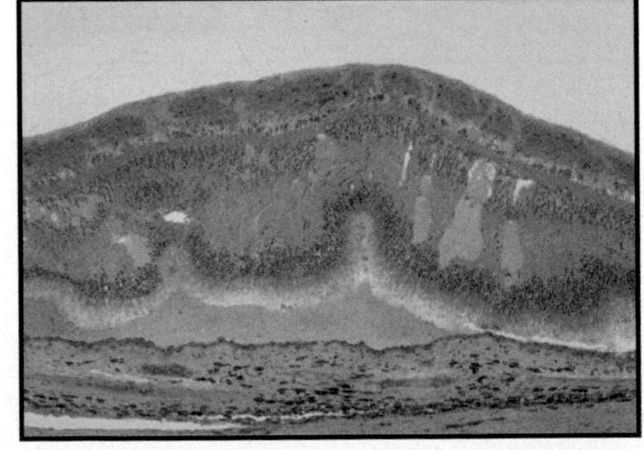

FIGURE 42.11 Histopathologic comparison of human and mouse uveitis. (Courtesy of Rachel Caspi, National Eye Institute, Bethesda, Maryland.) EAU, experimental autoimmune uveoretinitis.

SECTION II

Organization and Evolution of the Immune System

Chapter 2

Lymphoid Tissues and Organs

Eitan M. Akirav, Shan Liao, and Nancy H. Ruddle

INTRODUCTION

The mammalian immune system has evolved to provide defense against invading pathogens, taking advantage of the innate and adaptive systems. Although cells that can respond to pathogens are scattered in tissues throughout the body, the optimal structures for the response to antigens are organized, compartmentalized cellular aggregates that allow antigen concentration and presentation to a limited number of antigen-specific lymphocytes. The primary lymphoid organs are the sites where diverse populations of naïve, functionally mature lymphocytes are generated to disperse throughout the body and await foreign invaders. This remarkable differentiation process occurs in a foreign antigen-independent fashion. The secondary lymphoid organs and mucosal-associated lymphoid tissues are discrete sites in which naïve, antigen-specific T and B lymphocytes encounter invaders to generate an adaptive response. The lymph nodes and spleen, located in anatomically distinct sites, have traditionally been described as somewhat static structures. In fact, they are responsive to environmental influences and undergo remarkable changes in the course of antigenic challenge. The spleen, lymph nodes, Peyers patches, tonsils and adenoids, and the (mouse and rat) nose-associated lymphoid tissue (NALT) are controlled by precise developmental programs. Somewhat less anatomically restricted tissues that are even more sensitive to the environment include accumulations of lymphoid cells that are organized but less discretely defined: the bronchus associated lymphoid tissues (BALT) and isolated lymphoid follicles (ILF). Tertiary lymphoid organs, or more accurately, tertiary lymphoid tissues, are accumulations of lymphoid cells that arise ectopically in sites that are not anatomically restricted and are not regulated by developmental programs. Such chronic lymphoid-cell infiltrates into organs, such as the pancreas and joints, are not usually delimited by a capsule, as are the thymus and the majority of secondary lymphoid organs. They respond to environmental stimuli and arise during chronic inflammation subsequent to microbial infection, graft rejection, or autoimmunity by the process of lymphoid neogenesis (1,2). They are classified as tertiary lymphoid tissues because they resemble secondary lymphoid organs with regard to cellular composition and compartmentalization, chemokines, and vascular addressins. In this chapter, the structure, function, trafficking patterns, and developmental signals that regulate the hierarchy of lymphoid organs will be described.

PRIMARY LYMPHOID ORGANS

The primary lymphoid organs are the sites where pre-B and pre-T lymphocytes mature into naïve T and B cells in the absence of foreign antigen. Each T or B cell expresses a unique receptor that can recognize and respond to foreign antigens, and in most cases, discriminate between self and foreign antigens. Naïve cells leave the primary lymphoid organs having received and responded to developmental cues that result in the rearrangement of their genetic material to generate a repertoire capable of recognizing and responding to a wide variety of foreign antigens. In the course of maturation in the primary lymphoid organs, the naïve lymphocytes express various chemokine receptors and adhesion molecules that direct them to secondary lymphoid organs.

TABLE 2.1 Chemokines Implicated in Lymphoid Organ Development and Maintenance

Standard Name	*Common Names*	*Receptor*
CXCL12	SDF-1	CXCR4
CXCL13	BCA-1, BLC	CXCR5
CCL17	TARC	CCR4
CCL19	ELC, MIP-3β	CCR7
CCL20	MIP-3α	CCR6
CCL21	SLC, 6Ckine	CCR7
CCL25	TEC, TECK	CCR9
CCL28	MEC	CCR10

Fetal Liver

The earliest lymphoid cell precursors derive from self-renewing hematopoietic precursors called hematopoietic stem cells (HSCs). During ontogeny, these cells occupy several niches. In the fetal mouse, the first wave of hematopoiesis occurs in the yolk sac and aorta-gonad-mesonephros region at E10.5 (3). The placenta also contains HSC activity (4,5). Cells leave these tissues and migrate to the spleen and then the bone marrow under the influence of chemokines and adhesion molecules. The cells in the fetal liver CXCL12 (stromal cell derived factor, or SDF-1) (Table 2.1), in contrast to those in the bone marrow, also respond to the cytokine known as Steel factor (6). The fetal liver is the source of $CD4^+CD3^-$ lymphoid tissue inducer cells that express LTα and LTβ. The crucial importance of these cells in the development of secondary lymphoid organs is described later. Differentiation of HSC cells to B cells occurs in the fetal liver but does not require IL-7. Of the several different subsets of B cells, those generated by the fetal liver HSCs are somewhat limited and are of the B-1 subset (7). They do not give rise to CD5 B cells, predominately B1-B cells, and do not express terminal deoxynucleotidyl transferase and myosinlike light chain (7,8). It is not known whether these differences are intrinsic to the cells or are due to differences in the cytokine environment of fetal liver and bone marrow. P-selectin, E-selectin, and VCAM-1 are required for the cells to leave the fetal liver and move to the bone marrow (9,10).

Adult Bone Marrow

Functions

The bone marrow is the source of self-renewing populations of stem cells. These cells include precursors for HSCs and endothelial progenitor cells (ESC), which may derive from a single precursor (11). Bone marrow contains adult stem cells that can differentiate into adipocytes, chondrocytes, osteocyes, and myoblasts (12). The possibility that the bone marrow serves as a source of stem cells to, for example, repopulate the liver or that the stem cells residing in the bone marrow exhibit plasticity that allows them to develop into cells of other differentiated types has generated great interest in this organ (13). This chapter concentrates on the role of the bone marrow as an immunological organ, giving rise to B cells and T-cell precursors and serving as a repository for plasma cells. Prethymocytes leave the bone marrow and seed the thymus, where they undergo differentiation to naïve T cells. Bone marrow stromal cells secrete growth factors crucial for the development of HSCs. Additional factors enable the differentiation of immature B cells from HSC. The several stages of B cell differentiation that include Fraction A (pre-pro B cell), Fraction B/C (pro-B cell), and Fraction D (pre-B cell) are described in detail in Chapter 7 of this volume.

In addition to serving as a primary lymphoid organ where B cell differentiation and development occur, the bone marrow is also a home for antibody-secreting cells (14). After B cells have interacted with antigens in the secondary lymphoid organs, they enter the blood stream and travel to the marrow. Thus, this organ not only serves as a primary lymphoid organ, but also as a reservoir for fully differentiated plasma cells.

Architecture: Cellular and Functional Niches

The microenvironment of the bone marrow, contained in the central cavity of bone, is a complex three-dimensional structure with cellular niches that influence B cells during their development and later, as plasma cells, as they return to the bone marrow. The bone marrow has a rich blood supply with a nutrient artery that branches into ascending and descending arteries, which further divide into cortical capillaries, periosteal capillaries, and endosteal capillaries and finally merge into a sinus (15). Previously, the prevailing understanding of B cell differentiation in the bone marrow was that primitive HSCs were located in close contact with the endosteum near osteoblasts (the "endosteal niche"). During the course of differentiation into mature B cells, they moved into the central region of the bone marrow cavity (the "vascular niche") (16). The former niche was identified as the location of HSC; the latter, as the site of B cell differentiation (17). Recently, this anatomic concept has been challenged, because it has been reported that HSCs are found throughout the bone marrow. It has become clear that growth factors and cytokines produced by different stromal cells influence cells at certain stages in their differentiation. Thus, it is more appropriate to consider functional or cellular, rather than anatomical, niches (15,18). Once the HSCs differentiate into immature B cells expressing cell surface IgM, they undergo processes of negative selection and receptor editing, leave the bone marrow, and travel through the blood stream to the secondary lymphoid organs where they complete their differentiation.

Several cytokines and chemokines influence B cell differentiation in the bone marrow. Flt-3 ligand (also called Flk-2L) signals B cell differentiation and growth and synergizes with several other hematopoietic growth factors (19). Its receptor, Flt-3 (also known as Flk-2), expressed by primitive HSCs, is a member of the class II tyrosine kinase family. In contrast to fetal liver, HSCs from adult bone marrow do not respond to Steel factor. Chemokines contribute to B cell differentiation in the bone marrow and define the functional niches. Many of these factors affect other lymphoid cells, such as dendritic and T cells. For an excellent review of this topic, see Nagasawa (15). Several of these factors, whose functions have been identified in gene deletion studies in mice, in morphologic analysis, and in cell culture studies, play roles in multiple aspects of lymphoid organ development; their activities, though important in the bone marrow, are not limited to that organ. CXCL12, also known as SDF1, or stromal cell-derived factor-1, is a chemokine that is crucial for recruitment of HSCs to the bone marrow. It is widely expressed by osteoblasts, reticular cells (18) and endothelial cells (20). In fact, the interaction of HSCs expressing CXCR4, the receptor for CXCL12, with that chemokine on the endothelial surface is the first step in its exit from the circulation into the marrow (21). CXCL12 is also essential for the earliest stage of B cell development (pre-pro B cells). Its receptor, CXCR4, is expressed on early B cells and is down-regulated in pre-B cells. It remains at low levels in immature B cells and mature B cells in secondary lymphoid organs but is up-regulated after B cells interact with antigen and differentiate into plasma cells (14). This explains the propensity of antibody secreting cells to return to the bone marrow. Once a pre-pro B cell has interacted with CXCL12, it moves on to a different cell expressing IL-7. In B cell development, IL-7 acts later than CXCL12 in a narrow window between pro-B cells and immature B cells in the scheme proposed by Nagasawa (15).

Traffic In and Out: Chemokines and Adhesion Molecules

The extensive vascularization of the bone marrow allows the entrance of hematopoietic precursors and plasma cells and the egress of mature cells. Hematopoietic progenitor recruitment to the bone marrow in the mouse has been shown to be dependent on the interaction of a variety of chemokines, integrins, and selectins and their receptors, counter-receptors, and ligand vascular cell adhesion molecules. These include $\alpha4$ integrin (VLA4 or $\alpha4\beta1$) and VCAM-1 (22), P-selectin glycoprotein ligand-1 (PSGL-1) and E-selectin (23), and $\alpha4\beta7$ and mucosal addressin cell adhesion molecule (MAdCAM-1) (24). It has not been determined whether pre-B cells and precursor T cells in the bone marrow down-regulate one set of addressins and up-regulate another to enter into the secondary lymphoid organs and thymus. A small subpopulation of newly formed B cells in the bone marrow that expresses L-selectin has been described (25), suggesting a mechanism for entrance into lymph nodes.

In addition to the acquisition of immunoglobulin expression that occurs in the bone marrow under the control of stromal cells (see Chapter 7), B cells express various chemokine receptors and adhesion molecules in the process of differentiation. In a study of human bone marrow B cells, it was determined that pro-B and pre-B cells migrate toward CXCL12 but not toward a wide range of other chemokines, including CCL19 and CCL21, though they do express low levels of CCR7, the receptor for CCL19 and CCL21. However, mature bone marrow B cells do respond to CCL 19 and CCL 21 (26), CXCL13 (indicating a functional CXCR5), and CCL20 (MIP 3α). But CCR6 expression and responsiveness to CCL20 was only seen in mouse B cells after they had migrated into the periphery during the process of maturation in the circulating B cell pool (27).

Thymus

Function

The thymus is defined as a primary lymphoid organ due to its inimitable role in T cell development. Indeed, a mutant known as the "nude" (*nu/nu*) mouse, which lacks a normal thymus, is completely devoid of mature T cells (28). Recently, an additional, previously unappreciated thymus-like organ has been described in the mouse (29). This so-called "cervical thymus" is organized similarly to the main thymus and is capable of supporting T cell development. Although some studies suggest that T cells can develop extrathymically in organs such as the gut epithelium (30), the thymus remains the main site for T cell maturation, education, and selection. T cell precursors represent more than 95% of total cells in the thymus and give rise to mature T cells. These cells are crucial components of the adaptive immune system in that they are highly specific in their ability to recognize a nearly infinite number of antigens owing to their diverse repertoire (28,31).

The T cell repertoire is shaped during development in the thymus by the processes of positive and negative selection. Negative selection insures that T cells, which are capable of recognizing the organism's self-antigens presented on major histocompatibility complex (MHC) class I or II with high affinity, are eliminated prior to their export to the periphery. This process results in the deletion of approximately 95% of T cell precursors in the thymus (32). In contrast, positive selection allows for T cells recognizing self-antigen with low to medium affinity to leave the thymus and protect the organism against invading pathogens.

Although negative selection is highly efficient in eliminating the majority of self-reactive T cells, some cells do escape the thymus and exit to the periphery. These so-called "autoreactive cells" impose a serious threat to various organs, as their activation may result in the development of autoimmune diseases. The immune system has evolved several ways to prevent the activation of autoreactive T cells in the periphery. One mechanism that protects against autoimmunity is the generation of a T cell population capable of suppressing activation of self-reactive T cells. These thymus-derived protective T cells, known as regulatory or suppressive T cells, recognize self-antigens with relatively high affinity.

Thymic Architecture

The thymus in the mouse consists of two symmetric lobes located above the heart, while in humans the thymus is multilobed. Each lobe can be divided into three distinct regions: capsule, cortex, and medulla. The latter two regions harbor thymocytes at various maturation stages. Although maturing T cells constitute the majority of cells in the thymus, other cell types such as macrophages, dendritic cells, B cells, and epithelial cells are also present (33). Histological analysis of the thymus reveals a clear distinction between the thymic cortex and medulla, which are separated by a cortico-medullary border. The thymic cortex appears darker and more densely populated with T cell precursors, whereas the medulla appears considerably lighter and contains smaller numbers of T cells relative to other cell types (Figure 2.1, top panel). Blood vessels and small blood capillaries are found throughout the thymus. The fact that T cell progenitors are found in the more highly vascularized cortico-medullary border suggests that blood vessels in this region facilitate the entry of T cell progenitors into the thymic parenchyma (34). In the thymic medulla, the close association between medullary thymic epithelial cells and thymic blood vessels (35) suggests that these vessels may act as organizers of the medullary thymic compartment. Lymphatic vessel distribution coincides with that of blood vessels and capillaries (36). The majority of lymphatic vessels are located in the thymic medulla, though some can also be found in the cortex. The role of lymphatic vessels in thymic function remain unclear, although it has been proposed that these vessels may deliver extrathymic antigens into the thymus or export mature T cells from the thymus into the circulation.

Cellular Composition and Functions

T cell precursors at various stages of differentiation represent the majority of cells in the thymus. The education and selection of T cells in the thymus is mediated by antigen-presenting cells (APCs) of either hematopoietic or stromal origin. The different stages in T cell selection and maturation that take place in distinct regions of the thymus (Figure 2.1, bottom panel) are discussed at length

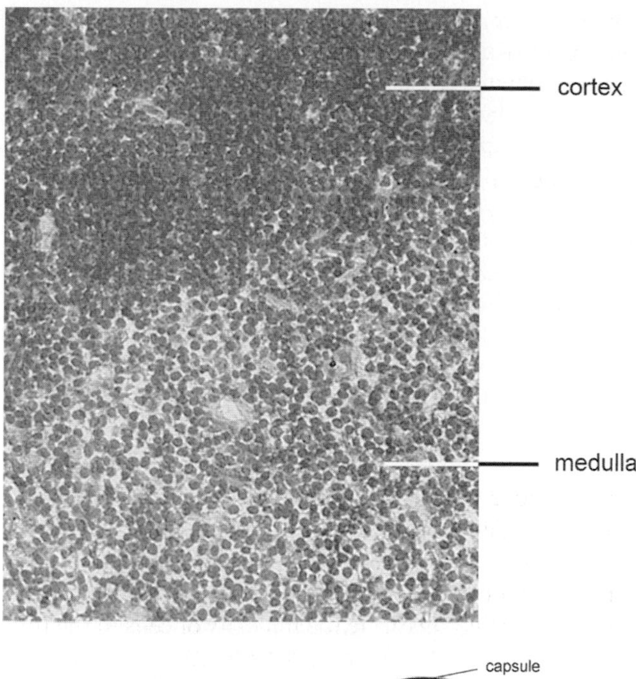

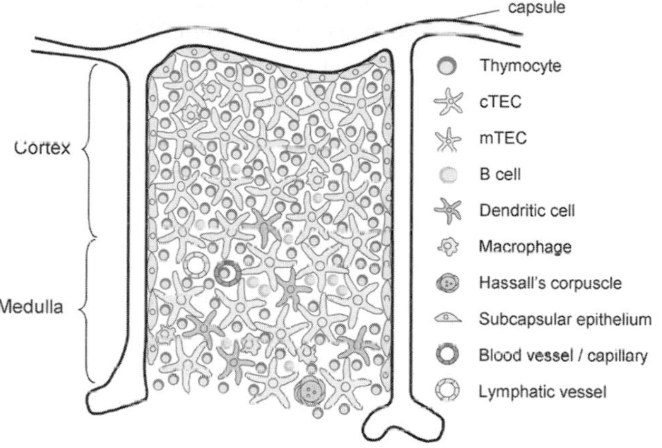

FIGURE 2.1 **Top panel:** Thymic structure. Low-power magnification of a Haematoxylin-stained frozen section of a mouse thymus. The cortex is well populated with lymphocytes; the medulla is less tightly packed and thus stains less intensely. **Bottom panel:** Thymic cellular populations. Diagram of a mouse thymus. Precursor T cells enter through blood vessels at the cortico-medullary junction. They progress to the medulla, where they undergo differentiation from double negative (DN) to double positive (DP) cells expressing T cell receptors. Thymic stromal cells provide growth factors. DP cells undergo positive selection, under the influence of cortical thymic epithelial cells (cTEC). Single positive (SP) CD4 or CD8 cells migrate into the medulla where they undergo negative selection, mainly through AIRE expressing mTECs and DCs. SP cells, having undergone differentiation, exit through blood vessels (not shown) to the periphery.

in Chapter 12. Briefly, lymphoid progenitors enter the thymus at the cortico-medullary border (34). Following their entry, these cells, identified as double negative (DN) T cells due to a lack of expression of the cell surface molecules CD4 and CD8, undergo four maturation steps termed DN1–DN4, which are distinguished by the expression of two additional cell surface molecules: CD25 and CD44 (37,38). DN3 cells migrate to the subcapsular zone while rearranging their T cell receptor (TCR) β chain and expressing it in combination with a surrogate α chain. Those cells that have successfully rearranged the genes for α and β chains of the TCR become double positive (DP) cells and express both CD4 and CD8 surface markers. In the cortex, DP cells undergo negative and positive selection (39,40). Positively selected DP cells further differentiate into single positive (SP) cells expressing either CD4 or CD8. Following their differentiation, SP cells relocate to the medulla, where they mature and undergo further rounds of deletion. SP cells that do survive are then exported out of the thymus (41). DN precursors can give rise to an additional T cell population expressing the $\gamma\delta$TCR. These T cells are distinct from TCR$\alpha\beta$ T cells in their tissue distribution and recognition of antigens. TCR$\alpha\beta$ DP cells control the development of TCR$\gamma\delta$ cells via the production of the cytokine, lymphotoxin β (LTβ) (42).

The thymic parenchyma consists of a complex three-dimensional structure supported by thymic epithelial cells (TECs). TECs in the thymic cortex and thymic medulla are phenotypically and functionally distinct and support different stages of T cell maturation. Several cell surface markers are used to distinguish medullary TECs (mTECs) from cortical TECs (cTECs) in the mouse. Among these markers are the cytokeratins K5 and K8, the adhesion molecule Ep-CAM, and the glycoprotein Ly-51. K8 and Ly-51 are expressed by cTECs, while K5 and Ep-CAM are expressed by mTECs (43,44). TECs are unique in that they express MHC II constitutively similarly to professional APCs. The role of TECs in T cell selection was recently elucidated by their expression of the transcription factor, autoimmune regulator (AIRE). This transcription factor plays an important role in T cell selection and prevention of autoimmunity as illustrated by the fact that humans with a mutated form of the AIRE gene exhibit polyendocrine autoimmunity due to inadequate T cell selection (45). It has become clear that AIRE controls the expression of certain tissue-specific antigens in the thymus, such as insulin, a protein that is unique to the β cells of the islets of Langerhans in the pancreas (44,46). The expression of tissue-specific antigens in the thymus facilitates the negative selection of maturing T cells, which would otherwise be allowed to leave the thymus. The thymic medulla includes distinct structures also known as Hassall's corpuscles. Originally described by Arthur Hill Hassall in 1849, this structure consists of concentric stratified keratinizing epithelium. Hassall's corpuscles are implicated in several processes of the thymus (47), including the expression of tissue-specific antigens, such as insulin (48), and serve as a prominent site for T cell apoptosis (49).

Dendritic cells (DCs) are professional antigen-presenting cells that are found in the thymus. Thymic DCs can be divided into two distinct populations. The first originates from a thymocyte precursor (50,51), whereas the second is derived from partially mature peripheral DCs that continuously enter the thymus from the circulation (52). DCs do not appear to be involved in positive selection but do contribute to negative selection (53–56). They have been recently implicated in the selection of regulatory T cells in humans (57). Activation of thymic DC can be mediated in part by the IL-7-like cytokine, known as thymic stromal lymphopoietin (TSLP). In the human thymus, TSLP is preferentially produced by Hassall's corpuscles, and TSLP-activated DCs can alter the fate of self-reactive T cell from deletion to positive selection of regulatory T cells (58). These findings highlight the heterogeneity of DCs and emphasize their ability to fulfill different roles during T cell development in the thymus.

Macrophages and B cells are additional hematopoietic-derived professional APCs in the thymus. In contrast to DCs, thymic macrophages are located throughout the thymus and do not play a significant role in T cell selection (59). B cells are detected in human and mouse thymus at relatively low numbers (60,61) and are characterized by the expression of the cell surface molecule CD5. They are capable of producing antibodies of several different isotypes (62). It has been suggested that thymic B cells induce negative selection in developing thymocytes (60), as B cell–deficient mice show a limited T cell repertoire when compared with normal mice (63).

Traffic In and Out: Adhesion Molecules and Chemokines

The extravasation of leukocytes from blood and lymphatic vessels into the thymus is mediated by adhesion molecules. These molecules also play an important role in facilitating lymphocyte homing into various regions of the thymus. Indeed, thymic blood vessels express the adhesion molecules ICAM-1, VCAM-1, CD34, peripheral node addressin (PNAd), and vascular adhesion protein-1 (VAP-1) (64). The expression of high levels of ICAM-1, VCAM-1, and VAP-1 on venules near the cortico-medullary border suggests that these molecules may play a role in the recruitment of thymocyte progenitors. More specifically, VAP-1, which is restricted to the venules surrounding the sites of progenitor homing, can mediate the extravasation of leukocytes. The regional distribution of these adhesion molecules further illustrates the importance of a distinct anatomical separation between cortex and medulla and represents their individual functions.

Chemokine-mediated T cell migration and traffic to and within the thymus is crucial for normal T cell selection. The compartmentalization of the thymus is orchestrated by a milieu of chemokines. The thymic cortex is involved in the maturation of DN cells to DP cells and in positive and negative selection of DP T cells, while the medulla acts as the site of negative selection and possibly positive selection of SP T cells and regulatory T cells, respectively. Various chemokines that are produced by the thymic cortex and medulla allow T cells expressing different chemokine receptors to home to specific regions of the thymus. This differential expression of chemokines is complemented by the fact that T cells at different maturation states express certain chemokine receptors. During development, the entry of the lymphoid progenitor into the thymus is highly dependent on CCL21 and CCL25, which bind the chemokine receptors CCR7 and CCR9, respectively. Mice lacking CCR7 or CCL21 (65,66) show a transient delay in thymus colonization by lymphocytes (day 14.5), and this delay is further extended (day 17.5) in mice lacking CCR9 (67). Lymphoid progenitors enter the thymus at the cortico-medullary border and commence their migration outward toward the subcapsular region of the cortex as DN3 cells. The expression of the chemokine receptors CXCR4 and CCR7 by DN cells is important in directing cell migration (68,69). In the subcapsular region, DN thymocytes that have successfully rearranged their TCR$\alpha\beta$ chains progress to the DP cell stage. Positively selected DP cells move inward toward the thymic medulla for further differentiation into SP cells. The ligands for CCR7 are crucial in mediating the migration of positively selected DP cells into the medulla, as illustrated by the fact that a deficiency in CCR7 or its ligands, CCL19 or CCL21, prevents DP cell relocation from the cortex to the medulla and results in abnormal central tolerance (70,71). The export of positively selected SP T cells out of the thymus is also dependent on chemokines. Chemokines involved in T cell emigration are CXCL12 and its receptor CXCR4, which repels SP cells out of the thymus (72), and CCL19, which promotes T cell emigration from the thymus of newborn mice (73). The chemoattractant, sphingosine 1-phosphate (S1P), is a additional mediator of T cell emigration. SP T cell express the S1P receptor ($S1P_1$) and are attracted to the high levels of S1P present in the serum promoting their egress (74,75).

While the role of different thymic compartments and chemokines in the maturation of naïve SP T cell has been extensively studied, the thymic regions and chemokines that control the selection of regulatory T cells remain largely unknown. Some studies suggest that cTECs are sufficient for mediating regulatory T cell development (76), while others implicate DCs as key APCs in regulatory T cell selection in the thymic medulla (57,77). It may be that chemokines produced by both cTECs and thymic DCs play a role in regulatory T cell selection, albeit during different stages of maturation.

Development

The initial development of the thymus at midgestation in the mouse is independent of vascularization or bone marrow–derived cells. In the mouse, the thymus rudiment is first evident on day 11 of gestation as it evolves from the endoderm of the third pharyngeal pouch (78). This gives rise to the thymic lobes as well as to the parathyroid gland. On day 12.5 of gestation, a separation of the primordium is observed, and by day 13.5 a distinct thymus is apparent. Evidence has suggested that not only the pharyngeal pouch endoderm, but also the ectoderm may also be involved in thymic development (79,80). More specifically, it was suggested that the pharyngeal pouch ectoderm contributes to the development cTECs, whereas the endoderm contributes solely to the development mTECs. This "dual origin" model was mainly supported by histological data, as well as data collected from thymi of *nu/nu* mice (81–83). Recently, it was shown that both thymic cortex and medulla are derived solely from the pharyngeal pouch endoderm (84) and that, although the endoderm and ectoderm are found in close proximity between gestational day 10.5 and 11, only the endoderm actively contributes to thymic development (85). These findings support the so-called "single origin" model of thymus development.

The contribution of lymphocytes to the normal development of thymic cortex and medulla is well recognized. In models of T cell deficiency, cTEC and mTEC development is halted at different stages depending on the stage of T cell arrest. If T cell development is arrested at the DN stage, as in the recombinase-activating gene (RAG)–deficient mouse, the thymic medulla is greatly reduced while the thymic cortex remains unaffected (86,87). A more severe phenotype is observed in transgenic mice that overexpress the human CD3-signaling molecule. In these mice, T cell arrest occurs earlier than in RAG-knockout mice, leading to a loss of both cortex and medulla and to a shift from a three- to a two-dimensional structure of the thymic epithelia (87).

Recently, two cytokines, LT α (also called tumor necrosis factor β) and LT β, have been identified as master regulators of mTEC development and expression of tissue-specific antigens. LT α and β are members of the tumor necrosis factor (TNF) superfamily and mediate the processes of secondary lymphoid organ development and inflammation (1,88). In the absence of LT, tissue-specific antigen and AIRE expression are reduced and certain mTEC subpopulations fail to develop (89,90). T cells appear to be the main source for LT production in the thymus (42), further highlighting the importance of lymphocytes in its development.

The development of the thymus in humans closely follows the model of thymic development in the mouse and bird. Similar to the mouse, thymic colonization by hematopoietic stem cells occurs relatively early, at week 8.2 of gestation. During this stage, the thymic medulla and cortex are organized, suggesting that thymocytes are required for normal thymic development. Between gestation week 9.5 and 10, the first signs of thymocyte negative selection are evident and by gestation week 10 to 12.75 the gradual onset of positive selection is detected (91).

SECONDARY LYMPHOID ORGANS AND TISSUES

Naïve cells express their receptors for specific antigens, leave primary lymphoid organs, circulate through the blood stream, migrate into the tissues, and lodge in secondary lymphoid organs. The frequency of naïve cells specific for an individual antigen is quite low (estimates range from 1 in 10^5 to 1 in 10^7). Thus, the chance that an individual T or B cell will encounter its specific antigen in the circulation is rather low. Secondary lymphoid organs are strategically located in anatomically distinct sites where foreign antigen and antigen-presenting cells efficiently concentrate and activate rare antigen-specific lymphocytes, thus leading to the initiation of adaptive immune responses and generation of long-lived protective immunity. These organs include highly organized, encapsulated, and compartmentalized tissues, such as lymph nodes, spleen, appendix, tonsils, murine NALT, and Peyers patches. Naïve cells are also primed in less discrete tissues throughout the body, including the BALT, cryptopatches, and ILF.

Lymph Nodes

Lymph nodes are yellowish, bean-shaped structures dispersed along lymphatic vessels. The lymphatic vessel system plays important roles in tissue-fluid balance, fat transport in the intestine, and the immune response. In contradistinction to blood vessels, which form a closed recirculating system, lymphatic vessels comprise a blind-end, unidirectional transportation system. The absorbing lymphatic vessels, or lymphatic capillaries, remove interstitial fluid and macromolecules from extracellular spaces and transport the collected lymph through the primary collector. The collected lymph and its cellular contents are transported into the thoracic duct and returned back to the blood circulation. In humans, lymph collected from the entire lower body region, the left head, and arm region accumulates in the thoracic duct and returns to blood circulation via the left subclavian vein; lymph collected from right head and arm region returns to blood via the right subclavian vein.

Lymph nodes, usually embedded in fat, are located at vascular junctions and are served by lymphatic vessels. Although most lymph nodes are classified as peripheral lymph nodes, a few (cervical, mesenteric, and sacral), termed mucosal nodes, express a slightly different complement of endothelial adhesion molecules, cooperate with the mucosal system, and are regulated somewhat differently in development (discussed later). Although all lymph nodes are vascularized and thus can receive antigens from the blood stream, they are also served by a rich lymphatic vessel system and are thus particularly effective in mounting responses to antigens that are present in tissues. These antigens may be derived from foreign invaders that are transported by antigen-presenting cells or can be derived from self-antigens. Thus, lymph nodes extend the role of the primary lymphoid organs and discriminate between dangerous foreign antigens and benign self-antigens. This capacity relies on the antigen-presenting cells and their state of activation in the lymph node and the recognition capacity of the naïve T and B cells.

Lymph nodes can also function as niches for generating peripheral tolerance, an additional mechanism to minimize the effects of those self-reactive T-cells that escape central tolerance in the thymus (92). DCs constitutively sample self-antigens and migrate to draining lymph nodes even in the steady state (93–95). Because most self-antigen–bearing DCs in lymph nodes are immature (96) and have low levels of costimulatory molecules, they are not effective at activating naïve cells. They regulate self-reactive T cells by inducing anergy, clonal deletion, and expanding regulatory T cells (95–99).

Structure and Organization

The highly compartmentalized lymph node is surrounded by a capsule derived from lymphatic vessels (Figure 2.2, top and bottom panels). The cortical region includes discrete clusters called primary follicles consisting of densely packed naïve B cells and follicular dendritic cells (FDCs). After B cells encounter their cognate antigen, they are activated and proliferate, and secondary follicles and germinal centers develop. T cells and DCs distribute in the paracortex. Macrophages reside in the subcortical zone and in the medullary area. Plasma cells are also concentrated in the medulla as they prepare to leave the lymph node and circulate to the bone marrow. FDCs, a population of mesenchymal origin, support B cell follicles or germinal centers under stimulation (1). In addition, a network composed of reticular fibers, fibrous extracellular matrix bundles, and fibroblastic reticular cells, support the entire lymph node (100). Compartmentalization of cells in the lymph node is orchestrated by lymphoid chemokines CCL19, CCL21, and CXCL13. CCL19 is made by stromal cells in the paracortical region and the protein is transported to the surface of high endothelial venules (HEVs) (101). CCL21 is encoded by several genes (102); CCL21-leu is expressed by lymphatic vessels outside the lymph node (103); CCL21-ser is made by stromal cells and HEVs in the lymph node. CCL19 and CCL21 recruit CCR7 expressing cells across the HEVs and direct T cells and dendritic cells to the paracortical region. CXCL13, produced by stromal cells in the B cell follicles, attracts CXCR5-expressing B cells (104). After naïve T and B cells encounter antigens, they undergo extensive changes in expression of chemokine receptors and adhesion molecules that result in their movement to different areas of the lymph node or leaving it all together (105,106). Sphingosine-1-phosphate receptor 1 ($S1P_1$) facilitates lymphocyte egress from lymph nodes as they move towards the ligand, S1P in the lymph (107,108).

Lymph Node Vasculature

Recirculating lymphocytes leave the bloodstream via HEVs, specialized vessels with a high cuboidal endothelium, and migrate into the lymph node parenchyma. After surveying antigens in the lymph nodes, lymphocytes leave those organs via efferent lymphatic vessels and finally return to blood circulation. Afferent lymphatic vessels allow entrance of soluble antigen and antigen-presenting cells into lymph nodes, and efferent lymphatic vessels return lymphocytes back to the blood (109–111). In this manner, HEVs and lymphatic vessels maintain lymph node lymphocyte homeostasis during the steady state.

Blood Vessels

Blood endothelial cells play a crucial role in lymphocyte trafficking in the lymph node. One or two arteries enter the lymph node at the hilus. These arteries branch and pass through the medulla area, enter the cortex, and sometimes continue in the subcapsular area. Beneath the subcapsular sinus, the branching capillaries form loops and some of them become arteriovenous communications (AVCs). AVCs become HEVs in the cortex area and occasionally extend from the subcapsular sinus to the medulla. HEVs constitute a specialized postcapillary network in the lymph node, playing a critical role in lymphocyte recirculation. Each main HEV trunk receives three to five branches lined with high endothelial cells and two or three branches lined with flat endothelial cells. The luminal diameters of HEVs progressively increase from cortex to medulla. Finally, HEVs merge into segmental veins in the medulla area and join larger veins in the hilus (109) (Figure 2.2, top panel). Intravital microscopy has revealed that the entire venular tree consists of five branching orders, with the higher orders in the paracortex and the lower orders in the medulla and hilus areas. Only the higher-order venules, located in the T cell area, are specialized into HEV and are recognized by the monoclonal antibody MECA-79 (110,111). Approximately one in four lymphocytes enters the lymph node via HEVs (112), whereas other capillaries and arterioles are normally nonadhesive. Peripheral node addressin (PNAd), defined by the MECA-79 antigen, is also known as an L-selectin ligand and is a characteristic HEV adhesion molecule. PNAd is composed of a variety of core glycoproteins, including GlyCAM-1, CD34, Sgp200, and podocalyxin; these proteins must be sialylated, sulfated, and fucosylated to become the functional L-selectin ligand (i.e., PNAd). These posttranslational modification events involve several enzymes, including FucT-IV, FucT-VII, and HEC-6ST. HEC-6ST (also called LSST, GST-3, HEC-GlcNAc6ST, GlcNAC6ST-2, gene name

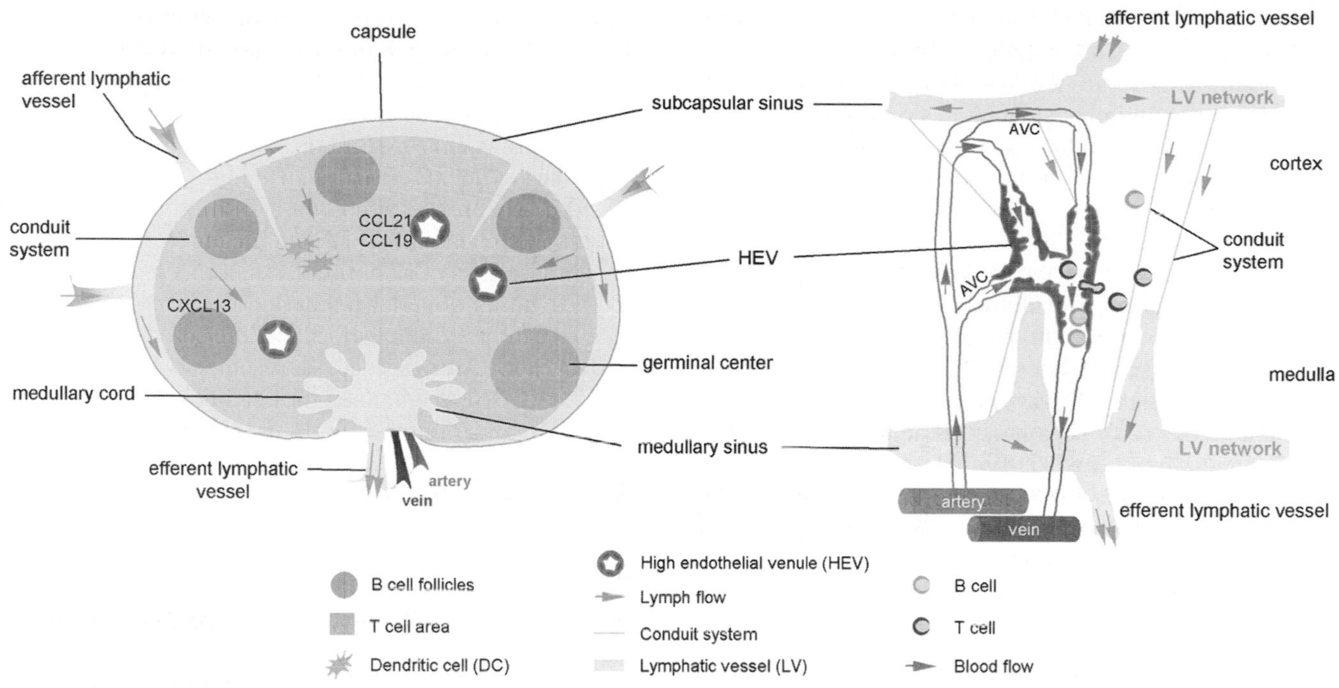

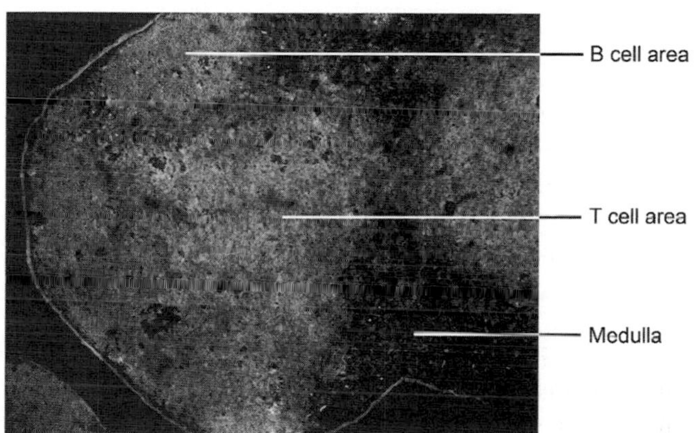

FIGURE 2.2 **Top panel:** Lymph node structure and functional regions. The lymph node is divided into an outer cortex and inner medulla surrounded by a capsule and lymphatic sinus. The cortex includes B cells and follicular dendritic cells. The paracortical region includes T cells and dendritic cells. Macrophages are found in the subcapsular sinus and medullary cord. Lymphocytes enter into the lymph node through an artery at the hilus region, and into the parenchyma through high endothelial venules (HEV) expressing PNAd and CCL19 and CCL21. These chemokines are also made by stromal cells. T cells and DCs are directed to the paracortical region by CCL19 and CCL21. B cells are directed to the cortex by CXCL13. After interaction with antigen and T cells, germinal centers develop. Antigen and DCs drain into the lymph node from the tissues through afferent lymphatic vessels. Antigen continues to percolate through the node via a conduit system. Activated cells leave through efferent lymphatic vessels. Diagram of the blood network of a rat lymph node (right) is adapted from Anderson et al. (109). Note the arteriovenous communications (AVC), the venous sphincters (VS), and cells leaving the HEVs into the parenchyma. **Bottom panel:** Lymph node compartmentalization. Immunofluorescent staining of B cells (anti-B220, green) in follicles in the cortex and T cells (anti-CD3, red) in the paracortical area. The medulla is unstained.

Chst4) (113–117), which is uniquely expressed in high endothelial cells, sulfates glycoproteins in the Golgi apparatus (118) to generate the MECA-79 epitope. PNAd, expressed on the endothelial surface, slows down (tethers) naïve L-selectin^{hi} lymphocytes in their progress through the blood vessels. After this initial interaction, CCL19 and CCL21 on the HEVs are instrumental in activating the lymphocyte integrin LFA-1. This results in tight binding of LFA-1 to ICAM-1 on the HEV, facilitating diapedesis of lymphocytes for transendothelial migration toward the chemokines located in the paracortical region (T cells, DCs) or cortex (B cells). Interestingly, the HEV-lymphocyte interaction is not random in different lymphoid tissues in the mouse (119,120). T lymphocytes adhere preferentially to peripheral lymph node HEVs, B cells prefer to adhere to HEVs in Peyers patches, and T and B cells exhibit an intermediate pattern of adhesion to mesenteric lymph node HEVs (32,119,121). The selective adhesion of naïve lymphocytes to HEVs is at least partially controlled by the differentially expressed adhesion molecules in different lymphoid organs. MAdCAM-1, the ligand for the integrin $\alpha_4\beta_7$, is expressed on HEVs of mesenteric lymph nodes and Peyers patches in adult mice; it is only apparent in early development on HEVs of peripheral lymph nodes and is thus a marker of immature HEVs in those nodes. MAdCAM-1 is rapidly replaced after birth by PNAd in mouse peripheral lymph nodes (122).

Lymphatic Vessels

Lymphatic vessels also play critical roles in the immune response. The collected lymph and cell contents enter the lymph node via several afferent lymphatic vessels and filter through the node. In this manner, soluble antigen and antigen-bearing antigen-presenting cells from peripheral tissues are efficiently concentrated in the draining lymph node and initiate an adaptive immune response. Lymphatic vessels are observed in the draining lymph node and concentrate in the subcapsular sinus and medullary area (109). Factors from afferent lymph can be either transported deep into the lymph node cortex or move via the subcapsular sinus and leave the lymph node through efferent lymphatic vessels (100). Several markers of human and murine lymphatic vessels including lymphatic vessel endothelial hyaluronan receptor (LYVE-1), Prox-1, podoplanin, the vascular endothelial growth factor receptor-3 (VEGFR-3), and CCL21 have recently been described (123).

Conduit System

A conduit system in the lymph nodes physically connects the lymphatic sinus with the walls of blood vessels and enables the incoming factor(s) from lymph to move rapidly deep into the paracortical area (100,109). The conduit system consists of four layers: (a) a core of type I and type III collagen bundles; (b) a microfibrillar zone composed largely of fibrillins; (c) a basement membrane abundant with laminins 8 and 10, perlecan, and type IV collagen that provides a supportive structure; and (d) fibroblastic reticular cells that embrace the entire conduit system (124,125). This conduit system enables incoming lymph to penetrate deep into the T cell area. In fact, soon after immunization, resident DCs quickly pinocytose and process soluble antigens draining into the regional lymph node (126). A special subset of immature DCs, called conduit associated DCs, can take up and process antigens moving along the conduit (125). In this manner, the conduit system probably provides a physical support for rapid initiation of adaptive immune responses after immunization.

The Intimate Relationship Between Lymph and HEVs

Incoming lymph is necessary for the maintenance of HEV phenotype and function. After afferent lymphatic vessels are severed, dramatic changes occur in HEVs. These include flattening of the endothelium, a decrease in the uptake of ^{35}S-sulphate (a functional marker of HEC-6ST) (127,128), a reduction of lymphocyte adherence to the vessels (129–131), and decreased expression of PNAd and HEV genes, *GlyCAM-1* and *Fuc-TVII* (130–132). However, an increase in MAdCAM-1 expression (130) suggests that these events are not simply due to a general down regulation of blood vessel gene expression, and indicates that continual accumulation of afferent lymph factor(s) in lymph nodes is necessary for HEV maintenance. The nature of such lymph factor(s) is unknown.

Topographic relations between HEVs and the lymphatic sinus have been described in the rat mesenteric lymph nodes. Some HEVs are located in the medulla area and positioned closely with the lymphatic sinus (109). Occasionally, HEVs are separated from an adjacent lymphatic sinus by only a thin layer of collagen bundles. The closely apposed HEV and lymphatic sinus in medulla provide the physical support for the intimate relationship between lymph and HEV. However, most HEVs are located in the paracortex area and are separated from lymphatic sinus by lymphocytes. The conduit system physically connects the subcapsular sinus and HEVs and allows incoming lymph factor(s) to migrate rapidly to the wall of HEVs (109,133,134). Low molecular weight fluorescent tracers (below 70kD) move rapidly via the conduit system and lead directly to the wall of HEVs. In this manner, low molecular weight tracers can migrate with lymph within minutes to HEVs and enter the HEV lumen (100). Lymph-borne chemokines likely adopt this route to regulate HEV function. IL-8 administration via afferent lymph increases lymphocyte HEV transmigration within minutes (109,135). In addition, lymph-borne chemokine MIP-1α also enters the conduit system and moves rapidly to HEVs (100). These data suggest that lymph factor(s) can quickly access and regulate HEVs.

Development

Despite their distinctions in the adult with regard to morphology and expressed genes, a close association of blood vessels and lymphatic vessels is seen during embryogenesis. The generation of embryonic lymphatic vessels from preexisting veins in pig embryos was first described in the early 1900s and has recently been molecularly defined (136–138). As early as mouse E9.5-10, upon the formation of vascular system, LYVE-1 is expressed in venous endothelial cells. In response to an unknown lymphatic vessel induction signal, these endothelial cells then polarize to become lymphatic-biased endothelial cells. At nearly the same time, PROX-1, expressed in a restricted subpopulation of endothelial cells in the cardinal vein, generates a feedback signal for the further maintenance of budding and migration of endothelial cells. At E11.5-12.0, CCL21 is expressed in these lymphatic-biased endothelial cells, as is VEGFR-3, which is reduced in blood endothelial cells. The endothelial cells expressing LYVE-1, PROX-1, VEGFR-3, and CCL21 become irreversibly committed towards a lymphatic pathway (139,140). The further separation of lymphatic endothelial cells from venous endothelium requires a Syk/SLP-76 signal (141). Thus, for a long period during early lymphangiogenesis, some endothelial cells express both blood vessel and lymphatic vessel markers, indicating the close association of these two vascular systems. Mesenchymal lymphangioblasts may also contribute to early lymphangiogenesis (142). Whether embryonic lymphatic vessels originate by budding from preexisting veins or from mesenchymal lymphangioblasts, a close association of lymphatic and venous endothelial cells is seen in the lymphatic and venous junction formation during early embryogenesis. The lymphatic venous junction remains in adults and plays an essential role in connecting the function of the two vascular systems.

Histologic studies in the rat reveal that popliteal and inguinal lymph node anlagen originally appear in a limited mesenchymal area along the vein wall at E17. The next day, lymphatic vessels form a sac running parallel to the vein. The lymph node anlage develops into a bulb-shaped structure with lymphatic vessels and the subcapsular sinus originating from the remaining lymphatic vessel. At the next stage, the lymph node divides into a primitive cortex, the basic network of reticular cells and medulla, and lymphocytes scatter in the lymph node anlage. Blood vessels branch into the lymph node and later develop into HEVs (143). The primary follicles appear at day 18 after birth, indicating that B cell migration into lymph nodes is a later event during lymphoid organogenesis. Later studies show that first lymphocytes invading the lymph node during lymphoid organogenesis are T cells; B cells become detectable only in the later stages (144–146).

Cytokines, Chemokines, and Transcription Factors in Lymphoid Organogenesis

The important roles of tumor necrosis factor/lymphotoxin-receptor (TNF/LT) family members in lymphoid organ development are well established. LTα3, signaling through TNFRI and TNFRII, and membrane-bound LT$\alpha_1\beta_2$, signaling through LTβ receptor (LTβR), have been implicated. Mice deficient in LTα lack all lymph nodes and Peyers patches and exhibit a disorganized spleen and severely disorganized NALT (discussed later) (147–149). Mice deficient in LTβ lack peripheral lymph nodes but retain mesenteric, sacral, and cervical lymph nodes (150–152). *Ltβr*$^{-/-}$ mice have a phenotype similar to that of *ltα*$^{-/-}$ mice (153). LTβR is also recognized by LTβ-related ligand, LIGHT, which also binds to the herpes virus entry mediator (HVEM). LIGHT-LTβR signaling does not appear to play an essential role during lymphoid organogenesis, because no significant defect is observed in *LIGHT*$^{-/-}$ mice (154); however, mice doubly deficient in LIGHT and LTβ have fewer mesenteric lymph nodes than mice deficient in LTβ alone, indicating a cooperative effect of the two LTβR ligands. Treatment of pregnant females with an inhibitory soluble protein of LTβR (LTβR and human IgG Fc fusion protein, LTβR-Ig) inhibits most lymph nodes in the developing embryos, depending on the time of administration. Mesenteric lymph nodes are not inhibited by this treatment. These studies indicate that individual lymph nodes differ in the nature and time of cytokine signaling during development (155). Several additional cytokine and chemokine-receptor pairs are crucial for lymphoid organogenesis. Mice deficient in IL-7 or IL-7R (156,157), TRANCE or TRANCER, also called RANKL and RANK (158,159), exhibit defects in lymph node development. CXCR5- or CXCL13-deficient mice (160,161) lack some lymph nodes and almost all Peyers patches (88).

The NF-κB signaling pathways, downstream of the TNF family, play important roles in lymphoid organ development (162). The alternative pathway, characterized by NF-κB-inducing kinase (NIK) and IKKα is particularly important. *aly/aly* mice, which have a point mutation in *nik*, lack all lymph nodes and Peyers patches (163,164). In these mice, LTβR, but not TNFR, mediated signaling between NIK and members the TRAF family appears to be disrupted (164–166). LTβR signaling induces gene expression via both the classical and alternative NF-κB pathways in mouse embryo fibroblasts. The classical pathway mediated by p50:p65 heterodimers induces expression of proinflammatory genes (*VCAM-1, MIP1b, MIP2*). Intraperitoneal injection of an agonistic LTβR antibody induces splenic chemokines (CCL19, CCL21, and CXCL13) and requires

NIK activity and subsequent p100 processing (167). IKKα is a critical component in alternative NF-κB pathway. Mice with a mutated form of the *ikkα* gene have reduced HEV expression of HEC-6ST and GlyCAM-1, further confirming that the LTβR signal regulates HEVs through the alternative NFκB pathway (168). Several other signaling pathways that contribute to lymphoid organogenesis include helix-loop-helix transcription factor inhibitor (Id2) and retinoic acid-related orphan receptors (RORs) RORγ and RORγt (169–171).

Studies of lymph node anlage formation reveal the mechanisms by which cytokines trigger and coordinate lymphoid organogenesis. The circulating CD4$^+$CD3$^-$ CD45$^+$ hematopoietic progenitor cells called lymphoid tissue-inducer cells, which are derived from fetal liver progenitors (88,170,172–174), provide crucial signals for inducing lymph node organogenesis. These lymphoid tissue-inducer cells, which express the integrin $\alpha_4\beta_7$ and interact with VCAM-1 positive stromal organizer cells, accumulate in the developing lymph node, forming clusters with resident stromal organizer cells, to initiate a cascade of intracellular and intercellular events that lead to the maturation of the primordial lymph node (1,88). During this early step, a positive feedback loop involves several signaling pathways, including LT$\alpha\beta$/LTβR, IL-7R/IL-7, CXCR5/CXCL13, and TRANCER/TRANCE expressed on the lymphoid tissue-inducer cells and the stromal organizer cells. The prolonged interaction between lymphoid tissue-inducer cells and stromal organizer cells promotes the development of HEVs, which support the entry of naïve lymphocytes (175). It is unclear how HEVs differentiate from the flat blood vessels during early lymphoid organogenesis. At birth, HEVs of all lymph nodes express MAdCAM-1, which is replaced in the first few days in peripheral lymph nodes by PNAd (176). Both MAdCAM-1 and PNAd are expressed in mucosal lymph nodes. LTα alone can induce MAdCAM-1, but PNAd requires LT$\alpha\beta$ (2,177,178). In the remaining mesenteric lymph nodes of $lt\beta^{-/-}$ mice, PNAd expression is impaired (178), indicating that optimal lymph node HEV PNAd expression requires LT$\alpha_1\beta_2$ signaling through the LTβR and the alternative NFκB pathway (168). Since the maturation of HEVs is coincident with further development of the lymph node (122,143), the homing of LT-expressing lymphocytes most likely contributes to HEV maturation.

Changes in Lymph Nodes after Immunization

Studies in rabbit, sheep, and rodents have revealed that lymph nodes undergo dramatic changes and remodeling after immunization. Early after a variety of immunogenic exposures, such as skin painting with oxazolone, injection of ovalbumin or sheep red blood cells in adjuvant, or bacterial or viral infection, remodeling occurs. This remodeling is apparent as a complex kinetics of changes in lymph flow, lymph cell content, blood flow, HEV gene expression, and lymphatic vessels (Figure 2.3). Afferent lymph flow and lymph cell content increase soon after initial inflammation and eventually return to a normal level (179–183). Lymph node lymphangiogenesis occurs, which eventually resolves (184,185). Blood flow and lymphocyte migration into lymph nodes peak at 72–96 hours (152,182,186,187), accompanied by an increase in HEV number and dilation (188,189), accounting for the significant lymph node enlargement apparent at 72–96 hours (186). After skin grafting, the permeability of rat lymph node HEVs is increased at 24–48 hours, and more branches form on HEVs at day 4. However, only 38% of the new HEV branches are lined by high endothelial cells, and the percentage is increased to 96% on day 10, indicating that the HEV matures progressively in the draining LN after antigen exposure (109). Efferent lymph flow also increases soon after immunization, but lymph cell content in the efferent lymph drops during the first several hours, indicating the first wave of accumulation of lymphocytes in the draining lymph node. The cell content of the efferent lymph later increases and peaks at 72–96 hours (190). These events, taken together, contribute to the significant enlargement of the draining LN at day 4 after immunization. During the early times after immunization, despite the increase in the number of HEVs, the expression of genes that contribute to L-selectin ligand, including FucT-VII, GlyCAM-1 and Sgp200, and HEC-6ST is initially down-regulated followed by a recovery (132,185,191). However, despite the down-regulation of chemokines CCL21 and CXCL12, some genes such as those encoding CXCL9, CCL3, and E-selectin are up-regulated (192), as is MAdCAM-1 (185), suggesting a reversion to an immature phenotype before the eventual recovery of the mature phenotype.

In rodents, HEV maturation is coincident with the continuing development of the lymph node and population of lymphocytes after birth, indicating that the mature HEV phenotype relies on the lymph node microenvironment (122,143). Plasticity of the mature lymph node is also seen after injection of LTβR-Ig. LTβR-Ig treatment reduces lymph node cellularity, reverts the HEV phenotype to the immature state, inhibits FDC function, and disrupts immune responses to foreign antigens (185,193,194). Thus, in addition to its critical role in lymphoid organogenesis, LTβR is essential in maintaining mature lymph node phenotype and function.

Spleen

Function

The spleen is a large reddish organ located beneath the diaphragm, close to the stomach and the pancreas. It is a crucial site for antigen clearance and presentation to T and B cells and is particularly important in responding to

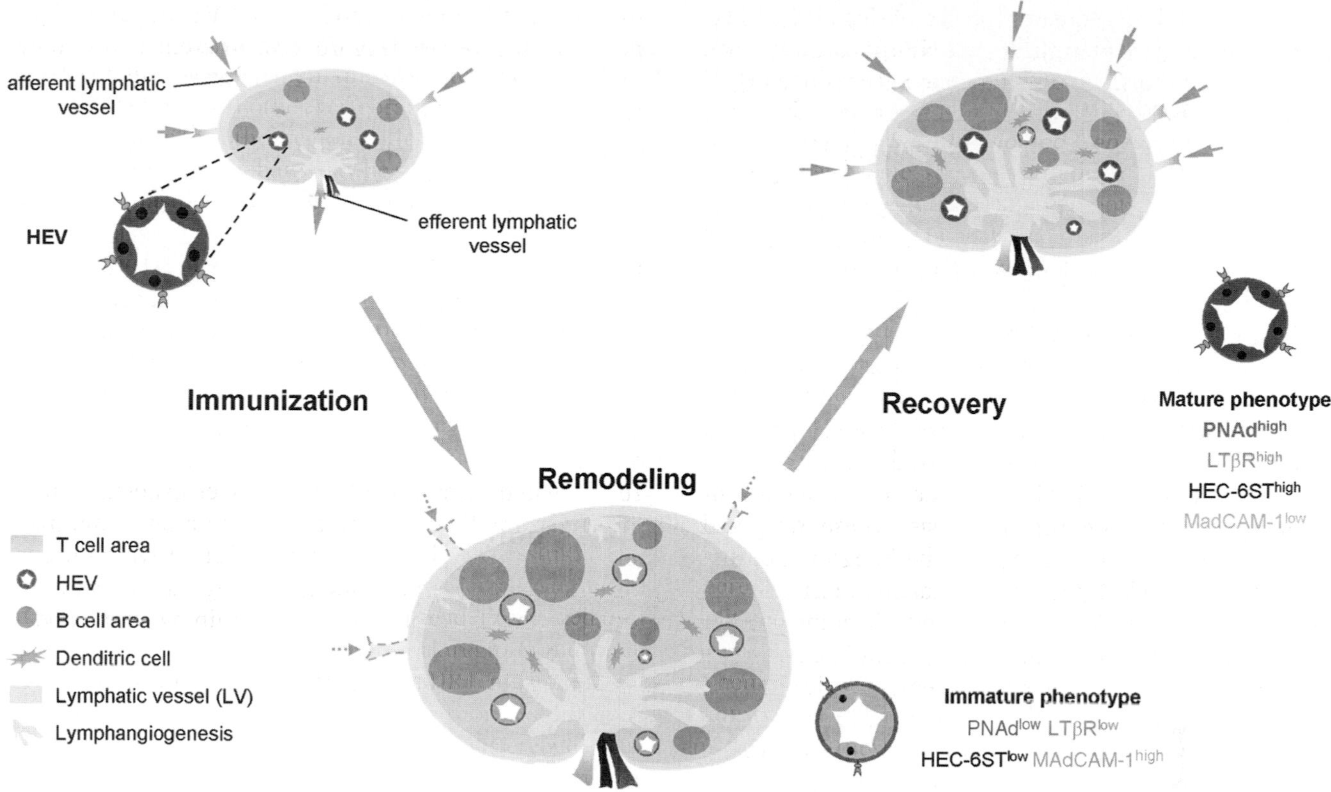

FIGURE 2.3 Plasticity of lymph nodes after immunization. Initially the lymph node enlarges due to increased blood flow and lymphocyte proliferation. Blood vessels proliferate and HEVs express markers typical of an immature phenotype. During the recovery period, HEVs recover to a mature phenotype. Lymphangiogenesis is induced during the remodeling period.

bloodborne antigens. In addition to its role as a secondary lymphoid organ, the spleen filters blood and removes damaged platelets, aged erythrocytes, and apoptotic cells. An additional function, consequent to its destruction of effete erythrocytes, is its role in iron recycling. In some species, such as the horse, the spleen stores blood that is released after stress. The spleen is particularly important in defense against bloodborne pathogens and contributes most significantly to defense against bacterial infections (195).

Architecture and Cellular Composition

The structure of the spleen is maintained by a fibrous capsule and trabeculae of fibrous connective tissue (Figure 2.4). The general principles of splenic organization are similar across species, though specifics may differ (196–200). Upon gross observation after slicing, the spleen can be divided into two areas: red pulp and white pulp. These compartments are anatomically and functionally distinct. The red pulp, in its activities as a hematogenous organ, removes damaged cells and acts as a site for iron storage and turnover. The white pulp is an organized lymphoid structure. The spleen is highly vascularized. The splenic artery, located immediately below the capsule is the source of cells and antigens. The artery branches into arterioles and cords in the red pulp where macrophages engulf antigen and remove it from the circulation. Blood then collects in venous sinuses that empty into the efferent splenic vein. Some blood reaches the marginal sinus and marginal zone (MZ), which demarcates the red and white pulp. Blood containing residual antigen then percolates through the MZ into the white pulp. The white pulp is surrounded by the MZ, a structure that differs somewhat between humans and rodents. The human MZ, which consists of inner and outer marginal zones, is surrounded by a perifollicular zone; the rodent MZ is a single structure and has no perifollicular zone. The MZ is an important transition between the innate and acquired immune systems, because it is the first region after the red pulp encountered by bloodborne antigens and is richly supplied with specialized phagocytic cells: the MZ macrophages and MZ metallophilic macrophages. The MZ macrophages express Toll-like receptors (TLRs) crucial for pattern recognition of bacteria and viruses and several other receptors that facilitate binding of pathogens. These include SIGNR1 and MARCO. SIGNR1, a C-type lectin in the mouse that is a homologue of human DC-SIGN (201), is also found in medullary and subcapsular macrophages in the lymph node. On splenic

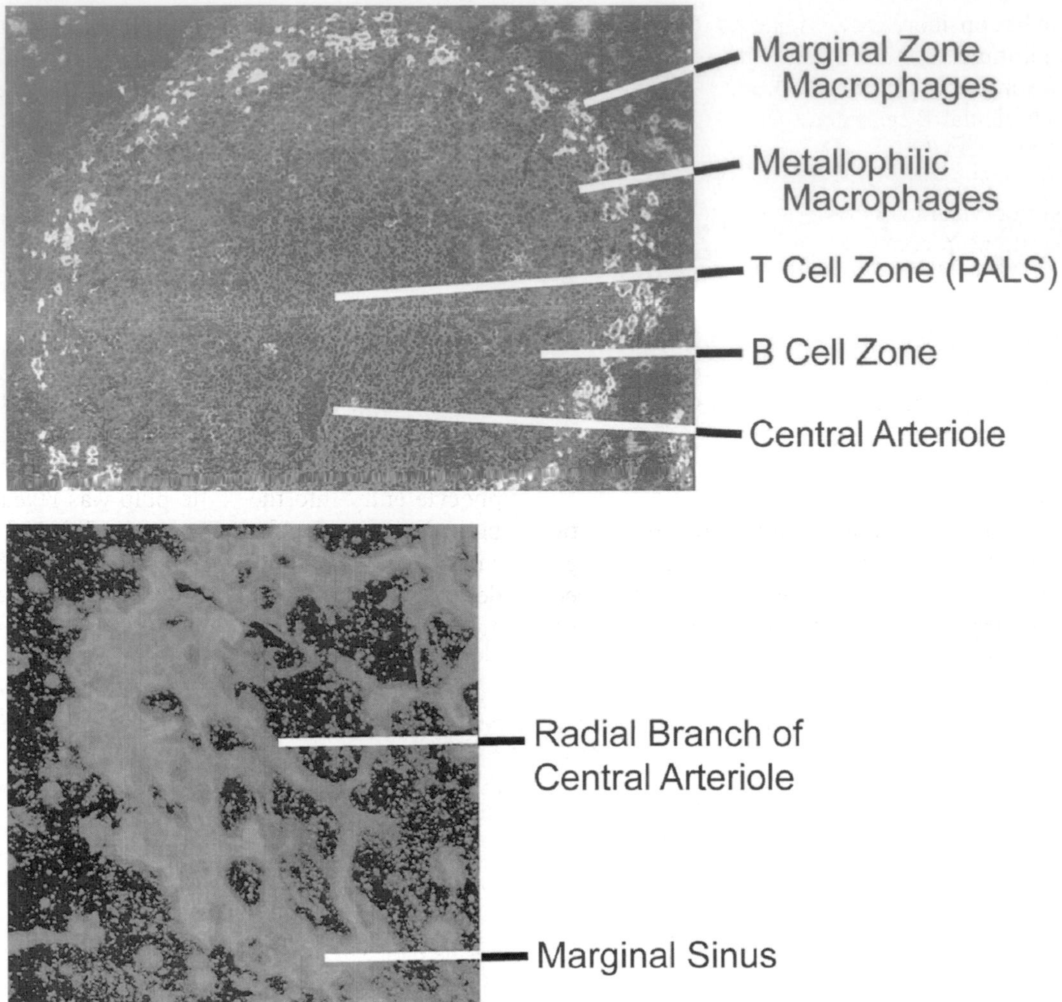

FIGURE 2.4 Organization of the spleen white pulp. **Top panel:** Immunofluorescent staining of a white pulp unit in the mouse spleen. T cells (anti-$CD4^{+}$anti-$CD8^{+}$, red) are localized around the central arteriole. B cells (anti-IgM, green) are localized in follicles around the T cell area, surrounded by a layer of metalophillic macrophages (labeled with monoclonal antibody-MOMA-1) and a more peripheral layer of marginal zone macrophages (labeled with monoclonal antibody ERTR9, orange). The marginal zone (MZ) is located between the metalophillic macrophage and the MZ macrophage layers (not shown) (307). **Bottom panel:** Structure of the marginal sinus in a thick (100 micrometer) frozen section of mouse spleen with targeted insertion of the *LacZ* gene into the ephrin B2 locus. Eprhrin B2 is expressed at high levels in the central arteriole, in radial branches of the central arteriole, and in the marginal sinus. LacZ is visualized by staining with FITC-labeled anti-LacZ antibody. Note the transition from discrete arteriolar vessels to a network of flattened vessels at the transition to the marginal sinus plexus (C. Zindl, University of Alabama at Birmingham, Birmingham, AL). From Chaplin (308), with permission. (See color insert.)

MZ macrophages, it appears to be crucial for the capture of a wide variety of pathogens, including yeast, bacteria, and viruses (202, 203). MARCO (macrophage-associated receptor with collaganeous structure), expressed constitutively on MZ macrophages (204), is a class-A scavenger pattern recognition receptor, which is a trimeric Type II protein. The TLR, SIGNR1, and MARCO receptors, which are all expressed on MZ macrophages, act synergistically to recognize, endocytose, and eliminate microorganisms (205). MZ metallophilic macrophages are located at the border of the MZ and differ from the MZ macrophages in that they express the sialic acid-binding Ig-like lectin sialoadhesin (Siglec-1), which binds to oligosaccharide ligands present on many cells. The ability of siglecs to interact with lipopolysaccharide on meningococcal bacteria (206) suggests that the metallophilic macrophages may also serve as an early line of defense. Lymphocytes express CD43, a counter receptor for Siglec-1 (207), suggesting that the metallophilic macrophages may use this pair of molecules to facilitate movement of lymphocytes into the white pulp. The MZ also contains a specialized subset of B cells that differ phenotypically and functionally from follicular B cells; they can be considered as a bridge between the innate and adaptive immune systems. They express higher levels of IgM and a somewhat limited B cell receptor repertoire compared to follicular B cells, and they express TLR9 and respond to CpG DNA (208). The organization of the remainder of the white pulp of the spleen is similar to that of the lymph node, compartmentalized into T and B cell areas. The white pulp consists of a central arteriole that is surrounded by T cells, also known as the periarteriolar lymphoid sheath (PALS), that are surrounded by B cells. As in the lymph node, T cells interact with DCs and B cells. B cells migrate to the follicles, where they interact with follicular DCs. At the T–B cell border, T cells interact with B cells. Germinal centers are the site of somatic hypermutation and Ig class switching. Plasma cells are found mainly in the red pulp.

Although the spleen does not have an afferent lymphatic system and initial antigen transport must occur through the blood vasculature, a conduit system has been described that allows antigens and chemokines to be transported through the white pulp in a manner similar to that described for the lymph node (209). This conduit differs with regard to the identity of the transported molecules by the fact that it contacts the blood, rather than the lymphatic system.

Traffic In and Out: Chemokines and Adhesion Molecules

Cell trafficking in the spleen is similar to that which occurs in the lymph node in some respects and differs from it in others. The lymphoid chemokines, CXCL13, CCL19, and CCL21 position cells in the splenic white pulp as they do in the lymph node. However, lymphoid chemokine production is limited to stromal cells, since the spleen has no HEVs. CXCL12 is expressed in the splenic red pulp (210). As B cells differentiate into plasma cells, they down-regulate CXCR5 and CCR7 and up-regulate CXCR4. As plasma cells, they migrate toward that chemokine, out of germinal centers and into the red pulp or return to the bone marrow.

The role of adhesion molecules with regard to lymphocyte traffic in the spleen is still unclear. Since the spleen lacks HEVs, the well-understood process by which lymphocytes leave the circulation and enter into the parenchyma of lymph nodes is not relevant, and there is no evidence for expression of PNAd (211). However, CD62L (L-selectin) is up-regulated in late transitional cells in the spleen, hinting at the possibility of an additional L-selectin ligand (212). Lymphocytes enter into the white pulp through the marginal sinus and MAdCAM-1 and ICAM-1 are expressed by cells lining that structure (213, 214). However, treatment with anti-MAdCAM-1 or anti-$\alpha 4\beta 7$ antibodies does not inhibit homing to the spleen, suggesting that this ligand-receptor pair is not required for lymphocyte entrance into the white pulp (213). Nolte et al. reported that several molecules associated with homing to lymph nodes, including L-selectin, CD44, PSGL-1, and $\alpha 4$ integrins, are not required for entry into the white pulp (214). Early studies indicating that treatment with an antibody that blocks the α_L-integrin chain of LFA-1 inhibits homing by only 20%, and that lymphocytes deficient in LFA-1 enter the white pulp (214), suggested that LFA-1 is not absolutely essential for entry of all cells into the white pulp. However, both $\alpha 4\beta 1$ and LFA-1 integrins are necessary for B cell retention in the MZ (215), indicating a role for VCAM-1 and ICAM-1. This effect is most pronounced with regard to MZ B cells; follicular B cells express lower levels of the integrins, and their entry into the spleen is not affected by treatment with antibodies that inhibit $\alpha 4$ or α_L. However, an important role for integrins in lymphocyte entry into the white pulp was revealed by combined treatment with antibodies to VCAM-1 and LFA-1, suggesting that entry into the white pulp is, in fact, integrin dependent (216). Once lymphocytes have encountered antigen, they most likely undergo changes in chemokine receptors and adhesion molecules similar to those noted in the lymph nodes, leave the white pulp, and enter the red pulp (plasma cells) or the circulation. $S1P_1$ plays a role in the spleen, but it appears to contrast with that in the lymph node. S1P receptors 1 and 3 are expressed by MZ B cells and $S1P_1$ is required for B cell localization in the MZ (217); MZ B cells from $S1P_1$-deficient mice are not found in the MZ but are found in the follicles. Further, MZ B cells down-regulate $S1P_1$ after activation, allowing their entrance into the white pulp. In contrast to the well-defined route of egress of activated lymphocytes from the lymph node through the efferent lymphatic vessels, the exit route from the spleen is not understood. The observation of channels that bridge into the marginal zone (218) suggests one route of egress.

Development

Because the spleen has characteristics of both a hematopoietic organ and a secondary lymphoid organ, the genes that regulate its development include, in addition to LT, other genes concerned with patterning and hematopoiesis. Several genes that contribute to the development of the spleen are also crucial for normal development of other nonlymphoid organs. The first sign of splenic development in the mouse occurs at E10.5-11, as progenitor cells begin to condense within the dorsal mesogastrium, adjacent to the stomach and dorsal pancreas. The spleen and pancreas are so intimately associated that it is difficult to distinguish between them at these early stages. In fact, many genes that affect splenic development also contribute to pancreatic development. Several of these are homeobox genes and transcription factors that are expressed in the spleno-pancreatic mesenchyme at E10.5 (summarized in 195). The effects of just one of these genes, *Hox11* (now called *Tlx1*; 195), are on the spleen.

The others affect multiple organs. *Tlx1* was originally described as an oncogene in T cell childhood acute leukemias (10,14) involving the translocation breakpoint (219). *Tlx1*-deficient mice are asplenic (220), and the product of this gene is a cell survival factor (221). Several additional genes that are important for development of lymph nodes, NALT, and Peyers patches also contribute to splenic development. Mice deficient in members of the LT/TNF ligand receptor family and their downstream signaling molecules in the classical and alternative pathways exhibit defects in splenic development. However, none of these molecules is necessary for the early splenic anlagen, as mice deficient in any of the chemokines or cytokines retain a spleen. The defects are mainly observed as an absence of particular cell populations or disorganized white pulp. The changes in organization are due in part to a reduction or near absence of lymphoid chemokines (CXCL13, CCL19, CCL21) (222). Lymphoid chemokine mRNA expression is reduced in the spleens of mice deficient in TNFR1, TNF, LTα, or LTβ, though CXCL12 mRNA levels are normal. However, treatment with an agonistic LTβR antibody induces expression of the lymphoid chemokines and CXCL12, suggesting that signaling through both the classical and alternative NFκB pathways are responsible for organization of splenic white pulp. Several cell populations are absent in mice deficient in genes signaled by the LT/TNF pathways (200). Mice deficient in LTα exhibit a disorganized white pulp with loss of T and B cell compartmentalization, loss of MZ macrophages, metallophilic macrophages, MZ B cells, MAdCAM-1 sinus lining cells, and germinal centers. $Lt\beta^{-/-}$ mice exhibit similar characteristics except that the disorganization is somewhat less pronounced. $Tnf^{-/-}$ and $Tnfr1^{-/-}$ mice show defects in all the above, with the exception of MZ B cells. The cytokines necessary for maintenance of splenic architecture are produced by T cells, B cells, and $CD4^+CD3^-$ cells (223,224).

Plasticity after Virus Infection

Though much is known regarding changes in the lymph node after immunization, the spleen has not been studied as extensively in this regard. However, after infection with cytomegalovirus, white pulp T–B compartmentalization is disrupted (225). The spleens of *lta*-deficient mice exhibit a marked reduction in expression of CCL21-ser. This is even further reduced in cytomegalovirus infection, indicating that, in the adult, LT-independent pathways can contribute to maintenance of expression of lymphoid chemokines.

MUCOSAL-ASSOCIATED LYMPHOID TISSUES

Mucosal-associated lymphoid tissues (MALT), though in some cases less structurally defined than the other secondary lymphoid tissues, quantitatively include the vast majority of lymphoid cells in the body. Because of their initial contact with the environment, they can be considered to be the body's gatekeepers. They are major producers of secreted IgA, allowing protection of epithelial surfaces. Further, the mucosal tissues play an important role in mounting defense against pathogens by generating cells that migrate to other sites. They are also responsible for inducing and maintaining tolerance to food antigens and commensal bacteria (226). The structure and organization of these tissues provide insight into their biological roles. Although the structure and location of some mucosal lymphoid tissues are predetermined, all are somewhat plastic and prone to induction and remodeling, because they are in intimate association with the external environment and under constant exposure to environmental antigens. The tonsils and adenoids in humans and the NALT in rodents have a capsule, a clear organization, and are in fixed locations. The Peyers patches are structurally defined and located in the intestine, but their number and location vary by species and antigen exposure. The BALT and ILF are located in fixed organs, the lung and the small intestine, but are even more plastic and subject to environmental influences.

Tonsils and Adenoids

The first defense against pathogens entering through the alimentary and respiratory portals is a group of lymphoid accumulations around the wall of the throat called Waldeyer's ring (227). Humans have one adenoid and several tonsils: two tubal, two palatine, and one lingual. These tissues have an extensive epithelial surface, which penetrates into the organ with a series of crypts. These provide additional surface area for the capture of pathogens. A specialized cell, called a mutifenestrated, microfold, or membranous (M) cell, is located in the epithelial surface of the tonsil, and, because of its high transcytotic capacity, transports antigens to the underlying lymphoid tissue. This tissue is compartmentalized and organized in a fashion similar to lymph nodes, with B cell follicles, FDCs, germinal centers, and interfollicular T cells and DCs (228). The tonsils contain a large complement of B cells, many of which are positive for IgA (227) and the polymeric IgA receptor, or secretory component (229), crucial for transport of that immunoglobulin across the epithelium. This secreted IgA provides an early form of defense against pathogens entering through the oral route. The cells in the tonsil are directed to their respective locations in that organ by chemokines similar to those in the lymph node, which include CCL19 and its receptor CCR7 (230). CCL25 and CCL28 and their receptors CCR9 and CCR10 are also detected in the tonsils (231). Tonsil HEVs express ICAM-1 (227) and, importantly, CD34, which, upon modification, is bound by the PNAd-defining MECA-79 antibody (211,

232). This allows entrance of L-selectin^{hi} naïve cells into the organ to interact with antigen. MAdCAM-1 is expressed weakly or not at all (233). Because the tonsils are frequently inflamed, they also express additional chemokines, cytokines, and adhesion molecules more typical of inflammatory sites, such as CCL19 (230), VCAM-1, and E- and P-selectin (151).

Nose-associated Lymphoid Tissue

The NALT, a pair of lymphoid organs above the soft palate in mice and rats, is considered analogous to human tonsils and adenoids due to its common embryonic origin from Waldeyer's ring (234). Its biologic importance lies not only in its immediate physical proximity to the external environment, but more important, its demonstrated crucial role with regard to generation of responses in the genitourinary track (235). After nasal immunization, IgA is detected in vaginal washes (149,236,237) and cytotoxic T cells are found in vaginal draining lymph nodes (238). The NALT drains into the cervical lymph node, and that node has been demonstrated to play a role in NALT activity and can even act as an inductive site in its absence (239). However, the NALT itself is clearly an inductive site for both humoral and cellular immune responses (240) and supports class switching to IgA (241). The NALT includes M cells and a large complement of B cells, surrounded by T cells. Lymphoid chemokines CCL19, CCL21, and CXCL13 define T and B cell areas in a manner similar to the lymph node. Both CCL19 and CXCL13 are made by stromal cells, whereas, in contrast to lymph nodes, CCL21 mRNA is detectable only in HEVs (149). NALT HEVs express high levels of luminal and abluminal PNAd and HEC-6ST (149). The major homing receptor-ligand pair to this organ involves L-selectin-PNAd interaction, rather than MAdCAM-1 (242).

Development

The NALT in the mouse and rat is hypocellular at birth and undergoes dramatic changes at the age of weaning. These changes include expression of LTα and LTβ and lymphoid chemokines, T and B cell compartmentalization, and HEV maturation (149). In fact, the fully developed NALT is not apparent until 6 weeks after birth. Although Id2 is required for initiation of the NALT (243), in contrast to lymph nodes, RORγT, LTα, and LTβ are not required for its initiation (148). However, the organ is hypocellular in mice deficient in the LTα, LTβ, IL7R, and NIK signaling pathways (149,168,244). CXCL13, CCL19, and CCL21 are also not required for initiation of the NALT structure; even in the absence of these chemokines, at 10 days of age, a small number of CD4$^+$CD3$^-$ cells are apparent. Nevertheless, chemokines and LT are required for NALT organization and function (148,149,245), and the alternative NFκB pathway is required for T and B cell compartmentalization, expression of chemokines, and the HEV genes *glycam-1* and *hec-6st* (168). The data concerning the continued maturation of NALT up to 6 weeks after birth strongly suggests that environmental influences are important for its maintenance and development.

Bronchus-associated Lymphoid Tissue

BALT is less organized but more environmentally regulated than Peyers patches or NALT. Some debate exists regarding whether BALT is a normal structure or whether it is entirely dependent on antigenic stimulation. If the former, it would be considered to be a secondary lymphoid organ; if the latter, a tertiary lymphoid organ (see discussion following). This varies by species in that it is common in rabbits and rats, less frequent in guinea pigs and pigs, and absent in cats and normal human lungs (246). It is not a prominent structure in the laboratory mouse, but its presence varies by strain and age (247). The BALT is highly dependent on immunological stimulation in that the number of lung lymphoid aggregates varies, at least in the pig, by the extent of exposure to microbes (248). The lung is capable of generating an immune response in splenectomized $lt\alpha^{-/-}$ mice that lack lymph nodes and Peyers patches (249), suggesting that an organized tissue is present or can be induced in the lung. An inducible form of the BALT (iBALT) develops in $lt\alpha^{-/-}$ mice upon infection with influenza virus (250). The iBALT has many characteristics of secondary lymphoid organs, including CXCL13 and CCL21 expression, T and B compartmentalization, FDCs, and PNAd$^+$ HEVs. Data obtained from mice that lack all other lymphoid organs indicate that memory can be generated in the iBALT (251). Similar structures have been described in humans with pulmonary complications of rheumatoid arthritis (245), though they were not apparent in the lungs of patients with several other forms of lung inflammation. Many of the infiltrates in the rheumatoid arthritis patients exhibit the characteristics of secondary lymphoid organs, including LTα, LTβ, lymphoid chemokines, T and B cell compartmentalization, germinal centers, DCs, PNAd, and a lymphatic vessel marker, M2A.

Peyers Patches

Peyers patches are lymphoid aggregates in the submucosa of the small intestine (Figure 2.5, top panel). They are present in most species, though their number and location vary. They have a single layer of epithelial cells, called the follicle-associated epithelium (FAE); interspersed in these follicles are M cells that lack surface microvilli and surface mucus, similar to those in the tonsil and NALT. Because the Peyers patches lack afferent lymphatic vessels, the M cells are critical transporters of antigen. As noted above, M cells are transcytotic. Further, they express receptors

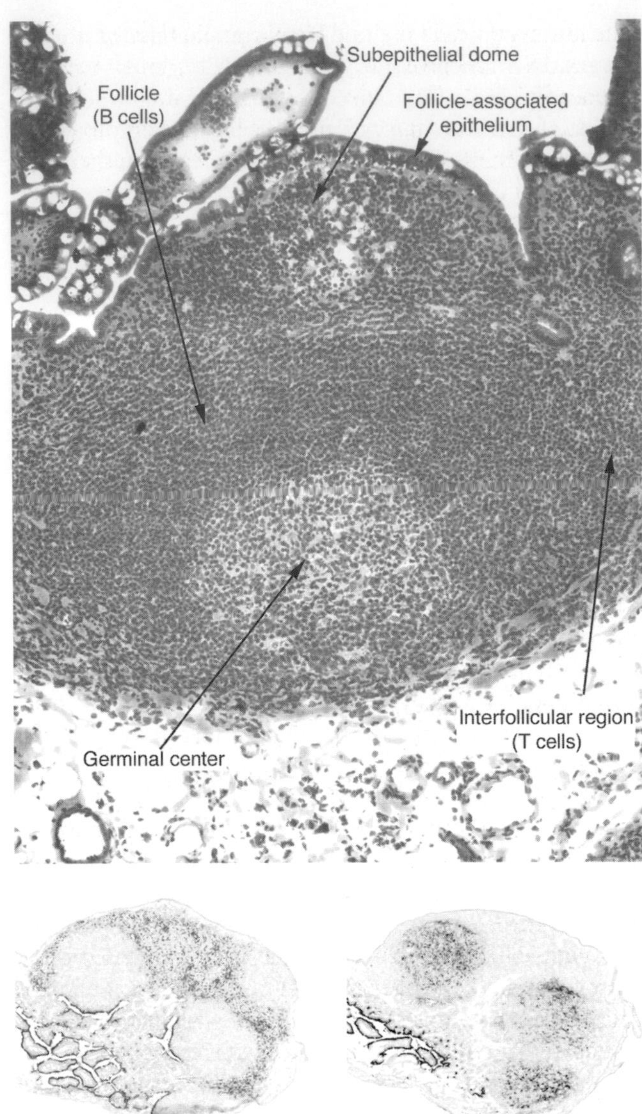

FIGURE 2.5 Organization of the Peyers patch. **Top panel:** Photomicrograph of Peyers patch. The Peyers patch is located in the intestine near intestinal villi. The follicle-associated epithelium (FAE) is in contact with the gut lumen. M cells (not shown) in the FAE transport antigen into the subepithelial dome, populated by DCs and T cells. The interfollicular T cell–rich region surrounds the B cell follicle and germinal center. Courtesy of A. Iwasaki (Yale University School of Medicine, New Haven, CT). **Bottom panel:** *In situ* hybridization of chemokine mRNAs. On the left, CCL21 mRNA defines the T cell zone and HEVs; on the right, CXCL13 defines the B cell zone.

for some pathogens, including HIV (252) and Salmonella (253), facilitating their uptake. Below the FAE is a diffuse area, the subepithelial dome, which includes DCs and lymphocytes. The Peyers patch organization is similar to that of the lymph node with compartmentalized B cell follicles, T cells, and antigen-presenting cells. T cells are found in the subepithelial dome, in the interfollicular region, and in germinal centers (Figure 2.5, bottom panel) (254). Although M cells transport antigen across the epithelial barrier, they are not believed to have a crucial role in processing or presenting antigen. Peyers patches are populated by several subsets of DCs (255,256) that produce various chemokines, important in generating either immunity or tolerance.

Traffic In and Out: Chemokines and Vasculature Adhesion Molecules

Cells enter the Peyers patches through HEVs, whose appearance is similar to those in lymph nodes. However, in contrast to peripheral lymph nodes, the HEVs of Peyers patches express MAdCAM-1 (257), and homing depends on $\alpha4\beta7$ interaction on lymphocytes. Luminal PNAd is rarely found in Peyers patch HEVs; only occasional abluminal expression is detected. This pattern is identical to that seen in lymph node HEVs in *hec-6st*$^{-/-}$ mice (113), suggesting that this modifying enzyme is not expressed in Peyers patch HEVs. However, lymphocytes from mice that lack in both L-selectin ligand and $\alpha4\beta7$ home less efficiently to Peyers patches than do lymphocytes from mice that lack only one or the other of the ligands (258,259), suggesting that an L-selectin ligand does contribute to homing to Peyers patches. Although P-selectin is expressed only weakly on Peyers patch HEVs, cells from mice deficient in that molecule show reduced rolling and adhesion in vivo, implicating P-selectin as well as MAdCAM-1 in homing to Peyers patches (258).

Lymphoid chemokines CCL19, CCL21, and CXCL13 are found in the T and B cell areas (260) (Figure 2.5, bottom panel). CXCL12 mRNA is made by stromal cells, but the protein is also found on HEVs (260), presumably transported in a manner similar to CCL19 (101). CXCL16 is constitutively produced by the FAE (254), even under germ-free conditions. $CD4^{+}$ and $CD8^{+}$ cells that express CXCR6 are found in the Peyers patches and require CXCL16 to home to the subepithelial dome, indicating a role for this chemokine receptor pair that has not been noted in lymph nodes. CCL20 and its receptor CCR6 are particularly important in Peyers patches. CCL20 is made by the intestinal epithelium, and it plays a crucial role in dendritic cell trafficking to Peyers patches (261). Peyers patch HEVs express CCL25, the ligand for CCR9, which has been defined as a mucosal homing chemokine receptor (67). Efferent lymphatic vessels from Peyers patches drain primed lymphocytes to the mesenteric lymph nodes.

Development

Models for Peyers patch organogenesis and maintenance have come from analysis of knock-out mice and from carefully phenotyping the cells in the anlagen during mouse embryonic development. Several cytokines and chemokines have been shown to be crucial for PP development. $lt\alpha^{-/-}$ and $lt\beta^{-/-}$ mice completely lack Peyers patches (147,262) as do mice that lack CXCR5, the receptor for CXCL13 (161). Since mice deficient in the LTβR also lack Peyers patches (263), these effects are mediated in large part through $LT\alpha_1\beta_2$. However, some $tnfr1^{-/-}$ mice lack organized Peyers patches, suggesting that either LTα3 or TNFα also influences generation or later stages in maintenance of Peyers patches (264). Similar to lymph nodes, mice deficient in IL-7 also lack PP (156). Mice deficient in CXCR5 or CXCL13 exhibit small or no Peyers patches (160,161,260), as do mice deficient in RORγt, Id2, NIK, and factors in the classical and alternative NFκB pathways (162,263). Peyers patch development differs from that of lymph nodes in the absence of a requirement for RANKL (158). A model for the embryonic development of Peyers patches, first proposed by Nishigawa and colleagues (265,266), has been experimentally substantiated (267). This model proposes stages that are similar to those described earlier for lymph node development and, in fact, provided the framework for studies in that organ. The first sign of Peyers patch development at E15.5 in the mouse is the appearance of regions on the small intestine that stain positively with antibodies to ICAM-1, VCAM-1, and LTβR. The cells in these aggregates are called the organizer cells. CXCL13, CCL19, and CCL21 are also apparent, as is IL-7. At E17.5, clusters of IL-7R$^+$CD4$^+$CD3$^+$ inducer cells are found. These express LTα and LTβ, CXCR5 and CCR7, Id2, and RORγ. They also express $\alpha4\beta1$ integrin activated by CXCR5 (268) that allows interaction with the VCAM-1$^+$ organizer cells. At E18.5, mature T and B cells enter through HEVs, CCL20 is produced by the FAE, and DCs expressing CCR7 and CCR6 are found. By day 4, the typical microarchitecture is apparent, with M cells and T and B cell compartmentalization (269).

Peyers patches are quite plastic in that they are affected by environmental influences, including bacterial flora. Their number and cellularity increase after immunization, and their lymphoid cell content decreases with aging (1,270). Lymphocytes also influence the maintenance of Peyers patches. Mice that lack mature T and B cells have either undetectable or small Peyers patches that lack follicles and germinal centers (271,272). B cell–deficient mice retain some M cells, suggesting that T cells may regulate M cell maintenance. When B cell–deficient mice are reconstituted by a membrane IgM transgene, FAE and M cells are found at levels comparable to those of normal mice (271), indicating that cells in addition to CD4$^+$CD3$^-$ inducer cells are crucial for the maintenance of mature, functioning Peyers patches.

Cryptopatches and Isolated Lymphoid Follicles

Even more environmentally regulated lymphoid tissues have been described in the adult gut. The cryptopatches in the lamina propria containing lymphoid tissue-inducer cells and DCs can give rise to ILF. The cryptopatches are composed of lin$^-$c-kit$^+$ cells, DCs, and VCAM-1$^+$ stromal cells with few or no mature T and B cells. The cryptopatch cells express RORγt, IL-7R, and CCR6 (273), and their development is dependent on IL-7, CCR6, and its receptor CCL20. Cryptopatches are quite plastic, and although the LT family is necessary for their development, they can be restored by administration of wild-type bone marrow to adult $lta^{-/-}$ mice.

After mice are exposed to microbes or during some forms of autoimmunity, cryptopatches give rise to ILFs (274,275), which resemble primitive lymph nodes. ILFs are found in the colon and small intestine in the mouse and serve as sites of mucosal immunity. ILFs include B cells and T cells, and, in fact, require B cells, but not T cells, expressing LT for their formation (270). In contrast to lymph nodes, they also require the TNFR1 (276). ILFs are quite plastic; they resolve completely after mice are treated with antibiotics or cytokine inhibitors (105,170,270,274,276).

TERTIARY LYMPHOID TISSUES

Similarities to Secondary Lymphoid Organs

Tertiary lymphoid tissues, also termed tertiary lymphoid organs, are ectopic accumulations of lymphoid cells that arise in nonlymphoid organs during chronic inflammation through a process termed lymphoid neogenesis (also lymphoid neoorganogenesis) (2). The iBALT could be considered as either a secondary or tertiary lymphoid tissue. This semantic issue epitomizes the plasticity of all lymphoid organs and the fact that lymphoid organ regulation represents a continuum from ontogeny through chronic inflammation. A notable difference between secondary lymphoid organs and tertiary lymphoid tissues is the fact that the latter can arise in almost any organ in the adult. Nonetheless, tertiary lymphoid tissues exhibit remarkable morphologic, cellular, chemokine, and vasculature similarities to secondary lymphoid organs. They exhibit T and B cell compartmentalization, naïve T and B cells, DCs, FDCs, plasma cells and lymphoid chemokines CCL19, CCL21, and CXCL13. Vessels with the morphological characteristics of HEVs have been detected in tertiary lymphoid tissues. In some cases, they express MADCAM-1. In others, they express PNAd and the enzymes and scaffold proteins necessary to generate that functional L-selectin ligand (118,178,277). Lymphatic vessels have been noted in tertiary lymphoid tissues (278,279), though it is not clear whether they function as afferent or efferent vessels.

Lymphoid neogenesis has been noted in humans in autoimmunity, microbial infection, and chronic allograft rejection (Table 2.2) (1). These accumulations occur in atherosclerotic plaques with expression of FDCs, organized B cell follicles, HEVs (HECA-452), and CCL19 and

TABLE 2.2 Lymphoid Neogenesis in Human Autoimmunity, Infectious Diseases, and Graft Rejection

Disease	Affected Tissue	Characteristics
Autoimmunity		
	Synovial membrane	T and B cells, plasma cells, GCs, FDCs, CXCL13, CCL21, HEVs (PNAd, HEC-6ST)
Sjögren's syndrome	Salivary glands	T and B cells, plasma cells, GCs, FDCs, CCL21, CXCL12, CXCL13 HEVs (PNAd)
Myasthenia gravis	Thymus	T and B cells, GCs, FDCs
Hashimoto's thyroiditis	Thyroid	T and B cells, GCs, FDCs CCL21, CXCL13, CXCL12, plasma cells, HEVs (PNAd)
Grave's disease	Thymus	T and B cells, GCs, FDCs, CCL21, CXCL13, CXCL12, HEVs (PNAd)
Multiple sclerosis	Brain	Lymphatic capillaries, B cell follicles and centroblasts, GCs, CCL19, CCL21, CXCL12, CXCL13
Ulcerative colitis	Colon	CXCL13
Inflammatory bowel disease (Crohn's disease)	Bowel	T cell-B compartments, LVs, HECA-452$^+$ HEV
Psoriatic arthritis	Joint	T cells and B cells, CXCL13, CCL19, CCL21, HEVs (PNAd)
Infectious diseases		
Borrelia burgdorferi/ Lyme Disease	Joints	T and B cells, FDCs, HEVs
Borrelia burgdorferi/ Neuroborreliosis	Central nervous system/ cerebrospinal fluid	CXCL13
Hepatitis C virus	Liver	T cell-B compartments, MAdCAM-1
Bartonella henselae/cat scratch disease	Granuloma	CXCL13
Graft rejection		
Organ		
Heart		Germinal centers
Kidney		Germinal centers, lymphatic vessels

Original references are in Drayton et al. (1).

CCL21 in addition to those chemokines more often associated with acute inflammation (280). Ectopic lymphoid tissues are also apparent in several animal models of autoimmune disease. The pancreatic infiltrates in early stages of diabetes in the nonobese diabetic (NOD) mouse express lymphoid chemokines (281) and HEVs expressing MAdCAM-1 (282,283), PNAd, and HEC-6ST (118). The brain in experimental autoimmune encephalomyelitis, a model of multiple sclerosis, has HEVs, CCL19, CCL21, CXCL13, and FDCs (284–286). The thyroid in the BB rat has T and B cell compartmentalization and DCs (287), and the gut in autoimmune gastritis in the mouse has HEVs and CXCL13 (288). Atherosclerotic plaques of apoprotein-E–deficient mice exhibit a marked increase in T and B cells and expression of CCL19 and CCL21 (289,290). Interestingly, although recruitment of T and B cells to the vessel wall depends in part on L-selectin, MECA-79–stained HEVs are not seen (289), suggesting the existence of an additional L-selectin ligand. Lymphoid neogenesis also occurs in chronic mouse heart allograft rejection (291). Tertiary lymphoid tissues have been induced in several transgenic mouse models with the use of tissue-specific promoters driving the expression of inflammatory cytokines or lymphoid chemokines (1). These murine models, in addition to serving as examples of autoimmunity, have provided invaluable insight into the regulation of secondary lymphoid organ development.

From Chronic Inflammation to Organized Lymphoid Microenvironments

Data generated from analyzing the cellular and molecular requirements for secondary lymphoid organ development have provided a paradigm for understanding the development of tertiary lymphoid tissues in chronic inflammation. This paradigm proposes that the processes and molecules governing secondary lymphoid organs are also the basis of tertiary lymphoid tissue development (2) and informs understanding of both secondary and tertiary lymphoid tissues. The physiologic event(s) that precipitate lymphoid neogenesis remain unclear. Data obtained from experiments in knockout and transgenic mice and clinical observations indicate that cooperative activities of TNF/LT family members and the lymphoid chemokines play central roles in this process.

Inflammation is a localized response to tissue injury, irritation, or infection often marked by tissue damage. Acute inflammation is an early innate immune response that is generally short-lived and self-limiting. However, in some situations, acute inflammation transitions to a chronic inflammatory response that is long-lived and self-perpetuating. Tertiary lymphoid tissues arise under conditions of constitutive cytokine or chemokine expression, but the precise signal(s) that initiates their development is unknown. By integrating studies of lymphoid neogenesis in human pathologies and in animal models, it is becoming clear that at least three critical events promote tertiary lymphoid tissue formation: inflammatory (e.g., TNF/LT) cytokine expression, lymphoid chemokine production by stromal cells, and HEV development. It is not known if lymphoid tissue inducer cells are necessary for lymphoid neogenesis, although such cells have been noted in the mouse models of lymphoid neogenesis (292).

Functions of Tertiary Lymphoid Tissues

Ectopic accumulation of lymphoid cells has been considered the hallmark of destructive inflammation. Indeed, some tertiary lymphoid tissues are accompanied by tissue damage. However, it is likely that tertiary lymphoid tissues in chronic inflammation have roles in addition to tissue destruction. In the case of microbial infection, it is likely that lymphoid neogenesis occurs as a way to sequester pathogens and prevent their access to the other parts of the body. This may represent a primitive form of immunity. Although local antigen presentation within the tertiary lymphoid tissue itself likely functions to prevent bacteremia or viremia, the propensity for tertiary lymphoid tissues to develop into lymphomas, and the ability of tertiary lymphoid tissues to serve as sites of prion accumulation, are obvious manifestations of possible detrimental functions (293). Further, the development of tertiary lymphoid tissues in autoimmunity may perpetuate disease.

Data from both human and murine studies provide compelling evidence that tertiary lymphoid tissues are permissive microenvironments for the induction of antigen-specific immune responses. Extensive immunohistochemical analyses of tertiary lymphoid tissues in autoimmunity and other chronic inflammatory states have established the presence of GCs and FDC networks in these tissues; several groups have demonstrated that tertiary lymphoid tissue GCs can support B cell differentiation. Microdissection of discrete lymphocytic foci and subsequent DNA sequence analysis of germinal center B cells from the inflamed synovial tissue of patients with rheumatoid arthritis revealed a restricted number of Vκ gene rearrangements, a result consistent with oligoclonal B cell expansion in the synovial tissue (294). Somatic hypermutation is apparent in synovial germinal center B cells (295). Further, synovial B cells exhibit a limited number of heavy and light chain gene rearrangements consistent with local clonal expansion of these cells. The molecular analysis of tertiary lymphoid tissue GCs from the salivary glands of patients with primary Sjögren's syndrome or the thymus of myasthenia gravis patients demonstrates oligoclonal B cell proliferation in these tissues in addition to somatic hypermutation of Ig variable genes (296–298). Together, these studies indicate that tertiary lymphoid tissue GCs in several autoimmune pathologies can support antigen-driven clonal expansion and extensive diversification.

Another important hallmark of antigen-driven B cell responses is the terminal differentiation of activated B cells into Ig-secreting plasma cells. Plasma cells have been detected in tertiary lymphoid tissues associated with GCs in rheumatoid arthritis (299) and in Sjögren's syndrome. Mice expressing LTα under the control of the insulin promoter (RIPLTα) exhibit tertiary lymphoid tissue at the sites of transgene expression (i.e., pancrease, kidney, and skin). After immunization with sheep red blood cells, evidence of isotype switching is apparent in these cellular infiltrates (2). Although the presence of plasma cells in tertiary lymphoid tissues is consistent with local antigen presentation, it is occasionally unclear whether these cells develop in the tertiary lymphoid tissues themselves or have migrated from canonical secondary lymphoid tissues. Nonetheless, when taken together, these studies indicate that tertiary lymphoid tissues in several human pathologies and animal models support antigen-driven B cell differentiation marked by somatic hypermutation of immunoglobulin variable genes, affinity maturation, isotype switching, and terminal differentiation into antibody-secreting plasma cells.

T cell priming occurs in tertiary lymphoid tissues, as suggested by the presence of isotype-switched plasma cells in the RIPLTα tertiary lymphoid tissues (2) and T cell epitope spreading in the central nervous system during experimental allergic encephalomyelitis (300). The restricted TCR repertoire in a melanoma-associated tertiary lymphoid tissue (301) further supports the concept that tertiary lymphoid tissues can act as priming sites. The demonstration of naïve T cell proliferation in the islets of NOD mice after surgical removal of pancreatic lymph nodes (302) suggests, together with evidence noted above, that tertiary lymphoid tissues present antigen to naïve cells at the local site and generate an immune response. Determinant or epitope spreading, a phenomenon that arises in several autoimmune diseases, occurs when epitopes other than the inducing antigen become major targets of an ongoing immune response. It is considered to occur subsequent to the tissue damage induced by the initiating autoreactive T cells and therefore is the result of the presentation of new antigens (303). Data generated in murine models of central nervous system inflammation support the possibility that intermolecular and intramolecular epitope spreading occurs in tertiary lymphoid tissues in the central nervous system (300).

Plasticity and Adaptability of Tertiary Lymphoid Tissues

Tertiary lymphoid tissues are the most plastic and adaptable of the lymphoid tissues. First, lymphoid neogenesis can be induced by a variety of stimuli. Their nimbleness in this regard suggests that they might represent the most primitive tissues in the immune system. Tertiary lymphoid tissues can be "turned off" (i.e., resolved) upon removal of the initial stimulus or after therapeutic intervention. The destruction of the islets of Langerhans β cells in Type I diabetes mellitus is an example of a situation in which removal of the antigen stimulus is accompanied by tertiary lymphoid tissue resolution. Antibiotic treatment results in the resolution of tertiary lymphoid tissues and even MALT lymphomas (304). Treatment has been shown to resolve some established tertiary lymphoid tissues, reversing insulitis and protecting against diabetes in NOD mice (305). Such treatment can also "turn off" established tertiary lymphoid tissues in a mouse model of collagen-induced arthritis (306). These studies are similar to those described earlier regarding the plasticity of lymph nodes after mice are immunized or treated with LTβR-Ig (185,193), again emphasizing the commonality of these tissues.

CONCLUSION

The immune system depends on a remarkable organization of tissues and cells. The organs have defined functions that include generation of an immune repertoire (primary lymphoid organs) and responding to antigens (secondary lymphoid organs and tertiary lymphoid tissues). Development of primary and secondary lymphoid organs depends on precisely regulated expression of cytokines, chemokines, and adhesion molecules. Similar signals regulate the transition from inflammation to tertiary lymphoid tissues. Chemokines and adhesion molecules regulate trafficking in and out of lymphoid organs. Secondary lymphoid organs are remarkably plastic in their response to antigenic assault and adapt with changes in expression of chemokines and adhesion molecules to maximize encounter of antigens with antigen-specific cells. Tertiary lymphoid tissues, characteristic of many pathologic states, may actually represent the most primitive form of lymphoid tissues in their even greater plasticity and ability to develop directly at the site of antigen exposure.

ACKNOWLEDGMENTS

The authors thank Myriam Hill for assistance in figure preparation. This work was supported National Institutes of Health grants CA16885 and DK57731.

REFERENCES

1. Drayton DL, Liao S, Mounzer RH, et al. Lymphoid organ development: from ontogeny to neogenesis. *Nat Immunol* 2006;7:344–353.
2. Kratz A, Campos-Neto A, Hanson MS, et al. Chronic inflammation caused by lymphotoxin is lymphoid neogenesis. *J Exp Med.* 1996;183:1461–1472.
3. Medvinsky AL, Samoylina NL, Muller AM, et al. An early pre-liver intraembryonic source of CFU-S in the developing mouse. *Nature.* 1993;364:64–67.
4. Gekas C, Dieterlen-Lievre F, Orkin SH, et al. The placenta is a niche for hematopoietic stem cells. *Dev Cell.* 2005;8:365–375.
5. Ottersbach K, Dzierzak E. The murine placenta contains hematopoietic stem cells within the vascular labyrinth region. *Dev Cell.* 2005;8:377–387.
6. Christensen JL, Wright DE, Wagers AJ, et al. Circulation and chemotaxis of fetal hematopoietic stem cells. *PLoS Biol.* 2004;2:E75.
7. Hardy RR, Hayakawa K. B cell development pathways. *Annu Rev Immunol.* 2001;19:595–621.
8. Li YS, Hayakawa K, Hardy RR. The regulated expression of B lineage associated genes during B cell differentiation in bone marrow and fetal liver. *J Exp Med.* 1993;178:951–960.
9. Frenette PS, Subbarao S, Mazo IB, et al. Endothelial selectins and vascular cell adhesion molecule-1 promote hematopoietic progenitor homing to bone marrow. *Proc Natl Acad Sci USA.* 1998;95:14423–14428.
10. Vermeulen M, Le Pesteur F, Gagnerault MC, et al. Role of adhesion molecules in the homing and mobilization of murine hematopoietic stem and progenitor cells. *Blood.* 1998;92:894–900.
11. Orkin SH, Zon LI. Hematopoiesis and stem cells: plasticity versus developmental heterogeneity. *Nat Immunol.* 2002;3:323–328.
12. Pittenger MF, Mackay AM, Beck SC, et al. Multilineage potential of adult human mesenchymal stem cells. *Science.* 1999;284:143–147.
13. Pauwelyn KA, Verfaillie CM. Transplantation of undifferentiated, bone marrow-derived stem cells. *Curr Top Dev Biol.* 2006;74:201–251.
14. Cyster JG. Homing of antibody secreting cells. *Immunol Rev.* 2003;194:48–60.
15. Nagasawa T. Microenvironmental niches in the bone marrow required for B-cell development. *Nat Rev Immunol.* 2006;6:107–116.
16. Jacobsen K, Osmond DG. Microenvironmental organization and stromal cell associations of B lymphocyte precursor cells in mouse bone marrow. *Eur J Immunol.* 1990;20:2395–2404.
17. Heissig B, Hattori K, Dias S, et al. Recruitment of stem and progenitor cells from the bone marrow niche requires MMP-9 mediated release of kit-ligand. *Cell.* 2002;109:625–637.
18. Tokoyoda K, Egawa T, Sugiyama T, et al. Cellular niches controlling B lymphocyte behavior within bone marrow during development. *Immunity.* 2004;20:707–718.
19. Banu N, Deng B, Lyman SD, et al. Modulation of haematopoietic progenitor development by FLT-3 ligand. *Cytokine.* 1999;11:679–688.
20. Heissig B, Ohki Y, Sato Y, et al. A role for niches in hematopoietic cell development. *Hematology.* 2005;10:247–253.
21. Lataillade JJ, Domenech J, Le Bousse-Kerdiles MC. Stromal cell-derived factor-1 (SDF-1)\CXCR4 couple plays multiple roles on

haematopoietic progenitors at the border between the old cytokine and new chemokine worlds: survival, cell cycling and trafficking. *Eur Cytokine Netw*. 2004;15:177–188.
22. Papayannopoulou T, Craddock C, Nakamoto B, et al. The VLA4/VCAM-1 adhesion pathway defines contrasting mechanisms of lodgement of transplanted murine hemopoietic progenitors between bone marrow and spleen. *Proc Natl Acad Sci U S A*. 1995;92: 9647–9651.
23. Katayama Y, Hidalgo A, Furie BC, et al. PSGL-1 participates in E-selectin-mediated progenitor homing to bone marrow: evidence for cooperation between E-selectin ligands and alpha4 integrin. *Blood*. 2003;102:2060–2067.
24. Katayama Y, Hidalgo A, Peired A, et al. Integrin alpha4beta7 and its counterreceptor MAdCAM-1 contribute to hematopoietic progenitor recruitment into bone marrow following transplantation. *Blood*. 2004;104:2020–2026.
25. Lindsley RC, Thomas M, Srivastava B, et al. Generation of peripheral B cells occurs via two spatially and temporally distinct pathways. *Blood*. 2007;109:2521–2528.
26. Honczarenko M, Glodek AM, Swierkowski M, et al. Developmental stage-specific shift in responsiveness to chemokines during human B-cell development. *Exp Hematol*. 2006;34:1093–1100.
27. Bowman EP, Campbell JJ, Soler D, et al. Developmental switches in chemokine response profiles during B cell differentiation and maturation. *J Exp Med*. 2000;191:1303–1318.
28. Pantelouris EM. Absence of thymus in a mouse mutant. *Nature*. 1968;217:370–371.
29. Terszowski G, Muller SM, Bleul CC, et al. Evidence for a functional second thymus in mice. *Science*. 2006;312:284–287.
30. Bubanovic IV. Crossroads of extrathymic lymphocytes maturation pathways. *Med Hypotheses*. 2003;61:235–239.
31. Cunliffe VT, Furley AJ, Keenan D. Complete rescue of the nude mutant phenotype by a wild-type Foxn1 transgene. *Mamm Genome*. 2002;13:245–252.
32. Scollay RG, Butcher EC, Weissman IL. Thymus cell migration. Quantitative aspects of cellular traffic from the thymus to the periphery in mice. *Eur J Immunol*. 1980;10:210–218.
33. Blackburn CC, Manley NR. Developing a new paradigm for thymus organogenesis. *Nat Rev Immunol*. 2004;4:278–289.
34. Lind EF, Prockop SE, Porritt HE,et al. Mapping precursor movement through the postnatal thymus reveals specific microenvironments supporting defined stages of early lymphoid development. *J Exp Med*. 2001;194:127–134.
35. Anderson M, Anderson SK, Farr AG. Thymic vasculature: organizer of the medullary epithelial compartment? *Int Immunol*. 2000;12:1105–1110.
36. Odaka C, Morisada T, Oike Y, et al. Distribution of lymphatic vessels in mouse thymus: immunofluorescence analysis. *Cell Tissue Res*. 2006;325:13–22.
37. Pearse M, Wu L, Egerton M, et al. A murine early thymocyte developmental sequence is marked by transient expression of the interleukin 2 receptor. *Proc Natl Acad Sci USA*. 1989;86:1614–1618.
38. Shinkai Y, Rathbun G, Lam KP, et al. RAG-2-deficient mice lack mature lymphocytes owing to inability to initiate V(D)J rearrangement. *Cell*. 1992;68:855–867.
39. Jameson SC, Hogquist KA, Bevan MJ. Positive selection of thymocytes. *Annu Rev Immunol*. 1995;13:93–126.
40. Kisielow P, Teh HS, Bluthmann H, et al. Positive selection of antigen-specific T cells in thymus by restricting MHC molecules. *Nature*. 1988;335:730–733.
41. Egerton M, Scollay R, Shortman K. Kinetics of mature T-cell development in the thymus. *Proc Natl Acad Sci USA*. 1990;87:2579–2582.
42. Silva-Santos B, Pennington DJ, Hayday AC. Lymphotoxin-mediated regulation of gammadelta cell differentiation by alphabeta T cell progenitors. *Science*. 2005;307:925–928.
43. Klug DB, Carter C, Crouch E, et al. Interdependence of cortical thymic epithelial cell differentiation and T-lineage commitment. *Proc Natl Acad Sci USA*. 1998;95:11822–11827.
44. Derbinski J, Gabler J, Brors B, et al. Promiscuous gene expression in thymic epithelial cells is regulated at multiple levels. *J Exp Med*. 2005;202:33–45.
45. Aaltonen J, Bjorses P, Sandkuijl L, et al. An autosomal locus causing autoimmune disease: autoimmune polyglandular disease type I assigned to chromosome 21. *Nat Genet*. 1994;8:83–87.
46. Anderson MS, Venanzi ES, Klein L, et al. Projection of an immunological self shadow within the thymus by the aire protein. *Science*. 2002;298:1395–1401.
47. Patel DD, Whichard LP, Radcliff G, et al. Characterization of human thymic epithelial cell surface antigens: phenotypic similarity of thymic epithelial cells to epidermal keratinocytes. *J Clin Immunol*. 1995;15:80–92.
48. Chentoufi AA, Palumbo M, Polychronakos C. Proinsulin expression by Hassall's corpuscles in the mouse thymus. *Diabetes*. 2004;53:354–359.
49. Douek DC, Altmann DM. T-cell apoptosis and differential human leucocyte antigen class II expression in human thymus. *Immunology*. 2000;99:249–256.
50. Ardavin C, Wu L, Li CL, et al. Thymic dendritic cells and T cells develop simultaneously in the thymus from a common precursor population. *Nature*. 1993;362:761–763.
51. Foss DL, Donskoy E, Goldschneider I. The importation of hematogenous precursors by the thymus is a gated phenomenon in normal adult mice. *J Exp Med*. 2001;193:365–374.
52. Donskoy E, Goldschneider I. Two developmentally distinct populations of dendritic cells inhabit the adult mouse thymus: demonstration by differential importation of hematogenous precursors under steady state conditions. *J Immunol*. 2003;170:3514–3521.
53. Anderson G, Owen JJ, Moore NC, et al. Thymic epithelial cells provide unique signals for positive selection of CD4+CD8+ thymocytes in vitro. *J Exp Med*. 1994;179:2027–2031.
54. Anderson G, Partington KM, Jenkinson EJ. Differential effects of peptide diversity and stromal cell type in positive and negative selection in the thymus. *J Immunol*. 1998;161:6599–6603.
55. Brocker T, Riedinger M, Karjalainen K. Targeted expression of major histocompatibility complex (MHC) class II molecules demonstrates that dendritic cells can induce negative but not positive selection of thymocytes in vivo. *J Exp Med*. 1997;185:541-550.
56. Heino M, Peterson P, Sillanpaa N, et al. RNA and protein expression of the murine autoimmune regulator gene (Aire) in normal, RelB-deficient and in NOD mouse. *Eur J Immunol*. 2000;30:1884–1893.
57. Watanabe N, Wang YH, Lee HK, et al. Hassall's corpuscles instruct dendritic cells to induce CD4+CD25+ regulatory T cells in human thymus. *Nature*. 2005;436:1181–1185.
58. Liu YJ, Soumelis V, Watanabe N, et al. TSLP: An epithelial cell cytokine that regulates T cell differentiation by conditioning dendritic cell maturation. *Annu Rev Immunol*. 2006;25:193–219.
59. Miyazaki T, Suzuki G, Yamamura K. The role of macrophages in antigen presentation and T cell tolerance. *Int Immunol*. 1993;5: 1023–1033.
60. Ferrero I, Anjuere F, Martin P, et al. Functional and phenotypic analysis of thymic B cells: role in the induction of T cell negative selection. *Eur J Immunol*. 1999;29:1598–1609.
61. Flores KG, Li J, Hale LP. B cells in epithelial and perivascular compartments of human adult thymus. *Hum Pathol*. 2001;32:926–934.
62. Fukuba Y, Inaba M, Taketani S, et al. Functional analysis of thymic B cells. *Immunobiology*. 1994;190:150–163.
63. Joao C, Ogle BM, Gay-Rabinstein C, et al. B cell-dependent TCR diversification. *J Immunol*. 2004;172:4709–4716.
64. Lepique AP, Palencia S, Irjala H, et al. Characterization of vascular adhesion molecules that may facilitate progenitor homing in the post-natal mouse thymus. *Clin Dev Immunol*. 2003;10:27–33.
65. Bleul CC, Boehm T. Chemokines define distinct microenvironments in the developing thymus. *Eur J Immunol*. 2000;30:3371–3379.
66. Liu C, Ueno T, Kuse S, et al. The role of CCL21 in recruitment of T-precursor cells to fetal thymi. *Blood*. 2005;105:31–39.
67. Wurbel MA, Malissen M, Guy-Grand D, et al. Mice lacking the CCR9 CC-chemokine receptor show a mild impairment of early T- and B-cell development and a reduction in T-cell receptor gammadelta(+) gut intraepithelial lymphocytes. *Blood*. 2001;98:2626–2632.
68. Misslitz A, Pabst O, Hintzen G, et al. Thymic T cell development and progenitor localization depend on CCR7. *J Exp Med*. 2004;200:481–491.

69. Plotkin J, Prockop SE, Lepique A, et al. Critical role for CXCR4 signaling in progenitor localization and T cell differentiation in the postnatal thymus. *J Immunol*. 2003;171:4521–4527.
70. Kurobe H, Liu C, Ueno T, et al. CCR7-dependent cortex-to-medulla migration of positively selected thymocytes is essential for establishing central tolerance. *Immunity*. 2006;24:165–177.
71. Ueno T, Saito F, Gray DH, et al. CCR7 signals are essential for cortex-medulla migration of developing thymocytes. *J Exp Med*. 2004;200:493–505.
72. Poznansky MC, Olszak IT, Evans RH, et al. Thymocyte emigration is mediated by active movement away from stroma-derived factors. *J Clin Invest*. 2002;109:1101–1110.
73. Ueno T, Hara K, Willis MS, et al. Role for CCR7 ligands in the emigration of newly generated T lymphocytes from the neonatal thymus. *Immunity*. 2002;16:205–218.
74. Edsall LC, Spiegel S. Enzymatic measurement of sphingosine 1-phosphate. *Anal Biochem*. 1999;272:80–86.
75. Slifka MK, Matloubian M, Ahmed R. Bone marrow is a major site of long-term antibody production after acute viral infection. *J Virol*. 1995;69:1895–1902.
76. Bensinger SJ, Bandeira A, Jordan MS, et al. Major histocompatibility complex class II-positive cortical epithelium mediates the selection of CD4(+)25(+) immunoregulatory T cells. *J Exp Med*. 2001;194:427–438.
77. Fontenot JD, Rasmussen JP, Williams LM, et al. Regulatory T cell lineage specification by the forkhead transcription factor foxp3. *Immunity*. 2005;22:329–341.
78. Manley NR. Thymus organogenesis and molecular mechanisms of thymic epithelial cell differentiation. *Semin Immunol*. 2000;12:421–428.
79. Gordon J, Bennett AR, Blackburn CC, et al. Gcm2 and Foxn1 mark early parathyroid- and thymus-specific domains in the developing third pharyngeal pouch. *Mech Dev*. 2001;103:141–143.
80. Manley NR, Blackburn CC. A developmental look at thymus organogenesis: where do the non-hematopoietic cells in the thymus come from? *Curr Opin Immunol*. 2003;15:225–232.
81. Kingston R, Jenkinson EJ, Owen JJ. Characterization of stromal cell populations in the developing thymus of normal and nude mice. *Eur J Immunol*. 1984;14:1052–1056.
82. Owen JJ, Jenkinson EJ. Early events in T lymphocyte genesis in the fetal thymus. *Am J Anat*. 1984;170:301–310.
83. Van Vliet E, Jenkinson EJ, Kingston R, et al. Stromal cell types in the developing thymus of the normal and nude mouse embryo. *Eur J Immunol*. 1985;15:675–681.
84. Le Douarin NM, Jotereau FV. Tracing of cells of the avian thymus through embryonic life in interspecific chimeras. *J Exp Med*. 1975;142:17–40.
85. Gordon J, Wilson VA, Blair NF, et al. Functional evidence for a single endodermal origin for the thymic epithelium. *Nat Immunol*. 2004;5:546–553.
86. Klug DB, Carter C, Gimenez-Conti IB, et al. Cutting edge: thymocyte-independent and thymocyte-dependent phases of epithelial patterning in the fetal thymus. *J Immunol*. 2002;169:2842–2845.
87. van Ewijk W, Hollander G, Terhorst C, et al. Stepwise development of thymic microenvironments in vivo is regulated by thymocyte subsets. *Development*. 2000;127:1583–1591.
88. Mebius RE. Organogenesis of lymphoid tissues. *Nat Rev Immunol*. 2003;3:292–303.
89. Boehm T, Scheu S, Pfeffer K, et al. Thymic medullary epithelial cell differentiation, thymocyte emigration, and the control of autoimmunity require lympho-epithelial cross talk via LTbetaR. *J Exp Med*. 2003;198:757–769.
90. Chin RK, Lo JC, Kim O, et al. Lymphotoxin pathway directs thymic Aire expression. *Nat Immunol*. 2003;4:1121–1127.
91. Haynes BF, Heinly CS. Early human T cell development: analysis of the human thymus at the time of initial entry of hematopoietic stem cells into the fetal thymic microenvironment. *J Exp Med*. 1995;181:1445–1458.
92. Bouneaud C, Kourilsky P, Bousso P. Impact of negative selection on the T cell repertoire reactive to a self-peptide: a large fraction of T cell clones escapes clonal deletion. *Immunity*. 2000;13:829–840.
93. Steinman RM. The dendritic cell system and its role in immunogenicity. *Annu Rev Immunol*. 1991;9:271–296.
94. von Andrian UH, Mempel TR. Homing and cellular traffic in lymph nodes. *Nat Rev Immunol*. 2003;3:867–878.
95. Wilson NS, El-Sukkari D, Belz GT, et al. Most lymphoid organ dendritic cell types are phenotypically and functionally immature. *Blood*. 2003;102:2187–2194.
96. Wilson NS, El-Sukkari D, Villadangos JA. Dendritic cells constitutively present self antigens in their immature state in vivo and regulate antigen presentation by controlling the rates of MHC class II synthesis and endocytosis. *Blood*. 2004;103:2187–2195.
97. Cavanagh LL, Von Andrian UH. Travellers in many guises: the origins and destinations of dendritic cells. *Immunol Cell Biol*. 2002;80:448–462.
98. Steinman RM, Hawiger D, Liu K, et al. Dendritic cell function in vivo during the steady state: a role in peripheral tolerance. *Ann N Y Acad Sci*. 2003;987:15–25.
99. Stoitzner P, Tripp CH, Douillard P, et al. Migratory Langerhans cells in mouse lymph nodes in steady state and inflammation. *J Invest Dermatol*. 2005;125:116–125.
100. Gretz JE, Norbury CC, Anderson AO, et al. Lymph-borne chemokines and other low molecular weight molecules reach high endothelial venules via specialized conduits while a functional barrier limits access to the lymphocyte microenvironments in lymph node cortex. *J Exp Med*. 2000;192:1425–1440.
101. Baekkevold ES, Yamanaka T, Palframan RT, et al. The CCR7 ligand elc (CCL19) is transcytosed in high endothelial venules and mediates T cell recruitment. *J Exp Med*. 2001;193:1105–1112.
102. Nakano H, Gunn MD. Gene duplications at the chemokine locus on mouse chromosome 4: multiple strain-specific haplotypes and the deletion of secondary lymphoid-organ chemokine and EBI-1 ligand chemokine genes in the plt mutation. *J Immunol*. 2001;166:361–369.
103. Vassileva G, Soto H, Zlotnik A, et al. The reduced expression of 6Ckine in the plt mouse results from the deletion of one of two 6Ckine genes. *J Exp Med*. 1999;190:1183–1188.
104. Cyster JG. Chemokines and cell migration in secondary lymphoid organs. *Science*. 1999;286:2098–2102.
105. Ebert LM, Schaerli P, Moser B. Chemokine-mediated control of T cell traffic in lymphoid and peripheral tissues. *Mol Immunol*. 2005;42:799–809.
106. Rodrigo Mora J, Von Andrian UH. Specificity and plasticity of memory lymphocyte migration. *Curr Top Microbiol Immunol*. 2006;308:83–116.
107. Cyster JG. Chemokines, sphingosine-1-phosphate, and cell migration in secondary lymphoid organs. *Annu Rev Immunol*. 2005;23:127–159.
108. Lo CG, Xu Y, Proia RL, et al. Cyclical modulation of sphingosine-1-phosphate receptor 1 surface expression during lymphocyte recirculation and relationship to lymphoid organ transit. *J Exp Med*. 2005;201:291–301.
109. Anderson AO, Anderson ND. Studies on the structure and permeability of the microvasculature in normal rat lymph nodes. *Am J Pathol*. 1975;80:387–418.
110. M'Rini C, Cheng G, Schweitzer C, et al. A novel endothelial L-selectin ligand activity in lymph node medulla that is regulated by alpha(1,3)-fucosyltransferase-IV. *J Exp Med*. 2003;198:1301–1312.
111. von Andrian UH, M'Rini C. In situ analysis of lymphocyte migration to lymph nodes. *Cell Adhes Commun*. 1998;6:85–96.
112. Hay JB, Hobbs BB. The flow of blood to lymph nodes and its relation to lymphocyte traffic and the immune response. *J Exp Med*. 1977;145:31–44.
113. Hemmerich S, Bistrup A, Singer MS, et al. Sulfation of L-selectin ligands by an HEV-restricted sulfotransferase regulates lymphocyte homing to lymph nodes. *Immunity*. 2001;15:237–247.
114. Hemmerich S, Butcher EC, Rosen SD. Sulfation-dependent recognition of HEV-ligands by L-selectin and MECA-79, an adhesion-blocking mAb. *J Exp Med*. 1994;180:2219–2226.
115. Hiraoka N, Kawashima H, Petryniak B, et al. Core 2 branching beta1,6-N-acetylglucosaminyltransferase and high endothelial venule-restricted sulfotransferase collaboratively control lymphocyte homing. *J Biol Chem*. 2004;279:3058–3067.
116. Hiraoka N, Petryniak B, Nakayama J, et al. A novel, high endothelial venule-specific sulfotransferase expresses 6-sulfo sialyl Lewis(x),

an L-selectin ligand displayed by CD34. *Immunity*. 1999;11: 79–89.
117. Homeister JW, Thall AD, Petryniak B, et al. The alpha(1,3)fucosyltransferases FucT-IV and FucT-VII exert collaborative control over selectin-dependent leukocyte recruitment and lymphocyte homing. *Immunity*. 2001;15:115–126.
118. Bistrup A, Tsay D, Shenoy P, et al. Detection of a sulfotransferase (HEC-GlcNAc6ST) in high endothelial venules of lymph nodes and in high endothelial venule-like vessels within ectopic lymphoid aggregates: relationship to the MECA-79 epitope. *Am J Pathol*. 2004;164:1635–1644.
119. Kraal G, Mebius RE. High endothelial venules: lymphocyte traffic control and controlled traffic. *Adv Immunol*. 1997;65:347–395.
120. Miyasaka M, Tanaka T. Lymphocyte trafficking across high endothelial venules: dogmas and enigmas. *Nat Rev Immunol*. 2004;4:360–370.
121. Butcher EC, Scollay RG, Weissman IL. Lymphocyte adherence to high endothelial venules: characterization of a modified in vitro assay, and examination of the binding of syngeneic and allogeneic lymphocyte populations. *J Immunol*. 1979;123:1996–2003.
122. Mebius RE, Streeter PR, Michie S, et al. A developmental switch in lymphocyte homing receptor and endothelial vascular addressin expression regulates lymphocyte homing and permits CD4+ CD3− cells to colonize lymph nodes. *Proc Natl Acad Sci USA*. 1996;93: 11019–11024.
123. Oliver G. Lymphatic vasculature development. *Nat Rev Immunol*. 2004;4:35–45.
124. Anderson AO, Shaw S. Conduit for privileged communications in the lymph node. *Immunity*. 2005;22:3–5.
125. Sixt M, Kanazawa N, Selg M, et al. The conduit system transports soluble antigens from the afferent lymph to resident dendritic cells in the T cell area of the lymph node. *Immunity*. 2005;22:19–29.
126. Itano AA, McSorley SJ, Reinhardt RL, et al. Distinct dendritic cell populations sequentially present antigen to CD4 T cells and stimulate different aspects of cell-mediated immunity. *Immunity*. 2003;19:47–57.
127. Drayson MT, Ford WL. Afferent lymph and lymph borne cells: their influence on lymph node function. *Immunobiology*. 1984;168:362–379.
128. Hendriks HR, Eestermans IL. Disappearance and reappearance of high endothelial venules and immigrating lymphocytes in lymph nodes deprived of afferent lymphatic vessels: a possible regulatory role of macrophages in lymphocyte migration. *Eur J Immunol*. 1983;13:663–669.
129. Hendriks HR, Duijvestijn AM, Kraal G. Rapid decrease in lymphocyte adherence to high endothelial venules in lymph nodes deprived of afferent lymphatic vessels. *Eur J Immunol*. 1987;17:1691–1695.
130. Mebius RE, Bauer J, Twisk AJ, et al. The functional activity of high endothelial venules: a role for the subcapsular sinus macrophages in the lymph node. *Immunobiology*. 1991;182:277–291.
131. Mebius RE, Breve J, Kraal G, et al. Developmental regulation of vascular addressin expression: a possible role for site-associated environments. *Int Immunol*. 1993;5:443–449.
132. Swarte VV, Joziasse DH, Van den Eijnden DH, et al. Regulation of fucosyltransferase-VII expression in peripheral lymph node high endothelial venules. *Eur J Immunol*. 1998;28:3040–3047.
133. Gretz JE, Anderson AO, Shaw S. Cords, channels, corridors and conduits: critical architectural elements facilitating cell interactions in the lymph node cortex. *Immunol Rev*. 1997;156:11–24.
134. Gretz JE, Kaldjian EP, Anderson AO, et al. Sophisticated strategies for information encounter in the lymph node: the reticular network as a conduit of soluble information and a highway for cell traffic. *J Immunol*. 1996;157:495–499.
135. Larsen CG, Anderson AO, Appella E, et al. The neutrophil-activating protein (NAP-1) is also chemotactic for T lymphocytes. *Science*. 1989;243:1464–1466.
136. Oliver G, Alitalo K. The lymphatic vasculature: recent progress and paradigms. *Annu Rev Cell Dev Biol*. 2005;21:457–483.
137. Sabin FR. On the origin of the lymphatic system from the veins, and the development of the lymph hearts and thoracic duct in the pig. *Am J Anat*. 1902;1:367–389.
138. Sabin FR. On the development of the superficial lymphatics in the skin of the pig. *Am J Anat*. 1904;3:183–195.
139. Wigle JT, Harvey N, Detmar M, et al. An essential role for Prox1 in the induction of the lymphatic endothelial cell phenotype. *Embo J*. 2002;21:1505–1513.
140. Wigle JT, Oliver G. Prox1 function is required for the development of the murine lymphatic system. *Cell*. 1999;98:769–778.
141. Abtahian F, Guerriero A, Sebzda E, et al. Regulation of blood and lymphatic vascular separation by signaling proteins SLP-76 and Syk. *Science*. 2003;299:247–251.
142. Scavelli C, Weber E, Agliano M, C et al. Lymphatics at the crossroads of angiogenesis and lymphangiogenesis. *J Anat*. 2004;204:433–449.
143. Eikelenboom P, Nassy JJ, Post J, et al. The histogenesis of lymph nodes in rat and rabbit. *Anat Rec*. 1978;190:201–215.
144. Groscurth P. Non-lymphatic cells in the lymph node cortex of the mouse. I. Morphology and distribution of the interdigitating cells and the dendritic reticular cells in the mesenteric lymph node of the adult ICR mouse *Pathol Res Pract*. 1980;169:212–234.
145. Nossal GJ, Pike BL. Studies on the differentiation of B lymphocytes in the mouse. *Immunology*. 1973;25:33–45.
146. Williams GM, Nossal GJ. Ontogeny of the immune response. I. The development of the follicular antigen-trapping mechanism. *J Exp Med*. 1966;124:47–56.
147. De Togni P, Goellner J, Ruddle NH, et al. Abnormal development of peripheral lymphoid organs in mice deficient in lymphotoxin. *Science*. 1994;264:703–707.
148. Harmsen A, Kusser K, Hartson L, et al. Cutting edge: organogenesis of nasal-associated lymphoid tissue (NALT) occurs independently of lymphotoxin-alpha (LT alpha) and retinoic acid receptor-related orphan receptor-gamma, but the organization of NALT is LT alpha dependent. *J Immunol*. 2002;168:986–990.
149. Ying X, Chan K, Shenoy P, et al. Lymphotoxin plays a crucial role in the development and function of nasal-associated lymphoid tissue through regulation of chemokines and peripheral node addressin. *Am J Pathol*. 2005;166:135–146.
150. Alimzhanov MB, Kuprash DV, Kosco-Vilbois MH, et al. Abnormal development of secondary lymphoid tissues in lymphotoxin beta-deficient mice. *Proc Natl Acad Sci USA*. 1997;94:9302–9307.
151. Andoh N, Ohtani H, Kusakari C, et al. Expression of E- and P-selectins by vascular endothelial cells in human tonsils. *Acta Otolaryngol Suppl*. 1996;523:52–54.
152. Soderberg KA, Linehan MM, Ruddle NH, et al. MAdCAM-1 expressing sacral lymph node in the lymphotoxin beta-deficient mouse provides a site for immune generation following vaginal herpes simplex virus-2 infection. *J Immunol*. 2004;173:1908–1913.
153. Futterer A, Mink K, Luz A, et al. The lymphotoxin beta receptor controls organogenesis and affinity maturation in peripheral lymphoid tissues. *Immunity*. 1998;9:59–70.
154. Scheu S, Alferink J, Potzel T, et al. Targeted disruption of LIGHT causes defects in costimulatory T cell activation and reveals cooperation with lymphotoxin beta in mesenteric lymph node genesis. *J Exp Med*. 2002;195:1613–1624.
155. Rennert PD, James D, Mackay F, et al. Lymph node genesis is induced by signaling through the lymphotoxin beta receptor. *Immunity*. 1998;9:71–79.
156. Adachi S, Yoshida H, Honda K, et al. Essential role of IL-7 receptor alpha in the formation of Peyers patch anlage. *Int Immunol*. 1998;10:1–6.
157. Cao X, Shores EW, Hu-Li J, et al. Defective lymphoid development in mice lacking expression of the common cytokine receptor gamma chain. *Immunity*. 1995;2:223–238.
158. Dougall WC, Glaccum M, Charrier K, et al. RANK is essential for osteoclast and lymph node development. *Genes Dev*. 1999;13:2412–2424.
159. Kim D, Mebius RE, MacMicking JD, et al. Regulation of peripheral lymph node genesis by the tumor necrosis factor family member TRANCE. *J Exp Med*. 2000;192:1467–1478.
160. Ansel KM, Ngo VN, Hyman PL, et al. A chemokine-driven positive feedback loop organizes lymphoid follicles. *Nature*. 2000;406:309–314.
161. Forster R, Mattis AE, Kremmer E, et al. A putative chemokine receptor, BLR1, directs B cell migration to defined lymphoid organs and

specific anatomic compartments of the spleen. *Cell*. 1996;87:1037–1047.

162. Weih F, Caamano J. Regulation of secondary lymphoid organ development by the nuclear factor-kappaB signal transduction pathway. *Immunol Rev*. 2003;195:91–105.
163. Miyawaki S, Nakamura Y, Suzuka H, et al. A new mutation, aly, that induces a generalized lack of lymph nodes accompanied by immunodeficiency in mice. *Eur J Immunol*. 1994;24:429–434.
164. Shinkura R, Kitada K, Matsuda F, et al. Alymphoplasia is caused by a point mutation in the mouse gene encoding Nf-kappa b-inducing kinase. *Nat Genet*. 1999;22:74–77.
165. Senftleben U, Cao Y, Xiao G, et al. Activation by IKKalpha of a second, evolutionary conserved, NF-kappa B signaling pathway. *Science*. 2001;293:1495–1499.
166. Yilmaz ZB, Weih DS, Sivakumar V, et al. RelB is required for Peyers patch development: differential regulation of p52-RelB by lymphotoxin and TNF. *Embo J*. 2003;22:121–130.
167. Dejardin E, Droin NM, Delhase M, et al. The lymphotoxin-beta receptor induces different patterns of gene expression via two NF-kappaB pathways. *Immunity*. 2002;17:525–535.
168. Drayton DL, Bonizzi G, Ying X, et al. I kappa B kinase complex alpha kinase activity controls chemokine and high endothelial venule gene expression in lymph nodes and nasal-associated lymphoid tissue. *J Immunol*. 2004;173:6161–6168.
169. Eberl G, Littman DR. The role of the nuclear hormone receptor RORgammat in the development of lymph nodes and Peyers patches. *Immunol Rev*. 2003;195:81–90.
170. Eberl G, Marmon S, Sunshine MJ, et al. An essential function for the nuclear receptor RORgamma(t) in the generation of fetal lymphoid tissue inducer cells. *Nat Immunol*. 2004;5:64–73.
171. Yokota Y, Mansouri A, Mori S, et al. Development of peripheral lymphoid organs and natural killer cells depends on the helix-loop-helix inhibitor Id2. *Nature*. 1999;397:702–706.
172. Mebius RE, Rennert P, Weissman IL. Developing lymph nodes collect CD4+CD3− LTbeta+ cells that can differentiate to APC, NK cells, and follicular cells but not T or B cells. *Immunity*. 1997;7:493–504.
173. Yoshida H, Honda K, Shinkura R, et al. IL-7 receptor alpha+ CD3(−) cells in the embryonic intestine induces the organizing center of Peyers patches. *Int Immunol*. 1999;11:643–655.
174. Yoshida H, Kawamoto H, Santee SM, et al. Expression of alpha(4)beta(7) integrin defines a distinct pathway of lymphoid progenitors committed to T cells, fetal intestinal lymphotoxin producer, NK, and dendritic cells. *J Immunol*. 2001;167:2511–2521.
175. Girard JP, Springer TA. High endothelial venules (HEVs): specialized endothelium for lymphocyte migration. *Immunol Today*. 1995;16:449–457.
176. Mebius RE, Schadee-Eestermans IL, Weissman IL. MAdCAM-1 dependent colonization of developing lymph nodes involves a unique subset of CD4+CD3− hematolymphoid cells. *Cell Adhes Commun*. 1998;6:97–103.
177. Cuff CA, Schwartz J, Bergman CM, et al. Lymphotoxin alpha3 induces chemokines and adhesion molecules: insight into the role of LT alpha in inflammation and lymphoid organ development. *J Immunol*. 1998;161:6853–6860.
178. Drayton DL, Ying X, Lee J, et al. Ectopic LT alpha beta directs lymphoid organ neogenesis with concomitant expression of peripheral node addressin and a HEV-restricted sulfotransferase. *J Exp Med*. 2003;197:1153–1163.
179. Hall JG, Hopkins J, Reynolds J. Studies of efferent lymph cells from nodes stimulated with oxazolone. *Immunology*. 1980;39:141–149.
180. Hall JG, Smith ME. Studies on the afferent and efferent lymph of lymph nodes draining the site of application of fluorodinitrobenzene (FDNB). *Immunology*. 1971;21:69–79.
181. Hay JB, Cahill RN, Trnka Z. The kinetics of antigen-reactive cells during lymphocyte recruitment. *Cell Immunol*. 1974;10:145–153.
182. He C, Young AJ, West CA, et al. Stimulation of regional lymphatic and blood flow by epicutaneous oxazolone. *J Appl Physiol*. 2002;93:966–973.
183. West CA, He C, Su M, et al. Stochastic regulation of cell migration from the efferent lymph to oxazolone-stimulated skin. *J Immunol*. 2001;166:1517–1523.
184. Angeli V, Ginhoux F, Llodra J, et al. B cell-driven lymphangiogenesis in inflamed lymph nodes enhances dendritic cell mobilization. *Immunity*. 2006;24:203–215.
185. Liao S, Ruddle NH. Synchrony of high endothelial venules and lymphatic vessels revealed by immunization. *J Immunol*. 2006;177:3369–3379.
186. Hay JB, Johnston MG, Vadas P, et al. Relationships between changes in blood flow and lymphocyte migration induced by antigen. *Monogr Allergy*. 1980;16:112–125.
187. Ottaway CA, Parrott DM. Regional blood flow and its relationship to lymphocyte and lymphoblast traffic during a primary immune reaction. *J Exp Med*. 1979;150:218–230.
188. Mebius RE, Breve J, Duijvestijn AM, et al. The function of high endothelial venules in mouse lymph nodes stimulated by oxazolone. *Immunology*. 1990;71:423–427.
189. Myking AO. Morphological changes in paracortical high endothelial venules to single and repeated application of oxazolone to mouse skin. *Virchows Arch B Cell Pathol Incl Mol Pathol*. 1980;35:63–71.
190. Cahill RN, Frost H, Trnka Z. The effects of antigen on the migration of recirculating lymphocytes through single lymph nodes. *J Exp Med*. 1976;143:870–888.
191. Hoke D, Mebius RE, Dybdal N, et al. Selective modulation of the expression of L-selectin ligands by an immune response. *Curr Biol*. 1995;5:670–678.
192. Yoneyama H, Matsuno K, Zhang Y, et al. Evidence for recruitment of plasmacytoid dendritic cell precursors to inflamed lymph nodes through high endothelial venules. *Int Immunol*. 2004;16:915–928.
193. Browning JL, Allaire N, Ngam-Ek A, et al. Lymphotoxin-beta receptor signaling is required for the homeostatic control of HEV differentiation and function. *Immunity*. 2005;23:539–550.
194. Mackay F, Browning JL. Turning off follicular dendritic cells. *Nature*. 1998;395:26–27.
195. Brendolan A, Rosado MM, Carsetti R, et al. Development and function of the mammalian spleen. *Bioessays*. 2007;29:166–177.
196. Blue J, Weiss L. Electron microscopy of the red pulp of the dog spleen including vascular arrangements, periarterial macrophage sheaths (ellipsoids), and the contractile, innervated reticular meshwork. *Am J Anat*. 1981;161:189–218.
197. Blue J, Weiss L. Periarterial macrophage sheaths (ellipsoids) in cat spleen—an electron microscope study. *Am J Anat*. 1981;161:115–134.
198. Snook T. A comparative study of the vascular arrangements in mammalian spleens. *Am J Anat*. 1950;87:31–77.
199. Waksman BH. *Atlas of Experimental Immunobiology and Immunopathology.* New Haven and London: Yale University Press; 1970; Figs. 5.3–5.5.
200. Mebius RE, Kraal G. Structure and function of the spleen. *Nat Rev Immunol*. 2005;5:606–616.
201. Geijtenbeek TB, Groot PC, Nolte MA, et al. Marginal zone macrophages express a murine homologue of DC-SIGN that captures blood-borne antigens in vivo. *Blood*. 2002;100:2908–2916.
202. Koppel EA, Wieland CW, van den Berg VC, et al. Specific ICAM-3 grabbing nonintegrin-related 1 (SIGNR1) expressed by marginal zone macrophages is essential for defense against pulmonary Streptococcus pneumoniae infection. *Eur J Immunol*. 2005;35:2962–2969.
203. Kraal G, Mebius R. New insights into the cell biology of the marginal zone of the spleen. *Int Rev Cytol*. 2006;250:175–215.
204. Ito S, Naito M, Kobayashi Y, et al. Roles of a macrophage receptor with collagenous structure (MARCO) in host defense and heterogeneity of splenic marginal zone macrophages. *Arch Histol Cytol*. 1999;62:83–95.
205. Mukhopadhyay S, Chen Y, Sankala M, et al. MARCO, an innate activation marker of macrophages, is a class A scavenger receptor for Neisseria meningitidis. *Eur J Immunol*. 2006;36:940–949.
206. Jones C, Virji M, Crocker PR. Recognition of sialylated meningococcal lipopolysaccharide by siglecs expressed on myeloid cells leads to enhanced bacterial uptake. *Mol Microbiol*. 2003;49:1213–1225.
207. van den Berg TK, Nath D, Ziltener HJ, et al. Cutting edge: CD43 functions as a T cell counterreceptor for the macrophage adhesion receptor sialoadhesin (Siglec-1). *J Immunol*. 2001;166:3637–3640.
208. Brummel R, Roberts TL, Stacey KJ, et al. Higher-order CpG-DNA stimulation reveals distinct activation requirements for marginal

zone and follicular B cells in lupus mice. *Eur J Immunol.* 2006;36:1951–1962.

209. Nolte MA, Belien JA, Schadee-Eestermans I, et al. A conduit system distributes chemokines and small blood-borne molecules through the splenic white pulp. *J Exp Med.* 2003;198:505–512.
210. Hargreaves DC, Hyman PL, Lu TT, et al. A coordinated change in chemokine responsiveness guides plasma cell movements. *J Exp Med.* 2001;194:45–56.
211. Puri KD, Finger EB, Gaudernack G, et al. Sialomucin CD34 is the major L-selectin ligand in human tonsil high endothelial venules. *J Cell Biol.* 1995;131:261–270.
212. Loder F, Mutschler B, Ray RJ, et al. B cell development in the spleen takes place in discrete steps and is determined by the quality of B cell receptor-derived signals. *J Exp Med.* 1999;190:75–89.
213. Kraal G, Schornagel K, Streeter PR, et al. Expression of the mucosal vascular addressin, MAdCAM-1, on sinus-lining cells in the spleen. *Am J Pathol.* 1995;147:763–771.
214. Nolte MA, Hamann A, Kraal G, et al. The strict regulation of lymphocyte migration to splenic white pulp does not involve common homing receptors. *Immunology.* 2002;106:299–307.
215. Lu TT, Cyster JG. Integrin-mediated long-term B cell retention in the splenic marginal zone. *Science.* 2002;297:409–412.
216. Lo CG, Lu TT, Cyster JG. Integrin-dependence of lymphocyte entry into the splenic white pulp. *J Exp Med.* 2003;197:353–361.
217. Cinamon G, Matloubian M, Lesneski MJ, et al. Sphingosine 1-phosphate receptor 1 promotes B cell localization in the splenic marginal zone. *Nat Immunol.* 2004;5:713–720.
218. Mitchell J. Lymphocyte circulation in the spleen. Marginal zone bridging channels and their possible role in cell traffic. *Immunology.* 1973;24:93–107.
219. Hatano M, Roberts CW, Minden M, et al. Deregulation of a homeobox gene, HOX11, by the t(10;14) in T cell leukemia. *Science.* 1991;253:79–82.
220. Roberts CW, Shutter JR, Korsmeyer SJ. Hox11 controls the genesis of the spleen. *Nature.* 1994;368:747–749.
221. Dear TN, Colledge WH, Carlton MB, et al. The Hox11 gene is essential for cell survival during spleen development. *Development.* 1995;121:2909–2915.
222. Ngo VN, Korner H, Gunn MD, et al. Lymphotoxin alpha/beta and tumor necrosis factor are required for stromal cell expression of homing chemokines in B and T cell areas of the spleen. *J Exp Med.* 1999;189:403–412.
223. Ngo VN, Cornall RJ, Cyster JG. Splenic T zone development is B cell dependent. *J Exp Med.* 2001;194:1649–1660.
224. Kim MY, McConnell FM, Gaspal FM, et al. Function of CD4+CD3− cells in relation to B and T zone stroma in spleen. *Blood.* 2007;109:1602–1610.
225. Benedict CA, De Trez C, Schneider K, et al. Specific remodeling of splenic architecture by cytomegalovirus. *PLoS Pathog.* 2006;2:e16.
226. Mowat AM. Anatomical basis of tolerance and immunity to intestinal antigens. *Nat Rev Immunol.* 2003;3:331–341.
227. Perry M, Whyte A. Immunology of the tonsils. *Immunol Today.* 1998;19:414–421.
228. van Kempen MJ, Rijkers GT, Van Cauwenberge PB. The immune response in adenoids and tonsils. *Int Arch Allergy Immunol.* 2000; 122:8–19.
229. Brandtzaeg P. Regionalized immune function of tonsils and adenoids. *Immunol Today.* 1999;20:383–384.
230. Dieu MC, Vanbervliet B, Vicari A, et al. Selective recruitment of immature and mature dendritic cells by distinct chemokines expressed in different anatomic sites. *J Exp Med.* 1998;188:373–386.
231. Meurens F, Whale J, Brownlie R, et al. Expression of mucosal chemokines TECK/CCL25 and MEC/CCL28 during fetal development of the ovine mucosal immune system. *Immunology.* 2007;120:544–555.
232. Berg EL, Mullowney AT, Andrew DP, et al. Complexity and differential expression of carbohydrate epitopes associated with L-selectin recognition of high endothelial venules. *Am J Pathol.* 1998;152:469–477.
233. Rebelatto MC, Mead C, HogenEsch H. Lymphocyte populations and adhesion molecule expression in bovine tonsils. *Vet Immunol Immunopathol.* 2000;73:15–29.
234. Goeringer GC, Vidic B. The embryogenesis and anatomy of Waldeyer's ring. *Otolaryngol Clin North Am.* 1987;20:207–217.
235. Wu HY, Russell MW. Induction of mucosal immunity by intranasal application of a streptococcal surface protein antigen with the cholera toxin B subunit. *Infect Immun.* 1993;61:314–322.
236. Balmelli C, Roden R, Potts A, et al. Nasal immunization of mice with human papillomavirus type 16 virus-like particles elicits neutralizing antibodies in mucosal secretions. *J Virol.* 1998;72:8220–8229.
237. Liu XS, Abdul-Jabbar I, Qi YM, et al. Mucosal immunisation with papillomavirus virus-like particles elicits systemic and mucosal immunity in mice. *Virology.* 1998;252:39–45.
238. Dupuy C, Buzoni-Gatel D, Touze A, et al. Nasal immunization of mice with human papillomavirus type 16 (HPV-16) virus-like particles or with the HPV-16 L1 gene elicits specific cytotoxic T lymphocytes in vaginal draining lymph nodes. *J Virol.* 1999;73:9063–9071.
239. Wiley JA, Tighe MP, Harmsen AG. Upper respiratory tract resistance to influenza infection is not prevented by the absence of either nasal-associated lymphoid tissue or cervical lymph nodes. *J Immunol.* 2005;175:3186–3196.
240. Zuercher AW, Coffin SE, Thurnheer MC, et al. Nasal-associated lymphoid tissue is a mucosal inductive site for virus-specific humoral and cellular immune responses. *J Immunol.* 2002;168:1796–1803.
241. Shikina T, Hiroi T, Iwatani K, et al. IgA class switch occurs in the organized nasopharynx- and gut-associated lymphoid tissue, but not in the diffuse lamina propria of airways and gut. *J Immunol.* 2004;172:6259–6264.
242. Csencsits KL, Jutila MA, Pascual DW. Mucosal addressin expression and binding-interactions with naive lymphocytes vary among the cranial, oral, and nasal-associated lymphoid tissues. *Eur J Immunol.* 2002;32:3029–3039.
243. Fukuyama S, Nagatake T, Kim DY, et al. Cutting edge: Uniqueness of lymphoid chemokine requirement for the initiation and maturation of nasopharynx-associated lymphoid tissue organogenesis. *J Immunol.* 2006;177:4276–4280.
244. Fukuyama S, Hiroi T, Yokota Y, et al. Initiation of NALT organogenesis is independent of the IL-7R, LTbetaR, and NIK signaling pathways but requires the Id2 gene and CD3(−)CD4(+)CD45(+) cells. *Immunity.* 2002;17:31–40.
245. Rangel-Moreno J, Hartson L, Navarro C, et al. Inducible bronchus-associated lymphoid tissue (iBALT) in patients with pulmonary complications of rheumatoid arthritis. *J Clin Invest.* 2006;116:3183–3194.
246. Pabst R, Gehrke I. Is the bronchus-associated lymphoid tissue (BALT) an integral structure of the lung in normal mammals, including humans? *Am J Respir Cell Mol Biol.* 1990;3:131–135.
247. Kolopp-Sarda MN, Bene MC, Massin N, et al. Immunohistological analysis of macrophages, B-cells, and T-cells in the mouse lung. *Anat Rec.* 1994;239:150–157.
248. Delventhal S, Hensel A, Petzoldt K, et al. Effects of microbial stimulation on the number, size and activity of bronchus-associated lymphoid tissue (BALT) structures in the pig. *Int J Exp Pathol.* 1992;73:351–357.
249. Constant SL, Brogdon JL, Piggott DA, et al. Resident lung antigen-presenting cells have the capacity to promote Th2 T cell differentiation in situ. *J Clin Invest.* 2002;110:1441–1448.
250. Moyron-Quiroz JE, Rangel-Moreno J, Kusser K, et al. Role of inducible bronchus associated lymphoid tissue (iBALT) in respiratory immunity. *Nat Med.* 2004;10:927–934.
251. Moyron-Quiroz JE, Rangel-Moreno J, Hartson L, et al. Persistence and responsiveness of immunologic memory in the absence of secondary lymphoid organs. *Immunity.* 2006;25:643–654.
252. Fotopoulos G, Harari A, Michetti P, et al. Transepithelial transport of HIV-1 by M cells is receptor-mediated. *Proc Natl Acad Sci USA.* 2002;99:9410–9414.
253. Jones BD, Ghori N, Falkow S. Salmonella typhimurium initiates murine infection by penetrating and destroying the specialized epithelial M cells of the Peyers patches. *J Exp Med.* 1994;180:15–23.
254. Hase K, Murakami T, Takatsu H, et al. The membrane-bound chemokine CXCL16 expressed on follicle-associated epithelium and M cells mediates lympho-epithelial interaction in GALT. *J Immunol.* 2006;176:43–51.
255. Iwasaki A, Kelsall BL. Localization of distinct Peyers patch dendritic cell subsets and their recruitment by chemokines macrophage

inflammatory protein (MIP)-3alpha, MIP-3beta, and secondary lymphoid organ chemokine. *J Exp Med*. 2000;191:1381–1394.
256. Iwasaki A, Kelsall BL. Unique functions of CD11b+, CD8 alpha+, and double-negative Peyers patch dendritic cells. *J Immunol*. 2001;166:4884–4890.
257. Williams MB, Butcher EC. Homing of naive and memory T lymphocyte subsets to Peyers patches, lymph nodes, and spleen. *J Immunol*. 1997;159:1746–1752.
258. Kunkel EJ, Ramos CL, Steeber DA, et al. The roles of L-selectin, beta 7 integrins, and P-selectin in leukocyte rolling and adhesion in high endothelial venules of Peyers patches. *J Immunol*. 1998;161:2449–2456.
259. Steeber DA, Tang ML, Zhang XQ, et al. Efficient lymphocyte migration across high endothelial venules of mouse Peyers patches requires overlapping expression of L-selectin and beta7 integrin. *J Immunol*. 1998;161:6638–6647.
260. Okada T, Ngo VN, Ekland EH, et al. Chemokine requirements for B cell entry to lymph nodes and Peyers patches. *J Exp Med*. 2002;196:65–75.
261. Cook DN, Prosser DM, Forster R, et al. CCR6 mediates dendritic cell localization, lymphocyte homeostasis, and immune responses in mucosal tissue. *Immunity*. 2000;12:495–503.
262. Koni PA, Sacca R, Lawton P, et al. Distinct roles in lymphoid organogenesis for lymphotoxins alpha and beta in lymphotoxi-beta deficient mice. *Immunity*. 1997;6:491–500.
263. Kiyono H, Fukuyama S. NALT- versus Peyers-patch-mediated mucosal immunity. *Nat Rev Immunol*. 2004;4:699–710.
264. Neumann B, Luz A, Pfeffer K, et al. Defective Peyers patch organogenesis in mice lacking the 55-kD receptor for tumor necrosis factor. *J Exp Med*. 1996;184:259–264.
265. Nishikawa S, Nishikawa S, Honda K, et al. Peyers patch organogenesis as a programmed inflammation: a hypothetical model. *Cytokine Growth Factor Rev*. 1998;9:213–220.
266. Nishikawa SI, Hashi H, Honda K, et al. Inflammation, a prototype for organogenesis of the lymphopoietic/hematopoietic system. *Curr Opin Immunol*. 2000;12:342–345.
267. Nishikawa S, Honda K, Vieira P, et al. Organogenesis of peripheral lymphoid organs. *Immunol Rev*. 2003;195:72–80.
268. Finke D, Acha-Orbea H, Mattis A, et al. CD4+CD3− cells induce Peyers patch development: role of alpha4beta1 integrin activation by CXCR5. *Immunity*. 2002;17:363–373.
269. Finke D, Kraehenbuhl JP. Formation of Peyers patches. *Curr Opin Genet Dev*. 2001;11:561–567.
270. Newberry RD, Lorenz RG. Organizing a mucosal defense. *Immunol Rev*. 2005;206:6–21.
271. Golovkina TV, Shlomchik M, Hannum L, et al. Organogenic role of B lymphocytes in mucosal immunity. *Science*. 1999;286:1965–1968.
272. Debard N, Sierro F, Browning J, et al. Effect of mature lymphocytes and lymphotoxin on the development of the follicle-associated epithelium and M cells in mouse Peyers patches. *Gastroenterology*. 2001;120:1173–1182.
273. Lugering A, Kucharzik T, Soler D, et al. Lymphoid precursors in intestinal cryptopatches express CCR6 and undergo dysregulated development in the absence of CCR6. *J Immunol*. 2003;171:2208–2215.
274. Lorenz RG, Newberry RD. Isolated lymphoid follicles can function as sites for induction of mucosal immune responses. *Ann N Y Acad Sci*. 2004;1029:44–57.
275. Eberl G. Inducible lymphoid tissues in the adult gut: recapitulation of a fetal developmental pathway? *Nat Rev Immunol*. 2005;5:413–420.
276. Lorenz RG, Chaplin DD, McDonald KG, et al. Isolated lymphoid follicle formation is inducible and dependent upon lymphotoxin-sufficient B lymphocytes, lymphotoxin beta receptor, and TNF receptor I function. *J Immunol*. 2003;170:5475–5482.
277. Pablos JL, Santiago B, Tsay D, et al. A HEV-restricted sulfotransferase is expressed in rheumatoid arthritis synovium and is induced by lymphotoxin-alpha/beta and TNF-alpha in cultured endothelial cells. *BMC Immunol*. 2005;6:6.
278. Kerjaschki D. Lymphatic neoangiogenesis in human neoplasia and transplantation as experiments of nature. *Kidney Int*. 2005;68:1967–1968.
279. Kerjaschki D, Regele HM, Moosberger I, et al. Lymphatic neoangiogenesis in human kidney transplants is associated with immunologically active lymphocytic infiltrates. *J Am Soc Nephrol*. 2004;15:603–612.
280. Reape TJ, Rayner K, Manning CD, et al. Expression and cellular localization of the CC chemokines PARC and ELC in human atherosclerotic plaques. *Am J Pathol*. 1999;154:365–374.
281. Hjelmstrom P, Fjell J, Nakagawa T, et al. Lymphoid tissue homing chemokines are expressed in chronic inflammation. *Am J Pathol*. 2000;156:1133–1138.
282. Hanninen A, Jaakkola I, Jalkanen S. Mucosal addressin is required for the development of diabetes in nonobese diabetic mice. *J Immunol*. 1998;160:6018–6025.
283. Yang XD, Sytwu HK, McDevitt HO, et al. Involvement of beta 7 integrin and mucosal addressin cell adhesion molecule-1 (MAdCAM-1) in the development of diabetes in obese diabetic mice. *Diabetes*. 1997;46:1542–1547.
284. Cannella B, Cross AH, Raine CS. Upregulation and coexpression of adhesion molecules correlate with relapsing autoimmune demyelination in the central nervous system. *J Exp Med*. 1990;172:1521–1524.
285. Columba-Cabezas S, Serafini B, Ambrosini E, et al. Lymphoid chemokines CCL19 and CCL21 are expressed in the central nervous system during experimental autoimmune encephalomyelitis: implications for the maintenance of chronic neuroinflammation. *Brain Pathol*. 2003;13:38–51.
286. Magliozzi R, Columba-Cabezas S, Serafini B, et al. Intracerebral expression of CXCL13 and BAFF is accompanied by formation of lymphoid follicle-like structures in the meninges of mice with relapsing experimental autoimmune encephalomyelitis. *J Neuroimmunol*. 2004;148:11–23.
287. Mooij P, de Wit HJ, Drexhage HA. An excess of dietary iodine accelerates the development of a thyroid-associated lymphoid tissue in autoimmune prone BB rats. *Clin Immunol Immunopathol*. 1993;69:189–198.
288. Katakai T, Hara T, Sugai M, et al. Th1-biased tertiary lymphoid tissue supported by CXC chemokine ligand 13-producing stromal network in chronic lesions of autoimmune gastritis. *J Immunol*. 2003;171:4359–4368.
289. Galkina E, Kadl A, Sanders J, et al. Lymphocyte recruitment into the aortic wall before and during development of atherosclerosis is partially L-selectin dependent. *J Exp Med*. 2006;203:1273–1282.
290. Damas JK, Smith C, Oie E, et al. Enhanced expression of the homeostatic chemokines CCL19 and CCL21 in clinical and experimental atherosclerosis. Possible pathogenic role in plaque destabilization. *Arterioscler Thromb Vasc Biol*. 2007;27:614–620.
291. Baddoura FK, Nasr IW, Wrobel B, et al. Lymphoid neogenesis in murine cardiac allografts undergoing chronic rejection. *Am J Transplant*. 2005;5:510–516.
292. Luther SA, Ansel KM, Cyster JG. Overlapping roles of CXCL13, interleukin 7 receptor alpha, and CCR7 ligands in lymph node development. *J Exp Med*. 2003;197:1191–1198.
293. Heikenwalder M, Zeller N, Seeger H, et al. Chronic lymphocytic inflammation specifies the organ tropism of prions. *Science*. 2005;307:1107–1110.
294. Gause A, Gundlach K, Zdichavsky M, et al. The B lymphocyte in rheumatoid arthritis: analysis of rearranged V kappa genes from B cells infiltrating the synovial membrane. *Eur J Immunol*. 1995;25:2775–2782.
295. Schroder AE, Greiner A, Seyfert C, et al. Differentiation of B cells in the nonlymphoid tissue of the synovial membrane of patients with rheumatoid arthritis. *Proc Natl Acad Sci USA*. 1996;93:221–225.
296. Dorner T, Hansen A, Jacobi A, et al. Immunglobulin repertoire analysis provides new insights into the immunopathogenesis of Sjogren's syndrome. *Autoimmun Rev*. 2002;1:119–124.
297. Sims GP, Shiono H, Willcox N, et al. Somatic hypermutation and selection of B cells in thymic germinal centers responding to acetylcholine receptor in myasthenia gravis. *J Immunol*. 2001;167:1935–1944.
298. Stott DI, Hiepe F, Hummel M, et al. Antigen-driven clonal proliferation of B cells within the target tissue of an autoimmune disease. The salivary glands of patients with Sjogren's syndrome. *J Clin Invest*. 1998;102:938–946.

299. Kim HJ, Krenn V, Steinhauser G, et al. Plasma cell development in synovial germinal centers in patients with rheumatoid and reactive arthritis. *J Immunol*. 1999;162:3053–3062.
300. McMahon EJ, Bailey SL, Castenada CV, et al. Epitope spreading initiates in the CNS in two mouse models of multiple sclerosis. *Nat Med*. 2005;11:335–339.
301. Schrama D, thor Straten P, Fischer WH, et al. Targeting of lymphotoxin-alpha to the tumor elicits an efficient immune response associated with induction of peripheral lymphoid-like tissue. *Immunity*. 2001;14:111–121.
302. Lee Y, Chin RK, Christiansen P, et al. Recruitment and activation of naive T cells in the islets by lymphotoxin beta receptor-dependent tertiary lymphoid structure. *Immunity*. 2006;25:499–509.
303. Kaufman DL, Clare-Salzler M, Tian J, et al. Spontaneous loss of T-cell tolerance to glutamic acid decarboxylase in murine insulin-dependent diabetes. *Nature*. 1993;366:69–72.
304. Wotherspoon AC, Doglioni C, Diss TC, et al. Regression of primary low-grade B-cell gastric lymphoma of mucosa-associated lymphoid tissue type after eradication of Helicobacter pylori. *Lancet*. 1993;342:575–577.
305. Wu Q, Salomon B, Chen M, et al. Reversal of spontaneous autoimmune insulitis in nonobese diabetic mice by soluble lymphotoxin receptor. *J Exp Med*. 2001;193:1327–1332.
306. Fava RA, Notidis E, Hunt J, et al. A role for the lymphotoxin/LIGHT axis in the pathogenesis of murine collagen-induced arthritis. *J Immunol*. 2003;171:115–126.
307. Martin F, Kearney JF. B-cell subsets and the mature preimmune repertoire. Marginal zone and B1 B cells as part of a "natural immune memory." *Immunol Rev*. 2000;175:70–79.
308. Chaplin DD. Lymphoid tissues and organs. In: Paul WE, editor. *Fundamental Immunology*. 5th ed: Lippincott Williams and Wilkins; 2003:419–453.

Chapter 3

Evolution of the Immune System

Martin F. Flajnik and Louis Du Pasquier

INTRODUCTION

Defense mechanisms are found in all living things, some surprisingly elaborate even in so-called "primitive" organisms. Although in recent years new adaptive or adaptive-like (somatically generated) immune systems have been discovered in invertebrates and the jawless fish, adaptive immunity-based on immunoglobulin (Ig), T cell receptors (TCR), and the major histocompatibility complex (MHC) is only present in jawed vertebrates (gnathostomes); because of clonal selection, positive and negative selection in the thymus, MHC-regulated initiation of all adaptive responses, etc., the major elements of the adaptive immune system are locked in a coevolving unit. In addition, a large cast of supporting players, including a considerable array of cytokines and chemokines, adhesion molecules, costimulatory molecules, and well-defined primary and secondary lymphoid tissues, evolved in the jawed vertebrates as well. This system was superimposed onto an innate system inherited from invertebrates, from which some innate molecules were coopted for the initial phase of the adaptive response and others for effector mechanisms at the completion of adaptive responses. In jawed vertebrates, fine-tuning or adaptations (or degeneration) in each taxon is observed and not a steady progression from fish to mammals as is seen—for example, in evolution of the telencephalon (forebrain) in the nervous system or in heart specialization. Given that all the basic adaptive immune system features are present in cartilaginous fish and none were lost (that we know of), variation on the theme (differential utilization) rather than progressive installation of new elements is the rule (1). In this chapter, there are only a few cases of increasing complexity in the adaptive system superimposed upon the vertebrate phylogenetic tree, but many examples of contractions/expansions of existing gene families; thus, on average "more (or less) of the same" rather than "more and more new features" is the rule. We observe a bush growing from a short stem rather than a tall tree with well-defined branches, and thus deducing primitive traits is not always easy.

Figure 3.1 displays the extant animal phyla ranging from the single-celled protozoa to the protostome and deuterostome lineages. It is often suggested or assumed that molecules or mechanisms found in living protostomes, like the well-studied *Drosophila,* are ancestral to similar molecules/mechanisms in mouse and human. While this is true in some cases, one should instead recognize that *Drosophila* and mouse/human have taken just as long (over 900 million years ago (MYA)) to evolve from a common ancestral triploblastic coelomate (an animal with three germ layers and a mesoderm-lined body cavity, features shared by protostomes and deuterostomes), and clearly *Drosophila* is not our ancestor (i.e., the manner by which flies and mouse/human utilize certain families of defense molecules may be quite different and both may be nothing like the common ancestor). Thus, understanding how model invertebrates and vertebrates perform certain immune tasks is always an important first step, but we only understand what is primordial or derived when we have examined similar immune mechanisms/molecules in species from a wide range of animal phyla. We will touch on all of the defense molecule families listed in Figures 3.1 and 3.2 and Table 3.1 and will emphasize those that have been conserved evolutionarily and those that have evolved rapidly.

GENERAL PRINCIPLES OF IMMUNE SYSTEM EVOLUTION

Rapid Evolution of Defense Mechanisms

Immune systems are often compared to the Red Queen in *Alice's Adventures in Wonderland,* (Red Queen's Hypothesis [2]), who must keep moving just to avoid falling behind: "Now, here, you see, it takes all the running you can do, to keep in the same place. If you want to get somewhere else, you must run at least twice as fast as that!" Because of the perpetual conflict with pathogens, the immune system is in constant flux. This is exemplified by great differences in the immune systems of animals that are even within the same phylogenetic group (e.g., mosquito and fruitfly, both arthropods). In fact, defense mechanisms are extremely diverse throughout the invertebrate phla, as Keppler et al. put it recently: "not homogeneous, not simple, not well understood" (3). In the vertebrate frame of reference, the most rapidly evolving system is natural killer (NK) cell recognition, governed by different classes (superfamilies) of receptors in mice and humans, but recently shown to be extremely plastic even within the same family (4). Rapid evolution of immune system molecules and mechanisms is a general rule, but we shall see that molecules functioning at different levels of immune defense (recognition, signaling, or effector) evolve at widely varying rates (5).

Convergent Evolution

As mentioned earlier, when our informational database was small, it was assumed that the same features appearing in different taxa proved that they were present in the common ancestor as well (i.e., divergent evolution). While this dictum still holds true and establishes one of the dogmas of comparative immunology, later we discovered, because of the aforementioned rapid evolution of immune systems, often convergence of similar function has occurred in evolution (i.e., the same function or molecular conformation has arisen in different organisms), sometimes in species that are relatively closely related. Although we will discuss several cases of convergent evolution throughout the

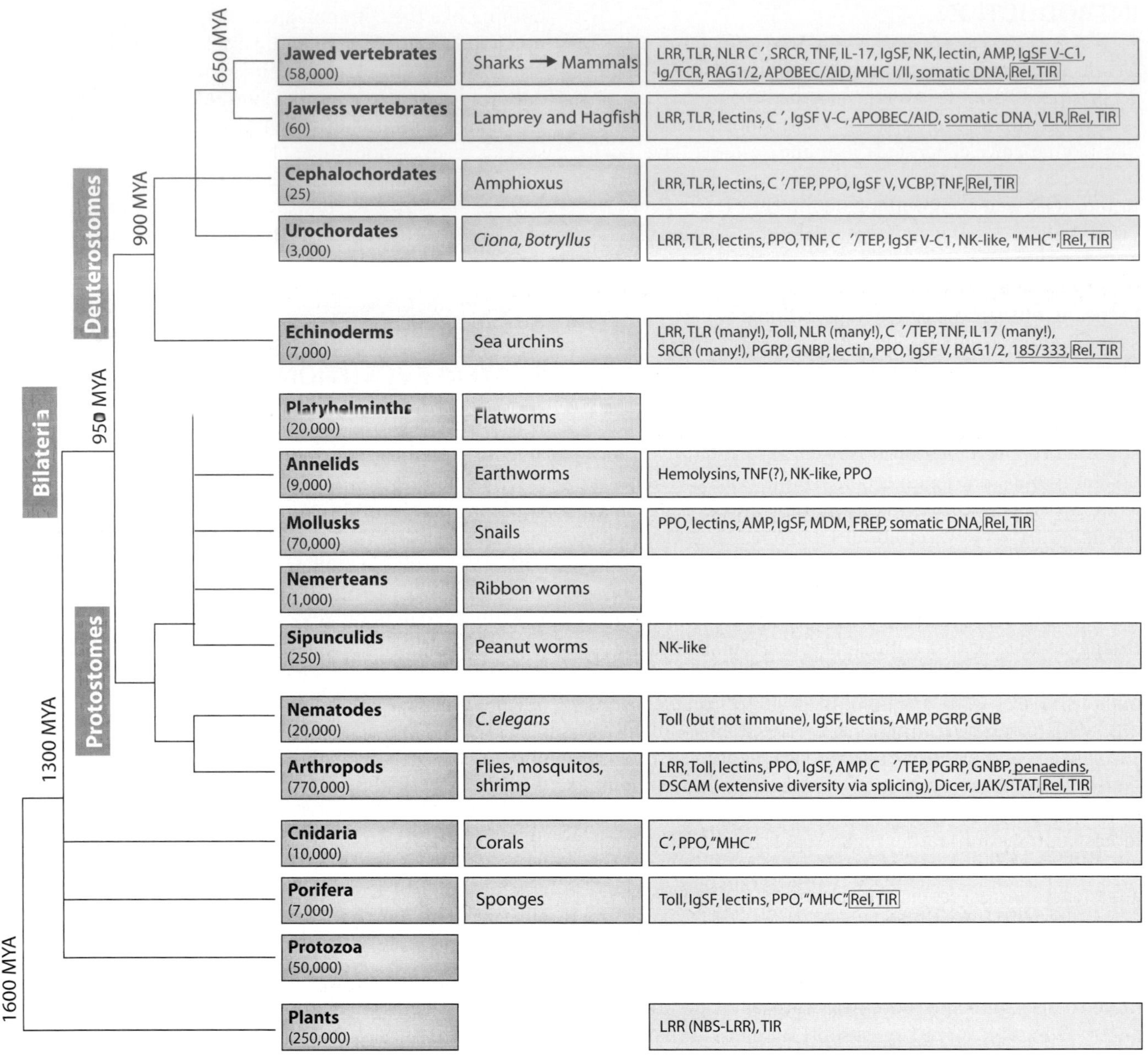

FIGURE 3.1 Major animal groups and immune mechanisms/molecules described to date in each group. The first box in each row describes the animal taxon and the approximate number of species in that group. The next box shows specific examples of species or subgroups. The third box lists molecules/mechanisms found in each group: Underlined terms indicate somatic changes to antigen receptors or secreted molecules. Figure modified from (20) and (32). See Table 3.1 for definition of the acronyms.

chapter, for frame of reference, the NK cells, which use different receptor families in primates and rodents to achieve precisely the same ends, are a striking example of convergence (4).

Multigene Families

Immune genes are often found in clusters, with extensive contraction and expansion via "birth and death" processes (6). It is well known that such clusters can change rapidly over evolutionary time due to unequal recombination and gene conversion (and not only in the immune system, but in any cis-duplicating gene family). Often, families of related immune genes—especially those involved in recognition events—are found near the telomeres of chromosomes, presumably to further promote gene-shuffling events. Nonclassical MHC class I loci and NK receptors are two conspicuous examples of this phenomenon, again believed to be a consequence of the race against pathogens. We will discuss many examples of how such multigene

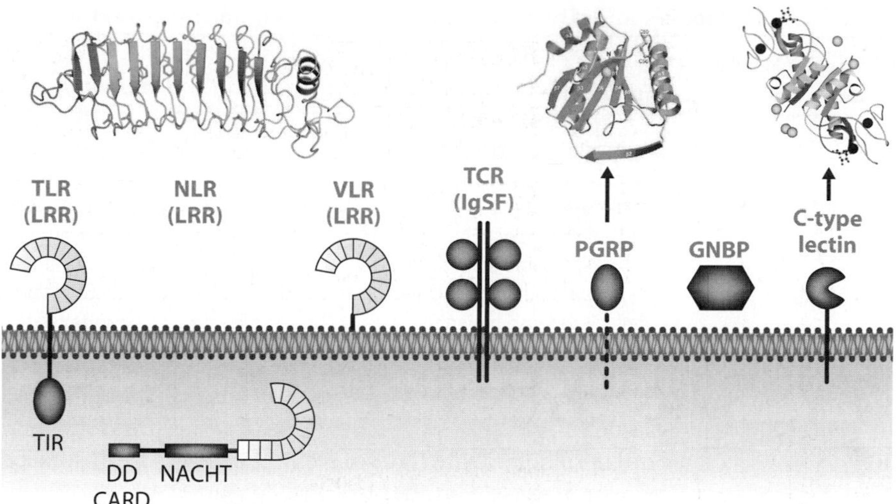

FIGURE 3.2 Major molecular families described in the text, and representatives of each family: Leucine-rich repeats (LRR), immunoglobulin superfamily (IgSF), peptidoglycan-recognition protein (PGRP), Gram negative–binding protein (GNBP), and C-type lectins. Representative structures are shown above for LRR (VLR, [104]), PGRP [306], and C-type lectin [307]). Other acronyms are defined in Table 3.1. For the NLR model, the echinoderms have N-terminal death domains (DD) while all other animals have CARDs. Figure modified from (32) with permission.

TABLE 3.1 Molecules and Abbreviations Found Throughout the Text

Acronym/Defense Molecule	*Full Name*	*Function*
AID	Activation-induced cytidine deaminase	SHM/gene conversion/CSR
APOBEC	Apolipoprotein B mRNA editing enzyme catalytic polypeptide	Innate immunity (antiviral)
AGM	Aorta/Gonad/Mesonephros	Embryonic origin of hematopoietic cells
AMP	Antimicrobial peptide	Innate immunity
APAR	Agnathan paired antigen receptor	Similarities to Ig/TCR and NK receptors
Bf	Factor B	Enzyme of C′ cascade
C′	Complement	Innate/adaptive immunity
CARD	Caspase-recruitment domain	Domain in intracellular defense molecules
CATERPILLER or CLR	CARD, transcription enhancer, R(purine)-binding, pyrin, lots of leucine repeats	Apoptosis/immunity/inflammation
CSR	Class-switch recombination	Adaptive humoral immunity
DSCAM	Down's syndrome cell-adhesion molecule	Insect immune (adaptive?) defense and neuron specification
ECM	Extracellular matrix	
FBA	F box associated domain	Intracellular domain
FcRN	Fc receptor neonatal	MHC-like FcR
FREP	Fibrinogen-related protein	Mollusk (adaptive?) defense
GALT	Gut-associated lymphoid tissue	
GNBP	Gram-negative binding protein	Response to gram-negative bacteria
GPI	Glycophosphatidylinositol	Lipid linkage to cell membrane (e.g., VLR)
Hemolysin		Cell lysis
ICE	Interleukin-converting enzyme	IL-1β processing
Ig	Immunoglobulin	Adaptive immunity
IgSF	Immunoglobulin superfamily	Innate/adaptive immunity
IFN	Interferon	Innate (type I)/adaptive (type II) immunity
IMD	Immune deficiency	Insect innate defense
IRF	Interferon regulatory factor	Innate (transcription factor)
ITAM	Immunoreceptor tyrosine-based activation motif	Signaling motif for NK and antigen receptors
ITIM	Immunoreceptor tyrosine-based inhibitory motif	Signaling motif for NK and antigen receptors
GC	Germinal center	
KIR	Killer IgSF receptor	NK cell receptor
Lectins	e.g., Galectin, C-type, S-type	Many (e.g., NK receptors, selectins)

(continued)

TABLE 3.1 Molecules and Abbreviations Found Throughout the Text (Continued)

Acroymym/Defense Molecule	*Full Name*	*Function*
LMP	Low-molecular-weight protein	Proteasome subunit
LRR	Leucine-rich repeat	Innate/adaptive immunity module
MAC	Membrane-attack complex	C′, pore-forming
MACPF	MAC-perforin domain	Potential pore former
MASP	MBP-associated serine protease	Lectin C′ pathway
MBP (or MBL)	Mannose-binding protein (lectin)	Lectin C′ pathway
MDM	Mollusk defense molecule	IgSF defense molecule
MHC	Major histocompatibility complex	T cell recognition; innate immunity
MIF	Macrophage inhibitory factor	Innate immunity; inflammation
MyD88 (also dMyD88)	Myeloid differentiation primary response gene 88	TLR adaptor
NK cell	Natural killer cell	Vertebrate innate cellular immunity
NALP	NACHT leucine-rich repeat and PYD-containing protein	Intracellular PRR
NBD-LRR	Nucleotide-binding domain LRR	Motif of intracellular defense molecules
NFκB	Nuclear factor-κ B (Rel homology domain)	Evolutionarily conserved transcription factor
NLR	NACHT leucine-rich repeat protein	Intracellular PRR
NOD	Nucleotide oligomerization domain protein	Intracellular PRR
NOS	Nitric oxide synthase	Intracellular killing innate defense molecule
PAMP	Pathogen-associated molecular pattern	Conserved target epitopes on Pathogens
PCD	Programmed cell death	Many pathways
Penaeidin		Defense molecule in shrimp
PGRP	Peptidoglycan-recognition protein	Gram-positive bacteria defense family; receptor and effector
PPO	Propolyphenol oxidase	Plant/invertebrate defense (melanization)
PRR	Pattern-recognition receptor	Recognize PAMP, innate/adaptive immunity
Polμ	DNA polymerase μ	Error-prone polymerase (related to TdT)
PYD	Pyrin domain	Domain in intracellular defense molecules
PPO	Prophenoloxidase	invertebrate defense molecule
RAG	Recombination-activating gene	Ig/TCR rearrangement
RFP-Y	Restriction Fragment Polymorphism-Y	Chicken nonclassical MHC gene cluster
RIG	Retinoic acid-inducible gene	Intracellular double-stranded RNA recognition
SHM	Somatic hypermutation	Adaptive humoral immunity
SPE	Spaetzle-processing enzyme	Insect defense molecule in Toll cascade
SRCR	Scavenger receptor cysteine-rich	Innate immunity recognition molecule
TAP (and TAP-L)	Transporter associated with antigen processing	Transports peptides from cytosol to ER lumen
TCR	T cell receptor	Adaptive defense
TdT	Terminal deoxynucleotidyl transferase	Involved in Ig/TCR rearrangement
TEP	Thioester-containing protein	Opsonization (like C3)
TGF	Transforming growth factor	Immunosuppressive cytokine
UPD	Unpaired	Protostome cytokine induced by viral infection
TNF	Tumor necrosis factor	Proinflammatory cytokine (and family)
V-, C1-, C2-, I-	Variable, constant 1 and 2, intermediate IgSF domain	IgSF domain types
VCBP	Variable domain chitin binding	Amphioxus defense molecule
VLR	Variable lymphocyte receptor	Agnathan adaptive defense molecule
XNC	*Xenopus* nonclassical	*Xenopus* class Ib cluster
185/333	Sea urchin defense molecule	(adaptive?) Defense

families have been exploited in different species throughout the chapter.

Gene duplication, either in the clusters mentioned above or as a consequence of *en bloc* duplications, certainly have been major features of immune system diversity and plasticity. The evidence is becoming clearer that two genomewide duplications (the so-called *2R hypothesis*) occurred early in vertebrate history, tracking very well with the emergence of the Ig/TCR/MHC-based adaptive immune system (7,8). This theory forms the basis for much that will be discussed concerning the development of the vertebrate adaptive immune response.

Polymorphism

Polymorphism (and polylocism) increases the diversity of recognition capacity in a population. It can be generated any time during the history of a gene family of either receptor or effector molecules: MHC, Toll-like receptors (TLR), Ig, TCR, NK receptors and related molecules, and AMPs are just a few examples. Polymorphism provides populations with flexibility in the face of the changing pathogenic environment. This subject, central to the studies on MHC, leukocyte receptor complex (LRC), and natural killer cell complex (NKC), is becoming well documented for immunity-related genes in insects as well. In *Drosophila,* polymorphism in signal transduction and pathogen recognition genes is significantly associated with variability in immunocompetence. Polymorphism in regulatory networks is indeed expected since parasites often target its elements (5).

Somatic Generation of Diversity

Somatic modifications can take place at multiple levels to generate immune system diversity. Long believed to be the sole domain of jawed vertebrates, modifications at the DNA level via somatic hypermutation (SHM), gene conversion, or rearrangement (primary and secondary [e.g., receptor editing]) irreversibly modify genes within an individual. The well-known V(D)J joining, class switch recombination (CSR), and SHM are examples of this processes in the Ig superfamily (IgSF) receptors of jawed vertebrates, but recent work has shown quite convincingly that modifications to genomic DNA can also occur in the jawless fish and some invertebrates (9). The list of organisms undergoing such diversity of germline immune genes will only grow as more organisms are examined and more genome and EST sequencing projects are undertaken (Figure 3.1).

Alternative splicing can be a source of tremendous diversity in some gene families encoding receptors involved in immunity in insects and crustaceans. The DSCAM (Down syndrome cell adhesion molecule) gene in several invertebrates (described in detail; see page 70) was shown to generate enormous diversity via RNA processing (10). In the vertebrate lineage, this mechanism is important in determining the function of different molecules, best known for the Igs (transmembrane [TM] versus secreted forms, as well as inflammatory versus neutralizing forms in nonmammalian vertebrates).

Further diversity can be obtained by the assembly of multichain receptors in which different components are combined. The classical example in the jawed vertebrate adaptive immune system is that of Ig light (L) and heavy (H) chains of antibodies, but similar combination can occur with insect peptidoglycan-recognizing proteins (PGRP), vertebrate TLR, and many other receptors in which all the components have not been discovered.

MAJOR GENE FAMILIES INVOLVED IN IMMUNITY

The involvement of relatively few gene families in the immune system probably reflects the fact that there were few evolutionary scenarios leading to recognition binding with reasonable affinities, and once invented those features were exploited in every niche where they were selectable (11,12). Some of the most common families (Figure 3.2) are IgSF, leucine rich repeat (LRR), C-type lectins, and the tumor necrosis family (TNF), and certain other domains in immune recognition (e.g., scavenger receptor cysteine-rich, SRCR; see Table 3.1). As a means of introduction, we describe in some detail two of these families, which are displayed prominently in this chapter.

Leucine-rich Repeats

The LRR family of receptors has a long evolutionary history (Figure 3.2) (13). LRR consist of 2 to 45 motifs of 20 to 30 amino acids in length XLXXLXLXXNX-HXXHXXXXFXXLX that fold into an arc shape, the concave part of which is well suited for protein-protein or protein-carbohydrate interactions. Molecular modeling suggests that the conserved pattern LxxLxL, which is shorter than the previously proposed LxxLxLxxN/CxL is sufficient to impart the characteristic horseshoe curvature to proteins with 20- to 30-residue repeats. LRR are often flanked by cysteine-rich domains. LRRs occur in proteins ranging from viruses to eukaryotes and include tyrosine kinase receptors, cell-adhesion molecules, resistance (R) factors in plants, and ECM-binding glycoproteins (e.g., peroxidasin) and are involved in a variety of protein-protein interactions: signal transduction, cell adhesion, DNA repair, recombination, transcription, RNA processing, disease resistance, apoptosis, and the immune response.

LRR-containing proteins can be associated with a variety of other domains, whether they are extracellular (LRR associated with IgSF or fibronectin type III [FN3]) or intracellular (caterpiller family LRR associated with a variety of effector domains, discussed later). In these chimeric molecules, the LRR moiety is involved in recognition, most likely due to its extraordinarily plastic structure. There are at least six families of LRR proteins, characterized by different lengths and consensus sequences of the repeats (14). Repeats from different subfamilies never occur simultaneously and have most probably evolved independently in different organisms.

LRR proteins are involved in immunity from plants to all metazoa. The functions they can exert in the immune systems range from control of motility of hemocytes and lymphocytes (15) to specific recognition of antigens via a novel system of gene rearrangement (the variable lymphocyte receptors, or VLR, described later). LRR can occur in soluble forms, the ECM, in the cytosol, or as TM forms, either integral membrane proteins or glycophoshatidylinositol (GPI)-anchored. The apparent lack of unity in evolution of some gene families, the change in commitment from one function to another is also well illustrated by the evolutionary fate of Toll and TLR. In triplobastic metazoans the structurally closely related members of this family range from not being involved in immunity (in several invertebrates) to becoming the equivalent of a cytokine receptor or a pathogen recognition receptor (PRR), like the vertebrate TLR (16).

Immunoglobulin Superfamily

IgSF domains are encountered in a very large number of molecules in the animal kingdom and constitute the most prevalent domain in defense molecules (17). They are found intracellularly (e.g., connectin), as cell adhesion molecules, many of which are in the nervous system (e.g., neural cell adhesion molecule (NCAM)), coreceptors and costimulatory molecules of the immune system (e.g., CD79, CD80), molecules involved in antigen presentation to lymphocytes (e.g., class I molecules), certain classes cytokine receptors (e.g., IL1R), and of course Ig and TCR, where they were first characterized and were bestowed with their name (Ig). They can be associated with other domains, such as fibronectin (FN; e.g., titin) and LRR, or they can be the sole constitutive elements of the polypeptide chain often linked to a TM segment and a cytoplasmic tail (or GPI-linked). The β barrel IgSF structure was adopted independently in other families such as cadherins, calycins, lipocalin, etc., and the superfamily has hundreds of members and has been selected for several different functions. These functions are somehow related, almost all involved with protein-ligand interactions. The vertebrate lymphocyte surface can express more than 30 different IgSF members (17).

IgSF domains are commonly classified according to different domain constitution in their β strands and loops (Figure 3.3). All conform to the stable shape of a β barrel consisting of two interfacing β sheets, usually linked by a disulfide bridge. There are three types of domains: variable (V) and two type of constant (C1 and C2); the so-called *I set domain* is intermediate between the C1 and C2. The V domain is most complex with more strands (C′ and C″), which make up complementarity determining region (CDR) 2 in conventional Igs and TCRs. C1 domains lack these strands entirely and C2/I domains have varying sizes in the C′/C″ region. V domains, either alone (e.g., the new antigen receptor, NAR) or in association with another V domain (e.g., Ig H/L), recognize the antigenic epitope, and are therefore the most important elements for recognition. Domains with the typical V fold, whether belonging to the true V set or the I set, have been found from sponges to insects (e.g., amalgam, lachesin and fascicilin), and even in bacteria. The mollusk FREPS (fibrinogen-related proteins, described; see page 70) have one or two V-like

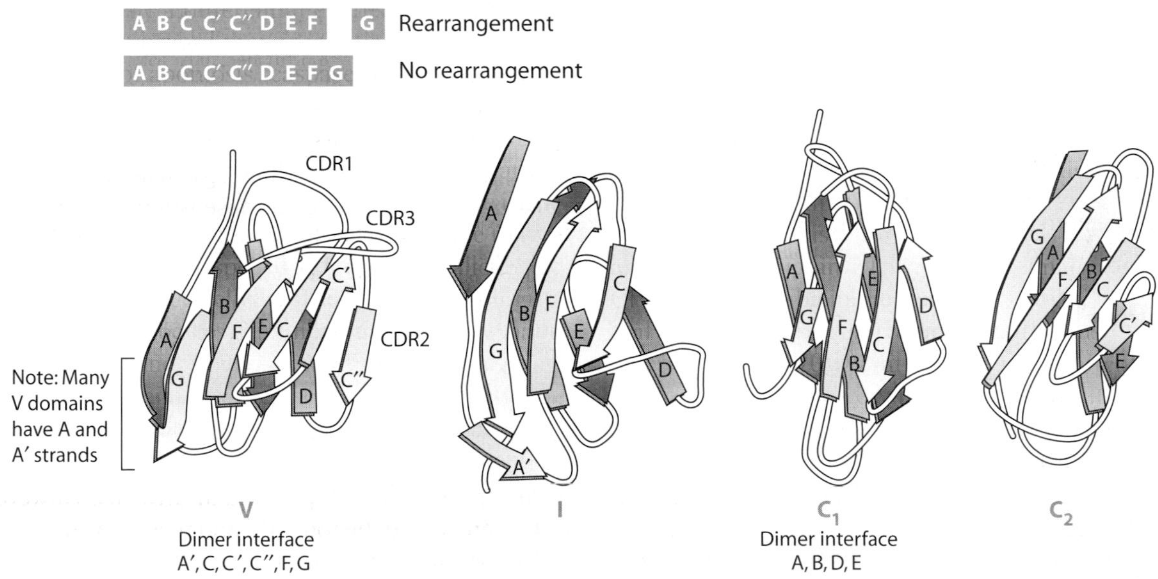

FIGURE 3.3 Major types of immunoglobulin superfamily (IgSF) domains (V, variable; I, intermediate; C1, constant domain-1; C2, constant domain-2). The domains are made up entirely of β strands that make up two sheets: A, B, D, E in one sheet and C, (C′, C″), F, and G in the other sheet. An intrachain disulfide bond is usually found that connects the two sheets (cys in the B and F strands). In Ig and TCR, the V exon encodes the A–F strands and the J segment encodes the G strand (a Gly-X-Gly tripeptide is encoded in the J segment of antigen receptors and in some non-rearranging domains of the "VJ-type"). Information taken from (11,17).

domains at their distal end, associated with a fibrinogen-like domain.

The binding capacities of a V domain can reside in different areas of the molecule (interstrand loops, A-A′ strand, F strand). In diversified molecules such as Ig/TCR, these regions are the targets for variation in shape and charge. The binding capacities can be modulated whether one domain acts as a single receptor unit (e.g., IgNAR), or whether it is associated with a contiguous domain (e.g., KIR, VCBP) or with another polypeptide chain (e.g., TCR, Ig). In the case of a dimer, the binding capacity can again be modulated by the presence or the absence in the G strand of a diglycine bulge, which can modify the space between the faces of the Ig domain. In several cases, the sites responsible for binding are known (KIR, Ig, TCR); in many other cases they are not known but inferred from crystal structures and/or variability plots (LITR, CHIR, FcRH, TREMs DSCAM, hemolin (11]).

IMMUNITY IN PLANTS AND INVERTEBRATES

Immune responses are often subdivided into recognition, signaling, and effector phases, which are subjected to different pressures defined by whether orthology is maintained and the relative divergence rates of the genes responsible for the various phases (5). Recognition molecules are from well-conserved families, but as described earlier, their genes are subjected to rapid duplication/deletion so that orthology is rarely maintained. By contrast, signaling pathways are well conserved (see Figure 3.6), despite the fact that the genes are often divergent in sequence. Effector molecules can either be extremely conserved (e.g., reactive oxygen intermediates) or extremely divergent to the point of being species-specific (e.g., antimicrobial peptides, AMP). Here, we break down the immune response into these three phases, beginning with the cells involved in recognition.

Recognition

Initiation of an immune reaction can theoretically involve either the recognition of non-self, altered self, or the absence of self. Non-self recognition can take place with receptors (PRR, pattern recognition receptors) for the so-called *pathogen-associated molecular patterns* (PAMP), which are defined as evolutionarily conserved epitopes expressed by molecules of pathogens but not host cells (18). The second mode, altered self, is typified by molecules that are induced in self-cells during infections and recognized by conserved defense molecules, similar to the SOS systems mentioned later in the MHC section, or by peptide presentation on MHC molecules. A third mechanism, "Am I still myself," depends on recognition of self-tags and their changes in expression (19)—for example, NK recognition of self-MHC molecules through KIR and C-type lectins. These latter two mechanisms have not been described in the invertebrates for immune defense against pathogens, but it would not be surprising if they were revealed in the future, considering the new features of invertebrate immune systems that have been discovered recently.

Whether the invader is related to an animal host (cells from individuals of the same species or cells from a parasitoid) or are very distant from the host (fungi and bacteria), there are different principles of recognition. Yet PAMP determinants have been identified on very different organisms—sugars such as β1,3 glucan of fungi, lipopolysaccharide (LPS) and peptidoglycans of bacteria, and phosphoglycan of some parasites—and they can trigger the same cascade of events. The foreign ligand can be bound by a molecule in solution that initiates an effector proteolytic cascade (e.g., clotting or the complement cascade). However, a proteolytic cascade can be initiated and result in the production of a self-ligand that interacts with a cell surface receptor. In this way there need not be a great diversity of cell surface receptors, an advantage in the absence of clonal selection.

Of the more than 1 million described species of animals (Figure 3.1) ~95% are invertebrates representing 33 phyla, some with one species (Placozoa, Cycliophora) and others with more than 1 million (Arthropoda). Since they have major differences in body plans, development, size, habitat, etc., wildly different types of immune systems in diverse species should be expected. Early studies of invertebrate immunology reached no consensus of how immunity should be examined, but because vertebrate immunity was often defined through transplantation reactions, attempts to reveal specific memory by allograft rejection as detailed in the following discussions was often used. After (mostly failed) attempts to demonstrate memory of such responses in the invertebrates (see following discussion) and after extensive molecular studies, a consensus was reached that an invertebrate adaptive immune system involving somatic generation of antigen receptors and their clonal expression was highly unlikely (however, now with caveats noted in following dicussion). Phagocytosis has long been cited as one example of such conservation, together with several proteins of the acute phase response and complement cascades. During innate responses in which memory to a particular antigen does not exist, selection is at the level of the species polymorphism and diversity. However, the term "innate" can be too rigid and masks the possibility of other somatic alterations of invertebrate immune system molecules, as will be discussed (20).

Invertebrate Cells

Examples of conservation of fundamental mechanisms of genetic control of developmental pathway between protostomes and deuterostomes, even in the absence of

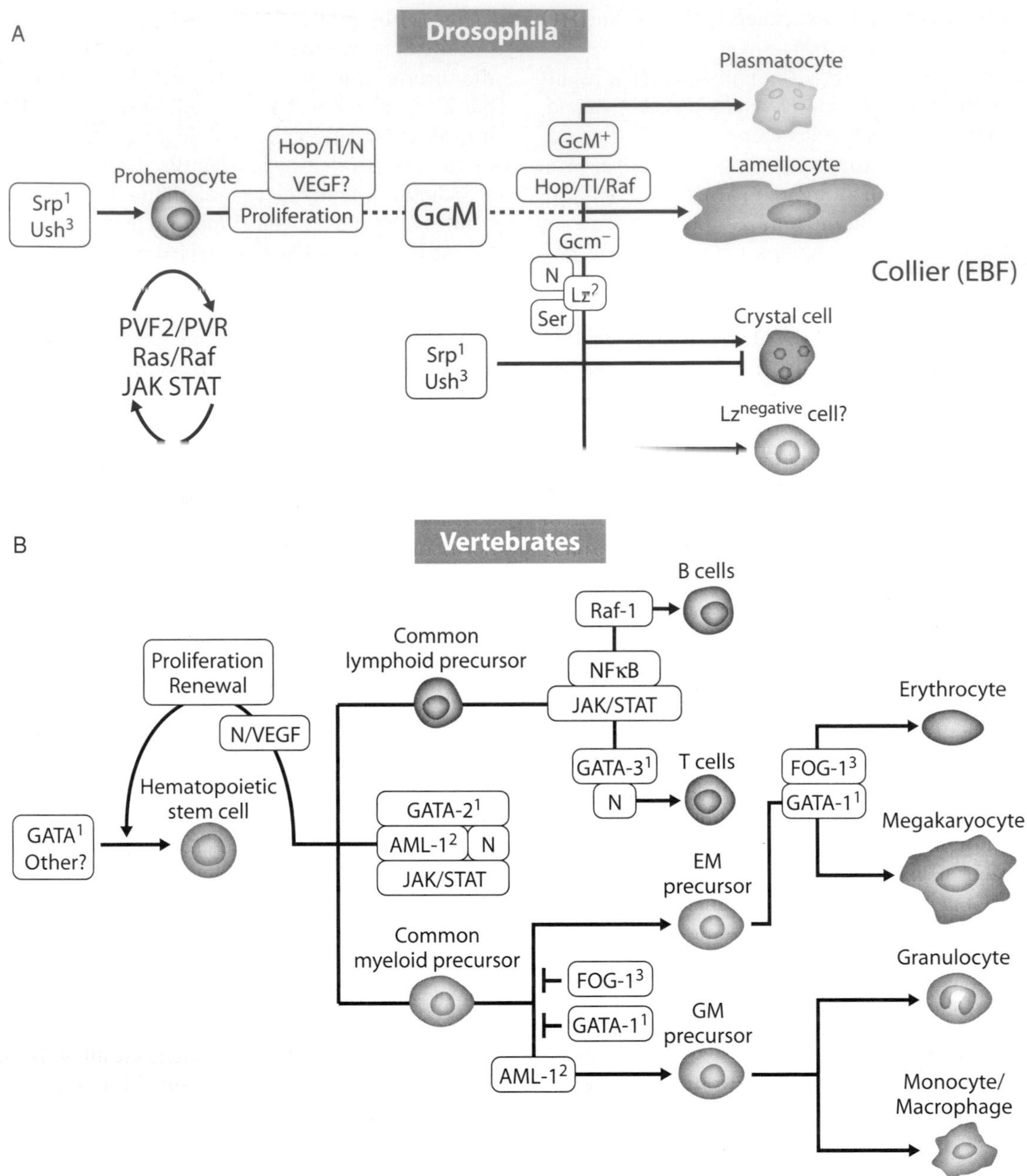

FIGURE 3.4 Comparison of blood cell differentiation in insects (*Drosophila*) and vertebrates. Homologous transcription factors are noted with superscripts: 1, Srp and GATA; 2, Lz and AML-1; 3, Ush and FOG-1. This figure was modified from (23,25); details in the text.

homology of the cells or organ considered, are accumulating: Wings are not homologous between *Drosophila* and birds, yet they follow a similar logic of development that includes a common network of genes. This applies also to the organization and expression of the homeotic gene clusters and eye formation through the function of a complex of proteins including Pax-6 (21,22). The cell types involved, besides direct interaction with the external layer of cells on the skin, or external teguments, are specialized cells of mesodermal origin devoted to defense. This is true for all coelomates where effector cells have been identified (Figure 3.4). The cells can be circulating or sessile, and often are found associated with the gut. Several morphologically distinct hemocyte types in insects cooperate in immune responses: They attach to invading organisms and isolate them, trapping larger organisms in nodules or forming large multicellular capsules around them. Indirect evidence for the role of hemocytes in immune responses can be derived by contrasting properties of such cells in healthy and parasitized

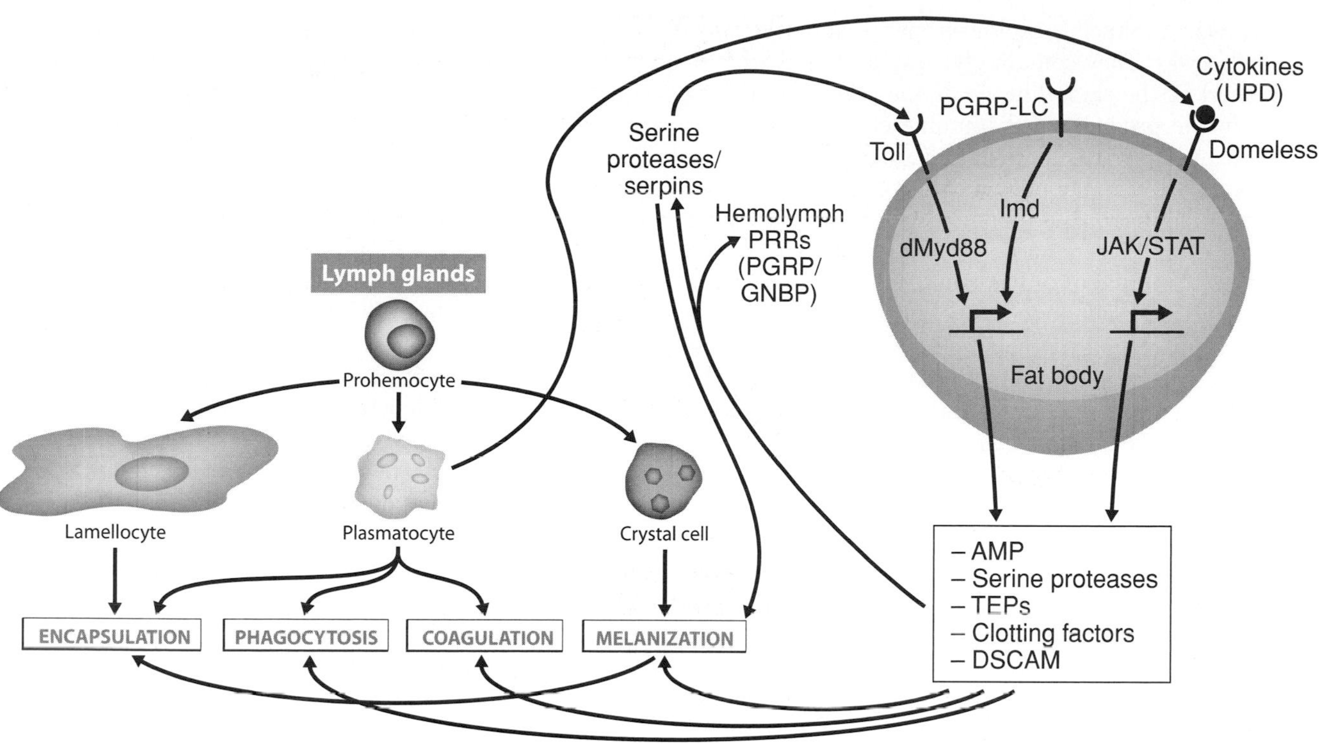

FIGURE 3.5 Types of immune responses in the insects, with *Drosophila* as the prototype. Secreted defense molecules are made by fat body cells in response to pathogens, which either act as direct effector molecules, or feed back on hemocytes to stimulate their defense functions. Unpaired (UPD) is produced after virus infection, stimulating defense molecule upregulation via the JAK/STAT pathway. Not shown is the RNAi pathway, also induced on virus infection. This figure was modified from (31,90) with permission. Details on stimulation of the Toll and Imd pathways.

animals (i.e., modifications in adherence and opsonic activity).

All eumetazoa show heterogeneity of the free circulating cells, generically called *hemocytes* (arthropods), *coelomocytes, amebocytes* (annelids, mollusks, and echinoderms), or *leukocytes* (Sipunculids). However, the repertoire of insect "blood cells" is clearly less heterogeneous than that of vertebrates. Basically three or four types of cell lineages can be identified in *Drosophila*: plasmacyte, crystal cells, and lamellocytes (Figures 3.4, 3.5) and an equivalent number in Lepidoptera (butterflies). They ultimately play important roles in development and in immunity. The functional roles they play consist of immune defense, disposing of apoptotic and other debris, contributing to the extracellular matrix (ECM), and modeling of the nervous system. The immunity role encompasses phagocytosis, encapsulation, and at time production of effector molecules (Figure 3.5). Both roles require recognition of PAMPS or self-derived defense molecules (i.e., opsonization) at the cell surface (23–25).

Only in a few organisms has the characterization of hemocyte lineages gone beyond morphological or basic physiological functions. Among these free circulating cells are always one or more types that can undergo phagocytosis. Different cells participate in encapsulation, pinocytosis, and nodule formation and can on stimulation produce a great variety (within an individual and among species) of soluble effector molecules that may eliminate the pathogen (Figure 3.5). In an attempt to integrate all of the data available in invertebrates, Hartenstein (23) has proposed a unified nomenclature of four basic types: prohemocytes, hyaline hemocytes (plasmatocytes or monocytes), granular hemocytes (granulocytes), and eleocytes (chloragocytes). These designations will be found in the following description of the blood cell types.

Although vertebrate blood cells are derived from mesoderm, free-moving cells with analogous and sometime homologous functions, and genes can be found in all metazoa including those that have no typical mesoderm (and obviously no coeloms). Porifera (sponges) remain perhaps the only metazoan completely without mesoderm and they have many motile amoebocytes (26). They apparently function for digestion, phagocytosis, and renewal of stem cells. Some archeocytes seem to be the phagocytic effectors. In triploblastic acoelomates like flatworms, motile cells can be observed in the parenchyma, perhaps corresponding to pluripotent cells—they can differentiate into many cell types of unknown immune function.

Earthworm (annelid) coelom-tropic coelomocytes are called *eleocytes*. They contain glycogen and lipid and are considered of the same lineage as the chloragocytes involved in the production of immune effector molecules such as fetidin or lysenin. The phagocytic cells of annelids are apparently granular "leukocytes" derived from the somatopleura and involved in wound healing, whereas the ones derived from the splanchnopleura participate in immunity. Heterogeneity of annelid coelomocytes is not encountered in primitive oligochaetes or in hirudinae (leeches). Phagocytic coelomocytes show an acid phosphatase activity and a beta glucoronidase activity (27). The large coelomocytes and free chloragocytes (eleocytes) in the typhlosole of *Eisenia foetida* appear to produce the bacteriolytic and cytolytic factor lysenin (28). Chloragocytes were also identified with plaque assays and produce fetidin (another name for lysenin). From electron microscopy (EM) studies, macrophagelike cells seem to be involved in graft rejection. In the closely related Sipunculid phylum, two main cell types can be identified in the blood, erythrocytes (a rare occurrence in invertebrates) and granular leukocytes. The latter are capable of cytotoxicity and even have dense granules reminiscent of vertebrate "NK cells" (29).

Two developmental series have been described in mollusks—the hyaline and granular cells—but cephalopods seem to have only one lineage. They participate in encapsulation, with hemocytes adhering around the foreign body like *Drosophila* lamellocytes. Phagocytosis is carried out by the wandering hemocytes (27). In oysters, EM revealed different types of circulating hemocytes, including granular hemocytes resembling the granulocytes of Sipunculus mentioned earlier (30). In crustaceans, the situation is similar to that in mollusks, with three main populations identified based again on the presence of granules in the cytoplasm. The hyaline cells are involved in the clotting process and the granular cells in phagocytosis, encapsulation, and the pro-phenoloxidase (PPO) pathway (Figure 3.5). The hematopoietic organ is located on the dorsal and dorsolateral regions of the stomach (24).

In insects, the so-called *prohemocytes* are believed to be the stem cells (Figures 3.4, 3.5). They are only found in the embryonic head mesoderm and the larval lymph glands but not in the hemolymph. However, prohemocytes are frequent in both the hemolymph and hematopoietic organs of the lepidopteran *Bombyx* (silkmoth). Plasmatocytes of *Drosophila* have a phagocytic function. This type of hemocyte is equivalent to the granulocytes of *Bombyx*, which play a key role in phagocytosis in normal larvae. Lamellocytes seem to be unique to *Drosophila*, but they are probably the equivalent of the Lepidopteran plasmacytoid cells. Their precursors reside in the larval lymph gland, where they differentiate in response to macroscopic pathogens, following a brief phase of mitosis linked to the presence of the pathogens and under hormonal control via ecdysone. The transcription factors (GATA, Friend-of-GATA, and Runx family proteins) and signal transduction pathways (Toll/NF-kappaB, Serrate/Notch, and Janus Kinase/Signal transduction activators of transcription (JAK/STAT)) that are required for specification and proliferation of blood cells during normal hematopoiesis, as well as during hematopoietic proliferation that accompanies immune challenge, have been conserved throughout evolution (Figure 3.4). The specific differentiation of lamellocytes requires the transcription factor Collier. The mammalian early B cell factor (EBF), an orthologue of Collier, is involved in B cell differentiation in mice. The *Drosophila* crystal cells are responsible for melanization through the PPO system (see later discussion). In silkworm oenocytoids, crystallike inclusions are also found, but they disappear later after bleeding (23,25,31).

Echinoderm coelomocytes express a diversity of effector functions, but no studies of lineages have been performed. In echinoderms, the number of different coelomocytes may vary according to the family. The sea urchin is endowed with at least four cell types, only one of which only is phagocytic and corresponds to the bladder or filiform forms. Another type is described as the round vibrating cell involved in clotting. Pigment cells (red spherule cells) have been detected ingesting bacteria; the morphology of phagocytic cells can vary enormously precluding any easy classification (32).

In tunicates, amoeboid cells circulate in the blood and are involved in a large number of processes, such as clotting, excretion, nutrition budding, and immunity. Large numbers of blood cells are present (avg. 10^7 per mL) in the blood of ascidians such as *Ciona*. Hemoblasts are considered to be undifferentiated cells, perhaps the equivalent of the prohemocytes of arthropods or the neoblasts of annelids. Blood cells in ascidians proliferate in the connective tissue next to the atrium. The pharyngeal hematopoietic nodule of this animal contains a large number of hyaline and granular cells called *leukocytes* with supposed intermediary forms of differentiation between blast and granular mature types. The granular form is likely to be involved in postphagocytic activity, like in the earthworms (33). Adoptive transfer of alloimmunity in the solitary tunicate *Styela* can be achieved via lymphocytelike cells (34).

In amphioxus, cells with phagocytic capacity have been identified in the coelom with a morphology resembling more the phagocytic echinoderm cells than urochordate blood cells, a fact that is consistent with the new systematic positions of amphioxus and echinoderms (35). Both free cells and the lining of the perivisceral coelom are able to phagocytose bacteria. Recently, cells with the morphological appearance of lymphocytes and expression of lymphocyte-specific genes were detected in this species; this is the earliest identification of such cells in phylogeny (36,37).

Hematopoietic Cell Origins: Hematopoiesis in Invertebrates

The history of the hemocytes cannot be dissociated from that of the mesoderm among the metazoa. The Bilaterian ancestor was most likely a small acoelomate or pseudocoelomate worm similar to extant platyhelminths (flatworms) or nemathelminths (Figure 3.1). A specialized vascular system or respiratory system was probably absent, although cells specialized for transport and excretions were likely present because they exist in most extant Bilaterian phyla. One can further assume that groups of mesoderm cells in the Bilaterian ancestor could have formed epithelial structures lining internal tubules or cavities (splanchopleura). In coelomates, the mesoderm transforms into an epithelial sac, the walls of which attach to the ectoderm (somatopleura) and the inner organs (splanchnopleura). Blood vessels are formed by tubular clefts bounded by the splanchnopleura. Excretory nephrocytes are integrated into those vascular walls, which also gives rise to blood cells circulating within the blood vessels (the pronephros of anurans and head kidney of teleost fish are important heneatopoietic organs in vertebrates, see Figure 3.14). Thus, further evolutionary changes separated the three systems, but there was a close original connection between them.

The origin of hemocytes has been investigated mainly in arthropods, particularly in *Drosophila* (Figure 3.4). When examining principles that govern hematopoietic pathways, similarities have been observed with vertebrates, raising interesting evolutionary issues (23,25). In jawed vertebrates, the yolk sac or its equivalent gives rise to blood precursors that are primarily erythroid in nature. In succession, definitive hematopoiesis occurs in the aorta/gonad/mesonephros (AGM) region of the embryo, encompassing all of the different cell types and multipotent progenitors (although this is controversial). Like in the vertebrates, hematopoiesis in insects is biphasic. One phase occurs in the embryo and the other during larval development. Additionally, these waves occur in distinct locations of the embryonic head mesoderm and the larval lymph gland. In the early embryo, expression of the GATA factor serpent (*Srp*) can be detected in the head mesoderm. This GATA family of zinc (Zn)-finger transcription factors is conserved from yeast to vertebrates where they are involved in various aspects of hematopoiesis. Blood cell formation in the head follows *Srp* expression, whereas in the lymph gland there is a long delay between *Srp* expression and the appearance of the lymph gland–derived hemocytes (38). Hematopoiesis in the head mesoderm and yolk sac may be related evolutionarily. A further similarity occurs at the AGM/lymph gland level in *Drosophila*. The lymph gland develops from a part of lateral mesoderm that also gives rise to vascular and excretory cells, much like the vertebrate AGM. The conserved relationship between blood precursors and vascular and excretory systems is intriguing.

Responses of Hemocytes

Proliferation of hemocytes on stimulation is an unresolved issue in the invertebrates; clearly, clonal selection resulting in extensive proliferation is not the rule. The turnover of cell populations has been the object of numerous, often unconvincing experiments. Still new data have emerged, and it is clear that in several invertebrate phyla, proliferation occurs in certain cell types following encounters with pathogens. Very little cell proliferation occurs in the circulation of crayfish, but cells in the hematopoietic tissue divide after an injection of the PAMP β1,3-glucan. New cells in the circulation developed into functional SGCs and GCs expressing the pro–phenol oxidase (PO) transcript. RUNT protein expression was upregulated prior to release of hemocytes. In contrast, pro-PO was expressed in these cells only after their release into the circulation (39).

By contrast to the study of transcription factors that regulate hematopoiesis, relatively little is known about cytokines that drive hematopoiesis among invertebrates. It was reported that differentiation and growth of hematopoietic stem cells *in vitro* from crayfish required the factor astakine, which contains a prokineticin domain (40); prokineticins are involved in vertebrate hematopoiesis, another case of conservation during the evolution of growth factors and blood cell development.

Parasitization of *Drosophila* by the wasp *Leptopilina boulardi* leads to an increase in the number of both lamellocytes and crystal cells in the *Drosophila* larval lymph gland. This is partially due a limited burst of mitosis, suggesting that both cell division and differentiation of lymph gland hemocytes are required for encapsulation. In genetic backgrounds where ecdysone levels are low (*ecdysoneless*) the encapsulation response is compromised, and mitotic amplification is absent. This ecdysone-dependent regulation of hematopoiesis is similar to the role of mammalian steroid hormones such as glucocorticoids that regulate transcription and influence proliferation and differentiation of hematopoietic cells (41).

Phagocytosis

To obtain phagocytosis at the site of microorganism invasion implies recruitment of cells via chemoattraction. In vertebrates, this can be done by several categories of molecules, such as chemokines like IL-8 or the complement fragments C3a and C5a (as mentioned later, C3a fragments as we know from mammals may be found in tunicates but not other nonvertebrates; yet, C3 may be cleaved in different ways in the invertebrates.) C3b, MBL, and many other lectins can function as opsonins, and recent studies of TEPs, DSCAMs, and eater have added to this

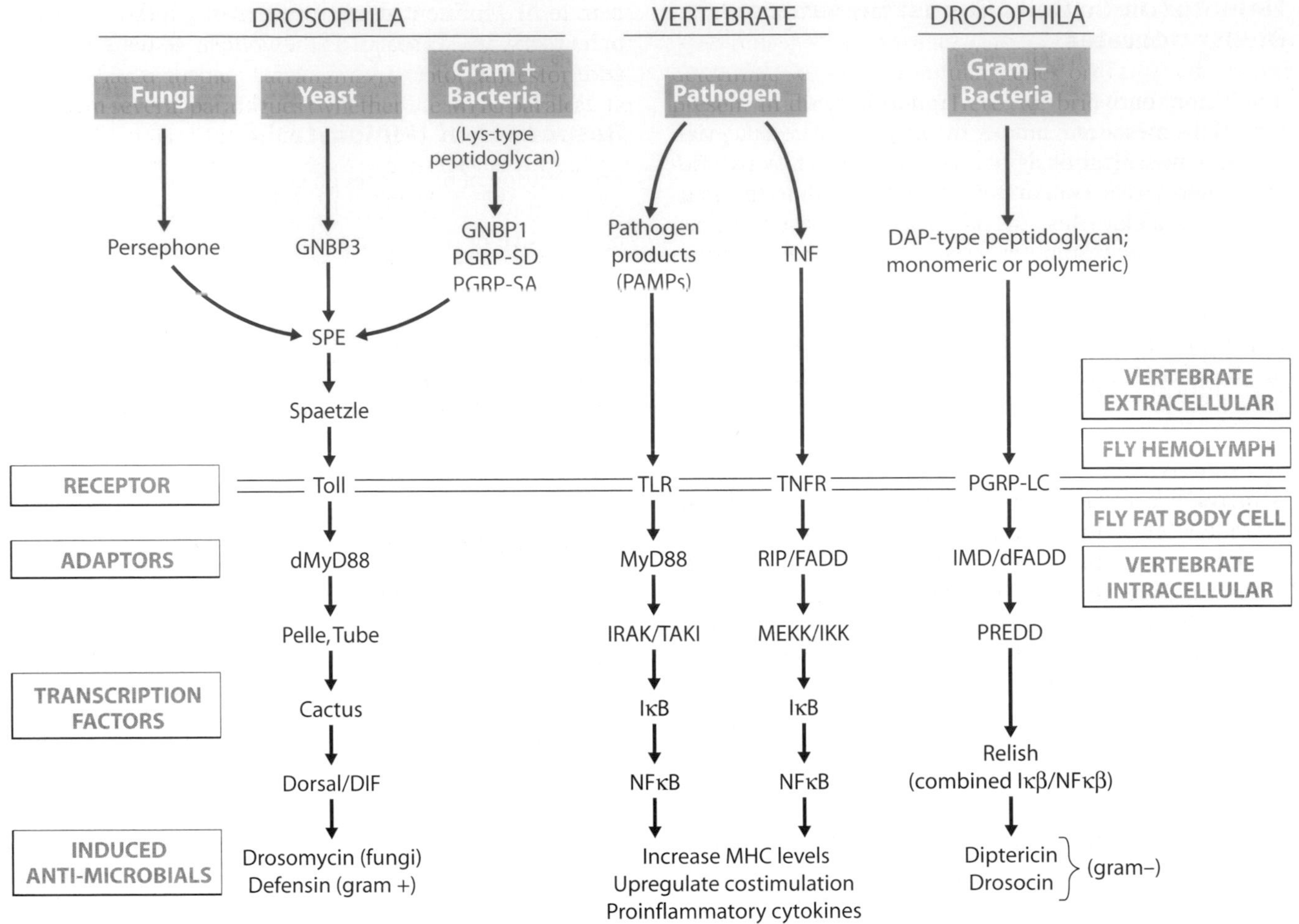

FIGURE 3.6 Comparison of immune response induction, intracellular pathways, and immune outcome in *Drosophila* and vertebrates. Note that the initiation of the response and the outcome(s) are quite different, but the intracellular signaling pathways are well conserved evolutionarily (details in the text). This figure was modified with permission from (31).

repertoire (Figure 3.5) (31). Ingestion follows phagocytosis, and then killing occurs by an oxidative mechanism with the production of reactive oxygen radicals and nitric oxide. These mechanisms are conserved in phylogeny, as described earlier. Unique to mammals and presumably all jawed vertebrates, the activation of phagocytes also leads to upregulation of the antigen processing machinery, costimulatory molecules, and proinflammatory cytokines that can enhance adaptive immunity (Figure 3.6) (42).

Melanization

A major defense system in invertebrates is the melanization of pathogens and damaged tissues (Figure 3.5) (43). The process is controlled by the circulating enzymes PPO and PO. The system is activated by GNBP, PGRP, LPS-binding proteins, and other proteins that can bind to various PAMPs (Figure 3.5). The complexes launch a cascade of serine protease activities resulting in cleavage of the pro-form of a prophenoloxidase-activating enzyme into the active form that in turn activates the PPO into PO. This leads to the production of quinones and finally melanin. Melanization can completely inhibit parasite growth, whereas concomitant with PPO activation, many other immune reactions are initiated, such as the generation of factors with antimicrobial, cytotoxic, opsonic, or encapsulation-promoting activities. The presence of specific proteinase inhibitors (of the serpin family) prevents unnecessary activation of the cascade and overproduction of toxic products. Phenoloxidase is the key enzyme responsible for the catalysis of melanization. It is a marker of the prophenoloxidase-activating system, and it can be an immune effector by itself as demonstrated in ascidians. It is therefore interesting to assess its conservation within all metazoa. A survey of the different organisms revealed the presence of phenoloxidase in many deuterostome and protostome phyla, and related molecules are also present in sponges. In arthropods, several PPO genes are present in the genome (nine in *Drosophila* and *Aedes*). Some may have different "immune" functions, such as injury repair. Several components that would maintain the role of melanization in immunity may be lacking in different phyla even if many elements are conserved, and so far the best examples of melanization associated with immunity are still found almost exclusively among arthropods and to a lesser extent in annelids. Despite the presence of molecules involved the pathway, the PPO cascade *per se* does not exist in vertebrates.

DEFENSE FAMILIES, BOTH RECOGNITION AND EFFECTOR

NOD and Intracellular Sensors

As mentioned earlier, proteins with the LRR motif are commonly found in defense molecules (Figure 3.2). One major family of intracellular sensors in animals is the NOD/NLR/CATERPILLER (CLR) group: (CARD (caspase-recruitment domain), Transcription Enhancer, R (purine)-binding, Pyrin, Lots of LEucine Repeats), which have an N-terminal CARD domain (a death domain [DD] in echinoderms), a central NBD (nucleotide-binding domain) or NACHT domain that regulates oligomerization, and C-terminal LRRs that provide the specificity for PAMPS (44) (Table 3.1, Figure 3.2). The composition of each member can vary drastically in structure and function. Several prominent members of the human CLR family include CIITA, CIAS1, and NOD2 and are linked to immunologic disorders that are hereditary, such as Crohn's disease. This indicates that these molecules not only are directly involved in defense but also regulate immune pathways (45), perhaps similar to new paradigms for how they function in plant defense. Thus far, the NLR have only been found in deuterostomes, which is somewhat surprising considering that plants have intracellular defense proteins with a similar structure.

The plant resistance (R) immune defense genes encode a NBD/LRR motif combined to other protein domains.

It has been proposed that the large number of NBD/LRR proteins in plants is due to gene-for-gene relationship for recognizing pathogen-specific products (46). The specificity of plant R proteins also depends principally on the LRR, and these are targets for diversifying selection, as described earlier for multigene families. Homo- and hetero-associations might generate further diversity to mediate appropriate responses. Recent evidence suggests that on recognition of pathogen effector molecules, the plant intracellular sensors derepress genes involved in basal defense by inactivating suppressor factors (47).

NLR are expressed by echinoderm coelomocytes, representing a highly diversified family (>200 members, similar to the TLR and SRCR, see later discussion) (Figures 3.1, 3.2). As mentioned, it is surprising that these genes do not seem to be represented in protostomes. On the contrary, in the vertebrates a search of the *Danio rerio* database did yield a large number of NBD/LRR sequences (32). NOD binds its ligand intracellularly, and the CARD domain associates with a kinase (RIP2) that activates the NFκB/MAP kinase cascade. In humans, most NLR genes are encoded in clusters on chromosomes 11p15, 16p12, and 19q13, where six sequences are found in a single region.

The retinoic acid-inducible gene-1 (RIG-1) is a newly described intracellular defense molecule that is unrelated to the NOD proteins, with N-terminal CARD and C-terminal helicase domains (48). With the helicase domain, RIG-1 binds to double-stranded RNA found in viruses or even to degraded cellular RNAs as a sign of distress (49). RIG genes are found in all vertebrates tested, and the family also has been expanded in the sea urchin.

PGRP and β1-3 Glucan Receptors

Numerous ligand-binding receptors have been recognized at the surface of invertebrate hemocytes (Figures 3.2, 3.5) or in solution. Insects have up to 19 PGRPs classified into short (S) and long (L) forms. S forms are soluble and found in the hemolymph, cuticle, and fat-body cells (31). L forms are mainly expressed in hemocytes as integral membrane proteins where their final structure depends on combinatorial association of different isoforms, modulated by alternative splicing. The expression of insect PGRPs is often upregulated by exposure to bacteria. They can activate the Toll or immune deficiency (Imd) signal transduction pathways or induce proteolytic cascades that generate antimicrobial products, melanization, or induce phagocytosis, and hydrolyze peptidoglycan (Figure 3.6). Homologues of PGRP are encountered in vertebrates, but they are only in soluble forms that display direct microbicidial activity (50). Both soluble and TM forms are present in sea urchins, some with potential catalytic function. Human PGRP genes are found on chromosomal paralogues 1q21 and 19q13/p13. In mice, a PGRP homologue (TagL) may be secreted as an inducible protein or retained on intracellular membranes. All detected splice-variant isoforms of TagL bind to bacteria and peptidoglycan. This binding was associated with the C-terminal portion of the polypeptides. Thus, this variety of isoforms of a single gene may play a role in circulating bacteria recognition in mammals.

Gram-negative binding proteins (GNBP, or beta 1-3 glucan receptors) are related to bacterial beta1-3 glucanases. They are found in insects and other arthropods (Figures 3.2, 3.5) where they bind gram-negative bacteria, fungal β-1, 3-glucans, LPS, or bacterial lipoteichoic acid (without necessarily showing glucanase activity.). An orthologue is present in the sea urchins, but not in vertebrates. Drosophila GNBP1, together with PGRP-SA, is required to activate the Toll pathway in response to infection (31). GNBPs have also been examined in both termites and

Daphnia. The *Daphnia* GNBP, like the *Drosophila* proteins, are under purifying selection. However, in termites, two *GNBP* genes showed some evidence of positive selection. It is possible that living in colonies exposes termites to higher pathogen pressures and more host-specific pathogens, resulting in stronger selection acting on their immunity genes (51).

Down Syndrome Cell Adhesion Molecule

DSCAM in *Drosophila* and other insects was described originally by neurobiologists as an axon-guidance protein, dependent on a large number of isoforms (>30,000) generated by alternative splicing of the Igsf domains and the TM segment. Recently, DSCAM was shown to be involved in insect immunity as well, expressed in cells of the hematopoietic lineage; like in the nervous system, a large number of splice variants are involved, clearly different from the ones expressed in neurons (10). DSCAM consists of nine Igsf domains and FN domains, present as either a membrane or soluble form (presumably generated by proteolysis of the membrane form). The membrane forms apparently signal through a known transduction pathway (DOC PAK) that has not yet been examined in detail. Each cell expresses only a fraction of the isoform repertoire.

Suppressing DSCAM (RNAi) and anti-DSCAM treatment significantly inhibit phagocytosis. Soluble DSCAM constructs with different exon combinations were found to have differential pathogen-binding properties. In addition, suppression of DSCAM in mosquitoes results in an impaired immunity to *Plasmodium*; exposure of hemocytes to different pathogens in culture gives rise to specific modifications and selection of alternative splicing patterns (52). The diversification of DSCAM seems to be specific for arthropods since neither flatworm nor sea urchin (nor vertebrate) DSCAM is diversified. The vertebrate DSCAM has only two forms, using two alternate TM exons. Human DSCAM is duplicated on chromosomes 21 and 11 but does not appear to be involved in immunity (53).

FREPs

Mollusk (genus *Biomphalaria*) FREPs are proteins found in the hemolymph with an IgSF moiety (one or two V-like domains) and a fibrinogen domain. FREP gene expression is upregulated following exposure to mollscan parasites such as schistosomes (54); a strain resistant to schistosomes shows an upregulation of the FREP 2 and 4 genes of up to 50-fold. The original discovery of FREPs followed the recovery of snail proteins that bound to worm antigens and thus this is one case in which the correlation between an invertebrate receptor and its ligand is clear. However, it is not known whether the IgSF or fibrinogen domain (or both) bind to the antigen or what effector functions are induced after FREP binding.

FREP diversity is remarkable in that many polymorphic genes as well as alternate mRNA splicing are used to generate the diversity. In addition, there appears to be a diversification mechanism that modifies the FREP genes, either via mutation or gene conversion in the region that encodes the IgSF domains (55). There are ~11 germline genes as suggested by Southern blotting with two to three members/gene subfamily. Therefore, finding 25 sequences within one individual for one member of a subfamily was strongly suggestive of somatic mutation.

185/333

There are a number of additional expanded gene families in the sea urchin genome that encode proteins with immune-related functions (Figure 3.1). The *185/333* genes were first noted because they are highly upregulated in coelomocytes after exposure to whole bacteria and LPS (56). Transcripts of the *185/333* genes constitute up to 6.5% of mRNA in activated coelomocytes. The *185/333* genes represent another family of linked and diverse genes that may be upregulated during immune responses. The encoded proteins have no detectable similarity to any other gene family, but they are highly diversified and are produced by a subset of coelomocytes. The mechanism by which diversity is generated is not known.

Variable Domain Chitin-binding Proteins

First discovered in amphioxus but present in *Ciona* as well, VCBP consist of two Ig domains of the V type but with a different folding motif when compared to Ig or TCR V domains followed by a chitin-binding domain (CBP). The CBP resembles chitinases found throughout the animal kingdom, and, like dedicated chitinases, VCBP are usually expressed in the gut. Apparently, there are no cell-surface expressed forms and thus all VCBP are likely to be effector molecules. Their diversity is enormous, apparently entirely because of polymorphism and polylocism. Each individual can carry up to five genes per haplotype, and in limited studies (11 individuals) an identical haplotype has not been encountered. While the general structure of the V domain is like that of the vertebrate rearranging antigen receptors (but with some unusual properties, including packing in a "head-to-tail" dimeric fashion, totally unlike Ig and TCR)(57). VCBP diversity does not reside in the Ig/TCR CDR resides but rather in the A, A′, and B strands, like in DSCAM.

Penaeidins

Another example of diverse defense molecules is the penaedins, present in crustaceans (shrimp). Penaeidins are AMPs consisting of a conserved leader peptide followed by an N-terminal proline-rich domain and a C-terminal cysteine-rich domain. Three classes of penaeidins, PEN2, PEN3, and PEN4, are expressed by shrimp hemocytes. A great diversity of isoforms is generated, with substitutions and deletions within the proline- and cysteine-rich domains, suggesting that this is a highly diverse gene family (58). Each penaeidin class is encoded by a unique gene and isoform diversity is generated by polymorphism.

Scavenger Receptors

The SRCR (SRCR) superfamily is an ancient and highly conserved group of cell surface and secreted proteins, some of which are involved in the development of the immune system as well as the regulation of both innate and adaptive immune responses. Group B SRCR domains usually contain eight regularly spaced cysteines that allow the formation of a well-defined intradomain disulfide-bond pattern. Scavenger receptors are best known for their housekeeping function of taking up lipids modified by oxidation or acetylation, but they have many other functions as well, such as uptake of apoptotic bodies (CD36 [59]).

SRCR have been studied mainly in the coleomocytes of echinoderms. Within six hours after bacterial injection, sea urchin coelomocytes upregulate a variety of genes, including an extremely diverse family of SRCR (60). A very large number of SRCR domains are present (~1,200), but each individual may express different groups of SRCR genes at different levels (and even with differential splicing). To assume that they are all involved in defense is premature, because SRCR genes can be both up- and downregulated after infection with bacteria. As mentioned, this high level of gene duplication is a general rule in the echinoderms. Recently, a new TM receptor in the SRCR family was discovered in *Drosophila* called *eater,* which, along with TEPS and DSCAM, is a major player in phagocytosis (61).

In mammals, the SRCR family as a whole is also poorly defined but is involved in endocytosis, phagocytosis, and adhesion, and some members act as PRR that bind to LPS or other bacterial components. One mammalian SRCR (gp340) is secreted into the saliva where it binds streptococci and helicobacter. SRCR are widespread in the human genome and participate as domains in the structure of numerous receptors (e.g., S4D-SRCRB, CD6, CD5-L, CD163), but without showing the high level of duplication seen in the echinoderm families.

C-type Lectins

Lectins were originally defined by their ability to bind carbohydrates, and some have been described previously (and throughout the chapter). They are found in many phyla in either membrane or secreted forms (62). C-type lectins, including CD94 and the Ly49 and NKG2 families, are encoded in the NKC and are central to NK cell function. A molecule resembling CD94 has been detected on a subset of hemocytes in *Botryllus* and *Ciona,* the functions of which are unknown (63). Effector cells of immunity probably also carry the receptors for the histocompatibility locus described recently (see below).

Another large gene family that is implicated in the response of the sea urchin to immune challenge includes 100 small C-type lectins, suggesting the existence of a complex immune system in the sea urchin (32). Diversity of immune receptors due to polymorphism within a population can be enormous. In some cases, polymorphism might be such that hardly two identical individuals are found within a population.

Peroxidasin

Among molecules containing LRR motifs and acting extracellularly, peroxidasin occupies a special place because of its involvement in hemocyte biology in insects and because of its homology to the LRR motifs in the agnathan VLR. *Drosophila* peroxidasin is an assembly of a cysteine-rich motif, six LRR, and four IgSF domains (64). The molecule is conserved in vertebrates although a role in immunity has not been reported. Another molecule called *peroxinectin,* with similarity at the level of the peroxidase region, has been described in crustaceans and shown to be associated with immunity via the PPO cascade (65). Its involvement in immunity is unlike any other effector so far described but illustrates the utility of LRR in many different types of molecules and processes. Pathogens bound by AMP can be phagocytosed or walled off by a barrier of flattened hemocytes and ECM. The ECM forms a basement membrane that becomes stabilized partly through peroxidases that generate tyrosine-tyrosine bonds. The combination of LRR and Ig structures suggests that peroxidasin may precisely mediate adhesion of cells to the ECM.

Defensins

Each metazoan phylum produces a variety of molecules with intrinsic antimicrobial activity (66). Some families are evolutionarily conserved, but generally they diverge rapidly and orthologous relationships are not apparent. There are numerous reviews at the following site: www.bbcm.univ.trieste.it/~tossi/pag4.htm#uno. The best-studied group of AMPs is the defensins, which are amphipathic cationic proteins; their positively charged surface allows them to associate with negatively charged membranes (more common in pathogens), and a hydrophobic surface that allows them to disrupt the membranes (either by disordering lipids or actually forming pores). Most of the molecules are proteins, but an antimicrobial lipid called squalamine, which also is modeled to have hydrophobic and positively charged surfaces, is found at very high levels in dogfish body fluids (67). Defensins can either be constitutively expressed (e.g., in respiratory epithelia in mammals), or inducible (e.g., see the following discussion for *Drosophila,* Figures 3.5, 3.6). Certain responses that seem systemic, like the production of *Drosophila* defensins, can also take place locally in the damaged tissues themselves; otherwise, a systemic response is initiated in organs distant from the site of infection, such as the fat body in *Drosophila* where induction of bactericidal peptide expression occurs. Defensins are the focus of great attention in commercially bred species such as oysters, mussels, and crustaceans, and it is hoped that they will be applied to medicine, whether they are derived from invertebrates or from vertebrates.

Toll and Toll-like Receptors (TLR)

Toll receptors were originally described in *Drosophila* as genes involved in early development. Later, they were also shown to be essential sensors of infection, initiating antimicrobial responses (68). This family was then revealed to be a major player in innate immunity in the vertebrates as well. As mentioned earlier, across the metazoa, structurally closely related members of the Toll family range from not being involved in immunity (in *C. elegans* and apparently in the horseshoe crab), to being the equivalent of a cytokine receptor (in *Drosophila*), to being pathogen recognition molecules in the vertebrates. Six spaetzlelike and eight Toll-like molecules have been identified in *Drosophila,* but only one or two of them are used in immunity. In jawed vertebrates, they belong to a multigene family of PRR specific for diverse PAMPs and exhibiting different tissue distributions and subcellular locations (69,70). In humans, many are on chromosome 4p and q (TLR 2, 1, 6, 10), but the others are distributed on chromosomes 9, 1, 3, and X.

Ectodomains of TLRs comprise 19 to 25 tandem repeats of LRR motifs made of 20 to 29 aa capped by characteristic N- and C-terminal sequences (Figure 3.2). All of the Toll receptors are homologous and appear similar in domain constitution among insects, echinoderms, and mammals. They also share the TIR domain, which is the intracellular segment shared with the IL1/18/33 receptors of vertebrates, as well as other molecules in plants. TIR domains associate with Myd88 to initiate signaling cascades culminating in the activation of NFκB/Rel (see further discussion later). The specificity of vertebrate TLR binding is concentrated in residues in the concave face of the receptor, which can be modified by various insertions after position 10 of the repeat (Figure 3.2). This feature is not present in the Tolls of invertebrates, which, as mentioned, are activated indirectly by pathogens. Thus, recognition within the Toll/TLR family is different in vertebrates and invertebrates, whereas the signaling cascades activated by Toll/TLR are remarkably conserved (31) (see below, Figure 3.6).

In *Drososphila,* Toll is triggered by an interaction with the unique ligand spaetzle, which is the product of a series of proteolytic cascades, with the most critical enzyme being recently identified (Spaetzle-processing enzyme or SPE [71]). Activation of the cascades triggers the production of AMPs (Figure 3.6). The specificity of recognition is not achieved at this receptor level but rather in solution via other intermediates (see below). In the horseshoe crab, Toll activation by coagulin could perhaps trigger the expression of wound healing proteins involved in restoration of tissues. *C. elegans* has only one Toll receptor, and rather than being antimicrobial, it promotes avoidance of a flatworm pathogen (72).

The arsenal of TLR in vertebrates is endowed with more specific and diverse capacities. Each vertebrate TLR has its range of specificities and, in addition, combinations of different TLR can create different binding specificities (e.g., the association of TLR2 with TLR6 or TLR1 and 2 [73]) This divergence in recognition function is well illustrated by the phylogenetic analysis of the Toll and Toll-related receptors in the different phyla, such as arthropods and vertebrates. Toll and related proteins from insects and mammals cluster separately in the analysis, indicating independent generation of the major families in protostomes and vertebrates (74). Consistent with the expansion of SRCR and NLR genes in sea urchins, hundreds of TLRs also were found in this species (32). TLR of the protostome-type are in small number (three members) while the vertebrate-type has been enormously amplified, all within a single family (222 members) and most without introns. Vertebrate TLRs do not diverge rapidly and evolve at about the same rate, and while there have been some duplications in amphibians and fish, they are not greatly expanded like in the echinoderms (no more than ~20 genes in any species).

PROTEOLYTIC AND SIGNALING CASCADES

Proteolytic cascades are initiated immediately following interaction of foreign material bound by preformed proteins in solution, and this principle is conserved throughout evolution. Indeed, the proteolytic cascade upstream of production of the Toll ligand spaetzle resembles the complement or clotting cascades. The PPO cascade of arthropods leading to melanization and the genesis of antibacterial products described above is another example in which peptidoglycans on microbial surfaces initiate a cascade resulting in the degranulation of hemocytes.

The best-studied immune proteolytic cascade that is (perhaps) surprisingly well conserved in the animal kingdom is complement (5,75). In contrast to the other defense molecules that we have discussed, orthologous complement genes can be detected in all of the deuterostomes without a great deal of expansion/contractions of the gene family (5). The three major functions of complement in jawed vertebrates are: (a) coating of pathogens to promote uptake by phagocytes (opsonization); (b) initiation of inflammatory responses by stimulating smooth muscle contraction, vasodilation, and chemoattraction of leukocytes;

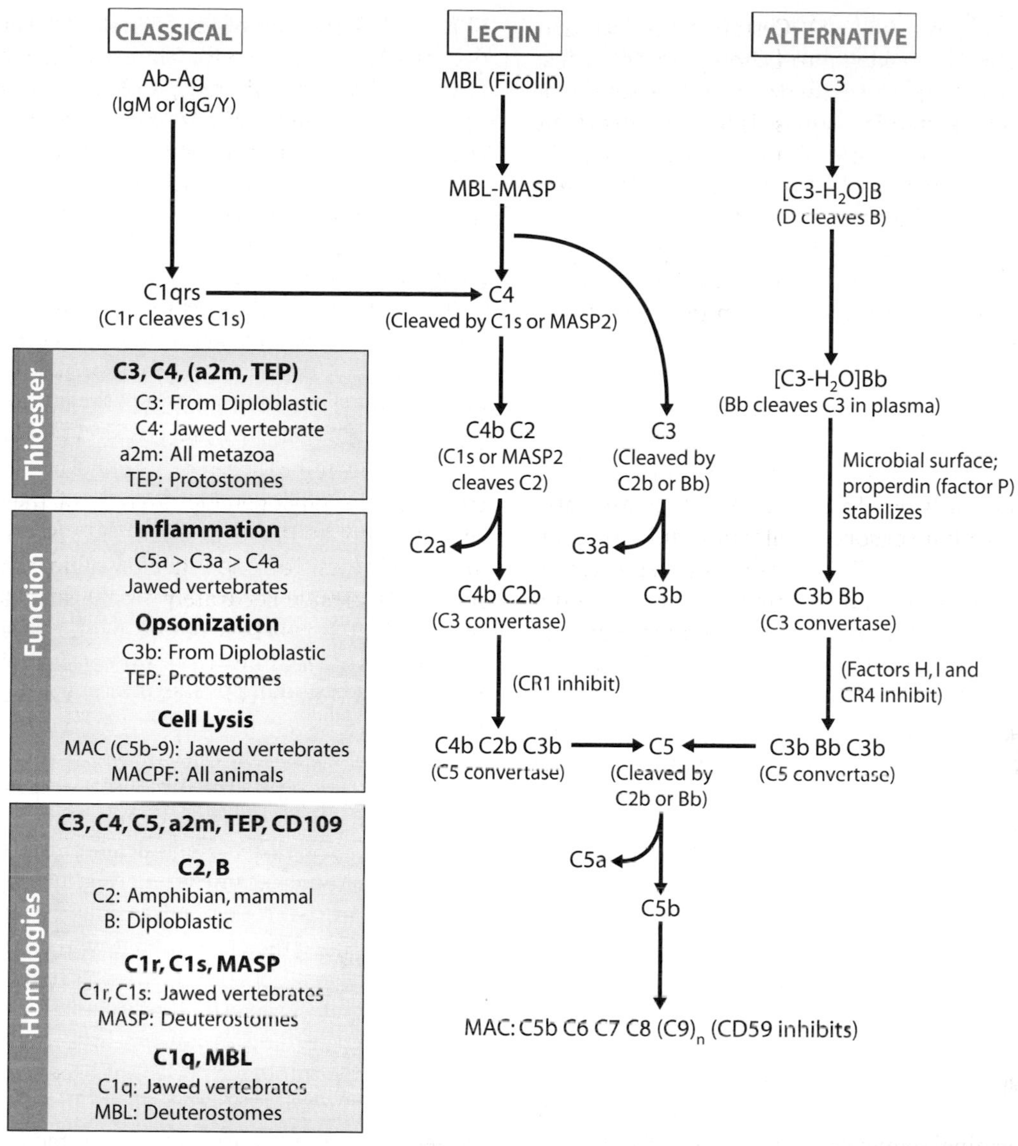

FIGURE 3.7 Evolution of the complement system. The general pathways and appearance of the various components in the phylogenetic tree are emphasized (75).

and (c) lysis of pathogens via membrane disruption (Figure 3.7). The focal point of complement is C3, which lies at the intersection of the alternative, classical, and lectin pathways of complement activation. It is the only known immune recognition molecule (besides its homologue C4) that makes a covalent bond with biologic surfaces. C3 has a nonspecific recognition function, and it interacts with many other proteins, including proteases, opsonic receptors, complement activators, and inhibitors. In the alternative pathway, C3 apparently exposes its thioester bond in solution, and in the presence of host cell surfaces lacking regulatory proteins that stop C3 in its tracks (by cleaving it into iC3b), it associates with the protease factor B (B or Bf). After binding to C3, B becomes susceptible to cleavage by the spontaneously active factor D, resulting in formation of the active protease Bb that in combination with the covalently attached C3 cleaves many molecules of C3 in an amplification step. Another nonadaptive recognition system, the lectin pathway, starts with the MBL (or the lectin ficolin), which is a PRR of the collectin family that binds mannose residues on the surface of pathogens and can act as an opsonin. MBL is analogous to C1q, with its high-avidity binding to surfaces by multiple interaction sites through globular C-terminal domains, but apparently it is not homologous to C1q. Like C1q, which associates with the serine proteases C1r and C1s, the MASP proteases (MBL-associated serine proteases) physically interact with MBL and not only activate the classical pathway of complement by splitting of C4 and C2 (the same function as C1s; MASP-2 appears to be the active protease), but also can activate the alternative pathway in ways that are not understood and thus completely bypass the classical pathway. Indeed MASP-1 and -2 are homologs of C1r and C1s. Both C1q and MBL can be involved in promoting the uptake of apoptotic bodies by phagocytes, via receptors that remain elusive. Recently, it has been shown that another lectin, ficolin, is also capable of initiating the MASP pathway (76), and it would not be surprising if other activators were discovered in the future. Finally, the classical pathway, which is dependent on antibody molecules bound to a surface, results in the same potential effector outcomes described earlier for the alternative pathway. Novel molecules initiating this pathway are C1q, C1r, C1s, C4, C2, as well as specific negative regulatory proteins.

C3 and MBL (and ficolin) are vital players in the immediate innate immune response in vertebrates, and both have been described in non vertebrate deuterostomes. Thus far, the best-studied invertebrate systems for investigation of C3 evolution are the sea urchin and the ascidians *Halocynthia* and *Ciona,* in which C3 and B molecules and genes have been analyzed in some detail (32,75). In contrast to the very high levels of C3 found in the plasma of jawed vertebrates, sea urchin C3 is not expressed at high levels but is induced in response to infection in coelomocytes. The C3 opsonic function clearly has been identified, but so far initiation of inflammatory or lytic responses (if they exist) has not been obvious. Receptors involved in the opsonization in echinoderms have not been identified, but in the ascidian gene fragments related to the C3 integrin receptor CR3 were identified, and antisera raised to one of the receptors inhibited C3-dependent opsonization.

Hagfish and lamprey C3-like genes were thought to be ancestral C3/C4 genes because the sequence predicts two processing sites (leading to a three-chain molecule), like C4, but a C3-like properdin-binding site is clearly present. However, like C3 in other animals the hagfish protein is composed of only two chains of 115 and 72 kDa, and sea urchin and ascidian C3 sequences predict only two chains (one proteolytic processing site). The lamprey, but not sea urchin C3, has a recognizable C3a fragment known from mammals to be involved in inflammation, so complement's role in inflammation may be a vertebrate invention (but see below).

Thioester-containing proteins (TEPs) have been isolated from *Drosophila* and the mosquito *Anopheles* (77). While the insect molecules function in a C3-like fashion (opsonization), phylogenetic analysis does not show them to be more related to C3 or α2-macroglobulin. TEPs in both these species function as opsonins, binding to parasites and promoting their phagocytosis or encapsulation. The evolution of multimember TEP families in these two insects followed independent evolutionary paths, perhaps as a result of specific adaptation to distinct ecological environments. The *Drosophila* genome encodes six TEPs (whereas there are 15 genes in *Anopheles*), three of which are upregulated after an immune challenge. Two of the *Drosophila* genes evolve rapidly (under positive selection), perhaps in response to certain parasites' capacity to block TEP activation.

Recently, C3-like genes were identified in the coral (78) and in the horseshoe crab *Limulus* (79). Good phylogenetic support was obtained for their relationship to C3, as compared to other members of the thioester-containing family like the TEPs. This suggests that the emergence of C3 as a defense molecule predates the split between protosomes and deuterostomes. A gene resembling the proteolytic enzyme Bf was discovered in these protostomes as well (and in sea anenomes), suggesting that the entire system was in place a billion years ago (Figure 3.1). The lack of C3 in many other protostomes suggests that the ancestral gene was lost and replaced by the TEPs in the majority of protostomes species (75).

In jawed vertebrates and some lower deuterostomes, certain species express more than one C3 gene, suggesting that the innate system might compensate in animals that do not optimally make use of their adaptive immune system. Changes in the amino acid composition of the C3-binding site are found that may somehow regulate the types of surfaces bound by the different isotypes. Likewise, in lower chordates such as *Ciona*, C3 and other complement components can be duplicated. Diversification of the carbohydrate recognition domains has been observed also in the *Ciona* MBL family (nine members).

Like Ig/TCR/MHC, the classical complement pathway and the terminal pathway membrane-attack complex (MAC) appear first in cartilaginous fish. However, because MBL can activate the classical pathway in mammals, it is possible that some portion of this pathway exists in pre-jawed vertebrates. Nevertheless, C4 and C2 genes have not been detected to date in jawless fish or invertebrates. A *bona fide* C2 homologue has only been identified to the level of amphibians, although duplicate B genes were isolated from cartilaginous fish and teleost fish that may function both in the classical and alternative pathways (75). The lytic or MAC pathway, which is initiated by the cleavage of C5 into C5a and C5b, also has not been described in taxa older than cartilaginous fish. Thus, opsonization and perhaps the induction of inflammatory responses were the primordial functions of the lectin/complement pathways. However, a cDNA clone for CD59, a molecule that inhibits MAC formation in self-cells, was identified from a hagfish library, and some of the terminal components of the pathway have been detected in lower deuterostomes with no described functions. Interestingly, proteins with the MAC/perforin (MACPF) domain have been detected throughout the animal kingdom, and some are even involved in cytotoxic reactions; however, it seems that only vertebrates have *bona fide* terminal C components that are highly evolved for targeted destruction of cell membranes (32,75).

C3, C4, C5, and α2m are members of the same small family. A new cell surface–expressed (GPI-linked) member of this family with unknown function, CD109, has been discovered (80). The protease inhibitor α2m, clearly present in invertebrates (protostomes and deuterostomes) and vertebrates, is thought to be the oldest, but obviously this must be viewed with caution considering the new data in coelenterates. Along with its ability to bind to and inactivate proteases of all known specificities through a "bait region," it has been shown to be opsonic as well in some situations. α2m, C3, and C4 have internal thioester sites, so this feature is primordial; C5 subsequently lost the site. The first divergence probably occurred between α2m and C3, with C5 and then C4 emerging later in the jawed vertebrates. Consistent with Ohno's vertebrate polyploidization scheme is the fact that C3, C4, and C5 genes are located on three of the four previously described paralogous clusters in mammals (see Figure 3.14), and this also fits with the absence of classical (no antibody) and lytic (no MAC) pathways in phyla older than cartilaginous fish. α2m is encoded at the border of the NK complex in mice and humans, and there are some tempting similarities between these regions and the other MHC paralogues. The C3a and C5a receptors that promote the inflammatory responses on complement activation have been identified in several vertebrates and (perhaps) some lower dueterostomes (81); they are G protein–coupled receptors whose genes may also be found on the Ohnologues (C3aR, chr 12p13; C5aR, chr 19q13). If indeed such receptors are found in the prejawed vertebrates, as suggested by recent pioneering experiments in *Ciona* (82) and *Styela* (83), it will be interesting to determine whether they are involved in some type of inflammation, thought to be the domain of the vertebrates (84).

Signaling Through Innate Surface Recognition Molecules

Four pathways of innate immunity triggering have conserved elements (if not the complete pathways) in eukaryotes: the Toll/TLR-like receptors, the TNFα/IMD receptors, the intracellular Nod, and the JAK/STAT (Figures 3.2, 3.5, 3.6). Although Toll receptors have been found in almost all triploblastic coelomates, most of the work and the elucidation of pathways has been accomplished in *Drosophila* because of the well known advantages of the model. The diversity of peptides that can be produced via the Toll/Imd pathways is substantial and classified in several categories depending on the type of pathogen that is recognized (e.g., gram [+], drosocin, gram (−), [−], diptericin; fungal, drosomycin) with different effector functions. *Drosophila* antimicrobial molecules were originally discovered by Hans Boman and colleagues in 1981, a seminal finding that heralded the molecular analyses of innate immunity in the invertebrates (85).

Toll and Imd Pathways

As described, invertebrate toll receptors are homologous to the vertebrate TLR in the sense that they are integral membrane proteins with an LRR binding regions. *Drosophila* Toll is activated after it binds spaetzle, the product of a proteolytic cascade activated in solution after the interaction of molecules produced by fungi or gram-positive bacteria with soluble PRR; as mentioned, the enzyme that mediates this cleavage has recently been identified (71). The Toll-interleukin 1 receptor (TIR) cytoplasmic domain of the Toll receptor then interacts with MyD88 (itself having a TIR domain) followed by Tube and Pelle, leading to activation of the homologous NFκB system (Cactus or Diff) that then induces transcription of various defense peptides (31,86,87). This is remarkably similar to the cascade of events following activation of mammalian TLRs where after their interaction with PAMPs at the cell surface, a cascade is induced through TLRs, including MyD88, IRAK, TRAF, TAK1, to NFκB via the IKK signalosome (Figure 3.6). Thus, infection-induced Toll activation in *Drosophila* and TLR-dependent activation in mammals reveal a common ancestry in primitive coelomates (or previous), in which defense genes under the control of a common signaling pathway lead to activation of Rel family transactivators.

The Imd pathway is employed for *Drosophila* responses to gram-negative bacteria (31,88). After interaction with a newly characterized cell surface receptor (the PRR PGRP-LC described earlier), in a cascade similar to the mammalian TNFαR signaling pathway, *Drosophila* tak1, an IKK signalosome, and a Relish-mediated (instead of Diff) NFκB step, results in transcription of antibacterial peptides like diptericin (Figure 3.6). The *Drosophila* intracellular pathway is like the mammalian TNFα receptor cascade, which also progresses via a death domain Mekk3, the signalosome, and NFκB resulting in cytokine production. In both cases, a link to pathways leading to programmed cell death is possible; overexpression of *Drosophila* Imd leads to apoptosis. When the activation of either the fly Toll or Imd pathway is considered, they are analogous to a mammalian cytokine/cytokine receptor system (e.g., TNFα) in which a soluble self-molecule activates cells via a surface receptor. Fitting with the recent paradigm put forward on recognition, signaling, and effector phases of the immune response, the diversity of external recognition systems is not matched by an equivalent diversity of intracellular signaling pathways (5). There are conserved signaling cascades coupled to the receptors, giving the impression of conservation of the innate immunity pathways; yet these pathways are also used in development, so which is primordial is an open question.

Responses to Viruses in the Invertebrates

Compared to responses to extracellular pathogens in the invertebrates, the study of responses to intracellular pathogens like viruses is in its infancy. First discovered in plants and in *C. elegans*, the RNAi pathway of defense against viruses is also operative in *Drosophila* and *Anopheles* (89). Double-stranded RNAs (dsRNA, viral or otherwise) are recognized by the enzyme Dicer 2, generating siRNAs that can associate with complementary RNAs and induce their degradation.

Viruses also induce an "interferonlike response" through a cytokine receptor (domeless) that is homologous to the IL6 receptor and signals through the JAK/STAT pathway. After viral infection, unknown signals (ds RNA?) induce the production of cytokines of the unpaired (Up) family that bind to domeless on neighboring cells and upregulate a large number of genes involved in defense (Figure 3.5). Nothing is known about the effector pathways of these responses, but mutants of one of the induced genes results in increased viral load.

In summary, arthropods (and presumably other invertebrates) use an RNAi pathway as well as a signaling pathway to combat viruses (90,91). As opposed to the systemic plant RNAi response, the same pathway in protostomes is rather cell autonomous. This response was lost in the vertebrates, presumably because: 1) Viruses have been able to effectively counter this response and render it ineffective, and 2) there have been remarkable evolutionary innovations in the vertebrate innate and adaptive immune systems to combat viruses. The discovery of a viral immune response quite like a type I interferon (IFN) response in vertebrates demonstrates that the three major signaling pathways of defense in Drosophila, Toll, Imd, and JAK/STAT, are similar to the vertebrate TLR/IL-1R, TNF, and IL6/IFN pathways, respectively (90).

Natural Killing Activity Across Metazoa

The word *cytotoxicity* encompasses vastly different protocols of cell killing by different cell types. It can be an effector function of cells of the adaptive (CTL or NKT cells) or of the innate arm (*bona fide* NK, see following discussion) of the jawed vertebrate immune system. Similarly the term *NK cells* covers different cell types and functions. NK cells of vertebrates can "recognize" missing self-MHC class I, but also ligands induced on stressed cells following virus infection, transformation, or stress. They can also have an immunoregulatory role by interactions with APCs. Many of these features obviously profit from a comparative approach.

In natural killing, the common denominator is the spontaneous reaction—that is, it does not require any (known) antigenic priming, but does require cell contact. Some form of natural killing can be observed from the earliest metazoans onward. Some marine sponge and corals avoid fusion with one another by the utilization of cytotoxic cells or induce apoptosis at the level of the teguments (92). Phenomena more similar to vertebrate NK killing are observed in sipunculid worms, where allorecognition among populations was shown to result in killing of allogeneic erythrocytes by lymphocytelike cells (93). Similar cases can be also encountered in annelids and molluscs (94). The role of IgSF and lectin receptors known to be involved as NK cell receptors in vertebrates has not been examined in these invertebrates, even though some candidate homologues have been identified.

When comparative morphology or function is not informative, searching for conservation of transcription factors or cell surface markers may be useful. Surveys of IgSF genes across databases have not yielded any promising candidates to date. Despite the presence of polymorphic IgSF members of the receptor tyrosine kinase (RTK) family in sponges, their role in allorecognititon or killing has not been demonstrated (95). As mentioned, similarities were found among the lectin families, especially in prochordates where cytotoxicity has been reported and associated with a discrete population of hemocytes, the granular amoebocytes. The urochordate genome (*Botryllus*, *Halocynthia*, *Ciona*) encodes many lectins with or without typical carbohydrate recognition signatures. Among them, a putative CD94 homologue has been cloned and its expression followed in *Botryllus*; this gene is differentially regulated during allorecognition, and a subpopulation of blood cells carries the corresponding receptor on its cell surface. An orthologue exists in *Ciona*. The function of urochordate CD94 is difficult to envisage, because these animals do not have the known ligand for the CD94 and NKG2 complex (i.e., MHC class I molecules). In addition, polymorphic receptors and ligands for the *Botryllus* histocompatibility reactions have been uncovered (see below), and CD94 does not seem to have any role in this process. However, CD94 is not an independent receptor, and finding it without its partner (NKG2 family members) that can be either activating or inhibiting does not reveal much. It can even be recruited in other cell types such as those in the nervous system, at least in *Ciona* (96).

Other C-type lectin homologs of CD209 and CD69 are linked to the CD94/L gene on *Ciona* chromosome 1 (LDP, personal observation). Could they be part of a "pre-NK complex"? Interestingly, all the human homologs of those lectin genes are present either in the NK complex on 12 p13 (CD94, CD69) or on an MHC paralogue 19p13 (CD209). Taken together with studies of the chicken MHC, which encodes some C-type lectins (see below), the data suggest that a conserved MHC-linked region containing several lectin genes was present before the emergence of MHC class I and II genes.

In addition, a number of genes encoding membrane proteins with extracellular C-type lectin and immunoreceptor tyrosine-based inhibitory motifs (ITIMs) or immunoreceptor tyrosine-based activation motifs (ITAMs), plus their associated signal transduction molecules, were identified in *Ciona*, which suggests that activating and inhibitory receptors have an MHC class I and II–independent function and an early evolutionary origin.

The ligands of these *Ciona* molecules are of great interest to uncover. ITIM- and ITAM-containing molecules have not been encountered in the protostomes (97).

VERTEBRATE ADAPTIVE IMMUNITY

Until recently, it was believed that only the jawed vertebrates had an adaptive immune system. From the discussion of invertebrate immune responses earlier, clearly there are mechanisms to generate high levels of diversity (apparently, even somatically), one of the hallmarks of an adaptive response (9). As described in the Introduction, we feel that the boundary between innate and adaptive immunity is artificial, and at times it is not a useful dichotomy when studying immune responses in diverse organisms (20). Despite this reluctance to exclusively categorize systems as innate or adaptive, some features clearly fall into the latter category, such as clonal expression of highly diverse receptors and specific memory. This condition is not fulfilled for the DSCAM, FREP, penaedin, or 185/333 invertebrate systems described earlier (to our knowledge), but of course we must be open to new mechanisms outside to the jawed vertebrate style of adaptive immunity.

Agnathan VLR

Long ago, the jawless vertebrates (hagfish and lampreys) were reported to mount humoral responses to sheep red blood cells (SRBC), keyhole limpet hemocyanin (KLH), bacteriophage, *Brucella*, and human RBC. For anti–group A streptococcal antigens, hagfish "antibodies" recognize predominantly rhamnose, while mammals recognize N acetylglucosamine. These "antibodies," or at least a proportion of them, were actually the complement component C3 (98). The alternative complement pathway was known in cyclostomes from earlier studies (see earlier discussion), and now most investigators believe that hagfish/lamprey have no rearranging Ig/TCR genes. Lamprey and hagfish do, however, possess cells resembling lymphocytes and plasma cells, with expression of lymphocyte- or at least leukocyte-specific genes, but the quest for RAG or *bona fide* Ig or TCR genes has been a miserable failure. Reports of specific memory in allograft rejection was difficult to reconcile with absence of the rearranging machinery and the possibility to generate specific lymphocyte clones (99).

Our view of the jawless fish immune system has been radically transformed over the past three years. Pancer et al. (100) prepared cDNA libraries of naïve lymphocyte RNA subtracted from lymphocyte RNA derived from lamprey larvae (ammocoetes) that had been immunized to a bacterial/PAMP mixture and found a highly diverse set of LRR sequences enriched in the immunized animals. The clones were not only diverse in sequence, but also in the number of LRR "cassettes" found between invariant 5′ (LRR NT) and 3′ (LRR CT) cassettes (Figure 3.8). Unlike what has been discussed earlier for immune genes in many species (especially the sea urchins), there were not a great number of the germline NT and CT cassettes, suggesting that a somatic recombination process, convergent with Ig/TCR rearrangement, occurred in the developing lamprey lymphocytes. The 5′ and 3′ LRR cassettes are separated by an intron in the genes encoding the germline VLR. Upstream and downstream of the invariant exons are a large number

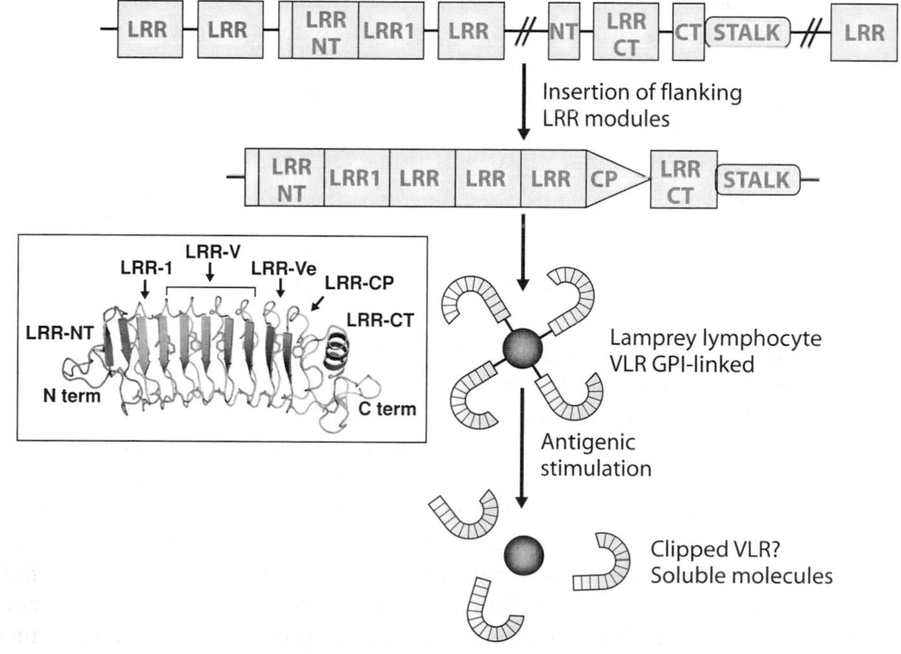

FIGURE 3.8 Genetics, generation of diversity, and speculative cell biology of the hagfish variable lymphocyte receptor (VLR) system (308). The top line shows an incomplete VLR gene (NT and CT, N-terminal and C-terminal cassettes, respectively). During lymphocyte ontogeny, upstream and downstream LRR cassettes are inserted between the NT and CT gene segments, resulting in an intronless, mature VLR gene (2nd line). VLR proteins are attached to the lymphocyte surface via a GPI linkage and may be released into the blood on antigenic stimulation. Boxed is a hagfish VLR protein, the structure of which was recently elucidated by Kasahara and colleagues (104).

of LRR, which become inserted between the 5′ and 3′ cassettes, presumably during differentiation of the lymphocyte (Figure 3.8). Individual lymphocytes apparently express a uniquely rearranged VLR gene in monoallelic fashion. The potential VLR repertoire may be as great as 10^{14}, vastly outnumbering the lymphocytes within an individual.

Fragments of homology between the LRR cassettes allow for joining and then priming of the synthesis of a copy of the particular transferred cassette. Because these small regions of homology are found throughout the cassettes, "hybrid" LRR can also be formed, further enhancing the diversity over a simple insertion of cassettes. This type of genomic change resembles the initial stage of gene conversion, but because there is not a complete transfer of genetic material between two homologous gene segments, but actually an addition of sequence, the assembly of the mature VLR is more similar to a recombinational mechanism described in yeast called "copy choice" (101). The enzymology of "copy choice" has not been examined; since a gene conversionlike process occurs, perhaps an APOBEC family member is involved. Indeed, APOBEC family members have been detected from the lamprey genome project and seem to be expressed in a lymphocyte-specific fashion (102). Because APOBEC family members are involved in repertoire building in jawless and jawed vertebrates, mutation/gene conversion may have predated RAG-mediated repertoire building of the repertoire.

VLR expressed on naïve lymphocytes are predicted to be associated via a GPI linkage, which has been proven in transfection experiments of mammalian cells. These receptors can also function as effectors in a soluble form: Lampreys immunized to anthrax spores responded with the production of soluble antigen-specific VLRs (103). Presumably, on stimulation, the lamprey lymphocyte either cleaves the GPI linkage, or there is a biosynthetic process that allows "plasma cells" to secrete the molecules. Such a type of recognition, activation, and "secretion" is obviously quite similar to the B cell system of the jawed vertebrates.

VLR homologs were found in two additional lamprey species (*Lampetra appendix* and *Ichthyomyzon fossor*), whereas two types of VLR genes A and B are expressed in hagfish, the only other order of contemporary jawless vertebrates. As in the sea lamprey, the incomplete hagfish germline VLR-A and -B generate somatically highly diverse repertoires. The presence of VLRs in both orders of extant agnathans lends additional molecular evidence favoring a monophyletic origin of cyclostomes. Across phyla, the comparison of the short LRR motifs can be misleading. VLR homologs have been identified in *Ciona* with 32% identity 47% similarity conservation, although without any demonstration of diversity or involvement in immunity. Interestingly the amphioxus genome harbors a large number of intronless VLR-like sequences. They might represent an alternative germline VLR diversity akin to the echinoderm gene families (TLR, SRCR) described earlier; one could even speculate that they are related to the ancestral VLR before invasion of its analogous "RAG transposon" (discussed later).

The crystal structures of three VLR have been determined (one VLR-A and two VLR-B). As expected for members of this family (see earlier discussion), the framework, or backbone, of the LRR is very similar between the cassettes. Diversity between cassettes is concentrated in the concave surface, presumably the region coming in contact with antigen. The first glance at these diverse receptors in consistent with the idea that VLR-based immunity is an anticipatory immune system, convergent with the Ig/TCR system of jawed vertebrates (104).

In sum, the VLR cell-surface receptors and the soluble molecules appear to be analogous to the jawed vertebrate membrane and secreted BCR, though much needs to be done to understand how VLR-bearing lymphocytes become stimulated. If there is only one type of lymphocyte in the lamprey, one would expect activation to be similar to T-independent pathways in jawed vertebrates (i.e., either direct stimulation through the surface VLR or surface VLR stimulation in combination with a PRR/PAMP interaction). Are VLR responsible for the graft rejections seen in the old experiments? It does not seem likely since MHC molecules have not been detected in the jawless fish. Grafting experiments should be repeated to study potential VLR involvement.

The independent development of two different strategies for receptor somatic diversification at the dawn of vertebrate evolution approximately 500 million years ago reveals the magnitude of the selective pressure applied on to the immune system and the emergence of individualized adaptive responses (99). Apparently, the elaborate innate and "semi-adaptive" immune responses that have evolved in several invertebrates were not sufficient for survival at particular times in evolution.

T Cell Receptors

Ig, TCR, and MHC class I and class II are all composed of IgSF domains (Figure 3.3). The membrane-proximal domains of each Ig/TCR/MHC chain are IgSF C1-set domains, while the N-terminal domains of Ig and TCR proteins are V-set domains encoded by genes generated via rearrangement of two or three gene segments during ontogeny (the membrane-distal domains of MHC are a special case; see later discussion). In all vertebrates studied to date, TCR are membrane-bound and never secreted, while almost all Ig proteins have TM and secreted forms (105).

α/β Constant Domains

Genes encoding the two types of TCR, α/β (which accounts for all known MHC-restricted regulatory and effector functions) and γ/δ (which to the best of our knowledge recognize antigens in an Ig-like manner and may play immunoregulatory or homeostatic roles during certain infections) existed in the earliest jawed vertebrates. cDNA sequences from species in the oldest vertebrate class (cartilaginous fish) revealed genes homologous to all four mammalian TCR chains. As mentioned, although many IgSF members exist in the invertebrates, thus far no *bona fide* Ig/TCR sequences (i.e., IgSF genes generated by somatic rearrangements) have been isolated from jawless vertebrates or invertebrates, a theme repeated throughout the chapter. Several genes from jawless fish and lower deuterostomes resemble antigen receptors, and they will be described in another section.

While TCR genes have been cloned from representatives of most vertebrate classes, few biochemical data are available, except in birds where α/β and γ/δ TCR have been identified with monoclonal antibodies (mAbs) (106). In amphibians, the *Xenopus* α/β TCR was coimmunoprecipitated with cross-reactive antibodies raised against human CD3ε chains (107). α chains from diverse vertebrates are poorly conserved, and the structure of the Cα IgSF domain itself is unusual: Only strands A, B, C, E, and F can be identified; strands E and F are shorter than those of mammals, and strand D is absent. The lack of conservation in this extracellular domain, as well as deletions found in bird and teleost fish TCR (especially in the connecting peptide), suggest that the coreceptor may be structurally distinct from mammalian CD3 complex components. Even within a class, the sequence divergence is great—for example, catfish Cα has only 44% and 29% amino acid identity to trout and pufferfish Cα, respectively.

Pre-Tα, which associates with TCR β chains during thymocyte development, has been identified only in mammals (108). The pre-Tα protein has no V domain, suggesting that the Vβ with which it associates acts as a single-chain binder. Unlike all of the other TCR chains, pre-Tα has a long cytoplasmic tail, which seems to be important for T cell differentiation. Interestingly, the pre-Tα gene is linked to the MHC in mammals, and phylogenetic studies should be performed to determine whether this linkage group is ancient (see later discussion).

The TM region and cytoplasmic tail of Cα are the most conserved parts of the molecule. Cα and Cβ TM segments in all species have the so-called *CART motif,* in which conserved amino acids form an interacting surface with the CD3 complex (109). Besides CART, the opposite TM face with conserved residues Ile-Lys-Leu interacts with other CD3 components. The cytoplasmic region is remarkably conserved among all vertebrates. TCR β genes have been sequenced from several species of cartilaginous and bony fish and two species of amphibians (axolotl and *Xenopus*). In addition to the typical IgSF domain features, there are several conserved regions among vertebrate TCRβ chains, especially at positions 81–86, probably involved in TCR dimerization. There are also remarkable differences: The solvent-exposed segment 98–120 in mammals is absent in all nonmammalian vertebrates. This loop has been shown in mouse TCR to be important for negative selection events in the thymus; perhaps the absence of this region in nonmammalian vertebrates results in subtle differences in tolerance induction as compared to mouse/human (110). The number of Cβ genes varies in different species: The horned shark has more TCR Cβ genes than the skate, but its genome size is largest of any elasmobranch so far studied. Unlike all other vertebrates, the axolotl has four Cβ genes as well as 4 DJCβ clusters that rearrange to the same collection of Vβs.

Like Cα, Cβ sequences are not well conserved in evolution (e.g., the *X. laevis* Cβ gene does not cross-hybridize with *X. tropicalis* genomic DNA, and catfish Cβ has only 41%–42% identity with other teleost Cβ and 26% identity with horned shark Cβ). Two different catfish Cβ cDNA sequences were identified, suggesting the existence of either two loci or allotypes, as is found in mammals. Indeed, the damselfish Cβ was shown to be encoded by two polymorphic genes, and this feature seems to extend to other teleosts. As the polymorphic sites are believed to interact with the associated CD3-signalling molecules, the authors suggested that signals might be transduced to T cells in different ways depending on the particular expressed Cβ allele. Also the damselfish Cα gene seems to be encoded by polymorphic alleles as well (111).

α/β Variable Domains

Because T cell recognition is MHC-restricted, TCR V regions have been evolutionarily selected for different properties as compared to Ig; indeed TCR V regions are much less similar to each other than are Ig V regions (105). Further, TCR Vs, unlike IgV$_H$, have conserved CDR3 lengths, suggesting that there is a restricted size for recognition of MHC-peptide complexes (112).Four Vα families were identified among only six skate cDNA clones, and six Vα families were identified in trout, and three in channel catfish. In the axolotl, five Vα and at least 14 Jα segments were identified, and 32 different trout Jαs have been sequenced. Thus, the α loci in all vertebrates examined have many J segments, and consistent with the mammalian paradigm, the absence of D and the large numbers of J segments favors the potential for receptor editing during thymic positive selection. A large number of Vβ gene families are another evolutionarily conserved feature. At least seven TCR Vβ families were isolated from horned sharks, and four to six in skate. at least four in trout (one with limited amino acid sequence similarity to the human Vβ 20 family), and 19 in *Xenopus*. In axolotls, Vβs are classified into nine categories, each with 75% or more nucleotide identity; since only 35 genes were cloned, there are probably more families, and several are related to mammalian Vβ genes (human Vβ13 and Vβ20). The D segment is encountered in all vertebrate classes, alone or in conjunction with other

Dβ. These segments usually encode glycines, suggesting a selection for flexibility in TCR CDR3 (112).

The *Fugu* α/δ locus suggests an organization similar to mouse/human, but with more rearrangement by inversion (interestingly, similar to the Ig L chain loci in teleosts; see discussion later in the chapter). The complete elucidation of the salmon α/δ TCR locus demonstrated extraordinary diversity of all gene segments, including the large number of Jα segments, and the flounder TCR loci are also highly diverse (105,113). Pulsed field gel analysis suggested that the horned shark α and δ TCR loci are closely linked (114).

The γ/δ TCR

cDNA sequences from the skate have significant identity with prototypic mammalian γ and δ TCR genes with extensive V region diversity, putative D segments in δ, and varying degrees of junctional diversity (114). Some of the six Vαs can associate with Cδ, and no specific Vδ has been detected, strongly suggesting that like mammals, the axolotl δ locus lies within the α locus. Vδ diversity was diminished in thymectomized animals, and TCR δ chains are expressed by cells in lymphoid organs, skin, and intestine. Chicken γ/δ T cells were identified long ago (106). Expression is found in thymus, spleen, and a γ/δ T cell line, but not in B cells or α/β T cell lines. Three V subfamilies, three J gene segments, and one C gene were identified at the TCR γ locus. All Vγ subfamilies participate in rearrangement during the first wave of thymocyte development, and the γ repertoire diversifies from embryonic day 10 onward, with random V-J recombination, nuclease activity, and P and N nucleotide addition. A new type of γ/δ TCR has been described in sharks and marsupials, which will be described in the IgNAR section that follows.

In ruminants and chickens (so-called *GALT species*—see discussion later in this chapter), the γ/δ repertoires are quite diverse, and there seems to be ligand-mediated selection of γ/δ cells during ontogeny. In sheep, where γ/δ TCR diversity is thymus dependent and follows a developmentally regulated progression, no invariant γ/δ TCRs are found. The degree of γ/δ expression is correlated with the evolution of the TCR V families in warm-blooded vertebrates. Indeed, mammals can be classified into "γ/δ low" (humans and mice, in which γ/δ T cells constitute limited portion of the T cell population) and "γ/δ high" (sheep, cattle, and rabbits, in which such γ/δ cells compose up to 60% of T cells). TCR V genes form subgroups in phylogenetic analyses, and humans and mice have representative loci in most subgroups whereas the other species appear to have lost some (115). Thus, γ/δ-low species have a high degree of TCR-V gene diversity, while γ/δ-high species have limited diversity. Interestingly this pattern is similar to that found for IgV$_H$ genes (see discussion later in this chapter).

Generally speaking, the γ/δ TCR can either be used for innate recognition (e.g., the cells in the skin of mice or the blood of humans) or adaptively with an enormous repertoire in ways we do not understand well—this will be discussed in more detail in the IgNAR and Conclusions sections.

Immunoglobulins

A typical Ig molecule is composed of four polypeptide chains (two heavy [H] and two light [L]) joined into a macromolecular complex via several disulfide bonds (Figure 3.9; note that an entire review issue has recently been devoted to the topic of comparative aspects of Igs, *Dev. Comp. Immunol.* 2006, Vol 30, issues 1 and 2). Each chain is composed of a linear combination of IgSF domains, much like the TCR, and almost all molecules studied to date can be expressed in secreted or TM forms.

Ig Heavy Chain Isotypes

Like all other building blocks of the adaptive immune system, Ig is present in all jawed vertebrates (Figures 3.1 and 3.9). Consistent with studies of most molecules of the immune system, the sequences of IgH chain C region genes are not well conserved in evolution, and insertions and deletions in loop segments occur more often in C than in V domains. As a consequence, relationships among non-μ isotypes (and even μ isotypes among divergent taxa) are difficult to establish. Despite these obstacles, recent work has allowed us to infer a working evolutionary tree among all of the isotypes.

IgM

IgM is present in all jawed vertebrates and has been assumed to be the primordial Ig isotype. It is also the isotype expressed earliest in development in all tetrapods; until recently it was believed to be the case in fish as well, but this view has changed recently (see discussion later in this chapter).The secretory μ H chain is found in all vertebrates and usually consists of one V and four C1 domains and is heavily glycosylated. H chains associate with each other and with L chains through disulfide bridges in most species, and IgM subunits form pentamers or hexamers in all vertebrate classes except teleost fish which form tetramers (116). The μ C$_H$4 domain is most evolutionarily conserved, especially in its C-terminal region. There are several μ-specific residues in each of the four C$_H$ domains among vertebrates, suggesting a continuous line of evolution, which is supported by phylogenetic analyses. Like TCR TM regions described earlier, μ TM regions are also well conserved among sharks, mammals, and amphibians, but the process by which the Ig TM mRNA is assembled varies in different species (117). In all vertebrate classes except teleosts, the μ TM region is encoded by separate exons that are spliced to a site on μ mRNA located ~30 bp from the end of the C$_H$4-encoding exon. In contrast, splicing of teleost fish μ mRNA takes place at the end of C$_H$3 exon. In holostean fish (gar and sturgeon), cryptic splice

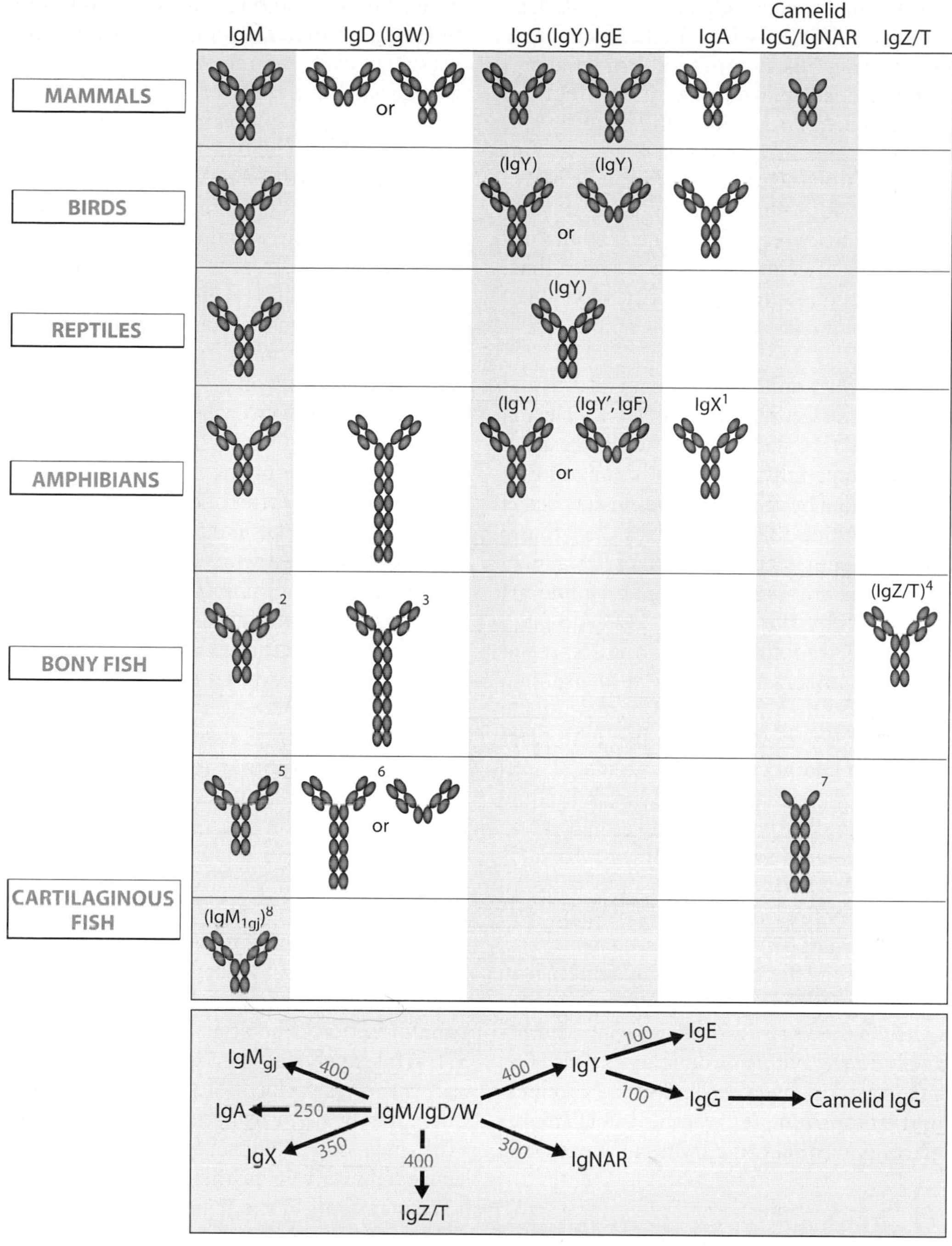

FIGURE 3.9 Ig isotypes in the jawed vertebrates. The bottom panel displays the approximate divergence times of all isotypes. IgM/D/W was found at the inception of adaptive immunity (160). **1:** IgX is in the IgA column because it is preferentially expressed in the intestine, but it is actually most similar in sequence to IgM; **2:** secreted IgM in teleost fish is a tetramer—the TM form only has three C domains; **3:** the teleost fish IgD H chains incorporate the μC1 domain via alternative splicing; **4:** the new bony fish isotype, IgZ/T, may not be found in all fish species; **5:** the secreted form of shark/skate IgM is present as a pentamer and monomer at ~equal levels; **6:** the TM form of IgW has 4 C domains; **7:** a major TM form of IgNAR has three C domains, and IgNAR is related to camelid IgG by convergent evolution; **8:** no TM form has been found (to date) for IgM_{1gj}.

donor sites are found in the C_H4 sequence that could lead to conventional splicing, but in the bowfin there is another cryptic splice donor site in C_H3. Some modifications apparently related to the particular environment were noticed in the Antarctic fish *Trematomus bernacchii*. There are two remarkable insertions, one at the V_H-C_H1 boundary and another at the C_H2-C_H3 boundary; the latter insertion results in a very long C_H2-C_H3 hinge region. Rates of nonsynonymous substitutions were high in the modified regions, suggesting strong selection for these modifications. These unusual features (also unique glycosylation sites) may permit flexibility of this IgM at very low temperatures (118).

It has been known for a long time that in all elasmobranchs, IgM is present at very high amounts in the plasma of cartilaginous fish and that it is found in two forms: multimeric (19S) and monomeric (7S) (119). It is unlikely that the two forms are encoded by different gene clusters since: 1) Peptide maps are identical; 2) early work by Clem found the sequences of the cysteine-containing tail of 19S and 7S H chains to be identical; and 3) all identified germline VH families are represented for the 19S form (116). Although most studies (but not all) reported that 19S and 7S are not differentially regulated during an immune response, in a recent study, the 19S response wanes over time and a stable 7S titer is maintained for periods of up to two years after immunization (120). In addition, antigen-specific 7S antibodies observed late in the response have a higher binding strength than those found early, suggesting a maturation of the response, also generally at odds with the previous literature. Finally, when specific antibody titers were allowed to drop, a memory response was observed that was exclusively of the 7S class. This work has shown that a "switch" indeed occurs in the course of an immune response; whether the "switch" is due to an induction of the 19S-producing cells to become 7S producers, or whether there are lineages of 19S- and 7S-producing B cells is an open question. One working hypothesis is that J chain expression is important for regulating whether a B cell makes 19S or 7S Ig, but of course that could be at the lineage level or the switch level.

IgM_{1gj}. Nurse shark *Ginglymostoma cirratum* expresses an IgM subclass in neonates (121). The V_H gene of this subclass underwent V-D-J rearrangement in germ cells ("germline-joined" or "gj"; see discussion later in this chapter). Expression of H_{1gj} is detected in primary and secondary lymphoid tissues early in life, but in adults only in the primary lymphoid tissue, the epigonal organ (see later discussion). H_{1gj} associates covalently with L chains and is most similar in sequence to IgM H chains, but like mammalian IgG, it has three rather than the typical four IgM constant domains; deletion of the ancestral IgM second domain thus defines both IgG and IgM_{1gj}. Because sharks are in the oldest vertebrate class known to possess antibodies, unique or specialized antibodies expressed early in ontogeny in sharks and other vertebrates were likely present at the inception of the adaptive immune system. It is suggested that this isotype interacts either with a common determinant on pathogens or a self-waste product.

IgNAR (Ig NAR) and NAR-TCR. A dimer found in the serum of nurse sharks and so far restricted to cartilaginous fish, IgNAR is composed of two H chains each containing a V domain generated by rearrangement and five constant C1 domains (122). IgNAR was originally found in sera, but TM forms exist as cDNA and cell-surface staining is detected with specific mAbs. The single V resembles a fraction of camel/llama (camelid) IgG that binds to antigen in a monovalent fashion with a single V region (116). In phylogenetic trees, NAR V domains cluster with TCR and L chain V domains rather with that V_H. A molecule with similar characteristics has also been reported in ratfish, although it was independently derived from IgM like the camelid molecule emerged from *bona fide* IgG. IgNAR V region genes accumulate a high frequency of somatic mutations (see later discussion).

The crystal structure of a Type I IgNAR V regions showed that, in contrast to typical V regions, they lacked CDR2 and had a connection between the two IgSF sheets much like an IgSF C domain (Figure 3.3, [123,124]). The domain wraps around its antigen (hen egg lysoszyme), with the CDR3 penetrating into the active site of the enzyme. The structure of a type II V region was revealed as well, showing a disulfide bond between CDR1 and CDR3 that forces the most diverse regions of the molecule to form a raised cap, similar to what has been described for camelid V domains (116,124). In total, the differential placement of disulfide bonds forces major changes in the orientations of CDR1 and CDR3 and provides two major conformations for antigen binding.

While analyzing the TCRVδ repertoire in nurse sharks, an entirely new form of this chain, which encodes three domains, V-V-C, was detected (125). The C is encoded by the single-copy Cδ gene, and the membrane-proximal V is encoded by a Vδ gene that rearranges to the DJδ elements. The membrane distal V domain is encoded by a gene in the NAR family, found in a rearranging VDJ cluster typical of all cartilaginous fish Ig clusters. The NAR-TCR V genes, unlike IgNAR V genes that have three D segments, only have a single D region in each cluster. The particular Vδ loci linked to each NAR-TCR gene—called *NAR-TCR-supporting Vδ*—encode a cysteine in CDR1 that likely makes a disulfide bridge with the NAR-TCR V domain. The J segment of the rearranged NAR-TCR V gene splices at the RNA level directly to the supporting Vδ segment, which has lost its leader exon. This organization likely arose from an IgNAR V cluster that translocated to the TCRδ locus upstream of a Vδ gene segment. After modifications of the supporting Vδ genes, this entire V-V gene set duplicated and diverged several times in different species of sharks. About 25% of the expressed nurse shark TCR δ repertoire is composed of this new type of TCR (encoded by 15-20 V-V genes in this species) and have proposed that the typical γ/δ TCR acts as a scaffold on which sits the single chain NAR V.

Our interpretation is that, true to the proposal that γ/δ TCRs interact with free antigen, the NAR V is providing a binding site that can interact with antigen in a different way than conventional heterodimeric Vs. Thus, this is the first case in which a particular V region family has been shown to be associated with a BCR and TCR; in the case of the BCR, the function likely resides within the Fc portion of IgNAR and for the TCR the function (cytokine secretion, killing) lies within the T cell itself. Interestingly, a second TCRδ chain locus has also been described in marsupials with properties similar to NAR-TCR (126). In this case, there are also two V domains, but one (proximal to the membrane) is germline-joined and only the membrane-distal domain undergoes rearrangement. This new TCRδ locus is preferentially expressed early in development. Discovery of two such antigen receptor loci in sharks and marsupials suggests that this type of receptor will be found in other vertebrates as well.

IgR/IgNARC/IgW/IgX/IgD

All elasmobranchs studied to date have another isotype called *IgW* (116). It was probably discovered long ago in skates as a non–IgM-secreted isotype called *IgR,* but no protein sequence of this molecule has been obtained for confirmation. Subsequently, an Ig gene was discovered in skates encoding a three-domain molecule with an unusual secretory tail that was named IgX (not to be confused with another isotype with that name in amphibians, Figure 3.9). A high molecular weight (MW) species detected by northern blotting with an IgW probe suggested that there might be a longer form of this isotype, subsequently shown to be true in the sandbar shark (IgW), nurse shark (IgNARC—it was so-named because the C domains had highest similarity to IgNAR C domains) and skate). It was originally believed that sharks only expressed the long (seven-domain) IgW form, but they were later shown to have both secretory forms); the reason for the discrepancy was shark-to-shark variation in expression of the short form, for unknown reasons (127). The major IgW TM form, like IgM, is composed of five domains, but variants with three domains—like the secretory forms—were also detected. Very little is known about the function of this isotype, as IgW-specific mAbs have not been generated as they have for IgM and IgNAR.

IgW was thought to be a dead-end isotype in the cartilaginous fish, but a homologue was found in the lungfish (128). It also is present in two secreted forms, one with eight domains and the other, like in the elasmobranchs, with three domains (unfortunately the secretory tail was not sequenced, and the TM form was not studied). Recently, an Ig isotype was found in *X. tropicalis* most related to the lungfish IgW (129,130). Computer searches of databases for the *X. tropicalis* genome project uncovered a new isotype flanked by the IgM and IgX genes at the IgH locus (Figure 3.10). The deduced amino acid sequence obtained from the exons on the genomic scaffold suggests a nine-domain molecule. The N-terminal C domains and the TM regions are most similar to mouse and human IgD regions, and its genomic location also suggests that it is an IgD equivalent. Thus, these new data reveal that like IgM, IgW/D is an isotype that was present at the emergence of all extant vertebrate taxa.

An interesting feature of this IgD/W locus is that it is highly plastic in evolution, both in terms of the number of domains in different fish species and the plethora of splice variants found, at least in cartilaginous fish (127). In sharks, two of the C domains were derived ~250 million years ago by a tandem duplication event, and there was a *Xenopus*-specific, two-domain tandem duplication event as well. Within teleost fish, the number of C exons for this isotype is different in various species, and the secreted and TM forms seem to be encoded by different loci in the catfish (Figure 3.10). In addition to the splice variants described earlier in the cartilaginous fish and lungfish, in teleosts, the IgM C1 domain exon is spliced into the IgD transcript (131). Even in mammals, there are different numbers of C domains in different species, and even exons that have emerged quite recently in evolution. It is our impression that this is the Ig locus that evolution "plays with," perhaps using it for different functions in vertebrate taxa. We are obviously at the beginning of our analysis of this system, but perhaps an evolutionary perspective of IgD/W will eventually lead to an understanding of the function of this ancient isotype.

IgZ/T

A third, novel bony fish isotype was uncovered in screens of the EST and genomic databases called *IgZ* in zebrafish and *IgT* in trout (132,133). Its genomic organization parallels the TCR α/δ locus in that the IgZ/T D, J, and C elements are found between the VH and Cζ/Cμ exons (Figure 3.10). IgZ/T is a five-domain H chain predicted to associate with L chains. The authors propose that lymphocytes bearing IgZ may be B1 cell equivalents, but a preliminary VH repertoire analysis does not suggest that unique sets of V regions are expressed on IgZ compared to IgM. IgT is not preferentially expressed over IgM early in trout development, and there is high expression in the spleen throughout ontogeny into adulthood. The effector function of IgZ/T is not known, but there may be species-specific differences in expression during ontogeny and in adult life among bony fishes.

Other Isotypes Related to IgG, IgE, IgA and the Switch. Other isotypes consist of four C domains in nonmammalian vertebrates, including *Xenopus* IgY and IgX, non-μ

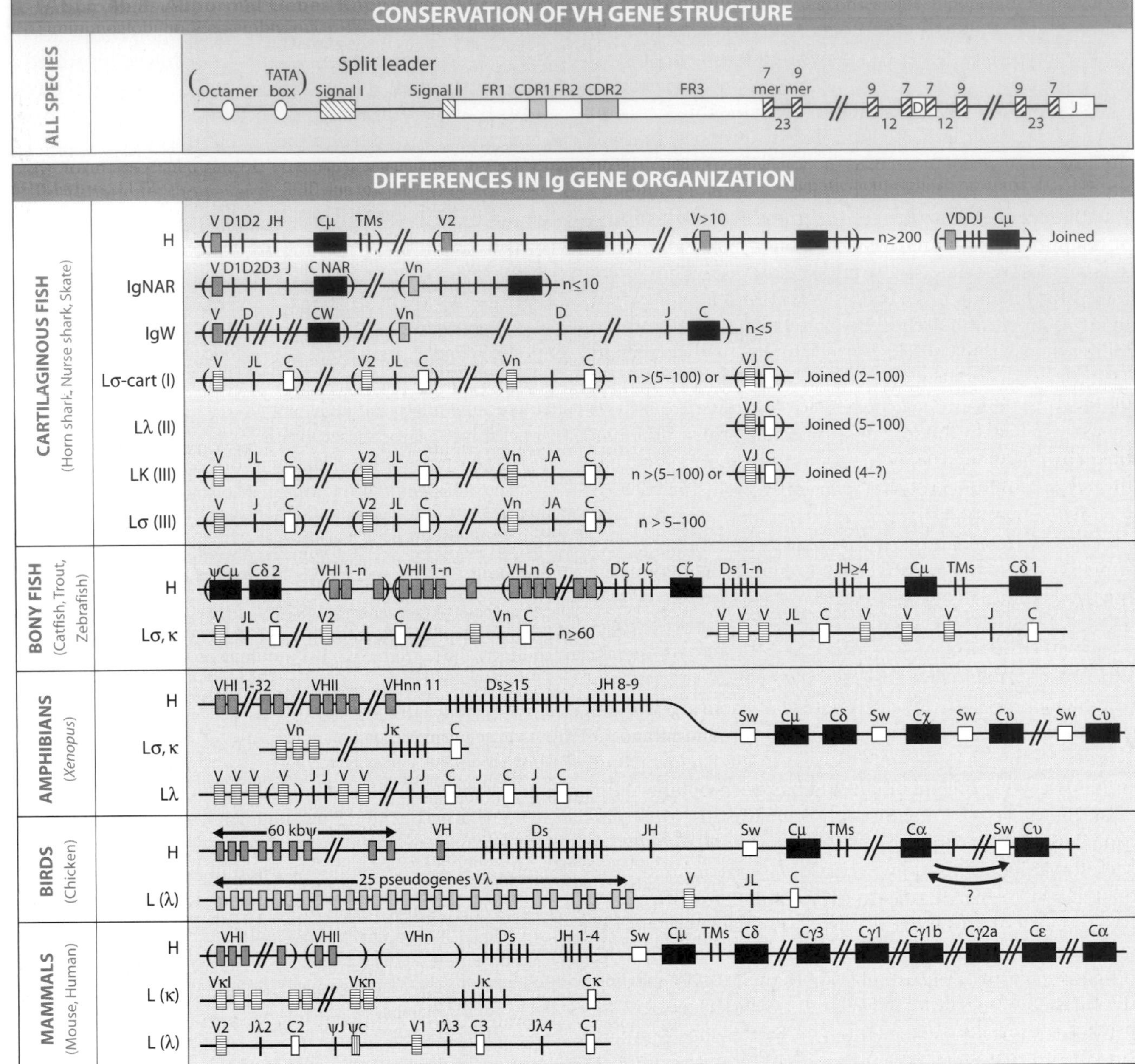

FIGURE 3.10 Organization of H and L chain genes in all jawed vertebrates. All cold-blooded gnathostomes except bony fish have three L chain isotypes, κ, λ, and σ; mammals have κ and λ; and birds have only λ. V_H genes, gray; C_H genes, black; V_L genes, horizontal lines; V_C genes, white. The top line shows a germline V, D, J gene with canonical RSS and promoter elements. Isotypes for each class are found in Figure 3.9. See text for details.

isotypes of *Rana*, IgY of axolotl, and IgA and IgY of birds (116,134). In *Xenopus*, IgY is thymus dependent; IgM and IgX are not, although thymectomy impacts specific IgM antibody production (i.e., antigen-specific IgM can be produced, but there is neither an increase in affinity after immunization nor elicitation of plaque-forming cells). IgM and IgX plasma cells are abundant in the gut, while IgY is expressed primarily in spleen. Axolotl IgM is present in the serum early during development and represents the bulk of specific antibody synthesis after antigenic challenge. In contrast to *Xenopus* IgY, the axolotl orthologue appears late in development and is relatively insensitive to immunization. From one to 7 months post-hatching, axolotl IgY is present in the gut epithelium, associated with a secretory component. IgY progressively disappears from the gut and is undetectable in the serum of 9-month-old animals. Thus, axolotl IgY, like *Xenopus* IgX, may be analogous to mammalian IgA. *Xenopus* IgX and IgY are not homologous (similar to sequence) to any mammalian non-μ Ig isotype and are most similar to IgM. The TM and cytoplasmic domains of *Xenopus* TM IgY, however, share residues with avian IgY and mammalian IgG and IgE, suggesting that mammalian/avian isotypes share a common ancestry with amphibian IgY (135). This homology is especially interesting, because a study in mice suggested that the IgG cytoplasmic tail is the central molecular element promoting rapid memory responses. Finally, another *Xenopus* isotype was discovered from the databases, called *IgF* (130) or *IgY′* (because it is closely related to IgY, probably duplicating within the *Xenopus* lineage). Like other isotypes described in this section, it only has two C domains, but rather than alternative splicing, the gene is organized in such a manner. There has been no biochemical identification of IgF to date.

Although cartilaginous and teleost fish have multiple Ig isotypes, CSR appears first in evolution in amphibians (134,136). CSR results from fusing switch regions upstream of the μ gene and another 3′ isotype gene, accompanied by the deletion of the intervening sequences. Among vertebrates, mammalian and bird class switch regions are GC-rich and contain tandem repeats in which certain motifs such as TGGGG, GGGGT, AGCT, GGCT are abundant. Because of the GC richness of these regions, transcription generates stable R loops that provide single-stranded substrates for AID activity. The first comparative studies on switch were done in the amphibian *Xenopus,* where the switch μ and χ region is not GC rich but AT-rich and cannot form R loops (137). Replacement in mouse of the switch region with the *Xenopus* switch μ showed that it mediated efficient CSR and that the junctions were associated with the short palindromic AGCT motifs, already recognized as the main component of the *Xenopus* switch μ region. As predicted from the absence of R loops, *Xenopus* switch μ supported recombination in both orientations. The breakpoints were located in the AGCT palindrome-rich region of the switch box. Other motifs have been identified in the other switch regions, such as in IgX and chicken isotypes; all of these correspond to the DGYW hotspot consensus. AID-mediated deamidation in the context of these motifs may be the conserved major event in the initiation of CSR.

As mentioned, a single gene can encode different Ig forms, such as for duck IgY, cartilaginous fish IgW, and camel IgG loci (116). It has been suggested that the two avian IgY short and long forms could be the functional equivalents of both IgE and IgG, respectively; the same may be true of the cartilaginous fish IgW short and long forms with two and six domains, respectively. As mentioned, IgF or IgY' also falls into this category but not through alternative splicing (130).

V_H Evolution

Diversity of the immune repertoire depends on the variety of V segments inherited in the germline and on the further diversification by rearrangement (CDR3 only) and SHM (all CDR). Early in life the repertoire depends chiefly on the inheritable genes as one finds little N-region diversity and somatic mutation (with exceptions; see discussion later in this chapter). A central question is how antibody germline V genes diversify CDR during evolution while they are subject to homogenizing forces operating in most multigene families. Perhaps environmental antigens have played a major role in shaping the germline repertoire and have selected some V_H/V_L germline sequences used by neonates. V_H families arose in a bony fish lineage and have been conserved for hundreds of millions of years (138). Conserved regions defining families are found on solvent-exposed faces of the V_H, at some distance from the antibody-combining site. Phylogenetic analyses show clustering of V_H into groups A, B, C, D, and E. All cartilaginous fish V_H belong to the monophyletic group E; bony fish V_H genes cluster into all groups (one group [D] unique only to them). By contrast, group C includes bony fish sequences as well as V_H from all other classes except cartilaginous fish. Another phylogenetic analysis classifies mammalian V_H genes in three "clans" (I, II, and III), which have coexisted in the genome for >400 million years. Only in cartilaginous fish does it appear that V_H gene families have been subjected to concerted evolution that homogenized member genes (except for the IgM_{1gj} V region described earlier). It has been debated whether Ig V genes could be under direct positive selection, because these genes hypermutate somatically. However several features (e.g., codon bias) and discovery of high-replacement/silent ratios in germline gene CDR codons indeed argue for positive selection during evolution (139,140).

In summary, much of the V_H germline repertoire has been conserved over extremely long periods of vertebrate evolution. The birds and some mammalian species that rely on gut-associated lymphoid tissue (GALT) to generate Ig diversity (see the discussion later in this chapter) are exceptions with a reduced germline repertoire (at least expressed repertoire), but as will be seen later in this discussion, gene conversion and SHM compensate for this situation in formation of the primary repertoire. Even in the cartilaginous fish where there is a single V_H family, there is nevertheless heterogeneity in CDR1 and CDR2 sequences (as well as hypermutation) that must boost diversity in the expressed repertoire.

Ig Light Chains

L chains can be classified phylogenetically not only by their sequence similarity, but also by the orientation of their V and J RSS, which differ for mammalian λ and κ. There has been much debate regarding the affiliations of

L chains in various vertebrates, but as sequences have accumulated, a picture starts to emerge (141). Contrary to what was believed, the κ and λ L chains emerged early in vertebrate evolution, probably in the cartilaginous fish or placoderms (Figure 3.10). In addition, a third L chain, σ, originally described in *Xenopus* as a dead-end isotype, appears to be the ancestral clade and is present in all cold-blooded vertebrates.

Elasmobranchs have four L chain isotypes (types I, II, III, and IV), and the combined data suggest that they are present in all elasmobranchs. Type IV seems to be the ancestral group and is the orthologue of the unusual *Xenopus* σ L chain, and type I is a dead-end variant of this isotype called *σ-cart* (for cartilaginous fish). Type II L chains are the λ of birds, *Xenopus*, and mammals and have been cloned from sharks and skates; all genes of this isotype are "germline-joined." The type III is clearly κ-like, at least in the V region (and RSS orientation). These relationships are more noticeable in the V sequences, which have some defining characteristics such as CDR length; while the C sequences also fall into the same clusters, they do so with much less phylogenetic support (141). Different elasmobranch species express the L chain isotypes preferentially—for example, κ in nurse sharks, σ in horned sharks, and λ in sandbar sharks. This pattern of expression may be due to expansions/contractions of the different isotype genes in various elasmobranch lineages (142).

Almost all of the L chains in bony fish can be categorized as either κ or σ, despite the large number of gene expansions and contractions. Genes in different species can be found either in the cluster type organization, translocon, or some intermediate type ([143]; discussed later in this chapter). In some species, mAbs were produced that distinguish L chain classes, such as the F and G L chains of the catfish, which are both of the κ type but are quite divergent in sequence.

MAb studies suggested the existence of three *Xenopus* L chain isotypes of 25, 27, and 29 kD with heterogeneous 2D gel patterns and preferential association of some L chain isotypes with IgY H chains (142). Indeed, three *Xenopus* L chains genes have been isolated: ρ (now κ), σ, and λ. Only one C gene is present in the ρ locus, and it encodes the most abundant L chain. The V and J RSS are of the κ-type, and the five identified J segments are nearly identical (Figure 3.10). The locus is deleted, like mammalian κ, when the other isotype genes are rearranged. Southern hybridizations with genomic DNA from different animals showed V_L sequences to be both diverse and polymorphic. The third *X. laevis* L chain isotype predicted from the biochemical studies is related to mammalian λ genes and consists of six distinct V_L families. In the σ locus, the J segment has an unusual replacement of the diglycine bulge by two serines. The *Rana* major L chain type has an unusual intrachain disulfide bridge that is seemingly precludes covalent association of its H and L chains (142).

Two L chain types were identified in reptiles. Chickens and turkeys only express one L chain (λ) with a single functional V and J gene, and the manner by which diversity is generated is likely responsible for this unusual evolutionarily derived arrangement (discussed later). Nonproductive rearrangements are not detected on the unexpressed L chain allele, and thus there is a strong pressure to generate functional joints (discussed later). Such a system probably rendered a second (or third) L chain locus superfluous. Within mammals (marsupial *Monodelphis domestica*), the Vλ repertoire is composed of at least three diverse families related to distinct placental families, suggesting the divergence of these genes before the separation of metatherians and eutherians more than 100 million years ago. Opossum λJC sequences are phylogenetically clustered, as if these gene duplications were recent and the complexity of the λ locus seems greater than that found at the H chain locus (144).

In summary, all vertebrate groups except the birds have two to four L chain isotypes, all of which can be categorized as κ, λ, or σ (and in cartilaginous fish, σ-cart) (141). However, we are still at a loss to understand the significance of possessing multiple isotypes, because there is scant evidence that L chains have any effector functions. It has been suggested that different isotypes may provide distinct CDR conformations in association with H chains, or there may be L chain/H chain preferences that provide some advantage that is not obvious (145). At least the differential CDR sizes for σ as compared to κ/λ suggest that the former rationale is plausible.

The J Chain

The joining (J) chain is a small polypeptide, expressed by mucosal and glandular plasma cells, that regulates polymer formation of IgA and IgM. J chain incorporation into dimeric IgA and pentameric IgM endows these antibodies with the ability to be transported across epithelial cell barriers. J chain facilitates creation of the binding site for poly-Ig receptor (spIgR, secretory component in the Ig polymers), not only by regulating the polymeric structure, but apparently also by interacting directly with the receptor. Therefore, both the J chain and the pIgR/SC are key proteins in secretory immunity (146). Mouse IgM is synthesized as hexamers in the absence of J chain and as pentamers in its presence. Since some *Xenopus* EM studies suggested the existence of Ig hexamers, it was of interest to examine J chain conservation over evolutionary time. J chain cDNAs have been reported in all jawed vertebrates. The existence of *Xenopus* J chain suggests that, unlike mouse IgM, *Xenopus* IgM forms hexamers with J chain; alternatively the previous EM studies identified IgX as the hexameric isotype (the χ chain has a stop codon before the Cys of C_{H4} domain and thus cannot make a covalent attachment to J chain) (134). The highest level of J chain expression was detected in frog and bird intestine, correlating well with a role for J chain in mucosal immunity (although obviously not for IgX secretion). Elasmobranch J chain shows high similarity to the N-terminal half of J chains from other vertebrates but is divergent or even missing in the other regions (146). This result suggests that the function of J chain may be solely for IgM polymerization in elasmobranchs, and the transporting function arose later in evolution; consistent with this idea, *Xenopus,* but not shark, J chain is capable if interacting with human IgA and poly-Ig receptor. There was a claim for J chain's presence in many protostomic invertebrates since a homologue was cloned in earthworms (147), but no J chain sequences have appeared in any of the protostomes or deuterostome invertebrate databases (e.g., *C. elegans, Drosophila*).

Antigen Receptor Gene Organization

V_H Regions

A rearranged V_H gene consists of a leader (encoded by a split exon) followed by four framework regions and three CDRs (Figure 3.10). Canonical V_H CDR1 nucleotide sequences are conserved in all jawed vertebrates, likely as targets for SHM (148). A major germline difference is the lack of conserved octamers and TATA box in the 5′ region of shark Vs. In all species, functional V genes are assembled by rearrangement and joining of germline V, D, and J elements. Cartilaginous fish H chains are encoded by large numbers of clusters (>100 in horned shark; ~15 in the nurse shark) (116,149). For IgNAR, there are only four V regions/haploid genome, and only a few IgW V genes are detected in nurse sharks (but a large number in skates). In teleosts, seven V_H families have been characterized in the catfish, each containing up to 7 to 10 genes (most with open reading frames), and in the trout, 11 V_H families were identified. *Xenopus* has at least 11 V families, three of which ($V_{H1\text{-}3}$) contain 20 to 30 members and ~10% to 30% pseudogenes; the other families are smaller (one to eight genes), so the total number of functional V_H elements is ~90 to 100. Reptiles have very large pools of V_H segments: The turtle *Pseudemys scripta* has four families, with ~700 V_H/haploid genome (10% to 20% pseudogenes), and at least 125 genes homologous to the mouse V_H S107 gene were detected in another turtle species, *Chelydra serpentine*. Importantly, the V_H complexity does not seem to limit diversity of the antibody repertoire in any ectothermic vertebrate studied to date. There are actually fewer functional human V_H (44 functional, 79 pseudogenes that fall into seven families) than in many ectotherms. Dynamic reorganization of the H chain V regions seems to have occurred at least eight times between 133 million and 10 million years ago (138). Perhaps species that utilize somatic mutation/selection "optimally" rely less on germline diversity, and therefore fewer functional genes are required. Only ~10% of *Xenopus* V_H are pseudogenes in the three families ($V_{H1\text{-}3}$) that have been exhaustively studied; thus, *Xenopus,* with fewer lymphocytes, has a greater number of functional V_H genes than humans.

Chondrichthyan Germline-joined Genes

In all vertebrate species, functional Ig genes are assembled by rearranging DNA segments scattered on the chromosome. However, in cartilaginous fish, some V genes are the products of V(D)J rearrangement in eggs/sperm (9,116,150). Type I L chain (σ) genes are all germline-joined in skates but split in horned sharks, and the piecemeal germline joins (e.g., VD, VDD, VDDJ) found in many horned shark H chain gene clusters and in nurse shark L chain type I (σ) clusters strongly suggest that the germline-joining is a derived feature (Figure 3.10). Definitive proof came from a study of a germline-joined nurse shark type III (κ) L chain gene, shown by phylogenetic analysis to have been joined within the past 10 million years (150). When there is a *mixture* of joined and conventional genes, the split genes are expressed in adults, while the joined genes are expressed at significant levels only early in ontogeny. When *all* of the genes in a particular family are joined (e.g., skate type I L chain genes and type II (λ) L chains in all elasmobranchs), they continue to be expressed into adult life at high levels. In mammals, what may appear like germline-rearranged V genes are in most cases processed pseudogenes (e.g., pseudo $V\kappa$ on chromosome 22 in human or in mouse). However, it is possible that the surrogate L chain gene VpreB is the product of a germline-joining event in the line leading to mammals.

Organization of Rearranging Genes

As mentioned, shark IgH chain genes are structured into perhaps hundreds of clusters, each consisting of V, D, J, and C elements (116); all evidence from studies in horned shark, nurse shark, skate, and sandbar shark (and holocephalan ratfish) suggest that V, D, and J genes rearrange only within one cluster (Figure 3.10). While there is extensive N-region diversity and sometimes usage of two D segments (three Ds in IgNAR), and there are V_H subfamilies having substantial CDR1/2 heterogeneity, diversity of the primary repertoire is lower than in other vertebrates since there is no (or infrequent) rearrangement between clusters. The special constitution of the shark H and L chain loci suggests an exclusion mechanism similar to that of mouse TCR γ loci, also in clusters. It appears that only one V_H transcript is expressed in each lymphocyte, consistent with isotypic exclusion, despite the many clusters (151). Bony fish (teleosts and chondrosteans, such as the sturgeon), frogs, reptiles, and mammals have very similar architectures of their H chain locus—the so-called *translocon configuration* (Figure 3.10). As described earlier, multiple families of V_H genes, each consisting of many apparently functional elements (1 to 30 per family), are separated from a smaller number of genomic D and

J elements. The possibility of combinatorial rearrangement enables more diversification than is possible with the cartilaginous fish clusters for a given number of segments. In birds, the organization is similar but all V genes except those most 3′ to the D elements are pseudogenes (discussed later in this chapter).

L chain gene organization is more variable. In elasmobranchs, the organization is the same (i.e., in clusters) as the H chain locus without the D segments. The prototypic horned shark type I (σ) L chain has a cluster organization in which V, J, and C segments are closely linked. As mentioned earlier, bony fish L chain genes have the shark cluster-type organization, but some species have multiple V genes in some clusters, demonstrating that there is rapid evolution of not only sequence, but also gene organization in this taxon (143). In *Xenopus,* there are multiple Vκ(ρ) presumably derived from one family, 5J and a single C gene segment (152). In cartilaginous fish and birds, there has been coevolution of Ig gene architecture for H and L loci, but the teleosts have shown that this is not a rule.

D Segments

D segments are always present in one of the two loci encoding an Ig/TCR heterodimer (IgH and TCR β,δ), and the pressure that maintains this asymmetry is unknown. Cartilaginous fish have one or two D genes/H chain clusters, and there are only minor variations among the clusters. In teleosts, amphibians, and reptiles, where the organization of the H chain locus is similar to humans, the number of Ds deduced from cDNAs ranges from 10 to 16. Two germline D segments have been identified in *Xenopus,* and their RSS follow the rules defined in mammals. In birds, there are 15 very similar D_H.

There are several reasons why D segments may have been preserved throughout evolution. Incorporation of D segments augments CDR3 diversity and size, obviously directly influencing the combining site (116,134). Three different Ds contribute to IgNAR CDR3, and besides generating great diversity, CDR3 length and amino acid composition fulfills special tertiary structure requirements: D-encoded cysteine residues bond with cysteine(s) in the body of the V domain, thereby stabilizing a loop involved in the antigen-binding of this unusual monomeric receptor (123). A similar situation has been reached by convergence in the monomeric variant of camel IgG. Finally, rearrangement of one locus "locks it in" and allows the second locus to undergo receptor editing, as is the case for negative selection of the B cell repertoire and positive selection of the T cell repertoire.

Major Histocompatibility Complex

T cells distinguish self from nonself through the presentation of small peptides bound to MHC class I and class II molecules (i.e., MHC restriction). The genetic restriction of T cell–APC collaboration, processing of antigen by professional APCs, and T cell education in the thymus described in mice hold true (or is assumed) for most vertebrate classes (153). No MHC-regulated T cell responses have been documented in cartilaginous fish, but the identification of polymorphic class I and II and rearranging TCRα/β genes (discussed earlier) strongly suggest that functional analyses will reveal MHC restriction of adaptive responses. Similarly, urodele amphibians are notorious for their poor immune responses (discussed later in this chapter), and biochemical and molecular evidence suggests that class II polymorphism is low in the axolotl. In addition, like the cod, axolotls have very high numbers of expressed class I loci, which might play into their poor adaptive immunity.

Class I/II Structure Through Evolution

The three-dimensional organizations of class I and class II are remarkably similar: The two membrane-distal domains of both molecules form a peptide-binding region (PBR) composed of two antiparallel α helices resting on a floor of eight β strands, and the two membrane-proximal domains are IgSF C1. Although sequence identity among class I and class II genes in vertebrates is low (like most other immune genes), the four extracellular domain organization and other conserved features are likely to be found in the ancestral class I/II gene (154). An intrachain disulfide bridge exists within the class I PBR α2 and class IIβ1 domains, but not the class I/II PBR α1 domains, and phylogenetic trees show that these respective domains are most similar (Figure 3.11). Bony fish class II α1 domains, like class II DMα molecules that are as old as the *bona fide* class II genes, do have a disulfide bridge. The exon/intron structure of class I and class II extracellular domains is also well conserved, but some teleosts have acquired an intron in the exon encoding the IgSF β2 domain. Other conserved features of class I genes include a glycosylation site on the loop between the α1 and α2 domains (shared with class II β chains), a Tyr, and one to three Ser in the cytoplasmic regions that can be phosphorylated in mammals, as well as several stabilizing ionic bonds. Class II, with its two TM regions, differs from class I with only one; conserved residues in the class II α and β TM/cytoplasmic regions facilitate dimerization. In summary, because sequence similarity is very low among MHC genes in different taxa, these conserved features are important for function and maintenance of structure (154).

β2m was the second IgSF molecule (C1-type) ever to be identified, originally found at high levels in the urine of patients with kidney disease. It associates with most class I molecules (discussed later in this chapter). Besides mammals, β2m genes have been cloned from representatives of all vertebrate classes except cartilaginous fish. The β2m gene is outside the MHC in all species tested and is a single-copy gene in all species except cod and trout, in which it

```
                     S1                S2           S3          S4    H1                H2
                  ---------          -----        ------      ----- ------ ----------------------------
PBR                  Y-7                                                    Y-59                    Y/R-84
HLA-A2a-1     --GSHSMRYFFTSVSRPGRGEPRFIAVGYVDDTQFVRFDSDAASGRMEPRAPWIEQEGPEYWDGETRKVKAHSQTHRVDLGTLRGYYNQSEA
DR1a-1        IKEEHVIIQAEFYLNPD----QSGEFMFDFDGDEIFHVDM------AKKETVWRLEEFGRFASFEAQGALANIAVDKANLEIMTKRSNYTPITN
                                                                            F S-53     N-62   N-69      ===

                        S1             S2            S3      S4            H1          H2            H3
                     ---------      ---------       ----    ----         ------    ----------  ----------------
PBR                    101#                                              T  KW-146,7        164#        Y-171
HLA-A2a-2     ----GSHTVQRMYGCDVGSDWRFLRGYHQYAYDGKDYIALKEDLRSWTAADMAAQTTKHKWEAA-HVAEQLRAYLEGTCVEWLRRYLENGKETLQRT
DR1b-1        GDTRPRFLWQLKFECHFFNGTERVRLLERCIYNQEESVRFDSDVGEYRAVTELGRPDAEYWNSQKDLLEQRRAAVDTYCRHNYGVGESFTVQRR
                        15#    ===                                       W-61                79# HN-81,2

                   S1(A)            S2(B)         S3(C             S4(D)        S5(E)          S6(F        S7(G)
                  -------          ---------      -----           -------      -------        -------      -----
C-1 Igsf             P                L C     FYP     W   NG                                P   Y C V H     P
HLA-A2a-3     --DAPKTHM--THHAVSDHEATLRCWALSFYPAEITLTWQRDGEDQTQDTELVETRPAGDGTFQKWAAVVVPSGQEQRYTCHVQHEGLPKPLTLR
DR1a-2        --VPPEVTVLTNSPVELREPNVLICFIDKFTPPVVNVTWLRNGKPVTTGVSETVFLPREDHLFRKFHYLPFLPSTEDVYDCRVEHWGLDEPLTKHW----
DR1b-2        --VHPKVTVYPSKTQPLQHHNLLVCSVSGFYPGSIEVRWFRNGQEEKTGVVSTGLIHNGDWTFQTLVMLETVPRSGEVYTCQVEHPSVTSPLTVEW----
b2m           IQRTPKIQVYSRHPAENGKSNFLNCYVSGFHPSDIEVDLLKNGERIEK-VEHSDLSFSKDWSFYLLYYTEFTPTEKDEYACRVNHVTLSQPKIVKWDRDM

TM/CYT        CON. PIECE      TRANSMEMBRANE              CYTOPLASMIC
HLA-A2        EPSSQPTIP       IVGIIAGLVLFGAVITGAVVAAV    MWRRKSSDRKGGSYSQAASSDSAQGSDVSLTACKV
DR1a          EFDAPSPLPETTE   NVVCALGLTVGLVGIIIGTIFII    KGVRKSNAAERRGP
DR1b          RARSESAQSK      MLSGVGGFVLGLLFLGAGLFI      YFRNQKGHSGLQPRGFLS
```

FIGURE 3.11 Amino acid residues conserved in classical class I and class II molecules in all jawed vertebrates. Displayed are sequences of HLA-A2 and DR1, for which crystal structures are available (309,310). Bold residues are found in the majority of classical class I/II sequences (or all but one class). Residues above the alignment for class I PBR a-1 and a-2 (Y-7, Y-59, Y/R-84, T-123, K-146, W-147, Y-171; note that Y-84 is invariant in mammals but R in all other vertebrates), and below the alignments for class II PBR a-1 and a-2 (Fa-53, Sa-55, Na-62, Na-69, Wb-61, Hb-78, Nb-82) are invariant residues that bind to mainchain atoms of acquired peptides. For the IgSF C1 domains, residues above the alignment are conserved in C1 set domains (17). Double-underlined residues are conserved glycosylation sites. Cysteines in the class I a-2 and class II b-1 that form conserved PBR disulfide bonds are indicated. Strands (S) and helices (H) for the PBR and strands for the IgSF domains are displayed. Figure modified from Kaufman et al (154).

has undergone multiple duplications. Based on the levels of similarity between the various domains of class I and class II, it is expected that β2m was originally encoded in the MHC and may still be present in some extant vertebrates (154).

Classical and Nonclassical Class I and Class II

Class Ia (classical) and class Ib (nonclassical) genes are found in all of the major groups of jawed vertebrates. Class Ia genes are defined by their ubiquitous expression, their presence in the MHC proper, and by high polymorphism. In addition, class Ia proteins almost always have eight conserved residues at both ends of the PBR that interact with "mainchain" atoms of bound peptides and constrain their size to eight or nine residues; this feature often distinguishes class Ia from class Ib (discussed later in this chapter). Thus, tight binding of peptides, a likely source of conformational changes in class I allowing transport through the ER and cell surface expression, is an evolutionarily conserved trait (155). In nonmammalian vertebrates, one of these residues at the C-terminus is lysine rather than tyrosine, the functional significance of which is unclear (154).

The class Ia/Ib distinction holds in most taxa: One to three polymorphic class Ia genes are expressed ubiquitously in most species, while other minimally polymorphic or monomorphic class Ib genes can be expressed in a tissue-specific fashion. The class Ib genes can be split into two major groups: one set that is most related to the class Ia genes within a taxon and thus recently derived, and one group that is ancient and emerged near the origin of the adaptive immune system. In mouse and human, the set most closely related to class Ia genes are closely linked within the MHC. In nonmammalian vertebrates, however, this first set are found in gene clusters on the same chromosome as the MHC proper but far enough away to segregate independently from MHC—for example, chicken (*Rfpy*) and *Xenopus* (*XNC*) (153). One *Xenopus* class Ib gene is expressed specifically in the lung and thus likely has a specialized function, and chicken Rfpy is associated with resistance to pathogens. Class Ib genes related but unlinked to the classical class I have also been found in bony and cartilaginous fish, and quite recently a lineage of class II–linked class I genes was discovered in bony fish (discussion later in this chapter for significance; (156). Thus, class Ib genes that arise in each taxon seem to have true class I–like functions, but perhaps have become specialized (sometimes the distinction between class Ia and class Ib is blurry; see the discussion later in the chapter) (157). The second set of older class Ib genes that predates divergence of taxa can have very different functions. For example, the neonatal Fc receptor (FCRN) is involved in binding and transport of IgG molecules across epithelia as well as protecting them from degradation (the Brambell receptor). Further, molecules only described so far in mouse/human are composed only of a PBR without IgSF domains; these unusual class I molecules do not bind peptides but rather are important for the regulation of NK and T cell function during infection. The paradigm for these SOS responses is the MIC class Ib molecule, which does have an IgSF domain but clearly does not bind peptides. Some teleost class Ib genes that fall outside the major cluster of fish class I genes may fit into this category (158,159). Finally, molecules like CD1 bind nonpeptidic antigens for presentation to innatelike NK-T cells. The phylogenetic analysis predicts that CD1 and FcRN are old class I genes, which may be present today in all vertebrates (however, discussion later in this chapter about CD1); the age revealed by the phylogenetic tree also correlates well with the hypothesis that ancient duplication events predating the emergence of jawed vertebrates resulted in the appearance of CD1, FcRN, and MHC-linked class I genes (see discussion later in this chapter). Was the original function of class I linked to antigen presentation (peptidic or otherwise), induction of an SOS response, or to housekeeping functions? We do not currently have the answer, because class Ia and class Ib molecules are just as ancient. The discovery of class I–like genes in animals derived from ancestors predating adaptive immunity (if such genes exist) will help resolve this question, but to date no recognizable MHC molecules or their kin have been detected in pre-jawed vertebrates (32).

Class II molecules also have nearly invariant residues that bind to main chain atoms of peptides, but these are in the center of the groove (Figure 3.11). Thus, tight binding to main chain peptide atoms occurs in the center of the class II PBR, and peptides are free to protrude from both ends (154). The only nonclassical class II molecules so far identified are the previously mentioned DM molecules that lack these residues. Thus far, DM molecules have been cloned only from tetrapods and have not been detected in any fish species, despite the large genomic and EST databases for the bony fish (160). Thus, they either had not emerged at the time fish arose or were lost in the bony fish lineage; phylogenetic trees suggest the latter and would be consistent with the rapid rate of genome evolution in the teleosts (161,162).

Polymorphism of MHC Class I and Class II Genes

High levels of polymorphism and genetic diversity are characteristic of most classical MHC genes, in fact the highest of any gene family studied to date. MHC variation among taxa has been derived via mutation, gene conversion, and recombination, and alleles are formed over evolutionary time. However, it is the retention of ancient allelic lineages through selection that accounts for the high levels of diversity observed within species (163). The repertoire of antigens recognized by MHC alleles is determined by the amino acids in the PBR, such that different MHC alleles recognize different sets of peptide derivatives. Although even minor alterations of the anchor residues in the PBR can drastically change the peptide binding capacity of an MHC molecule, in general, MHC alleles that differ by only a few amino acids can overlap considerably in their peptide binding repertoires, while highly divergent alleles bind unique sets of peptides. The differential binding capacities of MHC alleles form the basis of two models of balancing selection proposed to account for the extreme diversity observed at MHC. Overdominance, or heterozygote advantage, assumes that heterozygous individuals are capable of binding a wider array of pathogenic peptides than homozygous individuals; hence, they should be selectively favored (164). Alternately, negative frequency-dependent selection is based on the premise that a coevolutionary arms race between host MHC and pathogens exists, resulting in the development of escape mechanisms by pathogens to common MHC alleles and according an advantage to rare alleles (165). Although numerous individual studies exist providing support for one or the other of these selective mechanisms, from a population genetics standpoint, they give very similar theoretical results and are difficult to distinguish.

MHC Gene Organization

As mentioned earlier, because class I and class II proteins are structurally similar, it is no surprise that their genes are linked, a primordial trait subsequently lost only in bony fish. But why are structurally unrelated class I processing genes, including the immune proteasome components *lmp2* and *lmp7* and the *TAP* genes, also found in the MHC? There are two possible scenarios: primordial linkage of ancestral processing and presenting genes in the MHC or later recruitment of either the processing/presenting genes into a primordial MHC. Based on the presence of similar clusters of MHC genes on paralogous chromosomal regions in humans and mice, Kasahara et al. (7,166) proposed that ancestors of class I, class II, proteasome, transporter, and class III genes were already linked before the emergence of the adaptive immune system (Figures 3.12, 3.13). Genomewide duplications around the time of the origin of vertebrates (the 2R hypothesis), as proposed by Ohno (167), may have provided the raw material from which the immune system genes was assembled

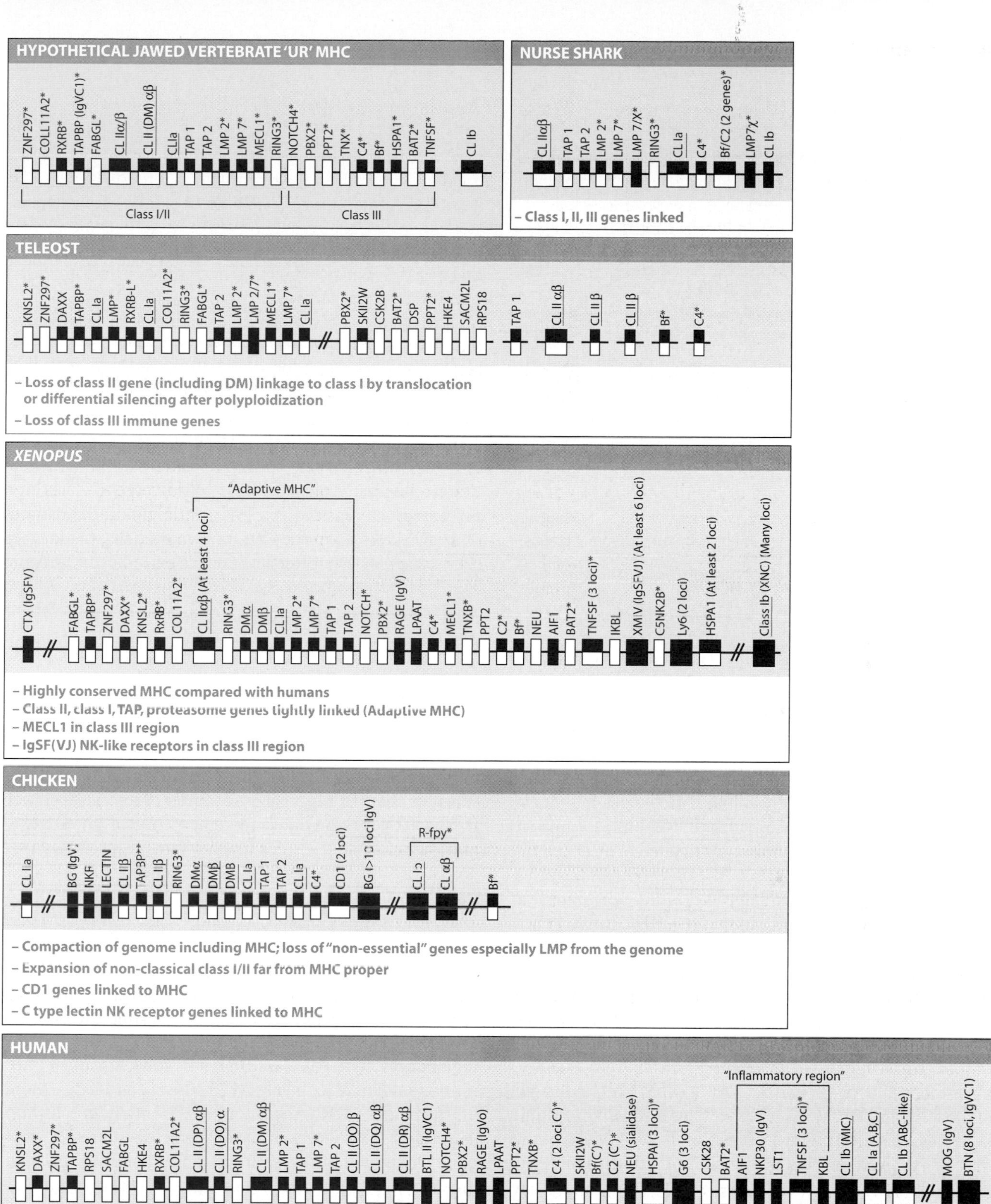

FIGURE 3.12 MHC evolution. White indicates that the gene is found in at least one other species besides human; black designates a gene with known or inferred immune function; asterisk indicates an ancestral gene found on at least two paralogous MHC regions in mammals; large box indicates at least two genes in the particular region; double slash indicates linkage far away on the same chromosome; space between lines indicates that the genes are on different linkage groups. The teleost MHC is a composite of the zebrafish, trout, *Fugu*, and medakafish maps. Extensively modified from (153,311).

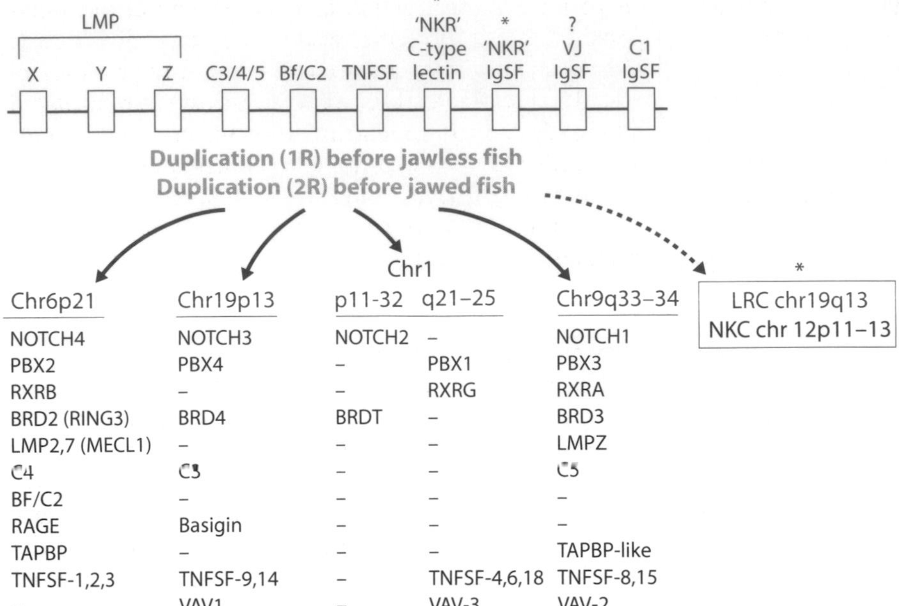

FIGURE 3.13 Genomewide duplication (2R) model of MHC evolution. Displayed are the MHC paralogous regions and their human chromosomal designations, first identified by Kasahara (7,166). Note that such paralogous regions have also been studied for chemokine receptors (259), TNF and TNF receptors (312), and IgSF molecules involved in cell-cell interactions and costimulation (11). Asterisks indicate that NK cell receptors (NKR) of the IgSF and C-type lectin categories from the NKC and LRC, respectively, are likely to have been in the Ur MHC based on linkages seen today in various taxa. VJ and C1 genes noted in the Ur MHC were likely related to the antigen receptor ancestor.

(discussed later in this chapter). As for all other adaptive immune genes described so far, neither class I/II nor immunoproteasome/TAP have been isolated from hagfish nor lampreys, and all of these genes as well as other genes involved in immunity could have emerged as a consequence of the duplications. Because class I genes are found on two or three of the clusters, class I–like molecules may have predated class II in evolution. Indeed, NK-like recognition of a class I or class I–like molecule encoded in an ancestral linkage group may have been at the origin of the adaptive immune system (discussed later in this chapter).

TAP is an interesting case in that the MHC-linked genes were clearly not part of the Ur MHC, but rather they were "recruited" to the MHC early in evolution. TAPs are members of the very large ABC transporter family and are most closely related to bacterial ABC transporters; this suggests that TAP1/2 were derived from a bacterial, or more likely a mitochondrial, gene, via horizontal transfer (168). Further, a close homologue of TAP1/2, TAP-L (TAP-like), unlike all of the other Ig/TCR/MHC genes we have discussed, is found in jawless fish (169). TAP-L's function is not known, but it may be involved in cross presentation (170). In summary, the TAP genes are not following any of the "rules" that seem to hold true for the other genes involved in adaptive immunity. This story will be exciting to monitor.

In all nonmammalian vertebrates, and even in marsupials (171), the imunoproteasome and TAP genes are closely linked to class I genes, not to class II, in a true "class I region." This result is most striking in bony fish (*Fugu*, zebrafish, medaka, trout), because class I/lmp/TAP/TAPBP and class II are found on different chromosomes (153,162; Figure 3.12). The class III region, historically defined by the innate immune genes such as Bf/C2, and C4 are also present in the *Xenopus* and elasmobranch MHC, showing that association of class I/II with such genes is ancient (160). If Kasahara's interpretation is correct—that is, that MHC syntenic groups found on different mammalian chromosomes resulted from ancient block duplications—it is expected that the physical association of ancestral class I, II, and III genes predated the emergence of jawed vertebrates, and such syntenies in ectothermic vertebrates are not surprising (Figures 3.12, 3.13). Indeed, linkage studies in nonvertebrates amphioxus and *Ciona* do support an ancient linkage of class I, II, and III genes (172). Taken together, the data reveal that lack of synteny of class I, class II, and class III genes in teleosts is a derived character (161). Independent assortment of class I and class II may allow these genes to evolve at different rates: In some telesots, class Ia alleles form ancient, slowly evolving lineages, whereas class II genes evolve at similar rates as mammalian MHC alleles (173,174).

The chicken MHC, the B complex, is on a microchromosome, and intron sizes and intergenic distances are both quite small so that the entire complex is only a few hundred kb as compared to more than 4,000 kb in humans and *Xenopus*. Class Ia (BF), class IIβ (BL and DM), and TAP genes are in the MHC, but there is no evidence for immunoproteasome genes, and almost all class III genes have been deleted except for C4 (175). The quail MHC is similar, although is somewhat expanded, especially in genes related to the C-type lectin NK receptors (176). Although most class III genes are found on other chromosomes, *lmp2/7* and *MECL1* genes are actually absent from the genome; indeed, peptides bound to chicken class I molecules sometimes have C-terminal glutamic acid or aspartic acid, which are rare after proteolysis by mammalian proteasomes containing lmp2 and lmp7. To explain the correlation of diseases with particular haplotypes, Kaufman proposed that the chicken has a minimal essential MHC composed of only those genes absolutely required to remain in the complex. This concept has been reenforced recently by an analysis of resistance to viral infection (Rous sarcoma virus) governed by classical class I molecules (177).

Surprisingly, CD1 genes are closely linked to the chicken MHC (178,179). As mentioned earlier, CD1 genes in mammals seem to be on one of the MHC paralogous regions, and it was suggested that it arose as a consequence of the *en bloc* duplication (see Figure 3.13). While this is still possible (i.e., there was differential silencing of CD1 and other class I genes on the two paralogous chromosomes), the more likely scenario is that CD1 arose by gene duplication within the MHC itself in an ancestor of warm-blooded vertebrates; no *bona fide* CD1 genes have been detected to date in any fish or amphibians.

In summary, in all animals except placental mammals, classical class I genes map closely to the *TAP* and *lmp* genes, suggesting that the processing, transport, and presenting genes were in an original "class I region" (153,180). The tight linkage of the functionally, but not structurally, related genes strongly suggests that such genes coevolve within particular MHC haplotypes. Indeed, in *Xenopus* there are biallelic lineages of class Ia, LMP7, and TAP that are always found as a set in wild-caught animals. Although teleosts underwent an explosive adaptive radiation 100 million years ago and primordial syntenies have been lost in many cases (162), there are deep lineages of class Ia genes in many species, also found for *Xenopus* and cartilaginous fish class Ia genes. A recent study in medaka suggests that divergent noncoding regions between the class I processing and presenting genes do not permit recombination between lineages, hence preserving the linkage disequilibrium (181). In (most) eutherian mammals, the class I region is not closely linked to lmp/TAP and is very unstable, with rapid duplications/deletions expected in a multigene complex; the same class I instability extends to the non-MHC linked class Ib genes in *Xenopus* species.

Class I/II Expression

In *Xenopus* species, immunocompetent larvae express high levels of class II on APCs such as B cells, but express only very low levels of class Ia molecules on hematopoietic cells until metamorphosis. Expression of the immunoproteasome element *lmp7* and all identified class Ib isotypes is also very low. Larval skin and gut, organs with epithelia in contact with the environment, appear to coexpress class I (transcripts) and class II (182). Such expression may provide immune protection during larval life; perhaps expression of class Ia is limited to organs that undergo massive destruction and remodeling at metamorphosis. Class II molecules also change their distribution after metamorphosis and are highly expressed by unstimulated T cells. Axolotl class II molecules are also regulated differentially during ontogeny, expressed in young animals on B cells and then expanding to all hematopoietic cells, including erythrocytes, later in life. Changes in MHC expression are not correlated with cryptic metamorphosis in axolotls, but class II expression by erythrocytes is correlated to the switch from larval to adult globins. Unlike *Xenopus*, class I transcripts isolated so far are expressed early in ontogeny, from hatching onward.

Carp class I and class II transcripts are detected in embryos 1 day after fertilization and reach a plateau at day 14. However, the suspected class Ia protein does not appear until week 13, whereas $\beta 2$m can be detected several weeks earlier (183). It was suggested that another class I molecule is expressed during early development of the carp hematopoietic system, perhaps one of the unusual nonclassical molecules that groups outside the teleost cluster. Interestingly, recent work has shown that class I is expressed in the brain of young, but not adult fish, suggesting that class I molecules may play a role in neurogenesis (184).

Lymphoid Tissues and Cells of Jawed Vertebrates

Hematopoisis and Transcription Factors

As mentioned earlier, transcription factors of the family PAX 2/5/8, GATA 1,2,3, ets/erg, and runt domain-containing factors have been cloned in several invertebrates (Figure 3.4). One plausible model to explain the genesis of true lymphocytes in vertebrates is that closely related members of transcription factor families are the result of a relatively late divergence in lineage pathways followed by specialization of duplicated genes (185). These duplications could be those that apparently occurred during the history of chordates (see MHC and "origins" section). Within deuterostomes, the generation of true GATA 2 and 3 probably occurred after echinoderms diverged from the chordate branch and the GATA, ets, EBF, Pax5 dependent pathways of T/B cell differentiation are thus specific to vertebrates. It is already known that lampreys express a member of the purine box 1 (PU.1)/spleen focus-forming virus integration-B (Spi-B) gene family that is critically and specifically involved in jawed vertebrate lymphocyte differentiation. Expression has been detected in the gut, which may be related to the fundamental nature of "GALT" as a lymphoid cell-producing organ (see Figure 3.14).

In vertebrates, the generation of T, B and NK lymphocyte lineages from pluripotent hematopoietic stem cells depends on the early and tissue-specific expression of *Ikaros* (and related loci), which by means of alternative splicing produces a variety of zinc finger DNA-binding

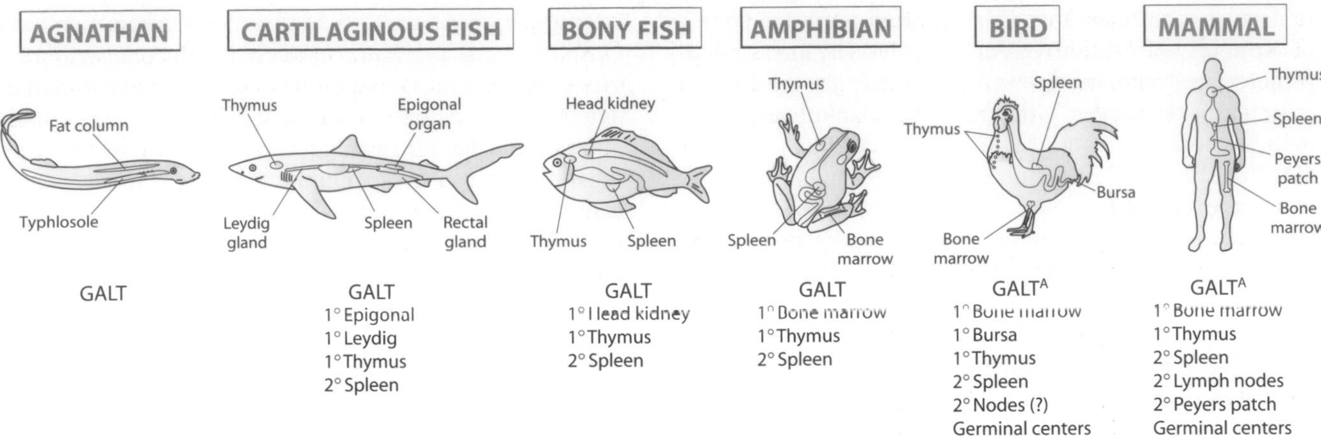

FIGURE 3.14 Evolution of lymphoid tissues in the vertebrates. All jawed vertebrates have a thymus and a spleen with demarcated T and B cell zones. Fish have different bone marrow equivalents (Epigonal, Leydig, head kidney), and amphibians are the oldest group with lymphopoietic bone marrow (also the fist to have a typical IgH chain class switch). Germinal centers are found only in warm-blooded vertebrates, see (134,189).

transcription factors. The orthologues of *Ikaros*, *Aiolos*, *Helios*, and *Eos* have been identified in the skate *Raja eglanteria*, where two of the four *Ikaros* family members are expressed in their specialized hematopoietic tissues (epigonal and Leydig organs; discussed later), like in mammals (186). An *Ikaros*-related gene has been identified in the lamprey *P. marinus*, in which neither Ig nor TCRs have been identified. In lower deuterostomes, single genes that seem to be related to the ancestor of the Ikaros and Ets family of transcription factors exist, further suggesting that the division of labor between the family members in the jawed vertebrates was a result of en bloc duplications (187,188). The conservation of *Ikaros* structure and expression reinforces its role as a master switch of hematopoiesis.

Lymphoid Tissues

In addition to the molecules and functions characteristic of adaptive immunity, primary (lymphocyte-generating) and secondary (immune response-generating) lymphoid tissues also define the specific immune system (134,189). The thymus is present in all jawed vertebrates, but not in the jawless fish, further solidifying the lack of (at least) conventional T cells outside the gnathostomes. *All* animals have hematopoietic cell-generating tissues (Figures 4.4, 4.14), and outside of the so-called *GALT species,* B cells develop in such bone marrow equivalents in all jawed vertebrates. With the advent of clonal selection, the accumulation and segregation of T and B cells in specialized organs for antigen presentation became necessary, and indeed the spleen is found in all jawed vertebrates, but not in agnathans or invertebrates. As mentioned earlier, if there is only one type of lymphocyte in agnathans that expresses VLR genes, then regulation by other cell types may not be required to initiate immune responses (i.e., the agnathans may be an example of a B cell–only system regulated cell autonomously through the antigen-specific receptor and costimulatory receptors).

All vertebrate species rearrange their antigen receptor genes (except the case mentioned earlier for some cartilaginous fish germline-joined genes [9,190]). Besides rearrangement, with combinatorial joining of gene segments and imprecision of the joins, there are two other sources of diversity to generate the repertoires: the TdT enzyme that modifies boundaries of rearranging gene segments, and somatic mutations, found exclusively in B cells usually introduced during immune responses (9,134). However, progression of rearrangement during B and T cell development and diversification follow different rules in different vertebrates. It is conceivable that species hatching early with just a few lymphocytes are under pressures to develop a rapid response and may not use the same mechanisms as species protected by the mother's uterine environment. It is also possible that immune systems of species with few offspring are under stronger pressures than species that have many offspring, and this could be reflected in the manner diversity is generated. Studies of B and T cell differentiation have been performed in many vertebrates. RAG and TdT genes have been cloned in representatives of many classes, probes that allow the monitoring of lymphocyte development (discussed later in the chapter). Reagents have become available, permitting an accurate monitoring of T cell appearance in the lymphoid organs of ectotherms (crossreactive anti-CD3 sera or TCR probes), as well as mAbs and gene probes specific for Ig H/L chains that allow examination of B cells. As a rule, the thymus is the first organ to become lymphoid during development. Another emerging rule is that development of the thymus-dependent MHC-restricted T cell repertoire is similar in all species, and this is reflected in the evolution of TCR gene organization described earlier; in contrast, B cell repertoire generation differs dramatically among different species, at times even within the same class of vertebrates (9,134).

Cartilaginous Fish

Like all other major adaptive immune system components, cartilaginous fish are the first in evolution to possess a thymus originating from pharyngeal pouches (191). As in mammals, it has a distinct cortex/medulla structure, and terminal deoxyribonucleotidyl transferase (TdT) expression was detected in thymocytes with crossreactive antisera and more recently by northern blotting. Interestingly, unlike all other vertebrates, age is not an indicator as to the size of the cartilaginous fish thymus; it can be small or large at any stage of development. GALT is also important in elasmobranchs, but lymphoid tissue in the spiral valve (intestine) does not have typical secondary lymphoid tissue structure; the spleen is the only tissue with compartmentalization of cells into discrete T cell and B cell zones (192). The Leydig and epigonal organs (associated with the gonads) are lymphopoietic and erythropoietic, producing mainly granulocytes and lymphocytes and there is high RAG expression in these tissues (discussed later). Lymphocytes form nodules in the epigonal organ, probably indicative of differentiative events.

During dogfish development, the liver is the first tissue to contain Ig^+ cells at 2 months, followed by the interstitial kidney at 3 months (193). The thymus, spleen, and Leydig organ appear at 4 months, and the epigonal organ and the GALT are the last tissues to differentiate. The hematopoietic/lymphoid nature of the kidney and thymus disappears after hatching, whereas the other lymphomyeloid tissues persist through adult life. At hatching, when embryos are exposed to waterborne antigens, structural development of the lymphomyeloid tissues is well advanced. In the nurse shark, neonatal spleen white pulp consists entirely of class II-negative B cells; by 5 months after birth, T cell zones containing class II dendritic–like cells appear adjacent to the B cell zones. Both the B cell and T cell zones are vascularized, and no detectable marginal zone separates red pulp from white pulp (192).

In the skate *Raja eglanteria,* Ig and TCR expression is sharply upregulated relatively late in development (8 weeks). At this age TCR and TdT expression is limited to the thymus; later, TCR gene expression appears in peripheral sites in hatchlings and adults (194). IgM expression is first detected in the spleen of young skates but IgW is expressed first in gonad, liver, Leydig organ, and thymus. In adults, Leydig organ and spleen are sites of the highest IgM and IgW expression. In nurse sharks, 19S IgM appears in the serum before 7S IgM and IgNAR, and this profile is reflected in the lack of $IgNAR^+$ cells in the spleen until 2 months after birth. RAG and TdT expression in the thymus and epigonal organ of the nurse shark suggests that lymphopoiesis is ongoing in adult life. In contrast to most other vertebrates, N-region diversity is detected in skate and nurse shark IgM and IgNAR CDR3 from the earliest stages analyzed, suggesting that a full-blown diverse repertoire is important for young elasmobranchs (192). As mentioned earlier, a subset of Ig genes is pre-rearranged in the germline of chondrichthyans, and many of those germline-joined genes are transcribed in the embryo and hatchling, but not in the adult. This pattern fits with the expression of the nurse shark IgM_{1gj} with its germline-joined V region and suggests that some germline-joined genes "take advantage" of their early transcriptional edge, and thus some clusters can be selected for specialized tasks in early development. With many gene clusters, it is not known how "clusteric exclusion" is achieved at the molecular level (and why the germline-joined gene expression is extinguished in adult life), but as mentioned earlier, preliminary experiments suggest that only one H chain cluster is expressed in each lymphocyte (151).

The architecture of cartilaginous fish Ig loci allows greatest diversity only in CDR3, because the CDR2 and CDR1 are always encoded in the germline and V segments do not combine with (D)J segments from other clusters. Yet the number of possible CDR3 is essentially limitless, and the number of germline clusters is also high (at least 15 genes in each species; and usually 3 rearrangement events take place since 2 D segments are in each cluster). Thus, the potential diversity is greater than the number of lymphocytes, a general rule for generation of diversity in the vertebrates.

Bony Fish

The teleost thymus gland originates from the pharyngeal pouches and can be uni-, bi-, or trilobed, depending on the species (195). It is the first organ to become lymphoid, and its structure may differ from species to species. The cortex/medulla architecture is not as precise in other vertebrate species, but the duality of the compartment is apparent. The spleen contains the basic elements seen in other vertebrates—blood vessels, red pulp, and white pulp—but the distinction between red and white pulp is less obvious (the white pulp being poorly developed). In the spleen, the ellipsoids, which are actually terminal capillaries, have a thin endothelial layer surrounded by fibrous reticulum and an accumulation of cells, mainly macrophages. Lymphocyte accumulations are often seen in their vicinity, especially during immune responses, which have been suggested to be primitive germinal centers, but they are not homologous. Red pulp is rich in melanomacrophage centers, groups of pigment-containing cells at bifurcations of large blood vessels, which may regulate immune responses. The other main lymphoid organ is head kidney, believed to function as mammalian bone marrow. The transparent zebrafish is being developed as a new model to study T cell differentiation (196).

In the sea bass *Dicentrarchus labrax,* a mAb detects differentiating T cells (perhaps pre-T cells) as well as mature T cells, as evidenced by the presence of TCR mRNA in the sorted populations. Cells seem to migrate from surrounding mesenchyme and subsequently mature in the thymus like in all vertebrates studied so far. T cells appear earlier in ontogeny (between 5 and 12 days after hatching) than cytoplasmic Ig^+ pre-B cells, which are detected only at 52 days post-hatching. Adult levels of T and B cells are reached between 137 and 145 days after hatching, quite a long time compared to young amphibians. In all teleosts examined, the thymus is the primary organ for T lymphocyte generation and head kidney the primary organ for B cell development (197).

RAG1 of the trout *Oncorhynchus mykiss* differs from mammalian RAG1 genes by the presence of an intron of 666 bp (an intron is also found in the sea urchin RAG1 gene in a similar position, [32]). Compared with other RAG1 sequences, trout RAG1 has a minimum of 78% similarity for the complete sequence and 89% similarity in the conserved region (aa 417-1042). RAG1 transcripts are detected chiefly in thymus, pronephros, mesonephros, spleen, and intestine starting at day 20 after fertilization. Trout TdT is highly expressed within the thymus and to a lesser extent in the pronephros beginning at 20 days post-fertilization, which correlates with the appearance of these two tissues. Because the H chain cluster is in the translocon configuration and there are many V_H families, it is assumed that diversity is generated in the mouse/human mode.

The best studies of mature B cell activation and homing have been done in trout (198,199). Immunization of animals results in the production of short-term Ig-secreting cells in the blood and spleen and long-lived plasma cells in the head kidney. Further analysis with B cell–specific transcription factors like PAX5 and BLIMP1 reinforced the previously noted functional studies and showed that the blood contains primarily "resting" B cells and the head kidney both plasma cells and B cell precursors. These last findings appear to be true of the cartilaginous fish as well, with the epigonal organ as the head kidney primary lymphoid tissue equivalent (Flajnik, unpublished). Interestingly, recent studies have shown trout (and other ectothermic) B cells to be quite efficient at phagocytosis, raising questions about myeloid/lymphoid lineage commitment in the vertebrates (200).

Amphibians

In anurans, the thymus develops from the dorsal epithelium of the visceral pouches (the number of pouches varies with species) and is the first tissue to become lymphopoietic (201). It is colonized from days 6/7 onward by precursors derived from lateral plate and ventral mesoderm through the head mesenchyme. Precursors proliferate *in situ* as the epithelium begins to express MHC class II molecules but not classical class I molecules. By day 8, thymic cortex/medulla architecture resembles that of other vertebrates. Amphibians possess a spleen with red and white pulp, GALT with no organized secondary lymphoid tissue, and many nodules (but no lymph nodes), with lymphopoietic activity in the kidney, liver, mesentery, and gills. The general morphology of lymphoid organs varies greatly according to species and changes with the season. In *Xenopus,* splenic white pulp is delineated by a boundary layer, and the central arteriole of the white pulp follicle terminates in the red pulp perifollicular area, a T-dependent zone. Anurans, like all ectothermic vertebrates lack germinal centers (Figure 3.14). In *Bufo calamita,* colloidal carbon particles injected via the lymph sac are trapped by red-pulp macrophages, which then move through the marginal zone to the white pulp. Giant, ramified, nonphagocytic cells found in both white and red pulp have been proposed to be dendritic cells. *Xenopus* bone marrow does not appear to be a major lymphoid organ from histologic observation, but high RAG expression in this tissue suggests lymphopoietic activity (202). The maintenance of RAG expression throughout adult life suggests that lymphocytes are continually produced.

Thymectomy decreases or abolishes allograft rejection capacity, mixed lymphocyte reaction (MLR) and phytobemagglutinin (PHA) responsiveness, IgY antibody synthesis, and all antibody responses that increase in affinity to classic thymus-dependent antigens. MLR reactivity matures before the ability to mount IgY responses in primary responses. Thymectomy at 7 days of age delays allograft rejection and abrogates specific IgY responses, whereas later in life it only abrogates antibody responses (201). Thymectomy performed later greatly affects the pool of peripheral T cells, as monitored with mAbs specific for molecules such as CD8. Early thymectomy results in the complete absence of T cells, but lymphocytes with T cell markers, perhaps corresponding to NK T cells, can still be detected. In *Xenopus,* thymocytes induce weak GVH reactions, whereas splenic T cells are good helpers and strong GVH inducers. The thymus contains some IgM-producing B cells and memory cells poised to switch to IgY synthesis, and *in vitro* responses are down-regulated by naïve thymus cells. Nitrosomethylurea (NMU) eliminates T cells and thereby abrogates alloreactivity, but rejection of xenografts is not abolished and thus may be controlled by thymus-independent mechanisms. *Xenopus* B cells respond *in vitro* to low doses of LPS not by proliferation, but rather by Ig synthesis and also respond to tumor-promoting agent (TPA). Old reports of B cell proliferation can be attributed to contaminants in LPS preparations (201).

Urodele embryos initially produce five pairs of thymic buds, the first two of which disappear (203). This results in a three-lobe thymus in *Ambystoma,* but in *Pleurodeles* and *Triturus* it forms one lobe. No cortex-medulla boundary is present, and the thymus generally resembles a canonical cortex. There are at least three types of stromal epithelial cells. There is no lymphopoietic activity in axolotl bone marrow, and hematopoeisis takes place in the spleen and in the peripheral layer of the liver. The spleen is not clearly divided into white and red pulp.

Axolotl lymphocytes proliferate in response to diverse mitogenic agents (204). In larval or adult axolotls, a population of B cells stimulated by LPS and can synthesize and secrete both IgM and IgY. T cell responses to mitogens or allogeneic determinants are allegedly poor, but adult (older than 10 months) splenocytes and thymocytes respond well to PHA when the medium is supplemented with 0.25% bovine serum albumin (BSA), rather than 1% fetal bovine serum. T cells are activated in these experiments, as shown by cell depletion with mAbs *in vitro,* and *in vivo* by thymectomy. Axolotl lymphocytes, like mammalian lymphocytes, proliferate *in vitro* when stimulated by staphylococcal enterotoxins A and B (SEA and SEB superantigens).

About 40% of TCRβ VDJ junctions in 2.5-month-old *Ambystoma* larvae have N additions, compared to about 73% in 10–25-month old animals. These VDJ junctions had ~30% defective rearrangements at all stages of development, which could be due to the slow rate of cell division in the axolotl lymphoid organs, and the large genome in this urodele. As mentioned earlier, many axolotl CDRβ3 sequences, deduced from in frame VDJ rearrangements, are the same in animals of different origins (105). In contrast, in *Xenopus,* rearrangement starts on day 5 after fertilization for the V_H locus, and within 9 days all V_H families are used. V_H1 rearranges first followed by V_H3, and by day 9–10 V_H 2, 6, 9, and 10 begin being rearranged, and then V_H 5, 7, 8, 11, on day 13. For VL, the κ locus is the first to rearrange on day 7 (two days after V_H), a situation similar to that found in mammals. During this early phase, B cells are present in the liver, where their number increases to ~500 cells (205). Later in larval life, rearrangement resumes at metamorphosis, as suggested by the low incidence of pre-B cells and by the reexpression of RAG during the second histogenesis of the lymphoid system. T cells show a similar type of RAG expression/cell renewal during ontogeny as the B cells, and the larval and adult Vβ T cell repertoires differ significantly. Even early in development, tadpoles express a highly variable TCR β repertoire despite the small number of lymphocytes (8,000–10,000 splenic T cells); little redundancy in TCR cDNA recovered from young larvae implies that clone sizes must be extremely small, unlike the axolotl situation.

In *Xenopus,* no lymphoid organ apart from the thymus is detectable until day 12 when the spleen appears and with it the ability to respond to antigen. For B cells, until this time, no selection occurs as suggested by the random ratio of productive/nonproductive VDJ rearrangements (2:1). After day 12, this ratio becomes 1:1 (i.e., the rearrangements have been selected). cDNA sequences on day 10–12 (when the number of B cells increases from 80 to 500) are not redundant as if each sequence was represented by one cell. RAG expression together with the detection of DNA rearrangement circles in the bone marrow suggests that rearrangement is ongoing throughout life and is not restricted to an early period like in birds. Tadpole rearrangements are characterized by a lack of N-region diversity, like in mammals but not axolotls or shark/skate (see earlier discussion), and thus very short CDR3. During ontogeny TdT appears in significant amounts in thymus of tadpoles at metamorphic climax, but little expression is detected at earlier stages, which correlates well with the paucity of N-region addition in larval IgH chain sequences. Studies of the ontogeny of the *Xenopus* immune system have revealed a less efficient tadpole immune response (skin graft rejection and Ig heterogeneity and affinity); the absence of TdT expression during tadpole life fits well with the findings of lower larval Ig (and TCR) diversity ([201], see discussion later in this chapter).

Reptiles. In all reptiles studied, the thymic cortex and medulla are clearly separated. The spleen has well-defined white and red pulp regions, but T and B cell zones have not been delineated with precision. In *C. scripta,* white pulp is composed of two lymphoid compartments: Lymphoid tissue surrounds both central arterioles and thick layers of reticular tissue called *ellipsoids* (206). Even after paratyphoid vaccine injection, splenic germinal centers are not formed, as in fish and amphibians. Splenic red pulp is composed of a system of venous sinuses and cords. In *Python reticulatus,* dendritic cells involved in immune complex trapping have been identified and may be related to mammalian follicular dendritic cells. GALT develops later than spleen during development, and it appears to be a secondary lymphoid organ (but does not seem to contain the equivalent of the bursa of Fabricius). Lymph node–like structures, especially in snakes (*Elaphe*) and lizards (*Gehyra*) have been reported.

Reptiles, the evolutionary precursors of both birds and mammals, are a pivotal group, but unfortunately the functional heterogeneity of reptile lymphocytes is poorly documented. There seems to be T/B cell heterogeneity because an antithymocyte antiserum altered some T cell–dependent functions in the viviparous lizard *Chalcides ocellatus*. Embryonic thymocytes responded in MLR at all stages, but Concanavalin A (ConA) responsiveness increased gradually during successive stages and declined at birth. In the alligator (*Alligator mississippiensis*), like in mammals after glass-wool filtration, nonadherent PBL responded to PHA and not to LPS, whereas adherent cells were stimulated by LPS.

Birds. The thymus, which develops in chickens from the third and fourth pharyngeal pouches, consists of two sets of seven lobes, each with definitive cortex/medulla. The thymus becomes lymphoid around day 11 of incubation. Splenic architecture is less differentiated than in mammals. It is not lymphopoietic during embryogenesis, as RAG-positive cells are found mainly in yolk sac and blood. Birds are the first vertebrate group where follicular germinal centers and T-dependent areas comprising the periarteriolar lymphatic sheath (PALS) are encountered. Plasma cells are located in the red pulp. γ/δ TCR^+ T lymphocytes are chiefly concentrated in sinusoids, whereas α/β T cells fill the PALS (106). Lymph nodes seem to be present in water and shore birds but not in chickens and related fowl.

The bursa of Fabricius is a primary lymphoid organ unique to birds in which B cells are produced (207). It arises at day 5 of development and involutes 4 weeks later (see B cell differentiation). T–B heterogeneity is obviously well defined in birds (indeed, the "B" in B cell stands for *bursa*.) The effects of thymectomy—T and B cell collaboration and generation of MHC-restricted helper and killer cells—are very similar to mammals, the other class of warm-blooded vertebrates.

During the embryonic period, chicken stem cells found in yolk sac and blood rearrange their IgH and L V genes simultaneously over a very restricted period of time, and very few cells colonize each bursal follicle (about 10^4 follicles). Three weeks after hatching, these cells have differentiated in the bursa and then seed the secondary lymphoid tissues, after which time B cells are no longer generated from multipotent stem cells; thus, only $\sim 2 \times 10^4$ productive Ig rearrangements occur in the life of the chicken (208). When an antiserum to chicken IgM is administered *in ovo* to block this early bursal immigration, there are no stem cells arising later in development that can colonize the bursa, and these chickens lack B cells for their entire lives (209). Although the general Ig locus architecture is similar to that of frogs and mammals, only one rearrangement is possible, as there is only one functional V_L or V_H on each allele. Diversity is created during bursal ontogeny by a hyperconversion mechanism in which a pool of pseudogenes (25 ψL and approximately 80 ψH) act as donors, and the unique rearranged gene acts as an acceptor during a proliferative phase in bursal follicles (Figure 3.10 [208,210]). For H chains, the situation is more complex, as there are multiple D elements. During ontogeny, selection of productive rearrangements parallels the selection of a single D reading frame, suggesting that the many D segments favor D–D joins to provide junctions that are diversified by gene conversion; the hyperconversion mechanism can also modify Ds because most donor pseudogenes are fused VD segments. The gene conversion process requires AID, which is also required for SHM and class switch (211).

Since diversification by gene conversion occurs after Ig rearrangement and cellular entry into bursal follicles, and there is only a single germline V_H and V_L expressed on all developing B cells, it was tempting to implicate a bursal ligand binding to cell surface IgM to initiate and sustain cellular proliferation and gene conversion. However, surface expression of IgM devoid of V regions permitted the typical B cell developmental progression, demonstrating that such receptor/ligand interactions are not required (212). Thus, currently we know little about how cells enter the bursa, which signals induce them to proliferate/convert, and how cells arrest their development and seed the periphery.

Mammals and Evolution of the Thymus

The discovery of a second (cervical) functional thymus in mice has raised some ontogenetic and immunological questions (213). Is this second thymus the result of an atavism, or does it correspond to what is seen in humans when a cervical thymus can form under certain pathogenic conditions during the migration of the thymus to its final mediastinal location? There are examples of cervical thymi in primitive mammals such as marsupials as well as in some prosimians. An "extra" thymus also is reminiscent of the multiple thymi encountered quite frequently in cold-blooded vertebrates.

As described, the thymus is promiscuous with regard to its precise developmental origin (206). The thymus arises from pouches 2–6 in cartilaginous fish, from the second pouch in frogs, the second and third in reptiles, and from the third or fourth in bony fish, birds, and mammals. The final number of thymi can also be variable. It ranges from five pairs of organs in sharks, to four in caecilian amphibians, to three in urodeles, and finally to one in many teleost fish species, anurans, and many mammals. The thymus of reptiles varies in terms of location and number of lobes reflecting variation in embryonic origin. The thymus may be found anywhere from the base of the heart to the neck. For example, in lizards and snakes there are two lobes on each side of the neck with no subdivision in lobules. The crocodilian thymus is an elongated chainlike structure, not unlike that of birds. In turtles, the thymus is a pair of lobes divided in lobules at the bifurcation of the common carotid associated with the parathyroids. The multilobed thymus in birds is not the equivalent of the multiple thymi found in sharks because the subdivision is secondary to primary organogenesis. Regardless of the underlying ontogenetic mechanism leading to the development the cervical thymus in mice, the result is suggestive of the secondary "thymus spreading" in birds, but it differs with regard to an uneven final size distribution. All marsupials, except koalas and some species of wombats that only have a cervical thymus, have a thoracic thymus similar to that of placentals. Some marsupials (kangaroos and possums) also have a cervical thymus; their thoracic thymus derives from the third and fourth pharyngeal pouches, whereas the cervical thymus arises mainly from the ectoderm of the cervical sinus with some participation from the second and third pouch (like in reptiles).

The second mouse thymus seems to show primitive characteristics such as the existence of a single lobe, a superficial location and a position compatible with an origin involving another pharyngeal pouch (presumably the second) that would be a marsupial and therefore perhaps a reptilian character (189). Embryology helps in determining the possible scenarios: During mouse ontogeny, the canonical thymus anlage can be recognized, beginning on day 11.5 in development, as a group of Foxn1-expressing cells located ventrally in the third pharyngeal pouch. If the cervical thymus were derived from an independent anlage, one would rather expect to detect Foxn1+ cells in the endoderm outside the third pouch. This argues for a common origin of thoracic and cervical thymi and against a second thymus anlage outside the third pouch, and, hence, against the above hypothesis that the cervical thymus represents an atavistic organ.

Generation of Diversity in Warm-blooded Vertebrates

Perhaps surprisingly, mechanisms leading to the generation of repertoire diversity vary among mammalian species. As data accumulate, categories can be made depending on the mode of B cell development: Rabbits, cattle, swine, and chickens (the so-called *GALT group*), unlike fish, amphibians, reptiles, and primates/rodents, use a single V_H family, of which only a few members (sometimes only one) are functional (134,214). This GALT group uses gene conversion or hypermutation in hindgut follicles early in life (rather than bone-marrow throughout life) to diversify their antibody repertoire. At the rabbit H locus, as in the chicken, a single V_H is expressed in most peripheral B cells. During development, B cells that have rearranged this particular V in the bone marrow (and other sites) migrate to the appendix where this rearranged gene is diversified by gene conversion using upstream donor V segments. This development of B cells in rabbits is dependent on the intestinal microflora (215), and efforts are being made to define the potential bacterial superantigens involved, as well as binding sites on IgM necessary for the differentiation. In ruminants, the ileal Peyer's patches (IPP) are the bursalike primary B cell–generating tissues. Although bursa, appendix, and sheep IPPs show morphological similarities, the mechanisms generating diversity are different: conversion in the chicken and hypermutation in sheep, and both in the rabbit (134). As described earlier, most of the GALT group also appears to lack IgD; thus IgD might serve some purpose in repertoire development in some groups of mammals and not others (216).

In summary, the organization of the lymphoid tissues is perhaps the only element of the immune system that shows increasing complexity that can be superimposed on the vertebrate phylogenetic tree (Figure 3.14). The absence of primary and secondary lymphoid tissues (thymus and spleen) is correlated with the absence of a rearranging or hypermutating receptor family in other animals, with the exception of the agnathan VLR in which the relevant lymphoid tissues (if they exist) are not yet defined. While all jawed vertebrates have a true secondary lymphoid tissue (spleen), ectotherms lack lymph nodes and organized GALT. In addition, while ectotherms clearly have B cell zones resembling follicles, and despite the clear ability for ectothermic B cells to undergo SMH and at least some degree of affinity maturation, germinal centers with follicular dendritic cells are not formed after immunization; clearly this was a major advance in the evolution of the vertebrate immune system (discussed later in this chapter).

The potential repertoire of Ig and TCR combining sites is enormous in all jawed vertebrates. The potential antigen receptor repertoire in all species for both T and B cells is far greater than could ever be expressed in an animal because of cell number limitations. Not all species or all gene families use combinatorial joining for repertoire building, but all species assemble V, (D), and J gene segments to generate their functional Ig genes during B cell ontogeny, and the imprecision of this assembly creates great somatic diversity. Thus, from this survey in various species, one could not predict that there would be major differences in immune responses in representatives of different vertebrate classes, and yet in the next section we shall see that mouse/human antibody responses are superior to those in many taxa.

Adaptive Immune Responses

The quality of T cell and B cell responses depends on the heterogeneity and diversity of the antigen receptor repertoires, the ability to select cells in secondary lymphoid tissues, and other undefined factors. As described, because of the indefinite and huge number of potential Ig/TCR V region sequences in most taxa, potential diversity exceeds the number of available lymphocytes. Yet, while potential repertoires are diverse in all vertebrate classes, and polymorphic MHC class I and II and TCR genes have been isolated from all classes, antibody diversity in nonmammalian vertebrates is relatively low (217,218). The expressed repertoire has been studied by indirect methods based on structural studies, affinity measurements during the maturation of the immune response, enumeration of antigen-binding Igs by isoelectrofocusing (IEF), and idiotypic analysis. Sequences of Ig and TCR genes expressed over the course of a response help to estimate diversity at another level, allowing studies of V genes diversified by gene conversion or somatic mutation during a response in a precise way. In the following survey, we describe studies of specific antibody synthesis, T cell responsiveness (T–B collaboration, MHC restriction). NK and NK-T cells will be considered in this section as well. Because of space limitation we focus on ectothermic vertebrates and birds.

Cartilaginous Fish

Natural antibodies binding many antigens have been detected at surprisingly high levels in chondrichthyans and in some teleosts. After immunization (for instance with 2-furyloxazolone-*Brucella*, or p-azobenzenearsonate), the horned shark mounts a low-affinity 19S IgM antibody response, which varies little among individuals and does not increase in affinity after prolonged immunization. Variation of L chains isolated from individuals is limited, with the major bands having identical isoelectric points. Nurse sharks immunized to heat-killed streptococcal A variant vaccine produced antibodies that among outbred individuals had very different L chain gel electrophoresis patterns (219).

The relative homogeneity and large number of V genes hindered somatic mutation studies until a single unique reference horned shark IgM V_H gene was found. Mutations in this gene were slightly more frequent than those in *Xenopus* (discussed later). Mutation rates could not be calculated, and no correlation with an immune response was attempted. The mutations were predominantly found at GC bases, and the frequency was rather low. Nevertheless, this work proved that somatic mutation preceded diversity obtained by combinatorial association of gene segments in evolution (220). In contrast to mutations in the horned shark IgM V_H genes, unusual patterns of somatic mutation were detected in nurse shark type II germline-joined L chains. Half of the mutations (338/631) occur in tandem without the G–C bias seen in *Xenopus* or shark H chain V genes. Tandem mutations and point mutations take place simultaneously and are unlikely to be generated by gene conversion, since there are no repeated patterns or potential donor genes (221). The germline-joined L chain genes can only diversify through SHM, perhaps like the hypothetical prototype V region gene prior to RAG-mediated rearrangement (i.e., SHM may have preceded gene rearrangement as the primordial somatic diversification mechanism; discussed later in the chapter). Lastly, a reappraisal of mutation at H chain loci in the nurse shark showed that the mutations were not so different from the L chains (222); the differences from the previous work were the different shark species and the analysis of all H chain loci in the species rather than only one unusual locus.

The small number of IgNAR genes also made it possible to analyze somatic mutation, and in the first experiments, random cDNAs were examined. The mutation frequency is about 10 times that of *Xenopus* and horned shark IgM, and even higher than in most studies in mammals. It is difficult to establish a pattern for the mutations due to their high frequency and because they are often contiguous, like in the L chain gene study described earlier; however, mutations are not targeted to GC bases, and analysis of synonymous sites suggested that the mechanism is similar to human/mouse (219). Mutations even in the randomly isolated clones appeared to be under positive selection in IgNAR secretory but not TM clones, strongly suggesting that mutations do not generate the primary repertoire like in sheep but arise only after antigenic stimulation.

Recent studies suggested that there is affinity (223) maturation and memory generation in nurse sharks. Soon after immunization with hen egg lysozyme (HEL) and IgM response can be detected, primarily of the pentameric class. Over time, 7S IgM and IgNAR responses develop, and the 7S antibodies have a higher binding strength than those of the 19S class (120). When titers are permitted to drop to baseline, a memory response can be induced by immunization of antigen without adjuvant. However, unlike responses in higher vertebrates, the titers do not increase over those in the primary response, suggesting a peculiar type of regulation of antigen-specific IgM and IgNAR. Nevertheless, these data strongly suggest that the hallmarks of an adaptive response occur in sharks. In another study, a family of HEL-specific IgNAR clones was followed over time after immuniczation, and a 10-fold increase in the affinity of an already high-affinity germline clone (10^{-9} M) was observed. These results suggest that affinity maturation, memory, and "switch" to the monomeric IgM isotype occurs, but it takes much longer to attain these adaptive hallmarks compared to mammals, perhaps a paradigm for ectotherms (218).

The role of T cells in shark immune responses has not been studied in detail. No thymectomy experiments have been performed, and T cells have not been monitored during an immune response. Shark MLR and graft rejection have been attempted—MLR with little success (probably for technical reasons), and grafts with the demonstration of a chronic type of rejection for which the genetics has not been analyzed. However, from the MHC and TCR studies, it is clear that all of the molecular components are available for proper antigen presentation in sharks and skates, and recent studies of splenic architecture suggestive of T cell zones containing class II^+ dendritic cells argue for a prominent T cell regulatory role in adaptive immunity (114,192). Further, an increase in binding strength and memory response also strongly suggest a T cell involvement in humoral immunity.

Bony Fish

There are high levels of low-affinity natural antibody (up to 11% of total Ig) to nitrophenylacetate (NP) in some bony fish. Natural antibodies in catfish have been correlated with resistance to virus infection or furonculosis. As a rule, and like in cartilaginous fish, little affinity maturation has been detected in fish, although some changes in fine specificities were noticed in the trout with a sensitive ELISA-based test. B cell and Ig heterogeneity was demonstrated in carp using mAbs, and DNP-specific antibody-secreting cells were identified with the ELISPOT assay in pronephros and spleen cell suspensions after immunization. The number of IEF antigen-specific bands per individual is small (up to 23), and there is little variation from one outbred individual to another. In sea bass, extremely low variability was reported in CDR1, and no variability in CDR2 or CDR3 in DNP-specific L chains, suggesting expression of dominant monospecific antibodies (217).

The mild increase in trout antibody affinity (similar to that found in *Xenopus*) is attributed to selection of either minor preexisting B cell populations or somatic mutants. In partially inbred self-fertilized or gynogenetic trout, variability of specific responses is even more restricted. Affinity measured by equilibrium dialysis was of the order of 2.0×10^{-6} M for TNP-specific antibodies. The percentage of L chains of the catfish "F" and "G" types can vary greatly in the course of a response (2 weeks versus 3 months). A large literature deals with vaccination attempts in teleost fish, due to their economic importance. The availability of catfish B cell, macrophage, and T cell lines have been instrumental in analyses of antibody production. There are puzzling differences in responses from different teleost groups, much like differences between urodeles and anurans (amphibians). Cod, for example, do not respond well to specific antigen and have very high levels of "natural antibodies."

Like the sharks, isolation of TCR genes and the existence of a polymorphic class I and class II molecules suggest that antigen presentation is operative in teleosts, but, unlike sharks, functional experiments examining mammalianlike T-APC interactions have been performed. TCR mRNAs are selectively expressed, and specific TCR rearrangements have been detected in catfish clonal cell lines, which produce factor(s) with leukocyte growth promoting activity. Modifications of the trout T cell repertoire during an acute viral infection have also been followed. In nonintentionally immunized trout, adaptation of the spectratyping technique for TCRβ CDR3 length revealed a polyclonal naïve T cell repertoire. After an acute infection with viral hemorrhagic septicemia virus (VHSV), CDR3 size profiles were skewed for several Vβ/Jβ combinations, corresponding to T cell clonal expansions. Both "public" and "private" T cell expansions were detected in the infected genetically identical individuals. The "public" response resulted in expansion of Vβ4/Jβ1-positive T cells that appeared first in the primary response and were boosted during the secondary response (224). Further work examined the fine specificity of the T cell response to the virus, which is a model for studies in cold-blooded animals (225).

We have seen that species living in extreme cold develop adaptive structural differences in their Igs. At the level of global immune response, temperature exerts a great influence in ectothermic vertebrates in general, low temperature generally being immunosuppressive. Lowering the water temperature from 23°C to 11°C over a 24-hour period suppresses both B and T cell functions of catfish for 3–5 weeks as assessed by *in vitro* responses. Virgin T cells are most sensitive to this cold-induced suppression, a property shared with mammals when tested appropriately. Fish have developed ways to adapt to the lack of fluidity of their B cell membranes by altering the composition of fatty acid by using more oleic acid at low temperatures. After appropriate *in vivo* acclimation, catfish T cells are better able to cap cell surface molecules at low assay temperatures than are B cells, suggesting that capping is not the low temperature–sensitive step involved in T cell immunosuppression in catfish (226).

Evidence that fish possess cytotoxic cells was derived from allograft rejections and graft versus host (GVH) reaction studies. *In vitro* studies have now shown that leukocytes from immunized fish specifically kill a variety of target cells (allogeneic erythrocytes and lymphocytes, hapten-coupled autologous cells); fish CTL of the $\alpha\beta$ (and perhaps $\gamma\delta$) lineages as well as NK cells were found. Naïve catfish leukocytes spontaneously kill allogeneic cells and virally infected autologous cells without sensitization, and allogeneic cytotoxic responses were greatly enhanced by *in vitro* alloantigen stimulation (227). Cloned cytotoxic cells contain granules and likely induce apoptosis in sensitive targets via a putative perforin/granzyme or by Fas/FasL-like interactions. An Fc receptor for IgM (FcμR) was detected on some catfish NK-like cells that appears to "arm" these cells with surface IgM (228). All catfish cytotoxic cell lines express a signal-transduction molecule with homology to the Fcγ chain of mammals. This chain with an ITAM motif is an accessory molecule for the activating receptor NKP46 on mammalian NK cells. Importantly, these cytotoxic cells do not express a marker for catfish nonspecific cytotoxic cells (NCC). NCC have been found in other fish species, including trout, carp, damselfish, and tilapia, and they spontaneously kill a variety of xenogeneic targets, including certain fish parasites and traditional mammalian NK cell targets. Unlike mammalian NK cells, NCCs are small agranular lymphocytes found in lymphoid tissues (pronephros and spleen), but rarely in blood. Recently, the gene for catfish NCCRP-1 was sequenced and found to be a novel type III membrane protein with no sequence homology to any known mammalian leukocyte receptor (229).

Amphibians

Differences in immune system features between urodele (axolotl) and anuran (*Xenopus*) amphibians, already discussed for MHC and Ig complexity, are also seen in immune responses. Rarely is such divergence seen within one vertebrate class (although the two groups diverged over 250 million years ago). Urodeles express a very restricted antibody repertoire in response to specific antigen that peaks at 40 days postimmunization and is entirely of the IgM class, even though the serum also contains IgY (230). They do not respond well to thymus-dependent antigens, which may be due to lack of T cell help, yet their expressed TCR diversity looks normal. A population of axolotl B cells proliferates specifically in response to LPS and also secretes both IgM and IgY. Moreover, a distinct lymphocyte subpopulation proliferates significantly in response to the T cell mitogens ConA. T cells from young axolotls (before 10 months) do not have this functional ability. As mentioned earlier, axolotl T cells also can be stimulated with to SEA/SEB known from mammalian studies to be superantigens.

Anuran larvae can respond specifically (with only 10^6 lymphocytes) to many antigens, with a modest affinity maturation of the IgM anti-DNP response. In adults, the number of different anti-DNP antibodies does not exceed 40, versus 500 in mammals. In secondary responses, the peak of the response is about 10-fold higher and is reached in 2 weeks; there are no major changes in affinity over this initial rise. Anti-DNP Abs, or even nonimmune Ig pools, yield easily interpretable sequences for the first 16 N-terminal residues of both H and L chain V regions. However, this simple view was challenged when a great heterogeneity of cDNA sequences could be detected in animals after immunization. Isogenic *Xenopus* produce homogenous antibodies to DNP, xenogenic RBC, or phosphorylcholine with identical or similar IEF spectrotypes and idiotypes, while outbred individuals differ (231). Both IEF spectrotypes and idiotypes are inheritable, suggesting that diversity is a reflection of the germline repertoire without a major contribution from somatic mutations. Thus, somatic mutations were followed during the course of an antigenspecific immune response at the peak of the modest affinity maturation in larvae and adults (232). The V_H genes, like their mammalian homologues, contain the sequence motifs described previously that target hypermutation. Of the 32 members of the V_H1 family involved in the anti-DNP response, expression of only five was detected, indicating that immunization was being monitored. Few mutations were detected (average: 1.6 mutations per gene, range: 1–5), and there was not a strong preference for mutations in CDR1 and 2 and virtually none in CDR3. Like in the shark IgM study noted earlier (but not IgNAR or type II L chains), the mutations were targeted to GC bases, and such a pattern has been suggested to be the first phase of SHM in mouse/human; perhaps *Xenopus* has lost the second phase of the process that results in an evening of mutation frequency for all bases (233). While the mutation frequency was lower than in mammalian B cells, the rates were only four- to seven-fold less in *Xenopus*. Thus, there is no shortage of variants, and the reasons for the low heterogeneity and poor affinity maturation may be due to less than optimal selection of the mutants. Indeed, because of a relatively low ratio of replacement to silent mutations in the CDRs, it was argued that there is no effective mechanism for selecting mutants, which in turn might be related to the absence of GC in *Xenopus*. In summary, the data from hypermutation, cDNA heterogeneity, and spectrotype dominance suggests that in the absence of refined modes of selection in late-developing clones, B cells producing somatic mutants may be out-competed by antibodies generated earlier in the response.

Essential T cell functions in anurans were shown with *in vitro* assays for T–B collaboration and MHC restriction, demonstrating the similarity of the role of MHC in *Xenopus* and mammals. Regulatory T cells have been shown indirectly in hematopoeitic/thymic chimaeras for control of CTL generation and in antibody responses. Ig synthesis can be enhanced following thymectomy in axolotl or *Xenopus,* again implying a role for thymic-dependent regulatory cells. As described previously, the class switch first occurs in amphibians, and thymectomy early in life totally prevents IgY, but not IgX synthesis; thus, T cells are absolutely required for the switch and also for high affinity IgM responses. Switching can also be induced in tadpoles, although one must hyperimmunize animals for this response, due to a paucity of T cells in larvae. The switch is also temperature-dependent, and as described earlier for channel catfish, ectotherm T cells are quite temperature-sensitive (201).

Similar to studies in mammals, the chaperone gp96 has been shown to shuttle peptides into target cells to make such cells targets for MHC-restricted CTL lysis. Immunization of frogs with gp96 from a thymic tumor results in the elicitation of CTL that display antitumor activity. Elegant experiments with gp96 vaccination have also shown that CTL activity against minor histocompatibility antigens is MHC-restricted. As mentioned earlier, NK cells have been characterized in *Xenopus* with mAbs that recognize non-B/T cells. Those cells kill MHC class I–negative target tumor cells but not class I^+ lymphocytes, and after thymectomy these cells are enriched in the spleen. More recently, $CD8^+$ cells expressing TCR were isolated with the same mAb suggesting the existence of amphibian NK-T cells. Expression of the mAb epitope on cells is induced by PMA/ionomycin and is also detected in CTL when MHC-dependent cytotoxicity is reduced.

Reptiles

Lack of an increase in affinity and homogeneity of IEF spectrotypes suggest low antibody heterogeneity in reptiles. In the turtle *Pseudemys scripta,* a number of genomic VH sequences, representing possibly four families, were isolated, as was a genomic $C\mu$, all shown to be encoded at a single locus. In Northern hybridizations, the $C\mu4$ probe detected two transcripts; of the four VH groups, only one was expressed, and multiple bands indicated the presence of at least two non-μ transcripts. Among 32 unique VDJ rearrangements from one animal, there were 22 sequence variants in FR4, suggesting either a large number of J segments or somatic modification (234). The latter interpretation is supported by point mutations found in FR3 and CDR3. For T cells, there are no data on T effector function, but there are studies on the behavior of T cell population changes due to seasonal and hormonal variations. Thymocytes from the turtle *Mauremys caspica* proliferate in response to PHA and ConA and can kill tumor target cells by both ADCC-mediated and NK-mediated cytotoxicity. Proliferative responses to PHA and ConA were higher for both sexes in spring and for females in winter than in the other seasons.

Birds and Mammals

Sequence data and L chains patterns on 2-D gel electrophoresis showed less antibody heterogeneity in chicken than in mouse. The poor increase in affinity of chicken anti-DNP and antifluorescein antibodies again indicates lower heterogeneity. Few changes occur after immunization, even if one waits one year after several injections. Perhaps similar to the trout study described earlier, a restricted population of high-affinity antibodies was found only after immunization in Freund's complete adjuvant (235). Hyperconversion and somatic mutation in Ig genes have been found in splenic germinal center B cells after immunization. The relatively poor affinity maturation of the chicken response may be due to a balance between gene conversion and somatic mutation. Indeed, modification of V genes with segments of DNA is not an optimal strategy for fine-tuning antibody responses. In the rabbit there is also conversion/mutation by B cells in germinal centers after immunization. Within mammals, large variations are found from marsupials with no obvious secondary response, to mice with 1,000-fold increases in affinity, but the basis for the relatively poor responses has not been established.

In conclusion, although all vertebrates have a very large potential for generating diverse antibodies after immunization, only some mammals studied to date make the most of this potential. Perhaps pressures on the immune system of cold-blooded vertebrates have been less intense due to a stronger innate immunity, and the architecture of their lymphoid system is not optimal for selecting somatic mutants, or the great rises in affinity detected in antihapten responses are not physiologically relevant. An immune system using somatic diversification at its "best" is well adapted to species where the value of single individuals is important (i.e., species with small progenies). Has that been the condition for the creation and selection of somatic rearrangement and of the optimal usage of somatic mutations? If this explanation provides a rationale for the utilization of somatic mechanisms in generating a repertoire and improving it, it does not tell us why it works so well in certain species and not in others. Perhaps the key is the organization of secondary lymphoid organs. Likely, a combination of factors (e.g., endothermy, secondary lymphoid tissues, mutation versus conversion, the hypermutation mechanism itself, rates of proliferation [pathogen and lymphocyte], etc.) are at work in the regulation of antibody responses (218).

NK AND NK-LIKE CELLS

NK cells express both activating and inhibitory cell surface receptors; in fact, the paradigm for positive and negative signaling via such receptors began with these cells; however, activating and inhibitory receptors (often paired) are conserved throughout vertebrates and invertebrate deuterostomes and are expressed in hematopoietic cell types of all types. In NK cells, stimulation of the activating receptors, which associate with proteins having an ITAM (DAP12 or DAP10 conserved at least to the level of bony fish [236]), results in killing of target cells. Inhibitory signaling receptors all possess cytoplasmic ITIMs, which recruit phosphatases and generally are dominant over the activating receptors. These receptors fall in two categories, IgSF and C-type lectin group V(II). In general, NK receptors recognize MHC class I molecules of either the classical or nonclassical type, the latter sometimes encoded by viruses.

Evolution of NK Receptor Families

As mentioned, NK cells in mammals can use different types of receptors, even encoded by different gene families. Some are conserved and others are highly variable even if one can group them into defined multigene families. Some families show conservation of domains throughout the jawed vertebrates. When dealing with the origin of these genes in invertebrates, one has to imagine under what pressures they evolved; pathogens come immediately to the mind rather than MHC class I molecules that appeared "simultaneously" with the RAG-mediated adaptive system. The most interesting phylogenetic information could come from future studies in deuterostomes such as echinoderms, protochordates, and agnathans. The question is whether NK cells, or NK-like cells, preceded the emergence of T and B lymphocytes.

As described in the Introduction, NK receptors are the most rapidly evolving molecular component of the gnathostome immune system (4). All known ligands for these diverse NK receptors are MHC class I molecules, or molecules of host or pathogen origin related to MHC class I. The KIR families are divergent, as very few genes are conserved even between chimpanzees and humans, and there are different numbers of genes in KIR haplotypes within a species. By contrast, CD94/NKG2 receptors are conserved throughout mammals. So whereas receptors for polymorphic class I molecules are divergent, those for nonpolymorphic class I molecules are conserved (despite the fact that their ligands Qa1 and HLA-E are not orthologous). Altogether, rapid evolution of NK cell receptor gene families distinguishes members of a species and causes substantial species-specific differences in NK cell receptor systems. NK cells play other important roles in other innate immune responses, for example in antiviral immunity. NK cell recognition of virus-infected cells engages the activating KIR and Ly49 receptors and NKG2D in this process. Thus, viruses are hypothesized to supply the evolutionary pressure on diversification of NK cell receptors. In fact, it has been shown in mice that inhibitory receptors can rapidly mutate into activating receptors when viral "decoy" class I molecules evolve to engage inhibitory receptors (237).

Comparative Studies of NK Function

NK cells were detected in *Xenopus* by *in vitro* ^{51}Cr assays. Splenocyte effectors from early thymectomized frogs spontaneously lyse allogeneic thymus tumor cell lines that lack MHC antigen expression. This activity is increased after the injection of tumor cells or after treating the splenocytes *in vitro* with mitogens, suggesting lymphokine activation of the killers. Splenocytes isolated with an anti-NK mAb revealed large lymphoid cells with distinct pseudopodia. Immunohistology indicated that each anti-NK mAb routinely labeled cells within the gut epithelium, but NK cells were difficult to visualize in spleen sections.

In amphibians. NK cell studies are especially interesting because of natural experiments done by nature (i.e., the absence or low levels of MHC classical class I during larval life of some species like *Xenopus* [238]). They are *bona fide* NK cells, distinct from T cells, since they fail to express TCR Vβ transcripts. NK cells emerge in late larval life, 7-weeks post-fertilization, about 2 weeks after the time when cell-surface class I can be detected. The proportion of splenic NK cells remains very low until 3–4 months of age, but by 1 year there is a sizeable population. Therefore, NK cells fail to develop prior to MHC class I protein normal expression (at least NK cells of the type that can be measured with these assays and with NK cell-specific mAbs) and do not contribute to the larval immune system, whereas they do provide an important backup for T cells in the adult frog by contributing to antitumor immunity. The molecules that govern killing in *Xenopus* have not been identified.

NK cells have also been described in a number of teleost fish with the most in-depth studies in catfish, in which there are clonal lines of cytotoxic cells (see earlier discussion).

Perforin and granzyme homologs are indeed found in birds, amphibians, and teleost fish (Ensembl). As mentioned earlier in the complement section, homologs with the MAC/perforin domains even exist in *C. elegans* and insects, with no functional evidence.

Phylogeny of NK Lectins

The phylogenetic appearance of NK lectins in the vertebrates has not been examined in detail. However, BLAST searches reveal possible homologues at least to the level of teleost fish, whereas no hits have been reported from cartilaginous fish or agnathans, but at least for the cartilaginous fish this may be due to a lack of sequence data. As mentioned previously, a CD94 homologue has been detected in lower deuterostomes, but its true orthology is dubious. A CD94/NKG2-like gene has been described in cichlid fish even though the orthology is not clear and no functional work has been done. Group II C-type lectin receptors, which are structurally similar to group V (NK) receptors, have been characterized in bony fish (239). A zebrafish multigene family of group II immune-related, lectinlike receptors (illrs) was identified from the databases with possible inhibiting or activating signaling motifs. These genes are differentially expressed in the myeloid and lymphoid cell lineages.

Given the apparent lack of MHC class I and class II in agnathans and their convergently acquired adaptive immune system (see earlier discussion), it is difficult to envisage how NK cells with receptors of any type might function in these animals. It should be mentioned, however, that sequence similarity might be difficult to detect for an MHC PBR, given the rapid rate of evolution of this gene family. Further, it would not be shocking if there were NK cells with ligands encoded by other gene families—in mammals, ligands for some activating NK receptors like NKp44 and NKp30 have not been identified. It would be of interest to study the non–VLR-expressing lymphocytes in agnathans (if such cells exist) for their killing potential or gene expression.

Interestingly, recent studies in mammals have shown that some of these NKC-encoded lectinlike receptors in the Nkrp-l family can recognize other lectinlike molecules, termed Clr, also encoded in the NKC (240). Having linked loci encoding receptor-ligand pairs suggests a genetic strategy to preserve this interaction; perhaps the CD94 homologues of invertebrates are genetically linked to genes encoding their ligands. In addition, as described later in this chapter, the close genetic linkage of receptor and ligand genes is a common theme in "histocompatibility reactions" throughout the animal and plant kingdoms.

Phylogeny of IgSF NK Receptors

IgSF activating receptors have been recognized as such from teleost fish onward with a relatively convincing NKP44 homologue in carp, but with no functional data. These sequences of the fish V domain NKP44 resemble the chicken CD300-L family as well as some skate molecules that could perhaps permit the extension of the lineage to the cartilaginous fish. NKp30 homologues have been detected in *Xenopus*; in addition, as described in the MHC section, there are V(J) genes within the frog MHC that are ancient homologues of NKp30 and may be NK receptors of both activating and inhibitory types (160). NITRs, seemingly specific of teleost fish, have one or two Ig domains with a charged residue in the TM and could therefore be associated (by analogy) to an ITAM DAP12 equivalent (discussed later [241]).

IgSF inhibitory receptors usually form larger families of molecules in comparison to activating receptors. This function can be devoted to two distinct families of receptors, giving another example of the extremely rapid evolution of these molecules. There are many ITIM-carrying IgSF integral membrane receptors across the classes of vertebrates, and they seem to have had independent histories since it is difficult to convincingly detect orthologous genes between species. This is especially true of multigene families in fish, with members equipped with possible ITIMs, including the teleost NITR and LITR, and bird CHIR and CD300L. Several members of these families can be expressed on NK cells, but expression studies are in their infancy in fish. It is sometimes difficult to distinguish FcRh families from NK KIR-like domains, and both FcR and KIR seem to stem from a same lineage. Given the role of the FcR binding to *bona fide* antibodies and conferring specificities to cells of the innate arms of the immune system, it is likely that these molecules will be restricted to jawed vertebrates. The KIR activity that can incorporate pathogen and virus recognition may be more primitive, but the ancestry of KIR is not well understood, and the *bona fide* KIR family seems to be restricted to primates.

Genes encoding the classical FcRs on the long arm of human chromosome 1 (1q21–23) are linked to other FcR-like genes. A large multigene family, which includes genes encoding the FcγR and the NK cell Ig-like receptors, is located in the LRC (human chromosome 19q13). This region could in fact be paralogous to 1q23 and may even have been originally associated with the MHC (discussed later). These families belong to a larger class of activating or inhibitory receptors. Their phylogenetic conservation in birds, amphibians, and bony fish suggests a biological importance even though the size of the families, their expression pattern, and the specific nature of the receptors vary greatly among species (242). In several cases, a commitment to a task in the immune system may not be conserved among homologous members and the evolutionary fate of the family will be probably affected. Comparison of key residues in the domains may suggest a possible common involvement in MHC recognition for the two families recently discovered in birds (CHIR [243]) and the teleosts (IpLITR [244]). Other families were generated within a single class or even within a single order of vertebrates (e.g., the KIR described earlier). The relationships of KIR with many other multigene families such as IpLITR or NITR remain to be explored. What was the scenario that led to the present mammalian situation? If the fish observation on potential MHC binding holds true, the KIR-type of receptor seems to be the most primitive NK cell receptor.

Other IgSF Families to Explore Further

Thymocytes express members of the IgSF TIM (T cell Ig and mucin domain-containing molecule) (245) corresponding to another independent amplification of nonrearranging V domains on chromosome 5, with 3 members, whereas the homologous locus on chromosome 11 in mice has 8. Nothing is known about relatives outside mammals.

In more primitive vertebrates, the physical or genetic linkage of relatively large IgSF families is well documented in the teleost NITR but not yet elucidated in the case of other interesting families in protochordates like the VCBP. In the sea urchin genome, many IgSF await a complete analysis and will certainly contribute to a better understanding of the evolution and origin of Ig/TCR. Among those, the discovery of leukocyte-expressed receptors APAR (agnathan paired receptors) in hagfish of what might have been a precursor of Ig or TCR (246). APARs resemble Ag receptors and are expressed in leukocytes and predicted to encode a group of membrane glycoproteins with organizations characteristic of paired Ig-like receptors. APAR-A molecules are likely to associate with an adaptor molecule with an ITAM and function as activating receptors. In contrast, APAR-B molecules with an ITIM motif are likely to function as inhibitory receptors Thus, the APAR gene family has features characteristic of paired Ig-like receptors. APAR V domains have a J region and are more closely related to those of TCR/BCR than any other V-type domain identified to date outside of jawed vertebrates. Thus, the extracellular domain of APAR may be descended from a V-type domain postulated to have acquired RSS in a jawed vertebrate lineage.

In jawed vertebrates, three such receptor families with VJ-type domains have been identified: a small family of mammalian proteins known as SIRP, a large family of the previously described teleost NITR, and MHC-linked XMIV in *Xenopus*. NITR were originally believed to be part of the LRC, but this is unlikely on further analyses. NITR encode a variable (V) region, a unique V-like C2 (V/C2) domain, a TM region (with or without a positively charged residue), and a cytoplasmic tail containing ITIM. They seem to form a teleost-specific family with no good homologue outside this class although they appear somewhat related to NKp30. NITRs can be expressed by cells of the hematopoietic lineage, presumably lymphocytes as judged from MLR. Eleven related genes encoding distinct structural forms have been identified in the channel catfish. In zebrafish, NITR genes group into 12 distinct families, including inhibitory and activating receptors. An extreme level of allelic polymorphism is apparent, along with haplotype variation, and family-specific isoform complexity (9).

CYTOKINES AND CHEMOKINES

Many cytokines/chemokines and their receptors, like most molecules of the immune system, evolve rapidly. However, consistent with the "Big Bang" theory, it is an emerging picture that the majority of cytokines and chemokines found in mouse and human are also found in the genome and EST projects of nonmammalian vertebrates, best studied in chickens (247) and certain bony fish (248). This suggests that whatever the initiating "force" in the evolution of the Ig/TCR adaptive immune system, the network of cytokines and chemokines emerged (practically) full blown early in evolution. While the overall picture is clear, the details are only starting to be understood, especially at the functional level. What is becoming apparent, however, is that some of the cyto/chemokine families in fish (and perhaps other groups) have been expanded or contracted in a species- or class-specific manner. This will clearly be a topic of interest in the future.

The Proinflammatory Cytokines, IL-1, IL-18, IL-6, IL-8, and TNFα

IL-1, IL-6, TNFα, and IL-8 are the prototypic cytokines associated with inflammatory responses, which are defined by induction of vasodilation and vascular permeability, and upregulation of innate immune system–specific molecules that have direct functions or that costimulate/attract T and B cells. Classically, many of these activities can be assayed in supernatants from LPS-stimulated phagocytes by determining whether thymocytes are stimulated to proliferate when one also adds suboptimal concentrations of T cell mitogens. It was reasonable to hypothesize that such cytokines, which act both at a distance as well as in a cognate fashion, might be found in the invertebrates. Indeed, IL-1-like *activities* have been described for echinoderm coelomocytes (either IL-1-like production by such cells, or the ability of the cells to respond to mammalian IL-1), but unfortunately no molecular data revealing the structures of the active invertebrate cytokine/cytokine receptor have been reported. In fact, no orthologue has been detected in the genome projects from protostomian invertebrates, and only IL-17 and TNF homologues have been detected in nonvertebrate deuterostomes (32,97), and IL-8 in agnathans (249); thus, we may consider these as primordial cytokines related to the vertebrate versions. A molecule from earthworms capable of activating the prophenoloxidase defense pathway cross-reacted with a mAb directed to mammalian TNFα (250). However, this molecule had no homology to TNFα on sequencing, but its activity is nonetheless quite interesting.

IL-1 activity as measured by costimulation assays or as a consequence of LPS (or other PAMPs) stimulation has been detected in all nonmammalian vertebrates. IL-1β upregulation has been detected after treatment of macrophages with LPS, consistent with its inflammatory function in mammals. In addition, injection of gram-negative bacteria into trout induced IL-1β expression in many tissues. Identity with the mammalian IL-1β gene in all other species ranges from 28% to 40% (identity between mammalian IL-1α and IL-1β is about 25%). In nonmammalian species, IL-1β lacks a so-called *ICE cleavage site,* important for function in mouse/human (251). IL-18 is an IL-1-related cytokine, and in contrast to IL-1 seems more focused in its function of potentiating TH1 responses. IL-18 has been detected in birds and fish, but the tissue distribution in fish seems to be expanded as compared to mammals. Additionally, IL-18 in nonmammalian vertebrates contain the ICE cleavage site, unlike its cousin IL-1β.

Both chicken IL-1β and the IL-1R were identified and have been expressed as recombinant proteins. The IL-1R homology to mammalian orthologues is quite high (61% identity), but the highest similarity is found in the cytoplasmic domains. In addition, there are four blocks of high similarity to the cytoplasmic tail of Toll/TLR proteins, and IL-1R and TLR use similar signal transduction cascades (see previous discussion). As mentioned, IL-8 has been identified in the jawless lamprey and in various gnathostomes such as trout, flounder, and perhaps chicken; a chicken CXC chemokine called *K*60 clusters with IL-8 in phylogenetic trees and is upregulated in macrophages stimulated with LPS, IL-1β, and IFN (247). Interestingly, Marek's disease virus expresses an IL-8 homologue (v-IL-8), which may be involved in inducing immune deviation.

The TNF family in mammals includes the canonical TNFα, lymphotoxin (LT)α, and LTβ, all encoded at the distal end of the MHC class III region, as well as a large number of other members with diverse immune functions (153). TNFα is the best studied of these cytokines, and it is one of the key regulators of innate and adaptive immunity. The other two cytokines have a more limited tissue distribution and function, especially in their roles in lymphoid tissue development. TNF homologues have been detected in sea urchin, *Ciona,* and amphioxus, consistent with the idea that such a multifunctional cytokine would predate the jawed vertebrate adaptive immune system. Homologues have also been cloned from several teleost species and TNFα expression in leukocytes is upregulated within 4 hours after treatment with LPS, IL-1β, and PMA. While there is good phylogenetic support for orthology of fish TNFα to that of mammals, the other TNF genes seem to be teleost-specific duplicates rather than the LT genes (252). Conversely, in *Xenopus,* the three TNF family members described above in mammals are closely linked in the class III region of the MHC (160). This is a bit of a surprising result, as all of these family members seem to be lacking in chickens, consistent (according to the authors) with a lack of lymph nodes in these animals (247); however, the unusual nature of the MHC in birds (e.g., the immunoproteasome genes are missing) rather is consistent with a loss of TNF genes in these animals, which is indeed surprising, especially for TNFα.

Interleukin-2/15

Costimulation assays of thymocytes, as described earlier for IL-1, and perpetuation of T cell lines with stimulated T cell supernatants are performed to detect IL-2 or "T cell growth factor" activities. Unlike IL-1, IL-2–like factors generally stimulate cells only from the same species, and it is a "cognate" cytokine, meant for release only between closely opposed cells, or as an autocrine factor. From teleost fish to mammals, stimulated T cell supernatants costimulate thymocyte proliferation or can maintain the growth of T cell blasts, and the orthologue has been detected in bony fish and birds. The chicken IL-2 protein is only 24% identical to human IL-2 and only 70% identical to a near cousin, the turkey. IL-2's relative IL15 has also been cloned in the chicken (253). A candidate IL-2R in chicken was identified by a mAb recognizing a 50-kDa molecule only on stimulated T cells (thus an IL-2Rα homologue). This mAb blocks costimulation by IL-2–like molecules in chicken T cell supernatants and also reduces the capacity of T cell blasts to absorb IL-2–like activity from supernatants. IL-2 has been studied in the bony fish *Fugu*. In both chicken and the deduced *Fugu* IL-2 protein, there is a second set of cysteine residues, which are found in IL-15 and thus is a primordial feature (254). Syntenic to the IL-2 gene in *Fugu* is the IL-2 relative IL-21.

The common γ chain (γC) is the signaling subunit of the IL-2, IL-4, IL-7, IL-9, IL-15, and IL-21 receptors; absence of this chain in mammals leads to major defects in lymphocyte development ("boy in the bubble"). A γC homologue was cloned in rainbow trout with unusually high identity (44%–46%) to mouse/human genes. IL-1β, but not LPS, upregulated the trout gene in macrophage cultures and a fibroblast cell line. Identification of this protein subunit should allow the biochemical isolation of several fish cytokine receptors.

In summary, similar phenomena described in mammals for IL-2 and IL-2R expression seem to exist in all jawed vertebrates. Future studies will lead not only to an understanding of IL-2 evolution at the structural level, but also insight into the seasonal changes in T cell stimulation in reptiles, the differential capacity of larval and adult amphibian T cells to produce or respond to T cell growth factors, and hyperstimulation of T cells in the mutant obese chicken strain.

Interferons

Type I IFN is expressed in leukocytes (IFN-α) and virus-infected fibroblasts (IFN-β) and induces inhibition of viral replication in neighboring cells, as well as molecules of the innate immune system such as iNOS and IRF-1. In contrast, type II IFN (IFN-γ or immune IFN) is synthesized by activated T cells, activates macrophages, and upregulates class I, class II, immune proteasome subunits, and TAP, and a large number of other genes. IFN has not been detected in the invertebrates, and in general cellular immunity in the invertebrates has lagged behind the explosion of data on humoral immunity. However, as described earlier, viral immunity does include a JAK/STAT response analogous to the IFN response of the deuterostomes (90).

Antiviral activity is detected in supernatants from virally infected fish fibroblasts, epithelial cell lines, and leukocytes. All of the biochemical properties of mammalian type I IFN (e.g., acid-stable, temperature-resistant) are present in these fish supernatants, and the putative IFN reduces viral cytopathic effects in homologous cell lines infected with virus. *In vivo,* passive transfer of serum from virally infected fish protects naïve fish from acute viral pathogenesis. There appears to be two lineages of type I IFNs in fish that are specific to this group. In chickens, there are up to 10 closely related, intronless type I IFN genes. Sequence identity to human type I IFN ranges from 25% to 80% with the apparent functional gene having highest similarity (255).

Type II IFN has been cloned in chickens and several teleosts. The chicken gene is 35% identical to human type II IFN and only 15% identical to chicken type I IFN. Recombinant chicken IFN stimulates nitric oxide production and class II expression by macrophages. The gene has been cloned in trout, *Fugu,* and zebrafish, and has been studied mostly in the trout where it has been shown to upregulate γIP10 and activate protein kinase C (PKC). Thus, at least in chickens and teleost fish, type II IFN seems to have the same function as in mammals, suggesting that the TH1-type responses emerged early in vertebrate evolution.

TH1 Cytokines Besides Type II IFNs

IL-12 is generally considered to be a proinflammatory cytokine produced by APC that promotes a TH1 response after exposure to intracellular pathogens. Consistent with the ancient derivation of TH1 responses, the two subunits of IL-12 p70 (p35 and p40) have been found in chickens and several teleost species. However, studies of *Fugu* suggest that the regulation of the two subunits is not the same as in mammals, which must be supplemented with functional studies and extension to other species (248).

The p40 subunit of IL-12 can also associate with p19 to form the cytokine IL-23, which is involved in the induction of TH17 cells. This subunit has yet to be found in any nonmammalian vertebrate. Similarly, whether the IL-12-related cytokine IL-27 is found in nonmammalian vertebrates is not known.

TH2 Cytokines: IL-4, IL-5, IL-9, and IL-13

Responses to extracellular pathogens are largely regulated by TH2 cytokines in mammals. IL-4 is the most pleiotropic cytokine in this regard, provoking the production of neutralizing cytokines, stimulation of eosinophils, and an antagonism of TH1 responses. IL-4, IL-5, and IL-13 are encoded in the so-called TH2 cytokine complex in mammals, and all of the genes are coordinately upregulated after stimulation of a nearby locus-control region. This same "TH2 complex" is found in chickens (256), but in *Xenopus* only the IL-4 gene has been identified to date, and it is controversial whether *any* of the genes are found in the teleost fish, although a candidate gene was detected in pufferfish that has a tissue distribution inconsistent with being genuine IL-4 (257).

Thus, at this stage of study, it may be that lower vertebrates do not have "full-blown" TH2 responses, consistent with the lack of canonical allergic responses in ectothermic vertebrates. On the other hand, we must be careful, because cytokine genes evolve rapidly and relying on synteny is not always dependable, especially in the teleost fish. It will be of interest to see whether IL-4 in nonmammalian vertebrates will promote switching to isotypes that are incapable of promoting inflammatory responses. In addition, further studies of this family and its receptors in teleost and cartilaginous fish will reveal whether this facet of the adaptive immune response is indeed a relative newcomer.

Transforming Growth Factor (TGF)β and IL-10

TGF forms a large family with pleiotropic effects in many developmental systems. For the immune system, TGF-β isoforms are best known for their capacity to suppress adaptive immune responses (even across species barriers), although they can also stimulate lymphocytes under certain conditions. TGF-β inhibits macrophage activation in trout and growth of T cell lines in *Xenopus* species. Trout TGF-β, most similar to mammalian TGF-β1 and -β5 (62%–66% identity), is expressed in lymphoid tissues and brain, but not in the liver. Two forms of TGF-β were isolated in *Xenopus* species, both of which act on embryonic ectoderm to induce mesoderm. Recombinant *Xenopus* TGF-β, like the mammalian form, also can inhibit IL-2-like dependent growth of splenic lymphoblasts. Four TGF-β isoforms were isolated from chickens, as opposed to three major forms in mammals. The three major forms of the cytokine have been isolated in several teleost species (248).

IL-10 is often considered along with TGF-β because it is mostly an immunosuppressive cytokine with multiple effects; both cytokines are expressed in subsets of "Treg" cells in mammals. This cytokine was originally discovered by its ability to suppress TH1 responses, but now is known to have a much-expanded role. IL-10 has been found in chickens and a large number of teleosts. As usual, functional experiments have lagged behind the molecular work, but recombinant chicken IL-10 can block IFNγ production by splenocytes. Of the cytokines related to IL-10, including IL-19, IL-20, and IL-24, only IL-20 was found to date in the *Fugu* genome.

Note that there have been no "Treg" experiments reported *per se* in the comparative literature, but many older experiments that suggest that such cells exist. More than 25 years ago, experiments in *Xenopus* showed that graft rejection could be delayed when lymphocytes from metamorphosing animals were adoptively transferred into adult frogs (258). This result suggested that a "wave" of suppressor cells emerged near the time of metamorphosis that evolved to protect animals from autoimmunity when adult-specific molecules were expressed. It is time to reexamine such experiments with modern tools.

IL-17

Recently, besides TH1 and TH2 cells, two new classes of CD4 cells, TH17 and the aforementioned Treg, have become popular among immunologists. TH17 is proposed to be a cell type important for inflammatory responses to extracellular bacteria via stimulation of neutrophils. Despite its late appearance on the scene in the general literature, this cytokine appears to be one of the oldest, with homologues in lower deuterostomes like amphioxus and extensively amplified in sea urchins (32). Even the different isoforms seem to be conserved among the jawed vertebrates, which should initiate many new avenues of study over the next few years.

The isolation of nonmammalian cytokines and cytokine receptor genes has followed molecular characterization of antigen receptors and MHC. However, with the advent of the genome and EST projects, we are rapidly acquiring a comparative view of this field, at least at the genetic and molecular level. Teleost fish and chickens have paved the way in this field, but amphibian and cartilaginous fish databases will soon be complete and provide the big picture. Already, it seems that cytokines like TNF and IL-17 are most primordial, with homologues in *Ciona*, amphioxus, and sea urchins. Conversely, *none* of the other so-called *adaptive cytokines* seem to be present in the lower deuterostomes, consistent with the Big Bang theory of adaptive immunity. If it is true that the jawless fish lack these genes as well, despite their convergent adaptive immune system, one can point to the evolution of lymphoid organs and the segregation of lymphocyte subsets into discrete areas to help to explain the explosion and recruitment of these genes.

Despite our "big picture" knowledge of the emergence of cytokines, obviously functional experiments have lagged behind. Further, is it true that TH2 responses are evolutionary latecomers, or are our early attempts at finding the genes in ectotherms because of some "missing pieces" in the databases (or our ability to find some of the genes)? Some genes may have been lost, as described earlier for the chicken—again, further studies of amphibians and cartilaginous fish should help in our understanding. In mammals, the LT TNF family members are important in the development of lymph nodes, and yet the three genes are present in lymph node–less *Xenopus*—what are their functions? If we can uncover these other roles in nonmammalian vertebrates, it could be quite informative to reinvestigate such functions in mammals. Finally, chickens and fish have evolved their own paralogues of some of the well-known cytokine genes; their study should reveal selection pressures on particular species that could also be quite informative in our understanding of the gestalt of the cytokine network.

General Evolution of Chemokines and Their Receptors

Chemokines and chemokine receptors are essential for many aspects of the immune system, including the differentiation of lymphoid tissues, trafficking of hematopoietic cells during ontogeny and immune responses, and even stimulation of cells under various conditions. With the advent of the genome and EST projects, a recent paper showed that, consistent with the Bing Bang theory of adaptive immune system evolution, all of the major classes of chemokines and their receptors emerged in the bony fish lineage (259) and probably will be found in cartilaginous fish as well when the genome is complete. In fact, bony fish have more chemokines/receptors than any other vertebrate, including amphibians and mammals.

Interestingly, no CC or CXC chemokines/receptors were detected in lower dueterstomes like *Ciona* and sea urchin. The chemokine receptors are members of the G protein-coupled receptor (GPCR) family, and of course such molecules are found in all animals. However, no members of the specialized family (GPCRγ) to which chemokine receptors belong were found in lower deuterostomes. The chemokine receptor genes are found on four chromosomes in mammals, each of which contain the HOX genes, one of the gene families that provided evidence for the 2R hypothesis early in the reawakening of this theory (7). The distribution of chemokine receptor genes on these chromosomes correlates very well with 2R and helps to account for the large-scale gene expansion of this family in the jawed vertebrates. Thus far, very few chemokines/receptors (e.g., IL-8 and CXCR4) have been detected in agnathans, but they are clearly present and likely required for movement of VLR-expressing cells throughout the body.

EVOLUTION OF ALLORECOGNITION

Histocompatibility Reactions in Plants and Invertebrates

Before the true role of MHC was discovered, histocompatibility reactions were the major means used to investigate evolutionary aspects of the immune system in comparative immunology. Scrutinizing specific memory in graft rejection assays across the animal kingdom demonstrated that allorecognition was almost universal among metazoa and led to speculations on the origins of vertebrate MHC (260). However, the mechanisms and molecular underpinnings of such alloreactions remained unsolved. With the new genome projects and functional analyses, a true picture starts to emerge when one examines these old experiments.

The prevention of self-fertilization has evolved several times in the plant kingdom (261). In one case, the molecular mechanism for the phenomenon has been elucidated in study of the highly polymorphic self-recognition (*S*) locus of crucifers. Genes encoding TM-receptor Ser/Thr kinases called SRK (*S*-locus receptor protein kinase) are expressed in the stigma and closely linked to genes for soluble SCR (*S*-locus cysteine-rich) proteins expressed by pollen. Both genes are highly polymorphic, and if a self-SCR is recognized by an SRK, pollen tube growth and hence self-fertilization is inhibited. SRKs are members of a plant gene family that have been recruited for this purpose, and the SCRs have structural similarities to the amphipathic defensins described earlier; thus, perhaps molecules involved in microbial pattern recognition were coopted for this new purpose. Here, the two very different linked genes must coevolve, in ways not understood, within each haplotype to ensure mutual binding of the self-gene products. Thus, while similar mechanisms at the genetic and population levels described earlier (e.g., balancing selection, ancient allelic lineages, coevolution of linked genes, etc.) are operational for *S* locus, MHC, and other recognition systems, clearly pressures can coopt quite different types of gene families for involvement in the recognition events. Close linkage of polymorphic receptor and ligand genes involved in all of the histocompatibility reactions outside of the jawed vertebrates is an inviolable rule.

The life histories of several aquatic invertebrates in the taxa Porifera, Cnidaria, Bryozoa, and Tunicata (Figure 3.1) are characterized by the sexual production of motile larvae that settle, metamorphose, and initiate asexual reproduction by budding. This results in the growth of a colony (polyps in Cnidaria or zooids in Tunicata). Colonies often compete for space and may develop histocompatibility reactions in the zone of contact. In addition, cell-lineage parasitism, in which the somatic or germ cell lineage of one partner replaces that of the other, may ensue if colonies fuse into a chimera (262). Thus, allorecognition also protects the genetic integrity of the individual. In some species, fusion is apparently restricted to tissues of the same individual (complete matching), in other species such as bryozoans, fusion also occurs between genetically distinct individuals if they share kinship (partial matching) (263). Two divergent invertebrate phyla have been studied in detail: Cnidaria and Tunicata (Figure 3.1). To preface this section, in no case does the genetic region responsible for the histocompatibility reactions resemble the vertebrate MHC, except by high polymorphism of all systems, and at times, analogous outcomes.

Porifera

Sponges (Porifera) are the phylogenetically oldest extant metazoan phylum. A surprising characteristic of sponges, considering their phylogenetic position, is that they possess a sophisticated histocompatibility system. Recently, elements of the sponge immune system have been analyzed at the molecular level. By differential display, two genes were identified in *S. domuncula,* the products of which are involved in a still undetermined manner in aggregation. Sponge cells associate in a species-specific process through multivalent calcium-dependent interactions of carbohydrate structures on a 200 kd extracellular membrane-bound proteoglycan called "aggregation factor." The glycan moiety is involved in cell adhesion and exhibits differences in size and epitope content among individuals, suggesting the existence of allelic variants. Therefore, strong carbohydrate-based cell adhesion evolved at the very start of metazoan history. Other genes involved in these reactions include one that is similar to the vertebrate MHC-linked allograft inflammatory factor (AIF-1, Figure 3.12) and another to the T cell factor transcription factor (TCF). AIF-1 and TCF genes are upregulated *in vivo* after tissue transplantation, and *in vitro* in mixed sponge cell reaction (MSCR). Polymorphic IgSF molecules are found on the surface of sponge cells, but their relationship to allorecognition events (if one exists) is not clear (264).

Allogeneic recognition *in vitro* led to apoptotic cell death in one partner and survival in the other. The process is controlled by a differential expression of the pro-apoptotic and pro-survival proteins that are characteristic for the initiation of apoptosis (caspase, MA3, ALG-2 protein) and the prevention of programmed cell death (2 Bcl-2 homology proteins, FAIM-related polypeptide and DAD-1-related protein). In an apoptotic mixed cell combination, characteristic apoptotic genes were expressed, while in the nonapoptotic aggregates the cell-survival genes are upregulated (265). In another species, *Microciona,* allogeneic interactions also induce cellular reactions involving gray cells (sponge immunocytes) and finally apoptosis. Analogous (but probably not homologous) to T cell responses, the response is inhibited by cyclosporin A (266).

Sponge genetics is in its infancy, but from observation of 50 pairs of larval grafts within one F1 progeny of the marine sponge *Crambe*, 75% could fuse, a proportion suggesting that the genetic control depends on one locus and sharing of one haplotype results in fusion; a 100% fusion between mother and offspring is consistent with this interpretation. Unfortunately, individuals from a given mother may not have the same father, complicating the issue. Still the few data available are consistent with a single or at least major histocompatibility locus (or region), the "rule" in other invertebrate phyla described in the following.

Cnidaria

The existence of highly polymorphic histocompatibility loci was demonstrated long ago in various corals or sea anemone, but the diploblastic colonial cnidarian *Hydractinia* was the only species to provide a model to analyze genetic control of such reactions. In 1950, Hauenschild noticed that allorecognition seemed to be under the control of a single genetic region with multiple alleles (267), and this system has been studied in great detail by Buss and his colleagues. Colonies of *Hydractinia* encrust the shells of hermit crabs, where they grow by elongation and branching of stolons. Embryos and larvae fuse indiscriminately. However, when two or more larvae are recruited to the same substratum, colonial forms may come into contact through their stolons. If the two colonies are histocompatible, stolon tips adhere and fuse, establishing gastrovascular connections and a permanent genetic chimera. If tips are incompatible, colonies fail to adhere. They swell (hyperplastic stolons) with the migration of nematocysts, which discharge and damage the tissues. In addition, transitory fusions can also occur in a few cases. Similar to the genetics of the sponge alloreactions discussed earlier (and in other invertebrates and plants), colonies fuse if they share one or two haplotypes, reject if they share no haplotypes, and display transitory fusion if they share only one allele at one haplotype and no alleles at the other. Examination of the polymorphic locus governing this reaction (*alr*) revealed that two closely linked polymorphic loci (likely encoding receptor and ligand) are involved (268). The *alr*-encoded receptors, as well as the effectors of the reaction (other than the nematocysts), are unkown.

Urochordates

Compared to Cnidaria, tunicates shared a recent common ancestor with the vertebrates and thus might be expected to have a histocompatibility system more related to MHC. Allorecognition has been studied in both colonial forms and solitary ascidians. The model originally developed by Oka and Watanabe in the tunicate *Botryllus* (269), a colonial ascidian, has been studied over the past 25 years by several groups (270). What attracted extra attention to this system was the discovery that the locus controlling histocompatibility was linked to, or was the same locus, as that controlling fertilization by preventing self-fertilization; in this case, the sperm must be genetically disparate from the egg.

Metamorphosis in *Botryllus* is followed by budding that eventually gives rise to a large colony of asexually derived genetically identical individuals (zooids), united through a vascular network. At the periphery of the colony, the vasculature ends in small protrusions called *ampullae,* which are the sites of interaction when two colonies meet during their expansion. The interaction results in either fusion of the two ampullae to form a single chimeric colony sharing a common blood supply, or a rejection reaction during which the interacting ampullae are destroyed, thus preventing vascular fusion. Hemocytes (morula cells) are involved in the reaction (271). Fusion or rejection is governed by a single highly polymorphic locus called the *FuHC* (for fusion/histocompatibility; 10 wild-type individuals collected from around the Monterey Bay area yielded 18 cFuHC alleles). When two colonies share one or both FuHC alleles, they will fuse; rejection occurs if no alleles are in common. The FuHC is highly polymorphic, with most populations containing tens to hundreds of alleles. However like in *Hydractinia,* the situation is not that straightforward since intermediary pathways have been reported in the past and have not been entirely elucidated.

The painstaking development of inbred lines of *Botryllus* homozygous for different FuHC alleles has resulted in a molecular characterization of the polymorphic FuHC locus (272). The deduced C-terminal region of the molecule consists of a nectinlike segment with 3 Ig domains, showing best homology to chicken IgSF4 and related members conserved in all vertebrates as well as to one of the *Ciona* nectins. Those members are found in a tetrad of paralogues in vertebrates but not linked to the tetrad of MHC paralogues ([11] discussed later). The N-terminal region contains an EGF domain and some other unrecognizable regions not conserved among ascidians. Any two alleles differ by an average of 4% at the nucleotide level. Unlike MHC class I and class II, polymorphic residues in FuHC alleles are not concentrated in particular regions.

Some 200 kb away from FuHC, on the same chromosome, is a second polymorphic (and polygenic) locus, *fester,* which is inherited in distinct haplotypes. Diversified through extensive alternative splicing, with each individual expressing a unique repertoire of splice forms, it potentially exists as both membrane-bound and secreted forms, all expressed in tissues intimately associated with histocompatibility. After *fester* knockdown, the histocompatibility reaction is blocked at the stage of initiation as if the colonies ignored each other. In contrast, when *fester* is blocked with specific mAbs, fusion reactions were unaffected, but rejection reactions were turned into fusions in an allele-dependent manner. These data combined with its genetic location suggest that *fester* encodes the FuHC ligand. *Fester* contains a short consensus repeat (SCR, or sushi domain) often found in vertebrate complement receptors (273).

Solitary Ascidians

In *Halocynthia roretzi,* a "polymorphism of color" has been observed, and histocompatibility reset by a mixed hemocyte technique *in vitro,* resulting in a melanization reaction likely to involve the PPO cascade (274). Depending on the strains, the percentage of positive reaction varied from ~55% to 70%, indicative of polymorphism. Grafting experiments had already shown the existence of allorecognition in solitary ascidians and investigation at the cellular level had demonstrated the occurrence of cytotoxic cells in such organisms (275). As mentioned earlier, in order to shed light on allorecognition in urochordates and on the molecules involved in preventing self-fertilization, gonadal cDNAs of three genetically unrelated *Ciona intestinalis* individuals were compared by suppression subtractive hybridization (SSH). This led to the discovery of the highly polymorphic VCLR1 (variable complement receptor–like 1) gene coding for a TM protein with several short consensus repeat domains (SCR/CCP), a motif shared with the variable fester receptor of *Botryllus* described earlier (276).

The Meaning and Selection of Histocompatibility Reactions

The association between allorecognition in *Botryllus* and fertilization led to the proposal that histocompatibility systems were selected during evolution to avoid inbreeding. The hypothesis made sense in the case of sessile colonial invertebrates that might have difficulty dispersing their gametes and therefore are susceptible to inbreeding depression. Indeed the partial matching mentioned earlier is a general characteristic of fusion compatibility in colonial invertebrates, perhaps driven by "selection operating on an error-prone genetic system for self-recognition that is perhaps constrained by derivation from a gametic function selected to reduce inbreeding." Further, even for mammals, there is a large literature suggesting a selection both at the mate-choice and pregnancy levels for preserving heterozygocity at the MHC (see Flajnik, Miller and Du Pasquier in the 5th edition of *Fundamental Immunology*). However, the possibility of a common genetic system, or linked systems, governing fusion and gametic compatibility awaits confirmation. Animals that are neither sessile nor unable to disperse their gametes can possess alloimmune responses, which is inconsistent with the general hypothesis. Moreover, inbreeding avoidance can only explain the selection of histocompatibility alleles if the histocompatibility loci are genetically linked to a large fraction of its genome (277). This is inconsistent with the tight linkage of histocompatibility genes to a single major locus, especially in invertebrates. So inbreeding avoidance is unlikely to contribute significantly to the selection of histocompatibility alleles, although in jawed vertebrates, selection for heterozygocity at the MHC itself has obvious advantages.

Another hypothesis is that alloimmunity was selected because it avoided intraspecific parasitism or competition for attachment sites (278). Indeed, after fusion of compatible colonies, bloodborne germline or totipotent stem cells are transferred between colonies and can expand

and differentiate in the newly arising, asexually derived individuals of the vascular partner (279). This can result in a situation where only one genotype is represented in the gametic output of the fused individuals. The FuHC polymorphism in *Botryllus* could function to restrict to compatible individuals the vascular fusion and the germline parasitism. The high allelic polymorphism characteristic of all invertebrate recognition systems may have evolved in response to selection for fusion with self rather than kin. Fusion with self will allow the development of a colony that benefits from fusion while eliminating the possible cost of somatic cell parasitism, and thus would be the *raison d'être* of the allorecognition mechanisms (280).

However, most animals are not sessile and thus are neither prone to intraspecific competition nor to competition for limited substrate attachment sites. Tunicates besides *Botryllus* have evolved differently—for example, in *Diplosoma*, large numbers of chimaeras are encountered in nature (281). In addition, the intraspecific competition hypothesis demands that individuals maintain expression of histocompatibility alleles, even when the expression of these alleles enables their own destruction during intraspecific competition. These considerations suggest that intraspecific competition might affect histocompatibility allele frequencies in some organisms under certain conditions but is unlikely to have broad relevance for the evolution of alloimmunity.

Both previous hypotheses are essentially based on observations made in colonial tunicates, but colony living has evolved several times independently. Urochordates are more ancient than the vertebrates, but the evidence argues against any of the systems being ancestral to MHC class I and class II. That all these studies show a general pressure for polymorphism is quite clear, but the evidence from all systems studied to date suggests strong pressures to evolve similar systems via convergence. However, as described earlier, genetic regions with homology to the vertebrate MHC have been detected in the invertebrates (282), yet are (most likely) unrelated to the reactions detailed here.

As described, in all of the allorecognition systems convergent mechanisms have been encountered to reach an analogous end, and thus it is unlikely that a unique "cause" arose for selecting them in diverse organisms. However in an attempt to find an ultimate and general explanation to the selection during evolution of highly polymorphic allorecognition systems, it has been suggested that pathogen and retroviruses are the force behind the selection of allopolymorphism (277). The hypothesis that places itself at the level of a general selection pressure exerted by pathogens has the advantage of not predicting one given genetic system but a general strategy of adaptation. It does not imply intimate phylogenetic relationships between the systems observed, but points to analogous solutions when facing similar pressures.

ORIGINS OF ADAPTIVE IMMUNITY

The immune system of vertebrates is unique because the antigen-specific receptor expressed by lymphocytes, which initiates cascades leading to activation of the adaptive immune system, is not the product of a complete germline inherited gene. Rather, receptors are generated somatically during lymphocyte ontogeny from gene segments scattered at a particular locus. As described earlier, jawed vertebrate are IgSF members composed of variable (V) and constant (C) domains, with the C domains being of the rare "C1" type, which is shared by MHC class II and class I molecules (Figure 3.3). There are many specific questions: 1) Did MHC class I or class II come first? 2) What is the origin of the MHC PBR? 3) Was the MHC involved with innate immunity before the emergence of adaptive immunity? 4) Did somatic rearrangement or somatic mutation come first to diversify antigen receptors? 5) Which of the extant antigen receptors, α/β TCR, γ/δ TCR, or IgH/L (if any) resembles the primordial receptor? The answers to these questions will always remain speculative, but deductions can be made based on the wealth of genetic data accrued over the past few years. We base many of our arguments on the large-scale duplications that were noticed for MHC by Kasahara in 1996 (Figure 3.13). The remarkable syntenies of paucicopy genes on the paralogous regions, and the recent finding that an animal that predated the duplications (Amphioxus and *Ciona*) has only single-copy genes in the same syntenic group orthologous to the four mammalian copies, make it incontrovertible that at least *en bloc* duplications were involved (282); recent evidence examining essentially all genes in the human genome strongly support the 2R hypothesis (161). Further analysis of this region in Amphioxus and other deuterostomes will begin to answer at least the first three questions in the preceding paragraph. Genetic analyses in protostome lineages have not been very informative, but we must have a second look once we piece together data from more deuterostome species.

MHC Origins

Class I and class II molecules have been found only on the jawed vertebrates—so far, painstaking screenings of the lower deuterostome or lamprey/hagfish databases have yielded no indication of these proteins. Based on phylogenetic analyses and thermodynamic arguments, most investigators believe that class II preceded class I in evolution. However, as stated earlier, class I is much more plastic than class II, as there are many different types of class I molecules, some that do not even bind to peptides. Because class I genes may be on two or three MHC paralogues, and they can have functions outside the immune system, this is evidence that the primordial PBR may not have even bound to anything. If this is true, and because class I and class II do bind peptides, it would suggest class I arose first.

Again, genome scans of jawless fish and lower deuterostomes should be informative on this point, but to date we have had no luck.

From the paralogue data, genes encoding the complement components C3 and Bf, TNFSF members, the signaling molecule Vav, and proteasome subunits, among other genes, should have been present in the proto-MHC before emergence of the adaptive immune system (Figure 3.13). Some of these genes were found in the Amphioxus MHC linkage groups, and C3 and Bf genes are linked in the sea urchin. A fifth paralogous region on human chr 12p13 contains the α2-macroglobulin gene (recall the C3/4/5 homologue), a tapasin homologue, the C3a-receptor, and this "complex" is linked to the NKC. Taken together, the data suggest that the proto MHC included vital nonhomologous genes of the innate immune system, which perhaps were linked to allow coordinate regulation of expression (283). After the *en bloc* duplications, Pontarotti has suggested that "functional restraints upon the complex were relaxed" and hence the duplicated members could evolve new functions, including features indispensable to the adaptive system (284). If indeed innate immunity genes were already linked to allow upregulation at times of infection, it is no surprise that the adaptive immune system piggybacked on such a gene complex. A final point: Why did the duplicate genes survive rather well over hundreds of millions of years? Cis duplicates have been shown to degenerate rapidly over evolutionary time. Evidence suggests that duplicates arising from polyploidy (and by inference large *en bloc* duplications) survive better than cis duplicates, most likely because they cannot be inactivated by unequal crossovers (285); the ability of the genes to survive over very long periods, perhaps combined with strong selection pressures, would allow for subspecialization.

Origins of Rearranging Receptors

The Rearranging Machinery

Most models propose that the generation of somatically rearranging receptors occurred abruptly in evolution via the generation of the RAG machinery made of two lymphocyte-specific proteins, RAG1 and RAG2. *RAG* genes have so far been isolated in all classes of jawed vertebrates, excluding reptiles, and have been quite conserved. In every case examined, *RAG1* and *RAG2* genes are closely linked and in opposite transcriptional orientation. Some regions of RAG1 and RAG2 are similar to bacterial recombinases or to molecules involved in DNA repair (e.g., RAD16), or the regulation of gene expression (e.g., rpt-1r). Similarities to prokaryotic proteins and the gene structure suggest that vertebrates acquired the RAG machinery by horizontal transfer and transposition from bacteria (286). Indeed, *RAG* genetic organization has some transposon characteristics: The RSS are reminiscent of sequences involved in targeting excision of transposons (287). A new class of transposons has been detected in several protostome and deuterostome invertebrate species that shows similarity to the catalytic domain of RAG1 (288). It is believed that RSS were derived from the terminal inverted repeats of this new transposon, called *transib*. In the sea urchin genome, there are many of such "RAG1 core regions," but only one has an open reading frame throughout the core and shows similarity to vertebrate RAG1 in other regions as well. Further, a *RAG2* homologue is adjacent to the urchin *RAG1* gene, in a similar orientation as is found in gnathostomes (289). This finding was a big surprise and suggests that both *RAG* genes were in place ~100 million years before the origin of the Ig/TCR system. Their precise tissue distribution and expression during ontogeny are not known; nor have there been any candidate genes recognized to date with RSS that might be recognized by the echinoderm homologues. It must be admitted that it is unclear how this new result fits into the puzzle of the origins of adaptive immunity.

Another source of somatic antigen receptor diversity shared by all gnathostomes characterized to date is a unique DNA polymerase, TdT, which diversifies CDR3 during Ig and TCR gene rearrangement through the addition of nucleotides in a template-independent fashion. Further, as detailed earlier, its expression serves as an unambiguous developmental marker for the sites of lymphopoiesis. TdT has been highly conserved in both sequence (> 70% aa similarity, >50% aa identity) and overall structure during vertebrate evolution (32). An amino acid alignment of all known TdT sequences reveals that some, but not all, structural motifs believed to be critical for TdT activity are particularly well conserved in all vertebrates studied. TdT protein alignments and the crystal structure for rat β-polymerase support the hypothesis that both evolved from a common ancestral DNA repair gene. In addition, four protein kinase C phosphorylation sites are conserved and hence may be involved in TdT regulation. Homologues related to the ancestor of polymerase β and TdT have been found in sea urchin and other lower deuterostomes. Thus, unlike RAG, TdT has evolved by gradual evolution from a polymerase family and was recruited for immune system function.

As described, somatic rearrangement is dependent on RAG1/2. It seems that a "horizontal" acquisition of a RAG-laden transposon occurred at some point during the history of the vertebrates. In principle, RAG activity is confined to lymphocytes, but the existence of germline rearrangements of shark Ig genes suggests that RAG can remain an active force, modifying the genome in some vertebrates (150). As the enzyme itself is not so informative for phylogenetic analysis of origins of the adaptive immune system, one must turn to the history of the substrate (i.e., the V(J)C IgSF domains, [discussed later]). Introduction of RAG genes from a unicellular organism would be a unique example of a modification of the primordial immune system by horizontal transfer. In this case, microorganisms that interacted with ancestral vertebrates (or lower deuterostomes) would not simply select the variation derived from the species on which it exerts its pressure, but it would introduce a new source of variation in the immune system. One must think of the cellular lineage in which somatic rearrangement was introduced. Such a dangerous innovation could not be tolerated under conditions where it would be ubiquitously expressed, because it might jeopardize the whole genome. Most likely the introduction was into a gene that controlled a lymphoid cell lineage where a mistake would not threaten the whole individual (perhaps one that already was part of an adaptive immune system governed by SHM; discussed later). Another scenario postulates that RAG was inactive until specific factors coevolved to permit lymphocyte-specific expression. The discovery that neighboring *RAG1/2* genes are controlled by a single switch in a small piece of DNA next to one end of the RAG2 gene may explain why, over the 450 million years since the genes first appeared, they have remained closely linked (290). What was important is that the original transposon became controlled by regulatory regions active in only specific cell types. Perhaps there were several "attempts" at transposition in evolution, resulting in catastrophes or in other activities such as translocation or deletions. An ideal candidate would be a locus control region regulating expression of activating receptors with VC1 domains in NK-like cells, perhaps in the proto MHC or the second set of paralogues (chr 1, 3, 11, 21) before the second duplication (11). The MHC paralogous region described earlier is near the NKC on chr 12p13 (Figure 3.13) and could be derived from the ancestral gene complex, and the *Xenopus* MHC-linked *XMIV* genes are also excellent candidates (160). In the same way as *RAG1/2* genes remain linked because of regulatory elements close to *RAG2,* an NK cell-specific region under the control of a regulatory region might have controlled expression of a set of genes.

Rearrangement or SHM First?

Since all antigen receptor genes use somatic rearrangement of V genes to generate diversity in CDR3 regions as well as to promote combinatorial diversity, there is no doubt that this mechanism is at the heart of adaptive immunity. Indeed, as described, most investigators believe that the introduction of the transposable element into a V gene was *the* driving force in the abrupt appearance of vertebrate adaptive immunity (291); the finding of the RAG genes in sea urchins challenges this notion at some level. However, it cannot be overemphasized that SHM is also at the origins of the immune system; further, all evidence to date suggests a gradual evolution of the hypermutation machinery (the AID/APOBEC family and associated polymerases/mismatch repair proteins) rather than the "hopeful monster" generated by the famous RAG transposon. Thus, diversity generated via SHM or gene conversion may have existed in an adaptive immune system prior to rearrangement, and V gene rearrangement was superimposed onto this already-existing system (217,221). The RAG-induced rearrangement break and subsequent repair provided something new, not only diversity in sequence but heterogeneity in size; this was a remarkable innovation and likely indeed heralded the sophistication of jawed vertebrate adaptive immunity. Perhaps it is no accident that the one gene discovered so far to be indispensable for SHM, AID, or activation-induced deaminase is encoded in the aforementioned chr 12p13 region. Further, the possibility that the VLR genes are pieced together under the influence of an APOBEC family member also suggests that conversion/mutation may have preceded rearrangement—a rare example of a homologous molecule functioning in an analogous system. If mutation indeed came first, we may find examples of it today in extant prochordates and invertebrates (though, as described earlier, no APOBEC family members have been found in the nonvertebrate deuterostomes to date.)

Which Antigen Receptor First?

Phylogenetic analyses have suggested that a γ/δ TCR-like ancestor may have predated α/β TCR and Ig H/L (292). This would suggest that direct antigen recognition, perhaps by a cell surface receptor, arose first in evolution followed by a secreted molecule and an MHC-restricted one. Hood and colleagues argue that phylogenetic analyses over such large evolutionary distances obscure true relationships among the antigen receptor genes (e.g., the relationships of the molecules in the phylogenetic trees has to impose multiple loss/gain of D segments in the different antigen receptor families) and suggests a model based on genomic organization, not so different from the Kasahara model (293). They propose an alternative phylogeny in which there exists an ancestral chromosomal region with linked genes encoding both chains of an ancestral antigen receptor heterodimer, one having D segments and one not. One *en bloc* duplication gave rise to the Ig and TCR divergence, and a second to the α/β and γ/δ TCR gene complexes. The α and δ loci are still closely linked in all vertebrates analyzed (human chr 14), and a pericentric inversion is suggested to have separated the TCR β and γ loci (linked on human chr 7). This model predicts that D segments only emerged once, and also explains the existence of inverted V elements in the TCR β and δ loci. This model does not predict which antigen receptor is oldest but does provide a "simple view" of receptor evolution, consistent with the Kasahara/Ohno model.

For the origin of the rearranging receptors, IgSF lineages have to be traced back through phylogeny, because such receptors generated by somatic rearrangement do not exist outside the jawed vertebrates. In a quest for molecules related to elusive ancestors, without focusing on genes expressed in the immune systems of various phyla (i.e., structure is more important than function in this case), the most homologous sequences and gene architectures in the various metazoan phyla must be scrutinized.

V(J) and C1 Domains

C1 domains are found in the antigen receptors, MHC class I and class II, and very few other molecules (Figures 3.3, 3.11). This IgSF domain is so far most prevalent in gnathostomes, as if C1 domains arose concurrently with the adaptive immune system and coevolved with it. What was the value of the C1 domain and why is it found almost exclusively in adaptive immune system-related molecules? All of these molecules interact with coreceptors such as CD3 (TCR), Igα and β chains (Ig on B cells), CD4, and CD8 (with MHC on opposing cells), and it is conceivable that in sections of IgSF domain in which C1 differs from the C2 there is a specific region favoring interaction with other molecules.

The G strand of Ig/TCR V domains is encoded by the J gene segment, separated from the V region-encoded A-F strands (Figure 3.3), and rearrangement is necessary to assemble a complete V gene. The primary structure of each Ig/TCR chain bears hallmarks of the dimeric nature of the receptor in which it participates. A diglycine bulge (Gly-X-Gly), present in all V domains, is thought either to be a beneficial adaptation, or to promote dimer formation by inducing a twist in the G strand that results in V domain pairing that appropriately orients the CDR. Monitoring this feature, therefore, might reveal genes that had the ability to form dimers similar to that of modern antigen specific receptors. In V genes that do not somatically rearrange, the G strand is an integral part of the V exon. In other remotely related IgSF genes, introns have invaded the V domain exon creating a variety of V gene families. Many examples of such events can be found in the history of the IgSF, for example in the genes encoding CD8 and CTX (294).

As described, no Ig/TCR genes have been isolated from hagfish or lampreys, although there are some tantalizing molecules potentially related to their ancestors (e.g., APAR, see earlier). Were Ig and TCR "invented" in a class of vertebrates now extinct (e.g., the placoderms, which are more primitive than cartilaginous fish but more advanced than agnathans)? It is not known whether agnathans have C1 domains, although from the study of the mammalian MHC paralogous regions, a relatively recent jawed vertebrate ancestor should have had such domains. The discovery of the three tapasin paralogues, all with C1 domains, suggests an origin prior to the full establishment of the vertebrate genome (11).

V domains, either alone (e.g., IgNAR) or in association with another V domain (e.g., Ig H/L), recognize the antigenic epitope and are therefore the most important elements for recognition. For this reason, they will be the first to be traced back in metazoan evolution by asking whether V domains exist in invertebrates. Domains with the typical V fold, whether belonging to the true V set or the I set, have been found from sponges to insects (although not necessarily involved in immune reactions; the first ones were discovered by nonimmunologists among molecules involved in nervous system differentiation in invertebrates—e.g., amalgam, lachesin, and fascicilin). Invertebrates also use IgSF members in immunity, but so far they are not V domains, but more I or C2 set (Figure 3.3, e.g., MDM, hemolin, DSCAM). However, the mollusk FREPS have a V domain at their distal end, associated with a fibrinogenlike domain. As described, they are involved in antiparasitic reactions and form a multigenic family with polymorphism (295).

Besides searching for VC1-encoding genes in nonvertebrates, surveying the human genome for such genes has been fruitful. Indeed, nonrearranging V-containing molecules, either VJ alone, VC1, or C1 alone, have been found in the human genome. Interestingly, many of them are present in the MHC class III region (human chromosome 6p21) or its paralogues (Figures 3.12, 3.13). Two MHC-linked gene segments stand out: a single V, NKP30, and a gene containing a VJC1 core, tapasin, involved in antigen processing. NKP30, made of a single Ig domain of the VJ type, is an NK cell activating receptor, and it may offer a link to cell types encountered (analogue or homologue?) in invertebrates. It could be a relative of an ancient receptor whose history is linked to the emergence of MHC class II and class I. To resemble an ancestor, the NKP30 V domain need only be associated with a C1 domain. In fact, a C1 single domain gene, pre-TCRα, is also encoded in the MHC. Besides Ig and TCR, tapasin is one of the rare cases, if not the only other case, of a gene segment with a VJC1 structure existing on several paralogous linkage groups (6, 9q33, 19q13). In other words, while this gene is related to the rearranging receptor structure, it is undoubtedly very old and probably predated the ancient block (genomewide) duplications. It could have acted as a donor of C1 to a V domain-containing gene in the MHC class III region (e.g., the XMIV), which then could have been the first substrate of the rearrangement. Another set of molecules with distal VJC1 segments, the signal-regulatory proteins (SIRPs, VJ C1 C1), and the poliovirus receptor (VJ C1 C2) could represent another group linked to the history of the Ig and TCR. For example, SIRPs may be involved in clearance of dead cells via binding to TREM1 and TREM2 receptors on monocytes/neutrophils involved in inflammatory responses that are composed of single VJ domains whose genes are MHC-linked. MOG and P0, two single V domains involved in the synthesis of myelin sheath, are encoded in the MHC paralogous region on chromosome 1. Chicken BG, which is related to MOG but probably having a different function, is encoded in the chicken MHC. Butyrophilin, CD83, and tapasin all have VJ domains, and butyrophilin also has a C1-type domain. More distant relatives with

VJC2-based architectures are also found in MHC (RAGE, CTX, lectin-related genes; Figure 3.12), and some of these genes related to the rearranging receptor ancestors are found on several paralogues (whether the MHC paralogues or other), suggesting that the V-C1 core was generated early in vertebrate evolution subsequent to the emergence of the chordate superphylum. Among all these molecules, butyrophilin is perhaps not on the direct track to antigen specific receptors. Its C domain, although proven to be C1 through its crystal structure, is more like a C2 at the primary sequence level and belongs to the CD80/86 family, rather than the TCR (296). Finally, tracing the VJ NITR gene family, described earlier, in evolution may lead us to an understanding of the original NKC/LRC/MHC, as well as identifying candidate genes related to the ancestral gene invaded by the RAG transposon (9).

Many invertebrate molecules not involved in immune responses are present as a distal V domain associated with one or more C2-type domains. In the vertebrates, many molecules have retained this feature, such as CD2 and CTX. Some members resemble "primitive" antigen receptors, and several of them map to the MHC or its paralogous regions. Many form dimers and are expressed in lymphocytes, where they form a family of adhesion molecules. A recent crystal structure analysis of a CTX-related molecule (JAM, or junctional-adhesion molecule) revealed a unique form of dimerization, suggesting that the diversity of ligand binding and domain-interactions used by different IgSF domains is extensive. Two JAM molecules form a U-shaped dimer with highly complementary interactions between the N-terminal domains. Two salt bridges are formed in a complementary manner by a novel dimerization motif, R (V, I, L) E. The RAGE gene (receptor for advanced glycosylation end products) has a rather "generic" receptor function, because it recognizes aged cells exposing particular carbohydrate motifs. CD47, another conserved IgSF member with a CTX-like V domain (297), suggests an ancient function. Perhaps such nonrearranging VJC1 genes that regulated cytotoxicity/phagocytosis were predecessors of the antigen receptors (298). Some molecules with VJ/C1 cores involved in cell-cell interactions often serve as ports of entry for viruses. In a move from "property to function," an arms race consequence could result in a virus receptor developing into an immune receptor. The best examples of such molecules are in the CTX/JAM family in which receptor interactions with viruses may trigger apoptosis, a primitive form of antiviral immunity (11,299).

CONCLUSIONS

Since the last edition of *Fundamental Immunology* was published 5 years ago, there have been several stunning findings, as well as other interesting discoveries and integrations, regarding the evolution of the structure and function of the immune system. Further, there have been many genome and EST projects that have allowed us to determine whether particular genes or gene families are present in different taxa. Here, we briefly describe these findings and discuss their broad relevance and relationship to future studies.

—As predicted in the previous edition, adaptive cytokines such as γIFN, IL-2, and IL-4 are not present outside of jawed vertebrates, nor are the vast array of chemokines seen in gnathostomes. However, at the moment it appears that almost all of the cytokines/chemokines discovered in mammals are also present in basal jawed vertebrates. IL-17, a cytokine garnering great attention in basic immunology, and TNF, a central cytokine in both innate and adaptive immunity, seem to be the first cytokines to have emerged in evolution based on studies of lower deuterostomes (32). If, as suggested from studies in mammals, IL-17 is important for responses to extracellular bacteria (300), nonvertebrate deuterostomes may hold the key to understanding the physiology of the entire system (i.e., in the absence of the competing TH1, TH2, and Treg cells, one may be able to study the dynamics of IL-17 development and function).

—A new defense system in *Drosophila*, previously recognized to be important for nervous system specialization by generating an enormous number of splice variants, is also used for immunity (with a different set of splice variants). A model for a primitive type of selection has been proposed to select for the splice variants that bind to particular invaders (301). This system is found in all insects studied to date, and importantly in parasitic vectors such as mosquitoes. Snail FREPs, shrimp penaedins, and sea urchin 185/333 have also shown that nonvertebrates can generate extraordinary levels of diversity in defense molecules. Studies of the mechanisms of diversity generation will not only provide new insights into how immune defense can be obtained (e.g., in economically important insects and agriculturally vital seafood), but also may permit new therapeutic strategies for certain diseases. In addition, "memory" or transfer of immunity from parent to offspring has been encountered in the invertebrates, without an understanding of the mechanisms involved.

—One of the great triumphs in the field of comparative immunology was the discovery that similar mechanisms are used to recognize extracellular pathogens and initiate immune responses (302). It has been ~10 years since the *Drosophila* Toll/IMD systems and their relationship to vertebrate TLR and TNFR was uncovered. By contrast, studies of viral and intracellular pathogen responses have lagged far behind in the protostomes (90,303). Now studies of viral responses in arthropods have shown that an IFN-like response working through a JAK/STAT pathway occurs (analogous, not homologous to IFN). Thus, the Toll/IMD/JAK/STAT pathways go back at least to the triploblastic ancestor about a billion years ago. Further, an RNAi-like system exists as well, consistent with previous studies of plants and other protostomes. Manipulating these defense pathways will be quite important in "immunization schedules" for commercially important aquatic species. In addition, the general breakthroughs in the study of intracellular recognition of all pathogens in eukaryotic systems, by NOD, TLR, RIG, etc., have changed our gestalt views of immune defense. Finally, similar basic strategies and gene members involved in hematopoiesis are encountered throughout the animal kingdom (23); it would be surprising if this knowledge did not permit a greater universal understanding of the differentiation and maintenance of pluripotent and restricted stem cells.

—The long-awaited molecular mechanisms of histocompatibility in nonvertebrates have been uncovered in *Botryllus* and several plants (and soon in *Hydractinia*). The common themes thus far are that the genes encoding the polymorphic receptors/ligands are closely linked and that the genes all appear to be unrelated to the vertebrate MHC. New theories have arisen concerning the physiological significance of these histocompatibility reactions (277), and in the next five years there may be some consensus on their origins and the selective pressures that maintain them.

—A totally unexpected, convergent system of adaptive, lymphocyte-based defense was discovered in jawless fish (100). While the stitching together of LRR cassettes to produce a functional VLR is definitely not RAG-based, it has been proposed that an AID/APOBEC family member is involved in the generation of diversity. If this is true, then either AID/APOBEC was recruited twice to generate diversity, or there are some cis-acting elements in both systems that were likely present in an ancestral antigen receptor gene (304).

—The sea urchin genome project exposed enormous expansions of many gene families involved in immune defense (32). The significance of these expansions is unclear; sea urchins are long-lived, and in the absence of adaptive immunity a large arsenal of defense molecules may have been selected for. Yet how an organism can use all of this innate diversity (and perhaps adaptive diversity with 185/333) is a conundrum for which we have no framework. The discovery of the Transib family in many invertebrates and of sea urchin RAG1/2 have modified our perception of the "RAG transposon," but the basic idea of an invasion of a VJ IgSF exon by such a transposon lives on.

—The central role of the complement factor and its partner C3 and Bf in the complement pathway, as well as in animal evolution, has been further emphasized by studies of protostomes and cnidarians over the past 5 years (75). The loss of C3 in many protostomes has been compensated by the emergence of the TEPs, which after all have quite similar (and apparently expanded) functions.

—The genomewide duplications early in the evolution of the vertebrates (the 2R hypothesis) have been confirmed in a variety of studies, and they were indeed important in the "Big Bang" emergence of the adaptive immune system (7). The 2R paradigm is useful for studying any gene family found on multiple chromosomes in the vertebrates; good examples of how it has aided in our understanding of immunity were the study of IgSF members involved in cell-cell interaction/costimulation (11) and the evolution/emergence of chemokines (259) and TNF family members (305). An emerging paradigm is the possibility that genes encoding NKC, LRC, and MHC, as well as the antigen receptors and costimulatory molecules (and other immune genes), were all linked at an early point in evolution.

—Finally, with the genome projects and advances in molecular biology, we have made strides in understanding old problems in vertebrate adaptive immunity (99), such as: 1) when did the L chains emerge and what is the significance of more than one isotype; 2) which antigen receptor (if any of the extant ones) came first, and how did all of them evolve to their present state; 3) when did IgD emerge and what is its function in different vertebrate phyla; and 4) how do γ/δ T cells recognize antigen? We propose that there are two arms of the γ/δ T cell lineage, one innate and the other adaptive, similar to B cells and α/β T cells.

In the next 5 years we will make inroads to answering all of these questions. Invariably, new, interesting molecules/mechanisms will be discovered, but we hope that this chapter makes card-carrying immunologists realize that we are nearing the end of the "gene-discovery period" in comparative immunology, and we are entering a new phase in which integration of mechanisms and pathways will open new doors to a comprehensive view of immunity.

ACKNOWLEDGMENTS

We thank Michael Criscitiello for help in text formatting; Katie Ris-Vicari for figure preparation; Christopher Secombes and Peter Kaiser for discussions of cytokine evolution; and Bruno Lemaitre and Jules Hofmann for permission to revise their figures on insect immunity. M. Flajnik is supported by NIH R01 grants AI027877 and RR006603.

REFERENCES

1. Pancer Z, Cooper MD. The evolution of adaptive immunity. *Annu Rev Immunol.* 2006;24:497–518.

2. Danilova N. The evolution of immune mechanisms. *J Exp Zoolog*. 2006;306(6):496–520.
3. Loker ES, Adema CM, Zhang SM, et al. Invertebrate immune systems—not homogeneous, not simple, not well understood. *Immunol Rev*. 2004;198:10–24.
4. Trowsdale J, Parham P. Mini-review: defense strategies and immunity-related genes. *Eur J Immunol*. 2004;34(1):7–17.
5. Waterhouse RM, Kriventseva EV, Meister S, et al. Evolutionary dynamics of immune-related genes and pathways in disease-vector mosquitoes. *Science*. 2007;316(5832):1738–1743.
6. Nei M, Gu X, Sitnikova T. Evolution by the birth-and-death process in multigene families of the vertebrate immune system. *Proc Natl Acad Sci USA*. 1997;94(15):7799–7806.
7. Kasahara M. The 2R hypothesis: an update. *Curr Opin Immunol*. 2007;19(5):547–552.
8. Abi-Rached L, Gilles A, Shiina T, et al. Evidence of *en bloc* duplication in vertebrate genomes. *Nat Genet*. 2002;31(1):100–105.
9. Litman GW, Cannon JP, Dishaw LJ. Reconstructing immune phylogeny: new perspectives. *Nat Rev Immunol*. 2005;5(11):866–879.
10. Watson FL, Puttmann-Holgado R, Thomas F, et al. Extensive diversity of Ig-superfamily proteins in the immune system of insects. *Science*. 2005;309(5742):1874–1878.
11. Du Pasquier L, Zucchetti I, De SR. Immunoglobulin superfamily receptors in protochordates: before RAG time. *Immunol Rev*. 2004;198:233–248.
12. Ortutay C, Siermala M, Vihinen M. Molecular characterization of the immune system: emergence of proteins, processes, and domains. *Immunogenetics*. 2007;59(5):333–348.
13. Enkhbayar P, Kamiya M, Osaki M, et al. Structural principles of leucine-rich repeat (LRR) proteins. *Proteins*. 2004;54(3):394–403.
14. Kajava AV, Kobe B. Assessment of the ability to model proteins with leucine-rich repeats in light of the latest structural information. *Protein Sci*. 2002;11(5):1082–1090.
15. Wong K, Park HT, Wu JY, et al. Slit proteins: molecular guidance cues for cells ranging from neurons to leukocytes. *Curr Opin Genet Dev*. 2002;12(5):583–591.
16. Akira S. Toll receptor families: structure and function. *Semin Immunol*. 2004;16(1):1–2.
17. Barclay AN. Membrane proteins with immunoglobulin-like domains–a master superfamily of interaction molecules. *Semin Immunol*. 2003;15(4):215–223.
18. Janeway CA, Jr., Medzhitov R. Innate immune recognition. *Annu Rev Immunol*. 2002;20:197–216.
19. Karre K. NK cells, MHC class I molecules and the missing self. *Scand J Immunol*. 2002;55(3):221–228.
20. Flajnik MF, Du Pasquier L. Evolution of innate and adaptive immunity: can we draw a line? *Trends Immunol*. 2004;25(12):640–644.
21. Kmita M, Duboule D. Organizing axes in time and space; 25 years of colinear tinkering. *Science*. 2003;301(5631):331–333.
22. Gehring WJ. New perspectives on eye development and the evolution of eyes and photoreceptors. *J Hered*. 2005;96(3):171–184.
23. Hartenstein V. Blood cells and blood cell development in the animal kingdom. *Annu Rev Cell Dev Biol*. 2006;22:677–712.
24. Jiravanichpaisal P, Lee BL, Soderhall K. Cell-mediated immunity in arthropods: hematopoiesis, coagulation, melanization and opsonization. *Immunobiology*. 2006;211(4):213–236.
25. Crozatier M, Meister M. *Drosophila* haematopoiesis. *Cell Microbiol*. 2007;9(5):1117–1126.
26. Wiens M, Korzhev M, Krasko A, et al. Innate immune defense of the sponge *Suberites domuncula* against bacteria involves a MyD88-dependent signaling pathway. Induction of a perforin-like molecule. *J Biol Chem*. 2005;280(30):27949–27959.
27. Engelmann P, Molnar L, Palinkas L, et al. Earthworm leukocyte populations specifically harbor lysosomal enzymes that may respond to bacterial challenge. *Cell Tissue Res*. 2004;316(3):391–401.
28. Prochazkova P, Silerova M, Felsberg J, et al. Relationship between hemolytic molecules in *Eisenia fetida* earthworms. *Dev Comp Immunol*. 2006;30(4):381–392.
29. Valembois P. Aims and methods in comparative immunology. *Dev Comp Immunol*. 1982;6(2):195–198.
30. Bachere E, Gueguen Y, Gonzalez M, et al. Insights into the antimicrobial defense of marine invertebrates: the penaeid shrimps and the oyster Crassostrea gigas. *Immunol Rev*. 2004;198:149–168.
31. Lemaitre B, Hoffmann J. The host defense of Drosophila melanogaster. *Annu Rev Immunol*. 2007;25:697–743.
32. Hibino T, Loza-Coll M, Messier C, et al. The immune gene repertoire encoded in the purple sea urchin genome. *Dev Biol*. 2006;300(1):349–365.
33. Wright RK. Protochordate immunity. I. Primary immune response of the tunicate *Ciona intestinalis* to vertebrate erythrocytes. *J Invertebr Pathol*. 1974;24(1):29–36.
34. Raftos DA, Cooper EL. Proliferation of lymphocyte-like cells from the solitary tunicate, Styela clava, in response to allogeneic stimuli. *J Exp Zool*. 1991;260(3):391–400.
35. Chourrout D, Delsuc F, Chourrout P, et al. Minimal ProtoHox cluster inferred from bilaterian and cnidarian Hox complements. *Nature*. 2006;442(7103):684–687.
36. Delsuc F, Brinkmann H, Chourrout D, et al. Tunicates and not cephalochordates are the closest living relatives of vertebrates. *Nature*. 2006;439(7079):965–968.
37. Huang G, Xie X, Han Y, et al. The identification of lymphocyte-like cells and lymphoid-related genes in amphioxus indicates the twilight for the emergency of adaptive immune system. *PLoS ONE*. 2007;2(2):e206.
38. Evans CJ, Hartenstein V, Banerjee U. Thicker than blood: conserved mechanisms in Drosophila and vertebrate hematopoiesis. *Dev Cell*. 2003;5(5):673–690.
39. Soderhall I, Bangyeekhun E, Mayo S, et al. Hemocyte production and maturation in an invertebrate animal; proliferation and gene expression in hematopoietic stem cells of Pacifastacus leniusculus. *Dev Comp Immunol*. 2003;27(8):661–672.
40. Soderhall I, Kim YA, Jiravanichpaisal P, et al. An ancient role for a prokineticin domain in invertebrate hematopoiesis. *J Immunol*. 2005;174(10):6153–6160.
41. Sorrentino RP, Carton Y, Govind S. Cellular immune response to parasite infection in the *Drosophila* lymph gland is developmentally regulated. *Dev Biol*. 2002;243(1):65–80.
42. Savina A, Amigorena S. Phagocytosis and antigen presentation in dendritic cells. *Immunol Rev*. 2007;219:143–156.
43. Cerenius L, Soderhall K. The prophenoloxidase-activating system in invertebrates. *Immunol Rev*. 2004;198:116–126.
44. Meylan E, Tschopp J, Karin M. Intracellular pattern recognition receptors in the host response. *Nature*. 2006;442(7098):39–44.
45. Ting JP, Davis BK. CATERPILLER: a novel gene family important in immunity, cell death, and diseases. *Annu Rev Immunol*. 2005;23:387–414.
46. Dangl JL, Jones JD. Plant pathogens and integrated defence responses to infection. *Nature*. 2001;411(6839):826–833.
47. Jones JD, Dangl JL. The plant immune system. *Nature*. 2006; 444(7117):323–329.
48. Yoneyama M, Fujita T. Function of RIG-I-like receptors in antiviral innate immunity. *J Biol Chem*. 2007;282(21):15315–15318.
49. Beutler B, Eidenschenk C, Crozat K, et al. Genetic analysis of resistance to viral infection. *Nat Rev Immunol*. 2007 Oct;7(10):753–766.
50. Xu M, Wang Z, Locksley RM. Innate immune responses in peptidoglycan recognition protein L-deficient mice. *Mol Cell Biol*. 2004;24(18):7949–7957.
51. Jiggins FM, Kim KW. Contrasting evolutionary patterns in Drosophila immune receptors. *J Mol Evol*. 2006;63(6):769–780.
52. Dong Y, Taylor HE, Dimopoulos G. AgDscam, a hypervariable immunoglobulin domain-containing receptor of the *Anopheles gambiae* innate immune system. *PLoS Biol*. 2006;4(7):e229.
53. Du Pasquier L. Immunology. Insects diversify one molecule to serve two systems. *Science*. 2005;309(5742):1826–1827.
54. Adema CM, Hertel LA, Miller RD, et al. A family of fibrinogen-related proteins that precipitates parasite-derived molecules is produced by an invertebrate after infection. *Proc Natl Acad Sci USA*. 1997;94(16):8691–8696.
55. Zhang SM, Adema CM, Kepler TB, et al. Diversification of Ig superfamily genes in an invertebrate. *Science*. 2004;305(5681):251–254.
56. Buckley KM, Smith LC. Extraordinary diversity among members of the large gene family, 185/333, from the purple sea urchin, *Strongylocentrotus purpuratus*. *BMC Mol Biol*. 2007;8:68.
57. Cannon JP, Haire RN, Mueller MG, et al. Ancient divergence of a complex family of immune-type receptor genes. *Immunogenetics*. 2006;58(5–6):362–373.

58. Cuthbertson BJ, Deterding LJ, Williams JG, et al. Diversity in penaeidin antimicrobial peptide form and function. *Dev Comp Immunol.* 2007 Aug 3.
59. Peiser L, Mukhopadhyay S, Gordon S. Scavenger receptors in innate immunity. *Curr Opin Immunol.* 2002;14(1):123–128.
60. Pancer Z. Dynamic expression of multiple scavenger receptor cysteine-rich genes in coelomocytes of the purple sea urchin. *Proc Natl Acad Sci USA.* 2000;97(24):13156–13161.
61. Kocks C, Cho JH, Nehme N, et al. Eater, a transmembrane protein mediating phagocytosis of bacterial pathogens in Drosophila. *Cell.* 2005;123(2):335–346.
62. Drickamer K, Fadden AJ. Genomic analysis of C-type lectins. *Biochem Soc Symp.* 2002;(69):59–72.
63. Zucchetti I, Marino R, Pinto MR, et al. ciCD94-1, an ascidian multipurpose C-type lectin-like receptor expressed in *Ciona intestinalis* hemocytes and larval neural structures. *Differentiation.* 2007 Oct 9.
64. Nelson RE, Fessler LI, Takagi Y, et al. Peroxidasin: a novel enzyme-matrix protein of *Drosophila* development. *EMBO J.* 1994;13(15):3438–3447.
65. Johansson MW, Lind MI, Holmblad T, et al. Peroxinectin, a novel cell adhesion protein from crayfish blood. *Biochem Biophys Res Commun.* 1995;216(3):1079–1087.
66. Selsted ME, Ouellette AJ. Mammalian defensins in the antimicrobial immune response. *Nat Immunol.* 2005;6(6):551–557.
67. Moore KS, Wehrli S, Roder H, et al. Squalamine: an aminosterol antibiotic from the shark. *Proc Natl Acad Sci USA.* 1993;90(4):1354–1358.
68. Imler JL, Hoffmann JA. Toll receptors in *Drosophila*: a family of molecules regulating development and immunity. *Curr Top Microbiol Immunol.* 2002;270:63–79.
69. Poltorak A, He X, Smirnova I, et al. Defective LPS signaling in C3H/HeJ and C57BL/10ScCr mice: mutations in Tlr4 gene. *Science.* 1998;282(5396):2085–2088.
70. Medzhitov R, Preston-Hurlburt P, Janeway CA, Jr. A human homologue of the *Drosophila* Toll protein signals activation of adaptive immunity. *Nature.* 1997;388(6640):394–397.
71. Jang IH, Chosa N, Kim SH, et al. A Spatzle-processing enzyme required for toll signaling activation in Drosophila innate immunity. *Dev Cell.* 2006;10(1):45–55.
72. Pradel E, Zhang Y, Pujol N, et al. Detection and avoidance of a natural product from the pathogenic bacterium *Serratia marcescens* by *Caenorhabditis elegans*. *Proc Natl Acad Sci USA.* 2007;104(7):2295–2300.
73. Triantafilou M, Gamper FG, Haston RM, et al. Membrane sorting of toll-like receptor (TLR)-2/6 and TLR2/1 heterodimers at the cell surface determines heterotypic associations with CD36 and intracellular targeting. *J Biol Chem.* 2006;281(41):31002–31011.
74. Luo C, Zheng L. Independent evolution of Toll and related genes in insects and mammals. *Immunogenetics.* 2000;51(2):92–98.
75. Nonaka M, Kimura A. Genomic view of the evolution of the complement system. *Immunogenetics.* 2006;58(9):701–713.
76. Endo Y, Matsushita M, Fujita T. Role of ficolin in innate immunity and its molecular basis. *Immunobiology.* 2007;212(4–5):371–379.
77. Blandin S, Levashina EA. Thioester-containing proteins and insect immunity. *Mol Immunol.* 2004;40(12):903–908.
78. Dishaw LJ, Smith SL, Bigger CH. Characterization of a C3-like cDNA in a coral: phylogenetic implications. *Immunogenetics.* 2005; 57(7):535–548.
79. Zhu Y, Thangamani S, Ho B, et al. The ancient origin of the complement system. *EMBO J.* 2005;24(2):382–394.
80. Solomon KR, Sharma P, Chan M, et al. CD109 represents a novel branch of the alpha2-macroglobulin/complement gene family. *Gene.* 2004;327(2):171–183.
81. Sunyer JO, Boshra H, Li J. Evolution of anaphylatoxins, their diversity and novel roles in innate immunity: insights from the study of fish complement. *Vet Immunol Immunopathol.* 2005;108(1–2): 77–89.
82. Melillo D, Sfyroera G, De SR, et al. First identification of a chemotactic receptor in an invertebrate species: structural and functional characterization of *Ciona intestinalis* C3a receptor. *J Immunol.* 2006;177(6):4132–4140.
83. Raftos DA, Robbins J, Newton RA, et al. A complement component C3a-like peptide stimulates chemotaxis by hemocytes from an invertebrate chordate-the tunicate, *Pyura stolonifera*. *Comp Biochem Physiol A Mol Integr Physiol.* 2003;134(2):377–386.
84. Yano K, Gale D, Massberg S, et al. Phenotypic heterogeneity is an evolutionarily conserved feature of the endothelium. *Blood.* 2007;109(2):613–615.
85. Steiner H, Hultmark D, Engstrom A, et al. Sequence and specificity of two antibacterial proteins involved in insect immunity. *Nature.* 1981;292(5820):246–248.
86. Sun SC, Faye I. Cecropia immunoresponsive factor, an insect immunoresponsive factor with DNA-binding properties similar to nuclear-factor kappa B. *Eur J Biochem.* 1992;204(2):885–892.
87. Lemaitre B, Nicolas E, Michaut L, et al. The dorsoventral regulatory gene cassette spatzle/Toll/cactus controls the potent antifungal response in Drosophila adults. *Cell.* 1996;86(6):973–983.
88. Lemaitre B, Kromer-Metzger E, Michaut L, et al. A recessive mutation, immune deficiency (imd), defines two distinct control pathways in the *Drosophila* host defense. *Proc Natl Acad Sci USA.* 1995;92(21):9465–9469.
89. Montgomery MK, Xu S, Fire A. RNA as a target of double-stranded RNA-mediated genetic interference in *Caenorhabditis elegans*. *Proc Natl Acad Sci USA.* 1998;95(26):15502–15507.
90. Beutler B, Eidenschenk C, Crozat K, et al. Genetic analysis of resistance to viral infection. *Nat Rev Immunol.* 2007;7(10):753–766.
91. Robalino J, Bartlett T, Shepard E, et al. Double-stranded RNA induces sequence-specific antiviral silencing in addition to nonspecific immunity in a marine shrimp: convergence of RNA interference and innate immunity in the invertebrate antiviral response? *J Virol.* 2005;79(21):13561–13571.
92. Theodor JL, Senelar R. Cytotoxic interaction between gorgonian explants: mode of action. *Cell Immunol.* 1975;19(2):194–200.
93. Boiledieu D, Valembois P. [In vitro study of the cytotoxic activity of sipunculid leukocytes towards allogeneic and xenogenic erythrocytes]. *C R Acad Sci Hebd Seances Acad Sci D.* 1976;283(3):247–249.
94. Nappi AJ, Ottaviani E. Cytotoxicity and cytotoxic molecules in invertebrates. *Bioessays.* 2000;22(5):469–480.
95. Pancer Z, Skorokhod A, Blumbach B, et al. Multiple Ig-like featuring genes divergent within and among individuals of the marine sponge *Geodia cydonium*. *Gene.* 1998;207(2):227–233.
96. Zucchetti I, Marino R, Pinto MR, et al. ciCD94-1, an ascidian multipurpose C-type lectin-like receptor expressed in *Ciona intestinalis* hemocytes and larval neural structures. *Differentiation.* 2007 Oct 9.
97. Azumi K, De SR, De TA, et al. Genomic analysis of immunity in a Urochordate and the emergence of the vertebrate immune system: "waiting for Godot". *Immunogenetics.* 2003;55(8):570–581.
98. Ishiguro H, Kobayashi K, Suzuki M, et al. Isolation of a hagfish gene that encodes a complement component. *EMBO J.* 1992;11(3):829–837.
99. Pancer Z, Cooper MD. The evolution of adaptive immunity. *Annu Rev Immunol.* 2006;24:497–518.
100. Pancer Z, Amemiya CT, Ehrhardt GR, et al. Somatic diversification of variable lymphocyte receptors in the agnathan sea lamprey. *Nature.* 2004;430(6996):174–180.
101. Nagawa F, Kishishita N, Shimizu K, et al. Antigen-receptor genes of the agnathan lamprey are assembled by a process involving copy choice. *Nat Immunol.* 2007;8(2):206–213.
102. Rogozin IB, Iyer LM, Liang L, et al. Evolution and diversification of lamprey antigen receptors: evidence for involvement of an AID-APOBEC family cytosine deaminase. *Nat Immunol.* 2007;8(6):647–656.
103. Alder MN, Rogozin IB, Iyer LM, et al. Diversity and function of adaptive immune receptors in a jawless vertebrate. *Science.* 2005;310(5756):1970–1973.
104. Kim HM, Oh SC, Lim KJ, et al. Structural diversity of the hagfish variable lymphocyte receptors. *J Biol Chem.* 2007;282(9):6726–6732.
105. Charlemagne J, Fellah JS, De Guerra A, et al. T-cell receptors in ectothermic vertebrates. *Immunol Rev.* 1998;166:87–102.
106. Chen CL, Bucy RP, Cooper MD. T cell differentiation in birds. *Semin Immunol.* 1990;2(1):79–86.
107. Gobel TW, Meier EL, Du Pasquier L. Biochemical analysis of the *Xenopus laevis* TCR/CD3 complex supports the "stepwise evolution" model. *Eur J Immunol.* 2000;30(10):2775–2781.
108. von BH. Unique features of the pre-T-cell receptor alpha-chain: not just a surrogate. *Nat Rev Immunol.* 2005;5(7):571–577.

109. Campbell KS, Backstrom BT, Tiefenthaler G, et al. CART: a conserved antigen receptor transmembrane motif. *Semin Immunol.* 1994;6(6):393–410.
110. Sasada T, Touma M, Chang HC, et al. Involvement of the TCR Cbeta FG loop in thymic selection and T cell function. *J Exp Med.* 2002; 195(11):1419–1431.
111. Criscitiello MF, Kamper SM, McKinney EC. Allelic polymorphism of TCRalpha chain constant domain genes in the bicolor damselfish. *Dev Comp Immunol.* 2004;28(7–8):781–792.
112. Rock EP, Sibbald PR, Davis MM, et al. CDR3 length in antigen-specific immune receptors. *J Exp Med.* 1994;179(1):323–328.
113. Nam BH, Hirono I, Aoki T. The four TCR genes of teleost fish: the cDNA and genomic DNA analysis of Japanese flounder (*Paralichthys olivaceus*) TCR alpha-, beta-, gamma-, and delta-chains. *J Immunol.* 2003;170(6):3081–3090.
114. Rast JP, Anderson MK, Strong SJ, et al. alpha, beta, gamma, and delta T cell antigen receptor genes arose early in vertebrate phylogeny. *Immunity.* 1997;6(1):1–11.
115. Su C, Jakobsen I, Gu X, et al. Diversity and evolution of T-cell receptor variable region genes in mammals and birds. *Immunogenetics.* 1999;50(5–6):301–308.
116. Hsu E, Pulham N, Rumfelt LL, et al. The plasticity of immunoglobulin gene systems in evolution. *Immunol Rev.* 2006;210: 8–26.
117. Bengten E, Wilson M, Miller N, et al. Immunoglobulin isotypes: structure, function, and genetics. *Curr Top Microbiol Immunol.* 2000;248:189–219.
118. Coscia MR, Morea V, Tramontano A, et al. Analysis of a cDNA sequence encoding the immunoglobulin heavy chain of the Antarctic teleost *Trematomus bernacchii. Fish Shellfish Immunol.* 2000;10(4):343–357.
119. Marchalonis J, Edelman GM. Polypeptide chains of immunoglobulins from the smooth dogfish (*Mustelus canis*). *Science.* 1966; 154(756):1567–1568.
120. Dooley H, Flajnik MF. Shark immunity bites back: affinity maturation and memory response in the nurse shark, *Ginglymostoma cirratum. Eur J Immunol.* 2005;35(3):936–945.
121. Rumfelt LL, Avila D, Diaz M, et al. A shark antibody heavy chain encoded by a nonsomatically rearranged VDJ is preferentially expressed in early development and is convergent with mammalian IgG. *Proc Natl Acad Sci USA.* 2001;98(4):1775–1780.
122. Greenberg AS, Avila D, Hughes M, et al. A NAR gene family that undergoes rearrangement and extensive somatic diversification in sharks. *Nature.* 1995;374(6518):168–173.
123. Stanfield RL, Dooley H, Flajnik MF, et al. Crystal structure of a shark single-domain antibody V region in complex with lysozyme. *Science.* 2004;305(5691):1770–1773.
124. Streltsov VA, Varghese JN, Carmichael JA, et al. Structural evidence for evolution of shark Ig new antigen receptor variable domain antibodies from a cell-surface receptor. *Proc Natl Acad Sci USA.* 2004;101(34):12444–12449.
125. Criscitiello MF, Saltis M, Flajnik MF. An evolutionarily mobile antigen receptor variable region gene: doubly rearranging NAR-TcR genes in sharks. *Proc Natl Acad Sci USA.* 2006;103(13):5036–5041.
126. Parra ZE, Baker ML, Schwarz RS, et al. A unique T cell receptor discovered in marsupials. *Proc Natl Acad Sci USA.* 2007;104(23):9776–97781.
127. Rumfelt LL, Diaz M, Lohr RL, et al. Unprecedented multiplicity of Ig transmembrane and secretory mRNA forms in the cartilaginous fish. *J Immunol.* 2004;173(2):1129–1139.
128. Ota T, Rast JP, Litman GW, et al. Lineage-restricted retention of a primitive immunoglobulin heavy chain isotype within the Dipnoi reveals an evolutionary paradox. *Proc Natl Acad Sci USA.* 2003;100(5):2501–2506.
129. Ohta Y, Flajnik M. IgD, like IgM, is a primordial immunoglobulin class perpetuated in most jawed vertebrates. *Proc Natl Acad Sci USA.* 2006;103(28):10723–10728.
130. Zhao Y, Pan-Hammarstrom Q, Yu S, et al. Identification of IgF, a hinge-region-containing Ig class, and IgD in *Xenopus tropicalis*. *Proc Natl Acad Sci USA.* 2006;103(32):12087–12092.
131. Wilson M, Bengten E, Miller NW, et al. A novel chimeric Ig heavy chain from a teleost fish shares similarities to IgD. *Proc Natl Acad Sci USA.* 1997;94(9):4593–4597.
132. Danilova N, Bussmann J, Jekosch K, et al. The immunoglobulin heavy-chain locus in zebrafish: identification and expression of a previously unknown isotype, immunoglobulin Z. *Nat Immunol.* 2005;6(3):295–302.
133. Hansen JD, Landis ED, Phillips RB. Discovery of a unique Ig heavy-chain isotype (IgT) in rainbow trout: Implications for a distinctive B cell developmental pathway in teleost fish. *Proc Natl Acad Sci USA.* 2005;102(19):6919–6924.
134. Flajnik MF. Comparative analyses of immunoglobulin genes: surprises and portents. *Nat Rev Immunol* 2002;2(9):688–698.
135. Mussmann R, Wilson M, Marcuz A, et al. Membrane exon sequences of the three Xenopus Ig classes explain the evolutionary origin of mammalian isotypes. *Eur J Immunol.* 1996;26(2):409–414.
136. Stavnezer J, Amemiya CT. Evolution of isotype switching. *Semin Immunol.* 2004;16(4):257–275.
137. Zarrin AA, Alt FW, Chaudhuri J, et al. An evolutionarily conserved target motif for immunoglobulin class-switch recombination. *Nat Immunol.* 2004;5(12):1275–1281.
138. Ota T, Sitnikova T, Nei M. Evolution of vertebrate immunoglobulin variable gene segments. *Curr Top Microbiol Immunol.* 2000;248:221–245.
139. Chang B, Casali P. The CDR1 sequences of a major proportion of human germline Ig VH genes are inherently susceptible to amino acid replacement. *Immunol Today.* 1994;15(8):367–373.
140. Hsu E. Canonical VH CDR1 nucleotide sequences are conserved in all jawed vertebrates. *Int Immunol.* 1996;8(6):847–854.
141. Criscitiello MF, Flajnik MF. Four primordial immunoglobulin light chain isotypes, including lambda and kappa, identified in the most primitive living jawed vertebrates. *Eur J Immunol.* 2007;37(10):2683–2694.
142. Lee SS, Greenberg A, Hsu E. Evolution and somatic diversification of immunoglobulin light chains. *Curr Top Microbiol Immunol.* 2000;248:285–300.
143. Hsu E, Criscitiello MF. Diverse immunoglobulin light chain organizations in fish retain potential to revise B cell receptor specificities. *J Immunol.* 2006;177(4):2452–2562.
144. Miller RD, Belov K. Immunoglobulin genetics of marsupials. *Dev Comp Immunol.* 2000;24(5):485–490.
145. Rast JP, Anderson MK, Ota T, et al. Immunoglobulin light chain class multiplicity and alternative organizational forms in early vertebrate phylogeny. *Immunogenetics.* 1994;40(2):83–99.
146. Braathen R, Hohman VS, Brandtzaeg P, et al. Secretory antibody formation: conserved binding interactions between J chain and polymeric Ig receptor from humans and amphibians. *J Immunol.* 2007;178(3):1589–1597.
147. Takahashi T, Iwase T, Takenouchi N, et al. The joining (J) chain is present in invertebrates that do not express immunoglobulins. *Proc Natl Acad Sci USA.* 1996;93(5):1886–1891.
148. Hsu E. Canonical VH CDR1 nucleotide sequences are conserved in all jawed vertebrates. *Int Immunol.* 1996;8(6):847–854.
149. Hinds KR, Litman GW. Major reorganization of immunoglobulin VH segmental elements during vertebrate evolution. *Nature.* 1986;320(6062):546–549.
150. Lee SS, Fitch D, Flajnik MF, et al. Rearrangement of immunoglobulin genes in shark germ cells. *J Exp Med.* 2000;191(10):1637–1648.
151. Eason DD, Litman RT, Luer CA, et al. Expression of individual immunoglobulin genes occurs in an unusual system consisting of multiple independent loci. *Eur J Immunol.* 2004;34(9):2551–2558.
152. Qin T, Ren L, Hu X, et al. Genomic organization of the immunoglobulin light chain gene loci in *Xenopus tropicalis*: Evolutionary implications. *Dev Comp Immunol.* 2007 Jun 26.
153. Kelley J, Walter L, Trowsdale J. Comparative genomics of major histocompatibility complexes. *Immunogenetics.* 2005;56(10):683–695.
154. Kaufman J, Salomonsen J, Flajnik M. Evolutionary conservation of MHC class I and class II molecules–different yet the same. *Semin Immunol.* 1994;6(6):411–424.
155. Hansen TH, Huang S, Arnold PL, et al. Patterns of nonclassical MHC antigen presentation. *Nat Immunol.* 2007;8(6):563–568.
156. Dijkstra JM, Katagiri T, Hosomichi K, et al. A third broad lineage of major histocompatibility complex (MHC) class I in teleost fish; MHC class II linkage and processed genes. *Immunogenetics.* 2007;59(4):305–321.

157. Hansen TH, Huang S, Arnold PL, et al. Patterns of nonclassical MHC antigen presentation. *Nat Immunol.* 2007;8(6):563–568.
158. Phillips RB, Zimmerman A, Noakes MA, et al. Physical and genetic mapping of the rainbow trout major histocompatibility regions: evidence for duplication of the class I region. *Immunogenetics.* 2003;55(8):561–569.
159. Shiina T, Dijkstra JM, Shimizu S, et al. Interchromosomal duplication of major histocompatibility complex class I regions in rainbow trout (*Oncorhynchus mykiss*), a species with a presumably recent tetraploid ancestry. *Immunogenetics.* 2005;56(12):878–893.
160. Ohta Y, Goetz W, Hossain MZ, et al. Ancestral organization of the MHC revealed in the amphibian *Xenopus*. *J Immunol.* 2006;176(6):3674–3685.
161. Jaillon O, Aury JM, Brunet F, et al. Genome duplication in the teleost fish *Tetraodon nigroviridis* reveals the early vertebrate protokaryotype. *Nature.* 2004;431(7011):946–957.
162. Sambrook JG, Figueroa F, Beck S. A genome-wide survey of Major Histocompatibility Complex (MHC) genes and their paralogues in zebrafish. *BMC Genomics.* 2005;6:152.
163. Klein J. Origin of major histocompatibility complex polymorphism: the trans-species hypothesis. *Hum Immunol.* 1987;19(3):155–162.
164. Hughes AL, Nei M. Pattern of nucleotide substitution at major histocompatibility complex class I loci reveals overdominant selection. *Nature.* 1988;335(6186):167–170.
165. Takahata N, Nei M. Allelic genealogy under overdominant and frequency-dependent selection and polymorphism of major histocompatibility complex loci. *Genetics.* 1990;124(4):967–978.
166. Kasahara M, Hayashi M, Tanaka K, et al. Chromosomal localization of the proteasome Z subunit gene reveals an ancient chromosomal duplication involving the major histocompatibility complex. *Proc Natl Acad Sci USA.* 1996;93(17):9096–9101.
167. Ohno S, Wolf U, Atkin NB. Evolution from fish to mammals by gene duplication. Hereditas 1968;59(1):169–187.
168. Hughes AL. Evolution of the ATP-binding-cassette transmembrane transporters of vertebrates. *Mol Biol Evol.* 1994;11(6):899–910.
169. Uinuk-ool TS, Mayer WE, Sato A, et al. Identification and characterization of a TAP-family gene in the lamprey. *Immunogenetics.* 2003;55(1):38–48.
170. Zhao C, Tampe R, Abele R. TAP and TAP-like–brothers in arms? *Naunyn Schmiedebergs Arch Pharmacol.* 2006;372(6):444–450.
171. Belov K, Deakin JE, Papenfuss AT, et al. Reconstructing an ancestral mammalian immune supercomplex from a marsupial major histocompatibility complex. *PLoS Biol.* 2006;4(3):e46.
172. Vienne A, Shiina T, bi-Rached L, et al. Evolution of the proto-MHC ancestral region: more evidence for the plesiomorphic organisation of human chromosome 9q34 region. *Immunogenetics.* 2003;55(7):429–36.
173. Shum BP, Guethlein L, Flodin LR, et al. Modes of salmonid MHC class I and II evolution differ from the primate paradigm. *J Immunol.* 2001;166(5):3297–3308.
174. Consuegra S, Megens HJ, Leon K, et al. Patterns of variability at the major histocompatibility class II alpha locus in Atlantic salmon contrast with those at the class I locus. *Immunogenetics.* 2005; 57(1–2):16–24.
175. Kaufman J, Milne S, Gobel TW, et al. The chicken B locus is a minimal essential major histocompatibility complex. *Nature.* 1999;401(6756):923–925.
176. Shiina T, Shimizu S, Hosomichi K, et al. Comparative genomic analysis of two avian (quail and chicken) MHC regions. *J Immunol.* 2004;172(11):6751–6763.
177. Wallny HJ, Avila D, Hunt LG, et al. Peptide motifs of the single dominantly expressed class I molecule explain the striking MHC-determined response to Rous sarcoma virus in chickens. *Proc Natl Acad Sci USA.* 2006;103(5):1434–1439.
178. Salomonsen J, Sorensen MR, Marston DA, et al. Two CD1 genes map to the chicken MHC, indicating that CD1 genes are ancient and likely to have been present in the primordial MHC. *Proc Natl Acad Sci USA.* 2005;102(24):8668–8673.
179. Miller MM, Wang C, Parisini E, et al. Characterization of two avian MHC-like genes reveals an ancient origin of the CD1 family. *Proc Natl Acad Sci USA.* 2005;102(24):8674–8679.
180. Nonaka M, Namikawa C, Kato Y, et al. Major histocompatibility complex gene mapping in the amphibian *Xenopus* implies a primordial organization. *Proc Natl Acad Sci USA.* 1997;94(11):5789–5791.
181. Tsukamoto K, Hayashi S, Matsuo MY, et al. Unprecedented intraspecific diversity of the MHC class I region of a teleost medaka, *Oryzias latipes*. *Immunogenetics.* 2005;57(6):420–431.
182. Salter-Cid L, Nonaka M, Flajnik MF. Expression of MHC class Ia and class Ib during ontogeny: high expression in epithelia and coregulation of class Ia and lmp7 genes. *J Immunol.* 1998;160(6):2853–2861.
183. Rodrigues PN, Hermsen TT, van MA, et al. Expression of MhcCyca class I and class II molecules in the early life history of the common carp (*Cyprinus carpio L.*). *Dev Comp Immunol.* 1998;22(5–6):493–506.
184. Fischer U, Dijkstra JM, Kollner B, et al. The ontogeny of MHC class I expression in rainbow trout (*Oncorhynchus mykiss*). *Fish Shellfish Immunol.* 2005;18(1):49–60.
185. Anderson MK, Pant R, Miracle AL, et al. Evolutionary origins of lymphocytes: ensembles of T cell and B cell transcriptional regulators in a cartilaginous fish. *J Immunol.* 2004;172(10):5851–5860.
186. Anderson MK, Pant R, Miracle AL, et al. Evolutionary origins of lymphocytes: ensembles of T cell and B cell transcriptional regulators in a cartilaginous fish. *J Immunol.* 2004;172(10):5851–5860.
187. Rothenberg EV, Pant R. Origins of lymphocyte developmental programs: transcription factor evidence. *Semin Immunol.* 2004;16: 227–238.
188. Schorpp M, Bialecki M, Diekhoff D, et al. Conserved functions of Ikaros in vertebrate lymphocyte development: genetic evidence for distinct larval and adult phases of T cell development and two lineages of B cells in zebrafish. *J Immunol.* 2006;177(4):2463–2476.
189. Boehm T, Bleul CC. The evolutionary history of lymphoid organs. *Nat Immunol.* 2007;8(2):131–135.
190. Lee SS, Fitch D, Flajnik MF, et al. Rearrangement of immunoglobulin genes in shark germ cells. *J Exp Med.* 2000;191(10):1637–1648.
191. Wyffels JT, Walsh CJ, Luer CA, et al. In vivo exposure of clearnose skates, *Raja eglanteria*, to ionizing X-radiation: acute effects on the thymus. *Dev Comp Immunol.* 2005;29(4):315–331.
192. Rumfelt LL, McKinney EC, Taylor E, et al. The development of primary and secondary lymphoid tissues in the nurse shark Ginglymostoma cirratum: B-cell zones precede dendritic cell immigration and T-cell zone formation during ontogeny of the spleen. *Scand J Immunol.* 2002;56(2):130–148.
193. Hart S, Wrathmell AB, Harris JE. Ontogeny of gut-associated lymphoid tissue (GALT) in the dogfish Scyliorhinus canicula L. *Vet Immunol Immunopathol.* 1986;12(1–4):107–116.
194. Miracle AL, Anderson MK, Litman RT, et al. Complex expression patterns of lymphocyte-specific genes during the development of cartilaginous fish implicate unique lymphoid tissues in generating an immune repertoire. *Int Immunol.* 2001;13(4):567–580.
195. Zapata A, Amemiya CT. Phylogeny of lower vertebrates and their immunological structures. *Curr Top Microbiol Immunol.* 2000;248:67–107.
196. Traver D, Herbomel P, Patton EE, et al. The zebrafish as a model organism to study development of the immune system. *Adv Immunol.* 2003;81:253–330.
197. Zapata A, Diez B, Cejalvo T, et al. Ontogeny of the immune system of fish. *Fish Shellfish Immunol.* 2006;20(2):126–136.
198. Bromage ES, Kaattari IM, Zwollo P, et al. Plasmablast and plasma cell production and distribution in trout immune tissues. *J Immunol.* 2004;173(12):7317–7323.
199. Zwollo P, Cole S, Bromage E, et al. B cell heterogeneity in the teleost kidney: evidence for a maturation gradient from anterior to posterior kidney. *J Immunol.* 2005;174(11):6608–6616.
200. Li J, Barreda DR, Zhang YA, et al. B lymphocytes from early vertebrates have potent phagocytic and microbicidal abilities. *Nat Immunol.* 2006;7(10):1116–1124.
201. Du Pasquier L, Schwager J, Flajnik MF. The immune system of *Xenopus*. *Annu Rev Immunol.* 1989;7:251–275.
202. Greenhalgh P, Olesen CE, Steiner LA. Characterization and expression of recombination activating genes (RAG-1 and RAG-2) in *Xenopus laevis*. *J Immunol.* 1993;151(6):3100–3110.
203. Zapata A, Amemiya CT. Phylogeny of lower vertebrates and their immunological structures. *Curr Top Microbiol Immunol.* 2000;248:67–107.

204. Koniski AD, Cohen N. Reproducible proliferative responses of salamander (Ambystoma mexicanum) lymphocytes cultured with mitogens in serum-free medium. *Dev Comp Immunol.* 1992;16(6):441–451.
205. Du Pasquier L, Robert J, Courtet M, et al. B-cell development in the amphibian *Xenopus*. *Immunol Rev*. 2000;175:201–13.
206. Phylogeny of lower vertebrates and their immunological structures. *Curr Top Microbiol Immunol*. 2000;248:67–107.
207. Cooper MD, Raymond DA, Peterson RD, et al. The functions of the thymus system and the bursa system in the chicken. *J Exp Med.* 1966;123(1):75–102.
208. Reynaud CA, Bertocci B, Dahan A, et al. Formation of the chicken B-cell repertoire: ontogenesis, regulation of Ig gene rearrangement, and diversification by gene conversion. *Adv Immunol.* 1994;57:353–378.
209. Ratcliffe MJ, Ivanyi J. Allotype suppression in the chicken. IV. Deletion of B cells and lack of suppressor cells during chronic suppression. *Eur J Immunol.* 1981;11(4):306–310.
210. Reynaud CA, Anquez V, Grimal H, et al. A hyperconversion mechanism generates the chicken light chain preimmune repertoire. *Cell.* 1987;48(3):379–388.
211. Arakawa H, Hauschild J, Buerstedde JM. Requirement of the activation-induced deaminase (AID) gene for immunoglobulin gene conversion. *Science.* 2002;295(5558):1301–1306.
212. Sayegh CE, Drury G, Ratcliffe MJ. Efficient antibody diversification by gene conversion in vivo in the absence of selection for V(D)J-encoded determinants. *EMBO J.* 1999;18(22):6319–6328.
213. Terszowski G, Muller SM, Bleul CC, et al. Evidence for a functional second thymus in mice. *Science.* 2006;312(5771):284–287.
214. Reynaud CA, Weill JC. Postrearrangement diversification processes in gut-associated lymphoid tissues. *Curr Top Microbiol Immunol.* 1996;212:7–15.
215. Rhee KJ, Sethupathi P, Driks A, et al. Role of commensal bacteria in development of gut-associated lymphoid tissues and preimmune antibody repertoire. *J Immunol.* 2004;172(2):1118–1124.
216. Butler JE. Immunoglobulin gene organization and the mechanism of repertoire development. *Scand J Immunol.* 1997;45(5):455–462.
217. Du Pasquier L, Wilson M, Greenberg AS, et al. Somatic mutation in ectothermic vertebrates: musings on selection and origins. *Curr Top Microbiol Immunol.* 1998;229:199–216.
218. Hsu E. Mutation, selection, and memory in B lymphocytes of exothermic vertebrates. *Immunol Rev*. 1998;162:25–36.
219. Dooley H, Flajnik MF. Antibody repertoire development in cartilaginous fish. *Dev Comp Immunol.* 2006;30(1-2):43–56.
220. Hinds-Frey KR, Nishikata H, Litman RT, et al. Somatic variation precedes extensive diversification of germline sequences and combinatorial joining in the evolution of immunoglobulin heavy chain diversity. *J Exp Med.* 1993;178(3):815–824.
221. Lee SS, Tranchina D, Ohta Y, et al. Hypermutation in shark immunoglobulin light chain genes results in contiguous substitutions. *Immunity.* 2002;16(4):571–582.
222. Malecek K, Brandman J, Brodsky JE, et al. Somatic hypermutation and junctional diversification at Ig heavy chain loci in the nurse shark. *J Immunol.* 2005;175(12):8105–8115.
223. Dooley H, Stanfield RL, Brady RA, et al. First molecular and biochemical analysis of in vivo affinity maturation in an ectothermic vertebrate. *Proc Natl Acad Sci USA.* 2006;103(6):1846–1851.
224. Boudinot P, Boubekeur S, Benmansour A. Rhabdovirus infection induces public and private T cell responses in teleost fish. *J Immunol.* 2001;167(11):6202–6209.
225. Boudinot P, Bernard D, Boubekeur S, et al. The glycoprotein of a fish rhabdovirus profiles the virus-specific T-cell repertoire in rainbow trout. *J Gen Virol.* 2004;85(Pt 10):3099–3108.
226. Bly JE, Quiniou SM, Clem LW. Environmental effects on fish immune mechanisms. *Dev Biol Stand.* 1997;90:33–43.
227. Shen L, Stuge TB, Zhou H, et al. Channel catfish cytotoxic cells: a mini-review. *Dev Comp Immunol.* 2002;26(2):141–149.
228. Shen L, Stuge TB, Evenhuis JP, et al. Channel catfish NK-like cells are armed with IgM via a putative FcmicroR. *Dev Comp Immunol.* 2003;27(8):699–714.
229. Jaso-Friedmann L, Peterson DS, Gonzalez DS, et al. The antigen receptor (NCCRP-1) on catfish and zebrafish nonspecific cytotoxic cells belongs to a new gene family characterized by an F-box-associated domain. *J Mol Evol.* 2002;54(3):386–395.
230. Charlemagne J. Antibody diversity in amphibians. Noninbred axolotls used the same unique heavy chain and a limited number of light chains for their anti-2,4-dinitrophenyl antibody responses. *Eur J Immunol*. 1987;17(3):421–424.
231. Wabl MR, Du Pasquier L. Antibody patterns in genetically identical frogs. *Nature.* 1976;264(5587):642–644.
232. Wilson M, Hsu E, Marcuz A, et al. What limits affinity maturation of antibodies in Xenopus–the rate of somatic mutation or the ability to select mutants? *EMBO J.* 1992;11(12):4337–4347.
233. Di Noia JM, Neuberger MS. Molecular mechanisms of antibody somatic hypermutation. *Annu Rev Biochem*. 2007;76:1–22.
234. Turchin A, Hsu E. The generation of antibody diversity in the turtle. *J Immunol.* 1996;156(10):3797–3805.
235. Du Pasquier L, Wilson M, Greenberg AS, et al. Somatic mutation in ectothermic vertebrates: musings on selection and origins. *Curr Top Microbiol Immunol.* 1998;229:199–216.
236. Wei S, Zhou JM, Chen X, et al. The zebrafish activating immune receptor Nitr9 signals via Dap12. *Immunogenetics.* 2007;59(10):813–821.
237. Voigt V, Forbes CA, Tonkin JN, et al. Murine cytomegalovirus m157 mutation and variation leads to immune evasion of natural killer cells. *Proc Natl Acad Sci USA*. 2003;100(23):13483–13488.
238. Horton TL, Stewart R, Cohen N, et al. Ontogeny of Xenopus NK cells in the absence of MHC class I antigens. *Dev Comp Immunol.* 2003;27(8):715–726.
239. Kikuno R, Sato A, Mayer WE, et al. Clustering of C-type lectin natural killer receptor-like loci in the bony fish *Oreochromis niloticus*. *Scand J Immunol.* 2004;59(2):133–142.
240. Plougastel BF, Yokoyama WM. Extending missing-self? Functional interactions between lectin-like NKrp1 receptors on NK cells with lectin-like ligands. *Curr Top Microbiol Immunol.* 2006;298:77–89.
241. Hawke NA, Yoder JA, Haire RN, et al. Extraordinary variation in a diversified family of immune-type receptor genes. *Proc Natl Acad Sci USA.* 2001;98(24):13832–13837.
242. Davis RS, Ehrhardt GR, Leu CM, et al. An extended family of Fc receptor relatives. *Eur J Immunol.* 2005;35(3):674–680.
243. Viertlboeck BC, Habermann FA, Schmitt R, et al. The chicken leukocyte receptor complex: a highly diverse multigene family encoding at least six structurally distinct receptor types. *J Immunol.* 2005;175(1):385–393.
244. Stafford JL, Bengten E, Du Pasquier L, et al. A novel family of diversified immunoregulatory receptors in teleosts is homologous to both mammalian Fc receptors and molecules encoded within the leukocyte receptor complex. *Immunogenetics.* 2006;58(9):758–773.
245. Kuchroo VK, Meyers JH, Umetsu DT, et al. TIM family of genes in immunity and tolerance. *Adv Immunol*. 2006;91:227–249.
246. Suzuki T, Shin I, Fujiyama A, et al. Hagfish leukocytes express a paired receptor family with a variable domain resembling those of antigen receptors. *J Immunol.* 2005;174(5):2885–2891.
247. Kaiser P, Poh TY, Rothwell L, et al. A genomic analysis of chicken cytokines and chemokines. *J Interferon Cytokine Res*. 2005;25(8):467–484.
248. Bird S, Zou J, Secombes CJ. Advances in fish cytokine biology give clues to the evolution of a complex network. *Curr Pharm Des.* 2006;12(24):3051–3069.
249. Uinuk-Ool T, Mayer WE, Sato A, et al. Lamprey lymphocyte-like cells express homologs of genes involved in immunologically relevant activities of mammalian lymphocytes. *Proc Natl Acad Sci USA.* 2002;99(22):14356–14361.
250. Bilej M, Joskova R, Van den BR, et al. An invertebrate TNF functional analogue activates macrophages via lectin-saccharide interaction with ion channels. *Int Immunol.* 2006;18(12):1663–1670.
251. Hong S, Zou J, Collet B, et al. Analysis and characterisation of IL-1beta processing in rainbow trout, *Oncorhynchus mykiss*. *Fish Shellfish Immunol.* 2004;16(3):453–459.
252. Glenney GW, Wiens GD. Early diversification of the TNF superfamily in teleosts: genomic characterization and expression analysis. *J Immunol*. 2007;178(12):7955–7973.
253. Kaiser P, Mariani P. Promoter sequence, exon:intron structure, and synteny of genetic location show that a chicken cytokine with

T-cell proliferative activity is IL2 and not IL15. *Immunogenetics.* 1999;49(1):26–35.
254. Bird S, Zou J, Kono T, et al. Characterisation and expression analysis of interleukin 2 (IL-2) and IL-21 homologues in the Japanese pufferfish, Fugu rubripes, following their discovery by synteny. *Immunogenetics.* 2005;56(12):909–923.
255. Kaiser P, Poh TY, Rothwell L, et al. A genomic analysis of chicken cytokines and chemokines. *J Interferon Cytokine Res.* 2005;25(8):467–484.
256. Avery S, Rothwell L, Degen WD, et al. Characterization of the first nonmammalian T2 cytokine gene cluster: the cluster contains functional single-copy genes for IL-3, IL-4, IL-13, and GM-CSF, a gene for IL-5 that appears to be a pseudogene, and a gene encoding another cytokinelike transcript, KK34. *J Interferon Cytokine Res.* 2004;24(10):600–610.
257. Li JH, Shao JZ, Xiang LX, et al. Cloning, characterization and expression analysis of pufferfish interleukin-4 cDNA: the first evidence of Th2-type cytokine in fish. *Mol Immunol.* 2007;44(8):2078–2086.
258. Du Pasquier L, Bernard CC. Active suppression of the allogeneic histocompatibility reactions during the metamorphosis of the clawed toad *Xenopus*. *Differentiation.* 1980;16(1):1–7.
259. DeVries ME, Kelvin AA, Xu L, et al. Defining the origins and evolution of the chemokine/chemokine receptor system. *J Immunol.* 2006;176(1):401–415.
260. Burnet FM. "Self-recognition" in colonial marine forms and flowering plants in relation to the evolution of immunity. *Nature.* 1971;232(5308):230–235.
261. Nasrallah JB. Recognition and rejection of self in plant self-incompatibility: comparisons to animal histocompatibility. *Trends Immunol.* 2005;26(8):412–418.
262. Poudyal M, Rosa S, Powell AE, et al. Embryonic chimerism does not induce tolerance in an invertebrate model organism. *Proc Natl Acad Sci USA.* 2007;104(11):4559–4564.
263. Hughes RN, Manriquez PH, Morley S, et al. Kin or self-recognition? Colonial fusibility of the bryozoan *Celleporella hyalina*. *Evol Dev.* 2004;6(6):431–437.
264. Muller WE, Krasko A, Skorokhod A, et al. Histocompatibility reaction in tissue and cells of the marine sponge *Suberites domuncula* in vitro and in vivo: central role of the allograft inflammatory factor 1. *Immunogenetics.* 2002;54(1):48–58.
265. Wiens M, Perovic-Ottstadt S, Muller IM, et al. Allograft rejection in the mixed cell reaction system of the demosponge *Suberites domuncula* is controlled by differential expression of apoptotic genes. *Immunogenetics.* 2004;56(8):597–610.
266. Sabella C, Faszewski E, Himic L, et al. Cyclosporin A Suspends Transplantation Reactions in the Marine Sponge *Microciona prolifera*. *J Immunol.* 2007;179(9):5927–5935.
267. Hauenschild C. Wilhelm Roux's Archives 147, 1–114. 1954. Ref Type: Generic.
268. Cadavid LF, Powell AE, Nicotra ML, et al. An invertebrate histocompatibility complex. *Genetics.* 2004;167(1):357–365.
269. Oka H, Watanabe H. Colony specificity in compound ascidians as tested by fusion experiments (a preliminary report). *Proceedings of the Japanese Academy of Sciences.* 1957;33:657–658.
270. Magor BG, De TA, Rinkevich B, et al. Allorecognition in colonial tunicates: protection against predatory cell lineages? *Immunol Rev.* 1999;167:69–79.
271. Cima F, Sabbadin A, Ballarin L. Cellular aspects of allorecognition in the compound ascidian *Botryllus schlosseri*. *Dev Comp Immunol.* 2004;28(9):881–889.
272. De Tomaso AW, Nyholm SV, Palmeri KJ, et al. Isolation and characterization of a protochordate histocompatibility locus. *Nature.* 2005;438(7067):454–459.
273. Nyholm SV, Passegue E, Ludington WB, et al. fester, A candidate allorecognition receptor from a primitive chordate. *Immunity.* 2006;25(1):163–173.
274. Ishii T, Sawada T, Sasaki K, et al. Study of color variation in the solitary ascidian *Halocynthia roretzi,* collected in the Inland Sea of Japan. *Zoolog Sci* 2004;21(8):891–898.
275. Raftos DA, Briscoe DA, Tait NN. The mode of recognition of allogeneic tissue in the solitary urochordate *Styela plicata*. *Transplantation.* 1988;45(6):1123–1126.
276. Kurn U, Sommer F, Hemmrich G, et al. Allorecognition in urochordates: identification of a highly variable complement receptor-like protein expressed in follicle cells of Ciona. *Dev Comp Immunol.* 2007;31(4):360–371.
277. Gould SJ, Hildreth JE, Booth AM. The evolution of alloimmunity and the genesis of adaptive immunity. *Q Rev Biol.* 2004;79(4):359–382.
278. Buss LW. Somatic cell parasitism and the evolution of somatic tissue compatibility. *Proc Natl Acad Sci USA.* 1982;79(17):5337–5341.
279. Laird DJ, De Tomaso AW, Weissman IL. Stem cells are units of natural selection in a colonial ascidian. *Cell.* 2005;123(7):1351–1360.
280. Hughes RN, Manriquez PH, Morley S, et al. Kin or self-recognition? Colonial fusibility of the bryozoan Celleporella hyalina. *Evol Dev.* 2004;6(6):431–437.
281. Sommerfeldt AD, Bishop JDD. Random amplified polymorphic DNA (RAPD) analysis reveals extensive natural polymorphism in a marine protochordate. *Molecular Ecology.* 1999;8:885–890.
282. Danchin E, Vitiello V, Vienne A, et al. The major histocompatibility complex origin. *Immunol Rev.* 2004;198:216–232.
283. Christova R, Jones T, Wu PJ, et al. P-STAT1 mediates higher-order chromatin remodelling of the human MHC in response to IFNgamma. *J Cell Sci.* 2007;120(Pt 18):3262–3270.
284. Abi RL, McDermott MF, Pontarotti P. The MHC big bang. *Immunol Rev.* 1999;167:33–44.
285. Lynch M, O'Hely M, Walsh B, et al. The probability of preservation of a newly arisen gene duplicate. *Genetics.* 2001;159(4):1789–1804.
286. Thompson CB. New insights into V(D)J recombination and its role in the evolution of the immune system. *Immunity.* 1995;3(5):531–539.
287. Sakano H, Huppi K, Heinrich G, et al. Sequences at the somatic recombination sites of immunoglobulin light-chain genes. *Nature.* 1979;280(5720):288–94.
288. Kapitonov VV, Jurka J. RAG1 core and V(D)J recombination signal sequences were derived from Transib transposons. *PLoS Biol.* 2005;3(6):e181.
289. Fugmann SD, Messier C, Novack LA, et al. An ancient evolutionary origin of the Rag1/2 gene locus. *Proc Natl Acad Sci USA.* 2006;103(10):3728–3733.
290. Yu W, Misulovin Z, Suh H, et al. Coordinate regulation of RAG1 and RAG2 by cell type-specific DNA elements 5′ of RAG2. *Science.* 1999;285(5430):1080–1084.
291. Bernstein RM, Schluter SF, Bernstein H, et al. Primordial emergence of the recombination activating gene 1 (RAG1): sequence of the complete shark gene indicates homology to microbial integrases. *Proc Natl Acad Sci USA.* 1996;93(18):9454–9459.
292. Richards MH, Nelson JL. The evolution of vertebrate antigen receptors: a phylogenetic approach. *Mol Biol Evol.* 2000;17(1):146–155.
293. Glusman G, Rowen L, Lee I, et al. Comparative genomics of the human and mouse T cell receptor loci. *Immunity.* 2001;15(3):337–349.
294. Chretien I, Robert J, Marcuz A, et al. CTX, a novel molecule specifically expressed on the surface of cortical thymocytes in Xenopus. *Eur J Immunol.* 1996;26(4):780–791.
295. Zhang SM, Adema CM, Kepler TB, et al. Diversification of Ig superfamily genes in an invertebrate. *Science.* 2004;305(5681):251–254.
296. Compte E, Pontarotti P, Collette Y, et al. Frontline: Characterization of BT3 molecules belonging to the B7 family expressed on immune cells. *Eur J Immunol.* 2004;34(8):2089–2099.
297. Sato A, Mayer WE, Klein J. A molecule bearing an immunoglobulin-like V region of the CTX subfamily in amphioxus. *Immunogenetics.* 2003;55(6):423–427.
298. van den Berg TK, Yoder JA, Litman GW. On the origins of adaptive immunity: innate immune receptors join the tale. *Trends Immunol.* 2004;25(1):11–16.
299. Barton ES, Forrest JC, Connolly JL, et al. Junction adhesion molecule is a receptor for reovirus. *Cell.* 2001;104(3):441–451.
300. Harrington LE, Mangan PR, Weaver CT. Expanding the effector CD4 T-cell repertoire: the Th17 lineage. *Curr Opin Immunol.* 2006;18(3):349–356.

301. Meijers R, Puettmann-Holgado R, Skiniotis G, et al. Structural basis of Dscam isoform specificity. *Nature.* 2007;449(7161):487–491.
302. Rudensky AS, Chervonsky AS. A goodbye to Charlie Janeway: Charles A. Janeway Jr (1943–2003). *Trends Immunol.* 2003;24(8):403.
303. Robalino J, Bartlett TC, Chapman RW, et al. Double-stranded RNA and antiviral immunity in marine shrimp: inducible host mechanisms and evidence for the evolution of viral counter-responses. *Dev Comp Immunol.* 2007;31(6):539–547.
304. Schatz DG. DNA deaminases converge on adaptive immunity. *Nat Immunol.* 2007;8(6):551–553.
305. Collette Y, Gilles A, Pontarotti P, et al. A co-evolution perspective of the TNFSF and TNFRSF families in the immune system. *Trends Immunol.* 2003;24(7):387–394.
306. Kim MS, Byun M, Oh BH. Crystal structure of peptidoglycan recognition protein LB from Drosophila melanogaster. *Nat Immunol.* 2003;4(8):787–793.
307. Poget SF, Legge GB, Proctor MR, et al. The structure of a tunicate C-type lectin from Polyandrocarpa misakiensis complexed with D -galactose. *J Mol Biol.* 1999;290(4):867–879.
308. Cooper MD, Alder MN. The evolution of adaptive immune systems. *Cell.* 2006;124(4):815–822.
309. Bjorkman PJ, Saper MA, Samraoui B, et al. Structure of the human class I histocompatibility antigen, HLA-A2. *Nature.* 1987;329(6139):506–512.
310. Brown JH, Jardetzky TS, Gorga JC, et al. Three-dimensional structure of the human class II histocompatibility antigen HLA-DR1. *Nature.* 1993;364(6432):33–39.
311. Flajnik MF, Kasahara M. Comparative genomics of the MHC: glimpses into the evolution of the adaptive immune system. *Immunity.* 2001;15(3):351–362.
312. Collette Y, Gilles A, Pontarotti P, et al. A co-evolution perspective of the TNFSF and TNFRSF families in the immune system. *Trends Immunol.* 2003;24(7):387–394.

SECTION III

Immunoglobulins and B Lymphocytes

Chapter 4

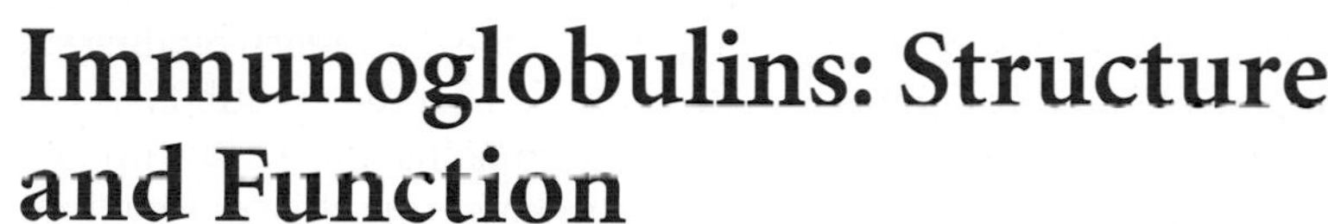

Immunoglobulins: Structure and Function

Harry W. Schroeder, Jr., David Wald, and Neil S. Greenspan

INTRODUCTION

Immunoglobulins (Igs) are marked by a duality of structure and function (1). They provide a polyclonal set of receptors for the B cell that permit the cell to produce a highly diverse range of ligand binding sites. This diversity allows Igs to recognize an almost unlimited array of self and nonself antigens, ranging from compounds as fundamental to life as DNA to manmade molecules that could not have played a role in the evolution of the immune system. Igs also provide the immune system with a conserved set of effector molecules. They can activate and fix complement, and they can bind to Fc receptors on the surfaces of granulocytes, monocytes, platelets, and other components of the immune response. Both activation of complement and binding to Fc receptors can contribute to the induction or maintenance of inflammation. The receptor and effector functions of each individual immunoglobulin can be localized to a separate region or domain of the molecule.

Immunoglobulins Are Heterodimers

Immunoglobulins are heterodimeric proteins, consisting of two heavy (H) and two light (L) chains (Figures 4.1, 4.2). The eponymous Ig domain serves as the basic building block for both chains. Each of the chains contains a single amino-terminal variable (V) Ig domain and one, three, or four carboxy-terminal constant (C) Ig domains. H chains contain three or four C domains. L chains contain only one. H chains with three C domains tend to include a spacer *hinge* region between the first (C_H1) and second (C_H2) domains (2). Each V or C domain consists of approximately 110–130 amino acids, averaging 12,000 kD–13,000 kD. A typical L chain will thus mass approximately 25 kD, and a three C domain $C\gamma$ H chain with its hinge will mass approximately 55 kD.

At the primary sequence level, immunoglobulins are marked by the interspersion of regions of impressive sequence variability with regions of equally impressive sequence conservation. The V domains demonstrate the greatest molecular heterogeneity, with some regions including near random variability and others exhibiting extensive conservation across 500 million years of evolution (3). The molecular heterogeneity of the V domains permits the creation of binding sites, or *paratopes,* which can discriminate between antigens that may differ by as little as one atom. Thus, it is the V domains that encode the receptor function and define the monovalent specificity of the antibody. The H chain C_H1 domain, which is immediately adjacent to the V, associates with the single L chain C domain. Together, the C_H1 and C_L domains provide a stable platform for the paired set of V_H and V_L domains, which together create the antigen binding site. The distal C_H2 and C_H3 domains, for those antibodies with a hinge, or the C_H3 and C_H4 domains, for those with an extra (C_H2) domain, typically encode the effector functions of soluble antibody. Each of these Ig C_H domains is encoded by a separate exon. Although the sequences of the individual C_H domains are constant within the individual (and nearly constant within a species), they can vary greatly across species boundaries. The carboxy-terminal C_H domain encodes a secretory tail, which permits the antibody to exit the cell.

Also encoded within the germline sequence of each C_H gene are two membrane/cytoplasmic tail domain exons, termed M1 and M2. Alternative splicing removes the secretory sequence typically encoded by the terminal C_H3 or C_H4 domain and replaces it with the peptides encoded by the M1 and M2 exons, converting a secretory antibody to a membrane-embedded receptor (4). The membrane/cytoplasmic tail region is the portion of the C_H domains that is most highly conserved between species, which befits its role as a link to the intracellular signal transduction pathways that ultimately regulate B cell function.

Paratopes and Epitopes

The immunoglobulin–antigen interaction takes place between the paratope, the site on the Ig at which the antigen binds, and the *epitope,* which is the site on the antigen that is bound. It is important to appreciate that antibodies do not recognize antigens, they recognize epitopes borne on antigens (5). This makes it possible for immunoglobulins to discriminate between two closely related antigens, each of which can be viewed as a collection of epitopes.

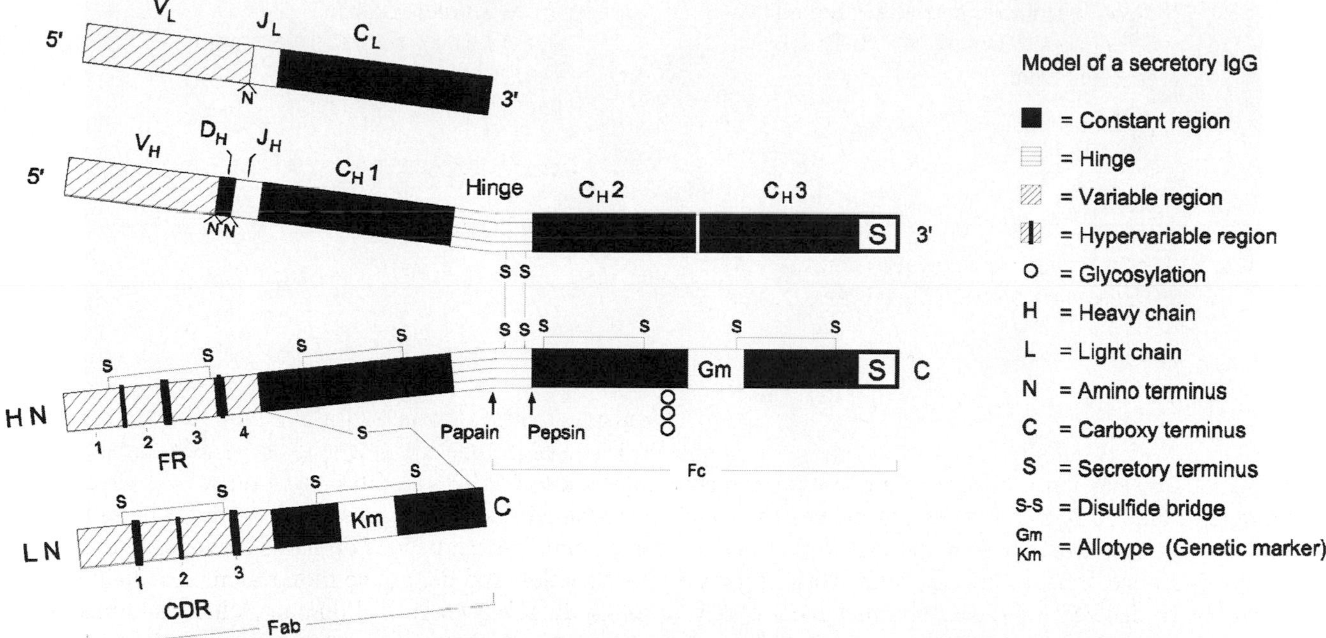

FIGURE 4.1 Model of a secretory IgG. The germline exonic derivation of the sequence is shown at the top, and the protein structure is shown at the bottom. The location of the various cysteine residues that help hold both the individual domains and the various Ig subunits together are illustrated. Papain digests IgG molecules above the cysteine residues in the hinge that holds the two H chains together, yielding two Fab molecules and an Fc, whereas pepsin digests below, releasing an $(Fab)'_2$ fragment and two individual Fcs (which are typically degraded to smaller peptide fragments). The location of some allotypic variants is illustrated. C_H2 domains can be variably glycosylated, which can also affect Ig protein structure and effector function.

It also is one scenario that permits the same antibody to bind divergent antigens that share equivalent epitopes, a phenomenon referred to as *cross-reactivity*.

It has been estimated that triggering of effector functions in solution typically requires aggregation of three or more effector domains, and thus tends to involve the binding of three or more epitopes (5). For antigens encoding repeating epitope structures such as polysaccharides or antigen aggregates, binding of a single polymeric Ig molecule carrying multiple effector domains, such as pentameric IgM, can be sufficient to induce effector function. For antigens encoding diverse epitopes, which is more typical of monodisperse single-domain molecules in solution, triggering of inflammatory effector functions may require the binding of a diverse set of Ig molecules, all binding the same antigen but at different epitopes (6).

Membrane and Secretory Immunoglobulin

Alternative splicing allows immunoglobulins to serve either as soluble antibodies or as membrane-bound antigen receptors. In their role as antibodies, Igs are released into the circulation from where they may traffic into the tissues and across mucosal surfaces. In their role as the B cell antigen receptor (BCR), they are anchored to the membrane by means of their M1:M2 transmembrane domain. However, soluble antibodies can also be pressed into service as heterologous cell surface antigen receptors by their attachment to membrane bound Fc receptors (7). This permits the power of antibody recognition to be extended to nonlymphoid cells such as Fc-expressing granulocytes, macrophages, and mast cells. The major difference between these two forms of cell surface receptors is that immunoglobulins as BCRs provide a monoclonal receptor for each B cell, whereas antibodies bound to Fc receptors endow the cell with a polyclonal set of antigen recognition molecules. This gives greater flexibility and increases the power of the effector cells to recognize antigens with multiple nonself epitopes.

Isotypes and Idiotypes

Immunoglobulins can also serve as antigens for other immunoglobulins. Immunization of heterologous species with monoclonal antibodies (or a restricted set of immunoglobulins) has shown that immunoglobulins contain both common and individual antigenic determinants. Epitopes recognized within the V portion of the antibodies used for immunization that identify individual determinants are termed *idiotypes* (Figure 4.3), whereas

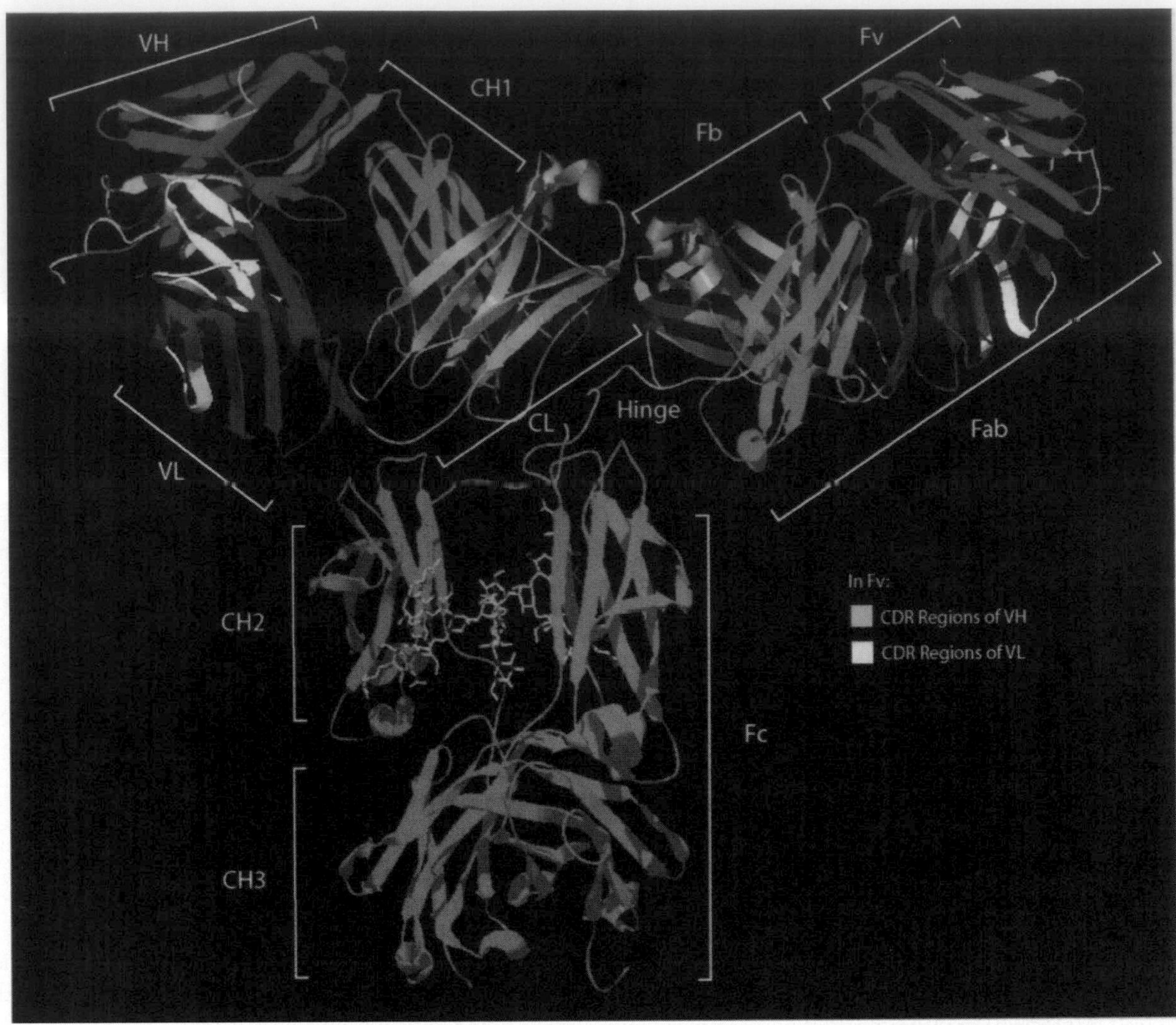

FIGURE 4.2 Ribbon diagram of a complete IgG1 crystal (1 hzh in PDB from data of Harris et al. [190]). The major regions of the immunoglobulin are illustrated. The heavy-chain constant regions (green) also include the hinge (yellow) between the first two domains. CH2 is glycosylated (also seen in yellow). The heavy- and light-chain variable regions (red and dark blue, respectively) are N terminal to the heavy-(green) and light-chain (light blue) constant regions. CDR loops in the heavy- and light-chain variable regions (yellow and white) are illustrated as well. (See color insert.)

epitopes specific for the constant portion are termed *isotypes*. Recognition of these isotypes first allowed grouping of immunoglobulins into recognized classes. Each class of immunoglobulin defines an individual set of C domains that corresponds to a single heavy chain constant region gene. For example, IgM utilizes μ H chain C domains and IgE utilizes ε C domains.

Some V domain epitopes derive from the germline sequence of V gene exons. These shared epitopes, commonly referred to as *public idiotopes* or *cross-reactive idiotypes* (Figure 4.3), are, from a genetic perspective, isotypic because they can be found on many immunoglobulins of different antigen binding specificities that derive from the same germline V region. Examples include the cross-reactive idiotypes found on monoclonal IgM rheumatoid factors derived from individuals with mixed cryoglobulinemia, each of which can be linked to the use of individual V gene segments (8).

Classes and Allotypes

Each of the various classes and subclasses of immunoglobulins has its own unique role to play in the immunologic defense of the individual. IgA, for example, is the major class of immunoglobulin present in all external secretions. It is primarily responsible for protecting mucosal surfaces. IgG subclasses bind Fc receptors differently, and thus vary in effector function (9). Determinants common to subsets

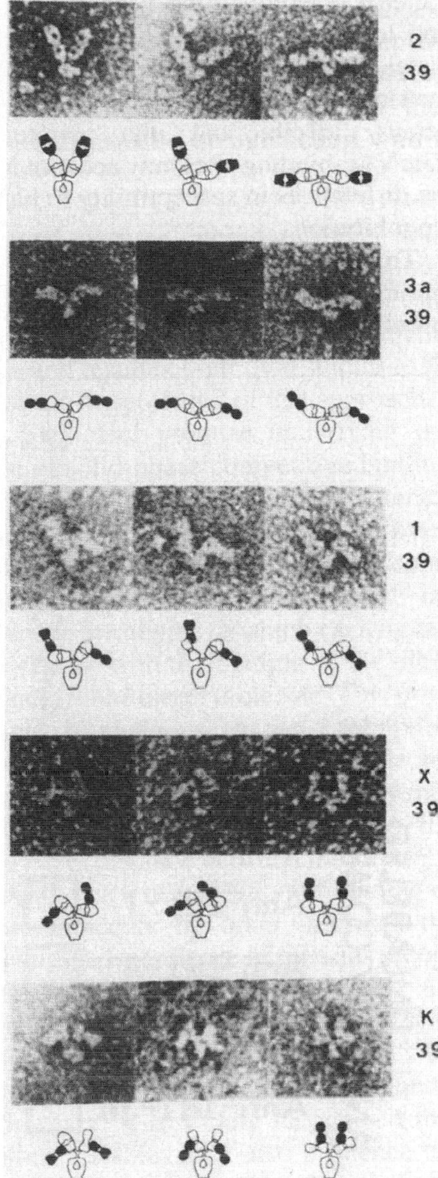

FIGURE 4.3 Electron micrographs (above; ×350,000) and interpretive diagrams (below) of murine mAb HGAC 39 (specific for the cell wall polysaccharide of *Streptococcus pyogenes*) in complex with antiidiotypic mAb Fab fragments. HGAC 39 is represented in the diagrams as an open figure and the Fab anti-Id probes are represented as solid figures. The Fab arms of the antibody targets and probes are drawn to indicate their rotational orientation as planar (oval with open center), intermediate (bone shape with or without central opening), or perpendicular ("dumbbell shaped"). Different complexes illustrate the range of Fab-Fab angles made possible by segmental flexibility. **Abbreviations:** 39, HGAC 39; 2, anti-IdI-2 Fab; 3a, anti-IdI-3a Fab; 1, anti-IdI-1 Fab; X, anti-IdX Fab; K, anti-Cκ Fab. IdI designates an individual idiotope, and IdX a crossreactive idiotope. Antibody complexes were stained with 2% uranyl formate as described Roux et al. (98). Reproduced from Proceedings of the National Academy of Sciences (from Roux et al. [98] with permission).

of individuals within a species, yet differing between other members of that species, are termed *allotypes* and define inherited polymorphisms that result from allelic forms of immunoglobulin C (less commonly, V) genes (10).

Glycosylation

N-linked carbohydrates can be found in all constant domains as well as in some variable domains (11). The structure of the attached N-linked carbohydrate can vary greatly, depending on the degree of processing. These carbohydrates can play a major role in Ig function. Human IgG molecules contain a conserved glycosylation site at Asn 297, which is buried between the C_H2 domains (12). This oligosaccharide structure is almost as large as the C_H2 domain itself. O-linked sugars are also present in some immunoglobulins (11). Human IgA1, but not IgA2, possesses a 13 amino acid hinge region that contains three to five O-linked carbohydrate moieties (13). A deficiency in proper processing of these O-glycans can contribute to IgA nephropathy, which is a disease that is characterized by the presence of IgA1-containing immune complexes in the glomerular mesangium (14).

A HISTORICAL PERSPECTIVE

The identification of immunoglobulin as a key component of the immune response began in the 19th century. This section describes the history of the identification of immunoglobulin and introduces fundamental terminology.

Antibodies and Antigens

Aristotle and his contemporaries attributed disease to an imbalance of the four vital humors: the blood, the phlegm, and the yellow and black biles (15). In 1890, Behring (later, von Behring) and Kitasato reported the existence of an activity in the blood that could neutralize diphtheria toxin (16). They showed that sera containing this humoral antitoxin activity would protect other animals exposed to the same toxin. Ehrlich, who was the first to describe how diphtheria toxin and antitoxin interact (17), made glancing reference to "Antikörper" in a 1891 paper describing discrimination between two immune bodies, or substances (18). The term *antigen* was first introduced by Deutsch in 1899. He later explained that antigen is a contraction of "Antisomatogen+Immunkörperbildner," or that which induces the production of immune bodies (antibodies). These operational definitions of antibody and antigen create a classic tautology.

Gamma Globulins

In 1939, Tiselius and Kabat immunized rabbits with ovalbumin and fractionated the immune serum by electrophoresis into albumin, alpha-goblulin, beta-globulin,

TABLE 4.1 Definitions of Key Immunoglobulin Structure Nomenclature

Fc	A constant region dimer lacking C_H1
Fab	A light chain dimerized to V_H-C_H1 resulting from papain cleavage; this is monomeric since papain cuts above the hinge disulfide bond(s)
F(ab)'$_2$	A dimer of Fab' resulting from pepsin cleavage below the hinge disulfides; this is bivalent and can precipitate antigen
Fab'	A monomer resulting from mild reduction of F(ab)'$_2$: an Fab with part of the hinge
Fd	The heavy chain portion of Fab (V_H-C_H1) obtained following reductive denaturation of Fab
Fv	The variable part of Fab: a V_H-V_L dimer
Fb	The constant part of Fab: a C_H1-C_L dimer
pFc'	A C_H3 dimer

From Carayannopoulos and Capra (188), with permission.

and gamma-globulin fractions (19). Absorption of the serum against ovalbumin depleted the gamma-globulin fraction, hence the terms *immunoglobulin* and *IgG*. "Sizing" columns were used to separate immunoglobulins into those that were "heavy" (IgM), "regular" (IgA, IgE, IgD, IgG), and "light" (light chain dimers) (1). Immunoelectrophoresis subsequently permitted identification of the various immunoglobulin classes and subclasses.

Fab and Fc

In 1949, Porter first used papain to digest IgG molecules into two types of fragments, termed Fab and Fc (Table 4.1) (20,21). Papain digested IgG into two Fab fragments, each of which could bind antigen, and a single Fc fragment. Nisonoff developed the use of pepsin to split IgG into an Fc fragment and a single dimeric F(ab)$_2$ that could cross-link antigens (22). Edelman broke disulfide bonds in IgG and was the first to show that IgG consisted of two H and two L chains (23).

Two Genes, One Polypeptide

The portion of the constant domain encoded by the Fc fragment was the first to be sequenced and then analyzed at the structural level. It could be readily crystallized when chilled. The heterogeneity of the V domain precluded sequence and crystallographic analysis of an intact Ig chain until Bence-Jones myeloma proteins were identified as clonal, isolated Ig light chains. These intact chains could be purified and obtained in large quantities, which finally permitted rational analysis of antibody structure and function (24). Recognition of the unique nature of a molecule consisting of one extremely variable V domain and one highly conserved C domain led to the then-heretical Dreyer-Bennett proposal of "two genes—one polypeptide" (25), which was subsequently and spectacularly confirmed by Tonegawa (26).

THE IG DOMAIN

The immunoglobulin domain is the core unit that defines members of the immunoglobulin superfamily (IgSF) (reviewed in Williams and Barclay [27] and Harpaz and Chothia [28]). This section describes the Ig domain in detail.

The Immunoglobulin Superfamily

Each Ig domain consists of two sandwiched β-pleated sheets "pinned" together by a disulfide bridge between two conserved cysteine residues (Figure 4.4). The structure of the β-pleated sheets in an Ig domain varies depending on the number and conformation of strands in each sheet.

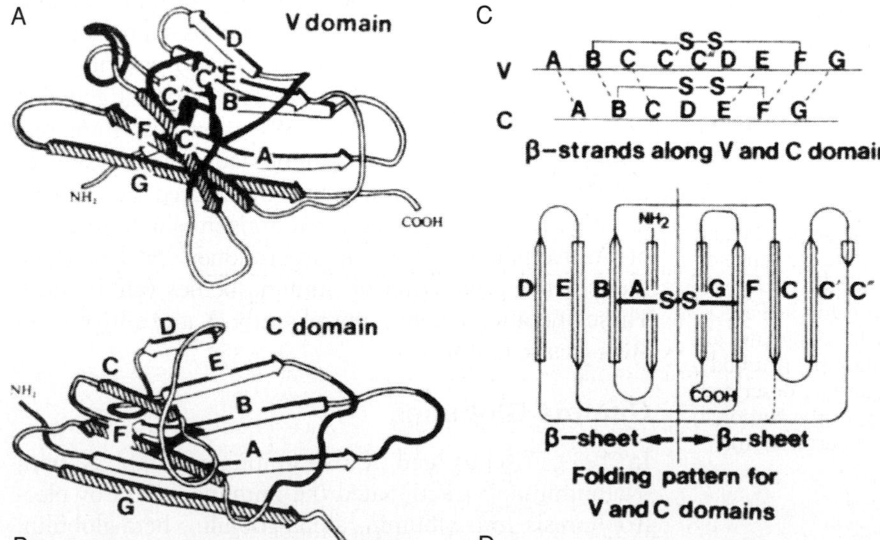

FIGURE 4.4 The Ig domain. **A:** A typical V domain structure. Note the projection of the C-C′ strands and loop away from the core. **B:** A typical compact C domain structure. **C:** The cysteines used to pin the two β-sheets together are found in the B and F strands. **D:** The folding pattern for V and C domains. From (27).

Two such structures, V and C, are typically found in immunoglobulins. C-type domains, which are the most compact, have seven antiparallel strands distributed as three strands in the first sheet and four strands in the second. Each strand has been given an alphabetical designation ranging from amino-terminal A to carboxy-terminal G. Side chains positioned to lie sandwiched between the two strands tend to be nonpolar in nature. This hydrophobic core helps maintain the stability of the structure to the point that V domains engineered to replace the conserved cysteines with serine residues retain their ability to bind antigen. The residues that populate the external surface of the Ig domain and the residues that form the loops that link strands can vary greatly in sequence. These solvent exposed residues offer multiple targets for docking with other molecules.

The V Domain

V-type domains add two additional antiparallel strands to the first sheet, creating a five strand–four strand distribution. Domain stability results from the tight packing of alternately inward-pointing residue side chains enriched for the presence of hydrophobic moieties to create a hydrophobic domain core. The H and L variable domains are held together primarily through noncovalent interaction between the inner faces of the β sheets (29,30).

Early comparisons of the primary sequences of the V domains of different antibodies identified four intervals of relative sequence stability, termed *framework regions,* or FRs, which were separated by three hypervariable intervals, termed *complementarity determining regions,* or CDRs (Figures 4.5, 4.6) (31). The exact location of these

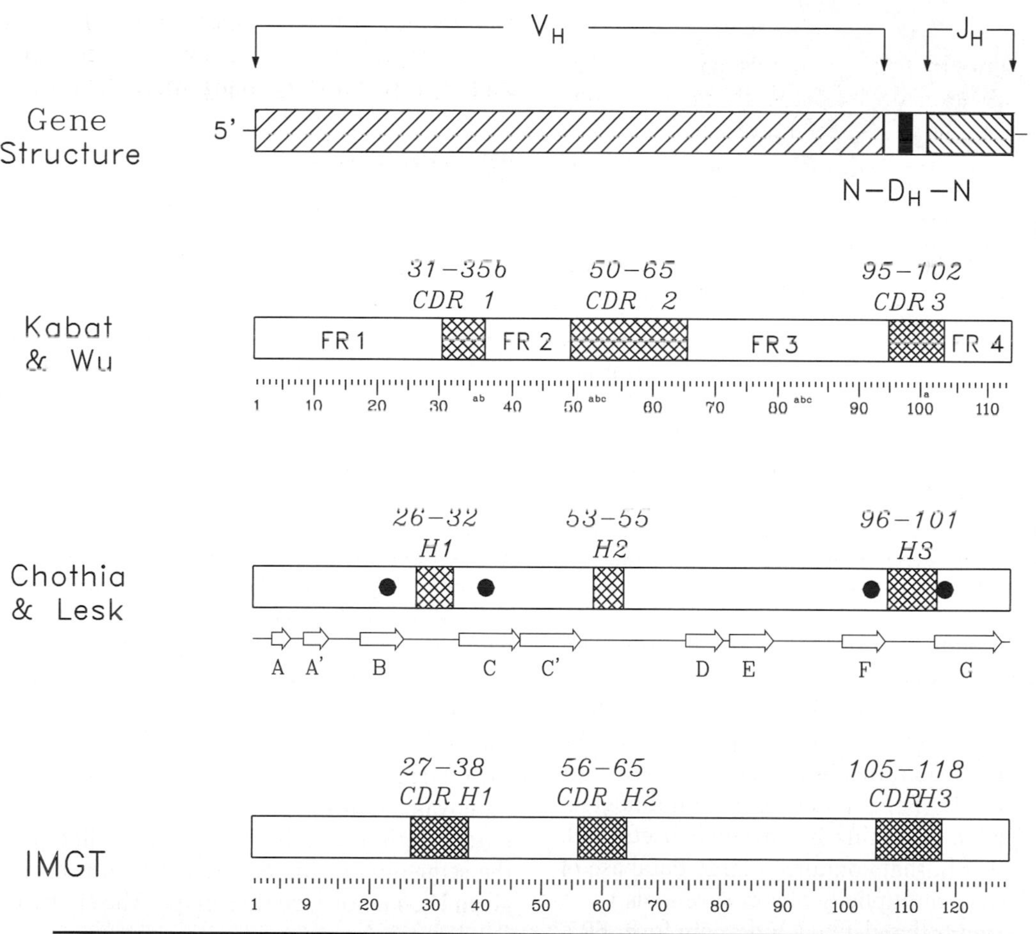

FIGURE 4.5 Sequence conservation and hypervariability within an H chain V domain. The primary sequence of the V domain can be divided into four regions of sequence conservation, termed *frameworks,* or FRs, and three regions of hypervariability, termed *complementarity determining regions,* or CDRs. A schematic of the genomic origin of the variable domain is shown at the top of the figure. The classic separation of the sequence into FR and CDR by Kabat and Wu (31) is shown below the gene structure. The letter designation for individual β strands is given beneath the Chothia and Lesk nomenclature (32), which focused more on structure. The positions of each of the four invariant residues of the V_H chain (FR1 Cys22, FR2 Trp36, FR3 Cys92, and FR4 Trp103) are shown as darkened circles on the Chothia and Lesk model. The IMGT designation has attempted to rationalize sequence variability with structure and is the current nomenclature of choice (33).

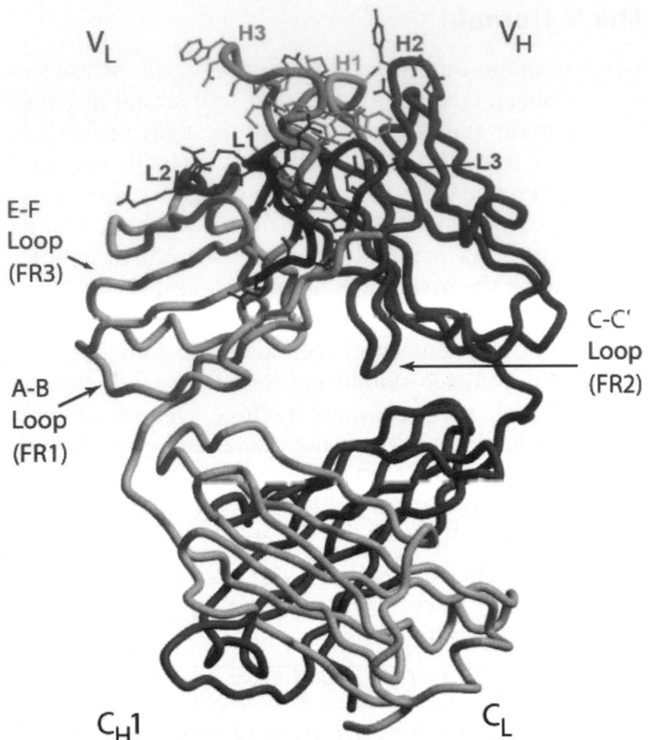

FIGURE 4.6 The structure of an Fab. The antigen binding site is formed by the H and L chain B-C, C′-C″, and F-G loops. Each loop encodes a separate complementarity determining region, or CDR. The location of CDRs H1, H2, H3, L1 L2, and L3 are shown. The opposing H and L chain C-C′ strands and loop help stabilize the interaction between VH and VL. This C-C′ structure is encoded by the second V framework region, FR2. The inclusion of this structure permits the V domains to interact in a head-to-head fashion. The E-F strands and loop are encoded by the FR3 region and lie directly below the antigen binding site. The A-B strands and loop encode FR1 and lie between the C_H1 and CL domains and the rest of the Vs. The beta sheet strands of the C_H1 and CL domains rest crosswise to each other. The illustration is modified from (191). (See color insert.)

intervals has been adjusted over the years, first by a focus on the primary sequence (31), then by a focus on the three-dimensional structure (32), and, more recently, by a consensus integration of the two approaches by the international ImMunoGeneTics information system®, or IMGT [33] (Figure 4.5). (For students of the immunoglobulin repertoire, IMGT maintains an extremely useful web site, http://imgt.cines.fr, that contains a large database of sequences as well as a multiplicity of software tools.)

The C and C′ strands that define a V domain form FR2. These strands project away from the core of the molecule (Figures 4.4 and 4.6), where they take on a conserved structure that is parallel and opposite to the FR2 of the companion V and adjacent to the FR4 of the complementary chain. Approximately 50% of the interdomain contacts in the hydrophobic core of the V domain are formed by contacts between the FR2 of one chain and the FR4 of the complementary chain (30). Another 30%–45% is contributed by contacts between the CDR3 and the FR2 or CDR3 of the complementary domain. The overall interdomain contact includes between 12 and 21 residues from the L chain V domain and 16–22 residues from H chain V domain, most of which are contributed by the FR2, CDR3, and FR4 regions.

There are approximately 40 crucial sequence sites that influence variable domain inter- and intradomain interactions (32,34). Four of these sites are relatively invariant—the two cysteines that form the disulphide bridge between the beta sheets, and two tryptophan (phenylalanine in Jκ) residues, one near the beginning of the C strand and the second near the beginning of the G strand, that pack against the bridge to add stability. Beyond these and other common core residues, Ig domains can vary widely in their primary amino acid sequences. However, a common secondary and tertiary structure characteristic of the core Ig V domain tends to be preserved.

FAB STRUCTURE AND FUNCTION

Introduction

It is the Fab domain that allows immunoglobulin to discriminate between antigens. Each developing B cell manufactures its own, largely unique, Fab. The Fab shows an amazing array of binding capabilities while maintaining a highly homologous scaffold. This section describes the characteristics of the Fab domain, its component V domains, and the paratope, which is the part of the Fab that actually binds antigen.

Fab, Fv, and Fb

The antigen-binding fragment (Fab) is a heterodimer that contains a light chain in its entirety and the V and C_H1 portions of the H chain (Figures 4.1, 4.6). In turn, the Fab can be divided into a variable fragment (Fv) composed of the V_H and V_L domains, and a constant fragment (Fb) composed of the C_L and C_H1 domains (Table 4.1). Single Fv fragments can be produced in the laboratory through genetic engineering techniques (35). They recapitulate the monovalent antigen-binding characteristics of the original parent antibody. Other than minor allotypic differences, the sequences of the constant domains do not vary for a given H chain or L chain isotype. The eponymous variable (V) domain, however, is quite variable.

Generation of Ig V Domains by Recombination

Ig variable domain genes are assembled in an ordered fashion by a series of recombination events (26,36–39). The elegant mechanisms used for the assembly of these genes and the Fvs they create are fully discussed in Chapter 6.

However, to understand the relationship between antibody structure and function, a brief review is in order.

In mice, immunoglobulin V assembly begins with the joining of one of 13 diversity (D_H) gene segments to one of four joining (J_H) gene segments. This is followed by the joining of one of 110 functional variable (V_H) gene segments (40–42). (These numbers come from common strains of laboratory mice. The number of gene segments often varies between strains.) Each D_H gene segment has the potential to rearrange in any one of six reading frames (RFs), three by deletion and three by inversion. Thus, these 127 gene segments can come together in 3.4×10^4 combinations. The V_H gene segment encodes FRs H1-H3 and CDRs H1 and H2 in their entirety (Figures 4.1, 4.5), and the J_H encodes FR-H4. CDR-H3 is created *de novo* in developing B cells by the joining process. CDR-H3 contains the D_H gene segment in its entirety, as well as portions of the V_H and J_H gene segments.

After a functional H chain has been created, light chain assembly begins. Mice contain two L chain loci, κ and λ. The κ locus includes five $J\kappa$ gene segments and 140 $V\kappa$ gene segments, of which 4 and 73 have been shown to be functional, respectively (43–45). This provides 292 combinations. There is only one $C\kappa$ (46). The λ locus contains 3 $V\lambda$, three functional $J\lambda$, and two or three functional $C\lambda$ chains (47,48). The λ–constant domains are functionally indistinguishable from each other. Due to gene organization, the λ repertoire provides at most seven combinations. Each V_L encodes FRs L1-L3, CDR L1 and L2, and two thirds of CDR-L3 (Figure 4.1). Each J_L encodes one-third of CDR-L3 and FR4 in its entirety. Any one H chain can combine with any one L chain, thus 211 V, D, and J gene segments can provide approximately 1×10^7 different H:L combinations.

At the V→D and D→J junctions, the potential for CDR-H3 diversity is amplified by imprecision in the site of joining, allowing exonucleolytic loss as well as palindromic (P junction) gain of terminal V_H, D_H, or J_H germline sequence. B cells that develop after birth express the enzyme terminal deoxynucleotidyl transferase (TdT) during the H chain rearrangement process (26,36). TdT catalyzes the relatively random incorporation of nongermline-encoded nucleotides between V_H and D_H, and between D_H and J_H. Each three nucleotides of N addition increase the potential diversity of CDR-H3 20-fold. Thus sequences with nine nucleotides of N addition each between the V→D and D→J junctions would enhance the potential for diversity by $(20)^6$, or by 6×10^7; sixfold greater than the potential diversity provided by VDJ gene segment combinations. These genomic gymnastics permit the length of CDR-H3 to vary from 5 to 20 amino acids among developing B cells in mouse bone marrow (49). Together, imprecision in the site of VDJ joining and N addition provides the opportunity to create nearly random CDR-H3 sequences, potentially freeing the CDR-H3 repertoire from germline sequence constraints. Although a limited amount of N addition is observed between V_L and J_L in human chains (50,51), N addition in murine L chains is distinctly uncommon. Moreover, the length of CDR-L3 appears to be under relatively strict control, greatly limiting the potential for somatic L chain junctional diversity (48,50). Thus, CDR-H3 represents the greatest focus for the initial somatic diversification of the antibody repertoire.

Segmental Conservation and Diversity within the V Domain

Although the large numbers of V gene segments might give the impression of a smooth incremental range of available diversity, multigene families are thought to evolve in concert through mechanisms of gene conversion, and V gene segments are no exception. Sequence relationships allow grouping them into families and clans of sequences that share nucleotide sequence homology (52), as well as structural features. Close inspection of the V_H gene repertoire has shown that these family relationships reflect segmental gene conversion coupled with selection for function (3,53,54).

Due to the need to maintain a common secondary and tertiary core Ig V domain structure capable of associating randomly with a complementary V chain to form a stable Fv, the core sequence of FR2, which is encoded by the V_H gene segment, and the core sequence of FR4, which is encoded by the J_H gene segment, are highly conserved among all Ig V domains. Conversely, the need to generate a diverse repertoire of antigen-binding sites has led to extensive diversity in the CDR1 and CDR2 intervals. One might presume that the FR1 and FR3 intervals, which form the external surface of the antibody, would not be under any particular constraints, but sequence comparisons would suggest otherwise.

Given the need to diversify the CDRs and the need to preserve FR2, it is not surprising that family identity, which might reflect ancestral relationships, can be assigned by the extent of FR1 and FR3 similarity (55). Of these, FR1 appears to be under the greatest constraints, with V_H gene segments belonging to different families both within and across species barriers exhibiting extensive similarities in FR1 sequence (Figure 4.7). Sequence similarities in FR1 and, to a lesser extent, FR3 allow grouping of V_H families into three clans of related sequences, presumably reflecting an early divergence in sequence from a primordial V_H gene sequence (Figure 4.8).

Constraints on the Sequence and Structure of V-Encoded CDRs

The antigen-binding site of an immunoglobulin is formed by the juxtaposition of the six hypervariable H and L chain V domain intervals: CDRs-H1, -H2, and -H3, and CDRs-L1, -L2, and -L3 (31). The CDR sequences of V gene

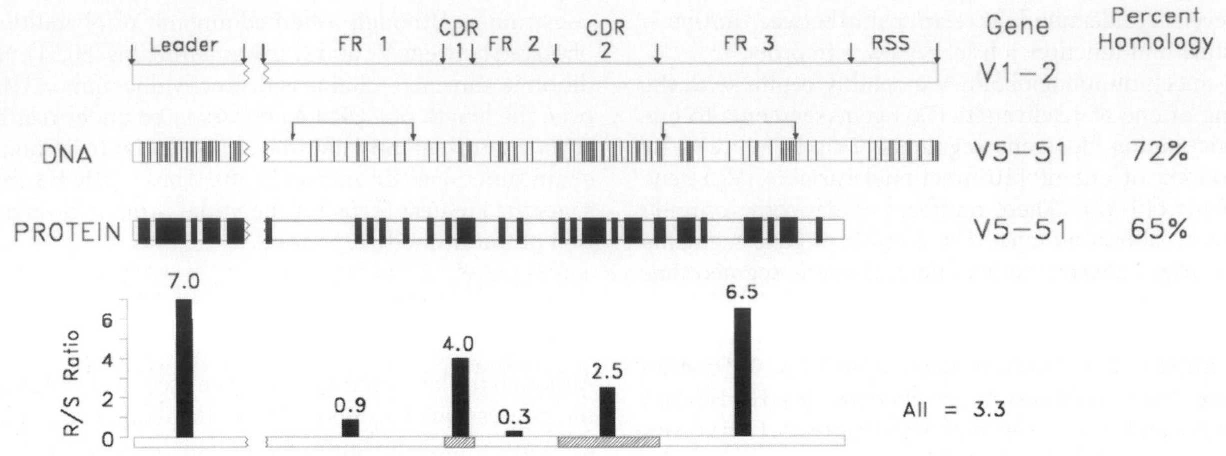

FIGURE 4.7 A comparison of two human Clan I V_H sequences that belong to different V_H families (modified from [3]). Shown is a comparison of the DNA and amino acid sequences of the V5-51 and V1-2 gene segments. Each line depicts a divergence in the identity of the nucleotide or amino acid at that position. Shown below is a replacement/silent site substitution analysis by interval. Random mutation tends to exhibit an R/S ratio of 2.9. The smaller the ratio, the greater the preservation of sequence. The intervals identified by the arrows predict the family and clan of origin.

segments tend to be enriched for codons where mutations maximize replacement substitutions (56). This includes the RGYW motif that facilitates somatic hypermutation (57,58). While evolution appears to favor CDR1 and CDR2 sequences that facilitate codon diversity, it also appears to preserve specific loop structures.

Although there is great variation in the sequences and sizes of these CDRs, it has been shown that five of them, CDR-H3 being the notable exception, possess one of a small set of main-chain conformations termed canonical structures (32,34,59,60). Each canonical structure is determined by the loop size and by the presence of certain residues at key positions in both the loop and framework regions. For example, three canonical structure types have been identified for CDR-H1, four for CDR-H2, five for CDR-L1, one for CDR-L2, and five for CDR-L3 (32,34,61). From

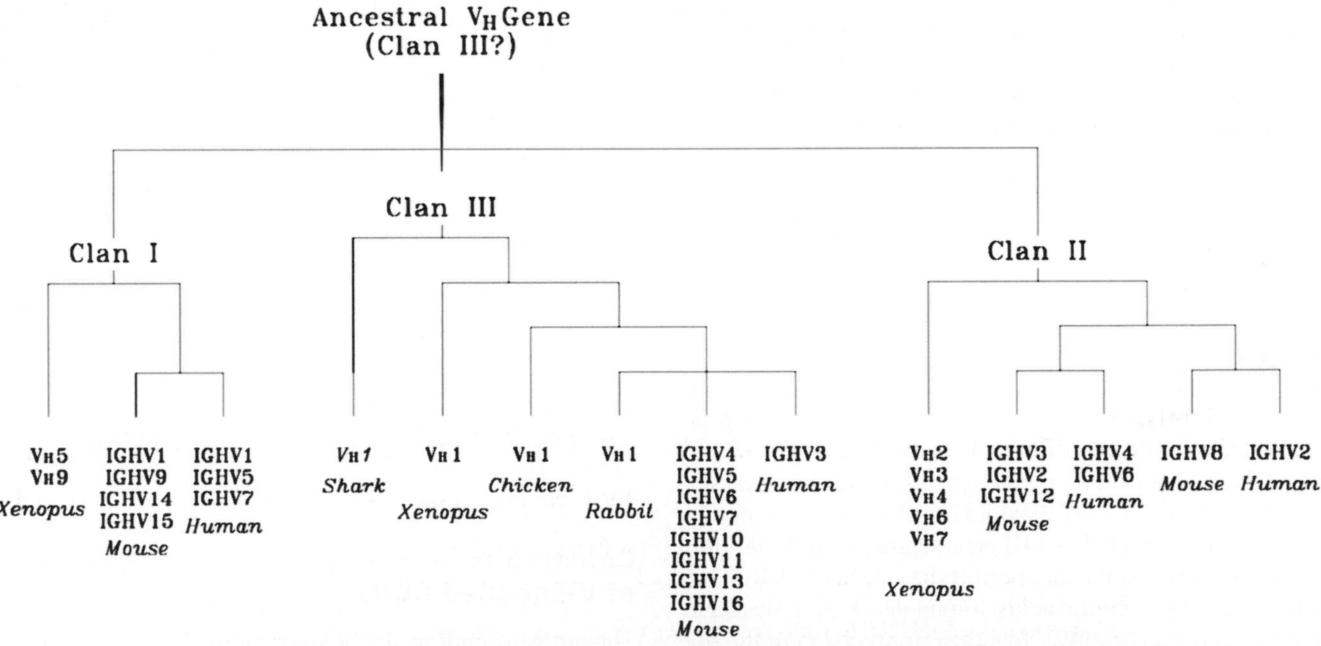

FIGURE 4.8 Evolutionary relationships among vertebrate V_H families. The sizes or relative placements of the evolutionary connecting lines are not to scale. V_H sequences from all mammalian species analyzed to date can be placed into one of these three clans. (Modified from [3].)

these types, it can be calculated that the total number of possible combinations of canonical structures, or structure classes, is 300 (62). However, only 10 of these combinations, or classes, are sufficient to describe seven-eighths of human and mouse Fab sequences. Of these, CDR-H1, -L2, and -L3 always appear with the same canonical structure type, and thus do not contribute to the variation in the structure of the most frequent classes of antigen binding sites. Only CDR-H2 and -L1 change from one class to another. Among specific classes, the lengths of CDR-H3 and -L1 appear to correlate with the type of recognized antigen. Antibodies with short loops in -H2 and -L1 appear to be preferentially specific for large antigens (proteins); whereas antibodies with long loops in -H2 and -L1 appear to be preferentially specific for small molecules (haptens) (62).

Given that the sequences and structures of the framework regions, which define families, influences the canonical structure of V_H-encoded CDRs, it is not surprising that the structure repertoire of canonical structures is both family- and clan-specific (63). This implies restrictions to the random diversification of the hypervariable loop structures (canonical structures) and their combinations within the same V_H gene segment (canonical structure classes). It further suggests evolutionarily- and structure imposed restrictions operating to counteract the random diversification of these CDRs.

Diversity and Constraints on the Sequence and Structure of CDR-H3

The combination of VDJ assortment, variation in the site of gene segment rearrangement, and N nucleotide addition makes CDR-H3 the most variable of the six hypervariable regions. Correspondingly, it has not yet been possible to define, much less assign, canonical structures to the CDR-H3 loops similar to those observed for the V-encoded CDRs. However, insight into a gradient of possible structures has been gained.

CDR-H3 can be separated into a base, which is adjacent to the frameworks, and a loop. The base tends to be stabilized by two common residues, an arginine at Kabat position 94 (IMGT 106) and an aspartic acid at Kabat 101 (IMGT 116) (32). These form a salt bridge that, together with the adjacent residues, tends to create one of three backbone conformations, termed *kinked, extra-kinked,* and *extended* (64). In approximately one-quarter of sequences with kinked or extra-kinked bases, it is also possible to predict whether an intact hydrogen-bond-ladder may be formed within the loop of the CDR-H3 region, or whether the hydrogen bond-ladder is likely to be broken (65). However, for the majority of CDR-H3 sequences, especially those that are longer, current tools do not allow prediction of potential structures.

In spite of the potential for totally random sequence provided by the introduction of N nucleotides, close inspection has shown that the distribution of amino acids in the CDR-H3 loop is highly biased for tyrosine and glycine (31,66) and relatively depleted of highly polar (charged) or nonpolar (hydrophobic) amino acids. This pattern of amino acid utilization is established early in B cell development, prior to the expression of immunoglobulin on the surface of the cell (Figure 4.9) (49,67,68) and reflects evolutionary conservation of J_H and D_H gene segment sequences. In particular, although the absolute sequence of the D_H is not the same, the pattern of amino acid usage by RF is highly conserved. Of the six potential RFs, RF1 by deletion is enriched for tyrosine and glycine. RF2 and RF3 by deletion are enriched for hydrophobic amino acids, as are RF2 and RF3 by inversion. RF1 by inversion tends to encode highly polar, often positively charged, amino acids (66). Various species use different mechanisms to

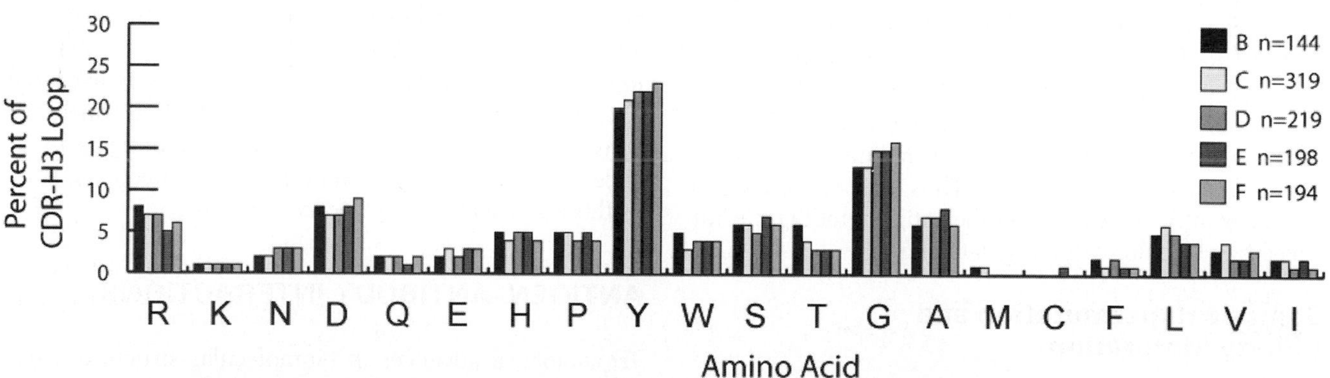

FIGURE 4.9 A preference for tyrosine and glycine in CDR-H3 begins early and intensifies with B cell development. V_H7183DJC transcripts were cloned and isolated from fractions B (pro-B cells) through F (mature B cells) from the bone marrow of 8 to 10 week-old BALB/c mice (49,67,68). The amino acids are arranged by relative hydrophobicity, as assessed by a normalized Kyte-Doolittle scale (186,187). Use is reported as the percent of the sequenced population. The number of unique sequences per fraction is shown.

bias for use of RF1 by deletion, to limit use of hydrophobic RFs, and to restrict or prevent use of RFs enriched for charged amino acids. Forced rearrangement into RFs with charged amino acids yields an altered repertoire enriched for charge and depleted of tyrosine and glycine (67). Mice forced to use a repertoire enriched for charged CDR-H3s exhibit disruptions in B cell development, reductions in serum IgG, and decreased responses to specific antigens.

The distribution of CDR-H3 lengths can also be regulated both as a function of differentiation and as a function of ontogeny (49,69). In association with long V-encoded CDRs, short CDR-H3s create an antigen binding cavity at the center of the antigen binding site, and CDRs of intermediate length can create an antigen binding groove. Each species appears to prefer a specific range of CDR-H3 lengths (70). Long CDR-H3s, which can create "knobs" at the center of the antigen binding site, are unevenly distributed between species and reflect both divergence in germline sequence and somatic selection.

The Antigen Binding Site Is the Product of a Nested Gradient of Regulated Diversity

The tension between the need to conserve essential structure and the need to emphasize diversity in an environment subject to unpredictable antigen challenge appears to create a gradient of regulated diversity in the Fv. The most highly conserved components of the Fv are FR2 and FR4, which form the hydrophobic core of the V_H:V_L dimer (Figures 4.4, 4.5). FR1, which in the H chain presents with three conserved structures, helps form the ball and socket joint between the V_H and C_H1. FR3, which in the H chain defines the family and provides 7 different structures in human versus 16 different structures in mouse, frames the antigen binding site (Figure 4.10). The V-encoded CDRs, -H1, -H2, -L1, -L2, and most of -L3, are programmed for diversity. However, conserved residues within these CDRs, which interact with V family-associated FR3 residues, constrain diversity within a preferred range of canonical structures. CDR-H3, the focus of junctional diversity, lies at the center of the antigen binding site. The conformation of its base tends to fit within three basic structures. The loop varies greatly in sequence, yet still maintains a bias for the use of tyrosine and glycine. Thus, diversity increases with proximity to the center of the antigen binding site but appears to be held within regulated limits.

Somatic Hypermutation and Affinity Maturation

Following exposure to antigen and T-cell help, the V domain genes of germinal center lymphocytes can undergo mutation at a rate of up to 10^{-3} changes per base pair per cell cycle (71), a process termed *somatic hypermutation*. Somatic hypermutation allows *affinity maturation* of the antibody repertoire in response to repeated immunization or exposure to antigen. Although affinity maturation often preserves the canonical structure of the CDR loops, the distribution of diversity appears to differ between the primary and antigen-selected repertoire (72). In the primary repertoire, diversity is focused at the center of the binding site in CDR-H3. With hypermutation, somatic diversity appears to spread to the V-encoded CDRs in the next ring of the binding site (Figure 4.10), enabling a more "custom-tailored" fit.

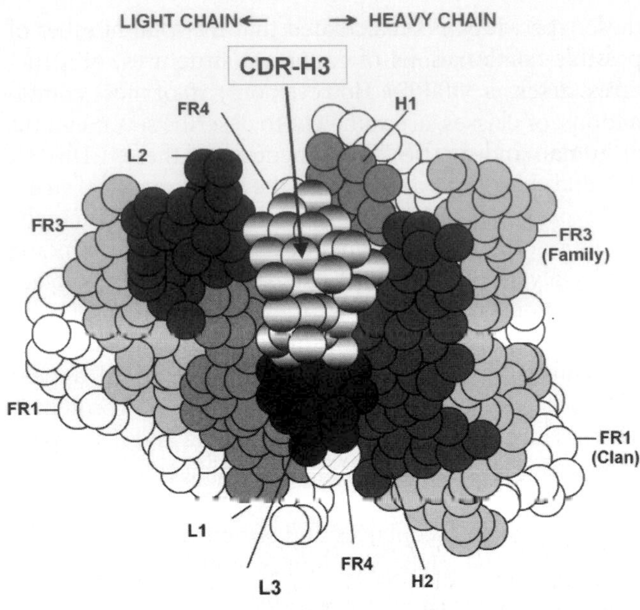

FIGURE 4.10 Location and generation of CDR-H3. A cartoon of the classic antigen binding site (modified from [3]). Due to its central location, most antigens bound to the antibody will interact with CDR-H3.

Binding of 'Superantigens' to Nonclassic V Domain Antigen Binding Sites

Not all antigens bind to the paratope created by the classic antigen binding site. Antigens that can bind to public idiotopes on V domain frameworks (73) and recognize large portions of the available repertoire are termed superantigens. There are indications that B cell superantigens influence the pathogenesis of some common infections, such as those caused by *Staphylococcus aureus*.

ANTIGEN–ANTIBODY INTERACTIONS

Technological advances in biomolecular structure determination, analysis of molecular dynamics, protein expression and mutagenesis, and biophysical investigation of receptor–ligand complex formation have facilitated significant advances in the understanding of antigen–antibody interactions. Particularly valuable has been the integration of high-resolution structural data with thermodynamic and kinetic analyses on a number of antigen–monoclonal antibody complexes. In this section, some of the key insights arising from these studies will be reviewed.

Molecular Flexibility

Like many other protein domains, V domains exhibit varying degrees and modes of molecular flexibility. Evidence suggests that some V modules (i.e., V_L-V_H pairs) can adopt two or more conformations with meaningful frequencies in the unbound state. Since these different conformational states can exhibit distinguishable binding proclivities, molecular flexibility provides monoclonal antibodies with a mechanism for polyspecificity (74). Molecular flexibility can also play a role in binding a single ligand, which, in such instances, may be better understood as a process of binding rather than as a simple event (75,76). The extent of conformational adjustment by antibody or antigen required for complex formation can influence both the thermodynamics and kinetics of that process.

Role of H_2O

A significant role for water molecules has become clear from the study of high-resolution structures and thermodynamic analyses of antigen–antibody complexes. Water molecules exhibit a broad range of association times with protein surfaces. Thus, some of the more tightly protein-associated of these solvent molecules effectively behave as parts of the protein (77). Water molecules found in the antigen–antibody interface, whether constitutively bound or newly recruited, can make important contributions to both the intrinsic (i.e., monovalent) affinity of the complex and to the differential affinities for different ligands (i.e., specificity) (78). Amino acid residues of antigen and antibody can interact, indirectly, through hydrogen bonds to one or more water molecules (78).

Thermodynamics and Antigen–antibody Interactions

Specific residues in the antibody V domains or the antigen can contribute to complex formation in different ways, and some residues can contribute in multiple ways (79). In addition to making van der Waals contact, residues can be important due to contributions to the free energy of complex formation or to the differential free energy of complex formation for two or more different ligands. Some residues may contribute primarily to modulation of the association rate, the "relaxation" of the forming complex, or the dissociation rate (75,80). Other contact residues contribute minimally to the energetics of complex formation, and yet other noncontact residues can be significant thermodynamic contributors (81,82).

Structural and thermodynamic/kinetic comparisons of antibodies possessing germline V domain sequences with somatically mutated V domain sequences have provided new insights into the structural and energetic bases for affinity maturation (81,82). Mutations in both contact and noncontact residues can have major consequences, positive or negative, for the affinity with which an antibody binds an antigen. They can also favor tighter binding by enhancing V domain rigidity, thereby reducing the entropic penalty associated with complex formation (82). Antibodies derived from secondary or later responses that have incorporated somatic mutations have been shown to exhibit less than absolute specificity. Even these "mature" antibodies can bind multiple ligands when screened on libraries of peptides or proteins (83,84), a lesson likely to be relevant to most biomolecules.

IMMUNOGLOBULIN 'ELBOW JOINTS' AND 'HINGES'

The structures of the constant domains can affect antibody–antigen interactions by influencing the range of molecular flexibility permitted between the two Fabs. In this section, the role of the immunoglobulin hinge will be discussed.

Elbow Joints

Individual Ig V and C domains tend to create rather rigid dimers. However, the antibody molecule as a whole, which consists of four or more such dimeric modules linked like beads on a string, can be viewed as a paradigm of molecular flexibility (85). Flexibility begins between the Fv and the Fb of the Fab at what is termed the *elbow bend* or *elbow angle* (86). This reflects both a ball and socket interaction between the FR1 of the H chain and the C_H1 domain (87) and the identity of the L chain (86). Five residues (three in V_H and two in C_H1) that are highly conserved in both antibodies and T-cell receptors make the key contacts that constitute this "joint." Elbow angles, assessed from crystal structures of homogeneous Fab fragments, range from 130° to 180°. λ light chains appear to permit an Fv to adopt a wider range of elbow angles than their κ chain counterparts.

Hinges

Some immunoglobulin isotypes contain a structural element that does not strictly correspond to the canonical structural motifs of IgSF V and C domains, which is termed the *hinge*. Where it occurs, it is located between the C-terminus of the C_H1 and the N-terminus of the C_H2 domains. In isotypes such as IgG and IgA, the hinge is encoded by one (or more) separate exon(s). In isotypes with four C_H domains (i.e., IgM and IgE), the C_H2 domain serves in place of a classical hinge.

The hinge, or the C_H2 domain in Igs that lack a hinge, permits a Fab arm to engage in an angular motion relative

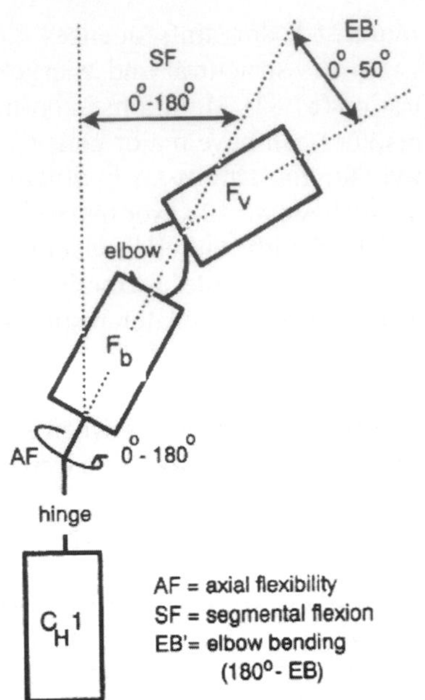

FIGURE 4.11 Illustration of the motions and flexibility of the immunoglobulin. Axial and segmental flexibility are determined by the hinge. The switch peptide (elbow) also contributes flexibility to the Fab. The measure of the elbow angle is defined with respect to the Fv and Fb axes of two-fold symmetry. (From Carayannopoulos and Capra [188] with permission.)

both to the other Fab arm and to its Fc stem (Figures 4.3, 4.11). This permits the two Fab arms to cover a range from maximal extension to an almost parallel alignment. The range of motion of the Fab arms reflects the nature of the hinge region, which in some C genes is rigid and in others, such as human IgA1, functions more as a tether than as a support for each individual Fab. This flexibility has major implications for antibody function, because it enables a bivalent antibody molecule to bind epitopes in a variety of relative spatial arrangements.

Among human IgG subclasses, the most unusual hinge region is that of IgG3. Unlike other human IgG hinge regions, the IgG3 hinge is encoded by a quadruplicated hinge exon, making it the longest hinge (62 amino acids) by far (see Table 4.2). The primary structure of this hinge has been divided into upper, core (or middle), and lower hinge regions with somewhat different functional associations. The upper hinge in particular has been associated with the magnitude of segmental flexibility as assessed by fluorescence emission anisotropy kinetics (88) and with the magnitude of Fab-Fab flexibility by immunoelectron microscopy (89). The core or middle hinge appears to serve, at least in part, a spacer function. The lower hinge functions primarily to facilitate C_H2-C_H2 interactions.

Segmental flexibility of the Ig molecule, conferred mainly by the hinge, permits or facilitates simultaneous binding through two or more Fab arms. Such monogamous bivalency or multivalency, which enhances overall binding (90,91), is a crucial factor permitting biosynthetically feasible antibody concentrations to offer adequate immunity against replicating pathogens. Although it is more speculative why the Fab-Fc geometry needs to vary, it may have to do with optimizing effector function activation when antigen is bound, such as maintaining antigen binding when Fc receptors are simultaneously engaged.

The attribution of flexibility control to the hinge is supported by protein engineering studies in which V domain-identical IgGs of different subclasses were analyzed (88,92). This basic conclusion is also supported by studies in which hinge regions have been selectively mutated or swapped among human or mouse IgG subclasses (93–95). One of these studies indicated that structural variation among subclasses in the C_H1 domain also influenced segmental flexibility as assessed by nanosecond fluorescence polarization measurements (93). Early suggestions that IgG subclass-related differences in activating the classical pathway of complement were explained by differences in segmental flexibility (88) were not confirmed by the studies in which mutant hinge regions were created (93–95).

TABLE 4.2 Properties of Hinges in Human IgG, IgA, and IgD

Ig Type	*Upper Hinge Length*	*Middle Hinge Length*	*Lower Hinge Length*	*Genetic Hinge Configuration (Amino Acids/Exon)*	*Susceptibility to Proteolysis*	*Special Features*
IgG1	4	10	6	15		
IgG2	3	8	6	12		
IgG3	12	49	6	17-15-15-15		
IgG4	7	4	6	12		
IgA1	1	23	2	19	high	Heavily O-linked glycosylation
IgA2	1	10	2	6		
IgD				34-24	high	Extensive charged amino acids; heavy O-linked glycosylation at N terminus

Note: Lengths represent amino acids.

There are several types of molecular motion attributable to the hinge region that contribute to overall segmental flexibility (see Figure 4.11). These include flexing between Fab arms (motion toward or away from one another in the same plane), Fab arms moving in and out of the same plane, Fab arms rotating along their long axes, and Fab arms moving in or out of the same plane as the Fc region (96,97). The inter-Fab angles observed by electron microscopy range from 0° to 180° (98,99). Similarly, Fab arm long-axis rotations can extend up to 180° (100).

Another key role of the hinge is the maintenance of the C_H2-C_H2 interaction (i.e., effectively constraining molecular mobility within the Fc region itself). The lower hinge stabilizes C_H2-C_H2 contacts by providing the key cysteine residues involved in inter-heavy chain disulfide bonds. Experiments in which IgG molecules were modified to eliminate the hinge region demonstrate that covalent linkage between the hinge regions just "upstream" of the two C_H2 domains is critical for the preservation of IgG effector function (101).

HEAVY CHAIN STRUCTURE AND FUNCTION

What might be termed *the fundamental strategy of humoral immunity* is a two-step process that begins with the identification by antibodies (of appropriate binding specificity) of the molecules or molecular complexes that should be eliminated. Following such identification (i.e., noncovalent complex formation), antibodies can then trigger other molecular systems (e.g., complement) or cells (e.g., phagocytes) to destroy or remove the antigenic material—guilt by association at the molecular level. Thus, antigen speci ficity, determined primarily by the V domains in the Fab arms, is physically and functionally linked to effector function, the activation of which is primarily attributable to the C domains of the Fc region. The effector functions associated with the humoral immune response primarily involve either complement or Fc receptor-bearing cells, such as neutrophils, macrophages, and mast cells. As might be expected, therefore, the Fc contains sites for noncovalently interacting with complement components, such as C1q, and with Fc receptors. This section focuses on the structures and functions of the Fc regions of the various Ig classes and subclasses.

Structure and Function of the Fc

The necessity for interacting effectively with relatively conserved molecules such as C1q and Fc receptors provides a selective basis for maintaining the primary structures of the Fc region, at least where changes would undermine such intermolecular contacts. The degeneracy possible in noncovalent molecular recognition events permits selected primary sequence variations without catastrophic alterations in function. However, there are allotypic differences in the heavy chain constant domains among both human and mouse immunoglobulins. In some cases, these allotypic differences are associated with variation in function, at least *in vitro*. For example, two recombinant V domain-identical IgG3 antibodies, of different allotypes, exhibited differential abilities to bind C1q or initiate antibody-dependent cell-mediated cytotoxicity (102). Nevertheless, the heavy chains of the human IgG subclasses are particularly well conserved, with >90% identity of amino acid sequences. In other mammalian species that have two or more IgG subclasses, they tend to exhibit less amino acid sequence identity than the human IgG subclasses.

By convention, the heavy chain constant domains are numbered from N-terminal to C-terminal, with C_H1 residing in the Fab arm and the remaining two (IgG, IgA, IgD) or three (IgM, IgE) C domains (C_H2, C_H3, and, if relevant, C_H4) residing in the Fc. In IgM and IgE, the C_H2 domain largely plays the role of the hinge region. The C domains of different isotypes and from different species share several key structural features. In distinction from V domains, which consist of four- and five-stranded β-pleated sheets linked through an intrachain disulfide bond, C domains consist of three- and four-stranded β-pleated sheets linked through an intrachain disulfide bond (Figure 4.4). Across isotypes amino acid sequence identity for CH domains is approximately 30%, while for subclasses (within an isotype), the amino acid sequence identity for C_H domains is in the range of 60%–90%. Important physical and biological properties of the human Ig isotypes are summarized in Table 4.3.

As alluded to earlier, the traditional and accepted functional anatomy of immunoglobulins attributes antigen binding (both specificity and affinity) to the V modules in the Fab arms and effector function activation to the Fc region. While this scheme is both well-supported and appealing, there is considerable (perhaps not widely appreciated) evidence that in some cases structural variations in heavy chain domains (i.e., C domains and hinge) can influence both the affinity of the antibody for antigen and the discrimination among antigens (103–108). Although these instances of C domain influence on ligand binding (through the V domains) primarily involve multivalent antigens, there are also reports that suggest C domain influence in instances of monovalent recognition (109–111). Mechanisms for these effects in the context of binding multivalent antigens include isotype-related differences in segmental flexibility, as well as the tendency for self-association. Results from a study comparing resistance to pneumococcal infection for IgG3-deficient and IgG3-producing mice are consistent with the notion that the cooperative binding permitted by murine IgG3 antibodies contributes to the effectiveness of humoral immunity (112).

TABLE 4.3 Properties of Immunoglobulin Isotypes

Class or Subclass Properties	*IgM*	*IgD*	*IgG1*	*IgG2*	*IgG3*	*IgG4*	*IgA1*	*IgA2*	*IgE*
Molecular weight of secreted form (kDa)[a]	950(p)	175	150	150	160	150	160(m), 300(d)	160(m), 350(d)	190
Sedimentation coefficient	19S	7S		6.6S			7S	11S	8S
Functional valency	5 or 10	2	2	2	2	2	2 or 4	2 or 4	2
Interheavy disulphide bonds per monomer	1	1	2	4	11	2	2	2	1
Membrane Ig cytoplasmic region	3	3	28	28	28	28	14	14	28
Secreted Ig tailpiece	20	9	2	2	2	2	20	20	2
Other chain	J chain (16 kDa)	—	—	—	—	—	J chain (16 kDa) secretory component (70 kDa)		—
N-glycosylation sites	5	3	1	1	2	1	2	4	7
O-glycosylation sites	0	7	0	0	0	0	8	0	0
Carbohydrate average (%)	10–12	9–14	2–3	2–3	2–3	2–3	7–11	7–11	12–13
Adult level range (age 16–60) in serum (mg/ml)[b]	0.25–3.1	0.03–0.4	5–12	2–6	0.5–1	0.2–1	1.4–4.2	0.2–0.5	0.0001–0.0002
Approximate % total Ig in adult serum	10	0.2	45–53	11–15	3–6	1–4	11–14	1–4	0.004
Synthetic rate (mg/kg weight/day)	3.3	0.2	33	33	33	33	19–29	3.3–5.3	0.002
Biological half-life (days)	5–10	2–8	21–24	21–24	7–8	21–24	5–7	4–6	1–5
Transplacental transfer	0	0	++	+	++	++	0	0	0
Complement activation classical pathway (C1q)	++++	0	+++	+	++++	0	0	0	0
Complement activation alternative pathway	0	0	0	0	0	0	+	0	0
Reactivity with protein A via Fc	0	0	++	++	+/−	++	0	0	0
Allotypes	—	—	G1m	G2m	G3m	—	—	A2m	Em
Biological properties	Primary antibody response, some binding to pIgR, some binding to phagocytes	Mature B cell marker	Placental transfer, secondary antibody for most responses to pathogen, binds macrophages and other phagocytic cells by FcγR				Secretory Ig, binds pIgR		Allergy and parasite reactivity, binds FcγR on mast cells and basophils

[a]Light chain, molecular weight is 25 kDa.
[b]Total = 9.5–21.7 mg/ml.
d, dimer; m, monomer; p, pentamer.
Compiled from Carayannopoulos and Capra [188], Lefranc and Lefranc [193], Kuby [194], and Janeway et al. [195], with permission.

Fc Glycosylation

All Igs contain N-linked oligosaccharides, and it is becoming increasingly clear that this glycosylation plays significant roles in Ig structure and function. Though the type and extent of glycosylation varies among isotypes, an N-linked oligosaccharide on ASN 297 in the C_H2 domain is conserved on all mammalian IgGs and homologous portions of IgM, IgD, and IgE. As the average serum IgG contains 2.8 oligosaccharides, there is often glycosylation present in the V domain as well (113). The consensus sequence for the V domain N-linked oligosaccharides is not present in the germline, but it can be created during somatic hypermutation (114). Glycosylation in the Fc region has been shown to be important for antibody half-life and effector functions (115–117). Glycosylation of the Fc domain influences complement activation as Ig hypoglycosylation influences affinity for C1q as well as Ig binding to the FcR, possibly due to its affects on Ig structure (118). Differential sialylation of the core Fc polysaccharide has recently been shown to have dramatic effects on the proinflammatory versus antiinflammatory activity of IgG (119). Further, IgD N-linked glycans are necessary for IgD to bind to the IgD receptor on T cells (120).

V domain glycosylation potentially affects the affinity for antigen, antibody half-life, antibody secretion, and organ targeting. Interestingly, glycosylation has been shown to be capable of both positively and negatively affecting antigen binding (121–124). The biologic significance of Ig glycosylation can be seen from studies demonstrating that IgG from patients with rheumatoid arthritis is galactosylated to a lesser extent (termed IgG G0) than IgG from normal controls. In some cases, hypogalactosylation correlates with disease activity (125). Hypogalactosylation of IgG has also been found to occur in other chronic inflammatory diseases such as Crohn's disease and systemic lupus erythematosus (126).

IgM

IgM is an isotype of firsts. It is ontogenetically primary, being expressed first on developing B lineage cells. IgM is also the isotype that initially dominates the primary humoral immune response. It is probably, along with IgD, a phylogenetically primitive isotype in jawed vertebrates (an almost first) and may be the most phylogenetically stable isotype (127).

IgM serves important immunological functions both on the surfaces of B lymphocytes and in the fluid phase in the blood and in the mucosal secretions. On the cell surface, IgM consists of two identical μ heavy chains and two identical light chains (μ_2L_2). It is initially expressed on B lineage cells in noncovalent association with surrogate light chains, and subsequently, following successful light chain gene rearrangement, with κ or λ light chains. On the mature B cell surface, IgM is noncovalently associated with two other polypeptide chains, Ig-α (CD79a) and Ig-β (CD79b) (128–130). These integral membrane proteins serve to transduce signals when surface IgM binds to and is cross-linked by cognate antigen.

In the secreted form, IgM can consist of either pentamers $(\mu_2L_2)_5$ or, less often, hexamers $(\mu_2L_2)_6$ (131). The μ_2L_2 monomers of the pentameric form are linked one to another by disulfide bonds in the C_H4 domains. Two of these monomers are, on one side, disulfide bonded not to another μ chain but to a 15,000 Da-polypeptide, called J chain. J chain is also found in polymeric IgA. There may be multiple patterns of such disulfide bonding, such that different cysteines participate in different monomeric units (132).

Application of electron microscopy to polymeric IgM molecules has suggested that IgM can adopt two different quaternary arrangements: star and staple (133,134). All of the antigen binding sites are arrayed in radial fashion, in the same plane as one another and the Fc regions, in the star arrangement. In the staple form, the Fab arms bend out of the plane of the Fc regions. It has been conjectured that the staple form is utilized in binding simultaneously to two or more epitopes on multivalent antigens, such as bacterial or viral surfaces.

A major pathway through which soluble IgM mediates immunity or immunopathology is the activation of the classical pathway of complement. On a per molecule basis, relative to other isotypes, IgM is highly effective at activating the classical pathway and can thereby opsonize bacterial pathogens. In select cases (e.g., *Neisseria meningitidis*), binding of IgM to bacterial surfaces, followed by complement activation, can cause direct lysis of the bacteria through the insertion of the membrane attack complex into the bacterial membrane (135). IgM, like polymeric IgA, can reduce the effective number of colony- or plaque-forming units for, respectively, bacteria and viruses, through agglutination. Significant physical and biological properties of IgM and the other Ig isotypes are shown in Table 4.3.

IgD

IgD is primarily of interest in its membrane form, as the soluble form of IgD is found in relatively modest concentrations in the blood and other body fluids. The cell surface form of IgD is found along with IgM on all mature, naïve B cells, where it appears capable of transducing activating and tolerizing signals (136). As is true for IgM, the membrane form of IgD associates noncovalently with Ig-α (CD79a) and Ig-β (CD79b). Simultaneous cell surface expression of two heavy chain isotypes expressing the same V_H domains and the same light chains occurs via differential RNA splicing (137).

IgD exhibits greater sensitivity to proteolytic cleavage than IgM, which is consistent with a relatively short serum half-life of only 2.8 days. The relatively long hinge region is a primary target for proteolysis. Little is known about the roles of serum IgD in immunity or immunopathology.

IgG

IgG is the predominant isotype (approximately 70%–75% of the total Ig) in the blood and extravascular compartments. The four human IgG subclasses (IgG1, IgG2, IgG3, and IgG4) are named in order of their relative serum concentrations, with IgG1 the most prevalent and IgG4 the least. There are differences in effector functions (e.g., complement activation and Fc receptor binding) and other biological properties (e.g., serum half-life) among these subclasses. However, there are also crucial functional commonalities, such as placental passage (see Table 4.3).

IgG antibodies are the hallmark of immunological memory in the humoral immune response. In addition to the isotype switch from IgM to IgG in a secondary antibody response, somatic hypermutation can lead to affinity maturation, a process by which the average affinity of antibody for the antigen eliciting the immune response can increase.

IgG antibodies contribute to immunity directly and through the activation of complement or FcR-bearing cells. Important examples of immunity mediated directly through antibody binding include neutralization of toxins (e.g., diphtheria toxin) and viruses (e.g., poliovirus). Medically important examples of IgG-induced complement activation include immunity to encapsulated bacterial pathogens leading either to opsonization and destruction within phagocytes (e.g., *Streptococcus pneumoniae*) or to direct complement-mediated lysis (e.g., *Neisseria meningitidis*). Activation of FcR-bearing cells by IgG antibodies has also been implicated in immunity to pathogens (e.g., *Cryptococcus neoformans*) (138). The consensus view is that human IgG1 and IgG3 isotypes are effective activators of the classical complement pathway. Although some older sources state that IgG2 and IgG4 are weak or nonactivators of the classical complement pathway, more recent evidence suggests that when epitope density is high, IgG2 is effective in activating complement (139,140). One possible source for the isotype-related variation in complement-activating ability is variation in affinity for C1q (IgG3>IgG1>IgG2>IgG4), the portion of the first component in the classical pathway that physically contacts the C_H2 domains of antibodies. However, isotype-associated differences in complement activation have also been found to occur at steps of the cascade subsequent to the binding of C1q to antibody (102,141). For example, in one study of chimeric monoclonal antibodies engineered to express identical V domains and representing all four human IgG subclasses, the IgG3 antibody fixed C1q better than the IgG1 antibody, but the IgG1 molecule was more effective in mediating complement-dependent cell lysis than the IgG3 molecule (141). Thus, it is probably not possible to rank the relative abilities of the IgG subclasses to activate complement in a single absolute hierarchy.

The affinities of IgG subclasses for Fc receptors vary from about 5×10^5 M^{-1} to about 10^8 M^{-1} (see Chapter 5). Recent studies in the mouse suggest that the relative contributions of IgG subclasses to various immunopathological processes depend on their relative affinities for the activating versus inhibiting isoforms of FcR (142).

A remarkable attribute of IgG (for three of the four subclasses) is its serum half-life of about 23 days. This property, attributable to the Fc region and its interaction with the neonatal Fc receptor (FcγRn), has been exploited for therapeutics through the genetic fusion of solubilized receptors (e.g., CTLA4) to IgG Fc regions (143).

IgA

Although IgG is the clearly predominant isotype in the blood, IgA is the dominant immunoglobulin isotype in the mucosal secretions, as well as in breast milk and colostrum (144).

In the blood, 10%–15% of the Ig is IgA (versus 65%–75% IgG). Moreover, IgA has a shorter half-life than IgG in serum. The predominant form of IgA in human serum or plasma is monomeric (i.e., α_2L_2), but there are small quantities of dimers $[(\alpha_2L_2)_2]$, and fewer still trimers and tetramers. Secretory IgA consists of dimers and lesser amounts of trimers and tetramers associated with one joining (J) chain (distinct from the J region in the heavy chain V domain) and one secretory component (SC) chain (see below). The latter is the extracellular portion of the polymeric Ig receptor (pIgR), which is expressed by mucosal epithelial cells and transfers polymeric IgA or IgM from basolateral to apical surfaces, thereby providing most of the Ig content of the mucosal secretions. The J chain is disulfide bonded to the tail pieces, short C-terminal extensions of the C_H3 domains, of the two IgA monomers of a dimer, while SC forms a disulfide bond to a cysteine in one C_H2 domain of one monomer.

The two α heavy chain constant region genes correspond to two IgA subclasses, IgA1 and IgA2. IgA1 is the predominant (>80%) IgA subclass in the serum. Although IgA2 is the major form in some human mucosal secretions, such as those in the large intestine and the female genital tract, there is variation in the relative proportion of IgA1 and IgA2 in different secretions. The shorter hinge region of IgA2 confers increased resistance to bacterial proteases that might be encountered in the mucosal environment. The extended hinge region of IgA1 is believed to permit molecules of this isotype to accommodate variable epitope spacings on multivalent antigens. Although the long hinge region of IgA1 molecules might be expected to confer relatively high susceptibility to proteolysis, relative protection against the activity of bacterial proteases is provided by

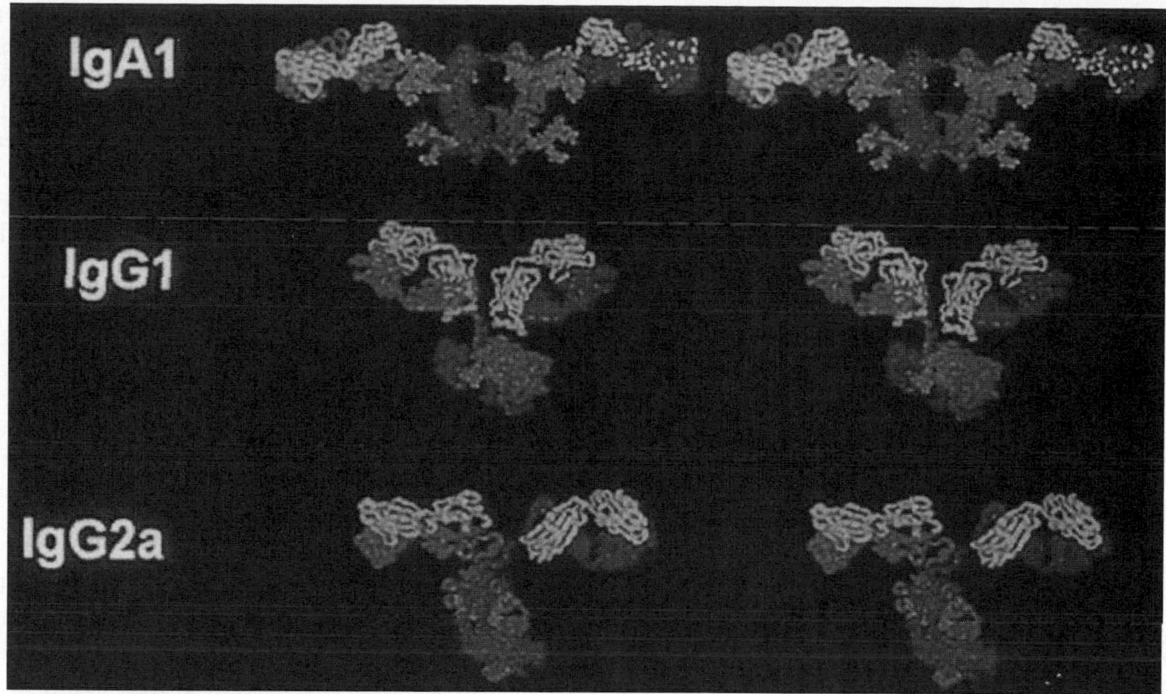

FIGURE 4.12 A comparison of an x-ray and neutron-solution-scattering theoretical model (human IgA1) and x-ray crystal (murine IgG1 and IgG2a) structures. Light chains (yellow), heavy chains (red and dark blue), and glycosylation (light blue) are illustrated. The extended length of IgA1 over that of IgG can be seen along with extensive glycosylation that characterizes this isotype. (From Boehm et al. [192], with permission. See color insert.)

heavy O-linked glycosylation in the hinge (see Figure 4.12). Nevertheless, the IgA1 hinge is uniquely susceptible to IgA proteases produced by certain pathogenic bacteria (145).

Secretory IgA (S-IgA) has been shown to participate in immunity against a range of viral, bacterial, and parasitic pathogens at mucosal surfaces. The relative absence of functional complement and phagocytes in mucosal secretions is consistent with a different mix of mechanisms for mediating immune effects associated with S-IgA versus, for example, serum IgG. Mechanisms associated with IgA are less dependent on inflammation-producing molecules or cells. Among these mechanisms are inhibition of microbial adherence through V module-mediated specific binding to microbial adhesins, agglutination of microbes, blocking of microbial receptors for cell surface carbohydrates with IgA-associated glycans, and mucus trapping (in which binding of S-IgA to bacteria makes them more adherent to host-generated mucus). There is also evidence that polymeric IgA can neutralize viruses in some circumstances by interfering with steps postattachment, such as internalization. In some cases, posttranslational modifications of viral surface molecules, related to proteolytic events associated with epithelial cell transit, lead to IgA antibodies expressing protection-related antigen specificities that have no parallel in the IgG pool (146,147). Some of the contributions of IgA to immunity are mediated through binding to FcαRI (CD89) on human neutrophils, monocytes/macrophages, and eosinophils. For example, cells bearing FcαRI on their plasma membranes can phagocytose IgA-antigen complexes. FcαRI binds to the IgA Fc region between the Cα2 and the Cα3 domains (148). Amino acid residues in the IgA Fc region critically involved in the interaction with FcαRI are indicated in Figure 4.13.

The ability of IgA to activate complement is controversial. At present, the preponderance of evidence suggests that IgA does not activate the classical complement pathway and only weakly, and under some pathophysiological circumstances, activates the alternative complement pathway. However, there is evidence suggesting that, *in vitro* at least, polymeric, but not monomeric, IgA can activate the complement pathway dependent on mannose-binding lectin (149).

Additional properties of the polymeric forms of IgM and IgA are considered in the following sections.

IgE

IgE is best known for its association with hypersensitivity reactions and allergy, but this isotype is also of interest in the context of immunity to parasites. In the blood, IgE is present at the lowest concentration of any of the immunoglobulin isotypes (with roughly five orders of

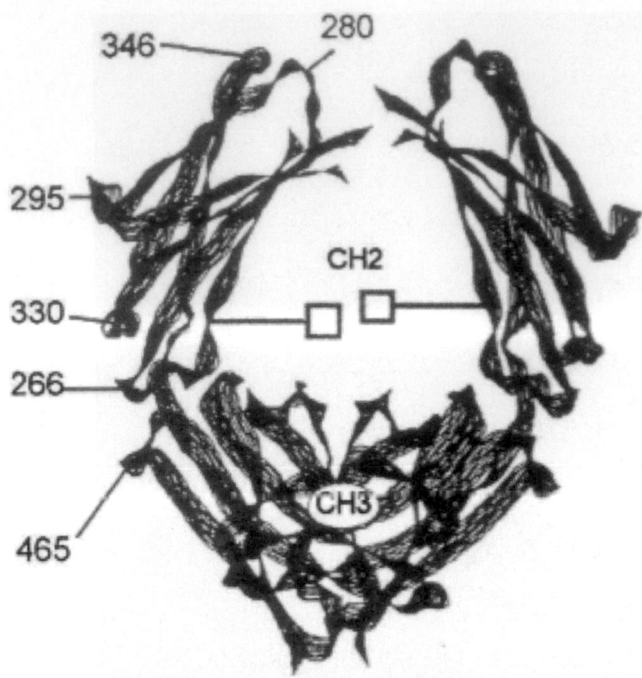

FIGURE 4.13 Illustration of the residues essential for the binding of IgA to FcαR (CD89). Residues represent mutations made in IgA C_H regions as mapped on an Fcγ fragment. Of the residues mutated, L465 and L266 were found to be important for binding to CD89. (From Carayannopoulos et al. [148] with permission.)

magnitude less IgE than IgG) and has the shortest half-life. The unimpressive quantitative representation of IgE in the blood is related to the high affinity of IgE antibodies for FcεRI, often referred to as the high-affinity Fc receptor for IgE. FcεRI is expressed on mast cells, basophils, Langerhans cells, and eosinophils. Due to the high affinity of FcεRI for its IgE ligand, mast cells and basophils are covered with relatively long-lived FcεRI-IgE complexes.

The interaction between IgE and FcεRI has an affinity of ~10^{10} L/M. It primarily involves contacts between FcεRI and amino acids in the C_H3 domains, with some contributions from amino acids in the C_H2 domains. Although each IgE potentially has two sites for interacting with the FcεRI, the stoichiometry has been shown to be 1:1. Further, it has been suggested that IgE binds to FcεRI in a kinked conformation (150).

Upon ligation with bivalent or multivalent antigens specifically recognized by the bound IgE molecules, the FcεRI molecules transduce signals that activate the mast cells or basophils to secrete potent mediators of inflammation, such as histamine. These mediators are responsible for the symptoms associated with asthma, allergic rhinitis, and anaphylaxis.

There is a second receptor for IgE. FcεRII (CD23), a type II membrane protein, is expressed on monocytes/macrophages, B lymphocytes, natural killer (NK) cells, follicular dendritic cells, Langerhans cells, eosinophils, activated epithelial cells, and platelets. It binds monomeric IgE with an affinity of ~10^7 L/M, roughly three orders of magnitude lower than the affinity of FcεRI for IgE. Functional consequences of FcεRII-IgE interaction on macrophages include secretion of mediators of immediate hypersensitivity, as well as cytokines and chemokines. There is also evidence suggesting that the FcεRII-IgE interaction can contribute to antigen capture and presentation to both B and T cells.

Fc Receptor Immunoglobulin Interactions

There are four receptors that bind the Fc regions of IgG molecules in humans and five such receptors in mice. Three of the human receptors are expressed primarily on hematopoietic cells directly involved in immune responses: FcγRI, FcγRII, and FcγRIII. Among the FcγR involved in antibody effector functions, there is important variation in affinity for IgG molecules. FcγRI binds IgG with relatively high affinity, permitting the binding of monomeric IgG. In contrast, FcγRII and FcγRIII bind to IgG with relatively low affinity. Consequently, these latter two receptors do not bind significant quantities of monomeric IgG but preferentially interact with IgG that has been effectively aggregated through interaction with bivalent or multivalent antigens (i.e., immune complexes). Key amino acid residues involved in the binding FcγRs and FcεR1 with their corresponding Ig can be seen in Figure 4.14. Allotypic variations in FcγRIIA can also influence affinity for IgG ligands and subsequent effector function (151).

There are different isoforms of FcγRII and FcγRIII. Of particular functional relevance, FcγRIIA is activating, whereas FcγRIIB is inhibiting. In mouse models, deficiency of FcγRIIB can be associated with an autoimmune syndrome similar to human lupus (152). Studies in mice have also suggested that the effectiveness of antibodies of the various murine IgG subclasses in mediating FcγR-dependent effector functions are correlated with the ratio of affinities of antibodies of those subclasses for activating versus inhibiting FcγR (142).

FcγRIIIA is expressed on NK cells, while FcγRIIIB is expressed on neutrophils. The former receptor is attached to the membrane by a standard transmembrane polypeptide, while the latter is attached via a glycophospholipid tail.

The fourth human receptor, the neonatal FcγR, or FcγRn (sometimes referred to as the *Brambell receptor*), transports IgG across the placenta. It also plays a crucial role in protecting IgG from proteolytic degradation, thereby prolonging serum half-life. While FcγRI, FcγRII, and FcγRIII are members of the immunoglobulin superfamily, FcγRn is structurally similar to MHC class I molecules, including noncovalent association with β_2-microglobulin. The interaction between FcγRn and IgG involves amino acid residues in the C_H2-C_H3 interface (153)

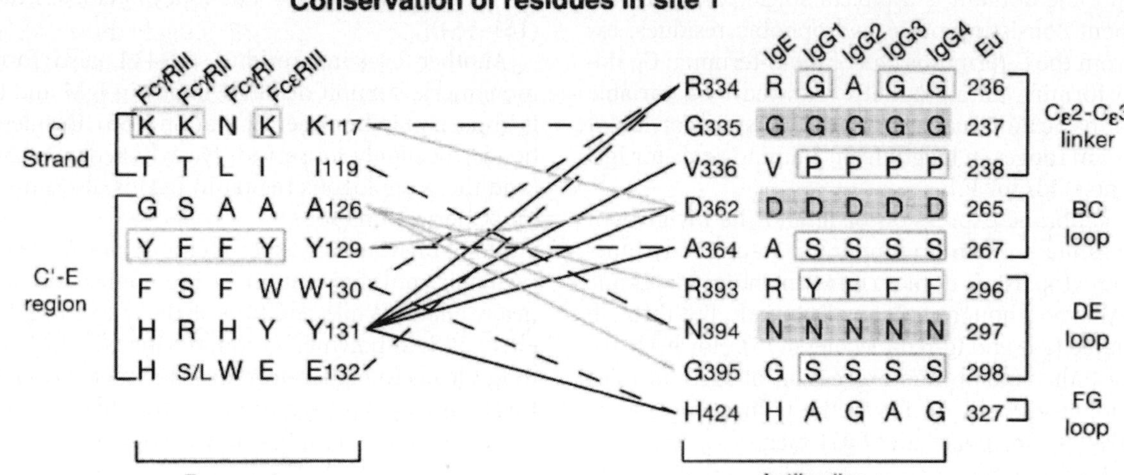

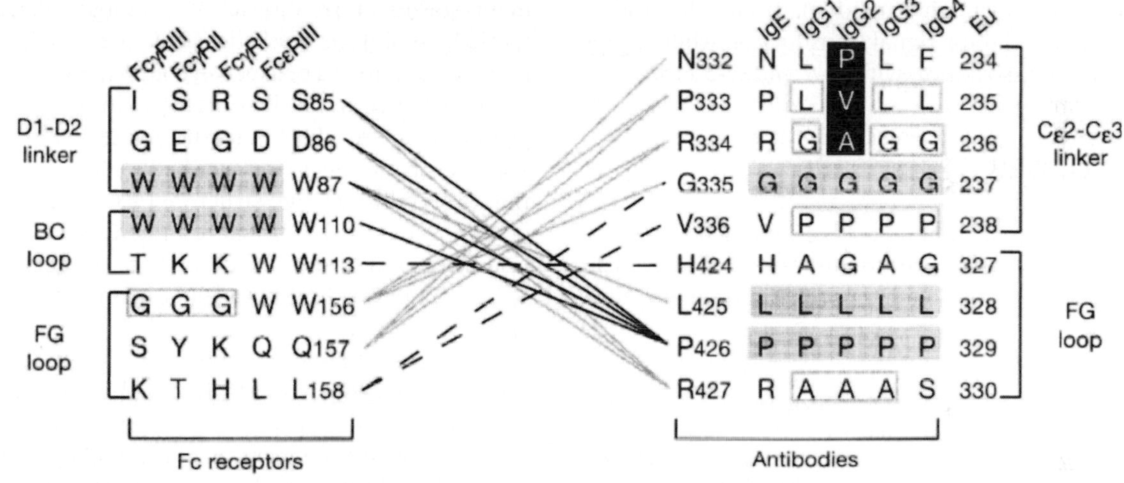

FIGURE 4.14 Certain residues are conserved between FcγRs and FcεRI as well as between IgG and IgE that facilitate binding. Two sites participate: site 1 in (a) and site 2 in (b). Heavy lines indicate the highest number of contacts and dashed lines indicate the least. Of considerable note are residues W87 and W110 in site 2 of the receptors and P426 in the immunoglobulin that form a core "praline sandwich" in the interaction between immunoglobulin and receptor. (From Garman [189] with permission.)

and is pH-sensitive. This latter property is consistent with the ability of FcγRn to bind IgG in acidic vesicular compartments and then release it into the neutral-pH environment of the blood. A crystallographic structure of the rat FcγRn in a 1:1 complex with a heterodimeric Fc (containing only one FcγRn-binding site) reveals that there are conformational changes in the Fc on binding to FcγRn (154). The investigators also identified three titratable salt bridges that confer pH-dependent binding of the IgG Fc to the FcγRn.

There are other FcR that interact with the non-IgG isotypes: IgM, IgD, IgA, and IgE. The FcR for IgA and IgE are covered in the respective sections devoted to the corresponding isotypes. An additional Fcα/μR binds both IgA and IgM. Functional attributes of this receptor and the FcRδ are in the process of being characterized in detail.

There are functional as well as structural parallels among FcR for IgG and non-IgG isotypes. Some of the features of Fc-FcR interaction that are conserved across isotypes are illustrated in Figure 4.14.

Transmembrane and Cytoplasmic Domains

Igs are expressed in both membrane and secreted forms. In contrast to the secreted form, the membrane Ig contains a transmembrane and a cytoplasmic domain. The transmembrane domain is a typical single-pass polypeptide segment consisting of 26 hydrophobic residues, extending from the C-terminus end of the C-terminal C_H domain and forming an alpha-helix followed by a variable number of basic amino acids. The cytoplasmic portion of the IgH chain ranges in length from 3 amino acids for IgG to 30 amino acids for IgE.

Both membrane expression of Ig and the integrity of the cytoplasmic domain are important in antibody function. As the cytoplasmic domain is rather short, membrane bound IgM is not thought to "signal" directly, but through the associated Ig-α and Ig-β molecules (155). However, disruption of either membrane expression of IgG1 in mice or the cytoplasmic tail results in the failure to generate an effective IgG1 response and IgG1 memory (156). Mice lacking IgE membrane expression exhibit significant impairment in IgE responses and have extremely low levels of secreted IgE (157). Thus, for those Igs with longer membrane:cytoplasmic tails, membrane Ig affects signaling beyond its association with Ig-α and Ig-β. Thus, specific residues in the transmembrane domain have been identified that are crucial for signal transduction while having no effect on the association with Ig-α and Ig-β (158).

HIGHER ORDER STRUCTURE

Many of the biological functions of IgA and IgM are dependent on their ability to form multimeric structures. This section will discuss the role of multimeric immunoglobulin in immune function.

Dimers, Pentamers, and Hexamers

The majority of multimeric IgA exists as dimers and, less commonly, trimers and tetramers, while IgM forms pentamers and occasionally hexamers. The polymeric structure of these antibodies enhances their functional affinity (avidity) for antigen, is essential for their active transport (both IgA and IgM) across epithelial cells to mucosal secretions, and, in the case of IgM, enhances the activation of the classical pathway of complement. Once multimerized, IgA or IgM in a complex with J chain can bind to pIgR and cross mucosal epithelial cells ([159], reviewed in [160]). Alhough IgM can undergo transcytosis to the mucosal secretions, its principal action is in the serum.

The ability of IgA and IgM to multimerize is due to a tailpiece (tp), an additional C-terminal segment of 18 amino acids in the secreted forms of the μ and α heavy chains. Tailpieces of both IgM and IgA contain a penultimate cysteine (residue 575 in IgM and 495 in IgA) that forms two different disulfide bonds important for multimer formation. In an Ig monomeric unit containing two identical heavy chains, one cysteine residue forms intermonomeric subunit bonds, while the remaining cysteine residue on the other heavy chain bonds to a cysteine on the J chain (161–164).

Another cysteine residue, Cys414, also forms intermonomeric subunit disulfide bonds in IgM and this bond is important in hexamer formation (165). Besides disulfide bonds, the highly conserved glycan linked to Asn563 in IgM (and the homologous region in IgA) is also important for multimerization (166).

Domain-swapping experiments demonstrate that the tp regulates multimerization in the context of the specific heavy chain. While addition of the α tp to IgM has little effect on IgM polymerization, the introduction of the μ tp to IgA leads to higher-order IgA polymers (167). Based on this finding, it has been proposed that IgM polymerization is more efficient than IgA polymerization.

The J Chain

The J chain, an evolutionarily conserved 137-amino-acid polypeptide produced by B lymphocytes, functions to regulate multimer formation and to promote linkage of multimeric Ig to pIgR on epithelial cells. The J chain consists of a single domain in a beta barrel conformation and does not show sequence similarity to Ig domains (168). It contains eight cysteine residues that participate in disulfide bonds with two tp cysteines, as described earlier, as well as function to stabilize its own structure through intramolecular bonds (167,169). The J chain influences the polymerization of the multimers, because in the absence of J chain, IgA forms fewer dimers and IgM forms fewer pentamers (170).

The J chain exists in all polymeric forms of IgA and is important in IgA polymerization and secretion across the mucosa. J chain is not required for IgM polymers, but is required for external secretion. While IgM pentamers contain J chain, hexamers almost always lack it. The makeup of IgM is biologically significant since IgM hexamers have about 20-fold greater ability to activate complement than IgM pentamers. The presence of increased levels of hexameric IgM has been postulated to play a role in the pathogenesis of Waldenstrom's macroglobulinemia and cold agglutinin disease (171).

Immunoglobulin Transport

Transport of dimeric IgA and pentameric IgM to the mucosal secretions occurs after binding to pIgR that is present on the basolateral surface of the lining epithelial cells. The J chain is essential for the secretion of IgA and IgM and, as described earlier, influences the polymeric structure of the Ig (159). pIgR is a transmembrane receptor synthesized by mucosal epithelial cells that contains seven domains, including five extracellular V-like domains, a transmembrane domain, and a cytoplasmic domain (172). Once bound to pIgR, polymeric Ig is endocytosed and transported to the apical surface of the cell. pIgR is then proteolytically cleaved between the fifth and sixth domains to release a complex (termed *secretory Ig*) containing the H, L and, J chains, and the secretory component (SC), which represents the cleaved extracellular portion of pIgR (173,174). As pIgR undergoes constitutive transcytosis in the absence of polymeric Ig, free SC is also released into the mucosal secretions. SC has several biological functions, including protecting the Ig from degradation by proteases and binding bacterial antigens such as the *Clostridium difficile* toxin A (175,176). SC also functions to localize sIgA to the mucus layer to help protect against invasion by pathogens (177). Results from pIgR-null mice demonstrate that alternate pathways exist to transport polymeric Ig to the mucosal secretions as some secretory Ig still crosses the epithelial cells in the absence of pIgR (178). Results from pIgR-null mice also demonstrate the importance of high levels of secretory antibodies, as these mice are more susceptible to mucosal infections with pathogens such as *Salmonella typhimurium* and *Streptococcus pneumoniae* (179,180).

The epithelial transcyotosis of polymeric Ig has several biological implications. First by delivering the Ig to the mucosal surface, it enables antibodies to bind to pathogenic agents and prevent them from penetrating the mucosa, a process termed *immune exclusion*. Second, transcytosing antibody can neutralize viruses intracellularly (181,182). Finally, polymeric Ig can bind to antigens in the mucosal lamina propria and excrete them to the mucosal lumen (where they can be removed from the body) by the same pIgR-mediated transcytosis process (183,184). Some pathogens can exploit the pIgR-mediated transcytosis process in reverse to penetrate the mucosa. For example, the pneumococcal adhesin, CbpA, can bind pIgR at the epithelial apical surface, leading to bacterial penetration of the mucosa (185).

CONCLUSION

Immunoglobulins are extremely versatile molecules that can carry out many biological activities at the same time. The need to be able to recognize unique antigen structures prior to any previous exposure, coupled with the need to maintain host cell receptor or complement recognition properties, presents a truly unique challenge for the system. As has been described, the system incorporates diversity within specific constraints. The precise biological niches may differ, but the overall design for these molecules is the same.

The flexibility and biologic properties of immunoglobulins have made them a major focus of molecular engineering. Immunoglobulins are being used as therapeutic agents, as well as for biotechnology applications. These opportunities have led to a resurgence of interest in the structure–function aspects of antibodies as we approach "designer antibodies." Both the variable and constant portions of these molecules are current substrates for engineering purposes, offering the potential for altering both receptor and effector function. The study of antibodies began with the need to understand how sera could neutralize toxins. It is likely that antibodies will continue to be a major focus for those who seek to take fundamental principles of protein chemistry to the bedside.

REFERENCES

1. Kolar GR, Capra JD. Immunoglobulins: Structure and function. In: Fundamental Immunology, 5th ed. Lippincott Williams & Wilkins, Philadelphia; 2003;47–68.
2. Sakano H, Rogers JH, Huppi K, et al. Domains and the hinge region of an immunoglobulin heavy chain are encoded in separate DNA segments. *Nature* 1979;277(5698):627–633.
3. Kirkham PM, Schroeder HW, Jr. Antibody structure and the evolution of immunoglobulin V gene segments. *Semin Immunol* 1994;6:347–360.
4. Rogers J, Early P, Carter C, et al. Two mRNAs with different 3′ ends encode membrane-bound and secreted forms of immunoglobulin mu chain. *Cell* 1980;20:303–312.
5. Cohn M. The immune system: a weapon of mass destruction invented by evolution to even the odds during the war of the DNAs. *Immunol Rev* 2002;185:24–38.
6. Cohn M. What are the commonalities governing the behavior of humoral immune recognitive repertoires? *Develop Comp Immunol* 2006;30:19–42.
7. Ravetch JV. Fc receptors. *Current Opinion in Immunology* 1997; 9(1):121–125.
8. Crowley JJ, Goldfien RD, Schrohenloher RE, et al. Incidence of three cross-reactive idiotypes on human rheumatoid factor paraproteins. *J Immunol* 1988;140:3411–3418.
9. Nimmerjahn F, Ravetch JV. Divergent immunoglobulin G subclass activity through selective Fc receptor binding. *Science* 2005;310(5753):1510–1512.
10. Jazwinska EC, Dunckley H, Propert DN, et al. GM typing by immunoglobulin heavy chain gene RFLP analysis. *Am J Hum Genet* 1988;43:175–181.
11. Wright A, Morrison SL. Effect of glycosylation on antibody function: implications for genetic engineering. *Trends in Biotechnology* 1997;15(1):26–32.
12. Jefferis R, Lund J, Goodall M. Recognition sites on human IgG for Fc gamma receptors: the role of glycosylation. *Immunology Letters* 1995;44(2–3):111–117.
13. Yoo EM, Morrison SL. IgA: an immune glycoprotein. *Clin Immunol* 2005;116(1):3–10.
14. Julian BA, Novak J. IgA nephropathy: an update. [Review] [85 refs]. *Current Opinion in Nephrology & Hypertension* 2004;13(2):171–179.
15. Silverstein AM. A history of immunology. 1–422. 1989. San Diego: Academic Press. Ref Type: Serial (Book, Monograph)
16. Behring E, Kitasato S. Ueber das Zustandekommen der Diphtherie-Immunitat und der Tetanus-Immunitat bei thieren. *Deutsche medizinsche Wochenschrift* 1890;16:1145–1148.
17. Ehrlich P. Die Wertbemessung des Diphtherieheilserums. Klinisches Jahrbuch 2006;6:299–326.
18. Lindenmann J. Origin of the terms 'antibody' and 'antigen.' *Scandinavian Journal of Immunology* 1984;19:281–285.
19. Tiselius A, Kabat EA. An electrophoretic study of immune sera and purified antibody preparations. *J Exp Med* 1939;69:119–131.
20. Porter RR. The formation of a specific inhibitor by hydrolysis of rabbit antiovalbumin. *Biochemical Journal* 1949;46:479–484.
21. Porter RR. Separation and isolation of fractions of rabbit gamma-globulin containing the antibody and antigenic combining sites. *Nature* 1958;182(4636):670–671.

22. Nisonoff A, Wissler FC, Lipman LN. Properties of the major component of a peptic digest of rabbit antibody. *Science* 1960;132:1770–1771.
23. Edelman GM, Poulik MD. Studies on the structural units of the gamma globulins. *J Exp Med* 1961;113:861–884.
24. Putnam FW. Immunoglobulin structure: variability and homology. *Science* 1969;163:633–644.
25. Dreyer WJ, Bennett JC. The molecular basis of antibody formation: a paradox. *Proc Nat Acad Sci USA* 1965;54:864–869.
26. Tonegawa S. Somatic generation of antibody diversity. *Nature* 1983;302:575–581.
27. Williams AF, Barclay AN. The immunoglobulin superfamily—domains for cell surface recognition. *Annu Rev Immunol* 1988;6:381–405.
28. Harpaz Y, Chothia C. Many of the immunoglobulin superfamily domains in cell adhesion molecules and surface receptors belong to a new structural set which is close to that containing variable domains. *J Mol Biol* 1994;238(4):528–539.
29. Chothia C, Novotny J, Bruccoleri R, et al. Domain association in immunoglobulin molecules. The packing of variable domains. *J Mol Biol* 1985;186:651–663.
30. Padlan EA: Anatomy of the antibody molecule. *Mol Immunol* 1994;31(3):169–217.
31. Kabat EA, Wu TT, Perry HM, et al. Sequences of proteins of immunological interest. ed 5, Bethesda, MD: U.S. Department of Health and Human Services, 1991.
32. Chothia C, Lesk AM. Canonical structures for the hypervariable regions of immunoglobulins. *J Mol Biol* 1987;196:901–917.
33. Lefranc MP, Giudicelli V, Kaas Q, et al. IMGT, the international ImMunoGeneTics information system. *Nucleic Acids Res* 2005;33(Database:issue):issue-7.
34. Chothia C, Lesk AM, Tramontano A, et al. Conformations of immunoglobulin hypervariable regions. *Nature* 1989;342:877–883.
35. Huston JS, McCartney J, Tai MS, et al. Medical applications of single-chain antibodies. *Int Rev Immunol* 1993;10(2-3):195–217.
36. Alt FW, Baltimore D. Joining of immunoglobulin heavy chain gene segments: Implications from a chromosome with evidence of three D-J heavy fusions. *Proc Nat Acad Sci USA* 1982;79:4118–4122.
37. Rajewsky K. Clonal selection and learning in the antibody system. *Nature* 1996;381(6585):751–758.
38. Hood L, Galas D. The digital code of DNA. *Nature* 2003;421:444–448.
39. Nossal GJV. The double helix and immunology. *Nature* 2003;421:440–444.
40. Ichihara Y, Hayashida H, Miyazawa S, et al. Only DFL16, DSP2, and DQ52 gene families exist in mouse immunoglobulin heavy chain diversity gene loci, of which DFL16 and DSP2 originate from the same primordial DH gene. *Eur J Immunol* 1989;19:1849–1854.
41. Feeney AJ, Riblet R: DST4: a new, and probably the last, functional DH gene in the BALB/c mouse. *Immunogenet* 1993;37(3):217–221.
42. Johnston CM, Wood AL, Bolland DJ, et al. Complete sequence assembly and characterization of the C57BL/6 mouse Ig heavy chain V region. *J Immunol* 2006;176(7):4221–4234.
43. Max EE, Seidman JG, Leder P. Sequences of five potential recombination sites encoded close to an immunoglobulin kappa constant region gene. *Proc Nat Acad Sci USA* 1979;76(7):3450–3454.
44. Sakano H, Huppi K, Heinrich G, et al. Sequences at the somatic recombination sites of immunoglobulin light-chain genes. *Nature* 1979;280(5720):288–294.
45. Thiebe R, Schable KF, Bensch A, et al. The variable genes and gene families of the mouse immunoglobulin kappa locus. *Eur J Immunol* 1999;29(7):2072–2081.
46. Seidman JG, Max EE, Leder P. A kappa-immunoglobulin gene is formed by site-specific recombination without further somatic mutation. *Nature* 1979;280(5721):370–375.
47. Selsing E, Miller J, Wilson R, et al. Evolution of mouse immunoglobulin lambda genes. *Proc Nat Acad Sci USA* 1982;79(15):4681–4685.
48. Sanchez P, Marche PN, Rueff-Juy D, et al. Mouse V lambda X gene sequence generates no junctional diversity and is conserveed in mammalian species. *J Immunol* 1990;144:2816–2820.
49. Ivanov II, Schelonka RL, Zhuang Y, et al. Development of the expressed immunoglobulin CDR-H3 repertoire is marked by focusing of constraints in length, amino acid utilization, and charge that are first established in early B cell progenitors. *J Immunol* 2005;174:7773–7780.
50. Lee SK, Bridges SL, Jr., Koopman WJ, et al. The immunoglobulin kappa light chain repertoire expressed in the synovium of a patient with rheumatoid arthritis. *Arthr Rheum* 1992;35:905–913.
51. Victor KD, Capra JD. An apparently common mechanism of generating antibody diversity: length variation of the VL-JL junction. *Mol Immunol* 1994;31(1):39–46.
52. Brodeur PH, Riblet RJ. The immunoglobulin heavy chain variable region (IgH-V) locus in the mouse. I. One hundred Igh-V genes comprise seven families of homologous genes. *Eur J Immunol* 1984;14:922–930.
53. Tutter A, Brodeur PH, Shlomchik MJ, et al. Structure, map position, and evolution of two newly diverged mouse Ig VH gene families. *J Immunol* 1991;147:3215–3223.
54. Perlmutter RM, Berson B, Griffin JA, et al. Diversity in the germline antibody repertoire: molecular evolution of the T15 VH gene family. *J Exp Med* 1985;162:1998–2016.
55. Kirkham PM, Mortari F, Newton JA, et al. Immunoglobulin VH clan and family identity predicts variable domain structure and may influence antigen binding. *EMBO J* 1992;11:603–609.
56. Chang B, Casali P. The CDR1 sequences of a major proportion of human germline Ig V_H genes are inherently susceptible to amino acid replacement. *Immunol Today* 1994;15:367–373.
57. Rogozin IB, Kolchanov NA. Somatic hypermutagenesis in immunoglobulin genes. II. Influence of neighbouring base sequences on mutagenesis. *Biochimica et Biophysica Acta* 1992;1171(1):11–18.
58. Dorner T, Brezinschek HP, Brezinschek RI, et al. Analysis of the frequency and pattern of somatic mutations within nonproductively rearranged human variable heavy chain genes. *J Immunol* 1997;158(6):2779–2789.
59. Tramontano A, Chothia C, Lesk AM. Framework residue 71 is a major determinant of the position and conformation of the second hypervariable region in the VH domains of immunoglobulins. *J Mol Biol* 1990;215:175–182.
60. Al Lazikani B, Lesk AM, Chothia C. Standard conformations for the canonical structures of immunoglobulins. *J Mol Biol* 1997;273(4):927–948.
61. Chothia C, Lesk AM, Gherardi E, et al. Structural repertoire of the human VH segments. *J Mol Biol* 1992;227:799–817.
62. Vargas-Madrazo E, Lara-Ochoa F, Almagro JC. Canonical structure repertoire of the antigen-binding site of immunoglobulins suggests strong geometrical restrictions associated to the mechanism of immune recognition. [Erratum appears in *J Mol Biol* 1996 May 24;258(5):893]. *J Mol Biol* 1995;254(3):497–504.
63. Almagro JC, Hernandez I, del Carmen RM, et al. The differences between the structural repertoires of VH germ-line gene segments of mice and humans: implication for the molecular mechanism of the immune response. *Mol Immunol* 1997;34(16–17):1199–1214.
64. Shirai H, Kidera A, Nakamura H: Structural classification of CDR-H3 in antibodies. *FEBS Letters* 1996;399(1–2):1–8.
65. Shirai H, Kidera A, Nakamura H: H3-rules: identification of CDR-H3 structures in antibodies. *FEBS Letters* 1999;455(1–2):188–197.
66. Ivanov II, Link JM, Ippolito GC, et al. Constraints on hydropathicity and sequence composition of HCDR3 are conserved across evolution; in: Zanetti M, Capra JD, (eds): *The Antibodies*. London, Taylor and Francis Group, 2002, vol 7, pp 43–67.
67. Ippolito GC, Schelonka RL, Zemlin M, et al. Forced usage of positively charged amino acids in immunoglobulin CDR-H3 impairs B cell development and antibody production. *J Exp Med* 2006;203(6):1567–1578.
68. Schelonka RL, Ivanov II, Jung D, et al. A single D_H gene segment is sufficient for B cell development and immune function. *J Immunol* 2005;175:6624–6632.
69. Schroeder HW, Jr., Zhang L, Philips JB, III. Slow, programmed maturation of the immunoglobulin HCDR3 repertoire during the third trimester of fetal life. *Blood* 2001;98(9):2745–2751.
70. Link JM, Larson JE, Schroeder HW, Jr. Despite extensive similarity in germline DH and JH sequence, the adult Rhesus macaque CDR-H3 repertoire differs from human. *Mol Immunol* 2005;42:943–955.

71. Shlomchik MJ, Marshak-Rothstein A, Wolfowicz CB, et al. The role of clonal selection and somatic mutation in autoimmunity. *Nature* 1987;328:805–811.
72. Tomlinson IM, Walter G, Jones PT, et al. The imprint of somatic hypermutation on the repertoire of human germline V genes. *J Mol Biol* 1996;256(5):813–817.
73. Goodyear CS, Silverman GJ. B cell superantigens: a microbe's answer to innate-like B cells and natural antibodies. *Springer Seminars in Immunopathology* 2005;26(4):463–484.
74. James LC, Roversi P, Tawfik DS. Antibody multispecificity mediated by conformational diversity. *Science* 2003;299(5611):1362–1367.
75. Li Y, Lipschultz CA, Mohan S, et al. Mutations of an epitope hot-spot residue alter rate limiting steps of antigen-antibody protein-protein associations. *Biochemistry* 2001;40(7):2011–2022.
76. Lipschultz CA, Yee A, Mohan S, et al. Temperature differentially affects encounter and docking thermodynamics of antibody—antigen association. *Journal of Molecular Recognition* 2002;15(1):44–52.
77. Levitt M, Park BH. Water: now you see it, now you don't. *Structure* 1993;1(4):223–226.
78. Bhat TN, Bentley GA, Boulot G, et al. Bound water molecules and conformational stabilization help mediate an antigen-antibody association. *Proc Nat Acad Sci USA* 1994;91(3):1089–1093.
79. Greenspan NS, Di Cera E. Defining epitopes: It's not as easy as it seems. *Nature* Biotechnology 1999;17(10):936–937.
80. Li Y, Urrutia M, Smith-Gill SJ, et al. Dissection of binding interactions in the complex between the anti-lysozyme antibody HyHEL-63 and its antigen. *Biochemistry* 2003;42(1):11–22.
81. Hawkins RE, Russell SJ, Baier M, et al. The contribution of contact and non-contact residues of antibody in the affinity of binding to antigen. The interaction of mutant D1.3 antibodies with lysozyme. *J Mol Biol* 1993;234(4):958–964.
82. Patten PA, Gray NS, Yang PL, et al. The immunological evolution of catalysis. *Science* 1996;271(5252):1086–1091.
83. Kramer A, Keitel T, Winkler K, et al. Molecular basis for the binding promiscuity of an anti-p24 (HIV-1) monoclonal antibody. *Cell* 1997;91(6):799–809.
84. Michaud GA, Salcius M, Zhou F, et al. Analyzing antibody specificity with whole proteome microarrays. *Nature Biotechnology* 2003;21(12):1509–1512.
85. Huber R, Bennett WS. Antibody-antigen flexibility. *Nature* 1987; 326(6111):334 335.
86. Stanfield RL, Zemla A, Wilson IA, et al. Antibody elbow angles are influenced by their light chain class. *J Mol Biol* 2006;357(5): 1566–1574.
87. Lesk AM, Chothia C. Elbow motion in immunoglobulins involves a molecular ball-and-socket joint. *Nature* 1988;335:188–190.
88. Dangl JL, Wensel TG, Morrison SL, et al. Segmental flexibility and complement fixation of genetically engineered chimeric human, rabbit and mouse antibodies. *EMBO J* 1988;7(7):1989–1994.
89. Roux KH, Strelets L, Brekke OH, et al. Comparisons of the ability of human IgG3 hinge mutants, IgM, IgE, and IgA2, to form small immune complexes: a role for flexibility and geometry. *J Immunol* 1998;161(8):4083–4090.
90. Gopalakrishnan PV, Karush F. Antibody affinity. VI. Synthesis of bivalent lactosyl haptens and their interaction with anti-lactosyl antibodies. *Immunochemistry* 1974;11(6):279–283.
91. Hornick CL, Karuch F. Antibody affinity. 3. The role of multivalance. *Immunochemistry* 1972;9(3):325–340.
92. Phillips ML, Oi VT, Schumaker VN. Electron microscopic study of ring-shaped, bivalent hapten, bivalent antidansyl monoclonal antibody complexes with identical variable domains but IgG1, IgG2a and IgG2b constant domains. *Mol Immunol* 1990;27(2):181–190.
93. Schneider WP, Wensel TG, Stryer L, et al. Genetically engineered immunoglobulins reveal structural features controlling segmental flexibility. *Proc Nat Acad Sci USA* 1988;85(8):2509–2513.
94. Tan LK, Shopes RJ, Oi VT, et al. Influence of the hinge region on complement activation, C1q binding, and segmental flexibility in chimeric human immunoglobulins. *Proc Nat Acad Sci USA* 1990;87(1):162–166.
95. Shopes B. A genetically engineered human IgG with limited flexibility fully initiates cytolysis via complement. *Mol Immunol* 1993;30(6):603–609.
96. Nezlin R. Internal movements in immunoglobulin molecules. *Adv Immunol* 1990;48:1–40.
97. Schumaker VN, Phillips ML, Hanson DC. Dynamic aspects of antibody structure. *Mol Immunol* 1991;28(12):1347–1360.
98. Roux KH, Monafo WJ, Davie JM, et al. Construction of an extended three-dimensional idiotope map by electron microscopic analysis of idiotope-anti-idiotope complexes. *Proc Nat Acad Sci USA* 1987;84(14):4984–4988.
99. Valentine RC, Green NM. Electron microscopy of an antibody-hapten complex. *J Mol Biol* 1967;27(3):615–617.
100. Wade RH, Taveau JC, Lamy JN. Concerning the axial rotational flexibility of the Fab regions of immunoglobulin G. *J Mol Biol* 1989;206(2):349–356.
101. Brekke OH, Michaelsen TE, Sandin R, et al. Activation of complement by an IgG molecule without a genetic hinge. Nature 1993;363(6430):628–630.
102. Bruggemann M, Williams GT, Bindon CI, et al. Comparison of the effector functions of human immunoglobulins using a matched set of chimeric antibodies. *J Exp Med* 1987;166(5):1351–1361.
103. Greenspan NS, Monafo WJ, Davie JM. Interaction of IgG3 anti-streptococcal group A carbohydrate (GAC) antibody with streptococcal group A vaccine: enhancing and inhibiting effects of anti-GAC, anti-isotypic, and anti-idiotypic antibodies. *J Immunol* 1987;138(1):285–292.
104. Cooper LJ, Robertson D, Granzow R, et al. Variable domain-identical antibodies exhibit IgG subclass-related differences in affinity and kinetic constants as determined by surface plasmon resonance. *Mol Immunol* 1994;31(8):577–584.
105. Cooper LJ, Shikhman AR, Glass DD, et al. Role of heavy chain constant domains in antibody-antigen interaction. Apparent specificity differences among streptococcal IgG antibodies expressing identical variable domains. *J Immunol* 1993;150(6):2231–2242.
106. Morelock MM, Rothlein R, Bright SM, et al. Isotype choice for chimeric antibodies affects binding properties. *Journal of Biological Chemistry* 1994;269(17):13048–13055.
107. Fulpius T, Spertini F, Reininger L, et al. Immunoglobulin heavy chain constant region determines the pathogenicity and the antigen-binding activity of rheumatoid factor. *Proc Nat Acad Sci USA* 1993;90(6):2345–2349.
108. Casadevall A, Scharff MD. The mouse antibody response to infection with Cryptococcus neoformans: VH and VL usage in polysaccharide binding antibodies. *J Exp Med* 1991;174(1):151–160.
109. Pritsch O, Hudry-Clergeon G, Buckle M, et al. Can immunoglobulin C(H)1 constant region domain modulate antigen binding affinity of antibodies? *J Clin Invest* 1996;98(10):2235 2243.
110. Pritsch O, Magnac C, Dumas G, et al. Can isotype switch modulate antigen-binding affinity and influence clonal selection? *Eur J Immunol* 2000;30(12):3387–3395.
111. Torres M, May R, Scharff MD, et al. Variable-region-identical antibodies differing in isotype demonstrate differences in fine specificity and idiotype. *J Immunol* 2005;174(4):2132–2142.
112. McLay J, Leonard E, Petersen S, et al. Gamma 3 gene-disrupted mice selectively deficient in the dominant IgG subclass made to bacterial polysaccharides. II. Increased susceptibility to fatal pneumococcal sepsis due to absence of anti-polysaccharide IgG3 is corrected by induction of anti-polysaccharide IgG1. *J Immunol* 2002;168(7):3437–3443.
113. Kinoshita N, Ohno M, Nishiura T, et al. Glycosylation at the Fab portion of myeloma immunoglobulin G and increased fucosylated biantennary sugar chains: structural analysis by high-performance liquid chromatography and antibody-lectin enzyme immunoassay using Lens culinaris agglutinin. *Cancer Research* 1991;51(21):5888–5892.
114. Dunn-Walters D, Boursier L, Spencer J. Effect of somatic hypermutation on potential N-glycosylation sites in human immunoglobulin heavy chain variable regions. *Mol Immunol* 2000;37(3–4):107–113.
115. Tao MH, Morrison SL. Studies of aglycosylated chimeric mouse-human IgG. Role of carbohydrate in the structure and effector functions mediated by the human IgG constant region. *J Immunol* 1989;143(8):2595–2601.
116. Wawrzynczak EJ, Cumber AJ, Parnell GD, et al. Blood clearance in the rat of a recombinant mouse monoclonal antibody lacking

the N-linked oligosaccharide side chains of the CH2 domains. *Mol Immunol* 1992;29(2):213–220.

117. Tsuchiya N, Endo T, Matsuta K, et al. Effects of galactose depletion from oligosaccharide chains on immunological activities of human IgG. *Journal of Rheumatology* 1989;16(3):285–290.
118. Krapp S, Mimura Y, Jefferis R, et al. Structural analysis of human IgG-Fc glycoforms reveals a correlation between glycosylation and structural integrity. *J Mol Biol* 2003;325(5):979–989.
119. Kaneko Y, Nimmerjahn F, Ravetch JV. Anti-inflammatory activity of immunoglobulin G resulting from Fc sialylation. *Science* 2006; 313(5787):670–673.
120. Amin AR, Tamma SM, Oppenheim JD, et al. Specificity of the murine IgD receptor on T cells is for N-linked glycans on IgD molecules. *Proc Nat Acad Sci USA* 1991;88(20):9238–9242.
121. Leibiger H, Wustner D, Stigler RD, et al. Variable domain-linked oligosaccharides of a human monoclonal IgG: structure and influence on antigen binding. *Biochem J* 1999;338(2):529–538.
122. Wright A, Tao MH, Kabat EA, et al. Antibody variable region glycosylation: position effects on antigen binding and carbohydrate structure. *EMBO J* 1991;10(10):2717–2723.
123. Coloma MJ, Trinh RK, Martinez AR, et al. Position effects of variable region carbohydrate on the affinity and in vivo behavior of an anti-(1–>6) dextran antibody. *J Immunol* 1999;162(4):2162–2170.
124. Gala FA, Morrison SL: V region carbohydrate and antibody expression. *J Immunol* 2004;172(9):5489–5494.
125. Parekh RB, Roitt IM, Isenberg DA, et al. Galactosylation of IgG associated oligosaccharides: reduction in patients with adult and juvenile onset rheumatoid arthritis and relation to disease activity. *Lancet* 1988;1(8592):966–969.
126. Tomana M, Schrohenloher RE, Koopman WJ, et al. Abnormal glycosylation of serum IgG from patients with chronic inflammatory diseases. *Arthr Rheum* 1988;31(3):333–338.
127. Ohta Y, Flajnik M. IgD, like IgM, is a primordial immunoglobulin class perpetuated in most jawed vertebrates. *Proc Nat Acad Sci USA* 2006;103(28):10723–10728.
128. Hombach J, Tsubata T, Leclercq L, et al. Molecular components of the B-cell antigen receptor complex of the IgM class. *Nature* 1990;343:760–762.
129. Venkitaraman AR, Williams GT, Dariavach P, et al. The B-cell antigen receptor of the five immunoglobulin classes. *Nature* 1991;352(6338):777–781.
130. Campbell MA, Sefton BM. Protein tyrosine phosphorylation is induced in murine B lymphocytes in response to stimulation with anti-immunoglobulin. *EMBO J* 1990;9(7):2519–2526.
131. Davis AC, Roux KH, Shulman MJ. On the structure of polymeric IgM. *Eur J Immunol* 1988;18(7):1001–1008.
132. Davis AC, Roux KH, Pursey J, et al. Intermolecular disulfide bonding in IgM: effects of replacing cysteine residues in the mu heavy chain. *EMBO J* 1989;8(9):2125–2131.
133. Feinstein A, Munn EA. Conformation of the free and antigen-bound IgM antibody molecules. *Nature* 1969;224(226):1307–1309.
134. Svehag SE, Bloth B, Seligmann M. Ultrastructure of papain and pepsin digestion fragments of human IgM globulins. *J Exp Med* 1969;130(4):691–705.
135. Griffiss JM, Jarvis GA, O'Brien JP, et al. Lysis of Neisseria gonorrhoeae initiated by binding of normal human IgM to a hexosamine-containing lipooligosaccharide epitope(s) is augmented by strain-specific, properdin-binding-dependent alternative complement pathway activation. *J Immunol* 1991;147(1):298–305.
136. Lutz C, Ledermann B, Kosco-Vilbois MH, et al. IgD can largely substitute for loss of IgM function in B cells. *Nature* 1998;393(6687):797–801.
137. Cheng HL, Blattner FR, Fitzmaurice L, et al. Structure of genes for membrane and secreted murine IgD heavy chains. *Nature* 1982;296(5856):410–415.
138. Yuan R, Clynes R, Oh J, et al. Antibody-mediated modulation of Cryptococcus neoformans infection is dependent on distinct Fc receptor functions and IgG subclasses. *J Exp Med* 1998;187(4):641–648.
139. Garred P, Michaelsen TE, Aase A. The IgG subclass pattern of complement activation depends on epitope density and antibody and complement concentration. *Scandinavian Journal of Immunology* 1989;30(3):379–382.
140. Michaelsen TE, Garred P, Aase A. Human IgG subclass pattern of inducing complement-mediated cytolysis depends on antigen concentration and to a lesser extent on epitope patchiness, antibody affinity and complement concentration. *Eur J Immunol* 1991;21(1):11–16.
141. Bindon CI, Hale G, Bruggemann M, et al. Human monoclonal IgG isotypes differ in complement activating function at the level of C4 as well as C1q. *J Exp Med* 1988;168(1):127–142.
142. Nimmerjahn F, Ravetch JV. Fcgamma receptors: old friends and new family members. *Immunity* 2006;24(1):19–28.
143. Gribben JG, Guinan EC, Boussiotis VA, et al. Complete blockade of B7 family-mediated costimulation is necessary to induce human alloantigen-specific anergy: a method to ameliorate graft-versus-host disease and extend the donor pool. *Blood* 1996;87(11):4887–4893.
144. Mestecky J, Lamm ME, Strober W, et al. Mucosal immunology. Mestecky J, Itaru M, Kerr MA, et al., eds. *Mucosal immunoglobulins.* 2005. Amsterdam, Elsevier. Ref Type: Serial (Book, Monograph)
145. Plaut AG, Wistar R, Jr., Capra JD. Differential susceptibility of human IgA immunoglobulins to streptococcal IgA protease. *J Clin Invest* 1974;54(6):1295–1300.
146. Sharpe AH, Fields BN. Pathogenesis of viral infections. Basic concepts derived from the reovirus model. *N Engl J Med* 1985;312(8):486–497.
147. Zhaori G, Sun M, Faden HS, et al. Nasopharyngeal secretory antibody response to poliovirus type 3 virion proteins exhibit different specificities after immunization with live or inactivated poliovirus vaccines. *J Infect Dis* 1989;159(6):1018–1024.
148. Carayannopoulos L, Hexham JM, Capra JD. Localization of the binding site for the monocyte immunoglobulin (Ig) A-Fc receptor (CD89) to the domain boundary between Calpha2 and Calpha3 in human IgA1. *J Exp Med* 1996;183(4):1579–1586.
149. Roos A, Bouwman LH, van Gijlswijk-Janssen DJ, et al. Human IgA activates the complement system via the mannan-binding lectin pathway. *J Immunol* 2001;167(5):2861–2868.
150. Zheng Y, Shopes B, Holowka D, et al. Conformations of IgE bound to its receptor Fc epsilon RI and in solution. *Biochemistry* 1991;30(38):9125–9132.
151. Sanders LA, van de Winkel JG, Rijkers GT, et al. Fc gamma receptor IIa (CD32) heterogeneity in patients with recurrent bacterial respiratory tract infections. *J Infect Dis* 1994;170(4):854–861.
152. Bolland S, Ravetch JV. Spontaneous autoimmune disease in Fc(gamma)RIIB-deficient mice results from strain-specific epistasis. *Immunity* 2000;13(2):277–285.
153. West AP, Jr., Bjorkman PJ: Crystal structure and immunoglobulin G binding properties of the human major histocompatibility complex-related Fc receptor. *Biochemistry* 2000;39(32):9698–9708.
154. Martin WL, West AP, Jr., Gan L, et al. Crystal structure at 2.8 A of an FcRn/heterodimeric Fc complex: mechanism of pH-dependent binding. *Molecular Cell* 2001;7(4):867–877.
155. Blum JH, Stevens TL, DeFranco AL. Role of the mu immunoglobulin heavy chain transmembrane and cytoplasmic domains in B cell antigen receptor expression and signal transduction. *Journal of Biological Chemistry* 1993;268(36):27236–27245.
156. Kaisho T, Schwenk F, Rajewsky K. The roles of gamma1 heavy chain membrane expression and cytoplasmic tail in IgG1 responses. *Science* 1997;276(5311):412–415.
157. Achatz G, Nitschke L, Lamers MC. Effect of transmembrane and cytoplasmic domains of IgE on the IgE response. *Science* 1997;276(5311):409–411.
158. Pleiman CM, Chien NC, Cambier JC. Point mutations define a mIgM transmembrane region motif that determines intersubunit signal transduction in the antigen receptor. *J Immunol* 1994;152(6):2837–2844.
159. Brandtzaeg P, Prydz H. Direct evidence for an integrated function of J chain and secretory component in epithelial transport of immunoglobulins. *Nature* 1984;311(5981):71–73.
160. Rojas R, Apodaca G. Immunoglobulin transport across polarized epithelial cells. *Nat Rev Mol Cell Biol* 2002;3(12):944–955.
161. Mestecky J, Schrohenloher RE. Site of attachment of J chain to human immunoglobulin M. *Nature* 1974;249(458):650–652.
162. Mestecky J, Schrohenloher RE, Kulhavy R, et al. Site of J chain attachment to human polymeric IgA. *Proc Nat Acad Sci USA* 1974;71(2):544–548.

163. Bastian A, Kratzin H, Fallgren-Gebauer E, et al. Intra- and interchain disulfide bridges of J chain in human S-IgA. *Advances in Experimental Medicine & Biology* 1995;371A:581–583.
164. Frutiger S, Hughes GJ, Paquet N, et al. Disulfide bond assignment in human J chain and its covalent pairing with immunoglobulin M. *Biochemistry* 1992;31(50):12643–12647.
165. Sorensen V, Sundvold V, Michaelsen TE, et al. Polymerization of IgA and IgM: roles of Cys309/Cys414 and the secretory tailpiece. *J Immunol* 1999;162(6):3448–3455.
166. de Lalla C, Fagioli C, Cessi FS, et al. Biogenesis and function of IgM: the role of the conserved mu-chain tailpiece glycans. *Mol Immunol* 1998;35(13):837–845.
167. Sorensen V, Rasmussen IB, Sundvold V, et al. Structural requirements for incorporation of J chain into human IgM and IgA. *Int Immunol* 2000;12(1):19–27.
168. Zikan J, Novotny J, Trapane TL, et al. Secondary structure of the immunoglobulin J chain. *Proc Nat Acad Sci USA* 1985;82(17):5905–5909.
169. Mole JE, Bhown AS, Bennett JC. Primary structure of human J chain: alignment of peptides from chemical and enzymatic hydrolyses. *Biochemistry* 1977;16(16):3507–3513.
170. Randall TD, Brewer JW, Corley RB. Direct evidence that J chain regulates the polymeric structure of IgM in antibody-secreting B cells. *Journal of Biological Chemistry* 1992;267(25):18002–18007.
171. Hughey CT, Brewer JW, Colosia AD, et al. Production of IgM hexamers by normal and autoimmune B cells: implications for the physiologic role of hexameric IgM. *J Immunol* 1998;161(8):4091–4097.
172. Mostov KE, Friedlander M, Blobel G. The receptor for transepithelial transport of IgA and IgM contains multiple immunoglobulin-like domains. *Nature* 1984;308:37–43.
173. Mostov KE, Blobel G. A transmembrane precursor of secretory component. The receptor for transcellular transport of polymeric immunoglobulins. *Journal of Biological Chemistry* 1982;257(19):11816–11821.
174. Kaetzel CS. The polymeric immunoglobulin receptor: bridging innate and adaptive immune responses at mucosal surfaces. *Immunol Rev* 2005;206:83–99.
175. Perrier C, Sprenger N, Corthesy B. Glycans on secretory component participate in innate protection against mucosal pathogens. *Journal of Biological Chemistry* 2006;281(20):14280–14287.
176. Dallas SD, Rolfe RD. Binding of Clostridium difficile toxin A to human milk secretory component. *J Med Microbiol* 1998;47(10):879–888.
177. Phalipon A, Cardona A, Kraehenbuhl JP, et al. Secretory component: a new role in secretory IgA-mediated immune exclusion in vivo. Immunity 2002;17(1):107–115.
178. Shimada S, Kawaguchi-Miyashita M, Kushiro A, et al. Generation of polymeric immunoglobulin receptor-deficient mouse with marked reduction of secretory IgA. *J Immunol* 1999;163(10):5367–5373.
179. Wijburg OL, Uren TK, Simpfendorfer K, et al. Innate secretory antibodies protect against natural Salmonella typhimurium infection. *J Exp Med* 2006;203(1):21–26.
180. Sun K, Johansen FE, Eckmann L, et al. An important role for polymeric Ig receptor-mediated transport of IgA in protection against Streptococcus pneumoniae nasopharyngeal carriage. *J Immunol* 2004;173(7):4576–4581.
181. Huang YT, Wright A, Gao X, et al. Intraepithelial cell neutralization of HIV-1 replication by IgA. *J Immunol* 2005;174(8):4828–4835.
182. Mazanec MB, Kaetzel CS, Lamm ME, et al. Intracellular neutralization of virus by immunoglobulin A antibodies. *Proc Nat Acad Sci USA* 1992;89(15):6901–6905.
183. Kaetzel CS, Robinson JK, Chintalacharuvu KR, et al. The polymeric immunoglobulin receptor (secretory component) mediates transport of immune complexes across epithelial cells: a local defense function for IgA. *Proc Nat Acad Sci USA* 1991;88(19):8796–8800.
184. Banks WA, Freed EO, Wolf KM, et al. Transport of human immunodeficiency virus type 1 pseudoviruses across the blood-brain barrier: role of envelope proteins and adsorptive endocytosis. *J Virol* 2001;75(10):4681–4691.
185. Zhang JR, Mostov KE, Lamm ME, et al. The polymeric immunoglobulin receptor translocates pneumococci across human nasopharyngeal epithelial cells. *Cell* 2000;102(6):827–837.
186. Kyte J, Doolittle RF. A simple method for displaying the hydropathic character of a protein. *J Mol Biol* 1982;157:105–132.
187. Eisenberg D. Three-dimensional structure of membrane and surface proteins. *Annu Rev Biochem* 1984;53:595–623.
188. Carayannopoulos L, Capra JD. Immunoglobulins: structure and function. In: Paul WE, (ed): *Fundamental Immunology*. New York: Raven Press, 1993, pp 283–314.
189. Garman SC, Wurzburg BA, Tarchevskaya SS, et al. Structure of the Fc fragment of human IgE bound to its high-affinity receptor Fc epsilonRI alpha. *Nature* 2000;406(6793):259–266.
190. Sarma VR, Davies DR, Labaw LW, et al. Crystal structure of an immunoglobulin molecule by x-ray diffraction and electron microscopy. *Cold Spring Harbor Symposia on Quantitative Biology* 1972;36:413–419.
191. Manivel V, Sahoo NC, Salunke DM, et al. Maturation of an antibody response is governed by modulations in flexibility of the antigen-combining site. *Immunity* 2000;13(5):611–620.
192. Boehm MK, Woof JM, Kerr MA, et al. The Fab and Fc fragments of IgA1 exhibit a different arrangement from that in IgG: a study by X-ray and neutron solution scattering and homology modelling. *J Mol Biol* 1999;286(5):1421–1447.
193. Lefranc M-P, Lefranc G. *The Immunoglobulin FactsBook*. San Diego: Academic Press, 2001.
194. Kuby J. *Immunology*. 3rd ed. New York: W.H. Freeman and Company, 1997.
195. Janeway CA, Jr., Travers P, Walport M, et al. *Immunobiology*, 4th ed. New York: Garland Publishing, 1999.

Chapter 5

Antigen–antibody Interactions and Monoclonal Antibodies

Jay A. Berzofsky, Ira J. Berkower, and Suzanne L. Epstein

INTRODUCTION

The basic principles of antigen–antibody interaction are those of any bimolecular reaction. Moreover, the binding of antigen by antibody can, in general, be described by the same theories and studied by the same experimental approaches as the binding of a hormone by its receptor, of a substrate by enzyme, or of oxygen by hemoglobin. There are several major differences, however, between antigen–antibody interactions and these other situations. First, unlike most enzymes and many hormone-binding systems, antibodies do not irreversibly alter the antigen they bind. Thus, the reactions are, at least in principle, always reversible. Second, antibodies can be raised, by design of the investigator, with specificity for almost any substance known. In each case, one can find antibodies with affinities as high as and specificities as great as those of enzymes for their substrates and receptors for their hormones. The interaction of antibody with antigen can thus be taken as a prototype for interactions of macromolecules with ligands in general. In addition, these same features of reversibility and availability of a wide variety of specificities have made antibodies invaluable reagents for identifying, quantitating, and even purifying a growing number of substances of biological and medical importance.

Another feature of antibodies that in the past proved to be a difficulty in studying and using them, compared to, say, enzymes, is their enormous heterogeneity. Even "purified" antibodies from an immune antiserum, all specific for the same substance and sharing the same overall immunoglobulin structure (see Chapter 4), will be a heterogeneous mixture of molecules of different subclass, affinity, and fine specificity and ability to discriminate among cross-reacting antigens. The advent of hybridoma monoclonal antibodies (1–3) has made available a source of homogeneous antibodies to almost anything to which antisera can be raised. Nevertheless, heterogeneous antisera are still in widespread use and even have advantages for certain purposes, such as precipitation reactions. Therefore, it is critical to keep in mind throughout this chapter, and indeed much of the volume, that the principles derived for the interaction of one antibody with one antigen must be modified and extended to cover the case of heterogeneous components in the reaction.

In this chapter, we examine the theoretical principles necessary for analyzing, in a quantitative manner, the interaction of antibody with antigen and the experimental techniques that have been developed to study these interactions and to make use of antibodies as quantitative reagents. Further, we discuss the derivation, use, and properties of monoclonal antibodies.

THERMODYNAMICS AND KINETICS

The Thermodynamics of Affinity

The basic thermodynamic principles of antigen–antibody interactions, as indicated earlier, are the same as those for any reversible bimolecular binding reaction. We review these as they apply to this particular immunological reaction.

Chemical Equilibrium in Solution

For this purpose, let S = antibody binding sites, L = ligand (antigen) sites, and SL = the complex of the two. Then for the reaction

$$S + L \rightleftharpoons SL \tag{1}$$

the mass action law states

$$K_A = \frac{[SL]}{[S][L]} \tag{2}$$

where K_A = association constant (or affinity) and square brackets indicate molar concentration of the reactants enclosed. The import of this equation is that, for any given set of conditions such as temperature, pH, and salt concentration, the ratio of the concentration of the complex to the product of the concentrations of the reactants at equilibrium is always constant. Thus, changing the concentration of either antibody or ligand will invariably change the concentration of the complex, provided neither reactant is limiting—that is, neither has already been saturated—and provided sufficient time is allowed to reach a new state of equilibrium. Moreover, because the concentrations of antibody and ligand appear in this equation in a completely symmetrical fashion, doubling either the antibody concentration or the antigen concentration results in a doubling of the concentration of the antigen–antibody complex, provided the other reactant is in sufficient excess. This proviso, an echo of the one just above, is inherent in the fact that $[S]$ and $[L]$ refer to the concentrations of free S and free L, respectively, in solution, not the total concentration, which would include that of the complex. Thus, if L is not in great excess, doubling $[S]$ results in a decrease in $[L]$ as some of it is consumed in the complex, so the net result is less than a doubling of $[SL]$. Similarly, halving the volume results in a doubling of the total concentration of both antibody and ligand. If the fraction of both reactants tied up in the complex is negligibly small (as might be the case for low-affinity binding), the concentration of the complex quadruples. However, in most practical cases, the concentration of complex is a significant fraction of the total concentration of antigen or antibody or both, so the net result is an increase in the concentration of complex, but by a factor of less than 4. The other important, perhaps obvious but often forgotten, principle to be gleaned from this example is that since it is concentration, not amount, of each reactant that enters into the mass action law (Equation 2), putting the same amount of antigen and antibody in a smaller volume will increase the amount of complex formed, and diluting them in a larger volume will greatly decrease the amount of complex formed. Moreover, these changes go approximately as the square of the volume, so volumes are critical in the design of an experiment.

The effect of increasing free ligand concentration $[L]$ at constant total antibody concentration on the concentration of complex $[SL]$ is illustrated in Figure 5.1. The mass action law (Equation 2) can be rewritten

$$[SL] = K_A[S][L] = K_A([S]_t - [SL])[L] \tag{3}$$

or

$$[SL] = \frac{K_A[S]_t[L]}{(1 + K_A[L])} \tag{3'}$$

where $[S]_t$ = total antibody site concentration; that is, $[S] + [SL]$. Initially, when the complex $[SL]$ is a negligible fraction of the total antibody $[S]_t$, the concentration of

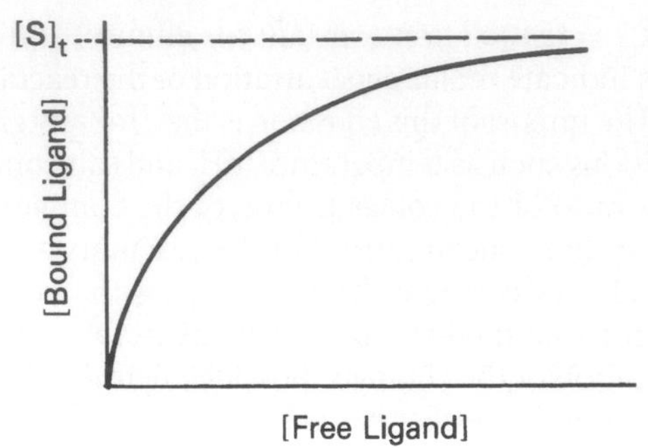

FIGURE 5.1 Schematic plot of bound ligand concentration as a function of free ligand concentration at a constant total concentration of antibody combining sites, $[S]_t$. The curve asymptotically approaches a plateau at which [bound ligand] = $[S]_t$.

complex increases nearly linearly with increasing ligand. However, as a larger fraction of antibody is consumed, the slope tapers off, and the concentration of complex, $[SL]$, asymptotically approaches a plateau value of $[S]_t$ as all the antibody becomes saturated. Thus, the concentration of antibody-binding sites can be determined from such a saturation-binding curve (Figure 5.1), taking the concentration of (radioactively or otherwise labeled) ligand bound at saturation as a measure of the concentration of antibody sites.[1] This measurement is sometimes referred to as *antigen-binding capacity*.

The total concentration of ligand at which the antibody begins to saturate is a function not only of the antibody concentration but also of the association constant, K_A, also called the *affinity*. This constant has units of M^{-1} or liters/mol, if all the concentrations in Equation 2 are molar. Thus, the product $K_A[L]$ is unitless. It is the value of this product relative to 1 that determines how saturated the antibody is, as can be seen from Equation 3′. For example, an antibody with an affinity of 10^7 M^{-1} will not be saturated if the ligand concentration is 10^{-8} M (product $K_A[L] = 0.1$), even if the total amount of ligand is in great excess over the total amount of antibody. From Equation 3′, the fraction of antibody occupied would be only 0.1/1.1, or about 9% in this example. These aspects of affinity and the methods for measuring affinity are analyzed in greater detail in the next section.

Free Energy

With regard to thermodynamics, the affinity, K_A, is also the central quantity, because it is directly related to the free energy, ΔF, of the reaction by the equations

$$\Delta F^\circ = -RT \ln K_A \quad (4)$$

$$K_A = e^{-\Delta F^\circ/RT} \quad (4')$$

[1] This point is strictly true only for univalent ligands, but most multivalent ligands behave as effectively univalent at large antigen excess, where this plateau is measured.

where R is the so-called gas constant (1.98717 cal/°K · mol), T is the absolute temperature (in degrees Kelvin), ln is the natural logarithm, and e is the base of the natural logarithms. The minus sign is introduced because of the convention that a negative change in free energy corresponds to positive binding. ΔF° is the standard free-energy change defined as the ΔF for 1 mol antigen + 1 mol antibody sites combining to form 1 mol of complex at unit concentration.

It is also instructive to note an apparent discrepancy in Equations 4 and 4′. As defined in Equation 2, K_A has dimensions of M^{-1} (i.e., liters/mol), whereas in Equation 4′ it is dimensionless. The reason is that for Equation 4′ to hold strictly, K_A must be expressed in terms of mole fractions rather than concentrations. The mole fraction of a solute is the ratio of moles of that solute to the total number of moles of all components in the solution. Because water (55 M) is by far the predominant component of most aqueous solutions, for practical purposes, one can convert K_A into a unitless ratio of mole fractions by dividing all concentrations in Equation 2 by 55 M. This transformation makes Equation 4′ strictly correct, but it introduces an additional term, $-RT \ln 55$ (corresponding to the entropy of dilution), into Equation 4. This constant term cancels out when one is subtracting ΔF values, but not when one discusses ratios of ΔF values.

An important rule of thumb can be extracted from these equations. Because ln 10 = 2.303, a 10-fold increase in affinity of binding corresponds to a free-energy change ΔF of only 1.42 kcal/mol at 37°C (310.15°K). (The corresponding values for 25°C and 4°C are 1.36 kcal/mol and 1.27 kcal/mol, respectively.) This is less than one-third the energy of a single hydrogen bond (about 4.5 kcal/mol). Looked at another way, a very high affinity of 10^{10} M^{-1} corresponds to a ΔF of only 14.2 kcal/mol, approximately the bonding energy of three hydrogen bonds. (Of course, since hydrogen bonds with water are broken during the formation of hydrogen bonds between antigen and antibody, the net energy per hydrogen bond is closer to 1 kcal/mol). It is apparent from this example that of the many interactions (hydrophobic and ionic as well as hydrogen bonding) that occur between the contact residues in an antibody-combining site and the contacting residues of an antigen (e.g., a protein), almost as many are repulsive as attractive. It is this small difference of a few kilocalories between much larger numbers corresponding to the total of attractive and the total of repulsive interactions that leads to net "high-affinity" binding. If ΔF were any larger, binding reactions would be of such high affinity as to be essentially irreversible. Viewed in this way, it is not surprising that a small modification of the antigen can result in an enormous change in affinity. A single hydrogen bond can change the affinity many-fold, and similar arguments apply to hydrophobic interactions and other forms of bonding. This concept is important when we discuss specificity and antigen structure later.

Effects of Temperature, pH, Salt Concentration, and Conformational Flexibility

It was mentioned earlier that K_A is constant for any given set of conditions such as temperature, pH, and salt concentration. However, it varies with each of these conditions. We have already seen that the conversion of free energy to affinity depends on temperature. However, the free energy itself is also a function of temperature

$$\Delta F^\circ = \Delta H^\circ - T\Delta S^\circ \quad (5)$$

where ΔH is change in enthalpy (the heat of the reaction)[2] and ΔS is the entropy (a term related to the change in disorder produced by the reaction),[2] and T is the absolute temperature (in degrees Kelvin).

It can be shown that the association constant K_A will thus vary with temperature, as follows:

$$\frac{d\ln K_A}{dT} = \frac{\Delta H^\circ}{RT^2} \quad (6)$$

or equivalently,

$$\frac{d\ln K_A}{d(1/T)} = \frac{-\Delta H^\circ}{R} \quad (6')$$

The derivation of these equations is beyond the scope of this book (see [4]). However, the practical implications are as follows: First, one can determine the standard enthalpy change ΔH° of the reaction from the slope of a plot of ln K_A versus $1/T$. Second, for an interaction that is primarily exothermic (i.e., driven by a large negative ΔH, such as the formation of hydrogen bonds and polar bonds), the affinity decreases with increasing temperature. Thus, many antigen–antibody interactions have a higher affinity at 4°C than at 25°C or 37°C, so maximum binding for a given set of concentrations can be achieved in the cold. In contrast, apolar or hydrophobic interactions are driven largely by the entropy term, $T\Delta S$, and ΔH° is near zero. In this case, there is little effect of temperature on the affinity.

As for the effects of pH and salt concentration (or ionic strength) on the affinity, these vary depending on the nature of the interacting groups. Most antigen–antibody reactions are studied near neutral pH and at physiologic salt concentrations (0.15 M NaCl). If the interaction is dominated by ionic interactions, high salt concentration lowers the affinity.

Conformational flexibility of an antigen can also affect the affinity by affecting the entropy term in Equation 5. An outstanding example comes from the thermodynamics of binding of a series of broadly neutralizing monoclonal antibodies to the HIV envelope protein gp120. The energetics of binding between HIV gp120 and its cellular receptor CD4 (5) or to a panel of monoclonal antibodies (6) has been studied in detail. The results provide insight into the ways protein flexibility can help the virus to evade antibody immunity. They may also explain part of the difficulty in eliciting antibodies of this type when immunizing with the native protein.

[2] For a more complete description of these concepts, see a physical chemistry text, such as Moore (4).

TABLE 5.1 Energetics of Antibody Binding to gp120 Core Structure (Based on [6])

Ligand	ΔF	ΔH	$-T\Delta S$
CD4	−10.4	−48.4	38.2
F105	−11.4	−30.0	18.6
b12	−12.3	−18.0	5.7
2G12	−7.8	−6.2	−1.6

Gp120 is a glycoprotein that exhibits at least two conformational states: One exists on the virus, and it changes to the other when it binds the CD4 receptor on the cell surface. Monoclonal antibodies F105 and b12 bind residues within the CD4 binding site on gp120, while monoclonal 2G12 binds the opposite surface. The CD4 binding site defines a neutralizing surface that is conserved among a broad range of HIV isolates.

As shown in Table 5.1, CD4 and each antibody demonstrated a strongly negative ΔF, corresponding to high-affinity binding. However, as shown by microcalorimetry, they arrived at the affinity in different ways. CD4 and F105 have a strong negative ΔH of binding, but they also have a large, negative entropy due to the conformational change required, as shown by strongly positive values for $-T\Delta S$. This entropy effect greatly reduces the overall ΔF of binding, so they depend on a very large negative ΔH to bind. In contrast, monoclonal b12 has moderate levels of both ΔH and $-T\Delta S$, resulting in a nearly identical ΔF. Monoclonal 2G12 binds gp120 with a less favorable ΔH but no entropy cost.

The two discrete conformations of gp120 may be called the open and closed forms. The excursion between these two conformations affects the entropy of binding. CD4 and F105 only bind the open form, which reduces randomness and creates an entropy barrier. Monoclonal b12 is less dependent on one conformation, so it binds with less entropy cost, and 2G12 is indifferent to the two forms, so it has no entropy effect at all.

The strong entropy effect observed for these monoclonals may illustrate one way for the virus to evade antibody binding through a mechanism called *conformational masking*. The randomness of gp120, as found on the virus, means that it is rarely in the open conformation, making it difficult for most antibodies like F105 to bind. Only the rare antibody that is b12-like can bind multiple forms and eventually pull gp120 into its most favorable conformation.

The same effect may explain the difficulty in eliciting antibodies to this site using native gp120. If it is rarely in the open form, it will be unable to trigger B cells to make antibodies that require this form, and it will deliver only a weak antigenic stimulus to those that bind partially to different conformations, such as b12. These considerations suggest that a more favorable vaccine antigen could be made if gp120 could be anchored in the open conformation, so it could stimulate B cells to make antibodies that require this form. The hallmark of this structure would be its ability to bind F105 and b12 with a good ΔH and reduced values of $-T\Delta S$.

Kinetics of Antigen–antibody Reactions

A fundamental connection between the thermodynamics and kinetics of antigen–antibody binding is expressed by the relationship

$$K_A = \frac{k_1}{k_{-1}} \quad (7)$$

where k_1 and k_{-1} are the rate constants for the forward (association) and backward (dissociation) reactions.

The forward reaction is determined largely by diffusion rates (theoretical upper limit 109 liters/mol·sec) and the probability that a collision will result in binding—that is, largely the probability that both the antigen and the antibody will be oriented in the right way to produce a good fit, as well as the activation energy for binding. The diffusive rate constant can be shown (7) to be approximated by the Smoluchowski equation

$$k_{\mathrm{dl}} = 4\pi a D(6 \times 10^{20}) \quad (7a)$$

where a is the sum of the radii in centimeters of the two reactants, D is the sum of the diffusion constants in $\mathrm{cm^2/sec}$ for the individual reactants, and the constant 6×10^{20} is necessary to convert the units to $\mathrm{M^{-1} \cdot sec^{-1}}$. For example, if $a = 10^{-6}$ cm and $D = 10^{-7}\ \mathrm{cm^2/sec}$, then $k_{\mathrm{dl}} \approx 7.5 \times 10^8\ \mathrm{M^{-1} \cdot sec^{-1}}$. Association rates will generally be slower for large protein antigens than for small haptens. This observation may be due to the smaller value of D, the orientational effects in the collision, and other nondiffusional aspects of protein–protein interactions. Therefore, association rates for protein antigens are more frequently on the order of 10^5 to $10^6\ \mathrm{M^{-1} \cdot sec^{-1}}$ (see below). However, this observation can also be partly understood from diffusion-limited rates alone. If the radii of hypothetically spherical reactants are r_1 and r_2, then in Equation 7a, $a = r_1 + r_2$, whereas D is proportional to $1/r_1 + 1/r_2$. The diffusive rate constant is, therefore, proportional to

$$(r_1 + r_2)\left(\frac{1}{r_1} + \frac{1}{r_2}\right) = \frac{(r_1 + r_2)^2}{r_1 r_2} \quad (7b)$$

From this result, it can be seen that if $r_1 = r_2 = r$, then r cancels out and the whole term in Equation 7b is simply equal to 4. Thus, for the interaction between two molecules of equal size, the diffusive rate constant is the same regardless of whether those molecules are large or small (8). However, if one molecule is large and the other small, the rate is greater than if both molecules are large. This difference occurs because reducing the radius r_1 while keeping r_2 constant (and larger than r_1) has a greater effect on increasing the diffusion constant term D, proportional to $(1/r_1 + 1/r_2)$, in which the smaller radius produces the larger term, than it has on the term a, which is still dominated by the larger radius r_2. For example, if $r_2 = r$ as above, but $r_1 = 0.1r$, then the numerator in Equation 7b is only reduced from $4r^2$ to $1.21r^2$, whereas the denominator is reduced from $1r^2$ to $0.1r^2$. Thus, the ratio is increased from 4 to 12.1. Viewed another way, the greater diffusive mobility of the small hapten outweighs its diminished target area relative to a large protein antigen, since the larger target area of the antibody is available to both.

The dissociation rate (or "off rate") k_{-1} is determined by the strength of the bonds (as it affects the activation energy barriers for dissociation) and the thermal energy kT (where k is Boltzmann's constant), which provides the energy to surmount this barrier. The activation energy for dissociation is the difference in energy between the starting state and the transition state of highest energy to which the system must be raised before dissociation can occur.

As pointed out by Eisen (9), if one compares a series of related antigens, of similar size and other physical properties, for binding to an antibody, the association rates are all very similar. The differences in affinity largely correspond to the differences in dissociation rates.

A good example is that of antibodies to the protein antigen staphylococcal nuclease (10). Antibodies to native nuclease were fractionated on affinity columns of peptide fragments to isolate a fraction specific for residues 99 to 126. The antibodies had an affinity of $8.3 \times 10^8\ \mathrm{M^{-1}}$ for the native antigen and an association rate constant, k_{on}, of $4.1 \times 10^5\ \mathrm{M^{-1} \cdot sec^{-1}}$. This k_{on} was several orders of magnitude lower than had been observed for small haptens (11), as discussed earlier. A value of k_{off} of $4.9 \times 10^{-4}\ \mathrm{sec^{-1}}$ was calculated using these results in Equation 7. This is a first-order rate constant from which one can calculate a half-time for dissociation (based on $t_{1/2} = \ln 2/k_{\mathrm{off}}$) of 23 minutes. These rates are probably typical for high-affinity ($K_A \approx 10^9\ \mathrm{M^{-1}}$) antibodies to small protein antigens such as nuclease ($MW \approx 17{,}000$). The dissociation rate is important to know in designing experiments to measure binding, because if the act of measurement perturbs the equilibrium, the time one has to make the measurement (e.g., to separate bound and free) is determined by this half-time for dissociation. For instance, a 2-minute procedure that involves dilution of the antigen–antibody mixture can be completed before significant dissociation has occurred if the dissociation half-time is 23 minutes. However, if the on rate is the same, but the affinity 10-fold lower, still a respectable $8 \times 10^7\ \mathrm{M^{-1}}$, then the complex could be 50% dissociated in the time required to complete the procedure. This caution is very relevant in the following discussion of methods of measuring binding and affinity below.

Because knowledge of the dissociation rate can be so important in the design of experiments, a word should be said about techniques to measure it. Perhaps the most widely applicable one is the use of radiolabeled antigen. After equilibrium is reached and the equilibrium concentration of bound radioactivity determined, a large excess of unlabeled antigen is added. Because any radioactive antigen molecule that dissociates is quickly replaced by an unlabeled one, the probability of a radioactive molecule associating again is very small. Therefore, one can measure the decrease in radioactivity bound to antibody with time to determine the dissociation rate.[3]

AFFINITY

It is apparent from our earlier discussion that a lot of information about an antigen–antibody reaction is packed into a single value: its affinity. In this section, we examine affinity more closely, including methods for measuring affinity and the heterogeneity thereof, the effects of multivalency of antibody and of antigen, and the special effects seen when the antigen–antibody interaction occurs on a solid surface (two-phase systems).

Interaction in Solution with Monovalent Ligand

The simplest case is that of the interaction of antibody with monovalent ligand. We may include in this category both antihapten antibodies reacting with truly monovalent haptens and antimacromolecule antibodies, which have been fractionated to obtain a population that reacts only with a single, nonrepeating site on the antigen.[4] In the latter case, the antigen behaves as if monovalent in its interaction with the particular antibody population under study. The proviso that the site recognized (antigenic determinant) be nonrepeating—that is, occur only once per antigen molecule—of course, is critical.

If the combining sites on the antibody are independent (i.e., display no positive or negative cooperativity for antigen binding), then for many purposes one can treat these combining sites, reacting with monovalent ligands, as if they were separate molecules. Thus many, but not all, of

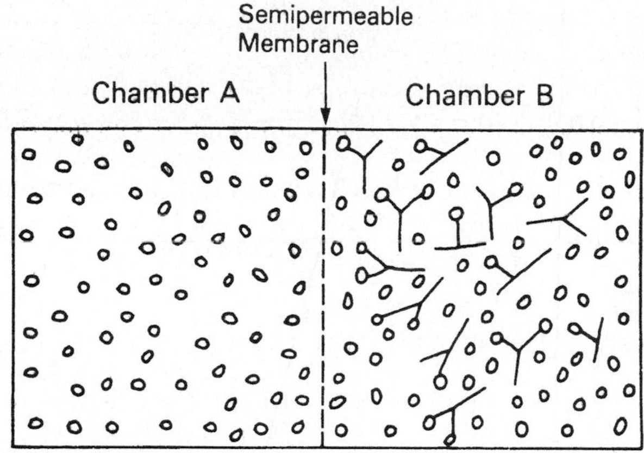

FIGURE 5.2 Equilibrium dialysis. Two chambers are separated by a semipermeable membrane that is freely permeable to ligand but not at all to antibody. Antibody is placed in one chamber (B), and ligand in one or both chambers. Regardless of how the ligand is distributed initially, after sufficient time to reach equilibrium, it will be distributed as follows: The concentration of free ligand will be identical in both chambers, but chamber B will have additional ligand bound to antibody. The concentration of bound ligand is thus the difference between the ligand concentration in the two chambers, whereas the free concentration is the concentration in chamber A. Since these concentrations must obey the mass action law, Equation 2, they can be used to determine the affinity K_A, from Equations 3 or 3′, by any of several graphical procedures, such as Scatchard analysis (described in the text).

the properties we discuss can be analyzed in terms of the concentration of antibody-combining sites, independent of the number of such sites per antibody molecule (2 for IgG and IgA, 10 for IgM).

To determine the affinity of an antibody, one generally determines the equilibrium concentrations of bound and free ligand at increasing total ligand concentrations but at constant antibody concentration. Alternatively, one can vary the antibody concentration, but then the analysis is slightly more complicated. Perhaps the theoretically most elegant experimental method to determine these quantities is equilibrium dialysis (12,13), depicted and explained in Figure 5.2, in which ligand (antigen) is allowed to equilibrate between two chambers, only one of which contains antibody, separated by a semipermeable membrane impermeable to antibody. The important feature of this method, as opposed to most others, is that the concentrations of ligand in each chamber can be determined without perturbing the equilibrium. The disadvantage of this method is that it is applicable only to antigens small enough to permeate freely a membrane that will exclude antibody. Another technical disadvantage is that bound antigen, determined as the difference between bound plus free antigen in one chamber and free antigen in the other, is not measured independently of free antigen.

Another category of method uses radiolabeled ligand in equilibrium with antibody and then physically separates

[3] This method assumes that all binding sites are independent, as is generally true for antibodies and monovalent ligands. If there were either negative or positive cooperativity in binding, then the change in receptor occupancy that occurs when a large excess of unlabeled antigen is added would probably perturb the dissociation rate of radiolabeled antigen molecules already bound to other sites.

[4] Such fractionated antibodies may contain mixtures of antibodies to overlapping sites within a domain on the antigen, but as long as no two antibody molecules (or combining sites) can bind to the same antigen molecule simultaneously, the antigen still behaves as effectively monovalent.

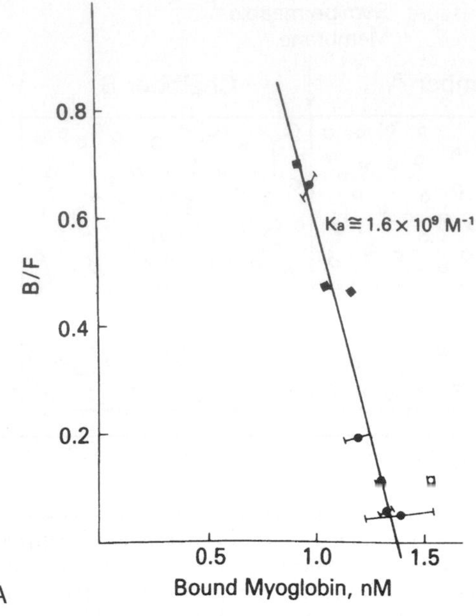

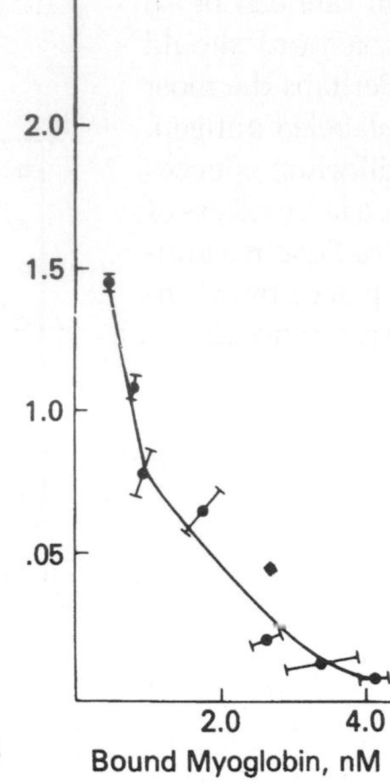

FIGURE 5.3 Scatchard analysis of the binding of [^{3}H]-sperm whale myoglobin by a monoclonal antibody to myoglobin (A) and by the serum antibodies from the same mouse whose spleen cells were fused to prepare the hybridoma (B). The monoclonal antibody (clone HAL 43-201E11, clone 5) produces a linear Scatchard plot, whose slope, -1.6×10^{9} M^{-1}, equals $-K_A$, and whose intercept on the abscissa gives the concentration of antibody-binding sites. In contrast, the serum antibodies produce a curved (concave up) Scatchard plot, indicative of heterogeneity of affinity. From (15), with permission.

free antigen from antigen bound to antibody and quantitates each separately. The methods used to separate bound and free antigen are discussed below in the section on radioimmunoassay. These methods generally allow independent measurement of bound and free antigen but may perturb the equilibrium.

Scatchard Analysis

Once data are obtained, there are a number of methods of computing the affinity; we shall discuss two. Perhaps the most widely used is that described by Scatchard (14) (Figure 5.3 [15]). The mass action equilibrium law is plotted in the form of Equation 3

$$[SL] = K_A([S]_t - [SL])[L] \tag{3}$$

and B is substituted for $[SL]$ and F for $[L]$, referring to bound and free ligand, respectively. Then the Scatchard equation is

$$\frac{B}{F} = K_A([S]_t - B) \tag{8}$$

Note that a very critical implicit assumption was made in this seemingly simple conversion. The $[SL]$ within the parentheses in Equation 3 was intended to be the concentration of bound antibody sites, so that $([S]_t - [SL]) =$ free $[S]$. However, in Equation 8, we have substituted B, the concentration of bound ligand. If the ligand behaves as monovalent, then this substitution is legitimate, since every bound ligand molecule corresponds to an occupied antibody site. However, if the ligand is multivalent and can bind more than one antibody site, then Equation 8 is valid only in ligand excess where the frequency of ligands with more than one antibody bound is very low. In this section we are discussing only monovalent ligands, but this proviso must be kept in mind when the Scatchard analysis is applied in other circumstances.

From Equation 8, we see that a plot of B/F versus B should yield a straight line (for a single affinity), with a slope of $-K_A$ and an intercept on the abscissa corresponding to antibody-binding site concentration (Figure 5.3). This is the so-called Scatchard plot. An alternative version that is normalized for antibody concentration is especially useful if the data were obtained at different values of total antibody concentration, $[A]_t$, instead of constant $[A]_t$. However, for this version one requires an independent measure of total antibody concentration, other than the intercept of the plot. Then one divides Equation 8 by the total concentration of antibody molecules (making no assumptions about the number of sites per molecule) to obtain

$$\frac{r}{c} = K_A(n - r) \tag{9}$$

where r is defined as the number of occupied sites per antibody molecule, n is defined as the total number of sites per antibody molecule, and c is free ligand concentration; that is, $c = F$. Thus,

$$r = \frac{B}{[\text{total antibody}]} = \frac{B}{[A]_t}$$

$$n = \frac{[\text{total sites}]}{[\text{total antibody}]} = \frac{[S]_t}{[A]_t}$$

where $[A]_t =$ total molar antibody concentration. In this form of the Scatchard plot, r/c versus r, the slope is still $-K_A$, and the intercept on the r axis is n. Thus, one can determine the number of sites per molecule. Of course, if one determines $[S]_t$ from the intercept of Equation 8, one can also calculate the number of sites per molecule by dividing $[S]_t$ by any independent measure of antibody concentration. Thus, the only advantage of normalizing all the data points first to plot the r/c form arises when the data were obtained at varying antibody concentrations. If the antibody concentration is unknown but held constant, then the B/F form is more convenient and actually provides one measure of antibody (site) concentration. Since today we know the value of n for each class of antibody (2 for IgG and serum IgA, 10 for IgM), the concentration of sites and that of antibody are easily converted in many cases.

Heterogeneity of Affinity

The next level of complexity arises when one is dealing with a mixture of antibodies of varying affinity for the ligand. This is the rule, rather than the exception, when one deals with antibodies from immune serum, even if they are fractionated to be monospecific—that is, all specific for the same site on the antigen. Contrast, for example, the linear Scatchard plot for a homogeneous monoclonal antibody to myoglobin (Figure 5.3A) with the curved Scatchard plot for the serum antibodies from the same mouse used to prepare the hybridoma monoclonal antibody (Figure 5.3B). This concave up Scatchard plot is typical for heterogeneous antibodies. In a system such as hormone receptor–hormone interaction in which negative cooperativity can occur between receptor sites (i.e., occupation of one site lowers the affinity of its neighbor), a concave up Scatchard plot can be produced by negative cooperativity in the absence of any intrinsic heterogeneity in affinity. However, in the case of antibodies, where no such allosteric effect has been demonstrated, a concave up Scatchard plot indicates heterogeneity of affinity.

Ideally, one would like to imagine that the tangents all along the curve correspond (in slope) to the affinities of the many subpopulations of antibodies. Mathematically, this is not strictly correct, but it is true that the steeper part of the curve corresponds to the higher-affinity antibodies and the shallower part of the curve to the lower-affinity antibodies. Graphical methods have been developed to analyze more quantitatively the components of such curves (16,17), and a very general and versatile computer program, LIGAND, has been developed by Munson and Rodbard (18) that can fit such curves using any number of subpopulations of different affinity. For purposes of this chapter, we discuss only the case of two affinities and then examine the types of average affinities that have been proposed when one is dealing with much greater heterogeneity. We also examine mathematical estimates of the degree of heterogeneity (analogous to a variance).

When an antibody population consists of only two subpopulations of different affinities, K_1 and K_2, then we can add the component Equations 3′ to obtain

$$r = r_1 + r_2 = \frac{n_1K_1c}{(1+K_1c)} + \frac{n_2K_2c}{(1+K_2c)} \tag{10}$$

so that

$$\frac{r}{c} = \frac{n_1K_1}{(1+K_1c)} + \frac{n_2K_2}{(1+K_2c)} \tag{10'}$$

where the subscripts correspond to the two populations. Then the graph of r/c versus r can be shown to be a hyperbola whose asymptotes are, in fact, the linear Scatchard plots of the two components (Figure 5.4). This situation has been analyzed graphically by Bright (19). Taking the limits as $c \to 0$ and as $c \to \infty$, it can easily be shown that the intercept on the abscissa is just $n_1 + n_2$ (or, in the form B/F versus B, the intercept is the total concentration of binding sites $[S]_t$), and the intercept on the ordinate is $n_1K_1 + n_2K_2$. Thus, one can still obtain the total value of

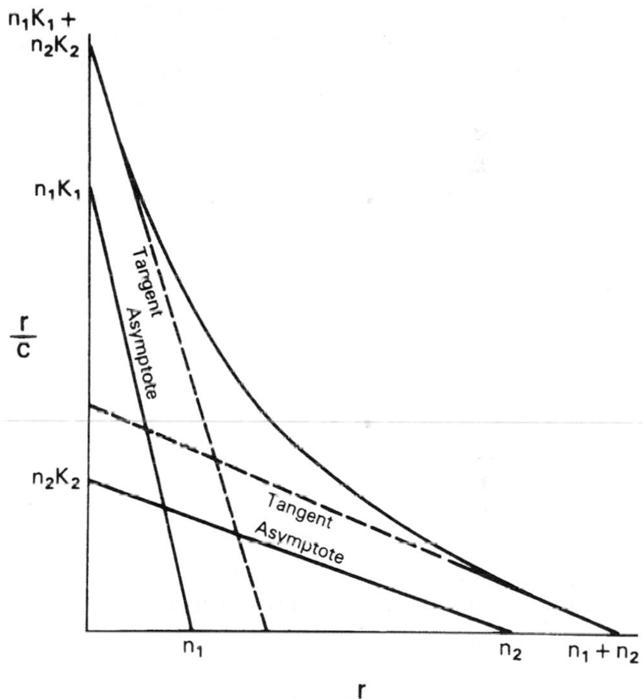

FIGURE 5.4 Analysis of a curved Scatchard plot produced by a mixture of two antibodies with different affinities. The antibodies have affinities K_1 and K_2 and have n_1 and n_2 binding sites per molecule, respectively. r is the concentration of bound antigen divided by the total antibody concentration (i.e., bound sites per molecule), and c is the free antigen concentration. The curve is a hyperbola that can be decomposed into its two asymptotes, which correspond to the linear Scatchard plots of the two components in the antibody mixture. The tangents to the curve at its intercepts only approximate these asymptotes, so that the slopes of the tangents estimate but do not accurately correspond to the affinities of the two antibodies. However, the intercept on the r axis corresponds to $n_1 + n_2$. Note that in this case n_1 and n_2 must be defined in terms of the total antibody concentration, not that of each component.

n or $[S]_t$ from the intercept on the abscissa. The problem is in obtaining the two affinities, K_1 and K_2, and the concentrations of the individual antibody subpopulations (corresponding to n_1 and n_2). If K_1 is greater than K_2, one can approximate the affinities from the slopes of the tangents at the two intercepts (Figure 5.4), but these will not, in general, be exactly parallel to the two asymptotes, which give the true affinities, so some error is always introduced, depending on the relative values of n_1 and n_2 and K_1 and K_2. A graphical method for solving for these exactly has been worked out by Bright (19) and computer methods by Munson and Rodbard (18).

Average Affinities

In practice, of course, one rarely knows that one is dealing with exactly two subpopulations, and most antisera are significantly more heterogeneous than that. Therefore, the previous case is more illustrative of principles than of practical value. When faced with a curved Scatchard plot, one usually asks what the average affinity is, and perhaps some measure of the variance of the affinities, without being able to define exactly how many different affinity populations exist.

Suppose one has m populations each with site concentration $[S_i]$ and affinity K_i, so that at free ligand concentration $[L]$, the fraction of each antibody that has ligand bound will be given by an equation of the form of Equation 3′:

$$B_i = \frac{K_i[S_i]_t[L]}{(1 + K_i[L])} \tag{11}$$

Then the bound concentrations sum to give

$$B = \sum_{i=1}^{m} B_i = \sum_{i=1}^{m} \frac{K_i[S_i]_t[L]}{(1 + K_i[L])} \tag{11′}$$

Substituting F for $[L]$ and dividing through by this quantity, one obtains

$$\frac{B}{F} = \sum_{i=1}^{m} \frac{K_i[S_i]_t}{(1 + K_i F)} \tag{12}$$

or equivalently

$$\frac{r}{c} = \sum_{i=1}^{m} \frac{K_i n_i}{(1 + K_i c)} \tag{12′}$$

These can be seen to be generalizations of Equations 10 and 10′. Taking the limits as $F \to 0$ and $F \to \infty$, one again sees that the

$$\text{intercept on ordinate} = \sum_{i=1}^{m} K_i[S_i]_t \tag{13}$$

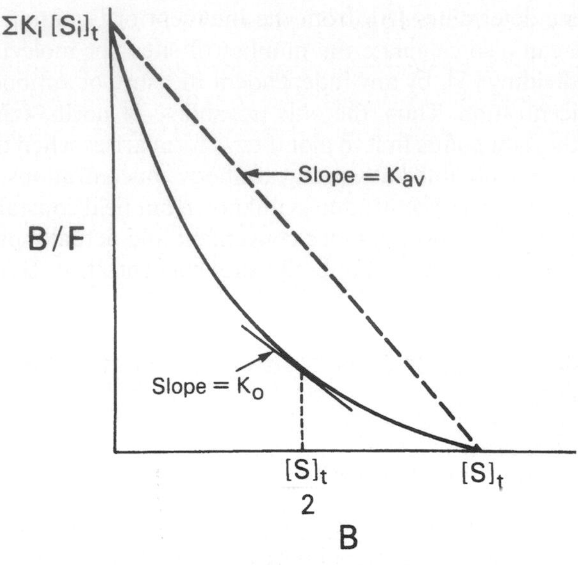

FIGURE 5.5 Types of average affinities for a heterogeneous population of antibodies, as defined on a Scatchard plot. K_0 is the slope of the tangent to the curve at a point where $B = [S]_t/2$, that is, where half the antibody sites are bound. Thus, K_0 corresponds to a median affinity. K_{av} is the slope of the chord between the intercepts and corresponds to a weighted average of the affinities, weighted by the concentrations of the antibodies with each affinity. Adapted from (20).

and the

$$\text{intercept on abscissa} = \sum_{i=1}^{m} [S_i]_t = [S]_t \tag{14}$$

Therefore, one can still obtain the total antibody site concentration from the intercept on the abscissa (Figure 5.5) (20).

Two types of average affinity can be obtained graphically from the Scatchard plot (20). Perhaps the more widely used K_0 is actually more accurately a median affinity rather than a mean affinity. It is defined as the slope of the tangent at the point on the curve where half the sites are bound—that is, where $B = [S]_t/2$ (Figure 5.5). A second type of average affinity, which we call K_{av}, is a weighted mean of the affinities, each affinity weighted by its proportional representation in the antibody population. Thus, we take the ratio

$$K_{av} = \sum_{i=1}^{m} \frac{K_i[S_i]_t}{[S]_t} \tag{15}$$

From Equations 13 and 14, it is apparent that K_{av} is simply the ratio of the two intercepts on the B/F and B axes—that is, the slope of the chord (Figure 5.5). This type of weighted mean affinity, K_{av}, is, therefore, actually easier to obtain graphically in some cases than K_0, and we shall see that it is useful in other types of plots as well.

Indices of Heterogeneity: The Sips Plot

For a heterogeneous antiserum, one would also like to have some idea of the extent of heterogeneity of affinity. For instance, if the affinities were distributed according to a normal (Gaussian) distribution, one would like to know the variance (21,22). More complex analyses have been developed that do not require as many assumptions about the shape of the distribution (23–25), but the first and most widely used index of heterogeneity arbitrarily assumes that the affinities fit a distribution, first described by Sips (26), that is similar in shape to a normal distribution. This was applied to the case of antibody heterogeneity by Nisonoff and Pressman (27) and is summarized by Karush and Karush (28). One fits the data to the assumed binding function

$$r = \frac{n(K_0c)^a}{(1 + (K_0c)^a)} \tag{16}$$

which is analogous to Equations 3′ and 11 (the Langmuir adsorption isotherm) except for the exponent a, which is the index of heterogeneity. This index, a, is allowed to range from 0 to 1. For $a = 1$, Equation 16 is equivalent to Equation 3, and there is no heterogeneity. As a decreases toward 0, the heterogeneity increases. To obtain a value for a graphically, one plots the algebraic rearrangement of Equation (16):

$$\log\left(\frac{r}{n - r}\right) = a \log c + a \log K_0 \tag{17}$$

so that the slope of $\log[r/(n - r)]$ versus $\log c$ is the heterogeneity index a.

C. DeLisi (personal communication) has derived the variance (second moment) of the Sips distribution in terms of the free energy $RT \ln K_0$, about the mean of free energy. The result (normalized to RT) gives the dispersion or width of the distribution as a function of a:

$$\frac{\sigma^2_{\text{Sips}}}{R^2T^2} = \frac{\pi^2(1 - a^2)}{3a^2} \tag{18}$$

This is useful for determining a quantity, σ_{Sips}, which can be thought of as analogous to a standard deviation, if one keeps in mind that this is not a true Gaussian distribution. In addition, as noted earlier, the use of the Sips distribution requires the assumption that the affinities (really the free energies) are continuously distributed symmetrically about a mean, approximating a Gaussian distribution. This assumption frequently is not valid.

The Plot of B/F versus F or T

Another graphical method that is useful for estimating affinities is the plot of bound/free versus free or total ligand concentration, denoted F and T, respectively (20) (Figure 5.6). To simplify the discussion, let us define the bound/free ratio, B/F, as R, and define R_0 as the intercept, or limit,

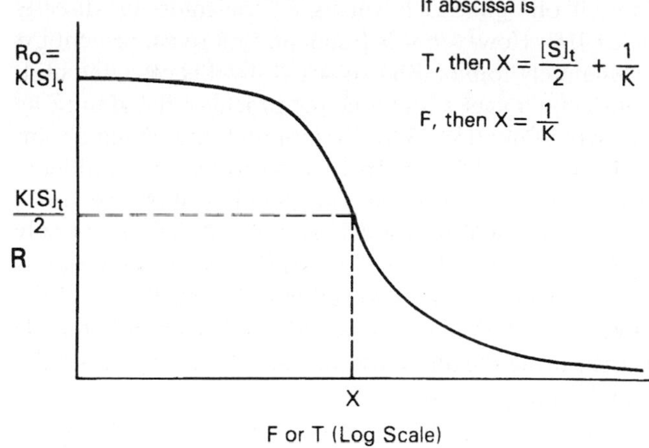

FIGURE 5.6 Schematic plot of R, the bound/free ratio, as a function of free (F) or total (T) antigen concentration. The curves have a similar sigmoidal shape, but the midpoint (where $R = R_0/2$) of the plot of R versus T has a term dependent on antibody site concentration ($[S]_t$), whereas the midpoint of the plot of R versus F is exactly $1/K$, independent of antibody concentration. Adapted from (20).

as free ligand $F \to 0$. First, for the case of a homogeneous antibody, from Equation 3′,

$$R = \frac{B}{F} = \frac{K[S]_t}{(1 + KF)} \tag{19}$$

and

$$R_0 = \lim_{F \to 0} \frac{B}{F} = K[S]_t \tag{20}$$

Let us define the midpoint of the plot (Figure 5.6) as the point at which R decreases to half its initial value, R_0—that is, at which $R = K[S]_t/2$. For the case of homogeneous antibody (i.e., a single affinity), simple algebraic manipulation (20), substituting $K[S]_t/2$ (i.e., $R_0/2$) for B/F in Equation 8, will show that at this midpoint[5]

$$F = \frac{1}{K} \tag{21}$$

and

$$B = \frac{[S]_t}{2} \tag{22}$$

so that the total concentration, T, is

$$T = B + F = \frac{[S]_t}{2} + \frac{1}{K} \tag{23}$$

[5] It is important to note that R_0 must be the limit of B/F as F truly approaches zero. In an RIA in which the concentration of tracer is significant compared to $1/K$, reducing the unlabeled ligand concentration all the way to zero will still not yield the true limit R_0. The tracer concentration must also be negligible. If not, R_0 will be estimated falsely low, and the affinity will also be underestimated.

Thus, if one plots B/F versus F, the midpoint directly yields $1/K$. However, it is frequently more convenient experimentally to plot B/F versus T. In this case, the midpoint is no longer simply the reciprocal of the affinity. As seen from Equation 23, the assumption that the midpoint is $1/K$ will result in an error equal to half the antibody-binding site concentration. Thus, in plots of B/F versus T, the midpoint will be a good estimate of the affinity only if $[S]_t/2 \ll 1/K$—that is, if the antibody concentration is low compared to the dissociation constant. In fact, if the affinity is so high that $1/K \ll [S]_t/2$, then one will merely be measuring the antibody concentration, not the affinity at all (20) (Figure 5.6).

In the case of a heterogeneous antiserum, we have already seen that

$$R_0 = \sum_i K_i[S_i]_t \qquad (13)$$

Therefore, at the midpoint, when $B/F = R_0/2$, it is easy to see that

$$K_{av} = \left(\frac{B}{F}\right)\left(\frac{2}{[S]_t}\right) = \frac{R_0}{[S]_t} \qquad (24)$$

Thus, one can still obtain the average affinity, as defined above (20).

Regardless of average affinities, the effect of affinity heterogeneity is to broaden the curve, or to make the slope shallower. This can be seen by visualizing the curve of B/F versus F as a step function. Each antibody subpopulation of a given affinity, K_i, will be titrated to 50% of its microscopic B/F at a free ligand concentration $F = 1/K_i$. The high-affinity antibodies will be titrated at low F, but the low-affinity antibodies will require much higher F to be titrated. The resulting step function is analogous to the successive transitions corresponding to different pK values in a pH titration.

Intrinsic Affinity

The affinity, K_A, that we have been discussing so far is what has been termed the *intrinsic affinity*—that is, the affinity of each antibody-combining site treated in isolation. We have been able to do this, regardless of the valence of the antibodies, by using the concentration of combining sites, $[S]$, in our equations rather than the concentration of antibody molecules, $[A]$, which may have more than one site. Even without any cooperativity between combining sites, there is a statistical effect that makes the actual affinity different from the intrinsic affinity if the antibody is multivalent and one uses whole antibody concentration rather than site concentration. The way this difference arises can best be seen by examining the case of a bivalent antibody, such as IgG. We assume that the two sites are equivalent and neither is affected by events at the other. The ligand, as in this whole section, is monovalent. Then there are two binding steps

$$A + L \overset{K_1}{\rightleftharpoons} AL, \qquad AL + L \overset{K_2}{\rightleftharpoons} AL_2 \qquad (25)$$

and the corresponding actual affinities are

$$K_1 = \frac{[AL]}{[A][L]}, \qquad K_2 = \frac{[AL_2]}{[AL][L]} \qquad (26)$$

If the intrinsic affinity of both equivalent sites is K, then K_1 will actually be twice K, because the concentration of available sites $[S]$ will be twice the antibody concentration when the first ligand is about to bind, in step 1. However, once one site is bound, the reverse (dissociation) reaction of step 1 can occur from only one site—namely, that which is occupied. Conversely, for the second step, the forward reaction has only one remaining available site; however, in the reverse reaction, $AL_2 \rightarrow AL + L$, either site can dissociate to go back to the AL state. The second site bound need not be the first to dissociate, and since the sites are identical, one cannot tell the difference. Thus, for step 2, the apparent concentration of sites for the reverse reaction is twice that available for the forward reaction, so the affinity K_2 for the second step will be only half the intrinsic affinity, K.

It is easy to see how this statistical effect can be extrapolated to an antibody with n sites (29):

$$K_1 = nK \qquad \text{and} \qquad K_n = \left(\frac{1}{n}\right)K \qquad (27)$$

For the steps in between, two derivations are available (9,29), which yield

$$K_i = \frac{(n - i + 1)}{i}K \qquad (28)$$

The actual affinity, rather than the intrinsic affinity, becomes important with monovalent ligands when one is interested in the effective affinity (based on a molar antibody concentration) under conditions where $[L]$ is so low that only one site can bind antigen. Then for IgG or IgM (with 2 or 10 sites per molecule, respectively), the apparent affinity will be theoretically 2 or 10 times the intrinsic affinity. For most purposes, it is easier to use site concentrations and intrinsic affinities. The analyses given earlier, such as B/F versus F or the Scatchard plot, whether B/F versus B or r/c versus r, will all yield intrinsic affinities. It is the intrinsic affinity that tells us something about the nature of the antibody–ligand interaction.

Once one enters the realm of multivalent ligands, the actual affinity or effective affinity involving multipoint binding between multivalent antibody molecule and multivalent ligand molecule can be much greater than the intrinsic affinity for binding at each site. This case is the subject of the next section.

Interaction with Multivalent Ligands

So far, we have discussed only situations in which the ligand is monovalent, or effectively monovalent with respect to the particular antibody under study. However, in many situations the ligand molecule has multiple repeating identical determinants, each of which can bind independently to the several identical combining sites on a divalent or multivalent antibody.[6] Although the intrinsic affinity for the interaction of any single antibody-combining site with any single antigenic determinant may be the same as that discussed in the preceding section, the apparent or effective affinity may be much higher, due to the ability of a single antibody molecule to bind more than one identical determinant of a multivalent antigen molecule. Karush (30) has termed this phenomenon "monogamous bivalency." Such monogamous binding can occur between two molecules in solution, or between a molecule in solution and one on a solid surface, such as a cell membrane or microtiter plate. We first discuss the situation in solution and then discuss the additional considerations that apply when one of the reactants is bound to a solid surface.

Monogamous Bivalency

Suppose a divalent antibody molecule reacts with antigen that has two identical determinants. This situation has been treated in detail by Crothers and Metzger (31) and by Karush (30). Let us call the two antibody sites S and S', and the antigenic determinants D and D', with the understanding that, in actuality, we cannot distinguish S from S' or D from D'. The interaction can be broken up into two steps, a bimolecular reaction

$$\begin{matrix} S \\ | \\ S' \end{matrix} + \begin{matrix} D \\ | \\ D' \end{matrix} \underset{}{\overset{K_1}{\rightleftharpoons}} \begin{matrix} S - D \\ | \quad\;\; | \\ S' \quad\; D' \end{matrix} \tag{29}$$

followed by an intramolecular reaction

$$\begin{matrix} S - D \\ | \quad\;\; | \\ S' \quad\; D' \end{matrix} \overset{K_2}{\rightleftharpoons} \begin{matrix} S - D \\ | \quad\;\; | \\ S' - D' \end{matrix} \tag{30}$$

The association constant for the first step, K_1, is related to the intrinsic affinity, K, simply by a statistical factor of 4 due to the degeneracy (equivalence) between S and S' and between D and D'. This is a typical second-order reaction between antigen and antibody. However, the second step (Equation 30) is a first-order reaction, since it is effectively an interconversion between two states of a single molecular complex, the reactants S' and D' being linked chemically (albeit noncovalently) through the S—D bond formed in the first step. Thus, the first-order equilibrium constant, K_2, is not a function of the concentrations of S—S and D—D in solution, as K_1 would be. Rather, the forward reaction depends on the geometry of the complex and the flexibility of the arms; in other words, the probability that S' and D' will encounter each other and be in the right orientation to react if they do come in contact depends on the distances and freedom of motion along the chain S'—S—D—D' rather than on the density of molecules in solution (i.e., concentration).

The reverse reaction for step 2, on the other hand, will have a rate constant similar to that for the simple monovalent $S\text{—}D \rightarrow S + D$ reaction, since the dissociation reaction depends on the strength of the S'—D' (or S—D) bond and is not influenced by the other S—D interaction unless there is strain introduced by the angles required for simultaneous bonds between S and D and S' and D'. Note that K_2 will inherently have a statistical factor of 1/2 compared to the intrinsic K'_2 for the analogous reaction if the S'—S—D—D' link were all covalent, since in the forward reaction of Equation 30 only one pair can react, whereas in the reverse reaction either S'—D' or S—D could dissociate to produce the equivalent result.

We would like to know the apparent or observed affinity for the overall reaction

$$\begin{matrix} S \\ | \\ S \end{matrix} + \begin{matrix} D \\ | \\ D \end{matrix} \overset{K_{obs}}{\rightleftharpoons} \begin{matrix} S - D \\ | \quad\;\; | \\ S - D \end{matrix} \tag{31}$$

Since the free energies, ΔF_1 and ΔF_2, for the two steps are additive, the observed affinity will be the product of K_1 and K_2

$$K_{obs} = K_1 K_2 \tag{32}$$

where we have defined K_1 and K_2 to include the statistical degeneracy factors.[7] The equilibrium constants K_1 and K_2 are each the ratios of forward and reverse rate constants, as in Equation 7. Of these four rate constants, all are directly related to the corresponding terms for the intrinsic affinity between S and D except for the intramolecular forward reaction of step 2, as noted above. Thus, the difficulty in predicting K_{obs} is largely a problem of analyzing the geometric (steric) aspects of K_2, assuming one already knows the intrinsic affinity. K. Crothers and Metzger (31) have analyzed this problem for particular situations. Qualitatively, we can say that whether K_2 will be larger or smaller than K will depend on factors such as the enforced proximity of S' and D' in step 2 and the distance between D and D' compared to the possible distances accessible between S and S', which in turn depends on the length of the antibody arms and the flexibility of the hinge between them (see Chapter 4).

6 If only the antigen is multivalent and the antibody monovalent, such as an Fab fragment, the situation can be analyzed using the same statistical considerations discussed earlier.

7 In some treatments where these statistical factors are not included in K_1 and K_2, the equivalent equation may be given as $K_{obs} = 2K_1K_2$.

Thus, since K_1 can be approximated by K, except for statistical factors, the apparent affinity for this "monogamous bivalent" binding interaction, K_{obs}, may range from significantly less than to significantly greater than K^2. If K_2 is of the same order of magnitude as K, then K_{obs} will be of the order of K^2, which can be huge (e.g., if $K \approx 10^9$ M^{-1}, K_{obs} could be $\approx 10^{18}$ M^{-1}). The half-time for dissociation would be thousands of years. It is easy to see how such monogamous bivalent interactions can appear to be irreversible, even though in practice the observed affinity is rarely more than a few orders of magnitude larger than the K for a single site, possibly due to structural constraints (32).

If apparent affinities this high can be reached by monogamous bivalency, even greater ones should be possible for the multipoint binding of an IgM molecule to a multivalent ligand. Although IgM is decavalent for small monovalent ligands, steric restrictions often make it behave as if pentavalent for binding to large multivalent ligands. However, even five-point binding can lead to enormously tight interactions. Therefore, even though the intrinsic affinity of IgM molecules tends to be lower than that of IgG molecules for the same antigen (30), the apparent affinity of IgM can be quite high.

Two-phase Systems

The same enhanced affinity seen for multipoint binding applies to two-phase systems. Examples include the reaction of multivalent antibodies with antigen attached to a cell surface or an artificial surface (e.g., Sepharose, or the plastic walls of a microtiter plate), the reaction of a multivalent ligand with antibodies on the surface of a B cell, a Sepharose bead, or a plastic plate, and the reaction of either component with an antigen–antibody precipitate. For the reasons outlined earlier, "monogamous" binding can make the apparent affinity of a multivalent antibody or antigen for multiple sites on a solid surface be quite large, to the point of effective irreversibility.

However, another effect also increases the effective affinity in a two-phase system. This effect applies even for monovalent antibodies (Fab fragments) or monovalent ligands. The effect arises from the enormously high effective local concentration of binding sites at the surface, compared to the concentration if the same number of sites were distributed in bulk solution (33). Looked at another way, the effect is due to the violation, at the liquid–solid interface, of the basic assumption in the association constants, K_A, discussed earlier, that the reactants are all distributed randomly in the solution. (To some extent, the latter is involved in the enhanced affinity of multivalency as well.) This situation has been analyzed by DeLisi (34) and DeLisi and Wiegel (35), who break the reaction down into two steps, the diffusive process necessary to bring the antigen and antibody into the right proximity and orientation to react, and the reactive process itself. The complex between antigen and antibody, when positioned but not yet reacted, is called the "encounter complex." The reaction can then be written

$$S + D \underset{k_-}{\overset{k_+}{\rightleftharpoons}} S \cdots D \underset{k_{-1}}{\overset{k_1}{\rightleftharpoons}} SD \quad (33)$$

where S is antibody site, D is antigenic determinant, k_+ and k_- are the forward and reverse diffusive rate constants, and k_1 and k_{-1} are the forward and reverse reactive rate constants once the encounter complex is formed. If the encounter complex is in a steady state, the overall rate constants will be given by

$$k_f = \frac{k_1 k_+}{(k_1 + k_-)} \quad (34)$$

$$k_r = \frac{k_{-1} k_-}{(k_1 + k_-)} \quad (35)$$

where subscripts f and r stand for forward and reverse (34). The association constant, according to Equation 7, is the ratio of these two, or

$$K_A = \frac{k_1 k_+}{k_{-1} k_-} \quad (36)$$

The relative magnitudes of k_1 and k_- determine the probable fate of the encounter complex. Is it more likely to react to form SD or to break up as the reactants diffuse apart?

Now suppose that k_- is slow compared to k_1. Then the SD bound complex and the encounter complex, $S \cdots D$, may interconvert many times before the encounter complex breaks up and one of the reactants diffuses off into bulk solution. If the surface has multiple antigenic sites, D, then even a monovalent antibody (Fab) may be much more likely, when SD dissociates to $S \cdots D$, to rereact with the same or nearby sites than to diffuse away into bulk solution, again depending on the relative magnitudes of these rate constants. This greater probability to rereact with the surface rather than diffuse away is the essence of the effect we are describing. A more extensive mathematical treatment of reactions with cells is given in DeLisi (34) and DeLisi and Wiegel (35).

A somewhat different, and very useful, analysis of the same or a very similar effect was given by Silhavy et al. (36). These authors studied the case of a ligand diffusing out of a dialysis bag containing a protein for which the ligand had a significant affinity. Once the ligand concentration became low enough that there was an excess of free protein sites, then the rate of exit of ligand from the dialysis bag was no longer simply its diffusion rate; nor was it simply the rate of dissociation of protein–ligand complex. These authors showed that under these conditions the exit of ligand followed quasi–first order kinetics, but with a half-life longer than the half-life in the absence of protein by a factor of $(1 + [P]K_A)$

$$t_+ = t_-(1 + [P]K_A) \quad (37)$$

where $[P]$ is the protein site concentration, K_A the affinity, and t_+ and t_- the half-lives in the presence and absence of protein in the bag.

In this case, the protein was in solution, so the authors could use the actual protein concentration and the actual intrinsic affinity, K_A. In the case of protein on a two-dimensional surface, it is harder to know what to use as the effective concentration. However, the high local concentration of protein compartmentalized in the dialysis bag can be seen to be analogous to the high local concentration attached to the solid surface. The underlying mechanism of the two effects is essentially the same and so are the implications. For instance, in the case of dialysis, a modest 10 μM concentration of antibody sites with an affinity of 10^8 M^{-1} can reduce the rate of exit of a ligand 1,000-fold. A dialysis that would otherwise take 3 hours would take 4 months! It is easy to see how this "retention effect" can make even modest affinities appear infinite (i.e., the reactions appear irreversible). This retention effect applies not only to immunological systems, but also to other interactions at a cell surface or between cell compartments where the local concentration of a protein may be high. In particular, these principles of two-phase systems should also govern the interaction between antigen-specific receptors on the surface of T cells and antigen–MHC molecule complexes on the surface of antigen-presenting cells, B cells, or target cells.

One final point is useful to note. Since these retention effects depend on a localized abundance of unoccupied sites, addition of a large excess of unlabeled ligand to saturate these sites will diminish or abolish the retention effect and greatly accelerate the dissociation or exit of labeled ligand. This effect of unlabeled ligand can be used as a test for the retention effect, although one must be aware that in certain cases the same result can be an indication of negative cooperativity among receptor sites.

RADIOIMMUNOASSAY AND RELATED METHODS

Since it was first suggested in 1960 by Yalow and Berson (37), radioimmunoassay (RIA) has rapidly become one of the most widespread, widely applicable, and most sensitive techniques for assessing the concentration of a whole host of biological molecules. Most of the basic principles necessary to understand and apply RIA have been covered earlier in this chapter. In this section, we examine the concepts and methodological approaches used in RIA. For a detailed methods book, we refer the reader to Chard (38), Rodbard (39), and Yalow (40).

The central concept of RIA is that the binding of an infinitesimal concentration of highly radioactive tracer antigen to low concentrations of a high-affinity, specific antibody is very sensitive to competition by unlabeled antigen and is also very specific for that antigen. Thus, concentrations of antigen in unknown samples can be determined by their ability to compete with tracer for binding to antibody. The method can be used to measure very low concentrations of a molecule, even in the presence of the many impurities in biological fluids. Accomplishment of this requires an appropriate high-affinity antibody and radiolabeled antigen, a method to distinguish bound from free-labeled antigen, optimization of concentrations of antibody and tracer-labeled antigen to maximize sensitivity, and generation of a standard curve, using known concentrations of competing unlabeled antigen, from which to read off the concentrations in unknown samples, as well as the best method for representing the data. We review all these steps and pitfalls in this procedure, except the preparation of antibodies and labeled antigens.

Separation of Bound and Free Antigen

Whatever parameter one uses to assess the amount of competition by the unlabeled antigen in the unknown sample to be tested, it will always be a function of bound versus free, radiolabeled antigen. Therefore, one of the most critical technical requirements is the ability to distinguish clearly between antibody-bound radioactive tracer and free radioactive tracer. This distinction usually requires physical separation of bound and free ligand. If the bound fraction is contaminated by free ligand, or vice versa, enormous errors can result, depending on the part of the binding curve on which the data fall.

Solution Methods

Solution RIA methods have the advantage that binding can be related to the intrinsic affinity of the antibody. However, bound and free antigen must be separated by a method that does not perturb the equilibrium. Three basic types of approaches have been used: precipitate the antibody with bound antigen, leaving free antigen in solution; precipitate the free antigen, leaving antibody and bound antigen in solution; or separate free from antibody-bound antigen molecules in solution on the basis of size by gel filtration. This last method is too cumbersome to use for large numbers of samples and is too slow, in general, to be sure the equilibrium is not perturbed in the process. Therefore, gel filtration columns are not widely used for RIA.

Methods that precipitate antibody are perhaps the most widely used. If the antigen is sufficiently smaller (MW <30,000) than the antibody that it will remain in solution at concentrations of either ammonium sulfate (41) or polyethylene glycol, MW 6,000 (10% W:W) (42), which will precipitate essentially all the antibody, then these two reagents are frequently the most useful. Precipitation with polyethylene glycol and centrifugation can be accomplished before any significant dissociation has occurred due to dilutional effects (43). However, if the antigen is much larger than about 30,000 MW to 40,000 MW, then these methods will produce unacceptably high background control values in the absence of specific antibody. If the antibody is primarily of a subclass of IgG that binds to staphylococcal protein A or protein G, one can take advantage of the high affinity of protein A or G for IgG by using either protein A (or G)-Sepharose or formalin-killed staphylococcal organisms (Cowan I strain) to precipitate the antibody (44). Finally, one can precipitate the antibody using a specific second antibody, an antiimmunoglobulin raised in another species. Maximal precipitation occurs not at antibody excess but at the "point of equivalence" in the middle of the titration curve where antigen (in this case, the first antibody) and the (second) antibody are approximately equal in concentration. Thus, one must add carrier immunoglobulin to keep the immunoglobulin concentration constant and determine the point of equivalence by titrating with the second antibody. Worse, the precipitin reaction is much slower than the antigen-antibody reaction itself, allowing re-equilibration of the antigen-antibody interaction after dilution by the second antibody. Some of these problems can be reduced by enhancing precipitation with low concentrations of polyethylene glycol.

The other type of separation method is adsorption of free antigen to an agent, such as activated charcoal or talc, that leaves antigen bound to antibody in solution. Binding of antigen by these agents depends on size and hydrophobicity. Although these methods are inexpensive and rapid, they require careful adjustment and monitoring of pH, ionic strength, and temperature to obtain reproducible results and to avoid adsorption of the antigen-antibody complex. Further, because these agents have a high affinity for antigen, they can compete with a low-affinity antibody and alter the equilibrium. Also, since charcoal quenches beta scintillation counting, it can be used only with gamma-emitting isotopes such as ^{125}I.

Solid-phase Methods

Solid-phase RIA methods have the advantages of high throughput and increased apparent affinity due to the effects at the solid-liquid interface noted earlier. However, they have the concomitant disadvantage that one is not measuring the true intrinsic affinity because of these same effects. The method itself is fairly simple. One binds the antibody in advance to a solid surface such as a Sepharose bead or the walls of a microtiter plate well. To avoid competition from other serum proteins for the solid phase, one must use purified antibody in this coating step. Once the wells (or Sepharose beads) are coated, one can incubate them with labeled tracer antigen with or without unlabeled competitor, wash, and count directly the radioactivity bound to the plastic wells or to the Sepharose. The microtiter plate method is particularly useful for processing large numbers of samples. However, because the concentration, or even the amount, of antibody coating the surface is unknown, and because the affinity is not the intrinsic affinity, one cannot use these methods for studying the chemistry of the antigen-antibody reaction itself. A detailed analysis of the optimum parameters in this method is given by Zollinger et al. (43).

A variation that does allow determination of affinity, based on the Enzyme-Linked Immunosorbant Assay (ELISA) described below, but equally applicable to RIA, was described by Friguet et al. (45). This uses antigen-coated microtiter wells and free antibody but measures competition by free antigen to prevent the antibody in solution from binding to the antibody on the plate (Figure 5.9B). Thus, the antibody bound to the plastic is antibody that was free in the solution equilibrium. The affinity measured is that between the antibody and antigen in solution, not that on the plastic, so it is not directly influenced by the multivalency of the surface. However, as pointed out by Stevens (46), the determination of affinity is strictly accurate only for monovalent Fab fragments, because a bivalent antibody with only one arm bound to the plastic and one bound by antigen in solution will still be counted as free. Therefore, there will be an underestimate of the ligand occupancy of the antibody combining sites, and thus an underestimate of affinity. Stevens also points out a method to correct for this error based on binomial analysis. Subsequently, Seligman (47) showed that the nature and density of the antigen on the solid surface can also influence the estimate of affinity.

Optimization of Antibody and Tracer Concentrations for Sensitivity

The primary limitations on the sensitivity of the assay are the antibody affinity and concentration, the tracer concentration, and the precision (reproducibility) of the data. In general, the higher the affinity of the antibody, the more sensitive the assay can be made. Once one prepares the highest affinity antibody available, this parameter limits the extent to which the other parameters can be manipulated. For instance, since the unlabeled antigen in the unknown sample is going to compete against labeled tracer antigen, the lower the tracer concentration, the lower the concentration of the unknown, which can be measured, up to a point. That point is determined by the affinity, K_A, as can be seen from the theoretical considerations earlier (38). The steepest part of the titration curve will occur in the range of concentrations around $1/K_A$. Concentrations of ligand much below $1/K_A$ will leave most of the antibody sites unoccupied, so competition will be less effective. Thus, there is no value in reducing the tracer concentration more than a few-fold lower than $1/K_A$. Therefore, although it is generally useful to increase the specific radioactivity of the tracer and reduce its concentration, it is important to be aware of this limit of $1/K_A$. Increasing the specific activity more than necessary can result in denaturation of antigen.

Similarly, lowering the antibody concentration will also increase sensitivity, up to a point. This limit also depends on $1/K_A$ and on the background "nonspecific binding." Decreasing the antibody concentration to the point that binding of tracer is too close to background will result in loss of sensitivity due to loss of precision. In general, the fraction of tracer bound in the absence of competitor should be kept greater than 0.2, and in general closer to 0.5 (see ref. 48).

A convenient procedure to follow to optimize tracer and antibody concentrations is first to choose the lowest tracer concentration that results in convenient counting times and counting precision for bound values of only one-half to one-tenth the total tracer. Then, keeping this tracer concentration constant, one dilutes out the antibody until the bound/free antigen ratio is close to 1.0 (bound/total = 0.5) in the absence of competitor. This antibody concentration in conjunction with this tracer concentration will generally give near-optimal sensitivities, within the limits previously noted. It is important to be aware that changing the tracer concentration will require readjusting the antibody concentration to optimize sensitivity.

Analysis of Data: Graphic and Numerical Representation

We have already examined the Scatchard plot (bound/free versus bound) and the plot of bound/free versus free or total antigen concentration as methods of determining affinity. The latter lends itself particularly to the type of competition curves that constitute a RIA. In fact, the independent variable must always be antigen concentration, because that is the known quantity one varies to generate the standard curve. Let us use B, F, and T to represent the concentrations of bound, free, and total antigen, respectively. Earlier, we saw that the plot of B/F versus F is more useful for determining the affinity, K_A, than the plot of B/F versus T. However, in RIA, the quantity one wants to determine is T, and, correspondingly, the known independent variable in generating the standard curve is T. Another difference between the situation in RIA and that discussed earlier is that, in RIA, one has both labeled and unlabeled antigen. The dependent variable, such as B/F, is the ratio of bound tracer over free tracer, because only radioactive antigen is counted. B/F for the unlabeled antigen will be the same at equilibrium, assuming that labeled and unlabeled antigen bind the antibody equivalently—that is, with the same K_A. This assumption is not always valid and requires experimental testing.

The sigmoidal shape of B/F versus F or T, when F or T (the "dose") is plotted on a log scale, can be seen in Figure 5.6. The shape for B/T versus F or T would be similar.

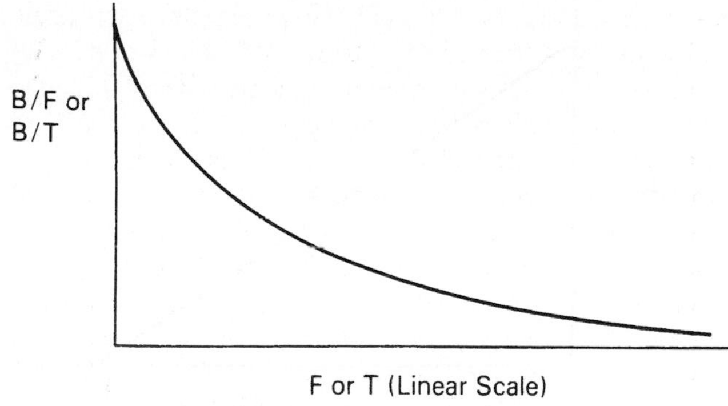

FIGURE 5.7 Schematic plot of B/F or B/T (the bound/free or total antigen concentration) as a function of free (F) or total (T) antigen concentration, when plotted on a linear scale. Contrast with similar plot on a log scale in Figure 5.6.

Note that since $B + F = T$,

$$\frac{B}{F} = \frac{B}{(T - B)} = \frac{B/T}{(1 - B/T)} \tag{38}$$

and

$$\frac{B}{T} = \frac{B/F}{(1 + B/F)} \tag{39}$$

These transformations can be useful. If one plots B/F or B/T versus F or T on a linear scale, then the shape is approximately hyperbolic, as in Figure 5.7. The plot of B/F versus T (log scale) was one of the first methods used to plot RIA data and is still among the most useful. The most sensitive part of the curve is the part with the steepest slope.

It has been shown by probability analysis that if the antigen has multiple determinants, each capable of binding antibody molecules simultaneously and independently of one another, then the more such determinants capable of being recognized by the antibodies in use, the steeper will be the slope (49). This effect of multideterminant binding on steepness arises because, in RIA, an antigen molecule is scored as bound whether it has one antibody molecule or several attached. It is scored as free only if no antibody molecules are attached. Thus, the probability that an antigen molecule is scored as free is the product of the probabilities that each of its determinants is free. The effect can lead to quite steep slopes and has been confirmed experimentally (49).

A transform that allows linearization of the data in most cases is the logit transform (50,51). To use this, one first expresses the data as B/B_0, where B_0 is the concentration of bound tracer in the absence of competitor. One then takes the logit transform of this ratio, defined as

$$\text{logit}\ (Y) = \ln\left[\frac{Y}{(1 - Y)}\right] \tag{40}$$

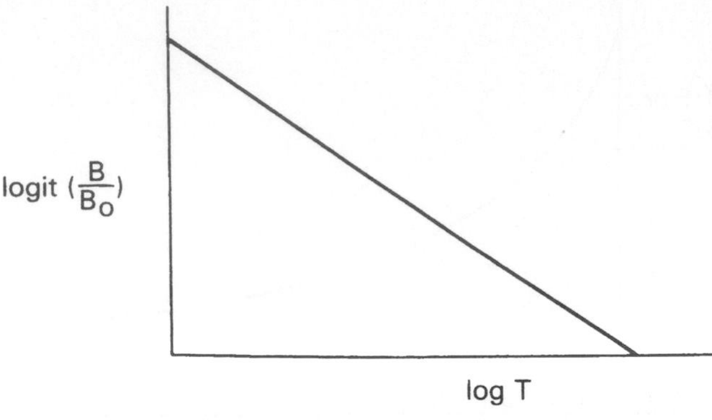

FIGURE 5.8 Schematic logit–log plot used to linearize RIA data. B and T are bound tracer and total antigen concentration, respectively, and B_0 is the value of B when no unlabeled antigen is added to tracer. The logit function is defined by Equation (40), logit $(Y) = \ln[Y/(1 - Y)]$.

where ln means the natural log (log to the base e). The plot of logit (B/B_0) versus ln T is usually a straight line (Figure 5.8). The slope is usually -1 for the simplest case of a monoclonal antibody binding a monovalent antigen. The linearity of this plot obviously makes it very useful for graphical interpolation, which one would like to do to read antigen concentration off a standard curve. One additional advantage is that linearity facilitates tests of parallelism. If the unknown under study is identical to the antigen used to generate the standard curve, then a dilution curve of the unknown should be parallel to the standard curve in this logit-log coordinate system. If not, the assay is not valid.

These and other methods of analyzing the data are discussed further by Feldman and Rodbard (52) and Rodbard (39), including statistical treatment of data. While a number of computer programs have become available for rapid analysis of RIA data without using manual plots of standard curves, they are all based on these and similar methods, and their accurate interpretation depends on an understanding of these concepts.

Corrections for B, F, and T

Before we leave this section on analysis of RIA data, we must point out a few controls and corrections to the data without which the results may be fallacious.

First, in any method that precipitates antibody and bound antigen (or uses a solid-phase antibody), there may always be a fraction of antigen that precipitates or binds nonspecifically in the absence of specific antibody. Thus, one must always run controls with normal serum or immunoglobulin to determine this background. The nonspecific binding usually increases linearly with antigen dose; that is, it does not saturate. This control value should be subtracted from B but does not affect F when measured independently, only F determined as T minus B. The total antigen that is meaningful is the sum of that which is specifically bound and that which is free. Nonspecifically bound antigen should be deleted from any term in which it appears.

A second correction is that for immunologically inactive radiolabel, either free radioisotope or isotope coupled to an impurity or to denatured antigen. The fraction of radioactive material that is immunologically reactive with the antibodies in the assay can be determined by using a constant, low concentration of labeled antigen and adding increasing concentrations of antibody. If there is no contamination with inactive material, all the radioactivity should be able to be bound by sufficient antibody. If the fraction of tracer bound reaches a plateau at less than 100% bound, then only this fraction is active in the assay. The importance of this correction can be seen from the example in which the tracer is only 80% active. Then, when the true B/F is 3 ($B/T = 0.75$), applying only to the active 80% of the tracer, the remaining 20%, which can never be bound, will mistakenly be included in the free tracer, doubling the amount that is measured as free. Thus, the measured B/F will be only 1.5 (i.e., 0.6/0.4) instead of the true value of 3 (i.e., 0.6/0.2). This factor of 2 will make a serious difference in the calculation of affinity, for instance, from a Scatchard plot. It will also result in a plateau in the Scatchard plot at high values of B/F, since with 20% of the tracer obligatorily free, B/F can never exceed 4 (i.e., 0.8/0.2). To correct for this potentially serious problem, the inactive fraction must always be determined subtracted from both F and T.

Nonequilibrium RIA

So far, we have assumed that tracer and unlabeled competitor are added simultaneously and sufficient incubation time is allowed to achieve equilibrium. To measure the affinity, of course, equilibrium must be assured. However, suppose one's sole purpose is to measure the concentration of competitor by RIA. Then one can actually increase the sensitivity of the assay by adding the competitor first, allowing it to react with the antibody, and then intentionally adding the tracer for too short a time to reach a new equilibrium. One is essentially giving the competitor a competitive advantage. It can be shown that the slope of the dose-response curve, B/T versus total antigen added, is increased in the low-dose range—a mathematical measure of increased sensitivity. A detailed mathematical analysis of this procedure may be found in Rodbard et al. (53). Note, however, that use of such nonequilibrium conditions requires very careful control of time and temperature.

Enzyme-linked Immunosorbent Assay (ELISA)

An alternative solid-phase readout system for the detection of antigen–antibody reactions is the ELISA assay (54). In principle, the only difference from RIAs is that antibodies

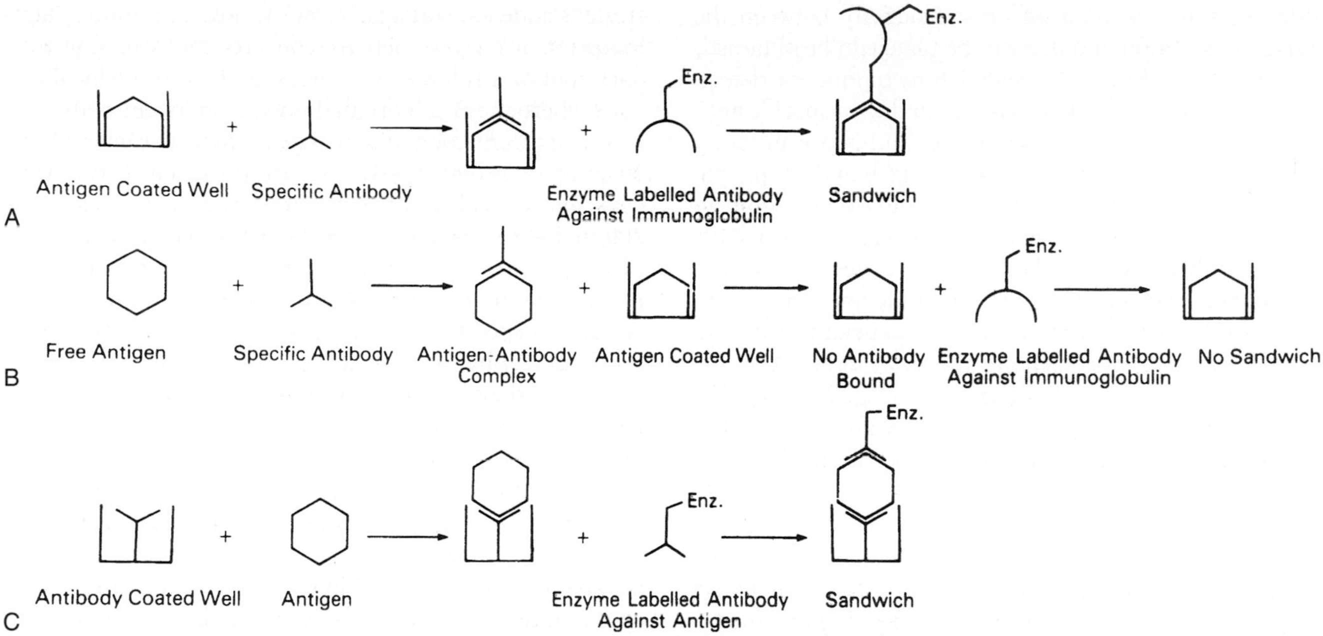

A

Enz.

Antigen Coated Well Specific Antibody Enzyme Labelled Antibody Against Immunoglobulin Sandwich

B

Enz.

Free Antigen Specific Antibody Antigen-Antibody Complex Antigen Coated Well No Antibody Bound Enzyme Labelled Antibody Against Immunoglobulin No Sandwich

C

Enz.

Antibody Coated Well Antigen Enzyme Labelled Antibody Against Antigen Sandwich

FIGURE 5.9 Three strategies for the detection of specific antibody–antigen reactions using the ELISA technique. **A:** Direct binding. **B:** Hapten inhibition. **C:** Antigen sandwich.

or antigen are covalently coupled to an enzyme instead of a radioisotope, so that bound enzyme activity is measured instead of bound cpm. In practice, the safety and convenience of nonradioactive materials and the commercial availability of plate readers that can measure the absorbance of 96 wells in a few seconds account for ELISA's widespread use. Since both ELISA and RIA are governed by the same thermodynamic constraints, and the enzyme can be detected in the same concentration range as commonly used radioisotopes, the sensitivity and specificity are comparable. We consider three basic strategies for using ELISA assays to detect specific antibody or antigen.

As shown in Figure 5.9A, the indirect antibody method is the simplest way to detect and measure specific antibody in an unknown antiserum. Antigen is noncovalently attached to each well of a plastic microtiter dish. For this purpose, it is fortunate that most proteins bind nonspecifically to plastic. Excess free antigen is washed off, and the wells are incubated with an albumin solution to block the remaining nonspecific protein binding sites. The test antiserum is then added, and any specific antibody binds to the solid-phase antigen. Washing removes unbound antibodies. Enzyme-labeled anti-immunoglobulin is added. This binds to specific antibody already bound to antigen on the solid phase, bringing along covalently attached enzyme. Unbound antiglobulin-enzyme conjugate is washed off, then substrate is added. The action of bound enzyme on substrate produces a colored product, which is detected as increased absorbance in a spectrophotometer.

Although this method is quick and very sensitive, it is often difficult to quantitate. Within a defined range, the increase in optical density is proportional to the amount of specific antibody added in the first step. However, the amount of antibody bound is not measured directly. Instead, the antibody concentration of the sample is estimated by comparing it with a standard curve for a known amount of antibody. It is also difficult to determine affinity by this method, since the solid-phase antigen tends to increase the apparent affinity. The sensitivity of this assay for detecting minute amounts of antibody is quite good, especially when affinity-purified antiglobulins are used as the enzyme-linked reagent. A single preparation of enzyme-linked antiglobulin can be used to detect antibodies to many different antigens. Alternatively, class specific antiglobulins can be used to detect how much of a specific antibody response is due to each immunoglobulin class. Obviously, reproducibility of the assay depends on uniform antigen coating of each well, and the specificity depends on using purified antigen to coat the wells.

Figure 5.9B shows the competition technique for detecting antigen. Soluble antigen is mixed with limiting amounts of specific antibody in the first step. Then the mixture is added to antigen-coated wells and treated as described in Figure 5.9A. Any antigen-antibody complexes formed in the first step will reduce the amount of antibody bound to the plate and hence will reduce the absorbance measured in the final step. This method permits the estimate of affinity for free antigen, which is related to the half-inhibitory concentration of antigen. Mathematical analysis of affinity by this approach was described by Friguet et al. (45), with modification by Stevens (46), as discussed earlier in the "RIA Solid-phase Methods" section. In addition, some estimate of cross-reactivity between the antigen in solution and that on the plate can be obtained.

Figure 5.9C shows the sandwich technique for detecting antigen. Microtiter plates are coated with specific antibody. Antigen is then captured by the solid-phase antibody. A second antibody specific for the antigen and coupled to enzyme is added. This binds to the solid-phase antigen-antibody complex, carrying enzyme along with it. Excess second antibody is washed off and substrate is added. The absorbance produced is a function of the antigen concentration of the test solution, which can be determined from a standard curve. Specificity of the assay depends on the specificity of the antibodies used to coat the plate and detect antigen. Sensitivity depends on the affinity as well as amount of the first antibody coating the well, which can be increased by using affinity-purified antibodies or monoclonal antibodies in this step. The sandwich method depends on divalency of the antigen, or else the two antibodies must be specific for different antigenic determinants on the same antigen molecule. When comparing two monoclonal antibodies to the same antigen, this technique can be used to ascertain whether they can bind simultaneously to the same molecule or whether they compete for the same site or sites close enough to cause steric hindrance (55).

When antibodies are serially diluted across a plate, the last colored well indicates the titer. Specificity of binding can be demonstrated by coating wells with albumin and measuring antibody binding in parallel with the antigen-coated wells. Because it can be used to test many samples in a short time, ELISA is often used to screen culture supernatants in the production of hybridoma antibodies. The sensitivity of the method allows detection of clones producing specific antibodies at an early stage in cell growth.

An important caution when using native protein antigens to coat solid-phase surfaces (Figure 5.9A) is that binding to a surface can alter the conformation of the protein. For instance, using conformation specific monoclonal antibodies to myoglobin, Darst et al. (56) found that binding of myoglobin to a surface altered the apparent affinity of some antibodies more than others. This problem may be avoided by using the solution phase methods of Figure 5.9B or 5.9C.

ELIspot Assay

The normal ELISA assay can be modified to measure antibody production at the single cell level. In this method, called the *ELIspot assay,* tissue culture plates are coated with antigen, and various cell populations are cultured on the plate for four hours. During that time, B cells settle to the bottom and secrete antibodies, which bind antigen nearby and produce a footprint of the antibody-secreting cell. The cells are then washed off, and a second antibody, such as enzyme labeled goat antihuman IgG, is added. Finally, unbound antibody is washed off, and enzyme substrate is added in soft agar. Over the next 10 minutes, each footprint of enzyme activity converts the substrate to a dark spot of insoluble dye, corresponding to the localized zone where the B cell originally secreted its antibody.

Using this method, it is possible to detect as few as 10 to 20 antibody-producing B cells in the presence of 10^6 spleen cells, and typical results for immunized mice range from 200 to 500 spot-forming cells per 10^6 spleen cells (57,58). Clearly, to work at all, this assay must be capable of detecting the amount of antibody secreted by a single immune B cell and be specific enough to exclude nonspecific antibodies produced by the vast majority of nonimmune B cells. Sensitivity depends on the affinity and amount of antibodies secreted and may be optimized by titering the amount of antigen on the plate.

This type of assay is useful in analyzing the cellular requirements for antibody production in vitro, because the number of responding B cells is measured directly. It can also be used to detect antibodies made in the presence of excess antigen. For example, during acute infections (59) and in autoimmunity (60), when antigen may be in excess over antibody, this assay makes it possible to measure antibody-producing B cells, even though free antibody may not be detectable in circulation. It can also be used to measure local production of self-reactive antibodies in a specific tissue, such as synovium. By using two detecting antibodies, each specific for a different immunoglobulin class and coupled to a different enzyme, and two substrates producing different colored dyes, cells secreting IgA and IgG simultaneously can be detected (61). In this way, ELIspot was used to show that bacterial DNA containing CpG sequences is a polyclonal B cell mitogen (62).

ELIspot can also detect secreted cytokines, as opposed to antibodies, by coating the plate with a capture antibody and detecting antigen with an enzyme-coupled second antibody (as in a sandwich ELISA, Figure 5.9C). For example, using plates coated with monoclonal antibody to IL-4, T cells secreting IL-4 could be detected (63), providing one measure of T helper 2 cells.

SPECIFICITY AND CROSS-REACTIVITY

The specificity of an antibody or antiserum is defined by its ability to discriminate between the antigen against which it was made (called the *homologous antigen,* or *immunogen*) and any other antigen one might test. In practice, one cannot test the whole universe of antigens, but only selected antigens. In this sense, specificity can only be defined experimentally within that set of antigens one chooses to compare. Karush (30) has defined a related term, *selectivity,* as the ability of an antibody to discriminate, in an all-or-none fashion, between two related ligands. Thus, selectivity depends not only on the relative affinity of the antibody for the two ligands, but also on the experimental lower limit for detection of reactivity. For instance, an anticarbohydrate antibody with an affinity of 10^5 M^{-1} for the immunogen may appear to be highly selective, because reaction with a related carbohydrate with a 100-fold lower affinity, 10^3 M^{-1}, may be undetectable. However, an antibody with an affinity of 10^9 M^{-1} for the homologous ligand may appear to be less selective because any reaction with a related ligand with a 100-fold lower affinity would still be quite easily detectable.

Conversely, cross-reactivity is defined as the ability to react with related ligands other than the immunogen. More usually, this is examined from the point of view of the ligand. Thus, one might say that antigen Y cross-reacts with antigen X because it binds to anti-X antibodies. Note that in this sense, it is the two antigens that are cross-reactive, not the antibody. However, the cross-reactivity of two antigens, X and Y, can be defined only with respect to a particular antibody or antiserum. For instance, a different group of anti-X antibodies may not react at all with Y, so that with respect to these antibodies, Y would not be cross-reactive with X. One can also use the term in a different sense, saying that some anti-X antibodies cross-react with antigen Y.

In most cases, cross-reactive ligands have lower affinity than the immunogen for a particular antibody. However, exceptions can occur, in which a cross-reactive antigen binds with a higher affinity than the homologous antigen itself. This phenomenon is called *heterocliticity,* and the antigen that has a higher affinity for the antibody than does the immunogen is said to be heteroclitic. Antibodies that manifest this behavior are also described as heteroclitic antibodies. A good example is the case of antibodies raised in C57BL/10 mice against the hapten nitrophenyl acetyl (NP). These antibodies have been shown by Mäkelä and Karjalainen (64) to bind with higher affinity to the cross-reactive hapten, nitroiodophenyl acetyl (NIP), than to the immunogen itself. Another example is the case of retro-inverso or retro-D peptides (65–69). By reversing the chirality from L to D amino acids and simultaneously reversing the sequence of amino acids, one can produce a peptide that is resistant to proteolysis and has its side chains approximately in the same position as the original L amino acid peptide, with the exception of some amino acids with secondary chiral centers, such as Thr and Ile. However, the backbone NH and CO moieties are reversed. Antibodies that interact with only the side chains might not distinguish these peptides, whereas antibodies that interact with the main chain as well as side chains might distinguish them and have potentially higher or lower affinity. In a study of monoclonal antibodies to a hexapeptide from histone H3, some bound the retro-D form with higher affinity than the native sequence and some did not (67,68). The former are an example of heterocliticity. In addition to greater binding affinity, the retro-D peptides may have even greater activity in vivo because of their resistance to proteolysis (65–69). This stability makes them more useful as drugs as well (65,66,70).

Cross-reactivity has often been detected by methods such as the Ouchterlony test, or hemagglutination (descriptions of both of these appear later) or similar methods, which have in common the fact that they do not distinguish well between differences in affinity and differences in concentration. This practical aspect, coupled with the heterogeneity of immune antisera, has led to ambiguities in the usage of the terms "cross-reactivity" and "specificity." With the advent of RIA and ELISA techniques, this ambiguity in the terminology, as well as in the interpretation of data, has become apparent.

For these reasons, Berzofsky and Schechter (71) have defined two forms of cross-reactivity and, correspondingly, two forms of specificity. These two forms of cross-reactivity are illustrated by the two prototype competition RIA curves in Figure 5.10. In reality, most antisera display both phenomena simultaneously.

Type 1 cross-reactivity, or true cross-reactivity, is defined as the ability of two ligands to react with the same site on the same antibody molecule, possibly with different affinities. For example, the related haptens dinitrophenyl (DNP) and trinitrophenyl (TNP) may react with different affinity for antibodies raised to dinitrophenyl hapten. In protein antigens, such differences could occur with small changes in primary sequence (e.g., the conservative substitution of threonine for serine), or with changes in conformation, such as the cleavage of the protein into fragments (Figure 5.11) (71–75). If a peptide fragment contained all the contact residues in an antigenic determinant (i.e., those which contact the antibody-combining site), it

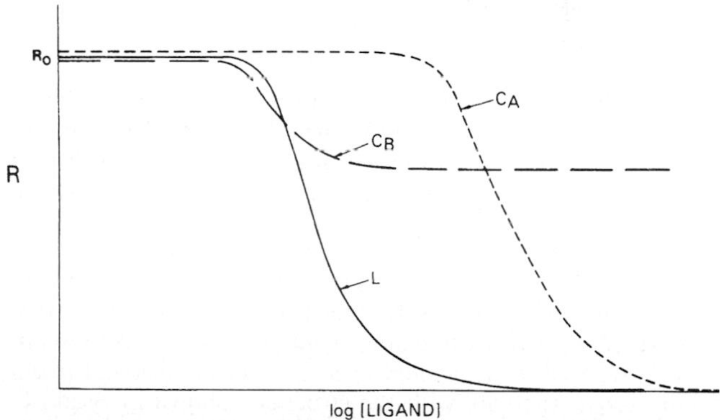

FIGURE 5.10 Schematic RIA binding curves for homologous ligand L and cross-reacting ligands. Cross-reacting ligand C_A manifests type 1 or true cross-reactivity demonstrated by complete inhibition of tracer ligand binding and a lower affinity. Ligand C_B displays type 2 cross-reactivity or determinant sharing, as recognized from the plateau at less than 100% inhibition, but not necessarily a lower affinity. The ordinate R is the ratio of bound/free radiolabeled tracer ligand, and R_0 is the limit of R as the concentration of all ligands, including tracer, approaches zero. From (71), with permission.

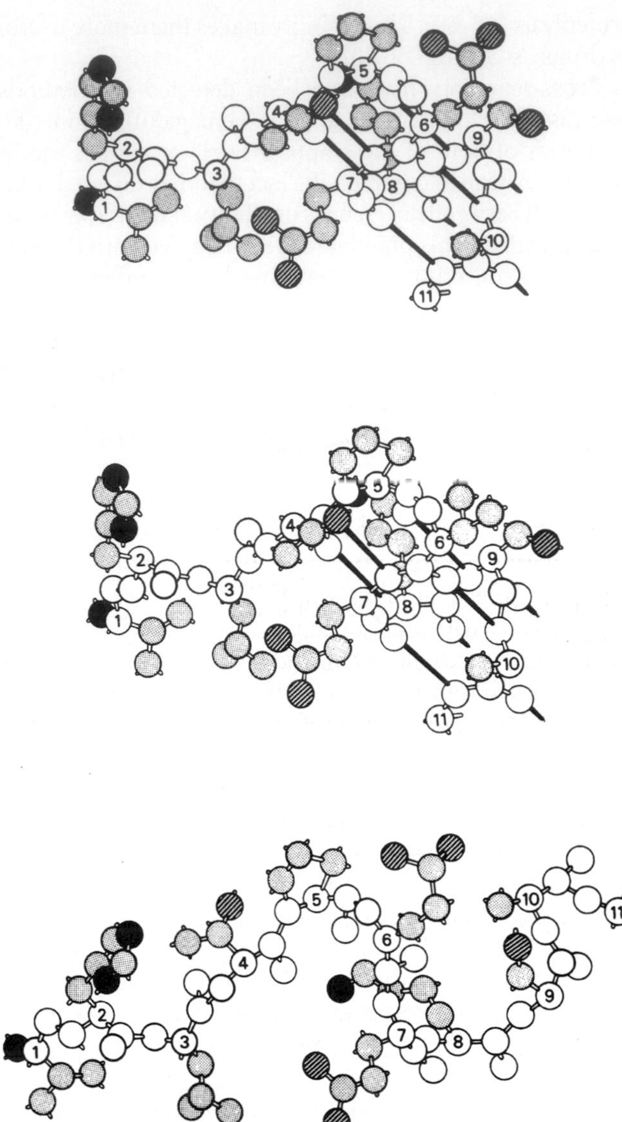

FIGURE 5.11 An artist's drawing of the amino terminal region of the ß chain of hemoglobin. **A:** The first 11 residues of the $ß^A$ chain. **B:** The comparable regions of the $ß^S$ chain. The substitution of valine for the normal glutamic acid at position 6 makes a distinct antigenic determinant to which a subpopulation of antibodies may be isolated (72,73). **C:** A schematic diagram of the sequence in A unfolded as occurs when the protein is denatured. This region may be cleaved from the protein, or the peptide synthesized (74), resulting in changed antigenic reactivity. An antiserum prepared to hemoglobin (or the ß chain thereof) might exhibit cross-reactivity with the structures shown in B and C, but the molecular mechanisms would be different. Polypeptide backbone atoms are in white in the side chains, oxygen atoms are hatched, nitrogen atoms are black, and carbon atoms are lightly stippled. Adapted from (71,75).

might cross-react with the native determinant for antibodies against the native form, but with lower affinity because the peptide would not retain the native conformation (see Chapter 21). This type of affinity difference is illustrated by competitor C_A in Figure 5.10, in which complete displacement of tracer can be achieved at high enough concentrations of C_A, but higher concentrations of C_A than of the homologous ligand, L, are required to produce any given degree of inhibition.

A separate issue from affinity differences is the issue of whether the cross-reactive ligand reacts with all or only a subpopulation of the antibodies in a heterogeneous serum. This second type of cross-reactivity, which we call *type 2 cross-reactivity* or *shared reactivity,* therefore, can occur only when the antibody population is heterogeneous, as in most conventional antisera. In this case, the affinity of the cross-reactive ligand may be greater than, less than, or equal to that of the homologous ligand for those antibodies with which it interacts. Therefore, the competition curve is not necessarily displaced to the right, but the inhibition will reach a plateau at less than complete inhibition, as illustrated by competitor C_B in Figure 5.10. As an example, let us consider the case of a protein with determinants X and Y and an antiserum against this protein containing both anti-X and anti-Y antibodies. Then a mutant protein in which determinant Y was so altered as to be unrecognizable by anti-Y, but determinant X was intact, would manifest type 2 cross-reactivity. It would compete with the wild-type protein only for anti-X antibodies (possibly even with equal affinity), but not for anti-Y antibodies.

Of course, both types of cross-reactivity could occur simultaneously. A classic example would be the peptide fragment discussed earlier in the case of type 1 cross-reactivity. Suppose the fragment contained the residues of determinant X, albeit not in the native conformation, but did not contain the residues of a second determinant, Y, which was also expressed on the native protein. If the antiserum to the native protein consisted of anti-X and anti-Y, the peptide would compete only for anti-X antibodies (type 2 cross-reactivity) but would have a lower affinity than the native protein even for these antibodies. Thus, the competition curve would be shifted to the right and would plateau before reaching complete inhibition.[8]

In the case of a homogeneous (e.g., monoclonal) antibody in which only type 1 or true cross-reactivity can occur, one can quantify the differences in affinity for different cross-reactive ligands by a method analogous to the *B*/*F* versus *F* method described earlier. Suppose that ligands X and Y cross-react with homologous ligand L for a monoclonal antibody. If one plots the bound/free ($B/F = R$)

[8] An ambiguous case could occur experimentally in which the distinction between the two types of cross-reactivity would be blurred. For example, in the case of antibodies that all react with determinant X but have a very wide range of affinities for X, some such antibodies may have such a low affinity for cross-reactive determinant X′ that they would appear not to bind X′ at all. Then a competition curve using X′ might appear to reach a plateau at incomplete inhibition even though all the antibodies were specific for X, and the only difference between X and X′ was affinity.

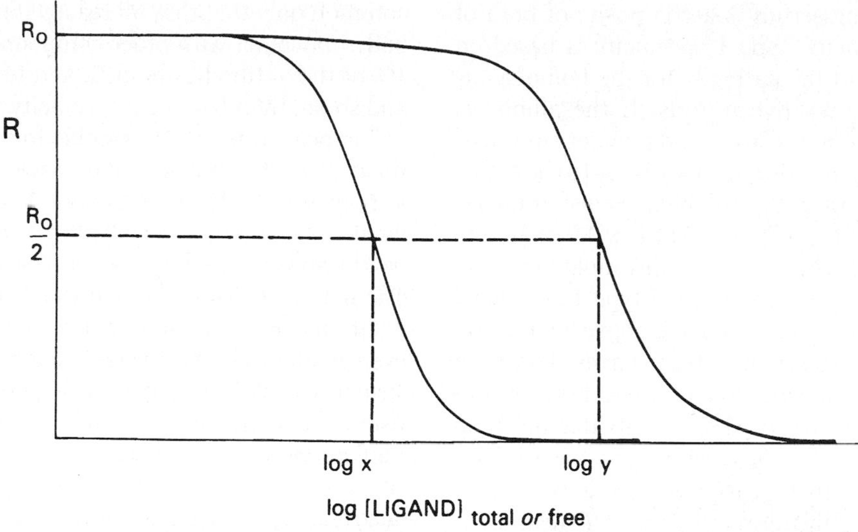

FIGURE 5.12 Schematic RIA binding curves showing the effect of affinity on the midpoint and the slope at the midpoint and the value of using free [ligand] rather than total [ligand]. Ordinate R is the ratio of bound/free radiolabeled tracer ligand, and R_0 the limit of R as all ligand concentrations approach zero. If x and y are the concentrations of ligands X and Y that reduce R to exactly $R_0/2$, then if the abscissa is total ligand concentration, $x = 1/K_X + [S]_t/2$ and $y = 1/K_Y + [S]_t/2$, where $[S]_t$ is the concentration of antibody binding sites and K_X and K_Y the affinities of the antibody for the respective ligands. However, if the abscissa is free ligand concentration, $x = 1/K_X$ and $y = 1/K_Y$ so that the ratio x/y (or the difference $\log x - \log y$ on a log plot) corresponds to the ratio of affinities K_Y/K_X. Note that the slopes at the midpoints are the same on a log scale, but that for Y would be only K_Y/K_X that for X on a linear scale. From (71), with permission.

ratio for radiolabeled tracer ligand L as a function of the log of the concentration of competitors X and Y, one obtains two parallel competition curves (Figure 5.12) (71), under the appropriate conditions (below). The first condition is that the concentration of free tracer be less than $1/K_L$, the affinity for tracer. In this case, it can be shown (71) that

$$K_X \approx \frac{1}{[X]_{\text{free}}} \qquad (41)$$

at the midpoint where $R = R_0/2$, where K_X is the affinity for X. This is analogous to Equation 21 for the case in which unlabeled homologous ligand is the competitor. Also, in analogy with Equation 23, it can be shown that if the total concentration of competitor, $[X]_t$, is used instead of the free concentration, $[X]_{\text{free}}$, an error term will arise, giving

$$[X]_t \text{ (at } R = R_0/2) = \frac{1}{K_X} + \frac{[S]_t}{2} \qquad (42)$$

Thus, with competitor on a linear scale, the difference in midpoint for competitors X and Y will correspond to the difference $1/K_X - 1/K_Y$, regardless of whether free or total competitor is plotted, but the ratio of midpoint concentrations will equal K_X/K_Y only if the free concentrations are used. This last point is important if one plots the log of competitor concentration, as is usually done, because the horizontal displacement between the two curves on a log scale corresponds to the ratio $[X]/[Y]$, not the difference (71).

If a second condition also holds, namely, that the concentration of bound tracer is small compared to the antibody site concentration $[S]_t$, then the slopes (on a linear scale) of the curves at their respective midpoints (where $R = R_0/2$) will be proportional to the affinity for that competitor, K_X or K_Y (71). (Both conditions can be met by keeping tracer L small relative to both K_L and $[S]_t$.) When $[X]_{\text{free}}$ and $[Y]_{\text{free}}$ are plotted on a log scale, the slopes will appear to be equal (i.e., the curves will appear parallel), since a parallel line shifted m-fold to the right on a log scale will actually be $1/m$ as steep, at any point, in terms of the antilog as abscissa.

When the antibodies are heterogeneous in affinity, the curves will be broadened and in general will not be parallel. When heterogeneity of specificity is present, and type 2 cross-reactivity occurs, it should be pointed out that the fractional inhibition achieved at the plateau in a B/F versus free competitor plot will not be proportional to the fraction of antibodies reacting with that competitor but will be proportional to a weighted fraction, where the antibody concentrations are weighted by their affinity for the tracer (71).

These two types of cross-reactivity lead naturally to two definitions of specificity (71). The overall specificity of a heterogeneous antiserum is a composite of both of these facets of specificity. Type 1 specificity is based on the relative affinities of the antibody for the homologous ligand and any cross-reactive ligands. If the affinity is much higher for the homologous ligand than for any cross-reactive ligand tested, then the antibody is said to be highly specific for the homologous ligand; that is, it discriminates very well between this ligand and the others. If the affinity for cross-reactive ligands is below the threshold for detection in an experimental situation, then type 1 specificity gives rise to selectivity, as was discussed above (cf. ref. 30). The specificity can even be quantitated in terms of the ratio of affinities for the homologous ligand and a cross-reactive ligand (cf. ref. 76). It is this type 1 specificity that most immunochemists would call true specificity, just as we have called type 1 cross-reactivity true cross-reactivity.

The common use of the term *cross-reactivity* to include type 2 or partial reactivity leads to a second definition of specificity, which applies only to heterogeneous populations of antibodies such as antisera. We call this type 2 specificity. If all the antibodies in the mixture react with the immunogen, but only a small proportion react with any single cross-reactive antigen, then the antiserum would be said to be relatively specific for the immunogen. Note that it does not matter whether the affinity of a subpopulation that reacts with a cross-reactive antigen is high or low (type 1 cross-reactivity). As long as that subpopulation is a small fraction of the antibodies, the mixture is specific. Thus, type 2 specificity depends on the relative concentrations of antibodies in the heterogeneous antiserum, not just on their affinities. Also note that one can use these relative concentrations of antibody subpopulations to compare the specificity of a single antiserum for two cross-reactive ligands. However, it would not be meaningful to compare the specificity of two different antisera for the same ligand by comparing the fraction of antibodies in each serum that reacted with that ligand. Although type 2 specificity may appear to some to be a less classic concept of specificity than type 1, it is type 2 specificity that one primarily measures in such assays as the Ouchterlony double immunodiffusion test, and it carries equal weight with type 1 specificity in such assays as hemagglutination, discussed later. Type 2 specificity also leads naturally to the concept of "multispecificity" described in the following section.

Multispecificity

The theory of multispecificity, introduced and analyzed by Talmage (77) and Inman (78,79) and discussed on a structural level by Richards et al. (80), suggests a mechanism by which the diversity and specificity of antisera can be expanded and also understood. The idea is that each antibody may actually bind, with high affinity, a variety of diverse antigens. When one immunizes with immunogen A, one selects for many distinct antibodies that have in common only that they all react with A. In fact, each antibody may react with other compounds, but if fewer than 1% of the antibodies bind B, and fewer than 1% bind C, and so on, then by type 2 specificity, the whole antiserum will appear to be highly specific for A. Note that the subpopulation that binds B may react with an affinity for B as high as or higher than that for A, so that the population would not be type 1 specific for A. This same population would presumably be selected if one immunized with B. The net result would be that the diversity of highly (type 2) specific antisera an organism could generate would be even greater than the diversity of B cell clones (or antibody structures). This principle can explain how polyclonal antisera can sometimes appear paradoxically more specific than a monoclonal antibody.

OTHER METHODS

We mention only a few of the other methods for measuring antigen–antibody interactions. Other useful techniques include quenching of the tryptophan fluorescence of the antibody by certain antigens on binding (81) (a sensitive method useful for such experiments as fast kinetic studies), antibody-dependent cellular cytotoxicity, immunofluorescence including flow cytometry, immunohistochemistry, and inhibition by antibody of plaque formation by antigen-conjugated bacteriophage (82) (a method as sensitive as RIA since inhibition of even a few phage virions can be detected).

Quantitative Precipitin

Among the earliest known properties of antibodies were their ability to neutralize pathogenic bacteria and their ability to form precipitates with bacterial culture supernatants. Both activities of each antiserum were highly specific for the bacterial strain against which the antiserum was made. The precipitates contained antibody protein and bacterial products. The supernatants contained decreased amounts of antibody protein and, under the right conditions, had lost the ability to neutralize bacteria. However, quantitation of the antibody precipitated was difficult, since the precipitate contained antigen protein as well as antibody protein. Heidelberger and Kendall (83,84) solved this problem when they found that purified pneumococcal cell wall polysaccharide could precipitate with antipneumococcal antibodies. In this case, the amount of protein nitrogen measured in the precipitate was entirely due to antibody protein, and the amount of reducing sugar was mostly due to the antigen. Plotting the amount of antibody protein precipitated from a constant volume of antiserum by increasing amounts of carbohydrate antigen gives the curve shown in Figure 5.13.

As shown in Figure 5.13A, the amount of antibody precipitated rises initially, reaches a plateau, and then

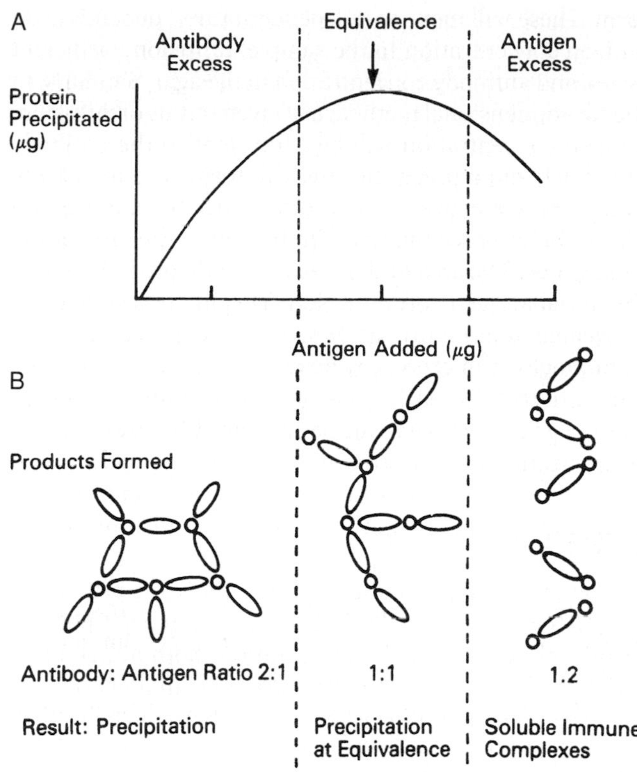

FIGURE 5.13 Quantitative immunoprecipitation. To a fixed amount of specific antibody are added increasing amounts of nonprotein antigen. The figure shows the amount of antibody protein (**A**) and the ratio of antibody to antigen (**B**) found in the precipitate. At antigen excess, soluble immune complexes are found in the supernatant, and the precipitate is decreased.

declines. The point of maximum precipitation was found to coincide with the point of complete depletion of neutralizing antibodies and is called the *equivalence point.* The amount of antibody protein in the precipitate at equivalence is considered to equal the total amount of specific antibody in that volume of antiserum. The rising part of the curve is called the *antibody excess zone* (antigen limiting), and the part of the curve beyond the equivalence point is called the *antigen excess zone.*

Supernatants and precipitates were carefully analyzed for each zone of antibody or antigen excess, as shown in Figure 5.13B. When antigen was limiting, the precipitate contained high ratios of antibody to antigen. The supernatant in this zone contained free antibody with no detectable antigen. As more antigen was added, the amount of antibody in the precipitate rose, but the ratio of antibody to antigen fell. At equivalence, no free antibody or antigen could be detected in the supernatant. As more antigen was added, the precipitate contained less antibody, but the ratio of antibody to antigen remained constant. The supernatant now contained antigen–antibody complexes, since the complexes at antigen excess were small enough to remain in solution. No unbound antibody was detected.

The lattice theory (83,84) is a model of the precipitation reaction that explains these observations. It assumes that antibodies are multivalent and antigens are bi- or polyvalent. Thus, long chains can form consisting of antibody linked to antigen linked to antibody, and so on. The larger the size of the aggregate, the less soluble the product, until a precipitate is formed. In the antibody excess zone, branch points can form whenever three antibodies bind to a single antigen, giving a large and insoluble product. For example, at the antibody to antigen ratio 2:1, every antigen molecule can bind three antibody molecules in a three-dimensional lattice structure. However, when equimolar amounts of antibody and antigen are mixed (the equivalence zone), the likelihood of more than two antibodies binding each antigen molecule decreases. The number of branch points decreases, and the product consists of longer chains of alternating antibody and antigen molecules. As the antigen concentration reaches excess, the precipitate approaches linear chains with molar ratio 1:1. At even higher antigen ratios, more antigen molecules will have 0 or 1 antibody bound. One antibody bound is equivalent to a chain termination, so shorter chain lengths are found, until the product is small enough to remain in solution. Such soluble antigen–antibody "immune complexes" are detectable in the antigen excess zone, where no free antibody is found.

Besides explaining the observed precipitation phenomena on a statistical basis, the lattice theory made the important prediction that antibodies are bivalent or multivalent. The subsequent structural characterization of antibodies (see Chapter 4) revealed their molecular weight and valency. Antibodies are indeed bivalent, except for IgM, which is functionally pentavalent and forms precipitates even more efficiently.

Antigens can be polyvalent either by having multiple copies of the same determinant or by having many different determinants, each of which reacts with different antibodies in a polyclonal antiserum. A good example of the former case, is described in Chapter 21. The predominant antigenic determinants of polysaccharides are often the nonreducing end of the chain. Branched chain polysaccharides have more than one end and are polyvalent. Nonbranched chains such as dextran (polymer of glucose) are monovalent for end-specific antidextran antibodies and do not precipitate them (85). However, a second group of antidextran antibodies is specific for internal glucose moieties. Since each dextran polymer consists of many of these internal units, it is polyvalent for internal $\alpha(1 \rightarrow A\ 6)$ linked glucose specific antibodies. Thus, unbranched dextran polymer can be used to distinguish between end-specific and internal-specific antibodies, as it will precipitate with the latter antibodies but not the former (85,86). Monomeric protein antigens, such as myoglobin (see Chapter 21) or lysozyme, are examples of the second case, because they behave as if they were polyvalent for heterogeneous antisera but monovalent for monoclonal antibodies. This results from the fact that each antigen molecule has multiple antigenic determinants but only one copy of each determinant. Thus, a polyspecific antiserum can bind more than one antibody to different determinants on the same molecule and form a lattice. However, using antibodies directed against a single determinant (e.g., a monoclonal antibody), no precipitate will form. In this case, antigen–antibody reactions must be measured by some other binding assay, such as RIA or ELISA.

Immunodiffusion and the Ouchterlony Method

One of the most useful applications of immunoprecipitation is in combination with a diffusion system (87). Diffusion could be observed by gently adding a drop of protein solution to a dish of water, without disturbing the liquid. The rate of migration of protein into the liquid is proportional to the concentration gradient times the diffusion coefficient of the protein according to Fick's law,

$$\frac{dQ}{dt} = -DA\frac{dc}{dx} \tag{43}$$

where Q is the amount of substance that diffuses across an area A per unit time t, D is the diffusion coefficient, which depends on the size of the molecule, and dc/dx is the concentration gradient. Since antibody molecules are so large, their diffusion coefficients are quite low, and diffusion often takes 1 day or more to cover the 5 mm to 20 mm required in most systems. In order to stabilize the liquid phase for such long periods of time, a gel matrix is added to provide support without hindering protein migration. In practice, 0.3% to 1.5% agar or agarose will permit migration of proteins up to the size of antibodies while preventing mechanical and thermal currents. By carefully adjusting the concentration of antibody and antigen, these systems can provide a simple analysis of the number of antigenic components and the concentration of a given component. By adjusting the geometry of the reactants entering the gel, immunodiffusion can provide useful information concerning antigenic identity or difference, or partial cross-reaction, as well as the purity of antigens and the specificity of antibodies.

In single diffusion methods (88–91), antibody is incorporated in the gel, and antigen is allowed to diffuse from one end of a tube gel or from a hole in a gel in a Petri dish in one or two dimensions, respectively. Over time, the antigen concentration reaches equivalence with the antibody in the gel, and a precipitin band forms. As more antigen diffuses, antigen excess is achieved at this position, so the precipitate dissolves and the boundary of equivalence moves farther. By integrating Fick's law, we find that the distance moved is proportional to the square root of time. If two species of antigen a and b are diffusing and the antiserum contains antibodies to both, two independent bands will form. These will move at independent rates, depending on antigen concentration in the sample, diffusion coefficient (size), and antibody concentration in the agar. Similarly, in the two-dimensional method, at a given radius of diffusion, antigen concentration will be equivalent to the antibody in the gel, and a precipitin ring will form. The higher the initial antigen concentration, the farther the antigen will diffuse before precipitating and the wider the area of the ring will be. The area of the ring is directly proportional to the initial antigen concentration. This method provides a convenient quantitative assay that can be used to measure immunoglobulin classes by placing test serum in the well and antiserum to each class of human immunoglobulin in the agar. Sensitivity can be increased by lowering the concentration of antiserum in the gel, giving wider rings, because the antigen must reach a lower concentration to be at equivalence. However, the antiserum cannot be diluted too far, or no precipitate will form.

The double diffusion methods use the same principles, except that instead of having one reactant incorporated in the gel at a constant concentration, both antigen and antibody are loaded some distance apart in a gel of pure agarose alone and allowed to diffuse toward each other. At some point in the gel, antigen diffusion and antibody diffusion will provide sufficient concentrations of both reactants for immunoprecipitation to occur. The line of precipitation becomes a barrier for the further diffusion of the reactants, so the precipitin band is stable. If the antigen preparation is heterogeneous and the antiserum is a heterogeneous mixture of antibodies, different bands will form for each pair of antigen and antibody reacting at positions dependent on concentration and molecular weight of each. The number of lines indicates the number of antigen–antibody systems reacting in the gel. The ability of immunodiffusion to separate different antigen–antibody systems gives a convenient estimate of antigen purity or antibody specificity.

In the most widely used Ouchterlony method of double diffusion in two dimensions (87), three or more wells are cut in an agarose gel in a dish in the pattern shown in Figure 5.14. Antigen a or b is placed in the upper wells, whereas antiserum containing anti-a or anti-b is placed in the lower well. Each antigen–antibody reaction system will form its own precipitin line between the wells. As shown in Figure 5.14A, this should extend an equal distance to the left and right of the wells. When different antigens are present in different wells (Figure 5.14C), the precipitating systems do not interact immunochemically, so the precipitin lines cross. However, when the same antigen is present in both wells (Figure 5.14B), each line of precipitation becomes a barrier preventing the antigen and antibody from diffusing past the precipitin line. This shortens the precipitin line on that side of the well. In addition, antigen diffusion from the neighboring wells shifts the zone of antigen excess, causing the equivalence line to deviate downward and meet between the two wells. Complete fusion

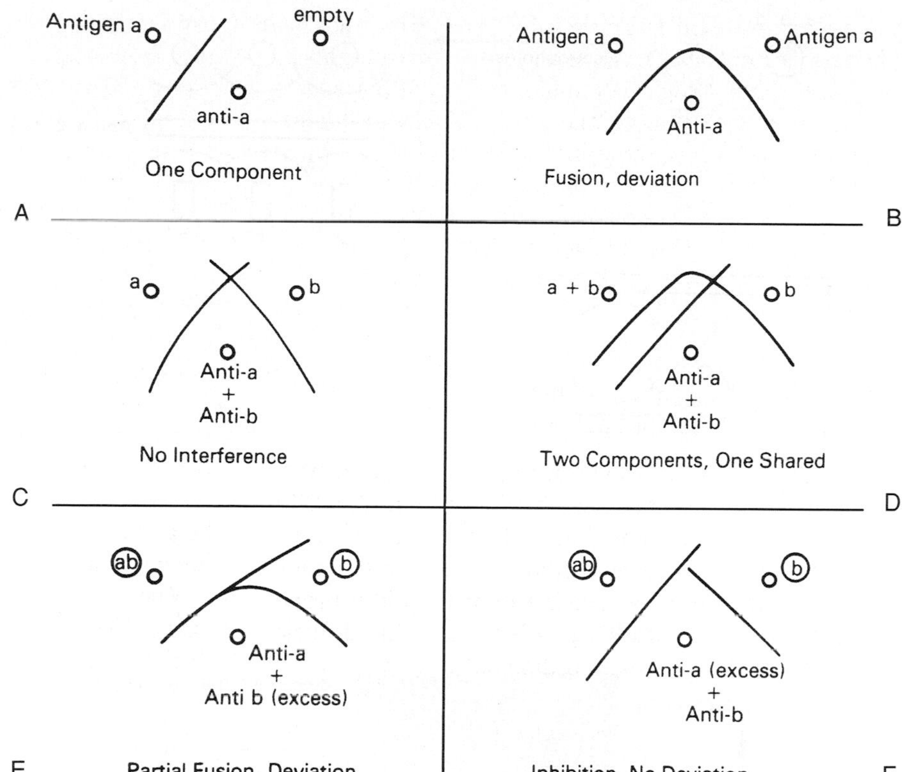

FIGURE 5.14 Immunodiffusion of two components in two dimensions. Cross-reactions produce inhibition (shortened bands) or deviation (curved bands). Lines of identity are shown in **B** and **D** (87).

of precipitin lines with no spurs is called a *line of identity,* indicating that the antigen in each well reacts with all antibody capable of reacting with antigen in the other well.

The analytical power of this method is shown in Figure 5.14D. When a mixed antigen sample is placed in one well, and pure antigen b is placed in the other well, antiserum to a plus b gives the pattern shown. Two precipitin lines form with the left well and one precipitin line with the right well. The line of complete fusion allows us to identify the second band as antigen b; the first band is antigen a. From their relative distance of migration, we can conclude that antigen a is in excess over antigen b, assuming their diffusion coefficients are comparable and both antibodies are present in equal amounts. Finally, since the precipitin line of antigen a-anti-a is not shortened at all, there is no contamination of the right sample with antigen a, and the two antigens do not cross-react.

The type of cross-reactivity detected by this Ouchterlony double immunodiffusion in agar is what we defined earlier as type 2 cross-reactivity. The method is not suitable for measuring affinity differences, required for quantitating type 1cross-reactivity. Sensitivity can be increased by use of radioactive antigen and detection of the precipitate by autoradiography.

Immunoelectrophoresis

Some antigen–antibody systems are too complex for double immunodiffusion analysis, either because there are too many bands or they are too close together. Immunoelectrophoresis combines electrophoresis in one dimension (Figure 5.15) with immunodiffusion in the perpendicular direction. In the first step, electrophoresis separates the test antigens according to charge and size, in effect separating the origin of diffusion of different antigens. This is equivalent to having each antigen start in a different well, as shown in the right-hand panel. A horizontal trough is then cut into the agar and filled with antiserum to all the components. Immunodiffusion occurs between the separated antigens and the linear source of antibody. The results for a mixture of three antigens approximate those shown for three antigens in separate wells (87). Fusion, deviation, and inhibition between precipitin lines can be analyzed as described earlier. The resolution of each band is somewhat decreased, due to widening of the origin of diffusion during electrophoresis. However, the immunodiffusion of unseparated human serum proteins, for example, is greatly facilitated by prior electrophoresis. Starting from a single well, only the heavier bands would be visible. However, prior electrophoresis makes it possible for each electrophoretic species to make its own precipitin line. Monospecific antiserum can be placed in a parallel horizontal trough, so that each band of precipitation can be identified. Immunoelectrophoresis is commonly used to diagnose myeloma proteins in human serum. The unknown serum is electrophoresed, followed by immunodiffusion against antibodies to human immunoglobulin heavy or light chains. A widening arc of IgG suggests the presence of an abnormal immunoglobulin species. At this same electrophoretic mobility, a precipitin line with

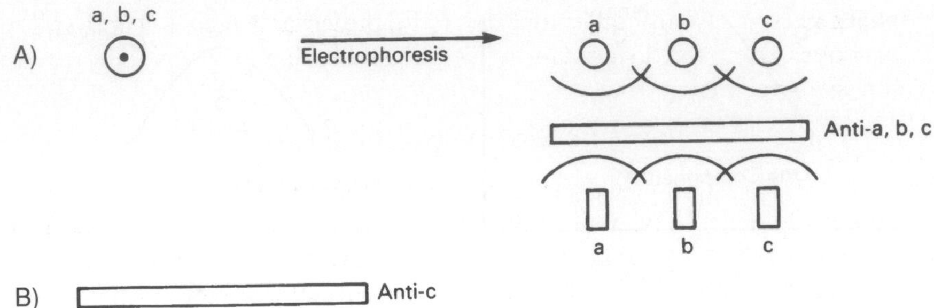

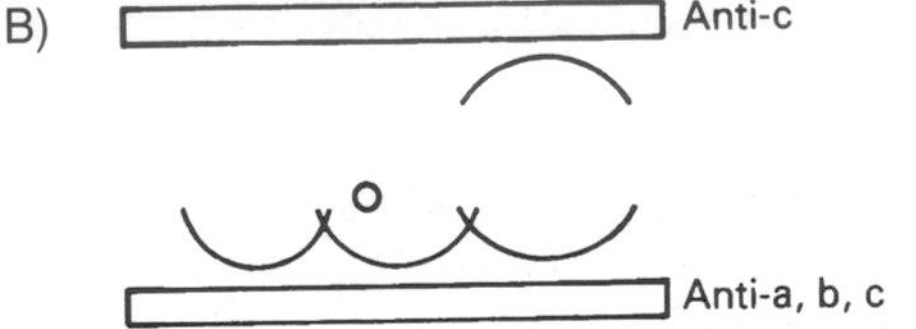

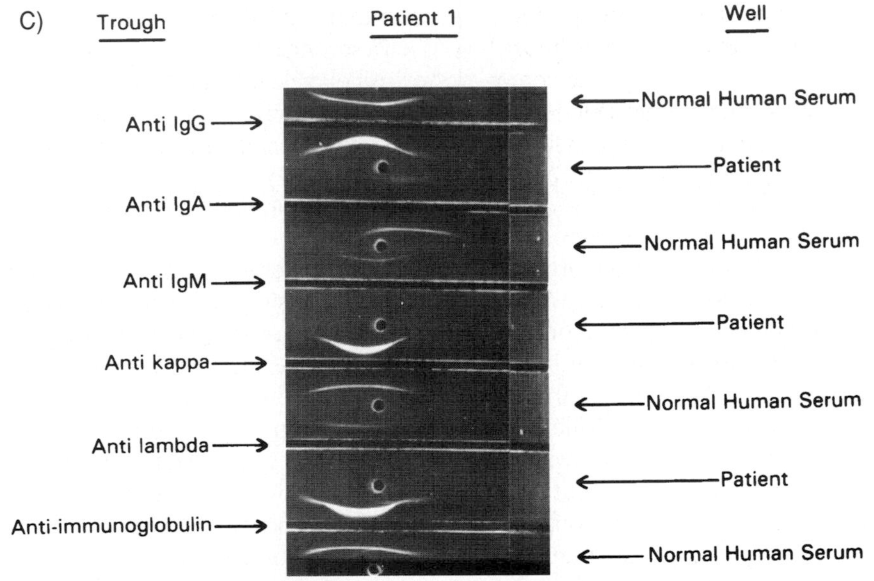

FIGURE 5.15 Immunoelectrophoresis. A sample containing multiple components is electrophoresed in an agarose gel, separating the antigens in the horizontal dimension. Then a horizontal trough is cut into the gel and antiserum is added. Immunodiffusion between the separated antigens and the trough is equivalent to having separate wells, each with a different antigen (87). This technique is used to identify a myeloma protein in human serum. Sera from the patient or normal individual were placed in the circular wells and electrophoresed. Antisera were then placed in the rectangular troughs and immunodiffusion proceeded perpendicular to the direction of electrophoresis. The abnormally strong reaction with anti-IgG and anti-κ, but no reaction with anti-λ antibodies, indicate a monoclonal protein (IgG,κ), because polyclonal Ig should react with both anti–light-chain antisera. Failure to form a band with anti-IgM and a reduced band with anti-IgA show typical reduction of normal immunoglobulins in this disease. Photographs courtesy of Theresa Wilson, NIH Clinical Chemistry Section.

anti-κ, but not anti-λ reactivity, strongly suggests the diagnosis of myeloma or monoclonal gammopathy, since these proteins arise from a single clone that synthesizes only one light chain. All normal electrophoretic species of human immunoglobulins contain both light chain isotypes, although κ exceeds λ by the ratio of 2:1 in humans. As shown in Figure 5.15C, the abnormal arc with γ mobility reacts with anti-IgG and anti-κ but not anti-λ antiserum. Thus, it is identified as an IgG-κ monoclonal protein.

Hemagglutination and Hemagglutination Inhibition

Hemagglutination

A highly sensitive technique yielding semiquantitative values for the interaction of antibody with antigen involves the agglutination by antibodies of red blood cells coated with the antigen (92). For exogenous antigens that are adsorbed to the red blood cell surface, the reaction is called *passive hemagglutination.* Untreated red blood cells are negatively charged, and electrostatic forces keep them apart. Following treatment with tannic acid (0.02 mg/ml for 10 minute at 37°C), however, they clump readily.

Untreated red blood cells are easily coated with polysaccharide antigens, which they adsorb readily. After tanning, the uptake of some protein antigens is good, giving a sensitive reagent, whereas for others it tends to be quite variable; coating red blood cells has been the limiting factor in the usefulness of this method for certain antigens. Apparently, slightly aggregated or partially denatured protein antigens are adsorbed preferentially (92).

The test for specific antibodies is done by serially diluting the antiserum in the U-shaped wells of a microtiter plate and adding antigen-coated red cells. When cross-linked by specific antibodies, agglutinated cells settle into an even carpet spread over the round bottom of the well. Unagglutinated red cells slide down the sides and form a much smaller button at the very bottom of the well. The titer of a sample is the highest dilution at which definite agglutination occurs. With hyperimmune antisera, inhibition of agglutination is observed at high doses of antibody, termed a *prozone effect.* Two interpretations have been offered: One is that, at great antibody excess, each cell is coated with antibody, so cross-linking by the same antibody molecule becomes improbable. The second interpretation is the existence of some species of inefficient or "blocking" antibodies that occupy antigen sites without causing aggregation of cells (9). To ensure antigen specificity, the antiserum should be absorbed against uncoated red cells prior to the assay, and an uncoated red cell control should be included with each assay. IgM is up to 750 times more efficient than IgG at causing agglutination, which may affect interpretation of data based on titration. The titer may vary by a factor of 2 simply due to subjective estimates of the endpoint.

Once the titer of an antiserum is determined, its interaction with antigen-coated red blood cells can be used as a sensitive assay for antigen. To constant amounts of antibody (diluted to a concentration twofold higher than the limiting concentration producing agglutination) are added varying amounts of free antigen. Agglutination will be inhibited when half or more of the antibody sites are occupied by free antigen. In a similar fashion, the assay can be used for the detection and quantitation of anti-idiotype antibodies that react with the variable region of antibodies and sterically block antigen binding.

Immunoblot (Western Blot)

A most useful technique in the analysis of proteins is polyacrylamide gel electrophoresis (PAGE), in which charged proteins migrate through a gel in response to an electric field. When ionic detergents such as sodium dodecyl sulfate are used, the distance traveled is inversely proportional to the logarithm of molecular weight. The protein components of complex structures, such as viruses, appear as distinct bands, each at its characteristic molecular weight. Because antibodies may be unable to diffuse into the gel, it is necessary to transfer the protein bands onto a nitrocellulose membrane support first, where they are exposed for antibody binding (93).

The immunoblot is often used to detect viral proteins with specific antibodies that bind these proteins on the nitrocellulose blot. Then a second antibody, which is either enzyme conjugated or radiolabeled, is used to detect the antigen–antibody band. Crude viral antigen preparations can be used, because only those bands that correspond to viral antigens will be detected.

Typical results are shown in Figure 5.16. Human immunodeficiency virus type 1 (HIV-1) was cultured in susceptible H9 cells. The viral proteins were separated by PAGE and detected by immunoblot, using the serum of infected patients. Each antigen band recognized by the antiserum has been identified as a viral component or

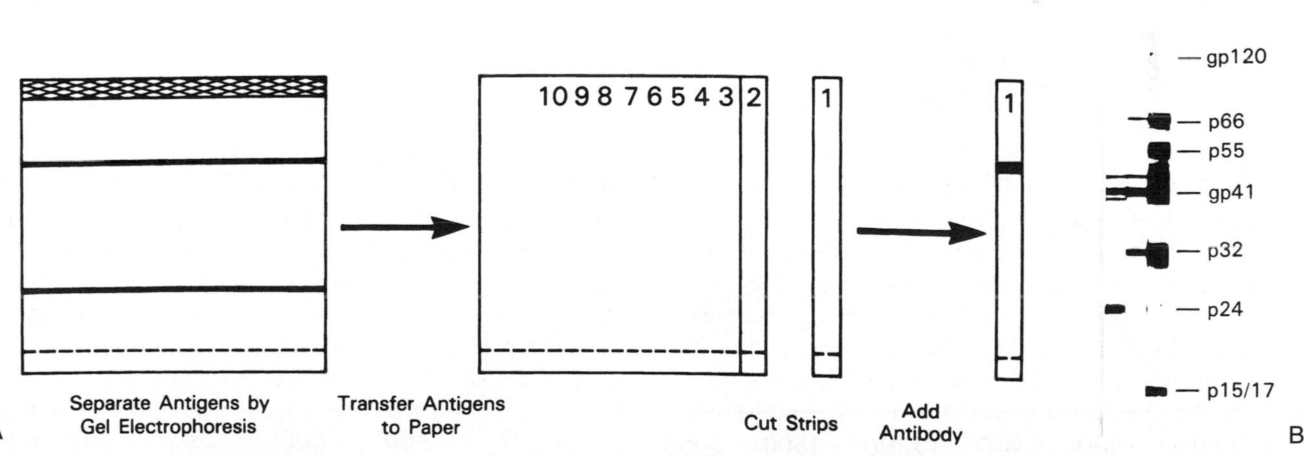

FIGURE 5.16 **A:** Western blot technique. The antigen preparation is run through a polyacrylamide gel, which separates its components into different bands. These bands are then transferred to paper by electrophoresis in the horizontal dimension. The paper is cut into strips. Each strip is incubated with test antibodies, followed by further incubation with enzyme-labeled second antibodies. If the test antibodies bind to the component antigens, they will produce discrete dark bands at the corresponding positions on the strip. **B:** Clinical specimens from AIDS patients tested on strips bearing HIV-1 viral antigens, showing antibodies to viral gag (p15/17, p24, and p55 precursor), pol (p66 and possibly p32), and env (gp41 and gp120) proteins. Lane 1 is the negative control, and lanes 2 to 4 are sera from three different patients.

precursor protein. The gp160 precursor is processed to mature gp120 and gp41 envelope proteins, while a p66 precursor is processed to the p51 mature form of reverse transcriptase, and a p55 precursor becomes the p24 and p17 gag and matrix proteins of the virus (94). The practical uses of the HIV western blot include diagnosing infection, screening blood units to prevent HIV transmission, and testing new vaccines.

Surface Plasmon Resonance (SPR)

SPR uses the electromagnetic properties of light to measure the binding affinity of a variety of biological molecules, including antigen–antibody pairs. In this method, polarized light passes through a glass plate coated on the back surface with a thin metal film, usually gold. Biological materials binding to the metal film behind the plate can alter its refractive index in ways that affect the angle and intensity of reflected light.

At angles close to perpendicular, light will pass through the glass, although it will bend at the interface due to differences in the refractive index of glass and what is behind it. Above a certain angle, called the *critical angle,* bending will be so great that total internal reflection will occur. Small changes in refractive index behind the glass can be detected as significant changes in the critical angle, where light reflection occurs, and in the intensity of reflected light at this angle. By reading the reflected light intensity in a diode array detector, the critical angle and intensity can be determined simultaneously. Due to the wave nature of light, the effect of refractive index in the gold film extends about one wavelength beyond the glass, or about 300 nm to 700 nm (95). Within this layer, if an antigen is covalently attached to the gold, then antibody binding can be detected as a change in refractive index, resulting in a different critical angle and intensity of the reflected light.

SPR systems have three essential features (96): an optical system that allows determination of the critical angle and light intensity at the same time; a coupling chemistry that links antigen or antibody to the gold surface; and a flow system that rapidly delivers the binding molecule in the mobile phase, so SPR can measure the rate of binding, rather than the rate of diffusion. Because binding causes a physical change in the gold film, there is no need to detect binding with radioactive labels or enzyme conjugates. Molecular binding interactions can be followed in real time.

A typical SPR experiment is shown in Figure 5.17. HIV gp120 of type IIIB (left panel) or MN (right panel) were fixed to the gold layer, and various concentrations of

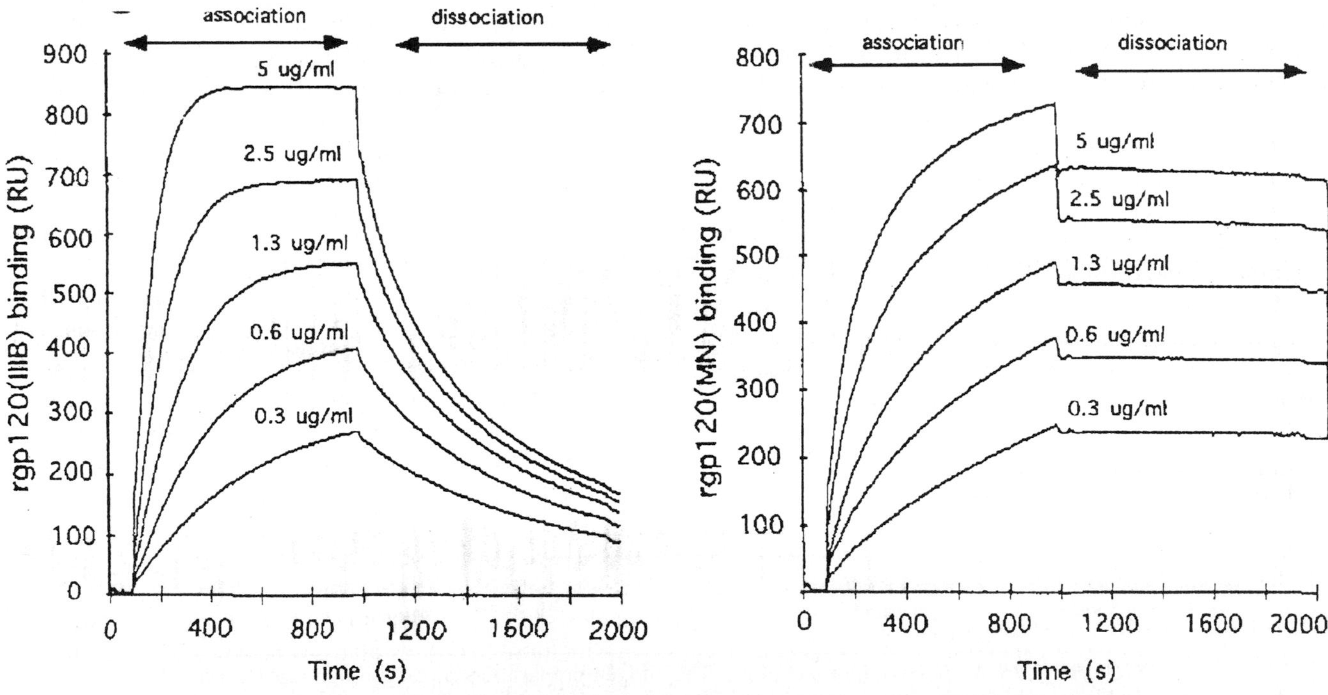

FIGURE 5.17 Monoclonal antibody to gp120 was introduced into the flow cell at time 0, and antibody binding was followed over time as a change in the critical angle, measured in response units. After 1,000 seconds, free antibody was washed out, and the release of bound antibody was measured as a decrease in refractive index. Lower-affinity binding to gp120 from the IIIB strain (left) was shown as a faster "off rate," as compared to the very slow rate of antibody release from the MN strain (right). These results, obtained under nonequilibrium conditions, provide direct measurement of the forward and reverse rate constants for antibody binding, and the ratio of these two gives the affinity constant. Modified from (97), with permission.

monoclonal antibody to gp120 were added to the flow cell (97). Over the first 1,000 seconds, antibody binding was measured as a change in reflected light (in response units), allowing a calculation of the rate constant for the forward reaction of antibody binding. Once the signal reached a plateau, antibody was washed out of the flow cell, and the decrease in SPR signal over time indicated the rate at which antibody came off the antigen. The "on rate" for antibody binding to IIIB gp120 (left) was about twice as fast as for MN (right) at each antibody concentration. However, the "off rate" was about 50-fold less for MN than for IIIB. Combining these kinetic results indicates much greater binding affinity for gp120 of MN type, which may explain the observation that MN type virus was 10-fold more sensitive to neutralization by this antibody than was the IIIB strain.

MONOCLONAL ANTIBODIES

Homogeneous immunoglobulins have long played important roles in immunological research. Starting in the 1950s, Kunkel and colleagues studied sera from human patients with multiple myeloma and recognized the relationship between abnormal myeloma proteins and normal serum globulins (98). Potter and colleagues characterized numerous mouse myeloma tumors and identified some of their antigenic specificities (99). Human and mouse myeloma proteins were studied as representative immunoglobulins and recognized for the advantages they had with proteins as diverse as antibodies, for studies of immunoglobulin structure, function, and genetics. It was not yet possible, however, to induce monoclonal immunoglobulins of desired specificity.

This goal was achieved by the introduction of hybridoma technology by Köhler and Milstein (1,100) and by Margulies and colleagues (101) in the 1970s. Since that time, monoclonal antibodies have come to play an enormous role in biological research and applications. They offer as advantages the relative ease of the production and purification of large quantities of antibody, the uniformity of antibody batches, and the ready availability of Ig mRNA and DNA from the hybrid cell lines.

Derivation of Hybridomas

Hybridomas producing monoclonal antibodies are generated by the somatic cell fusion of two cell types: antibody-producing cells from an immunized animal, which by themselves die in tissue culture in a relatively short time, and myeloma cells, which contribute their immortality in tissue culture to the hybrid cell. The myeloma cells are variants carrying drug selection markers, so only those myeloma cells that have fused with spleen cells providing the missing enzyme will survive under selective conditions. Initial work used myeloma cells that secreted their own immunoglobulin products, but later such fusion partners were replaced by myeloma variants that fail to express Ig (102,103), so that the fused cell secretes exclusively antibody of the desired specificity. Successful hybridoma production is influenced by the characteristics of the cell populations (immune lymphocytes and myeloma fusion partner), the fusion conditions, and the subsequent selection and screening of the hybrids. A diagrammatic version of the overall process of hybridoma derivation is presented in Figure 5.18.

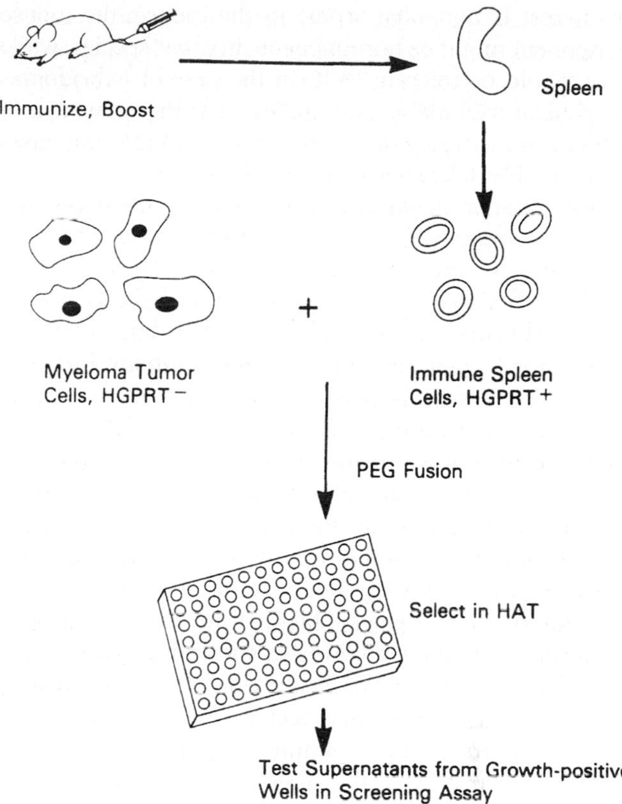

FIGURE 5.18 Production of hybridomas. Steps in the derivation of hybridomas can be outlined as shown. Spleen cells from immunized donors are fused with myeloma cells bearing a selection marker. The fused cells are then cultured in selective medium until visible colonies grow, and their supernatants are then screened for antibody production.

This section will not attempt to provide a detailed, step-by-step protocol for laboratory use. For that purpose, the reader is referred to monographs and reviews on the subject, including a detailed lab protocol with many hints and mention of problems to avoid (104).

Hybridomas Derived from Species Other than Mice

Laboratory mice are the most common species immunized for hybridoma production, but for a variety of reasons, other animal species often have advantages. If an antigen of interest is nonpolymorphic in the mouse, the mouse component might be immunogenic in other species, while mice would be tolerant to it. In the case of hybridomas for clinical use, mouse antibodies have the drawback of inducing anti–mouse immunoglobulin immune responses with possible deleterious effects.

Several approaches have been taken to the derivation of hybridomas in species other than mouse. First, interspecies hybridization can be performed using mouse myeloma fusion partners. The resulting hybrids are often unstable and throw off chromosomes, but clones can sometimes be selected that produce antibody in a stable fashion. Examples of this would be rat–mouse fusion to produce antibody to the mouse Fc receptor (105), and hamster–mouse fusion to produce antibody to the mouse CD3 equivalent (106). Rabbit–mouse hybridomas have also been described (107).

A second approach is the use of fusion partner cells from the desired species. Myeloma variants carrying drug selection markers are available in a number of species. A rat myeloma line adapted for this purpose, IR983F, was described by Bazin (108). Production of human hybridomas is of special importance, because their use in therapies would avoid the problem of human immune responses to Ig derived from other animal species, as discussed in detail in the later section on applications.

Use of Gene Libraries to Derive Monoclonal Antibodies

Monoclonal antibodies produced by hybridoma technology are derived from B cells of immunized animals. A recent alternative technology uses gene libraries and expression systems instead. This approach has the advantages of avoiding labor-intensive immunizations of animals and the screening of antibody-containing supernatants. Another advantage of the approach is circumventing tolerance. One can derive mAbs to antigens expressed in the animal species that donated the gene library, including highly conserved antigens for which there may be no available responder that does not express the antigen.

The first version of such an approach involved preparation of V_H and $V\kappa$ libraries and expression of the libraries in bacteria. Further development of the system led to use of V_H and V_L libraries made separately, and then preparation of a combinatorial library by cleaving, mixing, and religating the libraries at a restriction site (109,110). A linker can be used so that V_H and V_L can both be expressed on one covalent polypeptide; the flexibility of the linker allows association of the V_H and V_L in a normal three-dimensional configuration and thus formation of an antigen-binding site (110).

Another innovation involves expression of V_H and $V\kappa$ genes on the surface of bacteriophage as fusion proteins with a phage protein, to permit rapid screening of large numbers of sequences (110–112). Adsorption of antibody-bearing phage on antigen-coated surfaces allows positive selection of phage containing DNA encoding the desired variable region fragment (Fv) from combinatorial variable region gene libraries (111,112).

Human antibody gene sequences can be recovered by PCR from peripheral blood cells (113), bone marrow (114), or human cells reimmunized in SCID-hu mice (115). The phage display technique can then be used to select antigen-binding clones and derive human reagents of desired specificity, such as antibody to hepatitis surface antigen (113) or HIV envelope (114).

One limitation in the phage library technique initially was low affinity of the mAbs derived, because they were generated by a random process and not subject to further somatic mutation. Several approaches have now been used to improve affinities. Hypermutation and selection has now been achieved *in vitro* by a strategy using a bacterial mutator strain (116). The process involves multiple rounds of mutation followed by growth in nonmutator bacteria and then selection for high-affinity binding led to an overall 100-fold increase in affinity (116). Improved affinity has also been achieved by use of site-directed mutagenesis to alter residues in hypervariable regions affecting dissociation rates (117).

Applications of Monoclonal Antibodies

Since monoclonal antibodies can be made easily and reproducibly in large quantities, they allow many experiments that were not possible or practical before. Affinity chromatography based on monoclonal antibodies can be used as a step in purification of molecular species that are difficult to purify chemically. Homogeneous antibody can be crystallized and can also be crystallized together with antigen to permit the study of the structure of antibody and of antigen–antibody complexes by x-ray diffraction. Homogeneous antibodies are also very valuable in the study of antibody diversity. Such analyses have revealed much about the roles of somatic mutation, changes in affinity, and changes in clonal dominance in antibody responses.

Catalytic Antibodies

One area of recent interest is the use of antibody molecules to catalyze chemical reactions (118). In this role, antibodies serve as an alternative to enzymes, an alternative that can be customized and manipulated more easily in some cases.

The concept of antibodies as catalysts had been proposed a long time ago by D. W. Woolley (cited in ref. 118). Use of homogeneous antibodies permitted identification of some with significant catalytic effects; MOPC167 accelerates the hydrolysis of nitrophenyl-phosphorylcholine by 770-fold (119). Polyclonal antibodies have also been reported to possess detectable enzymatic activity (120). With the advent of hybridoma technology, purposeful selection of antibodies with potent enzymatic function became possible. Antibodies have been characterized that catalyze numerous chemical reactions, with rates nearing 10^8-fold above the spontaneous rate (reviewed in ref. 118). One common strategy for elicitation of such antibodies is immunization with transition state analogs (121), although there are other strategies (122). Antibodies function as catalysts in a stereospecific manner (123), a valuable property.

Molecular mechanisms of antibody-mediated catalysis vary, as do enzymatic reactions (122,124). To accelerate a reaction, an antibody has to lower the activation energy barrier to the reaction, which means lowering the energy of the transition state by stabilizing it. For this reason, an antibody that recognizes the transition state is favorable, and immunizations with analogs of the transition state have advantages.

Antibodies can serve as what has been termed an entropy trap (118); binding to the antibody "freezes out" the rotational and translational degrees of freedom of the substrate and thus makes a chemical reaction far more favorable energetically. Interactions with chemical groups on the antibody can neutralize charges or bury hydrophobic groups, thereby stabilizing a constrained transition state.

Discovery of such catalytic antibodies opens practical opportunities: antibodies can be customized for an application by appropriate selection and can be produced relatively cheaply and purified easily. Catalytic antibodies can be developed to perform chemical reactions for which no enzyme is available. They can shield intermediates from solvent—for example, allowing reactions that do not occur in aqueous solution (125). They can form peptide bonds (126), suggesting a new approach to polypeptide synthesis. Thus, catalytic antibodies will likely have many practical applications.

Bispecific and Bifunctional Antibodies

Antibodies produced naturally by a single B cell have only one binding site specificity, and their effector functions are determined by the structure of the Fc domain. The availability of monoclonal antibodies made possible the generation in quantity of artificial antibodies as cross-linking reagents, by linking binding sites of two specificities to form bispecific antibodies. A variety of techniques have been used to prepare such hybrid or bispecific antibodies, and they have been put to a variety of uses. In addition, antibody binding sites can be linked to other functional domains, such as toxins, enzymes, or cytokines, to create "bifunctional antibodies" (127).

One of the most powerful uses of hybrid antibodies is in redirecting cytolytic cells to targets of a defined specificity. In one early demonstration of this use (128), a monoclonal antibody specific for the Fcγ receptor and one specific for the hapten DNP were chemical cross-linked. In the presence of this hybrid antibody, FcγR-bearing cells were able to lyse haptenated target cells specifically. The FcγR played a critical role; antibody to MHC class I antigens on the cell could not be substituted. Antibody to the T cell receptor complex has also been used extensively to redirect T cell lysis to desired targets. For example, anti-CD3 was cross-linked to antitumor antibodies and mixed with effector cells. These "targeted T cells" were able to inhibit the growth of human tumor cells *in vivo* in nude mice (129). Bispecific antibodies have also been used recently to alter the tropism of a viral gene therapy vector to target specific cells (130).

Cumbersome cross-linking chemistry can now be replaced by genetic engineering for creation of designer antibodies (127). Bifunctional and bispecific antibodies can be engineered as single chain variable fragment (scFv) constructs or by specialized strategies using two chains. A wide variety of configurations are possible and can be used to make multivalent reagents as well as reagents with one site of each specificity. Tags can be built in by fusion of additional sequence such as streptavidin, or, as mentioned earlier, antibody domains can be combined with other functional domains, such as toxins, enzymes, or cytokines.

Clinical Applications

The possible clinical uses of monoclonal antibodies are many. *In vitro,* they are widely used in RIA and ELISA measurements of substances in biological fluids, from hormones to toxins. They are also extremely valuable in flow cytometric assays of cell populations using antibodies specific for differentiation antigens expressed on cell surfaces. Monoclonal antibodies plus complement or toxin-conjugated monoclonal antibodies have also been used to remove T cells from bone marrow prior to transplantation (131).

In vivo, although it took more than two decades for the original promise of hybridoma technology to be translated into widespread clinical applications, a number of monoclonal antibodies are now in use or in trials for a variety of purposes (reviewed in 132–134). Monoclonal antibody OKT3 directed to a marker on human T lymphocytes is used as a treatment for rejection reactions in kidney transplant patients (135). Other monoclonal antibodies, for example, ^{111}In-labeled CYT-103 referred to as *Oncoscint* (136), are used as diagnostic tumor-imaging reagents. Monoclonal antibodies are have now been approved for a variety of therapeutic uses (134,137). Cancer therapies use either unconjugated monoclonal antibody (132,138–142) or toxin-coupled (143,144) or radiolabeled monoclonal antibody (138,142,145). Molecules targeted in cancer therapies include CD25 (IL-2 receptor alpha chain) in adult T cell leukemia (132,134,142,146–148); CD20 in non-Hodgkin lymphoma using either unlabeled (141,149) or more recently, radionuclide-labeled anti-CD20 (150,151); the HER-2/neu oncoprotein in breast and ovarian cancer (139,140,152,153); CD22 in hairy cell leukemia (144); vascular endothelial growth factor to limit angiogenesis in diverse tumors, especially colorectal, renal, and non–small-cell lung cancer (154–159); antiepidermal growth factor receptor in colorectal carcinoma and others (160); anti-CD52 in chronic lymphocytic leukemia (161); and anti-CD33 in acute myelogenous leukemia (162). Other therapies studied include anti-LPS for treatment of sepsis, anti-IL-6 receptor for treatment of multiple myeloma, and anti-IgE for treatment of allergy (surveyed in 133), and anti-TNF for treatment of arthritis (163,164), anti-RSV for prevention of RSV morbidity and mortality in infants (165,166), and anti-IL-2 receptor (CD25) for prevention of graft rejection (142,167), as well as for treatment of autoimmune diseases such as uveitis (168) and multiple sclerosis (169).

In the specialized case of B cell lymphoma, monoclonal anti-idiotypes against the idiotype expressed by the patient's tumor have been tested as a "magic bullet" therapy (170). Active immunization of the patient with idiotype (171–175) has the advantage that escape mutants (176) are less likely to emerge because multiple idiotopes are recognized. Another approach under study is immunization using not idiotype as protein but plasmid DNA encoding patient idiotype (177). This approach would have additional advantages, such as ease of preparing customized reagents for each patient.

Production of Human or Humanized Monoclonal Antibodies

Many of the side effects of monoclonal antibodies in clinical use are due to the foreign Ig-constant regions. Recognition of foreign Ig epitopes can lead to sensitization and so preclude subsequent use in the same individual of different monoclonal antibodies. Thus, monoclonal antibodies with some or all structure derived from human Ig have advantages. Several approaches have been taken employing fusion of human cells with animal myelomas or with human tumor cells of various kinds (178,179), and use of Epstein-Barr virus to immortalize antibody-producing cells (180). Production of populations of sensitized human cells to be fused presents another special problem, since the donors cannot be immunized at will. In one example, *in vitro* stimulation of lymphocytes with antigen followed by fusion with mouse myeloma cells has been used to generate a series of antibodies to varicella zoster (181).

Another approach to production of monoclonal antibodies with human characteristics involves application of genetic engineering. The part of the antibody structure recognized as foreign by humans can be minimized by combining human constant regions with mouse variable regions (182,183) or even just mouse hypervariable segments (184) by molecular genetic techniques. Antigen-binding specificity is retained in some cases, and the "humanized" chimeric molecules have many of the advantages of human hybridomas.

Production of fully human mAbs in transgenic mice has now been achieved by multiple laboratories. The strategy has involved insertion into the mouse germline of constructs containing clusters of human Ig V, D, J, and C genes to generate one transgenic line, and targeted disruption of the mouse heavy chain and κ chain loci to generate another transgenic line. From these two lines, mice are then bred that express only human antibodies.

To show feasibility of this approach, cosmids carrying parts of the human heavy chain locus were used to make transgenic mice (185). The next step was to produce mice carrying human genes for both heavy and light chains to generate a functional human repertoire. Several groups using different technologies constructed heavy chain miniloci containing functional V segments representing several major V region families, D and J segments, constant and switch regions, and enhancers. κ chain constructs were made that contained multiple functional $V\kappa$ segments, the J segments, $C\kappa$, and enhancers (186,187). Mice were bred that were homozygous both for the transgene loci and for disruption of the mouse heavy chain and κ light chain loci; note that the mouse λ locus was left intact. The human Ig genes could rearrange in the mouse genome, and expression of human Ig resulted. If these mice were immunized with a fragment of tetanus toxin, resulting antibodies included some that were fully human (187). In one of the studies (186), serum contained human μ, $\gamma 1$, and κ, as well as mouse λ and γ. Immunization of such mice with various antigens led to class switching, somatic mutation, and production of human antibodies of affinities of almost 10^8 m^{-1}.

Ig expression in these mice demonstrates cross-species compatibility of the components involved in antibody gene rearrangement and diversification. The mice also provide a responder able to provide fully human antibodies to clinically important antigens, and they have the advantage that they are not tolerant to human antigens, such as the human IgE and human CD4 used by Lonberg, et al. (186).

Nucleotide Aptamers: An Alternative to mAbs

Antibodies are not the only biological macromolecules that have evolved to permit an enormous range of specific structures. Oligonucleotides selected for ability to bind a ligand with high affinity and specificity are termed *aptamers* and can be used in many of the ways antibodies have been used. Selection, properties, and uses of aptamers have been reviewed (188). Aptamers have the advantage that their production does not require animals or cell culture. These well-defined reagents may be used increasingly in diagnostic testing and are also being tested in clinical trials for use as imaging agents or therapeutics.

Specificity and Cross-reactivity

Specificity of Monoclonal Antibodies

Because all the molecules in a sample of monoclonal antibody have the same variable region structure, barring variants arising after cloning, they all have the same specificity. This uniformity has the advantage that batches of monoclonal antibody do not vary in specificity as polyclonal sera often do. The most obvious fact about cross-reactions of monoclonal antibodies is that they are characteristic of all molecules and cannot be removed by absorption without removing all activity. An exception would be an apparent cross-reaction due to a subset of denatured antibody molecules, which could be removed on the basis of that binding. The homogeneity of monoclonal antibodies allows refinement of specificity analysis that was not possible with polyclonal sera. A few examples follow.

First, one can use monoclonal antibodies to distinguish closely related ligands in cases where most antibodies in a polyclonal serum would cross-react and so absorption of a serum would not leave sufficient activity to define additional specificities. This ability is useful in designing clinical assays for related hormones, for example. Such fine discrimination also allows the definition of new specificities on complex antigens. When large numbers of monoclonal antibodies specific for class I and class II MHC antigens were analyzed, some defined specificities that could not be defined with existing polyclonal antisera (189–191).

However, monoclonal antibodies are also a powerful tool for demonstrating similarities rather than distinctions between two antigens. In some cases, only a minor portion of an antibody response detects a cross-reaction, and so it is not detected by polyclonal reagents. For example, determinants shared by the I-A and I-E class II MHC antigens in the mouse were demonstrated using monoclonal antibodies (191), while they had been suspected but were difficult to demonstrate using polyclonal sera.

Another type of fine specificity analysis possible only with monoclonal antibodies is the discrimination of spatial sites (epitope clusters) by competitive binding. In some cases, such epitope clusters correspond to specificities that are readily distinguished by other means. However, in other cases, the epitope clusters may not be distinguishable by any serologic or genetic means. An example is the splitting of the classical specificity Ia.7 into three epitope clusters by competitive binding with monoclonal antibodies (191). The epitopes cannot be distinguished genetically, because all three are expressed on cells of all Ia.7-positive mouse strains. Thus, polyclonal sera cannot be absorbed to reveal the different specificities. Only with the use of monoclonal antibodies were the epitopes resolved from each other.

The importance of this type of analysis is shown by another example—the definition of epitope clusters on CD4, a surface molecule on a subset of human T cells that also functions as the receptor for HIV. Monoclonal antibodies to CD4 can be divided into several groups based on competitive inhibition (192). The cluster containing the site recognized by OKT4A is closely related to virus infection, since antibodies to this site block syncytium formation. The cluster recognized by OKT4, however, is not related to infection because antibodies to it do not block syncytium formation (192), and cells expressing variant forms of the CD4 molecule lacking the OKT4 epitope can still be infected by HIV (193). This information about the sites on the molecule is important in understanding the molecular interactions of virus with its receptor and may be useful in designing vaccine candidates.

Although most antibodies are not MHC-restricted in their recognition of antigens, distinguishing them from T cell receptors, antibodies can be selected that recognize peptide-MHC complexes (MHC-restricted antipeptide antibodies or peptide-dependent anti-MHC class I antibodies) (194–196). Several monoclonal antibodies have been selected that require both a certain MHC class I antigen and a particular peptide for reactivity. Such mAbs are useful reagents capable of detecting cells presenting the appropriate peptide-MHC complexes on their surfaces (194). Such mAbs may also be useful in dissection of T cell responses. In one study, the mAbs could inhibit IL-2 secretion by a T cell hybridoma of corresponding specificity and could also block induction of CTL recognizing that epitope when given in vivo during priming (196). Such mAbs have been used to address structural questions about antigen recognition by T and B cells (195). Such antibodies also appeared to skew the repertoire of T cells for this particular HIV peptide–MHC complex to specific TCR Vβ types and T cell avidities (197). However, only very rare mAbs have this type of specificity, and they were purposely selected in the fusions, so they do not provide a general comparison of TCR and Ab characteristics.

Cross-reactions of Monoclonal Antibodies

Monoclonal antibodies display many type 1 cross-reactions, emphasizing that antibody cross-reactions represent real similarities among the antigens, not just an effect of heterogeneity of serum antibodies. Even antigens that differ for most of their structure can share one determinant, and a monoclonal antibody recognizing this site would then give a 100% cross-reaction. An example is the reactivity of autoantibodies in lupus with both DNA and cardiolipin (198).

It should be emphasized that sharing a "determinant" does not mean that the antigens contain identical chemical structures; instead, they bear a chemical resemblance that may not be well understood—for example, a distribution of surface charges. Antibodies to the whole range of antigens can react with immunoglobulins in idiotype anti-idiotype reactions, showing a cross-reactivity of the same antibodies with proteins (the anti-idiotypes) and with the carbohydrates, nucleic acids, lipids, or haptens against which they were raised.

Polyclonal versus Monoclonal Antibodies

When monoclonal antibodies first became available, some people expected that they would be exquisitely specific and would be superior to polyclonal sera for essentially all purposes. Further thought about the issues discussed here, however, suggests that this is not always the case and depends on the intended use of the antibodies. Not only do monoclonal antibodies cross-react, but when they do, the cross-reaction is not minor and cannot be removed by absorption. A large panel of monoclonal antibodies may be needed before one is identified with the precise range of reactivity desired for a study.

In polyclonal sera, however, each different antibody has a distinct range of reactivity, and the only common feature would be detectable reactivity with the antigen used for immunization or testing. Thus, the serum as a whole may show only a low-titered cross-reaction with any other particular antigen, and that cross-reaction can be removed by absorption, leaving substantial activity against the immunizing antigen. For the purposes of an experiment, a polyclonal serum may be "more specific" than any one of its clonal parts and may be more useful. This concept is the basis of the theory of multispecificity (see earlier discussion).

Polyclonal sera also have advantages in certain technical situations such as immunoprecipitation in which multivalency is important. Many antigens are univalent with respect to monoclonal antibody binding but display multiple distinct sites that can be recognized by different components of polyclonal sera. Thus, a greater degree of crosslinking can be achieved.

The ultimate serological reagent in many cases may well be a mixture of monoclonal antibodies that have been chosen according to their cross-reactions. The mixture would be better defined and more reproducible than a polyclonal antiserum and would have the same advantage of overlapping specificities.

CONCLUSION

In conclusion, antibodies, whether monoclonal or polyclonal, provide a unique type of reagent that can be made with high specificity for almost any desired organic or biochemical structure, often with extremely high affinity. These can be naturally divalent (e.g., in the case of IgG) or multivalent (e.g., in the case of IgM) or can be made as monovalent molecules, such as Fab or recombinant Fv fragments. They serve not only as a major arm of host defense, playing a major role in the protective efficacy of most existing antiviral and all antibacterial vaccines, but also as very versatile tools for research and clinical use. RIAs and ELISAs have revolutionized the detection of minute quantities of biological molecules, such as hormones and cytokines, and thus have become indispensable for clinical diagnosis and monitoring of patients, as well as for basic and applied research. Current solid-phase versions of these take advantage not only of the intrinsic affinity and specificity of the antibodies, but also of the implicit multivalency and local high concentration on a solid surface. Cross-reactivity of antibodies often provides the first clue to relationships between molecules that might not otherwise have been compared. Conversely, methods that use antigens to detect the presence of antibodies in serum have become widespread in testing for exposure to a variety of pathogens, such as HIV. Antibodies also provide specific reagents invaluable in the rapid purification of many other molecules by affinity chromatography. They have also become indispensable reagents for other branches of biology—for example, in histocompatibility typing and phenotyping of cells using a myriad of cell-surface markers that were themselves discovered with monoclonal antibodies, and for separating these cells by fluorescence activated cell sorting, panning, or chromatographic techniques. Monoclonal antibodies have also finally emerged as clinically important therapeutics in cancer, arthritis, organ graft rejection, and infectious diseases. Thus, antibodies are among the most versatile and widely used types of reagents today, and their use is constantly growing. Understanding the fundamental concepts in antigen–antibody interactions thus has become essential not only to an understanding of immunology, but also to the effective use of these valuable molecules in many other fields.

ACKNOWLEDGMENTS

We thank Drs. Charles DeLisi, Elvin A. Kabat, and Henry Metzger for their detailed critique of the manuscript, as well as many helpful discussions, and Dr. Fred Karush for valuable suggestions.

REFERENCES

1. Köhler G, Milstein C. Derivation of specific antibody-producing tissue culture and tumor lines by cell fusion. *Eur J Immunol* 1976;6: 511–519.
2. Melchers F, Potter M, Warner NC. *Lymphocyte hybridomas*. Berlin: Springer-Verlag, 1978.
3. Kennett RH, McKearn TJ, Bechtol KB. *Monoclonal Antibodies. Hybridomas: A New Dimension in Biological Analyses*. New York: Plenum Press, 1980.

4. Moore WJ. *Physical chemistry*. 3rd ed. Englewood Cliffs, NJ: Prentice-Hall, 1962.
5. Myszka DG, Sweet RW, Hensley P, et al. Energetics of the HIV gp120-CD4 binding reaction. *Proc Natl Acad Sci U S A* 2000;97: 9026–31.
6. Kwong PD, Doyle ML, Casper DJ, et al. HIV-1 evades antibody-mediated neutralization through conformational masking of receptor-binding sites. *Nature* 2002;420:678–82.
7. DeLisi C. The biophysics of ligand-receptor interactions. *Q Rev Biophys* 1980;13:201–230.
8. Fersht A. *Enzyme structure and mechanisms*. New York: Freeman, 1977.
9. Eisen HN. *Immunology*. 2nd ed. Baltimore: Harper & Row, 1980.
10. Sachs DH, Schecter AN, Eastlake A, et al. Inactivation of staphylococcal nuclease by the binding of antibodies to a distinct antigenic determinant. *Biochem* 1972;11:4268–4273.
11. Hammes GG. Relaxation spectrometry of biological systems. *Adv Protein Chem* 1968;23:1–57.
12. Eisen HN, Karush F. The interaction of purified antibody with homologous hapten. Antibody valence and binding constant. *J Am Chem Soc* 1949;71:363–364.
13. Pinckard RN. Equilibrium dialysis and preparation of hapten conjugates. 1978;1:1–17.
14. Scatchard G. The attractions of proteins for small molecules and ions. *Ann NY Acad Sci* 1949;51:660–672.
15. Berzofsky JA, Hicks G, Fedorko J, et al. Properties of monoclonal antibodies specific for determinants of a protein antigen, myoglobin. *J Biol Chem* 1980;255:11188–11191.
16. Rodbard D, Munson PJ, Thakur AK. Quantitative characterization of hormone receptors. *Cancer* 1980;46:2907–2918.
17. Thakur AK, Jaffe ML, Rodbard D. Graphical analysis of ligand-binding systems: evaluation by Monte Carlo studies. *Anal Biochem* 1980;107:279–295.
18. Munson PJ, Rodbard D. LIGAND: a versatile computerized approach for characterization of ligand-binding systems. *Anal Biochem* 1980;107:220–239.
19. Bright DS. *On interpreting spectrophotometric measurements of two quinoline- DNA complexes (Doctoral dissertation)*. Fort Collins, CO: Colorado State University, 1974.
20. Berzofsky JA. The assessment of antibody affinity from radioimmunoassay. *Clin Chem* 1978;24:419–421.
21. Pauling L, Pressman D, Grossberg AL. Serological properties of simple substances. VII. A quantitative theory of the inhibition by haptens of the precipitation of heterogeneous antisera with antigens, and comparison with experimental results for polyhaptenic simple substances and for azoproteins. *J Am Chem Soc* 1944;66:784–792.
22. Karush F. The interaction of purified antibody with optically isomeric haptens. *J Am Chem Soc* 1956;78:5519–5526.
23. Thakur AK, DeLisi C. Theory of ligand binding to heterogeneous receptor populations: characterization of the free-energy distribution function. *Biopolymers* 1978;17:1075–1089.
24. DeLisi C. Characterization of receptor affinity heterogeneity by Scatchard plots. *Biopolymers* 1978;17:1385–1386.
25. Thakur AK, Munson PJ, Hunston DL, et al. Characterization of ligand-binding systems by continuous affinity distributions of arbitrary shape. *Anal Biochem* 1980;103:240–254.
26. Sips R. On the structure of a catalyst surface. *J Chem Phys* 1948;16: 490–495.
27. Nisonoff A, Pressman D. Heterogeneity and average combining site constants of antibodies from individual rabbits. *J Immunol* 1958;80:417–428.
28. Karush F, Karush SS. Equilibrium dialysis. 3. Calculations. In: Williams CA, Chase MW, eds. *Methods in Immunology and Immunochemistry*. New York: Academic Press, 1971:389–393.
29. Klotz IM. Protein interactions. In: Neurath H, Bailey K, eds. *The Proteins*. New York: Academic Press, 1953:727–806.
30. Karush F. The affinity of antibody: range, variability, and the role of multivalence. 1978:85–116.
31. Crothers DM, Metzger H. The influence of polyvalency on the binding properties of antibodies. *Immunochemistry* 1972;9:341–357.
32. Hornick CL, Karush F. Antibody affinity - III. The role of multivalence. *Immunochemistry* 1972;9:325–340.
33. DeLisi C, Metzger H. Some physical chemical aspects of receptor-ligand interactions. *Immunol Commun* 1976;5:417–436.
34. DeLisi C. The effect of cell size and receptor density on ligand-receptor reaction rate constants. *Mol Immunol* 1981;18:507–511.
35. DeLisi C, Wiegel FW. Effect of nonspecific forces and finite receptor number on rate constants of ligand-cell bound-receptor interactions. *Proc Natl Acad Sci U S A* 1981;78:5569–5572.
36. Silhavy TJ, Szmelcman S, Boos W, et al. On the significance of the retention of ligand by protein. *Proc Natl Acad Sci U S A* 1975;72:2120–2124.
37. Yalow RS, Berson SA. Immunoassay of endogenous plasma insulin in man. *J Clin Invest* 1960;39:1157–1175.
38. Chard T. *An introduction to radioimmunoassay and related techniques*. Amsterdam: North Holland, 1978.
39. Rodbard D. Mathematics and statistics of ligand assays: an illustrated guide. In: Langan J, Clapp JJ, eds. *Ligand assay: analysis of international developments on isotopic and nonisotopic immunoassay*. New York: Masson, 1981:45–101.
40. Yalow R. Radioimmunoassay. *Rev Biophys Bioeng* 1980;9:327–345.
41. Farr RS. A quantitative immunochemical measure of the primary interaction between I*BSA and antibody. *J Infect Dis* 1958;103:239–262.
42. Desbuquois B, Aurbach GD. Use of polyethylene glycol to separate free and antibody-bound peptide hormones in radioimmunoassays. *J Clin Endocrinol Metab* 1971;33:732–738.
43. Zollinger WD, Dalrymple JM, Artenstein MS. Analysis of parameters affecting the solid phase radioimmunoassay quantitation of antibody to meningococcal antigens. *J Immunol* 1976;117:1788–1798.
44. Kessler SW. Rapid isolation of antigens from cells with a staphylococcal protein-A-antibody adsorbent: parameters of the interaction of antibody-antigen complexes with protein A. *J Immunol* 1975;115:1617–1624.
45. Friguet B, Chaffotte AF, Djavadi-Ohaniance L, et al. Measurements of the true affinity constant in solution of antigen-antibody complexes by enzyme-linked immunosorbent assay. *J Immunol Methods* 1985;77:305–319.
46. Stevens FJ. Modification of an elisa-based procedure for affinity determination: Correction necessary for use with bivalent antibody. *Mol Immunol* 1987;24:1055–1060.
47. Seligman SJ. Influence of solid-phase antigen in competition enzyme-linked immunosorbent assays (ELISAs) on calculated antigen-antibody dissociation constants. *J Immunol Methods* 1994;168:101–110.
48. Ekins RP. Basic principles and theory. *Br Med Bull* 1974;30:3–11.
49. Berzofsky JA, Curd JG, Schechter AN. Probability analysis of the interaction of antibodies with multideterminant antigens in radioimmunoassay: application to the amino terminus of the beta chain of hemoglobin S. *Biochemistry* 1976;15:2113–2121.
50. von Krogh M. Colloidal chemistry and immunology. *J Infect Dis* 1916;19:452–477.
51. Rodbard D, Lewald JE. Computer analysis of radioligand assay and radioimmunoassay data. *Acta Endocrinol* 1970;64:79–103.
52. Feldman H, Rodbard D. Mathematical theory of radioimmunoassay. In: Odell WD, Daughaday WH, eds. *Principles of competitive protein-binding assays*. Philadelphia: Lippincott, 1971:158–203.
53. Rodbard D, Ruder JH, Vaitukaitis J, et al. Mathematical analysis of kinetics of radioligand assays: improved sensitivity obtained by delayed addition of labeled ligand. *J Clin Endocrinol Metab* 1971;33:343–355.
54. Voller A, Bidwell D, Bartlett A. Enzyme-linked immunosorbent assay. In: Rose NR, Friedman H, eds. *Manual of Clinical Immunology*. Washington: American Society of Microbiology, 1980:359–371.
55. Kohno Y, Berkower I, Minna J, et al. Idiotypes of anti-myoglobin antibodies: shared idiotypes among monoclonal antibodies to distinct determinants of sperm whale myoglobin. *J Immunol* 1982;128:1742–1748.
56. Darst SA, Robertson CR, Berzofsky JA. Adsorption of the protein antigen myoglobin affects the binding of conformation-specific monoclonal antibodies. *Biophysical J* 1988;53:533–539.
57. Sedgwick J. A solid phase immunoenzymatic technique for the enumeration of specific antibody-secreting cells. *J Immunol Methods* 1983;57:301–309.

58. Czerkinsky CC, Nilsson L, Nygren H, et al. A solid-phase enzyme-linked immunospot (ELISPOT) assay for enumeration of specific antibody-secreting cells. *J Immunol Methods* 1983;65: 109–121.
59. Bocher WO, Herzog-Hauff S, Herr W, et al. Regulation of the neutralizing anti-hepatitis B surface (HBs) antibody response in vitro in HBs vaccine recipients and patients with acute or chronic hepatitis virus (HBV) infection. *Clin Exp Immunol* 1996;105:52–58.
60. Ronnelid J, Huang YH, Norrlander T, et al. Short-term kinetics of the humoral anti-C1q response in SLE using the ELIspot method: fast decline in production in response to steroids. *Scand J Immunol* 1994;40:243–250.
61. Czerkinsky C, Moldoveanu Z, Mestecky J, et al. A novel two colour ELISPOT assay I. Simultaneous detection of distinct types of antibody-secreting cells. *J Immunol Methods* 1988;115:31–37.
62. Krieg AM, Yi A, Matson S, et al. CpG motifs in bacterial DNA trigger direct B-cell activation. *Nature* 1995;374:546–549.
63. Ronnelid J, Klareskog L. A comparison between ELISPOT methods for the detection of cytokine producing cells: greater sensitivity and specificity using ELISA plates as compared to nitrocellulose membranes. *J Immunol Methods* 1997;200:17–26.
64. Mäkelä O, Karjalainen K. Inherited immunoglobulin idiotypes of the mouse. *Immunol Rev* 1977;34:119–138.
65. Jameson BA, McDonnell JM, Marini JC, et al. A rationally designed CD4 analogue inhibits experimental allergic encephalomyelitis. *Nature* 1994;368:744–746.
66. Brady L, Dodson G. Reflections on a peptide. *Nature* 1994;368:692–693.
67. Guichard G, Benkirane N, Zeder-Lutz G, et al. Antigenic mimicry of natural L-peptides with retro-inverso- peptidomimetics. *Proc Natl Acad Sci U S A* 1994;91:9765–9769.
68. Benkirance N, Guichard G, Van Regenmortel MHV, et al. Cross-reactivity of antibodies to retro-inverso peptidomimetics with the parent protein histone H3 and chromatin core particle. *J Biol Chem* 1995;270:11921–11926.
69. Briand J, Guichard G, Dumortier H, et al. Retro-inverso peptidomimetics as new immunological probes. *J Biol Chem* 1995;270: 20686–20691.
70. Häyry P, Myllärniemi M, Aavik E, et al. Stabile D-peptide analog of insulin-like growth factor-1 inhibits smooth muscle cell proliferation after carotid ballooning injury in the rat. *Faseb J* 1995;9:1336–1344.
71. Berzofsky JA, Schechter AN. The concepts of cross-reactivity and specificity in immunology. *Mol Immunol* 1981;18:751–763.
72. Young NS, Curd JG, Eastlake A, et al. Isolation of antibodies specific to sickle hemoglobin by affinity chromatography using a synthetic peptide. *Proc Natl Acad Sci U S A* 1975;72:4759–4763.
73. Young NS, Eastlake A, Schecter AN. The amino terminal region of the sickle hemoglobin beta chain. II. Characterization of monospecific antibodies. *J Biol Chem* 1976;251:6431–6435.
74. Curd JG, Young N, Schecter AN. Antibodies to an amino terminal fragment of beta globin. II. Specificity and isolation of antibodies for the sickle mutation. *J Biol Chem* 1976;251:1290–1295.
75. Dean J, Schecter AN. Sickle-cell anemia: molecular and cellular bases of therapeutic approaches. *N Engl J Med* 1978;299:752–763.
76. Johnston MFM, Eisen HN. Cross-reactions between 2,4-dinitrophenyl and nemadione (vitamin K3) and the general problem of antibody specificity. *J Immunol* 1976;117:1189–1196.
77. Talmage D. Immunological specificity. *Science* 1959;129:1643–1648.
78. Inman JK. Multispecificity of the antibody combining region and antibody diversity. In: Sercarz EE, Williamson AR, Fox CF, eds. *The immune system: genes, receptors, signals*. New York: Academic Press, 1974:37–52.
79. Inman JK. The antibody combining region: speculations on the hypothesis of general multispecificity. In: Bell GI, Perelson AS, Pimbley GH, Jr., eds. *Theoretical immunology*. New York: Marcel Dekker, 1978:243–278.
80. Richards FF, Konigsberg WH, Rosenstein RW, et al. On the specificity of antibodies. *Science* 1975;187:130–37.
81. Parker CW. Spectrofluorometric methods. In: Weir DM, ed. *Handbook of experimental immunology*. Oxford: Blackwell, 1978:18.1–18.25.
82. Haimovich J, Hurwitz E, Novik N, et al. Preparation of protein-bacteriophage conjugates and their use in detection of antiprotein antibodies. *Biochim Biophys Acta* 1970;207:115–124.
83. Heidelberger M, Kendall FE. The precipitin reaction between type III pneumococcus polysaccharide and homologous antibody. *J Exp Med* 1935;61:563–591.
84. Heidelberger M, Kendall FE. A quantitative theory of the precipitin reaction. II. A study of an azoprotein-antibody system. *J Exp Med* 1935;62:467–483.
85. Kabat EA. *Structural concepts in immunology and immunochemistry*. 2nd ed. New York: Hold, Rinehart, and Winston, 1976.
86. Cisar J, Kabat EA, Dorner MM, et al. Binding properties of immunoglobulin containing sites specific for terminal or nonterminal antigenic determinants in dextran. *J Exp Med* 1975;142:435–459.
87. Ouchterlony O, Nilsson LA. Immunodiffusion and immunoelectrophoresis. In: Weir DM, ed. *Handbook of experimental immunology*. Oxford: Blackwell, 1978:19.1–19.44.
88. Feinberg JG. Identification, discrimination and quantification in Ouchterlony gel plates. *Int Arch Allergy* 1957;11:129–152.
89. Tomasi TB, Jr., Zigelbaum S. The selective occurrence of gamma1A globulins in certain body fluids. *J Clin Invest* 1963;42:1552–1560.
90. Fahey JL, McKelvey EM. Quantitative determination of serum immunoglobulins in antibody-agar plates. *J Immunol* 1965;94:84–90.
91. Mancini G, Carbonara AO, Heremans JF. Immunochemical quantitation of antigens by single radial immunodiffusion. *Immunochem* 1965;2:235–254.
92. Herbert WJ. Passive haemagglutination with special reference to the tanned cell technique. In: Weir DM, ed. *Handbook of experimental immunology*. Oxford: Blackwell, 1978:20.1–20.20.
93. Towbin H, Staehelin T, Gordon J. Electrophoretic transfer of proteins from polyacrylamide gels to nitrocellulose sheets: Procedure and some applications. *Proc Natl Acad Sci U S A* 1979;76:4350–4354.
94. Schupbach J, Popovic M, Gilden RV, et al. Serological analysis of a subgroup of human T-lymphotropic retroviruses (HTLV-III) associated with AIDS. *Science* 1984;224:503–505.
95. Feynman RP, Leighton RB, Sands M. *The Feynman lectures on physics* Vol. II. Reading, MA: Addison-Wesley Publishing Co., 1964.
96. Mullett WM, Lai EP, Yeung JM. Surface plasmon resonance-based immunoassays. *Methods* 2000;22:77–91.
97. VanCott TC, Bethke FR, Polonis VR, et al. Dissociation rate of antibody-gp120 binding interactions is predictive of V3-mediated neutralization of HIV-1. *J Immunol* 1994;153:449–459.
98. Slater RJ, Ward SM, Kunkel HG. Immunological relationships among the myeloma proteins. *J Exp Med* 1955;101:85–108.
99. Potter M. Immunoglobulin-producing tumors and myeloma proteins of mice. *Physiol Rev* 1972;52:631–719.
100. Köhler G, Milstein C. Continuous cultures of fused cells secreting antibody of predefined specificity. *Nature* 1975;256:495–497.
101. Margulies DH, Kuehl WM, Scharff MD. Somatic cell hybridization of mouse myeloma cells. *Cell* 1976;8:405–415.
102. Shulman M, Wilde CD, Köhler G. A better cell line for making hybridomas secreting specific antibodies. *Nature* 1978;276:269–270.
103. Kearney JF, Radbruch A, Liesegang B, et al. A new mouse myeloma cell line that has lost immunoglobulin expression but permits the construction of antibody-secreting hybrid cell lines. *J Immunol* 1979;123:1548–1550.
104. Yokoyama WM. Production of monoclonal antibodies. In: Coligan JE, Kruisbeek AM, Margulies DH, Shevach EM, Strober W, eds. *Current Protocols in Immunology*. Vol. I. New York: John Wiley & Sons, Inc., 2001:2.5.1.
105. Unkeless JC. Characterization of monoclonal antibody directed against mouse macrophage and lymphocyte Fc receptors. *J Exp Med* 1979;150:580–596.
106. Leo O, Foo M, Sachs DH, et al. Identification of a monoclonal antibody specific for a murine T3 polypeptide. *Proc Natl Acad Sci U S A* 1987;84:1374–1378.
107. Yarmush ML, Gates FT, Weisfogel DR, et al. Identification and characterization of rabbit-mouse hybridomas secreting rabbit immunoglobulin chains. *Proc Natl Acad Sci U S A* 1980;77:2899–2903.

108. Bazin H. Production of rat monoclonal antibodies with the Lou rat non-secreting IR983F myeloma cell line. *Prot Biol Fluids* 1981;29:615–618.
109. Huse WD, Sastry L, Iverson SA, et al. Generation of a large combinatorial library of the immunoglobulin repertoire in phage lambda. *Science* 1989;246:1275–1281.
110. Clackson T, Hoogenboom HR, Griffiths AD, et al. Making antibody fragments using phage display libraries. *Nature* 1991;352: 624–628.
111. McCafferty J, Griffiths AD, Winter G, et al. Phage antibodies: filamentous phage displaying antibody variable domains. *Nature* 1990;348:552–554.
112. Kang AS, Barbas CF, Janda KD, et al. Linkage of recognition and replication functions by assembling combinatorial antibody Fab libraries along phage surfaces. *Proc Natl Acad Sci U S A* 1991;88:4363–4366.
113. Zebedee SL, Barbas CF, III, Hom Y, et al. Human combinatorial antibody libraries to hepatitis B surface antigen. *Proc Natl Acad Sci U S A* 1992;89:3175–3179.
114. Burton DR, Barbas CF, III, Persson MAA, et al. A large array of human monoclonal antibodies to type 1 human immunodeficiency virus from combinatorial libraries of asymptomatic seropositive individuals. *Proc Natl Acad Sci U S A* 1991;88:10134–10137.
115. Duchosal MA, Eming SA, Fischer P, et al. Immunization of hu-PBL-SCID mice and the rescue of human monoclonal Fab fragments through combinatorial libraries. *Nature* 1992;355:258–262.
116. Low NM, Holliger P, Winter G. Mimicking somatic hypermutation: Affinity maturation of antibodies displayed on bacteriophage using a bacterial mutator strain. *J Mol Biol* 1996;260:359–368.
117. Thompson J, Pope T, Tung J, et al. Affinity maturation of a high-affinity human monoclonal antibody against the third hypervariable loop of human immunodeficiency virus: use of phage display to improve affinity and broaden strain reactivity. *J Mol Biol* 1996;256:77–88.
118. Lerner RA, Benkovic SJ, Schultz PG. At the crossroads of chemistry and immunology: catalytic antibodies. *Science* 1991;252:659–667.
119. Pollack SJ, Jacobs JW, Schultz PG. Selective chemical catalysis by an antibody. *Science* 1986;234:1570–1573.
120. Shuster AM, Gololobov GV, Kvashuk OA, et al. DNA hydrolyzing autoantibodies. *Science* 1992;256:665–667.
121. Tramontano A, Janda KD, Lerner RA. Catalytic antibodies. *Science* 1986;234:1566–1570.
122. Shokat KM, Leumann CJ, Sugasawara R, et al. A new strategy for the generation of catalytic antibodies. *Nature* 1989;338:269–271.
123. Pollack SJ, Hsiun P, Schultz PG. Stereospecific hydrolysis of alkyl esters by antibodies. *J Am Chem Soc* 1989;111:5961–5962.
124. Wirsching P, Ashley JA, Benkovic SJ, et al. An unexpectedly efficient catalytic antibody operating by ping-pong and induced fit mechanisms. *Science* 1991;252:680–685.
125. Shabat D, Itzhaky H, Reymond J, et al. Antibody catalysis of a reaction otherwise strongly disfavoured in water. *Nature* 1995;374:143–146.
126. Hirschmann R, Smith AB, Taylor CM, et al. Peptide synthesis catalyzed by an antibody containing a binding site for variable amino acids. *Science* 1994;265:234–237.
127. Kriangkum J, Xu BW, Nagata LP, et al. Bispecific and bifunctional single chain recombinant antibodies. *Biomolecular Engineering* 2001;18:31–40.
128. Karpovsky B, Titus JA, Stephany DA, et al. Production of target-specific effector cells using hetero-cross-linked aggregates containing anti-target cell and anti-Fcγ receptor antibodies. *J Exp Med* 1984;160:1686–1701.
129. Titus JA, Garrido MA, Hecht TT, et al. Human T cells targeted with anti-T3 cross-linked to antitumor antibody prevent tumor growth in nude mice. *J Immunol* 1987;138:4018–4022.
130. Wickham TJ, Segal DM, Roelvink PW, et al. Targeted adenovirus gene transfer to endothelial and smooth muscle cells by using bispecific antibodies. *J Virol* 1996;70:6831–6838.
131. Vallera DA, Ash RC, Zanjani ED, et al. Anti-T-cell reagents for human bone marrow transplantation: Ricin linked to three monoclonal antibodies. *Science* 1983;222:512–515.
132. Waldmann TA. Monoclonal antibodies in diagnosis and therapy. *Science* 1991;252:1657–1662.
133. Berkower I. The promise and pitfalls of monoclonal antibody therapeutics. *Curr Opinion Biotech* 1996;7:622–628.
134. Waldmann TA. Immunotherapy: past, present and future. *Nat Med* 2003;9:269–277.
135. Ortho Multicenter Transplant Study G. A randomized clinical trial of OKT3 monoclonal antibody for acute rejection of cadaveric renal transplants. *N Eng J Med* 1988;313:337–342.
136. Collier BD, Abdel-Nabi H, Doerr RJ, et al. Immunoscintigraphy performed with In-111-labeled CYT-103 in the management of colorectal cancer: comparison with CT. *Radiology* 1992;185:179–186.
137. Ezzell C. Magic bullets fly again. *Scientific American* 2001;285: 34–41.
138. Sears HF, Herlyn D, Steplewski Z, et al. Effects of monoclonal antibody immunotherapy on patients with gastrointestinal adenocarcinoma. *J Biol Resp Mod* 1984;3:138–150.
139. Baselga J, Tripathy D, Mendelsohn J, et al. Phase II study of weekly intravenous recombinant humanized anti- p185HER2 monoclonal antibody in patients with HER2/neu-overexpressing metastatic breast cancer. *J Clin Oncol* 1996;14:737–744.
140. Baselga J, Norton L, Albanell J, et al. Recombinant humanized anti-HER2 antibody (Herceptin) enhances the antitumor activity of paclitaxel and doxorubicin against HER2/neu overexpressing human breast cancer xenografts. *Cancer Res* 1998;58:2825–2831.
141. Maloney DG, Grillo-Lopez AJ, Bodkin DJ, et al. IDEC-C2B8: results of a phase I multiple-dose trial in patients with relapsed non-Hodgkin's lymphoma. *J Clin Oncol* 1997;15:3266–3274.
142. Morris JC, Waldmann TA. Advances in interleukin 2 receptor targeted treatment. *Ann Rheum Dis* 2000;59 Suppl 1:i109–i114.
143. Frankel AE, Houston LL, Issell BF. Prospects for immunotoxin therapy in cancer. *Ann Rev Med* 1986;37:125–142.
144. Kreitman RJ, Wilson WH, Bergeron K, et al. Efficacy of the anti-CD22 recombinant immunotoxin BL22 in chemotherapy- resistant hairy-cell leukemia. *N Engl J Med* 2001;345:241–247.
145. Carrasquillo JA, Krohn JA, Beaumier P, et al. Diagnosis and therapy for solid tumors with radiolabeled antibodies and immune fragments. *Cancer Treat Rep* 1984;68:317–328.
146. Waldmann TA, Goldman CK, Bongiovanni KF, et al. Therapy of patients with human T-cell lymphotrophic virus I-induced adult T cell leukemia with anti-Tac, a monoclonal antibody to the receptor for interleukin-2. *Blood* 1988;72:1805–1816.
147. Waldmann TA. Multichain interleukin-2 receptor: a target for immunotherapy in lymphoma. *J Natl Cancer Inst* 1989;81:914–923.
148. Zhang M, Zhang Z, Garmestani K, et al. Activating Fc receptors are required for antitumor efficacy of the antibodies directed toward CD25 in a murine model of adult t-cell leukemia. *Cancer Res* 2004;64:5825–5929.
149. van Oers MH, Klasa R, Marcus RE, et al. Rituximab maintenance improves clinical outcome of relapsed/resistant follicular non-Hodgkin's lymphoma, both in patients with and without rituximab during induction: results of a prospective randomized phase III intergroup trial. *Blood* 2006;108:3295–3301.
150. Witzig TE, Gordon LI, Cabanillas F, et al. Randomized controlled trial of yttrium-90-labeled ibritumomab tiuxetan radioimmunotherapy versus rituximab immunotherapy for patients with relapsed or refractory low-grade, follicular, or transformed B-cell non-Hodgkin's lymphoma. *J Clin Oncol* 2002;20:2453–2463.
151. Gibson AD. Updated results of a Phase III trial comparing ibritumomab tiuxetan with rituximab in previously treated patients with non-Hodgkin's lymphoma. *Clin Lymphoma* 2002;3:87–89.
152. Robert N, Leyland-Jones B, Asmar L, et al. Randomized phase III study of trastuzumab, paclitaxel, and carboplatin compared with trastuzumab and paclitaxel in women with HER-2-overexpressing metastatic breast cancer. *J Clin Oncol* 2006;24:2786–2792.
153. Coudert BP, Arnould L, Moreau L, et al. Pre-operative systemic (neo-adjuvant) therapy with trastuzumab and docetaxel for HER2-overexpressing stage II or III breast cancer: results of a multicenter phase II trial. *Ann Oncol* 2006;17:409–414.

154. Yang JC, Haworth L, Sherry RM, et al. A randomized trial of bevacizumab, an anti-vascular endothelial growth factor antibody, for metastatic renal cancer. *N Engl J Med* 2003;349:427–434.
155. Hurwitz H, Fehrenbacher L, Novotny W, et al. Bevacizumab plus irinotecan, fluorouracil, and leucovorin for metastatic colorectal cancer. *N Engl J Med* 2004;350:2335–2342.
156. Rini BI, Halabi S, Taylor J, et al. Cancer and Leukemia Group B 90206: A randomized phase III trial of interferon-alpha or interferon-alpha plus anti-vascular endothelial growth factor antibody (bevacizumab) in metastatic renal cell carcinoma. *Clin Cancer Res* 2004;10:2584–2586.
157. Johnson DH, Fehrenbacher L, Novotny WF, et al. Randomized phase II trial comparing bevacizumab plus carboplatin and paclitaxel with carboplatin and paclitaxel alone in previously untreated locally advanced or metastatic non-small-cell lung cancer. *J Clin Oncol* 2004;22:2184–2191.
158. Starling N, Cunningham D. Monoclonal antibodies against vascular endothelial growth factor and epidermal growth factor receptor in advanced colorectal cancers: present and future directions. *Curr Opin Oncol* 2004;16:385–390.
159. Ferrara N, Hillan KJ, Gerber HP, et al. Discovery and development of bevacizumab, an anti-VEGF antibody for treating cancer. *Nat Rev Drug Discov* 2004;3:391–400.
160. Gibson TB, Ranganathan A, Grothey A. Randomized phase III trial results of panitumumab, a fully human anti-epidermal growth factor receptor monoclonal antibody, in metastatic colorectal cancer. *Clin Colorectal Cancer* 2006;6:29–31.
161. Wendtner CM, Ritgen M, Schweighofer CD, et al. Consolidation with alemtuzumab in patients with chronic lymphocytic leukemia (CLL) in first remission—experience on safety and efficacy within a randomized multicenter phase III trial of the German CLL Study Group (GCLLSG). *Leukemia* 2004;18:1093–1101.
162. Tsimberidou AM, Giles FJ, Estey E, et al. The role of gemtuzumab ozogamicin in acute leukaemia therapy. *Br J Haematol* 2006;132:398–409.
163. Lipsky PE, van der Heijde DM, St Clair EW, et al. Infliximab and methotrexate in the treatment of rheumatoid arthritis. Anti-Tumor Necrosis Factor Trial in Rheumatoid Arthritis with Concomitant Therapy Study Group. *N Engl J Med* 2000;343:1594–1602.
164. Pisetsky DS. Tumor necrosis factor blockers in rheumatoid arthritis. *N Engl J Med* 2000;342:810–811.
165. Johnson S, Oliver C, Prince GA, et al. Development of a humanized monoclonal antibody (MEDI-493) with potent in vitro and in vivo activity against respiratory syncytial virus. *J Infect Dis* 1997;176:1215–1224.
166. Group IRS. Palivizumab, a Humanized Respiratory Syncytial Virus Monoclonal Antibody, Reduces Hospitalization From Respiratory Syncytial Virus Infection in High-risk Infants. *Pediatrics* 1998;102:531–537.
167. Bumgardner GL, Hardie I, Johnson RW, et al. Results of 3-year phase III clinical trials with daclizumab prophylaxis for prevention of acute rejection after renal transplantation. *Transplantation* 2001;72:839–845.
168. Nussenblatt RB, Fortin E, Schiffman R, et al. Treatment of non-infectious intermediate and posterior uveitis with the humanized anti-Tac mAb: a phase I/II clinical trial. *Proc Natl Acad Sci U S A* 1999;96:7462–7466.
169. Bielekova B, Richert N, Howard T, et al. Humanized anti-CD25 (daclizumab) inhibits disease activity in multiple sclerosis patients failing to respond to interferon beta. *Proc Natl Acad Sci U S A* 2004;101:8705–8708.
170. Miller RA, Maloney DG, Warnke R, et al. Treatment of B-cell lymphoma with monoclonal anti-idiotype antibody. *N Eng J Med* 1982;306:517–522.
171. Kwak LW, Young HA, Pennington RW, et al. Vaccination with syngeneic, lymphoma-derived immunoglobulin idiotype combined with granulocyte/macrophage colony-stimulating factor primes mice for a protective T-cell response. *Proc Natl Acad Sci U S A.* 1996;93:10972–10977.
172. Hsu FJ, Caspar CB, Czerwinski D, et al. Tumor -specific idiotype vaccines in the treatment of patients with B-cell lymphoma—long-term results of a clinical trial. *Blood* 1997;89:3129–3135.
173. Timmerman JM, Czerwinski DK, Davis TA, et al. Idiotype-pulsed dendritic cell vaccination for B-cell lymphoma: clinical and immune responses in 35 patients. *Blood* 2002;99:1517–1526.
174. Davis TA, Hsu FJ, Caspar CB, et al. Idiotype vaccination following ABMT can stimulate specific anti-idiotype immune responses in patients with B-cell lymphoma. *Biol Blood Marrow Transplant* 2001;7:517–522.
175. Neelapu SS, Kwak LW, Kobrin CB, et al. Vaccine-induced tumor-specific immunity despite severe B-cell depletion in mantle cell lymphoma. *Nat Med* 2005;11:986–991.
176. Meeker T, Lowder J, Cleary ML, et al. Emergence of idiotype variants during treatment of B-cell lymphoma with anti-idiotype antibodies. *N Eng J Med* 1985;312:1658–1665.
177. Hakim I, Levy S, Levy R. A nine-amino acid peptide from IL-1á augments antitumor immune responses induced by protein and DNA vaccines. *J Immunol* 1996;157:5503–5511.
178. Cole RJ, Morrisey DM, Houghton AN, et al. Generation of human monoclonal antibodies reactive with cellular antigens. *Proc Natl Acad Sci USA* 1983;80:2026–2030.
179. Olsson L, Kaplan HS. Human-human monoclonal antibody-producing hybridomas: technical aspects. *Meth Enzymol* 1983;92: 3–16.
180. Seigneurin JM, Desgranges C, Seigneurin D, et al. Herpes simplex virus glycoprotein D: human monoclonal antibody produced by bone marrow cell line. *Science* 1983;221:173–175.
181. Sugano T, Matsumoto Y, Miyamoto C, et al. Hybridomas producing human monoclonal antibodies against varicella-zoster virus. *Eur J Immunol* 1987;17:359–364.
182. Morrison SL. Transfectomas provide novel chimeric antibodies. *Science* 1985;229:1202–1207.
183. Morrison SL, Johnson MJ, Herzenberg LA, et al. Chimeric human antibody molecules: mouse antigen-binding domains with human constant region domains. *Proc Natl Acad Sci USA* 1984;81:6851–6855.
184. Jones PT, Dear PH, Foote J, et al. Replacing the complementarity-determining regions in a human antibody with those from a mouse. *Nature* 1986;321:522–525.
185. Brüggemann M, Spicer C, Buluwela L, et al. Human antibody production in transgenic mice: expression from 100 kb of the human IgH locus. *Eur J Immunol* 1991;21:1323–1326.
186. Lonberg N, Taylor LD, Harding FA, et al. Antigen-specific human antibodies from mice comprising four distinct genetic modifications. *Nature* 1994;368:856–859.
187. Green LL, Hardy MC, Maynard-Currie CE, et al. Antigen-specific human monoclonal antibodies from mice engineered with human Ig heavy and light chain YACs. *Nature Genet* 1994;7:13–21.
188. Jayasena SD. Aptamers: An emerging class of molecules that rival antibodies in diagnostics. *Clinical Chemistry* 1999;45:1628–1650.
189. Klein J, Huang HS, Lemke H, et al. Serological analysis of H-2 and Ia molecules with monoclonal antibodies. *Immunogenetics* 1979;8:419–432.
190. Ozato K, Mayer N, Sachs DH. Hybridoma cell lines secreting monoclonal antibodies to mouse H-2 and Ia antigens. *J Immunol* 1980;124:533–540.
191. Pierres M, Devaux C, Dosseto M, et al. Clonal analysis of B and T-cell responses to Ia antigens. I. Topology of epitope regions on I-A^k and I-E^k molecules analyzed with 35 monoclonal alloantibodies. *Immunogenetics* 1981;14:481–495.
192. Sattentau QJ, Dalgleish AG, Weiss RA, et al. Epitopes of the CD4 antigen and HIV infection. *Science* 1986;234:1120–1123.
193. Hoxie JA, Flaherty LE, Haggarty BS, et al. Infection of T4 lymphocytes by HTLV-III does not require expression of the OKT4 epitope. *J Immunol* 1986;136:361–363.
194. Porgador A, Yewdell JW, Deng YP, et al. Localization, quantitation, and in situ detection of specific peptide MHC class I complexes using a monoclonal antibody. *Immunity* 1997;6:715–726.
195. Messaoudi I, LeMaoult J, Nikolic-Zugic J. The mode of ligand recognition by two peptide : MHC class I- specific monoclonal antibodies. *J Immunol* 1999;163:3286–3294.

196. Polakova K, Plaksin D, Chung DH, et al. Antibodies directed against the MHC-I molecule H-2D^d complexed with an antigenic peptide: Similarities to a T cell receptor with the same specificity. *J Immunol* 2000;165:5703–5712.
197. Chung DH, Belyakov IM, Derby MA, et al. Competitive inhibition *in vivo* and skewing of the T cell repertoire of antigen-specific CTL priming by an anti-peptide-MHC mAb. *J Immunology* 2001;167:699–707.
198. Koike T, Tomioka H, Kumagai A. Antibodies cross-reactive with DNA and cardiolipin in patients with systemic lupus erythematosus. *Clin Exp Immunol* 1982;50:298–302.

Chapter 6

Immunoglobulins: Molecular Genetics

Edward E. Max

INTRODUCTION

From the millions of naïve B cells circulating in an individual, a foreign antigen triggers a specific antibody response by activating the small fraction of B lymphocytes displaying antibody as a B cell receptor (BCR) that can bind the antigen; these B cells proliferate and mature into antibody-secreting cells, manufacturing large amounts of antibody specific for the triggering antigen. To be effective against a universe of diverse pathogens, this "clonal selection" mechanism requires that the diversity of immunoglobulin species expressed on naïve B cells prior to antigen exposure be huge enough so that virtually any antigen finds B cells displaying a cognate antibody (i.e., an antibody capable of binding that antigen). Indeed, in the 1960s the number of different antibody sequences in the repertoire of typical mouse was estimated in the millions; to encode this many sequences would seem to require an unreasonably high percentage of the mammalian genome (now estimated to contain only about 30,000 genes). Understanding the genetic source of immunoglobulin diversity—variable (V) region assembly recombination—was the first major challenge and achievement of the molecular biological investigations of antibody genes and will be discussed first in this chapter.

A week or so after antigen administration, the antibody response changes in two ways that generally improve the protective functions of antibodies. B cells initially express antibodies of the IgM isotype, but those cells that migrate into germinal centers receive stimuli that can induce them to switch to production of IgG, IgA, or IgE without changing the antigen specificity of the protein; this switch results from a DNA recombination event known as class switch recombination (CSR). In addition, over the course of an immune response, the affinity of antibody for antigen gradually improves as a result of somatic hypermutation (SHM) of antibody genes, with subsequent selection for B cells expressing high-affinity antibodies. CSR and SHM are discussed later in this chapter.

In this chapter, well-established facts about immunoglobulin genes are summarized concisely, while areas currently under investigation are considered in more detail, with particular attention to topics expected to interest immunologists.

OVERVIEW OF IMMUNOGLOBULIN V GENE ASSEMBLY

The three immunoglobulin gene loci—κ, λ, and heavy chain—each undergo similar V region assembly recombination during B lymphoid development, a novel form of DNA acrobatics that was initially discovered by Tonegawa's lab (1). The κ locus (murine or human) is conceptually the simplest, containing a single constant (C) region and a cluster of multiple upstream V region genes. During the development of an antibody-producing cell, one of the V region sequences rearranges to associate with the C region sequence, leading to a complete (V + C) gene, which the cell can then express. The difference between recombined DNA in a Ig-expressing B lymphocyte and the precursor "germline" DNA can be demonstrated by comparing these DNAs using Southern blotting or sequence analysis of cloned Ig genes (now often obtained by polymerase chain reaction [PCR]).

The general structures of the germline V genes are similar for the three Ig loci. Each V gene begins with sequence encoding a signal peptide of about 22 amino acids. Within codon –4 (numbering backward from the beginning of the mature protein sequence), the coding sequence is interrupted by an intron, usually roughly 0.1 kb to 0.3 kb long. Each V region gene as it exists in the germline is incomplete, and recombination is necessary to assemble a complete V gene as expressed in a B lymphocyte. For example, most murine κ chains have variable regions 108 amino acids in length, but murine germline Vκ genes encode only about 95 of these. The remaining 13 amino acids are encoded by segments known as J ("joining") regions that lie at some distance upstream of the Cκ gene. The murine κ locus contains four Jκ regions (plus an additional nonfunctional J sequence). An assembled Vκ gene thus results from recombination that joins one of many germline Vκ genes to one of four Jκ gene segments (Figure 6.1A). A similar recombination event is necessary to assemble a complete Vλ chain sequence from germline Vλ and Jλ genes. For heavy chains, recombination assembles a V region from three types of germline elements; between the residues encoded by germline VH and JH elements are extra amino acids—usually from two to eight residues—encoded by a D ("diversity") region. The assembly of a complete heavy chain V region occurs in two separate steps (Figure 6.1B): initially one of several germline DH regions joins with one

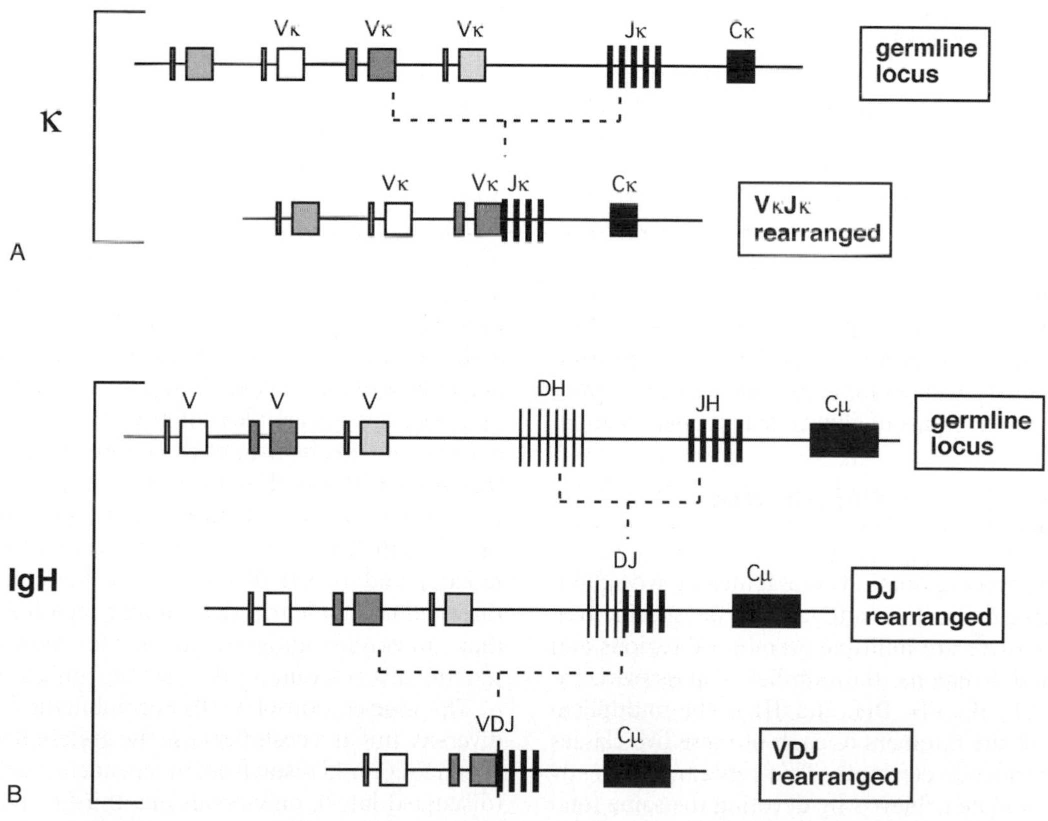

FIGURE 6.1 V assembly recombination. **A:** In the κ locus a single recombination event joins a germline Vκ region with one of the Jκ segments. **B:** In the IgH locus an initial recombination joins a D segment to a JH segment. A second recombination completes the V assembly by joining a VH to DJH.

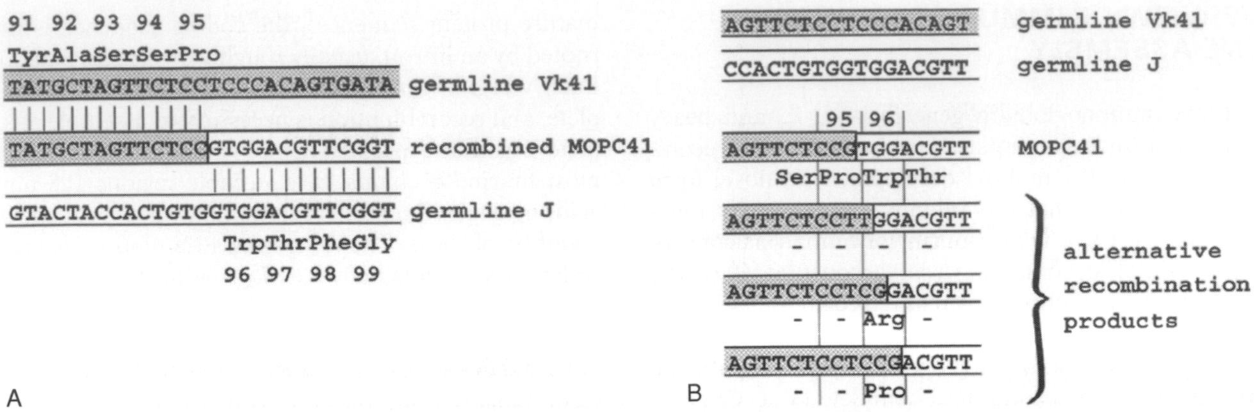

FIGURE 6.2 Vκ-Jκ recombination at single base resolution. **A:** The sequence of the recombined MOPC41 κ gene around the VJ junction is shown (center) with the sequences of the two germline precursors (Vκ41 and Jκ1) shown above and below. The germline origins of the recombined gene are indicated by the vertical lines and the shading of the V-derived sequence. **B:** The consequences of joining the same germline sequences (from part A) at four different positions are shown. Of the four alternative recombination products illustrated, the top one is that actually found in MOPC41. The second example has a single nucleotide difference but no change in encoded amino acid sequence. The third and fourth alternatives yield Arg or Pro at position 96; both of these amino acids have been found at this position in sequenced mouse κ chains.

of the JH regions; then a germline VH region is added to complete the assembled VDJ heavy chain gene.

Several PCR strategies can detect V(D)J recombination, depending on the needs of the experiment. An upstream sense primer can be specific to a particular V region or represent a consensus V primer (or primer mixture), while the downstream antisense primer may target the 3′-most J region. If the template DNA derives from a clonal B cell line, a single amplified band should result, or perhaps two bands if both alleles in the cell have undergone V(D)J rearrangement using different J regions. DNA from a mixed B cell population usually produces a "ladder" of bands, each corresponding to rearrangements of a different J region. No amplification product would be expected from germline DNA, because before recombination the primer sequences lie too far apart to allow efficient amplification.

How Recombination Contributes to Diversity

The V assembly recombination contributes in two significant ways to the diversity of antigen binding specificities. First, because there are multiple germline V regions and multiple D and J regions, the number of possible combinations of VL, JL, VH, DH, and JH is the multiplication product of the numbers of each of these five classes of germline sequence elements. This repertoire is vastly larger than could be achieved by devoting the same total lengths of DNA sequence to preassembled V regions. A second factor that increases diversity was recognized by comparing nucleotide sequences of various myeloma genes to their germline precursors. For example, as shown in Figure 6.2A, a comparison between the Vκ gene expressed in the murine myeloma MOPC41 and the corresponding germline Vκ and Jκ genes shows that the myeloma gene matches the germline precursor through the second nucleotide of codon 95; the VJ recombination junction occurs exactly at this point, because sequence beyond this position in the myeloma gene clearly derives from Jκ1. Similar analyses of other myelomas reveal that the recombination junctions can occur at several different positions within codon 95 or 96. As shown in Figure 6.2B, this "flexibility" of the position of the recombination junction increases the diversity of the affected codons. Heavy chain V regions exhibit this imprecision at both VD and DJ junctions. In addition, many heavy chain VDJ junctions (and a smaller percentage of light chain VJ junctions) contain insertions of a few extra nucleotides not present in the germline precursors; the mechanism of these insertions—known as N regions—is discussed later in this chapter. Significantly, the three-dimensional structure of immunoglobulins established from X-ray crystallography reveals that the VL-JL junction and the VH-DH-JH junction both form one of the three "complementarity determining region" loops (CDR3) that can contact antigen; thus this junctional diversity is functionally relevant for diversifying antigen binding.

The imprecision of V(D)J recombination increases Ig diversity, but at a cost. Because the precise boundaries between V, D, and J result from independent stochastic events (discussed later), only about one third of recombination events maintain the correct reading frame between V and J. In myelomas with rearrangements on both allelic copies of an immunoglobulin gene locus, the unexpressed recombination is generally out-of-frame or "nonproductive." For

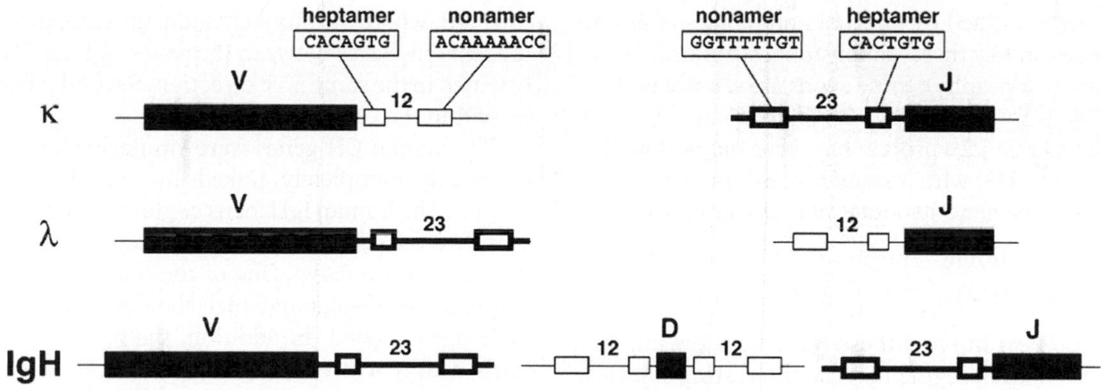

FIGURE 6.3 Conserved elements flank germline V, D, and J region genes. Conserved heptamer and nonamer RSSs lie adjacent to V, D, and J coding sequences and are important for targeting V(D)J recombination. The heptamer and nonamer elements are separated by spacer regions of about 12 bp (illustrated by thin lines in the figure) or 23 bp (thick lines). Depending on the locus, V regions may be flanked by 12 bp or 23 bp RSS, and similarly for J regions. But one of each type of element must be present for recombination to occur, a requirement that prevents futile recombination events (e.g., J to J).

heavy chain VDJ recombination, one could theoretically retain the correct reading frame between V and J while allowing the interposed D region segments to be used in all three reading frames; human B lymphocytes exploit this extra diversity *(2)*. In murine heavy chains, however, only a single D region reading frame is generally expressed, and several mechanisms prevent expression of antibodies with D regions in the other two reading frames (3).

Recombination Signal Elements

Analysis of DNA sequences flanking the germline V, D, and J region sequences revealed two conserved sequence elements that have subsequently been shown to define targets for V(D)J recombination: a heptamer adjacent to the coding sequence and a more distal nonamer. (These sequences are diagrammed in Figure 6.3.) For example, in the κ locus the consensus heptamer CACTGTG occurs 5′ of the Jκ coding sequences, with its (reverse) complement CACAGTG appearing 3′ to Vκ coding sequences. The consensus nonamer GGTTTTTGT appears about 23 nucleotides 5′ of the Jκ heptamer, and its complement ACAAAAACC appearing about 12 nucleotides 3′ of the Vκ heptamer. Similar sequences flank Vλ and Jλ, as well as VH, DH, and JH (as shown in Figure 6.3). These "recombination signal sequences" (RSSs) have been shown to be critical in the recombination, serving as recognition sequences for the recombination activating gene proteins RAG1 and RAG2, as discussed later in this chapter. Similar RSSs are present flanking light and heavy chain Ig genes throughout phylogeny, as well as in T cell receptor genes (see Chapter 8), which undergo similar V assembly recombinations. In all of these systems, the length of the spacer between the heptamer and nonamer (Figure 6.3) appears significant. Recombination apparently occurs almost exclusively between one coding sequence associated with a ~12 bp spacer and another coding sequence with a ~23 bp spacer, a requirement referred to as the "12/23" rule. This requirement may serve to prevent futile recombinations, such as between two Vκ or two Jκ gene segments. Although the heptamer and nonamer are the primary elements necessary for V(D)J recombination, a computerized alignment of several hundred spacer sequences has detected some preferred nucleotides at specific positions *(4)*, and different spacer sequences can affect recombination frequency *(5)*. For example, when T cells rearrange Vβ, Dβ, and Jβ regions, direct Vβ to Jβ rearrangements (omitting Dβ) would be consistent with the 12/23 rule, but are largely prevented by specific features of the Dβ RSS and spacer, a restriction known as "beyond 12/23" (reviewed in ref *[6]*).

After the DNA is cut by the RAG proteins, the two coding ends (e.g., V and J) undergo several processing steps and are eventually ligated together to create the assembled V gene; the two RSS ends are also joined, generally creating a circular DNA "excision product," as discussed later.

THE THREE IMMUNOGLOBULIN GENE LOCI

This section presents an overview of the three immunoglobulin loci (heavy chain, κ, and λ), mainly considering C regions. The V regions of these loci are described later in this chapter in the section on germline diversity.

Heavy Chain Genes

Murine and human genomic clones encoding constant region heavy chain (CH) genes include separate exons encoding the ~100 to 110 amino acid Ig domains that were independently identified by internal homologies of amino acid sequences and by three-dimensional structural analysis (X-ray crystallography); these exons are separated from each other by introns of roughly 0.1 kb to 0.3 kb. Thus, for example, the mouse γ2b protein has three major domains (CH1, CH2, and CH3) with a small hinge domain between CH1 and CH2. The gene structure may be summarized:

CH1	—intron—	**hinge**	—intron—	**CH2**	—intron—	**CH3**
(292)	(314)	(64)	(106)	(328)	(119)	(322)

where the numbers in parentheses represent the number of nucleotides in each segment. As an interesting contrast, the hinge region of the α gene is encoded contiguously with the CH2 domain with no intervening intron, while the unusually long human γ3 hinge is encoded by three or four hinge exons.

About 7 kb upstream from the murine Cμ gene lies a cluster of four JH segments that participate in VDJ recombination (the human locus has six JH segments). Further upstream lie 13 D segments (about 27 in human) and beyond them the VH regions.

Genomic Organization of CH Gene Loci

Each B lymphocyte initially produces IgM by expressing an assembled V region with Cμ, but may use CSR to replace Cμ with one of the several CH regions lying downstream, thereby allowing expression of IgG, IgA, or IgE (Figure 6.4A). These downstream CH genes were cloned by a variety of investigators, and all eight murine CH genes—spanning about 200 kb of DNA on chromosome 12—were linked by contiguous clones in 1982 (7) as shown in Figure 6.4B, where the numbers indicate the approximate distance in kilobases between the genes. All the CH genes are oriented in the same 5′-3′ direction. Several γ pseudogenes lie within the clustered γ genes *(8)*.

The human CH genes were similarly cloned, and then eventually completely linked by the Human Genome Project. The human IgH locus contains a large duplication, with two copies of a γ-γ-ε-α unit separated by a γ pseudogene (Figure 6.4B). One of the duplicated ε sequences is also a pseudogene in which the CH1 and CH2 domains have been deleted. In addition, the human genome contains a third closely homologous ε-related sequence—a "processed" pseudogene retroposed to chromosome 9. The map presented in Figure 6.4B also indicates several known deletions in the human heavy chain locus. The sequences of the entire human and mouse IgH loci are now available online at www.ncbi.nlm.nih.gov.

The IgH locus has also been examined in several other species besides mouse and human, and several notable differences have been observed. Rabbits, for example, have 13 Cα sequences and only a single Cγ gene *(9)*; this unusual expansion of genes contributing to mucosal immunity may be related to the peculiar habit of coprophagy in these animals. In contrast to the multiplicity of rabbit Cα genes, pigs have only one Cα gene and eight Cγ genes. Camels are unusual in having heavy chains that function in the absence of light chains *(10)*. Heavy chain Ig genes (VH or CH) have been cloned from a number of other species, including rat (which is highly homologous with mouse), cow, dog, chicken, horse, shark, bony fish, crocodile, frog, and axolotl.

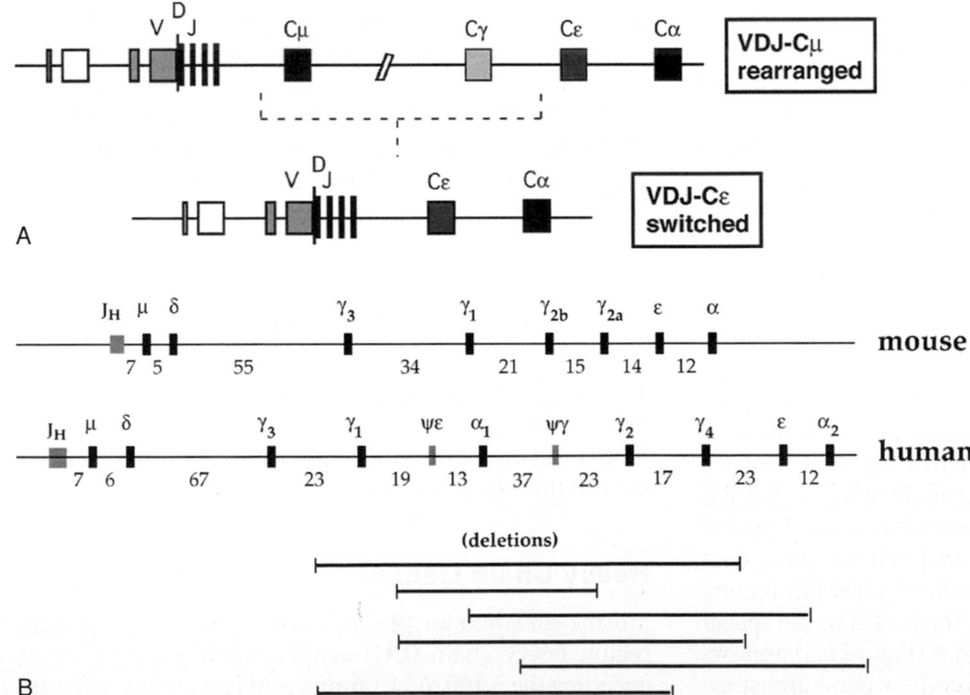

FIGURE 6.4 Deletional isotype switch recombination. **A:** The expression of "downstream" heavy chain genes is accomplished by a recombination event that replaces the Cμ gene with the appropriate heavy chain C gene (Cε is shown as an example), deleting the DNA between the recombination breakpoints. **B:** The murine and human heavy chain constant region genes are diagrammed with the approximate intergene distance indicated below (in kb); various literature values for these distances differ somewhat, possibly due to allelic polymorphisms. The human locus shows a large duplication of γ-γ-ε-α sequences. Deletions observed in various human alleles are shown below the map of the human locus.

Membrane vs. Secreted Ig

Studies of IgH gene and cDNA structure have provided an explanation for how a single heavy chain gene can encode both the soluble form of the H chain secreted by plasma cells and the alternative membrane-bound immunoglobulin displayed as BCR on the surface of B cells. The membrane-bound Ig H chains are slightly larger than the secreted forms owing to an additional C-terminal hydrophobic segment that anchors the protein in membrane lipids. In the case of the μ chain, the membrane and secreted forms are products of two different mRNAs of 2.7 kb and 2.4 kb, which can be separated by gel electrophoresis. Sequence comparisons between a genomic μ clone and μ cDNA clones corresponding to these two RNA species demonstrated that the two RNAs represent transcripts of the identical gene that have been spliced differently at their 3′ or C-terminal ends (Figure 6.5). The nucleotide sequence encoding the 20 C-terminal residues of the secretory (μs) form is derived from DNA contiguous with the CH4 domain of the μ gene, whereas in the membrane mRNA (μm), the sequence following CH4 derives from two exons (M1 and M2) lying about 2 kb further 3′. These membrane exons encode 41 residues, including a stretch of 26 uncharged residues that span the membrane to stabilize the Ig in the cell membrane. The same general gene structure has been found for the other CH genes, suggesting that the differential splicing mechanism accounts for the two forms of Ig of all isotypes.

Early B cells make roughly similar quantities of both μm and μs, whereas maturation to the plasma cell stage is associated with strong predominance of μs production, facilitating high-level secretion of circulating Ig. The balance between the two RNA splice forms of μ has been interpreted as a competition between CH4-M1 splicing versus the cleavage/polyadenylation at the upstream μs poly(A) addition site. These processes are mutually exclusive because CH4-M1 splice removes the μs poly(A) site, while cleavage at the μs poly(A) site removes the membrane exons. The cis elements influencing the balance between these processes have been studied by transfecting either early or late B cells (or nonlymphoid cells) with μ gene sequences or constructs in which the splice sites, coding exons, or cleavage/polyadenylation sites have been mutated, placed different distances apart, or replaced with other sequences.

The μm poly(A) site appears to be intrinsically more active than the μs poly(A) site when tested in separate plasmids, and some evidence suggests competition between these sites *(11,12)*. Their relative usage is influenced by cis-acting sequences near the μs poly(A) site of the RNA, including a hexamer polyadenylation signals (AAUAAA) upstream of the μs poly(A) addition site and GU-rich sequences downstream of the site *(12)*. The binding of a cleavage stimulator factor CstF64K to GU-rich sequences can apparently stimulate the strength of the μs poly(A) site, because the μs/μm ratio was increased when CstF64K was artificially increased in a B cell line (13). The binding of this protein to the μs GU-rich sequences may be suppressed prior to the secretory stage of B lymphoid development by inhibitory factors. One such inhibitor is the U1A protein, which binds to the RNA and prevents both CstF64K binding and μs poly(A) site cleavage *(14,15)*. A reduction in the level of free U1A fraction during maturation to secretory plasma cells apparently releases the μs poly(A) site from the block in CstF64K binding and allows RNA cleavage at that site *(16)*. The shift to μs expression has been found to require the activity of the "master regulator" of plasma cell differentiation Blimp-1 (B lymphocyte–induced maturation protein-1; discussed in Chapter 7) *(17)*. Cis-acting sequences affecting the ratio of alternative splice forms have been described for other isotypes besides Cμ, particularly Cα (18).

Membrane Ig serves as the antigen-specific component of the BCR that is critical for initiating the signal for lymphocyte activation following contact with antigen, as described in Chapter 8. The segments of membrane immunoglobulins (of all isotypes) that penetrate into the cytoplasm are too short to encode functional signal transduction domains. Instead, transduction is mediated by an associated protein dimer composed of the

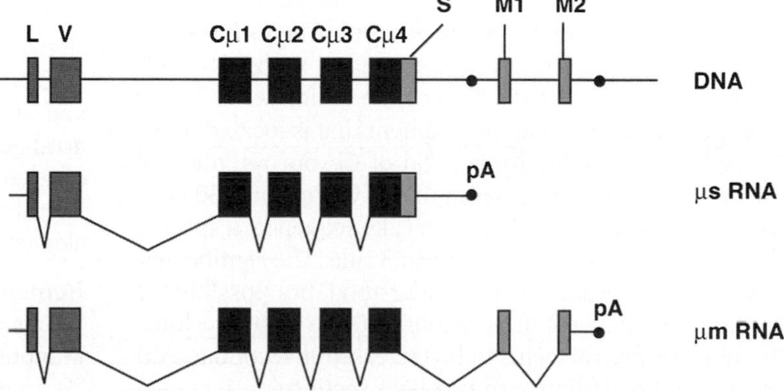

FIGURE 6.5 Two RNAs generated from the μ gene by alternative processing. The top line illustrates the exons of the μ gene (black rectangles) in an expressed, rearranged μ gene. A primary transcript including all the exons present in the DNA can be processed as shown to yield either μs RNA (containing a C-terminal "secreted" [S] sequence) or μm RNA (containing the two membrane [M] exons).

BCR components Ig-α and Ig-β (CD79a and CD79b) whose cytoplasmic domains contain immunoreceptor tyrosine-based activation motifs (ITAMs) similar to those found in the CD3 chains mediating T cell receptor (TCR) signaling. The Ig-α-Ig-β dimer also plays important signaling roles during B cell development before the mature BCR is assembled, as discussed later in this chapter.

Kappa Light Chain Genes

In comparison to the heavy chain genes, the κ locus is relatively simple. A single Cκ gene with a single exon and no reported alternative splice products is found in both mice and humans. Upstream of the murine Cκ gene lie the five Jκ gene segments mentioned earlier, spaced about 0.3 kb apart. The third of these Jκ segments encodes an amino acid sequence never observed in κ chains and is believed to be nonfunctional owing to a defect in the splice donor site that would join the corresponding RNA sequence to Cκ. The human locus is quite similar, with five functional Jκ regions upstream of Cκ. Upstream of the Jκ segments in both species are the Vκ genes, which will be described later in this chapter.

Apart from Vκ-Jκ rearrangement, an additional recombination event occurs uniquely in the κ locus, apparently mediated by the same heptamer/nonamer signal elements involved in V(D)J recombination. This event, which involves deletion of the Cκ gene segment, was initially suggested by the observation that Southern blots of DNA from λ-expressing human lymphoid cells generally show no detectable Cκ sequence *(19)*. Apparently in most B cells the Cκ genes are deleted from both chromosomes before λ gene rearrangement begins. When the boundaries of the deleted segment of DNA were examined in several human and mouse cell lines, a common sequence element was found at the downstream boundary; this element was designated RS (recombining sequence) in the mouse studies *(20)* and kde (kappa deleting element) in the human studies *(21)*. The human kde in germline DNA is located 24 kb downstream of the Cκ gene and is flanked by a heptamer/nonamer RSS similar to that found flanking the Jκ regions—that is, with a 23 bp spacer. The similar murine RS is about 25 kb downstream from murine Cκ. The kde element can apparently recombine either with a Vκ gene segment (leading to a deletion of the entire Jκ-Cκ locus) or with an isolated heptamer element that is located in the Jκ-Cκ intron (leading to deletion of Cκ but retention of the Jκ locus). The heptamer in the Jκ-Cκ intron is 30 bp 5′ from a poorly conserved nonamerlike sequence, a spacing that seems to violate the usual 12/23 rule. The significance of this unusual spacer is not understood, but possibly the heptamer in these recombinations is active without a functional nonamer, as seems to be the case for secondary VH recombinations (discussed in a later section).

Lambda Light Chain Genes

Murine λ Locus

In laboratory mouse strains, λ chains represent only about 5% of L chains, and this diminished abundance is associated with remarkably meager diversity. In contrast to the κ system with its multiple V region families, amino acid sequence analysis of monoclonal λ chains detected only two sequences that appeared to represent germline Vλ regions. Further, in contrast to the single mouse Cκ region, three nonallelic mouse Cλ isotypes are known from secreted λ chains; these are designated λ1, λ2, and λ3, in decreasing order of abundance.

Complete sequence analysis *(22)* (Figure 6.6) of the murine locus reveals four Cλ genes, each with its own Jλ region gene located about 1.3 kb 5′ of the C. The J-Cλ2 and J-Cλ4 genes are arranged in one cluster about 3 kb apart with the Vλ2 gene lying about 60 kb upstream. (At the 3′ end of Jλ4 a mutation has destroyed the "GT" found at almost all known "donor" splice sites, so that an RNA transcript of this gene would not be properly processed, reminiscent of the mouse Jκ3.) A second Cλ cluster lying about 110 kb downstream of the Cλ2-Cλ4 locus contains J-Cλ3 and J-Cλ1. The gene order (V2-Vx-JC2-JC4-V1-JC3-JC1) explains the common expression of Vλ2 (or Vx) in association with Cλ2, and Vλ1 with Cλ1 or Cλ3. The Vλ2 has been found in rare association with the Cλ1 locus, which lies 180 kb downstream in the germline; but the "backward" recombination of Vλ1 with Cλ2 has not been observed. The similarities between the four J-C genes suggest that the two clusters arose by a duplication of an ancestral V-J-Cλx-J-Cλy unit that in turn was the result of a prior J-Cλ duplication event. The ancestry of the Vx gene is uncertain, as this gene is rather dissimilar to the other Vλ genes; indeed it resembles Vκ as much as Vλ. Anti-Vλx antisera detect expression of this Vλ in all laboratory mice tested, but it may have a particular restricted function. Analyses of λ genes in wild mice by Southern blotting have indicated more complex and varied loci than that seen in typical laboratory strains.

The Jλ gene segments are all flanked on their 5′ side by sequences similar to the nonamer and heptamer signal elements observed in the heavy chain and κ system. The 12/23 rule discussed in relation to spacing between the signal elements applies as well to λ, but in the λ locus the RSS elements are spaced about 23 bp apart for V regions and about 12 bp apart for J regions (the opposite of the arrangement in κ genes) as shown in Figure 6.3. The decreased abundance of λ2 and λ3 relative to λ1 may be related to discrepancies between their nonamer homology elements and the consensus nonamer element.

Human λ Locus

Lambda L chains are much more abundant in man than in mouse (about 40% of human light chains versus about 5% in mouse). Four forms of human λ chains have been

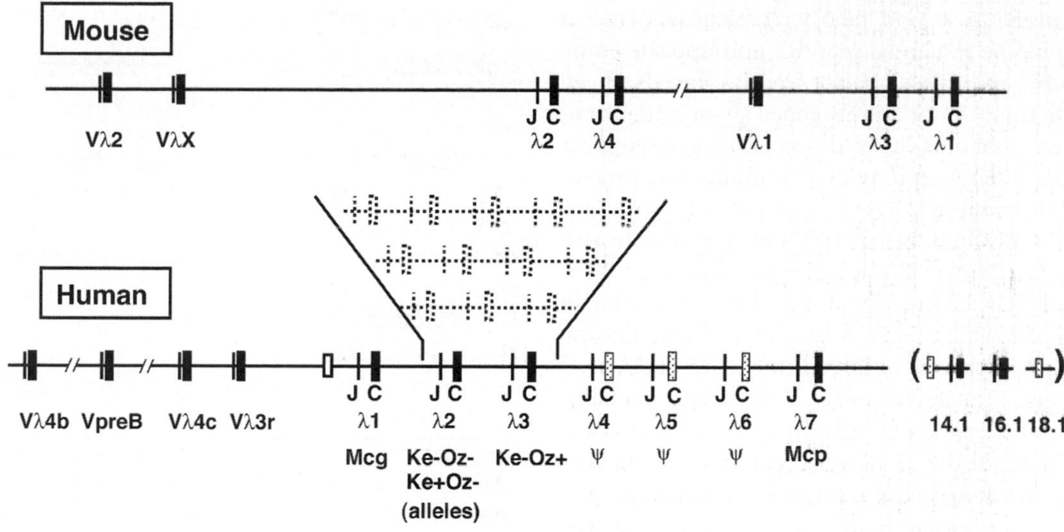

FIGURE 6.6 Germline λ genes. The maps in this figure are schematic, i.e., not to scale. A. The murine λ gene system includes four JC complexes and three V genes as shown. B. The human λ locus includes multiple V genes, of which only three are shown. The human VpreB "surrogate" light chain gene is located within the Vλ cluster. The Cλ locus includes a segment of seven JC complexes plus three additional unlinked sequences. The hatched JC complexes diagrammed above the seven linked λ sequences represent polymorphic variants with additional duplications of the JC unit. The 14.1 sequence—the human λ5 "surrogate" light chain homolog—lies downstream of the JC cluster. Exon 1 of the 14.1 gene is homologous to an exon upstream of Jλ1 (as indicated by the unlabeled white rectangle).

characterized serologically, with differences residing in a small number of amino acids in the constant region. The serological classification of Kern$^+$ depends on Gly at position 152 versus Ser in Kern$^-$. The Oz$^+$ designation depends on Lys at #190 vs. an Arg on Oz$^-$. And Mcg$^+$ λ chains (versus Mcg$^-$) have Asn112 (versus Ala), Thr114 (versus Ser) and Lys163 (versus Thr).

Seven human Jλ-Cλ segments are clustered within an approximately 33 kb region of DNA. As shown in Figure 6.6, genes for four major expressed human λ isotypes have been localized within the major cluster and correspond to JCλ1, JCλ2, JCλ3 and JCλ7. JCλ7 was originally interpreted as encoding the Kern$^+$Oz$^-$ serologic form of λ, but more recent data suggest that the latter is an allele of Cλ2, and that JCλ7 encodes an isotype provisionally designated Mcp (23). The other three homologous J-C segments found in most haplotypes are apparently pseudogenes, with either in-frame stop codons or frame-shifting deletions. However, JCλ6 may be functional in some individuals, and the common allele—which has a 4 bp insertion leading to a deletion of the C-terminal third of the Cλ region—can nevertheless undergo Vλ-Jλ recombination, encoding a truncated protein that can associate with heavy chains. A variety of polymorphic variants of the human λ locus have been detected, apparently the result of gene duplication; as shown in Figure 6.6, one to three extra λ segments have been detected on Southern blots of human DNA, and some have been sequenced (24).

Three Cλ-related sequences have been discovered near the major Jλ-Cλ cluster. One of these, designated λ14.1, represents the human homolog of the murine "surrogate" light chain λ5 (see below). Finally, an additional weakly hybridizing DNA segment outside the linked cluster has been characterized as a "processed" pseudogene. V genes of the human λ system have been completely characterized, as discussed in a later section.

λ-related "Surrogate" Light Chains

In mature B cells, Ig heavy chains cannot reach the cell surface if light chain synthesis is interrupted. However, immunoglobulin μ heavy chains can be detected on the surface of pre-B cells that do not make light chains. In these cells a "surrogate light chain" (SLC) composed of two smaller proteins facilitates the surface expression of μ protein. One component of SLC was identified as the product of a gene expressed exclusively in pre-B cells that showed high sequence similarity to the J and C regions of the λ locus. It was designated λ5, because four murine Cλ genes were already known *(25)*. The genomic λ5 gene includes three exons: exon 1, which appears to encode a signal peptide; exon 2, whose 3′ end is homologous to Jλ; and exon 3, homologous to Cλ. The second component of SLC was found as a transcribed segment about 4.7 kb 5′ of λ5 in the mouse genome. Sequence analysis of the latter region revealed similarities to both Vλ and Vκ; for this reason (and because of its expression in preB cells), it is called VpreB1. A second, nearly identical sequence in the mouse genome is named VpreB2 and appears to be functional *(26)*, and a less similar VpreB3 has also been described. Neither λ5 nor VpreB genes show evidence of gene rearrangement in B or pre-B cells. Both genes appear functional, and homologs have been found in every mammalian species examined.

The two SLC proteins have been found to associate with μ heavy chains to permit surface μ expression prior to the availability of light chains. Thus, when a μ heavy chain gene was transfected into an Ig-negative myeloma line, no surface μ expression was observed unless λ5 and VpreB genes were also transfected *(27)*. The surface μ chains were found to be covalently linked to the 22 kD product of the λ5 gene, while the 16 kD VpreB product was noncovalently associated. A similar complex is observed in pre-B cell lines and in normal bone marrow pre-B cells. The V-like VpreB gene product apparently associates with the Cλ-like λ5 product to form a light-chain-like heterodimer that is able to fulfill some functions of a true light chain.

One likely role for a μ-SLC complex is suggested by the observation that most Vκ-Jκ recombination occurs only in cells expressing a functional μ heavy chain; apparently μ-SLC expression on the cell surface can trigger the onset of Vκ-Jκ rearrangement. Evidence for this view comes from experiments in which a pre-B line that normally does not rearrange its κ locus was transfected with a construct encoding the membrane form of μ heavy chain (28); when the transfected μ gene was expressed in a complex containing VpreB and λ5, Vκ rearrangement was induced.

As mentioned earlier, three λ5-like sequences are located downstream of the human Cλ cluster on chromosome 22 (Figure 6.6), but only one—designated 14.1—appears to be functional, possessing the three-exon structure of λ5. The human VpreB homolog lies within the Vλ cluster *(29)*, in contrast to murine VpreB, which lies close upstream of λ5.

V GENE ASSEMBLY RECOMBINATION

The mechanism by which germline variable region constituents (VL and JL, or VH, D, and JH) assemble in the DNA to form a complete active V gene has been pursued ever since Ig gene recombination was first discovered. In this section we will address (1) the topology of the recombinations from a macro viewpoint, (2) the components of the recombinase machinery (a micro view), and (3) the regulation of that machinery in B cell development.

Topology of V Assembly Recombination

Deletion vs. Inversion

For V segments and J segments oriented in the same direction of transcription, the DNA between the recombining V and J segments can be simply deleted and religated as an excision circle, as described previously (and illustrated in Figure 6.7A). Such a DNA circle would not be attached to the main chromosome and, failing to replicate, it would be diluted out as cells divide after V(D)J recombination. Such circles are therefore generally absent in B lineage cell lines and in mature B lymphocytes that have undergone several rounds of proliferation after Ig expression. By isolating circular DNA from cells actively undergoing Vκ-Jκ rearrangement it has been possible to clone the predicted circular molecules bearing signal joints *(30)*. More recent experiments have used PCR to detect signal joints, especially those generated by V(D)J recombination of T cell receptor genes; a high content of TCR excision circles (TRECs) in a population has been interpreted as reflecting "recent" V(D)J recombination with relatively little subsequent proliferation (31).

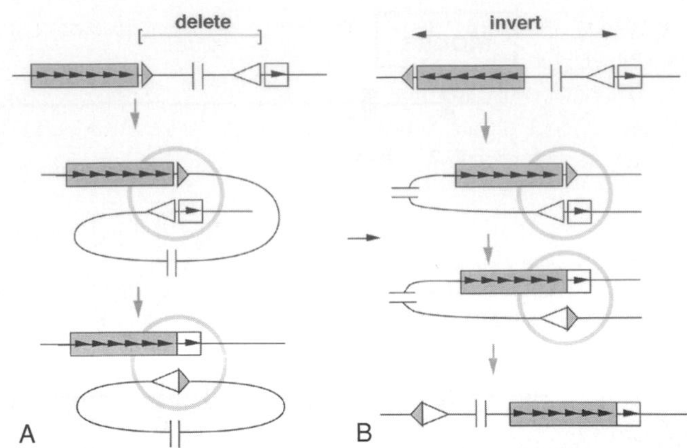

FIGURE 6.7 The same "micro" mechanism of recombination can join Vκ and Jκ by deletion or inversion, depending on the relative orientation of the two precursors in germline DNA. **A:** When V coding sequence (shaded rectangle) and J coding sequence (white rectangle) are oriented in the same 5′→3′ direction in germline DNA (as indicated by the internal arrowheads), the recombination yields a VJ coding joint plus a DNA circle containing the signal joint (apposed triangles). **B:** If V is oriented in the opposite direction in germline DNA then an identical recombination reaction at the "micro" level (inside shaded circle) leaves the signal joint linked to the recombined VJ coding joint.

However, some Vκ genes (both mouse and human) are oriented in the opposite direction from the Jκ-Cκ region, a topology that causes the VJ recombination to occur by an inversion of the DNA between the recombining V and J segments (Figure 6.7B), leaving both RSS heptamers retained on the chromosome. The same recombinase machinery can presumably rearrange the germline elements by either inversion or deletion—depending on the relative orientations of the sequences—because this enzymatic machinery "sees" only the DNA in the immediate vicinity of the recombination site (circled in Figure 6.7) and is insensitive to the topology of the DNA strands far from this site. Indeed retained "signal joints" (also known as "flank products" and "reciprocal joints") have been detected in several cell lines.

In contrast to the κ system, in the heavy chain or λ loci, there is no evidence for inverted V genes or retained signal joints, so these loci apparently recombine only by deletion (and this is also true for all the TCR gene loci).

Nonstandard Joints

Investigations of V(D)J recombination have documented several "nonstandard" recombination joints, which, though not contributing to physiological V gene assembly, may reflect features of the recombination mechanism *(32)*. These nonstandard joints can be understood by appreciating that there are three topologies in which DNA that has been cut twice—generating four ends—can be rejoined. If the four ends are coding (V), signal (V), signal (J), and coding (J), the three possibilities can be defined by considering the three different ends that may join to the coding (V) end (assuming that the remaining two ends must join to each other). The possibilities are

coding(V)-coding(J) plus signal(V)-signal(J)

This is the standard reaction product in which the coding(V)-coding(J) product encodes the assembled VJ gene and the signal(V)-signal(J) represents the signal joint.

coding(V)-signal(V) plus signal(J)-coding(J)

These products (i.e., open and shut joints) look like the starting DNAs, but can be distinguished from them if nucleotides have been added or deleted at the junctions so that they no longer hybridize to oligonucleotide probes specific for the coding/signal junction.

coding(V)-signal(J) plus signal(V)-coding(J)

These are "hybrid joints," in which the signal ends have switched places.

Hybrid and open and shut joints have been observed to form both in transfected plasmids bearing RSSs *(32)* and in endogenous immunoglobulin loci in vivo *(33)*.

Secondary Recombinations

As discussed in an earlier section, the imprecision of VJ or VDJ joining causes nonproductive, out-of-frame junctions in about two thirds of recombination products. A B lymphocyte that rearranged its κ genes nonproductively on both parental chromosomes might be thought to have no further avenue for making a functional light chain, but the availability of upstream Vκ genes and downstream Jκ segments could allow additional recombinations to occur as shown in Figure 6.8A. More complex events are possible as a consequence of the inverted orientation of some Vκ genes. The occurrence of such secondary recombinations has in fact been reported for κ genes and would be implied by the recovery of a chromosomal signal joint that is not reciprocal to a coding joint in the same cell. The preponderance of Jκ1-derived nonreciprocal flank products observed in myelomas may result from initial nonproductive recombinations between this J segment and inverted V genes, followed by successive recombinations involving more downstream J segments; by the time a productive rearrangement occurs, many myelomas will carry signal joint relics of earlier recombinations involving Jκ1. Secondary recombination may also occur in cells that have assembled a productive VκJκ joint if the resulting VH-VL pair recognizes an autoantigen. This type of secondary recombination, known as "receptor editing," is considered in more detail later in this chapter.

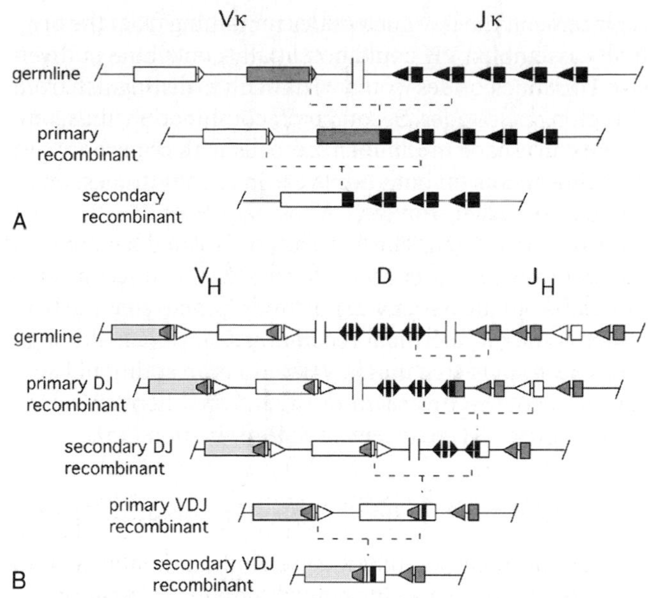

FIGURE 6.8 Secondary recombinations. **A:** In the κ light chain system, a primary recombination can be followed by recombination between an upstream V and a downstream J. **B:** Analogous secondary recombinations can occur in the heavy chain system between upstream D and downstream J segments. After VDJ recombination eliminates all "short spacer" signal elements from the chromosome, secondary recombination can still occur between VH (long spacer signal) and an internal heptamer within the VH coding sequence of the VDJ unit.

For H chain genes, secondary D-J rearrangements should be possible before VH-D recombination removes unrearranged upstream DH segments (Figure 6.8B), and indeed this has been shown to occur. Even though VDJ rearrangement must eliminate all the 12 bp-spaced signal elements from the VH locus, upstream germline VH genes can sometimes recombine with an established VDJ unit, displacing most of the originally assembled V gene *(34)*. This type of recombination (sometimes called *VH replacement*) is apparently mediated by a heptamerlike sequence that appears near the 3′ end of the coding region in about 70% of VH genes (Figure 6.8B). The internal heptamer is not generally found in light chain genes. After VH replacement, the few nucleotides remaining from the originally assembled VH could potentially contribute to diversity; such nucleotides would be difficult to distinguish from N-region nucleotides. Secondary recombination, thus, represents an escape mechanism for cells with nonproductive rearrangements on both heavy chain chromosomes, or, as alluded to earlier, for cells whose antibody can interact with an autoantigen. The fact that the isolated heptamer is apparently able to function in VH replacement recombinations without an associated nonamer implies that the heptamer is the more critical recombination signal, although it has been suggested that in VH regions an additional consensus sequence upstream of the internal heptamer may contribute to VH replacement recombination *(35)*.

Mechanism of V Assembly Recombination

As mentioned earlier, the same recombination machinery mediates all four types of immunoglobulin V gene assembly recombinations (Vκ-Jκ, Vλ-Jλ, VH-D and D-JH) as well as similar recombinations in the four TCR gene loci; this fact has allowed investigators to pool mechanistic knowledge from studies of B and T cell systems. However, the assumption of a common recombinase raises the question of how B cells preferentially rearrange Ig genes (and T cell TCR genes) when both gene systems are present in both cell lineages. This issue will be addressed later in this section.

Recombination Model Overview

A model for the detailed mechanism of the recombination event must account for the observed features of the recombination products—that is, the coding and signal joints—and of their germline precursors. In the germline precursors, the heptamer and nonamer RSS with appropriate spacing (12 bp and 23 bp) are necessary and sufficient to create efficient recombination targets; model substrates containing these elements are competent to undergo recombination even in the absence of normal V, D, or J coding regions. However, the efficiency of recombination can be influenced by features of the sequences replacing the coding regions. In the recombination products, the features of the signal joints are relatively simple: the RSS heptamers are joined "back-to-back," with only rare nucleotide additions or deletions. The features of the coding joints are more complex, due to the imprecision discussed earlier: (1) A variable number of bases are deleted from the ends of the coding regions (in comparison to the "complete" sequence in the germline precursor). (2) Nongermline nucleotides (N regions) unrelated to the germline precursor sequences are added in some coding joints; these are generally rich in G and C nucleotides. (3) Less frequently, extra bases are added that can be interpreted as "P" nucleotides; these are nucleotides that are joined to the end of an undeleted coding sequence and that form a palindrome (hence the P) with the end of that sequence (36). P nucleotides are generally only one or two base pairs, but they can be longer, especially in mice with the SCID (severe combined immunodeficiency defect) disorder.

The model shown in Figure 6.9 can serve as a framework for discussion of the recombination mechanism. The

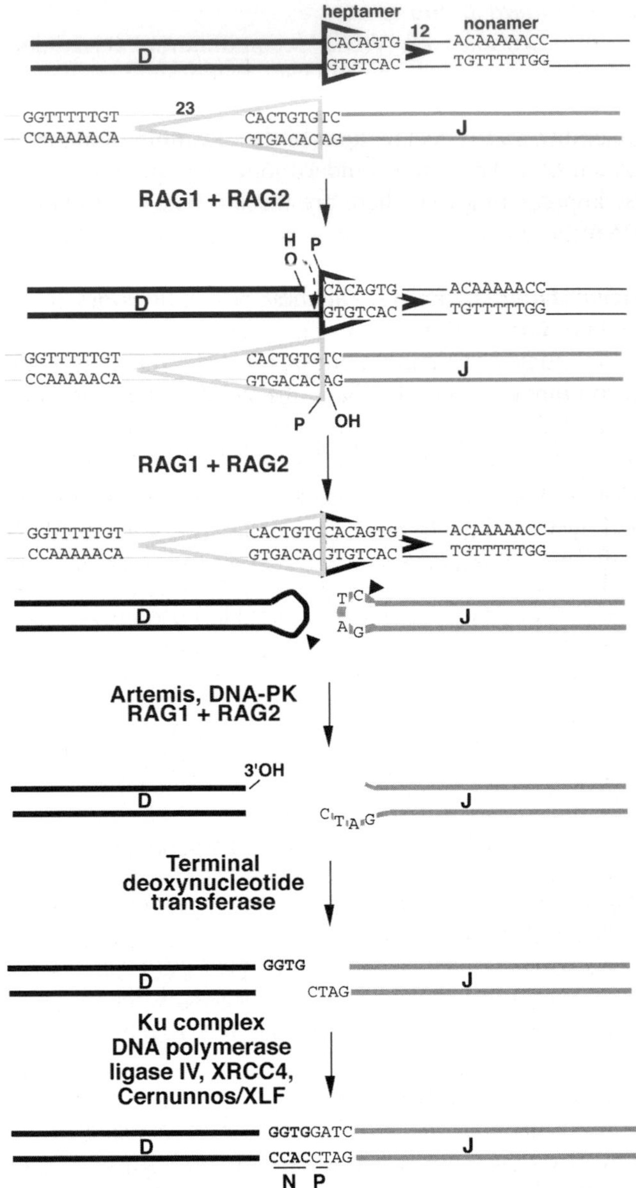

FIGURE 6.9 Model for V assembly recombinations. All V assembly recombination reactions (in Ig and TCR genes) may proceed by a common mechanism, illustrated here by D-J recombination. The RSS sequences are included in triangles, which is the conventionally used RSS graphic. Hairpin loops are created on coding ends dependent on the action of RAG1 and RAG2. After the opening of the hairpin loops the pictured D coding sequence shows the effects of "nibbling" by exonuclease but the J coding sequence is spared and shows P nucleotide generation; N region addition is pictured in this example as occurring only on the D region end. In reality, exonuclease digestion and N nucleotide addition can occur on either (or both) ends. The steps in the proposed mechanism are discussed in the text.

recombination is thought to begin with binding of the RAG1 and RAG2 proteins to the heptamer-nonamer RSS adjacent to the two segments to be recombined. Both DNA segments are then cleaved at the border of the two heptamers, and the two heptamer ends are joined together without modification. In contrast, the ends bearing the coding sequences form transient "hairpin" loops, which are then nicked open and digested to varying extents by an exonuclease activity. Recessed DNA strands may be lengthened with complementary nucleotides by a DNA polymerase, and a variable number of untemplated nucleotides may be added to the 3′ ends through the action of terminal deoxynucleotide transferase (TdT). Then the ends are ligated together, completing the recombination event.

Recombination Intermediates: Blunt Signal Ends, Hairpin Coding Ends

To study broken DNA ends as intermediates in V(D)J recombination, several labs have employed ligation-mediated PCR (LM-PCR) to detect signal ends. This technique involves ligating blunt genomic DNA ends with a double-stranded oligonucleotide, followed by amplification extending from a primer sequence near the genomic signal end to the ligated oligonucleotide sequence; amplified products can then be cloned and their sequence determined. LM-PCR analyses of both TCR and Ig genes have defined the signal ends as blunt-ended cuts, usually exactly at the heptamer border, leaving 5′ phosphate and 3′ hydroxyl groups *(37)*.

Even with less sensitive Southern blot assays, signal ends were detectable in cells undergoing intensive V(D)J recombination (e.g., thymus DNA rearranging TCR genes), but in these experiments the coding ends could not be visualized at all, perhaps because of rapid processing of these ends into coding joints. Based on the known defect of SCID lymphocytes in forming coding joints, Roth et al. (38) reasoned that SCID thymocytes might accumulate the cut coding ends that could not be visualized in normal thymocytes. Indeed, coding ends were detected in the SCID thymocyte DNA and, moreover, were found to have several properties suggestive of a hairpinlike structure. First, the coding ends in SCID thymocyte DNA were resistant to exonuclease treatment. Further, restriction fragments bearing these *in vivo*–generated ends on one side were found to move on a denaturing electrophoresis gel as if they were twice as long as predicted from the size of the double-stranded fragment before denaturation. Finally, LM-PCR experiments failed to detect the coding ends unless they were pretreated with a single strand–specific endonuclease, consistent with the impossibility of ligation to a hairpin unless it were first opened. The sequences of LM-PCR products obtained after endonuclease treatment suggested that the hairpins contained the entire sequence of the coding element, usually without loss or gain of a single nucleotide (39).

These hairpin ends apparently represent normal V(D)J recombination intermediates that—in wild-type cells—are opened at variable positions within the hairpin loop by an endonuclease activity that is dependent on the normal allele of the SCID gene. P nucleotides could then result from opening the loop at an asymmetric position (Figure 6.9); this model would explain the absence of P nucleotides from coding ends that have been "nibbled" after opening of the hairpin. Unusually long P nucleotide segments observed in the rare coding joints assembled in SCID mice might then be interpreted as resulting from resolution of hairpins by nonspecific nicking enzymes that—unlike the exonuclease activity dependent on the normal allele of the SCID gene—do not focus on the hairpin loops but nick in variable positions in the double-stranded hairpin "stem" (38). Hairpins have also been found in a non-SCID B lymphoid line engineered to sustain a high level of κ gene recombination *(40)*.

RAG Proteins: Mediators of Early Steps in V(D)J Recombination

A major advance in the investigation of V(D)J recombination was the identification of two genes whose products are critical for this process in B and T lineages. In the pioneering experiments, Schatz and Baltimore (41) stably transfected fibroblasts with a construct containing a selectable marker whose expression was dependent on V(D)J recombination; as expected, no measurable recombination occurred in this nonlymphoid cell. However, when either human or murine genomic DNA was transfected into these fibroblasts, a small fraction of recipient cells stably expressed recombinase activity, activating the selectable marker. This suggested that a single transfected genomic DNA fragment was able confer recombinase activity in a fibroblast. (Presumably the fibroblast contained endogenous copies of the same genes, but their expression was repressed by mechanisms that could not repress the transfected genes.) After successive rounds of transfection and selection for recombinase activity, the critical genomic fragment was identified. This fragment turned out to contain two genes, designated RAG1 and RAG2. Both RAG1 and RAG2 are required for recombination; therefore, these genes would not have been discovered by this transfection technique if they had chanced to lie too far apart in the genome for both to be transferred on a single DNA fragment. The genes are notable for having no introns in most species (certain fish are exceptions) and for their close association and opposite transcriptional orientation in all species examined.

A crucial role for the RAGs in V assembly recombination was supported by the conservation of these genes in a variety of Ig-producing vertebrate species from man through shark. RAG1 and RAG2 are expressed together in pre-B and pre-T cells, specifically at the stages expressing V(D)J recombinase activity. Moreover, mouse strains in which either gene has been eliminated by homologous recombination (gene "knockouts") have no mature B or T cells, as the result of abrogation of V(D)J recombination *(42,43)*. A subset of human patients with a SCID syndrome and no T or B lymphocytes have been found to have null mutations in RAGs *(44)*. Patients with less complete defects often have a complex of features (oligoclonal T cells, hepatosplenomegaly, eosinophilia, decreased serum immunoglobulin but elevated IgE) known as the Omenn syndrome, which can also be caused by defects in other genes involved in V(D)J recombination. The same RAG mutation can in different patients cause either Omenn syndrome or SCID, depending on unknown factors *(45)*.

Attempts to demonstrate activities of the RAG proteins on recombination substrates in vitro were initially hampered by poor solubility of the proteins, but functional analyses of truncated RAGs—using RAG expression vectors cotransfected into fibroblasts along with recombination substrate plasmids—revealed that surprisingly large segments of both proteins could be deleted without eliminating recombinase activity; and some of the remaining core regions were soluble and could be handled relatively easily as fusion proteins. This work allowed the demonstration that in a cell-free *in vitro* system core regions of the two RAG proteins together are capable of carrying out cleavage of substrate DNAs as well as hairpin formation on the coding end *(46)*.

Murine RAG1 is a 1040-residue protein, with a central core (residues 384 to 1008) that includes all the known enzymatic activities of the whole protein as well as a nuclear localization signal. The protein exists as a dimer, which shows intrinsic binding affinity for the RSS nonamer sequence in the absence of RAG2. This binding is dependent on residues 389 to 486, known as the nonamer-binding domain (NBD). Mutational analysis has revealed regions of the protein necessary for binding to RAG2, as well as three amino acids critical for enzymatic activity: D600, D708, and E962 *(47,48)*.

Murine RAG2 is a 527-residue protein, with a core (residues 1 to 382) sufficient for activity. This protein has little intrinsic binding affinity for RSS elements, but improves the strength and specificity of RAG1 binding *(49)*. The binding of RAG2 also extends the nucleotide sequence over which DNA-protein interactions can be detected (by DNA footprinting or ethylation interference experiments) beyond the nonamer and into the heptamer *(50)*. In the presence of divalent cations, the two RAG proteins can form a stable signal complex with an RSS having a 12 bp spacer (12-RSS), but efficient complex formation with a 23-RSS requires the addition of a high-mobility group (HMG) protein, either HMG1 or HMG2 *(51)*. These abundant and ubiquitous proteins are known to bind DNA in a non–sequence-specific manner and to cause a local bend in DNA. They apparently facilitate RAG1/2 binding by stabilizing bending induced by the RAG proteins themselves *(52)*.

The RAG-induced cleavage occurs in two steps: first a nick occurs on one strand adjacent to the heptamer—the top strand as drawn in Figure 6.9; then the 3′ hydroxyl created at the nick causes transesterification by nucleophilic attack on the phosphodiester bond adjacent to the heptamer on the bottom strand (Figure 6.9), yielding a hairpin on the coding end and a new 3′hydroxyl on the 3′ end of the bottom heptamer strand (53). RAG1 is apparently necessary for both steps, because some RAG1 mutants can nick at the heptamer efficiently but show impaired hairpin formation. After DNA cleavage, the RAG proteins remain in a complex with the DNA. RAG proteins likely facilitate steps beyond cleavage and hairpin formation, since mutant forms of RAG1 or RAG2 have been reported that are competent for cleavage but show impairment in coding or signal joint formation.

The activities of the RAG proteins are regulated by divalent ions in the medium *(54,55)*. In Mn^{++}, the RAG proteins catalyze cleavage of substrates with a single RSS, but in Mg^{++}, cleavage requires two RSSs and occurs most efficiently if the substrates conform to the 12/23 rule regarding the spacing between heptamer and nonamer elements. Thus, this rule may be enforced by the RAG proteins, though other proteins, including HMG1/2, seem to contribute to 12/23 specificity, perhaps by promoting an optimal molecular "architecture." *In vivo* experiments suggest that RAG proteins may bind to an RSS-12 and create a nick but do not complete DNA cleavage until an RSS-23 is captured (56). Further, experiments using thymocytes undergoing TCRβ V(D)J recombination indicate that cleavage at one signal end does not occur unless a "partner" DNA segment with a compatible RSS is available (57). These constraints would prevent creation of a potentially dangerous double-strand break (dsb) until DNA with a compatible RSS is present to complete the recombination.

In addition to the activities of RAG proteins on DNA segments containing RSSs, these proteins can act on several other "nonstandard" substrates:

(1) *In vitro,* core RAG proteins can catalyze the insertion of a DNA fragment with signal ends into foreign DNA, acting essentially like a transposase *(58,59)*. This transposase activity lends support to the early speculation that the V(D)J recombination system may have originated by insertion of transposonlike DNA fragment encoding RAG genes (and bearing RSSs at its ends) into a primordial V region, thereby separating J region sequence from the remainder of the V sequence upstream. This model is consistent with the many mechanistic similarities between V(D)J recombination and transposition (e.g., *[60]*), and the recent detection of RAG1 homologs in a transposon family found in of insect, echinoderm, helminth, coelenterate, and fungus genomes (61). (However, the recent finding of apparent homologs of both RAGs in a sea urchin genome complicates the view that the two RAGs entered the vertebrate genome via a transposon [62].) The transposase activity may also be the cause of certain oncogenic recombinations *(63,64)*.

(2) As mentioned earlier, VH replacement recombination utilizes a nonconsensus RSS heptamer within VH coding sequences. An *in vitro* model suggests that in VH replacement, the RAG proteins nick on both DNA strands without forming a hairpin coding end (65).

(3) The RAG complex also generates two nicks in cleaving within the major breakpoint region (Mbr) of the Bcl2 gene. This 150 bp segment is the target of a common RAG-catalyzed translocation between the IgH locus and the Bcl2 gene that occurs in most follicular lymphomas. In this segment, there are no RSSs, and the RAG proteins recognize an unusual sequence-dependent DNA conformation different from the normal B-form double helix (66).

Although the "core" RAG proteins have been useful for studying the biochemistry of V(D)J recombination, it is clear that the "noncore" portions of each protein confer important functions, as expected from their sequence conservation across species. These functions have been inferred by studying *in vivo* recombination in cells carrying core RAGs versus full-length copies, and by *in vitro* studies using full-length RAG proteins solubilized by various techniques. The N-terminal region of RAG1 is required *in vivo* for optimal RAG1 activity and for the formation of precise signal joints in D-J recombination (67). The C-terminal region of RAG2 has multiple functions, many of which are conferred by a PHD (plant homeo domain) finger structure (68). This region is required for precise signal joints in both D-J and V-D recombination (67), for achieving normal numbers of B and T lymphocytes *in vivo (69)* and to protect against RAG-mediated DNA transposition *(70,71)*. The RAG2 C-terminus binds directly to all four histones, and point mutations that disrupt this interaction inhibit V(D)J recombination (72). Finally the RAG2 C-terminus regulates RAG2 protein levels across the cell cycle to prevent double-strand breaks during DNA synthesis or mitosis, when such breaks could lead to chromosomal deletions *(37)*. Although the RAG1 protein and mRNA transcripts of both RAGs vary little across the cell cycle, a specific phosphorylation at Thr490 of RAG2 by a cyclin-dependent kinase mediates its destruction via ubiquitination and proteasomal degradation during S phase (73). In RAG2 knockout (KO) mice carrying a transgenic RAG2 gene with an alanine replacing the phosphorylatable threonine, RAG2 protein and double-stranded DNA breaks were found throughout the cell cycle, demonstrating the importance of the RAG2 degradation signal in cell-cycle control of V(D)J recombination *(74)*.

Apart from the obvious importance of the RAG proteins in understanding the initial steps of V(D)J recombination, knowledge of these proteins and their genes has allowed two major technical advances that have opened the way to many additional experiments. First, several nonlymphoid cell lines with known defects in various DNA repair genes have been transfected with the RAGs to see whether these gene defects impair V(D)J recombination; these experiments have revealed several other proteins required for V(D)J recombination, as described later. The second major technical fall-out from the RAGs has been the availability of the RAG1 and RAG2 KO mice. These mice have no functional B cells or T cells and are not "leaky" like SCID mice, which develop some functional B and T cells, especially as the animals age. The RAG KOs can be used to study the importance of the "innate" immune system (i.e., responses that occur in the absence of antigen-specific lymphocytes) in particular immune responses. The KOs can be used as recipients for various lymphocyte subsets to explore the roles of different cell types. They can be used to study the signals for B cell development by introducing transgenes with specific functionally recombined immunoglobulin genes and characterizing the phenotypes of lymphocytes that develop (as discussed later). Finally, they can be used in "RAG complementation" experiments designed to assess the phenotype—in lymphocytes—of various other gene KOs (75). In RAG complementation, embryonic stem (ES) cells in which the gene of interest has been knocked out by homologous recombination are injected into homozygous RAG KO (RAG $^{-/-}$) blastocysts. This procedure yields chimeric mice in which all B and T cells derive from the ES cells deleted for the gene of interest, because these are the only source of intact RAGs to support lymphocyte development. Such animals can be made more easily than a KO mouse line and can be used to study the effect of gene deletion in lymphocytes independent of effects the deletion may have in other cells. In particular, for cases where the gene KO causes embryonic lethality due to effects on nonlymphoid cells, RAG complementation allows the selective KO in lymphocytes to be studied in the background normal gene expression in nonlymphoid cells.

Nonhomologous End Joining Components

The RAGs are the critical lymphocyte-specific participants in the first steps in V(D)J recombination (recognition of RSS, cleavage, hairpin formation, and perhaps hairpin cleavage), but additional components are required to complete the reaction. The other known components function not only in V(D)J recombination but also in the ubiquitous DNA repair pathway known as nonhomologous end joining (NHEJ), which is the major pathway for repair of double-strand DNA breaks (e.g., those induced by ionizing radiation or reactive oxygen species) during the G0-G1 phases of the cell cycle. (In the S and G2 phases, the additional chromatid genome copy enables breaks to be repaired by homologous recombination.) There are six classical components of NHEJ—Ku70, Ku80, DNA-PK,

XRCC4, ligase IV, and artemis—but additional proteins play a role in some models of NHEJ. Presumably these nonlymphoid-specific proteins are engaged in the post-cleavage steps of V(D)J recombination.

The Ku Complex. The first gene for an NHEJ component to be recognized as participating in V(D)J recombination was the SCID gene described earlier. This mutation was originally identified in a mouse strain that was immunodeficient as a result of a marked impairment in V(D)J recombination of both immunoglobulin and T cell receptor genes. SCID lymphocytes are able to perform the RAG-mediated reactions of cleavage and hairpin formation and can form signal joints, but are markedly defective in coding joint formation. Subsequently it was found that the SCID mutation also impairs NHEJ, causing radiosensitivity.

The gene mutated in the mouse SCID model encodes DNA-PK, a DNA-dependent protein kinase that is part of a heterotrimer known as the Ku complex. Originally described as the autoantigen recognized by a patient antiserum, Ku is composed of an approximately 70 kD protein (Ku70) and an approximately 86 kD protein (Ku86, often called Ku80). Together these two very abundant proteins form a heterodimer that can bind to DNA. The DNA-Ku complex can then recruit DNA-PK. (In an alternative terminology, the Ku-DNA-PK complex is designated DNA-PK, and the protein kinase is designated $DNA\text{-}PK_{CS}$ [catalytic subunit].) Ku genes are conserved in drosophila, yeast, and even bacteria, consistent with a function in NHEJ not restricted to V(D)J recombination. Targeted DNA-PK murine KO strains show a phenotype resembling the original SCID mutation (i.e., defective coding but not signal joint formation *[76,77]*). Ku80 mutant cell lines are defective in both signal and coding joint formation, and mice with a KO of the Ku80 gene are severely impaired in B and T cell development *(78)*. Cells with homozygous disruption of Ku70 are also defective in V(D)J recombination induced by RAG gene transfection *(79)*.

The Ku complex had previously been studied as an activity with an unusual DNA binding specificity: rather than recognizing particular nucleotide sequences, it recognizes topological features of DNA, particularly double-stranded DNA ends such as might be generated by X-rays or by recombinases. Indeed, Ku may be the primary detector of broken DNA. Once bound to an end, Ku can translocate down the length of the DNA. These properties can be interpreted in light of the three-dimensional structure of the protein (80). DNA bound to the Ku heterodimer resembles a finger wearing two adjacent rings, with the negatively charged DNA "finger" contacting positive charges on the interior surface of the rings. Continuous unbroken DNA is topologically inaccessible to unbound Ku "rings," but a DNA end could be threaded into the ring, which could then slide along the DNA axis. How the Ku protein "ring" might be removed after a DNA break has been resealed is not known.

DNA-PK is a large protein (460 kD) with a domain near its C-terminus that is related to phosophoinositide-3-kinase (PI3K) and that contributes to activation and autophosphorylation of the protein. *In vitro* kinase activation of the DNA-PK in the presence of DNA fragments was found to be efficient when the DNA ends either were at high concentration or, if at low concentration, were on DNA fragments long enough to circularize readily; but when the DNA-PK was located on the ends of DNA fragments too short to circularize (and too dilute to interact efficiently with other DNA ends), the DNA-PK activation was much reduced. This implies that autophosphorylation, kinase activation, and exposure of DNA ends can only occur after two DNA ends are brought together by DNA-PK in "synapsis" (81,82). Further phosphorylation of DNA-PK inactivates the protein and may prepare it for removal once DNA ends have been sealed.

Ligase IV and XRCC4. An important role of activated Ku-DNA-PK complex is to recruit the additional components of NHEJ. One such component is DNA ligase IV, which is recruited to the Ku complex and activated by the protein XRCC4 *(83,84)*. The evidence suggests that ligase IV is the essential ligase that joins DNA ends in V(D)J recombination and NHEJ. Human patients with ligase IV deficiency have a severe phenotype including chromosomal instability, developmental and growth retardation, radiosensitivity and immunodeficiency with a $T^-B^-NK^+$ phenotype. The rare DH-JH junctions detected show extensive nucleotide deletion consistent with delayed ligation and prolonged exonuclease digestion (85). In mice, disruption of either the XRCC4 or the ligase IV genes causes embryonic lethality associated with neuronal apoptosis. Crossing these mice with p53 mutants does not improve V(D)J recombination but does rescue the mice from embryonic lethality, suggesting that neuronal cells may be unusually susceptible to p53-triggered apoptosis induced by normal low-level DNA damage (a similar mechanism may explain the severe human phenotype) (86). The importance of ligase IV for V(D)J recombination is supported by the ability of this protein to accomplish *in vitro* ligation of DNA ends. Indeed this is the only NHEJ component necessary to join compatible sticky DNA ends *in vitro*, though XRCC4 can stimulate this joining significantly *(84)*.

Recently two laboratories independently discovered a new protein required for V(D)J recombination and NHEJ. One group used yeast two-hybrid screening to search for proteins interacting with XRCC4 (87). The other group searched for the gene causing a syndrome of T^+B^- lymphocytopenia, increased radiosensitivity, and microcephaly in a Turkish family; these investigators used functional cDNA rescue of a patient's cell line from a radiomimetic drug to identify the gene (88). The protein identified by both groups is a 299 amino acid nuclear protein, which was named Cernunnos or XRCC4-like factor (XLF). The protein has a predicted secondary structure similar to that of XRCC4, to which it binds in cells *(89)* as expected from its isolation via two-hybrid screen. When Cernunnos/XLF-deficient fibroblasts were transfected with RAGs and a recombination substrate, imprecise signal joining was observed, similar to the defect in patients with hypomorphic ligase IV mutations. These experiments all suggest a role for Cernunnos/XLF linked to the function of XRCC4 and ligase IV.

Artemis. Since the coding ends generated by RAG cleavage are not directly ligatable because of their hairpin structure, V(D)J recombination requires a single-strand endonuclease activity to cleave the hairpins. This activity is conferred by the protein named Artemis, which was discovered through positional cloning in a group of human SCID patients carrying normal genes for the then-known V(D)J recombination proteins *(90)*. Patients with homozygous null mutations of Artemis survive (no embryonic lethality) and show radiosensitivity as well as defects in coding joint—but not signal joint—formation, similar to the phenotype of DNA-PK mutations. Hypomorphic Artemis mutations can cause features of the Omenn syndrome similar to those observed with hypomorphic RAG gene mutations (91). Purified recombinant Artemis protein has an intrinsic exonuclease activity *in vitro*; however, in the presence of DNA ends, it gains a single-strand endonuclease activity when it binds to DNA-PK and, in an ATP-dependent step, becomes phosphorylated at multiple sites in the C-terminal region of the protein (92,93). The Artemis endonuclease activity can cleave synthetic and RAG-generated hairpin ends as well as other single-strand DNA near a transition to double-strand DNA (94).

DNA Polymerase X Family Members

If hairpin opening leaves blunt ends or compatible sticky ends (like, the ends generated by restriction enzymes), *in vitro* joining experiments suggest that these ends can be joined by ligase IV without any additional processing (95). However, since Artemis opens hairpins at variable positions and may engage in exonuclease "nibbling" of opened DNA ends, further processing of DNA ends generally occurs before ligation completes the recombination. This processing may include further nuclease digestion and apparently also involves variable DNA extension by three DNA polymerases—polymerase λ, polymerase μ, and terminal deoxynucleotide transferase TdT—all of which are members of the polymerase X family. All three proteins contain a Brca1-C-terminus (BRCT) domain, which confers binding to Ku (96).

N Regions and TdT. Terminal deoxynucleotide transferase, the apparent source of untemplated "N region" additions in VDJ junctions, is an enzyme found in thymus and bone marrow; in the B lineage, it is expressed almost exclusively in pro-B cells. It catalyzes the addition of nucleotides onto the 3′ end of DNA strands. Though no template specificity determines the nucleotides added, the enzyme adds dG residues preferentially, consistent with N region sequences observed between V and D and between D and J. Both N region addition and TdT are characteristically absent from fetal lymphocytes *(97)*. N region addition is common in heavy chain genes (recombined in pro-B cells) but rare in murine light chain genes (recombined in pre-B cells), though perhaps somewhat less rare in human *(98)*.

As evidence that TdT is the primary source of N nucleotides, lymphocytes with engineered defects in their TdT genes produced rearranged immunoglobulin V regions with almost no N additions. Conversely, when TdT expression was engineered in cells undergoing κ or λ light chain rearrangement, the normally low level of N region insertion in these recombinations was dramatically increased. This result suggests that the low frequency of N region sequences in normal κ or λ recombinations is not due to the inability of these coding sequences to accept N region nucleotides, but to the loss of TdT as cells progress to the stage of light chain recombination; indeed, mice engineered to undergo premature Vκ-Jκ joining in pro-B cells show an increased frequency of N region nucleotides in their recombined Vκ genes *(99)*. In normal mice, the expression of a μ heavy chain may down-regulate TdT expression (100), contributing to the reduced level during the stage of light chain recombination.

In TdT mutant mice, as well as in normal fetal lymphocytes, which express minimal TdT activity, absence of N region addition is associated with an increase in the frequency of recombination junctions in which short stretches of nucleotides could have derived from either germline element because of an overlap of identical sequences at the coding ends. These junctions suggest a recombination intermediate in which the complementary single-stranded regions from the two coding ends hybridize to each other, much as "sticky ends" generated by restriction endonucleases can facilitate ligation of DNA fragments. Such "microhomology-mediated" recombination may restrict the diversity of neonatal antibodies; possibly the resulting antibodies are enriched in specificities for commonly encountered pathogens, or have broadened specificity, as has been reported for TCRs lacking N regions (101). Decreased N region nucleotides and a high incidence of homology-mediated recombination have also been found in the rare coding joints formed in Ku80 KO mice, consistent with a role for Ku in recruiting TdT or supporting its action *(102)*.

Polymerase μ and Polymerase λ. Pol μ and pol λ are ubiquitously expressed polymerases. Both readily fill in single-strand gaps in DNA and apparently participate in V(D)J recombination by filling in single-strand 3′ overhangs generated by asymmetric hairpin opening. Without this filling in, such overhangs might be destroyed by nucleases. Indeed, when *in vitro* NHEJ reconstitution experiments are performed using purified proteins and DNA fragments with overhanging ends, the omission of pol μ or pol λ increases the deletional trimming observed in recombined sequences (96). Similar excessive deletions at V(D)J junctions are observed in mice lacking pol μ or pol λ. Remarkably, however, pol μ KO mice show abnormalities only in their light chains (103), while the deletions in pol λ KOs are restricted to their heavy chains (104). This selectivity may be explained by corresponding changes in the relative mRNA levels for these two polymerases at different stages of B lineage maturation.

Other Possible Participants in V(D)J Recombination

Proteins that Bind to DNA Breaks. In eukaryotic cells, DNA breaks initiate signals that halt cell division, induce repair, and in some cases trigger apoptosis. Several proteins can be detected at dsbs induced by V(D)J recombination or irradiation, including: γ-H2AX, a phosphorylated form of the histone H2AX; ATM, the product of the gene mutated in the disease ataxia telangiectasia; and Nbs1 (or nibrin), the product of the gene mutated in Nijmegen breakage syndrome. The importance of these proteins in V(D)J recombination is not clear because defects in all three are compatible with near normal V(D)J recombination, possibly due to compensation by related proteins.

BSAP/Pax5. Pax5 (also known as B cell specific activator protein, or BSAP) is a transcription factor required for normal B cell development. Pax5$^{-/-}$ mice are able to complete DJH recombination, but VH to DJH recombination is impaired except for certain genes located proximal to the D regions. Surprisingly, 94% of human and mouse VH coding genes were found to have potential Pax5 binding sites. Pax5 was found to coimmunoprecipitate with RAG proteins, to potentiate *in vitro* cleavage of a VH gene RSS, and to enhance VH to DJH recombination in RAG-transfected fibroblasts; the latter enhancement required intact Pax5 binding sites in the VH sequence (105).

Regulation of V(D)J Recombination in B Cell Development

The recombination events that occur between immunoglobulin gene segments are carefully regulated so that most B cells expresses only one L chain isotype (isotype exclusion) and use only one of the two homologous chromosomal loci for H and L chain genes (allelic exclusion). Isotype and allelic exclusion ensure that each lymphocyte expresses a single H_2L_2 combination, and thus a single antigen binding specificity, a crucial feature of the clonal selection model of the immune response. Current evidence suggests that V(D)J recombination is controlled at two levels: regulation of the RAG protein levels and regulation of accessibility of the germline V, D, and J elements to the recombinase machinery. Both of these factors are affected by the stage of B cell development; and conversely, the expression of immunoglobulin provides a signal critical for regulating maturation of B cells. A brief scheme of B cell development is presented below as background; a detailed account is in Chapter 7.

As shown in Figure 6.10, B and T lymphocytes differentiate from pluripotent hematopoietic stem cells in the fetal liver and bone marrow. The primordial lymphoid progenitor has the potential to differentiate into B or T lymphocytes or natural killer (NK) cells. Among the earliest markers that indicate B lineage specificity are the non-immunoglobulin components of the pre-BCR: Ig-α, Ig-β and λ5. CD19, which functions as a coreceptor in signal transduction, first appears in large proliferating pro-B cells, which also express several other distinguishing surface markers including c-kit (receptor for the stem cell factor SCF), B220 (a B lineage form of the phosphatase CD45), TdT, and CD43 (a sialoglycoprotein known as leukosialin). In the absence of heavy chain protein, most of the SLC protein remains cytoplasmic, but some SLC is displayed on the surface membrane in association with a complex of glycoproteins (represented by a hook shape in Figure 6.10), which has sometimes been called a surrogate heavy chain. This includes a cadherin-related protein of 130 kD protein (p130 in Figure 6.10) *(106)*. RAG gene expression in these cells causes DJ rearrangements on both chromosomes. Subsequently, recombination with germline VH genes occurs; and, if the recombination is "productive" (i.e., yielding an "in-frame" VDJ junction), then μ heavy chain can be produced. The μ protein appears on the B cell surface along with SLC in a pre-BCR or μ-SLC complex that also includes Ig-α and Ig-β. The resulting large pre-B cells proliferate, with RAG gene expression down-regulated. After several rounds of division, the cells become smaller, stop dividing, turn up RAG gene expression once more, undergo light chain rearrangement, and express surface IgM ("immature B cells"), again turning down RAG expression. In IgM$^+$IgD$^-$ immature B cells, contact with autoantigens may up-regulate RAG expression again to facilitate receptor editing (discussed below). When immature B cells eventually also express surface IgD they become "mature B cells" and migrate into the periphery, ready to be triggered by antigen exposure.

Regulation of RAG Expression

A complete explanation of RAG gene expression would elucidate the mechanisms conferring lymphoid specificity, the two waves of RAG expression (during IgH and IgL rearrangements), and the autoantigen-induced up-regulation

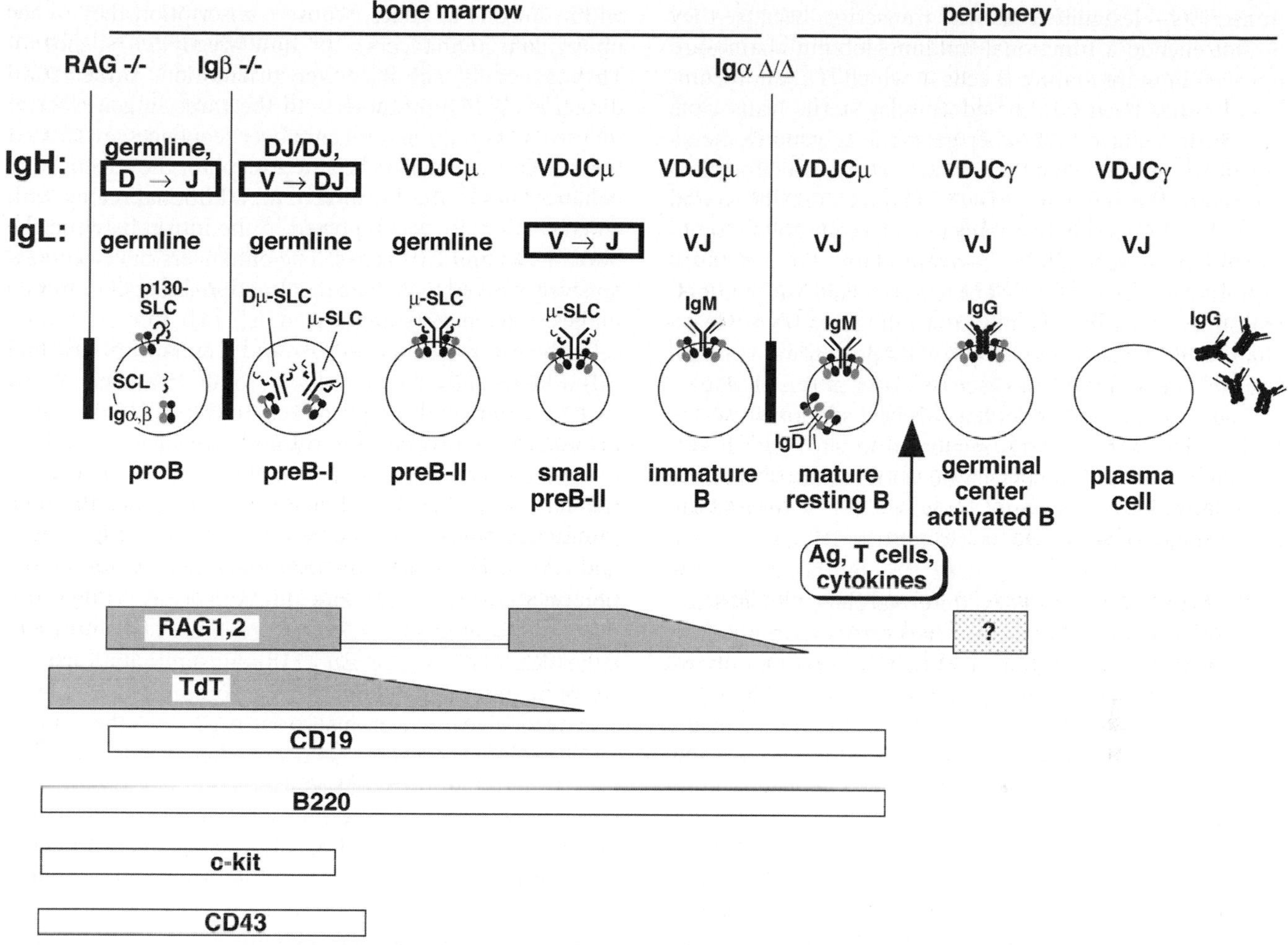

FIGURE 6.10 Ig gene recombination in B cell development. A simplified scheme of B cell development is presented as a background for discussion of Ig gene recombination. The stages occurring in the bone marrow vs. in the periphery (e.g., lymph nodes, spleen) are shown, along with the status of IgH and IgL genes at each stage. A graphic depicting the Ig-related proteins displayed on the surface at each stage is presented; and, at the bottom, the stage-dependent expression of RAGs and TdT—both important in V(D)J recombination—is schematically depicted, as well as the expression of several other marker proteins.

associated with receptor editing. Although current knowledge is incomplete, several cis elements involved in regulating RAG expression have been characterized. RAG1 and RAG2 are transcribed toward each other in opposite directions and are regulated by individual promoters and by two enhancers lying 5′ of the RAG2 genes. A RAG2 proximal enhancer designated Erag supports normal expression in B cells, and the more distal enhancer is required for expression in T cells (107,108). In addition, a silencer located between RAG1 and RAG2 inhibits expression of both RAGs in certain T cell subsets; this silencer is normally repressed by an antisilencer more than 70 kb 5′ of RAG2 (109). The B cell–specific function of many of these cis regulatory regions is explained by the intersecting specificities of transcription factors that interact with them, including Pax5, E2A, Runx, and Ikaros. Recently NFκB, which binds at several locations in the RAG enhancers, was found to be an important mediator of the up-regulation of RAG expression in cells undergoing receptor editing (110).

Parameters Affecting Recombinational Accessibility and Transcription

What maintains the locus specificity of V(D)J rearrangement in cells expressing RAG proteins—that is, why is Ig gene recombination confined to B cells, with heavy chain rearrangement before light chain, and why is TCR gene recombination exclusive to T cells? One clue is the observation that susceptibility to recombination seems to be correlated with transcriptional activity of germline gene elements. For example, many germline VH genes are transcribed at the pre-B cell stage, just at the time when these genes are targets for recombination (111); these transcripts—designated "sterile" transcripts because they do not encode a functional immunoglobulin chain—are not seen in more mature B cells in which H chain recombination has been terminated. Similar sterile transcripts have been reported for other germline Ig gene elements during the period when they are actively rearranging. Susceptibility of a segment of DNA to both transcription and recombination might be a reflection of a common chromosomal state—"accessibility"—required for both processes, or transcription itself might be a prerequisite for recombination, perhaps by partially unwinding the DNA. Heavy chain CSR is also associated with prerecombinational "sterile" transcription, as discussed later in this chapter.

The accessibility model has received support from the finding that RAG proteins incubated in vitro with nuclei from pro-B cells (which generate sterile transcripts in the IgH locus) were capable of cleaving DNA at an endogenous nuclear JH RSS, but not at a TCRδ RSS, while conversely in pro-T nuclei the TCRδ RSS but not an Ig gene RSS was cleaved (112). The differential chromatin accessibility of Ig versus TCR gene loci in B versus T lymphocytes appears to be regulated in part by the same regulatory regions that control transcription. For example, in the heavy chain locus, one enhancer (Eμ) is located in the intron between JH and Cμ. Deletion of this enhancer markedly decreased sterile transcription and V(D)J recombination *(113)*.

Ig gene expression and recombinational accessibility are regulated at several interrelated levels: (1) cis regulatory DNA sequences (e.g., promoters, enhancers and silencers) and the nuclear proteins that they recruit; (2) the chromatin context of the DNA, including covalent alterations of the histones in the nucleosomes associated with the immunoglobulin genes; (3) epigenetic DNA alterations, specifically methylation of CpG dinucleotides, which alters the binding of nuclear regulatory proteins; (4) movement of Ig genes to different subcompartments within the nucleus; (5) physical looping or contraction of the Ig loci prior to recombination; and (6) antisense transcription in the loci. A detailed account of the regulation of Ig gene expression and accessibility is beyond the scope of this chapter (see reviews, e.g., [114]), but topics will be outlined briefly to highlight recent developments.

Cis Control Sequences. Promoters, DNA regulatory regions that are generally located just upstream of the transcription initiation site, stimulate transcription in one direction—into the associated gene—by recruiting nuclear proteins that stimulate formation of a transcription complex. Each germline V gene has an upstream promoter, as do all other DNA segments that produce sterile transcripts, including DH regions, the Jκ and JH clusters, I regions (exons involved in CSR, as discussed later in this chapter), and the κ RS sequence. In contrast to promoters, enhancers and silencers may be located upstream, downstream, or within introns of genes, whose transcription they either up-regulate (enhancers) or down-regulate (silencers). They generally act in either orientation, rather than directionally like promoters. In the three Ig gene loci of mouse and human, several enhancer sequences are located downstream of each locus, and (except for the λ locus) one enhancer lies in the J-C intron. An additional region with enhancer activity was reported in the intron between the human Cδ3 and Cγ3 genes. The enhancers have been extensively studied to deduce the functional sequence motifs in these sequences (summarized in [114]). In κ-expressing cells, the κ intron enhancer (iEκ and 3′ enhancers 3′Eκ and Ed) were recently shown to loop around to associate with each other and with Vκ promoters in B cells (115); similar interactions may occur at the λ and heavy chain loci.

Although enhancers and promoters were originally discovered by placing them near reporter genes in transient transfection studies, recent experiments have used knockout or knockin replacement technologies to examine function of these elements more physiologically in their endogenous locations in the mouse genome. The deletion of either iEκ (116,117) or Eμ (118) substantially impaired germline transcription and V(D)J recombination in the respective loci. Moreover, insertion of Eμ into the κ locus in place of iEκ caused the κ locus to behave more like the heavy chain locus, in that VκJκ recombination now occurred in pro-B cells (when heavy chain VDJ recombination normally occurs) and occurred at reduced efficiency in pre-B cells, the normal stage for VκJκ recombination (119).

Sequences with silencer activity have been described upstream (120) and downstream (121) of the entire heavy chain locus, where they might play a role in insulating the locus from the regulation of neighboring genes. In the κ locus, a downstream silencer has been reported, as well as another silencer in the Vκ-Jκ intron (122).

The activity of all cis regulatory sequences depends on the nuclear content of specific transcription factors that bind to short motifs within these sequences; activities of these factors are in turn regulated by the developmental stage and the environmental milieu of the cell.

Histone Interactions. In mammalian nuclei, DNA is highly compacted at several levels, most fundamentally by being wrapped around a nucleosome composed of eight histone proteins. Several groups have shown that when purified DNA is reconstituted *in vitro* with histones, its susceptibility to RAG cleavage at RSSs is reduced *(123,124)*. Nucleosome reconstitution is also associated with decreased template activity for RNA transcription. *In vivo,* enhancer- or promoter-dependent acetylation of histones by histone acetyltransferases is associated with increased template activity of many genes, possibly because acetylation of histone tails loosens the association between DNA and the histones. In addition, methylation of specific residues in histone tails may, by providing binding targets for particular nuclear proteins, "mark" chromatin for silencing or activation. Experimentally, learning which covalent histone modifications are associated with a specific gene locus depends on the technique of chromatin immunoprecipitation (ChIP). In this technique, nucleosomes (with attached DNA) carrying a particular histone modification are precipitated with an antibody specific for that modification; DNA in the precipitate is then assayed for the presence of specific target sequences, commonly by PCR. Several groups have used ChIP to document the distribution of chromatin marks in Ig genes and have correlated changes with V(D)J recombination (e.g., 125,126).

For example, the extent of *in vivo* histone acetylation in the IgH (127) and κ (128) loci was found to correlate with developmentally regulated activation of susceptibility to V(D)J recombination, including a fall in acetylation as the IgH locus is deactivated during the κ locus recombination at the pre-B stage *(129)*. Trichastatin A, an inhibitor of the histone deacetylases (which remove the acetyl "marks" from chromatin), increased histone acetylation as well as VκJκ recombination in a pre-B cell line *(130)*. In an examination of *in vitro* (RAG + HMG1)–mediated cleavage of RSS-containing DNA, the inhibitory effect of nucleosome reconstitution was found to be relieved by acetylation of the histones and, additively, by adding ATP plus the ATP-dependent remodeling complex known as SWI/SNF; the inhibition was also relieved by complete removal of the histone tails *(131)*.

Apart from accessibility changes, V(D)J recombination has another link to histones through a direct interaction between the C-terminal domain of RAG2 and the histones. As described earlier, this interaction is required for efficient V(D)J recombination, but the mechanism is unknown (72).

DNA Methylation. Most cytosine residues within CpG dinucleotides are methylated in mammalian DNA, but genes that are actively expressed in a particular cell are generally relatively undermethylated in that cell type, suggesting that DNA methylation inhibits transcription. DNA methylation also seems to inhibit V(D)J recombination. Thus, the developmental maturation from pro-B cell to pre-B is associated with progression from a κ locus that is methylated, nontranscribed, and nonrearranging to one that is hypomethylated, transcribed, and rearranging *(132,133)*. Further, plasmid templates containing Ig RSSs were found to undergo V(D)J recombination when transfected into a recombination competent B cell line, but prior methylation of the DNA impaired recombination *(134)*, and V(D)J recombination of a transgenic construct occurred only when it was unmethylated *(135)*. Demethylation thus appears necessary for V(D)J recombination, though it is not sufficient. Methylation and histone acetylation are interrelated—for example, the methyl-CpG-binding protein MeCP2 recruits histone deacetylases, which reduce acetylation of histones.

Compartmentalization. Several studies using fluorescence in situ hybridization (FISH) have indicated that inactive genes tend to be located in the periphery of nuclei, while active genes are recruited to a more central nuclear location (*e.g., 136*). In multipotential progenitors and in T cells, most FISH signals of Ig genes were found in a peripheral region, but in a high percentage of pro-B cells both κ and IgH were in central nuclear positions, even though in pro-B cells, only the heavy chain and not the κ chain genes are being transcribed and rearranged (137). In addition, formerly active genes that are no longer being transcribed have been reported to localize near centromeric heterochromatin associated with the protein Ikaros *(138,139)*. In pre-B cells the nonfunctional IgH allele was found associated with centromeric heterochromatin and with deacetylated nucleosomes, a combination that might shut off VHDJH recombination of the nonfunctional IgH allele at a time when RAGs are rearranging the light chain genes (140). Similarly in pre-B cells, one κ allele is associated with centromeric heterochromatin and Ikaros, while the other allele appears open to transcription and VJ recombination (128), a mechanism that may contribute to allelic exclusion.

Locus Contraction. By FISH analysis with C-region probes of one color and distal V-region probes of another color, investigators using confocal microscopy have reported that in recombining cells, both the IgH and κ loci undergo a locus contraction that moves the fluorescence signals for V and C physically close to each other in the interphase nucleus (137,140,141). This contraction occurs in RAG$^{-/-}$ mice, and thus precedes recombination. Such contraction could facilitate recombination by looping together recombining segments that are quite distant in linear DNA. For both IgH and κ loci, contraction peaks at the stage when the respective genes are undergoing recombination: pro-B cells for IgH and pre-B cells for κ. Contraction requires Pax5 (142); in Pax5$^{-/-}$ pro-B cells no IgH contraction or V→DJ recombination occurs, although the locus moves normally to a central nuclear location and VH regions are transcriptionally active.

Antisense Transcription. Bidirectional RNA transcription is increasingly being recognized as a mechanism that can affect chromatin structure and function *(143)*. Recently an investigation of transcripts in the distal VH region in pro-B cells revealed abundant antisense transcripts including coding and noncoding segments between distal VH regions, but not from 3′ D through the Cμ region B. These transcripts were detected in RAG1$^{-/-}$ pro-B cells along with sense transcripts, so transcription from either strand does not depend on recombination. In a study of normal B lineage cells at different stages, the antisense transcripts were found almost exclusively in pro-B cells, fueling the speculation that they might be involved in preparing chromatin in the IgH locus for recombination. Further research will be necessary to clarify the relationship of these transcripts to V(D)J recombination.

Allelic Exclusion and Regulated V(D)J Recombination

A model to explain allelic exclusion first proposed by Alt and colleagues (145) suggests that the functional rearrangement of an L (or H) chain gene in a particular B cell would inhibit further L (or H) chain gene rearrangement in the same cell. If the inhibition occurred promptly after the first functional rearrangement, then two functional immunoglobulins could never be produced in the same cell. An initial nonproductive rearrangement would have no inhibitory effect, so recombination could continue until a functional product resulted or until the cell used up all its germline precursors. This model has received considerable experimental support.

In B lineage maturation, the first Ig gene rearrangements join D to JH segments (commonly on both chromosomes) in pro-B cells, when most κ and λ genes are in germline configuration. The next recombination step is VH→DJH. According to the model, if the initial VDJ junction is nonfunctional (e.g., out of frame), then H chain gene recombination can continue on the other chromosome. If the VDJ recombination on the second chromosome is also nonfunctional, then the cell may have reached a dead end leading to death by apoptosis. Indeed, mice transgenic for the apoptosis suppression gene *bcl-x*$_L$ harbor an expanded population of bone marrow pro-B cells with almost all nonproductive VDJ joints *(146)*. In normal mice, approximately 40% of mature B cells carry a nonproductive VDJ segment on the nonexpressed IgH allele, remnants of the initial recombination events in those cells.

In contrast, if the first VH→DJH recombination in a pro-B cell produces a functional VDJ gene, then its expression will lead to the synthesis of μ heavy chain. This heavy chain is expressed in the surface of pre-B cells as a pre-BCR in association with the "surrogate" light chains (SLC) VpreB and λ5 (as discussed earlier) and the Ig-α-Ig-β heterodimer. In the model, expression of this pre-BCR complex has two predicted regulatory consequences. The first is that it blocks further H chain recombination. Consistent with this prediction, functionally rearranged μ transgenes generally suppress the rearrangement of endogenous heavy chain genes in B lymphocytes, suggesting that the transgene-encoded protein can shut off V(D)J recombination of endogenous genes. A transgene encoding the membrane form of $\mu(\mu_m)$ can confer this suppression, but one encoding only the secreted form (μ_s) cannot, demonstrating that a membrane form of μ protein is required for allelic exclusion (147). The suppression signal is mediated by the Ig-α-Ig-β heterodimer *(148,149)* and includes the down-regulation of RAG gene expression *(150)*, as well as reduced target accessibility, as reflected in decreased VH gene transcription *(151)*. Continued inaccessibility of the IgH locus would prevent further VH→DJH recombination during the subsequent stage when RAG proteins are up-regulated to activate light chain recombination.

The second consequence of pre-BCR expression is that κ chain recombination is activated. This effect was originally deduced from the rarity of κ-expressing cells without H chain gene rearrangement, suggesting that H chain expression is required for κ expression. As additional evidence, a functional μ gene introduced into early B lineage cells can cause RAG gene expression, sterile κ gene transcription, and Vκ-Jκ rearrangement. (A few cells are apparently able to initiate light chain recombination in the absence of heavy chain synthesis *[152]*.)

When κ recombination begins in μ-expressing cells, the possibilities for functional and nonfunctional Vκ-Jκ rearrangements resemble those discussed earlier for the heavy chain. As soon as κ gene rearrangement leads to expression of a functional κ chain that can associate with μ to form a surface-expressed IgM molecule—that is, a mature BCR—then further κ rearrangement is suppressed. This regulatory influence would explain the observation of allelic exclusion in κ-expressing myelomas, and it has been supported by the finding that functional rearranged VJ-Cκ transgenes can suppress rearrangement of endogenous κ genes. This occurs in part by suppressing RAG gene expression *(153)*.

Although this scheme of regulatory pathways may seem sufficient to explain allelic exclusion, an additional level of control is suggested by the observation that in developing B cells only a single allele of the κ locus is initially demethylated, and that allele is the target for Vκ-Jκ recombination *(154)*. How demethylation might occur on only a single chromosome is unknown, but the mechanism may be similar to that causing monoallelic expression of other genes such as IL2, IL4 and odorant receptor genes (reviewed in *[155]*). The inactive methylated allele is the one associated with heterochromatin, as previously discussed.

Most B cells show isotypic exclusion—that is, express either κ or λ but not both. Further, κ rearrangement seems to occur before λ. Thus, in normal and malignant human B lymphoid cells, κ-expressing cells generally have their λ genes in germline configuration, while in λ-expressing cells, κ genes are either rearranged (rarely) or deleted (most commonly) *(19)*. The κ deletions reflect the RS recombination event discussed earlier in this chapter. It may be that λ gene recombination is suppressed until κ genes rearrange nonproductively or are deleted, but it is not clear how this suppression would be mediated. An alternative possibility is that κ and λ rearrangement occur independently, but in the B lineage developmental program κ is simply activated for recombination earlier than the λ locus *(156)*. Some overlap between the stages of κ and λ rearrangement might explain rare cells expressing both isotypes.

Regulation of B Cell Maturation by BCR and pre-BCR

The signals mediated by the pre-BCR (μ-SLC) and the mature BCR (IgM) are critical not only for regulating V(D)J recombination, but also for being checkpoints controlling other features of B lymphocyte differentiation. Thus, in the bone marrow of RAG or JH KO mice, the absence of BCR signaling leaves B lymphopoiesis blocked at the earliest pro-B stage—large cells staining positive for B220, CD43, and c-kit; and cells with surface markers typical of mature B cells are absent from the periphery. When a recombined VDJ-Cμ heavy chain transgene is introduced into a RAG KO background (157), the resulting μ protein allows the progression of B lineage cells to the stage of small pre-B-II cells where light chain recombination would normally occur (similar to the phenotype of a double KO of κ and λ loci [158]). RAG$^{-/-}$ pre-B cells cannot undergo VL→JL recombination in the absence of RAG proteins, but do show the up-regulation of sterile κ transcription discussed previously. If, in addition to the μ gene, a functional recombined light chain transgene is also added to the genome of the RAG KO mice, then B cell development is restored, with normal numbers of B cells in the periphery, expressing mature B cell surface markers. The permissive effect of the pre-BCR or BCR on developmental progression appears to be mediated by the Ig-α-Ig-β heterodimer, based on results with the mutant or chimeric μ transgenes linked to Ig-α or Ig-β cytoplasmic domains, as described earlier *(148,149)*. Indeed, when a chimeric molecule containing the cytoplasmic signaling domains of Ig-α and Ig-β without an extracellular domain was targeted to the inner leaflet of the plasma membrane, it was capable of driving developmental maturation beyond the pro-B stage, apparently through a basal unstimulated level of signaling (159). Even in mature circulating B cells the BCR apparently provides a tonic signal necessary for survival of B cells, since *in vivo* ablation of the BCR of adult mice by inducible Cre-lox gene targeting induces rapid B cell death (160). The BCR signal delivered by Ig-α-Ig-β thus can lead to the following outcomes: it permits progression from pro-B to pre-B or from pre-B to mature B; on ligation to an autoantigen the BCR, triggers anergy or receptor editing (discussed below); in mature cells, it prevents the cell death observed with BCR ablation; and on ligation to foreign antigen, induces proliferation and maturation to the plasma cell stage. How the same Ig-α-Ig-β can trigger such different outcomes is not completely understood (see Chapter 8), though the maturation stage, the strength of the BCR signal and the presence of other costimuli seem to contribute to selectivity of the response *(161,162)*.

Late RAG Expression: Receptor Editing and Receptor Revision

Although the RAGs are generally down-regulated by a signal mediated by the appearance of IgM at the end of the pre-B cell stage, RAG gene expression and V(D)J recombination can recur later during "receptor editing" of autoreactive B cells in the bone marrow. One estimate suggests that about 25% of immunoglobulin are products of receptor editing (163). After production of an initial IgM-κ protein, receptor editing by light chain rearrangement can take three forms: an initial VκJκ junction could be deleted by recombination between an upstream V and downstream J on the same chromosome; VκJκ recombination could occur on the other chromosome; or Vλ Jλ recombination could be activated.

Most replacement of productively rearranged light or heavy chain genes likely serves to extinguish an antibody that was autoreactive, thus complementing two other mechanisms to silence autoantibodies: anergization and cell deletion by apoptosis. Early studies with transgenic autoantibodies suggested that anergy or deletion were the main fates of self-reactive B cells, but these conclusions may have depended on the nonphysiologic inability of the cells to silence the transgenic autoantibody by receptor editing. More recent studies involving autoantibody genes "knocked in" to the physiological position in the IgH and Igκ loci have shown that receptor editing is the major mechanism for B cell tolerance (164,165). This conclusion was also supported by a study of mice expressing a transgenic antibody against the murine Cκ constant region, a model of a self-superantigen; these mice provided evidence of receptor editing leading to virtually 100% λ light chain expression (166).

As compared with light chain editing, V gene replacement of the heavy chain seems to occur less frequently, probably because it depends on an incomplete RSS, a lone heptamer embedded in the 3′ end of some VH coding regions, as described in an earlier section. An analysis of normal heavy chain sequences for "footprints" of VH replacement yielded an estimate that at least 5% of the sequences derived from VH replacement (167), possibly higher in autoimmune diseases *(168)*. Also, VH replacement was readily observed in mice engineered with a nonproductive VDJ gene knocked in at the physiological position in the heavy chain locus (169). However, one report has cautioned that some VHDJH genes that appear to have arisen by VH replacement may in fact be products of gene conversion mediated by activation-induced deaminase. This protein is known to participate in somatic hypermutation (SHM) in mammals and gene conversion in chickens, as discussed later in this chapter.

GERMLINE DIVERSITY

To understand the contribution of the germline V region repertoire to immunoglobulin diversity, several groups undertook cloning and sequence analysis of individual V region genes from the μ, κ, or λ loci of human or mouse. More recently, the complete sequences of all human and mouse Ig loci have been determined as part of the high-throughput genome sequencing projects for these two species, though annotation that describes function and refers to earlier literature is incomplete. Several Internet resources are devoted to providing convenient updated access to immunoglobulin germline gene sequences. The IMGT (international ImMunoGeneTics) database (http://imgt.cines.fr/), coordinated by Marie-Paule Lefranc, includes a database for Ig and T cell receptor genes from a variety of species and includes maps, sequences, lists of chromosomal translocations, and multiple helpful links. IgBLAST (http://www.ncbi.nlm.nih.gov/igblast/) is a service of the National Center for Biotechnology Information and allows a submitted sequence to be searched against germline V, D, and J sequences.

Germline Diversity of the Murine Igh Locus

VH Segments. The murine VH locus extends over about 2.5 megabases on chromosome 12 and includes 110 genes and 85 pseudogenes, all in the same transcriptional orientation as the D, JH and CH regions (170). These VH segments can be classified into related groups based on sequence similarity; two VH gene sequences are considered to be in the same group or family if they show more than about 80% nucleotide sequence identity and in different families if their sequences are less than 70% identical. (Empirically, few VH comparisons yield identities between 70% and 80%.) Sixteen families are now recognized, one of which (VH16) was discovered only when the complete nucleotide sequence of the VH locus revealed a single novel VH that did not match any recognized family (170). The largest and most upstream family, designated J558, contains 52 functional genes in the C56BL/6 strain, making up almost half of the repertoire, though this family is smaller in some other strains. The VH families have been further classified into three "clans" based on sequence conservation primarily in the framework I region (FR1; codons 6 to 24) and FR3 (codons 67 to 85). (Framework amino acids are the non-CDR parts of the Ig V region that hold the CDR loops in position to contact antigen.) The clans are conserved between man, mouse, and frog, suggesting that several fundamental steps in germline VH diversification preceded the amphibian-reptile divergence (171). Unlike the organization of the human VH locus, members of a given murine VH family tend to be clustered together on the chromosome, though some interdigitation of families occurs even in the mouse locus (Figure 6.11). The map order is of interest because the most proximal family cluster (designated 7183), and in particular its most proximal member (designated VH81X), were found to be significantly overrepresented in the VDJ rearrangements occurring in fetal liver pre-B cells of BALB/c mice, but this bias is not observed in C57BL/6, and its significance is uncertain. The VH RSS spacers are about 23 bp.

JH and D Segments. Four germline JH sequences were identified about 5 kb upstream of the murine Cμ gene. All appear to be functional in that the sequences they encode are found in secreted H chains. Upstream of each JH lies a typical RSS with 22 bp to 23 bp spacers.

D regions were initially hypothesized based on the highly diverse amino acid sequences in myeloma proteins between the V and J regions, as briefly discussed earlier in this chapter. The 13 murine D regions span about 80 kb upstream of the four JH segments. Eleven of the genes fall into two families: SP2 (nine Ds) and FL16 (two Ds). The most 3′ D region, DQ52 lies only 0.7 kb upstream of JH1. Although D regions could theoretically contribute to Ig diversity by being read in all three frames in different VDJ recombinants, the mouse has evolved mechanisms that strongly favor the reading frame known as RF1 (3). Rare rearranged VDJ sequences seem to be interpretable as V-D-D-J products, even though D-D recombination would violate the 12/23 rule *(172)*.

Germline Diversity of the Human Igh Locus

VH Segments. The human VH locus spans 1.1 Mb at the telomeric end of chromosome 14 (14q32.33). Essentially the entire locus (957 kb) was sequenced in 1998 (173) and more recently overlapping sequence has become available through the public database of the Human Genome Project. The original sequence includes 123 VH segments, including about 40 functional genes whose mRNA or protein products have been identified. Of the remaining sequences, 79 are clearly pseudogenes and 4 show no apparent defect but have not been documented to be expressed. The human VH sequences are all in the same orientation and fall into seven families, which are extensively interdigitated, in contrast to the family clusters characteristic of the murine locus (Figure 6.11). The families can be further classified into the same clans found in the murine VH locus. Some human VH sequences are polymorphic owing to VH insertions or deletions in different allelic chromosomes. In addition to the VH sequences on chromosome 14, 24 additional germline VH sequences have been mapped to chromosome 15 and 16 and represent nonfunctional "orphons" that were apparently duplicated from the functional locus on chromosome 14.

Human JH and DH Regions. Upstream of the human Cμ gene lie six functional JH regions interspersed with three JH pseudogenes. The pseudogenes encode amino acid sequences never found in human H chains and lack the RNA splice signal found at the 3′ end of all active JH genes. All of the JH segments and pseudogenes demonstrate ~23 bp RSS spacing (as in the mouse).

Most human D regions lie in a 92 kb region upstream of the JH segments *(2)*. One germline D gene is located in a position roughly homologous to that of the mouse DQ52—that is, 5′ to the human JHI. This human D gene, initially designated DHQ52, bears striking homology to

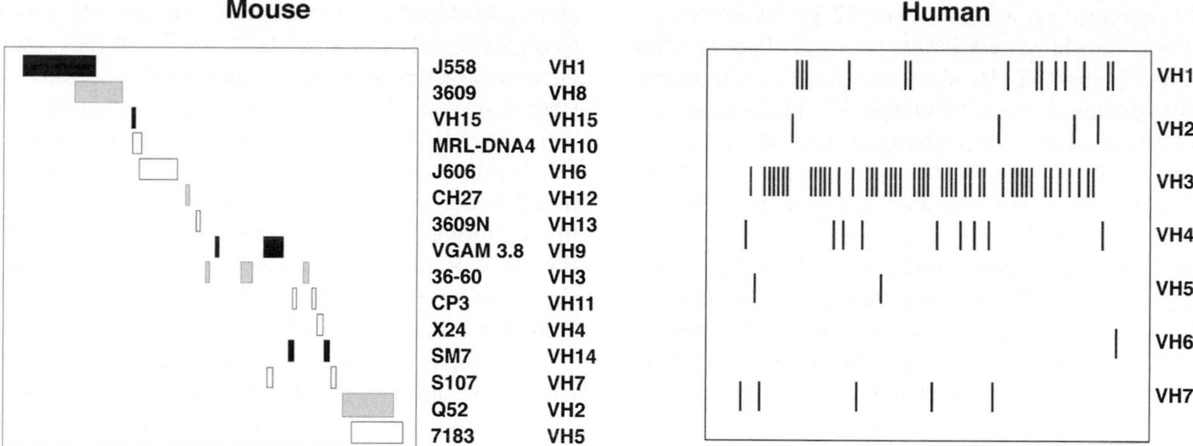

FIGURE 6.11 Maps of the murine and human VH loci. The fifteen known murine VH gene families are shown in their approximate map positions. Each rectangle represents a cluster of VH genes of the indicated family; the clan identification of the VH families is indicated by the color of the rectangle: black for clan I, gray for clan II, and white for clan III. Although some interdigitation is shown by overlapping families (e.g., the Q52 and 7183 families), the murine VH families are largely clustered. In contrast all human VH genes (vertical lines) of a prototypic haplotype are shown in the right panel; extensive interdigitation of families is apparent.

its murine counterpart, but is the only human D segment showing such human/mouse homology. All of the other human D regions fall into six families and lie in a cluster of duplicated domains beginning about 22 kb upstream of JH1. There are 27 D regions. Twenty-four of these are accounted for by four tandem approximate duplications of a 9.5 kb segment containing a representative of the six D families. Three D regions are apparently nonfunctional as a result of mutations in RSS heptamers, and there are two pairs of D regions with identical coding sequences (including one of the D segments with a heptamer mutation), so there are 23 distinct D regions that can contribute to human immunoglobulin diversity. All of these sequences appear in the expressed immunoglobulin VDJ regions, many in all three reading frames. In general, one reading frame encodes primarily hydrophilic residues, one encodes hydrophobic residues, and one includes frequent stop codons. Some D regions that contain stop codons can be used if these codons are removed by nuclease trimming before VDJ assembly is complete.

Germline Diversity of Light Chain Genes

Murine Germline κ Locus. The murine Vκ locus spans about 3.2 Mb upstream of the Cκ gene on chromosome 6 (174). Of the 140 Vκ sequences in the locus, 95 are potentially functional and 75 are known to be functional, as their mRNA or protein products have been detected. Of the remaining sequences, 44 are clearly pseudogenes, 21 are apparently defect-free but have not been demonstrated to be expressed, and the rest have minor defects that might not preclude function *(175)*. Of the 95 potentially functional genes, 61 lie in a transcriptional orientation opposite to that of the Jκ genes (174) and must recombine by inversion, as discussed earlier. A classification of the Vκ sequences by similarity (based on the criteria described above) recognizes about 20 Vκ families. As described for VH genes, some families are shared by human and mouse, suggesting that the family divisions preceded primate-rodent species divergence. Many related Vκ sequences within a family are found to lie clustered together in the locus, although some interspersion of families also exists. A few Vκ sequences have been localized to other chromosomes (chromosome 16 and 19), where they could not contribute to diversity and are thus considered orphons. As described previously, there are five Jκ regions, of which four are functional.

Human Germline κ Locus. The human Vκ locus is located on the short arm of chromosome 2 (2p11-2) within a sequence contig of about 1 Mb (10^6 bp) of DNA (176). This is comprised of a proximal segment including the Jκ-Cκ region and about 500 kb upstream and a distal segment of about 430 kb further upstream. These two segments are separated by a spacer of about 0.8 Mb that is apparently devoid of Vκ sequences. The distal and proximal segments represent a large inverted repeat, so most Vκ sequences on the proximal segment have duplicated copies in the opposite orientation on the distal segment. The average sequence similarity between the corresponding distal and proximal sequences is 98.9%, suggesting a duplication event less than 5 million years old. Consistent with this, the locus is not duplicated in chimpanzees, a species that is estimated to have diverged from the human lineage approximately 6 million years ago. About 5% of human alleles also lack the distal duplication.

The sequenced region contains 132 Vκ sequences, including 87 unambiguous pseudogenes and 46 open reading frames. Of these, 29 Vκ sequences have been found expressed in proteins; these 29 include 25 unique sequences plus four that derive from identical gene pairs. Among all examined B lymphoid cell lines, those with VκJκ rearrangements involving the distal inverted Vκ segments contained retained signal joints, consistent with Vκ-Jκ recombination by inversion. Outside the duplicated region, the two Jκ1-proximal Vκ genes are also in inverted orientation. The locus contains numerous insertions of retroposed elements (about 35% of the sequence) but no recognized interspersed non-Ig genes or pseudogenes. Multiple internal repeats suggest ancient duplications.

Apart from the Vκ sequences in the cluster near the Jκ-Cκ locus, at least 25 orphons have been identified. One orphon cluster is located in the long arm of chromosome 2; perhaps it was separated from the major locus—on the short arm of this chromosome—by a pericentric inversion (which must have occurred rather recently in evolution since it is absent from chimpanzee and gorilla). Other orphons are located on chromosomes 1 and 22, and at least one probably nonfunctional Vκ lies about 1.5 Mb downstream from Cκ.

Human Germline Vλ Locus

The human Vλ has also been characterized by intensive cloning, sequencing, and mapping of Vλ regions and ultimately by the complete sequence analysis of 1,025,415 bp covering the entire locus (177). The locus contains about 36 potentially functional Vλ genes (in 10 families), 56 pseudogenes, and 13 "relics," containing <200 bp of Vλ-like sequences. (As noted for other loci, exact numbers may differ depending on the haplotype and method of analysis.) Of the potentially functional genes, only about 30 have been documented to be expressed by comparison with cDNA sequences. Within the clustered Vλ sequences lies the human VpreB gene, as well as several genes and pseudogenes unrelated to the λ system. All the Vλ sequences (except a few pseudogenes) are in the same transcriptional orientation as the J-C cluster. Analysis of the ~1 Mb sequence reveals several segments of internal duplications, some including Vλ regions. The largest and most frequently expressed Vλ gene families lie relatively close to the J-C cluster, mostly within the proximal 400 kb.

Combinatorial Diversity Estimates

Before the era of recombinant DNA technology, the source of antibody diversity was so mysterious that it was whimsically referred to as "the problem of G.O.D." (generation of diversity). Knowledge of antibody genes gained over the past 20 years has elucidated the diversity inherent in the germline V repertoire plus the diversity contributed by recombinational mechanisms (combinatorial multiplication, "flexibility" of recombination site, N and P nucleotides) as already discussed. Together these diversity elements provide an immense potential repertoire, one so large that to some investigators it seemed sufficient to account for observed antibody diversity. As an exercise in estimating the contribution of germline and recombinational diversity in the human, consider the number of different antibodies that could be formed using the germline human V, D, and J sequences that are known to be functional. From 40 VH regions, 27 D regions, and 6 JH, regions we can obtain 6,480 combinations, but taking into account the three reading frames available for the D regions, the total comes to 19,440 combinations of amino acid sequences. For the light chain, we have the 145 κ combinations (29 Vκ × 5 Jκ) plus the 120 λ combinations (30 Vλ× 4Jλ), or 265 total light chain combinations. Assuming that H_2L_2 pairing occurs randomly, we can calculate a total of 19,440 × 265, or about 5 million combinations. This estimate has neglected additional sources of diversity that are substantial but difficult to quantitate: the variable "nibbling" of coding sequences and the insertion of N and P nucleotides. Yet even neglecting these factors the exercise demonstrates how nature has greatly enlarged the potential sequence diversity available from a limited number of total nucleotides by allowing flexible recombination between different sequence elements.

Although it is clear that these mechanisms imply a vast repertoire, it is worth considering some qualifications that tend to reduce the actual combinatorial diversity, especially early in ontogeny. It seems unlikely, for example, that every possible combination of L and H chains yields a functional antibody molecule, since in vitro L and H reassociation experiments show that certain hybrid molecules (formed from L and H chains derived from different antibodies) are relatively unstable. Similarly, association of V and J (or V, D, and J) is conceivably not completely random. Evidence of striking bias in the selection of VH genes in fetal pre-B hybridomas has been mentioned, and other biases have been reported in J usage. In addition, fetal and newborn VDJ junctions show a paucity of N nucleotides and a tendency to form VDJ junctions across short stretches of sequence identity between the recombining sequences ("homology mediated" recombination, discussed earlier in this chapter). Factors that reduce diversity in early VDJ recombination may facilitate the production of certain antibodies that are advantageous for young individuals.

IG GENE ALTERATIONS IN GERMINAL CENTERS

Several days after exposure to an antigen, B cells accumulate in local lymph nodes, gut-associated lymphoid tissue, and spleen and begin additional maturation steps in germinal centers (GC). During the GC response, antigen-driven B cells undergo cycles of proliferation and their Ig genes undergo two unique alterations: CSR and affinity maturation through SHM and selection. For many years, these two processes were considered to be mechanistically unrelated, but more recent evidence, although not completely clarifying either process, has suggested mechanistic similarities between them. These similarities will be discussed in more detail later, but can be briefly mentioned here. First, while double-strand DNA breaks are expected intermediates for DNA recombinations such as CSR, such breaks have also been detected as likely intermediates in SHM. Second (and conversely), in addition to the mutations occurring in V regions as part of SHM, mutations have also been observed surrounding the recombination junctions of CSR. Third, transcription is required for both processes. Fourth, some evidence suggests that palindromic DNA structures may be important for targeting both CSR and SHM to specific sequences.

Activation-induced Deaminase. A fifth and dramatic link between CSR and SHM was the discovery that both processes require the protein known as *activation-induced deaminase* (AID). The gene for AID (known as AICDA) was identified (178) by a subtractive strategy designed to screen for transcripts that were expressed in a murine B cell line when induced to undergo CSR, but that were not expressed when uninduced. AID is expressed almost exclusively in GC B cells and in B cells activated in vitro, though there are reports of expression in certain nonlymphoid cells *(179,180)*. Mice engineered with a targeted defect in the AICDA gene show profound defects in both CSR and SHM. The same defects are seen in patients with a homozygous defect in the human AICDA gene, a condition known as *hyper-IgM syndrome-2* (HIGM2) (181). These patients have elevated serum levels of IgM because their B cells are profoundly impaired in CSR. AID is not only necessary for CSR and SHM, but apparently sufficient (in a mammalian cell at least), because overexpression of AID in fibroblasts can confer transcription-dependent CSR of an artificial switch construct (182) and transcription-dependent SHM of a transfected model mutation target sequence (183). These experiments suggest that AID is the only B-cell-specific protein required for SHM and CSR. AID is also required for somatic gene conversion in those species (e.g., chicken) that use that process to somatically diversify Ig genes.

As translated from the cDNA, AID is a 198 amino acid protein that forms homodimers. AID shows 34% amino acid identity with the RNA editing enzyme APOBEC1, which catalyzes the deamination of a cytosine residue to uracil in a specific position in the mRNA encoding apolipoprotein B. (This change produces a UAA stop codon that shortens the translated protein to yield apoB48.) The human APOBEC1 and AICDA genes appear to be genetically linked, both lying at chromosome 12p13. Both are members of a cytidine deaminase family, including proteins (e.g., human APOBEC3G and AID itself) that destructively mutate unwelcome DNA sequences to protect against retroviral infection and against the spread of endogenous parasitic retroposons *(184–186)*. Like APOBEC1, recombinant AID protein has a cytidine deaminase activity in vitro, and it was initially proposed that, by analogy with APOBEC1, AID functions in vivo by editing specific RNAs to produce novel mRNA encoding one or more proteins required for CSR and SHM. Since a novel edited mRNA would need to be translated into protein before it could enable CSR, proponents of the RNA deamination model have found support in the observation that inhibitors of protein synthesis block CSR (187,188), though it is possible that this block reflects a requirement for a novel but unedited protein, or for maintenance of an existing protein with short half-life. In any case, no evidence of novel AID-dependent edited RNAs has been reported, nor does AID deaminate RNA cytidines *in vitro*.

An alternative hypothesis that has received considerable experimental support is that AID acts by deaminating cytidines in DNA to uracil—in V regions for SHM, and in Switch regions (discussed later) for CSR. The resulting uracil would be then recognized as an abnormal DNA base by the cell's genetic surveillance machinery, which might trigger error-prone repair of V regions to produce SHM, or DNA cleavage to mediate CSR. This DNA-deamination model for AID is consistent with various properties reported for this protein *in vitro* or in cells:

(1) AID is found by ChIP analysis to be associated with IgH genes *in vivo* in B cells undergoing CSR (189,190).
(2) AID can deaminate cytosines to uracil in single-strand DNA *in vitro* (191–193) or in double-strand DNA that is being transcribed *in vitro*, presumably because transcription causes localized regions of single-strandedness (193–195).
(3) Defective SHM and CSR are observed with inhibition or genetic inactivation of uracil-N-glycosylase (UNG), an enzyme that removes uracil residues from DNA (196,197), consistent with the idea that CSR and SHM require a step in which AID-produced uracil in DNA is removed by UNG.
(4) A DNA sequence motif WRC (where W is A or T and R [puRine] is A or G) that has been recognized as a hotspot target of SHM is also a preferred target for AID deamination *in vitro* (192,195). (Several related sequences have been proposed as the consensus hotspot, now generally recognized as WRCH [H = T/C/A] or its complement DGYW [D = A/G/T] [198].)
(5) In transfected E. coli cells, AID mutates cytosines to uracil in DNA, a result that would be unexpected by the RNA-deamination model because bacteria

presumably lack the specific mammalian RNA targets predicted by that model (199,200).

In light of these observations, most investigators accept the DNA-deamination model as a working hypothesis, but alternative interpretations of these observations consistent with the RNA-deamination model have been proposed (201).

Preparations of AID purified from transfected E. coli or nonlymphoid eukaryotic cells can deaminate single-strand DNA in vitro, as mentioned earlier, but deamination of transcribed double-strand DNA requires association of AID with replication protein A (RPA), a single-strand DNA binding protein (190). This association requires phosphorylation of AID by protein kinase A (PKA), a kinase activated by cAMP (202,203). When the AID gene was mutated by replacing the phosphorylated amino acids with alanine to prevent RPA association, the resulting protein could still deaminate cytosines on single-strand DNA but was impaired in deaminating transcribed double-strand DNA and in carrying out SHM and CSR in cells (202,204), indicating the physiologic relevance of the phosphorylation and RPA interaction. These results suggest that AID activity may be fine-tuned by cytokines and other mediators that regulate cAMP levels and thereby affect PKA activity, AID phosphorylation, and thus AID activity.

Regulation of AID activity is important because inappropriate mutations or DNA breakage could be dangerous. Indeed, constitutive expression of an AID transgene causes tumors in mice *(205)*, and even normal expression of AID in B cells may contribute to tumorigenic translocations and oncogenic mutations *(206)*. Early studies showed that AID expression in B cells is upregulated by IL4 and CD40 engagement. More recent investigations of AICDA regulatory regions have led to identification of a promoter, an enhancer lying within the first intron, and two other candidate regulatory regions showing patches of significant mouse/human sequence conservation *(207–209)*. Outside the B cell lineage, AID has been found only in embryonic germ cells and in spermatocytes, where it could play a role in the widespread deamination of methyl-cytosine to thymine, thereby causing the most frequent point mutation observed in mammals: the transition from CpG to TpG *(180)*.

Structure-function relationships of AID have been probed by examining cross-species sequence comparisons and the effects of natural and engineered mutations in the protein. Remarkably, mutations in the N-terminus of AID impaired SHM but not CSR, whereas mutations or deletion in the C-terminus selectively impaired CSR (210–212), suggesting the possibility that the N- and C-terminal regions of the protein contact specific cofactors required for SHM or CSR function. DNA-PK is a possible candidate for the latter cofactor; it is required for CSR but not SHM, and it has been found to bind to AID but not to C-terminal deletion mutants of AID (213). The C-terminus of AID also contains a conserved leucine/phenylalanine-rich nuclear export signal (NES), which mediates active transport of AID from the nucleus to the cytoplasm in association with exportin-1 *(214,215)*, but the CSR-specific function of the C-terminus requires more than an active NES *(216)*. Interestingly, agents causing nuclear DNA breaks were found to shift AID into the nucleus *(217)*. AID is highly conserved from fish to human, with all species having approximately 200 amino acids and sequence similarities throughout the protein. Sharks and bony fish show evidence of SHM but not CSR, while amphibians and all higher vertebrates are capable of both SHM and CSR. However, zebrafish AID expressed in murine cells can support CSR, implying that the lack of CSR in fish may be due to the structure of Ig genes rather than to a limitation in their AID *(218,219)*.

AID will be discussed further in the context of its function in SHM and CSR.

Somatic Hypermutation

The idea that antibody genes inherited in the germline might be subject to somatic mutation in lymphocytes during the life of an individual was suggested as an explanation for the diversity of antibodies several years before recombinant DNA technology became available and helped clarify the role of V(D)J recombination. Persuasive evidence for somatic mutation was reported in the 1970s: analyses of Vλ1 amino acid sequences of murine myeloma antibodies showed many instances of a particular prototype sequence, plus several variant sequences containing unique single amino acid substitutions that could be explained by single nucleotide changes. The prototype was interpreted as reflecting the germline sequence, with the variants arising by somatic mutation *(220)*. Subsequent investigations at the DNA level revealed myeloma V region sequences that deviated from their germline counterparts, verifying the principle of somatic mutation.

Somatic mutations are much rarer in IgM than in antibodies with "switched" isotypes (IgG, IgA, and IgE) made by B cells that have been exposed to AID in GCs, but they do occur; antibodies with "switched" isotypes without mutations are also found. These observations suggest that though both SHM and CSR normally occur in the same population of B cells in germinal centers, the two processes are unlinked.

It should be mentioned that, although SHM has been generally described as occurring in normal animals exclusively in germinal centers, some reports suggest that T cell–independent SHM may occur in a population of less mature cells, which may populate the splenic marginal zone and which may increase the repertoire of circulating lymphocytes prior to antigen exposure, especially in young individuals (221,222). Also, mice lacking histologically detectable GCs as a result of lymphotoxin-α-deficiency are capable of somatic hypermutation and affinity maturation *(223)*. T cell–independent antigens can undergo a low level of SHM (224).

Role of Hypermutation in Immune Responses

To understand the role of somatic mutation in the antibody response, several groups have studied the extent of somatic mutation at different times after the immunization of mice. Studies of the responses to p-azophenylarsonate (Ars), phosphorylcholine, influenza hemagglutinin, oxazalone, and several other antigens have all indicated that the initial response after primary immunization is contributed by antibodies showing no somatic mutation. About one week after immunization, mutated sequences begin to be observed, increasing during the next week or so. Booster immunizations yield sequences showing additional mutations.

Many hybridomas made late in the immune response produce mutated antibodies with a higher antigen affinity than the unmutated (sometimes loosely called "germline") antibodies made early after immunization. The shift to higher affinity is a phenomenon long recognized at the level of (polyclonal) antisera and has been termed *affinity maturation*. This phenomenon can now be explained as the result of an "evolutionary" mechanism selecting antibodies of progressively higher affinity from the pool of randomly mutated V sequences. According to this model, at the time of initial antigen exposure, an animal has a set of naïve B lymphocytes expressing IgM with germline (unmutated) versions of Ig variable regions resulting from gene rearrangements that occurred prior to immunization. Because of the diversity of available VH, D, JH, VL, and JL sequences as well as the impressive recombinational potential described earlier, some B cells will express Ig molecules capable of binding the antigen with modest affinity. These cells are stimulated by antigen binding—to proliferate, to secrete antibody and to move to lymphoid follicles, where they form germinal centers. In this environment, AID is expressed and somatic hypermutation machinery is activated, generating random mutations in the Ig genes of stimulated GC B cells. Many of these mutations reduce the resulting affinity of the encoded antibody for antigen *(225,226)*, and some may acquire autoantibody specificity *(227)*. As antigen clearance reduces antigen concentrations seen by the lymphocytes, only the cells displaying high affinity for antigen will be stimulated effectively; cells displaying lower-affinity antibodies or antibodies with affinity for self-antigens are subjected to programmed cell death (apoptosis) *(228,229)*. The preferential proliferation of the high-affinity cells and their maturation to secreting plasma cells will be reflected in an increase in the average affinity of the antibodies in the serum. These high-affinity cells will be left as the predominant population to be represented as memory cells when antigen exposure ceases; they thus can induce the rapid, high-affinity antibody response seen on secondary antigen exposure. In this model the driving force for affinity maturation—analogous to natural selection in the evolution of species—is selection for high antibody affinity in the face of falling antigen concentration. The importance of this selective force is suggested by the observation that affinity maturation can be inhibited by repeated injection of antigen (which removes the selective pressure for high affinity) *(230)* or by overexpression of the antiapoptotic protein Bcl-XL (which allows survival of B cells expressing low-affinity antibody) *(231)*.

Cellular Context of Somatic Mutation

Within the GC, SHM occurs in a subpopulation of B cells known as *centroblasts*. These cells proliferate in the "dark zone" of the germinal center and bear characteristic surface markers including IgD, CD38, and the receptor for peanut agglutinin *(232)*. Each GC appears to be populated by a small number of antigen-specific founder B cells *(233)* and an unusual Thy-1 negative T cell population, also antigen-specific *(234)*. The GC environment promotes contact between the B cell and follicular dendritic cells (FDCs)—which store, process and present antigen—and T lymphocytes, which activate somatic mutation in part via CD40-CD40L interaction *(235)*. Other critical signals promoting SHM have been investigated using *in vitro* systems, which implicate CD80:CD28 engagement *(236)* and cytokines *(237)*. Proliferating GC centroblasts give rise to centrocytes in the "light zone" of the GC; there, centrocytes are programmed for apoptosis unless they are rescued by FDC-presented antigen and T cell activation via CD40 engagement *(228,238)*. It is at this stage where positive selection for high-affinity antibodies occurs via apoptosis of cells expressing low-affinity antibodies, yet paradoxically apoptosis is also promoted by soluble antigen, perhaps functioning to select against autoantibodies *(239)*. As mentioned earlier, receptor editing may be another fate for autoantibody-producing cells in germinal centers. The features of antigen signaling that select for survival versus apoptosis or editing are not fully understood. Susceptibility of GC cell populations to apoptosis is correlated with their expression of Fas, Bax, p53, and c-myc, all of which promote apoptosis, and down-regulation of the apoptosis suppressors Bcl-2 and c-FLIP *(229)*. As mentioned previously, B cells of mice with engineered overexpression of Bcl-2 or Bcl-XL can escape selection against autoreactivity *(231)*.

SHM is apparently unusually active in $IgM^{-}IgD^{+}$ cells, as this subset of GC B cells from human tonsils was found to accumulate extremely high numbers of somatic mutations *(240)*. An important role for IgD in somatic mutation is also suggested by the observations that mice with a homozygous targeted disruption of their Cδ gene were impaired in affinity maturation *(241)* and that anti-IgD antiserum is an effective stimulant for triggering SHM *(242)*.

Germinal center B cells may undergo several successive cycles of mutation and proliferation followed by selection. Such a scheme has been supported by the sequence analysis of mutated Ig genes PCR-amplified from single cells microdissected from a histologic section of a germinal center *(243)* or from mutations in copies of an engineered transgene that is unusually susceptible to SHM *(244)*; in these and other systems, the mutated sequences can be organized into genealogical trees consistent with repeated mutation and selection cyles. Cyclical movement of the B cells from the dark zone to the light zone of the GC may be mediated by cyclically changing chemotactic responses to chemokines (245,246). A computer simulation has affirmed the high efficiency of alternating periods of somatic mutation and mutation-free selection as a strategy for generating high-affinity antibodies *(247)*.

Targeting and Distribution of Mutations

The mutation rate of Ig genes undergoing SHM may reach as high as 10^{-3} mutations/bp/generation, or about 10^6 times higher than the normal genomic mutation rate *(248,249)*, a rate that could be lethal if it were not carefully targeted specifically to Ig genes. The molecular nature of this targeting is a critical question closely related to understanding the molecular mechanism of SHM. However, it should be noted that some non-Ig genes that are transcribed in GC B cells (BCL6 and CD95) may be also subject to mutation, though several other genes expressed in GC B cells at comparable levels are not *(250)*. One possible interpretation is that some of the features that target SHM to Ig genes may be shared by a few other genes.

Exactly what feature of the V(D)J locus targets the hypermutation machinery to the expressed V(D)J gene is not understood. Unrearranged Vκ, VH regions and DJ regions are generally not mutated, suggesting that the V(D)J recombination generates a hypermutation target from elements contributed by both V and J, possibly by moving the V region promoters close to enhancers lying in the J-C intron. (In contrast to the κ and heavy chain loci, the λ locus lacks an enhancer between J and C; unrearranged Vλ regions are transcribed in B cells *[251]* and can be mutated *[252]*.) The specific chromosomal location of Ig genes does not seem to be necessary for hypermutation, since transgenic mice carrying a rearranged expressible Ig gene—presumably inserted randomly in the genome—show somatic mutations, as do stably transfected Ig genes in cell lines. Therefore investigators have been able to study the sequence requirements for SHM using transgenes and stable transfectants. More recent studies have examined the effects of altering gene structure at the endogenous Ig loci by homologous recombination (i.e. KOs and knock-ins).

The importance of transcription in targeting hypermutation is consistent with *in vitro* dependence of AID deamination on transcription of double-strand DNA targets. One striking confirmation of the correlation between transcription and SHM was reported in which a tetracycline-inducible reporter gene encoding Green Fluorescent Protein (GFP) was engineered with an internal stop codon. When this construct was stably transfected into a B cell line, the rate of reversion of the stop codon by SHM was found to be directly related to the transcription rate regulated by a tetracycline analog (253). A possible mechanistic explanation for the role of transcription is that DNA behind the advancing RNA polymerase complex becomes negatively supercoiled, which can facilitate access of the DNA to AID (254). The relationship between SHM and transcription is reinforced by studies showing that transgenes engineered with known transcriptional enhancers generally experienced more SHM than those without such enhancers. However, enhancers could theoretically regulate SHM independently of their transcriptional regulation, a possibility that is often hard to evaluate in these experiments. Further, recent studies have reported unexpected and sometimes conflicting differences in SHM effects of enhancer deletions in endogenous genes versus transgenes. For example, rearranged κ transgenes including intronic and 3′Eκ enhancers were more highly transcribed and better somatic mutation targets than similar constructs lacking these regions *(255)*. However, a targeted deletion of the endogenous 3′Eκ enhancer was found to minimally affect SHM in one study *(256)*, whereas another study reported greater effects from deletion of this enhancer than from the intronic enhancer (119). In another discrepancy, the downstream IgH enhancers HS3b and HS4 were found important for SHM in transgenes *(257)* but dispensible in the context of endogenous genes *(258)*. Even non–Ig enhancers could support SHM in a stably transfected cell line *(259)*, and so could non-Ig promoters such as the β-globin promoter *(260)*, though it cannot be concluded that every promoter or enhancer would have this property.

The V coding sequence can be replaced by a human β-globin gene or prokaryotic *neo* or *gpt* gene without affecting the hypermutation rate downstream of the promoter *(261)*. However, other constructs show little SHM despite high levels of transcription *(262,263)*. In studies probing differing SHM levels of similar transgene constructs, SHM was found to be enhanced by two repeats of the E box motif CAGGTG, the binding site for E2A transcription factors (264), even though transcription did not seem to be affected. Moreover, E2A proteins were found to strongly stimulate SHM of Ig genes in the chicken B cell line DT40 without significant effects on Ig gene (or AID) transcription (265). To summarize, it appears that transcription is necessary but not sufficient for targeting hypermutation, but the additional elements required for SHM have not been defined as of this writing (though E2A function seems likely to be among them).

A parameter related to transcription of Ig genes (–) their context in chromatin (–) has also been studied in relation to SHM targeting. Culture of a B cell line under conditions that upregulate SHM (in the presence of T cells and anti-IgM) led to increased acetylation of histone H3 and H4 at V region but not C region DNA, as assessed by ChIP analysis *(266)*, paralleling the distribution of mutations. The increased histone acetylation was not a consequence of AID action since it occurred when AID expression (and SHM) was inhibited by antisense treatment; moreover, when cells were treated with the deacetylase inhibitor trichostatin A, the C region was both acetylated and subjected to SHM. Another histone modification that may be even more tightly correlated with SHM is phosphorylation of histone H2B (267).

Within a specific V sequence, mutations seem to be targeted to a region beginning about 0.1 kb downstream of the transcription start site, peaking within the V region and tapering off downstream to define a mutation target domain of about 1.5 kb to 2 kb. Therefore, for VDJ units involving the downstream JH5 segment, mutations extend further towards the Cμ region than for units involving JH1. This distribution has suggested a model *(268)* in which a "mutator factor"—likely AID (269)—is loaded onto the transcription initiation complex as transcription elongation begins. The mutator factor then remains attached to the transcription machinery—and competent to induce mutations—for a period of time as this machinery moves downstream to extend the transcript; but eventually the mutator falls off, so that further transcription procedes without mutations. Consistent with this model, a VκJκ-Cκ transgene bearing a second Vκ promoter engineered upstream of the Cκ region was found to incur mutations over over a second domain extending into the Cκ region, in addition to the usual V region mutations *(268)*. Conversely, the insertion of an irrelevant 2 kb DNA fragment between a Vκ promoter and the leader (signal peptide) exon prevented mutation within the Vκ transgene, which now apparently was downstream of the mutational domain *(270)*. Remarkably, a similar envelope of AID-dependent cytidine deamination has been observed in an *in vitro* system, where AID binds to E. coli RNA polymerase transcribing a plasmid DNA *(271)*.

Mutations in V region genes observed in B cells *in vivo* may be highly selected for antigen-binding function of the expressed antibody. To better analyze the spectrum of mutations produced by SHM unbiased by selection, investigators have studied nonproductively rearranged VDJ alleles or "passenger" transgenes engineered with stop codons to prevent expression as a protein. In these genes, mutational "hot spots," as well as "cold spots," have been recognized, apparently due to local DNA features that may promote or suppress somatic mutation. The consensus sequence WRC (i.e., [A/T][G/A][C]) is the most consistent hotspot for mutation, presumably reflecting the predilection of AID for *in vitro* deamination of this sequence, and different triplet codons are mutation targets at differing but largely consistent frequencies. It is possible that evolution has concentrated mutational hotspot frequencies in CDR regions to enhance the potential for diversity generation in the parts of the protein critical for antigen contact *(272)*. All four nucleotides are targets for mutation, and all are found as products. Transitions (purine-purine and pyrimidine-pyrimidine interchanges) are somewhat more frequent than transversions (purine-pyrimidine interchanges), with some preferential targeting of G-C basepairs *(273)*. Small insertions and deletions occur rarely. In an unselected passenger Vκ transgene, A and G nucleotides were mutated more frequently on the coding strand than on the noncoding strand *(274)*. This "strand polarity" was also observed in human VH regions *(275)*, but is not universally found. Such polarity would suggest that the mutation mechanism may be affected by a process that can distinguish between the strands, such as transcription through the V region.

Molecular Mechanism of Hypermutation

A model of SHM has been formulated by Neuberger and colleagues (196) based on abnormalities in SHM that are observed in various mutant B cells (Figure 6.12). In brief, the model proposes that after AID-catalyzed deamination creates a uracil residue in the target DNA, there are several possible outcomes depending stochastically on which of several mechanisms engage the DNA and in what order they act. (1) The U:G mismatch may be replicated without correction, in which case the fact that uracil forms a Watson-Crick basepair with adenine means that the original C:G basepair will be mutated to T:A in progeny of the cell that receives the uracil-bearing DNA strand. These are referred to as *phase 1A mutations*. (2) The uracil base may be removed by UNG, creating an abasic site. As DNA is replicated, the strand with the abasic site may directly engage translesional polymerases (which are error-prone) to insert an unpaired nucleotide (i.e., any nucleotide) to replicate past the abasic lesion, creating phase 1B mutations. (3) The original U:G mismatch (or possibly the abasic site created by UNG action) may be recognized by the mismatch repair (MMR) system of the cell; MMR triggers nucleolytic digestion of the strand bearing the abasic site, and repair by error-prone polymerases, which create mutations (designated *phase 2*) near the position of the original U:G mismatch.

Role of Uracil-N-Glycosylase in SHM. The UNG gene encodes two proteins that differ in their N-termini as a result of alternative promoters that generate different initial coding exons. UNG1 is expressed ubiquitously in mitochondria, whereas UNG2 is specific to activated B cells. There are three other mammalian enzymes with uracil glycosylase activity, but they do not appear to contribute significantly to SHM or CSR. Hydrolytic deamination of cytosines to uracil occurs at a significant rate in all eukaryotic and prokaryotic cells, and misincorporation of dUTP

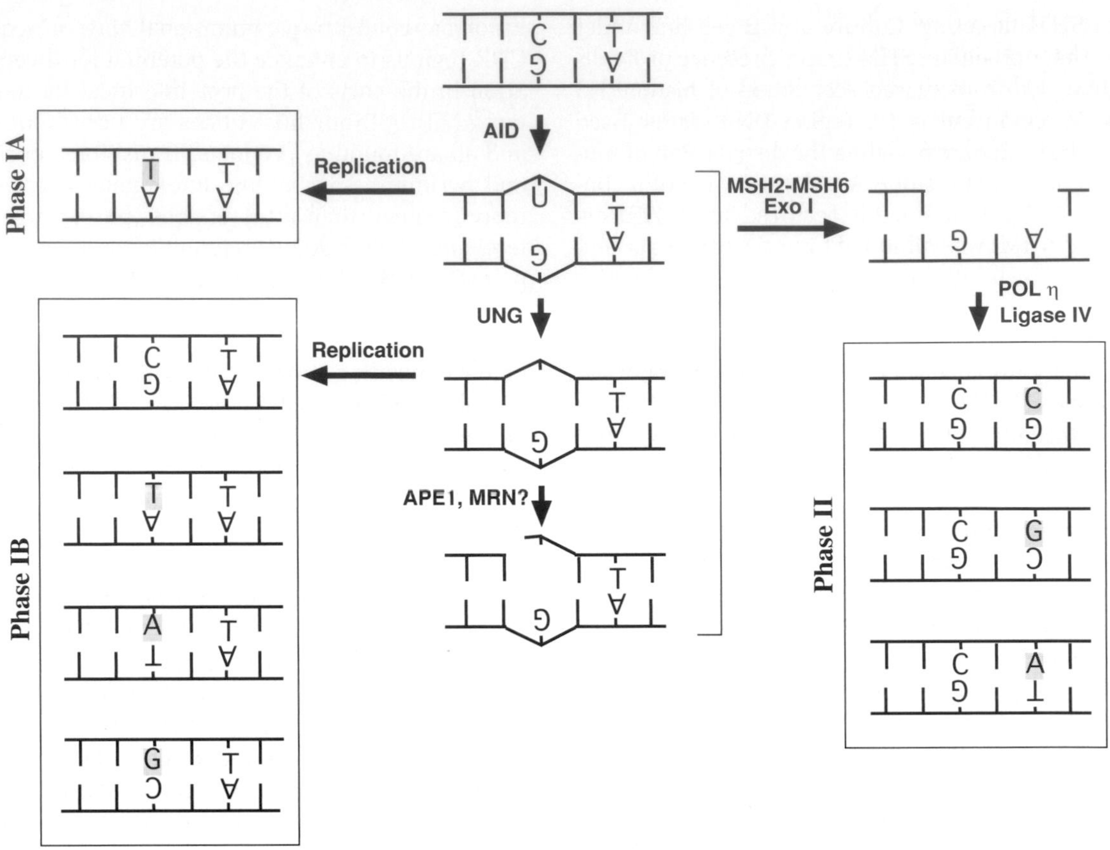

FIGURE 6.12 Mechanistic model of somatic hypermutation. The graphic depicts a small region in a VH gene showing a targeted C:G basepair and a nearby T:A pair. After AID-catalyzed deamination of a C residue, the DNA may be subjected to various modifications as shown, leading to mutations indicated by nucleotides in gray rectangles. The model is described in the text.

during replication further contributes to the load of uracil in DNA. UNG2 plays a major role in mitigating this load by initiating base excision repair (BER) in which the abasic site created by UNG2 activity is faithfully repaired to a cytosine by complex of recruited factors.

In SHM, the faithful repair of uracil is somehow subverted to introduce mutations. $UNG^{-/-}$ mice and human patients with a rare form of hyper-IgM immunodeficiency due to UNG mutations have similar immunological phenotypes. First, $UNG^{-/-}$ individuals are profoundly defective in CSR (discussed in more detail later), as expected if this process requires AID-catalyzed deamination of cytidine followed by UNG-catalyzed removal of uracil. Although SHM is roughly normal quantitatively, UNG-deficient individuals show a striking decrease in the frequency of transversions from C nucleotides (i.e., mutations at C are almost exclusively transitions to T). As suggested by Figure 6.12, $UNG^{-/-}$ individuals would not create the abasic sites that lead to C→G and C→ mutations by replication, though some mutations of these kinds could be produced by MMR. Indeed, the frequencies of mutations from the A, T, and G in these individuals are normal, apparently resulting from MMR engaged by the U:G mismatch in many cells.

Mismatch Repair in SHM. MMR is a highly conserved mechanism that detects abnormalities in DNA—including mispaired nucleotides and abnormal bases—and repairs them. The well-studied *E. coli* MMR system has three main components. MutS binds tightly and specifically to DNA defects. MutL then binds and recruits MutH (for which there is no mammalian homologue) and other components. The Mut complex then activates a latent nuclease activity to remove a segment of the DNA strand including the mismatched base; this gapped strand is then resynthesized by a DNA polymerase. Mammals have several MutS homologs, including three reported in somatic cells—MSH2, MSH3 and MSH6—which exist in the cell as heterodimers. MSH2-MSH6 (also known as MutSα) is the most abundant form and is specialized for recognizing single base gaps or mismatches, while MSH2-MSH3 (MutSβ) recognizes larger gaps and insertion/deletion loops. The mammalian homologs of MutL are heterodimers consisting of MLH1 paired with PMS1, PMS2, or MLH3. Apart from their effects on SHM and CSR, mutations in MMR genes, especially MSH2 and MLH1, underly hereditary nonpolyposis colorectal cancer. Recent efforts in several labs have led to *in vitro* reconstitution of mammalian MMR with purified components, enabling powerful analysis of this complex mechanism (reviewed in *[276]*). In addition to the MutS and MutL homologs, the system requires the following: Exo1 to excise the gap; RPA, which binds to the single strand DNA in the gapped region (and is known to bind to phosphorylated AID, as discussed earlier); PCNA (proliferating cell nuclear antigen), which promotes processivity by encircling DNA in a sliding ring clamp and recruiting other components; DNA polymerase δ; ligase 1; and several other proteins.

An early speculation that SHM might be caused by localized abrogation of MMR has been investigated by one group who found that GC centroblasts have an intact MMR system, as judged by an in vitro MMR assay and Western blot for MMR components *(277)*. If MMR normally operates to minimize mutations, KOs of MMR components might have been expected to increase mutation frequencies in immunoglobulin V regions, as they do in non-Ig genes. In fact, MMR KOs generally show normal or modestly decreased frequencies of mutation in SHM, but show interesting qualitative abnormalities in the spectrum of mutations observed.

KOs of MSH2 have been studied by several labs and show consistent decrease in SHM from A:T basepairs (with a corresponding increase in the percentage of mutations from G:C basepairs). KOs of MSH6 (but not MSH3) show similar decreased A:T mutation (278,279). These results, in the context of the model of Figure 6.12, suggest that MMR, triggered by the MSH2-MSH6 heterodimer, primarily introduces mutation at A:T basepairs. The predilection for mutating A:T basepairs matches the activity of polymerase η, as discussed in the next section, implying that this polymerase may by the one most frequently engaged by the MMR machinery in repairing AID-generated lesions. Indeed, MSH2-MSH6 is capable of binding to a U:G mismatch, MSH2 can bind to pol η in cell extracts, and MSH2-MSH6 can stimulate the activity of pol η *in vitro* (280).

Compared with the effects of MutS mutations, KOs of MutL homologs have shown less striking abnormalities in SHM, perhaps because of some redundancy in these proteins.

Exonuclease 1 is another important component of the MMR machinery. The human Exo1 protein interacts *in vitro* with human MSH2 and MutL homologs *(281)*, which may recruit Exo1 to Ig V regions. Exo1 KO mice were found to show a slight decrease in SHM frequency, with a significant decrease in mutation at A:T as seen in KOs of other MMR components (282). In addition, the protein was found by ChIP analysis to be strikingly enriched in VH region DNA, but not Cμ region, of a B cell line stimulated by anti-IgM and T cells to initiate SHM (282). The same study reported similar association of MLH1 with the VH region undergoing SHM.

These results are all consistent with the model of Figure 6.12, in which AID-catalyzed creation of a U:G mismatch has three possible fates. The DNA strand bearing U may be simply replicated, the U may be removed by UNG, or the U:G mismatch may be recognized by MMR, which is the only route for mutations at T:A or A:T positions. This model makes the strong prediction that a double KO UNG$^{-/-}$ MSH2$^{-/-}$ should only be capable of phase 1A transitions at C:G. In fact, SHM in this double KO was found to be limited almost exclusively to C:G→T:A transitions (283), although an alternative interpretation of these results has been proposed (201).

Error-prone Polymerases. Although avoidance of error is a high priority for most DNA replication, error-prone DNA synthesis served an important function long before SHM evolved to mutate Ig genes; indeed error-prone polymerases have been most thoroughly studied in E. coli and yeast. These polymerases are useful in all cells for replication of DNA containing focal lesions that would block replication of stringent high-fidelity polymerases. A panel of these polymerases has evolved, each specializing in different aspects of "translesion DNA synthesis" (TLS) and showing differing spectra of infidelity in replication of normal DNA. Evidence for participation of four specific TLS polymerases in SHM has come from comparing the known activities of a particular polymerase with the SHM abnormalities seen in mice or humans with mutations in the corresponding polymerase gene. Some polymerase KOs are homozygous lethals, requiring evaluation by gene knockdown or inhibition in B cells.

Polymerase η characteristically inserts mismatches at A or T nucleotides, and individuals lacking this polymerase show the predicted abnormality: decreased mutations at A:T basepairs. This was first demonstrated in patients with xeroderma pigmentosum variant (XP-V) disease, whose defects in pol η make them susceptible to sunlight-induced skin cancers (284); a similar defect in mutations from A:T basepairs was subsequently shown for pol η KO mice (285,286). Pol η binds to MSH2-MSH6, as mentioned earlier, and is up-regulated in cells undergoing SHM.

In addition to pol η, three other polymerases have been implicated in SHM by experiments in which their diminished expression was associated with abnormalities in SHM: pol ζ (287,288), pol θ (289), and REV1 (290). Several other polymerases have been studied and do not appear to play important roles in SHM; minor contributions might be difficult to detect unless tested in cells deficient in multiple other SHM components.

A fundamental question about the action of error-prone polymerases is how they are specifically engaged for SHM, given that most spontaneous cytosine deamination in nonlymphoid cells is accurately repaired. A recent investigation using the chicken B cell line DT40 showed that inactivation of RAD18, an E3 ubiquitin ligase of PCNA, inhibited SHM frequency by about 60%, and suggested that RAD18 may contribute to recruitment of error-prone TLS polymerases in SHM (291). Further work will be necessary to understand the upstream regulation of Rad18 in SHM and to clarify which MMR components are affected by PCNA ubiquitination.

DNA Breaks in V Regions. Brenner and Milstein proposed in 1966 that Ig V region genes might be cleaved by an endonuclease and that these defects might then be repaired by an error-prone polymerase that introduced mutations into the DNA *(292)*. Clearly error-prone polymerases participate importantly in SHM, but the role of double-strand breaks (dsbs) is less clear. DNA breaks are implied by the occurrence of insertions and deletions, which are found in about 5% of V regions undergoing SHM in normal human GC B cells isolated by flow cytometry *(293)*. Further, transfection of the SHM-competent human Burkitt lymphoma line Ramos with TdT was found to lead to many insertions in mutated immunoglobulin VH genes, insertions that were found (like typical somatic mutations) in the V but not C region *(294)*. These insertions are most easily interpreted as the result of TdT-catalyzed nucleotide addition at dsbs. Breaks are also suggested by the enrichment of phosphorylated histone H2B at V regions undergoing SHM (mentioned earlier), as this histone modification seems to be associated with dsbs *(295)*.

More direct evidence for such breaks has come from two laboratories using LM-PCR to amplify blunt DNA ends within Ig genes undergoing SHM *(296,297)*. However, the role of dsbs in SHM is unclear because both labs have subsequently reported that these V region dsbs were found at similar frequency in B cells from normal mice and from AID$^{-/-}$ mice, in which SHM does not occur *(298,299)*; this was surprising because it had been assumed that the V region dsbs were triggered by AID-catalyzed deamination, as has been reported for dsbs associated with CSR (discussed below). Perhaps dsbs play a role in only a small fraction of V region mutations, conceivably as low as the ~5% of mutations involving insertions or deletions. Consistent with a minimal contribution of dsbs to SHM is the observation that the variant histone H2AX, which rapidly accumulates in a phosphorylated form (γH2AX) at and near dsbs, was found to be enriched broadly in a heavy chain gene undergoing CSR and SHM, but not in a Vλ gene undergoing only SHM, as though dsbs may be widespread in CSR but not in SHM. Moreover, B cells lacking H2AX are impaired for CSR but undergo normal SHM (300), as are mice lacking Ku and DNA-PK.

Heavy Chain Switch

Switch Regions and Switch Junctions

As briefly mentioned earlier in this chapter, isotype switching involves removal of Cμ from downstream of the rearranged heavy chain VDJ gene and its replacement by a new downstream CH region. This occurs by a deletional recombination—CSR—between repetitive DNA sequences known as *switch* (or S) *regions* that lie 5′ of each CH region (except Cδ). While most switch breakpoints fall in the S regions, some are in nearby nonrepetitive DNA. The S region of the mouse μ gene, Sμ, is located about 1 kb to 2 kb 5′ to the Cμ coding sequence and is composed of numerous tandem repeats of sequences of the form $(GAGCT)_n(GGGGT)$, where n is usually 2 to 5 but can range as high as 17. All of the S regions of downstream isotypes include pentamers similar to GAGCT and GGGGT embedded in larger repeat units, rather than precisely tandemly repeated as in Sμ. The 10 kb murine Sγ1 region has an additional higher order structure: two direct repeat sequences flank each of two clusters of 49 bp tandem repeats. In support of the critical role of S regions for CSR, KO of Sγ1 by homologous recombination essentially abolished expression of IgG1 from that allele (301). However, mice with a complete deletion of the Sμ tandem repeats were still able to accomplish CSR, although at a reduced level (302). These mice still retained a few scattered G-rich pentamers flanking the tandem repeat region, and these may have supported CSR. Mice with a larger deletion removing most of the flanking G-rich pentamers had a more profound impairment in CSR (303).

A switch recombination between, for example, μ and ε genes produces a composite Sμ-Sε sequence (Figure 6.13). From a comparison between the sequence of an Sμ-Sε composite switch region and the sequences of the germline Sμ and Sε, one can localize the exact recombination sites between Sμ and Sε that occurred in each allele. Such comparisons have indicated that there is no specific site, either in Sμ or in any other S region, where the recombination always occurs, although clusters of recombination sites have been reported at two specific regions within the tandem repeats of murine Sγ3 region *(304)*. Thus, unlike the enzymatic machinery of VJ recombination, the switch machinery can join sequences in a broad target region. Often both IgH alleles in a single cell undergo switching to the same downstream isotype. Some alleles undergo sequential switching events; for example, a common pathway to IgE expression is an initial $\mu \rightarrow \gamma 1$ switch, followed by a CSR between the composite Sμ-Sγ1 region and the Sε region *(305)*. Although most CSR occurs as a deletion within a single IgH allele, switching between two allelic chromosomes can be detected at a frequency of roughly 7% to 10% in mouse and rabbit (306,307).

DNA fragments excised by switch recombination have been cloned from fractions of circular DNA isolated from cells actively undergoing isotype switch recombination. Thus, at least some of the excised DNA segments ligate their ends to form "switch circles," which contain composite switch junctions that are in theory reciprocal to the composite switch junction retained on chromosomal DNA (Figure 6.13). Because switch circles are not linked to centromeres and may not contain origins of replication, they are not efficiently replicated. Therefore, they are not found in cells that have divided many times after switching (e.g., in myelomas or hybridomas).

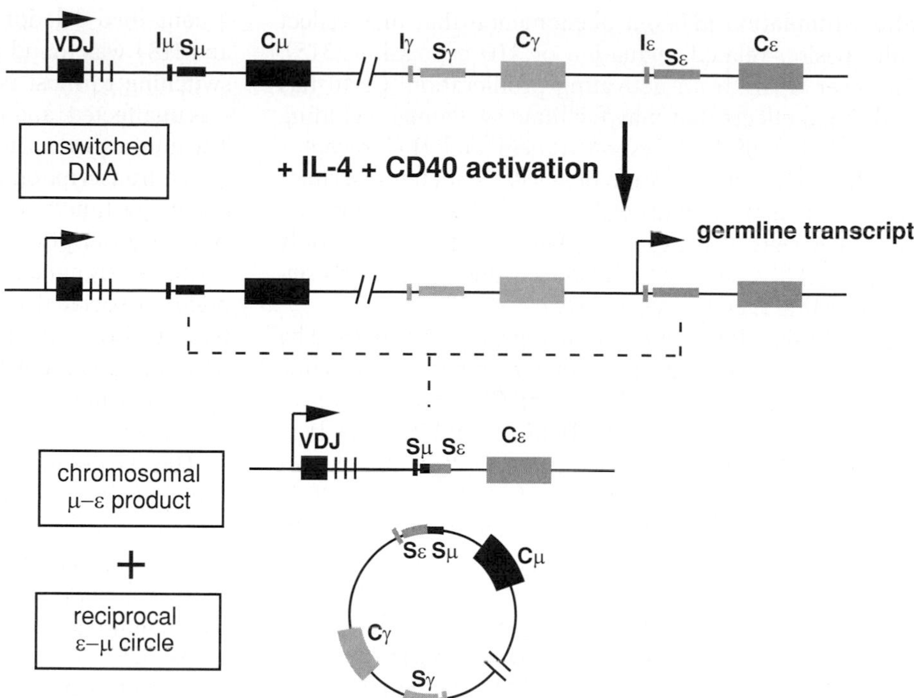

FIGURE 6.13 Switch regions and composite switch junctions. The recombination breakpoints in isotype switch recombination fall within repetitive "switch" (S) regions. Stimuli that activate switch recombination (IL-4 and CD40 activation in the example shown) generally promote transcription across the target S region, initiating just upstream at the "I" exon. Recombination between Sμ and Sε produces two composite switch junctions: an Sμ-Sε junction retained in chromosomal DNA, and a reciprocal Sε-Sμ junction found in fractions of circular DNA. PCR amplification across either composite junction can be used to study switch recombination.

Many composite switch junction sequences show mutations near the recombination breakpoint when compared to the corresponding germline switch sequences; these mutations have been interpreted as reflecting an error-prone DNA synthesis step that may be a component of the switch recombination mechanism *(308)*. Mutations are also observed in unrecombined Sμ regions in activated cells, but are much rarer in Sγ regions (309). Internal deletions also occur within individual S regions in cells undergoing CSR (310). Like functional CSR, both the mutations and internal deletions in the switch regions seem to be AID-dependent.

Regulation of Isotype Switching by CD40

Isotype switching occurs physiologically in animals about 1 week after immunization with T-dependent antigens, at about the same time that somatic mutation of Ig genes begins. Both processes normally occur in germinal centers of lymphoid organs—a location that facilitates interactions between B cells, T cells, and follicular dendritic cells presenting antigen. As demonstrated by *in vitro* switching experiments, T cells promote switching by secretion of cytokines (especially IL-4 and TGF-β), as well as by cell-to-cell contact.

A major component of the cell contact signal is mediated by an interaction between the B cell surface marker CD40 and its ligand—designated CD40L, CD154, or gp39—expressed on activated T cells (primarily CD4$^+$). CD40 is a member of the TNF-receptor family, while CD40L belongs to the TNF ligand family. The dependence of switching on the CD40-CD40L interaction is highlighted by the genetic disease known as the *X-linked hyper-IgM syndrome-1*, which was found to be caused by a defect in the human gene encoding the CD40L/gp39 (311). Like AID-deficient HIGM2 patients described earlier, patients with HIGM1 have elevated concentrations of IgM in their serum and almost no immunoglobulins of other isotypes. In addition, their antibodies fail to show affinity maturation or evidence of B cell memory responses. Similar defects are seen in humans with mutations in their CD40 gene, an autosomal recessive disease designated HIGM3 (312). CSR impairment may also be caused by abnormal function of CD40 signaling pathway components, including IKKγ (also known as *NEMO*), NFκB proteins, and c-Jun N-terminal kinase (JNK). Mouse strains with engineered defects in CD40 are defective in SHM and T-dependent CSR, but respond with normal isotype switching to T-independent antigens *(313)*; little is known about this T independent switching pathway.

The discovery of the importance of the of CD40-CD40L interaction has facilitated in vitro switching experiments in which B cells are incubated with stimuli designed to engage their CD40 molecules (i.e., with CD40L$^+$ T cells, with nonlymphoid cells engineered to display surface CD40L, or with antibodies to CD40).

One role of the CD40 engagement is to induce B cell proliferation. Indeed, other proliferative stimuli—for example, LPS or IgM or IgD crosslinking—can support cytokine-induced isotype switching in vitro in the absence of T cells and CD40 activation. The relationship of CSR to cell division is supported by evidence that switching is linked to the cell cycle *(313)* and to the number of cell divisions after stimulation *(314)*, a phenomenon that may reflect cell division–related regulation of AID expression (315). However, apart from activating proliferation, CD40 has additional effects that may facilitate switching, including upregulation of IL-4 responsiveness and IL-4 receptor number *(316)*, upregulation of sterile "switch transcripts" (discussed later), and upregulation of AID expression. Activated B cells also express CD40L, which can not only trigger CD40 signaling but also transduce a "reverse" signal affecting B cell function *(317)*.

The CD40-CD40L interaction appears to be opposed by an interaction between two other members of the same protein families: CD30 and its ligand CD153. CD30 expression on B cells is induced by CD40L, but inhibited by ligation of the BCR *(318)*. Engagement of CD30 by its ligand—CD30L—down-regulates several of the effects of CD40 ligation, apparently by inhibiting the action of NFκB *(319)*. This effect may represent a feedback mechanism to limit the activation of B cells that have not been stimulated effectively through their BCR by antigen. "Reverse" signaling by B cell-expressed CD30L has also been reported as an additional inhibitory influence on CSR *(320)*. Pathologic activation of CD30-CD153 signaling in chronic lymphocytic leukemia may contribute to the impairment in IgG and IgA production that leads to infection in these patients (321).

Isotype-specific Regulation of Germline Transcripts

Different isotypes are known to predominate in different immune responses depending on the antigen, route of antigen administration, and several other parameters. These different parameters act in part by influencing the cytokine milieu of the B cells. IL-4, for example, promotes the expression of IgE (and IgG1 in mouse), whereas TGFβ promotes switching to IgA. These lymphokines have been proposed to act by making the C region of the target isotype "accessible" to switch recombinase machinery that may be largely non–isotype-specific. The accessibility is associated with expression of a "sterile" or "germline" RNA transcript that initiates upstream of a target S region (Figure 6.13) and extends through the target C region. This transcript is spliced so that a noncoding upstream exon known as an *I* (or *intron*) *region* is joined to the first coding exon of the C region. The same experimental conditions—particularly the same cytokines—that favor the accumulation of sterile transcripts from a particular isotype generally also stimulate switch recombination involving the corresponding S region. In some cases, the signals transduced by the cytokine receptor have been elucidated. For example, IL-4 stimulates germline transcription by activating the transcription factor STAT6, which attaches to one of several nuclear protein binding motifs in the promoter region upstream of Iε and Iγ1. CD40 engagement also acts in part through NFκB-mediated binding to I region promoters *(322)*.

Apart from I region promoters, sterile transcription and isotype switching are also regulated by IgH enhancers. A combined deletion of the murine 3′α enhancers HS3b and HS4 was found to cause a significant impairment in switching to most isotypes, although switching to IgG1 was unaffected (and IgA only moderately decreased) (323). The diminished switching was associated with diminished sterile transcription of the same isotypes, suggesting that one major function of the enhancers in CSR is to increase sterile transcription. The relative independence of γ1 from regulation by enhancers may be related to the putative LCR region associated with that gene *(324)*. The intronic enhancer also seems to play a role in CSR, since IgH loci with a targeted deletion of the Eμ enhancer showed decreased switching when tested in RAG-complementation mice *(325)*.

The importance of sterile transcription for CSR has been highlighted by experiments in which an artificial switch substrate was constructed bearing an Sμ sequence, an Sα sequence whose transcription was driven by a tetracycline-regulatable promoter, and a GFP gene whose expression required recombination between the two S regions (326). When this plasmid was stably transfected into the switch-competent cell line CH12F3-2, and transcription across the Sα sequence was manipulated by adjusting the tetracycline concentration, higher transcription levels were associated with more CSR.

Although cytokines and CD40 ligation clearly affect CSR by regulating sterile transcription, it is likely that the B cell milieu regulates other aspects of the switching mechanism as well, because several examples have been reported of cytokines up- or down-regulating switch recombination without a parallel effect on sterile transcripts *(327)*. Further, when certain cell lines capable of switching their endogenous IgH loci to only one particular isotype were transfected with a panel of plasmid CSR substrates with different S regions, the isotype specificity of the cells for plasmid CSR matched that for their endogenous genes, even though all S regions of the engineered constructs were strongly transcribed; this observation suggests that the CSR machinery might show isotype specificity based on recognition of features specific to certain S region sequences (328). For example, *in vivo* footprinting demonstrated that NFκB p50 binds specifically to a motif in Sγ3, and this protein is required for efficient $\mu \rightarrow \gamma 3$ switching of both endogenous genes and plasmid substrates (329). In a related example, the protein Suv39h1, a histone methyltransferase, specifically increases $\mu \rightarrow \alpha$ CSR of plasmid substrates and endogenous genes, possibly by repressing a sequence-specific binding protein *(330)*. In principle the activity of isotype-specific switching factors could be regulated by the environment of the B cell.

Role of Transcription in the Mechanism of CSR

Gene targeting experiments have shown that mouse strains lacking the I region (and its promoter) of a particular isotype do not switch to that isotype, reinforcing the idea that sterile transcription is necessary for CSR (reviewed in ref *[331]*). The low extent of sequence conservation of the I exons and the lack of consistent open reading frames suggest that these transcripts do not encode a functional protein. Indeed, the exact sequence of the I region may be irrelevant since an I region can be replaced by an unrelated sequence and still support CSR *(332)*. However, the transcribed exon upstream of the S region may need a splice donor site allowing the S region to be removed from the transcript, because a targeted construct lacking such a splice donor site was reportedly unable to support CSR even though transcription through the S region occurred *(333)*.

One possible role for sterile transcripts in CSR involves the formation of an RNA:DNA complex known as an R loop, a structure in which RNA complementary to one strand of a DNA molecule binds to that strand with Watson-Crick base-pairing, displacing the other DNA strand, which forms a single-stranded loop. In support of the R loop model, cell-free transcription across switch regions was found to generate a stable association of the transcript RNA with the template DNA (334,335); significantly, no substantial association occurred when the switch region was transcribed in reverse orientation, leading to a C-rich transcript, or when the transcribed template was a DNA fragment other than an S region. The displaced DNA strand in S region R loops was susceptible to cleavage *in vitro* by nucleases that recognize single-strand DNA or junctions between single- and double-stranded DNA; *in vivo,* such cleavage could be a step in CSR. To probe whether R loops might exist *in vivo,* DNA was extracted (along with any R loops) from LPS-stimulated B cells switching to Sγ3 and was treated with sodium bisulfite, which efficiently deaminates cytosines to uracil only in unpaired single-strand DNA. The Sγ3 regions were then amplified from the genomic DNA by PCR and cloned. The clone sequences revealed long stretches in the upper strand where all the C residues were replaced by Ts (336,337), presumably marking regions of single-strand DNA that were displaced as stable R loops *in vivo*. In the lower DNA strand, only short patches of C→T mutations were found, suggesting short single-strand regions in that strand; such regions might be transiently created during transcription, or perhaps result from misalignment of repeats in the two strands when an R loop collapses. Regions of single-strand DNA on either strand might provide targets for deamination by AID *in vivo,* given that AID apparently deaminates only single-stranded DNA (or DNA regions transiently rendered single-stranded by transcription), as shown by *in vitro* experiments described earlier.

Apart from the formation of R loops, transcription may also facilitate access to AID by altering the supercoiling of the transcribed DNA, as previously discussed in the context of SHM (254).

A model in which AID loads onto an RNA polymerase complex and acts on DNA as the complex travels downstream was discussed earlier in the context of AID function in SHM. Some evidence consistent with a similar polymerase-loading model has been described in the context of CSR. Because uracils generated in S regions through AID-catalyzed deamination are apparently processed by UNG and MMR (as discussed below), double KO mice defective in both processes produce uracils that can by resolved only by replication, causing C:G → A:T mutations. A study of the distribution of such mutations in clones from these double KO B cells found that a domain of mutations began about 150 bp 3′ of the transcription start site of Iμ and extended 4 kb to 5 kb downstream, with diminishing mutation frequency near Cμ *(338)*. Within this domain, the overall frequency of C→T mutations was similar on the two strands, but individual sequences showed clustering of C→T mutations on one or the other strand, suggesting that AID may confine its action to one strand as the polymerase moves processively downstream. Cytokine conditions associated with sterile transcription of particular downstream isotypes increased the frequency of C:G→A:T mutations in the corresponding S regions. Another study supporting the concept of a promoter-initiated domain of CSR found that recombination breakpoints near Sμ extended further downstream than normal in mice with a deletion of the Sμ tandem repeats, as though a constant CSR domain length were maintained with a fixed upstream end (339).

Features that Target CSR to Switch Regions

Mammalian IgH switch regions have several notable properties: they are G rich on the nontranscribed "upper" strand, and they contain multiple repeated sequences, possibly including motifs that could serve as targets for the CSR machinery. To investigate which characteristics might be critical in targeting CSR, several laboratories have studied CSR in two main contexts: (1) in B cells transfected with model CSR targets, often containing reporter genes whose expression depends on a CSR event; or (2) in B cells of mice in which endogenous S regions have been modified by "knocking in" engineered constructs. In either context investigators can test how variant S regions affect CSR.

One study reported that replacement of a natural murine Sμ sequence with the chicken or frog Sμ sequences—neither of which are G rich—supported somewhat reduced but still substantial frequencies of CSR, while a randomly chosen sequence, even if G rich, did not support CSR *(340)*. These investigators proposed that palindromic sequences (which seem to be present in all S regions, including those of frogs) may contribute to CSR. In support of this, they reported that switch junctions tend to lie closer to boundaries of DNA stem-loops (which might be formed by palindromes) than statistically expected, an observation that has not been universally confirmed. However, they also tested the CSR potential of a synthetic palindrome-rich tandem repeat (derived from the multiple cloning site of a commercial Bluescript plasmid containing palindromic recognition sites for restriction enzymes) and found, surprisingly, that it supported a modest but clearly significant level of CSR.

In another study (mentioned earlier) homologous recombination was used to delete the endogenous ~10 kb Sγ1 region and replace it shortened versions. The efficiency of CSR to γ1 correlated well with length of the engineered Sγ1 region (301). When the Sγ1 region was inverted, it retained about 25% of the wild-type activity (341). Since this inverted, and now C-rich, DNA segment could not form an R loop, this result suggests that the R loop contributes to CSR, but other features of the S region that are preserved in the inverted sequence also play a role.

The nature of the other features is suggested by an analysis of switch junctions occurring between a knocked in frog Sμ and the endogenous murine Sγ1 (342). As mentioned earlier, the AT-rich frog S region is not prone to R-loop formation, but it was able to support efficient CSR when it was swapped into the position of the murine Sμ, and it functioned equally well in either orientation. Significantly, in either orientation the recombination junctions were clustered in a portion of the S region that is rich in repeats of the sequence AGCT, which is a special case of the WRCH/DGYW consensus sequence for AID targeting. Indeed, the AGCT-rich region was a good substrate for *in vitro* deamination by AID when transcribed in association with RPA. The AGCT motif is enriched in all mammalian S regions (and is also enriched in the Bluescript multiple cloning site). Among WRCH motifs, AGCT may be particularly effective as a target for CSR because of the potential for deamination on either strand, creating closely spaced nicks, or even a dsb with a single base overhang if the cytosines in same AGCT motif are targeted on both strands. The density of AGCT in S regions correlates with the location of switch junctions better than the density of WRC or the boundaries of G richness or R loops (337). These results all suggest that clusters of AGCT may represent a target for CSR that evolved in amphibians, with R-loop formation evolving later in mammals to further enhance AID accessibility to the "upper" G-rich strand of S regions.

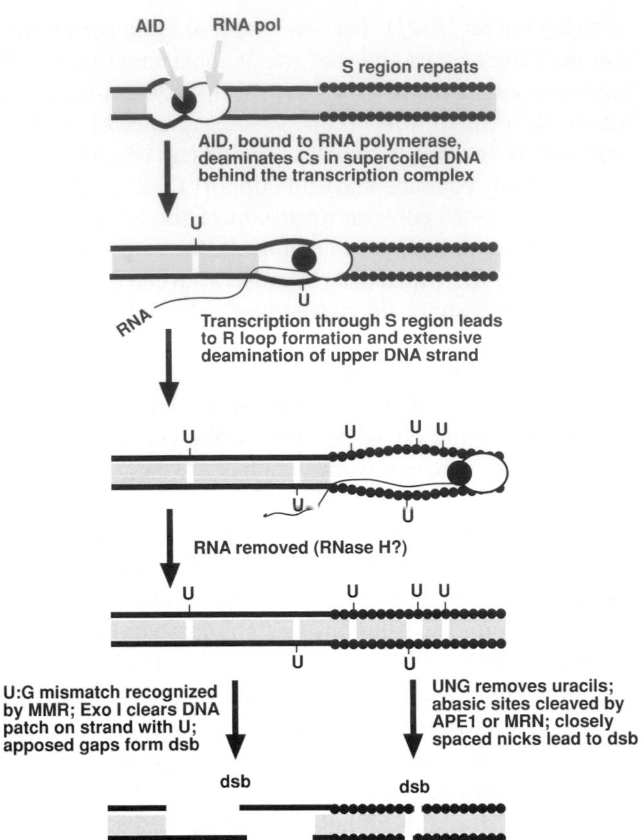

FIGURE 6.14 Mechanistic model of CSR. This figure incorporates features of the most widely accepted models, but some aspects are controversial at present. Two strands of DNA near the 5′ boundary of a Switch region are shown in black, with the S region repeats indicataed by dots. DNA with normal Watson-Crick base-pairing is indicated by the gray shading between the DNA strands. RNA Polymerase moves to the right, transcribing the sequence into an RNA strand; multiple other proteins accompany the RNA pol, but only AID (black circle) is shown. AID may deaminate C residues to U either in the negatively supercoiled DNA behind the transcription complex or in the single-strand R-looped DNA displaced by the RNA-DNA complex. Cleavage of the U-bearing DNA strand can lead to dsbs in pathways dependent or independent of MMR components as shown.

DNA Breaks in CSR

The recombination event that underlies isotype switching includes DNA breaks and rejoining events that must involve both strands of DNA. Although the RAG-induced DNA breaks that initiate V(D)J recombination occur at the corresponding position on the two strands (yielding a blunt end and a hairpin), the nature of the ends in the initial CSR cleavage is not clear. An early compilation of switch junctions *(308)* found only rare instances of microhomology at the junction. Because these microhomology examples would be consistent with invasion of one DNA strand from Sμ targeting a short homologous region in a downstream S region (or vice versa), the rarity of such junctions has been interpreted as an indication that CSR usually proceeds by ligation of blunt DNA ends rather than by strand invasion. However, DNA cuts with staggered—not blunt—ends would generally be the result of the widely discussed mechanism shown in Figure 6.14: a DNA break on one strand might result from AID-catalyzed cytosine deamination, removal of the resulting uracil by UNG, and cleavage 5′ to the abasic site by an endonuclease, possibly APE1 (apurinic-apyridinic endonuclease 1). The initial staggered ends could be converted to blunt ends through trimming of a 5′ or 3′ single-strand overhang, or through filling in the shorter strand by a DNA polymerase, or through a combination of both processes. Filling in by error-prone polymerases could explain the mutations commonly observed around the switch junction, mentioned previously.

Evidence supporting staggered DNA breaks in CSR was reported from the switch junctions observed in a model CSR substrate designed with two oppositely oriented S regions such that CSR would occur by inversion, preserving both recombination junctions on the same chromosome. Several duplications at the ends of inverted DNA after CSR suggested that complementary overhangs at dsbs had been filled in before joining (343). Additional evidence for staggered breaks has come from several investigators using LM-PCR to detect double-strand DNA ends at switch regions in cells undergoing CSR (344–346). LM-PCR protocols involving ligation of a blunt linker directly to blunt ends from genomic DNA was successful in amplifying blunt ends from DNA of B cells activated for CSR, but when the DNA was pretreated with T4 polymerase—which would convert staggered end cuts to blunt—the yield of amplified bands after LMPCR was significantly increased, suggesting that most of the ends in the isolated genomic DNA (before T4 polymerase treatment) were staggered.

As discussed earlier, SHM-associated dsbs in V regions occurred independently of AID. When the CSR-associated dsbs in Sμ were examined by LM-PCR in B cells from normal and AID$^{-/-}$ individuals, the dsbs were significantly fewer in AID$^{-/-}$ B cells, though not completely absent. Further, γH2AX foci (which mark dsbs, as mentioned earlier) were found at IgH genes marked by FISH in B cells undergoing CSR, and these foci were strikingly diminished in AID$^{-/-}$ B cells, consistent with AID-dependence of dsbs in CSR (347). However, a provocative recent report suggests that AID may play an additional role after dsbs have been created. Two unrelated human HIGM2 patients were observed to have a particular heterozygous mutation in AICDA: a premature stop codon replacing Arg190 (i.e., in the C-termininal region known to be important for CSR). Although other AICDA mutations cause an HIGM phenotype only when homozygous, this R190X mutation acted as a dominant negative for CSR; but significantly, there was no dramatic decrease in dsbs in the patients' activated B cells (348). This result suggests that after the creation of dsbs, the C-terminal residues of AID may be required for an additional step to complete CSR.

Ubiquitously Expressed Components of CSR Machinery

Role of Uracil-N-Glycosylase in CSR. The model of Figure 6.14 suggests that after AID-catalyzed deamination of a cytidine residue, the resulting uracil is removed by UNG, creating an abasic site that leads to a single-strand DNA break (nick), which can become double-stranded if there is a nearby nick on the opposite strand. This model predicts that both CSR and the creation of dsbs would be severely impaired in the absence of UNG. Indeed, B cells from UNG$^{-/-}$ mice showed almost complete inability to switch *in vitro* to IgG1and IgG3 secretion and significant impairment in IgA secretion (197). Double-strand breaks in UNG$^{-/-}$ B cells, as detected by LM-PCR, were also significantly impaired, but not abolished (346). Human patients with homozygous UNG deficiency due to mutations in both UNG alleles showed an HIGM phenotype, with a more profound defect than in UNG$^{-/-}$ mice: the patients showed essentially no IgG, IgE, or IgA secretion by stimulated B cells, and no dsbs (by LM-PCR) in Sμ (349). A role for UNG in CSR is also suggested by the fact that UNG expression was found to be upregulated in normal B cells stimulated for CSR (349).

These data support an important role for UNG in CSR as outlined in Figure 6.14, but several lines of evidence from Honjo's lab have challenged this model. First, mutant UNG proteins with profoundly impaired uracil deglycosylase enzymatic activity were able to rescue CSR in UNG$^{-/-}$ murine B cells (350); second, expression of the specific UNG inhibitor protein Ugi at concentrations sufficient to inhibit UNG enzymatic activity did not inhibit dsb formation in CSR as assessed by formation of γH2AX foci (351); and third, IgM$^+$ B cells from UNG$^{-/-}$ mice stimulated to undergo CSR showed a normal frequency of internal deletions in Sμ, deletions that depend on AID-induced recombination (352). These authors suggested that UNG may act in CSR by binding other CSR components rather than by removing uracils enzymatically, and that the step where UNG is required may be after, rather than before, DNA cleavage. One caveat is that a small residual amount of UNG activity remaining in the mutants or in the presence of Ugi might have confounded some results. A full reconciliation of the evidence on UNG function will require additional data.

Role of MMR in CSR. The complementary pathways of UNG and MMR action in SHM were discussed earlier (Figure 6.12); current evidence suggests a similar participation of both UNG and MMR in CSR. Although CSR was dramatically impaired in UNG$^{-/-}$ B cells (e.g., *in vitro* switching to IgG1 was reduced to about 6% of wild type), the double KO UNG$^{-/-}$, MSH2$^{-/-}$ caused significant further impairment (to 1.5% of wild type IgG1 switching) (283). Single KOs of MMR components (MSH2, PMS2 or MLH1) inhibit CSR efficiency by only two- to five-fold, but cause significant differences in the characteristics of switch junctions, including alterations in the extent of microhomology at the junctions *(353,354)*. Notably, Sμ junction breakpoints in MSH2$^{-/-}$ B cells were found to cluster in the Sμ tandem repeat sequences of Sμ (SμTR), with significantly fewer breakpoints upstream of the tandem repeats *(355)*. MSH2$^{-/-}$ B cells in which the Sμ tandem repeats were knocked out by homologous recombination (SμTRΔ), showed profoundly impaired CSR efficiency (to 0.6% of wild type) (356), whereas CSR efficiency in B cells carrying the SμTRΔ allele but wild type MSH2 was only modestly impaired (two- to three-fold reduced efficiency), as discussed earlier. These results suggest that MSH2 is primarily important for mediating CSR at positions outside the Sμ tandem repeats; presumably UNG can act without MSH2 to mediate the recombinations within the repeats. Perhaps the frequent AGCT motifs in the tandem repeats cause single-strand DNA nicks that lie close enough together to act as staggered double-strand breaks, able to participate in CSR with minimal further processing; whereas in the sparsely scattered hotspots flanking the tandem repeats, AID generates uracils that lie too far apart to engage in CSR without processing by MMR components.

As discussed previously, Exo1 is a component of MMR machinery that participates in SHM. Exo1 KO mice show a significantly decreased efficiency of CSR, from roughly 15% to 30% of normal (depending on isotype), with some decrease in microhomology at CSR junctions (282).

Nonhomologous End Joining Components in CSR. If AID triggers cleavage at switch regions, ubiquitous DNA repair and ligation enzymes may accomplish the subsequent DNA repair steps of CSR as in V(D)J recombination. This possibility has been tested for several proteins whose role in V(D)J recombination was discussed earlier in this chapter. Because KOs of NHEJ components are impaired in V(D)J recombination, investigators have studied NHEJ in CSR using mouse strains with "knock-ins" of recombined heavy and light chain genes, allowing normal B cell development up to the point of CSR. Whereas "knock-in" mice with intact Ku genes switched to downstream isotypes, the corresponding Ku-70– or Ku-80–deficient mice were dramatically impaired in CSR *(357,358)*. A role for the Ku complex in CSR is also suggested by the fact that incubation conditions favoring CSR (IL4 and CD40 engagement) increased the amount of Ku complex detectable in nuclear extracts of splenic B cells *(359)*.

Treatment with IL4 plus CD40 engagement also increased the level of nuclear DNA-PK, but the evidence for a role of this protein in CSR is complex. Although an early report indicated dramatically reduced CSR in pro-B cells from SCID mice—the classic DNA-PK mutant described earlier—more recent studies of conventional CSR in mature B cells of SCID mice with "knock-in" recombined Ig genes have found that the SCID mutation causes only modest (two- to three-fold) reductions CSR efficiency, differing for different isotypes *(360)*. In contrast, a null (KO) mutant of DNA-PK essentially abolished CSR to all isotypes except IgG1 (361). The reason for the more severe effect of KO versus the SCID mutation is not fully understood, but it is possible that the SCID mutant protein, while truncated and lacking kinase activity, may still retain a scaffolding function that facilitates switching by recruiting other CSR components, and that loss of this scaffolding function in the DNA-PK KO mouse accounts for the more severe phenotype. The sparing of CSR to IgG1 in the DNA-PK KO remains mysterious.

DNA Damage Response Proteins in CSR. Several additional proteins known to participate in the damage response to dsbs in DNA seem to participate in CSR. A complex of three proteins—Mre11, Rad50, and Nibrin (also known Nbs1, product of the abnormal gene in the human disease Nijmegen Breakage Syndrome, NBS)—is conserved in eukaryotes from yeast to mammals and has been implicated in telomere maintenance, cell cycle checkpoint signaling, meiotic recombination, and dsb repair. The Nibrin component binds rapidly to dsbs induced by irradiation and forms foci coincident with IgH gene FISH fluorescence in B cells undergoing CSR (347). Nibrin-deficient mouse B cells show impairments in CSR (to 30% to 50% of normal efficiency) (362,363), while human NBS patients show lower than normal concentrations of IgG and IgA in serum, consistent with a CSR defect *(364)*. The Mre11 protein has a nuclease activity and may contribute to dsb formation, since Mre11/RAD50 complex was found to cleave an AP site in *in vitro* experiments (365). Human patients with Mre11 deficiency (ataxia telangiectasia-like disorder, ATLD) also show evidence of decreased CSR efficiency and evidence of abnormal switch junctions, with increased microhomology and abnormal mutations (366).

An important function of the MRN complex is to recruit and activate ATM—product of the gene mutated in the human disease ataxia telengectasia (AT). ATM is a member of the phosphatidylinositol-3′-kinase family and participates in the DNA damage response by phosphorylating a number of critical protein targets including p53, Chk2, and Nibrin. Human AT patients have a complex disease similar to NBS, including an immunodeficiency with T cell abnormalities as well as variably low IgG and IgA levels. B cells from AT patients undergo $\mu \rightarrow \alpha$ *in vitro* switching at reduced efficiency, and the Sμ-Sα switch junctions formed show a very high frequency of microhomology with abnormally infrequent mutations near the junctions (367). ATM-deficient mouse B cells show impaired CSR with normal germline transcripts (368,369). One group reported an increase in microhomology at switch junctions, similar to that observed in human AT patients (368). While CSR between different S regions was impaired in the ATM KOs, internal deletions within Sμ occurred in IgM-secreting cells at a frequency similar to that in wild type, suggesting that the loss of ATM specifically impaired long-range joining; this may indicate a role for ATM in synapsis of DNA ends (369).

As discussed previously in the context of V(D)J recombination, γ-H2AX—the phosphorylated form of histone H2A—rapidly accumulates in foci at dsbs and may help assemble other proteins at dsbs to prevent the breaks from progressing to chromosome translocations. $H2AX^{-/-}$ B cells show a CSR defect very similar to that in $ATM^{-/-}$:

significantly decreased CSR efficiency with normal frequency of deletions within Sμ (300).

53BP1 (p53 binding protein 1) was originally discovered as a protein binding to the tumor suppressor p53 but was subsequently found to function in checkpoint control and to localize rapidly to DNA breaks *in vivo*. $53BP1^{-/-}$ murine B cells show significant impairment in CSR (to 5% to 25% of wild type) depending on isotype, without defects in cell proliferation, germline transcription in the IgH loci or V(D)J recombination (370,371).

Although the exact functions of ATM, the MRN complex, γ-H2AX and 53BP1 are unknown in dsb repair and specifically in CSR, the emerging evidence suggests that they have mutual interactions and distinct but related roles, so that the elimination of any one protein reduces CSR efficiency but permits residual CSR to occur by pathways that remain intact.

Other Possible CSR Components. Several other proteins implicated in CSR may be mentioned. Rare human patients lacking functional ligase IV have recently been described; they suffer a severe phenotype including immunodeficiency with dramatic decreases in T and B cell numbers, as discussed earlier in the context of their defect in V(D)J recombination. Abnormal Sμ-Sα switch junctions were amplified from patients' blood cells, suggesting that ligase IV normally participates in CSR (372). ERCC1-XPF is an endonuclease that nicks double-strand DNA several nucleotides 5′ of a gap in one strand. $ERCC1^{-/-}$ murine B cells showed slightly decreased CSR efficiency and subtle abnormalities in switch junctions, suggesting a possible role in CSR (373). Additional as yet unidentified components of CSR are suggested by reports of patients with an HIGM phenotype unexplained by defects in known components (374).

In summary, a consensus model for CSR would be that cytokines and CD40 ligation trigger AID expression and isotype-specific sterile transcription. As a result of transcription, DNA strands in S regions become separated (either by a helicase activity associated with transcription, or perhaps as a result of R-loop formation), allowing AID to deaminate cytosines on the exposed single-strand DNA. The resulting uracils serve as a target either for removal by UNG or for initiation of mismatch repair. If UNG removal creates an abasic site, that strand may be nicked by APE1 or by the MRN complex. Alternatively, MMR may be engaged and digest away several nucleotides surrounding the abasic site. Closely apposed single strand cuts on opposite strands may effectively become dsbs, as may more distant cuts after single-strand cuts are converted to single-strand gaps by MMR components. Dsbs quickly recruit repair factors of the MRN complex, ATM, 53BP1, γ -H2AX, and NHEJ components, which either seal internal gaps within one S region, or through synapsis with a dsb from a distant S region, complete a recombination event. This model leaves unanswered many questions about mechanisms that target these events to S regions and about the precise role of all the components; undoubtedly some of these questions will be clarified by future investigations.

CONCLUSION

Recombinant DNA technology has revolutionized the study of the antibody response. Initial investigations used powerful cloning and sequencing methods to define the structure of the Ig genes as they exist in the germline and in actively secreting B lymphocytes. Subsequent experiments have begun to shed light on the mechanisms of the processes unique to these genes: V(D)J recombination, CSR, and somatic hypermutation.

The knowledge of Ig genes gained so far has answered some of the most puzzling mysteries about antibody diversity, as discussed earlier, and has also led to many practical ramifications exploiting these genes that are beyond the scope of this chapter (reviewed in ref [375]). As one example, cloned Ig genes have allowed the production of recombinant monoclonal antibodies in bacteria and the bioengineering of Ig-fusion proteins that exploit the exquisite specificity of antibody V region binding (e.g., antibody-toxin fusions) or the ability of Ig constant region domains to extend serum half-life (e.g., immunoadhesins). Other engineered derivatives utilizing Ig genes include single-chain antibodies (e.g., *[376]*), bispecific antibodies (e.g., *[377]*), and "intrabodies" designed not to be secreted from a cell but rather to bind to intracellular targets (e.g., *[378]*. Ig V gene fragments cloned into bacteriophage so as to express single-chain V regions on the phage surface (phage display libraries) can be used to obtain specific monoclonal antibodies without immunization or use of mammalian cells, and *in vitro* mutation and selection protocols can mimic affinity maturation to yield high-affinity antibodies (reviewed in *[379]*). Even Ig gene regulatory regions have been exploited to achieve B cell–specific expression of oncogenes *(380)* and of intracellular toxins that could be used to target B lymphomas *(381)*. Apart from these biotechnology applications, Ig gene probes of Southern blots and library clones from lymphomas have led to the identification of numerous proto-oncogenes that become activated by translocation into Ig gene loci (reviewed in [382]). For instance, Bcl2 was initially discovered as the target of Ig heavy chain translocation in follicular lymphoma and provided an entrance into an entire family of apoptosis-related genes. A final example of medical benefit from Ig gene technology has been the amplification of unique Ig gene rearrangements by PCR to diagnose (or monitor minimal residual disease in) leukemias or lymphomas (383,384).

Further practical applications of Ig genes can be anticipated in the future, as well as a deeper scientific understanding of their molecular biology and their contribution to the immune system.

REFERENCES

1. Brack C, Hirama M, Lenhard SR, et al. A complete immunoglobulin gene is created by somatic recombination. *Cell.* 1978;15(1):1–14.
3. Gu H, Kitamura D, Rajewsky K. B cell development regulated by gene rearrangement: arrest of maturation by membrane-bound D mu protein and selection of DH element reading frames. *Cell.* 1991;65(47):47–54.
7. Shimizu A, Takahashi N, Yaoita Y, et al. Organization of the constant-region gene family of the mouse immunoglobulin heavy chain. *Cell.* 1982;28(3):499–506.
13. Takagaki Y, Seipelt RL, Peterson ML, et al. The polyadenylation factor CstF-64 regulates alternative processing of IgM heavy chain pre-mRNA during B cell differentiation. *Cell.* 1996;87(5):941–952.
18. Coyle JH, Lebman DA. Correct immunoglobulin alpha mRNA processing depends on specific sequence in the C alpha 3-alpha M intron. *J Immunol.* 2000;164(7):3659–3665.
23. Niewold TA, Murphy CL, Weiss DT, et al. Characterization of a light chain product of the human JC lambda 7 gene complex. *J Immunol.* 1996;157(10):4474–4477.
24. van der Burg M, Barendregt BH, van Gastel-Mol EJ, et al. Unraveling of the polymorphic C lambda 2-C lambda 3 amplification and the Ke+Oz- polymorphism in the human Ig lambda locus. *J Immunol.* 2002;169(1):271–276.
28. Tsubata T, Tsubata R, Reth M. Crosslinking of the cell surface immunoglobulin (mu-surrogate light chains complex) on pre-B cells induces activation of V gene rearrangements at the immunoglobulin kappa locus. *Int Immunol.* 1992;4(637):637–641.
31. Douek DC, McFarland RD, Keiser PH, et al. Changes in thymic function with age and during the treatment of HIV infection. *Nature.* 1998;396(6712):690–695.
36. McCormack WT, Tjoelker LW, Carlson LM, et al. Chicken IgL gene rearrangement involves deletion of a circular episome and addition of single nonrandom nucleotides to both coding segments. *Cell.* 1989;56(785):785–791.
38. Roth DB, Menetski JP, Nakajima PB, et al. V(D)J recombination: broken DNA molecules with covalently sealed (hairpin) coding ends in scid mouse thymocytes. *Cell.* 1992;70(6):983–991.
39. Zhu C, Roth DB. Characterization of coding ends in thymocytes of scid mice: implications for the mechanism of V(D)J recombination. *Immunity.* 1995;2(1):101–112.
41. Schatz DG, Baltimore D. Stable expression of immunoglobulin gene V(D)J recombinase activity by gene transfer into 3T3 fibroblasts. *Cell.* 1988;53(107):107–115.
53. van Gent DC, Mizuuchi K, Gellert M. Similarities between initiation of V(D)J recombination and retroviral integration [see comments]. *Science.* 1996;271(5255):1592–1594.
56. Curry JD, Geier JK, Schlissel MS. Single-strand recombination signal sequence nicks in vivo: evidence for a capture model of synapsis. *Nat Immunol.* 2005 Dec;6(12):1272–1279.
57. Tillman RE, Wooley AL, Hughes MM, et al. Restrictions limiting the generation of DNA double strand breaks during chromosomal V(D)J recombination. *J Exp Med.* 2002 Feb 4;195(3):309–316.
61. Kapitonov VV, Jurka J. RAG1 core and V(D)J recombination signal sequences were derived from Transib transposons. *PLoS Biol.* 2005;3(6):e181.
62. Fugmann SD, Messier C, Novack LA, et al. An ancient evolutionary origin of the Rag1/2 gene locus. *Proc Natl Acad Sci U S A.* 2006;103(10):3728–3733.
65. Rahman NS, Godderz LJ, Stray SJ, et al. DNA cleavage of a cryptic recombination signal sequence by RAG1 and RAG2. Implications for partial V(H) gene replacement. *J Biol Chem.* 2006;281(18):12370–12380.
66. Raghavan SC, Swanson PC, Ma Y, et al. Double-strand break formation by the RAG complex at the bcl-2 major breakpoint region and at other non-B DNA structures in vitro. *Mol Cell Biol.* 2005;25(14):5904–5919.
67. Talukder SR, Dudley DD, Alt FW, et al. Increased frequency of aberrant V(D)J recombination products in core RAG-expressing mice. *Nucleic Acids Res.* 2004;32(15):4539–4549.
68. Elkin SK, Ivanov D, Ewalt M, et al. A PHD finger motif in the C terminus of RAG2 modulates recombination activity. *J Biol Chem.* 2005;280(31):28701–28710.
72. West KL, Singha NC, De Ioannes P, et al. A direct interaction between the RAG2 C terminus and the core histones is required for efficient V(D)J recombination. *Immunity.* 2005;23(2):203–212.
73. Jiang H, Chang FC, Ross AE, et al. Ubiquitylation of RAG-2 by Skp2-SCF links destruction of the V(D)J recombinase to the cell cycle. *Mol Cell.* 2005;18(6):699–709.
75. Chen J, Lansford R, Stewart V, et al. RAG-2-deficient blastocyst complementation: an assay of gene function in lymphocyte development. *Proc Natl Acad Sci U S A.* 1993;90(10):4528–4532.
80. Walker JR, Corpina RA, Goldberg J. Structure of the Ku heterodimer bound to DNA and its implications for double-strand break repair. *Nature.* 2001;412(6847):607–614.
81. DeFazio LG, Stansel RM, Griffith JD, et al. Synapsis of DNA ends by DNA-dependent protein kinase. *Embo J.* 2002;21(12):3192–3200.
82. Weterings E, Verkaik NS, Bruggenwirth HT, et al. The role of DNA dependent protein kinase in synapsis of DNA ends. Nucleic Acids Res. 2003;31(24):7238–7246.
85. van der Burg M, van Veelen LR, Verkaik NS, et al. A new type of radiosensitive T-B-NK+ severe combined immunodeficiency caused by a LIG4 mutation. *J Clin Invest.* 2006;116(1):137–145.
86. Gao Y, Ferguson DO, Xie W, et al. Interplay of p53 and DNA-repair protein XRCC4 in tumorigenesis, genomic stability and development. *Nature.* 2000;404(6780):897–900.
87. Ahnesorg P, Smith P, Jackson SP. XLF interacts with the XRCC4-DNA ligase IV complex to promote DNA nonhomologous end-joining. *Cell.* 2006;124(2):301–313.
88. Buck D, Malivert L, de Chasseval R, et al. Cernunnos, a novel nonhomologous end-joining factor, is mutated in human immunodeficiency with microcephaly. *Cell.* 2006;124(2):287–299.
91. Ege M, Ma Y, Manfras B,et al. Omenn syndrome due to ARTEMIS mutations. *Blood.* 2005;105(11):4179–4186.
92. Drouet J, Frit P, Delteil C, et al. Interplay between Ku, Artemis, and the DNA-dependent protein kinase catalytic subunit at DNA ends. *J Biol Chem.* 2006;281(38):27784–27793.
93. Ma Y, Pannicke U, Lu H, et al. The DNA-dependent protein kinase catalytic subunit phosphorylation sites in human Artemis. *J Biol Chem.* 2005;280(40):33839–33846.
94. Ma Y, Schwarz K, Lieber MR. The Artemis:DNA-PKcs endonuclease cleaves DNA loops, flaps, and gaps. *DNA Repair (Amst).* 2005;4(7):845–851.
95. Budman J, Chu G. Processing of DNA for nonhomologous end-joining by cell-free extract. *Embo J.* 2005;24(4):849–860.
96. Ma Y, Lu H, Tippin B, et al. A biochemically defined system for mammalian nonhomologous DNA end joining. *Mol Cell.* 2004;16(5):701–713.
100. Wasserman R, Li YS, Hardy RR. Down-regulation of terminal deoxynucleotidyl transferase by Ig heavy chain in B lineage cells. *J Immunol.* 1997;158(3):1133–1138.
101. Gavin MA, Bevan MJ. Increased peptide promiscuity provides a rationale for the lack of N regions in the neonatal T cell repertoire. *Immunity.* 1995;3(6):793–800.
103. Bertocci B, De Smet A, Berek C, et al. Immunoglobulin kappa light chain gene rearrangement is impaired in mice deficient for DNA polymerase mu. *Immunity.* 2003;19(2):203–211.
104. Bertocci B, De Smet A, Weill JC, et al. Nonoverlapping functions of DNA polymerases mu, lambda, and terminal deoxynucleotidyltransferase during immunoglobulin V(D)J recombination in vivo. *Immunity.* 2006;25(1):31–41.
105. Zhang Z, Espinoza CR, Yu Z, et al. Transcription factor Pax5 (BSAP) transactivates the RAG-mediated V(H)-to-DJ(H) rearrangement of immunoglobulin genes. *Nat Immunol.* 2006;7(6):616–624.
107. Hsu LY, Lauring J, Liang HE, et al. A conserved transcriptional enhancer regulates RAG gene expression in developing B cells. *Immunity.* 2003;19(1):105–117.

108. Wei XC, Kishi H, Jin ZX, et al. Characterization of chromatin structure and enhancer elements for murine recombination activating gene-2. *J Immunol.* 2002;169(2):873–881.
109. Yannoutsos N, Barreto V, Misulovin Z, et al. A cis element in the recombination activating gene locus regulates gene expression by counteracting a distant silencer. *Nat Immunol.* 2004;5(4):443–450.
110. Verkoczy L, Ait-Azzouzene D, Skog P, et al. A role for nuclear factor kappa B/rel transcription factors in the regulation of the recombinase activator genes. *Immunity.* 2005;22(4):519–531.
111. Yancopoulos GD, Alt FW. Developmentally controlled and tissue-specific expression of unrearranged VH gene segments. *Cell.* 1985;40(2):271–281.
112. Stanhope-Baker P, Hudson KM, Shaffer AL, et al. Cell type-specific chromatin structure determines the targeting of V(D)J recombinase activity in vitro. *Cell.* 1996;85(6):887–897.
114. Calame K, Sen R. Transcription of Immunoglobulin Genes. In: Honjo T, Alt FW, Neuberger MS, ed. *Molecular Biology of B Cells.* Boston and others: Elsevier; 2004. p. 83–100.
115. Liu Z, Garrard WT. Long-range interactions between three transcriptional enhancers, active Vkappa gene promoters, and a 3′ boundary sequence spanning 46 kilobases. *Mol Cell Biol.* 2005;25(8): 3220–3231.
116. Xu Y, Davidson L, Alt FW, et al. Deletion of the Ig kappa light chain intronic enhancer/matrix attachment region impairs but does not abolish V kappa J kappa rearrangement. *Immunity.* 1996;4(4): 377–385.
117. Gorman JR, van der Stoep N, Monroe R, et al. The Ig(kappa) enhancer influences the ratio of Ig(kappa) versus Ig(lambda) B lymphocytes. *Immunity.* 1996;5(3):241–252.
118. Perlot T, Alt FW, Bassing CH, et al. Elucidation of IgH intronic enhancer functions via germ-line deletion. *Proc Natl Acad Sci U S A.* 2005;102(40):14362–14367.
119. Inlay MA, Lin T, Gao HH, et al. Critical roles of the immunoglobulin intronic enhancers in maintaining the sequential rearrangement of IgH and Igk loci. *J Exp Med.* 2006;203(7):1721–1732.
120. Pawlitzky I, Angeles CV, Siegel AM, et al. Identification of a candidate regulatory element within the 5′ flanking region of the mouse Igh locus defined by pro-B cell specific hypersensitivity associated with binding of PU.1, Pax5, and E2A. *J Immunol.* 2006;176(11):6839–6851.
121. Garrett FE, Emelyanov AV, Sepulveda MA, et al. Chromatin architecture near a potential 3′ end of the igh locus involves modular regulation of histone modifications during B-Cell development and in vivo occupancy at CTCF sites. *Mol Cell Biol.* 2005;25(4):1511–1525.
122. Liu Z, Widlak P, Zou Y, et al. A recombination silencer that specifies heterochromatin positioning and ikaros association in the immunoglobulin kappa locus. *Immunity.* 2006;24(4):405–415.
125. Espinoza CR, Feeney AJ. The extent of histone acetylation correlates with the differential rearrangement frequency of individual VH genes in pro-B cells. *J Immunol.* 2005;175(10):6668–6675.
126. Johnson K, Pflugh DL, Yu D, et al. B cell-specific loss of histone 3 lysine 9 methylation in the V(H) locus depends on Pax5. *Nat Immunol.* 2004;5(8):853–861.
127. Chowdhury D, Sen R. Stepwise activation of the immunoglobulin mu heavy chain gene locus. *Embo J.* 2001;20(22):6394–6403.
128. Goldmit M, Ji Y, Skok J, et al. Epigenetic ontogeny of the Igk locus during B cell development. *Nat Immunol.* 2005;6(2):198–203.
137. Kosak ST, Skok JA, Medina KL, et al. Subnuclear compartmentalization of immunoglobulin loci during lymphocyte development. *Science.* 2002;296(5565):158–162.
140. Roldan E, Fuxa M, Chong W, et al. Locus 'decontraction' and centromeric recruitment contribute to allelic exclusion of the immunoglobulin heavy-chain gene. *Nat Immunol.* 2005;6(1):31–41.
141. Sayegh C, Jhunjhunwala S, Riblet R, et al. Visualization of looping involving the immunoglobulin heavy-chain locus in developing B cells. *Genes Dev.* 2005 Feb 1;19(3):322–327.
142. Fuxa M, Skok J, Souabni A, et al. Pax5 induces V-to-DJ rearrangements and locus contraction of the immunoglobulin heavy-chain gene. *Genes Dev.* 2004;18(4):411–422.
144. Bolland DJ, Wood AL, Johnston CM, et al. Antisense intergenic transcription in V(D)J recombination. *Nat Immunol.* 2004 Jun;5(6): 630–637.
145. Alt FW, Enea V, Bothwell AL, et al. Activity of multiple light chain genes in murine myeloma cells producing a single, functional light chain. *Cell.* 1980;21(1):1–12.
147. Nussenzweig MC, Shaw AC, Sinn E, et al. Allelic exclusion in transgenic mice that express the membrane form of immunoglobulin mu. *Science.* 1987;236(4803):816–819.
157. Spanopoulou E, Roman CA, Corcoran LM, et al. Functional immunoglobulin transgenes guide ordered B-cell differentiation in Rag-1-deficient mice. *Genes Dev.* 1994;8(9):1030–1042.
158. Zou X, Piper TA, Smith JA, et al. Block in development at the pre-B-II to immature B cell stage in mice without Ig kappa and Ig lambda light chain. *J Immunol.* 2003;170(3):1354–1361.
159. Bannish G, Fuentes-Panana EM, Cambier JC, et al. Ligand-independent signaling functions for the B lymphocyte antigen receptor and their role in positive selection during B lymphopoiesis. *J Exp Med.* 2001;194(11):1583–1596.
160. Lam KP, Kuhn R, Rajewsky K. In vivo ablation of surface immunoglobulin on mature B cells by inducible gene targeting results in rapid cell death. *Cell.* 1997;90(6):1073–1083.
163. Casellas R, Shih TA, Kleinewietfeld M, et al. Contribution of receptor editing to the antibody repertoire. *Science.* 2001;291(5508):1541–1544.
164. Hippen KL, Schram BR, Tze LE, et al. In vivo assessment of the relative contributions of deletion, anergy, and editing to B cell self-tolerance. *J Immunol.* 2005;175(2):909–916.
165. Halverson R, Torres RM, Pelanda R. Receptor editing is the main mechanism of B cell tolerance toward membrane antigens. *Nat Immunol.* 2004;5(6):645–650.
166. Ait-Azzouzene D, Verkoczy L, Peters J, et al. An immunoglobulin C kappa-reactive single chain antibody fusion protein induces tolerance through receptor editing in a normal polyclonal immune system. *J Exp Med.* 2005;201(5):817–828.
167. Zhang Z, Zemlin M, Wang YH, et al. Contribution of Vh gene replacement to the primary B cell repertoire. *Immunity.* 2003;19(1):21–31.
169. Koralov SB, Novobrantseva TI, Konigsmann J, et al. Antibody repertoires generated by VH replacement and direct VH to JH joining. *Immunity.* 2006;25(1):43–53.
170. Johnston CM, Wood AL, Bolland DJ, et al. Complete sequence assembly and characterization of the C57BL/6 mouse Ig heavy chain V region. *J Immunol.* 2006;176(7):4221–4234.
171. Nei M, Gu X, Sitnikova T. Evolution by the birth-and-death process in multigene families of the vertebrate immune system [In Process Citation]. *Proc Natl Acad Sci U S A.* 1997;94(15):7799–7806.
173. Matsuda F, Ishii K, Bourvagnet P, et al. The complete nucleotide sequence of the human immunoglobulin heavy chain variable region locus. *J Exp Med.* 1998;188(11):2151–2162.
174. Brekke KM, Garrard WT. Assembly and analysis of the mouse immunoglobulin kappa gene sequence. *Immunogenetics.* 2004;56(7): 490–505.
176. Kawasaki K, Minoshima S, Nakato E, et al. Evolutionary dynamics of the human immunoglobulin kappa locus and the germline repertoire of the Vkappa genes. *Eur J Immunol.* 2001;31(4):1017–1028.
177. Kawasaki K, Minoshima S, Nakato E, et al. One-megabase sequence analysis of the human immunoglobulin lambda gene locus. *Genome Res.* 1997;7(3):250–261.
178. Muramatsu M, Sankaranand VS, Anant S, et al. Specific expression of activation-induced cytidine deaminase (AID), a novel member of the RNA-editing deaminase family in germinal center B cells. *J Biol Chem.* 1999;274(26):18470–18476.
181. Revy P, Muto T, Levy Y, et al. Activation-induced cytidine deaminase (AID) deficiency causes the autosomal recessive form of the Hyper-IgM syndrome (HIGM2). *Cell.* 2000;102(5):565–575.
182. Okazaki IM, Kinoshita K, Muramatsu M, et al. The AID enzyme induces class switch recombination in fibroblasts. *Nature.* 2002;416(6878):340–345.
183. Yoshikawa K, Okazaki IM, Eto T, et al. AID enzyme-induced hypermutation in an actively transcribed gene in fibroblasts. *Science.* 2002;296(5575):2033–2036.
187. Doi T, Kinoshita K, Ikegawa M, et al. De novo protein synthesis is required for the activation-induced cytidine deaminase function in class-switch recombination. *Proc Natl Acad Sci U S A.* 2003;100(5):2634–2638.

188. Begum NA, Kinoshita K, Muramatsu M, et al. De novo protein synthesis is required for activation-induced cytidine deaminase-dependent DNA cleavage in immunoglobulin class switch recombination. *Proc Natl Acad Sci U S A.* 2004;101(35):13003–13007.
189. Nambu Y, Sugai M, Gonda H, et al. Transcription-coupled events associating with immunoglobulin switch region chromatin. *Science.* 2003;302(5653):2137–2140.
190. Chaudhuri J, Khuong C, Alt FW. Replication protein A interacts with AID to promote deamination of somatic hypermutation targets. *Nature.* 2004;430(7003):992–998.
191. Bransteitter R, Pham P, Scharff MD, et al. Activation-induced cytidine deaminase deaminates deoxycytidine on single-stranded DNA but requires the action of RNase. *Proc Natl Acad Sci U S A.* 2003; 100(7):4102–4107.
192. Yu K, Huang FT, Lieber MR. DNA substrate length and surrounding sequence affect the activation-induced deaminase activity at cytidine. *J Biol Chem.* 2004;279(8):6496–6500.
193. Chaudhuri J, Tian M, Khuong C, et al. Transcription-targeted DNA deamination by the AID antibody diversification enzyme. *Nature.* 2003;422(6933):726–730.
194. Ramiro AR, Stavropoulos P, Jankovic M, et al. Transcription enhances AID-mediated cytidine deamination by exposing single-stranded DNA on the nontemplate strand. *Nat Immunol.* 2003;4(5):452–456.
195. Pham P, Bransteitter R, Petruska J,et al. Processive AID-catalysed cytosine deamination on single-stranded DNA simulates somatic hypermutation. *Nature.* 2003;424(6944):103–107.
196. Di Noia J, Neuberger MS. Altering the pathway of immunoglobulin hypermutation by inhibiting uracil-DNA glycosylase. *Nature.* 2002;419(6902):43–48.
197. Rada C, Williams GT, Nilsen H, et al. Immunoglobulin isotype switching is inhibited and somatic hypermutation perturbed in UNG-deficient mice. *Curr Biol.* 2002;12(20):1748–1755.
198. Rogozin IB, Diaz M. Cutting edge: DGYW/WRCH is a better predictor of mutability at G:C bases in Ig hypermutation than the widely accepted RGYW/WRCY motif and probably reflects a two-step activation-induced cytidine deaminase-triggered process. *J Immunol.* 2004;172(6):3382–3384.
199. Petersen-Mahrt SK, Harris RS, Neuberger MS. AID mutates E. coli suggesting a DNA deamination mechanism for antibody diversification. *Nature.* 2002;418(6893):99–103.
200. Sohail A, Klapacz J, Samaranayake M, et al. Human activation-induced cytidine deaminase causes transcription-dependent, strand-biased C to U deaminations. *Nucleic Acids Res.* 2003;31(12): 2990–2994.
201. Honjo T, Nagaoka H, Shinkura R, et al. AID to overcome the limitations of genomic information. *Nat Immunol.* 2005;6(7):655–661.
202. Basu U, Chaudhuri J, Alpert C, et al. The AID antibody diversification enzyme is regulated by protein kinase A phosphorylation. *Nature.* 2005;438(7067):508–511.
203. Pasqualucci L, Kitaura Y, Gu H, et al. PKA-mediated phosphorylation regulates the function of activation-induced deaminase (AID) in B cells. *Proc Natl Acad Sci U S A.* 2006;103(2):395–400.
204. McBride KM, Gazumyan A, Woo EM, et al. Regulation of hypermutation by activation-induced cytidine deaminase phosphorylation. *Proc Natl Acad Sci U S A.* 2006;103(23):8798–8803.
210. Ta VT, Nagaoka H, Catalan N, et al. AID mutant analyses indicate requirement for class-switch-specific cofactors. *Nat Immunol.* 2003;4(9):843–848.
211. Barreto V, Reina-San-Martin B, Ramiro AR, et al. C-terminal deletion of AID uncouples class switch recombination from somatic hypermutation and gene conversion. *Mol Cell.* 2003;12(2):501–508.
212. Shinkura R, Ito S, Begum NA, et al. Separate domains of AID are required for somatic hypermutation and class-switch recombination. *Nat Immunol.* 2004;5(7):707–712.
213. Wu X, Geraldes P, Platt JL, et al. The double-edged sword of activation-induced cytidine deaminase. *J Immunol.* 2005;174(2): 934–941.
221. Mao C, Jiang L, Melo-Jorge M, et al. T cell-independent somatic hypermutation in murine B cells with an immature phenotype. *Immunity.* 2004;20(2):133–144.
222. Weller S, Braun MC, Tan BK, et al. Human blood IgM "memory" B cells are circulating splenic marginal zone B cells harboring a prediversified immunoglobulin repertoire. *Blood.* 2004;104(12):3647–3654.
224. Toellner KM, Jenkinson WE, Taylor DR, et al. Low-level hypermutation in T cell-independent germinal centers compared with high mutation rates associated with T cell-dependent germinal centers. *J Exp Med.* 2002;195(3):383–389.
245. Casamayor-Palleja M, Mondiere P, Verschelde C, et al. BCR ligation reprograms B cells for migration to the T zone and B-cell follicle sequentially. *Blood.* 2002;99(6):1913–1921.
246. Allen CD, Ansel KM, Low C, et al. Germinal center dark and light zone organization is mediated by CXCR4 and CXCR5. *Nat Immunol.* 2004;5(9):943–952.
253. Bachl J, Carlson C, Gray-Schopfer V, et al. Increased transcription levels induce higher mutation rates in a hypermutating cell line. *J Immunol.* 2001;166(8):5051–5057.
254. Shen HM, Storb U. Activation-induced cytidine deaminase (AID) can target both DNA strands when the DNA is supercoiled. *Proc Natl Acad Sci U S A.* 2004;101(35):12997–13002.
264. Michael N, Shen HM, Longerich S, et al. The E box motif CAGGTG enhances somatic hypermutation without enhancing transcription. *Immunity.* 2003;19(2):235–242.
265. Schoetz U, Cervelli M, Wang YD, et al. E2A expression stimulates Ig hypermutation. *J Immunol.* 2006;177(1):395–400.
267. Odegard VH, Kim ST, Anderson SM, et al. Histone modifications associated with somatic hypermutation. Immunity. 2005;23(1):101–110.
269. Longerich S, Tanaka A, Bozek G, et al. The very 5′ end and the constant region of Ig genes are spared from somatic mutation because AID does not access these regions. *J Exp Med.* 2005;202(10):1443–1454.
278. Wiesendanger M, Kneitz B, Edelmann W, et al. Somatic hypermutation in MutS homologue (MSH)3-, MSH6-, and MSH3/MSH6-deficient mice reveals a role for the MSH2-MSH6 heterodimer in modulating the base substitution pattern. *J Exp Med.* 2000; 191(3): 579–584.
279. Martomo SA, Yang WW, Gearhart PJ. A role for Msh6 but not Msh3 in somatic hypermutation and class switch recombination. *J Exp Med.* 2004;200(1):61–68.
280. Wilson TM, Vaisman A, Martomo SA, et al. MSH2-MSH6 stimulates DNA polymerase eta, suggesting a role for A:T mutations in antibody genes. *J Exp Med.* 2005;201(4):637–645.
282. Bardwell PD, Woo CJ, Wei K, et al. Altered somatic hypermutation and reduced class-switch recombination in exonuclease 1-mutant mice. *Nat Immunol.* 2004;5(2):224–229.
283. Rada C, Di Noia JM, Neuberger MS. Mismatch recognition and uracil excision provide complementary paths to both Ig switching and the A/T-focused phase of somatic mutation. *Mol Cell.* 2004;16(2):163–171.
284. Zeng X, Winter DB, Kasmer C, et al. DNA polymerase eta is an A-T mutator in somatic hypermutation of immunoglobulin variable genes. *Nat Immunol.* 2001;2(6):537–541.
285. Martomo SA, Yang WW, Wersto RP, et al. Different mutation signatures in DNA polymerase eta- and MSH6-deficient mice suggest separate roles in antibody diversification. *Proc Natl Acad Sci U S A.* 2005;102(24):8656–8661.
286. Delbos F, De Smet A, Faili A, et al. Contribution of DNA polymerase eta to immunoglobulin gene hypermutation in the mouse. *J Exp Med.* 2005;201(8):1191–1196.
287. Zan H, Komori A, Li Z, et al. The translesion DNA polymerase zeta plays a major role in Ig and bcl-6 somatic hypermutation. *Immunity.* 2001;14(5):643–653.
288. Diaz M, Verkoczy LK, Flajnik MF, et al. Decreased frequency of somatic hypermutation and impaired affinity maturation but intact germinal center formation in mice expressing antisense RNA to DNA polymerase zeta. *J Immunol.* 2001;167(1):327–335.
289. Masuda K, Ouchida R, Hikida M, et al. Absence of DNA polymerase theta results in decreased somatic hypermutation frequency and altered mutation patterns in Ig genes. *DNA Repair (Amst).* 2006 Nov 8;5(11):1384–1391.
290. Jansen JG, Langerak P, Tsaalbi-Shtylik A, et al. Strand-biased defect in C/G transversions in hypermutating immunoglobulin genes in Rev1-deficient mice. *J Exp Med.* 2006 Feb 20;203(2):319–323.

291. Bachl J, Ertongur I, Jungnickel B. Involvement of Rad18 in somatic hypermutation. *Proc Natl Acad Sci U S A.* 2006 Aug 8;103(32): 12081–12086.
300. Reina-San-Martin B, Difilippantonio S, Hanitsch L, et al. H2AX is required for recombination between immunoglobulin switch regions but not for intra-switch region recombination or somatic hypermutation. *J Exp Med.* 2003 Jun 16;197(12):1767–1778.
301. Zarrin AA, Tian M, Wang J, et al. Influence of switch region length on immunoglobulin class switch recombination. *Proc Natl Acad Sci U S A.* 2005 Feb 15;102(7):2466–2470.
302. Luby TM, Schrader CE, Stavnezer J, et al. The mu switch region tandem repeats are important, but not required, for antibody class switch recombination. *J Exp Med.* 2001;193(2):159–168.
303. Khamlichi AA, Glaudet F, Oruc Z, et al. Immunoglobulin class-switch recombination in mice devoid of any S mu tandem repeat. *Blood.* 2004 May 15;103(10):3828–3836.
306. Reynaud S, Delpy L, Fleury L, et al. Interallelic class switch recombination contributes significantly to class switching in mouse B cells. *J Immunol.* 2005 May 15;174(10):6176–6183.
307. Kingzette M, Spieker-Polet H, Yam PC, et al. Trans-chromosomal recombination within the Ig heavy chain switch region in B lymphocytes. *Proc Natl Acad Sci U S A.* 1998 Sep 29;95(20):11840–11845.
309. Schrader CE, Bradley SP, Vardo J, et al. Mutations occur in the Ig Smu region but rarely in Sgamma regions prior to class switch recombination. *Embo J.* 2003 Nov 3;22(21):5893–5903.
310. Dudley DD, Manis JP, Zarrin AA, et al. Internal IgH class switch region deletions are position-independent and enhanced by AID expression. *Proc Natl Acad Sci U S A.* 2002 Jul 23;99(15):9984–9989.
311. Allen RC, Armitage RJ, Conley ME, et al. CD40 ligand gene defects responsible for X-linked hyper-IgM syndrome. *Science.* 1993;259(5097):990–993.
312. Ferrari S, Giliani S, Insalaco A, et al. Mutations of CD40 gene cause an autosomal recessive form of immunodeficiency with hyper IgM. *Proc Natl Acad Sci U S A.* 2001;98(22):12614–12619.
315. Rush JS, Liu M, Odegard VH, et al. Expression of activation-induced cytidine deaminase is regulated by cell division, providing a mechanistic basis for division-linked class switch recombination. *Proc Natl Acad Sci U S A.* 2005 Sep 13;102(37):13242–13247.
321. Cerutti A, Kim EC, Shah S, et al. Dysregulation of CD30+ T cells by leukemia impairs isotype switching in normal B cells. *Nat Immunol.* 2001;2(2):150–156.
323. Pinaud E, Khamlichi AA, Le Morvan C, et al. Localization of the 3′ IgH locus elements that effect long-distance regulation of class switch recombination. *Immunity.* 2001;15(2):187–199.
326. Lee CG, Kinoshita K, Arudchandran A, et al. Quantitative regulation of class switch recombination by switch region transcription. *J Exp Med.* 2001;194(3):365–374.
328. Ma L, Wortis HH, Kenter AL. Two new isotype-specific switching activities detected for Ig class switching. *J Immunol.* 2002;168(6): 2835–2846.
329. Kenter AL, Wuerffel R, Dominguez C, et al. Mapping of a functional recombination motif that defines isotype specificity for mu—>gamma3 switch recombination implicates NF-kappaB p50 as the isotype-specific switching factor. *J Exp Med.* 2004;199(5):617–627.
334. Tian M, Alt FW. Transcription-induced cleavage of immunoglobulin switch regions by nucleotide excision repair nucleases in vitro. *J Biol Chem.* 2000;275(31):24163–24172.
335. Daniels GA, Lieber MR. RNA:DNA complex formation upon transcription of immunoglobulin switch regions: implications for the mechanism and regulation of class switch recombination. *Nucleic Acids Res.* 1995;23(24):5006–5011.
336. Yu K, Chedin F, Hsieh CL, et al. R-loops at immunoglobulin class switch regions in the chromosomes of stimulated B cells. *Nat Immunol.* 2003;4(5):442–451.
337. Huang FT, Yu K, Hsieh CL, et al. Downstream boundary of chromosomal R-loops at murine switch regions: implications for the mechanism of class switch recombination. *Proc Natl Acad Sci U S A.* 2006;103(13):5030–5035.
339. Min IM, Rothlein LR, Schrader CE, et al. Shifts in targeting of class switch recombination sites in mice that lack mu switch region tandem repeats or Msh2. *J Exp Med.* 2005;201(12):1885–1890.
341. Shinkura R, Tian M, Smith M, et al. The influence of transcriptional orientation on endogenous switch region function. *Nat Immunol.* 2003;4(5):435–441.
342. Zarrin AA, Alt FW, Chaudhuri J, et al. An evolutionarily conserved target motif for immunoglobulin class-switch recombination. *Nat Immunol.* 2004;5(12):1275–1281.
343. Chen X, Kinoshita K, Honjo T. Variable deletion and duplication at recombination junction ends: implication for staggered double-strand cleavage in class-switch recombination. *Proc Natl Acad Sci U S A.* 2001;98(24):13860–13865.
344. Rush JS, Fugmann SD, Schatz DG. Staggered AID-dependent DNA double strand breaks are the predominant DNA lesions targeted to S mu in Ig class switch recombination. *Int Immunol.* 2004;16(4):549–557.
345. Catalan N, Selz F, Imai K, et al. The block in immunoglobulin class switch recombination caused by activation-induced cytidine deaminase deficiency occurs prior to the generation of DNA double strand breaks in switch mu region. *J Immunol.* 2003;171(5):2504–2509.
346. Schrader CE, Linehan EK, Mochegova SN, et al. Inducible DNA breaks in Ig S regions are dependent on AID and UNG. *J Exp Med.* 2005;202(4):561–568.
347. Petersen S, Casellas R, Reina-San-Martin B, et al. AID is required to initiate Nbs1/gamma-H2AX focus formation and mutations at sites of class switching. *Nature.* 2001;414(6864):660–665.
348. Imai K, Zhu Y, Revy P, et al. Analysis of class switch recombination and somatic hypermutation in patients affected with autosomal dominant hyper-IgM syndrome type 2. *Clin Immunol.* 2005;115(3):277–285.
349. Imai K, Slupphaug G, Lee WI, et al. Human uracil-DNA glycosylase deficiency associated with profoundly impaired immunoglobulin class-switch recombination. *Nat Immunol.* 2003;4(10):1023–1028.
350. Begum NA, Kinoshita K, Kakazu N, et al. Uracil DNA glycosylase activity is dispensable for immunoglobulin class switch. *Science.* 2004;305(5687):1160–1163.
351. Nagaoka H, Ito S, Muramatsu M, et al. DNA cleavage in immunoglobulin somatic hypermutation depends on de novo protein synthesis but not on uracil DNA glycosylase. *Proc Natl Acad Sci U S A.* 2005;102(6):2022–2027.
352. Begum NA, Izumi N, Nishikori M, et al. Requirement of non-canonical activity of uracil DNA glycosylase for class switch recombination. *J Biol Chem.* 2006.
356. Min IM, Schrader CE, Vardo J, et al. The Smu tandem repeat region is critical for Ig isotype switching in the absence of Msh2. *Immunity.* 2003;19(4):515–524.
361. Manis JP, Dudley D, Kaylor L, et al. IgH class switch recombination to IgG1 in DNA-PKcs-deficient B cells. *Immunity.* 2002;16(4):607–617.
362. Reina-San-Martin B, Nussenzweig MC, Nussenzweig A, et al. Genomic instability, endoreduplication, and diminished Ig class-switch recombination in B cells lacking Nbs1. *Proc Natl Acad Sci U S A.* 2005;102(5):1590–5.
363. Kracker S, Bergmann Y, Demuth I, et al. Nibrin functions in Ig class-switch recombination. *Proc Natl Acad Sci U S A.* 2005;102(5):1584–1589.
365. Larson ED, Cummings WJ, Bednarski DW, et al. MRE11/RAD50 cleaves DNA in the AID/UNG-dependent pathway of immunoglobulin gene diversification. *Mol Cell.* 2005;20(3):367–375.
366. Lahdesmaki A, Taylor AM, Chrzanowska KH, et al. Delineation of the role of the Mre11 complex in class switch recombination. *J Biol Chem.* 2004;279(16):16479–16487.
367. Pan Q, Petit-Frere C, Lahdesmaki A, et al. Alternative end joining during switch recombination in patients with ataxia-telangiectasia. *Eur J Immunol.* 2002;32(5):1300–1308.
368. Lumsden JM, McCarty T, Petiniot LK, et al. Immunoglobulin class switch recombination is impaired in Atm-deficient mice. *J Exp Med.* 2004;200(9):1111–1121.
369. Reina-San-Martin B, Chen HT, Nussenzweig A, et al. ATM is required for efficient recombination between immunoglobulin switch regions. *J Exp Med.* 2004;200(9):1103–1110.
370. Manis JP, Morales JC, Xia Z, et al. 53BP1 links DNA damage-response pathways to immunoglobulin heavy chain class-switch recombination. *Nat Immunol.* 2004 May;5(5):481–487.

371. Ward IM, Reina-San-Martin B, Olaru A, et al. 53BP1 is required for class switch recombination. *J Cell Biol.* 2004;165(4):459–464.
372. Pan-Hammarstrom Q, Jones AM, Lahdesmaki A, et al. Impact of DNA ligase IV on nonhomologous end joining pathways during class switch recombination in human cells. *J Exp Med.* 2005;201(2):189–194.
373. Schrader CE, Vardo J, Linehan E, et al. Deletion of the nucleotide excision repair gene Ercc1 reduces immunoglobulin class switching and alters mutations near switch recombination junctions. *J Exp Med.* 2004;200(3):321–330.
374. Imai K, Catalan N, Plebani A, et al. Hyper-IgM syndrome type 4 with a B lymphocyte-intrinsic selective deficiency in Ig class-switch recombination. *J Clin Invest.* 2003;112(1):136–142.
375. Carter PJ. Potent antibody therapeutics by design. *Nat Rev Immunol.* 2006;6(5):343–357.
382. Kuppers R. Mechanisms of B-cell lymphoma pathogenesis. *Nat Rev Cancer.* 2005;5(4):251–262.
383. van Dongen JJ, Langerak AW, Bruggemann M, et al. Design and standardization of PCR primers and protocols for detection of clonal immunoglobulin and T-cell receptor gene recombinations in suspect lymphoproliferations: report of the BIOMED-2 Concerted Action BMH4-CT98-3936. *Leukemia.* 2003;17(12): 2257–2317.
384. Campana D. Minimal residual disease studies in acute leukemia. *Am J Clin Pathol.* 2004;122 Suppl:S47–57.

Chapter 7

B Lymphocyte Development and Biology

Richard R. Hardy

INTRODUCTION

B lymphocytes constitute one of the major arms of the immune system, being responsible for humoral immunity. B cells in humans and mice are produced throughout life, primarily in the fetal liver before birth and in the bone marrow afterward. B lymphocytes development from hematopoietic stem cells has been extensively characterized in mice, and the generation of numerous gene-targeted and transgenic lines in many cases has provided crucial information about the role of transcription factors, cellular receptors, and interactions that are critical in their generation. The complexity of this process is now apparent, and their differentiation into multiple peripheral subsets with distinctive functions is also widely appreciated. This chapter will focus on B cell development and function in the mouse, touching more briefly on aspects of human B cells that are similar or distinctive with a focus on immunodeficiency. It will conclude with a brief description of novel aspects of B lymphocyte development in other species, highlighting differences from development in mouse and human.

B CELL DEVELOPMENT IN MICE

In mice, B cells are produced from hematopoietic stem cells through a complex process of differentiation that is gradually becoming understood. One of the goals of classical hematology is the delineation of differentiation pathways for different lineages of blood cells, and this is rapidly being achieved. Over the past decade, there has been considerable progress in utilizing the ordered expression of a diverse set of cell surface and internal proteins, some with known functions, others whose roles are only suspected, to construct a description of the intermediate stages that cells transit as they develop into B lymphocytes. A simplified example of such a description is presented in Figure 7.1. Thus, hematopoietic stem cells with the capacity to generate all the cell types in blood create progeny with a more restricted capacity, recognizable in this example by expression of the IL-7Rα. These in turn produce yet more restricted progenitor cells identified by expression of CD45R/B220 (and, importantly, by absence of CD19).

This kind of pathway is constructed based on isolation and short-term culture of intermediate stages, allowing progression to occur, which helps to define the order. This framework for development serves as a starting point for analysis of the effects of transcription factors, microenvironmental interactions, cytokines, and natural or engineered mutations. It can also be extended by analysis of gene or protein expression at distinct intermediate stages. Critical processes, such as D-J rearrangement and immunoglobulin (Ig) heavy chain expression, can also be mapped onto this framework. Progress in this work allows additional questions, such as key regulatory interactions,

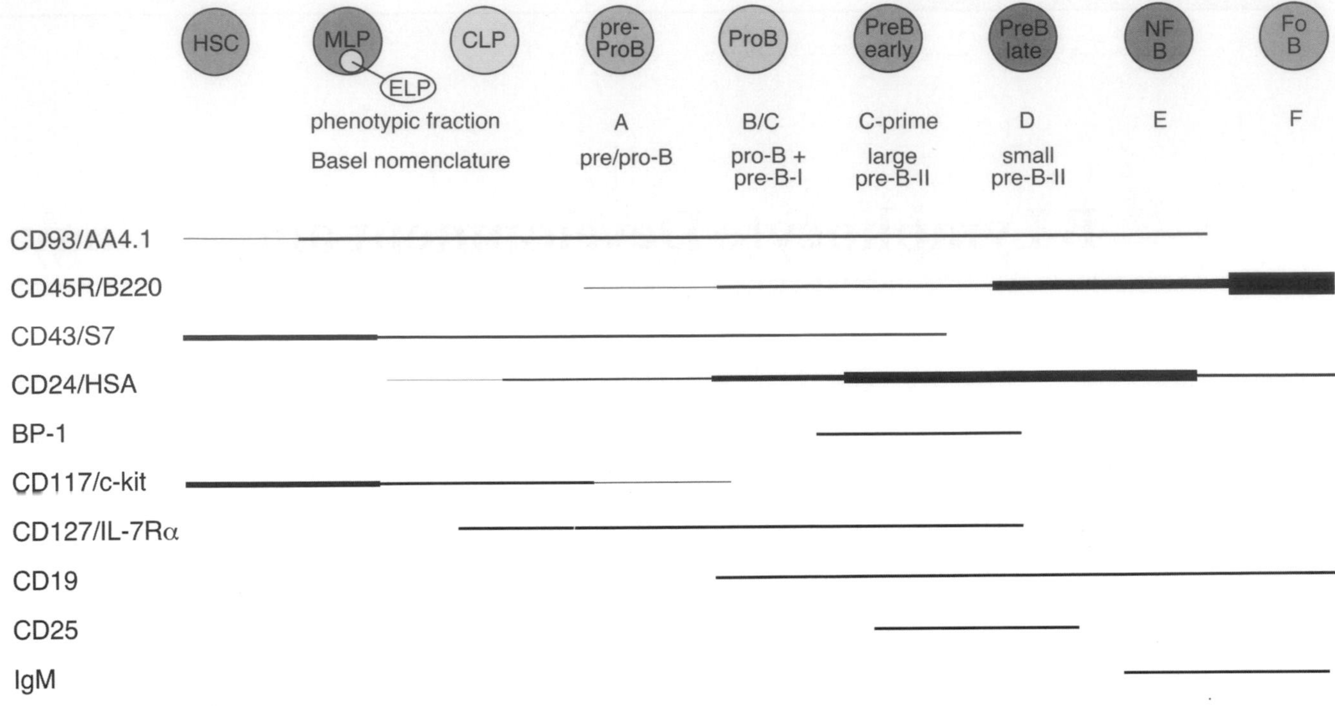

FIGURE 7.1 Differentiation diagram for development of B cells from hematopoietic stem cells. Expression of the each surface protein is indicated by a line. Changes in level of expression are indicated by line thickness. HSC, hematopoietic stem cell; MLP, multilineage progenitor; ELP, early lymphoid progenitor; CLP, common lymphoid progenitor; NF B, newly formed B cell; Fo B, follicular B cell.

developmental checkpoints, and the mechanism of B lineage commitment to be approached.

The following sections will cover the sites of B lineage development at different stages of ontogeny, then focus on what is known about their development in the bone marrow of adult mice, highlighting the function of the pre-B cell receptor and the crucial role of Ig heavy and light chains in guiding development. Later sections will consider their differentiation into various specialized peripheral populations and emphasize insights into B cell selection gained from various transgenic models of tolerance.

Early Development

Sites of B Lymphopoiesis During Ontogeny

In the mouse, hematopoiesis occurs predominantly in the fetal liver prior to birth, in the spleen just prior to and shortly after birth, and in the bone marrow thereafter. Prior to liver hematopoiesis, the blood islands of the yolk sack (YS) contain the first identifiable hematopoietic cells, nucleated erythrocytes with embryonic forms of hemoglobin *(1)*. However, these early YS precursors appear incapable of generating other blood cell lineages, and generation of all blood cell types, including lymphocytes (2,3), initiates at around 9 to 10 dpc in an embryonic region referred to as the *splanchnopleura/aorta-gonads mesonephros (AGM)* (or simply Sp/AGM). Cells from this site are capable of long-term repopulation of lethally irradiated adult recipients with all blood lineages (4,5). These cells colonize the fetal liver at about 11 dpc, initiating hematopoiesis there. Thus, there are two sites of very early hematopoietic precursors, with one in the YS largely limited to erythropoiesis and the other in the Sp/AGM capable of complete (referred to as *definitive*) hematopoiesis. However, it may be that precursors in the YS have a broader lineage potential in the fetal microenvironment, as when they are injected directly into the newborn liver (6).

Hematopoietic stem cells (HSC) capable of developing into all the blood cell types are produced in the Sp/AGM and migrate to the fetal liver at about d10. Thereafter, B lineage cells develop largely in a wave, with earlier stages present at earlier times and later stage predominating at later times, close to (and shortly after) birth (7,8). This progression with gestation day is easily visualized by staining with antibodies that delineate B cell development as shown in Figure 7.2. Early precursors can also be found in the fetal omentum *(9)*. In contrast with the bone marrow, cells at most differentiation stages in the fetal liver appear to be rapidly proliferating, so larger and larger numbers of B lineage cells are detected at progressive days of

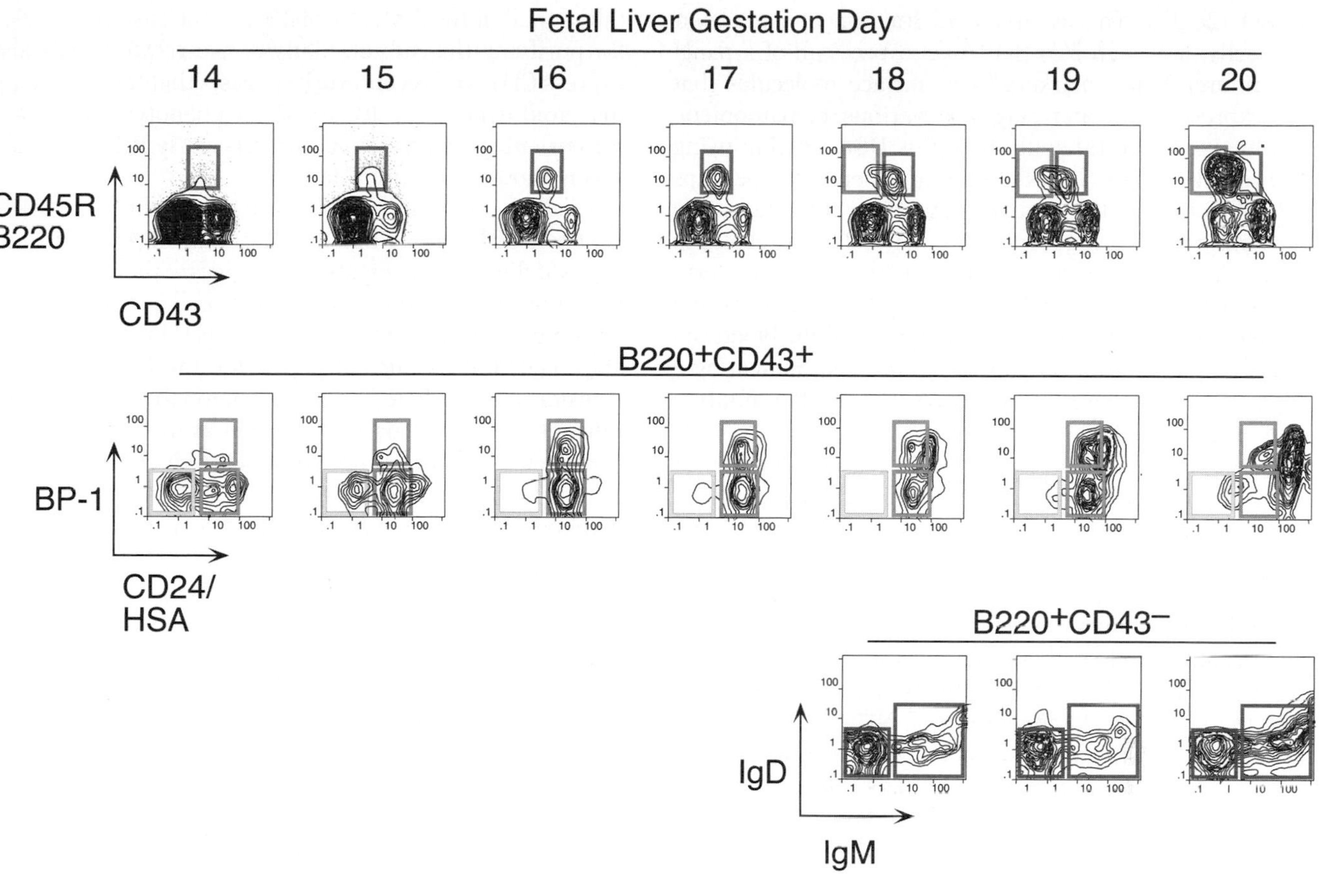

FIGURE 7.2 Phenotypic progression of developing B lineage cells in mouse fetal liver analyzed at different days of gestation. Note that B220$^+$CD43$^+$cells precede B220$^+$CD43$^-$cells and that within the B220$^+$CD43$^+$ fraction HSA$^-$ cells precede HSA$^+$ cells, and BP-1$^-$ cells precede BP-1$^+$ cells. Within the B220$^+$CD43$^-$ fraction, the IgM$^+$ percentage increases until birth (at about day 20).

gestation. Another distinction of fetal liver from bone marrow development in the adult is the absence of terminal deoxynucleotidyl transferase (TdT) (10,11), an enzyme that mediates nontemplated addition of nucleotides at the D-J and V-D junctions of Ig heavy chain *(12,*13,*14)*. Therefore, heavy chains produced during fetal development have little or no N-region addition, and CDR3 diversity is constrained even further by favoring of short stretches of homology at the V-D and D-J junctions (15,*16*). Rearrangement of certain V or D elements may also differ between fetal and adult development—such as, for example, the reported high utilization of the DFL16.1 segment in fetal liver *(17)*. Differential expression of genes other than TdT also distinguish B cell development during fetal life from that in the adult, including precursor lymphocyte regulated myosin light chain like PLRLC transcripts (11,*18*) and major histocompatibility complex (MHC) class II (19,*20*). Interestingly, while absence of the cytokine IL-7 completely eliminates bone marrow B linage development *(21)*, it nevertheless spares some fetal development (22), suggesting a difference in growth requirements. The B cell progeny of this early fetal wave may largely consist of B cell quite distinct from adult-derived cells, populating the B-1 subset (23).

At birth, B cell development can also be detected in spleen, but development at this site gradually decreases to very low levels by 2 to 4 weeks of age. Over this same period, B cell development shifts to the bone marrow, and thereafter it continues for the life of the animal. B lymphopoiesis decreases in aged mice, and this may be due to diminished responsiveness of precursors to IL-7 *(24,25)*.

Stem Cells, Commitment, and Early B Cell Progenitors in Bone Marrow

B cells are continually generated from HSCs in the bone marrow of adult mice. Considerable effort has focused on evaluating the functional capacity of fractions of bone marrow cells to repopulate different lineages of blood cells, and this work has progressed to the stage of defining a phenotype for such cells, with expression of c-KIT constituting an important marker in the so-called "lineage negative" subset (26,27). This is the small fraction of bone marrow cells (less than 5%) that lacks expression of a panel of "differentiation markers," cell surface molecules that are expressed on later stages of various hematopoietic cell lineages. Careful analysis of this HSC fraction using additional markers has shown that it represent perhaps 1/30,000 of nucleated bone marrow cells with as few as 10 mediating multilineage repopulation in cell transfer assays (28,*29,30*). An important capacity of "true" or "long-term repopulating" HSC is their ability to give rise to cells in a recipient mouse that can also repopulate all the blood cell lineages upon retransfer into a second host, indicating a capacity for extensive self-renewal without differentiation into more restricted progenitors.

In the past decade, a great deal of interest has focused on defining and characterizing lineage restricted progenitors, such as the common myeloid and common lymphoid progenitors (CLP) (31,32,*33*). The CLP cell fraction was identified by lack of a panel of "lineage markers," expression of the IL-7Rα chain, and distinctive intermediate levels of c-KIT, compared to higher levels on HSC. Initial characterization of these cells in various functional assays suggested that these cells could generate B, T, NK, and a subset of dendritic cells, but no other blood cell lineages. The reason for this restriction has been intensively studied, and down-regulation of the receptor for granulocyte-myeloid stimulating factor has been suggested to be a key event in this process (34). Cells with the phenotype of CLP constitute about 1/3,000 of bone marrow cells. Prior to the CLP stage, multipotent progenitors exhibit low-level expression of genes characteristic of diverse cell lineages, leading to the idea that such promiscuous expression indicates chromatin accessibility that facilitates flexibility in cell fate decisions (35).

CLP cells can give rise in short-term cultures to cells of the B lineage, naturally raising the issue of when cells become restricted to the B lineage. The majority of cells growing in stromal cultures give rise only to B cells upon transfer into mice, and the phenotype of these cells has been well characterized *(36)*. Most have at least some heavy chain rearrangement and bear the B lineage marker CD19 (*37*,38). There is less certainty concerning the cells isolated directly from primary lymphoid tissues, as such cells are quite rare, similar to the CLP and HSC. Most of the CD45R/B220$^+$ cells in bone marrow are also CD19$^+$, and such cells appear to be irreversibly committed to the production of B cells (39). However, a subset of B220$^+$ cells lacks detectable CD19 expression, and cells within this fraction can generate CD19$^+$ cells in short-term stromal culture with IL-7. Such cells are found within the CD43$^+$CD24^{low} fraction (Fr. A, 1% of bone marrow) of B220$^+$ cells in bone marrow, but this fraction also contains other cell types, including natural killer (NK)-lineage precursors (38,*40*). Thus, it is necessary to exclude cells lacking AA4.1 (about half [38]) and recent analysis *(41)* suggests that exclusion of Ly6c$^+$ cells (about half of the AA4.1$^+$ cells) is another useful criterion for purifying this subset. Many of these Ly6c$^+$ cells also express CD4, and recent work suggests that these are plasmacytoid dendritic cells *(42,43)*. A phenotypic approach for enriching and fractionating very early B lineage subsets is shown in Figure 7.3a.

Careful analysis of the LIN$^-$ (including CD19) IL7Rα^+c-KIT$^+$ CD45/B220$^-$ (CLP) and CD45/B220$^+$ (Fr. A), as delineated in Figure 7.3, suggests that our understanding of the earliest stages of B cell development in bone marrow needs some revision (44). First, while CLP stage cells fail to efficiently generate myeloid cells upon transfer into irradiated hosts, they nevertheless retain significant capacity to produce such cells in short-term cultures, likely due to continued (albeit reduced) expression of receptors for myeloid growth factors. In contrast, this myeloid capacity is greatly reduced as cells begin to express CD45R/B220 (i.e., become Fr. A), concomitant with reduced expression of receptors for myeloid growth factor receptors. Yet these Fr. A cells, while poorly reconstituting T cells in cell transfer assays, nevertheless retain the capacity to generate T lineage cells in culture, mediated by engagement of Notch by its ligand DL1 *(45)*. Thus, the loss of potential for alternate hematopoietic lineages appears to be lost somewhat later in progression down the B lineage pathway in mouse bone marrow than previously thought. However, it appears that initiation of Ig rearrangement is initiated earlier than some studies have indicated. Determination of the extent of germline DNA segments lost upon DJ rearrangement and the formation of such DJ segments in individual cells isolated by electronic cell sorting showed that 30% to 50% of cells in CLP and more than 80% of cells in Fr. A contained a DJ rearrangement on at least one chromosome (44). This is consistent with high-level expression of genes important in Ig rearrangement, including TdT, Rag-1, and Rag-2, in CLP (46) and Fr. A stage cells.

An emerging view of CLP (and possibly even the earlier multi lineage progenitor (MLP)) stage cells considers them to be early B lineage precursors, rather than branch points in the production of other hematopoietic cell lineages. Thus, analysis of CD4/CD8/CD3 "triple-negative" cells in thymus failed to identify cells with a surface phenotype comparable to CLP, and mutant mice lacking CLP in bone marrow nevertheless have relatively intact thymic development, leading to the suggestion of a distinct "early T progenitor" (ETP), different from CLP (47). It seems reasonable to hypothesize that MLP, CLP, and Fr. A stage cells occupy a distinctive microenvironmental niche in bone marrow, where they receive signals that guide them along the early stages of B lineage development, culminating in CD19$^+$ pro-B cells that are irreversibly committed to becoming B cells, due to expression of PAX-5 (39; and see following section). Identifying this niche and characterizing the key signals that lead to specification of the B cell fate are areas of continuing research.

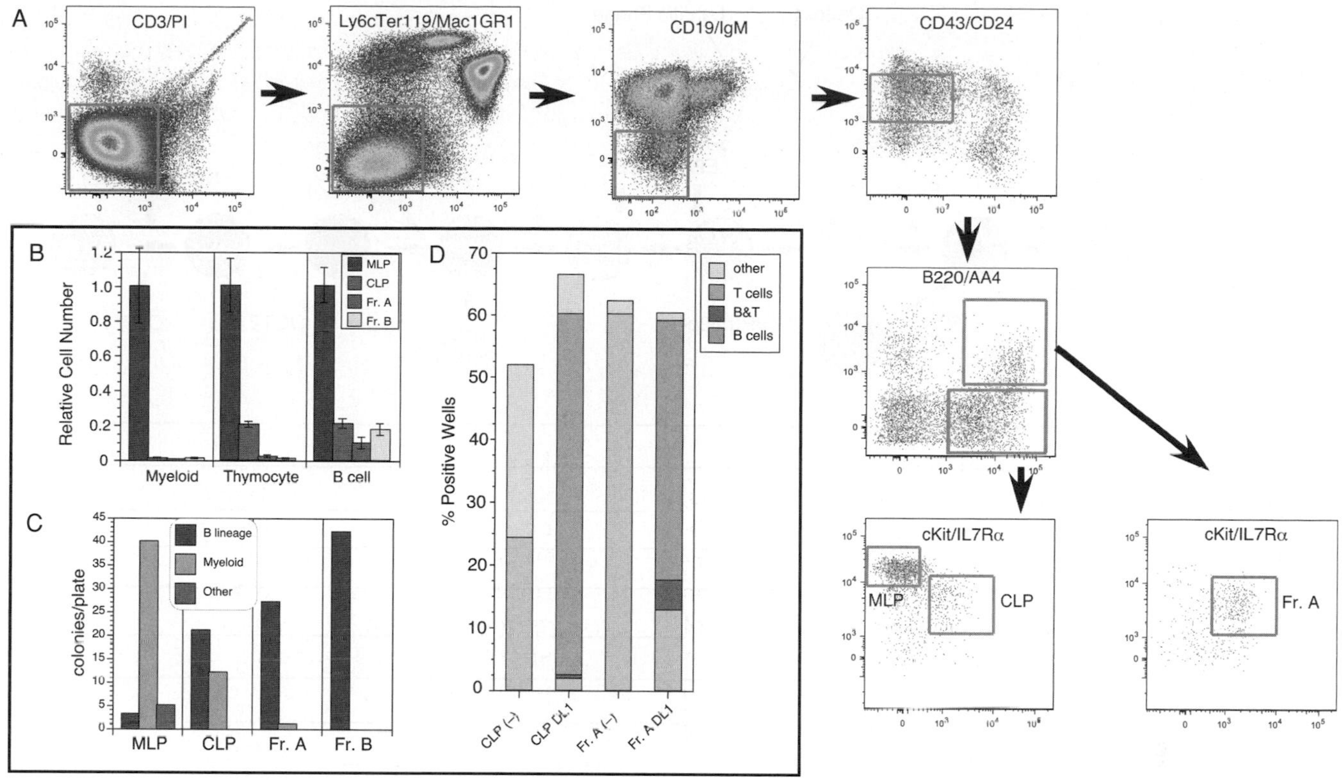

FIGURE 7.3 **A:** An approach for purifying the earliest stage of B lineage cells in mouse bone marrow. Bone marrow cells expressing cell surface proteins characteristic of differentiated stages of T, myeloid, erythroid, and B lineages are depleted sequentially by electronic gating in the first three panels. Cells with low-level expression of CD24/HSA and intermediate levels of CD43(S7) are selected in the fourth, and the distribution of Cd45R/B220 versus CD93/AA4 is shown in the fifth. AA4$^+$B220$^-$ cells contain MLP and CLP, resolved by analysis for cKit versus IL7Rα in panel six. AA4$^+$B220$^+$ cells, shown in the final panel, are enriched for cKit$^+$IL7Rα^+ cells, termed Fr. A. CLP stage cells resemble Fr. A, but lack detectable expression of CD45R/B220. In contrast with CLP and Fr. A, MLP stage cells have higher levels of cKit and lack IL7Rα expression. **B:** Functional analysis of early B lineage cells by *in vivo* competition assay, showing absence of myeloid or T lineage generation, but production of B lineage cells from Fr. A. In contrast, CLP stage cells generate B and T cells, whereas MLP repopulate B, T, and myeloid lineage cells. MLP, CLP, and Fr A as identified in A. Fr. B stage cells are DJ/DJ rearranged pro-B cells, identified as CD19$^+$CD43$^+$CD24(HSA)$^+$. **C:** Functional analysis of early B lineage cells by *in vitro* S17 stromal cell assay, showing predominant B lineage colony formation from Fr. A, but some myeloid generation from CLP stage cells. **D:** Functional analysis of early B lineage cells by *in vitro* DL1-OP9 stromal cell culture, revealing very significant T lineage potential in Fr. A stage cells.

Additional issues remain with regard to the lineage restriction of cells at these early stages in B cell development. For example, there is evidence that cells restricted to generating B and myeloid/macrophage (but not T) lineage may exist, in the fetal liver (48) and even in bone marrow *(49)*. There is also apparently a different dependence of fetal liver B lymphopoiesis on expression of the transcription factor BSAP compared to bone marrow, as determined by analysis of PAX-5 null mice *(50)*. Further comparison of B cell development in fetal liver with that in bone marrow is needed to clarify this point. Finally, the precise delineation and characterization of B cell precursors earlier than CLP, prior to IL-7 expression, remains imprecise. It seems likely that at least some of the MLP stage cells mentioned earlier are initiating a B lineage program, based on their expression of E2A, Rag-1, Rag-2, and TdT (44). However, potential heterogeneity in this fraction needs to be assessed. Determination of Rag-1 transcriptional activity at the single cell level by a GFP reporter, used for identification of the early lymphoid progenitor (ELP) fraction (51), may provide a key approach for such studies.

Transcription Factors Important in B Lineage Development (Figure 7.4)

The GATA-2 and Runx1/AML1 transcription factors are required for the development of hematopoietic stem cells that are the precursors of all the blood cell lineages,

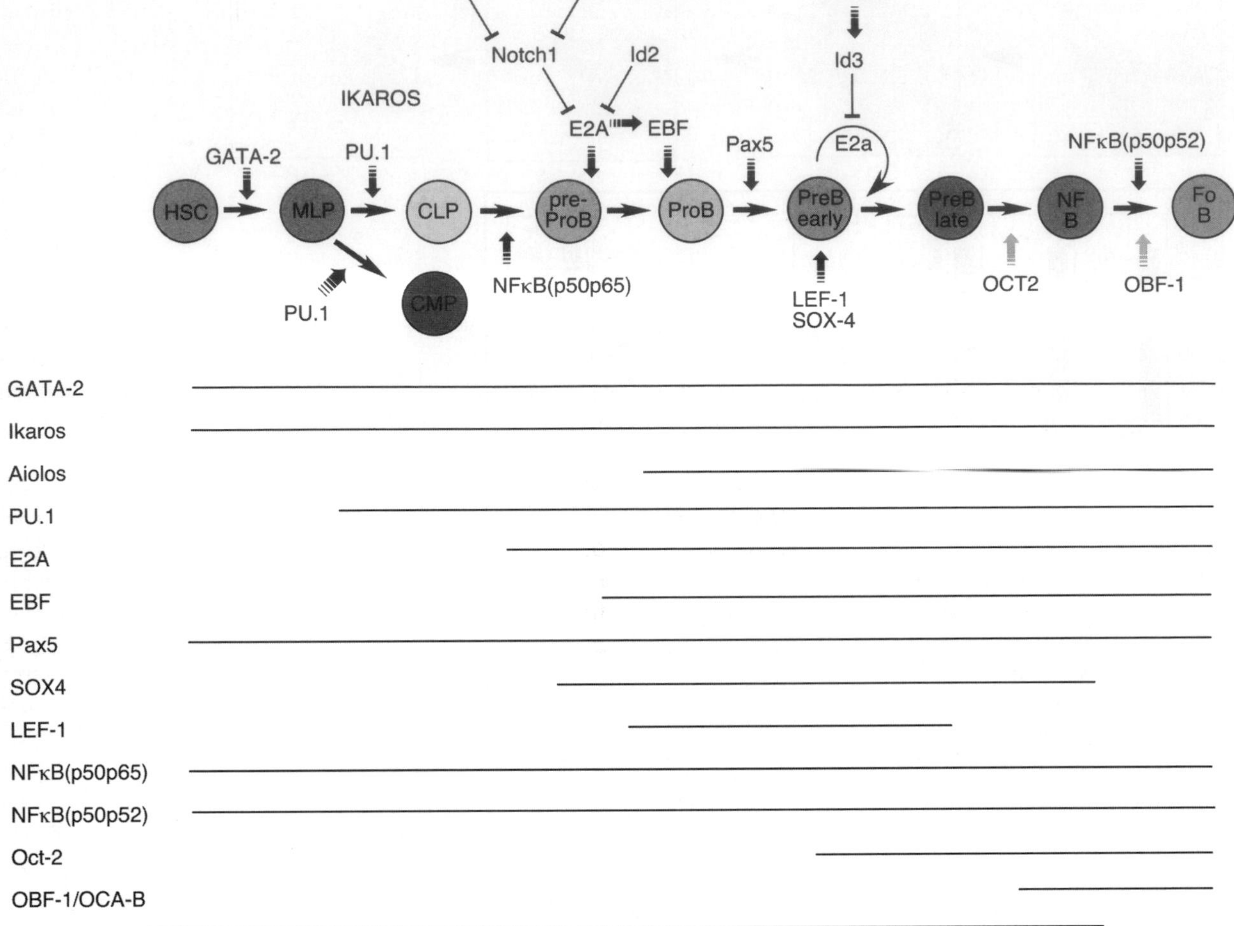

FIGURE 7.4 Transcription factors important at different stages in B cell development in mouse bone marrow. Some regulatory networks are also shown. Positive/activating activity is indicated by arrows, while negative or blocking activity is indicated by bars. The rapidly cycling stage, early pre-B, is also indicated. Predominant stages of expression are indicated below the diagram.

including B cells *(52–56)*. Somewhat later acting, but still very early in development, is the Ikaros transcription factor (57,*58*,59). Ikaros and the related transcription factor Aiolos (60) play important roles in lymphocyte development. Ikaros is expressed very early in hematopoietic precursors. Ikaros null mice lack B lineage cells (59) and a different Ikaros mutant that acts as a dominant negative completely blocks lymphoid development (57). Ikaros activates numerous early B lineage genes, including TdT, Rag-1, λ5, and VpreB. Aiolos is detected somewhat later in development, at about the stage of B lineage commitment, and its expression increases further at later stages.

PU.1, an ets family transcription factor, is critical for progression to the earliest stage of lymphoid development, as demonstrated by the inability of PU.1 null precursors to generate lymphocytes (61,62). An important target of PU.1 for B lineage development is the gene for Ig-β, known as MB-1. The level of PU.1 appears to be critical for development along the B lineage, as, while low-level expression induced in PU.1 null mice allowed B lineage development, high-level expression blocked this and fostered myeloid lineage development (63), likely due to differential induction of the IL-7Rα and M-CSF receptor chains *(64)*. In fact, retroviral mediated expression of the IL-7Rα chain complements defective B lymphopoiesis in PU.1 null bone marrow hematopoietic precursor cells (65). Surprisingly, recent work from several groups indicates that some B cell development can occur in the absence of PU.1 expression *(66)*. Further, analysis of conditional PU.1 knockout mice showed that expression of this transcription factor was not required after the pre-B cell stage *(67)*.

E2A codes for two proteins, E12 and E47, members of the basic helix-loop-helix family of transcription factors, and its induction is crucial from the earliest stages of B linage development, because all stages after CD19 expression are absent from E2A null mice (68,69). These mice lack detectable DJ rearrangements and, interestingly, such rearrangements can be induced in nonlymphoid cells by introduction of the Rag genes and ectopic expression of E2A *(70)*, implicating this transcription factor in the process of chromatin remodeling of the Ig heavy chain locus that permits accessibility by the recombinase machinery (71). The regulation of E2A is crucial for B lineage development, as negative regulators such as Notch1 and ID2 have been show to block this lineage and induce alternate cell fates, to the T and NK lineages (72,*73–75*). Consistent with this picture, ectopic expression of genes that negatively regulate Notch1, Lunatic Fringe, and Deltex1, induce the B cell fate (76,77,*78*).

Expression of the early B cell factor, EBF1, a member of the O/E protein transcription factor family, is requisite for progression of early B lineage progenitors to the DJ-rearranged pro-B stage (Fr B), as shown in EBF1 null mice (79). EBF1 and E2A act at a similar stage in early in B lineage development, and these two transcription factors can act together to up-regulate a family of early B lineage–specific genes, including Ig-α/β, VpreB/λ5, and Rag-1/2 (80,*81*). There is evidence that E2A up-regulates expression of EBF1, found by transfection of E2A in a macrophage cell line (82), suggesting an ordering of these two in development. Further, recent studies showed that there are two distinct promoters for EBF1 that are regulated differently (83). A distal promoter is activated by IL-7 signaling, E2A, and EBF1, whereas a proximal promoter is regulated by PAX5, Ets1, and PU.1. Such complex regulation indicates that B cell development occurs through the action of several feedback loops in a regulatory network that is gradually being uncovered (*84*,85).

BSAP, the product of the PAX5 gene, is expressed throughout B cell development until the plasma cell stage *(86)*. PAX5/BSAP transcriptional targets include CD19 and BLNK and expression of this transcription factor acts to up-regulate V to DJ heavy chain rearrangement *(50)*. Analysis of chromatin structure around the Ig heavy chain locus revealed that PAX5 induces V to DJ locus contraction, thereby promoting rearrangement *(87)*. PAX5 null mutant mice show an arrest in bone marrow development at the pro-B stage, likely due to the lack of complete heavy chain rearrangements and also due to the absence of the critical B cell adaptor protein BLNK that serves to link the pre-B cell receptor (BCR) to the intracellular signaling pathway via the tyrosine kinase syk *(88)*. BSAP/PAX5 also acts to repress alternate cell fates, because pro-B phenotype cells isolated from PAX5 null bone marrow can generate diverse hematopoietic cell lineages, in contrast with such cells from wild-type mice that are B lineage restricted (39,89). This occurs by repression of the myeloid growth factor receptor gene c-fms (90) and by repression of the Notch1 signaling pathway (91), critical for T cell fate specification (*45*,92). Finally, as mentioned earlier, in contrast with bone marrow, the absence of BSAP/PAX5 arrests B cell development prior to the B220$^+$ stage in fetal liver, suggesting a crucial difference in the early dependence on this transcription factor *(50)*.

Lymphoid enhancer binding factor (LEF-1) shows a pattern of expression restricted to the pro-B and pre-B stages of B cell development *(93)*. Targeted inactivation of the LEF-1 gene allows B cell development, but with reduced numbers (94). This is because LEF-1 regulates transcription of the Wnt/β-catenin signaling pathway whose activation increases proliferation and decreases apoptosis of early B lineage cells. In fact, exposure of normal pro-B cells to Wnt protein induces their proliferation (94). Interestingly, there is a counter-proliferative signal that can act at the pre-B proliferative stage, mediated by TGF-β1 (95). It appears that this occurs due to induction of the Id-3 inhibitor that negatively regulates the activity of E2A *(96)*. Another transcription factor whose expression is similar to LEF-1 is SOX-4 and its inactivation also results in the inability of normal early B lineage cell expansion and a block at the pro-B stage *(97)*.

Several forms of NF-κb subunits are expressed throughout B cell development, and this transcription factor can regulate kappa light chain expression and also growth factor signaling (98). Mice lacking the p65 subunit die before birth, and so development must be analyzed by transfer of fetal liver precursors into wild-type recipients. Such experiments showed diminished B lineage cell numbers, but the major defect was in mature B cell mitogenic responses (99). Mice lacking the p50 subunit showed relatively normal B cell development, but again poor response to mitogen by mature B cells (99). However, mice lacking both the p50 and p65 subunits failed to generate any B220$^+$ B lineage cells. Curiously, when mixed with wild-type fetal liver cells, normal numbers of mature B cells could be generated from the double-defective precursors, suggesting that the defect could be overcome by secreted or membrane-bound signals provided by the wild-type precursors. Another double mutant, p50p52, showed a late stage defect in B cell development, with a failure to generate mature B cells in spleen *(100)*.

Inactivation of the Oct-2 transcription factor results in neonatal lethality, but transfers of fetal precursors can reconstitute lymphoid cells in wild-type recipients, allowing assessment of effects on the B lineage. Such studies have shown that fewer mature follicular B cells are generated in these mice, and B-1 (CD5$^+$) B cells are completely eliminated *(101–103)*. Similarly, the Oct binding factor, OBF-1, also known as OCA-B and BOB-1, appears to function in the maturation of newly formed B cells in the bone marrow to become follicular B cells in the periphery, because inactivation of this gene resulted in a significant deficit in mature B cells *(104–106)*. Both of these transcription factors have been shown to regulate the follicular B cell chemokine receptor CXCR5, and this may explain at least part of the defect *(107)*. Curiously, unlike Oct-2 null mice, there was reportedly no deficit in B-1 B cells in OBF-1 null mice. Interestingly, when the OBF-1 mutant mouse is crossed with Bruton's tyrosine kinase (Btk)–deficient mice, then there is a complete lack of peripheral B cell generation *(108)*, suggesting that this transcription factor may function in the BCR-mediated selection of mature B cells.

Bone Marrow Developmental Stages

Functional Definition

Distinct stages of developing B lineage cells can be delineated based on their capacity for growth under different culture conditions. That is, the earliest precursors require cell contact with the stromal microenvironment, in addition to specific cytokines, notably IL-7 (95,109). This stromal cell/precursor adhesive interaction is mediated, at least in part, by binding of VLA-4 to ICAM-1 (*110*,111). Later stage cells do not require cell contact, but maintain a need for cytokines (112,113). Both cell types can undergo considerable cell proliferation in culture. Interestingly, the difference between cell contact requirement and independence is linked to the expression of heavy chain protein (112,*114*). A population of cytoplasmic heavy chain expressing B lineage cells later than either of these, the so-called *late* or *small pre-B cells,* does not proliferate in culture. These cells likely require different culture conditions for survival, as they usually do not persist for extended periods, but rather die with a half-life of less than 24 hours, unless protected from apoptosis by a Bcl-2 transgene *(115)*.

Phenotypic Definition

Further clarification of the heterogeneity in bone marrow can be achieved by analysis using fluorescent staining reagents and either microscopic or flow cytometric analysis. For example, the earliest determination that there were both heavy chain surface-positive B cell and cytoplasmic-positive pre-B cells was through microscopic examination using anti-Ig staining *(116,117)*. Later studies in mice showed that there were specific surface proteins or "markers" that could be useful in identifying these populations, notably a restricted isoform (CD45Ra) of the common leukocyte antigen, CD45 (118). This largely B lineage–restricted 200 kDa molecular mass isoform is often referred to as *B220*. Some highly B lineage–restricted monoclonal antibodies, such as RA3-6B2, recognize a specific glycosylation of the CD45Ra isoform *(119)*. However, as described earlier, even highly specific antibodies such as 6B2 may also recognize other cell types, such as particular differentiation stages or subsets of NK or dendritic cells.

The application of multiparameter/multicolor flow cytometry and additional monoclonal antibodies specific for other cell surface proteins differentially expressed during B lineage development has facilitated delineation of multiple additional intermediate stages in this pathway (113). For example, the B220$^+$ population in bone marrow can be further fractionated into an earlier subset expressing CD43 (about 3% to 5% of marrow cells) and a later fraction with much lower CD43 expression (20% to 30% of marrow). The precursor/progeny relationship of cells in these two fractions can be readily demonstrated by short-term culture, with CD43$^+$ cells giving rise to CD43$^-$ cells. These two populations can be further sub-fractionated based on additional developmentally regulated surface proteins, such as CD24/HSA (heat stable antigen), BP-1 (a zinc-dependent cell surface metallopeptidase also known as *aminopeptidase A [120]*), and the surface Ig molecules IgM and IgD (113). This is shown in Figure 7.5. Again, these cell populations can be isolated and short-term culture used to determine their order in the pathway. Alternative approaches based on other developmental markers can be correlated with this framework of cell stages, notably the system developed by Melchers' group using expression of CD45R/B220, CD19, c-KIT, and the IL-2 receptor

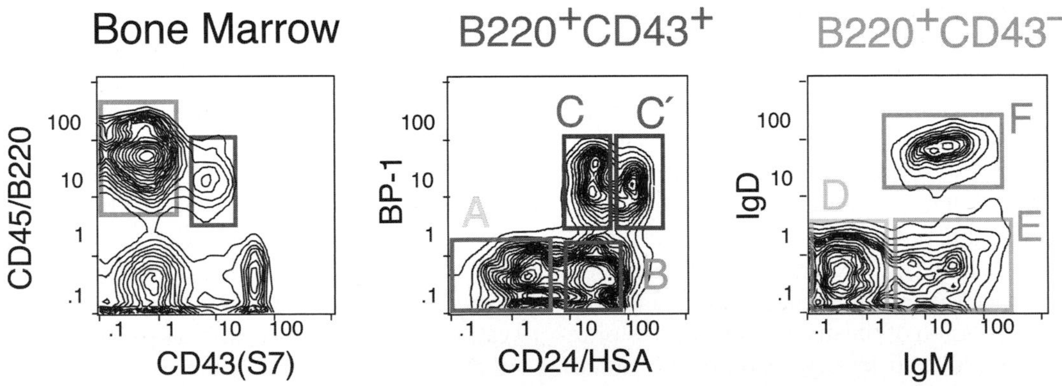

FIGURE 7.5 Flow cytometry approach for analyzing different stages of CD19$^+$ B cell development in mouse bone marrow. Note that the antibody used for CD24/HSA staining, 30F1, is important, as other monoclonal antibodies that recognize HSA do not resolve high from low-level expression as well. The cells expressing low levels of CD24/HSA, labeled "A," are CD19$^-$ and enriched for very early B lineage precursors, but also contaminated by other cell types that can be detected by staining for AA4, NK1.1, DX5, and Ly6c; early B lineage precursors are AA4$^+$NK1.1$^-$DX5$^-$Ly6c$^-$.

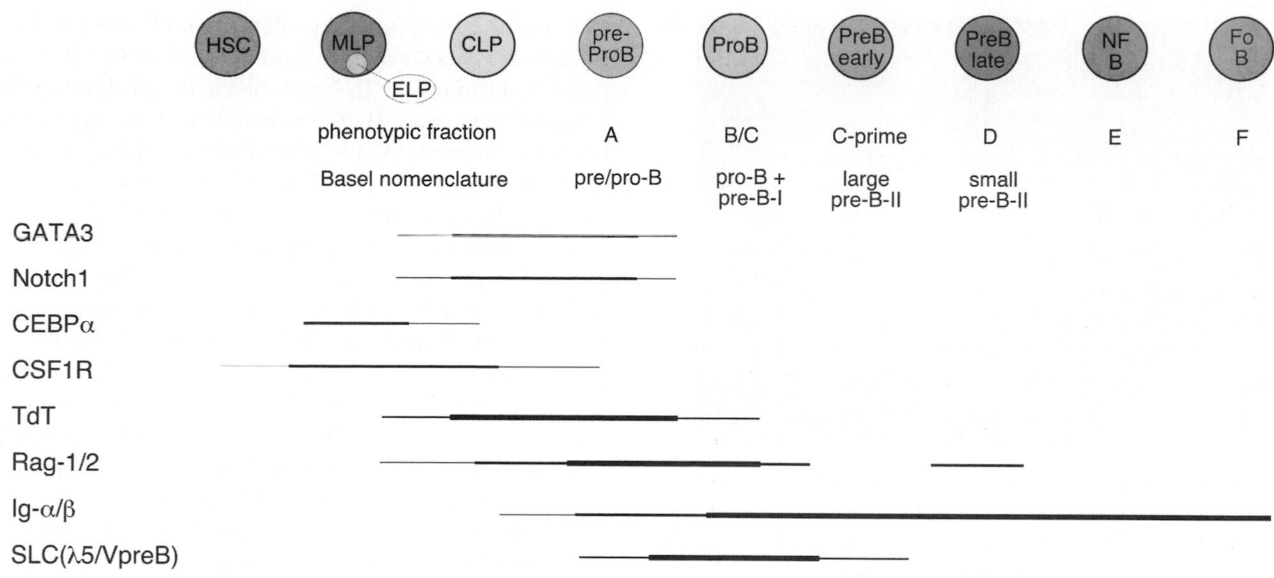

FIGURE 7.6 Diagram of distinct phenotypic stages and characterization of TdT, biphasic Rag expression, Ig-α/β, and surrogate light chain (SLC) expression. Genes characteristic of myeloid and T cell lineage are also shown. The cell type descriptions are cross-referenced to the alphabetic phenotypic fraction nomenclature and also to the Basel nomenclature. The early lymphoid progenitor (ELP) population is identified by activation of the Rag-1 locus in a GFP reporter mouse.

alpha chain *(121)*. A diagram summarizing this type of phenotypic subdivision and relating different nomenclatures is shown in Figure 7.6.

Culture Systems and Critical Microenvironmental Interactions

The combination of phenotypic characterization coupled with analysis of growth and differentiation in culture has provided a very powerful approach for the further under standing of B cell development, as employed by many different investigators. Bone marrow cultures developed by Whitlock and Witte (122,*123*,124) and fetal liver cultures developed by Melchers' group *(125,126)* have allowed determination of the critical cytokines and some of the cell adhesion molecules important in the *in vivo* development of these cells. Many of these are summarized in Table 7.1. A typical B lineage colony proliferating on S17 stromal cells in the presence of IL-7 is shown in Figure 7.7.

Survival and growth of the earliest stages of developing B lineage cells require cell contact with nonlymphoid-adherent cells that can be isolated from bone marrow, cells referred to generically as *stromal cells*. A number of lines

TABLE 7.1 Regulators of Growth of Early B Lineage Cells

Mediator	*Effect*	*Reference*
IL-7	Stimulates CLP and B precursor proliferation	95, 132, *133, 523*
TSLP	Alternate IL-7–like cytokine	140, *141*
IGF-1	Stimulates accumulation of cμ^+ cells in culture	168
FLT-3/FLK2-L	Critical for earliest stages of B lineage development	*151*, 155, *524, 525*
c-KIT-L	Synergizes in IL-7–induced proliferation	26, 149
IL-3	Substitute for IL-7–in proliferation of pre-B clones	159
CXCL12/CXCR4	Crucial chemokine interaction for early B-lineage precursors	177, *179*, 181, *182*
Hemokinin	Novel regulator of B lymphopoiesis	170
VLA4/VCAM-1	Adhesive interaction; antibodies to either block B lymphopoiesis	*110*, 111, 526
CD44/hyaluronate	Adhesive interaction; mediates association of B lineage/stromal cells	128, *130*
TGF-β	Inhibits proliferation stimulated by IL-7	95
Sex steroids	Decrease B lineage precursors in bone marrow	527, 528
Growth hormones	Required for normal B lymphopoiesis	171, *172, 529*
TLRs	Innate immune system regulation	173

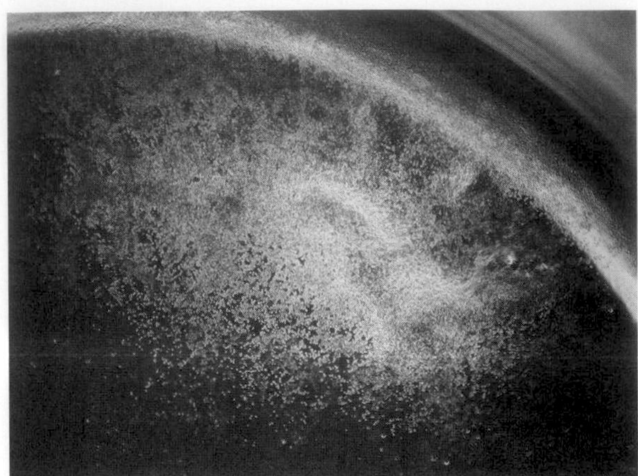

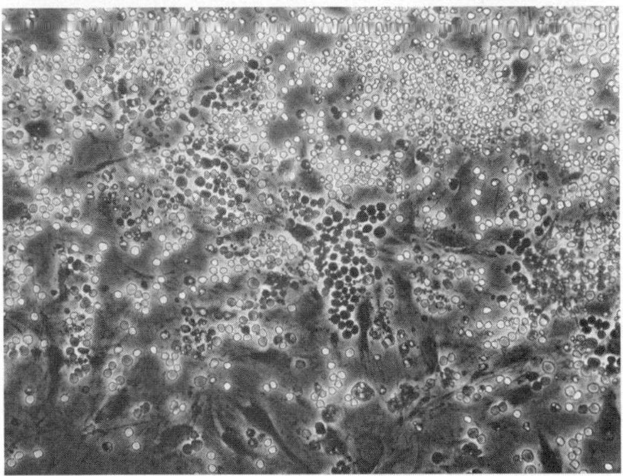

FIGURE 7.7 Photomicrographs of B lineage colony proliferating on S17 stromal layer (in the well of a 96 well microplate) in the presence of IL-7. Day 10 colony derived from a single Fr. A phenotype (Figure 7.3A) cell. Low- and high-power views. All of these cells now express CD19 and many have progressed to $BP\text{-}1^+$.

have been derived from primary cultures of bone marrow adherent cells and characterized in terms of their capacity to support B lymphopoiesis *in vitro* (127). This work has led to the discovery of adhesion molecules that play important roles in mediating the organization of clusters of developing B lineage cells on stromal layers, including CD44 interacting with hyaluronate and VLA-4 interacting with VCAM-1 (*110*,111,128,*129*). Both of these interactions could be disrupted by addition of blocking antibodies to CD44 and VLA-4 on B cell precursors, resulting in a disruption of normal pre-B proliferation *in vitro (130)*. Such adhesion interactions may serve to transmit signals directly to the stromal cells or B precursors or both. There is some evidence that stromal cells are induced to elaborate specific growth mediators after interaction with B cell precursors or soluble regulators *(131)*.

Another function of the stromal cells is to produce growth factors critical to B lineage survival, proliferation, and differentiation, and the most important of these for mouse B cell development is IL-7 (95,109,132,*133*). IL-7 promotes the survival and proliferation of pro-B and pre-B stage cells, both *in vivo* and *in vitro (134,135)*. Neutralizing antibody to IL-7 can block B cell development *in vitro* (113), and IL-7 expressed as a transgene can deregulate normal B cell development, leading to B cell lymphadenopathy *(136)*. The IL-7 receptor consists of a unique IL-7Rα chain *(137)* paired with the common gamma chain (γc) that is also found in the receptors for IL-2, IL-4, IL-9, IL-15, and IL-21 *(138)*. IL-7Rα null mice have a severe deficit of both B and T cells in the periphery and lack most B lineage cells in bone marrow (139). Mice with targeted inactivation of the γc or IL-7 do have some B lineage development, suggesting an alternate cytokine, and this appears to be TSLP. This protein was first identified as a pre-B cell growth factor produced by a thymic stromal line (140) and shows some of the same effects in culture as IL-7, although possibly inducing less proliferation and more differentiation *(141)*. Its receptor has been cloned and requires the IL-7Rα chain for function (142). It shares both sequence homology and genomic exon organization with the common gamma chain *(143)*. Signaling through the IL-7 receptor requires JAK3 and activates the transcription factor STAT5, whereas signaling through TSLP is JAK3 independent, but also activates STAT5 *(141,144)*. Unexpectedly, the growth response to TSLP requires synergy with the pre-BCR in bone marrow, but not in fetal liver (145), leading some to propose that this might be a marker for distinctive B-1 B cell development in bone marrow *(146)*.

The earliest precursors in the B lineage pathway, probably including cells that are not B lineage committed but that can efficiently give rise to B cells in a short time *in vitro,* have receptors for SCF/c-KIT-ligand (26,*27*,*147*,*148*,149,*150*) and FLK2/FLT3-ligand (*151–154*,155). Thus, the most permissive cultures for expanding precursors of B lineage cells will include these cytokines, in addition to IL-7 and a stromal adherent cell layer, such as S17 (156,*157*,158). IL-3 has also occasionally been suggested as playing a support role for pre-B cells *in vitro* (159), although its role *in vivo* may be at a much earlier stage. Although culture conditions have been reported that can support B lineage development in the absence of stromal cells *(160,161)*, the clear-cut alteration of contact dependence prior and post–heavy chain expression (112,113,*114*,*162*,163) argues that the most physiological model for early B lineage growth will include stromal cells. Besides providing important cell–cell contacts that may signal survival, proliferation, and differentiation, it is also likely that stromal cells bind at least some cytokines to their surface, providing higher local concentrations to the clusters of B lineage precursors that adhere *(164,165)*.

B lineage development may be modified by exposure to hormones and considerable interest has focused on sex steroids released during pregnancy that serve to depress B lymphopoiesis, particularly the pre-B cell pool (166).

This may be important to avoid autoimmune responses by the mother, but could have negative consequences due to possible transient immunodeficiency. Interestingly, fetal B lymphopoiesis is not similarly depressed, due to the absence of hormone receptors on fetal B lineage cells *(167)*. Insulinlike growth factor (IGF-1) has been reported to potentiate progression *in vitro* to the cμ^+ stage (168,*169*), and more recently, there is a report of a bioactive peptide, a type of tachykinin, that synergizes with IL-7 to enhance the growth of IL-7 dependent cultures (170). Besides IGF-1, other pituitary hormones, thyroxine and growth hormone (GH) have effects on B lymphopoiesis (171). For example, thyroxine treatment can restore normal B cell development in dwarf Pit-1 mutant mice with deficient pituitary function *(172)*. Recent work has highlighted the effect that activation of Toll-like receptors during infection may have on altering development (173). Thus, it is likely that more detail remains to be filled in to complete our picture of the growth requirements and modulating influences of B lineage cells in mouse bone marrow.

Another function of cell–cell interaction is cell fate determination during the lineage commitment stage, very early in development of B lineage cells. The Notch signaling pathway is implicated in cell fate determination in invertebrates and more recently has been shown to function in lymphoid lineage specification (*45*,72,174). Notch family transmembrane receptors regulate transcription by being cleaved upon ligand binding to release an intracellular cytoplasmic domain that translocates to the nucleus where it interacts with the transcriptional repressor CSL *(175)*. Recent studies have shown that Notch1 can play a pivotal role in commitment of common lymphoid progenitors to the T cell lineage (72). That is, expression of Notch1 by retroviral transduction has been shown to redirect B lineage differentiation in bone marrow along the T lineage. Further, a reciprocal result was found in conditional Notch1 null mice, blocking T cell development in the thymus, to be replaced by B cell development (92). Finally, altering the Notch1 modifier, Lunatic Fringe, by overexpressing this molecule under regulation of an lck promoter resulted in B cell development in the thymus (76). Differentiation of lymphoid precursors to NK or dendritic cell lineages was unaffected in Notch1 null CLP cells, so Notch apparently affects only the B/T lineage decision.

Role of Chemokines in Migration of B Cell Precursors

One of the most distinctive features of B cell development in bone marrow is the migration of developing precursors from early stages nearest the bone endosteum layer to latter stages progressively closer to the central arteriole, where they will eventually exit *(176)*. This migration is likely due to differential expression of specific adhesion molecules and also to expression of chemokine receptors. Analysis of B cell migration has identified a critical chemokine that is important in this process, SDF-1, now known as CXCL12 (177,*178*), and its receptor CXCR4 *(179)*. CXCL12 is expressed by fetal liver and bone marrow stromal cells, while CXCR4 is found on hematopoietic precursors and B cell progenitors *(180)*. Deletion of either the receptor or ligand results in severely impaired B lymphopoiesis (181,*182*,183). Interestingly, the critical defect appears to be failure to retain precursors in the primary lymphoid organ, as progenitors and precursors can be found in the blood of mutant mice *(184)*.

Gene Expression and Ig Rearrangement (Figure 7.8)

In addition to delineation of developmental stages based on changes in protein surface expression, B lineage cells can also be characterized for expression of internal proteins related to critical processes in their progression along this pathway, specifically those related to rearrangement and expression of the B cell antigen receptor. Thus, expression of μ heavy chain constant region, prior to Ig rearrangement, from a cryptic promoter generates a "sterile transcript" that likely reflects an open chromatin structure important for the onset of rearrangement *(185–187)*, and so analysis of sterile μ expression can be used to investigate very early stages of B cell development. Classical Northern analysis can be done with transformed lines, but much work analyzing RNA levels in B lineage cell fractions, whether directly isolated or cultured, has depended on PCR amplification of cDNA (38). For example, using this approach, sterile μ can be detected in a very early fraction of B220$^+$CD43$^+$CD19$^-$ (Fr. A) cells. Expression of the recombinase activating genes Rag-1 and Rag-2, that together make the double-strand breaks in DNA required for Ig rearrangement (188,*189,190*), also occurs in Fr. A stage cells, which also have high levels of TdT, the enzyme responsible for adding nontemplated nucleotides at the D-J and V-D junctions of the heavy chain (*12*,191).

The extent of heavy chain or light chain rearrangement can be quantitated, either in bulk-isolated populations (113) or in individual cells *(121,192,193)*. At the heavy chain locus, D-J rearrangement occurs prior to V-DJ rearrangement, and cells with extensive D-J but little V-DJ rearrangement can be detected at the B220$^+$CD43$^+$CD19$^-$ (Fr. A) stage, where Rag-1/2 and TdT are strongly expressed (44). V-DJ rearrangements are readily detected in the abundant B220$^+$CD43$^-$ (Fr. D) stage small pre-B cells, although productive rearrangement has already completed by the large pre–B (Fr. C-prime) stage (discussed later). Single cell sequence analysis of rearrangements in Fr. C stage cells shows a large proportion with nonproductive rearrangements on both chromosomes, suggesting that this may represent a dead-end fraction *(192)*. Some light chain rearrangement is detectable in early stage B220$^+$CD43$^+$

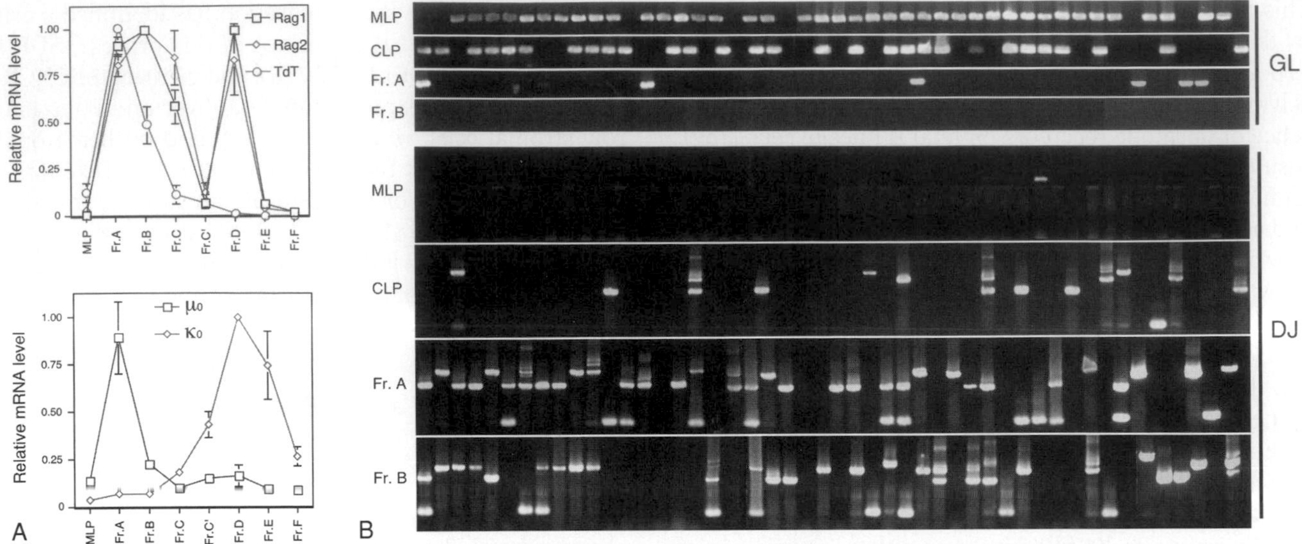

FIGURE 7.8 **A:** Profiles of Ig rearrangement-related gene expression. Cells isolated using fractionation scheme in Figure 7.3 for MLP and Fr. A; in Figure 7.5 for Fr. B through Fr. F. Relative mRNA levels assessed by performing semiquantitative RT-PCR using limited numbers of cycles, blotting, then probing and quantitating the probe signal. Note the biphasic expression of Rag genes and the early expression of sterile μ (labeled μ_0) during the first wave, where heavy chain rearranges, and the up-regulation of sterile kappa transcripts (κ_0) during the second Rag wave, when most light chain rearrangement takes place. **B:** Single cell PCR analysis of Ig heavy chain rearrangement in four early stages of developing B lineage cells. DNA prepared from individual cells isolated following the scheme shown in Figure 7.3 was divided into two aliquots and analyzed for retention of a DNA segment lost upon any DJ rearrangement (labeled GL, germline) and also for DJ rearrangement. Note that DJ rearrangement initiates at the CLP stage, where 30% to 50% of cells show a rearrangement.

(Fr. B) cells, and this is consistent with the observation that low-level kappa light chain rearrangement is detectable in bone marrow of mice where μ heavy chain has been crippled by deletion of the membrane exon *(194)*. However, much higher levels of kappa rearrangement can be detected in B220$^+$CD43$^-$ (Fr. D) stage cells, consistent with the finding of sterile kappa mRNA increase just prior to this stage likely induced by pre-BCR signaling (discussed later).

Role of Ig Heavy Chain and the pre-BCR

Careful analysis of SCID mouse (195) bone marrow revealed the presence of a population of B220$^+$ cells, all with a very early CD43$^+$ phenotype, suggesting a block in B cell development at this stage *(196)*. SCID mice have a defect in the catalytic subunit of the DNA-dependent protein kinase DNA-PKcs (197,*198*), and as a result B linage cells in these mice are very ineffective at completing even initial DJ rearrangements at the heavy chain locus. This block could be overcome by introduction of an Ig heavy chain transgene, supporting the model of a critical role for μ protein in progressing past an early developmental checkpoint *(199)*. An early gene targeting experiment eliminated the membrane exon of μ heavy chain (μ-mt), and such mice also showed a block at this stage (200,*201*).

μ heavy chain can be shown in coimmunoprecipitation experiments to associate with a set of B cell–specific peptides at the early pre-B cell stage (202), and this complex is referred to as the *pre-BCR,* or *pre-B cell receptor.* It seems clear that this complex mediates a type of signaling function, analogous to the BCR in mature B cells. Prior to light chain expression, two peptides known as λ5 and VpreB, originally isolated as B lineage–specific cDNAs (203,*204*), associate with heavy chain. λ5 shows homology to a lambda-constant region, and VpreB is so-termed because it has homology to a variable region domain, so together these peptides constitute a pseudo- or surrogate light chain (SLC). The critical role of λ5 was demonstrated unambiguously in gene-targeted mice, where B cell development was blocked at the B220$^+$CD43$^+$ stage (205). The production of some mature cells that accumulate in this mutant is likely due to early kappa rearrangement, with light chain substituting for SLC, as demonstrated in light chain transgenic experiments (206).

μ heavy chain has a very short cytoplasmic region consisting of only three amino acids, and an important finding has been that signal transduction through the BCR is mediated by accessory peptides, similar to the CD3

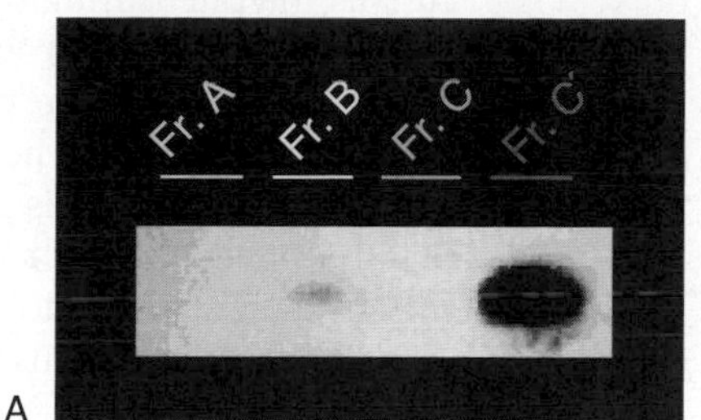

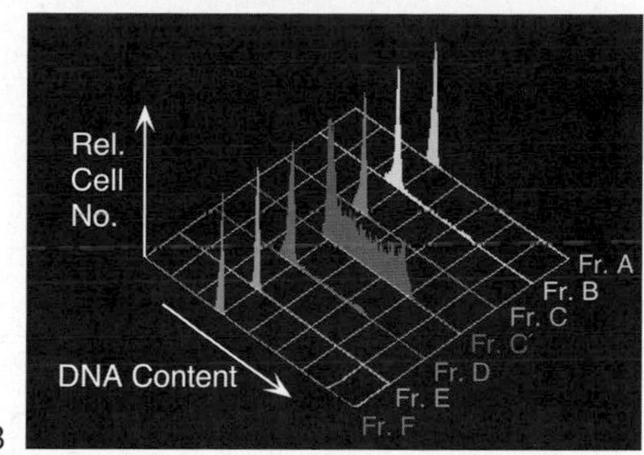

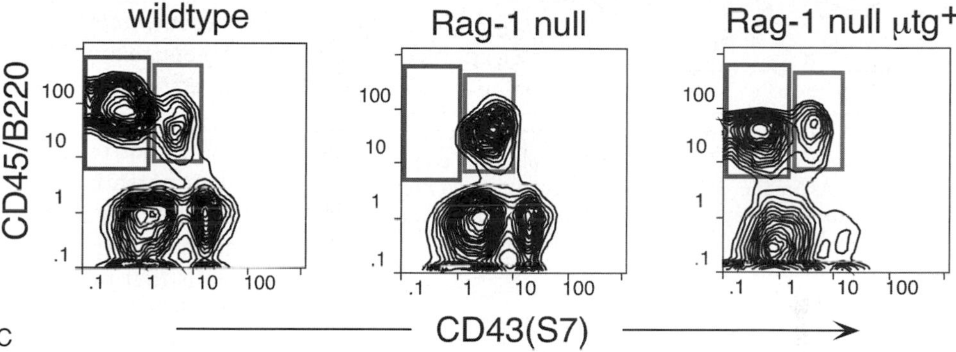

FIGURE 7.9 **A:** Western blot of Ig μ heavy chain expression showing high-level expression in Fr. C-prime. **B:** Cell cycle analysis of individual fractions shows most cells in Fr. C-prime are cycling. Propidium iodide staining of permeabilized sorted cells allows determination of DNA content per cell using flow cytometry. **C:** Block in B cell development in Rag-1–deficient mice can be overcome by introduction of an Ig μ heavy chain transgene.

components of the T cell receptor, known as Ig-α and Ig-β (207,208,*209,210*). As predicted by the pre-BCR signaling developmental checkpoint hypothesis, inactivation of Ig-β (211) results in a block at the B220$^+$CD43$^+$ stage in mouse bone marrow, similar to the μ-mt and λ5 null mice. Finally, the syc tyrosine kinase plays a critical role in transducing BCR cross-linking signals in mature B cells, and inactivation of this gene results in a "leaky" block at this same stage (212,*213*). Thus, any mutation that affects this pre-BCR complex (see the following section and Figure 7.10a) precludes efficient progression past the earliest stages of B cell development.

Careful examination of B cell development in normal mice shows that heavy chain is first expressed in a late fraction of B220$^+$CD43$^+$ stage cells, termed *Fr. C-prime* (Figure 7.9a). This fraction is also interesting because it shows a much higher proportion of cells in cycle (revealed by a high frequency of cells with greater than 2N DNA content; Figure 7.9b), compared with any other B220$^+$ stage in bone marrow (113). Mice unable to assemble a pre-BCR, due to inability to rearrange heavy chain (Rag-1 null) show a block in development at the CD43$^+$ stage that can be complemented by introduction of a functionally rearranged μ heavy chain as a transgene ([163] Figure 7.9c). Analysis of several types of pre-BCR defective mutant mice shows a complete absence of Fr. C-prime stage cells, suggesting that pre-BCR signaling results in the up-regulation of CD24/HSA and also entry into rapid cell proliferation. Thus, a model of pre-BCR function is that it signals the clonal expansion phase of pre-B cell development, amplifying cells with in-frame VDJ rearrangements capable of making heavy chain protein.

The precise nature of pre-BCR signaling remains to be completely understood. An early model suggested that crosslinking of heavy chain was mediated through interaction of SLC with a bone marrow–expressed ligand. However, subsequent experiments showed that normal light chain could substitute for SLC and that even a V_H truncated μ heavy chain could mediate progression past this stage. Further, intensive searches for the putative ligand over a 10-year period have been fruitless, leading to the model that pre-BCR signaling is more akin to "tonic" signaling in mature B cells (*214*,215,216). That is, simple assembly of the complex (or possibly some degree of multimerization fostered by the self-aggregating nature of SLC [*217*]) probably is sufficient for the cell to pass this developmental checkpoint (Figure 7.10b). One clear-cut finding is that pre-BCR signaling in a transformed pro-B cell model system can occur in the absence of any additional cell type, suggesting that if a ligand exists, it must be expressed on B lineage cells, rather than stromal cells (218).

Mutations in other molecules in the pre-BCR signaling pathway have been shown to affect B cell development and pre-B cell clonal expansion. While the Btk mutation is less severe in mouse than in human, there nevertheless is an alteration in pre-B cell expansion in Btk-deficient mice

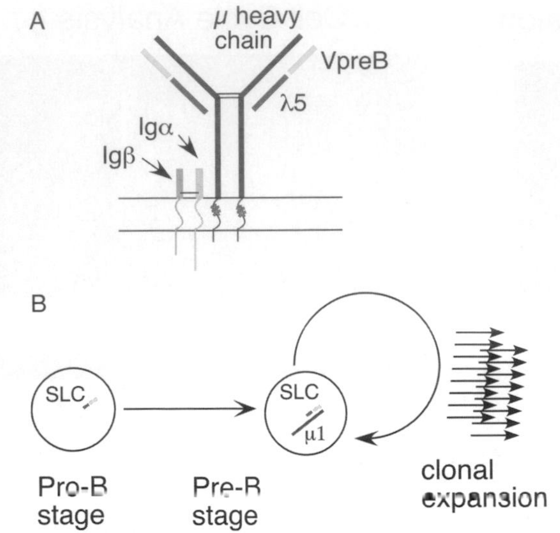

FIGURE 7.10 **A:** Diagram of the pre-BCR, μ heavy chain with surrogate light chain (λ5 and VpreB) in place of conventional light chain. As in the BCR, Ig-α and Ig-β serve to couple signals between the receptor and cytoplasmic components, such as BLNK and syk. Starred m transmembrane residues are important in mediating interaction with Ig-α/Ig-β, as mutation of these diminishes BCR function. **B:** Clonal expansion mediated by pre-BCR assembly. Association of newly generated μ heavy chain with preexisting surrogate light chain leads to a burst of proliferation at the pre-B stage.

(219). Also, xid B cells (deficient in Btk) have been reported to proliferate more in stromal cell cultures, possibly due to decreased differentiation to later nonproliferative stages *(220,221)*. The role of Btk is thought to modulate BCR signaling strength *(222)*, and this is probably also the case for pre-BCR signaling, allowing only strongly signaling pre-BCRs to progress in the mutant mice. BLNK serves to link the pre-BCR to the syk kinase, critical in BCR signaling (*223*,224). Mutant mice lacking BLNK show a partial block in B cell development at the pro-B to pre-B transition *(225)*. Curiously, while pre-BCR signaling is thought to mediate allelic exclusion (expression of a single heavy chain allele), this remains intact in BLNK-deficient mice (226). Syk deficient mice show a more severe block at the pro-B to pre-B transition and a lack of allelic exclusion (212,*213*,226).

Outcomes of pre-BCR signaling, in addition to pre-B proliferation, are down-regulation of the Rag genes (227), down-regulation of TdT (218), and transcriptional activation of the kappa locus, detected as up-regulation of sterile kappa transcripts (228). A control element for regulating Rag expression has been identified (*229*,230). Extinction of recombinase activity is probably important for chromosomal stability during the clonal burst period of B cell development (*231*,*232*,*233*) and is also at least a part of the mechanism that assures allelic exclusion, the expression of a single heavy chain by any given B cell *(234)*. There is evidence that pre-BCR selection requires low levels of IL-7 *(235)* and probably occurs naturally as the developing precursors migrate through different stromal cell microenvironments in bone marrow.

The function of the pre-BCR may be more complex than simply to sense whether an in-frame VDJ rearrangement has occurred. This possibility is suggested by the observation that heavy chains with different VDJ segments vary in their capacity to assembly with SLC components (*236*,237–239). V regions are classified into families based on sequence homology and many members of two of these families, the 7183 and Q52, appear to frequently generate heavy chains that assemble poorly with surrogate light chain (238). A consequence of this will likely be poor pre-BCR signaling and little clonal expansion, so such cells will become under-represented at later stages of B cell development relative to cells containing heavy chains that signal effectively. One explanation of the reason for this SLC assembly-mediated clonal expansion is that it serves a quality-control function to test heavy chain V regions for their potential to fold with real Ig light chain, a critical requirement if the cell is to express a complete BCR. An alternative (not necessarily mutually exclusive) explanation is that making pre-B cell proliferation dependent on pre-BCR expression provides a simple mechanism for regulating the extent of clonal expansion, since an immediate consequence of pre-BCR signaling is to terminate SLC expression. Thereafter, SLC protein levels decay and are diluted by cell division, so that after several rounds of proliferation, pre-BCR levels will decrease to below the threshold required to provide the signal to maintain the cell in cycle. Figure 7.11 illustrates a model for bone marrow B cell development, showing the pre-BCR checkpoint.

One of the most striking examples of pre-BCR selection is seen with the D-proximal V_H gene, V_H81X, where early precursors show biased over-utilization, due to preferential rearrangement of this V_H gene (11,*240*,*241*). V_H81X had also been identified as frequently rearranged in Abelson virus transformed pre-B cells (242), even though it was rarely seen in the mature B cell compartment. The demonstration of the decrease in representation of cells with V_H81X rearrangements at the pre-B clonal expansion phase in bone marrow (*243*,244), together with the demonstration that heavy chains utilizing V_H81X frequently fail to assemble functional pre-BCRs (*236*,237,*245*), explained this paradox. However, it is still curious that the most frequently rearranged V_H gene is so strongly selected *against* at the clonal expansion stage. A possible explanation may lie in comparisons of V_H utilization during fetal development. That is, in contrast with bone marrow precursor cultures, the ratio of productive/nonproductive V_H81X does not decrease during cultures of fetal precursors (*246*,247). Further, the proliferative burst that pre-BCR assembly provides to bone marrow pre-B cells may instead result in exit from cell cycle in fetal precursors (239), leading to

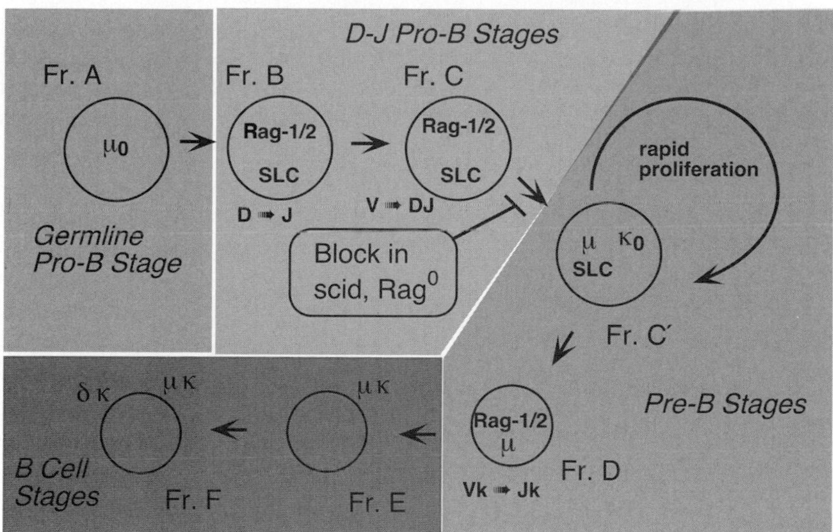

FIGURE 7.11 Model of mouse bone marrow B cell development showing relationship of Ig rearrangement with progression and proliferation.

selection of very different BCR repertoires during fetal and adult B lymphopoiesis. The possible significance of this is discussed below in the section on B-1 B cells.

Light Chain Rearrangement and Generation of Immature B Cells

Besides termination of TdT and SLC gene expression, pre-BCR signaling also results in the down-regulation of Rag-1 and Rag-2 expression, and protein levels rapidly drop as cells enter the rapidly cycling stage. However, as pre-BCR levels decrease and cells exit from cycle, the Rag genes are reexpressed at high levels. Sterile kappa transcripts become detectable during the cycling stage, likely reflecting chromatin remodeling to make the kappa light chain locus accessible (228), so induction of Rag expression together with the rest of the recombinase machinery will initiate kappa light chain V to J rearrangement. An interesting feature of the Vκ locus is that the approximately 100 genes are in both transcriptional orientations, and so these genes can rearrange either by deletion (generating an extrachromosomal excision circle) or by inversion *(248)*. The absence of intervening D segments also means that it is possible for upstream V kappa genes to rearrange to downstream J kappa segments, "leap-frogging" the initial rearrangement, assuming it was to any Jκ other than Jκ5. The successive association of different kappa chains with the same heavy chain in a B cell is referred to as BCR "editing" and was originally observed in the context of autoreactivity, which maintains Rag expression even at the B cell stage ([249,*250*]; see the following section on B cell tolerance). Since assembly and expression of a complete BCR (that is not self-reactive) terminates Rag expression, an additional reason for light chain editing in the bone marrow may be to replace an initial light chain that fails to assemble effectively with the particular heavy chain present in that pre-B cell. This is probably the explanation for multiple light chain rearrangements detected in single early B lineage cells *(251)*.

Newly formed B cells can be distinguished from mature B cells on the basis of their inability to proliferate in response to BCR cross-linking—that is, they are functionally immature. This is also the stage where negative selection is reported in transgenic models of autoreactivity (252,*253*). Cells at this stage have a short half-life, only a few days, compared to mature follicular B cells with a half-life measured in months. They can be distinguished by surface phenotype from other B cells based on expression of certain combinations of markers, such as IgM^+IgD^-, absence of CD23, and high-level expression of CD24/HSA (254). Recently, there are reports of single markers that are useful in distinguishing newly formed cells from any mature subset, such as the molecules recognized by monoclonal antibodies 493 (255) and AA4.1 (256). The AA4.1 target molecule has been cloned and identified as the mouse ortholog of a component of the human C1q receptor *(257)*.

Cells similar to newly formed B cells can be generated to varying extent during stromal cell culture of B cell precursors, although the more primitive cycling pre-B or pro-B cells are usually more abundant and tend to increase in frequency with prolonged culture. It is possible to induce differentiation of B cells in these cultures by withdrawing IL-7, which induces a wave of small pre-B and then newly formed B cell generation. Such cells do not persist for more than a day, unless the cultures are established from Bcl-2 transgenic mice *(115)*, suggesting that the short half-life of newly formed cells in these cultures, and possibly also *in vivo*, is due to their low level of antiapoptotic mediators. Both Bcl-2 and Bcl-X_L mRNA are present at only very low levels in these cells, in contrast with other B lineage stages where either one or the other predominates. Over-expression of Bcl-X_L from a transgene results in accumulation of a population of pro-B phenotype cells with nonfunctional rearrangements *(258)*, implicating this protein in the process of pre-BCR selection of cells with functional rearrangements.

Peripheral Maturation Stages and Functional Subsets

Transitional B Cells

Newly formed immature B cells migrate to the spleen where they either die or undergo further maturation to a mature B cell. These maturing B cells can be subdivided based on differential expression of several surface proteins, including CD21, CD23, CD24/HSA, and AA4.1. These subdivisions have been referred to as *transitional B cells* (259). One recent subdivision based on CD21, CD23, AA4.1, and IgM level has shown progression from an AA4.1^{+}CD21^{-}CD23^{-} T1 stage to an AA4.1^{+}CD21^{-}CD23^{+} T2 stage, followed by down-regulation of IgM as a T3 stage, and finally loss of AA4.1 with up-regulation of CD21 to yield the mature follicular phenotype (256). As shown in Figure 7.12, this approach also resolves two AA4.1^{-} subsets that lack CD23, the B-1 subset with low CD21 and the marginal zone (MZ) subset with very high CD21 (see following). The transitional stage cells are all short-lived, as shown by bromodeoxyuridine incorporation (256,*260*). They are also not functionally competent, as shown by inability to proliferate after BCR cross-linking (254,*261*). Another well-characterized functional distinction is that B cell tolerance, rather than an immune response, is induced by BCR cross-linking of immature B cells *(262–264)*. More recent studies with transgenic models of self-reactivity have shown that these B cells can be deleted, undergo receptor editing, or are rendered functionally unresponsive (anergic) by BCR signaling at the immature stage (249,252,265–269). One group has suggested that the "T3" stage is not an intermediate in production of follicular B cells, but rather a population of autoreactive anergic cells *(270)*, so clearly additional work needs to be done to

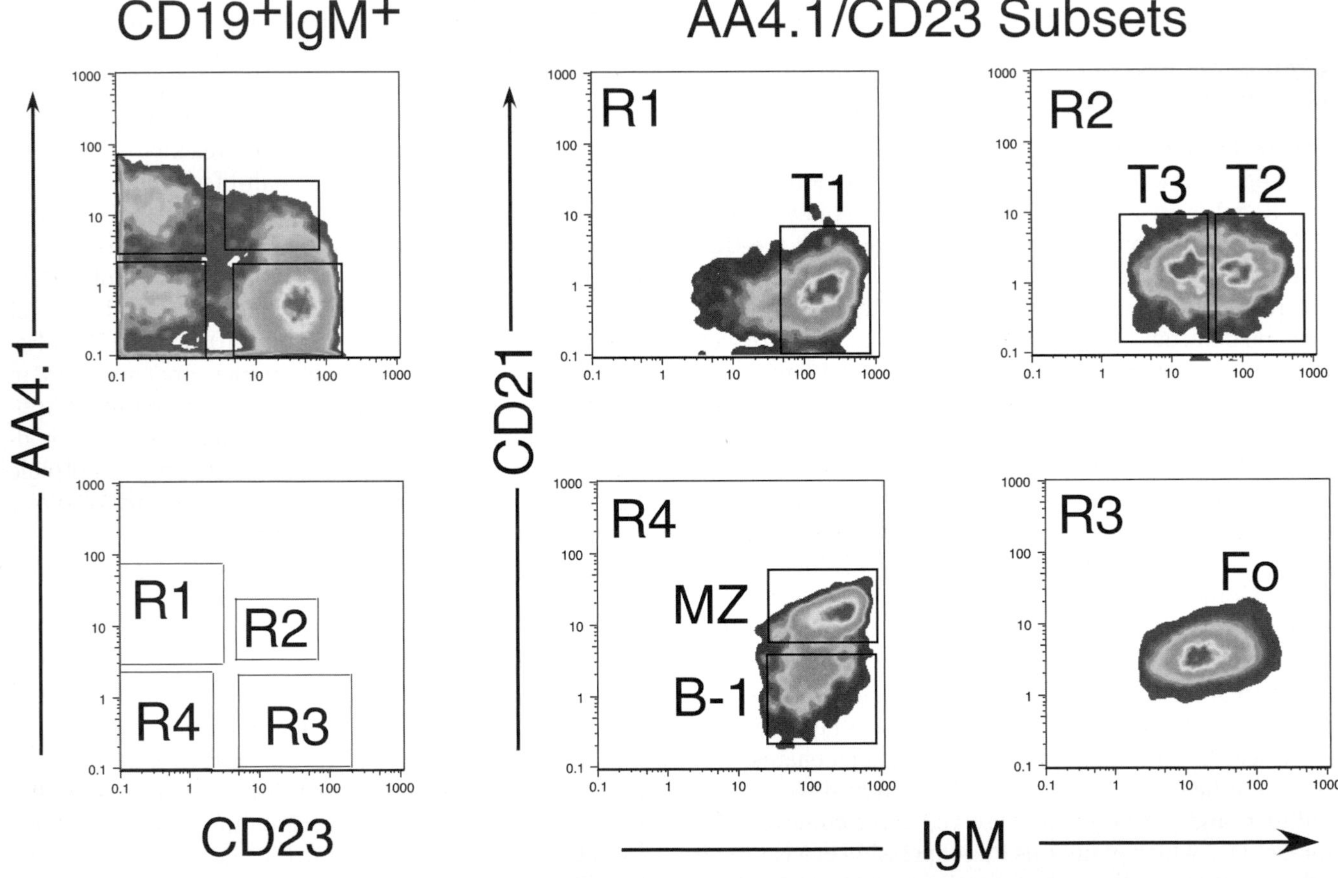

FIGURE 7.12 Flow cytometry approach for resolution of transitional (T1-T3) and mature (Fo, B-1, MZ) populations of B cells in mouse spleen. Left panels show the distribution of AA4.1 and CD23 on B cells (defined as CD19^{+}IgM^{+}). Cell in the boxed regions are then analyzed for correlated expression of CD21 and IgM, facilitating resolution of three AA4.1^{+} fractions (T1-T3), the follicular subset (AA4.1^{-}CD23^{+}CD21^{+}), the marginal zone subset (AA4.1^{-}CD23^{-}CD21^{++}), and the B-1 subset (AA4.1^{-}CD23^{-}CD21^{low}).

establish the identities of all the B cell subpopulations present in spleen.

It is not simply the inability to receive T cell help due to differences in microenvironment or receptor expression that makes immature B cells incapable of responding as mature B cells. Crosslinking the BCR on purified populations of immature, but not mature, B cells has been shown to induce apoptosis, suggesting distinctions in the signaling pathways between these two stages (271,*272*). Studies with transgenic mice suggest that this apoptosis is not mediated through the Fas/Fas-ligand pathway, because central deletion is intact in Fas-mutant mice (273,274). Prior to induction of apoptosis, immature B cells have been shown to complete some of the early events associated with entry into cell cycle, while failing to complete this program *(275)*. Distinct stages in maturation appear more or less capable of responding to BCR cross-linking by reinduction (or maintenance) of Rags to facilitate receptor editing *(253)*. Further, it appears that immature B cells are more sensitive to smaller changes in intracellular free calcium, compared to mature B cells (276). It is possible that the capacity to up-regulate antiapoptotic molecules, such as A1, may play a critical role in the inability of immature B cells to survive and complete a normal response *(277,278)*. The characterization of signaling pathways in different immature stages of developing B cells is ongoing and should eventually provide insights into the detailed mechanism for immature B cell tolerance.

Analyses of various normally occurring or engineered mutant mice have provided approaches for investigation of the process of progressing from a newly formed B cell to a mature follicular B cell. B cell populations and B cell function has been studied for many years in CBA/N mice, bearing the x-linked immunodeficiency (xid) mutation. This mouse has a mutation in the Btk gene that produces a milder phenotype than the complete absence of peripheral B cells seen in humans. The Btk gene likely plays a role at several stages of B cell development and activation which complicates the analysis, but it appears clear that one major consequence is altered BCR signaling that has a profound effect on progression through the various transitional stages in spleen. A likely consequence of diminished strength of BCR signaling is a compensatory requirement for higher surface BCR expression that eventually produces at decreased frequency a type of "mature" B cell that is still functionally handicapped *(279,280)*. Several groups have produced xid mice on a nu/nu T cell–less background that results in a more profound absence of mature B cells, suggesting a requirement for T cells or T cell–produced factors in the maturation of xid B cells *(281,282)*. A more recent variation of this type of investigation is the production of xid/CD40 deficient mice that show a similar deficit in mature B cells, suggesting a role for the CD40/CD40L interaction in the generation of mature B cells from transitional B cells, particularly when the BCR is handicapped by defective Btk (283).

Lyn is a src family protein kinase that is associated with the BCR and functions in signaling in mature B cells (284). Lyn-deficient mice exhibit defects in maturation of immature cells, suggesting a positive role for BCR/Lyn signaling at this stage, but these mice also develop a severe autoimmune condition, suggesting an additional negative regulatory role for Lyn in maintaining tolerance in mature B cells *(285,286)*.

CD72 is a predominantly B lineage restricted C-type lectin, and ligating this molecule was recognized for many years (when it was known as Lyb2) as having functional consequences *(287)*. Recent analyses of a CD72 null mouse has clarified its function in B cell development and activation *(288)*. CD72 has been shown to recruit SHP-1 to the BCR, supporting a negative regulatory role in BCR activation *(289)*. Consistent with this model for CD72 function, null gene-targeted mice have been shown to produce B cells that are hyper-responsive *(288)*. Interestingly, late stages of B cell development are affected, with fewer mature B cells and relatively normal numbers of immature B cells in spleen *(288)*. Thus, too intense signaling may also delay maturation of immature B cells.

Follicular B Cells

The major population of mature recirculating B cells in the spleen is located in the B cell follicle region, hence the term *follicular B cells*. Entry into this anatomical site appears to constitute a final stage in maturation for developing bone marrow B cells, as competition for this site is compromised in several transgenic models of B cell tolerance (290,*291*,*292*,293). Cells in this compartment do not proliferate, but persist in the resting state for several months. A conditional knockout study, eliminating expression of the BCR (by deleting the V region), revealed that expression of the BCR is required for cell survival (215,216). It is not yet established whether this is due to "tonic signaling" (simple assembly of the BCR signaling complex), or instead reflects signaling by low-affinity binding to cross-reactive self-determinants, a kind of "positive selection." It is interesting to note that ablation of heavy chain from the immature B cell, thereby eliminating any possibility of pre-BCR or BCR tonic signaling, results in a "reversion" of cell phenotype to an earlier developmental stage *(294)*. Finally, the maintenance of follicular B cells has been found to depend on the function of the c-Myb transcription factor, due to its role in BAFF signaling ([295] see following section).

The repertoire of the follicular B cell pool appears to differ from the earlier immature splenic B cell population, as assessed by sequence analysis of the light chain repertoire in heavy chain transgenic mice *(296)*. The approach of fixing the heavy chain and then examining the light chain repertoire simplifies the analysis, and the results of this study were interpreted to indicate that BCR-mediated antigen selection is indeed operating. However, the resolution of the analysis probably could not have rigorously excluded populations known to show V gene biases, such as B-1 or MZ B cells (see following sections), so further work will be required to provide convincing evidence of antigenic selection in the follicular B cell pool.

B Cell Migration and Maintenance

Newly formed B cells migrate from the bone marrow to the spleen, undergo further maturation in the red pulp, and eventually enter the follicle where they constitute the mature B cell pool that recirculates. Their migration is dependent on chemokines/receptor interactions, notably the SLC(CCL21)/CCR7 interaction, as demonstrated by the inability of mature B cells to be retained normally in spleens of CCR7 null mice *(297)*. The role of the CXCR5 receptor on B cells in homing to the lymphoid follicle due a gradient of the B lymphocyte chemoattractant CXCL13 is also well known and additionally CXCL13 can directly induce Ltα1β2 on the recruited cells (298). Finally, it is also possible that the SDF1(CXCL12)/CXCR4 interaction, critical for normal B lymphopoiesis, may also be important at this later stage, although investigation of this issue is complicated by the early defect. This is an ongoing area of investigation and may eventually be clarified by developmentally regulated gene targeting studies.

Recently, considerable interest has focused on the role of a TNF family member cytokine known variously as BAFF, BLyS, TALL-1, zTNF4, or THANK in the process of peripheral B cell maturation *(299)*. BAFF is a TNF family member found to enhance survival of B cells or even produce autoimmunity in transgenic mice constitutively expressing it *(300,301)*. Initially two receptors defined for BAFF, BCMA and TACI, provided a complex picture, as targeted inactivation of BCMA yielded no B cell defect and deletion of TACI had increased B cell numbers (suggesting that TACI might be a negative regulator). This puzzle was resolved by identification of a third receptor, BAFF-R/BR3 (302,*303*), that was mutated in the A/WySnJ strain of mice, known to lack most mature B cells (304). A second ligand, APRIL, can bind to BCMA and TACI, but not to BAFF/BR3, and this binding is proliferative rather than survival-promoting *(305)*. Thus, the critical interaction for maintenance of follicular B cells is BAFF/BLyS with its receptor. B-1 cells are not deficient in A/WySnJ mice (304), suggesting that their maintenance does not depend on this pathway, but instead is more BCR-dependent.

B Cell Turnover

It is estimated that 10 million to 20 million B cells are produced in bone marrow of the mouse each day *(306)*, yet it appears that only about 10% of this number reach the periphery *(260)*. Thus, there is considerable loss at this bone marrow emigration stage/spleen entry stage, possibly due to elimination of autoreactive cells (B cell tolerance) or to homeostatic regulation. The latter possibility is supported by the observation that depletion of the mature B cell population results in a relatively rapid recovery of this pool, suggesting that most of the immature B cell population can enter the mature follicular subset in this situation *(307)*.

Once functionally mature B cells are generated, it has been difficult to unambiguously determine their half-life, although accumulating data from several laboratories using bromodeoxyuridine labeling has led to the idea that follicular B cells have a relatively long half-life, on the order of months (*260*,308). A recent elegant study provided definitive confirmation of this by conditional elimination of Rag-2 expression, allowing termination of B cell development in adult mice (309). This study showed that follicular B cells have a half-life of about 4.5 months. This same analysis showed that two other subsets of B cells, B-1 and MZ B cells, did not diminish over time, consistent with their well-known capacity for self-renewal and life-long persistence.

Germinal Center B Cells

T cell dependent immune responses usually give rise to anatomically distinctive structures in spleen and lymph nodes that are referred to as germinal centers (GC) containing large numbers of rapidly cycling B cells (310,*311*). These cells can be recognized in stained sections of spleen by binding of high levels of peanut agglutinin (PNA) and by the absence of IgD (312,*313*). Many of the B cells with this phenotype have down-regulated-BCL-2/upregulated-Fas expression and, in the absence of strong BCR signaling, will likely die by apoptosis (*314*,315,*316*,317). The termination of IgD expression means that surface BCR expression decreases at least 10-fold and so limiting amounts of antigen will favor the cells with increased affinity for antigen, generated by a process termed *somatic hypermutation*, or SHM. The molecular details of this mechanism are still unclear, but a major advance has been the recent discovery that activation-induced cytidine deaminase (AID), a putative DNA or RNA-editing enzyme that can induce class switch recombination in fibroblasts (318,*319,320*), is also a key player in the process of hypermutation (321,*322*). In fact, a third means for Ig gene diversification used in nonmammalian species, V gene conversion, is also dependent on AID *(323,324)*.

A potential means for repertoire diversification in the GC, distinct from SHM, has been suggested by the finding that the Rag genes are induced in at least some GC B cells *(325–328)*. Receptor editing is a potential consequence of this induction, but to date, it is unclear that there is any physiological relevance for the induction of

Rag in the periphery. Considering the important role that the pre-BCR and BCR play in regulating Rag expression in bone marrow development, it seems quite possible that the reexpression of Rag may be a consequence of hypermutation of the heavy or light chain (or both), resulting in generation of nonfunctional receptor genes. This could occur either from truncation by stop codons or by less severe alterations that result in an inability of Ig HL pairing. Consistent with this notion, it appears that much of the Rag expression by GC B cells is coincident with apoptotic cells in the GC *(329)*. Recent Rag-reporter approaches have failed to indicate significant Rag reinduction in mature B cells *(330,331)*. An alternative explanation for some peripheral Rag expression may be an influx of immature cells into the spleen induced as a consequence of immunization (332).

The precise mechanism of selection for higher affinity B cells generated by hypermutation of the BCR V regions remains to be fully understood, but regulation of pro- and antiapoptotic genes likely plays a major role. B cells able to bind antigen with high affinity can present antigen to $CD4^+$ T cells that then signal the B cell through a CD40/CD40L interaction, resulting in the up-regulation of Bcl-X_L (*314*,315,*316*). Most GC B cells have sharply down-regulated levels of Bcl-2 and up-regulated levels of Fas (*316*,317), and so in the absence of rescue by expression of the alternative antiapoptotic mediator Bcl-X_L, cell death by apoptosis will be the fate of most B cells in the GC. Careful regulation of selection is critical to affinity maturation, and elimination of self-reactive cells that potentially could be generated during this process must also occur efficiently to avoid the potential of autoimmune disease. This is an active area of investigation, and more players in this selection process are continuing to be identified *(333)*.

Memory B Cells

Memory B cells were initially defined functionally as cells that could respond rapidly by production of high-affinity antibody when challenged in a host reconstituted with B cells and T cells from a primed animal (*334–338*,339). Subsequently, such cells have been purified based on their antigen-binding properties *(340)* and shown to consist primarily of isotype-switched (IgG^+) B cells that continue to express CD45R/B220 and have distinctively lower levels of cell surface BCR (341). They arise during the T cell–dependent immune response, probably only from follicular B cells, in the GC. They are very long-lived or self-regenerating, as cell transfer assays have shown that memory responses can be detected for long periods after the primary immunization (341,*342*).

It is not clear whether all B cells are capable of giving rise to memory B cells. Memory or "secondary" B cells were originally described as expressing distinctively low levels of CD24/HSA, recognized by the monoclonal antibody J11d *(343)*. Some years later, fractionation of naïve spleen B cell precursors into J11d^{low} and J11d^{high} subsets in a spleen focus assay system showed that while rapid antibody secretion derived from J11d^{high} cells, memory came largely from the J11d^{low} subset *(344)*. Subsequent experiments demonstrated that GCs (the sites where most memory B cells are generated) were only produced in cell transfers of J11d^{low} B cells and not with J11d^{high} or $CD5^+$ B cells *(345)*. Considering the rapid Ig secretory response of B-1 B cells and MZ B cells, both contained in the CD24/HSA^{high} fraction, and the fact that most other CD24/HSA^{high} cells are immature (transitional) B cells, likely to be highly susceptible to apoptosis, it seems quite reasonable that memory B cells would not be a major product of this fraction. Rather, the most likely candidate for the memory B cell precursor is the follicular B cell subset (Fo), which has variable, but lower expression of CD24/HSA. Whether there is heterogeneity for GC formation or memory B cell generation within the Fo population remains to be determined.

Whether the maintenance of memory requires periodic restimulation by antigen has been a longstanding, controversial issue. On the one hand, transfer of B cells and T cells into irradiated recipients usually required simultaneous challenge with antigen to elicit the full response and maintain B cell memory in recipients *(346)*. Antigenic fragments can persist for very extended periods on follicular dendritic cells, very potent antigen-presenting cells, and so in this model the memory B cells are periodically triggered to self-renew by interaction with antigen on FDC. However, on the other hand, memory B cells can be maintained in the apparent absence of T cells or FDCs *(347,348)*. Further, analysis by bromodeoxyuridine labeling of memory B cell populations showed that they were nondividing *(342)*. This issue has recently been addressed in elegant experiments that used the inducible cre recombinase system to switch the BCR on memory cells away from the immunizing antigen (349). Such antigen-negative memory cells still persisted for extended periods, clearly demonstrating that this was a physiological property of the cell type, independent of the presence of antigen.

B-1 B Cells

B-1 B cells, initially described as Ly-1/$CD5^+$ B cells, are distinguished from follicular B cells by phenotype, anatomical distribution, and function (23,*350*). The B-1 B cell phenotype encompasses both $CD5^+$ and $CD5^-$ B cells that are IgM^{high}, $IgD^{low/-}$, $CD23^-$, and $CD43^+$. They constitute a large proportion of the B cells found in the peritoneal and pleural cavities (30% to 50% of B cells, around 10^6 cells), but are also found in spleen where they are present at numerically similar levels, but constitute a much lower proportion of the total B cell pool (2% of B cells, around 10^6 cells). The B-1 B cells in the peritoneal cavity are also CD11b/Mac-1^+, unlike those in spleen. They appear early in ontogeny, representing 30% or more of the B cells in spleen of 1-week-old animals. They also have a distinctively higher frequency of λ light chain usage compared to follicular B cells (20% versus 5%). Also, unlike follicular B cells, they maintain their population in adult animals largely by self-renewal (possibly dependent on periodic stimulation by self-antigen, discussed later), rather than by input from precursor cells, as shown in cell transfer studies *(351)*.

Perhaps the most distinctive feature of $CD5^+$/B-1 B cells is their enrichment of certain self-reactive specificities, notably for branched carbohydrates, glycolipids, and glycoproteins, including phosphorylcholine, phosphatidylcholine (PtC), the Thy-1 glycoprotein, and bacterial cell wall constituents (352,*353*,354,*355*). These antibodies, while autoantibodies, are not pathogenic, but rather referred to as *natural autoantibodies* whose existence has been recognized in serum for several decades *(356–358)*. Their function is still under active investigation, but at least some natural autoantibodies are thought to function in clearance of senescent cells or proteins and to provide an initial immunity to common bacterial or viral pathogens, serving as a kind of "hard-wired" memory B cell population (359,360,*361*,362).

Under physiologic conditions in normal mice, most of the $CD5^+$ B cells in the B-1 population (so called *B-1a B cells*) arise from precursors in fetal liver, as cell transfer studies showed many years ago that B cells with this phenotype were inefficiently generated from bone marrow precursors in adult mice, compared to fetal or neonatal precursors (363). This is very clearly shown by repopulation of SCID mice by pro-B stage cells isolated from fetal liver and adult bone marrow (Figure 7.13). Part of the reason for this difference may be that novel BCRs are enriched by distinctive mechanisms of fetal B lymphopoiesis, including recombination in the absence of TdT (thereby favoring rearrangement of certain D-J and V-D junctions possessing short regions of homology [16]) and distinctive pre-BCR selection (239,247,*364*). It is also possible, although not yet tested, that the threshold for elimination of self-reactive B cells at the newly formed stage may be less stringent during fetal development. Forced expression of transgenic BCRs cloned from $CD5^+$ B cells can give rise to $CD5^+$ B cells from bone marrow of adult animals, but the physiological relevance of this remains to be carefully assessed. The development of B cells in bone marrow of such transgenic mice often appears handicapped, and the precise reason for this requires further study.

The development of B-1/$CD5^+$ B cells is thought to be more dependent on antigenic selection compared to follicular B cells. This idea was first suggested by the finding of particular specificities enriched in this population and strengthened by the observation of repeated occurrences of particular V_H/V_L pairs *(365)*. Thus, for example, the anti-PtC specificity is predominantly encoded by $V_H11V_\kappa9$ and $V_H12V_\kappa4$, utilizing two V_H genes rarely found in conventional T-dependent immune responses *(353,366)*. These cells appear to participate in T-independent responses, but in normal physiology may in fact provide an initial low-affinity "first wave" response to many pathogens that eventually will also elicit a T-dependent response (362,367).

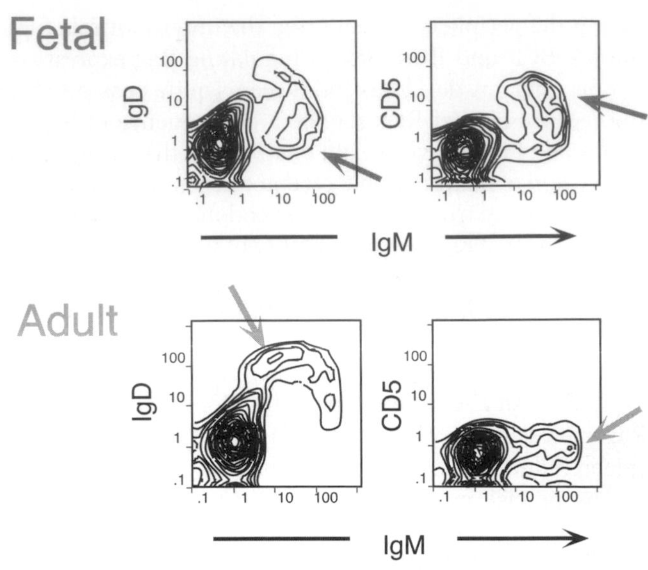

FIGURE 7.13 Generation of B cells in SCID mice shows the distinctive phenotypes produced from fetal and adult pro-B cells. Similar numbers of pro-B cells, isolated as in Figure 7.5, Fr. B/C, were injected i.v. into sublethally irradiated adult SCID mice, then recipients were analyzed 3 weeks later for spleen cell lymphocytes by staining as shown in the figure.

The observation of their self-reactive bias, their capacity for self-renewal, and their restricted repertoire of distinctive BCRs all are consistent with an important role for BCR–antigen interaction in generation and maintenance of this population. This has been formally confirmed recently by studying mice bearing a BCR transgene specific for a glycosylation present only on the Thy-1 membrane protein *(368)*. In these mice, transgene-encoded serum anti-Thy-1 autoantibody (354) was readily detected, and there was a corresponding accumulation of a population of $CD5^+$ transgene BCR^+ B cells in the peritoneal cavity. Importantly, in Thy-1 null mice generated by gene targeting, neither serum autoantibody nor the B cell population was found, demonstrating the critical role for antigen in selection of this B cell population (369).

Consistent with the importance of antigen selection in the generation and maintenance of these cells, this population is often severely affected in mice bearing mutations that alter BCR signaling intensity. The loss of negative mediators such as PTP1C/SHP-1 in "motheaten" mice *(370)*, of CD72 that recruits this phosphatase *(370)*, and of the CD22 co-receptor *(371,372)*, all result in an increased frequency of B-1/$CD5^+$ B cells relative to follicular B cells. However, the loss of critical BCR signaling components or positive mediators in this pathway such as an Ig-α tail mutant *(373)*, Btk deficiency (in xid or btk null mice [374,375]), CD19 null mice (*376*,377), CD21 null mice *(378)*, CD45 null mice (367), and vav null mice *(379)* all negatively affect this B cell population. A further indication of a signal-dependent selection model is the accumulation of B-1 type B cells with high-level expression of a BCR surrogate, LMP2A, but only B-2 B cells and MZ B cells with low level expression (380).

Marginal Zone B Cells

MZ B cells are localized in a distinct anatomical region of the spleen that represents the major antigen-filtering and scavenging area (by specialized macrophages resident there). It appears that they are preselected to express a BCR repertoire similar to B-1 B cells, biased toward bacterial cell wall constituents *(381)* and senescent self-components (e.g., oxidized low density lipoprotein (LDL) [*382,383*]). Similar to B-1 B cells, they respond very rapidly to antigenic challenge, likely independently of T cells, but participating in the early phase of T-dependent responses (*384*,385,*386*). Uniquely, among all populations of B cells, MZ B cells are dependent on Notch2 signaling for their development (387,*388*).

There are similarities and differences in the cell surface phenotype of MZ and B-1 B cells. Thus, they both are $IgM^{+++}IgD^{-/+}$, $CD23^{-}$, and $CD9^{+}$ *(389)*. However, while B-1/$CD5^{+}$ B cells express CD5 and CD43, MZ B cells do not, and MZ B cells express distinctively high levels of CD21, while B-1 cells have distinctively low levels (Figure 7.12). Also, MZ B cells have high levels of CD1, while B-1 B cells do not *(390)*. Certain mutant mice show similar effects on MZ and B-1 B cells, distinct from Fo B cells. For example, most of the mutations described for B-1 B cells that alter BCR signaling have similar consequences for MZ B cells (391), although cells that resemble MZ B cells are present in xid/Btk-deficient mice, leading to some controversy in their origins (392). Both are decreased by a mutation in the Ig-α tail that weakens overall BCR signaling *(393)*. They are also both decreased in the Aiolos transcription factor null mouse (60). Interestingly, deletion of the Pyk-2 tyrosine kinase results in elimination of MZ B cells, while B-1 cells are still found *(394)*.

MZ B cell development can be studied in a heavy chain transgenic mouse model system where large numbers of such cells are produced (*381*,395). In this V_H81X heavy chain mouse, B cells with a specific light chain accumulate with a marginal zone phenotype. This MZ population is eliminated by deletion of CD19, Btk, or CD45, all genetic changes that weaken BCR signaling (391).

B Cell Tolerance and Receptor Editing (Table 7.2)

The past decade has seen the development of several transgenic models for the study of B cell tolerance. In two of these systems, high-affinity BCRs are expressed as IgM-IgD transgenes, one specific for the antigen hen eggwhite lysozyme (HEL), the other for a specific polymorphic determinant on MHC class I (249,265–267,*396*,*397*,398). The advantage of these systems is that they utilize antigens that can be regulated: Transgenic B cells can develop in either the presence or absence of antigen, and cell transfer experiments can be employed to alter the B cell's antigenic milieu. These have been used initially to confirm ideas on B cell tolerance that originated in work with nontransgenic B cells, namely that exposure to antigen is generally deleterious to developing B cells, resulting in their elimination or failure to mature (instead entering an "anergic" state). However, the resolution of these systems, coupled with advances in gene targeting and other molecular technologies have uncovered important new details regarding the way that self-reactive B cells develop (or fail to develop). For example, studies in the anti-H-2 model uncovered an alternative to deletion in response to immature B cell encounter with antigen, BCR editing to escape autoreactivity (249).

In the HEL system, differences have been uncovered in immature B cell responses to soluble versus membrane-bound antigen, suggesting that differences in the extent of BCR cross-linking can influence cell fate (266). Further, studies with this system on different mutant backgrounds that shift BCR signaling thresholds up or down has shown that such alterations can result in striking alterations in selection outcomes (399,400). More recently, work in this system has shown that one consequence of B cell tolerance may be arrest of B cell migration, so that follicular entry is inefficient (290,*291*). Presumably, failure to reach such follicular niches contributes to handicapping the autoreactive B cells, resulting in their relatively speedy elimination.

Another major line of investigation has focused on a more "physiologic" example of pathogenic autoreactivity, the anti-DNA antibodies produced in lpr (Fas-deficient) mice that are generally considered to model the human disease of systemic lupus erythematosus (SLE). Analysis of transgenic mice bearing a heavy chain transgene known to be capable of generating anti-dsDNA reactivity with numerous light chains showed that only light chains with ssDNA activity were tolerated in the periphery, and even these did not contribute to the serum antibody pool (268). Follow-up work uncovered receptor editing in this model (269,*401–403*) and also showed that when such editing was blocked, the B cells were eliminated in the bone marrow at an immature stage (252). More recent work analyzing transgenic B cells expressing lambda light chain (or in kappa null mice) where B cells have dsDNA binding, has shown the failure of follicular entry previously described in the HEL system (*292*,293). Interestingly, similar analyses on an "autoreactive" (Fas-deficient) background have shown that this follicular exclusion is lost and production of pathogenic autoantibodies ensues, providing a powerful model for the further characterization of the development of autoimmunity due to breakdown of B cell tolerance.

TABLE 7.2 Transgenic Models of B cell Tolerance

Ig Transgene	*Antigen*	*Background*	*Effect*	*Reference*
3-83 $\mu\kappa$	MHC class I H-2Kk,b	H-2Kk H2-Kd	Deletion, receptor editing Normal development	249, 267, 398
3-83 $\mu\kappa$	""	H-2Kk lpr autoimmune-prone	Deletion unaffected	274
anti-HEL $\mu\delta$	HEL	sHEL-Tg Wildtype	Anergy Normal development	265, *396, 397*
anti-HEL $\mu\delta$	""	mHEL-TG	Deletion	266
anti-HEL $\mu\delta$	""	HEL-Tg lpr autoimmune-prone	Deletion unaffected	273
anti-HEL $\mu\delta$	HEL	sHEL-Tg CD45 null	Self-antigen promoted development	400
anti-HEL $\mu\delta$	HEL	sHEL-Tg motheaten	Deletion by lower-valency autoantigen	399
3H9 μ-only	ssDNA with many light chains	BALB/c	No anti-DNA autoantibodies	268
3H9 μ-only	""	lpr autoimmune-prone	Anti-DNA autoantibodies	530
3H9 $\mu\kappa$	dsDNA	BALB/c	Deletion, editing	269
3H9 $\mu\kappa$	dsDNA	J_H^-/J_κ^-	Deletion	252
3H9 $\mu\lambda$	""	Wild-type and lpr autoimmune-prone	Anergy	*292*, 293
3H9-R/Vκ4-R 3H9-R/Vκ8-R	dsDNA ssDNA	BALB/c	Deletion, editing anergy	531
3H9-R/Vκ4-R 3H9-R/Vκ8-R	dsDNA, ssDNA	Rag-2$^-$	Deletion, activation	532
3H9/56R 3H9/56R76R	dsDNA, ssDNA	BALB/c	Deletion, editing	533
anti-erythrocyte	Red blood cell		Tg$^+$ cells only in peritoneal cavity	404, *405, 406*
$V_H11\mu$, $V_H12\mu$	PtC, BrMRBC	Wildtype	Increased number of B-1 B cells	534, 535
6C10μ	ATA determinant (glycosylation of Thy-1)	Wildtype Thy1 null	ATA B cells ATA serum Normal development; no ATA	369
ATA $\mu\kappa$ (6C10μVκ21c)	ATA determinant	Wildtype	Receptor editing or development block in BM; ATA in serum	409, 410
		Thy1 null	Normal development	

A different model of a pathogenic anti–erythrocyte autoantibody has shown another possible mechanism whereby self-reactive B cells may escape deletion or receptor editing, by sequestration from self-antigen (404,*405*). In this system, the transgenic B cells are largely absent from spleen, but instead survive in the peritoneal cavity, where exposure to the distinctive microenvironment may also contribute to the persistence of these cells. Eventual activation of the B cells by mitogen or antigen can lead to an autoimmune condition in these mice *(406)*.

A common thread in all of the studies described earlier is the negative impact that the B cell experiences upon interaction with self-antigen, an expected result for systems that model the regulation of pathogenic autoantibodies. However, a class of autoantibodies is produced in healthy individuals, and these "natural autoantibodies" may play a role in early responses to certain classes of pathogens (359,360,362,*407*). Such a natural autoantibody has been used to construct a transgenic model system where the self-antigen can be regulated. Most natural self-antigens are common glycosylations or cell constituents such as PtC that cannot be eliminated, but a class of natural autoantibodies binds to thymocytes (antithymocyte autoantibody, ATA), and many of these recognize a glycolylation that is only present on the abundant thymocyte cell surface glycoprotein CD90/Thy-1 (369). Thy-1 null mice have already been generated *(408)*, so production of ATA-BCR μ-only transgenic mice enabled the study of the role of antigen in the generation of this natural autoantibody. Interestingly, both production of serum ATA and accumulation of B cells with the appropriate light chain (by rearrangement of endogenous Ig light chain locus) for the ATA BCR required the presence of Thy-1 self-antigen (369). Thus, at least some B cells are selected for binding to self-antigen,

transcriptional repressor that is linked to both GC B cells and to B lymphomas that likely derive from GC B cells *(441,442)*. Bcl-6 expression is high in GC B cells and is required for formation of the GC *(443)*. Strikingly, its 5′ regulatory region is mutated as a consequence of hypermutation in GC B cells, the first example of hypermutation targeted outside the Ig regions *(441,442)* and links this process to deregulated cell growth and lymphomagenesis. Subsequently, mutations have also been found, albeit at a lower level, in CD95/Fas, suggesting this as another potential cause for lymphomas of GC origin *(444)*.

Abnormalities of Development

A key discovery in the past decade has been the finding that a well-known immunodeficiency, X-linked immunodeficiency (XLA), characterized by inability to respond to bacterial infections and a severe deficit in peripheral B cells *(445)*, is due to mutations in Btk, or Bruton's tyrosine kinase (446). Shortly after this finding, the mouse ortholog of Btk was shown to be the cause of murine xid, an extensively studied mutation originally identified in CBA/N mice (447). Btk deficiency in humans is more severe than xid, with little B cell development past the early B cell stage, in contrast with an absence of normal peripheral B cell development in mouse and inability to respond to certain types of T-independent antigens *(448)*. This difference is not simply due to specific difference in the mutations, as a complete null mutation in mouse is indistinguishable from xid (375). Thus, human B cell development, likely at the pre-BCR signaling stage, is much more dependent on Btk.

While XLA is by far the most common B cell deficiency, amounting to more than 80% of those identified, non X linked mutations have also been observed. These correspond to mutations in the pre-BCR signaling complex, and in most cases similar effects had been observed in the mouse. For example, deletions or mutations in the μ constant regions accounted for another 5% *(439)*. Examples have been found of mutations in the 14.1 gene, the human ortholog of the mouse surrogate light chain $\lambda 5$ protein (437) and also in Ig-α *(438)*. In both of these cases, early B lineage cells, identified as $CD19^{+}CD34^{+}$, were present in normal numbers in bone marrow, but $CD19^{+}CD34^{-}$ $c\mu^{+}$ cells (pre-B cells) and all later stages were absent. Finally, a patient with a mutation in BLNK, an adaptor protein that links pre-BCR signaling from syk to the rest of the signaling cascade, showed a similar phenotype (449).

Very few peripheral B cells are detected in any of these disorders, which suggests that pre-BCR signaling is more critical in human than in the mouse, where mutations in $\lambda 5$ and BLNK allow the generation of variable numbers of peripheral B cells. The reason for this difference is not yet understood. Interestingly, common variable immunodeficiency has been shown to result from mutations in the common gamma chain *(138)* or in the JAK3 gene *(450)*, consistent with IL-7 playing a much less critical role in human pre-B cell growth than in mouse, as had already been determined from culture studies *(429,430)*, B cell development is relatively intact, whereas T cells are ablated. The reverse is true for mouse *(451,452)*.

New Insights into Treatment of B Cell Malignancies

One of the principle reasons for studying the regulation of B cell development is that defects in this process may result in lymphoma. Human B lineage neoplasias can be viewed as transformed counterparts of normal B cell developmental stages, such as pro-B, pre-B, immature B, mature B, or plasma cell, based on rearrangement status and surface phenotype (433). In some cases, transformed cells may even retain growth characteristics of the normal counterpart. This type of classification scheme, correlating features of neoplasias with their normal counterparts, has been useful in diagnosis and prognosis of B lineage neoplasias. For example, B precursor acute lymphoblastic leukemia (ALL), the most common type of ALL in children (ALL accounts for 25% of childhood cancer), is a clonal expansion of a cell defined by surface phenotype and Ig rearrangement status as representing the pro-B stage *(453–455)*. Recent analyses of B precursor ALL suggests that it can be subdivided into a pro-B type, predominant in pediatric patients, and a pre-B type, more frequent in adults *(456)*.

Whereas traditional chemotherapeutic agents typically target proliferating cells without specificity for malignant cells, the identification of molecular abnormalities that result in the abnormal survival and proliferation of leukemic cells may lead to the design of novel therapies that specifically target these cells. For example, the successful treatment of mice carrying human B precursor leukemias with antisense strategies and tyrosine kinase inhibitors holds promise for efficacy in humans *(457,458)*. The identification of novel translocations in B-precursor ALL also holds promise in understanding this disease at the molecular level *(459–462)*.

Another therapeutic approach makes use of knowledge of the surface phenotype of the transformed cell, as in the recent development of anti-CD20 therapy for several types of B lymphomas *(463)*. CD20 is a 33 kDa phosphoprotein expressed highly on the surface of mature B cells *(464–466)*. Antibodies to CD20, originally called *B*1, were initially characterized by their stimulatory and inhibitory effects on human B cells, indicating the importance of CD20 in regulating B cell proliferation and differentiation *(467–469)*. Therapeutic anti-CD20, called *Rituximab*, is a chimeric antibody derived by fusing the V regions of a mouse antibody to the human IgG1 constant segment *(470)*. The precise mechanism of depletion is not yet fully understood but likely includes contributions from antibody-dependent cell-mediated cytotoxicity, complement mediated cytotoxicity, and direct antibody binding effects, including sensitization to apoptosis *(463)*.

As most of the cells in many indolent B cell neoplasms, such as non-Hodgkin's lymphoma or chronic lymphocytic leukemia (CLL), are not predominantly in cycle, the problem may be more a failure to die appropriately, rather than a failure to regulate proliferation. A greater understanding of the growth and sensitivity to apoptosis of different types of lymphomas and leukemias may allow more specific targeting using this approach *(471)*. For example, while CLL cells express relatively low levels of CD20, likely requiring higher doses of anti-CD20 for a response, a combination with another antibody recognizing a molecule that is highly expressed on CLL, CD52, has shown promise *(472)*. Alternatively, treatment with anti-CD20 may render the cells generally more sensitive to apoptosis, so that use in combination with more conventional chemotherapeutic agents will be efficacious. These combination therapies are already in clinical trials. Finally, new insights into distinctive growth properties of transformed B cells, such as the role of Wnt signaling in CLL (473), may suggest new approaches to treat such disorders.

Novel technologies may revolutionize our understanding of B cell development and the relationship between normal and transformed cells. For example, recent gene profiling analysis suggests that CLL can be subdivided into two types of diseases, with different severity and different response to therapies (474). This analysis also challenges the earlier classification of the disease as a transformation of normal CD5$^+$ B cells, since there are more similarities with normal memory B cells. It is likely that advances in our understanding of the growth and differentiation of cells that represent transformed counterparts of normal developmental stages will suggest novel therapeutic approaches. In the case of CLL, the development of gene therapy has allowed introduction of a gene product, CD40, into patient leukemia cells that can then serve as stimulators for induction of antitumor responses (475). Analysis of the V gene repertoire of CLL has also revealed recurrent BCR usage, reminiscent of mouse B-1 B cells, potentially a therapeutic target for anti-idiotypic antibodies (476).

ALTERNATIVE STRATEGIES FOR B CELL DEVELOPMENT

The broad outlines, and even many of the details of B cell development are quite similar in mouse and man, but there are striking differences in other species. There is a notable common alternative approach that involves generation of Ig$^+$ cells during fetal/neonatal development with a relatively restricted repertoire that is then diversified by novel approaches (gene conversion or SHM) in specialized lymphoid organs that are associated with the gut. In these species, most development from Ig$^-$ precursors appears to cease by birth, and the B cell population is maintained by self-renewal of mature B cells. Here we consider the development and diversification of B cells in chicken and rabbit.

Chicken

B cell development in the avian occurs in the bursa of Fabricius *(477,478)*. In fact, the term *B cell* refers to "bursa-derived," reflecting the historical origins of research in lymphocyte development. That is, removal of the bursa just after hatching eliminated the ability to mount an antibody response, demonstrating the importance of this organ in generating cells capable of antibody formation *(477)*. In contrast with the bone marrow, the bursa, being associated with the gut *(479)*, facilitates exposure of developing cells to external antigens and bacterial flora. B cell development in chicken is usually divided into three stages: pre-bursal, bursal, and post-bursal (480).

During pre-bursal development, at day E5, early precursors can be identified in the para-aortic foci *(481)*, likely corresponding with similar precursor stages localized in this anatomic site in mammals *(2)*. B lineage commitment, as indicated by DJ rearrangements, is detected in the YS at day E5/6, and V gene rearrangement is found 3 days later *(482)*. Unlike mammalian ordered development, light chain rearrangement is detected at about the same time as heavy chain and light chain can precede heavy chain *(483)*. This means that there is no pre-B stage, per se, and also probably no requirement for surrogate light chain. Rearranging B lineage precursors migrate into the bursal mesenchyme at about day E12, and thereafter these cells begin to proliferate in bursal epithelial buds. This proliferation selectively expands cells that have BCR. These receptors have very limited diversity, since the heavy chain is formed by rearrangement of a single VH, several Ds and a single JH pairing with a light chain generated by rearrangement of a single VL with a single JL (*484*,485). As in mouse fetal development, there is no TdT-mediated N-region addition at the junctions (485).

This "pre-bursal" receptor is diversified by gene conversion by a set of V pseudo-genes during this proliferative phase. At about hatching, these cells become exposed to the contents of the bursal lumen that is connected to the gut lumen via the bursal duct, similar to the appendix. Thus, these proliferating B cells are exposed to the contents of the digestive tract, and there is also reverse peristalsis at the end of the gut that transports external antigens into the bursal duct *(479)*. At about this time, the level of apoptosis increases dramatically, and it is possible that only 5% of the cells generated in the bursa eventually emerge *(486)*. This death may be due to generation of nonfunctional receptors during the course of gene conversion or it may reflect antigenic selection.

At hatching, emigration of B cells from the bursa increases, but most of these cells constitute a population with a relatively short half-life, measured in days (487). The long-lived pool colonizes the peripheral lymphoid organs over several weeks as the bursa atrophies. By 3 weeks after hatching bursectomy no longer results in agammaglobulinemia, indicating that the post-bursal phase has become established.

Rabbit

B cell development in rabbit is similar to chicken, in that B cells initially are produced with a limited BCR diversity (488,489,490) during fetal life, with little new production after birth (491,492). This repertoire is then expanded through gene conversion (488,493) and SHM (493,494) in a specialized gut-associated organ, the appendix (495). However, unlike chicken, this diversification process is dependent on antigen availability (496–498).

Pre-B cells can be found in rabbit before birth in the liver, bone marrow, and omentum (491,499–501), but B lymphopoiesis decreases at birth and is negligible in adult animals (492). Ig rearrangement during fetal and neonatal times is dominated by usage of the most D-proximal V_H gene paired with multiple V_L genes in the light chain (489,490,502–505). In contrast with chicken and mouse, there is significant N-addition (490,504). From 4 to 8 weeks after birth, there is a striking increase in the diversity of this primary repertoire that occurs during proliferation of B cells in the gut-associated lymphoid tissues (GALT) (492, 493). V genes are diversified by both gene conversion (488) and also by SHM (493,494). Importantly, surgical removal of GALT organs, appendix, sacculus rotundus, and the Peyer's patch, from neonatal rabbits led to unresponsiveness to many antigens, suggesting that this diversification was crucial for normal immune function (506). This finding has been confirmed by sequence analysis, demonstrating that removal of the GALT blocks diversification (495).

Considering the relatively late diversification in rabbit compared to the chicken, these gut areas will provide a milieu of microbial antigens, and this appears to be a critical aspect of the diversification process (507). For example, surgery to prevent access of intestinal flora to the appendix blocked diversification in this organ (508,509) that could be restored by reversing the ligation (508). Further, analysis of rabbits reared in germ-free conditions revealed abnormal cellular development in the GALT (497) and a lack of responsiveness to certain antigens (496). The dependence of V gene diversification on antigen has been directly demonstrated in animals where the sacchus rotundus and Peyer's patches were removed at birth and the appendix ligated. Testing the peripheral blood B cell V gene repertoire showed an absence of diversification, in contrast to controls (498). Although the mechanism for this stimulation remains to be established, possibilities include B cell activation by a BCR superantigen (510,511,512) or through a B cell Toll-like receptor (513).

Two B Cell Developmental Pathways?

The similarities of chicken and rabbit B cell development with that in other species, such as sheep, swine, and cow, suggests that the initial production of a limited BCR repertoire during fetal/neonatal life, diversification at a later time, and maintenance of the B cell pool in adult life by self-renewal (rather than *de novo* generation from unrearranged precursors) is a major pattern in the design of the immune system (Figure 7.15). This pattern contrasts with that described for mouse and man, where ordered heavy and light chain rearrangement, pre-BCR selection, and replacement of senescent B cells by newly generated B cells are major aspects of development. This raises the interesting question of whether there is an analogous B cell development pathway in humans or mouse, perhaps as a vestige.

The idea of two pathways in bone marrow development was suggested previously, based on the observation that heavy and light chain ordering is not absolute: Light chain rearrangements are detected in mice incapable of making heavy chain rearrangements and can be detected in cells early in B cell development (514). In one pathway, heavy chains rearrange first, the pre-BCR is assembled and signals down-regulation of Rag-1/2 expression (ending heavy chain rearrangement), clonal expansion, and accessibility of the kappa locus. Cessation of proliferation is coincident with reinduction of Rag-1/2 and light chain rearrangement. Expression of a complete BCR signals a final termination of Rag expression. In this model, pre-BCR and BCR mediates allelic exclusion by a feedback mechanism regulating Rag expression. Thus, most B cells have DJ or even VDJ rearrangements on both alleles. In the alternative pathway, heavy and light chains rearrange stochastically and allelic exclusion is mediated by relative inaccessibility of the loci (and thereby low frequency of rearrangement). If this is the major pathway in chicken and rabbit, it is consistent with the observation that most chicken B cells have only one allele rearranged (485,515,516). Further, the careful ordering of TdT expression, being down-regulated at the light chain rearranging stage, is apparently not the case for rabbit, where a large percentage of light chains have N-regions (505).

Most rabbit B cells express CD5 (517). In mouse, much of the $CD5^+$ B cell population is generated during fetal/neonatal development and persists in the adult through self-renewal (351). Further, these cells express a relatively restricted BCR repertoire that is dependent on antigen selection (23). Finally, the pre-BCR selection phase of several heavy chains abundant in CD5 B cells appears to follow different rules than classical pre-BCR mediated expansion (239). In fact, the process of development in mouse fetal

Human/Mouse Primary Pathway Bone Marrow B Cell Development

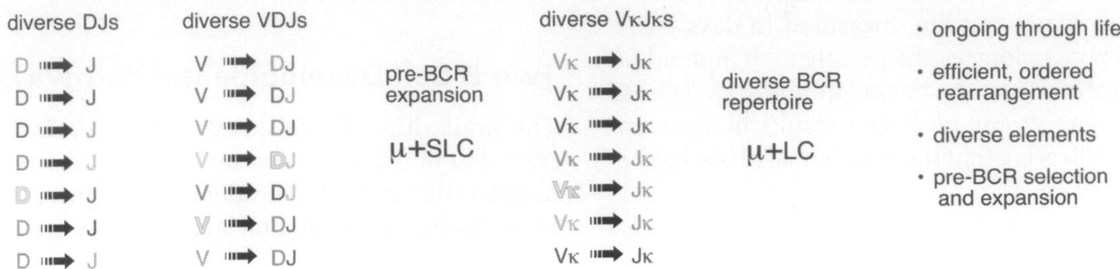

Chicken/Rabbit Alternate Pathway B Cell Development

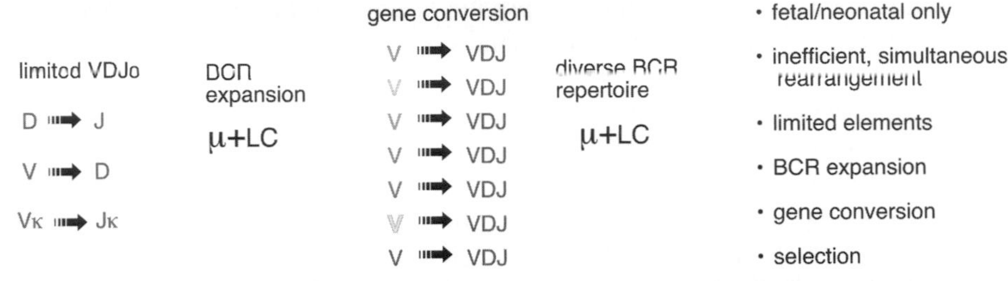

FIGURE 7.15 Alternative strategies of repertoire diversification and B cell development. In both mouse and human bone marrow B cell development, ordered rearrangement predominates, with a pre-BCR selection phase dividing heavy and light chain rearrangement. The eventual outcome is a population of newly formed B cells with a diverse set of BCRs, produced throughout life. In chicken and rabbit, Ig rearrangement appears less efficient (usually the other allele is germline) and much less diverse, with a single BCR for chicken. However, these cells proliferate and undergo gene conversion during fetal/neonatal life, followed by selection, eventually generating a set of B cells with a more diverse repertoire that persist for the life of the animal.

liver may predominantly follow this alternative pathway *(364)*. Thus, in mouse, fetal development, culminating in production of B-1 B cells, may represent a type of alternative or "primitive" B cell development, as has been proposed previously *(518)*. It is less clear whether a similar distinction exists in human B cell development, as data are lacking. Nevertheless, one can envision a primordial pathway, randomly combining heavy and light chains and simply selecting cells that express BCRs with weak reactivity to self- or environmental antigens as an alternative to ordered rearrangement, pre-BCR selection, and BCR selection, an elaborate process fine tuned to generate more variation.

CONCLUSION

There has been considerable progress over the past decade in understanding the mechanisms that regulate B cell development, with important insights coming from application of the novel genetic approaches of transgenesis and gene targeting. In a sense, this has allowed progression from research with simple model systems using cell lines to analysis of "normal B cells" in whole animals. The use of such mutant mouse "reagents," together with much higher resolution of normal development made possible by multiparameter flow cytometry, has proven a powerful combination for unraveling much of the complexity of this process. It is daunting to attempt to predict where new advances in the field will come, but undoubtedly the completion of the genome sequence for both mouse and human will provide impetus to large-scale gene profiles of B cell development, as have already begun (519,520). A complementary approach to gene targeting based on such profiling will involve characterizing new mutant mice generated by chemical mutagenesis (521,*522*). Considering the recent unanticipated discoveries of AID in isotype switching and BAFF in peripheral B cell development, it seems likely that the coming decade will provide many surprises. A goal will be to eventually understand how the interplay of the innate and adaptive immune systems generates protective responses, while avoiding autoimmune pathologies, at the organism level.

ACKNOWLEDGMENTS

Work in my laboratory is supported by grants from the NIH, CA06927, AI26782, and AI40946, and by an appropriation from the Commonwealth of Pennsylvania.

REFERENCES

3. Medvinsky AL, Samoylina NL, Muller AM, et al. An early pre-liver intraembryonic source of CFU-S in the developing mouse. *Nature.* 1993;364:64–67.
4. Muller AM, Medvinsky A, Strouboulis J, et al. Development of hematopoietic stem cell activity in the mouse embryo. *Immunity.* 1994;1:291–301.
6. Yoder MC, Hiatt K, Dutt P, et al. Characterization of definitive lymphohematopoietic stem cells in the day 9 murine yolk sac. *Immunity.* 1997;7:335–344.
8. Strasser A, Rolink A, Melchers F. One synchronous wave of B cell development in mouse fetal liver changes at day 16 of gestation from dependence to independence of a stromal cell environment. *J Exp Med.* 1989;170:1973–1986.
10. Gregoire KE, Goldschneider I, Barton RW, et al. Ontogeny of terminal deoxynucleotidyl transferase-positive cells in lymphohemopoietic tissues of rat and mouse. *J Immunol.* 1979;123:1347–1352.
11. Li YS, Hayakawa K, Hardy RR. The regulated expression of B lineage associated genes during B cell differentiation in bone marrow and fetal liver. *J Exp Med.* 1993;78:951–960.
13. Desiderio SV, Yancopoulos GD, Paskind M, et al. Insertion of N regions into heavy-chain genes is correlated with expression of terminal deoxytransferase in B cells. *Nature.* 1984;311:752–755.
15. Feeney AJ. Lack of N regions in fetal and neonatal mouse immunoglobulin V-D-J junctional sequences. *J Exp Med.* 1990;172: 1377–1390.
19. Hayakawa K, Tarlinton D, Hardy RR. 1994. Absence of MHC class II expression distinguishes fetal from adult B lymphopoiesis in mice. *J Immunol.* 1994;152:4801–4807.
22. Carvalho TL, Mota-Santos T, Cumano A, et al. Arrested B lymphopoiesis and persistence of activated B cells in adult interleukin 7(−/−) mice. *J Exp Med.* 2001;194:1141–1150.
23. Hardy RR, Hayakawa K. B cell development pathways. *Annu Rev Immunol.* 2001;19:595–621.
26. Ogawa M, Matsuzaki Y, Nishikawa S, et al. Expression and function of c-kit in hemopoietic progenitor cells. *J Exp Med.* 1991;174:63–71.
28. Spangrude GJ, Heimfeld S, Weissman IL. Purification and characterization of mouse hematopoietic stem cells. *Science.* 1988;241: 58–62.
31. Kondo M, Weissman IL, Akashi K. Identification of clonogenic common lymphoid progenitors in mouse bone marrow. *Cell.* 2000;91: 661–672.
32. Akashi K, Traver D, Miyamoto T, et al. A clonogenic common myeloid progenitor that gives rise to all myeloid lineages. *Nature.* 2000;404:193–197.
34. Kondo M, Scherer DC, Miyamoto T, et al. Cell-fate conversion of lymphoid-committed progenitors by instructive actions of cytokines. *Nature.* 2000;407:383–386.
35. Miyamoto T, Iwasaki H, Reizis B, et al. Myeloid or lymphoid promiscuity as a critical step in hematopoietic lineage commitment. *Dev Cell.* 2002;3:137–147.
38. Li YS, Wasserman R, Hayakawa K, et al. Identification of the earliest B lineage stage in mouse bone marrow. *Immunity.* 1996;5:527–535.
39. Nutt SL, Heavey B, Rolink AG, et al. Commitment to the B-lymphoid lineage depends on the transcription factor Pax5. *Nature.* 1999;401:556–562.
44. Rumfelt LL, Zhou Y, Rowley BM, et al. Lineage specification and plasticity in CD19- early B cell precursors. *J Exp Med.* 2006;203: 675–687.
46. Borghesi L, Hsu LY, Miller JP, et al. B lineage-specific regulation of V(D)J recombinase activity is established in common lymphoid progenitors. *J Exp Med.* 2004;199:491–502.
47. Allman D, Sambandam A, Kim S, et al. Thymopoiesis independent of common lymphoid progenitors. *Nat Immunol.* 2003;4:168–174.
48. Cumano A, Paige CJ, Iscove NN, et al. Bipotential precursors of B cells and macrophages in murine fetal liver. *Nature.* 1992;356:612–615.
51. Igarashi H, Gregory SC, Yokota T, et al. Transcription from the RAG1 locus marks the earliest lymphocyte progenitors in bone marrow. *Immunity.* 2002;17:117–130.
57. Georgopoulos K, Bigby M, Wang JH, et al. The Ikaros gene is required for the development of all lymphoid lineages. *Cell.* 1994;79:143–156.
59. Wang JH, Nichogiannopoulou A, Wu L, et al. Selective defects in the development of the fetal and adult lymphoid system in mice with an Ikaros null mutation. *Immunity.* 1996;5:537–549.
60. Wang JH, Avitahl N, Cariappa A, et al. Aiolos regulates B cell activation and maturation to effector state. *Immunity.* 1998;9:543–553.
61. Scott EW, Simon MC, Anastasi J, et al. Requirement of transcription factor PU.1 in the development of multiple hematopoietic lineages. *Science.* 1994;265:1573–1577.
62. McKercher SR, Torbett BE, Anderson KL, et al. Targeted disruption of the PU.1 gene results in multiple hematopoietic abnormalities. *Embo J.* 1996;15:5647–5658.
63. DeKoter RP, Singh H. Regulation of B lymphocyte and macrophage development by graded expression of PU.1. *Science.* 2000;288:1439–1441.
65. DeKoter RP, Lee HJ, Singh H. PU.1 regulates expression of the interleukin-7 receptor in lymphoid progenitors. *Immunity.* 2002;16:297–309.
68. Bain G, Maandag EC, Izon DJ, et al. E2A proteins are required for proper B cell development and initiation of immunoglobulin gene rearrangements. *Cell.* 1994;79:885–892.
69. Bain G, Robanus Maandag EC, te Riele HP, et al. Both E12 and E47 allow commitment to the B cell lineage. *Immunity.* 1997;6:145–154.
71. Espinoza CR, Feeney AJ. The extent of histone acetylation correlates with the differential rearrangement frequency of individual VH genes in pro-B cells. *J Immunol.* 2005;175:6668–6675.
72. Pui JC, Allman D, Xu L, et al. Notch1 expression in early lymphopoiesis influences B versus T lineage determination. *Immunity.* 1999;11:299–308.
76. Koch U, Lacombe TA, Holland D, et al. 2001. Subversion of the T/B lineage decision in the thymus by lunatic fringe- mediated inhibition of Notch-1. *Immunity.* 15:225–236.
77. Izon DJ, Aster JC, He Y, et al. Deltex1 redirects lymphoid progenitors to the B cell lineage by antagonizing Notch1. *Immunity.* 2002;16:231–243.
79. Lin H, Grosschedl R. Failure of B-cell differentiation in mice lacking the transcription factor EBF. *Nature.* 1995;376:263–267.
80. O'Riordan M, Grosschedl R. Coordinate regulation of B cell differentiation by the transcription factors EBF and E2A. *Immunity.* 1999;11:21–31.
82. Kee BL, Murre C. Induction of early B cell factor (EBF) and multiple B lineage genes by the basic helix-loop-helix transcription factor E12. *J Exp Med.* 1998;188:699–713.
83. Roessler S, Gyory I, Imhof S, et al. Distinct promoters mediate the regulation of ebf1 gene expression by interleukin-7 and pax5. *Mol Cell Biol.* 2007;27:579–594.
85. Singh H, Medina KL, Pongubala JM. Contingent gene regulatory networks and B cell fate specification. *Proc Natl Acad Sci U S A.* 2005;102:4949–4953.
90. Tagoh H, Ingram R, Wilson N, et al. The mechanism of repression of the myeloid-specific c-fms gene by Pax5 during B lineage restriction. *Embo J.* 2006;25:1070–1080.
91. Souabni A, Cobaleda C, Schebesta M, et al. Pax5 promotes B lymphopoiesis and blocks T cell development by repressing Notch1. *Immunity.* 2002;17:781–793.
92. Wilson A, MacDonald HR, Radtke F. Notch 1-deficient common lymphoid precursors adopt a B cell fate in the thymus. *J Exp Med.* 2001;194:1003–1012.
94. Reya T, O'Riordan M, Okamura R, et al. Wnt signaling regulates B lymphocyte proliferation through a LEF-1 dependent mechanism. *Immunity.* 2000;13:15–24.
95. Lee G, Namen AE, Gillis S, et al. Normal B cell precursors responsive to recombinant murine IL-7 and inhibition of IL-7 activity by transforming growth factor-beta. *J Immunol.* 1989;142: 3875–3883.
98. Lenardo MJ, Baltimore D. NF-kappa B: a pleiotropic mediator of inducible and tissue-specific gene control. *Cell.* 1989;58:227–229.
99. Horwitz BH, Scott ML, Cherry SR, et al. Failure of lymphopoiesis after adoptive transfer of NF-kappaB-deficient fetal liver cells. *Immunity.* 1997;6:765–772.

109. Hayashi S, Kunisada T, Ogawa M, et al. Stepwise progression of B lineage differentiation supported by interleukin 7 and other stromal cell molecules. *J Exp Med.* 1990;171:1683–1695.
111. Miyake K, Weissman IL, Greenberger JS, et al. Evidence for a role of the integrin VLA-4 in lympho-hemopoiesis. *J Exp Med.* 1991;173:599–607.
112. Era T, Ogawa M, Nishikawa S, et al. Differentiation of growth signal requirement of B lymphocyte precursor is directed by expression of immunoglobulin. *Embo J.* 1991;10:337–342.
113. Hardy RR, Carmack CE, Shinton SA, et al. Resolution and characterization of pro-B and pre-pro-B cell stages in normal mouse bone marrow. *J Exp Med.* 1991;173:1213–1225.
118. Johnson P, Greenbaum L, Bottomly K, et al. Identification of the alternatively spliced exons of murine CD45 (T200) required for reactivity with B220 and other T200-restricted antibodies. *J Exp Med.* 1989;169:1179–1184.
122. Whitlock CA, Witte ON. Long-term culture of B lymphocytes and their precursors from murine bone marrow. *Proc Natl Acad Sci U S A.* 1982;79:3608–3612.
124. Whitlock C, Denis K, Robertson D, et al. In vitro analysis of murine B-cell development. *Annu Rev Immunol.* 1985;3:213–235.
127. Pietrangeli CE, Hayashi S, Kincade PW. 1988. Stromal cell lines which support lymphocyte growth: characterization, sensitivity to radiation and responsiveness to growth factors. *Eur J Immunol* 18:863–872.
128. Miyake K, Underhill CB, Lesley J, et al. Hyaluronate can function as a cell adhesion molecule and CD44 participates in hyaluronate recognition. *J Exp Med.* 1990;172:69–75.
132. Namen AE, Lupton S, Hjerrild K, et al. Stimulation of B-cell progenitors by cloned murine interleukin-7. *Nature.* 1988;333:571–573.
139. Peschon JJ, Morrissey PJ, Grabstein KH, et al. Early lymphocyte expansion is severely impaired in interleukin 7 receptor-deficient mice. *J Exp Med.* 1994; 180:1955–1960.
140. Ray RJ, Furlonger C, Williams DE, et al. Characterization of thymic stromal-derived lymphopoietin (TSLP) in murine B cell development in vitro. *Eur J Immunol.* 1996;26:10–16.
142. Park LS, Martin U, Garka K, et al. Cloning of the murine thymic stromal lymphopoietin (TSLP) receptor: Formation of a functional heteromeric complex requires interleukin 7 receptor. *J Exp Med.* 2000;192:659–670.
145. Vosshenrich CA, Cumano A, Muller W, et al. Thymic stromal-derived lymphopoietin distinguishes fetal from adult B cell development. *Nat Immunol.* 2003;4:773–779.
149. Tsuji K, Lyman SD, Sudo T, et al. Enhancement of murine hematopoiesis by synergistic interactions between steel factor (ligand for c-kit), interleukin-11, and other early acting factors in culture. *Blood.* 1992;79:2855–2860.
155. Veiby OP, Lyman SD, Jacobsen SE. Combined signaling through interleukin-7 receptors and flt3 but not c- kit potently and selectively promotes B-cell commitment and differentiation from uncommitted murine bone marrow progenitor cells. *Blood.* 1996;88:1256–1265.
156. Billips LG, Petitte D, Dorshkind K, et al. Differential roles of stromal cells, interleukin-7, and kit-ligand in the regulation of B lymphopoiesis. *Blood.* 1992;79:1185–1192.
158. Cumano A, Dorshkind K, Gillis S, et al. The influence of S17 stromal cells and interleukin 7 on B cell development. *Eur J Immunol.* 1990;20:2183–2189.
159. Winkler TH, Melchers F, Rolink AG. Interleukin-3 and interleukin-7 are alternative growth factors for the same B-cell precursors in the mouse. *Blood.* 1995;85:2045–2051.
163. Spanopoulou E, Roman CA, Corcoran LM, et al. Functional immunoglobulin transgenes guide ordered B-cell differentiation in Rag-1-deficient mice. *Genes Dev.* 1994;8:1030–1042.
166. Kincade PW, Medina KL, Payne KJ, et al. Early B-lymphocyte precursors and their regulation by sex steroids. *Immunol Rev.* 2000;175:128–137.
168. Landreth KS, Narayanan R, Dorshkind K. Insulin-like growth factor-I regulates pro-B cell differentiation. *Blood.* 1992;80:1207–1212.
170. Zhang Y, Lu L, Furlonger C, et al. Hemokinin is a hematopoietic-specific tachykinin that regulates B lymphopoiesis. *Nat Immunol.* 2000;1:392–397.
171. Montecino-Rodriguez E, Clark RG, Powell-Braxton L, et al. Primary B cell development is impaired in mice with defects of the pituitary/thyroid axis. *J Immunol.* 1997;159:2712–2719.
173. Nagai Y, Garrett KP, Ohta S, et al. Toll-like receptors on hematopoietic progenitor cells stimulate innate immune system replenishment. *Immunity.* 2006;24:801–812.
174. Allman D, Karnell FG, Punt JA, et al. Separation of Notch1 promoted lineage commitment and expansion/transformation in developing T cells. *J Exp Med.* 2001;194:99–106.
177. Bleul CC, Fuhlbrigge RC, Casasnovas JM, et al. A highly efficacious lymphocyte chemoattractant, stromal cell-derived factor 1 (SDF-1). *J Exp Med.* 1996;184:1101–1109.
181. Nagasawa T, Hirota S, Tachibana K, et al. Defects of B-cell lymphopoiesis and bone-marrow myelopoiesis in mice lacking the CXC chemokine PBSF/SDF-1. *Nature.* 1996;382:635–638.
183. Zou YR, Kottmann AH, Kuroda M, et al. Function of the chemokine receptor CXCR4 in haematopoiesis and in cerebellar development. *Nature.* 1998;393:595–599.
188. Oettinger MA, Schatz DG, Gorka C, et al. RAG-1 and RAG-2, adjacent genes that synergistically activate V(D)J recombination. *Science.* 1990;248:1517–1523.
191. Desiderio SV, Yancopoulos GD, Paskind M, et al. Insertion of N regions into heavy-chain genes is correlated with expression of terminal deoxytransferase in B cells. *Nature.* 1984;311:752–755.
195. Bosma GC, Custer RP, Bosma MJ. A severe combined immunodeficiency mutation in the mouse. *Nature.* 1983;301:527–530.
197. Blunt T, Finnie NJ, Taccioli GE, et al. Defective DNA-dependent protein kinase activity is linked to V(D)J recombination and DNA repair defects associated with the murine scid mutation. *Cell.* 1995;80:813–823.
200. Kitamura D, Roes J, Kuhn R, et al. A B cell-deficient mouse by targeted disruption of the membrane exon of the immunoglobulin mu chain gene. *Nature.* 1991;350:423–426.
202. Karasuyama H, Kudo A, Melchers F. The proteins encoded by the VpreB and lambda 5 pre-B cell-specific genes can associate with each other and with mu heavy chain. *J Exp Med.* 1990;172:969–972.
203. Sakaguchi N, Melchers F. Lambda 5, a new light-chain-related locus selectively expressed in pre- B lymphocytes. *Nature.* 1986;324:579–582.
205. Kitamura D, Kudo A, Schaal S, et al. A critical role of lambda 5 protein in B cell development. *Cell.* 1992;69:823–831.
206. Papavasiliou F, Jankovic M, Nussenzweig MC. Surrogate or conventional light chains are required for membrane immunoglobulin mu to activate the precursor B cell transition. *J Exp Med.* 1996;184:2025–2030.
207. Sakaguchi N, Kashiwamura S, Kimoto M, et al. B lymphocyte lineage-restricted expression of mb-1, a gene with CD3- like structural properties. *Embo J.* 1988;7:3457–3464.
208. Hermanson GG, Eisenberg D, Kincade PW, et al. B29: a member of the immunoglobulin gene superfamily exclusively expressed on beta-lineage cells. *Proc Natl Acad Sci U S A.* 1988;85:6890–6894.
211. Gong S, Nussenzweig MC. Regulation of an early developmental checkpoint in the B cell pathway by Ig beta. *Science.* 1996;272:411–414.
212. Cheng AM, Rowley B, Pao W, et al. Syk tyrosine kinase required for mouse viability and B-cell development. *Nature.* 1995;378:303–306.
215. Lam KP, Kuhn R, Rajewsky K. In vivo ablation of surface immunoglobulin on mature B cells by inducible gene targeting results in rapid cell death. *Cell.* 1997;90:1073–1083.
216. Kraus M, Alimzhanov MB, Rajewsky N, et al. Survival of resting mature B lymphocytes depends on BCR signaling via the Igalpha/beta heterodimer. *Cell.* 2004;117:787–800.
218. Wasserman R, Li YS, Hardy RR. Down-regulation of terminal deoxynucleotidyl transferase by Ig heavy chain in B lineage cells. *J Immunol.* 1997;158:1133–1138.
219. Middendorp S, Dingjan GM, Hendriks RW. Impaired precursor B cell differentiation in Bruton's tyrosine kinase-deficient mice. *J Immunol.* 2002;168:2695–2703.
224. Kurosaki T. Genetic analysis of B cell antigen receptor signaling. *Annu Rev Immunol.* 1999;17:555–592.

226. Xu S, Wong SC, Lam KP. Cutting edge: B cell linker protein is dispensable for the allelic exclusion of immunoglobulin heavy chain locus but required for the persistence of CD5+ B cells. *J Immunol.* 2000;165:4153–4157.
227. Grawunder U, Leu TM, Schatz DG, et al. Down-regulation of RAG1 and RAG2 gene expression in preB cells after functional immunoglobulin heavy chain rearrangement. *Immunity.* 1995;3:601–608.
228. Schlissel MS, Baltimore D. Activation of immunoglobulin kappa gene rearrangement correlates with induction of germline kappa gene transcription. *Cell.* 1989;58:1001–1007.
230. Hsu LY, Lauring J, Liang HE, et al. A conserved transcriptional enhancer regulates RAG gene expression in developing B cells. *Immunity.* 2003;19:105–117.
232. Li Z, Dordai DI, Lee J, et al. A conserved degradation signal regulates RAG-2 accumulation during cell division and links V(D)J recombination to the cell cycle. *Immunity.* 1996;5:575–589.
237. Kline GH, Hartwell L, Beck-Engeser GB, et al. Pre-B cell receptor-mediated selection of pre-B cells synthesizing functional mu heavy chains. *J Immunol.* 1998;161:1608–1618.
238. ten Boekel E, Melchers F, Rolink AG. Changes in the V(H) gene repertoire of developing precursor B lymphocytes in mouse bone marrow mediated by the pre-B cell receptor. *Immunity.* 1997;7:357–368.
239. Wasserman R, Li YS, Shinton SA, et al. A novel mechanism for B cell repertoire maturation based on response by B cell precursors to pre-B receptor assembly. *J Exp Med.* 1998;187:259–264.
242. Yancopoulos GD, Desiderio SV, Paskind M, et al. Preferential utilization of the most JH-proximal VH gene segments in pre-B-cell lines. *Nature.* 1984;311:727–733.
244. Decker DJ, Kline GH, Hayden TA, et al. Heavy chain V gene-specific elimination of B cells during the pre-B cell to B cell transition. *J Immunol.* 1995;154:4924–4935.
247. Marshall AJ, Paige CJ, Wu GE. V(H) repertoire maturation during B cell development in vitro: differential selection of Ig heavy chains by fetal and adult B cell progenitors. *J Immunol.* 1997;158:4282–4291.
249. Tiegs SL, Russell DM, Nemazee D. Receptor editing in self-reactive bone marrow B cells. *J Exp Med.* 1993;177:1009–1020.
252. Chen C, Nagy Z, Radic MZ, et al. The site and stage of anti-DNA B-cell deletion. *Nature.* 1995;373:252–255.
254. Allman DM, Ferguson SE, Cancro MP. Peripheral B cell maturation. I. Immature peripheral B cells in adults are heat-stable antigenhi and exhibit unique signaling characteristics. *J Immunol.* 1992;149:2533–2540.
255. Rolink AG, Andersson J, Melchers F. Characterization of immature B cells by a novel monoclonal antibody, by turnover and by mitogen reactivity. *Eur J Immunol.* 1998;28:3738–3748.
256. Allman D, Lindsley RC, DeMuth W, et al. Resolution of three nonproliferative immature splenic B cell subsets reveals multiple selection points during peripheral B cell maturation. *J Immunol.* 2001;167:6834–6840.
259. Carsetti R, Kohler G, Lamers MC. Transitional B cells are the target of negative selection in the B cell compartment. *J Exp Med.* 1995;181:2129–2140.
265. Goodnow CC, Crosbie J, Adelstein S, et al. Altered immunoglobulin expression and functional silencing of self-reactive B lymphocytes in transgenic mice. *Nature.* 1988;334:676–682.
266. Hartley SB, Crosbie J, Brink R, et al. Elimination from peripheral lymphoid tissues of self-reactive B lymphocytes recognizing membrane-bound antigens. *Nature.* 1991;353:765–769.
267. Nemazee DA, Burki K. Clonal deletion of B lymphocytes in a transgenic mouse bearing anti-MHC class I antibody genes. *Nature.* 1989;337:562–566.
268. Erikson J, Radic MZ, Camper SA, et al. Expression of anti-DNA immunoglobulin transgenes in non-autoimmune mice. *Nature.* 1991;349:331–334.
269. Gay D, Saunders T, Camper S, et al. Receptor editing: an approach by autoreactive B cells to escape tolerance. *J Exp Med.* 1993;177:999–1008.
271. Norvell A, Mandik L, Monroe JG. Engagement of the antigen-receptor on immature murine B lymphocytes results in death by apoptosis. *J Immunol.* 1995;154:4404–4413.
273. Rathmell JC, Goodnow CC. Effects of the lpr mutation on elimination and inactivation of self-reactive B cells. *J Immunol.* 1994;153:2831–2842.
274. Rubio CF, Kench J, Russell DM, et al. Analysis of central B cell tolerance in autoimmune-prone MRL/lpr mice bearing autoantibody transgenes. *J Immunol.* 1996;157:65–71.
276. Benschop RJ, Melamed D, Nemazee D, et al. Distinct signal thresholds for the unique antigen receptor-linked gene expression programs in mature and immature B cells. *J Exp Med.* 1999;190:749–756.
283. Oka Y, Rolink AG, Andersson J, et al. Profound reduction of mature B cell numbers, reactivities and serum Ig levels in mice which simultaneously carry the XID and CD40 deficiency genes. *Int Immunol.* 1996;8:1675–1685.
284. Clark MR, Campbell KS, Kazlauskas A, et al. The B cell antigen receptor complex: association of Ig-alpha and Ig-beta with distinct cytoplasmic effectors. *Science.* 1992;258:123–126.
290. Cyster JG, Hartley SB, Goodnow CC. Competition for follicular niches excludes self-reactive cells from the recirculating B-cell repertoire. *Nature.* 1994;371:389–395.
293. Mandik Nayak L, Seo SJ, Sokol C, et al. MRL-lpr/lpr mice exhibit a defect in maintaining developmental arrest and follicular exclusion of anti-double-stranded DNA B cells. *J Exp Med.* 1999;189:1799–1814.
295. Thomas MD, Kremer CS, Ravichandran KS, et al. c-Myb is critical for B cell development and maintenance of follicular B cells. *Immunity.* 2005;23:275–286.
298. Ansel KM, Ngo VN, Hyman PL, et al. A chemokine-driven positive feedback loop organizes lymphoid follicles. *Nature.* 2000;406:309–314.
302. Thompson JS, Bixler SA, Qian F, et al. BAFF-R, a newly identified TNF receptor that specifically interacts with BAFF. *Science.* 2001;293:2108–2111.
304. Lentz VM, Cancro MP, Nashold FE, et al. Bcmd governs recruitment of new B cells into the stable peripheral B cell pool in the A/WySnJ mouse. *J Immunol.* 1996;157:598–606.
308. Forster I, Rajewsky K. The bulk of the peripheral B cell pool in mice is stable and not rapidly renewed from the bone marrow. *Proc Natl Acad Sci U S A.* 1990;87:4781–4784.
309. Hao Z, Rajewsky K. Homeostasis of peripheral B cells in the absence of B cell influx from the bone marrow. *J Exp Med.* 2001;194:1151–1164.
310. MacLennan IC. Germinal centers. *Annu Rev Immunol.* 1994;12:117–139.
312. Butcher EC, Rouse RV, Coffman RL, et al. Surface phenotype of Peyer's patch germinal center cells: implications for the role of germinal centers in B cell differentiation. *J Immunol.* 1982;129:2698–2707.
315. Tuscano JM, Druey KM, Riva A, et al. Bcl-x rather than Bcl-2 mediates CD40-dependent centrocyte survival in the germinal center. *Blood.* 1996;88:1359–1364.
317. Takahashi Y, Ohta H, Takemori T. Fas is required for clonal selection in germinal centers and the subsequent establishment of the memory B cell repertoire. *Immunity.* 2001;14:181–192.
318. Muramatsu M, Kinoshita K, Fagarasan S, et al. Class switch recombination and hypermutation require activation-induced cytidine deaminase (AID), a potential RNA editing enzyme. *Cell.* 2000;102:553–563.
321. Martin A, Bardwell PD, Woo CJ, et al. Activation-induced cytidine deaminase turns on somatic hypermutation in hybridomas. *Nature.* 2002;415:802–806.
332. Nagaoka H, Gonzalez-Aseguinolaza G, Tsuji M, et al. Immunization and infection change the number of recombination activating gene (RAG)-expressing B cells in the periphery by altering immature lymphocyte production. *J Exp Med.* 2000;191:2113–2120.
339. Herzenberg LA, Black SJ, Tokuhisa T. Memory B cells at successive stages of differentiation. Affinity maturation and the role of IgD receptors. *J Exp Med.* 1980;151:1071–1087.
341. Hayakawa K, Ishii R, Yamasaki K, et al. Isolation of high-affinity memory B cells: phycoerythrin as a probe for antigen-binding cells. *Proc Natl Acad Sci U S A.* 1987;84:1379–1383.

349. Maruyama M, Lam KP, Rajewsky K. Memory B-cell persistence is independent of persisting immunizing antigen. *Nature.* 2000;407:636–642.
352. Hayakawa K, Hardy RR, Honda M, et al. Ly-1 B cells: functionally distinct lymphocytes that secrete IgM autoantibodies. *Proc Natl Acad Sci U S A.* 1984;81:2494–2498.
354. Hayakawa K, Carmack CE, Hyman R, et al. Natural autoantibodies to thymocytes: origin, VH genes, fine specificities, and the role of Thy-1 glycoprotein. *J Exp Med.* 1990;172:869–878.
359. Ochsenbein AF, Fehr T, Lutz C, et al. Control of early viral and bacterial distribution and disease by natural antibodies. *Science.* 1999;286:2156–2159.
360. Macpherson AJ, Gatto D, Sainsbury E, et al. A primitive T cell-independent mechanism of intestinal mucosal IgA responses to commensal bacteria. *Science.* 2000;288:2222–2226.
362. Baumgarth N, Herman OC, Jager GC, et al. B-1 and B-2 cell-derived immunoglobulin M antibodies are nonredundant components of the protective response to influenza virus infection. *J Exp Med.* 2000;192:271–280.
363. Hardy RR, Hayakawa K. A developmental switch in B lymphopoiesis. *Proc Natl Acad Sci U S A.* 1991;88:11550–11554.
367. Martin F, Kearney JF. B-cell subsets and the mature preimmune repertoire. Marginal zone and B1 B cells as part of a "natural immune memory." *Immunol Rev.* 2000;175:70–79.
369. Hayakawa K, Asano M, Shinton SA, et al. Positive selection of natural autoreactive B cells. *Science.* 1999;285:113–116.
374. Hayakawa K, Hardy RR, Parks DR, et al. The "Ly-1 B" cell subpopulation in normal immunodefective, and autoimmune mice. *J Exp Med.* 1983;157:202–218.
375. Khan WN, Alt FW, Gerstein RM, et al. Defective B cell development and function in Btk-deficient mice. *Immunity.* 1995;3:283–299.
377. Rickert RC, Rajewsky K, Roes J. Impairment of T-cell-dependent B-cell responses and B-1 cell development in CD19-deficient mice. *Nature.* 1995;376:352–355.
380. Casola S, Otipoby KL, Alimzhanov M, et al. B cell receptor signal strength determines B cell fate. *Nat Immunol.* 2004;5:317–327.
385. Martin F, Oliver AM, Kearney JF. Marginal zone and B1 B cells unite in the early response against T- independent blood-borne particulate antigens. *Immunity.* 2001;14:617–629.
387. Saito T, Chiba S, Ichikawa M, et al. Notch2 is preferentially expressed in mature B cells and indispensable for marginal zone B lineage development. *Immunity.* 2003;18:675–685.
391. Martin F, Kearney JF. Positive selection from newly formed to marginal zone B cells depends on the rate of clonal production, CD19, and btk. *Immunity.* 2000;12:39–49.
392. Cariappa A, Tang M, Parng C, et al. The follicular versus marginal zone B lymphocyte cell fate decision is regulated by Aiolos, Btk, and CD21. *Immunity.* 2001;14:603–615.
395. Martin F, Chen X, Kearney JF. Development of VH81X transgene-bearing B cells in fetus and adult: sites for expansion and deletion in conventional and CD5/B1 cells. *Int Immunol.* 1997;9:493–505.
398. Russell DM, Dembic Z, Morahan G, et al. Peripheral deletion of self-reactive B cells. *Nature.* 1991;354:308–311.
399. Cyster JG, Goodnow CC. PTP1C negatively regulates antigen receptor signaling in B lymphocytes and determines thresholds for negative selection. *Immunity.* 1995;2:13–24.
400. Cyster JG, Healy JI, Kishihara K, et al. Regulation of B-lymphocyte negative and positive selection by tyrosine phosphatase CD45. *Nature.* 1996;381:325–328.
404. Murakami M, Tsubata T, Okamoto M, et al. Antigen-induced apoptotic death of Ly-1 B cells responsible for autoimmune disease in transgenic mice. *Nature.* 1992;357:77–80.
409. Hayakawa K, Asano M, Shinton SA, et al. Positive selection of anti-thy-1 autoreactive B-1 cells and natural serum autoantibody production independent from bone marrow B cell development. *J Exp Med.* 2003;197:87–99.
410. Wen L, Brill-Dashoff J, Shinton SA, et al. Evidence of marginal-zone B cell-positive selection in spleen. *Immunity.* 2005;23:297–308.
414. Carroll MC. The role of complement in B cell activation and tolerance. *Adv Immunol.* 2000;74:61–88.
415. Inaoki M, Sato S, Weintraub BC, et al. CD19-regulated signaling thresholds control peripheral tolerance and autoantibody production in B lymphocytes. *J Exp Med.* 1997;186:1923–1931.
425. LeBien TW, Wormann B, Villablanca JG, et al. Multiparameter flow cytometric analysis of human fetal bone marrow B cells. *Leukemia.* 1990;4:354–358.
427. Ghia P, ten Boekel E, Sanz E, et al. Ordering of human bone marrow B lymphocyte precursors by single-cell polymerase chain reaction analyses of the rearrangement status of the immunoglobulin H and L chain gene loci. *J Exp Med.* 1996;184:2217–2229.
431. LeBien TW. Fates of human B-cell precursors. *Blood.* 2000;96:9–23.
433. Bauer SR, Kubagawa H, Maclennan I, et al. VpreB gene expression in hematopoietic malignancies: a lineage- and stage-restricted marker for B-cell precursor leukemias. *Blood.* 1991;78:1581–1588.
437. Minegishi Y, Coustan-Smith E, Wang YH, et al. Mutations in the human lambda5/14.1 gene result in B cell deficiency and agammaglobulinemia. *J Exp Med.* 1998;187:71–77.
446. Tsukada S, Saffran DC, Rawlings DJ, et al. Deficient expression of a B cell cytoplasmic tyrosine kinase in human X- linked agammaglobulinemia. *Cell.* 1993;72:279–290.
447. Rawlings DJ, Saffran DC, Tsukada S, et al. Mutation of unique region of Bruton's tyrosine kinase in immunodeficient XID mice. *Science.* 1993;261:358–361.
449. Minegishi Y, Rohrer J, Coustan-Smith E, et al. An essential role for BLNK in human B cell development. *Science.* 1999;286:1954–1957.
473. Lu D, Zhao Y, Tawatao R, et al. Activation of the Wnt signaling pathway in chronic lymphocytic leukemia. *Proc Natl Acad Sci U S A.* 2004;101:3118–3123.
474. Rosenwald A, Alizadeh AA, Widhopf G, et al. Relation of gene expression phenotype to immunoglobulin mutation genotype in B cell chronic lymphocytic leukemia. *J Exp Med.* 2001;194:1639–1647.
475. Wierda WG, Cantwell MJ, Woods SJ, et al. CD40-ligand (CD154) gene therapy for chronic lymphocytic leukemia. *Blood.* 2000;96:2917–2924.
476. Widhopf GF, 2nd, Rassenti LZ, Toy TL, et al. Chronic lymphocytic leukemia B cells of more than 1% of patients express virtually identical immunoglobulins. *Blood.* 2004;104:2499–2504.
480. McCormack WT, Tjoelker LW, Thompson CB. Avian B-cell development: generation of an immunoglobulin repertoire by gene conversion. *Annu Rev Immunol.* 1991;9:219–241.
485. Reynaud CA, Dahan A, Anquez V, et al. Somatic hyperconversion diversifies the single Vh gene of the chicken with a high incidence in the D region. *Cell.* 1989;59:171–183.
488. Becker RS, Knight KL. Somatic diversification of immunoglobulin heavy chain VDJ genes: evidence for somatic gene conversion in rabbits. *Cell.* 1990;63:987–997.
492. Crane MA, Kingzette M, Knight KL. Evidence for limited B-lymphopoiesis in adult rabbits. *J Exp Med.* 1996;183:2119–2121.
495. Vajdy M, Sethupathi P, Knight KL. Dependence of antibody somatic diversification on gut-associated lymphoid tissue in rabbits. *J Immunol.* 1998;160:2725–2729.
507. Mage RG, Lanning D, Knight KL. B cell and antibody repertoire development in rabbits: the requirement of gut-associated lymphoid tissues. *Dev Comp Immunol.* 2006;30:137–153.
512. Silverman GJ, Cary SP, Dwyer DC, et al. A B cell superantigen-induced persistent "Hole" in the B-1 repertoire. *J Exp Med.* 2000;192:87–98.
515. Reynaud CA, Anquez V, Grimal H, et al. A hyperconversion mechanism generates the chicken light chain preimmune repertoire. *Cell.* 1987;48:379–388.
516. McCormack WT, Tjoelker LW, Barth CF, et al. Selection for B cells with productive IgL gene rearrangements occurs in the bursa of Fabricius during chicken embryonic development. *Genes Dev.* 1989;3:838–847.
519. Glynne R, Akkaraju S, Healy JI, et al. How self-tolerance and the immunosuppressive drug FK506 prevent B-cell mitogenesis. *Nature.* 2000;403:672–676.
520. Hoffmann R, Seidl T, Neeb M, et al. Changes in gene expression profiles in developing B cells of murine bone marrow. *Genome Res.* 2002;12:98–111.
521. Nelms KA, Goodnow CC. Genome-wide ENU mutagenesis to reveal immune regulators. *Immunity.* 2001;15:409–418.
526. Funk PE, Kincade PW, Witte PL. Native associations of early hematopoietic stem cells and stromal cells isolated in bone marrow cell aggregates. *Blood.* 1994;83:361–369.

527. Medina KL, Kincade PW. Pregnancy-related steroids are potential negative regulators of B lymphopoiesis. *Proc Natl Acad Sci U S A.* 1994;91:5382–5386.
528. Smithson G, Couse JF, Lubahn DB, et al. The role of estrogen receptors and androgen receptors in sex steroid regulation of B lymphopoiesis. *J Immunol.* 1998;161:27–34.
530. Roark JH, Kuntz CL, Nguyen KA, et al. Breakdown of B cell tolerance in a mouse model of systemic lupus erythematosus. *J Exp Med.* 1995;181:1157–1167.
531. Chen C, Prak EL, Weigert M. Editing disease-associated autoantibodies. *Immunity.* 1997;6:97–105.
532. Xu H, Li H, Suri-Payer E, et al. Regulation of anti-DNA B cells in recombination-activating gene- deficient mice. *J Exp Med.* 1998; 188:1247–1254.
533. Li H, Jiang Y, Prak EL, et al. Editors and editing of anti-DNA receptors. *Immunity.* 2001;15:947–957.
534. Chumley MJ, Dal Porto JM, Kawaguchi S, et al. A VH11V kappa 9 B cell antigen receptor drives generation of CD5+ B cells both in vivo and in vitro. *J Immunol.* 2000;164:4586–4593.
535. Arnold LW, Pennell CA, McCray SK, et al. Development of B-1 cells: segregation of phosphatidyl choline-specific B cells to the B-1 population occurs after immunoglobulin gene expression. *J Exp Med.* 1994;179:1585–1595.

Chapter 8

B Lymphocyte Signaling Mechanisms and Activation

Anthony L. DeFranco

OVERVIEW

During an immune response, the B cell antigen receptor (BCR) plays a critical role in the activation of the B cell and in this way ensures that only B cells recognizing antigen are induced to become antibody-secreting cells. The BCR also plays an essential role in the development of B cells, in the maturation of newly generated B cells into long-lived mature B cell subtypes, in the survival of B lineage cells at various stages, and in a variety of mechanisms promoting tolerance in the B cell compartment. Most of these biological effects are mediated by signaling events generated by the BCR, some of which may be generated at a low level by expression of the BCR on the cell surface, a process called *tonic signaling,* and others of which require oligomerization of the BCR to enhance its signaling. This chapter focuses primarily on the mechanisms of signaling and what is known about the biological relevance of this signaling. In addition, the BCR serves as an endocytic receptor for uptake of antigen, allowing efficient presentation of antigenic peptide-major histocompatability complex (MHC) complexes to helper T cells, which is essential to T-dependent antibody responses.

In addition to responding to soluble proteins and small particulate antigens derived from degraded virus particles and microbes, B cells may recognize and respond to antigen bound to other immune cells, such as dendritic cells, macrophages, and follicular dendritic cells (1). Such antigens or fragments of microbes may be held on the immune cell surface by Fc receptors, complement receptors, and innate immune receptors such as C-type lectin receptors. Such means of presentation likely influence the nature of activation signals the B cell receives from antigen contact, although little is understood about this aspect of B cell activation. Some of these cells secrete BAFF (B cell activating factor of the tumor necrosis factor (TNF) family), which is a strong survival signal for unstimulated mature B cells and may also promote B cell activation through the BCR (2).

B cells can mount some antibody responses without helper T cells, and these have been divided into two subgroupings, called *T-independent type I* and *T-independent type II* antibody responses. This distinction is generally based on the responsiveness of a mutant mouse strain, the *xid* mouse. Mice with this mutation have a complete loss of function of the Btk protein tyrosine kinase, which plays an important role in BCR signaling, as is described below. These mice still make antibody responses to T-independent type I antigens, which include molecules containing Toll-like receptor (TLR) ligands and highly polymeric structures such as certain types of virus particles (3), but fail to make responses to T-independent type II antigens, which typically are polysaccharide antigens (4). Recent work demonstrates that B cell TLRs are likely to have importance for many antibody responses, not just the T-independent type I responses (5–7). Polysaccharide antigens induce robust and sustained BCR signaling, probably due to their multimerization of epitopes on a flexible backbone (4). Interestingly, capsular polysaccharides of certain bacterial pathogens have been purified for use as vaccines, and these vaccines behave as T-independent type II antigens. The vaccines are often poorly efficacious in young children, younger than the age of 2, and in addition they generate relatively little memory. As a response to these limitations, in the early 1990s, conjugate vaccines were developed in which capsular polysaccharides are chemically coupled to protein antigens (e.g., tetanus toxoid, etc.). These vaccines have the property that they can promote antibody responses by both T-independent type II and T-dependent mechanisms.

T-independent antibody responses are typically quite rapid and serve the purpose of generating a rapid IgM response to provide early protection against infection, whereas T-dependent antibody responses, as described in more detail in the next chapter, can lead to vigorous germinal center responses that generate high-affinity isotype-switched antibody, and also generate long-lived plasma cells and memory B cells, both of which are of great value for protection from infection at a later date.

BCR signaling participates in T cell-dependent antibody responses in multiple ways. BCR signaling changes the responsiveness of the B cell to chemokine signals that position the B cell within secondary lymphoid organs and, in this way, the antigen-recognizing B cell is induced to move to the edge of the T cell areas, where T cells are scanning B cells for peptide-MHC complexes (8). BCR signaling also changes the adhesive properties of the B cell, enhancing its binding to T cells, and it induces expression of molecules the B cell needs to activate T cells. In particular, BCR signaling increases the expression of MHC class II molecules and induces expression of costimulatory molecules, particularly B7-2 (CD86). BCR signaling also protects B cells from Fas-mediated killing, which can be induced by activated helper T cells, by the action of FasL, in combination with CD40L (9,10).

BCR FUNCTION AND B CELL DEVELOPMENT

Although the focus of this chapter is on B cell activation, defects in B cell development often result from genetic alterations in mice of BCR components or individual BCR signaling components (11). This is because BCR-signaling reactions play multiple roles in the development of B cells. The first of these reactions occurs following the successful rearrangement of the Ig heavy chain locus, when the resulting heavy chain protein assembles with two proteins, $\lambda 5$ and VpreB, called *surrogate light chain,* and the signaling chains Ig-α and Ig-β to form the pre-BCR, which is structurally similar to the BCR. Pre-BCR signaling promotes development from the pro-B cell stage to the pre-B cell stage. Subsequent successful rearrangement of one of the Ig light chain loci promotes the next developmental step, to the immature B cell stage in the bone marrow. If a bone marrow immature B cell is not self-reactive, it can leave the bone marrow and transit to the spleen, where it is called a transitional 1 (T1) B cell (12). T1 cells mature further to the T2 developmental stage and eventually to either of two mature B cell types, the marginal zone B cell or the follicular B cell. This choice is also influenced by BCR signaling, with low signaling in response to weak reactivity to self-antigens probably favoring development to the follicular B cell type and even lower signaling favoring development to the marginal zone B cell (13), although some investigators have argued for the opposite relationship between signaling and choice between follicular and marginal zone B cells. Selection of T2 cells into the long-lived follicular B cell population on the basis of a low level of self-reactivity may resemble positive selection of thymocytes in T cell development. Notch-2 signaling also influences the long-lived choice of cell type between follicular and marginal zone B cell, promoting development of marginal zone B cells.

In fetal life and immediately after birth, B cell precursors access a third type of mature B cell, the B1 cell. B1 cells reside primarily in the peritoneal and plural cavities, where they make rapid T-independent antibody responses to microbes that enter these locations (14). In addition, early in life, B1 cells spontaneously secrete polyreactive IgM antibodies, called *natural antibody,* and this antibody has been shown to be protective in the case of several infections in mice (15). B1 cells appear to require a higher level of self-reactivity to enter and survive in this compartment than what is needed to develop into a follicular B cell (14,16). Indeed, some signaling defects that do not greatly affect development of marginal zone or follicular B cells result in loss of B1 cells (13,14).

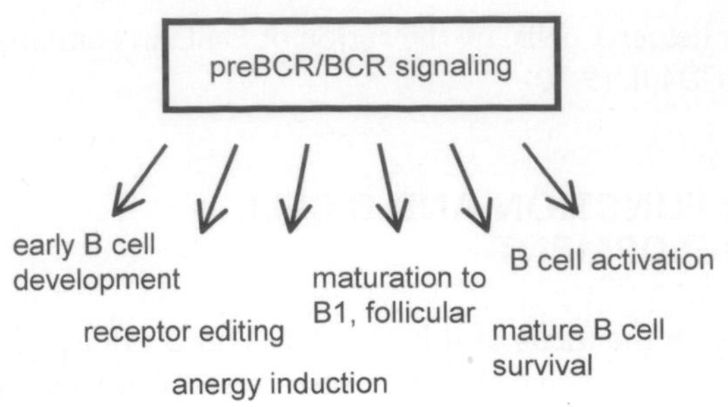

FIGURE 8.1 Functions of signaling by the BCR and pre-BCR. BCR signaling regulates the development and maturation of B cells, B cell survival, B cell activation, and B cell tolerance.

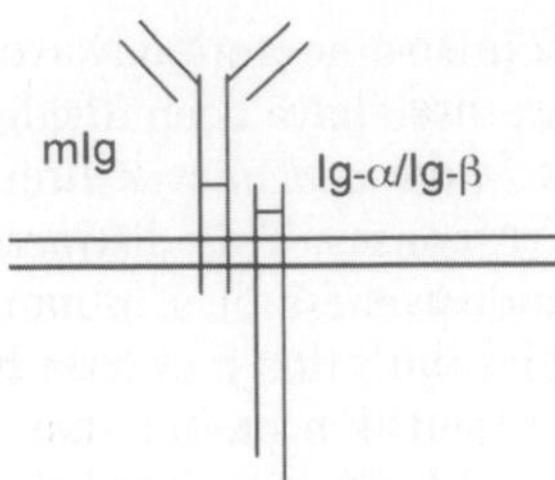

FIGURE 8.2 Structure of the BCR. The BCR consists of two moieties, the antigen binding membrane immunoglobulin, consisting of a two heavy chain, two light chain structure, and the signal transducing Ig-α/Ig-β heterodimer. The two component parts are weakly associated with one another through hydrophilic amino acid side chains in their transmembrane domains and probably also through interactions of heavy chain Ig domains with Ig domains of Ig-α or Ig-β. Surprisingly, experimental evidence indicates that only one Ig-α/Ig-β heterodimer pairs with a H_2L_2 membrane immunoglobulin.

B cells with reactivity to self antigens generate moderate to high levels of BCR signaling, which induce biological responses promoting immunological tolerance in the B cell compartment. The response varies depending on the developmental stage of the B cell when it contracts self antigen. If immature B cells bind well to self antigens, then the resulting BCR signaling causes maturation arrest and further Ig light chain rearrangements, which may replace the first light chain with a new one, in which case self-reactivity may be erased. This process is called *receptor editing,* and it appears to occur in at least 25% of B cells (17). Self-reactive T1 cells begin the receptor editing process like immature B cells in the bone marrow but die due to lack of protective signals provided to immature B cells by bone marrow stromal cells (18).

BCR signaling above the level that promotes follicular B cell development induces T2 or follicular B cells to enter a tolerized but alive state referred to as *anergy* (19). In most cases, anergic B cells are characterized by chronic low-level BCR signaling (20). This level of signaling is sufficient to induce relocalization from the follicles to the T cell zone (8), but is insufficient to protect from Fas-mediated killing (21). In addition, the lifespan of anergic B cells is shorter than that of follicular B cells due to an increased requirement for BAFF (22). Analysis of normal mice indicates that anergic B cells are present in substantial numbers (23), so anergy likely represents an important mechanism for establishing and maintaining tolerance in the B cell compartment.

The functions of the pre-BCR and BCR in B cell development, choice of mature cell type, tolerance, and activation are summarized in Figure 8.1.

STRUCTURE OF THE B CELL ANTIGEN RECEPTOR

The BCR is a multimeric complex containing membrane Ig (mIg) of any of the five isotypes noncovalently associated with a disulfide-linked heterodimer of two signaling chains called Ig-α and Ig-β, also known as CD79a and CD79b, respectively (Figure 8.2). Ig-α and Ig-β are the products of the *mb-1* and *B29* genes (24). Ig-α and Ig-β have structures similar to those of the CD3 chains that pair with the T cell receptor (TCR)—namely, they each have an N-terminal Ig-like domain, a single hydrophobic transmembrane domain, and a C-terminal cytoplasmic domain of 61 and 48 amino acid residues in length. These cytoplasmic domains each contain an amino acid sequence motif referred to as the *Immunoreceptor Tyrosine-based Activation Motif* (*ITAM*), which is also present in the CD3 and ζ chains of the TCR and in several other polypeptides of activating Fc receptors of myeloid cells and activating natural killer cell receptors. The ITAM plays a central role in BCR signaling, as described in the next section.

The association between mIgM and Ig-α/Ig-β is rather weak and is maintained if B cell membranes are solubilized in very gentle, nonionic detergents such as digitonin, but is disrupted by more commonly used nonionic detergents such as NP-40 and Triton X-100. There is a striking number of hydrophilic amino acid residues within the Ig heavy chain transmembrane domains, particularly serine, threonine, and tyrosine residues. Mutagenesis data indicates that these –OH-containing side chains contribute importantly to the association between mIgM and Ig-α/Ig-β (25,26). This association is probably also stabilized by interactions of extracellular Ig domains of the different components.

Given that membrane forms of Ig are composed of two heavy chains and two light chains, symmetry considerations originally led to the proposal that the BCR would contain two dimers of Ig-α and Ig-β. Co-immunoprecipitation experiments using two distinct epitope tags, however, indicate that a single BCR complex contains only one Ig-α/Ig-β heterodimer (Figure 8.2). Fluorescence resonance energy transfer (FRET) studies in intact B cells have supported this conclusion (27) and, moreover, have indicated that the BCR complexes are single units (H_2L_2 + 1 Ig-α/Ig-β dimer) rather than higher order structures.

Although most evidence favors the view of BCRs as independent units dispersed in the plasma membrane, one study (28) suggested the possibility that BCRs may form into a lattice in the membrane that has tonic signaling properties that are perturbed by binding to antigen to induce the stronger signaling seen upon acute stimulation. Fluorescence imaging studies have not supported the idea of large preformed lattices of BCRs in the membranes of B cells, but the possibility of small microclusters cannot be ruled out by light microscopic techniques. The FRET studies mentioned earlier also did not find evidence for clustering of BCRs prior to cross-linking. In addition, electron microscopy studies have supported the view that BCRs are dispersed in the plasma membrane (29). As will be discussed later, tonic signaling is a feature of the BCR and is important for promoting B cell survival (30,31), but it seems likely that this low-level signaling in the absence of ligand results from the equilibrium between protein tyrosine kinases and protein tyrosine phosphatases acting on the BCR and its signaling components, rather than by formation of multimeric complexes in the absence of antigen.

INITIATION OF SIGNALING

Cross-linking of the BCR by antigen or experimentally by anti-Ig antibodies induces rapid and robust signaling, including activation of protein tyrosine kinases, elevation of intracellular free calcium, activation of mitogen-activated protein (MAP) kinases, and activation of several transcription factors, including NF-κB. The magnitude of signaling is generally related to the extent of BCR clustering achieved. The signaling reactions are all dependent upon the ITAM sequences in the cytoplasmic domains of Ig-α and Ig-β. An ITAM has two tyrosines in a conserved sequence context and with a conserved spacing (D/E XXYXXL/IX$_7$YXXL/I). Tyrosine kinase-based signaling systems typically involve phosphorylation-induced assembly of multiprotein complexes (32), and this is also true for BCR signaling. Each half of the ITAM (YXXL/I) is, when phosphorylated, a binding site for several signaling proteins containing Src-homology 2 (SH2) domains, especially tyrosine kinases involved in the early steps of BCR signaling, the Src-family tyrosine kinases, and Syk (Figure 8.3).

The BCR contains two ITAMs, one each in the cytoplasmic domains of Ig-α and Ig-β. These ITAMs are largely redundant: Mice in which either the Ig-α or the Ig-β ITAM is ablated by tyrosine to phenylalanine mutations have defects that are subtle, but mice in which both ITAMs are ablated have a strong block in B cell development at the stage where pre-BCR signaling is required for progression (33).

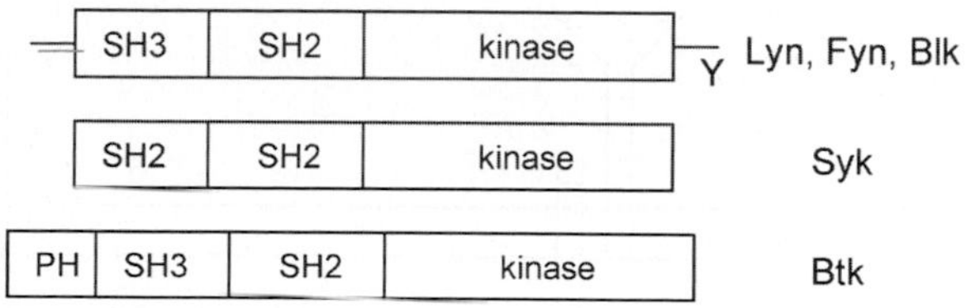

FIGURE 8.3 Three families of intracellular protein tyrosine kinases are involved in BCR signaling. The Src-family kinases Lyn, Fyn, and Blk each have an N-terminal unique region that has fatty acid addition sites, myristic acid in all cases and an additional palmitic acid in the case of Lyn and Fyn. The former fatty acid targets these kinases to membranes, whereas the latter additionally targets them to lipid raft membrane subdomains. Blk is also preferentially localized to lipid rafts, but this is achieved by a different mechanism. In addition, Src-family kinases all have three conserved domains, called Src-homology 1 (the kinase domain), Src-homology 2 (SH2), and Src-homology 3 (SH3) domains and also have a negative regulatory tyrosine phosphorylation site near the C-terminus. Syk lacks lipid modifications and has two SH2 domains and a kinase domain. Btk has an architecture similar to Src-family kinases, but lacks the lipid modification and negative regulatory tyrosine and instead at the N-terminus has a pleckstrin homology (PH) domain, which can bind to PIP_3.

In addition, Ig-α has two tyrosines outside of its ITAM, and one of these (Y204) has been shown to be important for downstream signaling reactions, as is described later.

The first step in the BCR signaling cascade is tyrosine phosphorylation of the Ig-α and Ig-β ITAM tyrosines by Src-family tyrosine kinases. B cells express primarily three members of the Src family, Lyn, Fyn, and Blk. These three tyrosine kinases function redundantly for ITAM phosphorylation, as indicated by analysis of development between the pro-B cell stage and the pre-B cell stage in single, double and triple knockout (KO) mice (34): triple KO mice exhibit a strong block at this early stage of development, presumably reflecting a defect in pre-BCR signaling, whereas the single and double KO mice exhibit normal B cell development. The strong block in B cell development in these mice suggests that pre-BCR signaling requires Lyn, Fyn, or Blk acting redundantly to initiate pre-BCR signaling.

Exactly how antigen binding to the BCR leads to ITAM tyrosine phoyphorylation and initiation of signaling is not fully understood. Three explanations have been proposed. Originally, it was proposed that Src-family tyrosine kinases were noncovalently associated with Ig-α/Ig-β cytoplasmic domains prior to stimulation in a way that did not allow them to efficiently phosphorylate the ITAMs of the Ig-α and Ig-β to which they were associated, but allowed them to phosphorylate ITAMs of other BCRs brought nearby by antigen-induced clustering. Although attractive in its simplicity, this model has little experimental support. Immunoprecipitation of BCRs from unstimulated B cells does bring down Lyn, Fyn, and Blk, but the amounts are quite small, a few percent of the amount of these kinases present in the cell. Immunoprecipitation of the BCR from B cell lines expressing transfected mIgM demonstrated

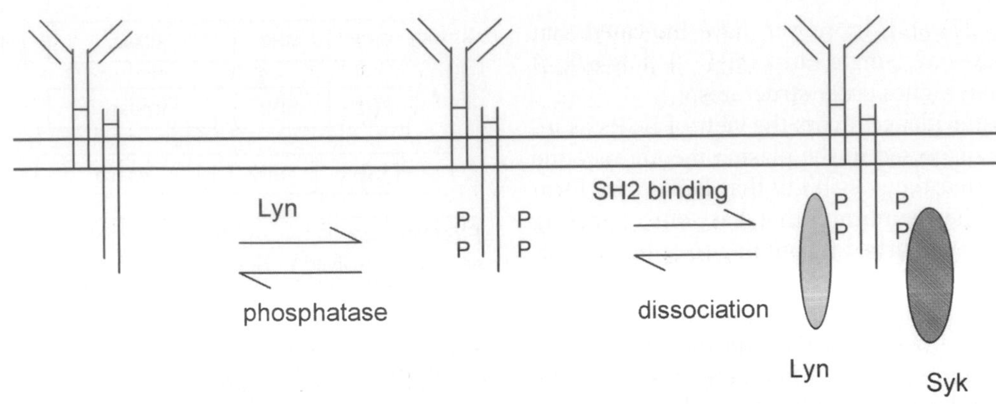

FIGURE 8.4 Model for BCR tonic signaling mediated by equilibrium between tyrosine kinases and protein tyrosine phosphatases. According to the model shown, Src-family tyrosine kinases are responsible for phosphorylating BCR ITAM tyrosines, which creates a binding site for Syk (via its tandem SH2 domains) and also for Src-family kinases (via their single SH2 domain) to bind to the receptor and initiate a low level of signaling. Dissociation of Syk or Src family SH2 domains from ITAM phosphorylated tyrosines exposes them to allow phosphatases (SHP1, CD45, or others) to dephosphorylate the ITAMs and terminate tonic signaling from that receptor.

that a small amount of Fyn is specifically associated with mIgM, but the amounts of Lyn or Blk detected were not above the negative control (35). Since Fyn KO mice have no defect in BCR signaling (36), it seems likely that pre-association of Src kinases with the BCR is not important for BCR signaling. It should be noted, however, that Lyn and Fyn were found to associate specifically with the BCR after cross-linking (35), possibly reflecting an association between the SH2 domains of Lyn and Fyn and one half of one of the ITAMs, since phosphorylated YXXL/I represents a consensus sequence for binding of Src-family SH2 domains. Although Lyn and Fyn bound in this way would presumably not be responsible for initiating BCR signaling, they could function to amplify it.

A second hypothesis is that the initiation of BCR signaling involves a change in location of the BCR within the plasma membrane that takes it from the nonlipid raft region of the membrane to the lipid raft region, which is highly enriched in the Src-family kinases. Indeed, cross-linked BCRs have been shown by both biochemical means (37) and by fluorescent microscopy (38) to associate with lipid rafts after antigen– or anti–Ig-induced BCR clustering, but not before. Originally, it was argued that this change in location occurred independently of signaling reactions (37), although not all data are consistent with this possibility, and more recent data has suggested that this change of localization may occur after signaling has initiated (39), in which case its function may be to amplify signaling or allow efficient association with adaptor molecules required for downstream signaling. Another problem with the hypothesis that BCR signaling is initiated by a movement of the BCR into lipid rafts is that, in immature B cells, this movement appears not to occur and yet clearly BCR cross-linking induces signaling in immature B cells, although perhaps not as robustly as in mature B cells (40,41). The relationship of BCR signaling to lipid rafts is discussed additionally in the next section.

Finally, a third hypothesis for how ITAM signaling is initiated is that cross-linking alters the equilibrium between kinases phosphorylating the ITAMs and phosphatases dampening signaling by removing phosphates from ITAM tyrosines (Figure 8.4). According to this view, dispersed BCR complexes in the plasma membrane are being phosphorylated by Src-family tyrosine kinases frequently, and this allows some recruitment of Syk and downstream signaling, as described below. This tonic signaling is maintained at a low level by the action of tyrosine phosphatases (perhaps SHP-1 or CD45) that remove phosphates from phosphorylated ITAMs, attenuating signaling. Interesting in this regard is the observation that addition of inhibitors of tyrosine phosphatases (e.g., pervanadate) results in a pattern of signaling reactions that closely mimics what is seen upon treatment of B cells with anti-Ig antibodies (42). Moreover, it is likely that antigen-induced clustering of BCRs changes the dynamic equilibrium between tyrosine kinases and protein tyrosine phosphatases, because when BCRs are clustered, Src-family tyrosine kinases and Syk bound to phosphorylated ITAMs are now close to other ITAMs and can efficiently phosphorylate them and in that way promote sustained signaling.

Evidence that Syk can propagate signaling of cross-linked BCRs comes from studies of ITAM signaling in the absence of Src-family kinases. For example, Lyn-deficient DT-40 chicken B cells, which apparently lack other Src-family kinases, exhibit substantial BCR signaling upon treatment with anti-Ig, although the calcium response is somewhat delayed compared to parental cells (43). Similarly, mouse macrophages genetically lacking Src-family kinases have greatly delayed ITAM signaling through their activating Fc receptors, but once signaling is initiated, it is sufficient to mediate internalization of antibody-coated red blood cells (44). These observations have been interpreted as indicating that Syk is sufficient to mediate ITAM signaling in the absence of Src-family tyrosine kinases, but it is inefficient at doing so due to inefficient initiation of signaling. Signaling ability of the BCR expressed with Syk in an epithelial cell line that has endogenous Fyn (45) or of the BCR expressed with Lyn and Syk in Drosophila S2 cells (46) support these conclusions.

The ability of Syk to promote ITAM signaling in the absence of Src-family tyrosine kinases is in contrast to ZAP-70, which is primarily expressed in T cells and NK cells. ZAP-70 absolutely requires a Src-family kinase to become activated (47). Thus, the ITAM signaling machinery in B cells and myeloid cells is more flexible than its counterpart in T cells, perhaps to accommodate the greater variety of antigen types that B cells must respond to in contrast to T cells, which primarily respond to MHC-peptide ligands.

LIPID RAFTS AND BCR SIGNALING

BCR signaling in mature B cells is probably enhanced by compartmentalization into subdomains of the plasma membrane, called *lipid rafts* or *glycolipid-enriched membrane microdomains* (GEMMs). Lipid rafts are highly dynamic self-assembling lipid structures within membranes. They contain glycosphingolipids, cholesterol, and various lipid-modified proteins. The lipids in these structures pack together more closely than do the lipids in the rest of the plasma membrane, giving these structures a "liquid-ordered" structure, as opposed to the more fluid structure of the other parts of the plasma membrane. It should be emphasized that lipid rafts, particularly in unstimulated cells, are very small, highly dynamic structures in which individual components, both lipid and protein molecules, are continually exchanging between the rafts and the surrounding membrane.

Another point that should be emphasized about lipid rafts is that some of the methods for analyzing them have significant limitations, and hence there is some disagreement about their importance for immunoreceptor signaling (48,49). The association of molecular components with lipid rafts is typically assessed by extraction of cellular membranes with nonionic detergents such as NP-40 or Triton X-100 at 0°C, a condition that solubilizes the majority of the plasma membrane, but not glycosphingolipids, GPI-linked proteins, or many lipid-modified membrane proteins, and hence is believed not to solubilize lipid rafts. These unsolubilized structures are typically isolated by sucrose density gradient centrifugation, as the unsolubilized membranes are of lighter density than are detergent-solubilized proteins. This approach is less than perfect, as the concentration of detergent used can affect the spectrum of proteins obtained in the lipid raft fraction, perhaps because some membrane proteins are less tightly associated with lipid rafts, and hence are more easily extracted, than others. It is also theoretically possible that some proteins in the nonraft part of the membrane join the lipid raft structures after extraction, although there is not strong evidence for this possibility. Lipid rafts can also be studied by fluorescence microscopy of intact cells, but this approach has the limitation that, in unstimulated cells, most lipid rafts are sufficiently small as to be below the resolution limit of light microscopy. However, in lymphocytes, as in many other cell types, receptor stimulation causes lipid rafts to come together into larger structures, such that in stimulated B cells, distinguishable lipid rafts become increasing prominent within several minutes of BCR ligation, and the association of particular proteins with these structures can readily be visualized (38).

With regard to addressing the biological significance of lipid rafts for particular cellular events, there are two methods that have been used to disrupt lipid rafts. There are antifungal components such as filipin that intercalate into membranes and disrupt lipid rafts, and it is also possible to extract cholesterol from membranes of cells with methyl β-cyclodextrin, and this is believed to cause the remaining lipid raft components to disperse in the plasma membrane. Although interesting data have been collected with these methods, it is possible that some functions of the non-lipid raft plasma membrane are perturbed as well, so the specificity of these effects is not entirely clear. Finally, in some cases, it is possible to convert a lipid raft resident membrane protein to a nonlipid raft distribution by mutating it to remove lipid addition sites. In this case, the role of lipid raft localization of a particular protein within the membrane can be assessed. For example, this has been done with the T cell adaptor protein LAT (linker for activation of T cells), which is necessary for TCR signaling. LAT function is greatly decreased by mutations that prevent its palmitoylation, which is the modification that targets it to lipid rafts (50,51). This observation argues strongly that TCR signaling occurs primarily in lipid rafts, and it is likely that BCR signaling is similar.

Among components involved in BCR signaling, the Src-family tyrosine kinases are enriched in lipid rafts. The BCR itself is not detectably associated with lipid rafts prior to ligation, but once cross-linked by antigen, it rapidly associates with lipid rafts. The mechanism by which this occurs is not well established, but one possibility is that this is the result of association between phosphorylated ITAMs of the BCR and the SH2 domain of Src-family tyrosine kinases (39). Alternatively, the association of the BCR with lipid rafts may be favored by the coalescence of lipid rafts from smaller structures into larger ones that become visible in the light microscope. This coalescence is facilitated by BCR signaling induced dephosphorylation of ezrin (52). Prior to stimulation, ezrin binds to both lipid raft–associated proteins (PAG1 and possibly others) and to the cortical actin cytoskeleton. This linkage of lipid raft proteins to the cytoskeleton may keep lipid rafts in a dispersed state by limiting their mobility. Dephosphorylation of ezrin causes it to release from actin and from lipid rafts and, preventing this release by expressing a mutant form of ezrin that is constitutively linked to lipid rafts and to actin, attenuates the coalescence of lipid rafts that is otherwise observed following BCR cross-linking (52).

Interestingly, stimulation-dependent association of the BCR with lipid rafts occurs in mature B cells but not in immature B cells (40,41). This difference appears to be due to changes in the cholesterol content of the membranes of immature versus mature B cells (53). The functional significance of this change is not well established, but it is striking that BCR engagement of immature B cells in the spleen leads to rapid cell death, whereas engagement of the BCR of mature B cells promotes their activation. It may be that one or more signaling reaction is particularly dependent upon localization to lipid rafts and that this signaling reaction is required for production of prosurvival or proliferative signals. Activation of the transcription factor NF-κB is an attractive candidate for such a signaling event, as described later, although further studies will be required to address this point.

TONIC SIGNALING BY THE BCR

Expression of the BCR and the pre-BCR result in a constitutive low level of "tonic" signaling even without interaction with a ligand (33). This conclusion is supported by a number of experimental strategies. For example, plasma membrane expression of chimeric proteins containing the ITAMs of Ig-α and/or Ig-β is sufficient to drive several of the B lineage developmental transitions that require the pre-BCR or the BCR. This tonic signaling could be the result of an equilibrium between, on the one hand, ITAM phosphorylation, recruitment of Syk, and activation of some downstream signaling reactions (described below), and, on the other hand, dissociation of Syk, dephosphorylation of ITAM tyrosines, and inactivation of signaling reactions. In the absence of ligand binding, this equilibrium favors the dephosphorylations and, therefore, the amount of signaling is low. Nonetheless, this low-level tonic signaling may be sufficient to mediate some biological effects, including promotion of the pro-B cell to pre-B cell transition or export of immature B cells from the bone marrow. It should be noted that there is evidence both for ligands for the pre-BCR and for surrogate light chain-induced oligomerization of the pre-BCR, so pre-BCR signaling may not rely solely on low-level tonic signaling (33). Similarly, chronic low-level BCR signaling is required for survival of mature B cells (31), but whether this signaling is truly independent of ligand or is stimulated by a low degree of reactivity to one or more self-antigens is not known. Thus, the significance of tonic signaling for normal B cell biology remains unclear at this time, although it is likely to be important in some contexts.

AMPLIFICATION OF SIGNALING

The association of Syk and Src-family tyrosine kinases with phosphorylated ITAMs and the ability of these tyrosine kinases to phosphorylate adjacent ITAMs on antigen-clustered BCRs represents a positive feedback loop that can convert tonic BCR signaling to ligand-induced amplified signaling. This is only one of several amplification mechanisms that promote robust, high-level signaling by cross-linked BCRs.

A second amplification mechanism may result from the association of clustered BCRs with lipid rafts, which occurs in mature B cells but not in immature B cells (33). Src-family kinases are highly enriched in lipid rafts by virtue of their N-terminal lipid modifications, particularly the palmitate groups present in Lyn and Fyn, so localization of the BCR to lipid rafts presumably increases the amount of phosphorylation of BCR ITAM tyrosines. In addition, the assembly of the CARMA1/Bcl-10/MALT1 complex, which is necessary for activation of the transcription factor NF-κB, occurs primarily in lipid rafts, and this may be enhanced by localization of the BCR to lipid rafts. Thus, a key function of lipid rafts for BCR signaling may be to concentrate together key signaling components to enhance the efficiency of signal propagation from the receptor to downstream events.

A third mechanism for amplifying signaling has recently been proposed in which reactive oxygen species such as H_2O_2 are generated and transiently inactivate tyrosine phosphatases near the signaling BCRs, further tipping the balance between the tyrosine kinases, which are not inhibited, and the tyrosine phosphatases, which are inhibited (42,54). In this regard, it is noteworthy that protein tyrosine phosphatases have highly reactive cysteine residues in their active sites, which are selectively oxidized in a reversible fashion with low levels of reactive oxygen species generated at the plasma membrane (55). Thus, the generation of low levels of reactive oxygen species may be a novel mode of receptor signaling with highly selective effects that amplify BCR signaling.

DOWNSTREAM SIGNALING REACTIONS

Signaling by the BCR and the pre-BCR mediates a remarkable diversity of cellular responses, including developmental progression or arrest, change in location within peripheral lymphoid tissues, survival or apoptosis, and

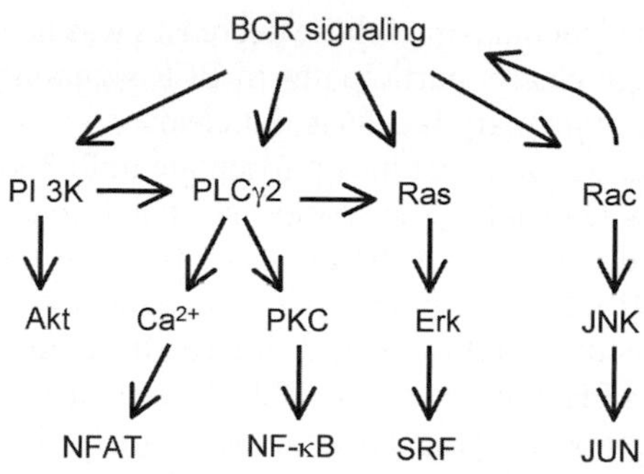

FIGURE 8.5 Activation of multiple signaling reactions by the BCR. BCR signaling activates the signaling pathways shown, which are each described in detail in the text.

PI ⇄ PI4P ⇄ PI4,$5P_2$ ⇄ (PI 3K / PTEN) PIP_3 → (SHIP) PI3,$4P_2$
PI4,$5P_2$ → (PLCγ2) IP_3 DAG

FIGURE 8.6 Phosphatidylinositol lipid signaling reactions. Phosphatidylinositol (PI) is a major lipid found on the cytoplasmic side of the plasma membrane. The inositol head group is a cyclic hexose sugar that can be phosphorylated on any of the six positions other than the 1 position, which is connected to diacylglycerol. Enzymes within the cell convert a small fraction of PI to PI4,$5P_2$ by adding phosphates to the 4 position and then to the 5 position of the inositol ring. The second step is positively regulated downstream of Vav signaling, which serves to keep PI4,$5P_2$ levels high in the context of phospholipase C (PLC) action to hydrolyze this lipid. PIP_2 hydrolysis generates the second messengers inositol 1,4,5-trisphosphate (IP_3), which induces opening of calcium channels in the endoplasmic reticulum, and diacylglycerol, which activates protein kinase C isoforms, and which promotes activation of Ras via RasGRP3. BCR signaling activates PLCγ2. PI4,$5P_2$ can also be converted to PIP_3 by the action of PI 3-kinase, which is activated by BCR signaling. PIP_3 is a membrane-bound phospholipid that activates the protein kinase Akt and aids in the activation of PLCγ2. PIP_3 phosphates are removed by two phosphatases, PTEN, which removes the 3 phosphate, and SHIP, which removes the 5 phosphate, creating a new second messenger PI3,$4P_2$, which serves as a membrane-recruiting ligand for some signaling proteins via their PH domains.

proliferation. Which particular response ensues depends on the developmental stage of the B lineage cell and the context of other signals coming from TLRs, cytokines, or helper T cells. Therefore, it is not surprising that the BCR triggers a wide variety of intracellular signaling events. Interactions with helper T cells are promoted by upregulation of integrin adhesion, changes in chemokine responsiveness, regulation of intracellular organelle function promoting antigen presentation, and changes in the transcription of many genes. Key signaling reactions triggered by the BCR or pre-BCR that mediate one or more of these cellular responses include activation of phosphoinositide 3-kinase (PI 3-kinase), hydrolysis of phosphatidylinositol 4,5-bisphosphate (PIP_2) resulting in elevation of intracellular free calcium and production of diacylglycerol (DAG), activation of small molecular weight GTP-binding proteins including Ras, Rac and Rap, activation of the Erk MAP kinase, and to a lesser extent the JNK and p38 MAP kinases, and activation of transcription factors including NFAT, AP-1, and NF-κB (Figure 8.5). In this regard, BCR signaling closely resembles signaling by other ITAM-containing receptors, including the TCR, and also signaling by many transmembrane tyrosine kinase receptors, such as the platelet-derived growth factor receptor and epidermal growth factor receptor.

To connect with these signaling reactions, the BCR and its associated intracellular tyrosine kinases require adaptor proteins that efficiently connect the kinases to the targets that mediate particular signaling reactions (56,57).

The PI 3-Kinase Pathway

Activation of PI 3-kinase is an early signaling event that promotes many of the other BCR-induced signaling events and also promotes B cell survival. PI 3-kinases are a diverse family of enzymes, but the isoform activated downstream of the BCR is a dimeric enzyme composed of a regulatory subunit, p85α, which contains an SH2 domain that recruits PI 3-kinase to tyrosine-phosphorylated adaptor molecules, and a catalytic domain, p110δ. Mice with targeted mutations in the genes encoding either of these subunits have a loss of B1 cells and also a substantial decrease in the number of mature follicular B cells or of marginal zone B cells (11). Low-level expression of other isoforms of these subunits may attenuate the defects seen in the knockout mice, allowing some B cell development.

The product of PI 3-kinase, PIP_3 (Figure 8.6), serves as a membrane-bound ligand for a subset of signaling proteins with pleckstrin homology (PH) domains. PH domains often mediate interactions with phosphorylated phosphatidylinositols and in that way contribute to signaling reactions. Thus, elevation of PIP_3 in the membrane adjacent to signaling receptors aids in the recruitment to this location of other signaling molecules and, in that way, promotes signaling. Key signaling molecules with PIP_3-binding PH domains include Btk, PLCγ2, and Akt (58). Btk and PLCγ2 are discussed in more detail in the next section. Akt is a serine-threonine protein kinase that is activated by PI 3-kinase action to promote enhanced protein synthesis, which is a preparation for proliferation, and to promote cell survival. Akt is both recruited to the plasma membrane by binding PIP_3 and is activated by phosphorylation by an upstream protein kinase, called PDK1 (phosphoinositide-dependent protein kinase 1), which is itself activated by PIP_3. The growth promoting actions of Akt involve activation of mTOR (mammalian target of rapamycin), which regulates protein synthesis (59), and phosphorylation and inactivation of the transcription factors of the FoxO family, which promote quiescence (60). In addition, Akt promotes cell cycle progression by blocking GSK3 (glycogen synthase kinase 3), which is an inhibitor of cell cycle regulators cyclin D and Myc. Akt promotes cell survival by phosphorylating and inactivating the BH3-only pro-apoptotic regulator Bad and probably also by other, less understood mechanisms. Thus, Akt is a key regulator in B cells as well as in many other cell types.

Activation of PI 3-kinase by the BCR is thought to occur by the participation at least three adaptor molecules: CD19, BCAP, and Gab-1. The most important of these is the transmembrane coreceptor molecule CD19, which is present in a complex with the CR2 complement receptor (also called CD21) and the tetraspan protein CD81 (61). The cytoplasmic tail of CD19 has 9 conserved tyrosines, two of which are consensus sites for binding by p85α of PI 3-kinase (YXXM). These sites are required for CD19 to mediate the activation of PI 3-kinase and are the primary sites responsible for CD19 signaling function (62,63). The CR2/CD19 complex greatly potentiates BCR signaling when an antigen has C3b-derived fragments attached to it, as is described later, but CD19 clearly participates in BCR signaling even when the antigen has not been decorated with C3 fragments. Mice deficient in CD19 exhibit a complete defect in B1 cell development and also lack marginal zone B cells. There also appears to be a partial deficiency in maturation of follicular B cells. T-independent type 2 antibody responses are highly deficient, perhaps due to the lack of B1 and marginal zone B cells. T cell-dependent antibody responses are also partially defective in germinal centers, and this deficiency is also seen in mice expressing CD19 with the two PI 3-kinase binding sites mutated (63).

Despite the striking defects in CD19-deficient mice, there are stronger defects in mice lacking the p85α component of PI 3-kinase (58). This observation suggests that there are alternative mechanisms by which the BCR activates PI 3-kinase, perhaps to a lesser degree than CD19. Two cytoplasmic adaptors, BCAP (B cell adaptor for PI3K) and Gab-1 (Grb2-associated binder 1), may promote activation of PI 3-kinase downstream of BCR ligation, but this is not clearly established in primary mammalian B cells. Disruption of the gene encoding BCAP in the DT-40 chicken B cell line ablates PI 3-kinase signaling, leading to the view that a primary function of BCAP is to mediate activation of PI 3-kinase. In mice, mutation of the BCAP gene results in clear B cell defects, including loss of B1 cells, an increase in the number of immature B cells in the spleen, a corresponding decrease in the number of follicular B cells, and a strong defect in T-independent type 2 antibody responses (64). Surprisingly, biochemical studies failed to reveal a clear defect in PI 3-kinase activation or in activation of Akt, which is dependent upon PIP_3 but not other signaling reactions. In contrast, there was a partial decrease in PIP_2 hydrolysis and calcium elevation, although the mechanism of these decreases was not defined. Thus, BCAP clearly participates in BCR signaling, but its exact role in primary B cells is not clear.

Another adaptor that may participate in PI 3-kinase activation is Gab-1 (or the closely related Gab-2) (65,66). Gab-1 and Gab-2 have PH domains that are thought to bind to PIP_3. BCR stimulation leads to Gab-1 recruitment to the plasma membrane, and this recruitment is dependent on its PH domain and on PIP_3. Once recruited, Gab-1 becomes phosphorylated and associates with PI 3-kinase and also with the SH2-domain-containing protein tyrosine phosphatase SHP-2. It has been proposed that Gab-1 may represent a positive feedback loop that amplifies PIP_3 production, but genetic evidence has suggested that primary effect of Gab 1 is to attenuate BCR signaling via SHP-2.

PI 3-kinase signaling is countered by two enzymes that remove phosphates from PIP_3, PTEN, which removes the phosphate that PI 3-kinase adds, and SHIP (SH2-containing polyphosphoinositide 5 phosphatase), which removes the 5-phosphate, generating phosphatidylinositol 3,4 bis-phosphate (Figure 8.6). This molecule does bind to some PH domains, including that of an adaptor involved in BCR signaling, Bam32 (see below), so it may continue to promote certain signaling reactions, although Akt and PLCγ2 action both require PIP_3. SHIP is recruited to sites of BCR signaling via SH2-domain interactions and is particularly important for inhibitory coreceptor function, as described below.

The Phospholipase Cγ2 Pathway

Phospholipase Cγ (PLCγ) is the second major BCR-stimulated signaling enzyme that generates second messengers of importance for B cell responses to antigen (Figure 8.6) and most biological responses to the BCR require this signaling reaction. PLCγ1 and PLCγ2 are the primary isoforms of PLC that are activated by tyrosine phosphorylation-based signaling receptors, including the BCR, and of these PLCγ2 is the major form expressed in B cells. PLCs hydrolyze PIP_2 to generate two second messengers, inositol 1,4,5- trisphosphate (IP_3) and diacylglycerol (DAG). The former second messenger is a soluble molecule that diffuses to the endoplasmic reticulum (ER), where there are IP_3 receptors that release calcium stores (67). This is responsible for the initial elevation of intracellular free calcium released upon BCR stimulation. Maintenance of elevated intracellular calcium in response to sustained generation of IP_3 is mediated by poorly understood signals released from the ER when its calcium stores are depleted. These signals act upon plasma membrane calcium channels to cause them to open to keep intracellular free calcium high. Recently some of the components of this system have been identified in T cells (68,69), and a similar system probably operates in B cells. Elevated intracellular free calcium activates NFAT (nuclear factor of activated T cells) through removal of inhibitory phosphate by the calmodulin-regulated protein phosphatase, calcineurin. Elevation of intracellular free calcium also can stimulate calcium-activated protein kinases, such as CaM kinase 2 (calmodulin-regulated protein kinase 2).

The other second messenger generated by PLCγ2 action is the lipid DAG, which activates isozymes of the protein kinase C (PKC) family, often in conjunction with elevated intracellular calcium, and also activates Ras-activating proteins of the RasGRP family, as is discussed in more detail below. PKCβ participates positively in signaling to Ras and to NF-κB, whereas another isoform, PKCδ appears to be critical for signaling in anergic cells and mice lacking PKCδ exhibit loss of self tolerance, suggesting that PKCδ generates signals that establish or maintain the anergic state of B cells (70–72).

Activation of PLCγ2 by the BCR is largely dependent on the signaling scaffold molecule BLNK (B cell linker), which is also called SLP-65 (SH2-containing leukocyte protein of 65kDa) and BASH (B cell adaptor containing SH2 domain). BLNK is required for B cell development in humans (73), probably reflecting a role for this molecule in pre-BCR signaling. Mouse B cells lacking BLNK exhibit a substantial but less complete block at the pro-B cell to pre-B cell stage and exhibit a further block at the immature to mature B cell stage (74).

BLNK has an N-terminal region containing a short putative leucine-zipper structure, a central region with at least five tyrosines that become phosphorylated upon BCR stimulation, and a C-terminal SH2 domain. Although BLNK appears to be a soluble cytoplasmic protein, a fraction of the molecules associate with the plasma membrane of B cells prior to antigen stimulation via the leucine zipper (75), and this association appears to be important for BLNK function. Full BLNK function also requires its SH2 domain, which binds to phosphorylated Y204 in Ig-α and thereby localize BLNK to the signaling BCRs (Figure 8.7). Mice in which Ig-α contains a Y204F mutation exhibit clear defects, including decreased BCR-induced proliferation and decreased T-independent type II antibody responses in vivo (76).

Recruitment of BLNK to the BCR leads to phosphorylation of 5 tyrosines that are important for signaling function (77). Three of these (Y84, Y178, and Y189 in human BLNK) are responsible for recruiting PLCγ2 via an SH2 domain in the latter, perhaps reflecting an amplification mechanism (one BLNK molecule attracting three PLCγ2 molecules). Recruitment to the membrane of PLCγ2 is also promoted by its PH domain binding to PIP_3, generated by PI 3-kinase. Once recruited to BLNK, PLCγ2 becomes tyrosine phosphorylated by Syk, but this is insufficient for PLCγ2 enzymatic activation. Additional tyrosine phosphorylation of PLCγ2 on two sites (Y753 and Y759) is required for enzymatic activity, and these phosphorylations are provided by a third type of intracellular protein tyrosine kinase, Btk.

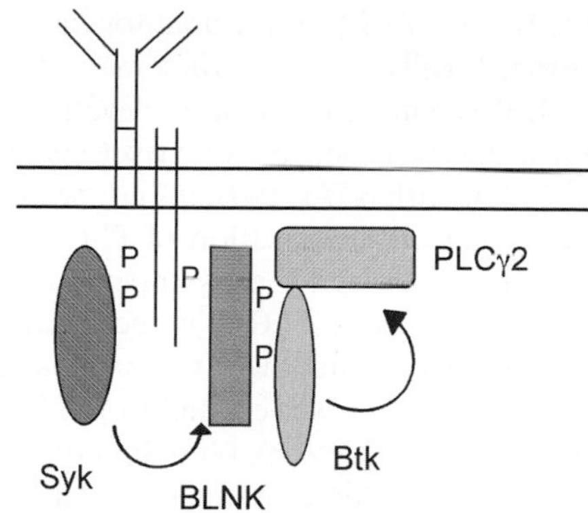

FIGURE 8.7 Adaptor molecules involved in PLCγ2 signaling in B cells. BLNK binds via its SH2 domain to phosphorylated Y204 of Igα. BLNK then becomes phosphorylated on tyrosines, which allows it to bind to PLCγ2 and Btk and thereby scaffold a complex for activation of PIP_2 hydrolysis. Syk phosphorylates BLNK; Btk is necessary to activate PLCYγ2.

Btk is recruited to BLNK by binding to a distinct tyrosine (Y96 in human BLNK) from those that recruit PLCγ2. Interestingly, for BLNK to be functional for inducing calcium signaling, it must have an intact Btk recruitment site, as well as at least one PLCγ2 recruitment site. Expression of two mutant forms of BLNK, one lacking the Btk-binding site and the other lacking the PLCγ2-binding sites, is insufficient for restoring function (77), indicating that BLNK must scaffold a complex between Btk and PLCγ2 (Figure 8.7) to promote the activation of the latter. The fifth tyrosine site on BLNK appears to recruit Vav and Nck, which may also contribute to PIP_2 breakdown and are discussed below.

Mice deficient in Btk, PLCγ2, or BLNK all exhibit significant defects in B cell development, probably reflecting defects in pre-BCR or BCR signaling, although the severity of the defects differ to some degree. There may be some redundancy between Btk and other Tec family kinases, and similarly there could be some redundancy between PLCγ2 and PLCγ1, accounting for small differences in phenotypes. Mice expressing the Y204F mutant form of Ig-α, which is responsible for recruiting BLNK to the signaling BCR, have some defects, but they are clearly lesser defects than those that are seen in mice deficient in Btk, PLCγ2 or BLNK, so it seems likely that either membrane localization of BLNK mediated by the leucine zipper motif is sufficient for some function, or there is another molecule that can recruit BLNK to the vicinity of signaling BCRs. The latter possibility has been suggested by analogy with SLP-76, which is similar to BLNK in some ways. Recruitment of SLP-76 is mediated by the transmembrane lipid raft-associated protein LAT (linker for activation of T cells). B cells express a molecule similar to LAT, called NTAL (non-T cell activation linker) or LAB (linker for activation of B cells), but genetic evidence argues against it playing a necessary role in the activation of BLNK in B cells (78).

Mice lacking this transmembrane adaptor molecule have close to normal B cells, although they may have a slight increase in BCR signaling to calcium elevation and in T-independent antibody responses. Moreover, convincing association of BLNK with NTAL/LAB has not been reported.

Thus, surprisingly, the activation of PLC by the antigen receptors of B cells and T cells appears to be significantly different: In B cells, PLCγ2 is recruited to a scaffold (BLNK) that is recruited directly to signaling BCRs, whereas in T cells PLCγ1 is recruited to the LAT-SLP-76 complex, which is not believed to bind directly to the TCR. It may be that the signaling architecture in T cells has greater potential for amplification, since many LAT/SLP-76 complexes can be phosphorylated, bind and activate PLCγ1, even if only a small number of TCRs are engaged. Such an amplification may explain how T cells can generate a robust calcium elevation when only 1 to 10 TCRs are engaged with foreign peptide-MHC ligands (79). In contrast, the recruitment of BLNK directly to the BCR suggests that the calcium response would be more nearly proportional to the number of BCRs engaged. Thus, B cells may only be able to generate a biologically meaningful calcium signal if many antigen receptors are engaged and signaling.

The Ras-Raf-Erk Pathway

The Ras-Raf-Erk signaling pathway controls several steps in the developmental progression of B cell and is also critical for BCR-stimulated proliferation of mature B cells. Receptor stimulation activates guanine-nucleotide exchange factors (GEFs) that convert Ras from the inactive GDP-bound form to the active GTP-bound form by inducing it to release bound GDP and thereby allowing GTP to bind. GEFs are countered in the cell by GTPase-activating factors (GAPs) that induce Ras to hydrolyze the bound GTP and release phosphate, leaving GDP bound to Ras in the inactive conformation (Figure 8.8). Active Ras binds to and activates a series of Ras effectors, of which the best understood is the serine-threonine protein kinase Raf, which activates MEK1 and MEK2, which in turn activate the Erk1 and Erk2 MAP kinases (80). Among the major functions of Erk is phosphorylation and activation of various transcription factors. For example, in B cells, the Ras pathway activates Ets-family transcription factors acting at Serum Response Elements (SREs) in the Egr1 gene to induce its expression, which in turn promotes expression of adhesion molecules ICAM-1 and CD44 (81–84). Also, in mature B cells, MEK1 and MEK2 inhibitors strongly interfere with anti-Ig-induced B cell proliferation (84). Transgenic expression in B lineage cells of dominant negative forms of Ras block developmental progression to the pre-B cell and immature B cell stages (85,86), demonstrating that Ras also has developmental roles in developing B cells, probably via Erk activation.

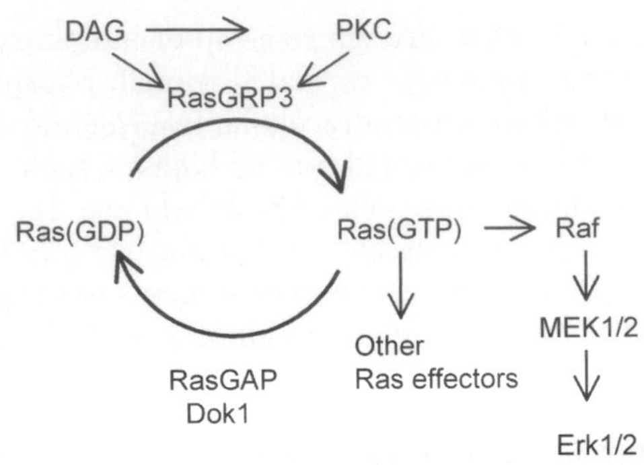

FIGURE 8.8 Control of Ras activity in B cells. Ras exists in two conformations, an inactive conformation bound to GDP and an active conformation bound to GTP. Conversion from the inactive to the active conformation is achieved by guanine nucleotide exchange factors (GEFs) that induce release of GDP, allowing GTP to bind and induce the active conformational. The most important GEF for BCR regulation of Ras is Ras guanine nucleotide releasing factor 3 (RasGRP3), which is activated by diacylglycerol (DAG) and by phosphorylation by protein kinase C. Ras is inactivated by GTPase activating factors (GAPs), neurofibromin, which acts constitutively, and RasGAP, which is controlled by signaling reactions, including those downstream of the negative coreceptor FcγRIIb, which recruits RasGap via SHIP and the adaptor Dok1. Ras effectors include the serine-threonine protein kinase Raf, which activates the Erk MAP kinase, and other effectors of unknown function in B cells.

BCR-induced activation of Ras primarily results from activation of RasGEFs and, in particular, RasGRP3 (Ras guanine nucleotide releasing protein 3), and to a lesser extent RasGRP1 (87,88). RasGRPs have domains structurally related to the C1 DAG-binding domains found in protein kinase C (PKC) isoforms, and their activation is correspondingly dependent on DAG, which is generated by PLC action. Indeed, BCR activation of Ras is highly dependent on PLCγ2. RasGRP3 is found in the cytoplasm of unstimulated B cells, and it is recruited to the membrane in response to PLCγ2 action (87). However, forced recruitment to the membrane of RasGRP3 only activates Ras to a small degree. Recent studies have identified BCR-induced phosphorylation of T133 of RasGRP3 as a key regulatory step in full activation of Ras. It appears that conventional isoforms of PKC (which in B cells would be PKCα or PKCβ) are responsible for this phosphorylation (89,90), which means that DAG acts in two ways to promote RasGRP3 activation and also that calcium elevation contributes importantly to Ras activation, because conventional PKCs are dependent on both calcium and diacylglycerol for their activation (Figure 8.8).

Ras-Raf-Erk signaling is attenuated in several ways following BCR signaling. One mechanism by which this pathway is attenuated is by the recruitment of RasGAP to the membrane by the formation of a tyrosine phosphorylation/SH2-based multiprotein complex including SHIP, Dok1 (downstream of kinase 1), and RasGAP (19). This complex likely also contains the adaptor Shc (91,92). This pathway is strongly engaged by the inhibitory coreceptor FcγRIIb (93,94) and is discussed further below. In addition, among the early response genes induced by BCR signaling is a MAP kinase phosphatase, MKP1, which can directly inactivate Erk and other MAP kinases (95).

The Vav-Rac Pathway

Rac is a small molecular weight GTP-binding protein related to Ras, but more closely related to Rho, Cdc42, and a handful of other Rho family members. Rho family members function in the regulation of actin polymerization, which is important for cell shape and cell migration. Rho family members also are important for activation of two types of MAP kinases, JNK (c-Jun N-terminal kinase) and p38 MAP kinase. BCR signaling activates Rac through the Vav family of GEFs, which are recruited into signaling complexes via BLNK and CD19 (Figure 8.9). B cells express all three members of this family (Vav1, Vav2, and Vav3), and the phenotypes of mice lacking one or more forms of Vav suggests that all three of these Vav isoforms participate in B cell function, largely in nonredundant ways (96). Rac appears to enhance PIP_2 hydrolysis by activation of a PIP 5-kinase, which replenishes PIP_2 to allow its hydrolysis to continue at a high level (97). Rac also activates production of reactive oxygen species to amplify BCR signaling at an early stage as described earlier. Rac also promotes activation of a protein kinase called HPK1 (hematopoietic progenitor kinase 1), which appears to be upstream of JNK activation. JNK in turn phosphorylates and activates the c-Jun transcription factor, promoting transcription of early response genes. An adaptor Bam32 (B lymphocyte adaptor molecule of 32kDa) also contributes to this pathway (98). B cells from mice genetically ablated for this adaptor exhibit defects in BCR-induced activation of HPK1 and JNK, as well as MEKK1, which is likely an intermediate in this signaling cascade (Figure 8.9). These B cells also exhibit decreased anti-Ig-induced proliferation in vitro. Bam32-deficient mice have normal development of follicular and marginal zone B cells, but had defective development of B1 cells in one study and an inability to make antibodies in response to T-independent type II antigens (98).

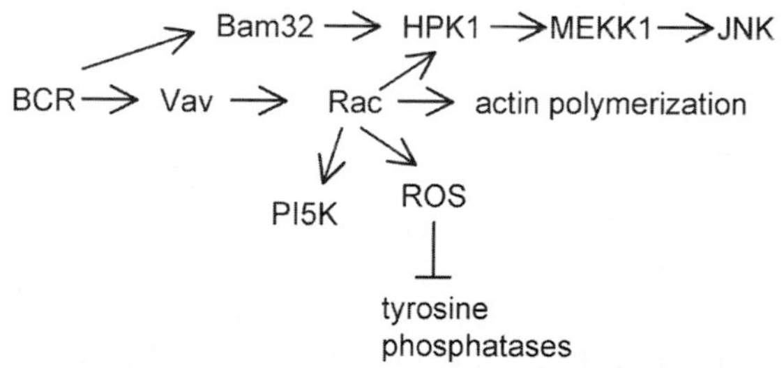

FIGURE 8.9 The Vav-Rac pathway activated by BCR signaling. BCR signaling results in recruitment to the membrane and activation of Vav, which is a guanine nucleotide exchange factor for Rac. Rac promotes actin polymerization, JNK activation, and probably production of reactive oxygen species (ROS) that amplify BCR signaling in general. Rac also activates PIP 5-kinase, which replenishes $PI4,5P_2$ levels, promoting high-level generation of second messengers from this compound. HPK1: hematopoietic progenitor kinase 1; MEKK1: MAPK/Erk kinase kinase 1.

The Rap-Integrin Pathway

BCR stimulation leads to increased binding by integrins expressed on B cells, particularly LFA-1 ($\alpha L\beta 2$), which binds to ICAM-1, and $\alpha 4\beta 1$ which binds to VCAM-1 and to fibronectin. Integrins promote adhesion between the B cell and a variety of immune cells that may have antigen bound to their surface (1) or to helper T cells and, therefore, likely promote the prolonged recognition and response to antigen in many circumstances. The ability of integrins to promote adhesion is controlled both by conformational changes between a low-affinity state and one or more higher affinity states (99) and by release from the actin cytoskeleton, which gives integrins the freedom to cluster and more efficiently bind to ligands fixed in the extracellular matrix or on the surface of another cell. The former is referred to as *affinity regulation*, whereas the latter is sometimes called *avidity regulation*, although more properly, the term *avidity* refers to the combination of the effects of affinity and multivalency on binding strength. In the case of BCR activation of integrins, there may be regulation of either or both integrin conformation and integrin mobility within the membrane.

A key regulator of integrin activation in B cells, as well as in other cells is the Rap family of Ras-like small GTP-bindings proteins (100,101). Both BCR and chemokine receptor stimulation of B cells induce activation of Rap1 and Rap2 and blocking this activation by overexpressing a highly specific Rap GTPase-activating protein blocks the increase in integrin adhesion (101). Recent evidence demonstrates that two adaptor proteins, ADAP (adhesion and degranulation-promoting adaptor protein) and SKAP55 (Src kinase-associated phosphoprotein of 55kD) are required for the TCR to induce integrin activation in T cells and suggests that this is mediated by targeting of activated Rap to the correct location at the plasma membrane (102). B cells likely use related but distinct molecules, as gene knockouts for these two molecules do not exhibit clear B cell defects, but B cells from mice lacking SKAP-HOM, which is closely related to SKAP55, do show a strong defect in BCR-induced integrin activation (103). Recent evidence suggests that Rap may act by promoting the binding of talin to the cytoplasmic domains of integrin β chains,

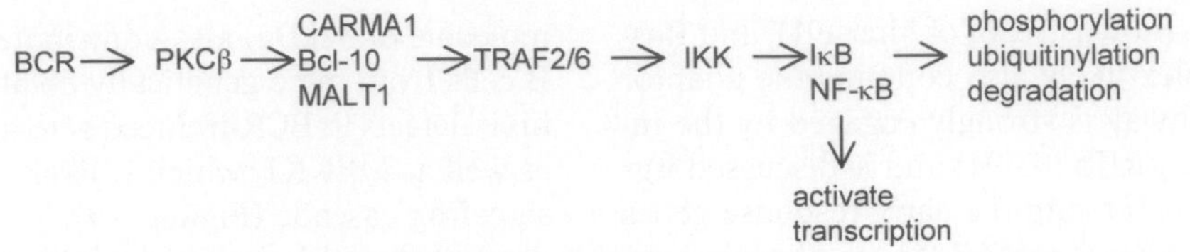

BCR → PKCβ → CARMA1 Bcl-10 MALT1 → TRAF2/6 → IKK → IκB NF-κB → phosphorylation ubiquitinylation degradation

↓ activate transcription

FIGURE 8.10 Activation of the NF-κB pathway downstream of the BCR. BCR signaling induces phosphorylation and oligomerization of the scaffold molecule CARMA1 and its association with adaptors Bcl-10 and MALT1, which then activate TNF receptor–associated factors TRAF2 and TRAF6. TRAFs activate the IκB kinase (IKK) complex to phosphorylate IκB. Phosphorylated IκB is then ubiquitinylated and degraded, freeing NF-κB to enter the nucleus and induce transcription.

which promotes their unfolding into the higher affinity conformation (104).

The NF-κB Pathway

The transcription factor NF-κB is central to inflammatory, innate immune, and adaptive immune responses. In B cells, NF-κB is activated by the BCR, by TNF receptor family members, including CD40 and BAFF receptor, and by TLRs (105). In mature B cells, BCR-induced survival and proliferation pathways are particularly dependent on NF-κB signaling, and mice genetically defective for signaling components that connect the BCR (but not TLRs or cytokine receptors) to NF-κB activation have a severe defect in lymphocyte activation (105,106).

NF-κB is a family of transcription factors originally discovered as binding to a site in the Ig κ intronic enhancer and is composed of homo- and heterodimers of five different related members, called p50 (NFKB1), p52 (NFKB2), p65 (RelA), c-Rel, and RelB (105). NF-κB can be held in an inactive form in the cytoplasm by an inhibitor called IκB, of which there are several isoforms. The activation of NF-κB generally follows phosphorylation, ubiquitination, and proteasome-mediated degradation of IκBs (Figure 8.10). Although different types of receptors activate NF-κB via distinct mechanisms, in most cases, referred to as the *classical* or *canonical pathway,* activation occurs via the IκB kinase (IKK) complex, which is a high molecular weight complex of multiple copies of three different subunits, called IKKα, IKKβ and IKKγ (or NEMO). IKKα and IKKβ are serine/threonine protein kinases and in this pathway IKKβ is essential for the phosphorylation and subsequent ubiquitination and degradation of IκB, IKKα plays a less important role and IKKγ is a scaffold that holds together the IKK complex and mediates its association with upstream activators. A second pathway of NF-κB activation, the *alternative* or *noncanonical pathway,* is mediated primarily by IKKα downstream of a subset of TNF receptor family members including BAFF receptor (105).

Antigen receptors utilize a unique set of signaling components to activate the IKK complex, although they ultimately use components from the TNF receptor, IL-1 receptor, and TLR pathways in the terminal steps leading to IKK activation. BCR signaling induces the assembly of a plasma membrane lipid raft–associated complex between the scaffold molecule CARMA1 and two adaptor proteins, Bcl-10 and MALT1, which then binds to TRAF2 (TNF receptor associated factor 2) or TRAF6. In the pathway connecting the BCR to IKK activation, TRAF2 and TRAF6 are thought to be alternative and equivalent components, although there are subtle mechanistic differences (106). TRAF2 also participates in NF-κB signaling downstream of TNF receptor family members, whereas TRAF6 also participates in NF-κB signaling from TLRs, IL-1 receptor family members, and CD40 (107). TRAFs are E3 ubiquitin ligases that catalyze ubiquitinylation reactions forming K63-linked polyubiquitin chains on themselves (TRAF6) or on associated proteins (RIP1 in the case of TRAF2). The K63-polyubiquitin chains are recognized by ubiquitin-binding domains on IKKγ and on the adaptor proteins TAB2 (TAK1-binding protein 2) or TAB3, and in this way TRAF action nucleates formation of a larger signaling complex that includes TRAF2 or TRAF6, the IKK complex and the TAK1 (TGFβ-activated protein kinase 1) complex with TAB1 and TAB2 or TAB3 (Figure 8.10). Once this complex forms, IKKγ also becomes decorated with a K63-polyubiquitin chain that appears to be necessary for IKK enzymatic activation, as is phosphorylation of IKKβ by TAK1.

How antigen receptors trigger this sequence of signaling reactions leading to IKK complex activation is not completely understood, but a key event is phosphorylation of CARMA1 by PKCβ in B cells (108) and PKCθ in T cells (Figure 8.10). PKCβ is a conventional PKC that is activated by calcium and DAG, both of which are generated downstream of PLCγ2 action. In contrast, PKCθ is activated by DAG alone, without a requirement for calcium elevation. The significance of this difference in signaling to NF-κB in B cells versus T cells is not known at this time. Phosphorylation of CARMA1 has been proposed to promote its multimerization and binding to Bcl-10, which in turn multimerizes MALT1 and TRAF2 or TRAF6, which appears to be how TRAFs become activated. CARMA1 multimerization occurs at the plasma membrane in areas of coalesced lipid rafts (108,109). CARMA1 is mostly cytosolic in resting lymphocytes, so its multimerization at the plasma membrane likely reflects binding to an unknown membrane protein. The significance of CARMA1 lipid raft localization is also not known, although it may reflect the localization of the putative binding protein. In any case, it is clear that NF-κB is triggered by PKCβ activation in B cells (106), possibly with involvement of additional signaling reactions.

CORECEPTORS FOR BCR SIGNALING

The term "coreceptors" has been given to CD4 and CD8 in T cells because these molecules also bind to the peptide-MHC ligand that is bound by the TCR. As described in Chapters 10 and 11, CD4 and CD8 aid T cell activation by promoting the binding between TCR and peptide-MHC and also by cooperation of their intracellular domains with the intracellular domains of the TCR subunits, particularly with the ITAMs in the CD3 and ζ chains. The cytoplasmic tails of CD4 and CD8 bind to the Src-family tyrosine kinase Lck, so the simultaneous binding of a TCR and CD4 or CD8 to the same peptide-MHC complex results in juxtaposition of Lck with ITAMs, promoting efficient ITAM phosphorylation. Thus, CD4 and CD8 effectively tell the T cell that the TCR has bound to the correct type of ligand.

Analogously, the B cell expresses at least three different molecules that can bind to the same molecular complex bound by the BCR and, if this happens, modulate BCR signaling. These B cell coreceptors provide additional information about the nature of the antigen that is relevant to B cell activation. One of these B cell coreceptors, the complement receptor 2 (CR2) complex, functions positively to promote B cell activation, whereas two of these coreceptors, FcγRIIb and CD22, function negatively to inhibit B cell activation (Figure 8.11). Complement deposited on an antigen provides an indication to the B cell that the innate immune system or preexisting antibody has tagged the molecular complex as foreign, whereas the presence of antigen in an IgG-containing immune complex is an indication that sufficient antibody has already been made to counter the threat. The logic of the coreceptor role for CD22 is less well established, but this molecule binds to α2, 6-linked sialic acid oligosaccharides, which are expressed on most host cells but less commonly on microbe surfaces, so this coreceptor may act to decrease antibody responses to cell surface self-antigens (110,111).

Complement receptor 2 (CR2, also called CD21) is found in a complex with CD19 and the tetraspanin protein CD81 (61). When CR2 is coligated with the BCR, CD81 promotes prolonged association of the BCR with lipid rafts, which may enhance its signaling (111a). CD19, the other component of the CR2 complex, is a major adaptor molecule for activation of PI 3-kinase signaling, as described above, and it is thought to be responsible for the major coreceptor signaling function of the CR2 complex. Lyn binds to CD19 after the latter becomes activated, so this association may amplify signaling. Genetic studies indicate that the PI 3-kinase binding sites in the cytoplasmic tail of CD19 (Y482, Y513) are responsible for most of the signaling function of CD19 (62,63). Curiously, in its signaling mechanism, CD19 is more closely analogous to signaling by the T cell costimulatory receptor CD28 than to signaling by the T cell coreceptors CD4 and CD8. For both CD28 and the CR2 complex, the ligands are molecules related to innate immune recognition: In T cells, the B7 ligands for CD28 can be induced on dendritic cells by TLR signaling, and in B cells, the fragments of C3 may be deposited on antigenic particles due to the alternative or lectin pathways of complement, or due to complement activation by weak reactivity to preexisting

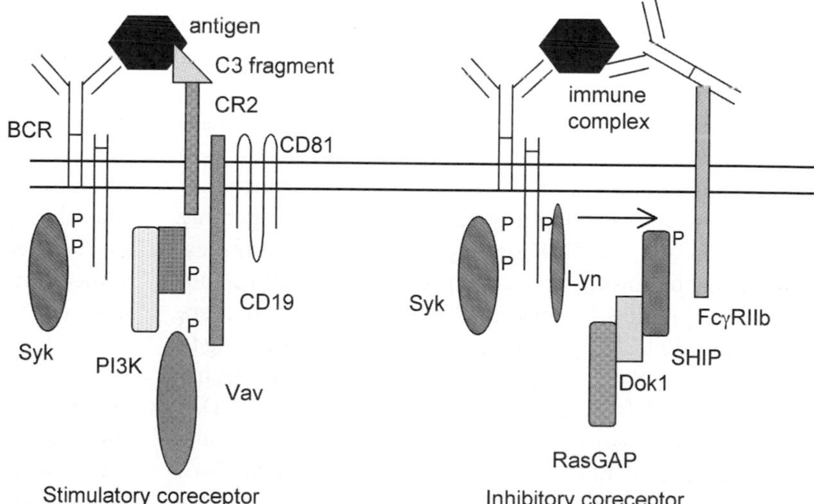

FIGURE 8.11 Coreceptors and BCR signaling. The complement receptor 2 (CR2) complex with CD19 and CD81 serves as a positive coreceptor for BCR signaling (left). When an antigen is coated with C3b-derived complement fragments, CR2 is brought adjacent to the BCR, where the cytoplasmic tail of CD19 can be phosphorylated on several tyrosines. Phosphorylated CD19 serves as a binding site for signaling proteins including PI 3-kinase and Vav. CD19 also participates in BCR signaling in the absence of complement activation, although less efficiently. FcγRIIb is a negatively acting coreceptor (right). If the antigen has IgG bound to it, then FcγRIIb is recruited adjacent to the BCR. Lyn associated with the BCR phosphorylates the ITIM tyrosine of FcγRIIb, which attracts SHIP, which counters PI 3-kinase. SHIP also recruits RasGAP via the adaptor Dok1, resulting in inactivation of Ras.

IgM. Thus, whether one considers the CR2 complex to be more analogous to T cell coreceptors or T cell costimulatory receptors is a matter of choice. In either case, juxtaposition of the signaling BCR with CR2 strongly promotes B cell activation (112).

The inhibitory coreceptors of B cells are part of an extensive family of immune inhibitory receptors characterized by the presence in their cytoplasmic tails of an immunoreceptor tyrosine-based inhibitory motif (ITIM) (113). These inhibitory receptors play critical roles in restraining activation of all immune cells, including B cells. Indeed, in addition to FcγRIIb and CD22, B cell express a variety of other inhibitory receptors whose function is less well understood but that clearly serve to inhibit BCR signaling, including CD72 (114,115), PIR-B (116), and CD5 (117,118).

When a B cell binds to antigen that is in an immune complex with specific IgG, then it engages FcγRIIb as well as the BCR, and this juxtaposition promotes phosphorylation of the ITIM tyrosine in the cytoplasmic tail of FcγRIIb. The phosphorylated ITIM serves as a high-affinity binding site for SHIP (SH2-containing polyphosphoinositide 5 phosphatase), which removes the 5 phosphate from PIP_3 (Figure 8.6), thereby countering most of the actions of PI 3-kinase, because the resulting lipid, PI 3,4P_2, does not activate Akt or promote activation of PLCγ2, although it does serve as a ligand for some PH domains, including the PH domain of the adaptor Bam32 (98). SHIP also recruits to this inhibitory complex the adaptor Dok-1 and RasGAP, which inactivates Ras (93,94). Thus, coligation of the BCR and FcγRIIb results in some signaling but attenuation of the most important downstream signaling events. Presumably, an antigen with a small amount of IgG bound could still induce B cell activation, whereas soluble antigen in an extensive IgG-containing immune complex or present on a cell surface covered with IgG would likely not induce an immune response from naïve B cells. It should be noted, however, that FcγRIIb on follicular dendritic cells plays a positive role in promoting germinal center B cell responses, so the role of FcγRIIb in antibody responses is complex and depends on the stage of the response.

The role of CD22 in the regulation of antibody responses is less well understood, but a major function of CD22 is to inhibit BCR signaling via its ITIMs (111). In contrast to FcγRIIb, which is thought to only inhibit BCR signaling if coligated with the BCR by a specific immune complex, some CD22 on the cell surface is preassociated with a subset of mIgM molecules on naïve B cells. Alternatively, there is evidence that CD22 function is regulated by it binding to ligands on the B cell surface, perhaps reflecting a mechanism for tuning BCR signaling (119). In either case, CD22 and its ITIM appear to attenuate BCR signaling in a tonic way (111,120). In addition, it has been proposed that CD22 binding to sialic acid-containing glycoproteins on the antigen or antigen-bearing particle would increase the amount of CD22 coligated with the BCR and thereby attenuate signaling (110). CD22-deficient mice do exhibit some autoantibody production, but it appears to be modest compared to what is seen in mice lacking other molecules involved in these inhibitory pathways, as discussed below. BCR crosslinking leads to phosphorylation of CD22 and recruitment of SHP-1 (SH2-containing tyrosine protein phosphatase 1) and of SHIP (121). Other inhibitory receptors on B cells, including CD72, PIR-B, and CD5 (on B1 cells), also have ITIMs and bind SHP-1 and so likely provide some redundancy that may compensate to some degree for the loss of CD22 in the knockout mice. SHP-1 probably attenuates BCR signaling by dephosphorylating early components in the signaling cascade, including BLNK (122). CD22 also appears to directly regulate calcium influx induced by the BCR (123).

Phosphorylation of the ITIM tyrosines of FcγRIIb, CD22, and other inhibitory receptors of B cells is heavily dependent on the Src-family tyrosine kinase Lyn (124). In contrast, BCR ITAM tyrosine phosphorylation is mediated by all three of the most highly expressed Src-family tyrosine kinases of B cells, Lyn, Fyn, and Blk (34), and probably once started is maintained in part by Syk, as described earlier. The mechanism for the heavy dependence of inhibitory receptor function on Lyn is not understood in detail, although in the case of CD22, Lyn binds to a tyrosine phosphorylation site in the cytoplasmic domain of CD22 distinct from the ITIM, and it has been proposed that Lyn binds and then efficiently phosphorylates the ITIM (125). In any case, the heavy dependence of inhibitory receptor function in B cells on Lyn has made it interesting to examine the effects of Lyn-defeciency on B cell function (124,126). Lyn-deficient mice exhibit elevated levels of serum IgM and IgG, suggesting enhanced activation of B cells during immune responses. In addition, these mice make high levels of antinuclear antibodies and anti–double-stranded DNA antibodies and develop lupus nephritis and kidney disease, which is eventually fatal on a mixed genetic background (127). Autoantibody production in Lyn-deficient mice is attenuated on either a C57BL/6 background or a Balb/c background but still occurs (Gross, A. J. and DeFranco, A. L., unpublished observations). Mice deficient in other elements of the inhibitory receptor pathway in B cells also exhibit autoantibody production, although to variable degrees. Thus, FcγRIIb-deficient mice exhibit autoimmunity, even on some nonautoimmune genetic backgrounds (128), CD22-deficient mice exhibit some autoreactivity, but to a lower degree than that seen in Lyn-deficient or FcγRIIb-deficient mice (126). Finally, SHP-1-deficient mice were originally isolated as motheaten mice, which have a severe autoimmune and inflammatory disease that is fatal early in life. The severe nature of this disease may reflect important roles for SHP-1 in inhibitory receptor function in all lymphocytes and leukocytes, compared to the less dramatic effects of mutations that affect only B cells or B cells and a few other cell types.

ANTIGEN PRESENTATION BY B CELLS

In addition to being a signaling receptor, the BCR is an endocytic receptor that takes up antigens for presentation to T cells, which in turn promote activation of B cells, as described in detail in the next chapter. Internalization of the BCR is achieved via tyrosine-containing sequences found in the cytoplasmic domains of Ig-α and Ig-β (129,130). Uptake is primarily via a clathrin-mediated pathway, although a second pathway involving lipid rafts also is active (131,132). Studies with chimeric molecules in which the cytoplasmic tails of Ig-α or Ig-β have been fused to heterologous proteins indicate that both cytoplasmic tails can mediate uptake and that they function in a complementary fashion to promote antigen presentation (129,133). In particular, the Ig-β cytoplasmic domain is responsible for targeting the BCR/antigen complex to late endosomes, where antigenic peptide loading onto MHC class II molecules occurs. Recently, internalization of the BCRs have been examined in a more physiological context by the use of targeted gene mutations and analysis of B cells from mice with these targeted mutations (130). B cells in which the Ig-α cytoplasmic tail has been modified to change the two ITAM tyrosines to phenylalanine or in which the Ig-β cytoplasmic tail has been modified to change its two ITAM tyrosines to alanines were examined. B cells with either alteration showed a profound loss of constitutive BCR internalization and clearly slower BCR-cross-linking induced internalization. B cells with mutant Ig-β showed the greater delay in ligand-stimulated internalization and also a decrease in the final extent of internalization, whereas B cells with mutant Ig-α had decreased internalization but to a smaller degree. B cells from both mice had elevated levels of cell surface IgM and IgD, in agreement with decreased constitutive BCR internalization.

In addition to the role of the Ig-α ITAM tyrosines in BCR internalization, there is also evidence for a role for Ig-α Y204 in BCR internalization (133). Y204 is the tyrosine that when phosphorylated binds to BLNK (76,134,135). Interestingly, phosphorylation of Ig-α Y204 appears to block internalization (133). Given the central role of BLNK in BCR signaling, as described earlier, this observation suggests that ligand-engaged BCRs can either signal or be internalized as alternative contributions to B cell activation. Mathematical modeling indicates that a feature of competition between the two BCR functions is that the difference in the amounts of signaling resulting from ligands that bind to the BCR with higher avidity versus those that bind with lower avidity is less than would occur in a situation where signaling and internalization are not antagonistic (133). In other words, antagonism between signaling and internalization is predicted to allow B cells to respond to a wide variety of ligands of different avidity by promoting signaling at low avidity where there is a low degree of internalization.

Although individual BCRs may signal or be internalized, BCR signaling in the cell contributes positively to antigen presentation and interactions with T cells in multiple ways. BCR signaling induces migration of follicular B cells from the follicles to the boundary of the T cell zone and also induces migration of marginal zone B cells to promote their interactions with helper T cells (8). BCR signaling induces increased adhesion of a B cell's LFA-1 integrin molecules, as described earlier, which promotes binding to helper T cells. In addition, BCR-stimulated B cells induce expression of the costimulatory molecule B7-2 (CD86) and also increase their expression of MHC class II molecules, both of which would promote activation of helper T cells recognizing peptides contained in the antigen internalized via the BCR. BCR signaling also promotes acidification of endosomes, which is important for antigen processing and loading onto class II MHC molecules (129).

LINKAGE OF ANTIGEN PRESENTATION TO ITAM SIGNALING IN B CELLS

Activation of B cells either through the BCR or via IL-4 leads to association of MHC class II molecules with Ig-α/Ig-β heterodimers (136). Subsequent clustering of MHC molecules by anti-MHC antibodies or by recombinant soluble TCRs induces strong ITAM signaling, which promotes B cell activation in vitro. Although the physiological relevance of this pathway is not clearly established, it is striking that in cell-cell conjugates between antigen-presenting B cells and antigen-specific T cells, there is a strong concentration of B cell MHC class II molecules at the interface, suggesting that they are engaged and are likely signaling. Moreover, it is interesting that the association of Ig-α/Ig-β with the class II MHC molecules requires prior B cell stimulation, which may promote antigen specificity of the response, as would the fact that B cell–T cell conjugates generally are only stable if T cells are recognizing cognate peptide-MHC complexes. Thus, although further work is required, the possibility that this signaling process is important for B cell activation in many circumstances is an attractive one.

CONCLUSION

B cells make antibodies in response to a rich diversity of physical forms of antigens, implying the existence of a considerable flexibility in the mechanisms that control B cell activation. In addition, B cells make a wide variety of cellular responses to BCR stimulation, including promotion or arrest of developmental progression, choice of lineage between marginal zone and follicular types of mature B cells, promotion of survival or of apoptosis, migration to particular places within secondary lymphoid tissues, and entry into cell cycle. This flexibility and variety may explain why BCR signaling employs a large number of signaling pathways and why there is overlap between some of these pathways and signaling pathways induced by other key regulators of B cells, including TLRs and CD40. Clearly we have come a long way in the past two decades in understanding in detail how B cell activation is regulated. Just as clearly, much more needs to be learned to reduce this complexity to a clearer and more complete understanding of how the molecular mechanisms described in this chapter combine to regulate B cell activation in a way that generates rapid and useful antibody responses but largely avoids destructive autoantibody production.

REFERENCES

1. Carrasco YR, Batista FD. B cell recognition of membrane-bound antigen: an exquisite way of sensing ligands. *Curr Opin Immunol.* 2006;18:286–291.
2. Bossen C, Schneider P. BAFF, APRIL and their receptors: structure, function and signaling. *Semin Immunol.* 2006;18:263–275.
3. Hangartner L, Zinkernagel RM, Hengartner H. Antiviral antibody responses: the two extremes of a wide spectrum. *Nat Rev Immunol.* 2006;6:231–243.
4. Mond JJ, Lees A, Snapper C. T cell-independent antigens type 2. *Ann Rev Immunol.* 1995;13:655–692.
5. Ruprecht CR, Lanzavecchia A. Toll-like receptor stimulation as a third signal required for activation of human naive B cells. *Eur J Immunol*. 2006;36:810–816.
6. Pasare C, Medzhitov R. Control of B-cell responses by Toll-like receptors. *Nature.* 2005;438:364–368.
7. Lau CM, Broughton C, Tabor AS, et al. RNA-associated autoantigens activate B cells by combined B cell antigen receptor/Toll-like receptor 7 engagement. *J Exp Med.* 2005;202:1171–1177.
8. Okada T, Cyster JG. B cell migration and interactions in the early phase of antibody responses. *Curr Opin Immunol.* 2006;18:278–285.
9. Foote LC, Schneider TJ, Fischer GM, et al. Intracellular signaling for inducible antigen receptor-mediated Fas resistance in B cells. *J Immunol*. 1996;157:1878–1885.
10. Rathmell JC, Cooke MP, Ho WY, et al. CD95 (Fas)-dependent elimination of self-reactive B cells upon interaction with CD4+ T cells. *Nature.* 1995;376:181–184.
11. Niiro H, Clark EA. Regulation of B-cell fate by antigen-receptor signals. *Nat Rev Immunol.* 2002;2:945–956.
12. Carsetti R, Kohler G, Lamers MC. Transitional B cells are the target of negative selection in the B cell compartment. *J Exp Med.* 1995;181:2129–2140.
13. Pillai S, Cariappa A, Moran ST. Marginal zone B cells. *Annu Rev Immunol.* 2005;23:161–196.
14. Hardy RR. B-1 B cells: development, selection, natural autoantibody and leukemia. *Curr Opin Immunol.* 2006;18:547–555.
15. Baumgarth N, Tung JW, Herzenberg LA. Inherent specificities in natural antibodies: a key to immune defense against pathogen invasion. *Springer Semin Immunopathol.* 2005;26:347–362.
16. Berland R, Wortis HH. Origins and functions of B-1 cells with notes on the role of CD5. *Annu Rev Immunol*. 2002;20:253–300.
17. Pelanda R, Torres RM. Receptor editing for better or for worse. *Curr Opin Immunol.* 2006;18:184–190.
18. Sandel PC, Monroe JG. Negative selection of immature B cells by receptor editing or deletion is determined by site of antigen encounter. *Immunity.* 1999;10:289–299.
19. Gauld SB, Merrell KT, Cambier JC. Silencing of autoreactive B cells by anergy: a fresh perspective. *Curr Opin Immunol.* 2006;18:292–297.
20. Dolmetsch RE, Lewis RS, Goodnow CC, et al. Differential activation of transcription factors induced by Ca^{2+} response amplitude and duration. *Nature.* 1997;386:855–858.
21. Rathmell JC, Townsend SE, Xu JC, et al. Expansion or elimination of B cells in vivo: dual roles for CD40- and Fas (CD95)-ligands modulated by the B cell antigen receptor. *Cell.* 1996;87:319–329.
22. Lesley R, Xu Y, Kalled SL, et al. Reduced competitiveness of autoantigen-engaged B cells due to increased dependence on BAFF. *Immunity.* 2004;20:441–453.
23. Merrell KT, Benschop RJ, Gauld SB, et al. Identification of anergic B Cells within a wild-type repertoire. *Immunity.* 2006;25:953–962.
24. Venkitaraman AR, Williams GT, Dariavach P, et al. The B cell antigen receptor of the five immunoglobulin classes. *Nature.* 1991;352:777–781.
25. Blum JH, Stevens TL, DeFranco AL. Role of the m immunoglobulin heavy chain transmembrane and cytoplasmic domains in B cell antigen receptor expression and signal transduction. *J Biol Chem.* 1993;268:27238–27247.
26. Grupp SA, Campbell K, Mitchell RN, et al. Signaling-defective mutants of the B lymphocyte antigen receptor fail to associate with Ig-α and Ig-β/γ. *J Biol Chem*. 1993;268:25776–25779.
27. Tolar P, Sohn HW, Pierce SK. The initiation of antigen-induced B cell antigen receptor signaling viewed in living cells by fluorescence resonance energy transfer. *Nat Immunol.* 2005;6:1168–1176.
28. Schamel WW, Reth M. Monomeric and oligomeric complexes of the B cell antigen receptor. *Immunity.* 2000;13:5–14.
29. Kim JH, Cramer L, Mueller H, et al. Independent trafficking of Ig-α/Ig-β and μ heavy chain is facilitated by dissociation of the B cell antigen receptor complex. *J Immunol*. 2005;175:147–154.
30. Lam K-P, Kuhn R, Rajewsky K. In vivo ablation of surface immunoglobulin on mature B cells by inducible gene targeting results in rapid cell death. *Cell.* 1997;90:1073–1083.
31. Kraus M, Alimzhanov M, Rajewsky N, et al. Survival of resting mature B lymphocytes on BCR signaling via the Ig-α/β heterodimer. *Cell.* 2004;117:787–800.
32. Pawson T. Protein modules and signalling networks. *Nature.* 1995; 373:573-80.
33. Monroe JG. ITAM-mediated tonic signalling through pre-BCR and BCR complexes. *Nat Rev Immunol.* 2006;6:283–294.
34. Saijo K, Schmedt C, Su IH, et al. Essential role of Src-family protein tyrosine kinases in NF-κB activation during B cell development. *Nat Immunol*. 2003;4:274–279.
35. Law DA, Chan VWF, Datta SK, et al. B-cell antigen receptor motifs have redundant signalling capabilities and bind the tyrosine kinases PTK72, Lyn and Fyn. *Curr Biol.* 1993;3:645–657.
36. Gauld SB, Cambier JC. Src-family kinases in B-cell development and signaling. *Oncogene.* 2004;23:8001–8006.
37. Dykstra M, Cherukuri A, Sohn HW, et al. Location is everything: lipid rafts and immune cell signaling. *Annu Rev Immunol.* 2003;21:457–481.
38. Gupta N, DeFranco AL. Visualization of lipid raft dynamics and early signaling events during antigen receptor-mediated B cell activation. *Mol Biol Cell.* 2003;14:432–444.
39. Sohn HW, Tolar P, Jin T, et al. Flourescence resonance energy transfer in living cells reveals dynamic membrane changes in the initiation of B cell signaling. *Proc Natl Acad Sci U S A.* 2006;103:8143–8148.
40. Sproul TW, Malapati S, Kim J, et al. Cutting edge: B cell antigen receptor signaling occurs outside lipid rafts in immature B cells. *J Immunol*. 2000;165:6020–6023.
41. Chung JB, Baumeister MA, Monroe JG. Cutting edge: differential sequestration of plasma membrane-associated B cell antigen receptor in mature and immature B cells into glycosphingolipid-enriched domains. *J Immunol*. 2001;166:736–740.
42. Reth M, Brummer T. Feedback regulation of lymphocyte signaling. *Nat Rev Immunol.* 2004;4:269–277.
43. Takata M, Sabe H, Hata A, et al. Tyrosine kinases Lyn and Syk regulate B cell receptor-coupled Ca^{2+} mobilization through distinct pathways. *EMBO J.* 1994;13:1341–1349.

44. Fitzer-Attas CJ, Lowry M, Crowley MT, et al. Fcγ receptor-mediated phagocytosis in macrophages lacking the Src family tyrosine kinases Hck,Fgr, and Lyn. *J Exp Med.* 2000;191:669–682.
45. Richards JD, Gold MR, Hourihane SL, et al. Reconstitution of B cell antigen receptor-induced signaling events in a nonlymphoid cell line by expressing the Syk protein-tyrosine kinase. *J Biol Chem.* 1996;271:6458–6466.
46. Rolli V, Gallwitz M, Wossning T, et al. Amplification of B cell antigen receptor signaling by a Syk/ITAM positive feedback loop. *Mol Cell.* 2002;10:1057–69.
47. Kolanus W, Romeo C, Seed B. T cell activation by clustered tyrosine kinases. *Cell.* 1993;74:171–183.
48. Munro S. Lipid rafts: elusive or illusive? *Cell.* 2003;115:377–388.
49. Shaw AS. Lipid rafts: now you see them, now you don't. *Nat Immunol.* 2006;7:1139–1142.
50. Zhang W, Irvin BJ, Trible RP, et al. Functional analysis of LAT in TCR-mediated signaling pathways using a LAT-deficient Jurkat cell line. *Int Immunol.* 1999;11:943–950.
51. Lin J, Weiss A, Finco TS. Localization of LAT in glycolipid-enriched microdomains is required for T cell activation. *J Biol Chem.* 1999;274:28861–28864.
52. Gupta N, Wollscheid B, Watts JD, et al. Quantitative proteomic analysis of B cell lipid rafts reveals that ezrin regulates antigen receptor-mediated lipid raft dynamics. *Nat Immunol.* 2006;7:625–633.
53. Karnell FG, Brezski RJ, King LB, et al. Membrane cholesterol content accounts for developmental differences in surface B cell receptor compartmentalization and signaling. *J Biol Chem.* 2005;280:25621–25628.
54. Singh DK, Kumar D, Siddiqui Z, et al. The strength of receptor signaling is centrally controlled through a cooperative loop between Ca+2 and an oxidant signal. *Cell.* 2005;121:281–293.
55. Tonks NK. Redox redux: revisiting PTPs and the control of cell signaling. *Cell.* 2005;121:667–670.
56. Jordan MS, Singer AL, Koretzky GA. Adaptors as central mediators of signal transduction. *Nat Immunol.* 2003;4:110–116.
57. Horejsi V, Zhang W, Schraven B. Transmembrane adaptor proteins: organizers of immunoreceptor signaling. *Nat Rev Immunol.* 2004;4:603–616.
58. Fruman D. Phosphoinositide 3-kinase and its targets in B-cell and T-cell signaling. *Curr Opin Immunol.* 2004;3:314–320.
59. Wullschleger S, Loewith R, Hall MN. TOR signaling in growth and metabolism. *Cell.* 2006;124:471–484.
60. Chen J, Yusuf I, Andersen H, et al. FOXO transcription factors cooperate with delta EF1 to activate growth suppressive genes in B lymphocytes. *J Immunol.* 2006;5:2711-21.
61. Carroll MC. The complement system in regulation of adaptive immunity. *Nat Immunol.* 2004;5:981–986.
62. Wang Y, Brooks S, Li X, et al. The physiologic role of CD19 cytoplasmic tyrosines. *Immunity.* 2002;17:501–514.
63. Wang Y, Carter R. CD19 regulates B cell maturation, proliferation, and positive selection in the FDC zone of murine splenic germinal centers. *Immunity.* 2005;22:749–761.
64. Yamazaki T, Takeda K, Gotoh K, et al. Essential immunoregulatory role for BCAP in B cell development and function. *J Exp Med.* 2002;195:535–545.
65. Ingham RJ, Santos L, Dang-Lawson M, et al. The Gab1 docking protein links the B cell antigen receptor to the phosphatidylinositol 3-kinase/Akt signaling pathway and to the SHP2 tyrosine phosphatase. *J Biol Chem.* 2001;276:12257–12265.
66. Sarmay G, Angyal A, Kertesz A, et al. The multiple function of Grb2 associated binder (Gab) adaptor/scaffolding protein in immune cell signaling. *Immunol Lett.* 2006;104:76–82.
67. Hikida M, Kurosaki T. Regulation of phospholipase C-γ2 networks in B lymphocytes. *Adv Immunol.* 2005;88:73–96.
68. Feske S, Gwack Y, Prakriya M, et al. A mutation in Orai1 causes immune deficiency by abrogating CRAC channel function. *Nature.* 2006;441:179–185.
69. Prakriya M, Feske S, Gwack Y, et al. Orai1 is an essential pore subunit of the CRAC channel. *Nature.* 2006;443:230–233.
70. Guo B, Su TT, Rawlings DJ. Protein kinase C family functions in B cell activation. *Curr Opin Immunol.* 2004;16:367–373.
71. Mecklenbrauker I, Saijo K, Zheng NY, et al. Protein kinase Cδ controls self-antigen-induced B-cell tolerance. *Nature.* 2002;416:860–865.
72. Miyamoto A, Nakayama K, Imaki H, et al. Increased proliferation of B cells and auto-immunity in mice lacking protein kinase Cδ. *Nature.* 2002;416:865–869.
73. Minegishi Y, Rohrer J, Coustan-Smith E, et al. An essential role for BLNK in human B cell development. *Science.* 1999;286:1954–1957.
74. Pappu R, Cheng AM, Li B, et al. Requirement for B cell linker protein (BLNK) in B cell development. *Science.* 1999;286:1949–1954.
75. Kohler F, Storch B, Kulathu Y, et al. A leucine zipper in the N terminus confers membrane association to SLP-65. *Nat Immunol.* 2005;6:204–210.
76. Patterson H, Kraus M, Kim Y, et al. The B cell receptor promotes B cell activation and proliferation through a non-ITAM tyrosine in the Igalpha. *Immunity.* 2006;25:55–65.
77. Chiu C, Dalton M, Ishiai M, et al. BLNK: molecular scaffolding through 'cis'-mediated organization of signaling proteins. *EMBO J.* 2002;21:6461–6472.
78. Wang Y, Horvath O, Hamm-Baarke A, et al. Single and combined deletions of the NTAL/LAB and LAT adaptors minimally affect B cell development and function. *Mol Cell Biol.* 2005;25:4455–65.
79. Irvine DJ, Purbhoo MA, Krogsgaard M, et al. Direct observation of ligand recognition by T cells. *Nature.* 2002;419:845–849.
80. Cantrell DA. GTPases and T cell activation. *Immunol Rev.* 2003;192:122–130.
81. McMahon SB, Monroe JG. A ternary complex factor-dependent mechanism mediates induction of egr-1 through selective serum response elements following antigen receptor cross-linking in B lymphocytes. *Mol Cell Biol.* 1995;15:1086–1093.
82. Maltzman J, Monroe JG. Transcriptional regulation of the Icam-1 gene in antigen receptor and phorbol ester stimulated B lymphocytes: Role for transcription factor EGR1. *J Exp Med.* 1996;183:1747–1759.
83. Maltzman J, Monroe JG. A role for EGR1 in regulation of stimulus-dependent CD44 transcription in B lymphocytes. *Mol Cell Biol.* 1996;16:2283–2294.
84. Richards JD, Dave SH, Chou CH, et al. Inhibition of the MEK/ERK signaling pathway blocks a subset of B cell responses to antigen. *J Immunol.* 2001;166:3855–3864.
85. Iritani BM, Forbush KA, Farrar MA, et al. Control of B cell development by Ras-mediated activation of Raf. *EMBO J.* 1997;16:7019–7031.
86. Nagaoka H, Takahashi Y, Hayashi R, et al. Ras mediates effector pathways responsible for pre-B cell survival, which is essential for the developmental progression to the late pre-B cell stage. *J Exp Med.* 2000;192:171–182.
87. Oh-hora M, Johmura S, Hashimoto A, et al. Requirement for Ras guanine nucleotide releasing protein 3 in coupling phospholipase C-gamma2 to Ras in B cell receptor signaling. *J Exp Med.* 2003;198:1841–1851.
88. Coughlin JJ, Stang SL, Dower NA, et al. RasGRP1 and RasGRP3 regulate B cell proliferation by facilitating B cell receptor-Ras signaling. *J Immunol.* 2005;175:7179–7184.
89. Aiba Y, Oh-hora M, Kiyonaka S, et al. Activation of RasGRP3 by phosphorylation of Thr-133 is required for B cell receptor-mediated Ras activation. *Proc Natl Acad Sci U S A.* 2004;47:16612–16617.
90. Zheng Y, Liu H, Coughlin J, et al. Phosphorylation of RasGRP3 on threonine 133 provides a mechanistic link between PKC and Ras signaling systems in B cells. *Blood.* 2005;105:3648–3654.
91. Harmer SL, DeFranco AL. The src homology domain 2-containing inositol phosphatase SHIP forms a ternary complex with Shc and Grb2 in antigen receptor-stimulated B lymphocytes. *J Biol Chem.* 1999;274:12183–12191.
92. Coggeshall KM. Inhibitory signaling by B cell FcγRIIb. *Curr Opin Immunol.* 1998;10:306–313.
93. Yamanashi Y, Tamura T, Kanamori T, et al. Role of the rasGAP-associated docking protein p62dok in negative regulation of B cell receptor-mediated signaling. *Genes Dev.* 2000;14:11–16.
94. Tamir I, Stolpa JC, Helgason CD, et al. The RasGAP-binding protein $p62^{dok}$ is a mediator of inhibitory FcγRIIB signals in B cells. *Immunity.* 2000;12:347–358.

95. Mittelstadt PR, DeFranco AL. Induction of early response genes by cross-linking membrane Ig on B lymphocytes. *J Immunol.* 1993;150:4822–4832.
96. DeFranco AL. Vav and the B cell signalosome. Nature Immunol. 2001;2:482–4.
97. O'Rourke LM, Tooze R, Turner M, et al. CD19 as a membrane-anchored adaptor protein of B lymphocytes: costimulation of lipid and protein kinases by recruitment of Vav. *Immunity.* 1998;8:635–645.
98. Niiro H, Clark EA. Branches of the B cell antigen receptor pathway are directed by protein conduits Bam32 and Carma1. *Immunity.* 2003;19:637–640.
99. Carman CV, Springer TA. Integrin avidity regulation: are changes in affinity and conformation under-emphasized? *Curr Opin Cell Biol.* 2003;15:547–556.
100. McLeod SJ, Ingham RJ, Bos JL, et al. Activation of the Rap1 GTPase by the B cell antigen receptor. *J Biol Chem.* 1998;273:29218–29223.
101. McLeod SJ, Shum AJ, Lee RL, et al. The Rap GTPases regulate integrin-mediated adhesion, cell spreading, actin polymerization, and Pyk2 tyrosine phosphorylation in B lymphocytes. *J Biol Chem.* 2004;279:12009–12019.
102. Kliche S, Breitling D, Togni M, et al. The ADAP/SKAP55 signaling module regulates T-cell receptor-mediated integrin activation through plasma membrane targeting of Rap1. *Mol Cell Biol.* 2006;26:7130–7144.
103. Togni M, Swanson KD, Reimann S, et al. Regulation of in vitro and in vivo immune functions by the cytosolic adaptor molecule SKAP-HOM. *Mol Cell Biol.* 2005;25:8052–8063.
104. Campbell ID, Ginsberg MH. The talin-tail interaction places integrin activation on FERM ground. *Trends Biochem Sci.* 2004;29: 429–435.
105. Sen R. Contol of B lymphocyte apoptosis by the transcription factor NF-κB. *Immunity.* 2006;25:871–883.
106. Rawlings DJ, Sommer K, Moreno-Garcia ME. The CARMA1 signalosome links the signalling machinery of adaptive and innate immunity in lymphocytes. *Nat Rev Immunol.* 2006;6:799–812.
107. Bishop GA, Hostager BS, Brown KD. Mechanisms of TNF receptor-associated factor (TRAF) regulation in B lymphocytes. *J Leukoc Biol.* 2002;72:19–23.
108. Su TT, Guo B, Kawakami Y, et al. PKC-β controls IκB kinase lipid raft recruitment and activation in response to BCR signaling. *Nat Immunol.* 2002;3:780–786.
109. Gaide O, Favier B, Legler DF, et al. CARMA1 is a critical lipid raft-associated regulator of TCR-induced NF-κB activation. *Nature Immunol.* 2002;3:836–843.
110. Lanoue A, Batista FD, Stewart M, et al. Interaction of CD22 with alpha2,6-linked sialoglycoconjugates: innate recognition of self to dampen B cell autoreactivity. *Eur J Immunol.* 2002;32:348–355.
111. Nitschke L. The role of CD22 and other inhibitory co-receptors in B-cell activation. *Curr Opin Immunol.* 2005;17:290–397.
111a. Cherukuri A, Shoham T, Sohn HW, et al. The tetraspanin CD81 is necessary for partititioning of coligated CD19/CD21-B cell antigen receptor complexes into signaling-active lipid rafts. *J Immunol.* 2004;172:270–280.
112. Dempsey PW, Allison MED, Akkaraju S, et al. C3d of complement as a molecular adjuvant: Bridging innate and acquired immunity. *Science.* 1996;271:348–350.
113. Ravetch JV, Lanier LL. Immune inhibitory receptors. *Science.* 2000;290:84–89.
114. Kumanogoh A, Shikina T, Watanabe C, et al. Requirement for CD100-CD72 interactions in fine-tuning of B-cell antigen receptor signaling and homeostatic maintenance of the B-cell compartment. *Int Immunol.* 2005;17:1277–1282.
115. Li DH, Tung JW, Tarner IH, et al. CD72 down-modulates BCR-induced signal transduction and diminishes survival in primary mature B lymphocytes. *J Immunol.* 2006;176:5321–5328.
116. Ho LH, Uehara T, Chen CC, et al. Constitutive tyrosine phosphorylation of the inhibitory paired Ig-like receptor PIR-B. *Proc Natl Acad Sci U S A.* 1999;96:15086–15090.
117. Sen G, Bikah G, Venkataraman C, et al. Negative regulation of antigen receptor-mediated signaling by constitutive association of CD5 with the SHP-1 protein tyrosine phosphatase in B-1 B cells. *Eur J Immunol.* 1999;29:3319–3328.
118. Ochi H, Watanabe T. Negative regulation of B cell receptor-mediated signaling in B-1 cells through CD5 and Ly49 co-receptors via Lyn kinase activity. *Int Immunol.* 2000;12:1417–1423.
119. Collins BE, Smith BA, Bengtson P, et al. Ablation of CD22 in ligand-deficient mice restores B cell receptor signaling. *Nat Immunol.* 2006;7:199–206.
120. Nadler MJ, McLean PA, Neel BG, et al. B cell antigen receptor-evoked calcium influx is enhanced in CD22-deficient B cell lines. *J Immunol.* 1997;159.
121. Poe JC, Fujimoto M, Jansen PJ, et al. CD22 forms a quaternary complex with SHIP, Grb2, and Shc. A pathway for regulation of B lymphocyte antigen receptor-induced calcium flux. *J Biol Chem.* 2000;275:17420–17427.
122. Mizuno K, Tagawa Y, Mitomo K, et al. Src homology region 2 (SH2) domain-containing phosphatase-1 dephosphorylates B cell linker protein/SH2 domain leukocyte protein of 65 kDa and selectively regulates c-Jun NH2-terminal kinase activation in B cells. *J Immunol.* 2000;165:1344–1351.
123. Chen J, McLean PA, Neel BG, et al. CD22 attenuates calcium signaling by potentiating plasma membrane calcium-ATPase activity. *Nat Immunol.* 2004;5:651–657.
124. Xu Y, Harder KW, Huntington ND, et al. Lyn tyrosine kinase: accentuating the positive and the negative. *Immunity.* 2005;22: 9–18.
125. Fujimoto M, Fujimoto Y, Poe JC, et al. CD19 regulates Src family protein tyrosine kinase activation in B lymphocytes through processive amplification. *Immunity.* 2000;13:47–57.
126. Yu CCK, Mamchak AA, DeFranco AL. Signaling mutations and autoimmunity. *Curr Dir Autoimmun.* 2003;6:61–88.
127. Yu CCK, Yen TSB, Lowell CA, et al. Lupus-like kidney disease in mice deficient in the Src-family tyrosine kinases Lyn and Fyn. *Curr Biol.* 2001;11.
128. Bolland S, Yim YS, Tus K, et al. Genetic modifiers of systemic lupus erythematosus in FcγRIIB($-/-$) mice. *J Exp Med.* 2002;195: 1167–1174.
129. Clark MR, Massenburg D, Siemasko K, et al. B-cell antigen receptor signaling requirements for targeting antigen to the MHC class II presentation pathway. *Curr Opin Immunol.* 2004;16: 382–387.
130. Gazumyan A, Reichlin A, Nussenzweig MC. Igβ tyrosine residues contribute to the control of B cell receptor signaling by regulating receptor internalization. *J Exp Med.* 2006;203:1785–1794.
131. Stoddart A, Dykstra ML, Brown BK, et al. Lipid rafts unite signaling cascades with clathrin to regulate BCR internalization. *Immunity.* 2002;17:451–462.
132. Stoddart A, Jackson AP, Brodsky FM. Plasticity of B cell receptor internalization upon conditional depletion of clathrin. *Mol Biol Cell.* 2005;16:2339–2348.
133. Hou P, Araujo E, Zhao T, et al. B cell antigen receptor signaling and internalization are mutually exclusive events. *PLOS Biology.* 2006;4:1147–1158.
134. Kabak S, Skagg BJ, Gold MR, et al. The direct recruitment of BLNK to Ig-α couples the B-cell antigen receptor to distal signaling pathways. *Mol Cell Biol.* 2002;22:2524–2535.
135. Engels N, Wollscheid B, Wienands J. Association of SLP-65/BLNK with the B cell antigen receptor through a non-ITAM tyrosine of Ig-α. *Eur J Immunol.* 2001;31:2126–2134.
136. Mills D, Cambier JC. B lymphocyte activation during cognate interactions with CD4+ T lymphocytes: molecular dynamics and immunologic consequences. *Sem Immunol.* 2003;15:325–329.

Chapter 9

B Lymphocyte Biology

Michael McHeyzer-Williams

OVERVIEW

Preexisting diversity in the antigen receptor repertoire is the central feature of the adaptive immune system. Foreign antigen triggers clonal selection mechanisms that regulate the quantity and quality of adaptive immunity. This chapter will focus on mature B lymphocyte biology and consider the cellular and molecular processes that promote antibody production and the development of high-affinity B cell memory in response to foreign antigen exposure *in vivo*.

There are at least three major subsets of mature B cells that can participate in the adaptive response to foreign antigen, each with different developmental life histories, survival needs, and activation requirements upon antigen receptor triggering. The innate immune system participates in rapid early antigen clearance and communicates the nature of the foreign antigen assault to the adaptive immune system. Dendritic cells (DC) are the most efficient antigen-presenting cells (APC) of innate immunity and will be discussed in some detail. DCs exist in multiple forms that can present antigen to specific B cells and pMHCII complexes to specific helper T (Th) cells. Th cell independent B cell responses will be discussed; however, emphasis remains on antigen-specific mechanisms of Th cell regulated B cell immunity.

In the past few years, experimental access to immune response biology has dramatically shifted with the advent of multiphoton laser–based intravital imaging techniques. These studies provide direct access to the mechanics and cell dynamics of antigen-specific cognate regulation *in vivo*. This information serves to integrate existing knowledge in the field using a real-time scaffold for the developmental progression *in vivo*. This chapter will be broadly organized across the four major checkpoints in the evolution of high-affinity B cell memory. The first checkpoint defines contact between antigen-experienced pMHCII$^+$ DC and naïve pMHCII-specific Th cells. Clonal selection within the Th cell compartment underpins effector Th cell differentiation required for regulating B cell fate in this pathway. Cognate control of antigen-primed pMHCII-expressing B cells defines the second major checkpoint in this pathway. Commitment to antibody class switch, short-lived plasma cell (PC) development and entry into the germinal center (GC) reaction to memory B cell development occurs at this stage of the immune response. The GC reaction underpins memory B cell evolution and is discussed in detail. The interaction of the B cell receptor (BCR) and antigen followed by the cognate control of GC B cell fate by GC-Th cells defines the third major checkpoint, determining entry of high-affinity GC B cells into the memory B cell compartment. Little is understood about the cellular heterogeneity within the memory B cell compartment and the memory Th cell compartment and how such heterogeneity affects the response to antigen recall. The fourth major checkpoint defines cognate control of antigen recall responses and is central to the consolidation of antigen-specific B cell responses in all vaccine regimes.

This chapter mainly focuses on what is known of the antigen-specific immune response in mouse models, with reference to work conducted in humans. Further, there is an emphasis on the response to model hapten-protein antigens that is pertinent to our understanding and manipulation of adaptive immunity for preventive vaccination but may not provide a full appreciation of the immune response to infection.

MATURE B CELL SUBSETS

Mature peripheral B cells subdivide into at least three major compartments based on cell surface phenotype, cellular ontogeny and tissue distribution. B1 B cells, marginal zone (MZ) B cells, and follicular (FO) B cells respond characteristically to different sets of foreign antigens, creating a broad subdivision of function in the mature B cell compartment. Differences in BCR repertoire and helper T cell requirements for antigen responsiveness underscore this functional divide and further distinguish the mature B cell subsets. More recently, the identification of separable precursors for B1 and FO B cells support the existence of distinct B cell lineages and provide a mechanism for their differential development *in vivo*. All three subsets are also found in humans with some notable distinctions in overall organization and cellular composition.

B1 B Cells

The B1 B cell subset was first identified by differential expression of CD5, phenotypic similarity to a set of B cell lymphomas and expansion of the CD5$^+$ (Ly-1$^+$) B cells in autoimmune-prone mice strains (1,2). B-1 B cells characteristically express high levels of sIgM, demonstrable CD11b, and low levels of sIgD, CD21, CD23, and the B cell isoform of CD45R (B220). In adult mice, B1 B cells constitute a minor fraction of the spleen and secondary lymphoid tissues but are enriched in the pleural and peritoneal cavities (3,4). B1 B cells were shown to arise from precursors in the fetal liver and neonatal but not adult bone marrow and constitute the earliest wave of mature peripheral B cells.

B1 B cells express a separable BCR repertoire (5). Sequence analysis indicates antibodies with restricted sets of V region genes, no evidence for somatic hypermutation (SHM), and few nontemplated nucleotide (N) sequence insertions, a pattern typical of neonatal B cells. BCR transgenic B cells of known B1 B cell specificities differentially assort into this mature B cell subcompartment (6–8). Further, efficient B1 B cell development appears to be dependent on positive regulators of BCR signaling and the loss of negative regulators promotes greater accumulation of B1 B cells (1,2,9). Hence, there appears to be a role for self or foreign antigen in shaping the repertoire of the B1 B cell compartment (10).

In contrast, the differential propensity of fetal and adult hematopoietic tissue to promote B1 B cells suggests the existence of developmentally separate precursors (11). Recent studies identify a novel CD45R$^{low/-}$ CD19$^+$ B1 B cell precursor whose developmental potential is limited to B1 B cell development (12). These B1 B precursors reach peak levels around day 17 of gestation and rapidly decline postnatally. FO B cell precursors differentially express CD138 and MHC II and dominate the adult bone marrow pro–B cell pool (13). Hence, subspecialization in the mature B cell compartment is also preprogrammed during development due to the distinct attributes of the separable B cell progenitors.

Adoptively transferred B1 B cells self-renew and spontaneously secrete IgM and IgG3 serum antibodies. These natural serum antibodies display extensive polyreactivity and demonstrable self-reactivity and bind to many common pathogen-associated carbohydrates (5). Natural serum antibodies play an important early role in the immune response to many bacteria and viruses but require complement fixation for effective antigen clearance. B1 B cells are the key responders to type II thymus-independent antigens with characteristic repetitive epitopes such as bacterial capsular polysaccharides (8,9). Innate sensing mechanisms can rapidly mobilize B1 B cells regardless of specificity highlighting the innatelike activity of this separate B cell compartment. Peritoneal B1 B cells are also responsible for large numbers of the IgA PCs found in mucosal and intestinal tissue, an important early innatelike defense mechanism.

B1 B cells can be further subdivided into B1a (CD5$^+$) and B1b (CD5$^-$) subtypes. Unlike B1a B cells, the B1b subtype can be generated from precursors in the adult bone marrow. The B1a and B1b precursors have been reported to differ in the expression levels of CD138 (13). Recent functional studies indicate a further subdivision of labor assigning B1a cells as the precursors of natural serum antibody (14). In contrast, B1b cells appear to be the primary source of dynamic T cell independent (TI) antibody production and long-term protection after bacterial infection such as *B. hermsii* (15) and *S. pneumonia* (14). These studies indicate preexisting subset differences in BCR specificity and antigen-driven B cell fate that remain important unresolved features of the system.

Marginal Zone B Cells

MZ B cells are noncirculating mature B cells that segregate anatomically into the MZ of the spleen (16). The MZ is located at the perimeter of splenic white pulp beginning with the marginal sinus and bordering the red pulp. This region contains multiple subtypes of macrophages, dendritic cells, and the MZ B cells and is not fully formed until 2 to 3 weeks after birth in rodents and 1 to 2 years in humans (17). The MZ B cells within this region typically express high levels of sIgM, CD21, CD1, CD9 with low to negative levels of sIgD, CD23, CD5, and CD11b that help to distinguish them phenotypically from FO B cells and B1 B cells (Figure 9.1).

Similar to B1 B cells, MZ B cells can be rapidly recruited into the early adaptive immune responses in a TI manner. The MZ B cells are especially well positioned as a first line of defense against systemic blood-borne antigens that enter the circulation and become trapped in the spleen (18). MZ B cells also display a lower activation threshold than their FO B cell counterparts with heightened propensity for PC differentiation that contributes further to the accelerated primary antibody response (19).

	B1a	B1b	MZ B	FO B
IgM	+++	+++	+++	++
IgD	+	+	+	+++
CD21	+	+	+++	++
CD23	+	+	+	+++
CD45R	++	++	++	+++
CD5	+++	-	-	-
CD11b	+	+	-	-
CD43	++	++	-	-

High +++ Intermediate ++ Low + Negative -

FIGURE 9.1 Cell surface phenotype of mature B cell subsets.

In rodents, the MZ B cell compartment expresses largely germline-encoded BCRs supporting the TI status of MZ B cell development. In contrast, MZ B cells from humans express somatically diversified receptors suggesting a difference in the development that results in their resembling IgM^+ memory B cells following foreign antigen encounter (20). Further to this thinking, $CD27^+IgM^+IgD^-$ memory B cells in human peripheral blood display higher levels of CD21 and lower CD23, similar to their MZ counterparts in the spleen. Nevertheless, it is also clear from adoptive transfer experiments in mouse models that MZ B cells can be recruited into typical Th cell dependent (TD) antiprotein responses, diversify their BCR in germinal centers, and be selected into the high-affinity memory B cell compartment (21). Hence, MZ B cells express rapid TI B cell functions resembling B1 B cells but have a capacity for TD responses that overlaps with FO B cells.

The vast majority of IgM^+IgD^{lo} B cells exported from the adult bone marrow will not enter the long-lived mature peripheral B cell compartment (22). There is evidence for positive selection of these B cells based on the repertoire of their expressed BCR (23). As discussed for B1 B cells, the specificity of the BCR can impact the propensity of B cells to develop into MZ B cells. However, enlarged MZ B cell compartments are also found in single-chain BCR transgenic animals of diverse specificities, suggesting that specificity may not be the major influence in MZ B cell development. Decreased MZ B cell development is found in the absence of CD79a signaling, CD19, Btk, CD45, PI3K, PKCβ all associated with BCR signal integration. Thus, strength of the positive selecting BCR signal appears to play a role in mature B cell subset assortment.

Earlier alterations in B cell development can preprogram mature B cell fate. There are proportionately enlarged MZ B cell compartments in the absence of IL7, IL7Rα, lambda-5, and Rag-1, all of which also truncate the total peripheral B cell compartment (16). Differential sensitivity of mature B cell subsets to growth factors also regulates the compartment size. While BAFF-deficient mice lack MZ and FO B cells with some sparing of B1 B cells, over-expression of BAFF favors MZ B cells and enlarges the size of this compartment. Disorganized splenic architecture in the absence of LTα, LTβ and LTβR and decreased chemokine responsiveness in the absence of Pyk2, Dock2, and Lsc also leads to reduced MZ B cell numbers in the spleen. Hence, differential access to specialized environmental niches may play an important role in the development and maintenance of mature B cell subsets.

Follicular B Cells

The majority of mature B cells in the spleen express high levels of IgM, IgD, and CD23; lower C21; and no CD1 or CD5, readily distinguishing this FO B cell compartment from B1 B cells and MZ B cells. As the name implies, FO B cells organize into the primary follicles of B cell zones focused around follicular dendritic cells in the white pulp of the spleen and the cortical areas of peripheral lymph nodes. Multiphoton-based live imaging of lymph nodes indicate continuous movement of FO B cells within these follicular areas at velocites of ~6 μm per min (24). Recent studies indicate movement along the processes of FDC as a guidance system for mature resting B cells in peripheral lymph nodes (25). Unlike their MZ counterpart, FO B cells freely recirculate, comprising >95% of the B cells in peripheral lymph nodes.

The BCR repertoire of the FO B cell compartment also appears under positive selection pressures during final maturation in the spleen; however, diversity is substantially broader than B1 B and MZ B cell compartments. Most important, FO B cells require CD40-CD40L dependent T cell help to promote effective primary immune responses and antibody isotype switch and establish high-affinity B cell memory (26).

INITIATING B CELL IMMUNITY

The initial antibody response to many infectious agents is largely based on the rapid TI expansion of B cells and their subsequent differentiation into PCs. The B1 and MZ B cells are largely responsible for these rapid TI humoral responses, suggesting that some level of "natural memory" function resides in these B cell subsets and may be predetermined in an evolutionarily conserved manner. TI antigens can be separated into two broad categories based on their ability to polyclonally activate B cells (TI-1) or require BCR recognition of multivalent epitopes to induce B cell differentiation in the absence of T cell help (TI-2). TI-2 antigens can activate BCR signaling but require accessory signals to promote the development of antigen-specific PCs.

In contrast, monovalent protein antigens require antigen-specific helper T cell regulation to promote high titer antibody responses and the development of B cell memory. These TD antibody responses take longer to emerge and display a spectrum of affinities and isotypes and engage multiple strategies for antigen-specific clearance *in vivo*. Immune responses to model protein antigens provide experimental access to the complex cascade of cellular and molecular events that underpin long-term protective immunity. The recruitment and behavior of antigen-experienced APCs initiate this program of development and shapes the quality and quantity of peptide-MHCII (pMHCII) specific Th cell responses.

Preexisting Dendritic Cell Diversity

DCs are essential APCs for initiating adaptive immunity and preexist antigen challenge in multiple cellular subsets. Different phenotypic schemes can be used to characterize DC subsets with the origins and developmental relatedness of different DC subsets still subject to debate (27,28). In the murine system, three main bone marrow–derived DC subsets enter via the blood to reside at different levels in all secondary lymphoid organs (Figure 9.2). These blood-derived DC all express CD11c and are distinguishable as CD11b^{high} CD8α^{neg} DC, CD8α^{high} DC, and 6B2^{high} plasmacytoid DC (pDC). In lymph nodes (LN) draining the skin, there are at least two further CD11c^{+} DC subsets, Langerhans cells (LC) and dermal DC (dDC), that emigrate from the skin, even at homeostasis (29). Thus, before antigen challenge, multiple subsets of DC are available to differentially process and present antigen to the adaptive immune compartment.

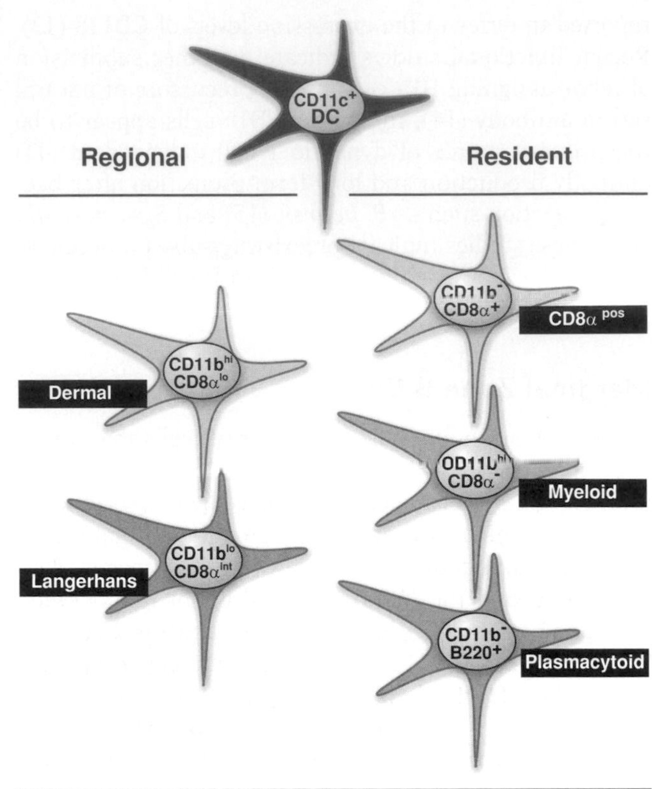

FIGURE 9.2 Regional and lymphoid resident dendritic cell subsets in mice.

pMHCII^{+} DC

Protein antigen administration without inflammation induces immune tolerance. In contrast, coadministration of immune adjuvant activates facets of innate immunity, induces inflammation, and primes antigen-specific adaptive immunity. Sensing pathogens involves pattern recognition receptors such as the evolutionarily conserved toll-like receptors (TLR) (30,31) and the more recently described nod-like receptors (NLR) (32). Both families of receptors recognize different types of microbial components initiating programs of DC maturation and promote immediate local inflammation and innate effector clearance mechanisms.

The processing and presenting of antigenic peptides in the MHC II pathway of DC is also an elaborate and highly regulated cellular activity that can be influenced by the inflammatory context of antigen stimulus (33). Hence, both the inflammatory context of the immune assault and antigen specificity can be rapidly imprinted on the local innate immune system. While the mechanisms remain poorly resolved, differential activation of DC subtypes provides a powerful means for controlling cell fate decisions in the development of adaptive immunity (34). In this manner, pMHCII$^+$ DC expressing an appropriate spectrum of costimulatory molecules become the critical regulators of antigen-specific adaptive immunity.

Temporal and spatial constraints on DC maturation provide another layer of regulation for the innate system that can impact adaptive immunity. In the steady-state, DCs form dense networks at the T-B borders of LNs. Interestingly, motile lipopolysaccharide (LPS)–activated DC immigrants will rapidly coalesce with this preexisting network *in vivo* (35). In separate studies using genetically tagged LC, the emigrants of LC and dDC were shown to emerge separately in time and colonize separate regions of the T-B border (36). A similar temporal regulation was seen using antibodies to specific pMHCII complexes with resident DC presenting an early wave of pMHCII and dDC emerging later in a second wave (37). In each of these studies, the immune stimulus was varied and the coordinated response of the innate system was also qualitatively and quantitatively different.

Antigen Presentation to B Cells

Categorizing an antigen as TI-I was originally based on the ability to elicit an antibody response in immunocompromised mice with defects in Btk function and BCR signaling. Many such polyclonal activators are compounds of bacterial cell wall, such as LPS, peptidoglycans (PGN), and lipoteichoic acid (LTA) that activate B cell–expressed TLRs (38). In contrast, TI-2 antigens trigger the BCR and are typically repetitive polymers, such as bacterial capsular polysaccharides or repetitive epitopes found in many viral particles. Studies using antigen coupled to polyacrylamide determined that a minimum of 12 to 16 haptens (small chemical antigens) per molecule were required to induce a strong TI-2 antibody response (39). The size of the epitope array indicates the aggregate BCR cluster required to initiate signal transduction at the cellular level.

The backbone flexibility or the density of accessible epitope is also a factor in antigenicity. A high ratio of hapten conjugated to protein molecules still requires T cell help to induce antibody production. Dextran molecules have been used to conjugate anti-IgM and -IgD into potent TI-2 reagents that can stimulate phosphoinositde breakdown and intracellular Ca^{2+} responsiveness at 1,000-fold lower concentrations than the soluble antibody alone. Many TI-2 antigens can also fix complement and thereby co-cross-link the BCR complex and CD21/CD19 molecules.

TI-2 antigens require accessory signals to drive B cell proliferation and PC development. While B cells can recognize soluble antigen, forms of antigen directly conjugated to complement components potently induce B cell immunity. APC-associated bacterial antigen also drives rapid MZ B cell activation in the spleen that appears dependent on the TNF family member, TACI (18). DC can internalize and recycle IgG-opsonized antigen in an FcγRIIB- and complement-dependent manner (40). This nondegradative processing of antigen can activate MZ B cells in the spleen and promote a TI B cell response. In general, B cell recognition of cell-associated antigen can be influenced by the costimulatory factors expressed by the APC that may regulate the outcome of the initial B cell priming event.

Antigen-presenting DC can also drive TD B cell immunity. Injection of DC pulsed with protein antigen can induce isotype switch and promote efficient B cell responses. B cells can form synapselike interactions with antigen pulsed DC (41,42). More recently, two-photon imaging revealed that naïve B cells entering local LNs surveyed protein antigen-pulsed DC before entering the follicular areas (43). In this model, engagement of BCR led to calcium flux, migration arrest, and the local accumulation of the antigen-specific B cells. Further, there is a reticular network of collagen fibers that physically connects the subcapsular and paracortical sinuses of LNs to blood vessels and separates these regions from T and B cell areas (44). This organization facilitates the efficient delivery of soluble antigen toward the lumen of high-endothelial venules (HEV) without it entering the LN parenchyma. While resident DCs can access this conduit transport system, FO B cells may have difficulty accessing soluble antigen.

Nevertheless, in the context of TD protein antigens, B cells must recognize their cognate antigen and internalize, process, and present peptides from this antigen in the context of MHCII to receive pMHCII-specific T cell help. If the TD antigen is cell associated, in the presence of adequate costimulation, some aspects of the B cell response can proceed in a TI manner. B cell proliferation and PC development can occur in the absence of CD40-CD40L interactions with some residual isotype switch induced by the action of TACI and BAFF-R (45). Thus, FO B cells can respond in a TI manner to TD antigens but do not express the characteristic range of outcomes and the full extent of protective immunity that is found with cognate regulation and T cell help.

ANTIGEN-SPECIFIC HELPER T CELL DIFFERENTIATION

Following initial protein immunization, pMHCII$^+$ DC appear in the lymph nodes that drain the site of antigen administration in patterns that depend on the quality of

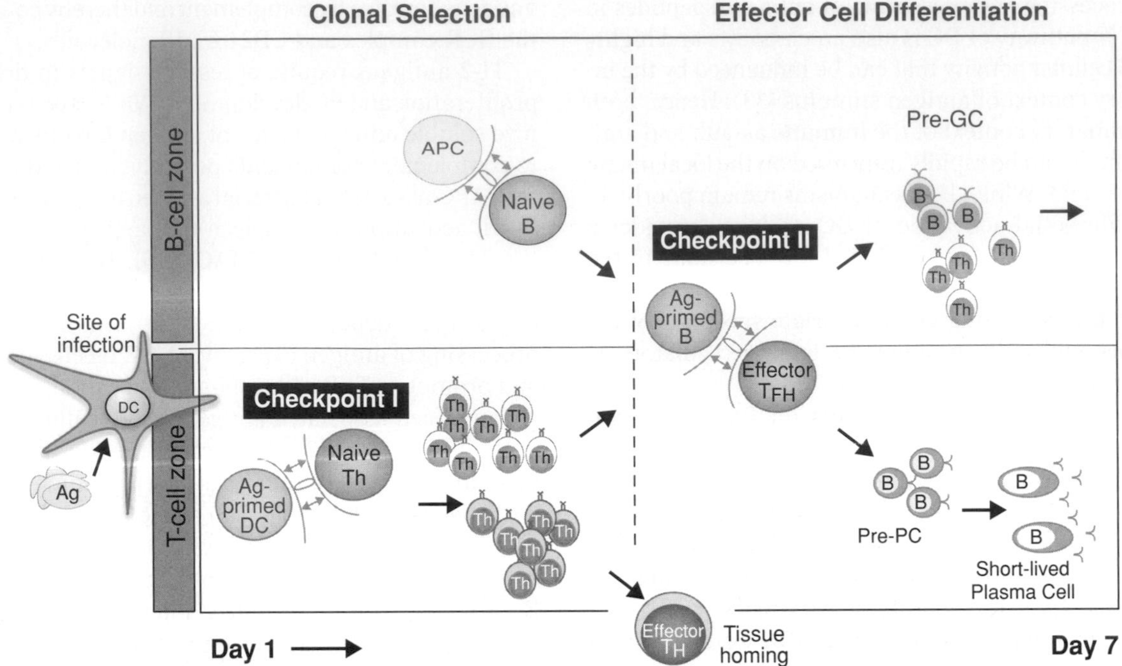

FIGURE 9.3 Initial helper T cell regulated checkpoints in memory B cell evolution. Protein vaccination induces antigen uptake, processing and presentation of pMHCII complexes and local DC maturation and migration to draining secondary lymphoid tissues. In the T cell zones, pMHCII$^+$ DC will make contact with naïve pMHCII-specific naïve Th cells to define the first major checkpoint in the development of Th cell regulated B cell immunity. Subsets of antigen-specific effector Th cells destined to migrate to the site of initial antigen contact will exit after clonal expansion. Antigen-specific Th clonal expansion and migration of effector T_{FH} cells to the T-B borders will make contact with antigen-primed pMHCII$^+$ B cells at checkpoint II. Antigen-specific B cell then either progress in an extra-FO pathway to switch antibody isotype and become short-lived PCs or pre-GC B cells to enter the GC pathway to memory B cell development.

immune stimulus (Figure 9.3). The antigen-experienced pMHCII$^+$ DC populations then sample the naïve Th cell compartment for clonotypes that express pMHCII-specific TCR. While there are many "bystander" influences in the outcome of adaptive responses, the "cognate" regulation of cell fate focuses primarily on the TCR of the Th cells that bind complexes of foreign peptide in MHC II molecules (pMHCII). These critical recognition events control antigen-specific development *in vivo* and are modified by a multitude of molecular interactions. Importantly, regulation occurs at the cellular interface between antigen-experienced cells as critical checkpoints to the ongoing developmental process that is adaptive immunity.

Priming pMHCII-specific Th Cells

DC maturation proceeds at the site of antigen challenge. Levels of total MHC II and the costimulatory molecules CD40, CD80, and CD86 increase substantially from the immature or resting state (27,28,46). Specific pMHCII levels also increase; however, the capacity for antigen uptake is rapidly truncated as maturation proceeds. Activated DCs also up-regulate CCR7, a chemokine receptor that facilitates their migration via afferent lymphatics to the T cell zones of draining LNs (47). The concentrations of the CCR7 ligands CCL19 and CCL21 in the T cell zones provide the means to draw these antigen-experienced pMHCII$^+$ DC to the appropriate microenvironment (48). Integrins such as LFA-1 ($\alpha_L\beta_2$) and the expression of matrix metalloproteinase MMP2 and MMP9 also play a role in mature DC migration to LNs.

The recognition of pMHCII complexes by the TCR of specific Th cells is central to the development of adaptive immunity (49–51). Successful cognate interactions occur through organized rearrangement of cell surface molecules at the cellular interface, now commonly referred to as the *immunological synapse* (52,53). Specific TCR-pMHCII interactions cluster toward the center of the immune synapse surrounded by complementary adhesion molecule interactions and excluding negative regulators of TCR signaling. *In vitro,* at least 2h conjugate formation is necessary to promote Th cell proliferation (54) with antigen-specific signaling evident up to 10 h (55). Direct imaging provides outstanding clarity to the dynamic nature of conjugate formation (24,56), resolving the timescale and quality of APC-T cell interactions *in vivo* (57). Two-photon imaging of labeled DCs and Th cell contacts indicates an early phase of short-lived contacts lasting ~10 min with dendrites of DCs (24). Subsequent altered patterns of T cell motility promote serial engagement with several different DCs that lead to clustering and swarming behavior that precedes cell division (58,59). These three phases of initial activation are also found in CD8 T cell responses with transient contacts that precede long-lasting contacts before resumption of dynamic movement (57). Interestingly, early activation and tolerance induction appear broadly similar in this early antigen-specific DC contact (60).

In the draining LNs, chemo-attraction and intercellular adhesion helps to initiate first contact with naïve pMHCII-specific Th cells. Differential expression of Notch ligands, DC production of cytokines, other growth factors, and the expression of a multitude of surface molecules can impact and alter antigen-specific Th cell fate. Recent studies that genetically manipulate cellular expression of pMHCII emphasize the role of persistent antigen in the complete activation of CD4 T cells (61). Two-photon imaging also suggested that there are at least two separate and successive contacts with APC in the activation of CD4 T cells *in vivo* (62). In models of virus infection, activating depots of antigen can be shown to persist for >3 weeks in draining lymphoid tissue (63,64). These elegant sets of studies indicate multiple levels of innate to adaptive control in the earliest phases of an immune response that regulate Th cell fate and function.

Clonal Selection in Th Cells

The central and defining outcome for pMHCII$^+$ DC interactions with naïve Th cells is TCR-driven clonal selection. Helper T cell responses in which a set of dominant TCR are utilized provide access to the mechanisms that underpin Th clonal selection (65–67). Earlier studies indicate the importance of TCR-pMHCII affinity in determining Th cell fate (65,68–70). In this model, selective expansion of clonotypes expressing higher affinity TCR would rely on competition for pMHCII complexes on APC. Alternatively, *in vitro* studies using altered peptide ligands suggested that the duration of TCR-pMHCII contact is critical to cell fate and therefore defined "best fit" *in vivo* (71–74). In support of this model, Th cells expressing TCRs with fast off-rates were lost over time *in vivo* (75). Further, there is evidence for different peptides stabilizing the pMHCII to create a hierarchy of dominant peptides (76). Each and all of these variables would impact what is considered "best fit" and influence the outcome of clonal selection.

More recently, we provide evidence for a model of Th clonal selection that is based on a TCR affinity threshold (77). These studies place emphasis back on overall TCR affinity and define a level of TCR-pMHCII binding above which there was no further skewing of clonal expansion due to TCR affinity. As depicted, multiple affinity-based thresholds underpin cell fate and clonal expansion (Figure 9.4). Importantly, we noted that varying the antigen dose until clonal expansion was compromised did not alter

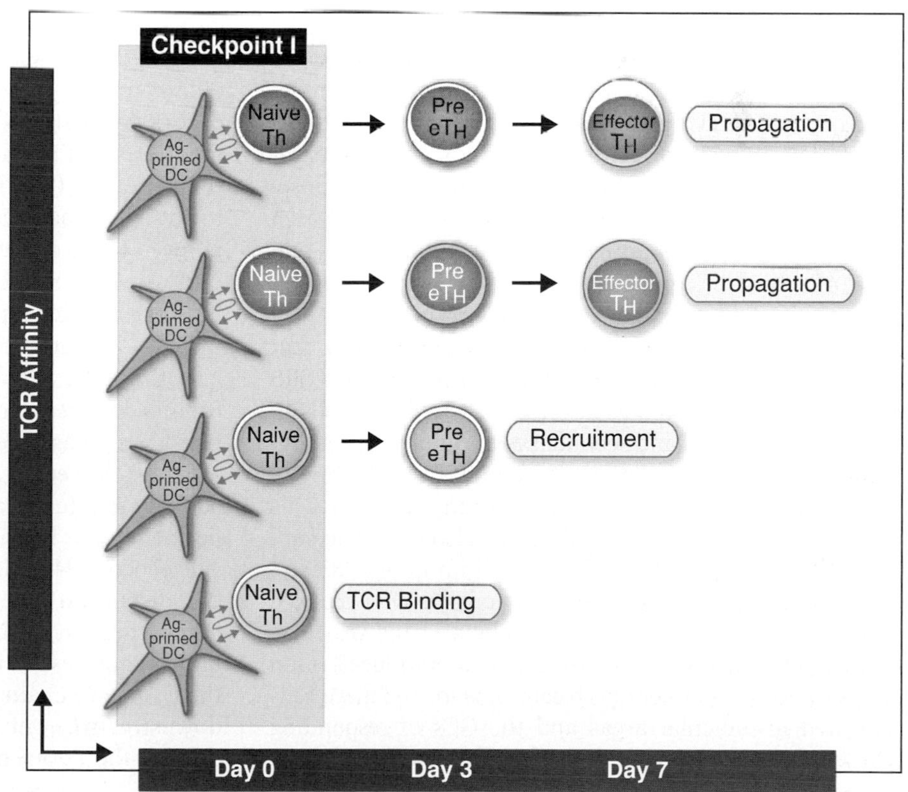

FIGURE 9.4 Multiple TCR-pMHCII affinity thresholds regulate Th cell fate *in vivo*. Following adoptive transfer of oligoclonal antigen-specific Th cells and priming *in vivo*, Th cells with the lowest affinity TCR bind pMHCII tetramers but do not get recruited into the immune response. Clonotypes expressing the next lowest affinity TCR are recruited into the early phase of the response with substantial clonal expansion but are not found at the peak of the primary response. The final set of clonotypes expressing the highest affinity TCR are recruited to the early response and fully propagated to the peak of the local primary response. Interestingly, based on clonal expansion, above the high-affinity threshold there was no skewing toward clonotypes that expressed even higher affinity TCR and the numbers of antigen-specific Th cells after propagation was directly proportional to the precursor frequency upon transfer. We have labeled checkpoint I as involved in the early selection activity and predict that checkpoint II impacts full propagation of antigen-specific T_{FH} cells *in vivo*.

clonal diversity. These data suggested interclonal competition was not part of the selection process and that TCR recognition and signal strength was a more intrinsic attribute of "good fit." Hence, establishing and perhaps modifying selection thresholds *in vivo* provides another important mechanism for generating antigen-specific clonal diversity that may impact effector Th cell function.

Regulation of B Cell Immunity

Antigen-activated B cells rapidly relocate to the T/B cell interface of secondary lymphoid organs. These earliest events in B cell activation are difficult to access experimentally in nontransgenic animals with polyclonal BCR due to the extremely low preimmune precursor frequency for any known antigens. Adoptive transfer of BCR transgenic B cells and TCR transgenic Th cells allow direct visualization of cognate interactions at these T-B borders (78). Activated B cells up-regulate CCR7 expression to drive them toward T cell areas, while maintaining CXCR5 allows them the appropriate counterbalance for this migration event to the T-B border (79). Two-photon imaging of antigen-specific contact indicates long-lasting 10 min to 60 min interactions (80). Interestingly, the Th-B conjugates appear highly motile, displaying extensive migration lead by the B cells at this early stage of the B cell response.

The range of cognate effector Th cell functions defines a broad spectrum of activities that is still not fully appreciated. B cell expansion in the T cell zones is the prelude to short-lived PC development, while expansion in the follicular regions forms secondary follicles as the precursor to GCs. We recently identified subpopulations of naïve Th cells based on the expression of Ly6C that have a greater propensity to promote PC formation after antigen priming *in vivo* (81). The Ly6C^{high} subset of Th cells also expressed separable TCR repertoires, arguing that the differential capacity to promote PCs was preprogrammed as a consequence of thymic development. Antibody isotype switch occurs in both arms of antigen-driven B cell response and is also likely to be imprinted in a cognate manner by Th cells at this early juncture of B cell development.

There have also been reports of effector Th cells that are specialized to regulate B cell responsiveness. CXCR5 expression was first reported on CD4$^+$CD45RO$^+$ cells in the peripheral blood and secondary lymphoid tissue in humans (82). Gene ablation studies emphasized the role of CXCR5 and CCR7 in the correct positioning of T and B cells in secondary lymphoid tissue that was also needed to support effective Th cell dependent B cell immunity (83,84). Blocking CD28 and OX40 interactions *in vivo* blocked the development of CXCR5$^+$ Th cells and the GC reaction (85). Further, CXCR5 expression was induced in an antigen-specific manner on Th cells *in vivo,* and these cells relocated to follicular areas and the GCs of responding lymphoid tissue (86). CXCR5$^+$ Th cells were sorted from human tonsil and shown to support antibody production *in vitro* (87,88). The tonsillar CXCR5$^+$ Th cells express high levels of CD40L and ICOS and are found in both the follicular mantle and GC. Adoptive transfers distinguish CXCR5$^+$ B cell helper activity (T_{FH}) from P-selectin ligand^{high} tissue homing inflammatory mediators (DTH-promoting Th) that emerge together from the same set of precursors *in vivo* (89). The term *follicular B helper T cells* (T_{FH}) was coined to categorize this functionally and phenotypically distinct effector Th cell compartment (87,88).

T_{FH} have also been detected in studies of human tonsil focusing on a subset of CXCR5$^+$ Th cells that also express CD57 and CD69 in the GC (90). These GC-localized T_{FH} exhibit gene expression programs distinct from the more typical Th1 and Th2 type effector Th cells and will be discussed in more detail in a later section. While the nomenclature and identity of the cells under analysis remains somewhat confusing, these studies begin to access the range of specialized effector Th cell activities focused on controlling TD B cell immunity *in vivo*. Figure 9.5 depicts the functional divisions that are predicted to exist within this broad category of T_{FH} cells that will be discussed in detail in the following sections.

Controlling Antibody Class Switch

The initial delivery of cognate T cell help to antigen-experienced pMHCII$^+$ B cells defines the second major checkpoint in the evolution of B cell immunity (Figure 9.3). At this developmental juncture, primed and helped B cells either remain in the T cell zone in a pathway to short-lived PC production or enter the GC pathway toward high-affinity memory B cell development. Antibody class switch occurs synchronously in both pathways of B cell development (91) and requires multiple rounds of cell division in the target cell (92). Thus, it is likely that the commitment to antibody class switch occurs at this critical early checkpoint in B cell differentiation.

Class switch recombination (CSR) is an intrachromosonal deletional process between the switch (S) regions that reside 5′ of each constant region gene in B cells (except Cδ) (93). Signaling through CD40 and cytokine receptors induces germline transcription through the targeted S regions. The Sμ region and the targeted S region are then cleaved by a putative DNA-cleaving enzyme. The activation-induced deaminase (AID) is required and sufficient for the initiation of the CSR reaction in the activated locus (94). AID-deficient animals (95) and humans (96) display no CSR or SHM of the Ig genes. Repair and ligation through nonhomologous end joining completes the process and results in the looping-out and replacement of the Cμ heavy chain constant region gene (C_H) with other downstream C_H genes. Isotype switch can proceed without SHM in the T zone pathway; however, SHM within the GC

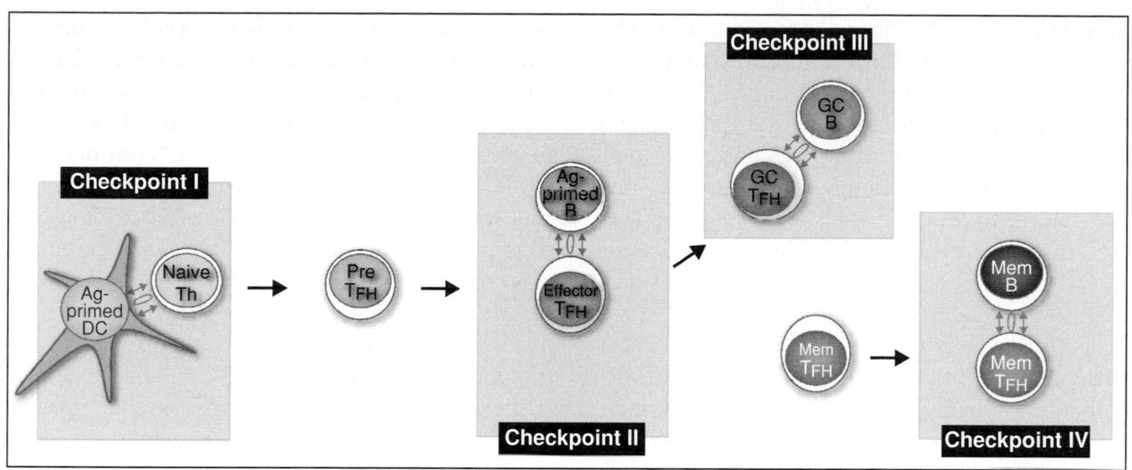

FIGURE 9.5 Checkpoints in antigen-specific T_{FH} cell development. Recognition of pMHCII complexes initiates naïve Th cell activation, expansion and development of effector Th precursors. The quantity of pMHCII expressed by mature DC and the coexpressed modifiers of Th cell activation can induce multiple cellular outcomes for the Th cells, one of which will be the effector T_{FH} precursor. Movement to the T-B borders accompanies development of antigen-specific effector T_{FH} functions to allow contact with antigen-primed pMHCII$^+$ B cells. There is evidence indicating that pMHCII B cell contact promotes further T_{FH} expansion at this developmental juncture. We also propose that checkpoint II events precede T_{FH} movement into the GC reaction and may be required for the development of antigen-specific GC T_{FH} cells. There is scant evidence for memory T_{FH} cells or information on the pathway of their development *in vivo*. Nevertheless, we propose that antigen-specific memory T_{FH} cells are related to the primary response T_{FH} compartment and are the regulators of local memory B cell responses that proceed in lymphoid tissues after re-exposure to the same antigen.

reaction is thought to use the same molecular machinery and will be discussed in a later section.

Induced CD40L on effector Th cells and the receipt of this signal through CD40 on B cells is required for antibody class switch (97,98). Animals and humans lacking CD40 display a hyper-IgM syndrome with profound defects in class switch, GC formation, and the development of affinity-matured B cell memory (98). ICOS is an inducibly expressed homologue to CD28 with a distinct ligand-binding motif and cytoplasmic tail and no detectable CD80 or CD86 binding. ICOS expression on activated Th cells is thought to act upstream of CD40L in this temporally orchestrated set of events (99). ICOS-deficient animals also have clear defects in antibody class switch, GC formation, and the development of B cell memory (100–102). Some residual class switch in the absence of CD40/CD40L interactions may be explained by the action of TACI and BAFF-R (45). OX40/OX40L interactions also quantitatively impact class switch, while CD27-CD70 interactions promote PC production (103). Thus, the range of molecules expressed at the effector Th cell surface influences the quality of TCR-pMHCII contact on antigen-primed B cells.

Considering the range of antibodies that can be produced, there must be multiple subtypes of effector T_{FH} that control class switch commitment. Different classes of effector T_{FH} would vary in production of Th cell–derived cytokines to control antibody isotype. IL-4 and IFN-γ are reciprocal regulators of IgG1 and IgG2a production (104). Animals lacking IL-4 or Stat 6 have decreased IgG1 levels and no IgE (105,106). IL-4 also acts together with IL-21 to control IgG subtypes and IgE levels (107). In contrast, TGFβ is implicated in the induction IgA, while IL-2 and IL-5 augment IgA production(108). Similarly, IL-6 may selectively support IgG2a and IgG2b expressing B cells *in vivo* (109). Each of these factors can exert their effects *in vitro* or in a bystander manner *in vivo*. However, it is thought that the directed delivery of these soluble molecules toward points of TCR-pMHCII contact allows soluble signals to focus locally in an antigen-specific cognate manner.

SHORT-LIVED PLASMA CELL DEVELOPMENT

Under the cognate regulation of effector T_{FH} cells, a cohort of antigen-primed B cells clonally expand within the T cell zones of secondary lymphoid organs and rapidly give rise to short-lived PCs. Within the first few days after antigen exposure, small foci of B cell blasts can be seen within the T cell zones (91). The B cell blasts that have committed to the short-lived PC pathway are depicted as non-GC pre-PCs (Figure 9.3). This plasmablast stage in short-lived

PC development appears transitional and defines pre-PCs that may secrete antibody but also retain the capacity to proliferate. In contrast, PCs are typically considered terminally differentiated and in a postmitotic state. PCs display a marked increase in IgH and IgL mRNA and prominent amounts of rough endoplasmic reticuluum (ER) to accommodate translation and secretion of abundant Ig. They have reduced or lost numerous cell surface molecules including MHC II, B220, CD19, CD21, and CD22 with an increase in the proteoglycan syndecan-1 (CD138), often used as a distinguishing marker for PCs.

In mice deficient for SLAM-associated protein (SAP), the extra-follicular pathway to short-lived PC development remains largely intact, but the GC pathway is blocked (110). Recent studies indicate that SAP deficient Th cells exhibit heightened CD40L expression but decreased ICOS induction that alone can account for this defect (111). It will be important to dissect the separable signals and cellular subsets of effector T_{FH} cells that regulate the rapid but short-lived effector B cell response *in vivo*.

Heterogeneity within the PC Compartment

Short-lived PCs have half-lives of 3 to 5 days (112) and express germline-encoded antigen-specific antibodies (113,114). Newly formed PCs migrate via the MZ bridging channels into the red pulp of the spleen and into the medullary cords of lymph nodes. Migration patterns *in vivo* appear controlled by increased responsiveness to the CXCR4 ligand CXCL12 and decreased expression of CXCR5 and CCR7 (115). There is evidence for BCR affinity-based selection even at this early stage in the response (114). In some studies, B cells expressing low-affinity BCR remain non-GC and high-affinity B cells preferentially enter the GC pathway (116). The converse can also be seen with high-affinity B cells preferentially entering the non-GC short-lived PC pathway (117). While seemingly contradictory, these different outcomes *in vivo* may reflect the plasticity of intercellular control at the Th-B point of contact. Under some circumstances, the capacity to promote the highest germline affinity rapid antibody response may be favored over the development of high-affinity memory B cells. Nevertheless, variations in the strength of initial BCR engagement can also direct B cell fate at this second checkpoint in antigen-specific B cell development.

Currently, there are no phenotypic differences between short-lived and long-lived PCs. Long-lived PCs, as discussed in a later section, are distinguished as the cellular products of the GC reaction that contribute to long-lasting humoral memory. The polyclonal activation of naïve B cells induces short-lived PC that die rapidly *in vitro*. Similarly, the rapid emergence after antigen priming *in vivo* provides one operational means for isolating short-lived PCs (118,119). The expression of germline BCR in these PC provides genotypic support that these cells remain outside the GC in an extra-follicular pathway of development. However, non-GC B cells and B cells in TI responses can also give rise to long-lived PC (120,121). Similarly, it is possible that the precursors of long-lived PC in TD immune responses exit the GC reaction without diversifying their BCR. Hence, longevity itself provides the best distinguishing attribute for these two types of PC and the basis for this physiological difference remains an important issue to resolve.

Microenvironment is also a key factor controlling longevity in PC populations. The right growth factor niche can potentially convert a short-lived PC into a long-lived PC. Differential migration patterns associated with production of antibodies of different isotype may also contribute to variation and functional subspecialization among the antigen-specific PC compartment. The short-term production of antibody represents different antigen clearance mechanisms, while the deployment of long-lived PCs is a function of B cell memory and a strategy for long-term humoral protection. What controls expansion of particular precursors, migration patterns of progeny, or survival across PC subsets expressing different antibody isotypes remains an important area of research with potentially high impact on the field of vaccine design.

Molecular Regulation of PC Development

The transcriptional control of PC development also exists in multiple layers controlling a cascade of developmental change. The transcriptional repressor prdm-1 (encoding Blimp-1) plays a central role in the regulation of PC development (122). B cells lacking Blimp-1 do not differentiate into short- or long-lived PC, with TI and TD antibody responses profoundly diminished *in vivo* (123). These Blimp-1–deficient animals also display defective levels of serum antibody, suggesting that spontaneous production of antibody by B1 B cells also requires Blimp-1 expression. Structure function analysis indicates the modular action of Blimp-1 integrating a variety of environmental cues that lead to PC development (124,125). Blimp-1 represses proliferation through c-myc as one direct target among many others involved in cell cycle control. Blimp-1 also induces antibody secretion by repressing the transcription factor Pax-5, thereby de-repressing Xbp-1. The transcription factor Xbp-1 controls the unfolded protein response (UPR) and many facets of the cellular secretory mechanism that are critical to PC function and survival (126–128).

The transcriptional coactivator, OBF-1 also appears important for B cells to complete the PC program (129). In the absence of OBF-1, Bcl-6, Pax-5, and AID are not repressed, blocking the induction of Blimp-1 and PC development. In contrast, ablation of the transcription factor MitF leads to the spontaneous development of PC that appears independent of antigen stimuli (130). Interestingly, reexpression of bcl-6 and its cofactor MTA3 reactivates the B cell program and increases CD19 and MHC II and decreases CD138 in PC cell lines (131). This remarkable study suggests that PC fate is not as terminal and passive as it has been thought to be and that the PC fate remains subject to dynamic gene expression programs.

THE GERMINAL CENTER REACTION

Movement of antigen-primed B cells into the follicular regions of lymphoid organs after effector T_{FH} cell contact initiates the GC pathway to memory B cell development. These pre-GC B cells expand rapidly within the follicular region to form areas of $B220^{+}IgD^{low}$ antigen-specific B cells referred to as secondary follicles. Secondary follicles polarize into T cell proximal dark zones of cycling centroblasts and opposing light zones of largely noncycling centrocytes among the dense processes of follicular dendritic cells (FDC) and sparse presence of GC Th cells (132,133). This broad anatomical distribution of the GC reaction orients the activities of clonal expansion, BCR diversification, and clonal variant selection that underpin the evolution of high-affinity memory B cells in this pathway (depicted in Figures 9.6 and 9.7).

Under normal physiological conditions the GC reaction emerges as the most efficient means to control affinity maturation and memory B cell development. However, in the disorganized or absent preimmune lymphoid subcompartments of mice lacking LTα, LTβ, TNFRI, and LTβR, the activities of the GC reaction remain disorganized but largely intact (134–137). Vestiges of the GC or small cell aggregates manage the expansion, diversification, and selection steps required for affinity maturation and memory B cell development. Selective reexpansion of high-affinity variants upon antigen recall appears to continue the selection of the best memory B cell compartment in these less than ideal priming conditions.

Memory B Cell Evolution

The GC reaction requires T cell help, as it is absent in athymic nude mice and CD40- and CD40L-deficient mice and is diminished using reagents that block or deplete Th cell function, such as anti-CD4, anti-CD40, and anti-CD28 (138–140). Mice deficient in ICOS also display profound defects in all aspects of TD B cell responses (100–102). Conversely, mice deficient in Roquin, an inhibitor of ICOS expression, produce excessive numbers of T_{FH} cells and

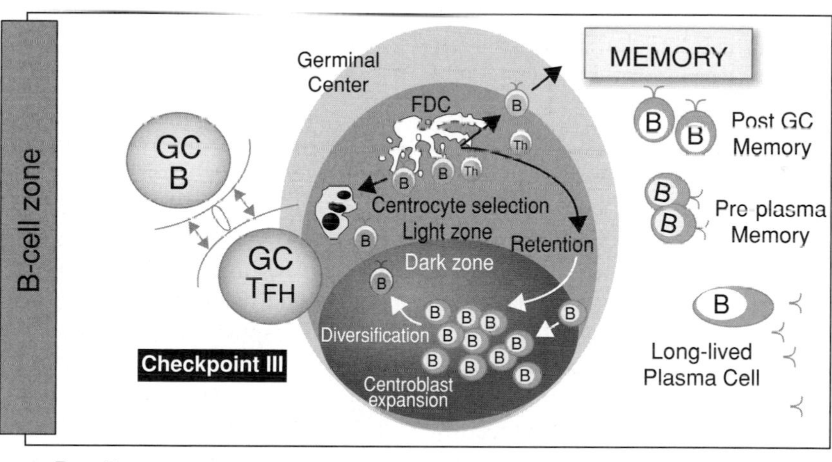

FIGURE 9.6 The GC pathway to memory B cell development. The GC pathway for B cells involves clonal expansion, BCR diversification and antigen-driven selection for high-affinity variants. Antigen-specific contact with GC T_{FH} cells at this developmental juncture defines a critical checkpoint in the survival and export of high affinity GC B cells into the memory B cell compartment. Importantly, the unique cellular outcomes at each checkpoint are driven by the quality of TCR-pMHCII interactions and the presence of molecular comodifiers that differ substantially at each progressive stage of development. Multiple subsets of memory B cells emerge from the GC reaction of the primary immune response. $6B2^{high}$ post-GC memory B cells are the first cellular product that exits the GC. We propose that these cells can give rise to $6B2^{low}$ pre-plasma memory B cells that are phenotypically and functionally distinct non-secreting memory response precursors. Further, the $6B2^{low}$ pre-plasma memory B cells appear to be the immediate cellular precursors of long-lived plasma cells that are a terminally differentiated antibody secreting memory B cell compartment. Both pre-plasma memory B cells and the long-lived plasma cells can be found in the spleen but preferentially home to the bone marrow.

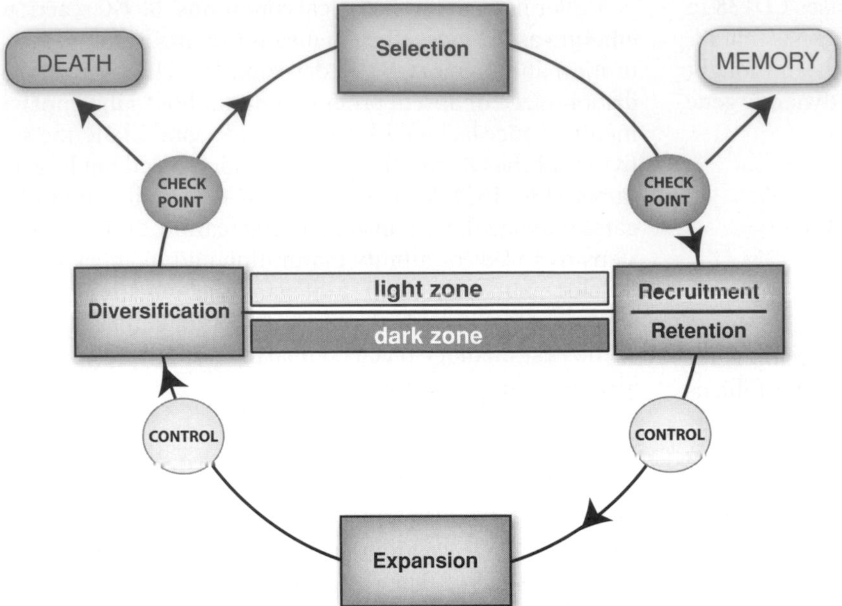

FIGURE 9.7 The GC cycle of activity. Antigen-specific B cells enter the follicular area and rapidly expand into secondary follicles that polarize into the light and dark zones of the GC reaction. Clonal expansion is accompanied by somatic diversification of antibody variable region genes in the dark zone. Exit from cell cycle and expression of variant BCR allows for antigen-specific selection of centrocytes in the light zones. Negative selection leads to apoptosis while positive selection of high affinity variants results in GC cycle reentry or exit from the GC into the memory B cell compartment under the cognate control of GC Th cells.

GCs and are prone to autoimmunity (141). However, TI antigens can also promote GC reactions, but they collapse within the first week after priming with no evidence of BCR diversification (142). In contrast, MZ B cells can be recruited into TD responses and form GCs that diversify and affinity mature (21). Interestingly, in these studies, the MZ B cells responding to antigen challenge expressed a distinctive preimmune BCR repertoire to the FO B cells responding in the same animals. Hence, there is some redundancy to the control of GC formation and flexibility to the origins of the B cells recruited into the GC reaction.

The transcriptional repressor Bcl6 is highly expressed in the GC and is necessary for GC formation (143). However, IgM and IgG1 antigen-specific memory B cells can develop in the absence of Bcl6 (144). These studies were based on direct labeling with antigen and their capacity to respond to soluble low-dose antigen recall. However, there were no GCs formed, and the memory B cells expressed no SHM or evidence for affinity maturation. Bcl6 has been recently shown to repress p53, the tumor-suppressor gene that controls DNA damage–induced apoptosis (145). Regulation of p53 in this manner may protect GC B cells to allow for the DNA breaks that are necessary intermediates in SHM and CSR. Bcl6 also directly represses Blimp-1 (146) and hence must be lost at some point during the GC reaction to allow subsequent development of pre-plasma memory B cells and long-lived PC *in vivo* (123).

The GC cycle of activity regulates clonal evolution within antigen-primed B cell responders. All pre-GC B cells express some measure of antigen specificity and appear preselected into the memory B cell pathway based on germline BCR expression. Massive and rapid clonal expansion with doubling times of 6 h to 8 h underpins secondary follicle formation and drives clonal expansion in the GC reaction. It is now clear that GC B cells in the light zone also have the capacity to proliferate (147). Further, recent studies using two-photon imaging of established GC *in situ* demonstrate in real-time that GC B cells in the light zone can also reenter the dark zone of GCs (148,149). These studies also emphasize the more open nature of the GC itself, demonstrating the capacity of naïve B cells to traverse the follicular region occupied by the antigen-responsive GC (149). Importantly, antigen-specific B cells could also be recruited into ongoing GCs if they expressed sufficiently high-affinity BCR. While these studies use high frequencies of BCR transgenic B cells pulsed into the ongoing response, it is intriguing to consider the ramifications of such an open network of affinity-based selection and its impact on the composition of the memory B cell compartment.

Somatic Hypermutation

Upon expansion in the GC reaction, antigen-specific B cells down-regulate their germline BCR and diversify their variable region genes through SHM. Single base substitutions, rare insertions, and deletions are introduced into a region spanning 1.5 kb to 2.0 kb downstream of the transcription initiation site; however, activity peaks within the V(D)J region and decreases within the J-C intronic region of IgH and IgL V genes (150). The mutation rate approaches 10^{-3} per base pair per generation, which is $\sim$ 6 orders of magnitude greater than spontaneous mutation frequencies. Approximately one mutation is introduced with each cell division. Analysis of mutation in "passenger" Ig transgenes that are not under selection pressure indicate intrinsic sequence hotspots for the mutator mechanism (151). Hence,

BCR diversification accompanies extensive clonal expansion within the GC reaction generating progeny that express variant antigen-binding BCR.

AID is the central component of the SHM mechanism. Originally discovered through cDNA subtraction focused on novel genes in GC B cells (152), it was then found to be the defect associated with an autosomal recessive form of hyper-IgM syndrome (96). Mice deficient in AID were able to form the GC reaction but were unable to undergo CSR or SHM (95). AID deaminates cytidine to uracil in single-stranded DNA that can be processed by a mutagenic repair pathway (93,153). The processing of these mutagenic changes creates the double-stranded breaks required for CSR and the mutagenic substrate for SHM. AID is the only B cell–specific enzyme that guides this phase of the diversification mechanism. However, distinct DNA damage response and histone modifications may discriminate SHM and CSR targets in this system (154).

Cell Cycle Arrest and Apoptosis

The control of cell cycle in the GC environment is of fundamental importance to the evolution of high-affinity B cell memory. Variant GC B cells exit cell cycle and move toward the light zone to undergo selection. Dysregulated cell cycle arrest promotes enlarged GCs in situ. This phenotype is found in multiple genetic knockout models that also influence the composition of the memory B cell compartment. Large GCs form in the absence of AID and are thought to indicate a negative feedback mechanism that follows SHM or CSR (95). The absence of the CDK inhibitor p18^{INK4c} more directly impacts GC size through blocking cell cycle arrest and also decreases the formation of long-lived PCs (155). The large GCs in the absence of Blimp-1 (123) may also be related to the lack of cell cycle control that may contribute to the pre-plasma memory cell and long-lived PC defect in these mice. The absence of the main regulatory subunit of calcineurin CnB1 results in the large GC phenotype, the loss of late-stage antibody production, and diminution of the memory B cell response to antigen recall (156). It will be important to assess whether these putative cell cycle defects directly impact high-affinity memory B cell evolution or indirectly modifies GC B cell fate and the onset of apoptosis.

It is generally believed that the majority of GC B cells expressing variant BCR will die *in situ*. Extensive local apoptosis is characteristic of the GC reaction. Further, overexpression of antiapoptotic molecules such as Bcl-2 or Bcl-xL prolongs survival of GC B cells without improving selection efficiency (157). In the absence of CD95 (Fas), there is also a dilution of high-affinity clonotypes in the memory B cell compartment (158). Mutations in the comodifiers of BCR signal also impact GC B cell dynamics. Unlike the CnB1 mutation, defects in CD45 and CD19 reduce proliferation and survival of GC B cells, arguing for a more global impact of these molecules on BCR signal integration (147,159,160). Initiation of the GC development program may also be altered to differing degrees in these animal models in ways that are difficult to dissect. Driving the expression of Cre recombinase at a stage in development when germline Cγ1 transcript provides access to later-stage antigen-responsive B cells and GC B cells without interfering with the early antigen specific events. (161). This model allows the conditional deletion of alleles at a late stage in antigen-driven B cell development that occurs after the first Th-B cell checkpoint in development.

Affinity Maturation

Affinity maturation requires the positive selection of GC B cells expressing high-affinity variant BCRs. The details of this process are still poorly understood. Receipt and integration of signals through the BCR are clearly involved in positive selection and must be based on the affinity for antigen. Ablating BCR signals such as calcineurin-dependent signals and CD19 signaling mutants and loss of CD45 interferes with positive selection and memory B cell development (147,156,159,160). However, as discussed earlier, it is difficult to dissect the GC BCR interactions with antigen from the initial BCR triggers that recruited naïve B cells into the primary response. Most models suggest immune complex (IC) trapping on FDCs as the most likely means for variant BCRs to receive a rescuing signal from native antigen. Antigen appears rapidly in this location and can persist for extended periods of time focused to FDC in lymphoid tissue draining the site of antigen administration (162). In support of this notion, complement receptors CD21/CD35 on FDC are needed to generate long-term serum antibody response (163). However, animals that do not secrete antibody and therefore cannot form IC can still support affinity maturation (164). In the absence of inhibitor of nuclear factor (NF)-κB kinase 2 (IKK2)–dependent activation of the NF-κB pathway, FDCs can still capture ICs but are not stimulated to up-regulate vascular cellular adhesion molecule-1 (VCAM-1) and intercellular adhesion molecule-1 (ICAM-1) (165). In the absence of these adhesion molecules, GC B cells appear more susceptible to apoptosis with evidence for altered gene expression and decreased affinity maturation.

Polarity in the GC microenvironment is partly controlled by the differential expression of chemokines and their receptors (166). Higher expression of CXCL12 in the dark zone assorts CXCR4-expressing centroblasts, while higher CXCL13 in the light zone attracts CXCR5-expressing centrocytes. These studies use flow cytometry and cell cycle status to identify GC B cell subsets and demonstrate the aberrant behavior of GC B cells from various genetically modified host animals. Recent two-photon analysis reveals the movement of GC B cells along FDC processes within the GC (148). These studies emphasize the lack of dwell time for GC B cells on FDC processes with little change in GC B cell velocity upon FDC contact. Therefore, if antigen binding is associated with GC B cell-FDC contact, there appears to be no evidence for interclonal competition between different GC B cells. In contrast, there was prolonged contact between antigen-specific GC Th cells and GC B cells. As there are also very few GC Th cells in the light zone of GCs, the Th cells create a rate limiting stage within the GC pathway. Thus, competition for cognate GC Th cell interaction may provide a final selection mechanism for the pMHCII-expressing GC B cells and constitutes a third major checkpoint in memory B cell development. These direct imaging strategies provide important clues to the dynamic facets of antigen-driven selection in the GC microenvironment and, importantly, begin to identify the central function of GC Th cells.

As with all *in vivo* studies, there are substantial influences associated with the choice of models, affinities of BCR, type of antigen, and method of immunization that will impact the observations presented in the studies. The issues of antigen receptor monoclonality are self-evident in BCR transgenic models in the context of repertoire studies but less clearly understood in association with the expression of diverse effector functions *in vivo*. More important, in the context of T cell responses, it is now apparent that elevated precursor frequency deviates the dynamics of clonal expansion (167,168) and can alter the development of T cell memory *in vivo* (169). Changing the balance or affinity of regulator populations will impact cell fate of the target populations in ways that remain difficult to assess. Nevertheless, new insights offered by dynamic imaging continue to buttress our appreciation for the workings of the immune system and serve to challenge existing dogma in powerful and productive ways.

GC T_{FH} Cells

In contrast to pre-GC effector T_{FH} cells discussed earlier, $CXCR5^+$ Th in GC will be referred to as "germinal center" T_{FH} cells (Figures 9.5 and 9.6). Many $CXCR5^+$ T_{FH} cells were found very early in the immune response (day 3), at the T-B borders and within follicular regions of LNs (86). These studies also provide further evidence for a circulating compartment of $CXCR5^+$ Th cells. Hence, it is clear that CXCR5 expression is not a reliable marker of GC Th cells only. Further, the expected function of GC T_{FH} cells would be broadly different from those described for pre-GC effector T_{FH} cells. The presence of GC T_{FH} cells among the dense follicular dendritic cell networks of the GC light zone predict a role in the propagation of high-affinity variant GC B cells into the long-lived memory B cell compartment (166).

During antiprotein immune responses, the Th cells within the light zone of the GC express pMHCII-specific TCRs. There appears to be sequential movement of antigen-specific Th cells from the T cell zones into the GC microenvironment (66,170) with evidence that suggests GC Th cells can also move between different GCs (171). Interestingly, all antigen-specific Th cells responding to a protein antigen are not represented within the GC reaction, indicating pre-GC functional differentiation for responding Th cells (172). Further, non-GC Th cells can reemerge in a memory response, indicating that the GC is not required for memory Th cell development (66). Downregulation of CD90 (Thy-1) has been used as a marker of GC Th cells in the mouse, although when this occurs and how well it discriminates only GC Th cells is not clear (171). Interfering with CD40L-CD40 interactions disrupts the GC reaction, while blocking B7-2 interaction impairs memory B-cell development (173). Hence, the cognate control of GC B cell fate appears to be modified by the cellular and molecular context of pMHCII presentation.

The more recent work on human T_{FH} cells use expression of CD57, as well as CXCR5, to define T_{FH} cells that are contained within the GC of tonsils (174,175). Microarray analysis highlights the distantly related functional programs of $CD57^+$ GC T_{FH} cells as compared to naïve Th cells, central memory Th cells (T_{CM}), and effector memory Th cells (T_{EM}) from the peripheral blood (175). Differences in adhesion molecules, chemokine receptors, cytokines, and transcription factors appear as distant as different lineages. Interestingly, the CXCR5 ligand, CXCL13, is highly expressed in GC T_{FH} cells. *In vitro* derived Th1 and Th2 effector Th cells also appear distant in gene expression program to GC T_{FH} cells (174). This analysis associates CD84, CD200, IL-21, and BCL6 with $CD57^+$ GC T_{FH} cells. A separate analysis of T_{FH} cells by function and gene expression demonstrates that T_{FH} activity in human tonsil is independent of CD57 expression (176). These studies highlight $ICOS^{high}CXCR5^{high}$ T_{FH} as CXCL13 secretors and the most potent inducers of antibody production *in vitro*. Therefore, it is clear *in situ* that all GC T_{FH} cells express CXCR5, and many express CD57; however, these molecules are not exclusively expressed on GC T_{FH} cells nor expressed on all T_{FH} cells in the tonsil. Nevertheless, it remains important to clarify GC T_{FH} phenotype so that the details of their function can be pursued *in vivo*.

B CELL MEMORY

It is now clear that centrocytes can undergo proliferation in the light zone (160), and there is direct evidence for movement of centrocytes back into the dark zone of GCs (148,149). Thus, it appears that one outcome of GC B cell-GC T_{FH} interactions is reentry into the GC cycle and reiterative rounds of expansion, diversification, and selection (Figure 9.7). In this model, each subsequent round of clonal expansion and BCR diversification is applied to GC B cell variants that have been positively selected based on

	FO B	Short lived PC	GC B	PostGC Mem	Pre Plasma Mem	Long lived PC
(s)Ig	+++	+/-	+/-	++	++	+/-
(ic)Ig	+	+++	+	+	+	+++
CD79b	+++	++/-	++	+++	+/++	++/-
CD19	+++	++/-	++	++	+/++	++/-
CD45R	+++	+/+	+++	+++	+/-	+/-
GL7	-	-	+++	-/+	-	-
CD38	+++	-	-/+	+++	+++	-
CD43	+	+++	-	-/+	++	+++
CD138	-	+++	-	-	-	+++

High +++ Intermediate ++ Low + Negative -

FIGURE 9.8 Cell surface phenotype of antigen-response B cells in Th cell regulated development of B cell memory.

increased BCR affinity. Hence, the introduction of a few mutations in each clonal progeny of selected variants is less likely to destroy BCR specificity and leaves room for further increases in an already high-affinity variant BCR.

The second major outcome of checkpoint III is exit from the GC cycle and entry into the memory B cell compartment (Figures 9.6, 9.8). The GC reaction produces at least two broad categories of affinity-matured memory B cells (26). The most typical memory B cells are the precursors for a memory response to antigen recall. These memory B cells are easily distinguished functionally from the second cellular compartment of memory, the long-lived PCs (177). The long-lived PCs are terminally differentiated cells that continually produce high-affinity antibody and will not be drawn into a secondary response. In both categories of memory B cells, the expression of antibody isotype distinguishes separable memory B cell compartments. By definition, these subsets differ in the antibody they can produce and hence their developmental program and cellular function is distinct. However, these "isotype-specific" memory B cell subsets may also differ in migration patterns, survival needs, and the requirements for reactivation at the time of antigen recall. These issues define a level of heterogeneity that have received very little attention at the current time and remain important features in the organization of B cell memory *in vivo*.

Memory B Cell Subsets

Memory response precursors are affinity-matured BCR^+ post-GC cells that have often isotype-switched and can still respond, in a Th-cell-dependent manner, to low-dose soluble antigen recall. The long-term persistence *in vivo* of antigen-binding BCR^+ B cells, after the decline of the primary response, provides the single best indicator for all memory response precursors. Beyond this particular attribute, antibody isotype and stage of development within the memory B cell compartment introduces a level of cellular heterogeneity that is only recently being appreciated.

As soluble antigen is the ligand for the BCR, most experimental approaches use variations of labeled antigen to identify antigen-specific B cells. While panning techniques used gel-associated antigen (178,179), flow cytometry provided the most reliable access to antigen-specific B cells (180,181). These earliest studies (180,181) coupled cell sorting technology and direct labeling to enrich antigen-specific B cells for adoptive transfer. These early studies helped to demonstrate that B cells with receptors for antigen were the precursors for antibody-forming cells. This approach has been adopted by many groups (182–185) with the subsequent evaluation of specificity and purity demonstrated by the frequency for antibody-forming cells or the enrichment for production of antigen-specific antibodies *in vitro*.

Early studies indicated antigen-binding B cell populations of long-lived cells with slow or no turnover *in vivo* (186). These memory B cells can survive independent of their expressed BCR specificity and hence do not require persistent antigen depots *in vivo* (187). Loss of membrane IgM/IgD and expression of downstream isotype are also indicative of antigen experience but are not required for memory cell development (181,183,188). Further, the expression of mutated BCRs with evidence for affinity increasing changes is the most useful molecular marker for the memory B cell compartment (114,189–191). However, there are also abundant examples of germline-encoded

BCRs expressed by memory response precursors. Location has also been a reliable means for isolating memory B cells from the blood very soon after intentional priming (189). The combination of location, phenotype, genotype, and time after intentional priming has many elements of a comprehensive definition for memory B cells.

Memory response precursors have been typically defined as $IgM^{-}IgD^{-}6B2^{high}$ antigen-binding B cells (183,191–193) that do not secrete antibody until expansion and differentiation into PC after re-challenge with antigen. These $6B2^{high}$ memory B cells express mutated receptors and can be found in late primary and secondary responses to antigen (114,191,194). There is now evidence for a second subset of antigen-binding memory B cells that down-regulates the CD45 glycoform B220, displaying reduced levels of 6B2 binding (195–197). Upon adoptive transfer, both $6B2^{high}$ and $6B2^{low}$ memory B cell subsets give rise to antigen-specific memory responses (197). The pattern of cellular expansion, conversion of cell surface phenotype, and extent of PC development suggests that the $6B2^{high}$ "post-GC" memory B cells lie developmentally upstream from the $6B2^{low}$ "pre-plasma" memory B cell compartment.

The $6B2^{low}$ pre-plasma memory B cells have been seen across a number of different antigen systems following a variety of immunization regimes. Following hapten-protein immunizations, $6B2^{low}$ memory B cells are found with high-dose antigen (400 μg) using the Ribi adjuvant system (118) but not with low-dose (40 μg) using alum as the adjuvant (189). There is clear evidence of $6B2^{low}$ antigen-experienced B cells across multiple regimes of BCR transgenic transfer using the B cells from the QM mouse model that express germline-encoded and hapten-specific BCR (195,196). The QM B cells also produce a phenotypically distinct B cell subset of $6B2^{low}$ pre-plasma cells that can differentiate into plasma cells in an antigen-independent manner (198). This change can be induced upon adoptive transfer into naïve recipients but requires some level of clonal expansion. Cells with a similar $6B2^{low}$ pre-plasma cell phenotype have been recently described in a mouse model of bacteriophage capsid immunization (199). The 6B2 antibody also recognizes a similar determinant on human B cells with the majority of $CD27^{+}$ IgM and non-IgM memory B cells in the blood displaying a $6B2^{low}$ phenotype (200). Hence, the $6B2^{high}$ and $6B2^{low}$ memory B cells represent separable subsets of the memory B cell compartment that may describe a linear progression of development as the cellular products of the GC reaction and immediate precursors of high-affinity plasma cells upon antigen recall.

Long-lived Plasma Cells

Long-lived antibody-secreting B cells can also be considered part of the memory B cell compartment. The long-lived PCs do not replenish through turnover, but do secrete isotype-switched antibody and display evidence of SHM with affinity increasing mutation patterns (177,201,202). This post-GC antigen-specific B cell compartment appears during the second week after initial antigen exposure (114) and preferentially homes to the BM for growth factor support of stromal cells (203). Based on gene ablation studies, these cells use a variety of redistribution mechanisms such as up-regulation of CXCR4, $\alpha4\beta1$ integrin binding to its ligand VCAM-1 (115) to get to the BM, where they can persist for the life of the animal (112,204–208). In the BM, long-lived PCs need signals through the TNFR family member, BCMA for survival (209). It has also been proposed that a pre-PC precursor (198) or memory cells themselves (210) produce PCs in a non–antigen-dependent manner as a means of maintaining serum antibody levels for extended periods.

The extended longevity of the long-lived PC can be demonstrated using BrdU incorporation and adoptive transfer (205–208). The extinguished gene programs associated with PC development (128,211,212) support a terminally differentiated end-stage cell that needs to arrest cell cycle progression (155) and will not be reactivated on antigen recall. Nevertheless, based on the evidence of a GC phase in development, the extended longevity of these PCs and the continued production of high-affinity antibody, it is reasonable to consider these end-stage B cells to belong to the memory B cell compartment.

Based on variability in memory B cell formation across different antigen models, it appears likely that different sets of initiating stimuli modify the balance of cells within the different memory B cell compartments. The memory cell balance may be a quantitative "interpretation" of the quality of the initial immunizing signals. Ultimately, memory B cell fate is likely to be controlled by checkpoint III interactions in the GC itself. The strength of BCR signal and costimulatory context serve to select variant BCRs and initiate changes in memory B cell development. Cognate interactions with GC T_{FH} cells may consolidate these functional outcomes. Understanding the role of the different memory B cell subsets in long-term protection and the rules that govern their development *in vivo* remain important unresolved areas in this field.

Memory Response to Recall

Persistent high-affinity serum antibody provides the first layer of protection against a secondary challenge. While antibody binding to antigen is a clearance mechanism, it also serves to increase the efficiency of antigen presentation to memory B cells through rapid IC formation and binding to FcR or complement receptors on cells of the innate system. In this manner, antibody may amplify the sensitivity of the memory B cell response to secondary antigen challenge. Furthermore, antigen re-challenge also seems necessary to establish adequate long-term protection following protein vaccination. The cognate cellular dynamics and molecular regulation of the memory response boost are important factors in the consolidation of B cell memory that remain poorly understood and inadequately optimized in most vaccine regimes.

Primary response GC persists for around three weeks after initial priming, but this timing may vary substantially depending on the immune stimuli (132,133). There is evidence for continued selection in the memory B cell compartment even after the demise of the GC reaction (202). This selection process represents more typical interclonal competition without further BCR diversification (213). Where this secondary selection occurs and how it relates to the selection mechanisms in the GC remains to be determined. Nevertheless, secondary selection events appear capable of reshaping the memory compartment toward higher affinity clonotypes that can substantially influence the quality of the secondary response and consolidation of the memory compartment (210).

Using priming doses of antigen and adjuvant, antigen-specific memory Th cell responses (66,67,214) and memory B cell response (215) emerge more rapidly than their naïve response counterparts. Memory Th cell responses reach peak levels more rapidly but to similar levels as the primary response. In contrast, memory B cells display accelerated kinetics but reach substantially higher maximal levels compared to the primary response. Even in the presence of priming doses of antigen and adjuvant, the memory responders dominate the recall response (66,197), out-competing naïve lymphocytes that may express specific Ag-R.

Memory Th Cells

Memory B cell response to TD antigens require antigen-specific T cell help (26). Under normal physiological circumstances, this secondary T cell help must be antigen-specific and is most likely delivered by memory Th cells that are specific to the immunizing antigen. Under typical low-dose antigen re-challenge regime in the absence of immune adjuvant, antigen-specific B cells are likely to be the APC for the memory response. Hence, the cognate interactions of pMHCII$^+$ memory B cells and antigen-specific memory Th cells define a fourth developmental checkpoint in the evolution of long-term immune protection (Figure 9.9). Alternately, circulating antibody and innate immune activation induce an accelerated memory response due to increased frequencies and heightened responsiveness of memory response precursors. In this scenario, the memory Th cell-memory B cell checkpoint may be preceded by an independent series of antigen presentation events prior to checkpoint IV.

The major cellular outcome of the secondary boost is rapid and exaggerated memory B cell expansion and the production of large numbers of high-affinity PCs. While high-affinity B cells can be drawn into GC reactions (149), it is not clear that the GC pathway is operative at the time of the secondary boost. Regardless, there is clear evidence for secondary selection events upon antigen re-challenge that are more likely to be driven by cellular selection without somatic BCR diversification (26). The nature of the selection mechanism for B cells at this stage of the response is also poorly understood. In contrast, the accelerated local reexpansion of antigen-specific memory Th cells occurs with little change in the expressed TCR repertoire (216) or cytokine-secreting potential (214). Hence, the antigen-specific memory Th cell compartment appears to conserve and reexpress many of the functions associated with the initial primary immune response.

There is evidence for a division of labor in the memory T cell compartment that involves the migratory capacity of memory Th cell subsets (217). Recirculating central

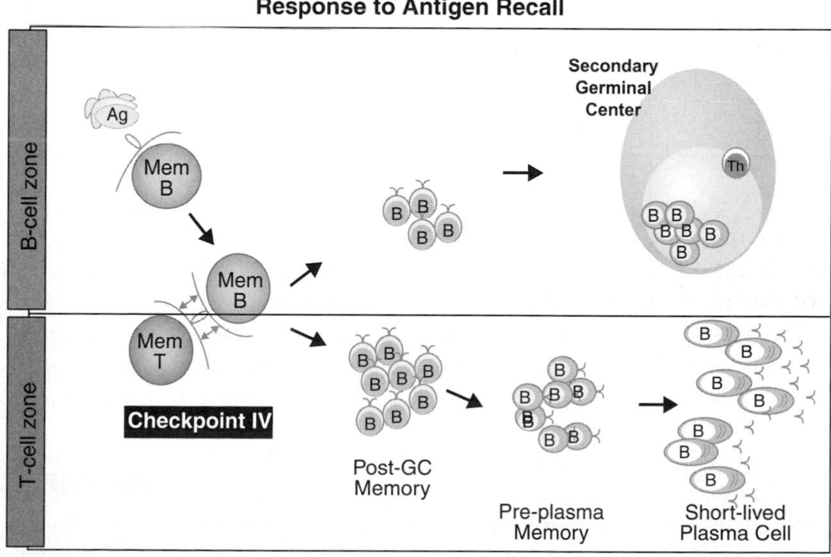

FIGURE 9.9 The response to antigen recall. Low-dose soluble antigen in the absence of adjuvant can induce a rapid and exaggerated humoral immune response. Hence, antigen-specific B cells are the most likely APC for pMHC II complexes at checkpoint IV interactions between memory Th cells and memory B cells are the critical developmental checkpoint for the memory response. Memory cell expansion is vigorous to produce large numbers of high-affinity memory response plasma cells as the dominant cellular outcome. Secondary GC reactions are also part of the memory response, although more a minor outcome than seen in the primary response.

memory T cells (T_{CM}) and tissue-homing effector memory T cells (T_{EM}) further divide on their readiness to reexpress effector function upon reexposure to antigen. It is reasonable to propose that each antigen-specific effector Th cell subset will produce a memory Th cell counterpart (214). However, the range of Th memory effector attributes required to control antigen-specific memory B cell responses is not well understood. Compartments of tissue-localized memory Th cells provide rapid "reactive" immune protection that is antigen-specific (217). For example, the focal placement of T_{EM} cell subsets at sites of original antigen entry preempts the life history of the pathogen. In this manner, location provides an opportunity to accelerate the recall response, enhancing the capacity of the immune system to block overt infection. As the precursors of the memory response to antigen recall, high-affinity memory B cells belong to a similar "reactive" set of memory cells. However, in contrast to local hypersensitivity responses by Th cells, antigen reexposure promotes rapid and exaggerated memory B cell responses in the lymphoid tissue that drains the site of re-challenge. In this context, we can refer to the memory Th cell compartment that controls memory B cell responses as memory T_{FH} cells.

It is not clear whether memory T_{FH} cells would necessarily express $CXCR5^+$ like their primary response T_{FH} compartment. Further, it is not clear whether both effector T_{FH} and GC T_{FH} produce memory T_{FH} counterparts. Nevertheless, it will be important to unravel the programs of cognate control used by antigen-specific memory T_{FH} to regulate the memory B cell response to antigen re-challenge. It is plausible that manipulating cellular and molecular interactions at checkpoint IV can alter the shape of antigen-specific B cell memory.

Antigen Persistence *in vivo*

Unlike CD8 T cells, CD4 Th cells appear to require continued presence of antigen to reach maximal clonal expansion *in vivo*. The conditional induction and abrogation of pMHCII molecules demonstrate that as soon as a lower threshold level of antigen is breached, Th cell cease to divide (61). Surprisingly, this model induces no form of inflammation and would otherwise be considered a model of tolerance induction. Recent intravital imaging studies also indicate that antigen-responsive Th cells engage multiple DCs at successive early stages after priming (62). These multiple DC-Th cell contacts also impact the development of effector Th cell function *in vivo*. Most surprisingly, there is evidence for persistent depots of pMHCII complexes up to 3 weeks after viral infection (63). These pMHCII depots are present at times after viral clearance *in vivo*. The same persistent depots can be demonstrated for pMHCI with the capacity for local activation of viral-specific naïve CD8 cells (64). While persistent antigen is not required for the maintenance of antigen-specific T cell memory (218,219), there may be a role for persistent depots of pMHC complexes as local guidance cues for antigen-specific memory T cells.

CONCLUSION

Understanding the cellular and molecular control of memory B cell development remains a high priority for fundamental research with important application to the field of immunotherapeutics and vaccine design. There has been substantial progress in our understanding of this complex developmental cascade *in vivo,* with many of the cellular processes being more carefully defined in their most relevant *in vivo* context. The sophisticated manipulation of mouse genetics provides a powerful set of tools that begin to unravel the regulatory mechanisms operative across each developmental checkpoint controlling cell fate *in vivo*. Real-time intravital imaging provides a major advance to our appreciation of cell dynamics and intercellular communication as it proceeds in the crowded confines of secondary lymphoid tissue.

Clonal selection underpins all adaptive immune activities with significant differences emerging between Th cells and B cells in the antigen-specific pathway to immune memory. Effector Th cell function remains somewhat convoluted and still difficult to fathom *in vivo,* although we are beginning to appreciate the extraordinary heterogeneity that resides among these antigen-specific regulators of adaptive immunity. Antigen-driven B cell development is less divergent than its Th cell counterpart; however, the organization of the antigen-responsive B cell compartment is still difficult to access experimentally *in vivo*. Nevertheless, the progression of cellular and molecular events that underpin immune memory are rapidly coming into focus. Many new antigen-specific models provide high resolution to the nature of effector B cell function and antigen-specific B cell memory that may unravel the rules of immune control and substantially impact the redesign of vaccine formulations.

ACKNOWLEDGMENTS

I would like to acknowledge Louise McHeyzer-Williams in the collaborative unfolding of the ideas that structure this chapter and the images that illustrate the flow of ideas presented here. There has been immeasurable input from the members of my laboratory and collaborators over the years that helped to shape and reshape the nature of our understanding of these fascinating processes *in vivo*.

REFERENCES

1. Berland R, Wortis HH. Origins and functions of B-1 cells with notes on the role of cd5. *Annu Rev Immunol.* 2002;20:253–300.

2. Hardy RR, Hayakawa K. B cell development pathways. *Annu Rev Immunol.* 2001;19:595–621.
3. Hayakawa K, Hardy RR, Herzenberg LA, et al. Progenitors for Ly-1 B cells are distinct from progenitors for other B cells. *J Exp Med.* 1985;161(6):1554–1568.
4. Lalor PA, Stall AM, Adams S, et al. Permanent alteration of the murine Ly-1 B repertoire due to selective depletion of Ly-1 B cells in neonatal animals. *Eur J Immunol.* 1989;19(3):501–506.
5. Kantor AB, Herzenberg LA. Origin of murine B cell lineages. *Annu Rev Immunol.* 1993;11:501–538.
6. Arnold LW, Pennell CA, McCray SK, et al. Development of B-1 cells: segregation of phosphatidyl choline-specific B cells to the B-1 population occurs after immunoglobulin gene expression. *J Exp Med.* 1994;179(5):1585–1595.
7. Clarke SH, Arnold LW. B-1 cell development: evidence for an uncommitted immunoglobulin (Ig)M+ B cell precursor in B-1 cell differentiation. *J Exp Med.* 1998;187(8):1325–1334.
8. Martin F, Oliver AM, Kearney JF. Marginal zone and B1 B cells unite in the early response against T-independent blood-borne particulate antigens. *Immunity.* 2001 May;14(5):617–629.
9. Martin F, Kearney JF. B1 cells: similarities and differences with other B cell subsets. *Curr Opin Immunol.* 2001;13(2):195–201.
10. Bendelac A, Bonneville M, Kearney JF. Autoreactivity by design: innate B and T lymphocytes. *Nature Rev Immunol.* 2001;1(3):177–186.
11. Hardy RR, Hayakawa K. A developmental switch in B lymphopoiesis. *Proc Natl Acad U S A.* 1991;88(24):11550–11554.
12. Montecino-Rodriguez E, Leathers H, Dorshkind K. Identification of a B-1 B cell-specified progenitor. *Nat Immunol.* 2006;7(3): 293–301.
13. Tung JW, Mrazek MD, Yang Y, et al. Phenotypically distinct B cell development pathways map to the three B cell lineages in the mouse. *Proc Natl Acad U S A.* 2006;103(16):6293–6298.
14. Haas KM, Poe JC, Steeber DA, et al. B-1a and B-1b cells exhibit distinct developmental requirements and have unique functional roles in innate and adaptive immunity to S. pneumoniae. *Immunity.* 2005;23(1):7–18.
15. Alugupalli KR, Leong JM, Woodland RT, et al. B1b lymphocytes confer T cell-independent long-lasting immunity. *Immunity.* 2004;21(3):379–390.
16. Martin F, Kearney JF. Marginal-zone B cells. *Nat Rev Immunol.* 2002;2(5):323–335.
17. MacLennan IC, Bazin H, Chassoux D, et al. Comparative analysis of the development of B cells in marginal zones and follicles. *Adv Exp Med Biol.* 1985;186:139–144.
18. Balazs M, Martin F, Zhou T, et al. Blood dendritic cells interact with splenic marginal zone B cells to initiate T-independent immune responses. *Immunity.* 2002;17(3):341–352.
19. Lopes-Carvalho T, Foote J, Kearney JF. Marginal zone B cells in lymphocyte activation and regulation. *Curr Opin Immunol.* 2005; 17(3):244–250.
20. Weller S, Braun MC, Tan BK, et al. Human blood IgM "memory" B cells are circulating splenic marginal zone B cells harboring a prediversified immunoglobulin repertoire. Blood. 2004;104(12): 3647–3654.
21. Song H, Cerny J. Functional heterogeneity of marginal zone B cells revealed by their ability to generate both early antibody-forming cells and germinal centers with hypermutation and memory in response to a T-dependent antigen. *J Exp Med.* 2003;198(12):1923–1935.
22. Meffre E, Casellas R, Nussenzweig MC. Antibody regulation of B cell development. *Nat Immunol.* 2000;1(5):379–385.
23. Tsuiji M, Yurasov S, Velinzon K, et al. A checkpoint for autoreactivity in human IgM+ memory B cell development. *J Exp Med.* 2006;203(2):393–400.
24. Miller MJ, Wei SH, Parker I, et al. Two-photon imaging of lymphocyte motility and antigen response in intact lymph node. *Science.* 2002;296(5574):1869–1873.
25. Bajenoff M, Egen JG, Koo LY, et al. Stromal cell networks regulate lymphocyte entry, migration, and territoriality in lymph nodes. *Immunity.* 2006;25(6):989–1001.
26. McHeyzer-Williams LJ, McHeyzer-Williams MG. Antigen-specific memory B cell development. *Annu Rev Immunol.* 2005;23:487–513.
27. Banchereau J, Steinman RM. Dendritic cells and the control of *Immunity. Nature.* 1998 Mar 19;392(6673):245–252.
28. Shortman K, Liu YJ. Mouse and human dendritic cell subtypes. *Nat Rev Immunol.* 2002;2(3):151–161.
29. Itano AA, Jenkins MK. Antigen presentation to naïve CD4 T cells in the lymph node. *Nat Immunol.* 2003;4(8):733–739.
30. Aderem A, Ulevitch RJ. Toll-like receptors in the induction of the innate immune response. *Nature.* 2000;406(6797):782–787.
31. Janeway CA, Jr., Medzhitov R. Innate immune recognition. *Annu Rev Immunol.* 2002;20:197–216.
32. Inohara N, Nunez G. NODs: intracellular proteins involved in inflammation and apoptosis. *Nat Rev Immunol.* 2003;3(5):371–382.
33. Trombetta ES, Mellman I. Cell biology of antigen processing *in vitro* and *in vivo*. *Annu Rev Immunol.* 2005;23:975–1028.
34. Dudziak D, Kamphorst AO, Heidkamp GF, et al. Differential antigen processing by dendritic cell subsets *in vivo*. *Science.* 2007;315(5808):107–111.
35. Lindquist RL, Shakhar G, Dudziak D, et al. Visualizing dendritic cell networks *in vivo*. *Nat Immunol.* 2004;5(12):1243–1250.
36. Kissenpfennig A, Henri S, Dubois B, et al. Dynamics and function of Langerhans cells *in vivo* dermal dendritic cells colonize lymph node areas distinct from slower migrating Langerhans cells. *Immunity.* 2005;22(5):643–654.
37. Itano AA, McSorley SJ, Reinhardt RL, et al. Distinct dendritic cell populations sequentially present antigen to CD4 T cells and stimulate different aspects of cell-mediated immunity. *Immunity.* 2003;19(1):47–57.
38. Beutler B. Innate immunity: an overview. *Mol Immunol.* 2004; 40(12):845–859.
39. Dintzis HM, Dintzis RZ, Vogelstein B. Molecular determinants of immunogenicity: the immunon model of immune response. *Proc Natl Acad U S A.* 1976;73(10):3671–3675.
40. Bergtold A, Desai DD, Gavhane A, et al. Cell surface recycling of internalized antigen permits dendritic cell priming of B cells. *Immunity.* 2005;23(5):503–514.
41. Batista FD, Iber D, Neuberger MS. B cells acquire antigen from target cells after synapse formation. *Nature.* 2001;411(6836):489–494.
42. Batista FD, Neuberger MS. Affinity dependence of the B cell response to antigen: a threshold, a ceiling, and the importance of off-rate. *Immunity.* 1998;8(6):751–759.
43. Qi H, Egen JG, Huang AY, et al. Extrafollicular activation of lymph node B cells by antigen-bearing dendritic cells. *Science.* 2006;312(5780):1672–1676.
44. Sixt M, Kanazawa N, Selg M, et al. The conduit system transports soluble antigens from the afferent lymph to resident dendritic cells in the T cell area of the lymph node. *Immunity.* 2005 Jan 22(1): 19–29.
45. Castigli E, Wilson SA, Scott S, et al. TACI and BAFF-R mediate isotype switching in B cells. *J Exp Med.* 2005;201(1):35–39.
46. Pulendran B. Modulating vaccine responses with dendritic cells and Toll-like receptors. *Immunol Rev.* 2004;199:227–250.
47. Sallusto F, Mackay CR, Lanzavecchia A. The role of chemokine receptors in primary, effector, and memory immune responses. *Annu Rev Immunol.* 2000;18:593–620.
48. Cyster JG. Chemokines and cell migration in secondary lymphoid organs. *Science.* 1999;286(5447):2098–2102.
49. Bromley SK, Burack WR, Johnson KG, et al. The immunological synapse. *Annu Rev Immunol.* 2001;19:375–396.
50. Iezzi G, Karjalainen K, Lanzavecchia A. The duration of antigenic stimulation determines the fate of naïve and effector T cells. *Immunity.* 1998;8(1):89–95.
51. Norcross MA. A synaptic basis for T-lymphocyte activation. *Ann Immunol (Paris).* 1984;135D(2):113–134.
52. Grakoui A, Bromley SK, Sumen C, et al. The immunological synapse: a molecular machine controlling T cell activation. *Science.* 1999;285(5425):221–227.
53. Monks CR, Freiberg BA, Kupfer H, et al. Three-dimensional segregation of supramolecular activation clusters in T cells. *Nature.* 1998;395(6697):82–86.
54. Lee KH, Holdorf AD, Dustin ML, et al. T cell receptor signaling precedes immunological synapse formation. *Science.* 2002;295(5559): 1539–1542.

55. Huppa JB, Gleimer M, Sumen C, et al. Continuous T cell receptor signaling required for synapse maintenance and full effector potential. *Nat Immunol*. 2003;4(8):749–755.
56. Stoll S, Delon J, Brotz TM, et al. Dynamic imaging of T cell-dendritic cell interactions in lymph nodes. *Science*. 2002;296(5574):1873–1876.
57. Mempel TR, Henrickson SE, Von Andrian UH. T-cell priming by dendritic cells in lymph nodes occurs in three distinct phases. *Nature*. 2004;427(6970):154–159.
58. Miller MJ, Hejazi AS, Wei SH, et al. T cell repertoire scanning is promoted by dynamic dendritic cell behavior and random T cell motility in the lymph node. *Proc Natl Acad USA*. 2004;101(4):998–1003.
59. Miller MJ, Safrina O. Imaging the single cell dynamics of CD4+ T cell activation by dendritic cells in lymph nodes. *J Exp Med*. 2004;200(7):847–856.
60. Shakhar G, Lindquist RL, Skokos D, et al. Stable T cell-dendritic cell interactions precede the development of both tolerance and immunity *in vivo*. *Nat Immunol*. 2005.
61. Obst R, van Santen HM, Mathis D, et al. Antigen persistence is required throughout the expansion phase of a CD4(+) T cell response. *J Exp Med*. 2005;201(10):1555–1565.
62. Celli S, Garcia Z, Bousso P. CD4 T cells integrate signals delivered during successive DC encounters *in vivo*. *J Exp Med*. 2005;202(9):1271–1278.
63. Jelley-Gibbs DM, Brown DM, Dibble JP, et al. Unexpected prolonged presentation of influenza antigens promotes CD4 T cell memory generation. *J Exp Med*. 2005;202(5):697–706.
64. Zammit DJ, Turner DL, Klonowski KD, et al. Residual antigen presentation after influenza virus infection affects CD8 T cell activation and migration. *Immunity*. 2006;24(4):439–449.
65. Malherbe L, Filippi C, Julia V, et al. Selective activation and expansion of high-affinity CD4+ T cells in resistant mice upon infection with Leishmania major. *Immunity*. 2000;13(6):771–782.
66. McHeyzer-Williams LJ, Panus JF, Mikszta JA, et al. Evolution of antigen-specific T cell receptors *in vivo*: Preimmune and antigen-driven selection of preferred complementarity-determining region 3 (CDR3) motifs. *J Exp Med*. 1999;189(11):1823–1837.
67. McHeyzer-Williams MG, Davis MM. Antigen-specific development of primary and memory T cells *in vivo*. *Science*. 1995;268:106–111.
68. Alam SM, Travers PJ, Wung JL, et al. T-cell-receptor affinity and thymocyte positive selection. *Nature*. 1996;381(6583):616–620.
69. Busch DH, Pamer EG. T cell affinity maturation by selective expansion during infection. *J Exp Med*. 1999;189(4):701–710.
70. Fasso M, Anandasabapathy N, Crawford F, et al. T cell receptor (TCR)-mediated repertoire selection and loss of TCR vbeta diversity during the initiation of a CD4(+) T cell response *in vivo*. *J Exp Med*. 2000;192(12):1719–1730.
71. Kedl RM, Rees WA, Hildeman DA, et al. T cells compete for access to antigen-bearing antigen-presenting cells. *J Exp Med*. 2000;192(8):1105–1113.
72. Kedl RM, Schaefer BC, Kappler JW, et al. T cells down-modulate peptide-MHC complexes on APCs *in vivo*. *Nat Immunol*. 2002;3(1):27–32.
73. Lyons DS, Lieberman SA, Hampl J, et al. A TCR binds to antagonist ligands with lower affinities and faster dissociation rates than to agonists. *Immunity*. 1996;5(1):53–61.
74. Matsui K, Boniface JJ, Steffner P, et al. Kinetics of T-cell receptor binding to peptide/I-Ek complexes: correlation of the dissociation rate with T-cell responsiveness. *Proc Natl Acad U S A*. 1994;91(26):1286212866.
75. Savage PA, Boniface JJ, Davis MM. A kinetic basis for T cell receptor repertoire selection during an immune response. *Immunity*. 1999;10(4):485–492.
76. Lazarski CA, Chaves FA, Jenks SA, et al. The kinetic stability of MHC class II:peptide complexes is a key parameter that dictates immunodominance. *Immunity*. 2005;23(1):29–40.
77. Malherbe L, Hausl C, Teyton L, et al. Clonal selection of helper T cells is determined by an affinity threshold with no further skewing of TCR binding properties. *Immunity*. 2004;21(5):669–679.
78. Garside P, Ingulli E, Merica RR, et al. Visualization of specific B and T lymphocyte interactions in the lymph node. *Science*. 1998;281(5373):96–99.
79. Reif K, Ekland EH, Ohl L, et al. Balanced responsiveness to chemoattractants from adjacent zones determines B-cell position. *Nature*. 2002;416(6876):94–99.
80. Okada T, Miller MJ, Parker I, et al. Antigen-engaged B cells undergo chemotaxis toward the T zone and form motile conjugates with helper T cells. *PLoS Biol*. 2005;3(6):e150.
81. McHeyzer-Williams LJ, McHeyzer-Williams MG. Developmentally distinct Th cells control plasma cell production *in vivo*. *Immunity*. 2004;20(2):231–242.
82. Forster R, Emrich T, Kremmer E, et al. Expression of the G-protein–coupled receptor BLR1 defines mature, recirculating B cells and a subset of T-helper memory cells. *Blood*. 1994;84(3):830–840.
83. Forster R, Mattis AE, Kremmer E, et al. A putative chemokine receptor, BLR1, directs B cell migration to defined lymphoid organs and specific anatomic compartments of the spleen. Cell. 1996;87(6):1037–1047.
84. Forster R, Schubel A, Breitfeld D, et al. CCR7 coordinates the primary immune response by establishing functional microenvironments in secondary lymphoid organs. *Cell*. 1999;99(1):23–33.
85. Walker LS, Gulbranson-Judge A, Flynn S, et al. Compromised OX40 function in CD28-deficient mice is linked with failure to develop CXC chemokine receptor 5-positive CD4 cells and germinal centers. *J Exp Med*. 1999;190(8):1115–1122.
86. Ansel KM, McHeyzer-Williams LJ, Ngo VN, et al. *In vivo*-activated CD4 T cells upregulate CXC chemokine receptor 5 and reprogram their response to lymphoid chemokines. *J Exp Med*. 1999;190(8):1123–1134.
87. Breitfeld D, Ohl L, Kremmer E, et al. Follicular B helper T cells express CXC chemokine receptor 5, localize to B cell follicles, and support immunoglobulin production. *J Exp Med*. 2000;192(11):1545–1552.
88. Schaerli P, Willimann K, Lang AB, et al. CXC chemokine receptor 5 expression defines follicular homing T cells with B cell helper function. *J Exp Med*. 2000;192(11):1553–1562.
89. Campbell DJ, Kim CH, Butcher EC. Separable effector T cell populations specialized for B cell help or tissue inflammation. *Nat Immunol*. 2001;2(9):876–881.
90. Vinuesa CG, Tangye SG, Moser B, et al. Follicular B helper T cells in antibody responses and autoimmunity. *Nat Rev Immunol*. 2005;5(11):853–865.
91. Jacob J, Kassir R, Kelsoe G. In situ studies of the primary immune response to (4-hydroxy-3-nitrophenyl)acetyl. I. The architecture and dynamics of responding cell populations. *J Exp Med*. 1991;173(5):1165–1175.
92. Hasbold J, Corcoran LM, Tarlinton DM, et al. Evidence from the generation of immunoglobulin G-secreting cells that stochastic mechanisms regulate lymphocyte differentiation. *Nat Immunol*. 2004;5(1):55–63.
93. Honjo T, Kinoshita K, Muramatsu M. Molecular mechanism of class switch recombination: linkage with somatic hypermutation. *Annu Rev Immunol*. 2002;20:165–196.
94. Okazaki IM, Kinoshita K, Muramatsu M, et al. The AID enzyme induces class switch recombination in fibroblasts. *Nature*. 2002;416(6878):340–345.
95. Muramatsu M, Kinoshita K, Fagarasan S, et al. Class switch recombination and hypermutation require activation-induced cytidine deaminase (AID), a potential RNA editing enzyme. *Cell*. 2000;102(5):553–563.
96. Revy P, Muto T, Levy Y, et al. Activation-induced cytidine deaminase (AID) deficiency causes the autosomal recessive form of the Hyper-IgM syndrome (HIGM2). *Cell*. 2000;102(5):565–575.
97. Armitage RJ, Fanslow WC, Strockbine L, et al. Molecular and biological characterization of a murine ligand for CD40. *Nature*. 1992;357(6373):80–82.
98. Banchereau J, Bazan F, Blanchard D, et al. The CD40 antigen and its ligand. *Annu Rev Immunol*. 1994;12:881–922.
99. Sharpe AH, Freeman GJ. The B7-CD28 superfamily. *Nat Rev Immunol*. 2002;2(2):116–126.
100. Dong C, Juedes AE, Temann UA, et al. ICOS co-stimulatory receptor is essential for T-cell activation and function. *Nature*. 2001;409(6816):97–101.

101. McAdam AJ, Greenwald RJ, Levin MA, et al. ICOS is critical for CD40-mediated antibody class switching. *Nature.* 2001;409(6816):102–105.
102. Tafuri A, Shahinian A, Bladt F, et al. ICOS is essential for effective T-helper-cell responses. *Nature.* 2001;409(6816):105–109.
103. Bishop GA, Hostager BS. B lymphocyte activation by contact-mediated interactions with T lymphocytes. *Curr Opin Immunol.* 2001;13(3):278–285.
104. Snapper CM, Paul WE. Interferon-gamma and B cell stimulatory factor-1 reciprocally regulate Ig isotype production. *Science.* 1987;236(4804):944-7.
105. Kuhn R, Rajewsky K, Muller W. Generation and analysis of interleukin-4 deficient mice. *Science.* 1991;254(5032):707–710.
106. Takeda K, Tanaka T, Shi W, et al. Essential role of Stat6 in IL-4 signalling. *Nature.* 1996;380(6575):627–630.
107. Ozaki K, Spolski R, Feng CG, et al. A critical role for IL-21 in regulating immunoglobulin production. *Science.* 2002;298(5598):1630–1634.
108. Cazac BB, Roes J. TGF-beta receptor controls B cell responsiveness and induction of IgA *in vivo*. *Immunity.* 2000;13(4):443–451.
109. Kopf M, Herren S, Wiles MV, et al. Interleukin 6 influences germinal center development and antibody production via a contribution of C3 complement component. *J Exp Med.* 1998;188(10):1895–1906.
110. Crotty S, Kersh EN, Cannons J, et al. SAP is required for generating long-term humoral immunity. *Nature.* 2003;421(6920):282–287.
111. Cannons JL, Yu LJ, Jankovic D, et al. SAP regulates T cell-mediated help for humoral immunity by a mechanism distinct from cytokine regulation. *J Exp Med.* 2006;203(6):1551–1565.
112. Ho F, Lortan JE, MacLennan ICM, et al. Distinct short-lived and long-lived antibody-producing cell populations. *Eur J Immunol.* 1986;16:1297–1301.
113. Jacob J, Kelsoe G. In situ studies of the primary immune response to (4-hydroxy-3-nitrophenyl)acetyl. II. A common clonal origin for periarteriolar lymphoid sheath-associated foci and germinal centers. *J Exp Med.* 1992;176(3):679–687.
114. McHeyzer-Williams MG, McLean MJ, Lalor PA, et al. Antigen-driven B cell differentiation *in vivo*. *J Exp Med.* 1993;178(1):295–307.
115. Hargreaves DC, Hyman PL, Lu TT, et al. A coordinated change in chemokine responsiveness guides plasma cell movements. *J Exp Med.* 2001;194(1):45–56.
116. Shih TA, Meffre E, Roederer M, et al. Role of BCR affinity in T cell dependent antibody responses *in vivo*. *Nat Immunol.* 2002;3(6):570–575.
117. Paus D, Phan TG, Chan TD, et al. Antigen recognition strength regulates the choice between extrafollicular plasma cell and germinal center B cell differentiation. *J Exp Med.* 2006;203(4):1081–1091.
118. Driver DJ, McHeyzer-Williams LJ, Cool M, et al. Development and maintenance of a B220- memory B cell compartment. *J Immunol.* 2001;167(3):1393–1405.
119. McHeyzer-Williams LJ, Black MY, McHeyzer-Williams MG. Antigen-specific memory B cell development *in vivo*. 1999.
120. Hsu MC, Toellner KM, Vinuesa CG, et al. B cell clones that sustain long-term plasmablast growth in T-independent extrafollicular antibody responses. *Proc Natl Acad U S A.* 2006;103(15):5905–5910.
121. Sze DM, Toellner KM, Garcia de Vinuesa C, et al. Intrinsic constraint on plasmablast growth and extrinsic limits of plasma cell survival. *J Exp Med.* 2000;192(6):813–821.
122. Turner CA Jr., Mack DH, Davis MM. Blimp-1, a novel zinc finger-containing protein that can drive the maturation of B lymphocytes into immunoglobulin-secreting cells. *Cell.* 199;77(2):297–306.
123. Shapiro-Shelef M, Lin KI, McHeyzer-Williams LJ, et al. Blimp-1 is required for the formation of immunoglobulin secreting plasma cells and pre-plasma memory B cells. *Immunity.* 2003;19(4):607–620.
124. Calame K. Transcription factors that regulate memory in humoral responses. *Immunol Rev.* 2006;211:269–279.
125. Calame KL, Lin KI, Tunyaplin C. Regulatory mechanisms that determine the development and function of plasma cells. *Annu Rev Immunol.* 2003;21:205–230.
126. Iwakoshi NN, Lee AH, Vallabhajosyula P, et al. Plasma cell differentiation and the unfolded protein response intersect at the transcription factor XBP-1. *Nat Immunol.* 2003;4(4):321–329.
127. Reimold AM, Iwakoshi NN, Manis J, et al. Plasma cell differentiation requires the transcription factor XBP-1. *Nature.* 2001;412(6844):300–307.
128. Shaffer AL, Shapiro-Shelef M, Iwakoshi NN, et al. XBP1, Downstream of Blimp-1, expands the secretory apparatus and other organelles, and increases protein aynthesis in plasma cell differentiation. *Immunity.* 2004;21(1):81–93.
129. Corcoran LM, Hasbold J, Dietrich W, et al. Differential requirement for OBF-1 during antibody-secreting cell differentiation. *J Exp Med.* 2005;201(9):1385–1396.
130. Lin L, Gerth AJ, Peng SL. Active inhibition of plasma cell development in resting B cells by microphthalmia-associated transcription factor. *J Exp Med.* 2004;200(1):115–122.
131. Fujita N, Jaye DL, Geigerman C, et al. MTA3 and the Mi-2/NuRD complex regulate cell fate during B lymphocyte differentiation. *Cell.* 2004;119(1):75–86.
132. MacLennan IC. Germinal centers. *Annu Rev Immunol.* 1994;12:117–139.
133. MacLennan ICM, Gray D. Antigen-driven selection of virgin and memory B cells. *Immunol Rev.* 1986;91:61–85.
134. Matsumoto M, Mariathasan S, Nahm MH, et al. Role of lymphotoxin and the type I TNF receptor in the formation of germinal centers. *Science.* 1996;271(5253):1289–1291.
135. Matsumoto M, Lo SF, Carruthers CJ, et al. Affinity maturation without germinal centres in lymphotoxin-alpha-deficient mice. *Nature.* 1996;382(6590):462–466.
136. Koni PA, Sacca R, Lawton P, et al. Distinct roles in lymphoid organogenesis for lymphotoxins alpha and beta revealed in lymphotoxin beta-deficient mice. *Immunity.* 1997;6(4):491–500.
137. Futterer A, Mink K, Luz A, et al. The lymphotoxin beta receptor controls organogenesis and affinity maturation in peripheral lymphoid tissues. *Immunity.* 1998;9(1):59–70.
138. Jacobson EB, Caporale LH, Thorbecke GJ. Effect of thymus cell injections on germinal center formation in lymphoid tissues of nude (thymusless) mice. *Cell Immunol.* 1974;13(3):416–430.
139. Kawabe T, Naka T, Yoshida K, et al. The immune responses in CD40-deficient mice: impaired immunoglobulin class switching and germinal center formation. *Immunity.* 1994;1(3):167–178.
140. Renshaw BR, Fanslow WC 3rd, Armitage RJ, et al. Humoral immune responses in CD40 ligand-deficient mice. *J Exp Med.* 1994;180(5):1889–1900.
141. Vinuesa CG, Cook MC, Angelucci C, et al. A RING-type ubiquitin ligase family member required to repress follicular helper T cells and autoimmunity. *Nature.* 2005;435(7041):452–458.
142. de Vinuesa CG, Cook MC, Ball J, et al. Germinal centers without T cells. *J Exp Med.* 2000;191(3):485–494.
143. Dent AL, Shaffer AL, Yu X, et al. Control of inflammation, cytokine expression, and germinal center formation by BCL-6. *Science.* 1997;276(5312):589–592.
144. Toyama H, Okada S, Hatano M, et al. Memory B cells without somatic hypermutation are generated from Bcl6-deficient B cells. *Immunity.* 2002;17(3):329–339.
145. Phan RT, Dalla-Favera R. The BCL6 proto-oncogene suppresses p53 expression in germinal-centre B cells. *Nature.* 2004;432(7017):635–639.
146. Tunyaplin C, Shaffer AL, Angelin-Duclos CD, et al. Direct repression of prdm1 by Bcl-6 inhibits plasmacytic differentiation. *J Immunol.* 2004;173(2):1158–1165.
147. Wang Y, Carter RH. CD19 regulates B cell maturation, proliferation, and positive selection in the FDC zone of murine splenic germinal centers. *Immunity.* 2005;22(6):749–761.
148. Allen CD, Okada T, Tang HL, et al. Imaging of germinal center selection events during affinity maturation. *Science.* 2007;315(5811):528–531.
149. Schwickert TA, Lindquist RL, Shakar G, et al. *In vivo* imaging of germinal center reveals a dynamic open structure. *Nature.* 2007;446(7131):83–87.
150. Neuberger MS, Milstein C. Somatic hypermutation. *Curr Opin Immunol.* 1995;7(2):248–254.
151. Jolly CJ, Wagner SD, Rada C, et al. The targeting of somatic hypermutation. *Semin Immunol.* 1996;8(3):159–168.
152. Muramatsu M, Sankaranand VS, Anant S, et al. Specific expression of activation-induced cytidine deaminase (AID), a novel member of

the RNA-editing deaminase family in germinal center B cells. *J Biol Chem*. 1999;274(26):18470–18476.
153. Larson ED, Cummings WJ, Bednarski DW, et al. MRE11/RAD50 cleaves DNA in the AID/UNG-dependent pathway of immunoglobulin gene diversification. *Mol Cell*. 2005;20(3):367–375.
154. Odegard VH, Kim ST, Anderson SM, et al. Histone modifications associated with somatic hypermutation. *Immunity*. 2005;23(1):101–110.
155. Tourigny MR, Ursini-Siegel J, Lee H, et al. CDK inhibitor p18(INK4c) is required for the generation of functional plasma cells. *Immunity*. 2002;17(2):179–189.
156. Winslow MM, Gallo EM, Neilson JR, et al. The calcineurin phosphatase complex modulates immunogenic B cell responses. *Immunity*. 2006;24:141–152.
157. Smith KG, Light A, O'Reilly LA, et al. bcl-2 transgene expression inhibits apoptosis in the germinal center and reveals differences in the selection of memory B cells and bone marrow antibody-forming cells. *J Exp Med*. 2000;191(3):475–484.
158. Takahashi Y, Cerasoli DM, Dal Porto JM, et al. Relaxed negative selection in germinal centers and impaired affinity maturation in bcl-xL transgenic mice. *J Exp Med*. 1999;190(3):399–410.
159. Huntington ND, Xu Y, Puthalakath H, et al. CD45 links the B cell receptor with cell survival and is required for the persistence of germinal centers. *Nat Immunol*. 2006;7(2):190–198.
160. Wang Y, Brooks SR, Li X, et al. The physiologic role of CD19 cytoplasmic tyrosines. *Immunity*. 2002;17(4):501–514.
161. Casola S, Cattoretti G, Uyttersprot N, et al. Tracking germinal center B cells expressing germ-line immunoglobulin gamma1 transcripts by conditional gene targeting. *Proc Natl Acad U S A*. 2006;103(19):7396–7401.
162. Mitchell J, Abbot A. Ultrastructure of the antigen-retaining reticulum of lymph node follicles as shown by high-resolution autoradiography. *Nature*. 1965;208(9):500–502.
163. Fearon DT, Carroll MC. Regulation of B lymphocyte responses to foreign and self-antigens by the CD19/CD21 complex. *Annu Rev Immunol*. 2000;18:393–422.
164. Hannum LG, Haberman AM, Anderson SM, et al. Germinal center initiation, variable gene region hypermutation, and mutant B cell selection without detectable immune complexes on follicular dendritic cells. *J Exp Med*. 2000;192(7):931–942.
165. Victoratos P, Lagnel J, Tzima S, et al. FDC-specific functions of p55TNFR and IKK2 in the development of FDC networks and of antibody responses. *Immunity*. 2006;24(1):65–77.
166. Allen CD, Ansel KM, Low C, et al. Germinal center dark and light zone organization is mediated by CXCR4 and CXCR5. *Nat Immunol*. 2004;5(9):943–952.
167. Ford ML, Koehn BH, Wagener ME, et al. Antigen-specific precursor frequency impacts T cell proliferation, differentiation, and requirement for costimulation. *J Exp Med*. 2007 Jan 29.
168. Hataye J, Moon JJ, Khoruts A, et al. Naïve and memory CD4+ T cell survival controlled by clonal abundance. *Science*. 2006;312(5770):114–116.
169. Marzo AL, Klonowski KD, Le Bon A, et al. Initial T cell frequency dictates memory CD8+ T cell lineage commitment. *Nat Immunol*. 2005;6(8):793–799.
170. Gulbranson-Judge A, MacLennan I. Sequential antigen-specific growth of T cells in the T zones and follicles in response to pigeon cytochrome c. *Eur J Immunol*. 1996;26(8):1830–1837.
171. Zheng B, Han S, Kelsoe G. T helper cells in murine germinal centers are antigen-specific emigrants that downregulate Thy-1. *J Exp Med*. 1996;184(3):1083–1091.
172. Mikszta JA, McHeyzer-Williams LJ, McHeyzer-Williams MG. Antigen-driven selection of TCR *In vivo*: related TCR alpha-chains pair with diverse TCR beta-chains. *J Immunol*. 1999;163(11):5978–5988.
173. Han S, Hathcock K, Zheng B, et al. Cellular interaction in germinal centers. Roles of CD40 ligand and B7-2 in established germinal centers. *J Immunol*. 1995;155(2):556–567.
174. Chtanova T, Tangye SG, Newton R, et al. T follicular helper cells express a distinctive transcriptional profile, reflecting their role as non-Th1/Th2 effector cells that provide help for B cells. *J Immunol*. 2004;173(1):68–78.
175. Kim CH, Lim HW, Kim JR, et al. Unique gene expression program of human germinal center T helper cells. *Blood*. 2004;104(7):1952–1960.
176. Rasheed AU, Rahn HP, Sallusto F, et al. Follicular B helper T cell activity is confined to CXCR5(hi) ICOS(hi) CD4 T cells and is independent of CD57 expression. *Eur J Immunol*. 2006;36(7):1892–1903.
177. McHeyzer-Williams MG, Ahmed R. B cell memory and the long-lived plasma cell. *Curr Opin Immunol*. 1999;11(2):172–179.
178. Nossal GJ, Pike BL, Battye FL. Sequential use of hapten-gelatin fractionation and fluorescence-activated cell sorting in the enrichment of hapten-specific B llymphocytes. *Eur J Immunol*. 1978;8(3):151–157.
179. Noelle RJ, Snow EC, Uhr JW, et al. Activation of antigen-specific B cells: role of T cells, cytokines, and antigen in induction of growth and differentiation. *Proc Natl Acad U S A*. 1983;80(21):6628–6631.
180. Bonner WA, Hulett HR, Sweet RG, et al. Fluorescence activated cell sorting. *Rev Sci Instrum*. 1972;43(3):404–409.
181. Julius MH, Masuda T, Herzenberg LA. Demonstration that antigen-binding cells are precursors of antibody-producing cells after purification with a fluorescence-activated cell sorter. *Proc Natl Acad U S A*. 1972;69(7):1934–1938.
182. Greenstein JL, Leary J, Horan P, et al. Flow sorting of antigen-binding B cell subsets. *J Immunol*. 1980;124(3):1472–1481.
183. Hayakawa K, Ishii R, Yamasaki K, et al. Isolation of high-affinity memory B cells: phycoerythrin as a probe for antigen-binding cells. *Proc Natl Acad U S A*. 1987;84(5):1379–1383.
184. Gray D, Skarvall H. B-cell memory is short-lived in the absence of antigen. *Nature*. 1988;336(6194):70–73.
185. Kodituwakku AP, Jessup C, Zola H, et al. Isolation of antigen-specific B cells. *Immunol Cell Biol*. 2003;81(3):163–170.
186. Schittek B, Rajewsky K. Maintenance of B-cell memory by long-lived cells generated from proliferating precursors. *Nature*. 1990;346(6286):749–751.
187. Maruyama M, Lam KP, Rajewsky K. Memory B-cell persistence is independent of persisting immunizing antigen. *Nature*. 2000;407(6804):636–642.
188. McHeyzer-Williams MG, Nossal GJ, et al. Molecular characterization of single memory B cells. *Nature*. 1991;350(6318):502–505.
189. Blink EJ, Light A, Kallies A, et al. Early appearance of germinal center-derived memory B cells and plasma cells in blood after primary immunization. *J Exp Med*. 2005;201(4):545–554.
190. Jacob J, Kelsoe G, Rajewsky K, et al. Intraclonal generation of antibody mutants in germinal centres. *Nature*. 1991;354(6352):389–392.
191. McHeyzer-Williams MG, Nossal GJV, Lalor PA. Molecular characterization of single memory B cells. *Nature*. 1991;350(6318):502–505.
192. Black SJ, van der Loo W, Loken MR, et al. Expression of IgD by murine lymphocytes. Loss of surface IgD indicates maturation of memory B cells. *J Exp Med*. 1978;147(4):984–996.
193. Herzenberg LA, Black SJ, Tokuhisa T. Memory B cells at successive stages of differentiation. Affinity maturation and the role of IgD receptors. *J Exp Med*. 1980;151(5):1071–1087.
194. Lalor PA, Nossal GJV, Sanderson RD, et al. Functional and molecular characterization of single, (4-hydroxy-3-nitrophenyl)acetyl (NP)-specific, IgG1+ B cells from antibody-secreting and memory B cell pathways in the C57BL/6 immune response to NP. *Eur J Immunol*. 1992;22(11):3001–3011.
195. Cascalho M, Ma A, Lee S, et al. A quasi-monoclonal mouse. *Science*. 1996;272(5268):1649–1652.
196. Cascalho M, Wong J, Brown J, et al. A B220(-), CD19(-) population of B cells in the peripheral blood of quasimonoclonal mice. *Int Immunol*. 2000;12(1):29–35.
197. McHeyzer-Williams LJ, Cool M, McHeyzer-Williams MG. Antigen-specific B cell memory: expression and replenishment of a novel $B220^-$ memory b cell compartment. *J Exp Med*. 2000;191(7):1149–1166.
198. O'Connor BP, Cascalho M, Noelle RJ. Short-lived and long-lived bone marrow plasma cells are derived from a novel precursor population. *J Exp Med*. 2002;195(6):737–745.
199. Gatto D, Pfister T, Jegerlehner A, et al. Complement receptors regulate differentiation of bone marrow plasma cell precursors expressing transcription factors Blimp-1 and XBP-1. *J Exp Med*. 2005;201(6):993–1005.

200. Bleesing JJ, Fleisher TA. Human B cells express a CD45 isoform that is similar to murine B220 and is downregulated with acquisition of the memory B-cell marker CD27. *Cytometry.* 2003;51B(1):1–8.
201. Smith KG, Light A, Nossal GJV, et al. The extent of affinity maturation differs between the memory and antibody-forming cell compartments in the primary immune response. *Embo Journal.* 1997;16(11):2996–3006.
202. Takahashi Y, Dutta PR, Cerasoli DM, et al. In situ studies of the primary immune response to (4-hydroxy-3-nitrophenyl)acetyl. V. Affinity maturation develops in two stages of clonal selection. *J Exp Med.* 1998;187(6):885–895.
203. Minges Wols HA, Underhill GH, Kansas GS, et al. The role of bone marrow-derived stromal cells in the maintenance of plasma cell longevity. *J Immunol.* 2002;169(8):4213–4221.
204. Benner R, Hijmans W, Haaijman JJ. The bone marrow: the major source of serum immunoglobulins, but still a neglected site of antibody formation. *Clin Exp Immunol.* 1981;46(1):1–8.
205. Manz RA, Thiel A, Radbruch A. Lifetime of plasma cells in the bone marrow. *Nature.* 1997;388(6638):133–134.
206. Manz RA, Lohning M, Cassese G, et al. Survival of long-lived plasma cells is independent of antigen.*International Immunol.* 1998;11:1703–1711.
207. Slifka MK, Matloubian M, Ahmed R. Bone marrow is a major site of long-term antibody production after acute viral infection. *J Virol.* 1995;69(3):1895–1902.
208. Slifka MK, Antia R, Whitmire JK, et al. Humoral immunity due to long-lived plasma cells. *Immunity.* 1998;8(3):363–372.
209. O'Connor BP, Raman VS, Erickson LD, et al. BCMA is essential for the survival of long-lived bone marrow plasma cells. *J Exp Med.* 2004;199(1):91–98.
210. Bernasconi NL, Traggiai E, Lanzavecchia A. Maintenance of serological memory by polyclonal activation of human memory B cells. *Science.* 2002;298(5601):2199–2202.
211. Shaffer AL, Lin KI, Kuo TC, et al. Blimp-1 orchestrates plasma cell differentiation by extinguishing the mature B cell gene expression program. *Immunity.* 2002;17(1):51–62.
212. Underhill GH, George D, Bremer EG, et al. Gene expression profiling reveals a highly specialized genetic program of plasma cells. *Blood.* 2003;101(10):4013–4021.
213. Furukawa K, Akasako-Furukawa A, Shirai H, et al. Junctional amino acids determine the maturation pathway of an antibody. *Immunity.* 1999;11(3):329–338.
214. Panus JF, McHeyzer-Williams LJ, McHeyzer-Williams MG. Antigen-specific T helper cell function: differential cytokine expression in primary and memory responses. *J Exp Med.* 2000;192(9):1301–1316.
215. McHeyzer-Williams LJ, McHeyzer-Williams MG. Analysis of antigen-specific B-cell memory directly ex vivo. *Methods Mol Biol.* 2004;271:173–188.
216. McHeyzer-Williams LJ, Panus JF, Mikszta JA, et al. Evolution of antigen-specific T cell receptors *in vivo*: preimmune and antigen-driven selection of preferred complementarity-determining region 3 (CDR3) motifs. *J Exp Med.* 1999;189(11):1823–1838.
217. Sallusto F, Geginat J, Lanzavecchia A. Central memory and effector memory T cell subsets: function, generation, and maintenance. *Annu Rev Immunol.* 2004;22:745–763.
218. Lau LL, Jamieson BD, Somasundaram T, et al. Cytotoxic T-cell memory without antigen. *Nature.* 1994;369(6482):648–652.
219. Swain SL, Hu H, Huston G. Class II-independent generation of CD4 memory T cells from effectors. *Science.* 1999;286(5443):1381–1383.

SECTION IV

T Lymphocytes

Chapter 10

T Cell Antigen Receptors

Mark M. Davis and Yueh-Hsiu Chien

INTRODUCTION

T lymphocytes expressing $\alpha\beta$ or $\gamma\delta$ T cell receptors (TCRs) are found together with B lymphocytes in all but the most primitive vertebrate animals. These three cell types are the only ones that use random V, D, J, gene rearrangement to generate diverse antigen receptors. During the past two decades, there has been a great deal of progress in identifying the molecules and genes of TCRs, and there is considerable information on their biochemistry and structure. Although TCRs share structural and genetic similarities with B cell receptors (BCRs) (immunoglobulins [Igs]), they also possess a number of unique features pertinent to their specific functions. The first major difference was suggested by the experiments of Zinkernagel and Doherty, who found that the cytotoxic cells could only lyse infected cells expressing certain major histocompatibility complex (MHC) haplotype (1,2). This phenomenon of "MHC restricted recognition" is in marked contrast to the recognition of intact antigens by Igs *(3,4)*. In fact, antigen recognition by T cells has helped to define their functions.

$\alpha\beta$ TCRs are expressed on classical helper and cytotoxic T cells, which predominate in most lymphoid compartments (90%–95%) of humans and mice *(5)*. $\alpha\beta$ TCRs are also expressed on natural killer (NK) T cells *(6)*, regulatory T cells *(7)*, and T cells in the mucosal sites such as the intestinal epithelial compartment (IELs) (8). In most cases, the $\alpha\beta$ TCR ligand is a peptide antigen bound to a class I or class II MHC molecule; but in the case of NKT cells, the antigen is a glycolipid bound to a nonclassical class I MHC molecule, CD1d *(6)*.

T cells bearing $\gamma\delta$ TCRs are less numerous than the $\alpha\beta$ type in most cellular compartments of humans and mice (less than 5%). However, they make up a substantial fraction of T lymphocytes in cows, sheep, and chickens *(9)*. $\gamma\delta$ T cells coexist with $\alpha\beta$ T cells but seem to be better represented in the mucosal compartments (9,10). Although $\alpha\beta$ T cells perform most of the functions classically attributed to T cells, mice lacking $\gamma\delta$ T cells clearly have compromised immune systems, indicating that $\gamma\delta$ and $\alpha\beta$ T cells contribute to host immune defense differently (10,11). $\gamma\delta$ TCRs also have distinct antigen recognition requirements in that no antigen processing is required (12). During the past few years, there have been considerable advances in our understanding of antigen recognition by $\gamma\delta$ T cells. This should lead to a better understanding of how $\gamma\delta$ T cells contribute to host immune competence.

TCR POLYPEPTIDES

The search for the molecules responsible for T cell recognition first focused on deriving antisera or monoclonal antibodies specific for molecules on T cell surfaces. Ultimately, a number of groups identified "clonotypic" sera (13) or monoclonal antibodies (14–18). Several of these antibodies were able to block antigen-specific responses by the T cells they were raised against or, when coated on a surface, could activate the T cells for which they are specific. They were also able to immunoprecipitate 85 to 90,000 MW disulfide-bonded heterodimers from different T cell clones or hybridomas consisting of two 40,000 MW to 50,000 MW glycosylated subunits referred to as α and β. Peptide mapping studies showed that there was a striking degree of polymorphism between heterodimers isolated from T cells of differing specificity, thus suggesting that these antigen recognition molecules might be akin to Igs (19,20).

Work in parallel to these serological studies exploited the small differences (~2%) observed between B and T cell gene expression (21) and isolated both a mouse (22,23) and a human (24) T cell–specific gene that had antibody-like V, J, and C region sequences and could rearrange in T lymphocytes (23). This molecule was identified as TCRβ by partial sequence analysis of immunoprecipitated materials (25). Subsequent subtractive cloning work rapidly identified two other candidate T cell receptors cDNAs identified as TCRα (26,27) and TCRγ (28). It was quickly established that all antigen-specific helper or cytotoxic T cells expressed TCR $\alpha\beta$ heterodimers. Where TCRγ fit in remained a puzzle until work by Brenner et al. (29) showed that it was expressed on a small (5%–10%) subset of peripheral T cells together with another polypeptide, TCRδ. The nature of TCRδ remained unknown until it was discovered within the TCRα locus, between the V_α and J_α regions (30). Formal proof that the TCR α and β subunits were sufficient to transfer antigen/MHC recognition from one T cell to another came from gene transfection experiments (31,32) and equivalent experiments have also been done with $\gamma\delta$ TCRs (33).

As shown in Figure 10.1, all TCR polypeptides have a similar primary structure, with distinct variable (V), diversity (D) in the case of TCR β and δ, joining (J), and constant (C) regions exactly analogous to their Ig counterparts. They also share many of the amino acid residues thought to be important for the characteristic variable and constant domains of Igs *(34)*. The C_β region is particularly homologous, sharing 40% of its amino acid sequences with C_K and C_λ. The TCR polypeptides all contain a single C region domain (versus up to four for Igs) followed by a connecting peptide. These usually contain the cysteine for the disulfide linkage that joins the two chains of the heterodimer (some human TCR $\gamma\delta$ isoforms lack this cysteine and consequently are not disulfide-linked; ref. [35]). N-linked glycosylation sites vary from two to four for each polypeptide, with no indications of O-linked sugar addition. C-terminal to the connecting peptide sequences are the hydrophobic transmembrane regions. These have no similarity to those of the *IgH* genes, but instead have one (TCRβ and γ) or two (TCRα and δ) positively charged residues. As discussed later, these charged residues are critical for the association of the ligand binding TCR polypeptides with the CD3

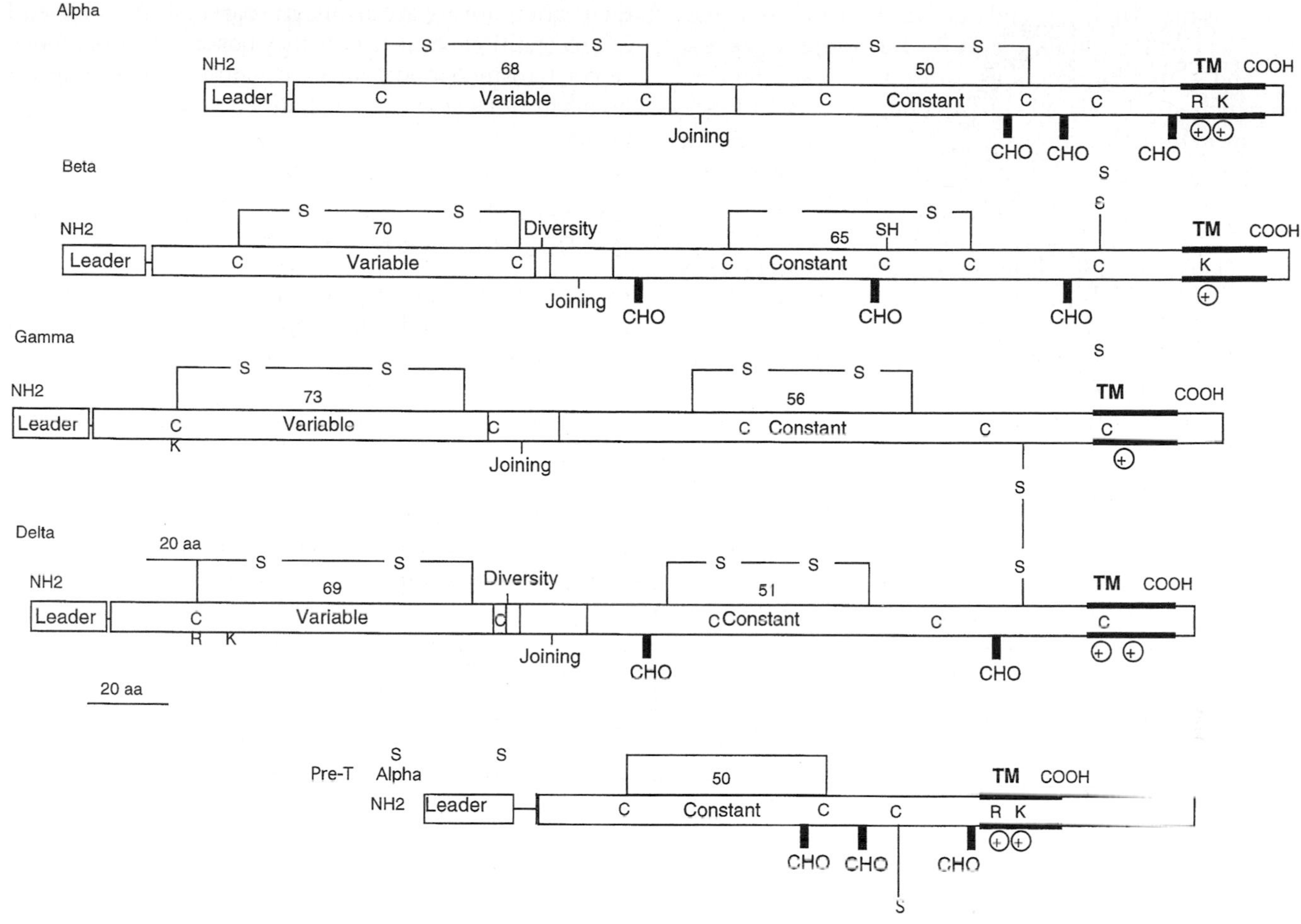

FIGURE 10.1 Structural features of T cell receptors and pre-T α polypeptides. Leader (L), variable (V), diversity (D), joining (J), and constant region (C) gene segments are indicated. TM and bold horizontal lines delineate the putative transmembrane regions; CHO indicates potential carbohydrate addition sites; C and S refer to cystein residues that form interchain and intrachain disulfide bonds; R and K indicate the positively charged amino acids (arginine and lysine, respectively) that are found in the transmembrane regions.

signaling polypeptides. This is important because the TCR polypeptides themselves have very short cytoplasmic regions with no known role in signaling.

A more recent member of the TCR polypeptide family is the pre–T α chain, which serves as a chaperone for TCRβ in early thymocytes, similar to the role of λ5 in pre-B cells. It was first identified and cloned by von Boehmer and colleagues (*36*,37). It has an interesting structure that consists of a single Ig constant region-like domain followed by a cysteine-containing connecting peptide, a transmembrane region containing two charged residues—an arginine and a lysine spaced identically to the TCRα transmembrane region. The cysteine in the connecting peptide is presumably what allows heterodimer formation with TCRβ, and the similarity to TCRα in the transmembrane region is most likely to accommodate the CD3 polypeptides. In both the mouse and humans, the cytoplasmic tail is much longer than any of the TCR chains (37 and 120 amino acids, respectively) and the murine sequence contains two likely phosphorylation sites and sequences homologous to an SH3 domain binding region. These are not present in the human sequence, however, and so their functional significance is questionable (37). Thus, the pre–Tα molecule could function as signaling intermediate independent of the CD3 polypeptides, and it has recently been shown that at least one CD3 component ($\delta\varepsilon$, discussed later) is not required for it to function normally in early thymocyte differentiation (*38*).

CD3 POLYPEPTIDES

Immunoprecipitation of the human TCR with anti-idiotypic antibodies after solubilization with the nonionic detergent, noniodet P-40 (NP-40), initially revealed only the α- and β-chain heterodimer. However, the use of other detergents, such as digitonin or Triton-X100, revealed four other proteins (as reviewed in (39,*40*,41). These are known as the CD3γ, δ, ε, and ζ. γ and δ form distinct heterodimers with ε within the TCR/CD3 complex ($\gamma\varepsilon$ and $\delta\varepsilon$), and ζ usually occurs as a disulfide-linked homodimer. In mouse T cells, NP-40 does not dissociate TCR heterodimers from CD3 molecules *(42,43)*. In some cases, the ζ-chain can be part of a heterodimer in at least two forms. In mouse T cells, the ζ-chain can disulfide bond with a minor variant called the η (eta) chain *(44,45)*. This latter chain is an alternate splicing variant of the ζ-chain gene *(46)*. This alternatively spliced species of the ζ-chain is not found in significant quantities in human T cells *(47)*. The second type of ζ-chain containing heterodimer contains the γ-chain associated with the $F_c\varepsilon RI$ ($F_c\varepsilon RI\ \gamma$) and $F_c\gamma RIII$ (CD16) receptors *(48)*. These CD3 subunits, in their various forms, are an integral part of TCR-mediated T cell recognition because only they possess the immunoreceptor tyrosine-based activation motifs (ITAMs) that are necessary for cellular activation when the TCR engages ligand.

Characterization and Structural Features of the CD3 Polypeptides

Figure 10.2 illustrates the principal structural features of the CD3 γ-, δ-, ε-, and ζ- polypeptides as derived from gene cloning and sequencing (as reviewed in refs *40*,49) and more recently by protein crystal structures of the extracellular domains of γ, δ, and ε (50–52,*53*). The extracellular

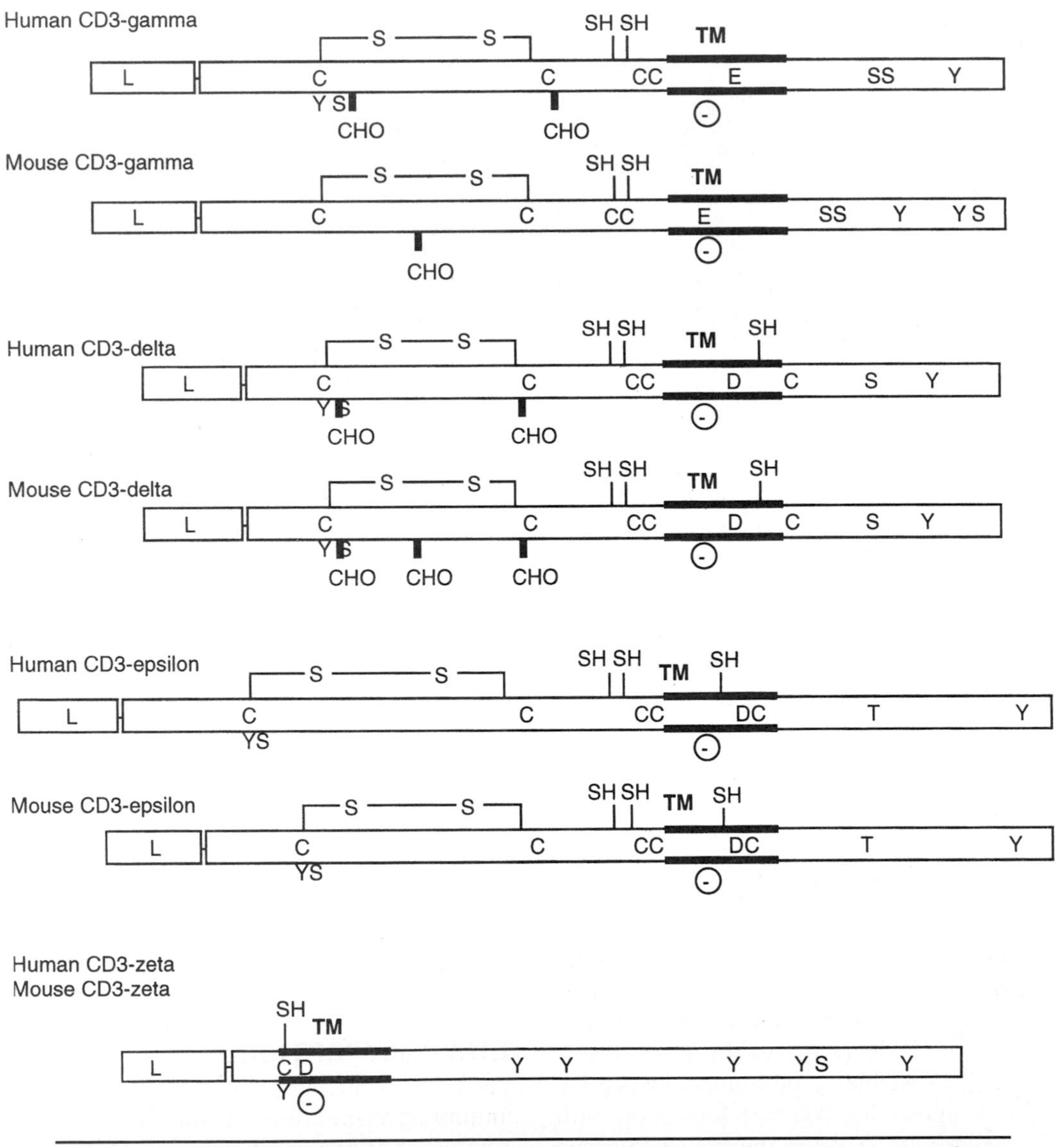

FIGURE 10.2 Structural features of the CD3 molecules. As in Figure 10.1, transmembrane regions (TM), carbohydrate addition sites (CHO), and cysteine residues (C) are indicated. In addition, negatively charged transmembrane residues (D for aspartic acid and E for glutamic acid) and putative phosphorylation sites are shown.

domains of the γ-, δ-, and ε-chains show a significant degree of similarity to one another. These domains retain the cysteines that have been shown to form intrachain disulfide bonds, and each consists of a single Ig superfamily domain. The spacing of the cysteines in these domains produces a compact Ig-fold, similar to a constant region domain. The γ and δ subunits form distinct heterodimers with ε via highly conserved residues at the dimerizing interface (50–52,*53*). The connecting peptides of the CD3 γ-, δ-, and ε-chains all contain highly conserved, closely spaced cysteines just before the membrane-spanning regions. These residues are likely candidates for the formation of intrachain disulfide bonds and appear to play a role in the assembly of the CD3 and TCR polypeptides *(50,54)*. The extracellular domain of the ζ-chain consists of only nine amino acids and contains the only cysteine, which is responsible for the disulfide linkage of the $\zeta\zeta$ homodimer or the $\zeta F_c\varepsilon RI\gamma$ heterodimer. Each of the γ-, δ-, ε-, and ζ-polypeptides contain a conserved, negatively charged amino acids in their transmembrane region complementary to the positive charges seen in the TCR TM regions (55,*56*,*57*,58).

The cytoplasmic regions of the γ-, δ-, ε-, and ζ-chains are the intracellular signaling "domains" of the TCR heterodimer. Each of these molecules contains one or more amino acid sequence motifs that can mediate cellular activation *(59)*. The intracellular sequences responsible for this activation are contained within an 18 amino acid conserved ITAM motif (60) with the sequence $X_2YX_2L/IX_7YX_2L/I$. Both of the tyrosines in this motif are absolutely required to mediate signal transduction because mutation of either completely prevents the mobilization of free Ca^{++} or cytolytic activity *(61)*. This sequence occurs three times in the ζ-chain, and once in each of the CD3 γ-, δ-, ε-, and F_cRI γ-chains. There are also pairs of tyrosines present in the cytoplasmic domains of the γ-, δ-, ε-, and ζ-chains. This sequence motif is also present in the mβ-1 and B29 chains associated with the (Ig) β-cell receptor and in the $F_c\varepsilon RI$ β-chain, but there are many more *(9)* in TCR/CD3 than in any other receptors that use ITAMS. The tyrosines in these cytoplasmic sequences are substrates for the tyrosine phosphorylation that is one of earliest steps in T cell signaling *(59)* and is thought to occur aberrantly in nonproductive T cell responses (e.g., antagonism, discussed later). Serine phosphorylation of the CD3γ also occurs upon antigen or mitogenic stimulation of T cells *(62)* and may play a role in T cell activation as well.

Assembly and Organization of the TCR/CD3 Complex

The assembly of newly formed TCR α- and β-chains with the CD3 γ-, δ-, ε-, and ζ-chains and their intracellular fate have been studied in detail (39,*40*,41,*61*,63). Early studies have focused on mutant hybridoma lines, which fail to express TCR on their cell surface and on transfection studies using cDNA for the different chains in the receptor; but recently, Wucherpfennig and colleagues have developed an elegant *in vitro* translation and assembly system that has clarified a number of important issues (55,54).

Experiments in a nonlymphoid cell system *(64)* have shown that TCRα can assemble with CD3 δ and ε but not CD3 γ and ζ. In contrast, the TCR β-chain can assemble with any of the CD3 chains except the ζ-chain. When the ζ-chain was transfected with either α- or β-chain genes, or any of the three CD3 chains, no pairwise interaction occurred. Only when all six cDNA's were cotransfected was it shown that the ζ-chain could be coprecipitated with the other chains *(64)*. Based on these data, a model has been proposed that suggests that TCRα- pairs with CD3 δ- and ε-chains and that TCRβ-pairs with the CD3 γ- and ε-chains in the completed molecule. The ζ-chain is thought to join the TCR and other CD3 polypeptides in that last stage of assembly.

Pulse-chase experiments have shown that all six chains are assembled in the ER, transported to the Golgi apparatus, and then transferred to the plasma membrane. It also appears that the amount of ζ-chain is rate limiting, as it is synthesized at only 10% the level of the other chains. This results in the vast majority of newly synthesized α-, β-, or CD3 components being degraded within four hours of their synthesis. The remaining nondegraded chains are long lived due to the formation of complete TCR/CD3 complexes with the limiting ζ-chain *(65)*. TCR/CD3 lacking CD3 ζ-chains migrate through the ER and Golgi intact but then are transported to and degraded in the lysosomes and degraded. The immunological significance of this pre-Golgi degradation pathway is most evident in $CD4^+CD8^+$ thymocytes, where, despite high levels of synthesis of both mRNA and protein for all the TCR, CD3, and ζ-chains, surface expression is relatively low. The TCR chains in immature thymocytes seem to be selectively degraded *(65)*. Thus posttranslation regulation appears to be an important means of controlling the cell surface expression of TCR heterodimers.

The TCR and CD3 γ-, δ-, and ε-chains contain ER retention signals *(65,66)*. If the γ and δ signals are removed, then the chains are transported through the Golgi and rapidly degraded in the lysosomes. In contrast, removal of the CD3 ε ER retention signal allows this chain and any associated chains to be transported to the cell surface. Thus, association of the TCR and other CD3 chains with ε renders their ER retention signals inoperative. However, the ε ER retention signal remains functional. This prevents the surface expression of partial complex intermediaries until CD3 ζ is incorporated into the complex, which then masks the ε ER retention signal and allows the transport of mature complexes to the cell surface.

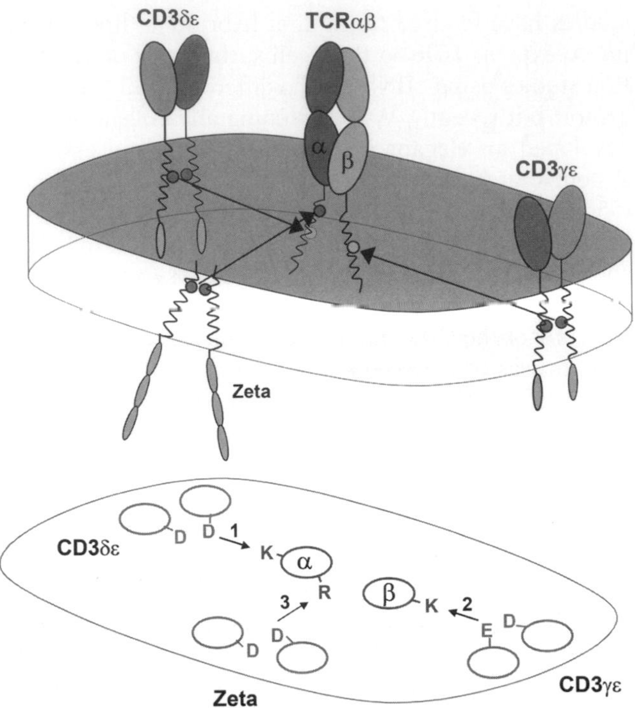

FIGURE 10.3 A model of the $\alpha\beta$ T cell receptor (TCR)–CD3 complex. This shows the approximate positions of the $\alpha\beta$ TCR chains and the CD3α, δ, ε, and ζ chains based on the membrane reconstitution and mutagenesis experiments of Call and Wucherpfennig (55). More recent experiments suggest that the CD3 polypeptides may be somewhat more clustered on the side of the TCR heterodimer (299).

The overall stoichiometry of the $\alpha\beta$ TCR/CD3 complex is controversial. The work of Call and Wucherpfennig (55) has shown the relationships between different CD3 dimers ($\gamma\varepsilon$, $\delta\varepsilon$, and $\zeta\zeta$) and a single TCR $\alpha\beta$ heterodimer (as shown in Figure 10.3). Using mutagenesis, they found very specific interactions based on the positive charges in each TCR transmembrane domain with complementary negative charges in the transmembrane domains of the different CD3 components. The two positively charged residues of TCRα mediate interactions with the negatively charged residues of the of CD3$\delta\varepsilon$ and CD3$\zeta\zeta$ dimers, while the single positively charged residue of TCRβ mediate interactions with the negatively charged resiudes of CD3$\gamma\varepsilon$. In addition, their data suggest a highly ordered assembly process as they found that the TCR/CD3$\delta\varepsilon$ association facilitates the assembly of CD3$\gamma\varepsilon$ into the complex and that the association of the TCR and CD3 heterodimers was a prerequisite for incorporation of CD3$\zeta\zeta$ into the complex. Importantly, the data show that there is only one TCR heterodimer per nascent TCR/CD3 complex in their in vitro expression system.

In contrast, a number of groups have found evidence that there can be two TCR heterodimers in a given TCR/CD3 cluster on T cell surfaces. In particular, Terhorst and colleagues (as reviewed in ref. *[40]*) showed that in a T–T hybridoma, a monoclonal antibody against one TCR$\alpha\beta$ pair could comodulate a second $\alpha\beta$ heterodimer. In addition, sucrose gradient centrifugation of TCR/CD3 showed a predicted molecular weight of 300 kDa, more than 100 kDa larger than expected from a minimal δ subunit complex ($\alpha,\beta,\gamma,\delta,\varepsilon_2,\zeta_2$) *(67)*. Another study suggesting that there are least two TCRs in a given CD3 complex is Scatchard analysis indicating that the number of CD3ε molecules on a T cell surface equals the number of $\alpha\beta$ TCRs *(68,69)*. Finally, there is the work of Fernandez-Miguel et al. (70), who showed that in T cells that have two transgenic TCRβ chains, antibodies to one Vβ can immunoprecipitate the other. It was also found that they are often close enough to allow fluorescence energy transfer, meaning that the two TCRβs in a cluster are within approximately 50 Angstroms of each other (70). Interestingly, it appears that the TCR complexes with CD3 either have CD3 γ or CD3δ, but not both, and these two receptor types are expressed in different ratios in different cells. These data may not be irreconcilable; because while the initial TCR/CD3 assembly may involve only one TCR, these may dimerize or multimerize later on the cell surface (50,71).

The composition of TCR/CD3 complexes on $\gamma\delta$ T cells is distinct from that of $\alpha\beta$ T cells and changes with the activation state of the cell. Biochemical analysis showed that most murine $\gamma\delta$ TCRs contain only CD3$\gamma\varepsilon$ dimers. Interestingly, a differentially glycosylated form of CD3γ was found to associate with $\gamma\delta$ TCRs dependent on the activation state of the cells (72). In addition, while C3$\zeta\zeta$ is incorporated into the complexes of naïve cells, activation results in the expression and incorporation of $F_c\varepsilon R1$ γ into the $\gamma\delta$TCR complex (72). Using quantitative immunofluorescence, Hayes and Love have suggested a model of murine $\gamma\delta$TCR stoichiometry in which there are two CD3$\gamma\varepsilon$ dimers, as well as one CD3ζ dimer in each TCR complex (73). This strongly suggests that signal transduction through the TCR will occur differently in $\gamma\delta$ versus $\alpha\beta$ T cells.

TCR GENES

As shown in Figure 10.4, TCR gene segments are organized similarly to those of Igs, and the same recombination machinery is responsible for joining separate V and D segments to a particular J and C. This was initially indicated by the fact that the characteristic seven and nine nucleotide conserved sequences adjacent to the V, D, and J regions with the 12 or 23 nucleotide spacing between them, first described for Ig genes, are also present in TCRs (74). The most conclusive evidence of this common rearrangement mechanism is that both a naturally occurring recombination-deficient mouse strain (severe combined immune deficiency, SCID; ref. 75) and mice engineered to

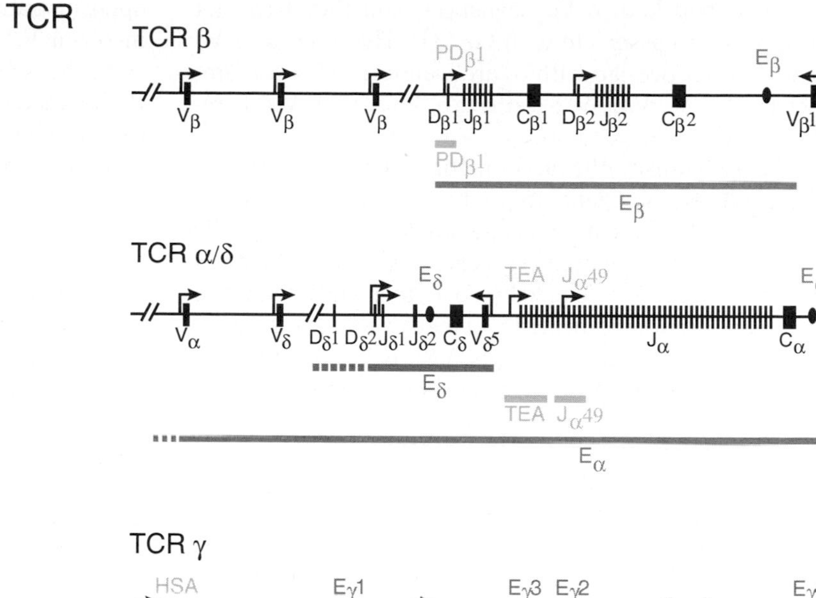

FIGURE 10.4 T cell receptor gene organization in mice and humans. Schematic of V, D, J, and C elements of the T cell receptor genes. Transcriptional orientation is from left to right, except where noted. The overall size of each locus is as indicated to the right. **E** designates enhancer elements, and **S** are silencer elements.

lack recombinase activating genes (RAG) 1 *(76)* or 2 *(77)* are unable to rearrange either TCR or Ig gene segments properly. Many of the other molecules involved in Ig gene rearrangement serve the same function in TCRs as well (78). As with Igs, if the V region and J region gene segments are in the same transcriptional orientation, the intervening DNA is deleted during recombination. DNA circles of such material can be observed in the thymus (79,80), the principal site of TCR recombination (see below). In the case of TCRβ and TCRδ, there is a single V region 3′ to the C in the opposite transcriptional orientation to J and C. Thus rearrangement to these gene segments occurs via an inversion. Variable points of joining are seen along the V, D, and J gene segments as well as random nucleotide addition (N regions) in postnatal TCRs. The addition of several nucleotides in an inverted repeat pattern, referred to a P element insertion, at the V–J junction of the TCRγ chains has also been observed (81).

Organization of the TCR α/δ Locus

In humans and in mice there is a single α-chain C-region gene that is composed of four exons encoding: 1) the constant region domain, 2) 16 amino acids, including the cysteine that forms the interchain disulfide bond, 3) the transmembrane and intracytoplasmic domains, and 4) the 3′ untranslated region (Figure 10.4). The entire α/δ locus spans about 1.1 MB in both mice and humans. There are 50 different J-region gene segments upstream of the C-region in the murine locus. At least eight of these J-regions are nonfunctional because of in-frame stop codons or rearrangement and splicing signals that are likely to be defective. A similar number of α-chain J-regions are present in the human locus. This very large number of J-regions compared to the Ig loci may indicate that the functional diversity contributed by the J segment of the TCR (which constitutes a major portion of the CDR3 loop) makes an important contribution to antigen recognition (discussed later).

Both the murine and human Cδ, Jδ, and two Dδ gene segments are located between the Vα and Jα gene segments. In the murine system there are two Jδ and two Dδ gene segments on the 5′ side of Cδ, and the Cδ gene is approximately 75 kb upstream of the Cα gene, but only approximately 8 kb upstream of the most 5′ known Jα gene segments. The human organization is similar, with three Dα gene segments and two Jδ. Surprisingly, in both species, all of the D elements can be used in one rearranged gene rather than alternating as is the case with TCRβ or IgH. That is, in mice one frequently finds Vδ D_1, D_2, Jδ rearrangements (82), and in humans Vδ, D_1, D_2, D_3, Jδ (83). This greatly increases the junctional or CDR3 diversity that is available, especially because of the potential for N-region addition in between each gene segment. This property makes TCRδ the most diverse of any of the antigens receptors known, with approximately 10^{12} to 10^{13} different amino acid sequences in a relatively small (10 to 15aa) region (82). The implications for this and comparisons with other antigen receptor genes are discussed later.

The location of Dδ, Jδ, and Cδ genes between Vα and Jα gene segments suggests that TCR δ and α could share the same pool of V gene segments. Although there is some overlap in V gene usage, in the murine system, four of the commonly used Vδ genes (Vδ1, Vδ2, Vδ4, Vδ5) are very different than known Vα sequences, and they have not been found to associate with Cα (84). The other four Vδ gene families overlap with or are identical to Vα subfamilies (Vδ3, Vδ6, Vδ7, Vδ8 with Vα6, Vα7, Vα4, Vα11, respectively).

The mechanisms that account for the preferential usage of certain gene segments to produce δ versus α chain are not known. While some Vδ genes are located closer to the Dδ and Jδ fragments than Vα genes (e.g., Vδ1), other Vδs (e.g., Vδ6) are rarely deleted by Vα Jα rearrangements and thus seem likely to be located 5′ of many Vα gene segments.

One of the Vδ gene segments, Vδ5, is located approximately 2.5 kb to the 3′ of Cδ in the opposite transcriptional orientation and rearranges by inversion. Despite its close proximity to Dδ Jδ gene segments, Vδ5 is not frequently found in fetal γδ T cells. Instead, the Vδ5→DJδ rearrangement predominates in adult γδ T cells.

An implicit characteristic of the α/δ gene locus is that a rearrangement of Vα to Jα deletes the entire D-J-C core of the δ-chain locus. In many αβ T cells, the α-chain locus is rearranged on both chromosomes and thus no TCR δ could be made. In most cases this is due to Vα →Jα rearrangement, but evidence suggesting an intermediate step in the deletion of TCRδ has been reported (85). This involves rearrangements of an element termed T early alpha (*TEA*) to a pseudo-Jα 3′ of Cδ. The rearrangement of TEA to this psuedo Jα would eliminate the δ-chain locus in αβ T cells. Gene targeting of the TEA element resulted in normal levels of αβ and γδ T cells but usage of the most Jαs was severely restricted (86), suggesting that its function is to govern the accessibility of the most proximal 5′ Jαs for recombination.

Organization of the TCR β Locus

The entire human 685 kb β-chain gene locus was originally sequenced by Hood and coworkers *(87)* (Figure 10.5). One interesting feature is the tandem nature of J_β-C_β in the TCRβ locus. This arrangement is preserved in all higher vertebrate species that have been characterized thus far (mouse, human, chicken, frog). The two C_β coding sequences are identical in the mouse and nearly so in humans and other species. Thus it is unlikely that they represent two functionally distinct forms of C_β. However, the J_β clusters have relatively unique sequences, and thus this may be a mechanism for increasing the number of J_β gene segments. Together with the large number of Jα gene segments, there is far more combinatorial diversity ($J\alpha \times J\beta = 50 \times 12 = 600$) provided by J regions in αβ TCR's than in Igs.

Most of the V-regions are located upstream of the joining and constant regions, and in the same transcriptional orientation as the D and J gene element and rearrange to DβJβ gene via deletion. Similar to the case of Vδ5, a single Vβ gene, Vβ14 is located 3′ to C-regions and in the opposite transcriptional orientation, thus rearrangements involving Vβ14 occur via inversion.

In the NZW strain of mouse, there is a deletion in the β chain locus that spans from Cβ1, up to and including the Jβ 2 cluster *(88)*. In SJL, C57BR, and C57L mice, there is a large deletion (89) in the V-region locus from Vδ5-Vβ9. These mice also express a V gene, Vβ17, that is not expressed in other strains of mice. Deletion of about half of the V genes (in SJL, C57BR, and C57L mice) does not seem to have any particular effect on the ability of these mice to mount immune responses, whereas mice which have deleted the $J_\beta 2$ cluster show impaired responses (90).

Organization of the TCR γ Locus

The organization of the mouse and human γ-chain loci are shown in Figure 10.4. The human γ genes span about 150 kb (81) and are organized in a fashion similar to that of the β chain locus with two JγCγ regions. The mouse locus is much smaller, encompassing only about 36 κb (91). There is more than one commonly used nomenclature used to describe the γ chain genes (81,92,93,*94*). Here, we use that of Lefranc and Rabbitts (95) and Tonegawa and colleagues (81)—for the human and mouse γ chains respectively. An array of Vγs, in which at least six of the V-regions are pseudogenes, is located 5′ to these JγCγ clusters, and each of the V genes is potentially capable of rearranging to any of the five J-regions. The sequences of the two human Cγ regions are very similar overall and only differ significantly in the second exon. In Cγ2, this exon is duplicated two to three times, and the cysteine that forms the interchain disulfide bond is absent. Thus, Cγ2 bearing human T cells have an extra large γ-chain (55,000 MW) that is not disulfide bonded to its δ-chain partner.

The organization of the murine γ chain genes is very different than that of the human genes in that there are three separate rearranging loci that span about 205kb (96,97). Of four murine Cγ genes, Cγ3 is apparently a pseudogene in BALB/c mice, and the Jγ3 Cγ3 region is deleted in several mouse strains including C57 Bl/10. Cγ1 and Cγ2 are very similar in coding sequences. The major differences between these two genes is in the 5 amino acid deletion in the Cγ2 gene that is located in the C II exon at the amino acid terminal of the cysteine residue used for the disulfide formation with the δ chain. The Cγ4 gene differs significantly in sequences from the other Cγ genes (in 66% overall amino acid identity). In addition, the Cγ4 sequences contain a 17 amino acid insertion (compared to Cγ1) in the C II exon located at similar position to the 5 amino acid deletions in the Cγ2 gene (G. Kershard, S.M. Hedrick, unpublished results). Each Cγ gene is associated with a single Jγ gene segment. The sequences of Jγ1 and Jγ2 are identical at the amino acid level, whereas Jγ4 differs from Jγ1 and Jγ2 at 9 out of 19 amino acid residues.

The murine Vγ genes usually rearrange to the Jγ Cγ gene that is most proximal and in the same transcription orientation. Thus Vγ1 rearranges to Jγ4, Vγ1 to Jγ2 and Vγ4, Vγ5, Vγ6, and Vγ7 to Jγ1. Interestingly, some Vγ genes are rearranged and expressed preferentially during $\gamma\delta$ T cell ontogeny and in different adult tissues as well (97). The reasons for this are not understood at this time.

Control of Transcription and Rearrangement

It has become increasingly apparent that transcriptional accessibility and rearrangement of TCR and Ig loci are closely linked, following the early work of Alt and colleagues (98). Factors governing accessibility and rearrangement include histone methylation (*99,100*,101,102), DNA methylation, and the presence of enhancer and specific promoter elements (103). Even specific variations in the recombination signal sequence (RSS) have been shown to elicit specific biases in V (D)- J joining (78). With respect to enhancer elements in the TCR loci, these were first identified in the TCRβ locus, 3′ of Cβ2 (104,105) and subsequently for the other TCR loci as well (103), as indicated in Figure 10.4. These TCR enhancers all share sequence similarities with each other. Some of the transcriptional factors that bind to the TCR genes are also found to regulate Ig gene expressions. It has been shown that TCRα enhancer (Eα) is not only important for normal rearrangement and expression for the α chain locus, but is also required for the normal expression level of mature TCRδ transcripts *(106)*. Also interesting is the work of Lauzurica and Krangel *(107,108)*, who have shown that a human TCR δ enhancer-containing minilocus in transgenic mice is able to rearrange equally well in $\alpha\beta$ T cells as in $\alpha\delta$ T cells, but that an Eα-containing construct was only active in $\alpha\beta$ lineage T cells. Similar to Ig genes, promoter sequences are located 5′ to the V gene segments. Although, D$\rightarrow J_\beta$ rearrangement and transcription occur fairly often in B cells, and in B cell tumors *(109)*, V_β rearrangement and transcription appears highly specific to T cells. In addition to enhancers, there also appear to be "silencer" sequences 3′ of Cα (110,111) and in the Cγ1 locus (112). It has been suggested that these "repressor sites" could turn off the expression of either of these genes, influencing T cell differentiation toward either the $\alpha\beta$ or the $\gamma\delta$ T cell lineage.

The murine TCR Cγ1 gene cluster comprises four closely linked Vγ gene segments, in the order Vγ7, 4, 6, and 5, which rearrange to a single common downstream J gene segment, Jγ1 (Figure 10.4). In early fetal thymocytes, rearrangements of Vγ5 and Vγ6 genes predominate, and the resulting V$\gamma3^+$ and Vg4$^+$ cells migrate to the skin or reproductive tissue, respectively. Later in ontogeny, Vγ4 and Vγ7 rearrangements predominate, and cells expressing these V regions migrate from the adult thymus to the secondary lymphoid organs (96,97). At least two *cis*-acting, enhancer/LCR elements are present in the Cγ1 cluster. One is a T cell–specific transcriptional enhancer, 3γEγ, located 3 kb downstream of the Cγ1 gene segment (113). A second element, has, was found between the Vγ7 and Vγ4 genes, based on Dnase I hypersensitivity (114). Similar enhancers have also been found to be associated with the Cγ2 and Cγ3 genes (91). Experiments suggest that simultaneous deletion of has and 3γEγ in Cγ1 cluster severely diminishes TCRγ transcription, selectively impairs development of $\gamma\delta$ thymocyte subsets, but only modestly reduces TCRγ gene rearrangement, while deletion of each element separately has little effect (115). In contrast to these results in thymocytes, deletion of has alone reduces transcription of one Vγ gene, specifically in peripheral $\gamma\delta$ T cells. Thus, the two elements not only exhibit functional redundancy in thymocytes but also have unique functions in other settings.

Allelic Exclusion

In Igs, normally only one allele of the heavy chain locus and one of the light chain alleles is productively rearranged and expressed, a phenomenon termed *allelic exclusion*. With respect to $\alpha\beta$ TCR expression, while TCRβ exhibits allelic exclusion (116), TCRα seems much less constrained (*117*,118), and many mature T cells express two functional TCRα chains. As the chances of forming an in-frame joint with any antigen receptor is only one in three, the probability that a T cell would have two productively rearranged TCRαs is only $1/3 \times 1/3 = 1/9$ or 11%. However, even when this happens, the two TCRα chains may not form heterodimers equally well with the single TCRβ that is expressed; and, thus, only one heterodimer may be expressed.

There also appears to be an important role for the pre-TCR heterodimer (e.g., pre–Tα:TCRβ) in blocking further TCRβ rearrangement and thus ensuring allelic exclusion at that locus (119,120). In particular, pre–Tα deficient mice had a significant increase in the number of cells with two productive TCRβ rearrangements, compared with wild-type mice (119).

TCR Diversity

Although the basic organization and V(D)J recombination machinery are shared between TCR loci and Igs, there are a number of striking differences. One of these is somatic hypermutation. In antibodies, this form of mutation typically raises the affinities of antigen-specific Igs several order of magnitude, typically from the micromolar (10^{-6}M) to the nanomolar (10^{-9}M) range (121,122). We now know that most cell surface receptors that bind ligands on other cell surfaces, including TCRs, typically have affinities in the micromolar range (see later section), but that they compensate for this relatively low affinity by engaging multiple receptors simultaneously (e.g., increasing the valency) and by functioning in a confined, largely two-dimensional volume (e.g., between two cells). Cells employing such receptors require weak but highly specific interactions so that they can disengage quickly (123,*124*). The rapid off-rates seen with TCRs (see later section) may even amplify the effects of small numbers of ligands (125,126).

There has also been no enduring evidence for a naturally secreted form of either an $\alpha\beta$ or $\gamma\delta$ TCR. Here again, it can be argued that such a molecule would have no obvious use, as the affinities are too low to be very useful in solution. Thus, for most TCRs, the concentration of protein would have to be extremely high in order to achieve an effect similar to soluble antibodies (in the milligram/mL range).

A third mechanism seen in antibodies but not TCRs is C_H switching, which allows different Ig isotypes to maintain a given V region specificity and associate it with different constant regions that have different properties in solution (e.g., complement fixation, basophil binding, etc.). As there is no secreted form of the TCR, this feature would also lack any obvious utility.

Where TCRs are equal—and in fact generally superior—to Igs is in the sheer number of possible receptors that can be generated through recombination alone. Table 10.1 summarizes the potential V region diversity that TCRs are capable of when the number of V region gene segments is multiplied by D, J, and N region diversity. It can be seen from this table that while the V region number is generally lower in murine TCRs, particularly TCR δ and TCR γ, this is more than compensated for by the degree of junctional diversity (where V and J or V, D, and J come together) and chain combinations, such that overall TCRs have orders of magnitude greater potential diversity than Igs. This junctional region corresponds to complementarity-determining region 3 (CDR3) as originally defined by Kabat and Wu for Igs *(127)*. With respect to $\alpha\beta$ TCRs, the concentration of diversity in this region (in both chains) can be explained by the key role that these sequences play in recognizing diverse peptides in MHC molecules (see later section), as supported by mutagenesis and structural studies. For $\gamma\delta$ TCRs and Igs, however, the diversity is almost all in just one chain (TCRδ and IgH, respectively) and the implications of this are discussed later.

The CDR3 Length Distributions of $\gamma\delta$ TCRs Are More Similar to Those of Ig than to Those of $\alpha\beta$ TCRs

Because CDR regions are loops between different β strands of an Ig or TCR V region (see later section), the configurations they adopt are generally very sensitive to their length, such that a difference of even one amino acid may produce a significant change in the overall structure *(3,128)*. A comparison of CDR3 length distributions between the different TCRs and Igs (Figure 10.5) (129,*130*) showed that those of TCR α and β have a very constrained distribution of lengths and that these are nearly identical in size. These length constraints may reflect a requirement for both the α and β chains of TCRs to contact both the MHC molecules and bound peptides on the same plane, as borne out by structural studies (see later section). In contrast, the CDR3s of Ig heavy chains are long and variable,

TABLE 10.1 Sequence Diversity in T-cell Receptor and Immunoglobulin Genes

	Immunoglobulin		*TCR α/β*		*TCR γ/δ*	
	H	κ	α	β	γ	δ
Variable segments	250–1,000	250	100	25	7	10
Diversity segments	10	0	0	2	0	2
Ds read in all frames	Rarely	—	—	often	—	often
N-region addition	V-D, D-J	none	V-J	V-D, V-J	V-J	V-D1, D1-D2, D1-J
Joining segments	4	4	50	12	2	2
Variable region combinations	62,500–250,000		2,500		70	
Junctional combinations	~10^{11}		~10^{15}		~10^{18}	

Calculated potential amino acid sequence diversity in TCR and immunoglobulin genes without allowance for somatic mutation. The approximate number of V gene segments are listed for the four TCR polypeptides and contrasted with immunoglobulin heavy and light chains. CDR1 and CDR2 are encoded within the V gene segments. The pairing of random V regions generates the combinatorial diversity listed as "variable region combinations." Because there are fewer TCR V gene segments than immunoglobulin V gene segments, the combinatorial diversity is lower in TCRs than in immunoglobulins. Estimates for the number of unique sequences possible within the junctional region are contrasted for TCRs and immunoglobulins. Amino acids within CDR3 are encoded almost entirely within the D and/or J region gene segments. (The last few amino acids encoded by a TCR V gene segment can contribute to diversity within the TCR CDR3-equivalent region, but the effects of these residues on junctional diversity are not included in these calculations.) The mechanisms for generation of diversity within the junctional region that are used for this calculation include usage of different D and J gene segments. N region addition up to six nucleotides at each junction, variability in the 3′ joining position in V and J gene segments, and translation of D region in different reading frames. Numbers are corrected for out-of-frame joining codon redundancy and N-region mimicry of germ-line sequences. Modified from Elliott JF, Rock EP, Patten PA, et al. The adult T-cell receptor delta-chain is diverse and distinct from that of fetal thymocytes. *Nature.* 1988;331(6157):627–631.

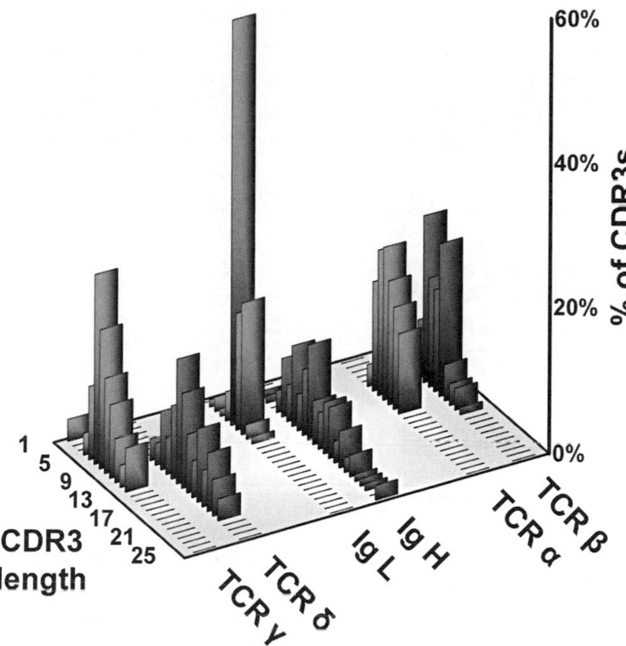

FIGURE 10.5 CDR3 length analysis of T cell receptor (TCR) polypeptides versus immunoglobulin (Ig) heavy and light chains. These data, modified from Rock et al. (129), show that whereas TCR α and β CDR3 regions are relatively uniform with respect to each other, the other antigen receptor pairs show a marked asymmetry. Specifically, both Ig light chains (κ and λ) show very short CDR3s, as do TCR γ chains. In contrast, both IgH and TCR δ TCRs are quite heterogeneous and tend to be longer. These data suggests that $\gamma\delta$ TCRs have a more antibodylike structure and binding properties. This has been borne out by subsequent analysis (see text).

while those of Ig light chains are short and constrained. This may reflect the fact that Igs recognize both very small molecules (e.g., haptens) as well as very large ones (e.g., proteins). Surprisingly, $\gamma\delta$ TCR CDR3 length distributions are similar to those of Igs in that the CDR3 lengths of TCR δ chains are long and variable, while those of the TCR γ chains are short and constrained. Thus, on the basis of this measure of ligand recognition, one might expect $\gamma\delta$ TCRs to be more similar to Igs than to $\alpha\beta$ TCRs. This has been validated in subsequent biochemical and structural studies (see later sections).

Chromosomal Translocations and Disease

The chromosomal locations of the different TCR loci have been delineated in both mouse and humans, and the results are summarized in Table 10.2. One significant factor in cancers of hematopoietic cells are chromosomal translocations that result in the activation of genes normally turned off or the inactivation of genes that are normally turned on. Thus, B or T lymphocyte neoplasia is frequently associated with inter- or intra-chromosomal rearrangements of Ig or TCR loci, and in some cases both *(131,132)*.

TABLE 10.2 Chromosomal Locations of T-cell Receptor, Immunoglobulin, and Related Loci in Mouse and Human

	Mouse Chromosome	*Human Chromosome*
TCR-α	14	14(q11–q12)
TCR-δ	14	14(q11–q12)
IgH	12	14(qter)
TCR-β	6	7(q35)
CD4	6	12
CD8	6	2(p11)
Ig*k*	6	2(p12)
TCR-γ	13	7(p14)
CD3-γ	9	11(q23)
CD3-δ	9	11(q23)
CD3-ε	9	11(q23)
CD3-ζ	1	1
Thy-1	9	11(q23)
Ig-λ	16	22(q11.2)
MHC	17	6(p21)
Pre-Tα	17	6

Ig, immunoglobulin; IgH, heavy chain immunoglobulin; MHC, major histocompatibility complex; TCR, T-cell receptor.

These translocations seemed to be mediated by the V(D)J recombinase machinery, indicating the inherent danger and need for tight regulation of this pathway. Such rearrangements are particularly common in the α/δ locus, perhaps because this locus spans the longest developmental window in terms of gene expression, with TCRδ being the first and TCRα the last gene to rearrange during T cell ontogeny (as discussed in more detail later). In addition, the α/δ locus is in excess of 1 Mb in size, and this provides a larger target for rearrangement than either TCRβ or TCRγ. Interestingly, in humans, TCRα/δ is on the same chromosome as the IgH locus, and $V_H \rightarrow J_\alpha$ rearrangements (by inversion) have been observed in some human tumor material *(133,134)*. The functional significance of this is not known.

Particularly frequent is the chromosome 8–14 translocation (t(8;14) (q24;q11)) that joins the α/δ locus to the c-myc gene, analogous to the c-myc$\rightarrow$IgH translocation in many mouse myeloma tumors and in Burkitt's lymphomas in humans. In one cell line, a rearrangement occurred between the Jα-region coding sequences, and a region 3′ of c-myc *(135)*. In both B and T cell malignancies, the translocation of c-myc into IgH or TCR α/β appears to increase the expression of c-myc and may be a major factor in the unregulated cell growth that characterizes cancerous cells. Other putative protooncogenes that have been found translocated into the TCR α/β locus are the LIM domain containing transcription factors Ttg-1 *(136)*, and Ttg-2 *(137,138)* which are involved in neural development; the helix-loop-helix proteins Lyl-1 *(139)* and Scl *(140)*, which are involved in early hematopoietic development; and the homeobox gene Hox 11 *(141)*, which is normally active in the liver. How these particular translocations contribute to malignancy is unknown, but they presumably causes aberrations in gene expression that contribute to cell growth or escape from normal regulation. In T cell leukemia patients infected with the HTLV-I virus, there are large numbers of similar translocations, and here it is thought that HTLV-I itself is not directly leukemogenic, but acts by causing aberrant rearrangements in the T cells that it infects, some of which become malignant.

Another disorder that frequently associates with TCR and Ig locus translocation is ataxia telangiectasia (AT), an autosomal recessive disorder characterized by ataxia, vascular telangiectasis, immunodeficiency, increased incidence of neoplasia, and an increased sensitivity to ionizing radiation. Peripheral blood lymphocytes (PBL) from patients with AT have an especially high frequency of translocations involving chromosomes 7 and 14 *(142)*. These sites correspond to the TCR γ, β, and α loci, and the Ig heavy chain locus. Thus, it appears as though one of the characteristics of Ataxia Telangiectasia patients is a relatively error-prone rearrangement process that indiscriminately recombines genes that have the TCR and Ig rearrangement signals *(143)*.

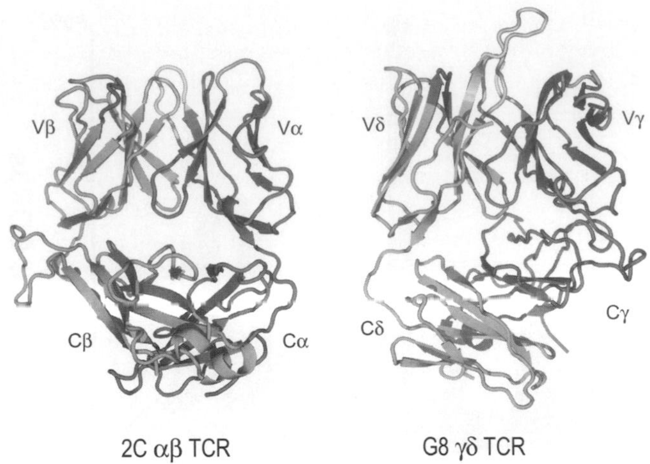

FIGURE 10.6 Ribbon diagrams of the T cell receptor (TCR) structures. This shows the structures of the 2C$\alpha\beta$TCR (150) versus the G8$\gamma\delta$ TCR (153). The TCRβ and the TCRγ chains are in cyan, and the TCRα and γ chains are in vermillion. The CDRs of both are in yellow. The very long TCRδCDR3 in G8, which binds the T10/T22 ligands, is very apparent here but is shorter in most other $\gamma\delta$ TCRs. Note the different C region interactions with these TCRs and the deviations from the classic "β barrel" structure in both Cα and Cδ. The prominent Cβ loop to the left is also unusual and may mediate interactions with CD3 or other molecules on the T cell surface. (Figure courtesy of Dr. K. C. Garcia) (See color insert.)

THE STRUCTURE OF $\alpha\beta$ AND $\gamma\delta$ TCRs

As discussed earlier, the sequences of TCR polypeptides show many similarities to Igs, and thus it has long been suggested that both $\alpha\beta$ and $\gamma\delta$ heterodimers would be antibody-like in structure (23,24,*144*). The similarities between TCRs and Igs include the number and spacing of specific cysteine residues within domains, which in antibodies form intrachain disulfide bonds. Also conserved are many of the inter-and intra-domain contact residues, and, in addition, secondary structure predictions are largely consistent with an Ig-like "β barrel" structure. This consists of three to four antiparallel β strands on one side of the "barrel" facing a similar number on the other side, with a disulfide bridge (usually) connecting the two β "sheets" (sets of β strands in the same plane). All Ig variable and constant region domains have this structure, with slight variations in the number of β strands in variable region domains (by convention including V, D, and J sequences) compared with constant domains.

$\alpha\beta$ TCR Structure

Efforts to derive x-ray crystal structures of TCR heterodimers and fragments of heterodimers presented many technical hurdles (as summarized in [145]). One difficulty is that structure determination required engineering the molecules into a soluble form. A second problem is that many of the TCRs are heavily glycosylated, and it was necessary to eliminate most or all of the carbohydrates on each chain to achieve high-quality crystals. An alternative is to express soluble TCRs in insect cells, where they have compact N-linked sugars, or in E. coli, where they are unglycosylated. The first successes in TCR crystallization come from the laboratory of Mariuzza and collaborators who solved the structure of first a Vβ Cβ polypeptide (146), and then a Vα fragment (147). In the following year, the first complete $\alpha\beta$ TCR structures were solved (*148*,149). The structure of the 2C TCR by Garcia and colleagues is shown in Figure 10.6 (from *[148]*). In general, as predicted from sequence homologies, these domains are all Ig-like, with the classical β-barrel structure in evidence in all three domains. At each end of the barrel in each V region-domain there are four loops between the β sheets, three of which form the CDRs of Igs, which are numbered in Figure 10.6. The fourth loop, between the D and E strands has been implicated in superantigen binding. The six CDR loops from the two variable domains form the antigen-binding surface in both Igs and TCRs. The major anomaly in terms of similarity of TCRs to Igs is the structure of the Cα (150). Cα consists of one half of the classical β-barrel—that is, one set (or "sheet") of β strands—while the rest of the partially truncated domain exhibits random coils. This type of structure is unprecedented in the Ig gene family. The functional significance of such a variant structure is unknown, but it has been suggested that this incompletely formed Ig-like domain may be responsible for the observed lability of TCR α, and this may allow greater flexibility in the regulation of its expression. Another possible explanation is that this configuration is designed to accommodate one or more of the CD3 molecules.

The now large number of solved $\alpha\beta$ TCR structures can be compared to the two $\gamma\delta$ heterodimers (discussed in more detail later), and although these also resemble the Fab fragment of an antibody, there are several features that are unique to the $\alpha\beta$ molecules, which may be significant. These include: 1) In one structure (150), four out of seven N-linked sugars diffracted to high resolution, indicating that they are not free to move very much and thus are likely to play a structural role, particularly in $C\alpha$:$C\beta$ interactions. This correlates with mutagenesis data indicating that certain $C\alpha$ sugars cannot be eliminated without abolishing protein expression *(151)* and the disordered state of a $C\alpha$ domain in the structure of a TCR lacking glycosylation (149). 2) There is significantly more contact between $V\beta$ and $C\beta$ and between $V\alpha$ and $C\alpha$ than in the equivalent regions of antibodies. 3) The geometry of the interaction of $V\alpha$ and $V\beta$ more closely resembles that of the C_H3 domains of antibodies than V_HV_L. 4) Between the CDR3 loops of $V\alpha$ and $V\beta$, there is a pocket that can (and does in at least one case [150]) accommodate a large side chain from the peptide bound to an MHC.

$\gamma\delta$ TCR Structure

There are now two $\gamma\delta$ heterodimer structures: a $\gamma\delta$ TCR from a human T cell clone G115 (152), which can be activated by natural or synthetic pyrophosphomonoesters, and a $\gamma\delta$ TCR from the murine T cell clone G8 together with its ligand, the nonclassical MHC class I molecule T22 (153). The G8 structure is shown in Figure 10.6, alongside the 2C $\alpha\beta$ TCR. The structure of a single human $V\delta3$ domain also has been determined (154). The $V\delta2$ domain of the G115 structure is similar to the isolated $V\delta3$ domain, and the quaternary structure of G8 is similar to that of G115 (153).

The most distinctive feature of both the G115 and the G8 TCR, when compared with $\alpha\beta$ TCRs and Igs, is that the C domains "swing out" from under the V domains. This unusual shape is highlighted by both a small elbow angle of 110°, defined as the angle between the pseudo two-fold symmetry axes that relate V to V and C to C, and a small V-C inter-domain angle. This contrasts with an average of 149° for $\alpha\beta$ TCR structures (Adams and Garcia, unpublished communication). The small angle between the $V\gamma$ and $C\gamma$ domains shifts both $C\delta$ and $C\gamma$ to one side. Moreover, the molecular surfaces of the constant domains are different than those of $\alpha\beta$TCRs with no clear similarities either in the shape or the nature of the $C\alpha C\beta$ and $C\gamma C\delta$ surfaces; there are only a few solvent-exposed residues that are conserved in both $C\beta$ and $C\gamma$ domains as well. Thus, it is unclear where or how the extracellular domains of the CD3 subunits interact with the extracellular portions of $\gamma\delta$ TCRs compared with $\alpha\beta$ TCRs. This may explain why the CD3 components of $\alpha\beta$TCRs are so different from those of $\gamma\delta$TCRs.

In terms of ligand binding surfaces, we note that although the CDR3 lengths of the G8 and G115 TCR are similar to those of $\alpha\beta$ TCRs, the $V\delta$ CD3 of G8 protrudes significantly away from the other CDRs, as shown in Figure 10.6. This has significance in that this is the major region of contact with the T10 ligand (see later section). In the case of G115, both $V\delta$ and $V\gamma$ CDR3 loops protrude from the rest of the putative binding surface and create a cleft between them. Portions of the CDR1γ and δ and CDR2γ combine with the clefts between the CDR3 loops to form a pocket, which is surrounded by positively charged amino acid residues contributed by CDR2γ, δ, and CDR3γ. The jagged surface of this TCR resembles the surface of an antibody that binds a small-molecule antigen. Although this would be consistent with the supposition that this TCR binds the negatively charged phosphate compounds (155), direct binding between the TCR and phospho-antigen-binding experiments including crystal-soaking and co-crystallization experiments have not been successful. Instead, a soluble G115 was found to bind a soluble form of ATP synthase F1 and Apolipoprotein A-1 *(156)*.

$\alpha\beta$ TCR-LIGAND RECOGNITION

Binding Characteristics

Although it has long been established that T cells recognize a peptide in association with an MHC molecule, a formal biochemical demonstration showing that this was due to TCR binding to a peptide/MHC complex took many years to establish. Part of the difficulty in obtaining measurements of this type has been the intrinsically membrane-bound nature of MHC and TCR molecules. Another major problem is that the affinities are relatively low, in the micromolar range, which is too unstable to measure by conventional means.

The problem of membrane-bound molecules can be circumvented by expressing soluble forms of TCR and MHC, which is also essential for structural studies (discussed earlier). For TCRs, many successful strategies have been described, including replacing the transmembrane regions with signal sequences for glycolipid linkage (157), expressing chains without transmembrane regions in either insect or mammalian cells *(158)*, or a combination of cysteine mutagenesis and E. coli expression (149). Unfortunately, no one method seems to work for all TCR heterodimers, although the combination of insect cell expression and leucine zippers at the c-terminus to stabilize heterodimer expression has been successful in many cases *(159)*. The production of soluble forms of MHC molecule has a much longer history, starting with the enzymatic cleavage of detergent solubilized native molecules *(160)* as well as some of the same methods employed for TCR such as GPI-linkage *(161)*, E. coli expression and refolding *(162,163)*, and insect cell expression of truncated (or leucine-zippered) molecules *(164)*. One interesting variant that seems necessary for the stable expression of some class II MHC molecules in insect cells has been the addition of a covalent peptide to the N-terminus of the β chain (165).

The first measurements of TCR affinities binding to peptide/MHC complexes were performed by Matsui et al. (166) and Weber et al. (167). Matsui and colleagues used a high concentration of soluble peptide/MHC complexes to block the binding of a labeled anti-TCR Fab fragment to T cells specific for those complexes, obtaining an equilibrium binding affinity (K_d) value of $\sim 50 \mu M$ for several different T cells and two different cytochrome peptide/I-E^kcomplexes (as shown in Table 10.3). Weber and colleagues (167) used a soluble TCR to inhibit the recognition of a flu peptide/I-E^d complex by a T cell and obtained a K_D value of $\sim 10 \mu M$. While these measurements were an important start in TCR biochemistry, they gave no direct information about the kinetics of TCR-ligand interactions. Fortunately the development of surface plasmon resonance instruments, particularly the BIAcore[TM] (Pharmacia Biosensor), with its remarkable sensitivity to weak macromolecular interactions *(168)*, has allowed rapid progress in this area. In this technique, one component is covalently cross-linked to a surface, and then buffer containing the ligand is passed in solution over it. The binding of even ~5% of the surface-bound material is sufficient to cause a detectable change in the resonance state of gold electrons on the surface. This method allows the direct measurement of association and dissociation rates—that is, kinetic parameters—and has the advantage of requiring neither cells nor radioactive labels. Recently, microcalorimetry has also been used to measure some TCR ligand affinities, and these analyses have confirmed the SPR values (169) but do not allow kinetic measurements. These and other data (reviewed in [*124*,145]) showed definitively that TCR and peptide-loaded MHC molecules alone are able to interact and that expression in a soluble form has not altered their ability to bind to each other. As shown in Table 10.3, SPR measurements show that while the on-rates of TCRs binding to peptide/MHC molecules vary from very slow (1,000 M sec) to moderately fast (200,000 M sec) their off-rates fall in a relatively narrow range (0.5 to .01 sec^{-1}) or a $t_{1/2}$ of 12 to 30 seconds at 25°C. This is in the general range of other membrane-bound receptors that recognize membrane molecules on other cells (123), but it has been noted that most TCRs have very slow on-rates *(124)*, which reflects a flexibility in the binding site that might help to foster cross-reactivity (discussed later). In the case of a class I MHC-restricted TCR, 2C, this relatively fast off-rate may be stabilized (10-fold) if soluble CD8 is introduced (150), but this result is

TABLE 10.3 T-cell Receptor – Ligand Binding

T Cell	Ligand	K_D (mM)	k_{on} ($M^{-1}s^{-1}$)	K_{off} (s^{-1})	Method	Reference
T_H Cells						
5C.C7	MCC/E^k	50	—	—	anti-TCR comp.	166
2B4	MCC/E^k	50	—	—	anti-TCR comp.	166
2B4	MCC/E^k	30	—	—	anti-P/MHC comp.	166
2B4	MCC/E^k	90	600	0.057	BIA1	166
228.5	MCC 99E/E^k	50	—	—	anti-TCR comp.	166
14.3d	Flu H1N1/E^d	~10	—	—	sol. TCR	167
14.3d	SEC 1,2,3	5.4–18.2	>100,000	>0.1	BIA1	251
HA1.7	HA/DR1	>25	—	—	BIA1	*300*
HA1.7	SEB	0.82	13,000	0.001	BIA1	*300*
Tc cells						
2C	p2Ca/L^d	0.5	11,000	0.0055	anti-TCR comp.	*176*
2C	p2/Ca/L^d	0.1	21,000	0.026	BIA1	*301*
2C	OL9/L^d	0.065	53,000	0.003	Labeled MHC	*176*
4G3	pOV/L^d	0.65	22,000	0.02	Labeled MHC	*176*
42.12	OVA/K^b	6.5	3,135	0.02	BIA4	179
2C	p2Ca/L^d	3.3	8,300	0.027	BIA1	208
HY	M80/D^b	23.4	6,200	0.145	BIA1	208
HY	CD8 α/β + M8/D/^{b}	2.0	5,100	0.01	BIA1	208
2/C	CD8 α/β + p2Ca/L^d	0.32	1,200	0.0038	BIA1	208
$T\gamma\delta$ cells						
G8	T10/T22	0.13	65,000	0.0081	BIA1	*274*

BIA1, TCR amine coupled; BIA2, TCR cysteine coupled; BIA3, MHC-peptide amine coupled in competition experiment; BIA4, TCR coupled by using H57 antibody and MHC coupled via amine chemistry; Comp. MHC, major histocompatibility complex; sol., soluble; TCR, T-cell receptor.

controversial *(170)*. CD8 stabilization of TCR binding has been seen by Luescher et al. in cell-based TCR labeling assay *(171)*; however, no enhancement of TCR binding has been seen using soluble CD4 *(172)*. Although most of the SPR measurements cited earlier were performed at 25°C due to instrument limitations, the actual dissociation rates are likely to be much faster (10 to 20×) at 37°C (173). One major caveat is that thus far all of these measurements have been made in solution, and it remains to be seen how the peculiar conditions of binding in between two cell membranes will influence the actual values in situ.

To what extent are we now able to predict a T cell response based on the binding characteristic of its TCR to a ligand? One of the most intriguing discoveries concerning T cell reactivity has been the phenomenon of altered peptide ligands. These are single amino acid variants of antigenic peptides that either change the nature or degree of the T cell response (partial agonists) or prevent a response to a normally stimulating ligand (antagonists) *(174,175)*. Discussions concerning the mechanism of these "altered peptide" responses have centered on whether they are due to some conformational phenomenon involving TCRs and/or CD3 molecules or to affinity or kinetic characteristics. With the data now available, we can say that most, but not all, T cell responses correlate well with the binding characteristics of their T cell receptors. In particular, Sykulev et al. *(176)* first noted that higher affinity peptide variants elicited more robust T cell responses. Subsequently Matsui et al. (177) found that in a series of three agonist peptides, increasing dissociation rates correlated with decreasing agonist activity. Lyons et al. (178) found that this correlation extended to antagonist peptides in the same antigen system (moth cytochrome c/I-E^k). They also showed that while an antagonist peptide might differ only slightly in affinity compared with the weakest agonist, its dissociation rate differed by 10-fold or more. This data in a class II MHC-restricted system is largely supported by the studies of Alam et al. in a class I MHC system (179), which also saw a drop-off in affinities and an increase in off-rates (with one exception as noted in Table 10.2) with antagonist versus agonist ligands. In the cell-based TCR labeling system of Luescher, a survey of related peptide ligands of varying potency also found a general, but not absolute, correlation between receptor occupancy and stimulatory ability (180). Thus, while there is a general trend toward weaker T cell responses and faster off rates and lower affinities, this does not seem to be an absolute rule, and thus other factors may be important in some cases. Alternatively, Holler et al. (181) have suggested that some or all of the discrepancies may derive from differences in peptide stability (in the MHC) between the relatively short (minutes) time scale of BIAcore analysis at 25°C compared with the much longer (days) cellular assays at 37°C. But this explanation probably only applies to a fraction of the anomalous cases in which TCR ligands fail to adhere to the "$t_{1/2}$ rule." In particular, Krogsgaard et al. *(182)* performed a very comprehensive survey of both known and newly derived cytochromic peptide antigens and found that almost half of the peptide-MHC ligands analyzed failed to exhibit a linear relationship between $t_{1/2}$ and T cell stimulatory ability (Figure 10.7). Extensive thermodynamic analyses of these ligands showed that one particular parameter, the change in heat capacity ($-\Delta Cp$), which reflects changes in conformation or flexibility upon binding, seems to be synergistic with $t_{1/2}$ in enhancing a ligand's stimulatory capacity. In fact, as shown in Figure 10.7, when ΔCp values are combined with $t_{1/2}$ the x axis, values for the range of ligands correlate much better with T cell stimulation. This suggests that ΔCp may be the "missing" variable in correlating ligand binding to stimulation.

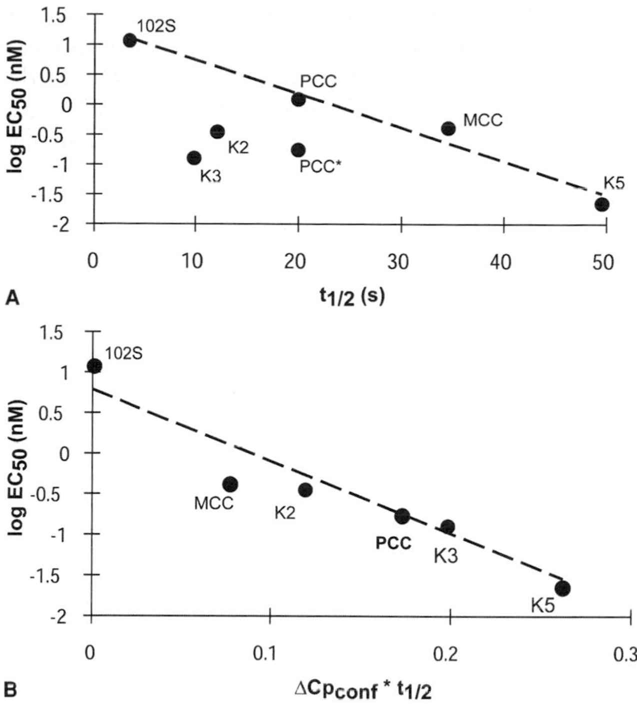

FIGURE 10.7 Dissociation rate and heat capacity with peptide–major histocompatibility complex (MHC) ligands both influence T cell activation. Data from Krogsgaard et al. show that where deviations from the general dependence of T cell activation on dissociation rate occur, they may be compensated for by another factor, namely the heat capacity (ΔC_p) of the T cell receptor (TCR)–pMHC interaction (169). This is a measure of changes in mobility or conformation during the binding interaction and suggests that other binding parameters can influence TCR-mediated activation besides half-life (184). **A:** The relationship between the half-maximal peptide concentration needed for T cell activation (EC_{50}) and the half-life ($t_{1/2}$) of the TCR binding to that particular ligand. In this series, three of the seven peptides tested (K2, K3, and PPC) do not seem as dependent on $t_{1/2}$ as the others (PCC* represents a correction for a lack of stability when bound to the MHC at 37°C). **B:** When ΔC_p is factored in, all of the peptides can be plotted on a line.

How could a negative change in heat capacity synergize with the stability of binding? One possibility is that large conformational changes at the binding surface of a TCR that can occur when it engages pMHC ligands (as shown by structural studies; see later discussion) can translocate the TCR deeper into the membrane—as suggested by the "piston (50,183) and twist cap"(169) models—and trigger conformational changes in the CD3 signaling domains. Chakraborty and colleagues recently suggested another possibility for how conformational changes at the binding surface might exert their effect (184). They found that in the context of membrane–membrane interactions, conformational changes in the surfaces of relatively rigid proteins (e.g., as TCRs are thought to be) would act to increase the effective half-life of TCR–pMHC interactions. Thus $t_{1/2}$ and ΔCp may be equivalent in the unique environment in between two cell surfaces.

How might the relatively small differences in the binding characteristics of the ligands cause such different T cell signaling outcomes as agonism or antagonism? As McKeithan (185) and Rabinowitz (186) have noted, a multistep system such as T cell recognition has an inherent ability to amplify small differences in signals that are received on the cell surface to much larger differences at the end of the pathway, in this case gene transcription in the nucleus. Thus antagonism may occur at one threshold and an agonist response at another. Alternatively, an antagonist ligand may traverse the activation pathway just far enough to use up some critical substrate, as proposed by Lyons et al. (178). Yet another possibility that has also been suggested is that some antagonists may act even earlier, by blocking TCR clustering at the cell surface *(187)*. Lastly, Germain and colleagues have found evidence that a feedback loop involving the phosphatase SHP-1 may act as an alternative pathway to inactivate TCR signaling of insufficient strength (188,189).

Another controversy that relates to TCR binding characteristics is the "serial engagement" model of Lanzavecchia and colleagues (190), which proposed that one way that a small number of peptide/MHC complexes can initiate T cell activation is by transiently binding many TCRs in a sequential fashion. While the dissociation rates reviewed here show that TCR binding is likely to be very transient, they do not in fact, support the statement that more interactions are better. This is because, in most cases, improvements in TCR-peptide/MHC stability within any one system result in a more robust T cell response. This has been shown most eloquently in the work of Kranz and colleagues (191), who selected a nanomolar affinity TCR from a mutagenized library expressed in yeast. With a ~100-fold slower off-rate than the original, this TCR should have been only poorly stimulatory based on the serial engagement model. Instead, T cells bearing it are considerably more sensitive to antigen, which casts considerable doubt on this model. But the concept that the rapid dissociation rates of TCRs for peptide-MHC liquids could serve to amplify signaling has reemerged in the context of the "pseudodimer" model (126,192), as discussed later.

Topology and Cross-reactivity

As discussed earlier, TCR sequence diversity resides largely in the region between the V and J region gene segments, which corresponds to the CDR3 regions of antibodies (193). This has led to models in which the CDR3 loops of Vα and Vβ make the principal contacts with the antigenic peptide bound to the MHC (193). Support for this model has come from many studies that have shown that the CDR3 sequences of TCRs are important predictors of specificity (as reviewed in ref. [193]), as well as elegant mutagenesis studies that have shown that a single CDR3 point mutation could alter the specificity of a TCR (194), and a CDR3 "transplant" could confer the specificity of the donor TCR onto the recipient (195). In addition, a novel approach to TCR–ligand interactions was developed by Jorgensen et al. (196), who made single amino acid changes in an antigenic peptide at positions that affect T cell recognition but not MHC binding. These variant peptides are then used to immunize mice that express either α or β chain of a TCR that recognizes the original peptide, and the responding T cells are analyzed. Using these "hemi-transgenic" mice allows the resulting T cells to keep one half of the receptor constant, while allowing considerable variation in the chain that pairs with it. The results from this study and work in another system by Sant'Angelo et al. (197) are very similar in that every mutation at a TCR sensitive residue triggered a change in the CDR3 sequence of Vα, Vβ, or both, and in some cases, changed the Vα or Vβ gene segment as well (as summarized in Figure 10.8). One of the more striking examples of a CDR3-peptide interaction occurred in the cytochrome c system, where a Lys→Glu change in the central TCR determinant on the peptide triggered a Glu→Lys charge reversal in the Vα

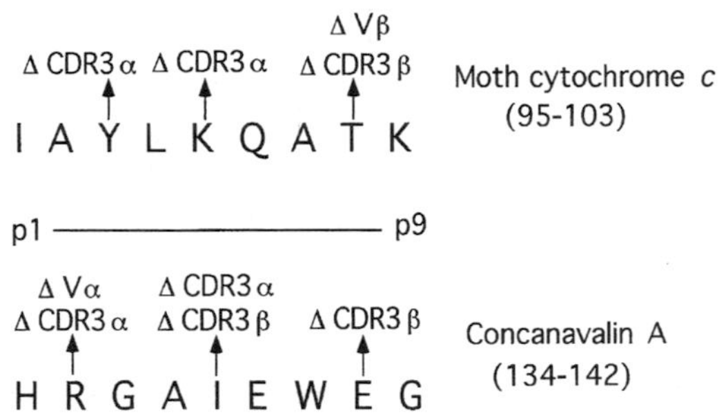

FIGURE 10.8 Sensitivity of T cell receptor (TCR) complementarity-determining region 3 (CDR3) sequences and Vα/Vβ usage to changes in the antigen peptide. This figure summarizes the data of Jorgensen et al. (196,198) and Sant'Angelo et al. (197), who immunized single-chain transgenic mice (TCRα or TCRβ) with antigenic peptides (MCC or CVA) altered at residues that influence T cell recognition but not major histocompatibility complex binding. These data show that such changes invariably affect the CDR3 sequences of Vα or Vβ or both and that there appears to be a definite topology in which Vα governs the N-terminal region and Vβ seems more responsible for the C-terminal portion of the peptide.

CDR3 loop, arguing for a direct Lys→Glu contact between the two molecules (196).

Another interesting finding was the order of Vα→Vβ preference going from the N-terminal to the C-terminal residues of the peptides. This led Jorgensen to a proposed "linear" topology of TCR-peptide/MHC interaction in which the CDR3 loops of Vα and Vβ line up directly over the peptide (196,198). Sant'Angelo et al. (197) proposed an orientation of the TCR in which the CDR3 loops are perpendicular to the peptide. This was partially based on intriguing data they found suggesting an interaction between the CDR1 of Vα and an N-terminal residue of the peptide. A third orientation was proposed by Sun et al. (188) based on the analysis of a large number of class I MHC mutants and their effect on TCR reactivity. This produced a roughly, diagonal footprint of TCRs over the MHC compared to the two previous models. On the other hand, an extensive class II MHC mutagenesis study failed to reveal a consistent "footprint" of TCR interaction and, furthermore, found the pattern of TCR sensitivity was remarkably labile and highly dependent on sequences in the TCR CDR3 region or the peptide (199).

This controversy regarding orientation has been largely resolved by the numerous crystal structures of TCR-pMHC complexes (145). These studies show that TCRs bind in roughly diagonal to 90° configurations, ranging over 30°.

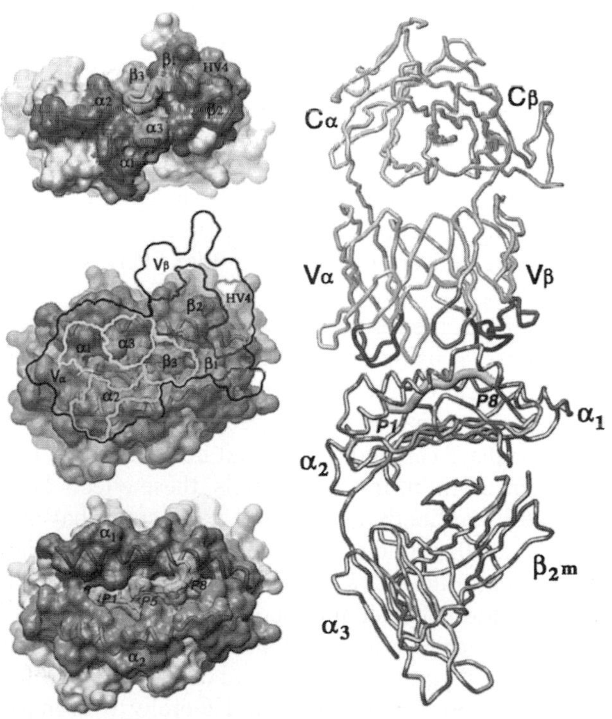

FIGURE 10.9 T cell receptor (TCR)-peptide/major histocompatibility complex (MHC) crystal structure of a TCR-peptide/MHC complex. Peptide and complementary-determining regions are portrayed in different colors (150). (See color insert.)

In these structures, one of which is shown in Figure 10.9 (150), the CDR3 loops are centrally located over the peptide, but the Vα CDR1 and the Vβ CDR1 are also in a position to contact the N-terminal and C-terminal peptide residues, respectively. Such a contact between Vα CDR1 and an N-terminal residue has now been seen in other structures as well *(200)*. The confined nature of TCR recognition constitutes a major departure from antibody–antigen interactions and may reflect a need to accommodate other molecules into a particular configuration that is optimal for signaling, such as CD4, CD8, or CD3 components.

As αβ T cell receptor heterodimers are first selected in the thymus for reactivity to self-peptides bound to MHC molecules, all foreign-peptide reactive TCRs could be considered to be inherently cross-reactive. Indeed a number of T cells have reactivity to very different peptide sequences, as shown by Nanda and Sercarz (201). It has also been argued by Mason (202) that the universe of peptides is so large that each T cell must on average be cross-reactive to $\sim 10^6$ different peptides (although many of the differences in peptide sequence in this calculation would not be accessible to the TCR, being buried in the MHC binding groove). Several large-scale screens of a random 9-mer peptide library with different T cells did turn up a great many stimulatory peptides, but very few have changes in the 2-4 key TCR sensitive residues (203,204). This lead Garcia and colleagues to conclude that cross-reactivity to different agonist peptides may not be a general feature of T cell specificity (203). Instead, the major requirement for cross-reactivity may be in thymic selection (205) or in the use of endogenous peptide-MHC's to augment T cell sensitivity to agonist ligands (192,206). Analyses of a T cell hybridoma that could recognize either a lysine or a glutamic acid residue in the center of a cytochrome c peptide on a panel of MHC mutants revealed that a different MHC "footprint" was evident, depending on which peptide was recognized (199,207). This suggests a plasticity of TCR binding to particular pMHC complexes. More direct evidence of TCR plasticity was first obtained by Garcia et al. (208), who in comparing the x-ray crystal structures of the same TCR bound to two different peptide-MHC ligands found a large conformational change in the CDR3 loop and a smaller one in the CDR1α loop. An even larger conformational change (15 Å) has been found in the CDR3β residue of another TCR as it binds to a pMHC complex (209), as shown in Figure 10.10. That each TCR may have many different conformations of its CDR3 loops is suggested by the 2D NMR studies of Reinherz and Wagner and colleagues, who found that the CDR3 regions of a TCR in solution were significantly more mobile than the rest of the structure (210). That this may be a general feature of most TCRs is supported by thermodynamic analyses of various TCRs binding to their peptide/MHC ligands, both class I and class II. Here the binding is often

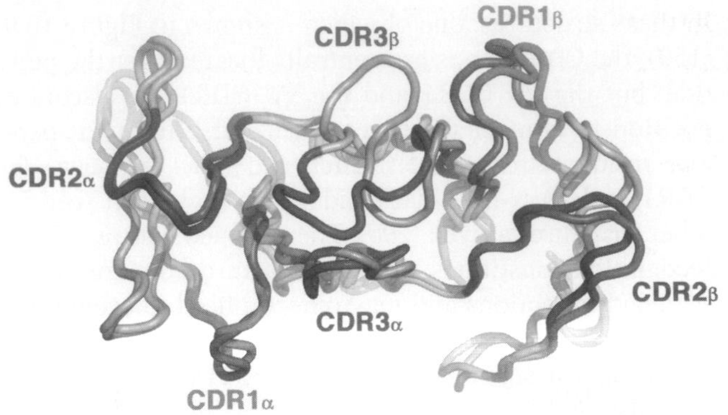

FIGURE 10.10 CDR3 movement in $\alpha\beta$ T cell receptor (TCR) binding. In most cases where there is a structure for an $\alpha\beta$ TCR as well as for one (or more) for that TCR in complex with a peptide-MHC, there is a marked movement of one or the other of the Vα or Vβ CDR3s. This example from Mallissen et al. (209) shows a particularly large (14 Å) movement of CDR3β with binding. This meshes well with thermodynamic data showing an "induced fit" binding mechanism for most TCRs (173,211). (See color insert.)

accompanied by a substantial loss of entropy (Table 10.4) and, in most cases, an "induced fit" mechanism (169,173,211). This seems to be a situation where an inherently flexible binding site achieves greater order upon binding. This is a mechanism that is also employed by DNA recognition proteins, and Boniface et al. (173) have suggested that it might represent a common mechanism of "scanning" an array of very similar molecular structures (MHCs or DNA) rapidly for those few that "fit" properly. We have seen previously that the association rates are often remarkably slow, with K_as ranging from 1,000 to 10,000 $M^{-1}s^{-1}$ (Table 10.3). This indicates that either a multistep process is occurring before stable binding can be achieved or that only a fraction of the TCRs in solution have the correct conformation. Just how such a scanning mechanism might work for TCRs is seen in the analysis of Wu and colleagues (212), who found that a cytochrome c/MHC II–specific TCR derived most of its stability of binding from antigenic peptide residues, but very little of its initial activation energy from these residues. In contrast, MHC residues contributed by far the most of the initial binding, but had relatively modest effects on stability. This indicates that "scanning" may be a process (as shown in Figure 10.11) that first involves contact with (and orientation by) the α-helices of the MHC, and then a "fitting" process with and stabilization by peptide residues that involves a substantial loss of entropy. This model of TCR binding might help to explain the striking efficiency and sensitivity of T cell recognition with the MHC helices guiding the TCR into the correct orientation. It might also be the structural basis for cross reactivity in which structurally different peptides bind to the same TCR, as the CDR3 regions of TCR could "fold" into the peptide in many possible configurations. While attractive, there remain caveats about this "two-step binding" model; one is the existence of some important human class I MHC antigens that "bulge" out of the binding groove, creating a barrier to "scanning" as a mechanism of binding to those antigens (213). A second issue is that one would expect a reproducible "footprint" for MHC binding of particular TCR V regions, which until recently has been elusive. But recently, Garcia and colleagues have documented such specific footprints that correlate to particular Vβ usage, although it does seem that there are multiple ways way in which a particular V region can contact a particular MHC (203).

Role of CD4 and CD8

What is the role of CD4 and CD8 with respect to the T cell response to agonist and antagonist peptides? In the case of a T helper cell response, the presence of CD4 greatly augments the amount of cytokine produced and, in some cases, determines whether there is a response at all (as reviewed in [214]). Much of the effect of CD4 seems to come from the recruitment of lck to the TCR/CD3 complexes. In addition, there is also a significant positive effect even with CD4 molecules that are unable to bind lck, and thus there appears to be an effect on TCR–ligand interaction as well. Nonetheless, while a weak binding of CD4 to class II MHC has been observed *(172)*, there is no apparent cooperativity with respect to TCR binding to peptide-MHC, unlike the case of CD8 and class I–specific TCRs (discussed later). Together with the recent low-resolution structure of CD4-class II MHC *(215)*, the classical model of CD4 binding to the same MHC as a TCR that it is associated with (104) seems untenable. And yet there is abundant evidence that CD4 molecules do associate with TCRs, especially on previously activated T cells *(216)*. Thus models in which CD4 cross-linking to MHC II indirectly supports TCR binding to peptide-MHCs and potentiates signaling through the delivery of lck seem more likely (discussed later).

In addition, the results of Irvine et al. (217) and Purbhoo et al. (218) using a single-peptide labeling technique, found appreciable T cell responses to even one agonist peptide in all four T cells analyzed, resulting in a "stop" signal for the T cell and a small but detectable rise in intracellular calcium. In CD4$^+$ T cells, these effects are attenuated by antibody blockade of CD4, such that many more (25 to 30) peptides are required to elicit a stop signal and a calcium flux (217). How could CD4 be facilitating the recognition of small numbers of peptides? Irvine et al. (217) have proposed a "psuedodimer" model, which suggests that a CD4 molecule associated with a TCR binding to an agonist peptide-MHC could bind laterally to an endogenous peptide-MHC complex that is also being bound by an adjacent TCR. This takes advantage of the apparent abundance of endogenous pMHCs that can be bound by a given TCR (219) and uses two weak interactions (CD4 $\rightarrow$ MHC

TABLE 10.4 Thermodynamic and Structural Parameters for TCR Peptide-MHC Interactions

TCR	pMHC	ΔG° (kcal/mol)	ΔH° (kcal/mol)	ΔCp (kcal/mol)	TCR Conformational Change	pMHC Conformational Change	Reference
2C	dEV8-H2-K^b	−6.3	−22.7	−1.1	CDR3α (6 Å)	None[a]	169,208
2C	p2Ca-H2-K^b	−6.1	−29	−1.5	ND	ND	169
2C	SIYR- H2-K^b	−7.2	−8.4	−1.1	CDR3α (3.9 Å)	None	169,208
2C	dEV8-H2-K^{bm3}	−5.8	ND	ND	CDR3α (6 Å)	None	305,308
JM22z	MP(58-66)-HLA-A2	−7.1	−23	ND	—	Q155-A2 (2.4 Å)	211,307
KB5-C20	PKB1-H2-K^b	ND	ND	ND	CDR3β (15 Å)	None	209
LC13	EBNA3A-HLA-B8	−6.8	ND	ND	CDR3α (2.5 Å); CDR1α(1.9 Å): Cα	(Q155)-HLA-B8	304
A6	Tax-HLA-A2	−8.2	ND	ND	CDR3β(4.4 Å)	A2-α2 (1.4 Å)	149,209
BM3.3	VSV8-H2-K^b	−5.4	ND	ND	CDR3α (5.3 Å)	None	303
D10	CA-I-A^k	−7.0	ND	ND	CDR3β	None	172,210
F5z	AM9-H2-K^b	−6.7	−19	ND	ND	ND	211
2B4	MCC-I-E^k	−6.9	−13	−0.6	ND	ND	169,173
2B4	K2-I-E^k	−6.9	−9.4	−2.1	ND	ND	169
2B4	K3-I-E^k	−6.1	−30.5	−4.0	ND	ND	169
2B4	K5-I-E^k	−7.5	−8.0	−1.2	ND	ND	169
2B4	102S-I-E^k	−5.6	−13.2	−0.3	ND	ND	169
2B4	PCC-I-E^k	−6.1	13.3	−1.8	ND	ND	169
2B4	PCC-103K-I-E^k	−7.0	−8.4	−1.0	ND	ND	169
172.10	MBP(1-11)-I-A^u	−6.9	−21.2	−0.16	ND	None	305
1934.4	MBP(1-11)-I-A^u	−8.0	−15.7	−1.2	ND	ND	305
D3	SL9-HLA-A2	−7.5	−10.4	0.4	ND	ND	309

The ΔG values were derived from the equation $\Delta G = -RT \ln(K_A)$ where R = 0.001987 kcal/mol/K. ND, not determined.
[a]No major conformational change observed after ligand recognition.

II and TCR → endogenous peptide-MHC) to help create a dimeric "trigger" for activation. CD8 also greatly augments the response of class I MHC–specific T cells (214) and binds to class I MHC in much the same fashion as CD4 *(220)*. $CD8^+$ T cells have the same sensitivity to antigen as $CD4^+$ T cells (219), but the data of Gascoigne and colleagues suggests that they are not sensitive to particular endogenous pMHCs (206). Overall, it seems likely that each of these coreceptor molecules has two roles: to stabilize TCR–ligand interactions physically and to aid in signaling by recruiting lck. Consistent with this is data showing CD4 can convert an antagonist peptide into a weak agonist *(221,222)*, although CD4 has no apparent effect on antagonism (223,224). This situation with CD8 is less clear, but there are clearly some differences in how it synergizes with TCR versus CD4, some of which may relate to its much higher affinity for its MHC (~10μM for CD8-MHC1 *[148,170]* versus >250μM for CD4-MHCII *[172]*).

Superantigens

One of the most interesting and unexpected areas to emerge from the study of αβ T cell reactivities is the discovery of "superantigens." Whereas a particular antigenic peptide might only be recognized by one in 100,000 or fewer T cells in a naïve organism, a given superantigen might stimulate 1% to 20% of the T cells (as reviewed in [225,226]). As will be discussed in more detail later, the physical basis for this is that the superantigen binds to a Vβ domain of the TCR on T cells while simultaneously binding to an MHC class II molecule on an antigen presenting cell (although not in the peptide-binding groove). This allows a single superantigen, such as SEA in Table 10.5, to stimulate virtually every murine T cell bearing Vβ 1, 3, 10, 11, 12, or 17 (about ~15% of all αβ T cells), in most cases regardless of what Vα it is paired with or what CDR3 sequence is expressed. Clearly this is a very unique class of T cell stimulatory molecule.

The first indication of a superantigen effect was the discovery of minor lymphocyte stimulating (MIS) determinants by Festenstein in the early 1970s (227). Many years later, Kappler and Marrack and their colleagues characterized a mouse strain-specific deletion of T cells expressing specific TCR Vβs that were attributable to these loci (228). It emerged that these effects were due to endogenous retroviruses of the mouse mammary tumor virus family (229–233). Different family members bind different TCR Vβ domains (as shown in Table 10.5) and

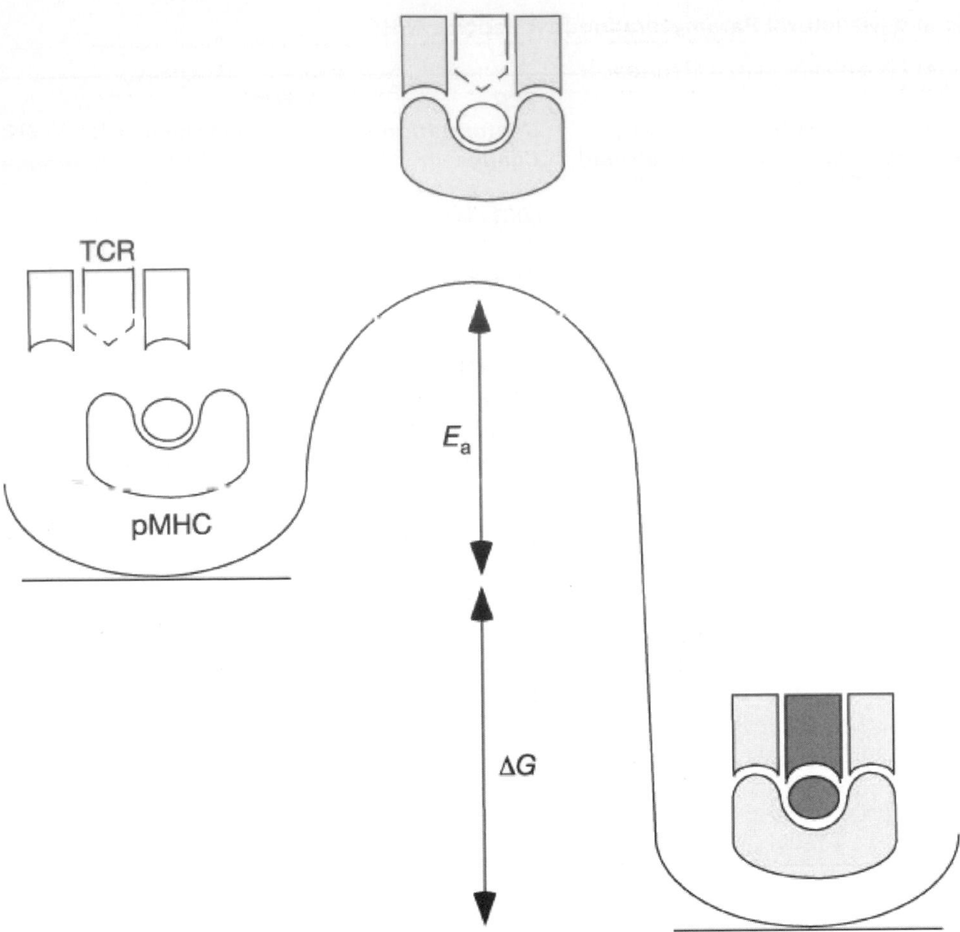

FIGURE 10.11 As shown by Wu et al. (212), mutational analysis of T cell receptor (TCR)-peptide/major histocompatibility complex (MHC) binding indicates that the TCR first contacts MHC residues (in the transition state), and the peptide has very little influence. Subsequently, however, the peptide residues contribute greatly to the stability of the complex. Thus, we have proposed that the transition state largely involves TCR–MHC contact followed by stabilization of mobile complementarity-determining region 3 residues into a stable state, usually involving significant conformational change and loss of entropy.

stimulate T cells expressing them. Meanwhile, Janeway and colleagues (234) had shown earlier that staphylococcus enterotoxins could polyclonally active naïve T cells in a Vβ-specific manner without a requirement for antigen processing. Many of these enterotoxins have been characterized extensively (225,226,235,236). Unlike the MMTV proteins, which are type II membrane proteins, the enterotoxins are secreted. Subsequently, proteins having similar properties have been isolated from other bacteria specifically (Yersinia pseudotuberculosis *[237,238])*, streptococcus *(239)*, and from mycoplasma *(240,241)*. There is also evidence of superantigen-like activities in other mammalian viruses such as rabies *(242)*, cytomeglovirus *(243)*, herpes virus *(244)*, Epstein-Barr virus *(245)*, and also in the toxoplasma gondii *(246)*. Because so many pathogenic or parasitic organisms possess these molecules, apparently by convergent evolution, there must be some selective advantage, but in most cases there is no conclusive evidence as to what this might be. The one exception is the case of the MMTV superantigens, where it has been shown that polyclonal T cell stimulation allows the virus to more efficiently infect the B lymphocytes that are activated by the T cells (247,248). This may be a special case, however, and most authors have suggested that superantigens primarily serve to confuse and occupy the immune system while the pathogen escapes specific targeting and elimination. Large doses of superantigens have also been implicated in various "shock" syndromes, such as food poisoning or "toxic shock" (225), but this is probably not their everyday purpose, as it would violate the general rule that the host and parasite should coexist.

It has also been suggested that superantigens might be involved in triggering autoimmune diseases (249). Here the hypothesis is that a large number of T cells bearing a particular Vβ are activated by a pathogenic superantigen and that subsequently self-reactive T cells within those activated cells are more easily stimulated by a particular tissue antigen. That this may occur in some cases is supported by the work of Stauffer et al. on a human endogenous retrovirus that specifically stimulates Vβ7 T cells and is implicated in the initiation of type I diabetes *(220)*. Another report implicates a superantigen in Crohn's disease, another autoimmune disorder (250).

Although the biochemistry of superantigen binding to TCR and MHC is similar to that of TCR peptide/MHC interactions (251), mutagenesis, and particularly x-ray structural data, has shown that the topology is both quite

TABLE 10.5 Vβ Specificity of Exogenous and Endogenous Superantigens

Bacterial Superantigen	*Human Vβ Specificity*	*Reference*	*Murine Vβ Specificity*	*Reference*
				(as referenced in 235, 314)
SEA	ND		1, 3, 10, 11, 12, 17	*310,311*
SEB	3, 12, 14, 15, 17, 20	*315,316*	(3), 7, 8.1, 8.3, (11), (17)	*310,311,312*
SEC_1	12	*316*	7, 8.2, 8.3, 11	*310*
SEC_2	12, 13, 14, 15, 17, 20	*315,316*	8.2, 10	*310*
SEC_3	5, 12	*316*	(3), 7, 8.2	*310*
SED	5, 12	*316*	3, 7, (8.2), 8.3, 11, 17	*310*
SEE	5.1, 6.1–6.3, 8, 18	*315,316*	11, 15, 17	*310*
TSST-1	2	*316*	15, 16	*310*
ExFT	2	*315*	10, 11, 15	*310*
Strep M	2, 4, 8	*239*	ND	
Endogenous Proviruses	***Vβ Specificity***	***Mls Type***[a]	***Chromosome***	***Reference***
				(as referenced in 235, 236)
Mtv-1	3	c, 4a	7	
Mtv-2	14	NA	18	
Mtv-3	3, 17	c	11	
Mtv-6	3, 17	c, 3a	16	
Mtv-7	6, 7, 8.1, 9	a, 1a	1	
Mtv-8	11, 12	f, Dvbll.1	6	
Mtv-9	5, 11, 12	f, Etc-1	12	
Mtv-11	11, 12	f, Dvbll.3	14	
Mtv-13	3	c, 2a	4	
Mtv-43	6, 7, 8.9, 9	Mls-like	ND	
Exogenous Viruses	***Vβ Specificity***	***Mls Type***	***Chromosome***	***Reference***
MMTV-C3H	14, 15	NA		*231*
MMTV-SW	6, 7, 8.1, 9	Mls-like		*247*
Rabies	ND			*242*
EBV	ND	HERV-K18		*245*
CMV	ND			*243*
Herpiovirus				*244*
Other Pathogens	***Vβ Specificity***	***Name***	***Chromosome***	***Reference***
Mycoplasma arthritidis	h17, 6, 8.1, 8.3	MAM		*240,241*
Toxoplasma gondii	5			*246*
Yersinia enterocolitica	ND			*237*
Yersinia pseudotuberolosis	ND			*238*

Vβ in parentheses are reactive with commercial but not recombinant enterotoxins.
CMV, cytomegalovirus; EBV, Epstein-Barr virus; MMTV, mouse mammary tumor virus; NA, not applicable; ND, not determined.
[a]The nomenclature in use before the discovery that the phenotype resulted from endogenous retroviruses.

different and variable (226). In particular, it has been found that Mls-la presentation to T cells is most affected by mutations on the "outside" surface of the Vβ domain, which do not affect peptide/MHC recognition (147). In contrast, the CDR1 and CDR2 of regions of Vβs are involved in bacterial superantigen reactivity (252).

An example of the structural data is shown in Figure 10.12, which shows how a model TCR-SAg-MHC complex (derived from separate structures) would displace the TCR somewhat (but not entirely) away from the MHC binding groove (253), thus making the interaction largely insensitive to the TCR/peptide specificity. Other TCR-SAg-MHC complexes have very different geometries (254–256).

Why do all the many independently derived superantigens interact only with the TCR β-chain? One possibility is that the β-chain offers the only accessible "face" of the TCR, perhaps because the CD4 molecules hinders access to the Vα side (as suggested by the antibody blocking studies of Janeway and colleagues *[257]*).

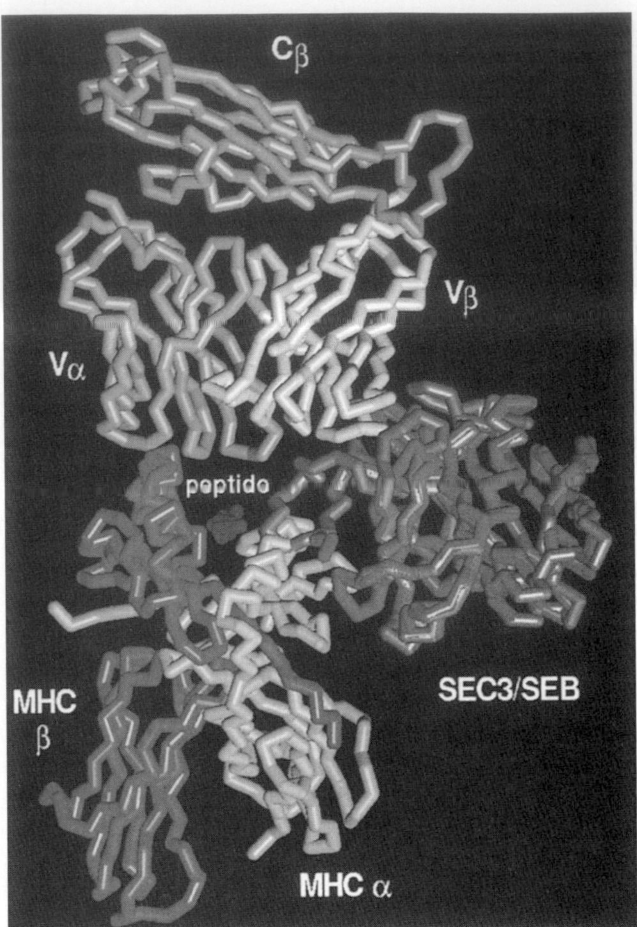

FIGURE 10.12 Crystal structure of a T cell receptor (TCR) β/superantigen (SAg) complex. Fields et al. (253) crystallized TCR-SAg complexes and from the structure of the same superantigens with a class II major histocompatibility complex (MHC) molecule and were able to deduce the relative spatial arrangement of the three molecules. This model suggests that TCR does not contact the MHC very strongly, which is consistent with the relative peptide insensitivity of SAg activation. (See color insert.)

ANTIGEN RECOGNITION BY γδ T CELLS

Antigen Recognition Requirements

Because the study of γδ T cells is relatively recent and does not stem from any knowledge of their biological function, experiments designed to characterize their specificity and function had drawn heavily on our knowledge of αβ T cells. Because αβ T cell recognition requires antigen presentation by MHC and related molecules, it was assumed that γδ T cell recognition would also follow the same rules. Even in cases where classical MHCs are clearly not involved, it has been suggested that nonclassical MHC molecules or some yet-to-be-identified surface molecules might play a similar role. These possibilities are difficult to test experimentally. Thus, analysis of γδ T cells specific for MHC molecules were carried out to determine the antigen recognition requirement of γδ TCRs. This approach asks the following questions: When γδ T cells recognize MHC molecules, what kind of antigen processing is required? Is any of the specificity conferred by bound peptide? Which part of the MHC molecule is recognized? This approach takes advantage of the detailed knowledge of the molecular structure of MHC class I (258,259) and MHC class II molecules (260), thus making T cell epitope mapping feasible and interpretable. In addition, and more important, the biosynthetic pathways and antigen processing requirements for both MHC class I and MHC class II molecules had been extensively studied. Mutant cell lines defective in either pathway were readily available and could be transfected with various MHC class I and MHC class II genes. Therefore, potential antigen processing and presentation requirements for alloreactive γδ T cells could be studied with precision and compared with those of αβ T cells.

The γδ T cell LBK5 *(261,262)* recognizes I-$E^{b,k,s}$, but not I-E^{d}. An analysis of the fine specificities of LBK5 showed that the peptide bound to the I-E molecules does not confer specificity and that no known antigen processing pathways were required in the recognition of I-E by LBK5. All variations in the ability of different stimulator cells to activate LBK5 can be attributed solely to their level of surface I-E expression and are independent of their species origin (mouse, hamster, human) and cell type (B cells, T cells, fibroblasts). Modifications of the repertoire of peptides loaded onto MHC molecules also showed no effect because native I-E^{k}, GPI-linked I-E^{k}, I-E^{k} expressed with or without invariant chains, and the presence or absence of functional MHC class I or class II antigen processing pathways all stimulated LBK5 similarly (263). Thus, LBK5 recognizes native I-E^{k} molecules with a variety of different bound peptides or in the case of GPI-linked I-E^{k}, which most likely does not complex with a peptide. In addition, LBK5 recognizes *E. coli*-produced I-E^{k} α and β chains folded with a single peptide *(264)*.

The functional epitope on IE for LBK5 recognition maps to the β67 and β70 residues *(264)*. This explains why LBK5 recognizes I-$E^{b,k,s}$ but not I-E^{d} and why peptide bound to IEk does not confer the specificity. Surprisingly, IEk mutants with an altered carbohydrate structure on the α84 position are not recognized by LBK5 *(264)*. Although the binding interface of the LBK5 γδ TCR and I-E has yet to be determined, it is reasonable to assume that it will not deviate much from those reported for antibodies, αβ TCRs and the G8 γδ TCR. From the coordinates of a published crystal structure of I-E^{k} *(265)*, the distance between β67 to 70 (the LBK5 epitope) and the carbohydrate attachment site at position α82 was estimated to be around 28 to 33Å. Hence, it is likely that the carbohydrate structure is peripheral to the core of the LBK5/I-E interaction.

This type of interaction may be similar to that described for human growth hormone and the extracellular domain of its receptor *(266)*, where a central hydrophobic region at the contact site, which is dominated by two tryptophan residues, accounts for more than three quarters of the binding free energy and where peripheral electrostatic contacts contribute substantially to the specificity of binding but not to the net binding energy. This type of protein–protein interaction has been postulated to ensure the specificity of an interaction without requiring a high affinity *(267)*.

Two independently derived $\gamma\delta$ T cell clones, KN6 *(268)* and G8 *(269)*, are found to recognize T10 and T22, two closely-related, nonclassical MHC class I molecules that have 94% amino acid identity. T22 appears to be expressed constitutively on a variety different cell types, while the expression of T10 is inducible on cells of the immune system. Among strains of mice tested so far, all express T10. However, mice of the H-2^d or H-2^k MHC haplotypes (e.g., BALB/c and C3H, respectively) lack functional T22 molecules (*[268]* and MP Crowley, thesis) (Figure 10.13). T10 and T22 have also been identified as natural ligands for murine $\gamma\delta$ T cells and ~0.2 to 1% of the $\gamma\delta$. T cells in normal, unimmunized mice are T10/T22 specific *(269)*.

The primary sequences of T10 and T22 suggest that the necessary structural features that enable classical MHC

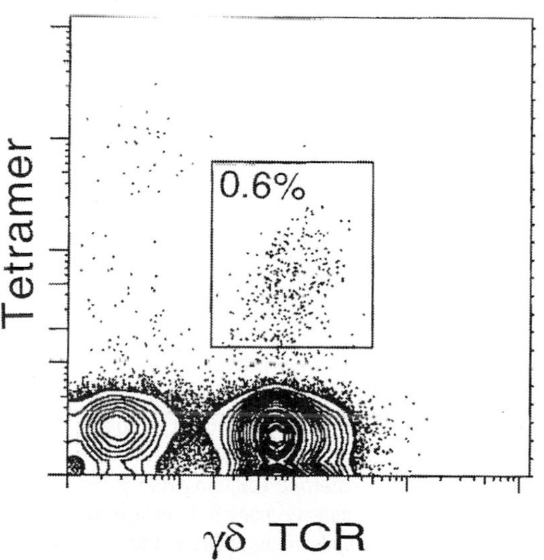

FIGURE 10.13 T10/T22-specific $\gamma\delta$ T cells can be detected in normal mice through use of a tetrameric T22 staining reagent. As shown by Crowley et al. (274), a T22 reagent that was generated by similar methods as tetrameric peptide/major histocompatibility complex reagents stained approximately 0.6% of splenic $\gamma\delta$ T cells in normal animals. More than 90% of these cells are $CD4^-CD8^-$; the rest are either CD4 or CD8 single positive (about 3% to 4% each). A similar frequency of tetramer-positive $\gamma\delta$ T cells was also found in the intestinal intraepithelial lymphocyte (IEL) population (data not shown).

class I molecules to bind peptides are absent. Indeed, X-ray crystallography has shown that T10 and T22 adopt a severely modified MHC-like fold that lacks a classical peptide-binding groove and exposes part of the β sheet "floor" of the $\alpha 1/\alpha 2$ platform (270,271). Consistent with the structural data, no endogenous peptides can be eluted from chimeric T10/L^d molecules that are expressed by transfected cells (*[272]* and H. Schild, Y-h. Chien, and H. Rammensee, unpublished results). This indicates that these molecules can reach the cell surface devoid of peptide. Importantly, the *E. coli*–produced, *in vitro*–folded T10/β_2m and T22/β_2m molecules can stimulate the G8 $\gamma\delta$ T cell *(273)*, which provides unequivocal evidence that these peptide-free molecules retain their immunological function.

Direct binding between soluble G8 $\gamma\delta$ TCRs and T10/β_2m and T22/β_2m complexes has been measured (274). Surface plasmon resonance showed that the dissociation rates for the interaction between G8 and $T10^b$ and $T22^b$ were similar ($k_d = 8.1 \pm 2.3 \times 10^{-3}\ s^{-1}$) and slower than those that had been observed for most interactions between $\alpha\beta$ TCRs and peptide/MHC complexes. The association rates ($k_a = 6.53 \pm 1.73 \times 10^4\ M^{-1}s^{-1}$) are among the fastest that had been reported for $\alpha\beta$ TCRs and their ligands. Therefore, compared to $\alpha\beta$ TCRs, the affinity between G8 $\gamma\delta$ TCRs and their ligand is rather high ($K_D = 0.13 \pm 0.05\ \mu M$). A Scatchard analysis of equilibrium binding generated a similar affinity of 0.11 ± 0.07 μM for this interaction (274).

As summarized in Table 10.6, the recognition of I-E, T10/T22 (263,275), herpes simplex virus glycoprotein gI (276), MICA and MICB (277), and the recently described recognition of the F1-ATPase and the apoliprotein A-I complex specific $\gamma\delta$ T cells *(156)* indicates that the molecular nature of $\gamma\delta$ T cell antigen recognition is fundamentally different than that of $\alpha\beta$ T cells. In all cases, the antigens are recognized directly. This suggests that many (and perhaps all) $\gamma\delta$ T cells can function without a requirement for antigen processing. While MHC and MHC-related molecules are recognized by $\gamma\delta$ T cells, $\gamma\delta$ T cell antigens need not be MHC or MHC-related molecules. Thus, pathogens and damaged tissues can be recognized directly, and cellular immune responses can be initiated by $\gamma\delta$ T cells without a requirement for antigen degradation and specialized antigen presenting cells, such as B cells, macrophages, and dendritic cells. This would allow for greater flexibility than is present in classical $\alpha\beta$ T cell responses. T10, I-E, as well as MICA and MICB expression can be induced under certain physiological/pathological conditions *(278)*. ATP synthase F1 is normally localized in the membranes of mitochondria, but it has also been found on the surfaces of tumors, hepatocytes, and endothelial cells *(279–281)*. Thus, $\gamma\delta$ T cell activation may be regulated through the level of protein expression. In addition, the recognition of I-E by LBK5 is acutely sensitive

TABLE 10.6 Partial List of $\gamma\delta$ T Cell Reactivities

Name (referred to as)	Source	Reported Reactivities	Comments	Reference
Murine				
DGT3	Lymph node cells from DBA2 mouse primed with poly($Glu^{50}Tyr^{50}$)	Qa-1/($Glu^{50}Tyr^{50}$)		317
KN6	Double-negative thymocytes from C57Bl/6	T10/T22*b*,*k* not *d*		318
Tgl4.4	Lymph node of HSV infected C3H mouse and restimulated with L cells transfected with HSV-gl	HSV-gl	Can be stimulated by gl protein alone	319,320
G8	BALB/c nu/nu immunized with B10.BR APCs	T10/T22*b*,*k* not *d*	Direct binding and co-crystal structure have been shown	153,274,323
LBK5	C57Bl/10 nu/nu immunized with B10.BR splenocytes	I-E*k*,*s*,*r* not *d*	Can be stimulated by I-E proteins alone; reactivity is not peptide-specific	322,323
LKD1	B10.BR immunized with B10.D2 splenocytes	I-A*d*		322
69BAS-122	C57Bl/10, adult splenocyte	HSP-60 peptide, cardiolipin, b2-glycoprotein 1	Transferring TCR transfers reactivity	324,325
BNT-19.8.12	C57Bl/10, newborn thymocyte	Mycobacterium PPD, cardiolipin, b2-glycoprotein 1	Transferring TCR transfers reactivity	325,326
7–17 and other dendritic epidermal T cells	$\gamma\delta$ T cells from murine epidermis	Keratinocytes	Transferring TCR transfers reactivity	33
Human				
Panels of T cell clones expressing Vγ9Vδ2	PBMC stimulated with irradiated PBMCs and PHA	Tumor cells (e.g., Molt-4), M. tuberculosis extracts (MT), metabolites in the mevalonate pathway	20% of Vg9Vd2 clones do not react to MT; only slightly more than 50% of MT- or Molt-4-specific clones recognize the other specificities	327,328
Panels of T cell clones expressing Vγ9Vδ2 including G42 and G115	$\gamma\delta$ T cells from PBM cultured with irradiated PBLs and lymphoblastoid cells	phosphoAg, tumor cells (e.g., Daudi), AS/ApoA-I (G115 TCR)	Close correlation between Daudi and mycobacterial reactivity; direct binding between AS/ApoA-I; heterogenous reactivity to ApoA-I	156,329,330
DG.SF13 (Vγ9Vδ2)	$\gamma\delta$ T cells isolated from RA synovial fluid stimulated with sonicate of M. tuberculosis	Daudi cells, M. tuberculosis, MEP	Transferring TCR transfers reactivity	331
Panels of T cell clones expressing Vγ9Vδ2 including CP1.15 and DG.SF68	PBMC $\gamma\delta$ T cells stimulated with M. tuberculosis extract	phosphoAg, alkylamines, aminobisphosphonates	Reactivities require cell-cell contact	332,333
Clones 1, 2, 3, 4, 5 (Vδ1)	Lymphocytes extracted from human intestinal epithelial tumors cultured with irradiated CIR-MICA and CIR-MICB cells	MICA, MICB	Transferring TCR transfers reactivity; Vδ1-Jδ1 with diverse CDR3 are used; not all Vδ1-Jδ1 cells are MIC-specific	334,335
JR.2 and XV.1 (Vδ1)	PBL stimulated with autologous $CD1^{+}$ DC and M. tuberculosis extract	CD1c expressing cells	Transferring TCR transfers reactivity; many Vd1 positive gd T cells are not CD1c-reactive	335
Vγ1.3Vδ2 expressing BW5147	gd TCR chains PCR'd from muscle-infiltrating T cells of a polymyositis patient and transfected into TCR-deficient BW5147	Muscle cell extract and E. coli extract		336,337
4-29 and 5-3 (Vδ2 negative)	PBMC from CMV-infected transplant recipients stimulated with irradiated PBMC and PHA	CMV-infected fibroblasts, Hela, HT-29, Caco-2		338

The names of the T cells, the way they are generated and their reported reactivities.

to changes in the glycosylation of the I-E molecule. This suggests a novel way by which antigen recognition by $\gamma\delta$ T cells can be regulated. Changes in the posttranslational modifications of surface glycoproteins often indicate that tissues have become infected, have undergone neoplastic transformations, or have experienced other types of cellular stress. For example, it has been shown that the infection of mice with *Listeria monocytogenes* impairs the addition of sialic acid to host cell glycoproteins that include MHC molecules (282). Additionally, whereas the surface glycoprotein mucin is heavily glycosylated in normal cells, it is under-glycosylated in breast, ovarian, and pancreatic carcinomas, such that the peptide backbone is unmasked *(283)*. Thus, both the quantity and the quality of the ligand could contribute significantly to the specificity of $\gamma\delta$ TCR recognition.

$\gamma\delta$ TCR Ligands

Despite intense efforts, the identification of $\gamma\delta$ TCR ligands has been difficult and confusing. Few "agents" are known to activate $\gamma\delta$ T cells (Table 10.6). Even fewer are known to be both necessary and sufficient to trigger T cell responses through the $\gamma\delta$ TCR and are therefore $\gamma\delta$ TCR antigens. These include the murine MHC class Ib molecules T10 and T22 that are the ligands for 0.2 to 1% of $\gamma\delta$ T cells (274), the human MHC class I–like molecules MICA and MICB (277), and an ATP synthase F1/apolipoprotein A-I (AS/ApoA-I) complex *(156)*.

Significantly, the same human $\gamma\delta$ T cell clones that recognize AS/ApoA-I complexes are activated by a set of nonpeptidic pyrophosphomonoesters that are collectively referred to as *phosphoantigens* (phosphoAgs) (reviewed in [155]). It has been observed for well over a decade that human peripheral blood Vγ9Vδ2 cells can be stimulated by phosphoAgs such as isopentenyl pyrophosphate (IPP) and dimethylallyl pyrophosphate (DMAPP). These cells show *in vitro* responses to tumors, phosphoAgs produced by eukaryotes and prokaryotes, natural and synthetic alkylamines, and aminobisphosphonates. However, repeated attempts to show interactions between phosphoAgs and Vγ9Vδ2 TCRs have failed. The identification of AS/ApoA-I complexes as antigens of some of these T cells further challenges this notion.

As indicated in Table 10.6 *(130)*, other than phosphoAgs, the reactivities of Vγ9Vδ2-expressing T cells to other challenges such as tumors and AS/ApoA-I are far from homogeneous. Further, these cells mount a much more robust response to phosphoAgs than to CD3 crosslinking. Thus, it is possible that IPP and other isoprenoid intermediates enhance antigen-specific responses of Vγ9Vδ2 cells without being TCR antigens themselves. IPP and DMAPP are metabolites of the mevalonate pathway that regulates the biosynthesis of cholesterol, as well as of isoprenoids that mediate the membrane association of certain GTPases. The addition of isoprenoid intermediates has been shown to augment antigen-specific $\alpha\beta$ T cell responses and to alter their cytokine profiles *(284)*.

Antigen Recognition Determinants of $\gamma\delta$ TCRs: V Genes Versus CDR3 Regions in $\gamma\delta$ TCR Ligand Recognition

In part because $\gamma\delta$ T cells from different anatomical sites show preferential V gene expression, $\gamma\delta$ T cells are commonly divided into subsets based on V gene usage *(285,286)*. Numerous studies have also reported that $\gamma\delta$ T cell functions segregate with Vγ, or VγVδ usage *(285–288)*. These observations have led to suggestions that the bias in V gene usage enables $\gamma\delta$ T cells to respond to antigens that are specific to their resident tissues (10,*286*,289). If this were the case, then $\gamma\delta$ TCRs would function like innate immune receptors even though VDJ recombination of the TCR δ chain leads to orders of magnitude higher potential junctional (CDR3 region) diversity than is found in Ig and $\alpha\beta$ TCRs (as discussed previously).

To resolve this issue, it is essential to understand the basis of $\gamma\delta$ TCR antigen recognition. Based on the analysis of T22 specific $\gamma\delta$ T cells isolated from normal mice, the majority of T22-specific $\gamma\delta$ TCRs use Vγ1 and Vγ4 in the spleen and a sizeable number use Vγ7 in the IEL compartment (290). Thus, at least for T22 specificity, Vγ usage reflects tissue origin and not antigen specificity. Consistent with this, it has been demonstrated that the preferential usage of Vγ7 by $\gamma\delta$ T cells that can migrate into the IEL compartment primarily results from IL15-driven control of Vγ7 accessibility during thymic VJ rearrangement (291).

While different Vγs and Vδs were associated with T22-specific TCR sequences, there is one defining feature that is common among them (290). This is a prominent CDR3δ motif shown in Figure 10.14 that consists of a Vδ or Dδ1-encoded Trp (W), a Dδ2-encoded sequence of Ser, Glu, Gly, Tyr, and Glu (SEGYE) and a P-nucleotide-encoded Leu (L). Gene transfer experiments established that TCRs with the W-(S)EGYEL motif bound T22, while those lacking the motif did not ([290] and Table 10.6).

Proof that the W-(S)EGYEL motif is the antigen contact site came from the crystal structure of the G8 $\gamma\delta$ TCR bound to T22 (153). As discussed in the previous section, T22 has an MHC class I–like fold, but one side of what would normally be a peptide-binding groove is severely truncated and exposes the β-sheet "floor" (270). G8 binds T22 at a tilted angle that contrasts with the essentially parallel alignments of the long axes of the $\alpha\beta$ TCR and the peptide/MHC when in complex (Figure 10.15). The majority of the contact residues are contributed by theβ-sheet floor and the α1 helix of T22 and the fully-extended CDR3d loop with Trp anchoring at the N-terminal end and residues Gly,

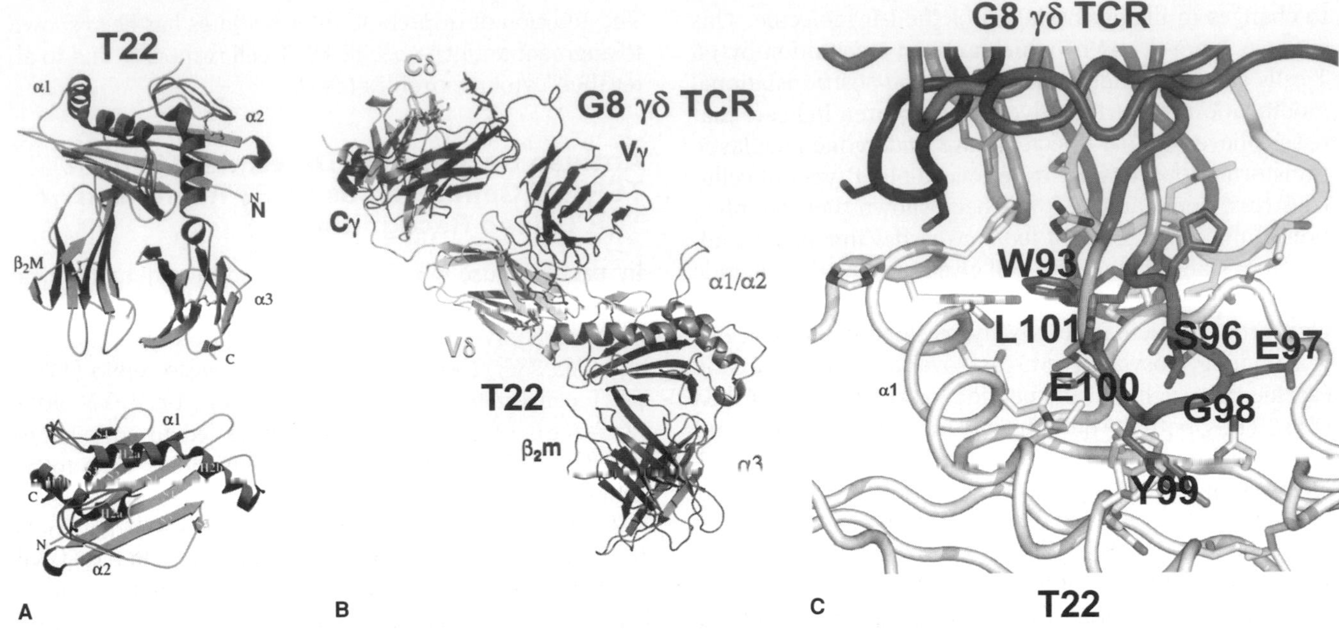

FIGURE 10.14 The T22 structure and the interaction with the G8 $\gamma\delta$ TCR. **A:** The structure of a T22 molecule, a nonclassical class I MHC that is missing half of an alpha helix and does not bind peptides (270). **B, C:** The intersection with the G8 TCR, where the long TCR δ CDR3 accounts for almost all of the contact residues (153). (See color insert.)

	Vδ	P/N	Dδ1 (GTGGCATATCA)	P/N	Dδ2 (ATCGGAGGGATACGAG)	P/N	Jδ1 (CTACCGACAAACTC)
G8	TGT GCT GCT GA C A A D	C AC T	G TGG CAT AT W H I		A TCG GAG GGA TAC GAG S E G Y E	CTC GG L G	T ACC GAC AAA CTC T D K L
KN6	TGT GCC TCG GGG C A S G		TAT Y	TG W	G GAG GGA TAC GAG E G Y E	CTG L	ACC GAC AAA CTC T D K L
Vδ6	TGT GCT CTC TGG GAG CTG C A L W E L	GAG E			TCG GAG GGA TAC GAG S E G Y E	CTC G L A	CC GAC AAA CTC D K L
	TGT GCT CTC TGG GAG CTG C A L W E L	GTT A V M	TG GC A		A TCG GAG GGA TAC GAG S E G Y E	CTA L	ACC GAC AAA CTC T D K L
	TGT GCT CTC TGG GAG CTG C A L W E L		AT I		A TCG GAG GGA TAC GAG S E G Y E	CTA L	ACC GAC AAA CTC T D K L
Vδ4	TGT GCT CTC ATG GAG C A L M E	GGT ATA G I	TGG CAT AT W H I		A TCG GAG GGA TAC GAG S E G Y E	CTT G L A	CT ACC GAC AAA CTC T D K L
	TGT GCT CTC ATG GAG CG C A L M E R	A	AT I		A TCG GAG GGA TAC GAG S E G Y E	CTG GA L D	C GAC AAA CTC D K L
Vδ5	TGT GCC TCG GGG T C A S G S	CC CCC P	CAT AT H I	A TGG CTC GG W L G	A TCG GAG GGA TAC GAG S E G Y E	CTC CTC G L L A	CT ACC GAC AAA CTC T D K L
	TGT GCC TCG GGG TAT C A S G Y	AT M	G TGG W	AGC AT S I	A TCG GAG GGA TAC GAG S E G Y E	CTT G L A	CT ACC GAC AAA CTC T D K L

A

Vγ1	Vδ6	$t_{1/2}$ (min)	K_D (nM)
CAVWI LS GTSWVKIF	CALWEL E SEGYEL A DKL	64 ± 7	12.0 ± 0.5
CAVWI P GTSWVKIF	CALWEL VMA SEGYEL T DKL	86 ± 22	17.2 ± 2.8
CAVWI T GTSWVKIF	CALWEL I SEGYEL T DKL	109 ± 19	13.8 ± 2.8

B

FIGURE 10.15 Conserved TCRδCDR3 sequences correlate with T10/T22 specificity in $\gamma\delta$ T cells. Sequence data from Shin et al. (290) showing that both established cell lines (G8 and KNG) and $\gamma\delta$ T cells from clonal cultures that are specific for the T10/T22 share highly conserved TCRδCDR3 sequences. These are largely derived from the Dδ2 gene segment and from the structural data (Adams et al., color plate 4, 153). These conserved sequences constitute the main interaction between these $\gamma\delta$ T cell receptors and their ligand. (See color insert.)

Tyr, Glu, and Leu together with a Thr residue encoded in the J region anchoring the loop at its C-terminal end. This is similar to Ig, where antigen specificity in nonsomatically mutated antibodies resides predominantly in the CDR3 of the heavy chain (292). This mode of antigen recognition also fits well with analyses of CDR3 length distributions of all immune receptor chains that first suggested that $\gamma\delta$ TCRs bind antigens more similar to Igs than to $\alpha\beta$ TCRs (129).

There are two G8/T22 complexes in the asymmetric unit (153). While the contact residues are similar at the interface of the CDR3/T22 β sheet, the two complexes differ by a relative rotation between the G8 TCRs. This shift alters the contacts formed between the CDR1, CDR2, HV4, and CDR3 loops and T22 in each TCR, suggesting that the CDR3 loop acts as a pivot point for G8 binding, with some flexibility in the interaction between the other CDR loops and T22. The hinge-like flexibility around this pivot point stands in stark contrast to interactions seen in antibody/antigen and $\alpha\beta$ TCR/pMHC complexes. In those cases, the relatively straight-on docking mode results in multipoint (i.e., multi-CDR) attachment of the receptor to the ligand, essentially rigidifying the intermolecular orientations between the two binding partners. In most cases, the $\alpha\beta$ TCR CDR1 and CDR2 loops provide a perimeter of contacts with the MHC helices surrounding the CDR3 loops, and so far, no variation has been seen in the docking angle of TCR to MHC in cases where multiple complexes exist in the asymmetric unit. Thus, the CDR3 motif of G8 and other $\gamma\delta$ TCRs may be thought of as a somewhat autonomous binding entity that is presented by a variety of germline-encoded variable domain scaffolds without strong preference for particular CDR1 and 2 sequences. It would be interesting to see whether these features are present in other examples of $\gamma\delta$ TCR/ligand binding.

CDR3 regions were found to be important for $\gamma\delta$ T cell recognition of MICA/MICB. In this case, the reactivity correlates only with a junction between Vδ1 and Jδ1. Aside from the W-(S)EGYEL motif, the T22-specific CDR3$\gamma\delta$ sequences were diverse and were encoded by various Vδs, N- and P-nucleotides and Dδ1 of different lengths and reading frames. Importantly, it was shown that sequence variations in the CDR3 regions around this motif modulated the affinity and the kinetics of T22 binding (290). In fact, the T22-specific repertoire in normal mice covers a range of affinities, as is evident by the large range of T22 tetramer staining intensities (274,290). This allows for the selection of T cells with the "most optimal" antigen binding capabilities during an immune response, which is a hallmark of the adaptive immune response.

Nonetheless, such a repertoire that is created mainly by V, D, and J region–derived germline-encoded nucleotides, despite requiring VDJ recombination, would be "innate" in character, because the antigen specificities would be predetermined and the repertoire would be much less variable among individuals of the same species.

Analysis of the formation of T10/T22-reactive repertoire indicates that biases linked to the recombination machinery influence the generation of a $\gamma\delta$ T cell repertoire toward certain specificities. A repertoire that is generated by recombination but conferred by a limited set of germline or germline-like residues at the CDR3 region will be created at a much higher frequency than one whose specificity is conferred primarily by N-nucleotide additions, as is the case with that of $\alpha\beta$ TCRs. Indeed, the one in 100 frequency of T22-specific $\gamma\delta$ T cells in normal mice is much higher than the estimated one in 10^5 to 10^6 frequency of naïve peptide/MHC-specific $\alpha\beta$ T cells (293,294,295). This could provide a solution to the apparent paucity of $\gamma\delta$T cells and could allow for a significant response without an initial need for clonal expansion as is required for most $\alpha\beta$ T cell responses. It was shown that rearrangements at the TCR δ locus are biased toward full-length Dδ2 sequences rather than extensive D region nucleotide deletion, as is the case for the TCRβ locus (290). Thus, different reading frames of Dδ2 may contribute to the recognition of other ligands by $\gamma\delta$ TCRs in a manner similar to that of T22-specific $\gamma\delta$ TCRs and would lead to a repertoire that is biased toward a relatively small number of ligands, more on the order of hundreds to thousands versus millions as estimated for $\alpha\beta$ T cells, but with highly variable antigen binding affinities. A repertoire of this type would allow more flexible and efficient responses to changes in ligand expression. These are testable hypotheses, especially once more $\gamma\delta$TCR ligands have been identified.

GENERAL FEATURES OF TCR AND Ig DIVERSITY

A Dominant Role for Diverse CDR3 Regions in Antigen Specificity

One interesting observation that emerges from a detailed analysis of the gene rearrangements that create both T cell receptor and Igs is how the diversity of the CDR3 loop region in one or both of the chains in a given TCR is so much greater than that available to the other CDRs. A schematic of this skewing of diversity is shown in Figure 10.16 for human Igs and for $\alpha\beta$ and $\gamma\delta$ TCR heterodimers. In the case of $\alpha\beta$ TCRs, this concentration of diversity occurs in both Vα and Vβ CDR3 loops, and numerous TCR-pMHC structures (145) have confirmed that these loops sit largely over the center of the antigenic peptide (see previous section). While this concentration of diversity in $\alpha\beta$ TCRs in the regions of principal contact with the many possible antigenic peptides seems reasonable, it is much harder to explain for Ig or $\gamma\delta$ TCRs. Clearly, there must be some chemical or structural "logic" behind this phenomenon. A clue as to what this might be comes from the elegant

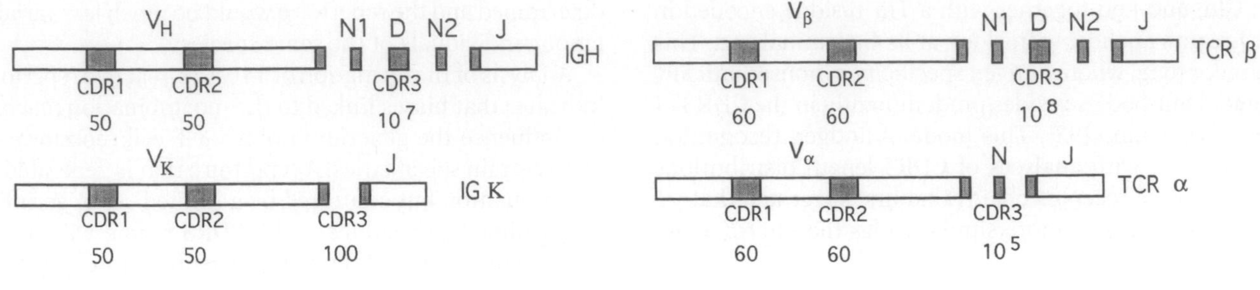

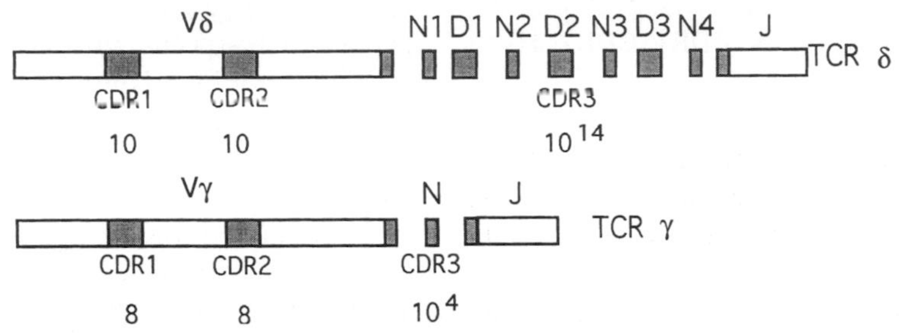

FIGURE 10.16 Diversity "map" of immunoglobulins and T cell receptors; calculated potential for sequence diversity in human antigen receptor molecules (Adams et al., 153). The N region addition is assumed to contribute zero to six nucleotides to the junction of each gene segment, except for immunoglobulin K chains, in which this form of diversity is seldom used.

work of Shin et al. (290) in the demonstration that for at least one $\gamma\delta$ T cell specificity, the antigen recognition determinants are encoded by germline V or D region residues, with remaining sequence diversity modulating the affinity (Figure 10.15). While this may be a feature of some or many $\gamma\delta$ TCRs, it could not explain the much broader repertoire of Igs. Instead, one possible explanation comes from the studies of Wells and colleagues *(266)*, who systematically mutated all of the amino acids (to alanine) at the interface of human growth hormone and its receptor as determined by x-ray crystallography. Interestingly, only a quarter of the 30 or so mutations on either side had any effect on the binding affinity, even in cases where the x-ray structural analysis showed that the amino acid side chains of most of the residues were "buried" in the other. This study illustrates an important caveat to the interpretation of protein crystal structures, which is that although they are invaluable for identifying which amino acids could be important in a given interaction, they rarely show which ones are the most important. This is presumably because the "fit" at that many positions is not "exact" enough to add significant binding energy to the interaction. In this context, we have proposed a new model (296,297) in which the principle antigen specificity of an Ig or TCR is derived from its most diverse CDR3 loops. In the case of antibodies, we imagine that most of the specific contacts (and hence the free energy) with antigen are made by the V_H CDR3 and that the other CDR's provide "opportunistic" contacts that make generally only minor contributions to the energy of binding and specificity. Once antigen has been encountered and clonal selection activates a particular cell, somatic mutation would then "improve" the binding of the CDR1s and 2s to convert the typically low-affinity antibodies to the higher affinity models as observed by Berek and Milstein (121) and also by Patten et al. (122,*298*). As a test of this model, Xu et al. (292) analyzed mice, which have a severely limited Ig V region repertoire, consisting of one V_H and effectively two V_Ls ($V\lambda_1$ and $V\lambda_2$). These mice are able to respond to a wide variety of protein and haptenic antigens, even with this very limited complement of V regions. In several cases, hybridomas specific for very different antigens (e.g., ovalbumin versus DNP) differ only in the V_H CDR3. A limited V region repertoire also seemed no barrier to deriving high-affinity antibodies with somatic mutation, as repeated immunizations produced IgG monoclonals with very high affinities (10^9 to 10^{-10}M). The major immune deficit in these mice was in their inability to produce antibodies to carbohydrates, which may require a special type of binding site or specific V region. Thus, while these experiments only involved one V_H, the results are highly suggestive about the inherent malleability ofV_HV_L in general, at least with respect to protein and haptenic epitopes. With respect to $\alpha\beta$ TCRs we expect that most of the energy of the interaction with a typical ligand will reside in the CDR3-peptide contacts, and here again the CDR1 and 2 regions will make less energetically important contacts. For $\gamma\delta$ TCRs, it is not yet clear whether the T10/T22 specificity (290) is an isolated case or the general rule. From the hypothesis discussed here, if there are $\gamma\delta$ TCRs that use the very large inherent diversity in the Vδ CDR3 directly for antigen recognition, it may be that the lack of somatic mutation forces it to provide more diversity in the initial repertoire (versus Igs).

CONCLUSION

Since T cell receptor genes were first identified in the early 1980s, information about their genetics, biochemistry, structure, and function has accumulated to become a field unto itself. Despite this very real progress, many issues still remain unsolved, such as: What do $\gamma\delta$ T cells normally "see" and what function do they serve? What do superantigens actually do during the course of a normal response and how is this of benefit to the pathogen/parasite? What is the structural/chemical basis of TCR specificity? What rearrangements or conformational charges occur in the TCR/CD3 molecular ensemble upon ligand engagement? These and other questions will require many more years of effort.

ACKNOWLEDGMENTS

We are grateful to M. Call, K. Wucherpfennig, M. Krangel, M. Krogsgaard, and K. C. Garcia for providing some of the figures and tables used here. We also thank M. Kuhns, M. Krogsgaard, Qi-jing Li, and K. C. Garcia for invaluable help with the manuscript, and B. Whyte for expert secretarial assistance. This work was supported by grants from the National Institutes of Health (to MMD and YC) and from the Howard Hughes Medical Institute (to MMD).

REFERENCES

1. Zinkernagel RM, Doherty PC. Immunological surveillance against altered self components by sensitised T lymphocytes in lymphocytic choriomeningitis. *Nature.* 1974;251(5475):547–548.
8. Cheroutre H. IELs: enforcing law and order in the court of the intestinal epithelium. *Immunol Rev*. 2005;206:114–131.
10. Hayday AC. gamma.delta. cells: a right time and a right place for a conserved third way of protection. *Annu Rev Immunol.* 2000;18:975–1026.
11. Havran WL, Jameson JM, Witherden DA. Epithelial cells and their neighbors. III. Interactions between intraepithelial lymphocytes and neighboring epithelial cells. *Am J Physiol Gastrointest Liver Physiol.* 2005;289(4):G627–G630.
12. Chien YH, Jores R, Crowley MP. Recognition by gamma/delta T cells. *Annu Rev Immunol.* 1996;14:511–532.
13. Infante AJ, Infante PD, Gillis S, et al. Definition of T cell idiotypes using anti-idiotypic antisera produced by immunization with T cell clones. *J Exp Med.* 1982;155(4):1100–1107.
14. Allison JP, McIntyre BW, Bloch D. Tumor-specific antigen of murine T-lymphoma defined with monoclonal antibody. *J Immunol.* 1982;129(5):2293–2300.
15. Meuer SC, Fitzgerald KA, Hussey RE, et al. Clonotypic structures involved in antigen-specific human T cell function. Relationship to the T3 molecular complex. *J Exp Med.* 1983;157(2):705–719.
16. Haskins K, Kubo R, White J, et al. The major histocompatibility complex-restricted antigen receptor on T cells. I. Isolation with a monoclonal antibody. *J Exp Med.* 1983;157(4): 1149–1169.
17. Kaye J, Porcelli S, Tite J, et al. Both a monoclonal antibody and antisera specific for determinants unique to individual cloned helper T cell lines can substitute for antigen and antigen-presenting cells in the activation of T cells. *J Exp Med.* 1983;158(3): 836–856.
18. Samelson LE, Germain RN, Schwartz RH. Monoclonal antibodies against the antigen receptor on a cloned T-cell hybrid. *Proc Natl Acad Sci U S A.* 1983;80(22):6972–6976.
19. McIntyre BW, Allison JP. Biosynthesis and processing of murine T-cell antigen receptor. *Cell.* 1984;38(3):659–665.
20. Kappler J, Kubo R, Haskins K, et al. The major histocompatibility complex-restricted antigen receptor on T cells in mouse and man: identification of constant and variable peptides. *Cell.* 1983;35(1):295–302.
21. Davis M, Cohen EA, Nielsen AL, et al. The isolation of B and T cell-specific genes. New York: Academic Press 1982.
22. Hedrick SM, Cohen DI, Nielsen EA, et al. Isolation of cDNA clones encoding T cell-specific membrane-associated proteins. *Nature.* 1984;308(5955):149–153.
23. Hedrick SM, Nielsen EA, Kavaler J, et al. Sequence relationships between putative T-cell receptor polypeptides and immunoglobulins. *Nature.* 1984;308(5955):153–158.
24. Yanagi Y, Yoshikai Y, Leggett K, et al. A human T cell-specific cDNA clone encodes a protein having extensive homology to immunoglobulin chains. *Nature.* 1984;308(5955):145–149.
25. Acuto O, Fabbi M, Smart J, et al. Purification and NH2-terminal amino acid sequencing of the beta subunit of a human T-cell antigen receptor. *Proc Natl Acad Sci U S A.* 1984;81(12):3851–3855.
26. Chien Y, Becker DM, Lindsten T, et al. A third type of murine T-cell receptor gene. *Nature.* 1984;312(5989):31–35.
27. Saito H, Kranz DM, Takagaki Y, et al. A third rearranged and expressed gene in a clone of cytotoxic T lymphocytes. *Nature.* 1984;312(5989):36–40.
28. Saito H, Kranz DM, Takagaki Y, et al. Complete primary structure of a heterodimeric T-cell receptor deduced from cDNA sequences. *Nature.* 1984;309(5971):757–762.
29. Brenner MB, McLean J, Dialynas DP, et al. Identification of a putative second T-cell receptor. *Nature.* 1986;322(6075):145–149.
30. Chien YH, Iwashima M, Kaplan KB, et al. A new T-cell receptor gene located within the alpha locus and expressed early in T-cell differentiation. *Nature.* 1987;327(6124):677–682.
31. Dembic Z, Haas W, Weiss S, et al. Transfer of specificity by murine alpha and beta T-cell receptor genes. *Nature.* 1986;320(6059): 232–238.
32. Saito T, Weiss A, Miller J, et al. Specific antigen-Ia activation of transfected human T cells expressing murine Ti alpha beta-human T3 receptor complexes. *Nature.* 1987;325(7000):125–130.
33. Havran WL, Chien YH, Allison JP. Recognition of self antigens by skin-derived T cells with invariant gamma delta antigen receptors. *Science.* 1991;252(5011):1430–1432.
35. Brenner MB, McLean J, Scheft H, et al. Two forms of the T-cell receptor gamma protein found on peripheral blood cytotoxic T lymphocytes. *Nature.* 1987;325(6106):689–694.
37. Saint-Ruf C, Ungewiss K, Groettrup M, et al. Analysis and expression of a cloned pre-T cell receptor gene. *Science.* 1994;266(5188): 1208–1212.
39. Call ME, Wucherpfennig KW. THE T CELL RECEPTOR: Critical Role of the Membrane Environment in Receptor Assembly and Function. *Annu Rev Immunol.* 2005;23:101–125.
41. Klausner RD, Lippincott-Schwartz J, Bonifacino JS. The T cell antigen receptor: insights into organelle biology. *Annu Rev Cell Biol.* 1990;6:403–431.

49. Clevers H, Alarcon B, Wileman T, et al. The T cell receptor/CD3 complex: a dynamic protein ensemble. *Annu Rev Immunol.* 1988;6:629–662.
50. Sun ZJ, Kim KS, Wagner G, et al. Mechanisms contributing to T cell receptor signaling and assembly revealed by the solution structure of an ectodomain fragment of the CD3 epsilon gamma heterodimer. *Cell.* 2001;105(7):913–923.
51. Sun ZY, Kim ST, Kim IC, et al. Solution structure of the CD3epsilondelta ectodomain and comparison with CD3epsilon-gamma as a basis for modeling T cell receptor topology and signaling. *Proc Natl Acad Sci U S A.* 2004;101(48):16867–16872.
52. Kjer-Nielsen L, Dunstone MA, Kostenko L, et al. Crystal structure of the human T cell receptor CD3 epsilon gamma heterodimer complexed to the therapeutic mAb OKT3. *Proc Natl Acad Sci U S A.* 2004;101(20):7675–7680.
54. Xu C, Call ME, Wucherpfennig KW. A Membrane-proximal Tetracysteine Motif Contributes to Assembly of CD3{delta}{epsilon} and CD3{gamma}{epsilon} Dimers with the T Cell Receptor. *J Biol Chem.* 2006;281(48):36977–36984.
55. Call ME, Pyrdol J, Wiedmann M, et al. The organizing principle in the formation of the T cell receptor-CD3 complex. *Cell.* 2002;111(7):967–979.
58. Alarcon B, Ley SC, Sanchez-Madrid F, et al. The CD3-gamma and CD3-delta subunits of the T cell antigen receptor can be expressed within distinct functional TCR/CD3 complexes. *Embo J.* 1991;10(4):903–912.
60. Reth M. Antigen receptor tail clue. *Nature.* 1989;338(6214):383–384.
63. Kuhns MS, Davis MM, Garcia KC. Deconstructing the Form and Function of the TCR/CD3 Complex. *Immunity.* 2006;24(2):133–139.
70. Fernández-Miguel G, Alarcón B, Iglesias A, et al. Multivalent structure of an alphabetaT cell receptor. *Proc Natl Acad Sci U S A.* 1999;96(4):1547–1552.
71. Schamel WW, Risueno RM, Minguet S, et al. A conformation- and avidity-based proofreading mechanism for the TCR-CD3 complex Trends Immunol. 2006;27(4):176–182.
72. Hayes SM, Laky K, El-Khoury D, et al. Activation-induced modification in the CD3 complex of the gammadelta T cell receptor. *J Exp Med.* 2002;196(10):1355–1361.
73. Hayes SM, Love PE. Stoichiometry of the murine {gamma}{delta} T cell receptor. *J Exp Med.* 2006.
74. Chien YH, Gascoigne NR, Kavaler J, et al. Somatic recombination in a murine T-cell receptor gene. *Nature.* 1984;309(5966):322–326.
78. Krangel MS. Gene segment selection in V(D)J recombination: accessibility and beyond. *Nat Immunol.* 2003;4(7):624–630.
79. Fujimoto S, Yamagishi H. Isolation of an excision product of T-cell receptor alpha-chain gene rearrangements. *Nature.* 1987;327(6119):242–243.
80. Okazaki K, Davis DD, Sakano H. T cell receptor beta gene sequences in the circular DNA of thymocyte nuclei: direct evidence for intramolecular DNA deletion in V-D-J joining. *Cell.* 1987;49(4):477–485.
81. Heilig JS, Tonegawa S. Diversity of murine gamma genes and expression in fetal and adult T lymphocytes. *Nature.* 1986;322(6082):836–840.
82. Elliott JF, Rock EP, Patten PA, et al. The adult T-cell receptor delta-chain is diverse and distinct from that of fetal thymocytes. *Nature.* 1988;331(6157):627–631.
83. Hata S, Satyanarayana K, Devlin P, et al. Extensive junctional diversity of rearranged human T cell receptor delta genes. *Science.* 1988;240(4858):1541–1544.
84. Raulet DH. The structure, function, and molecular genetics of the gamma/delta T cell receptor. *Annu Rev Immunol.* 1989;7:175–207.
85. de Villartay JP, Lewis D, Hockett R, et al. Deletional rearrangement in the human T-cell receptor alpha-chain locus. *Proc Natl Acad Sci U S A.* 1987;84(23):8608–8612.
86. Villey I, Caillol D, Selz F, et al. Defect in rearrangement of the most 5′ TCR-J alpha following targeted deletion of T early alpha (TEA): implications for TCR alpha locus accessibility. *Immunity.* 1996;5(4):331–342.
89. Chou HS, Nelson CA, Godambe SA, et al. Germline organization of the murine T cell receptor beta-chain genes. *Science.* 1987;238(4826):545–548.
90. Woodland DL, Kotzin BL, Palmer E. Functional consequences of a T cell receptor D beta 2 and J beta 2 gene segment deletion. *J Immunol.* 1990;144(1):379–385.
91. Vernooij BT, Lenstra JA, Wang K, et al. Organization of the murine T-cell receptor gamma locus. *Genomics.* 1993;17(3):566–574.
92. Garman RD, Doherty PJ, Raulet DH. Diversity, rearrangement, and expression of murine T cell gamma genes. *Cell.* 1986;45(5):733–742.
93. LeFranc MP, Forster A, Baer R, et al. Diversity and rearrangement of the human T cell rearranging gamma genes: nine germ-line variable genes belonging to two subgroups. *Cell.* 1986;45(2):237–246.
95. Lefranc MP, Forster A, Rabbitts TH. Genetic polymorphism and exon changes of the constant regions of the human T-cell rearranging gene gamma. *Proc Natl Acad Sci U S A.* 1986;83(24):9596–9600.
96. Raulet DH. The structure, function, and molecular genetics of the gamma/delta T cell receptor. *Annu Rev Immunol.* 1989;7(1):175–207.
97. Havran WL, Allison JP. Developmentally ordered appearance of thymocytes expressing different T-cell antigen receptors. *Nature.* 1988;335(6189):443–445.
98. Yancopoulos GD, Alt FW. Regulation of the assembly and expression of variable-region genes. *Annu Rev Immunol.* 1986;4:339–368.
101. Hawwari A, Krangel MS. Regulation of TCR delta and alpha repertoires by local and long-distance control of variable gene segment chromatin structure. *J Exp Med.* 2005;202(4):467–472.
102. Hawwari A, Bock C, Krangel MS. Regulation of T cell receptor alpha gene assembly by a complex hierarchy of germline Jalpha promoters. *Nat Immunol.* 2005;6(5):481–489.
103. Abarrategui I, Krangel MS. Regulation of T cell receptor-alpha gene recombination by transcription. *Nat Immunol.* 2006;7(10):1109–1115.
104. McDougall S, Peterson CL, Calame K. A transcriptional enhancer 3′ of C beta 2 in the T cell receptor beta locus. *Science.* 1988;241(4862):205–208.
105. Krimpenfort P, de Jong R, Uematsu Y, et al. Transcription of T cell receptor beta-chain genes is controlled by a downstream regulatory element. *Embo Journal.* 1988;7(3):745–750.
110. Winoto A, Baltimore D. Alpha beta lineage-specific expression of the alpha T cell receptor gene by nearby silencers. *Cell.* 1989;59(4):649–655.
111. Diaz P, Cado D, Winoto A. A locus control region in the T cell receptor alpha/delta locus. *Immunity.* 1994;1(3):207–217.
112. Ishida I, Verbeek S, Bonneville M, et al. T-cell receptor gamma delta and gamma transgenic mice suggest a role of a gamma gene silencer in the generation of alpha beta T cells. *Proc Natl Acad Sci U S A.* 1990;87(8):3067–3071.
113. Spencer DM, Hsiang YH, Goldman JP, et al. Identification of a T-cell-specific transcriptional enhancer located 3′ of C gamma 1 in the murine T-cell receptor gamma locus. *Proc Natl Acad Sci U S A.* 1991;88(3):800–804.
114. Baker JE, Kang J, Xiong N, et al. A novel element upstream of the Vgamma2 gene in the murine T cell receptor gamma locus cooperates with the 3′ enhancer to act as a locus control region. *J Exp Med.* 1999;190(5):669–679.
115. Xiong N, Kang C, Raulet DH. Redundant and unique roles of two enhancer elements in the TCRgamma locus in gene regulation and gammadelta T cell development. *Immunity.* 2002;16(3):453–463.
116. Uematsu Y, Ryser S, Dembic Z, et al. In transgenic mice the introduced functional T cell receptor beta gene prevents expression of endogenous beta genes. *Cell.* 1988;52(6):831–841.
118. Malissen M, Trucy J, Jouvin-Marche E, et al. Regulation of TCR alpha and beta gene allelic exclusion during T-cell development. *Immunology Today.* 1992;13(8):315–322.
119. Aifantis I, Buer J, von Boehmer H, et al. Essential role of the pre-T cell receptor in allelic exclusion of the T cell receptor beta locus published erratum appears in Immunity 1997 Dec;7(6):following 895. *Immunity.* 1997;7(5):601–607.
120. O'Shea CC, Thornell AP, Rosewell IR, et al. Exit of the pre-TCR from the ER/cis-Golgi is necessary for signaling differentiation, proliferation, and allelic exclusion in immature thymocytes. *Immunity.* 1997;7(5):591–599.
121. Berek C, Milstein C. The dynamic nature of the antibody repertoire. *Immunol Rev.* 1988;105:5–26.

122. Patten PA, Gray NS, Yang PL, et al. The immunological evolution of catalysis. *Science*. 1996;271(5252):1086–1091.
123. van der Merwe PA, Barclay AN. Transient intercellular adhesion: the importance of weak protein-protein interactions. Trends in Biochemical. Sciences. 1994;19(9):354–358.
125. Valitutti S, Muller S, Cella M, et al. Serial triggering of many T-cell receptors by a few peptide-MHC complexes. *Nature*. 1995;375(6527):148–51.
126. Davis MM, Huse M, Lillemeier BF. T Cells as a Self-Referential Sensory Organ. *Annu Rev Immunol*. 2007;25:681–695
129. Rock EP, Sibbald PR, Davis MM, CDR3 length in antigen-specific immune receptors. *J Exp Med*. 1994;179(1):323–328.
145. Rudolph MG, Stanfield RL, Wilson IA. How TCRs bind MHCs, peptides, and coreceptors. *Annu Rev Immunol*. 2006;24:419–466.
146. Bentley GA, Boulot G, Karjalainen K, et al. Crystal structure of the beta chain of a T cell antigen receptor see comments. *Science*. 1995;267(5206):1984–1987.
147. Fields BA, Ober B, Malchiodi EL, et al. Crystal structure of the V alpha domain of a T cell antigen receptor. *Science*. 1995;270(5243):1821–1824.
149. Garboczi DN, Ghosh P, Utz U, et al. Structure of the complex between human T-cell receptor, viral peptide and HLA-A2. *Nature*. 1996;384(6605):134–141.
150. Garcia KC, Degano M, Stanfield RL, et al. An alphabeta T cell receptor structure at 2.5 A and its orientation in the TCR–MHC complex see comments. *Science*. 1996;274(5285):209–219.
152. Allison TJ, Winter CC, Fournie JJ, et al. Structure of a human gammadelta T-cell antigen receptor. *Nature*. 2001;411(6839):820–824.
153. Adams EJ, Chien YH, Garcia KC. Structure of a gamma delta T cell receptor in complex with the nonclassical MHC T22. *Science*. 2005;308(5719):227–231.
154. Li H, Lebedeva MI, Llera AS, et al. Structure of the Vdelta domain of a human gammadelta T-cell antigen receptor. *Nature*. 1998;391(6666):502–506.
155. Bonneville M, Fournie JJ. Sensing cell stress and transformation through Vgamma9Vdelta2 T cell-mediated recognition of the isoprenoid pathway metabolites. *Microbes Infect*. 2005;7(3):503–509.
157. Lin AY, Devaux B, Green A, et al. Expression of T cell antigen receptor heterodimers in a lipid-linked form. *Science*. 1990;249(4969):677–679.
165. Kozono H, White J, Clements J, et al. Production of soluble MHC class II proteins with covalently bound single peptides. *Nature*. 1994;369(6476):151–154.
166. Matsui K, Boniface JJ, Reay PA, et al. Low affinity interaction of peptide-MHC complexes with T cell receptors. *Science*. 1991;254(5039):1788–1791.
167. Weber S, Traunecker A, Oliveri F, et al. Specific low-affinity recognition of major histocompatibility complex plus peptide by soluble T-cell receptor. *Nature*. 1992;356(6372):793–796.
169. Krogsgaard M, Prado N, Adams EJ, et al. Evidence that structural rearrangements and/or flexibility during TCR binding can contribute to T cell activation. *Mol Cell*. 2003;12(6):1367–1378.
173. Boniface JJ, Reich Z, Lyons DS, et al. Thermodynamics of T cell receptor binding to peptide-MHC: evidence for a general mechanism of molecular scanning. *Proc Natl Acad Sci U S A*. 1999;96(20):11446–11451.
177. Matsui K, Boniface JJ, Steffner P, et al. Kinetics of T-cell receptor binding to peptide/I-Ek complexes: correlation of the dissociation rate with T-cell responsiveness. *Proc Natl Acad Sci U S A*. 1994;91(26):12862–12866.
178. Lyons DS, Lieberman SA, Hampl J, et al. A TCR binds to antagonist ligands with lower affinities and faster dissociation rates than to agonists. *Immunity*. 1996;5(1):53–61.
179. Alam SM, Travers PJ, Wung JL, et al. T-cell-receptor affinity and thymocyte positive selection. *Nature*. 1996;381(6583):616–620.
180. Kessler BM, Bassanini P, Cerottini JC, et al. Effects of epitope modification on T cell receptor-ligand binding and antigen recognition by seven H-2Kd-restricted cytotoxic T lymphocyte clones specific for a photoreactive peptide derivative. *J Exp Med*. 1997;185(4):629–640.
181. Holler PD. CD8(−) T cell transfectants that express a high affinity T cell receptor exhibit enhanced peptide-dependent activation. *J Exp Med*. 2001;194(8):1043–1052.
183. Aivazian D, Stern LJ. Phosphorylation of T cell receptor zeta is regulated by a lipid dependent folding transition. *Nat Struct Biol*. 2000;7(11):1023–1026.
184. Qi S, Krogsgaard M, Davis MM, et al. Molecular flexibility can influence the stimulatory ability of receptor-ligand interactions at cell-cell junctions. *Proc Natl Acad Sci U S A*. 2006;103(12):4416–4421.
185. McKeithan TW. Kinetic proofreading in T-cell receptor signal transduction. *Proc Natl Acad Sci U S A*. 1995;92(11):5042–5046.
186. Rabinowitz JD, Beeson C, Lyons DS, et al. Kinetic discrimination in T-cell activation. *Proc Natl Acad Sci U S A*. 1996;93(4):1401–1405.
188. Stefanova I, Hemmer B, Vergelli M, et al. TCR ligand discrimination is enforced by competing ERK positive and SHP-1 negative feedback pathways. *Nat Immunol*. 2003;4(3):248–254.
189. Altan-Bonnet G, Germain RN. Modeling T cell antigen discrimination based on feedback control of digital ERK responses. *PLoS Biol*. 2005;3(11):e356.
190. Viola A, Lanzavecchia A. T cell activation determined by T cell receptor number and tunable thresholds. *Science*. 1996;273(5271):104–106.
191. Holler PD, Lim AR, Cho BK, et al. CD8(−) T cell transfectants that express a high affinity T cell receptor exhibit enhanced peptide-dependent activation. *J Exp Med*. 2001;194(8):1043–1052.
192. Krogsgaard M, Li QJ, Sumen C, et al. Agonist/endogenous peptide-MHC heterodimers drive T cell activation and sensitivity. *Nature*. 2005;434(7030):238–243.
193. Davis MM, Bjorkman PJ. T-cell antigen receptor genes and T-cell recognition published erratum appears in Nature 1988 Oct 20;335(6192):744. *Nature*. 1988;334(6181):395–402.
194. Engel I, Hedrick SM. Site-directed mutations in the VDJ junctional region of a T cell receptor beta chain cause changes in antigenic peptide recognition. *Cell*. 1988;54(4):473–484.
195. Katayama CD, Eidelman FJ, Duncan A, et al. Predicted complementarity determining regions of the T cell antigen receptor determine antigen specificity. *Embo J*. 1995;14(5):927–938.
196. Jorgensen JL, Esser U, Fazekas de St Groth B, et al. Mapping T-cell receptor-peptide contacts by variant peptide immunization of single-chain transgenics. *Nature*. 1992;355(6357):224–230.
197. Sant'Angelo DB, Waterbury G, Preston-Hurlburt P, et al. The specificity and orientation of a TCR to its peptide-MHC class II ligands. *Immunity*. 1996;4(4):367–376.
198. Jorgensen JL, Reay PA, et al. Molecular components of T-cell recognition. *Annu Rev Immunol*. 1992;10(6357):835–873.
199. Ehrich EW, Devaux B, Rock EP, et al. T cell receptor interaction with peptide/major histocompatibility complex (MHC) and superantigen/MHC ligands is dominated by antigen. *J Exp Med*. 1993;178(2):713–722.
201. Nanda NK, Arzoo KK, Geysen HM, et al. Recognition of multiple peptide cores by a single T cell receptor. *J Exp Med*. 1995;182(2):531–539.
202. Mason D. A very high level of crossreactivity is an essential feature of the T-cell receptor. *Immunol Today*. 1998;19(9):395–404.
203. Maynard J, Petersson K, Wilson DH, et al. Structure of an autoimmune T cell receptor complexed with class II peptide-MHC: insights into MHC bias and antigen specificity. *Immunity*. 2005;22(1):81–92.
204. Wilson DB, Pinilla C, Wilson DH, et al. Immunogenicity. I. Use of peptide libraries to identify epitopes that activate clonotypic CD4+ T cells and induce T cell responses to native peptide ligands. *J Immunol*. 1999;163(12):6424–6434.
205. Huseby ES, Crawford F, White J, et al. Interface-disrupting amino acids establish specificity between T cell receptors and complexes of major histocompatibility complex and peptide. *Nat Immunol*. 2006;7(11):1191–1199.
206. Yachi PP, Ampudia J, Gascoigne NR, et al. Nonstimulatory peptides contribute to antigen-induced CD8-T cell receptor interaction at the immunological synapse. *Nat Immunol*. 2005;6(8):785–792.
207. Chien YH, Davis MM. How alpha beta T-cell receptors "see" peptide/MHC complexes. *Immunol Today*. 1993;14(12):597–602.
208. Garcia KC, Degano M, Pease LR, et al. Structural basis of plasticity in T cell receptor recognition of a self peptide-MHC antigen. *Science*. 1998;279(5354):1166–1172.

209. Reiser JB, Gregoire C, Darnault C, et al. A T cell receptor CDR3beta loop undergoes conformational changes of unprecedented magnitude upon binding to a peptide/MHC class I complex. *Immunity*. 2002;16(3):345–354.
210. Reinherz EL, Tan K, Tang L, et al. The crystal structure of a T cell receptor in complex with peptide and MHC class II. *Science*. 1999;286(5446):1913–1921.
211. Willcox BE, Gao GF, Wyer JR, et al. TCR binding to peptide-MHC stabilizes a flexible recognition interface. *Immunity*. 1999;10(3): 357–365.
212. Wu LC, Tuot DS, Lyons DS, et al. Two-step binding mechanism for T-cell receptor recognition of peptide MHC. *Nature*. 2002; 418(6897):552–556.
213. Tynan FE, Burrows SR, Buckle AM, et al. T cell receptor recognition of a 'super-bulged' major histocompatibility complex class I-bound peptide. *Nat Immunol*. 2005;6(11):1114–1122.
214. Janeway CA, Jr. The T cell receptor as a multicomponent signalling machine: CD4/CD8 coreceptors and CD45 in T cell activation. *Annu Rev Immunol*. 1992;10:645–674.
217. Irvine DJ, Purbhoo MA, Krogsgaard M, et al. Direct observation of ligand recognition by T cells. *Nature*. 2002;419(6909):845–849.
218. Purbhoo MA, Irvine DJ, Huppa JB, et al. T cell killing does not require the formation of a stable mature immunological synapse. *Nat Immunol*. 2004;5(5):524–530.
219. Wulfing C, Sumen C, Sjaastad MD, et al. Costimulation and endogenous MHC ligands contribute to T cell recognition. *Nat Immunol*. 2002;3(1):42–47.
223. Hampl J, Chien YH, Davis MM. CD4 augments the response of a T cell to agonist but not to antagonist ligands. *Immunity*. 1997;7(3):379–385.
224. Madrenas J, Chau LA, Smith J, et al. The efficiency of CD4 recruitment to ligand-engaged TCR controls the agonist/partial agonist properties of peptide-MHC molecule ligands. *Journal of Experimental Medicine*. 1997;185(2):219–229.
225. Marrack P, Kappler J. The staphylococcal enterotoxins and their relatives. *Science*. 1990;248(4959):1066.
226. Sundberg EJ, Li Y, Mariuzza RA. So many ways of getting in the way: diversity in the molecular architecture of superantigen-dependent T-cell signaling complexes. *Curr Opin Immunol*. 2002;14(1): 36–44.
227. Festenstein H. Immunogenetic and biological aspects of in vitro lymphocyte allotransformation (MLR) in the mouse. *Transplant Rev*. 1973;15:62–88.
228. Kappler JW, Staerz U, White J, et al. Self-tolerance eliminates T cells specific for Mls-modified products of the major histocompatibility complex. *Nature*. 1988;332(6159):35–40.
229. Woodland DL, Happ MP, Gollob KJ, et al. An endogenous retrovirus mediating deletion of alpha beta T cells? *Nature*. 1991;349(6309): 529–530.
230. Marrack P, Kushnir E, Kappler J. A maternally inherited superantigen encoded by a mammary tumour virus. *Nature*. 1991;349(6309):524–526.
231. Choi Y, Kappler JW, Marrack P. A superantigen encoded in the open reading frame of the 3′ long terminal repeat of mouse mammary tumour virus. *Nature*. 1991;350(6315):203–207.
232. Dyson PJ, Knight AM, Fairchild S, et al. Genes encoding ligands for deletion of V beta 11 T cells cosegregate with mammary tumour virus genomes. *Nature*. 1991;349(6309):531–532.
233. Frankel WN, Rudy C, Coffin JM, et al. Linkage of Mls genes to endogenous mammary tumour viruses of inbred mice. *Nature*. 1991;349(6309):526–528.
234. Janeway CA, Jr., Yagi J, Conrad PJ, et al. T-cell responses to Mls and to bacterial proteins that mimic its behavior. *Immunol Rev*. 1989;107:61–88.
235. McDonald KR, Acha-Orbea H. Superantigens of mouse mammary tumor virus. *Annu Rev Immunol*. 1995;13:459.
236. Li H, Llera A, Malchiodi EL, et al. The structural basis of T cell activation by superantigens. *Annu Rev Immunol*. 1999;17:435–466.
247. Held W, Waanders GA, Shakhov AN, et al. Superantigen-induced immune stimulation amplifies mouse mammary tumor virus infection and allows virus transmission. *Cell*. 1993;74(3):529–540.
248. Golovkina TV, Chervonsky A, Dudley JP, et al. Transgenic mouse mammary tumor virus superantigen expression prevents viral infection. *Cell*. 1992;69(4):637–645.
249. Stauffer Y, Marguerat S, Meylan F, et al. Interferon-induced endogenous superantigen: a model linking envionment and autoimmunity. *Immunity*. 2001;15:591–601.
250. Dalwadi H, Wei B, Kronenberg M, et al. The Crohn's disease-associated bacterial protein I2 is a novel enteric t cell superantigen. *Immunity*. 2001;15(1):149–158.
251. Malchiodi EL, Fields BA, Ohlendorf DH, et al. Superantigen binding to a T cell receptor of known three-dimensional structure. *J Exp Med*. 1995;182:1833.
252. Patten PA, Sonoda T, Fazekas de St. Groth B, et al. Transfer of putative CD$ loops of T cell receptor V domains confers toxin reactivity, but not peptide specificity. *J Immunol*. 1993;150:2281–2294.
253. Fields BA, Malchiodi EL, Li H, et al. Crystal structure of a T-cell receptor beta-chain complexed with a superantigen. *Nature*. 1996;384(6605):188–192.
254. Li Y, Li H, Dimasi N, et al. Crystal structure of a superantigen bound to the high-affinity, zinc-dependent site on MHC class II. *Immunity*. 2001;14(1):93–104.
255. Petersson K, Nilsson H, Forsberg G, et al. Crystal structure of a superantigen bound to MHC class II displays zinc and peptide dependence. *EMBO*. 2001;20:3306–3312.
256. Fields BA, Li HM, Ysern X, et al. Crystal structure of the β chain of a T-cell receptor complexed wth a superantigen. *Nature*. 1996;384: 188.
258. Bjorkman PJ, Saper MA, Samraoui B, et al. Structure of the human class I histocompatibility antigen, HLA-A2. *Nature*. 1987;329(6139):506–512.
260. Brown JH, Jardetzky TS, Gorga JC, et al. Three-dimensional structure of the human class II histocompatibility antigen HLA-DR1. *Nature*. 1993;364(6432):33–39.
263. Schild H, Mavaddat N, Litzenberger C, et al. The nature of major histocompatibility complex recognition by gamma delta T cells. *Cell*. 1994;76(1):29–37.
270. Wingren C, Crowley MP, Degano M, et al. Crystal structure of a gammadelta T cell receptor ligand T22: a truncated MHC-like fold. *Science*. 2000;287(5451):310–314.
271. Rudolph MG, Wingren C, Crowley MP, et al. Combined pseudo-merohedral twinning, non-crystallographic symmetry and pseudo-translation in a monoclinic crystal form of the gammadelta T-cell ligand T10. *Acta Crystallogr D Biol Crystallogr*. 2004;60(Pt 4):656–664.
274. Crowley MP, Fahrer AM, Baumgarth N, et al. A population of murine gammadelta T cells that recognize an inducible MHC class Ib molecule. *Science*. 2000;287(5451):314–316.
275. Weintraub BC, Jackson MR, Hedrick SM. Gamma delta T cells can recognize nonclassical MHC in the absence of conventional antigenic peptides. *J Immunol*. 1994;153(7):3051–3058.
276. Sciammas R, Bluestone JA. HSV-1 glycoprotein I-reactive TCR gamma delta cells directly recognize the peptide backbone in a conformationally dependent manner. *J Immunol*. 1998;161(10):5187–5192.
277. Wu J, Groh V, Spies T. T cell antigen receptor engagement and specificity in the recognition of stress-inducible MHC class I-related chains by human epithelial gamma delta T cells. *J Immunol*. 2002;169(3):1236–1240.
282. Villanueva MS, Beckers CJ, Pamer EG. Infection with Listeria monocytogenes impairs sialic acid addition to host cell glycoproteins. *J Exp Med*. 1994;180(6):2137–2145.
289. Janeway CA, Jr., Jones B, Hayday A. Specificity and function of T cells bearing gamma delta receptors. *Immunol Today*. 1988;9(3): 73–76.
290. Shin S, El-Diwany R, Schaffert S, et al. Antigen recognition determinants of gammadelta T cell receptors. *Science*. 2005;308(5719):252–255.

291. Zhao H, Nguyen H, Kang J. Interleukin 15 controls the generation of the restricted T cell receptor repertoire of gamma delta intestinal intraepithelial lymphocytes. *Nat Immunol*. 2005;6(12):1263–1271.
292. Xu JL, Davis MM. Diversity in the CDR3 region of V(H) is sufficient for most antibody specificities. *Immunity*. 2000;13(1):37–45.
294. McHeyzer-Williams MG, Altman JD, Davis MM. Enumeration and characterization of memory cells in the TH compartment. *Immunol Rev*. 1996;150:5–21.
296. Davis MM, Lyons DS, Altman JD, et al. T cell receptor biochemistry, repertoire selection and general features of TCR and Ig structure. *Ciba Found Symp*. 1997;204:94–100; discussion 4.
297. Davis MM. The evolutionary and structural 'logic' of antigen receptor diversity. *Semin Immunol*. 2004;16(4):239–243.
299. Kuhns MS, Davis MM. Disruption of extracellular interactions impairs T Cell Receptor-CD3 complex stability and signaling. *Immunity*. 2007;26:357–369.

Chapter 11

T Lymphocyte Signaling Mechanisms and Activation

Gary A. Koretzky

INTRODUCTION

Protection of the host from the universe of potential pathogens requires a rapid, dynamic, and flexible immune system capable of responding to organisms that are evolving to escape immune detection. The most rapid responders are cells of the innate immune system that recognize patterns commonly present on pathogens but absent on host cells. Cells of the adaptive immune system (T and B lymphocytes) are generally slower to respond but are equally essential for host protection, as lymphocytes are uniquely able to recognize subtle differences between self and non-self. This chapter focuses on how T cells sense their environment and mount the appropriate response when challenges are detected. Several essential tenets of T cell biology are discussed, including how T cells recognize antigen, the biochemical consequences of this recognition event, what signals beyond antigen recognition are required for T cells to be stimulated to respond, how the T cell response is terminated once the pathogenic challenge has been met, how an appropriate T cell response might go awry, and how knowledge regarding these critical processes has led to therapeutic modalities to treat immune-mediated disorders.

THE ANTIGEN-BINDING COMPONENT OF THE T CELL ANTIGEN RECEPTOR COMPLEX

Similar to immunoglobulin (Ig) (see Chapters 4 and 6), the antigen-binding component of the receptor expressed on T cells (T cell antigen receptor, or TCR) is composed of the products of rearranging gene segments (1). In most T cells, these proteins are present as an $\alpha\beta$ disulphide-linked heterodimer; however, a minority of T cells express instead a related dimer that is the product of rearranged γ and δ genes (see Chapter 10). The combinatorial rearrangement of multiple gene segments, the error-prone process of joining these different DNA segments, and the various combinations of α with β or γ with δ lead to tremendous diversity of the TCRs, enabling these receptors to respond to the universe of antigens that pathogens present.

Much more is understood about the biology of $\alpha\beta$ T cells compared to their $\gamma\delta$ T cell counterparts; however, it is clear that there are major differences in where these cell types reside in the body and in the antigens that stimulate their activation. As described more fully in Chapter 10, $\gamma\delta$ T cells respond most often to lipid antigens presented by CD1 (a major histocompatibility complex [MHC]–like molecule), while classical $\alpha\beta$ T cells respond to peptide antigens presented within MHC. $\gamma\delta$ T cells are found largely in epithelial and mucosal barriers and to a lesser extent in secondary lymphoid organs, where $\alpha\beta$ T cells reside. The remainder of this chapter focuses on $\alpha\beta$ T cells. For a fuller description of the biology of $\gamma\delta$ T cells, see Chapters 12 and 13 and reference (2).

T cell precursors arise in the bone marrow and then home to and mature in the thymus (3). Early in T cell ontogeny (at the double-negative three [DN3] stage in the thymus; see Chapter 12), the gene segments of the β chain of the TCR rearrange. Because this is a stochastic event and will often lead to a nonfunctional protein, the cell must pass a checkpoint (β selection) to move forward through development. β selection requires that the newly rearranged gene product indicate that it is correctly assembled by stimulating a biochemical change in the cell. It is not known precisely what this biochemical signal is; however, many of the key signaling proteins discussed later in this chapter have been demonstrated to be required for β selection to occur. It appears that at this stage in T cell development, the β chain is only signaling its appropriate formation and conformation and is not tested for antigen reactivity, as the ligand-binding region of the receptor is not essential for β selection to proceed (4). Successful β selection leads to silencing of the other TCR β allele (allelic exclusion), protection of the cell from apoptosis, cell division, and differentiation into CD4/CD8 double-positive thymocytes. Failed signaling results in rearrangement of the other allele, testing of that β chain, and either developmental progression, if productively rearranged, or cell death.

THE CD3 CHAINS ARE CRITICAL FOR SURFACE EXPRESSION OF THE TCR

Cells that move beyond the DN3 stage in the thymus rearrange their TCR α chains as they become double-positive thymocytes preparing for positive and negative selection. For development beyond this checkpoint, appropriate antigen recognition is required; therefore, the $\alpha\beta$ heterodimers must be transported to the cell surface. This surface expression cannot occur without coexpression of the CD3 chains (5), a collection of protein dimers ($\gamma\varepsilon$, $\delta\varepsilon$, and $\zeta\zeta$) that associate with α and β. Neither the CD3 nor $\alpha\beta$ dimers can be expressed on the cell surface in isolation, because the partner proteins are needed to mask charged residues or sequences that target the isolated proteins for degradation (6). It is this same $\alpha\beta$-CD3 complex (henceforth referred to as the *TCR complex*) that is essential for antigen recognition and signal transduction by mature T cells in the periphery (Figure 11.1A).

Once the components of the TCR complex were discovered, a great deal of work was undertaken to determine the roles of the α and β chains versus the CD3 molecules. Given that α and β arise from Ig-like rearranging gene segments, it seemed plausible that these components of the TCR complex were responsible for antigen recognition. This role was proven formally by the transfection of cDNAs encoding α and β chains from one T cell clone into another, resulting in transfer of reactivity to both peptide antigen and MHC sequences (7). Not only did this experiment demonstrate the role of the $\alpha\beta$ heterodimer, but it also cemented the notion that there is a single receptor for antigen plus MHC, ending a long controversy in the field of T cell biology.

Understanding the role of the CD3 molecules was more difficult. It seemed likely that these proteins were responsible for signal transduction—that is, informing the inside of the cell that an antigen recognition event (mediated by the α and β chains) had taken place. This notion was suggested by the observation that antibodies directed against CD3 proteins elicited the same T cell activation events as did stimulation of T cells with peptide antigen plus MHC. Additionally, it was known that the $\alpha\beta$ proteins

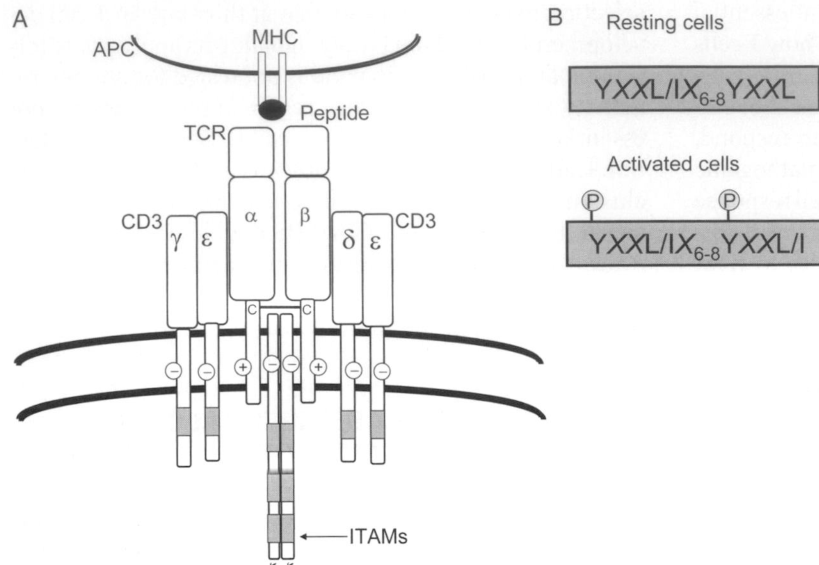

FIGURE 11.1 Structure of the T cell antigen receptor/CD3 complex and the immunoreceptor tyrosine-based activation motifs. **A:** The T cell antigen receptor (TCR) is a complex of proteins that includes a disulfide-linked dimer ($\alpha\beta$) that binds peptide antigen and MHC. There is an obligatory, noncovalent association of $\alpha\beta$ with a series of protein dimers ($\gamma\varepsilon$, $\delta\varepsilon$, and $\zeta\zeta$) collectively known as CD3. The association between $\alpha\beta$ and CD3 is mediated in part by charged residues within the transmembrane domains of each receptor component. Adapted from Janeway CA, et al. *Immunobiology*. 6th ed. New York: Garland Science, 2005. **B:** Within the cytoplasmic domains of the CD3 molecules are stretches of amino acids known as ITAMs (immunoreceptor tyrosine-based activated motifs) that are critical for signal transduction. In resting cells, the tyrosines within the ITAMs are nonphosphorylated; however, following TCR engagement, these residues become phosphorylated and then are able to bind to other proteins.

possess very short cytoplasmic tails, making it difficult to imagine how signals could be initiated by ligation of these molecules, whereas the CD3 proteins each possess a large number of cytoplasmic amino acids. However, it was difficult to prove the role for CD3, given that these molecules could not be expressed in isolation, without α and β. Investigators turned to cell line model systems (in particular the Jurkat T cell leukemic and BW5147 mouse T cell lymphoma lines) as an initial approach to unravel the biochemical events that occurred when the TCR complex was engaged. These cell lines were particularly useful, because they can be grown in large numbers and are genetically stable (eliminating donor to donor variation), yet can be genetically manipulated for both loss and gain of function experiments. Although the precise antigen specificity of the TCRs expressed on these cell lines was not known, it was possible to stimulate T cell responses using agonistic monoclonal antibodies, directed against the TCR complex. Importantly, the lessons learned about the molecular and biochemical signals critical for receptor ligation to be translated into downstream biologic functions from these cell line studies (with rare but notable exceptions) have been confirmed using primary cells from murine or human sources (8).

Critical tools for the earliest studies that deciphered the role of the CD3 chains were variants of the Jurkat and BW5147 cell lines that lacked surface expression of the TCR complex. Once it became clear that the impediment for cell surface expression of the CD3 molecules in the absence of $\alpha\beta$ was due to sequences that targeted the incomplete complexes for degradation, it was possible to engineer CD3 mutants that could be transported to the membrane without other TCR components. Several groups created artificial receptors that were constructed by fusing irrelevant extracellular domains and transmembrane domains (e.g., from the CD8 protein) to the cytoplasmic domain of one of the CD3 molecules, enabling stable expression without other elements of the TCR. When such chimeric receptors were expressed on T cells lacking the TCR, it was shown that binding the extracellular domains of these molecules was sufficient to activate the same biochemical second messengers that are stimulated when the intact TCR binds antigen (9,10). These model systems led to a subsequent series of structure/function studies, demonstrating conclusively that the signal transduction capacity of the TCR rests within specialized domains within the cytoplasmic domains of the CD3 molecules, the immunoreceptor tyrosine-based activation motifs, or ITAMs (Figure 11.1B).

ITAMS AND PROXIMAL SIGNALS MEDIATED BY THE TCR

ITAMs were first discovered as signature sequences that appeared in cell surface molecules on immune cells (11). ITAM-containing proteins that regulate immune responses include the CD3 chains and similar proteins associated with the B cell antigen receptor (the Ig-α [CD79α] and Ig-β [CD79β] molecules), different classes of Fc receptors, and adapter proteins (e.g., DAP10 or DAP12) associated with MHC recognition molecules on natural killer (NK) cells. ITAMs are defined by the presence of a tyrosine residue followed by two amino acids, then a leucine or isoleucine, followed again by a spacer of 6 to 8 unspecified amino acids, then another tyrosine, a 2 amino acid spacer, followed by a leucine or isoleucine ($YXXL/IX_{6-8}YXXL/I$) (12). Each of the CD3 γ, δ, and ε molecules contain a single ITAM, while each ζ chain possesses three ITAMs in tandem. Mutagenesis of the CD3 molecules prior to transfection into the TCR-deficient cell lines revealed that the most critical features of the ITAMs are the two tyrosines and the spacing between them (13).

As the CD3 complex is composed of two ζ chains (each with three ITAMS), two ε chains, one γ chain, and one δ chain (each with a single ITAM), there are 10 ITAMs associated with each TCR complex. The reason for this large collection of signaling modules associated with the receptor is unclear. It has been proposed that the various ITAMs couple differentially to unique biochemical pathways or that the multiple ITAMs are necessary for signal amplification. To date, however, there is no definitive evidence to support these or other models for the role of the large number of signaling modules associated with the TCR. Although ITAMs are found in all hematopoietic cell types, this strategy for coupling receptors to signaling pathways is not widespread in other nonhematopoietic lineages. Although ITAMs are found in ERM (ezrin, radixin, moesin) proteins, which are expressed not only in immune cells but also in most other tissues, the role of the motif in the function of this family of proteins has not yet been established (14). Additionally, ITAMs have been reported to be expressed in neuronal tamalin, a cytoplasmic protein that is recruited to the membrane in activated cells (15). ITAMs also appear in proteins of pathogenic viruses that infect cells of the immune system, allowing these viruses to coopt the signaling machinery of their target cells (16).

Concurrent with the studies that identified the different roles of the various components of the TCR complex were other experiments designed to uncover the biochemical signals elicited by TCR engagement that are critical for T cell activation. Biochemical, genetic, and pharmacologic approaches established that the most proximal event associated with TCR ligation is the activation of protein tyrosine kinases (PTKs), including the following: fyn and lck, two members of the src PTK family (17); ZAP-70 (ζ chain-associated protein of 70 kDa), a syk (spleen tyrosine kinase) family PTK (18); and at least two members of the tec family, ITK (interleukin [IL]-2-induced tyrosine kinase) and RLK (receptor-like kinase) (19). As the importance of PTKs for T cell activation became clear, attention refocused on the CD3 ITAMs and their essential tyrosines. Studies revealed that upon TCR engagement, the CD3 ITAM tyrosines rapidly become phosphorylated. It was shown further that once phosphorylated, these tyrosines become docking sites for proteins that possess src homology 2 (SH2) domains (canonical sequences found in a wide spectrum of proteins that allow for phosphotyrosine binding) and that the critical binder to the phospho-ITAMs is ZAP-70, a PTK critical for T cell activation. These studies and others led to a model (20) suggesting that upon binding of antigen/MHC to the TCR, a conformational change occurs making the CD3 ITAMs susceptible to phosphorylation by lck and/or fyn, allowing for recruitment of activated ZAP-70 to the complex (Figure 11.2). Exactly how ligand binding induces such a conformational change and the precise character of this change have not yet been established, but it is clear that an essential event in initiating a T cell response is for the TCR complex to be converted from an enzymatically inactive structure to one that is associated with active PTK function.

Ample evidence now exists for the essential role played by src, syk, and tec family PTKs in signal transduction mediated via the TCR complex and in subsequent T cell development and/or activation. This evidence has come from experiments making use of cell lines (in particular, variants of the Jurkat line) that have been selected for TCR signaling abnormalities (21,22), mice in which genes for these PTKs have been targeted for deletion or mutation (23,24), and naturally arising mutations in humans that lead to severe immune disorders (25). Loss of fyn has a more minor phenotype than loss of lck in both cell line models and in deficient mice, as lck loss results in a severe block in thymocyte development *in vivo*, whereas peripheral T cells appear in nearly normal numbers in fyn-deficient animals, suggesting that T cell development can occur in the absence of this PTK. Inducible lck deletion in peripheral T cells leads to T cells that fail to be activated upon TCR engagement, similar to what is seen in an lck-deficient Jurkat variant (26). In contrast, fyn-deficient T cells can transduce signals via their TCR, and early reports suggested that only minor functional defects were present (23). More recently, though, rigorous studies of fyn-deficient mice have revealed abnormalities in effector T cell functions, including skewing of T helper (Th) subsets and cytokine production (27,28). Double deficiency of both lck and fyn leads to a complete block of T cell development in mice, with the absence of any cells beyond the DN3 stage in the thymus (29,30), indicating that Fyn can compensate, albeit suboptimally, for the absence of Lck.

ZAP-70 deficiency also results in a severe TCR signaling block in cell lines (nearly all second messenger cascades normally stimulated by the TCR are absent [22]), and ZAP-70–deficient mice demonstrate a block in T cell development at the CD4/CD8 double-positive stage in the thymus (31). Interestingly, the defect in ZAP-70–deficient mice is not as pronounced as that in the fyn/lck double-deficient animals, suggesting that another PTK can compensate, at least partially, in the absence of ZAP-70 prior to the DP stage. Follow-up studies suggest that syk, the other member of this PTK family, is present in developing thymocytes and that mice lacking both syk and ZAP-70 phenocopy the lck/fyn double-deficient animals (32).

The importance of these PTKs for development and function of human T cells has been documented with the description of patients with mutations in lck or ZAP-70. One individual with virtually no T cell function has been identified as having a mutation in lck (33). A number of individuals deficient in ZAP-70 have also been described. These patients have no peripheral $CD8^+$ T cells. Although $CD4^+$ T cells are present, they fail to respond to TCR engagement (34). It is intriguing that the same genetic

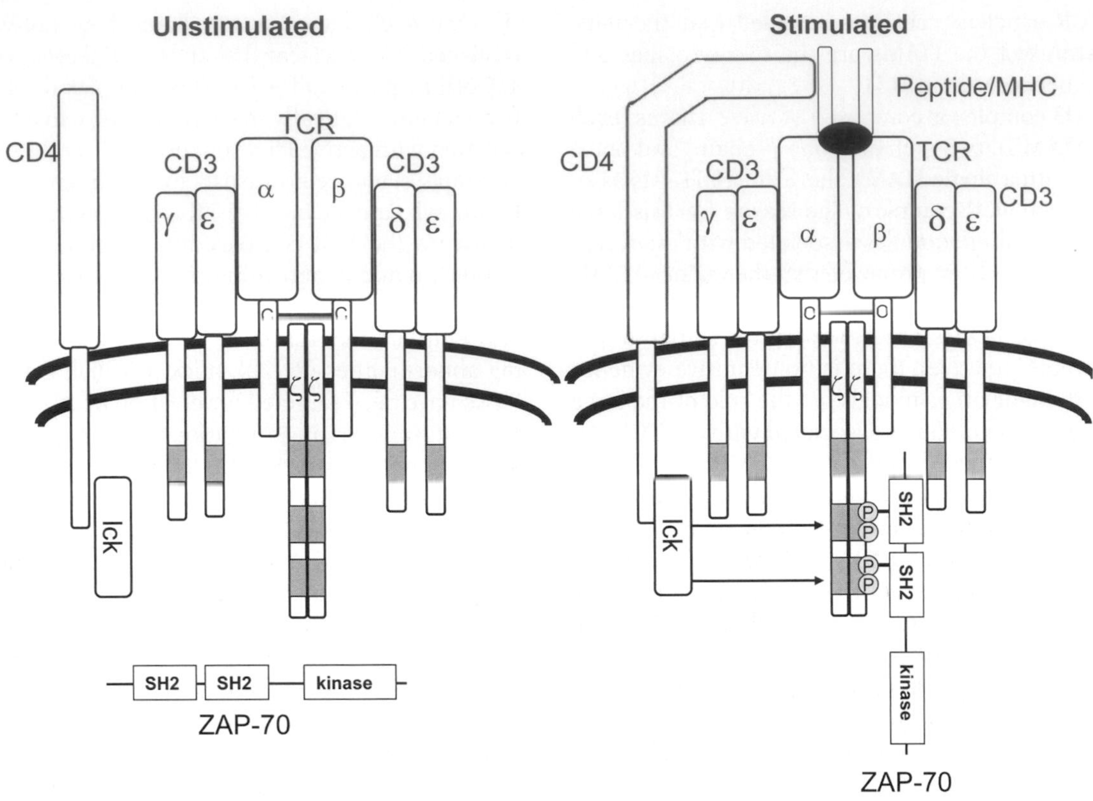

FIGURE 11.2 TCR complex stimulation induces tyrosine phosphorylation of the CD3 ITAMs and recruitment of effector molecules. In unstimulated T cells, the ITAMs within the CD3 chains are not phosphorylated, and ZAP-70 is present in the cytosol. The CD4 coreceptor (bound to lck) is present at the membrane, but not in close proximity to the CD3 ITAMs. Upon engagement of the TCR with peptide/MHC, CD4/lck is brought into the vicinity of the bound TCR due to the interaction of CD4 with nonpolymorphic residues of MHC. This results in the tyrosine phosphorylation of the CD3 ITAMs by lck and recruitment of ZAP-70 to the engaged receptor via the ZAP-70 SH2 domains. The enzymatically inactive receptor on the resting T cell is thus converted to an active PTK (protein tyrosine kinase).

alteration (ZAP-70 deficiency) in mice and humans does not result in the exact same T cell phenotype, underscoring the idea that, although often excellent model systems, studies of mice can only suggest but not conclusively prove mechanisms by which human T cells function. The importance of ZAP-70 expression in human disease has recently been demonstrated further with studies profiling gene expression in malignant cells from patients with chronic lymphocytic leukemia (CLL). The expression of ZAP-70 is a marker of a more aggressive form of the disease (35,36). Experiments are currently underway to determine the molecular basis for why ZAP-70 expression in these B cell leukemias leads to more severe disease.

As both src and syk family PTKs function in the most proximal step of the TCR signaling pathway (i.e., phosphorylation of and recruitment of ZAP-70 to the CD3 ITAMs), it is not surprising that deficiency of these proteins has a marked effect on TCR complex function. In contrast, the tec family PTKs (ITK and RLK) function later in the TCR complex signaling cascade (discussed later) and therefore have a more subtle effect on T cell development. As such, in the absence of ITK or RLK, secondary lymphoid organs are populated with nearly normal numbers of T cells, and assays of T cell activation, while showing mild impairment, are much closer to normal than what is seen in the absence of lck or ZAP-70 (37,38). However, when ITK- or RLK-deficient (and even more so when ITK/RLK double-deficient) mice are challenged with pathogens *in vivo,* the T cell response is markedly abnormal, most obviously in responses that require differentiation of $CD4^+$ T cells into Th1 versus Th2 subsets (19). It is virtually certain that as mice deficient in tec kinases are examined with greater scrutiny, additional defects in T cell function will be revealed.

THE REGULATION OF TCR-STIMULATED PTK ACTIVITY

The simplest model for how the TCR makes use of src, syk, and tec family PTKs for T cell activation is that upon TCR engagement, lck or fyn are activated and phosphorylate the CD3 ITAMs. Both lck and fyn are positioned strategically to enable them to act upon the CD3 molecules. Fyn co-immunoprecipitates with CD3, suggesting a close association even in resting cells (39), and lck is associated with the cytoplasmic domains of both CD4 and CD8 (40). CD4 binds to conserved residues of MHC class II, and CD8 binds similarly to MHC class I (see Chapter 20). Thus, as the TCR comes into contact with an antigen/MHC complex, both fyn and lck are available to catalyze ITAM phosphorylation. This phosphorylation allows for the recruitment of ZAP-70, which in turn phosphorylates multiple substrates, eventually recruiting a number of key signaling molecules, including ITK and RLK, into a larger activation complex.

While there is a great deal of experimental evidence to support this model of sequential activation of PTKs, additional data suggest that while this general scheme is correct, there is also considerable cross-talk between the PTKs that makes their regulation more complex. Hence, it appears that the PTKs are substrates of each other and that kinases originally thought to act only downstream of particular activation events may also influence their upstream activators. There is a great deal of current work examining the tyrosines of the src, syk, and tec PTKs that are phosphorylated, as mounting evidence points to phosphorylation of specific residues having significant effects (positive or negative) on PTK function and the ultimate T cell response (41,42). Ongoing studies, again using cell lines with mutations in the PTKs and mice in which specific residues have been altered within the genome, will certainly shed light into the intricate regulation of each of these critical signaling molecules.

As the importance of tyrosine phosphorylation for TCR-induced T cell activation was becoming appreciated, additional work was focusing on other T cell proteins. One of the most abundant surface antigens present on all immune cells is CD45, a transmembrane molecule that was shown to have potent protein tyrosine phosphatase activity (43). With this discovery, the notion developed that CD45 most likely functioned as a negative regulator of TCR signaling, as it was reasoned that CD45 would reverse the TCR-stimulated tyrosine phosphorylation events. CD45-deficient cell lines were established, with the expectation that these cells would exhibit uninhibited TCR function. The CD45-deficent cells were examined, and the result of these experiments was exactly the opposite of the predictions: T cells without CD45 failed to signal via their TCR (44,45). These studies indicated that CD45 was, in fact, a required positive regulator of T cell activation. An explanation for this surprising result came from studies demonstrating that a key substrate for CD45 is a tyrosine residue in the carboxyl-terminal region of src family kinases (46), a tyrosine that, when phosphorylated, diminishes the ability for the PTK to function. Thus, the model arose for CD45 being permissive for TCR-stimulated lck or fyn activation by dephosphorylating a tyrosine that would otherwise impede src family PTK function (Figure 11.3).

Although there is a single gene for CD45, there are multiple isoforms expressed on the surface of immune cells, due to alternative splicing of exons that comprise the extracellular domain of this transmembrane phosphatase (47). The importance of these alternative forms of CD45 is suggested by the fact that their expression is highly regulated and that different forms of CD45 predominate in cells with different functions (e.g., resting versus activated or memory T cells). The appreciation of the regulated expression of the different isoforms led to an intensive search for ligands that are specific for the different CD45 splice variants, the results of which remain elusive. It was suggested that the extracellular domains of CD45 contain signals important for dimerization of the phosphatase, an event that is speculated to alter the ability of CD45 to dephosphorylate substrates (either through changing enzymatic activity or substrate availability) (48). Support for this notion comes from a study of mice with a mutation of CD45 knocked into the locus that is predicted to interrupt CD45

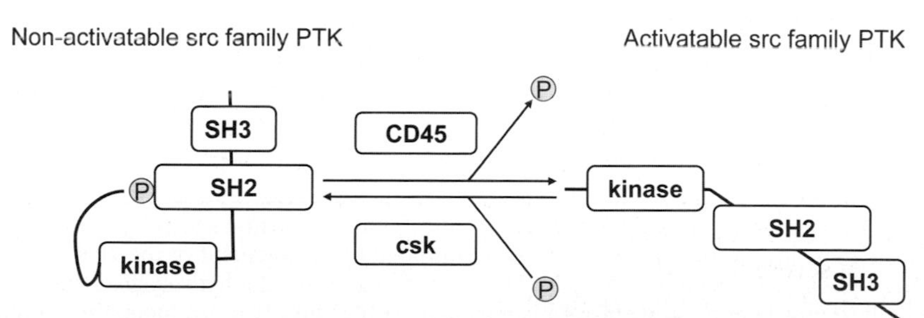

FIGURE 11.3 Dynamic regulation of src family PTKs by a kinase and a phosphatase. Src family PTKs possess a carboxyl-terminal tyrosine that, when phosphorylated, mediates an intramolecular interaction that diminishes enzymatic activity. Phosphorylation of this tyrosine is highly regulated, being mediated by the kinase csk (carboxy-terminal Src kinase) and its dephosphorylation by the phosphatase CD45. When dephosphorylated, src PTKs adopt a more open conformation that is permissive for their activation. This feature of src PTK control makes CD45 an essential positive regulator of T cell activation and csk an effective inhibitor.

dimerization (49). Mice expressing this CD45 mutant exhibit autoimmunity, suggesting unimpeded activation of immune cells. This idea has been extended to human immune-mediated diseases with the recent description of polymorphisms of the CD45 gene being correlated with multiple sclerosis, autoimmune hepatitis, and other autoimmune disorders (50). Exactly how these alterations in the gene translate into abnormal CD45 function remains to be determined.

Given the importance of the carboxyl-terminal tyrosine of src family PTKs as a controller of kinase activity, it is not surprising that phosphorylation (in addition to dephosphorylation) of this residue is a regulated event. Csk (carboxyl-terminal src kinase) opposes the action of CD45 by catalyzing the phosphorylation of this inhibitory tyrosine (51) (Figure 11.3). Thus, one means to control the likelihood that engagement of the TCR will result in T cell activation is how csk versus CD45 action is balanced. Exactly how this balance is accomplished appears to rest in large part on where in the cell CD45 and csk reside and which enzyme is found in proximity to the src PTKs. This subcellular localization of the src PTK regulators is a complex process that involves a chaperone protein for csk (discussed later) and regulated movement of CD45 before and during TCR engagement.

SIGNALS DOWNSTREAM OF THE PTKs

The discovery of the essential role played by PTKs for T cell activation was followed by a search for substrates of these PTKs in an effort to understand how activation of these kinases leads ultimately to T cell effector function. Among these substrates are key components of several signal transduction pathways known to be essential for activation of multiple cellular lineages. One of the critical second messenger cascades is initiated when the TCR-stimulated PTKs phosphorylate and activate phospholipase C $\gamma 1$ (PLC$\gamma 1$), an enzyme that hydrolyzes the membrane phospholipid phosphatidylinositol-1,4-bisphosphate (PIP_2) into a soluble sugar, inositol-1,4,5-trisphosphate (IP_3), and the lipid diacylglycerol (DAG) (52) (Figure 11.4). IP_3

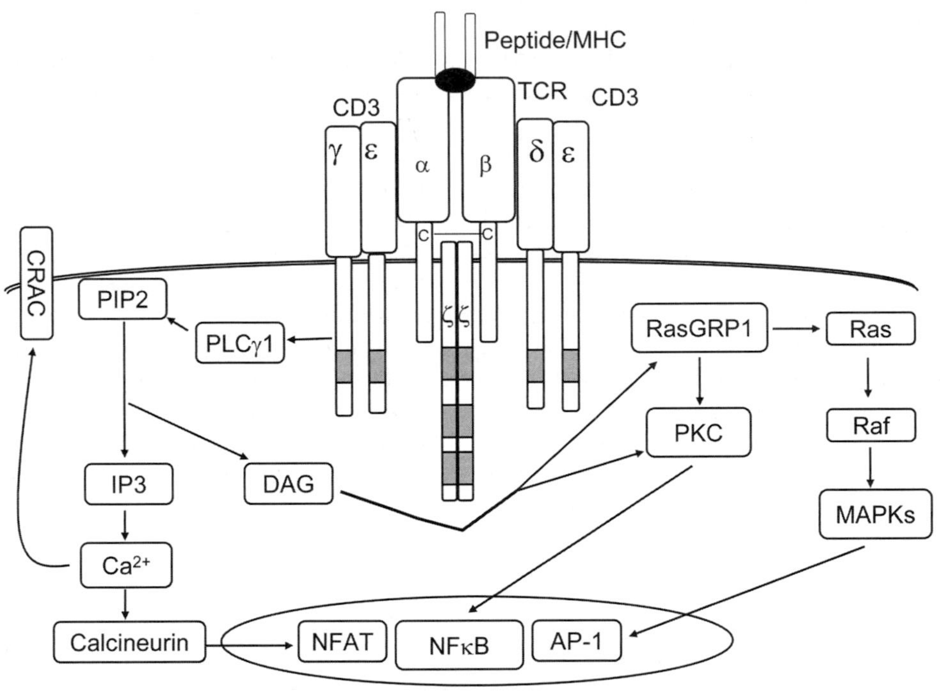

FIGURE 11.4 Binding of the TCR initiates the phosphatidyl inositol second messenger cascade. One of the most important signaling pathways initiated by engagement of the TCR begins by activation of phospholipase c $\gamma 1$ (PLC$\gamma 1$). This enzyme catalyzes the hydrolysis of the membrane phospholipid phosphatidylinositol-1,4-bisphosphate (PIP2) into two products, the soluble sugar inositol-1,4,5-triphosphate (IP3) and the lipid diacylglycerol (DAG). IP3 interacts with its receptor on the endoplasmic reticulum causing a release of intracellular calcium. Increased cellular calcium activates a calcium-regulated calcium channel (CRAC) and calcium-dependent enzymes such as calcineurin, a phosphatase that dephosphorylates nuclear factor of activated T cells (NFAT), allowing this transcription factor to enter the nucleus. DAG activates members of the protein kinase C (PKC) family and the Ras signaling pathway via the Ras exchange factor, RasGRP1. PKCs activate the NFκB transcription factor, and a Ras-stimulated kinase cascade including Raf and members of the mitogen-activated protein kinase (MAPK) family activates activator protein-1 (AP-1).

binds to its receptor on the endoplasmic reticulum (ER), causing a release of calcium from this organelle.

The increase in cytosolic free calcium in TCR-stimulated cells occurs in two phases. The initial burst in calcium release from the ER (mediated by the interaction between IP_3 and its receptor) is followed by a more sustained increase in calcium that is mediated by activation of a calcium-regulated membrane channel designated *CRAC* (calcium release-activated calcium channel) (53). While it was clear that such a channel existed and that its function was essential for T cell activation to occur and be sustained, the identity of this channel until recently was a mystery. Studies of a patient with severe combined immunodeficiency coupled with a novel genetic screen demonstrated that at least one CRAC component critical for T cell activation is the product of the *orai1* gene, a transmembrane protein found in multiple cell lineages (54). This discovery is one of many examples of how investigators, studying human immune disorders, have added to our fundamental knowledge of the mechanisms by which immune cells translate antigen receptor occupancy to an effector immune response. Experiments are now underway to determine the molecular nature of the entire channel and its mode of regulation.

TCR-mediated increases in cellular calcium activate several calcium-dependent enzymes, including the serine phosphatase calcineurin (55). When activated, calcineurin dephosphorylates nuclear factor of activated T cells (NFAT), allowing NFAT to leave the cytosol and enter the nucleus, where it cooperates with other transcription factors to stimulate expression of key T cell activation-associated genes (56). NFAT activation is terminated by kinases in the nucleus that phosphorylate the transcription factor, leading to its nuclear export back to the cytosol (57,58). In the cytosol, it can again be dephosphorylated by calcineurin and transported back to the nucleus, if the appropriate activation conditions are still in place. The key role that calcineurin and the NFAT pathway play in T cell activation is underscored by the efficacy of cyclosporine, a pharmacologic inhibitor of this pathway, as a clinically important immunosuppressive agent (59).

The other hydrolysis product of PIP_2, DAG, is also critical for T cell activation (Figure 11.4). DAG functions by binding to specialized motifs on several other proteins, including members of the protein kinase C (PKC) family and RasGRP1, a guanine nucleotide exchange factor (GEF) for the small molecular weight GTP-binding protein Ras (60). DAG binding activates the PKCs and promotes the ability of RasGRP1 to allow Ras to release GDP and bind GTP (61). PKCs phosphorylate several key substrates (discussed later), while activated Ras stimulates yet another series of kinases. These kinases include Raf and different members of the mitogen-activated protein kinase (MAPK) family (62). Collectively these signals are integrated, leading to the activation of other transcription factors critical for initiating the genetic program for T cell activation. Among these key transcription factors are the AP-1 (activator protein-1) complex (that cooperates with NFAT) and members of the NFκB family (63).

Although much has been learned about TCR signal transduction, many of the details regarding the molecular events critical for its activation remain unknown. For example, although it has been shown that the src family PTK fyn associates directly with CD3 components and that the src PTK lck is brought into the activation complex via the association of lck with the important coreceptors CD4 and CD8, exactly how ligand binding to the TCR α and β chains is translated into increased enzymatic activity of the src PTKs is unclear. Additionally, it is not known if activation of the src PTKs is sufficient for CD3 ITAM phosphorylation or if other TCR-mediated events are required. For example, it has been argued that ligand binding to the TCR induces a conformational change in the entire TCR complex, making the CD3 ITAMs susceptible to phosphorylation by lck and/or fyn; however, a detailed explanation of this conformational change has not yet been provided and remains an important area for future discovery.

HEMATOPOIETIC-SPECIFIC ADAPTER PROTEINS ARE CRITICAL FOR T CELL ACTIVATION

Insights into how TCR-stimulated PTK activation initiates the PLC signaling cascade arose from the discovery of two adapter proteins: linker of activated T cells (LAT) (64) and SH2 domain-containing leukocyte-specific phosphoprotein of 76 kDa (SLP-76) (65) (Figure 11.5). Adapter proteins are molecules that possess no intrinsic catalytic activity but act as scaffolds to create multimolecular complexes, bridging receptors with their downstream effector molecules. LAT is a transmembrane protein that resides largely in lipid rafts, membrane microdomains enriched in cholesterol, due to palmitoylation of two cytoplasmic cysteines within the juxtamembrane region of LAT (66). Upon TCR ligation, LAT becomes tyrosine phosphorylated on multiple residues, providing docking sites for other proteins that possess SH2 domains. Among the proteins that bind to phosphorylated LAT are effector molecules (e.g., PLCγ1) and phosphatidylinositol 3-kinase (PI3K), a lipid kinase that activates a cascade of important second messengers. While TCR engagement appears to simulate the PI3K pathway, ligation of coreceptors on T cells, in particular CD28, is much more effective at initiating this signaling cascade and is discussed in more detail later in this chapter. Phosphorylated LAT also associates with the SH2 domain of growth factor receptor binding protein 2 (Grb2), an adapter molecule that binds constitutively to son of sevenless (SOS), a GEF that allows Ras to bind to GTP. Although Grb2/Sos appears less important than RasGRP1

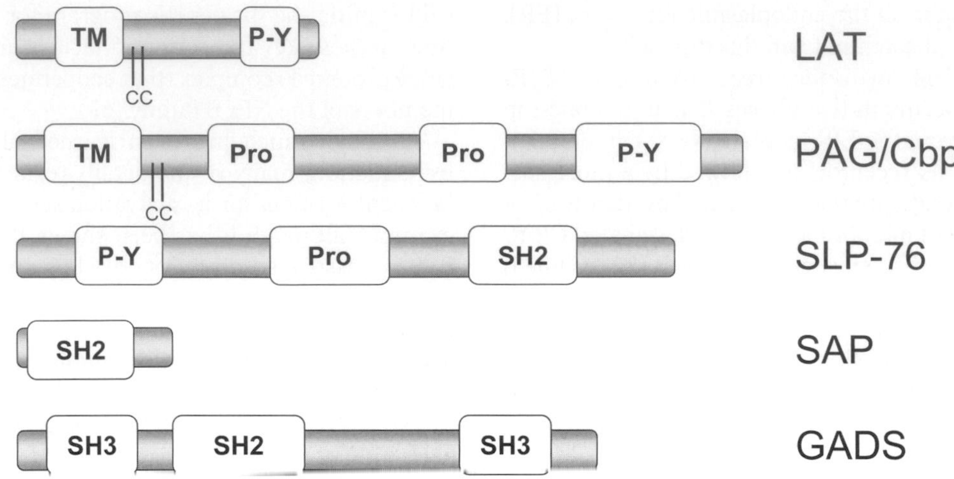

FIGURE 11.5 Adapter molecules are proteins that contain modular domains that function by mediating interactions with other molecules in the cell. Shown here are several adapters (not drawn to scale) mentioned in the text, containing some but not all of the possible protein interaction domains. Src homology 2 (SH2) domains mediate interactions with other proteins phosphorylated on tyrosine residues, SH3 domains associate with other proteins that are rich in proline residues, proline-rich regions (Pro) bind to other proteins with SH3 domains, and residues that are themselves substrates of protein tyrosine kinases (P-Y) allow for interactions with other proteins that possess SH2 domains. Some adapters are cytosolic, while others possess transmembrane domains (TM), allowing their insertion into the plasma membrane. These adapters may also possess juxtamembrane cysteines (C) that are posttranslationally modified for targeting to lipid rafts within the membrane (see text for details). LAT, linker for activated T cells; PAG/Cbp, phosphoprotein associated with glycosphingolipid-enriched domains/csk-binding protein; SLP-76, SH2 domain-containing leukocyte-specific phosphoprotein of 76 kDa; SAP, SLAM-associated protein; GADS, Grb2-related adapter downstream of Shc.

for Ras activation in T cells, genetic studies indicate that this pathway is important for optimal T cell function (67). When phosphorylated, LAT inducibly associates with another member of the Grb2 family, Grb2-related adapter downstream of Shc (Gads) (68). The LAT/Gads interaction is critical, because Gads binds constitutively to SLP-76 (69).

Like LAT, SLP-76 is a hematopoietic-specific adapter molecule. SLP-76 possesses three functional domains: an amino-terminal region that becomes phosphorylated upon TCR engagement and inducibly binds to other proteins with SH2 domains, a central proline-rich region allowing it to bind to proteins with src homology 3 (SH3) domains constitutively, and a carboxyl-terminal SH2 domain allowing SLP-76 to bind to other proteins that are themselves phosphorylated on tyrosines (70). In resting cells, SLP-76 associates with Gads in the cytosol. Upon TCR engagement and LAT phosphorylation, the SLP-76/Gads complex is recruited to LAT (and lipid rafts). Because both SLP-76 and LAT bind independently to PLCγ1, the association between SLP-76 and LAT (mediated by Gads) stabilizes the recruitment of this critical enzyme, enhancing its ability to interact with PIP_2 within the membrane (71). PLCγ1 function is enhanced further, because SLP-76 associates also with ITK, a tec family PTK that phosphorylates PLCγ1. In addition to recruiting PLCγ1 and ITK to LAT and lipid rafts, SLP-76 binds to Vav, a GEF critical for TCR-induced changes in the cytoskeleton, Nck, an adapter that cooperates in this same pathway, and adhesion- and degranulation-promoting adapter protein (ADAP), an adapter that coordinates TCR signaling to integrins (72,73) (Figure 11.6).

In addition to stimulation of the PLCγ1-dependent pathway, TCR complex engagement results in numerous other downstream signals that are essential for full T cell activation. As alluded to earlier, TCR ligation results in an alteration of the cytoskeleton characterized by polymerization of actin and T cell shape change (74). This process requires Vav, a protein with adapter domains and a region that enhances the exchange of GDP for GTP on members of the Rac and Rho family of small molecular weight GTPases (75). Tyrosine phosphorylation of Vav leads to both enhancement of its GEF function as well as its binding to a number of other proteins in the T cell activation pathway. Vav is critical as a regulator of the T cell cytoskeleton and as a modulator of T cell migration and adhesion after activation. This requires the GEF activity of Vav acting on Rac proteins and another GTP-binding protein, Cdc42, to increase actin polymerization at the leading edge as T cells migrate. Vav also is necessary for the redistribution of

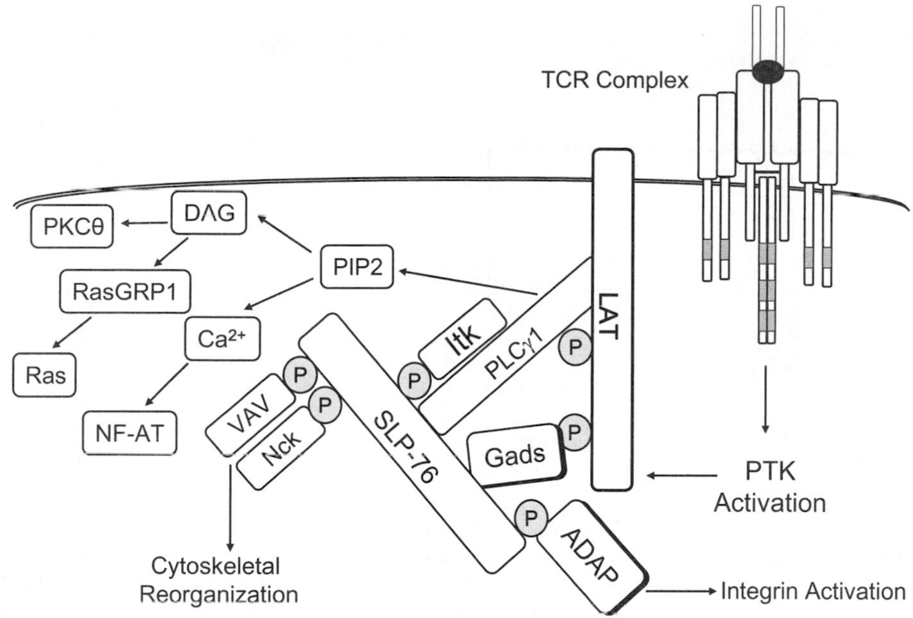

FIGURE 11.6 TCR binding results in the formation of a multimolecular signaling complex critical for initiating several signaling pathways. Following TCR engagement, inducible tyrosine phosphorylation of the two adapters linker of activated T cells (LAT) and SH2 domain-containing leukocyte-specific phosphoprotein of 76 kDa (SLP-76) results in a multimolecular complex that couples protein tyrosine kinase (PTK) activation to downstream signaling events. Activation of lck, fyn, and ζ-associated protein of 70 kDa (ZAP-70) leads to phosphorylation of LAT. SLP-76, which binds constitutively to Gads, is recruited to phospho-LAT, because the Gads SH2 domain has affinity for several of the LAT phosphorylation sites. Phospholipase Cγ1 (PLCγ1) binds to both SLP-76 and LAT, bringing this enzyme into the complex. PLCγ1 is activated when it is phosphorylated by a series of PTKs, including ITK, a tec family PTK that is also recruited by SLP-76. Activated PLCγ1 then initiates the calcium and DAG signaling pathways described for Figure 11.4. In addition to binding the effectors of this signaling pathway, SLP-76 also recruits adhesion- and degranulation-promoting adapter protein (ADAP) to the complex, enhancing integrin activation. The LAT/SLP-76 complex also promotes alterations in the cytoskeleton by recruiting Vav and Nck to the site of TCR engagement.

molecules on the surface of T cells, most notably integrins, during T cell activation (76). Analyses of mice deficient in Vav reveal that this protein has additional effects, including modulation of TCR-stimulated increases in calcium mobilization and activation of ERK (77). Expression of Vav mutants on the background of Vav-null T cells will provide insights into how the various domains of this molecule function, allowing it to have its multiplicity of effects on T cell activation.

Another important regulator of actin polymerization in activated T cells is the Wiskott-Aldrich syndrome protein (WASP), a protein that is either absent or mutated in an immunodeficiency syndrome that is characterized by defective B and T cell immunity and platelet function (78). WASP is brought into the TCR-stimulated activation complex by its association with Nck, but it is activated through its association with Vav (79,80). These two pathways are linked, as both Vav and Nck bind to phosphorylated SLP-76. Biochemical and genetic studies have shown that WASP functions as a regulator of the cytoskeleton by activating the Arp2/3 complex that is critical for initiating actin polymerization, directed T cell migration, and T cell adhesion (81) (Figure 11.7). However, this mechanism is not the only one by which TCR engagement promotes alteration in the cytoskeleton, as T cells with mutations in these signaling components still manifest actin polymerization, albeit with less efficiency.

T CELL ACTIVATION OF SERINE/THREONINE KINASES

One of the earliest observations made in the study of signaling events that occur following TCR engagement was that treatment of T cells with phorbol esters (DAG-like molecules) plus calcium ionophores could recapitulate the activation events seen with receptor binding (82). This work led quickly to the notion that PKC (as the target of phorbol esters) was an important component of the TCR signaling cascade. As studies began to uncover the

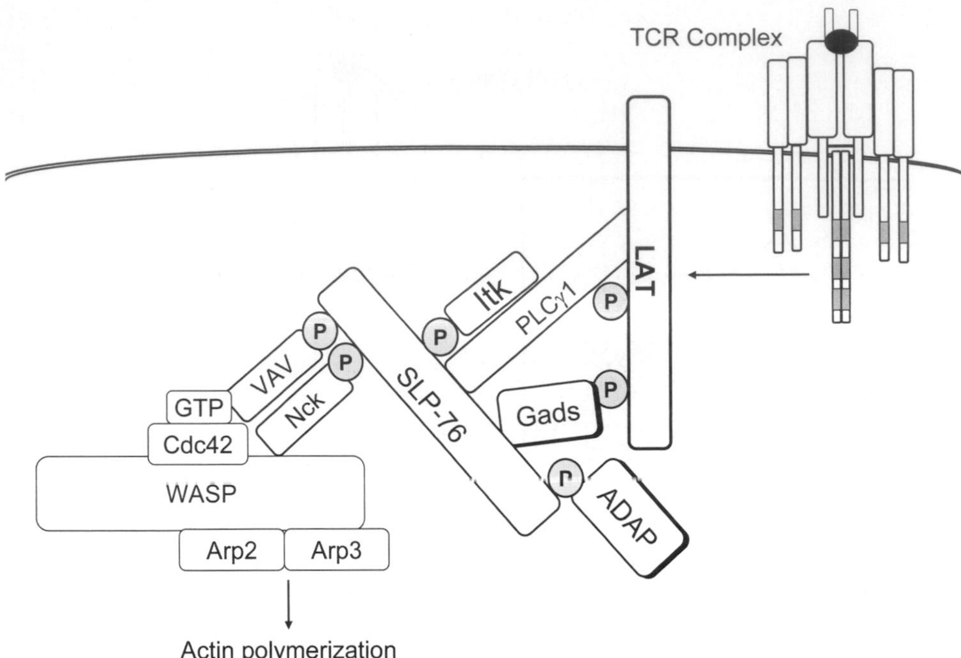

FIGURE 11.7 The LAT/SLP-76 complex stimulates cytoskeletal changes by recruiting the WASP signaling complex. Recruitment of SH2 domain-containing leukocyte-specific phosphoprotein of 76 kDa (SLP-76) to linker of activated T cells (LAT) via Grb2-related adapter downstream of Shc (GADS) (described in detail for Figure 11.6) initiates changes in the cytoskeleton by localizing active Vav, Cdc42, Wiskott-Aldrich syndrome protein (WASP), and the Arp2/3 complex, resulting in actin polymerization. This is one of several ways in which the TCR engagement causes alterations in the cytoskeleton, a key step for T cell migration and effector function.

importance of PTKs in T cell activation, experiments examining particular PKC family members and the potential role of other serine/threonine kinases lagged. Recently, however, there have been numerous reports of the importance of these second messengers for effective T cell responses.

Understanding the role of PKC in T cell activation is complicated by the fact that there are multiple members of the PKC family (83). The PKC isoform that has received the most attention as a regulator of T cell function is PKCθ, an enzyme that exhibits an intriguing subcellular localization pattern. In resting T cells, PKCθ is found in the cytosol; however, upon engagement of the TCR complex, it quickly translocates to the site of the engaged receptor (84). Following this observation, investigators generated mice targeted for PKCθ deletion and discovered a requirement for this enzyme in TCR-induced activation of the NFκB pathway (85) (Figure 11.8). The signaling pathway downstream of PKCθ is becoming clear, as mounting evidence has shown that PKCθ phosphorylates CARMA1 (caspase-recruitment domain [CARD] membrane–associated guanylate kinase [MAGUK] protein 1), an adapter protein that when phosphorylated nucleates a molecular complex including two other signaling proteins, MALT1 (mucosa-associated-lymphoid-tissue lymphoma-translocation gene 1) and Bcl10 (B cell lymphoma 10) (86). The resultant complex recruits yet another serine kinase, IKK (inhibitor of NFκB [IκB] kinase) that,

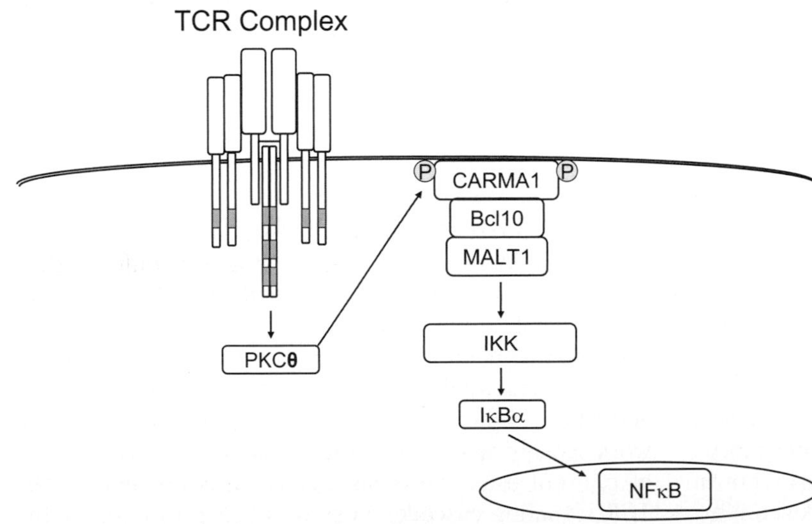

FIGURE 11.8 Engagement of the TCR results in PKC-mediated activation of the NFκB pathway. Following TCR stimulation, protein kinase C θ (PKCθ) becomes activated, in part via the generation of diacylglycerol (DAG) (see Figure 11.4). PKCθ then phosphorylates caspase-recruitment domain (CARD) membrane–associated guanylate kinase (MAGUK) protein 1 (CARMA1), which forms a complex with two other proteins, B cell lymphoma 10 (Bcl10) and mucosa-associated-lymphoid-tissue lymphoma-translocation gene 1 (MALT1). Together, these proteins activate inhibitor of NFκB (IκB) kinase (IKK), which phosphorylates IκB, a negative regulator of NFκB. Upon its phosphorylation, IκB is degraded, allowing NFκB to escape the cytosol and enter the nucleus. Adapted from Matthews SA, Cantrell DA. *Current Opinion in Immunology.* 2006;18:314–320.

when activated, leads to the degradation of IκB, a negative regulator of the NFκB transcription factor (87). Loss of IκB allows NFκB to escape the cytosol and enter the nucleus, where it can transactivate genes critical for T cell activation, including the gene for IL2, a cytokine essential for T cell proliferation.

Recent studies have embarked on the difficult task of unraveling the roles of the other members of the PKC family in the regulation of T cell activation. Investigators have made use of mice with targeted deletion of genes for particular isoforms and pharmacologic inhibitors or activators that are relatively selective for different PKC enzymes. The collective results of these studies indicate that PKC enzymes other than PKCθ are also essential for T cell function, in particular to mediate T cell adhesion and migration, both critical steps to position T cells appropriately to respond to antigenic challenges (60). To add to the complexity of how PKC functions in T cells, it appears that members of the PKC family may serve as negative regulators of immune cell function, a finding that has important implications when one considers PKC as a potential therapeutic target (88).

One difficult but useful approach to decipher the role of PKC in T cell activation has been to search for substrates of the kinases. Antibodies have now been developed that are able to detect signature sequences of phosphorylated residues that are targets for PKC enzymes. These reagents have been used to identify protein kinase D (PKD) as a protein that is inducibly phosphorylated by PKC following TCR engagement (89). Multiple PKC isoforms have been shown to be capable of phosphorylating PKD. The consequences of PKC phosphorylation of PKD have been described best in nonlymphoid cells; however, there is considerable evidence that PKD plays a role regulating the activity of small molecular weight GTPases in T cells (90,91), which are critical for inside-out signaling from the TCR to integrins (see later discussion). Additional work has shown that subcellular localization of PKD is also a key determinant in its function and that PKD phosphorylation likely plays a role in its trafficking within the cell. Other serine/threonine kinases and their substrates have been identified recently as important for T cell function, including AMPK (5′AMP-activated protein kinase), a regulator of glucose metabolism and cellular bioenergetics (92). It is anticipated that with the advent of improved reagents, additional serine kinases will be identified that are critical for T cell development and function.

INSIDE-OUT SIGNALS FROM THE TCR TO INTEGRINS

In addition to activation of genes important for T cell effector function, TCR engagement primes the cell to respond to other activating stimuli. One mechanism for this priming is a TCR-inducible increase in avidity of integrins for their ligands. Integrins are cell surface receptors that mediate interactions between other cells or the extracellular matrix (93). Increased adhesion of T cells to antigen presenting cells (APCs) via integrins increases the stability of the association between the TCR and antigen/MHC (also present on the APCs), thus potentiating the ability of the TCR to transduce its activating signals. The process of TCR-induced changes in integrin avidity is known as "inside-out" signaling, as intracellular signals initiated by the TCR feed back onto the integrins to change their surface properties (Figure 11.9). The biochemical basis of inside-out signaling requires many of the same components as signals leading to transcriptional activation of cytokine genes, including the src PTKs, ZAP-70, LAT, SLP-76, and Vav. However, it appears that an additional set of adapter proteins is essential to translate TCR engagement into increased integrin avidity. These proteins include ADAP, src kinase–associated phosphoprotein of 55 kDa (SKAP55), and Rap1-GTP interacting adapter molecule (RIAM) (94,95). Recent data suggest that for maximal integrin function, it is necessary to form a complex of SLP-76/ADAP/SKAP55/RIAM to bring the Rap1 GTPase to the cell surface. Active Rap1, when expressed as a transgene in T cells, increases T cell adhesion by stimulating clustering of LFA-1 (leukocyte function-associated antigen 1), making it a better binder to its ligand, ICAM-1 (intercellular adhesion molecule-1) (96). A potential link between Rap1 and integrin function has been provided by the observation that for active Rap1 to function as an enhancer of integrin avidity, it must bind one additional protein, RAPL (regulator of adhesion and cell polarization enriched in lymphoid tissues), which has been shown to bind directly to LFA-1 (97). Collectively, these studies, making use of biochemical and imaging approaches in cell lines and genetically altered mice, have revealed an intricate pathway that at least partially explains how inside-out signaling couples the TCR complex to integrins.

The pathway described results in clustering of integrins on the T cell surface, thus increasing their avidity for ligands. It is known additionally that engagement of the TCR complex results in a change in the integrins themselves, so that their binding affinity for ligand is increased. The structural basis for the change in affinity has been described in a series of elegant experiments that have captured and visualized integrins in their resting state, in a transitional state, and in their most active conformation (98). It is not clear exactly what biochemical event is the most critical for inducing these conformational changes, but possibilities include posttranslational modifications of the integrin cytoplasmic domains (e.g., by PKC). The entire spectrum of the signals downstream of the TCR that are necessary for integrin clustering and avidity changes remain unknown, but considerable work has implicated Vav and other cytoskeletal regulators (76).

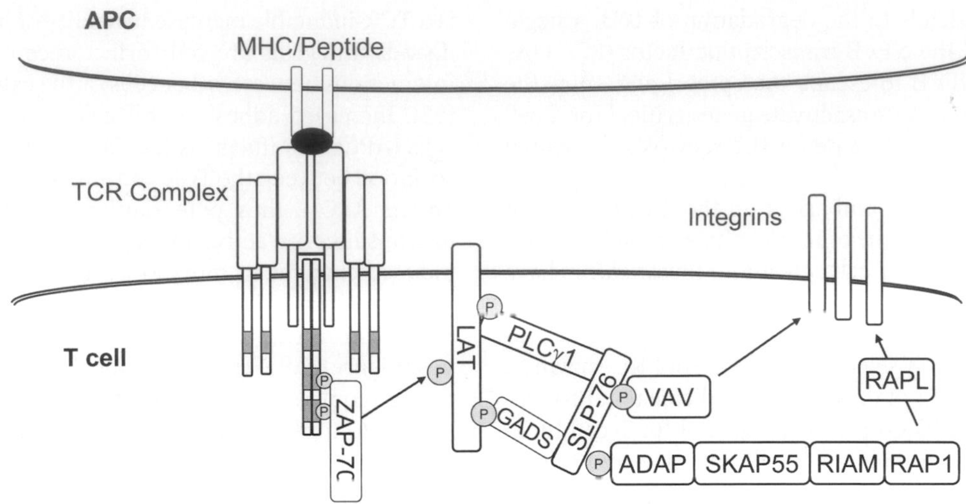

FIGURE 11.9 TCR engagement leads to increased avidity of integrins. The signaling complex described in Figure 11.4 recruits another series of adapter proteins including adhesion- and degranulation-promoting adapter protein (ADAP), src kinase-associated phosphoprotein of 55 kDa (SKAP-55), and Rap1-GTP interacting adapter molecule (RIAM). Together, these molecules allow the activated form of the GTPase Rap1 to be recruited to the membrane in the vicinity of integrins. Active Rap1 (likely via effector molecules such as regulator of adhesion and cell polarization enriched in lymphoid tissues [RAPL]) stimulates clustering of integrins, hence increasing their avidity for ligand. Genetic experiments have also implicated Vav in this process. In addition to increasing integrin clustering, TCR stimulation also activates a signaling pathway that causes alterations in integrin conformation resulting in increased affinity for ligand.

T CELL COSTIMULATION

One of the most striking features of T cell activation is that engagement of the TCR complex alone, while stimulating multiple second messenger cascades, is not sufficient to activate a mature peripheral T cell. In fact, such stimulation often results not only in failed activation but also in a long-lived state of T cell unresponsiveness known as anergy (see Chapter 30 and ref [99]). Effective T cell activation therefore requires two signals: signal 1 initiated by engagement of the TCR complex, and signal 2 initiated by binding of one of several costimulatory receptors that transduce independent signals or enhance the signaling cascades initiated by engagement of the TCR complex (Figure 11.10). Although there are no conclusive data to explain the need for two signals to drive full T cell activation, one attractive model is that such a system allows for an extremely sensitive antigen receptor that is "held in check" by the requirement for a second signal to ensure that activation occurs only at the right time and place. This model predicts that the second signal should require an interaction between the T cell and the appropriate APC, a prediction that has been born out by experimental data.

Although there are a number of costimulatory receptors on T cells that are able to provide the essential second signal in various experimental models, CD28 appears to be the most physiologically relevant. CD28, a cell surface homodimer, is present on virtually all $CD4^+$ T cells and the majority of $CD8^+$ T cells (100). It is bound by members of the B7 family of ligands (predominantly B7-1 [also known as CD80] and B7-2 [now designated CD86]) that are present, as would be predicted, on APCs. In fact, members of the B7 family are only expressed at low levels on resting APCs (e.g., quiescent macrophages or immature dendritic cells [DCs]), but as innate immune cells begin to signal the presence of pathogens, one important response is the induction of both MHC class II and the CD28 ligands, making APCs better able to deliver both signals 1 and 2 (see Chapter 15 and ref [101]). The importance of CD28 has been established *in vivo* through analysis of mice made deficient in the gene. Although these animals are still able to mount immune responses, they occur much less efficiently than in wild type mice (102).

Since the identification of CD28 as a major inducer of signal 2, many studies have been performed to determine the critical biochemical event initiated by CD28 that prevents T cells from becoming anergic and instead initiates activation (100) (Figure 11.11). As is the case for other costimulatory receptors on T cells, one consequence of CD28 ligation is more efficient signal transduction by the TCR complex, resulting in enhanced as well as prolonged activation of downstream pathways (100). Exactly how CD28 engagement results in enhanced TCR signaling remains obscure, but mechanisms that have been hypothesized include stabilization of the TCR/APC interaction, decreased turnover of the receptor, or synergistic recruitment of effector molecules.

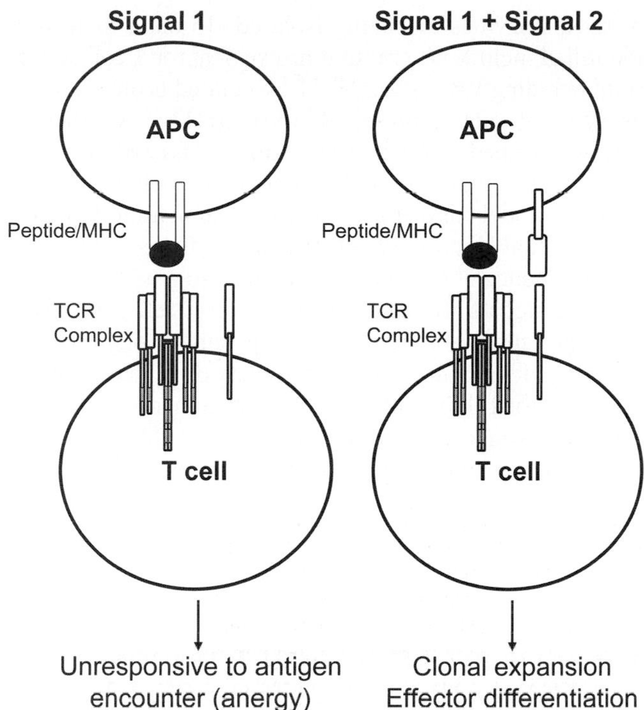

FIGURE 11.10 Two signals are required for productive T cell activation. Engagement of the TCR by peptide/MHC results in activation of multiple second messenger pathways. These signals by themselves, however, are not sufficient to stimulate T cell proliferation or differentiation into effector cells. In fact, delivery of signal 1 alone results in T cells becoming unresponsive to antigen encounter, in some model systems, exhibiting long term "anergy." When signal 1 is delivered concurrently with a costimulatory signal (signal 2), instead of being rendered anergic, T cells are stimulated to expand and develop effector function. There are many molecules that can deliver signal 2 to activate a T cell, the prototype being CD28 when bound by members of the B7 family of ligands present on APCs.

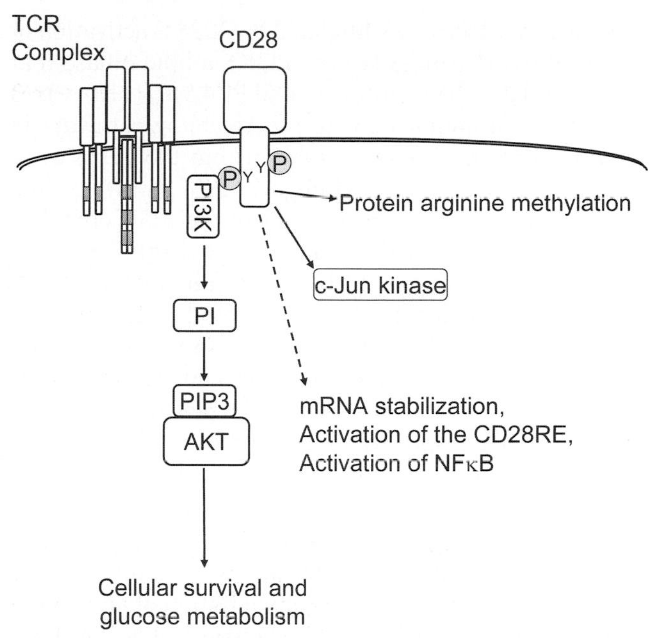

FIGURE 11.11 Costimulation of T cells by CD28 activates numerous signaling events. Stimulation of CD28 by its ligands on APCs results in enhanced signaling via the TCR as well as stimulation of additional second messengers. One such signaling pathway is activation of the phosphatidyl inositol-3 kinase (PI3K) pathway that leads to increased enzymatic activity of AKT, a serine kinase that promotes cellular survival and glucose metabolism. CD28 engagement potentiates cytokine production both by inducing mRNA stability and by stimulating transcription through unique promoter elements (e.g., the CD28 response element [CD28RE]). Additionally, CD28 stimulation results in activation of c-Jun kinase and several protein arginine methyltransferases. Adapted from Alegre ML, et al. *Nature Reviews Immunology.* 2001;1:220–228.

Although microarray analysis to date has not revealed qualitative changes in gene transcription during T cell costimulation (103,104), there is compelling evidence that in addition to augmenting TCR signals, CD28 engagement results in unique second messenger signaling events. The first demonstration of such a unique CD28 signal came from mutagenesis studies demonstrating that within the promoter for the IL2 gene is a specific sequence, designated the CD28 RE (response element), that when altered abrogates CD28-mediated transcriptional up-regulation of the IL2 promoter while leaving TCR-mediated activation largely intact (105). The CD28RE acts in conjunction with the adjacent AP-1 site to form a unique composite element, RE/AP, whose activation absolutely requires two signals for stimulation, in contrast to other transcriptional elements from the IL2 promoter, such as NFAT, which can be activated by TCR stimulation alone (106). In addition, CD28 clearly relies on signals that are different from those induced by the TCR, since CD28 signaling leading to the up-regulation of RE/AP and IL2 is cyclosporine insensitive, in contrast to TCR-stimulated signals (106,107). However, it remains unclear exactly what biochemical signals are necessary to uniquely activate this region of the *Il2* promoter.

In addition to increasing the transcription of the *Il2* gene, CD28 has been shown to enhance IL2 production by stabilizing mRNA for this cytokine (108). This outcome of CD28 signaling is not unique to the *Il2* gene, as compelling data exist for the ability of CD28 to significantly enhance mRNA half-life of multiple other cytokine genes. The transcripts that respond to CD28 in this manner are alike, in that they have stretches with many adenosine and uracil bases (so-called *AU-enriched sequences*) 3′ to the translational stop codons. Again, the precise biochemical mechanism for the CD28-stimulated mRNA stability remains unclear; however, there is evidence to suggest that one important signal is activation of c-Jun kinase, a pathway stimulated strongly by CD28 engagement (ref [109]; discussed later).

Many laboratories have searched for the unique signal(s) initiated by CD28 engagement separate from those seen following stimulation of the TCR complex. One pathway critical for effective T cell responses that appears to be relatively selectively stimulated by CD28 is activation of phosphatidyl inositol-3 kinase (PI3K), a lipid kinase that phosphorylates the membrane lipid PI(4,5)P_2 (110). CD28 appears to communicate with this signaling pathway via phosphorylation of a key residue within the CD28 cytoplasmic tail (the tyrosine within a YMNM motif), leading to recruitment of the p85 subunit of the PI3K complex. The result is an altered lipid composition of the membrane in the vicinity of engaged CD28 with subsequent recruitment of other molecules containing pleckstrin homology (PH) domains, such as the tec family kinases and a serine/threonine kinase, AKT (111). The concurrent recruitment of PDK1, PDK2, and AKT to the plasma membrane results in dual phosphorylation of AKT by PDK1 and PDK2 at two key regulatory sites, resulting in AKT activation, which in turn stimulates a cascade of signaling events leading to enhanced cell survival. Mounting evidence supports the notion that activation of this pathway is important for effective T cell costimulation and inhibition of an apoptosis program.

The finding that CD28 potentiates cell survival has led to the investigation of other signals stimulated by CD28 binding, but not by engagement of the TCR, that lead ultimately to protection from apoptosis. Experiments in other cellular systems have shown that the balance between various members of the MAPK family of enzymes, in particular the relative activation of the ERK (extracellular signal-regulated kinase) versus Jun kinase pathways, is a critical determinant of cell survival. These findings led to a series of studies in T cells demonstrating that engagement of CD28 is a potent activator of c-Jun kinase, whereas ERK activation appears to be driven mainly by TCR ligation (109). It remains unclear, however, whether this is the pivotal difference in the cell signaling program that dictates survival of stimulated cells. Regardless of whether ERK versus Jun kinase activation is the critical step, many experiments have now shown that CD28 engagement does up-regulate important anti-apoptotic genes, including Bcl2 family member proteins (112–114).

Several intriguing reports suggest other possible mechanisms for CD28 to deliver its unique signals. Like phosphorylation of serine, threonine, or tyrosine residues, protein methylation appears to be an important posttranslational modification that modulates function, although in most cases the mechanism for altered function is not known. With the advent of improved detection approaches and the cloning of genes encoding protein arginine methyltransferases, it has become apparent that arginine methylation of proteins is important in many biologic systems, most often to regulate activity of transcription factors. Recent work has shown that TCR engagement has only a minor effect on protein arginine methyltransferase activity in T cells; however, costimulation via the TCR with CD28 (and even CD28 engagement alone) results in potent activation of the methyltransferases (115). Substrates of these enzymes are being isolated. To date, molecules identified include several that are critical for T cell activation including Vav and an NFAT-associated protein known as NFAT-interacting protein 45 (NIP45) (116). Another recently described model for CD28 function is costimulation-dependent changes in cellular energy metabolism. This intriguing model has attracted a great deal of attention, as it suggests that glucose uptake and utilization is a cause not a consequence of enhanced T cell activation (117).

CD28 signals are major costimuli for T cells, and CD28 has many functions. It is likely that only through a combination of its many described effects on signaling pathways can the full impact of CD28 engagement be realized. Many investigators continue to work on CD28, anticipating that understanding the molecular basis for how CD28 contributes to T cell activation will provide new opportunities to modulate immune cell function for therapeutic purposes.

THE CD28-RELATED RECEPTOR ICOS COSTIMULATES ACTIVATED T CELLS

CD28 is expressed at high levels on resting T cells and plays a critical role in the initial activation of cells once they encounter antigen/MHC on an activated APC. More recent studies have identified another member of the CD28 family, inducible costimulator or ICOS (118). In contrast to CD28, ICOS expression is low on naïve cells but up-regulated on cells stimulated via their TCR (119). Although CD28 stimulation is not absolutely required for ICOS induction, engagement of CD28 promotes ICOS expression, further suggesting that these two related proteins function sequentially during T cell activation. ICOS does not bind to either B7-1 or B7-2, but instead it interacts with a novel member of the B7 family known as ICOS ligand (120). ICOS ligand is expressed more broadly than B7-1 or B7-2, as it is found on nonhematopoietic cells following stimulation with inflammatory cytokines. This expression provides one likely explanation for how activated, ICOS-bearing T cells can be stimulated in tissues that may be deficient in professional APCs but that have been induced to express ICOS ligand.

ICOS is a disulfide-linked homodimeric glycoprotein that, like CD28, contains a binding site for the p85 subunit of PI3K in its cytoplasmic domain. When engaged, ICOS stimulates greater PI3K activity than does CD28, but some of the other CD28 effectors (e.g., Ras and Jun kinase) are not activated upon the binding of ICOS to its ligand. As expected based on these differences, there are overlapping but also distinct consequences of stimulating T cells via ICOS versus CD28. Both enhance T cell–mediated cytokine production; however, ICOS does not up-regulate IL2. ICOS appears to be more important in regulating the ability of T cells to provide help to B cells, both for Ig class switching and for formation of mature germinal centers (121).

Because of its expression and role on activated T cells, many investigators have considered ICOS blockade as an attractive target to interfere with ongoing, unwanted immune responses. Interruption of the interaction between ICOS and its ligand has been shown to ameliorate immune-mediated disorders such as collagen-induced arthritis or experimental allergic encephalomyelitis, two well-studied models of autoimmunity in mice (122).

ADDITIONAL RECEPTORS THAT MODULATE T CELL RESPONSES

In addition to CD28 and ICOS, other cell surface receptors have been identified that, when engaged, either augment the efficiency of TCR signaling or provide additional signals that potentiate T cell activation. These receptors include integrins that when bound to ligands on APCs stabilize the contact between APCs and T cells, thus allowing for more effective interactions between the TCR complex and MHC/peptide. In addition to inside-out signaling that links TCR engagement to integrin function, integrins are also known to transduce signals when they are engaged by ligand, a process known as *outside-in signaling*. Many studies have shown that at least some integrin-mediated signaling occurs independently of the TCR but, interestingly, makes use of many of the same biochemical intermediates including src and syk PTKs and the adapter protein SLP-76 (but not LAT) (123). Among the major downstream effects of integrin stimulation are T cell spreading and adhesion, two events that require activation of Vav and alterations in the cytoskeleton. Integrin interactions with their ligands are also important for creation of the immunological synapse (see later discussion), a structure that is thought to correctly position the TCR and its effector machinery. Other cell surface receptors have also been shown to provide costimulatory signals for T cell activation. Most of these receptors have been identified in experiments where cross-linking that particular receptor together with the TCR significantly enhances the known signaling events, cytokine production, and T cell effector function. One important group of such receptors belongs to the tumor necrosis factor (TNF) family and includes CD137 (4-1BB), CD27, CD30, HVEM (herpes virus entry mediator), GITR (glucocorticoid-induced TNF receptor), and CD134 (OX40) (124). Some of these proteins are present on resting cells, while others in this group are found only on cells that have already been activated and function primarily downstream of initial T cell activation to sustain immune responses. These receptors transduce their signals in a way similar to other TNF receptors that are better known as inducers of apoptosis (see the discussion of CD95 [Fas] later in this chapter).

Another family of costimulatory receptors for T cells was identified that makes use of a novel signaling pathway. This second messenger cascade appears to be particularly important, as mutations in one critical component lead to a rare but devastating immune disorder known as X-linked lymphoproliferative syndrome (XLP) (125). SLAM (signaling lymphocytic activating molecule) was the first identified member of a family of T cell costimulatory receptors that function by homotypic interactions, leading to signaling cascades that are also initiated by activation of src family PTKs (126). In studies designed to unravel how SLAM signals, experiments were performed to identify molecules that interact with the receptor. These experiments converged with studies by other groups attempting to identify the causal gene for XLP, leading to the identification of a novel adapter molecule known as SLAM-associated protein or SAP. SAP is a small cytosolic adapter that consists only of an SH2 domain and a short cytoplasmic tail. It appears to function by serving as a bridge between SLAM (and other SLAM family receptors) and fyn (127,128). Recent studies have suggested that the SAP/Fyn interaction is critical for optimal activation of PKCθ and NFκB during T cell activation (129) (Figure 11.12). Loss of SAP severely

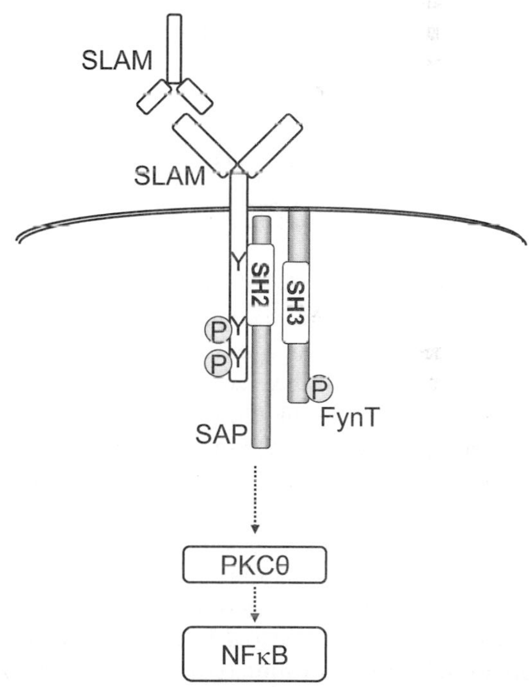

FIGURE 11.12 The adapter protein SAP links the TCR to a fyn PTK signaling pathway important for directing T cell effector differentiation. SAP (SLAM [signaling lymphocytic activating molecule]–associated protein) is a small cytosolic molecule that associates with tyrosine (in some cases nonphosphorylated and in other cases phosphorylated) residues in the cytoplasmic domains of SLAM family receptors, T cell costimulatory molecules that are stimulated by homotypic interactions. SAP bridges SLAM family receptors to the fyn PTK via a unique interaction with the fyn SH3 domain. The SLAM/SAP/Fyn module has been shown to function in the PKC/NFκB pathway to direct cytokine production in activated T cells.

impacts multiple immune cell lineages (including T cells, NK cells, and NKT cells), suggesting that loss of this single adapter impairs normal function of multiple receptors (130). The consequence of SAP deficiency in the T cell compartment is severe perturbation of cytokine responses, in particular after Epstein-Barr virus infection, leading to an uncontrolled inflammatory response, ultimately causing death in many affected children (125). Studies in several laboratories are underway, using mice deficient in SAP as well as mice in which mutations have been introduced into the SAP gene, to investigate the molecular basis for SAP function in the various lineages in which this adapter protein is expressed.

In addition to SLAM (CD150), which is expressed on T cells, B cells, DCs, macrophages, platelets, and hematopoietic stem cells, other SLAM family members include 2B4 (CD244), NTBA (Ly108), Ly9 (CD229), CD84, and CRACC (CD319, CS1) (131). Studies performed thus far indicate that deletion of any particular SLAM family member impairs immune cell function but only to a moderate extent, indicating that the various family members may be able to at least partially compensate for each other. As more data accumulate, the unique importance of each of the individual members of this family of costimulatory receptors will become apparent.

THE IMMUNOLOGICAL SYNAPSE, CONCENTRATING SIGNALING MOLECULES, AND LIPID RAFTS

As the components most critical for TCR signaling became known, efforts were made to uncover where in the cell these molecules reside, both under resting and stimulating conditions. These studies have made use of biochemical approaches to fractionate the cell and then separate proteins using typical electrophoresis techniques, as well as imaging modalities to visualize molecules in either fixed samples or in real time in living cells. Early work in this area led to the interesting observation that molecules important for T cell activation appear to cluster as the TCR is engaged. One seminal series of experiments described several structures that appeared in a temporally defined fashion during T cell activation (132).

In model systems where T cells are engaged by an APC or are stimulated by antigen/MHC on a planar bilayer that also includes the integrin ligand ICAM-1, the first event that can be seen is the recruitment of LFA-1 (the integrin receptor for ICAM-1) to the point of contact between the T cell and stimulating surface. This engagement is followed closely by the migration of LFA-1 away from the central contact site to a more peripheral location and the replacement of LFA-1 at the center by the TCR complex (133). The larger structure has been designated the supramolecular activation cluster (SMAC), with a central region (cSMAC), enriched quickly for the TCR, and peripheral region (pSMAC), where LFA-1 resides. As these structures were first being described, additional imaging approaches making use of cytoplasmic staining techniques and expression of molecules tagged directly with fluorochromes followed by three-dimensional reconstruction indicated that as the cSMAC is formed, molecules known to be critical for transducing TCR-dependent signals (e.g., PKCθ) appeared at the site of the engaged TCR. These findings led to the notion of an "immunological synapse," reminiscent of the contact site between neurons or neurons and muscle cells, where a concentrated stimulus interacts with aggregated receptors to initiate a cellular response (Figure 11.13).

These early findings led to the hypothesis that formation of the immunological synapse was a necessary step in T cell activation, as signaling efficiency would be enhanced by localizing the receptor and its effector molecules to the point of contact of the TCR with antigen (134). Subsequent experiments have demonstrated that this simple model of creating the synapse to initiate TCR signaling is unlikely to be correct, as careful kinetic analyses have documented effective TCR signaling prior to synapse formation (135). Further, as reagents have been developed to detect molecules that are active in the TCR signaling pathway (e.g., phospho-site–specific antibodies that can distinguish active ZAP-70 molecules from ZAP-70 molecules that have not been stimulated to increase PTK function), a surprising observation has emerged that there is a relative paucity of active signaling molecules within the synapse. These observations have led to the suggestion that the role of the immunological synapse is not to initiate TCR signaling but instead to terminate activation events, perhaps by providing a site for collecting and degrading signaling molecules (136). Another model speculates that the immunological synapse is not critical for signaling but is necessary to direct activated T cells to secrete either cytotoxic materials, in the case of CD8$^+$ T cells, or cytokines, in the case of CD4$^+$ T cells, that will influence other cells of the immune system. It is likely that the immunological synapse plays multiple roles (almost certainly including some that have not yet been proposed) in the biology of T cell activation. A complete understanding of the importance of this structure will require additional experiments that make use of improved reagents for real time imaging of living cells.

The description of the immunological synapse instigated another controversy related to how receptors and their effector molecules position themselves within the plasma membrane. In contrast to the longstanding fluid mosaic model that described membranes as a sea of homogenous lipids in which proteins floated randomly, recent studies have demonstrated clearly that cell membranes are quite heterogeneous and that they contain large and small islands of proteins (137). The protein islands are not uniform; their constituents differ. Additionally, the lipid regions of the membrane are also heterogeneous, as

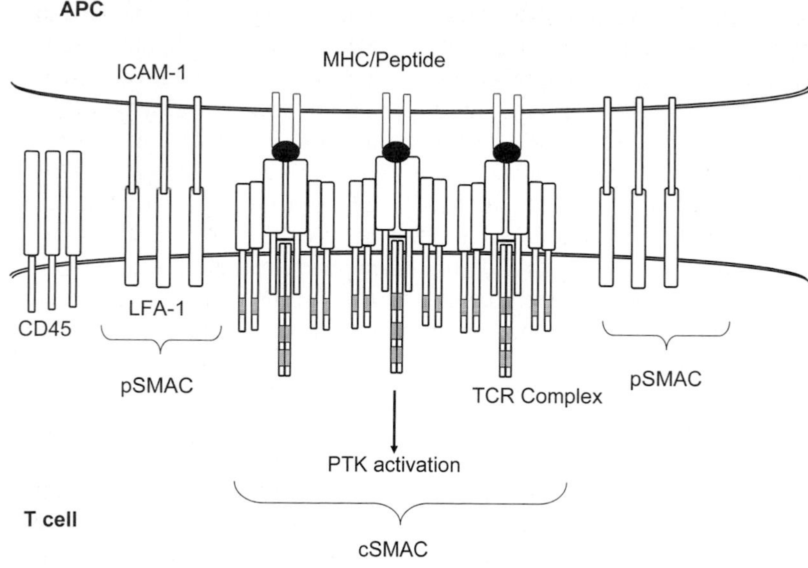

FIGURE 11.13 The immunological synapse appears at the site of the engaged TCR. The first intermolecular interaction to occur upon encounter between an APC and T cell is the binding of intercellular adhesion molecule-1 (ICAM-1) to its receptor leukocyte function-associated antigen-1 (LFA-1). If there is also recognition between the TCR and MHC/peptide present on the APC, LFA-1 moves from the center of the recognition domain to its periphery, while the TCR, bound to peptide/MHC, aggregates within the center of the complex. Other molecules—for example, the tyrosine phosphatase CD45—are excluded from the developing synapse. Although intracellular signaling molecules also appear at the synapse, the kinetics of their appearance and activation suggests that the synapse does not form to initiate T cell activation. Models for the biologic role of the synapse are presented in the text. pSMAC, peripheral supramolecular activation cluster; cSMAC, central supramolecular activation cluster. Adapted from Koretzky GA. T-cell activation and inactivation. In: Rich R, et al., eds. *Clinical Immunology*. London: Mosby, 2001.

there are discreet domains that differ greatly in lipid composition, with some regions rich in cholesterol and others where this lipid is less abundant. The cholesterol-rich regions are designated lipid (or membrane) rafts, as these domains float to the top of a sucrose gradient when disrupted and subjected to ultracentrifugation. These lipid rafts are also enriched in a subset of proteins that are posttranslationally modified to contain lipid species (e.g., palmitoyl groups) that insert preferentially into the cholesterol-rich domains.

The role of lipid rafts in receptor signaling and how these structures relate, if at all, to the immunological synapse is an area of intense investigation. There is compelling evidence demonstrating that in resting cells, the TCR is found either outside of lipid rafts or in rafts that are of very small size, whereas upon antigen encounter, the TCR is easily found within these domains (138). The potential importance of this localization was shown when disruption of lipid raft integrity by pharmacologic cholesterol depletion abrogated the ability of the TCR to signal (139). Other evidence for the importance of lipid rafts in TCR function is that some molecules essential for TCR-mediated signal transduction (e.g., LAT) are targeted to lipid rafts due to posttranslational palmitoylation. Mutation of the raft-targeting sequences abrogates the ability of these proteins to support TCR-mediated signal transduction (140). In addition to certain proteins being restricted to lipid rafts, others seem to function normally only if they are excluded from these membrane domains. In these circumstances, forced expression of these molecules within rafts interferes with TCR signaling events.

It is recognized that the experiments described earlier, where molecules are artificially relocalized, while consistent with a role for lipid rafts in TCR function, do not prove causality. Similarly, the effect of pharmacologic disruption of lipid rafts is suggestive of their importance; however, the agents that are used may have other effects on the cell. A number of laboratories are now combining imaging and signaling assays at the single cell level to probe the importance of these membrane domains for T cell activation.

T CELL PROLIFERATION REQUIRES SIGNALING VIA THE HIGH AFFINITY RECEPTOR FOR IL2

In addition to the acquisition of effector function by T cells, combating pathogenic challenges also requires the number of antigen-specific T cells to expand so that a critical mass of responding cells is achieved. This proliferative response requires the signaling pathways described earlier, both to stimulate production of IL2, an essential growth factor for T cell proliferation (via the TCR/CD28 signaling pathways detailed earlier) and to make the stimulated T cells responsive to this cytokine. Prior to stimulation, naïve T cells express a moderate affinity receptor for IL2 consisting of two components, the β and γ chains. One of the outcomes of TCR engagement is the inducible expression of a third IL2 receptor component, the α chain (CD25), that together with the β and γ chains results in a receptor with substantially higher affinity. Binding of IL2 secreted by activated T cells to the trimeric high-affinity receptor initiates a series of biochemical signals that drive the proliferative response to expand the number of antigen-reactive cells. The details of the signaling pathways stimulated by IL2 and other cytokines are detailed in Chapter 24.

PREVENTING T CELL ACTIVATION: THE BIOCHEMICAL BASIS FOR ANERGY

The material presented in this chapter thus far has focused on how T cells become activated when an antigenic challenge has been detected. As noted earlier, an effective T cell response only occurs when the TCR is engaged and costimulatory receptors are bound. This dual signaling allows for highly responsive TCRs but ensures that T cells only respond in the appropriate setting—that is, when the TCR stimulus is associated with an activated APC. Stimulation of the TCR alone, presumably indicating that the TCR has been engaged aberrantly, leads not to cellular activation but instead to a state of unresponsiveness or anergy. Even more striking is the observation that anergy may be maintained long after the TCR stimulus in the absence of a costimulatory receptor signal has occurred (see Chapter 30). This property of T cell biology has attracted a great deal of attention by investigators, as understanding the biochemical basis of anergy will likely provide insights into how it may be possible to disable T cell responses in an antigen-specific fashion. Such knowledge would be extremely useful in the design of novel therapeutics directed toward selectively turning off T cell responses to particular antigens—for example, antigens presented by an allograft in a transplant patient or self-antigens that are inappropriately stimulating a T cell response in an individual with autoimmunity. Studies examining the biochemistry of anergy have been informative but have also suggested that the biology of anergy versus activation is extremely complex. There are likely multiple mechanisms by which this decision is made.

Some of the earliest studies investigating the molecular basis of anergy were spawned by the finding that effective T cell stimulation correlates with activation of both the calcium pathway, leading to NFAT translocation to the nucleus, and the Ras pathway, leading to the MAPK cascade and stimulation of the AP-1 family of transcription factors. When experiments were performed that selectively activated the calcium pathway without concomitant Ras stimulation (initially with the use of calcium ionophores as a pharmacologic means to stimulate only calcium increases), T cell anergy ensued (141). These studies suggested a model that T cell activation required a balance between Ras and calcium signals and that conditions that created an imbalance in these events would fail to activate T cells, leading to long-term unresponsiveness (142). A number of experimental systems have provided support for this model, including those that have used pharmacological approaches or genetically altered mice to manipulate one or the other of these two key signaling pathways.

A series of recent experiments using different approaches has converged on the idea that costimulation may be critical for determining whether a T cell will adopt an activated or anergic phenotype, at least in part by regulating the balance between calcium and Ras signaling. One consequence of costimulation of T cells via the TCR plus CD28 is enhanced DAG production, which is greater than that seen when cells are stimulated via the TCR alone (143). This increased DAG production presumably results in enhanced Ras activation via more potent stimulation of RasGRP1. Concordant with this finding was the observation that transcription of a member of the diacylglycerol kinase (DGK) family (DGKα) is markedly up-regulated in anergic cells. DGKs act by phosphorylating DAG, leading to the production of phosphatidic acid, thus terminating the ability of DAG to stimulate RasGRP1 (and hence Ras) or members of the PKC family (144). Thus, it was suggested that anergic cells display decreased signaling relative to calcium responses because of rapid loss of DAG. Subsequent studies revealed that in contrast to anergic cells, T cells that have been productively activated reveal marked decreases in DGK isoform gene expression, suggesting a means to maintain high levels of Ras signaling (143). Concordantly, overexpression of DGK in T cells leads to failed activation and enhanced anergy (145), while loss of expression due to targeted deletion of DGK isoform genes leads to failed anergy induction in both *in vitro* assays and *in vivo* (140).

Further studies have indicated that although modulation of DAG signaling is an effective means to alter anergy induction, there are other biochemical events (that may or may not converge on the Ras pathway) that can affect whether stimulation of the TCR without a costimulus will result in effector cell function or anergy. The T cell hyperactivity and failed anergy observed in DGK-deficient animals is phenocopied quite closely in mice in which the gene for the PTEN (phosphatase and tensin homolog deleted on chromosome 10) phosphatase is targeted for deletion (146). PTEN is a lipid phosphatase that dephosphorylates phosphatidylinositol 3,4,5-trisphosphate (PIP_3), the product of PI3K activity, the enzyme system that appears critical for effective CD28-mediated costimulation. Several recent studies have shown that loss of PTEN in the T cell compartment results in enhanced TCR function (147). It has been reported further that loss of PTEN allows T cells to be effectively stimulated via signal 1 alone, presumably because the requirement for CD28 engagement is obviated, since the product of low levels of PI3K activity is maintained in the absence of the phosphatase (146).

Additional studies have focused on yet other mechanisms of anergy induction. A large series of experiments has implicated control of the half-life of particular signaling molecules as a major determinant of outcome following receptor engagement. Many of these studies have focused on the biology of E3 ubiquitin ligases in the control of T cell effector versus anergic fate. Ubiquitin ligases form part of the complex that targets proteins for degradation. Genetic studies have implicated several ubiquitin ligases as key controllers of T cell fate following receptor engagement; these include c-Cbl, Cbl-b, GRAIL, Itch, and Nedd4 (148). Each of these proteins appears to negatively regulate T cell activation, in most cases by targeting key activators (including the TCR itself, as well as important components of the TCR-stimulated signaling cascades) for degradation. Loss of these proteins results in unchecked TCR function that, in animal models, leads to failed central or peripheral tolerance and lymphoproliferation, frequently leading to overt autoimmunity. Further work to clarify precisely the substrates of the individual E3 ubiquitin ligases will provide additional insights into the mechanisms by which T cell anergy is induced to control undesired outcomes of T cell effector function.

There are many mechanisms that have evolved to hold T cell responses in check. While failure to adequately costimulate T cells results in the inability of the adaptive immune system to clear invading pathogens, defects in anergy induction lead to devastating, inappropriate immune responses. It is only by carefully titrating activating and inhibitory signals that the host can mount a vigorous immune response to combat pathogens yet protect itself from the potential danger of T cells that are allowed to respond in an uncontrolled fashion.

NEGATIVE REGULATION OF T CELL RESPONSES

The TCR complex has evolved to possess exquisite sensitivity to antigen/MHC, enabling the host to respond to subtle differences between self and foreign proteins. When stimulated to become effectors, T cells are extremely potent at perpetuating inflammatory responses and directly destroying host cells that have been infected by a pathogen. This is necessary to combat invading organisms; however, whenever T cells are stimulated, there is a risk that bystander host tissue (not affected by the pathogen) may be injured as well. Further, to maintain the sensitivity of the TCR, it is also necessary to have mechanisms in place to thwart a T cell response that has been initiated inappropriately. The immune system has developed a number of critical, overlapping approaches to hold T cell responses in check and to eliminate stimulated T cells once a pathogenic challenge has been met.

IMMUNORECEPTOR TYROSINE-BASED INHIBITORY MOTIF–CONTAINING PROTEINS AND OTHER INHIBITORS OF T CELL ACTIVATION

One potent means to terminate T cell responses is to activate biochemical pathways that interdict the stimulatory events associated with a productive T cell response. This mechanism involves engagement of cell surface receptors that signal T cell inhibition. Among these receptors are those that contain immunoreceptor tyrosine-based inhibitory motifs (ITIMs) instead of ITAMs (Figure 11.14). ITIMs are recognized by their signature sequence (S/I/V/L*X*Y*XX*I/V/L) (149). Like ITAMs, the tyrosines of ITIMs are inducibly phosphorylated (most often by src PTKs), but instead of recruiting activating molecules (e.g., ZAP-70), the inhibitory receptors recruit enzymes that counter the pathways required for T cell activation. Examples of such inhibitors are the tyrosine phosphatases SH2 domain-containing phosphatase 1 (SHP-1) and SHP-2 (150) and the lipid phosphatase SH2 domain-containing inositol phosphatase (SHIP) (151). Physiologically important ITIM-expressing receptors include killer inhibitory receptors (KIRs) that are best known for inhibiting the cytotoxicity of NK cells (see Chapter 16). KIRs are also present on activated cytotoxic T cells and appear to have this same inhibitory function.

SHP-1 and SHP-2 are cytosolic protein tyrosine phosphatases that possess a catalytic domain carboxyl-terminal to two tandem SH2 domains. Upon tyrosine phosphorylation of the ITIMs of the inhibitory receptors, the SH2 domains of SHP-1 or SHP-2 are recruited to the ITIMs and convert the receptor complex into an active tyrosine phosphatase. It is presumed that because the ITIM-bearing receptors are present in close proximity to the TCR-stimulated activation complex, SHP-1 and SHP-2 can then oppose the action of src and syk PTKs by dephosphorylating the kinases themselves (thus rendering them less active) or key proximal substrates of the PTKs. In this regard, a number of experiments have shown that SHP-1 and SHP-2 are able to dephosphorylate Vav, PLCγ1, and SLP-76. SHIP does not act on substrates of the TCR-stimulated PTKs but instead dephosphorylates key lipid second messengers that are critical for cellular activation.

One area of intense current investigation involves studies designed to unravel the circumstances that favor

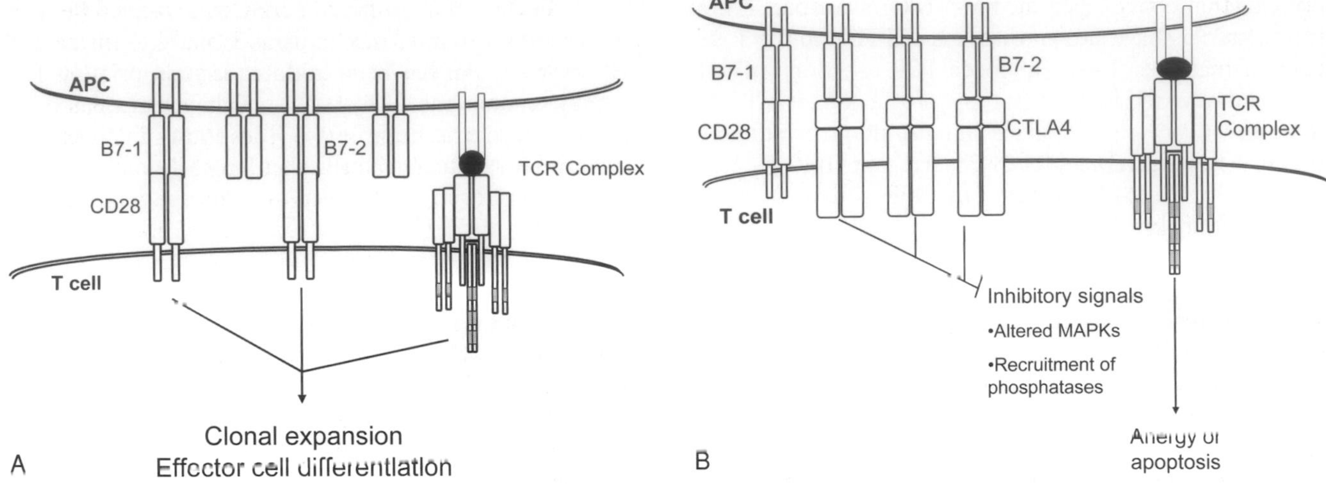

FIGURE 11.14 CTLA4 inhibits T cell activation. **A:** Stimulation of T cells via the TCR (by peptide/MHC) and CD28 (by B7-1 and B7-2) results in numerous biochemical signaling events, leading ultimately to clonal expansion and effector cell function. **B:** CTLA4, present on activated T cells, competes for binding to B7-1 and B7-2 precluding CD28-mediated activating signals. Engagement of CTLA4 also induces inhibitory signals, including changes in the spectrum of MAPKs that are activated and recruitment of phosphatases that counteract the effects of the TCR-stimulated PTKs. Failed costimulation in the setting of continued TCR signals may lead to apoptosis or anergy.

inhibitory versus stimulatory responses when the TCR complex encounters antigen/MHC. One intriguing notion is that the quality of the antigen itself plays a large part in this determination, and a number of studies have revealed the existence of so-called *altered peptide ligands* (APLs). APLs are antigens that bind the TCR, but instead of activating a response (even in the presence of costimulation), APLs induce no response or even induce anergy (152). Some experiments indicate that whether a peptide induces full T cell activation or blocks T cell responses depends upon the affinity of interaction with the TCR complex. How this translates into altered signaling remains controversial. Some studies have provided evidence that APLs stimulate some but not all of the TCR signals required for activation (e.g., partial phosphorylation of the ζ chain and other CD3 ITAMs with failed recruitment of ZAP-70 [153]). Other proposed models for APL function are that the APLs may activate ITIM-bearing receptors out of proportion to what is seen when fully agonistic peptides encounter the TCR complex or that APLs stimulate a different spectrum of MAPKs than do agonistic peptides. Additional studies are required to evaluate these models further.

ADAPTER PROTEINS ARE ALSO NEGATIVE REGULATORS OF T CELL ACTIVATION

Adapter proteins, such as LAT and SLP-76, play critical roles in integrating signaling pathways that are essential for T cell activation. Adapter proteins have also been identified that function to regulate the inhibition of these signaling cascades. Examples of such molecules include the transmembrane adapter proteins LAX (linker for activation of X cells) and SIT (SHP-2–interacting transmembrane adapter protein) (154,155). Data from mice made deficient in these proteins suggest that these proteins do not play as central a role as LAT or SLP-76, but they do appear to modulate the ability of the TCR to become activated and potentially keep autoimmunity in check.

Another transmembrane adapter protein, PAG (phosphoprotein associated with glycosphingolipid-enriched domains) or Cbp (csk-binding protein), has attracted considerable attention by investigators studying signaling events important for T cell activation (156,157). PAG/Cbp was identified as a binder of csk. The adapter is present in lipid rafts due to posttranslational modifications and is basally phosphorylated on a key tyrosine residue that is an excellent docking site for the SH2 domain of csk. Thus, PAG/Cbp is thought to position csk in lipid rafts to maintain src family PTKs in their inactive state (by phosphorylating their regulatory carboxyl-terminal tyrosines). Upon TCR stimulation, PAG/Cbp becomes dephosphorylated (by an as yet unknown tyrosine phosphatase), thus losing its ability to bind csk. Csk leaves the lipid rafts, allowing lck and fyn to exert their positive effect on the TCR signaling machinery. While there are considerable data from cell lines and transgenic mice to support this model of PAG/Cbp action (158), mice engineered to be deficient in the adapter protein show no overt T cell phenotype (159). This result suggests that either there are additional proteins that can compensate for PAG/Cbp function or that the notion for how these proteins function needs to be reconsidered.

INTERFERING WITH COSTIMULATION, THE ROLE OF CTLA4 IN INHIBITING T CELL RESPONSES

A critical tenet in T cell biology is that stimulation of the TCR without costimulation leads to failed T cell activation and in many cases to T cell anergy. Thus, interfering with the ability of CD28 to transduce its signals is a logical means to inhibit T cell responses. As might be predicted, interfering with CD28 signaling has been shown to be an extremely potent (and physiologically crucial) means to regulate T cell function.

One of the most effective ways to prevent CD28 signaling is the coexpression of CTLA4 (CD152), a cell surface receptor expressed once an initial T cell response has begun (160). Although CTLA4 is only one of a number of negative regulators of T cell activation, its physiologic importance sets it apart from the others. Mice in which the gene for CTLA4 has been eliminated suffer from a uniformly fatal lymphoproliferative syndrome characterized by massive enlargement of secondary lymphoid organs (161,162). Although these mice are born with an apparently normal repertoire of T cells (both in numbers and antigen reactivity), implying that CTLA4 is not critical for thymic development, within several weeks of birth, the animals demonstrate markedly enhanced T cell mass and severe autoimmunity. These observations led to tremendous interest in the mechanisms by which CTLA4 modulates T cell responses. Evidence has emerged indicating that CTLA4 engagement may lead to inactivation of T cell responses and, in some cases, death of effector T cells, both important ways in which this surface molecule terminates T cell function.

CTLA4 is in the CD28 family, but it has much greater affinity for B7 family members than does CD28 itself. Thus, expression of high levels of CTLA4 on an activated T cell provides a "sink" for CD28 ligands, thereby prohibiting the activating costimulatory receptor from stimulating a T cell effector response (163). Lack of CD28 costimulation prevents further T cell activation and terminates additional expansion of antigen-specific clones. This observation has been turned into a new and extremely effective therapeutic tool. A soluble fusion protein consisting of CTLA4 covalently linked to the Fc region of antibody (CTLA4-Ig) was administered first to mice and then to human patients suffering from transplant rejection or autoimmune diseases (164,165). CTLA4-Ig binds the B7 ligands with high affinity, thus depriving antigen-specific T cells from receiving a CD28 signal, abrogating the unwanted *in vivo* immune response.

CTLA4 does not function merely in a passive fashion by competing with CD28 for ligand binding. Instead, it appears that CTLA4 also transduces signals of its own to actively dampen T cell responses. This activity has been shown in two ways. First, studies show that CTLA4 expression is effective at blocking activation of T cells that lack CD28 (166). Second, other experiments show that a mutant of CTLA4 lacking the cytoplasmic tail but still able to bind with high affinity to B7 ligands only partially ameliorates the autoimmune phenotype of CTLA4-deficient mice (167). Although it is clear that the ability of CTLA4 to interfere with T cell activation directly requires the CTLA4 cytoplasmic domain, the precise molecular mechanism of this action is unclear. Several models, each of which is supported by experimental evidence, have been put forth.

In one scenario, CTLA4 has been shown to modulate signaling pathways downstream of the TCR that are critical for activation. In a number of these studies, engagement of CTLA4 affects various members of the MAPK family, most prominently ERK and c-Jun kinase (168). The relative effect on the various kinases is not consistent from study to study, underscoring the complexity of the system and the potential differences one may uncover when different model systems are studied. It is unclear also whether the effects of CTLA4 on MAPK activation are direct or whether these findings represent the ability of CTLA4 engagement to interfere with TCR-mediated events upstream of MAPK stimulation. One mechanism for how CTLA4 may manipulate membrane proximal events stimulated by the engaged TCR came from studies demonstrating that the complement of proteins that associate with the cytoplasmic domain of CTLA4 changes upon engagement of this receptor by B7 ligands. One such experiment suggested a regulated interaction between CTLA4, the protein tyrosine phosphatase SHP-2, and the ζ chain of the TCR (169); however, the molecular basis for these associations and whether they control CTLA4 function remain controversial. In fact, although there are several phosphorylated tyrosines within the CTLA4 cytoplasmic domain, a number of investigators have provided compelling evidence that phosphorylation of these residues is not critical for the inhibitory effects of CTLA4 on T cell activation (170,171).

Several groups have suggested another mechanism by which the CTLA4 cytoplasmic region may control its ability to regulate T cell activation. In this scenario, in productively activated cells, the cytoplasmic tail of CTLA4 associates with the clathrin adapter, AP50, leading to CTLA4 endocytoses and degradation (172). Stimulation of CTLA4 abrogates its association with AP50, retaining CTLA4 on the cell surface (173). Still other groups have provided complementary evidence suggesting that the function of CTLA4 is regulated most precisely by where in the cell CTLA4 is localized, being sequestered away from the TCR contact site as cells are stimulated and being directed toward the activation complex to terminate T cell responses.

Thus, while it is clear from genetic, biochemical, and molecular studies that CTLA4 is a major negative regulator of T cell activation, details regarding how it exerts its essential functions remain obscure.

OTHER INHIBITORY RECEPTORS THAT BIND TO B7 LIGANDS

PD-1 (programmed death-1) belongs to the same family as CD28 and CTLA4, but PD-1 exists as a monomer on the cell surface, as it lacks the cysteine required for dimerization (174,175). It contains two phosphorylatable tyrosines within its cytoplasmic domain, at least one of which forms a partial ITIM and therefore has negative regulatory functions. PD-1 binds to two members of the B7 family of ligands, PD-L1 and PD-L2. Evidence for a negative role of PD-1 in T cell function comes from mice made deficient in the gene for this molecule; these mice exhibit lymphoproliferation early in life and overt autoimmunity as they age (176). More recent studies have shown that the interaction between PD-L1 and PD-1 results in failed clearance of viral pathogens, providing one mechanism for the development of chronic viral infection, such as is seen after exposure to human immunodeficiency virus (HIV) (177). This finding has resulted in a great deal of excitement about the potential of blocking PD-1 in the setting of chronic infection as a means to generate a maximal effector T cell response. It is not yet clear how PD-1 interferes with T cell function, as preliminary studies have failed to reveal any defects in TCR-mediated signaling when PD-1 is engaged. It does appear that PD-1 interferes with expression of T cell survival genes, and the costimulatory receptor has been shown to associate with SHP-2 (but not SHP-1 or SHIP), suggesting a possible mechanism of action.

Additional members of the CD28 family have been identified as binders to other newly identified members of the B7 family of ligands (178). Biochemical and genetic studies suggest that these ligand/receptor pairs will also play important costimulatory roles for T cell activation, indicating that we do not yet appreciate the full complexity of this process. It is likely that each of these receptors will play its most essential role under particular circumstances (e.g., in naïve versus memory cells or in T cells that are fated to particular *in vivo* functions), but it is also likely that these molecules will have overlapping functions and compensate, at least partially, for each other during immune responses.

ELIMINATING THE EXPANDED T CELL POPULATION

Interfering with the activation of resting or antigen-stimulated T cells is not sufficient for homeostasis of the T cell compartment. The normal T cell response to a pathologic challenge is massive clonal expansion of antigen-specific cells, so that the number of effector cells is sufficient to eliminate the pathogen. As described earlier, it is essential that once the antigenic challenge has been met, the responding T cells stop dividing and discontinue their effector functions to prevent damage to tissue unaffected by the pathogen. Additionally, it is necessary to resolve the increased mass of T cells to prevent progressive enlargement of the secondary lymphoid organs and eliminate any T cells that may have been inadvertently stimulated (as bystanders) as the immune response developed. Thus, the vast majority of T cells that participated in the effector response must be removed, leaving only a small number of previously activated antigen-specific T cells that will be retained to provide a memory response, should that particular pathogen be encountered again in the future.

At the completion of an immune response, T cells are eliminated via apoptosis, otherwise known as programmed cell death. There are several mechanisms by which this death occurs (179). Some T cells die because factors necessary for their growth (e.g., IL2) are no longer being produced. This results in the failed production of anti-apoptotic proteins, such as members of the Bcl2 family. In addition to this passive means of apoptosis, T cell death following an effector immune response occurs actively in a process designated *AICD* (activation-induced cell death) that results from the orchestration of signaling events initiated by engagement of specific cell surface receptors (Figure 11.15).

An extremely important pathway for *in vivo* AICD was revealed by a confluence of observations made by different teams of investigators, some studying basic receptor biology *in vitro*, others investigating spontaneously arising mutations in mice, and yet another group interested in understanding the molecular basis of a rare but severe lymphoproliferative disorder. The receptor biologists were interested in the question of how T cell numbers are controlled, and they reasoned that if T cell loss is regulated, it was likely that this process is mediated by cell surface receptors. These investigators generated monoclonal antibodies directed against cell surface proteins present on activated T cells in the hope that some of these antibodies would serve as agonists that, when incubated with activated T cells, would lead to cell death. Such antibodies were identified that were potent inducers of apoptosis in activated but not resting T cells (180). As this work progressed and Fas (now known as CD95), the receptor that was recognized by the death-inducing antibodies, was being characterized, other investigators were examining mice that carried spontaneously occurring mutations that led to massive lymphoproliferation and autoimmune events. Careful examination of the mice revealed that two strains of animals existed with identical phenotypes but clearly different genotypes. Follow up

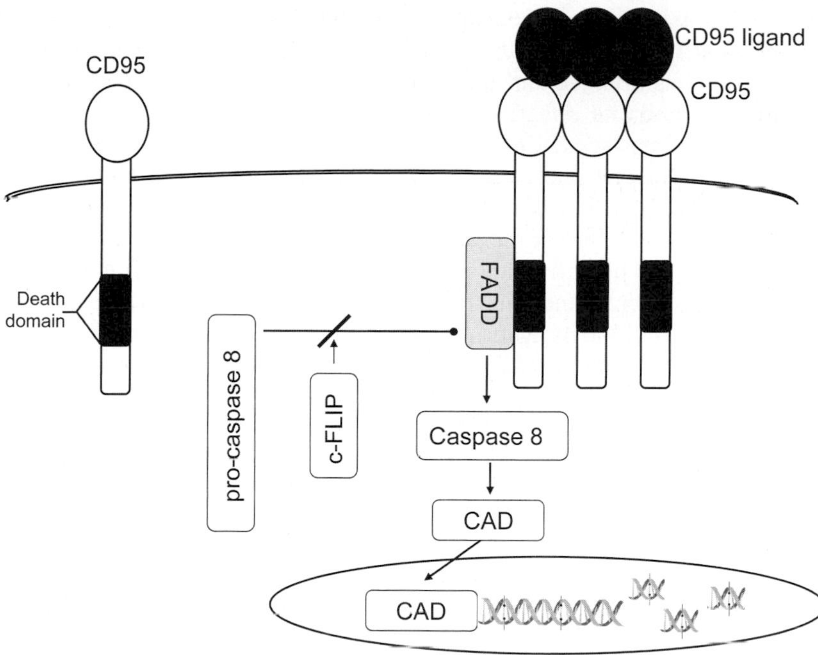

***FIGURE 11.15* Stimulation of CD95 by its ligand results in AICD.** One consequence of T cell activation is the up-regulation of the surface receptor CD95 (Fas) and its ligand. Engagement of CD95 leads to the recruitment of the adapter protein Fas-associated death domain (FADD) that nucleates the formation of a molecular complex, activating pro-caspase 8, leading to a cascade of cysteine-directed proteases that ultimately leads to DNA cleavage by Caspase-activatable DNAse (CAD). The resultant apoptosis eliminates the majority of activated T cells once an antigenic challenge has been cleared. CD95-mediated apoptosis is a highly regulated process and can be inhibited by endogenous inhibitors, such as c-FLIP (cellular FLICE [FADD-like interleukin-1β converting enzyme] inhibitory protein) that functions by preventing the activation of the proenzyme form of Caspase 8. Adapted from Koretzky GA. T-cell activation and inactivation. In: Rich R, et al., eds. *Clinical Immunology*. London: Mosby, 2001.

studies demonstrated that one of the strains (designated *lpr*) carried a mutation in a molecule that likely served as a receptor expressed on T cells, while the second strain (designated *gld*) was mutated in the ligand for that receptor (181). As these studies were being performed, clinical immunologists were identifying patients with immune system dysfunction that resembled that of the *lpr* and *gld* mice. Although these patients appeared normal at birth and had no difficulty with early childhood illnesses, as they aged they demonstrated significant lymphadenopathy, and their peripheral T cells lacked both CD4 and CD8. The constellation of these findings plus the propensity of these patients to develop autoimmune syndromes led to the description of autoimmune lymphoproliferative syndrome (ALPS) (182). Eventually, it became clear that all three investigations were examining the same phenomenon and that CD95 was the causal gene for the *lpr* strain (183), CD95 ligand was the causal gene for the *gld* strain (184), and that mutations in CD95, CD95 ligand, or the signaling pathway stimulated by this receptor ligand pair were responsible for ALPS (182).

Follow-up molecular experiments, further examination of the mice, and additional studies of the patient samples have led to considerable insight into the biochemistry of AICD. CD95 is present at low levels on the surface of resting T cells. One of the consequences of TCR stimulation is up-regulation of this key death receptor. Another consequence of the signaling pathways stimulated by engagement of the TCR is inducible expression of CD95 ligand. Thus, in addition to stimulating all of the steps necessary for cellular activation, TCR ligation also results in up-regulation of the machinery critical for AICD (185). In fact, it appears that one other control point that prevents inappropriate T cell activation is that effective costimulation is required to interdict the AICD pathway.

CD95 exists as a trimer on the cell surface. When bound to CD95 ligand (also a trimer, either present on other activated T cells, other cell types, or secreted), a signaling pathway is initiated that involves the recruitment of an adapter protein named FADD (Fas-associated death domain protein), which in turn brings the proenzymatic form of Caspase 8 into the complex (186). This results in activation of Caspase 8, which initiates a sequence of enzymatic events leading to activation of a series of additional caspases that eventually stimulates a DNAse, designated CAD for Caspase-activatable DNAse. Active CAD enters the nucleus and cleaves cellular DNA into the nucleosome pattern characteristic of apoptosis. A critical step in the apoptotic process is loss of mitochondrial membrane integrity, leading to the leakage of cytochrome C from this organelle into the cytosol. In the cytosol, cytochrome C binds to Apaf-1 (apoptosis protease activating factor-1), forming a complex that participates in Caspase activation leading eventually to DNA cleavage within the nucleus (187).

AICD is a carefully regulated process. In addition to control of expression of both CD95 and CD95 ligand, there are cytoplasmic inhibitors of the apoptosis pathway. One such example is FLIP (FLICE [FADD-like IL-1β converting enzyme] inhibitory protein), a protein that inhibits formation of the FADD-mediated death-inducing complex (188). FLIP expression is modulated in T cells and has been found to be up-regulated in T cells that have received effective costimulation in addition to engagement of the TCR. Other cytoplasmic regulators of AICD include members of the Bcl2 family (e.g., Bcl-XL and Bcl2), which preserve mitochondrial membrane integrity, as well as *in vivo* modulators of the Caspases (I-CADs or inhibitors of Caspase-activatable DNase), which are critical for prevention of cell death (189,190). To make matters even more complex, there are also members of the Bcl2 family (most notably Bax and Bak) that potentiate apoptosis by destabilizing the mitochondrial membrane (191).

Although CD95 and its ligand have attracted a great deal of attention as regulators of AICD, other TNF receptor family members are also important in the control homeostasis of the T cell compartment. These receptors work by similar mechanisms; however, the identities of the signal transducers are different. Thus, TNF receptors cooperate with other adapter proteins including TRADD (TNF receptor 1–associated death domain protein) and members of the TRAF (TNF receptor–associated factor) family, leading to activation of signaling pathways that overlap with those stimulated by CD95. In addition to TNF receptors that activate the apoptosis pathway, other so-called *decoy receptors* are present on the cell surface that appear to serve as a sink for death receptor ligands. Engagement of these receptors fails to initiate apoptosis and is thought to deprive the activating death-inducing receptors from interacting with ligands. Abnormalities in the signaling pathways initiated by engagement of CD95 and the other TNF family receptors have been described, not only in immune disorders, but also in other diseases associated with abnormalities in cell death, most notably in malignancy. Thus, understanding the basic mechanisms by which these receptors function normally has become an important goal of many laboratories with far-ranging interests.

SIGNALING MOLECULES ARE IMPORTANT TARGETS FOR IMMUNOMODULATORY THERAPY

There are a number of clinical circumstances during which it is important to dampen T cell responses. Among these are autoimmune disorders, which are spontaneously arising diseases characterized by inappropriate immune responses against self tissues, and Iatrogenic conditions, where it is necessary to abrogate an otherwise normal immune response—for example, protecting a transplant from rejection. Because T cells play a central role in mediating both autoimmunity and transplant rejection, molecules critical for T cell activation are important targets for therapeutic intervention. Initially, such drugs were identified empirically, by screening compounds in assays designed to detect inhibitors of T cell activation using a very distal event (e.g., cellular proliferation or cytokine production) as a readout. This strategy was required, because the molecular identity of the key signaling molecules was not yet known. Even so, extremely effective drugs were developed. Among these is cyclosporine, a natural (fungal) product that is one of the most important immunosuppressive agents in clinical use today (192). Cyclosporine acts by inhibition of the calcineurin pathway, thus preventing NFAT dephosphorylation and translocation to the nucleus. This drug was used for decades before its molecular mode of action was discovered. In fact, much of what we know about calcineurin and NFAT came from studies undertaken to explain why cyclosporine is such an effective immunosuppressant. Rapamycin is another clinically important immunosuppressive agent that was identified originally in a search for bacteria-derived products that could potentially serve as anti-fungal agents (193). Further testing of this drug revealed potent immunosuppressive effects (as well as antiproliferative effects that are now being exploited to combat various cancers [194]). Like cyclosporine, in addition to being a clinically useful immunosuppressant, studies of rapamycin have provided a great deal of basic knowledge about how immune cells transduce signals—in this case, the biochemical basis for IL2 receptor function.

As knowledge about particular signaling molecules was gained, drug discovery became directed toward validated biologic targets in the hope that more effective and specific therapies could be developed. OKT3, a monoclonal antibody directed against the CD3 proteins, is now a mainstay in the clinical armamentarium for therapy against transplant rejection (195). Similarly, monoclonal antibodies directed against the receptor for IL2 have found an important place in the clinic (196). As mentioned earlier, one very recent example of a novel therapeutic agent that has been introduced into the clinic based on our understanding of the biology of T cell activation is soluble CTLA4-Ig, an agent that was developed as an inhibitor of CD28 function (197). Although early in its clinical use, CTLA4-Ig has shown outstanding promise as an inhibitor of unwanted T cell activation. Numerous other agents are now being developed and tested based on what we have learned over the past few years. Intriguing candidates are drugs directed toward modifying functions of other receptors, such as ICOS, activity of enzymes, such as ZAP-70 and PKCθ, and key transcription factors, such as members of the NFκB family. The next decade is also likely to see yet another class of immunomodulatory agents, in this case drugs that will augment rather than inhibit T cell responses. One of the limitations of T cell immune responses in the setting of chronic viral infections is early termination of T cell responses, an event known as T cell exhaustion. Recent work has implicated key receptors (e.g., PD-1) and signaling molecules (e.g., SHP-1) in T cell exhaustion. Agents are now being developed that are designed to interfere with this inhibition of T cell responses in the hope that better therapies can be developed for chronic viral illnesses.

CONCLUSION

The past two decades have seen an explosion in our knowledge regarding the molecular and biochemical basis of T cell activation. Prior to the early 1980s, the identity of the TCR, the receptor that initiates the T cell response to antigen, was unknown. In fact, it was then unclear whether T cells responded to peptide antigen via one receptor and MHC proteins via a second cell surface protein or whether a single receptor was capable of binding to both antigen and MHC. Since the discovery of the TCR and its obligatory relationship with the CD3 molecules, an intricate cascade of signaling networks has been described. These pathways are now known to be critical for T cell activation as well as termination of T cell responses. We have learned how these signal transduction cascades intersect with others initiated by other receptors on T cells and what the biochemical consequences are of signaling via some receptors in isolation versus signaling via multiple receptors simultaneously. Studies of how T cells respond to activating and inhibitory stimuli have made great use of new knowledge gained by investigators in other fields but have also informed scientists studying other biologic systems about ways in which their work should proceed. Most importantly, however, investigations into how T cells are programmed to respond have provided crucial insights into the basic mechanisms of multiple human disorders and have given us important clues to help develop novel therapeutic modalities that promise to significantly diminish the morbidity and mortality of immune system diseases.

Initial insights into the molecular events associated with T cell activation utilized malignant cell lines that represent either developing thymocytes or mature T cells. While there are limitations to this approach (malignant cell lines are transformed and thus may not faithfully recapitulate the situation of a normal primary cell), results of studies using these reagents have been remarkably predictive of what is seen in more physiological settings. Especially during the early days of study, before the important molecules themselves were known, the availability of a stable source of cells that could be manipulated genetically provided outstanding experimental tools. Now, as may of the critical modulators of immune cell signaling have been identified, more physiologically relevant experiments are performed routinely using mice in which genes for these key regulators are modified within the genome.

The next generation of studies will continue to make use of such genetically altered mice. An important new direction for these investigations is generating mice in which mutations in signaling molecules can be selectively expressed in a temporal and lineage-specific manner. This control is particularly important, since mutations in signaling molecules often have dramatic effects on T cell development. It is often impossible to ascertain if abnormalities detected in peripheral T cell function are a result of altered development or because that particular molecule is also essential for transducing signals in mature T cells. The advent of mice in which wild type genes can be switched to genes with targeted mutations after T cell development is complete will soon allow studies to proceed that will selectively probe the importance of signaling pathways for thymocyte development versus mature T cell activation.

Advances in imaging will also markedly impact our ability to take studies of T cell activation to the next level of rigor and sophistication. A key advantage of modern image analysis approaches is that such studies make it possible to study individual cells, in contrast to most of our current methodologies that analyze thousands to millions of cells concurrently for any single data point. Clearly, much information is lost under these circumstances. To this end, techniques are also being developed to analyze posttranslational modifications of cytoplasmic molecules on a single cell basis. Reagents are now becoming available that can detect activation of particular signal transduction pathways using antibodies that can distinguish resting versus activated enzymes and substrates by flow cytometry.

Although most of the receptors and signaling molecules described in this chapter are designated as either positive or negative regulators, recent data have demonstrated that many of these proteins appear to function as activators under some circumstances and as inhibitors under others. For example, mice deficient in FADD, a key component of the pathway leading to AICD, demonstrate developing thymocytes and mature T cells that are resistant to activation, suggesting that FADD may be an essential positive regulator of T cell function. Similarly, PD-1, described initially as an inhibitor of T cell activation, appears essential for function in some model systems. Even the best-established negative regulators, such as CTLA4, have been shown to have positive regulatory function under some experimental conditions. Thus, similar to all other biologic systems, the more we learn about the biology of T cell activation, the more we realize we have yet to learn and that future experiments will continue to require an unbiased assessment of data as they emerge.

The importance of combining *in vitro* studies, experiments using model organisms, and learning from human patients cannot be underestimated. While valuable insights into the basic functioning of the human immune system have been elucidated in the laboratory utilizing cell lines and animal models, it has been shown time and again that these findings are not always recapitulated identically in humans. Additionally, many of the features of how T cells are stimulated to respond or to terminate their effector functions have been learned directly from careful analysis of patients afflicted with immune-mediated disorders. As new therapies based on our understanding of basic immune mechanisms are being brought into the clinic, it will be increasingly important for clinical and basic immunologists to work closely together so that these novel agents can be used for optimal advantage. Without doubt, the use of these new drugs will yield some surprising results that will require an adjustment to our thinking of how T cell function is regulated *in vivo*. These new insights will then be translated into the next generation of agents that will hopefully have even greater efficacy.

REFERENCES

1. Meuer SC, Acuto O, Hercend T, et al. The human T-cell receptor. *Annu Rev Immunol.* 1984;2:23–50.
2. Pennington DJ, Vermijlen D, Wise EL, et al. The integration of conventional and unconventional T cells that characterizes cell-mediated responses. *Adv Immunol.* 2005;87:27–59.
3. Bhandoola A, Sambandam A. From stem cell to T cell: one route or many? *Nat Rev Immunol.* 2006;6(2):117–126.
4. Irving BA, Alt FW, Killeen N. Thymocyte development in the absence of pre-T cell receptor extracellular immunoglobulin domains. *Science.* 1998;280(5365):905–908.
5. Weiss A, Stobo J. Requirement for the coexpression of T3 and the T cell antigen receptor on a malignant human T cell line. *J Exp Med.* 1984;160(5):1284–1299.
6. Manolios N, Letourneur F, Bonifacino JS, et al. Pairwise, cooperative and inhibitory interactions describe the assembly and probable structure of the T-cell antigen receptor. *EMBO J.* 1991;10(7):1643–1651.
7. Dembic Z, Haas W, Weiss S, et al. Transfer of specificity by murine alpha and beta T-cell receptor genes. *Nature.* 1986;320(6059):232–238.
8. Abraham RT, Weiss A. Jurkat T cells and development of the T-cell receptor signalling paradigm. *Nat Rev Immunol.* 2004;4(4):301–308.
9. Wegener AM, Letourneur F, Hoeveler A, et al. The T cell receptor/CD3 complex is composed of at least two autonomous transduction modules. *Cell.* 1992;68(1):83–95.
10. Irving BA, Weiss A. The cytoplasmic domain of the T cell receptor zeta chain is sufficient to couple to receptor-associated signal transduction pathways. *Cell.* 1991;64(5):891–901.
11. Reth M. Antigen receptor tail clue. *Nature.* 1989;338:383–384.
12. Flaswinkel H, Barner M, Reth M. The tyrosine activation motif as a target of protein tyrosine kinases and SH2 domains. *Semin Immunol.* 1995;7(1):21–27.
13. Cambier JC. Antigen and Fc receptor signaling. The awesome power of the immunoreceptor tyrosine-based activation motif (ITAM). *J Immunol.* 1995;155(7):3281–3285.
14. Ivetic A, Ridley AJ. Ezrin/radixin/moesin proteins and Rho GTPase signalling in leucocytes. *Immunology.* 2004;112(2):165–176.
15. Hirose M, Kitano J, Nakajima Y, et al. Phosphorylation and recruitment of Syk by immunoreceptor tyrosine-based activation motif-based phosphorylation of tamalin. *J Biol Chem.* 2004;279(31):32308–32315.
16. Grande SM, Ross SR, Monroe JG. Viral immunoreceptor-associated tyrosine-based activation motifs: potential players in oncogenesis. *Future Oncol.* 2006;2(2):301–310.
17. Weiss A, Littman DR. Signal transduction by lymphocyte antigen receptors. *Cell.* 1994;76(2):263–274.
18. Chan AC, Iwashima M, Turck CW, et al. ZAP-70: a 70 kd protein-tyrosine kinase that associates with the TCR zeta chain. *Cell.* 1992;71(4):649–662.
19. Schaeffer EM, Debnath J, Yap G, et al. Requirement for Tec kinases Rlk and Itk in T cell receptor signaling and immunity. *Science.* 1999;284(5414):638–641.
20. Iwashima M, Irving BA, van Oers NS, et al. Sequential interactions of the TCR with two distinct cytoplasmic tyrosine kinases. *Science.* 1994;263(5150):1136–1139.
21. Straus DB, Weiss A. Genetic evidence for the involvement of the lck tyrosine kinase in signal transduction through the T cell antigen receptor. *Cell.* 1992;70(4):585–593.
22. Williams BL, Schreiber KL, Zhang W, et al. Genetic evidence for differential coupling of Syk family kinases to the T-cell receptor: reconstitution studies in a ZAP-70-deficient Jurkat T-cell line. *Mol Cell Biol.* 1998;18(3):1388–1399.
23. Stein PL, Lee HM, Rich S, et al. pp59fyn mutant mice display differential signaling in thymocytes and peripheral T cells. *Cell.* 1992;70(5):741–750.
24. Molina TJ, Kishihara K, Siderovski DP, et al. Profound block in thymocyte development in mice lacking p56lck. *Nature.* 1992;357(6374):161–164.
25. Roifman CM. Studies of patients' thymi aid in the discovery and characterization of immunodeficiency in humans. *Immunol Rev.* 2005;203:143–155.
26. Lovatt M, Filby A, Parravicini V, et al. Lck regulates the threshold of activation in primary T cells, while both Lck and Fyn contribute to the magnitude of the extracellular signal-related kinase response. *Mol Cell Biol.* 2006;26(22):8655–8665.
27. Sugie K, Jeon MS, Grey HM. Activation of naive CD4 T cells by anti-CD3 reveals an important role for Fyn in Lck-mediated signaling. *Proc Natl Acad Sci U S A.* 2004;101(41):14859–14864.
28. Davidson D, Shi X, Zhang S, et al. Genetic evidence linking SAP, the X-linked lymphoproliferative gene product, to Src-related kinase FynT in T(H)2 cytokine regulation. *Immunity.* 2004;21(5):707–717.
29. Groves T, Smiley P, Cooke MP, et al. Fyn can partially substitute for Lck in T lymphocyte development. *Immunity.* 1996;5(5):417–428.
30. van Oers NS, Lowin-Kropf B, Finlay D, et al. alpha beta T cell development is abolished in mice lacking both Lck and Fyn protein tyrosine kinases. *Immunity.* 1996;5(5):429–436.
31. Negishi I, Motoyama N, Nakayama K, et al. Essential role for ZAP-70 in both positive and negative selection of thymocytes. *Nature.* 1995;376(6539):435–438.
32. Cheng AM, Negisihi I, Anderson SJ, et al. The Syk and ZAP-70 SH2-containing tyrosine kinases are implicated in pre-T cell receptor signaling. *Proc Natl Acad Sci U S A.* 1997;94(18):9797–9801.
33. Goldman FD, Ballas ZK, Schutte BC, et al. Defective expression of p56lck in an infant with severe combined immunodeficiency. *J Clin Invest.* 1998;102(2):421–429.
34. Elder ME. SCID due to ZAP-70 deficiency. *J Pediatr Hematol Oncol.* 1997;19(6):546–550.
35. Orchard J, Ibbotson R, Best G, et al. ZAP-70 in B cell malignancies. *Leuk Lymphoma.* 2005;46(12):1689–1698.
36. Rosenwald A, Alizadeh AA, Widhopf G, et al. Relation of gene expression phenotype to immunoglobulin mutation genotype in B cell chronic lymphocytic leukemia. *J Exp Med.* 2001;194(11):1639–1647.
37. Liao XC, Littman DR. Altered T cell receptor signaling and disrupted T cell development in mice lacking Itk. *Immunity.* 1995;3(6):757–769.
38. Lucas JA, Miller AT, Atherly LO, et al. The role of Tec family kinases in T cell development and function. *Immunol Rev.* 2003;191:119–138.
39. Samelson LE, Phillips AF, Luong ET, et al. Association of the fyn protein-tyrosine kinase with the T-cell antigen receptor. *Proc Natl Acad Sci U S A.* 1990;87(11):4358–4362.
40. Rudd CE. CD4, CD8 and the TCR-CD3 complex: a novel class of protein-tyrosine kinase receptor. *Immunol Today.* 1990;11(11):400–406.
41. Pelosi M, Di Bartolo V, Mounier V, et al. Tyrosine 319 in the interdomain B of ZAP-70 is a binding site for the Src homology 2 domain of Lck. *J Biol Chem.* 1999;274(20):14229–14237.
42. Kong G, Dalton M, Wardenburg JB, et al. Distinct tyrosine phosphorylation sites in ZAP-70 mediate activation and negative regulation of antigen receptor function. *Mol Cell Biol.* 1996;16(9):5026–5035.
43. Tonks NK, Diltz CD, Fischer EH. Purification and assay of CD45: an integral membrane protein-tyrosine phosphatase. *Methods Enzymol.* 1991;201:442–451.
44. Pingel JT, Thomas ML. Evidence that the leukocyte-common antigen is required for antigen- induced T lymphocyte proliferation. *Cell.* 1989;58(6):1055–1065.
45. Koretzky GA, Picus J, Thomas ML, et al. Tyrosine phosphatase CD45 is essential for coupling T-cell antigen receptor to the phosphatidyl inositol pathway. *Nature.* 1990;346(6279):66–68.
46. Trowbridge IS, Thomas ML. CD45: an emerging role as a protein tyrosine phosphatase required for lymphocyte activation and development. *Annu Rev Immunol.* 1994;12:85–116.

47. Hathcock KS, Laszlo G, Dickler HB, et al. Expression of variable exon A-, B-, and C-specific CD45 determinants on peripheral and thymic T cell populations. *J Immunol.* 1992;148(1):19–28.
48. Xu Z, Weiss A. Negative regulation of CD45 by differential homodimerization of the alternatively spliced isoforms. *Nat Immunol.* 2002;3(8):764–771.
49. Majeti R, Xu Z, Parslow TG, et al. An inactivating point mutation in the inhibitory wedge of CD45 causes lymphoproliferation and autoimmunity. *Cell.* 2000;103(7):1059–1070.
50. Tchilian EZ, Beverley PC. Altered CD45 expression and disease. *Trends Immunol.* 2006;27(3):146–153.
51. Chow LM, Veillette A. The Src and Csk families of tyrosine protein kinases in hemopoietic cells. *Semin Immunol.* 1995;7(4):207–226.
52. Nishibe S, Wahl MI, Hernandez-Sotomayor SM, et al. Increase of the catalytic activity of phospholipase C-gamma 1 by tyrosine phosphorylation. *Science.* 1990;250(4985):1253–1256.
53. Lewis RS. Calcium signaling mechanisms in T lymphocytes. *Annu Rev Immunol.* 2001;19:497–521.
54. Feske S, Gwack Y, Prakriya M, et al. A mutation in Orai1 causes immune deficiency by abrogating CRAC channel function. *Nature.* 2006;441(7090):179–185.
55. Winslow MM, Neilson JR, Crabtree GR. Calcium signalling in lymphocytes. *Curr Opin Immunol.* 2003;15(3):299–307.
56. Hogan PG, Chen L, Nardone J, et al. Transcriptional regulation by calcium, calcineurin, and NFAT. *Genes Dev.* 2003;17(18):2205–2232.
57. Beals CR, Sheridan CM, Turck CW, et al. Nuclear export of NF-ATc enhanced by glycogen synthase kinase-3. *Science.* 1997; 275(5308):1930–1934.
58. Zhu J, Shibasaki F, Price R, et al. Intramolecular masking of nuclear import signal on NF-AT4 by casein kinase I and MEKK1. *Cell.* 1998;93(5):851–861.
59. Hemenway CS, Heitman J. Calcineurin. Structure, function, and inhibition. *Cell Biochem Biophys.* 1999;30(1):115–151.
60. Spitaler M, Cantrell DA. Protein kinase C and beyond. *Nat Immunol.* 2004;5(8):785–790.
61. Ebinu JO, Bottorff DA, Chan EY, et al. RasGRP, a Ras guanyl nucleotide- releasing protein with calcium- and diacylglycerol-binding motifs. *Science.* 1998;280(5366):1082–1086.
62. Rincon M. MAP-kinase signaling pathways in T cells. *Curr Opin Immunol.* 2001;13(3):339–345.
63. Schulze-Luehrmann J, Ghosh S. Antigen receptor signaling to nuclear factor kappa B. *Immunity.* 2006;25(5):701–715.
64. Zhang W, Sloan-Lancaster J, Kitchen J, et al. LAT: the ZAP-70 tyrosine kinase substrate that links T cell receptor to cellular activation. *Cell.* 1998;92(1):83–92.
65. Jackman J, Motto D, Sun Q, et al. Molecular cloning of SLP-76, a 76kDa tyrosine phosphoprotein associated with Grb2 in T cells. *J Biol Chem.* 1995;270:7029–7032.
66. Zhang W, Sommers CL, Burshtyn DN, et al. Essential role of LAT in T cell development. *Immunity.* 1999;10(3):323–332.
67. Gong Q, Cheng AM, Akk AM, et al. Disruption of T cell signaling networks and development by Grb2 haploid insufficiency. *Nat Immunol.* 2001;2(1):29–36.
68. Zhang W, Samelson LE. The role of membrane-associated adaptors in T cell receptor signalling. *Semin Immunol.* 2000;12(1):35–41.
69. Liu SK, Fang N, Koretzky GA, et al. The hematopoietic-specific adaptor protein gads functions in T-cell signaling via interactions with the SLP-76 and LAT adaptors. *Curr Biol.* 1999;9(2):67–75.
70. Koretzky GA, Abtahian F, Silverman MA. SLP76 and SLP65: complex regulation of signalling in lymphocytes and beyond. *Nat Rev Immunol.* 2006;6(1):67–78.
71. Deng L, Velikovsky CA, Swaminathan CP, et al. Structural basis for recognition of the T cell adaptor protein SLP-76 by the SH3 domain of phospholipase Cgamma1. *J Mol Biol.* 2005;352(1):1–10.
72. Peterson EJ, Woods ML, Dmowski SA, et al. Coupling of the TCR to integrin activation by Slap-130/Fyb. *Science.* 2001;293(5538):2263–2265.
73. Griffiths EK, Krawczyk C, Kong YY, et al. Positive regulation of T cell activation and integrin adhesion by the adapter Fyb/Slap. *Science.* 2001;293(5538):2260–2263.
74. Acuto O, Cantrell D. T cell activation and the cytoskeleton. *Annu Rev Immunol.* 2000;18:165–84.
75. Tybulewicz VL. Vav-family proteins in T-cell signalling. *Curr Opin Immunol.* 2005;17(3):267–274.
76. Krawczyk C, Oliveira-dos-Santos A, Sasaki T, et al. Vav1 controls integrin clustering and MHC/peptide-specific cell adhesion to antigen-presenting cells. *Immunity.* 2002;16(3):331–343.
77. Fujikawa K, Miletic AV, Alt FW, et al. Vav1/2/3-null mice define an essential role for Vav family proteins in lymphocyte development and activation but a differential requirement in MAPK signaling in T and B cells. *J Exp Med.* 2003;198(10):1595–1608.
78. Rosen FS, Cooper MD, Wedgwood RJ. The primary immunodeficiencies. *N Engl J Med.* 1995;333(7):431–440.
79. Bubeck Wardenburg J, Pappu R, Bu JY, et al. Regulation of PAK activation and the T cell cytoskeleton by the linker protein SLP-76. *Immunity.* 1998;9(5):607–616.
80. Zeng R, Cannon JL, Abraham RT, et al. SLP-76 coordinates Nck-dependent Wiskott-Aldrich syndrome protein recruitment with Vav-1/Cdc42-dependent Wiskott-Aldrich syndrome protein activation at the T cell-APC contact site. *J Immunol.* 2003;171(3):1360–1368.
81. Badour K, Zhang J, Siminovitch KA. The Wiskott-Aldrich syndrome protein: forging the link between actin and cell activation. *Immunol Rev.* 2003;192:98–112.
82. Truneh A, Albert F, Golstein P, et al. Early steps of lymphocyte activation bypassed by synergy between calcium ionophores and phorbol ester. *Nature.* 1985;313(6000):318–320.
83. Mellor H, Parker PJ. The extended protein kinase C superfamily. *Biochem J.* 1998;332 (Pt 2):281–292.
84. Monks CR, Kupfer H, Tamir I, et al. Selective modulation of protein kinase C-theta during T-cell activation. *Nature.* 1997;385(6611): 83–86.
85. Sun Z, Arendt CW, Ellmeier W, et al. PKC-theta is required for TCR-induced NF-kappaB activation in mature but not immature T lymphocytes. *Nature.* 2000;404(6776):402–407.
86. Thome M. CARMA1, BCL-10 and MALT1 in lymphocyte development and activation. *Nat Rev Immunol.* 2004;4(5):348–359.
87. Matsumoto R, Wang D, Blonska M, et al. Phosphorylation of CARMA1 plays a critical role in T Cell receptor-mediated NF-kappaB activation. *Immunity.* 2005;23(6):575–585.
88. Mecklenbrauker I, Saijo K, Zheng NY, et al. Protein kinase Cdelta controls self antigen-induced B-cell tolerance. *Nature.* 2002;416(6883):860–865.
89. Spitaler M, Emslie E, Wood CD, et al. Diacylglycerol and protein kinase D localization during T lymphocyte activation. *Immunity.* 2006;24(5):535–546.
90. Medeiros RB, Dickey DM, Chung H, et al. Protein kinase D1 and the beta 1 integrin cytoplasmic domain control beta 1 integrin function via regulation of Rap1 activation. *Immunity.* 2005;23(2): 213–226.
91. Mullin MJ, Lightfoot K, Marklund U, et al. Differential requirement for RhoA GTPase depending on the cellular localization of protein kinase D. *J Biol Chem.* 2006;281(35):25089–25096.
92. Tamas P, Hawley SA, Clarke RG, et al. Regulation of the energy sensor AMP-activated protein kinase by antigen receptor and Ca2+ in T lymphocytes. *J Exp Med.* 2006;203(7):1665–1670.
93. Pribila JT, Quale AC, Mueller KL, et al. Integrins and T cell-mediated immunity. *Annu Rev Immunol.* 2004;22:157–180.
94. Kliche S, Breitling D, Togni M, et al. The ADAP/SKAP55 signaling module regulates T-cell receptor-mediated integrin activation through plasma membrane targeting of Rap1. *Mol Cell Biol.* 2006;26(19):7130–7144.
95. Ménaschí G, Kliche S, Chen EJ, et al. RIAM links the ADAP/SKAP-55 signaling module to Rap 1, facilitating T-cell-receptor-mediated integrin activation. *Mol Cell Biol.* 2007;27(11): 4070–4081.
96. Sebzda E, Bracke M, Tugal T, et al. Rap1A positively regulates T cells via integrin activation rather than inhibiting lymphocyte signaling. *Nat Immunol.* 2002;3(3):251–258.
97. Katagiri K, Maeda A, Shimonaka M, et al. RAPL, a Rap1-binding molecule that mediates Rap1-induced adhesion through spatial regulation of LFA-1. *Nat Immunol.* 2003;4(8):741–748.
98. Takagi J, Springer TA. Integrin activation and structural rearrangement. *Immunol Rev.* 2002;186:141–163.
99. Schwartz RH. T cell anergy. *Annu Rev Immunol.* 2003;21:305–334.
100. Acuto O, Michel F. CD28-mediated co-stimulation: a quantitative support for TCR signalling. *Nat Rev Immunol.* 2003;3(12):939–951.

101. Sharpe AH, Freeman GJ. The B7-CD28 superfamily. *Nat Rev Immunol.* 2002;2(2):116–126.
102. Shahinian A, Pfeffer K, Lee KP, et al. Differential T cell costimulatory requirements in CD28-deficient mice. *Science.* 1993;261(5121):609–612.
103. Riley JL, Mao M, Kobayashi S, et al. Modulation of TCR-induced transcriptional profiles by ligation of CD28, ICOS, and CTLA-4 receptors. *Proc Natl Acad Sci U S A.* 2002;99(18):11790–11795.
104. Diehn M, Alizadeh AA, Rando OJ, et al. Genomic expression programs and the integration of the CD28 costimulatory signal in T cell activation. *Proc Natl Acad Sci U S A.* 2002;99(18):11796–11801.
105. Fraser JD, Irving BA, Crabtree GR, et al. Regulation of interleukin-2 gene enhancer activity by the T cell accessory molecule CD28. *Science.* 1991;251(4991):313–316.
106. Shapiro VS, Truitt KE, Imboden JB, et al. CD28 mediates transcriptional upregulation of the interleukin-2 (IL-2) promoter through a composite element containing the CD28RE and NF-IL-2B AP-1 sites. *Mol Cell Biol.* 1997;17(7):4051–4058.
107. June CH, Ledbetter JA, Gillespie MM, et al. T-cell proliferation involving the CD28 pathway is associated with cyclosporine-resistant interleukin 2 gene expression. *Mol Cell Biol.* 1987;7(12):4472–4481.
108. Lindstein T, June CH, Ledbetter JA, et al. Regulation of lymphokine messenger RNA stability by a surface-mediated T cell activation pathway. *Science.* 1989;244(4902):339–343.
109. Su B, Jacinto E, Hibi M, et al. JNK is involved in signal integration during costimulation of T lymphocytes. *Cell.* 1994;77(5):727–736.
110. Pages F, Ragueneau M, Rottapel R, et al. Binding of phosphatidylinositol-3-OH kinase to CD28 is required for T-cell signalling. *Nature.* 1994;369(6478):327–329.
111. Kane LP, Andres PG, Howland KC, et al. Akt provides the CD28 costimulatory signal for up-regulation of IL-2 and IFN-gamma but not TH2 cytokines. *Nat Immunol.* 2001;2(1):37–44.
112. Boise LH, Minn AJ, Noel PJ, et al. CD28 costimulation can promote T cell survival by enhancing the expression of Bcl-XL. *Immunity.* 1995;3(1):87–98.
113. Okkenhaug K, Wu L, Garza KM, et al. A point mutation in CD28 distinguishes proliferative signals from survival signals. *Nat Immunol.* 2001;2(4):325–332.
114. Burr JS, Savage ND, Messah GE, et al. Cutting edge: distinct motifs within CD28 regulate T cell proliferation and induction of Bcl-XL. *J Immunol.* 2001;166(9):5331–5335.
115. Blanchet F, Schurter BT, Acuto O. Protein arginine methylation in lymphocyte signaling. *Curr Opin Immunol.* 2006;18(3):321–328.
116. Mowen KA, Schurter BT, Fathman JW, et al. Arginine methylation of NIP45 modulates cytokine gene expression in effector T lymphocytes. *Mol Cell.* 2004;15(4):559–571.
117. Frauwirth KA, Riley JL, Harris MH, et al. The CD28 signaling pathway regulates glucose metabolism. *Immunity.* 2002;16(6):769–777.
118. Hutloff A, Dittrich AM, Beier KC, et al. ICOS is an inducible T-cell co-stimulator structurally and functionally related to CD28. *Nature.* 1999;397(6716):263–266.
119. Yoshinaga SK, Whoriskey JS, Khare SD, et al. T-cell co-stimulation through B7RP-1 and ICOS. *Nature.* 1999;402(6763):827–832.
120. Coyle AJ, Gutierrez-Ramos JC. The expanding B7 superfamily: increasing complexity in costimulatory signals regulating T cell function. *Nat Immunol.* 2001;2(3):203–209.
121. Coyle AJ, Lehar S, Lloyd C, et al. The CD28-related molecule ICOS is required for effective T cell-dependent immune responses. *Immunity.* 2000;13(1):95–105.
122. Dong C, Nurieva RI. Regulation of immune and autoimmune responses by ICOS. *J Autoimmun.* 2003;21(3):255–260.
123. Judd BA, Myung PS, Leng L, et al. Hematopoietic reconstitution of SLP-76 corrects hemostasis and platelet signaling through alpha IIbbeta 3 and collagen receptors. *Proc Natl Acad Sci U S A.* 2000;97(22):12056–12061.
124. So T, Lee SW, Croft M. Tumor necrosis factor/tumor necrosis factor receptor family members that positively regulate immunity. *Int J Hematol.* 2006;83(1):1–11.
125. Nichols KE, Ma CS, Cannons JL, et al. Molecular and cellular pathogenesis of X-linked lymphoproliferative disease. *Immunol Rev.* 2005;203:180–199.
126. Cocks BG, Chang CC, Carballido JM, et al. A novel receptor involved in T-cell activation. *Nature.* 1995;376(6537):260–263.
127. Chan B, Lanyi A, Song HK, et al. SAP couples Fyn to SLAM immune receptors. *Nat Cell Biol.* 2003;5(2):155–160.
128. Latour S, Roncagalli R, Chen R, et al. Binding of SAP SH2 domain to FynT SH3 domain reveals a novel mechanism of receptor signalling in immune regulation. *Nat Cell Biol.* 2003;5(2):149–154.
129. Cannons JL, Yu LJ, Hill B, et al. SAP regulates T(H)2 differentiation and PKC-theta-mediated activation of NF-kappaB1. *Immunity.* 2004;21(5):693–706.
130. Ma CS, Nichols KE, Tangye SG. Regulation of Cellular and Humoral Immune Responses by the SLAM and SAP Families of Molecules. *Ann Rev Immunol.* 2007;25:337–379.
131. Veillette A. Immune regulation by SLAM family receptors and SAP-related adaptors. *Nat Rev Immunol.* 2006;6(1):56–66.
132. Monks CR, Freiberg BA, Kupfer H, et al. Three-dimensional segregation of supramolecular activation clusters in T cells. *Nature.* 1998;395(6697):82–86.
133. Bromley SK, Burack WR, Johnson KG, et al. The immunological synapse. *Annu Rev Immunol.* 2001;19:375–396.
134. Dustin ML, Shaw AS. Costimulation: building an immunological synapse. *Science.* 1999;283(5402):649–650.
135. Lee KH, Holdorf AD, Dustin ML, et al. T cell receptor signaling precedes immunological synapse formation. *Science.* 2002;295(5559):1539–1542.
136. Lee KH, Dinner AR, Tu C, et al. The immunological synapse balances T cell receptor signaling and degradation. *Science.* 2003;302(5648):1218–1222.
137. Simons K, Ikonen E. Functional rafts in cell membranes. *Nature.* 1997;387(6633):569–572.
138. Montixi C, Langlet C, Bernard AM, et al. Engagement of T cell receptor triggers its recruitment to low-density detergent-insoluble membrane domains. *Embo J.* 1998;17(18):5334–5348.
139. Xavier R, Brennan T, Li Q, et al. Membrane compartmentation is required for efficient T cell activation. *Immunity.* 1998;8(6):723–732.
140. Zhang W, Trible RP, Samelson LE. LAT palmitoylation: its essential role in membrane microdomain targeting and tyrosine phosphorylation during T cell activation. *Immunity.* 1998;9(2):239–246.
141. Heissmeyer V, Macian F, Varma R, et al. A molecular dissection of lymphocyte unresponsiveness induced by sustained calcium signalling. *Novartis Found Symp.* 2005;267:165–174; discussion 174–9.
142. Fields PE, Gajewski TF, Fitch FW. Blocked Ras activation in anergic CD4+ T cells. *Science.* 1996;271(5253):1276–1278.
143. Olenchock BA, Guo R, Carpenter JH, et al. Disruption of diacylglycerol metabolism impairs the induction of T cell anergy. *Nat Immunol.* 2006;7(11):1174–1181.
144. Macian F, Garcia-Cozar F, Im SH, et al. Transcriptional mechanisms underlying lymphocyte tolerance. *Cell.* 2002;109(6):719–731.
145. Zha Y, Marks R, Ho AW, et al. T cell anergy is reversed by active Ras and is regulated by diacylglycerol kinase-alpha. *Nat Immunol.* 2006;7(11):1166–1173.
146. Buckler JL, Walsh PT, Porrett PM, et al. Cutting edge: T cell requirement for CD28 costimulation is due to negative regulation of TCR signals by PTEN. *J Immunol.* 2006;177(7):4262–4266.
147. Hagenbeek TJ, Naspetti M, Malergue F, et al. The loss of PTEN allows TCR alphabeta lineage thymocytes to bypass IL-7 and Pre-TCR-mediated signaling. *J Exp Med.* 2004;200(7):883–894.
148. Mueller DL. E3 ubiquitin ligases as T cell anergy factors. *Nat Immunol.* 2004;5(9):883–890.
149. Barrow AD, Trowsdale J. You say ITAM and I say ITIM, let's call the whole thing off: the ambiguity of immunoreceptor signalling. *Eur J Immunol.* 2006;36(7):1646–1653.
150. Unkeless JC, Jin J. Inhibitory receptors, ITIM sequences and phosphatases. *Curr Opin Immunol.* 1997;9(3):338–343.
151. Lioubin MN, Algate PA, Tsai S, et al. p150Ship, a signal transduction molecule with inositol polyphosphate-5-phosphatase activity. *Genes Dev.* 1996;10(9):1084–1095.
152. Nicholson LB, Kuchroo VK. T cell recognition of self and altered self antigens. *Crit Rev Immunol.* 1997;17(5-6):449–462.
153. Sloan-Lancaster J, Shaw AS, Rothbard JB, et al. Partial T cell signaling: altered phospho-zeta and lack of zap70 recruitment in APL-induced T cell anergy. *Cell.* 1994;79(5):913–922.
154. Simeoni L, Posevitz V, Kolsch U, et al. The transmembrane adapter protein SIT regulates thymic development and peripheral T-cell functions. *Mol Cell Biol.* 2005;25(17):7557–7568.

155. Zhu M, Granillo O, Wen R, et al. Negative regulation of lymphocyte activation by the adaptor protein LAX. *J Immunol.* 2005;174(9):5612–5619.
156. Brdicka T, Pavlistova D, Leo A, et al. Phosphoprotein associated with glycosphingolipid-enriched microdomains (PAG), a novel ubiquitously expressed transmembrane adaptor protein, binds the protein tyrosine kinase csk and is involved in regulation of T cell activation. *J Exp Med.* 2000;191(9):1591–1604.
157. Kawabuchi M, Satomi Y, Takao T, et al. Transmembrane phosphoprotein Cbp regulates the activities of Src-family tyrosine kinases. *Nature.* 2000;404(6781):999–1003.
158. Torgersen KM, Vang T, Abrahamsen H, et al. Release from tonic inhibition of T cell activation through transient displacement of C-terminal Src kinase (Csk) from lipid rafts.*J Biol Chem.* 2001;276(31):29313–29318.
159. Davidson D, Bakinowski M, Thomas ML, et al. Phosphorylation-dependent regulation of T-cell activation by PAG/Cbp, a lipid raft-associated transmembrane adaptor. *Mol Cell Biol.* 2003;23(6):2017–2028.
160. Perkins D, Wang Z, Donovan C, et al. Regulation of CTLA-4 expression during T cell activation. *J Immunol.* 1996;156(11):4154–4159.
161. Tivol EA, Borriello F, Schweitzer AN, et al. Loss of CTLA-4 leads to massive lymphoproliferation and fatal multiorgan tissue destruction, revealing a critical negative regulatory role of CTLA-4. *Immunity.* 1995;3(5):541–547.
162. Waterhouse P, Penninger JM, Timms E, et al. Lymphoproliferative disorders with early lethality in mice deficient in Ctla-4. *Science.* 1995;270(5238):985–988.
163. Carreno BM, Bennett F, Chau TA, et al. CTLA-4 (CD152) can inhibit T cell activation by two different mechanisms depending on its level of cell surface expression. *J Immunol.* 2000;165(3):1352–1356.
164. Abrams JR, Lebwohl MG, Guzzo CA, et al. CTLA4Ig-mediated blockade of T-cell costimulation in patients with psoriasis vulgaris. *J Clin Invest.* 1999;103(9):1243–1252.
165. Genovese MC, Becker JC, Schiff M, et al. Abatacept for rheumatoid arthritis refractory to tumor necrosis factor alpha inhibition. *N Engl J Med.* 2005;353(11):1114–1123.
166. Lin H, Rathmell JC, Gray GS, et al. Cytotoxic T lymphocyte antigen 4 (CTLA4) blockade accelerates the acute rejection of cardiac allografts in CD28-deficient mice: CTLA4 can function independently of CD28. *J Exp Med.* 1998;188(1):199–204.
167. Masteller EL, Chuang E, Mullen AC, et al. Structural analysis of CTLA-4 function in vivo. *J Immunol.* 2000;164(10):5319–5327.
168. Calvo CR, Amsen D, Kruisbeek AM. Cytotoxic T lymphocyte antigen 4 (CTLA-4) interferes with extracellular signal-regulated kinase (ERK) and Jun NH2-terminal kinase (JNK) activation, but does not affect phosphorylation of T cell receptor zeta and ZAP70. *J Exp Med.* 1997;186(10):1645–1653.
169. Marengere LE, Waterhouse P, Duncan GS, et al. Regulation of T cell receptor signaling by tyrosine phosphatase SYP association with CTLA-4. *Science.* 1996;272(5265):1170–1173.
170. Baroja ML, Luxenberg D, Chau T, et al. The inhibitory function of CTLA-4 does not require its tyrosine phosphorylation. *J Immunol.* 2000;164(1):49–55.
171. Nakaseko C, Miyatake S, Iida T, et al. Cytotoxic T lymphocyte antigen 4 (CTLA-4) engagement delivers an inhibitory signal through the membrane-proximal region in the absence of the tyrosine motif in the cytoplasmic tail. *J Exp Med.* 1999;190(6):765–774.
172. Shiratori T, Miyatake S, Ohno H, et al. Tyrosine phosphorylation controls internalization of CTLA-4 by regulating its interaction with clathrin-associated adaptor complex AP-2. *Immunity.* 1997;6(5):583–589.
173. Baroja ML, Vijayakrishnan L, Bettelli E, et al. Inhibition of CTLA-4 function by the regulatory subunit of serine/threonine phosphatase 2A. *J Immunol.* 2002;168(10):5070–5078.
174. Shinohara T, Taniwaki M, Ishida Y, et al. Structure and chromosomal localization of the human PD-1 gene (PDCD1). *Genomics.* 1994;23(3):704–706.
175. Zhang X, Schwartz JC, Guo X, et al. Structural and functional analysis of the costimulatory receptor programmed death-1. *Immunity.* 2004;20(3):337–347.
176. Nishimura H, Okazaki T, Tanaka Y, et al. Autoimmune dilated cardiomyopathy in PD-1 receptor-deficient mice. *Science.* 2001;291(5502):319–322.
177. Day CL, Kaufmann DE, Kiepiela P, et al. PD-1 expression on HIV-specific T cells is associated with T-cell exhaustion and disease progression. *Nature.* 2006;443(7109):350–354.
178. Greenwald RJ, Freeman GJ, Sharpe AH. The B7 family revisited. *Annu Rev Immunol.* 2005;23:515–548.
179. Lenardo M, Chan KM, Hornung F, et al. Mature T lymphocyte apoptosis–immune regulation in a dynamic and unpredictable antigenic environment. *Annu Rev Immunol.* 1999;17:221–253.
180. Yonehara S, Ishii A, Yonehara M. A cell-killing monoclonal antibody (anti-Fas) to a cell surface antigen co-down-regulated with the receptor of tumor necrosis factor. *J Exp Med.* 1989;169(5):1747–1756.
181. Cohen PL, Eisenberg RA. Lpr and gld: single gene models of systemic autoimmunity and lymphoproliferative disease. *Annu Rev Immunol.* 1991;9:243–269.
182. Puck JM, Sneller MC. ALPS: an autoimmune human lymphoproliferative syndrome associated with abnormal lymphocyte apoptosis. *Semin Immunol.* 1997;9(1):77–84.
183. Watanabe-Fukunaga R, Brannan CI, Copeland NG, et al. Lymphoproliferation disorder in mice explained by defects in Fas antigen that mediates apoptosis. *Nature.* 1992;356(6367):314–317.
184. Ramsdell F, Seaman MS, Miller RE, et al. gld/gld mice are unable to express a functional ligand for Fas. *Eur J Immunol.* 1994;24(4):928–933.
185. Arnold R, Brenner D, Becker M, et al. How T lymphocytes switch between life and death. *Eur J Immunol.* 2006;36(7):1654–1658.
186. Muzio M, Chinnaiyan AM, Kischkel FC, et al. FLICE, a novel FADD-homologous ICE/CED-3-like protease, is recruited to the CD95 (Fas/APO-1) death—inducing signaling complex. *Cell.* 1996;85(6):817–827.
187. Green DR, Droin N, Pinkoski M. Activation-induced cell death in T cells. *Immunol Rev.* 2003;193:70–81.
188. Irmler M, Thome M, Hahne M, et al. Inhibition of death receptor signals by cellular FLIP. *Nature.* 1997;388(6638):190–195.
189. Marrack P, Kappler J. Control of T cell viability. *Annu Rev Immunol.* 2004;22:765–87.
190. Nagata S. Apoptotic DNA fragmentation. *Exp Cell Res.* 2000;256(1):12–18.
191. Lindsten T, Ross AJ, King A, et al. The combined functions of proapoptotic Bcl-2 family members bak and bax are essential for normal development of multiple tissues. *Mol Cell.* 2000;6(6):1389–1399.
192. Stahelin HF. The history of cyclosporin A (Sandimmune) revisited: another point of view. *Experientia.* 1996;52(1):5–13.
193. Pritchard DI. Sourcing a chemical succession for cyclosporin from parasites and human pathogens. *Drug Discov Today.* 2005;10(10):688–691.
194. Easton JB, Houghton PJ. mTOR and cancer therapy. *Oncogene.* 2006;25(48):6436–6446.
195. Chatenoud L. CD3-specific antibody-induced active tolerance: from bench to bedside. *Nat Rev Immunol.* 2003;3(2):123–132.
196. Vincenti F, Kirkman R, Light S, et al. Interleukin-2-receptor blockade with daclizumab to prevent acute rejection in renal transplantation. Daclizumab Triple Therapy Study Group. *N Engl J Med.* 1998;338(3):161–165.
197. Vincenti F, Larsen C, Durrbach A, et al. Costimulation blockade with belatacept in renal transplantation. *N Engl J Med.* 2005;353(8):770–781.

Chapter 12

Development of T Cells

Ellen V. Rothenberg and Mary A. Yui

INTRODUCTION

T cell development is a composite of overlapping processes in the domains of developmental biology, immunology, and cell biology. It starts with purely hematopoietic developmental mechanisms leading to T lymphoid lineage commitment; then gradually, the basis for subsequent developmental choices becomes dominated by the immunology of T cell receptor (TCR) repertoire selection. The underlying mechanisms by which these later choices are made can be understood only in terms of a richly complex cell biology of checkpoint enforcement, defining the two TCR-dependent fate-determination processes of β selection and positive/negative selection. Repertoire selection is crucial for establishing a functionally competent, mostly self-tolerant population of peripheral T cells, and it has attracted a great deal of interest in isolation from other aspects of T cell development. In this chapter, we show how this cellular process occurs, on the basis of mechanisms that emerge from a unique and fascinating developmental program. A recurrent theme is how the signals from various TCR complexes come to intertwine with underlying developmental mechanisms to control cell fate at a succession of distinct checkpoints and lineage choices.

To begin, this chapter introduces the broad map of T cell developmental events. The subsequent sections focus in on the mechanisms involved in a few of its most interesting watersheds.

OVERVIEW OF T CELL DEVELOPMENT

In mammals, most circulating T cells develop in the thymus. Bone marrow precursors in small numbers enter the thymus from the blood and undertake a course of proliferation, differentiation, and selection, which converts them into T cells. In an adult mouse, this takes 3 to 4 weeks (faster in fetal animals). The mature cells then emigrate from the thymus and take up their surveillance roles in the body. Precursors seed the thymus and differentiate into T cells continuously from midgestation throughout adult life. An additional site of development may be the intestinal epithelium, in which certain T cells that mostly remain associated with the gut epithelium may also be generated. In either case, T cells distinguish themselves from most hematopoietic cell types by migrating away from the bone marrow to carry out their differentiation. It is in the thymus that most TCR gene rearrangement occurs and the cells first acquire their clonal recognition properties. The thymus not only promotes maturation but also rigorously screens each cohort of developing cells to eliminate those with either useless or dangerous TCRs in a process called *repertoire* selection.

Key Molecules: Cell Stage Markers and TCR Genes

At any one time after birth, the thymus contains cells in all stages of development, from the earliest precursors to cells that are virtually mature. Understanding of the process of T cell differentiation has been possible because cells in different stages can be distinguished, and cells of each type can be isolated preparatively without being killed. At least seven developmental stages can be distinguished on the basis of their expression of useful surface molecules. These are introduced in Figure 12.1. Key markers for subdividing the majority of thymocytes are TCR$\alpha\beta$, TCR$\gamma\delta$, and the coreceptors CD4 and CD8 (Figure 12.1A). These help to identify cells in the later half of intrathymic differentiation. The majority of thymocytes, approximately 80%, express both CD4 and CD8 and low levels of surface TCR$\alpha\beta$ complexes, a constellation of markers that is not seen in general on peripheral T cells (Figure 12.1A). This distinctive population, called *double positive* (DP), is a key developmental intermediate that undergoes TCR repertoire selection, the complex process that eliminates cells with either useless or autoreactive TCR specificities. The unique properties of DP cells make TCR repertoire selection possible. Minorities of the cells are CD4$^+$CD8$^-$ TCR$\alpha\beta^{high}$ or CD4$^-$CD8$^+$ TCR$\alpha\beta^{high}$, and these single positive (SP) thymocytes are the most mature cells.

Cells in the earlier 2 weeks of differentiation in the thymus lack any TCR expression as well as any expression of CD4 or CD8. Nevertheless, different stages can be distinguished in this double negative (DN) or triple negative population. In mice, they can be subdivided, on the basis of expression of the interleukin (IL)–2 receptor α-chain CD25, the adhesion molecule CD44, and the stem cell growth factor receptor c-Kit (CD117), into progressive developmental stages termed DN1, DN2, DN3, and DN4 (or TN1, TN2, and so forth) (Figure 12.1B). Two other useful markers for these stages are up-regulated with CD25: the small phospholipid-linked heat-stable antigen (HSA, CD24), which remains on until the late stages of thymocyte maturation, and Thy-1, which once activated is expressed on all T cells. In the human system, different markers are useful for distinguishing corresponding stages, and they are described later. An outline of the progression of mouse precursor cells through these stages is shown in Figure 12.2 as a framework for this narrative.

TCR gene rearrangement plays a pivotal role in thymocyte fate. Ultimately, thymocytes can survive to maturity only if they successfully carry out combinations of gene rearrangements that will give them in-frame α and β chains or γ and δ chains, to be assembled into TCR$\alpha\beta$/CD3 or TCR$\gamma\delta$/CD3 complexes. The rules of the rearrangement process are, therefore, worth reviewing (see Chapters 6, 10). There are four TCR gene loci, each consisting of the constant region exons and multiple variable (V), joining (J), and sometimes diversity (D) segments of the TCRα, β, γ, and δ chain genes (see Chapter 10). The TCRβ and TCRδ loci have D segments as well as V and J segments to be rearranged, whereas the TCRα and TCRγ loci do not. Also note that the TCRδ locus is embedded in the middle of the TCRα locus in such a way that any V-Jα rearrangement automatically deletes the TCRδ locus entirely, regardless of whether it had undergone rearrangement before. These features are important for the regulation of rearrangement and, as described later, for understanding the choice between becoming a TCR$\alpha\beta$- or a TCR$\gamma\delta$-lineage thymocyte. The rearrangement process is ordered, with D-Jβ rearrangements occurring before V-D-Jβ and V-Dδ rearrangements occurring before V-D-Jδ.

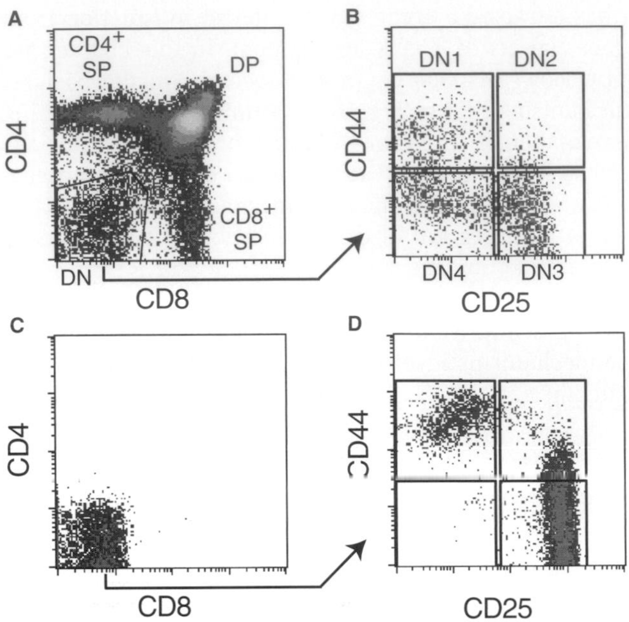

FIGURE 12.1 Subsets of T cell precursors: normal development versus development without TCR gene rearrangement. The major subsets of cells discussed in this chapter are shown in a typical flow cytometric analysis. Top panels (**A** and **B**) show normal thymocytes, and bottom panels (**C** and **D**) show thymocytes from RAG-deficient mice, which cannot rearrange any TCR genes. Cells are stained with fluorescent antibodies against CD4 and CD8 (**A** and **C**), and the DN cells (boxed in **A**) are further analyzed with fluorescent antibodies against CD44 and CD25 (**B** and **D**). The axes show increasing levels of these surface molecules on a 4-decade logarithmic scale (10^4-fold range) of staining intensity. The main populations discussed in Figure 12.2 are indicated (DN, DP, CD4 SP, CD8 SP) (**A**), and the DN cells are subdivided into DN1, DN2, DN3, and DN4 (**B**). The recombinase-deficient thymocytes are developmentally arrested in the DN stages (**C**; cf. **A**), and these DN cells accumulate in the DN3 state and are blocked from progressing forward to the DN4 state (**D**; cf. **B**). RAG-deficient thymocytes also accumulate to only about 1/100 as many cells per thymus as wild-type ($\sim 4 \times 10^6$ versus $\sim 3 \times 10^8$). (See color insert.)

Narrative of T Cell Development

Figure 12.2 traces the progress of cells through the best-known stages of mouse T cell development.

The cells that enter the thymus are capable of giving rise to all subsets of T cells plus natural killer (NK) cells and dendritic cells. As discussed later, they may be able to give rise to macrophages and B cells, too. These cells are initially c-Kit$^+$, Thy-1^{low}, CD44^{high}, CD25$^-$, and CD24^{low}. At this stage, the TCR genes are not yet rearranged. These precursor cells form the key component of the subset called DN1 or TN1.

Once in the thymus, these cells undergo a major transition, losing much of their ability to give rise to anything but T cells, turning on the expression of multiple T cell genes, and starting to proliferate. They begin to express Thy-1, CD25, and CD24, and CD44 and c-Kit continue to be expressed on the cell surface, although at declining levels. The stage marked by this new phenotype is classified as DN2 (TN2) (Figures 12.1B, 12.2). This is the stage when TCR gene rearrangement begins. TCRγ, TCRδ, and the D-J segments of TCRβ all appear to become accessible to rearrangement during this initial period, but TCRα is not. Proliferative expansion in the DN1 and DN2 stages is considerable, approximately 6 to 10 rounds of division.

During the next stage, DN3, CD44 and c-Kit are fully down-regulated, most cell proliferation stops, and rearrangement of the TCRβ, γ, and δ genes occurs with maximum efficiency. The DN3 stage (Thy-1$^+$ c-Kit$^-$ CD44$^-$ CD25$^+$ CD24$^+$ cells) is a landmark because, in both adult and fetal thymocytes, it is the first stage at which the cells appear to have lost the ability to develop into anything but T cells. It is also the first stage when the protein products of rearranged TCR genes are detected in the cytoplasm. Beyond this stage, the proliferation and survival of the cells depend essentially on interactions mediated by TCR proteins. If they rearrange their TCR genes correctly, they can proceed, often with a burst of proliferation. If they fail, they die.

The exact path that the cells follow from this point depends on whether the cells succeed in making D-Jβ and V-D-Jβ rearrangements to form a productive TCRβ open-reading frame before they have completed productive rearrangements of both the γ and δ loci. In the first case, they develop into $\alpha\beta$ T cells; in the second case, they develop into $\gamma\delta$ T cells. The $\gamma\delta$ cells mature with modest additional proliferation and with few known changes to their surface phenotype other than down-regulation of CD25 and CD24. Cells that rearrange β, on the other hand, undergo a complex succession of events known as β selection. These cells proliferate in a rapid burst; down-regulate the DN2/DN3 marker CD25; turn on expression of CD4 and CD8; stop TCRβ, TCRγ, and TCRδ rearrangements; begin rearranging TCRα; and undergo profound functional transformations. Through this cascade of events, the cells are converted from DN3 to DP cells, through proliferating intermediates called *DN4* and *immature single positive* (ISP) cells, usually CD8$^+$CD4$^-$CD3$^-$ (Figure 12.2). DP cells are physiologically peculiar, and their peculiarities make them uniquely poised for TCR-dependent repertoire selection. They are, therefore, key intermediates in the production of a self-tolerant T cell population. As a rule, the DP cell fate is part of the $\alpha\beta$ program and not part of the $\gamma\delta$ program. Thus, although the choice of $\alpha\beta$ versus $\gamma\delta$ fate

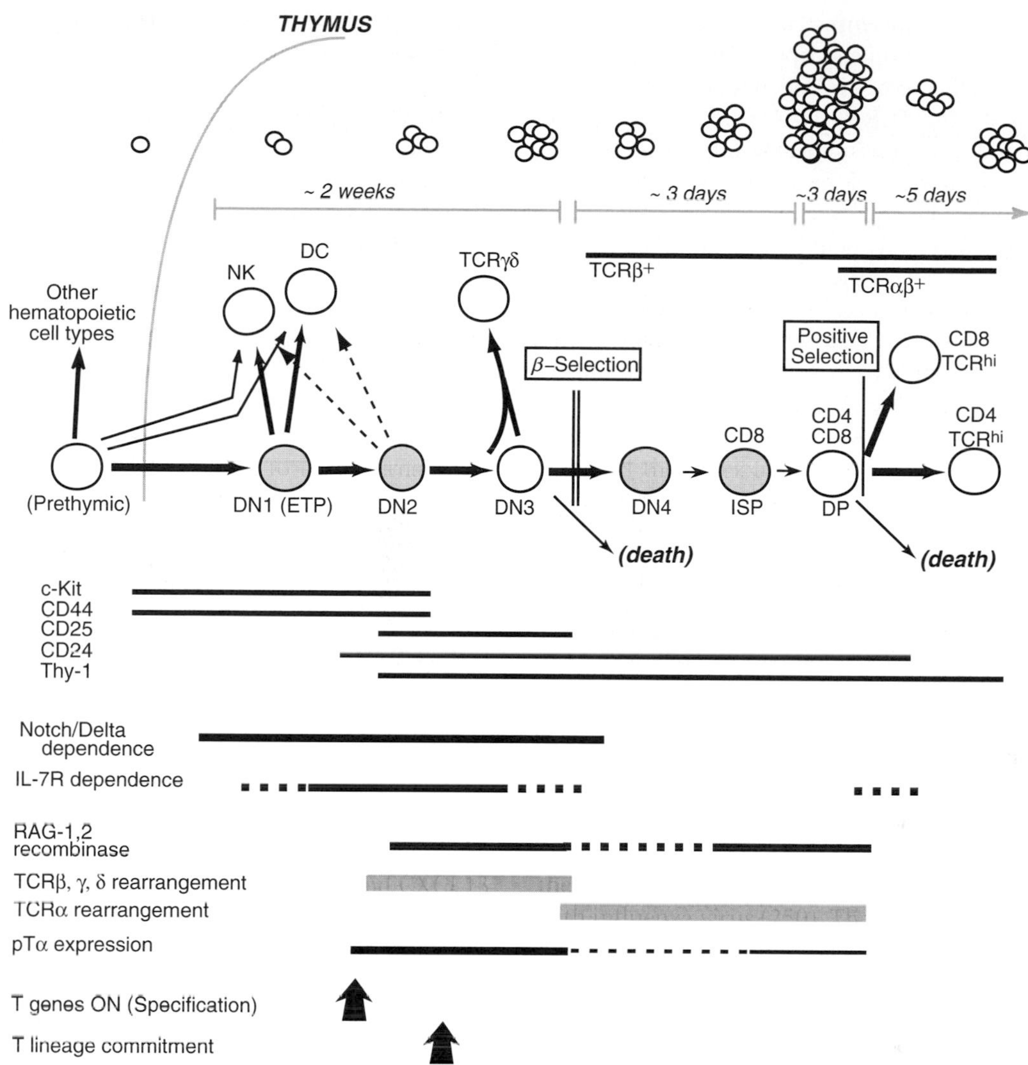

FIGURE 12.2 Outline of events in T cell development. Summary of the events occurring in normal mouse T cell development, including developmental branch points, changes in growth and survival requirements, CD4 and CD8 expression, other key changes in gene expression, and TCR gene rearrangement status. The approximate time taken in each set of transitions is also indicated. Developmental branch points taken rarely are indicated *by broken-line arrows*. The two major checkpoints discussed in the chapter, β selection and positive selection, are indicated. The alternative to positive selection, death, includes both negative selection and death by "neglect," as discussed in the text. Additional branch points, to NKT, CD8$\alpha\alpha$, and T_{reg} cells, also exist but are not depicted. Stages of development in which a majority of cells are proliferating are indicated by *gray filled circles*. Cells expressing rearranged TCRγ and TCRδ genes (TCR$\gamma\delta$) and cells expressing rearranged TCRβ genes either alone or together with rearranged TCRα genes are indicated above the main diagram. Below the main diagram, *bars* show the extents of expression of major cell-surface markers and growth factor receptors. Periods of recombinase expression, specific gene rearrangement, and key developmental events are also indicated by *horizontal bars. Broken bars* show reduced levels of expression. Common abbreviations of cell stages are given in the text. ETP = early T cell precursor, c-Kit-high CD44$^+$ CD25$^-$ DN1 cells. ISP = immature single positive, a transitional stage between DN and DP.

is based at least partly on the stochastic success or failure of rearrangements, it results in a real choice between developmental programs.

Cells that fail to complete any productive TCRβ or TCRγ and δ gene rearrangements die within a few days. In mutant mice that cannot make rearrangements at all, development cannot proceed beyond the DN3 stage (Figure 12.1C,D), and death of cells blocked at that point results in a thymus that is only about 1% of the normal cellularity. Besides the choice of TCR$\alpha\beta$ versus TCR$\gamma\delta$, the

DN3 stage, therefore, represents a rigorous developmental checkpoint. The "β selection checkpoint" is the first of two checkpoints at which survival is dependent on the TCR.

For cells taking the TCRβ^+ CD4$^+$CD8$^+$ path, rescue from death at the β selection checkpoint is only a temporary, conditional reprieve. In these DP cells, TCRβ rearrangement must be followed by a successful TCRα gene rearrangement within about 3 days after the proliferative burst subsides, or else the cells die of "neglect." The selection for cells that have made an acceptable TCR$\alpha\beta$ complex defines the second TCR-dependent checkpoint in T cell development: "positive selection." The criteria for rearrangement success here are more stringent than for β selection. Any TCRβ gene rearrangement that generates a translatable protein coding sequence is adequate for β selection, but the TCRα rearrangement is evaluated both on the basis of a translatable protein coding sequence and on the basis of the recognition specificity that emerges from the new combination of TCRα chain with the previously fixed TCRβ chain. The cells must be able to interact with major histocompatibility complex (MHC) molecules in the microenvironment, but not too well, or else the cells die. The criterion is set so that individual CD4$^+$CD8$^+$ TCRβ^+ cells have less than a 5% chance of satisfying it. As a result, about 30% of this population dies each day in the young mouse thymus (more than 90% die without maturing in the whole 3- to 4-day lifetime of each cell cohort) and must be replaced as a fresh cohort of CD4$^+$CD8$^+$ cells enters the selection pool.

DP cells are actually put through two tests. The first determines whether the newly expressed TCR$\alpha\beta$ can make sufficiently strong interactions with MHC molecules to be useful, and the second assesses whether the interactions of this TCR with self-antigens in the thymus are weak enough to reduce the danger of autoimmunity. These thresholds are tested in two separable processes: positive selection and negative selection. Cells exceeding the minimum affinity threshold are positively selected, initiating a new cascade of phenotypic changes and enhancing the viability and functional responsiveness of the cells. Cells that exceed the maximum affinity threshold can be stripped of their receptors or negatively selected by induced apoptosis. Key changes that help trace progress through positive selection are the transient up-regulation of the activation marker CD69, the stepwise increase in TCR$\alpha\beta$ surface expression from low to intermediate to high, a parallel up-regulation of CD5 and MHC class I molecules, and ultimately the down-regulation of the immature cell marker CD24. Cells remain susceptible to negative selection for several days after the initiation of positive selection, however. They may even encounter the most potent negative selection stimuli in the period after positive selection. Only cells escaping both death by neglect and death by negative selection can complete their maturation and emigrate to the peripheral lymphoid system.

Positive selection also appears to drive a choice of maturation fates. The molecular mechanisms activated in positive selection determine whether a cell will be a CD4$^+$ helper cell, a CD8$^+$ killer cell, or a specialist in other functions such as an NKT cell. As described further later, detailed aspects of the TCR–ligand receptor interactions during this process guide or select cells to develop into one type of effector or the other. Cells with TCRs that recognize MHC class II molecules tend to develop as CD4$^+$ cells, whereas those with TCRs that recognize MHC class I molecules develop as CD8$^+$ cells. The basis of this profound differentiation choice begins with subtle quantitative and kinetic aspects of TCR/coreceptor interaction with MHC, which trigger distinctive regulatory gene expression cascades. The exact maturation pathway followed also depends on the type of cell that interacts with the developing thymocyte for TCR/MHC interaction. Most dramatically, there is even an alternative maturation pathway that rescues some high-affinity interacting cells from negative selection, by converting them into tolerance-enforcing "regulatory T cells" (T_{reg}).

Regulated Proliferation in T Cell Development

TCR-dependent selection is draconian. To supply enough TCR$^+$ "input" cells to leave a diverse TCR repertoire among the survivors of selection, the T cell development program needs to include proliferation as an integral part. As a result, in steady state, the thymus always contains far fewer cells in the earliest stages than in the later stages. All the DN stages together, representing approximately 2 weeks of developmental change, contribute only approximately 2% to 4% of the cells in a typical young adult thymus. The earliest precursors in the DN population have been estimated to be less than 1 one-hundredth of that frequency. In other words, a thymus that turns over approximately 5×10^7 cells per day, through negative selection and death by neglect, may be resupplied continuously with an input averaging only 50 to 100 cells per day.

During T cell development, phases of intense proliferation alternate with phases of little or no cycling. The differences in cell cycle activity are dramatic. As shown in Figure 12.2, DN1 and DN2 cells are cycling, DN3 cells halt, and then, after β selection, cells appear to go through six to eight rounds of division in about 3 days (1,2). After positive selection, in contrast, maturing cells appear to reside in the medulla for almost a week with little if any significant proliferation (2a). Each phase of proliferation tends to be driven by a different mechanism (3). The growth controllers used at various stages include many genes that are essential for progression through the T cell developmental pathway (4).

In the first DN1 precursors, the initiation of cell division may be controlled by c-Kit signaling (5). In the DN1-DN2 states, proliferation is mostly driven by signals from the interaction of IL-7, a cytokine secreted by the thymic stroma, with IL-7 receptor complexes, composed of IL-7Rα (CD127) and γc chains (CD132) (Figure 12.2) (6–8). The cells also depend on interactions with stromal ligands that signal to them through the Notch receptor throughout these early stages. During β selection, population expansion is driven by signaling through the pre-TCR (TCRβ complex), which is discussed later in detail. The later events of positive selection and maturation do not involve significant proliferation; however, they completely depend on TCR$\alpha\beta$ for survival signaling. These sequential requirements for survival have overlapping critical periods, so that the mutant phenotypes are slightly leaky but still have powerful quantitative effects (9). After export from the thymus, mature T cell proliferation depends on TCR$\alpha\beta$ triggering and signals through the IL-2, IL-4, IL-7, or IL-15 receptors. The shift from one kind of proliferative stimulus to another is caused, at least in part, by intrinsic developmental changes in the cells. It is an important factor contributing to the one-way polarity of developmental change.

The proliferative bursts are vital for setting up the large excess of precursors that makes it possible to use stringent selection at the checkpoints in T cell development. The huge losses that occur in these selection processes seem shocking, except that the developmental program also provides for more than 10^5-fold clonal expansion from each precursor. Harsh selection against useless or autoreactive cells is a price the adaptive immune system pays for its somatic generation of diversity in recognition structures. This suggests that the mechanisms used by lymphoid precursors to drive developmental proliferation are evolutionarily old and likely to have coevolved with the mechanisms generating clonal diversity.

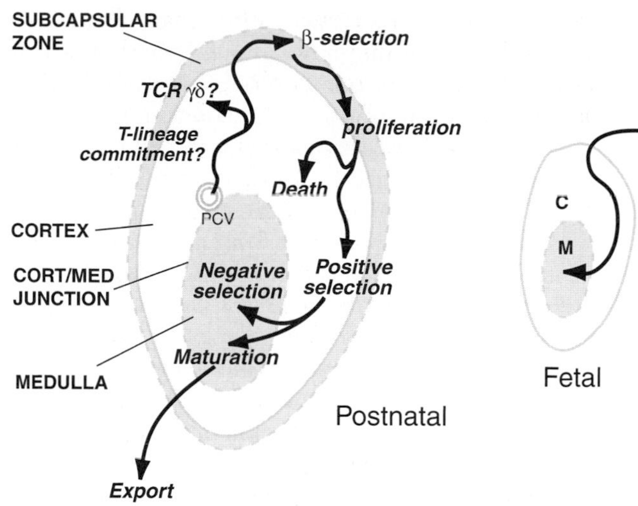

FIGURE 12.3 Summary of migration pathways of thymocytes through the postnatal and fetal thymic microenvironments. The pathway of migration of adult thymocytes from the postcapillary venule (PCV) through the cortex, subcapsular zone, cortex, and medulla is shown on the **left.** For comparison, the entry and migration through the fetal thymus is shown on the **right.**

Anatomical Path of T Cell Development

The thymus is made up of lobes, each of which is divided into distinct zones with different stromal cells making up their microenvironments (10). The largest domain is the cortex, which is packed mostly with DP thymocytes. The cortex surrounds an inner domain called the medulla, where the more advanced, SP thymocytes are found. The outermost rim of the cortex (i.e., the subcapsular region) and the region defining the cortical/medullary junction are also specialized in some ways. The organization of the thymus is diagrammed schematically in Figure 12.3.

It is now clear that the cells migrate through this organ in a hairpinlike path as they differentiate (10a). Blood-borne precursors enter the parenchyma of the postnatal thymus from the medium-size blood vessels (postcapillary venules) at the cortical/medullary junction. These cells, in an early DN1 state, initially proliferate in the deep cortex. They then make their way outward toward the subcapsular zone over the next 2 weeks, differentiating through the DN2 and DN3 states as they go. The subcapsular zone is where the cells audition for β selection and where proliferation of the successful cells resumes. Numerous, rapidly cycling blasts can be seen in the outer cortex; they represent the DN4, ISP, and early DP cells that have just passed this test. As they gradually stop proliferating, the DP thymocytes in profusion fall back into the cortex, reversing direction from before. The cells continue to sink inward during their 3 days of postmitotic life, while new generations of precursors on their way to the subcapsular zone continue to work their way up through the crowd. Even if the DP cells fall back to the cortical/medullary junction, however, they are not allowed to enter the medulla unless they have passed positive selection. Those that do not succeed die in the cortex and are rapidly engulfed by resident macrophages. Those few that are positively selected, along with mature $\gamma\delta$ cells, cross over from the cortex to the medulla (Figure 12.3) (11).

Maturation of the surviving cells occurs in the medulla over the following week (2a), if they can avoid negative selection. The medullary epithelial cells are distinct from the cortical epithelial cells. One remarkable property of these cells is that they express a very wide range of self-antigens that are otherwise expressed only in some other particular organ of the body. In effect, they present an "immunological homunculus" in molecular terms, which is valuable in negative selection or the programming of T_{reg} cells (12). Dendritic cells, which are also specifically located in the medulla, present self-antigen to the new SP cells in the most efficient way for the most stringent form of negative selection. It is only if they survive these encounters that the SP cells complete their maturation, changing their response physiology so that high-affinity interactions with antigen can lead to activation instead of paralysis or death.

The compartmentalization of functions in the thymus probably helps guide certain developmental transitions (10). As the cells change in intrinsic responsiveness to different proliferative signals, their migration may carry them from a zone rich in early stimuli (e.g., IL-7) (13) to a zone that may be rich in a distinct set of stimuli. Certain transitions from proliferation to G_1 arrest, such as from DN2 to DN3 or from β selection to a resting DP state, could result from migration of the cells into a zone where the most recent proliferative stimulus is no longer present. Also, the change in direction of migration of precursors through the cortex, from outbound to inbound, is likely to be a result of a change in the expression of adhesion molecules and chemokine receptors in the DN3 state or during β selection (4). At least one adhesion molecule, CD44, is expressed very highly in the DN1 cells but then clearly turned off between the DN2 and DN3 state; this could be a participant in the early homing or guidance mechanisms or both. Later, at least one new chemokine receptor is turned on at β selection, and this may help attract DP cells back toward the interior (14,15). Migration between domains with different kinds of stromal cells allows a separation between positive and negative selection events in space and time.

Variations in Thymocyte Development in Ontogeny

The general outlines of thymocyte development are similar in postnatal and fetal mice, but there are many differences (16). The mouse fetal thymic stroma develops from the outpocketing of third pharyngeal pouch endoderm, between 10 and 12.5 days of gestation (E10 to E12.5) (reviewed in refs. 17,18). It may undergo some inductive interaction with the overlying ectoderm and neural crest cells of the third branchial arch. The thymic epithelium establishes a distinctive structure and gene expression pattern before any lymphoid precursors arrive. Starting at about E12, hematopoietic precursors migrate directly across the mesenchyme from the subclavian vessels to the tiny, nonvascularized epithelial rudiment; they collect around the thymus and then enter it directly from the outside (Figure 12.3, right panel).

Lymphoid precursors proliferate exponentially in the fetal murine thymus, increasing from about 10^4 cells at E14.5 to about 5×10^5 at E18. In contrast to the postnatal thymus, in the fetal thymus the first TCR$\alpha\beta$ DP cells are generated at about E16, the first SP CD4 cells about 2 days later, and CD8 cells a day after that, followed by birth at day 20. The first emigrants are exported to the periphery within 3 days after birth. Thus, the times spent in the DN state and in the medulla are cut from approximately 14 days and 7 days in the postnatal ("adult") thymus to less than 3 days each in the fetal thymus.

The precursors that initially seed the fetal thymus from fetal liver are qualitatively different from any that enter it later. Radiation chimera experiments establish that they can generate the same types of T cells that are made from adult bone marrow–derived precursors, but they also have a capacity that adult precursors do not. The first thymic immigrants are uniquely capable of generating two classes of $\gamma\delta$ T cells that seed the skin, tongue, and reproductive organ epithelia in late fetal life but are not produced at all after birth (19). These "early-wave" $\gamma\delta$ cells express directed, predetermined V(D)J rearrangements without junctional diversification, so that their recognition specificities are completely invariant. They are, in fact, the first wave of TCR$^+$ thymocytes made in the mouse at all, maturing by E15.5 to E16.5, and they have a number of distinctive properties, including growth factor requirements and transcription factor profiles (20,21).

The thymus continues to be seeded by precursors in discrete waves, around birth and then throughout postnatal life (22). In the meantime, the properties of the major populations of hematopoietic precursors themselves continue to change not only in site of origin but also in molecular programming (23–25). Certain gene disruptions have sharply different effects on T cell development in fetal, postnatal, and adult mice, because of intrinsic differences in different precursor cohorts.

Thymocyte Development in Species Other than Mouse

The overall organization of thymic lobes is conserved from mammals to cartilaginous fish (26). The overall roles of cortex and medulla for T cell development seem to have been established early in vertebrate evolution. In chickens and *Xenopus*, there is also strong evidence for development of distinctive T cell populations in the tadpole or embryo, unlike those made after hatching. Chicken thymocyte developmental studies have actually provided some of the first evidence for the distinctiveness of early-wave $\gamma\delta$ cells (27). However, relatively few markers are available to distinguish developmental stages in these animals, and much remains to be learned about homology or lack of homology of their T cell developmental pathways with those in mice.

Thymocyte development has been studied in much more detail in rats and humans. Surprisingly, the detailed patterns of surface marker expression have not been well conserved, even over the short phylogenetic distances among mammals. The Thy-1 surface glycoprotein is not expressed in rat or human mature T cells, and CD25, which is distinctively up-regulated in murine DN2 and DN3 stages, is not up-regulated at a corresponding stage in human (28).

TABLE 12.1 Comparison of Markers in Human and Murine T-Cell Development

Stage	Mouse Phenotype	Human Phenotype
Intrathymic T/DC/NK precursor	$CD44^+$ c-kit^+ $CD25^-$	$CD34^+$ $CD38^{lo}$ $CD1a^-$ $CD44^+$
Intrathymic T/NK precursor	(Fetal only) $NK1.1^+$ $CD122^+$ $CD44^+$ c-kit^+ $CD25^-$	$CD34^+$ $CD38^+$ $CD1a^-$
Committed T precursor	$CD44^-$ c-kit^- $CD25^+$ $CD24^+$	$CD34^+$ $CD38^+$ $CD1a^+$
TCRδ, TCRγ, TCRβ rearrangement	$CD44^{+/-}$ c-$kit^{+/-}$ $CD25^+$	$CD34^+$ $CD38^+$ $CD1a^+$ $CD4^-$ (possibly earlier) to $CD4^+$
β-selection*	$CD25^+$ $CD4^-$ $CD8^-$ (DN3)	$CD34^+$ $CD38^+$ $CD1a^+$ $CD4^{+/-}$ $CD8^-$ to $CD4^+$ $CD8\alpha^+\beta^-$ (CD4 ISP, early DP)
TCRα rearrangement	$CD25^-$ $CD4^{+/-}$ $CD8\alpha\beta^+$ (ISP, DP)	$CD4^+$ $CD8\alpha^+\beta^-$ (possibly earlier) to $CD4^+$ $CD8\alpha^+\beta^+$ (early DP to DP)
Mature cells	TCR/$CD3^{hi}$ and $CD4^+$ or $CD8\alpha\beta^+$	$CD1a^-$ TCR/$CD3^{hi}$ and $CD4^+$ or $CD8\alpha\beta^+$

TCR, T-cell receptor; T/DC/NK, T cells/dendritic cells/natural killer cells.
Human data from Blom and Spits (262) and Dik et al. (31).
*The position of β-selection may not be as sharply defined by CD4 and CD8 phenotype in human as in the mouse, and data for pre-TCR deficient mutant human cells are not available for confirmation.

Rat and human differ from mouse also in their expression patterns of MHC class II molecules and CD2, and in the fine timing of CD4 and CD8 expression. Homologous surface markers cannot always be assumed to mark homologous developmental stages in these three mammalian species.

Against this background of evolutionary variation, however, the central framework of T cell development appears to be highly conserved between mouse and human, as listed stage by stage in Table 12.1 (28–30). The human pathway starts with an uncommitted precursor ($CD34^+CD38^{lo}$) that enters the thymus with a range of developmental potentials that is similar or identical to that of its mouse counterpart. Although the markers useful for distinguishing stages are different (Table 12.1), the basic sequence of lineage commitment, TCR gene rearrangements, CD4 and CD8 expression, selection, and postselection maturation is the same.

EARLY LINEAGE CHOICES: CLUES TO MOLECULAR MECHANISMS

Developmental Potential of Earliest Intrathymic Precursors

The cells that enter the thymus in either fetal or postnatal life are not committed to the T cell pathway yet (30a,30b). They can be removed from the thymus, purified, and reintroduced *in vivo* or in any of a variety of *in vitro* culture systems, and these experiments reveal that they are still multipotent. Not only the same populations, but even the same individual cells, when assayed under clonal conditions, can efficiently give rise to innate immune system cells, especially dendritic cells, NK cells, and macrophages, as well as T cells. Thus commitment to the T cell lineage is an event that occurs only after the cells have entered the thymus and only under the influence of the thymic microenvironment.

A striking feature of the commitment process is that the precursor cells in the thymus with T cell potential demonstrate little or no B cell potential, even when they continue to show ability to generate nonlymphoid cell types. The data are particularly emphatic on this point for immigrants to the fetal thymus (31,32). This result is surprising because it is a natural expectation that B and T cells should be closely related in developmental lineage, as they are the two main cell types of the adaptive immune system and the only two cell types known to use recombination activating gene (RAG)–mediated recombination. There has been a great deal of experimental analysis and discussion about what this means (33–42), but a few general points emerge. First, the thymic cortex provides a microenvironment in which any B cell potential of sensitive precursors can rapidly be extinguished. Second, cells can enter the thymus from any of a range of developmental states, from stem cell through various kinds of partially restricted hematopoietic precursors, and still be sucked into the vortex of T cell development. There are some exceptions that escape the T cell fate—there are even some nests of B cells within the thymus, and both NK and dendritic cells are also generated by intrathymic precursors, but the thymus can make T cells out of a variety of starting materials. Third, commitment to the T cell fate occurs at a late stage in the thymus relative to most of the proliferation and early differentiation events (30b). The most clear evidence of this is the ability of some thymocytes to reverse course and differentiate into dendritic cells and macrophages, simply by being removed from the thymic microenvironment, even after they have undergone some TCR gene rearrangements (37,43). Actual commitment to a T cell fate does not appear to become complete and irreversible until the cells reach the DN3 stage—that is, closely associated with the proliferation arrest at that point.

Dominant Role of Notch Ligands in the Thymic Environment

From the time of entry into the thymus through β selection, T cell development is guided by Notch signaling and totally dependent on interaction of thymocyte Notch molecules with Delta-family Notch ligands in the thymic microenvironment. This was first revealed to be a major control mechanism for blocking B cell development while enabling and promoting T cell development (44). The transcription factor that is the agent of many Notch signaling effects (called *RBP-Jκ* or *CSL*) is also indispensable for early T cell development and for the suppression of the B cell fate (45). Subsequent work has shown that Delta-type ligand expression is a unique requirement that defines a T lineage–promoting microenvironment (4). A stromal cell line expressing the DL1 or DL4 Notch ligand has now been shown to support early T cell development from stem cells all the way through the DP stage in monolayer culture, and this has opened the way to remarkably accelerated progress (46). In fact, until commitment, recurrent, high-dose Notch/Delta interactions are needed to keep cells within the T cell pathway and away from the NK and dendritic cell pathways, as well as away from the B cell pathway (30b,47–53). In addition to instructively activating and maintaining the T cell program (54–56), Notch signaling is needed to maintain viability, especially at the DN3 stage, as the cells become poised for β-selection (57). There is evidence that other receptor/ligand systems, such as the canonical Wnt pathway, also play a role in thymic epithelial effects on lymphoid precursors (58), but the role of Notch appears to be paramount through these early stages.

Successful β selection, though not $\gamma\delta$-selection, depends on continued Notch signaling (59–63). Interestingly, though, after β selection, Notch-dependent transcription appears to become dispensable for T cell maturation (59,64). Thus, the Notch-dependent phase of T cell development gives way to the TCR-dependent phase.

Transcription Factor Requirements for T Lineage Specification

The Notch signal impinges on a complex regulatory state in the developing thymocytes. Prethymic cells competent to respond to Notch/Delta interaction already express a large number of cell-intrinsic transcription factors, many of which continue to be required for T cell development. The Notch/Delta signal induces the expression of more of these factors, setting in motion a richly combinatorial regulatory cascade. The full progress to successful T lineage commitment and passage through β selection or $\gamma\delta$-selection depends on Ikaros, PU.1, c-Myb, GATA-3, Gfi1, Bcl11b, and factors of the T cell factor (TCF)/lymphoid enhancer factor (LEF) family, the Runx family, and the basic helix-loop-helix E protein family (65–67,78–80). The exact regulatory relationships between these factors and their target genes still need to be worked out in detail. But it is interesting that some of the key factors in T cell development appear to have important roles as repressors, suggesting that one necessary aspect of early T cell development is to silence previously active stem cell genes.

Ikaros, PU.1, c-Myb, and GATA-3 are critical for the earliest T cell precursor generation. An additional phase of transcription factor action is during the specification and expansion events in the DN2 and DN3 stage. The "E proteins" E2A and HEB are prominent here (66). Expressed in overlapping patterns and working as homo- or heterodimers, they collectively provide a vital regulatory input that combines with Notch-activated transcription factors to turn on many components of the T cell program (54,68). Also, E2A seems to be important for the proliferative arrest in the DN3 state that makes TCR gene rearrangement possible (66).

The high-mobility group (HMG) box transcription factors TCF-1 and LEF, have important roles in β selection and before. TCF-1 and LEF mediate Wnt signaling through the canonical β-catenin-dependent pathway, and they also can affect gene regulation in a Wnt-independent way through "architectural" roles in enhanceosome assembly (69,70). TCF-1 and LEF are not needed until β selection in fetal and young postnatal thymocytes, but the later cohorts of precursors that populate the adult thymus also need TCF-1 for the initial stages of T cell development, at the DN1-to-DN2 transition (58,71–75). In fact TCF-1 and GATA-3 are two of the earliest T lineage genes induced in hematopoietic precursors in response to Notch signaling (55).

These regulatory factors that are essential for T lineage differentiation are not themselves T cell specific. Ikaros, c-Myb, and Runx1 are all required for mature hematopoietic stem cell function, the E proteins are crucial for B cell development as well as for T cell development, and factors such as PU.1 have the potential to divert cells completely from the T lineage fate to various myeloid fates (reviewed in ref. 65). Even GATA-3 can have lineage-diversionary effects at high levels (65a). The two things that make T cell development emerge from this mixture of regulatory inputs seem to be, first, the quantitative balance among the levels of expression of different regulators at each stage, and, second, the dominant modulating influence of Notch signaling on the activities of individual transcription factors (48,65a,65b).

The regulatory factors involved in early T cell development do not act in a simple, sequential way limited to particular stages. Although none of these factors appear to be "master regulators" of T cell identity, the regulatory genes that drive initial T lineage differentiation are used repeatedly throughout T cell development (65). Only PU.1 is an exception, playing a hit-and-run function confined to the earliest stage. Like the TCF family factors, GATA-3, Myb, and Runx1 are all required again at β selection as well as for initial specification. Notch family genes may participate in as many as three lineage choices within the T cell pathway. E2A family and Id genes act in β selection and positive selection (66). GATA-3 influences not only the CD4/CD8 choice but also the postthymic differentiation of T_H1 and T_H2 effector subsets of helper T cells (65,76). Even Ikaros recurs in specific roles in later T cell development. Thus, early T cell specification sets up an interplay of developmentally potent factors that becomes a permanent feature of the T cell regulatory apparatus. Shifting combinations of these factors may help to give mature T cells some of their richly nuanced repertoire of responses to their environment.

β SELECTION AND $\gamma\delta$-SELECTION

A Regulatory Upheaval: Transition from TCR–Independent to TCR–Dependent T Cell Development

The β selection checkpoint is a watershed in T cell development that marks the change from events dominated by hematopoietic-like mechanisms to events dominated by TCR interactions with the microenvironment. After 2 weeks of TCR-independent growth, this checkpoint suddenly polarizes the fates of cells that have succeeded or failed at TCR gene rearrangement. A novel criterion of viability is imposed on the cells: The successful ones are rewarded with proliferation and differentiation, and the failures die. In mice that can assemble neither TCR$\gamma\delta$ complexes nor TCRβ-containing "pre-TCR" complexes, such as RAG-1 or RAG-2 knockout animals, all the cells die at this point. There are two related but divergent pathways through this checkpoint, β selection and $\gamma\delta$ selection. Both β selection and $\gamma\delta$-selection trigger distinct programs of sweeping regulatory change.

The β selection checkpoint is encountered by developing DN3 cells as they reach the subcapsular cortex. More than a differentiation arrest, this is a survival and growth arrest (77). Inappropriate passage through the checkpoint appears to be a hotspot for T lineage leukemias and lymphomas. Functions known to be required for checkpoint enforcement also act as T lineage tumor suppressors, including p53, E2A, Ikaros, and correctly regulated Notch signaling (78–86). There are sharp discontinuities in regulatory gene expression when the cells first enter the resting DN3 stage, including a transient burst of Notch response gene expression, which may reflect checkpoint functions. Gene expression dramatically shifts again during β selection itself (61,87,88). This suggests that specific regulatory changes in the DN3 stage are needed to separate the cells from their uncommitted, "hematopoietic" past, before they can safely pass through β selection.

β selection, the escape from checkpoint arrest, is important both because of the special form of TCR complex signaling that it involves and because of its dramatic impact on cell physiology (62,89–93). In murine DN3 cells, β selection causes the cells to shut off CD25 gene expression and to turn on CD4 and CD8 for transition to the DP stage. DN3 cells just beginning selection rapidly enlarge and increase their expression of the cell-surface receptor CD27 (61,94). TCR gene rearrangement temporarily halts as the cells surge into proliferation, and the TCRβ, γ, and δ loci convert to a conformation that is inaccessible to future rearrangement, causing allelic exclusion of TCRβ. The ability of a pre-rearranged TCRβ transgene to cause precocious β selection explains why it blocks endogenous TCRβ gene rearrangement. Under normal circumstances, though, the particularly intense proliferation triggered by β selection expands each cell into a large clone so that each successful TCRβ rearrangement can be tested later for the recognition specificity it confers in association with multiple different TCRα rearrangements. This mitotic burst may also include some of the last cell cycles that T cell precursors undergo, in adults, before they finish development and emerge to the periphery. The transition to the DP stage through β selection confers unusual properties on the cells that optimize them for TCR repertoire selection, described later.

Triggering Requirements for β Selection

β selection is triggered when a TCRβ gene rearrangement generates a sequence that can be translated into a β chain protein. For example, Figure 12.4A (middle right) shows that RAG-deficient thymocytes can be triggered to undergo β selection *in vitro* if they are transfected with a productively rearranged β chain gene. The β chain assembles into a pre-TCR complex with the surrogate α chain pTα, the CD3 components γ, δ, and ε, and TCRζ_2, which are already being expressed in DN2 and DN3 cells, and the complex enters the traffic to the plasma membrane. pTα, a key component of this complex, is an invariant transmembrane glycoprotein that is encoded by a nonrearranging immunoglobulin superfamily gene and expressed very specifically in DN and DP thymocytes (90). The TCRβ/pTα/CD3/TCRζ_2 complexes associate very efficiently into cholesterol-rich lipid microdomains (lipid rafts) on the cell membrane, and they oligomerize with each other and spontaneously initiate signaling (90,95,96). Artificial crosslinking of CD3 complexes on the DN3 thymocytes of RAG-knockout mice is also sufficient to drive the full β selection response. The DN3 thymocytes

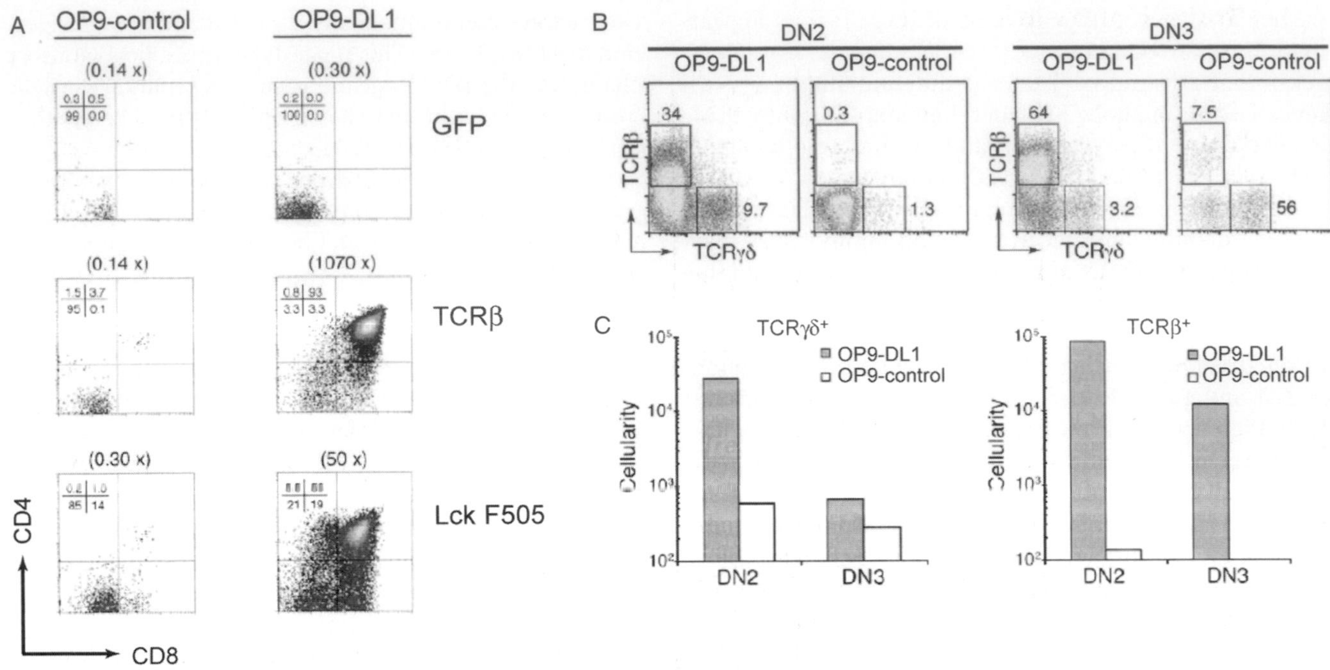

FIGURE 12.4 Triggering requirements for β selection and $\gamma\delta$ selection. **A:** DN to DP transition induced in RAG-deficient thymocytes by introduction of a rearranged TCRβ transgene or activated Lck (LckF505): proliferation and differentiation depend on Notch/DL1 interaction. Left panels show RAG-knockout thymocytes cultured on OP9 stromal cells that do not express the Notch ligand DL1 (OP9-control); right panels show the same populations of cells cultured on OP9 stromal cells that do express DL1 (OP9-DL1). Numbers in parentheses above panels show the change in cell number recovered from each culture relative to input. Note that DN to DP transition and proliferation require both an Lck-activating stimulus (pre-TCR assembly or LckF505) and an interaction between cellular Notch and its DL1 ligand. From ref. (253), with permission. **B:** Wild-type DN3 thymocytes can generate $\gamma\delta$ cells, but not TCRβ^+ cells, in the absence of Notch/DL1 interaction. Here cells were pre-fractionated into DN2 and DN3 subsets and only then cultured on OP9-control or OP9-DL1. DL1 is needed for both kinds of TCR$^+$ cells to be generated from DN2 cells, but once the cells reach DN3 stage, DL1 is no longer needed for $\gamma\delta$ cell development. **C:** Cell counts for cultures shown in panel **B.** Panels **B, C** from ref. (62), with permission.

themselves may be particularly responsive to any kind of CD3 complex signaling.

The pre-TCR signaling cascade launches the complex β selection response by activating the kinase Lck, engaging the adaptors SLP-76 and linker of activated T cells (LAT), and thus activating protein kinase C, Ras, and MAP kinases. All these mediators are essential, and protein kinase C is particularly important for TCRβ allelic exclusion (97,98). Artificial activation of Lck or the Ras/Raf, PI3-kinase, or protein kinase C pathways is sufficient to cause a burst of DP cells to be generated even in RAG-knockout mutants, which cannot rearrange their TCR genes and so cannot undergo β selection legitimately (99) (reviewed in 91–93). Figure 12.4A (lower right) shows the dramatic effect of constitutively activated Lck, comparable to a rearranged TCRβ itself. Similarly, Lck can be activated constitutively by mutation of the *csk* gene, and this also enables cells without pre-TCR to differentiate spontaneously to DP cells (100).

These details imply that β selection is activated by a signaling cascade that is strikingly similar to the one that is triggered by the mature $\alpha\beta$ TCR in later stages of T cell development, during positive selection, as well as in mature T cell responses to antigen. Indeed, β selection serves as the "maiden voyage" in development for the multicomponent TCR signaling apparatus that will govern all future interactions of the T cell with its environment.

The TCRα locus under normal conditions is neither rearranged nor transcribed appreciably until β selection. However, already-rearranged TCRα transgenes can be expressed in DN cells to make TCR$\alpha\beta$ complexes as well as pTα:TCRβ pre-TCR complexes. To a limited extent, rearranged TCRα can replace pTα to mediate β selection. However, TCR$\alpha\beta$ complexes are less effective than pre-TCR complexes in triggering the major proliferative expansion that normally occurs at β selection, due to intrinsic differences in signaling capability (101,102).

Constituent Events in the β Selection Cascade

Gene disruption and overexpression experiments show that once triggered, successful β selection consists of components under partially separable control: (a) early proliferation, with short-term protection from apoptosis (DN→ISP); (b) later proliferation (ISP→DP); (c) CD4, CD8, TCRα transcriptional activation; (d) transcriptional repression of CD25 and a variety of Notch response genes; (e) transient down-regulation of RAG1, RAG2, and pTα; (f) allelic exclusion (i.e., long-term shutoff of Vβ and Vγ rearrangement); (g) antiapoptotic functions for ISP→DP cells; and (h) transcriptional silencing of the TCRγ genes, whether or not they are rearranged, once the cells reach the DP stage. These phases are regulated discontinuously by a variety of factors with dynamically shifting roles. E protein (E2A/HEB) function is required for TCR rearrangement but must be counteracted to allow the initial burst of proliferation. This occurs through a transient increase in expression of the E protein inhibitor, Id3, which then subsides to allow differentiation (66,103). Factors of the Egr family are sharply induced by pre-TCR signaling and important for many of the initial transcriptional responses, but become antagonistic if their expression is not subsequently shut off (104–107). The HMG box transcription factors TCF-1 and LEF have a substantial role, later in making β selection effective overall, at least by promoting proliferation in the ISP to DP stage and viability of emergent DP cells (30,71,108). Transitions in viability support functions are particularly complex, involving shifts in Bcl-2 family member expression (87,94,109), NF κB activation (94,110), induction of the DP-specific orphan nuclear receptor RORγt (111–113). The roles of death-domain containing signaling adaptors such as FADD also shift between pro-apoptotic and pro-proliferative effects (82,114).

Perhaps surprisingly, the phenotypic differentiation from CD4$^-$ CD8$^-$ DN to CD4$^+$ CD8$^+$ DP may be the aspect of β selection that is closest to a default program. RAG-knockout DN3 thymocytes can begin to differentiate spontaneously if the mice are recovering from irradiation, if the p53 checkpoint control function is absent, or if they are expressing a dominant-negative allele of FADD (82,84,86), in spite of their lack of pre-TCR. These are manipulations that are unlikely to "instruct" the DP developmental program. Instead, they presumably remove a barrier to it. Further, in RAG-knockout mice with a diabetes-prone NOD genetic background, although the thymocytes cannot express any form of TCR, an age-dependent breakthrough of the checkpoint occurs that generates DP cells at a high penetrance (87). DN3 cells thus appear to be developmentally primed for DP cell differentiation, but restrained by the β selection checkpoint machinery. One major thing that the pre-TCR and Lck signaling cascade appears to do is to lift this barrier.

In these violations of the β selection checkpoint, however, what fails is the normal level of proliferation. Also correlated with the poor proliferation in these cases is a failure to complete the down-regulation of DN3-specific genes such as CD25. In the NOD case, which has been analyzed most closely, the breakthrough cells demonstrably fail to extinguish expression of the IL-7Rα (CD127) and c-Kit (CD117) genes as well as a series of DN3-specific transcription factors including the Notch-response transcription factor HES1 (87). Proliferation is also required to terminate expression of the TCRγ genes in the DP cells emerging from β selection (115). These results suggest that the extensive proliferation normally triggered during β selection is functionally linked with the ability to "clear the decks" developmentally and to relinquish the gene expression patterns of the pre-selection state.

Choices of Fate within the T Cell Lineage: Differences between $\alpha\beta$ and $\gamma\delta$ T Cells

At every point in T cell development at which TCR complex signaling affects cell fate, the outcome is affected by quantitative details of the strength and duration of signaling. The choice at these checkpoints is not just whether the cells will be allowed to survive, but also a choice between at least two developmental programs to follow by the cells that succeed. This is true of positive and negative selection based on TCR$\alpha\beta$ interactions with MHC and self-peptide, and somewhat surprisingly, it also appears to be true of the generation of $\alpha\beta$ or $\gamma\delta$ T cells by DN3 thymocytes.

Mature TCR$\gamma\delta$ cells differ in many respects from TCR$\alpha\beta$ cells. Their program of gene expression generally does not include expression of CD4 or CD8β, in contrast to TCR$\alpha\beta$ cells. Because the cytoplasmic tails of CD4 and CD8 are the major known docking sites for Lck, their absence probably alters the way mature TCR$\gamma\delta$ cells can recruit Lck to lipid rafts with the TCR during antigen recognition. TCR$\gamma\delta$ cells can express conventional immune cytokines such as IL-2, but with distinctive features of their regulation (116). In the periphery, TCR$\gamma\delta$ cells home to different sites and carry out different surveillance assignments from those of TCR$\alpha\beta$ cells, including wound healing and epithelial maintenance (117). These functions reflect TCR$\gamma\delta$-specific programming for expression of insulinlike growth factor I and keratinocyte growth factor (FGF-7), which act on the epithelial cells.

Intracellular expression of TCRγ and δ proteins is first detectable in a subset of DN3 cells (118), and a variety of staining and reporter gene knock-in techniques visualize TCR$\gamma\delta$ cells emerging from the DN3 population (61,62,119). $\gamma\delta$-selection causes the cells to shift to a CD25$^-$ CD44$^{+/-}$ phenotype, with relatively high CD5 expression. Emerging $\gamma\delta$-selected cells diverge from β-selected cells immediately in their expression levels of survival and regulatory genes, including Bcl2, Runx3, Aiolos,

Egr family, and HEB genes (61,120). Direct comparisons between β selection and $\gamma\delta$ selection show that $\gamma\delta$ selection triggers fewer rounds of proliferation (61,63). The question has been how developing thymocytes can tell the difference.

TCR$\gamma\delta$ cells are usually defined by their success in making both V-Jγ and V-D-Jδ gene rearrangements productively before they either die or undergo complete β selection. The TCR$\gamma\delta$ receptor is both their main distinguishing feature and their most apparent cause of divergence from the TCR$\alpha\beta$ path. TCRγ and nondeleted δ genes may also be rearranged in TCR$\alpha\beta$ cells, but these are usually out of frame for protein translation. On the other hand, the correlation between TCR rearrangement and fate is imperfect. There are some in-frame TCRβ rearrangements in $\gamma\delta$ cells, so the commitment to the $\gamma\delta$ fate can occur sometimes in spite of TCRβ expression (121,122). In some circumstances, a TCR$\gamma\delta$ receptor can even promote development to a DP fate, or a TCR$\alpha\beta$ complex can drive differentiation toward a $\gamma\delta$-lineage-like fate (123–125), Therefore, the unique structural properties of the $\gamma\delta$ and pTα:TCRβ complexes cannot be the only things that determine developmental fate.

Factors Influencing Commitment to the $\alpha\beta$ or $\gamma\delta$ Lineage

Tantalizing evidence has shown that the generation of TCR$\gamma\delta$ lineage cells depends on different balances of regulatory inputs than the generation of TCR$\alpha\beta$ cells via β selection. For example, IL-7 signaling is crucial for the development of almost all subtypes of $\gamma\delta$ cells, and this is due to direct effects of the IL-7R–activated transcription factor STAT5 on TCRγ locus rearrangement and expression (126–132). IL-7 also influences generation of $\alpha\beta$-lineage cells, mostly in the degree of proliferative expansion before β selection, but for $\gamma\delta$ cell generation the effect is all or nothing. Accordingly, at stages before TCR rearrangement is complete and before any TCRγ or δ protein is detectable in the cells (133), subsets of DN2 cells with the highest levels of IL-7R expression show more competence to develop into TCR$\gamma\delta$ cells than those with lower IL-7R surface expression (134). Conversely, there are genetic circumstances under which TCR$\gamma\delta$ cells can develop and $\alpha\beta$-lineage cells cannot. For example, loss of function of various genes, ranging from E proteins to the Notch transcription factor RBP-Jκ (CSL) to a DNA methyltransferase, can each block generation of DP cells while leaving TCR$\gamma\delta$ cell numbers unchanged (59,135–137). Conceivably, then, the precursors of $\alpha\beta$ and $\gamma\delta$ cells could diverge at a regulatory gene level before reaching the first TCR-dependent selection point. But even if such differences exist before TCR rearrangement, it turns out that differential strength of signaling through the $\gamma\delta$ TCR and pre-TCR is sufficient to control which developmental program the cells actually choose (reviewed by 138,139).

The strength of the signal transduced by a fully assembled $\gamma\delta$ complex appears normally to be stronger than that transduced by the TCRβ:pTα pre-TCR complex (96). Remarkably, in elegant transgenic systems, the same TCR$\gamma\delta$ complex can promote either β-selection or $\gamma\delta$-selection with high efficiency, depending on the strength of the signal that it is allowed to deliver (120,140). A great deal of ingenuity was used to determine this, because in general the ligands for TCR$\gamma\delta$ and their roles in $\gamma\delta$-selection are not known. One study took advantage of a rare TCR$\gamma\delta$ transgene that is known to be positively selected by interaction with a nonclassical class I MHC protein. In this transgenic, the availability of the ligand could be controlled separately by mutation of the essential MHC class I component β_2-microglobulin (120). Where the ligand was present, the TCR$\gamma\delta$ transgene-expressing cells developed into $\gamma\delta$ lineage cells; where it was not, they proliferated more and developed into DP cells instead. In another study, a different TCR$\gamma\delta$ transgene with an unknown ligand was used, but signaling through this receptor was manipulated by separate mutations that affected the intrinsic signaling efficiency of the TCRζ chains that transduce signals from the TCR complex. Here any TCR$\gamma\delta$–ligand interaction would be exactly the same as in the normal case. However, as the competence of the TCR$\gamma\delta$ signaling complex was reduced, the cells again generated increasing numbers of thymocytes in steady state and increasingly developed into DP cells instead of TCR$\gamma\delta$ cells (140). Thus, not only the presence or absence of an assembled TCR complex but also the quantitative details of its signaling determine the future differentiation of cells confronting the β-selection checkpoint.

Differential Notch Requirements for TCR$\alpha\beta$ vs. TCR$\gamma\delta$ Cell Production

As signal strength appears to favor the TCR$\gamma\delta$ lineage, one of the most important factors favoring TCR$\alpha\beta$ lineage development now appears to be Notch signaling. The first TCR-dependent checkpoint is the stage when developing T lineage cells graduate from Notch dependence to TCR dependence. Once selection has begun, Notch signaling is not strictly needed for either β or $\gamma\delta$ selection to finish successfully (59,64). The down-regulation of Notch target gene HES1 (49,141) and many others including Notch1 and Notch3 themselves, is an early feature of both types of selection (61). However, Notch/Delta signaling remains vital for cells beginning to undergo β selection even as it becomes dispensable for $\gamma\delta$ selection.

The clearest demonstration of this specific requirement has been revealed by *in vitro* culture of sorted DN3 cells with stromal cells that do or do not express the Notch ligand DL1 (46). As shown in Figure 12.4A, ongoing

Notch/Delta signaling (OP9-DL1 stromal culture) is absolutely required for DN3 cells to start β selection; this is true no matter what kind of TCR they have (61–63,89,142). In contrast, eligible DN3 cells can undergo $\gamma\delta$ selection without these signals (Figure 12.4B,C: OP9-DL1 versus OP9-control samples). There is even evidence that the strength of the pre-TCR signal may need to be offset by the intensity of Notch signaling in order to generate DP thymocytes (63,89). These results imply that Notch signaling is an integral part of a balance of signals that determines the choice between $\alpha\beta$ and $\gamma\delta$ developmental programs.

The essential role of Notch pathway regulation in β selection illuminates a grim side of its role. Hyperactivity of the Notch pathway at β selection, or a failure to turn it off once β selection begins, appears to be a key precipitating factor for T lineage acute lymphoblastic leukemia, with or without other predisposing mutations in Ikaros, E2A, or other genes (78–80,143–145). The explosive proliferation that β selection entails mobilizes other proto-oncogenes, such as c-Myb and Pim-1 (146–149), and the cells can be imagined to come close to the brink of oncogenic transformation in every generation. The mechanism leading to down-regulation of the Notch pathway during β selection is not well understood yet, but if it allows DP cells to come to a resting state, it may be critical for the health of the organism.

CD4+ CD8+ DOUBLE-POSITIVE THYMOCYTES AND THYMIC HOMEOSTASIS

Impacts of β Selection on Later T Cell Differentiation

As a developmental event, β selection is momentous. The approximately 10^2-fold proliferation at β selection effectively erases the developmental alternatives for TCR$\alpha\beta$ cells, consummating not only T lineage commitment but the separation of $\alpha\beta$ and $\gamma\delta$ cell fates. In adult mammals, this is the last significant proliferation that T cell precursors undergo before being exported to the periphery. Thus, the form in which cells emerge from the various stages of β selection dictates the defaults for their responses to positive and negative selection signals for most of the rest of their residence in the thymus.

β selection causes an immediate impact on the cells that in certain ways is the reverse of the impact of positive selection (see later discussion). In particular, there are changes in Bcl-2, Bcl-X_L, NF-κB, and AP-1 activation, RORγt expression, glycoprotein sialylation, and signaling thresholds that will all be reversed when the cells are positively selected, as summarized in Figure 12.5. Nevertheless, many of the triggering functions used in β selection are the same as those used in positive selection. The signals

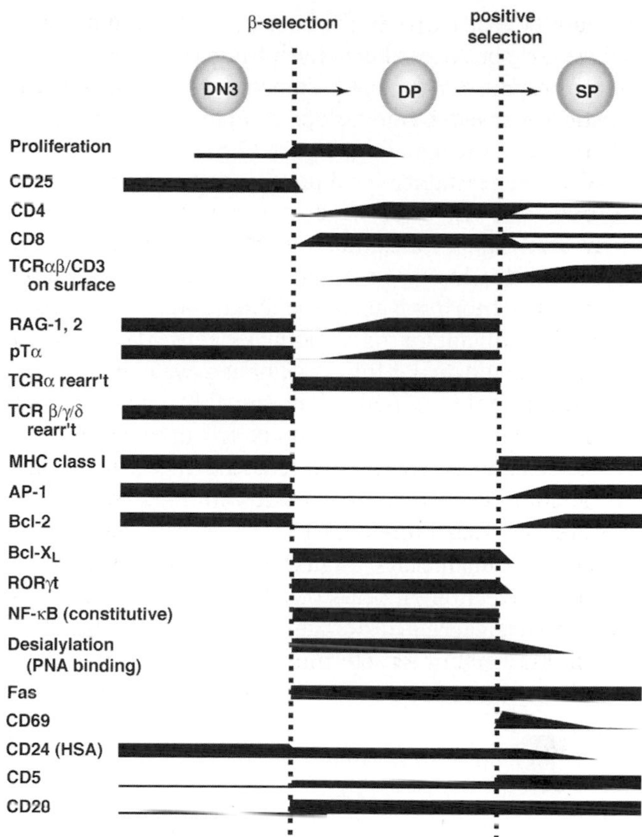

FIGURE 12.5 Transformations of cell phenotype during β selection in mouse thymocytes: comparison with later transformations during positive selection. The changes in gene expression, rearrangement accessibility, and cell-surface phenotype at the transition from DN3 cells to DP are shown, compared with changes that occur later during positive selection. Changes in cell-surface phenotype where several distinct levels of marker expression are useful to distinguish among developmental states are depicted by sloping or stepped forms, whereas others are simplified as all-or-none changes. For discussion, see text. CD4 and CD8 expression patterns are shown bifurcating at positive selection to represent the CD4/CD8 SP lineage split. Proliferation between the DN3 and DP stages extends through the DN4 and immature SP stages (not marked here) and into the beginning of the DP stage. RAG1 and RAG2 and pTα are transiently shut off during proliferation after β selection and then expressed again in DP thymocytes. Expression of RORγt in DP cells correlates with alterations in functional responsiveness. AP-1 loss of function in DP thymocytes is a loss of inducibility of deoxyribonucleic acid (DNA) binding and transactivation activity, leading to broad defects in effector gene inducibility. The up-regulation shown for NF-κB in the DP stage refers only to constitutive nuclearization of DNA-binding activity: NF-κB is also inducible by stimulation at other stages of development. The expression of surface glycoproteins deficient in sialic acid is detected by a sharp increase in binding to the lectin peanut agglutinin (PNA). Fas is a TNF receptor family death receptor. CD69, CD24 (HSA), CD5, and CD28 are cell-surface receptors with potential roles in modulating or costimulating TCR signaling activity.

may not be instructive in themselves, therefore, but more like a toggle between alternative physiological states.

The responses to pre-TCR signaling include changes in expression of other cell-surface receptors that can themselves affect TCR signaling (Figure 12.5). An important one is CD5, which is induced in direct proportion to TCR signal strength, but which also acts as an inhibitor of subsequent TCR signal transduction (150,151). The stable conversion of developing thymocytes from CD5-low to CD5-intermediate during β selection should make signaling a little more difficult for the resulting DP cells. Most provocatively, it should make future signaling weaker, in direct proportion to the strength of the signal by which the cells were selected. CD5 is even more strongly up-regulated during $\gamma\delta$ selection, as already noted, in agreement with the model that TCR$\gamma\delta$ complexes signal more strongly than pre-TCR. It is also interesting that the transcription factor Ikaros, which plays a checkpoint-enforcement function in β selection, appears to act as a brake on spontaneous TCR triggering in later development (152). Signaling thresholds can thus be determined and fixed for individual cells through the balance of regulators that triggered their β selection.

The threshold-setting functions mobilized in β selection may turn out to be an important immunological legacy of the process. Conceivably, the levels of threshold-setting functions such as CD5, Csk, and Ikaros could be maintained from β selection through proliferation and into the DP population. If so, then the later positive/negative selection thresholds for individual DP cells could depend on the strength of the pre-TCR signals that triggered their β selection initially.

Uniqueness of DP Thymocytes

The CD4$^+$CD8$^+$DP thymocytes produced through β selection are physiologically specialized for undergoing selection on the basis of TCR recognition (Figure 12.5). These cells are a paradoxical combination of extreme sensitivity to TCR ligands and, by some criteria, extreme functional paralysis. Unable to turn on any of the functional response genes of mature T cells in response to stimulation, they nevertheless do recognize TCR ligands with ultrasensitive dose–response relationships. Antigenic peptides presented on conventional antigen-presenting cells can trigger apoptosis of DP thymocytes with median effective dose values that are substantially lower ($\sim$10-fold) than those needed to trigger responses of mature T cells with the same TCR (109–111). This is especially surprising because the cell-surface density of TCR on DP thymocytes, even after productive TCRα rearrangement, is about 10-fold lower than on SP thymocytes. Operationally, this means that DP thymocytes can make responses to peptide/MHC complexes that are low-affinity ligands for their TCR, too low to be stimulatory for mature cells with the same TCR.

One important mechanism contributing to this ultrasensitivity is the distinctive glycosylation state of many DP thymocyte surface molecules. These are strikingly deficient in terminal sialylation in comparison with surface glycoproteins of mature T cells and immature DN cells alike, reducing the electrostatic repulsion between DP thymocytes and other cells with a more typically strong negative surface charge. This reduced repulsion apparently lowers the affinity threshold for TCR signaling (153). Another feature enhancing the sensitivity of DP cells is the fact that they still express a relatively low level of CD5, the negative regulator of TCR signaling (150,151), as compared to mature cells. For these or additional reasons, immunological synapses formed by DP thymocytes with thymic epithelial cells are distinct in organization from those that mature T cells form with professional antigen-presenting cells (154,155).

DP thymocytes have other features that bear on their eventual fates. Because of the regulatory changes that generate them during β selection, these cells are extremely sensitive to death induced by glucocorticoids, and, even without perturbation, they die quickly outside of the thymic microenvironment. These properties are especially pronounced in the mouse; human and rat DP thymocytes are somewhat more robust. Thymocyte glucocorticoid sensitivity exactly coincides with the cell-surface carbohydrate changes (peanut agglutinin–binding phenotype) and the lack of class I MHC and is tightly developmentally regulated; it can be used as an efficient method to deplete DP cells specifically. Even mildly elevated physiological levels of glucocorticoids *in vivo* shrink the thymus dramatically through loss of DP cells. It is widely assumed that normal circulating levels of glucocorticoids play a major role in setting the three- or four-day deadline for DP thymocyte selection or death. However, DP cells are not just death-row inmates awaiting a reprieve. Throughout their few days of passage, they maintain their own antiapoptotic functions by expressing Bcl-xL and Bcl2A1 (109,111). Further, the regulatory molecule that turns on these DP-specific antiapoptotic molecules is the orphan nuclear receptor RORγt, and this is the same regulatory molecule that appears to shut off the ability of DP cells to make conventional effector responses (111,112,156). Thus, in the DP stage, developing thymocytes exchange one kind of response program for another (Figure 12.5).

DP Thymocyte Impact on the Thymic Microenvironment

Most interestingly, recent work has shown that part of this DP cell program is to take an active role in shaping the thymic environment. There is a long history of evidence for cross-talk between DP cells and the thymic stroma, which affects the state of the epithelium, its ability to maintain thymocyte viability through β selection, and indirectly the carrying capacity of the thymus (77,157,158). The presence of DP cells causes a polarization of the cortical structure, with IL-7 production compartmentalized in the inner regions close to the cortical-medullary junction (13). DP cells also act to control the programming of new waves of precursors through a more direct route. As they emerge from β selection, DP cells turn on lymphotoxin-β, a tumor necrosis factor (TNF)–family secreted molecule that is used by embryonic lymphoid tissue-inducing cells to initiate lymph node development. RORγt is also important for making this possible (159). The cells that receive the lymphotoxin-β signal are not just other DP cells or thymic epithelial cells, but also the immature DN cells migrating past them in the bidirectional traffic of the cortex. DP-derived lymphotoxin-β has a remarkable effect on the gene expression patterns in these immature precursors and even on the maturation of TCR$\gamma\delta$ cells from those precursors (159). Thus, the presence of normally developed DP cells may be important even for the maturation of cells that took an alternative pathway.

There are two other features of DP cells that are increasingly seen to be important for thymic function. One is that as they take up most of the cellular volume of the thymic cortex, DP cells may buffer outwardly migrating DN cells against the effects of competition for Notch ligands. This is possible because DN but not DP cells express high levels of Lunatic Fringe, a modifying enzyme that greatly enhances the efficiency with which a cell can engage with Delta-family Notch ligands. It is now clear that the amount of Delta presented by thymic stroma is limited, and T cell development can be deranged or blocked when there is excessive competition (160–162). By their "self-denying" downregulation of Lunatic Fringe, the DP cells provide a neutral neighborhood for DN cells. In this role, DP cells could be analogous to the control rods in a nuclear reactor. At the same time, it is possible to imagine such a mechanism helping to regulate the carrying capacity of the thymus.

A last important feature of the DP cells is that they may themselves be the antigen-presenting cells for certain kinds of positive selection. The DP cells themselves express neither classical class I nor class II MHC: The lack of class II is normal for murine T cells, and the shutoff of conventional class I MHC expression is another unique feature of the DP state (Figure 12.5). However, DP cells in several mammalian species express nonclassical class I MHC antigens, such as TL or CD1, which are the restricting elements for antigen recognition by specific subsets of $\alpha\beta$-T cells such as NKT cells with an invariant TCRα (iNKT) and epithelial-associated T cells using CD8$\alpha\alpha$ homodimers. The importance of these minority T cell lineages is suddenly becoming appreciated, as these cells have some characteristics of innate immune cells and play a role in the regulation of peripheral immune responses. Both cell types undergo thymic development, pass through a DP stage, and appear to be positively selected on high-affinity agonists presented in the context of the nonconventional MHC molecules (163–165). Thus, DP cells may themselves take the place of thymic epithelium for selection of cells that will mature in these particular lineages.

POSITIVE SELECTION AND CHOICE OF CD4 OR CD8 CELL FATE

Positive selection is the canonical example demonstrating that quantitative differences in TCR signaling can elicit wholly different developmental outcomes. Transgenes encoding pre-rearranged TCRα and TCRβ genes impose a predictable recognition specificity on developing T cells, blocking most endogenous TCR gene rearrangement and diversity by allelic exclusion. From the earliest such experiments, it has been evident that the recognition specificity also imposes a predictable developmental fate. Transgenes encoding a receptor that recognizes some foreign peptide antigen in the context of the same MHC allelic forms expressed in the thymus give thymocytes a greatly increased chance of survival (positive selection). Transgenes encoding a receptor that recognizes both self-MHC and a self-peptide expressed in the thymus generally cause the transgenic TCR^{+} cells to be eliminated (negative selection). Further, the nature of the ligand recognized controls the developmental programming of two major effector classes of T cells. Transgenes encoding a receptor for peptide complexes with class II MHC direct the cells to mature into CD4 SP cells, whereas transgenes encoding a receptor for peptide complexes with class I MHC direct development to a CD8 SP lineage. Although details of the expression of TCR transgenes *in vivo* are not normal (they are expressed at an earlier stage, typically, than normal TCR that depend on TCRα rearrangement), they have revealed the overwhelming importance of details of TCR signaling for thymocyte fate determination. Clever experimental strategies have now made it possible to tease out how the cells distinguish between interactions with different ligands and how they translate these features of a transient interaction into an irreversible choice of developmental program.

Positive Selection and the TCR Recognition Repertoire

Positive selection ensures that only thymocytes expressing a useful TCR can survive the DP stage and mature beyond it. *Useful* here means capable of mediating interactions with either class I or class II MHC, but not with such high affinity as to cause autoreactivity. In practice, this usually involves a weak interaction with MHC complexes that include thymic self-peptide, as some other "foreign" antigenic peptide in the same MHC is likely to exist that has much stronger interaction with such a receptor in the periphery. Positive selection and its importance for repertoire selection are discussed in detail in many reviews (166–169). It is important to note that positive selection does not need to be precise in terms of antigen specificity. After all, the thymus only expresses self-antigens. Therefore, it cannot positively select for a particular foreign antigenic peptide specificity, but only for the competence to contribute to a useful TCR repertoire. The process can also afford to be permissive, because any positively selected cells that turn out to have too high an affinity for self-antigen will still have time to be negatively selected or diverted to a T_{reg} fate in the thymic medulla (170). It is the superimposition of the positive selection window and the more stringent negative selection window that selects the useful, self-tolerant T cell repertoire.

The TCR-ligand interactions that trigger positive selection appear to be low affinity and fairly promiscuous. As a result, a single peptide/MHC complex can positively select DP cells with any of numerous different TCR specificities, as long as they cross-react weakly with that complex (171). The heightened sensitivity of DP cells to certain weak TCR interactions means that the peptide/MHC complex that actually triggers positive selection may bind with an affinity that becomes undetectable, or detectable only as competitive antagonism, once the cell has matured into a peripheral T cell. However, mature T cells continue to recognize other peptides in association with the same class I or class II MHC molecule that mediated their positive selection.

Triggering of Positive Selection

The receptors that are important for positive selection include not only the newly expressed TCR$\alpha\beta$ complexes, but also the CD4 and CD8 coreceptors (especially in the form of CD8$\alpha\beta$ heterodimers), which interact with Lck through their cytoplasmic tails. CD4 co-engages class II MHC, and CD8 co-engages class I MHC. Because the DP cells express both CD4 and CD8, one or the other coreceptor can be engaged to bring Lck to the vicinity of the engaged TCR, whether the MHC that is being recognized is class II or class I. In either case, this triggers a TCR signaling cascade including activation of Lck, ZAP70, Ras, Vav, Itk, calcineurin, and protein kinase C. These events have been extensively studied and validated by knockout mutations in various signaling components (reviewed in refs. 127,166,167,172–174). Structural features of the TCR$\alpha\beta$ complex, as opposed to the pre-TCR, may cause positive selection signaling to differ qualitatively from β selection signaling: There are hints that a particular subdomain of TCRα and the presence of CD3δ in the TCR$\alpha\beta$ complexes may be crucial for activating the MAP kinases ERK1, 2 (175,176). Distinctively, positive selection elicits sustained ERK activation, which depends on calcineurin B (177) and activates a cascade of SAP-1 (Elk4), Egr1, and Id3 (178;179). CD8$\alpha\beta$ coreceptor complexes bring less Lck to the immunological synapse than CD4 coreceptor complexes, but both trigger seemingly similar response pathways.

Time Window for Positive Selection

Positive selection occurs in the cortex. DP thymocytes in the cortex have only a three-day lifespan on average before they die "by neglect," and throughout this time they actively carry on V-J rearrangement of the TCRα locus. This starts as soon as RAG expression resumes after β selection and sometimes even before the cells finish proliferating (see Figure 12.2). There is no allelic exclusion of TCRα gene rearrangement; the process is terminated either by positive selection, which finally shuts off RAG expression, or by cell death. Individual cells can rearrange the α-chain genes on both chromosomes, not only once but many times, because the locus offers more than 50 possible Jα segments as well as Vα segments in a permissive topology (180). Expression of an in-frame TCRα chain replaces pTα in complexes with TCRβ, enabling the cells to be auditioned for positive selection immediately based on the interaction with ligands on the cortical epithelial cells. The cortical epithelium provides a rich source of MHC class I and class II surface complexes with a notable lack of costimulatory molecules for T cells. This is important because at the DP stage, costimulation causes not activation but negative selection (reviewed in ref. 166; see next section). Thus, the cortical epithelial microenvironment provides a uniquely forgiving testing ground for newly generated TCR recognition specificities.

The sequence of events triggered by positive selection includes little if any proliferation, in contrast to β selection. CD69 is up-regulated, RAG genes are turned off permanently, CD5 levels increase, and TCR/CD3 complexes are stabilized so that their surface expression increases in parallel. Concomitantly, expression of the chemokine receptor CCR7 is turned on. This enables the cells to migrate from the cortex to the medulla, starting another multiple-day maturation process (181). Glycoprotein processing is altered back to a more "normal" pattern, so that new glycoproteins are once again fully sialylated. The cells regain the Bcl-2 and class I MHC expression that they had lost at β selection, and they begin to recover the functional responsiveness that had disappeared at that time (Figure 12.5). As this proceeds, the cells eventually become resistant to negative selection, and they down-regulate CD24 (HSA) as TCR/CD3 levels rise even higher and CD69 expression finally subsides. Eventually, the cells are enabled to leave the medulla and migrate out to the periphery through a process dependent on a G protein–coupled receptor for the glycolipid sphingosine 1-phosphate (182). The TCR up-regulation, rescue from death by neglect, release to the medulla, and functional maturation events appear to be common to all positively selected thymocytes.

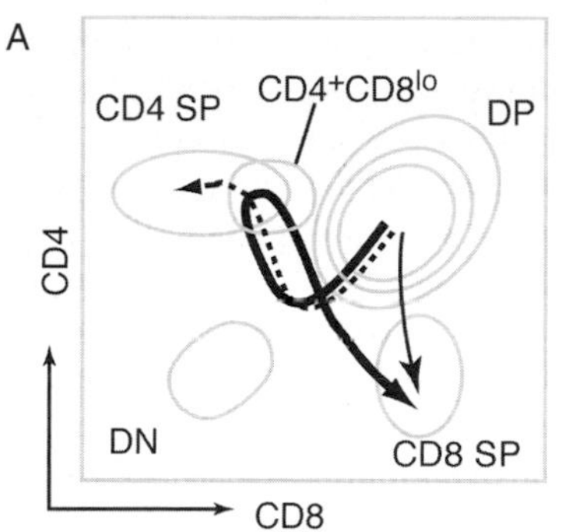

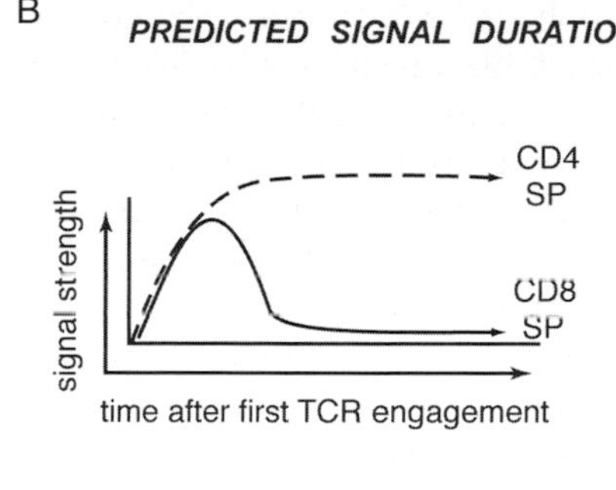

FIGURE 12.6 CD4/CD8 developmental regulation and signal kinetics in positive selection. **A:** Observed paths of phenotypic change through which DP thymocytes differentiate into CD4 SP (broken arrow) or CD8 SP (solid arrows) cells. Some CD8 SP cells can develop by immediate loss of CD4 (thin arrow), but the majority transiently lose CD8 expression and go through a CD4$^+$ CD8^{low} intermediate (thick arrow). **B:** Implications of the initial CD8 loss for the duration of Lck signaling during positive selection of CD4 SP (broken line) and CD8 SP cells (solid line). See text for details.

The process of positive selection is more than the initial contact with MHC ligand, therefore, and the interesting fact is that TCR signaling must continue for several days for the process to be completed (183,184). This has been shown elegantly *in vivo* by genetically engineering mice so that the expression of the crucial TCR signaling mediator, ZAP70, is tightly limited to the DP stage and turned off by the first flashes of positive selection signaling (185). In these mice, positive selection can begin, and a first wave of phenotypic changes is seen, but the cells cannot complete the process. This requirement for ongoing or repeated TCR signaling after the first responses to positive selection signals now appears to be a crucial element of the mechanism that determines the CD4/CD8 lineage choice.

Duration and Strength of Signal Control CD4/CD8 Lineage Choice

The problem of what determines whether $\alpha\beta$ T cell lineage cells will differentiate into CD4$^+$ helper T cells or CD8$^+$ cytotoxic T cells was passionately debated for years (127,186–190), though a consensus is now emerging. The basic questions were whether the signals through the TCR and CD4 versus CD8 coreceptors alone could provide a sufficiently informative difference to instruct the choice between divergent differentiation programs for CD4 helper cells and CD8 killer cells, and whether any other signaling pathway played a major role. Candidates for other pathways were widely discussed. In fact, a skewing of CD4/CD8 differentiation was one of the first aspects of thymocyte development observed to be affected by Notch signaling (191). This was historically critical in bringing Notch to the attention of the T cell development field, although the mechanism of this Notch effect is now thought to be indirect (192).

There are two differences between the positive selection signals experienced by cells selected on class II MHC and those experienced by cells selected on class I MHC. The first difference is quantitative: TCR/class I MHC/CD8 complexes, on average, induce less Lck activation than TCR/class II MHC/CD4 complexes, because Lck is bound less efficiently to CD8 cytoplasmic tails than to CD4. The second difference is kinetic: The time course of Lck signaling in the case of class I recognition is more interrupted, while Lck signaling induced by class II recognition is sustained. This is because the initial response to positive selection includes asymmetrical changes in the surface expression of the two coreceptors, even before any sign that the cell can distinguish a class I ligand from a class II ligand. Figure 12.6A shows the pathways the cells take from DP to CD4 SP or CD8 SP. There is a relatively straight path from DP to CD4 SP by CD8 down-regulation and silencing. In contrast, the major pathway to the CD8 fate is a sinuous loop as the cells initially down-regulate CD8—the wrong coreceptor—so that they are first intermixed with the cells undergoing CD4 selection, and only afterward do they reverse phenotype by reexpressing CD8 and silencing CD4 ("coreceptor reversal"). Reexpression of CD8 then makes use of different cis-regulatory elements and different transcription factors than prior expression of CD8 in the DP stage (193). This makes a qualitative difference because the cell is not finished being selected when it first downregulates CD8 (186). Cells that used CD4/TCR coengagement to bring Lck to the immunological synapse at the start of positive selection still have plenty of CD4 to provide an equally strong signal the next time its TCR engages. Cells that used CD8/TCR coengagement for a signal of equal initial strength, however, have far less CD8 available to mobilize Lck the second time, and they experience a sharp time-dependent falloff in Lck signal intensity (Figure 12.6B).

Signal intensity in the aggregate can have a powerful effect on the lineage choice. Lck especially has been implicated by transgenic manipulations that modestly increase or reduce Lck activity levels in developing thymocytes. Although the effect is not visible in a normal thymocyte population with diverse receptors, there is a dramatic effect on thymocytes with a fixed TCR specificity (194). Cells expressing a class II–restricted TCR transgene can be switched from CD4, helper-lineage positive selection to CD8, cytotoxic-lineage positive selection, through low-level expression of a dominant negative form of Lck. Cells expressing a class I-restricted transgene, conversely, can be switched from CD8 to CD4 lineage by low-level expression of activated Lck. It is interesting to note that an important design feature in this experimental system was the expression of the modified Lck transgenes from a promoter that is expressed mostly *after* positive selection begins—that is, affecting the duration of the Lck signal as well as the initial amplitude. Downstream of Lck, ERK activity levels have also been shown to affect CD4/CD8 lineage choice in a similar way (168,173,188,195,196).

The importance of signal duration has emerged from increasing evidence that differences in initial signaling intensity are not required for the CD4/CD8 choice. Strikingly, the same signal through the same TCR can result in positive selection of CD4 cells, if sustained, while it results in positive selection of CD8 cells, if interrupted (197–199). To control the timing of the signal in these experiments, both elegant transgenic designs and extremely high-resolution fetal thymic organ culture approaches have been used, and these give dramatic and concordant results *in vivo* and *in vitro*. An example in a two-stage fetal thymus organ culture system is illustrated in Figure 12.7 (199). To rule out any remaining question about special signaling capabilities of the CD4/TCR/MHC class II complex as opposed

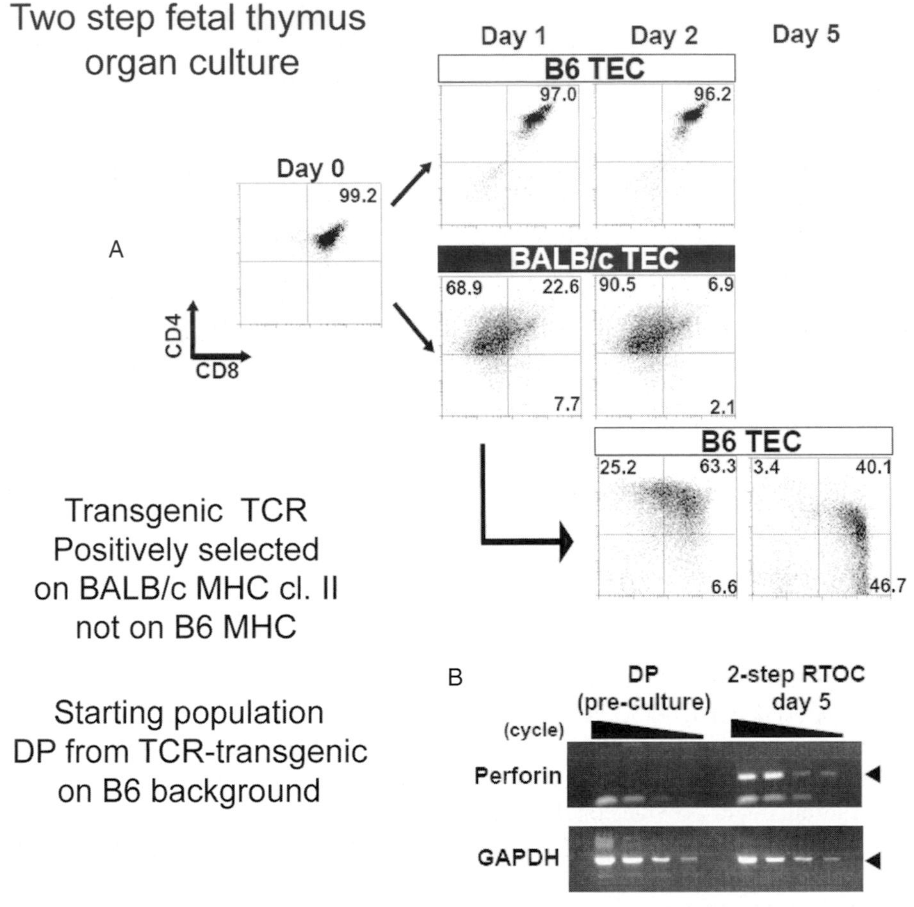

FIGURE 12.7 Signaling through TCR-class II MHC interaction can drive either CD4 or CD8 SP development depending on duration of signal. The figure shows a two-step fetal thymic organ culture system in which cells can be exposed to the same positively selecting ligands for longer or shorter periods. **A:** Fetal thymocytes with an MHC class II–restricted TCR transgene would normally develop into CD4 SP cells if exposed to the correct MHC haplotype. However, in the B6 genetic background, the right MHC class II product is not expressed. Therefore, in the thymus of a TCR transgenic on the B6 background, the thymocytes cannot progress beyond the DP stage in spite of their expression of a good TCR (left panel). These DP cells can be rescued into differentiation toward CD4 SP within 1–2 days if they are transferred to a reaggregate fetal thymic organ culture (RTOC) with TECs from a BALB/c mouse (middle panels), but they remain arrested at DP in RTOC with TEC from a B6 mouse (upper panels). However, if they are aggregated with the BALB/c TEC for just one day, and then are reisolated and reassociated with B6 TEC, they turn on CD8 again and begin differentiating into CD8 SP cells instead (lower panels). Note that transient exposure to selecting signals, followed by return to nonselecting conditions, has distinct effects from a continuous exposure to either nonselecting or selecting conditions. **B:** RT-PCR analysis of gene expression in cells derived from two-step RTOC, showing that the cells not only differentiate toward the CD8 SP phenotype but also turn on expression of the CD8-lineage associated gene, perforin. From ref. (199), with permission.

to CD8/TCR/MHC class I, targeted mutation experiments have now been done to place CD4 itself under the control of regulatory elements in the CD8 locus, so that CD4 is expressed with a transient down-regulation during positive selection like CD8 instead of its normal stable expression (200). In these mice, class II MHC interaction with TCR and CD4 now selects CD8 cells instead of CD4 cells. Thus, the different kinetic profiles of signaling via TCR-CD4 interaction and via TCR-CD8 interaction in DP thymocytes turn out to be fully sufficient to determine the paths the cells will take.

Molecular Regulators that Control CD4/CD8 Lineage Divergence

That a sustained signal and a discontinuous signal might activate different downstream regulatory cascades is not biologically novel. The general phenomenon of receptor desensitization, for example, or habituation, is based on the need to discriminate between these two kinds of stimuli. However, kinetic discrimination of this kind usually involves not just a pathway, but a control network—for example, by use of a signal-activated feedback inhibitor with a short half-life. The challenge in CD4/CD8 discrimination has been to identify the members of the regulatory network that are responsible for converting a difference in transient activation experiences into the execution of two divergent developmental programs. Since 2002, a small group of transcription factors have emerged as major players in these programs. Their identification is a huge stride toward defining the actual mechanisms that operate during the lineage choice itself (199,201–204).

The regulatory gene with the most remarkable effects on CD4/CD8 lineage choice is a zinc finger, BTB/POZ[1] domain transcription factor called variously Th-POK, cKrox, Zfp-67, or Zbtb7b. This gene was discovered by two completely independent kinds of approach that converged on the same target. It was identified by the Kappes group (201) as the site of a spontaneous point mutation that caused a dramatic "helper-independent" phenotype: In spite of normal TCR interaction with MHC class II, mice with this mutation could not make helper T cells but generated CD8 cells instead (205) (Figure 12.8A). The same gene was also discovered in the Bosselut group as one of the top few genes that were most differentially expressed between developing CD4 SP cells and CD8 SP cells (202). The Zbtb7b gene is normally turned on only in the later half of CD4 cell positive selection, not as an initial response to TCR signaling. Complete loss of its expression, like the point mutation, completely blocks CD4 cell development, while forced expression of this gene in thymocytes diverts class I MHC–restricted cells completely to the CD4 cell lineage. This is illustrated in Figure 12.8. The converted cells have not just changed expression of surface CD4 and CD8 molecules, but have adopted the whole gene expression program that goes with the new phenotype (201) (Figure 12.8C). This transcription factor thus can duplicate the effect of sustained TCR-CD4-Lck signaling in positive selection, imposing the CD4 helper fate in a dominant way, and it is likely that the sustained signal is required especially to induce this factor's expression (206).

CD4 cell development also depends on GATA-3, the same factor that is essential for early T cell development, as shown by experiments where it is deleted or down-regulated in DP thymocytes (204,207). Surprisingly, GATA-3 is normally down-regulated at the DP stage and virtually shut off in CD8 SP cells, but it can reactivated by strong TCR signals consistent with CD4 positive selection. Forced expression of GATA-3 blocks CD8 cell selection, but it does not have the power on its own to cause redirection of CD8 cells to a CD4 fate (204). This suggests that GATA-3 is not sufficient to activate Zbtb7b expression in the absence of sustained TCR signaling, in contrast with Zbtb7b, which may help to activate or sustain GATA-3 expression.

The drivers of CD8 cell development most prominently include the transcription factor Runx3, with assistance from Ikaros and an HMG-box transcription factor named TOX (199,208,209). Runx3 in particular is probably a general driver of the CD8 cell fate. It is seen to cause the repression of CD4 (210), as well as participating with Ikaros in CD8 upregulation, and it must be activated as CD8 cells finally make the "coreceptor reversal" turn and become $CD4^- CD8^+$. In the two-step culture system shown in Figure 12.7, CD8 cell development cannot occur when Runx3 is antagonized (199). There has been some controversy about whether forced expression of Runx3 can actually impose the CD8 fate on cells with a class II MHC–specific receptor (211,212); it is possible that this depends on the level at which Runx3 is expressed. Similarly, the roles of Ikaros and TOX in positive selection seem to be more complex than the simple fate-determining activity seen with Zbtb7b. The reported activities of these factors have to be considered in light of the evidence that CD8 cell fate is likely to be a default fate, one that can be overridden by sustained TCR/Lck signaling, as discussed earlier. If the CD4/CD8 lineage choice is inherently asymmetrical like this, then a true CD8-promoting factor need not work as dominantly as Zbtb7b. CD8 cell programming could even begin in the majority of positively selected cells regardless of selecting ligand, only to be repressed by Zbtb7b in cases where Lck signaling is sustained (206).

The positive selection process thus provides a developmental cascade in which evolving transcription factor expression states are confronted repeatedly with TCR and Lck signals over a period of days. Many if not all of the

[1] A protein interaction domain found in some transcription factors and chromatin remodeling proteins. Abbreviation stands for Bric-a-brac, Tramtrack, Broad complex/POxvirus-and-Zinc Finger domain.

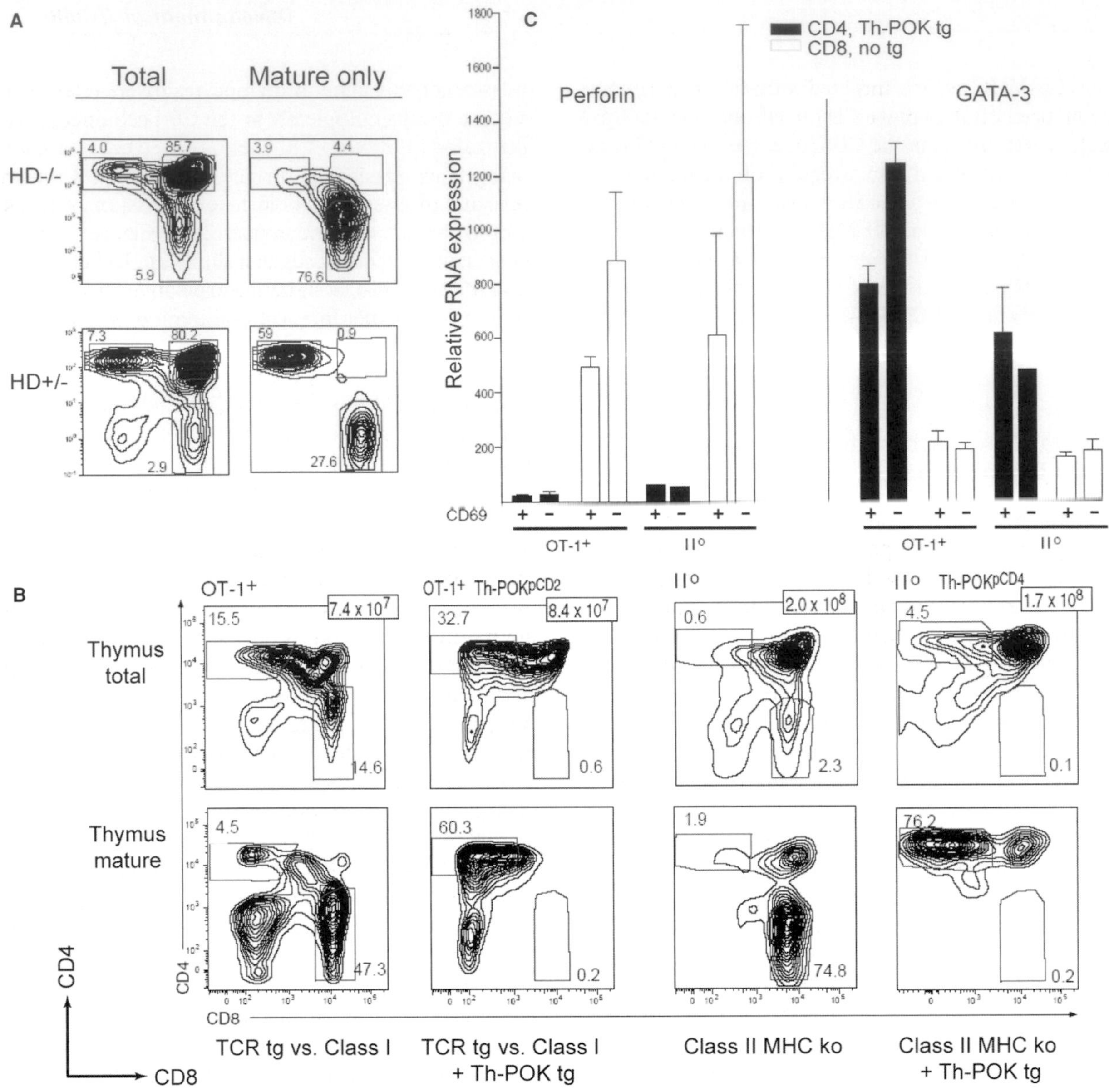

FIGURE 12.8 Zbtb7b (Th-POK) is necessary for CD4 SP maturation and can override TCR–MHC interactions that normally promote CD8 development to direct thymocytes into CD4 SP maturation instead. From ref. (201), with permission. **A:** Lack of normal Zbtb7b (Th-POK) function in $HD^{-/-}$ mice causes a specific absence of mature CD4 SP cells in the thymus. Mutant phenotype: top panels. Wild-type phenotype: lower panels. Mature thymocytes here are the subset defined by low expression of CD24 (HSA) and high expression of the marker CD62L. Note that there are some $CD4^{+}$ $CD8^{low}$ cells in the mutant (left upper panel), but these are transitional cells that are not fully mature (right upper panel). **B:** Forced expression of Zbtb7b (Th-POK) from either of two T cell–specific transgenes (Th-POK^{pCD2}, Th-POK^{pCD4} = Th-POK tg) can force cells that would otherwise develop into CD8 SP cells to become CD4 SP cells instead. Normally only CD8 SP cells mature in mice with a class I MHC-restricted TCR transgene (OT-I), or with a genetic deficiency of class II MHC expression (II°) (lower panels, "TCR tg vs. Class I," "Class II MHC ko"). Combining these mutations with Th-POK transgenes overrides CD8 cell programming to drive maturation to the CD4 SP fate instead (lower panels). Numbers in boxes in upper panels show total thymocyte cellularity in each transgenic. These results imply that the Th-POK transgenes cause redirection of cells without gross changes in survival. **C:** Cells converted to CD4 phenotype by Th-POK transgenes up-regulate the CD4-associated transcription factor GATA-3 and downregulate the CD8-associated effector gene perforin, even if they were positively selected by a class I-restricted TCR transgene (OT-I) or in the absence of class II MHC (II°). RNA expression levels are shown for the CD8 SP cells that would normally be selected in each of these conditions (open bars), compared with those for the CD4 SP cells that are selected instead when a Th-POK transgene is present (black bars). The figure confirms that the change occurs during positive selection itself, as similar effects are seen in subsets of each population that are enriched for cells just undergoing selection ($CD69^{+}$) and subsets that are fully mature ($CD69^{-}$).

critical regulators of the lineage choice are now in hand, and good preliminary guesses can be made about the ways through which they regulate each other to guide the cells to two distinct developmental fates. These linkages can be directly tested, and then the way positive selection guides the choice between helper and killer fates will be truly understood.

CENTRAL TOLERANCE

An inevitable outcome of the random generation of TCR diversity and the relatively promiscuous positive selection process is the survival of cells that can be highly reactive to both foreign and self-peptides bound by self-MHC. TCR-positive cells go through an additional checkpoint in the thymus, which shapes the final TCR repertoire by pruning out or altering self-reactive cells. Positively selected cells continue to mature for several additional days in the thymic medulla during which time they not only acquire effector function but also undergo "central tolerance" mechanisms. In the process, they repetitively test their TCRs for self-reactivity through interactions with medullary epithelial cells (mTECs) and dendritic cells (DCs) expressing a huge range of self-peptide–MHC complexes (Figure 12.9). The outcome of these selective processes is a final TCR repertoire that is self-tolerant. The first of these mechanisms, negative selection or clonal deletion, results in the apoptotic death of cells with high affinity TCRs for at least one of the self-antigen–MHC complexes. Another thymic selection mechanism has been elucidated only in recent years with the discovery of regulatory T cells (T_{reg}) that are potent dominant suppressors of autoimmune T cells, which also arise in the thymus. These T cells, whose TCRs also recognize high-affinity self-antigen–MHC, are not induced to undergo apoptosis, but instead survive in an altered state from conventional positively selected CD4 and CD8 SP cells. Failure of either of these central tolerance mechanisms can result in systemic autoimmune disease in humans and mice. What intrinsic and extrinsic factors, in addition to TCR specificity and affinity, determine these very different alternative fate choices made by developing $\alpha\beta$-T cells, are areas of very active research.

Negative Selection

The phenomenon of negative selection of self-reactive T cells in the thymus was first demonstrated in response to endogenous superantigens and self-MHC (213), and studies using transgenic TCRs over the past two decades have shown that T cells with high-affinity TCRs to self-antigen–MHC complexes are induced to undergo apoptotic death (reviewed by 214,215). Using these transgenic model systems, deletion was found to occur at a range of stages from the DN or DP stage of T cell development in the thymic cortex to the SP stage in the medulla. The exact stage of T cell development and thymic location in which negative selection normally occurs is controversial because of the early timing and high level of transgenic TCR expression relative to normal T cells (215,216). However, several lines of evidence suggest that under normal conditions, negative selection may be predominantly separated from positive selection, both developmentally and spatially, as shown in Figure 12.9. In a transgenic TCR model system where the TCR was expressed with normal timing, deletion was found to predominantly occur in SP cells in the medulla (217). In addition, the medulla is the specific site of two kinds of antigen-presenting cells, which are potent inducers of negative selection: mTECs and dendritic cells (DCs). These cells express high levels of MHC and costimulatory molecules, both of which greatly facilitate negative selection and are highly specialized for the presentation of a large array of peripheral self-antigens acquired by several unique mechanisms. Finally, the critical importance of the thymic medulla to central tolerance, but not SP cell maturation, was demonstrated in experiments showing that when T cells are prevented from migrating from the cortex to the medulla by the lack of the chemokine receptor CCR7 or its ligand, cells undergo normal maturation and export from the thymus, but the animals develop autoimmunity (218). The autoimmune phenotype resembles a failure of negative selection, although faulty regulatory T cell development (see later discussion) has not been ruled out. This shows that central tolerance is, at least in part, dependent upon T cell passage through the medulla and interactions with medullary cells.

Long after negative selection was discovered, it was unknown whether the thymus could express and present the vast array of protein peptides found throughout the body for negative selection at a sufficient level to maintain self-tolerance and to avoid autoimmunity, and if so what mechanism could allow for such expression. In the absence of such a mechanism, and with evidence that self-reactive T cells can be found in the circulation of even normal healthy animals, it was debated whether negative selection was necessary or sufficient to prevent autoimmune disease. The discovery of the transcription factor gene, *Aire*, which causes a rare autoimmune disease, APECED (autoimmune polyendocrinopathy-candidiasis-ectodermal dystrophy) syndrome, when mutated in humans and mice, has now confirmed the critical importance of negative selection in the maintenance of self-tolerance and has contributed greatly to our understanding of this process (219–223). Central to this mechanism are the mTECs. *Aire* plays a unique, though as yet poorly understood, role in inducing the expression in mTECs of clusters of genes that are normally highly restricted in their tissue specificity or timing of expression. Genes from tissues throughout the body are expressed in the mTECs, and each mTEC expresses

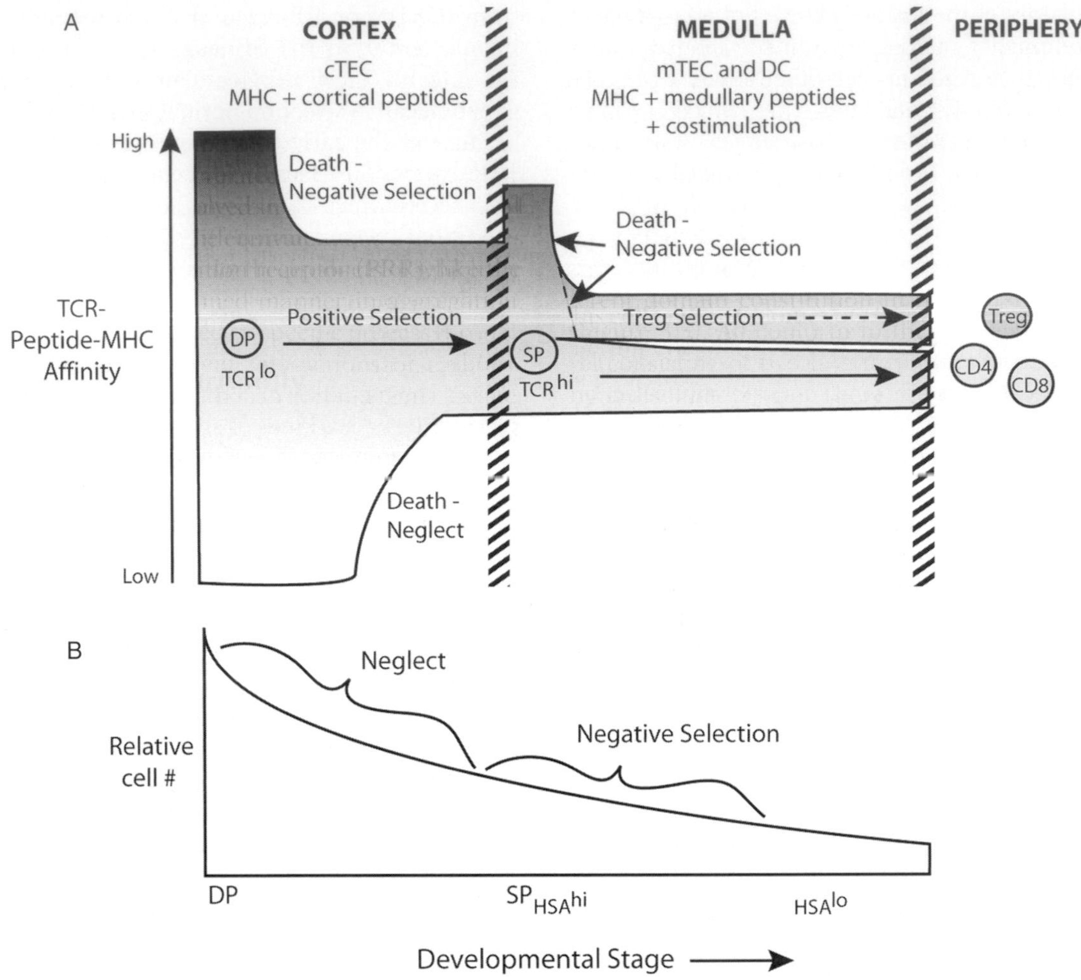

FIGURE 12.9 Progressive narrowing of the $\alpha\beta$-TCR repertoire during development based upon affinity to self-peptide–MHC complexes, leading to MHC restriction and self-tolerance. **A:** TCR^{lo} $CD4^{+}CD8^{+}$ DP cells in the thymic cortex test their newly generated TCRs against self-peptide–MHC complexes presented by cortical cells with three major outcomes: those unable to bind self-MHC die by "neglect," those binding self-peptide–MHC with high affinity die by negative selection, and those with weak affinities to self-peptide–MHC are positively selected to undergo differentiation to CD4 or CD8 lineages. The TCRs of these positively selected cells are restricted to self-MHC and migrate to the medulla for further selection and maturation. TCR^{hi} CD4 or CD8 SP cells in the thymic medulla pass through a new network of different antigen-presenting cells expressing a larger subset of peptide antigens plus costimulatory molecules. Self-reactive T cells, those with high-affinity interactions with self-peptide–MHC, are either induced to die by negative selection (arrow) or are positively selected into the T_{reg} lineage, upregulating Foxp3 and CD25. The cells with highest affinity interactions in the cortex are not necessarily those with the highest affinity for antigens expressed in the medulla due to the changes in cell properties and antigen presentation. Note that the affinity range for T_{reg} selection overlaps with the affinity range for negative selection. These selective mechanisms establish the level of T cell central tolerance in the individual. T cells with TCRs of weak affinity to the constellation of presented self-peptides undergo maturation, downregulation of CD69 and CD24 (HSA), and they eventually emigrate into the periphery as naïve $CD4^{+}$ or $CD8^{+}$ T cells. Hatched lines indicate compartment boundaries. Gradient shading indicates the range of TCR affinities, on surviving cells, for ligands within the relevant compartment. **B:** The relative numbers of $\alpha\beta$-T cells decline precipitously during development from the DP to mature SP stages due to neglect and negative selection in the thymus.

and presents peptides from a subset of these genes to T cells in the medulla. Although *Aire* is responsible for this promiscuous expression of peripheral antigens in mTECs, not all tissue-specific genes are dependent upon *Aire* for expression in mTECs. However, even in cases where antigens are expressed in mTECs in the absence of *Aire*, negative selection of specific T cells is still impaired even though levels of MHC and costimulatory molecules are not different (224,225). Thus, in addition to its novel transactivating activity, *Aire* clearly plays an additional critical role in mediating negative selection by mTECs.

DCs are more abundant in the thymic medulla than in the cortex and are very potent mediators of negative selection, even more so than mTECs. They do not express *Aire* and and so do not express the huge range of tissue-specific genes that mTECs do. However, DCs have the capability to cross-present antigens obtained from various other cells. It has been demonstrated that that medullary DCs can cross-present antigens expressed by mTECS, possibly acquiring these antigens from the short-lived mTECs as they die (226). In addition, DCs have been shown to be capable of acquiring antigens from the periphery, migrating to the thymic medulla for antigen presentation to developing T cells, and inducing apoptosis in antigen-specific T cells (227). Thus, DCs in the medulla have access to antigens obtained in the periphery and indirectly from promiscuous gene expression by mTECs, as well as those they express themselves, for presentation to T cells.

In addition to their extraordinary capacity for acquiring and presenting self-antigens, mTECS and DCs also express costimulatory molecules such as B7 and CD40. CD28/B7 or possibly CD40/40L interactions appear to play an important role in negative selection, although neither is absolutely required for deletion (228) (reviewed in 166). It is possible that in the absence of these molecules very strong TCR signals or other costimulatory molecules may be able to provide the additional signal.

Negative selection triggers apoptosis that appears to be mediated by up-regulation or phosphorylation of a proapoptotic Bcl-2 family member, Bim (229), in collaboration with Bax and Bak (230). Up-regulation of the orphan steroid receptor, Nur77, also plays a role in this apoptosis (231). Distinctive signaling pathways from TCR and costimulatory molecules that may activate these mediators are under intense investigation. In knockdown experiments using small interfering (si)-RNA, the serine-threonine kinase MINK has recently been reported to be involved in negative selection specifically, potentially linking TCR signals with JNK and p38, as well as Bim, activation (232).

Negative vs. Positive Selection

What are the molecular mechanisms that developing T cells use to distinguish between positive and negative selection signals from the TCR? Once again, TCR signal strength helps to determine the outcome of TCR engagement by antigen-MHC complexes: Weaker signals result in survival and differentiation, while stronger signals trigger cell death. How these signals give such different outcomes is still not well understood, and conflicting results have been obtained using different models of selection (reviewed in 214,215). Both modes of selection use the Lck proximal signaling pathway, but signals transduced during positive selection appears to be particularly dependent upon calcineurin and ERK, while negative selection depends upon JNK and p38 activation, although ERK also appears to be activated. One model for how T cells distinguish between weak and strong TCR signals predicts that positive selection results from low, sustained ERK activation, while negative selection results from a transient burst of ERK activation and JNK and p38 activation. A recent study showed that differences in the subcellular compartmentalization of Ras/MAPK signaling intermediates, in response to variants of agonist peptides giving differing TCR signal strengths, may determine the thresholds for positive versus negative selection (233).

The difference may not simply be based on signal strength. The physiological context changes between positive selection, occurring in the more immature DP cells in the thymic cortex, and negative selection, occurring typically, but not exclusively, in more mature positively selected SP T cells in the thymic medulla (Figure 12.9). Not only do the SP T cells pass through a network of mTECs and DCs expressing an expanded array of self-peptides and MHC complexes as well as costimulatory molecules, but also, as a result of positive selection, these SP T cells have undergone major changes in differentiation programming as CD4 or CD8 cells (Figure 12.5). The higher levels of surface TCR and other changes as a result of positive selection, such as up-regulation of CD5 and restored sialylation of surface glycoproteins, are likely to change sensitivity of SP cells to high-affinity TCR signals. Thus, the different developmental states (DP versus SP), levels of surface TCR and other signaling components, gene expression programs, and microenvironment of the T cells, as well as the differing arrays of presented antigens in the cortex versus medulla, are all factors that likely to contribute to the different outcomes of high- versus low-affinity TCR-peptide–MHC interactions leading to negative versus positive selection.

Development of Regulatory T Cells

Negative selection of autoimmune cells was originally thought to be the major mechanism of tolerance in the thymus. However, recently, a very potent and critically important T cell population which mediates active suppression of immunity, including autoimmunity, was found to develop in the thymus. They are known as regulatory T cells or T_{reg} cells (see Chapter 30). This specialized lineage of highly immune suppressive

T cells was first characterized by surface expression of CD4 and CD25, having a dependence upon exogenously supplied IL-2, and uniquely expressing the transcription factor *Foxp3* (*Scurfin*) (234,235). *Foxp3* is a lineage-determining factor for T_{reg} cells and retroviral transduction of this gene into peripheral *Foxp3*$^-$ T cells can induce them to adopt a regulatory T cell phenotype and function. This factor is absolutely required for the development of T_{reg} cells as shown in mixed bone marrow chimera experiments (236). *Foxp3,* a forkhead winged-helix transcription factor family member, was initially identified as the mutated gene causing a severe autoimmune disease in humans, immunodysregulation, polyendocrinopathy and enteropathy, X-linked (IPEX) syndrome, and a similar disease in *scurfy* mice (reviewed by 234,237). These mutations, along with *Foxp3*-gene knockouts, result in complete loss of T_{reg} cells, demonstrating their vital importance in the maintenance of self-tolerance.

The first evidence that a population of suppressive T cells might arise as a separate lineage from the thymus came from experiments in which neonatal mice thymectomized 2–3 days after birth were not only lymphopenic as expected, but also surprisingly developed autoimmune disease (238). The missing population was eventually identified and characterized as CD4$^+$CD25$^+$T cells which first appear in the thymus around 2–3 days after birth (239). These thymic T cells were found to be capable of dominantly suppressing the activation and proliferation of antigen-activated T cells similarly to the peripheral CD4$^+$CD25$^+$ regulatory T (T_{reg}) cells. Using mice with the marker green fluorescent protein (GFP), knocked into the *Foxp3* locus to study the development of T_{reg} cells, it was confirmed that *Foxp3* expression can begin in the thymus. The majority of the GFP$^+$ cells in the thymus are CD4 SP cells in the medulla, although some DP cells are also positive, and there is evidence that they develop within the thymus (240). In fact, regulatory T cells make up approximately 5% of thymic CD4$^+$ cells and the TCRs expressed by T_{reg} cells have a comparable range of diversity to conventional T cells (241). Mice with various rearranged transgenic TCRs also contain CD4$^+$CD25$^+$ regulatory T cells, in a process that requires the presence of the cognate antigen for their development (242,243).

Overall it appears that commitment to the T_{reg} lineage and negative selection occur in the same developmental stages and thymic regions, and are dependent on similar or at least overlapping sets of TCR-ligand affinities (Figure 12.9). Several lines of evidence suggest that selection for T_{reg} cells, like negative selection, can be a response to high-affinity TCR-peptide-MHC interactions (235,244). Using a model system with influenza virus hemagglutinin (HA) expressed as a neo–self-antigen and transgenic TCRs with varying affinities to HA, the proportion of regulatory T cells that was generated declined with decreased TCR affinity (245). Indeed, the affinity range permissive for T_{reg} development overlaps considerably with the range promoting negative selection. When *Foxp3* is mutated so that T_{reg} cannot develop, the same TCR as used by suppressive T_{reg} cells can be used by pathogenic autoimmune cells instead, demonstrating that there is overlap in these two self-reactive TCR repertoires (246). In double transgenic systems, regulatory T cell development is accompanied by deletion of T cells sharing the same rearranged TCR genes. However, the relative proportions of cells undergoing these two modes of central tolerance change with alterations in amount or mode of antigen expression. Careful analysis of transgenic TCR with graded doses of agonist peptide/MHC resulted in dramatic changes in the numbers of cells undergoing negative selection, while the numbers of T_{reg} cells changed only modestly (247). Taken together, these results show that, above a certain minimum TCR-ligand affinity, the choice between apoptosis due to negative selection and differentiation and survival as a regulatory T cell may be due to differences in the intrinsic state of the T cell, conferred by earlier developmental events, or due to extrinsic factors rather than the precise affinity of the TCR.

Although it is currently unknown what intrinsic and extrinsic factors distinguish these two central tolerance mechanisms, recent studies are just beginning to provide insights (reviewed in ref. 247a). One possibility is that *Foxp3* induction depends on a special kind of stimulatory experience. CD28 constimulatory molecules appear to be necessary for T_{reg} development and can play a role in the upregulation of *Foxp3* in T cells (248,249), although CD28 may also be important in negative selection, suggesting that the cell response to CD28 or additional signals distinguish these fates. It also appears that earlier developmental events may in fact determine a subpopulation of cells that is more likely to respond to high-affinity TCR engagement in the thymus with survival rather than death. Two recent studies have shown that pT$\alpha^{-/-}$ mice, which generate few DP and mature T cells due to an incomplete block at β selection, have a relative enrichment of T_{reg} cells in the thymus and periphery (250,251). This effect may be due to the atypical β selection experience these cells undergo, or due to the reduced exposure of their DN precursors to an intercellular mediator produced by DP cells (159). If confirmed, these findings suggest that immature thymocytes undergoing selective events are intrinsically diverse in their ability to respond to TCR ligation and costimulation due to as yet uncharacterized variations in their developmental history.

Autoimmunity as a Result of Failures of Central Tolerance

Overall, positive and negative selection processes in the thymus act to narrow the TCR repertoire of an individual to be responsive to self-MHC molecules but not responsive to high-affinity self-peptides when presented by self-MHC, in principle allowing survival of only TCRs that can respond to non–self-peptides presented by self-MHC (Figure 12.9). Not all T cells with high affinity to self-peptide–MHC are deleted, but this "exception proves the rule": Many are diverted to the T_{reg} lineage, which in the periphery can dominantly suppress any surviving autoreactive T cells that avoided negative selection. This process of selection and passage through TCR-mediated events during T cell development results in major changes in overall repertoire sensitivity to self-antigens. Autoimmunity may result from several failures of central tolerance: (1) a failure to present specific self-antigens in the thymus, (2) the failure of clonal deletion of conventional T cells with TCRs of high self-reactivity due to intrinsic or extrinsic factors, or (3) a failure of T_{reg} cell generation due to intrinsic or extrinsic factors. The human diseases APECED syndrome and IPEX, and their mouse counterparts with mutations in *Aire* and *Foxp3*, emphasize the critical importance of negative selection and generation of T_{reg} cells respectively in preventing autoimmune reactions. Understanding the different means by which central tolerance is achieved, and determining what mechanisms can lead to its failure and autoimmunity, is a major challenge in the study of T cell development and lineage choices.

CONCLUSION

We have focused in depth on several aspects of intrathymic T cell development that are particularly significant in terms of developmental mechanisms or immunological impact. These are areas in which work since 2000 has offered new glimpses of understanding how a momentous developmental choice or transition will be made. But it is worth returning to the larger picture of T cell development sketched in Figures 12.2 and 12.9. In overview, it is striking how much functional diversity and lineage choice remain with cells after they have undergone T lineage commitment. The cells take advantage of the intricate architecture of the thymus to migrate from one domain to another, using a core group of signaling molecules, carefully modulated interactions with environmental ligands, and a few newly induced transcription factors that interact with another, more persistent set of transcription factors, to refine progressively what kind of T cell their initial T lineage commitment will produce. T cell development begins in the thymus as we have seen, but the ultimate working-out of a T cell's destiny extends through many rounds of differentiative response to TCR-mediated signals, not only in the thymic medulla but also long after they have left the thymus, in the periphery.

ACKNOWLEDGMENTS

The authors thank the investigators who kindly allowed their work to be reproduced for this chapter. We apologize to our many colleagues whose work and thoughtful interpretations have contributed greatly to the background of this chapter, yet which we could not discuss adequately because of space limitations. Related work in the authors' laboratory was supported by grants from the U.S. Public Health Service (R01CA90233, R01CA98925, R01AI64590).

REFERENCES

1. Hoffman ES, Passoni L, Crompton T, et al. Productive T cell receptor β-chain gene rearrangement: coincident regulation of cell cycle and clonality during development in vivo. *Genes & Dev.* 1996;10:948–962.
2. Penit C, Lucas B, Vasseur F. Cell expansion and growth arrest phases during the transition from precursor ($CD4^-8^-$) to immature ($CD4^+8^+$) thymocytes in normal and genetically modified mice. *J Immunol.* 1995;154:5103–5113.

2a. McCaughtry TM, Wilken MS, Hogquist KA. Thymic emigration revisited. *J Exp Med.* 2007;204:2513–2520.

3. Di Santo JP, Rodewald H-R. *In vivo* roles of receptor tyrosine kinases and cytokine receptors in early thymocyte development. *Curr Opin Immunol.* 1998;10:196–207.
4. Schmitt TM, Zuniga-Pflucker JC. Thymus-derived signals regulate early T-cell development. *Crit Rev Immunol.* 2005;25:141–160.
5. Massa S, Balciunaite G, Ceredig R, et al. Critical role for c-kit (CD117) in T cell lineage commitment and early thymocyte development in vitro. *Eur J Immunol.* 2006;36:526–532.
6. Candéias S, Muegge K, Durum SK. IL-7 receptor and VDJ recombination: trophic versus mechanistic actions. *Immunity.* 1997;6:501–508.
7. Maraskovsky E, O'Reilly LA, Teepe M, et al. Bcl-2 can rescue T lymphocyte development in interleukin-7 receptor-deficient mice but not in mutant *rag-1*$^{-/-}$mice. *Cell.* 1997;89:1011–1019.
8. von Freeden-Jeffry U, Solvason N, Howard M, et al. The earliest T lineage-committed cells depend on IL-7 for Bcl-2 expression and normal cell cycle progression. *Immunity.* 1997;7:147–154.
9. Di Santo JP, Aifantis I, Rosmaraki E, et al. The common cytokine receptor γ chain and the pre-T cell receptor provide independent but critically overlapping signals in early α/β T cell development. *J Exp Med.* 1999;189:563–573.
10. Petrie HT. Cell migration and the control of post-natal T-cell lymphopoiesis in the thymus. *Nat Rev Immunol.* 2003;3:859–866.

10a. Petrie HT, Zuniga-Pflucker JC. Zoned out: functional mapping of stromal signaling microenvironments in the thymus. *Annu Rev Immunol.* 2007;25:649–679.

11. Lind EF, Prockop SE, Porritt HE, et al. Mapping precursor movement through the postnatal thymus reveals specific microenvironments supporting defined stages of early lymphoid development. *J Exp Med.* 2001;194:127–134.
12. Derbinski J, Schulte A, Kyewski B, et al. Promiscuous gene expression in medullary thymic epithelial cells mirrors the peripheral self. *Nat Immunol.* 2001;2:1032–1039.
13. Zamisch M, Moore-Scott B, Su DM, et al. Ontogeny and regulation of IL-7-expressing thymic epithelial cells. *J Immunol.* 2005;174:60–67.
14. Norment AM, Bogatzki LY, Gantner BN, et al. Murine CCR9, a chemokine receptor for thymus-expressed chemokine that is up-regulated following pre-TCR signaling. *J Immunol.* 2000;164:639–648.
15. Uehara S, Song K, Farber JM, et al. Characterization of CCR9 expression and CCL25/thymus-expressed chemokine responsiveness during T cell development: $CD3^{high}$ $CD69^+$ thymocytes and $\gamma\delta TCR^+$ thymocytes preferentially respond to CCL25. *J Immunol.* 2002;168:134–142.
16. David-Fung ES, Yui MA, Morales M, et al. Progression of regulatory gene expression states in fetal and adult pro-T cell development. *Immunol Rev.* 2006;209:212–236.
17. Anderson G, Jenkinson WE, Jones T, et al. Establishment and functioning of intrathymic microenvironments. *Immunol Rev.* 2006;209:10–27.
18. Holländer G, Gill J, Zuklys S, et al. Cellular and molecular events during early thymus development. *Immunol Rev.* 2006;209:28–46.
19. Ikuta K, Kina T, NacNeil I, et al. A developmental switch in thymic lymphocyte maturation potential occurs at the level of hematopoietic stem cells. *Cell.* 1990;62:863–874.

20. Bain G, Romanow WJ, Albers K, et al. Positive and negative regulation of V(D)J recombination by the E2A proteins. *J Exp Med.* 1999;189:289–300.
21. Leclercq G, Debacker V, De Smedt M, et al. Differential effects of interleukin-15 and interleukin-2 on differentiation of bipotential T/natural killer progenitor cells. *J Exp Med.* 1996;184:325–336.
22. Foss DL, Donskoy E, Goldschneider I. The importation of hematogenous precursors by the thymus is a gated phenomenon in normal adult mice. *J Exp Med.* 2001;193:365–374.
23. Dzierzak E. The emergence of definitive hematopoietic stem cells in the mammal. *Curr Opin Hematol.* 2005;12:197–202.
24. Dzierzak E, Medvinsky A, de Bruijn M. Qualitative and quantitative aspects of haematopoietic cell development in the mammalian embryo. *Immunol Today.* 1998;19:228–236.
25. Bonifer C, Faust N, Geiger H, et al. Developmental changes in the differentiation capacity of haematopoietic stem cells. *Immunol Today.* 1998;19:236–241.
26. Miracle AL, Anderson MK, Litman RT, et al. Complex expression patterns of lymphocyte-specific genes during the development of cartilaginous fish implicate unique lymphoid tissues in generating an immune repertoire. *Int Immunol.* 2001;13:567–580.
27. Cooper MD, Chen CL, Bucy RP, et al. Avian T cell ontogeny. *Adv Immunol.* 1991;50:87–117.
28. Spits H. Development of $\alpha\beta$ T cells in the human thymus. *Nat Rev Immunol.* 2002;2:760–772.
29. Dik WA, Pike-Overzet K, Weerkamp F, et al. New insights on human T cell development by quantitative T cell receptor gene rearrangement studies and gene expression profiling. *J Exp Med.* 2005;201:1715–1723.
30. Staal FJT, Weerkamp F, Langerak AW, et al. Transcriptional control of T lymphocyte differentiation. *Stem Cells.* 2001;19:165–179.
30a. Bhandoola A, von Boehmer H, Petrie HT, et al. Commitment and developmental potential of extrathymic and intrathymic T cell precursors: plenty to choose from. *Immunity.* 2007;26:678–689.
30b. Rothenberg EV. Negotiation of the T lineage fate decision by transcription-factor interplay and microenvironmental signals. *Immunity.* 2007;26:690–702.
31. Masuda K, Itoi M, Amagai T, et al. Thymic anlage is colonized by progenitors restricted to T, NK, and dendritic cell lineages. *J Immunol.* 2005;174:2525–2532.
32. Harman BC, Jenkinson WE, Parnell SM, et al. T/B lineage choice occurs prior to intrathymic Notch signalling. *Blood.* 2005;106:886–892.
33. Krueger A, Garbe AI, von Boehmer H. Phenotypic plasticity of T cell progenitors upon exposure to Notch ligands. *J Exp Med.* 2006;203:1977–1984.
34. Jenkinson EJ, Jenkinson WE, Rossi SW, et al. The thymus and T-cell commitment: the right niche for Notch? *Nat Rev Immunol.* 2006;6:551–555.
35. Wu L. T lineage progenitors: the earliest steps en route to T lymphocytes. *Curr Opin Immunol.* 2006;18:121–126.
36. Weerkamp F, Pike-Overzet K, Staal FJT. T-sing progenitors to commit. *Trends Immunol.* 2006;27:125–131.
37. Balciunaite G, Ceredig R, Rolink AG. The earliest subpopulation of mouse thymocytes contains potent T, significant macrophage, and natural killer cell but no B-lymphocyte potential. *Blood.* 2005;105:1930–1936.
38. Zediak VP, Maillard I, Bhandoola A. Closer to the source: notch and the nature of thymus-settling cells. *Immunity.* 2005;23:245–248.
39. Petrie HT, Kincade PW. Many roads, one destination for T cell progenitors. *J Exp Med.* 2005;202:11–13.
40. Pelayo R, Welner R, Perry SS, et al. Lymphoid progenitors and primary routes to becoming cells of the immune system. *Curr Opin Immunol.* 2005;17:100–107.
41. Rothenberg EV, Dionne CJ. Lineage plasticity and commitment in T-cell development. *Immunol Rev.* 2002;187:96–115.
42. Katsura Y, Kawamoto H. Stepwise lineage restriction of progenitors in lympho-myelopoiesis. *Int Rev Immunol.* 2001;20:1–20.
43. Weerkamp F, Baert MR, Brugman MH, et al. Human thymus contains multipotent progenitors with T/B lymphoid, myeloid, and erythroid lineage potential. *Blood.* 2006;107:3131–3137.
44. Pear WS, Radtke F. Notch signaling in lymphopoiesis. *Semin Immunol.* 2003;15:69–79.
45. Han H, Tanigaki K, Yamamoto N, et al. Inducible gene knockout of transcription factor recombination signal binding protein-J reveals its essential role in T versus B lineage decision. *Int Immunol.* 2002;14:637–645.
46. Schmitt TM, Zúñiga-Pflücker JC. Induction of T cell development from hematopoietic progenitor cells by Delta-like-1 in vitro. *Immunity.* 2002;17:749–756.
47. Schmitt TM, Ciofani M, Petrie HT, et al. Maintenance of T cell specification and differentiation requires recurrent Notch receptor-ligand interactions. *J Exp Med.* 2004;200:469–479.
48. Franco CB, Scripture-Adams DD, Proekt I, et al. Notch/Delta signaling constrains re-engineering of pro-T cells by PU.1. *Proc Natl Acad Sci U S A.* 2006;103:11993–11998.
49. Tan JB, Visan I, Yuan JS, et al. Requirement for Notch1 signals at sequential early stages of intrathymic T cell development. *Nat Immunol* 2005;6:671–9.
50. De Smedt M, Hoebeke I, Reynvoet K, et al. Different thresholds of Notch signaling bias human precursor cells toward B-, NK-, monocytic/dendritic-, or T-cell lineage in thymus microenvironment. *Blood.* 2005;106:3498–3506.
51. van den Brandt J, Voss K, Schott M, et al. Inhibition of Notch signaling biases rat thymocyte development towards the NK cell lineage. *Eur J Immunol.* 2004;34:1405–1413.
52. Lehar SM, Dooley J, Farr AG, et al. Notch ligands Delta1 and Jagged1 transmit distinct signals to T cell precursors. *Blood.* 2005;105:1440–1447.
53. Dallas MH, Varnum-Finney B, Delaney C, et al. Density of the Notch ligand Delta1 determines generation of B and T cell precursors from hematopoietic stem cells. *J Exp Med.* 2005;201:1361–1366.
54. Ikawa T, Kawamoto H, Goldrath AW, et al. E proteins and Notch signaling cooperate to promote T cell lineage specification and commitment. *J Exp Med.* 2006;203:1329–1342.
55. Taghon TN, David E-S, Zúñiga-Pflücker JC, et al. Delayed, asynchronous, and reversible T-lineage specification induced by Notch/Delta signaling. *Genes Dev.* 2005;19:965–978.
56. Höflinger S, Kesavan K, Fuxa M, et al. Analysis of Notch1 function by in vitro T cell differentiation of *Pax5* mutant lymphoid progenitors. *J Immunol.* 2004;173:3935–3944.
57. Ciofani M, Zúñiga-Pflücker JC. Notch promotes survival of pre-T cells at the β-selection checkpoint by regulating cellular metabolism. *Nat Immunol.* 2005;6:881–888.
58. Weerkamp F, Baert MR, Naber BA, et al. Wnt signaling in the thymus is regulated by differential expression of intracellular signaling molecules. *Proc Natl Acad Sci U S A.* 2006;103:3322–3326.
59. Tanigaki K, Tsuji M, Yamamoto N, et al. Regulation of $\alpha\beta/\gamma\delta$ T cell lineage commitment and peripheral T cell responses by Notch/RBP-J signaling. *Immunity.* 2004;20:611–622.
60. Wolfer A, Wilson A, Nemir M, et al. Inactivation of Notch1 impairs VDJβ rearrangement and allows pre-TCR-independent survival of early $\alpha\beta$ lineage thymocytes. *Immunity.* 2002;16:869–879.
61. Taghon T, Yui MA, Pant R, et al. Developmental and molecular characterization of emerging β- and $\gamma\delta$-selected pre-T cells in the adult mouse thymus. *Immunity.* 2006;24:53–64.
62. Ciofani M, Knowles GC, Wiest DL, et al. Stage-specific and differential Notch dependency at the $\alpha\beta$ and $\gamma\delta$ T lineage bifurcation. *Immunity.* 2006;25:105–116.
63. Garbe AI, Krueger A, Gounari F, et al. Differential synergy of Notch and T cell receptor signaling determines $\alpha\beta$ versus $\gamma\delta$ lineage fate. *J Exp Med.* 2006;203:1579–1590.
64. Wolfer A, Bakker T, Wilson A, et al. Inactivation of Notch 1 in immature thymocytes does not perturb CD4 or CD8 T cell development. *Nat Immunol.* 2001;2:235–241.
65. Rothenberg EV, Taghon T. Molecular genetics of T cell development. *Annu Rev Immunol.* 2005;23:601–649.
65a. Taghon T, Yui MA, Rothenberg EV. Mast cell lineage diversion of T lineage precursors by the essential T-cell transcription factor GATA-3. *Nat Immunol.* 2007;8:845–855.
65b. Laiosa CV, Stadtfeld M, Xie H, et al. Reprogramming of committed T cell progenitors to macrophages and dendritic cells by C/EBPα and PU.1 transcription factors. *Immunity.* 2006;25:731–744.
66. Murre C. Helix-loop-helix proteins and lymphocyte development. *Nat Immunol.* 2005;6:1079–1086.

67. Inoue J, Kanefuji T, Okazuka K, et al. Expression of TCR$\alpha\beta$ partly rescues developmental arrest and apoptosis of $\alpha\beta$ T cells in Bcl11b$^{-/-}$ mice. *J Immunol.* 2006;176:5871–5979.
68. Schwartz R, Engel I, Fallahi-Sichani M, et al. Gene expression patterns define novel roles for E47 in cell cycle progression, cytokine-mediated signaling, and T lineage development. *Proc Natl Acad Sci U S A.* 2006;103:9976–9981.
69. Staal FJT, Clevers HC. WNT signalling and haematopoiesis: a WNT-WNT situation. *Nat Rev Immunol.* 2005;5:21–30.
70. Giese K, Kingsley C, Kirshner JR, et al. Assembly and function of a TCRα enhancer complex is dependent on LEF-1-induced DNA bending and multiple protein-protein interactions. *Genes Dev.* 1995;9:995–1008.
71. Goux D, Coudert JD, Maurice D, et al. Cooperating pre-T cell receptor and TCF-1-dependent signals ensure thymocyte survival. *Blood.* 2005;106:1726–1733.
72. Gounari F, Aifantis I, Khazaie K, et al. Somatic activation of β-catenin bypasses pre-TCR signaling and TCR selection in thymocyte development. *Nat Immunol.* 2001;2:863–869.
73. Ioannidis V, Beermann F, Clevers H, et al. The β-catenin–TCF-1 pathway ensures CD4$^+$CD8$^+$ thymocyte survival. *Nat Immunol.* 2001;2:691–697.
74. Schilham MW, Wilson A, Moerer P, et al. Critical involvement of Tcf-1 in expansion of thymocytes. *J Immunol.* 1998;161:3984–3891.
75. Verbeek S, Izon D, Hofhuis F, et al. An HMG-box-containing T-cell factor required for thymocyte differentiation. *Nature.* 1995;374: 70–74.
76. Murphy KM, Reiner SL. The lineage decisions of helper T cells. *Nat Rev Immunol.* 2002;2:933–944.
77. Petrie HT, Tourigny M, Burtrum DB, et al. Precursor thymocyte proliferation and differentiation are controlled by signals unrelated to the pre-TCR. *J Immunol.* 2000;165:3094–3098.
78. Dumortier A, Jeannet R, Kirstetter P, et al. Notch activation is an early and critical event during T Cell leukemogenesis in Ikaros-deficient mice. *Mol Cell Biol* 2006;26:209–220.
79. Reschly EJ, Spaulding C, Vilimas T, et al. Notch1 promotes survival of E2A-deficient T cell lymphomas through pre-T cell receptor-dependent and -independent mechanisms. *Blood.* 2006;107:4115–4121.
80. Campese AF, Garbe AI, Zhang F, et al. Notch1-dependent lymphomagenesis is assisted by but does not essentially require pre-TCR signaling. *Blood.* 2006;108:305–310.
81. Engel I, Murre C. E2A proteins enforce a proliferation checkpoint in developing thymocytes. *EMBO J.* 2004;23:202–211.
82. Newton K, Harris AW, Strasser A. FADD/MORT1 regulates the pre-TCR checkpoint and can function as a tumour suppressor. *EMBO J.* 2000;19:931–941.
83. Winandy S, Wu L, Wang J-H, et al. Pre-T cell receptor (TCR) and TCR-controlled checkpoints in T cell differentiation are set by Ikaros. *J Exp Med.* 1999;190:1039–1048.
84. Haks MC, Krimpenfort P, van den Brakel JHN, et al. Pre-TCR signaling and inactivation of p53 induces crucial cell survival pathways in pre-T cells. *Immunity.* 1999;11:91–101.
85. Guidos CJ, Williams CJ, Grandal I, et al. V(D)J recombination activates a p53-dependent DNA damage checkpoint in *scid* lymphocyte precursors. *Genes & Dev.* 1996;10:2038–2054.
86. Jiang D, Lenardo MJ, Zúñiga-Pflücker JC. p53 prevents maturation to the CD4$^+$CD8$^+$ stage of thymocyte differentiation in the absence of T cell receptor rearrangement. *J Exp Med.* 1996;183:1923–1928.
87. Yui MA, Rothenberg EV. Deranged early T cell development in immunodeficient strains of nonobese diabetic mice. *J Immunol.* 2004;173:5381–5391.
88. Engel I, Johns C, Bain G, et al. Early thymocyte development is regulated by modulation of E2A protein activity. *J Exp Med.* 2001;194:733–746.
89. Guidos CJ. Synergy between the pre-T cell receptor and Notch: cementing the $\alpha\beta$ lineage choice. *J Exp Med.* 2006;203:2233–2237.
90. von Boehmer H. Unique features of the pre-T-cell receptor α-chain: not just a surrogate. *Nat Rev Immunol.* 2005;5:571–577.
91. Michie AM, Zuniga-Pflucker JC. Regulation of thymocyte differentiation: pre-TCR signals and β-selection. *Semin Immunol.* 2002;14:311–323.
92. Borowski C, Martin C, Gounari F, et al. On the brink of becoming a T cell. *Curr Opin Immunol.* 2002;14:200–206.
93. Kruisbeek AM, Haks MC, Carleton M, et al. Branching out to gain control: how the pre-TCR is linked to multiple functions. *Immunol Today.* 2000;21:637–644.
94. Voll RE, Jimi E, Phillips RJ, et al. NF-κB activation by the pre-T cell receptor serves as a selective survival signal in T lymphocyte development. *Immunity.* 2000;13:677–689.
95. Yamasaki S, Ishikawa E, Sakuma M, et al. Mechanistic basis of pre-T cell receptor-mediated autonomous signaling critical for thymocyte development. *Nat Immunol.* 2006;7:67–75.
96. Hayes SM, Shores EW, Love PE. An architectural perspective on signaling by the pre-, $\alpha\beta$ and $\gamma\delta$ T cell receptors. *Immunol Rev.* 2003;191:28–37.
97. Gärtner F, Alt FW, Monroe R, et al. Immature thymocytes employ distinct signaling pathways for allelic exclusion versus differentiation and expansion. *Immunity.* 1999;10:537–546.
98. Iritani BM, Alberola-Ila J, Forbush KA, et al. Distinct signals mediate maturation and allelic exclusion in lymphocyte progenitors. *Immunity.* 1999;10:713–722.
99. Hagenbeek TJ, Naspetti M, Malergue F, et al. The loss of PTEN allows TCR $\alpha\beta$ lineage thymocytes to bypass IL-7 and Pre-TCR-mediated signaling. *J Exp Med.* 2004;200:883–894.
100. Schmedt C, Tarakhovsky A. Autonomous maturation of α/β T lineage cells in the absence of COOH-terminal Src kinase (Csk). *J Exp Med.* 2001;193:815–826.
101. Lacorazza HD, Tucek-Szabo C, Vasovic LV, et al. Premature TCR$\alpha\beta$ expression and signaling in early thymocytes impair thymocyte expansion and partially block their development. *J Immunol.* 2001;166:3184–3193.
102. Borowski C, Li X, Aifantis I, et al. Pre-TCRα and TCRα are not interchangeable partners of TCRβ during T lymphocyte development. *J Exp Med.* 2004;199:607–615.
103. Greenbaum S, Zhuang Y. Regulation of early lymphocyte development by E2A family proteins. *Semin Immunol.* 2002;14: 405–414.
104. Xi H, Schwartz R, Engel I, et al. Interplay between RORγt, Egr3, and E proteins controls proliferation in response to pre-TCR signals. *Immunity.* 2006;24:813–826.
105. Xi H, Kersh GJ. Sustained early growth response gene 3 expression inhibits the survival of CD4/CD8 double-positive thymocytes. *J Immunol.* 2004;173:340–348.
106. Carleton M, Haks MC, Smeele SA, et al. Early growth response transcription factors are required for development of CD4$^-$CD8$^-$ thymocytes to the CD4$^+$CD8$^+$ stage. *J Immunol.* 2002;168:1649–1658.
107. Miyazaki T. Two distinct steps during thymocyte maturation from CD4$^-$CD8$^-$ to CD4$^+$CD8$^+$ distinguished in the Early Growth Response (Egr)-1 transgenic mice with a Recombinase-activating Gene-deficient background. *J Exp Med.* 1997;186:877–885.
108. Yu Q, Erman B, Park JH, et al. IL-7 receptor signals inhibit expression of transcription factors TCF-1, LEF-1, and RORγt: impact on thymocyte development. *J Exp Med.* 2004;200:797–803.
109. Mandal M, Borowski C, Palomero T, et al. The BCL2A1 gene as a pre-T cell receptor-induced regulator of thymocyte survival. *J Exp Med.* 2005;201:603–614.
110. Aifantis I, Gounari F, Scorrano L, et al. Constitutive pre-TCR signaling promotes differentiation through Ca^{2+} mobilization and activation of NF-κB and NFAT. *Nat Immunol.* 2001;2: 403–409.
111. Sun Z, Unutmaz D, Zou YR, et al. Requirement for RORγ in thymocyte survival and lymphoid organ development. *Science.* 2000;288:2369–2373.
112. He Y-W, Beers C, Deftos ML, et al. Down-regulation of the orphan nuclear receptor RORγt is essential for T lymphocyte maturation. *J Immunol.* 2000;164:5668–5674.
113. Villey I, de Chasseval R, de Villartay JP. RORγT, a thymus-specific isoform of the orphan nuclear receptor RORγ/TOR, is up-regulated by signaling through the pre-T cell receptor and binds to the TEA promoter. *Eur J Immunol.* 1999;29:4072–4080.
114. Kabra NH, Kang C, Hsing LC, et al. T cell-specific FADD-deficient mice: FADD is required for early T cell development. *Proc Natl Acad Sci U S A.* 2001;98:6307–6312.

115. Ferrero I, Mancini SJ, Grosjean F, et al. TCRγ silencing during $\alpha\beta$ T cell development depends upon pre-TCR-induced proliferation. *J Immunol.* 2006;177:6038–6043.
116. Yui MA, Sharp LL, Havran WL, et al. Preferential activation of an IL-2 regulatory sequence transgene in TCR$\gamma\delta$ and NKT cells: subset-specific differences in IL-2 regulation. *J Immunol.* 2004; 172:4691–4699.
117. Komori HK, Meehan TF, Havran WL. Epithelial and mucosal $\gamma\delta$ T cells. *Curr Opin Immunol.* 2006;18:534–538.
118. Wilson A, Capone M, MacDonald HR. Unexpectedly late expression of intracellular CD3ε and TCR $\gamma\delta$ proteins during adult thymus development. *Int Immunol.* 1999;11:1641–1650.
119. Prinz I, Sansoni A, Kissenpfennig A, et al. Visualization of the earliest steps of $\gamma\delta$ T cell development in the adult thymus. *Nat Immunol.* 2006;7:995–1003.
120. Haks MC, Lefebvre JM, Lauritsen JP, et al. Attenuation of $\gamma\delta$ TCR signaling efficiently diverts thymocytes to the $\alpha\beta$ lineage. *Immunity.* 2005;22:595–606.
121. Wilson A, MacDonald HR. A limited role for β-selection during $\gamma\delta$ T cell development. *J Immunol.* 1998;161:5851–5854.
122. Burtrum DB, Kim S, Dudley EC, et al. TCR gene recombination and $\alpha\beta$-$\gamma\delta$ lineage divergence: productive TCR-β rearrangement is neither exclusive nor preclusive of $\gamma\delta$ cell development. *J Immunol.* 1996;157:4293–4296.
123. Terrence K, Pavlovich CP, Matechak EO, et al. Premature expression of T cell receptor (TCR)$\alpha\beta$ suppresses TCR$\gamma\delta$ gene rearrangement but permits development of $\gamma\delta$ lineage T cells. *J Exp Med.* 2000;192:537–548.
124. Kang J, Coles M, Cado D, et al. The developmental fate of T cells is critically influenced by TCR$\gamma\delta$ expression. *Immunity.* 1998;8:427–438.
125. Bruno L, Fehling HJ, von Boehmer H. The $\alpha\beta$ T cell receptor can replace the $\gamma\delta$ receptor in the development of $\gamma\delta$ lineage cells. *Immunity.* 1996;5:343–352.
126. Yao Z, Cui Y, Watford WT, et al. Stat5a/b are essential for normal lymphoid development and differentiation. *Proc Natl Acad Sci U S A.* 2006;103:1000–1005.
127. Berg LJ, Kang J. Molecular determinants of TCR expression and selection. *Curr Opin Immunol.* 2001;13:232–241.
128. Schlissel MS, Durum SD, Muegge K. The interleukin 7 receptor is required for T cell receptor gamma locus accessibility to the V(D)J recombinase. *J Exp Med.* 2000;191:1045–1050.
129. Ye S-K, Maki K, Kitamura T, et al. Induction of germline transcription in the TCRγ locus by Stat5: implications for accessibility control by the IL-7 receptor. *Immunity.* 1999;11:213–223.
130. Kang J, Coles M, Raulet DH. Defective development of γ/δ T cells in interleukin 7 receptor- deficient mice is due to impaired expression of T cell receptor γ genes. *J Exp Med.* 1999;190:973–982.
131. Durum SK, Candéias S, Nakajima H, et al. Interleukin 7 receptor control of T cell receptor γ gene rearrangement: role of receptor-associated chains and locus accessibility. *J Exp Med.* 1998;188:2233–2241.
132. Moore TA, von Freeden-Jeffry U, Murray R, et al. Inhibition of $\gamma\delta$ T cell development and early thymocyte maturation in IL-7 $-/-$ mice. *J Immunol.* 1996;157:2366–2373.
133. Wilson A, Capone M, MacDonald HR. Unexpectedly late expression of intracellular CD3ε and TCR $\gamma\delta$ proteins during adult thymus development. *Int Immunol.* 1999;11:1641–1650.
134. Kang J, Volkmann A, Raulet DH. Evidence that $\gamma\delta$ versus $\alpha\beta$ T cell fate determination is initiated independently of T cell receptor signaling. *J Exp Med.* 2001;193:689–698.
135. Lee PP, Fitzpatrick DR, Beard C, et al. A critical role for Dnmt1 and DNA methylation in T cell development, function, and survival. *Immunity.* 2001;15:763–774.
136. Barndt RJ, Dai M, Zhuang Y. Functions of E2A-HEB heterodimers in T-cell development revealed by a dominant negative mutation of HEB. *Mol Cell Biol.* 2000;20:6677–6685.
137. Blom B, Heemskerk MHM, Verschuren MCM, et al. Disruption of $\alpha\beta$ but not of $\gamma\delta$ T cell development by overexpression of the helix-loop-helix protein Id3 in committed T cell progenitors. *EMBO J.* 1999;18:2793–2802.
138. Lauritsen JP, Haks MC, Lefebvre JM, et al. Recent insights into the signals that control $\alpha\beta/\gamma\delta$-lineage fate. *Immunol Rev.* 2006;209:176–190.
139. Pennington DJ, Silva-Santos B, Hayday AC. $\gamma\delta$ T cell development—having the strength to get there. *Curr Opin Immunol.* 2005;17:108–115.
140. Hayes SM, Li L, Love PE. TCR signal strength influences $\alpha\beta/\gamma\delta$ lineage fate. *Immunity.* 2005;22:583–593.
141. Choi JW, Pampeno C, Vukmanovic S, et al. Characterization of the transcriptional expression of Notch-1 signaling pathway members, Deltex and HES-1, in developing mouse thymocytes. *Dev Comp Immunol.* 2002;26:575–588.
142. Maillard I, Tu L, Sambandam A, et al. The requirement for Notch signaling at the β-selection checkpoint in vivo is absolute and independent of the pre-T cell receptor. *J Exp Med.* 2006;203:2239–2245.
143. Weng AP, Millholland JM, Yashiro-Ohtani Y, et al. c-Myc is an important direct target of Notch1 in T-cell acute lymphoblastic leukemia/lymphoma. *Genes Dev.* 2006;20:2096–2109.
144. Weng AP, Ferrando AA, Lee W, et al. Activating mutations of NOTCH1 in human T cell acute lymphoblastic leukemia. *Science.* 2004;306:269–271.
145. Screpanti I, Bellavia D, Campese AF, et al. Notch, a unifying target in T-cell acute lymphoblastic leukemia? *Trends Mol Med.* 2003;9:30–35.
146. Bender TP, Kremer CS, Kraus M, et al. Critical functions for c-Myb at three checkpoints during thymocyte development. *Nat Immunol.* 2004;5:721–729.
147. Pearson R, Weston K. c-Myb regulates the proliferation of immature thymocytes following β-selection. *EMBO J.* 2000;19:6112–6120.
148. Jacobs H, Krimpenfort P, Haks M, et al. PIM1 reconstitutes thymus cellularity in interleukin 7- and common γ chain-mutant mice and permits thymocyte maturation in Rag- but not CD3γ-deficient mice. *J Exp Med.* 1999;190:1059–1068.
149. Schmidt T, Karsunky H, Rodel B, et al. Evidence implicating Gfi-1 and Pim-1 in pre-T-cell differentiation steps associated with β-selection. *EMBO J.* 1998;17:5349–5359.
150. Azzam HS, DeJarnette JB, Huang K, et al. Fine tuning of TCR signaling by CD5. *J Immunol.* 2001;166:5464–5472.
151. Tarakhovsky A, Kanner SB, Hombach J, et al. A role for CD5 in TCR-mediated signal transduction and thymocyte selection. *Science.* 1995;269:535–537.
152. Urban JA, Winandy S. Ikaros null mice display defects in T cell selection and CD4 versus CD8 lineage decisions. *J Immunol.* 2004;173:4470–4478.
153. Starr TK, Daniels MA, Lucido MM, et al. Thymocyte sensitivity and supramolecular activation cluster formation are developmentally regulated: a partial role for sialylation. *J Immunol.* 2003;171:4512–4520.
154. Richie LI, Ebert PJ, Wu LC, et al. Imaging synapse formation during thymocyte selection: inability of CD3ζ to form a stable central accumulation during negative selection. *Immunity.* 2002;16:595–606.
155. Hailman E, Burack WR, Shaw AS, et al. Immature CD4$^+$CD8$^+$ thymocytes form a multifocal immunological synapse with sustained tyrosine phosphorylation. *Immunity.* 2002;16:839–848.
156. He Y-W, Deftos ML, Ojala EW, et al. RORγt, a novel isoform of an orphan receptor, negatively regulates Fas ligand expression and IL-2 production in T cells. *Immunity.* 1998;9:797–806.
157. Shores EW, Sharrow SO, Uppenkamp I, et al. T cell receptor-negative thymocytes from SCID mice can be induced to enter the CD4/CD8 differentiation pathway. *Eur J Immunol.* 1990;20:69–77.
158. van Ewijk W, Wang B, Hollander G, et al. Thymic microenvironments, 3-D versus 2-D? *Semin Immunol.* 1999;11:57–64.
159. Silva-Santos B, Pennington DJ, Hayday AC. Lymphotoxin-mediated regulation of $\gamma\delta$ cell differentiation by $\alpha\beta$ T cell progenitors. *Science.* 2005;307:925–928.
160. Visan I, Tan JB, Yuan JS, et al. Regulation of T lymphopoiesis by Notch1 and Lunatic fringe-mediated competition for intrathymic niches. *Nat Immunol.* 2006;7:634–643.
161. Koch U, Lacombe TA, Holland D, et al. Subversion of the T/B lineage decision in the thymus by lunatic fringe-mediated inhibition of Notch-1. *Immunity.* 2001;15:225–236.

162. Hicks C, Johnston SH, di Sibio G, et al. Fringe differentially modulates Jagged1 and Delta1 signalling through Notch1 and Notch2. *Nat Cell Biol.* 2000;2:515–520.
163. Baldwin TA, Hogquist KA, Jameson SC. The fourth way? Harnessing aggressive tendencies in the thymus. *J Immunol.* 2004;173:6515–6520.
164. Kronenberg M. Toward an understanding of NKT cell biology: progress and paradoxes. *Annu Rev Immunol.* 2005;23:877–900.
165. Gangadharan D, Lambolez F, Attinger A, et al. Identification of pre- and postselection TCR$\alpha\beta^+$ intraepithelial lymphocyte precursors in the thymus. *Immunity.* 2006;25:631–641.
166. Starr TK, Jameson SC, Hogquist KA. Positive and negative selection of T cells. *Annu Rev Immunol.* 2003;21:139–176.
167. Love PE, Chan AC. Regulation of thymocyte development: only the meek survive. *Curr Opin Immunol.* 2003;15:199–203.
168. Hogquist KA. Signal strength in thymic selection and lineage commitment. *Curr Opin Immunol.* 2001;13:225–231.
169. Sebzda E, Mariathasan S, Ohteki T, et al. Selection of the T cell repertoire. *Annu Rev Immunol.* 1999;17:829–874.
170. Anderson G, Partington KM, Jenkinson EJ. Differential effects of peptide diversity and stromal cell type in positive and negative selection in the thymus. *J Immunol.* 1998;161:6599–6603.
171. Ignatowicz L, Rees W, Pacholczyk R, et al. T cells can be activated by peptides that are unrelated in sequence to their selecting peptide. *Immunity.* 1997;7:179–186.
172. Zamoyska R, Lovatt M. Signalling in T-lymphocyte development: integration of signalling pathways is the key. *Curr Opin Immunol.* 2004;16:191–196.
173. Alberola-Ila J, Hernández-Hoyos G. The Ras/MAPK cascade and the control of positive selection. *Immunol Rev.* 2003;191:79–96.
174. Broussard C, Fleischecker C, Horai R, et al. Altered development of CD8+ T cell lineages in mice deficient for the Tec kinases Itk and Rlk. *Immunity.* 2006;25:93–104.
175. Delgado P, Fernandez E, Dave V, et al. CD3δ couples T-cell receptor signalling to ERK activation and thymocyte positive selection. *Nature.* 2000;406:426–430.
176. Werlen G, Hausmann B, Palmer E. A motif in the $\alpha\beta$ T-cell receptor controls positive selection by modulating ERK activity. *Nature.* 2000;406:422–426.
177. Neilson JR, Winslow MM, Hur EM, et al. Calcineurin B1 is essential for positive but not negative selection during thymocyte development. *Immunity.* 2004;20:255–266.
178. Costello PS, Nicolas RH, Watanabe Y, et al. Ternary complex factor SAP-1 is required for Erk-mediated thymocyte positive selection. *Nat Immunol.* 2004;5:289–298.
179. Bain G, Cravatt CB, Loomans C, et al. Regulation of the helix-loop-helix proteins, E2A and Id3, by the Ras-ERK MAPK cascade. *Nat Immunol.* 2001;2:165–171.
180. Krangel MS, Carabana J, Abbarategui I, et al. Enforcing order within a complex locus: current perspectives on the control of V(D)J recombination at the murine T-cell receptor alpha/delta locus. *Immunol Rev.* 2004;200:224–232.
181. Takahama Y. Journey through the thymus: stromal guides for T-cell development and selection. *Nat Rev Immunol.* 2006;6:127–135.
182. Rosen H, Goetzl EJ. Sphingosine 1-phosphate and its receptors: an autocrine and paracrine network. *Nat Rev Immunol.* 2005;5:560–570.
183. Yasutomo K, Lucas B, Germain RN. TCR signaling for initiation and completion of thymocyte positive selection has distinct requirements for ligand quality and presenting cell type. *J Immunol.* 2000;165:3015–3022.
184. Wilkinson RW, Anderson G, Owen JJ, et al. Positive selection of thymocytes involves sustained interactions with the thymic microenvironment. *J Immunol.* 1995;155:5234–5240.
185. Liu X, Adams A, Wildt KF, et al. Restricting Zap70 expression to $CD4^+CD8^+$ thymocytes reveals a T cell receptor-dependent proofreading mechanism controlling the completion of positive selection. *J Exp Med.* 2003;197:363–373.
186. Singer A. New perspectives on a developmental dilemma: the kinetic signaling model and the importance of signal duration for the CD4/CD8 lineage decision. *Curr Opin Immunol.* 2002;14:207–215.
187. von Boehmer H. T-cell lineage fate: instructed by receptor signals? *Curr Biol.* 2000;10:R642–R645.
188. Basson MA, Zamoyska R. The CD4/CD8 lineage decision: integration of signalling pathways. *Immunol Today.* 2000;21:509–514.
189. Chan S, Correia-Neves M, Benoist C, et al. CD4/CD8 lineage commitment: matching fate with competence. *Immunol Rev.* 1998;165:195–207.
190. Robey EA, Fowlkes BJ, Gordon JW, et al. Thymic selection in CD8 transgenic mice supports an instructive model for commitment to a CD4 or CD8 lineage. *Cell.* 1991;64:99–107.
191. Robey E, Chang D, Itano A, et al. An activated form of Notch influences the choice between CD4 and CD8 T cell lineages. *Cell.* 1996;87:483–492.
192. Laky K, Fleischacker C, Fowlkes BJ. TCR and Notch signaling in CD4 and CD8 T-cell development. *Immunol Rev.* 2006;209:274–283.
193. Kioussis D, Ellmeier W. Chromatin and *CD4*, *CD8A* and *CD8B* gene expression during thymic differentiation. *Nat Rev Immunol.* 2002;2:909–919.
194. Hernandez-Hoyos G, Sohn SJ, Rothenberg EV, et al. Lck activity controls CD4/CD8 T cell lineage commitment. *Immunity.* 2000;12:313–322.
195. Fischer AM, Katayama CD, Pages G, et al. The role of erk1 and erk2 in multiple stages of T cell development. *Immunity.* 2005;23:431–443.
196. Adachi S, Iwata M. Duration of calcineurin and Erk signals regulates CD4/CD8 lineage commitment of thymocytes. *Cell Immunol.* 2002;215:45–53.
197. Yasutomo K, Doyle C, Miele L, et al. The duration of antigen receptor signalling determines $CD4^+$ versus $CD8^+$ T-cell lineage fate. *Nature.* 2000;404:506–510.
198. Liu X, Bosselut R. Duration of TCR signaling controls CD4-CD8 lineage differentiation in vivo. *Nat Immunol.* 2004;5:280–288.
199. Sato T, Ohno S, Hayashi T, et al. Dual functions of Runx proteins for reactivating CD8 and silencing CD4 at the commitment process into CD8 thymocytes. *Immunity.* 2005;22:317–328.
200. Sarafova SD, Erman B, Yu Q, et al. Modulation of coreceptor transcription during positive selection dictates lineage fate independently of TCR/coreceptor specificity. *Immunity.* 2005;23:75–87.
201. He X, He X, Dave VP, et al. The zinc finger transcription factor Th-POK regulates CD4 versus CD8 T-cell lineage commitment. *Nature.* 2005;433:826–833.
202. Sun G, Liu X, Mercado P, et al. The zinc finger protein cKrox directs CD4 lineage differentiation during intrathymic T cell positive selection. *Nat Immunol.* 2005;6:373–381.
203. Aliahmad P, Kaye J. Commitment issues: linking positive selection signals and lineage diversification in the thymus. *Immunol Rev.* 2006;209:253–273.
204. Hernández-Hoyos G, Anderson MK, Wang C, et al. J. GATA-3 expression is controlled by TCR signals and regulates CD4/CD8 differentiation. *Immunity.* 2003;19:83–94.
205. Keefe R, Dave V, Allman D, et al. Regulation of lineage commitment distinct from positive selection. *Science.* 1999;286:1149–1153.
206. Liu X, Taylor BJ, Sun G, et al. Analyzing expression of perforin, Runx3, and Thpok genes during positive selection reveals activation of CD8-differentiation programs by MHC II-signaled thymocytes. *J Immunol.* 2005;175:4465–4474.
207. Pai SY, Truitt ML, Ting CN, et al. Critical roles for transcription factor GATA-3 in thymocyte development. *Immunity.* 2003;19:863–875.
208. Aliahmad P, O'Flaherty E, Han P, et al. TOX provides a link between calcineurin activation and CD8 lineage commitment. *J Exp Med.* 2004;199:1089–1099.
209. Harker N, Naito T, Cortes M, et al. The CD8α gene locus is regulated by the Ikaros family of proteins. *Mol Cell.* 2002;10:1403–1415.
210. Taniuchi I, Osato M, Egawa T, et al. Differential requirements for Runx proteins in *CD4* repression and epigenetic silencing during T lymphocyte development. *Cell.* 2002;111:621–633.
211. Kohu K, Sato T, Ohno S, et al. Overexpression of the Runx3 transcription factor increases the proportion of mature thymocytes of the CD8 single-positive lineage. *J Immunol.* 2005;174:2627–2636.
212. Grueter B, Petter M, Egawa T, et al. Runx3 regulates Integrin αE/CD103 and CD4 expression during development of $CD4^-/CD8^+$ T cells. *J Immunol.* 2005;175:1694–1705.

213. Kappler JW, Roehm N, Marrack P. T cell tolerance by clonal elimination in the thymus. *Cell.* 1987;49:273–280.
214. Palmer E. Negative selection–clearing out the bad apples from the T-cell repertoire. *Nat Rev Immunol.* 2003;3:383–391.
215. Hogquist KA, Baldwin TA, Jameson SC. Central tolerance: learning self-control in the thymus. *Nat Rev Immunol.* 2005;5:772–782.
216. von Boehmer H, Kisielow P. Negative selection of the T-cell repertoire: where and when does it occur? *Immunol Rev.* 2006;209:284–289.
217. Baldwin TA, Sandau MM, Jameson SC, et al. The timing of TCRα expression critically influences T cell development and selection. *J Exp Med.* 2005;202:111–121.
218. Kurobe H, Liu C, Ueno T, et al. CCR7-dependent cortex-to-medulla migration of positively selected thymocytes is essential for establishing central tolerance. *Immunity.* 2006;24:165–177.
219. Nagamine K, Peterson P, Scott HS, et al. Positional cloning of the APECED gene. *Nat Genet.* 1997;17:393–398.
220. Anderson MS, Venanzi ES, Klein L, et al. Projection of an immunological self shadow within the thymus by the Aire protein. *Science.* 2002;298:1395–1401.
221. Liston A, Lesage S, Wilson J, et al. Aire regulates negative selection of organ-specific T cells. *Nat Immunol.* 2003;4:350–354.
222. Villasenor J, Benoist C, Mathis D. AIRE and APECED: molecular insights into an autoimmune disease. *Immunol Rev.* 2005;204:156–164.
223. Kyewski B, Klein L. A central role for central tolerance. *Annu Rev Immunol.* 2006;24:571–606.
224. Kuroda N, Mitani T, Takeda N, et al. Development of autoimmunity against transcriptionally unrepressed target antigen in the thymus of Aire-deficient mice. *J Immunol.* 2005;174:1862–1870.
225. Anderson MS, Venanzi ES, Chen Z, et al. The cellular mechanism of Aire control of T cell tolerance. *Immunity.* 2005;23:227–239.
226. Gallegos AM, Bevan MJ. Central tolerance to tissue-specific antigens mediated by direct and indirect antigen presentation. *J Exp Med.* 2004;200:1039–1049.
227. Bonasio R, Scimone ML, Schaerli P, et al. Clonal deletion of thymocytes by circulating dendritic cells homing to the thymus. *Nat Immunol.* 2006;7:1092–1100.
228. Punt JA, Osborne BA, Takahama Y, et al. Negative selection of CD4+CD8+ thymocytes by T cell receptor-induced apoptosis requires a costimulatory signal that can be provided by CD28. *J Exp Med.* 1994;179:709–713.
229. Bouillet P, Purton JF, Godfrey DI, et al. BH3-only Bcl-2 family member Bim is required for apoptosis of autoreactive thymocytes. *Nature.* 2002;415:922–926.
230. Rathmell JC, Lindsten T, Zong WX, et al. Deficiency in Bak and Bax perturbs thymic selection and lymphoid homeostasis. *Nat Immunol.* 2002;3:932–939.
231. Calnan BJ, Szychowski S, Chan FKM, et al. A role for the orphan steroid receptor Nur77 in apoptosis accompanying antigen-induced negative selection. *Immunity.* 1995;3:273–282.
232. McCarty N, Paust S, Ikizawa K, et al. Signaling by the kinase MINK is essential in the negative selection of autoreactive thymocytes. *Nat Immunol.* 2005;6:65–72.
233. Daniels MA, Teixeiro E, Gill J, et al. Thymic selection threshold defined by compartmentalization of Ras/MAPK signalling. *Nature.* 2006; 444:724–729.
234. Sakaguchi S. Naturally arising Foxp3-expressing CD25+CD4+ regulatory T cells in immunological tolerance to self and non-self. *Nat Immunol.* 2005;6:345–352.
235. Kim JM, Rudensky A. The role of the transcription factor Foxp3 in the development of regulatory T cells. *Immunol Rev.* 2006;212:86–98.
236. Fontenot JD, Gavin MA, Rudensky AY. Foxp3 programs the development and function of $CD4^+CD25^+$ regulatory T cells. *Nat Immunol.* 2003;4:330–336.
237. Wildin RS, Freitas A. IPEX and FOXP3: clinical and research perspectives. *J Autoimmun.* 2005;25 Suppl:56–62.
238. Nishizuka Y, Sakakura T. Thymus and reproduction: sex-linked dysgenesia of the gonad after neonatal thymectomy in mice. *Science.* 1969;166:753–755.
239. Asano M, Toda M, Sakaguchi N, et al. Autoimmune disease as a consequence of developmental abnormality of a T cell subpopulation. *J Exp Med.* 1996;184:387–396.
240. Fontenot JD, Rasmussen JP, Williams LM, et al. Regulatory T cell lineage specification by the forkhead transcription factor Foxp3. *Immunity.* 2005;22:329–341.
241. Itoh M, Takahashi T, Sakaguchi N, et al. Thymus and autoimmunity: production of $CD25^+CD4^+$ naturally anergic and suppressive T cells as a key function of the thymus in maintaining immunologic self-tolerance. *J Immunol.* 1999;162:5317–5326.
242. Apostolou I, Sarukhan A, Klein L, et al. Origin of regulatory T cells with known specificity for antigen. *Nat Immunol.* 2002;3:756–763.
243. Picca CC, Larkin J, III, Boesteanu A, et al. Role of TCR specificity in CD4+ CD25+ regulatory T-cell selection. *Immunol Rev.* 2006;212:74–85.
244. Picca CC, Caton AJ. The role of self-peptides in the development of CD4+ CD25+ regulatory T cells. *Curr Opin Immunol.* 2005;17:131–136.
245. Caton AJ, Cozzo C, Larkin J, III, et al. CD4+ CD25+ regulatory T cell selection. *Ann NY Acad Sci.* 2004;1029:101–114.
246. Hsieh CS, Zheng Y, Liang Y, et al. An intersection between the self-reactive regulatory and nonregulatory T cell receptor repertoires. *Nat Immunol.* 2006;7:401–410.
247. van Santen HM, Benoist C, Mathis D. Number of T_{reg} cells that differentiate does not increase upon encounter of agonist ligand on thymic epithelial cells. *J Exp Med.* 2004;200:1221–1230.
247a. Liston A, Rudensky AY. Thymic development and peripheral homeostasis of regulatory T cells. *Curr Opin Immunol.* 2007;19:179–185.
248. Salomon B, Lenschow DJ, Rhee L, et al. B7/CD28 costimulation is essential for the homeostasis of the CD4+CD25+ immunoregulatory T cells that control autoimmune diabetes. *Immunity.* 2000; 12:431–440.
249. Tai X, Cowan M, Feigenbaum L, et al. CD28 costimulation of developing thymocytes induces Foxp3 expression and regulatory T cell differentiation independently of interleukin 2. *Nat Immunol.* 2005;6:152–162.
250. Bosco N, Agenes F, Rolink AG, et al. Peripheral T cell lymphopenia and concomitant enrichment in naturally arising regulatory T cells: the case of the pre-Tα gene-deleted mouse. *J Immunol.* 2006;177:5014–5023.
251. Pennington DJ, Silva-Santos B, Silberzahn T, et al. Early events in the thymus affect the balance of effector and regulatory T cells. *Nature.* 2006;444:1073–1077.
252. Blom B, Spits H. Development of human lymphoid cells. *Annu Rev Immunol.* 2006;24:287–320.
253. Ciofani M, Schmitt TM, Ciofani A, et al. Obligatory role for cooperative signaling by pre-TCR and Notch during thymocyte differentiation. *J Immunol.* 2004;172:5230–5239.

Chapter 13

Peripheral T Lymphocyte Responses and Function

Steven L. Reiner

INTRODUCTION

After a thymus-derived T lymphocyte enters the peripheral circulation, it constantly, albeit indirectly, samples the body for evidence of its cognate foreign antigen via encounters with dendritic cells (DCs) in secondary lymphoid organs. Once activated in secondary lymphoid organs, a naïve T cell undergoes a regulated process of division and differentiation, leading to alterations in gene expression of its migrating progeny, allowing them to mediate the functional properties associated with T cell–dependent immunity at sites of infection and inflammation. After an immune response has ended, a system for preserving the T cell with useful antigen specificity is hard-wired into the differentiation process, leaving behind a remnant of memory T cells. This chapter will provide an overview of the milestones in the lives of T cells as they function in anticipation of, during, and after an immune response.

THE FUNCTIONAL IMPLICATIONS OF T CELL DEVELOPMENT

Prior to their entry into the thymus, progenitors of the T cell lineage develop in the bone marrow. T cells are born in the thymus, which together with the bone marrow, are considered the primary lymphoid organs. After expression of α-β T cell antigen receptors and coexpression of CD4 and CD8, so-called *double positive thymocytes* undergo a matchmaking process to determine their suitability for specific functions in the periphery. Among the first major criteria being assessed is whether the T cell receptor is of too high an affinity for self-peptide/major histocompatibility complex (MHC). Such cells should undergo negative selection through trigger of T cell receptor (TCR) signaling–dependent apoptosis. To ensure that self-peptides are adequately foreshadowed in the restricted confines of the thymus, the putative transcription factor *Aire* mediates expression of numerous nonthymic genes in thymic medullary epithelial cells (1). Thymocytes that sample their way through hematopoietic-derived DCs and this "self-shadow" on epithelial cells are thereby screened for virtual whole-body reactivity (2). Mutation of *Aire* results in the autoimmune polyendocrinopathy candidiasis ectodermal dystrophy (APECED) syndrome (1,3).

Cells that seem to fall just short of the critical threshold for negative selection but are in some ways still self-reactive undergo an unusual differentiation process to become natural regulatory T (Treg) cells (4). This likely occurs in the thymic medulla when DCs receive a signal from epithelial cells expressing thymic stromal lymphopoietin (5). The differentiation of Treg cells involves induction of the forkhead transcription factor, FoxP3, which specifically marks and specifies the major attributes of the Treg lineage (6–9). Natural Treg cells do not undergo typical antigen-induced proliferation and effector differentiation; their behavior, instead, is likened to an anergic state (10). These cells are far from functionless, however, as they mediate critical inhibitory activity of other autoreactive T cells and, potentially, of T cells engaged in immune responses against pathogens. Their mode of suppression or inhibition is not fully understood but may involve actions directly on T cells or indirectly through antigen-presenting cells. Mutation of FoxP3 results in immune dysregulation, polyendocrinopathy, enteropathy, X-linked (IPEX) syndrome (11).

Double-positive thymocytes with a TCR of too weak an affinity to have signaling engaged by self-peptide–MHC will subsequently die from this neglect. In contrast, thymocytes with a TCR of a suitably weak affinity to have some (but not too much) signaling elicited by self-peptide–MHC undergo positive selection, their licensure for eventual export to the peripheral lymphoid system. In general, thymocytes with TCRs recognizing self-peptide–MHC class I become $CD8^+$ ($CD4^-$) single positive thymocytes and then naïve $CD8^+$ (or cytotoxic) T cells when they exit the thymus and populate the periphery. Thymocytes with TCRs recognizing self-peptide–MHC class II become $CD4^+$ ($CD8^-$) single positive thymocytes and then naïve $CD4^+$ (or helper) T cells when they exit the thymus and populate the periphery.

Expressing CD4 versus CD8 has significant functional bearing on helper and cytotoxic T cell function, respectively. Nonetheless, these coreceptors are not sufficient to specify all of the attributes specific to helper or cytotoxic T cells. How coreceptor (CD4 versus CD8) and lineage (helper versus cytotoxic) choices could be coupled has been a central enigma of T lymphocyte development and function (12,13). Recently, there has been increasing evidence that a key transcriptional regulator can coordinately activate and silence one coreceptor versus the other while also imparting essential differences on the helper versus cytotoxic potential of the single positive thymocyte (14,15). In developing $CD4^+$ thymocytes, ThPOK is necessary for *Cd4* gene expression, induction of several molecules that are helper T cell–specific, including Gata3, a transcriptional activator implicated in $CD4^+$ T cell positive selection and function. In addition, ThPOK can repress *Cd8* gene expression and inhibit other essential aspects of the cytotoxic lineage. More information about this can be found in the chapter Development of T Cells.

The discovery that a single factor can coerce developing thymocytes to adopt the helper fate and abandon the cytotoxic fate provides a satisfying mechanism for coupling coreceptor and lineage choice. It also raises some new questions about the evolution of effector diversity in adaptive immunity. Whether this means that the cytotoxic T cell lineage is a more ancestral lineage or more of the default pathway of thymic development than the helper T cell lineage is uncertain. In terms of peripheral functions, however, a $CD8^+$ T cell bears closer resemblance to a natural killer (NK) cell than does a $CD4^+$ T cell (16).

NAÏVE T CELLS

Transitioning to the Periphery: New Place, New Name

After positive selection, mature single positive thymocytes are licensed to leave the thymus and dwell in secondary lymphoid tissues. An essential signaling pathway for thymic exit, or egress, to the periphery involves sphingosine 1-phosphate receptor-1 (S1P1), which will also turn out to be dually critical for the ability of peripheral T cells to leave lymph nodes (17). The transcriptional regulator KLF2 is likely to be an essential activator of this receptor (18). The secondary (or peripheral) lymphoid tissues include the spleen, lymph nodes, and mucosal-associated lymphoid tissues (gut and bronchial, among the best studied). Gut-associated lymphoid tissues include Peyer's patches and other organs such as tonsils and adenoids. Their detailed anatomy is covered in the chapter on lymphoid tissues and organs.

After its birth and export from the thymus, what was once the most mature of thymocytes from the perspective of the primary lymphoid organs (a single positive $CD4^+$ or $CD8^+$ cell) is now considered to be the most immature lineage from the perspective of the secondary lymphoid organs and T cell functioning. The nomenclature for the continued T cell development that occurs during peripheral function is, however, slightly different than the terminology of thymopoiesis. Instead of calling a nascent peripheral T cell immature, it is referred to as a naïve CD4$^+$ or CD8$^+$ T cell, the operative term designating that the T cell has yet to encounter antigenic foreign peptide/MHC ligands. After being engaged by antigenic foreign peptide–MHC ligands, naïve T cells are then considered to be antigen-experienced. Antigen experience, however, represents a considerable variety of maturational states and fates including, but not limited to, acutely activated but not fully differentiated, abortively differentiated (or anergic) and fully differentiated effector and memory cells. The distinctions between these conditions will be discussed later in this chapter.

How Naïve T Cells Live

Naïve T cells have often been described as "resting," owing to the fact that they are not actively dividing. A naïve T cell that has not yet been activated by antigen is, however, far from physically inactive (Figure 13.1). Instead, naïve T cells undergo a relentless process of migration through blood, entry into lymph node, extensive sampling of self-peptide/MHC, exit through lymph, return to blood, and re-entry into another lymph node that repeats incessantly for many months—this is the lifespan of naïve cells (19–21). Among the concerns in life of a bona fide naïve T cell that is suited to undergo an immune response are survival, migration, and surveillance. These essential processes are geographically united by secondary lymphoid

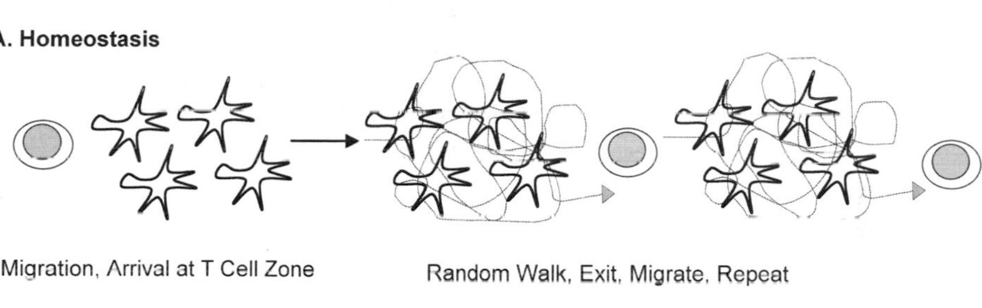

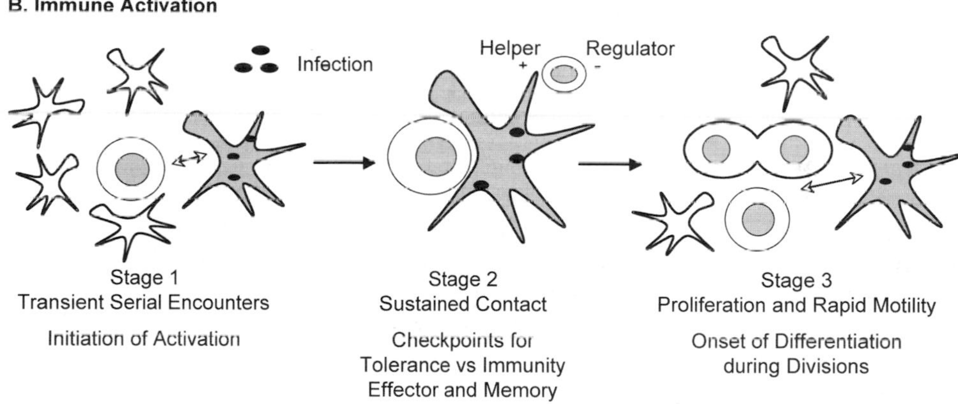

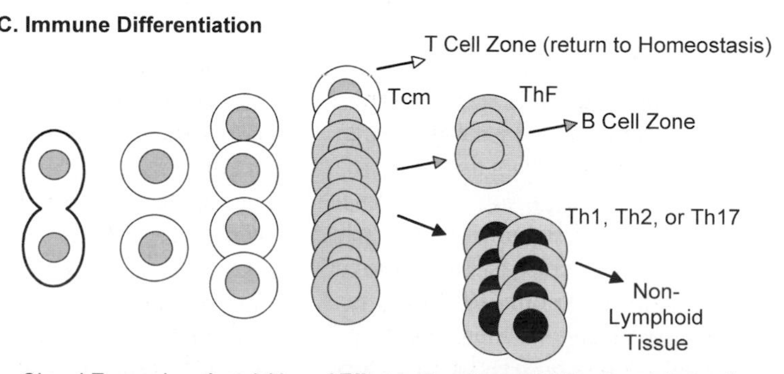

FIGURE 13.1 T cells during homeostasis and immunity. **A:** A naïve T cell circulating through the blood enters a secondary lymphoid tissue and quickly arrives at the T cell–rich zone. It undergoes random migration through the T cell zone for many hours. After exiting the lymph node, it reenters the circulation briefly before arriving at another lymph node and repeating the process. The lengthy stopovers in secondary lymphoid tissue provide survival signals for the long-lived, nondividing cell. **B:** Upon encounter with foreign pathogen-associated antigen, random motion changes to purposeful but brief contacts with DCs during the first several hours, followed by sustained contact lasting for hours, followed by the first cell division and resumption of brief encounters. During the second stage, sustained contact is augmented by several factors, including inflammatory signaling received by the DC and, for CD8$^+$ T cells, the presence of CD4$^+$ T cells. The presence of Treg cells, conversely, limits the degree of sustained contact for newly activated CD4$^+$ T cells. Correlates to immunity emerging from these variations suggest that the sustained contact is a key checkpoint in the activation process. **C:** After the first division, still in the secondary lymphoid tissue, further division coincides with acquisition of new effector (or memory) potency and migratory instructions, for relocating to other zones in the lymph node or nonlymphoid tissue.

organs, which contain attractants to lure T cell entry, survival signals to license their nourishment, and the relevant display of peptide/MHC complexes that would reflect the likelihood (or not) that foreign invaders are violating innate defense mechanisms (22,23).

Naïve T cells arrive at each surveillance stopover in a secondary lymphoid organ via the bloodstream (22). In the case of lymph nodes and Peyer's patches, the high endothelial venules (HEVs), which are specialized blood vessels, serve as the nidus of attraction for the T cell to enter the tissue. HEVs express a unique set of ligands that interact with the receptors characteristic of naïve T cells. Among the most critical attractant molecules on HEVs are the chemokine CCL21 that engages CCR7 and vascular addressins that engage CD62L, or L selectin. From a functional perspective, the expression of high levels of CCR7 and CD62L are important T cell markers used to identify populations such as naïve cells, newly activated cells that have not yet been licensed for tissue migration, and a subset of memory cells with migration patterns similar to naïve cells, with preference for secondary lymphoid organs. Extravasation of the naïve lymphocyte through HEVs relies on intercellular adhesion molecules (ICAMs) that engage the integrin LFA-1. Entry into the spleen differs from entry into lymph node and mucosal lymphoid tissue. Naïve T cells enter the spleen through terminal arterioles, not HEVs, and this does not require CD62L. Subsequent migration to the white pulp, however, does require integrins and chemokine receptor signaling.

Secondary lymphoid organs are composed of distinct zones enriched with T or B lymphocytes (22). In the lymph node, the paracortical T cell zone contains T cells and the critical supplier of peptide/MHC complexes, DCs. By virtue of their location, migration, and function, DCs are assumed to be a specialized cell that exists to supply the demands of T cells and ensure that they remain quiescent during homeostasis or alert and educate T cells during an attack. In the spleen, T cells and DCs primarily reside in the periarteriolar lymphoid sheath (PALS) within the white pulp. Once inside the secondary lymphoid organs, naïve T cells are lured and retained in the T cell–rich zones by CCL21 and CCL19 produced by stromal cells, which signal to CCR7 on naïve T cells. DCs also express CCR7, thereby insuring colocalization of T cells and DCs in these tissues. Naïve T cells dwell in the T cell–rich zones for several hours before exiting the secondary lymphoid organs (Figure 13.1).

Coupling Survival and Surveillance

Within the T cell–rich zones of secondary lymphoid organs, naïve T cells gain access to the ligands of their antigen receptor, peptide/MHC complexes, presented primarily on the surface of resident or newly arrived DCs. For a naïve T cell that does not encounter antigenic foreign peptide/MHC complexes, it receives critical survival signals from self-peptide/MHC complexes (24–27). In addition to a survival signal, this periodic engagement of the TCR may offer refinement or validation of the suitability of the TCR for eventual antigenic peptide/MHC engagement. It is thought that naïve $CD8^+$ T cells may show greater dependence than naïve $CD4^+$ T cells for continual low-level, or "tonic," signaling through the TCR. Nonetheless, the long life span of nondividing naïve T cells of both subsets is dependent on receipt of the peptide/MHC signal.

The other major survival signal for both subsets of naïve T cells is IL-7 (28–33). Although it has not been well visualized, it is presumed that IL-7 will also be accessed in the secondary lymphoid organs, probably expressed by stromal cells, analogous to its provision in the primary lymphoid organs. Loss of IL-7 signaling results in fairly rapid disappearance of naïve T cells. Although deprivation of cytokine and TCR signals impairs survival of naïve T cells, it is probably not the only reason these signals are embedded in the T cell zones. Without them, T cells also undergo atrophy, decreased metabolic activity, and become sluggish in response to proliferative signals (28,29). Secondary lymphoid tissues, thus, seem to provide the necessary cues to elicit T cell entry, survival, and health while focusing the attention of T cells in the event of an invading pathogen.

Because T cells and secondary lymphoid tissue evolved for host defense, their major function could be thought of as surveillance and reaction against pathogens. This is accomplished by continuous scanning of the peptide/MHC complexes on DCs and the intrinsic capacity to rapidly mobilize growth and proliferation when antigenic foreign peptide/MHC is encountered (34). It can thus be imagined that T cells, as they are tending to their most primitive need of finding trophic signals to license their metabolism and survival, have their functioning thrust upon them. This conveniently occurs by virtue of the fact that secondary lymphoid tissues not only provide survival signals but also antigenic foreign peptides/MHC complexes.

When Not Encountering Pathogen

Our understanding of the time spent in the T cell zone of secondary lymphoid tissues is getting progressively more detailed, in large part owing to technical advances in fluorescence microscopic imaging of *in vivo* or *ex vivo* tissues (19,35–43). Naïve T cells move rapidly (12 micrometers/minute) through the T cell zone in a pattern termed *random walk*. It is estimated that hundreds ($CD8^+$) to thousands ($CD4^+$) of naïve T cells can interact with a single DC in an hour (Figure 13.1). After thoroughly sampling DCs for several hours without encountering antigen, naïve T cells exit the lymph node through the efferent lymphatic vessels and then return to the bloodstream via the thoracic duct. Exit from the spleen probably occurs through migration from white pulp to red pulp and entry into venous sinuses then bloodstream. Naïve T cells will only spend short intervals in the blood before rapidly finding a new secondary lymphoid organ to enter, repeating the cycle of migration and surveillance, then exiting.

Exit from the secondary lymphoid tissues, like exit from the thymus, is dependent on signaling through the S1P1 on T cells (22,44). The ligand, sphingosine 1-phosphate, is found in high concentrations in plasma and lymph. A working model for egress from secondary lymphoid tissue, therefore, entails that an S1P gradient at exit vessels of the secondary lymphoid tissues counterbalances the chemokine gradients that retain naïve T cells as they move through the T cell zones. In the event that the T cell does encounter foreign antigen, as will be discussed later, the egress process must be temporarily dampened in favor of prolonged retention in secondary lymphoid tissues (45).

T CELLS IN THE IMMUNE RESPONSE

When Encountering Pathogen

Secondary lymphoid tissues are the focal point of an adaptive immune response because they unite anticipatory naïve lymphocytes with the arrival of foreign antigens (46). At least two routes exist to bring antigen to secondary lymphoid organs (47). Free antigen can travel by blood to the spleen, or by lymph via the afferent lymphatic vessels to lymph nodes. Productive foreign peptide/MHC complexes on resident DCs can form in the lymph node by this soluble route of antigen delivery within a few hours of antigen injection into tissue and quickly result in the initial T cell activation to jumpstart an immune response.

More slowly, from several hours to a few days, antigen-bearing, CCR7-expressing DCs will migrate from infected tissues through the lymphatic vessels in a CCL21-dependent process (47). This wave of antigen presentation may be important for sustaining responses, because CD4^{+} T cells may need extended antigen presentation for effective expansion and differentiation (48,49). Generally, DCs resident in nonlymphoid tissue will undergo maturation and migrate to lymph nodes because of pathogen-associated inflammatory signals (22,47,50). In addition to influx of antigen-bearing DCs from tissues, resident DCs and macrophages can also rearrange locations within secondary lymphoid tissues in response to inflammation (22). The ontogeny, activation, maturation, migration, and functioning of myeloid, lymphoid, plasmacytoid, and follicular DCs can be found in earlier chapters. This chapter will, instead, focus on the immune response from the perspective of the T cell as it encounters a mature DC in the lymph node.

If a pathogen breaches the innate defense mechanisms, this will result in inflammatory signaling to DCs in the form of a combinatorial variety of pathogen- and host-associated ligands. Pathogen-associated ligands interact with intracellular and extracellular Toll-like receptors and other classes of intracellular (NOD) and extracellular (C-type lectin) pattern recognition receptors on DCs that will be discussed in detail in the chapter covering innate immunity. Together pathogen-associated signals refine the gene expression pattern of the activated DCs. Depending on the type of pathogen that is encountered, the DC provides quantitatively and qualitatively distinct soluble and membrane-bound signals to the newly activated T cell (34,51–54). The specific ligands that are made by DCs to inform T cells of each class of pathogens are not yet fully understood, but are an area of active investigation.

Host cells, especially innate immune cells such as macrophages or the initially activated T cells themselves, will provide other critical signals for DCs that contribute to the ability to successfully trigger a T cell–mediated immune response. TNF-α and IL-1 made by a neighboring parasitized macrophage or IFN-γ and CD40L expressed by a recently activated T cell will contribute to the ability of a mature DC to support productive clonal expansion and differentiation of the antigen-specific T cells. Pathogen and host-associated signaling to the DC contribute to its stabilized expression of foreign peptide/MHC complexes and induction of CD80, CD86 (the ligands for CD28), and other so-called *costimulatory* molecules (34).

The net effect of infection is to load the DC with novel peptide/MHC complexes, which by virtue of being foreign, should be bound by one of the many anticipatory TCRs with high affinity (54). Inflammation from infection allows DCs to simultaneously deliver abundant ligation of CD28, which together with sufficient foreign peptide/MHC initiates mitogenic signaling in the naïve T cell, triggering a clonal burst of division. Mature DCs must, therefore, provide sufficient amount of proliferative information (through peptide/MHC and costimulatory ligands) to kick-start the division of naïve T cells. But mature DCs must also convey, through a set of specific signals that may involve a combinatorial code (costimulatory receptors, cytokines, Notch ligands), information about the class of invading pathogen to the newly activated T cell (53). During an immune challenge, DCs alert T cells about the presence of infection and the type of pathogen. The latter information is especially useful to helper T cells that have several fates they can adopt during immune response differentiation, each of them well-suited to orchestrate elimination of different classes of pathogens (Figure 13.2).

Dynamic T Cell–DC Interactions During Immune Response

Activation of a naïve T cell during the immune response involves physical contact between the T cell and a mature DC presenting specific foreign peptide/MHC complex. When T cells are activated *in vitro* they undergo a

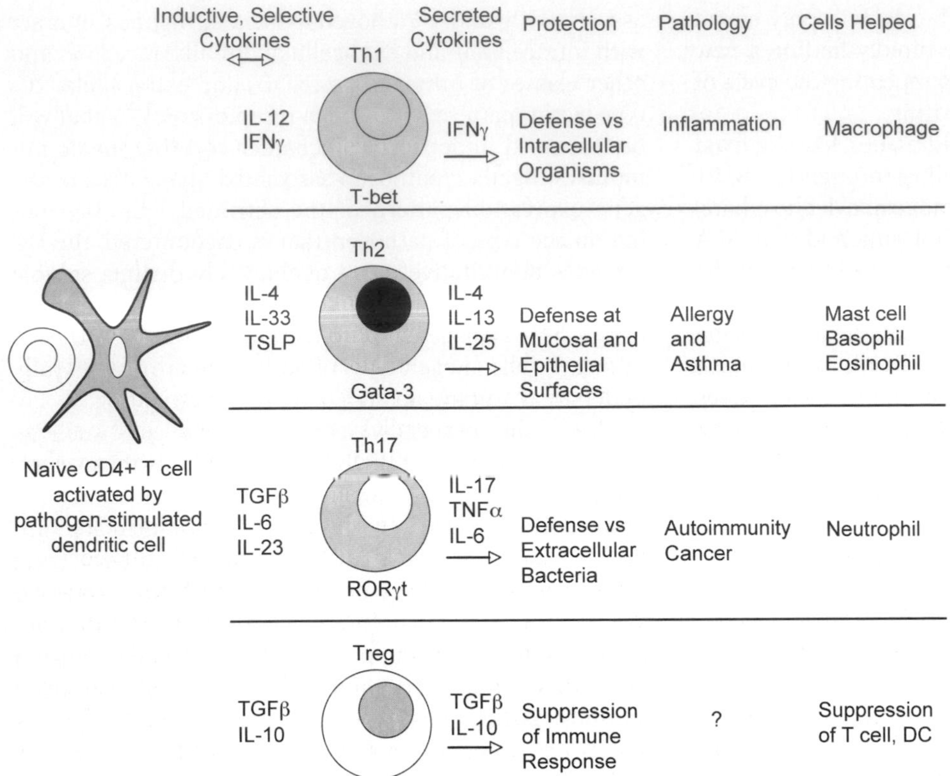

FIGURE 13.2 Lineage choices of effector CD4+ T cells. The progeny of antigen experienced CD4+ T cells exposed to specific pathogen-associated signals, especially cytokines (listed), can develop into Th1, Th2, and Th17 effector cells that can migrate to tissue. Hypothetically, some may become adaptive Treg cells and exert intraclonal control over the magnitude of the response. Some effector cells will develop into follicle-homing helpers of B cells ThF cells, probable variants of Th1, Th2, or Th17 (not shown). The critical transcription factor directing lineage commitment of each subset is listed below the cell. Roles in host defense, pathological processes, and mobilization of other cell types are listed.

signature reorganization during this attachment, which has been called the *immunological synapse* (55). The immunological synapse will be discussed in greater detail in the chapter on T cell signal transduction. The stereotyped features of the immunologic synapse are a cluster of T cell signaling molecules (including TCR, CD28) encircled by adhesion molecules (LFA-1) at the site of contact with an antigen-bearing cell. In addition, chemokine and cytokine receptors have also been shown to colocalize at the immunological synapse (56,57). Other molecules move to the distal pole of the T cell, away from the contact. Another characteristic of the immunological synapse is that the organizing center of microtubules, called the *centrosome* or *MTOC,* is pointing toward the site of contact at or near the cortex beneath the immunological synapse. Located between the MTOC and the nucleus, the Golgi apparatus is also polarized toward the site of contact. It is believed that this latter feature facilitates the directional or polarized secretion of IL-2 and IFN-γ into the contact zone between T cell and DC (58,59). Although this has not all been documented to occur with precise subcellular resolution *in vivo,* there is reason to postulate that such reorganization occurs during an immune response when newly activated T cells are engaged by mature DCs. T cell–DC conjugates have been observed *in vivo* within the first 18 hours of the immune response, and they appear to exhibit characteristic accumulation of TCR and IL-2 at the side of DC contact, with exclusion of distal markers from the site of contact (37,59).

In contrast to the random walk of naïve T cells exposed to immature DCs that are presenting self-peptide/MHC, movement of the T cell changes to purposeful but brief (less than 10 minutes in duration) serial encounters with those DCs that specifically display foreign peptide/MHC complexes (19,37–39,41,60). Even if the DC is inflamed and presenting antigen, the interactions are primarily brief but specific serial contacts in the initial 8 to 10 hours of the immune response *in vivo* (Figure 13.1). This phase of T cell activation *in vivo* is followed by a period of approximately 15 to 20 hours in which the T cell has prolonged interactions (up to several hours or more) with the antigen-presenting DCs (Figure 13.1). In this phase, T cells exhibit characteristic markers of activation and are starting to secrete early response cytokines such as IL-2 in a polarized manner and TNFα in a nonpolarized fashion (58,59). At approximately 25 to 30 hours after initial antigen presentation, the quality of the interactions again changes to rapid motion with brief interactions (39). Importantly, the onset of this stage is coincident with the first T cell division of the immune response (Figure 13.1).

The foregoing behavior, as chronicled by time-lapsed fluorescence imaging within intact and explanted lymph nodes, was largely similar in the hands of several investigators. Nonetheless some differences emerged that could either be due to intrinsic differences in CD4+ versus CD8+ T cells, or experimental nuances such as the immunization or adoptive T cell transfer system employed. In this vein, it is important to note that many experimental approaches upon which the field relies may inevitably have confounding features.

One potential pitfall of a modeled antigen-specific response *in vivo* relates to the fundamental nature of how adaptive immunity protects the host. According to the clonal selection theory of lymphocyte biology, an adaptive immune response might be initiated by the response of very few, or perhaps one, cell(s). In essence, immunologists seek to determine the cellular and subcellular composition of a clonal burst that emanated from a single cell under the circumstance where only a single cell is responding (Figure 13.1). The only experimentally tractable approaches to model this behavior, however, are often reliant on observations made when tens of thousands of cells respond in unison. Although all of the T cells in an experiment may have the identical antigen receptor, there is increasing evidence to postulate that they may behave differently as group than they might as individuals because of their competition for rare ligands (61–65). The very similarity that makes it useful to employ transgenic T cells carrying a fixed TCR may also make them behave in a way that might not occur if only a small few were able to respond.

When Encountering Self-antigen

How does the initial encounter of naïve T cell with antigenic peptide/MHC appear if the antigen is not a derivative of foreign life, but rather a component of self? In this situation, vigorous clonal expansion and effector differentiation on the part of a T cell would not be desirable. Instead, there seem to be peripheral mechanisms to deal with highly self-reactive cells that escaped the screening of negative selection in the thymus (10). Their net effect is to abort the incipient program of clonal expansion and effector differentiation on the part of the self-reactive T cell. Some of these mechanisms involve cell intrinsic negative regulators of T cell activation, so-called mediators of "recessive tolerance." Emerging as an essential and increasingly well-characterized mechanism is the counterregulation in *trans* by natural Treg cells, so-called mediators of "dominant tolerance." These principles will be discussed in greater detail in the chapters on tolerance and suppression.

The aforementioned scenario describing rapid motion/brief contact, then sustained contact, followed by rapid motion and cell division is primarily the behavior associated with productive immune responses when antigenic peptide/MHC is presented in an inflammatory context. In parallel with the realization that there is stereotyped sustained contact between the newly activated T cell and antigen-presenting DCs prior to the first division of the immune response, another set of findings, discussed later in this chapter, pointed to an important function of this newly appreciated phase of initial T cell activation. The phase of sustained contact is, thus, emerging as a key checkpoint in the ability of the T cell undergoing mitogenic signaling to proceed through successful versus abortive activation (Figure 13.1).

Several lines of evidence support the functional importance of the signaling that might occur during the sustained, premitotic interaction that occurs *in vivo*. There is a positive relationship between productive immunity, DC inflammation, and the duration of contact in that phase of T cell activation occurring prior to the first division (41,60). CTLA4, an intrinsic negative regulator of T cell activation, negatively influences the sustained contact phase (66). Consistent with these findings, there is an inverse relationship between the presence of natural Treg cells and the duration of the sustained contacts between self-antigen–specific T cell and DCs (35,36). Finally, the activation of Toll-like receptors on DCs can disarm the suppressive effect of Treg cells to promote successful immune activation (67). In this manner, integrity of the sustained contact appears to have an essential role in arming the nascent progeny of the T cell for further division, appropriate effector differentiation and function (Figure 13.1). By contrast, disruption of the sustained contact is associated with unproductive immunity, or tolerance. An emerging subtext of these and other new findings that will be discussed later in this chapter is that the dynamics of intercellular communication will be a critical component in illuminating the inside of the "black-box" of initial T cell activation and differentiation *in vivo*. In addition to preventing newly activated cells from becoming armed, Treg cells may also act at later stages of the immune response to disarm effector cells (68). This will be discussed in greater detail in the following sections and in the chapters on tolerance and suppression.

Before and After the First T Cell Division

The first day of the immune response looks largely similar for a pathogen-specific CD8+ and CD4+ T cell in terms of the general dynamics of initial T cell interaction with and activation by DCs as outlined earlier. Although each subset is activated by a different class of MHC molecule presenting foreign peptide, the initial activation of the two cell types can be physically united by a cross-presenting DC (69). This mode of presentation of exogenous antigens to CD8+ T cells will be discussed in the chapter on antigen presentation and the section on immunity to infectious agents. *In vivo* imaging studies suggest that the initial interaction between CD8+ T cell and DC is promoted by a CD4+ T cell interacting with the same DC (42,43). This may play a role in both effector (43) and memory (42) differentiation of CD8+ T cells. Of note, this enhanced response by $CD8^+$ T cells is accompanied by more sustained contact between T cell and DC (Figure 13.1). The ability of $CD4^+$ T cells to enhance contact appears to involve secretion of the chemokines CCL3 and CCL4 (42) and ligation of CD40 on the DC, but without necessarily imposing greater maturation on the DC (43). Thus, the phase of sustained contact prior to the first division is emerging as an important quality-control checkpoint for $CD8^+$ T cell–mediated immunity (Figure 13.1).

There are, however, some differences between the $CD4^+$ and $CD8^+$ T cell responses to antigen. The degree of clonal expansion is one well-characterized difference. As mentioned earlier, it is generally assumed that the response to infection will involve very few initially responding cells. For instance, it is estimated that there are 2 million different antigen-specific clones in the spleen, with approximately10 duplicate cells of each specificity (70). A naïve mouse has five cells specific for the Db/gp33 epitope of lymphocytic choriomeningitis virus (LCMV) per million $CD8^+$ T cells, or about 100 cells per mouse. These cells can expand 100,000-fold, suggesting that 15 or more rounds of division can occur (71). For $CD4^+$ T cells, clonal expansion has been estimated to be a few to several orders of magnitude lower than for virus-specific $CD8^+$ T cells, depending on the class of pathogen (72,73). Likewise, there are some $CD8^+$ T cell responses with lesser expansion than seen following LCMV infection.

After the first day of the immune response, a newly activated T cell begins to divide, and its resulting progeny begin to acquire the properties of more mature effector cells. $CD8^+$ T cells seem capable of undergoing substantial division and differentiation without the daughter cells needing to reconnect with antigen-bearing cells, although such experiments do not rule out important potential contributions from such interactions (74,75). In contrast, $CD4^+$ T cells seem to be dependent on more persistent antigen presentation for full expansion and differentiation, and renewed contact between daughter cells and antigen-bearing DCs has been documented (48,49). It is not yet known, however, after which daughter generation antigen may no longer be required. The possibility for continued education of the T cell's progeny on antigen-loaded cells is afforded when the S1P1 on activated T cells becomes temporarily repressed, in part due to inflammatory cytokines that act via induction of CD69 (45). Thus, the initial clonal burst of T cell progeny in response to a pathogen is sequestered temporarily in the lymph node, perhaps to ensure appropriate exposure to differentiation signals (Figure 13.1).

Division and Beyond: Instructions and Directions

A response of 10 or so naïve T cells by itself would be unlikely to muster the "fire power" necessary to eradicate a typical infection, even if those cells could differentiate into fully armed effector cells. Clonal expansion thereby serves at least one purpose of providing a sufficiently large armamentarium for host defense (Figure 13.1). With the advent of dyes that allow analysis of cell division, it has become increasingly appreciated that the newly activated antigen-specific cell (the "parent," if you will) does not itself undergo effector/memory differentiation. Instead, it is its daughter cells or, more accurately, even later cell generations that are the real participants in clearance of the pathogen (48,76). Examination of the timing or division number required to achieve effector cytokine expression, induction of homing molecules that permit access to infected tissue, loss of lymph node homing/retention molecules, and reacquisition of exit receptors all point to a concerted division-dependent mechanism that licenses the later cell generation progeny to mature and migrate for immune reactions at the site of infection (45,48,76–78).

In the first few days after activation, T cells have transiently down-regulated the egress molecule, S1P1 (45). After re-expression of the receptor and recovering their ability to exit the secondary lymphoid organs, the newly minted mature effector T cells must additionally migrate to the appropriately inflamed or infected tissue to exert their function (79,80). This is partly promoted by the loss of homing receptors for the secondary lymphoid organs, such as CD62L and CCR7. In addition, a new set of homing molecules is acquired, such as PSGL-1, CD44, CCR5, and CXCR3, which bind ligands in inflamed tissue. Much in the same manner that the character of their effector differentiation choice is instructed by their environment to be matched with the type of pathogen encountered, so too are their directions and "ZIP codes" for migration to specific tissues imprinted from the history of their antigen-presenting cell's experiences (79). DCs that arose in the gut induce intestinal homing receptors, while DCs from cutaneous sites induce skin-homing receptors on effector T cells (81,82). Some antigen-experienced $CD4^+$ T cells, called *follicular helper T cells* (ThF), however, are fated to stay in the lymph nodes and migrate to B cell follicles to perform their helper functions (83,84).

Like entry of a naïve T cell into secondary lymphoid organs, the entry of an effector T cell into inflamed or uninflamed nonlymphoid tissues proceeds through characteristic multistep adhesion cascades of tethering, rolling, integrin activation, and firm adhesion (80). This involves specific patterns of expression of ligands for selectins, chemokine receptors, and integrins on the T cell. Skin-homing effector T cells or regulators of atopic skin inflammation would express cutaneous leukocyte antigen (or other ligands for P- and E-selectin), CCR4 (receptor for CCL17), or CCR10 (receptor for CCL27). Small bowel-homing effector T cells or mediators of Crohn's disease would express PSGL-1 (ligand for P-selectin), $\alpha4\beta7$ integrin (receptor for MAdCAM), and chemokine receptors CCR9 (receptor for CCL25) and CXCR3 (receptor for

CXCL9). More details can be found in other chapters of this book. Although some differences in tissue homing receptors between mature effector CD4+ and CD8+ T cells are evident, the overall strategy for both activated subsets is similar: to coordinate the acquisition of specific nonlymphoid tissue migratory information with the acquisition of specific effector function (Figure 13.1). The DC and the rest of the cellular/soluble milieu of the secondary lymphoid organ are responsible for this coordinated imprinting process, although the specific signals are not fully understood (85,86).

EFFECTOR T CELLS

Differences Between Effector CD4+ and CD8+ T Cells

Armed effector CD4+ T cells must move to sites of infection or inflammation to perform their function, which is primarily orchestration of other immune cells and nonimmune cells to eradicate a pathogen (Figure 13.2). In addition, a subset of CD4+ effector T cells will remain in the lymph node to provide help for B cells (83,84). The most influential function of effector CD4+ T cells is not the direct elimination of pathogen but instead the mobilization and activation of other cells. An effector CD4+ T cell is truly a helper cell more than it is an effector cell. The term *effector* is used here (and elsewhere) primarily to imply that the cell is competent to immediately express maximal levels of its signature gene products, usually cytokines. In this regard, effector CD4+ T cells differ greatly from effector CD8+ effect T cells, which by themselves are the mediators of pathogen clearance. Thus, as used in this chapter, the term *effector CD4+ T cell* implies full functional maturation following antigen experience for helper T cells, while effector CD8+ T cell implies full functional maturation following antigen experience for cytotoxic T cells. As will be discussed later, CD4+ and CD8+ T cells differ greatly in the spectrum of effector fates they can adopt.

Effector Choice for CD4+ T Cells

After naïve helper T cells become activated and begin to divide and differentiate, they adopt different patterns of gene expression or fates that correspond to a division of labor designed for the eradication of pathogens with diverse life cycles and evasion strategies (Figure 13.2). One of the most remarkable aspects of the differentiation process of helper T cells is how environmentally sensitive is the selection of lineage choices (87–89). The newly activated T cell and its daughters or granddaughters integrate signals from DCs, which already reflect an imprint of the type of pathogen that was encountered by the combinatorial ligation of pattern recognition receptors (34). The DCs take their impression of the class of pathogen and transmit this information to the T cell by the elaboration of distinct cytokines or costimulatory molecules and Notch ligands. In addition, other innate and noninnate cells that bear a reflection of the type of pathogen contribute other cytokines or membrane-bound ligands that will influence the differentiation decisions of the maturing helper T cell progeny.

The combinatorial signaling that the newly activated T cell receives is somehow processed to create a dominant subset for many immune responses (53). In some immune responses, however, there is more of a mixed-lineage differentiation pattern of the maturing helper T cells. The degree of polarization or heterogeneity may vary according to the chronicity of the infection and the complexity of the pathogen's life cycle. Chronic infestations with intestinal worms are often characterized by polarized Th2 responses (90–93), yet IL-4-producing cells are also evident early in the Th1 response against *Leishmania* (73). Organisms that have intracellular and extracellular stages might be capable of evoking a mixed response of helper T cell subsets so that diverse effector mechanisms can be mobilized. Several important themes have emerged concerning effector CD4+ T cell lineage choice during the immune responses. Many of these principles are specific to CD4+ T cells, but others apply broadly to CD8+ T cells and atypical T cell subsets.

Division of Labor

At least three subsets of effector CD4+ T cells are now recognized (Figure 13.2), Th1, Th2, and Th17 (87,94,95). Th1 cells are characterized by the secretion of IFN-g and are important activators of macrophages, NK cells, and CD8+ T cells (96). Th1 cells are thought to be involved in systemic immunity, in particular the defense against intracellular pathogens. Th2 cells secrete IL-4, IL-13, and IL-25 and are important for barrier defense at mucosal and epithelial surfaces. Th2 cells mobilize and activate eosinophils, basophils, mast cells, and alternatively activated macrophages (97). Th17 cells produce IL-17A, IL-17F, IL-6, and TNFα and are responsible for regulating acute inflammation (98). Th17 cells act in concert with neutrophils and are important for defense against extracellular bacteria (99,100).

Antibody responses are quite likely to be mediated by subsets of effector CD4+ T cells with specialized homing properties and function. Follicular helper T cells, or ThF cells, are antigen-experienced CD4+ T cells found in the lymph node and are identified as being PSGL-1− and CXCR5+ (83,84,101). ThF cells are found at the periphery of B cell follicles and appear to mediate naïve B cell activation and germinal center formation, probably through the expression of ligand for CD40 and the secretion of Th1- and Th2-like cytokines. It is possible that ThF cells might arise as branches in the Th1 and Th2 differentiation pathways, veritable ThF1 or ThF2 cells, but their precise lineage relationship to the other effector CD4+ T cell subsets is still uncertain.

Good Can Be Bad: Division of Damage

Effector CD4+ T cell subsets, thus, provide a division of labor in mobilizing the immune armamentarium to combat the diversity in the microbial world. An additional theme relating to the diverse but unique protective role played by each subset is that each subset contributes to pathological conditions mediated by T cells (Figure 13.2). Th1 cells cause tissue damage in response to inflammation and infection and may mediate some forms of autoimmunity (102,103). Th2 cells mediate allergic disease and asthma (104). Th17 cells are responsible for some forms of organ-specific autoimmunity, notably experimental arthritis and multiple sclerosis, and may contribute to cancerous states (98,105–107). Finally, dysregulated ThF cells can cause systemic autoimmunity and auto-antibody production or contribute to T cell–mediated organ-specific autoimmunity (108). One of the costs associated with adaptive host defense is the extra burden of inflammatory and autoimmune diseases for the species. An emerging theme in immune response regulation is that collateral damage mediated by cytokines is often limited by other cytokines. IL-27, TGF-β, and IL-10 have been particularly implicated to varying degrees as signals that dampen Th1-, Th2-, and Th17-associated inflammation (99,102,109–115).

Inductive and Selective Signals

The critical signaling pathways for eliciting distinct helper T cell subsets are still not completely resolved. Several potent positive and negative regulators, however, have been defined. Curiously, among the most prominent positive regulators of subset induction are the products of that subset itself. IFN-γ promotes Th1 induction, IL-4 promotes Th2 induction, and IL-6 (together with TGFβ) promotes Th17 induction (87,89,95,96,112,113,116). This chameleon-like property of the helper T cell lineages may contribute to fortification of a particular subset if progeny are dividing in spatially restricted niches. For example, complex instructions received by the newly activated helper T cell from a DC could be relayed from daughter to granddaughter in a simpler form via the paracrine actions of these cytokines, especially if the clonal burst is expanding away from the original DC.

Other cytokines are also critical during and after lineage commitment (Figure 13.2). IL-12 acts selectively to promote the survival, proliferation, and enhanced gene expression of Th1 cells. Combinatorial TLR signaling to DCs can synergistically induce IL-12 and a Th1-associated Notch ligand pattern (53). Thymic stromal lymphopoietin (TSLP) can seemingly act on DCs to cause them to induce Th2 responses (117–120). A signature set of pathogen-associated receptors for helminths has not yet been found on DCs, raising the possibility that Th2 skewing results from the absence of Th1-associated ligands plus receipt of the TSLP signal. IL-4, IL-25, and IL-33 may augment the survival, proliferation, and action of Th2-committed cells and counter the development of Th1 cells (92,93,121,122). IL-23 is a critical signal for Th17 cells, but primarily for maintenance and not induction (99,112,113,123). Other inductive signals that have recently emerged are Notch signaling pathways and costimulatory ligands (124–127). For ThF cells, ICOS has proven to be a particularly critical signal, although it is not clear if that role is in induction or progressive maturation (101,108).

Key Transcriptional Regulators

For each of the well-characterized helper T cell lineages, there is a key transcription factor that is essential for their lineage commitment (Figure 13.2). T-bet is a critical regulator of Th1 cells (96,128,129). It acts to promote the IL-12 responsiveness of activated cells by enhancing expression of IL-12Rβ2, and it directly promotes IFN-γ expression (130–133). Gata-3 is the central transcription factor for lineage commitment of Th2 cells, although it also plays some essential roles in various stages of thymopoiesis (134–136). Gata-3 functions directly to activate the Th2 cytokine cluster, containing IL-4, IL-13, and IL-5, and it may promote the selective growth of Th2 cells in response to IL-4 signaling (137–139). T-bet and Gata-3 gene expression is induced by TCR signaling, specific cytokine signals, specific Notch ligand signaling, and by their own gene products (124,125,127,130,132,133,140–142). T-bet and Gata-3 are negatively regulated by cytokines from opposing subsets and TGFβ. T-bet is able to physically interact with Gata-3, which may contribute to the counter-dominance observed between Th1 and Th2 subsets (143–145). Factors that may provide additional transcriptional control of Th1 and Th2 cells during their maintenance phase include c-maf and Hlx, respectively (133,146).

RORγt has been identified as a critical lineage commitment factor for the Th17 cells (123). IL-6 and TGFβ seem to synergistically induce RORγt. Both IL-6 and TGFβ contribute to the induction of IL-23 receptor expression, which would allow IL-23 to promote maintenance of Th17 cells, although it is not known if IL-23R expression is dependent on RORγt (99,123). Bcl-6 is factor identified in ThF cells, but it may have roles that extend beyond this subset, because it has been implicated in memory CD8+ T cell development (147,148). Blimp-1, an important factor for plasma cell differentiation, is an emerging intrinsic regulator of T cell function, because its loss leads to severe dysregulation of effector and memory T cell subsets (149,150). Yet to be determined is whether Bcl-6 and

Blimp-1 will act in a counter-regulatory loop against one another in peripheral T cell differentiation, as they have been proposed to function during memory B cell homeostasis versus plasma cell differentiation.

Slow to Learn but Quick to Remember

In the differentiation of effector CD4$^+$ T cell subsets, several peculiar demands are placed on the signaling and transcriptional networks needed to achieve the end results of mature Th1, Th2, Th17, and ThF cells. Although the naïve (parent) T cell is the cell that first receives a critical set of instructions from the DC, within one day the parent cell does not formally exist, having become two daughters. After the first division, subsequent divisions proceed even faster, perhaps occurring every 6 hours, such that daughters and granddaughters may not be present shortly. In addition, it is evident that parents, daughters, and granddaughters do not typically exhibit effector maturity—that is, being fully armed to secrete maximal amounts of their signature cytokine. There must, therefore, be a mechanism for progressive learning and imprinting of the type of effector function being taught in the draining lymph node so that it can eventually reach maximal productivity and be remembered by the ensuing progeny as they migrate to follicle or tissue, temporally and spatially removed from the inductive signal (Figure 13.1).

It is thought that one of the ways in which the signaling events are amplified and remembered by the progeny of the T cell as they divide and move to tissue is the result of so-called epigenetic effects (87–89,151,152). The term *epigenetic* has at least two connotations: (1) the mediators of this effect are not alterations in primary nucleotide sequence (genetic material), but instead covalent modifications of histones and CpG dinucleotides, and (2) the consequence of a signaling pathway (genetic circuit) is still manifest after the initiating signal has disappeared, either on account of cell division, migration, or temporal decay. The epigenetic aspect of effector CD4$^+$ T cell differentiation involves a progressive dismantling of condensed chromatin structure at the signature cytokine loci expressed by effector CD4$^+$ T cells. Chromatin remodeling involves feed-forward cascades of cytokine signals and transcription factors that, by building in concerted potency, eventually unfurl the repressed structure of the gene so that it is readily activated (within minutes) by general and lineage-specific factors. This progressive de-repression is occurring in tandem with cell divisions, making it a matter of cellular inheritance (76). Once fully unfurled, the remodeled state is capable of being locked in, in such a way that the cytokine signals and transcription factors used to create the remodeled active state are not always required to maintain its activity in a mature cell or one of its subsequent daughter cells (153). For example, the Th2 cytokine cluster containing IL-4, IL-5, and IL-13 cannot be activated and remodeled during Th2 differentiation without signaling through the IL-4 receptor or the transcription factor Gata-3. Yet both are dispensable to maintain the ability of mature Th2 cell or their subsequent daughters to rapidly secrete copious amounts of IL-4 upon reencountering antigen (134,136).

Epigenetic repression of the cytokine genes in CD4$^+$ T cells seems to play an additional role in the proper functioning of an immune response. The appropriate repression of the forbidden cytokines within a maturing lineage is enforced by gene silencing mechanisms that operate to further dampen the multipotential state of gene activity that is necessary for the naïve T cell to be able to make multiple choices, but deleterious for mature Th1 or Th2 cells with restricted functional repertoires (137,154–158). The epigenetic effects that operate during effector CD4$^+$ T cell differentiation, therefore, help to pace the progress of effector maturation, restrict the potential options of the progenitor as discrete subsets emerge, and help the signaling pathways that are ignited in the parent cell move through division, space, and time, so that a distant progeny knows exactly what to secrete upon arrival at the site of infection.

Other Subsets

In an idealized immune response, the critical players are the naïve T cell, the DC, and other cells that have encountered pathogen. It is likely that some regional immune responses may have more complex interactions. The intestines, for example, exhibit an active interplay between pro- and antiinflammatory regulators. Within various intestinal tissues, there are previously activated, constitutively cytokine-expressing (IL-10, TGF-β, IL-17, IL-25) T cell subsets (92,123). In a site with constitutive inflammatory mediators and counter-reactive suppressive factors, the shaping of Th1, Th2, Th17, and regulatory responses might be expected to follow distinct rules.

CD4$^+$ T cell subsets with atypical differentiation patterns have also been induced *in vitro* and *in vivo,* such as IL-10-producing regulatory T cells that do not express FoxP3, and so-called *adaptive Treg cells* that are the progeny of conventional naïve T cells activated by antigen plus TGFβ or low doses of antigen and that express FoxP3 like their thymically derived cousins (114,115). It is yet unknown whether these cells have physiological roles in the response to self- or foreign antigens and, if so, under what circumstances. It is tempting to speculate that an adaptive Treg cell could regulate the magnitude and degree inflammation of its kindred (sharing the same TCR) effector CD4$^+$ T cells in the response to foreign antigen. This has not yet been visualized, however, in the responses to pathogens that have thus far been interrogated (9). As mentioned earlier, there remain many uncertainties about whether suppressive action of thymically derived Treg cells during an immune response is likely to be at the site of induction (secondary lymphoid tissue) or infection (peripheral tissue), or both. Indeed whether control of immune response against pathogens is primarily the responsibility of another T cell (dominant mechanism) or owing to cell-intrinsic negative regulators within the effector cell itself (recessive mechanism) is not fully resolved (35,36,66,68,159).

Effector CD8+ T Cells

During the immune response to viruses and some intracellular microbes, naïve CD8+ T cells are activated to undergo a program of massive clonal expansion, with acquisition of new effector functions in the resulting progeny (16). The primary effector products of CD8+ T cells are IFN-γ and the contents of cytotoxic granules, notably perforin and granzymes. Unlike effector CD4+ (helper) T cells, effector CD8+ (cytotoxic) T cells make limited choices in their repertoire of effector genes. Primarily type 1 or Tc1 effector cells predominate *in vivo*. Also contrasting with effector CD4+ T cells, which migrate to infected sites to orchestrate the actions of other cells, effector CD8+ T cells are the direct executioners of pathogen-infected cells. The pro-inflammatory and toxic products of effector CD8+ T cells are themselves regulators of the magnitude of expansion and contraction of the T cell response, and loss of certain effector proteins alters the dynamics of effector and memory cell generation (160).

The induction of effector CD8+ T cells is dependent on many of the same classes of signals as for effector CD4+ T cells, antigenic peptide/MHC, pathogen-related inflammatory signals including costimulators, and cytokine signals. CD4+ T cell help has become recognized as an important component of the activation of antigen-specific CD8+ T cells. Although CD4+ T cell help may be imparted early in the response and influence effector function (43), its effects may be more manifest in memory CD8+ T cells (42,161–165). T-bet, the transcription factor responsible for Th1 lineage commitment, is expressed in CD8+ T cells and may play a similar role inducing effector gene expression in both cell types (166,167). Another transcription factor that is highly homologous to T-bet, called Eomesodermin (Eomes), is also expressed in antigen-specific CD8+ T cells. It is thought that T-bet and Eomes may play some redundant and nonredundant roles in the spectrum of cytotoxic effector and memory cell programming (166–169).

MEMORY T CELLS

After migration to inflamed tissues, T cells mediate their function by the secretion of cytokines or cytotoxic granules. Following successful clearance of a pathogen, there is a phase of massive cell death, which results in elimination of most effector T cells (Figure 13.3). The basis for the demise is not completely understood but may involve some combination of cytokine withdrawal, receptor-mediated death signaling, or toxicity from effector products. After the elimination of approximately 90 percent of effector cells, a group of memory T cells persist, often for the life of the host (Figure 13.3). For example, if one naïve T cell expands 10,000-fold in response to a pathogen, and 90 percent of effectors are eliminated after the resolution, then the original clone has seeded 1,000 memory cells to deal with subsequent reinfections. Thus, the remnant population of memory T cells is typically orders of magnitude higher in frequency than the pre-immune state. Some general features of memory cells will be discussed later, but more information can be found in the chapter on T cell memory.

Virtually Indestructible but Not Always Faster and Better

After an acute infection, it is highly unusual for the host to be left without a remnant of antigen-experienced memory T cells (Figure 13.3). If the naïve T cell pool that is specific for a pathogen is small in number, and all such cells are recruited into the effector response, there would seem to be a hard-wired mechanism associated with T cell activation that ensures the generation of an indestructible subpopulation. From an evolutionary perspective, this would likely be advantageous, so that a host retains an armamentarium against a pathogen that has now been validated as an actual, rather than simply a potential, threat. In fact, without robust insurance that all clonal bursts leave some memory cells behind, there would routinely be a selective T cell immunodeficiency (temporary or permanent) for the pathogen subsequent to the resolution of infection. In dealing with pathogens requiring cellular defense, where antibodies may serve no benefit, a temporary hole in the T cell repertoire might be an unacceptable state for the host. Despite the near-invariant appearance of antigen-experienced, or memory, T cells following resolution of infection, however, the host is not always left with heightened state of resistance to reinfection, as one might expect from a successful vaccination. This has raised some fundamental issues about the nature of memory T cells, including their purpose and their lineage relationship to naïve and effector T cells (170,171).

Two Models for Memory Formation

One way to think about memory cells is that they are simply effector cells that escaped clonal deletion and have entered a resting, rather than activated, state (Figure 13.3). This sort of model for memory T cell formation is considered a linear or progressive form of differentiation, because it implies that memory cells are derived from effector cells (170,171). An alternative theory suggests that, at some point after initial activation, a subset of antigen-specific

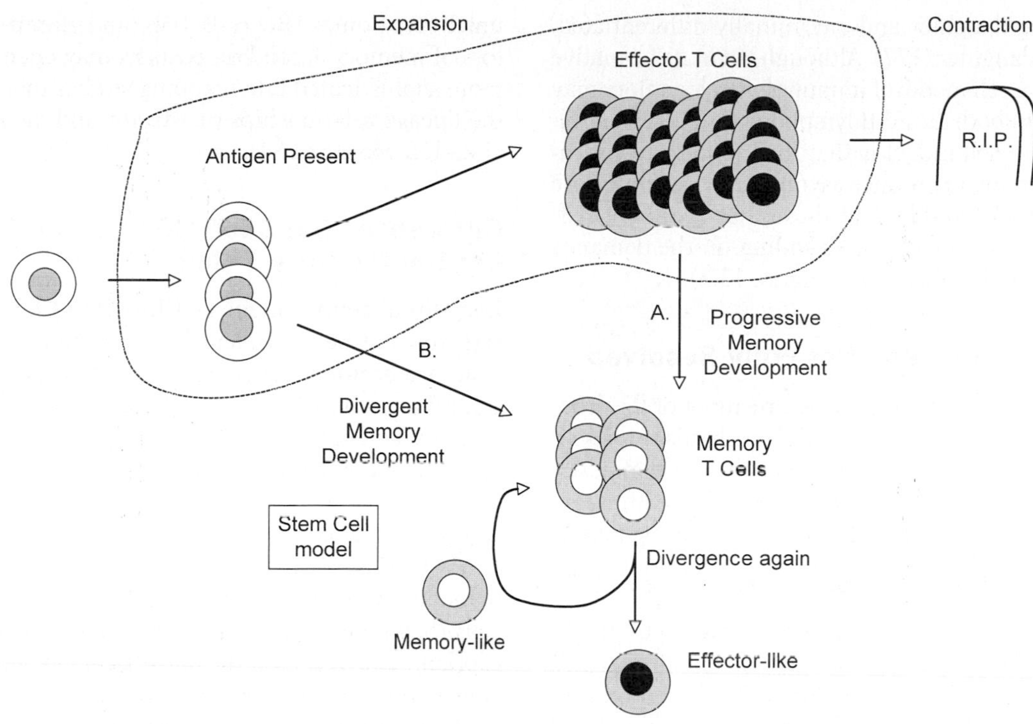

FIGURE 13.3 Models for memory T cell formation. Pathogen-derived antigen exposure causes clonal expansion and effector differentiation. Clearance of pathogen results in cell death of the majority of effector cells (clonal contraction). Clonal elimination is typically incomplete, leaving a remnant of memory cells. Scenario A places memory T cells as posteffector cells that underwent progressive development. Scenario B places memory T cells as being committed to the lineage without becoming an effector cell. The pathway of memory cells arising in scenario B and their subsequent ability to have self-renewing and terminally differentiated progeny has been likened to the behavior of stem cells.

progeny split off before the effector pathway of differentiation and instead become memory cells. This type of model is considered a branching or divergent form of differentiation because two clonally related T cells adopt different cell fates. The relative contribution of each of these models of memory T cell formation during various immune responses has not yet been resolved (46,64,172–174).

Two Memory Habitats

Analysis of memory T cells has demonstrated that antigen-experienced T cell populations can exhibit two distinct patterns of migration after infection and during homeostasis, those that migrate through lymphoid tissues and those that migrate through nonlymphoid and inflamed tissue. Memory cells that express the lymph node homing molecules CCR7 and CD62L are termed *central memory cells,* because of their access to primary and secondary lymphoid tissue, including the bone marrow (46,64,173–176). In contrast, memory cells with loss of CCR7 and CD62L expression but displaying inflammation-associated chemokine receptors are called *effector memory T cells* because of their immediate expression of effector genes upon reactivation and their ability to access nonlymphoid tissue. Thus, central memory cells can continually be sampling secondary lymphoid tissue alongside the parade of naïve cells, while effector memory cells may be patrolling peripheral tissues for a heightened level of security.

A Stem Cell Model

The original concept of central memory cells represented one of the first concrete challenges to the linear paradigm of memory differentiation that had considered memory cells as effector cells that had transitioned to a resting, long-lived state (173). Instead, these central memory cells seemed to be the early byproduct of antigen experience, representing a cell that dropped out of the normal path of effector-bound cells that progressively divide and differentiate. As progeny of the newly activated T cell, the less terminally differentiated central memory daughter is, in a sense, a closer approximation of its naïve parent cell than its siblings that go on to be full-fledged, terminally differentiated effector cells (Figure 13.3). This way of looking at the clonal burst is reminiscent of the paradigm of a stem cell, which is capable of dividing and giving rise to a self-renewing daughter and a terminally differentiated, nonrenewing daughter (177). Although yet in its formative stages, the stem cell model of immunological memory may be applicable to both T and B lymphocytes (178). A corollary to the stem cell model is that the memory cell is capable of continuing to produce asymmetric progeny, those that are more effector-like and those that are more self-renewing to varying degrees, depending on the demands of rechallenge and homeostasis (Figure 13.3).

Lineage Relationships Not Fully Resolved

Whether memory cells represent the precursor or the product of effector cells, there must be a mechanism for self-renewal to maintain a steady number during homeostasis that will offset the attrition owing to a finite life span. Central memory CD8$^+$ T cells undergo slow cytokine-dependent, peptide/MHC-independent proliferation in response to basal IL-7 and IL-15 signaling (32,179–181). Slow proliferation has also been suggested to occur in central memory CD4$^+$ T cells, although it is not clear which signals are necessary to achieve this (182). For both CD4$^+$ and CD8$^+$ T cells, then, central memory T cells may carry the burden of durability in the absence of antigen, the defining property of a memory cell. Nonetheless, there has not been direct quantitative comparison of the proliferative capacity and turnover of CD4$^+$ versus CD8$^+$ central memory T cells. It, thus, remains possible that memory CD8$^+$ T cells are more stable than memory CD4$^+$ T cells in the absence of antigen (72).

The precise role of the effector memory cell and from whence it arises is not yet resolved. Effector memory T cells might be the byproduct of central memory T cells. This could be akin to another type of stem cell behavior, such that during homeostasis a central memory cell could periodically give rise to central memory daughters with potential to renew, and effector memory daughters that are not self-renewing but are continually generated for heightened security to explore even more peripherally than secondary lymphoid tissue (Figure 13.3). On the other hand, effector memory cells might simply be a direct descendant of a recently generated effector cell, which escaped clonal deletion.

Even for central memory T cells, lineage relationships have not been resolved. For CD4$^+$ T cells, there are well-characterized instances where the central memory T cell appears to have bifurcated or diverged prior to effector maturation (171,173,183). Central memory CD8$^+$ T cells have been alternatively suggested to arise sequentially from effector/effector memory T cells or as a branch distinct from the effector pathway (64,172,174). It remains possible that more than one pathway may lead to each lineage in physiological circumstances. Indeed, many uncertainties about memory cell programming remain. The discovery of several critical transcription factors, including T-bet, Eomes, Bcl-6, Bcl-6b, and Blimp-1 as regulators of memory T cell homeostasis may open avenues for more sophisticated fate mapping studies that could refine the lineage relationships of effector and memory subsets (148–150,166–168,184).

Differences Between CD4$^+$ and CD8$^+$ Central Memory T Cells

Long-lived, central memory CD4$^+$ and CD8$^+$ T cell subsets may not be equivalent in their ability to protect the host. In a prototypical cytotoxic response (against LCMV), central memory CD8$^+$ T cells function as highly effective, long-lived memory cells, capable of mediating vaccine-like protection upon reinfection, and in a manner superior to effector-like memory cells (174). In the CD4$^+$ Th1 response against *Leishmania*, complete elimination of parasite (which is not the norm) leaves the host with a residual, long-lived central memory CD4$^+$ T population. Such cells, however, function according to their original conception, as a reservoir of not-yet-effector cells, some of which will achieve effector status in the event of reinfection (183). By themselves, the central memory CD4$^+$ T cells afford protection to their host, but not at the level of immunity achieved when effector-like cells are present. In essence, central memory cells seem to share the property of durability in the absence of antigen across both the CD4$^+$ and CD8$^+$ lineages, perhaps with some quantitative differences (72). In regard to mediating highly effective heightened immunity, there may be greater disparity between the two central memory lineages. Determining whether this is strictly a CD4$^+$ versus CD8$^+$ difference will, however, require interrogation of a great variety of immune responses.

If Pathogen Is Not Eliminated

Previously activated T cells that exist in a host with chronic infection or nonsterile immunity have been difficult to categorize. If infection, and hence antigen, is not cleared, then remnant T cells are not necessarily memory cells, possibly being overly activated or recently generated effector cells. In LCMV infection, inability to eliminate virus completely results in a persistent population of CD8$^+$ T cells that fails to acquire the characteristics of highly effective central memory cells (185). These cells do not seem to behave like freshly minted effector cells and instead have been considered "exhausted" by overexposure to antigen. Their suboptimal functional properties can be partially reversed by blocking the negatively acting costimulatory family receptor, PD-1 (186,187).

Persistent infection has also been associated with enhanced protection by T cells. The phenomenon in which the nonsterile state is essential for heightened protection is called concomitant immunity. In such a situation, a host that harbors continual low-level infections is more protected than a host that has eliminated the pathogen. In *Leishmania* infection, for example, incomplete clearance of parasite is an essential requirement for optimal immunity to secondary challenge (159,183). In this case, central memory $CD4^+$ T cells that persist after pathogen eradication are long-lived in the absence of antigen but afford less protection from rechallenge than the continual stream of short-lived effector cells being generated by exposure to persisting parasite antigen. Optimal, or vaccine-like, protection afforded by nonsterile immunity is, therefore, not mediated solely by bona fide antigen-independent central memory $CD4^+$ T cells, but instead requires their continual conversion to effector cells owing to persistence of the parasite.

THE FUTURE

The past decade has seen tremendous advances in developing *in vivo* techniques that allow for a better understanding of the actual sequence of events that occur when a naïve T cell is born, undergoes migration, becomes activated, and gives birth to differentiating progeny. These *in vivo* techniques are on the verge of achieving subcellular resolution. Models of activation and differentiation during the immune response often regard the newly activated T cell as adopting a new fate and having similarly fated progeny. If differentiation decisions are delayed until at least the first cell division or two, the formal possibility remains that one newly activated T cell can have progeny with diverse fates. It is still uncertain if, for example, effector cells arise from the first antigen-specific naïve cell to arrive on the scene, while central memory cells are derived from a second naïve cell that arrived later. It might be the case, instead, that central memory $CD4^+$ T cells represent a minority subset of progeny within the clonal burst of a single naïve cell, in which the majority of the progeny were destined to be effector cells. If true intraclonal heterogeneity were possible, that is one single cell having daughters with different fates, it is unclear whether the mechanism for such a diversification event would be a stochastic or instructed process. Recent evidence suggests daughtee T cell diversity could be achieved in a non-random fashion through a mechanism known as asymmetric cell division (188). One of the main challenges facing the field of peripheral T cell differentiation in the coming years will be to visualize some of these fundamental uncertainties about the initial stages of peripheral T cell maturation during the immune response.

ACKNOWLEDGEMENTS

I am grateful to Terri Laufer, Richard Locksley, Jonathan Maltzman, and Phillip Scott for critical suggestions. I apologize to colleagues whose work was omitted due to space limitations.

REFERENCES

1. Anderson MS, Venanzi ES, Klein L, et al. Projection of an immunological self shadow within the thymus by the aire protein. *Science.* 2002;298:1395–1401.
2. Bousso P, Bhakta NR, Lewis RS, et al. Dynamics of thymocyte-stromal cell interactions visualized by two-photon microscopy. *Science.* 2002;296:1876–1880.
3. Villasenor J, Benoist C, Mathis D. AIRE and APECED: molecular insights into an autoimmune disease. *Immunol Rev.* 2005;204:156–164.
4. Hsieh CS, Zheng Y, Liang Y, et al. An intersection between the self-reactive regulatory and nonregulatory T cell receptor repertoires. *Nat Immunol.* 2006;7:401–410.
5. Watanabe N, Wang YH, Lee HK, et al. Hassall's corpuscles instruct DCs to induce CD4+ CD25+ regulatory T cells in human thymus. *Nature.* 2005;436:1181–1185.
6. Fontenot JD, Gavin MA, Rudensky AY. Foxp3 programs the development and function of CD4+CD25+ regulatory T cells. *Nat Immunol.* 2003;4:330–336.
7. Hori S, Nomura T, Sakaguchi S. Control of regulatory T cell development by the transcription factor Foxp3. *Science.* 2003;299:1057–1061.
8. Khattri R, Cox T, Yasayko SA, et al. An essential role for Scurfin in CD4+ CD25+ T regulatory cells. *Nat Immunol.* 2003;4:337–342.
9. Fontenot JD, Rasmussen JP, Williams LM, et al. Regulatory T cell lineage specification by the forkhead transcription factor foxp3. *Immunity.* 2005;22:329–341.
10. Shevach EM. From vanilla to 28 flavors: multiple varieties of T regulatory cells. *Immunity.* 2006;25:195–201.
11. Ziegler SF. FOXP3: of mice and men. *Annu Rev Immunol.* 2006;24:209–226.
12. He X, Kappes DJ. CD4/CD8 lineage commitment: light at the end of the tunnel? *Curr Opin Immunol.* 2006;18:135–142.
13. Robey EA. Immunology: guide for a cell-fate decision. *Nature.* 2005;433:813–814.
14. Sun G, Liu X, Mercado P, et al. The zinc finger protein cKrox directs CD4 lineage differentiation during intrathymic T cell positive selection. *Nat Immunol.* 2005;6:373–381.
15. He X, He X, Dave VP, et al. The zinc finger transcription factor Th-POK regulates CD4 versus CD8 T-cell lineage commitment. *Nature.* 2005;433:826–833.
16. Glimcher LH, Townsend MJ, Sullivan BM, et al. Recent developments in the transcriptional regulation of cytolytic effector cells. *Nat Rev Immunol.* 2004;4:900–911.
17. Matloubian M, Lo CG, Cinamon G, et al. Lymphocyte egress from thymus and peripheral lymphoid organs is dependent on S1P receptor 1. *Nature.* 2004;427:355–360.
18. Carlson CM, Endrizzi BT, Wu J, et al. Kruppel-like factor 2 regulates thymocyte and T-cell migration. *Nature.* 2006;442:299–302.
19. Miller MJ, Wei SH, Parker I, et al. Two-photon imaging of lymphocyte motility and antigen response in intact lymph node. *Science.* 2002;296:1869–1873.
20. Miller MJ, Hejazi AS, Wei SH, et al. T cell repertoire scanning is promoted by dynamic dendritic cell behavior and random T cell motility in the lymph node. *Proc Natl Acad Sci U S A.* 2004;101:998–1003.
21. Cahalan MD, Parker I. Imaging the choreography of lymphocyte trafficking and the immune response. *Curr Opin Immunol.* 2006;18:476–482.
22. Cyster JG. Chemokines, sphingosine-1-phosphate, and cell migration in secondary lymphoid organs. *Annu Rev Immunol.* 2005;23:127–159.
23. Catron DM, Itano AA, Pape KA, et al. Visualizing the first 50 hr of the primary immune response to a soluble antigen. *Immunity.* 2004;21:341–347.

24. Labrecque N, Whitfield LS, Obst R, et al. How Much TCR Does a T Cell Need? *Immunity.* 2001;15:71–82.
25. Dorfman JR, Stefanova I, Yasutomo K, et al. CD4+ T cell survival is not directly linked to self-MHC-induced TCR signaling. *Nat Immunol.* 2000;1:329–335.
26. Clarke SR, Rudensky AY. Survival and homeostatic proliferation of naive peripheral CD4+ T cells in the absence of self peptide:MHC complexes. *J Immunol.* 2000;165:2458–2464.
27. Polic B, Kunkel D, Scheffold A, et al. How alpha beta T cells deal with induced TCR alpha ablation. *Proc Natl Acad Sci U S A.* 2001;98:8744–8749.
28. Cinalli RM, Herman CE, Lew BO, et al. T cell homeostasis requires G protein-coupled receptor-mediated access to trophic signals that promote growth and inhibit chemotaxis. *Eur J Immunol.* 2005;35:786–795.
29. Rathmell JC, Farkash EA, Gao W, et al. IL-7 enhances the survival and maintains the size of naive T cells. *J Immunol.* 2001;167:6869–6876.
30. Vella A, Teague TK, Ihle J, et al. Interleukin 4 (IL-4) or IL-7 prevents the death of resting T cells: Stat6 is probably not required for the effect of IL-4. *J Exp Med.* 1997;186:325–330.
31. Tan JT, Dudl E, LeRoy E, et al. IL-7 is critical for homeostatic proliferation and survival of naive T cells. *Proc Natl Acad Sci U S A.* 2001;98:8732–8737.
32. Schluns KS, Kieper WC, Jameson SC, et al. Interleukin-7 mediates the homeostasis of naive and memory CD8 T cells in vivo. *Nat Immunol.* 2000;1:426–432.
33. Vivien L, Benoist C, Mathis D. T lymphocytes need IL-7 but not IL-4 or IL-6 to survive in vivo. *Intl Immunol.* 2001;13:763–768.
34. Reis e Sousa C. Activation of dendritic cells: translating innate into adaptive immunity. *Curr Opin Immunol.* 2004;16:21–25.
35. Tang Q, Adams JY, Tooley AJ, et al. Visualizing regulatory T cell control of autoimmune responses in nonobese diabetic mice. *Nat Immunol.* 2006;7:83–92.
36. Tadokoro CE, Shakhar G, Shen S, et al. Regulatory T cells inhibit stable contacts between CD4+ T cells and dendritic cells in vivo. *J Exp Med.* 2006;203:505–511.
37. Stoll S, Delon J, Brotz TM, et al. Dynamic imaging of T cell-dendritic cell interactions in lymph nodes. *Science.* 2002;296:1873–1876.
38. Bousso P, Robey E. Dynamics of CD8+ T cell priming by dendritic cells in intact lymph nodes. *Nat Immunol.* 2003;4:579–585.
39. Mempel TR, Henrickson SE, Von Andrian UH. T-cell priming by dendritic cells in lymph nodes occurs in three distinct phases. *Nature.* 2004;427:154–159.
40. Miller MJ, Safrina O, Parker I, et al. Imaging the single cell dynamics of CD4 T cell activation by dendritic cells in lymph nodes. *J Exp Med.* 2004;200:847–856.
41. Hugues S, Fetler L, Bonifaz L, et al. Distinct T cell dynamics in lymph nodes during the induction of tolerance and immunity. *Nat Immunol.* 2004;5:1235–1242.
42. Castellino F, Huang AY, Altan-Bonnet G, et al. Chemokines enhance immunity by guiding naive CD8 T cells to sites of CD4 T cell-dendritic cell interaction. *Nature.* 2006;440:890–895.
43. Beuneu H, Garcia Z, Bousso P. Cutting edge: Cognate CD4 help promotes recruitment of antigen-specific CD8 T cells around dendritic cells. *J Immunol.* 2006;177:1406–1410.
44. Schwab SR, Pereira JP, Matloubian M, et al. Lymphocyte sequestration through S1P lyase inhibition and disruption of S1P gradients. *Science.* 2005;309:1735–1739.
45. Shiow LR, Rosen DB, Brdickova N, et al. CD69 acts downstream of interferon-alpha/beta to inhibit S1P1 and lymphocyte egress from lymphoid organs. *Nature.* 2006;440:540–544.
46. Reinhardt RL, Khoruts A, Merica R, et al. Visualizing the generation of memory CD4 T cells in the whole body. *Nature.* 2001;410: 101–105.
47. Itano AA, McSorley SJ, Reinhardt RL, et al. Distinct dendritic cell populations sequentially present antigen to CD4 T cells and stimulate different aspects of cell-mediated immunity. *Immunity.* 2003;19:47–57.
48. Celli S, Garcia Z, Bousso P. CD4 T cells integrate signals delivered during successive DC encounters in vivo. *J Exp Med.* 2005;202:1271–1278.
49. Obst R, van Santen HM, Mathis D, et al. Antigen persistence is required throughout the expansion phase of a CD4(+) T cell response. *J Exp Med.* 2005;201:1555–1565.
50. Bonasio R, von Andrian UH. Generation, migration and function of circulating dendritic cells. *Curr Opin Immunol.* 2006;18:503–511.
51. Reinhardt RL, Hong S, Kang SJ, et al. Visualization of IL-12/23p40 in vivo reveals immunostimulatory dendritic cell migrants that promote Th1 differentiation. *J Immunol.* 2006;177:1618–1627.
52. Aggarwal S, Ghilardi N, Xie M-H, et al. Interleukin-23 promotes a distinct CD4 T cell activation state characterized by the production of interleukin-17. *J Bio Chem.* 2003;278:1910–1914.
53. Napolitani G, Rinaldi A, Bertoni F, et al. Selected Toll-like receptor agonist combinations synergistically trigger a T helper type 1-polarizing program in dendritic cells. *Nat Immunol.* 2005;6:769–776.
54. Blander JM, Medzhitov R. Toll-dependent selection of microbial antigens for presentation by dendritic cells. *Nature.* 2006;440:808–812.
55. Cemerski S, Shaw A. Immune synapses in T-cell activation. *Curr Opin Immunol.* 2006;18:298–301.
56. Maldonado RA, Irvine DJ, Schreiber R, et al. A role for the immunological synapse in lineage commitment of CD4 lymphocytes. *Nature.* 2004;431:527–532.
57. Molon B, Gri G, Bettella M, et al. T cell costimulation by chemokine receptors. *Nat Immunol.* 2005;6:465–471.
58. Huse M, Lillemeier BF, Kuhns MS, et al. T cells use two directionally distinct pathways for cytokine secretion. *Nat Immunol.* 2006;7:247–255.
59. Reichert P, Reinhardt RL, Ingulli E, et al. Cutting edge: in vivo identification of TCR redistribution and polarized IL-2 production by naive CD4 T cells. *J Immunol.* 2001;166:4278–4281.
60. Shakhar G, Lindquist RL, Skokos D, et al. Stable T cell-dendritic cell interactions precede the development of both tolerance and immunity in vivo. *Nat Immunol.* 2005;6:707–714.
61. Catron DM, Rusch LK, Hataye J, et al. CD4+ T cells that enter the draining lymph nodes after antigen injection participate in the primary response and become central-memory cells. *J Exp Med.* 2006;203:1045–1054.
62. Hataye J, Moon JJ, Khoruts A, et al. Naive and memory CD4+ T cell survival controlled by clonal abundance. *Science.* 2006;312:114–116.
63. Kedl RM, Rees WA, Hildeman DA, et al. T cells compete for access to antigen-bearing antigen-presenting cells. *J Exp Med.* 2000;192:1105–1113.
64. Marzo AL, Klonowski KD, Le Bon A, et al. Initial T cell frequency dictates memory CD8+ T cell lineage commitment. *Nat Immunol.* 2005;6:793–799. Epub 2005 Jul 17.
65. Smith AL, Wikstrom ME, Fazekas de St Groth B. Visualizing T cell competition for peptide/MHC complexes: a specific mechanism to minimize the effect of precursor frequency. *Immunity.* 2000;13:783–794.
66. Schneider H, Downey J, Smith A, et al. Reversal of the TCR Stop Signal by CTLA-4. *Science.* 2006;313:1972–1975.
67. Pasare C, Medzhitov R. Toll pathway-dependent blockade of CD4+ CD25+ T cell-mediated suppression by dendritic cells. *Science.* 2003;299:1033–1036.
68. Rudensky AY, Campbell DJ. In vivo sites and cellular mechanisms of T reg cell-mediated suppression. *J Exp Med.* 2006;203:489–492.
69. Shen L, Rock KL. Priming of T cells by exogenous antigen cross-presented on MHC class I molecules. *Curr Opin Immunol.* 2006;18:85–91.
70. Casrouge A, Beaudoing E, Dalle S, et al. Size estimate of the alpha beta TCR repertoire of naive mouse splenocytes. *J Immunol.* 2000;164:5782–5787.
71. Blattman JN, Antia R, Sourdive DJ, et al. Estimating the precursor frequency of naive antigen-specific CD8 T cells. *J Exp Med.* 2002;195:657–664.
72. Homann D, Teyton L, Oldstone MB. Differential regulation of antiviral T-cell immunity results in stable CD8+ but declining CD4+ T-cell memory. *Nat Med.* 2001;7:913–919.
73. Stetson DB, Mohrs M, Mallet-Designe V, et al. Rapid expansion and IL-4 expression by Leishmania-specific naive helper T cells in vivo. *Immunity.* 2002;17:191–200.

74. Kaech SM, Ahmed R. Memory CD8+ T cell differentiation: initial antigen encounter triggers a developmental program in naive cells. *Nat Immunol.* 2001;2:415–422.
75. van Stipdonk MJ, Lemmens EE, Schoenberger SP. Naive CTLs require a single brief period of antigenic stimulation for clonal expansion and differentiation. *Nat Immunol.* 2001;2:423–429.
76. Bird JJ, Brown DR, Mullen AC, et al. Helper T cell differentiation is controlled by the cell cycle. *Immunity.* 1998;9:229–237.
77. Langenkamp A, Messi M, Lanzavecchia A, et al. Kinetics of dendritic cell activation: impact on priming of TH1, TH2 and nonpolarized T cells. *Nat Immunol.* 2000;1:311–316.
78. Reinhardt RL, Bullard DC, Weaver CT, et al. Preferential accumulation of antigen-specific effector CD4 T cells at an antigen injection site involves CD62E-dependent migration but not local proliferation. *J Exp Med.* 2003;197:751–762.
79. Mora JR, von Andrian UH. T-cell homing specificity and plasticity: new concepts and future challenges. *Trends in Immunology.* 2006;27:235–243.
80. Luster AD, Alon R, von Andrian UH. Immune cell migration in inflammation: present and future therapeutic targets. *Nat Immunol.* 2005;6:1182–1190.
81. Mora JR, Bono MR, Manjunath N, et al. Selective imprinting of gut-homing T cells by Peyer's patch dendritic cells. *Nature.* 2003;424: 88–93.
82. Mora JR, Cheng G, Picarella D, et al. Reciprocal and dynamic control of CD8 T cell homing by dendritic cells from skin- and gut-associated lymphoid tissues. *J Exp Med.* 2005;201:303–316.
83. Campbell DJ, Kim CH, Butcher EC. Separable effector T cell populations specialized for B cell help or tissue inflammation. *Nat Immunol.* 2001;2:876–881.
84. Okada T, Miller MJ, Parker I, et al. Antigen-Engaged B Cells Undergo Chemotaxis toward the T Zone and Form Motile Conjugates with Helper T Cells. *PLoS Biology.* 2005;3:e150.
85. Johansson-Lindbom B, Svensson M, Pabst O, et al. Functional specialization of gut CD103+ dendritic cells in the regulation of tissue-selective T cell homing. *J Exp Med.* 2005;202:1063–1073.
86. Iwata M, Hirakiyama A, Eshima Y, et al. Retinoic acid imprints gut-homing specificity on T cells. *Immunity.* 2004;21:527–538.
87. Reinhardt RL, Kang SJ, Liang HE, et al. T helper cell effector fates—who, how and where? *Curr Opin Immunol.* 2006;18:271–277.
88. Ansel KM, Lee DU, Rao A. An epigenetic view of helper T cell differentiation. *Nat Immunol.* 2003;4:616–623.
89. Murphy KM, Reiner SL. The lineage decisions of helper T cells. *Nat Rev Immunol.* 2002;2:933–944.
90. Voehringer D, Shinkai K, Locksley RM. Type 2 immunity reflects orchestrated recruitment of cells committed to IL-4 production. *Immunity.* 2004;20:267–277.
91. Shinkai K, Mohrs M, Locksley RM. Helper T cells regulate type-2 innate immunity in vivo. *Nature.* 2002;420:825–829.
92. Owyang AM, Zaph C, Wilson EH, et al. Interleukin 25 regulates type 2 cytokine-dependent immunity and limits chronic inflammation in the gastrointestinal tract. *J Exp Med.* 2006;203:843–849.
93. Fallon PG, Ballantyne SJ, Mangan NE, et al. Identification of an interleukin (IL)-25-dependent cell population that provides IL-4, IL-5, and IL-13 at the onset of helminth expulsion. *J Exp Med.* 2006;203:1105–1116.
94. Tato CM, O'Shea JJ. Immunology: what does it mean to be just 17?*Nature.* 2006;441:166–168.
95. Harrington LE, Mangan PR, Weaver CT. Expanding the effector CD4 T-cell repertoire: the Th17 lineage. *Curr Opin Immunol.* 2006;18:349–356.
96. Szabo SJ, Sullivan BM, Peng SL, et al. Molecular mechanisms regulating Th1 immune responses. *Annu Rev Immunol.* 2003;21:713–758.
97. Voehringer D, Reese TA, Huang X, et al. Type 2 immunity is controlled by IL-4/IL-13 expression in hematopoietic non-eosinophil cells of the innate immune system. *J Exp Med.* 2006;203:1435–1446.
98. Langrish CL, Chen Y, Blumenschein WM, et al. IL-23 drives a pathogenic T cell population that induces autoimmune inflammation. *J Exp Med.* 2005;201:233–240.
99. Mangan PR, Harrington LE, O'Quinn DB, et al. Transforming growth factor-beta induces development of the T(H)17 lineage. *Nature.* 2006;441:231–234.
100. Happel KI, Dubin PJ, Zheng M, et al. Divergent roles of IL-23 and IL-12 in host defense against Klebsiella pneumoniae. *J Exp Med.* 2005;202:761–769.
101. Akiba H, Takeda K, Kojima Y, et al. The role of ICOS in the CXCR5 follicular B helper T cell maintenance in vivo. *J Immunol.* 2005;175:2340–2348.
102. Villarino A, Hibbert L, Lieberman L, et al. The IL-27R (WSX-1) is required to suppress T cell hyperactivity during infection. *Immunity.* 2003;19:645–655.
103. Bettelli E, Sullivan B, Szabo SJ, et al. Loss of T-bet, but not STAT1, prevents the development of experimental autoimmune encephalomyelitis. *J Exp Med.* 2004;200:79–87.
104. Ziegler SF, Liu YJ. Thymic stromal lymphopoietin in normal and pathogenic T cell development and function. *Nat Immunol.* 2006;7:709–714.
105. Murphy CA, Langrish CL, Chen Y, et al. Divergent pro- and antiinflammatory roles for IL-23 and IL-12 in joint autoimmune inflammation. *J Exp Med.* 2003;198:1951–1957.
106. Park H, Li Z, Yang XO, et al. A distinct lineage of CD4 T cells regulates tissue inflammation by producing interleukin 17. *Nat Immunol.* 2005;6:1133–1141.
107. Langowski JL, Zhang X, Wu L, et al. IL-23 promotes tumour incidence and growth. *Nature.* 2006;442:461–465.
108. Vinuesa CG, Cook MC, Angelucci C, et al. A RING-type ubiquitin ligase family member required to repress follicular helper T cells and autoimmunity. *Nature.* 2005;435:452–458.
109. Stumhofer JS, Laurence A, Wilson EH, et al. Interleukin 27 negatively regulates the development of interleukin 17-producing T helper cells during chronic inflammation of the central nervous system. *Nat Immunol.* 2006;7:937–945.
110. Artis D, Villarino A, Silverman M, et al. The IL-27 receptor (WSX-1) is an inhibitor of innate and adaptive elements of type 2 immunity. *J Immunol.* 2004;173:5626–5634.
111. Batten M, Li J, Yi S, et al. Interleukin 27 limits autoimmune encephalomyelitis by suppressing the development of interleukin 17-producing T cells. *Nat Immunol.* 2006;7:929–936.
112. Veldhoen M, Hocking RJ, Atkins CJ, et al. TGF[beta] in the context of an inflammatory cytokine milieu supports de novo differentiation of IL-17-producing T cells. *Immunity.* 2006;24:179–189.
113. Bettelli E, Carrier Y, Gao W, et al. Reciprocal developmental pathways for the generation of pathogenic effector TH17 and regulatory T cells. *Nature.* 2006;441:235–238.
114. Chen W, Jin W, Hardegen N, et al. Conversion of peripheral CD4+ CD25− naive T cells to CD4+ CD25+ regulatory T cells by TGF-beta induction of transcription factor Foxp3. *J Exp Med.* 2003;198:1875–1886.
115. Vieira PL, Christensen JR, Minaee S, et al. IL-10-secreting regulatory T cells do not express Foxp3 but have comparable regulatory function to naturally occurring CD4+ CD25+ regulatory T cells. *J Immunol.* 2004;172:5986–5993.
116. Tato CM, Laurence A, O'Shea JJ. Helper T cell differentiation enters a new era: le roi est mort; vive le roi! *J Exp Med.* 2006;203:809–812.
117. Zhou B, Comeau MR, De Smedt T, et al. Thymic stromal lymphopoietin as a key initiator of allergic airway inflammation in mice. *Nat Immunol.* 2005;6:1047–1053.
118. Al-Shami A, Spolski R, Kelly J, et al. A role for TSLP in the development of inflammation in an asthma model. *J Exp Med.* 2005;202: 829–839.
119. Wang YH, Ito T, Wang YH, et al. Maintenance and polarization of human TH2 central memory T cells by thymic stromal lymphopoietin-activated dendritic cells. *Immunity.* 2006;24:827–838.
120. Ito T, Wang YH, Duramad O, et al. TSLP-activated dendritic cells induce an inflammatory T helper type 2 cell response through OX40 ligand. *J Exp Med.* 2005;202:1213–1223.
121. Fort MM, Cheung J, Yen D, et al. IL-25 Induces IL-4, IL-5, and IL-13 and Th2-Associated Pathologies In Vivo. *Immunity.* 2001;15:985–995.
122. Schmitz J, Owyang A, Oldham E, et al. IL-33, an Interleukin-1-like Cytokine that Signals via the IL-1 Receptor-Related Protein ST2 and Induces T Helper Type 2-Associated Cytokines. *Immunity.* 2005;23:479–490.

123. Ivanov, II, McKenzie BS, Zhou L, et al. The orphan nuclear receptor RORgammat directs the differentiation program of proinflammatory IL-17(+) T helper cells. *Cell.* 2006;126:1121–1133.
124. Amsen D, Blander JM, Lee GR, et al. Instruction of Distinct CD4 T Helper Cell Fates by Different Notch Ligands on Antigen-Presenting Cells. *Cell.* 2004;117:515–526.
125. Tu L, Fang TC, Artis D, et al. Notch signaling is an important regulator of type 2 immunity. *J Exp Med.* 2005;202:1037–1042.
126. Tacchini-Cottier F, Allenbach C, Otten LA, et al. Notch1 expression on T cells is not required for CD4 T helper differentiation. *Euro J Immunol.* 2004;34:1588–1596.
127. Minter LM, Turley DM, Das P, et al. Inhibitors of gamma-secretase block in vivo and in vitro T helper type 1 polarization by preventing Notch upregulation of Tbx21. *Nat Immunol.* 2005;6:680–688.
128. Szabo SJ, Kim ST, Costa GL, et al. A novel transcription factor, T-bet, directs Th1 lineage commitment. *Cell.* 2000;100:655–669.
129. Szabo SJ, Sullivan BM, Stemmann C, et al. Distinct effects of T-bet in TH1 lineage commitment and IFN-gamma production in CD4 and CD8 T cells. *Science.* 2002;295:338–342.
130. Afkarian M, Sedy JR, Yang J, et al. T-bet is a STAT1-induced regulator of IL-12R expression in naive CD4+ T cells. *Nat Immunol.* 2002;3:549–557.
131. Avni O, Lee D, Macian F, et al. T(H) cell differentiation is accompanied by dynamic changes in histone acetylation of cytokine genes. *Nat Immunol.* 2002;3:643–651.
132. Mullen AC, High FA, Hutchins AS, et al. Role of T-bet in commitment of TH1 cells before IL-12-dependent selection. *Science.* 2001;292:1907–1910.
133. Mullen AC, Hutchins AS, High FA, et al. Hlx is induced by and genetically interacts with T-bet to promote heritable T(H)1 gene induction. *Nat Immunol.* 2002;3:652–658.
134. Pai SY, Truitt ML, Ho IC. GATA-3 deficiency abrogates the development and maintenance of T helper type 2 cells. *Proc Natl Acad Sci U S A.* 2004;101:1993–1998.
135. Zheng W, Flavell RA. The transcription factor GATA-3 is necessary and sufficient for Th2 cytokine gene expression in CD4 T cells. *Cell.* 1997;89:587–596.
136. Zhu J, Min B, Hu-Li J, et al. Conditional deletion of Gata3 shows its essential function in TH1-TH2 responses. *Nat Immunol.* 2004;5:1157–1165.
137. Hutchins AS, Mullen AC, Lee HW, et al. Gene silencing quantitatively controls the function of a developmental trans-activator. *Mol Cell.* 2002;10:81–91.
138. Lee DU, Rao A. Molecular analysis of a locus control region in the T helper 2 cytokine gene cluster: A target for STAT6 but not GATA3. *Proc Natl Acad Sci U S A.* 2004;101:16010–16015.
139. Lee GR, Fields PE, Griffin TJ, et al. Regulation of the Th2 cytokine locus by a locus control region. *Immunity.* 2003;19:145–153.
140. Lighvani AA, Frucht DM, Jankovic D, et al. T-bet is rapidly induced by interferon-gamma in lymphoid and myeloid cells. *Proc Natl Acad Sci U S A.* 2001;98:15137–15142.
141. Mullen AC, Hutchins AS, Villarino AV, et al. Cell cycle controlling the silencing and functioning of mammalian activators. *Curr Biol.* 2001;11:1695–1699.
142. Ouyang W, Lohning M, Gao Z, et al. Stat6-independent GATA-3 autoactivation directs IL-4-independent Th2 development and commitment. *Immunity.* 2000;12:27–37.
143. Hwang ES, Hong JH, Glimcher LH. IL-2 production in developing Th1 cells is regulated by heterodimerization of RelA and T-bet and requires T-bet serine residue 508. *J Exp Med.* 2005;202:1289–1300.
144. Hwang ES, Szabo SJ, Schwartzberg PL, et al. T helper cell fate specified by kinase-mediated interaction of T-bet with GATA-3. *Science.* 2005;307:430–433.
145. Usui T, Preiss JC, Kanno Y, et al. T-bet regulates Th1 responses through essential effects on GATA-3 function rather than on IFNG gene acetylation and transcription. *J Exp Med.* 2006;203:755–766.
146. Kim JI, Ho IC, Grusby MJ, et al. The transcription factor c-Maf controls the production of interleukin-4 but not other Th2 cytokines. *Immunity.* 1999;10:745–751.
147. Chtanova T, Tangye SG, Newton R, et al. T follicular helper cells express a distinctive transcriptional profile, reflecting their role as non-Th1/Th2 effector cells that provide help for B cells. *J Immunol.* 2004;173:68–78.
148. Ichii H, Sakamoto A, Hatano M, et al. Role for Bcl-6 in the generation and maintenance of memory CD8+ T cells. *Nat Immunol.* 2002;3:558–563.
149. Kallies A, Hawkins ED, Belz GT, et al. Transcriptional repressor Blimp-1 is essential for T cell homeostasis and self-tolerance. *Nat Immunol.* 2006;7:466–474.
150. Martins GA, Cimmino L, Shapiro-Shelef M, et al. Transcriptional repressor Blimp-1 regulates T cell homeostasis and function. *Nat Immunol.* 2006;7:457–465.
151. Reiner SL. Epigenetic control in the immune response. *Hum Mol Genet.* 2005;14 Spec No 1:R41–R46.
152. Wilson CB, Merkenschlager M. Chromatin structure and gene regulation in T cell development and function. *Curr Opin Immunol.* 2006;18:143–151.
153. Martins GA, Hutchins AS, Reiner SL. Transcriptional activators of helper T cell fate are required for establishment but not maintenance of signature cytokine expression. *J Immunol.* 2005;175:5981–5985.
154. Ansel KM, Greenwald RJ, Agarwal S, et al. Deletion of a conserved Il4 silencer impairs T helper type 1-mediated immunity. *Nature Immunology.* 2004;5:1251–1259.
155. Grogan JL, Mohrs M, Harmon B, et al. Early transcription and silencing of cytokine genes underlie polarization of T helper cell subsets. *Immunity.* 2001;14:205–215.
156. Hutchins AS, Artis D, Hendrich BD, et al. Cutting edge: a critical role for gene silencing in preventing excessive type 1 immunity. *J Immunol.* 2005;175:5606–5610.
157. Makar KW, Perez-Melgosa M, Shnyreva M, et al. Active recruitment of DNA methyltransferases regulates interleukin 4 in thymocytes and T cells. *Nat Immunol.* 2003;4:1183–1190.
158. Makar KW, Wilson CB. DNA methylation is a nonredundant repressor of the Th2 effector program. *J Immunol.* 2004;173:4402–4406.
159. Belkaid Y, Piccirillo CA, Mendez S, et al. CD4+ CD25+ regulatory T cells control Leishmania major persistence and immunity. *Nature.* 2002;420:502–507.
160. Badovinac VP, Tvinnereim AR, Harty JT. Regulation of antigen-specific CD8+ T cell homeostasis by perforin and interferon-gamma. *Science.* 2000;290:1354–1358.
161. Janssen EM, Lemmens EE, Wolfe T, et al. CD4+ T cells are required for secondary expansion and memory in CD8+ T lymphocytes. *Nature.* 2003;421:852–856.
162. Shedlock DJ, Shen H. Requirement for CD4 T cell help in generating functional CD8 T cell memory. *Science.* 2003;300:337–339.
163. Sun JC, Bevan MJ. Defective CD8 T cell memory following acute infection without CD4 T cell help. *Science.* 2003;300:339–342.
164. Sun JC, Williams MA, Bevan MJ. CD4+ T cells are required for the maintenance, not programming, of memory CD8+ T cells after acute infection. *Nat Immunol.* 2004;5:927–933.
165. Janssen EM, Droin NM, Lemmens EE, et al. CD4+ T-cell help controls CD8+ T-cell memory via TRAIL-mediated activation-induced cell death. *Nature.* 2005;434:88–93.
166. Juedes AE, Rodrigo E, Togher L, et al. T-bet controls autoaggressive CD8 lymphocyte responses in type 1 diabetes. *J Exp Med.* 2004;199:1153–1162.
167. Sullivan BM, Juedes A, Szabo SJ, et al. Antigen-driven effector CD8 T cell function regulated by T-bet. *Proc Natl Acad Sci U S A.* 2003;100:15818–15823.
168. Intlekofer AM, Takemoto N, Wherry EJ, et al. Effector and memory CD8+ T cell fate coupled by T-bet and eomesodermin. *Nat Immunol.* 2005;6:1236–1244.
169. Pearce EL, Mullen AC, Martins GA, et al. Control of effector CD8+ T cell function by the transcription factor Eomesodermin. *Science.* 2003;302:1041–1043.
170. Intlekofer AM, John Wherry E, Reiner SL. Not-so-great expectations: re-assessing the essence of T-cell memory. *Immunol Rev.* 2006;211:203–213.
171. Moulton VR, Farber DL. Committed to memory: lineage choices for activated T cells. *Trends Immunol.* 2006;27:261–267.
172. Manjunath N, Shankar P, Wan J, et al. Effector differentiation is not prerequisite for generation of memory cytotoxic T lymphocytes. *J Clin Invest.* 2001;108:871–878.

173. Sallusto F, Lenig D, Forster R, et al. Two subsets of memory T lymphocytes with distinct homing potentials and effector functions. *Nature.* 1999;401:708–712.
174. Wherry EJ, Teichgraber V, Becker TC, et al. Lineage relationship and protective immunity of memory CD8 T cell subsets. *Nat Immunol.* 2003;4:225–234.
175. Becker TC, Coley SM, Wherry EJ, et al. Bone marrow is a preferred site for homeostatic proliferation of memory CD8 T cells. *J Immunol.* 2005;174:1269–1273.
176. Mazo IB, Honczarenko M, Leung H, et al. Bone marrow is a major reservoir and site of recruitment for central memory CD8+ T cells. *Immunity.* 2005;22:259–270.
177. Fearon DT, Manders P, Wagner SD. Arrested differentiation, the self-renewing memory lymphocyte, and vaccination. *Science.* 2001;293:248–250.
178. Luckey CJ, Bhattacharya D, Goldrath AW, et al. Memory T and memory B cells share a transcriptional program of self-renewal with long-term hematopoietic stem cells. *Proc Natl Acad Sci U S A.* 2006;103:3304–3309.
179. Becker TC, Wherry EJ, Boone D, et al. Interleukin 15 is required for proliferative renewal of virus-specific memory CD8 T cells. *J Exp Med.* 2002;195:1541–1548.
180. Goldrath AW, Sivakumar PV, Glaccum M, et al. Cytokine requirements for acute and basal homeostatic proliferation of naive and memory CD8+ T cells. *J Exp Med.* 2002;195:1515–1522.
181. Tan JT, Ernst B, Kieper WC, et al. Interleukin (IL)-15 and IL-7 jointly regulate homeostatic proliferation of memory phenotype CD8+ cells but are not required for memory phenotype CD4+ cells. *J Exp Med.* 2002;195:1523–1532.
182. Macallan DC, Wallace D, Zhang Y, et al. Rapid turnover of effector-memory CD4(+) T cells in healthy humans. *J Exp Med.* 2004;200:255–260.
183. Zaph C, Uzonna J, Beverley SM, et al. Central memory T cells mediate long-term immunity to Leishmania major in the absence of persistent parasites. *Nat Med.* 2004;10:1104–1110.
184. Manders PM, Hunter PJ, Telaranta AI, et al. BCL6b mediates the enhanced magnitude of the secondary response of memory CD8+ T lymphocytes. *Proc Natl Acad Sci U S A.* 2005;102:7418–7425.
185. Wherry EJ, Barber DL, Kaech SM, et al. Antigen-independent memory CD8 T cells do not develop during chronic viral infection. *Proc Natl Acad Sci U S A.* 2004;101:16004–16009.
186. Barber DL, Wherry EJ, Masopust D, et al. Restoring function in exhausted CD8 T cells during chronic viral infection. *Nature.* 2006;439:682–687.
187. Day CL, Kaufmann DE, Kiepiela P, et al. PD-1 expression on HIV-specific T cells is associated with T-cell exhaustion and disease progression. *Nature.* 2006;443:350–354.
188. Chang JT, Palanivel VR, Kinjyo I, et al. Asymmetric T lymphocyte division in the initiation of adaptive immune responses. *Science* 2007;315:1687–1691.

SECTION V

The Intersection of Innate and Adaptive Immunity

Chapter 14

The Innate Immune System

Ruslan Medzhitov

INTRODUCTION

Host defense against microbial infection is mediated by a variety of mechanisms that fall into two categories: innate and adaptive (or acquired). The adaptive immune system is found only in jawed vertebrates and apparently developed as a result of the acquisition of the recombinase activating gene (RAG) by common ancestors of the vertebrate lineage (1). Accordingly, the adaptive immune system exists only in the context of vertebrate physiology and relies on the function of the RAG genes for somatic recombination of gene segments that encode antigen receptors. Clonal distribution and selection of antigen receptors from a randomly generated and highly diverse repertoire of specificities are the two unifying principles of the adaptive immune system. Innate immunity, however, is an evolutionarily ancient and universal form of host defense found in all multicellular organisms studied.

The vast majority of metazoan species (>98%) rely exclusively on the innate immune system for their defense against microbial infections. The main distinction between innate and adaptive immune systems is in their mechanisms and targets of recognition. The adaptive immune system can recognize an almost unlimited universe of antigens using a somatically generated repertoire of antigen receptors. The innate immune system, however, relies on germline-encoded receptors to detect a limited set of microbial structures that are uniquely associated with microbial infection. Another important distinction is that innate immunity is not a function of a single defined physiologic system; rather, it is a product of multiple and diverse defense mechanisms as discussed in more detail next.

MODULES OF THE INNATE IMMUNE SYSTEM

The innate immune system consists of multiple distinct subsystems, or modules, that perform different functions in host defense. The following is a list of some of the major modules and the immune functions associated with them:

Surface epithelium is an ancient and universal module of innate immunity found in all metazoans. The surface epithelium generally represents the main site of interaction with the microbial world, both pathogenic and commensal, and plays many important functions in protecting the host from pathogen entry as well as in establishing a mutualistic coexistence with commensal microbiota. Accordingly, some types of surface epithelia, notably mucosal epithelium, evolved with specialized functions essential for antimicrobial defense, including the production of mucins that help prevent the attachment and entry of pathogens, and the production of antimicrobial peptides and other microbicidal products that limit the viability and multiplication of pathogens.

The *phagocyte system* is an essential component of innate immunity, particularly in complex metazoans where specialized (or professional) phagocytes (macrophages and neutrophils) perform various host defense functions that rely on phagocytic uptake of pathogens. Phagocytes are equipped with multiple antimicrobial mechanisms that become activated upon the initial contact with pathogens. The phagocyte system is critical for the defense against both intracellular and extracellular bacteria as well as fungal pathogens. The functions of phagocytes are greatly aided by opsonins—secreted proteins that bind to microbial cell walls and facilitate phagocytosis through cell surface receptors specific for them. Opsonins are products of the acute phase response and complement systems.

The *acute phase response and complement* are part of a module consisting of a variety of secreted proteins that function in the circulation and in tissue fluids. These proteins are secreted by hepatocytes in response to the inflammatory cytokines IL-1 and IL-6, and their concentration rises dramatically soon after infection. Acute phase proteins and complement products opsonize pathogens for phagocytic uptake, recruit phagocytes to the site of infection, and have direct antimicrobial activities.

Natural killer (NK) cells are specialized in the elimination of infected host cells and in aiding defense against viral and other intracellular infections through production of cytokines, particularly IFN-γ. The activity of NK cells is regulated by type I interferons (IFN-α/β) either directly or through the induction of IL-15.

Type I IFNs and IFN-induced proteins play a critical role in defense against viral infections. Type I interferons are produced in response to viral infections and trigger the expression of more than a hundred so-called IFN-induced genes, many of which are either known or presumed to have antiviral functions. There are two major modes of IFN-α/β production and action: First, virtually any virally infected cell can produce IFNs-α/β, which act in an autocrine or paracrine fashion to induce an antiviral state in the local site of infection. Second, IFN-α/β can be produced by specialized IFN-producing cells known as *plasmacytoid dendritic cells* (pDC). pDCs produce large amounts of IFN-α/β that can act systemically, and this production does not necessarily require that the pDCs are virally infected themselves. In addition to inducing the antiviral state, IFN-α/β has many other functions in host defense, including the control of NK cell functions.

Mast cells, eosinophils, and basophils are specialized in defense against multicellular parasites, such as helminthes. Although mast cells reside in mucosal and connective tissues, eosinophils and basophils are recruited to the sites of infection from the circulation. These cells play multiple important functions in host defense against parasites through their effects on vasculature and mucosal epithelium to limit parasite spread and to facilitate their excretion from the host organism. They also produce proteins that are toxic to parasites. The function of this module is regulated by several cytokines, including IL-4, IL-5, IL-9, and IL-13.

Importantly, some of the modules of the innate immune system evolved independently from each other and appeared at different stages of phylogeny. For example, surface epithelium and antimicrobial peptides are evolutionarily ancient modules that exist in all metazoans, whereas NK cells and type I interferons are only found in higher vertebrates. NK-mediated killing of virally infected cells is presumably a viable host defense mechanism in complex metazoans with renewable tissues, but not in most invertebrates that are made up of postmitotic cells that do not self-renew. Similarly, mast cells, eosinophils, and basophils and the host defense functions associated with them exist only in vertebrates.

Another important aspect of the modular organization of innate immunity is that some modules are functionally linked with each other, while others are not. The phagocyte system and the acute phase proteins are functionally linked through the inflammatory cytokines (IL-1 and IL-6) produced by phagocytes that stimulate the acute phase response. In turn, many acute phase proteins function as opsonins that facilitate phagocytosis by macrophages and neutrophils.

Another example of functionally coupled modules are NK cells and type I interferons, which cooperate in host defense against viral infections. However, type I interferons and eosinophils/basophils are not functionally linked, presumably because they never become coinduced by the same infection.

Finally, different modules are activated by different sets of receptors of the innate immune system. In fact, different strategies of innate immune recognition have evolved to activate different modules of the innate immune system with their distinct mechanisms of defense from infection.

INNATE IMMUNE RECOGNITION

Strategies of Innate Immune Recognition: Microbial Nonself and Missing Self

The innate immune system uses at least two distinct strategies of immune recognition: recognition of *microbial nonself* and recognition of *missing self*. The first strategy, often referred to as *pattern recognition,* is based on the recognition of molecular structures that are unique to microorganisms and that are not produced by the host (2,3). Recognition of these microbial products directly leads to the activation of immune responses. The second strategy is based on the recognition of molecules expressed only on normal, uninfected cells of the host (4). These molecules function as molecular "flags" of normal (i.e., healthy) self because they are not produced by micro-organisms, and their expression is lost on infected cells. These flags are recognized by inhibitory receptors (e.g., on NK cells), or by proteins that inhibit activation of innate immune effector mechanisms (e.g., factor H of complement). Recognition of missing self plays an important role in the function of NK cells and complement and is discussed in the context of NK and complement biology in Chapters 16 and 34, respectively.

Targets of Innate Immune Recognition

The pattern recognition strategy is based on the detection of conserved molecular structures produced by microbial pathogens, but not by the host organism (3). There are multiple differences between the metabolic pathways of prokaryotic and eukaryotic cells, as well as of protozoan pathogens and multicellular hosts. Some of the pathways that are unique to microbial metabolism have essential physiologic functions and are, therefore, found in all micro-organisms of a given class. The products of these metabolic pathways, as well as some individual gene products, are referred to as *pathogen-associated molecular patterns* (PAMPs) and represent targets of innate immune recognition. The receptors of the innate immune system that evolved to recognize PAMPs are called *pattern-recognition receptors* (PRRs) (2,5). The best-known examples of PAMPs include lipopolysaccharide (LPS) of gram-negative bacteria; lipoteichoic acids (LTA) of gram-positive bacteria; peptidoglycan; lipoproteins generated by palmitylation of the N-terminal cysteines of many bacterial cell wall proteins; lipoarabinomannan of mycobacteria; double-stranded RNA (dsRNA), which is produced by most viruses during the infection cycle; and β-glucans and mannans found in fungal cell walls. All these structures are produced by different classes of microbial pathogens, but importantly, not by the host organisms. Therefore, they function as "molecular signatures" of microbial metabolism, and their recognition by the innate immune system signals the presence of infection. PAMPs derived from different species of pathogens may differ from one another in the details of their chemical structure, but they always share a common molecular pattern. For example, the lipid A region of LPS is highly conserved across a wide range of gram-negative bacteria and is responsible for the pro-inflammatory activity of LPS, whereas the core region and the O side chain can be variable even among closely related strains and are not recognized by the innate immune system. Although different PAMPs are not structurally related to each other, they all share several features that reflect the evolutionary strategy of innate immune recognition (2,5). First, all PAMPs are produced by microbes, but not by the host organism. This is the basis of self/nonself discrimination, a key aspect of innate immune recognition that enables innate and adaptive immune responses to be mounted only against microbial cells and antigens. Second, PAMPs are invariant among pathogens of a given class. This allows a limited number of germline-encoded PRRs to detect any microbial infection. For example, recognition of the conserved lipid-A portion of LPS allows a single PRR to detect the presence of almost any gram-negative bacterial infection. Third, PAMPs often perform physiologic functions that are essential for microbial survival, which means that loss or mutational change of PAMPs would be lethal or at least highly disadvantageous for the micro-organism. Therefore, microbial pathogens are limited in their ability to either mutate or lose expression of PAMPs in order to avoid recognition by the innate immune system. It is important to note that while PAMPs are unique to micro-organisms, they are not unique to pathogens. Indeed, all the known PAMPs are produced by both pathogenic and nonpathogenic (e.g., commensal) micro-organisms. For example, LPS derived from commensal gram-negative bacteria is as potent in inducing host macrophages as LPS derived from pathogenic species of bacteria. This means that the receptors of the innate immune system cannot distinguish between pathogens and nonpathogenic microbes. This distinction, however, clearly has to be made by the innate immune system, because all multicellular organisms live in close and continuous contact with commensal microflora. Failure to tolerate or ignore PAMPs derived from commensal microbes would have disastrous consequences to the host. The mechanisms that allow the innate immune system to distinguish between pathogens and commensals are not well understood. However, anti-inflammatory cytokines (such as IL-10 and TGF-β) and compartmentalization (confinement of the commensals to the apical side of the surface epithelia) play an important role in preventing the inappropriate triggering of innate immune responses.

THE RECEPTORS OF THE INNATE IMMUNE SYSTEM

The innate immune system detects infection using a variety of PRRs that recognize PAMPs and trigger various effector responses (6). Several classes of PRRs that evolved to perform these functions differ in expression profile, localization (cell surface, cytosolic, secreted into serum and tissue fluids), and function. All PRRs can be broadly categorized into three functional classes (Figure 14.1):

1. PRRs that signal the presence of infection. These can be expressed on the cell surface or intracellularly. In either case, recognition of PAMPs by these receptors leads to the activation of "pro-inflammatory" signaling pathways, typically NFκB, interferon regulatory factors (IRFs), Jun N-terminal kinase (JNK), and p38 MAP kinase. Activation of these evolutionarily conserved signaling pathways by PRRs leads to the induction of numerous genes. There are three categories of gene products induced by PRRs: (a) proteins and peptides that have direct antimicrobial effector functions (e.g., antimicrobial peptides and lysozyme); (b) inflammatory cytokines and chemokines (e.g., TNF, IL-1, IL-8) that induce multiple physiologic reactions aimed at optimizing conditions to combat the infection); and (c) gene products that control activation of the adaptive immune response (e.g., MHC, CD80/CD86, IL-12). The best-known receptors of this class are the family of Toll-like receptors (TLRs), Dectin-1, NOD proteins, and RIG-I and MDA-5 proteins.
2. Phagocytic (or endocytic) PRRs. These receptors are expressed on the surface of macrophages, neutrophils, and dendritic cells (DCs). As the name implies, these PRRs recognize PAMPs on pathogen surfaces and mediate their uptake into the phagocytes. Phagocytosed micro-organisms are delivered into lysosomal compartments where they are killed by several effector mechanisms available in phagocytes. In DCs and macrophages, phagocytosis is followed by processing of pathogen-derived proteins and their presentation by MHC molecules for recognition by T cells. PRRs of this class include the macrophage mannose receptor (MR) and MARCO (macrophage receptor with collagenous structure).
3. Secreted PRRs. PRRs of this class perform three types of functions: They activate complement, opsonize microbial cells to facilitate their phagocytosis, and, in the case of some PRRs, function as accessory proteins for PAMP recognition by transmembrane receptors, such as TLRs. Some PRRs are secreted by macrophages and epithelial cells into tissue fluids. Most, however, are secreted into the serum by the liver; many of these are acute phase proteins, as their production is increased dramatically during the acute phase response. Examples of secreted PRRs are the mannan-binding lectin (MBL) and peptidoglycan-recognition proteins (PGRPs).

Toll-like Receptors

The Toll-like receptors play a unique and essential role in innate immune recognition. TLRs comprise a family of type I transmembrane receptors that are characterized by leucine rich repeats (LRRs) in the extracellular portion and an intracellular TIR (Toll/IL-1 receptor) domain, which is homologous to the intracellular domain of IL-1 receptor family members (7,8). LRRs are found in many functionally distinct proteins where they appear to be involved in protein interactions and ligand recognition (9). The TIR domain is a conserved signaling module found in a number of cytoplasmic proteins

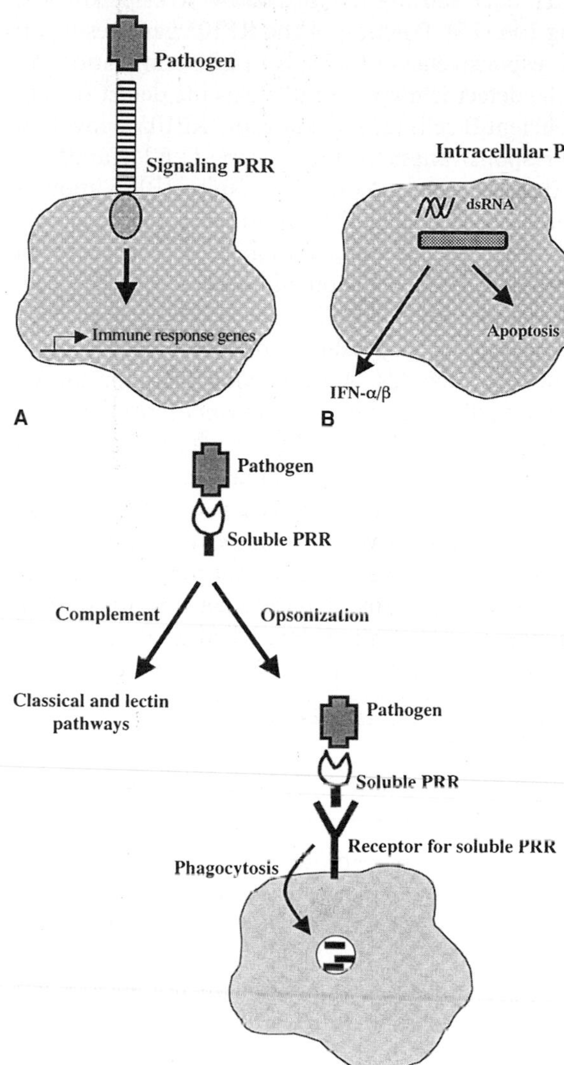

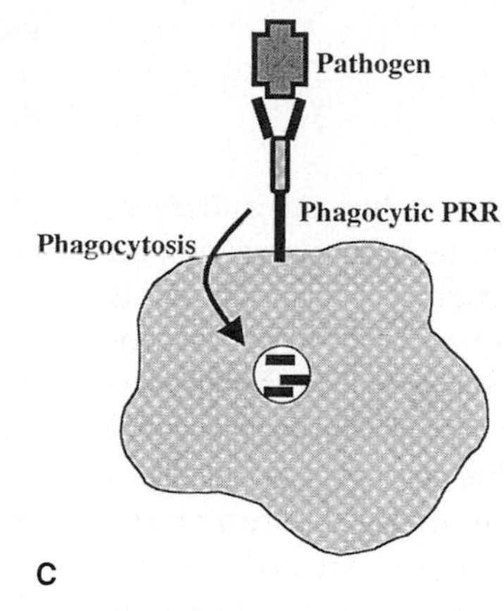

FIGURE 14.1 Functional classes of pattern recognition receptors. **A:** Signaling PRRs recognize pathogens and pathogen-derived products and initiate signaling pathways that induce inflammatory responses. In specialized professional antigen-presenting cells, PRR-triggered signaling pathways also induce the expression of accessory molecules necessary for the induction of adaptive immune responses. **B:** Intracellular PRRs. These receptors recognize intracellular pathogens and pathogen-derived products (e.g., viral dsRNA) and induce production of IFN-α/β, which in turn induces an antiviral state in the infected cell as well as in neighboring cells. In some cases, recognition of an intracellular pathogen can induce apoptosis of the infected cell, thus preventing the pathogen from spreading to other cells of the host. **C:** Phagocytic PRRs bind to pathogens directly, without the aid of opsonins. Binding is followed by phagocytosis and delivery of pathogens or pathogen-derived products into lysosomal compartments. In specialized professional antigen-presenting cells, pathogen-derived proteins are degraded and presented on the cell surface on MHC molecules for recognition by T cells. **D:** Secreted PRRs, upon binding to pathogen cell walls, activate complement and function as opsonins. Both the classical and the lectin pathways of complement can be induced, depending on the PRR. Opsonization is followed by phagocytosis, which is mediated by a receptor expressed on phagocytes that binds to the PRR complexed with the pathogen.

in animals and plants in addition to Tolls and IL-1 receptors. Interestingly, most, if not all, TIR domain–containing proteins in animals and plants are involved in host defense pathways. The number of functional TLRs in mammalian species varies, because of species-specific gene loss. Thus, TLR10 is a pseudogene in mice, but appears to be intact in humans. TLRs 11, 12, and 13, however, are pseudogenes in humans but are intact in mice (10). The reasons for this lineage-specific gene loss are currently unknown. Unlike Drosophila Tolls, all mammalian TLRs function as receptors of the innate immune system. TLRs differ from one another in their expression pattern, their ligand specificities, the signaling pathways they utilize, and the cellular responses they induce. Most TLRs have at least one known ligand (the exceptions are human TLR10 and mouse TLRs 12 and 13). All well-defined TLR ligands are conserved microbial products (PAMPs) derived from all the major classes of pathogens—bacterial, viral, fungal, and protozoan. It is not yet known if any of the TLRs can recognize molecular products associated with multicellular parasites. The PAMPs that are known to signal through TLRs are structurally quite diverse and, importantly, lack any common chemical features. The exact mechanism of PAMP recognition by TLRs is not yet known, but the available information suggests that TLRs either directly recognize their ligands, or at least contribute to direct recognition and, therefore, may function as *bona fide* PRRs (11–13). It is interesting in this regard that at least some of the TLRs can recognize more than one ligand, and again, these ligands can be structurally unrelated to each other (10). Another important feature of TLR-mediated recognition and function is that at least some TLRs use accessory proteins for ligand recognition.

TLRs can be grouped into two classes based on their subcellular localization, signaling mechanisms, and the nature of the ligands they recognize: TLRs 1, 2, 4, 5, and 6 are expressed on the plasma membrane and detect bacterial and fungal cell wall components. TLRs 3, 7, and 9 are expressed in endosomal compartments and recognize viral nucleic acids.

TLR4

TLR4 is expressed on many cell types in humans and mice, most predominantly in the cells of the immune system, including macrophages, DCs, neutrophils, mast cells, and B cells (14). TLR4 is also expressed on various nonhematopoetic cell types, including endothelial cells, fibroblasts, surface epithelial cells, and muscle cells. TLR4 is the signal transducing receptor for LPS. This was discovered by positional cloning of the *Lps* gene in the LPS-unresponsive C3H/HeJ mouse strain (15,16) and by a targeted deletion of the *Tlr4* gene in mice (17). In C3H/HeJ mice, TLR4 fails to signal in response to LPS due to a point mutation in the TIR domain that results in the substitution of proline for histidine at position 712 (15–17). Analysis of C3H/HeJ mice and TLR4 knockout mice demonstrated that TLR4 is absolutely crucial for LPS recognition and responsiveness by macrophages, DCs cells, and B cells. *In vivo* responses to LPS (e.g., endotoxic shock) are also completely abrogated in TLR4-deficient mice (17). The mechanism of LPS recognition by TLR4 is quite complex and requires several accessory proteins. LPS first binds to LBP (LPS-binding protein), a serum protein that binds LPS monomers and transfers them to CD14 (18). CD14 is a GPI-linked protein expressed on the surface of macrophages and some subsets of DCs. CD14 also exists as a soluble protein in the serum. Both forms of CD14 bind LPS with high affinity (18). The mechanism of CD14 function is unknown but appears to be important for LPS recognition, as demonstrated by the profound defect in LPS responsiveness in CD14-deficient mice (19). The ectodomain of TLR4 is associated with another accessory protein called MD-2. MD-2 is a small protein that lacks a transmembrane domain but is expressed on the cell surface in a complex with TLR4 (20). The function of MD-2 is not known except that it is required for LPS recognition by TLR4 (21). Several experimental approaches have indicated that TLR4 and MD-2 make a direct contact with LPS (11–13), although much remains to be learned about the composition of the TLR4 complex and the mechanism of LPS recognition. The issue of LPS recognition is complicated even further by the discovery of another cell-surface receptor that appears to cooperate with TLR4 in LPS recognition in B cells. This protein, called RP105 (22), is expressed on B cells and some subsets of DCs and has an ectodomain closely related to that of TLR4. Similar to TLR4, RP105 is associated through its ectodomain with an accessory protein called MD-1, which is a homolog of MD-2 (23,24). Unlike TLR4, RP105 lacks a TIR domain, and instead has a short cytoplasmic tail that contains the tyrosine phosphorylation motif, YXXI (22). Cross-linking of RP105 leads to B cell proliferation and upregulation of CD80/CD86 costimulatory molecules, similar to the effect of LPS stimulation (23). RP105 is also known to induce activation of Src-family tyrosine kinases, including Lyn (25). Deletion of the RP105 gene results in reduced responsiveness of B cells to LPS stimulation, although the defect is not as complete as the defect seen in TLR4-deficient B cells (26). In addition, RP105 is involved in B cell responsiveness to at least some TLR2 ligands, including bacterial lipoproteins (27). Thus, RP105 appears to cooperate with TLR2 and TLR4 in lipoprotein and LPS recognition by B cells, but the molecular mechanism of this cooperation in recognition and signaling remains unknown.

In addition to LPS, TLR4 is involved in recognition of several other ligands. A heat-sensitive factor associated with the cell walls of *Mycobacterium tuberculosis* was shown to signal through TLR4, but the chemical nature of the ligand is not yet known (28). TLR4 along with CD14 was also shown to mediate responsiveness to the fusion (F) protein of respiratory syncytial virus (RSV) (29). However, it is not clear yet whether TLR4 recognizes some feature of the F protein that is shared with other viral fusion proteins. In other words, it is not clear whether TLR4 evolved to recognize the F protein, or if the F protein evolved to bind to TLR4 and trigger its activation because it provides some unknown benefit to RSV.

TLR2, TLR1, and TLR6

TLR2 is involved in recognition of a surprisingly broad range of microbial products. These include lipoteichoic acids (LTA) and peptidoglycan from gram-positive bacteria (30,31), bacterial lipoproteins (32–34), mycoplasma lipoprotein (34,35), mycobacterial lipoarabinomannan (28,36), a phenol-soluble modulin from *Staphylococcus epidermidis* (37), zymosan of yeast cell walls (38), and glycosylphosphotidylinositol from *Trypanosoma cruzi* (39). TLR2 was also shown to mediate recognition of two kinds of atypical LPS, one derived from *Leptospira interrogans* (40) and the other from *Porphyromonas gingivitis* (41). In terms of their structure, most of these ligands are completely distinct from each other. It is puzzling, then, how all these different microbial products can signal through the same receptor. Although the answer to this question is unknown at the moment, there are at least two factors that can help explain the broad range of ligands recognized by TLR2. One is the use of accessory proteins. Indeed, recognition of some TLR2 ligands (e.g., peptidoglycan) requires CD14 (18), and recognition of lipoproteins requires CD36 (42). As mentioned earlier, RP105 is also involved in recognition of some TLR2 ligands. It is quite possible that recognition of other TLR2 ligands may be assisted by additional accessory proteins. Different accessory proteins could conceivably recognize structurally distinct PAMPs and then bind to and trigger TLR2. The second factor that contributes to the diversity of TLR2 ligands is the cooperation of TLR2 with two other TLRs, TLR1 and TLR6, such that the TLR2/TLR1 heterodimer recognizes one set of ligands, whereas the TLR2/TLR6 heterodimer recognizes a different set of ligands (35,43). These observations were made using mice with targeted deletions in either the TLR2 or TLR6 genes: While both triacylated (tripalmitylated) bacterial lipopeptides and MALP-2 (mycoplasmal macrophage-activating lipopeptide 2kD) failed to signal in TLR2 knockout cells, only MALP-2 (but not tripalmitylated bacterial lipopeptides) required TLR6 for cellular responsiveness (35). Recognition of tripalmitylated lipopeptides, however, requires the TLR2 and TLR1 heterodimer (10). *In vitro* studies, which showed that TLR2 can heterodimerize and signal cooperatively with TLR1 and TLR6 (43), are also consistent with these observations. Interestingly, the only relevant difference between the two ligands is that bacterial lipopeptides have a third palmityl chain attached to the amino group of their N-terminal cysteine, while MALP-2 does not. It is not yet known if any of the other TLRs can heterodimerize for ligand recognition and signaling, but *in vitro* studies suggest that at least TLR4 and TLR5 may function as homodimers (43). TLR2 is expressed constitutively on macrophages, DCs, and B cells and can be induced in some other cell types, including epithelial cells. TLR1 and TLR6, however, are expressed almost ubiquitously (44). In human DCs, expression of TLR2 and TLR4 is restricted to monocyte-derived DCs. Accordingly, this subtype of DCs, but not plasmocytoid DCs, respond to TLR2 and TLR4 ligands (LPS and peptidoglycan, respectively) by producing IL-12 and other inflammatory cytokines (45–47).

TLR3

TLR3 functions as a receptor for dsRNA (48). dsRNA is a molecular pattern associated with viral infections, as most viruses produce dsRNA at some point of their infection cycle. dsRNA and its synthetic analog, poly(IC), have long been known to activate inflammatory responses. As discussed in the next sections, dsRNA is also recognized by the intracellular recognition systems that mediate antiviral responses in infected cells. TLR3 can mediate responses to poly(IC), and TLR3 knockout mice and cells are deficient in their responsiveness to poly(IC) and viral dsRNA (48). TLR3 is expressed on DCs, macrophages, and surface epithelial cells, including intestinal epithelium. In the mouse, TLR3 is expressed in $CD8^+$ DCs, which are known to be particularly efficient in cross-presentation of antigens by MHC class I molecules. $CD8^+$ DCs have also been demonstrated to present antigens derived from virally infected apoptotic cells. Interestingly, viral dsRNA present in apoptotic cells is recognized by TLR3 expressed by $CD8^+$ DCs, and this recognition is important for cross-presentation of viral antigens to CD8 T cells (49). These findings strongly suggest that TLR3 is involved in viral recognition, although the contribution of TLR3 to antiviral immunity remains to be demonstrated.

TLR5

TLR5 is the receptor for flagellin, the protein that polymerizes to form bacterial flagella (50). An interesting aspect of this TLR ligand is that, unlike most other PAMPs, flagellin does not undergo any posttranslational modifications that would distinguish it from cellular proteins. However, flagellin is extremely conserved at its amino- and carboxyl-termini, which presumably explains why it can be a target for innate immune recognition. TLR5 is expressed on epithelial cells as well as on macrophages and DCs, particularly the DCs present in the lamina propria (51). Interestingly, expression of TLR5 on intestinal epithelium is polarized such that TLR5 is expressed only on the basolateral side of the cell (52). Since pathogenic but not commensal microbes cross the epithelial barrier, confining TLRs to the basolateral side may help the host to distinguish between pathogenic and commensal microbes, although this notion has not yet been experimentally proven.

TLR7

TLR7 shares many functional properties with TLR9. Both receptors are involved in viral recognition and both detect nucleic acids. TLR7 recognizes viral ssRNA (derived from RNA viruses), whereas TLR9 recognizes unmethylated DNA derived from DNA viruses (discussed later) (10). Consistent with their function in viral recognition, both receptors are expressed primarily by plasmacytoid dendritic cells (pDC) and utilize similar signal transduction pathways for the induction of type-I interferons. TLR7 was first shown to be activated by small antiviral compounds, such as imiquimod (10). Subsequent studies have shown that TLR7 is responsible for recognition of ssRNA from a variety of RNA viruses, including Sendai virus and influenza virus (53–55). Endocytosis of viruses by pDCs leads to uncoating of viral RNA genomes, which are recognized by TLR7 in the acidic environment of late endoseomes and lysosomes. This recognition generally does not require viral infection and replication in pDC. Interestingly, however, in the case of some viruses, including vesicular stomatitis virus (VSV), TLR7-mediated recognition of viral RNA and IFN-α production were found to require viral infection and replication in pDC. Viral replication and production of viral RNA occurs in the cytosol whereas TLR7-mediated recognition takes place inside the late lysosomes; therefore, the viral RNA somehow has to gain access to lysosomes. It was found that the delivery of viral RNA to lysosomes occurs via autophagy—a process whereby cellular constituents, including organelles and portions of cytosol, become engulfed by internal membranes into specialized vesicles (autophagosomes) that fuse with and deliver their content to the lysosomes (56).

Interestingly, TLR7 appears to be able to recognize ssRNA regardless of its origin (cellular or viral). Normally only viral RNA is efficiently delivered to lysosomes through endocytosis of virions or autophagy of viral RNA. Whether and how the autophagic process can discriminate between viral and cellular RNAs is unclear. Self-RNA, usually in the form of RNA-protein complexes, can be released into the extracellular space from dying cells. However, the concentration of self-RNA in extracellular fluids is normally very low due to efficient removal of apoptotic cells by macrophages and due to activity of RNAses that degrade extracellular RNA. However, when removal of apoptotic cells is compromised (e.g., due to genetic defects in phagocytic pathways), the amount of self-RNA can rise to the levels sufficient to activate TLR7 in pDC and B cells. This can result in activation of autoreactive B cell responses directed at self-RNA–protein complexes and can lead to the development of systemic autoimmune diseases such as lupus (57).

TLR9

DNA that contains unmethylated CpG dinucleotides has long been known for its immunostimulatory properties (58,59). Oligonucleotides that contain unmethylated CpG motifs strongly induce B cell proliferation and cytokine production by dendritic cells and murine macrophages (58,59). Permutation of a single nucleotide or methylation of the CpG motif results in a complete loss of activity (58,59). The stimulatory property of CpG DNA is due to its ability to trigger TLR9 (60). TLR9 knockout mice are completely unresponsive to CpG DNA, demonstrating that all the known effects of CpG DNA are mediated by this TLR (60). Signaling by CpG DNA requires its internalization into late endosomal/lysosomal compartments (59,61). Optimal responsiveness to CpG DNA by mouse versus human cells requires a slightly different sequence motif flanking the CpG dinucleotide (58). Interestingly, the CpG motifs that preferentially stimulate mouse cells also induce a much stronger activation of transfected mouse TLR9, and correspondingly, the CpG motif that elicits optimal responsiveness in human cells preferentially activates transfected human TLR9. This observation suggests that TLR9 itself can distinguish between the two CpG motifs and, therefore, that it presumably recognizes CpG DNA directly (62). Similar to TLR7, expression of TLR9 in humans is restricted to B cells and plasmocytoid dendritic cells, whereas in the mouse, TLR9 is also expressed in macrophages and conventional DCs. Expression of TLR9 in type I INF–producing plasmacytoid DCs (45–47) suggested that TLR9 may be involved in antiviral host defense. Indeed, it was demonstrated that TLR9 is involved in recognition of DNA viruses, such as herpes simplex virus (HSV). Viral genomic DNA becomes accessible to TLR9 in acidified lysosomes following endocytosis and uncoating of virions (63).

While more prevalent in bacterial and viral genomes, unmethylated CpG DNA is present in the mammalian genomes and can trigger TLR9 activation under certain conditions. Similar to the situation with TLR7 and self-RNA–protein complexes, chromatin complexes containing immunostimulatory CpG DNA can be found in the extracellular environment when the removal of apoptotic cells (the major source of self-nucleic acids) is compromised in some way. Indeed, it has been shown that chromatin fragments derived from apoptotic cells can efficiently stimulate B cell activation via TLR9, provided that B cell receptors can recognize and internalize these complexes, whether directly or through recognition of immune complexes containing chromatin fragments (64). The requirement for B cell receptor involvement is presumably due to its ability to deliver CpG DNA to TLR9 in lysosomal compartment. Other receptors capable of delivering chromatin complexes to lysosomes (e.g., Fc receptors) can also promote TLR9 activation in DCs.

Activation of TLR9 by chromatin complexes was initially thought to contribute to the development of pathogenic autoantibodies and the development of lupus. Interestingly, however, TLR9-induced antibodies, particularly of IgM class, can actually contribute to protection from lupus, because these antibodies help to clear chromatin complexes from the circulation. Why this is not the case for TLR7 and its ligands is not yet clear. Currently available evidence in the mouse model indicates that TLR7 and TLR9 play distinct (and perhaps even opposite) roles in promoting or protecting from lupus development, respectively (57).

TLR11

TLRs 11, 12, and 13 are found in mice but not in humans. Mouse TLR11 was found to play a role in defense against uropathogenic infections (65). In addition, TLR11 was found to play a critical role in immunity against a parasitic protozoan *Toxoplasma Gondii* (66). *T. gondii* infection results in the induction of a robust Th1 immune response in mice, which is required for protection from infection. The major immunostimulatory activity was found to be present in the soluble antigen extract of *T. gondii* tachyzoites (STAg). The active component of STAg was found to be profilin—a cytoskeletal protein. Profilin, in turn, was shown to be a potent activator of TLR11. Activation of TLR11 by profilin leads to the production of IL-12 and other cytokines by CD8α DCs, which results in the induction of protective Th1 immune responses. Profilin is also a major immunodominant antigen of recognition of *T. gondii*, and this property was shown to be due to its ability to stimulate TLR11.

TLR Signaling Pathways

Activation of TLRs by microbial products leads to the induction of numerous genes that function in inflammatory and immune responses. These include cytokines, (e.g., TNF, IL-1, IL-6, and IL-12), inflammatory chemokines (e.g., the neutrophil chemoattractant IL-8), antimicrobial effector molecules (e.g., inducible nitric oxide synthase and antimicrobial peptides), and MHC and costimulatory molecules (7,8,14). Stimulation of TLRs activates several signaling pathways, including the NF-κB pathway, as well as three MAP kinase signaling pathways, JNK, p38, and ERK (7,8,14). In addition, TLRs induce the activation of several members of the IRF family of transcription factors.

Specificity of signaling pathways activated by TLRs is controlled by four receptor-proximal adaptor proteins: MyD88, TIRAP, TRAM, and TRIF. All four adaptors contain TIR domains that are involved in homophilic TIR–TIR interactions with each other and with TIR domains of TLRs. MyD88 controls a canonical TLR signaling pathway and is utilized by all TLRs with the exception of TLR3, as well as by the members of the IL-1 receptor family. In addition to the TIR domain, MyD88 contains a death domain, which is also involved in homophilic interactions. In response to receptor activation, MyD88 is recruited to the receptor complex and initiates the downstream signaling cascade. The components of the MyD88 signaling pathway include serine/threonine protein kinases of the IRAK family (IRAK1 and IRAK4), the ubiquitin ligase TRAF6 (TNF receptor–associated factor 6), and several members of the MAP3K family, including TAK1, ASK1, and MEKKs, which are responsible for activation of NF-κB and three MAP kinase cascades: JNK, p38, and ERK (10).

In addition to IRAKs 1 and 4, two closely related kinases, IRAK2 and IRAKM, have also been identified and have been reported to function in the TLR and IL-1R signaling pathways (67,68). While function of IRAK2 is currently unknown, IRAKM is a negative regulator of MyD88-dependent signaling. Recruitment of IRAKs 1 and 4 to the receptors results in IRAK4 activation and phosphorylation of IRAK1, followed by their dissociation from the receptor complex. Once IRAK1 is phosphorylated, it interacts with and activates TRAF6 (69,70). TRAF6 is a member of the TRAF family of RING-finger E3 ubiquitin ligases (71). Other members of the TRAF family mediate signal transduction by receptors of the TNF receptor superfamily (72). Activation of TRAF6 is thought to be triggered by oligomerization induced by interaction with phosphorylated IRAK. Once activated, TRAF6 functions in concert with the noncanonical E2 ubiquitin–conjugating enzymes, Ubc13 and Uev1A, to conjugate polyubiquitin chains onto itself (and perhaps other as yet unidentified targets) (71). Unlike the polyubiquitin chains that target substrates for degradation by the 26S proteasome, which are linked through K48 of ubiquitin, TRAF6 catalyzes conjugation of noncanonical K63-linked polyubiquitin chains (71). In *in vitro* reconstitution systems, this ubiquitination event is necessary and sufficient for subsequent activation of the IκB kinase (IKK) complex by the kinase TAK1 (73). As TAK1 does not seem to be a target of ubiquitination, how autoubiqutination of TRAF6 activates TAK1 is not yet clear. Nevertheless, TRAF6-activated TAK1 phosphorylates IKK-β, which leads to activation of the NF-κB pathway (see later discussion) (73). In addition, TRAF6-activated TAK1 also phosphorylates the MAP kinase MKK6, which in turn phosphorylates the MAPK JNK. Therefore, activation of TAK1 by a TRAF6-catalyzed ubiquitination reaction leads to activation of both the NF-κB and AP-1 pathways (73). The NF-κB family of transcription factors plays a crucial role in innate immunity. In flies as well as mammals, most inducible host defense genes are critically regulated, at least in part, by the NF-κB pathway (74,75). NF-κB is usually composed of a heterodimer of two Rel/NF-κB family transactivators (most commonly p50 and p65) bound to an inhibitory subunit called IκB (inhibitor of κB). In unstimulated cells, IκB masks the nuclear localization signal on NF-κB and thus blocks its nuclear translocation. Upon stimulation by TLR ligands and IL-1 (as well as other signals), IκB is rapidly phosphorylated and degraded by the 26S proteasome. Freed of its cytosolic inhibitor, NFκB can then translocate to the nucleus, where it turns on expression of target genes (74,75). Phosphorylation-dependent degradation of IκB, a pivotal checkpoint in activating NFκB, is controlled by the IKK complex (76). The IKK complex consists of two kinases, IKK-α and IKK-β, and a third noncatalytic subunit, IKK-γ. Mutagenesis studies have established serines 32 and 36 of IκB as the targets of IKK β phosphorylation (76). Phosphorylation at these sites enables recognition of IκB by the F-box/WD protein, β-TrCP, the receptor subunit of a multisubunit SCF ubiquitin ligase complex that subsequently ubiquitinates IκB, thereby targeting IκB for degradation (74,75).

While all TLRs (except TLR3) and IL-1R family members use the MyD88 dependent signaling pathways described earlier, in the case of some TLRs, MyD88 engages additional components for signal transduction. Thus, activation of MyD88 signaling downstream of TLR2 and TLR4 requires an additional adaptor called TIRAP. In addition to a TIR domain, TIRAP contains a phosphoinositide (2,5) biphosphate (PIP2) binding domain. TIRAP associates with the plasma membrane through its PIP2 binding region and recruits MyD88 to TLR2 and TLR4 receptor complexes.

In addition to the recruitment and activation of IRAKs, MyD88 associates with and activates several members of the IRF family. Specifically, MyD88 recruits IRF1 and IRF5. These IRFs in turn play a critical role in transcription of target genes, including inflammatory cytokines and chemokines. IRF1 is an IFN-γ–inducible gene and induction of IRF1 by IFN-γ provides an important mechanism of synergy between IFN-γ and TLR ligands in the induction of multiple genes in macrophages. IRF4 can also associate with MyD88 but plays an inhibitory role by competing with IRF1 and IRF5 for MyD88 binding. Finally, TLR7 and TLR9, but not other TLRs, can induce activation of IRF7 in a MyD88-dependent fashion. Downstream of these receptors, MyD88 associates with and activates IRF7, which plays a critical role in induction of IFN-α genes by these TLRs in pDCs. Activation of IRF7 depends on ubiquitination by TRAF6, as well as on phosphorylation. Three kinases, IRAK1, IRAK4, and IKK-α, have been demonstrated to be responsible for IRF7 phosphorylation (77). The mechanism responsible for TLR-specific activation of IRF7 is currently unknown.

In addition to the MyD88-dependent signaling pathway described earlier, TLR4 and TLR3 signal through a distinct signaling pathway via the adaptor called *TRIF*. TRIF can directly bind to TLR3 and indirectly to TLR4 via another adaptor called *TRAM*. Activation of TRIF leads to the induction of the IKK-related kinases TBK-1 and IKK-ε. TBK-1 in particular plays a critical role in phosphorylation and activation of IRF3, a transcription factor involved in the induction of type I IFNs in most cell types. In addition to IRF3 activation, TRIF induces NF-κB and MAP kinases via TRAF6 and RIP1. These pathways synergize with IRF3 in the induction of IFN-β and other target genes (77).

The diversity of signaling pathways activated by TLRs presumably reflects their differential role in defense against different classes of pathogens. With the exception of TLRs 3, 7, and 9, which are all involved in viral recognition and induction of type I IFNs, it is not yet clear why some of the other differences in signaling pathways exist. For example, it is not yet obvious why TLR4, but not TLR2, can activate the IRF3 signaling pathway. These questions will likely be answered by the future analyses of TLR signaling and function in host defense.

Phagocytic Receptors

Scavenger Receptors

Scavenger receptors (SRs) are cell-surface glycoproteins that are defined by their ability to bind to modified low-density lipoprotein (LDL) (78). There are six classes of structurally unrelated SRs (79). The class A SRs include the macrophage SR (SR-A), the founding member of the SR family, and MARCO (macrophage receptor with collagenous structure). Both SR-A and MARCO are type II transmembrane glycoproteins that contain a collagenous region and a so-called scavenger receptor cysteine-rich (SRCR) domain. The SR-A isoforms generated by alternative splicing are referred to as SR-AI and SR-AII. SR-AII is the shorter isoform that lacks the C-terminal SRCR domain. Both SR-A and MARCO are homotrimeric proteins. SR-A also contains an α-helical–coiled coil region that is absent in MARCO. SR-A is expressed in most macrophage subtypes, as well as in endothelial cells. This receptor has an unusually broad ligand specificity and has been reported to bind, in addition to oxidized and acetylated LDL, a variety of microbial ligands, including gram-negative and gram-positive bacteria, LPS, LTA, and poly(IC) (78). Interestingly, SR-AI and SR-AII have almost identical ligand-binding specificities, suggesting that the SRCR domain is not required for ligand binding. Indeed, binding of the polyanionic ligands has been shown to be mediated by the collagenous domain (78). The role of SR-A in host defense is demonstrated by the increased susceptibility of SR-A–deficient mice to *Listeria monocytogenes*, HSV, and malaria infection (80). SR-A–deficient mice are also more susceptible to endotoxic shock than wild-type mice, suggesting that SR-A may be involved in the clearance of LPS from the circulation (81). MARCO is expressed predominantly in the macrophages of the marginal zone of the spleen, but its expression can be induced in other macrophage subsets by LPS and inflammatory cytokines (82,83). MARCO binds gram-positive and gram negative bacteria but not yeast zymosan (82,83) and mediates phagocytosis of bound bacteria (82,84). Unlike SR-A, MARCO binds its ligands through the SRCR domain (85). A definitive demonstration of the role of MARCO in host defense will have to await the generation of MARCO-deficient mice.

Macrophage Mannose Receptor

The MR is a 175-kD type I transmembrane protein expressed primarily in macrophages (86). The MR contains cysteine-rich and fibronectin type 2 domains at the N-terminus followed by eight carbohydrate recognition domains (CRD) of the C-type lectin family (86,87). Individual CRDs of the MR appear to have different carbohydrate specificities, with CRD4 being primarily responsible for mannose specificity (88). Although the MR has been implicated in the recognition of microbial carbohydrates, it can also recognize oligo-mannoses found in host-derived, high-mannose asparagine-linked carbohydrates. Indeed, in addition to microbial ligands, the MR has been shown to endocytose several host-derived, high-mannose glycoproteins (89). Although the MR appears to be a multiligand receptor and may have several physiologic roles, the main function of MR is thought to be in phagocytosis of micro-organisms (86,89). Indeed, the MR has been implicated in the phagocytosis of a variety of pathogens. Many of these studies are based on the inhibition of MR-mediated phagocytosis by soluble carbohydrate ligands, such as mannan. As micro-organisms contain multiple carbohydrate ligands that presumably engage several receptors on the host cell, some of these analyses are inconclusive and will need to be confirmed using MR-deficient macrophages. A combination of inhibition and transfection studies demonstrated that MR is involved in phagocytosis of bacterial (*M. tuberculosis, Pseudomonas aeruginosa, Klebsiella pneumoniae*), fungal (*Saccharomyces cerevisiae, Candida albicans*), and protozoan pathogens (*Pneumocystis carinii*) (86,89). Upon recognition of microbial ligands, the MR presumably delivers them to the late endosome/lysosome. Thus, the MR was shown to deliver mycobacterial lipoglycan lipoarabinomannan (LAM) into the late endosomal compartment where LAM binds to CD1b for subsequent presentation to T cells (90). While the MR clearly can mediate phagocytosis of micro-organisms, the outcome of MR-mediated phagocytosis is not well defined and appears to depend on several factors, including the activation and differentiation status of the macrophage. At least some carbohydrate structures recognized by the MR on micro-organisms (e.g., α-linked branched oligo-mannoses) are similar to mammalian high-mannose oligosaccharides. However, these structures may be present as particulate ligands (in the context of a microbial cell), or as soluble ligands (in host glycoproteins). As the mechanism of uptake differs for particulate and soluble ligands, the effect of MR ligation may be distinct depending on the origin of the carbohydrate that is bound. The most important factor influencing the outcome of MR ligation by microbial versus host-derived ligand, however, is the co-ligation of the microbial cell by other cell-surface receptors, in particular the TLRs. Some of the results implicating the MR in inducing cytokine production may be due to the co-engagement of TLRs by complex microbial structures, such as yeast cell walls. The MR is structurally related to DEC205, a member of the C-type lectin family expressed preferentially on dendritic cells (91). Although the binding of DEC205 to microbial cell walls has not yet been demonstrated, this protein is very likely to function as a PRR, given the high degree of similarity between the CRD domain structures of the MR and DEC205. Moreover, DEC205 has been shown to direct bound material into antigen-processing compartments in DCs (91), supporting the notion that it may function as a phagocytic PRR.

Dectin-1

Dectin-1 is a type II transmembrane receptor that contains one CRD at the C-terminal portion of the protein and an atypical ITAM motif in the N-terminal, cytoplasmic region (92). The CRD of dectin-1 belongs to the C-type lectinlike subfamily of the CTL domain. Unlike the classical CTL domain, the C-type lectinlike domain lacks amino acid residues required for calcium binding and, therefore, binds its ligands in a calcium-independent manner. Dectin-1 was first identified as a DC-specific lectin, but was later found to be expressed on macrophages as well (93). An expression-cloning approach led to the identification of dectin-1 as a β-glucan receptor (93). Dectin-1 is specific for β-1,3–linked and β-1,6–linked glucans, which are PAMPs found in fungal and other microbial cell walls. Dectin-1 binds and phagocytoses β-glucan–rich zymosan and functions as a phagocytic PRR on macrophages and DCs (93).

Zymosan recognition is mediated by both TLR2 and Dectin-1, and analysis of macrophage responses to zymosan revealed that the two receptors cooperate to induce unique TLR2 and Dectin-1–dependent responses. Importantly, the ITAM motif of Dectin-1 was found to be tyrosine phosphorylated upon receptor ligation. This phosphorylation results in the recruitment of Syk-27 tyrosine kinase, which initiates downstream signal transduction (94,95). The Dectin-specific signaling pathway was dissected using the β-glucan, curdlan, which activates Dectin but not TLR2. Interestingly, the Dectin-induced signaling pathway is remarkably similar to the antigen receptor–induced signaling pathway. Indeed, in addition to Syk-72 kinase, both antigen receptors and Dectin-1 utilize CARD-coiled-coil adaptor proteins to link to the Bcl10-Malt1 complex and activate NF-κB and MAP kinases (96,97). Antigen receptors employ the adaptor Carma1, whereas Dectin-1 uses CARD9. In addition, activation of Syk-72 leads to Ca^{+2} mobilization and activation of the transcription factor NFAT. The target genes induced by Dectin-1 include IL-2 and IL-10, as well as inflammatory cytokines. Importantly, Dectin-1 induces expression of IL-23, but not IL-12 through the selective induction of the p19 and p40 subunits of IL-23, and the lack of induction of the p35 subunit of IL-12. Analysis of Dectin-1–deficient mice demonstrated that Dectin plays a critical role in antifungal defense. Specifically, Dectin-1 was found to be required for host defense against *Candida albicans* (94,95).

Secreted Pattern-recognition Molecules

Secreted pattern-recognition receptors (or pattern-recognition molecules, PRMs), similar to PRRs expressed on the cell surface, are specific to microbial PAMPs, but their physiologic roles in host defense are different. The two main functions of secreted PRMs are activation of complement and opsonization of microbial cells for phagocytosis. In addition, some secreted PRMs have direct bactericidal effects on bound bacteria. Soluble PRMs are produced and secreted into the circulation mainly by the liver (primarily by hepatocytes), and to a lesser degree by several other cell types, including phagocytes. The serum concentration of these PRMs increases dramatically during the acute-phase response, a systemic inflammatory response induced by inflammatory cytokines such as IL-6, IL-1, and TNF-α. Secreted PRMs, therefore, are sometimes referred to as *acute-phase proteins*. Depending on their domain composition, secreted PRMs fall into four major structural classes: collectins, pentraxins, lipid transferases, and PGRPs. The function of each of these classes will be discussed next.

Collectins

Collectins comprise a group of structurally related PRMs characterized by the presence of a carbohydrate recognition domain of the C-type lectin family at the C-terminus, and a collagenous domain at the N-terminus (98). The CRD domains of the collectins are engaged in ligand recognition, whereas the collagenous portions are responsible for the effector functions, such as activation of the complement cascade. All collectins form multimers in solution, which permits higher avidity interactions with their cognate ligands (99). Multimerization is also responsible for orienting the CRD domains such that they match the spatial arrangement of their carbohydrate ligands on the microbial surface, thereby allowing the collectins to distinguish microbial carbohydrates from mannose residues on self-glycoproteins (100). MBL is the best-characterized member of the collectin family. MBL binds to terminal mannose and fucose residues in a calcium-dependent manner and has been reported to recognize a broad range of pathogens, including gram-positive (*Staphylococcus aureus, Streptococcus pneumonia*) and gram-negative (*P. aeruginosa, K. pneumonia, Escherichia coli, Salmonella enteritidus*) bacteria; mycobacteria (*M. tuberculosis*); yeast (*Cryptococcus neoformans, C. albicans, S. cerevisiae*); viruses (influenza A, HSV, HIV); and protozoan pathogens (*T. cruzi, P. carinii*) (101). The main function of MBL is to activate the lectin pathway of complement. MBL is associated with two serine proteases, MASP-1 and MASP-2 (MBL-associated serine proteases). Upon binding to microbial cells, MBL induces a conformational change in the associated MASPs that leads to MASP activation, similar to the activation of C1r and C1s by antibody-bound C1q. Activated MASPs then cleave C2 and C4 complement components, thus initiating the complement cascade. In addition to the triggering of the lectin pathway of complement, MBL can function as an opsonin. MBL bound to pathogen cell walls promotes phagocytosis by interacting with C1qRp, a receptor for C1q and MBL expressed on phagocytes (101). Surfactant proteins A and D (SP-A and SP-D) are collectins expressed in the lung and secreted by airway epithelial cells into the alveolar fluid. Both SP-A and SP-D interact with a variety of pathogens, including gram-positive and gram-negative bacteria, fungi, and several viruses (102). Similar to MBL, SP-A and SP-D recognize terminal mannose, fucose, and N-acetyl glucosamine residues expressed on microbial surfaces. SP-A and SP-D proteins function as opsonins and bind to several macrophage receptors that mediate the phagocytosis of the bound micro-organism (99). SP-A, similar to MBL and C1q, binds C1qRp expressed on macrophages. SP-D binds to Gp340 (also known as hensin), a receptor expressed in macrophages and epithelial cells (102). It is not yet clear if Gp340 plays any role in phagocytosis (102). SP-A–deficient mice show increased susceptibility to infection with a number of bacterial, fungal, and viral pathogens—for example, *Group B streptococci, S. aureus, P. aeruginosa, K. pneumoniae, P. carinii,* and respiratory syncytial virus (RSV) (102). SP-D–deficient mice are also compromised in their resistance to several pathogens; however, this defect is difficult to interpret because deletion of SP-D leads to abnormalities of alveolar macrophages and surfactant homeostasis (102).

Pentraxins

C-reactive protein (CRP) and serum amyloid P (SAP) are two structurally related proteins that belong to the pentraxin family (103). Both CRP and SAP are acute-phase proteins in humans and mice, respectively. They are produced primarily by hepatocytes in response to inflammatory cytokines, particularly IL-6. CRP and SAP bind to bacterial surfaces, in part through recognition of phosphorylcholine (104). These PRRs function as opsonins and can activate the classical pathway of complement by binding to and activating C1q (103,105). All pentraxins form multimeric (usually pentameric) structures. CRP and SAP are referred to as short pentraxins, as opposed to long pentraxins that, in addition to the conserved pentraxin domain, have an additional long N-terminal sequence. PTX3 is a prototypical long pentraxin that plays an important role in antibacterial and antifungal defense (106). PTX3 is expressed by a variety of cell types, most notably by DCs, macrophages, and neutrophils. PTX3 can be induced directly by TLR engagement on these cells, or indirectly, through inflammatory cytokines. Like CRP and SAP, PTX3 binds directly to microbial cell walls, activates complement, and facilitates phagocytosis (106).

LBP and BPI

LBP and bactericidal permeability-increasing protein (BPI) are members of a lipid transferase family that also includes cholesteryl ester transfer protein (CETP) and phospholipid transfer protein (PLTP). All four proteins are related to each other in primary structure, which suggests a common origin; however, unlike LBP and BPI, CETP and PLTP do not play any role in host defense, but rather function as lipid carriers in the serum. Both LBP and BPI are components of the acute-phase response, although BPI can also be produced by activated phagocytes. Given that BPI functions as a bactericidal protein, it will be discussed later, along with other effector mechanisms of innate immunity. LBP functions as a transfer protein for LPS and various host-derived lipids. In this sense, LBP is not a true pattern recognition receptor. However, LBP does play a role in LPS recognition by monomerizing LPS from aggregates or micelles and transferring it onto CD14, the high-affinity LPS receptor (18,107). LBP can also function as an opsonin—LBP bound to LPS or gram-negative bacteria was shown to bind to CD14 expressed on the macrophage plasma membrane (107). This binding can subsequently lead to endocytosis of the bound bacteria or LPS. The physiologic significance and mechanism of LBP-mediated phagocytosis are currently unknown. The function of LBP in LPS recognition may be redundant as LBP-deficient mice exhibit normal responsiveness to LPS injection *in vivo* (18).

PGRPs

PGRPs comprise a family of recently discovered PRRs that function as receptors for peptidoglycan in evolutionarily distant organisms, including insects and mammals (108–110). All PGRPs contain a highly conserved peptidoglycan binding domain. Some PGRPs have putative transmembrane regions and presumably function as cell surface receptors, whereas other PGRPs are secreted proteins (109,110). There are four known PGRPs in humans, but more are likely to exist. Human PGRPs are differentially expressed, with one gene predominantly expressed in the liver, one in neutrophils, and one in the esophagus (109). The function of mammalian PGRPs is unknown, but one mammalian PGRP was shown to inhibit bacterial growth, suggesting that at least some PGRPs may function as bactericidal effector molecules (111). Surprisingly, one PGRP that has been analyzed so far inhibited phagocytosis of gram-positive bacteria by macrophages (111). This PGRP also blocked peptidoglycan-induced cytokine production and oxidative burst in macrophages. These effects were presumably due to competition for peptidoglycan binding between PGRP and PGN-binding cell-surface receptors such as TLR2. Since PGRPs were shown to trigger a serine protease cascade in insects in response to bacterial infection, it is likely that at least some mammalian PGRPs may have a similar role—for example, in inducing the complement cascade—to the way in which the lectin pathway is activated by MBL upon microbial recognition (18,107).

Intracellular Recognition Systems

Although most of the initial recognition of microbial infection occurs outside the host cell, many pathogens, and in particular, viruses, gain access to intracellular compartments such as the cytosol. Several intracellular recognition systems have evolved to detect pathogens in the cytosol of infected cells. In addition to the typical outcomes of innate immune recognition—induction of microbicidal effector mechanisms and production of cytokines that activate effector cells— intracellular immune recognition often leads to apoptosis of the infected cell. This is true for both innate and adaptive immune systems (compare NK and CD8 T cell functions). Apoptosis of the infected cell can be cell autonomous or can be triggered by specialized effectors.

Several receptor families are involved in the intracellular recognition of viral and bacterial pathogens. Some are involved in the initial detection of intracellular infections, and others play a role in effector responses. These pathways and their role in innate host defense are described next.

RIG-I/MDA-5

Intracellular recognition of viral dsRNA has long been known to result in a potent induction of IFN-β in infected cells. The identity of the receptors responsible for the initial detection of viral RNA has recently been discovered. Two proteins, called RIG-I and MDA-5, are responsible for detection of two forms of viral RNAs—ssRNA containing 5′ triphosphate and dsRNA, respectively. Most cellular RNAs either contain short hairpin structures with a limited stretch of dsRNA (e.g., tRNAs and rRNAs), or in the case of mRNA, a 5′ cap structure. In contrast, viral RNAs have extended double-stranded structures recognized by MDA-5, or they have 5′ triphosphate ss RNAs, which are detected by RIG-I (113). Thus, structural differences allow for self-/nonself discrimination by these intracellular sensors of viral RNA.

RIG-I and MDA-5 have similar structures, with two N-terminal CARD domains followed by a DEAD family helicase domain. The helicase domain is responsible for RNA recognition, while CARD domains activate downstream signaling pathways leading to IFN production Recent studies have demonstrated that the CARD domain of RIG-I, but not MDA-5, is K63 ubiquitinated by a RING finger E3 ligase, TRIM25. Further, TRIM25 was found to be essential for virus-induced, RIG-I–mediated IFN production (112). Both RIG-I and MDA-5 signal through a downstream adaptor, MAVS (also known as IPS-1, CARDIF and VISA). MAVS is associated with the mitochondrial membrane through a C-terminal hydrophobic region. This mitochondrial attachment is essential for MAVS signaling. Interestingly, hepatitis C virus–encoded protein NS3/4A is a protease that specifically cleaves MAVS off the mitochondrial membrane and thus effectively shuts off RIG-I–mediated induction of the antiviral response. Downstream of MAVS is the serine/threonine kinase TBK-1, which is the kinase responsible for IRF3 phosphorylation and activation. TBK-1 also induces NF-κB and AP1 activation resulting in activation of the IFN-β gene (113).

The role of RIG-I and MDA-5 in antiviral defense has been established using mice deficient in these receptors. Interestingly, RIG-I was found to be essential for the recognition of paramyxoviruses, including influenza virus and Japanese encephalitis virus. MDA5, on the other hand is critical for the detection of picornaviruses, including encephalomyocarditis virus. Accordingly RIG-I$^{-/-}$ and MDA5$^{-/-}$ mice are highly susceptible to infection with these respective RNA viruses compared to control mice (114). MAVS/IPS-1–deficient mice, as expected, are highly susceptible to infection with both classes of RNA viruses, consistent with its role as a critical mediator of RIG-I and MDA-5 signaling (114).

PKR

PKR is a serine/threonine protein kinase that contains three double-stranded RNA (dsRNA) binding domains at the N-terminal part of the protein and a C-terminal kinase domain. PKR can be activated by dsRNA and thus may function as an intracellular sensor of viral infection, as dsRNA of the length that is sufficient to activate PKR is produced by many viruses, but not by host cells. PKR is expressed ubiquitously, and its expression can be further induced by interferons. Activated PKR phosphorylates the translation initiation factor eIF-2α on Ser 51, which results in a block of cellular and viral protein synthesis (115). PKR can also induce apoptosis in infected cells, thus preventing the further spread of the virus.

2′-5′-Oligoadenylate Synthase and RNaseL. 2′-5′-Oligoadenylate synthases (OAS) are a family of IFN-inducible enzymes that synthesize an unusual polymer—2′-5′-oligoadenylate (116,117). Activation of OAS requires dsRNA and, therefore, is triggered by viral infection. 2′-5′-Oligoadenylate produced by activated OAS then induces dimerization and activation of a dormant endonuclease, RNaseL. Once activated, RNaseL degrades viral and cellular RNA, including ribosomal RNA, which leads to a block of mRNA translation and to apoptosis (116,117) (Figure 14.2). There are at least three genes encoding OAS proteins, and one of them can induce apoptosis through an additional pathway—by binding the anti-apoptotic proteins Bcl2 and BclXL via the C-terminal BH3 domain of the OAS. Sequestration of Bcl2 and BclXL then results in apoptosis of virally infected cells. Interestingly, the dsRNA-binding specificity of OAS evolved independently of that of PKR, as the dsRNA-binding domains in OAS and PKR are not related to each other. The importance of the OAS/RNaseL system in antiviral defense is demonstrated by the increased susceptibility of RNaseL-deficient mice to ECMV infection (117).

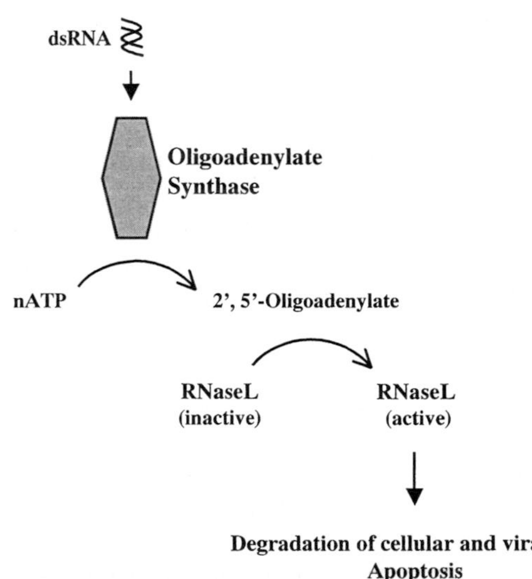

FIGURE 14.2 Recognition of viral infection by oligoadenylate synthase (OAS). OAS is activated by viral dsRNA and generates 2′, 5′-oligoadenylate, which functions as a second messenger to activate a dormant ribonuclease, RNaseL. Once activated by 2′5′-oligoadenylate, RNaseL degrades cellular and viral RNA, which results in an inhibition of viral replication. Activated RNase L can also trigger pathways that lead to apoptosis of the infected cell. Some OAS proteins can induce apoptosis more directly by additional pathways that involve the sequestration of the anti-apoptotic members of the Bcl2 family.

NOD-like Receptors

The NOD-like receptor (NLR) family of proteins is a large group of intracellular proteins named after the prototypical family members NOD1 and NOD2. There are approximately 20 different NLRs in humans and mice with a characteristic arrangement of a C-terminal LRR and a central nucleotide binding and oligomerization domain. Three NLR subfamilies can be defined by the identity of the N-terminal protein–protein interaction domain. Thus, the NOD subfamily contains a CARD domain, the NALPs contain a pyrin domain, and the NAIPs contain a Bir domain (118). In all cases studied, the N-terminal domain is responsible for interaction with adaptor proteins or kinases, whereas the LRR region is presumably responsible for ligand recognition (although direct ligand recognition has not yet been demonstrated for any of the NLRs).

Although a number of NLRs have yet to be functionally characterized, available information indicates that NLRs have diverse functions in the immune system. Some NOD proteins, including NOD1, NOD2, and NOD10—all of which contain CARD domains—activate NFκB and MAP-kinase signaling pathways (119–122). The N-terminal CARD domains of these NODs interact with and activate the serine/threonine protein kinase RIP2, which in turn induces the NFκB and MAP-kinase signaling pathways (119–121).

Nod1 and Nod2 are involved in intracellular bacterial recognition. Both proteins detect different structures derived from bacterial peptidoglycan. Specifically, Nod2 detects muramyl dipeptide, the conserved molecular structure common to gram-negative and gram-positive bacteria. In contrast, Nod1 is involved in the recognition of peptidoglycan fragments containing *meso*-diaminopimelic acid (*meso*-DAP), which is more characteristic of gram-negative bacterial peptidoglycan (118). It is not yet known whether NOD proteins recognize peptidoglycan directly, or via some accessory protein. Regardless of the mechanism, detection of peptidoglycan by NOD1 and NOD2 leads to induction of inflammatory cytokines and chemokines and the recruitment of neutrophils to the site of infection (118). In addition, NOD proteins contribute to the initiation of the adaptive immune responses. Importantly, mutations in NOD2 proteins have been implicated in the pathogenesis of Crohn's disease (123,124).

The NALP subfamily of NLRs includes 14 members, and at least some of them play an important role in the regulation of inflammatory responses mediated by the IL-1 family of cytokines (125–127). The IL-1 family members,

IL-1β, IL-18, and IL-33 are produced as inactive precursors that have to be processed in the cytosol by the inflammatory caspases, caspase-1 and caspase-5/caspase-11. Recent studies have demonstrated that activation of caspases occurs in a mutisubunit complex named the *inflammasome* (125–127). There are several different types of inflammasomes, depending on their composition and the involvement of a particular NALP protein. The two best characterized are the NALP3 inflammasome and the IPAF inflammasome. Both of these contain a critical adaptor protein known as *ASC* that couples the pyrin domain of NALP3 or IPAF to the CARD domain of caspases (125–127). There are several pathways of inflammasome activation triggered by bacterial or endogenous stimuli. The NALP3 inflammasome can be activated by TLR ligands together with ATP. ATP induces K^+ efflux through the P2X7 receptor. Bacterial pore-forming toxins, such as nigericine and maitotoxin, can also induce K^+ efflux and thus bypass the requirement for ATP and P2X7. The NALP1 inflammasome can be activated by the anthrax lethal toxin, while Salmonella virulence factor SipB activates the IPAF inflammasome. In addition, *Legionella pneumophila* infection induces caspase-1 activation via NAIP5, which presumably forms yet another type of inflammasome. Both *Legionella* and *Salmonella* can induce IPAF-dependent caspase-1 activation (125–127).

Interestingly, several endogenous products have been shown to activate the inflammasome. Crystals of monosodium urate (MSU) and calcium pyrophosphate dihydrate (CPPD), the causative agents of gout and pseudogout, respectively, induce the NALP3 inflammasome and consequently IL-1 production. Because MSU, CPPD, and extracellular ATP can all be produced by stressed or damaged cells, it is possible that the NALP3 inflammasome induces inflammatory responses to tissue damage.

Importantly, several gain-of-function mutations associated with inflammatory diseases have been identified in NALP3, also known as *cryopyrin*. These occur in Muckle-Wells syndrome, familial cold autoinflammatory syndrome, and neonatal onset multisystem inflammatory disease. In addition, similar mutations in NALP1 (also known as *pyrin*) are responsible for the Mediterranean fever syndrome. Characterization of the pathways of inflammasome activation has revealed the molecular basis for these inflammatory diseases and suggested novel forms of therapy, including the blockade of IL-1 by IL-1 receptor antagonist (128).

THE CELLS OF THE INNATE IMMUNE SYSTEM

Unlike antigen receptors of the adaptive immune system, which are expressed exclusively on lymphocytes, the receptors of the innate immune system are expressed on many cell types. In fact, some of these receptors, most notably the intracellular receptors involved in the detection of viral infections, are expressed in almost every cell type. In this sense, innate host defense is not a function of a few specialized cell types. However, several cell types do have specialized functions related to innate immunity, although some of these cell types have other functions unrelated to immunity as well. Among these cells are macrophages, neutrophils, NK cells, mast cells, basophils, eosinophils, and surface epithelial cells. These cells are specialized to function at different stages of infection and to deal with different types of pathogens.

Macrophages

Macrophages have the most central and essential functions in the innate immune system, and have multiple roles in host defense. Mature, resident macrophages differentiate from circulating monocytes and occupy peripheral tissues and organs where they are most likely to encounter pathogens during the early stages of infection. Upon encounter with infectious agents, macrophages can employ a broad array of antimicrobial effector mechanisms, including phagocytosis of the pathogen and the induction of microbicidal effector systems, such as reactive oxygen and nitrogen intermediates and antimicrobial proteins and peptides. In addition, interaction of macrophages with pathogens leads to the induction of a plethora of inflammatory mediators, such as TNF-α, IL-1, and IL-6, and chemokines, such as KC-1 (and IL-8 in humans). TNF-α and IL-1 induce a local inflammatory response, and at higher concentrations, these cytokines (along with IL-6) induce the acute-phase response by triggering the expression of acute-phase genes in the liver. IL-8, a neutrophil chemoattractant produced by resident macrophages, recruits neutrophils to the site of infection. Production of antimicrobial effector genes, cytokines, and chemokines is mediated primarily by TLRs, whereas phagocytosis is mediated by multiple phagocytic PRRs. Many of the effector functions of macrophages are strongly augmented by IFN-γ, which comes from either NK cells or Th1 T cells. IFN-γ also induces the antigen-presenting functions of macrophages by turning on the expression of a battery of genes involved in antigen processing and presentation.

In addition to their roles in host defense, macrophages have multiple "housekeeping functions," the most appreciated of which is their function as the body's scavengers. Macrophages phagocytose apoptotic cells, cell debris, oxidized lipoproteins, and other byproducts of the normal physiology of multicellular organisms. Kupffer cells (liver macrophages) remove from circulation senescent cells and desialated glycoproteins through phagocytosis mediated by asialoglycoprotein receptors (100). Similarly, macrophages located in the red pulp of the spleen phagocytose and remove from circulation senescent erythrocytes. Thus, in addition to the recognition of microbial nonself by PRRs, macrophages are equipped with a separate set of receptors for the recognition of "altered self" (desialated self-glycoproteins and phosphotidylserine exposed on apoptotic cells) and missing self (e.g., the lack of expression of CD47 on senescent erythrocytes) (129–131). It is important to note that, unlike the phagocytosis of pathogens, which is mediated by PRRs and is followed by the induction of inflammatory mediators, phagocytosis of apoptotic and senescent cells is immunologically "silent" in that it does not lead to the induction of inflammatory responses. In fact, recognition and phagocytosis of apoptotic cells result in the production of the antiinflammatory cytokine TGF-β (132). This phagocytosis pathway is mediated by the recently characterized macrophage receptor specific for phosphatidylserine (133). Thus, functionally distinct receptors expressed on macrophages determine the functional outcome of phagocytosis mediated by these versatile cells.

Neutrophils

Neutrophils are short-lived cells (average life span is about 24 to 48 hours) equipped with numerous antimicrobial effector mechanisms. Unlike resident macrophages, mast cells, and immature dendritic cells, neutrophils do not reside in peripheral tissues prior to infection. Rather, neutrophils are recruited from the circulation to the site of infection by cytokines and chemokines produced by resident macrophages and mast cells that have encountered pathogens. Recruited neutrophils accumulate at the site of infection and phagocytose and kill pathogens using several microbicidal mechanisms. In addition to reactive oxygen and nitrogen intermediates, neutrophils employ a number of antimicrobial proteins and peptides that are stored in neutrophil granules. Neutrophils contain several types of granules, including primary (or azurophil) granules, and secondary (or specific) granules that are specialized for the storage and secretion of antimicrobial products. Neutrophils are capable of both extracellular and intracellular killing of micro-organisms, depending on the type of granules used. The content of primary granules is predominantly secreted into the extracellular space, whereas antimicrobial peptides of the secondary granules are predominantly released into the phagolysosome for the intracellular killing of pathogens.

Mast Cells

Although mast cells are best known as effectors of allergic responses, they are also an important component of innate immunity. Mature mast cells reside in connective and mucosal tissues, where they encounter and phagocytose infecting micro-organisms and produce inflammatory mediators that play an important role in leukocyte recruitment (134–136) The role of mast cells in innate host defense has been addressed using Kit^{W}/Kit^{W-v} mice, which carry an inactivating mutation in the c-kit gene and are essentially mast cell-deficient. Experiments carried out in these mice demonstrated that mast cells play an essential role in antibacterial defense in a model of acute septic peritonitis (137,138). Moreover, the protective role of mast cells is mediated mainly by the rapid production of TNF-α and leukotriene B4, which in turn are responsible for neutrophil recruitment to the site of infection (135,137,138). The dramatic effect of mast cell deficiency revealed in the acute septic peritonitis experiments performed on Kit^{W}/Kit^{W-v} mice reflects the unique ability of mast cells to store preformed TNF-α that can be quickly secreted upon interaction with pathogens (139). Mast cells also produce lipid mediators of inflammation and a vast array of cytokines, including the "type II cytokines" IL-4, IL-5, and IL-13 (134,135).

Eosinophils

Mature eosinophils are found mainly in tissues, primarily in the respiratory, intestinal, and genitourinary tracts. Eosinophils, similar to mast cells, are rich in granules and produce a variety of cytokines and lipid mediators. In addition, eosinophil granules contain several cationic effector proteins that have potent toxic effects against parasitic worms (140). Unlike neutrophils and macrophages, eosinophils are poor phagocytes and consequently release the content of their granules into the extracellular space. The production of various cationic antiparasitic proteins (which include major basic protein, eosinophil cationic protein, and eosinophil-derived neurotoxic protein), as well as the fact that eosinophilia is induced in several model parasitic infections, implicate this cell type as an effector involved in host defense against parasite infections.

Dendritic Cells

Immature DCs reside in peripheral tissues and are highly active in macropinocytosis and receptor-mediated endocytosis (141). DCs express a number of PRRs, including phagocytic receptors and TLRs. DCs are best known for their role in the initiation of adaptive immune responses, but these cells can also contribute to direct antimicrobial responses (141). Thus, stimulation of DCs with microbial products leads to the induction of several antimicrobial effector responses, such as nitric oxide production. The role of DCs in the initiation of the adaptive immune responses is discussed later in this chapter. The biology of DCs is described in more detail in Chapter 15.

Surface Epithelium

The epithelial cells that line the mucosal surfaces of the intestinal, respiratory, and genitourinary tracts provide an important physical barrier that separates the host from the environment. Mucins, which are highly glycosylated glycoproteins expressed on the surface of these cells, help to prevent pathogen attachment and invasion. In addition to providing physical separation of the host from the microbial environment, surface epithelial cells produce antimicrobial effectors, such as β-defensins and lysozyme, and secrete a number of cytokines and chemokines that contribute to the local inflammatory response and to the recruitment of leukocytes to the site of pathogen entry (142).

THE EFFECTOR MECHANISMS OF THE INNATE IMMUNE SYSTEM

The innate immune system possesses a wide variety of antimicrobial effector mechanisms that differ in inducibility, site of expression, mechanism of action, and activity against different pathogen classes. The major categories of antimicrobial effectors are as follows:

1. Enzymes that hydrolyze components of microbial cell walls (lysozyme, chitinases, phospholipase A2)
2. Antimicrobial proteins and peptides that disrupt the integrity of microbial cell walls (BPI, defensins, cathelicidins, complement, eosinophil cationic protein)
3. Microbicidal serine proteases (serprocidins)
4. Proteins that sequester iron and zinc (lactoferrin, NRAMP, calprotectin)
5. Enzymes that generate toxic oxygen and nitrogen derivatives (phagocyte oxidase, nitric oxide synthase, myeloperoxidase)

The major sites of expression of antimicrobial effectors are granulocytes (especially neutrophils), macrophages, and surface epithelium. It is worth pointing out that the antimicrobial activities of most of these effectors were demonstrated *in vitro*; physiologic roles in *in vivo* host defense have only been demonstrated for a few of these gene products.

Lysozyme

Lysozyme (also known as *muramidase*) and its antimicrobial properties were first described by Alexander Fleming in 1921. Lysozyme is a 14-kD enzyme that degrades the peptidoglycan of some gram-positive bacteria by cleaving the β-1,4-glycosidic linkage between N-acetylmuramic acid and N-acetylglucosamine. Disruption of the peptidoglycan layer leads to the osmotic lysis of the bacteria. Some gram-positive pathogens with highly cross-linked peptidoglycans are resistant to the action of lysozyme, and gram-negative bacteria are also generally protected from lysozyme by their outer membrane. Lysozyme is highly concentrated in secretions such as tears and saliva. In humans, there is a single lysozyme gene that is expressed in neutrophils and macrophages. In the mouse there are two lysozymes: lysozyme M, which is expressed in macrophages, and lysozyme P, which is expressed by Paneth cells of the small intestine.

Chitinases

Chitinases comprise a family of enzymes that degrade chitin, a structural polysaccharide that forms the cell wall of fungi and the exoskeleton of insects. Chitinases are secreted by activated macrophages and presumably play a role in antifungal defense, although direct evidence for this function is lacking (143). Several members of the chitinase family are enzymatically inactive due to amino acid substitutions in their catalytic sites. Some of them are expressed in human neutrophils, but their physiologic role is not known.

Phospholipase A2

Phospholipase A2 (PLA2) belongs to a family of disulfide rich enzymes that share similar structures and catalytic mechanisms, but differ in substrate preferences and disulfide arrangements. Group II PLA2 is a 14-kD enzyme that hydrolyses the ester bonds at the 2-acyl position in the phospholipids of bacterial membranes. PLA2 is found in primary granules of neutrophils (and, therefore, is secreted upon degranulation), Paneth cells, and epithelial secretions (e.g., in tear fluid) and is produced by the liver as an acute-phase protein. The bactericidal activity of PLA2 is strongly potentiated by other antimicrobial products of neutrophils and by complement (144). PLA2 is particularly efficient against gram-positive bacteria (145). Killing of gram-negative bacteria is potentiated by antimicrobial effectors that disrupt the outer membrane, such as BPI. The important role of PLA2 in innate host defense is demonstrated by the finding that PLA2-deficient mice are more susceptible to infection with *S. aureus* than their wild-type controls (145–147).

BPI

BPI is a cationic 55-kD protein that has several effector activities against gram-negative bacteria but is inactive against gram-positive bacteria (148). BPI is structurally related to the acute-phase reactant LBP and, similar to LBP, binds to the conserved lipid-A portion of LPS. BPI exerts its bactericidal activity by disrupting the integrity of the outer and inner membranes of gram-negative bacteria, thereby increasing their permeability and susceptibility to the action of other antimicrobial proteins, such as PLA2. BPI can also function as an opsonin by binding to gram-negative bacteria and facilitating their uptake by neutrophils. Unlike LBP, which functions by potentiating LPS recognition by CD14/TLR4, BPI neutralizes free LPS and inhibits LPS signaling (148). BPI is expressed predominantly in neutrophils, where it is found in large quantities in the primary granules and is secreted into inflammatory fluids upon neutrophil activation (148).

Defensins

Defensins are small (3 kD to 4 kD) cationic peptides with a broad spectrum of antimicrobial activities. Defensins are active against gram-positive and gram-negative bacteria, fungi, parasites, and some enveloped viruses (140,149). Defensins kill micro-organisms by forming multimeric voltage–dependent pores in their membranes. The selective toxicity of defensins toward microbial cells can be explained in part by the differences in phospholipid composition between microbial and mammalian cell membranes and by the presence of cholesterol in mammalian but not bacterial membranes (150). Defensins are characterized by a common structural feature—a hydrophobic β sheet stabilized by three disulfide bonds. Depending on the pattern of disulfide bond formation between the six conserved cysteines, vertebrate defensins fall into two classes—α-defensins and β-defensins (140,149,150). The α-defensins are generally presynthesized and stored in granules of neutrophils (in humans but not in mice) and Paneth cells of the small intestine. The β-defensins, in contrast, are produced by epithelial cells and in most cases are not stored in cytoplasmic granules (140,149,150). The secretion of β-defensins is controlled primarily at the level of gene transcription and is inducible by microbial products (through TLRs) and by inflammatory cytokines (140,149,150). Like all known antimicrobial peptides, defensins are synthesized as inactive precursors that contain a prodomain (which includes a leader sequence) and an acidic region that neutralizes and inactivates the cationic mature peptide. Processing of defensins results in the generation of active peptides. In neutrophils, active (processed) defensins are stored in the granules, whereas the epithelial defensins are secreted as propeptides and are processed in the lumen of the crypt (140,149,150). For mouse α-defensins, the lumenal processing enzyme has been shown to be the matrix metalloprotease matrilysin (151). Matrilysin-deficient mice do not contain active α-defensins in their intestinal crypts and consequently are susceptible to intestinal infection (151).

Cathelicidins

Cathelicidins comprise a family of antimicrobial peptides that contain a conserved N-terminal prodomain called *cathelin* and a C-terminal peptide that becomes active after cleavage from the cathelin domain. The C-terminal peptide is highly divergent between different cathelicidins within and between mammalian species (152,153). In the single human member of the cathelicidin family, the C-terminal peptide is 37 amino acids long and lacks cysteines but can form an amphipathic α helix that allows it to interact with microbial membranes. Cathelicidins are active against gram-positive and gram-negative bacteria and fungi and can act synergistically with other antimicrobial proteins (152,153). Cathelicidins are produced in neutrophils and stored as inactive proproteins in the secondary granules. Activation of cathelicidins occurs when the neutrophil protease elastase cleaves off the cathelin domain. Interestingly, elastase is stored in the primary granules of neutrophils and gains access to cathelicidin precursors only when the primary and secondary granules fuse with the phagosomes of activated neutrophils (140,152).

Serprocedins

Serprocedins comprise a family of 25- to 35-kD cationic serine proteases with antimicrobial activity and include neutrophil elastase, proteinase 3, cathepsin G, and azurocidin/CAP37 (140,154). Unlike other members of the family, azurocidin/CAP37 is catalytically inactive. Serprocedins are localized in the primary granules of neutrophils and are structurally related to the granzymes of NK cells and CD8 T cells. Serprocedins exert their antimicrobial activity either by direct perturbation of microbial membranes, or by proteolysis (140,154). Neutrophil elastase, as discussed earlier, converts cathelicidin precursors into active bactericidal peptides. Mice deficient for neutrophil elastase are more susceptible to gram-negative and fungal infections (155).

Lactoferrin, NRAMP, and Calprotectin

The antimicrobial activities of lactoferrin, NRAMP, and calprotectin are due to their ability to sequester iron and zinc, which are essential for microbial metabolism and replication. Lactoferrin is an 80-kD iron-chelating protein of the transferrin family that contains two iron-binding sites. Lactoferrin is found in the secondary granules of neutrophils, in epithelial secretions such as breast milk, in the intestinal epithelium of infants, and in airway fluids. Lactoferrin has two mechanisms of antimicrobial activity: bacteriostatic and microbicidal. The bacteriostatic effect is due to iron sequestration (156). Pathogens depend on iron provided by the host, and iron deprivation is an efficient strategy to block microbial metabolism, as iron is critically required for both oxidative and anaerobic pathways of ATP generation. In addition, lactoferrin can be processed by limited proteolysis to yield a cationic microbicidal peptide called *lactoferricin* (157). The bactericidal effect of lactoferricin is not dependent on iron sequestration and is thought to be due to a perturbation of microbial membranes (157). NRAMP (natural resistance–associated macrophage protein) is a 65-kD integral membrane protein that functions as an ion pump in the phagocytic vacuoles of macrophages and neutrophils (158). NRAMP is thought to function by pumping out iron from phagocytic vacuoles that harbor mycobacteria and other such bacteria that can persist in these vacuoles. Indeed, the gene encoding NRAMP is mutated in mouse strains that are highly susceptible to mycobacterial infections (155). NRAMP is inducible by IFN-γ. Calprotectin, a member of the S-100 family of calciumbinding proteins, is composed of 8- and 14-kD subunits and is found in large amounts in the cytoplasm of neutrophils. The antimicrobial activity of this protein resides in its histidine-rich regions, which chelate and sequester zinc ions (159).

Phagocyte Oxidase, Myeloperoxidase, and Nitric Oxide Synthase

Phagocytes (granulocytes and macrophages) are equipped with an enzymatic machinery that generates highly toxic reactive oxygen and nitrogen intermediates that have potent antimicrobial activities (160). The induction of these antimicrobial effector responses is tightly regulated and is triggered upon interaction of phagocytes with pathogens (160,161). Phagocyte oxidase (also known as NADPH oxidase) is responsible for the mitochondria-independent respiratory burst induced in phagocytes during the phagocytosis of micro-organisms. NADPH oxidase is a multicomponent enzymatic complex that consists of three cytosolic subunits (p40phox, p47phox, and p67phox) and a membrane-associated flavocytochrome complex (p22phox and p91phox). Assembly of the subunits into a functional NADPH complex is induced by phagocyte activation through a Rac GTPase–dependent pathway. Once the complex is assembled, it produces superoxide anions (a primary product) and hydrogen peroxide (a secondary product), which are released into phagocytic vacuoles or outside the cell where they exert their direct and potent microbicidal effect. Mice deficient for various components of the NADPH complex are susceptible to multiple microbial infections (160,161). Superoxide and hydrogen peroxide, in addition to their own antimicrobial activity, can also be used as substrates for another neutrophil enzyme called *myeloperoxidase* (160,161). Myeloperoxidase is stored in the primary granules of neutrophils and is also expressed in monocytes. Using the products of the NADPH oxidase as substrates, myeloperoxidase generates hypochlorous acid and chloramines as well as other reactive oxygen intermediates, all of which have potent microbicidal activities. Myeloperoxidase-deficient mice are highly susceptible to infection with *Candida albicans* (160,161). Inducible nitric oxide synthase (iNOS) is expressed in neutrophils and macrophages and generates large amounts of nitric oxide (NO). NO is toxic to bacteria, although the exact mechanism(s) of its toxicity is not yet known (162). iNOS is inducible by IFN-γ and TLR ligands such as LPS (in mouse but not in human macrophages) (162). The role of iNOS and NO in the innate immune resistance to infection has been demonstrated in mice deficient for this enzyme. INOS knockout mice are more susceptible than their wild-type counterparts to infection with multiple bacterial, viral, and protozoan pathogens (161,162). Interestingly, mice deficient for both NADPH oxidase and iNOS are severely immunocompromised and are highly susceptible not only to infection with pathogens, but also to commensal microorganisms (163).

The Antiviral Effector Mechanisms of the Innate Immune System

NK cells, which play a major role in the innate antiviral host defense, are discussed in depth in Chapter 16. Therefore, the discussion here is focused on cell-autonomous effector mechanisms that appear to be unique to antiviral defense. These mechanisms include the induction of apoptosis in virally infected cells and the inhibition of the viral life cycle by IFN-α/β–inducible gene products. Apoptosis of infected cells is an efficient way to prevent viral spread and can be induced either by cell-autonomous mechanisms (e.g., through PKR and OAS pathways, as discussed earlier in this chapter), or with the help of NK or CD8 T cells. The best-characterized IFN-inducible gene products with intrinsic antiviral activity are members of the Mx protein family (164). The Mx protein and the closely related GBP (guanylate-binding protein) are members of the dynamin family of GTPases. The antiviral function of Mx proteins was discovered by the demonstration that the mouse Mx-1 gene confers resistance to influenza virus infection in A2G mice, whereas most other mouse strains carry a defective allele of Mx-1 and consequently are highly susceptible to influenza infection (164). Mx-1 appears to block transcription of the viral genome by inhibiting the influenza-virus polymerase complex (164–167). The second mouse Mx protein, Mx-2, is also mutated in most inbred strains of mice, except in the feral mouse strains NJL and SPR. In these mice, IFN-inducible Mx-2 protein confers resistance to VSV infection. Unlike the Mx-1 protein, which functions in the nucleus, the Mx-2 protein is cytoplasmic (168). In human cells, there are two IFN-inducible Mx proteins, Mx-A and Mx-B. Mx-A is a cytoplasmic protein that inhibits replication of several viruses, including influenza, measles virus, and VSV. Transgenic expression of the Mx-A protein in mice deficient for the IFN-α receptor protects these mice from lethal viral infections and demonstrates that Mx-A has intrinsic antiviral activity independently of other IFN-inducible genes (165,169). GBP proteins are structurally related to Mx proteins and likewise are inducible by IFN-α/β and confer resistance to some viral infections (170). Not all the mechanisms of the antiviral function of Mx and GBP are known. Cytoplasmic Mx and GBP proteins may interfere with viral infection by blocking viral assembly, as suggested by the similarity of these proteins to other members of the dynamin family that play a role in vesicular trafficking and fusion.

CONTROL OF ADAPTIVE IMMUNITY BY THE INNATE IMMUNE SYSTEM

In addition to directly activating antimicrobial effector responses, innate immune recognition plays a critical role in controlling the activation of adaptive immunity. Many aspects of innate control of adaptive immunity are covered in detail elsewhere in this book. Discussion here will be limited to an overview of some general concepts.

As noted earlier, there are several classes of PRRs in the mammalian innate immune system. PRRs that signal the presence of infection (e.g., TLRs, Dectins, RIG-I/MDA-5, NODs, etc.) not only induce the inflammatory and antimicrobial responses, but also activate the adaptive immune system. Innate immune recognition is required for the activation of adaptive immune responses in part because the innate immune system can determine the origin of the antigen (2,3,5). Adaptive immune recognition relies on two types of antigen receptors—the T cell receptor and the B cell receptor. The specificities of these receptors are generated by random processes such as gene rearrangement and, therefore, are not predetermined to recognize pathogen-derived antigens. Receptors of the innate immune system, on the other hand, are specific for microbial structures and thus their activation can signal the origin of the associated antigens. The translation of the innate, nonclonal recognition into signals that activate adaptive immune responses is mediated in part by antigen presenting cells, particularly DCs (171).

Immature DCs are located in peripheral tissues where they are likely to encounter invading pathogens (141). Interaction of DCs with pathogens leads to the activation of signaling PRRs, such as TLRs or Dectins, and the phagocytosis of pathogens by phagocytic PRRs, such as DEC205 and the mannose receptor. Once activated through PRRs, DCs begin to express high levels of MHC class II and costimulatory molecules and migrate to the T cell zone in the draining lymph nodes where they present pathogen derived antigens to T lymphocytes (7,8,141). In addition, PRRs induce expression by DCs of cytokines that control T cell differentiation into different effector lineages. Thus, TLRs induce production of IL-12 and IL-23 in response to intracellular and extracellular pathogens favoring Th1 and Th17 differentiation, respectively. Dectin-1 selectively induces expression of IL-23 and thus enhances Th17 differentiation in response to extracellular fungal pathogens. RIG-I/MDA-5 induces high levels of IFN-α/β, which are important for CD8 T cell activation and differentiation. Helminths induce production of IL-4 and TSLP in an unknown cell type through an unknown mechanism, and these cytokines lead in turn to Th2 differentiation and IgE production. Thus, different classes of PRRs detect different types of infection and induce the appropriate effector response of the adaptive immune system.

It should be noted that although the basic principles of innate immune recognition and induction of adaptive immunity, as originally proposed by Janeway, have now been confirmed, little is known about the mechanisms of adaptive immune activation. The key signals that are induced by PRRs and required for induction of adaptive immune responses are arguably unknown. The molecular mechanisms that couple innate immune sensing with activation of T cells and their differentiation into the appropriate effector type are also unknown. Although cytokines that play an essential role in inducing T helper cell differentiation have been characterized, it is not yet clear what are the relevant features of the pathogens that are detected by the PRRs and translated into the appropriate set of effector cytokines. Likewise, it is not clear why self-/nonself discrimination by the innate immune system is not sufficient to ensure peripheral tolerance, as evidenced by the severe autoimmune phenotype of mice and humans deficient in regulatory T cells.

These and many other exciting questions await elucidation in the near future.

CONCLUSION

Innate immunity is an evolutionarily ancient and universal system of host defense. Innate immunity is a function of multiple cell types, receptors, signaling systems, and effector mechanisms. Innate immune recognition is directed at conserved molecular patterns unique to micro-organisms, which allows the innate immune system to distinguish self from microbial nonself. Recognition of infectious micro-organisms by the innate immune system leads to the induction of antimicrobial effector mechanisms and thus provides the first line of host defense. In addition, the innate immune system plays an essential role in the initiation of adaptive immune responses and in the control of the effector responses of the adaptive immune system.

ACKNOWLEDGMENTS

This work is supported by the Howard Hughes Medical Institute and by the National Institutes of Health.

REFERENCES

1. Agrawal A, Eastman QM, Schatz DG. Transposition mediated by RAG1 and RAG2 and its implications for the evolution of the immune system. *Nature.* 1998;394(6695):744–751.
2. Janeway CA Jr. Approaching the asymptote? Evolution and revolution in immunology. *Cold Spring Harb Symp Quant Biol.* 1989;54Pt1:1–13.

3. Janeway CA Jr. The immune system evolved to discriminate infectious nonself from noninfectious self. *Immunol Today.* 1992;13(1):11–16.
4. Karre K. How to recognize a foreign submarine. *Immunol Rev.* 1997;155:5.
5. Medzhitov R, Janeway CA Jr. Innate immunity: the virtues of a non-clonal system of recognition. *Cell.* 1997;91(3):295–298.
6. Medzhitov R, Janeway Jr CA. Innate immunity: impact on the adaptive immune response. *Curr Opin Immunol.* 1997;9(1):4–9.
7. Akira S, Takeda K, Kaisho T. Toll-like receptors: critical proteins linking innate and acquired immunity. *Nat Immunol.* 2001;2(8):675–680.
8. Medzhitov R. Toll-like receptors and innate immunity. *Nat Rev Immunol.* 2001;1(2):135–145.
9. Kobe B, Deisenhofer J. Proteins with leucine-rich repeats. *Curr Opin Struct Biol.* 1995;5(3):409–416.
10. Akira S, Uematsu S, Takeuchi O. Pathogen recognition and innate immunity. *Cell.* 2006;124(4): 783–801.
11. da Silva Correia J, et al. Lipopolysaccharide is in close proximity to each of the proteins in its membrane receptor complex. Transfer from cd14 to tlr4 and md-2. *J Biol Chem.* 2001;276(24):21129–21135.
12. Lien E, et al. Toll-like receptor 4 imparts ligand-specific recognition of bacterial lipopolysaccharide. *J Clin Invest.* 2000;105:497.
13. Poltorak A, et al. Physical contact between lipopolysaccharide and Toll-like receptor 4 revealed by genetic complementation. *Proc Nat'l Acad Sci U S A.* 2000;97:2163.
14. Medzhitov R, Preston-Hurlburt P, Janeway CAJ. A human homologue of the Drosophila Toll protein signals activation of adaptive immunity. *Nature.* 1997;(388):394–397.
15. Poltorak A, et al. Defective LPS signaling in C3H/HeJ and C57BL/10ScCr mice: mutations in Tlr4 gene. *Science.* 1998;282(5396):2085–2088.
16. Qureshi ST, et al. Endotoxin-tolerant mice have mutations in Toll-like receptor 4 (Tlr4). *J Exp Med.* 1999;189:615.
17. Hoshino K, et al. Cutting edge: Toll-like receptor 4 (TLR4)-deficient mice are hyporesponsive to lipopolysaccharide: evidence for TLR4 as the Lps gene product. *J Immunol.* 1999;162(7):3749–3752.
18. Wright SD. Innate recognition of microbial lipids. In *Inflammation: basic principles and clinical correlates.* J.I. Gallin and R. Snyderman, eds. Philadelphia: Lippincott, Williams & Wilkins. 1999;525.
19. Haziot A, et al. Resistance to endotoxin shock and reduced dissemination of gram-negative bacteria in CD14-deficient mice. *Immunity.* 1996;4(4):407–414.
20. Shimazu R, et al. MD-2, a molecule that confers lipopolysaccharide responsiveness on Toll-like receptor. *J Exp Med.* 1999;189:1777.
21. Schromm AB, et al. Molecular genetic analysis of an endotoxin nonresponder mutant cell line: a point mutation in a conserved region of MD-2 abolishes endotoxin-induced signaling. *J Exp Med.* 2001;194(1):79–88.
22. Miyake K, et al. RP105, a novel B cell surface molecule implicated in B cell activation, is a member of the leucine-rich repeat protein family. *J Immunol.* 1995;154(7):3333–3340.
23. Miura Y, et al. RP105 is associated with MD-1 and transmits an activation signal in human B cells. *Blood.* 1998;92:2815.
24. Miyake K, et al. Mouse MD-1, a molecule that is physically associated with RP105 and positively regulates its expression. *J Immunol.* 1998;161(3):1348–1353.
25. Chan VW, et al. The molecular mechanism of B cell activation by toll-like receptor protein RP-105. *J Exp Med.* 1998;188(1):93–101.
26. Ogata H, et al. The toll-like receptor protein RP105 regulates lipopolysaccharide signaling in B cells. *J Exp Med.* 2000;192(1):23–29.
27. Nagai Y, et al. The radioprotective 105/MD-1 complex links TLR2 and TLR4/MD-2 in antibody response to microbial membranes. *J Immunol.* 2005;174(11):7043–7049.
28. Means TK, et al. Human toll-like receptors mediate cellular activation by Mycobacterium tuberculosis. *J Immunol.* 1999;163(7):3920–3927.
29. Kurt-Jones EA, et al. Pattern recognition receptors TLR4 and CD14 mediate response to respiratory syncytial virus. *Nat Immunol.* 2000;1(5):398–401.
30. Schwandner R, et al. Peptidoglycan- and lipoteichoic acid-induced cell activation is mediated by toll-like receptor 2. *J Biol Chem.* 1999;274(25):17406–17409.
31. Takeuchi O, et al. Differential roles of TLR2 and TLR4 in recognition of gram-negative and gram-positive bacterial cell wall components. *Immunity.* 1999;11(4):443–451.
32. Aliprantis AO, et al. Cell activation and apoptosis by bacterial lipoproteins through Toll-like receptor-2. *Science.* 1999;285(5428):736–739.
33. Brightbill HD, et al. Host defense mechanisms triggered by microbial lipoproteins through toll-like receptors. *Science.* 1999;285(5428):732–736.
34. Takeuchi O, et al. Cutting edge: preferentially the R-stereoisomer of the mycoplasmal lipopeptide macrophage-activating lipopeptide-2 activates immune cells through a Toll-like receptor 2- and MyD88-dependent signaling pathway. *J Immunol.* 2000;164(2):554–557.
35. Takeuchi O, et al. Discrimination of bacterial lipoproteins by Toll-like receptor 6. *Int Immunol.* 2001;13(7):933–940.
36. Means TK, et al. The CD14 ligands lipoarabinomannan and lipopolysaccharide differ in their requirement for Toll-like receptors. *J Immunol.* 1999;163(12):6748–6755.
37. Hajjar AM, et al. Cutting edge: functional interactions between Toll-like receptor (TLR)2 and TLR1 or TLR6 in response to phenol-soluble modulin. *J Immunol.* 2001;166:15.
38. Underhill D, et al. The Toll-like receptor 2 is recruited to macrophage phagosomes and discriminates between pathogens. *Nature.* 1999;401:811.
39. Campos MA, et al. Activation of Toll-like receptor-2 by glycosylphosphatidylinositol anchors from a protozoan parasite. *J Immunol.* 2001;167(1):416–423.
40. Werts C, et al. Leptospiral lipopolysaccharide activates cells through a TLR2-dependent mechanism. *Nat Immunol.* 2001;2(4):346–352.
41. Hirschfeld M, et al. Signaling by toll-like receptor 2 and 4 agonists results in differential gene expression in murine macrophages. *Infect Immun.* 2001;69(3):1477–1482.
42. Hoebe K, et al. CD36 is a sensor of diacylglycerides. *Nature.* 2005;433(7025):523–527.
43. Ozinsky A, et al. The repertoire for pattern recognition of pathogens by the innate immune system is defined by cooperation between toll-like receptors. *Proc Natl Acad Sci U S A.* 2000;97(25):13766–13771.
44. Muzio M, et al. Differential expression and regulation of toll-like receptors (TLR) in human leukocytes: selective expression of TLR3 in dendritic cells. *J Immunol.* 2000;164(11):5998–6004.
45. Jarrossay D, et al. Specialization and complementarity in microbial molecule recognition by human myeloid and plasmacytoid dendritic cells. *Eur J Immunol.* 2001;31(11):3388–3393.
46. Kadowaki N, et al. Subsets of human dendritic cell precursors express different toll-like receptors and respond to different microbial antigens. *J Exp Med.* 2001;194(6):863–869.
47. Krug A, et al. Toll-like receptor expression reveals CpGDNA as a unique microbial stimulus for plasmacytoid dendritic cells which synergizes with CD40 ligand to induce high amounts of IL-12. *Eur J Immunol.* 2001;31:3026.
48. Alexopoulou L, et al. Recognition of doublestranded RNA and activation of NF-kappaB by Toll-like receptor 3. *Nature.* 2001;413:732.
49. Schulz O, et al. Toll-like receptor 3 promotes cross-priming to virus-infected cells. *Nature.* 2005;433(7028):887–892.
50. Hayashi F, et al. The innate immune response to bacterial flagellin is mediated by Toll-like receptor 5. *Nature.* 2001;410(6832):1099–1103.
51. Uematsu S, et al. Detection of pathogenic intestinal bacteria by Toll-like receptor 5 on intestinal CD11c+ lamina propria cells. *Nat Immunol.* 2006;7(8):868–874.
52. Gewirtz AT, et al. Cutting edge: bacterial flagellin activates basolaterally expressed TLR5 to induce epithelial proinflammatory gene expression. *J Immunol.* 2001;167(4):1882–1885.
53. Diebold SS, et al. Innate antiviral responses by means of TLR7-mediated recognition of single-stranded RNA. *Science.* 2004;303(5663):1529–1531.
54. Heil F, et al. Species-specific recognition of single-stranded RNA via toll-like receptor 7 and 8. *Science.* 2004;303(5663):1526–1529.
55. Lund JM, et al. Recognition of single-stranded RNA viruses by Toll-like receptor 7. *Proc Natl Acad Sci U S A.* 2004;101(15):5598–5603.

56. Lee HK, et al. *Autophagy-dependent viral recognition by plasmacytoid dendritic cells. Science.* 2007;315(5817):1398–1401.
57. Christensen SR, et al. Toll-like receptor 7 and TLR9 dictate autoantibody specificity and have opposing inflammatory and regulatory roles in a murine model of lupus. *Immunity.* 2006;25(3):417–428.
58. Krieg AM. The role of CpG motifs in innate immunity. *Curr Opin Immunol*. 2000;12(1):35–43.
59. Krieg AM, et al. CpG motifs in bacterial DNA trigger direct B-cell activation. *Nature*. 1995;374(6522):546–549.
60. Hemmi H, et al. A Toll-like receptor recognizes bacterial DNA. *Nature*. 2000;408(6813):740–745.
61. Hacker H, et al. CpG-DNA-specific activation of antigen-presenting cells requires stress kinase activity and is preceded by non-specific endocytosis and endosomal maturation. *Embo J.* 1998;17:6230.
62. Bauer S, et al. Human TLR9 confers responsiveness to bacterial DNA via species-specific CpG motif recognition. *Proc Natl Acad Sci U S A.* 2001;98(16):9237–9242.
63. Lund J, et al. Toll-like receptor 9-mediated recognition of Herpes simplex virus-2 by plasmacytoid dendritic cells. *J Exp Med.* 2003;198(3):513–520.
64. Leadbetter EA, et al. Chromatin-IgG complexes activate B cells by dual engagement of IgM and Toll-like receptors. *Nature.* 2002;416(6881):603–607.
65. Zhang D, et al. A toll-like receptor that prevents infection by uropathogenic bacteria. *Science.* 2004;303(5663):1522–1526.
66. Yarovinsky F, et al. TLR11 activation of dendritic cells by a protozoan profilin-like protein. *Science*. 2005;308(5728):1626–1629.
67. Muzio M, et al. IRAK (Pelle) family member IRAK-2 and MyD88 as proximal mediators of IL-1 signaling. *Science*. 1997; 278(5343):1612–1615.
68. Wesche, H, et al. IRAK-M is a novel member of the Pelle/interleukin-1 receptor-associated kinase (IRAK) family. *J Biol Chem.* 1999;274: 19403.
69. Cao Z, Henzel WJ, Gao X. IRAK: a kinase associated with the interleukin-1 receptor. *Science*. 1996;271(5252):1128–1131.
70. Cao Z, et al. TRAF6 is a signal transducer for interleukin-1. *Nature.* 1996;383:443.
71. Deng L, et al. Activation of the IkappaB kinase complex by TRAF6 requires a dimeric ubiquitin-conjugating enzyme complex and a unique polyubiquitin chain. *Cell.* 2000;103(2):351–361.
72. Arch RH, Gedrich RW, Thompson CB. Tumor necrosis factor receptor-associated factors (TRAFs)—a family of adapter proteins that regulates life and death. *Genes Dev.* 1998;12(18):2821–2830.
73. Wang C, et al. TAK1 is a ubiquitin-dependent kinase of MKK and IKK. *Nature*. 2001;412:346.
74. Ghosh S, May MJ, Kopp EB. NF-kappa B and Rel proteins: evolutionarily conserved mediators of immune responses. *Annu Rev Immunol.* 1998;16:225–260.
75. Silverman N, Maniatis T. NF-kappaB signaling pathways in mammalian and insect innate immunity. *Genes Dev.* 2001;15(18):2321–2342.
76. Karin M, Delhase M. The I kappa B kinase (IKK) and NF-kappa B:key elements of proinflammatory signalling. *Semin Immunol.* 2000;12:85.
77. Honda K, Taniguchi T. IRFs: master regulators of signalling by Toll-like receptors and cytosolic pattern-recognition receptors. *Nat Rev Immunol.* 2006;6(9):644–658.
78. Krieger M, Herz J. Structures and functions of multiligand lipoprotein receptors: macrophage scavenger receptors and LDL receptor-related protein (LRP). *Annu Rev Biochem*. 1994;63:601–637.
79. Pearson AM. Scavenger receptors in innate immunity. *Curr Opin Immunol.* 1996;8(1):20–28.
80. Suzuki H, et al. A role for macrophage scavenger receptors in atherosclerosis and susceptibility to infection. *Nature*. 1997; 386(6622):292–296.
81. Haworth R, et al. The macrophage scavenger receptor type A is expressed by activated macrophages and protects the host against lethal endotoxic shock. *J Exp Med.* 1997;186(9):1431–1439.
82. Kraal G, et al. The macrophage receptor MARCO. *Microbes Infect.* 2000;2(3):313–316.
83. van der Laan LJ, et al. Macrophage scavenger receptor MARCO: in vitro and in vivo regulation and involvement in the anti-bacterial host defense. *Immunol Letter.* 1997;57:203.
84. Palecanda A, et al. Role of the scavenger receptor MARCO in alveolar macrophage binding of unopsonized environmental particles. *J Exp Med.* 1999;189(9):1497–1506.
85. Elomaa O, et al. Structure of the human macrophage MARCO receptor and characterization of its bacteria-binding region. *J Biol Chem*. 1998;273(8):4530–4538.
86. Fraser IP, Koziel H, Ezekowitz RA. The serum mannose-binding protein and the macrophage mannose receptor are pattern recognition molecules that link innate and adaptive immunity. *Semin Immunol.* 1998;10(5):363–372.
87. Taylor ME, et al. Primary structure of the mannose receptor contains multiple motifs resembling carbohydrate-recognition domains. *J Biol Chem*. 1990;265(21):12156–12162.
88. Taylor ME, Bezouska K, Drickamer K. Contribution to ligand binding by multiple carbohydrate-recognition domains in the macrophage mannose receptor. *J Biol Chem*. 1992;267(3):1719–1726.
89. Linehan SA, Martinez-Pomares L, Gordon S. *Macrophage lectins in host defense. Microbes Infect.* 2000;2:279.
90 Prigozy TI, et al. The mannose receptor delivers lipoglycan antigens to endosomes for presentation to T cells by CD1b molecules. *Immunity.* 1997;6(2):187–197.
91. Jiang W, et al. The receptor DEC-205 expressed by dendritic cells and thymic epithelial cells is involved in antigen processing. *Nature*. 1995;375(6527):151–155.
92. Ariizumi K, et al. Identification of a novel, dendritic cell-associated molecule, dectin-1, by subtractive cDNA cloning. *J Biol Chem.* 2000;275(26):20157–20167.
93. Brown GD, Gordon S. Immune recognition. A new receptor for beta-glucans. *Nature.* 2001;413(6851):36–37.
94. Brown GD. Dectin-1: a signalling non-TLR pattern-recognition receptor. *Nat Rev Immunol.* 2006;6(1):33–43.
95. Lee MS, Kim YJ. Signaling pathways downstream of pattern-recognition receptors and their cross talk. *Annu Rev Biochem.* 2007;(76):447–480.
96. Gross O, et al. Card9 controls a non-TLR signalling pathway for innate anti-fungal immunity. *Nature*. 2006;442(7103):651–656.
97. Leibundgut-Landmann S, et al. Syk- and CARD9-dependent coupling of innate immunity to the induction of T helper cells that produce interleukin 17. *Nat Immunol*. 2007;(6):630–638.
98. Holmskov U, et al. Collectins: collagenous C-type lectins of the innate immune defense system. *Immunol Today.* 1994;15(2):67–74.
99. Clark HW, Reid KB, Sim RB. Collectins and innate immunity in the lung. *Microbes Infect*. 2000;2(3):273–278.
100. Weis WI, Drickamer K. Structural basis of lectin-carbohydrate recognition. *Annu Rev Biochem.* 1996;65:441–473.
101. Fraser I, Ezekowitz RAB. Receptors for microbial products: carbohydrates. In: *Inflammation basic principles and clinical correlates*. J.I. Gallin and R. Snyderman, eds. Philadelphia: Lippincott, Williams & Wilkins. 1999;515.
102. Crouch E, Wright JR. Surfactant proteins a and d and pulmonary host defense. *Annu Rev Physiol.* 2001;63:521–554.
103. Gewurz H, et al. C-reactive protein and the acute phase response. *Adv Intern Med.* 1982;27:345–372.
104. Schwalbe RA, et al. Pentraxin family of proteins interact specifically with phosphorylcholine and/or phosphorylethanolamine. *Biochemistry*. 1992;31(20):4907–4915.
105. Agrawal A, et al. Topology and structure of the C1q-binding site on C-reactive protein. *J Immunol*. 2001;166(6):3998–4004.
106. Garlanda C, et al. Pentraxins in innate immunity and inflammation. *Novartis Found Symp*. 2006;279:80–86; discussion 86–91, 216–219.
107. Ulevitch RJ, Tobias PS. Receptor-dependent mechanisms of cell stimulation by bacterial endotoxin. *Annu Rev Immunol.* 1995;13:437–457.
108. Kang D, et al. A peptidoglycan recognition protein in innate immunity conserved from insects to humans. *Proc Natl Acad Sci U S A.* 1998;95(17):10078–10082.
109. Liu C, et al. Peptidoglycan recognition proteins: a novel family of four human innate immunity pattern recognition molecules. *J Biol Chem*. 2001;276(37):34686–34694.
110. Werner T, et al. A family of peptidoglycan recognition proteins in the fruit fly Drosophila melanogaster. *Proc Natl Acad Sci U S A.* 2000;97(25):13772–13777.

111. Liu C, et al. Mammalian peptidoglycan recognition protein binds peptidoglycan with high affinity, is expressed in neutrophils, and inhibits bacterial growth. *J Biol Chem*. 2000;275(32):24490–24499.
112. Gack MU, et al. TRIM25 RING-finger E3 ubiquitin ligase is essential for RIG-I-mediated antiviral activity. *Nature*. 2007;446(7138):916–920.
113. Meylan E, Tschopp J. Toll-like receptors and RNA helicases: two parallel ways to trigger antiviral responses. *Mol Cell*. 2006;22(5):561–569.
114. Seth RB, Sun L, Chen ZJ. Antiviral innate immunity pathways. *Cell Res*. 2006;16(2):141–147.
115. Williams BR. PKR; a sentinel kinase for cellular stress. *Oncogene*. 1999;18(45):6112–6120.
116. Kumar M, Carmichael GG. Antisense RNA: function and fate of duplex RNA in cells of higher eukaryotes. *Microbiol Mol Biol Rev*. 1998;62(4):1415–1434.
117. Samuel CE. Antiviral actions of interferons. *Clin Microbiol Rev*. 2001;14(4):778–809, table of contents.
118. Fritz JH, et al. Nod-like proteins in immunity, inflammation and disease. *Nat Immunol*. 2006;7(12):1250–1257.
119. Bertin J, et al. Human CARD4 protein is a novel CED-4/Apaf-1 cell death family member that activates NF-kappaB. *J Biol Chem*. 1999;274:12955.
120. Inohara N, et al. Nod1, an Apaf-1-like activator of caspase-9 and nuclear factor-kappaB. *J Biol Chem*. 1999;274(21):14560–14567.
121. Ogura Y, et al. Nod2, a Nod1/Apaf-1 family member that is restricted to monocytes and activates NF-kappaB. *J Biol Chem*. 2001; 276(7):4812–4818.
122. Wang L, et al. Card10 is a novel caspase recruitment domain/membrane-associated guanylate kinase family member that interacts with BCL10 and activates NF-kappa B. *J Biol Chem*. 2001; 276:21405.
123. Cho JH. The Nod2 gene in Crohn's disease: implications for future research into the genetics and immunology of Crohn's disease. *Inflamm Bowel Dis*. 2001;7(3):271–275.
124. Hampe J, et al. Association betwween insertion mutation in NOD2 gene and Crohn's disease in German and British populations. *Lancet*. 2001(357):1925.
125. Mariathasan S, Monack DM. Inflammasome adaptors and sensors: intracellular regulators of infection and inflammation. *Nat Rev Immunol*. 2007;7(1):31–40.
126. Martinon F, Tschopp J. Inflammatory caspases: linking an intracellular innate immune system to autoinflammatory diseases. *Cell*. 2004;117(5):561–574.
127. Tschopp J, Martinon F, Burns K. NALPs: a novel protein family involved in inflammation. *Nat Rev Mol Cell Biol*. 2003;4(2):95–104.
128. Ferrero-Miliani L, et al. Chronic inflammation: importance of NOD2 and NALP3 in interleukin-1beta generation. *Clin Exp Immunol*. 2007;147(2):227–235.
129. Fadok VA, et al. Loss of phospholipids asymmetry and surface exposure of phosphatidylserine is required for phagocytosis of apoptotic cells by macrophages and fibroblasts. *J Biol Chem*. 2001;276:1071.
130. Fadok VA, et al. Exposure of phosphatidylserine on the surface of apoptotic lymphocytes triggers specific recognition and removal by macrophages. *J Immunol*. 1992;148(7):2207–2216.
131. Oldenborg PA, et al. Role of CD47 as a marker of self on red blood cells. *Science*. 2000;288:2051.
132. Henson PM, Bratton DL, Fadok VA. Apoptotic cell removal. *Curr Biol*. 2001;11(19):R795–805.
133. Fadok VA, et al. A receptor for phosphatidylserine-specific clearance of apoptotic cells. *Nature*. 2000;405(6782):85–90.
134. Galli SJ. Mast cells and basophils. *Curr Opin Hematol*. 2000;7(1): 32–39.
135. Ramos BF, et al. Mast cells are critical for the production of leukotrienes responsible for neutrophil recruitment in immune complex-induced peritonitis in mice. *J Immunol*. 1991;147(5):1636–1641.
136. Zhang Y, Ramos BF, Jakschik BA. Neutrophil recruitment by tumor necrosis factor from mast cells in immune complex peritonitis. *Science*. 1992;258(5090):1957–1959.
137. Echtenacher B, Mannel DN, Hultner L. Critical protective role of mast cells in a model of acute septic peritonitis. *Nature*. 1996;381(6577):75–77.
138. Malaviya R, et al. Mast cell modulation of neutrophils influx and bacterial clearance at sites of infection through TNF-alpha. *Nature*. 1996;381:77.
139. Gordon JR, Galli SJ. Mast cells as a source of both preformed and immunologically inducible TNF-alpha/cachectin. *Nature*. 1990;346:274.
140. Levy O. Antimicrobial proteins and peptides of blood: templates for novel antimicrobial agents. *Blood*. 2000;96(8):2664–2672.
141. Banchereau J, Steinman RM. Dendritic cells and the control of immunity. *Nature*. 1998;392(6673):245–252.
142. Kagnoff MF, Eckmann L. Epithelial cells as sensors for microbial infection. *J Clin. Invest*. 1997;100:6.
143. Boot RG, et al. Cloning of a cDNA encoding chitotriosidase, a human chitinase produced by macrophages. *J Biol Chem*. 1995;270(44):26252–26256.
144. Wright GC, et al. Bacterial phospholipid hydrolysis enhances the destruction of Escherichia coli ingested by rabbit neutrophils. Role of cellular and extracellular phospholipases. *J Clin Invest*. 1990;85(6):1925–1935.
145. Qu XD, Lehrer RI. Secretory phospholipase A2 is the principal bactericide for staphylococci and other gram-positive bacteria in human tears. *Infect Immun*. 1998;66:2791.
146. Laine VJ, Grass DS, Nevalainen TJ. Protection by group II phospholipase A2 against Staphylococcus aureus. *J Immunol*. 1999;162(12):7402–7408.
147. Laine VJ, Grass DS, Nevalainen TJ. Resistance of transgenic mice expressing human group II phospholipase A2 to Escherichia coli infection. *Infect Immun*. 2000;68(1):87–92.
148. Elsbach P, Weiss J. Role of the bactericidal/permeability-increasing protein in host defence. *Curr Opin Immunol*. 1998;10(1):45–49.
149. Martin E, Ganz T, Lehrer RI. Defensins and other endogenous peptide antibiotics of vertebrates. *J Leukoc Biol*. 1995;58(2):128–136.
150. Boman HG. Peptide antibiotics and their role in innate immunity. *Annual Rev Immunol*. 1995;13:61.
151. Wilson CL, et al. Regulation of intestinal alpha-defensin activation by the metalloproteinase matrilysin in innate host defense. *Science*. 1999;286(5437):113–117.
152. Zanetti M, Gennaro R, Romeo D. Cathelicidins: a novel protein family with a common proregion and a variable C-terminal antimicrobial domain. *FEBS Lett*. 1995;374(1):1–5.
153. Zanetti M, Gennaro R, Romeo D. The cathelicidin family of antimicrobial peptide precursors: a component of the oxygen-independent defense mechanisms of neutrophils. *Ann NY Acad Sci*. 1997;832:147–162.
154. Gabay JE, Almeida RP. Antibiotic peptides and serine protease homologs in human polymorphonuclear leukocytes: defensins and azurocidin. *Curr Opin Immunol*. 1993;5(1):97–102.
155. Belaaouaj A, et al. Mice lacking neutrophils elastase reveal impaired host defense against gram negative bacterial sepsis. *Nat Med*. 1998;4:615.
156. Jurado RL. Iron, infections, and anemia of inflammation. *Clin Infect Dis*. 1997;25(4):888–895.
157. Hoek KS, et al. Antibacterial activity in bovine lactoferrin-derived peptides. *Antimicrob Agents Chemother*. 1997;41(1):54–59.
158. Vidal SM, et al. Natural resistance to infection with intracellular parasites: isolation of a candidate for Bcg. *Cell*. 1993;73(3):469–485.
159. Loomans HJ, et al. Histidine-based zinc-binding sequences and the antimicrobial activity of calprotectin. *J Infect Dis*. 1998;177(3):812–814.
160. Klebanoff, S.J. Oxygen metabolites from phagocytes. In *Inflammation: Basic Principles and Clinical Correlates*. Gallin JI, Snyderman R, eds. Philadelphia: Lippincott, Williams & Wilkins. 1999;721.
161. Bogdan C, Rollinghoff M, Diefenbach A. Reactive oxygen and reactive nitrogen intermediates in innate and specific immunity. *Curr Opin Immunol*. 2000;12(1):64–76.
162. MacMicking J, Xie QW, Nathan C. Nitric oxide and macrophage function. *Annu Rev Immunol*. 1997;15:323–350.
163. Shiloh MU, et al. Phenotype of mice and macrophages deficient in both phagocyte oxidase and inducible nitric oxide synthase. *Immunity*. 1999;10(1):29–38.
164. Arnheiter, H, et al. Transgenic mice with intracellular immunity to influenza virus. *Cell*. 1990;62(1):51–61.

165. Pavlovic J, et al. Enhanced virus resistance of transgenic mice expressing the human MxA protein. *J Virol.* 1995;69(7):4506–4510.
166. Pavlovic J, et al. Mx proteins: GTPases involved in the interferon-induced antiviral state. *Ciba Found Symp.* 1993;176:233–243; discussion 243–247.
167. Pavlovic J, Staeheli P. The antiviral potentials of Mx proteins. *J Interferon Res*. 1991;11(4):215–219.
168. Landolfo S, et al. Mechanisms of vial inhibition by interferons. *Pharmacol Ther.* 1995;65:415.
169. Hefti HP, et al. Human MxA protein protects mice lacking a functional alpha/beta interferon system against La crosse virus and other lethal viral infections. *J Virol*. 1999;73(8):6984–6991.
170. Anderson SL, et al. Interferon-induced guanylate binding protein-1 (GBP-1) mediates an antiviral effect against vesicular stomatitis virus and encephalomyocarditis virus. *Virology*. 1999;256(1):8–14.
171. Iwasaki A, Medzhitov R. Toll-like receptor control of the adaptive immune responses. *Nat Immunol*. 2004;5(10):987–995.

Chapter 15

Dendritic Cells

Muriel Moser

DISCOVERY AND DEFINITION

In the 1960s, several research groups demonstrated that a population of adherent cells was required for the induction of B and T cell responses *in vitro* and *in vivo*. Most immunologists believed at that time that macrophages were the critical "accessory" cells, on the basis of their adherent properties *(1)*.

In 1973, during the course of observations of murine splenic cells that adhere to glass and plastic surfaces, Steinman and Cohn (2) noticed large stellate cells whose cytoplasm was arranged in pseudopods of varying length and form. These authors reported that these cells, named *dendritic cells (DCs)* because of their branchlike projections (from δενδρεον, tree), undergo characteristic movements, do not exhibit the endocytic capacities of macrophages, and adhere to glass. The function of DCs was elucidated 5 years later when it was reported that these cells were the most potent stimulators of the primary mixed leukocyte reaction in mice, which led to the suggestion that DCs instead of macrophages could be the accessory cells required in the generation of many immune responses (3). This hypothesis was amply demonstrated in the years that followed.

The dendritic family includes many members located throughout the body that share phenotypic and functional properties:

- Dendritic morphology (at least at some stage) and low buoyant density
- Elevated expression of major histocompatibility complex (MHC) molecules (class I and class II) and intermediate to high expression of costimulatory molecules
- Motility
- Specialization of function over time—that is, a shift from an antigen-capturing mode to a T cell sensitizing mode

The hallmark of the DC family is the conversion of these cells from immature sentinels to mature immunostimulatory cells, a phenomenon called *maturation.*

Figure 15.1 illustrates the development of DCs *in vivo* at the precursor, immature, and mature stages. The right column corresponds to the induction of DC maturation by a "danger signal" (pathogen invasion), and their subsequent migration to lymphoid organs. The left column describes the movement of (presumably immature) DCs at the steady state. These pathways are described in the following chapters.

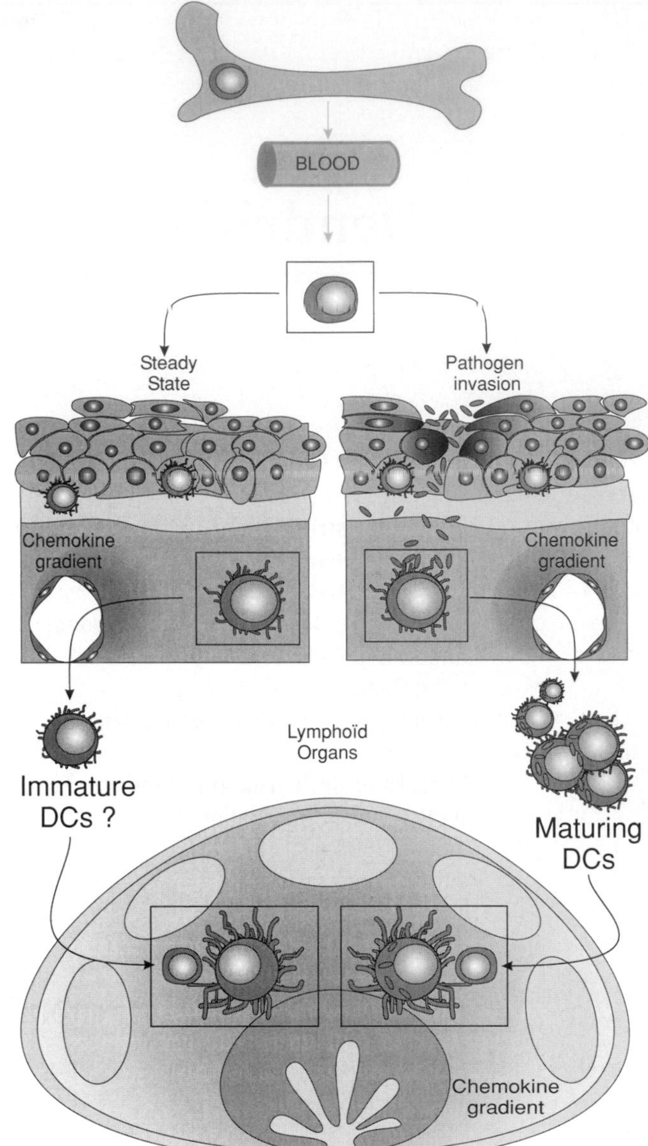

FIGURE 15.1 Developmental stages of DCs *in vivo.* The generation of DC precursors in the bone marrow, the recruitment of immature DCs in peripheral tissues, and the migration of DCs into the lymphoid organs are illustrated. The maturation of DCs into potent APCs in case of infection or inflammation and their migration have been amply documented (right), but there is also evidence that in the "steady state"—that is, in the absence of a "danger signal"—these immature DCs may migrate into the lymphoid organs while remaining at the immature stage (left). The phenotype of the DC migrating in baseline conditions is still unclear. The movement of maturing DCs and the "constitutive" migration of immature DCs have been shown to depend on chemokine gradients.

ORIGIN AND DISTRIBUTION OF DENDRITIC CELLS *IN VIVO:* A MULTIMEMBER FAMILY

Interstitial Dendritic Cells

DCs are found as immature cells in virtually all organs (except the brain) within the interstitial spaces that are drained by afferent lymphatic vessels. DCs have been isolated from the heart, kidney, dermis, liver, and other organs.

DCs are found in mucosal surfaces, such as those of the lung and intestine. In the lung, the network of airway DCs is particularly well developed to capture inhaled antigens *(4).* Its location above the basement membrane of the airway epithelium ensures accessibility to inhaled antigens. There is some evidence that these DCs are maintained in an immature state by an inhibitory mechanism that may involve macrophages *(5,6).* In the intestine, DCs from Peyer's patches have been characterized and are known to contain three populations that differ by their phenotype and function *(7,8).*

In the mouse, all splenic DCs express similar amounts of CD11c, class II MHC, and costimulatory molecules CD80, CD86, and CD40. Two major subtypes can be found: The first is positive for the CD8α marker and the C-type lectin CD205 (CD8α^+ DEC205$^+$), and the second lacks CD8α and expresses the antigen recongnized by the 33D1 monoclonal antibody CD8$^-$ 33D1$^+$ (9). The subsets also differ by their localization: The majority of DCs in the marginal zone are CD8α^-, whereas most DCs in the T cell areas express the

CD8α homodimer (ref. [9], and our own observations). The DC populations in lymph nodes appear to be even more complex. In addition to the populations present in the spleen, two DC subtypes that likely correspond to dermal- and epidermal-derived DCs *(10)* have been described. The mouse thymus *(11)* has been shown to contain two DC types that differ at the level of CD8α expression.

Precursors of DC Populations

Geissmann et al. have recently identified a clonogenic bone marrow progenitor specific for macrophages and DCs (12). A mouse bone marrow population that expresses CD117 (c-kit, the receptor for stem cell factor) and the chemokine receptor CX3CR1 but not markers of lineage-committed precursors (Lin-) gives rise to monocytes, several subsets of macrophages, and steady state CD11c$^+$ CD8α^+ and CD11c$^+$ CD8α^- DCs *in vivo*. In contrast, this progenitor is devoid of lymphoid, erythroid and megakaryocytic potential. No plasmacytoid DC was detected in the progeny of this bone marrow progenitor, suggesting that this DC subset may originate from a distinct lineage.

Several reports have suggested that monocytes are capable of generating DCs in mice. Randolph et al. *(13)* investigated the differentiation and trafficking *in vivo* of inflammatory monocytes that phagocytosed subcutaneously injected fluorescent microspheres. They found that most of the monocytes became macrophages in the subcutaneous tissue, but that 25% of latex$^+$ cells migrated to the T cell area of draining lymph nodes several days later, where they expressed DC-restricted markers and high levels of costimulatory molecules. In another report, some monocytes transferred into animals with experimentally induced peritonitis were shown to infiltrate the peritoneal cavity and acquire CD11c and MHCII expression, suggestive of differentiation into DC *(14)*. A third study demonstrates *(15)* that monocytes can generate DCs on extravasation from the bloodstream during homing to the spleen when adoptively transferred in irradiated recipients.

Whether monocytes can differentiate into DC in noninflammatory conditions is less clear. A recent study (16) suggests that monocytes from spleen, blood, or bone marrow generate few if any conventional DCs. However, when systemic inflammation was induced, transferred monocytes in the spleen upregulated both CD11c and MHC II and could be classed as DCs, They express intermediate levels of CD11c and high levels of CD11b, a phenotype distinct from the resident steady state DCs (CD11c^{hi}CD11b^{int}). Of note, monocytes remained as monocytes in the blood, bone marrow, and peritoneum in the same inflammatory conditions (16). Varol et al. *(17)* similarly concluded from their adoptive transfer experiments in WT and mononuclear phagocyte-depleted recipient mice that monocytes appear to be dedicated to DC replenishment of nonlymphoid organs, such as the intestinal lamina propria, whereas splenic DCs seem to arise from local precursors without a monocytic intermediate. Collectively, these data suggest that monocytes give rise to inflammatory DCs but not to classical steady-state subset resident in lymphoid organs (Figure 15.2).

Another form of inflammatory DCs, which produces TNFα and iNOS, was identified in spleens of *Listeria monocytogenes*–infected mice *(18)*. It is interesting that this subset is not essential for T cell priming but, as the major producer of TNF and iNOS during the first 48 hours of bacterial infection, mediates the innate defense and is critical to clear the infection. The TNF/iNOS-producing DCs are not present in an uninfected spleen but are recruited following systemic infection through a mechanism dependent on CCR2 (a chemokine receptor known to target monocytes to sites of inflammation) signaling. Similar cells have recently been found to be the dominant DC and the dominant source of TNFα in the human skin disease psoriasis *(19)*, which is treated by blockade of TNFα.

A splenic precursor population was identified [16] that produces all splenic CD8$^+$ and CD8$^-$ conventional DCs (but not plasmacytoid DCs or other lineages), suggesting that the spleen contains a substantial reservoir of immediate DC precursors. They comprise 0.05% of splenocytes and expressed a CD11c^{int}CD45RA^{lo}CD43^{int}SIRP-a^{int}CD4$^-$CD8$^-$MHC$^-$ phenotype. This population accounts for most of the total conventional DC precursor activity. There is evidence that precommitment to the separate CD8$^+$ versus CD8$^-$ DC subtypes can be found in the splenic precursor population (differing by CD24 expression), suggesting that these subsets are separate sublineages.

The origin of plasmacytoid DCs is less clear. Based on the observation that FLT3 ligand is a growth factor for hemopoietic progenitors and can promote the expansion of both conventional and plasmacytoid DCs, D'Amico and Wu *(20)* examined the expression of Flt3 on the surface of bone marrow cells. They found that the majority of Flt3$^+$ cells were within the Lin- c-kit fraction of bone marrow that contains the common lymphoid precursor (CLP) and the common myeloid precursor (CMP). Of note, the DC precursor activity for both conventional and plasmacytoid DCs was strongly enriched in the CMP and CLP Flt3$^+$ fractions. These observations suggest that early precursors for all DC subtypes are within the bone marrow Flt3$^+$ precursor population. The separation of the pathways leading to conventional or plasmacytoid-restricted DC precursors at some point downstream the bone marrow Flt3$^+$ precursor is yet to be defined.

Langerhans Cells

Cells with a dendritic structure were visualized in the skin by Paul Langerhans in 1868. They were described as cells displaying long processes and were considered to belong to

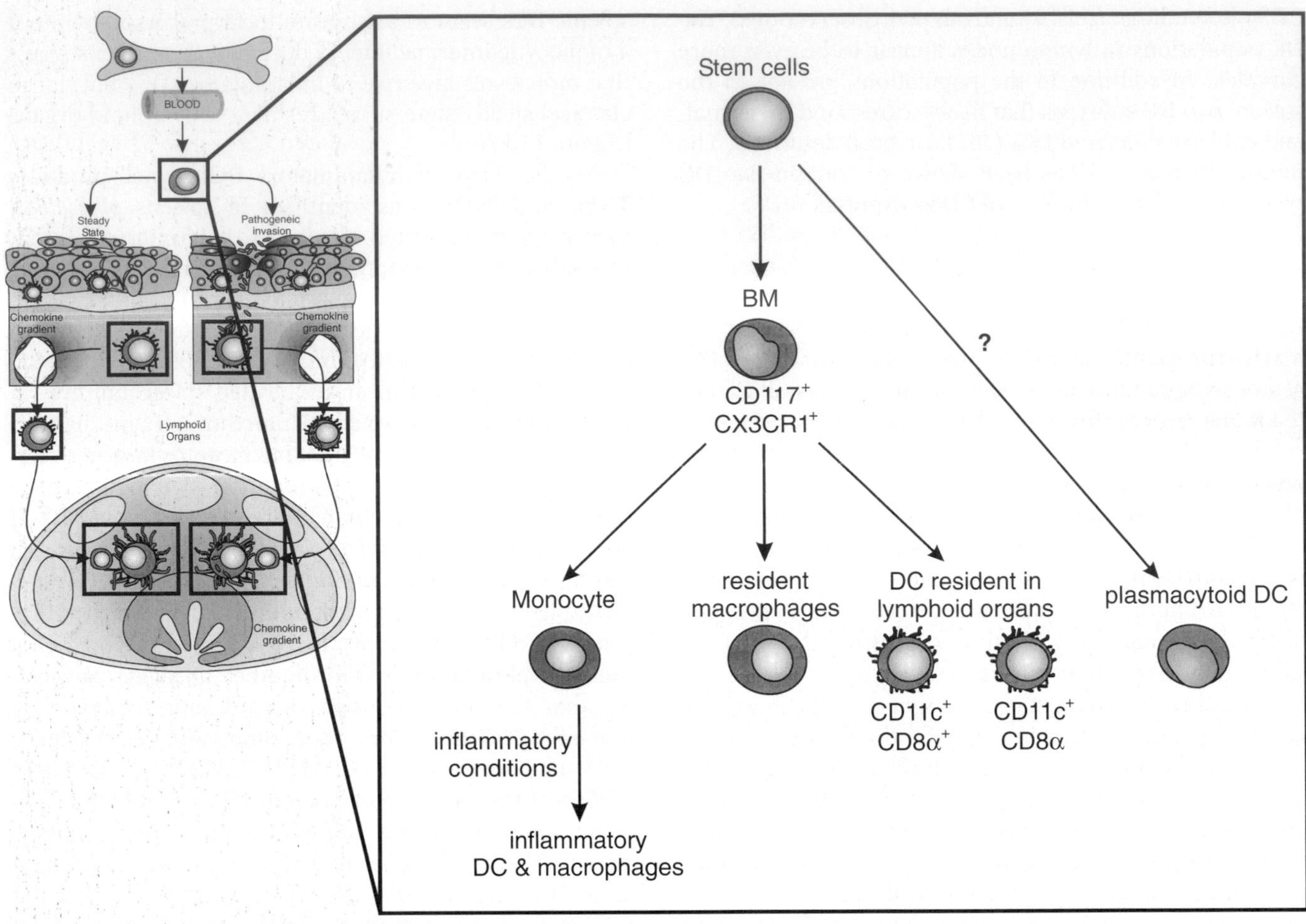

FIGURE 15.2 DC development. A clonogenic bone marrow progenitor specific for macrophages and DCs was recently identified (12). Cells expressing CD117 (c-kit, the receptor for stem cell factor) and the chemokine receptor CX3CR1 give rise to monocytes, some macrophages, and $CD11c^+$ $CD8\alpha^+$ and $CD11c^+$ $CD8\alpha^-$ DCs in lymphoid organs. No plasmacytoid DC was detected in the progeny of this progenitor. Recent data suggest that monocytes give rise to inflammatory DCs but not to classical subsets resident in lymphoid organs.

the nervous system. The nature of these so-called Langerhans cells remained obscure until they were shown to be derived from bone marrow and to express class II MHC and were identified as the active cells in epidermis for presenting antigen to T cells (*21–22*,23) The relationship of these epidermal Langerhans cells to DCs was established by the observations that murine epidermal Langerhans cells mature into potent immunostimulatory DCs *in vitro* (24).

Ultrastructurally, Langerhans cells are characterized by a unique pentalamellar cytoplasmic organelle: the Birbeck granule. Valladeau et al. (25) identified a type II Ca^{2+}–dependent lectin displaying mannose-binding specificity, exclusively expressed by Langerhans cells. This lectin was called *langerin* (now CD207) and is constitutively associated with Birbeck granules. Although the role of Birbeck granules remains enigmatic, they are attractive candidate receptors for nonconventional antigen routing in Langerhans cells.

Distinctly present in the epidermis, but also found in other stratified squamous epithelia in the pharynx, upper esophagus, vagina, and external cervis, LCs are distributed in a network fashion (although cell–cell contacts have yet to be described) that covers the entire body surface, constituting the first immunological barrier against the external environment. LC migrate to draining lymph nodes at a low rate in the steady state and at an accelerated rate in the context of inflammation. Whether migrating LCs simply carry the antigen (26) to DC resident in the lymph node or whether they directly prime or tolerize antigen-specific T cells is still under investigation.

Merad et al. (27) recently identified the immediate circulating LC precursor that repopulates LC *in vivo*. They exposed skin to ultraviolet irradiation, leading to strong decrease in Langerhans cell numbers, and monitored the repopulation of Langerhans cells in skin with ultraviolet irradiation injury. They used chimeric mice (i.e, lethally irradiated recipient mice) reconstituted 3 weeks earlier with mixed hematopoietic precursors expressing or not expressing the CSF-1 receptor (*Csf1r*$^{-/-}$ and *Cfs1r*$^{+/+}$). Analysis of chimeric mice 3 weeks after ultraviolet irradiation showed that *Csf1r*$^{-/-}$ Langerhans cells were absent, showing that *Csf1r*$^{-/-}$ hemopoietic cells are unable to differentiate into Langerhans cells in inflamed skin. Of note, the requirement for CSF-1R appears restricted to LCs as mutant and wild-type splenic DCs were similarly reconstituted. The authors further confirmed that the GR-1^{hi} monocytes were the direct circulating Langerhans cells precursors using monocyte tagging *in vivo* with fluorescent latex beads and adoptive transfer.

Veiled Cells

Typical DCs are found in afferent lymphatic vessels and are called *veiled cells* because of their sheetlike cell processes, or lamellipodia. Early studies underscored the crucial role of the afferent lymphatics during cell-mediated immunity: Priming to skin transplants was shown to be blocked by lymphatic ablation *(28)*. In contrast, efferent lymphatic vessels seem to lack DCs, which suggests that they do not leave the lymph nodes. Indeed, there is evidence that mature DCs undergo apoptosis in the lymphoid organ *(29)* and can be widely processed by other DCs in the node to form peptide MHC complexes *(30)*.

Plasmacytoid derived Dendritic Cells

CD4$^+$CD11c$^-$ DC precursors with the appearance of plasma cells have been identified in human blood and are identical to natural interferon (IFN) α/β–producing cells, which secrete high amounts of IFN-α/β in response to viruses. These plasmacytoid cells can give rise to DCs *in vitro* in the presence of IL-3 or during viral infection. IFN-α/β and TNFα produced by virus-activated plasmacytoid cells act as an autocrine survival factor and a DC differentiation factor, respectively (31). These cells appear, therefore, to play a role in innate immune responses as IFN-α producers and in adaptive immune responses as antigen-presenting cells (APCs).

The equivalent murine type of type I IFN-producing cells (mIPCs), described in 2001, consists of a population of immature DCs Ly6C/Gr-1$^+$, B220$^+$, CD11c^{lo}, and CD4$^+$ *(32,33)*, showing a homogeneous plasmacytoid structure—that is, a round shape, a smooth surface, and an eccentric nucleus. Upon activation, these cells display a more irregular shape, up-regulate their immunostimulatory properties, and produce IFN-α, IL-12, or both, depending on the stimulus.

HALLMARKS OF CELLS FROM THE DENDRITIC FAMILY

Among the populations of APCs, which include DCs, B lymphocytes, and macrophages, DCs display some unique properties aimed at sensitizing T lymphocytes specific for dangerous antigens encountered earlier in periphery. Indeed, pathogens often invade peripheral tissues, whereas the immune response is initiated in lymphoid structures in which T and B lymphocytes reside *(34)*. DCs appear to form a physical link between the periphery and the secondary lymphoid organs: They act as sentinels for "dangerous" antigens in the peripheral tissues and then migrate to the areas where T cells are located to transmit information about the nature of the pathogen and the infected tissues. To efficiently perform these different tasks, most DCs have a specialization of function over time and location, with a possible exception for plasmacytoid DCs.

During the process of maturation, often associated with their migration from the periphery to the lymphoid organs, DCs shift from an antigen-capturing mode to a T cell–sensitizing mode. The maturation process is induced by microbial products and inflammatory chemokines, thereby favoring the sensitization of T lymphocytes specific for non–self-infectious antigens (Figure 15.3). The following sections review the properties of DCs that confer on them the capability to focus the adaptive immune response on pathogens, avoiding autoimmunity.

The Process of Maturation

The relationship of Langerhans cells to DCs isolated from lymphoid organs was provided in 1985 by Schuler and Steinman (24). The authors showed that fresh Langerhans cells are weak stimulators of T cell proliferation but undergo a progressive increase in stimulatory capacity *in vitro*. The development of enhanced stimulatory activity during culture was called *maturation* (Figure 15.3) and could not be ascribed only to an increase in the level of class II MHC molecules. The authors suggested that functioning DCs, present in lymphoid organs, may be derived from less mature precursors located in nonlymphoid tissues. By comparing the efficacy of fresh and cultured DCs to present a protein to T cell clones, Romani et al. (35) showed that the capacity of DC populations to present proteins varies inversely with stimulating activity in the mixed leukocyte reaction (MLR). Freshly isolated Langerhans cells are very active in presenting proteins, whereas cultured spleen DCs and epidermal Langerhans cells present native protein weakly. These observations suggested that DCs in nonlymphoid tissues such as skin act as sentinels for presenting antigens *in situ,* whereas DCs in lymphoid organs have the capacity to sensitize naïve T cells. This hypothesis was further confirmed, although many DCs in spleen can be found at the immature state (36,37).

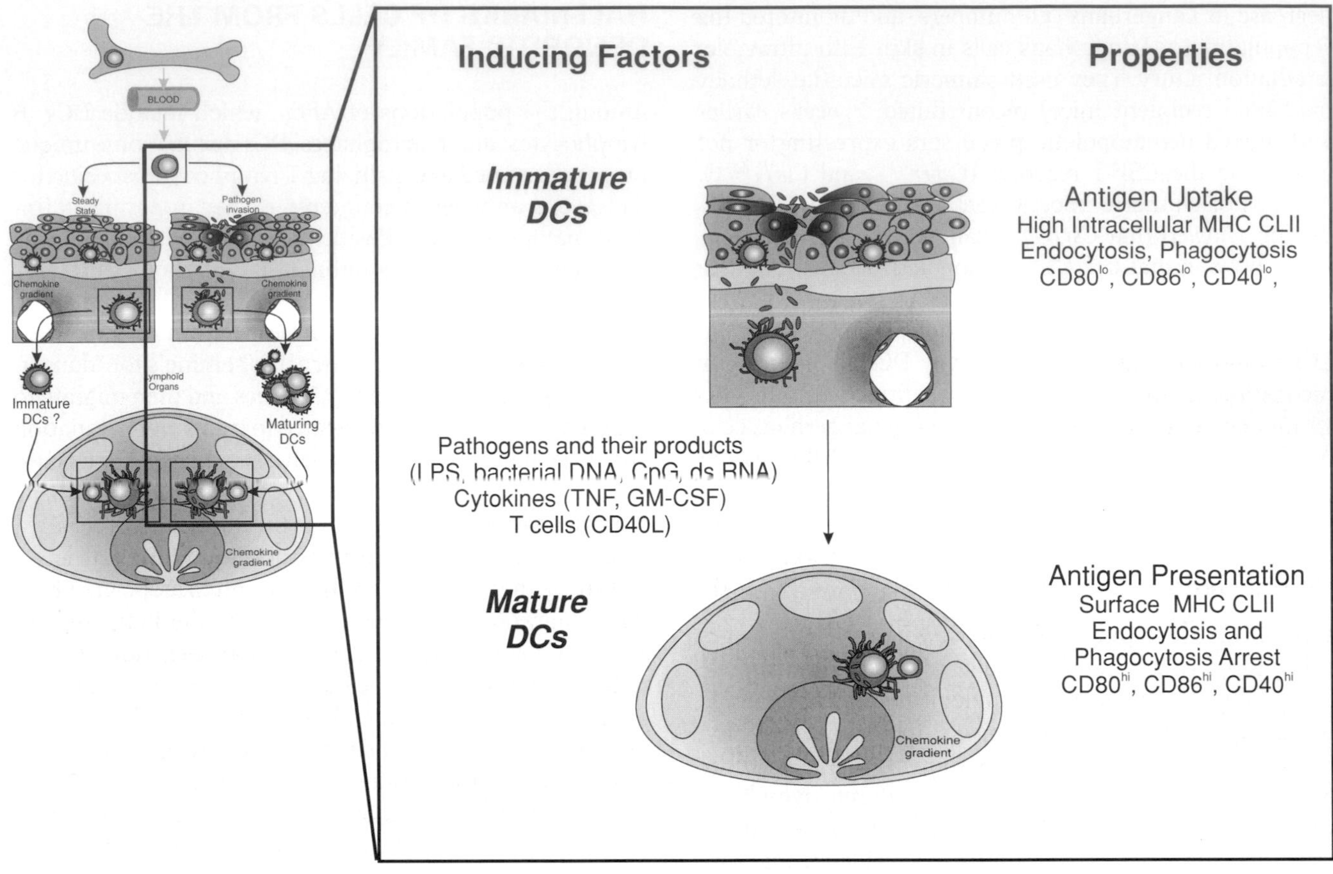

FIGURE 15.3 The phenomenon of maturation. In the presence of inflammatory cytokines, microbial products or antigen-activated T lymphocytes, DCs undergo a phenomenon of maturation—that is, they shift from an antigen-capturing mode to a T cell–sensitizing mode. The phenotypic and functional changes are associated with their migration into the T cell area of lymphoid organs.

Therefore, cells of the dendritic family have a specialization of function over time, as they shift from an antigen-capturing mode to a T cell–sensitizing mode during a process called *maturation* (Figure 15.3). DC maturation induces multiple alterations in the function and intracellular transport of class II MHC molecules, leading to the redistribution of class II MHC from intracellular compartments to the plasma membrane (see later discussion). Importantly, the type of maturation stimulus determines the type of DC differentiation pathway and then the type of T cell response (e.g, exposure of human blood DCs to thymic stromal lymphopoietin yields a mature DC that induces an inflammatory type of Th2 cell, while exposure to CD40L yields a mature DC that induces a Th1 type response *[38]*). To recognize antigen, T cells need to establish contact with APCs. The two cell types form an immunological synapse, in which T cell receptors (TCRs) and costimulatory molecules are congregated in a central area surrounded by a ring of adhesion molecules (see later discussion). In particular, the B7 family has been shown to contain six members, which positively or negatively regulate the expansion or function of T cells, or both (for review, see Coyle and Gutierrez-Ramos *[39]*). The CD80 and CD86 molecules, the first CD28 ligands to be described, have been shown to promote clonal expansion of resting T cells through CD28 and inhibit T cell expansion through interactions with CTLA-4. Expression of ligands for the CTLA-4/CD28 molecules was shown to be up-regulated on epidermal Langerhans cells *(40)* and splenic DCs *(41,42)* during their functional maturation *in vitro*. The process of maturation also occurs *in vivo:* Systemic administration of endotoxin (lipopolysaccharide [LPS]) induces the migration of most splenic DCs from the marginal zone between the red and white pulp to the T cell area in the white pulp (43,44). This movement parallels a maturation process, as assessed by down-regulation of processing capacity and up-regulation of immunostimulatory properties (43).

Maturation can be mediated by inflammatory cytokines (TNF-α, IL-1), T cells (through CD40/CD40L interaction), microbial constituents (LPS, CpG oligonucleotides), and stress (necrosis, transplantation). DC maturation has been shown to involve signaling cascades initiated by the

Toll/interleukin-1 receptor homology domains of Toll-like receptor (TLR) family that can lead to activation of nuclear factor κB (NF-κB) and mitogen-activated protein kinase (MAPK). TLR4 is the mammalian homolog of *Drosophila* Toll, which is involved in dorsoventral patterning and in host defense against fungal infection. To date, more than 10 members have been reported to belong to the TLR family in mammals and seem involved in recognizing pathogen-associated molecular patterns (for review, see Kaisho and Akira *[45]*). Other pathways that induce powerful stimulatory DCs involve interaction with innate natural killer (NK) *(46)* and NKT lymphocytes *(36,47)* and selective triggering through activating Fcγ receptors *(48,49)*.

Antigen Uptake

At the immature stage, DCs exhibit some endocytic activity. To sample their environment in peripheral tissues, they can take up extracellular fluid and concentrate the macrosolutes in the endocytic compartment. The fluid volume taken up per hour by a single cultured monocyte derived DC has been estimated to be 1,000 to 1,500 μm^3, a volume that is close to that of the cell itself, but similar levels of uptake have yet to be documented *in vivo (50)*.

In addition, DCs express various receptors mediating endocytosis and phagocytosis of antigens, pathogens, and dying cells: crystallized fragment (Fc) receptors for IgE and IgG, which internalize immune complexes receptors for heat shock proteins; receptors, such as CD36 and $\alpha v\beta 5$, which bind and phagocytose apoptotic bodies; and C-type lectins, such as macrophage mannose receptor and DEC-205 *(51)*, which contain 8 and 10 contiguous C-type lectin domains, respectively *(52)*. Whereas most receptors, including the macrophage mannose receptor, internalize and recycle through early endosomes, the DEC-205 cytosolic domain mediates a unique recycling pathway through late endosomes or lysosomes, rich in antigen-presenting class II MHC products, and greatly enhances antigen presentation relative to the mannose receptor tail *(53)*.

Antigen uptake is down-modulated during the process of maturation *(50)*. Most receptors are expressed at lower levels on mature DCs, except DEC-205 in the mouse, which is expressed at higher levels. In addition, endocytosis and macropinocytosis are down-regulated. Garrett et al. *(54)* found that endocytic down-regulation reflects a decrease in endocytic activity controlled by Rho family guanosine triphosphatase Cdc42. Blocking Cdc42 function in immature DCs abrogates endocytosis, whereas injection of active Cdc42 in mature DCs reactivates endocytosis *(54)*, which suggests that the regulation of endocytosis during maturation is at least partly controlled by the levels of active Cdc42. Another report, however, demonstrates that the Rho family guanosine triphosphatases Cdc42 and Rac are required for constitutive macropinocytosis by DCs but do not control its regulation *(55)*.

The differential expression of innate receptors that sense microbial products on the human and mouse DC subsets could form the basis of a selective response to different pathogens. TLRs are highly conserved from *Drosophila* to humans and recognize molecular patterns specific to microbial pathogens. Different TLRs are triggered by a distinct set of microbial compounds (e.g, TLR4 is triggered by lipopolysaccharide, TLR9 by unmethylated oligonucleotide, TLR3 by double-stranded RNA), are coupled to distinct signal transduction pathway (all TLRs except TLR3 are coupled to the MyD88 adaptor, and TLR3 and TLR4 couple to the adaptor TRIF), are localized in different compartments (most TLRs are present on the cell surface, TLRs 7, 8, and 9 are in the endosomal compartement, and TLR3 is intracellular) and are expressed in a constitutive or induced way in different cell types. DCs express the broadest repertoire of TLRs: Freshly isolated human plasmacytoid DCs express TLR7 and TLR9, whereas CD11c$^+$ human myeloid cells express TLR1, TLR2, TLR3, TLR5, TLR6, and TLR8. In mice, all splenic subsets express TLRs 1, 2, 4, 6, 8, and 9. TLR3 is expressed on CD8$^+$ and CD4$^-$CD8$^-$ DCs, TLR5 and TLR7 are expressed on all subsets except CD8$^+$(for review see *[56]*). Similarly, C-type lectins appear differentially expressed on DCs, depending on the subset, activation state, and tissue localization *(52)*.

Recent reports have identified the pathways involved in the recognition of various pathogens. Plasmacytoid DCs have been shown to produce high levels of IFN-α in response to the influenza virus, and this requires endosomal recognition of influenza genomic RNA and signaling by means of TLR7 *(57)*. Murine CD8α^+ DCs, which are the principal cross-presenting APCs *in vivo*, are activated by double-stranded RNA present in virally infected cells. DC activation requires phagocytosis of infected material, followed by signaling through the double-stranded RNA receptor TLR-3 *(58)*. Thus, TLR-3 is crucial for cross-priming of CTL against viruses that do not directly infect DCs. Another important class of receptors is the C-type lectin receptor family, which is involved in the recognition and uptake of glycan structures. The β-glucan receptor Dectin-1 is a yeast binding C-type lectin, which has been shown to synergize with TLR-2 to induce TNF-α and IL-12. A second pathway involving Syk has been identified that induces IL-2 and IL-10 and seems to take place in DCs, but not in macrophages. DEC-205 is a DC-specific lectin receptor in mice and humans but its natural ligands have yet to be characterized. Studies using anti-DEC-205 antibodies have demonstrated its efficacy to mediate adsorptive uptake and presentation by DCs *in vivo (59)*. This was determined by selective *in vivo* targeting of antigens to DEC-205 using the corresponding monoclonal antibody. The SIGN (specific ICAM-3-grabbing nonintegrin) family consists of three members (DC-SIGN, L-SIGN, LSECtin) in human and five homologues (mDC-SIGN and mSIGNR1-to-4) in mice. DC-SIGN is specifically expressed by DCs.

Notably, DC-SIGN recognizes and internalizes a number of viruses (e.g, HIV-1, Dengue virus, HCMV, Ebola), bacteria, and protozoa. Pathogen interactions with DC-SIGN result in infection of DCs in the case of Dengue virus *(60)* and transmission—in the absence of infection from DCs—to permissive cells in the case of HIV (61). It is thought that, after capture of HIV-1 by DC-SIGN or other receptors, DCs migrate to lymphoid organs and present HIV-1 (which survives in the nonlysosomal compartment) to T cells leading to transinfection. The mannose receptor binds a range of bacteria, yeasts and viruses through interactions between a mannose-type carbohydrate recognition domain and pathogen-associated high mannose structures. The significance of the mannose receptor contribution in microbial uptake *in vivo* is still unclear. Lee et al. *(62)* used mannose receptor–deficient mice to examine the role of this receptor in immune response during disseminated candidiasis and found that mannose receptor was not required for host defense or for the phagocytosis of Candida albicans.

Interestingly, Yarovinsky et al. (63) have recently shown that TLR recognition may affect the antigen presentation *in vivo* and regulate immunodominance in an antimicrobial CD4$^+$ T cell response. They showed that the immunogenicity of profilin, a TLR11 ligand present in the parasite, was entirely dependent on both TLR11 recognition and signaling through the adaptor MyD88 at the level of the DC.

Antigen Processing

Class II MHC–restricted Presentation

Stimulation of naïve T and B lymphocytes is likely to occur in primary lymphoid organs, which are organized to favor cellular interactions. Because DCs are posted as sentinels in peripheral organs, an initial step of the immune response most probably requires the migration of DCs to the zone where lymphocytes reside. Of importance is that DCs have the unique capability to present antigens encountered earlier in periphery after they have migrated to lymphoid organs (Figure 15.4). This property, a form of "antigenic memory," results from (a) a shift in class II MHC half-life in mature versus immature DCs, (b) the sequestration of class II MHC/peptide combinations intracellularly in immature DCs, and (c) a blockade of the peptide-loading step in immature DCs. A discussion of each follows.

A Shift in Class II Half-life in Mature versus Immature Dendritic Cells

Class II MHC molecules of immature DCs are expressed at low levels at the plasma membrane but are abundant in endocytic compartments. In contrast, mature DCs express high levels of class II MHC loaded with peptides at the surface. The mechanism that controls class II MHC expression in DCs has remained elusive until recently. Two models were proposed that involved the modulation of cathepsin S activity or the rate of endocytosis. According to the first model, cathepsin S activity is inhibited by the presence of protease inhibitor cystatin C in the class II MHC compartments of immature DCs, thereby preventing the full degradation of the invariant chain. The complexes formed by the class II MHC and partly degraded invariant chain would be transported to lysosomes and degraded. In mature DCs, cystatin C would be down-regulated, thereby enabling cathepsin S to fully degrade the invariant chain and class II MHC to bind antigenic peptides and shuttle to the cell surface *(64)*. However, the similar regulation of class II MHC expression for cathepsin S–independent class II MHC allotypes and in cathepsin S–deficient mice *(65)* argues against this hypothesis. The second model suggests that class II MIIC expression is regulated in murine *(65)* and human *(66)* DCs by controlling the rate of endocytosis and subsequent degradation of peptide-loaded class II MHCs. In immature DCs, class II MHC molecules are rapidly internalized and recycled, turning over with a half-life of about 10 hours, whereas in mature DCs, there is a rapid and transient boost of class II MHC synthesis, and the half-life of class II MHC molecules increases over 100 hours. Indeed, in immature DCs, biotinylated Fab fragments of an anti-DR antibody bound to surface class II molecules are rapidly internalized and recycled back to the cell surface, whereas the pool of recycling class II molecules progressively disappears after maturation *(66)*. Thus, delivery of class II MHC/peptide combinations to the cell surface would proceed similarly in immature and mature DCs, but immature DCs would reendocytose and degrade the complexes much faster than the mature DCs. A recent report by Mellman et al. strongly supports the second model (67). They show that MHC II β-chain cytoplasmic tail is ubiquitinated in mouse immature DCs. The ubiquitination has an important role in endocytosis and enhances the rate of MHC II degradation in lysosomes, thus decreasing its accumulation at equilibrium. Notably, ubiquitination of MHC II ceases upon maturation, resulting in the accumulation of MHC II at the cell surface.

The Sequestration of Class II/Peptide Combinations Intracellularly in Immature Dendritic Cells

There is evidence that immature DCs exhibit a phenotype in which most class II MHC molecules are intracellular and localized to lysosomes. Upon maturation, these cells progressively differentiate into cells in which intracellular class II MHC molecules are found in peripheral nonlysosomal vesicles and then into mature DCs that express almost all of their class II MHC molecules on the plasma membrane *(68,69)*. Of note, although early DCs do not present antigen immediately after uptake, they efficiently present previously internalized antigen after maturation. By delaying antigen presentation, DCs retain the memory of antigens encountered in the periphery.

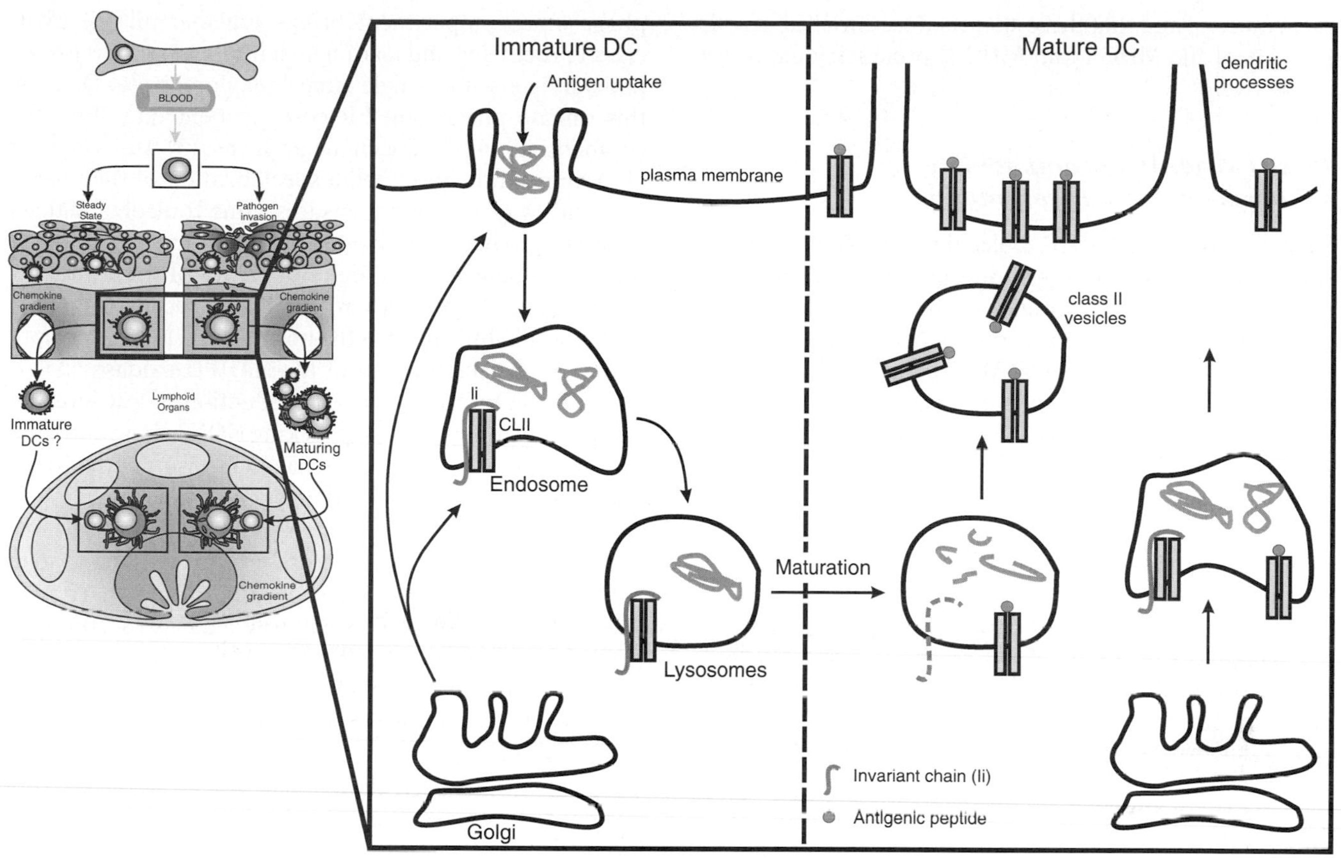

FIGURE 15.4 Antigen handling and class II MHC expression in immature and mature DCs. The maturation of DCs is associated with a redistribution of class II MHC molecules from intracellular compartments to the plasma membrane. In immature DCs (left), class II MHC molecules are associated mainly with invariant chain and are sequestered intracellularly in lysosomes. Indeed, the activity of cathepsin S (which has a major role in the cleavage of the class II MHC–associated invariant chain) remains low, thereby slowing the processing of the invariant chain, which contains a lysosomal targeting signal in its cytoplasmic domain. Although the majority of new class II MHC molecules are targeted directly to endosomes and lysosomes upon exit from the trans-Golgi network, some class II MHC molecules also seem to reach lysosomes after endocytosis from the plasma membrane. Maturation (right) has been shown to enhance the peptide loading of class II MHC molecules that have accumulated in lysosomes before maturation. The peptide/MHC combinations are then transported to the class II MHC vesicles and reach the cell surface as small clusters, partly associated with CD86 (not shown). In addition, the activity of cathepsin S is enhanced, allowing a greater fraction of new class II MHC molecules to avoid lysosomes and reach the cell surface after antigen loading in endosomes. Redrawn from Mellman and Steinman *(319)*, with permission.

Blockade of the Peptide-loading Step in Immature Dendritic Cells

There is evidence that DCs also regulate the intracellular formation of immunogenic class II MCH/peptide combinations. Indeed, although a protein antigen has been shown to colocalize with class II MHC products in late endosomes and lysosomes, class II MHCs do not form unless the DCs are exposed to maturation agents. These observations suggest an arrest to antigen presentation at the peptide-loading step at the immature stage *(70,71)*.

Of importance is that the down-regulation of antigen processing may help avoid induction of autoimmune reactions. Indeed, by turning off endocytosis, a mature DC arriving in the lymph node with pathogenic peptides would be unable to pick up self-antigens and would present only epitopes generated at sites of infection. Of note, adjacent DCs in the T cell area in the steady state may present self-antigens and contribute to peripheral tolerance (see later discussion).

Dudziak et al. recently reported (9) that DC subsets differentially processed antigen *in vivo*. To examine antigen processing and presentation, they specifically targeted antigens to the CD8α^+DEC205$^+$ or to the CD8α^-33D1$^+$ subset using chimeric monoclonal antibodies. They found that CD8α^+DEC205$^+$ were biased for MHC I presentation, whereas CD8α^-33D1$^+$ were biased for MHC II presentation, and that these subsets were enriched in components of the MHC I and MHC II processing pathways, respectively.

Class I Major Histocompatibility Complex–restricted Presentation

In most cells, class I MHC molecules associate exclusively with peptides derived from endogenous cytosolic proteins, such as virus-encoded proteins or tumor antigens. In contrast, peptides derived from internalized exogenous antigens associate not with class I MHC molecules but, instead, with class II MHC molecules. The class I MHC–restricted presentation of endogenous but not exogenous antigens should prevent cytotoxic T cell (CTL) lysis of noninfected neighboring cells that have phagocytosed infected cells.

The class I MHC–restricted presentation of antigens in DCs is similar to that seen in other cells, except for three features:

1. There is a marked increase in class I MHC synthesis during maturation, and half-life is increased *(72)*.
2. Several proteasome subunits characteristic of the immunoproteasome are induced during maturation (73).
3. DCs appear very efficient in presenting exogenous cell–associated antigens in the context of class I MHC molecules, a processed referred to as *cross-presentation.* Albert et al. (74) demonstrated that human DCs have the capability to efficiently present antigens derived from apoptotic, influenza-infected cells and to stimulate class I MHC–restricted $CD8^+$ cytotoxic T lymphocytes. Regnault et al. *(75)* showed that Fcγ receptors induce the maturation of DCs and mediate efficient internalization of immune complexes. This process requires proteasomal degradation and is dependent on functional peptide transporters associated with antigen processing (TAP) 1 and 2. Glycoprotein 96–associated antigens can be cross-presented on class I MHC by DCs *(76)* as well as foreign proteins expressed by bacteria *(72)*. There is evidence that internalized antigens may access the cytosol for processing by the proteasome and loading in the endoplasmic reticulum (ER).

Crosspresentation requires antigen transit through endosomes or phagosomes and eventually partial proteolysis. The antigen is then transported to the cytosol, degraded by the proteosome, and the resulting peptides translocated into ER or ER-phagosome compartments and loaded on MHC class I molecules. Three unique features have been described: (1) DCs have developed a unique membrane transport pathway for the export of exogenous antigens from endocytic compartments to the cytosol. Endosome-to-cytosol transport is restricted to DCs and allows internalized antigens to gain access to the cytosolic antigen-processing machinery and to the conventional class I MHC antigen-presentation pathway (77). (2) A mix ER-phagosome compartment brings together all the MHC class I processing and loading machinery as well as exogenous antigens in a single subcellular organelle. Of note, this unique phagosome/ER compartment may limit the competition with endogenous antigens. (3) Amigorena et al. have recently described a specialization of the phagocytic pathway of DCs that ensures a fine control of antigen processing. They have shown that the phagosomes of DCs maintain a neutral, even slightly alkaline, pH in contrast to macrophage phagosomes, which become acidified rapidly (78). The alkalinization of the phagosomal lumen is maintained by the recruitment of the NADPH oxidase NOX2, which mediates the sustained production of low levels of reactive oxygen species. DCs lacking NOX2 show impaired cross presentation, revealing that NOX2 is involved in the control of adaptive immunity in addition to its role in microbe killing in innate immune responses.

Of importance is that the cross-presentation can lead to the generation of cytotoxic responses to viruses that do not infect DCs themselves. This pathway may also account for the *in vivo* phenomenon of cross-priming, whereby antigens derived from tumor cells or transplants are presented by host APCs. Cross-priming of antigen via DCs would allow nonreplicating vaccines to prime for $CD8^+$ T cell immunity. It has been shown that DCs are able to cross-present HIV gag proteins across a spectrum of MHC haplotypes *(79)*.

A potentially critical role of cross-presentation could be to allow DCs in the steady state to present self-antigens on class I MHC and thereby to induce tolerance (see later discussion). This process would be essential to prevent the induction of autoimmunity when DCs capture dying infected cells *(80)*.

Migratory Properties

The trafficking events that bring together T cells, B lymphocytes, and DCs involve chemokines, which are small basic proteins that engage seven transmembrane receptors on responsive cells and promote chemotaxis *(81)*.

Chemokines and their receptors regulate the movement and interaction of APCs such as DCs and T cells. CC chemokine receptor (CCR) 2 has been shown to be required for Langerhans cell migration to the lymph nodes and is also an important determinant of splenic DC migration, especially in the localization of CD8α^+ cells (see later discussion) *(82)*. Two other chemokines have been suggested to serve a homing function in the T cell compartment: the secondary lymphoid tissue chemokine (SLC)/6Ckine and the Epstein-Barr virus–induced molecule 1 ligand chemokine (ELC)/macrophage inflammatory protein (MIP)-3β. SLC and ELC are structurally related chemokines, and both bind the receptor CCR7. Immature DCs express CCR6 and respond to MIP-3α, whereas maturing DCs down-regulate expression of

CCR6, up-regulate expression of CCR7, and chemotactically respond to ELC/MIP-3β (83). SLC appears to be needed for efficient passage of DCs from lymphatic vessels into the T cell zone of lymph nodes *(84)*. Interaction of CXCR4 on DCs with stromal cell factor might also contribute to the localization of DCs into the T cell area.

The tight regulation of chemokine receptors allows DCs to be recruited to inflammatory sites and to leave these sites after antigen capture to reach secondary lymphoid organs. Mature DCs have been shown to produce ELC/MIP-3β, an observation that correlates with their unique capacity to organize the structure of T cell areas within the lymph nodes by attracting antigen-carrying DCs as well as naïve T cells *(85)*.

The DC migration to the draining lymph node has a strong impact on T cell priming. Indeed, Martin-Fontecha et al. (86) have reported that the magnitude and quality of CD4$^+$ T cell response was proportional to the number of antigen-carrying DCs that reach the lymph nodes. Lack of CCR7 prevented the migration of DCs, whereas preinjection of inflammatory cytokines, which increased the expression of the CCR7 ligand CCL21 in lymphatic endothelial cells, strongly increased DC migration. These results delineate an additional level at which inflammation acts to increase T cell responses: Inflammatory stimuli promote recruitment of immature DCs into tissues, initiate the DC maturation process, and boost recruitment of mature DCs into lymphatics.

Migration In Situ

The capability of DCs to transport antigen has been illustrated in several models *in situ*. Larsen et al. (87) showed that, when mouse skin is transplanted, the DCs enlarge, express higher levels of class II MHC, and begin to migrate. Xia et al. *(88)* showed that primary sensitization of naïve T cells after an airway challenge occurs predominantly within local lymph nodes and not in the lung- or bronchial-associated lymphoid tissues and that antigen presentation by DCs shifts from lung to lymph node during the response to inhaled antigen. Antigen transport from the airway mucosa to the thoracic lymph nodes was studied by intratracheal instillation of fluorescein isothiocyanate (FITC)–conjugated macromolecules (ovalbumin). After instillation, FITC$^+$ cells with stellate structure were found in the T cell area of thoracic lymph nodes. The FITC signal was detected only in migratory airway-derived lymph node DCs, which display a mature phenotype and present ovalbumin to TCR transgenic T cells specific for an ovalbumin peptide (89). In the intestine, Huang et al. (90) identified a DC subset that constitutively endocytoses and transports apoptotic epithelial cells to T cell areas of mesenteric lymph nodes *in vivo*.

The importance of DC recruitment in the induction or maintenance of immune responses has been recently demonstrated: Lauterbach et al. *(91)* have reported that adoptive immunotherapy of exogenously derived pathogen-specific memory T cells to mice burdened with a persistent lymphocytic choriomeningitis virus (LCMV) infection resulted in eradication of the pathogen from all tissues, including the central nervous system. As a consequence of immunotherapy, a substantial number of DCs were recruited in the brain parenchyma and were required for TNF-α production and successful viral clearance. These results underline the dependence of memory T cells on DCs and the importance of DC migration for successful immunotherapeutic clearance.

Whether plasmacytoid DCs, like classical DCs, migrate from peripheral mucosal tissues via afferent lymph is still unclear. To determine whether plasmacytoid DCs migrate in lymph, Yrlid et al. removed intestine- or liver-draining lymph nodes and collected thoracic leukocytes in rats *(92)*. They found that intestinal and hepatic lymph were devoid of plasmacytoid DCs under both steady-state conditions and after TLR7/8 stimulation. These observations suggest that the antigen-presenting capacity of plasmacytoid DCs may not result from peripheral antigen capture followed by migration to the lymph nodes. How these cells in lymph nodes do acquire peripheral antigens remains an open question. Another report suggests, however, that plasmacytoid DCs migrate from the lung to the draining lymph nodes under steady-state conditions, as inhaled antigens were found to be associated with this subset in the lungs and the draining lymph nodes *(93)*.

Cytokine Release

Interleukin-12

In 1995, Macatonia et al. (94) demonstrated that murine splenic DCs produce IL-12 and direct the development of Th1 cells *in vitro*. Similar observations were reported by Koch et al. *(95)*, who further showed that ligation of either CD40 or class II MHC molecules independently triggered IL-12 production in splenic DCs and that IL-12 production was down-regulated by IL-4 and IL-10. Biedermann et al. *(96)* found, however, that IL-4, when present during the initial activation of bone marrow–derived DCs, could instruct these cells to produce bioactive IL-12.

Although previous *in vitro* studies had suggested that the macrophage was a major source of the IL-12 produced on microbial stimulation, DCs but not macrophages were shown to be the initial cells to synthesize IL-12 in the spleens of mice exposed *in vivo* to an extract of *Toxoplasma gondii* or to LPS (44). The major producers of IL-12 are CD8α^+ DCs in response to bacterial or intracellular parasite infection (44,97), whereas plasmacytoid DCs can produce IL-12 in response to various viruses, to CpG oligodeoxynucleotides, and *in vivo* to mouse cytomegalovirus (MCMV) *(32)*. Iwasaki and Kelsall *(7,8)* demonstrated that CD11b$^-$CD8α^+ Peyer's patch DCs but not CD11b$^+$CD8α^- or double-negative subset produce IL-12 p70 on stimulation *in vitro*.

Although the CD8α^+ DC subset seems to have the greatest capacity for IL-12 production, different stimuli can change the balance. *Escherichia coli* LPS induces IL-12 p70 in the CD8α^+ DC subset, presumably through TLR4, whereas *Porphyromonas gingivalis* LPS does not. Both LPSs activate the two DC subsets to up-regulate costimulatory molecules and produce IL-6 and TNF-α *(98)*. Of note, all splenic populations respond with increased IL-12 p70 production *in vitro* when IL-4 is present during stimulation, whereas only CD8α^+ DCs produce IL-12 in the absence of IL-4 *(99)* (for review, see Maldonado-López and Moser *[100]*). Both subsets have the capacity to produce IL-12 after *in vivo* priming with *Toxoplasma* extracts *(97)*. CD8α^- DCs from IL-10–deficient animals have an increased capacity to produce IL-12, in comparison with DCs from wild-type animals, which suggests that IL-12 release is tightly controlled in this subset *(101)*.

In humans, Langerhans cells, particularly after maturation, have been shown to release functional IL-12 heterodimer *in vitro (102)*. Rissoan et al. (103) reported that CD40L activation up-regulates the expression of mRNA for IL-12 p40 in human monocyte–derived but not plasmacytoid-derived DCs *in vitro*.

IL-12 exerts a powerful positive regulatory influence on the development of Th1 helper T cell immune responses and is a potent inducer of IFN-γ production and cytotoxic differentiation and function, which suggests that DCs could dictate the class selection of the subsequent adaptive response (see later discussion).

The release of heterodimeric IL-12 p70, which is potentially harmful, appears tightly regulated *in vivo*. The production of IL-12 has been shown to depend on two signals: initial APC activation by a microbial stimulus and an amplifying signal through DC–T interaction *(104)*. Numerous negative regulatory mechanisms have been described *(105)*: IL-10 has been shown to down-regulate the production of IL-12 by murine splenic DCs *(101)*; IL-12 production by DCs is rapid and intense but relatively short-lived *(97,106)*. This paralysis of DC IL-12 production is likely to prevent infection-induced immunopathology *(97)*. In addition, IL-12 inhibition can be achieved by the engagement of G-protein–coupled receptors, by a mechanism mediated by activation of the phosphatidylinositol 3-kinase-protein 3 kinase B/Akt pathway and JNK *(105,107)*.

IL-12 is a disulfide-like 70-kD heterodimer composed of 35-kD (p35) and 40-kD (p40) subunits, each of which is encoded by a distinct gene. Although the regulation of IL-12 expression may be largely focused on p40 in other cell types, one report demonstrated that the regulation of IL-12 p70 expression at the transcriptional level by Rel/NFκB is controlled through both the p35 and p40 genes in CD8α^+ DCs *(108)*.

IL-23

In 2000, it was discovered that p40 can also dimerize with p19 to form IL-23. Like IL-12, IL-23 is primarily secreted by activated DCs, monocytes and macrophages, and transgenic mice constitutively overexpressing IL-23p19 develop fatal multiorgan inflammation *(109)*.

IL-23 was first thought to activate adaptive Th17 cells only. However, Kullberg et al. provided evidence that IL-23 induce both Th1 and Th17 cells (110). Using two models of Helicobacter hepaticus-triggered T cell–dependent colitis, they showed that IL-23, and not IL-12, was essential for the development of maximal intestinal disease. Their results support a model in which both Th1 and Th17 may be overactivated by IL-23 and synergize to trigger severe intestinal inflammation. Another study showed that depletion of IL-23 was associated with decreased proinflammatory responses in the intestine but had little impact on systemic T cell inflammatory responses (111). In a CD40-induced colitis, a strong increase in IL-12 and mainly IL-23 expression was found in both DCs and monocytes/macrophages, with the highest amount of IL-23 p19 found among colonic DCs *(112)*.

Interferon-α

In the mouse, a population of plasmacytoid cells has been shown to produce IFN-α when cultured with inactivated influenza virus. These cells were detected in low numbers in the spleen, bone marrow, thymus, lymph nodes, blood, lungs, and liver. *In vivo* activated CD8α^+Ly6G/C$^+$CD11b$^-$ DCs appear to be the major producers of IFN-α/β during MCMV but not LCMV infection, and they probably derive from plasmacytoid CD11c$^+$CD8α^-Ly6G/C$^+$CD11b$^-$ immature APCs *(32,113)*. Interestingly, IFN-α/β appear to regulate DC cytokine production by enhancing their own expression while inhibiting IL-12 synthesis during MCMV infection *(113)*. Another report demonstrates that among the splenic DCs, only the CD4$^-$CD8$^+$ DCs produced IFN-α in culture when stimulated by a combination of CpG and polyinosine:polycytidylic acid poly(I:C) *(99)*. The relationship between both IFN-α–producing populations requires further study, especially because a proportion of plasmacytoid APCs has been shown to express CD8α *(32)*. In humans, plasmacytoid-derived DCs release IFN-α during viral infection or inflammation *(31,114)*.

Interleukin-2

The analysis of genes that are differentially expressed upon maturation induced by exposure to gram-negative bacteria revealed that IL-2 mRNA was transiently up-regulated at early time points (4 to 6 hours) after bacterial encounter (115). The same authors showed that DC-derived IL-2 mediates T cell activation, inasmuch as the ability of IL-2$^{-/-}$

DCs to induce proliferation of allogeneic CD4+ and CD8+ T cells was severely impaired. Of note, DC-derived IL-2 and type I interferons have been shown to promote the IFN-γ production and cytotoxic function of NK cells *(116)*.

In addition, DCs have been shown to produce IL-6 *(117)*, IL-10, and IFN-γ *(118,119)*. Mature DCs, predominantly of CD8α phenotype, appear to constitutively produce small amounts of IL-12, which induces the secretion of IFN-γ, leading to up-regulation of IL-12 production. Liver-derived DC progenitors *(120)* and freshly isolated Peyer's patch DCs *(7)* have the capacity to produce IL-10.

EXPRESSION AND FUNCTION OF ACCESSORY MOLECULES

There are many molecules that are constitutively or potentially expressed in almost all T cells and whose deficiencies or expression anomalies affect the balance between effector and regulatory function. The critical positive costimulatory molecules are the immunoglobulin (Ig) superfamily molecules CD28 and ICOS (inducible costimulator), which bind the B7 family ligands B7-1/B7-2 and B7h, respectively. The negative costimulatory receptors include cytotoxic T lymphocyte antigen (CTLA)-4, which also binds to B7-1 and B7-2; programmed death (PD)-1, which binds PD-1 ligand (PD-L1 or B7-H1) and PD-L2 (also known as B7-DC); and B and T lymphocyte attenuator, which binds herpes virus entry mediator. Other B7 family ligands have been identified (B7-H3 and B7-H4), but their receptors on T cells are not yet known. More recently, members of the TNF-R family have been shown to display costimulatory fucntion.

The B7:CD28 Superfamily

The expression of B7-1 (CD80) and B7-2 (CD86) is restricted to professional APCs, suggesting that these molecules are mainly involved in initial priming in lymph nodes. By contrast, other B7 family members are widely expressed in many different tissues by both hematopoietic and nonhematopoietic cells. For example, PD-L1 is expressed in the placenta during gestation and is involved in fetomaternal tolerance.

The members of the CD28 family (including ICOS, CTLA-4, BTLA, PD-1) have a single extracellular Ig variablelike domain followed by a short cytoplasmic tail (Figure 15.5). The cytoplasmic domains of CD28, ICOS, and CTLA-4 have a common Tyr-Xaa-Met motif that binds to the SH2 domain of the p85 subunit of phosphatidylinositol 3-kinase.

Common to all three coreceptors is the recruitment of PI3K and the downstream regulation of proteins with pleckstrin-homology domains, such as PDK1 and PKB, that leads to the regulation of events as diverse as cytokine production, cell death and cellular metabolism (for review, see [121]).

CD28

CD28 is a type I transmembrane glycoprotein expressed constitutively on all murine T cells, all human CD4 T cells, and 50% of CD8 T cells. Ligation of CD3 and CD28

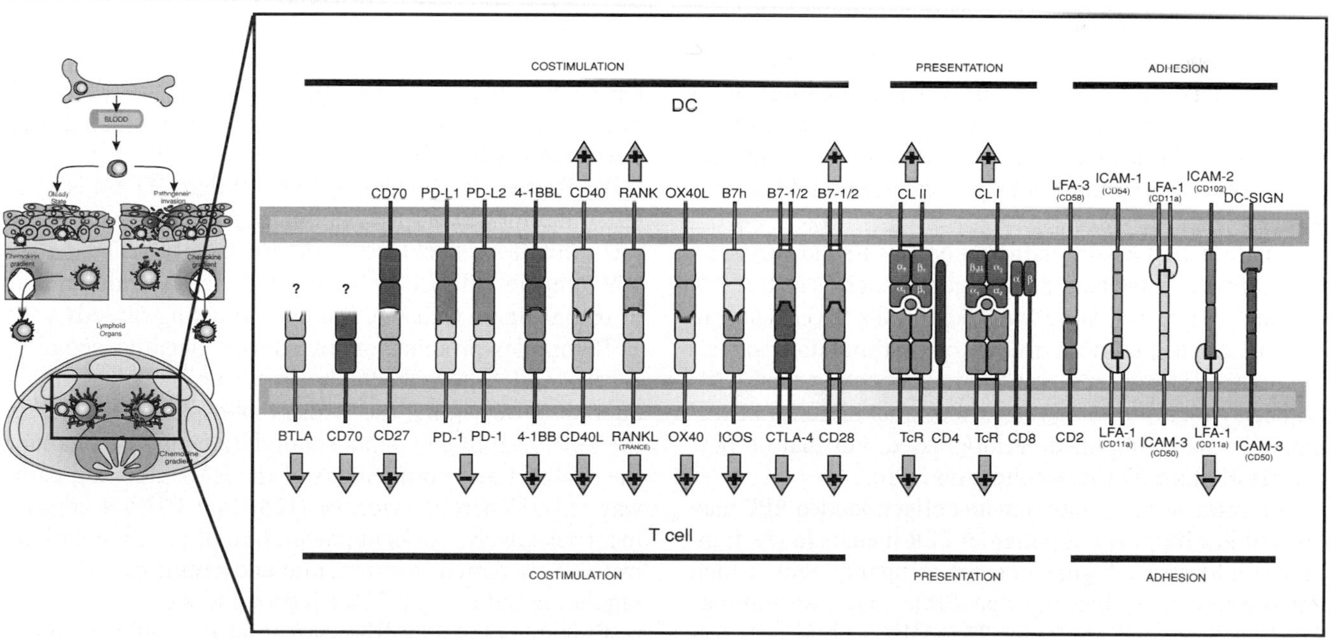

FIGURE 15.5 Molecules involved in the T cell/DC synapse. The interaction between DCs and T lymphocytes involves several ligand/receptor pairs that include MHC, adhesion, and costimulatory molecules.

promotes increases in glucose metabolism, high levels of cytokine/chemokine expression, resistance to apoptosis, and long-term expansion of T cells.

Upon interaction with its ligand, CD28 becomes phosphorylated on tyrosines. One tyrosine (Y170 in mouse CD28, Y173 in human CD28) permits CD28 to recruit SH2-containing signaling molecules, including phosphoinositide 3 kinase, Grb2, and Gads. Okkenhaug et al. (122) built a CD28 mutant that uncouples these SH2-mediated interactions from CD28. This mutant was unable to upregulate expression of the prosurvival protein Bcl-xL, but still promoted T cell proliferation, IL-2 secretion, and prevented the induction of anergy. Another report confirms that the ability of CD28 to regulate proliferation and induction of Bcl-X(L) maps to distinct motifs: Indeed, mutation of C-terminal proline residues abrogated the proliferative and cytokine regulatory features of CD28 costimulation, while preserving Bcl-X(L) induction. Conversely, mutation of residues important in phosphatidylinositol 3-kinase activation partially inhibited proliferation but prevented induction of Bcl-X(L) *(123)*.

The signals generated from CD28 ligation seem to modify the gene regulation induced by TCR stimulation rather than turning on the expression of a separate subset of genes. Indeed, Diehn et al. *(124)* have shown that the principal effect of simultaneous engagement of CD28 was to increase the amplitude of the CD3 transcriptional response. They showed that CD28 signaling promotes phosphorylation, and thus inactivation, of the NFAT nuclear export kinase glycogen synthase kinase-3 (GSK3), leading to decreased nuclear export of NFAT. This decreased nuclear export and the increased nuclear import induced by increased calcium flux *(125)* lead to increased NFAT activation and transcription of genes such as IL-2. These observations suggest a critical role of NFAT in the integration of the TCR and CD28 signals. In addition, CD28 has been shown to favor accumulation and activation of signaling components, and amplify PLCγ1 activation and Ca^{2+} responses *(125)*.

Finally, CD28 costimulation enhances the downregulation of transcripts of suppressor genes, such as genes coding for factors whose role is to keep T cells in G_0. A strong support for a quantitative view of costimulatory signaling comes from microarray analysis showing that TCR-induced expression of several thousands of genes in primary T cells is amplified or suppressed, but that no new gene is induced by CD28 coligation (126).

It is interesting to note that an antigen-loaded APC may present low numbers of potential TCR ligands (a few hundred?) and much higher density of ligands with which CD28 interacts, suggesting that CD28 may also stabilize APC/T cell contact and favor TCR/MHC peptide engagement. Of note, the CD86 costimulatory molecule is not only abundant on DCs but also associates with antigen-presenting MHC products in stable patches on the DC surface. The polyvalent configuration may facilitate the activation of quiescent T cells *(69)*.

Further, Viola et al. (127) proposed that CD28 may induce a reorganization of the signaling machinery. They stimulated human resting T cells with surrogate APCs, consisting of beads coated with antibody to CD3 in the presence or absence of CD28. They tested whether CD28 engagement affected the distribution of rafts, which concentrate various molecules involved in signal transduction such as Lck, LAT, Ras. Using a fluorescent marker that binds the GM1 glycosphingolipids, they showed that rafts segregated in the zone of contact only when CD3 and CD28 were simultaneously engaged. In unstimulated T lymphocytes, the surface distribution of GM1 was homogeneous, and this pattern did not change when the cells were stimulated with anti-CD3–coated beads.

CTLA-4

CTLA-4 (CD152) was discovered by screening for genes differentially expressed in cytotoxic T lymphocytes. CTLA-4 expression is merely detectable on resting T cells and undergoes complex intracellular trafficking mediated by its binding to the clathrin-adaptor molecules AP-1 and AP-2. Upon T cell activation, CTLA-4 trafficks to the sites of TCR engagement *(128)* and is rapidly upregulated on $CD4^+$ and $CD8^+$ T cells.

A crucial Met-Tyr-Pro-Pro-Pro-Tyr loop in the CD28 and CTLA-4 Ig-like domain provides a structural specificity for the interaction with CD80 and CD86, but the increased strength of this binding by CTLA4 is mediated by nonconserved residues in the CDR1- and CDR3-analogous regions *(129)*. CD28 has been shown to interact with a single binding domain, whereas each CTLA-4 dimer binds two independent bivalent B7 molecules in the formation of a zipperlike matrix *(130)*. This observation suggests that B7-1 interactions with CTLA-4 may be markedly favored over interactions with CD28.

While there is a general agreement that CTLA-4 is a potent inhibitor of T cell activation, the mechanism by which this inhibition is achieved remains unclear. CTLA-4 may out-compete with CD28 for their shared ligands, inhibit proximal signal transduction by interacting directly with TCR complex proteins, or transduce a negative signal to T cells. CTLA-4 has been shown to inhibit signal transduction by recruiting the tyrosine phosphatase SHP-2 to the TCR, resulting in dephosphorylation of the ζ chain of the complex and components of the RAS signaling pathway *(131)*. There is evidence *(126)* that CTLA-4 engagement selectively blocks augmentation of gene regulations by CD28-mediated costimulation and does not ablate gene regulation induced by TCR triggering alone.

Chikuma et al. have shown that, after T cell activation, CTLA-4 is induced and translocates from the intracellular vesicles to the immunological synapse where it associates with TCR ζ in the lipid rafts attenuating T cell signaling

(132). Two phosphatases, SHP-1 and SHP-2, have been suggested to mediate CTLA-4-mediated inhibition either directly by dephosphorylating TCRζ or indirectly through dephosphorylation of the regulatory tyrosine of ZAP-70. A recent study has shown that CTLA-4 signaling may also inhibit Akt directly by activation of the type II serine/threonine phosphatase (PP2A) (133).

CTLA-4 not only regulates TCR and CD28 signals in T cells but also delivers signals via B7 into APC. Grohmann et al. have shown that B7 can transmit suppressive signals into DCs, following engagement of CTLA-4: engagement of B7-1/B7-2 on murine DCs by CTLA-4Ig activates a signaling pathway that stimulates DCs to produce IFN-γ, which in turn induces indoleamine 2, 3-dioxygenase (IDO). CTLA-4 on mouse $CD4^{+}CD25^{+}$ Treg can mediate the same IDO-inducing effect *in vitro* (*134–136*,137) in DCs by interacting with their CD80/CD86.

Although most of the evidence establishes that CTLA-4 is a key negative regulator of T cell responses, it may also act as a positive regulator of T cell activation. Linsley et al. *(138)* have shown that CTLA-4 and CD28 could act synergistically to enhance T cell proliferation. Ligation of CTLA-4 with mutant B7-1 that had lost its ability to bind CD28 also resulted in T cell clonal expansion.

$CD4^{+}CD25^{+}$ natural Tregs in the thymus and the periphery constitutively express CTLA-4 *(139,140)*. There is evidence that CTLA-4 may actively contribute to Treg suppression, although the presence of functional Tregs in CTLA-4 deficient mice suggest that CTLA-4 may be dispensable in some conditions.

PD-1

PD-1 (CD279) was isolated as a gene upregulated in a T cell hybridoma undergoing apoptotic cell death and was thus named *programmed death 1*. PD-1 has an extracellular domain with a single Ig domain and a cytoplasmic domain with two tyrosines, one that constitutes an immunoreceptor tyrosine-based inhibitory motif. The broad expression of PD-1 contrasts with the T cell–restricted expression of CD28 and CTLA-4. Indeed, PD-1 is inducibly expressed on CD4 and CD8 T cells, NKT cells, B cells, and monocytes upon activation. PD-1 transduces a signal only when engaged in combination with TCR ligation.

PD-L1 expression can be induced by IFN-γ (its promoter region contains several IFN-γ–responsive elements) in several tissues including tumor cells where it can facilitate tumor evasion *(141)*. Keir et al. have recently reported a greater increase in IL-2 and IFN-γ production in doubly deficient mice (lacking PD-L1 and PD-L2), suggesting that PD-L1 and L2 synergistically inhibit T cell activation. Double-deficient NOD mice develop early and fulgurant diabetes, with 100% penetrance in males and females (142). Of note, PD-L1 is the main factor preventing autoimmune attack at the islet level, and PD-L1 expressed by parenchyma cells seems to play a more important role in preventing diabetes than PD-L1 expressed by APCs. B7-H4 is expressed in multiple nonlympoid tissues and in human breast and ovarian cancers. Krycez et al. report *(143)* the intracellular expression of B7-H4 in ovarian tumor cells and the cell surface expression on macrophages isolated from the tumor. B7-H4 is the critical immunosuppressive molecule expressed by macrophages as blocking B7-H4, but not arginase-inducible nitric oxide synthase, or B7-H1 restored the T cell stimulatory capacity of the macrophages and contributed to tumor regression *in vivo*. This finding adds a new level of regulation of tumor-specific immunity by macrophages that have been shown to promote angiogenesis and secrete matrix metalloproteinases and epidermal growth factor that promote the escape of the tumor cells. Iwai et al. showed that liver nonparenchymal cells and Kuppfer cells constitutively expressed PD-L1 and that the blockade of the PD-1 pathway could augment antiviral immunity *(144)*. Recent studies have shown that PD-1 is highly expressed by CD8 T cells during chronic LCMV infection and that *in vivo* PD-1-PD-L blockade may reverse CD8 exhaustion and reduce tumor load *(145)*. Three recent studies show that PD-1 expression is elevated on HIV-specific CD8 T cells and that blocking this pathway leads to increased T cell proliferation and effector functions, including cytokine production and cytolysis *(146–148)*.

Parry et al. (133) have shown that PD-1 and CTLA-4 blocked CD3/CD28–mediated up-regulation of glucose metabolism and Akt activity, using distinct mechanisms. PD-1 signaling inhibits Akt phosphorylation by preventing CD28-mediated activation of phosphatidylinositol 3-kinase (PI3K), whereas CTLA-4 preserves the activity of PI3K. These observations suggest that CTLA-4 and PD-1 may control T cell activation through additive or synergistic mechanisms.

ICOS

The CD28 homolog ICOS is upregulated on T cells after activation. Like CD28 and CTLA-4, ICOS is a glycosylated disulfide-linked homodimer. The ICOS cytoplasmic tail contains a YMFM motif that binds to the p85 subunit of PI3K, similar to the YMNM motif of CD28. Riley et al. (126) compared gene expression triggered by CD28 and ICOS costimulation. They showed that gene regulations induced by ICOS and CD28 costimulation were very similar, although a few genes (IL-2, ICOS, IL-9, . . .) were more regulated by CD28 than ICOS stimulation.

While CD28 costimulation is crucial for priming the immune response, ICOS seems more important for maintaining a T cell response and for the effector function. ICOS does not stimulate T cell expansion. The level of expression of ICOS has been shown to correlate with the type of cytokines produced, with $ICOS^{high}$ T cells linked to IL-10 production, $ICOS^{medium}$ T cells with IL-4, IL-5 and IL-13 (320) secretion, and $ICOS^{low}$ with IL-2, IL-6, IFN-γ production. Studies in $ICOS^{-/-}$ and $ICOSL^{-/-}$ mice have revealed a critical role for ICOS in T cell–dependent B cell responses: Mice lacking ICOS exhibit reduced germinal centers in response to primary immunization and defects in IgG class switching *(321)*.

ICOS has been shown to be involved in the suppressive function of regulatory T cells *in vivo*. Herman et al. have reported (149) that Tregs and T effector cells coexist within the pancreatic lesion before type 1 diabetes onset. These $CD4^+CD25^+$ Tregs express higher levels of IL-10 and ICOS than their lymph node counterparts. Of note, blockade of ICOS rapidly converts early insulitis into diabetes.

ICOS and ICOS-L appear to be a monogamous pair, as mice deficient for ICOS or ICOS-L display similar phenotypes. ICOS-L has been detected on the surface of B cells, macrophages, DCs, and other nonlymphoid cell types, including endothelial cells and epithelial cells.

BTLA

B and T lymphocyte attenuator (BTLA), the most recently recognized member of the CD28 family, is expressed in activated B and T cells. BTLA is preferentially expressed on CD4 Th1 cells *(150)*, while ICOS may more dedicated for Th2 and Treg cells.

BTLA contains a single IgV domain and two intracellular immunoreceptor tyrosine-based inhibitory motifs that are phosphorylated after BTLA coligation to antigen receptors, resulting in recruitment of protein tyrosine phosphatases SHP-1 and SHP-2 and inhibition of T cell activation.

BTLA, as the other CD28-like proteins, does not interact with members of the B7 family but instead interacts with the TNFR family member HVEM (herpes virus entry mediator). The interaction between BTLA and HVEM is the only receptor-ligand interaction that directly bridges the two families of receptors. There is evidence that engagement of HVEM with its endogenous ligand (LIGHT) from the TNF family induces a powerful immune response, whereas HVEM interactions with BTLA negatively regulate T cell responses *(151)*.

Tumor Necrosis Factor Receptor Superfamily

Several members of the TNF receptor family, including CD27 and its close relatives 4-1BB (CD137) and OX40 (CD134) have been shown to display the function of costimulatory receptors.

CD27

The TNF-receptor family member, CD27, acts as a costimulatory molecule to elicit T and B cell responses. Its activity is governed by the transient availability of its TNF-like ligand CD70 on lymphocytes and DCs. CD27 is found on a large proportion of NK cells and on most $CD4^+$ and $CD8^+$ T cells and is induced on B cells upon priming. CD27 determines the magnitude of primary and memory T cell responses to influenza virus. Hendriks et al. *(152)* have examined the relative contributions of CD27 and CD28 to generation of the virus-specific effector T cell pool and its establishment at the site of infection (the lung). They reported that, in contrast to CD28, CD27 does not affect cell cycle entry but rescues activated T cells from death from the onset of TCR/CD3 stimulation, throughout successive divisions. Although the antigen-specific $CD8^+$ T cell response to intranasal influenza virus is reduced in $CD28^{-/-}$ mice, significant accumulation of virus-specific $CD8^+$ T cells in the lung still occurred, which was dependent on CD27.

Of note, persistent delivery of costimulatory signals via CD27-CD70 interactions, as may occur during chronic active viral infections, has been shown to exhaust the T cell pool, leading to lethal immunodeficiency *(153)*. In particular, Matter et al. have analyzed the role of CD27 signaling in the virus control after infection with LCMV. They recently showed that, during LCMV infection, CD27 signaling on $CD4^+$ T cells enhances the secretion of interferon-γ and TNF-α. These inflammatory cytokines lead to the destruction of splenic architecture and immunodeficiency with reduced and delayed virus-specific neutralizing antibody responses. Blocking the CD27-CD70 interaction reduced immunopathology, improved antibody responses, and prevented chronic infection (154). Interestingly, CD70 is overexpressed on B cells and T cells in active HIV infection, suggesting a possible role for this costimulatory pathway in the induction of suppression.

OX40

OX40 is expressed very transiently on T cells. $OX40^{-/-}$CD8 cells become activated and expand relatively normally, but fail to sustain their numbers over time. OX40 signaling has been shown to selectively promote TNF secretion in CD4 and CD8 T cells and cytotoxicity in CD8 T cells. Recent data using human DCs activated by thymic stromal lymphopoietin (TSLP) have demonstrated a critical role of OX40/OX40L interaction in driving Th2 cell responses but only in the absence of IL-12. By contrast, OX40L has the ability to promote IL-12–mediated Th1 autoimmunity by enhancing TNF-α and IFN-γ production while inhibiting IL-10 production. These observations suggest that the development of a Th2 cell response depends on a Th2 cell-polarizing signal OX40L, as well as a default mechanim of no IL-12. Of note, only TSLP seem to stimulate DCs to provide both (155,156).

4-1BB

4-1BB is expressed on activated $CD4^+$ and $CD8^+$ T cells, activated NK cells, and DCs. Its ligand 4-1BBL is expressed on resting B cells and can be regulated on activated APCs. Agonist anti-4-1BB can lead to opposite effects: Anti-4-1BB can augment CTL generation and improve immunity against tumors and viruses, but it can also inhibit immune responses in autoimmune models. Treatment with an agonistic monoclonal antibody to 4-1BB blocks lymphadenopathy and spontaneous autoimmune diseases in Fas-deficient mice and prolongs their survival. This treatment rapidly augments IFN-γ production and induces the depletion of autoreactive B cells and abnormal double-negative T cells, probably by increasing their apoptosis *(157)*. Similarly, lupus-prone NZB × NZW F1 mice given three injections of anti-4-1BB mAb can reverse acute disease and block chronic disease. The suppression of IgG autoantibody production may be attributed to the suppression of B cell maturation in germinal centers due to the lack of CD4$^+$ T cell help. The authors hypothesize that the antibody acts at the T cell–DC interface during antigen priming, at a time when DC, but not yet T cells, express 4-1BB.

4-1BB and OX40 appear to be closely related in terms of their inducible expression patterns and their apparent signaling capacity (e.g, they recruit TNFR-associated factors [TRAF] and activate Pi3K-Akt-NF-kB pathways). Lee et al. compared the role of OX40 and 4-1BB in generating effector CD8 T cells to Ag delivered by adenovirus. They demonstrated that OX40 and 4-1BB physiologically operate in an opposing manner during initial priming of CD8 effector cells: OX40-deficient CD8 T cells had multiple defects in expression of effector cell surface markers, the synthesis of cytokines and in cytotoxic activity, whereas 4-1BB–deficient CD8 T cells displayed hyper-responsiveness, expanding more than wild-type cells. These results suggest that OX40 can positively regulate effector function and survival, whereas 4-1BB can initially operate in a negative manner to limit primary CD8 responses.

Collectively, these observations suggest that several TNFR family molecules, originally thought to play overlapping and potentially redundant roles, might function as a positive manner (OX40, CD27), whereas others might function positively and negatively (4-1BB, HVEM) depending on either the stage of the T cell response or the availability of multiple opposing ligands.

CD40-L (CD154)

The CD40-CD154 pathway is required for effective T and B cell responses. Activated CD4$^+$ T cells express CD154 and bind to APCs expressing CD40. Engagement of CD40 provides critical signals for B cell expansion, Ig production, and isotype class switching. There is evidence that CD154 binding on APCs enhances B7-1 and B7-2 and the secretion of cytokines, suggesting that CD154 indirectly promotes T cell differentiation. CD40 (a 40-45 kD type I membrane protein) is expressed on B cells, activated macrophages, DCs, thymic epithelium, and endothelial cells, whereas CD154 (a 39 kD type II intramembrane protein) is expressed on activated CD4$^+$ T cells, some CD8$^+$ cells, eosinophils, basophils, and NK cells. CD40/CD154 interactions are critical for the development of a protective immune response against an intracellular parasite, bacterial, and viral infections. Conversely, blocking this interaction has been shown to prevent autoimmune disease and transplant rejection. A model of NKT cell–mediated DC maturation *in vivo,* using α-galactoceramide as activator, demonstrated that antigenic and costimulatory signals do not induce immunity and that a distinct CD40/CD40L signal is required to generate CD4$^+$ T helper cells and CD8$^+$ cytolytic T lymphocytes (36).

Adhesion Molecules

In addition to costimulatory moleules, adhesion molecules seems to play a major role in strengthening the early interaction between DC and T lymphocytes. Early studies indicated that DC and T cells tend to form clusters in an antigen-dependent manner *(2)*. Exploiting a flow cytometric adhesion assay, Figdor et al. tested the capacity of DC and monocytes to bind to fluorescent beads coated with ICAM-3-Fc. ICAM-3 was studied because of its extremely high expression on resting T cells. Whereas ICAM-3 binding by monocytes was found essentially LFA-1 mediated, binding of ICAM-3 by DC was completely LFA-1 independent. The authors found that a novel ICAM-3 binding C-type lectin, exclusively expressed by DC, mediated strong adhesion between DC to ICAM-3 on resting T cells and was essential for DC-induced T cell proliferation (61). DC-SIGN not only functions as a cell-adhesion receptor that regulates DC migration (through its interaction with ICAM-2 *[158]*) and DC–T cell interaction (via ICAM-3 binding), but is implicated in the recognition of multiple pathogens. DC-SIGN recognizes the viral envelope glycoproteins that contain a large number of N-linked carbohydrates, such as HIV-1, Ebola, Dengue, cytomegalovirus, hepatitis C, etc. In addition, nonviral pathogens interact with DC-SIGN, and in particular Mycobacterium tuberculosis, and parasites such as Leishmania amastigotes and Schistosoma mansoni.

DENDRITIC CELLS AND T CELL–MEDIATED IMMUNITY

Immunostimulatory Properties *In Vitro*

The first evidence that DCs have a potent capacity to activate T cells was provided in 1978 by Steinman and Witmer (3), who showed that these cells are at least 100 times more effective as MLR stimulators than are other splenic cells. Selective removal of DCs dramatically reduced stimulation of the primary MLR, whereas populations enriched in DCs were potent stimulators *(159)*. DCs have been shown to activate both CD4$^+$ and CD8$^+$ T lymphocytes in various models *(160–162)*. Although DCs have the capacity to directly sensitize CD8$^+$ T cells, differentiation of CD8$^+$ T cells into killer cells requires help from CD4$^+$ T lymphocytes.

The classical model suggests that T helper and T killer cells recognize their specific antigens simultaneously on the same APC and that cytokines (e.g., IL-2) produced by the activated T helper cells facilitate the differentiation of the killer cell. The three-cell interaction seems unlikely, inasmuch as all cell types are rare and migratory. According to an alternative theory, proposed by P. Matzinger and demonstrated by three independent groups (*163*,164,*165*), the interaction could occur in two steps: The helper cell can first engage and condition the APC and in particular the DC (164), which then becomes empowered to stimulate a killer cell.

Immunostimulatory Properties *In Vivo*

DCs were further shown to be powerful stimulators of immune responses *in vivo* after adoptive transfer. Injection of epidermal Langerhans cells *(166)* or splenic DCs *(166)*, coupled to trinitrophenyl, was shown to activate effector T cells in mice, in contradiction with other coupled cells. In a model of rat kidney allograft, Lechler and Batchelor *(167)* found that injection of small numbers of donor strain DCs triggers an acute rejection response, which suggests that intrarenal DCs provide the major stimulus of a kidney allograft. The *in vivo* priming capacity of DCs has been documented in several CD4$^+$ *(117,168)* and CD8$^+$ T cell responses in rodents and in humans (see later section on tumor immunity). In addition, adoptive transfer of syngeneic DCs, pulsed extracorporeally with an antigen, induces a primary humoral response characterized by the secretion of IgG1 and IgG2a antibodies (169).

Whether the very same DCs that have captured antigen migrate to the T cell areas in lymphoid organs and directly sensitize T lymphocytes is still a matter of speculation. Direct priming by injected antigen-pulsed DCs has been suggested by studies showing that, in F1 recipient mice, parental DCs prime only T cells restricted to the MHC of the injected DCs *(168,170)*. In addition, migratory DCs (which may be apoptotic) can be processed, distributing their peptides widely and efficiently to other DCs to form MHC/peptide combinations *(30)*. Surprisingly, a protein from phagocytosed cells can be presented 1,000 to 10,000 times better than preprocessed peptide. DCs that have captured the antigen may also transfer their antigen through the release of antigen-bearing vesicles (exosomes) (171).

In favor of an indirect priming, Knight et al. *(172)* have provided evidence for a transfer of antigen between DCs in the stimulation of primary T cell proliferation. *In vivo* studies by Inaba et al. *(30)* demonstrated that short-lived migrating DCs could be processed by most of the recipient DCs in the lymph node. More recently, Allan et al. (26) have shown that after skin infection with HSV, CTL activation required CD8$^+$ DCs rather than skin-derived DCs. Their observations suggest that initial transport of antigen by migrating DCs is followed by its spreading over a wider DC pool, thereby increasing priming efficiency. Whether this inter-DC antigen transfer is a general phenomenon or is restricted to skin infection with HSV will require further investigation.

Dendritic Cells as Physiological Adjuvant

Several observations suggest that DCs play a major role in the initiation of immune responses in physiological situations *in situ*. DCs are the major cell type transporting the antigen in an immunogenic form for T cells. Rat intestinal DCs have been shown to acquire antigen administered orally, can stimulate sensitized T cells *in vitro*, and can prime popliteal lymph node CD4$^+$ T cells *in vivo* after footpad injection *(170)*. DCs but not B cells present antigenic complexes to class II MHC–restricted T cells after administration of protein in adjuvants *(173)*. Pulmonary DCs are able to present a soluble antigen shortly after it is introduced into the airways *(88)*. In spleens of mice injected with protein antigens, DCs are the main cell type that carry the protein in a form that is immunogenic for T cells *(174)*. DCs have been shown to migrate rapidly out of mouse cardiac allografts into recipients' spleen, where they home to the peripheral white pulp and associate predominantly with CD4$^+$ T lymphocytes. This movement probably represents the initiation of the graft rejection (175). The essential role of DCs in the activation of T cells *in vivo* has been demonstrated in a model of asthma. Lambrecht et al. (176) used conditional depletion of airway DCs by treatment of thymidine kinase–transgenic mice with the antiviral drug ganciclovir to deplete DCs during the second exposure to ovalbumin. The depletion of DCs before challenge with inhaled antigen results in a decrease in the number of bronchoalveolar CD4 and CD8 T lymphocytes and B lymphocytes and prevents the Th2 cytokine–associated eosinophilic airway inflammation (176).

DCs are presented as nature's adjuvant as they function to initiate immune responses *in vivo*. In line with this hypothesis, DCs are activated by endogenous signals received from cells that are stressed, virally infected, or killed necrotically *(177)*.

T Cell/Dendritic Cell Synapses

The concept of synapse proposes a central contact zone between APCs and T cells and is characterized by the large-scale segregation of cell surface molecules into concentric zones. Synapse formation has been shown to follow and depend on T cell antigen receptor signaling and may fulfill several roles: It participates in sustained TCR signaling, facilitates costimulation, polarizes the T cell secretory apparatus toward the APC, and may play a role in the late signaling. The zone contains multiple copies of molecular couples: the TCR and peptide/MHC molecules and the adhesion and costimulatory molecules (Figure 15.5).

Observations made *in vitro* have suggested that a large number of productive interactions (5,000 to 20,000) are needed for T cell activation. According to the serial triggering model, proposed by Valitutti et al. (178), the threshold could be reached by serial engagement of a limited number of MHC molecules loaded by the cognate peptide on each APC. The immunological contact appears dynamic, as, when offered another APC displaying ligands in greater quantities, T cells that have been activated by encounter with a first APC can form a new synapse within minutes *(179)*. The time of commitment of naïve CD4$^+$ cells varies from 6 hours (high antigen and costimulatory APCs) to more than 30 hours (low antigen or absence of costimulation). In contrast, primed CD4$^+$ cells respond rapidly, within 0.5 hours to 2 hours *(180)*. Some results suggest that CD8$^+$ T cells might achieve commitment more rapidly than CD4$^+$ T cells *(181)*. Indeed, naïve CTLs become committed after as little as 2 hours of exposure to APCs, and their subsequent division and differentiation can occur without the need for further antigenic stimulation, whether priming is *in vitro* or *in vivo*.

An elegant study explored the *in vivo* significance of the number of molecules engaged and the duration of engagement in transgenic mice expressing TCRs in a quantitatively and temporally controlled manner *(182)*. Very few surface TCR molecules were found to be needed for T cells to respond to immunization *in vivo* (100 or less). These results would be compatible with models in which TCR:MHC/peptide combinations form on a one-to-one basis and persist for a long time, rather than forming serial engagements. Whether *in vivo* T cell differentiation requires stimulation by a single DC or by continuously recruited DCs is still a matter of speculation.

Zell et al. *(183)* analyzed signaling events in individual CD4 T cells after antigen recognition *in vivo*. Phosphorylation of c-jun and p38 MAPK was detected within minutes in virtually all antigen-specific CD4 T cells in secondary lymphoid organs after injection of peptide antigen into the bloodstream. The rapidity of signaling correlates with the finding that about 60% to 70% of the naïve DO11.10 T cells are constantly interacting with class II$^+$ MHC CD11c$^+$ (presumably DCs) in the T cell zones of lymphoid organs. Contrary to predictions from *in vitro* experiments, the rate and magnitude of c-jun phosphorylation appears independent of CD28 signals. Collectively, these observations highlight the efficiency of T cell sensitization under physiological conditions *in vivo,* in comparison with *in vitro* models.

Dynamics of Dendritic Cell–T Cell Interaction *In Vivo*

A few reports have examined the dynamics of the contact between antigen-bearing DC and antigen-specific T. In intact explanted lymph nodes, Stoll et al. (184) have reported cell–cell contact and prolonged interactions between DC and T cells, followed by the activation, dissociation and rapid migration of T cells away from the antigenic stimulus. A similar sequence of events was observed *in vivo* in lymph nodes where antigen-specific stable DC–T cell interactions were observed during the induction of priming of CD4$^+$ (*185*,186) and CD8$^+$ *(187–189)* T cells. Whether the duration of interaction is associated with commitment to immunity or tolerance is still unclear. Hugues et al. (190) have shown that, in tolerogenic conditions, naïve CD8 T cells remained motile and established serial brief contacts with multiple DCs, whereas Shakhar et al. have reported that tolerance and immunity were similarly characterized by an early arrest and stable CD4 T cell–DC interaction followed by restoration of mobility (186).

Adjuvants

The induction of immune response *in vivo* is typically performed with antigens administered in external adjuvants. The presence of adjuvants has been shown to increase the level of antibodies and the duration of the immune response, to modify the Th1/Th2 balance, and to induce an anamnestic response. The mechanism by which adjuvants coinitiate an immune response is still poorly understood. Their role could be to provide a signal of "danger" that is necessary to turn on the immune system and could be detected by DCs *(177)*. In favor of this hypothesis, it was shown that the adjuvant monophosphoryl lipid A provokes the migration and maturation of DCs *in vivo (191)*. LeBon et al. *(192)* demonstrated that type I interferons, the major ones of which are IFN-α and IFN-β, potently enhance humoral immunity and can promote isotype switching by stimulating DCs *in vivo*. Adjuvants such as poly(I:C) or complete Freund's adjuvant (containing heat-killed mycobacteria) may act through the induction of endogenous type I IFN production and the subsequent stimulation of DCs by type I IFN *(192)*. Although TLR were considered as key contributors of enhancing effects of vaccine adjuvants, Gavin et al. recently reported that mice deficient in the critical signaling components for TLR mounted robust antibody responses to T cell–dependent antigen given in classical adjuvants (193). These observations suggest that TLR signaling does not account for the action of alum, Freund's complete and incomplete adjuvants.

Immune Escape

Viruses and parasites have developed various means to evade the immune response. MCMV infects and productively replicates in DCs and strongly impairs their endocytic and stimulatory capacities *(194)*. Of note, infected DCs appear incapable of transducing the "danger" signals required to induce antiviral immune responses. DCs appear to be the major target of measles virus proteins, which is related to the profound defect in lymphocyte priming.

The capacity of DCs to stimulate T cells was shown to be impaired after measles virus infection *in vitro,* and their production of IL-12 was down-regulated *in vitro* and *in vivo (195).* Schistosomes have been shown to inhibit Langerhans cell migration *in vivo,* probably through the production of prostaglandin D2 *(196).*

DENDRITIC CELLS AND THE POLARIZATION OF THE IMMUNE RESPONSE

There is evidence that the onset of an immune response may not be sufficient to eliminate all pathogens but that the character of the response (the Th1/Th2/Th17 balance) determines its efficiency. Of importance is that an inadequate immune response may even be deleterious and result in tissue damage, allergic reactions, or disease exacerbation. Th1 cells, by their production of IFN-γ and lymphotoxin, are responsible for the eradication of intracellular pathogens, but they may also cause organ-specific autoimmune diseases if dysregulated. Th2 cells, by their production of IL-4 and IL-5, can activate mast cells and eosinophils and induce humoral immune responses, but they can also provoke atopy and allergic inflammation. The recently described Th17 subset exhibits proinflammatory cytokines such as IL-1β and TNF-α and mediates protective cellular immunity against bacterial infection, but in addition appears to be responsible for tissue inflammation in various autoimmune disorders. The identification of the factors that affect T helper subset development is therefore a prerequisite for the development of effective vaccination strategies.

Role of Antigen-presenting Cells

Several observations suggest that APCs may govern the development of T helper cell populations:

1. The development of Th1 versus Th2 cells seems to be determined early on, at the stage of antigen presentation. Indeed, T cell proliferation and up-regulation of mRNA for interferon-γ in response to Swiss-type murine mammary tumor virus and IL-4 in response to haptenated protein has been shown to start on the third day after immunization *(197).*
2. APCs release cytokines (IL-12, IL-23, IFN-γ, IL-10), which play a central role in Th1/Th2/Th17 differentiation.
3. The strength of interaction mediated through the TCR and MHC/peptide combination or the dose of antigen appears to affect lineage commitment (198). The number of TCR molecules engaged has also been correlated with the outcome (for review, see Lanzavecchia et al. *[199]*).
4. Membrane-bound costimulators, as CD80 or CD86, may influence Th development *in vitro* and *in vivo.*

In favor of this notion, it was shown that the nature of the cell presenting the antigen *in vitro* and *in vivo (117)* strongly influences the development of Th1 versus Th2 cells.

Polarizing Dendritic Cell–derived Cytokines

IL-12 plays a major role in immunity to intracellular pathogens by governing the development of IFN-γ–dependent host resistance (for review, see O'Garra *[200]*). IL-12 receptor–deficient patients display severe mycobacterial and *Salmonella* infections, which indicates an essential role of IL-12 and type 1 cytokine pathway in resistance to infections by intracellular bacteria *(201).*

DCs appear to be the initial cells to synthesize IL-12 in the spleens of mice exposed to microbial stimulants. The production of IL-12 in mice exposed to an extract of *T. gondii* or to LPS occurs very rapidly, is independent of signals from T-lymphocytes, and is associated with DC redistribution to the T cell areas, which suggests that DCs function simultaneously as APCs and as initiators of the Th1 response (44). It was subsequently shown that CD40 ligation induces a significant increase in IL-12 p35 and IL-12 p70 heterodimer production *(104).* Thus, production of high levels of bioactive IL-12 appears to be dependent on two signals: a microbial priming signal and a T cell–derived signal.

There is strong evidence that the Th1-prone capacity of murine DCs is dependent on its IL-12 production, although the role of IL-23 (a combination of p19 and the p40 subunit of IL-12 *[202]*) and IL-18 *(203)* has not been clearly assessed *in vivo.* The role of IL-12 in Th1 priming by DCs has been demonstrated by the correlation between IL-12 production and Th1-prone capacity (204). In parallel with the loss of IL-12 production, human DCs appear to switch from a Th1- to a Th2-inducing mode *(106).* An important determinant of Th1 development in CD4$^+$ T cells is STAT4 activation by IL-12 *(205),* although a STAT4-independent pathway has been reported. Among the transcription factors selectively expressed in Th1 cells, T-bet seems to play a crucial role, and its overexpression by retroviruses in T cells increases the frequency with which Th1 and Th2 cells that produce IFN-γ develop *(206).*

There is no evidence so far that indicates that DCs produce a Th2-prone cytokine. In contrast to IL-12, IL-4 has been shown to skew the development of naïve T cells toward an IL-4–producing Th2 phenotype *(207).* Activated CD4$^+$ T cells themselves may provide the IL-4 required for Th2 differentiation. Other sources of IL-4 or IL-13 include mast cells and basophils (for rev see [208]). The contribution of DCs to Th2 development does not appear to require APC-derived IL-4, inasmuch as injection of DCs from wild-type or IL-4–deficient mice induces similar Th2-type responses in wild-type recipients *(101).* Also, in humans, activated plasmacytoid-derived DCs do not seem to produce detectable amounts of IL-4, and blocking IL-4 at the beginning of culture does not prevent generation of IL-4–producing cells *(103)*. This view is, however, still controversial *(209,210)*. The costimulatory molecule CD86 has been shown to be required for Th2 development *in vitro* and *in vivo (117,211)*, whereas CD80 is a more neutral costimulatory molecule. Of note, CD28 signaling alone appears to induce the pro-Th2 transcription factor GATA-3 and the presence of IL-12 has been shown to repress Th2 development *in vivo*. Indeed, CD8α^+ DCs from IL-12p40–deficient mice prime for Th2, whereas the same subset from wild-type animals primes for Th1 (204). It is, therefore, conceivable that Th2 is a default pathway—that is, that type II T cells would develop spontaneously in the absence of IL-12. The hypothesis that Th2 is a default pathway suggests that IL-12 has a greater opportunity to drive naïve T cells to polarize to Th1 than Th2-prone stimuli such as IL-4. In favor of this notion, TCR ligation has been shown to transiently desensitize IL-4R by inhibiting STAT6 phosphorylation *(212)*. The mechanism by which IL-12 would prevent Th2 priming is still unclear, but it involves inhibition of GATA-3 expression by IL-12 signaling through STAT4, indirect inhibition through IFN-γ production, or both. The requirements for Th2 induction may, therefore, be less stringent and may require only priming and relief from Th1 induction.

Neutralization of IL-4 has been shown to prevent the differentiation of Th2 responses, and IL-4 acts as antagonist of Th1-induced inflammatory responses. However, it has been clearly demonstrated that, paradoxically, IL-4 may promote Th1 development and induce IL-12 production by DCs. These contradictory observations were resolved by a report showing that IL-4 has opposite effects on DC development versus T cell differentiation. When present during the initial activation of DCs by infectious agents, IL-4 instructs DCs to produce IL-12 *(213–215)* and favor Th1 development, but when present later, during the period of T cell priming, IL-4 includes Th2 differentiation. These opposing effects correlate with resistance/sensitivity to *Leishmania major in vivo (96)*.

Unlike murine T cells, human T cells respond to type I interferons by inducing Th1 development. The basis of selective Th1 induction by IFN-α in human T cells appears to be a difference in IFN-α signaling between the mice and humans *(216)*. In particular, IFN-α has been shown to activate STAT4 in human but not mouse T cells. Of note, it has been reported that the COOH-terminal region of human and murine STAT2, which acts as an adapter for STAT4, are widely divergent, because of the insertion of a minisatellite region in mouse exon 23 (which encodes this region).

It has recently been recognized that in many of the mouse autoimmune disease models that have been attributed to Th1 cells, disease severity was in fact increased in the absence of these cells. The characterization of a third subset of T helper cells that secrete IL-17 and expand in response to IL-23 has helped to resolve the paradox. Within tissues, Th17 effector cells stimulate production of a variety of inflammatory chemokines, cytokines, metallopreoteases, and other proinflammatory mediators and promote recruitment of granulocytes. Although IL-23 has a clear role in Th17-mediated inflammation *in vivo*, recent studies have demonstrated that *in vitro* polarization of naïve CD4$^+$ T cells to the Th17 lineage requires a combination of TCR stimulation and the cytokines TGF-β and IL-6, but seems independent of IL-23 *(217,218)*. Instead, IL-23 may be required for promoting survival or maintaining the Th17 phenotype. Therefore, TGF-β at the steady state will induce regulatory T cells, whereas, on infection or inflammation, IL-6 produced by the activated immune system (and in particular by DCs) will suppress the generation of TGF-β–induced regulatory T cells and induce a proinflammatory response of Th17-type (217).

Ivanov et al. recently showed that the nuclear receptor RORγt directs the differentiation program of Th17$^+$ T helper cells. RORγt induces transcription of genes encoding IL-17 in naïve CD4$^+$ T cells and is required for their expression in response to IL-6 and TGF-β, the cytokines known to induce IL-17 (219).

Mechanisms of Dendritic Cell Polarization

Kalinski et al. *(220)* suggested that migrating DCs not only provide an antigen-specific signal 1 and a costimulatory signal 2, but also carry an additional signal 3, contributing to the initial commitment of naïve T helper cells into Th1 or Th2 subsets. This would allow the efficient induction of T helper cells with adequate cytokine profiles during early infections without requirement for a direct contact between antigen-specific T cells and the pathogens *(220)*.

Reports in the literature are consistent with three models through which DCs may control T cell polarization: (a) subclasses of DCs, (b) the nature of the stimuli that activate DCs, and (c) the kinetics of DC activation.

Dendritic Cell Subclasses

In the mouse, three *in vivo* studies have demonstrated that DC subsets differed in the cytokine profiles that they induce in T cells. In one study (221), TCR transgenic T cells from DO11.10/SCID mice were adoptively transferred into Balb/c recipients. CD11c$^+$CD11b$^{dull/-}$ (mainly CD8α^+) or CD11c$^+$CD11b^{bright}CD8α^- cells were loaded with ovalbumin peptide *in vitro* and injected into the footpads of transferred animals. Both DC subpopulations induced antigen-specific proliferation *in vivo* and *in vitro* upon restimulation with the antigen. Assessment of cytokine production revealed that both subsets induced IFN-γ and IL-2 production but that the CD11c$^+$CD11b^{bright}CD8α^- subset induced much greater levels of IL-10 and IL-4 production. The differences in the cytokine profiles of T cells correlated with class-specific differences in the antibody profiles. In the second study (204), antigen-pulsed CD8α^+ and CD8α^- DCs were injected into the footpads of syngeneic recipients. Administration of CD8α^- DCs induced a Th2-type response, whereas injection of CD8α^+ DCs led to Th1 differentiation. In a third study, CD11b$^+$CD8α^- DCs from murine Peyer's patch have been shown to prime naïve T cells to secrete high levels of IL-4 and IL-10 *in vitro,* whereas the CD11b$^-$CD8α^+ and double-negative subsets from the same tissue primed for IFN-γ production *(8)*. The role of murine DC subsets in the regulation of Th1/Th2 balance *in vivo* has been more directly assessed by the targeting of antigens to receptors that are DC subset-restricted. Steinman et al. have shown that injection of 33D1 mAb-coupled to an antigen targeted CD8α^- DCs and induced the development of T cells producing IL-4 and little IFN-γ, whereas the same antigen coupled to anti-DEC-205 mAb was presented by CD8α^+ DCs and led to the secretion of higher levels of IFN-γ and no IL-4 *(322)*.

In humans, monocyte-derived DCs were found to induce Th1 differentiation, whereas DCs derived from plasmacytoid cells favor Th2 development of allogeneic T cells (23). Subsequent work has demonstrated, however, that the T cell stimulatory function of plasmacytoid-derived DCs was regulated by the environment: Virus-induced plasmacytoid DCs stimulate naïve T cells to produce IFN-γ and IL-10, whereas IL-3 induced plasmacytoid DCs stimulate naïve T cells to produce Th2-type cytokines (IL-4, IL-5, and IL-10) *(31)*. Cella et al. *(114)* reported that blood plasmacytoid DCs represent the principal source of type I interferon during inflammation and participate in antiviral Th1-type responses.

There is evidence that DC subsets express distinct pattern-recognition and presentation receptors that differentially regulate the production of cytokines known to direct the T helper cell differntation (see previous discussion, antigen uptake).

Little is known on the nature of the DCs which produce IL-12 versus IL-23. Like IL-12, IL-23 is expressed predominantly by activated DCs and phagocytic cells, and both cytokines may induce IFN-γ by T cells. The discovery that IL-23, but not IL-12, is essential in some models of chronic inflammation led to a model in which IL-12 is required to induce IFN-γ–producing Th1 cells, whereas IL-23 mediates Th1 effector functions. In favor of this notion: (1) IL-23 has been shown to be the effector cytokine in two models of intestinal inflammation (110,111) and in an experimental model of autoimmune encephalitis. (2) Vaknin-Dembinsky et al. have quantified the expression of IL-23 in monocyte-derived DCs in multiple sclerosis patients and found that DCs from these patients secrete elevated amounts of IL-23 (222). They reported increased IL-17 production by CD4$^+$ T cells, but no differences in IFN-γ secretion. (3) IL-23 appears as an essential promoter of end-stage collagen-induced arthritis in mice, whereas IL-12 paradoxically mediates protection from autoimmune inflammation *(223)*. Other reports, however, suggest that the IL-23/IL-17 axis may display suppressive functions. Mice deficient for IL-23 appear highly susceptible for the development of experimental T cell–mediated TNBS colitis (224). The authors reported an over-expression of IL-12 by DCs from lamina propria in the absence of IL-23, suggesting that IL-23 inhibits IL-12 secretion. Similarly, IL-17 has a dual role: It is essential during antigen sensitization to establish allergic asthma and attenuates the allergic response in sensitized mice by inhibiting DCs and chemokine synthesis *(225)*.

Morelli et al. *(226)* have analyzed the APC function of different subsets of human DCs that migrate spontaneously from human skin explants. Langerhans cells and dermal DCs induced Th1 memory cells, and this function depended on their ability to produce IL-23.

Nature of the Stimuli

Vieira et al. *(227)* showed that the Th1- and Th2-inducing function of human monocyte-derived DCs is not an intrinsic attribute but depends on environmental instruction. DCs that matured in the presence of IFN-γ induce Th1 responses, whereas DCs that matured in the presence of prostaglandin E_2 induce Th2 responses. Similarly, the presence of IL-10 during maturation has been shown to lead to the development of DCs with Th2-driving function, whereas incubation of DC subsets with IFN-γ favors the priming of Th1 cells to the detriment of Th2 cell development *(101,220,228)*. This provides evidence for the adaptation of DC function to the conditions that they encounter in the pathogen-invaded tissue.

The antigen itself has been shown to regulate DC function. DCs have the capacity to discriminate between yeasts and hyphae of the fungus *Candida albicans* and release distinct cytokines *(209)*. Using oligonucleotides microarrays, Huang et al. (229) measured gene expression profiles of DCs in response to *E. coli, C. albicans,* and influenza virus. The data show that a common set of 166 genes, as well as particular subsets of genes, is regulated by each pathogen, which demonstrates that DCs discriminate between diverse pathogens and elicit tailored pathogen-specific immune responses.

TLRs have been shown to translate the information regarding the nature of the pathogens into differences in the cytokines and the chemokines produced by DCs: Re et al. have reported that activation of DCs by microbial agonists of TLR2 and TLR4 led to comparable activation of NF-kB and MAPK family members but that only the TLR4 agonist promoted the production of IL-12 p70 and the chemokine IP-10, which is associated with Th1 responses (230) (see also earlier discussion, antigen uptake).

It is interesting that synergic TLR stimulation appears to increase the production of IL-12 and IL-23 as well as the Delta-4/Jagged-1 ratio, leading to DCs with enhanced Th1-polarizing capacity (231).

Sporri and Reis e Sousa have tested whether inflammatory mediators produced in physiological amounts *in vivo* can substitute for direct PAMP recognition in DC activation and T cell priming (230). Interestingly, they have shown that indirectly activated DCs upregulate MHC molecules and costimulation and drive T cell proliferation, but not their differentiation in cytokine-producing T helper cells. They conclude that direct PAMP recognition is required for T helper–polarizing signals (of Th1- or Th2-types).

Kinetics of Dendritic Cell Activation

In addition to the nature of the maturation stimulus, the kinetics of activation may influence the capacity of DCs to induce different types of T cell responses. Recent *in vitro* observations suggest that, indeed, DCs produce IL-12 during a narrow time window and afterward become refractory to further stimulation. The exhaustion of cytokine production has been shown to affect the T cell polarizing process: DCs taken at early times after induction of maturation (active DCs) prime strong Th1 responses, whereas the same cells taken at later times ("exhausted" DCs) preferentially prime Th2 and nonpolarized cells *(106)*. These observations, although made *in vitro,* suggest a dynamic regulation of the generation of effector and memory cells during the immune response.

Two subsets of memory T lymphocytes with distinct homing potentials and effector functions have been described *(232)*. Expression of CCR7, a chemokine receptor that controls homing to secondary lymphoid organs, divides memory T cells into $CCR7^-$ effector memory cells, which migrate to inflamed tissues and display immediate effector function, and $CCR7^+$ central memory cells, which home in the lymph nodes and lack immediate effector function. Both subsets may persist for years, and the central memory cells give rise to effector memory upon secondary stimulation.

It has been proposed that the nature of DCs bearing antigen and costimulatory molecules, as well as the amount and duration of TCR triggering, determines whether effector memory or central memory cells are generated. A short TCR stimulation may expand nonpolarized T cells that home to lymph nodes and respond promptly to antigenic stimulation. In contrast, a prolonged stimulation in the presence of polarizing cytokines may drive differentiation of Th1 or Th2 effector cells that home to inflamed peripheral tissues.

DENDRITIC CELLS AND T CELL TOLERANCE

Central Tolerance

The normal development of T cells in the thymus requires both positive and negative selection. During positive selection, thymocytes mature only if their TCRs react with some specificity to host MHC and host peptides. Laufer et al. *(233)* used the keratin promoter to reexpress a class II MHC antigen in class II–negative mice and showed that autoimmunity develops in transgenic mice in which class II MHC products are expressed only by epithelial cells and not by bone marrow–derived APCs. Autoreactive cells that constitute up to 5% of the peripheral CD4 T cells were generated.

During negative selection, developing T cells reacting strongly to self-peptide/self-MHC combinations are eliminated. Brocker et al. (234) demonstrated that thymic DCs are sufficient to mediate negative selection *in vivo.* Using a CD11c promoter, they targeted the expression of an MHC class II I-E transgene to DCs and showed that tolerance to I-E was induced. These observations demonstrate that thymocyte development is a sequential process: Positive selection occurs on thymic cortical epithelium independently of negative selection, which is mediated by thymic DCs.

Of note, a report demonstrates that the level of class I MHC protein is 10-fold higher on thymic DCs than on thymic epithelial cells and that an increase in the level of a particular cognate peptide/MHC ligand may be sufficient to result in negative rather than positive selection. This finding suggests a role for the quantitative differences in the level of MHC expression in thymic selection *(235)*.

Mathis et al. have emphasized the crucial role of the transcription factor AIRE (autoimmune regulator gene) in the "central" tolerance. They showed that AIRE regulates autoimmunity by promoting the ectopic expression of peripheral tissue-restricted antigens in thymic medullary epithelial cells (apparently not in DCs) (236). They recently reported that AIRE exerts its tolerance-promoting function not by positive selection of regulatory T cells, but rather by negative selection of T effector cells. It is interesting that, in addition, AIRE appears to enhance the antigen-presentation capability of medullary epithelial cells by a mechanism still unknown. Very recent data have confirmed the link between aire-driven regulation of tissue specific expression in the thymus and the development of a spontaneous autoimmune disease in mice. It was shown that autoimmune eye disease in aire-deficient mice develops as a result of loss of thymic expression of a single eye antigen, interphotoreceptor retinoid-binding protein (IRBP). In addition, lack of IRBP expression solely in the thymus, even in the presence of aire expression, is sufficient to trigger spontaneous eye-specific autoimmunity *(237)*.

Peripheral Tolerance

Many proteins, however, may not have access to the thymus during development, and a significant proportion of self-reactive T cells has been shown to escape negative selection, which suggests that a mechanism must be able to silence autoreactive T cells in the periphery. Bouneaud et al. *(238)* studied a peptide-specific T cell repertoire in the presence and absence of the deleting ligand. The authors used mice transgenic for the TCR-β chain of an anti-HY T cell clone and compared the preimmune repertoire reactive to the male-specific peptide in male and female animals. Interestingly, their results showed that a large proportion of $CD8^+$ T cells specific for the male-specific peptide persist in male animals, as detected by MHC/peptide tetramer staining and functional assays. Of note, male T cells (specific to the male peptide) that escape clonal deletion do not react with the endogenous male peptide, as predicted by the observation that the threshold of antigenic stimulation is lower for negative selection that for activation of mature cells, but those cells are still capable of functional reactivity with self-peptides when facing high doses of antigen.

There is evidence that, besides their immunostimulatory functions, DCs may also maintain and regulate T cell tolerance in the periphery. This control function may be exerted by certain maturation stages, specialized subsets, or cells influenced by immunomodulatory agents such as IL-10.

Immature Dendritic Cells

In the periphery, immature DCs are specialized for antigen capture but display weak stimulatory properties for naïve $CD4^+$ and $CD8^+$ T cells. Several observations *(65,66)* show that immature DCs express MHC/peptide combinations, albeit at low levels. On the basis of *in vitro* studies showing that TCR engagement in the absence of costimulation may lead to anergy of T cell clones *(239)*, it was postulated that immature DCs may induce a state of unresponsiveness in antigen-specific T lymphocytes. This hypothesis would be in agreement with several observations: (a) Both immature and mature DCs are constantly acquiring peptide cargo, although immature DCs clearly display lower levels of antigen/MHC combinations; (b) immature DCs are in close contact with T lymphocytes in lymphoid organs; and (c) immature DCs present self-antigens *(240)*.

Consistent with tolerogenic properties of DCs, several reports suggest a major flux of tissue antigens via DCs migrating to the lymph nodes. Huang et al. (90) have identified in rat a DC subset ($OX41^-$) that constitutively transports apoptotic bodies derived from the intestinal epithelium to T cell areas of mesenteric lymph nodes *in vivo*. $OX41^-$ DCs are weak APCs despite expressing high levels of B7 molecules and may play a role in inducing and maintaining self-tolerance. In addition, rat intestinal lymph contains another subset of $OX41^+$ DCs that are strong APCs but may not reach the T cell area in the absence of inflammation. Specific migratory DCs rapidly transport antigen from the airways to the thoracic lymph nodes in baseline conditions (89). These observations suggest that DC internalize potential self-antigens from tissues and from noninfectious environmental proteins. It is important to note that exposure of DCs to primary tissue cells or apoptotic cells do not induce their maturation *(241)*. These observations led to the hypothesis *(242)* that immature DCs phagocytose tissue cells undergoing normal cell turnover by apoptosis, leading to unresponsiveness of self-reactive T cells in the draining lymph node.

Hawiger et al. (243) examined the function of murine DCs in the steady state, using as antigen delivery system a monoclonal antibody to a DC-restricted endocytic receptor DEC-205. Targeting the antigen on DCs resulted in transient antigen-specific T cell activation, followed by T cell deletion and unresponsiveness. T cells initially activated by DCs in these conditions could not be reactivated when the mice were challenged with the same antigen in complete Freund's adjuvant. In contrast, coinjection of the DC-targeted antigen and anti-CD40 agonistic antibody resulted in prolonged T cell activation and immunity. These observations suggest that, in the steady state, the primary function of DCs may be to maintain peripheral tolerance. Consistently, an initial burst of $CD8^+$ T cell proliferation followed by deletion was observed when antigen was expressed as transgene in pancreatic β cells, in kidney proximal tubular cells, and in the testes of male mice. The antigen was shown to be presented not by pancreatic β cells, but by bone marrow–derived APCs in the draining lymph nodes (244). Similar results were obtained by Morgan et al. *(245)*, who further demonstrated a direct correlation between the amounts of antigen expressed in the periphery and the rate of tolerance of specific $CD8^+$ T cells. Another study showed that administration of immature DCs may prolong cardiac allograft survival in nonimmunosuppressed recipients *(246)*. Probst et al. used an elegant system to demonstrate that resting DCs induced peripheral $CD8^+$ T cell tolerance (247). Injection of double-transgenic DIETER (DC-specific inducible expression of T cell epitopes by recombination) mice with tamoxifen induced the presentation of three transgenic CTL epitopes by 5% of all DCs. Of note, this presentation resulted in peripheral tolerance if the DCs are resting and in protective immunity if DCs are activated *in vivo* by coinjection of agonistic CD40 antibodies. The authors further reported that $CD8^+$ T cell tolerance depended on signaling via the costimulatory molecule PD-1 (248). Collectively, these observations support the hypothesis that activation of T cells in a noninflammatory environment, presumably by immature DCs, could be part of a normal mechanism of peripheral tolerance.

In humans, Dhodapkar et al. *(249)* analyzed the immune response induced after injection of immature DCs pulsed with influenza matrix peptide and keyhole limpet hemocyanin (KLH) in two healthy subjects. A decline in matrix peptide–specific IFN-γ–producing T cells was observed, whereas such cells were detected in both subjects before immunization as expected, because most adults have been exposed to the influenza virus. Of note, the decline in IFN-γ production was associated with the appearance of IL-10–producing cells specific for the same antigen. KLH priming was much greater when mature DCs were used and KLH-specific, IFN-γ–secreting cells were detected. *In vitro* studies *(250)* have shown that repetitive stimulation with immature human DCs induced nonproliferating, IL-10–producing CD4$^+$ T cells. These T cells, in co-culture experiments, have been shown to inhibit the antigen-driven proliferation of Th1 cells in a contact- and dose-dependent but antigen-nonspecific manner.

The Existence of Specialized Subsets of Dendritic Cells

The existence of these cells, which would display tolerogenic properties, is still a matter of speculation. Initial *in vitro* studies by Suss and Shortman *(251)* demonstrated that splenic CD8α^- DCs induced a vigorous proliferative response in CD4$^+$ T cells, whereas CD8α^+ DCs induced a lesser response that was associated with T cell apoptosis. The tolerogenic capacity of CD8α^+ DCs was demonstrated *in vivo* in one report, but the negative regulatory effect appears restricted to tumor/self-peptide P815AB and was not observed with other antigens *(252)*. The potential role of CD8α^+ DCs in peripheral tolerance was challenged by numerous reports showing that these DCs are the major producers of IL-12 and induce the development of IFN-γ–producing T cells *in vivo* (see earlier discussion).

There is evidence that DC subsets may display tolerogenic functions. De Heer et al. have shown that lung plasmacytoid DCs had an essential role in preventing asthmatic reactions in mice (253). Depletion of pDCs during inhalation of normally inert antigens led to cardinal features of asthma, whereas adoptive transfer of plasmacytoid DCs before sensitization prevented disease. Recently, plasmacytoid DCs were identified as phagocytic APCs essential for tolerance to vascularized cardiac allografts in mice (254). These cells acquire and process MHC class II–derived donor allopeptide in allografts, migrate to peripheral lymph nodes across high endothelial venules, and induce the peripheral development of CD4$^+$CD25$^+$FoxP3$^+$ Treg. Depletion of plasmacytoid DCs or prevention of their lymph node homing inhibited peripheral regulatory T cell development. In humans, herpes virus–stimulated plasmacytoid DCs have been shown to induce allogeneic naïve CD4$^+$ T cells to differentiate into cytotoxic regulatory T cells that inhibit proliferation of coexisting naïve CD4$^+$ T cells *(255)*. Similarly, human CD40$^-$activated plasmacytoid DCs induce the differentiation of CD8 T cells into IL-10–producing anergic CD8 T cells that suppress the allospecific proliferation of naïve CD8 T cells.

A recent report by Kaplan et al. (256) examined the functional requirement of LCs in skin immunity and generated mice with a constitutive and durable absence of epidermal Langerhans cells. Unexpectedly, they found that Langerhans cells were dispensable for contact hypersensitivity but regulated the response.

Powrie et al. (257) have identified a subpopulation of DC at mucosal sites that expresses CD103 (the α_E integrin) and is crucial to allow CD4$^+$ CD25$^+$ Treg cells to dominate and suppress the colitogenic effector cell response. They showed that CD103$^+$DCs, but not their CD103$^-$ counterparts, promoted expression of the gut-homing receptor CCR9 on T cells. Although the mechanism by which CD103 regulates the balance of effector and regulatory responses in the intestine is still unknown, it may involve TGF-β, which has been shown to induce CD103 on T cells *(258)*. A minor population of murine splenic CD19$^+$ DCs (distinct from plasmacytoid DCs) appears to acquire potent IDO-dependent T cell suppressive functions following CpG oligonucleotide treatment *(259)*.

A population of CD11c^{low}CD45RB^{high} DCs has been described in the spleen and lymph node of normal mice, which displays plasmacytoid morphology, secretes high levels of IL-10 after activation, and induces tolerance through the differentiation of Tr1 cells (260). Finally, Svensson et al. (261) reported that spleen-derived stromal cells promote the development of CD11c^{lo}CD45RB$^+$ IL-10–producing regulatory DC from lineage-negative c-kit$^+$ progenitor cells. These DCs have the capacity to suppress T cell responses and induce IL-10–producing Treg. Stromal cells from Leishmania donovani–infected mice are more efficient in supporting their development, suggesting that regulatory DCs may have an impact on the outcome of parasitic disease.

Interleukin-10

IL-10 has been shown to suppress multiple activities of the immune response. The immunosuppressive properties of IL-10 on DCs are caused by a reduction in the upregulation of expression of class II MHC, costimulatory, and adhesion molecules, as well as an inhibition of the production of inflammatory cytokines (IL-1, IL-6, TNF-α, and IL-12). Of note, IL-10 modulates the function of immature DCs but has little effect on mature DCs (for review, see Jonuleit et al. *[262]*). Human DCs generated from peripheral progenitors and exposed to IL-10 for the last 2 days of culture were shown to induce a state of antigen-specific anergy in T cells *(263)*. The tolerogenic properties of these IL-10–treated DCs correlate with a reduced expression of class II MHC molecules, CD58 and CD86 costimulatory molecules, and the DC-specific antigen CD83. The role of IL-10–producing DCs has been illustrated in the lung (264). Pulmonary DCs from mice exposed to respiratory antigen transiently produce IL-10 and induce antigen unresponsiveness in recipient mice. Although they are phenotypically mature, these DCs stimulate the development of CD4$^+$ T regulatory cells that also produce high amounts of IL-10. Upon transfer, these pulmonary DCs induce antigen unresponsiveness in recipient mice.

DENDRITIC CELLS AND REGULATORY T CELLS

The mechanims responsible for peripheral T cell tolerance can be divided into those acting directly on the responding T cells, such as inactivation or deletion of specific T cells (T cell intrinsic), and those that act through additional cells or factors, such as regulatory T cells or suppressive cytokines (T cell extrinsic).

Interest in Treg cells has exploded since the discovery by Sakaguchi et al. of a minor population of CD4$^+$ CD25$^+$ T cells that plays a central role in the prevention of autoimmune reactions *in vivo* (for review see *[265]*). "Natural Treg" develop in the thymus, are present in naïve animals, and their depletion causes the development of a spectrum of autoimmune diseases.

By contrast, "adaptive or induced" Treg develop in peripheral lymphoid tissues under partcular conditions of antigen stimulation. In particular, TGF-β seems to be involved in the conversion of CD4$^+$ CD25$^-$ T cells into CD4$^+$ CD25$^+$ FoxP3$^+$ (317). Another factor is the mode of antigen presentation: Regulatory T cell populations can be induced in subimmunogenic conditions and expanded by delivery of antigen in immunogenic conditions (266), suggesting that a limited antigen dose and the delivery of antigen to unactivated DC may be a strategy to develop adaptive Treg.

The role of CD8$^+$ T cells as Treg cells is still poorly documented. Of note, a few reports *(267,268)* have shown that plasmacytoid DC could induce antigen-specific CD8$^+$ IL-10–producing cells.

The respective role of thymic-derived versus peripherally generated FoxP3$^+$ Treg still needs to be established. The molecular mechanism(s) underlying their suppressive activity is (are) still elusive and may involve cell-contact pathway, suppressor cytokines, or killing. A recent report (269) suggests that mast cells are critical in Treg-dependent allograft tolerance and would be recruited and activated through IL-9, which is produced by all categories of Treg cells, Therefore, Treg through the production of IL-9, IL-10, and TGF-β may interact with cells of the innate system (mast cells, macrophages, and DCs) leading to inhibition of the immune responses.

Bidirectional Dendritic Cell-T Signaling: Role of CD28 and CTLA-4

It is interesting that tolerogenic DCs not only display antigens in a way that makes T cells tolerate that antigen, but that the Treg cells can modulate DC function, so that they are no longer able to alert the adaptive cells to danger. Grohmann et al. have identified a reverse signaling through B7 molecules in tolerogenic DCs, which leads to cytokine-dependent tryptophan catabolism. Thus, exposure of DCs to CTLA-4-Ig *in vitro* and *in vivo* induces IDO protein expression and promotes a tolerant state and long-term allograft survival (137). Of note, Munn et al. have identified the GCN2 kinase as a downstream mediator for the immunoregulatory action of IDO in T cells *(270)*. GCN2 is a stress-response kinase that can be activated by elevations in uncharged tRNA. In addition, *in vivo* studies have demonstrated that regulatory T cells can modify DCs to down-regulate expression of costimulatory molecules *(271,272)*. In particular, CD4$^+$ CD25$^+$ FoxP3$^+$ T cells appear in the airway mucosa and regional lymph nodes within 24 hours of initiation of aerosol exposure and inhibit subsequent T helper–mediated upregulation of resident airway mucosal DC functions *(272)*.

DENDRITIC CELLS AND B CELL ACTIVATION

Several observations have underscored the role of DCs in the induction of humoral responses. Inaba et al. (273,274) demonstrated that DCs were required for the development of T cell–dependent antibody responses by murine and human lymphocytes *in vitro*. Injection of syngeneic DCs, which have been pulsed *in vitro* with soluble protein antigen, induced a strong antibody response in mice that were boosted with soluble antigen (169). Antigen-specific antibodies of isotypes similar to the Ig classes produced after immunization with the same antigen in complete Freund's adjuvant were detected in treated animals. In particular, IgG1 and IgG2a antibodies were produced, which suggests that Th1 and Th2 cells are activated and a memory response was induced.

The classical view of DC function in antibody formation was that these cells activate CD4$^+$ T helper cells, which in turn interact directly with B cells to provide help. However, more recent findings have suggested a role for direct DC–B cell interaction. CD40-activated DCs have been shown to enhance both the proliferation and IgM secretion of CD40-activated B lymphocytes *(275)* and to switch naïve IgD$^+$ cells to become IgA secretors in the presence of IL-10 *(276)*.

Further, Grouard et al. (277) identified a population of DCs capable of stimulating T cells in the germinal center. This population of germinal center DCs is distinct from the follicular DCs, which retain immune complexes and promote the activation and selection of high-affinity B cells. Germinal center DCs express CD11c and CD4 and represent 0.5% to 1% of all germinal center cells in human tonsils, spleen, and lymph nodes. Germinal center DCs display much stronger T cell stimulatory function than do germinal center B cells and were found in close association with memory T cells *in situ*, which suggests that they may maintain the germinal center reaction by sustaining the activation state of germinal center memory T cells.

DENDRITIC CELLS AND CELLS OF THE INNATE SYSTEM

In addition to their major role in the induction or adaptative immune responses, DCs appear to activate the innate arm of antitumor immunity; that is, NK and NKT effector cells.

NK cells participate in the innate response against transformed cells *in vivo (278)*. Murine DCs have been shown to enhance proliferation, cytotoxicity properties, and IFN-γ production by NK cells *in vitro (279)*. Moreover, in mice with class I MHC–negative tumors, DCs promote NK-dependent antitumor effects *in vivo*. The activation depends on direct DC–NK cell contact and on secreted factors that include IL-12, IL-18, and possibly IL-15. In addition, IL-2 released by DCs *(115)* could play a role in the activation of NK functions by DCs.

Gerosa et al. *(46)* analyzed the interaction between human peripheral blood NK cells and monocyte-derived DCs. Fresh NK cells were activated, and their cytolytic activity was strongly augmented by contact with mature DCs. Reciprocally, fresh NK cells cultured with immature DCs strongly enhance DC maturation and IL-12 production. A recent study shows, however, that immature NK cells may suppress DC functions during the development of leukemia in a mouse model *(280)*.

NKT cells are TCRα/β^+ CD4$^+$ or CD4$^-$CD8$^-$ T cells that display distinctive phenotypic and functional properties *(281–283)*. They can be distinguished from conventional T cells by their expression of the NK cell locus-encoded C-type lectin molecule NK1.1. Another hallmark of murine NKT cells is their restricted TCR repertoire: The great majority express an invariant TCR-α chain structure. NKT cells are relevant in innate antitumor immunosurveillance. Both mouse and human NKT cells rapidly secrete cytokines associated with both Th1 (IFN-γ) and Th2 (IL-4) responses upon TCR engagement or stimulation with the synthetic CD1d ligand, the α-galactosylceramide. This ligand induces IL-12 production by DCs and IL-12 receptor expression on NKT cells, thereby activating NKT cells for production of IFN-γ (284). Injection of the α-galactosylceramide has been shown to stimulate the full maturation of DCs *in situ*, by a mechanism dependent on NKT cells, and to induce T helper CD4$^+$ and CD8$^+$ T cell immunity to a coadministered protein *(285)*.

Neutrophils are also able to communicate with DCs. Neutrophils not only instantly kill pathogens when they invade tissues, but they can also travel from the site of infection to the nearest lymph node to directly or indirectly present antigen. Neutrophils can induce DCs to mature and to produce IL-12, thereby favoring a Th1-type response. Of note, DCs and neutrophils are found in close proximity in the mucosa of patients with Crohn's disease (a Th1-type inflammation) (286).

DENDRITIC CELL–BASED IMMUNOTHERAPY FOR CANCER

The first experimental evidence that lack of immunogenicity could be caused by the tumor's inability to activate the immune system rather than the absence of tumor antigens was provided by Boon and Kellerman in 1977 (287). This observation was confirmed in various tumor models and paved the way for a vaccination therapy of cancer.

As a complement to other less specific therapies, the immunotherapy may be highly beneficial to tumor patients because it would ideally induce an antigen-specific, widespread, long-term protection. DCs are currently under active clinical investigation, mostly for their immunostimulatory properties in cancer.

A large body of literature involves animal models showing that DCs loaded with tumor-associated antigens are able to induce a protective immune response, even to established tumors. In mice, successful protection against a B cell lymphoma was achieved by immunization with idiotype-pulsed splenic DCs *(288)*. Naïve mice injected with bone marrow–derived DCs pulsed with tumor-associated, class I–restricted peptides were protected against a subsequent lethal tumor challenge and against preestablished C3 sarcoma cells or 3LL lung carcinoma cells *(289)*.

In addition, immunity has been induced against unidentified antigens by injecting DCs pulsed with tumor cell membranes, RNA from tumors, peptides eluted from class I MHC molecules, or DC/tumor cell hybrids. The fusion of DCs with tumor cells has been shown to generate hybrid cells that display the functional properties of DCs and present one or more tumor antigens. Administration of hybrid cells prevents the growth of preimplanted tumor cells in various models, induces long-lasting tumor resistance *in vivo (290–292)*, and can reverse unresponsiveness to a tumor-associated antigen *(293)*. Another strategy is to expand DCs *in vivo* through administration of Fms-like tyrosine kinase 3 (FLT-3) ligand, which results in mobilization of DC precursors from the bone marrow and induction of antitumor immunity. FLT-3 ligand and CD40L synergize in the generation of immune response against two poorly immunogenic tumors, leading to complete rejection in a high proportion of mice and long-lasting protection *(294)*.

Although animal studies provided the proof of principle for antigen-pulsed DC vaccination against cancer, this approach is still in an early stage in humans, due to numerous variables to be tested that are pertinent to DC function and induction of innate and adaptive immune responses against cancer.

The use of DCs as adjuvants for immunotherapy of cancer has been possible because of the discovery that DCs might be generated from peripheral monocytes or CD34 bone marrow precursors, in the presence of certain cytokines such as GM-CSF, IL-4, and TNF-α (295).

DCs loaded with tumor antigens have been used in a number of trials in humans (for review, see Fong and Engelman *[296]* and Gunzer and Grabbe *[297]*). It was initially demonstrated that DCs can be used to vaccinate B cell lymphoma patients with the induction of antigen-specific T cells, and clinical responses were achieved in two of four patients *(298)*. DCs were further used to treat melanoma, prostate cancer, and bladder cancer (for review, see Nestle *[299]*). Nestle et al. *(300)* injected the DC preparation directly under ultrasound control in a normal inguinal lymph node. KLH was added as a CD4 helper antigen and immunological tracer molecule. DC vaccination induced delayed-type hypersensitivity reactivity toward KLH in all 16 patients and toward peptide-pulsed DCs in 11 patients. Objective clinical responses were obtained in five patients. In another trial *(301)*, injection of mature monocyte-derived DCs, pulsed with a MAGE-3 peptide and a recall antigen, was shown to enhance circulating MAGE-3–specific cytotoxic effectors in patients with melanoma and lead to regression of individual metastases in 6 of 11 patients. Antigen-specific immune response was induced after intradermal injection but decreased after intravenous injection *(301)*. In another study, Banchereau et al. *(302)* used DCs derived from $CD34^+$ cells that consist of two phenotypically and functionally distinct populations: Langerhans cells and the interstitial/dermal DCs (similar to those derived from blood monocytes). Patients with metastatic melanoma received subcutaneous injections of CD34 progenitor–derived autologous DCs, pulsed with peptides derived from four melanoma antigens, as well as control antigens (influenza matrix peptide and KLH). The long-term outcomes in vaccinated patients showed that patients who have survived longer are those in whom vaccination with CD34-DCs elicited T cell immunity to at least two melanoma peptides *(303)*.

It is still unclear whether the rates of tumor regression are clearly different in the trials involving DCs from those observed with other vaccine modalities. Of note, the analysis of the clonal diversity of CTL responses in patients vaccinated with DCs pulsed with the HLA-A1–restricted MAGE-3 peptide showed that several CTL clones were amplified *(304)*. This polyclonality contrasts with the monoclonality of the CTL responses observed in patients vaccinated with MAGE-3.A1 peptide or with ALVAC recombinant virus coding for this antigenic peptide.

A critical aspect of immunotherapy is the identification of immunologic markers that will permit prediction of clinical efficacy. The analysis of immune responses in melanoma patients vaccinated with antigens encoded by MAGE genes revealed a possible involvement of T cells directed against tumor antigens other than the vaccine antigen (305,306). T. Boon, P. Coulie, et al. found a low frequency of antivaccine T cells and a high frequency of antitumor CTLs with high enrichment in regressing metastases, suggesting that the antivaccine CTLs are not the effectors that kill the tumor cells, but that their interaction with the tumor induces activation of competent tumor-specific CTL.

Although promising, DC vaccination is in an early stage, and several parameters that may be critical for the immunological and clinical outcome need to be defined: the DC type, antigen loading, site of injection, DC dosage, and frequency of injections. Labeling studies with radioactive tracers have demonstrated significant differences in the distribution of DCs administered by different routes, although only a minor fraction of the injected DCs can be recovered in the draining lymph nodes in mouse and human experiments *(307,308)*. A more direct and less laborious strategy would be to target antigens *in vivo* via specific surface receptors. DEC-205 and DC-SIGN (DC-specific intercellular adhesion molecule 3-grabbing nonintegrin) were identified as target molecules. Steinman, Nussenzweig, et al. found that proteins delivered to DCs by antibodies to DEC-205 receptor in combination with a maturation stimulus were higly effective in inducing cellular *(59)* and humoral *(309)* immune responses. Figdor et al. developed a humanized antibody directed against the C-type lectin DC-SIGN, which was crosslinked to an antigen. They demonstrated delivery of antigen to DCs via DC-SIGN, resulting in naïve as well as recall responses by T cells *(309)*. Steinman et al. introduced the HIV p24 gag protein into a mAb that targets DEC-205 and assessed the processing of noreplicating internalized antigens onto MHC class I (cross-presentation) for recognition by $CD8^+$ T cells *(79)*. They found that αDEC205-gag stimulated proliferation and IFN-γ production by $CD8^+$ T cells isolated from blood of HIV-infected donors. αDEC205 was found more effective than αDEC209/DC-SIGN.

There is clear evidence that, although immunity can be induced in cancer patients, mechanisms may exist that impair effective tumor rejection. Suppressive cell populations have been described and include myeloid suppressor cells, natural or induced regulatory T cells, NKT cells, etc. Therefore, novel therapeutic approaches are envisaged that combine vaccination and treatment(s) to overcome tolerance.

"Killer" Dendritic Cells

Two recent reports have identified a novel subset of cells coexpressing DC and NK cell markers, which kills tumor cells through a predominantly TRAIL-dependent pathway (310). The infiltration of activated NK/DCs into the tumor mass was induced by a combination of IL-2 and Gleevec (imatinib mesylate), and the NK/DCs recognize and kill tumor cells *in vitro* and *in vivo*. These cells produce substantial amounts of IFN-γ and were termed interferon-producing killer DCs (IKDC). There is evidence that their cytolytic capacity is inversely regulated with their antigen-presenting activity (311), suggesting that these cells provide a link between innate and adaptive immunity. It is still unclear whether a human equivalent exists and whether immunosurveillance is a normal function of IKDC (i.e, in mice not treated with Gleevec and IL-2). Further studies are needed to determine whether the IKDC are indeed a form of antigen-presenting DC or a form of NK cell.

DENDRITIC CELLS AND THE DEVELOPMENT AUTOIMMUNITY

An interesting question is whether cells of the dendritic family are implicated in the onset and the pathogenesis of autoimmune diseases. Indeed, these cells produce inflammatory cytokines, play a key role in immunity and peripheral tolerance, and express TLRS, which appear to have an important role in triggering disease onset in experimental models of arthritis, multiple sclerosis, and diabetes (for review see *[312]*).

Nonobese Diabetic Mouse Model

Studies of autoimmune diabetes are facilitated by mouse models such as nonobese diabetic (NOD) mice, which develop diabetes spontaneously. This disease is biphasic: in the first stage, named *insulitis*, the islets are invaded by DCs, macrophages, and B and T cells, but this is followed by a benign interlude. Progression to diabetes occurs only at a second stage, when the islet infiltrate converts to a destructive process, resulting in destruction of β cells, and eventually loss of insulin and glucose homeostasis. There is evidence that $CD4^+$ or $CD8^+$ T cells, specific for β cell epitopes in the context of self-MHC, are first sensitized in pancreatic lymph nodes at 15 days of age. Turley et al. have tested whether changes in APCs may underlie the initiation of antigen exposure. Interestingly, they found that the stimulus initiating insulitis was a ripple of β cell death that occurs physiologically and that the APC that ferries β cell debris from the pancreas to the draining lymph nodes is a DC of $CD11b^+CD8\alpha^-$ phenotype (313).

The reason why this sequence of events leads to immunity and not tolerance (as apoptotic cells are considered as tolerogenic) is still unknown, but could involve the loss of the balance between effector and regulatory T cells. Of note, a recent report (314) visualized islet-specific regulatory T cells and helper T cells *in vivo* in the lymph nodes of NOD mice. It was found that regulatory T cells can dampen the stability of T helper–DC interactions, possibly preventing T helper cells from receiving optimal activation signals from DCs.

Recent studies have shown that DCs are active APCs for expanding natural Treg, as well as differentiating or inducing Treg from Foxp3 and CD25 negative, $CD4^+$ precursors. These treg exhibit efficacy in treating recent onset diabetes in NOD mice *(315)*.

Human Diseases

There is some evidence that DCs may also play a role in the induction of autoimmune diseases in humans. Jego et al. (316) underscored the role of two DC subsets in patients suffering from systemic lupus erythematosus. They found that the sustained overproduction of IFN-α produced by plasmacytoid DCs, contributes to peripheral tolerance breakdown through the activation of immature conventional DCs, leading to expansion of autoreactive B cells and sensitization of cytotoxic $CD8^+$ T cells. Plasmacytoid DCs were also found to massively infiltrate the skin of psoriatic patients and become activated to produce IFN-I during disease formation. Howard et al. have shown that two retinal antigens, S-antigen and interphotoreceptor retinoid-binding protein, which are associated with uveitis, can attract immature DCs and lymphocytes, suggesting that DCs may be involved in the early steps of autoimmune uveitis *(317)*. Similarly, the autoantigen PR3, which is involved in the pathogenesis of autoimmune-mediated vasculitis in Wegener granulomatosis, is increased in the extracellular space and induces phenotypic and functional maturation of a fraction of blood monocyte–derived iDCs, leading to increased expression of interferon-γ (IFN-γ), which favors the development of a granulomatous inflammation. Of note, PR3-maturated DCs derived from WG patients induce a higher IFN-γ response of PR3-specific $CD4^+$ T cells compared with healthy controls *(318)*.

CONCLUSION

DCs perform several tasks with high efficiency. They present the antigenic sample at the time of danger through evolutionary conserved pattern-recognition systems and sensitize lymphocytes specific for these dangerous antigens. They also seem to play an active role in central and peripheral tolerance by silencing autoreactive T cells generated by the stochastic recombination of the T cell variable pattern-recognition receptors. There is indeed evidence that DCs constitutively present self-antigens and that tolerogenic DCs that directly or indirectly prevent the activation of T cells specific to self may exist. Regulatory DCs may also control and dampen immune responses to foreign antigens to avoid excessive inflammatory responses that are deleterious to the organism. This dual role—ensuring tissue integrity through activation of adaptive reactions and maintenance of privileged microenvironment—seems to be a general feature of innate cells, as illustrated for mast cells (269), and macrophages.

The immune system is confronted with the difficult task of combining the detection of potential pathogens in the periphery with the ability of adequately instructing cells of the adaptative immune system often located in lymphoid organs distant from the infection site. In general, when distant cells of a multicellular organism must communicate with one another, they secrete chemicals (hormones) that travel in the bloodstream to reach their target cells (endocrine communication). The immune system has developed a unique form of cell–cell communication, implying the migration of DCs carrying the biological information gathered at the site of infection (signals 1, 2, and 3) to the lymphoid organ, where they establish immunological synapses with lymphoid cells, exchanging information through locally secreted (paracrine communication) or membrane-bound molecules. This unique form of cell communication (which may be referred to as *motocrine communication*), combines long-distance communication between the periphery and the lymphoid organs, with the confidentiality and specificity of a short-range synapse.

ACKNOWLEDGMENTS

I am grateful to Ralph Steinman for careful review and excellent suggestions; Oberdan Leo for interesting discussions; and Guillaume Oldenhove and Roberto Maldonado-López for drawing the figures.

REFERENCES

2. Steinman RM, Cohn ZA. Identification of a novel cell type in peripheral lymphoid organs of mice. I. Morphology, quantitation, tissue distribution. *J Exp Med* 1973;137:1142–1162.
3. Steinman RM, Witmer MD. Lymphoid dendritic cells are potent stimulators of the primary mixed leukocyte reaction in mice. *Proc Natl Acad Sci U S A* 1978;75:5132–5136.
9. Dudziak D, Kamphorst AO, Heidkamp GF, et al. Differential antigen processing by dendritic cell subsets in vivo. *Science* 2007;315:107–111.
12. Fogg DK, Sibon C, Miled C, et al. A clonogenic bone marrow progenitor specific for macrophages and dendritic cells. *Science* 2006;311:83–87.
16. Naik SH, Metcalf D, van Nieuwenhuijze A, et al. Intrasplenic steady-state dendritic cell precursors that are distinct from monocytes. *Nat Immunol* 2006;7:663–671.
23. Rowden G, Lewis MG, Sullivan AK. Ia antigen expression on human epidermal Langerhans cells. *Nature* 1977;268:247–248.
24. Schuler G, Steinman RM. Murine epidermal Langerhans cells mature into potent immunostimulatory dendritic cells in vitro. *J Exp Med* 1985;161:526–546.
25. Valladeau J, Ravel O, Dezutter-Dambuyant C, et al. Langerin, a novel C-type lectin specific to Langerhans cells, is an endocytic receptor that induces the formation of Birbeck granules. *Immunity* 2000;12:71–81.
26. Allan RS, Waithman J, Bedoui S, et al. Migratory dendritic cells transfer antigen to a lymph node-resident dendritic cell population for efficient CTL priming. *Immunity* 2006;25:153–162.
27. Ginhoux F, Tacke F, Angeli V, et al. Langerhans cells arise from monocytes in vivo. *Nat Immunol* 2006;7:265–273.
31. Kadowaki N, Antonenko S, Lau JY, et al. Natural interferon alpha/beta-producing cells link innate and adaptive immunity. *J Exp Med* 2000;192:219–226.
35. Romani N, Koide S, Crowley M, et al. Presentation of exogenous protein antigens by dendritic cells to T cell clones. Intact protein is presented best by immature, epidermal Langerhans cells. *J Exp Med* 1989;169:1169–1178.
36. Fujii S, Liu K, Smith C, et al. The linkage of innate to adaptive immunity via maturing dendritic cells in vivo requires CD40 ligation in addition to antigen presentation and CD80/86 costimulation. *J Exp Med* 2004;199:1607–1618.
43. De Smedt T, Pajak B, Muraille E, et al. Regulation of dendritic cell numbers and maturation by lipopolysaccharide in vivo. *J Exp Med* 1996;184:1413–1424.
44. Reis e Sousa C, Hieny S, Scharton-Kersten T, et al. In vivo microbial stimulation induces rapid CD40 ligand-independent production of interleukin 12 by dendritic cells and their redistribution to T cell areas. *J Exp Med* 1997;186:1819–1829.
61. Geijtenbeek TB, Kwon DS, Torensma R, et al. DC-SIGN, a dendritic cell-specific HIV-1-binding protein that enhances trans-infection of T cells. *Cell* 2000;100:587–597.
63. Yarovinsky F, Kanzler H, Hieny S, et al. Toll-like receptor recognition regulates immunodominance in an antimicrobial CD4+ T cell response. *Immunity* 2006;25:655–664.
67. Shin JS, Ebersold M, Pypaert M, et al. Surface expression of MHC class II in dendritic cells is controlled by regulated ubiquitination. *Nature* 2006;444:115–118.
73. Morel S, Levy F, Burlet-Schiltz O, et al. Processing of some antigens by the standard proteasome but not by the immunoproteasome results in poor presentation by dendritic cells. *Immunity* 2000;12:107–117.
74. Albert ML, Sauter B, Bhardwaj N. Dendritic cells acquire antigen from apoptotic cells and induce class I- restricted CTLs. *Nature* 1998;392:86–89.
77. Rodriguez A, Regnault A, Kleijmeer M, et al. Selective transport of internalized antigens to the cytosol for MHC class I presentation in dendritic cells. *Nat Cell Biol* 1999;1:362–368.
78. Savina A, Jancic C, Hugues S, et al. NOX2 controls phagosomal pH to regulate antigen processing during crosspresentation by dendritic cells. *Cell* 2006;126:205–218.
83. Dieu MC, Vanbervliet B, Vicari A, et al. Selective recruitment of immature and mature dendritic cells by distinct chemokines expressed in different anatomic sites. *J Exp Med* 1998;188:373–386.
86. Martin-Fontecha A, Sebastiani S, Hopken UE, et al. Regulation of dendritic cell migration to the draining lymph node: impact on T lymphocyte traffic and priming. *J Exp Med* 2003;198:615–621.
87. Larsen CP, Steinman RM, Witmer-Pack M, et al. Migration and maturation of Langerhans cells in skin transplants and explants. *J Exp Med* 1990;172:1483–1493.
89. Vermaelen KY, Carro-Muino I, Lambrecht BN, et al. Specific migratory dendritic cells rapidly transport antigen from the airways to the thoracic lymph nodes. *J Exp Med* 2001;193:51–60.
90. Huang FP, Platt N, Wykes M, et al. A discrete subpopulation of dendritic cells transports apoptotic intestinal epithelial cells to T cell areas of mesenteric lymph nodes. *J Exp Med* 2000;191:435–444.
94. Macatonia SE, Hosken NA, Litton M, et al. Dendritic cells produce IL-12 and direct the development of Th1 cells from naive CD4+ T cells. *J Immunol* 1995;154:5071–5079.
97. Reis e Sousa C, Yap G, Schulz O, et al. Paralysis of dendritic cell IL-12 production by microbial products prevents infection-induced immunopathology. *Immunity* 1999;11:637–647.
103. Rissoan MC, Soumelis V, Kadowaki N, et al. Reciprocal control of T helper cell and dendritic cell differentiation. *Science* 283: 1183–1186.
110. Kullberg MC, Jankovic D, Feng CG, et al. IL-23 plays a key role in Helicobacter hepaticus-induced T cell-dependent colitis. *J Exp Med* 2006;203:2485–2494.
111. Hue S, Ahern P, Buonocore S, et al. Interleukin-23 drives innate and T cell-mediated intestinal inflammation. *J Exp Med* 2006;203:2473–2483.
115. Granucci F, Vizzardelli C, Pavelka N, et al. Inducible IL-2 production by dendritic cells revealed by global gene expression analysis. *Nat Immunol* 2001;2:882–888.
121. Rudd CE, Schneider H. Unifying concepts in CD28:ICOS and CTLA4 co-receptor signalling. *Nat Rev Immunol* 2003;3:544–556.
122. Okkenhaug K, Wu L, Garza KM, et al. A point mutation in CD28 distinguishes proliferative signals from survival signals. *Nat Immunol* 2001;2:325–332.
126. Riley JL, Mao M, Kobayashi S, et al. Modulation of TCR-induced transcriptional profiles by ligation of CD28, ICOS, and CTLA-4 receptors. *Proc Natl Acad Sci U S A* 2002;99:11790–11795.
127. Viola A, Schroeder S, Sakakibara Y, et al. T lymphocyte costimulation mediated by reorganization of membrane microdomains. *Science* 1999;283:680–682.
132. Chikuma S, Imboden JB, Bluestone JA. Negative regulation of T cell receptor-lipid raft interaction by cytotoxic T lymphocyte-associated antigen 4. *J Exp Med* 2003;197:129–135.

133. Parry RV, Chemnitz JM, Frauwirth KA, et al. CTLA-4 and PD-1 receptors inhibit T-cell activation by distinct mechanisms. *Mol Cell Biol* 2005;25:9543–9553.
137. Grohmann U, Orabona C, Fallarino F, et al. CTLA-4-Ig regulates tryptophan catabolism in vivo. *Nat Immunol* 2002;3:1097–1101.
142. Keir ME, Liang SC, Guleria I, et al. Tissue expression of PD-L1 mediates peripheral T cell tolerance. *J Exp Med 2006;* 203: 883–895.
149. Herman AE, Freeman GJ, Mathis D, et al. CD4+CD25+ T Regulatory Cells Dependent on ICOS Promote Regulation of Effector Cells in the Prediabetic Lesion. *J Exp Med* 2004;199:1479–1489.
154. Matter M, Odermatt B, Yagita H, et al. Elimination of chronic viral infection by blocking CD27 signaling. *J Exp Med* 2006;203:2145–2155.
155. Ito T, Wang YH, Duramad O, et al. OX40 ligand shuts down IL-10–producing regulatory T cells. *Proc Natl Acad Sci U S A* 2006;103: 13138–13143.
156. Ito T, Wang YH, Duramad O, et al. TSLP-activated dendritic cells induce an inflammatory T helper type 2 cell response through OX40 ligand. *J Exp Med* 2005;202:1213–1223.
164. Ridge JP, Di Rosa F, Matzinger P. A conditioned dendritic cell can be a temporal bridge between a CD4+ T- helper and a T-killer cell. *Nature* 1998;393:474–478.
169. Sornasse T, Flamand V, De Becker G, et al. Antigen-pulsed dendritic cells can efficiently induce an antibody response in vivo. *J Exp Med* 1992;175:15–21.
171. Thery C, Regnault A, Garin J, et al. Molecular characterization of dendritic cell-derived exosomes. Selective accumulation of the heat shock protein hsc73. *J Cell Biol* 1999;147:599–610.
175. Larsen CP, Morris PJ, Austyn JM. Migration of dendritic leukocytes from cardiac allografts into host spleens. A novel pathway for initiation of rejection. *J Exp Med* 1990;171:307–314.
176. Lambrecht BN, Salomon B, Klatzmann D, et al. Dendritic cells are required for the development of chronic eosinophilic airway inflammation in response to inhaled antigen in sensitized mice. *J Immunol* 1998;160:4090–4097.
178. Valitutti S, Muller S, Cella M, et al. Serial triggering of many T-cell receptors by a few peptide-MHC complexes. *Nature* 1995;375:148–151.
184. Stoll S, Delon J, Brotz TM, et al. Dynamic imaging of T cell-dendritic cell interactions in lymph nodes. *Science* 2002;296:1873–1876.
186. Shakhar G, Lindquist RL, Skokos D, et al. Stable T cell dendritic cell interactions precede the development of both tolerance and immunity in vivo. *Nat Immunol* 2005;6:707–714.
190. Hugues S, Fetler L, Bonifaz L, et al. Distinct T cell dynamics in lymph nodes during the induction of tolerance and immunity. *Nat Immunol* 2004;5:1235–1242. Epub 2004 Oct 31.
193. Gavin AL, Hoebe K, Duong B, et al. Adjuvant-enhanced antibody responses in the absence of toll-like receptor signaling. *Science* 2006;314:1936–1938.
198. Constant SL, Bottomly K. Induction of Th1 and Th2 CD4+ T cell responses: the alternative approaches. *Annu Rev Immunol* 11997;5:297–322.
204. Maldonado Lopez R, De Smedt T, Michel P, et al. CD8alpha+ and CD8alpha– subclasses of dendritic cells direct the development of distinct T helper cells in vivo. *J Exp Med* 1999;189: 587–592.
208. Kalinski P, Moser M. Consensual immunity: success-driven development of T-helper-1 and T-helper-2 responses. *Nat Rev Immunol* 2005;5:251–260.
217. Bettelli E, Carrier Y, Gao W, et al. Reciprocal developmental pathways for the generation of pathogenic effector TH17 and regulatory T cells. *Nature.* 2006;441:235–238. Epub 2006 Apr 30.
219. Ivanov II, McKenzie BS, Zhou L, et al. The orphan nuclear receptor RORgammat directs the differentiation program of proinflammatory IL-17+ T helper cells. *Cell* 2006;126:1121–1133.
221. Pulendran B, Smith JL, Caspary G, et al. Distinct dendritic cell subsets differentially regulate the class of immune response in vivo. *Proc Natl Acad Sci U S A* 1999;96:1036–1041.
222. Vaknin-Dembinsky A, Balashov K, Weiner HL. IL-23 is increased in dendritic cells in multiple sclerosis and down-regulation of IL-23 by antisense oligos increases dendritic cell IL-10 production. *J Immunol* 2006;176:7768–7774.
224. Becker C, Dornhoff H, Neufert C, et al. Cutting edge: IL-23 cross-regulates IL-12 production in T cell-dependent experimental colitis. *J Immunol* 2006;177:2760–2764.
229. Huang Q, Liu do N, Majewski P, et al. The plasticity of dendritic cell responses to pathogens and their components. *Science* 2001;294:870–5.
230. Spörri R, Reise Sousa C. Inflammatory mediators are insufficient for full dendritic cell activation and promote expansion of CD4+ T cell populations lacking helper function. *Nat Immunol.* 2005;6(2):125–126.
231. Napolitani G, Rinaldi A, Bertoni F, et al. Selected Toll-like receptor agonist combinations synergistically trigger a T helper type 1-polarizing program in dendritic cells. *Nat Immunol* 2005;6: 769–776.
234. Brocker T, Riedinger M, Karjalainen K. Targeted expression of major histocompatibility complex (MHC) class II molecules demonstrates that dendritic cells can induce negative but not positive selection of thymocytes in vivo. *J Exp Med* 1997;185:541–550.
236. Anderson MS, Venanzi ES, Klein L, et al. Projection of an immunological self shadow within the thymus by the aire protein. *Science* 2002;298:1395–1401.
243. Hawiger D, Inaba K, Dorsett Y, et al. Dendritic cells induce peripheral T cell unresponsiveness under steady state conditions in vivo. *J Exp Med* 2001;194:769–779.
244. Kurts C, Kosaka H, Carbone FR, et al. Class I-restricted cross-presentation of exogenous self-antigens leads to deletion of autoreactive CD8(+) T cells. *J Exp Med* 1997;186:239–245.
247. Probst HC, Lagnel J, Kollias G, et al. Inducible transgenic mice reveal resting dendritic cells as potent inducers of CD8(+) T cell tolerance. *Immunity* 2003;18:713–20.
248. Probst HC, McCoy K, Okazaki T, et al. Resting dendritic cells induce peripheral CD8+ T cell tolerance through PD-1 and CTLA-4. *Nat Immunol* 2005;6:280–286.
253. de Heer HJ, Hammad H, Soullie T, et al. Essential role of lung plasmacytoid dendritic cells in preventing asthmatic reactions to harmless inhaled antigen. *J Exp Med* 2004;200:89–98.
254. Ochando JC, Homma C, Yang Y, et al. Alloantigen-presenting plasmacytoid dendritic cells mediate tolerance to vascularized grafts. *Nat Immunol* 2006;7:652 662.
256. Kaplan DH, Jenison MC, Saeland S, et al. Epidermal langerhans cell-deficient mice develop enhanced contact hypersensitivity. *Immunity* 2005;23:611 620.
257. Annacker O, Coombes JL, Malmstrom V, et al. Essential role for CD103 in the T cell-mediated regulation of experimental colitis. *J Exp Med* 2005;202:1051–1061.
260. Wakkach A, Fournier N, Brun V, et al. Characterization of dendritic cells that induce tolerance and T regulatory 1 cell differentiation in vivo. *Immunity* 2003;18:605–617.
261. Svensson M, Maroof A, Ato M, et al. Stromal cells direct local differentiation of regulatory dendritic cells. *Immunity* 2004;21: 805–816.
264. Akbari O, DeKruyff RH, Umetsu DT. Pulmonary dendritic cells producing IL-10 mediate tolerance induced by respiratory exposure to antigen. *Nat Immunol* 2001;2:725–731.
266. Kretschmer K, Apostolou I, Hawiger D, et al. Inducing and expanding regulatory T cell populations by foreign antigen. *Nat Immunol* 2005;6:1219–1227.
269. Lu LF, Lind EF, Gondek DC, et al. Mast cells are essential intermediaries in regulatory T-cell tolerance. *Nature* 2006;442:997–1002.
273. Inaba K, Steinman RM, Van Voorhis WC, et al. Dendritic cells are critical accessory cells for thymus-dependent antibody responses in mouse and in man. *Proc Natl Acad Sci U S A* 1983;80:6041–6045.
274. Inaba K, Witmer MD, Steinman RM. Clustering of dendritic cells, helper T lymphocytes, and histocompatible B cells during primary antibody responses in vitro. *J Exp Med* 1984;160:858–876.
277. Grouard G, Durand I, Filgueira L, et al. Dendritic cells capable of stimulating T cells in germinal centres. *Nature* 1996;384:364–367.
284. Kitamura H, Iwakabe K, Yahata T, et al. The natural killer T (NKT) cell ligand alpha-galactosylceramide demonstrates its immunopotentiating effect by inducing interleukin (IL)-12 production by dendritic cells and IL-12 receptor expression on NKT cells. *J Exp Med* 1999;189:1121–1128.

286. van Gisbergen KP, Sanchez-Hernandez M, Geijtenbeek TB, et al. Neutrophils mediate immune modulation of dendritic cells through glycosylation-dependent interactions between Mac-1 and DC-SIGN. *J Exp Med* 2005;201:1281–1292.
287. Boon T, Kellermann O. Rejection by syngeneic mice of cell variants obtained by mutagenesis of a malignant teratocarcinoma cell line. *Proc Natl Acad Sci U S A* 1977;74:272–275.
295. Sallusto F, Lanzavecchia A. Efficient presentation of soluble antigen by cultured human dendritic cells is maintained by granulocyte/macrophage colony-stimulating factor plus interleukin 4 and downregulated by tumor necrosis factor alpha. *J Exp Med* 1994;179:1109–1118.
305. Germeau C, Ma W, Schiavetti F, et al. High frequency of antitumor T cells in the blood of melanoma patients before and after vaccination with tumor antigens. *J Exp Med* 2005;201:241–248.
306. Lurquin C, Lethe B, De Plaen E, et al. Contrasting frequencies of antitumor and anti-vaccine T cells in metastases of a melanoma patient vaccinated with a MAGE tumor antigen. *J Exp Med* 2005;201:249–257.
310. Taieb J, Chaput N, Menard C, et al. A novel dendritic cell subset involved in tumor immunosurveillance. *Nat Med* 2006;12:214–219.
311. Chan CW, Crafton E, Fan HN, et al. Interferon-producing killer dendritic cells provide a link between innate and adaptive immunity. *Nat Med* 2006;12:207–213.
313. Turley S, Poirot L, Hattori M, et al. Physiological beta cell death triggers priming of self-reactive T cells by dendritic cells in a type-1 diabetes model. *J Exp Med* 2003;198:1527–1537.
314. Tang Q, Adams JY, Tooley AJ, et al. Visualizing regulatory T cell control of autoimmune responses in nonobese diabetic mice. *Nat Immunol* 2006;7:83–92.
316. Jego G, Palucka AK, Blanck JP, et al. Plasmacytoid dendritic cells induce plasma cell differentiation through type I interferon and interleukin 6. *Immunity* 2003;19:225–234.
317. Maynard CL, Harrington LE, Jamowski KM, et al. Regulatory T cells expressing interleukin 10 develop from Foxp3+ and Foxp3 – precursor cells in the absence of interleukin 10. *Nat Immunol.* 2007;8(9):931–941.

Chapter 16

Natural Killer Cells

Wayne M. Yokoyama

GENERAL DESCRIPTION

Natural killer (NK) cells were initially described as such because they spontaneously kill certain tumor targets (1,2,*3*,*4*). Morphologically, NK cells are typically large lymphocytes containing azurophilic granules (5). However, the large granular lymphocyte (LGL) morphology is not invariably associated with NK cells because small, agranular lymphocytes may display natural killing (6) and activated cytotoxic T lymphocytes (CTLs) can display this morphology *(7)*. Indeed, human LGL leukemias are now recognized to contain NK and T cell variants (8).

Recent studies have provided strong evidence that NK cells belong to the lymphocyte lineage (discussed in detail later). Although NK cells express B220 (CD45R) that is often used as a B cell–specific marker indicating that CD19 rather than B220 is more reliable to distinguish B cells from NK cells *(9)*, NK cells more closely resemble T cells than B cells. Indeed, before the molecular description of the T cell receptor/CD3 (TCR/CD3) complex, NK cells were frequently confused with T cells. Thus, it is useful to compare and contrast these two lymphocyte populations as well as consider another enigmatic cell termed "lymphokine activated killer" (LAK) cell.

NK Cells versus T Cells

NK cells are most often confused with T cells because they may have similar morphologies, express several cell surface molecules in common *(10,11)*, and share functional capabilities, including responses to target cells, such as cytotoxicity and cytokine production (described in greater detail later). However, mature NK cells are clearly not T cells by several criteria (12). NK cells do not require a thymus for development and are normal in athymic nude mice. NK cells do not express the TCR on the cell surface, do not produce mature transcripts for TCR chains, and do not rearrange TCR genes (13,*14*). Mice with the *scid* mutation or deficiencies in *Rag1* or *Rag2* lack TCR gene rearrangements and mature T cells but possess NK cells with apparently normal function (15,16,*17,18*). Several CD3 components may be found in the cytoplasm of NK cells, particularly immature NK cells, but they are not displayed on the cell surface *(19)*, with the exception of CD3ζ. But CD3ζ is expressed in association with FcγRIII (CD16) and other NK cell activation receptors instead of the TCR/CD3 complex (20,*21*). Whereas mice lacking CD3ζ lack most T cells, NK cell number and function are minimally affected *(22)*. However, NK cells are completely absent in mice with only partial defects in T cell subsets, such as in mice lacking components of the IL-15R (discussed later). Finally, in an important functional distinction from CD8$^+$ major histocompatibility complex (MHC) I–restricted T cells, NK cells do not require the presence of MHC class I molecules on their targets for lysis. Instead, NK cells kill more efficiently when their targets lack MHC-I expression. Thus, NK cells can be clearly distinguished from T cells.

NK Cells and LAK Cells

Another area of overlap between NK and T cells concerns responses to high concentrations of IL-2 (800 U/mL to 1,000 U/mL) that induce robust lymphocyte proliferation *in vitro* (i.e., generation of LAK cells) (23–25,*26*). Although most are CD3$^-$ NK cells, TCR/CD3$^+$ T cells are also found. To distinguish NK cells within this population, they are sometimes called "CD3$^-$ LAK" cells or "IL-2-activated NK cells." In a related phenomenon, NK cells are activated when mice are injected with polyinosinic-polycytidylic acid (poly I:C) or other agents that trigger through Toll-like receptors (TLRs), often on plasmacytoid dendritic cells (pDCs) *(27)*. NK cells can also be activated *in vitro* with IFNα/β, IFNγ or low concentrations of IL-2 that are insufficient to induce proliferation *(3,4,28)*. NK cells activated in these various ways display enhanced killing of typical NK-sensitive targets.

Activated NK cells also kill a broader panel of targets, including those that are generally resistant to freshly isolated NK cells, such as the murine P815 mastocytoma cells, and freshly explanted tumors. Many agents that enhance killing by NK cells may also activate T cells, such that even T cell clones may display promiscuous killing of targets that is no longer MHC-restricted (29). This phenomenon was a source of confusion between NK cells and T cells during the initial characterization of both cell types.

Why IL-2-activated NK or T cells display enhanced killing is not completely understood. Cytokines enhance expression of perforin and granzymes that presumably contribute to more lytic capacity *(30)*. The activated cells express additional receptors that may deliver stimulatory signals (31,*32*), but their contribution to the LAK phenomenon is as yet unclear. Recent studies implicate a receptor termed *NKG2D* (discussed later), although how much this applies to conventional NK cells is not understood (33). Enhanced killing may also be due to adhesion molecules on targets and their appropriate counterreceptors on the effector cells *(34,35)*.

It seems unlikely that high concentrations of IL-2 can be achieved, even locally, to stimulate NK cells *in vivo*. Further, NK cells tend to be early responders in immune responses, whereas the prime reservoir of IL-2 is the activated T cell that produces it somewhat later. Although recent studies suggest that dendritic cells (DCs) can produce IL-2 to enhance NK lytic activity *(36)*, whether such IL-2 concentrations is sufficient to generate LAK cells is unclear. Interestingly, NK cells are apparently normal in mice with a targeted mutation in the IL-2 gene or the IL-2Rα chain *(37,38)*, indicating that IL-2 itself is not required for normal NK cell development.

Paradoxically, NK cells are deficient in mice with a mutation in either IL-2Rβ or IL-2Rγ (39,40,*41*). In brief, the high-affinity IL-2 receptor (IL-2R) is a heterotrimeric receptor complex comprised of α (p55), β (p75), and γ (p64) chains *(42)*. Although individual components may bind IL-2 with low affinity, only the intermediate-affinity $\beta\gamma$ receptor ($K_d \sim$1nM) and the high-affinity $\alpha\beta\gamma$ receptor ($K_d \sim$10 pM) are capable of signaling. Resting NK cells constitutively express IL-2R$\beta\gamma$ *(42,43)* and, upon activation, may induce α and further up-regulate γ chain expression *(42)*. In contrast, resting T cells generally do not express any functional IL-2 receptors, and most naïve T cells do not respond to high concentrations of IL-2 *(44)*.

The discrepancy in NK cell dependence on IL-2 versus IL-2R may be best understood when considering that the IL-2Rγ chain is also termed the *common γ subunit* (γc) because it is a required component of the multimeric receptor complexes for other cytokines, including IL-4, IL-7, IL-9, IL-15, and IL-21 *(45)*, with IL-15 having special relevance to NK cells. IL-15 does not bind to IL-2Rα but instead utilizes a unique IL-15Rα chain to form a high-affinity complex with IL-2R$\beta\gamma$ *(46,47)*. The IL-15Rα chain does not directly signal. Its distribution is widespread on numerous cell and tissue lineages, including NK cells. IL-15 is required for NK cell development and also has antiapoptotic effects on NK cells (48–50). Interestingly, IL-15 is expressed at very low levels and is difficult to detect *in vivo (51)*. The IL-15Rα chain can present IL-15 in *trans* to NK cells that can respond through IL-2/15R$\beta\gamma$ *(52)*. For example, IL-15Rα–deficient NK cells develop in bone marrow (BM) chimeric mice in which IL-15Rα–deficient BM was used to reconstitute IL-15Rα–sufficient animals *(53)*. It remains to be established whether *trans* presentation of IL-15 is physiologically important to NK cell function. When NK cells are transferred to NK cell–deficient mice, there is "homeostatic" proliferation *(54,55)*, akin to T cell homeostatic proliferation *(56)*. Like memory CD8$^+$ T cell homeostasis, NK cell homeostasis is IL-15-dependent *(54,55)*, to a more or less degree *(57)*, consistent with the role of IL-15 as a proliferative and anti-apoptotic factor (50). Finally, LAK cells can be generated with IL-15 (58). These studies strongly suggest that LAK cells are generated because high-dose IL-2 acts through the IL-2R$\beta\gamma$ that is expressed with IL-15Rα as components of the constitutively expressed IL-15 receptor complex on resting NK cells. Thus, the LAK cell phenomenon has helped illustrate the importance of IL-15 and its receptor in NK cell biology.

SELECTIVE NK CELL SURFACE MARKERS

The constitutive expression on NK cells of IL-15R complex with IL-2Rβ has practical usefulness because anti–IL-2Rβ (CD122) is sometimes used to identify naïve CD3$^-$ NK cells or deplete them in mice *(59)*. (Anti–IL-15Rα antibodies are not widely available at this time.) Other markers have also proven to be useful for analysis of NK cells.

The NK1.1 molecule is especially important as a marker on mouse NK cells in C57BL strains (12). NK1.1 is encoded by *Nkrp1c* (60), a member of the *Nkrp1* gene family (discussed later). In FACS sorting experiments, the NK1.1$^+$ fraction contained all of the natural killing activity in the spleen (61). *In vivo* administration of the anti–NK1.1 mAb PK136 *(62)* abrogated natural killing but did not affect adaptive immune responses (63). (mAb PK136 is available from the American Type Culture Collection [ATCC], Manassas, VA [HB-191] and is an IgG2a isotype [ATCC, and data not shown], not IgG2b as originally described *[62]*.) Unfortunately, mAb PK136 recognizes an epitope on NK1.1 that is confined to C57BL/6, C57BL/10, and a few other strains *(62)*. Moreover, in Swiss.NIH and SJL/J mice, mAb PK136 recognizes another NKRP1 family member, NKRP1B *(64,65)*. However there are now available NK1.1$^+$ congenic strains, such as BALB.B6-*Cmv1^r* (catalogued as C.B6-*Klra8^{Cmv1-r}*/UwaJ, stock number 002936 at The Jackson Laboratory, Bar Harbor, ME) in which the C57BL/6 allele of NK1.1 has been genetically bred onto the BALB/c background which otherwise lacks the NK1.1 epitope.

A subpopulation of T cells expresses NK1.1 *(66)*. These so-called *NKT cells* express the TCR/CD3 complex and typically are restricted by the nonclassical MHC-I molecule, CD1, which presents glycolipid antigens to NKT cells. NKT cells respond early during the course of an immune response and may potently activate conventional NK cells (67). NKT cells are described in detail in Chapter 17; they can be distinguished from conventional NK cells by expression of TCR/CD3 complex (i.e., conventional NK cells are NK1.1$^+$ CD3$^-$).

The mAb DX5 recognizes a molecule that is coexpressed on most NK1.1$^+$ CD3$^-$ cells and on small populations of splenocytes in NK1.1$^-$ strains, consistent with identification of NK cells in all strains. However, mAb DX5 recognizes the α2 integrin that is widely expressed on other leukocytes, not just NK cells (68,69), and its expression is regulated (70). Nevertheless, the DX5 mAb is helpful in identifying NK cells, especially in mouse strains that do not express the NK1.1 epitope, especially when coupled with other nonpolymorphic markers, such as NKG2D or CD122.

The glycolipid determinant asialo-GM$_1$ is expressed by most if not all murine NK cells and a subpopulation of T cells *(71–73)*. Although the functional significance of this molecule is unknown, polyclonal rabbit anti–asialo-GM$_1$ (Wako Chemicals USA, Richmond, VA) has been used to effectively deplete NK cells. In more recent studies, the anti–NK1.1 mAb PK136 has become the reagent of choice for NK cell depletion because of an available defined mAb and its more restricted reactivity with NK cells (12,61,*62*,63). However, anti–asialo-GM$_1$ remains useful when mAb PK136 cannot be used due to absence of the NK1.1 allele *(62)*.

Human NK cells selectively express CD56. Although it is also found on neural tissues and some tumors, CD56 is generally not expressed by other hematopoietic cells or lymphocytes (*74*,75,*76*). This 140 kDa molecule is derived from alternative splicing of the gene encoding neural cell adhesion molecule (NCAM) involved in nervous system development and cell–cell interactions *(77,78)*. CD56 may be involved in adhesion between NK cells and their targets *(79)*, but this function is controversial. Curiously, mouse CD56 is not expressed on hematopoietic cells *(80)*, suggesting that its functional role on NK cells is not conserved. Nevertheless, CD56 is particularly useful as a pan-NK cell marker in humans.

Recent data suggest that human NK cells can be functionally divided according to the level of CD56 expressed (75,*81*). Most human peripheral blood NK cells are CD56^{dim}, a phenotype associated with more cytotoxicity and less cytokine production than a smaller subset of NK cells that express CD56 at higher levels (CD56^{bright}). These cells also tend to differentially express receptors involved in target recognition as well as CD16. The CD56^{bright} cells may undergo a different maturation process than the CD56^{dim} subpopulation (82).

Additional specific markers on NK cells are more thoroughly discussed later under the general topic of NK cell receptors because they are molecularly defined and their ligands are known.

A MOLECULAR DEFINITION OF NK CELLS?

A precise molecular definition of NK cells has been elusive. There are no known molecules that are exclusively expressed on NK cells and are responsible for critical functions only displayed by NK cells. The NK cell is therefore still defined by function to the exclusion of other cells, a concept first articulated 20 years ago (12).

The defining functional feature of NK cells remains their intrinsic ability to perform natural killing—that is, they spontaneously lyse certain tumor cells in a perforin-dependent manner. Unlike other lymphocytes, NK cells do not express surface immunoglobulin (Ig) or the TCR/CD3 complex and generally do not require MHC-I expression on targets for lysis. Therefore, a current working definition is that an NK cell is a sIg^-, TCR/$CD3^-$ lymphocyte that can mediate perforin-dependent natural killing against targets that may lack MHC-I expression.

It is noteworthy that T cells were historically defined by an awkward functional definition (thymus-derived, sIg^- lymphocytes responsible for cell mediated immunity) *(83)*. With the molecular definition of the TCR and coexpressed CD3 molecules, immunologists can now define a T cell as a cell expressing the TCR/CD3 complex *(84)*. The availability of molecular probes and mAbs directed against this complex provides precise definition even in pathologic tissue sections, without the need for functional analysis (cell mediated immunity, thymus dependence). Similarly, a molecular definition should permit unequivocal identification of NK cells to define their role in normal immune responses and pathologic settings.

Presumably such a definition will require further knowledge of the molecular basis for NK cell function, such as the receptors involved in natural killing. On the other hand, one difficulty is that the function that is most attributed to NK cells, natural killing, can be displayed by other cells, such as cytokine-treated T cells. Moreover, NK cells can utilize more than one receptor for target recognition, and individual NK cells can simultaneously express several of these receptors. Thus, there is, as yet, no consensus on the elusive "NK cell receptor" analogous to the TCR.

Meanwhile, most investigators consider the following phenotypes to be surrogate markers of bona fide NK cells. Mouse NK cells are typically $NK1.1^+$ (in appropriate strains), $Fc\gamma RIII^+$ (CD16), $CD122^+$, and $CD3^-$. Human NK cells are generally $CD56^+$ and $CD3^-$. Note that these markers are generally correlated with cells having natural killing capacity, but the markers themselves are not required for target recognition. Nevertheless, these markers have helped shape our current concepts of NK cell biology and elaborate their effector functions.

EFFECTOR FUNCTIONS OF NK CELLS

Cytotoxicity

"Natural killing" does not require prior host exposure to the target cells and is mediated by granule exocytosis. Like CTLs, NK cells possess preformed cytoplasmic granules that resemble secretory lysosomes with properties of both secretory granules and lysosomes *(85)*. Granule formation is affected by Lyst, the molecule defective in beige (*bg*) mice and humans with Chediak-Higashi syndrome *(86,87)*. The granules contain perforin and granzymes (granule enzymes). Perforin, a pore-forming protein, is rendered inactive by association with calreticulin and serglycin, and is activated by a cysteine protease (reviewed in [88]). Granzymes are first produced as inactive pro-enzymes that are activated by N-terminal cleavage by dipeptidyl peptidase I (DPPI), also known as cathepsin C. However, granzymes are rendered inactive by the acidic pH of the granules. Upon activation by a sensitive target, NK and T cells are triggered to polarize the granules and reposition the microtubule organizing center (MTOC) and Golgi apparatus toward the target *(89,90)*. By a process requiring Rab27a, a GTPase in the Ras superfamily, the granule membrane ultimately fuses with the plasma membrane and externalizes, releasing granule contents. Ca^{++}-dependent polymerization of perforin results in "perforation" of the target cell plasma membrane, leading to apoptosis. This exocytic process can be initiated by specific activation receptors for target cell ligands and is blocked by inhibitory receptors (described in more detail later).

Human T and NK cells also express another pore-forming molecule, granulysin, that is related to a family of saposin-like proteins that includes NK-lysin, found in porcine T and NK cells *(91)*. Based on crystallographic studies, these molecules appear to be active against bacteria, fungi, and tumor cells by charge association with target membranes and subsequent disruption, leading to target cell lysis *(92)*. Granulysin, however, is not expressed in mouse cytotoxic lymphocytes.

Natural killing was first assessed with a simple *in vitro* assay for target membrane integrity that is still used today, the standard ^{51}Cr-release assay (93). The prototypical NK-sensitive tumor target for mouse NK cells is YAC-1 (TIB-160 from ATCC), a thymoma derived from Moloney virus–infected A strain mice, whereas the standard human target is K-562 (CCL-243 from ATCC), an erythroleukemic cell line derived from a human patient with chronic myelogenous leukemia in blast crisis *(94)*. Although a small amount of label is released spontaneously, much larger amounts are released into the supernatant when membrane integrity is disrupted during the killing process. In most experiments, the data are represented according to a standard formula that takes into account spontaneous and maximal release of ^{51}Cr from labeled targets. Varying numbers of effector cells are often used as indicated by effector-to-target (E:T) ratios. Maximal killing by enriched, activated NK cells usually occurs with E:T ratios of $<$10:1, whereas unfractionated, freshly isolated peripheral blood or splenocyte preparations usually require E:T ratios of $>$100:1. Even at high E:T ratios, not all targets are killed, with % specific cytotoxicity typically ranging from ~10% with fresh NK cells to ~80% with activated NK cells. Note that perforin-dependent leakage of ^{51}Cr is mostly complete at about one hour; 4-hour assays are standard. Longer periods may assess other apoptotic processes, such as Fas-induced apoptosis.

While ^{51}Cr-release is still the standard assay, there are also numerous nonradioactive tests for perforin-dependent killing, including release of intracellular enzymes or use of fluorochromes for target labeling *(95–97)*. The release of granule components, including granzymes, into the supernatant can be determined by conversion of an appropriate substrate, such as granzyme A–mediated cleavage of alpha-N-benzyloxy-carbonyl-L-lysinethiobenzyl ester (BLT) (also known as *BLT-esterase activity*) *(98)*. New assays have been developed that exploit the association of cytotoxic granules with lysosomal-associated membrane protein-1 (LAMP-1, CD107a) on the luminal side. During granule exocytosis, the granule fuses with the plasma membrane, resulting in externalization of the granule membrane and exposing CD107a on the surface as an indicator of NK cell activation (99,*100*,*101*). By contrast to other assays, the CD107a assay provides the opportunity for measuring individual NK cell responses, isolating triggered NK cells *(102)*, and possibly simultaneously assessing other NK cell functions.

Activated NK cells and CTLs also induce perforin-independent target cell killing by expressing Fas ligand (TNF superfamily 6, TNFSF6) that binds Fas (TNF receptor SF 6, TNFRSF6) on the target, triggering apoptosis *(103–108)*. Similarly, other tumor necrosis factor (TNF) superfamily members, such as TNF-related apoptosis-inducing ligand (TRAIL, TNFSF10), can be involved in related processes *(109)*. However, mice deficient in TNF family members or their receptors may manifest significant alterations in lymphoid organogenesis and splenic architecture, and NK cell number and function *(110–112)*, such that the relative contributions of these pathways to NK cell function are incompletely understood. On the other hand, NK cells from mice deficient in perforin, granzymes, or molecules involved in granule formation or exocytosis (Lyst, Rab27a) demonstrate profound defects in natural killing *in vitro* (113,*114*,115). Similar defects have been found with NK cells derived from patients lacking these components *(116)*. Thus, the available data strongly suggest that granule exocytosis is the predominant mechanism for natural killing.

Cytokine Production

When exposed to NK-sensitive targets or cross-linking of receptors, NK cells also produce cytokines, including interferon-γ (IFNγ), TNF-α, and granulocyte-macrophage colony stimulating factor (GM-CSF) (*117*,118,119). They can also be similarly triggered to produce chemokines, such as RANTES, lymphotactin, MIP-1α and MIP-1β (120). NK cells also produce a similar repertoire of cytokines in response to other cytokines. For example, in response to IL-12, NK cells produce IFNγ (121). Similarly, NK cells respond to type I IFNs (IFN$\alpha\beta$), which are generated by *in vivo* administration of poly-I:C and other TLR ligands. Cytokine-stimulated responses tend to be independent of expression of target recognition receptors such that they may obscure detection of specific activation *in vivo* (120).

In immune responses, NK cell production of cytokines should occur relatively early and may thereby influence the subsequent adaptive immune response. Moreover, their responses to cytokines are regulated by complex interacting pathways *(122)*. A more in-depth description of NK cell cytokine responses and production is discussed in the upcoming sections on NK cell responses during infections and interactions with DCs.

NK CELL RECOGNITION OF TARGETS

Intense interest in the past two decades devoted to delineation of the receptors responsible for target recognition and activation yielded several surprises. In contrast to CTL recognition: 1) The NK cell receptors are germline-encoded, and the receptors are not strictly "clonotypic" as defined in terms of clonotypic TCRs (unique receptor only expressed by the rare effector clone and its progeny.) 2) Individual NK cells express both inhibitory and activation receptors for target recognition and often simultaneously express several different receptors of each type. 3) The receptors are often promiscuous and frequently have overlapping specificities. 4) NK cell receptors specifically bind MHC-I molecules, but they are functionally and structurally distinct from other receptors that bind MHC-I (i.e., TCR and CD8). In the following sections, we will discuss NK cell receptors involved in target recognition by first considering the relationship between target susceptibility to natural killing and expression of MHC-I.

Target Cell MHC-I and NK Cells: The "Missing-Self" Hypothesis

Whereas initial studies suggested that natural killing was "MHC-unrestricted" (12), substantial progress in understanding NK cell recognition began with ascertaining the role of MHC-I molecules in natural killing (Figure 16.1).

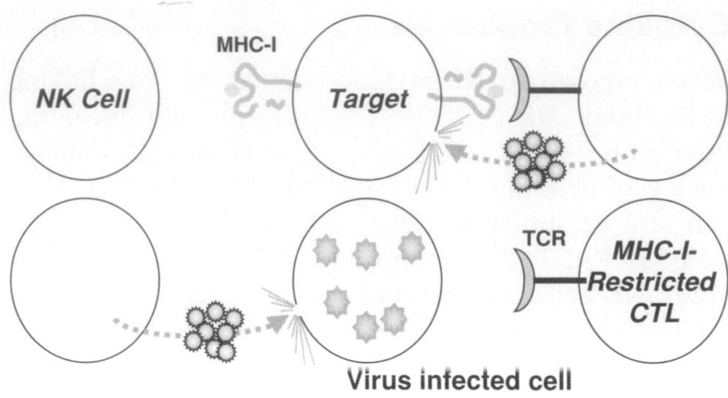

FIGURE 16.1 MHC-I expression on targets is inversely related to natural killing. Targets expressing MHC-I are more resistant to lysis by NK cells than targets lacking MHC-I expression, such as following viral infection. This is the exact opposite of the requirements for MHC-I–restricted CTLs that recognize foreign peptides presented by MHC-I. As depicted, viruses may evade T cells by down-regulating MHC-I, but infected cells should then become more susceptible to NK cells.

Kärre and colleagues discovered that MHC-I–deficient tumors remained susceptible to *in vivo* rejection, apparently by NK cells (123). Conversely, target cell expression of MHC-I molecules appeared to have a protective effect against NK cell–mediated lysis *in vitro*. A number of methods, such as IFNγ treatment, to upregulate MHC-I correlated with target protection, but other effects could not be excluded *(124)*. There was significant variability in capacity of specific MHC-I molecules to protect targets (125,126), *in vitro* culture conditions could influence NK cell specificities (127), and the specificities of individual human NK cell clones were not easily assignable to specific MHC-I alleles (128). Thus, the MHC-I effect on natural killing was controversial for some time.

Several groups, however, observed that MHC-I–expressing parental targets were resistant to natural killing, whereas mutants selected for absence of MHC-I expression became susceptible (Figure 16.1). The parental (resistant) phenotype could be restored by reconstitution of MHC-I expression by transfected expression of molecules to correct the defect, such as β_2-microglobulin (β2m) (129) or transporter associated with processing (TAP) *(130,131)*. Studies utilizing mice with a targeted mutation in the β2m gene added substantial support to the MHC-I protective effect, because normal expression of MHC-I heavy chains requires β2m (132,*133*). β2m-deficient lymphoblasts were susceptible to lysis by normal NK cells. Moreover, $\beta 2m^{-/-}$ BM transplanted into otherwise syngeneic normal hosts was rejected by recipient NK cells (*133*,134). These results resembled hybrid resistance, whereby NK cells in irradiated F_1 hybrid mice reject parental BM transplants (135). Hybrid resistance is regulated by parental determinants that are genetically linked to the MHC-I region, H-2D *(136)*. Thus, in several distinct NK cell recognition systems, the target cell expression of certain MHC-I molecules correlated with resistance to natural killing, whereas absence of MHC-I was associated with susceptibility to NK cells.

NK cells, therefore, have a different relationship to target cell MHC-I molecules than MHC-I–restricted CTLs (Figure 16.1). Strictly speaking, NK cell lysis is "MHC-unrestricted" (12), at least as far as MHC restriction is precisely defined for T cells having a requirement for specific self-MHC molecules presenting a given peptide antigen *(137)*. However, the term *MHC-unrestricted* (and its synonyms) is now somewhat outdated because it implies, when defined in a broader sense, that MHC plays no role in NK cell cytotoxicity. Avoidance of these terms will minimize confusion concerning the relationship of target cell MHC-I molecules with NK cell specificity.

As initially observed and discussed by Kärre in the "missing-self" hypothesis, the relationship between target expression of MHC-I and resistance to natural killing highlights a fundamental distinction between NK and T cells (138) (Figure 16.1). Whereas T cells are triggered by detection of "foreign" epitopes, Kärre proposed that NK cells are equipped to detect the absence of "self" epitopes. The "missing self" hypothesis suggests that NK cells survey tissues for expression of MHC-I molecules that are normally ubiquitously expressed and that chronically prevent NK cell activity. If MHC-I molecules are down-regulated or mutated, NK cells are released to lyse the target. The generally opposite requirements of NK and T cells for target cell MHC-I expression may be physiologically important. Several pathogens, including herpes viruses, possess mechanisms that prevent the normal expression of MHC-I molecules on infected cells, providing means to avoid MHC-I-restricted T cells *(139)*. Moreover, tumorigenesis is frequently associated with alterations in MHC molecules, either mutation in structural genes or decreased expression, again leading to escape from T cell surveillance *(140–142)*. In either case, however, the MHC-I–deficient cells should become more susceptible to natural killing. The host therefore is endowed with two components (T and NK cells) with opposing requirements for self–MHC-I expression. This fail-safe system should eliminate pathologic processes that might otherwise evade immune responses by any alteration of MHC-I expression (either increased to avoid NK cells or decreased to avoid T cells). The missing-self hypothesis thus provided a teleological explanation for MHC-I–associated resistance, creating a framework for initial attempts to define NK cell recognition of their targets.

Current Principles of Target Recognition by NK Cells

The MHC-I–associated resistance to natural killing inspired a panoply of models and their variants to explain not only resistance but also natural killing (125). The *target interference* or *masking* model predicted that a single NK cell receptor activates natural killing when it engages its putative target cell ligand (138). MHC-I molecules mask the putative target cell ligand and block its recognition by the NK cell receptor. This hypothesis was initially favored because it was the simplest *(143)*. Moreover, it made the most sense if one considered that NK cells should have only one defined receptor analogous to the TCR. The *effector inhibition* or *inhibitory receptor* model suggested that NK cells are inhibited from natural killing by an NK cell receptor that binds MHC-I on the target and delivers negative signals overriding a default pathway of activation (138).

Although the target interference model has not been refuted, it is now known that NK cells express inhibitory receptors specific for MHC-I (144) (Figure 16.2). All known inhibitory receptors contain cytoplasmic immunoreceptor tyrosine-based inhibitory motifs (ITIMs) consisting of V/I/L/SxYxxL/V (single amino acid code where x is any amino acid) *(145)*. Ligand engagement leads to phosphorylation of the ITIM, presumably by a Src family tyrosine kinase. Two phosphorylated ITIMs are generally required for recruitment of the intracellular tyrosine phosphatase, SHP (SH2-containing protein tyrosine phosphatase)-1 (also known as SHP; hematopoietic cell phosphatase, HCP; protein tyrosine phosphatase 1C, PTP1C; and protein-tyrosine phosphatase, nonreceptor-type, 6, PTPN6). Other phosphatases, such as SHP-2, and SHIP (SH2-containing inositol polyphosphate 5-phosphatase) can also be recruited to phosphorylated ITIMs, depending on the receptor and cell, but the predominant phosphatase recruited by the NK cell inhibitory receptors appears to be SHP-1, which is activated by ITIM recruitment, leading to inhibition of NK cell activation.

MHC-I inhibitory receptors on NK cells have either of two general structures *(146)*: (a) C-type lectinlike receptors that are disulfide-linked dimers with type II transmembrane topology (extracellular carboxyl termini); these receptors are encoded in the NK gene complex (NKC) and were first described in mice. (b) Ig-superfamily receptors that have type I transmembrane orientation. These molecules are encoded in a different genetic region, termed the *leukocyte receptor complex* (LRC), and were first described in humans. Although ongoing studies indicate that both structural types of receptors are expressed on mouse and human NK cells, the lectinlike receptors (Ly49 receptors) are the major MHC-specific inhibitory receptors in mouse, whereas the Ig-like receptors (killer Ig-like receptors, KIRs) predominate in human.

The absence of MHC-I does not always result in killing, indicating that release from inhibition does not result in activation by default (Figure 16.2B). Instead, it was suggested that NK cells express two functionally different receptors for target cell ligands *(147,148)*. In this *two receptor model,* one receptor would be capable of interacting with a target cell ligand for activation (Figure 16.2C) whereas

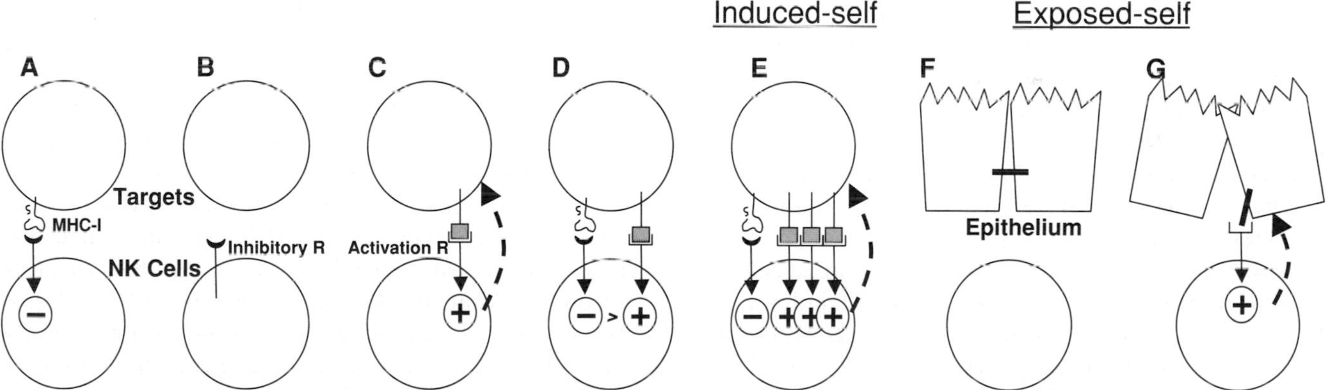

FIGURE 16.2 Current principles of target recognition by NK cells. Pictured are several scenarios of interactions between ligands on targets (top row) and receptors on NK cells (bottom row). Successful activation of NK cells is shown by the dashed upward line. **A:** Targets expressing MHC-I are resistant to lysis by NK cells because of MHC-I–specific inhibitory receptors. **B:** The absence of MHC-I (or lack of receptors specific for target MHC-I, not depicted) does not automatically result in target killing. **C:** Activation receptor engagement is required to trigger target killing. **D:** In the situation where both inhibitory and activation receptors are engaged, the inhibitory receptor effect often dominates and no killing occurs. **E:** In the induced-self model, induced expression of NKG2D ligands can overcome the inhibitory influence of MHC-I, resulting in NK cell activation. **F:** Normal epithelium masks ligands for NK cell activation receptors at the tight junctions. **G:** Under pathologic situations, the epithelial architecture may be disrupted, leading to ligand exposure. (Not depicted are inhibitory ligands at the epithelial tight junctions, which may inhibit NK cells when they transmigrate through epithelial barriers.) NK cells can also recognize pathogen encoded ligands on infected cells (not shown but similar to C or E).

MHC-I–specific receptor inhibits activation by negative signaling. In many circumstances, the inhibitory receptor effect dominates over the activation receptor (Figure 16.2D), but the outcome is likely to reflect the integration of signals from both types of receptors that can be affected by ligand expression or affinities (not shown).

Many NK cell activation receptors are encoded in the NKC and LRC, having similar structural properties as their inhibitory receptor counterparts except for absence of cytoplasmic ITIMs. The activation receptors typically do not have signaling motifs in their cytoplasmic domains but contain charged transmembrane residues that facilitate association with reciprocally charged residues in the transmembrane domains of signaling chains having immunoreceptor tyrosine-based activation motifs (ITAMs) analogous to ITAMs in TCR and BCR complexes (D/ExxYxxL/Ix$_{6-8}$YxxL/I). NK cells express three ITAM-containing signaling chains: CD3ζ, FcεRIγ, and DAP12 (DNAX associated protein of 12 kDa, also known as killer activating receptor associated protein, KARAP; Ly83; tyrosine kinase binding protein, Tyrobp). NK cells also express DAP10 (hematopoietic cell signal transducer, Hcst) that lacks ITAMs and instead contains a motif for recruitment of phosphatidylinositol 3-kinase (PI3K). The signaling chains typically endow the activation receptors with two major functions, capacity for cell surface expression, and signal transduction.

To date, the ligands for activation receptors fall into several major groups. One group is encoded by the host and expressed normally. Presumably, NK cell attack against cells expressing these ligands is limited by inhibitory receptors (Figure 16.2D). Another group of ligands is characterized by their relatively low expression on normal tissues and is induced expression under "stress" conditions (Figure 16.2E). Other ligands become exposed when tissue architecture is altered (Figure 16.2F,G). Because the ligands are encoded in the normal host genome, they would be recognized by the NK cell as indicators of pathologic conditions, either as "induced-self" or "exposed-self," respectively. Another group of ligands is found on infected cells and is encoded by the pathogen (not shown but similar to Figure 16.2C or E).

Finally, many other NK cell receptors have been discovered that do not fall neatly into the categories described here. Some appear to have similar inhibitory function as the MHC-specific inhibitory receptors but bind non-MHC ligands, strongly suggesting MHC-independent self-recognition. The function of these and other receptors remain under intense investigation.

In the following sections, we will describe the major receptors on NK cells in detail by first discussing the MHC-specific inhibitory receptors, which helped elucidate NK recognition paradigms, before delving into MHC-independent inhibitory receptors, activation receptors, and other receptors found on NK cells.

NK CELL RECEPTORS

Inhibitory NK Cell Receptors Specific for MHC-I Molecules

Mouse Ly49

The Ly49A receptor was the first inhibitory MHC-I–specific receptor to be described in molecular terms (144,*149*). Ly49A was originally identified as a molecule of unknown function on a T cell tumor *(150,151)*. It is a disulfide-linked homodimer (44 kDa subunits), with type II membrane orientation, and has C-type lectin superfamily homology (152,153). Previously termed *Ly49,* it is now appreciated that Ly49A (Klra1) belongs to a family of highly related molecules (*148,154,155*,156). Indeed, genetic analysis revealed that the genes for Ly49A and NK1.1 are linked in the NKC (Figure 16.3), leading to studies indicating that Ly49A is constitutively expressed on a distinct subpopulation (20%) of NK cells in C57BL/6 mice (156).

Multiple lines of evidence indicate that Ly49A is an inhibitory receptor specific for MHC-I, particularly H2D^d: 1) Functional analysis: The Ly49A$^+$ NK cell subset could not lyse a large panel of targets that were lysed by Ly49A$^-$ NK cells; this phenotype was related to MHC-I expression of certain H2 haplotypes (144,*157,158*). Transfected expression of H-2D^d selectively rendered a susceptible target resistant to natural killing by Ly49A$^+$ NK cells. Moreover, killing through disparate stimuli by Ly49A$^+$ NK cells was also inhibited. 2) Cell binding: Ly49A$^+$ tumor cells bound specifically to immobilized MHC-I molecules *(159)* and to H-2D^d-transfectants *(160)*. 3) Antibody blocking: F(ab')$_2$ fragments of mAb directed against either Ly49A or the $\alpha 1/\alpha 2$ (but not the $\alpha 3$ domain) of H-2D^d reversed resistance in killing experiments (permitted lysis) and blocked the cell binding assay (144,*157,159,160*). 4) *In vivo* expression: The apparent level of Ly49A expressed per NK cell was down-regulated in MHC congenic and transgenic (Tg) mice expressing H-2D^d (161,*162,163*). This was not due to negative selection because the percentage of Ly49A$^+$ NK cells was unchanged. 5) Gene transfer: Primary NK cells and T cells expressing a Ly49A transgene and a Ly49A-transfected NK cell line were specifically inhibited by H-2D^d (164,165). 6) Inhibition by Ly49A is ITIM-dependent, based on gene transfer of mutant Ly49A molecules (165). 7) H2D^d tetramers bind Ly49A transfectants (166). 8) Ly49A tetramers bind H2D^d on transfected cells (167,*168*). 9) Biophysical studies: Recombinant Ly49A binds recombinant H2D^d in surface plasmon resonance (SPR) studies with $K_D = \sim 2.0\ \mu M$ *(169)*. 10) Crystallography: The structure of Ly49A complexed with H2D^d was determined (170). 11) Less extensive studies also indicate that Ly49A recognizes H-2D^k and H2D^p (144,161,166,*171*). Therefore, Ly49A is an MHC-I–specific receptor for H-2D^d, H-2D^k and H2D^p.

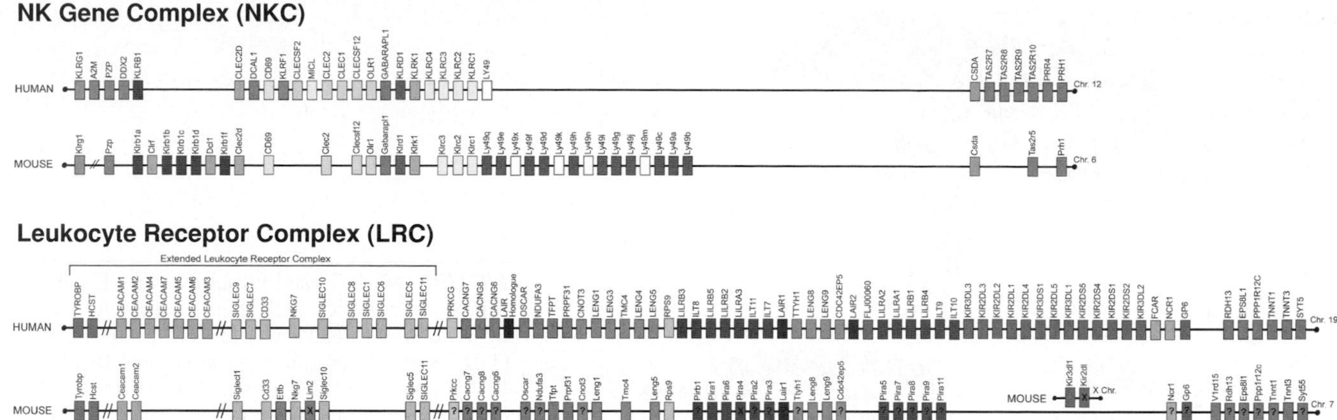

FIGURE 16.3 The genomic organization of the NKC and LRC in humans and mice. The figures are not drawn to scale, but the organization is accurate. The grey shading is coordinated to represent related genes. Question marks indicate genes whose precise location is not known. An "X" indicates genes not homologous to other aligned genes. Double slashes represent large genomic distances. Note that most but not all genes are expressed on NK cells. Many remain orphan genes because the functions of their gene products have not been determined. Modified from (246).

The nature of the Ly49A interaction with MHC-I, however, is fundamentally different from TCR/MHC-I interactions because the former appears to be independent of the specific peptide bound by H2D^d (172,*173*). However, bound peptides are required for appropriately folded MHC-I molecules that can be recognized. Despite its structural homology to C-type lectins that are carbohydrate-binding proteins *(174,175)*, Ly49A does not have the residues for coordinate binding to Ca^{++} that is required for lectin binding. Notwithstanding initial studies to the contrary *(176–178)*, Ly49A binding to its MHC ligands is not carbohydrate-dependent because Ly49A functionally interacts with H2D^d molecules with mutations in all of its Asn-linked residues *(179)*. Further, SPR reveals binding between bacterially produced H2D^d (lacking carbohydrates) and Ly49A *(169)*. Although carbohydrates could still affect receptor-ligand interactions, such as their affinities or kinetic parameters, this has not been studied in depth.

The x-ray crystallographic structure of lectinlike domain of Ly49A complexed to H2D^d was solved to 2.3Å resolution (170) (Figure 16.4). Two interaction sites were seen: site 1 involving the "left" side of the peptide-binding cleft of H2D^d and a wedgelike site 2 involving the undersurface of the peptide-binding cleft. The residues in Ly49A involved in binding either ligand site are overlapping. Mutational analysis revealed that Ly49A binds site 2, where it contacts $\alpha1$, $\alpha2$, and $\alpha3$ of H2D^d and β2m (167,*169,180*). This site is near Asn80, an Asn-linked glycosylation site conserved in all MHC-I molecules, leaving open the issue of whether carbohydrates could affect the interaction. These studies also provide a structural explanation for species-specific β2m requirements *(181)* as revealed by functional studies. Thus, Ly49A recognizes site 2 in the MHC molecule in terms of *trans* recognition between the NK cell receptor and target cell MHC-I molecule.

Recent studies strongly suggest that Ly49 molecules also bind MHC in a *cis* interaction between receptor and ligand on the NK cell itself (182,183). For example, an MHC ligand for Ly49A or Ly49C on the same cell prevents binding of MHC tetramer (182,183). If the cells are briefly exposed to mild acidic conditions, MHC-I expression is lost (due to disruption of the noncovalently linked MHC-I heterotrimer), and Ly49A binding to cognate MHC-tetramers is restored. This *cis* interaction is dependent on site 2 residues in the MHC molecule. These findings may help explain the observation that the presence of self-MHC ligands leads to "down-regulation" of Ly49 expression, as previously noted on primary NK cells in MHC congenic mice (161,*162,163*). *Cis* interactions may also explain functional differences in NK cells that do or do not express MHC ligands in Tg mice that are mosaic for MHC expression (184,*185*). At the moment, however, the physiologic importance of *cis* interactions is incompletely understood but may be relevant because NK cells do express MHC-I molecules (as well as MHC-specific receptors).

Other Ly49 receptors are also MHC-I-specific inhibitory receptors, although they have been less well studied than Ly49A. First noted by Southern blot analysis and cDNA cloning, genome sequence analysis now reveals 16 complete Ly49 genes in C57BL/6 mice (152,153,*154,155,186*). Notably, Ly49C has broad specificity for H2 alleles as revealed by tetramer staining and is the only known receptor specific for an H2^b haplotype allele (H2K^b) in C57BL/6 mice (166,183,*187*). It is recognized by two mAbs, 5E6 which also binds Ly49I and 4LO3311 which has exquisite specificity for Ly49C *(188–190)*. Ly49G2 (also known as

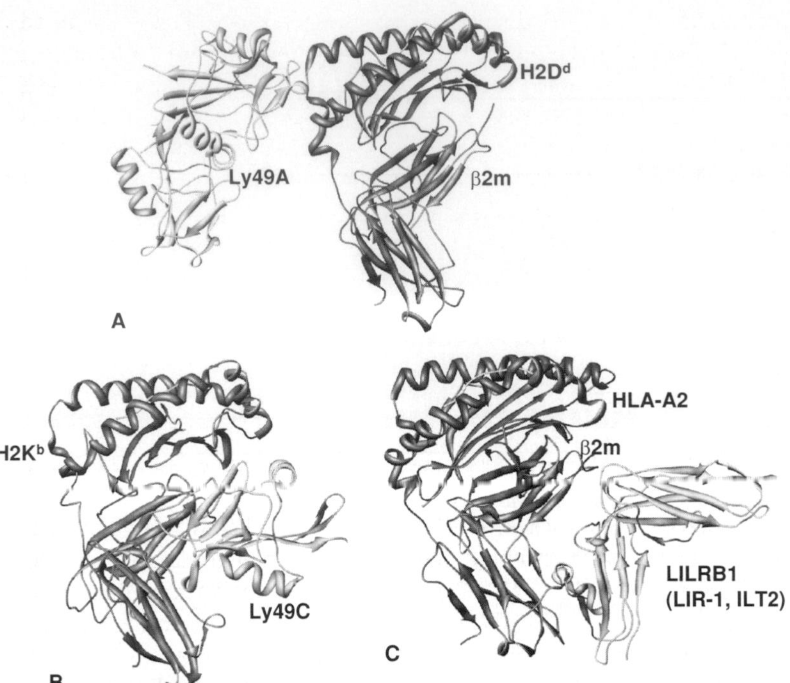

FIGURE 16.4 Crystal structures of NK cell receptors in complex with their ligands. **A:** Mouse Ly49A bound to H2D^d at site 1 (PDB ID = 1QO3) (170). Site 2 interaction is not shown. **B:** Mouse Ly49C bound to H2K^b at site 2 (PDB ID = 1P1Z) (193). Ly49A interaction with site 1 of H2D^d is very similar (170). **C:** Human LILRB1 (LIR1, ILT2) bound to HLA-A2 (PDB ID = 1P7Q) (266). Figures were produced using the UCSF Chimera package from the Resource for Biocomputing, Visualization, and Informatics at the University of California, San Francisco (www.cgl.ucsf.edu/chimera) *(776)*. The structures are viewed from the side with the NK cell positioned at the top of the figure and the target cell surface at the bottom. The MHC molecules are oriented similarly. (See color insert.)

LGL-1, recognized by mAb 4D11) binds H2D^d in tetramer binding experiments, and conversely, H2D^d binds several different Ly49 receptors, indicating the overlapping and promiscuous specificities (166,*191*). Finally, there is evidence for alternative splicing of the Ly49 genes *(155,192)*, though their importance has not been elucidated.

X-ray crystallographic studies have indicated that Ly49C binds H2K^b in a manner similar to Ly49A interaction with H2D^d (193) (Figure 16.4). Only a site 2 interaction was seen with the contact residues showing a similar but distinct topology to the Ly49A-H2D^d interaction. Interestingly, however, peptides bound to H2K^b clearly affect functional interactions with Ly49C (194) and affinities as measured by SPR (193). However, Ly49C does not directly engage the peptide, indicating long-range effects. Thus, Ly49 receptors bind their MHC ligands in a structurally related manner.

Individual NK cells may express multiple Ly49 receptors simultaneously *(163,190,195)*, often (but not always) two or more Ly49s, suggesting that individual NK cells may be inhibited by more than one MHC-I molecule. Detailed ontogenetic studies demonstrate that the total repertoire of Ly49 expression does not reach adult levels until sometime after 3 weeks of age, concomitant with attainment of full NK cell cytolytic activity (196). Thereafter the expression of Ly49 receptors is generally thought to be fixed and stable on an individual NK cell.

The expression of Ly49 receptors appears to occur in a stochastic manner. There is evidence for monoallelic expression of Ly49 receptors (expression from one chromosome), initially described as *allelic exclusion,* a term that has fallen out of favor because it has a specific meaning and mechanism for TCRs and B cell receptors *(197)*. Recent studies indicate that Ly49 genes possess bidirectional, overlapping promoters, directed in opposite orientations (198). Factors driving transcription in one direction prevent binding of other factors driving transcription in the opposite direction. Directionality and monoallelic expression may also be controlled by DNA methylation *(199)*. A "probabilistic" model has been proposed to explain these findings, and it may also explain the stochastic expression of Ly49 genes and their stable expression.

The description of the Ly49 receptors thus far is based on analysis of the C57BL/6 alleles, but the Ly49 receptors display extensive polymorphism. The Ly49 family is encoded in the NKC located on mouse chromosome 6 with the syntenic human region being chromosome 12p13.2 (*148*,156,200,*201*) (Figure 16.3). Although the NKC also contains genes for other lectinlike receptors, the Ly49 genes are clustered with the exception of *Ly49b*. Corresponding to restriction fragment length polymorphic (RFLP) variants originally detected with the Ly49A cDNA (156), there is significant allelic polymorphism of the Ly49 cluster between inbred mouse strains with differences in gene number as well as alleles for the *Ly49* genes *(186,202–205)*. Genomic sequence analysis shows 8 putative *Ly49* genes in BALB/c mice, and 19 potential *Ly49* genes in 129S6 mice (of which at least 9 appear to be pseudogenes), in contrast to C57BL/6 mice. There are also multiple alleles for individual *Ly49* family members *(186,197,204–206)*. Thus, there is significant polymorphism of the *Ly49* molecules.

The polymorphisms raise practical issues when studying NK cells. mAbs specific for one Ly49 allele may bind another molecule with a different function or specificity in another mouse strain *(207,208,209)*. Perhaps the profound allelic differences are to be expected because the Ly49 molecules bind highly polymorphic MHC molecules.

Human Killer Immunoglobulinlike Receptors (KIRs)

In contrast to mouse NK cells, human NK cells can be cloned by limiting dilution in the presence of irradiated feeder cells, phytohemagglutinin, and IL-2, leading to establishment of short-term NK cell clones that have differences in target killing and surface molecules. mAbs were isolated that reacted specifically with these clones; reactivity correlated with the capacity of the clones to kill certain tumors, and the mAbs affected cytotoxicity. This general approach led to the identification of the human NK cell receptors.

A series of studies, for example (210,211,*212*), showed that the mAbs GL183 and EB6 identify serologically distinct 55 kDa or 58 kDa molecules, initially termed *p*58. These molecules had several features: 1) Selective expression on overlapping NK cell subsets. 2) Expression on NK cell clones correlated with expression of certain HLA class I alleles on resistant targets. 3) A target susceptible to a given NK cell clone bearing p58 molecules reactive with either mAb was made resistant by transfection of cDNAs encoding certain HLA-C molecules. 4) The otherwise resistant HLA-C-transfected targets could be lysed in the presence of the appropriate anti-p58 mAbs. The mAb effect occurred with $F(ab')_2$ fragments, suggesting that the interaction between p58 and an HLA class I molecule on the target cell inhibits the NK cell. Thus, the p58 molecules displayed features consistent with a role as inhibitory human NK cell receptors specific for MHC-I, analogous to the mouse Ly49A receptor that was being studied in parallel as described earlier.

Other studies noted that NK cell specificity was skewed when the NK cells were grown in the presence of cells bearing allo-MHC determinants (213,*214*). This specificity correlated with reactivities that mapped to paired residues at position 77 and 80 in the $\alpha 1$ domain of HLA-C. All known HLA-C molecules could be divided into two groups, one with Asn77-Lys80 (HLA-Cw2, Cw4, -Cw5, -Cw6) and the other with Ser77-Asn80 (HLA-Cw1, -Cw3, -Cw7, -Cw8). Indeed, transfection analysis showed that p58 specificity for HLA-C molecules was related to expression of the EB6 epitope for the former (specificity 1), whereas the latter was related to the GL183 epitope (specificity 2) on the NK cell clones (213,*215,216*). Thus, human NK cell receptors showed promiscuous specificity that was dependent on residues 77 and 80 in HLA-C.

The NKB1 (p70) molecule was serologically similar to p58 molecules with regard to subset expression and correlation of expression on NK cell clones to specificity for HLA class I (217,*218*). In contrast to p58 molecules, however, NKB1 had a distinct M_r (70 kDa) and specificity for HLA-B. The NKB1$^+$ clones were specifically inhibited by targets expressing transfected HLA-Bw4 molecules, and the anti-NKB1 mAb reversed the inhibition. Analysis of informative HLA-B alleles showed that this specificity was conferred by a region in the $\alpha 1$ domain overlapping the area on HLA-C recognized by p58 molecules *(219)*. Finally, HLA-A3, -A11-specific receptors have similar properties to p58 and NKB1 except that they appear to be disulfide-linked dimers termed p140 *(220)*, whereas others have found that a monomeric HLA-A3–specific receptor resembles NKB1 *(221)*. Thus, representative alleles of all classical HLA class I loci are capable of inhibiting NK cells through p58/NKB1/p140 receptors, although HLA-B and -C alleles dominate human NK cell specificities, and it is not yet known whether there are receptors reactive with *each* HLA allele.

When the cDNAs for the p58 and NKB1 molecules were cloned, they were surprisingly found to encode type I integral membrane proteins with Ig-like domains (222,223,*224*) rather than features similar to the lectinlike Ly49 family of type II receptors. Subsequently, multiple cDNAs were identified *(212,214,218,225–229)*.

The Ig-like receptors are now collectively known as killer Ig-like receptors (KIRs) or CD158 *(230)*. The KIR nomenclature is based on whether the receptor has two or three Ig-like external domains (KIR2D or KIR3D, respectively), and possession of a long (L) or short (S) cytoplasmic domain. In general, the L forms are inhibitory because they contain ITIMs, whereas the S forms appear to be activation receptors (discussed later). Each distinct receptor is also designated by a number. The KIR2DL1 (CD158a, p58.1) molecule thus bears the original EB6 epitope and is specific for HLA-C (Asn77-Lys80), whereas KIR2DL2 (CD158b, p58.2) has the GL183 epitope and is specific for HLA-C (Ser77-Asn80). KIR3DL1, originally named NKB1, is specific for HLA-Bw4. KIR3DL2 was originally named p140 and has HLA-A specificity.

There is unequivocal evidence that the KIR2DL and KIR3DL molecules are inhibitory HLA class I–specific receptors. In addition to the data with NK cell clones and mAbs mentioned earlier, the following have been described: 1) KIR bind directly to HLA class I: Soluble KIR2DL-Fc fusion proteins bind cells expressing the appropriate transfected HLA class I alleles (231,*232*). In addition, a soluble KIR2DL molecule containing only the extracellular domain bind specifically to its HLA-C ligand in solution *(233)*. 2) Gene transfer of KIR: KIR2DL specificity and inhibitory function were transferred when KIR2DL cDNAs were transiently expressed with vaccinia constructs in human NK cell clones (231). Similarly, Tg expression of KIR2DL2 conferred inhibition of rejection of BM expressing Tg HLA-Cw3 *(234)*. 3) SPR measurements indicate that the KIRs bind their HLA ligands with $K_d = \sim 10\ \mu M$ (235,236,*237*). Binding is affected by peptide bound by HLA molecule (*237*). Through histidine-rich domains, the KIRs bind Zn^{++}, which affects KIR multimerization and binding kinetics to HLA ligands (*238,239*). 4) Crystallographic studies demonstrate KIR2DL1 (2.8 Å resolution) and KIR2DL2 (3.0 Å resolution) interactions with their cognate HLA ligands (236,240). Thus, KIR molecules are clearly MHC-I–specific inhibitory receptors on NK cells.

Interestingly, the KIR molecules bind HLA class I molecules in a manner analogous to recognition of MHC by TCRs (Figure 16.5). In particular, both KIR2DL1 and KIR2DL2 use surface loops near their interdomain hinge regions to bind their cognate HLA-C ligands (Cw4 and Cw3, respectively) with a footprint overlying the "right" side of the peptide-binding cleft (when viewed from the "top" in standard depictions of MHC-I molecules) (236,240). The receptors bind both $\alpha1$ and $\alpha2$ helices with interactions between KIR2DL1 and Lys80 of HLA-Cw4 and between KIR2DL2 and Asn80 of HLA-Cw3. These interactions with residue 80 of the HLA-C molecules would be lost if the reciprocal residues were swapped, accounting for the previously described HLA-C groupings and KIR specificities in functional studies (213,*214*) and mutational analysis indicating that residue 80 is more significant for KIR interaction than residue 77 *(241–244)*. Although neither KIR2DL molecule has extensive contacts with peptides bound to HLA-C, KIR2DL interactions with HLA-C imposes physical constraints on the p8 position of the peptide, accounting for observed peptide preferences in functional studies *(245)*. Thus, KIRs and Ly49s bind their MHC ligands in markedly different ways, despite their analogous functions as MHC-specific inhibitory receptors.

Also unlike the Ly49s, the KIRs are encoded in the leukocyte receptor complex (LRC) on human chromosome 19q13.4 that encodes many other Ig-like receptors (Figure 16.3); the KIR genes are clustered toward the telomeric end of the LRC (246). Interestingly, the mouse LRC on chromosome 7qA1 does not include genes for KIR-like molecules that instead are encoded on the X chromosome *(247,248)*. However, like the Ly49s, the KIRs display remarkable polymorphism (249,250). (See http://www.ebi.ac.uk/ipd/kir/index.html for updated database.) The human KIR complex demonstrates considerable haplotype diversity (249,250). Two major types of haplotypes have been described. Haplotype A contains nine genes that appear to be fixed but may display extensive allelic polymorphism. Haplotype B shows more widespread variation in gene content, with more than 20 different haplotypes described. Regardless, the *3DL3*, *3DP1*, *2DL4*, and *3DL2* genes (P designates pseudogene) and possibly *2DL2* (or *2DL3*) and *3DL1* (or *3DS1*) have been termed *framework loci* because they appear to be present in all haplotypes described thus far. With such extensive polymorphism, a large number of different KIR genotypes have already been described, and they are distributed differently in the various ethnic populations. Studies of these genetic variants have not only provided clues to new receptors and ligand specificities, but also valuable links to the role of NK cells and their

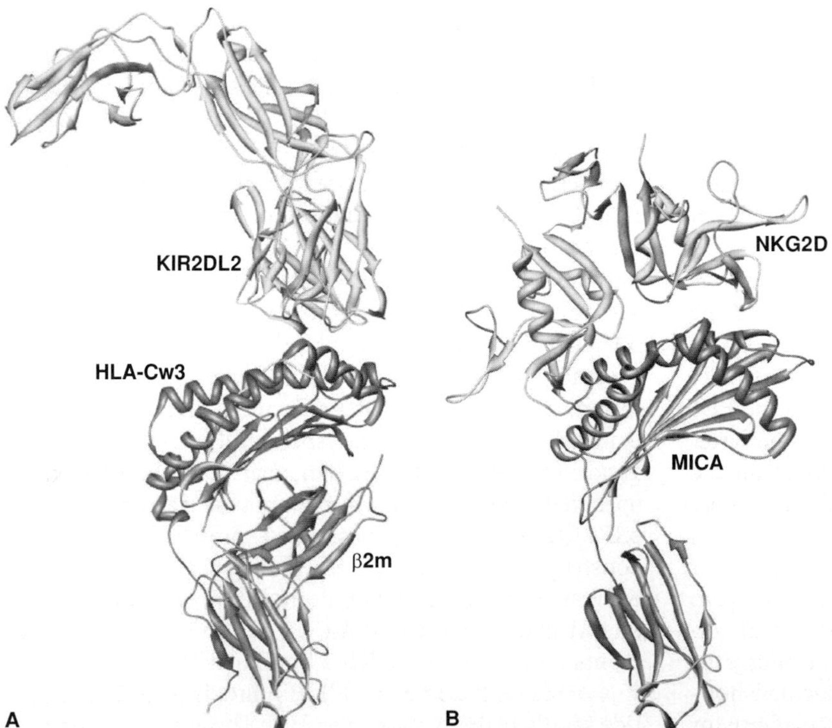

FIGURE 16.5 Additional structures of NK cell receptors in complex with their ligands. **A:** Human KIR2DL2 with HLA-Cw3 (PDB ID = 1EFX) (236). Two KIR molecules are apparent in the crystal structure with only one molecule (KIR A) contacting the HLA molecule. In this view, the D2 domain of the KIR A obscures the D1 domain behind it. **B:** Human NKG2D with MICA (PDB ID = 1HYR) (412). The figures were produced and oriented as described in Figure 16.4. (See color insert.)

receptors in disease pathogenesis and, more broadly, human evolution.

Recent studies also suggest that understanding of KIR specificities may be clinically useful. For example, in BM transplantation for leukemia, donor NK cells may help provide an anti-leukemia effect against residual malignant cells in the recipient if there is a mismatch between the donor and recipient HLA alleles (251). However, this observation has not been uniformly observed in other transplant centers (252,*253*,254). It is possible that differences in transplantation protocols may influence this effect or that there are additional parameters affecting NK cell tolerance (255).

Combinations of KIR and HLA genotypes may affect clinical outcomes (250,*256*,257,*258*,*259*). For example, hepatitis C virus (HCV) can cause a chronic, persistent infection in some patients, whereas other patients resolve the infection. Interestingly, patients who are homozygous for a KIR gene (KIR2DL3) are more likely to clear HCV if they are also homozygous for the HLA-C alleles recognized by KIR2DL3 (257). In papillomavirus infections that can go on to produce cervical carcinomas, resistance to developing neoplasia is similarly associated with genotypes encoding certain KIR-HLA receptor-ligand pairs *(258)*. While the means by which certain KIR-HLA combinations lead to protection is a topic under current investigation, the emerging data nonetheless demonstrate the importance of NK cells and KIR specificities in human disorders and treatments.

Other Human Ig-like Receptors Specific for MHC

The human LILR (leukocyte Ig-like receptor) family is encoded in the LRC (Figure 16.3), just centromeric to the KIR genes. In contrast to the highly polymorphic KIR genes, the LILR genes appear to be much more stable *(260)*. There are two general forms of these receptors: subfamily A, which appear to be activation receptors, and subfamily B, which have the ITIMs characteristic of inhibitory receptors. At least two members, LILRB1 (also known as CD85, Ig-like transcript 2 [ILT2] or leukocyte Ig-like receptor 1 [LIR1]) and LILRB2 (ILT4 or LIR2), recognize HLA class I molecules (261,262,*263*). LILRB1 is broadly expressed, whereas LILRB2 is not expressed on NK cells but is expressed by myelomonocytic cells, including DCs and monocytes, and can bind HLA-G tetramers *(264)*. Interestingly, a human cytomegalovirus (CMV) protein, UL18, binds LILRB1 with 1,000-fold higher affinity than HLA molecules, implicating a role for LILRB1 in host defense *(265)*.

LILRB1 has four Ig-like domains and binds a conserved region in the $\alpha 3$ domain of most, if not all, classical and nonclassical HLA class I molecules (HLA-A, -B, -C, -E, -F, and -G) *(265)*. Interestingly, the crystal structure of LILRB1 bound to HLA-A2 (3.4 Å resolution) reveals that it binds MHC molecule under the peptide-binding domain where it contacts $\alpha 3$ and $\beta 2$m, more akin to Ly49 engagement of MHC than KIR (266) (Figures 16.4, 16.5).

Human and Mouse CD94/NKG2

The analysis of CD94 (Klrd1) and NKG2 (Klrc, excluding NKG2D [Klrk1]) family of molecules was especially challenging and required insightful investigations. Identified by subtractive hybridization, the human NKG2 molecules are type II integral membrane proteins with external C-type lectin domains (267) encoded in the NKC *(268)* (Figure 16.3). Initial attempts to express NKG2 molecules on the cell surface were thwarted. Meanwhile, mAb reactivity suggested that CD94 was variably expressed on human NK cells as a disulfide-linked dimer (70 kDa NR, 43 kDa R) (269), and both activation and inhibition functions for CD94 were described *(270–273)*. Surprisingly, cDNA cloning revealed that CD94 has a short 7 amino acid cytoplasmic domain, suggesting that it cannot signal on its own *(272)*. Further, anti-CD94 immunoprecipitates were not detectable from radiolabeled CD94 transfectants, despite easily detectable expression on FACS analysis with the same mAbs (274,*275*). These apparent discrepancies were resolved when it became clear that CD94 heterodimerizes with NKG2 molecules (274); NKG2A is the 43 kDa molecule previously identified as Kp43 with anti-CD94 mAbs (276,*277*). (NKG2B is an alternatively spliced form of NKG2A. The rest of the NKG2 family is discussed later.) Although CD94 may be expressed as a homodimer, the NKG2 partner provides the signaling motif, whether activation (discussed later) or inhibition (276,*278*).

The ligand specificity for NKG2/CD94 receptors was also initially thought to be promiscuous as interactions with many classical (class Ia) and nonclassical (class Ib) HLA molecules had been described (*271*,274,276, *279–282*). However, human CD94/NKG2 receptors directly recognize HLA-E, a MHC-Ib molecule homologous to mouse Qa-1 (*283*,284,*285*). HLA-E (and Qa-1) is widely expressed with limited polymorphism (*286–288*). While HLA-E heavy chain is expressed with $\beta 2$m and a peptide occupying its peptide-binding cleft, its peptide repertoire is largely derived from the leader sequences of MHC-Ia molecules, as previously noted for mouse Qa-1 (*289,290*). HLA-E (or Qa-1) expression thus requires normal production of HLA-E (or Qa-1) and synthesis of certain MHC-Ia molecules. Mouse CD94/NKG2 recognizes Qa-1 that shares many features with HLA-E (291,*292*). These findings need to be considered in the context of the prevailing view at the time that mouse and human NK cells use structurally different receptors to recognize MHC-I molecules *(293)*. Clearly, the studies on CD94/NKG2 receptors and their ligands in humans and mice indicate the conservation of this receptor-ligand pair.

Despite its conservation, the role of CD94/NKG2 receptors in NK cell function is still incompletely understood.

For example, viruses encode peptides that bind and enhance expression of HLA-E, providing a CD94/NKG2A-dependent mechanism to avoid NK cell attack (294,*295*). However, human NK cells expressing CD94/NKG2C (an activation receptor) expand in response to CMV-infected targets (296). When a large number of human NK cell clones were obtained from two normal individuals, CD94/NKG2 seemed to account for the majority of self-MHC–specific receptors on clones from one individual, whereas KIRs dominated the self-specific receptors on clones from the other individual, suggesting that some individuals may depend on CD94/NKG2 for self-tolerance (297). Qa-1 and HLA-E can present peptides derived from other molecules, including the signal sequence of heat shock protein 60 (Hsp60) that is induced by a number of stimuli *(298,299)*, a multidrug resistance transporter *(300)*, or blastocyst MHC expressed in embryonic tissues *(301)*. This may result in loss or gain of recognition by the inhibitory CD94/NKG2A receptor, suggesting intrinsic mechanisms to perturb inhibition by CD94/NKG2A in certain circumstances. Yet CD94 appears to be dispensable in certain strains of mice, such as DBA/2J, that do not appear to have any untoward NK cell phenotype *(302)*.

CD94/NKG2 molecules may be important in T cell function. CD94/NKG2A is rapidly induced on antigen-specific $CD8^+$ T cells during polyoma virus and other infections (303,*304,305*), and $CD8^+$ T cells expressing CD94/NKG2A preferentially proliferate during persistent infection, suggesting that CD94/NKG2 receptors may play a role in memory T cell responses *(306)* and that TCR specificity is correlated with CD94/NKG2A expression by human CTL *(307)*. Indeed, CD94/NKG2A inhibits antigen-specific cytotoxicity in polyoma virus responses although this effect is pathogen-dependent. Thus, CD94/NKG2 receptors may regulate T cell responses.

Convergent Evolution of MHC-Specific Receptors

More than a decade has passed since the mouse Ly49s and human KIRs and LILRs were first cloned and identified. Detailed genome sequence information is available on the NKC and LRC in mice and humans and other species. In the mouse, MHC-specific NK cell receptors with Ig-like domains have not yet been described, although there is conservation of several genes in the broader LRC on mouse chromosome 7 (246) (Figure 16.3). Activated mouse NK cells do express gp49b (Lilrb4), an Ig-like inhibitory receptor also expressed on other leukocytes, including mast cells *(308–311)*. However, it is not expressed by resting NK cells and is not specific for MHC. Instead it binds the integrin $\alpha v\beta 3$ and appears more important in terms of neutrophil and inflammatory responses (312,*313,314*). A mouse molecule is closely related to human KIR3DL1 (*247,248*). It is encoded on the X chromosome (Figure 16.3) and expressed in NK and T cells, but its function and ligand are not known. The Ly49 locus in humans consists only of LY49L (KLRA1), which is a pseudogene because of a point mutation that gives rise to a splicing abnormality *(315)*. Perhaps further investigation may reveal additional human or mouse NK cell receptors for MHC-I ligands that are orthologues to Ly49 or KIR, respectively, because genomic sequencing has revealed a multitude of candidate orphan receptors in the LRC and NKC that have yet to be studied.

The alternative view is that mice and humans independently evolved analogous receptors to serve the same function. While both human and mouse NK cells express a conserved lectinlike receptor, CD94/NKG2, it does not possess many of the features that are shared by mouse Ly49 and human KIRs: 1) Both are constitutively and selectively expressed on naïve, unstimulated NK cells (with exceptions for rare populations of T cells). 2) Both bind MHC-I molecules with intermediate affinity ($K_D = \sim 2$ to 10 μM). 3) Binding to MHC is promiscuous. 4) MHC-bound peptides have only a modest effect, if at all, on recognition. 5) Both use ITIMs to inhibit NK cell activation. 6) They are expressed in a stochastic fashion on overlapping subsets of NK cells. 7) A single NK cell simultaneously expresses one or more of either type of inhibitory receptor; each may be functional. 8) Once they are expressed, their expression appears to be stable. 9) Both are germline encoded by small families of genes that are clustered in the genome. 10) Both display impressive polymorphism, in terms of gene number and alleles for each gene. 11) Both are related to molecules that lack ITIMs and instead are activation receptors. Thus, the mouse Ly49 receptors and human KIRs are analogous receptors in a striking example of convergent evolution *(316)*.

In other species, Ly49 and KIR genes have been analyzed primarily with respect to sequence and gene number. For example, the LY49L gene in baboons appears to be functional, but the putative polypeptide lacks an ITIM *(317)*. In rats, the Ly49 cluster appears to have markedly expanded with at least 25 genes *(318,319)*, demonstrating one of the most rapid rates of gene expansion *(320)*. Dog, cat, and pig appear to have only one Ly49, whereas the horse represents the only known nonrodent mammal with several Ly49 genes *(321)*. However, multiple KIR genes have been described in primates and cattle *(322–325)*. In rat, a KIR-like sequence has been reported *(248)*. Studies on the expression and functions of these putative receptors should be forthcoming.

Additional studies of the Ly49- and KIR-like molecules and their specificities will be of interest to evolutionary biologists, especially when considered in the context of MHC genes that are co-evolving *(326)* and the possibility that these molecules may have evolved other functions. In a somewhat broader context, the NKC, not just Ly49, has been described in other species and a number of genes are conserved, suggesting that the NKC is conserved in all placental species (327). Evolutionary consideration of the NKC also demonstrates complexity and heterogeneity at several levels. More distantly, the chicken genome has several lectinlike receptor genes, and at least some are genetically linked to the MHC (327,*328,329*). In teleost fish, a large number of novel immune-type receptors (NITRs) with Ig-like domains have been described with sequence homology to mammalian LRC-encoded receptors *(330)*. Interestingly, genes for these molecules are clustered with genes for putative lectinlike receptors *(331)*.

MHC-independent NK Cell Inhibitory Receptors

As already mentioned, NK cells also express inhibitory receptors for non-MHC ligands, such as mouse gp49b, which binds the $\alpha v\beta 3$ integrin (312), and there is a growing list of other molecules (332). Some of these receptors (2B4, Nkrp1, Klrg1, and CEACAM1) will be discussed in a more appropriate context in the following sections. Most of these receptors contain cytoplasmic ITIMs, so their inhibitory function can be predicted even if not directly tested, though some caution is required because the motifs may be involved in other signaling processes.

Human and mice NK cells express the ITIM-bearing LAIR-1 (leukocyte associated Ig-like receptor 1), which is an Ig-like molecule broadly expressed by most leukocytes *(333,334)*. Initial reports indicating that LAIR-1 binds epithelial cellular adhesion molecule (Ep-CAM) were proven to be irreproducible (335,*336*). A recent report suggests that LAIR-1 binds multiple forms of collagen *(337)*. Although the *in vivo* context for functional interaction awaits further characterization, it is reminiscent of the broader reactivity of the Siglecs.

The Siglecs (sialic acid binding Ig-like lectins) are CD33-related type I receptors with varying numbers of Ig-like domains expressed on a broad array of cells and encoded in the "extended" LRC (246,*338*) (Figure 16.3). Despite having sialic acid recognition in common, the Siglecs appear to show differences in carbohydrate recognition, depending on the specific glycan context *(338)*. Human NK cells express Siglec-7 (p75, adhesion inhibitory receptor 1, or AIRM1)(339), Siglec-9, and Siglec-11, whereas mouse NK cells express a related Siglec-E *(338,340,341)*. Siglec-7 has been most extensively studied. As expected, its cytoplasmic ITIM can recruit SHP-1 and inhibit NK cell functions (339,*342*). Moreover, expression of its ligand on targets inhibits NK cells in a Siglec-dependent manner *(343)*. However, the effects appear to be modulated by *cis* interactions between the Siglec receptor and its carbohydrate ligands on the NK cell itself *(338,343,344)*.

Thus, NK cells (and other leukocytes) express multiple inhibitory receptors that are capable of MHC-independent recognition. How they participate in NK cell responses is beginning to be elucidated, and some appear to play a specific role in the context of activation receptors, as discussed later.

NK Cell Activation Receptors

Despite evidence for MHC-independent inhibitory receptors, NK cells clearly kill MHC-I-deficient targets more efficiently than MHC-I-sufficient targets. However, this enhanced killing does not occur simply because a nonspecific default pathway is released when MHC-I is absent. Instead, evidence indicates that susceptible targets express ligands for NK cell activation receptors. These receptors and their ligands have been under intense investigation during the past few years.

Approaches to Identification of Activation Receptors

Initial progress in elucidating NK cell activation receptors was difficult. The approaches that yielded the molecular definition of the TCR, such as subtractive hybridization, mutagenesis of T cell tumors, and anticlonotypic mAbs *(345–347)*, were of limited success *(348,349)*. Indeed, there was incomplete understanding of what principle governed NK cell activation by targets, unlike the working paradigm of MHC-restriction that guided the molecular identification of the TCR. Breakthroughs in identifying NK cell activation receptors thus required other approaches.

Some receptors were recognized because they were first identified on other cells, such as FcγRIII. Other activation receptors were identified by genetic means, such as cDNA clones for molecules resembling the inhibitory receptors but lacking cytoplasmic ITIMs. Others were identified by a genetic positional cloning approach. The ability to induce specific stimulation of NK cells through mAbs proved to be extremely useful for the initial identification of candidate activation receptors and for validating the activation function of receptors identified by other means.

NK cells can be stimulated to mediate antibody-dependent cellular cytotoxicity (ADCC) through the FcγRIII (CD16) receptor which binds the Fc portion of IgG coating a target. In a related way, anti-FcγRIII can also trigger through CD16 in a process termed *redirected lysis* or *reverse ADCC*, because the antibody binds in the opposite orientation to ADCC. Several mAbs can activate NK cells in the redirected lysis assay, highlighting a relatively unique functional property of the recognized molecules, since activation does not occur when most NK cell surface molecules are cross-linked. First popularized for analysis of anti-TCR antibodies *(350)*, redirected lysis occurs when IgG reacts specifically with the NK cell receptor and its Fc portion binds a target cell Fc receptor (FcγR) that apparently provides bridging and cross-linking effects *(350)*. Target lysis does not occur if FcγR binding on the target is prevented with FcγR-deficient targets, F(ab')$_2$ fragments of the anti-NK cell receptor antibody, or anti-target cell FcγR Ab blockade. In the latter case, Fc regions must be removed to prevent inadvertent triggering of conventional ADCC via CD16 on the NK cell. Thus, the redirected lysis assay is a very helpful experimental tool.

Gene transfer studies have been helpful adjuncts to study NK cell receptors. NK cells are difficult to transfect, and there are few useful tumors with the notable exception of RNK-16, a rat NK tumor line *(351)*. Viral vectors, such as vaccinia virus, have been useful for gene transfer with the caveat that functional experiments have to be performed within a small time frame *(352)*.

Recent studies have exploited reporter cell assay systems similar to those used to identify TCR ligands *(353)*. ITAM-mediated signaling leads to inducible, NFAT (nuclear factor of activated T cells)–dependent expression of a reporter molecule, such as β-galactosidase or green fluorescent protein (GFP). Even an inhibitory receptor can be used to activate the reporter cell by fusion of its extracellular domain to a suitable transmembrane and cytoplasmic domain containing ITAMs. Such reporter cells can then be used to detect ligands on other cells (354–356).

In the following sections, we will describe NK cell activation receptors with an emphasis on those with known ligands.

Activation Receptors Related to MHC-specific Inhibitory Receptors

Despite initial characterization as inhibitory receptors for MHC-I, other members of the Ly49 family—that is, Ly49D and Ly49H in C57BL/6 mice—do not contain cytoplasmic ITIMs. Instead, they are activation receptors associated with DAP12 *(357–360)*. Although Ly49H will be considered later in the context of viral infection, Ly49D has no known role in viral defense. A positional cloning approach indicated that Ly49D is the product of the *Chok* locus, which controls NK cell specificity for killing of a xenogeneic target, Chinese hamster ovary (CHO) cells *(361,362)*, due to recognition of a Chinese hamster MHC-I molecule *(363)*. Interestingly, when Ly49D was transfected into RNK-16 cells, Ly49D can recognize $H2D^d$ *(351)*, but $H2D^d$ tetramers do not bind Ly49D for unclear reasons (166,*207*). Several other Ly49 receptors have been identified in other mouse strains that have properties of activation receptors (charged transmembrane residues, no ITIMs), but they have been less well characterized *(204,205)*. Finally, the available anti-Ly49 mAbs show cross-reactivity with inhibitory and activation receptors, depending on the allele and mouse strain *(207,364)*. Thus, some members of the Ly49 family are activation receptors involved in recognition of MHC-I molecules on targets.

Molecular cloning of the KIR family also led to the identification of two domain receptors (also known as p50) or three domain Ig-like receptors with short cytoplasmic domains lacking the ITIM (365,*366*). These molecules are now known as the KIR2DS or KIR3DS, respectively, and can be recognized by anti-p58 mAbs for the KIR2DL inhibitory receptors, making it sometimes difficult to distinguish activating from inhibitory receptors by mAb reactivity alone. KIR2DS2 and KIR2DS4 can associate with DAP12 and can activate NK cells in the redirected lysis assay. Also, T cell clones constitutively express p50 that are costimulatory with concomitant activation through the TCR/CD3 complex *(367)*. For example, KIR2DS4-Ig binds HLA-Cw4–expressing cells and not HLA-Cw6–expressing cells, and it binds less well than KIR2DL1-Ig proteins *(368)*. KIR2DS1 binds HLA-Cw7, but much weaker than KIR2DL1 *(369)*, and KIR2DS2 did not bind any HLA allele tested *(370)*. Thus, the activating forms of KIRs apparently bind HLA alleles less well than the inhibitory receptors, perhaps providing an explanation for the dominance of inhibition over activation (Figure 16.2D), although ligand information for the activating KIRs is limited.

Alternatively, the activating forms of the Ly49s and KIRs have other ligands, and perhaps their MHC specificities are misleading or cross-reactive. Indeed, this has been demonstrated for Ly49H that recognizes a virus-encoded ligand with a putative MHC-I-like fold (354,356). Moreover, KIR2DS4 may recognize a non-MHC ligand *(371)*. However, rat Ly49 activation receptors can recognize MHC allodeterminants *(372,373)*, providing an explanation for genetic analysis showing that MHC-linked allorecognition is stimulatory for NK cells *(374)*. Thus, further analysis is required for understanding the role of Ly49 and KIR activation receptors in MHC recognition, particularly with respect to their inhibitory counterparts.

In addition to NKG2A, the NKG2 family also contains NKG2C, NKG2E, and NKG2F, which are products of different genes (267,*375*). (NKG2H is an alternatively spliced isoform of NKG2E). NKG2C and NKG2E lack cytoplasmic ITIMs and contain charged transmembrane residues for association with DAP12 (376). Although the role of NKG2F is unknown because it lacks an external domain and remains inside the cell, associated with DAP12 but not with CD94 *(377)*, NKG2C and NKG2E form functional heterodimers with CD94 (276). Like NKG2A/CD94 receptors, these heterodimers recognize HLA-E or Qa-1, but unlike NKG2A/CD94 receptors, they activate NK cells (*378*,379). Interestingly, the inhibitory form appears to bind with higher affinity to HLA-E than the activating form *(380)*. There also appears to be some peptide preference between the different functional forms *(381)* that may be relevant in certain stress situations. Thus, perhaps unlike the activating and inhibitory forms of the Ly49s and KIRs, the CD94/NKG2 receptors may discriminate between subtle differences in their MHC-Ib ligands.

FcγRIII (CD16)

Frequently overlooked but perhaps the first molecularly defined activation receptor on NK cells is FcγRIII (CD16), through which NK cells mediate ADCC against

IgG-coated targets *(382,383)*. Unlike other Fcγ receptor-bearing effector cells, NK cells are generally thought to express only one of the known Fcγ receptors that binds IgG with low affinity *(384)*, although others suggest that human NK cells may express FcγRII isoforms *(385)*. There are two human FcγRIII isoforms with identical extracellular domains *(384)*. Human NK cells express only FcγRIIIA, which is a transmembrane molecule, whereas FcγRIIIB has a glycosylphosphatidyl-inositol (GPI) linkage and is expressed by neutrophils. In mice, only the transmembrane isoform (FcγRIII) is present *(386)* and displays 95% sequence conservation with muFcγRII. There are species differences in CD16 binding to mouse IgG isotypes; mouse IgG3 mAbs bind human CD16 the most efficiently (3>2a>2b>>1), while they bind mouse CD16 with the lowest affinity (2b>2a>1>>3) *(384)*. In the laboratory, a rabbit anti-mouse Ig polyclonal Ab, which binds strongly to both human and mouse CD16, could be added to facilitate Fc receptor binding.

The transmembrane FcγRIII molecules are physically associated with FcεRIγ and less commonly with CD3ζ *(387)*. FcγRIII can also associate with γ–ζ heterodimers. The associated chains are required for optimal cell surface expression of FcγRIII and for signal transduction. After cross-linking, FcγRIII activates biochemical events that are reminiscent of T cell activation, leading to granule exocytosis and cytokine production (118,388,*389–391*). *In vivo,* ADCC may be useful in host defense against pathogens or infected cells if Abs are bound to their surface, triggering not only killing but also cytokine production and other NK cell responses. Although NK cells are generally thought to participate early in a primary immune response (discussed later), the delay required for isotype switching to IgG production suggests that CD16 cross-linking on NK cells plays a role in secondary immune responses *in vivo*.

Regardless, ADCC is remarkably similar to natural killing and was important for the initial establishment of the concept of NK cell activation receptors (118). Yet CD16 is not required for NK cell target recognition because human CD16$^-$CD3$^-$ lymphocytes can still mediate natural killing *(392)*. Moreover, CD3ζ is phosphorylated upon CD16 ligation, but not when NK cells are exposed to NK-sensitive targets. Deficiency of γ chain abrogated ADCC but not natural killing *(382)*. Thus, CD16 is not involved in natural killing.

CD16-related artifacts must be considered when studying NK cells. Flow cytometry experiments may be flawed if CD16 binding is not taken into account. To eliminate this possibility, F(ab')$_2$ fragments should be used. Alternatively, blockade of FcγRIII binding may be sufficient with protein A or G (that bind Fc region on Ig) or anti-FcγRIII mAbs, such as unlabeled mAb 2.4G2 (ATCC HB 197) that reacts with both mouse FcγRII and FcγRIII *(386)*. Similarly, as discussed earlier, antibody blockade experiments should be done with caution if the antibody specifically reacts with the target because ADCC may be stimulated.

NKG2D

NKG2D (KLRK1) was first cloned from human NK cells as a cDNA related to NKG2A and C (267). However, NKG2D is distinct from other NKG2 molecules for several reasons. There is only limited sequence homology between NKG2D and other NKG2 molecules (28% amino acid identity for the lectinlike domain), whereas other NKG2 molecules are closely related to each other (70% identity). Rather than heterodimerizing with CD94, NKG2D is expressed as a disulfide-linked homodimer on all NK cells in humans and mice. In humans, NKG2D is also expressed on all $\gamma\delta$TCR$^+$ and CD8$^+$ T cells, whereas in mice, NKG2D is expressed on most NKT and $\gamma\delta$TCR$^+$ T cells, but not on resting CD8$^+$ T cells (393–395). However, essentially all activated mouse CD8$^+$ T cells express NKG2D. In both humans and mice, CD4$^+$ T cells do not normally express NKG2D, but it is found on a subset CD4$^+$CD28$^-$ T cells in rheumatoid arthritis patients (396). Finally, NKG2D has functional properties and ligand specificities that distinguish it from the other NKG2 molecules, indicating that NKG2D should not be considered as a member of the NKG2 family.

NKG2D does not have any known cytoplasmic motif and was first shown in humans to preferentially associate with a signaling chain termed *DAP10*, encoded by a gene localized 130 bp away from the gene for DAP12 (397). DAP10 does not have any ITAMs; instead it contains a YxxM motif for recruitment of PI3K (397) (similar to CD28), and initial functional studies suggested that NKG2D acts as a costimulatory molecule on human T cells (398).

Other studies have suggested that NKG2D functions as a primary activation (triggers alone) rather than costimulatory receptor (does not stimulate unless it synergizes with another receptor) on NK cells *(399,400)*. Such studies will need to be reconsidered now that several factors that have come to light: 1) Many studies of NKG2D function use targets that are poorly killed by NK cells. When transfected with NKG2D ligands, killing is enhanced in an NKG2D-dependent manner. However, such studies do not distinguish whether NKG2D functions as a primary activation receptor or as a costimulatory receptor (analogous to CD28 requirement for full activation of T cells) because the same experimental outcome is anticipated in either case. When cross-linking is done with immobilized mAbs alone, NKG2D functions as a costimulatory receptor on mouse IL-2-activated NK cells *(400)*. 2) In mice but not humans, there are two alternatively spliced isoforms of NKG2D (401,*402*). A long form (NKG2D-L) contains a 13 amino acid extension at the amino terminus (cytoplasmic domain) as compared to the short form (NKG2D-S). Resting NK cells predominantly express NKG2D-L that preferentially associates with DAP10. However, activation of NK cells with cytokines causes a transient increase in NKG2D-S that associates with DAP12 as well as DAP10. These latter two points, however, appear to be unresolved, as others have found that NKG2D-L can associate with DAP12, albeit to a lesser degree, and that both isoforms are present in resting NK cells (403). Regardless, in the absence of DAP10, mouse NKG2D can associate with DAP12 (404), allowing it to signal akin to a primary activation receptor. Thus, mouse NKG2D is an unusual example of a receptor with the same extracellular domain (and presumably ligand specificity) but with potentially different functional outcomes (primary activation versus co-stimulation), depending on its associated partner chain (DAP12 versus DAP10, respectively).

Human NKG2D ligands are MICA and MICB (MHC-I chain-related) encoded on chromosome 6p21.3), and the ULBP (UL16 binding protein) family encoded on chromosome 6q24.2-q25.3 (393,405). The ULBPs are also known as being encoded by genes in the 10 member *RAET1* gene family (official HUGO nomenclature) discovered by genomic mining. ULBP1 (RAET1I), ULBP2 (RAET1H), ULBP3 (RAET1N), ULBP4 (RAET1E), and RAET1G have been most extensively studied as ligands for NKG2D (405,*406,407*), whereas *RAET1F*, *RAET1J*, *RAET1K*, and *RAET1M* are pseudogenes *(408)*. Mouse NKG2D interacts with H-60, the retinoic acid early inducible gene-1 (RAE-1) family, consisting of RAE-1α, β, γ, δ, and ε, and murine ULBP-like transcript (MULT1) (394,395,409,*410*). There are reciprocal strain-specific differences in ligand expression—BALB/c mice express H60, RAE-1α, β, and γ, whereas C57BL/6 mice do not express these molecules and express RAE-1δ and ε *(411)*. Finally, there is remarkable plasticity for NKG2D in that it can bind many apparently disparate ligands that are only superficially related to each other by sequence alignment (only ~20% to 25% amino acid identity in pairwise comparison), and mouse NKG2D can bind human ligands and vice-versa.

Where studied, all NKG2D ligands have structural relatedness to MHC-I, although they do not associate with β2m or bind peptides (412,413,*414,415*). Many contain only the $\alpha 1/\alpha 2$ platforms and many are GPI-linked to the plasma membrane. The ligands display binding to NKG2D in two ways based on affinity (*410*,412,*416*,417). RAE1α, β, γ, and δ demonstrate a low-affinity interaction with mouse NKG2D, similar to MICA to human NKG2D (K_D = ~300 to 1,000 nM). In contrast, RAE1ε, H60, and MULT1 show a much higher-affinity interaction (K_D = 6 to 30 nM). Thus, closely related molecules may display wide disparity in affinities, whereas distantly related molecules can show high affinity with NKG2D.

Structural studies indicate that NKG2D binds its ligands more analogous to TCR docking on MHC (Figure 16.5) and unlike Ly49 recognition (Figure 16.4), despite the relationship of NKG2D and Ly49 receptors as NKC-encoded, lectinlike homodimers that bind MHC-related molecules (412,*418,419*). Moreover, NKG2D uses largely nonoverlapping patches to engage a similar orthogonal footprint on its disparate ligands. Two mechanisms have been proposed to account for this binding, induced fit where NKG2D has conformational flexibility (413) and rigid adaptation in which NKG2D has a rigid binding site *(419)*, an important issue in the context of multispecific immune receptors *(420)*. Thermodynamic studies support the rigid adaptation mechanism to explain how one receptor can bind disparate ligands *(421,422)*. However, structures of NKG2D complexed with other ligands may yield other information.

NKG2D function has been described in the "induced-self" model (Figure 16.2E) because the expression of many of its ligands appears to be inducible and can override inhibitory influences of MHC-I (*423*,424,*425*). Human MICA and MICB expression is markedly enhanced on epithelial tissues in inflammatory bowel disease (426). In mice, RAE-1 transcripts are induced by retinoic acid treatment or by phorbol ester stimulation (409). Moreover, TLR signaling and ionizing irradiation and other DNA-damaging agents can induce NKG2D ligand expression (*427*,428). Recent studies also indicate that NKG2D ligand expression can be regulated by the transcription factor JunB *(429)*. Thus, while transcripts for the ULBP and MULT1 molecules are readily detectable in normal tissues (405,*410*), the function of NKG2D is generally thought to trigger immune cells in the context of inflammatory reactions which lead to stress-induced expression of self-molecules *(430)*.

Chronic exposure to NKG2D ligands results in down-regulation of NKG2D expression and lower functional responsiveness *(431–433)*. Soluble forms of NKG2D ligands can also mediate these effects. Patients with tumors expressing MIC frequently contain soluble MIC in their peripheral blood, presumably as a result of proteolytic cleavage of membrane-expressed ligands *(431)*. Localized ligand expression can also result in impotent NKG2D responses in mice *(434)*. These findings may explain why tumors frequently express NKG2D ligands which otherwise would enhance their susceptibility to NK cell attack, supporting a role for NKG2D in tumor surveillance.

Additional studies support a role for NKG2D in tumor surveillance. For example, mice are more sensitive to developing methylcholanthrene-induced fibrosacromas when NKG2D is neutralized *(435)*. Moreover, mice lacking $\gamma\delta$T cells are more susceptible to carcinogenesis apparently due to an NKG2D-dependent effect (409). IFNγ is a known host mediator that shapes the tumor phenotypes in a broader process known as "immunoediting" *(436,437)*, and IFNγ also mediates down-regulation of H60 expression on tumors *(438)*. Thus, NKG2D and its ligands are important in the host response (or lack thereof) to tumors.

A role for NKG2D in antiviral responses is indicated by studies indicating that viruses encode molecules that interfere with ligand recognition by NKG2D. This was first noted when the human CMV protein UL16 was found to bind ULBPs (405). In infected cells, UL16 retains some (MICB, ULBP1, and ULBP2) but not all NKG2D ligands in the endoplasmic reticulum and cis-Golgi, preventing their expression on the cell surface and protecting from NK cell lysis (*439,440*,441). In mice, murine CMV (MCMV) encodes gp40 from the *m152* open reading frame (ORF) that down-regulates all five RAE-1 ligands but has no effect on H60 or MULT1 (*411*,442). However, H60 is down-regulated by the product of the *m155* ORF at a post-Golgi level, perhaps by targeting H60 for proteasomal degradation *(443,444)* and MULT1 expression is affected by *m145 (445)*. Recent studies also indicate that H60 and MULT1 are down-regulated by the herpesvirus Fc receptor (fcr-1), the product of the *m138* ORF *(446)*. Thus, the multitude of CMV proteins that affect NKG2D ligands strongly suggest that NKG2D plays an important role in the host response to CMV infections.

Finally, emerging data suggest that NKG2D may play a role in autoimmune disorders. There is an unusual population of $CD4^+$ $CD28^-$ T cells that is expanded in human patients with inflammatory syndromes, such as rheumatoid arthritis (RA), Wegener's granulomatosis, and unstable angina *(447–449)*. NKG2D may provide a missing costimulatory signal, at least in RA (396). NKG2D expression is upregulated by TNFα and IL-15 and RA synovium expresses NKG2D ligands. IL-15 also induces NKG2D expression on intestinal epithelial T lymphocytes, which then display a LAK cell-like promiscuous killing capacity against enterocytes, which upregulate NKG2D ligands from gliadin exposure, suggesting that NKG2D may play a pathogenic role in celiac sprue (33,*450,451*). Finally, NKG2D ligands are expressed in the prediabetic NOD mouse pancreas, and anti-NKG2D blockade prevents autoimmune diabetes mellitus *(452)*. Thus, NKG2D may play a pathogenic role in several autoimmune disorders in humans and mouse models.

Nkrp1 and Clr (LLT1)

First identified in redirected lysis assays with mAb 3.2.3, rat Nkrp1 is expressed as a disulfide-linked homodimer with 30 kDa subunits *(453)*. Expression is relatively selective for NK cells, although in rats and mice, Nkrp1 molecules are also expressed by NKT cells *(454,455)* (see Chapter 17). Nkrp1 (Klrb1) is now known to belong to a family of lectinlike molecules with type II orientation encoded in the mouse and rat NKC (60,200,*456–458*) (Figure 16.3). However, there is only a single gene (*NKRP1A*) in humans that is expressed on a subpopulation of NK cells *(459)*. The continuing allure of the Nkrp1 family stems from observations that NK1.1 (the best serologic marker of NK cells) is encoded by *Nkpr1c* (*Klrb1c*) in C57BL/6 mice (60), Nkrp1 receptors are conserved, and they have interesting genetics with respect to their ligands.

Initial functional studies indicated that rodent Nkrp1 molecules can activate NK cells through redirected lysis (31,*453,460–462*), which can be prevented by inhibitory Ly49 receptor engagement *(98)*. Mouse Nkrp1c (NK1.1) is functionally associated with FcεRIγ, although its deficiency does not affect NK1.1 expression (463). An Nkrp1a loss mutant of rat RNK-16 cells failed to kill certain targets; transfection restored killing capacity, suggesting that rat Nkrp1a is an activation receptor specific for target determinants *(464)*. Thus, Nkrp1 molecules were among the first described NK cell-specific activation receptors.

Inasmuch as Nkrp1 molecules are homologous to C-type lectins, the ligands for Nkrp1 molecules were presumed to be carbohydrates, but Nkpr1 molecules lack residues for coordinate binding of Ca^{++} that is required for authentic C-type lectin recognition of carbohydrates *(174)*. While the ligands for Nkrp1c have not yet been identified, Nkrp1f recognizes C-type lectin-related g (Clrg, also known as Clec2i, Dcl1) (355,*465,466*). Nkrp1f is presumed to be an activation receptor, because it has a charged transmembrane residue and no cytoplasmic signaling motifs. The inhibitory receptor, Nkrp1d, is expressed on all NK cells in C57BL/6 mice and is specific for Clrb (Clec2d; osteoclast inhibitory lectin, Ocil). Thus, the Nkrp1 family is an MHC-independent system that is presumably involved in self-tolerance and is the first example of a lectinlike receptor recognizing a lectinlike ligand unlike MHC-like ligands for other NKC-encoded receptors.

Recent genome sequence analysis suggests that *Nkrp1d* in other mouse strains is represented by *Nkrp1b*, an inhibitory receptor (*64,65,457,467*). The Nkrp1b molecule from SJL and SW mice was discovered to be reactive with the anti-NK1.1 mAb, highlighting the close similarities of these molecules and serologic cross-reactivity. Whereas the older literature suggested that there are also strain differences in transcript expression with markedly lower expression in BALB/c NK cells *(468)*, more recent data demonstrate abundant expression of Nkrp1 transcripts *(467)*. Moreover, the BALB/c allele of Nkpr1b also reacts with Clrb, indicating conserved specificity and function.

The Clr molecules belong to a small NKC-encoded family with type II orientation and C-type lectin homology *(469)*. They are most closely related to the CD69 molecule encoded by an adjacent gene. In C57BL/6 mice, seven Clr genes have been identified at the genomic level. RT-PCR analysis indicates that *Clrb* is broadly expressed, whereas *Clrg* and *Clrf* genes are present in restricted and nonoverlapping tissues, including NK cells, and *Clra* and *Clrc* transcripts have not yet been identified. *Clre,* a probable pseudogene, demonstrates numerous stop codons in its expected open reading frame. Genomic analysis indicates the existence of a rat *Clr* family *(458)*, whereas in humans, three genes, *LLT1 (470)*, *AICL (471)*, and *DCAL-1 (472)* are localized next to CD69 and are related to the Clr family of genes. Indeed, human NKRP1A binds LLT1, indicating that at least human LLT1 is a functional homologue of mouse Clr *(473,474)*. Thus, the Clr family consists of conserved molecules that are ligands for Nkrp1 receptors.

The genetics of the *Nkrp1* and *Clr* loci is especially interesting from several viewpoints. 1) These loci are comingled in the NKC, from rodents to humans (355,*458,467,473–475*) (Figure 16.3). 2) There is limited allelic polymorphism, with conservation of gene order and content, despite genetic proximity to the highly polymorphic *Ly49* cluster (355,*467*). 3) The *Nkpr1* alleles appear to be much less divergent than the corresponding *Ly49* alleles in the same inbred mouse strains (*204*,355,*467*). 4) The *Nkpr1-Clr* interval of the NKC appears to be genetically protected with suppression of recombination *(476,477)*. Genetic linkage of Nkrp1 and its ligands thus resembles the tight genetic linkage of receptor and ligand genes and recombinational suppression of the self-incompatibility (SI) loci in plants to prevent self-fertilization and related mating loci in other species *(478,479)*. Further, the coevolution of such linked genes for receptors and ligands also represents an interesting issue in evolutionary biology because reciprocal mutations in both receptor and ligand genes are simultaneously needed to generate new specificities *(478)*. Nevertheless, the genetic pressure to conserve the *Nkrp1-Clr* gene order and coding sequences may therefore reflect a critical role for Nkrp1 and Clr molecules in innate immune cell interactions and functions.

2B4, CD2, and Related Receptors

The 2B4 (CD244) molecule was originally identified on mouse NK cells with a mAb that perturbed mouse NK cell function (480). 2B4 is a type I integral membrane protein that belongs to the family of Ig-like molecules homologous to CD2, including CD48, CD58, signaling lymphocytic activation molecule (SLAM) (CD150), CD84, NTBA (NK, T, and B cell antigen; also known as SLAMF6, or Ly108), CD229 (Ly9), CD319 (CRACC, CD2-like receptor activating cytotoxic cells), and B lymphocyte activator macrophage expressed (BLAME) (*481,482*,483).

Although these receptors may be broadly expressed, 2B4, CD2, NTBA, and CRACC are expressed on NK cells. Whereas NTBA and CRACC are involved in homophilic interactions, 2B4 recognizes CD48, a GPI-linked molecule expressed on hematopoietic cells (483,*484*). CD48 itself is also recognized by CD2, albeit at a 9-fold lower affinity than by 2B4 ($K_d = \sim 16\,\mu M$). Anti-CD2 mAbs can stimulate NK cells in the redirected lysis assay *(485)* and granule exocytosis *(486)*, but $CD2^-$ NK cells can still mediate natural killing (10). The cytoplasmic domains of 2B4, NTBA, and CRACC as well as SLAM, CD84, and CD229 contain a motif with sequence similarity to the ITIM, termed the *immunoreceptor tyrosine-based switch motif* (ITSM) consisting of TxYxxV/I consensus sequence *(487)*. The ITSMs allow interactions with a signaling adapter, SLAM-associated protein (SAP, also known as SH2D1A). The importance of SAP and its associated receptors is highlighted by the X-linked lymphoproliferative syndrome (XLP, also known as Duncan's disease), a human immunodeficiency involving abnormal proliferation of T and B cells during Epstein-Barr virus infections due to mutations in SAP *(488)*.

SAP is related to Ewing's sarcoma–associated transcript (EAT2, also known as SH2D1B) and EAT2-related transducer (ERT, also known as SH2D1C) in rodents (483). SAP and the SAP-related molecules contain a single Src homology 2 (SH2) domain for interaction with the ITSM. 2B4 and NTBA can recruit SAP, whereas CRACC does not *(489,490)*. Instead, CRACC recruits EAT2, which functionally substitutes for SAP *(482)*. Subsequently, the SAP-related proteins appear to recruit a Src-family tyrosine kinase for downstream activation events.

The complexities of this receptor-ligand signaling pathway are still being unraveled. 2B4 can apparently inhibit as well as activate mouse NK cells (480). These outcomes may depend on spatial distribution, 2B4 isoforms, or differential recruitment of SAP or its related molecules (483). However, a 2B4-deficient mouse primarily displays effects consistent with 2B4 being primarily an inhibitory receptor *(491)*, although the inhibitory effect of 2B4 is more apparent in mice than humans (483). CRACC recruitment of EAT2 can promote signaling *(482)*, whereas in other studies recruitment leads to inhibition *(492)*. These differences may be species specific due to presence of Tyr residues in mouse but not human EAT2 that are required for inhibition *(482)*. Analysis of these discrepancies should enlighten NK cell function and signaling because 2B4 and related receptors demonstrate MHC-independent regulation of NK cells, mediate inhibition in a functionally distinct manner from the MHC-specific inhibitory receptors, and can activate NK cells.

Natural Cytotoxicity Receptors (NCRs)

A series of mAbs that redirected lysis of human NK cell clones lacking KIRs led to the identification of the "natural cytotoxicity receptors" (NCRs), NKp46 (NCR1, CD335), NKp44 (NCR2, CD336), and NKp30 (NCR3, CD337) (493,*494–497*). These molecules are selectively expressed on NK cells, although NKp44 is expressed only upon activation. Whereas NKp46 is encoded in the LRC (Figure 16.3), NKp44 and NKp30 are encoded in the class III region of the MHC on human chromosome 6 *(498,499)*. cDNA cloning revealed that they are type I integral proteins with one (NKp30, NKp44) or two (NKp46) Ig-like extracellular domains. They contain charged transmembrane residues for association with ITAM-signaling chains—that is, ζ–γ heterodimers (NKp46, NKp30) or DAP12 (NKp44). They appear to play a role in cytotoxicity against tumors of varying origins because anti-NCR antibodies block target killing *(500)*. However, NKp46 fusion proteins do not bind well to targets that appear to be recognized by NCRs (501), and a ligand for NKp44 appears to be up-regulated on $CD4^+$ T cells during HIV infection *(502)*, implying complex interactions that require further investigation.

In the mouse, only the gene for NKp46 is present in the syntenic region of chromosome 7, with the genes for other NCRs being absent (NKp44) or a pseudogene (NKp30) *(503)*. A mouse NKp46-Ig fusion protein binds RMA-S targets, and deficiency of NKp46 leads to impaired *in vivo* clearance of RMA-S cells *(504)*. Interestingly, human NCRs apparently recognize mouse tumors and vice versa, suggesting conservation of these receptor-ligand pairs across species but their tumor target ligands have remained elusive *(500)*.

Human NKp46 appears to recognize influenza hemagglutinin on infected cells (501). The interaction is dependent on sialic acid residues on oligosaccharides on NKp46 itself, but this specificity is difficult to explain due to the ubiquitous expression of sialylated saccharides. Conversely, NKp30 and NKp46 may recognize heparan sulfate proteoglycans on their cellular targets, although this is also controversial *(505,506)*. Nevertheless, a NKp46-deficient mouse is susceptible to influenza, consistent with a role for NKp46 in defense against influenza *(504)*, albeit possibly in an indirect manner *(507)*. These studies may provide important clues to understanding of a conserved receptor (NKp46) and other NCRs.

Other Activation Receptors

Several other NK cell-expressed molecules can activate cytolysis. For example, mAbs against mouse CD69 and Ly-6 and rat gp42 can trigger killing (31,*32*). CD69 is encoded in the NKC and is structurally related to other NKC-encoded receptors. Interestingly, CD69 expression is upregulated upon stimulation *(311)*, and its expression is not confined to NK cells *(508)*. CD69 is functionally active on a large variety of hematopoietic cells when cross-linked by anti-CD69 mAbs. Ly-6 belongs to a large family of small (15 to 18 kDa) GPI-anchored molecules that can activate lymphocytes when cross-linked *(509,510)*. Rat gp42 is a GPI-anchored protein with two Ig-like domains that was originally identified on IL-2-activated NK cells and the rat RNK-16 NK cell line *(32)*. Anti-gp42 can activate RNK-16 but not IL-2–activated NK cells. However, CD69, Ly-6 and gp42 are not expressed on freshly isolated NK cells and are expressed only after activation through other pathways, and are therefore not involved in triggering natural killing by freshly isolated NK cells. Although their physiological role is unknown, their activation potential and enhanced killing by IL-2–activated NK cells suggest that these molecules may contribute to this phenotype.

Receptors Involved in Recognition of Epithelial Tissues

Recent studies indicate that NK cells possess receptors that are specific for ligands expressed at cell–cell junctions in epithelial tissues. Interestingly, ligands, such as cadherins, carcinoembryonic antigen (CEA)–related adhesion molecules (CEACAMs), nectins, and nectinlike proteins (necls), are involved in forming adherens junctions and are engaged in homotypic or heterotypic interactions, and thus, are not normally exposed *(511)*. KLRG1 (also known as mast cell–associated function antigen, MAFA) is a lectinlike receptor with cytoplasmic ITIMs *(512–514)*. Unlike human *KLRG1*, mouse *Klrg1* resides relatively distant and centromeric from the rest of the NKC, consistent with gene duplication and chromosomal inversion events. First discovered on rat mast cells, it has a broader distribution in human and mouse, including NK and T cells, but not mast cells. Expression of KLRG1 on NK cells is down-regulated in MHC-I-deficient mice, unlike the Ly49s, which are upregulated, but no MHC binding has been observed for KLRG1 *(515)*. Recently, mouse KLRG1 was found to bind the "classical" cadherins, E-, N-, and R-cadherin (516,517). E-cadherin recognition by KLRG1 led to inhibition of NK lysis. Similarly, the human CEACAMs appear to be involved in MHC-independent inhibition of NK cell activity. In particular, CEACAM1 contains a cytoplasmic ITIM and can directly bind CEA, thereby potentially regulating NK cell activities in human MHC-I-deficient patients and during pregnancy (518,*519,520*). Thus, NK cells express inhibitory receptors for ligands normally expressed at adherens junctions.

NK cells also express activation receptors for molecules at the adherens junction—that is, nectins and necls. Specifically, they express CD226 (DNAM-1, DNAX accessory molecule-1), an LFA-1–associated receptor that recognizes necl-5 (CD155, poliovirus receptor, PVR) and nectin-2 (CD112) *(521)*. NK cells also express CD96 (tactile) that binds necl-5, and CRTAM (class I–restricted T cell–associated molecule), a receptor that recognizes necl-2 (522,*523,524*).

These studies suggest that these receptors may affect different NK cell functions as related to epithelial tissues (*511*,516). For example, the inhibitory receptors may regulate NK cell transmigration across an epithelial barrier or prevent NK cell attack against normal tissues (516,*525*). While the activation receptors could also affect NK cell transmigration (516,*525,526*), the activation receptors could be poised to attack cells that have disordered cell–cell junctions, such as tumors, which typically lose cadherin expression and expose nectins and necls, potentially making them more susceptible to NK attack, consistent with an "exposed-self" model for NK cell activation (Figure 16.2F, G). However, tumors may be become resistant to NK cells by altering expression of these molecules. Current evidence provides some support to these complex scenarios that will require further investigation *(511)*.

Accessory Molecules

The role of accessory molecules in NK cell activation has been difficult to address without knowledge of the "NK cell (activation) receptor." Nevertheless, NK cell function is critically dependent on classical accessory and adhesion molecules, such as LFA-1 *(527,528)*. Insect cells expressing ICAM-1, a ligand for LFA-1, can be killed by human NK cells through an LFA-1–dependent process, suggesting that LFA-1 alone is sufficient to trigger killing *(529)*. However, the insect cell targets could express ligands for unknown NK cell receptors. Recent studies also indicate that LFA-1 cross-linking does not lead to granule polarization, suggesting that it may be insufficient for triggering the killing process by itself *(101)*. How LFA-1 or other "accessory" molecules contribute to each activation receptor on NK cells remains to be systematically determined.

SIGNAL TRANSDUCTION IN NK CELLS

In general, the signal transduction pathways stimulated by NK cell activation receptors coupled to ITAM-containing signaling chains resemble those of TCR and B cell receptor (BCR) signaling (530). Activation receptor cross-linking leads to ITAM phosphorylation by Src family tyrosine kinases, recruitment and activation of Syk family tyrosine kinases, and subsequent downstream activation events. Inasmuch as TCR and BCR signaling is covered in detail in other chapters, we will highlight here some notable differences with TCR and BCR signaling.

In addition to difficulties in dissecting NK cell activation because of differences due to species (mouse, human), and cell origin (freshly isolated, activated, NK cell clones), there are additional complexities. 1) Like CTLs, NK cells form discrete protein clusters at the site of contact with their targets, termed the *immunological synapse* (*531*,532), although obviously the TCR is not involved. The NK immunological synapse (NKIS) is formed in discrete stages whereby CD2, f-actin, LFA-1, and Mac-1 accumulate in the peripheral supramolecular activation complex (pSMAC) whereas granules (perforin) accumulate centrally (cSMAC) (533). Inhibitory receptor engagement results in early KIR and SHP-1 recruitment to areas surrounded by LFA-1 *(534)*. Other pSMAC and cSMAC patterns are found depending on whether or not the contacts lead to cytolysis (532,535). Also, there is emerging data on the contribution of NKG2D/DAP10 and Vav1 to the NKIS *(536)*. 2) Individual NK cells may simultaneously express multiple activation receptors, each of which may associate with different ITAM-signaling chains that could be phosphorylated by different Src family tyrosine kinases. 3) NK cells express multiple Src kinases, including Lck, Fyn, Src, Yes, Lyn, and Fgr *(537)*, with redundancies in their contributions to ITAM phosphorylation. For example, Fyn is activated following Ly49D (DAP12) cross-linking, but NK cells deficient in Fyn, Lck, or both still kill in a Ly49D-dependent manner (538). 4) NK cells express both Syk family tyrosine kinases, ZAP-70 and Syk itself, whereas T and B cells express either, respectively, but not both. Further, deficiency of either ZAP-70, Syk, or both has only minimal effects on NK cell killing *(539)*, suggesting other pathways for transmitting NK activation signals. 5) NK cells express many adapter molecules found in T and B cells, but their contributions to NK signal transduction is less well defined. For example, SLP-76 is dispensable for NK cell signaling, although it is required for T cell signaling *(540)*. 6) Different isoforms of signal transduction molecules are responsible for NK cell activation. For example, mouse NK cells utilize phospholipase C-γ2 (PLCγ2) as a critical signaling mediator *(541)*, more like B cells than T cells *(542)*. 7) Finally, most studies have been performed on bulk populations of NK cells or NK cell clones, which may not be representative of pathways triggered in individual NK cells that may express only some but not all signaling molecules detected in the entire NK cell population. Taken together, these data strongly suggest multiple pathways for signal transduction in NK cells that may be dependent on which activation receptor (and associated signaling chain) is triggered *(543)*.

Reinforcing this concept are recent studies on the Vav family of guanine nucleotide exchange factors, Vav1, Vav2, and Vav3, which are all expressed in NK cells (544). Vav2 and Vav3 are required for FcRγ and DAP12 signaling, whereas Vav1 is required for DAP10 signal transduction. Additionally, NK cell number and differentiation are not apparently affected by Vav deficiencies even when they are required for NK cell activation. In contrast, deficiencies in Vav family members leads to T and B cell development defects *(545)*. Similarly, NK cells are not deficient in number or maturation state in PLCγ2-deficient mice, unlike B cells, which require PLCγ2 for development *(541,542)*. These observations suggest that signal transduction through NK cell activation receptors is generally not required for NK cell development, unlike T and B cells, or that there is redundancy in the pathways that contribute to NK cell development.

Recruitment and activation of PI3K appears to be critical to NK cell activation for target killing (546). How PI3K is activated depends on proximal signal transduction events. In the case of NKG2D, the YxxM motif in DAP10 is phosphorylated and recruits PI3K directly (547) that appears to be sufficient to activate NK cell killing in the absence of DAP12 or Syk family tyrosine kinases *(548)*. The pathway may be more complex in human NK cells, where recent evidence suggests that DAP10 also recruits a Grb2-Vav1 intermediate for activation *(549)*. For other activation receptors, Syk activation is upstream of PI3K *(550)* and may directly recruit PI3K *(551)*. PI3K in turn activates a mitogen-activated protein kinase (MEK) for stimulation of extracellular signal-regulated kinase (ERK) (546). Ultimately, actin polymerization occurs, and a large molecular weight complex is formed containing actin binding proteins *(552)*. Granules become polarized toward the target and exocytosis occurs, resulting in target apoptosis. Thus, the complexities of NK cell activation remain under investigation.

Biochemical Mechanism of Inhibition by NK Cell Receptors

A typical human KIR molecule has two ITIMs separated by ~24 residues. In contrast, Ly49A has only one ITIM per chain, but Ly49 molecules are normally expressed as homodimers. Each ITIM can be phosphorylated upon receptor cross-linking (difficult to visualize) or tyrosine phosphatase inhibition (165,553,*554–556*), presumably by a Src family tyrosine kinase as in B cells *(557)*, although redundant expression and function have precluded identification of a single kinase required for ITIM phosphorylation in NK cells. In studies of KIR transfectants of human Jurkat T cells, the KIR ITIM is phosphorylated by Lck *(558)*, but it is not known if this tyrosine kinase is responsible for phosphorylation of all inhibitory receptors in primary NK cells, especially because NK cells express multiple Src family tyrosine kinases. ITIM phosphorylation results in SHP-1 recruitment and activation (165,553,*554,555,559*). Two ITIMs are required for sequential binding of the two Src homology-2 (SH2) domains in SHP-1 *(560)*. The NK cell inhibitory receptors preferentially recruit SHP-1 rather than SHIP, although they may occasionally bind SHP-2 (553,*561,562*). However, a SHIP-deficient mouse demonstrates abnormalities in NK cell function and receptor expression (563). Nevertheless, available data strongly support an inhibitory mechanism consisting of receptor cross-linking followed by ITIM phosphorylation and recruitment of SHP-1, and that this mechanism operates with both structural types of inhibitory receptors.

The downstream target of the ITIM-recruited tyrosine phosphatase appears to be Vav1 in human NK cells (564). However, in view of the differential role of Vav2 and Vav3 but not Vav1 in murine NK cell activation by ITAM-signaling chains (544), this observation will need further evaluation. Moreover, other studies suggest earlier events in NK cell activation are blocked by inhibitory receptors, such as formation of the NKIS *(534,565,566)*. However, KIR phosphorylation occurs within clusters at the NKIS, which may serve to focus inhibition on downstream targets (567), such as Vav1, which is recruited into the mature synapse during NKG2D/DAP10 signaling *(536)*. Future studies should clarify these relationships.

Finally, investigators have observed that Ly49 receptors on NK cells can acquire their cognate MHC-I ligands from surrounding cells, resulting in display of both molecules on the NK cells *(568,569)*. Whether this contributes to *cis* effects on inhibitory receptor function or is physiologically important requires further evaluation.

NK CELL DEVELOPMENT

Early evidence indicated that the complete phenotypic and functional maturation of NK cells occurs in the BM and requires an intact microenvironment because BM ablation or congenital BM defects lead to abnormal NK cells *(570–574)*. Indeed, certain aspects of NK cell development are regulated by direct interactions between developing NK cells and stromal elements, such as interactions between membrane lymphotoxin-α (LTα)–expressing NK cell precursors and LTα-responsive stromal cells that are necessary for normal development *(112,575)*. *In vitro*, NK cells can be generated from early hematopoietic cells (*576–580*) in a cytokine cocktail consisting of stem cell factor (c-kit ligand), IL-7, flt-3 ligand (FL), and IL-15 (*581*,582). However, direct contact with stromal cells is required for acquisition of Ly49 receptors by developing NK cells. Recent evidence implicates the Tyro3 family of receptors (Tyro3, Mer, Axl) on NK cells and their ligands (Gas6, protein S) on stromal cells as being critical for expression of NK cell receptors and functional differentiation *in vitro* and *in vivo* (583). Thus, NK cell development requires certain cytokines and direct stromal cell contact.

A model has been proposed for the developmental process of mouse NK cells in the BM that is divided into several major steps (reviewed) in *[584,585]*). The earliest step involves the commitment of hematopoietic stem cells (HSC) in the BM to the common lymphoid progenitor (CLP) that can give rise to NK, T, and B cells, but not to myeloid cell lineages *(586,587)*. Mice deficient in various transcription factors, including Ikaros and PU.1, display severe defects in the development of all lymphoid cells, including NK cells, while myeloid and erythroid lineages are less affected (588,*589–592*). Thus, the earliest step of NK cell development appears to share a common pathway with other lymphocytes, providing evidence that NK cells belong to the lymphocyte lineage.

The CLP differentiates to a bipotential T/NK progenitor (T/NKP), reflecting the close resemblance of T and NK cell effector functions. T/NKP can give rise to T and NK cells, but not to other lineages, depending on culture conditions (593,*594–597*). Consistent with this bipotentiality, CD3ε and FcεRIγ Tg mice exhibit selective defects in both NK and T cell development *(598,599)*. More recently, in *in vitro* studies using BM stromal cell monolayers, T or NK cells can be generated from precursor populations, including undifferentiated thymocytes, depending on whether Notch signaling occurs (*594,600*,601).

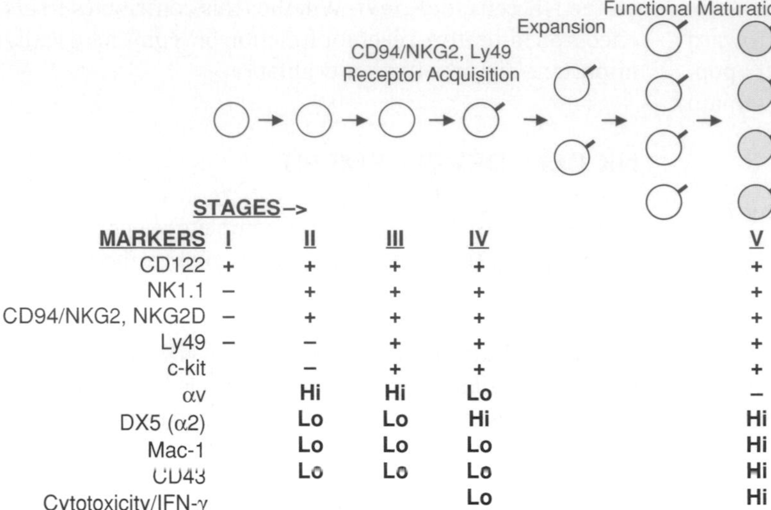

FIGURE 16.6 Developmental stages of committed mouse NK cells. During development in BM, informative surface markers characterize distinct stages from the NK cell progenitor to mature NK cells. After acquisition of NK cell receptors (NKG2 and Ly49), significant proliferation occurs while the cells are still immature. The licensing process may affect the proliferation phase (183). Modified from *(584)*.

The acquisition of IL-2/15Rβ subunit (CD122) marks the transition from T/NKP to a committed NKP *(596,602)* (Figure 16.6). In Ets1- or Id2-deficient mice, NK cell development appears to be blocked here because NK cells fail to develop while T and B cells develop normally (*603*,604). The committed NKP appears to become responsive to IL-15 at this stage because IL-15 or IL-15Rα–targeted mutations produce a relatively selective NK cell deficiency with effects only on relatively rare T cell subsets, such as NKT cells (48,49). Not surprisingly, mice deficient in other components of the IL-15R complex and its signaling pathway (IL-2Rβ, Jak3 and STAT5α/β) exhibit similar defects in NK cell development (39,*605–607*). IRF-1 (interferon regulatory factor 1)–deficient mice lack NK cells, and this defect can be overcome by the addition of IL-15, suggesting that stromal cells produce IL-15 in an IRF-1-dependent manner (608). Deficiency in T-bet, a T-box transcription factor involved in T helper development, also results in a defect in NK and NKT cell maturation *(609)*, further supporting a close developmental relationship between NK and NKT cells.

NKPs next differentiate into mature NK cells in a series of putative developmental intermediate stages that occur in the BM (70,*602*). The CD122$^+$ NK1.1$^-$ NKP has been denoted as intermediate Stage I (Figure 16.6) (70) and has also been isolated from fetal thymus (579,*596*). Thereafter, NK1.1 (Nkrp1c) is expressed (Stages II to V), comparable to studies of *in vitro* differentiation of human NK cells where NKR-P1A molecule is one of the earliest markers expressed *(610)*. Among the mouse CD3$^-$ CD122$^+$ NK1.1$^+$ population, there is an integrin αv$^+$ c-kit$^-$ population (Stage II) that can express CD94/NKG2 and NKG2D but not Ly49 (70). Subsequently, Ly49s are expressed along with both αv and c-kit (Stage III). The acquisition of CD94/NKG2 and Ly49 receptor expression on immature adult BM NK cells recapitulates their expression on fetal and neonatal NK cells in which CD94/NKG2 receptors are first expressed, then the cells acquire Ly49 expression in an ordered manner (196,611,*612*).

At Stage IV, integrin α2 (DX5) expression is increased and developing NK cells undergo vigorous proliferation (70) (Figure 16.6). Thereafter, as NK cells acquire high-level expression of Mac-1 (αMβ1) and CD43 (Stage V), proliferation markedly decreases unless challenged by pathogens such as viruses that can stimulate mature NK cell proliferation (70,613). NK cells at Stage V become fully capable of functional activities associated with mature peripheral NK cells. A selective NK cell deficiency in a Tg is manifested by a failure to generate mature, functional Mac-1^{high} cells *(614,615)*, consistent with this terminal differentiation step.

The aforementioned models suggest that developing murine NK cells expand at a phenotypically distinct stage and that NK cell development is characterized by a dynamic process involving changes in surface receptors for cytokines, extracellular matrix, and self- and target-recognition. Whether expression of these receptors represent functionally important, rate-limiting steps needs to be determined. Nevertheless, current models provide guidance for future investigation.

Like developing mouse NK cells, human NK cells display regulated *in vitro* development *(610,616–618)*, but there are some differences with mouse NK cell development. For example, IL-12 is important in human NK cell development *in vitro* (619), whereas mouse NK cells do not require IL-12 *(620–622)*. Human NK cell development also appears to be dependent on IFN-γ or IL-18, but there is no NK cell defect with deficiencies of IFN-γ or IL-18 *(623)*. Therefore, there may be *in vitro* versus *in vivo* or species effects to explain these differences in NK cell development.

ACQUISITION OF NK CELL TOLERANCE

Influence of Host MHC-I Environment

Although the MHC-specific inhibitory receptors explain the influence of MHC expression on NK cell effector functions against target cells, how these receptors are related to self-tolerance *in vivo* has been a challenging issue. Several hypotheses have been considered. An individual NK cell can simultaneously express multiple inhibitory receptors, but some may not recognize self-MHC. The "at least one receptor model" suggests tolerance is achieved as long as each NK cell expresses at least one receptor with self-MHC-specificity (297,*624*). There are changes in the repertoire of MHC-I-specific inhibitory receptors, depending on the MHC haplotype, but these differences are modest, regardless of whether the receptor is self-specific (297,*624*,625,*626*). As determined by antibody reactivity, the expression level of an NK receptor on an individual NK cell decreases when the host expresses the MHC ligand for that receptor (161,*162,627*). Functional analyses of NK cells with "down-regulated" receptor expression suggest that such NK cells are more sensitive to small changes in MHC ligand expression on the target, as explained by the "receptor calibration" model (625,*628*). However, these studies involved *in vitro* conditions that could alter their intrinsic functional capacities. Thus, several hypotheses based on the MHC-specific inhibitory receptors were proposed to account for NK cell self-tolerance.

There are several observations that need explanation when considering the role played by MHC-specific inhibitory receptors in NK cell self-tolerance. The "missing self" hypothesis implies that there should be overt NK cell autoreactivity in MHC-I–deficient hosts, but this was not observed in humans or mice (132,*133,1*34, 629,*630–632*). Instead, NK cells from MHC-I–deficient mice demonstrate poor killing of MHC-I-deficient targets or rejection of MHC-I–deficient BM, even though they appear normal in number, tissue distribution, and expression of activation receptors. Another very difficult issue is related to hybrid resistance whereby host NK cells in an F_1 hybrid animal can reject BM grafts from either inbred parent *(633,634)*. It was difficult to understand how NK cells discriminate between cells expressing the full complement of self-MHC alleles versus those otherwise normal cells expressing only some self-MHC molecules. NK cell–mediated rejection of MHC-I–sufficient BM grafts also depends on which host MHC-I allele is present (635,*636*). Thus, NK cells are regulated by host MHC environment, not just by the target cell in effector responses.

Also unexplained was the pairing of polymorphic inhibitory receptors with their highly polymorphic cognate MHC ligands (*202*,249). The genes for the receptors and their ligands are located on different chromosomes (i.e., the receptor and ligand genes segregate independently). Thus, there must be mechanisms to provide NK cells with the appropriate inhibitory receptors with specificity for self-MHC because the appropriate pairs are not inherited together, unlike the closely linked *Nkpr1-Clr* gene pairs (355).

The Licensing Hypothesis

Recent studies with target cell-free stimulation and single cell assays of NK cell responsiveness have been revealing (183,637). Freshly explanted, resting murine NK cells from MHC-I-deficient mice were functionally defective in triggering by immobilized antiactivation receptor antibodies (183). Conversely, in wild-type mice, functional competence correlated with expression of a Ly49 inhibitory receptor for self-MHC-I (183). Moreover, NK cells without expression of known self-receptors were hyporesponsive (637). Particularly informative were studies with a single chain trimer (SCT) MHC-I molecule, consisting of antigenic peptide-linker-β2m-linker-H2K^b as a single polypeptide that binds only Ly49C (183). In Tg mice expressing only this MHC-I molecule, only Ly49C$^+$ NK cells were functionally competent. Thus, NK cells normally acquire the competence to be triggered through their activation receptors by their MHC-specific receptors interacting with host MHC-I (Figure 16.7), a process termed *licensing*.

Licensing thus leads to appropriate pairing of inhibitory receptors with self-MHC and strongly suggests that there are two types of self-tolerant NK cells (Figure 16.7). Regardless of the MHC-I environment, licensed NK cells are tolerant because they have inhibitory receptors for self-MHC, the same receptors involved in licensing. Unlicensed NK cells are also tolerant because they are not functionally competent and have no need for inhibition by self-MHC under steady-state conditions. In hosts heterozygous for MHC alleles, each MHC allele could potentially license different NK cell populations. This aspect of licensing is relevant to hybrid resistance because an $(A \times B)F_1$ hybrid animal should have NK cells that are separately licensed on different MHC alleles. F_1 hybrid NK cells that were licensed by MHC alleles from parent A should be inhibited by A alleles but not B alleles and thus reject BM from parent B. The converse should also be true. In the F_1 animal itself, NK cells are licensed by either parental allele, so all NK cells should be inhibited by normal tissues that codominantly express both MHC alleles. Licensing potentially explains how NK cells distinguish cells expressing the full complement of MHC-I from those expressing only some alleles.

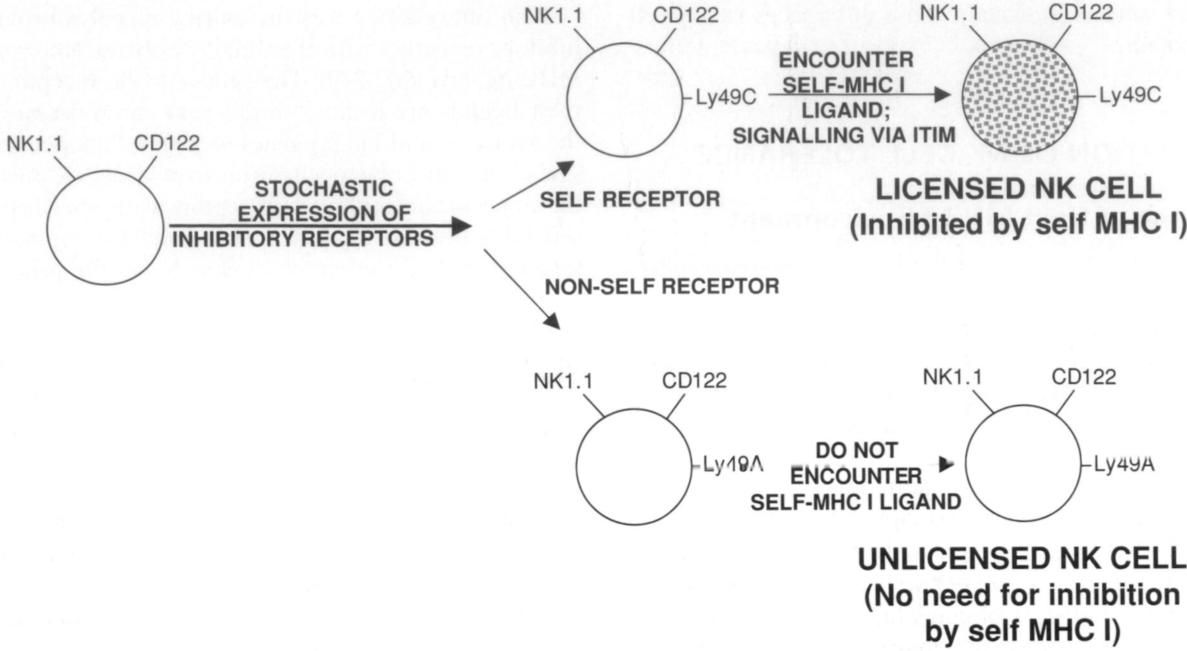

FIGURE 16.7 Licensing of NK cells by host MHC-I. Depicted is the situation in a mouse expressing only $H2K^b$ that is a ligand for Ly49C but not Ly49A. Cells expressing Ly49C therefore have a self-specific receptor whereas those expressing Ly49A do not. Ly49C engagement by self-MHC-I results in a licensed NK cell that has functional competence to be triggered through its activation receptors. These cells can be inhibited by self-MHC through the same receptor that conferred licensing. $Ly49A^+$ NK cells remain self-tolerant because they are unlicensed. For clarity, only one MHC allele and cells expressing one Ly49 receptor are shown. Normally, the host has multiple MHC alleles, each of which could license different NK cells, and individual NK cells express multiple Ly49s simultaneously. Each NK cell is likely to be licensed separately, potentially by different MHC alleles, and through different Ly49s. Taken from (183).

Although licensing is a positive outcome (i.e., the acquisition of functional competence), it requires the ITIM of the self-specific Ly49 receptor to deliver signals that ultimately result in a licensed NK cell (183) (Figure 16.7). Although this appears to occur in the BM, the nature of such signals is not yet known. At least two qualitatively different models are being considered. The MHC-specific receptor could confer licensing in a positive way (stimulatory model) by delivery of signals that directly induce a differentiation process and license NK cells. In the inhibitory model, the MHC-specific receptors may act to decrease the effect of a putative, as yet uncharacterized, self-specific activation receptor. When unimpeded by self-MHC-I, NK cells may become hyporesponsive due to overstimulation through the activation receptor. This model is somewhat akin to T cell anergy. Both models are similar to those previously proposed *(638)*, but engagement of the MHC-specific receptor with self-MHC is now known to be a required key step (183) and is common to both models. Also, the models are not mutually exclusive and either could be affected by co-receptors or adhesion molecules. Thus, studies of these tolerance mechanisms should be forthcoming.

Recent studies suggest that human NK cells are also subjected to a similar process involving KIR and self-HLA ligands (639). These effects may be relevant to the increasing awareness that the outcome of human disorders is associated with certain combinations of KIR and HLA genotypes (250). Such KIR-HLA relationships frequently involve pairs with high affinities and resolution of chronic infections (257) and are difficult to explain when only considering effector inhibitory function of the KIRs. Thus, licensing may be clinically relevant.

ROLE OF NK CELLS IN IMMUNE RESPONSES

Mature NK cells in the periphery are involved in rapid innate defense. However, they constitute only a small population of cells (about 2.5% of splenic leukocytes in C57BL/6 mice). How can this small population quickly respond with enough of a critical mass to effect significant innate defense? One mechanism involves the expression of multiple activation receptors by individual NK cells *(359)*. In contrast to clonally distributed TCRs endowing the individual

T cell with the ability to respond only to one antigen, an individual NK cell appears capable of responding to multiple activation receptor ligands. Further, the naïve T cell population contains only rare cells with a TCR for the relevant antigen, whereas large percentages of the NK cell population express any given activation receptor in an overlapping fashion. This multiple activation receptor expression on sizeable subpopulations would allow a substantial number of NK cells to quickly respond to a given specific insult. Another mechanism is related to their constitutive expression of cytokine receptors that permit many NK cells to be stimulated by pro-inflammatory cytokines produced early in the course of an immune response. Thus, large numbers of NK cells can rapidly respond to a particular stimulus through their activation or cytokine receptors.

Another issue in NK cell immune responses concerns their tissue location. Mature peripheral NK cells are found primarily in the blood, spleen, and liver. The homing of NK cells to these locations is not well characterized, but NK cells appear to have developmentally regulated expression of a number of integrins that may play a role in their localization as well as effector functions (70,*640*). In addition, several chemokines, including CXCL12 and MIP1α, have been implicated in NK cell localization to other tissues during immune responses (*641*,642–*646*).

Interestingly, immunohistochemical *in situ* staining has shown that NK cells are localized to the red pulp of the spleen *(647,648)*. In the liver, they are in the sinusoidal regions rather than the parenchyma, and few NK cells are present in other solid organs. Surprisingly, there are relatively few NK cells in naïve lymph nodes *(647,649)*. Injection of tumor targets leads to NK cell accumulation if the targets are sensitive to natural killing *in vitro (650)*. In viral infections, NK cells infiltrate the liver parenchyma in the vicinity of infected foci *(644,647)*. Although NK cells may be less effective in killing when they migrate into parenchymal tissues *(651)*, others have not recapitulated tissue-specific differences in NK effector function *(652)*. Thus, NK cells seem best suited for surveying the blood for transformed or infected cells and pathogens though interactions with DCs support additional roles (discussed later).

NK Cells and Tumor Surveillance

Abundant literature supports a role for NK cells in resisting tumor growth and metastasis *(3)*. In addition, LAK cells have been infused into patients with cancers refractory to conventional therapy *(653)*. Several cases of complete remission were reported, but the treatment required intravenous administration of high doses of IL-2 that has significant toxicity.

Most prior work on NK cells and anti-tumor effects utilized experimental protocols involving adoptive transfer of tumor cells into mice where NK cells can eliminate >90% of tumor cells within the first 24 hours *(654)*. Several long term assays of*in vivo* tumor clearance are available, such as survival or lesion size. However, T cell immune responses need to be excluded even in syngeneic hosts due to the possibility of tumor-specific peptides. Clearance of intravenous-administered radiolabeled tumor cells can be measured with radioactivity of the lung as an index of tumor burden. Because this lung clearance assay can be performed as early as 4 hours after tumor inoculation, it is relatively confined to innate NK cell responses in the unimmunized host (16,*614*). With these assays, perforin-deficient mice are unable to clear tumors *(655)*, and augmentation of NK cell activity with various agents increases the capacity of the hosts to eliminate tumors *(654)*.

However, few studies are available on control of primary tumor formation by NK cells—that is, tumor surveillance—that have only recently garnered attention (656). Probably the most systematic studies in a single experimental model involve fibrosarcoma development after subcutaneous methylcholanthrene challenge *(657–659)*. In brief, NK cells collaborate with NKT cells in preventing fibrosarcomas through mechanisms involving perforin, TRAIL, and IFNγ. There is also evidence for involvement of NKG2D *(435)* and its ligands with respect to the immunoediting of tumors by NK cells *(437,438)*.

NK Cells in Host Defense Against Pathogens

Although NK cells reportedly respond to a wide variety of microorganisms *(660)*, the role of NK cells in infections is probably best illustrated by human patients with selective NK cell deficiencies (661,*662*,*663*,664). Although the molecular basis for most human NK cell deficiencies is unknown, several points can be gleaned: 1) NK cell deficiency is associated with a propensity for severe or recurrent virus infections, particularly herpes viruses. 2) Difficulty with tumors is not a common feature, except for virus-related lesions. 3) The disorder is rare, perhaps because patients succumb to overwhelming infection before the syndrome is recognized. 4) Defective NK cells can be found in other genetic and acquired immunodeficiency disorders that affect other immune components. For example, NK cell activity is significantly diminished in AIDS *(665,666)*. NK cell infection with herpesvirus 6 induces *de novo* expression of CD4 rendering susceptibility to HIV-1 infection *(667)*, perhaps accounting, in part, for increased susceptibility of AIDS patients to opportunistic infections, such as severe CMV (668). Immature NK cell number and function in the developing fetus may be clinically relevant to the classic "TORCH" syndrome, birth defects associated with maternal Toxoplasma, rubella, CMV, and herpesvirus infections *(669–671)*. Thus, NK cells appear to be especially important in controlling infections, especially from herpes viruses.

In mouse models, detailed and ongoing evaluation of mouse NK cell responses, especially against viral and Listeria infections, have been especially revealing (summarized in *[672,673]*). For example, beige mice are susceptible to MCMV infections (674). *In vivo* antibody depletion of NK cells results in marked viral replication in internal organs (spleen, liver), and lethality with MCMV, vaccinia virus, or mouse hepatitis virus (675,*676,677*). A similar phenotype was observed in Tg mice lacking NK cells *(652,678)*. Interestingly, if depleting antibody was given to wild-type mice later in the infection, there was no untoward effect *(676)*. Thus, NK cells are significant in early, innate immunity to infections.

NK Cell Cytokine Responses and Production During Infection

During infection, NK cells can respond to several different cytokines resulting in production of other cytokines. In Listeriosis, the classic model for T cell–dependent resistance, *scid* mice achieve acute control of infection despite absence of T cells *(679)*, due to early NK cell production of IFNγ *(680)*. However, NK cells do not appear to respond directly to Listeria. Rather, macrophages produce IL-12 that then stimulate NK cell secretion of IFNγ and infection control (121,*681*). Further, TNF-α can synergize with IL-12 to induce NK cell production of IFNγ, whereas IL-10 is antagonistic (121). The increased susceptibility of mice lacking IL-12 receptor, IFNγ, or the IFNγ receptor signaling pathway *(682–685)* are consistent with macrophage production of IL-12 that stimulates NK cells to secrete IFNγ in Listeriosis.

While a similar IL-12-IFNγ pathway is also operational in MCMV infections (*673,678,*686), IL-18 also contributes somewhat to NK cell control of MCMV *(687)*. However IL-12 appears to be more critical than IL-18 because uniform lethality was observed in IL-12p35$^{-/-}$ mice challenged with MCMV, while all IL-18$^{-/-}$ mice survived *(687)*. On the other hand, neutralization of IL-18 is a common feature of orthopoxviruses *(688)*. For example, ectromelia virus (EV, mousepox) contains an ORF for an IL-18 binding protein (IL18BP) that effectively neutralizes the effects of IL-18 on NK cells *(689)*. In addition to augmented IFNγ production, IL-18 enhances perforin-dependent cytotoxicity *(623,690,691)*.

Importantly, not all viral infections are controlled by NK cells. For example, NK cell depletion has little effect on lymphocytic choriomeningitis virus (LCMV) infections (*673*,675,*692*). Yet many NK cell activities are stimulated by LCMV infection.

During infections, even with LCMV, cytotoxicity of NK cells is enhanced, and proliferation ensues. These events constitute systemic effects directly or indirectly mediated by cytokines, such as IL-12, IL-18, and IFNα/β *(693)*. However, IFNγ production is not seen in LCMV infections (*678*,694). This apparent paradox is due to an inhibitory effect of IFNα/β on IL-12–dependent IFNγ production (694). Inhibition by IFNα/β is mediated through the STAT1 signaling pathway. In the absence of STAT1, IL-12 responsiveness is restored and IFNα/β induces IFNγ production. Although it remains to be determined how the IFNα/β response to LCMV differs from MCMV, these studies indicate that the NK cell cytokine response to infection varies with the pathogen even though many responses may appear to be similar.

A challenging area of investigation is the role of IL-15 in NK cell responses *in vivo (695)* because IL-15 and IL-15Rα–deficient mice lack NK cells (48,49). Nevertheless, NK cells can be stimulated during infection by IL-15 and control viral replication during *in vitro* cultures *(695–699)*. Moreover, IL-15 can provide protection to *Herpes simplex* viral infections *(699)*. Finally, IFNα/β can stimulate IL-15 production that can drive NK cell proliferation *(700)*.

NK cell responses to cytokines are also regulated by other innate lymphocytes. For example, in TCR$\delta^{-/-}$ mice, Listeria infection is enhanced compared to TCR$\beta^{-/-}$ mice and is associated with diminished production of IFNγ by NK cells, suggesting that γ/δT cells regulate NK cell responses *(701)*. Similarly, NKT cells can regulate NK cells because administration of α-galactosylceramide, a potent ligand for the TCR on NKT cells, results in nearly concomitant activation of NK cells, possibly due to release of IFNγ by the NKT cell (67). Inasmuch as NKT cells can recognize glycolipid antigens in Mycobacteria *(702,703)*, these studies indicate a potential physiologically important mechanism for NK cell activation in innate immunity to these organisms.

NK Cell Activation Receptors in Infection

There are several observations from studies of viral evasion indicating the importance of NK cell activation receptors in infection. Because viruses have evolved numerous strategies to down-regulate MHC-I molecules on infected cells to avoid MHC-I-restricted cytotoxic T lymphocytes *(139)*, virally infected cells should have enhanced susceptibility to NK cell lysis. However, viruses also encode proteins that interfere with natural killing (for recent review, see [704]).

In many cases, viral interference of natural killing is related to enhanced function of inhibitory MHC-I-specific NK cell receptors. For example, murine and rat CMV contain ORFs *m144* and *r144*, respectively, which encode molecules with sequence homology to MHC-I and enhance *in vivo* virulence, presumably by interacting with as yet unidentified NK cell inhibitory receptors (705,*706–708*). Human CMV (HCMV) encodes an MHC-I-like molecule (UL18) that interacts with LIR1 (ILT2), an Ig-like inhibitory receptor on NK cells (261,709). HCMV also encodes a peptide that binds and enhances expression of HLA-E that in turn binds CD94/NKG2A, a lectinlike NK cell inhibitory receptor (294,710). Another example is the selective down-regulation of MHC-I by the human immunodeficiency virus, HIV-1 *(711)*. In this case, the virus down-regulates HLA-A and B but not HLA-C or E; the former HLA molecules tend to be restricting elements for MHC-I-restricted CTLs, while the latter are selectively recognized by human KIRs and CD94/NKG2A. Therefore, viruses have evolved mechanisms to selectively engage inhibitory receptors that presumably prevent the action of NK cell activation receptors.

Viruses can also directly block triggering of NK cell activation receptors. For example, both human and mouse CMV block NKG2D recognition of its ligands with functional consequences *in vitro* and *in vivo* (discussed in greater detail earlier in this chapter) (405,*411*,442,*443–446,712*). More generally, the Kaposi's sarcoma–associated herpesvirus (KSHV) avoids NK cell activation through K5 that down-regulates expression of ICAM-1 and B7-2, ligands for NK cell coreceptors involved in target-induced stimulation *(713)*. Indeed, the interaction of LFA-1 on the NK cell with target ICAM-1 is critical for NK cell killing of targets *(714)*. Thus, viruses encode multiple proteins to specifically thwart NK cell responses through their activation receptors.

The viral evasion strategies implicate NK cell activation receptors that specifically recognize infected cells; these receptors are just beginning to be identified. Human NKp46 binds hemagglutinin of influenza virus and hemagglutinin-neuraminidase of parainfluenza virus, suggesting it may be involved in resistance to these viruses (501). However, this interaction is dependent on sialic acid residues that are widely expressed, and the *in vivo* significance of these findings is difficult to assess in humans. Nevertheless, recent studies in NKp46–deficient mice corroborate these findings *(504)*.

The autosomal dominant *Cmv1* gene in the NKC is responsible for resistance of certain mouse strains to MCMV (*476,477*,715,*716*); MCMV-resistant C57BL/6 mice are susceptible when depleted of NK cells *(717)*. Extensive genetic and immunological evidence established that *Ly49h* is responsible for genetic resistance to MCMV (*359,717*,718–720). A DAP12 signaling mutant mouse could not resist MCMV *(721)*, consistent with *in vitro* signaling studies showing that Ly49H signals through DAP12 (*358*,718). Thus, Ly49H is an NK cell activation receptor responsible for genetic resistance to MCMV.

The ligand for Ly49H is encoded by the *m157* ORF in MCMV (354,356). M157 has a predicted MHC-I fold, among 11 other MCMV molecules. Interestingly, in mice lacking adaptive immunity, m157 mutant MCMV clones emerge during MCMV infection, indicating selection pressure from Ly49H$^+$ NK cells result in escape mutant viruses (722). The reasons for maintenance of *m157* in the MCMV genome are still under investigation, but several observations suggest *m157* may be advantageous to the virus under certain circumstances: 1) m157 binds to an inhibitory Ly49 receptor in certain mouse strains (356). 2) *m157*-deletion viruses cause a modest decrease in viral titers in mice lacking Ly49H, suggesting another immune evasion role *(723)*. 3) Host-virus coevolution often results in attenuated viruses *(724)*, and other MCMV proteins have positive effects on host responses *(725)*. 4) Finally, a unique aspect of herpesvirus biology is the capacity to become latent. If the virus kills the host during the acute viral replicative phase during which Ly49H mediates its control, then there will be no latent phase. Additional studies of m157 will be required to fully understand its biology.

Loci for resistance to other pathogens, such as mouse pox (ectromelia) virus and HSV, have also been genetically mapped to the NKC *(726,727)*. These loci are termed *Rmp1* and *Rhs1*, respectively, and C57BL/6 mice are resistant. However, recent studies have reported that *Rhs1* independently segregates from *Cmv1 (727)*. Nevertheless, the parallel phenotypes with *Cmv1* suggest that other NKC encoded NK cell activation receptors may be involved in NK cell–mediated resistance to other viruses.

In addition to target killing, NK cell activation receptors also trigger cytokine production *in vitro*. Although the relative contribution of this pathway of cytokine secretion to NK cell function in infection is currently unknown, Ly49H$^+$ NK cells can be selectively activated to produce IFNγgnd chemokines within 6 to 8 hours after coincubation *in vitro* with MCMV-infected macrophages or m157 transfectants (354,*728*), and m157 itself is expressed soon after infection *(729)*, indicating that competent NK cells can respond within hours of recognizing virus-infected cells.

These findings, however, contrast with the relative "nonspecific" stimulation of NK cells found during early MCMV infection *in vivo* where IFNγ production was not confined to the Ly49H$^+$ NK cell subset (613). Moreover, while direct assessment of NK cell proliferation by FACS analysis of *in vivo* BrdU (bromo-deoxyuridine) incorporation (613) confirmed that infection stimulates NK cell proliferation *(730,731)*, it also revealed that early (days 1 to 2 postinfection) *in vivo* NK cell proliferation was nonse lective with respect to Ly49H expression. This proliferation resembled the cytokine-driven "bystander proliferation" observed in T cells in response to viral infections or stimulation with IFNα/β *(732)*, suggesting that the initial phase of viral-induced NK cell proliferation represents a nonspecific response to pro-inflammatory cytokines (IL-12, IFNα/β) and proliferative cytokines such as IL-15. The nonselective proliferation phase was followed by a period of preferential proliferation of Ly49H$^+$ NK cells peaking at days 4 to 6 of MCMV infection (613). The selective phase of NK cell proliferation reflected the augmentation of pro-proliferative cytokine stimulation by Ly49H signaling mediated via DAP12 *(733)*. In vaccinia infection, the initial phase of nonspecific NK cell proliferation was found but the later specific proliferation of Ly49H$^+$ NK cells was not (613). Thus, initial virus-specific NK cell responses may be masked by generic cytokine responses and only later are detectable.

NK AND DC INTERACTIONS

Given that both NK and DCs, when separately studied, are critical early responders in host immune defense, it is not surprising that these cells communicate in a bidirectional manner (734). In this "cross-talk," NK cells can respond to signals derived from DCs and vice versa (735,736,*737*, *738*). Data support both cell contact-independent and -dependent pathways.

contact independent pathways are perhaps better understood. Activated DCs can produce cytokines, including IFNα/β, IL-12, IL-15, and apparently IL-2 *(27,739–742)*. As mentioned previously, all of these cytokines can stimulate NK cell production of other cytokines, such as IFNγ. Moreover, these cytokines enhance NK cell cytotoxicity by increasing expression of perforin and granzymes as well as perforin-independent cytotoxic pathways. The cytokines can also enhance signaling through ITAM-signaling chain-associated receptors *(743)*. A variety of stimuli, such as certain TLR ligands (*27,741*,744), can activate DCs to produce cytokines that activate NK cells, although it remains to be established whether all DC stimuli are capable of similar effects. Nevetheless, TLR9-dependent activation of pDCs in MCMV infections is critical for appropriate NK cell control of infection (744).

Direct NK–DC cell–cell contact can also enhance NK cell activation (734). Several molecules have been implicated in this process, including cytokine-induced DC expression of ligands for human or mouse NKG2D *(745,746)*. Human DCs can also activate resting NK cells via the NKp30 receptor *(747)*. Other studies indicate that mouse NK cells can be activated by DCs in a TREM-2–dependent manner through the DAP12 signaling pathway *(748)*.

Conversely, NK–DC interactions can induce DC maturation *(738)*. For example, MHC-I-deficient targets can activate NK cells, which then induce DC maturation (749). NK–DC interactions also enhance TH1 polarization apparently through NK cell production of IFNγ (750). During MCMV infections, recognition of virus-infected cells by NK cells is critical for maintenance of DC subsets in the spleen *(751)*. NK cells can also prime DCs to stimulate protective memory T cell responses against lymphomas (749). While NK–DC cell contact is also subject to inhibitory effects and even killing of DCs by NK cells *(752,753)*, the capacity of NK–DC interactions to induce T cell responses (*746*,749,750,*754*) has led to interest in exploiting these interactions for therapeutic vaccines *(755)*.

Although a hallmark of DC maturation is migration to a draining lymph node (LN), very few NK cells are present in the resting LN *(647)*. Interestingly, however, deliberate introduction of DCs into the lymphatics leads to robust recruitment of activated NK cells (750). Real-time imaging indicates that NK cells contact DCs in the superficial regions of the LNs, where they are less motile and their interactions with DCs are more extensive than T cell motility and contacts with DCs *(756)*. Leishmania infection led to NK cell secretion of IFNγ and migration to the paracortex where CD4 T cell activation occurred, indicating dynamic interactions in the LN not previously appreciated.

Recent evidence also suggest differences in LN NK cells in terms of capacity to be activated as compared to NK cells from conventional sources (peripheral blood, spleen) *(740,757)*. For example in humans, nearly all NK cells in the LN are CD56^{bright}, whereas only ~10% of peripheral blood NK cells are CD56^{bright} *(649)*. Since CD56^{bright} NK cells have greater capacity to produce cytokines and lower cytotoxic capacity as compared to CD56^{dim} NK cells that dominate peripheral blood, LN NK cell populations appear to be particularly poised to stimulate subsequent immune responses. Moreover, LN NK cells appear to differ in capacity to respond to DCs *(758)*.

Finally, NK cells express markers associated with DCs, such as CD11b (Mac-1, αM/β2, CD11b/CD18) and CD11c (p150/95, CD11c/CD18), that led to recent descriptions of cells with dual NK and DC phenotypes *(759–761)*. However, whether such NK/DC cells are truly a distinct or overlapping lineage of cells, separable from conventional NK cells, remains to be established. In this regard, it is notable that NK cells frequently express markers originally thought to be exclusively found on other cells, such as B220 on B cells *(9)* and Mac-1.

NK CELLS AND MATERNAL–FETAL INTERACTIONS

One enigmatic area of continuing interest concerns NK cells in maternal–fetal interactions (summarized in [*762,763*,764]). Several observations are related: 1) Initially described as granulated metrial gland cells, maternal NK cells accumulate in the uterus, near the fetal trophoblast layer, in all mammalian species examined thus far. 2) Accumulation is related to local production of IL-15 *(765)*. 3) Uterine NK cells more closely resemble CD56^{high} subpopulation, but there are still phenotypic differences, including expression of activation markers and different repertoire of MHC-specific receptors. 4) Human trophoblasts express the nonclassical MHC-I molecule, HLA-G, *(766)* but not other MHC-I or -II molecules. 5) Trophoblasts are sensitive to NK cells *(767)*, but deficiencies of mouse NK cells are not associated with significant changes in fecundity. 6) Mice lacking NK cells show defects in placental blood vascular remodeling that appears to be IFNγ-dependent (768). 7) There are significant differences in the anatomy of the maternal–fetal interface that may limit extrapolation of experimental results from one species to another (764). Nevertheless, uterine NK cells may provide important clues to understanding maternal–fetal interactions.

NK CELLS IN HUMAN DISEASE

Throughout this chapter, we have used human disorders involving NK cells to help illustrate their biology. In addition, NK cells are associated with autoimmune disorders *(769)*, such as multiple sclerosis, where they may regulate pro-inflammatory cells *(770)*. Interestingly, NK cell proliferative disorders are associated with both chronic viral infections (Epstein-Barr virus) and autoimmune phenomenon (8,*771*). NK cell malignancies can appear as lethal midline granuloma due to the propensity of NK lymphomas to present in the sinus and nasopharyngeal passages and be especially destructive *(772)*. NK cells are also associated with hydroa vacciniforme and hypersensitivity to mosquito bites *(773)*. Dysfunctional NK cells are found in patients with familial perforin deficiency *(774)* who typically demonstrate hemophagocytic lymphohistiocytosis that is also found in the macrophage activation syndrome and systemic-onset juvenile rheumatoid arthritis *(775)*.

Thus, as immunologists and physicians gain more appreciation for the molecular basis for NK cell biology, the future holds promise for insight into a number of enigmatic and unusual human diseases as well as common disorders, such as HCV and HIV infections, and exploitation of NK cells for immunotherapy.

ACKNOWLEDGMENTS

I thank members of my laboratory and our collaborators for their continued interest in dissecting the molecular basis for NK cell activities and tolerance. I thank Marco Colonna, Tony French, and Sungjin Kim for their review of the manuscript. Investigations in the author's laboratory are supported by the NIH, the Barnes-Jewish Hospital Research Foundation, and the Howard Hughes Medical Institute.

REFERENCES

1. Kiessling R, Klein E, Wigzell H. Natural killer cells in the mouse. I. Cytotoxic cells with specificity for mouse Moloney leukemia cells: Specificity and distribution according to genotype. *European J Immunol.* 1975;5:112–117.
2. Herberman RB, Nunn ME, Lavrin DH. Natural cytotoxic reactivity of mouse lymphoid cells against syngeneic and allogeneic tumors. I. Distribution of reactivity and specificity. *International Journal of Cancer.* 1975;16:216.
5. Timonen T, Ortaldo JR, Herberman RB. Characteristics of human large granular lymphocytes and relationship to natural killer and K cells. *J Exp Med.* 1981;153(3):569–582.
6. Inverardi L, Witson JC, Fuad SA, et al. CD3 negative "small agranular lymphocytes" are natural killer cells. *J Immuno.* 1991;146:4048–4052.
8. Lamy T, Loughran TP, Jr. Clinical features of large granular lymphocyte leukemia. *Semin Hematol.* 2003;40(3):185–195.
12. Lanier LL, Phillips JH, Hackett J, Jr., et al. Natural killer cells: definition of a cell type rather than a function. *J Immunol.* 1986; 137(9):2735–2739.
13. Ritz J, Campen TJ, Schmidt RE, et al. Analysis of T-cell receptor gene rearrangement and expression in human natural killer clones. *Science.* 1985;228:1540.
15. Dorshkind K, Pollack SB, Bosma MJ, et al. Natural killer (NK) cells are present in mice with severe combined immunodeficiency (scid). *J Immunol.* 1985;134:3798–3801.
16. Hackett J, Jr., Bosma GC, Bosma MJ, et al. Transplantable progenitors of natural killer cells are distinct from those of T and B lymphocytes. *Proc Natl Acad Sci U S A.* 1986;83(10):3427–3431.
20. Anderson P, Caligiuri M, Ritz J, et al. CD3-negative natural killer cells express zeta TCR as part of a novel molecular complex. *Nature.* 1989;341(6238):159–162.
23. Grimm EA, Mazumder A, Zhang HZ, et al. Lymphokine-activated killer cell phenomenon. Lysis of natural killer-resistant fresh solid tumor cells by interleukin 2-activated autologous human peripheral blood lymphocytes. *J Exp Med.* 1982;155(6):1823–1841.
24. Trinchieri G, Matsumoto-Kobayashi M, Clark SC, et al. Response of resting human peripheral blood natural killer cells to interleukin 2. *J Exp Med.* 1984;160(4):1147–1169.
25. Phillips JH, Lanier LL. Dissection of the lymphokine-activated killer phenomenon. Relative contribution of peripheral blood natural killer cells and T lymphocytes to cytolysis. *J Exp Med.* 1986;164(3): 814–825.
29. Brooks CG, Holscher M, Urdal D. Natural killer activity in cloned cytotoxic T lymphocytes: regulation by interleukin 2, interferon, and specific antigen. *J Immunol.* 1985;135(2):1145–1152.
31. Karlhofer FM, Yokoyama WM. Stimulation of murine natural killer (NK) cells by a monoclonal antibody specific for the NK1.1 antigen. IL-2-activated NK cells possess additional specific stimulation pathways. *J Immunol.* 1991;146(10):3662–3673.
33. Meresse B, Chen Z, Ciszewski C, et al. Coordinated induction by IL15 of a TCR-independent NKG2D signaling pathway converts CTL into lymphokine-activated killer cells in celiac disease. *Immunity.* 2004;21(3):357–366.
39. Suzuki H, Duncan GS, Takimoto H, et al. Abnormal development of intestinal intraepithelial lymphocytes and peripheral natural killer cells in mice lacking the IL-2 receptor beta chain. *J Exp Med.* 1997;185(3):499–505.
40. DiSanto JP, Muller W, Guy-Grand D, et al. Lymphoid development in mice with a targeted deletion of the interleukin 2 receptor gamma chain. *Proc Natl Acad Sci U S A.* 1995;92(2):377–381.
48. Lodolce JP, Boone DL, Chai S, et al. IL-15 receptor maintains lymphoid homeostasis by supporting lymphocyte homing and proliferation. *Immunity.* 1998;9(5):669–676.
49. Kennedy MK, Glaccum M, Brown SN, et al. Reversible defects in natural killer and memory CD8 T cell lineages in interleukin 15-deficient mice. *J Exp Med.* 2000;191(5):771–780.
50. Cooper MA, Bush JE, Fehniger TA, et al. In vivo evidence for a dependence on interleukin 15 for survival of natural killer cells. *Blood.* 2002;100(10):3633–3638.
58. Carson WE, Giri JG, Lindemann MJ, et al. Interleukin (IL) 15 is a novel cytokine that activates human natural killer cells via components of the IL-2 receptor. *J Exp Med.* 1994;180(4):1395–1403.
60. Ryan JC, Turck J, Niemi EC, et al. Molecular cloning of the NK1.1 antigen, a member of the NKR-P1 family of natural killer cell activation molecules. *J Immunol.* 1992;149(5):1631–1635.
61. Hackett J, Jr., Tutt M, Lipscomb M, et al. Origin and differentiation of natural killer cells. II. Functional and morphologic studies of purified NK-1.1$^+$ cells. *J Immunol.* 1986;136(8):3124–131.
63. Seaman WE, Sleisenger M, Eriksson E, et al. Depletion of natural killer cells in mice by monoclonal antibody to NK-1.1. Reduction in host defense against malignancy without loss of cellular or humoral immunity. *J Immunol.* 1987;138(12):4539–4544.
67. Carnaud C, Lee D, Donnars O, et al. Cutting edge: Cross-talk between cells of the innate immune system: NKT cells rapidly activate NK cells. *J Immunol.* 1999;163(9):4647–4650.

68. Arase H, Saito T, Phillips JH, et al. Cutting edge: the mouse NK cell-associated antigen recognized by DX5 monoclonal antibody is CD49b (alpha 2 integrin, very late antigen-2). *J Immunol*. 2001; 167(3):1141–1144.
70. Kim S, Iizuka K, Kang HS, et al. In vivo developmental stages in murine natural killer cell maturation. *Nature Immunol*. 2002;3(6): 523–528.
75. Lanier LL, Le AM, Civin CI, et al. The relationship of CD16 (Leu-11) and Leu-19 (NKH-1) antigen expression on human peripheral blood NK cells and cytotoxic T lymphocytes. *J Immunol*. 1986;136: 4480.
82. Freud AG, Becknell B, Roychowdhury S, et al. A human CD34(+) subset resides in lymph nodes and differentiates into CD56bright natural killer cells. *Immunity*. 2005;22(3):295–304.
88. Lieberman J. The ABCs of granule-mediated cytotoxicity: new weapons in the arsenal. *Nat Rev Immunol*. 2003;3(5):361–370.
93. Brunner KT, Mauel J, Cerottini JC, et al. Quantitative assay of the lytic action of immune lymphoid cells on 51Cr-labelled allogeneic target cells in vitro; inhibition by isoantibody and by drugs. *Immunology*. 1968;14:181.
99. Betts MR, Brenchley JM, Price DA, et al. Sensitive and viable identification of antigen-specific CD8$^+$ T cells by a flow cytometric assay for degranulation. *J Immunol Methods*. 2003;281(1–2):65–78.
113. Kagi D, Ledermann B, Burki K, et al. Cytotoxicity mediated by T cells and natural killer cells is greatly impaired in perforin-deficient mice. *Nature*. 1994;369(6475):31–37.
115. Pham CT, Ley TJ. Dipeptidyl peptidase I is required for the processing and activation of granzymes A and B in vivo. *Proc Natl Acad Sci U S A*. 1999;96(15):8627–8632.
118. Anegon I, Cuturi MC, Trinchieri G, et al. Interaction of Fc receptor (CD16) ligands induces transcription of interleukin 2 receptor (CD25) and lymphokine genes and expression of their products in human natural killer cells. *J Exp Med*. 1988;167(2):452–472.
119. Cuturi MC, Anegon I, Sherman F, et al. Production of hematopoietic colony stimulating factors by human natural killer cells. *J Exp Med*. 1989;169:569.
120. Dorner BG, Scheffold A, Rolph MS, et al. MIP-1alpha, MIP-1beta, RANTES, and ATAC/lymphotactin function together with IFN-gamma as type 1 cytokines. *Proc Natl Acad Sci U S A*. 2002;99(9): 6181–6186.
121. Tripp CS, Wolf SF, Unanue ER. Interleukin 12 and tumor necrosis factor alpha are costimulators of interferon gamma production by natural killer cells in severe combined immunodeficiency mice with listeriosis, and interleukin 10 is a physiologic antagonist. *Proc Natl Acad Sci U S A*. 1993;90(8):3725–3729.
123. Karre K, Ljunggren H-G, Piontek G, et al. Selective rejection of H-2-deficient lymphoma variants suggests alternative immune defence strategy. *Nature*. 1986;319(6055):675–678.
125. Ljunggren HG, Karre K. In search of the 'missing self': MHC molecules and NK cell recognition. *Immunology Today*. 1990;11(7): 237–244.
126. Storkus WJ, Salter RD, Alexander J, et al. Class I-induced resistance to natural killing: identification of nonpermissive residues in HLA-A2. *Proc Natl Acad Sci U S A*. 1991;88(14):5989–5992.
127. Colonna M, Brooks EG, Falco M, et al. Generation of allospecific natural killer cells by stimulation across a polymorphism of HLA-C. *Science*. 1993;260(5111):1121–1124.
128. Litwin V, Gumperz J, Parham P, et al. Specificity of HLA class I antigen recognition by human NK clones: evidence for clonal heterogeneity, protection by self and non-self alleles, and influence of the target cell type. *J Exp Med*. 1993;178(4):1321–1336.
129. Quillet A, Presse F, Marchiol-Fournigault C, et al. Increased resistance to non-MHC-restricted cytotoxicity related to HLA A,B expression. Direct demonstration using beta 2-microglobulin-transfected Daudi cells. *J Immunol*. 1988;141:17–20.
132. Liao NS, Bix M, Zijlstra M, et al. MHC class I deficiency: susceptibility to natural killer (NK) cells and impaired NK activity. *Science*. 1991;253(5016):199–202.
134. Bix M, Liao NS, Zijlstra M, et al. Rejection of class I MHC-deficient haemopoietic cells by irradiated MHC-matched mice. *Nature*. 1991;349(6307):329–331.
135. Yu YYL, Kumar V, Bennett M. Murine natural killer cells and marrow graft rejection. *Ann Rev Immunol*. 1992;10:189–213.
138. Kärre K. Role of target histocompatibility antigens in regulation of natural killer activity: A reevaluation and a hypothesis. In: Herberman RB, Callewaert DM, eds. *Mechanisms of cytotoxicity by NK cells*. Orlando: Academic Press; 1985:81–103.
144. Karlhofer FM, Ribaudo RK, Yokoyama WM. MHC class I alloantigen specificity of Ly-49$^+$ IL-2-activated natural killer cells. *Nature*. 1992;358(6381):66–70.
152. Chan PY, Takei F. Molecular cloning and characterization of a novel murine T cell surface antigen, YE1/48. *J Immunol*. 1989;142:1727.
153. Yokoyama WM, Jacobs LB, Kanagawa O, et al. A murine T lymphocyte antigen belongs to a supergene family of type II integral membrane proteins. *J Immunol*. 1989;143(4):1379–1386.
156. Yokoyama WM, Kehn PJ, Cohen DI, et al. Chromosomal location of the Ly-49 (A1, YE1/48) multigene family. Genetic association with the NK 1.1 antigen. *J Immunol*. 1990;145(7):2353–8.
161. Karlhofer FM, Hunziker R, Reichlin A, et al. Host MHC class I molecules modulate in vivo expression of a NK cell receptor. *J Immunol*. 1994;153(6):2407–2416.
164. Held W, Cado D, Raulet DH. Transgenic expression of the Ly49A natural killer cell receptor confers class I major histocompatibility complex (MHC)-specific inhibition and prevents bone marrow allograft rejection. *J Exp Med*. 1996;184(5):2037–2041.
165. Nakamura MC, Niemi EC, Fisher MJ, et al. Mouse Ly-49A interrupts early signaling events in natural killer cell cytotoxicity and functionally associates with the Shp-1 tyrosine phosphatase. *J Exp Med*. 1997;185(4):673–684.
166. Hanke T, Takizawa H, McMahon CW, et al. Direct assessment of MHC class I binding by seven Ly49 inhibitory NK cell receptors. *Immunity*. 1999;11(1):67–77.
167. Matsumoto N, Mitsuki M, Tajima K, et al. The functional binding site for the C-type lectinlike natural killer cell receptor Ly49A spans three domains of its major histocompatibility complex class I ligand. *J Exp Med*. 2001;193(2):147–158.
170. Tormo J, Natarajan K, Margulies DH, et al. Crystal structure of a lectinlike natural killer cell receptor bound to its MHC class I ligand. *Nature*. 1999;402(6762):623–631.
172. Correa I, Raulet DH. Binding of diverse peptides to MHC class I molecules inhibits target cell lysis by activated natural killer cells. *Immunity*. 1995;2(1):61–71.
182. Doucey MA, Scarpellino L, Zimmer J, et al. Cis association of Ly49A with MHC class I restricts natural killer cell inhibition. *Nat Immunol*. 2004;5(3):328–336.
183. Kim S, Poursine-Laurent J, Truscott SM, et al. Licensing of natural killer cells by host major histocompatibility complex class I molecules. *Nature*. 2005;436(7051):709–713.
184. Johansson MH, Bieberich C, Jay G, et al. Natural killer cell tolerance in mice with mosaic expression of major histocompatibility complex class I transgene. *J Exp Med*. 1997;186(3):353–364.
193. Dam J, Guan R, Natarajan K, et al. Variable MHC class I engagement by Ly49 natural killer cell receptors demonstrated by the crystal structure of Ly49C bound to H-2K(b). *Nat Immunol*. 2003;4(12):1213–1222.
194. Franksson L, Sundback J, Achour A, et al. Peptide dependency and selectivity of the NK cell inhibitory receptor Ly-49C. *Eur J Immunol*. 1999;29(9):2748–2758.
196. Dorfman JR, Raulet DH. Acquisition of Ly49 receptor expression by developing natural killer cells. *J Exp Med*. 1998;187(4):609–618.
198. Saleh A, Davies GE, Pascal V, et al. Identification of probabilistic transcriptional switches in the Ly49 gene cluster: a eukaryotic mechanism for selective gene activation. *Immunity*. 2004;21(1):55–66.
200. Yokoyama WM, Ryan JC, Hunter JJ, et al. cDNA cloning of mouse NKR-P1 and genetic linkage with Ly-49. Identification of a natural killer cell gene complex on mouse chromosome 6. *J Immunol*. 1991;147(9):3229–3236.
210. Moretta A, Tambussi G, Bottino C, et al. A novel surface antigen expressed by a subset of human CD3- CD16$^+$ natural killer cells. Role in cell activation and regulation of cytolytic function. *J Exp Med*. 1990;171:695.
211. Moretta A, Bottino C, Pende D, et al. Identification of four subsets of human CD3-CD16$^+$ natural killer (NK) cells by the expression of clonally distributed functional surface molecules: Correlation between subset assignment of NK clones and ability to mediate specific alloantigen recognition. *J Exp Med*. 1990; 172(6):1589–1598.

213. Colonna M, Borsellino G, Falco M, et al. HLA-C is the inhibitory ligand that determines dominant resistance to lysis by NK1- and NK2-specific natural killer cells. *Proc Natl Acad Sci U S A*. 1993; 90(24):12000–12004.
217. Litwin V, Gumperz J, Parham P, et al. NKB1: a natural killer cell receptor involved in the recognition of polymorphic HLA-B molecules. *J Exp Med*. 1994;180:537–543.
222. Wagtmann N, Biassoni R, Cantoni C, et al. Molecular clones of the p58 NK cell receptor reveal immunoglobulin-related molecules with diversity in both the extra- and intracellular domains. *Immunity*. 1995;2(5):439–449.
223. Colonna M, Samaridis J. Cloning of immunoglobulin-superfamily members associated with HLA-C and HLA-B recognition by human natural killer cells. *Science*. 1995;268(5209):367–368.
231. Wagtmann N, Rajagopalan S, Winter CC, et al. Killer cell inhibitory receptors specific for HLA-C and HLA-B identified by direct binding and by functional transfer. *Immunity*. 1995;3(6):801–809.
236. Boyington JC, Motyka SA, Schuck P, et al. Crystal structure of an NK cell immunoglobulin-like receptor in complex with its class I MHC ligand. *Nature*. 2000;405(6786):537–543.
240. Fan QR, Long EO, Wiley DC. Crystal structure of the human natural killer cell inhibitory receptor KIR2DL1-HLA-Cw4 complex. *Nat Immunol*. 2001;2(5):452–460.
246. Kelley J, Walter L, Trowsdale J. Comparative genomics of natural killer cell receptor gene clusters. *PLoS Genet*. 2005;1(2):129–139.
249. Vilches C, Parham P. KIR: diverse, rapidly evolving receptors of innate and adaptive immunity. *Annu Rev Immunol*. 2002;20: 217–251.
250. Bashirova AA, Martin MP, McVicar DW, et al. The Killer Immunoglobulin-like Receptor Gene Cluster: Tuning the Genome for Defense. *Annu Rev Genomics Hum Genet*. 2006.
251. Ruggeri L, Capanni M, Urbani E, et al. Effectiveness of donor natural killer cell alloreactivity in mismatched hematopoietic transplants. *Science*. 2002;295(5562):2097–2100.
252. Davies SM, Ruggieri L, DeFor T, et al. Evaluation of KIR ligand incompatibility in mismatched unrelated donor hematopoietic transplants. Killer immunoglobulin-like receptor. *Blood*. 2002;100(10):3825–3827.
254. Hsu KC, Keever-Taylor CA, Wilton A, et al. Improved outcome in HLA-identical sibling hematopoietic stem-cell transplantation for acute myelogenous leukemia predicted by KIR and HLA genotypes. *Blood*. 2005;105(12):4878–4884.
255. Yokoyama WM, Kim S. How do natural killer cells find self to achieve tolerance? *Immunity*. 2006;24(3):249–257.
257. Khakoo SI, Thio CL, Martin MP, et al. HLA and NK cell inhibitory receptor genes in resolving hepatitis C virus infection. *Science*. 2004;305(5685):872–874.
261. Cosman D, Fanger N, Borges L, et al. A novel immunoglobulin superfamily receptor for cellular and viral MHC class I molecules. *Immunity*. 1997;7:273–282.
262. Colonna M, Navarro F, Bellon T, et al. A common inhibitory receptor for MHC class I molecules on human lymphoid and myelomonocytic cells. *J Exp Med*. 1997;186(11):1809–1818.
266. Willcox BE, Thomas LM, Bjorkman PJ. Crystal structure of HLA-A2 bound to LIR-1, a host and viral major histocompatibility complex receptor. *Nat Immunol*. 2003;4(9):913–919.
267. Houchins JP, Yabe T, McSherry C, et al. DNA sequence analysis of NKG2, a family of related cDNA clones encoding type II integral membrane proteins on human natural killer cells. *J Exp Med*. 1991;173(4):1017–1020.
269. Aramburu J, Balboa MA, Izquierdo M, et al. A novel functional cell surface dimer (Kp43) expressed by natural killer cells and gamma/delta TCR+ T lymphocytes. II. Modulation of natural killer cytotoxicity by anti-Kp43 monoclonal antibody. *J Immunol*. 1991; 147(2):714–721.
274. Phillips JH, Chang CW, Mattson J, et al. CD94 and a novel associated protein (94ap) form a NK cell receptor involved in the recognition of HLA-A, HLA-B, and HLA-C allotypes. *Immunity*. 1996;5(2):163–172.
276. Lazetic S, Chang C, Houchins JP. Human natural killer cell receptors involved in MHC class I recognition are disulfide-linked heterodimers of CD94 and NKG2 subunits. *J Immunol*. 1996;157(11): 4741–4745.
284. Braud VM, Allen DSJ, O'Callaghan CA, et al. HLA-E binds to natural-killer-cell receptors CD94/NKG2A, B and C. *Nature*. 1998; 391(6669):795–799.
291. Vance RE, Kraft JR, Altman JD, et al. Mouse CD94/NKG2A is a natural killer cell receptor for the nonclassical major histocompatibility complex (MHC) class I molecule Qa-1(b). *J Exp Med*. 1998;188(10):1841–1848.
294. Tomasec P, Braud VM, Rickards C, et al. Surface expression of HLA-E, an inhibitor of natural killer cells, enhanced by human cytomegalovirus gpUL40. *Science*. 2000;287(5455):1031.
296. Guma M, Budt M, Saez A, et al. Expansion of CD94/NKG2C+ NK cells in response to human cytomegalovirus-infected fibroblasts. *Blood*. 2006;107(9):3624–3631.
297. Valiante NM, Uhrberg M, Shilling HG, et al. Functionally and structurally distinct NK cell receptor repertoires in the peripheral blood of two human donors. *Immunity*. 1997;7(6):739–751.
303. Moser JM, Gibbs J, Jensen PE, et al. CD94-NKG2A receptors regulate antiviral CD8+ T cell responses. *Nat Immunol*. 2002;3(2):189–195.
312. Castells MC, Klickstein LB, Hassani K, et al. gp49B1-alpha(v)beta3 interaction inhibits antigen-induced mast cell activation. *Nat Immunol*. 2001;2(5):436–442.
327. Hao L, Klein J, Nei M. Heterogeneous but conserved natural killer receptor gene complexes in four major orders of mammals. *Proc Natl Acad Sci U S A*. 2006;103(9):3192–3197.
332. Kumar V, McNerney ME. A new self: MHC-class-I-independent natural-killer-cell self-tolerance. *Nat Rev Immunol*. 2005;5(5):363–374.
335. Meyaard L, van der Vuurst de Vries AR, de Ruiter T, et al. The epithelial cellular adhesion molecule (Ep-CAM) is a ligand for the leukocyte-associated immunoglobulin-like receptor (LAIR). *J Exp Med*. 2001;194(1):107–112.
339. Falco M, Biassoni R, Bottino C, et al. Identification and molecular cloning of p75/AIRM1, a novel member of the sialoadhesin family that functions as an inhibitory receptor in human natural killer cells. *J Exp Med*. 1999;190(6):793–802.
354. Smith HR, Heusel JW, Mehta IK, et al. Recognition of a virus-encoded ligand by a natural killer cell activation receptor. *Proc Natl Acad Sci U S A*. 2002;99(13):8826–8831.
355. Iizuka K, Naidenko OV, Plougastel BF, et al. Genetically linked C-type lectin-related ligands for the NKRP1 family of natural killer cell receptors. *Nat Immunol*. 2003;4(8):801–807.
356. Arase H, Mocarski ES, Campbell AE, et al. Direct recognition of cytomegalovirus by activating and inhibitory NK cell receptors. *Science*. 2002;296(5571):1323–1326.
365. Moretta A, Sivori S, Vitale M, et al. Existence of both inhibitory (p58) and activatory (p50) receptors for HLA-C molecules in human natural killer cells. *J Exp Med*. 1995;182(3):875–884.
376. Wu J, Cherwinski H, Spies T, et al. DAP10 and DAP12 form distinct, but functionally cooperative, receptor complexes in natural killer cells [In Process Citation]. *J Exp Med*. 2000;192(7):1059–1068.
379. Vance RE, Jamieson AM, Raulet DH. Recognition of the class Ib molecule Qa-1(b) by putative activating receptors CD94/NKG2C and CD94/NKG2E on mouse natural killer cells. *J Exp Med*. 1999;190(12):1801–1812.
388. Cassatella MA, Anegon I, Cuturi MC, et al. Fc gamma R(CD16) interaction with ligand induces Ca2+ mobilization and phosphoinositide turnover in human natural killer cells. Role of Ca2+ in Fc gamma R(CD16)-induced transcription and expression of lymphokine genes. *J Exp Med*. 1989;169(2):549–567.
393. Bauer S, Groh V, Wu J, et al. Activation of NK cells and T cells by NKG2D, a receptor for stress-inducible MICA. *Science*. 1999; 285(5428):727–729.
394. Cerwenka A, Bakker ABH, McClanahan T, et al. Retinoic acid early inducible genes define a ligand family for the activating NKG2D receptor in mice. *Immunity*. 2000;12:721–727.
395. Diefenbach A, Jamieson AM, Liu SD, et al. Ligands for the murine NKG2D receptor: expression by tumor cells and activation of NK cells and macrophages. *Nat Immunol*. 2000;1(2):119–126.
396. Groh V, Bruhl A, El-Gabalawy H, et al. Stimulation of T cell autoreactivity by anomalous expression of NKG2D and its MIC ligands in rheumatoid arthritis. *Proc Natl Acad Sci U S A*. 2003;100(16):9452–9457.

397. Wu J, Song Y, Bakker AB, et al. An activating immunoreceptor complex formed by NKG2D and DAP10. *Science*. 1999;285(5428):730–732.
398. Groh V, Rhinehart R, Randolph-Habecker J, et al. Costimulation of CD8ab T cells by NKG2D via engagement by MIC induced on virus-infected cells. *Nat Immunol*. 2001;2(3):255–260.
401. Diefenbach A, Tomasello E, Lucas M, et al. Selective associations with signaling molecules determine stimulatory versus costimulatory activity of NKG2D. *Nat Immunol*. 2002;3(12):1142–1149.
403. Rabinovich B, Li J, Wolfson M, et al. NKG2D splice variants: a reexamination of adaptor molecule associations. *Immunogenetics*. 2006;58(2–3):81–88.
404. Gilfillan S, Ho EL, Cella M, et al. NKG2D recruits two distinct adapters to trigger natural killer cell activation and costimulation. *Nature Immunol*. 2002;3(12):1150–1155.
405. Cosman D, Mullberg J, Sutherland CL, et al. ULBPs, novel MHC class I-related molecules, bind to CMV glycoprotein UL16 and stimulate NK cytotoxicity through the NKG2D receptor. *Immunity*. 2001;14(2):123–133.
409. Girardi M, Oppenheim DE, Steele CR, et al. Regulation of cutaneous malignancy by gd T Cells. *Science*. 2001;294(5542):605–609.
412. Li P, Morris DL, Willcox BE, et al. Complex structure of the activating immunoreceptor NKG2D and its MHC class I-like ligand MICA. *Nat Immunol*. 2001;2(5):443–451.
413. Radaev S, Rostro B, Brooks AG, et al. Conformational plasticity revealed by the cocrystal structure of NKG2D and its class I MHC-like ligand ULBP3. *Immunity*. 2001;15(6):1039–1049.
417. Carayannopoulos LN, Naidenko OV, Kinder J, et al. Ligands for murine NKG2D display heterogeneous binding behavior. *Eur J Immunol*. 2002;32(3):597–605.
424. Diefenbach A, Jensen ER, Jamieson AM, et al. Rae1 and H60 ligands of the NKG2D receptor stimulate tumour immunity. *Nature*. 2001;413(6852):165–171.
426. Groh V, Bahram S, Bauer S, Herman et al. Cell stress-regulated human major histocompatibility complex class I gene expressed in gastrointestinal epithelium. *Proc Natl Acad Sci U S A*. 1996;93(22):12445–12450.
428. Gasser S, Orsulic S, Brown EJ, et al. The DNA damage pathway regulates innate immune system ligands of the NKG2D receptor. *Nature*. 2005;436(7054):1186–1190.
441. Dunn C, Chalupny NJ, Sutherland CL, et al. Human cytomegalovirus glycoprotein UL16 causes intracellular sequestration of NKG2D ligands, protecting against natural killer cell cytotoxicity. *J Exp Med*. 2003;197(11):1427–1439.
442. Krmpotic A, Busch DH, Bubic I, et al. MCMV glycoprotein gp40 confers virus resistance to CD8$^+$ T cells and NK cells in vivo. *Nat Immunol*. 2002;3(6):529–535.
463. Arase N, Arase H, Park SY, et al. Association with FcR-g is essential for activation signal through NKR-P1 (CD161) in natural killer (NK) cells and NK1.1$^+$ T cells. *J Exp Med*. 1997;186(12):1957–1963.
480. Garni-Wagner BA, Purohit A, Mathew PA, et al. A novel function-associated molecule related to non-MHC-restricted cytotoxicity mediated by activated natural killer cells and T cells. *J Immunol*. 1993;151(1):60–70.
483. Veillette A. Immune regulation by SLAM family receptors and SAP-related adaptors. *Nat Rev Immunol*. 2006;6(1):56–66.
493. Sivori S, Vitale M, Morelli L, et al. p46, a novel natural killer cell-specific surface molecule that mediates cell activation. *J Exp Med*. 1997;186(7):1129–1136.
501. Mandelboim O, Lieberman N, Lev M, et al. Recognition of haemagglutinins on virus-infected cells by NKp46 activates lysis by human NK cells. *Nature*. 2001;409(6823):1055–1060.
516. Ito M, Maruyama T, Saito N, et al. Killer cell lectinlike receptor G1 binds three members of the classical cadherin family to inhibit NK cell cytotoxicity. *J Exp Med*. 2006;203(2):289–295.
518. Stern N, Markel G, Arnon TI, et al. Carcinoembryonic antigen (CEA) inhibits NK killing via interaction with CEA-related cell adhesion molecule 1. *J Immunol*. 2005;174(11):6692–6701.
522. Fuchs A, Cella M, Giurisato E, et al. Cutting edge: CD96 (tactile) promotes NK cell-target cell adhesion by interacting with the poliovirus receptor (CD155). *J Immunol*. 2004;172(7):3994–3998.
530. MacFarlane AWt, Campbell KS. Signal transduction in natural killer cells. *Curr Top Microbiol Immunol*. 2006;298:23–57.
532. Davis DM, Dustin ML. What is the importance of the immunological synapse? *Trends Immunol*. 2004;25(6):323–327.
533. Orange JS, Harris KE, Andzelm MM, et al. The mature activating natural killer cell immunologic synapse is formed in distinct stages. *Proc Natl Acad Sci U S A*. 2003;100(24):14151–14156.
535. Vyas YM, Mehta KM, Morgan M, et al. Spatial organization of signal transduction molecules in the NK cell immune synapses during MHC class I-regulated noncytolytic and cytolytic interactions. *J Immunol*. 2001;167(8):4358–4367.
538. Mason LH, Willette-Brown J, Taylor LS, et al. Regulation of Ly49D/DAP12 signal transduction by Src-family kinases and CD45. *J Immunol*. 2006;176(11):6615–6623.
544. Cella M, Fujikawa K, Tassi I, et al. Differential requirements for Vav proteins in DAP10- and ITAM-mediated NK cell cytotoxicity. *J Exp Med*. 2004;200(6):817–823.
546. Jiang K, Zhong B, Gilvary DL, et al. Pivotal role of phosphoinositide-3 kinase in regulation of cytotoxicity in natural killer cells. *Nat Immunol*. 2000;1(5):419–425.
547. Wu J, Song Y, Bakker AB, et al. An activating immunoreceptor complex formed by NKG2D and DAP10. *Science*. 1999;285(5428):730–732.
553. Burshtyn DN, Scharenberg AM, Wagtmann N, et al. Recruitment of tyrosine phosphatase HCP by the killer cell inhibitor receptor. *Immunity*. 1996;4(1):77–85.
563. Wang JW, Howson JM, Ghansah T, et al. Influence of SHIP on the NK repertoire and allogeneic bone marrow transplantation. *Science*. 2002;295(5562):2094–2097.
564. Stebbins CC, Watzl C, Billadeau DD, et al. Vav1 dephosphorylation by the tyrosine phosphatase SHP-1 as a mechanism for inhibition of cellular cytotoxicity. *Mol Cell Biol*. 2003;23(17):6291–6299.
567. Treanor B, Lanigan PM, Kumar S, et al. Microclusters of inhibitory killer immunoglobulin-like receptor signaling at natural killer cell immunological synapses. *J Cell Biol*. 2006;174(1):153–161.
579. Williams NS, Moore TA, Schatzle JD, et al. Generation of lytic natural killer 1.1$^+$, Ly-49- cells from multipotential murine bone marrow progenitors in a stroma-free culture: definition of cytokine requirements and developmental intermediates. *J Exp Med*. 1997;186(9):1609–1614.
582. Roth C, Carlyle JR, Takizawa H, et al. Clonal acquisition of inhibitory Ly49 receptors on developing NK cells is successively restricted and regulated by stromal class I MHC. *Immunity*. 2000;13(1):143–153.
583. Caraux A, Lu Q, Fernandez N, et al. Natural killer cell differentiation driven by Tyro3 receptor tyrosine kinases. *Nat Immunol*. 2006;7(7):747–754.
588. Georgopoulos K, Bigby M, Wang JH, et al. The Ikaros gene is required for the development of all lymphoid lineages. *Cell*. 1994; 79(1):143–156.
593. Rodewald HR, Moingeon P, Lucich JL, et al. A population of early fetal thymocytes expressing Fc gamma RII/III contains precursors of T lymphocytes and natural killer cells. *Cell*. 1992;69(1): 139–150.
601. Zuniga-Pflucker JC. T-cell development made simple. *Nat Rev Immunol*. 2004;4(1):67–72.
604. Yokota Y, Mansouri A, Mori S, et al. Development of peripheral lymphoid organs and natural killer cells depends on the helix-loop-helix inhibitor Id2. *Nature*. 1999;397(6721):702–706.
608. Ogasawara K, Hida S, Azimi N, et al. Requirement for IRF-1 in the microenvironment supporting development of natural killer cells. *Nature*. 1998;391(6668):700–703.
611. Sivakumar PV, Gunturi A, Salcedo M, et al. Cutting edge: expression of functional CD94/NKG2A inhibitory receptors on fetal NK1.1$^+$Ly-49- cells: a possible mechanism of tolerance during NK cell development. *J Immunol*. 1999;162(12):6976–6980.
613. Dokun AO, Kim S, Smith HR, et al. Specific and nonspecific NK cell activation during virus infection. *Nat Immunol*. 2001;2(10):951–956.
619. Bennett IM, Zatsepina O, Zamai L, et al. Definition of a natural killer NKR-P1A(+)/CD56(-)/CD16(-) functionally immature human NK cell subset that differentiates in vitro in the presence of interleukin 12. *J Exp Med*. 1996;184(5):1845–1856.
625. Sentman CL, Olsson MY, Karre K. Missing self recognition by natural killer cells in MHC class I transgenic mice. A "receptor

calibration" model for how effector cells adapt to self. *Semin Immunol.* 1995;7(2):109–119.

629. Furukawa H, Yabe T, Watanabe K, et al. Tolerance of NK and LAK activity for HLA class I-deficient targets in a TAP1-deficient patient (bare lymphocyte syndrome type I). *Hum Immunol.* 1999;60(1): 32–40.
635. Ohlen C, Kling G, Hoglund P, et al. Prevention of allogeneic bone marrow graft rejection by H-2 transgene in donor mice. *Science.* 1989;246(4930):666–668
637. Fernandez NC, Treiner E, Vance RE, et al. A subset of natural killer cells achieves self-tolerance without expressing inhibitory receptors specific for self-MHC molecules. *Blood.* 2005;105(11):4416–4423.
639. Anfossi N, Andre P, Guia S, et al. Human NK cell education by inhibitory receptors for MHC class I. *Immunity.* 2006;25(2):331–342.
642. Salazar-Mather TP, Orange JS, Biron CA. Early murine cytomegalovirus (MCMV) Infection induces liver natural killer (NK) cell inflammation and protection through macrophage inflammatory protein 1-alpha (MIP-1-alpha)-dependent pathways. *J Exp Med.* 1998;187(1):1–14.
656. Smyth MJ, Dunn GP, Schreiber RD. Cancer immunosurveillance and immunoediting: the roles of immunity in suppressing tumor development and shaping tumor immunogenicity. *Adv Immunol.* 2006;90:1–50.
661. Biron CA, Byron KS, Sullivan JL. Severe herpesvirus infections in an adolescent without natural killer cells. *New England Journal of Medicine.* 1989;320(26):1731–1735.
664. Orange JS. Human natural killer cell deficiencies and susceptibility to infection. *Microbes Infect.* 2002;4(15):1545–1558.
668. Fauci AS, Mavilio D, Kottilil S. NK cells in HIV infection: paradigm for protection or targets for ambush. *Nat Rev Immunol.* 2005;5(11):835–843.
674. Shellam GR, Allan JE, Papadimitriou JM, et al. Increased susceptibility to cytomegalovirus infection in beige mutant mice. *Proc Natl Acad Sci U S A.* 1981;78:5104–108.
675. Bukowski JF, Woda BA, Habu S, et al. Natural killer cell depletion enhances virus synthesis and virus-induced hepatitis in vivo. *J Immunol.* 1983;131(3):1531–1538.
686. Orange JS, Wang B, Terhorst C, et al. Requirement for natural killer cell-produced interferon gamma in defense against murine cytomegalovirus infection and enhancement of this defense pathway by interleukin 12 administration. *J Exp Med.* 1995;182(4):1045–1056.
694. Nguyen KB, Cousens LP, Doughty LA, et al. Interferon a/b-mediated inhibition and promotion of interferon-g: STAT1 resolves a paradox. *Nat Immunol.* 2000;1(1):70–76.
704. Orange JS, Fassett MS, Koopman LA, et al. Viral evasion of natural killer cells. *Nat Immunol.* 2002;3(11):1006–1012.
705. Farrell HE, Vally H, Lynch DM, et al. Inhibition of natural killer cells by a cytomegalovirus MHC class I homologue in vivo. *Nature.* 1997;386(6624):510–514.
709. Reyburn HT, Mandelboim O, Vales-Gomez M, et al. The class I MHC homologue of human cytomegalovirus inhibits attack by natural killer cells. *Nature.* 1997;386(6624):514–517.
715. Scalzo AA, Fitzgerald NA, Simmons A, et al. Cmv-1, a genetic locus that controls murine cytomegalovirus replication in the spleen. *J Exp Med.* 1990;171(5):1469–1483.
717. Scalzo AA, Fitzgerald NA, Wallace CR, et al. The effect of the Cmv-1 resistance gene, which is linked to the natural killer cell gene complex, is mediated by natural killer cells. *J Immunol.* 1992;149(2):581–589.
718. Brown MG, Dokun AO, Heusel JW, et al. Vital involvement of a natural killer cell activation receptor in resistance to viral infection. *Science.* 2001;292(5518):934–937.
720. Daniels KA, Devora G, Lai WC, et al. Murine cytomegalovirus is regulated by a discrete subset of natural killer cells reactive with monoclonal antibody to ly49h. *J Exp Med.* 2001;194(1):29–44.
722. French AR, Pingel JT, Wagner M, et al. Escape of mutant double-stranded DNA virus from innate immune control. *Immunity.* 2004;20(6):747–756.
734. Fernandez NC, Lozier A, Flament C, et al. Dendritic cells directly trigger NK cell functions: cross-talk relevant in innate anti-tumor immune responses in vivo. *Nat Med.* 1999;5(4):405–411.
735. Gerosa F, Baldani-Guerra B, Nisii C, et al. Reciprocal activating interaction between natural killer cells and dendritic cells. *J Exp Med.* 2002;195(3):327–333.
736. Degli-Esposti MA, Smyth MJ. Close encounters of different kinds: dendritic cells and NK cells take centre stage. *Nat Rev Immunol.* 2005;5(2):112–124.
744. Krug A, French AR, Barchet W, et al. TLR9-dependent recognition of MCMV by IPC and DC generates coordinated cytokine responses that activate antiviral NK cell function. *Immunity.* 2004;21(1):107–119.
749. Mocikat R, Braumuller H, Gumy A, et al. Natural killer cells activated by MHC class I(low) targets prime dendritic cells to induce protective CD8 T cell responses. *Immunity.* 2003;19(4): 561–569.
750. Martin-Fontecha A, Thomsen LL, Brett S, et al. Induced recruitment of NK cells to lymph nodes provides IFN-gamma for T(H)1 priming. *Nat Immunol.* 2004;5(12):1260–1265.
764. Moffett A, Loke C. Immunology of placentation in eutherian mammals. *Nat Rev Immunol.* 2006;6(8):584–594.
768. Ashkar AA, Di Santo JP, Croy BA. Interferon gamma contributes to initiation of uterine vascular modification, decidual integrity, and uterine natural killer cell maturation during normal murine pregnancy. *J Exp Med.* 2000;192(2):259–270.

Chapter 17

NKT Cells and Other Innatelike T and B Lineages

Albert Bendelac

INTRODUCTION AND DEFINITION OF INNATELIKE LYMPHOCYTES

Characteristic features oppose innate and adaptive immunity in vertebrates. Innate immunity is an evolutionarily primitive, rapid arm of the immune response that relies on a set of germline-encoded receptors, some of which are conserved in plants and insects. These receptors are broadly expressed in body fluids, tissue cells, or mobile hemopoietic cells, and they generally recognize conserved self or pathogen structures to trigger effector mechanisms that are more or less tailored to the pathogen. In contrast, adaptive immunity evolved in vertebrates as a delayed arm of the response that relies on the expansion of rare lymphocytes expressing highly diverse, clonally restricted, antigen-specific receptors arising through random rearrangement of large families of gene segments encoded in specialized genetic loci. These receptors include leucine-rich-repeat domain receptors (variable lymphocyte receptor, VLR) in primitive fish and, in other vertebrates, the immunoglobulin domain receptors immunoglobulin (Ig) H/L, T-cell receptor (TCR) α/β or TCR γ/δ. Lymphocytes expanded after antigen encounter persist to form the basis of memory responses, another hallmark of adaptive immunity.

Some subsets of T and B lymphocytes, however, straddle the boundaries between innate and adaptive immunity. These "innatelike" lymphocytes express canonical

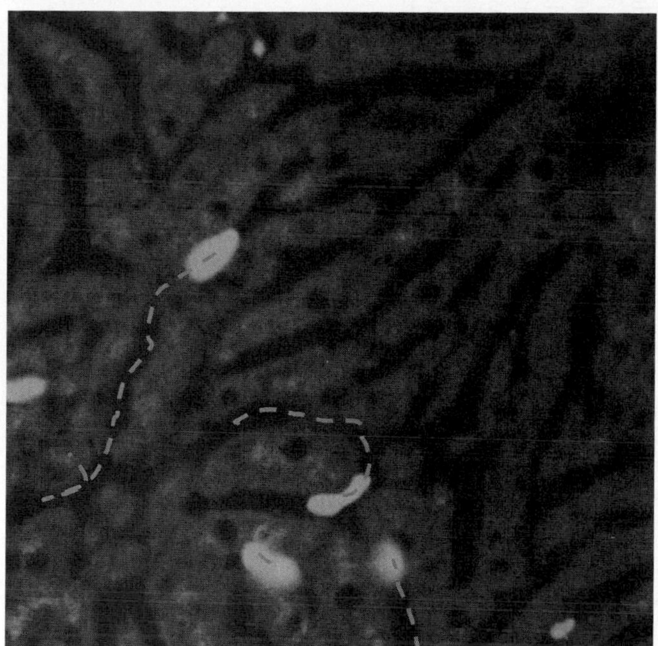

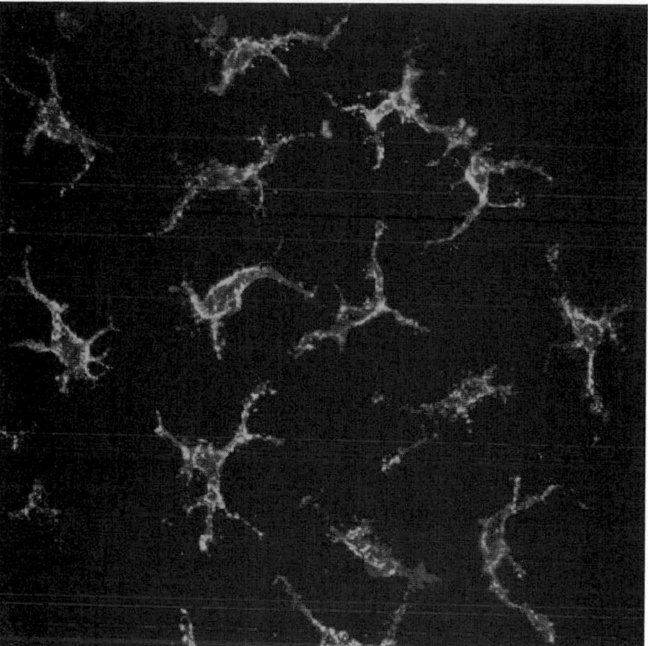

FIGURE 17.1 Specialized tissue niches and their resident innatelike lymphocytes. Left: Fluorescent NKT cells in CXCR6-GFP "knock-in" mice are "patrolling" the liver sinusoids. Dashed lines show their path over a period of 10 min in a live imaging study. (Courtesy of Frederic Geissmann, Hopital Necker, Paris, France, and Dan Littman, New York University, New York, NY, USA.) Right: DETC labeled with GL3 anti-$\gamma\delta$TCR antibody in whole epidermal sheet. Note the dendritic shape adopted by these skin-resident T cells. (Courtesy of Jessica Strid and Adrian Hayday, King's College, London, UK.)

germline-encoded antigen receptors that are specific for conserved self- and microbial ligands and are present at high frequency in specific tissues, suggesting that they function as immunologic sentinels and first line of defense in various strategic locations (Figure 17.1). With their memory/effector differentiation, they appear poised to mediate innatelike functions, which have been documented in a surprisingly broad range of conditions, from the regulation of autoimmunity and inflammation to antimicrobial defense and cancer rejection, as well as in homeostasis.

Innatelike lymphocytes include so-called B-1 B cells and a subset of marginal-zone B (MZB) cells; a fraction of $\gamma\delta$ T cells; subsets of $\alpha\beta$ T cells such as CD1d-restricted "NKT" cells and MR1-restricted mucosal-associated innate T cells ("MAIT cells") (Table 17.1). Studies have revealed common themes and principles in their development, antigen specificity, and function, although variations are found with individual subsets. Innatelike lymphocyte subsets are variably represented in different mammalian species. They represent a distinct host defense strategy, perhaps corresponding to an early phase of evolution of adaptive T- and B-cell immunity. With a particular focus on the well-studied NKT cell subset, this chapter will treat them as a group, using specific examples that illustrate similarities and differences.

CANONICAL GERMLINE-ENCODED ANTIGEN RECEPTORS

Antigen Receptor Structure

The most characteristic feature of innatelike lymphocytes is the expression by relatively large numbers of lymphocytes of so-called canonical and germline-encoded B- or T-cell receptors that are specific for conserved self- or foreign antigens. "Canonical" sequences are invariant sequences or motifs in the CDR3 regions of one or the two receptor chains, which are involved in antigen contact. The "germline" nature of these canonical receptors arises from nucleotide sequences that are entirely encoded in the genome, and do not require nontemplated N-nucleotide addition or mutation. Thus, these genetic elements could have been naturally selected for their protective value during the evolution of the immune system. For each of these canonical sequences, there are individual examples exhibiting nucleotide trimming and N additions. Because these changes are conservative—that is, they preserve the canonical amino acid sequence—they illustrate another important aspect of the biology of innatelike lymphocytes, which will be discussed later: antigen-driven cellular selection.

TABLE 17.1 Examples of Innatelike B and T Cell Subsets

Lineage	*BCR/TCR*	*Ontogeny*	*Antigen*	*Tissue*	*Effector Properties*	*Proposed in vivo Function*	*Species*
B-1	mVHS107/Vκ22 (T15 idiotype)	Fetal	PC, oxLDL, apoptotic cell mb	Peritoneum	IgM secretion	Antimicrobial defense	Mouse
	mVH11/Vκ9, mVH12/Vκ4	Adult	PtC, oxLDL, apoptotic cell mb	Peritoneum	IgM secretion	Antimicrobial defense	Mouse
	mVH3609/Vκ21C	Fetal	Thy-1	Peritoneum	IgM secretion	?	Mouse
MZ B	mVHS107/Vκ24 (M167 idiotype)	Fetal?	PC, oxLDL apoptotic cell mb	Marginal zone	IgM secretion	Antimicrobial defense	Mouse
$\gamma\delta$ T	mVγ5/Vδ1	Fetal	Unknown	Skin	KGF, cytolysis	Wound healing, tumor rejection anti-inflammatory	Mouse
	mVγ6/Vδ1	Fetal	Unknown	Uterovaginal mucosa	?	?	Mouse
	mVγ1/Vδ6*	Perinatal	Unknown	Liver	IL-4, IL-10, IFN-γ	?	Mouse
	mDδ_2	Fetal/adult	T10/T22	Spleen, IEL	?	?	Mouse
	hVγ9/Vδ_2	Fetal/adult	Phosphoantigens, F1-ATPase	Fetal liver, adult PBL	INF-γ, TNFα, cytolysis	Antimicrobial defense, tumor rejection	Human
CD1d-restricted NKT	mVα14/Vβ2, 7, 8 hVα24/Vβ11	Fetal/adult	CD1d + lipid (self iGb3, microbial αGalCer)	Liver, spleen, mesenteric LN	IL-4, IL-13, IL-10, IFN-γ	Antimicrobial defense, tumor rejection, inflammation autoimmunity	Mouse Human Rat
MR1-restricted MAIT	mVα19/Vβ6 ,8 hVα7.2/Vβ2, 13	Fetal/adult	MR1$^+$ unidentified ligand	Gut lamina propria	IL-4, IL-10, IFN-γ	Mucosal immunity	Mouse Human Cow

Nomenclature of murine Vγ gene segments is according to Heilig JS, Tonegawa S. Diversity of murine gamma genes and expression in fetal and adult T lymphocytes. *Nature.* 1986;322(6082):836–840.

*We refer here to a subset of Vγ1/Vδ6 cells that is Thy-1dull and NK1.1$^+$. Not listed, because of the apparent absence of canonical sequence motifs and their naïve phenotype are human Vδ1 T cells, a prominent subset in the intestinal epithelium, which have been associated with recognition of various antigens, including CD1c and MHC class I (MIC). OxLDL, oxidized low-density lipoprotein; KGF, keratinocyte growth factor; MZ B, marginal zone B cell; NKT, natural killer T cell; PC, phosphorylcholine, PtC, phosphatidylcholine.

TABLE 17.2 Invariant BCR of T-15 Idiotype+ B-1 Cells

	IGKV7	TAT CTT CT		IGHV7	GCA AGA GAT
	IGKJ5	CTC ACG TTC		IGHD1	AT TAC TAC GGT AGT AGC TAC
				IGHJ1	TAC TGG
Canonical mVκ122		TAT CTT CTC ACG TTC	Canonical mV_HS107		GCA AGA GAT TAC TAC GGT AGT AGC TAC TGG
		Y L L T F			A R D Y Y G S S Y W

Regions of short homology between V, D, and J segments, which guide the rearrangement process, are underlined.

Some canonical receptors, such as the T15 antiphosphatidylcholine BCR (Table 17.2) and the Vγ5 [nomenclature according to Heilig and Tonegawa (1)] dendritic epidermal T-cell (DETC) TCR (Table 17.3) are made of invariant H/L or γ/δ pairs, and their production is generally limited to the fetal or neonatal period (2,3). Others appear to be "semi-invariant," as only one chain is invariant whereas the other exhibits diversity. For example, CD1d-restricted NKT cells express a canonical Vα14-Jα18 TCR α chain paired with β chains that use a limited set of Vβ8, Vβ7, Vβ2 families joined to variable DβJβ (4) (Table 17.4). Similarly, antiphosphatidylcholine-specific B1 B cells use invariant VH11 and VH12 heavy chains, with Vκ9 or Vκ4 light chains that are diverse in their Jκ usage (5,6). Other receptors exhibit relatively limited areas of sequence conservation or "motifs." In the case of γδ T cells specific for the MHC class I–like molecule T10/T22, a canonical sequence was not apparent until multiple T-cell clones were obtained and sequenced to suggest the importance of a W-(S)EGYEL motif, where W could be contributed by a Vδ or by Dδ1, SEGYE was from a Dδ2 segment, and L was encoded by a P nucleotide (7). The crystal structure of the TCR bound to T22 directly demonstrated that this canonical sequence contacts the antigen (8).

Ultimately, the canonical BCRs and TCRs functionally resemble innate receptors such as Toll-like receptors (TLR), for example, by their germline specificity for conserved antigens. Like TLRs, they can be monospecific or multispecific, recognizing related antigens or antigens of vastly different structure. The variable parts of these canonical receptors can modulate the affinity of antigen recognition, as shown for NKT cells (9–11) and for T10/T22-specific γδ T cells (7), perhaps affording greater plasticity for functional responses and for recognition of variant antigens.

Achieving a high frequency of canonical rearrangements is a prerequisite to contribute to innate responses. Depending on the canonical receptor, this requirement is met by diverse genetic strategies, by cellular selection, and, in some cases, by clonal expansion.

Genetic Mechanisms That Produce Canonical Antigen Receptors

Some genetic mechanisms operate early in fetal and newborn life, revealing distinct intrinsic properties of fetal progenitors, whereas others operate throughout newborn and adult life.

Programmed Rearrangements

In the fetal and neonatal periods, B and T lymphocytes show conspicuous tendencies to rearrange and express particular V(D)J gene segments encoding the canonical antigen receptors of some γδ T cells and B-1 B cells. This is particularly well illustrated for the sequential rearrangements that give rise to waves of TCR γδ T cells colonizing the skin and the other mucosal tissues in mice (2,12) and for the B-1 B cells that express the so-called T-15 idiotype (corresponding to the canonical portion of the antibody structure) (3). The molecular basis of these ordered rearrangements involves local as well as large-scale changes in chromatin structure that are still poorly understood (13). Nevertheless, signaling through the cytokine receptors for interleukin-7 (IL-7) or IL-15 involving Stat5 was shown to be essential for the expression of various B-1 and γδ TCR canonical receptors (14–17). IL-7 receptor signaling regulated histone acetylation and transcriptional activation of V_H558 genes through Stat5 binding the transcription factor Oct-1 (18). Interestingly, thymic

TABLE 17.3 Invariant γδ TCR of Dendritic Epidermal T Cells

	TRGV5	TGC TGG GAT		TRDV1	GAT AT
	TRGJ1	AT AGC TCA		TRDD2	*AT* ATC GGA GGG A
				TRDJ2	*GG A*GC TCC
Canonical mVγ5		TGC TGG GAT AGC TCA	Canonical mVδ1		GAT ATC GGA GGG AGC TCC
		C W D S S			D I G G S S

Vγ nomenclature according to Heilig JS, Tonegawa S. Diversity of murine gamma genes and expression in fetal and adult T lymphocytes. *Nature.* 1986;322(6082):836–840.
P nucleotides, palindromic to the first nucleotides at the end of germline V, D and J elements, are in italics. Regions of short homology between V, D, and J segments, which guide the rearrangement process, are underlined.

TABLE 17.4 Semi-invariant TCRs of CD1d-Restricted NKT and MR1-Restricted MAIT Cells

	TRAV10	GTG GTG AGC G	
	TRAJ18	C GAC AGA	
Canonical hVα24		GTG GTG AGC GAC AGA	Variable hVβ11
		V V S D R	
	TRAV19	GTG AGG GAT	
	TRAJ33	G GAT AGC	
Canonical mVα19		GTG AGG GAT AGC	Variable mVβ6, mVβ8
		V R D S	

Regions of short homology between V, D, and J segments, which guide the rearrangement process, are underlined.

stromal-derived lymphopoietin (TSLP) can substitute for IL-7 and signal through IL-7Rα in fetal but not adult B-cell ontogenesis (19,20). These differences might explain intrinsic differences in BCR repertoire and possibly also other lineage characteristics of B cells produced in early life as compared to adult life.

Terminal Deoxynucleotidyl Transferase (TdT)

Low-level expression of TdT in the fetal and neonatal period favors germline canonical sequences by decreasing the frequency of nontemplated nucleotide addition (N diversity) at the joining end of the rearranging segments. Thus, genetic overexpression of TdT impairs, whereas abrogation favors, canonical rearrangements (21,22).

Short-Nucleotide-Homology-Mediated Rearrangements

The formation of canonical sequences is enhanced by regions of short homology that guide the recombination process (Tables 17.2 through 17.5). These short-homology regions are contributed sometimes by P nucleotides palindromic to the nucleotides at the end of V, D, or J elements (Tables 17.3 and 17.5). Suggested initially for the formation of T-15 antibody rearrangement (3), this general mechanism has been demonstrated *in vivo* for the fetal TCR $\gamma\delta$ rearrangements that generate DETC cells (21).

Several canonical antigen receptors are produced continuously over the lifespan of the animal. This is the case, for example, for CD1d-restricted NKT cells, MR1-specific MAIT cells, phosphoantigen-specific Vγ9 T cells, and phosphatidylcholine-specific B-1 B cells. Because the Vα14 and Jα18 segments are distal, their recombination depends on the prolonged lifespan of double-positive thymocytes, which requires the induction of the antiapoptotic Bcl-xL protein by the transcription factor RORγt expressed at the double-positive stage of thymocyte development (23,24).

Antigen-driven Cellular Selection of Canonical Antigen Receptors

Although they were debated initially, there are now converging findings indicating that many innatelike lymphocyte subsets, including those that rely on programmed fetal rearrangements, undergo a phase of cellular selection driven by specificity for their self-ligand. Furthermore, as will be discussed in the section on lymphocyte development, these antigen-recognition events appear to be essential to initiate the peculiar signaling pathways that drive lineage differentiation.

Transgenic expression models have been generated for several canonical receptors and have usually demonstrated that receptor expression instructed the corresponding lineage differentiation for NKT cells (25,26) (Figure 17.2), DETC (27) and liver $\gamma\delta$ T cells (28), B-1 B cells (29–32) (33), and MZB cells (34). Conversely, expression of

TABLE 17.5 Invariant $\gamma\delta$ TCR of Human Vγ9 Peripheral Blood Lymphocytes

	TRGV9	TGG GAG GTG *CA*		TRDV2	GAC A
	TRGJP	G CAA GAG		TRDD3	*TA* CTG GGG GAT AC
				TRDJ1	ACC GAT
Canonical hVγ9		TGG GAG GTG CAA GAG	Canonical hVδ2		GAC ATA CTG GGG GAT ACC GAT
		W E V Q E			D I L G D T D

P nucleotides, palindromic to the first nucleotides at the end of germline V, D, and J elements, are in italics. Regions of short homology between V, D, and J segments, which guide the rearrangement process, are underlined.

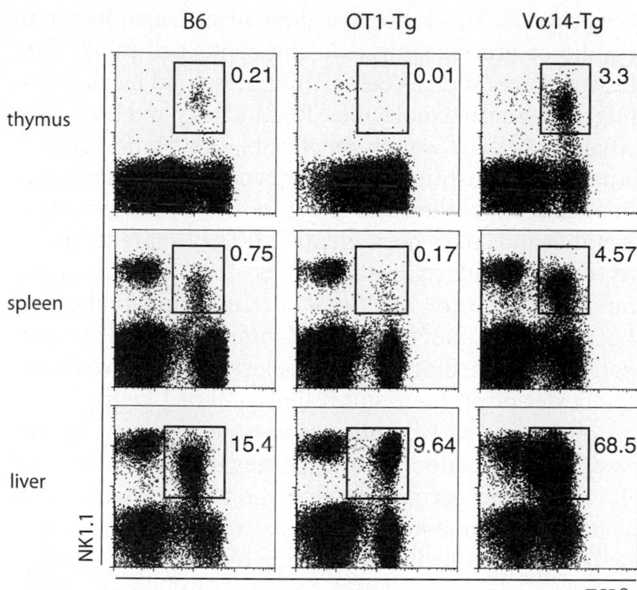

FIGURE 17.2 Developmental instruction of the NKT lineage by transgenic expression of the Vα18-Jα18 TCR α chain. In C57BL/6 mice, NKT cells labeled by anti-TCRβ and -NK1.1 are found in thymus and spleen but predominate among liver lymphocytes. Transgenic (Tg) mice expressing the Vα14-Jα18 Tg TCR α chain have increased NKT cell frequency, whereas mice expressing the MHC class I–restricted ovalbumin-specific TCR OT-1 are deprived of NKT cells. The NK1.1$^-$ T cells in Vα14-Jα18 Tg mice include cells that express inappropriate Vβ families. The NK1.1$^+$ T cells in OT-1 mice include cells that express endogenous Vα14-Jα18 TCR alpha chains.

"mainstream" αβ TCRs or BCRs prevented the development of NKT cells, B-1 B cells, and MZB cells, respectively. In cases where the self-ligand is known and could be deleted, development was interrupted, indicating that selection is based on antigen receptor/ligand interactions. Thus, ablation of CD1d (35–37), MR1 (38) specifically abrogated the development of TCR αβ NKT or MAIT cells, respectively. Beta 2-microglobulin–deficient mice did not support the development of T10/T22-specific KN6 γδ transgenic cells (39). B-1 B cells expressing an antibody specific for a carbohydrate determinant on the glycoprotein Thy-1 were not found in Thy1-deficient mice (40).

In the presence of a rearranged Vα14-Jα18 TCR α chain, TCRs using a Vβ8, Vβ7, or Vβ2 chain are the only ones that recognize the endogenous NKT ligand iGb3. This bias, which contrasts with the ability of Vα14-Jα18 to pair broadly with the entire Vβ repertoire, precisely matches the set of Vβs used by NKT cells, consistent with the notion of positive selection by this antigen (10).

Detailed analysis of the nucleotide sequences of canonical antigen receptors provide further unambiguous examples of antigen-driven selection. For example, a subset of the Vα14-Jα18 sequences of CD1d-restricted NKT cells exhibit variations in nucleotides, but these variations preserve the canonical amino acid sequence (4). In the case of MR1-specific MAIT cells, the mouse Vα19-Jα33 nucleotide sequence is largely invariant, probably owing to a long stretch of nucleotide homology between Vα19 and Jα33 (Table 17.4), but the human Vα7.2-Jα33 sequences show junctional variations with N nucleotides. The length of the CDR3 loop and its canonical amino acid motif are well preserved, however (38,41). Similar examples of antigen-driven selection have been found for the VH11 and VH12 heavy chains of phosphatidylcholine-specific B1 B cells (31,42).

T10/T22specific γδ TCRs have a canonical CDR3δ motif W-(S)EGYEL that includes a W variably originating from Vδ6, Dδ1, or even P/N elements (7). Although this T10/T22-specific sequence is found at relatively high frequency among peripheral γδ T cells, it is unclear whether the corresponding cells have undergone antigen-driven selection *in vivo*, because the specificity is still expressed at high frequency in β2-microglobulin–deficient mice and a large fraction of the T10/T22-specific cells exhibit a naïve phenotype. However, memory-type cells do require T10/T22 expression.

In the case of DETC cells with tightly programmed Vγ5/Vδ1 rearrangements, Vγ5 gene-ablation experiments demonstrated that only select Vγ/Vδ TCRs could substitute for Vγ5/Vδ1. These substitutes exhibited reactivity to a skin-derived epidermal cell line, shared a conformational epitope (idiotype) with Vγ5/Vδ1 as detected by a monoclonal antibody, or used select Vδs, suggesting selection by the same self-ligand (43,44), perhaps expressed by thymic stromal cells (45).

Vγ9/Vδ2 TCRs exhibit a changing pattern of formation with age (46–48). Thus, canonical germline sequences are found in nearly all the Vγ9Vδ2 cells of the human fetal liver (Table 17.5). These cells already express a memory CD45RO$^+$ phenotype. Later, in the perinatal period, substantial N-diversification is observed and a majority of the cells have a naïve phenotype, likely because they have lost specificity for self-antigen. Ultimately, antigen-driven selection becomes evident as the sequences accumulating in the adult repertoire retain the specificity of the germline fetal TCR and are associated with a memory phenotype. These observations illustrate both the importance of genetic mechanisms to increase the production of canonical sequences early in life and the presence of self-antigen–mediated selection at all stages of life.

Other, non–antigen-driven selection mechanisms have been proposed to narrow the antigen-receptor repertoire of future innatelike B-1 lymphocytes during early development. These include altered pairing with the surrogate light chain for pre-BCR signaling, which may have different consequences in fetal and adult precursors, or biased pairing with light chains (31,49,50).

Cellular Expansion of Innatelike Lymphocytes

Another mechanism contributing to the high frequency of some innatelike lymphocyte subsets is illustrated by the massive clonal expansion undergone by NKT cells during thymic development (51). Rounds of cell divisions occur in the thymus just after positive selection and before NKT cells emigrate to the periphery. These divisions, which increase the NKT cell frequency from $<10^{-4}$ among recently selected thymocytes to 2% to 5% among thymic emigrants, is independent of exposure to microbial or environmental antigens, as it is reproduced in fetal thymic organ culture *in vitro* and as NKT cell frequency is conserved in germ-free mice (52). It is not clear at present whether this expansion phase also applies to other subsets of innatelike lymphocytes. The "self-renewing" capacity ascribed to Ig-expressing B-1 B cells (53) may reflect the property of expansion post–BCR expression and/or increased survival compared with other B cells. This expansion is associated with the acquisition of a memory/effector phenotype that is a hallmark of many innatelike lymphocytes.

CONSERVED SELF- AND MICROBIAL ANTIGENS

General Considerations about Self- and Microbial Ligand Reactivities

The conservation of the invariant or semi-invariant BCRs and TCRs and their germline-encoded specificities are reminiscent of other innate immune receptors such as TLRs. Like TLRs, innatelike BCRs and TCRs appear to be monospecific or to recognize a restricted set of self- and microbial structures of particular evolutionary significance.

Autoreactivity

A quasi-universal feature of innatelike lymphocytes that has dominated the search for their ligands is their autoreactivity in various *in vitro* or *in vivo* assays against normal or transformed cells, or against soluble ligands. For example, NKT hybridomas or clones can be activated to secrete cytokines by fresh thymocytes, by DCs, and by various tumor cell lines (54–58), and $\gamma\delta$ T-cell clones kill stressed or transformed cells (59–62). TCR transfection or transgenic expression have established that these reactivities are linked to the TCR (25,63–65), although they could also be modulated by additional receptors such as NKG2D, for example (65,66). Many B-1- and MZB-cell–derived antibodies recognize senescent or apoptotic cell membranes (67–69); others recognize thymocytes (70).

Molecular identification of the self-ligands involved has been generally difficult and, in many cases, is still debated or in progress. This is because these ligands are often nonpeptidic or are recognized in the context of more complex structures such as cell membranes, lipid particles, or antigen-presenting molecules. Redundancy and broad disturbances associated with genetic ablation of their synthesis pathways constitute further impediments to a definitive understanding of the basis of autoreactivity. Nevertheless, several ligands have been identified. They share the property of being full agonists, that is, they activate proliferation and effector functions of mature innatelike lymphocytes. They, therefore, differ from the "partial agonist" peptides that mediate positive selection of conventional thymocytes or promote survival of mature T cells.

How innatelike lymphocytes use these agonist ligands for positive selection yet escape negative selection, and how they avoid permanent activation and exhaustion in the periphery, are issues that have generally not been fully answered. It is also becoming apparent that the developmental signals initiated by encounter of these agonist ligands may be central to the instruction of innatelike lymphocyte commitment. Another emerging theme is that autoreactivity can be the basis of their activation during some of the antimicrobial immune responses in which innatelike lymphocytes are involved. Thus, autoreactivity constitutes a central feature of innatelike lymphocyte biology, and it appears to be by design rather than by accident (71). These aspects will be further addressed in the sections on development and function.

Dual Reactivity for Self- and Microbial Ligands

Systematic screening for responses to microbial extracts *in vitro* or studies of mutant mice lacking individual innatelike subsets *in vivo* have led to the discovery of microbial antigen targets and the demonstration that, at least in some conditions, innatelike lymphocytes can contribute substantially to the clearance of the corresponding pathogens. Two models have emerged to integrate the dual reactivity against self- and microbial ligands, each of which has received some support in different systems. In one model, microbial and mammalian cells express structurally related ligands, but the microbial ligands are recognized with very high affinity while the low affinity mammalian ligands require overexpression during transformation or infection to induce the full activation of innatelike lymphocytes. This is the proposed scenario for the microbial and mammalian phosphorylated isoprenoid metabolites recognized by human Vγ9 cells (72,73). A similar scenario governs the dual recognition of phosphorylcholine residues on Streptococcus *pneumoniae* carbohydrates by natural B-1 B-cell antibodies and of phosphatidylcholine in altered cell membranes or oxidized LDL (68,74). In another model illustrated by NKT cells, self- and microbial ligands are structurally very distinct (75–77) but they are also recognized with different affinities by the canonical receptor.

Nonclassical MHC-like Ligands of Innatelike T Lymphocytes

The evolutionary significance and the functions of nonpolymorphic MHC class I–like molecules remained mysterious (78) until recent studies established that they function as ligands for multiple receptors, including those expressed by NK cells, which are true innate lymphocytes, or by the TCRs of innatelike $\alpha\beta$ and $\gamma\delta$ T cells. The MHC-like ligands of innatelike lymphocytes identified so far include CD1d (54) (NKT cells), MR1 (MAIT cells) (38), T10/T22 (79), CD1c (80), and MIC (65, 81) ($\gamma\delta$ T cells) (Figure 17.3).

CD1d

CD1d is a member of the CD1 family of β2-microglobulin–associated MHC class I–like molecules, which comprises five isotypes, CD1a–e (82). Although the mammalian CD1 genes are encoded in a locus outside the MHC, studies in chicken have suggested that they evolved from a precursor in the MHC locus (83,84). CD1a, b, c, and d are expressed on the cell surface of most antigen-presenting cells, including dendritic cells, macrophages, and B cells, as well as on cortical thymocytes (85,86). They bind lipid alkyl chains within hydrophobic channels buried in their groove and present their polar head to the TCR. Examples of CD1a-, b-, or c-restricted T cells include autoreactive or microbial lipid specific human clones generated *in vitro*, whose $\gamma\delta$ or $\alpha\beta$ TCRs appear to be diverse. In contrast, CD1d, the only isotype found in mice and rats, is recognized by a prominent subset of T cells in both rodents and humans. These T cells are dominated by innatelike NKT cells with canonical mVα14-Jα18/hVα24-Jα18 TCRs (87).

Vα14 NKT cells are autoreactive to CD1d-expressing cells in a manner that depends on CD1d endosomal trafficking (88,89), suggesting recognition of endosomal/lysosomal lipid antigens. Several glycolipid antigens require endosomal trafficking of CD1d for processing by glycosidases (90) or loading by glycolipid transfer proteins such as saposins (91–93) before recycling to the plasma membrane. Search for a lysosomally loaded self-ligand recognized by NKT cells has identified a trihexosylceramide, iGb3, first synthesized in the Golgi as an intermediate in the biosynthetic pathway of iGb4. In the lysosome, iGb4 is degraded into iGb3 by β-hexosaminidase AB, and then further degraded into LacCer, following established pathways of glycosphingolipid degradation. Mice that lacked β-hexosaminidase B lacked 95% of their NKT cells, a defect associated with the impaired ability of their thymocytes to stimulate autoreactive NKT hybridomas. Direct stimulation of mouse and human NKT cells with natural and synthetic iGb3, but not with any other known mammalian glycosphingolipids, indicated that iGb3 is a universal ligand of mouse and human NKT cells (75). Studies of Vα14-Jα18 transgenic T cells expressing a diverse Vβ repertoire showed that only those expressing the biased set of Vβ8, Vβ7 and Vβ2 chains normally found in mature NKT cells responded to iGb3 (10). The general functions of iGb3, like those of most glycosylceramides, remain largely unknown, and the regulation of iGb3 expression in different cell-types has not been studied yet. Thus, it is not clear why iGb3 may have been coopted by the NKT cell system.

Search for microbial ligands uncovered an interesting family of gram-negative lipopolysaccharide (LPS)-negative bacteria that use novel α-branched

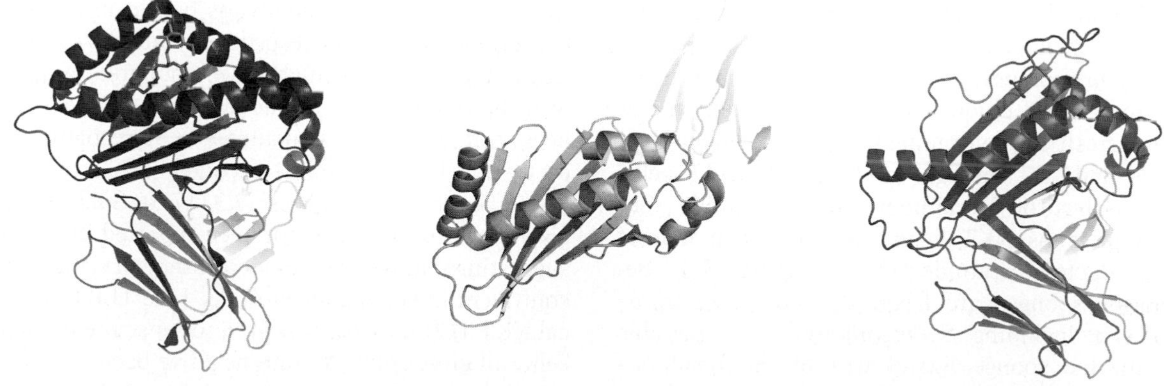

FIGURE 17.3 MHC class I–like ligands of innatelike T lymphocytes. Ribbon-diagram structures of CD1d in complex with αGalCer (left), of MICA (center), and of H-2T22 (right). These MHC class I–like molecules serve as ligands of NKT cells, some Vδ1 T cells, and Dδ2 $\gamma\delta$ T cells, respectively. Note that the unliganded MICA has a disordered α2 helix. (Courtesy of Erin Adams, University of Chicago, Chicago, IL, USA.)

αGC (KRN7000)

GSL-1

iGb3

BbGL-IIc

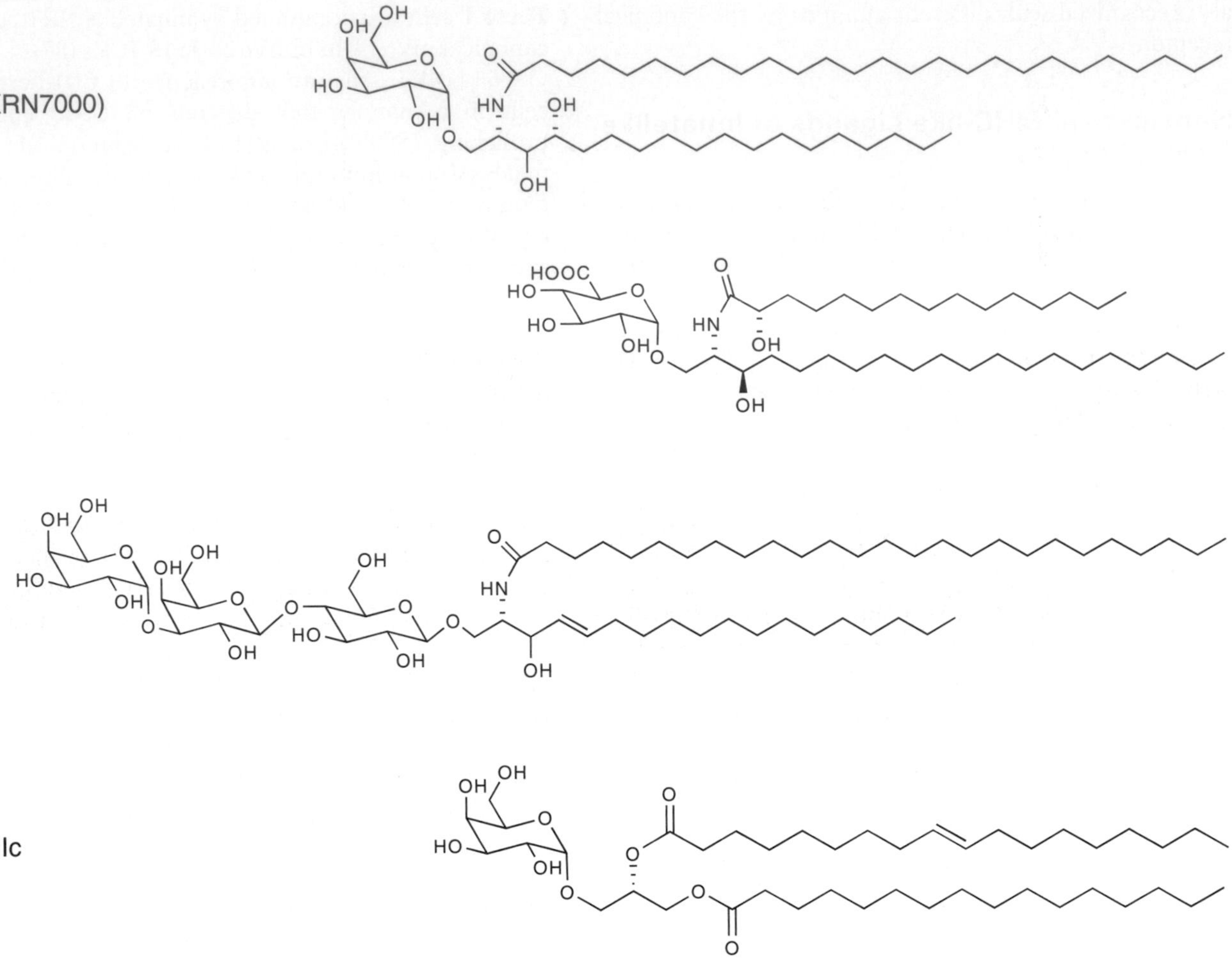

FIGURE 17.4 Lipid ligands of NKT cells. Note the structural similarities among foreign α-galactosylceramide (αGC) (derived from marine sponge), the *Sphingomonas* cell wall glycosphingolipid (GSL)-1, and *Borrelia burgdorferi* BbGl-IIc. All three lipids have a single carbohydrate with an α-anomeric linkage to the lipid. In contrast, the endogenous ligand iGb3 has a Galα1,3Galβ1,4Glc in a β-anomeric linkage to ceramide.

glycuronylceramides as substitute for LPS in the outer membrane of their cell wall (94). The best-studied example is *Sphingomonas*, a member of the class of α-proteobacteria and a ubiquitous bacterium found in marine and terrestrial environment that can infect dendritic cells and macrophages and activate NKT cells. Microbial α-glycuronylceramides are structurally very close to a previous NKT ligand isolated from marine sponge, α-galactosylceramide (95,96) (Figure 17.4). Because marine sponges are frequently colonized by α-proteobacteria including *Sphingomonas*, it is possible that the marine sponge ligand was of microbial origin. Another structurally related α-glycosylated lipid, α-galactosyldiacylglycerol, found in *Borrelia burgdorferi*, the agent of Lyme disease, was shown to activate mouse and human NKT cells (97).

The crystal structure of the α-branched glycosylceramide complexed to CD1d has been elucidated, showing the acyl and sphingosine chains buried in the A′ and F′ hydrophobic channels, respectively, and the carbohydrate sitting flat on top of the groove, anchored by a network of hydrogen bonds to amino acids on the α1 and α2 helices to form a rigid structure that is recognized nearly exclusively by the germline-encoded CDR3α of the canonical TCR (98–99a) (Figures 17.3, 17.5). Such α-branched glycosylceramides have not been reported in vertebrates, suggesting that they represent a pathogen signature that is equivalent in significance to LPS. Like TLR4, the canonical NKT TCR may have evolved to sense the predominant cell wall glycolipids of gram-negative bacteria. Indeed, α-glycosylceramide ligands can activate NKT cells at subnanomolar concentrations, and their Kd for the canonical TCR has been measured around 100 nM in mouse and 7 μM in human. In contrast, iGb3 is active at 100-fold higher concentration, and its affinity for the TCR appears to be lower than that of α-galactosylceramide (3).

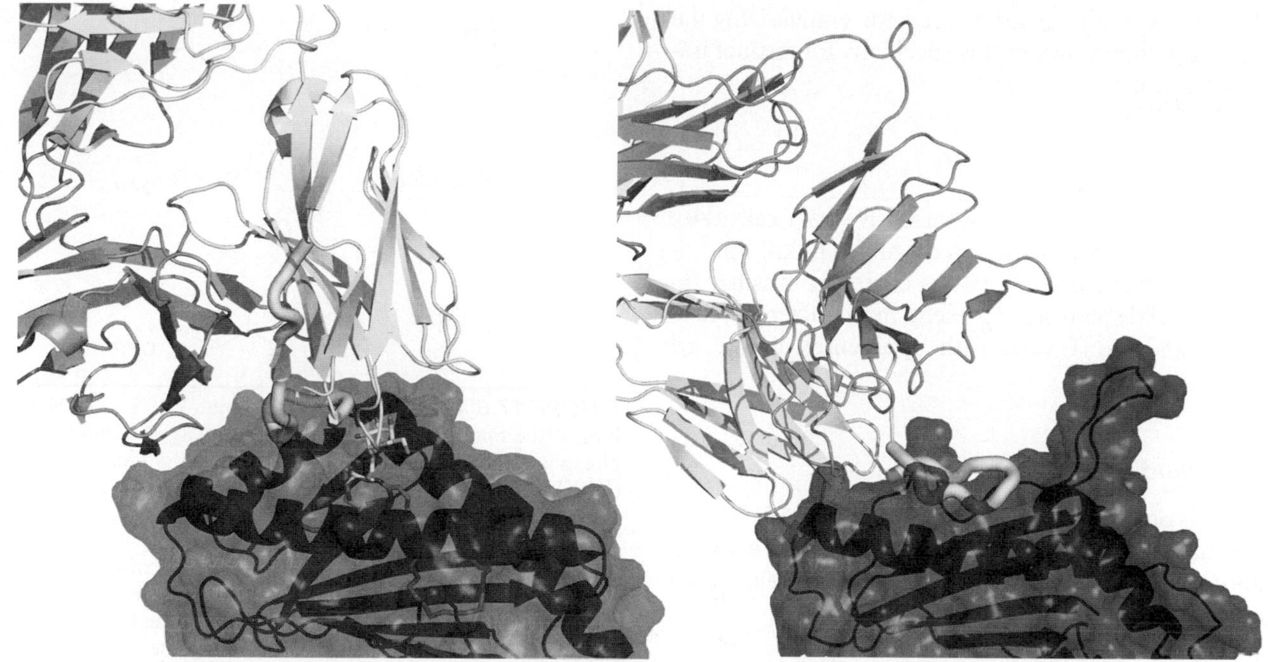

FIGURE 17.5 Structural determinants of ligand recognition. Left: The rearranged TCR α chain of NKT cells exclusively use Jα18, shown as a thick tube in the structure of the human Vα24-Jα18/Vβ11 TCR. The CDR3α of the NKT TCRs are nearly identical in amino acid sequence between mouse and human and provide most of the contact points with CD1d complexed with an α-galactosylceramide ligand (99a). Right: $\gamma\delta$ T cells specific for the H-2T22 MHC class I molecule use a conserved amino acid motif (W.EGYEL) in their CDR3δ loop, shown as a thick tube in the structure of the G8 $\gamma\delta$ TCR in complex with H-2T22. These amino acids, which are encoded by the germline V region and D segments, contribute most of the contact points with H-2T22 (7). (Courtesy of Erin Adams, University of Chicago, Chicago, IL, USA.) (See color insert.)

T10/T22

$\gamma\delta$ T cells that are specific for the T10/T22 molecules constitute another well-studied system. T10 and T22 are β2-microglobulin–associated nonpolymorphic MHC class Ib molecules that are found in mouse, but not rat or human, and are upregulated by LPS or concanavalin A (79). Tetramers of empty T22 molecules stain 1% to 2% of $\gamma\delta$ T cells. Interestingly their TCRs appeared quite diverse until extensive sequence analysis uncovered a canonical sequence motif encoded mainly by the Dδ2 gene segment. A crystal structure of the G8 TCR complexed with T22 was generated (7), demonstrating that G8 binds empty T22 at a tilted angle through extensive, nearly exclusive contacts of Dδ with the exposed β-sheet floor and the α1 helix of T22 (Figure 17.5). Although residues flanking the canonical motif could influence the binding, the Kd of TCR/ligand interactions could be as high as the 10 nM range.

MR1

MR1 is a non–MHC-encoded, β2-microglobulin–associated MHC class I–like molecule conserved in mouse, human, and cow that is recognized by a subset of mucosal-associated invariant T (MAIT) lymphocytes that express a canonical hVα7.2/mVα19 Jα33 chain combined with diverse β chains (38). Although MR1 has yet to be detected at the cell surface of normal cells *in vivo*, it can be expressed upon transfection. Mutagenesis of residues putatively involved in peptide binding (based on modeling) influenced recognition by MR1-autoreactive hybridomas, suggesting ligand presentation rather than recognition of empty MR1 (100). The nature of these putative ligands remains mysterious. Selection of MAIT cells in mouse is independent of TAP or the invariant chain.

MIC

MICA and MICB are MHC-encoded glycoproteins expressed in conditions of stress by various epithelial and hemopoietic cells (101). Their MHC-like structure does not associate with β2-microglobulin and harbors the remnant of a peptide-binding groove reduced to a small, empty cavity (102) (Figure 17.3). MIC proteins can be recognized by the Vδ1 TCRs of some human T-cell clones (65,81), suggesting the possibility that dedicated TCR sequences akin to the ones associated with T10/T22 recognition may be involved. Interestingly, these $\gamma\delta$ T cells coexpress NKG2D, another MIC-specific activating receptor, emphasizing the evolutionary importance of this specificity for distinct immune cell lineages.

CD1c

CD1c is recognized by some autoreactive $\gamma\delta$ T cells (80), but information on canonical recognition motif, lipid ligands, or the structure of CD1c is currently missing. Interestingly, CD1c can also present mycobacterial phosphoisoprenoids to T cells with apparently diverse $\alpha\beta$ TCRs (103).

DETC Ligand

The ligands of intraepithelial $\gamma\delta$ T cells such as DETC cells have remained totally elusive, although there is a strong likelihood that some unidentified MHC-like proteins could be involved.

Phosphorylated Metabolites of the Isoprenoid Pathway

The prominent subset of Vγ9 T cells found in human peripheral blood show broad antimicrobial and antitumoral reactivities that have been ascribed to the recognition of metabolites of the isoprenoid biosynthetic pathways of microorganisms (1-deoxy-D-xylulose-5-phosphate [DOXP] pathway) and mammalian cells (mevalonate pathway) (72,73,104,105). These are small nonpeptidic phosphorylated compounds, with the microbial hydroxy-dimethyl-allyl-pyrophosphate (HDMAPP) being active at 0.1 nM concentrations and the mammalian isopentenylpyrophosphate (IPP) at 10,000-fold higher concentrations (Figure 17.6). Other activators such as aminobiphosphonates and alkylamines probably mediate their effect indirectly through inhibition of the mevalonate pathway leading to accumulation of IPP, whereas statins downregulate IPP levels (106,107). The requirement for cell–cell interactions in Vγ9 T-cell activation and the lack of direct binding of these phosphoantigens to the TCR have suggested the existence of a more complex structure at the target cell surface. Recently, F1-ATPase, a mitochondrial enzyme that is translocated to the plasma membrane of hepatocytes and some tumor cell lines, was shown to be the target of $\gamma\delta$ T cells based on antibody-blocking experiments and direct binding to soluble TCR (108). Apolipoprotein A1 bound F1-ATPase and enhanced recognition. These findings could constitute a challenge to the previous model that phosphoisoprenoids are relevant or exclusive $\gamma\delta$ T-cell antigens. Conversely, they may indicate some interaction between the two pathways—for example, F1-ATPase may present the phosphoantigens to the $\gamma\delta$ TCR.

IPP — OPP

HDMAPP — OH, OPP

DMAPP — OPP

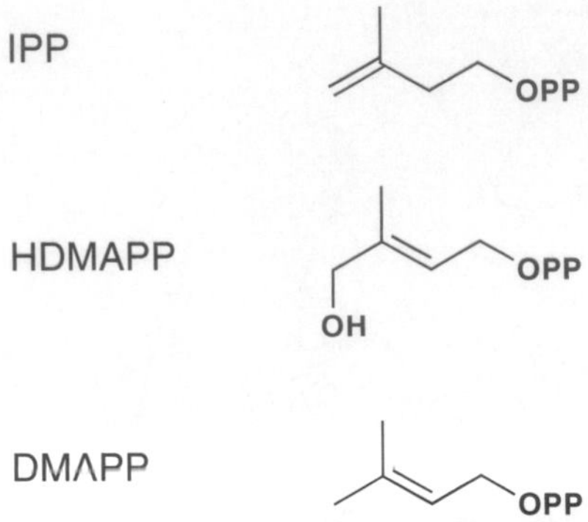

FIGURE 17.6 Phosphoantigens of human Vγ9 T cells. Metabolites of the mammalian mevalonate pathway, isopentenyl-pyrophosphate (IPP), or of the microbial deoxyxylulose-phosphate (DOXP) pathway, hydroxydimethylallyl PP (HDMAPP), and dimethylallyl-PP (DMAPP). Microbial HDMAPP activates Vγ9 T cells at picomolar concentrations, whereas mammalian IPP requires 10,000-fold higher concentrations. Because Vγ9 stimulation requires cell–cell contact and the Vγ9 TCR does not bind these phosphoantigens in solution, it is assumed that the phosphoantigens are presented by some unidentified molecule, possibly F1-ATPase translocated at the plasma membrane.

B-1 and MZB Cell Ligands

B-1 and MZB cells produce a fraction of the so-called natural IgM antibodies that are present in unimmunized animals (109). Although some canonical recurrent antibodies have been ascribed to B cells of the B-1 or MZB lineages, the diversity and origins of other natural antibodies remain to be further investigated. For example, several natural antibodies against carbohydrate sequences (e.g., blood group) are elicited in a T-independent manner by the gut commensal flora from conventional B cells without germline canonical BCRs.

Membrane Phospholipids, Lipid Particles, Apoptotic Membranes, Microbial Cell Wall

One recurrent specificity group appears to be directed at phospholipids exposed in altered cell membranes or lipid particles. A significant fraction of B-1- or MZB-derived natural antibodies bind to apoptotic cells (34,68,110,111), a specificity shared by many other soluble membrane-bound innate receptors. Phosphorylcholine-specific T15 idiotype–bearing cells were found to be expanded in apolipoprotein E–deficient mice accumulating oxidized LDL particles. The B-1 cell–derived VH11/Vκ9, VH12/Vκ4 and the T15 idiotype–bearing antibodies, as well as the MZB-derived M167 idiotype–bearing antibodies all bind apoptotic cells and the phospholipid phosphatidylcholine, particularly after processing into lysophosphatidylcholine (lysoPC) by phospholipase A2 (110). LysoPC, by virtue of lacking one of the two acyl chains that normally anchor phosphatidylcholine in the plasma membrane, is thought to expose its PC headgroup for recognition by natural antibodies. Natural IgM against autologous bromelain-treated red blood cells mainly include the VH11/Vκ9 and VH12/Vκ4 antibodies whose corresponding B-1 cells represent up to 10% of the peritoneal B-cell population based on staining with fluorescent liposome enriched in phosphatidylcholine (67). These antibodies cross-react onto lipoteichoic acid, a glycolipid component of the gram-positive bacterial cell wall of *Streptococcus pneumoniae,* whose carbohydrates are heavily decorated with PC headgroups (22,74).

Thymocyte Antigen

A minor subset of B-1 B cells uses VH3609 to produce natural antithymocyte antibodies (70). These B-1 BCRs are specific for a glycosylated epitope present on Thy1, a glycoprotein expressed by T cells and neural cells. Although the function of these antibodies is unknown, the system has been elegantly used to elucidate the role of self-antigen in development (40,112).

FUNCTIONS OF INNATELIKE LYMPHOCYTES

Functional Properties of Innatelike Lymphocytes

Many innatelike lymphocytes are memory/effector cells that reside or traffic in specific tissues and are endowed with specialized functional properties.

B-1 B cells, like MZB cells, express high-surface IgM and low IgD, a pattern that is characteristic of activated B cells. They are thought to be a major, though not exclusive, source of the natural IgM antibodies found in unimmunized mouse serum, which are produced in a T-independent manner (109). MZB cells respond faster and more strongly to stimulation than do conventional B cells (113). In addition, MZB cells express high levels of the complement receptor CD21, which considerably enhances their ability to detect and respond to blood-borne pathogens (114,115).

By virtue of their autoreactivity, NKT cells can reciprocally activate immature dendritic cells through CD40 ligand/CD40 interactions (76,116,117). This property can be further exploited by administering *in vivo* synthetic agonist ligands of NKT cells (α-galactosylceramide), which are efficiently presented by immature DCs to initiate a powerful cellular and molecular inflammatory network (118,119). Thus, after injection of 1 μg of the NKT ligand αGalCer, mice show an early and transient IL-4 response peaking in the first hour and a delayed but prolonged IFNγ and TNFα as well as various chemokines. DCs upregulate CD40, B7.1, B7.2, and IL12p40, which enhance NKT-cell activation and cytokine production. NK cells are also activated to release IFNγ and acquire cytolytic properties (120,121). These effects explain the superior effects of NKT ligands over TLR ligands as adjuvants of adaptive B- and T-cell responses, which is particularly important for CTL responses against nonreplicating, cross-presented antigens (122–124). Interestingly, synthetic phosphoantigens of Vγ9 T cells also elicit DC activation and exhibit adjuvant properties (125,126).

Massive Th1 and Th2 cytokine production within minutes of TCR activation (127), potent cytolytic functions mediated by granzyme and perforin as well as FasL/Fas that can be augmented by NKG2D cosignaling, help for B cell have been reported for both NKT and $\gamma\delta$ T cells. Human Vγ9 $\gamma\delta$ T cells can upregulate MHC class II and have been suggested to present antigen to CD4 T cells in some conditions (128). Th1 and Th2 properties have also been identified in unimmunized MAIT cells (129).

In line with their peculiar "sentinel" association with specific tissues, $\gamma\delta$ T cells secrete growth factors such as keratinocyte growth factor-1 and insulin growth factor-1, which promote wound healing at mucosal barriers (130,131).

Natural Functions of Innatelike Lymphocyte Subsets in Physiology and Disease

Despite a very large body of literature dedicated to their functions in the context of host defense, inflammation and allergy, autoimmunity, and cancer rejection, the precise role of individual innatelike subsets is still partially understood and sometimes controversial.

NKT Cells

Microbial Infections. The best-characterized functions of NKT cells are related to antimicrobial immunity. Many micro-organisms elicit various networks of cellular and molecular interactions that involve NKT cells. Recent advances in identifying endogenous and exogenous NKT ligands have suggested the existence of two distinct pathways of antimicrobial defense (Figure 17.7).

A direct pathway is specifically recruited upon infection by micro-organisms that express NKT ligands in their cell wall. This is illustrated by the α-proteobacterium *Sphingomonas*. Though it is not a common pathogen in humans, *Sphingomonas* can cause severe infections, particularly in immunocompromised patients, and it is found

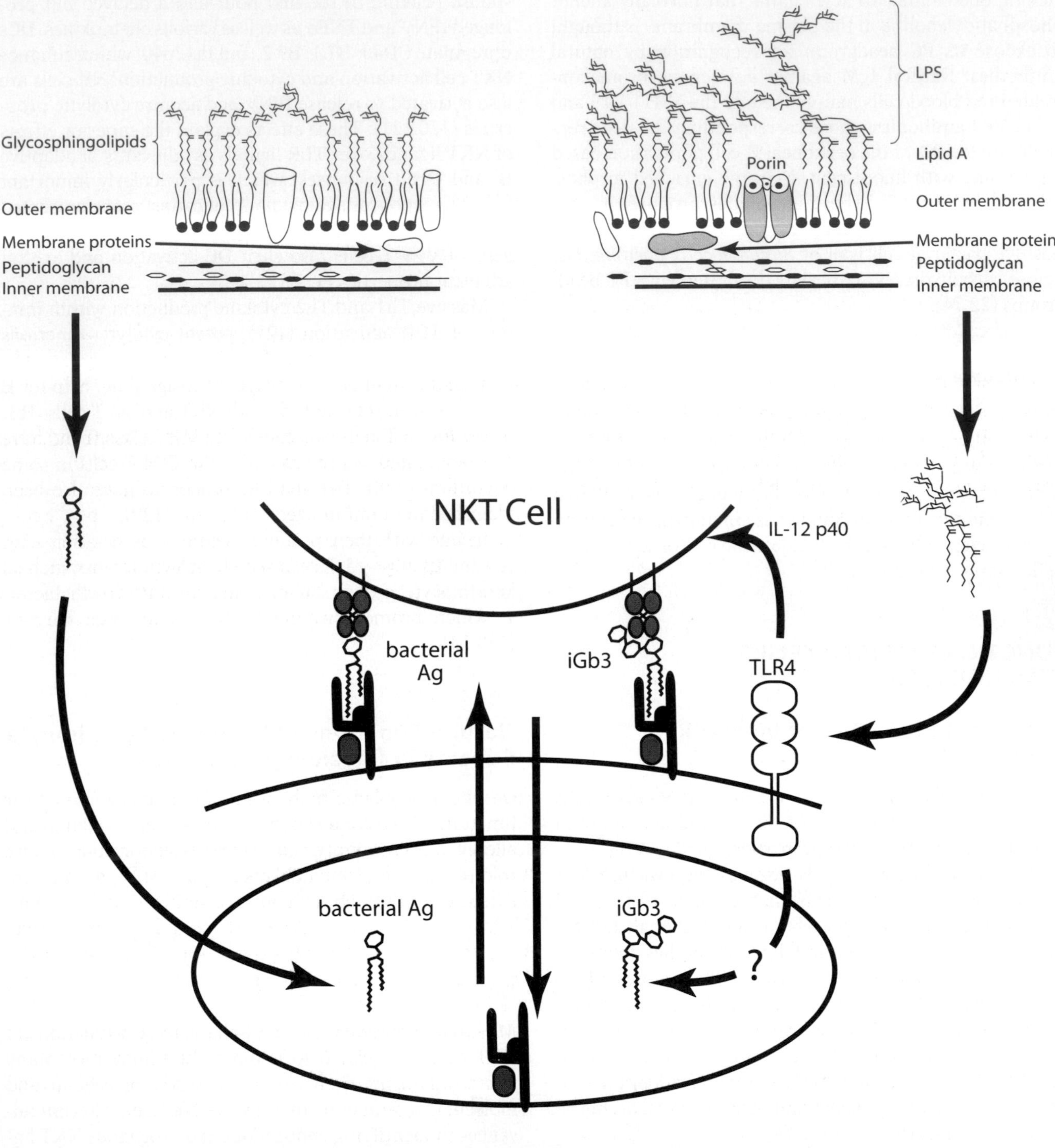

FIGURE 17.7 Dual recognition of self- and foreign ligands by NKT cells. The gram-negative, LPS-negative cell wall of Sphingomonas activates NKT cells directly, through loading of glycosphingolipids onto CD1d in the lysosome and presentation at the plasma membrane. In contrast, the gram-negative, LPS-positive cell wall of *Salmonella* activates NKT cells indirectly, through TLR-mediated activation of DC and presentation of endogenous ligand iGb3 along with IL-12. It is unclear whether TLR signaling upregulates endogenous NKT ligands or only amplifies the consequences of basal TCR signaling by induction of IL-12, IL-15 or NK ligands.

by polymerase chain reaction (PCR) in the feces of healthy subjects (132). NKT cells are directly activated by infected antigen-presenting cells and function as an immediate innate source of help in a Toll-like receptor-independent manner, resulting in the rapid clearance of the pathogen (76,77). Thus, NKT cells substitute for TLR in the same way as their α-glycuronylceramide ligands substitute for LPS in the bacterial cell wall. A similar pathway appears to be elicited by another gram-negative, LPS-negative α-proteobacterium, *Ehrlichia muris*, a tick-borne intracellular pathogen member of the *Rickettsiales* (76), although the chemical nature of the NKT ligands involved is unknown. Both *Sphingomonas* and *Ehrlichia* activate NKT cells after cellular infection in a CD1d-dependent and TLR-independent manner, and their clearance is severely impaired in CD1d$^{-/-}$ and Jα18$^{-/-}$ NKT-deficient mice (76,77). *Borrelia burgdorferi* expresses α-glycosyldiacylglycerols that can be recognized by mouse and human NKT cells (77). However, unlike *Sphingomonas* or *Ehrlichia*, antigen presenting cells exposed to *Borrelia* have not been shown to stimulate NKT cells, and the effect of NKT cell deficiency on bacterial clearance was modest (133).

Seropositivity against *Sphingomonas* proteins was specifically found in nearly all patients with primary biliary cirrhosis (PBC) (132). PBC is a chronic liver disease characterized by the destruction of small intrahepatic bile ducts and the presence of diagnostic antimitochondrial antibodies (134). In fact, these antimitochondrial antibodies were found to cross-react against an identical epitope on the homologous *Sphingomonas* enzyme PDC-E2 (132). Mitochondria are evolutionarily related to α-proteobacteria–like *Sphingomonas*, suggesting that PBC may be triggered or promoted by aberrant NKT cell responses to *Sphingomonas* infection. This intriguing hypothesis is supported by a report that NKT cells are increased in the liver of PBC patients and depleted in their blood (135).

Another, indirect pathway of NKT-cell activation is frequently elicited in many bacterial, viral, and parasitic infections. For example, in the presence of *Salmonella*, NKT cells produce substantial quantities of IFNγ, in a manner dependent on the IL-12 secreted by TLR-activated DCs (76,117). Contrary to initial beliefs, however, IL-12 is not sufficient to activate IFNγ secretion by NKT cells. Interactions with CD1d are required, as demonstrated by the interruption of NKT-cell activation in the presence of anti-CD1d antibody or CD1d-deficient DCs. Furthermore, contrasting with the direct activation pathway, NKT-cell activation was impaired in β-hexosaminidase B–deficient-mice with impaired lysosomal iGb3 production or by blocking with the lectin *Griffonia simplicifoliam,* specific for the terminal Galα1,3Gal of iGb3 alone or bound to CD1d (76). These findings suggest that NKT-cell responses can be based on the autoreactivity of NKT cells rather than on the recognition of specific microbial ligands. It is unclear at present whether iGb3 is induced in these conditions, or whether it is constitutive and low-level TCR signaling is amplified through activating NK lineage receptors such as NKG2D, the presence of IL-12, or the removal of influences from inhibitory NK lineage receptors, leading to IFNγ production. As might be expected from the diversity of cell types recruited to produce IFNγ early after this type of microbial infection, including NK cells and $\gamma\delta$ T cells, ablation of NKT cells does not detectably change the outcome. However, delayed clearance and alterations in granuloma formation have been reported for particular pathogens and in specific tissue locations. For example, NKT-deficient mice exhibited a transient but marked defect in secretion of macrophage inflammatory protein-2, attraction of neutrophils, and clearance of *Pseudomonas aeruginosa* in lungs (136).

Cancer Rejection. A role of NKT cells in cancer rejection has been suggested by studies in CD1d$^{-/-}$ and Jα18$^{-/-}$ NKT-deficient mice. The most striking observation reported an increased incidence of spontaneous fibrosarcomas after subcutaneous injection of methylcholanthrene (MCA) and also demonstrated a requirement for IL-12 and IFNγ (137). This report, however, has remained isolated, and other studies have examined the role of NKT cells in the setting of tumor transplants. NKT cells, particularly CD4$^-$CD8$^-$ cells, contributed to the prevention of liver metastasis after intravenous injection of fibrosarcoma cells. CD1d expression by host rather than tumor cells was essential, and the production of IFNγ by both NKT cells and other cell types, likely NK cells and CD8 T cells, was required. However, perforin expression was required only from non-NKT cells. These results suggested that activation of NKT cells was triggered by host-derived antigen-presenting cells, initiating a Th1 cascade involving NK cells and CD8 killer cells, and resulting in tumor elimination (138,139). In contrast, NKT cells suppressed the rejection of RMA/S transfected with CD1d (140). NKT cells may therefore recognize some undefined ligands either directly on the tumor or on antigen-presenting cells. Although Vα14 NKT cells represent ~80% CD1d-restricted T cells in mice, non-Vα14 T cells exist and, based on the differential phenotypes of CD1d$^{-/-}$ and Jα18$^{-/-}$ mice, have been implicated in the IL-13-mediated suppression of other tumors.

MAIT Cells

MAIT cells accumulate in the lamina propria and the mesenteric lymph nodes of mouse and human (38,129). Their requirement for B cells, their dependence on the gut bacterial flora, and their ability to secrete various Th1 and Th2 cytokines have suggested a role in intestinal immunity, perhaps in controlling IgA secretion.

$\gamma\delta$ T Cells

Consistent with the autoreactivity of the canonical DETC TCR against keratinocytes undergoing stress and transformation (59,63) TCR$\delta^{-/-}$ and V$\gamma 5^{-/-}$ mice exhibited a greater frequency of chemically induced skin cancer, which was reduced upon transfer of Vγ5 T cells (66,141). Mice lacking DETC cells also exhibited greater susceptibility to spontaneous or irritant-induced dermatitis (142,143). The secretion of keratinocyte growth factor-1 (130) and insulin growth factor-1 (131) and the induction of hyaluronan by neighboring epidermal cells (144) underlie a role in skin homeostasis and repair in mouse. Gut $\gamma\delta$ T cells perform similar functions as well (145). Interestingly, DETC responses to stress and transformed keratinocytes is augmented by their expression of NKG2D, a NK lineage receptor specific for Rae1 ligands, which are also induced by stress and transformation (66).

Other subsets of $\gamma\delta$ T cells, such as the human Vγ9 T cells, are likely to contribute to the rejection of primary and secondary cancers (146), but their importance and the precise mechanism involved have remained somewhat elusive. Likewise, there is abundant suggestion that $\gamma\delta$ T cells are recruited in various infections, but their precise functions remain to be clarified (147).

B-1 and MZB Cells

Unlike NKT cells, MAIT cells and subsets of $\gamma\delta$ T cells which have been specifically targeted by ablation of their ligands or of their TCR genes, B-1, and MZB cells, have not been properly "knocked out" of the mouse system.

Nevertheless, convergent findings suggest important functions for B-1 cell–derived natural IgM antibodies that share germline-encoded specificity to phosphatidylcholine, phosphorylcholine, oxidized LDL, and apoptotic cells. Through recognition of phosphorylcholine residues on microbial cell walls, such IgM antibodies can provide natural protection against infection by *Streptococcus pneumoniae* upon transfer into X-linked immunodeficiency (*Xid*) CBA/N mice (74). *Xid* mice have a missense mutation in the Bruton tyrosine kinase gene (*Btk*), which is essential for B-1 B cell development, but also for T-independent activation of conventional B cells. Thus, they do not represent a pure model of B-1 B cell deficiency. By virtue of their location in the marginal sinus of the splenic B-cell follicles and their expression of high levels of the complement receptor CD21, MZB cells can promptly detect and respond to blood-borne pathogens.

Natural IgM antibodies more generally provide protection at the early phase of infection by various bacterial, viral, and parasitic organisms (148,149). It is not always clear, however, whether the natural antibodies involved in particular conditions have germline-encoded specificities and originate from B-1 or MZB cells, or whether they have diverse non-germline–encoded sequences and originate from ongoing T-independent responses to various microbial polysaccharides (e.g., blood group or Galα1,3Gal epitopes). Conversely, natural antibodies and complement aggravate reperfusion injury after ischemia, likely through recognition of self-determinants exposed upon tissue ischemia (150).

DEVELOPMENT OF INNATELIKE LYMPHOCYTES

Innatelike lymphocytes comprise multiple lineages and sublineages that share a memory/effector differentiation but express quite diverse phenotypes, functional properties, and tissue locations. A cardinal principle underlying the diversity of these lineages is that they are instructed by the corresponding canonical antigen receptor during development, as a result of interaction with self-antigen. These self-antigens are often agonists that can fully activate the mature product of the lineage, explaining the autoreactive phenotype. The tight relationship between antigen receptor and lineage differentiation is abundantly illustrated by antigen-receptor transgenic experiments where each antigen receptor instructed differentiation according to the lineage of origin, including NKT cells (25,26) (Figure 17.2), DETC (27) and liver $\gamma\delta$ T cells (28), B-1 B cells (29,30,32,33) and MZB cells (34). The production and selection of these canonical receptors have been examined in detail in the section on canonical germline-encoded antigen receptors. This section will therefore examine the cellular and molecular events driving lineage differentiation downstream of the expression of these receptors, using different examples in the NKT cell, mucosal $\gamma\delta$ T cell, and B-1 B cell lineages.

One possible exception to this general scheme of production of differentiated memory/effector lineages is represented by the T10/T22-specific Dδ2 $\gamma\delta$ T cells. T10/T22 are MHC-encoded β2-microglobulin–associated class Ib molecules that are expressed only in some MHC haplotypes. Self-ligand recognition is largely encoded in their Dδ2 segment, whose random usage in the absence of antigen (i.e., in β2-microglobulin—deficient mice) can explain the high frequency of reactivity to T10/T22 among naïve $\gamma\delta$ T cells (7). However, there is also evidence of antigen selection for the KN6 TCR in transgenic mice, where the cells express a memory/effector differentiation in the presence of their ligand (151) and also depend on β2-microglobulin expression for development (39). Thus, antigen-independent naïve and antigen-experienced memory-type cells might coexist in this lineage.

Development of NKT Cells

Developmental Stages

The use of tetramers of CD1d-αGalCer specific for the canonical mVα14-Jα18/hVα24-Jα18 TCRs has revealed a previously unsuspected sequence of selection, expansion, and differentiation events preceding the terminally differentiated NK1.1$^+$ stage (51,152). As illustrated in Figure 17.8, NKT cells originate from mainstream thymocyte precursors that transit through the pre-TCRα/TCRβ stage to reach the CD4$^+$CD8$^+$ double-positive (DP) stage, where stochastic Vα-Jα rearrangements lead to expression of canonical Vα14-Jα18/Vβ8, Vβ7, or Vβ2 TCRs (153). These rearrangements involve distal gene segments and require prolonged cell survival mediated by RORγt and Bcl-xL (23,24). Studies of Vα14-Jα18 transgenic mice have demonstrated that whereas all Vβ families could pair with Vα14-Jα18, only the biased set of Vβs conferred specificity for the endogenous iGb3 ligand (10). The NKT precursors that are first detected are rare CD4$^+$CD8$^+$ double-positive and CD4$^+$ cells, both expressing high levels of CD24, a marker of immature cortical thymocytes, as well as CD69, a marker of positive selection (153). Early DP thymocytes that have not yet undergone positive selection are beyond the limits of detection because of the low frequency of Vα14-Jα18 rearrangements. As CD24^{high}CD4$^+$cells mature into the next CD24^{low}CD4$^+$ stage, they undergo several rounds of cell divisions (51). This lineage expansion after thymic positive selection ensures the high copy number that is critical for innatelike functions. During this phase, a fraction of CD4$^+$ cells downregulates CD4 to become CD4$^-$CD8$^-$ double-negative (DN) T cells (153), which differ from CD4 cells by their more restricted Th1 and chemokine profile and their enhanced ability to reject tumors. Dividing cells acquire a CD44^{high} memory phenotype and sequentially activate their IL-4 and IFN-γ loci, which enables them to produce these cytokines explosively upon TCR triggering (51,152,154). Thus, unlike other $\alpha\beta$ T cells, NKT lineage cells undergo a sequence of events that is reminiscent of the antigen-driven activation, expansion, and effector differentiation of mature T cells but is independent of exposure to environmental or microbial antigens (52). Because this sequence immediately follows positive selection, it is presumably driven in part by the same set of TCR signals and cosignals involved in positive selection, as discussed in the following.

NKT lineage cells emigrate from the thymus to seed peripheral tissues as dividing, memory/effector-type cells. They represent 3% to 5% of recent thymic emigrants in the mouse spleen (51,155). Recent emigrants activate a program of expression of NK lineage receptors, including activating NK1.1 and NKG2D and inhibitory CD94/NKG2A, Ly49 A, C/I, and G2. A fraction of NKT thymocytes remains as permanent residents in the thymus, where they undergo the same terminal maturation program. These thymic residents appear to be absent in humans (156), and their role is unknown. NKT cells are found in the spleen but are most abundant in the liver, where they exhibit a dynamic pattern of patrolling the vascular sinusoid space with sudden arrest upon exposure to NKT ligand (157). This pattern is consistent with an intravascular function of NKT cells at sites of filtration of blood-borne pathogens. Although the factors controlling the specific migration and anatomic location of NKT cells are still unknown, their expression of CXCR6 was found to be critical for survival in the CXCL16-expressing sinusoid environment (157).

Cellular Interactions

Because TCR expression instructs NKT lineage commitment, the thymic cell types involved in presenting NKT ligands have been thoroughly investigated. Consistent with the prominent expression of CD1d, but not MHC class I or class II, on cortical thymocytes, and with the ability of cortical thymocytes to stimulate NKT hybridomas (55), bone marrow chimera experiments have demonstrated that NKT-cell development required CD1d expression by cortical thymocytes but not radioresistant stromal cells (158–160). This is radically different from conventional T-cell development, which is driven by MHC expression on thymic epithelial cells. Transgenic experiments using promoters for Lck, MHC class I, or MHC class II to redirect the expression of CD1d to various cell compartments in CD1d-deficient hosts have shown thymocyte expression to be necessary and sufficient for lineage development (161–164). Mixed-chimera experiments using pLck-CD1d transgenic TCR Cα-deficient bone marrow (where thymocyte development is arrested at the DP stage) as the sole source of CD1d expression demonstrated that recognition of CD1d on cortical thymocytes was sufficient for the long-range differentiation of NKT cells, including acquisition of NK-lineage receptors in the periphery (162). Peripheral expression of CD1d, however, significantly enhanced the transition between NK1.1-negative and -positive stages (155,162).

Signaling

The signals driving NKT cell lineage commitment are expected to differ from those involved in mainstream T-cell development. First, the autoreactive response of NKT hybridomas to cortical thymocytes (55), which is a result of the agonist nature of their iGb3 ligand (75), indicates that the TCR signals must differ from those of mainstream thymocytes seeing partial agonist MHC/peptide ligands. Second, the homotypic (DP-DP) cellular interactions involved in the presentation of the NKT ligand during development may recruit a different set of receptor/ligand interactions (162). In line with these expectations, various signaling mutants have demonstrated differential requirements for the development of NKT *versus* mainstream T lineages. In

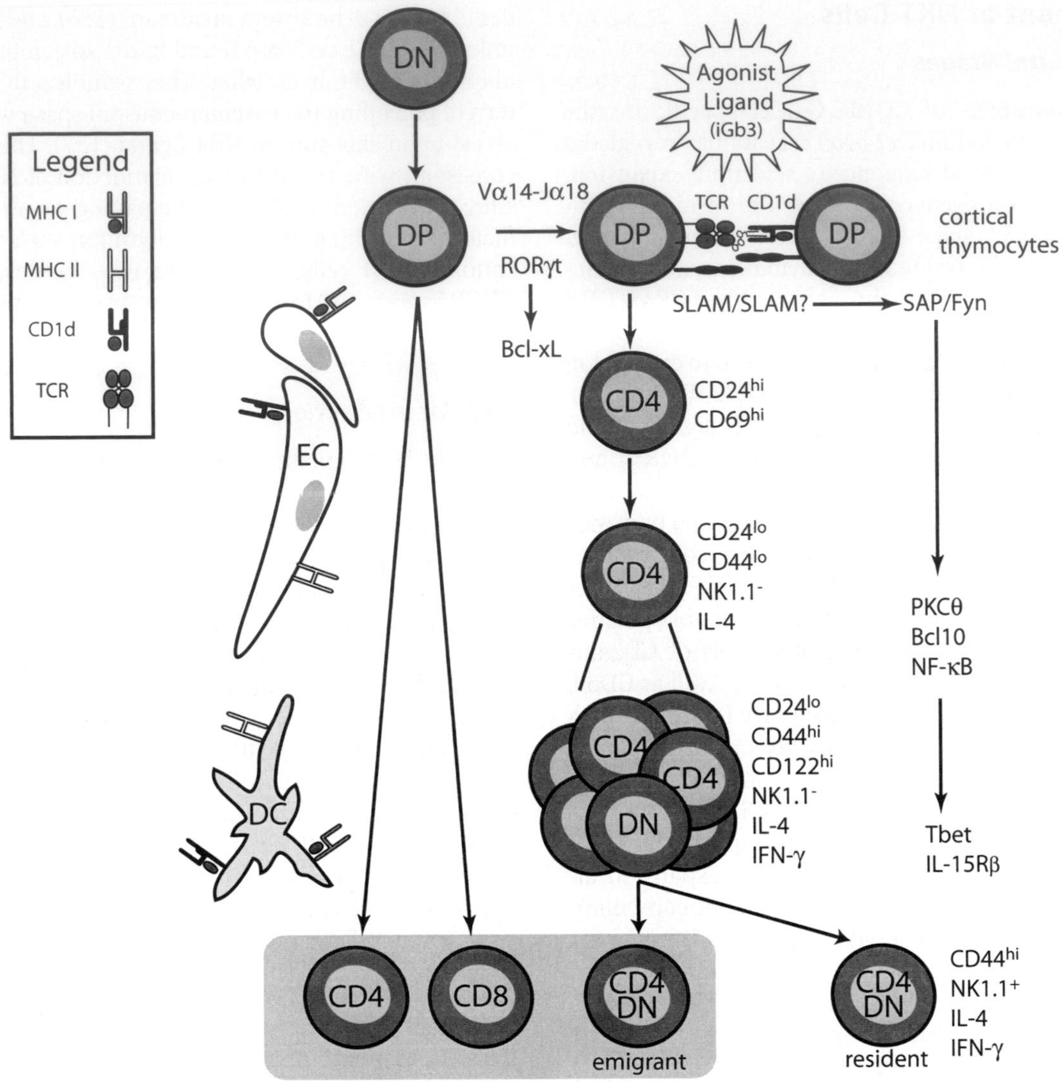

FIGURE 17.8 Development of NKT cells. Lineage bifurcation between conventional T cells and NKT cells occurs at the double-positive (DP) thymic stage. Stochastic expression of the canonical Vα14-Jα18 TCR α chain at the DP stage requires prolonged survival through Bcl-xL induced by RORγt. Upon pairing with appropriate Vβ8, 7, or 2, a CD1d-reactive TCR is formed that interacts with other DP-expressing agonist ligands, such as iGb3 presented by CD1d. These homotypic DP–DP interactions enable the homophilic association of members of the SLAM family of receptors, such as SLAM and Ly108, resulting in signaling through the SLAM-associated protein (SAP) adaptor-mediated recruitment of the Src kinase Fyn. Because of the reciprocal pattern of expression of SLAM receptors and MHC molecules in the thymus, these homophilic signals are not available to conventional MHC-restricted thymocytes during positive selection by MHC ligands. Thus, a combination of agonist TCR signaling and SLAM-family receptor signaling defines the NKT lineage. After positive selection, and as they mature, NKT lineage cells undergo a massive expansion, acquire memory/effector differentiation, including expression of Tbet that induces IL-15Rβ, and sequential epigenetic changes in their *IL-4* and *IFN-γ* loci. Terminal NK differentiation occurs after emigration to peripheral tissues or, for a minor fraction of NKT cells that become thymic residents, directly in the thymus. NF-κB signaling is critical for survival of NKT cells during their expansion phase and may be elicited through TCR- and/or Fyn-mediated signaling and recruitment of PKCθ and Bcl-10.

particular, ablation of the Src kinase Fyn and its adaptor SLAM adaptor protein (SAP) severely impaired NKT-cell but not T-cell development (165–168). SAP associates with the cytoplasmic tail of several members of the SLAM family of homotypic self-associating receptors (169), which are prominently expressed on cortical thymocytes, suggesting that one or several SLAM family receptors may be recruited during the homotypic DP-DP interactions required for NKT-cell development. Signaling downstream of SAP and Fyn involves activation of the canonical NF-κB pathway and may account, in conjunction with TCR signaling, for the defective NKT-cell development in mice expressing a dominant negative IκBα transgene and those lacking NF-κBp50 (170,171). Development was arrested at the CD44^{high}NK1.1^{-} stage and partially rescued by a Bcl-xL transgene, suggesting a survival role for NF-κB. Further, ablation of PKCθ and Bcl-10, which have been implicated in the signaling pathways downstream of SLAM and the TCR leading to NF-κB activation, induced partial defects in NKT-cell development (172,173). Thus, the current scenario suggests the importance of differential signaling through agonist ligand recognition by the TCR combined with SLAM family signaling for the bifurcation of the NKT lineage from mainstream T-cell development.

The downregulation of CD8β after exit from the DP stage remains a puzzling observation. One possible explanation in line with current models of CD4/CD8 coreceptor choice may be that strong, coreceptor-independent signaling maintains CD4 expression (174). Another, nonexclusive possibility is that CD8 binds CD1d and its persistence results in negative selection (158).

The induction of an NK program after the phase of clonal expansion constitutes a highly intriguing aspect of NKT-cell development. The transcription factor T-bet induces expression of the IL2Rβ component of the IL-15 receptor, which is critical for the survival of NKT cells during their expansion phase (175,176). A similar role was reported for CD8 T cells and NK cells. Whether Tbet exerts a more general role in the NK differentiation program remains to be investigated. Interestingly, studies have suggested that the Tec family kinases Itk and Rlk downstream of the TCR play a central role in regulating the decision between conventional and "NKT-like" lineages (177,178). Thus, conventional CD8 T cells lacking these kinases upregulated both eomesodermin, a Tbet homolog, and the IL15 receptor to differentiate into NKT-like T cells. Like true NKT cells, these NK-like T cells recognized their ligand on bone marrow–derived cells rather than epithelial cells. These findings suggest that Tec kinases are critical to transduce the positive selection signals mediated by partial agonist antigens. In their absence, cells that can see ligands on bone marrow–derived cells and induce eomesodermin would differentiate into NK-like T cells, perhaps with critical signaling from the SLAM/SAP/Fyn pathway.

Together, these observations suggest that a fundamental bifurcation between T cells and NKT cells may occur as a result of ligand recognition expressed on different cell types, namely, epithelial cells and thymocytes. Conventional T cells require Tec kinases to undergo positive selection by partial agonists, whereas NKT cells require agonist recognition and SLAM family member interactions. The coexpression of high levels of SLAM family members and CD1d on bone marrow–derived cells favors the NKT lineage, whereas the restricted expression of MHC class I or II on epithelial cells ensures their development in the absence of "cognate" SLAM signaling.

Development of MAIT Cells

The rarity of MAIT cells in mouse, which contrasts with their relative abundance in humans, has impeded studies of their development. MAIT cells are thymus-dependent, CD4^{-}CD8^{-} double-negative T cells with a memory phenotype that coexpress their invariant mVα19/hVα7.2 TCR α chain with variable Vβ6 and Vβ8 in mouse, Vβ2 and Vβ13 in human. They require MR1 expression by bone marrow–derived cells rather than thymic epithelium for thymic development (38). Thus, they resemble mVα14/hVα24 NKT cells in many respects. They exhibit considerably different properties, however, which are recapitulated in a TCRα transgenic model (129). MAIT cells express the $\alpha 4\beta 7$ intestinal homing integrin receptor and selectively accumulate in the lamina propria in mouse and human (38). Importantly, JH$^{-/-}$ mice lacking the immunoglobulin heavy-chain joining region and therefore B cell–deficient also lacked MAIT cells in the gut lamina propria. In contrast, μMT$^{-/-}$ mice lacking the transmembrane region of immunoglobulin μ, which harbor IgA-expressing B cells in their intestine, have lamina propria B cells. Strikingly, unlike any other innatelike lymphocyte studied to date, MAIT cells were undetectable in germ-free mice. Together, these findings have suggested a role of the commensal flora and IgA-secreting intestinal B cells in MAIT cell expansion or survival (38).

Development of Skin $\gamma\delta$ T Cells

Developmental Stages

The development of antibodies specific for the canonical Vγ5Vδ1 TCR has allowed the analysis of the stages of DETC development in the fetal thymus (Figure 17.9). Like Vα14-Jα18 NKT cells, Vγ5/Vδ1 thymocytes undergo a thymic activation process whereby CD122, the IL15 receptor β chain that is essential for survival (179), is induced along with several NK receptors including inhibitory CD94/NKG2 and Ly49E as well as activating NKG2D (44,180) and with CCR10, a skin-homing chemokine receptor. Because there is evidence of antigen-driven selection

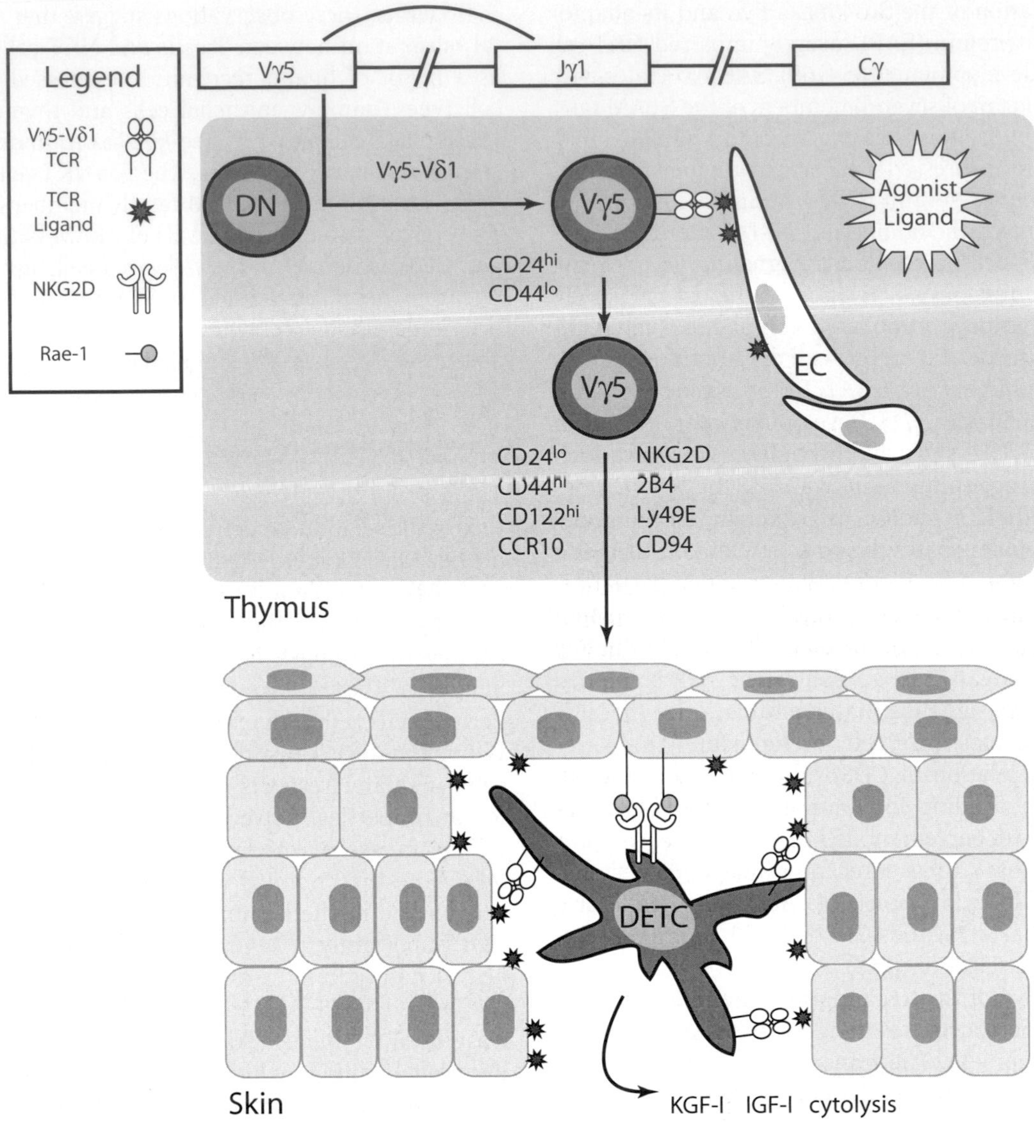

FIGURE 17.9 Development of DETC cells. Genetically programmed rearrangements in the fetal thymus lead to expression of canonical Vγ5-Jγ1/Vδ1-Dδ2-Jδ2 TCRs. As the CD24^{high} DETC precursors mature to become CD24^{low}, they undergo cellular activation leading to memory/effector differentiation, expression of NK lineage receptors, and the skin-homing receptor CCR10. Intrathymic activation requires interaction with epithelial stromal cells, perhaps involving recognition of an as yet unidentified agonist ligand (depicted as black star). In the skin epidermis, DETC cells are activated upon induction of an unidentified agonist ligand of their Vγ5/Vδ1 TCR (possibly identical to the thymic ligand) on stressed or transformed keratinocytes to release cytokines and growth factors that contribute to wound healing. Additional signals through NKG2D and its inducible Rae1 ligands contribute to the DETC response.

of the DETC TCR (27,44), these findings suggest the existence of an as yet unidentified selecting antigen recognized by DETC in the thymus.

Cellular Interactions

Consistent with this antigen-mediated activation hypothesis, a recent study identified a substrain of FVB mice in which Vγ5/Vδ1 thymocytes were arrested at a naïve, preactivation stage and failed to colonize the skin (45). Genetic analysis suggested a single recessive gene, whereas fetal thymic reaggregation cultures demonstrated that the defect resided at the level of stromal, nonhemopoietic cells. These findings are therefore compatible with the notion that Vγ5/Vδ1 thymocytes recognize a self-antigenic ligand on thymic stromal cells, which may be identical to their ligand expressed on stressed or transformed keratinocytes. The nature of this self-antigen, possibly a nonclassical MHC-like molecule independent of β2-microglobulin, remains to be characterized. Because previous studies had indicated that stromal cells of adult thymus could not sustain the development of DETCs from fetal hemopoietic precursors (181), this ligand may be downmodulated in the adult period. An unexpected level of crosstalk between the development of $\gamma\delta$ T cells and that of $\alpha\beta$ T cells was recently uncovered with the observation that lymphotoxin/lymphotoxin β–receptor interactions between $CD4^+CD8^+$ double-positive (DP) cortical thymocytes (mainly $\alpha\beta$ lineage) and stromal cells shaped the functional differentiation of $\gamma\delta$ T cells (182). Absence of this crosstalk in the fetal period when DP cells are absent could be a determining factor of DETC functional differentiation (183).

These recent findings have revealed a sequence of cellular and molecular interactions triggered by ligand recognition and resulting in the instruction of a highly specialized effector differentiation and tissue migration program. This appears to be a central theme of innatelike lymphocyte development, as previously illustrated in the case of NKT cells and their endogenous ligand iGb3. Unlike NKT cells, however, in which the presence of CD1d ligands is absolutely required for development, both Vγ5Vδ1 T cells in mouse and Vγ9Vδ2 T cells in humans may be able to develop and survive in the absence of TCR engagement by self-antigen, i.e., in the absence of positive selection, although they fail to acquire the cardinal differentiation and migration features of their antigen-selected memory/effector-type counterparts.

Development of B-1 B Cells and Marginal-Zone B Cells

Although there are intrinsic features of the fetal B-cell precursors and their environment that favor the expression of canonical B-cell receptors and the development of B-1 B cells (184), as reviewed in the section on canonical germline-encoded antigen receptors, adult precursors also give rise to B-1 cells expressing canonical germline-encoded BCRs, although their phenotypes may be somewhat different from their fetal counterparts, for example, by lacking CD5 expression (so-called B-1b cells).

Signaling the B-1 and MZB Fates

This section focuses on the mechanisms instructing the bifurcation between B-1 and conventional B-2 cells that revolve around signaling through the BCR and other pathways as a consequence of self-ligand recognition. The compelling rationale for these studies is that transgenic expression of a BCR derived from B-1 cells usually recapitulates B-1 B cell development, whereas transgenic expression of a B-2 BCR excludes B-1 development (29–33). Further, removal of the B-1 B cell ligand Thy1 abrogated the development of B-1 cells of the corresponding specificity (40).

Thus, the transitional B-cell stage is thought to represent the bifurcation point where BCR signaling and other factors instruct innatelike differentiation. The agonist nature of the self-antigens has been noted and, in experiments in which the density of the B-1 BCR was decreased by dilution with a second BCR transgene, reversion to the conventional B-2 phenotype was observed, suggesting that exquisite signaling thresholds regulate lineage differentiation (29,30,33).

In direct support of a contribution of BCR signaling, genetic alterations of components of the BCR signaling complex selectively perturbed the development of B1 B cells. Thus, *motheaten* mice with defective SHP-1 phosphatase, a negative regulator of BCR signaling, had increased frequency of $CD5^+$ B-1–like cells, but their repertoire excluded canonical B-1 BCRs such as the phosphatidylcholine-specific VH11 and VH12 BCRs, suggesting a general shift in the BCR avidity threshold of B-1 development leading to the negative selection of canonical BCRs and positive selection of other conventional B-2 BCRs (67). Likewise, mice lacking the negative regulators Lyn (185) and CD22 (186) exhibited hyperreactive B cells and increased B-1 B–like cells. *Xid* mice with a missense mutation of *Btk* or $Btk^{-/-}$ mice selectively lacked natural IgM antibodies and B-1 B cells (74,187) and mice lacking CD19 (188,189) also exhibited a striking reduction of B-1 B cells. A more precise evaluation of Btk in the context of a B-1 BCR transgene revealed differentiation toward the conventional B-2 lineage in the absence of Btk, further supporting a BCR signaling instruction model at a common precursor stage (190). Low level expression of LMP2a, an Epstein–Barr virus gene, allowed BCR-independent generation of mature $CD19^+$ cells resembling follicular and marginal-zone B cells, whereas high-level expression converted all cells to the B1 lineage (191,192).

Together, these observations have suggested a generally accepted model whereby a higher level of BCR signaling nearing the threshold of negative selection is an essential component of the instructive mechanisms leading to the B-1 B cell fate (Figure 17.10). With some exceptions (193), there is evidence that differentiation toward conventional B-2 B cells, marginal-zone B cells and B-1 B cells is determined by an increasing level of BCR signaling during development (34,69). Such a model is elegantly supported by transgenic experiments in which changing the level of autoantigen from absent to moderate to high induced development into B-2, MZB, and B-1 B cells, respectively (112).

Differentiation into the various B-cell lineages also involves differences in chemokine receptor and integrin expression that dictate residence in the follicle, marginal zone, or peritoneum. B1 B cells require CXCL13 for

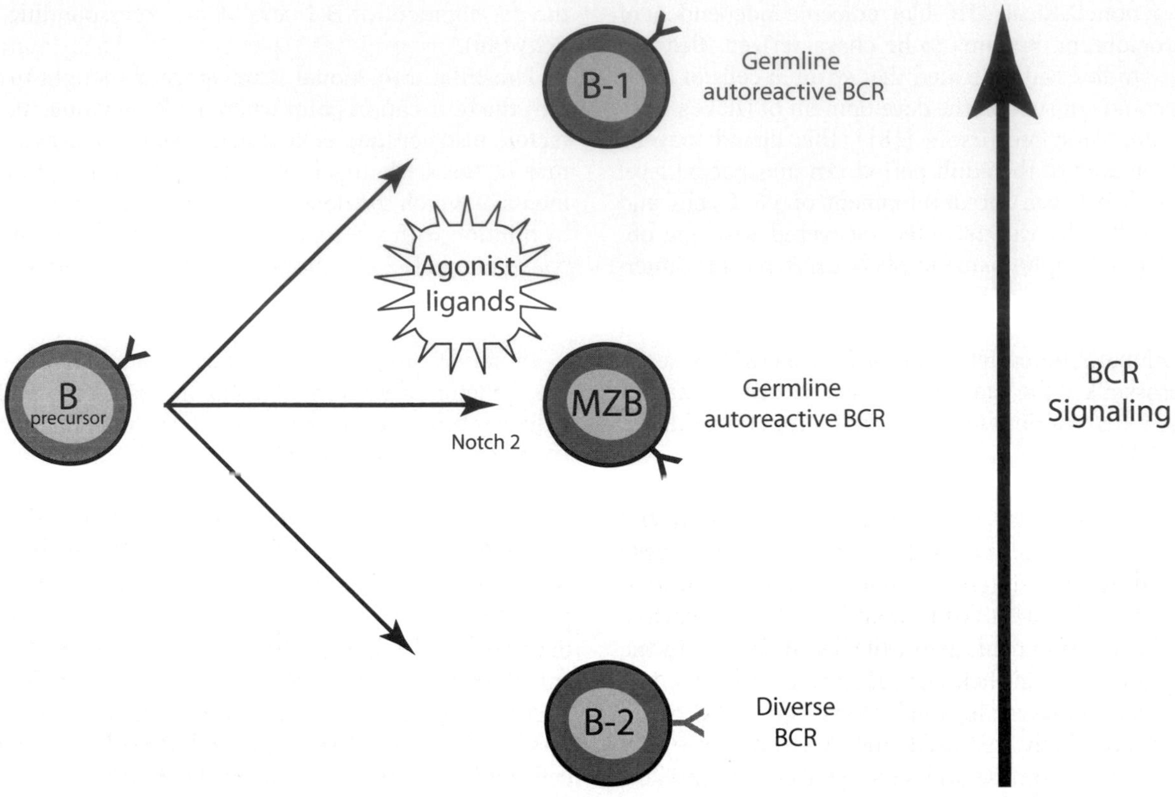

FIGURE 17.10 A signal-strength model of B-1 and MZB cell development. Interactions between germline-encoded canonical BCR sequences and endogenous agonist ligands such as apoptotic membrane phospholipids lead to the development of MZB and B-1 B cells. Exquisite signaling thresholds set by the affinity and the density of BCR and antigen and by signaling components such as Btk and SHP-1 are essential for proper lineage commitment. Additional differentiation signals are involved in this complex lineage decision scheme, including age-associated factors for some B-1 B cells and Notch2 for MZB cells.

peritoneal homing and natural antibody production (194), whereas MZB cells are retained in the marginal zone through high-level expression of the integrins LFA1 and $\alpha4\beta1$ and signaling through the S1P receptor to overcome CXCL13-mediated recruitment to the follicules (195,196). How chemokine receptor induction is coordinated with BCR signaling during development remains to be determined. Nevertheless, the process is reminiscent of the specialized induction of skin-homing or liver-homing properties of DETC and NKT cells, respectively, during development. Additional signals involving Notch2 for MZB cells have been demonstrated (197), perhaps indicative of microenvironmental interactions with cellular partners that remain to be elucidated.

In conclusion, the exquisite role of BCR signaling for the development of B-1 and MZB cells is now well established. Further studies combining individual BCR transgenes with various mutations are warranted to develop a more precise understanding of signaling in B-cell lineage development. Current knowledge, however, strongly supports the notion that the B-1 and MZB cell fates are specified primarily through their evolutionarily selected germline-encoded specificity and affinity for a select group of conserved self-ligands.

CONCLUSION

Harnessing Autoreactivity

The demonstrated autoreactivity of nearly all canonical antigen receptors and their germline nature support the notion that autoreactivity is by evolutionary design rather than by accident (71). Indeed, the type of agonist signaling associated with autoreactivity appears to be essential both for lineage commitment and, in many cases, for function as well.

It is envisioned that reactivity to self-ligands may serve to form an expanded pool of memory/effector cells with innate protective value against cross-reactive microbial pathogens. However, there are also examples of conditions in which recognition of the self-ligands themselves, whether constitutive or inducible, serves a protective function. More generally, dual reactivity to self- and foreign ligands is a hallmark of nearly all innate receptor systems, from soluble C-reactive protein to surface-bound scavenger receptors and TLRs. This may reflect the evolutionary advantage of receptors that detect multiple components of the same aggression event, for example, antigenic structures associated with the pathogen, as well as consequences of pathogenic aggression such as tissue damage.

This autoreactivity raises several issues. First, are innatelike lymphocytes resistant to negative selection? Several experiments suggest that this is not the case. Rather, the affinities of canonical antigen receptors are precisely tuned to their self-antigens. For example, the endogenous ligand iGb3 exclusively activates the Vα14-Jα18 TCRs that use Vβ7, Vβ8, and Vβ2, the biased Vβ set normally expressed by mature NKT cells with a Vβ7>Vβ8>Vβ2 hierarchy of affinity that precisely matches the relative enrichment of these Vβs after thymic selection (10). Transgenic overexpression of CD1d decreased the relative frequency of the high-affinity Vβ7$^+$ cells, likely through negative selection, whereas very low CD1d levels increased their relative representation (9,10,163,198). These observations suggest that the levels of ligand expression and TCR affinity are naturally set for optimal selection of NKT cells.

Second, how is autoreactivity controlled to prevent overt reactivity and exhaustion of innatelike lymphocytes? One possibility is that endogenous ligands are only induced under some conditions in the periphery. This could be the case for the apoptotic material that stimulates B-1 B cells, for example, or for the T10/T22 ligands of γδ T cells. Another possibility is that endogenous ligands are constitutively expressed but autoreactivity is controlled by a balance of inhibitory and activating receptors. Thus, inhibitory and activating NK receptors expressed by NKT cells and γδ T cells have been shown to control autoreactive TCR responses (199–201). In addition, induction of NKG2D ligands such as Rac1 family members by transformed epidermal cells triggered NKG2D signaling to promote cytolysis by DETCs (66). There are also indications that CD5 may have inhibitory functions on BCR signaling (202). Importantly, B-1 B cells have not been found to engage naturally in antigen-driven somatic hypermutation, which could lead to uncontrollable autoimmunity, perhaps because their phospholipid antigens do not elicit concomitant T-cell help or, alternatively, because of intrinsic inhibition.

Finally, the dual reactivity to self- and microbial antigens exhibited by various canonical antigen receptors raises issues of specificity and sensitivity of recognition. In the case of Vγ9Vδ2 T cells, endogenous isoprenoid antigens are 10,000-fold less stimulatory than their microbial counterparts. In the case of NKT cells, iGb3 also appears to be much less stimulatory than the microbial α-glycuronylceramides. Thus, it may be that self-antigens alone seldom stimulate innatelike lymphocytes but will do so only when combined with factors associated with infection or inflammation that activate costimulatory pathways, for example, IL-12 released by TLR-activated DCs or NKG2D induced by IL-15.

Evolving Canonical B- and T-Cell Receptors

Genetic Basis of Specificity

Because each TCR or BCR is made of the pairing of chains that themselves originate from several gene segments, the evolution of these canonical specificities is difficult to understand. Of note, the specificities of several canonical antigen receptors rely largely on one rather than two canonical chains, as is the case for the Vα14-Jα18 invariant chain combined with a set of variable Vβ chains, or the VH11 heavy chain combined with variable Vκ9. Recent observations further suggest that a single junctional segment can confer most of the specificity to antigen. For example, low-affinity clones specific for the NKT ligand αGalCer were found to use the canonical Jα18 combined with Vαs other than Vα24 (203,204). The T10/T22-specific γδ T cells also illustrate at the structural level the predominant contribution of the Dδ2 segment to antigen binding (7,8). It is possible, therefore, to envision that, starting from one low-affinity gene segment, a higher-affinity canonical receptor can be built over evolutionary time through the selection of additional V, D, or J gene segments.

Inter- and Intraspecies Variations

Whereas some canonical antigen receptors and their corresponding innatelike lymphocyte subsets are represented in multiple mammalian species, others appear to be restricted. For example, NKT cells have been identified in humans, mice, and rats (86) and MAIT cells in humans, mice, and cows (38). Skin DETCs, however, are not found in humans, and phosphoantigen-specific Vγ9Vδ2 T cells are absent in mice (205). From an evolutionary standpoint, these findings suggest that different canonical specificities may have different protective value in different species and thus may have been independently added or removed from the mammalian genome during evolution.

Intriguingly, there is also a wide polymorphism of expression of these innatelike lymphocyte subsets within species. For example, NKT-cell frequencies vary widely among humans, in which high expressors can express up to 100 times more NKT cells than low expressors (206). These frequencies are under tight genetic control, as shown by identical-twins studies (206). Similarly, there are up to 10-fold variations in NKT-cell frequencies among common inbred mouse strains (127,207). Some mouse substrains, such as FVB/tac, have lost expression of skin DETCs and, as a consequence, show heightened responses to inflammatory stimuli (45). Thus, while the genetic basis of these extraordinary variations is under investigation, it is tempting to speculate that such balanced polymorphism could reflect the "ying and yang" of innatelike lymphocytes, which serve protective functions in some conditions or environments but may be deleterious in others.

Other "Innatelike" Lymphocytes

This chapter has focused on expanded lymphocyte subsets that carry *germline-encoded specificities* and are endowed with functional innatelike properties. There are, however, additional populations of T and B lymphocytes that do not express canonical germline-encoded receptors, yet share some features of innatelike lymphocytes. For example, exposure to gut-flora carbohydrate antigens is thought to trigger the production of the natural IgM antibodies that cause rejection of incompatible red blood cells. Likewise, natural IgM antibodies against Galα1,3Galβ1,4GlcNAc epitopes probably derived from the gut flora, are found in the human species because humans lack Galα1,3 transferase and are therefore not tolerant of Galα1,3Galβ1,4GlcNAc. These antibodies are the basis of the abrupt rejection of xenotransplants carrying this carbohydrate epitope on their glycoproteins (208). Although they are absent in wild-type mice, which express the Galα1,3Galβ1,4GlcNAc epitopes on their glycoproteins, the antibodies are observed in "humanized" Galα1,3 transferase knockout mice, in which they are found mainly in the spleen and express an intermediate $IgM^{high}CD5^{-}Mac1^{-}CD43^{+}$ phenotype partially overlapping with B-1 cells (209,210). Importantly, however, neither anti-Gal nor anti–blood group antibodies have been reported to express canonical receptors.

CD8$\alpha\alpha$ TCR$\alpha\beta$ intraepithelial lymphocytes are found in the mouse intestine (though they are absent in humans) and are often referred to as "innate" based on their effector differentiation with transcriptionally active *IFN*γ gene (154,211), their expression of NK-lineage receptors (212), and their specificity for unidentified, nonclassical MHC class I–like ligands (213,214). Exposure to agonist antigens in a fetal thymic reaggregation culture system recapitulated the CD8$\alpha\alpha$ lineage (215). However, although the population is made of expanded clones, their $\alpha\beta$ TCRs are diverse and noncanonical (216).

Like CD1d-restricted NKT and MR1-restricted MAIT cells, MHC class Ib–restricted T cells acquire a memory/effector phenotype in the thymus by interaction with bone marrow–derived rather than epithelial cells (217). These properties enable H-2M3–restricted T cells, for example, to jump-start the CTL response to *Listeria monocytogenes* infection (218). However, studies so far have not documented the presence of recurrent canonical or germline-encoded TCRs among these cells.

Future Challenges

Comparative Immunology

Studies are needed to search for additional canonical germline-encoded receptors in B-1 and MZB populations of mice and humans. Likewise, comparative studies in more distant species should provide a broader picture of the array of innatelike BCRs and TCRs selected over evolutionary time and their species- or environment-specific protective value.

Antigens and Functions of Innatelike Lymphocytes

Several gaps remain in our knowledge of the antigen specificity of innatelike lymphocytes. The nonpeptidic nature of many ligands hinders their identification and complicates the interpretation of genetic ablation experiments. The functional redundancy of individual subsets prevents a definitive assessment of their role in physiologic and pathologic conditions. Thus, future identification of the self-ligand of DETCs, clarification of the respective roles of F1-ATPase and small phosphoantigens in Vγ9-cell activation, understanding of the regulation of iGb3 and other NKT ligands, and elucidation of the MAIT ligands associated with MR1 will be needed, along with new strategies for specific ablation of ligands and receptors. Novel approaches such as live imaging microscopy should prove particularly useful in studying the specialized functions of innatelike lymphocytes in their tissue context, for example, in the liver for NKT cells (157), skin for DETCs, peritoneum for B-1 B cells, and marginal zone for MZB cells.

Structural Biology of Innate Immune Recognition

As suggested by the unusual mode of recognition of T10/T22 by the $\gamma\delta$ TCR, the crystal structures of other innatelike receptor/ligand complexes will provide important information about the structural basis of innatelike receptor recognition. The phospholipidic and glycolipidic nature of several ligands, and their association with the membrane lipid bilayer or with proteins such as CD1d, complicate the studies, but their recognition by antibodies and TCRs likely involve novel structural solutions of great immunologic interest.

Lymphocyte Lineage Decisions

The instructional mechanisms involved in the differentiation of conventional and innatelike lineage differentiation are based on specific sets of receptors that signal the transcriptional and epigenetic control of lineage commitment. Current studies indicate that, in addition to the strength of antigen, additional cofactors recruited through the topology and the timing of antigen expression contribute essential steps in the differentiation of specialized lineage subsets. Because these signals underlie a developmental bifurcation between "conventional" and "innatelike" B- and T-cell lineages, their studies should provide important insights into a general understanding of lymphocyte lineage development.

Therapeutics

As a follow-up to basic studies investigating the conserved antigens of innatelike lymphocytes, several synthetic NKT- and $\gamma\delta$ T-cell ligands have now been designed, and some have shown promising value in preclinical trials, particularly for their effects as adjuvants in anticancer and microbial vaccines (122,124,219). The interplay among these and other adjuvant pathways mediated by TLRs, NODs, and NALPs provides exciting new avenues of research and development.

ACKNOWLEDGMENTS

Albert Bendelac is supported by the Howard Hughes Medical Institute and by National Institutes of Health grants. I thank Erin Adams, Marc Bonneville, Yueh-Hsiu Chien, Adrian Hayday, John Kearney, Richard Locksley, David Raulet, and Robert Tigelaar for discussions and insights; Luc Teyton, Paul Savage, and current and past members of my laboratory for providing innumerable ideas, stimulating discussions and collaborations, and dedicated research; and Erin Adams, Klaus Griewank, Seth Scanlon, and Omita Trivedi for help with the figures.

REFERENCE

1. Heilig JS, Tonegawa S. Diversity of murine gamma genes and expression in fetal and adult T lymphocytes. *Nature.* 1986;322(6082):836–840.
2. Havran WL, Allison JP. Developmentally ordered appearance of thymocytes expressing different T-cell antigen receptors. *Nature.* 1988;335(6189):443–445.
3. Feeney AJ. Predominance of the prototypic T15 anti-phosphorylcholine junctional sequence in neonatal pre-B cells. *J Immunol.* 1991;147(12):4343–4350.
4. Lantz O, Bendelac A. An invariant T cell receptor α chain is used by a unique subset of MHC class I-specific $CD4^+$ and $CD4^-8^-$ T cells in mice and humans. *J Exp Med.* 1994;180:1097–1106.
5. Hardy RR, Carmack CE, Shinton SA, et al. A single VH gene is utilized predominantly in anti-BrMRBC hybridomas derived from purified Ly-1 B cells. Definition of the VH11 family. *J Immunol.* 1989;142(10):3643–3651.
6. Pennell CA, Mercolino TJ, Grdina TA, et al. Biased immunoglobulin variable region gene expression by Ly-1 B cells due to clonal selection. Eur *J Immunol.* 1989;19(7):1289–1295.
7. Shin S, El-Diwany R, Schaffert S, et al. Antigen recognition determinants of gammadelta T cell receptors. *Science.* 2005;308(5719):252–255.
8. Adams EJ, Chien YH, Garcia KC. Structure of a gammadelta T cell receptor in complex with the nonclassical MHC T22. *Science.* 2005;308(5719):227–231.
9. Schumann J, Voyle RB, Wei BY, et al. Cutting edge: influence of the TCR V beta domain on the avidity of CD1d:alpha-galactosylceramide binding by invariant V alpha 14 NKT cells. *J Immunol.* 2003;170(12):5815–5819.
10. Wei DG, Curran SA, Savage PB, et al. Mechanisms imposing the Vbeta bias of Valpha14 natural killer T cells and consequences for microbial glycolipid recognition. *J Exp Med.* 2006;203(5):1197–1207.
11. Schumann J, Mycko MP, Dellabona P, et al. Cutting edge: influence of the TCR Vbeta domain on the selection of semi-invariant NKT cells by endogenous ligands. *J Immunol.* 2006;176(4):2064–2068.
12. Itohara S, Mombaerts P, Lafaille J, et al. T cell receptor d gene mutant mice: independent generation of ab T cells and programmed rearrangements of gd TCR genes. *Cell.* 1993;72:337.
13. Jackson AM, Krangel MS. Turning T-cell receptor beta recombination on and off: more questions than answers. *Immunol Rev.* 2006;209:129–141.
14. Kang J, Coles M, Raulet DH. Defective development of gamma/delta T cells in interleukin 7 receptor-deficient mice is due to impaired expression of T cell receptor gamma genes. *J Exp Med.* 1999;190(7):973–982.
15. Schlissel MS, Durum SD, Muegge K. The interleukin 7 receptor is required for T cell receptor gamma locus accessibility to the V(D)J recombinase. *J Exp Med.* 2000;191(6):1045–1050.
16. Ye SK, Agata Y, Lee HC, et al. The IL-7 receptor controls the accessibility of the TCRgamma locus by Stat5 and histone acetylation. *Immunity.* 2001;15(5):813–823.
17. Zhao H, Nguyen H, Kang J. Interleukin 15 controls the generation of the restricted T cell receptor repertoire of gamma delta intestinal intraepithelial lymphocytes. *Nat Immunol.* 2005;6(12):1263–1271.
18. Bertolino E, Reddy K, Medina KL, et al. Regulation of interleukin 7-dependent immunoglobulin heavy-chain variable gene rearrangements by transcription factor STAT5. *Nat Immunol.* 2005;6(8):836–843.
19. Vosshenrich CA, Cumano A, Muller W, et al. Thymic stromal-derived lymphopoietin distinguishes fetal from adult B cell development. *Nat Immunol.* 2003;4(8):773–779.
20. Vosshenrich CA, Cumano A, Muller W, et al. Pre-B cell receptor expression is necessary for thymic stromal lymphopoietin responsiveness in the bone marrow but not in the liver environment. *Proc Natl Acad Sci U S A.* 2004;101(30):11070–11075.
21. Zhang Y, Cado D, Asarnow DM, et al. The role of short homology repeats and TdT in generation of the invariant gamma delta antigen receptor repertoire in the fetal thymus. *Immunity.* 1995;3(4):439–447.
22. Benedict CL, Kearney JF. Increased junctional diversity in fetal B cells results in a loss of protective anti-phosphorylcholine antibodies in adult mice. *Immunity.* 1999;10(5):607–617.
23. Bezbradica JS, Hill T, Stanic AK, et al. Commitment toward the natural T (iNKT) cell lineage occurs at the CD4+8+ stage of thymic ontogeny. *Proc Natl Acad Sci U S A.* 2005;102(14):5114–5119.
24. Egawa T, Eberl G, Taniuchi I, et al. Genetic evidence supporting selection of the Valpha14i NKT cell lineage from double-positive thymocyte precursors. *Immunity.* 2005;22(6):705–716.
25. Bendelac A, Hunziker RD, Lantz O. Increased interleukin 4 and immunoglobulin E production in transgenic mice overexpressing NK1 T cells. *J Exp Med.* 1996;184:1285–1293.
26. Skold M, Faizunnessa NN, Wang CR, et al. CD1d-specific NK1.1+ T cells with a transgenic variant TCR. *J Immunol.* 2000;165(1):168–174.
27. Ferrero I, Wilson A, Beermann F, et al. T cell receptor specificity is critical for the development of epidermal gammadelta T cells. *J Exp Med.* 2001;194(10):1473–1483.
28. Gerber DJ, Azuara V, Levraud JP, et al. IL-4-producing gamma delta T cells that express a very restricted TCR repertoire are preferentially localized in liver and spleen. *J Immunol.* 1999;163(6):3076–3082.

29. Lam KP, Rajewsky K. B cell antigen receptor specificity and surface density together determine B-1 versus B-2 cell development. *J Exp Med.* 1999;190(4):471–477.
30. Watanabe N, Nisitani S, Ikuta K, et al. Expression levels of B cell surface immunoglobulin regulate efficiency of allelic exclusion and size of autoreactive B-1 cell compartment. *J Exp Med.* 1999;190(4):461–469.
31. Tatu C, Ye J, Arnold LW, et al. Selection at multiple checkpoints focuses V(H)12 B cell differentiation toward a single B-1 cell specificity. *J Exp Med.* 1999;190(7):903–914.
32. Chumley MJ, Dal Porto JM, Kawaguchi S, et al. A VH11V kappa 9 B cell antigen receptor drives generation of CD5+ B cells both in vivo and in vitro. *J Immunol.* 2000;164(9):4586–4593.
33. Kenny JJ, Rezanka LJ, Lustig A, et al. Autoreactive B cells escape clonal deletion by expressing multiple antigen receptors. *J Immunol.* 2000;164(8):4111–4119.
34. Martin F, Kearney JF. Positive selection from newly formed to marginal zone B cells depends on the rate of clonal production, CD19, and btk. *Immunity*. 2000;12(1):39–49.
35. Smiley ST, Kaplan MH, Grusby MJ. Immunoglobulin E production in the absence of interleukin-4 secreting CD1-dependent cells. *Science.* 1997;275:977–979.
36. Mendiratta SK, Martin WD, Hong S, et al. CD1d1 mutant mice are deficient in natural T cells that promptly produce IL-4. *Immunity*. 1997;6:469–477.
37. Chen Y-H, Chiu NM, Mandal M, et al. Impaired NK1+ T cell development and early IL-4 production in CD1-deficient mice. *Immunity*. 1997;6:459–467.
38. Treiner E, Duban L, Bahram S, et al. Selection of evolutionarily conserved mucosal-associated invariant T cells by MR1. *Nature.* 2003;422(6928):164–169.
39. Pereira P, Zijlstra M, McMaster J, et al. Blockade of transgenic gamma delta T cell development in beta 2-microglobulin deficient mice. *EMBO J.* 1992;11(1):25–31.
40. Hayakawa K, Asano M, Shinton SA, et al. Positive selection of natural autoreactive B cells. *Science.* 1999;285(5424):113–116.
41. Tilloy F, Treiner E, Park SH, et al. An invariant T cell receptor alpha chain defines a novel TAP-independent major histocompatibility complex class Ib-restricted alpha/beta T cell subpopulation in mammals. *J Exp Med.* 1999;189(12):1907–1921.
42. Carmack CE, Shinton SA, Hayakawa K, Hardy RR. Rearrangement and selection of VH11 in the Ly-1 B cell lineage. *J Exp Med.* 1990;172:371–374.
43. Mallick-Wood CA, Lewis JM, Richie LI, et al. Conservation of T cell receptor conformation in epidermal gammadelta cells with disrupted primary Vgamma gene usage. *Science.* 1998;279(5357):1729–1733.
44. Xiong N, Kang C, Raulet DH. Positive selection of dendritic epidermal gammadelta T cell precursors in the fetal thymus determines expression of skin-homing receptors. *Immunity*. 2004;21(1):121–131.
45. Lewis JM, Girardi M, Roberts SJ, et al. Selection of the cutaneous intraepithelial gammadelta+ T cell repertoire by a thymic stromal determinant. *Nat Immunol.* 2006;7(8):843–850.
46. McVay LD, Carding SR. Extrathymic origin of human gamma delta T cells during fetal development. *J Immunol.* 1996;157(7):2873–2882.
47. Parker CM, Groh V, Band H, et al. Evidence for extrathymic changes in the T cell receptor gamma/delta repertoire. *J Exp Med.* 1990;171(5):1597–1612.
48. Davodeau F, Peyrat MA, Hallet MM, et al. Peripheral selection of antigen receptor junctional features in a major human gamma delta subset. Eur *J Immunol.* 1993;23(4):804–808.
49. Wasserman R, Li YS, Shinton SA, et al. A novel mechanism for B cell repertoire maturation based on response by B cell precursors to pre-B receptor assembly. *J Exp Med.* 1998;187(2):259–264.
50. Ye J, McCray SK, Clarke SH. The majority of murine VH12-expressing B cells are excluded from the peripheral repertoire in adults. Eur *J Immunol.* 1995;25(9):2511–2521.
51. Benlagha K, Kyin T, Beavis A, et al. A thymic precursor to the NKT cell lineage. *Science.* 2002;296:553–555.
52. Park SH, Benlagha K, Lee D, et al. Unaltered phenotype, tissue distribution and function of Valpha14(+) NKT cells in germ-free mice. Eur *J Immunol.* 2000;30(2):620–625.
53. Hayakawa K, Hardy RR, Stall AM, et al. Immunoglobulin-bearing B cells reconstitute and maintain the murine Ly-1 B cell lineage. Eur *J Immunol.* 1986;16(10):1313–1316.
54. Bendelac A, Lantz O, Quimby ME, et al. CD1 recognition by mouse NK1+ T lymphocytes. *Science.* 1995;268:863–865.
55. Bendelac A. Positive selection of mouse NK1+ T cells by CD1-expressing cortical thymocytes. *J Exp Med.* 1995;182:2091–2096.
56. Park S-H, Roark JH, Bendelac A. Tissue specific recognition of mouse CD1 molecules. *J Immunol*. 1998;160:3128–3134.
57. Behar SM, Podrebarac TA, Roy CJ, et al. Diverse TCRs recognize murine CD1. *J Immunol.* 1999;162(1):161–167.
58. Couedel C, Peyrat MA, Brossay L, et al. Diverse CD1d-restricted reactivity patterns of human T cells bearing "invariant" AV24BV11 TCR. Eur *J Immunol.* 1998;28(12):4391–4397.
59. Havran WL, Chien YH, Allison JP. Recognition of self- antigens by skin-derived T cells with invariant gamma-delta antigen receptors. *Science.* 1991;252:1430–1432.
60. Fisch P, Malkovsky M, Kovats S, et al. Recognition by human V gamma 9/V delta 2 T cells of a GroEL homolog on Daudi Burkitt's lymphoma cells. *Science.* 1990;250(4985):1269–73.
61. De Libero G, Casorati G, Giachino C, et al. Selection by two powerful antigens may account for the presence of the major population of human peripheral gamma/delta T cells. *J Exp Med.* 1991;173(6):1311–1322.
62. Malkovska V, Cigel FK, Armstrong N, et al. Antilymphoma activity of human gamma delta T-cells in mice with severe combined immune deficiency. *Cancer Res*. 1992;52(20):5610–5616.
63. Jameson JM, Cauvi G, Witherden DA, et al. A keratinocyte-responsive gammadelta TCR is necessary for dendritic epidermal T cell activation by damaged keratinocytes and maintenance in the epidermis. *J Immunol.* 2004;172(6):3573–3579.
64. Gui M, Li J, Wen LJ, et al. TCR beta chain influences but does not solely control autoreactivity of V alpha 14J281T cells. *J Immunol.* 2001;167(11):6239–6246.
65. Wu J, Groh V, Spies T. T cell antigen receptor engagement and specificity in the recognition of stress-inducible MHC class I-related chains by human epithelial gamma delta T cells. *J Immunol.* 2002;169(3):1236–1240.
66. Girardi M, Oppenheim DE, Steele CR, et al. Regulation of cutaneous malignancy by gammadelta T cells. *Science.* 2001;294(5542):605–609.
67. Mercolino TJ, Arnold LW, Hawkins LA, et al. Normal mouse peritoneum contains a large population of Ly-1+ (CD5) B cells that recognize phosphatidyl choline. Relationship to cells that secrete hemolytic antibody specific for autologous erythrocytes. *J Exp Med.* 1988;168(2):687–698.
68. Shaw PX, Horkko S, Chang MK, et al. Natural antibodies with the T15 idiotype may act in atherosclerosis, apoptotic clearance, and protective immunity [see comments]. *J Clin Invest*. 2000;105(12):1731–1740.
69. Lopes-Carvalho T, Kearney JF. Development and selection of marginal zone B cells. *Immunol Rev.* 2004;197:192–205.
70. Hayakawa K, Carmack CE, Hyman R, et al. Natural autoantibodies to thymocytes: origin, VH genes, fine specificities, and the role of Thy-1 glycoprotein. *J Exp Med.* 1990;172(3):869–878.
71. Bendelac A, Bonneville M, Kearney JF. Autoreactivity by design: innate B and T lymphocytes. *Nat Rev Immunol*. 2001;1(3):177–186.
72. Jomaa H, Feurle J, Luhs K, et al. Vgamma9/Vdelta2 T cell activation induced by bacterial low molecular mass compounds depends on the 1-deoxy-D-xylulose 5-phosphate pathway of isoprenoid biosynthesis. *FEMS Immunol Med Microbiol.* 1999;25(4):371–378.
73. Tanaka Y, Morita CT, Tanaka Y, et al. Natural and synthetic nonpeptide antigens recognized by human gamma delta T cells. *Nature.* 1995;375(6527):155–158.
74. Briles DE, Nahm M, Schroer K, et al. Antiphosphocholine antibodies found in normal mouse serum are protective against intravenous infection with type 3 Streptococcus pneumoniae. *J Exp Med.* 1981;153(3):694–705.
75. Zhou D, Mattner J, Cantu C 3rd, et al. Lysosomal glycosphingolipid recognition by NKT cells. *Science.* 2004;306(5702):1786–1789.

76. Mattner J, DeBord KL, Ismail N, et al. Both exogenous and endogenous glycolipid antigens activate NKT cells during microbial infections. *Nature.* 2005;434:525–529.
77. Kinjo Y, Wu D, Kim G, et al. Recognition of bacterial glycosphingolipids by natural killer T cells. *Nature.* 2005;434(7032): 520–525.
78. Stroynowski I. Molecules related to class-I major histocompatibility complex antigens. *Ann Rev Immunol.* 1990;8:501–530.
79. Crowley MP, Fahrer AM, Baumgarth N, et al. A population of murine gammadelta T cells that recognize an inducible MHC class Ib molecule. *Science.* 2000;287(5451):314–316.
80. Spada FM, Grant EP, Peters PJ, et al. Self-recognition of CD1 by gamma/delta T cells: implications for innate immunity [see comments]. *J Exp Med.* 2000;191(6):937–948.
81. Groh V, Steinle A, Bauer S, et al. Recognition of stress-induced MHC molecules by intestinal epithelial gammadelta T cells. *Science.* 1998;279(5357):1737–1740.
82. Martin LH, Calabi F, Milstein C. Isolation of CD1 genes: a family of major histocompatibility complex-related differentiation antigens. Proc. *Natl Acad Sci U S A.* 1986;83:9154–9158.
83. Miller MM, Wang C, Parisini E, et al. Characterization of two avian MHC-like genes reveals an ancient origin of the CD1 family. *Proc Natl Acad Sci U S A.* 2005;102(24):8674–8679.
84. Salomonsen J, Sorensen MR, Marston DA, et al. Two CD1 genes map to the chicken MHC, indicating that CD1 genes are ancient and likely to have been present in the primordial MHC. *Proc Natl Acad Sci U S A.* 2005;102(24):8668–8673.
85. Brigl M, Brenner MB. CD1: antigen presentation and T cell function. *Annu Rev Immunol.* 2004;22:817–890.
86. Bendelac A, Savage PB, Teyton L. The biology of NKT cells. *Annu Rev Immunol.* 2007;25:297–336.
87. Park SH, Weiss A, Benlagha K, et al. The mouse CD1d-restricted repertoire is dominated by a few autoreactive t cell receptor families. *J Exp Med.* 2001;193(8):893–904.
88. Chiu YH, Jayawardena J, Weiss A, et al. Distinct subsets of CD1d-restricted T cells recognize self-antigens loaded in different cellular compartments [in process citation]. *J Exp Med.* 1999;189(1):103–110.
89. Chiu YH, Park SH, Benlagha K, et al. Multiple defects in antigen presentation and T cell development by mice expressing cytoplasmic tail-truncated CD1d. *Nat Immunol.* 2002;3(1):55–60.
90. Prigozy TI, Naidenko O, Qasba P, et al. Glycolipid antigen processing for presentation by CD1d molecules. *Science.* 2001;291(5504):664–667.
91. Zhou D, Cantu C 3rd, Sagiv Y, et al. Editing of CD1d-bound lipid antigens by endosomal lipid transfer proteins. *Science.* 2004;303(5657):523–527.
92. Kang SJ, Cresswell P. Saposins facilitate CD1d-restricted presentation of an exogenous lipid antigen to T cells. *Nat Immunol.* 2004;5(2):175–181.
93. Winau F, Schwierzeck V, Hurwitz R, et al. Saposin C is required for lipid presentation by human CD1b. *Nat Immunol.* 2004;5(2):169–14.
94. Kawahara K, Moll H, Knirel YA, et al. Structural analysis of two glycosphingolipids from the lipopolysaccharide-lacking bacterium Sphingomonas capsulata. *Eur J Biochem.* 2000;267(6):1837–1846.
95. Kobayashi E, Motoki K, Uchida T, et al. KRN7000, a novel immunomodulator, and its antitumor activities. *Oncol Res.* 1995;7(10–11):529–534.
96. Morita M, Motoki K, Akimoto K, et al. Structure-activity relationship of alpha-galactosylceramides against B16-bearing mice. *J Med Chem.* 1995;38(12):2176–2187.
97. Kinjo Y, Tupin E, Wu D, et al. Natural killer T cells recognize diacylglycerol antigens from pathogenic bacteria. *Nat Immunol.* 2006;7(9):978–986.
98. Zajonc DM, Cantu C 3rd, Mattner J, et al. Structure and function of a potent agonist for the semi-invariant NKT cell receptor. *Nat* Immunol. 2005;6:810–818.
99. Koch M, Stronge VS, Shepherd D, et al. The crystal structure of human CD1d with and without alpha-galactosylceramide. *Nat Immunol.* 2005;6(8):819–826.
99a. Borg NA, Wun KS, Kjer-Nielsen L, et al. CD1d-lipid-antigen recognition by the semi-invariant NKT T-cell receptor. *Nature.* 2007;448(7149):44–49.
100. Huang S, Gilfillan S, Cella M, et al. Evidence for MR1 antigen presentation to mucosal-associated invariant T cells. *J Biol Chem.* 2005;280(22):21183–21193.
101. Bahram S, Bresnahan M, Geraghty DE, et al. A second lineage of mammalian major histocompatibility complex class I genes. *Proc Natl Acad Sci U S A.* 1994;91:6259–6263.
102. Li P, Willie ST, Bauer S, et al. Crystal structure of the MHC class I homolog MIC-A, a gammadelta T cell ligand. *Immunity.* 1999;10(5):577–584.
103. Moody DB, Ulrichs T, Muhlecker W, et al. CD1c-mediated T-cell recognition of isoprenoid glycolipids in Mycobacterium tuberculosis infection. *Nature.* 2000;404(6780):884–888.
104. Begley M, Gahan CG, Kollas AK, et al. The interplay between classical and alternative isoprenoid biosynthesis controls gammadelta T cell bioactivity of Listeria monocytogenes. *FEBS Lett.* 2004;561(1–3):99–104.
105. Gober HJ, Kistowska M, Angman L, et al. Human T cell receptor gammadelta cells recognize endogenous mevalonate metabolites in tumor cells. *J Exp Med.* 2003;197(2):163–168.
106. Thompson K, Rojas-Navea J, Rogers MJ. Alkylamines cause Vgamma9Vdelta2 T-cell activation and proliferation by inhibiting the mevalonate pathway. *Blood.* 2006;107(2):651–654.
107. Bukowski JF, Morita CT, Brenner MB. Human gamma delta T cells recognize alkylamines derived from microbes, edible plants, and tea: implications for innate immunity. *Immunity.* 1999;11(1): 57–65.
108. Scotet E, Martinez LO, Grant E, et al. Tumor recognition following Vgamma9Vdelta2 T cell receptor interactions with a surface F1-ATPase-related structure and apolipoprotein A-I. *Immunity.* 2005;22(1):71–80.
109. Forster I, Rajewsky K. Expansion and functional activity of Ly-1+ B cells upon transfer of peritoneal cells into allotype-congenic, newborn mice. *Eur J Immunol.* 1987;17(4):521–528.
110. Kim SJ, Gershov D, Ma X, et al. I-PLA(2) activation during apoptosis promotes the exposure of membrane lysophosphatidylcholine leading to binding by natural immunoglobulin M antibodies and complement activation. *J Exp Med.* 2002;196(5):655–665.
111. Shaw PX, Goodyear CS, Chang MK, et al. The autoreactivity of anti-phosphorylcholine antibodies for atherosclerosis-associated neo-antigens and apoptotic cells. *J Immunol.* 2003;170(12):6151–6157.
112. Wen L, Brill-Dashoff J, Shinton SA, et al. Evidence of marginal-zone B cell-positive selection in spleen. *Immunity.* 2005;23(3):297–308.
113. Oliver AM, Martin F, Gartland GL, et al. Marginal zone B cells exhibit unique activation, proliferative and immunoglobulin secretory responses. *Eur J Immunol.* 1997;27(9):2366–2374.
114. Dempsey PW, Allison ME, Akkaraju S, et al. C3d of complement as a molecular adjuvant: bridging innate and acquired immunity. *Science.* 1996;271(5247):348–350.
115. Guinamard R, Okigaki M, Schlessinger J, et al. Absence of marginal zone B cells in Pyk-2 deficient mice defines their role in the humoral response. *Nat* Immunol. 2000;1:31–36.
116. Vincent MS, Leslie DS, Gumperz JE, et al. CD1-dependent dendritic cell instruction. *Nat Immunol.* 2002;3(12):1163–1168.
117. Brigl M, Bry L, Kent SC, et al. Mechanism of CD1d-restricted natural killer T cell activation during microbial infection. *Nat Immunol.* 2003;4(12):1230–1237.
118. Kitamura H, Iwakabe K, Yahata T, et al. The natural killer T (NKT) cell ligand alpha-galactosylceramide demonstrates its immunopotentiating effect by inducing interleukin (IL)-12 production by dendritic cells and IL-12 receptor expression on NKT cells. *J Exp Med.* 1999;189(7):1121–1128.
119. Tomura M, Yu WG, Ahn HJ, et al. A novel function of Valpha14+CD4+NKT cells: stimulation of IL-12 production by antigen-presenting cells in the innate immune system. *J Immunol.* 1999;163(1):93–101.
120. Eberl G, MacDonald HR. Selective induction of NK cell proliferation and cytotoxicity by activated NKT cells. *Eur J Immunol.* 2000;30(4):985–92.
121. Carnaud C, Lee D, Donnars O, et al. Cross-talk between cells of the innate immune system: NKT cells rapidly activate NK cells. *J Immunol [Cutting Edge].* 1999;163:4647–4650.
122. Fujii S, Shimizu K, Smith C, et al. Activation of natural killer T cells by alpha-galactosylceramide rapidly induces the full maturation of

dendritic cells in vivo and thereby acts as an adjuvant for combined CD4 and CD8 T cell immunity to a coadministered protein. *J Exp Med.* 2003;198(2):267–279.

123. Fujii S, Liu K, Smith C, et al. The linkage of innate to adaptive immunity via maturing dendritic cells in vivo requires CD40 ligation in addition to antigen presentation and CD80/86 costimulation. *J Exp Med.* 2004;199(12):1607–1618.

124. Gonzalez-Aseguinolaza G, Van Kaer L, Bergmann CC, et al. Natural killer T cell ligand alpha-galactosylceramide enhances protective immunity induced by malaria vaccines. *J Exp Med.* 2002;195(5):617–624.

125. Conti L, Casetti R, Cardone M, et al. Reciprocal activating interaction between dendritic cells and pamidronate-stimulated gammadelta T cells: role of CD86 and inflammatory cytokines. *J Immunol.* 2005;174(1):252–260.

126. Collins C, Wolfe J, Roessner K, et al. Lyme arthritis synovial gammadelta T cells instruct dendritic cells via fas ligand. *J Immunol.* 2005;175(9):5656–5665.

127. Yoshimoto T, Bendelac A, Watson C, et al. Role of NK1.1+ T cells in a TH2 response and in immunoglobulin E production. *Science.* 1995;270:1845–1847.

128. Brandes M, Willimann K, Moser B. Professional antigen-presentation function by human gammadelta T Cells. *Science.* 2005;309(5732):264–268.

129. Kawachi I, Maldonado J, Strader C, et al. MR1-restricted V alpha 19i mucosal-associated invariant T cells are innate T cells in the gut lamina propria that provide a rapid and diverse cytokine response. *J Immunol.* 2006;176(3):1618–1627.

130. Boismenu R, Havran WL. Modulation of epithelial cell growth by intraepithelial gamma delta T cells. *Science.* 1994;266:1253–1255.

131. Sharp LL, Jameson JM, Cauvi G, et al. Dendritic epidermal T cells regulate skin homeostasis through local production of insulin-like growth factor 1. *Nat Immunol.* 2005;6(1):73–79.

132. Selmi C, Balkwill DL, Invernizzi P, et al. Patients with primary biliary cirrhosis react against a ubiquitous xenobiotic-metabolizing bacterium. *Hepatology.* 2003;38(5):1250–1257.

133. Kumar H, Belperron A, Barthold SW, et al. Cutting edge: CD1d deficiency impairs murine host defense against the spirochete, Borrelia burgdorferi. *J Immunol.* 2000;165(9):4797–4801.

134. Kaplan MM, Gershwin ME. Primary biliary cirrhosis. *N Engl J Med.* 2005;353(12):1261–1273.

135. Kita H, Naidenko OV, Kronenberg M, et al. Quantitation and phenotypic analysis of natural killer T cells in primary biliary cirrhosis using a human CD1d tetramer. *Gastroenterology.* 2002;123(4):1031–1043.

136. Nieuwenhuis EE, Matsumoto T, Exley M, et al. CD1d-dependent macrophage-mediated clearance of Pseudomonas aeruginosa from lung. *Nat Med.* 2002;8(6):588–593.

137. Smyth MJ, Thia KY, Street SE, et al. Differential tumor surveillance by natural killer (NK) and NKT cells. *J Exp Med.* 2000;191(4):661–668.

138. Crowe NY, Smyth MJ, Godfrey DI. A critical role for natural killer t cells in immunosurveillance of methylcholanthrene-induced sarcomas. *J Exp Med.* 2002;196(1):119–127.

139. Crowe NY, Coquet JM, Berzins SP, et al. Differential antitumor immunity mediated by NKT cell subsets in vivo. *J Exp Med.* 2005;202(9):1279–1288.

140. Renukaradhya GJ, Sriram V, Du W, et al. Inhibition of antitumor immunity by invariant natural killer T cells in a T-cell lymphoma model in vivo. *Int J Cancer.* 2006;118(12):3045–3053.

141. Girardi M, Glusac E, Filler RB, et al. The distinct contributions of murine T cell receptor (TCR)gammadelta+ and TCRalphabeta+ T cells to different stages of chemically induced skin cancer. *J Exp Med.* 2003;198(5):747–755.

142. Girardi M, Lewis JM, Filler RB, et al. Environmentally responsive and reversible regulation of epidermal barrier function by gammadelta T cells. *J Invest Dermatol.* 2006;126(4):808–814.

143. Girardi M, Lewis J, Glusac E, et al. Resident skin-specific gammadelta T cells provide local, nonredundant regulation of cutaneous inflammation. *J Exp Med.* 2002;195(7):855–867.

144. Jameson JM, Cauvi G, Sharp LL, et al. Gammadelta T cell-induced hyaluronan production by epithelial cells regulates inflammation. *J Exp Med.* 2005;201(8):1269–1279.

145. Chen Y, Chou K, Fuchs E, et al. Protection of the intestinal mucosa by intraepithelial gamma delta T cells. *Proc Natl Acad Sci U S A.* 2002;99(22):14338–14343.

146. Bonneville M, Fournie JJ. Sensing cell stress and transformation through Vgamma9Vdelta2 T cell-mediated recognition of the isoprenoid pathway metabolites. *Microbes Infect.* 2005;7(3):503–509.

147. Born WK, Reardon CL, O'Brien RL. The function of gammadelta T cells in innate immunity. *Curr Opin Immunol.* 2006;18(1):31–38.

148. Ochsenbein AF, Fehr T, Lutz C, et al. Control of early viral and bacterial distribution and disease by natural antibodies. *Science.* 1999;286(5447):2156–2159.

149. Paciorkowski N, Porte P, Shultz LD, et al. B1 B lymphocytes play a critical role in host protection against lymphatic filarial parasites. *J Exp Med.* 2000;191(4):731–736.

150. Weiser MR, Williams JP, Moore FD Jr, et al. Reperfusion injury of ischemic skeletal muscle is mediated by natural antibody and complement. *J Exp Med.* 1996;183(5):2343–2348.

151. Bonneville M, Ishida I, Itohara S, et al. Self tolerance to transgenic gamma delta T cells by intrathymic inactivation. *Nature.* 1990;344(6262):163–165.

152. Pellicci DG, Hammond KJ, Uldrich AP, et al. A natural killer T (NKT) cell developmental pathway involving a thymus-dependent NK1.1(−)CD4(+) CD1d-dependent precursor stage. *J Exp Med.* 2002;195(7):835–844.

153. Benlagha K, Wei DG, Veiga J, et al. Characterization of the early stages in thymic NKT cell development. *J Exp Med.* 2005;202:485–492.

154. Stetson DB, Mohrs M, Reinhardt RL, et al. Constitutive cytokine mRNAs mark natural killer (NK) and NK T cells poised for rapid effector function. *J Exp Med.* 2003;198(7):1069–1076.

155. McNab FW, Berzins SP, Pellicci DG, et al. The influence of CD1d in postselection NKT cell maturation and homeostasis. *J Immunol.* 2005;175(6):3762–3768.

156. Berzins SP, Cochrane AD, Pellicci DG, et al. Limited correlation between human thymus and blood NKT cell content revealed by an ontogeny study of paired tissue samples. *Eur J Immunol.* 2005;35(5):1399–1407.

157. Geissmann F, Cameron TO, Sidobre S, et al. Intravascular immune surveillance by CXCR6+ NKT cells patrolling liver sinusoids. *PLoS Biol.* 2005;3(4):e113.

158. Bendelac A, Killeen N, Littman D, et al. A subset of CD4+ thymocytes selected by MHC class I molecules. *Science.* 1994;263:1774–1778.

159. Ohteki T, MacDonald HR. Major histocompatibility complex class I related molecules control the development of CD4+8- and CD4-8- subsets of natural killer 1.1+ T cell receptor-a/b+ cells in the liver of mice. *J Exp Med.* 1994;180:699–704.

160. Coles MC, Raulet DH. NK1.1+ T cells in the liver arise in the thymus and are selected by interactions with class I molecules on CD4+CD8+ cells. *J Immunol.* 2000;164(5):2412–2418.

161. Forestier C, Park SH, Wei D, et al. T cell development in mice expressing CD1d directed by a classical MHC class II promoter. *J Immunol.* 2003;171(8):4096–4104.

162. Wei DG, Lee H, Park SH, et al. Expansion and long-range differentiation of the NKT cell lineage in mice expressing CD1d exclusively on cortical thymocytes. *J Exp Med.* 2005;202(2):239–248.

163. Xu H, Chun T, Colmone A, et al. Expression of CD1d under the control of a MHC class Ia promoter skews the development of NKT cells, but not CD8+ T cells. *J Immunol.* 2003;171(8):4105–4112.

164. Zimmer MI, Colmone A, Felio K, et al. A cell-type specific CD1d expression program modulates invariant NKT cell development and function. *J Immunol.* 2006;176(3):1421–1430.

165. Gadue P, Morton N, Stein PL. The Src family tyrosine kinase Fyn regulates natural killer T cell development. *J Exp Med.* 1999;190:1189.

166. Eberl G, Lowin-Kropf B, MacDonald HR. Cutting edge: NKT cell development is selectively impaired in Fyn-deficient mice. *J Immunol.* 1999;163(8):4091–4094.

167. Pasquier B, Yin L, Fondaneche MC, et al. Defective NKT cell development in mice and humans lacking the adapter SAP, the X-linked lymphoproliferative syndrome gene product. *J Exp Med.* 2005;201(5):695–701.

168. Nichols KE, Hom J, Gong SY, et al. Regulation of NKT cell development by SAP, the protein defective in XLP. *Nat Med*. 2005;11(3):340–345.
169. Veillette A. Immune regulation by SLAM family receptors and SAP-related adaptors. *Nat Rev Immunol*. 2006;6(1):56–66.
170. Sivakumar V, Hammond KJ, Howells N, et al. Differential requirement for Rel/nuclear factor kappa B family members in natural killer T cell development. *J Exp Med*. 2003;197(12):1613–1621.
171. Stanic AK, Bezbradica JS, Park JJ, et al. NF-kappa B controls cell fate specification, survival, and molecular differentiation of immunoregulatory natural T lymphocytes. *J Immunol*. 2004;172(4):2265–2273.
172. Schmidt-Supprian M, Tian J, Grant EP, et al. Differential dependence of CD4+CD25+ regulatory and natural killer-like T cells on signals leading to NF-kappaB activation. *Proc Natl Acad Sci U S A*. 2004;101(13):4566–4571.
173. Stanic AK, Bezbradica JS, Park JJ, et al. Cutting edge: the ontogeny and function of Va14Ja18 natural T lymphocytes require signal processing by protein kinase C theta and NF-kappa B. *J Immunol*. 2004;172(8):4667–4671.
174. Sarafova SD, Erman B, Yu Q, et al. Modulation of coreceptor transcription during positive selection dictates lineage fate independently of TCR/coreceptor specificity. *Immunity*. 2005;23(1):75–87.
175. Intlekofer AM, Takemoto N, Wherry EJ, et al. Effector and memory CD8+ T cell fate coupled by T-bet and eomesodermin. *Nat Immunol*. 2005;6(12):1236–1244.
176. Matsuda JL, Zhang Q, Ndonye R, et al. T-bet concomitantly controls migration, survival, and effector functions during the development of Valpha14i NKT cells. *Blood*. 2006;107(7):2797–2805.
177. Broussard C, Fleischecker C, Horai R, et al. Altered development of CD8(+) T cell lineages in mice deficient for the tec kinases itk and rlk. *Immunity*. 2006;25(1):93–104.
178. Atherly LO, Lucas JA, Felices M, et al. The tec family tyrosine kinases itk and rlk regulate the development of conventional CD8(+) T cells. *Immunity*. 2006;25(1):79–91.
179. De Creus A, Van Beneden K, Stevenaert F, et al. Developmental and functional defects of thymic and epidermal V gamma 3 cells in IL-15-deficient and IFN regulatory factor-1-deficient mice. *J Immunol*. 2002;168(12):6486–6493.
180. Van Beneden K, De Creus A, Stevenaert F, et al. Expression of inhibitory receptors Ly49E and CD94/NKG2 on fetal thymic and adult epidermal TCR V gamma 3 lymphocytes. *J Immunol*. 2002;168(7):3295–3302.
181. Ikuta K, Kina T, MacNeil I, et al. A developmental switch in thymic lymphocyte maturation potential occurs at the level of hematopoietic stem cells. *Cell*. 1990;62:863–874.
182. Silva-Santos B, Pennington DJ, Hayday AC. Lymphotoxin-mediated regulation of gammadelta cell differentiation by alphabeta T cell progenitors. *Science*. 2005;307(5711):925–928.
183. Pennington DJ, Silva-Santos B, Silberzahn T, et al. Early events in the thymus affect the balance of effector and regulatory T cells. *Nature*. 2006;444:1073–1078.
184. Hardy RR. B-1 B cell development. *J Immunol*. 2006;177(5):2749–2754.
185. Chan VW, Meng F, Soriano P, et al. Characterization of the B lymphocyte populations in Lyn-deficient mice and the role of Lyn in signal initiation and down-regulation. *Immunity*. 1997;7(1):69–81.
186. O'Keefe TL, Williams GT, Davies SL, et al. Hyperresponsive B cells in CD22-deficient mice. *Science*. 1996;274(5288):798–801.
187. Hayakawa K, Hardy RR, Herzenberg LA. Peritoneal Ly-1 B cells: genetic control, autoantibody production, increased lambda light chain expression. *Eur J Immunol*. 1986;16(4):450–46.
188. Rickert RC, Rajewsky K, Roes J. Impairment of T-cell-dependent B-cell responses and B-1 cell development in CD19-deficient mice. *Nature*. 1995;376(6538):352–355.
189. Haas KM, Poe JC, Steeber DA, et al. B-1a and B-1b cells exhibit distinct developmental requirements and have unique functional roles in innate and adaptive immunity to S. pneumoniae. *Immunity*. 2005;23(1):7–18.
190. Clarke SH, Arnold LW. B-1 cell development: evidence for an uncommitted immunoglobulin (Ig)M+ B cell precursor in B-1 cell differentiation. *J Exp Med*. 1998;187(8):1325–1334.
191. Casola S, Otipoby KL, Alimzhanov M, et al. B cell receptor signal strength determines B cell fate. *Nat Immunol*. 2004;5(3):317–327.
192. Ikeda A, Merchant M, Lev L, et al. Latent membrane protein 2A, a viral B cell receptor homologue, induces CD5+ B-1 cell development. *J Immunol*. 2004;172(9):5329–5237.
193. Pillai S, Cariappa A, Moran ST. Positive selection and lineage commitment during peripheral B-lymphocyte development. *Immunol Rev*. 2004;197:206–218.
194. Ansel KM, Harris RB, Cyster JG. CXCL13 is required for B1 cell homing, natural antibody production, and body cavity immunity. *Immunity*. 2002;16(1):67–76.
195. Cinamon G, Matloubian M, Lesneski MJ, et al. Sphingosine 1-phosphate receptor 1 promotes B cell localization in the splenic marginal zone. *Nat Immunol*. 2004;5(7):713–720.
196. Lu TT, Cyster JG. Integrin-mediated long-term B cell retention in the splenic marginal zone. *Science*. 2002;297(5580):409–412.
197. Cariappa A, Liou HC, Horwitz BH, et al. Nuclear factor kappa B is required for the development of marginal zone B lymphocytes. *J Exp Med*. 2000;192(8):1175–1182.
198. Chun T, Page MJ, Gapin L, et al. CD1d-expressing dendritic cells but not thymic epithelial cells can mediate negative selection of NKT cells. *J Exp Med*. 2003;197(7):907–918.
199. Ikarashi Y, Mikami R, Bendelac A, et al. Dendritic cell maturation overrules H-2D-mediated natural killer T (NKT) cell inhibition. Critical role for b7 in cd1d-dependent nkt cell interferon gamma production. *J Exp Med*. 2001;194(8):1179–1186.
200. Exley M, Garcia J, Balk SP, et al. Requirements for CD1d recognition by human invariant Va24+CD4-CD8- T cells. *J Exp Med*. 1997;186:109–120.
201. Halary F, Peyrat MA, Champagne E, et al. Control of self-reactive cytotoxic T lymphocytes expressing gamma delta T cell receptors by natural killer inhibitory receptors. *Eur J Immunol*. 1997;27(11):2812–2821.
202. Bikah G, Carey J, Ciallella JR, et al. CD5-mediated negative regulation of antigen receptor-induced growth signals in B-1 B cells. *Science*. 1996;274(5294):1906–1909.
203. Gadola SD, Koch M, Marles-Wright J, et al. Structure and binding kinetics of three different human CD1d-alpha-galactosylceramide-specific T cell receptors. *J Exp Med*. 2006;203(3):699–710.
204. Brigl M, van den Elzen P, Chen X, et al. Conserved and heterogeneous lipid antigen specificities of CD1d restricted NKT cell receptors. *J Immunol*. 2006;176(6):3625–3634.
205. Hayday AC. [gamma][delta] cells: a right time and a right place for a conserved third way of protection. *Annu Rev Immunol*. 2000;18:975–1026.
206. Lee PT, Putnam A, Benlagha K, et al. Testing the NKT cell hypothesis of human IDDM pathogenesis. *J Clin Invest*. 2002;110(6):793–800.
207. Gombert JM, Herbelin A, Tancrede-Bohin E, et al. Early quantitative and functional deficiency of NK1+-like thymocytes in the NOD mouse. *Eur J Immunol*. 1996;26:2989–2998.
208. Galili U. Evolution and pathophysiology of the human natural anti-alpha- galactosyl IgG (anti-Gal) antibody. *Springer Semin Immunopathol*. 1993;15(2-3):155–171.
209. Ohdan H, Swenson KG, Kruger Gray HS, et al. Mac-1-negative B-1b phenotype of natural antibody-producing cells, including those responding to Gal alpha 1,3Gal epitopes in alpha 1,3-galactosyltransferase-deficient mice. *J Immunol*. 2000;165(10):5518–5529.
210. Kawahara T, Ohdan H, Zhao G, et al. Peritoneal cavity B cells are precursors of splenic IgM natural antibody-producing cells. *J Immunol*. 2003;171(10):5406–5414.
211. Shires J, Theodoridis E, Hayday AC. Biological insights into TCRgammadelta+ and TCRalphabeta+ intraepithelial lymphocytes provided by serial analysis of gene expression (SAGE). *Immunity*. 2001;15(3):419–434.
212. Guy-Grand D, Cuenod-Jabri B, Malassis-Seris M, et al. Complexity of the mouse gut T cell immune system: identification of two distinct natural killer T cell intraepithelial lineages. Eur *J Immunol*. 1996;26(9):2248–2256.
213. Park SH, Guy-Grand D, Lemonnier FA, et al. Selection and expansion of CD8alpha/alpha(1) T cell receptor alpha/beta(1) intestinal intraepithelial lymphocytes in the absence of both classical major

histocompatibility complex class I and nonclassical CD1 molecules. *J Exp Med.* 1999;190(6):885–890.

214. Gapin L, Cheroutre H, Kronenberg M. Cutting edge: TCR alpha beta+ CD8 alpha alpha+ T cells are found in intestinal intraepithelial lymphocytes of mice that lack classical MHC class I molecules. *J Immunol.* 1999;163(8):4100–4104.
215. Yamagata T, Mathis D, Benoist C. Self-reactivity in thymic double-positive cells commits cells to a CD8 alpha alpha lineage with characteristics of innate immune cells. *Nat Immunol.* 2004;5(6): 597–605.
216. Regnault A, Cumano A, Vassalli P, et al. Oligoclonal repertoire of the CD8 alpha alpha and the CD8 alpha beta TCR-alpha/beta murine intestinal intraepithelial T lymphocytes: evidence for the random emergence of T cells. *J Exp Med.* 1994;180(4):1345–1358.
217. Urdahl KB, Sun JC, Bevan MJ. Positive selection of MHC class Ib-restricted CD8(+) T cells on hematopoietic cells. *Nat Immunol.* 2002;3(8):772–779.
218. Xu H, Chun T, Choi HJ, et al. Impaired response to Listeria in H2-M3-deficient mice reveals a nonredundant role of MHC class Ib-specific T cells in host defense. *J Exp Med.* 2006;203(2):449–459.
219. Sicard H, Ingoure S, Luciani B, et al. In vivo immunomanipulation of V gamma 9V delta 2 T cells with a synthetic phosphoantigen in a preclinical nonhuman primate model. *J Immunol.* 2005;175(8):5471–4580.

Chapter 18

Macrophages and Phagocytosis

Siamon Gordon

INTRODUCTION

Macrophages (Mϕ) represent a family of mononuclear leukocytes that are widely distributed throughout the body within and outside of lymphohemopoietic organs. They vary considerably in life span and phenotype, depending on their origin and local microenvironment. Mature Mϕ are highly phagocytic, relatively long-lived cells that are adaptable in their biosynthetic responses to antigens and microbial stimuli. The functions of Mϕ within tissues are homeostatic, regulating the local and systemic milieu through diverse plasma membrane receptors and varied secretory products. They react to, and themselves generate, signals that influence growth, differentiation, and death of other cells, recognizing and engulfing senescent and abnormal cells. These activities contribute substantially to recognition and defense functions against invading microorganisms, foreign particulates, and other immunogens. Innate immune functions of Mϕ complement their contributions to acquired humoral and cellular immunity, in which they regulate activation of T and B lymphocytes; this is achieved in part through their specialized derivatives, dendritic cells (DCs) of myeloid origin. Mϕ, with or without DCs, process and present antigen, produce chemokines and cytokines such as interleukin-1 (IL-1), IL-6, IL-12, IL-18, IL-23, tumor necrosis factor-α (TNFα), and IL-10, and phagocytose apoptotic and necrotic cells. Acting directly or under the influence of other immune cells, Mϕ capture extra- and intracellular pathogens, eliminate invaders, and deliver them to appropriate subcompartments of lymphoid organs. As key regulators of the specific as well as the natural immune response, Mϕ boost as well as limit induction and effector mechanisms of the specific immune response by positive and negative feedback.

The properties and roles of DCs are described in detail elsewhere in this volume. Here we focus on other members of the Mϕ lineage, consider their interrelationship, and outline specialized properties that underlie their roles in the execution and regulation of immune responses. A number of books deal with the history and broad aspects of Mϕ immunobiology (1–10).

SOME LANDMARKS IN THE STUDY OF MACROPHAGES

Our understanding of Mϕ developed in parallel with the growth of immunology as an experimental science. Metchnikoff, a comparative developmental zoologist, is widely credited for his recognition of phagocytosis as a fundamental host defense mechanism of primitive, as well as highly developed, multicellular organisms (1–3). He clearly stated the link between capture of infectious microorganisms by the spleen and subsequent appearance of reactive substances (antibodies) in the blood, although mistakenly ascribing their production to the phagocytes themselves. The importance of systemic clearance of particles by Mϕ, especially Kupffer cells in liver and other endothelial cells, was enshrined in the term reticuloendothelial system (RES). Although it was rejected by influential investigators in the field in favor of the term mononuclear phagocyte system (MPS), the appreciation that sinus-lining Mϕ in liver and elsewhere share common properties with selected endothelial cells is worth preserving (4). Earlier studies by Florey and his students, including Gowans, established that circulating monocytes give rise to tissue Mϕ. Van Furth and his colleagues investigated the life history of Mϕ by kinetic labeling methods; subsequently, the development of membrane antigen markers facilitated a more precise definition of specialized Mϕ subpopulations in tissues such as brain (5). The appearance and potential importance of Mϕ during development also became evident as a result of sensitive immunocytochemical methods. Morphologic and functional studies by Humphrey and many others drew attention to striking diversity among Mϕ-like cells in secondary lymphoid organs, especially within the marginal zone of the spleen, where complex particulates and polysaccharides are captured from the circulation (6,7).

The era of modern cell biology impinged on Mϕ studies following the studies of Cohn, Hirsch, and their colleagues (8). Their work touched on many aspects of cell structure and function, including phagocytosis (the zipper mechanism of Silverstein), fluid- and receptor-mediated endocytosis, secretion, and antimicrobial resistance. Isolation and *in vitro* culture systems became available for cells from mice and humans, especially after the identification of specific growth and differentiation factors such as colony-stimulating factor-1 (CSF-1; M-CSF) (9). It is perhaps fitting that the earliest known natural knockout (ko) affecting macrophages, a natural mutation in the op gene in the osteopetrotic mouse, should involve CSF-1 (9,10). Cell lines retaining some but not all features of mature Mϕ have been useful for many biochemical and cellular studies (11). Macrophages and dendritic cells can be readily derived from embryonic stem (ES) cells by growth in appropriate culture conditions.

The role of Mϕ as antigen-processing cells able to initiate adaptive immune responses had false trails ("immunogenic RNA" was thought to be involved at one time) and encompassed early genetic strategies (Mϕ of mice selected for high anti–sheep erythrocyte antibody responses by Biozzi and colleagues displayed enhanced degradative properties; adherent cells from defined guinea pig strains were shown to play an important role in major histocompatibility complex (MHC) Ia–restricted antiinsulin responses. For many years the antigen presenting cell (APC) functions of adherent cells were highly controversial as promoted by Unanue, who concentrated on intracellular processing by Mϕ, and Steinman, who discovered the specialized role of "dendritic cells" in antigen presentation to naive T lymphocytes. The importance of Mϕ as effector cells in immunity to intracellular pathogens such as *Mycobacterium tuberculosis* was recognized early by Lurie and Dannenberg. Mackaness used *Listeria monocytogenes* and bacille Calmette-Guérin (BCG) infection in experimental models and developed the concept of Mϕ activation as an antigen-dependent but immunologically nonspecific enhancement of antimicrobial resistance. The subsequent delineation of T lymphocyte subsets and characterization of interferon-γ (IFNγ) (12) as the major cytokine involved in macrophage activation, including MHC II induction, merged with increasing knowledge of the role of reactive oxygen and, later, nitrogen metabolites as cytotoxic agents (13). The role of virus-infected Mϕ as MHC I–restricted targets for antigen-specific CD8$^+$ killer cells was part of the initial characterization of this phenomenon by Zinkernagel and Doherty. D'Arcy Hart was an early investigator of the intracellular interactions between Mϕ and invaders of the vacuolar system, especially mycobacteria, which survive within Mϕ by inhibiting acidification and phagosome–lysosome fusion, thus evading host resistance mechanisms (14). Mouse breeding studies by several groups defined a common genetic locus involved in resistance to BCG, *Leishmania*, and *Salmonella* organisms. The host phenotype was shown to depend on expression in Mϕ and, many years later, the gene (termed N-ramp for natural resistance-associated membrane protein) was identified by positional cloning by Skamene, Gros, and their colleagues (15). Positional cloning by Beutler and associates led to the identification of the gene responsible for lipopolysaccharide (LPS) resistance in particular mouse strains (16). Together with studies by Hoffmann and his colleagues on the Toll pathway in *Drosophila* (17), this work resulted in an explosion of interest in the identification of mammalian Toll-like receptors (TLRs) and their role in innate immunity to infection (18,19). At the same time it became apparent that some malignant tumors contain macrophage populations that may favor their growth (20).

This brief survey concludes with the identification of Mϕ as key target cells for infection, dissemination, and persistence of HIV (21), tropic for macrophages by virtue of their expression of CD4, chemokine coreceptors, and DC-SIGN, a C-type lectin also expressed by DCs (22). Although Mϕ had been implicated by earlier workers such as Mims as important in antiviral resistance generally, their role in this regard was neglected before the emergence of HIV as a major pathogen.

Many molecules have been identified as important in Mϕ functions in immunity and serve as valuable markers to study their properties in mice and humans. These include Fc (23) and complement (24) receptors, which are important in opsonic phagocytosis, killing, and immunoregulation; scavenger receptors implicated in foam cell formation and atherogenesis by Brown and Goldstein (25); nonopsonic lectin receptors, such as the mannose receptor (MR) (26) and β-glucan receptor (BGR) (27); and secretory products such as lysozyme (28), neutral proteinases, TNFα (29), chemokines, and many other cytokines. A range of membrane antigens (ag) expressed by human and rodent mononuclear phagocytes has been characterized and reagents made available for further study of Mϕ in normal and diseased states (5). Recently, the role of DNA-binding transcription factors including members of the nuclear factor (NF)-κB and ETS (Pu-1) families has received increased attention in the study of differential gene expression by Mϕ (30,31). Gene inactivation has confirmed the important role of many of these molecules within the intact host, and use has been made of cell-specific or conditional ko to uncover the role of Mϕ in immunologic processes (32). Naturally occurring inborn errors in humans such as the leukocyte adhesion deficiency syndrome and chronic granulomatous disease have contributed to the analysis of important leukocyte functions, including those of Mϕ, in host resistance to infection. Mutations in a monocyte-expressed gene (NOD-2), involved in cytosolic sensing of microbial products and NF-κB activation, have been implicated in a subset of individuals with an enhanced susceptibility to Crohn's disease (33). The validity of murine ko models for human genetic deficiencies has been confirmed for key molecules involved in Mϕ activation, such as IFNγ and IL-12 (34). *N*-Ethyl *N*-nitrosourea mutagenesis has begun to reveal new macrophage innate immune functions (35).

PROPERTIES OF MACROPHAGES AND THEIR RELATION TO IMMUNE FUNCTIONS

Introduction

Mϕ participate in the production, mobilization, activation, and regulation of all immune effector cells. They interact reciprocally with other cells while their own properties are modified to perform specialized immunologic functions. As a result of cell surface and auto- and paracrine interactions, Mϕ display marked heterogeneity in phenotype (5,36,37), a source of interest and considerable confusion to the investigator. Increasing knowledge of cellular and molecular properties of Mϕ bears strongly on our understanding of their role in the immune response. These will be reviewed briefly, with emphasis on functional significance, and draw attention to unresolved and controversial issues.

Growth and Differentiation: Life History and Turnover

In contrast with T and B lymphocytes, monocytes from blood give rise to terminally differentiated Mϕ that cannot recirculate or reinitiate DNA replication except in a limited way; DCs may represent specialized migratory derivatives of mononuclear cells. Unlike other myeloid granulocytic cells, Mϕ can be long lived and retain the ability to synthesize RNA and protein to a marked extent, even when in a relatively quiescent state, as "resident" cells. These are distributed throughout the tissues of the body and constitute a possible alarm-response system, but they also mediate poorly understood trophic functions. Following inflammatory and immune stimuli, many more monocytes can be recruited to local sites and give rise to "elicited" or "immunologically activated" Mϕ with altered surface, secretory, and cytotoxic properties. The origins of Mϕ from precursors are well known; from yolk sac (and possibly earlier paraaortic progenitors), migrating to fetal liver, then spleen and bone marrow, before and after birth (38). In the fetus, mature Mϕ proliferate actively during tissue remodeling in developing organs. In the normal adult, tissue Mϕ do not self-renew extensively except in specialized microenvironments such as lung epidermis or, the pituitary; after injury there can be considerable further replication at local sites of inflammation. Growth and differentiation are tightly regulated by specific growth factors and their receptors (e.g., IL-3, CSF-1, granulocyte-macrophage [GM]-CSF, IL-4, IL-13) and inhibitors (e.g., IFNα/β, transforming growth factor-β [TGFβ], leukemia inhibitory factor), which vary considerably in their potency and selectivity. These processes are modulated by interactions with adjacent stromal and other cells (e.g., through c-kit/ligand and Flt-3/ligand interactions). The growth-response of the target cell to an extrinsic stimulus decreases progressively and markedly (from 10^8 or more to 10^0) during differentiation from stem cell to committed precursor to monoblast, monocyte, and Mϕ, yet even the most terminally differentiated Mϕ such as microglial cells can be "reactivated" to a limited extent by local stimuli (39). Elicited/activated Mϕ respond more vigorously than resident Mϕ to growth stimuli *in vivo* and *in vitro*, but the molecular basis for their enhanced proliferation is unknown.

Although the general picture of blood monocyte-to-tissue Mϕ differentiation has been clear for some time as a result of parabiosis, adoptive transfer, and irradiation-reconstitution experiments, there are still major unsolved issues. Are all "monocytes" equivalent, or is there heterogeneity in the circulating mononuclear cell pool corresponding with the ultimate tissue localization of their resident, constitutively distributed progeny? Our understanding of DCs and osteoclast differentiation is compatible with a relatively simple model (Figure 18.1) in which major Mϕ populations in tissues can be characterized by selected ag

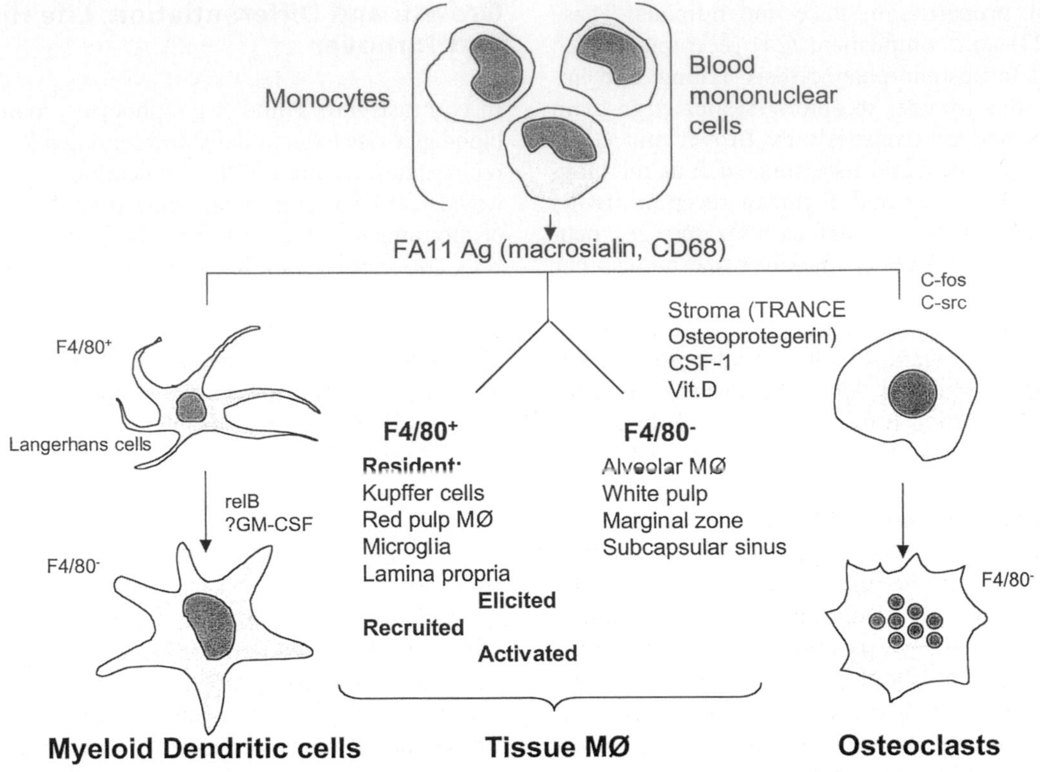

FIGURE 18.1 Differentiation of mononuclear phagocytes based on antigen markers FA-11 (macrosialin, murine CD68) and F4/80. See text for detailed discussion.

markers such as F4/80 (Emr1, a member of a new family of EGF-TM7 molecules) (40) and macrosialin (CD68), a pan-Mϕ endosomal glycoprotein related to the lysosome-associated membrane protein (LAMP) family (41). The DCs of myeloid origin (see elsewhere in this volume) can be viewed as products of Langerhans-type cells in nonlymphoid organs such as skin and airway epithelium, which may undergo further differentiation and migrate to secondary lymphoid organs in response to an antigenic stimulus (42). Circulating precursors of DCs and recirculating progeny are also normally present in the mononuclear fraction of blood in small numbers and may be already "marked" for distribution to peripheral sites as Langerhans cells. Monocytes that have crossed the endothelium may be induced to "reverse migrate" into the circulation by selected stimuli in tissues (43).

Circulating mononuclear precursors for osteoclasts are less defined and differentiate into mononucleate cells in bone and cartilage, where they fuse to form multinucleate bone-resorbing osteoclasts (44). Local stromal cells, growth factors such as CSF-1, steroids (vitamin D metabolites), and hormones (e.g., calcitonin, for which osteoclasts express receptors) all contribute to local maturation. Osteoprotegerin, a naturally occurring secreted protein with homology to members of the TNF-receptor family, interacts with TRANCE, a TNF-related protein, to regulate osteoclast differentiation and activation *in vitro* and *in vivo*.

Use of ag markers such as CD34 on progenitors, CD14 and CD16 (45) on monocytes, and chemokine receptors (46) and multichannel fluorescein-activated cell sorter (FACS) analysis makes it possible to isolate leukocyte subpopulations and study their progeny and differential responses (see later discussion). The mononuclear fraction of blood may contain precursors of other tissue cells, including "fibrocytes" (47) thought to be hemopoietic yet able to synthesize matrix proteins such as collagen, and some endothelial cells. Perhaps the mysterious follicular dendritic cells (FDCs) with mixed hemopoietic and mesenchymal properties fall in this category.

The large-scale production of immature and mature DC-like cells from bulk monocytes in cytokine-supplemented culture systems (IL-4, GM-CSF, TNFα) has revolutionized the study of these specialized APCs (48,49). Individually, the same cytokines give rise to Mϕ-like cells, and early during *in vitro* differentiation, the cellular phenotype is reversible. Later, when mature DCs with high MHC II, APC function, and other characteristic markers are formed, differentiation is irreversible. This process is independent of cell division, although earlier progenitors in bone marrow and G-CSF–mobilized blood mononuclear cells can be stimulated to multiply, as well as differentiate, *in vitro*. These examples of terminal differentiation observed with DCs and osteoclasts may extend to other specialized, more obvious Mϕ-like cells. Mature Mϕ

can be derived by growth and differentiation in steroid-supplemented media in Dexter-type long-term bone marrow cultures that contain stromal fibroblasts and hemopoietic elements. These Mϕ express adhesion molecules responsible for divalent cation–dependent cluster formation with erythroblasts (EbR) (50). This receptor, possibly related to V-CAM, cannot be induced on terminally differentiated peritoneal Mϕ if these are placed in the same culture system. This contrasts sharply with the ready adaptation of many tissue Mϕ to conventional cell culture conditions, when the cells often adopt a common, standard phenotype. Irreversible stages of Mϕ differentiation may therefore occur in specialized microenvironments *in vitro* or *in vivo*.

Little is known about determinants of Mϕ longevity and turnover. Growth factors such as CSF-1 enhance Mϕ survival and prevent induction of an apoptotic program. The expression of Fas-L and Fas on Mϕ has been less studied than on lymphocytes; they and other members of the TNF and its receptor family may play a major role in determining Mϕ survival, especially in induced populations, where cell turnover is markedly enhanced. Tissue Mϕ vary greatly in their life span, from days to months. Apart from inflammatory and microbial stimuli, local and systemic environmental factors such as salt loading and hormones, including estrogen, are known to influence Mϕ turnover.

Tissue Distribution and Phenotypic Heterogeneity of Resident Macrophages in Lymphoid and Nonlymphoid Organs

The use of the F4/80 plasma membrane ag made it possible to detect mature Mϕ in developing and adult murine tissues and define their anatomic relationship to other cells in endothelium, epithelium, and connective tissue, as well as the nervous system (5,51). Subsequently, other membrane antigens (52) [macrosialin (41), sialoadhesin (53,54)] were identified as useful markers for Mϕ *in situ* (Table 18.1). Mϕ subpopulations in different tissues display considerable heterogeneity in expressing these and selected receptor antigens, for example, CR3 (55) and SR-A (56), drawing attention to unknown mechanisms of homing, emigration, and local adaptation to particular microenvironments. From the viewpoint of immune responses, a few aspects deserve comment.

Fetal Liver and Bone Marrow

Mature Mϕ form an integral part of the hemopoietic microenvironment and play a key role in the production, differentiation, and destruction of all hemopoietic cells (57). The fetal liver is a major site of definitive erythropoiesis from midgestation. The bone marrow becomes

TABLE 18.1 Selected Differentiation Antigens Used to Study Murine Macrophage Heterogeneity

Ab	Ag	Structure	Ligands	Cellular Expression	Function	Comment
F4/80	F4/80 (EMR1)	EGF-TM7	?	Mature Mϕ, absent T areas	Peripheral tolerance	Useful marker development, CNS
FA-11	Macrosialin (CD68)	Mucin-LAMP	OX-LDL	Pan-Mϕ, DC	Late endosomal	Glycoforms regulated by inflammation and phagocytosis
5C6	CR3 (CD11b, CD18)	β2-integrin	iC3b, ICAM	Monocytes, microglia, PMN, NK cells	Phagocytosis, adhesion	Important in inflammatory recruitment, PMN apoptosis
2F8	SR-A (I, II)	Collagenous, type II glycoprotein	Polyanions, LTA, LPS, bacterial proteins		Adhesion, endocytosis	Protects host against LPS-induced shock
		Isoforms differ, cysteine-rich domain	Modified proteins β-amyloid Apolipoprotein A, E	Mϕ, sinusoidal Endothelium	Phagocytosis of apoptotic cells and bacteria	Promotes atherosclerosis
SER-4 3D6	Sn (Siglec-1)	Ig superfamily	Sialyl glycoconjugates e.g., CD43	Subsets Tissue Mϕ	Lectin	Strongly expressed Marginal zone metallophils in spleen and subcapsular sinus of lymph nodes

Ab, antibody; Ag, antigen; CNS, central nervous system; DC, dendritic cells; ICAM, intercellular adhesion molecule; Ig, immunoglobulin; LAMP, lysosome-associated membrane protein; LPS, lipopolysaccharide; LTA, lipoteichoic acid; Mϕ, macrophages; NK, natural killer cells; PMN, Sn, sialoadhesin; SR-A, type A scavenger receptor.

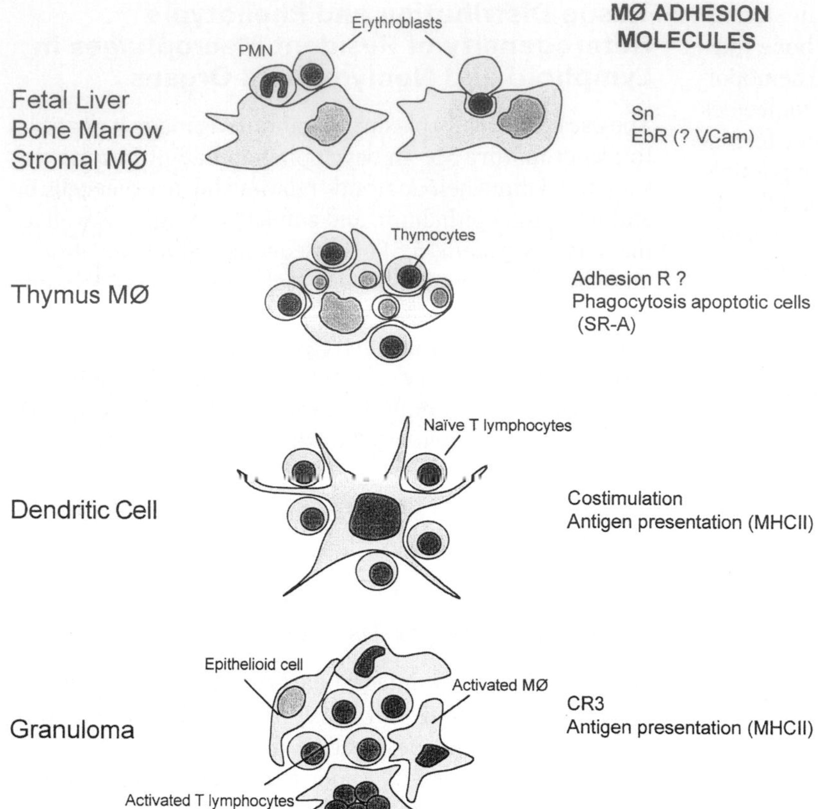

FIGURE 18.2 Associations of tissue macrophages with other hemopoietic cells to illustrate variations on a common theme. See text for details.

active in the production of hemopoietic cells from shortly before birth, and Mϕ are a prominent component of the hemopoietic stroma throughout adult life. Mature "stromal" Mϕ in fetal liver and adult bone marrow express nonphagocytic adhesion molecules such as sialoadhesin (Sn), an immunoglobulin (Ig)-superfamily sialic acid–binding lectin (53,54) (Table 18.1), and the EbR referred to previously (50), which is also involved in adhesion of developing myeloid and possibly lymphoid cells (Figure 18.2). VLA-4 has been implicated as a ligand for EbR. Ligands for Sn include CD43 on developing granulocytes (58) and on lymphocyte subpopulations. Sialoadhesin clusters at sites of contact between stromal Mϕ and myeloid but not erythroid cells. Chemokines are able to induce polarized expression of adhesion molecules such as intercellular adhesion molecules (ICAMs) and CD43 in leukocytes, but the significance of altered ligand distribution for interactions between Mϕ and bound hemopoietic cells is unknown. Adhesion of immature cells to stromal Mϕ may play a role in regulating their intermediate stages of development before release into the bloodstream, whereas fibroblasts in the stroma associate with earlier progenitors, as well as with Mϕ. Discarded nuclei of mammalian erythroid cells are rapidly engulfed by stromal Mϕ, but the receptors involved in their binding and phagocytosis are unknown. Mϕ also phagocytose apoptotic hemopoietic cells generated in bone marrow, including large numbers of myeloid and B cells. We know little about the plasma membrane molecules and cytokine signals operating within this complex milieu, but it is clear that stromal Mϕ constitute a neglected constituent within the hemopoietic microenvironment.

Thymus

Apart from their remarkable capacity to remove apoptotic thymocytes, the possible role of Mϕ in positive and negative selection of thymocytes has been almost totally overlooked; more attention has been given to local DCs and their specialized properties. Mature Mϕ with unusual features are also present in cortex and medulla. Clusters of viable thymocytes and Mϕ can be isolated from the thymus of young animals by collagenase digestion and adherence to a substratum (Figure 18.2). The nonphagocytic adhesion receptors responsible for cluster formation are more highly expressed by thymic than other Mϕ, but their nature is unknown (N. Platt, unpublished observations). These Mϕ also express MHC class II antigens and other receptors such as the class A scavenger receptor (SR-A) (see later discussion), which contributes to phagocytosis of apoptotic thymocytes *in vitro* (59) but is redundant *in vivo* (60); other markers, such as the F4/80 ag, are poorly expressed *in situ* but can be readily detected after cell isolation. A striking difference between thymic and several other tissue

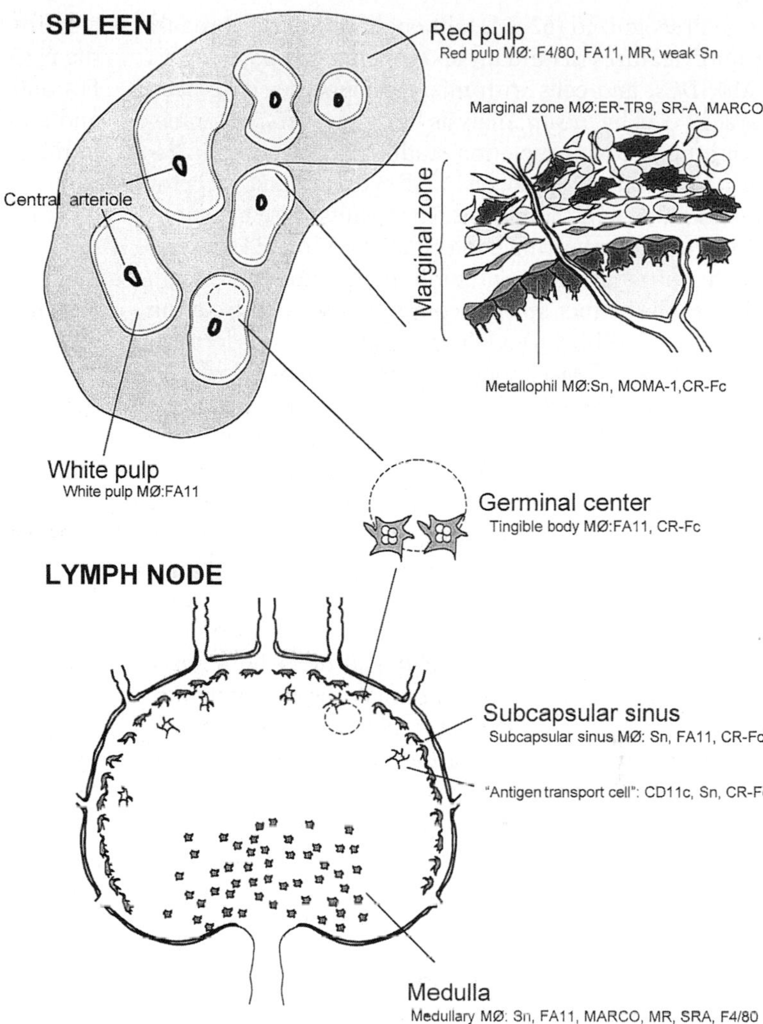

FIGURE 18.3 Microheterogeneity of macrophages in spleen, resting, and antigen-stimulated lymph nodes. See text for markers and details.

Mϕ subpopulations is their independence of CSF-1; the CSF-1–deficient *op/op* mouse lacks osteoclasts and some Mϕ populations, including monocytes, peritoneal cells, and Kupffer cells, but contains normal numbers of thymic Mϕ, as well as DCs and selected Mϕ in other sites (61). Factors involved in constitutive recruitment of thymic Mϕ are unknown; following death of thymocytes induced by ionizing radiation or glucocorticoids, intensely phagocytic Mϕ appear in large numbers; it is not known what proportion arises locally and by recruitment.

Spleen

From the viewpoint of the Mϕ, the spleen is perhaps the most complex organ in the body (6,7). It contributes to hemopoiesis, which persists postnatally in some species or can be induced by increased demand, and to the turnover of all blood elements at the end of their natural life span. In addition, the spleen filters a substantial proportion of total cardiac output, captures particulate and other antigenic materials from the bloodstream, and plays an important role in natural and acquired humoral and cellular immunity. The organ is rich in subpopulations of Mϕ that differ in microanatomic localization, phenotype, life history, and functions (Figure 18.3). Mϕ are central to antigen capture, degradation, transport, and presentation to T and B lymphocytes and contribute substantially to antimicrobial resistance. Because other hemopoietic and secondary lymphoid organs can replace many of these functions after maturation of the immune system, the unique properties of the spleen have been mainly recognized in the immature host and in immune responses to complex polysaccharides. Splenectomy in the adult renders the host susceptible to infection by pathogenic bacteria such as pneumococci that contain saccharide-rich capsular antigens; the marginal zone of the spleen in particular may play an essential role in this aspect of host resistance.

The properties of Mϕ in the unstimulated mature mouse spleen are very different according to their localization in red or white pulp and the marginal zone. Mϕ are intimately associated with the specialized vasculature. Species differences in splenic anatomy and phenotype are well recognized (62–64), although Mϕ display broadly common features in humans and rodents. Subpopulations of Mϕ, DCs, and cells with mixed phenotypes have been characterized by *in situ* analysis by ag markers, liposome- or diphtheria toxin–depletion studies, various immunization and infection protocols, and cytokine and receptor gene ko models in the mouse. The results raise questions about the dynamics and molecular basis of cell production, recruitment, differentiation, emigration, and death within each distinct splenic compartment. Cell isolation methods are still primitive in correlating *in vitro* properties with those of Mϕ subpopulations *in vivo* and remain an important challenge. Detailed aspects of splenic architecture, DC origin and function, and T and B lymphocyte induction and differentiation are described elsewhere in this volume. Here I highlight some features of Mϕ in the normal and immunoreactive organ.

Marginal Zone Macrophages

The marginal zone of spleen consists of a complex mixture of resident cells (reticular and other fibroblasts, endothelium), Mϕ, DCs, and lymphoid cells, including subpopulations of B lymphocytes (7). It constitutes an important interface with the circulation that delivers cells, particulates, or soluble molecules directly into the marginal sinus or via the red pulp. Resident Mϕ are present as specialized metallophilic cells in the inner marginal zone, and other Mϕ are found in the outer zone; the latter may be more phagocytic. Sialoadhesin is very strongly expressed by the marginal metallophils, compared with only weak expression in red pulp and virtual absence in the white pulp (65). Sialoadhesin-positive cells appear in this zone 2 to 4 weeks postnatally in the mouse as the white pulp forms (66). Liposomes containing clodronate, a cytotoxic drug, can be delivered systemically and deplete Sn^+ cells and other Mϕ; regeneration of different Mϕ subpopulations in spleen occurs at different times, and this procedure has been used to correlate their reappearance with distinct immunologic functions. Marginal zone Mϕ lack F4/80 but may express an undefined ligand for F4/80 on circulating activated DCs, which mediates peripheral tolerance to anterior chamber or gut-derived antigens (67). Marginal zone Mϕ express phagocytic receptors, such as SR-A (68), which is more widely present on tissue Mϕ, as well as MARCO, a distinct collagenous scavenger receptor (69), which is almost exclusively present on these Mϕ in the normal mouse (70). The structures and possible role of these pattern recognition receptors in uptake of microbes are discussed later. *In vivo* studies have shown that a Mϕ lectin, the MR, may be involved in transfer of mannosylated ligands to the site of an immune response in the white pulp (26,71–73). The MR contains a highly conserved cysteine-rich domain, not involved in mannosyl recognition, that reacts strongly with ligands on a subset of marginal metallophilic Mϕ (73a), sulfated glycoforms of Sn, and CD45, among others; this has been demonstrated with a chimeric probe of the cysteine-rich domain of the MR and human Fc (CR-Fc) and by immunochemical analysis of tissue sections and affinity chromatography of spleen ligands. After immunization, this probe additionally labels undefined cells in the FDC network of germinal centers, as well as tingible body Mϕ. It is possible that marginal zone Mϕ can be induced to migrate into white pulp as described after LPS injection; alternatively, they may shed complexes of soluble MR-glycoprotein ligand for transfer to other $CR\text{-}Fc^+$ cells, which may be resident, or newly recruited mononuclear cells. Finally, the marginal metallophilic Mϕ population depends on CSF-1 for its appearance (61) and on members of the TNF receptor family (74), as shown with *op/op* and experimentally produced ko mice.

White Pulp Macrophages

The F4/80 ag is strikingly absent on murine white pulp Mϕ, which do express FA-11 (macrosialin), the murine homolog of CD68. Actively phagocytic Mϕ express this intracellular glycoprotein in abundance compared with DCs. After uptake of a foreign particle (e.g., sheep erythrocytes or an infectious agent, such as BCG or *Plasmodium yoellii*), white pulp Mϕ become more prominent, although it is not known whether there is migration of cells into the white pulp or transfer of phagocytosed material and reactivation of previous resident Mϕ. Tingible body Mϕ appear to be involved in uptake and digestion of apoptotic B lymphocytes.

Red Pulp Macrophages

These express F4/80 ag and MR (75) strongly and in the mouse include stromal-type Mϕ involved in hemopoiesis. Extensive phagocytosis of senescent erythrocytes results in accumulation of bile pigments and ferritin. The role of various phagocytic receptors in clearance of host cells and pathogens by red pulp Mϕ requires further study.

There is no evidence that Mϕ, other than interdigitating DCs, associate directly with $CD4^+$ T lymphocytes in the normal spleen. Following infection by BCG, for example, or by other microorganisms such as *Salmonella*, there is massive recruitment and local production of Mϕ, many of which associate with T lymphocytes. Newly formed granulomata often appear first in the marginal zone (focal accumulations of activated Mϕ and activated T cells. As infections spread into the white and red pulp, the granulomata become confluent and less localized, obscuring and/or disrupting the underlying architecture of the spleen. The possible role of activated Mϕ in T cell apoptosis and clearance in spleen has not been defined.

Lymph Nodes

F4/80 ag is relatively poorly expressed in lymph node (Figure 18.3), but many macrosialin $(CD68)^+$ cells are present. The subcapsular sinus is analogous to the marginal zone and contains strongly Sn^+ cells; this is the site where afferent lymph enters, containing antigen and migrating DCs derived from Langerhans cells. The medulla contains Sn^+, $CD68^+$ Mϕ, which also express high levels of SR-A. As in the spleen marginal zone, subcapsular sinus Mϕ are strongly labeled by the CR-Fc probe. Following primary or secondary immunization, the staining pattern moves deeper into the cortex and eventually becomes concentrated in germinal centers. The kinetics of this process strongly suggests a transport process by Mϕ-related cells resembling antigen transport cells described previously. CR-Fc^+ cells can be isolated by digestion of lymph nodes and form clusters with CR-Fc^- lymphocytes. Adoptive transfer has shown that FACS-isolated CR-Fc^+ cells resemble DCs in their ability to home to T cell areas and to present antigen to naive T and B cells (76). Overall, there is considerable heterogeneity in the population of migratory APCs involved in antigen capture, transport, and delivery to T and B cells, and it may turn out that specialized tissue Mϕ as well as myeloid-type DCs can migrate in response to immunologic stimuli, especially TLR ligands (73).

Peyer's Patch

Although less studied, the Mϕ in Peyer's patch resemble the $CD68^+$, $F4/80^-$ cells described in spleen and white pulp and in other T cell–rich areas. They are well placed to interact with gut-derived antigens and pathogens taken up via specialized epithelial M cells in the dome, and deliver antigens to afferent lymphatics, as myeloid DCs. These cells are distinct from abundant $F4/80^+$ cells in the lamina propria found all the way down the gastrointestinal tract and may play a role in the induction of mucosal immunity.

Nonlymphoid Organs

Regional $F4/80^+$ and $CD68^+$ Mϕ are well described in liver (Kupffer cells), dermis, neuroendocrine and reproductive organs, and serosal cavities, where they are able to react to systemic and local stimuli. In the lung, alveolar Mϕ are strongly $CD68^+$ but only weakly $F4/80^+$ and are distinct from interstitial Mϕ and intraepithelial DCs. In the lamina propria of the intestine, macrophages display a downregulated phenotype, ascribed to TGFβ of local origin (77). In addition, resident Mϕ are found throughout connective tissue and within the interstitium of organs, including heart, kidney, and pancreas. These cells vary greatly depending on their local microenvironment; for example, in the central nervous system, microglia within the neuropil differ strikingly from Mϕ in the meninges or choroid plexus. Perivascular Mϕ in the brain can be distinguished from resident microglia by their expression of endocytic receptors, for example, the SR-A and MR, and of MHC I and II antigens. Microglia are highly ramified, terminally differentiated cells of monocytic origin, and many Mϕ markers are downregulated; their phenotype is influenced by the blood–brain barrier, normally absent in circumventricular organs, and disrupted by inflammatory stimuli. Microglia can be reactivated by local LPS and neurocytotoxins, and they are then difficult to distinguish from newly recruited monocytes, which acquire microglial features once they enter the parenchyma of the brain (51). Resting microglia are unusual among many tissue Mϕ in that they constitutively express high levels of CR3 and respond to CR3 ligands, such as mAb, by induced DNA synthesis and apoptosis (39). In other sites, such as lung and liver, CR3 expression is a feature of recent myeloid recruitment, including monocytes. Resident Kupffer cells lack constitutive CR3 but express a novel CR implicated in clearance function (78).

Enhanced Recruitment of Monocytes by Inflammatory and Immune Stimuli: Activation *in vivo*

In response to local tissue and vascular changes, partly induced by resident Mϕ during (re)activation by inflammatory and immunologic stimuli, monocytes are recruited from marrow pools and blood in increased numbers; they diapedese and differentiate into Mϕ with altered effector functions as they enter the tissues. These Mϕ are classified as "elicited" when cells are generated in the absence of γ-interferon and as "immunologically activated" after exposure to γ-interferon. Enhanced recruitment can also involve that of other myeloid or lymphoid cells; selectivity of the cellular response depends on the nature of the evoking stimulus (immunogenic or not), the chemokines produced, and the receptors expressed by different leukocytes. Mϕ and other cells produce a range of different chemokines and express multiple seven-transmembrane, G protein–coupled chemokine receptors. The chemokines can also act in the marrow compartment, especially if anchored to matrix and glycosaminoglycans, may display other growth regulatory functions, and can control egress. Locally bound or soluble chemokines induce the surface expression and activity of adhesion molecules on circulating white cells, as well as directing their migration through and beyond endothelium. Feedback mechanisms from periphery to central stores and within the marrow stroma may depend on cytokines and growth factors such as macrophage inflammatory protein-1α and GM-CSF, which inhibit or enhance monocyte production, respectively. The adhesion molecules involved in recruitment of monocytes, originally defined by studies in humans with inborn errors and by use of inhibitory antibodies in experimental animal models, overlap with those of polymorphonuclear neutrophils (PMNs) and lymphocytes and include L-selectin, β_2-integrins, especially CR3, CD31, an Ig-superfamily molecule, and CD99 (79); additional

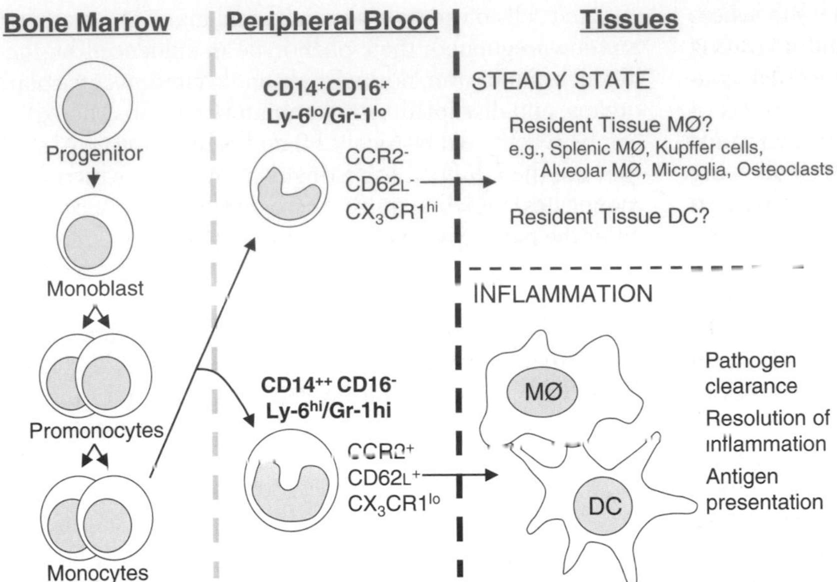

FIGURE 18.4 Distinct monocyte subsets give rise to inflammatory and resident macrophages and dendritic cells. The origin of different resident subpopulations is not clear. See text for further details.

monocyte adhesion molecules for activated endothelium include CD44, vascular cell adhesion molecules, β_1-integrins, and newly described receptors such as EMR2 and CD97, members of the EGF-TM7 family (37,40). The mechanisms of constitutive entry of monocytes into developing and adult tissues, in the absence of an inflammatory stimulus, are unknown.

By contrast with the uncertain precursors of resident Mϕ and DC populations, distinct monocyte subsets have been implicated in the enhanced mobilization and turnover in response to inflammatory, infectious, and metabolic stimuli (37,46,80) (Figure 18.4). Differential expression of fractalkine receptor, CCR2, and other chemokine receptors, together with antigen markers (Gr-1 in mouse and CD14 in human), have made it possible to define monocyte heterogeneity (81,82). Although such subsets seem to be conserved across several species, their properties may reflect stages of cell activation along a continuous spectrum rather than true differentiation.

The migration and differentiation of newly recruited monocytes once they have left the circulation are poorly understood. They are able to enter all tissues, undergoing alterations in membrane molecules and secretory potential under the influence of cytokines and surface interactions with endothelial cells, leukocytes, and other local cells. Phenotypic changes mentioned in the following section have been characterized by a range of *in vitro* and *in vivo* studies. Well-studied examples include murine peritoneal Mϕ—resident, elicited by thioglycollate broth or biogel polyacrylamide beads, and immunologically activated by BCG infection. The latter provides a useful model of granuloma formation in solid organs but does not fully mimic the human counterpart associated with *M. tuberculosis* infection. Granuloma Mϕ vary in their turnover and immune effector functions and display considerable heterogeneity; lesions contain recently recruited monocytes, mature, epithelioid Mϕ (described as secretory cells), and Langhans giant cells. Interactions with T lymphocytes, other myeloid cells, DCs, fibroblasts, and microorganisms yield a dynamic assembly of cells as the granuloma evolves, heals, and resolves (Figure 18.2). Apoptosis and necrosis of Mϕ and other cells contribute to the balance of continued recruitment and local proliferation. The emigration of Mϕ rather than DCs from sites of inflammation is less evident, although it has become clear that elicited Mϕ within the peritoneal cavity, for example, migrate actively to draining lymph nodes.

Gene ko models have confirmed the role of molecules previously implicated in recruitment, activation, and granuloma formation. These include the adhesion molecules listed previously, their ligands, such as ICAM-1, and key cytokines such as γ-interferon, IL-12, and TNFα, as well as their receptors. Antimicrobial resistance and Mϕ cytotoxicity resulting from production of reactive oxygen and nitrogen metabolites are now accessible to study in knockouts of the phagocyte oxidase and inducible nitric oxide synthase (iNOS) (83). Knockouts of membrane molecules of immunologic interest expressed by Mϕ and other cells include MHC class II and I, CD4, and CD40L, other accessory molecules such as B7-1 and B7-2, and the Mϕ-restricted intracellular molecule N-ramp.

The use of knockouts and/or antibodies or soluble receptors has brought insight into essential, nonredundant contributions of molecules that regulate Mϕ activation, immunopathology syndromes such as septic shock, and autoimmunity. Examples include myeloid antigens such as TREM-1 (84), associated with DAP-12, receptor–ligand pairs such as CD200/CD200 receptor (85,86), and suppressors of cytokine signaling (SOCS) proteins (87). TNFα is essential for host resistance to infection (88), and also contributes to immunopathology. Highly effective anti-TNFα therapy for chronic inflammatory diseases such as rheumatoid arthritis (89) can result in reactivation of latent tuberculosis.

The potential for Th1- and Th2-type regulation of Mϕ demonstrated *in vitro*, and discussed later, can result in highly complex, often coexistent, heterogeneity of Mϕ phenotype *in situ* (90) (Figure 18.4). Although almost all granuloma Mϕ express lysozyme (28), only minor subpopulations express cytokines such as IL-1β, IL-6, and TNFα. Pro- and antiinflammatory cytokines, IL-12, IL-18, IL-10, and TGFβ, produced by Mϕ themselves and other cells, modulate the phenotype of Mϕ *in vivo*.

Apart from the local interactions outlined, Mϕ regulate systemic host reactions to immune and infectious stimuli by producing circulating cytokines such as IL-6 and arachidonate- and other lipid-derived metabolites, including resolvins, that contribute to the resolution of acute inflammation (91). These also act on neural and endocrine centers, crossing the blood–brain barrier, or are generated locally by reactive microglia and Mϕ. Glucocorticosteroids are powerful immunomodulators (92) and form part of a network that regulates monocyte recruitment and Mϕ functions through circulating mediators such as MIF (migration inhibition factor). Mϕ contain potent enzymes involved in steroid biosynthesis and catabolism.

Although the immunologic relevance of Mϕ-induced responses may seem evident, many aspects remain unclear. For example, do Mϕ actively suppress or destroy activated T lymphocytes, thus contributing to regulation of immune responses and peripheral tolerance, or are Mϕ only passive removers of dying cells; do Mϕ contribute to recruitment, differentiation, and death of DCs at sites of inflammation before their migration to secondary lymphoid organs; do adjuvant-stimulated Mϕ interact with B lymphocytes, directing their migration into germinal centers; are interactions of activated Mϕ with antibody and complement, through different Fc and complement receptors, implicated in fine-tuning humoral responses; are activated Mϕ themselves cytocidal for infected host cells, and to what extent do they in turn interact with and provide targets for attack by natural killer (NK) cells and cytotoxic T lymphocytes? Study of a range of experimental models and disease processes *in vivo* should yield new insights, as well as extend and confirm mechanisms already defined *in vitro*.

Phagocytic Recognition and Intracellular Infection

The initiation and localization of an immune response depend on recognition by Mϕ and other cells of particulate agents or soluble proteins that are foreign or modified-self. Phagocytic and endocytic recognition by Mϕ and DCs depends on opsonic (mainly antibody, complement) and nonopsonic pattern recognition receptors that interact with a range of related ligands (93–95). Innate and acquired responses are thus interlinked. Different FcR are involved in uptake and destruction of targets as well as in negative regulation of effector functions (23). Complement receptors are also heterogeneous; CR3 interacts with C3-derived ligands formed by activation of the classical, alternate, or lectin pathways and mediate phagocytosis, cell migration, and cell activation. Other ligands include I-CAM. CR3 functions are modulated by fibronectin, via integrins, other adhesion molecules, and inflammatory stimuli. FcR ligation and cross-linking activates tyrosine kinases such as syk that are essential for phagocytosis (96); CR3 signaling is less defined and may not trigger a respiratory burst or arachidonate release, unlike FcR, thus favoring pathogen entry (97). Antibody-mediated uptake targets an organism or soluble antigen to a different, degradative compartment (Figure 18.6A) and usually results in its neutralization and destruction, although enhancement of infection can also occur in Mϕ. For example, flavivirus infection in the presence of specific antibody can result in the Dengue hemorrhagic shock syndrome (98). Immune complexes, with or without complement, localize antigens to FDCs and other FcR$^+$ CR$^+$ cells (99). Mϕ themselves are able to produce all components of the complement cascade in significant amounts at local sites, which may be less accessible to circulating proteins made by hepatocytes.

Nonopsonic receptors reacting directly with ligands on microorganisms (95) include CR3, lectins, especially the MR (26) and β-glucan receptor (27), the scavenger receptors SR-A (100) and MARCO, and the family of TLRs (19). MRs are present on Mϕ, DCs, and sinusoidal endothelium. They mediate phagocytosis and endocytosis, including macropinocytosis, and structurally resemble another multilectin, Dec 205, present on DCs as well as tissue Mϕ and epithelial cells in thymus; carbohydrate recognition by the latter has not been demonstrated (101). The MR has eight C-type lectin domains, homologous to the mannose-binding protein (MBP), a circulating hepatocyte-derived, acute-phase reactant. MBP, also known as mannose-binding lectin (MBL), contains a single lectin domain per polypeptide, which oligomerizes like other collectins to achieve multivalent interactions and activate complement via associated serine proteases. MR expression on Mϕ is selectively down- and upregulated by IFNγ and IL-4/13 (90,102), respectively. The possible role of the cysteine-rich domain in transport of immunogenic glycopeptides within secondary lymphoid organs has been noted.

The β-glucan receptor, previously reported as Dectin 1, is related to C-type lectins and is responsible for phagocytic recognition of unopsonized zymosan and for Mϕ activation (103). It contains an ITAM-like motif in its cytoplasmic domain that is essential for phagocytosis and induced secretory responses (e.g., TNFα). It cooperates with TLR2 and synergizes with other TLRs in cell activation.

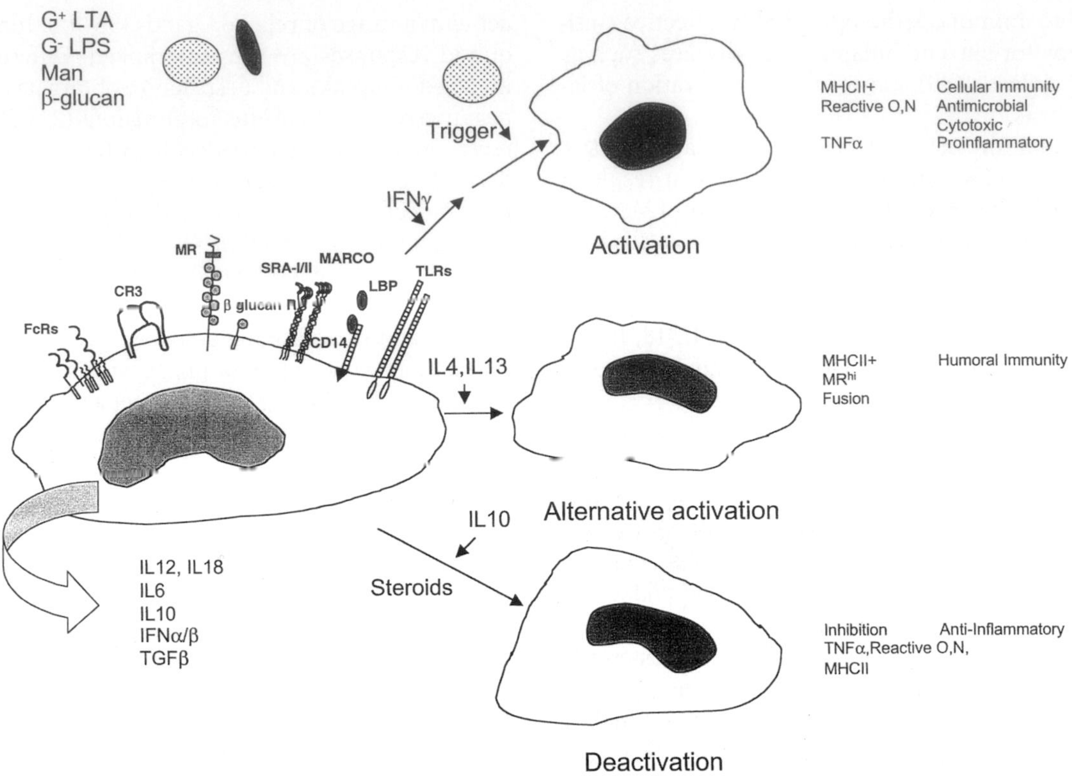

FIGURE 18.5 Macrophage activation. Role of microbial stimuli and cytokines. See text for details.

It is essential for resistance to a range of fungal particles *in vivo*, as shown by studies with knockout mice (104). The SR-A mediates endocytosis of modified proteins (e.g., acetylated lipoproteins) and selected polyanions, such as LPS and lipoteichoic acid (LTA). In addition, it can serve as an adhesion molecule (56) and contributes to phagocytic clearance of apoptotic thymocytes (59) and gram-negative as well as gram-positive bacteria (105). MARCO, a related collagenous receptor, mediates cell adhesion and phagocytosis of bacteria but is independently regulated (106), as discussed later. The report of a phosphatidylserine (PS) receptor implicated in the recognition of novel lipid ligands expressed on the surface of apoptotic cells has not been confirmed (107). CD36 (thrombospondin receptor) (108), vitronectin receptors, CD91, and CD44 have all been implicated in the uptake of senescent PMNs by Mϕ. Other opsonins for apoptotic cell clearance include milk fat globule protein (lactadherin) (109). A role for Mϕ SR-A in immune induction has not been demonstrated, but studies in SR-A ko mice have revealed an important inhibitory role in limiting TNFα production by immunologically activated Mϕ (109a). Wild-type, BCG-primed mice produce granulomata rich in SR-A$^+$ Mϕ; SR-A ko mice restrict growth of this organism and form normal granulomata containing activated, MHC II$^+$ Mϕ; on additional challenge with LPS, the ko mice die approximately 10-fold more readily than wild-type animals. TNFα levels in the circulation rise markedly because of unopposed triggering via CD14, a receptor for the LPS-binding protein, and contribute to septic shock, because blocking anti-TNF mAb protects these mice (110).

TABLE 18.2 Toll-Like Receptors and Their Selected Ligands

Receptor	*Ligands*
TLR2/6 or unknown	Peptidoglycan (gram-positive), LPS (*Leptospira, Porphyromonas gingivalis*)
	Bacterial lipoprotein, lipoarabinomannan, zymosan, GPI anchor (*Trypanosoma cruzi*)
TLR3	Double-stranded RNA
TLR4	LPS (gram-negative), taxol (plant), F protein (respiratory syncytial virus), heat shock protein 60 (host), fibronectin fragments
TLR5	Flagellin
TLR9	CpG DNA

GPI, glycosylphosphatidylinisotol; LPS, lipopolysaccharide; TLR; Toll-like receptor.

The family of TLRs consists of homo- or heterodimeric transmembrane molecules related to the IL-1 receptor, which are involved in innate immunity to microbial

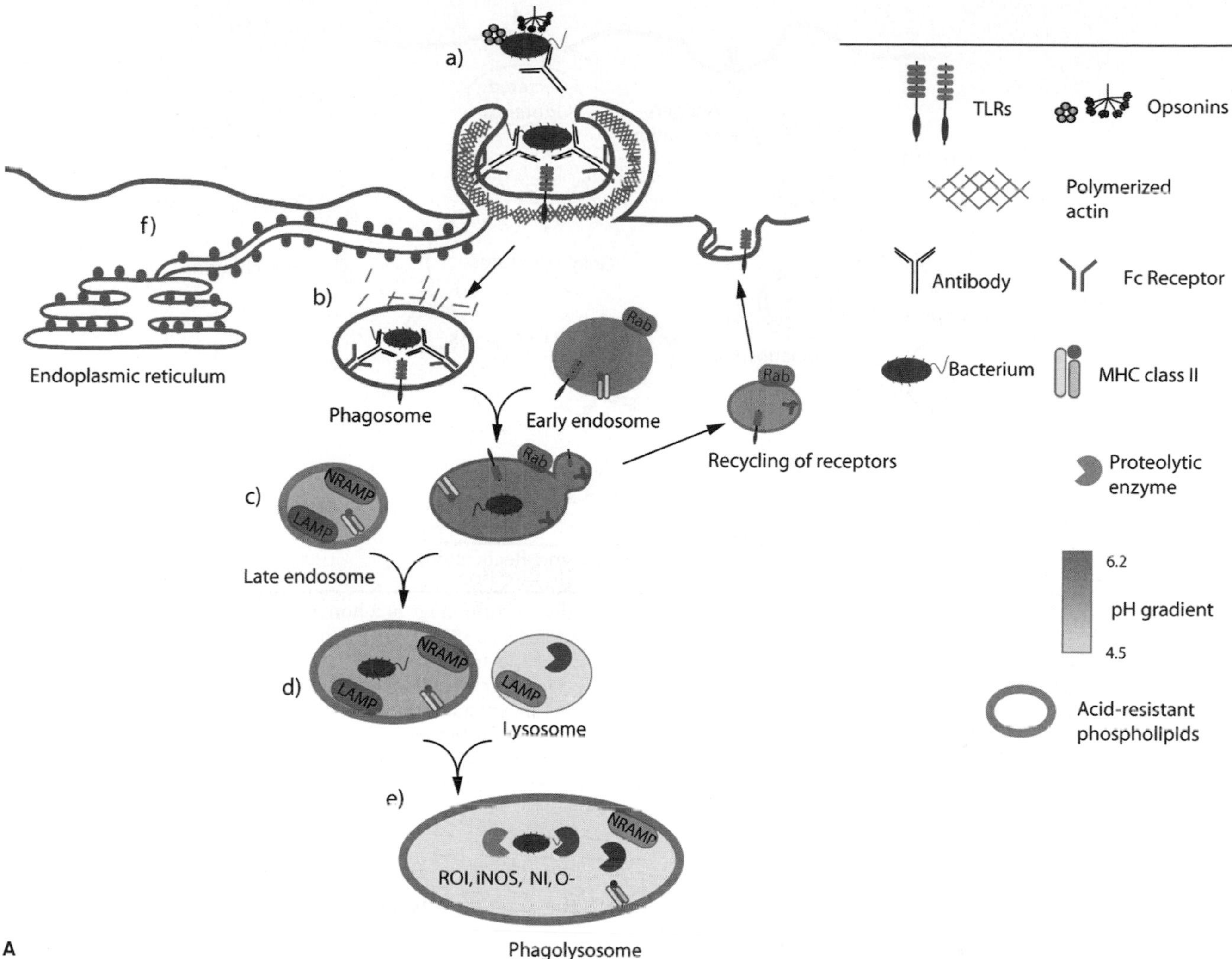

A

FIGURE 18.6 Phagocytic pathway in macrophages. **A:** Heterophagy. Fc receptor mediated phagocytosis. (a) Microbes are coated with a variety of opsonins, including complement, pentraxin 3, and antibodies. A number of receptors are involved in initial recognition of microbes and induction of proinflammatory signaling (e.g., the Toll-like receptors [TLRs], and especially TLRs 2, 4, and 5), but these receptors are not phagocytic. Receptors involved in phagocytosis include the complement receptors, Fc receptors, and others. (b) Fc receptor ligation initiates a signaling cascade that results in actin polymerization and extension of the plasma membrane. Phagocytosis mediated by this method occurs via the "zipper" mechanism (i.e., sequential binding between the Fc receptors and their ligands along the length of the microbe). (c) Fusion with the early endosome results in a slight drop in pH that results in the uncoupling of receptors with their ligands. Receptor recycling is facilitated by the Rab proteins, which also confer the ability to undergo subsequent fusion. The developing phagosome now contains MHC class II and TLRs, including those that signal from within the developing endosome (e.g., TLR9). (d) Fusion with the late endosome results in the addition of the LAMP proteins, the accumulation of acid-resistant phospholipids, and a subsequent drop in pH. (e) On fusion with lysosomes the low pH results in the activation of a number of proteolytic enzymes. These are necessary for both direct antimicrobial activity and the creation of peptides for presentation via MHC class II. The phagolysosome is a highly oxidative environment, exposing the pathogen to destructive reactive oxygen and reactive nitrogen intermediates. (f) Under certain circumstances the phagosome may contain markers specific for the endoplasmic reticulum (ER). The ER may contribute directly to the creation of the phagocytic membrane in some circumstances (e.g., phagocytosis of latex beads), or ER-derived vacuoles may contribute MHC class I and other molecules to the endosomes or the developing phagolysosome. For further information see refs. 97, 121, 122, and 138. *(continued)*

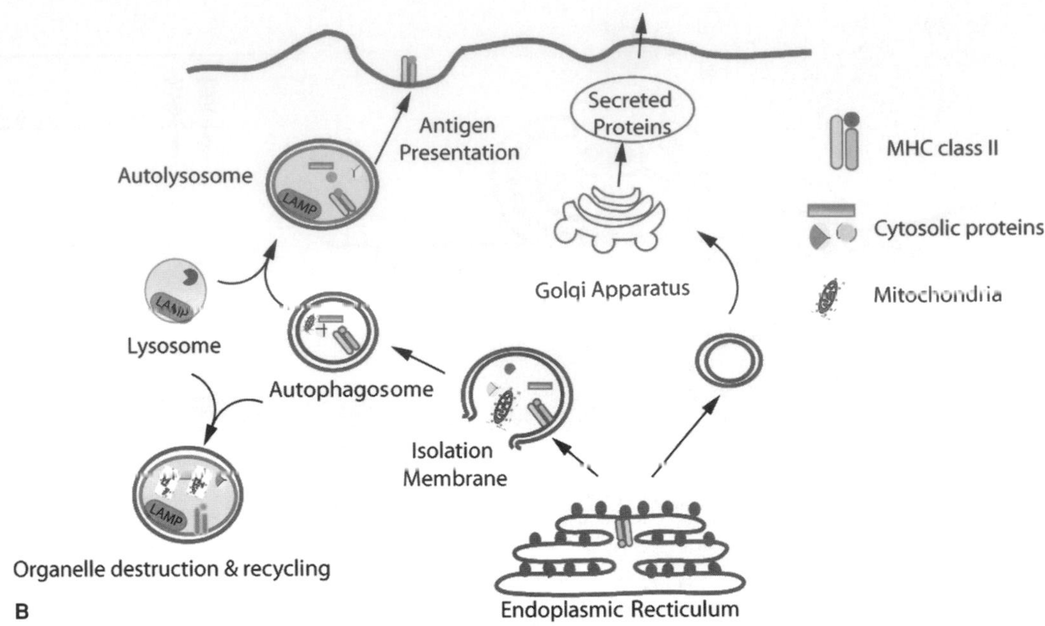

FIGURE 18.6 *(CONTINUED)* **B:** The autophagy pathway. Autophagy is a homeostatic process that can be further enhanced in macrophages in the presence of interferons or by starvation. Cytosolic proteins and organelles are found in ER-derived cytoplasmic vesicles. These vesicles fuse with lysosomes, and the proteins and organelles are degraded and recycled. Conventional wisdom states that endogenous and cytoplasmic proteins are presented by MHC class I molecules, whereas exogenous peptides are presented by MHC class II molecules; however, it has become clear that peptide presentation is altered considerably on induction of autophagy. The presentation of peptides from intracellular and lysosomal source proteins is increased on MHC-II. For further information see refs. 139–141.

constituents and activation of Mϕ responses (Table 18.2) (19,111–113). Downstream signaling depends on association with other soluble and membrane molecules, as well as with intracellular proteins. MyD88, for example, has been implicated in many but not all TLR-induced signaling resulting in transcription factor regulation, cell activation, or apoptosis.

Naturally occurring microbial ligands for these nonopsonic receptors are still poorly defined; individual receptors mediate microbial binding and uptake of microorganisms, although each contributes only part of total binding (Figure 18.6A) (105). Particle uptake involves the cytoskeleton, bulk membrane flow, and remodeling, as well as multiple plasma membrane receptors (97). Phagosome formation and maturation resemble endocytic uptake, initiating Mϕ vesicle trafficking and recirculation, fusion with lysosomes, acidification, ion fluxes, and digestion. Table 18.3 lists immunologic and other markers used to identify intracellular compartments (114). GTP-binding proteins and complex signaling cascades play an important role in these dynamic events. A key issue that needs to be resolved is how cell and receptor functions are modulated so that microbial phagocytosis or invasion induces inflammatory responses, unlike the uptake of apoptotic cells (115). The MHC II biosynthesis and subcellular localization and proteolytic processing of peptide antigens in

TABLE 18.3 Membrane or Content Markets Used to Identify Phagosomes as Resembling a Given Endocytic Compartment or the Endoplasmic Reticulum

Compartment	*Markers*
Early endosome	Membrane markers: TfR, Rab5, annexins, I, II, and III Proteases: immature cathepsin D
Late endosome	Membrane markers: M6PR, Rab7, LAMP1, LAMP2, CD63, CD68 Hydrolases: acid phosphatase, aryl sulfatase, trimetaphosphatase Proteases: cathepsin B, D, H, dipeptidyl peptidase I and II Phospholipid: LBPA
Lysosome	Membrane markers: LAMP1, LAMP2, CD63 Hydrolases: acid phosphatase, aryl sulfatase, trimetaphosphatase Proteases: cathepsin B, D, H, dipeptidyl peptidase I and II
ER	Membrane markers: calnexin, calreticulin Enzyme: glucose-6-phosphatase

LAMP, lysosome-associated membrane protein; LBPA, lysobisphosphatidic acid; M6PR, mannose-6-phosphate receptor; TfR, transferrin receptor.
From de Chastellier C. Electron microscopy. In: Cossart P, Boquet P, Normark, et al., eds. *Cellular microbiology*, 2nd ed. Washington, DC: ASM Press, 2005:451, with permission.

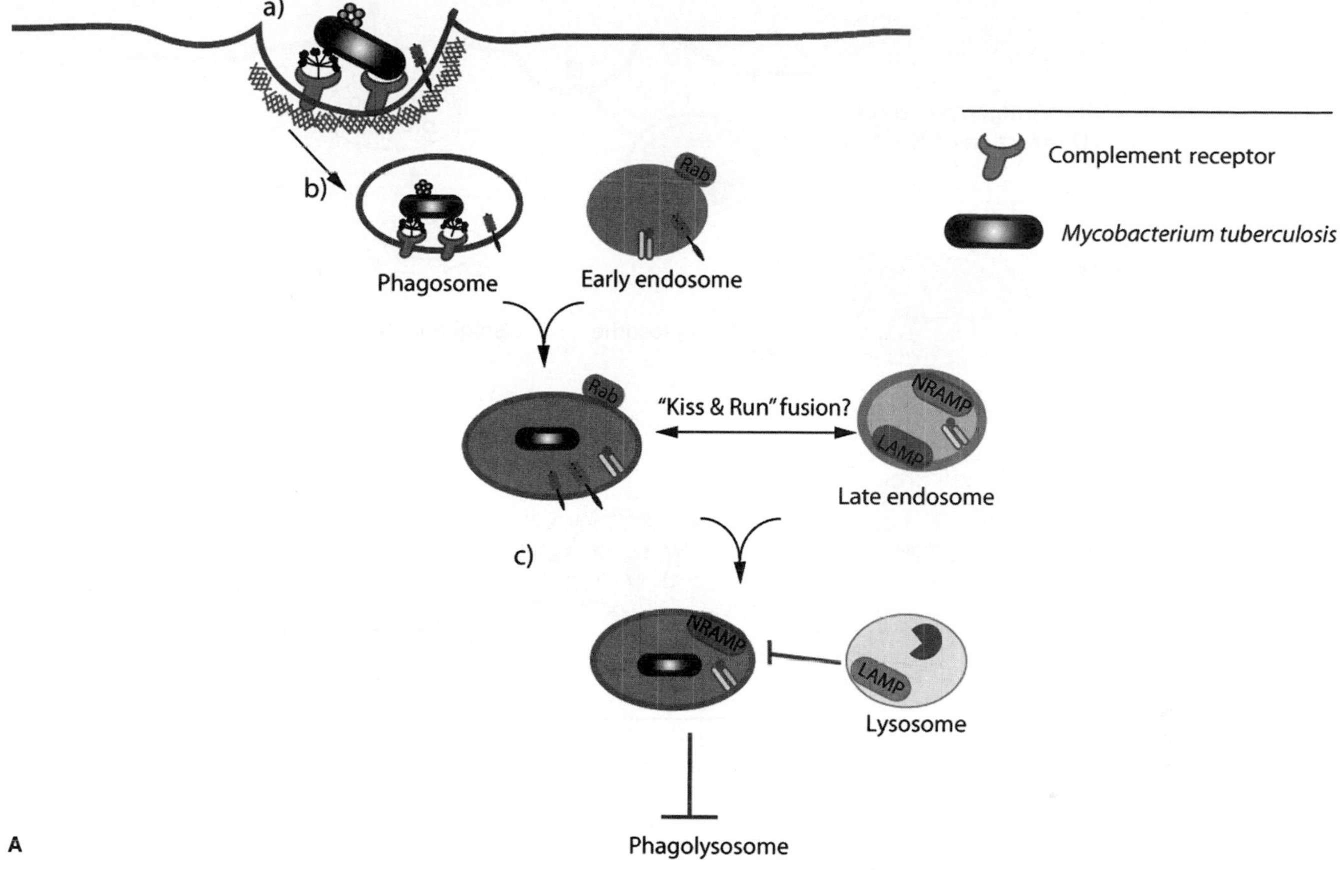

FIGURE 18.7 Interactions of selected intracellular pathogens with the phagocytic pathway. **A:** *Mycobacterium tuberculosis* evades destruction by subverting normal phagolysosome maturation. (a) Phagocytosis of *M. tuberculosis* occurs via the complement pathway (although it may not require direct binding of complement to the bacterium) and is characterized by (b) "sinking" phagocytosis (i.e., very little filopodia formation or actin polymerization. (c) The *M. tuberculosis*–containing vacuoles contain markers of the early and late endosomes such as Rab5 and Nramp1 but are devoid of most lysosomal markers, including the LAMP proteins, and do not undergo normal acidification. It has been proposed that the colocalization of some but not the normal allotment of endosomal markers can be explained by the concept of "Kiss & Run" fusion. This implies that the early and late endosomes may have transient contact with the *M. tuberculosis*–containing vacuoles, and there may be a selective transfer of markers rather than a complete fusion. The high pH of the *M. tuberculosis*–containing vacuole (pH 6.2) does not allow optimum loading of major histocompatibility complex class II molecules, and thus they remain loaded with nonmycobacterial peptides. Elevated pH also inhibits production of inducible nitric oxide synthase, which is required for killing. In the presence of interferon-γ (IFNγ), normal acidification may be restored, resulting in destruction of the pathogen (142). *(continued)*

vacuolar and cytosolic compartments of APC are discussed elsewhere in this volume. Cytokines, especially IL-4/13, IL-10, and IFNγ, influence endocytosis via MR-dependent and -independent pathways and selectively alter vesicle dynamics.

Pathogens vary in using Mϕ plasma membrane molecules for entry and modify the composition of the resultant phagosome membrane (Figure 18.7) (116). Mycobacteria, for example, employ a range of mechanisms to evade killing by Mϕ, including delayed maturation of phagosomes and inhibition of fusion with lysosomes and acidification (Figure 18.7A). *Listeria monocytogenes* escapes into the cytosol by disruption of the phagosome membrane, whereas *Leishmania* multiplies in phagolysosomes. Humoral (antibody, complement) and cellular (γ-interferon) mechanisms overcome parasitization of Mϕ by diversion to lysosomes or induce killing via O/N-dependent and other mechanisms.

Entry of microbial constituents such as muramyldipeptide from vacuolar compartments to the cytosol can result in sensing by NOD-like receptors (NLRs), inflammasome assembly, activation of caspase-1, and processing and release of IL-1β (117). Nucleic acid recognition results in cytoplasmic and mitochondrial-associated protein signaling

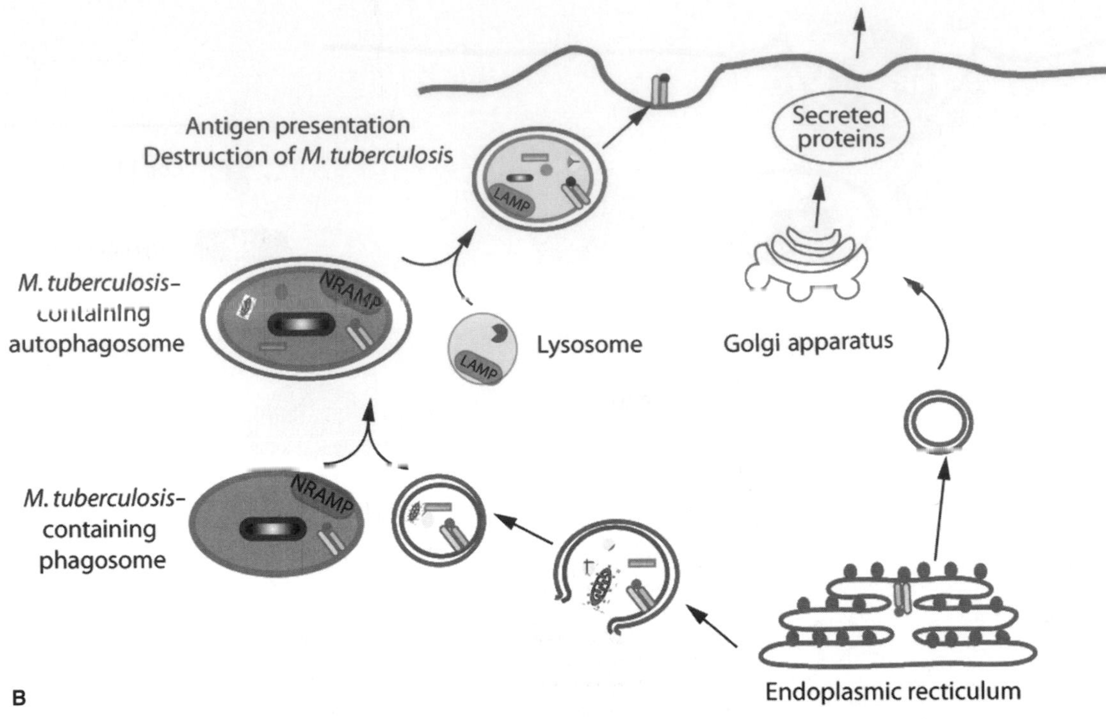

FIGURE 18.7 (*CONTINUED*) **B:** *Mycobacterium tuberculosis*–containing phagosomes are targeted to the autophagy pathway on treatment with IFNγ. IFNγ treatment can both restore the normal process of acidification and alter the expression of a number of endoplasmic reticulum proteins, the result of which is the targeting of *M. tuberculosis*–containing phagosomes to the autophagosomes. The fusion between the *M. tuberculosis*–containing phagosomes and lysosomes results in an autolysosome with low pH that destroys *M. tuberculosis* and results in *M. tuberculosis* peptides being presented via MHC class II (143).

responsible for type 1 interferon gene expression (118). It has recently become clear that induction of autophagy and apoptosis by intracellular pathogens, including *Mycobacterium tuberculosis*, provides important host-protective responses (119,120) (Figures 18.6B, 18.7A, B).

Although the "canonical" entry pathway described here and illustrated in Figure 18.6A is used and modified by many pathogens, recent evidence has shown that organisms such as *Legionella pneumophila* (Figure 18.7C, D) and *Brucella abortus* induce vacuoles with novel membrane components or colonize compartments derived from the Golgi apparatus and the endoplasmic reticulum (121). The relative contributions of plasma membrane and endoplasmic reticulum (Figure 18.6A) to vacuole formation can thus vary considerably, depending on the nature of the phagocytic cargo or invading pathogen (122–124). Opsonins such as antibody are able to divert the cargo to lysosomes. Interferon-γ can induce GTP-binding proteins that associate with vacuoles inhabited by a range of intracellular pathogens (e.g., *Toxoplasma gondii*), thus marking them for destruction within the macrophage (125).

Clearance of proteinase–inhibitor complexes (e.g., by CD91) and of haptoglobin–hemoglobin complexes by the Mϕ-receptor CD163 are essential homeostatic functions of tissue Mϕ, limiting potentially injurious extracellular molecules (126).

Major unsolved questions remain concerning phagocytosis, intracellular infection, and immune responses. How do particulate antigens and microbial agents induce T cell responses, and what are the relative contributions to this process of Mϕ and DCs, abundant and sparser professional phagocytes, respectively; what is the role of the receptors mediating entry in subsequent adaptive immunity? Does TLR engagement within vacuoles determine the kinetics of phagosome maturation as well as induce local intracellular responses? What determines the balance between total antigen degradation and loading of MHC molecules; what interactions take place between intracellular pathogens and host Mϕ, especially in regard to nutritional requirements of the organism; what is the role of pathogen-derived secretory products in the vacuolar milieu, in recruitment of organelles such as endoplasmic reticulum and mitochondria, and in effects on host cell biosynthesis; what are the intracellular killing mechanisms, and how can organisms survive, or become latent, within Mϕ? Finally what receptor-mediated signals induce the secretion of Mϕ molecules such as IL-12 and IL-23 that direct the resultant specific immune response?

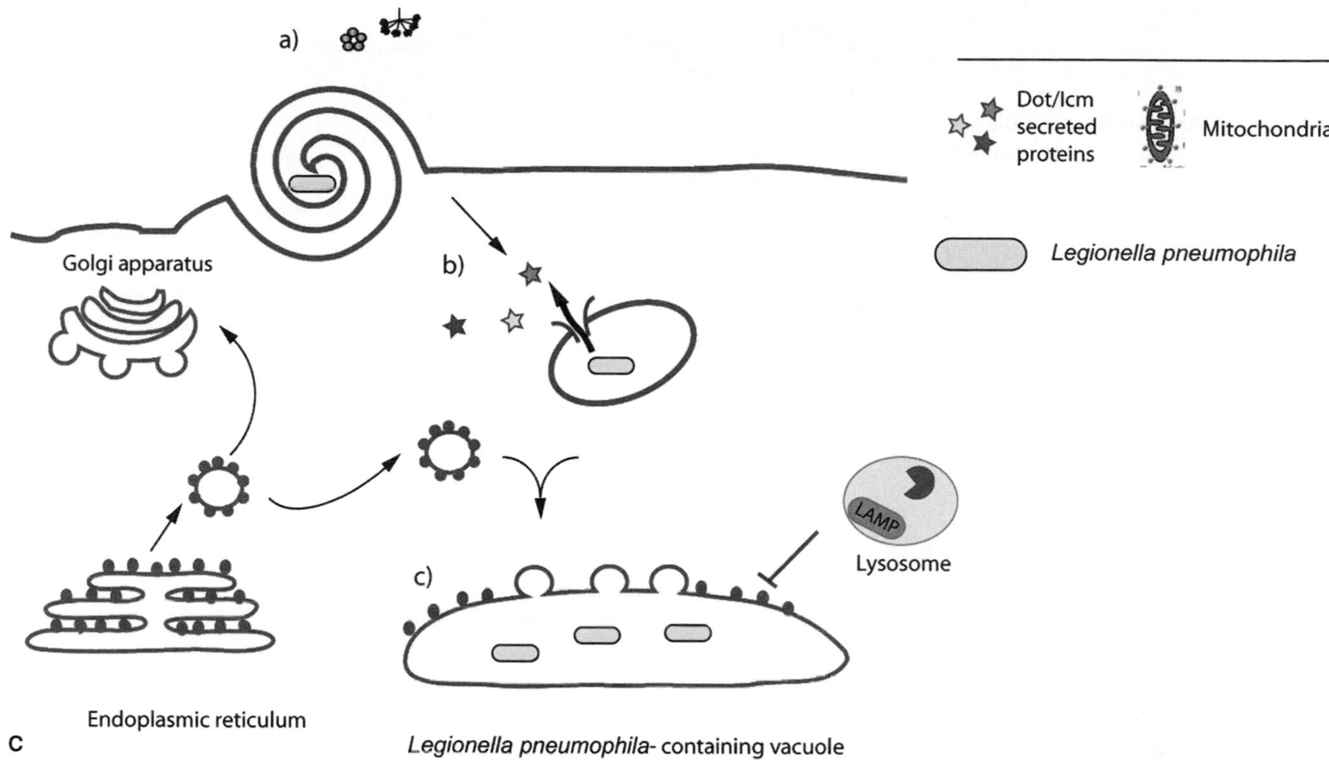

FIGURE 18.7 (CONTINUED) **C:** *Legionella pneumophila* survives intracellularly by subverting phagosome maturation at an early stage. (a) The recognition and uptake of *L. pneumophila* are not well characterized, but phagocysis occurs via a "spiral" mechanism. (b) Once inside the cell, *L. pneumophila* uses a specialized secretion system (i.e., Dot/Icm secretion system) to secrete proteins directly into the cytosol. These proteins alter the morphology of the vacuole in a number of ways, for example, by actively recruiting vesicles in transit from the ER to the Golgi apparatus and inhibiting the fusion of lysosomes. (c) The *L. pneumophila*–containing vacuole thus has many similarities to the Golgi apparatus and ER and is rich in peptides, the primary carbon source for *L. pneumophila*. (*continued*)

Gene Expression and Secretion

Knowledge of Mϕ gene expression and protein synthesis is growing rapidly from the application of gene array and proteomic technologies (e.g., 127,128). After surface and endocytic stimulation the mature Mϕ is able to secrete a very large range of high– and low–molecular weight products. These include enzymes involved in antimicrobial resistance (lysozyme), neutral proteinases and arachidonate metabolites that contribute to inflammation and tissue repair, cytokines such as IL-1 and TNFα that modulate the activities of other leukocytes and endothelium, and reactive oxygen and nitrogen intermediates implicated in host defense (129). Proinflammatory cytokines account for part of the effects of immune adjuvants in promoting, broadening, and sustaining humoral responses. The ability to release these products depends on the prior history of the Mϕ—whether resident, recruited, or activated (primed), its encounters with microbial wall products, including LPS acting via TLR, or with apoptotic cells, and exposure to cytokines and other immunomodulatory molecules in its immediate environment. Ligation of specific receptors induces various signaling pathways and is able to alter gene expression in the Mϕ selectively. Transcription factors such as the NF-κB, Pu-1, and interferon regulatory factor families contribute to Mϕ-restricted or activation-dependent changes in gene expression. Product expression depends further on translational regulation, posttranslational modification such as proteolytic processing, intracellularly or at the cell surface, and coexpression of inhibitors such as IL-10. mRNA turnover varies greatly for different products due to the presence or absence of specific 3′ instability sequences. Many Mϕ products are labile and act close to the cell surface; overproduction results in tissue catabolism and systemic effects associated with widespread infection or chronic inflammation, often as a result of an immunologically driven disease process.

Whereas most bioactivities have been defined *in vitro*, there is evidence that expression of Mϕ secretory activities may be quite different *in situ*; lysozyme production is characteristic of all Mϕ in culture but is downregulated on most resident cells *in vivo*, and its expression by

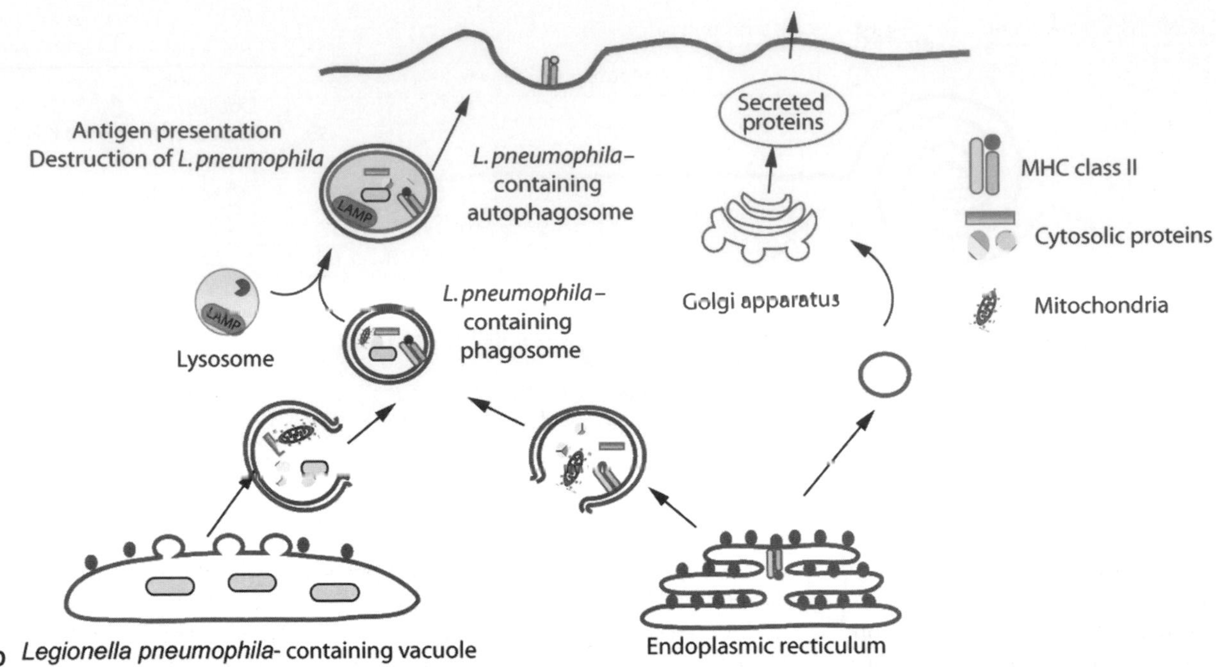

FIGURE 18.7 *(CONTINUED)* **D:** Macrophages enhance autophagy in response to *Legionella pneumophila*. A consequence of residing in a vacuole that so closely resembles the ER is that it is subject to autophagy. *L. pneumophila*–containing phagosomes fuse with lysosomes, resulting in destruction of the pathogen and antigen presentation. Factors secreted from *L. pneumophila* cause macrophages to increase the number of autophagosomes, although autophagosomes containing *L. pneumophila* mature more slowly, and thus it is believed that the bacteria encode factors to delay normal progression. For more information see ref. 144.

granuloma Mϕ, for example, depends on induction by immune or phagocytic stimuli (28). 5′ promoter sequences of human lysozyme (130) and CD68 (131) transgenes have been used to target tissue- and Mϕ activation-specific expression of reporter molecules *in vivo*. The promoters of these and other Mϕ-restricted molecules may, in due course, make it possible to direct Mϕ biosynthetic activities precisely, to boost or inhibit immune responses.

Modulation of Macrophage Activation *in vitro*

Our understanding of Mϕ activation derives from studies of induction of MHC II and costimulatory antigens of effector functions such as proteinase, TNFα, reactive oxygen intermediate and reactive nitrogen intermediate release, expression of membrane receptors such as MRs, and resistance to infectious agents, for example, *Mycobacteria*, *Listeria*, *Candida*, and HIV. Generalizations can be made, but it must be remembered that organisms vary considerably in their ability to evade or survive Mϕ restriction mechanisms, and they interact with Mϕ in individual ways. Various inhibitory cell surface molecules (e.g., CD200 and SIRPα) (132) are known to regulate Mϕ activation through interactions with other activating plasma membrane receptors. Receptors including FcRγ (23) and C-type lectins (133) use paired ITAM and ITIM intracellular signaling motifs.

Figure 18.4 and Table 18.4 illustrate various pathways and markers of Mϕ activation that result from microbial, cellular, and cytokine interactions. Knowledge is based mainly on *in vitro* experiments and *in vivo* challenge of selected animal models. Innate activation depends on direct stimulation by microbial products, independent of cytokines, although often enhanced by concomitant stimulation (e.g., by IFNγ). Newly discovered markers of innate activation of mouse peritoneal macrophages include upregulation of MARCO, a type A SR, via a TLR pathway, and of CD200, a more widely expressed IgSF membrane glycoprotein. Induction of MARCO, a phagocytic receptor for a range of bacteria, represents an adaptive innate immune response to microbial contact (106). Analysis of the actions of individual cytokines (IFNγ, IL-10, IL-4/13) on defined Mϕ targets (murine peritoneal Mϕ and human monocyte–derived Mϕ) reveals three characteristic and distinctive *in vitro* phenotypes across a spectrum of activation. IFNγ and its production and amplification via IL-12, IL-23, or IL-18 play a central role in MHC II induction, enhanced antimicrobial resistance, and proinflammatory cytokine production, characteristic of Th1-type responses; conversely, IL-10 suppresses markers of activation while inducing selective expression of other Mϕ genes. A

TABLE 18.4 Modulation of Macrophage Phenotype

Category	*Stimulus*	*Selected Marker Changes*	*Function*
Innate activation	Microbial products (e.g., LPS, other TLR ligands)	Costimulatory molecule expression, MARCO upregulation	Phagocytosis Adaptive immunity,
Classic activation	Interferon γ	MHC II upregulation, proinflammatory cytokine secretion, inducible NO synthase	Cell-mediated immunity, e.g., intracellular pathogens
Alternative activation	IL-4/IL-13	Upregulation of MHC II, arginase, mannose receptor, Ym1, FIZZ1 (resistin-like), production of selected chemokines, macrophage fusion	Parasitic and allergic immunity, repair
Innate and acquired deactivation	Apoptotic cells, IL-10, glucocorticoids, TGFβ, PGE2	Various surface and secretory markers, e.g., anti-TNFα actions	Antiinflammatory and altered immunity

IL, interleukin; LPS, lipopolysaccharide; MHC, major histocompatibility complex; NO, nitric oxide; PGE2, prostaglandin E2; TGFβ, transforming growth factor-β; TLR, Toll-like receptor; TNFα, tumor necrosis factor-α.

comparable link between Mϕ/APC and the induction of Th2-type responses has proved elusive to identify. IL-4/IL-13 have closely overlapping functions and induce an alternative activation phenotype in Mϕ consistent with increased APC function and humoral responses in allergy and parasitic infection as well as giant cell formation (Table 18.3) (134). It is important to distinguish modulation of Mϕ immunologic properties by IL-4/IL-13 from marked deactivation and inhibition of proinflammatory and cytotoxic functions by IL-10 and glucocorticosteroid (92). Immune complexes are also able to induce an analogous alternative activation pathway, which overlaps with but differs from IL-4/IL-13– and IL-10–induced phenotypes. By extension, M-CSF, glucocorticosteroids, TGF-β, and type I IFN all modulate Mϕ gene expression with individual signatures.

The interplay of cytokines derived from Mϕ themselves, from activated T and B lymphocytes, and from other cells (NK, endothelial cells) results in reciprocal positive or negative interactions and time-dependent changes in activating and inhibitory signals. Some predictions from *in vitro* studies can be extended to the intact host. For example, IFNγ, IL-12, and IL-23 deficiency results in inability to restrict opportunistic organisms in murine models and in humans, and i-NOS is important for resistance to a range of infectious agents. IL-10 deficiency, on the other hand, results in overactive Th1-dependent inflammation, for example, in gut (135). IL-4 deficiency by itself has little effect on Mϕ phenotype *in vivo* because IL-13 mimics many of its actions. These cytokines share a common receptor subunit, and its targeted genetic ablation makes it possible to study Mϕ that lack the ability to respond to both IL-4 and IL-13 (32).

The foregoing analysis is oversimplified. Combinations of cytokines *in vitro* have different effects on Mϕ than the sum of the parts. For example, the combination of IL-4 and GM-CSF induces differentiation of human monocytes into immature DCs, whereas each alone induces cells with distinctive Mϕ properties. Furthermore, a particular "Th2-type" cytokine such as IL-10 can display radically different effects on antimicrobial (i-NOS dependent) killing, which is markedly suppressed, and anti-HIV activities of Mϕ, which are enhanced (136). Whereas IFNγ and IL-4 may have opposing actions on MR expression and phagocytosis of yeasts, in combination they synergize to enhance uptake markedly. Other combinations of cytokines, such as IFN$\alpha\beta$ and IFNγ, can antagonize each other, presumably by competition for signaling pathways. Although extrapolations with predictive value can be made in some situations, a great deal remains to be learned about Mϕ behavior in complex immune environments *in vivo*.

CONCLUSIONS AND SOME REMAINING ISSUES

Mϕ influence and respond to all other cells involved in immunity, during both the afferent and efferent limbs. Many of the molecules that mediate particular functions are now defined, but their role within the Mϕ and in intercellular interactions is often poorly understood. Mϕ developed during the evolution of multicellular organisms before immunologically specific, clonotypic responses of B and T lymphocytes emerged. Mϕ themselves diversified in parallel with T helper lymphocytes, generating DCs as specialized APCs for naïve T lymphocytes and yielding a range of effector cell phenotypes in response to diverse activated T cells, both CD4$^+$ and CD8$^+$. Mϕ and their derivatives cluster with differentiating hemopoietic cells in fetal liver and bone marrow, with developing thymocytes, with naïve CD4$^+$ T lymphocytes and antigen during immune induction, and with activated T cells and microbial pathogens in granuloma formation (Figure 18.2). In addition, they associate with antigen-stimulated B lymphocytes during cell expansion, diversification, and apoptosis. A major challenge will be to define the role of specific and accessory surface molecules by which Mϕ discriminate between live and dying cells and to uncover the intrinsic and extrinsic factors that control Mϕ activities within these diverse immune cell interactions.

Our understanding of the multiple roles of Mϕ and DCs in immunoregulation is also evolving as we better appreciate their specializations and adaptations. Central issues in the immunobiology of Mϕ remain obscure and interesting topics for further investigation. These include the following.

Mϕ display broad functions in homeostasis, beyond host defense and immunity, which may be special instances of a more general role in preserving host integrity, comparable to that of the central nervous and endocrine systems. Their dispersion, plasticity, and responsiveness raise obvious questions for the biologist. In particular, what are their roles in development and in trophic interactions within different organs?

The Mϕ lies at the heart of the classic immunologic question of recognition of altered or non-self, especially of particulates. What are the actual ligands recognized by the diverse range of plasma membrane receptors capable of direct discrimination, and what determines whether uptake of a target is immunologically silent or productive? How can this information be harnessed for vaccine development?

The delineation of further subsets of CD4^{+} T lymphocytes (TH17, regulatory T cells) suggests that it will be useful to define the effects on the Mϕ phenotype of contact- and cytokine-dependent interactions with these cells. It is likely that further distinctive type 2 activation pathways of Mϕ will be discovered by microarray and protein analysis.

Once activated, Mϕ change their ability to recognize and destroy targets, directly or in concert with antibody, complement, and other less-defined opsonins. Can Mϕ directly kill virus-infected and other immunologically activated cells? If so, do they use MHC matching, even in a limited way, and do they contribute to tolerance and, by implication, autoimmunity by failure to perform such a suppressive function?

A special case in which Mϕ are present in large numbers at a site of "failure" to respond immunologically is the fetoplacental unit. CSF-1 is produced locally at high levels; does this deactivate Mϕ or make them switch to perform a trophic role? Do tumors that are rich in Mϕ adopt a similar strategy? Catabolism of tryptophan by Mϕ enzymes has been put forward as another mechanism for preventing local destruction of an allogeneic fetus (137).

Although Mϕ express a large number of genes involved in household functions and share expression of others with a limited range of cell types, they also express highly restricted molecules responsible for unique functions. Can these be harnessed for Mϕ-specific gene targeting at selected microanatomic sites to deliver functionally precise signals at predetermined times? Techniques are becoming available for at least part of this fantasy, and they should provide new insights into the multiple roles of the Mϕ an immunity.

ACKNOWLEDGMENTS

I thank the members of my laboratory for discussions, Dr. Luisa Martinez-Pomares and Dr. Dawn Bowdish for illustrations, and Christine Holt for preparing the manuscript. Research in the author's laboratory is supported by grants from the Medical Research Council, UK, the Wellcome Trust, the Arthritis and Rheumatism Research Council, and the British Heart Foundation.

REFERENCES

1. Metchnikoff E. *Immunity in infective disease*. Cambridge: Cambridge University Press, 1905.
2. Bolis MCKL, ed. *Phagocytosis—past and future*. New York: Academic Press, 1982.
3. Chernyak AITL. *Metchnikoff and the origins of immunology: from metaphor to theory*. Oxford: Oxford University Press, 1991.
4. van Furth ER. *Mononuclear phagocytes: biology of monocytes and macrophages*. Dordrecht, Netherlands: Kluwer, 1992.
5. Gordon S, Lawson L, Rabinowitz S, et al. *Antigen markers of macrophage differentiation in murine tissues*. Berlin: Springer-Verlag, 1992.
6. Kraal G. Cells in the marginal zone of the spleen. *Int Rev Cytol.* 1992;132:31.
7. Kraal G, Mebius R. New insights into the cell biology of the marginal zone of the spleen. *Int Rev Cytol.* 2006;250:175.
8. Steinman RM, Moberg CL. Zanvil Alexander Cohn 1926–1993. *J Exp Med.* 1994;179(1):1.
9. Gordon S. The macrophage. *Bioessays.* 1995;17(11):977.
10. Wiktor-Jedrzejczak W, Gordon S. Cytokine regulation of the macrophage (M phi) system studied using the colony stimulating factor-1–deficient op/op mouse. *Physiol Rev.* 1996;76(4):927.
11. Gordon S, ed. *The myeloid system*, 5th ed. Oxford: Blackwell Scientific, 1997.
12. Dalton DK, Pitts-Meek S, Keshav S, et al. Multiple defects of immune cell function in mice with disrupted interferon-gamma genes. *Science*. 1993;259(5102):1739.
13. MacMicking J, Xie QW, Nathan C. Nitric oxide and macrophage function. *Annu Rev Immunol.* 1997;15:323.
14. Gordon AH, D'Arcy-Hart P, Young MR. Ammonia inhibits phagosome-lysosome fusion in macrophages. *Nature.* 1980;296:79.
15. Gruenheid S, Pinner E, Desjardins M, et al. Natural resistance to infection with intracellular pathogens: the Nramp1 protein is recruited to the membrane of the phagosome. *J Exp Med.* 1997;185(4):717.
16. Poltorak A, He X, Smirnova I, et al. Defective LPS signaling in C3H/HeJ and C57BL/10ScCr mice: mutations in Tlr4 gene. *Science.* 1998;282(5396):2085.
17. Lemaitre B, Nicolas E, Michaut L, et al. The dorsoventral regulatory gene cassette spatzle/Toll/cactus controls the potent antifungal response in *Drosophila* adults. *Cell.* 1996;86(6):973.
18. Medzhitov R, Preston-Hurlburt P, Janeway CA Jr. A human homologue of the *Drosophila* Toll protein signals activation of adaptive immunity. *Nature.* 1997;388(6640):394.
19. Akira S, Takeda K. Toll-like receptor signalling. *Nat Rev Immunol.* 2004;4(7):499.
20. Balkwill F, Mantovani A. Inflammation and cancer: back to Virchow? *Lancet.* 2001;357(9255):539.
21. Zink W, Ryan L, Gendelman H. Macrophage-virus interactions. In Burke, B and Lewis, C. (Eds). *The Macrophage*. 2nd Edition. OUP, Oxford 2002, pp. 138–209.

22. Geijtenbeek TB, Engering A, Van Kooyk Y. DC-SIGN, a C-type lectin on dendritic cells that unveils many aspects of dendritic cell biology. *J Leukoc Biol.* 2002;71(6):921.
23. Nimmerjahn F, Ravetch JV. Fcgamma receptors: old friends and new family members. *Immunity*. 2006;24(1):19.
24. Barrington R, Zhang M, Fischer M, et al. The role of complement in inflammation and adaptive immunity. *Immunol Rev.* 2001;180:5.
25. Brown MS, Goldstein JL. Lipoprotein metabolism in the macrophage: implications for cholesterol deposition in atherosclerosis. *Annu Rev Biochem.* 1983;52:223.
26. Taylor PR, Gordon S, Martinez-Pomares L. The mannose receptor: linking homeostasis and immunity through sugar recognition. *Trends Immunol.* 2005;26(2):104.
27. Brown GD, Gordon S. Immune recognition. A new receptor for beta-glucans. *Nature.* 2001;413(6851):36.
28. Keshav S, Chung P, Milon G, et al. Lysozyme is an inducible marker of macrophage activation in murine tissues as demonstrated by in situ hybridization. *J Exp Med.* 1991;174(5):1049.
29. Kindler V, Sappino AP, Grau GE, et al. The inducing role of tumor necrosis factor in the development of bactericidal granulomas during BCG infection. *Cell.* 1989;56(5):731.
30. Anderson KL, Smith KA, Conners K, et al. Myeloid development is selectively disrupted in PU.1 null mice. *Blood.* 1998;91(10):3702.
31. Wells CA, Ravasi T, Sultana R, et al. Continued discovery of transcriptional units expressed in cells of the mouse mononuclear phagocyte lineage. *Genome Res.* 2003;13(6B):1360.
32. Herbert DR, Holscher C, Mohrs M, et al. Alternative macrophage activation is essential for survival during schistosomiasis and downmodulates T helper 1 responses and immunopathology. *Immunity.* 2004;20(5):623.
33. Fritz JH, Ferrero RL, Philpott DJ, et al. Nod-like proteins in immunity, inflammation and disease. *Nat Immunol.* 2006;7(12):1250.
34. Casanova JL, Abel L. The human model: a genetic dissection of immunity to infection in natural conditions. *Nat Rev Immunol.* 2004;4(1):55.
35. Beutler B, Hoebe K, Georgel P, et al. Genetic analysis of innate immunity: identification and function of the TIR adapter proteins. *Adv Exp Med Biol.* 2005;560:29.
36. Gordon S, Hughes, DA. *Macrophages and their origins: heterogeneity in relation to tissue microenvironment*. New York: Marcel Dekker, 1997.
37. Gordon S, Taylor PR. Monocyte and macrophage heterogeneity. *Nat Rev Immunol.* 2005;5(12):953.
38. Morris L, Graham CF, Gordon S. Macrophages in haemopoietic and other tissues of the developing mouse detected by the monoclonal antibody F4/80. *Development.* 1991;112(2):517.
39. Reid DM, Perry VH, Andersson PB, et al. Mitosis and apoptosis of microglia *in vivo* induced by an anti-CR3 antibody which crosses the blood–brain barrier. *Neuroscience.* 1993;56(3):529.
40. Stacey M, Lin HH, Gordon S, et al. LNB-TM7, a group of seven-transmembrane proteins related to family-B G-protein-coupled receptors. *Trends Biochem Sci.* 2000;25(6):284.
41. Holness CL, da Silva RP, Fawcett J, et al. Macrosialin, a mouse macrophage-restricted glycoprotein, is a member of the lamp/lgp family. *J Biol Chem.* 1993;268(13):9661.
42. Shortman K, Liu YJ. Mouse and human dendritic cell subtypes. *Nat Rev Immunol.* 2002;2(3):151.
43. Tacke F, Randolph GJ. Migratory fate and differentiation of blood monocyte subsets. *Immunobiology.* 2006;211(6–8):609.
44. Quinn JM, Gillespie MT. Modulation of osteoclast formation. *Biochem Biophys Res Commun*. 2005;328(3):739.
45. Ziegler-Heitbrock L. The CD14+ CD16+ blood monocytes: their role in infection and inflammation. *J Leukoc Biol.* 2007;81:584.
46. Geissmann F, Jung S, Littman DR. Blood monocytes consist of two principal subsets with distinct migratory properties. *Immunity.* 2003;19(1):71.
47. Quan TE, Cowper SE, Bucala R. The role of circulating fibrocytes in fibrosis. *Curr Rheumatol Rep.* 2006;8(2):145.
48. Inaba K, Steinman RM, Pack MW, et al. Identification of proliferating dendritic cell precursors in mouse blood. *J Exp Med.* 1992;175(5):1157.
49. Sallusto F, Lanzavecchia A. Efficient presentation of soluble antigen by cultured human dendritic cells is maintained by granulocyte/macrophage colony-stimulating factor plus interleukin 4 and downregulated by tumor necrosis factor alpha. *J Exp Med.* 1994;179(4):1109.
50. Morris L, Crocker PR, Gordon S. Murine fetal liver macrophages bind developing erythroblasts by a divalent cation-dependent hemagglutinin. *J Cell Biol.* 1988;106(3):649.
51. Perry VH, Andersson PB, Gordon S. Macrophages and inflammation in the central nervous system. *Trends Neurosci.* 1993;16(7):268.
52. Taylor PR, Martinez-Pomares L, Stacey M, et al. Macrophage receptors and immune recognition. *Annu Rev Immunol.* 2005;23:901.
53. Crocker PR, Mucklow S, Bouckson V, et al. Sialoadhesin, a macrophage sialic acid binding receptor for haemopoietic cells with 17 immunoglobulin-like domains. *EMBO J.* 1994;13(19):4490.
54. Crocker PR. Siglecs in innate immunity. *Curr Opin Pharmacol.* 2005;5(4):431.
55. Rosen H, Gordon S. Monoclonal antibody to the murine type 3 complement receptor inhibits adhesion of myelomonocytic cells *in vitro* and inflammatory cell recruitment in vivo. *J Exp Med.* 1987;166(6):1685.
56. Fraser I, Hughes D, Gordon S. Divalent cation-independent macrophage adhesion inhibited by monoclonal antibody to murine scavenger receptor. *Nature.* 1993;364(6435):343–346.
57. Crocker PR, Kelm S, Morris L, et al. *Cellular interactions between stromal macrophges and haematopoietic cells*. Dordrecht, Netherlands: Kluwer, 1992.
58. Crocker PR, Freeman S, Gordon S, et al. Sialoadhesin binds preferentially to cells of the granulocytic lineage. *J Clin Invest.* 1995;95(2):635.
59. Platt N, Suzuki H, Kurihara Y, et al. Role for the class A macrophage scavenger receptor in the phagocytosis of apoptotic thymocytes in vitro. *Proc Natl Acad Sci U S A.* 1996;93(22):12456.
60. Platt N, Suzuki H, Kodama T, et al. Apoptotic thymocyte clearance in scavenger receptor class A-deficient mice is apparently normal. *J Immunol.* 2000;164(9):4861.
61. Witmer-Pack MD, Hughes DA, Schuler G, et al. Identification of macrophages and dendritic cells in the osteopetrotic (op/op) mouse. *J Cell Sci.* 1993;104 (Pt 4):1021–9.
62. Mebius RE, Kraal G. Structure and function of the spleen. *Nat Rev Immunol.* 2005;5(8):606.
63. Steiniger B, Barth P, Hellinger A. The perifollicular and marginal zones of the human splenic white pulp: do fibroblasts guide lymphocyte immigration? *Am J Pathol.* 2001;159(2):501.
64. Martinez-Pomares L, Hanitsch LG, Stillion R, et al. Expression of mannose receptor and ligands for its cysteine-rich domain in venous sinuses of human spleen. *Lab Invest.* 2005;85(10):1238.
65. Martinez-Pomares L, Kosco-Vilbois M, Darley E, et al. Fc chimeric protein containing the cysteine-rich domain of the murine mannose receptor binds to macrophages from splenic marginal zone and lymph node subcapsular sinus and to germinal centers. *J Exp Med.* 1996;184(5):1927.
66. Morris L, Crocker PR, Hill M, et al. Developmental regulation of sialoadhesin (sheep erythrocyte receptor), a macrophage-cell interaction molecule expressed in lymphohemopoietic tissues. *Dev Immunol.* 1992;2(1):7.
67. Lin HH, Faunce DE, Stacey M, et al. The macrophage F4/80 receptor is required for the induction of antigen-specific efferent regulatory T cells in peripheral tolerance. *J Exp Med.* 2005;201(10):1615.
68. Hughes DA, Fraser IP, Gordon S. Murine macrophage scavenger receptor: *in vivo* expression and function as receptor for macrophage adhesion in lymphoid and non-lymphoid organs. *Eur J Immunol.* 1995;25(2):466.
69. Elomaa O, Kangas M, Sahlberg C, et al. Cloning of a novel bacteria-binding receptor structurally related to scavenger receptors and expressed in a subset of macrophages. *Cell.* 1995;80(4):603.
70. van der Laan LJ, Dopp EA, Haworth R, et al. Regulation and functional involvement of macrophage scavenger receptor MARCO in clearance of bacteria *in vivo*. *J Immunol.* 1999;162(2):939.
71. Martinez-Pomares L, Crocker PR, Da Silva R, et al. Cell-specific glycoforms of sialoadhesin and CD45 are counter-receptors for the cysteine-rich domain of the mannose receptor. *J Biol Chem.* 1999;274(49):35211.

72. Taylor PR, Zamze S, Stillion RJ, et al. Development of a specific system for targeting protein to metallophilic macrophages. *Proc Natl Acad Sci U S A.* 2004;101(7):1963.
73. McKenzie EJ, Taylor PR, Stillion RJ, et al. Mannose receptor expression and function define a new population of murine dendritic cells. *J Immunol.* 2007;178:4975.
73a. Martinez-Pomares L, Kosco-Vilbois M, Darley E, et al. F_c chimeric protein containing the cysteine-rich domain of the murine mannose receptor binds to macrophages from splenic marginal zone and lymph node subcapsular sinus and to germinal centers. *J Exp Med.* 1996 Nov;184(5):1927–37.
74. Yu P, Wang Y, Chin RK, et al. B cells control the migration of a subset of dendritic cells into B cell follicles via CXC chemokine ligand 13 in a lymphotoxin-dependent fashion. *J Immunol.* 2002;168(10):5117.
75. Linehan SA, Martinez-Pomares L, Stahl PD, et al. Mannose receptor and its putative ligands in normal murine lymphoid and nonlymphoid organs: in situ expression of mannose receptor by selected macrophages, endothelial cells, perivascular microglia, and mesangial cells, but not dendritic cells. *J Exp Med.* 1999;189(12):1961.
76. Berney C, Herren S, Power CA, et al. A member of the dendritic cell family that enters B cell follicles and stimulates primary antibody responses identified by a mannose receptor fusion protein. *J Exp Med.* 1999;190(6):851.
77. Smythies LE, Sellers M, Clements RH, et al. Human intestinal macrophages display profound inflammatory anergy despite avid phagocytic and bacteriocidal activity. *J Clin Invest.* 2005;115(1):66.
78. Helmy KY, Katschke KJ Jr, Gorgani NN, et al. CRIg: a macrophage complement receptor required for phagocytosis of circulating pathogens. *Cell.* 2006;124(5):915.
79. Schenkel AR, Mamdouh Z, Chen X, et al. CD99 plays a major role in the migration of monocytes through endothelial junctions. *Nat Immunol.* 2002;3(2):143.
80. Gordon S. Macrophage heterogeneity and tissue lipids. *J Clin Invest.* 2007;117(1):89.
81. Fogg DK, Sibon C, Miled C, et al. A clonogenic bone marrow progenitor specific for macrophages and dendritic cells. *Science.* 2006;311(5757):83.
82. Varol C, Landsman L, Fogg DK, et al. Monocytes give rise to mucosal, but not splenic, conventional dendritic cells. *J Exp Med.* 2006;204:171.
83. Shiloh MU, MacMicking JD, Nicholson S, et al. Phenotype of mice and macrophages deficient in both phagocyte oxidase and inducible nitric oxide synthase. *Immunity.* 1999;10(1):29.
84. Klesney-Tait J, Turnbull IR, Colonna M. The TREM receptor family and signal integration. *Nat Immunol.* 2006;7(12):1266.
85. Barclay AN, Wright GJ, Brooke G, et al. CD200 and membrane protein interactions in the control of myeloid cells. *Trends Immunol.* 2002;23(6):285.
86. Hoek RM, Ruuls SR, Murphy CA, et al. Down-regulation of the macrophage lineage through interaction with OX2 (CD200). *Science.* 2000;290(5497):1768.
87. Elliott J, Johnston JA. SOCS: role in inflammation, allergy and homeostasis. *Trends Immunol.* 2004;25(8):434.
88. Havell EA. Production of tumor necrosis factor during murine listeriosis. *J Immunol.* 1987;139(12):4225.
89. Feldman M, Nagase H, Saklatvala J, et al., eds. The scientific basis of rheumatology. *Arthritis Res.* 2002;4(Suppl 3):51.
90. Gordon S. Alternative activation of macrophages. *Nat Rev Immunol.* 2003;3(1):23.
91. Bannenberg GL, Chiang N, Ariel A, et al. Molecular circuits of resolution: formation and actions of resolvins and protectins. *J Immunol.* 2005;174(7):4345.
92. Yona S, Gordon S. Glucocorticoids turn the monocyte switch. *Immunol Cell Biol.* 2007;85(2):81.
93. Janeway CA Jr, Medzhitov R. Innate immune recognition. *Annu Rev Immunol.* 2002;20:197.
94. Gordon S. Pattern recognition receptors: doubling up for the innate immune response. *Cell.* 2002;111(7):927.
95. Pluddemann A, Mukhopadhyay S, Gordon S. The interaction of macrophage receptors with bacterial ligands. *Expert Rev Mol Med.* 2006;8(28):1.
96. Crowley MT, Costello PS, Fitzer-Attas CJ, et al. A critical role for Syk in signal transduction and phagocytosis mediated by Fcgamma receptors on macrophages. *J Exp Med.* 1997;186(7):1027.
97. Aderem A, Underhill DM. Mechanisms of phagocytosis in macrophages. *Annu Rev Immunol.* 1999;17:593.
98. Halstead SB, Heinz FX, Barrett AD, et al. Dengue virus: molecular basis of cell entry and pathogenesis, 25-27 June 2003, Vienna, Austria. *Vaccine.* 2005;23(7):849.
99. Taylor PR, Pickering MC, Kosco-Vilbois MH, et al. The follicular dendritic cell restricted epitope, FDC-M2, is complement C4; localization of immune complexes in mouse tissues. *Eur J Immunol.* 2002;32(7):1888.
100. Peiser L, Mukhopadhyay S, Gordon S. Scavenger receptors in innate immunity. *Curr Opin Immunol.* 2002;14(1):123.
101. East L, Isacke CM. The mannose receptor family. *Biochim Biophys Acta.* 2002;1572(2–3):364.
102. Stein M, Keshav S, Harris N, et al. Interleukin 4 potently enhances murine macrophage mannose receptor activity: a marker of alternative immunologic macrophage activation. *J Exp Med.* 1992;176(1):287.
103. Brown GD. Dectin-1: a signalling non-TLR pattern-recognition receptor. *Nat Rev Immunol.* 2006;6(1):33.
104. Taylor PR, Tsoni SV, Willment JA, et al. Dectin-1 is required for beta-glucan recognition and control of fungal infection. *Nat Immunol.* 2007;8(1):31.
105. Peiser L, Makepeace K, Pluddemann A, et al. Identification of Neisseria meningitidis nonlipopolysaccharide ligands for class A macrophage scavenger receptor by using a novel assay. *Infect Immun.* 2006;74(9):5191.
106. Mukhopadhyay S, Chen Y, Sankala M, et al. MARCO, an innate activation marker of macrophages, is a class A scavenger receptor for *Neisseria meningitidis*. *Eur J Immunol.* 2006;36(4):940.
107. Henson PM, Bratton DL, Fadok VA. Apoptotic cell removal. *Curr Biol.* 2001;11(19):R795.
108. Ren Y, Silverstein RL, Allen J, et al. CD36 gene transfer confers capacity for phagocytosis of cells undergoing apoptosis. *J Exp Med.* 1995;181(5):1857.
109. Savill J, Dransfield I, Gregory C, et al. A blast from the past: clearance of apoptotic cells regulates immune responses. *Nat Rev Immunol.* 2002;2(12):965.
109a. Haworth R, Platt N, Keshav S, et al. The macrophage scavenger receptor type A is expressed by activated macrophages and protects the host against lethal endotoxic shock. *J Exp Med.* 1997;186(9):1431–9.
110. Haziot A, Ferrero E, Kontgen F, et al. Resistance to endotoxin shock and reduced dissemination of gram-negative bacteria in CD14-deficient mice. *Immunity.* 1996;4(4):407.
111. Ozinsky A, Underhill DM, Fontenot JD, et al. The repertoire for pattern recognition of pathogens by the innate immune system is defined by cooperation between toll-like receptors. *Proc Natl Acad Sci U S A.* 2000;97(25):13766.
112. Schnare M, Barton GM, Holt AC, et al. Toll-like receptors control activation of adaptive immune responses. *Nat Immunol.* 2001;2(10):947.
113. Underhill DM, Ozinsky A, Hajjar AM, et al. The Toll-like receptor 2 is recruited to macrophage phagosomes and discriminates between pathogens. *Nature.* 1999;401(6755):811.
114. De Chastellier C. Electron microscopy. In: Cossart P, Boquet, P, Normark, S, eds. *Cellular microbiology*, 2nd ed. Washington, DC: ASM Press, 2005:451.
115. Freire-de-Lima CG, Nascimento DO, Soares MB, et al. Uptake of apoptotic cells drives the growth of a pathogenic trypanosome in macrophages. *Nature.* 2000;403(6766):199.
116. Russell DG. Where to stay inside the cell: a homesteader's guide to intracellular parasitism. In Cossart P, Boquet P, Normark S, et al., eds. *Cellular microbiology*, 2nd ed. Washington, DC: ASM Press, 2005:131.
117. Meylan E, Tschopp J, Karin M. Intracellular pattern recognition receptors in the host response. *Nature.* 2006;442(7098):39.
118. Honda K, Taniguchi T. IRFs: master regulators of signalling by Toll-like receptors and cytosolic pattern-recognition receptors. *Nat Rev Immunol.* 2006;6(9):644.

119. Deretic V. Autophagy in innate and adaptive immunity. *Trends Immunol.* 2005;26(10):523.
120. Gutierrez MG, Master SS, Singh SB, et al. Autophagy is a defense mechanism inhibiting BCG and *Mycobacterium* tuberculosis survival in infected macrophages. *Cell.* 2004;119(6):753.
121. Roy CR, Salcedo SP, Gorvel JP. Pathogen–endoplasmic-reticulum interactions: in through the out door. *Nat Rev Immunol.* 2006;6(2):136.
122. Stuart LM, Ezekowitz RA. Phagocytosis: elegant complexity. *Immunity.* 2005;22(5):539.
123. Desjardins M. ER-mediated phagocytosis: a new membrane for new functions. *Nat Rev Immunol.* 2003;3(4):280.
124. Touret N, Paroutis P, Terebiznik M, et al. Quantitative and dynamic assessment of the contribution of the ER to phagosome formation. *Cell.* 2005;123(1):157.
125. Feng CG, Collazo-Custodio CM, Eckhaus M, et al. Mice deficient in LRG-47 display increased susceptibility to mycobacterial infection associated with the induction of lymphopenia. *J Immunol.* 2004;172(2):1163.
126. Kristiansen M, Graversen JH, Jacobsen C, et al. Identification of the haemoglobin scavenger receptor. *Nature.* 2001;409(6817):198.
127. Ehrt S, Schnappinger D, Bekiranov S, et al. Reprogramming of the macrophage transcriptome in response to interferon-gamma and *Mycobacterium* tuberculosis: signaling roles of nitric oxide synthase-2 and phagocyte oxidase. *J Exp Med.* 2001;194(8):1123.
128. Martinez FO, Gordon S, Locati M, et al. Transcriptional profiling of the human monocyte-to-macrophage differentiation and polarization: new molecules and patterns of gene expression. *J Immunol.* 2006;177(10):7303.
129. Nathan CF. Secretory products of macrophages. *J Clin Invest.* 1987;79(2):319.
130. Clarke S, Greaves DR, Chung LP, et al. The human lysozyme promoter directs reporter gene expression to activated myelomonocytic cells in transgenic mice. *Proc Natl Acad Sci U S A.* 1996;93(4).1434.
131. Lang R, Rutschman RL, Greaves DR, et al. Autocrine deactivation of macrophages in transgenic mice constitutively overexpressing IL-10 under control of the human CD68 promoter. *J Immunol.* 2002;168(7):3402.
132. Barclay AN, Brown MH. The SIRP family of receptors and immune regulation. *Nat Rev Immunol.* 2006;6(6):457.
133. Marshall AS, Willment JA, Lin HH, et al. Identification and characterization of a novel human myeloid inhibitory C-type lectin-like receptor (MICL) that is predominantly expressed on granulocytes and monocytes. *J Biol Chem.* 2004;279(15):14792.
134. Helming L, Gordon S. Macrophage fusion induced by IL-4 alternative activation is a multistage process involving multiple target molecules. *Eur J Immunol.* 2007;37(1):33.
135. Duchmann R, Schmitt E, Knolle P, et al. Tolerance towards resident intestinal flora in mice is abrogated in experimental colitis and restored by treatment with interleukin-10 or antibodies to interleukin-12. *Eur J Immunol.* 1996;26(4):934.
136. Montaner LJ, Griffin P, Gordon S. Interleukin-10 inhibits initial reverse transcription of human immunodeficiency virus type 1 and mediates a virostatic latent state in primary blood-derived human macrophages *in vitro*. *J Gen Virol.* 1994;75 (Pt 12):3393.
137. Mellor AL, Sivakumar J, Chandler P, et al. Prevention of T cell-driven complement activation and inflammation by tryptophan catabolism during pregnancy. *Nat Immunol.* 2001;2(1):64.
138. Gagnon E, Duclos S, Rondeau C, et al. Endoplasmic reticulum-mediated phagocytosis is a mechanism of entry into macrophages. *Cell.* 2002;110(1):119.
139. Dorn BR, Dunn WA Jr, Progulske-Fox A. Bacterial interactions with the autophagic pathway. *Cell Microbiol.* 2002;4(1):1.
140. Schmid D, Dengjel J, Schoor O, et al. Autophagy in innate and adaptive immunity against intracellular pathogens. *J Mol Med.* 2006;84(3):194.
141. Dengjel J, Schoor O, Fischer R, et al. Autophagy promotes MHC class II presentation of peptides from intracellular source proteins. *Proc Natl Acad Sci U S A.* 2005;102(22):7922.
142. Russell DG. *Mycobacterium* tuberculosis: here today, and here tomorrow. *Nat Rev Mol Cell Biol.* 2001;2(8):569.
143. Deretic V, Singh S, Master S, et al. *Mycobacterium* tuberculosis inhibition of phagolysosome biogenesis and autophagy as a host defence mechanism. *Cell Microbiol.* 2006;8(5):719.
144. Amer AO, Swanson MS. A phagosome of one's own: a microbial guide to life in the macrophage. *Curr Opin Microbiol.* 2002;5(1):56.

Chapter 19

Major Histocompatibility Complex (MHC) Molecules: Structure, Function, and Genetics

David H. Margulies, Kannan Natarajan, Jamie Rossjohn, and James McCluskey

INTRODUCTION

Not only because of their profound immunologic importance as cell surface receptors that mediate recognition of infected, tumor, or foreign cells by T lymphocytes, but also because they are encoded by the immunoregulatory genes identified first, the set of molecules commonly referred to as the major histocompatibility complex or MHC molecules is central to understanding both the phenomenon and mechanism of immune recognition. The sophistication of our knowledge of MHC molecules and their function reflects the steady improvement of our understanding of the details of molecular mechanism and also outlines a conceptual framework for appreciating the elegance of nature's solutions to complicated cellular and ultimately molecular problems. MHC molecules play a crucial role in defense of the host against bacterial and viral pathogens and recognition of tumors. Our approach in this chapter will be first to give a cursory view of function and then to explore the structural solutions to functional requirements posed by the complexities of immune recognition. We will consider key features of the molecular skeletons, subunit organization, and surface shape and charge of representative members of the MHC family and correlate these structures with their known functions. We will progress to a more critical investigation of the role of these molecules with respect to their cellular biosynthesis and assembly, and their contribution to immunologic cell communication. We will continue with a status report on the genetics of MHC molecules, focused on both mouse and human, and will conclude with a contemporary view of the evolution of this broad gene family. Speculation on the coevolution of these molecules with their host ligands as well as viral homologs will finish the chapter, providing the reader with a factual and conceptual foundation with which to address current literature. Along the way, important structural and functional aspects of MHC molecules as they relate to human disease will be discussed. The story of MHC molecules is incomplete, not only because our database is incomplete, but also because the pathogens and tumors with which both the adaptive and innate immune systems wrestle continue to change. Like human families, the MHC gene family expands, contracts, and adapts to changing environments and to emerging requirements and opportunities.

We cannot, in the allotted space, provide a complete historical background and the didactic aspects of mouse genetics offered in earlier editions of this book. We can only strongly suggest that the student explore the important history of the development of inbred mouse strains and the contemporary view of detailed genetic analysis that has been previously summarized elsewhere. The power of Internet Web sites for seeking some of this information should not be overlooked, but we raise a necessary note of caution because such sources of information may not be expertly curated and may be erroneous or inaccurate.

The molecular focus of the immune system consists of MHC molecules—those cell surface receptors that govern, by interaction with membrane-expressed molecules on crucial cells of the innate and adaptive immune systems, the initiation, perpetuation, and regulation of cellular activation in response to infection and neoplasia. MHC molecules are not static surface receptors that merely bind another set of receptors to indicate their presence and number, but are structurally and conformationally dynamic—they modulate their structure by incorporating peptides derived from degraded self- and foreign proteins expressed in the same cell; and they sense the presence of proteins from viruses and other cellular pathogens that affect the nature or efficiency of the MHC molecules' cell surface expression. Molecules encoded by the major histocompatibility complex (*Mhc*) represent a microcosm of complex molecular, cellular, and organismic biology. Members of the family of *Mhc*-encoded molecules interact extensively with a number of other molecules, during both their biosynthesis and intracellular trafficking. When poised at the cell surface as ligands for specific molecules on T cells and natural killer (NK) cells, they control the response of these immunoeffectors. MHC genes have also been purloined by some viruses that have exploited these to encode immunoevasins—molecules that either counterregulate host MHC expression or that deceptively bind NK receptors to allow viral escape from the immune response. Understanding the MHC molecules in detail, then, provides a foundation for comprehending the layers of complex regulation to which the immune system is servant. The genetics of the *Mhc* offers a groundwork for understanding immunologic selection, and also reveals living footprints of molecular genetic evolution.

Although an earlier view was that the *Mhc*-encoded molecules were uniquely involved as recognition elements for T cells, it is now overwhelmingly clear that MHC molecules interact with receptors on NK cells as well. As the strict definitions of MHC molecules based purely on the location of their encoding genetic loci have given way to looser groupings based on similarities of the protein structures or on functional relationships, we now appreciate that a larger family of genes, molecules, and functions should be included in this chapter. The *Mhc* provides a genetic link from immune responsiveness to autoimmune disease—those well-known strong associations of particular *Mhc* genes with particular human diseases, and we will outline the molecular basis for some such associations.

The *Mhc* is a set of linked genes, located on chromosome 6 of the human, chromosome 17 of the mouse, chromosome 20 of the rat, and cluster I of the chicken, that was first identified by its effects on tumor or skin transplantation and control of immune responsiveness (1,*2*,3). More recently, in part because of evolutionary interest and in part because of the importance of *Mhc* loci in species that serve as models for human disease, particularly human immunovirus (HIV) infection, extensive information has been gathered on the *Mhc* genes of several primate species (*4*). The *Mhc* also plays a role in resistance to infection. Early observations indicated an *Mhc*-linked control of immune responsiveness (5–8,*9*) and have culminated in a molecular understanding of the critical details of genetically encoded cellular recognition in the immune system. The control of transplantation and the immune response are the phenotypic consequences of the function of molecules encoded in the *Mhc*. Therefore, we gain a deeper understanding of the *Mhc* as we explore it in molecular and cellular terms. MHC molecules are cell surface receptors that bind antigen fragments and display them to various cells of the immune system, T cells that bear $\alpha\beta$ receptors (*10*,11,*12*), NK cells (13–15), T cells that express $\gamma\delta$ receptors (*16*), and NKT cells (17–19,*20*). Molecules that are structurally similar to MHC-I molecules but are encoded beyond the strict genetic bounds of the *Mhc*, and in some cases lacking the full complement of MHC-I domains, are now known to be expressed on particular subsets of somatic cells, some tumors, and cells of the placenta. Thus, we have witnessed a transition in knowledge from that of mysterious genetic entities with ill-defined mechanisms but distinct immunologic functions and genetic locations to a biochemical understanding of specific molecules with known structures, biosynthetic pathways, biophysical parameters of interaction, and temporal expression that convey specific signals between and within cells, and that map precisely to defined regions of the chromosome. The study of the *Mhc* has also made a transition, from that of genetics and cellular immunology to detailed molecular mechanisms.

The focus of this chapter is the *Mhc*, and our primary goal will be to outline the general principles of molecular organization and function both of the genetic regions that encode MHC molecules as well as of the functional cell surface molecules themselves. Human disease associations, molecular typing of MHC molecules and *Mhc* genes, and relevant functional polymorphisms will complete our explication of these markers of immunologic function.

A Note on Nomenclature

Students have frequently been confused by *Mhc* nomenclature. Like language, nomenclature evolves, and our attempts at standardization are inevitably only partially successful. Current usage differs from species to species, journal to journal, and writer to writer, although there are standards of which the informed scientist should be aware. For the mouse and rat *Mhc*, these have been set down by an international committee and are available at the Jackson Laboratory home page (www.informatics.jax.org/mgihome/nomen). For the human *Mhc*, there is a standard World Health Organization (WHO) nomenclature that is periodically evaluated and revised (17). By convention, genes or genetic loci are indicated in italics and the encoded protein products or phenotypic descriptions are shown in a standard font. For the genes of the human *Mhc* this convention is often overlooked, whereas for those of the mouse and other species it is frequently followed. The mouse *Mhc* is referred to as *H2* because it was the second genetic locus involved in control of expression of erythrocyte antigens to be identified by Gorer (18,19). Now, the *Mhc* is known to consist of many loci, and the extended genetic region is referred to as the complex; thus, the general term used for all species is the *Mhc* or *MHC*. The *Mhc* in the rat is known as *RT1*, the human locus is known as *HLA* (for Human Leucocyte Antigen). *DLA* for the dog, *GPLA* for the guinea pig, *SLA* for the swine, and *RLA* for the rabbit are the common usages. For other species, the taxonomic name forms the basis for the designation, contributing the first two letters of the genus and the first two of the species to name the locus. Thus we have *Patr* for the chimpanzee, *Pan troglodytes*, *Gogo* for the gorilla, *Gorilla gorilla*, *Mamu* for the Rhesus macaque, *Macacca mulatta*, and *Papa* for the Bonobo, *Pan paniscus*.

We now know of over 400 genes that map to the human or mouse *Mhc*, and though technically they are all "*Mhc*" genes, the "MHC" molecules refer specifically to the MHC class I (MHC-I) or MHC class II (MHC-II) molecules that are related in structure and function. Other *Mhc*-encoded molecules with distinct structure and function are referred to by their more specific names.

Particular *Mhc* genes are designated by a letter (or letters) for the locus (e.g., *H2K*, *H2D*, *H2L*, *H2IA*, in the mouse; and *HLA-A*, *HLA-B*, *HLA-C*, *HLA-E*, *HLA-F*, *HLA-G*, *HLA-H*, *HLA-J*, *HLA-K*, *HLA-L*, *HLA-DR*, *HLA-DQ*, *HLA-DO*, and *HLA-DP* in the human). *HLA-H*, *-J*, *-K*, and *-L* are pseudogenes. Allelic genes (and their expressed cell surface protein products) have been denoted in the mouse by the addition of a superscript (e.g., $H2K^b$ and $H2K^d$ are distinct alleles at the same locus). In the human, a letter and a number distinguish serologically defined MHC allotypes (*HLA-A2* and *HLA-A3* are allotypes of *HLA-A*; whereas *HLA-B8* and *HLA-B27* are allotypes of *HLA-B*). Precise designation of human genes uses a nomenclature including a four-digit (or longer) number following the locus (e.g., HLA-A*0101 and HLA-A*0201 are alleles of *HLA-A*; see Table 19.1 for clarification of the nomenclature of the HLA alleles). Clarity in understanding the human designations requires a conversion table to align the older allotype nomenclature based on definition of gene products by serology (often encompassing families of allelic gene products) with the more recent one based on DNA typing (Tables 19.2, 19.3).

For the *Mhc* class II genes, the designation in the human is *HLA-D* (including *-DM*, *-DO*, *-DP*, *-DQ*, and *-DR*), whereas in the mouse *H2-IAa*, *H2-IAb*, *H2-IEa*, and *H2-IEb* are used, frequently shortened to *IAa*, *IAb*, *IEa*, and *IEb*, respectively. *a* and *b* refer to the *a*- or α- (alpha) and *b*- or β-) chain encoding genes, respectively. Current usage tends to employ the Roman letter for the gene designation and the Greek for the encoded protein chain. The MHC-II molecules are often referred to as IA or IE with a superscript denoting the haplotype (i.e., IA^b, IA^d, or IE^d). Several murine MHC-II–like genes, originally named *H2-Ma*, *H2-Mb1*, and *H2-Mb2*, which are homologs of the human *HLA-DMA* and *HLA-DMB* genes, are now called *H2-DMA*, *H2-DMB1*, and *H2-DMB2* in an effort to emphasize their structural and functional similarity to the human *HLA-DMA* and *-DMB* genes, as well as to distinguish them from the *H2-M* genes that lie most distal on chromosome 17 (*20*). Another complication that demands the precise use of gene and encoded protein names is that the number of genes in a particular homologous genetic region can differ between strains or between individuals. In the mouse, whereas some strains have only a single gene at the MHC-I *H2-D* locus ($H2\text{-}D^b$, for instance), other strains may have as many as five genes in the homologous regions ($H2\text{-}D^d$, $H2\text{-}D2^d$, $H2\text{-}D3^d$, $H2\text{-}D4^d$, and $H2\text{-}L^d$ (*21*).

An important description commonly used is "haplotype," which refers to the linked constellation of particular alleles at distinct loci that occur as a group on a parental chromosome (*22*). The concept of haplotype is important in typing the *HLA* loci in the human, where the linked *Mhc* genes of one chromosome of one parent will generally segregate as a linkage group to the children. When alleles at linked loci segregate more commonly together than

TABLE 19.1 Nomenclature of HLA Loci and Alleles[a]

Nomenclature	*Definition*
HLA	The HLA (human leukocyte antigen) region and prefix for an HLA gene
HLA-DRB1	A particular HLA locus, i.e., DRB1
HLA-DRB1*13	A group of alleles that encode the DR13 antigen defined serologically by microlymphocytotoxicity or by mixed lymphocyte reactivity (MLR)
HLA-DRB1*1301	A specific HLA allele
HLA-DRB1*1301N	A null allele (i.e., nonexpressed)
HLA-DRB1*130102	An allele that differs by a synonymous mutation (i.e., identical amino acid encoded by a different codon)
HLA-DRB1*13010102	An allele that contains a mutation outside the coding region
HLA-A*2409N	A null allele
HLA-A*3014L	An allele encoding a protein with significantly reduced or "low" cell surface expression
HLA-A*24020102L	An allele encoding a protein with significantly reduced or "low" cell surface expression, where the mutation is found outside the coding region
HLA-B*44020102S	An allele encoding a protein that is expressed as a "secreted" molecule only
HLA-A*3211Q	An allele that has a mutation that has previously been shown to have a significant effect on cell surface expression, but for which this has not been confirmed and its expression remains "questionable"

[a] In addition to the unique allele number, there are additional optional suffixes that may be added to an allele to indicate its expression status. Alleles that have been shown not to be expressed, "null" alleles, have been given the suffix "N." Those alleles that have been shown to be alternatively expressed may have the suffix "L," "S," "C," "A," or "Q." The suffix "L" is used to indicate an allele that has been shown to have "low" cell surface expression when compared to normal levels. The "S" suffix is used to denote an allele specifying a protein that is expressed as a soluble "secreted" molecule but is not present on the cell surface. A "C" suffix indicates an allele product that is present in the "cytoplasm" but not on the cell surface. An "A" suffix indicates "aberrant" expression, where there is some doubt as to whether a protein is expressed. A "Q" suffix is used when the expression of an allele is "questionable," given that the mutation seen in the allele has previously been shown to affect normal expression levels.
Source: Adapted from IMGT Web site, www.ebi.ac.uk/imgt/hla/nomenclature/index.html.

predicted by chance, this is called linkage disequilibrium, a phenomenon that leads to the presence of well-recognized MHC haplotypes in unrelated individuals. Individual haplotypes of the *Mhc* in the mouse are referred to by a lowercase letter superscript as $H2^b$, $H2^d$, or $H2^k$. Thus, the $H2^k$ haplotype refers to the full set of linked genes, $H2\text{-}K^k$, $H2\text{-}IA^k$, $H2\text{-}IE^k$, $H2\text{-}D^k$, and extends to the genes of the *Q* and *T* regions as well (23,24). (Some haplotype designations, such as $H2^a$, refer to natural recombinants and thus have some of the linked genes from one haplotype and some from another). Table 19.4 summarizes the haplotypes of common mouse strains.

In parallel with the genetic nomenclature system, a system has developed that focuses on the expressed proteins rather than on the genes, and by its use emphasizes both structural and functional differences. The main distinction of MHC molecules is between the MHC class I (MHC-I) and MHC class II (MHC-II) molecules. (MHC class III molecules have also been included in a group originally characterized as serum molecules involved in the complement system (C4/C2/Bf) but now also include products of the genetically linked loci mapping between the class I and class II regions of the *Mhc*). MHC-I molecules all consist of a heavy chain (also called an α chain), which is noncovalently assembled with a monomorphic (genetically invariant, or almost so) light chain known as β2-microglobulin (β2m), encoded by the *B2m* gene. MHC-I molecules are subclassified into the MHC class Ia and MHC class Ib groups, distinctions made based on amino acid sequence differences as well as gene location (*25,26*). Recently, genes of members of the herpesvirus families have been shown to encode proteins that are structurally related to MHC-I molecules and are designated "MHC-Iv," as virus-encoded molecules (27). MHC-II molecules are heterodimeric, consisting of noncovalently assembled α and β chains. The bulk of the serologically defined differences in HLA-DR molecules reside in the β chain. The heterodimers usually consist of the assembled products of the linked genes encoding the two chains. In the mouse the products of the *IAa* (also known as $IA\alpha$) and *IAb* (or $IA\beta$ genes) assemble to form the IA heterodimer, and similarly, the products of the *IEa* ($IE\alpha$) and *IEb* ($IE\beta$ genes assemble to form IE. IA and IE are often referred to as "isotypes." The allelic forms are usually referred to as IA^b, IA^d, or IA^k. Under some circumstances, mixed heterodimers, which may be of immunologic importance, are observed (*28–33*). Thus, when one refers to a mixed heterodimer consisting of the α chain of IE^d and the β chain of IA^d, one must use the more precise but cumbersome description $IA\beta^dE\alpha^d$ (IAb^dEa^d). In the human, particularly in referring to MHC-II molecules,

TABLE 19.2 HLA Class I Alleles[a]

HLA-A		HLA-B		HLA-C	
Serology	Alleles	Serology	Alleles	Serology	Alleles
A1	A*0101–0125	B7	B*0702–0755	Cw1	Cw*0102–0118
A2	A*0201–0299	B8	B*0801–0833	Cw2	Cw*0202–0218
	A*9201–9216	B13	B*1301–1318	Cw3	Cw*0302–0340
A3	A*0301–0329	B14	B*1401–1407N	Cw4	Cw*0401–0427
A11	A*1101–1130	B15	B*1501–1599	Cw5	Cw*0501–0516
A23(9)	A*2301–2315		B*9501–9529	Cw6	Cw*0602–0618N
A24(9)	A*2402–2476	B18	B*1801–1826	Cw7	Cw*0701–0748
A25(10)	A*2501–2506	B27	B*2701–2737	Cw8	Cw*0801–0814
A26(10)	A*2601–2634	B35	B*3501–3575	—	Cw*1202–1221
A29(19)	A*2901–2916	B37	B*3701–3713	—	Cw*1402–1408
A30(19)	A*3001–3021	B38(16)	B*3801–3816	—	Cw*1502–1520
A31(19)	A*3101–3117	B39(16)	B*3901–3941	—	Cw*1601–1609
A32(19)	A*3201–3215	B40	B*4001–4075	—	Cw*1701–1704
A33(19)	A*3301–3310	B41	B*4101–4108	—	Cw*1801–1803
A34(10)	A*3401–3408	B42	B*4201–4209		
A36	A*3601–3604	B44(12)	B*4402–4453		
A43	A*4301	B45(12)	B*4501–4507		
A66	A*6601–6606	B46	B*4601–4610		
A68(28)	A*6801–6838	B47	B*4701–4705		
A69(28)	A*6901	B48	B*4801–4816		
A74(19)	A*7401–7412	B49(21)	B*4901–4905		
	A*8001	B50(21)	B*5001–5004		
		B51(5)	B*5101–5148		
		B52(5)	B*5201–5211		
		B53	B*5301–5312		
		B54(22)	B*5401–5413		
		B55(22)	B*5501–5526		
		B56(22)	B*5601–5620		
		B57(17)	B*5701–5712		
		B58(17)	B*5801–5815		
		B59	B*5901–5902		
		B67	B*6701–6702		
		B73	B*7301		
		B78	B*7801–7805		
		—	B*8101–8102		
		—	B*8201–8202		
		—	B*8301		

HLA-E	HLA-F	HLA-G
E*0101–0104	F*0101–0104	G*0101–0108

[a]This table summarizes the designations of the human MHC-I HLA gene products as they are known based on serology, and as they have been assigned by nucleotide (and thus inferred amino acid) sequences. Current serologic designations are given in the "Serology" column, with older (broader) serologic assignments listed in parentheses. Serologic assignments are usually based on reactivity with alloantisera in a microlymphocytotoxicty assay. Some of the most recently identified HLA polymorphisms and products of nonclassical loci (e.g., HLA-E and HLA-G) have no historical serologic designation. Note that the serologically defined HLA B15 antigen comprises some 128 allelic members (B*1501–1599 and B*9501–9529), and HLA A2 comprises 115 members (A*0201–0299 and A*9201–9216) as of April 2007. The table is based on a listing of alleles maintained by the WHO Nomenclature Committee for Factors of the HLA System. All new and confirmatory sequences are generally submitted directly to the committee via the IMGT/HLA Database using the sequence submission tool provided. The IMGT/HLA Database may be accessed via the World Wide Web at: www.ebi.ac.uk/imgt/hla.

TABLE 19.3 HLA Class II Alleles[a]

HLA-DR		HLA-DQ		HLA-DP		HLA-DM and HLA-DO	
Serology	*Alleles*	*Serology*	*Alleles*	*Serology*	*Alleles*	*Serology*	*Alleles*
α-Chain		*α-Chain*		*α-Chain*		*α-Chain*	
DRA		DQA1		DPA1		DMA	DMA*0101-0104
—	DRA*0101-010202	—	DQA1*010101-0107	—	DPA1*010301-0109	DOA	DOA*010101-0104N
			DQA1*0201		DPA1*020101-0203		
			DQA1*030101-0303		DPA1*0301-0303		
			DQA1*040101-0404		DPA1*0401		
			DQA1*050101-0509				
			DQA1*060101-0602				
β-Chain		*β-Chain*		*β-Chain*		*β-Chain*	
DRB1		DQB1		DPB1		DMB	DMB*0101-0107
DR1	DRB1*010101-0116	DQ5(1)	DQB1*050101-0505	DPw1	DPB1*010101-010103	DOB	DOB*01010101-01040102
DR15(2)	DRB1*150101-1522	DQ6(1)	DQB1*060101-0630	DPw2	DPB1*020102-020106		
DR16(2)	DRB1*160101-1611	DQ2	DQB1*020101-0205	DPw3	DPB1*030101-030102		
DR3	DRB1*030101-0335	DQ3(7,8,9)	DQB1*030101-0320	DPw4	DPB1*040101-040102		
DR4	DRB1*040101-0464	DQ4	DQB1*0401-0402	DPw5	DPB1*0501		
DR11(5)	DRB1*110101-1163			DPw6	DPB1*0601		
DR12(5)	DRB1*120101-1215				DPB1*0801		
DR13(6)	DRB1*130101-1379				DPB1*0901		
DR14(6)	DRB1*140101-1466				DPB1*1001		
DR7	DRB1*070101-0712				DPB1*110101-110102		
DR8	DRB1*080101-0832				DPB1*1301-4101		
DR9	DRB1*090102-0906				DPB1*4401-9901		
DR10	DRB1*100101-100102				DPB1*0102-2002		
DRB3							
DR52	DRB3*01010201-0111						
	DRB3*0201-0222						
	DRB3*030101-0303						
DRB4							
DR53	DRB4*01010101-0107						
	DRB4*0201N						
	DRB4*0301N						
DRB5							
DR51	DRB5*010101-0113						
	DRB5*0202-0205						
DRB6	DRB6*0101						
	DRB6*0201-0202						
DRB7	DRB7*010101-010102						
DRB8	DRB8*0101						
DRB9	DRB9*0101						

[a]The table is based on a listing of alleles maintained by the WHO Nomenclature Committee for Factors of the HLA System as of April 2007. All new and confirmatory sequences are generally submitted directly to the committee via the IMGT/HLA Database using the sequence submission tool provided. The IMGT/HLA Database may be accessed at www.ebi.ac.uk/imgt/hla. Note that the serologic assignments of HLA class II molecules do not always correlate with the DNA nomenclature. This is particularly true for some of the DRB1*11/12/13/14 alleles. Serologicl assignment of HLA-DR molecules is largely determined by the DRB1 gene product, whereas assignment of DQ molecules reflects serologic contributions from both DQA1 and DQB1 gene products. As new alleles of DR and DQ have been identified, original assignments have been "split," and these relationships are indicated in brackets. Thus DR15 and DR16 are splits of DR2, DR11 and DR12 are splits of DR5, and DQ3 includes the serologically determined DQ7, DQ8, and DQ9 antigens. The "w" designations (for HLA-C and HLA-DP) are "workshop" assignments because serologic and cellular assignments are sometimes imprecise. The DPw cellular assignments (e.g., DPw1, etc) generally, but not always, correlate with the same numbers used for allele assignments (e.g., DPB1*0101). Some null alleles and alleles with synonymous mutations are omitted. In addition to those serologic designations listed in the table, Bw4 and Bw6 specificities group the following: Bw4: B5, B5102, B5103, B13, B17, B27, B37, B38(16), B44(12), B47, B49(21), B51(5), B52(5), B53, B57(17),B58(17), B59, B63(15), B77(15), and A9, A23(9), A24(9), A2403, A25(10), A32(19); Bw6: B7, B703, B8, B14, B18, B22, B2708, B35, B39(16), B3901, B3902, B40, B4005, B41, B42, B45(12), B46, B48, B50(21), B54(22), B55(22), B56(22), B60(40), B61(40), B62(15), B64(14), B65(14), B67, B70, B71(70), B72(70), B73, B75(15), B76(15), B78, B81 (www.anthonynolan.org.uk/HIG/data.html).

TABLE 19.4 Commonly Used Mouse Strains: *H2* Haplotypes[a]

		H2 Complex							
Strain	***Haplotype***	*K*	*Ab*	*Aa*	*Eb*	*Ea*	*D*	*Qa1*	*Tla*
Common strains									
129/J	*bc*	*b*	*b*	*b*	*b*	—	*b*	*b*	*f*
AKR/J	*k*	*k*	*k*	*k*	*k*	*k*	*k*	*b*	*b*
ASW/Sn	*s*	*s*	*s*	*s*	*s*	—	*s*	*b*	*b*
BALB/c	*d*	*d*	*d*	*d*	*d*	*d*	*d*	*b*	*c*
C3H/HeJ	*k*	*k*	*k*	*k*	*k*	*k*	*k*	*h*	*h*
CBA/J	*k*	*k*	*k*	*k*	*k*	*k*	*k*	*b*	*b*
C57BL/6	*b*	*b*	*b*	*b*	*b*	—	*b*	*b*	*b*
C57BL/10	*b*	*b*	*b*	*b*	*b*	—	*b*	*b*	*b*
C57BR	*k*	*k*	*k*	*k*	*k*	*k*	*k*	*a*	*a*
DBA/2J	*d*	*d*	*d*	*d*	*d*	*d*	*d*	*b*	*c*
NOD/LtJ	*y7*	*d*	*y7*	*d*	—	—	*b*		
NON/LtJ	*nb1*	*b*	*nb1*	?	*k*	*k*	*b*		
NZB/BINJ	*d2*	*d*	*d*	*d*	*d*	*d*	*d*	*a*	*a*
NZW/LacJ	*z*	*u*	*u*	*u*	*u*	*u*	*z*		
P/J	*p*	*p*	*p*	*p*	*p*	*p*	*p*	*a*	*e*
PL/J	*u*	*u*	*u*	*u*	*u*	*u*	*d*		
RIII	*r*	*r*	*r*	*r*	*r*	*r*	*r*	*c*®	*b*
SJL	*s2*	*s*	*s*	*s*	*s*	—	*s*	*a*	*a*
Congenic strains									
B10.BR	*k2*	*k*	*k*	*k*	*k*	*k*	*k*		
B10.D2	*d*	*d*	*d*	*d*	*d*	*d*	*d*		
B10.S	*s*	*s*	*s*	*s*	*s*	—	*s*		
BALB.B	*b*		*b*	*b*	*b*	*b*	—	*b*	
BALB.K	*k*	*k*	*k*	*k*	*k*	*k*	*k*		
C3H.SW	*b*	*b*	*b*	*b*	*b*	—	*b*		
Recombinant strains									
A	*a*	*k*	*k*	*k*	*k*	*k*	*d*		
A.TL	*t1*	*s*	*k*	*k*	*k*	*k*	*d*		
B10.A	*a*	*k*	*k*	*k*	*k*	*k*	*d*		
B10.A(1R)	*h1*	*k*	*k*	*k*	*k*	*k*	*b*		
B10.A(2R)	*h2*	*k*	*k*	*k*	*k*	*k*	*b*		
B10.A(3R)	*I3*	*b*	*b*	*b*	*b/k*	*k*	*d*		
B10.A(4R)	*h4*	*k*	*k*	*k*	*k/b*	—	*b*		
B10.A(5R)	*I5*	*b*	*b*	*b*	*b/k*	*k*	*d*		
B10.T(6R)	*y2*	*q*	*q*	*q*	*q*	—	*d*		
B10.S(7R)	*t2*	*s*	*s*	*s*	*s*	—	*d*		
B10.S(8R)	*as1*	*k*	*k*	*k*	*k/s*	—	*s*		
B10.S(9R)	*t4*	*s*	*s*	*s*	*s/k*	*k*	*d*		
B10.HTT	*t3*	*s*	*s*	*s*	*sd/k*	*k*	*d*		

[a]A dash indicates abnormal gene expression, although the precise mechanism may differ in different strains (*475*). Blanks indicate insufficient data for characterization.
Source: Adapted from (*473*) and (*474*).

the distinctions between molecules identified by antibodies and those identified by DNA sequence typing must be made (Tables 19.2, 19.3).

The Immunologic Functions of MHC Molecules

MHC molecules are a molecular reflection of the health of either the cell that synthesizes them (for MHC-I molecules) or of the local environment in which the cell resides (for MHC-II). The structure of the MHC molecule reflects not only the amino acid sequence of the two polypeptide chains (α and β for MHC-II; and heavy [or α] and β2m for MHC-I) that form the bulk of the complex, but also of a variable bound peptide (generally from 8 to 15 amino acids in length) that forms an integral part of the trimer. The MHC molecule, governed by the sequence of the encoding structural genes for *Mhc-I* heavy chain and the *Mhc-II*

α and β chains, as well as other genes involved in antigen processing and presentation that map to the *Mhc*, must satisfy at least two distinct recognition functions: the binding of peptides or in some cases nonpeptidic molecules, and the interaction with either T or NK cells via their respective receptors. The T-cell receptor (TCR) may augment its interaction with the MHC molecule by virtue of interaction of a T-cell–expressed coreceptor (CD8 for MHC-I and CD4 for MHC-II). Evidence now suggests that some NK receptors, when expressed on T cells, may also serve as coreceptors (*34*). The binding of peptides by an MHC-I or MHC-II molecule is the initial selective event that permits the cell expressing the MHC molecule (the antigen-presenting cell, APC) to sample fragments derived either from its own proteins (for MHC-I–restricted antigen presentation) or from those proteins ingested from the immediate extracellular environment (for the case of MHC-II).

In particular, cell surface MHC class I glycoproteins gather from the cell's biosynthetic pathway fragments of proteins derived from infecting viruses, intracellular parasites, or self-molecules, either expressed normally or in a dysregulated fashion as a result of tumorigenesis, and then display these molecular fragments, in complex with the mature MHC-I molecule, at the cell surface (*12*,35,36,*37*,*38*). Here, the cell-bound MHC-I/β2m/peptide complex on the APC is exposed to the extracellular milieu and is available for interaction with T cells or NK cells. A T cell bearing an $\alpha\beta$ receptor recognizes the particular MHC/peptide complex (MHC/p) by virtue of a specific physical binding interaction. Each mature T cell bears a unique TCR encoded by somatically rearranged TCR genetic elements. T cells bearing $\alpha\beta$ receptors are first selected for weak reactivity with one or other self-MHC/p complexes in the thymus (a process known as positive selection), and then TCRs that bind strongly are deleted (negative selection) so that only a small proportion of T cells that develop in the thymus ultimately reach peripheral lymphoid organs such as lymph nodes and spleen. A particular TCR is therefore selected to bind only a limited set of MHC/p complexes based on this bias for self-recognition. The recognition by T cells is thus described as "MHC-restricted" in that TCR interact preferentially with self-MHC molecules. However, T cells are also "antigen-specific" in that a particular T cell sees a particular peptide. For any given T-cell clone, single amino acid substitutions of either the MHC or the peptide may severely diminish, or even obliterate, TCR recognition of the MHC/p complex. The MHC-I system draws its spectrum of peptides from proteins in the cytosol that are degraded by the multiproteolytic proteasome complex. These peptides that are transported from the cytosol to the endoplasmic reticulum via the intrinsic membrane peptide transporter, the transporter associated with antigen processing (TAP), are then trimmed at their amino terminus and cooperatively folded within the peptide loading complex to form an intrinsic component of the newly synthesized MHC-I molecule (*39*).

MHC-II molecules, in contrast to MHC-I, are expressed on a more limited set of somatic cells—B cells, macrophages, dendritic cells, activated but not resting T cells in the human—and have a somewhat more specific function in peptide selection and presentation. In general, they bind peptides derived from the degradation of proteins ingested by the antigen-presenting cell (APC), as well as endogenous cytosolic and endosomal proteins. They then sort their MHC-II molecules into endosomal cellular compartments, where the degraded peptides are generated and catalytically transferred to the binding site of the MHC-II. The MHC-II antigen-presentation pathway is based on the initial assembly of the MHC-II $\alpha\beta$ heterodimer with a dual-function molecule, the invariant chain (Ii). Ii serves as both a chaperone to direct the $\alpha\beta$ heterodimer to an endosomal, acidic protein-processing location, where it encounters antigenic peptides, and also protects the antigen-binding site of the MHC-II molecule so that it will be preferentially loaded with antigenic peptides in this endosomal/lysosomal location (40,*41*–*43*). The loading of the MHC-II molecule with antigenic peptide, a process dependent on the release of the Ii-derived "CLIP" (class II–associated invariant chain peptide), in part dependent on the MHC-II–like molecules, HLA-DM and HLA-DO in the human, and H2-DM and H2-DO in the mouse (*44*,*45*), then leads to the cell surface expression of MHC-II peptide complexes. HLA-DM functions by interacting directly with an acidic face of the MHC-II molecule (*46*) to catalyze the exchange of the CLIP peptide with an antigenic peptide in the endosomal compartment. HLA-DO modulates HLA-DM function by altering the repertoire of MHC-II/peptide complexes observed in DO-expressing cells (*47*,*48*). The MHC-II–recognizing T cells then secrete lymphokines and may also be induced to proliferate or to undergo programmed cell death. Such MHC-restricted lymphokine production that facilitates and augments the recruitment of additional inflammatory cells as well as antigen-presenting cells and antibody-producing cells is a key component of what was historically referred to as "T-cell help."

Distinct from the recognition of MHC molecules by TCRs, a number of activating and inhibitory NK cell receptors bind MHC-I molecules, whereas several NK receptors interact with MHC-I–like molecules (49). In general, the NK/MHC-I interaction, as compared to the TCR/MHC interaction, shows considerably less peptide specificity, although the interaction is peptide-dependent, and in some cases may exhibit clear-cut peptide preferences (13,50,*51*,*52*). The functional purpose of the MHC-I or MHC-I–like molecule in NK-cell recognition appears to be more subtle than that in T-cell recognition. The NK cell is tuned by a balance of inhibitory and activating signals conveyed to it via MHC interaction, and in its resting state the inhibitory signals predominate. MHC-I is a sensor of the biosynthetic and metabolic state of the cell in which it is synthesized—when dysregulated by tumorigenesis or viral infection, the altered level of MHC-I can be detected by the NK cell. This ability of the NK cell to sense altered levels of MHC-I on target cells is the basis of the "missing-self hypothesis," which explains that NK cells detect and lyse those cells that are defective in MHC-I expression as a result of the loss of the inhibitory signal that results from engagement of NK receptors by MHC I (53–55). The prototype NK receptor is the mouse NK inhibitory receptor, Ly49A, a C-type lectinlike molecule that delivers an inhibitory signal to the cell, expressing it as a result of its interaction with normally expressed MHC-I molecule, H2-D^d (56). Distinct clones of NK cells differ in the combinatorial expression of different NK receptors that have different MHC preferences. Thus, in the mouse, each distinct NK clone may express a different combination of NK-inhibitory receptors such as Ly49A, Ly49C, Ly49G2, and Ly49I (*57*). Because each inhibitory molecule may exhibit slight differences in its MHC-I and/or peptide preference and specificity, this kind of combinatorial variation of NK activity provides a breadth of specificity toward different potential target cells. The interaction of MHC-I on the NK cells themselves with an NK inhibitory receptor, such as Ly49A or Ly49C (i.e., a "cis" interaction), plays an important role in the priming of NK cells (*58*). The interaction of the NK-activating receptor, NKG2D, with MHC-I–like molecules induced by stress in the target cell results in the activation of the NK cell and follows distinct molecular rules of recognition (*34*).

MHC-I and MHC-II molecules, because of differences in the cellular compartments that they traverse from biosynthesis to maturation, reveal strong preferences for the origin of the proteins that they sample for antigen presentation (*59*,60). The MHC-I antigen-presentation pathway in nondendritic cells is most easily thought of as an "inside-out" pathway by which protein fragments of molecules synthesized by the cell are delivered to and bound by the MHC-I molecule during its biosynthesis. Certain specialized dendritic cells can acquire exogenous antigen and present this via the MHC-I pathway. In contrast, the MHC-II antigen-presentation pathway is best visualized as both an "inside-out" pathway and an "outside-in" one, in which endogenous and ingested proteins are degraded by enzymes in the endosomal/lysosomal system and are delivered to MHC-II molecules in that degradative compartment (*12,38,61–64*). The processes of antigen processing and presentation are described in more detail elsewhere in this volume. The biochemical steps involved in the production of antigen fragments from large molecules are known collectively as "antigen-processing," whereas those that concern the binding of antigen fragments by MHC molecules and their display at the cell surface are known as "antigen-presentation."

Our understanding of the complexities of antigen processing and presentation continues to improve. Not only do we now recognize the importance of proteasome components in controlling the specificity of the degradation of proteins in the cytoplasm (*37*), we also are aware of contributions made by the chaperone tapasin (*48,65*), by ubiquitination (*37,66*), by amino-terminal trimming of peptides in the endoplasmic reticulum (ER) (67), and the role of disulfide interchange as controlled by the resident ER proteins ERp57 and/or protein disulfide isomerase (PDI) in peptide loading during MHC-I assembly (68,*69*). MHC-II peptide loading is controlled in part by the multifunctional chaperone/groove protector, Ii, as well as by the important catalytic machinery of the endosomes, molecules known as HLA-DM and -DO in the human, and H2-DM and H2-DO in the mouse (*48*).

In addition to showing preference for distinct pathways of antigen presentation, the MHC-I and MHC-II molecules also show preferential presentation to T cells of the CD8- or CD4-bearing subsets, respectively. This is related to the observation that CD8 binds to the nonpolymorphic $\alpha 3$ domain of MHC-I molecules (*70–72*,73), whereas CD4 interacts with membrane proximal domains of MHC-II (*74*,75,*76*,77,78). The CD8 and CD4 molecules serve as "coreceptors" on the surface of the T lymphocyte, providing both adhesion (avidity increase) and specific activating signals that modulate the avidity of the T cell in a time-dependent manner (*79,80*). The precise location of the site of interaction of the CD8$\alpha\alpha$ homodimer with the MHC-I $\alpha 3$ domain has been determined crystallographically for both human and murine molecules (81,82). The CD8$\alpha\beta$ molecule, expressed on peripheral T cells bearing $\alpha\beta$-TCR and on thymocytes, presumably has a similar site of interaction, but has not yet been directly visualized by structural methods. In addition, the amino-terminal two immunoglobulinlike domains of human CD4 complexed with a murine MHC-II molecule, IA^k, have been visualized crystallographically (78). The numerous interactions of MHC molecules with other cellular components as well as with the wide variety of peptides and of various immunologic receptors reflect the robust potential of the MHC structure as a molecular sensor and as a master regulator of immune responses. These molecular interactions then orchestrate different cell trafficking and signaling functions. Table 19.5 summarizes some of these interactions, emphasizing the similarities and differences between MHC-I and MHC-II molecules.

THE MAJOR HISTOCOMPATIBITY COMPLEX

Mhc Genetic Maps

The major histocompatibility complex is an extended region of the genome that spans some 4 million base pairs (Mb) on the short arm of human chromosome 6 in the

TABLE 19.5 Comparison of MHC-I and MHC-II Molecules

	MHC-Ia, Ib, and Iv	*MHC-II*
Genetics	Multiple heavy-chain loci, many linked to the MHC. Light chain, β2-m, is genetically unlinked.	Several heavy and light chain loci, α- and β-chain genes linked to each other.
Polymorphism	Highly polymorphic MHC-Ia heavy chain. Few alleles of β2m. Polymorphism of MHC-Ib and Iv variable.	β chain most polymorphic. α chain shows some allelic diversity.
Tissue-specific expression	MHC-Ia, ubiquitous. MHC-Ib on various cell subsets. MHC-Iv encoded by viruses.	MHC-II on B cells, macrophages. In human, also found on T cells and many activated cell types.
Molecular structure	Heavy chain/light chain form heterodimer. Obligate cell surface molecule. Heavy chain has three extracellular domains, α1, α2, and α3. α1/α2 form peptide-binding site. α3 and β2-m are Ig-like. Only heavy chain is membrane bound; β2-m is noncovalently assembled. (Some MHC-Ib, like MICA, not β2-m–associated; MHC-Iv may or may not be β2-m–associated.) Some MHC-Ib and MHC-Iv, unique disulfide bonds.	α and β chains form heterodimer of four domains; α1/β1 form peptide-binding site; α2 and β2 are Ig-like. Both chains are membrane-bound. Association of nascent MHC-II with invariant chain.
Site of peptide acquisition	In endoplasmic reticulum during biosynthesis. Role of Erp57 oxidoreductase in peptide loading. At cell surface when exposed to exogenous peptides.	In endosome or lysosome, where degraded products of ingested proteins are encountered; assistance of DO and DM for peptide exchange and loading.
Nature of peptides bound	MHC-Ia Preference for 8- to 10-mers; though longer peptides can be bound. "Motif" residues for particular MHC I molecules. MHC-Ib CD1 capable of binding lipid antigens. MICA, RAE-1, HL-60, MULT1, FcRn, no peptide-binding cleft. MHC-Iv m144, m153, no peptide-binding cleft.	Longer peptides are acceptable.
Rules for peptide binding	Defined termini. Anchor residues crucial.	Core motif of 9 residues may be extended variably at either N or C terminus. Anchors more subtle. Role for backbone interactions.
T-cell recognition	Primarily CD8$^+$.	Primarily CD4$^+$.
NK-cell recognition	Interaction with both NK-activating and NK-inhibitory receptors.	No known binding by NK receptors.
Associated molecules	β2-microglobulin. TAP. Tapasin. Calnexin.	Ii—invariant chain. H2-DM, (HLA-DM), H2-DO, HLA-DO.

region of 6p21.3. A recent analysis (*83*) suggests that the extended *Mhc* covers as much as 8 Mb. Although *Mhc* genes were among the first to be mapped here, it is now clear that many genes with function unrelated to immune recognition also reside in this region. The interested reader is referred to the continually updated maps and linkages available at various Web sites, including www.ebi.ac.uk/imgt/hla, and the MHC haplotype project at www.sanger.ac.uk/HGP/Chr6.

Figure 19.1 shows schematically a map of some of the major genes of the human (*84*), mouse, and rat *Mhc*, which includes those that encode MHC-I and MHC-II proteins. These comparative maps are not drawn to scale and do not show every gene identified in the region. Three markers, *Ke2*, *Bat1*, and *Mog*, serve to define the gross collinearity of the MHC of the three species (*85*), though there are clearly major differences between strains and even detectable differences between individuals within a species. *Bat1* and *Mog* define the boundaries of the MHC-I regions in all three species. The mapping and sequence information now available for the human MHC is more extensive than that available for the mouse and the rat, though

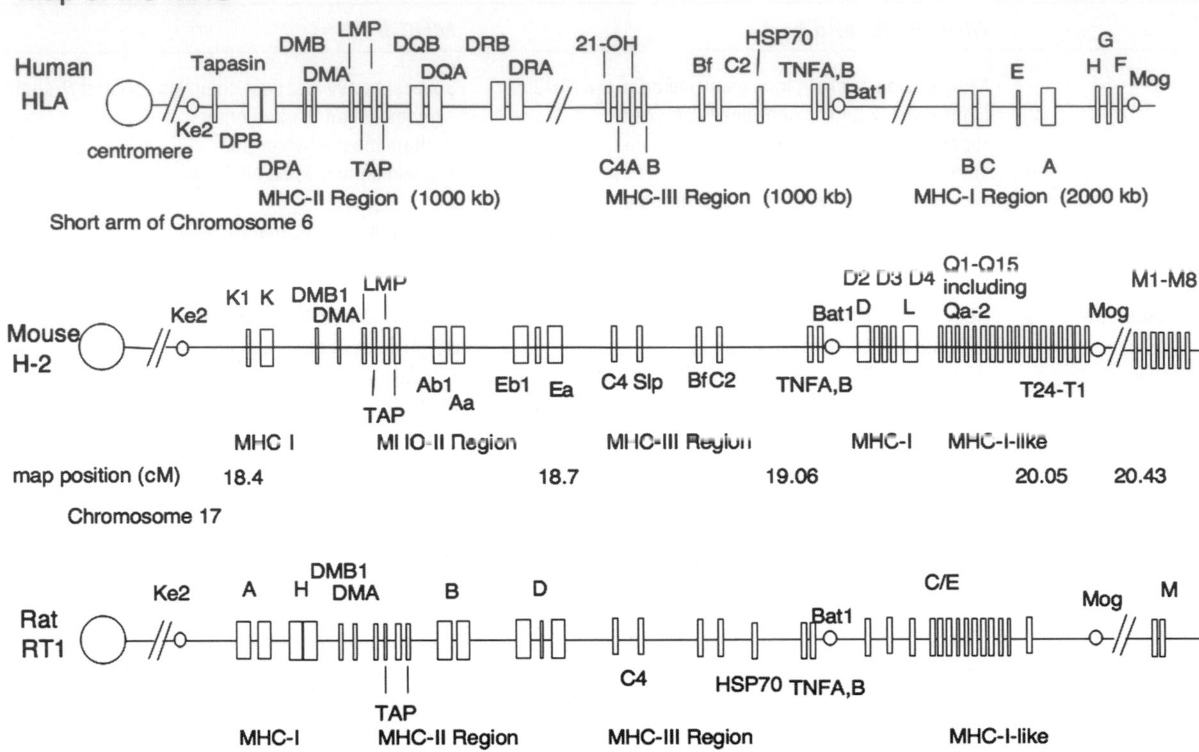

FIGURE 19.1 Genetic maps of the *Mhc*. Comparative map of the human, mouse, and rat *Mhc*. This schematic map is not complete, nor drawn to scale, and is derived from maps available elsewhere (*85,86,141,151,502–505*). The centromere and major genes are indicated.

data on these are improving rapidly. A database of the human *Mhc* is available (www.hgmp.mrc.ac.uk) (*86*). The homology of the *Mhc* region of mouse chromsome 17 to that region on human chromosome 6 can be found at www.ncbi.nlm.nih.gov/Homology, and extensive maps of syntenic regions of the human and mouse are available there.

The human MHC map reveals clusters of genes grouped roughly into an *Mhc* class II region covering about 1,000 kilobases (kb), an *Mhc* class III region of about 1,000 kb, and an *Mhc* class I region spanning 2,000 kb (Figure 19.1). *HLA-DP* genes (*DPA* encoding the α chain and *DPB* encoding the β chain) are proximal to the centromere on the short arm of the chromosome and are linked to the genes encoding the related HLA-DM molecule (*DMB* and *DMA*). Between these and the *DQ* genes lie *LMP* [for low-molecular-weight proteins (*87–90*)] and *TAP* (*91*,92–94,*95,96*) genes. *LMP* and *TAP* genes encode molecules that are involved in peptide generation in the cytosol and peptide transport across the endoplasmic reticulum membrane, respectively. LMPs are subunits of the multicatalytic proteolytic proteasome complex that regulate the specificity of cleavage of proteins and thus modulate the repertoire of peptides available for MHC-I–restricted antigen presentation (*97–100*). The *TAP* genes encode a two-chain intrinsic membrane protein that resides in the endoplasmic reticulum of all cells and functions as an ATP-dependent transporter that pumps peptides generated in the cytosol into the lumen of the ER (*101,102*). The selective transport of cytoplasmically generated peptides by different TAP proteins in the rat demonstrates that the spectrum of MHC/peptide complexes expressed at the cell surface can be significantly altered by differences in the antigen-presentation pathway (*103*,104,*105*), although there is little evidence for this phenomenon in humans (106).

The major *Mhc-II* genes of the human are *HLA-DRA* and *HLA-DRB*, which encode the chains that form the HLA-DR molecule, a major antigen-presentation element. Genetic mapping of the human DRB region now indicates that several alternative arrangements of DRB loci explain the varied serotypes and genotypes observed among different individuals (Figure 19.2). Because these are carried as sets of genes in linkage disequilibrium, they are frequently referred to as "haplotypes." The *Mhc-III* region is important in immunologic terms for several reasons—the structural genes for several complement components map here, as well as the structural genes for 21-hydroxylase (CYP21A2) (*107,108*), an enzyme that is critical to the biosynthesis of glucocorticoids, a deficiency of which can lead to the

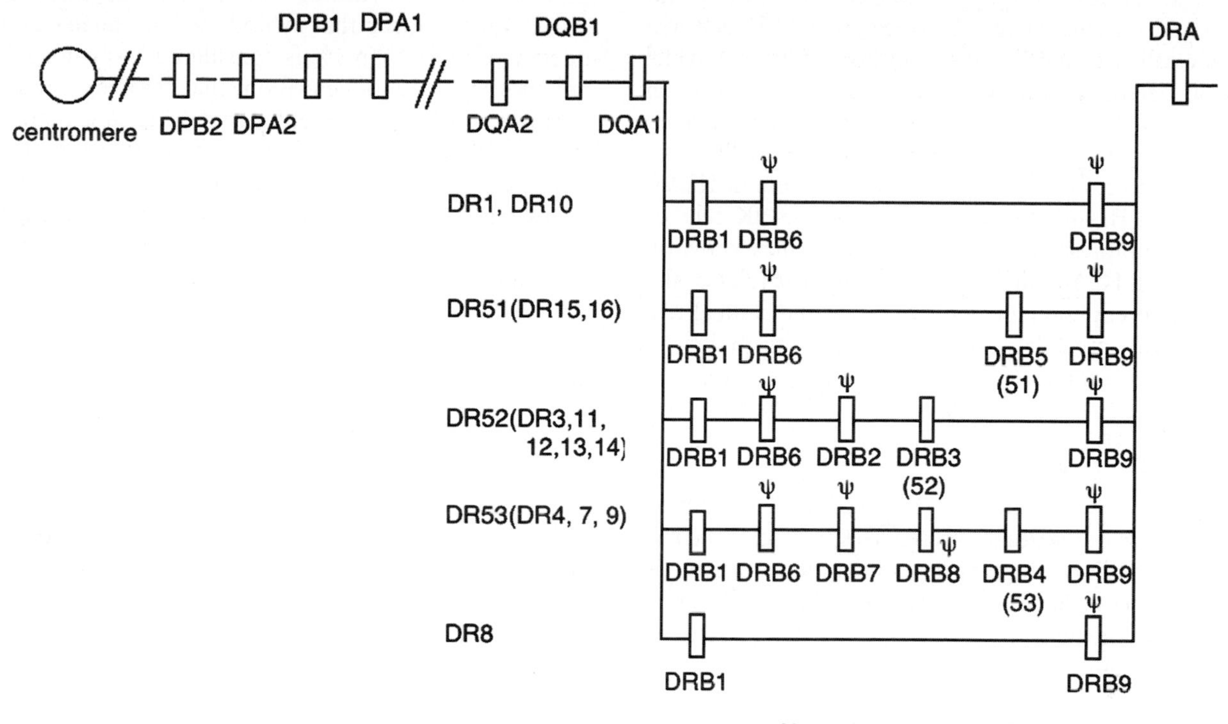

FIGURE 19.2 Genetic basis of structural variation in HLA class II haplotypes. All HLA class II haplotypes contain DPA1, DPB1, DQA1, DQB1, DRA, and DRB1 loci; however, there is variation in the number of additional DRB loci found on different haplotypes. The DRB9 pseudogene (labeled with a ψ) is common to all haplotypes; however, a DRB3 locus product is also expressed on halotypes containing any of the serologic DRB1 specificities DR3, DR5 (11,12) or DR6 (13,14). The DRB3 β chain forms a cell surface heterodimer with the DRA α-chain and creates the serologic specificity DR52. These haplotypes also contain DRB6 and DRB2 loci that are pseudogenes. The DRB5 locus is found on most haplotypes containing the serologic DRB1 specificity, DR2, but occasionally this gene product is also expressed on other DRB1 haplotypes (*506*).

genetic disease congenital adrenal hyperplasia. Also located in the *Mhc-III* region are the structural genes for tumor necrosis factors A and B (TNF-A and TNF-B), which are lymphokines made by activated T cells (*109–111*). TNF-B is also known as lymphotoxin α.

The more distal region of the *Mhc* encodes other MHC molecules. In humans, the cluster of the major *Mhc-I* genes lies here, spanning 2 Mb, including the genes encoding HLA-B, HLA-C, HLA-E, and HLA-A, as well as HLA-H, HLA-G, and HLA-F. HLA-A, HLA-B, and HLA-C are the major MHC-I molecules of humans. (A summary of the serologic and genetic identification of these is in Table 19.2). Serologic identification of HLA-C molecules has been difficult and imprecise, however, HLA-C molecules interact directly with NK receptors of the KIR2D family. Direct binding studies have analyzed the kinetics of the interaction of the KIR2 Ig-like NK receptors (*112*,113,*114*), and three-dimensional structures of KIR2DL2 in complex with HLA-Cw3 and KIR2DL1 complexed with HLA-Cw4 have been published (115,116). The precise functions of HLA-E, HLA-F, and HLA-G are not yet clear. HLA-E and its murine analog Qa-1 bind the hydrophobic leader peptides derived from some MHC-I molecules, forming a complex that is recognized by the C-type lectinlike NK receptor CD94/NKG2 (*117–121*). This implies an important function for HLA-E, because these molecules are expressed on placental trophoblast cells and would be expected to bind the inhibitory NK receptor, CD94/NKG2A, preventing NK-mediated rejection of the fetus (*122,123*). HLA-E has been shown to serve as a recognition element for some T cells as well, so it seems capable of a classical as well as a unique functional role (*120,124,125*). Some evidence now also supports an antigen-presentation function of HLA-F, and -G l (*126,127*), and the tissue-restricted expression of HLA-G as well as the observation that a soluble form leads to apoptosis of $CD8^+$ T cells suggest that this molecule may be involved in the mother's immunologic tolerance of the fetus (*128*). *HLA-H* (*129*) is a pseudogene that maps to this region. This should not be confused with the more distantly related *HLA-HFE*, an *Mhc-Ib* gene erroneously called *HLA-H* by some authors (*130,131*), which controls hereditary hemochromatosis by virtue of the interaction of its encoded protein with the transferrin receptor (*132–137*). The observations that extravillous trophoblast cells express an unusual combination of HLA-C, HLA-E, and HLA-G molecules, that uterine NK cells express NK-inhibitory receptor (KIR) molecules known to interact with HLA-C allelic products, and the relationship among different complex genotypes and the clinical relationship with pre-eclampsia all raise the possibility that not only this complex medical condition, but also important aspects of fetal rejection and clinical infertility, may be related to MHC recognition by NK cells in the placenta (138).

Comparison of the mouse, rat, and human *Mhc* maps reveals several interesting differences (*139–142*). The *Mhc* genes proximal to the centromere of the mouse and rat belong to the *Mhc-I* family, rather than to the *Mhc-II* family, as they do in the human. This mapping has suggested that an intrachromosomal recombination event that occurred in some common rodent ancestor relocated some of the *Mhc-I* genes from a more distal location to the proximal site (143). Inspection of the current human, mouse, and rat maps clearly indicates similarities in the relative locations and organization of *Mhc-II*, *Mhc-III*, and the distal *Mhc-I* genes (*141*). Various genetic expansions and contractions (144) are obvious as well. In particular, the mouse *Q* and *T* regions have expanded the pool of *Mhc-I* genes, of which there are relatively few in the human and the rat. Early studies of congenic mouse strains mapped multiple genes to the *Q* and *T* regions (145,146,*147*), and recent evidence suggests significant differences in the number of genes of this region in different strains. The mouse has some *MHC-Ib* genes that seem to be relatively unique in function. In particular, the *H2-M3* gene (not to be confused with the *Mhc-II H2-Ma* and *H2-Mb* genes, which encode the homologs of the human HLA-DMA and HLA-DMB proteins), which maps distal to the *Q* and *T* regions, encodes a protein that exhibits a preference for binding peptides that have N-formyl amino-terminal modifications. This antigen-presentation function may be geared to bacterial, protozoal, and mitochondrial antigens (*148–150*). Rat homologs of the mouse *H2-M3* and *H2-M2* genes have also been identified (*151*).

Mhc Polymorphism

The *Mhc*'s function in immune responsiveness is also reflected in its genetic polymorphism. Polymorphism is the presence at any given time of a larger than expected number of genetic variants in a population. As populations change and evolve, we expect that genetic variants should arise, but because of the selection exerted on most gene products, relatively few of these genetic variants will persist. A genetic locus that exhibits variant alleles at a frequency of more than 1% is considered "polymorphic." A polymorphic locus or gene is one that has a high frequency (not raw number) of genetic variants (1). A genetic locus that is relatively invariant is often referred to as "monomorphic," even if more than one allele is recognized. *HLA* genes exhibit a high degree of polymorphism, and a number of different mechanisms may contribute to the generation and maintenance of polymorphism. Among these are the selective advantage of a heterozygous pool of antigen-presenting elements in a given individual that might allow the binding and presentation of antigenic peptides derived from a wide variety of environmental pathogens. Limited polymorphism would make the entire population susceptible to a chance infectious agent for which all individuals would be unable to respond, whereas widespread polymorphism would be expected to allow the antigen-presenting cells of at least a proportion of the population to bind and present antigens derived from invading pathogens effectively (*152,153*). Although such a view was originally based on HLA molecules as presenting elements for pathogen-derived peptide fragments to T cells and their antigen-specific T-cell receptors, recent studies suggest an additional role for MHC-I–related resistance to viral infection via NK cell–mediated recognition (*154*,155) and altered antigen-presentation pathway (156).

The human *Mhc-I* and *Mhc-II* genes are clearly polymorphic, with more than 100 alleles at each of the *HLA-A*, *HLA-B*, and *HLA-DRB* loci identified (17,*157*) (Tables 19.2, 19.3). It is more difficult to demonstrate polymorphism in terms of population genetics in experimental animals, although typing of wild mice has confirmed the existence of natural polymorphism predicted from the analysis of inbred strains and their mutants (*158*,159). The polymorphism of *Mhc-I* and *Mhc-II* genes, so evident in human and mouse, has also been documented in analyses of cichlid fishes, animals that diverged from the line leading to mammals at least several hundred million years ago (*160–163*).

Mhc Evolutionary Mechanisms

As both an extended genetic region and a group of genes with many belonging to the immunoglobulin supergene family (164,165), the *Mhc* has served as a prototype for elucidating mechanisms that contribute to the evolution of a multigene family and that add to the polymorphism that is such a dominant characteristic of the classical MHC molecules (*142*). The analysis of mutations in the mouse, mostly those of *Mhc-I* genes, has led to the understanding of the mechanisms that give rise to polymorphism. The mutations have been identified in mice based on screening of large numbers of animals by skin grafting among siblings. Both induced and spontaneous mutations affecting skin-graft acceptance or rejection have been identified, and many of these have been mapped to the *Mhc*. Gross recombinational events have been documented in the *Mhc* (*166,167*), as well as more subtle mutations, many of which are multiple amino acid substitutions in a relatively small part of the protein that seem to derive from nonreciprocal recombinational events. Such recombination that occurs over short sequences is known as "gene conversion" because of its similarity to the phenomenon that occurs in yeast (*166,167*,168,*169,170*,171,*172,173*).

The mechanism of gene conversion in mice is now better understood because nucleotide sequence analysis and oligonucleotide-specific hybridization have been used to characterize the mutations that have occurred and the genes that serve as donors of the mutant sequences. Although the precise enzymatic details are not clear, we now understand gene conversion as a genetic event that allows the copying or transposition of short sequences from a donor gene to a recipient. Some of the polymorphisms of *Mhc* genes that have been identified clearly reflect point mutations (17). Recently, structural studies have shown that the profound immunologic effects of mutations of the *H2* genes $H2K^{bm1}$ and $H2K^{bm8}$ result from minimal detectable changes that may affect thermostability (*174*). In addition to such mouse mutants, a number of somatic cell variants and mutants, some resulting from major deletions or regulatory defects, others clearly point mutants of structural genes, have been described (*175*). An effort to identify the donor gene for the $H2K^{bm3}$, $H2K^{bm23}$, and $H2D^{bm23}$ mutations leads to the conclusion that these complex mutations must have arisen by the contribution of at least two different donor genes acting either in sequence or in synergy (*175*).

The *Mhc* and Transplantation

Although the early description of the genes of the *Mhc* was based on identification of loci involved in tumor and allograft rejection (the rejection of grafts from genetically disparate donors of the same species), and although these genes clearly play a role in such complex phenomena, a contemporary understanding of the function of *Mhc* genes in immunology requires little understanding of the rules of transplantation. The early history of transplantation is chronicled extensively in several books (1,3) and reflects a developing interest in tumor immunology and congenic mouse strains. The most extensively studied species for tumor, tissue, and organ transplantation has been the mouse, so a brief description of some relevant principles is in order. Comprehensive manuals and reviews are available (176). Propagation of a mouse strain by repeated matings of brothers and sisters leads to the establishment of an inbred strain, a group of animals that is genetically identical at all loci. More complete descriptions of the process by which brother–sister mating leads to homozygosity at all loci are given elsewhere (1,3). The probability of fixation of all loci (P_{fix}) as a function of the number of generations, n, is given by $P_{fix} = 1 - (7/8)^{n-1}$. Thus, after five generations of brother × sister matings, the probability of all loci being identical is 0.414; after 10 generations it is 0.7, after 15 generations ir is 0.85, and after 20 generations it is 0.91.

"Congenic" mouse strains, also known as "congenic resistant" or "CR" strains, are those derived by first crossing two inbred strains that differ in a histocompatibility phenotype such as resistance to a transplantable tumor or ability to reject a skin graft. These are then successively backcrossed to one parental strain, and the resistance phenotype is preserved. Following at least 10 backcross generations (N10), a point at which $(1/2)^9 = 0.002$, of the genes of the selected strain should be present, the new strain is propagated by brother × sister mating. From such breeding schemes, a number of strains critical to genetic studies of the *Mhc* have been derived. Several relevant inbred and congenic mouse strains are listed in Table 19.4 along with their *H2* designations.

The availability of numerous polymerase chain reaction (PCR)–based genetic markers throughout the mouse genome allows the direct identification of those progeny that have a greater proportion of the desired background at each generation. Selective backcrossing, taking advantage of the genotype of a large number of such genetic markers distributed widely throughout the genome, a process known as "speed congenics," can hasten the process of establishing a homogeneous background for a particular mutant or knock-in trait (*177–179*). Because strains obtained by brother × sister matings may reveal genetic drift as spontaneous mutations accumulate in the strain, it is crucial to keep track of the stock from which the animals were derived and the number of generations that they have been propagated without backcrossing to founder stock. This has been of particular concern in recent years as various lines of embryonic stem cells derived from different lines of strain 129 have been used for genetic manipulation (gene knockout experiments) (*180*), and there are clearly differences in histocompatibility (*181*).

The early rules of transplantation were determined by observation of the ability of either transplantable tumors or of allografts (usually from skin) to survive in a particular inbred mouse-strain host. The graft-rejection phenomenon is an extremely sensitive and specific bioassay that permits the detection of genetic differences as small as a single amino acid in an MHC protein. It has been particularly valuable in assessing spontaneous and induced mutants (see earlier discussion) and remains the absolute experimental discriminator of "histocompatibility."

In addition to the *Mhc* genes, we should not overlook the genes that encode minor histocompatibility antigens.

In the mouse, these were originally identified as genetic loci responsible for graft rejection after extended periods of time. More recently, several minor histocompatibility loci have been identified as those that encode polymorphic proteins that give rise to peptides presented by MHC molecules (*182–186*), and we now can understand the complexities of transplantation tolerance not only in terms of *Mhc* genes but also in terms of numerous proteins that may give rise to variant peptides for T-cell recognition. Not only can peptides derived from polymorphic genes throughout the genome serve as minor histocompatibility antigens, also defective translation products, or peptides resulting from transcription of introns or alternate coding strands of DNA may also produce immunologically significant peptides that, bound by self-MHC molecules, may stimulate T cells (187,188). Whether such defective newly synthesized proteins seve as a major source of MHC-I–bound peptides remains controversial (189). Minor antigens that are confined to hematopoietic cells can be recognized as targets by antitumor cytolytic cells and may explain the lower incidence of relapse in hematopoietic stem cell (HSC) transplant recipients who experience graft-versus-host disease (*190*).

The *Mhc* and Clinical Transplantation

Processed foreign antigen complexed to HLA class I or class II molecules is recognized by a specific clonally distributed TCR for antigen on the surface of T lymphocytes. The T cell bearing an $\alpha\beta$ receptor is capable of recognizing the unitary structure of the HLA molecule itself coordinately with the exposed parts of the peptide antigen. Corecognition of HLA and peptide antigen means that TCRs are highly specific and genetically restricted to recognizing HLA molecules of the individual from which they were derived. Thus, a killer (cytotoxic) T cell raised against an influenza virus peptide in an individual expressing HLA-A2 will not recognize influenza-infected HLA-A1. This concept is known as "MHC restriction" and was first described by Shevach and Rosenthal for recognition of alloantigens (7), by Zinkernagel and Doherty (8) for recognition of viral antigens, and by Shearer for recognition of altered self-ligands (6). Given that T cells are MHC-restricted, it is difficult to understand why they should ever recognize a foreign HLA type. However, in practice they do, and data indicate that such alloreactive T cells arise with remarkably high frequency. Estimates of between 1/10 to 1/1,000 activated clonally distinct T cells are capable of responding to any random allogeneic HLA molecule (*191–194*). Given the number of T cells in the human lymphoid system, this represents a striking tendency for T cells that are normally restricted to recognizing self-HLA molecules complexed to foreign peptides to cross-react on allogeneic HLA molecules. This cross-reaction can arise from direct recognition of the allogeneic HLA/peptide complex, which usually depends on the peptide antigen as well as the allogeneic HLA molecule. Alternatively, allorecognition by T cells can occur indirectly (*195,196*). In such cases, peptides derived from the allogeneic HLA molecules are presented as nominal antigen after processing by the host cells bearing self-HLA molecules. In the normal course of events, T-cell alloreactivity is an in vitro curiosity, although it is still not entirely clear why the fetal "allograft" does not stimulate the maternal immune system. However, it is the clinical transplantation of organs and hematopoietic stem cells across HLA compatibility barriers that produces graft rejection or graft-versus-host disease due to T-cell alloreactivity. Fully allogeneic transplants theoretically expose the recipient immune system to up to 12 non–self-HLA allele products expressed by the allograft. Moreover, the "self-peptides" constitutively presented by allogeneic HLA molecules are likely to be quite distinct from those presented by syngeneic HLA molecules, because the polymorphisms of the peptide antigen-binding cleft of the MHC-I molecule that distinguish HLA alleles alter the spectrum of selected peptides. Allogeneic HLA/peptide complexes probably stimulate powerful T-cell responses because of the high density of unusual determinants and the diversity of new peptide ligands presented by the allogeneic HLA/peptide complexes. Because there are many MHC-linked genes encoding a host of proteins, many lacking known immunologic function, it is likely that polymorphisms in these molecules contribute significantly to the alloresponse (see earlier discussion of *Mhc* genetic maps). Accordingly, many studies have demonstrated an incremental improvement in long-term graft survival with progressively higher levels of HLA matching at HLA-A, -B, and -DR loci. For this reason, HLA matching is essential in allogenic HSC transplantation, and highly desirable in solid-organ transplantation. The degree of HLA matching usually required for renal transplantation is shown in Figure 19.3 and for bone marrow transplantation in Table 19.6. The effect of HLA matching on solid-organ transplantation has been monitored by the Collaborative Transplant Study since 1982 (see www.ctstransplant.org/public/introduction.html).

In addition to the allogeneic cellular response, the antibody response to HLA molecules and ABO blood groups can also cause rejection of certain grafts, especially where these antibodies are preformed and therefore present at the time of organ transplantation. Antibodies to ABO blood-group antigens react with these determinants on vascular endothelium, and therefore ABO-incompatible solid organs can be rapidly rejected by humoral mechanisms. In patients who have been transfused or previously transplanted, or in multiparous females, exposure to allogeneic HLA molecules can also result in the production of anti-HLA class I antibodies. These preformed antibodies can lead to acute and hyperacute rejection of grafts expressing the particular HLA molecules recognized by these

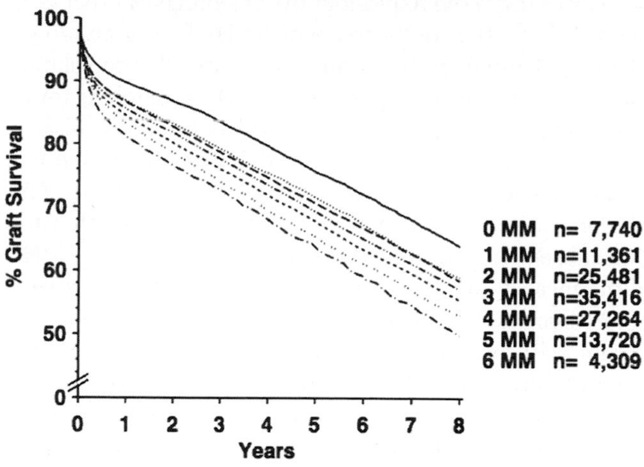

FIGURE 19.3 Renal graft survival improves with fewer HLA mismatches. Cumulative data for graft survival are plotted as a function of time. Curves represent those groups with the indicated number of mismatches. From the Collaborative Transplant Study, www.ctstransplant.org/public/introduction.html.

antibodies. Therefore for solid-organ transplants, individuals are not only matched as closely as possible for their HLA types to avert cellular rejection, it is also necessary to ensure ABO compatibility and to exclude preformed antidonor HLA antibodies in the host.

Paradoxically, some patients who have received multiple blood transfusions prior to transplantation appear to develop some form of T-cell tolerance to allogeneic donor HLA alleles, and renal graft survival is actually enhanced in these individuals. This is known as the "transfusion effect," and in some centers, pretransplant transfusion and even donor-specific transfusions are routinely carried out. Transfusion of potential renal transplant recipients carries the risk, however, of inducing undesirable anti-HLA antibodies in the patient.

Testing for anti-HLA antibodies is known as the "crossmatch." In practice, many laboratories crossmatch only for anti-HLA class I antibodies. Crossmatch compatibility to exclude anti-HLA class I antibodies is essential in renal transplantation and is widely practiced in heart/lung transplantation. Crossmatching for liver transplantation is practiced at only some centers, and the evidence that a positive crossmatch predicts allogeneic liver graft rejection has not convinced everyone of its importance in routine matching. Patients awaiting renal transplantation are usually monitored regularly for anti-HLA class I antibodies, because the level and specificity of these antibodies can change with time. This monitoring involves regular crossmatching of patient serum against a panel of randomly selected cells bearing different HLA types. The percentage of positively reacting cells is known as the "panel reactivity." When carrying out a crossmatch between a patient's serum and donor cells, many centers test the current as well as "historical peak" serum from the patient. The "historical peak" is defined as the patient serum sample giving the highest panel reactivity throughout the monitoring period and is thought to be a sensitive reflection of previous HLA sensitization. Many centers now prescreen patients on transplant waiting lists for anti-HLA antibodies using MHC-coated beads as a source of antigen and a highly sensitive flow cytometry technology for their detection. In highly sensitized patients with multiple host antidonor antibodies, these unwanted antibodies can sometimes be functionally eliminated using B-cell ablation therapies (anti-CD20 mAb), plasmapharesis, and intravenous gamma-globulin infusions, thus allowing successful transplantation.

The role of antibody crossmatching in allogeneic HSC transplantation is less clear, and many centers do not take the class I or class II crossmatch into account when

TABLE 19.6 MHC Matching versus Success of Bone Marrow Transplantation

MHC Compatibility	*Risk of Graft Rejection (%)*	*Risk of Acute Graft-versus-Host-Disease (%)*	*Survival (3 y) (%)*
Share two haplotypes (HLA-identical sibling)	2	40	50
Share one haplotype plus:			
Phenotypically identical	7	40	50
1 HLA mismatch	9	70	50
>2 HLA mismatches	21	80	15
Share zero haplotypes (unrelated):			
"Matched"	3	80	35
"Mismatched"	5	95	35

Source: From (*476*).

identifying a bone marrow transplant donor. On the other hand, some large centers place considerable importance on a positive crossmatch as a predictor of bone marrow rejection, and it is therefore advisable to crossmatch bone marrow donor–recipient pairs when there is a high risk of rejection (e.g., aplastic anemia). Crossmatching is also used to detect anti-HLA antibodies that caused refractoriness to platelet transfusion with random platelets.

Family Studies in Histocompatibility Testing

The linkage of HLA loci on chromosome 6 means that individuals will usually inherit a set of nonrecombined HLA alleles encoded at linked HLA loci from each parent. This set of genes (the haplotype) is often identifiable in family studies, where all the alleles present on one chromosome cosegregate. In identifying donors for hematopoietic stem cell transplantation, testing of family members is essential to determine haplotypes accurately (*197,198*). This is because sharing of HLA antigens from different haplotypes is quite common in families, so mismatches within HLA subtypes (i.e., allele-level mismatches) are easily overlooked as a result of mistaken haplo-identity of siblings or other family members. Because unrecognized HLA mismatching is poorly tolerated in hematopoietic stem cell transplantation, high-resolution sequence-based DNA matching (or its equivalent) is required to avoid graft-versus-host disease (*199–201*). Although allogeneic HSC transplantation can be carried out across single-locus mismatches, there is little correlation with the magnitude of a given mismatch and the subsequent immune response. Donor–recipient MHC differences of just a single amino acid can provoke strong alloresponses comparable to reactions between vastly different MHC products (*202*). An example of haplotyping in a family study is shown in Figure 19.4. Added complexity of the kinds of cell surface molecules that are expressed as a result of the codominant expression of molecules encoded by the human MHC-I and MHC-II loci is illustrated in Figure 19.5.

The role of HLA-DP in allogeneic stem cell transplantation is still unclear, so testing for this locus is not

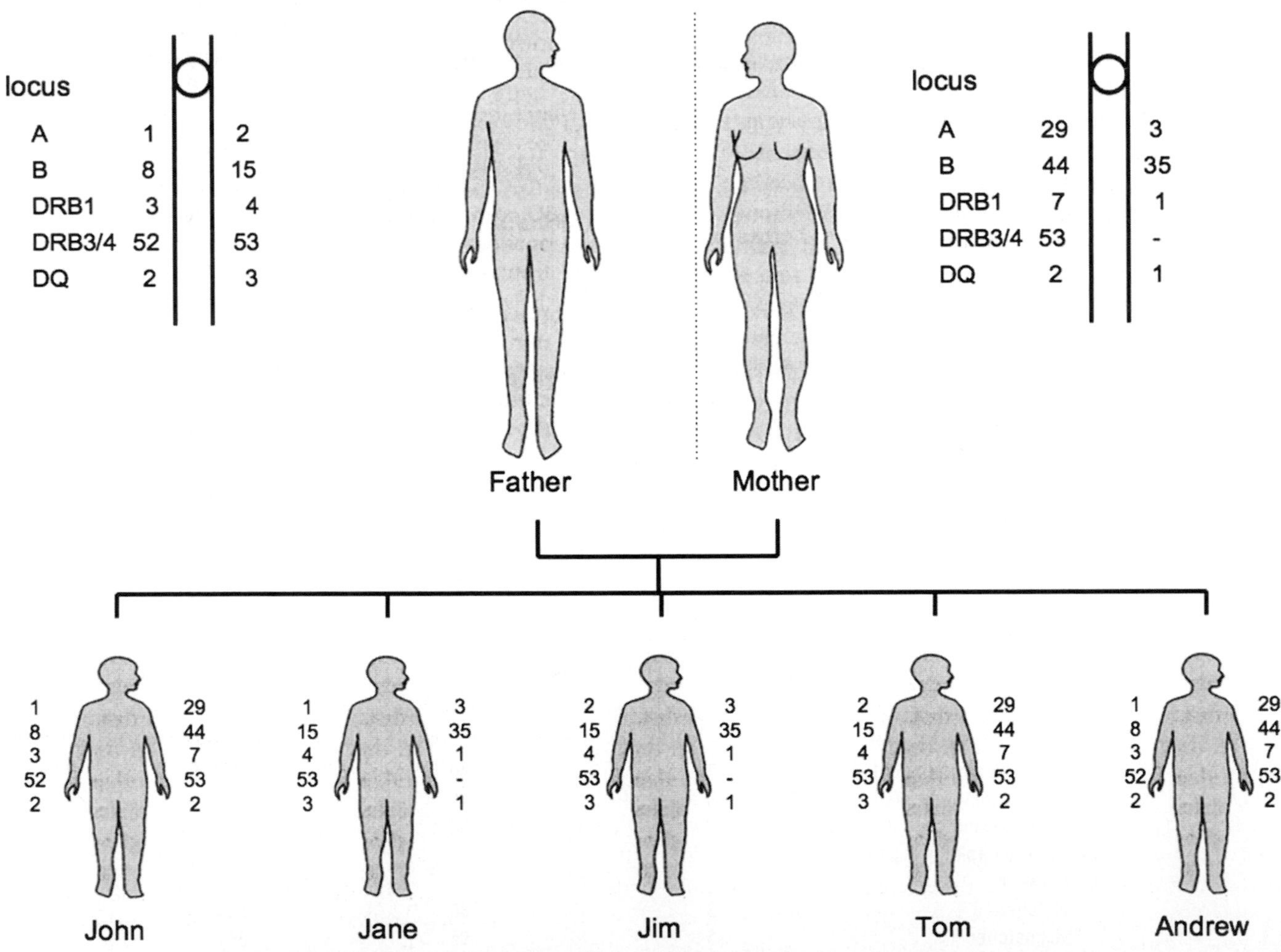

FIGURE 19.4 Segregation of HLA haplotypes in a family. From (*507*), with permission.

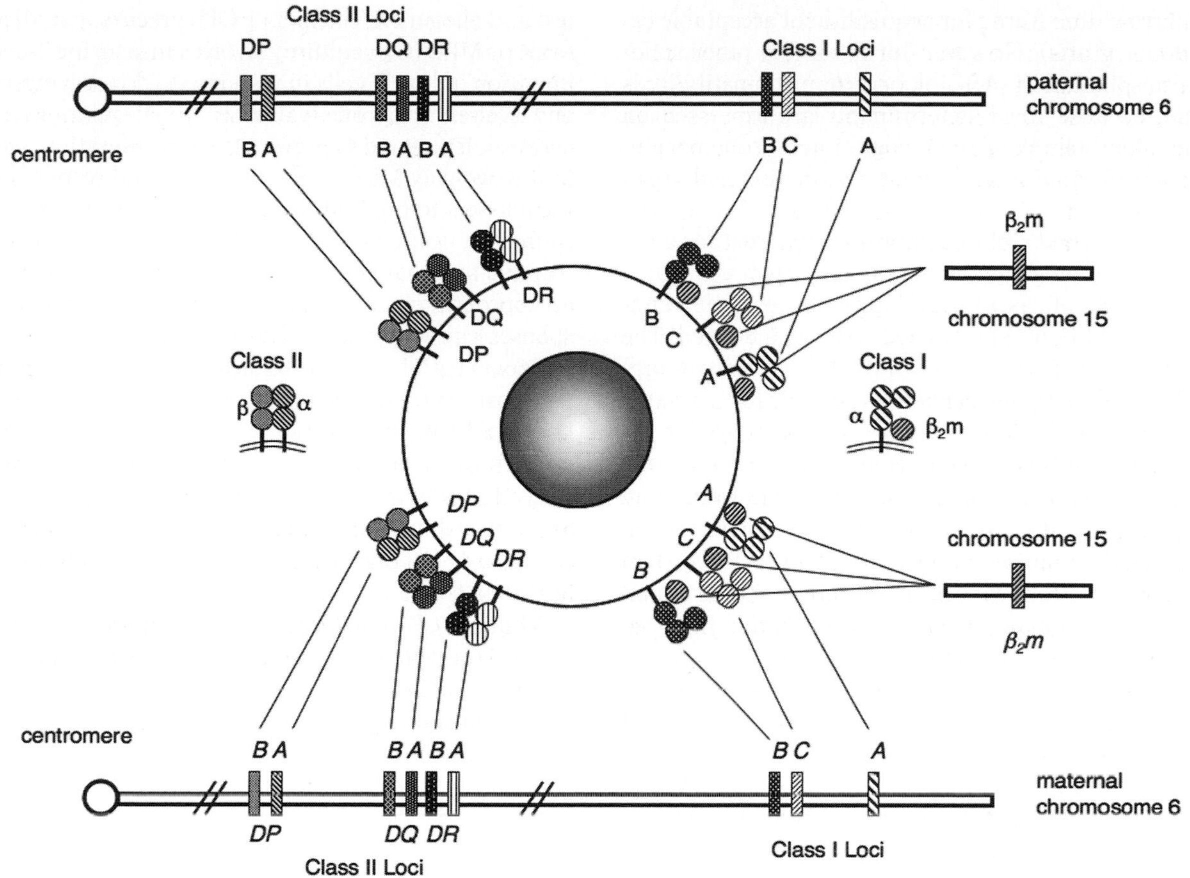

FIGURE 19.5 Codominant expression of HLA gene products encoded by the major histocompatibility complex. The *HLA-A, -B,* and *-C* class I loci, and the linked *HLA-DR, -DQ,* and *-DP* class II loci are located the short arm of chromosome 6 (6p21), and the class I light-chain locus, *β2M,* is encoded on chromosome 15. HLA genes and their respective proteins are shaded to reflect the different loci encoding these proteins and the inheritance of different alleles from the two parental chromosomes. The separate HLA class II α- and β-chain loci are also shown. The products of both maternal and paternal chromosomes are codominantly expressed on the surface of antigen-presenting cells, resulting in expression of up to six distinct class I allotypes. The number of expressed class II gene products can be even greater, because some haplotypes have extra DRB loci that produce additional β chains capable of assembling with DRα. In addition, pairing of certain DQα molecules from the DQA locus encoded on one chromosome, with DQβ chains derived from the other chromosome, can result in expression of new DQ cis–trans isotypes. The HLA class I and class II loci are separated by the class III region of the major histocompatibility complex (not shown). HLA class II molecules are constitutively expressed only on B cells, macrophages, and dendritic cells, whereas class I molecules are found on nearly all nucleated cell types.

routinely carried out clinically except when several donors are available and a rational choice of the best donor has to be made (*203,204*). [Note that some recent studies suggest a contribution of HLA-DP to graft success in both stem cell and renal transplantation (*205,206*)]. Typically, an HLA typing laboratory will test for HLA-A, -B, -DRB1, -DRB3, -DRB4, -DRB5, and -DQ loci (207). In the family study shown in Figure 19.4, the mother and father are mismatched at both haplotypes. Among the children, John and Andrew are haploidentical (and therefore phenotypically identical). Jane and Jim share a single haplotype, as do Tom and Jim. Jane's paternal haplotype is a recombinant involving a crossover event between HLA-A and -B. Recombination is observed between HLA-A/B and HLA-B and HLA-DR in about 1% of meiotic events. The implications of this family study are that Andrew and John would be ideal bone marrow donors for each other. However, none of the other siblings would be suitable as a donor for these brothers. Even though there is sharing of a single haplotype between Tom and both Andrew and John, the complete mismatch in the second haplotype would make Tom unsuitable as a donor for hematopoietic stem cell transplantation, which requires very close matching of HLA. On the other hand, haplotype mismatching is common in renal transplantation, in which perfect HLA matching is not absolutely required or routinely achievable (because of the narrow time frame for acquisition of acceptable cadaver donor grafts). However, for renal and other solid-organ transplantation, ABO blood group compatibility is essential, because these determinants are expressed on vascular endothelium, where recognition by isohemagglutinins leads to rapid intravascular coagulation and organ failure.

When a matched sibling donor does not exist for a patient requiring allogeneic hematopoietic stem cell transplantation (70% of cases), searching of the extended family or unrelated bone marrow registries is indicated. The National Marrow Donor Panel (NMDP; www.marrow.org) has several million potential donors suitable for unrelated stem cell transplantation, and these donors are used in the United States and worldwide. Bone marrow donor registries also exist in Europe, Australia, Hong Kong, and Japan, and these registries often provide donors for patients in other parts of the world. Mobilization of stem cells in the blood following administration of hematopoietic growth factors is now widely used to avoid the need for marrow collections from donors.

Cord blood banks have also been established around the world (*208,209*,210). However, cord blood donation of stem cells is often unsuitable for adult transplantation because of limitations in the volume of cord blood collections. Cord bloods offer the advantage of finding donors faster than adult unrelated registries (*211*) and theoretically providing banked stem cells from ethnic minority groups that are not well represented in bone marrow donor registries (*212*). Cord blood transplants induce less graft-versus-host disease than bone marrow or peripheral blood stem cell transplants, but posttransplant engraftment is slower (*213*).

Functional Tests of HLA Compatibility

Testing for HLA identity at all HLA loci is a daunting task for most laboratories because of the very large number of alleles present in the population. Moreover, in renal transplantation, some mismatches appear to be well tolerated and are associated with long-term graft survival, whereas other mismatches of similar genetic disparity are poorly tolerated and are associated with early rejection (*214*). Reliable methods for predicting these "taboo" mismatches are not readily available. Similarly, high-resolution HLA typing does not predict all graft-versus-host disease (GVHD) when selecting suitable unrelated donors for hematopoietic stem cell transplantation (*200,215*). Therefore, there has been a great deal of interest in developing functional or in vitro cellular tests of overall donor–recipient compatibility. Unfortunately, none of the tests so far developed provides convincing predictability of impending graft rejection or, more important, GVHD. Among the tests used historically for assessing functional compatibility are the mixed lymphocyte reactivity (MLR) test and allogeneic T-helper or CTL precursor studies. The MLR or MLC (C = culture) involves measuring T-cell proliferation of host T cells in response to donor lymphocytes and vice versa. In a one-way MLR, the stimulating lymphocytes are irradiated to prevent their proliferation; whereas in the two-way MLR, both stimulator and responder cells are allowed to proliferate. In MLR studies, it is necessary to include controls showing that responder cells can all respond and that stimulator cells can all stimulate across an appropriate barrier such as third-party donor cells. Responses can vary widely, and individual laboratories use their own cutoff values to define negative (i.e., nonreactive) and positive (reactive) MLR results (*215*). Unfortunately, known HLA mismatches can be present in a negative MLR, and a positive MLR can be obtained between phenotypically HLA-identical individuals. Because the MLR is biased toward measuring HLA class II discrepancies and is notoriously irreproducible (*215*), many laboratories have abandoned this test in favor of implementation of high-resolution PCR-based HLA class II typing.

Measurement of allogeneic CTL or helper T-cell precursor frequencies is carried out at specialized bone marrow transplant centers but is not universally accepted as being predictive of GVHD (*216,217*). The test is labor-intensive and requires a skilled technician for reproducibility. Precursor frequencies are estimated by limiting dilution analysis or Elispot of donor-versus-host lymphocytes (i.e., T cells expected to cause GVHD). High precursor frequencies (up to 1 in 10^4 cells) are thought to be associated with a greater risk of acute GVHD (*218*). It is possible that precursor studies detect major and minor incompatibilities and so, theoretically, they might give a broad measure of the transplant barrier, but technical improvements will be required before this test is widely adopted in clinical practice (*219*).

The *Mhc* and Disease

In addition to the control of transplant acceptance or rejection and immune responsiveness, the *Mhc* in the human plays an important role in the etiology of a number of diseases, many of which are autoimmune in nature (144,220–222). Several human diseases are associated with the *Mhc* class III genes, because some of the structural genes for enzymes involved in the adrenal steroid biosynthetic pathway (i.e., 21-hydroxylase, CYP21A2) map to this region. More than 40 diseases have well-established genetic linkages to the *Mhc* (144,221,222,*223*); the most important are summarized in Table 19.7. Recent genome-wide association studies confirm the importance of the HLA-DRB1 locus in rheumatoid arthritis and type 1 diabetes (224). The precise mechanisms underlying the association of most of these diseases with the particular *Mhc* haplotypes are unknown, but several models have been proposed, including the cross-reactivity of antimicrobial antibodies

TABLE 19.7 Some HLA Disease Associations

Disease	MHC-I	Strength of Association[a]
Ankylosing spondylitis	HLA-B27	+++
Reiter disease	HLA-B27	++
Psoriasis	HLA-Cw6	+
Abacavir drug hypersensitivity	HLA-B*5701	+++
Behcet disease	HLA-B51	+
Birdshot retinopathy	HLA-A29	+++
	MHC-II	
Narcolepsy	HLA-DQB1*0602	++
Insulin-dependent diabetes mellitus	HLA-DQ8	++
	HLA-DQ2	+
	HLA-DR2	−
Rheumatoid arthritis	HLA-DR4	+
Celiac disease	HLA-DQ2	+++
	HLA-DQ8	+
Multiple sclerosis	HLA-DR2	+

[a] +++ = very strong association that is clinically useful as a diagnostic tool.
++ = strong association with likely primary involvement in disease pathogenesis.
+ = clear association with likely role in disease pathogenesis.
− = negative or protective influence on disease probability.
For a more detailed summary of MHC and disease associations, see (144).

with particular MHC molecules (*225*) and the molecular mimicry of viral antigens that might induce T-cell responses to self-antigens (226,*227–232*). The very high incidence of some diseases associated with certain *HLA* genes assists in the diagnosis as well as the counseling of patients and their families. Several of these diseases are of particular note. Because virtually 100% of patients with narcolepsy have *HLA-DQB1*0602* (associated with *HLA-DR2*) (*233,234*), HLA typing can be used as a test of disease exclusion. Thus, a diagnosis of narcolepsy can be excluded with reasonable certainty if the patient does not have HLA-DQB1*0602. On the other hand, the presence of HLA-DQB1*0602 is of little predictive value in diagnosis of narcolepsy, because this HLA type is relatively common in many populations and occurs frequently in the absence of disease.

Ankylosing spondylitis is so strongly associated with the *Mhc-I* allele *HLA-B27* and the presence of some bacterial pathogens that it is a popular hypothesis that ankylosing spondylitis is due to the stimulation of particular T cells by HLA-B27–presented bacterial antigens that cross react on self-tissues. These T cells are then thought to initiate an inflammatory cascade. Despite the strong association of HLA with spondyloarthropathy, critical evaluation of the literature brings a postinfectious etiology into question, and certainly more studies are indicated (*235*). The tendency of HLA-B27 to form disulfide-linked covalent dimers raises the question whether the resulting cellular pathology related to poor cell surface expression of this MHC-I molecule may be related to the inflammation of joints that is characteristic of this disease (236,*237*).

Hereditary hemochromatosis (HH) is one of the most common genetic disorders in Caucasian populations (with a prevalence of 1/300 to 1/400), and the gene controlling this condition (HFE) is MHC-linked, mapping approximately 3Mb telomeric to the HLA-A locus (*134*). The HFE protein is a class I–like molecule, the structure of which is now solved (*238*,239). The HFE protein assembles with β2m and is expressed in the intestinal mucosa and placenta, where it plays a role in regulating iron uptake and transport (*240,241*). Mice that are homozygous for an induced defect of β2m as well as those with targeted inactivation of the *HFE* gene suffer from iron overload, hemochromatosis (*242*) (*515–517*), although there are mutations at loci other than β2m or *HFE* that also lead to the same disease phenotype (*137*). HFE regulates the affinity of the transferrin receptor for transferrin, resulting in an alteration of the efficiency of iron transport. The most common molecular defect associated with hereditary hemochromatosis involves a point mutation that results in a Cys282Tyr substitution in the α3 domain of this class I–like molecule (*134*). This mutation accounts for >80% of patients with hereditary hemochromatosis (*243*). The disruption of the disulfide bond in the α3 domain at this site prevents efficient folding of the molecule and impairs assembly with β2m, resulting in improper HFE protein expression. This leads to a failure to downregulate the affinity of the transferrin receptor for its ligand, transferrin, presumably causing increased iron uptake by cells and tissue damage as a result of iron overload. A second common *HFE* mutation, 187G, results in a His63Asp substitution and a very slight increase in susceptibility to developing hereditary hemochromatosis, depending on the genotype of the individual (*244*). Incomplete penetrance of even the high-risk Cys282Tyr *HFE* genotypes can be partly explained by natural iron deficiency from limited dietary intake and menstrual losses in women.

As summarized in Table 19.7 and discussed earlier, there are a number of autoimmune diseases associated with particular alleles of HLA class II loci, especially with DR and DQ (*245*). These diseases include type 1 (insulin dependent) diabetes mellitus, rheumatoid arthritis, multiple sclerosis, systemic lupus erythematosus, thyrogastric autoimmunity, Sjogren syndrome, and many others. Rheumatoid arthritis is strongly associated with HLA-DR4 subtypes that share a common sequence motif within the DRβ chain (*246*), suggesting preferential antigen presentation of self-epitopes by these molecules. The relative risk of severe rheumatoid arthritis is increased in DR4 homozygotes, particularly compound heterozygotes with high-risk alleles (*247,248*), indicating a gene dose effect in susceptibility to autoimmune inflammation.

Although the number of different *HLA* class I and class II alleles that are associated with insulin-dependent diabetes mellitus (type 1 diabetes) clearly indicates that this relatively common disease has a complex etiology, the identification of a novel *Mhc-II* haplotype in the mutant NOD (nonobese diabetic) mouse (*249–253*), and the recognition that particular TCRs can mediate disease (*254*), suggest that a cross-reactive response to a common self- or environmental antigen may play an important role in the etiology of this disease as well. In human type 1 diabetes, the incidence of disease is significantly increased in Caucasians with *HLA-DR3-DQ2* and *DR4-DQ8* haplotypes (*255,256*). These haplotypes impart a synergistically increased relative risk when they occur as a heterozygous combination compared to the risk of disease conferred by either haplotype alone (*245,255,256*). This raises the possibility of trans-complementation of *HLA-DQ* gene products producing new molecules involved in antigen presentation (*257*). Analysis of large cohorts of patients in genome-wide marker studies offers a promising approach to identify additional genetic factors that act synergistically with HLA-allelic linkages in raising the odds of disease susceptibility (224). Online genomic maps and correlations of associations with particular loci further augments our ability to understand the relative contributions of MHC-linked and unlinked genes in autoimmune diseases such as type 1 diabetes (*258*).

In addition to recent progress in recognizing *Mhc* associations with a variety of autoimmune and immune deficiency conditions, further analysis has identified relationships of HLA-linked markers with susceptibility and prognosis in a number of infectious diseases. Among the most striking has been the recognition that delayed progression of HIV infection to acquired immunodeficiency syndrome (AIDS) correlates with possession of HLA-B Bw4 alleles that express a molecule with isoleucine at position 80 along with a gene for the NK-cell receptor KIR3DS1. This observation suggested that KIR3DS1 offered protection early in HIV infection for those patients bearing the appropriate Bw4 allele (155). More recent observations indicate that patients with such a KIR3DS1/Bw4 ile80 genotype also exhibit resistance to late opportunistic infections (*259*). Other studies now show that particular *HLA-DRB* alleles as well as *MHC-I* alleles significantly influence hepatitis B and C virus susceptibility, persistence, and response to treatment (*260*).

Mutations at the *H2* Locus

Mutations at the *H2* locus have been identified in animals screened by skin grafting in extensive experiments carried out over a 25-year period (*261,262*). By grafting tail skin of siblings to and from each other, spontaneous or induced mutant animals that displayed either a "gain," "loss," or "gain plus loss" transplantation phenotype were identified. Gain mutants are those that express a new transplantation antigen—thus, their skin is rejected by their nonmutant siblings; loss mutants have lost a transplantation antigen—thus, they recognize the skin of their siblings as foreign and reject that graft. Gain-plus-loss mutations give effects in both directions—they reject the skin of their siblings, and their skin is rejected by their siblings as well. In a classic series of experiments over an extended period of time, Melvold, Kohn, and their colleagues screened a large number of mouse progeny. Both homozygous inbred and F1 animals were examined, yielding a total of 25 *H2* mutations identified at *K*, *D*, *L*, and *Ab* loci, and an additional 80 mutations of non-*H2* histocompatibility genes. Although earlier studies suggested that all *H2* genes might be hypermutable, a more complete retrospective evaluation of the available data suggests that with the exception only of the $H2K^b$ gene, the spontaneous mutation rate for *H2* genes was comparable to that for non-*H2* genes. The characterization of these mutant animals, first based on peptide maps and amino acid sequences of the H2 proteins (*263,264*,265,266), later based on the nucleotide sequences of the cloned cDNAs or genes (171), provided some of the basic biochemical information on which later studies of structure and function and mechanism of gene evolution were based. Recently, x-ray structure determination of the H2-K^{bm1} and H2-K^{bm8} mutants suggest explanations for the differences in T-cell recognition that result from what might appear to be subtle amino acid substitutions (*174*).

Expression of MHC Molecules

MHC molecules, synthesized in the endoplasmic reticulum and destined for cell surface expression, are controlled at many checkpoints before their final disposition as receptors available for interaction with either T cells or NK cells. The MHC-I molecules should be viewed as trimers, consisting of the polymorphic heavy chain, the light-chain β2m, and the assembled self-peptide. A number of steps in biosynthesis and expression are inhibited by virus-encoded proteins. The first level of control of MHC-I expression is genetic; that is, the genes for a particular chain or key components of the peptide loading complex must be present for the trimer to be expressed. This is particularly relevant for β2m, which is the obligate light chain for the complex. Induced β2m-defective animals (*B2m*$^{o/o}$) (267,268) lack normal levels of MHC-I expression. The next level of MHC-I expression control is transcriptional, and interferon-γ (IFN-γ)-dependent regulation is particularly important (*269*). For the most part, MHC-Ia molecules are ubiquitously expressed, and expression is dependent on a complex trans-regulatory process that coordinately controls the transcription of both MHC-I and β2m (*270–272*). The basis of the more limited tissue-specific expression of MHC-Ib molecules is of interest because of the potential importance in the role of some of the MHC-Ib molecules in tolerance to the placenta. HLA-E and HLA-G, expressed on placenta, and HLA-F, another MHC-Ib with limited tissue-specific expression, have been examined in considerable detail (*273–277*). The rest of the MHC-I biosynthetic pathway is dependent on proper generation of cytosolic peptides by the proteasome and delivery to the endoplasmic reticulum by TAP, appropriate core glycosylation in the ER, transport through the Golgi, and arrival at the plasma membrane (*278*). A number of persistent viruses have evolved mechanisms for subverting this pathway of expression (*279*). The herpes simplex virus encodes a protein, infected cell peptide 47 (ICP47) (*280–282*), that blocks the activity of the peptide transporter TAP (*283*). Several proteins encoded by the human cytomegalovirus (HCMV), unique short-region proteins 2 and 11 (US2 and US11), cause rapid protein degradation of MHC-I molecules (*284*). Another HCMV protein, unique long-region protein 18 (UL18), which has sequence similarity to MHC-I molecules, may affect normal MHC-I function by limiting β2m availability. The biologic effect may be related to functional inhibition of NK recognition of viral-infected cells (*285–288*). Other molecules that assist the large DNA viruses in evading either the T-cell or NK-cell immune response include HCMV UL142 (*289*). Murine cytomegalovirus (290) encodes a number of open reading frames considered MHC-I homologs that may function to deceive NK cells into the perception of normal MHC-I expression (291,*292,293*). Adenovirus 2 (*294,295*) also has genes that function in blocking the transfer of folded assembled MHC-I molecules from the ER to the Golgi.

MHC-II molecules are also susceptible to regulation at multiple steps. The clear-cut tissue dependence of MHC-II expression—MHC-II molecules are generally found on cells that have specific antigen-presentation functions, such as macrophages, dendritic cells, Langerhans cells, thymic epithelial cells, and B cells, and can also be detected on activated T cells of the human and rat—suggests that transcriptional regulation plays an important role. Extensive studies of the promoter activities of *Mhc-II* genes have defined a number of specific transcriptional regulatory sequences (*296*), and one transcriptional activator, MHC class II transcriptional activator (CIITA) clearly plays a major role (*270,296–298*). Considerations of differential expression of MHC-II molecules in different tissues, MHC-II deficiency diseases known as "bare lymphocyte syndromes" (*298,299*,300,*301,302*,303), and current views of the role of the balance of Th1 and Th2 T-lymphocyte subsets, have led to a provocative hypothesis that suggests that the contribution of MHC-II differential expression and the resulting balance of Th1- and Th2-derived lymphokines are critical in the control of autoimmune disease (159,304,*305,306*).

A unique aspect of MHC-II regulation is the need to protect its peptide-binding site from loading of self-peptides in the ER, and the requirement to traffic to an acidic endosomal compartment where antigenic peptides, the products of proteolytic digestion of exogenous proteins, can be obtained. These two functions are provided by the type II membrane protein, invariant chain, Ii (40,*307–309*), which forms a nine-subunit complex (consisting of three Ii and three $\alpha\beta$ MHC-II heterodimers). The region of Ii that protects the MHC-II peptide-binding groove, CLIP, is progressively trimmed from Ii, and is ultimately released from the MHC-II by the catalytic action of HLA-DM in the endosome to allow exchange for peptides generated there. HLA-DO regulates the repertoire of bound peptides, presumably by modulating the catalytic activity of the DM exchange reaction. The important role of Ii in regulating MHC-II expression has been emphasized by the behavior of induced mutant mice lacking normal Ii (*310–312*), which exhibit a profound defect in MHC-II function and expression.

STRUCTURE OF MHC MOLECULES

There is nothing that living things do that cannot be understood from the point of view that they are made of atoms acting according to the laws of physics.

RICHARD FEYNMAN (*313*)

So central are *Mhc* genes and their encoded molecules to both the regulation and the effector function of the immune system that it has been apparent almost since their discovery that an understanding of their structure and structural interactions would be fundamental to a comprehension of their physiologic effects. Structural relationships of MHC molecules came first from understanding serologic differences, then from cellular immunologic analysis, and subsequently from biochemical studies of the MHC-I and MHC-II chains. Amino acid sequence comparisons suggested a domain structure for the MHC-I molecules. With the identification of first cDNA and then genomic clones of those genes encoding MHC molecules, it became routine to determine the encoded protein sequences of a large number of molecules. We now have available high-resolution three-dimensional structures of >200 different MHC/peptide, MHC/peptide/TCR, MHC/peptide/coreceptor, and MHC/peptide/NK receptor complexes that allow an understanding of the function of these molecules in a detailed structural context (314). The details of these structures also pose a number of questions that may only be addressed by additional functional experiments in whole animals complemented by biophysical methods applied in vitro. The molecular biologic, functional, and structural studies have led to the development of the use of MHC multimers as extremely powerful tools for imaging specific T cells as well as NK cells. The goal of this section of this chapter is to summarize these developments with an eye toward explanation of function by structure, and in hopes of revealing some of the current quandaries that continue to confound our understanding of the function of the *Mhc*.

Amino Acid Sequences—Primary Structure

Before the cloning of *Mhc* genes, the biochemical purification and amino acid sequence determination of the human MHC-I molecules, HLA-A2 and HLA-B7, and of the mouse molecule H2-K^b (*315*,316) indicated that the MHC molecules showed similarities to immunoglobulins in their membrane proximal regions. Early concerns were to identify the differences between allelic gene products as well as the differences between MHC proteins encoded at different loci. With the cloning of cDNAs and genomic clones for MHC-I molecules (168,317,*318,319*) and then for MHC-II molecules (*320–322*), the encoded amino acid sequences of a large number of MHC molecules of a number of species quickly became available. The comparison of gene and cDNA structures gave an indication of the exon/intron organization of the genes and explained the evolution of the MHC molecules as having been derived from primordial single-domain structures of a unit size of a single Ig domain (such as the light chain β2m), which duplicated to form the basic unit of the MHC-II chains (two extracellular domains) and the MHC-I chain (three extracellular domains) (*142*). The canonical MHC-I molecule has a heavy chain that is an intrinsic type I integral membrane protein with amino-terminal domains called α1, α2, and α3, is embedded in the cell membrane by a hydrophobic transmembrane domain, and extends into the cytoplasm of the cell with a carboxyl-terminal tail. The light chain of the MHC-I molecule, β2m, is a single-domain soluble molecule.

The MHC-II molecule consists of two chains inserted in the membrane, an α chain and a β chain. The α and β chains consist of two major extracellular domains, α1 and α2, and β1 and β2, respectively, each linked to a transmembrane domain and cytoplasmic sequences. Thus, both MHC-I and MHC-II molecules are noncovalently assembled heterodimers consisting of four extracellular domains, the two membrane proximal domains (α3 and β2m for MHC-I and α2 and β2 for MHC-II) of each molecule are Ig-like, while the two amino terminal domains (α1 and α2 of MHC-I and α1 and β1 of MHC-II) are not. The α1 domains of both MHC-I and MHC-II lack the intradomain disulfide-bond characteristic of the other extracellular domains. The cytoplasmic domain of MHC-I molecules can be regulated by splicing and differential phosphorylation or other modification, and is likely to play a role in cell surface stability and cycling between the cell surface and other intracellular compartments (*323–327*). However, analysis of directed mutants of MHC-I in some systems indicates that the cytoplasmic domain is not required for cytoskeletal association or surface recycling (*328*). The MHC-II transmembrane and cytoplasmic domains have clear effects on the level of cell surface expression, the efficiency of antigen presentation, and the rate of lateral diffusion of the molecules in the cell membrane (*329,330*). Amino acid sequence alignments of MHC-I and MHC-II proteins, particularly of the human molecules, are available in a number of databases, such as www.ebi.ac.uk/imgt/hla and www.ebi.ac.uk/ipd/mhc. Both *Mhc-I* and *Mhc-II* genes, like many other mammalian genes, reflect the protein structure by an exon/domain correspondence (331).

Identification of Peptides Bound by MHC Molecules

Many different lines of evidence coalesced over a short period of time to demonstrate that MHC molecules function by binding peptides. From functional experiments, MHC-II–restricted T-cell responses to protein antigens were shown to be dependent on peptide fragments (332). The first direct evidence of MHC–peptide interactions came from the demonstrations that purified MHC-II proteins could bind synthetic peptides in a specific, saturable, and stable manner (333,334) with measurable affinity, and remarkably slow dissociation rate (334). For MHC-I molecules, the results were at first less clear, but the realization that some cell lines defective in MHC-I surface expression could be induced to express higher levels of surface MHC-I molecules by exposure to the appropriate peptides (*335*,336) led the way for direct measurement of MHC-I peptide binding (*337*).

Several laboratories succeeded in developing methods for the partial purification and identification of the peptides that copurified with MHC molecules. One approach for identifying the peptide derived from a virus that was bound by the MHC-I molecule H2-K^b involved recovering

TABLE 19.8 Peptide-Binding Motifs for Some MHC-I Molecules[a]

Position	*1*	*2*	*3*	*4*	*5*	*6*	*7*	*8*	*9*
HLA-A1		(TS)	DE				(L)		Y
HLA-A*0201		LM				(V)			VL
HLA-A*0301									K
HLA-A*1101		VIFY	MLFYIA				LIYVF		KR
HLA-A*3		LVM	FY			IMFVL	ILMF		KYF
HLA-B*07		P	®						LF
HLA-B*0801			K						LF
HLA-B*2705		R							LFYRHK
HLA-B*3501		P							YFMLI
HLA-B*5301		P							WFL
H2-Kb			(Y)		FY			LMIV	
H2-Kd		YF							ILV
H2-Kk		E							IV
H2-Db					N				MIL
H2-Dd		G	P		(RK)				LIF
H2-Ld		PS							FLM
Qa-2		(MLQ)	(NI)		(VI)	(KMI)	H		LIF
H2M3	N-formyl-met								
RT1.A1		(ASV)	FY						YFLM

[a] Peptide-binding motifs for the indicated MHC-I molecules are shown in the single amino acid code. Position refers to the amino acid position of the peptide from the amino terminus. Only the most common residues are shown. Assignments in parentheses are less common than the others. These motifs are taken from the more extensive summary of http://syfpeithi.bmi-heidelberg.com/ and from the extensive description (*477*). Also see www.cancerimmunity.org/peptidedatabase/differentiation.htm and www.immuneepitope.org/home.do.

MHC molecules from infected cells, fractionating the bound peptides chromatographically, identifying a peak of functional biological activity in a cytotoxic T-cell assay, and determining the amino acid sequence of the recovered peptide by radiochemical techniques (338). Another method that was useful for identifying both viral-derived peptides as well as the "motif" of self-peptides by particular MHC-I molecules involved first the isolation of a large amount of detergent-solubilized MHC-I using appropriate antibodies, the elution of the bound peptides, their partial purification as pools by reverse-phase high-pressure liquid chromatography, and the determination of the amino acid sequence of the bound peptides by classic Edman degradation of the peptide pools (339,*340,341*). The unpredictable and surprising result obtained from these studies of MHC-I–derived peptides was that specific amino acid residues were favored at particular positions of the sequence, depending on the MHC-I molecule from which the peptides were obtained, and that the length of the bound peptides was well defined and short, ranging from 8 to 10 amino acids. From such experiments, a number of peptide "motifs" of peptides bound to particular MHC-I molecules and allelic products were identified. Often, specific amino acids were identified at particular Edman degradation steps, indicating a common, highly preferred residue at the same spacing from the amino terminus of the peptide. Thus, the peptide "motif" could be determined even from heterogeneous pools of peptides eluted from particular MHC-I molecules. Further refinements in methodology included the application of mass spectrometry to the identification of individual peptides and their sequencing (*342*,343). Alternative approaches for identifying peptide motifs include the use of soluble analogs of MHC-I molecules to ease the purification (*344,345*) or the use of peptide display libraries to identify those peptides that can bind the MHC (*346,347*). A summary of MHC-I peptide motifs is given in Table 19.8. An online database that is regularly maintained is available (http://syfpeithi.bmi-heidelberg.com) (*348*). Antigenic peptides that represent those observed as tumor antigens, and available for recognition by T cells, are summarized at www.cancerimmunity.org/peptidedatabase/differentiation.htm. In addition, the immune epitope database (www.immuneepitope.org) (*349*) offers a regularly updated and curated Web site that describes MHC motifs, allows evaluation of new proteins for MHC epitopes, and provides new computational tools for such evaluation. An algorithm that allows the prediction of candidates for MHC-I–restricted peptides based on the amino acid sequence of the protein of interest is also available (www-bimas.dcrt.nih.gov/molbio/hla_bind/index.html) (*350*). The distinction between "motif" residues of an MHC-restricted peptide and "anchor" residues is an important one. "Motif" refers to those amino acid residues that are identified based on the sequences of self- or antigenic peptides that have been demonstrated to bind or copurify with

TABLE 19.9 Peptide-Binding Motifs for Some MHC-II Molecules[a]

Position[b]	i (P1)	i + 1	i + 2	i + 3 (P4)	i + 4	i + 5 (P6)	i + 6	i + 7	i + 8 (P9)	i + 9
DRB1*0101	YVLFIAMW			LAIVMNQ		AGSTCP			LAIVMFY	
DRB1*0301(DR17)	LIFMV			D		KRHEQN			YLF	
DRB1*0401(DR4Dw4)	FYWILVM			PWILVADE		NSTQHR	Many		Many	
DRB1*0405(DR4Dw15)	FYWVILM			VILMDE		NSTQKD			DEQ	
DQA1*0501/B1*0301(DQ7)	WYAVM			A		ANTS			QN	
IAb(H2-Ab)[c]										
IAd(H2-Ad)	STYE (+)			VLIA		AV				
IAg7(H2-Ag7)	KHSAV			L		VA			DSE	
IAs(H2-As)[c]										
IEb(H2-Eb)[d]	WFYILV			LIFSA		QNASTHRE			KR	
IEd(H2-Ed)	WYFILV			KRIV		ILVG			KR	
IEg7(H2-Eg7)	ILVFWM			DESMV		QNASTED (+)			RKMF	
IEk(H2-Ek)	ILVFYW			ILVFSA		QNASTHRE			KRG	

[a]MHC-II peptide-binding motifs. These are drawn from the more extensive summary of (*477*) and from http://syfpeithi.bmi-heidelberg.com.

[b]As indicated, the peptide positions are relative, with i being the amino acid residue that is thought to be situated in pocket P1, I + 1, P2, and so forth.

[c]No motif assigned because of great variation in alignment possibilities.

[d]Motif assigned based on structural similarity to IEd and IEk (*478*).

a particular MHC molecule. "Anchor" implies a biophysical function of the particular amino acid residue as interacting specifically with a particular part of the MHC molecule itself. The designation of a residue as an anchor residue may be inferred by analysis of binding to peptide variants in the context of the parental peptide. Alternatively, anchors can be defined from a knowledge of the x-ray structure of the peptide complexed to the MHC-I molecule, and predictions of likely peptide motifs for MHC molecules whose sequence is known but whose structure has not yet been determined can be made by comparison to known structures.

The identification of MHC-II–bound self- or antigenic peptides by biochemical methods similar to those employed for MHC-I molecules has proved more difficult, because the MHC-II molecules do not have the rigorous requirement for a defined amino terminus or the restricted length that MHC-I molecules need. Whereas MHC-I molecules bind peptides with a particular motif residue at a specific position as defined by the amino terminus, resulting in the ability to identify the dominant residue at a particular step in the Edman degradation, even amidst a pool of peptides, MHC-II molecules bind peptides with "ragged ends," and little information is obtained from the sequencing of pools of peptides (*351–354*). Identification of MHC-II peptide-binding motifs by bacteriophage display is also possible (*355*). In accord with the view that MHC-II molecules present peptides derived from an "outside-in" pathway, many of the peptides that copurify with MHC-II molecules represent molecules derived from the extracellular milieu of the medium in which the cells were grown. Analysis of MHC-II/peptide complexes with cloned T cells and monoclonal antibodies with MHC/peptide specificity reveals that, in part because of the ability of MHC-II molecules to accommodate peptides with extensions at their amino and carboxyl termini, and in part because of the smaller role that anchor residues seem to play in peptide binding by MHC-II molecules, occasionally even a unique peptide can bind a particular MHC-II molecule in more than one frame (*356–358*). As a result of structural studies (summarized later) and compilation of peptide sequences of those peptides bound by particular MHC-II molecules, the general conclusion is that MHC-II molecules all have binding pockets identifiable for the particular allelic product. For some alleles, such as HLA-DR1 and IA^d, these pockets are spaced at position P1, P4, P6, and P9 (or i, i + 3, i + 5, i + 9). Because of the complexity and potential degeneracy of peptide motifs for MHC-II molecules, more elaborate schemes have been devised for prediciting those peptides that may bind to particular MHC-II molecules (359). A summary of identified peptide-binding motifs for MHC-II molecules is given in Table 19.9.

High-Resolution Crystallographic Structures

MHC-I Molecules

The most graphic description of the relationship of form and function of the MHC molecule was first made by Bjorkman and colleagues, who determined the three-dimensional structure of the human MHC-I molecule, HLA-A2, by x-ray crystallography (360,361). The extracellular, soluble portion of the membrane-associated molecule was cleaved from the surface of tissue culture cells by papain and further purified. At the time, there was not a clear appreciation of the role of peptide either in the assembly of the molecule or of the nature of the recognition of the MHC molecule by TCRs or, for that matter, NK receptors. Despite the fact that the first purified HLA-A2 molecules possessed a heterogeneous mixture of bound peptides, protein from these preparations crystallized readily, and electron density maps calculated from the diffraction data were interpretable, allowing modeling of the backbone molecular structure. The most important insight in the interpretation of the electron density map derived was that part of the density, and thus part of the structure, was due to a heterogeneous collection of peptides bound tightly by the molecule, and that this density could not be modeled based on the known amino acid sequence of HLA-A2.

This first MHC-I structure clarified several important aspects of the mechanism by which the MHC-I molecule carries out its peptide-binding function. The amino-terminal domains ($\alpha 1$ and $\alpha 2$) form a unitary binding site for peptide. This domain unit consists of a floor of eight strands of antiparallel β-pleated sheet, which supports two α-helices, one contributed from the $\alpha 1$ domain and one from the $\alpha 2$ domain, aligned in an antiparallel orientation. The membrane-proximal $\alpha 3$ domain has an immunoglobulin C-type fold (27), and pairs asymmetrically with the other immunoglobulin domain of the molecule contributed by β2m. The nature of recognition by T cells was suggested by comparing the location of those amino acid residues that had been characterized as being strong elements in T-cell recognition, residues that distinguished closely related allelic gene products and amino acid residues that had been identified as those that were responsible for the transplant rejection of the mutants of the *H2-K*^{b} series (361). Amino acid residues of the MHC-I molecule responsible for T-cell recognition were most clearly classified into one of two categories, or an overlapping set: those residues that were "on the top of the molecule," exposed to solvent and available for direct interaction with the TCR, and those residues whose side chains pointed into the peptide-binding groove and might be considered crucial in the peptide-binding specificity of the particular MHC molecule. The original publications, based on a structure determined to a resolution of 3.5 Å, focused mainly on the structural outline of the molecule. More recent structures have been determined of HLA-A2 complexed with specific peptides at higher resolutions. Ribbon diagrams of HLA-A2 as seen from the side (Figure 19.6A) and from the top (Figure 19.6B) indicate how the entire structure of the molecule is designed; the peptide-binding site is supported by the β-sheet floor, and the floor in turn is supported by the two

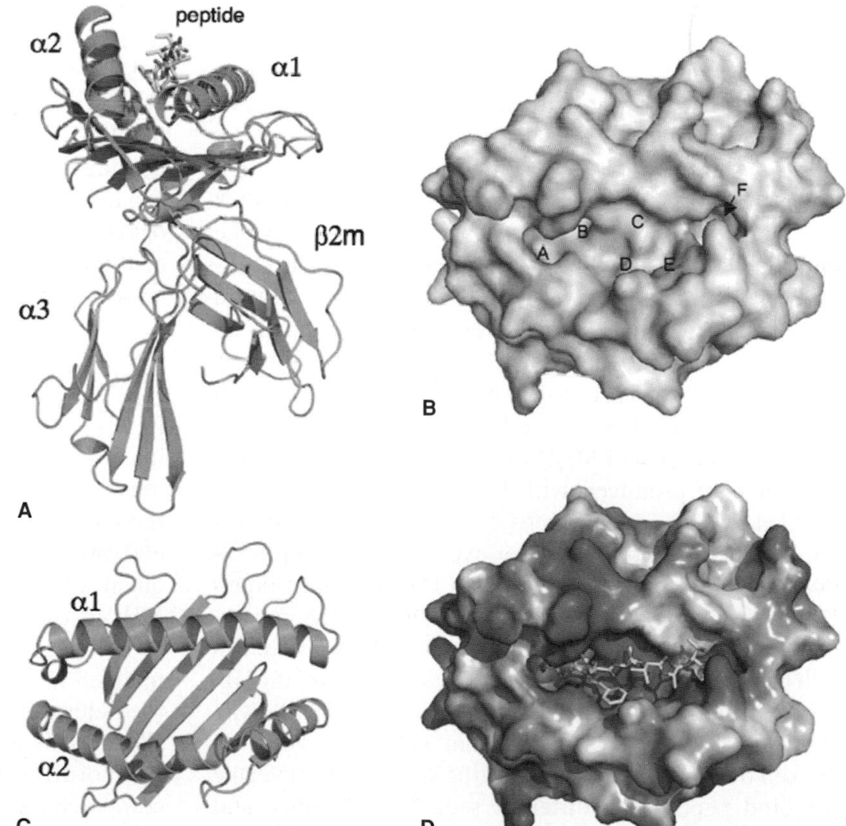

FIGURE 19.6 Structure of HLA-A*0201. **A:** Ribbon representation of HLA-A2 heavy chain (green), β2m light chain (cyan), and bound peptide (yellow). **B:** Ribbon representation of the peptide-binding groove. **C:** Surface representation of the binding groove, with pockets labeled. **D:** Surface representation of binding groove with peptide shown in stick illustration. Figure generated from protein data bank (*508*) structure 2BSV using PyMol (*509*). (See color insert.)

immunoglobulinlike domains, the $\alpha 3$ domain of the heavy chain and the $\beta 2m$ light chain.

The comparison of this structure and higher-resolution refinement of it to that of the closely related human MHC-I molecule, HLA-Aw68 (now known as HLA-A68 or, more accurately, HLA-A*68011; see Table 19.2), suggested that surface depressions in the groove of the MHC-I molecule, now known as pockets A through F, would be available for interactions with some of the side chains of the bound peptide (*362,363*). These six pockets are illustrated in Figure 19.6C and with bound peptide in Figure 19.6D. These MHC-I structures were determined of molecules purified from tissue culture cells and containing a heterogeneous spectrum of self-peptides. Concurrently with the structural studies, a number of laboratories developed methods to identify the motifs of peptides bound by particular MHC-I molecules (see earlier discussion of MHC-bound peptides). Concomitant with the determination of the x-ray structure of the human MHC-I molecule, HLA-B*2705 (*364*), the motif of the peptides that were recovered from this molecule was determined, permitting the more precise modeling of the bound peptide in the cleft of the MHC-I (365). For HLA-B27 this was of particular interest because the bound peptides had a strong overrepresentation of arginine at position 2, and scrutiny of the HLA-B27 structure suggested that the amino acid residues lining the B pocket, particularly glutamic acid at position 45 as well as cysteine 67, were complementary to the long, positively charged arginine side chain of the peptide amino acid at that position (*364*). These structural studies supported a view of MHC-I/peptide binding in which the side chain of the carboxyl-terminal residue of the bound peptide sits deep in the F pocket. In addition, the amino-terminal amino group forms strong hydrogen bonds with the hydroxyl groups of conserved amino acids tyrosine 59 and tyrosine 171. A hydrogen bond from the amino group of conserved tryptophan 147 to the backbone carbonyl oxygen of the penultimate peptide amino acid (usually position 8) also seems to be important, as do charge interactions and hydrogen bonds of the free carboxyl group at the carboxyl terminus of the peptide with tyrosine 84, threonine 143, and lysine 146.

Other structures of MHC-I molecules were determined of complexes produced with homogeneous peptide, assembled either in vitro from bacterially expressed proteins with synthetic peptide (*366*), or exploiting MHC proteins expressed in insect cells (367,*368*). The structures determined with homogeneous peptide confirmed the impression obtained from the structures obtained from molecules with heterogeneous self-peptides. The structures of the H2-K^b molecule complexed with synthetic peptides derived either from Sendai virus, vesicular stomatitis virus, or chicken ovalbumin revealed that the same MHC molecule can bind peptides of different sequences, lengths, and structures by virtue of their conserved motif residue side chains. Although small conformational changes of the MHC are detectable on binding the different peptides, the main distinction in the recognition of different peptides bound by the same MHC molecule is a result of the location, context, size, and charge of amino acid side chains of the peptide displayed when bound by the MHC molecule.

The most consistent rule learned from the first x-ray structures and complemented by peptide recovery and early binding studies was that MHC-I–bound peptides were required to embed the side chain of their carboxyl-terminal amino acid into the F pocket. However, with further studies, it became clear that MHC-I molecules could bind longer peptides that extended beyond the residue anchored in the F pocket (*369*), a view that was confirmed by a crystallographic structure (*370*). More recently, the lack of an absolute requirement for a free C-terminal amino acid has been exploited in the engineering of a single-chain peptide, $\beta 2m$, H2-K^b molecule that shows unusual stability and is an effective MHC/peptide immunogen (371). An additional variation on the theme of MHC-I–binding peptides based on particular anchor residues includes the demonstration that glycopeptides, bound to the MHC-I via amino acid side chains and termini, can expose their carbohydrate moieties to solvent and be available for TCR interaction (*372–374*). An example of a 13-residue peptide bound to its MHC-I–presenting element, the rat MHC-I molecule, RT1-Aa, was crystallized and shown to produce a peptide/MHC complex with a large central bulge. Two different complexes consisting of the same MHC and peptide reveal significantly different conformations in this central bulge region (*375*). Bulged viral peptides have also been characterized in complex with human MHC-I structures of HLA-B35 allotypes complexed with 13-mer and 11-mer peptides (*376*,377). TCR recognition of "bulged" peptides can involve conformational adjustments of the TCR in recognizing fairly rigid bulged peptide (*378*) or "crumplings" of the bound peptide by a largely rigid face of the TCR upon binding the MHC-I/p complex (*379*).

MHC-II Structures

Before any MHC-II structure had been determined experimentally, a model was constructed based on the alignment of amino acid sequences and the available MHC-I three-dimensional structure (*380*). This model made several valid predictions that were borne out by the subsequent x-ray structure determination of HLA-DR1 (*381*). MHC-II clearly showed similarity to MHC-I and formed its binding groove by the juxtaposition of the $\alpha 1$ and β domains. The position of the electron density representing the heterogeneous peptide that copurified with the HLA-DR1 was identified. Figures 19.7A and C show a ribbon diagram of HLA-DR1 with a homogeneous bound peptide. In comparison to the MHC-I structure (Figure 19.6), the peptides bound to the MHC-II molecule extend through the

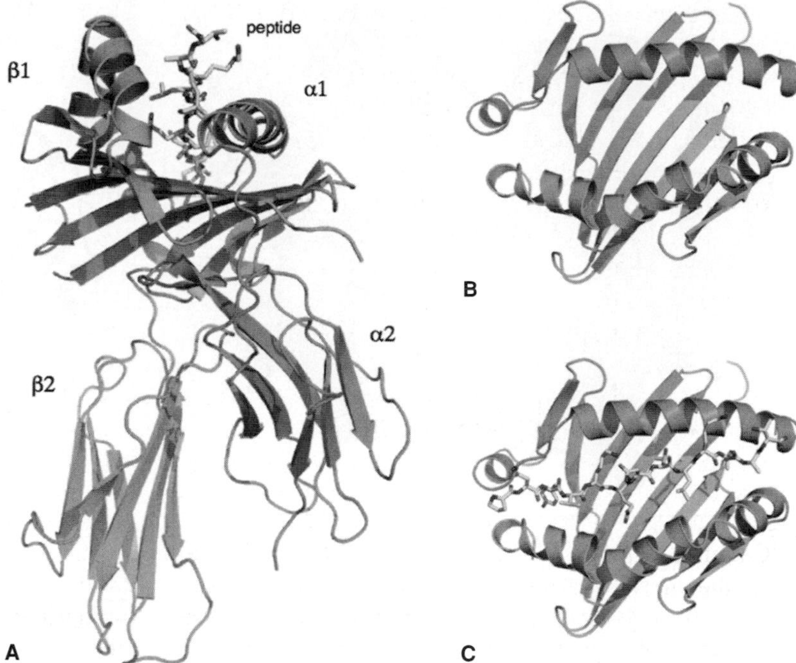

FIGURE 19.7 Color ribbon representation of HLA-DR1. **A:** Side view; *α* chain is in green, *β* chain is in blue, peptide in stick representation is in yellow. **B:** Top view. **C:** Top view with bound peptide (PKYVKQNTLKLAT) visualized. The illustration was made with PyMol (*509*) based on the protein data bank (*508*) coordinates of 1DLH. (See color insert.)

binding groove, rather than being anchored in it at both ends.

A comparison of the *α*-carbon backbone of the peptide-binding region of an MHC-I structure with that of an MHC-II structure is shown in Figure 19.8. It is remarkable that the structures are so similar, whether the binding domain is built of the *α*1 and *α*2 domains from the same chain (for MHC-I) or of the *α*1 and *β*1 domains that derive from two chains (for MHC-II). The location of polymorphic residues can be determined by variability plots based on multiple sequence alignments as originally suggested by Kabat and Wu (*382*). Comparative ribbon diagrams (Figure 19.9), in which the locations of the amino acid residues that are polymorphic for the human MHC-I and MHC-II chains are indicated, show that the bulk of the polymorphism derives from amino acid variability in regions that line the peptide-binding groove. This suggests that MHC polymorphism is required to allow the MHC molecules, and as a result, the organism and its species, to respond to a changing antigenic environment.

As with MHC-I, a further understanding of the details of the interactions of peptides with the MHC-II molecule came from crystallographic studies of molecules prepared

FIGURE 19.8 Superposition of the *α*-carbon backbones of an MHC-I [PDB (*508*)], 3HLA (*363*), and an MHC-II [1DLH (383)] molecule. The backbone tracings were displayed and superposed with QUANTA 97 (Molecular Simulations, Inc). MHC-I is shown in blue, MHC-II in red. Amino termini are labeled N. (See color insert.)

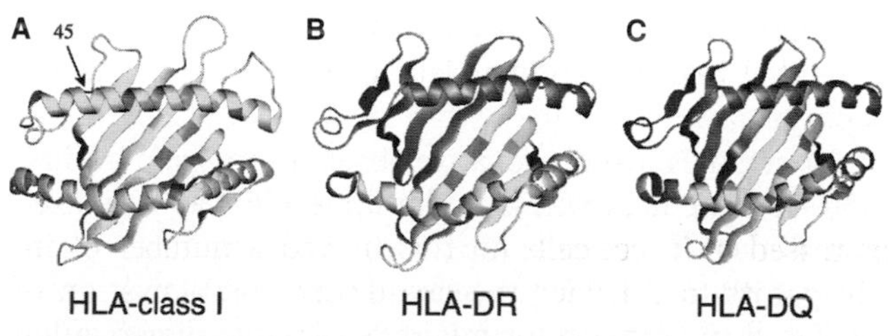

FIGURE 19.9 Location of polymorphic amino acid residues in MHC-I and MHC-II molecules. Variability plots were calculated according to the method of Kabat and Wu (*382*) and the level of variability illustrated on ribbon diagrams. Generated in QUANTA 2000 (Accelrys) of 3HLA (*363*) (HLA-class I), 1DLH (383) (HLA-DR), and 1JK8 (*510*) (HLA-DQ), where greatest variability is red, intermediate is green, and least is blue. (See color insert.)

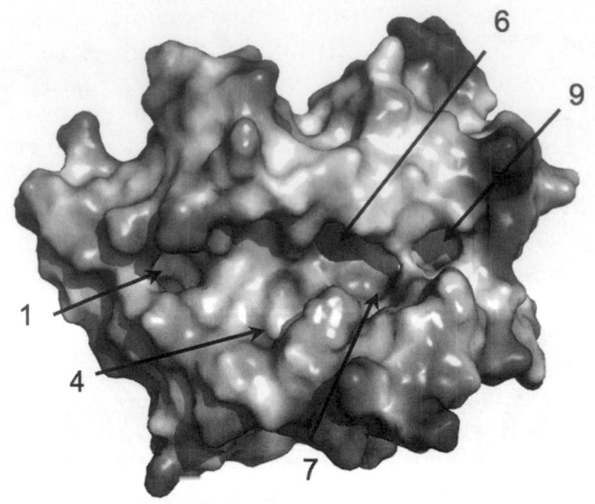

FIGURE 19.10 Location of pockets in HLA-DR1 based on the cocrystal of HLA-DR1 with a peptide derived from the influenza hemagglutinin. The surface representation of the molecule, looking into the cleft, is shown colored based on electrostatics—red, acidic; blue, basic. Numbering of the major binding pockets of HLA-DR1 is according to (383). (See color insert.)

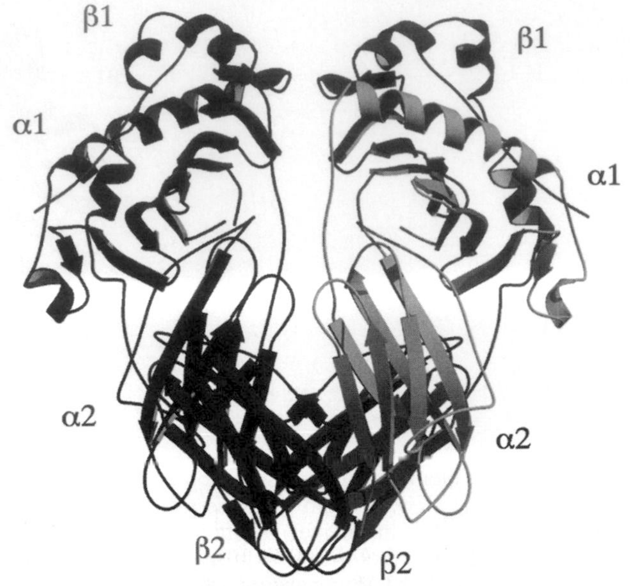

FIGURE 19.11 Ribbon diagram of the structure of HLA-DR1 showing the dimer of dimers and the individual domains of the protein. α chains are in blue and I, β chains are in red and green. Peptide is in red. The illustration was generated from 1DLH (383) in MOLSCRIPT (*511*) and rendered in RASTER3D (*512*). (See color insert.)

with homogeneous peptide, in the first case HLA-DR1 complexed with an antigenic peptide derived from the hemagglutinin of influenza virus (383). Figure 19.7 shows side (panel A) and top (panels B and C) views of HLA-DR1 bound to an influenza peptide. Based on this structure, a set of pockets was initially designated, numbered for the peptide position that is bound. For the influenza peptide studied in this example, the major interactions were from peptide positions 1, 4, 6, 7, and 9, which are indicated in Figure 19.10. The deep P1 pocket accommodates the tyrosine (the third position of the peptide PKYVKQNTLKLAT) and the pockets indicated by 4, 6, 7, and 9 fit the Q, T, L, and L residues, respectively. The MHC-II is similar in its mode of binding to MHC-I but reveals key differences: the lack of requirement for free amino and carboxyl termini of the peptide, the binding of the peptide in a relatively extended conformation (like that of a type II polyproline helix), and a number of hydrogen bonds between conserved amino acids that line the binding-cleft main-chain atoms of the peptide.

Among the most provocative observations from the first MHC-II structures was that the molecule was visualized as a dimer of dimers, and this moved a number of investigators to consider the possibility that activation of the T cell via its receptor might require the dimerization or multimerization of the TCR, an event thought to be dependent on the propensity of the MHC/peptide complex to self-dimerize. The simple elegance of this dimer of dimers is illustrated in Figure 19.11. Several arguments support the dimerization hypothesis: the finding of a dimer of dimers in the crystals of HLA-DR that formed in several different space groups (*381*,383), the observation that a TCR Vα domain formed tight dimers and in its crystals formed dimers of the dimers (*384*), the demonstration of the ability to immunoprecipitate MHC-II dimers from B cells (*385*), the apparent requirement for purified MHC-I dimers for stimulation of a T cell in an in vitro system (*386*), and the finding that MHC-II/peptide/TCR complexes could form higher-order multimers in solution as detected by quasi-elastic light scattering (*387*). However, a number of strong counterarguments draw this hypothesis into question. MHC-II molecules other than HLA-DR1 that have been crystallized do not seem to form the same kind of dimer of dimers in their crystals (*388,389*). None of the MHC-I molecules that have been examined by x-ray crystallography shows dimers in the same orientation as the MHC-II ones reported. A different Vα domain fails to dimerize even at high concentration (*390*). The reported x-ray structures of TCR/MHC/peptide complexes (391,392,*393,394*) fail to show dimerization. Despite the simple elegance of the dimer hypothesis, it is clear that additional experimentation will be required to understand the topologic requirements for T-cell activation through the $\alpha\beta$ TCR.

Recent additions to the library of MHC-II structures include the I-A^{g7} molecule, a unique MHC-II that provides one link in the susceptibility to insulin-dependent diabetes in the mouse model (*395,396*). Although the structure fails to provide direct evidence to explain the linkage to diabetes, it suggests that the novel repertoire of peptides bound by this MHC-II molecule reflects unique features of its wider peptide-binding groove and resulting relatively low-affinity interaction with peptide.

MHC-Ib Molecules

H2-M3

To this point, our description of MHC-I molecules has focused on the classical molecules, represented by HLA-A, HLA-B, and HLA-C in the human and by H2-K, H2-D, and H2-L in the mouse. Several MHC-Ib molecules, for which three-dimensional structures have been determined, are of particular interest: the CD1 molecules (*397,398*), H2-M3 (*399,400*), MICA (*401,402*), nFcR (*403*), Rae-1 (*404*), H-60 (*186*), MULT1 (*405*), and MR1 (406). H2-M3 is of particular note because of its ability to bind and present peptide antigens that contain amino-terminal N-formyl groups. H2-M3 was originally identified as the MHC-Ib molecule that presents an endogenous peptide derived from the mitochondrially encoded protein ND1 that has been called MTF (maternally transmitted factor) (*150,407*). Thus, it was of interest to understand in structural terms how this molecule binds such N-formylated peptides (*400*,408). The crystal structure of H2-M3 complexed with an N-formylated nonamer peptide, fMYFINILTL, revealed that the structure of the A pocket, highly conserved among MHC-Ia molecules, which have tyrosine 7, tyrosine 59, tyrosine 159, tryptophan 167, and tyrosine 171, is quite different, so that it can accommodate the N-formyl group in the A pocket. In particular, H2-M3 has hydrophobic residues, leucine at 167 and phenylalanine at 171, and because of the side chain orientation of leucine 167, the A pocket is dramatically reduced in size, causing the amino-terminal nitrogen of the formylated peptide to be positioned where the peptide position 2 amino nitrogen would lie in a MHC-Ia molecule. Thus, the unique peptide selectivity of H2-M3 is explained in structural terms.

CD1

Another MHC-Ib molecule of great interest is CD1, representative of a class of MHC-I molecules that map outside of the MHC, that have limited tissue specific expression, and that seem capable of interaction with both $\alpha\beta$ and $\gamma\delta$ T cells (*409*). In the human, there are two clearly distinct groups of CD1 molecules: one consisting of CD1a, CD1b, CD1c, and CD1e; and another of CD1d alone (*410*). CD1a, CD1b, and CD1c are capable of binding and presenting various nonpeptidic mycobacterial cell wall components such as mycolic acid–containing lipids and lipoarabinomannan lipoglycans (*411,412*). A minor subset of $\alpha\beta$-bearing T cells, believed to be an independent lineage, and defined by the expression of the NK1.1 marker and known as NKT cells, is restricted to CD1 recognition (*413*). The crystal structure of mouse CD1d1, which corresponds to human CD1d, has been determined (*397*), revealing a classic MHC-I structure with a basic α-carbon fold and β2m association quite similar to that of the MHC-Ia molecules. Remarkably, this molecule was purified without the addition of either exogenous lipid or peptidic antigen, but the crystallographic structure revealed some poorly defined electron density in the binding-cleft region. Consistent with its apparent biologic function of binding hydrophobic lipid-containing molecules, its binding groove is somewhat narrower and deeper than that of either MHC-Ia molecules or MHC-II molecules. The backbone configuration of the $\alpha 1\ \alpha 2$ domain structure of CD1 is shown in Figure 19.12, where it is compared to the homologous region of H2-K^b, HLA-DR1, and another MHC-Ib molecule, FcRn, a neonatal Fc receptor. To get a three-dimensional understanding of the shape and charge distribution of the peptide-binding grooves of several examples of MHC-Ia, MHC-Ib and MHC-II molecules, Zeng et al. (*397*) displayed a surface representation of the binding regions with electrostatic potentials mapped to that surface (Figure 19.13). Despite the narrowness of the entrance to the groove resulting from the distance between the α helices, the CD1-binding groove, because of its depth, has the largest volume. The depth of the groove results from the merging of pockets to form what have been termed the A′ and F′ pockets in place of the MHC-Ia A through F pockets (see Figure 19.6C). This A′ pocket is about the size of the binding site of a nonspecific lipid-binding protein. For comparison, the groove of H2-M3, with a small charged A pocket, and deep B and F pockets, is shown. An example of an MHC-Ia molecule, H2-D^b (*414*), shows how different charge distribution occurs in molecules of this group, and the depiction of HLA-DR1 reveals the depth of side-chain pockets there. The very narrow groove of FcRn (see later) appears to lack sufficient space to accommodate a conventional peptide antigen.

In an effort to understand more precisely how CD1 molecules bind lipid antigens, Gadola et al. crystallized human CD1b complexed with either phosphatidylinositol (PI) or ganglioside GM2 (GM2) and determined their x-ray structures (*398*). The structures were essentially identical for the CD1b heavy chain and β2m in the two complexes and revealed a network of four hydrophobic channels at the core of the $\alpha 1\ \alpha 2$ domain, which accommodates four hydrocarbon chains of length from 11 to 22 carbon atoms. These channels are called A′, C′, and F′ for the three analagous to the A, C, and F pockets of the MHC-Ia molecules, and a fourth, termed T′, which is a distinct tunnel. An illustration of the binding groove with the bound alkyl chains is given in Figure 19.14, which shows orthogonal views of the binding pocket of CD1b (panel A) and compares these with the pocket of CD1d with the hydrocarbon chains superposed (panel B). These features illustrate quite elegantly how the binding site of a classical MHC-I molecule may have evolved from (or to) the binding site of a molecule such as CD1 to provide antigen selectivity for

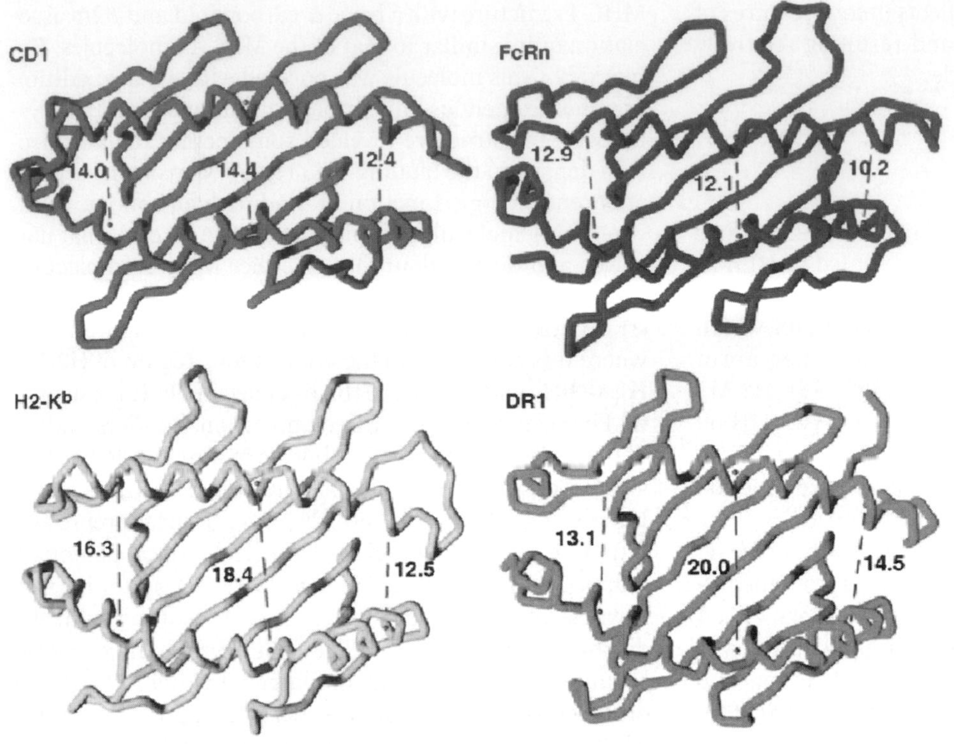

FIGURE 19.12 Comparison of the α-carbon backbone tracings and size of the potential peptide-bindng cleft of MHC-I molecule H2-K^b, MHC-II HLA-DR1, and MHC-Ib molecules CD1d, and FcRn. (From (*397*), with permission.) (See color insert.)

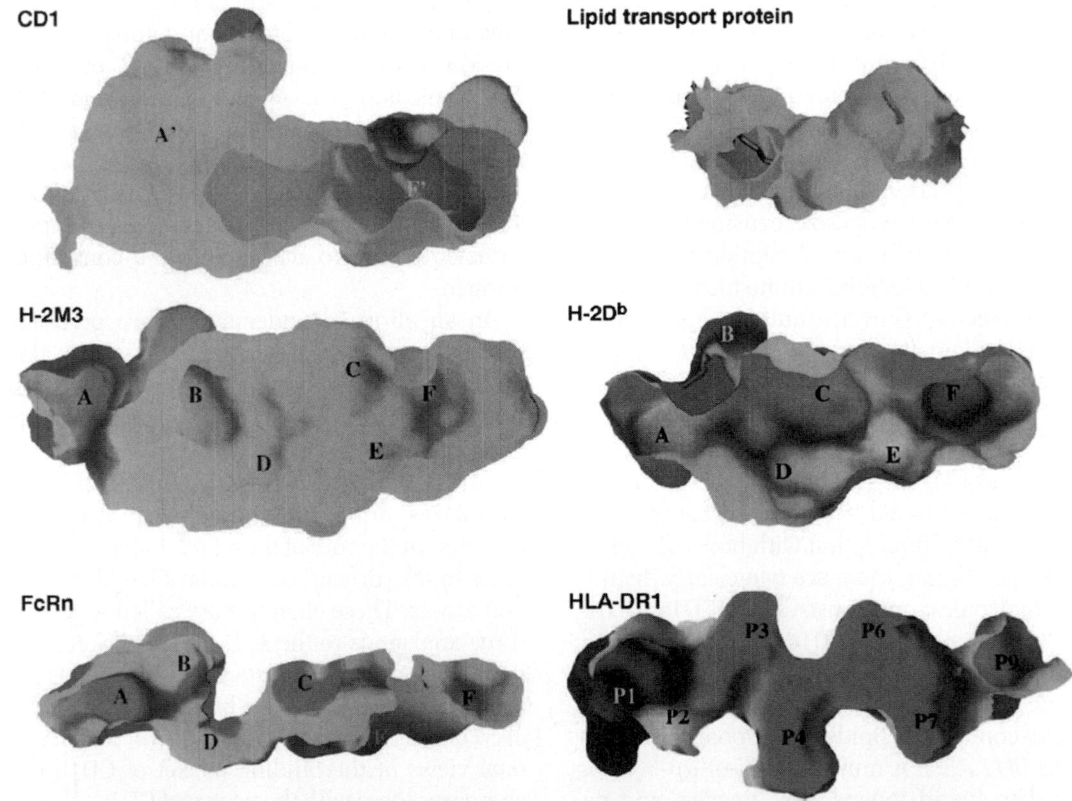

FIGURE 19.13 Shape, size, and charge of the binding groove of CD1d compared with those of several other MHC molecules and with a lipid-transport protein. Surface representation of the ligand-bindng cleft is displayed with acidic regions in red, basic regions in blue, and hydrophobic regions in green. (From (*397*), with permission.) (See color insert.)

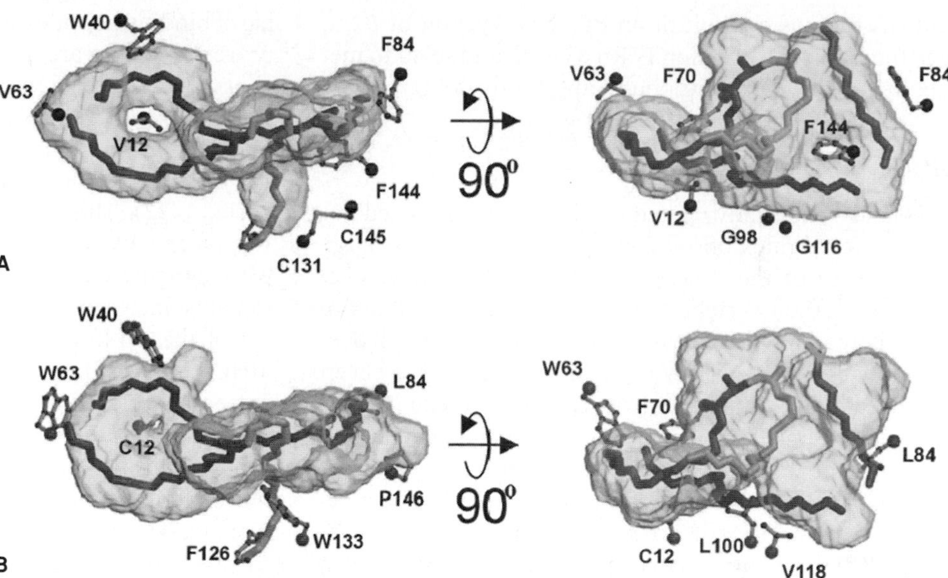

FIGURE 19.14 Structural differences between the binding grooves of CD1b and CD1d. **A:** Orthogonal views for CD1b. **B:** Orthogonal views for CD1d. The hydrophobic groove and key side chains for CD1b and CD1d are in blue and green, respectively. Position of alkyl chains and detergent visualized in CD1b are colored with respect to the binding channels they occupy: A′ (red), C′ (yellow), F′ (pink), and T′ (violet). (From *(398)*, with permission.) (See color insert.)

a distinct set of molecules that would be common to a set of important mycobacterial pathogens.

FcRn

Another example of an MHC-Ib molecule, noteworthy because it serves as an example of a novel function of MHC molecules, is the neonatal Fc receptor. Originally described in the rat as a molecule of the intestinal epithelium that is involved in the transport of colostral immunoglobulin from the lumen to the bloodstream *(415,416)*, homologs in the mouse and human have also been described *(417–419)*, and the structure of the rat molecule has been determined crystallographically *(403)* (Figure 19.15). As suggested by the amino acid sequence similarity of the FcRn to MHC-I proteins, the three-dimensional structure revealed considerable similarity to MHC-Ia molecules *(403)*. Specifically, $\alpha 1$ and $\alpha 2$ domains have similar topology to the MHC-I molecule, although, as we discussed earlier, what would be the peptide-binding groove in the MHC-Ia molecules is closed tightly and lacks space sufficient for a ligand. The most provocative feature of the structure of the FcRn/Fc complex is that the MHC-I–like FcRn interacts with the Fc through contacts from the $\alpha 2$ and $\beta 2$m domains to interact with the Fc $C\gamma 2$–$C\gamma 3$ interface. As compared to the structure of the unliganded Fc, the complex reveals both conformational changes in the Fc and the presence of several titratable groups in the interface that must play a role in the pH-dependent binding and release of Ig molecules from the FcRn. The FcRn has taken the MHC-I fold and diverted its function to an interaction with the Fc of the immunoglobulin. Amino acids at what would classically be considered the "right-hand side" of the peptide-binding groove make contact with the Fc interface that lies between the $C\gamma 2$ and $C\gamma 3$ domains. The FcRn serves as an excellent example of similar structures in the immune system being diverted for an alternative purpose. The importance of the FcRn has been underscored by the recent observations of differences in the serum half-life of immunoglobulin in

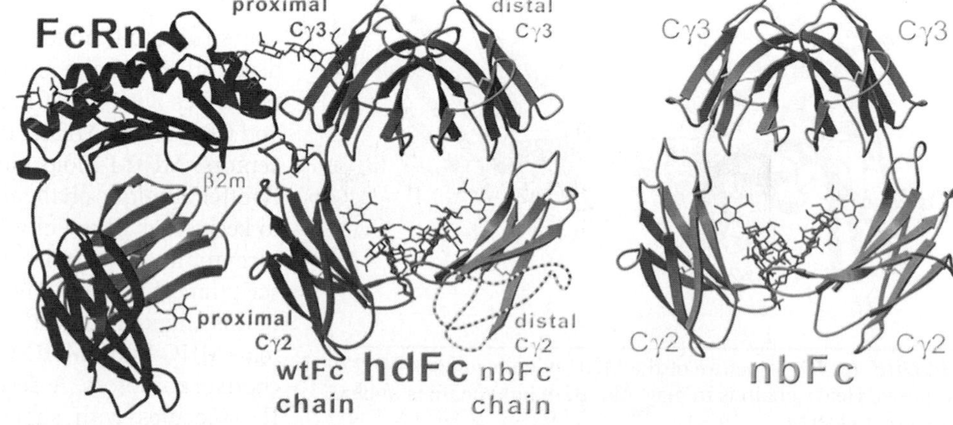

FIGURE 19.15 Structure of the FcRn complexed with Fc. Ribbon diagram of the FcRn (purple), $\beta 2$m (green) interacting with the Fc (magenta and brown) heterodimer consisting of the wild-type (wt) and nonbinding (nb) engineered chain. For comparison, the homodimer of the nbFc is shown on the right. These are PDB *(508)* files, 1I1A and 1I1C *(513)*, respectively. (From *(513)*, with permission.) (See color insert.)

animals that, as a result of an induced deletion of β2m, lack the normal expression FcRn as well, and seem to metabolize serum immunoglobulin aberrantly (*420*).

MHC-Iv Molecules

MHC and structurally related molecules are produced not only by vertebrates but also by cytomegaloviruses, large DNA viruses of the β-herpesvirus family that have coevolved with their vertebrate hosts over millennia and are exquisitely adapted to survive and persist in the face of host immune responses. Viral MHC-I–like molecules have been identified bioinformatically from amino acid sequences of the open reading frames predicted from genome sequence data. In some cases, such as the UL18 protein of human cytomegalovirus (HCMV) and the m144 protein of mouse cytomegalovirus (MCMV), the sequence homology to bona-fide MHC-I molecules is sufficiently strong to identify them unambiguously as MHC-I–like. However, in most cases, such as with the m145 family of MCMV, the sequence homology to MHC-I is very weak and relatedness to MHC-I is based on structure prediction algorithms alone. We term these virally encoded MHC-I–like molecules MHC-Iv to reflect their distinct evolutionary history, their structural deviation from typical MHC-I molecules in some cases, and their role in evading host immune responses. A survey of DNA sequences of 11 genes obtained from 26 wild murine cytomegalovirus isolates and laboratory strains indicated that several of the *MHC-Iv* genes (m144, m145, and m155) revealed significant sequence variation, consistent with the view that this variation may offer some immune-evasive benefit to the virus (421).

Structural characterization of MHC-Iv molecules begins with an evaluation of the requirement for β2m and/or peptide for stable expression. UL18 is associated with both β2m and peptide, whereas m144 is associated only with β2m. The structure of m144 has been reported (27), revealing the preservation of all structural elements of the MHC-I fold (Figure 19.16). The cleft of m144 does not seem capable of binding peptides, as the groove is narrow and critical tyrosine residues are not conserved. A unique disulfide anchors the α1 helix to the β sheet. Recently, the structure of m157, a cytomegalovirus MHC-I–like immunoevasin that binds the Ly49H activation receptor of C57BL/6 mice and the Ly49I inhibitory receptor of 129/J mice, has been reported (422). This β2m-independent, peptide-free MHC-Iv molecule reveals the major features of the MHC-I fold with some unique aspects. How it binds its Ly49 ligands remains unclear. The m153 protein of MCMV, also a member of the m145 family, reveals novel adaptations of the MHC-I fold (*423*). The m153 protein does not require β2m or peptide and, in contrast to other MHC-I molecules, is a noncovalent dimer. The monomers are associated in a head to tail fashion. An extended unstructured N terminus contains a unique disulfide that anchors it to the α3 domain. The m153 structure hints tantalizingly of more surprises to come as structures of other MHC-Iv molecules become available.

In those cases where functions have been elucidated, MHC-1v molecules have been shown to act as immunoevasins that inhibit NK cells to enable virus survival and persistence in the host. Both UL18 and UL142 inhibit human NK function, the former by binding to the inhibitory receptor LIR-1. The mode of action of UL142 remains to be determined. The m157 binds to the inhibitory receptor Ly49I in mouse strains that are susceptible to viral infection. The m144 protein has also been shown to inhibit NK activation, but the ligand remains to be identified.

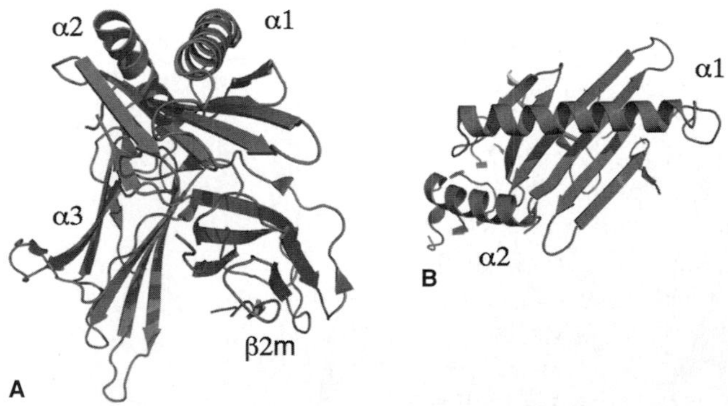

FIGURE 19.16 Structure of the MHC-Iv molecule, m144 (27), is shown. Heavy chain is in magenta, β2m light chain is in blue. (See color insert.)

Mill MHC–like Molecules

A novel set of MHC-Ib–like genes designated *Mill* (MHC class I–like located near the leukocyte receptor complex) has recently been identified in both mice and rats (*424–426*). These encode MICA/B-like glycophosphatidylinsollinked cell surface molecules that are associated with β2m and do not require TAP for cell surface expression. Their function remains unclear.

Complexes of MHC Molecules with Ligands

Our structure/function survey will be completed by brief descriptions of the interactions of MHC-I and MHC-II molecules with $\alpha\beta$ TCRs, with the T-cell coreceptors CD8 and CD4, and of MHC-I molecules interacting with NK receptors. MHC-I molecules, MHC-Ia, MHC-Ib, and MHC-Iv, offer a unique challenge to the student and investigator to keep track of which MHC molecule binds which other receptor and with what function. Although a complete description of these many interactions is beyond the scope of this chapter, Table 19.10 offers a compilation of the human MHC-I and MHC-I–like molecules and their known cognate receptors. A description of interactions of MHC-II molecules with superantigen follows. Each of these structural studies complements a host of biologic experiments that have led to an appreciation of the importance of understanding the structural basis of these immune reactions.

MHC/TCR Interactions

Perhaps the most exciting of the recent structural observations has been the solution of x-ray structures of MHC molecules complexed with both specific peptides and TCR. This has been accomplished in several systems (391,392,*393,427,428*). The first examples were of MHC-I–restricted TCR, one from the mouse (392) and one from the human (391). The mouse MHC-I molecule H2-K^b was analyzed in complex with a self-peptide, dEV8, and a TCR known as 2C (392,429), and the human HLA-A2 complexed with the Tax peptide was studied with its cognate TCR derived from a cytolytic cell known as A6 (391). These structures offered a consistent first glimpse at the orientation of the TCR on the MHC/peptide complex, but additional structures, including one involving a murine MHC class II–restricted TCR, suggest that more molecular variations may exist. As a canonical example of the MHC/peptide/TCR complex, we include an illustration of the H2-K^b/dEV8/2CTCR complex (429) (Figure 19.17). Another view of this mouse TCR as mapped onto its cognate MHC/peptide complexes is illustrated in Figure 19.18. This illustration shows that the complementarity-determining regions (CDRs) of the TCR (labeled $1\alpha 2\alpha 3\alpha$ for CDRs of Vα and $1\beta 2\beta$ and 3β for the CDRs of Vβ, respectively) sit symmetrically on the MHC/peptide complexes. For the 2C/H2-K^b/dEV8 complex (Figure 19.18), the region contacted by the CDRs of the Vα domain of the TCR lies to the left and that contacted by the CDRs of the Vβ domain lies to the right. The regions contacted by CDR3, labeled 3α and 3β, are at the center of the bound peptide, while the regions contacted by CDR1 and CDR2 of both Vα and Vβ lie peripherally. Footprints of other TCRs have been reviewed elsewhere (314).

With the publication of additional MHC/peptide/TCR structures (314), several additional points have emerged: (a) There is considerable variability in the orientation of the TCR Vα and Vβ domains with respect to the MHC/peptide complex. Although the first MHC-II/peptide/TCR structure suggested that an orthogonal disposition, in which Vβ makes the great majority of contacts with the MHC-II $\alpha 1$ domain and the Vα interacts predominantly with the $\beta 1$ domain, might be the preference for MHC-II/TCR interactions (*393*), additional MHC-II/peptide/TCR structures (*394,427*) suggest that this disposition is not indicative of MHC-I as compared to MHC-II but rather reveals the wide variety of possibilities. (b) Considerable plasticity in the conformation of the CDR loops of the TCR, particularly long CDR3 loops, is observed in the comparison of TCRs free or bound to their cognate MHC/peptide ligands (429,*430*). A striking example of this is illustrated by the structure of the KB5-C20 TCR alone as compared to its complex with H2-K^b/peptide (Figure 19.19).

Recent Structural Insights into Alloreactivity

During T-cell development, TCRs destined to be useful to the host are selected for weak reactivity with one or more self-peptides complexed with cell surface host major histocompatibility (MHCp) molecules. TCR selection is customized in each individual because of extensive polymorphism in MHC molecules that is designed to diversify peptide repertoire and optimize immune responsiveness. Thymic selection and MHC polymorphism combine to generate antimicrobial T-cell responses that are genetically restricted to recognizing host MHC molecules while retaining Ag specificity. MHC-restriction has been a central paradigm of T-cell immunity and was the basis for the 1996 Nobel Prize awarded to Peter Doherty and Rolf Zinkernagel.

Unfortunately for transplant clinicians and their patients, the rule of MHC restriction is violated when T cells are exposed to allogeneic MHC/p complexes. Remarkably, up to 10% of naive T cells react strongly against allogeneic MHC/p in vitro (mixed lymphocyte reaction) and in vivo, leading to allograft rejection and graft-versus-host disease. This reaction, known as T-cell alloreactivity, is why MHC molecules were initially called transplantation or histocompatibility molecules and has puzzled immunologists for decades.

There are two main historical theories to explain the high frequency of alloreactive T cells. The first, proposed in 1977 by Matzinger and Bevan, postulated that a single allogeneic MHC molecule could give rise to multiple binary complexes with cell surface molecules, creating "neoantigenic" determinants recognized by clonally distinct T cells. This has been reinterpreted in a "peptide-centric" hypothesis whereby a single MHC molecule presents disparate peptides recognized by multiple different T-cell clones. The "multiple binary complex" model implies that the TCR interacts with a set of amino acids shared by self- and allogeneic MHC molecules, so the cross-reaction depends crucially on the peptide antigen. However, Bevan later suggested that alloreactive T cells might focus on polymorphic residues exposed on the allogeneic MHC molecule itself, the "high determinant density" model in which the TCR focus is "MHC-centric" and the peptide is largely irrelevant.

Recently, Garcia and colleagues have solved the structure of the 2C TCR in complex with its known allogeneic ligand, H2-L^d-QL9 and then compared it to the structure of 2C in complex with its positively selecting ligand, H2-K^b-dEV8, and thus were able to provide important insight into the structural basis of alloreactivity (431). These two TCR footprints were typical of known TCR-MHC/p structures but differed from each other in a number of ways. For instance, each chain of 2C made contact with one MHC

TABLE 19.10 Human MHC-Ia and MHC-Ib Molecules and Their Ligands

	$\alpha\beta$ TCR	$\gamma\delta$ TCR	KIR2DL1	KIR2DL2/3	KIR2DL4	KIR3DL1	KIR3DL2
MHC-1a							
HLA-A	a						a HLA-A3, A11 peptide-dependent (*479*)
HLA-B	a					a Bw4 group (40% of B-allotypes) (*480,481*)	
HLA-C	a		a C2-group (C^{Lys80}) Younger & stronger (*482*,483)	a C1-group (C^{Asn80}) Older & weaker (*482*,483)			
MHC-1b							
HLA-E	a HLA-context-dependent (125)						
HLA-F	?						
HLA-G	?				a Soluble HLA-G (*491,492*)		
MHC-1–like							
MIC-A		? $V\gamma 1V\delta 1$ Costimulus role not excluded (*494*)					
MIC-B							
CD1	a (*497,498*)	aCD1c ($V\delta 1$) (*499*)					
MR1	a (406)						
Hfe	? (*500*)						
RAET-I (ULBP)							
UL18							

α-helix of H2-L^d-QL9, whereas both chains contacted both α helices in H2-K^b-dEV8. The geometry of 2C adopted a more perpendicular orientation on H2-L^d-QL9 and there was a relative rotation of H2-K^b-dEV8 by 20 degrees. The alloreactive complex reveals that both peptide-centric and MHC-centric interactions underpin direct T-cell allorecognition by the 2C receptor, but with a heavy emphasis on MHC-centric interactions. Most surprising, however, was the small number of shared contacts between the two structures, implying a limited role for mimicry between cognate and allogeneic MHC/p. H2-K^b and H2-L^d have 31 amino acid differences and there is no sequence similarity between the H2-K^b–restricted octamer self-peptide dEV8 and the H2-L^d–restricted nonamer QL9. Given these differences, it was a fair bet that the cross-reactivity of 2C on H2-K^b-dEV8 and H2-L^d-QL9 would depend on plasticity in the CDR3 regions of the TCR as documented in comparisons of bound and free TCRs, including 2C. Surprisingly, this was not the case, as the TCR actually adopted very similar conformations in the two structures.

KIR2S1	***KIR2S2***	***KIR2S4***	***NKG2A CD94/159a***	***NKG2C CD94/159c***	***NKG2D CD94/159d***	***BY55 (CD160)***	***LIR1 (LILRB1/ ILT2/ CD85j)***	***LIR2 (LILRB2/ ILT4/ CD85d)***
C2-group (C^{Lys80}) Weak (*484*)	C1-group (C^{Asn80}) Weak (*484*)	a not Cw6 but some non–MHC-1a ligands (*485,486*)				a (*487,488*)		
			a complexed with MHC-I or viral leader peptides (117,*489,490*)	a complexed with MHC-I viral leader peptides (117,*490*)				
								a (*493*)
					a (*495,496*)			
					a (*495*)			
					a (*495*)			
							a (*501*)	

The role of molecular mimicry and the relative importance of "peptide-centric" versus "MHC-centric" bias in T-cell allorecognition is likely to vary in different systems. Hence, it is likely that the nature of the polymorphisms between cognate and allogeneic MHC allotypes will affect TCR focus. Thus, closely related MHC allotypes that differ by as little as one amino acid (e.g., H2-K^b mutants in mice; HLA-A2, B44, and B27 families in humans) are set up for MHC mimicry to be a key component of T-cell allorecognition, where *specificity* is likely to be "peptide-centric." For example, HLA-B*4402 and B*4403 allotypes differ by only a single amino acid and yet stimulate strong mutual allogeneic T-cell responses. Indeed, the potency of T-cell alloresponses between closely related MHC allotypes probably occurs because positive selection of host T cells is purposely designed to create a repertoire responsive to subtle changes in peptide display. Therefore, closely related MHC allotypes, with differences in both peptide repertoire and MHC/p conformation of a shared repertoire, play straight into nature's design for T-cell recognition.

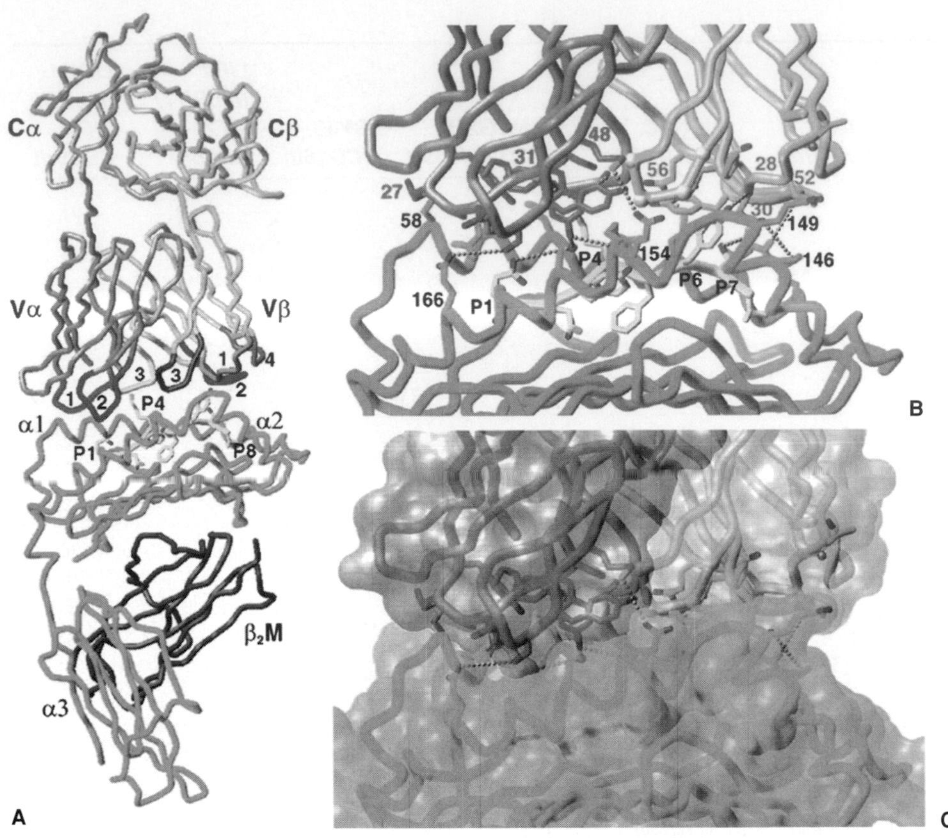

FIGURE 19.17 Structure of an MHC-I/peptide/TCR complex. H2-K^b bound to the peptide dEV8 (EQYKFYSV) in complex with the 2C TCR is shown. The TCR α and β chains (magenta and light blue) as well as H2-K^b (green) and peptide (yellow) are shown. Complementarity-determining regions (CDRs) of the TCR, colored in contrasting colors, and labeled 1, 2, and 3, are also indicated. (From (429), with permission.) (See color insert.)

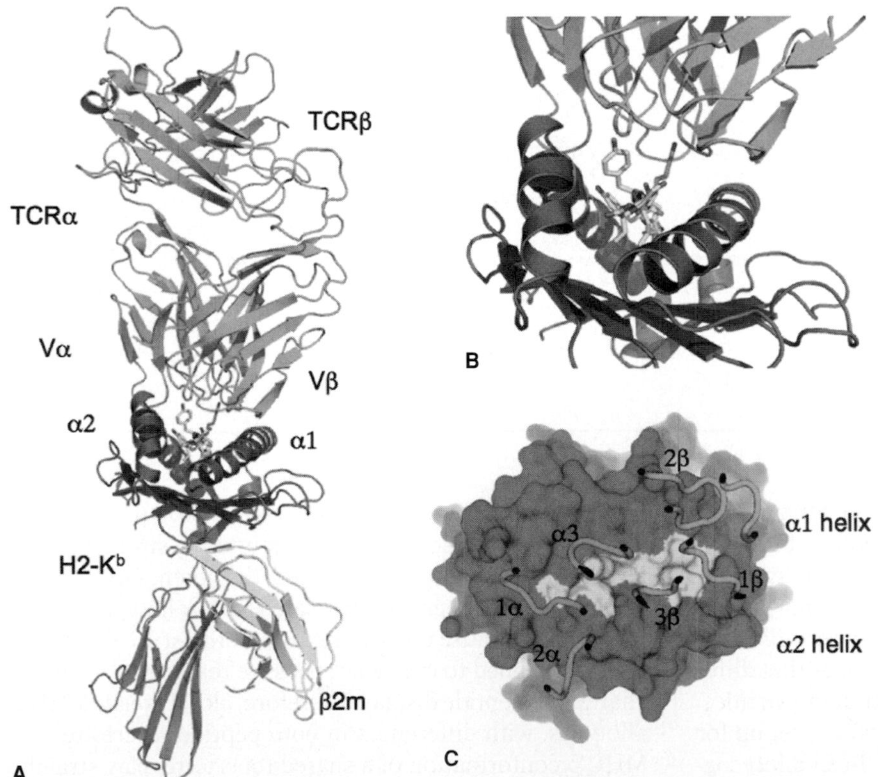

FIGURE 19.18 Footprint of CDRs. The structure of the H2-K^b/dEV8/2CTCR complex (2TCR) was displayed in PyMol (*509*). **(A)** shows the full complex, **(B)** a close-up of the TCR/MHC/peptide interface, and **(C)** shows the surface of the MHC (magenta)/peptide (yellow) complex with the CDR loops of the TCR Vα (green) and Vβ (blue) shown and labeled. (See color insert.)

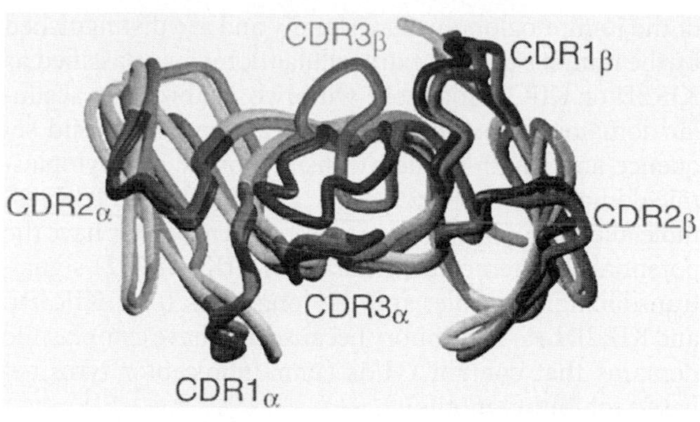

FIGURE 19.19 CDR3 plasticity. Backbone tracings of the KB5-C20 TCR CDR loops free or bound to the MHC/peptide complex are superposed. The unliganded forms are in lighter colors. (From (*430*), with permission.) (See color insert.)

MHC/Coreceptor Interactions

The major coreceptors for recognition by $\alpha\beta$ TCRs are CD8, which interacts with MHC-I molecules, and CD4, which interacts with MHC-II. Coreceptor function likely plays a role in signaling the T cell in addition to or distinct from any contribution the coreceptor MHC interaction may provide in increasing apparent avidity between the MHC/peptide and the TCR complexes. CD8, the coreceptor on MHC-I–restricted $\alpha\beta$ T cells, exists as a cell surface homodimer of two α chains or a heterodimer of α and β chains and plays an important role both in the activation of mature peripheral T cells as well as in the thymic development of MHC-I–restricted lymphocytes (*432,433*). The three-dimensional structures of human and mouse MHC-I/CD8$\alpha\alpha$ complexes have been reported (81,82). These structures have localized the binding site of the CD8 immunoglobulinlike $\alpha\alpha$ homodimer to a region beneath the peptide binding platform of the MHC, focusing an antibodylike combining site on an exposed loop of the MHC-I α3 domain. This interaction is illustrated in Figure 19.20, which shows the flexible loop of residues 223 to 229 clamped into the CD8 combining site.

The T-cell coreceptor associated with cells restricted to MHC-II antigens, CD4, has also been the subject of detailed structural studies, in part because of its role as a receptor for attachment and entry of the human immunodeficiency virus, HIV (*434*). The x-ray structure determination of the complete extracellular portion of the molecule (domains D1 through D4) indicates that there is segmental flexibility between domains D2 and D3, and both crystallographic and biochemical data suggest that dimerization of cell surface CD4 occurs (*435*). These results have been interpreted to support a role for CD4-mediated, MHC-II–dependent dimerization in facilitating TCR dimerization and signaling. The geometry that facilitates the CD4/MHC–II/TCR interaction has been suggested by a crystal structure of an MHC-II/CD4 D1D2 complex and the superposition modeling of this with both a TCR/MHC structure and the full structure of the D1–D4 homodimer (78) (Figure 19.21).

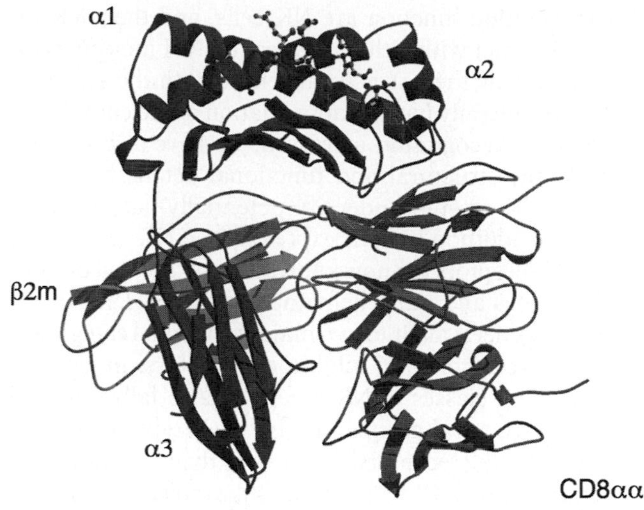

FIGURE 19.20 MHC-I–binding site for CD8$\alpha\alpha$ homodimer lies beneath the peptide-binding groove. HLA-A2 heavy chain, red, β2m, orange, and peptide (ball-and-stick) are shown in complex with the CD8$\alpha\alpha$ homodimer (red and blue). MOLSCRIPT (*511*) illustration based on the PDB (*508*) file 1AKJ (82). (See color insert.)

MHC/NK Receptor

A cellular system that parallels T cells in recognition of cells altered by oncogenesis or pathogens is that of the innate immune system. The crucial cells that perform

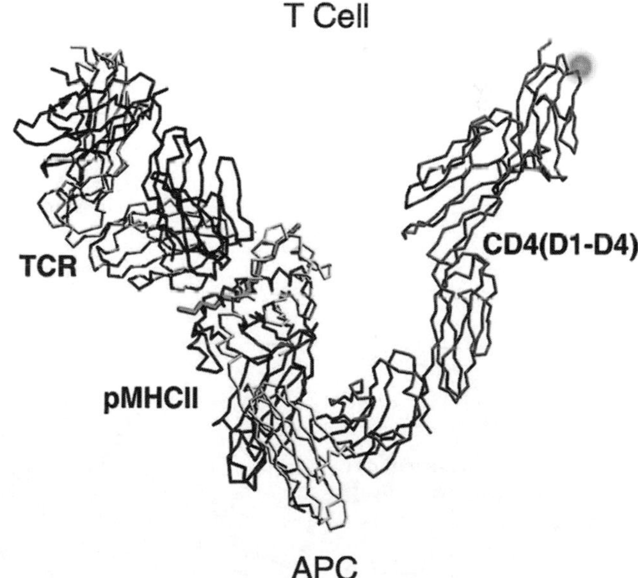

FIGURE 19.21 Model of TCR/MHC-II/peptide complex interacting with CD4. Superposition of MHC-II/CD4 D1D2 structure with that of a complete D1-D4 CD4 structure results in this model suggesting how MHC-II may contribute to multimerization of a TCR/CD4 complex. (From (78), with permission.) (See color insert.)

this recognition function are NK cells, and their NK receptors interact with either classical MHC-I molecules on their targets or their structural relatives. In the past several years, not only has our appreciation of the complexity of NK/MHC recognition increased, we have also learned some of the structural and functional details by which different NK receptors identify potentially harmful cells (13,49). In addition to their expression on NK cells, some of the NK receptors are now known to be expressed on subsets of T cells and other hematopoietic cells. The NK receptors in general fall into two major functional categories, activating receptors and inhibitory receptors. In general, each of these classes of NK receptors also falls into two different structural groups, the Ig-like receptors and the C-type lectinlike receptors. Because of their functional interactions with MHC-I and MHC-I–like molecules, and because several different systems have evolved to recognize MHC-I molecules differently, it is worthwhile to examine the recently determined structures of several MHC-I/NK receptor complexes.

In the human, the major NK receptors are known as KIRs, for killer-cell immunoreceptors. These molecules are of the immunoglobulin superfamily and are distinguished by the number of their extracellular domains (classified as KIR2D or KIR3D for those with two or three extracellular domains, respectively), as well as the amino acid sequence and length of their transmembrane and cytoplasmic domains. The short KIRs (e.g., KIR3DS and KIR2DS molecules) are considered activating because they have the potential to interact with the DAP12 (KARAP12) signal-transducing molecule, and the long KIRs (e.g., KIR3DL and KIR2DL) are inhibitory because they have cytoplasmic domains that contain ITIMs (immunoreceptor tyrosine-based inhibitory motifs).

The KIR2DL1 and KIR2DL2 molecules have been studied extensively. They interact with the human MHC-I molecules HLA-Cw4 and HLA-Cw3, respectively, and show some preferences for MHC-I molecules complexed with particular peptides. Among the polymorphic amino acid residues that distinguish HLA-Cw3 and HLA-Cw4 are Asn80 of -Cw3 and Lys80 of -Cw4. Thus, it was of interest when the structures of KIR2DL2/HLA-Cw3 (115) and KIR2DL1/HLA-Cw4 complexes were reported (116). These structures are illustrated in Figure 19.22. The important

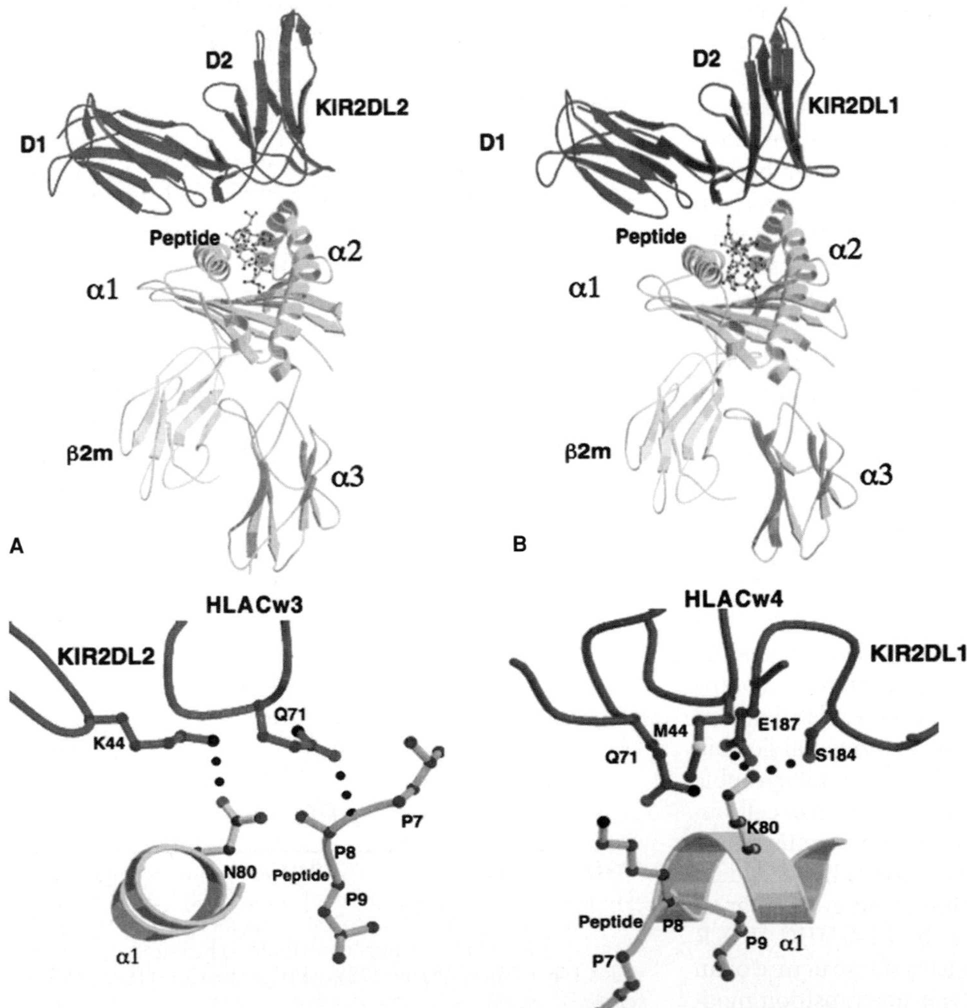

FIGURE 19.22 Interactions of KIR2D molecules with their HLA-Cw ligands. KIR2DL2 **(A, C)** and KIR2DL1 **(B, D)** are shown (magenta) in complex with their respective HLA-Cw3 and HLA-Cw4 ligands. (From (13), with permission.) (See color insert.)

conclusions from these structures is that the recognition of the MHC-I is via amino acid residues of the elbow bend joining the two immunoglobulinlike domains of the KIR and that residues that vary among different KIRs determine the molecular specificity of the interaction with the particular allelic product of HLA-C. In addition, the interaction of the KIR with the HLA-C is also modulated by the particular bound peptide, explaining the results of binding/peptide specificity studies.

The mouse exploits a set of NK receptors of a different structural family to provide the same function. In particular, the predominant, and best studied, mouse NK receptors are those of the Ly49 family, and Ly49A is the best studied. Functional experiments had demonstrated that Ly49A interacts with the MHC-I molecule, H2-D^d, and also that, for appropriate interaction, the H2-D^d needs to be complexed with a peptide. In contrast to human NK recognition, however, surveys of H2-D^d–binding peptides reveal little if any peptide preference or specificity. This would explain the function of the NK-inhibitory receptor, in that they are at baseline chronically stimulated by normal MHC-I on somatic cells, turning off the NK cell. When MHC-I is dysregulated by tumorigenesis or by pathogenic infection, the lower level of surface MHC-I diminishes the NKIR-mediated signal, and the NK cell is activated. The structure of the mouse Ly49A–inhibitory receptor in complex with its MHC-I ligand, H2-D^d (Figure 19.23), reveals several crucial features of the interaction: (a) the Ly49A C-type lectinlike molecule is a homodimer; (b) the Ly49A molecule makes no direct contact with residues of the MHC-bound peptide; and (c) in the x-ray structure, there are two potential sites for Ly49A interaction with the MHC molecule—site 1 at the end of the α1 and α2 helices, and site 2, an extensive region making contact with the floor of the peptide binding groove, the α3 domain of the MHC-I molecule, and the β2m domain as well. The ambiguity suggested by the x-ray structure has been resolved by extensive mutagenesis studies that are consistent with the view that site 2 is functionally significant (*436*,437). Recently, several other NK receptors have been studied structurally. These include the Ly49I inhibitory receptor, which interacts functionally with H2-K^b, which has been crystallized without a ligand, revealing a basic fold similar to that of Ly49A, but with a somewhat different dimeric arrangement (438). Ly49C, another murine NK-inhibitory receptor, has been examined in complex with its H2-K^b ligand (439). Differences between H2-K^b/Ly49C and H2-D^d/Ly49A suggest different modes of NK-receptor binding to MHC-I, depending on whether the interaction is "cis" (i.e., between the NK receptor and the MHC-I on the same NK cell) or "trans" (between the NK receptor on the NK cell and the MHC-I on its target). Both human and mouse NKG2D C-type lectinlike activation receptors have been examined by crystallography as well. The human NKG2D molecule forms a complex with an MHC-I–like molecule, MICA, which is expressed on epithelial cells and a wide variety of epithelial tumors (*401*). The murine NKG2D molecule has been crystallized in complex both with RAE-1β (*404*), a distantly related MHC-I–like molecule that lacks the α3 and β2m domains of the classical MHC-I molecules, and with another MHC-I–like α1 α2-domain molecule, ULBP3 (*440*). The general lesson learned from the studies of NKG2D interactions are that: (a) this C-type lectinlike receptor, unlike Ly49A, binds to MHC-like molecules spanning the α1 and α2 domains of the MHC-I like ligands; and (b) NKG2D has considerable plasticity in its ability to interact with several different molecules while maintaining the same general docking orientation (441).

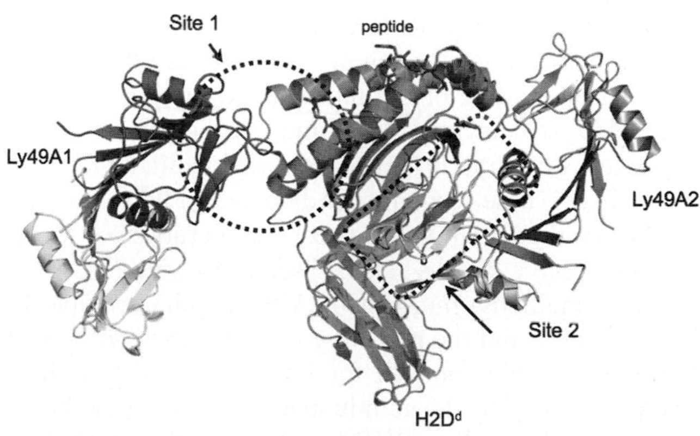

FIGURE 19.23 H2-D^d interactions with the C-type lectinlike receptor, Ly49A. The crystallographic determination of two distinct sites of H2-D^d interacting with the Ly49A homodimer is shown. Extensive mutagenesis and binding studies suggest that the functional site of interaction is site 2. (From (13), with permission.) (See color insert.)

MHC-II Superantigen

Superantigens are molecules, frequently toxic products of bacteria, that bind MHC molecules on the cell surface and are then presented to a large subset of T cells, usually defined by the expression of a particular family of TCR V regions (*442*). Most of the known superantigens bind MHC-II molecules, though one, the agglutinin from *Urtica dioica*, the stinging nettle, can be bound by both MHC-I and MHC-II molecules and presented to T cells of the Vβ8.3 family (*443*). Its structure in complex with carbohydrate ligand has been reported (*444,445*). MHC-II interactions with superantigens, such as those derived from pathogenic bacteria, are the first step in the presentation of the multivalent array of the APC-bound superantigen to T cells bearing receptors of the family or class that can bind the superantigen (*442*). A number of structural studies examining the interaction of superantigen, both with their MHC-II ligands and with TCRs, have been reported (*446*). Structural analysis of crystals derived from staphylococcal enterotoxin B (SEB) complexed with HLA-DR1 (*447*) and from toxic shock syndrome toxin-1 (TSST-1) complexed with HLA-DR1 (*448*) revealed that the two toxins bind to an overlapping site, primarily on the MHC-II α chain, and

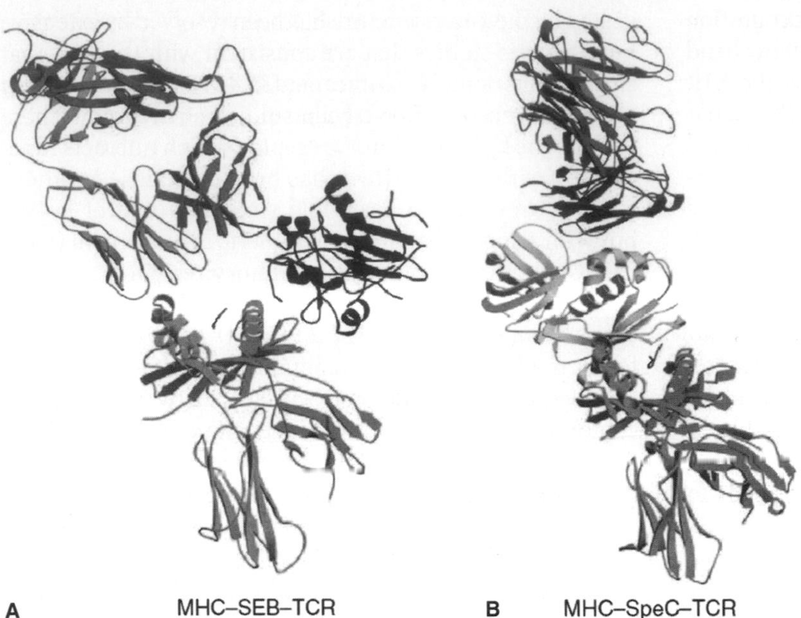

FIGURE 19.24 Different superantigens, **(A)** SEB and **(B)** SpeC, interact differently with TCR and MHC-II. (From (*514*), with permission.)

indicated that the SEB site would not be expected to be influenced by the specific peptide bound by the MHC, although the TSST-1 site would. Recently, the view that superantigens exert their biologic effects by interaction with conserved regions of the MHC-II molecule as well as conserved regions of the TCR has been challenged by the determination of two structures, that of *Staphylococcus aureus* enterotoxin H complexed with HLA-DR1 (*449*), and that of streptococcal pyrogenic toxin C in complex with HLA-DR2a (*450*). Both of these studies indicate that these superantigens can interact with the MHC-II β chain through a zinc-dependent site that includes superantigen contacts to bound peptide. Looking at models for the complete complex of MHC-II/SEB/TCR and MHC-II/SpeC/TCR based on these structures, a sense of the biologic variety available for superantigen presentation to TCRs was developed. These models are shown in Figure 19.24.

MOLECULAR INTERACTIONS OF MHC MOLECULES

Physical Assays

Whereas the crystal stuctures provide a vivid static illustration of the interactions of MHC molecules with their peptide, FcRn, CD8, CD4, superantigen, NK receptor, and TCR ligands, the dynamic aspects of these binding steps can be approached by a variety of biophysical methods (451). It is important to note that affinities and kinetics of interaction of MHC/peptide complexes for TCR have been determined by several methods in a variety of systems (*452–454*,455,*456–459*). In addition, MHC interactions with NK receptors (*112*,113,460,*461*) have been quantified by similar techniques. Although there are clear differences in the affinity and kinetics of binding of different TCR and NK receptors for their respective cognate MHC/peptide complexes, the generally consistent findings are that the affinities are low to moderate (i.e., $K_d = 5 \times 10^{-5}$ to 10^{-7} M) and are characterized by relatively rapid dissociation rates (i.e., $k_d = 10^{-1}$ to 10^{-3} s^{-1}).

Multivalent MHC/Peptide Complexes

A major development in the past several years has been the engineering and application of multivalent MHC/peptide complexes for the identification, quantification, purification, and functional modulation of T cells with particular MHC or MHC/peptide specificity. Two general approaches have been exploited: one based on the enzymatic biotinylation of soluble MHC/peptide molecules generated in bacterial expression systems that are then multimerized by binding of the biotinylated molecules to the tetravalent streptavidin (*462*); and another based on the engineering of dimeric MHC/immunoglobulin fusion proteins (*463*). These reagents can be used in flow cytometric assays that permit the direct enumeration of MHC/peptide-specific T cells taken directly ex vivo. In either of these methods, multivalent MHC/peptide complexes are generated and the relatively weak intrinsic affinity of the MHC/peptide complex for its cognate TCR is effectively magnified by the gain in avidity obtained by the increase in valency. For MHC-I molecules, the technology has been so reliable in producing multivalent (tetrameric) molecules loaded homogeneously with synthetic peptides that a wide variety of specific peptide/MHC-I multimers are available either from a resource facility sponsored by the National Institute of Allergy and Infectious Diseases (www.niaid.nih.gov/reposit/tetramer/index.html) or from commercial suppliers that offer either the tetramer or the immunoglobulin multimer. The MHC-I/peptide multimers have also been exploited for identification of specific populations of NK cells and for assignment of various NK-receptor specificities (*117,464–466*). For some MHC-II molecules, similar success has been achieved in the production of such multimers, using insect cell or mammalian cell expression systems for molecules produced by either the tetramer or the immunoglobulin chimera strategy (*467–471*). Despite many reports of successful application of these MHC class II multimers for identification of specific MHC-II/peptide–directed T cells, the technology at the present time seems less predictable than for MHC-I molecules. No doubt, further methodologic improvements will be needed (*472*).

CONCLUSION

We have surveyed the *Mhc* as a genetic region and a source for molecules that are crucial to immune regulation and immunologic disease. These genes reflect the panoply of mechanisms involved in the evolution of complex systems and encode cell surface proteins that interact via a complex orchestration with small molecules, including peptides and glycolipids, as well as with receptors on T cells and NK cells. The MHC-I molecules provide the immune system with a window for viewing the biologic health of the cell in which they are expressed, and MHC-II molecules function as scavengers to taste and display the remnants of the cellular environment. Viruses and bacterial pathogens contribute enormously to the genetic dance—they modulate and compete in the control of MHC expression—and the host, by adjusting its T-cell and NK-cell repertoire on the time scale of both the individual organism and the species, resists the push to extinction. The immune system, dynamically, resourcefully, creatively, provides, through the concerted action of its MHC molecules, TCR, NK receptors, and antibodies, as well as a host of other regulatory molecules, an organ system that is vital not only to the survival of the individual but to the success of the species. As we understand better the molecular functions of the MHC, we should better understand rational approaches to manipulating the immune system in the prevention, diagnosis, and treatment of immunologic and infectious diseases.

ACKNOWLEDGMENTS

We wish first to accept responsibility for any errors of fact and citation throughout this review. We ask our colleagues to forgive our shortcomings in the proper crediting of their work, either in terms of priority or of importance, and thank the members of our laboratories, for their comments and criticism, and our families for their encouragement and forbearance.

REFERENCES

1. Klein J. *Natural History of the Major Histocompatibility Complex*. New York: Wiley-Interscience; 1986.
3. Snell GD, Dausset J, Nathenson S. *Histocompatibility*. New York: Academic Press; 1976.
5. Benacerraf B, McDevitt HO. Histocompatibility-linked immune response genes. *Science*. 1972;175(19):273–279.
6. Shearer GM, Rehn TG, Garbarino CA. Cell-mediated lympholysis of trinitrophenyl-modified autologous lymphocytes. Effector cell specificity to modified cell surface components controlled by H-2K and H-2D serological regions of the murine major histocompatibility complex. *J Exp Med*. 1975;141(6):1384–1364.
7. Shevach EM, Rosenthal AS. Function of macrophages in antigen recognition by guinea pig T lymphocytes. II. Role of the macrophage in the regulation of genetic control of the immune response. *J Exp Med*. 1973;138(5):1213–1229.
8. Zinkernagel RM, Doherty PC. Restriction of in vitro T cell-mediated cytotoxicity in lymphocytic choriomeningitis within a syngeneic or semiallogeneic system. *Nature*. 1974;248(450):701–702.
11. Germain RN. MHC-dependent antigen processing and peptide presentation: providing ligands for T lymphocyte activation. *Cell*. 1994;76(2):287–299.
13. Natarajan K, Dimasi N, Wang J, et al. Structure and function of natural killer cell receptors: multiple molecular solutions to self, nonself discrimination. *Annu Rev Immunol*. 2002;20:853–885.
14. Yokoyama WM, Daniels BF, Seaman WE, et al. A family of murine NK cell receptors specific for target cell MHC class I molecules. *Semin Immunol*. 1995;7(2):89–101.
15. Hoglund P, Sundback J, Olsson-Alheim MY, et al. Host MHC class I gene control of NK-cell specificity in the mouse. *Immunol Rev*. 1997;155(Feb):11–28.
17. Marsh SG. Nomenclature for factors of the HLA system, update January 2007. *Tissue Antigens*. 2007;69(6):623–625.
18. Gorer PA. Studies in antibody response of mice to tumour inoculation. *Br J Cancer*. 1950;4:372–379.
19. Gorer P. The detection of antigenic differences in mouse erythrocyte by the employment of immune sera. *Br J Exp Pathol*. 1936;17:42–50.
27. Natarajan K, Hicks A, Mans J, et al. Crystal structure of the murine cytomegalovirus MHC-I homolog m144. *J Mol Biol*. 2006;358(1):157–171.
35. Germain RN, Margulies DH. The biochemistry and cell biology of antigen processing and presentation. *Annu Rev Immunol*. 1993;11:403–450.
36. Yewdell JW, Bennink JR. Cell biology of antigen processing and presentation to major histocompatibility complex class I molecule-restricted T lymphocytes. *Adv Immunol*. 1992;52:1–123.
40. Cresswell P. Invariant chain structure and MHC class II function. *Cell*. 1996;84(4):505–507.
49. Lanier LL. NK cell receptors. *Annu Rev Immunol*. 1998;16:359–393.
50. Correa I, Raulet DH. Binding of diverse peptides to MHC class I molecules inhibits target cell lysis by activated natural killer cells. *Immunity*. 1995;2(1):61–71.
53. Karre K. How to recognize a foreign submarine. *Immunol Rev*. 1997;155:5–9.
54. Karre K. NK cells, MHC class I molecules and the missing self. *Scand J Immunol*. 2002;55(3):221–228.
55. Ljunggren HG, Karre K. In search of the "missing self": MHC molecules and NK cell recognition. *Immunol Today*. 1990;11(7):237–244.
56. Karlhofer FM, Ribaudo RK, Yokoyama WM. MHC class I alloantigen specificity of Ly-49+ IL-2-activated natural killer cells. *Nature*. 1992;358(6381):66–70.

60. Germain RN. Immunology. The ins and outs of antigen processing and presentation. *Nature*. 1986;322(6081):687–689.
67. Shastri N, Schwab S, Serwold T. Producing nature's gene-chips: the generation of peptides for display by MHC class I molecules. *Annu Rev Immunol*. 2002;20:463–493.
68. Dick TP, Bangia N, Peaper DR, et al. Disulfide bond isomerization and the assembly of MHC class I-peptide complexes. *Immunity*. 2002;16(1):87–98.
73. Salter RD, Norment AM, Chen BP, et al. Polymorphism in the alpha 3 domain of HLA-A molecules affects binding to CD8. *Nature*. 1989;338(6213):345–347.
75. Doyle C, Strominger JL. Interaction between CD4 and class II MHC molecules mediates cell adhesion. *Nature*. 1987;330(6145):256–259.
77. Konig R, Fleury S, Germain RN. The structural basis of CD4-MHC class II interactions: coreceptor contributions to T cell receptor antigen recognition and oligomerization-dependent signal transduction. *Curr Top Microbiol Immunol*. 1996;205:19–46.
78. Wang JH, Meijers R, Xiong Y, et al. Crystal structure of the human CD4 N-terminal two domain fragment complexed to a class II MHC molecule. *Proc Natl Acad Sci U S A*. 2001;98(19):10799–10804.
81. Kern PS, Teng MK, Smolyar A, et al. Structural basis of CD8 coreceptor function revealed by crystallographic analysis of a murine CD8alphaalpha ectodomain fragment in complex with H-2Kb. *Immunity*. 1998;9(4):519–530.
82. Gao GF, Tormo J, Gerth UC, et al. Crystal structure of the complex between human CD8alpha(alpha) and HLA-A2. *Nature*. 1997;387(6633):630–634.
92. Spies T, Cerundolo V, Colonna M, et al. Presentation of viral antigen by MHC class I molecules is dependent on a putative peptide transporter heterodimer. *Nature*. 1992;355(6361):644–646.
93. Powis SJ. Major histocompatibility complex class I molecules interact with both subunits of the transporter associated with antigen processing, TAP1 and TAP2. *Eur J Immunol*. 1997;27(10):2744–2747.
94. Hill A, Ploegh H. Getting the inside out: the transporter associated with antigen processing (TAP) and the presentation of viral antigen. *Proc Natl Acad Sci U S A*. 1995;92(2):341–343.
104. Livingstone AM, Powis SJ, Diamond AG, et al. A trans-acting major histocompatibility complex-linked gene whose alleles determine gain and loss changes in the antigenic structure of a classical class I molecule. *J Exp Med*. 1989;170(3):777–795.
106. McCluskey J, Rossjohn J, Purcell AW. TAP genes and immunity. *Curr Opin Immunol*. 2004;16(5):651–659.
113. Vales-Gomez M, Reyburn HT, Erskine RA, et al. Differential binding to HLA-C of p50-activating and p58-inhibitory natural killer cell receptors. *Proc Natl Acad Sci U S A*. 1998;95(24):14326–14331.
115. Boyington JC, Motyka SA, Schuck P, et al. Crystal structure of an NK cell immunoglobulin-like receptor in complex with its class I MHC ligand. *Nature*. 2000;405(6786):537–543.
116. Fan QR, Long EO, Wiley DC. Crystal structure of the human natural killer cell inhibitory receptor KIR2DL1-HLA-Cw4 complex. *Nat Immunol*. 2001;2(5):452–460.
138. Moffett A, Hiby SE. How does the maternal immune system contribute to the development of pre-eclampsia? *Placenta*. 2007;28 (suppl A):S51–S56.
143. Bodmer WF. HLA structure and function: a contemporary view. *Tissue Antigens*. 1981;17(1):9–20.
144. Shiina T, Inoko H, Kulski JK. An update of the HLA genomic region, locus information and disease associations: 2004. *Tissue Antigens*. 2004;64(6):631–649.
145. Steinmetz M, Minard K, Horvath S, et al. A molecular map of the immune response region from the major histocompatibility complex of the mouse. *Nature*. 1982;300(5887):35–42.
146. Margulies DH, Evans GA, Flaherty L, et al. H-2-like genes in the Tla region of mouse chromosome 17. *Nature*. 1982;295(5845): 168–170.
155. Martin MP, Gao X, Lee JH, et al. Epistatic interaction between KIR3DS1 and HLA-B delays the progression to AIDS. *Nat Genet*. 2002;31(4):429–434.
156. Zernich D, Purcell AW, Macdonald WA, et al. Natural HLA class I polymorphism controls the pathway of antigen presentation and susceptibility to viral evasion. *J Exp Med*. 2004;200(1):13–24.
159. Mitchison NA, Mayer W. A survey of H2 gene sequences, including new wild-derived genes. *Int J Immunogenet*. 2007;34(1):3–12.
164. Williams AF. Immunoglobulin-related domains for cell surface recognition. *Nature*. 1985;314(6012):579–580.
165. Hood L, Steinmetz M, Malissen B. Genes of the major histocompatibility complex of the mouse. *Annu Rev Immunol*. 1983;1:529–568.
168. Evans GA, Margulies DH, Camerini-Otero RD, et al. Structure and expression of a mouse major histocompatibility antigen gene, H-2Ld. *Proc Natl Acad Sci U S A*. 1982;79(6):1994–1998.
171. Nathenson SG, Geliebter J, Pfaffenbach GM, et al. Murine major histocompatibility complex class-I mutants: molecular analysis and structure-function implications. *Annu Rev Immunol*. 1986;4:471–502.
176. Silver LM. *Mouse Genetics: Concepts and Applications*. New York: Oxford University Press; 1995.
187. Schwab SR, Li KC, Kang C, et al. Constitutive display of cryptic translation products by MHC class I molecules. *Science*. 2003;301(5638):1367–1371.
188. Yewdell JW, Anton LC, Bennink JR. Defective ribosomal products (DRiPs): a major source of antigenic peptides for MHC class I molecules? *J Immunol*. 1996 Sep 1;157(5):1823–1826.
189. Eisenlohr LC, Huang L, Golovina TN. Rethinking peptide supply to MHC class I molecules. *Nat Rev Immunol*. 2007;7(5):403–410.
207. Rubinstein P. HLA matching for bone marrow transplantation—how much is enough? *N Engl J Med*. 2001;345(25):1842–1844.
210. Rubinstein P. Why cord blood? *Hum Immunol*. 2006;67(6):398–404.
220. Nepom GT, Erlich H. MHC class-II molecules and autoimmunity. *Annu Rev Immunol*. 1991;9:493–525.
221. Thomson G. HLA disease associations: models for the study of complex human genetic disorders. *Crit Rev Clin Lab Sci*. 1995;32(2):183–219.
222. Lechler R, Warrens A. *HLA in Health and Disease*. 2nd ed. San Diego: Academic Press; 2000.
224. Wellcome-Trust-Case-Control-Consortium. Genome-wide association study of 14,000 cases of seven common diseases and 3,000 shared controls. *Nature*. 2007;447(7145):661–678.
226. von Herrath MG, Oldstone MB. Virus-induced autoimmune disease. *Curr Opin Immunol*. 1996;8(6):878–885.
236. Bird LA, Peh CA, Kollnberger S, et al. Lymphoblastoid cells express HLA-B27 homodimers both intracellularly and at the cell surface following endosomal recycling. *Eur J Immunol*. 2003;33(3):748–759.
239. Bennett MJ, Lebron JA, Bjorkman PJ. Crystal structure of the hereditary haemochromatosis protein HFE complexed with transferrin receptor. *Nature*. 2000;403(6765):46–53.
265. Ewenstein BM, Uehara H, Nisizawa T, et al. Biochemical studies on the H-2K antigens of the MHC mutants bm3 and bm11. *Immunogenetics*. 1980;11(4):383–395.
266. Yamaga KM, Pfaffenbach GM, Pease LR, et al. Biochemical studies of H-2K antigens from a group of related mutants. II. Identification of a shared mutation in B6-H-2bm6, B6.C-H-2bm7, and B6.C-H-2bm9. *Immunogenetics*. 1983;17(1):31–41.
267. Zijlstra M, Li E, Sajjadi F, et al. Germ-line transmission of a disrupted beta 2-microglobulin gene produced by homologous recombination in embryonic stem cells. *Nature*. 1989;342(6248):435–438.
268. Koller BH, Smithies O. Inactivating the beta 2-microglobulin locus in mouse embryonic stem cells by homologous recombination. *Proc Natl Acad Sci U S A*. 1989;86(22):8932–8935.
290. Koszinowski UH, Reddehase MJ, Del Val M. Principles of cytomegalovirus antigen presentation in vitro and in vivo. *Semin Immunol*. 1992;4(2):71–79.
291. Scalzo AA, Corbett AJ, Rawlinson WD, et al. The interplay between host and viral factors in shaping the outcome of cytomegalovirus infection. *Immunol Cell Biol*. 2007;85(1):46–54.
300. Reith W, Mach B. The bare lymphocyte syndrome and the regulation of MHC expression. *Annu Rev Immunol*. 2001;19:331–373.
303. Mach B. MHC class II regulation—lessons from a disease. *N Engl J Med*. 1995;332(2):120–122.
304. Mitchison NA, Schuhbauer D, Muller B. Natural and induced regulation of Th1/Th2 balance. *Springer Semin Immunopathol*. 1999;21(3):199–210.
314. Rudolph MG, Stanfield RL, Wilson IA. How TCRs bind MHCs, peptides, and coreceptors. *Annu Rev Immunol*. 2006;24:419–466.

316. Coligan JE, Kindt TJ, Uehara H, et al. Primary structure of a murine transplantation antigen. *Nature*. 1981;291(5810):35–39.
317. Steinmetz M, Frelinger JG, Fisher D, et al. Three cDNA clones encoding mouse transplantation antigens: homology to immunoglobulin genes. *Cell*. 1981;24(1):125–134.
331. Margulies DH, McCluskey J. Exon shuffling: new genes from old. *Surv Immunol Res*. 1985;4(2):146–159.
332. Schwartz RH. Immune response (Ir) genes of the murine major histocompatibility complex. *Adv Immunol*. 1986;38:31–201.
333. Babbitt BP, Allen PM, Matsueda G, et al. Binding of immunogenic peptides to Ia histocompatibility molecules. *Nature*. 1985;317 (6035):359–361.
334. Buus S, Sette A, Colon SM, et al. Isolation and characterization of antigen-Ia complexes involved in T cell recognition. *Cell*. 1986;47(6):1071–1077.
336. Townsend A, Ohlen C, Bastin J, et al. Association of class I major histocompatibility heavy and light chains induced by viral peptides. *Nature*. 1989;340(6233):443–448.
338. Van Bleek GM, Nathenson SG. Isolation of an endogenously processed immunodominant viral peptide from the class I H-2Kb molecule. *Nature*. 1990;348(6298):213–216.
339. Rotzschke O, Falk K, Deres K, et al. Isolation and analysis of naturally processed viral peptides as recognized by cytotoxic T cells. *Nature*. 1990;348(6298):252–254.
343. Hunt DF, Henderson RA, Shabanowitz J, et al. Characterization of peptides bound to the class I MHC molecule HLA-A2.1 by mass spectrometry. *Science*. 1992;255(5049):1261–1263.
359. Chang KY, Suri A, Unanue ER. Predicting peptides bound to I-Ag7 class II histocompatibility molecules using a novel expectation-maximization alignment algorithm. *Proteomics*. 2007;7(3):367–377.
360. Bjorkman PJ, Saper MA, Samraoui B, et al. The foreign antigen binding site and T cell recognition regions of class I histocompatibility antigens. *Nature*. 1987;329(6139):512–518.
361. Bjorkman PJ, Saper MA, Samraoui B, et al. Structure of the human class I histocompatibility antigen, HLA-A2. *Nature*. 1987;329 (6139):506–512.
365. Jardetzky TS, Lane WS, Robinson RA, et al. Identification of self peptides bound to purified HLA-B27. *Nature*. 1991;353(6342):326–329.
367. Fremont DH, Matsumura M, Stura EA, et al. Crystal structures of two viral peptides in complex with murine MHC class I H-2Kb. *Science*. 1992;257(5072):919–927.
371. Lybarger L, Yu YY, Miley MJ, et al. Enhanced immune presentation of a single-chain major histocompatibility complex class I molecule engineered to optimize linkage of a C-terminally extended peptide. *J Biol Chem*. 2003;278(29):27105–27111.
377. Tynan FE, Borg NA, Miles JJ, et al. High resolution structures of highly bulged viral epitopes bound to major histocompatibility complex class I. Implications for T-cell receptor engagement and T-cell immunodominance. *J Biol Chem*. 2005;280(25):23900–23909.
383. Stern LJ, Brown JH, Jardetzky TS, et al. Crystal structure of the human class II MHC protein HLA-DR1 complexed with an influenza virus peptide. *Nature*. 1994;368(6468):215–221.
391. Garboczi DN, Ghosh P, Utz U, et al. Structure of the complex between human T-cell receptor, viral peptide and HLA-A2. *Nature*. 1996;384(6605):134–141.
392. Garcia KC, Degano M, Stanfield RL, et al. An alphabeta T cell receptor structure at 2.5 A and its orientation in the TCR-MHC complex. *Science*. 1996;274(5285):209–219.
406. Treiner E, Duban L, Bahram S, et al. Selection of evolutionarily conserved mucosal-associated invariant T cells by MR1. *Nature*. 2003;422(6928):164–169.
408. Wang CR, Castano AR, Peterson PA, et al. Nonclassical binding of formylated peptide in crystal structure of the MHC class Ib molecule H2-M3. *Cell*. 1995;82(4):655–664.
421. Smith LM, Shellam GR, Redwood AJ. Genes of murine cytomegalovirus exist as a number of distinct genotypes. *Virology*. 2006;352(2):450–465.
422. Adams EJ, Juo ZS, Venook RT, et al. Structural elucidation of the m157 mouse cytomegalovirus ligand for Ly49 natural killer cell receptors. *Proc Natl Acad Sci U S A*. 2007;104(24):10128–10133.
429. Garcia KC, Degano M, Pease LR, et al. Structural basis of plasticity in T cell receptor recognition of a self peptide-MHC antigen. *Science*. 1998;279(5354):1166–1172.
431. Colf LA, Bankovich AJ, Hanick NA, et al. How a single T cell receptor recognizes both self and foreign MHC. *Cell*. 2007;129(1):135–146.
437. Wang J, Whitman MC, Natarajan K, et al. Binding of the natural killer cell inhibitory receptor Ly49A to its major histocompatibility complex class I ligand. Crucial contacts include both H-2Dd AND beta 2-microglobulin. *J Biol Chem*. 2002;277(2):1433–1442.
438. Dimasi N, Sawicki MW, Reineck LA, et al. Crystal structure of the Ly49I natural killer cell receptor reveals variability in dimerization mode within the Ly49 family. *J Mol Biol*. 2002;320(3):573–585.
439. Dam J, Guan R, Natarajan K, et al. Variable MHC class I engagement by Ly49 natural killer cell receptors demonstrated by the crystal structure of Ly49C bound to H-2K(b). *Nat Immunol*. 2003;4(12):1213–1222.
441. Strong RK. Asymmetric ligand recognition by the activating natural killer cell receptor NKG2D, a symmetric homodimer. *Mol Immunol*. 2002;38(14):1029–1037.
451. Fremont DH, Rees WA, Kozono H. Biophysical studies of T-cell receptors and their ligands. *Curr Opin Immunol*. 1996;8(1):93–100.
455. Corr M, Slanetz AE, Boyd LF, et al. T cell receptor-MHC class I peptide interactions: affinity, kinetics, and specificity. *Science*. 1994;265(5174):946–949.
460. Natarajan K, Boyd LF, Schuck P, et al. Interaction of the NK cell inhibitory receptor Ly49A with H-2Dd: identification of a site distinct from the TCR site. *Immunity*. 1999;11(5):591–601.
483. Parham P. MHC class I molecules and KIRs in human history, health and survival. *Nat Rev Immunol*. 2005;5(3):201–214.

Chapter 20

Cell Biology of Antigen Processing and Presentation

Lélia Delamarre and Ira Mellman

To be recognized by T lymphocytes, antigens must be bound to antigen-presenting molecules, which are displayed at the cell surface. Classically, antigen-presenting molecules—class I and class II major histocompatibility complex (MHC) molecules—bind peptides derived from intracellular proteins and from proteins captured by the antigen-presenting cells (APCs), respectively, whereas CD1 MHC-like molecules bind lipid antigens. Antigen recognition by T lymphocytes primarily depends on the ability of APCs to process protein antigens into peptides, load them onto MHC molecules, and finally display the MHC–peptide complexes at the cell surface. In this chapter we begin by giving a brief overview of the different types of APCs, concentrating on their properties that both facilitate and modulate the processing and presentation of antigens. We then discuss the mechanisms of antigen processing and loading onto MHC molecules, and transport of the MCH–antigen complexes to the cell surface for each of the major antigen-presenting molecules MHC I, MHC II, and CD1.

ANTIGEN-PRESENTING CELLS

Almost all nucleated cells constitutively display at their surface MHC I molecules presenting peptides derived from intracellular proteins. This process is called the classic MHC I presentation pathway, and it allows $CD8^+$ T cells to monitor the contents of the cells, identify and eliminate cells infected by viruses or intracellular pathogens, and possibly tumor cells. In contrast, MHC II and CD1 molecules present respectively peptides and lipids derived primarily from captured exogenous antigens to $CD4^+$ T cells and natural killer T cells. MHC II and CD1 molecules are expressed mainly on a limited subset of cells, called professional APCs (pAPCs), which are to varying degrees involved in the initial presentation of antigens to naive T cells. pAPCs include B lymphocytes, macrophages (Mϕ), and especially dendritic cells (DCs). As we discuss later, pAPCs can also present peptides derived from exogenous antigens on MHC I to activate naive $CD8^+$ T cells and prime an immune response by a process called cross-presentation. pAPCs vary in their capacity to capture, process, and present antigens on MHC molecules. They also differ in the level expression of the costimulatory molecules and released cytokines required for activating naive T cells.

B Lymphocytes

The ability of B cells to internalize antigen is very limited because they do not exhibit a marked capacity for endocytosis. For example, B cells are generally not capable of phagocytosis of large particles, and therefore they are unable to capture and present antigens derived from invading microorganisms. B cells do, however, efficiently bind and internalize soluble antigens that bind specifically to their unique surface immunoglobulins. Because they express high levels of MHC II and costimulatory molecules, B cells are highly efficient at presenting only their cognate antigens, generating peptide–MHC class II complexes that are presented to $CD4^+$ T cells. Not only does presentation by B cells serve to stimulate T cell proliferation, $CD4^+$ T cells return the favor and facilitate the proliferation and differentiation of B cells into antibody-secreting B cells and plasma cells (see Chapters 8 and 9).

Macrophages

Macrophages exhibit an exceptional capacity for endocytosis and thus have the ability to capture a broad spectrum of antigens by fluid-phase endocytosis, receptor-mediated endocytosis (e.g., via Fcγ receptors, various lectins such as mannose receptor), and phagocytosis of large particles (see Chapter 18). However, Mϕ express relatively low levels of MHC and costimulatory molecules. Upon activation by inflammatory stimuli, Mϕ upregulate the expression of MHC II and costimulatory molecules, although their level of expression is still substantially lower than in B cells and DCs. On the other hand, Mϕ exhibit an exceptional capacity for lysosomal digestion, unlike B cells or DCs (1). This allows for a rapid clearance of the captured antigens but may limit the generation of antigenic peptides by premature destruction and thus affect MHC presentation. Together, these results suggest that although Mϕ can initiate innate immune responses and were once thought to be essential for initiating adaptive immunity, they are suboptimal for efficient MHC presentation.

Dendritic Cells

DCs are believed to play a primary role in priming T cell–mediated immune responses (2,3) (see also Chapter 15). Their efficiency stems not only from their location in tissues, high endocytic capacities, migratory properties in response to inflammatory stimuli, and high surface expression of MHC and costimulatory molecules, but also from their capacity to developmentally regulate these functions (4). Immature DCs mainly reside in peripheral tissues, where they act as sentinels, capturing a wide spectrum of antigens via various mechanisms. Like Mϕ, DCs have a capacity for multiple forms of endocytosis. While in their immature state, however, DCs are poor at antigen presentation, expressing low levels of surface MHC and costimulatory molecules. MHC II molecules accumulate inside lysosomal compartments together with internalized intact antigens. After receiving an inflammatory stimulus, peripheral DCs begin to mature and migrate to secondary lymphoid organs, where they present processed antigens to T cells. DC maturation is accompanied by a dramatic structural reorganization of the cells. DCs acquire the capacity to process captured antigens, load immunogenic peptides onto MHC II molecules, and selectively transfer the MHC II/peptide complexes from lysosomes to the plasma membrane together with costimulatory molecules. Not all mature DCs, however, are functionally equivalent. It is now clear that different maturation stimuli produce mature DCs with different abilities for T cell stimulation and other functions (5). In addition, several DC subsets have been identified that appear to have distinct abilities to prime immune responses (6,7).

MHC I PRESENTATION

To protect the host effectively, the immune system must be constantly surveying for signs of infection. Because many pathogens have evolved to enter a host's cells and replicate intracellularly, the immune system has developed the means to detect the presence of not only extracellular but also intracellular infections. This is the primary function of the MHC I system. Peptides derived from intracellular antigens (both pathogen encoded and host derived) are loaded onto MHC I molecules, which then traffic to the plasma membrane for recognition by $CD8^+$ T cells (Figure 20.1). It has been estimated that any given cell presents hundreds of thousands of such peptides. All nucleated cells express MHC I products.

Classic Pathway of MHC I Antigen Processing

Source of Antigenic Peptides for MHC I Presentation

It had long been thought that proteins at the end of their life span were the source of peptides for MHC I presentation, probably because inhibitors of the proteasome altered protein turnover as well as antigen presentation by MHC I molecules (8). More recently, however, it has been shown that most antigenic peptides (approximately 70%) originate from newly synthesized polypeptides. These are likely to largely consist of premature termination products and misfolded full-length proteins, called defective ribosomal products (DRIPs) (9–11). Thus, peptide presentation on MHC I molecules appears to depend on the rate of protein translation rather than the rate of protein turnover or the total amount of the protein. This process favors the rapid presentation of newly synthesized viral proteins early during viral infection.

Soon after the induction of DC maturation, DRIPs transiently accumulate as aggregates in the cytosol, suggesting that the generation of antigenic peptides and their presentation by MHC I might be regulated (12).

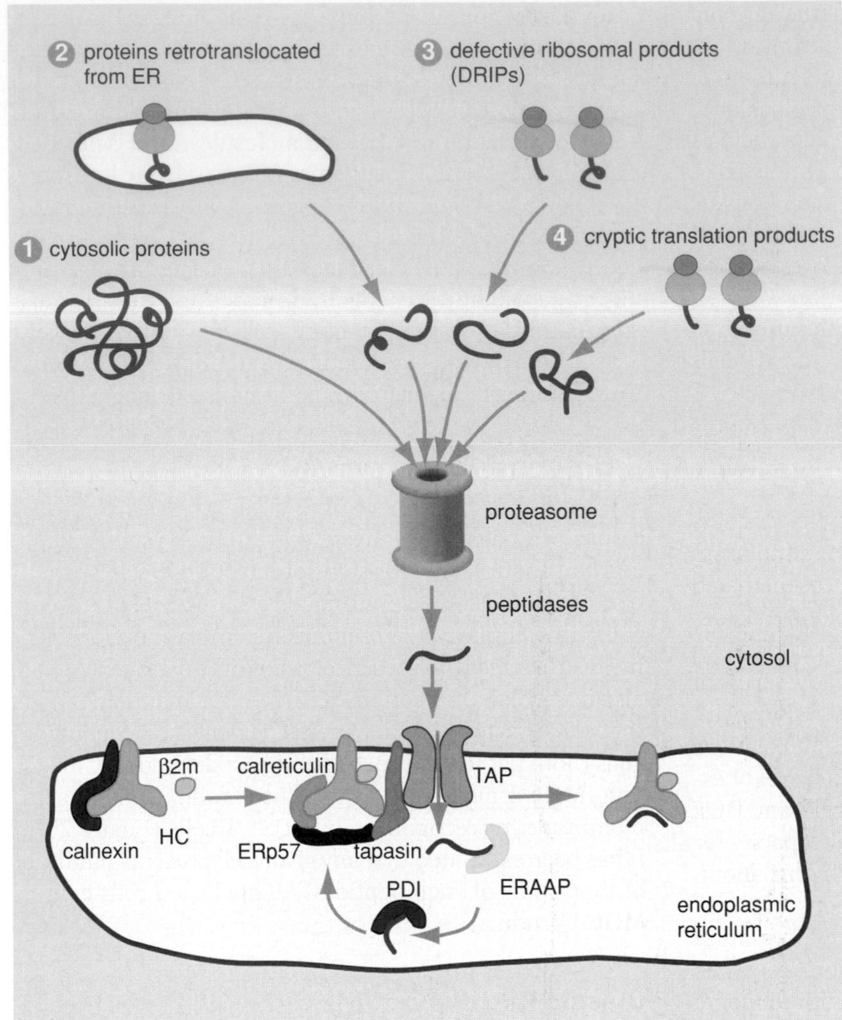

FIGURE 20.1 Overview of the major histocompatibility complex (MHC) I classic pathway. MHC I peptides derive from various sources of endogenous proteins, including (1) cytosolic proteins, (2) proteins retrotranslocated from the endoplasmic reticulum (ER), (3) defective ribosomal products, and (4) cryptic translation products. Polyubiquinated polypeptides are degraded by the proteasome in the cytosol and further processed by cytosolic proteases. The resulting peptides are then translocated into the ER by the transporter associated with antigen processing (TAP), where further trimming by the ER aminopeptidase associated with antigen processing (ERAAP) can occur. The newly synthesized MHC I heavy chain (HC) initially associates with the chaperone calnexin, which assists its folding and binding to β_2-microglobulin (β_2m) in the endoplasmic reticulum. The HC–β_2m complex is then incorporated into the loading complex composed of TAP, tapasin, calreticulin, ERp57, and protein disulfide isomerase (PDI). The role of the loading complex is to help the binding of HC–β_2m complexes to high-affinity peptides and enhance HC–β_2m–peptide complex stability. The peptide-loaded MHC I complexes then leave the ER and are transported to the cell surface via the Golgi apparatus. (Adapted from Trombetta ES and Mellman I. Cell biology of antigen processing in vitro and in vivo. *Annu Rev Immunol* 2005;23:975, with authorization)

In addition to conventional translation products, a small fraction of antigenic peptides can also be generated from cryptic translation products, including introns, intron/exon junctions, untranslated regions, and alternate reading frames (13,14).

Peptide Generation

Peptides presented on MHC I molecules are generated primarily by the ubiquitin-proteasome pathway in the cytosol, whose primary function is to rapidly degrade proteins to amino acids (15). Indeed the peptides produced by this pathway range in size from 2 to 25 amino acids, most of which (approximately 70%) are too short to bind to MHC I molecules (16,17). To be recognized by the degradation machinery, most substrate proteins must be first conjugated to ubiquitin (18). This process is adenosine triphosphate (ATP) dependent and requires multiples enzymes (19). How protein substrates are recognized by the ubiquitin machinery, however, remains elusive. It has been proposed that the same chaperones that usually promote the folding of nascent polypeptides and misfolded proteins can also facilitate polyubiquitination if folding is unsuccessful. It has recently been shown that the knockdown of the chaperone Hsp90 and CHIP, a ubiquitin ligase E3 that interacts with heat shock proteins and ubiquitinates their bound substrates, results in the reduced presentation of MHC I–peptide complexes (20).

The ubiquitinated proteins are then targeted to the proteasome for degradation. The 26S constitutive proteasome is composed of the 20S-core particle responsible for substrate proteolysis and the 19S-regulator complex responsible for substrate recognition and access to the 20S core (21). The 20S core is a cylindrical structure made up of 28 subunits arranged in four stacked heptameric rings. The two inner rings are each composed of homologous but distinct β-subunits, which surround a central chamber where proteolysis occurs. Eukaryotic proteasomes contain two sites that cleave after hydrophobic residues, two after acidic residues, and two after basic residues; thus they can cut most types of peptide bonds, although with different efficiencies depending on the residues that flank the cleavage sites. The two outer rings are each composed of homologous but distinct α-subunits and are arranged to form a central gate that controls the access of substrates to the catalytic chamber. This gate is normally closed, and access is controlled by the 19S particle. The 19S particle consists of two functionally distinct entities: the base and the lid. The base contains ATPases that have the ability to unfold the substrate and to open the gate and thus promote its translocation into the inner chamber of the 20S core, whereas the lid binds and deubiquitinates protein substrates before they access the 20S core.

On interferon γ (IFNγ) stimulation, as occurs during inflammation, new catalytic subunits are incorporated into the proteasome to generate the immunoproteasome (β1, β2, and β5 of the constitutive proteasome are replaced by the IFNγ-inducible homologs LMP2 [β1i], MECL-1 [β2i], and LMP7 [β5i], respectively) (22). The replacement of the three catalytic subunits in the immunoproteasome does not affect the rate at which proteins are degraded, but it alters the cleavage specificity, favoring cleavage behind basic and hydrophobic residues that preferentially bind MHC I molecules, and thus it often enhances the generation of antigenic peptides (23,24). In rare cases, immunoproteasome can also destroy MHC I epitopes normally generated by the constitutive proteasome (25). Of interest, *in vitro* studies have suggested that compared to the constitutive proteasome, the immunoproteasome produces greater amounts of N-extended versions of a dominant antigenic peptide derived from ovalbumin. Thus, antigenic peptides can be generated by further trimming by peptidases in the cytosol and/or the endoplasmic reticulum (ER) rather than being completely degraded to amino acids (26). However, studies with other protein substrates are needed to determine whether this is a general feature of the immunoproteasome.

IFNγ also stimulates the expression of an additional regulator complex called PA28 that can bind both ends of the 20S proteasome (27). Its function in antigen processing is unclear. Although PA28 modifies the profile of peptides produced by the proteasome *in vitro* (28), it does not seem to be essential for MHC I presentation of most antigens *in vivo* (29).

As mentioned earlier, although the proteasomes can generate peptides 8 to 10 amino acids in length that are capable of stably binding MHC I molecules (see Chapter 19), they more frequently produce longer peptides requiring further trimming to potentially become MHC I epitopes (28,30). *In vivo* studies using proteasome inhibitors have shown that additional proteases can be involved in peptide processing (31–33). However, the proteasome must generate the final C-terminus of MHC I–binding peptides. In contrast, N-extended precursors generated by the proteasome can be further processed by aminopeptidases and endopeptidases in the cytosol (34–37,37a). Further trimming can also occur in the ER. The ER aminopeptidase associated with antigen processing (ERAAP/ERAP1) has been recently identified as being a major player in this process (38,39). In ERAAP/ERAP1-deficient mice, cell surface expression of some but not all MHC I alleles is significantly decreased. The presentation of peptides also appears to be differentially affected, with expression of some peptides unchanged, whereas expression of others is either enhanced or absent (40,41). Furthermore, ERAAP-deficient cells present many peptides with N-terminal extensions (42). This suggests that a significant amount of N-extended peptides are translocated from the cytosol into the ER. As for the proteasome, one has to keep in mind that the major role of most these proteases is most likely to hydrolyze peptides to amino acids for cellular homeostasis, a process that would normally contribute to the destruction of MHC I epitopes, although clearly they can sometimes also favor their production (43,44).

Peptides derived from signal sequences of proteins translocated into the ER have also been shown to bind MHC I in an antigen-processing defective cell line (45). How and where these peptides are generated, in the ER or in the cytosol in a proteasome-dependent manner, and whether this phenomenon occurs under normal conditions remain to be determined. The same applies to MHC I–binding peptides that are derived from the membrane anchors of integral membrane proteins.

Peptide Transport into the Endoplasmic Reticulum

As mentioned, peptides generated in the cytosol must be translocated across the ER membrane in order to bind MHC I molecules. This is achieved by the *transporter associated with antigen processing* (TAP) localized in the ER and *cis*-Golgi (46). TAP belongs to the large family of ATP-binding cassette (ABC) transporters, which translocate a variety of solutes across membranes in an ATP-dependent fashion (47). TAP is a heterodimer composed of two subunits, TAP1 and TAP2, both of which are essential and sufficient for peptide translocation (48,49). Each subunit comprises an N-terminal transmembrane domain containing the peptide-binding pocket and a C-terminal cytosolic domain containing the ATP-binding and hydrolysis sites. Peptide transport into the ER lumen is a multistep process: (a) ATP and peptide binding, (b) ATP hydrolysis, and (c) peptide translocation. TAP most efficiently binds and transports peptides 8 to 12 amino acids in length. The binding affinity depends on the three N-terminal and the C-terminal residues (50). Of interest, it is the C-terminal residue preferentially produced by the immunoproteasome that also binds preferentially TAP and MHC I molecules, suggesting a coevolution of these molecules. However, the TAP preferences for the three N-terminal residues and the length of the peptides does not always correspond to those of MHC I molecules confirming that further trimming might be required for some peptides in the ER (see previous section). Nevertheless, it is clear that the TAP affinity for peptides has a substantial impact on the range of peptides presented by MHC I (51,52).

MHC I/Peptide Assembly

MHC I/peptide assembly occurs in the ER. This complex process requires a number of chaperones, which help with the folding of the MHC I heavy chain (HC), its binding to β_2-microglobulin (β_2m), and the peptide loading (53–55). Once formed, the MHC I complexes are transported to the cell surface to present peptides to CD8$^+$ T cells.

The HC is cotranslationally translocated into the ER; it is glycosylated and associates successively with the chaperones BIP and calnexin (56,57), which assist HC folding and the recruitment of disulfide isomerase ERp57 to facilitate disulfide bond formation (58). Toward the end of the folding process, HC binds to β_2m and dissociates from calnexin (56,59); the newly formed complex HC–β_2m is incorporated into an ensemble of accessory molecules called the loading complex, composed of TAP, the transmembrane protein tapasin (TAP-associated glycoprotein), calreticulin, ERp57, and the protein disulfide isomerase (PDI) (59–62). In mice, the loading complex also contains calnexin. Most HC–β_2m complexes are held in association with the loading complex until they stably assemble with a peptide (63,64). The peptide-loaded MHC I complexes then leave the ER and are transported to the cell surface via the Golgi apparatus.

Although it is clear that the role of the loading complex is to help the binding of HC–β_2m complexes with high-affinity peptides and enhance HC–β_2m–peptide complex stability, the precise function of each of the components of the peptide-loading complex is far from completely understood. Each of the components is essential to the MHC I pathway. Deficiency in any of them leads to a similar phenotype, although with various degrees of severity: impaired peptide association with MHC I molecules and reduced MHC I surface expression (48,49,62,65–69). TAP is indispensable for peptide transport into the ER, as mentioned in the previous section. Tapasin appears to have multiple critical roles: (a) stabilizing TAP and thus enhancing peptide translocation in the ER (70,71), (b) recruiting MHC I molecules to the peptide-loading complex by forming a bridge between TAP and HC–β_2m (65), and (c) facilitating and optimizing peptide loading (72,73). ERp57 is also crucial for the recruitment of MHC I molecules into the peptide-loading complex (69). PDI stabilizes a peptide-receptive site by regulating the oxidation state of the disulfide bond in the MHC peptide-binding groove. In addition, PDI binds efficiently to peptides and thus could also help peptide delivery (62). Calreticulin appears to be important in the optimization of peptide loading. but its precise contribution remains to be determined (68).

Cross-presentation: Presentation of Exogenous Antigens by MHC I Molecules

Although MHC I molecules classically present peptides derived from proteins of endogenous origin, exogenous antigens can also enter the MHC I pathway in a process called "cross-presentation" (74,75) (Figure 20.2). This process is likely to be crucial in the initial phase of an immune response because naive CD8$^+$ T cells can only be stimulated by antigens presented on the MHC I molecules of pAPCs. If the pAPC does not synthesize a given antigen, then it must acquire the antigen exogenously. The resulting stimulation of the CD8$^+$ T cell response *in vivo* is called cross-priming.

Cross-presenting APCs

In vitro, Mϕ and DCs are the principal cells able to present peptides derived from exogenous antigens on MHC I molecules, although DCs do it far more efficiently (76). Recently it has also been suggested that B cells can cross-present antigens (76a,76b). By contrast, *in vivo*, DCs seem to be the key players in cross-priming CD8-dependent responses: Ablation of CD11$^+$ DCs in mice abrogates T cell cross-priming (77).

In addition, a new mechanism of antigen transfer has been identified and suggests that cross-presentation might not be limited to pAPCs. Peptides can be transferred through gap junctions from the cytosol of one cell directly into the cytosol of neighboring cells, either innocent bystander cells or pAPCs (78). The physiologic role of this mechanism remains to be elucidated.

Source and Nature of the Cross-presented Antigens

In vitro, virtually any form of antigen (soluble, particulate, aggregated, cell associated, bacterial, protozoan) can be cross-presented. However, under physiologic conditions, it is possible that cross-presented peptides are most often generated from cell-associated antigens captured by phagocytosis.

Cell remnants contain three potential pools of peptides for cross-presentation by MHC I molecules—stable proteins, chaperone-associated peptides, and MHC I–associated peptides. Which of these sources actually contributes to cross-presentation remains controversial. Using different approaches, recent reports showed that stable intact proteins derived from dying cells are the predominant source of cross-presented antigens *in vivo* (79–81), whereas others suggested that fully processed peptides can also be transferred to pAPCs and directly cross-presented

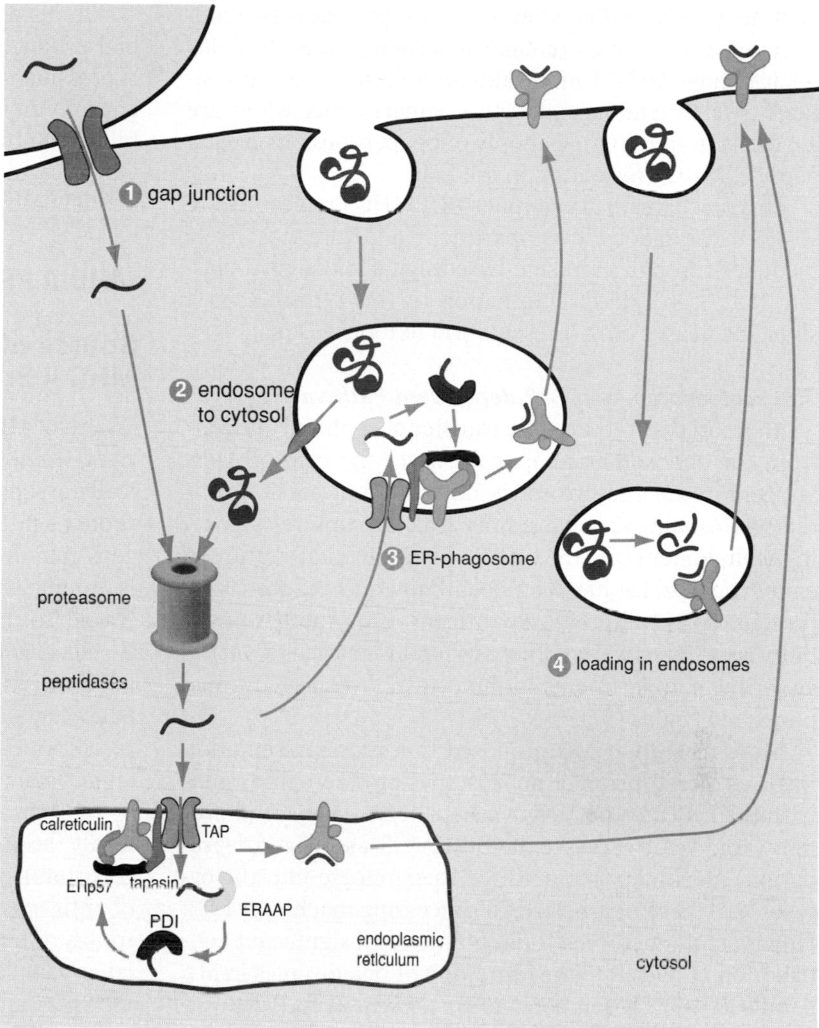

FIGURE 20.2 Mechanisms of cross-presentation of exogenous antigens by major histocompatibility complex (MHC) I molecules. Exogenous antigens enter the classic MHC I pathway through various potential routes: (1) Peptides are transferred through gap junctions from the cytosol of one cell directly into the cytosol of neighboring cells. (2) Antigens can gain access to the classic MHC I pathway after endocytosis. This process requires their transfer from the endosomal compartments to the cytosol. How antigens reach the cytosol is unclear. One possibility is that endosomal vesicles simply leak or rupture, delivering their content into the cytosol. Alternatively, internalized antigens are selectively transported from the endocytic compartments to the cytosol via specific transporter molecules. (3) It was recently suggested that cross-presentation could involve direct fusion of phagosomes or macropinosomes with the endoplasmic reticulum (ER). As a consequence, endocytosed proteins would gain access to the ER-associated degradation machinery required for their release into the cytosol. Once in the cytosol, the exogenous antigens are degraded by the proteasome, and the resulting peptides are transported by the transporter associated with antigen processing (TAP) into the ER or the ER/phagosome and loaded onto MHC I molecules. (4) Some endocytosed antigens appear to be processed and loaded onto MHC I molecules in endocytic compartments independent of the proteasome and TAP. ERAAP, ER aminopeptidase associated with antigen processing; PDI, protein disulfide isomerase.

on MHC I (82). The use of different antigens might be the explanation for these discrepancies, although it is certainly possible that both mechanisms contribute. Notably, these results suggest that the requirements for proteins to be presented by MHC I in the classic pathway and in the cross-presentation pathway are different, and thus the repertoire of peptides presented by MHC I might be influenced by the pathway that is followed.

Mechanisms of Cross-presentation

How the antigens captured by APCs reach the MHC I pathway for cross-presentation is the subject of intense debate (83). Two major mechanisms have been described based on their sensitivity to proteasome inhibitors and their dependence on TAP molecules. One pathway involves antigen proteolysis and peptide loading on MHC I molecules in the endocytic compartments and is thus proteasome and TAP independent. Alternatively, captured antigens are transferred (by an as-yet-unknown mechanism) to the cytosol for proteasomal proteolysis and therefore reach the MHC I via the classic pathway. The choice of the pathway might depend on the nature of the antigen and its intracellular fate after capture. For example, soluble or latex bead-bound ovalbumin is cross-presented in a proteasome- and TAP-dependent manner. The same antigen incorporated into microsphere composed of biodegradable copolymer, however, is cross-presented by a TAP-independent pathway (84). It is important to note that the use of proteasome inhibitors or TAP-deficient cells also directly affects the expression of MHC I molecules, which strongly relies on both TAP and proteasome activities. It is thus likely that the proteasome- and TAP-independent cross-presentation pathway has been largely underestimated.

The Proteasome- and TAP-independent Pathway

The precise mechanism of this pathway, also called the vacuolar pathway, is poorly understood and has been largely characterized as being insensitive to proteasome inhibitors and independent of TAP. Recent work, both *in vitro* and *in vivo*, has shown that the lysosomal protease cathepsin S is required for the generation of the antigenic peptides (84). Whether other lysosomal proteases also contribute to this pathway remains to be determined. It is also unclear how MHC I molecules sample or bind the peptides generated in the endocytic compartments, which are generally devoid of the panoply of chaperones involved in peptide–MHC I formation in the ER.

This mechanism also implies that MHC I molecules are sorted to the endocytic compartment, a feature most likely mediated through a tyrosine-based signal in their cytoplasmic tail (85). Indeed, elimination of this tyrosine-based signal decreases cross-presentation in mouse DCs.

The Proteasome- and TAP-dependent Pathway

This pathway requires the transfer of captured antigens from the endosomal compartments to the cytosol. How antigens reach the cytosol is unclear. One possibility is that endosomal vesicles simply leak or rupture, delivering their content into the cytosol. Experimental rupture of endocytic vesicles has long been known to induce cross-presentation of internalized antigens (86). Another possibility is the selective export of exogenous antigens from the endocytic compartments to the cytosol via specific transporter molecules (87).

More recently it was proposed that cross-presentation involves direct fusion of phagosomes or macropinosomes with the ER (88–91). As a consequence, endocytosed proteins would gain access to the ERAD (ER-associated degradation) machinery required for their release into the cytosol, and therefore the MHC I processing machinery (92). However, other studies could not detect a significant contribution of the ER to the formation of phagosomes in Mϕ or DCs (93). If ER components are present in endocytic organelles, they are therefore present in trace amounts relative to the ER proper, making it difficult to understand how they might work. Alternatively, it is possible that small amounts of internalized antigen reach the lumen of the ER proper. That this can occur has been demonstrated by the fact that endocytosis in caveolae can lead to direct delivery to the ER, avoiding conventional endosomes and lysosomes (94).

Internalized antigens have to survive the harsh environment of endosomes/lysosomes before being delivered to the cytosol. Lysosomes contain proteases the primary function of which is to degrade proteins to amino acids. Indeed, limiting lysosomal protease activity by artificially reducing acidification of the endosomal compartments increases the transfer of endocytosed antigens to the cytosol and enhances their cross-presentation (95). Similarly, it has been recently shown in DCs that phagosomes recruit the nicotinamide adenine dinucleotide phosphate oxidase NOX2 to neutralize the phagosomal pH and promote cross-presentation (96). Antigen targeting to protease-poor recycling endosomes also may favor cross-presentation, probably by sequestering antigens away from lysosomal degradation (97).

After exposure to inflammatory stimuli, such as microbial products or inflammatory cytokines, surface MHC I expression increases in pAPCs. In DCs, this reflects at least partially an increase in synthesis and posttranslational stability (98–100). In addition, the cross-presentation pathway is regulated in DCs independently of the endogenous MHC I pathway (100–102).

MHC II PRESENTATION

Source of Antigenic Peptides for MHC II Presentation

Whereas MHC I molecules present mainly peptides derived from endogenous proteins, MHC II molecules typically associate with peptides generated from exogenous proteins internalized by the APCs. B cells internalize antigens mainly through their B cell receptor. Although this is an efficient mechanism of capture, it essentially limits B cells to the internalization of a single type of antigen. B cells also express Fcγ receptors that in principle could allow any immune complex to be taken up and presented. However, alternative mRNA splicing ensures that the Fcγ receptors expressed by B cells are incapable of efficient endocytosis for antigen presentation (103,104).

In contrast, both Mϕ and immature DCs endocytose avidly through a wide array of mechanisms (including Fcγ receptors), allowing them to internalize a broad spectrum of antigens (105). Different types of antigens use different routes of internalization, which determine the intracellular organelles to which antigens are delivered, which in turn may affect their processing and loading onto MHC II molecules.

Endocytosis falls into two major categories: phagocytosis and pinocytosis (106,107). Phagocytosis involves the capture of large particles, such as bacteria or cell debris, and is likely to be the most physiologically relevant mode of antigen uptake *in vivo* (107a) (see also Chapter 18). Phagocytosis is typically triggered by the binding of particulate antigens to specific surface receptors, which in turn transduce the signals for particle engulfment. Pinocytosis includes fluid-phase uptake by macropinocytosis and receptor-mediated endocytosis. In most DC subsets (Langerhans cells being a notable exception), macropinocytosis plays a major role in internalization of soluble antigen, at least *in vitro*. Greater efficiency of endocytosis can be achieved when antigens are captured by specific high-affinity receptors, such as the mannose receptor, which binds glycosylated ligands, Fcγ receptors, which bind immunoglobulin G–antigen complexes, or scavenger receptors, which bind a wide variety of ligands.

In DCs macropinocytosis is regulated during maturation. Immediately after receiving maturation stimuli, there is a brief increase in macropinocytosis, followed by its complete downregulation. This is believed to boost the capture of the pathogens responsible for inducing maturation (108–111). Paradoxically, because macropinocytosis is largely responsible for endocytosis *in vitro*, it is commonly believed that all forms of endocytosis are shut down in mature DCs. However, this question has never been properly addressed, and the various mechanisms involved in antigen endocytosis may not be affected in the same way during DC maturation. Indeed, the number of clathrin-coated structures is unchanged in immature and mature mouse bone marrow–derived DCs, suggesting that receptor-mediated endocytosis still occurs in mature DCs (109).

MHC II molecules can also present peptides derived from endogenous proteins. How cytoplasmic and nuclear proteins gain access to this antigen presentation pathway remained elusive until recently. Autophagy is now believed to be the main mechanism responsible for the delivery of cytoplasmic proteins to lysosomes (112). Two main autophagic pathways have been identified—macroautophagy and chaperone-mediated autophagy. In macroautophagy, aggregate-prone, long-lived cytosolic and nuclear proteins get preferentially incorporated into autophagosomes, which then fuse with endosomal/lysosomal compartments. Proteins from the autophagosome are then degraded by lysosomal proteases and the generated peptides loaded onto MHC II molecules (113,114). Macroautophagy is a constitutive pathway in DCs and B cells *in vitro* (114). In chaperone-mediated autophagy, cytosolic proteins are believed to be directly translocated into late endosomes/lysosomes by a process somehow dependent on the lysosomal membrane glycoprotein Lamp-2a (115). This process is facilitated by the chaperone protein hsc70. The efficiency of the autophagic pathways in the presentation of cytosolic proteins by MHC II molecules in primary APCs remains to be established.

MHC II Assembly in the ER and Transport to the Endosomal Pathway

Unlike MHC I molecules, the assembly of MHC II molecules and peptide association occurs in two distinct and independent steps (Figure 20.3). The initial assembly of the MHC II molecules with the chaperone-invariant chain (Ii) takes place in the ER. The MHC II–Ii complexes are then targeted through the Golgi apparatus to the endosomal compartment, where the Ii chain is degraded and peptide loading occurs. The newly formed MHC II–peptide complexes are then transported to the cell surface.

MHC II molecules are heterodimers of two variable-transmembrane glycoproteins–α chain and β chain. They are synthesized and assembled in the ER with the help of the chaperone Ii chain and form a nine-chain structure consisting of three α–β dimers associated with an Ii chain trimer (116). The Ii chain is a transmembrane type II glycoprotein. In mice, two splicing forms of the Ii chain have been identified—p33 and p41—based on their molecular weight. p41 contains an additional domain that can bind the lysosomal protease cathepsin L, although its physiologic significance is unclear (117). In humans, there are two additional forms of Ii chain—p35 and p43—resulting from alternative initiation of translation. As a consequence, p35 and p43 possess an additional 15 amino acids containing an ER retention signal (118).

MHC II association with Ii chain has multiple functions. The ER retention signal prevents premature transport of the MHC II molecules before they are properly assembled and folded. This signal is overridden when the MHC II–Ii chain assembly is complete, allowing the export of the complex to the Golgi apparatus (119). The second function of Ii chain is to prevent premature peptide loading of MHC II in the ER (120,121). The Ii chain contains a domain called MHC II–associated invariant chain peptide (CLIP) that protects the peptide-binding groove until the MHC II–Ii complex enters the endocytic pathway. Finally, targeting signals contained in the cytoplasmic domain of Ii chain drive the MHC II–Ii complexes into the endosomal pathway where the peptide loading occurs (122–124).

MHC II–Peptide Assembly

Two major steps take place in the endocytic pathway: The Ii chain is degraded, liberating the peptide-binding site of MHC II molecules, and antigens are processed into peptides associating with MHC II molecules. Newly formed MHC II–peptide complexes are then transported to the cell surface. This process is believed to occur largely in late endosomes/lysosomes–like structures where proteases are the most active and intracellular MHC II molecules accumulate (125). However, lysosomes have classically been considered a degradative dead end, from which very few proteins escape. This consideration led to the idea that APCs might have developed specialized MHC II–containing compartments (MIICs) devoted to antigen processing and peptide loading. However, recent studies instead suggest that DCs have developed the unique capacity to modify the features of otherwise conventional late endosomes/lysosomes to overcome their inherent limitations of strictly degradative organelles, as discussed later.

Ii Degradation

As they progress through the endocytic pathway toward lysosomes, MHC II–Ii complexes are exposed to increasingly acidic environments, causing the activation of endosomal/lysosomal proteases. Perhaps as a result, Ii chain undergoes cleavages directionally from the C-terminus to the N-terminus involving multiple proteases after delivery to late endocytic compartments, although the process may well begin even in early compartments (117). *In vitro* studies have suggested the participation of several endosomal/

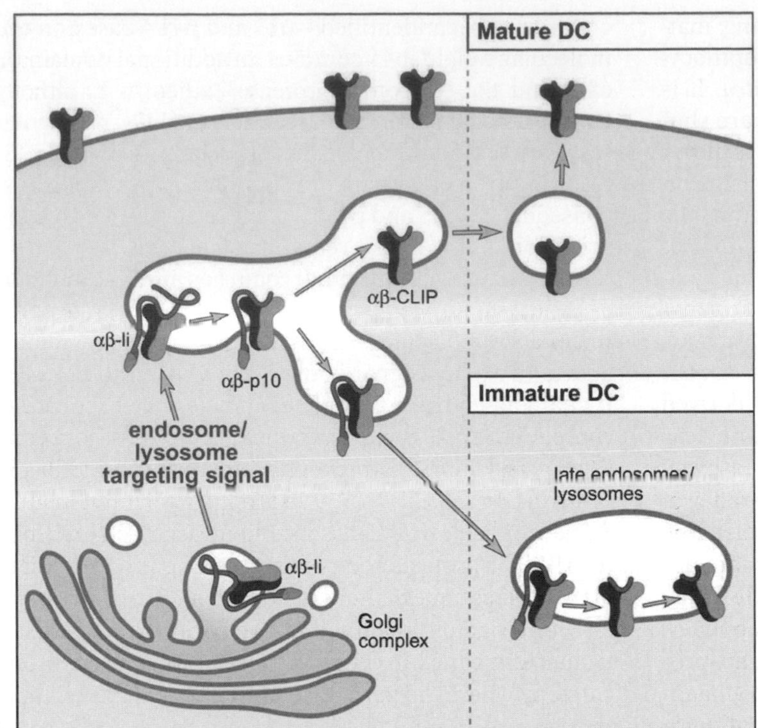

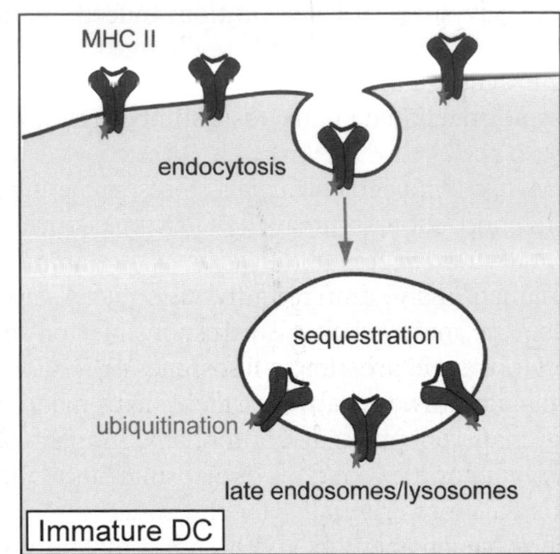

FIGURE 20.3 Overview of the major histocompatibility complex (MHC) II pathway in dendritic cells. **A:** MHC II peptides are mainly derived from exogenous proteins endocytosed by dendritic cells (DCs) through a wide array of mechanisms, including phagocytosis, macropinocytosis, and receptor-mediated endocytosis. The captured antigens eventually reach endosomal/lysosomal compartments. Endogenous proteins can also be imported into lysosomes by autophagy for loading onto MHC II molecules. Newly synthesized MHC II molecules associate with the invariant chain (Ii) in the ER. The MHC II–li complexes are then targeted through the Golgi apparatus to the endosomal/lysosomal compartments. In immature DCs, internalized antigens and Ii chain are poorly degraded, and MHC II–peptide complex generation is thus relatively inefficient. Upon DC maturation, some lysosomal proteases are converted into their active mature forms, expression of protease inhibitors is downregulated, and, perhaps most important, there is acidification of the endosomes/lysosomes, which induces nonspecific activation of most proteases. As a result, Ii chain removal, antigen processing, and peptide loading onto MHC II are enhanced. The newly formed MHC II–peptide complexes are then transported to the cell surface. (From Trombetta ES, Mellman I. Cell biology of antigen processing *in vitro* and *in vivo*. *Annu Rev Immunol* 2005;23:975, with permission.) **B:** Another mechanism for regulating surface expression of MHC class II molecules in DCs is polyubiquination. In immature DCs, ubiquitination of the cytoplasmic tail of MHC II-β chain limits surface expression of MHC II molecules by inducing their clearance from the cell surface by endocytosis and possibly their sequestration in the endosomal/lysosomal compartments. In mature DCs, ubiquitination of MHC II molecules is suppressed.

lysosomal proteases in Ii degradation, but the use of protease-deficient mice largely failed to confirm a critical role for most proteases tested. This suggests that there may be large redundancy among these proteases. However, the terminal stages of Ii processing seem to be differentially dependent on the cysteine protease cathepsin S, at least in some MHC II haplotypes. Cathepsin S–deficient B cells and DCs show accumulation of the processing intermediate p10 (126–128).

Ultimately, only the end product, CLIP, remains in the MHC II peptide groove. CLIP is subsequently exchanged for antigenic peptides in a reaction favored by acidic pH and facilitated by the MHC II–like chaperone DM (also called HLA-DM in humans and H2-DM or H2-M in mice) (129). The current model is that the association of DM with the MHC II–CLIP complex induces a conformational change of the peptide-binding groove, decreasing its affinity for CLIP and thus facilitating its dissociation (130,131). DM also catalyzes the dissociation of any peptide from MHC II molecules. Thus, by enhancing the rate of peptide exchange, DM favors the presentation of high-affinity peptides with slower intrinsic rates of dissociation (132–134).

In B cells and some DC subsets, there is an additional MHC II–like molecule DO (also called HLA-DO in humans and H2-O in mice) (135). Its intracellular trafficking is dependent on DM, with which DO is tightly associated. In human B cells, DO inhibits DM activity. DO-transfected cells express increased surface levels of MHC II-CLIP (136).

However, after antigen internalization via the B cell receptor (BCR), DO dissociates from DM (135). These results suggest that DO promotes MHC II presentation of antigens recognized by the BCR while it inhibits the presentation of antigens from endogenous origin or those taken up nonspecifically.

Antigen Processing

Antigenic peptides presented on MHC II molecules are produced by endosomal/lysosomal proteases (117,137). However, a requirement for specific proteases in the processing of most antigens has been difficult to establish. Some proteases may regulate MHC II presentation by exerting a dual effect on both protein antigen processing and Ii-chain degradation. In addition, most endosomal/lysosomal proteases have redundant activities, with few exceptions. The IFNγ-induced lysosomal thiol reductase (GILT) is the only lysosomal reductase known, and it does play a role in the degradation of protein antigens containing disulfide bonds (138); however, even GILT is dispensable. An example in which a single enzyme does play a unique and necessary role is the asparaginyl cysteine endoprotease (AEP) (also called legumain), which controls the processing of tetanus toxoid (139). Conversely, AEP limits the presentation of myelin basic protein (MBP) by destroying its immunodominant peptide (140). Cathepsin L and cathepsin S expression can also positively or negatively affect the generation of some antigenic peptides (141). In conclusion, it is likely that the redundancy of degradative activities in late endosomes and lysosomes ensures that a single protease is rarely required for antigen processing in general.

The late endosomal/lysosomal compartment is a hostile environment for proteins. Its primary function is to degrade proteins into amino acids. How antigenic peptides survive such an environment remains elusive. It has been suggested that intact or partially processed protein antigens rapidly bind the MHC II groove before destruction and that processing happens on each side of the groove after binding (142). Consistent with this idea, it was found that large protein fragments are associated with MHC II molecules (143–149).

Another way in which to reduce epitope destruction is to limit protease activity. DCs and B cells contain low levels of proteases, resulting in a limited capacity for antigen degradation (1). DCs further limit proteolysis by expressing protease inhibitors (150,151). Limited proteolysis also allows DCs to sequester captured antigens for up to several days, providing a source of antigens for sustained processing and presentation by DCs within secondary lymphoid organs. Conversely, limiting susceptibility to lysosomal proteolysis enhances protein antigen presentation by MHC II molecules and antigen immunogenicity (152). In contrast to DCs and B cells, Mϕ express exceptionally high levels of lysosomal proteases and rapidly degrade captured proteins. These low protease levels, together with relatively low MHC II expression, help to explain why, compared to DCs and B cells, Mϕ are better adapted for the clearance of the captured pathogens than for their presentation to T cells.

Regulation of Antigen Processing and MHC II Pathway in DCs

In response to inflammatory and microbial stimuli, DCs enhance their capacity to form and present MHC II–peptide complexes (4,153,154), in part by controlling their lysosomal proteolytic activities through multiple mechanisms. In immature DCs, internalized antigens are degraded slowly, with MHC II–peptide complex generation or accumulation thus being relatively inefficient (155,156). Upon DC maturation, the lysosomal proteases AEP and cathepsin L are converted into their active mature forms (157,158), expression of cystatin C, a cathepsin S/B inhibitor, is downregulated (150), and, perhaps most important, there is acidification of the endosomes/lysosomes, which induces nonspecific activation of most proteases (158,159). DC maturation enhances activation of vacuolar proton ATPase, which lowers endosomal/lysosomal pH and favors antigen processing and the formation of MHC II–peptide complexes (158).

DCs also control MHC II presentation by tightly regulating MHC II trafficking during maturation. In immature DCs, MHC II molecules accumulate in late endosomes/lysosomes, whereas in mature DCs, MHC II molecules accumulate at the cell surface (160,161). In immature DCs, most of the newly synthesized MHC II–Ii complexes are targeted from the Golgi apparatus to the endosomal pathway (161). As discussed earlier, in immature DCs the attenuated activity of endosomal/lysosomal proteases limits Ii degradation and the generation of antigenic peptides, thus leading to the retention and eventually the degradation of MHC II molecules in the lysosomes. There is also a significant portion of MHC II molecules that reach endosomes/lysosomes following endocytosis from the plasma membrane. Recent data indicate that MHC II clearance from the surface of immature DCs is triggered by ubiquitination of the cytoplasmic tail of MHC II-β chain (162–164). Upon maturation, general endosomal/lysosomal proteolytic activity increases, resulting in the rapid maturation and peptide loading of the newly synthesized MHC II molecules, which are then targeted to the plasma membrane. Ubiquitination of MHC II molecules no longer occurs, causing their accumulation at the cell surface (163,164).

It is remarkable that MHC II–peptide complexes can escape the late endosomal/lysosomal compartments in DCs, because lysosomes are conventionally considered inefficient sites of membrane recycling to the plasma membrane. DC maturation elicits the formation of lysosomal tubules, which move in a retrograde manner to fuse directly with the plasma membrane (165–167). In the presence of specific T cells, the tubules may even be selectively targeted to the DC–T cell interface (166), thus facilitating antigen presentation to T cells.

MHC II molecules exhibit a unique distribution at the surface of DCs. They appear to be organized into clusters (156). The discontinuous distribution is at least in part mediated by lateral association of MHC II molecules with the tetraspan molecule CD9 and could facilitate T cell recognition (168).

CD1 PRESENTATION

CD1 molecules are MHC-like proteins that bind and present lipid antigens (169,170). Compared to the MHC I and MHC II presentation pathways, little is known about the intracellular pathways leading to lipid presentation by CD1 molecules. In humans, five CD1 isoforms have been identified, and two classes can be distinguished: The first group, containing CD1a, CD1b, and CD1c molecules, presents bacterial lipid antigens to conventional $\alpha\beta$ T cells. The second group, composed of CD1d molecules, mainly presents self-lipid antigens to a specialized population of T cells, named NKT cells, expressing an invariant TCR α chain. The function of CD1e molecules is poorly understood. CD1e molecules appear to remain intracellular, apparently never reaching the plasma membrane, which would exclude a direct role in lipid antigen presentation to T cells (171). It was recently proposed that CD1e might instead be involved in lipid antigen processing, as discussed later. In mice, only the CD1d isoform is expressed. CD1a, b, c, e isoforms are expressed mainly by DCs, whereas the CD11d isoform is also expressed in other tissues. Like MHC I molecules, CD1 molecules consist of one transmembrane heavy chain that associates with β_2m. Unlike MHC I molecules, however, CD1 molecules are targeted to the endocytic pathway, where they bind lipid antigens.

Source and Nature of Antigens for CD1 Presentation

A wide variety of lipid antigens from microbial and self-origin have been found to bind CD1 molecules. Most of the identified foreign lipid antigens are constituents derived from the cell wall of mycobacteria. Some of these are shed and might therefore be readily available for loading onto CD1 molecules. Others are covalently attached to the bacterial cell wall and require processing in the endosomal pathway before association to CD1 molecules. The characterized self-lipids capable of binding CD1 molecules include glycolipids, phospholipids, and lipopeptides (172,173).

A comparison of the structures of the known CD1 ligands has revealed a large flexibility both in the type of hydrophobic tail that can bind the CD1 molecules and in the hydrophilic region that interacts with TCR (174).

The mechanisms of exogenous lipid antigen capture have been poorly scrutinized. It is likely that protein antigens and lipid antigens, both associated with bacteria or cell debris, are internalized through the same routes (see section on MHC II presentation). In addition, pathways specific to lipid antigen recognition and internalization have been developed by APCs. The lipid transporter apolipoprotein E mediates the delivery of serum-borne lipid antigens to the endocytic pathway in a receptor-dependent manner, leading to their efficient presentation (175).

Assembly and Intracellular Trafficking of the CD1 Molecules

CD1 molecules are synthesized in the ER, where they assembled with β_2m in a process requiring the chaperones calnexin, calreticulin, and ERp57, analogous to MHC I molecules (176) (Figure 20.4). The CD1b and CD1d molecules, and probably the other CD1 isoforms, associate with the self antigen phosphatidylinositol (PI) in the ER (177), suggesting that PI plays a role similar to the Ii in the MHC II pathway by facilitating CD1 assembly and possibly protecting the binding groove until the CD1 molecules enter the endocytic pathway. This hypothesis has yet to be verified. Microsomal triglyceride transfer protein (MTP), an ER-resident protein, associated with CD1d *in vitro*, is essential to lipid antigen presentation, and was proposed to assist in loading of lipids onto nascent CD1d proteins (178,179). However, recent studies suggest instead a distal role of MTP at a later stage in the recycling of CD1d from the lysosomes to the plasma membrane (180). CD1d has also been shown to associate with Ii chain alone or in complex with MHC II molecules *in vitro*, suggesting that the intracellular trafficking of CD1d may be altered in presence of Ii and MHC II molecules (181,182). However, a potential role of the Ii chain in the intracellular trafficking of CD1d was not confirmed *in vivo* (183).

The newly assembled CD1 complexes are transported from the ER to the cell surface via the Golgi apparatus, although an endosomal intermediate remains possible. In any event, targeting signals contained in the cytosolic tails of the various CD1 isoforms induce their internalization via diverse mechanisms and their traffic through different portions of the endocytic pathway (184–188). CD1a molecules traffic only within the recycling early endosomes, whereas CD1b and CD1d molecules accumulate in the late endosomes/lysosomes. CD1c molecules are equally distributed in the early endosomes and the late endosomes/lysosomes at steady state.

During DC maturation, intracellular distribution and trafficking of the CD1a, b, c isoforms does not appear to be dramatically affected (189). However, certain features

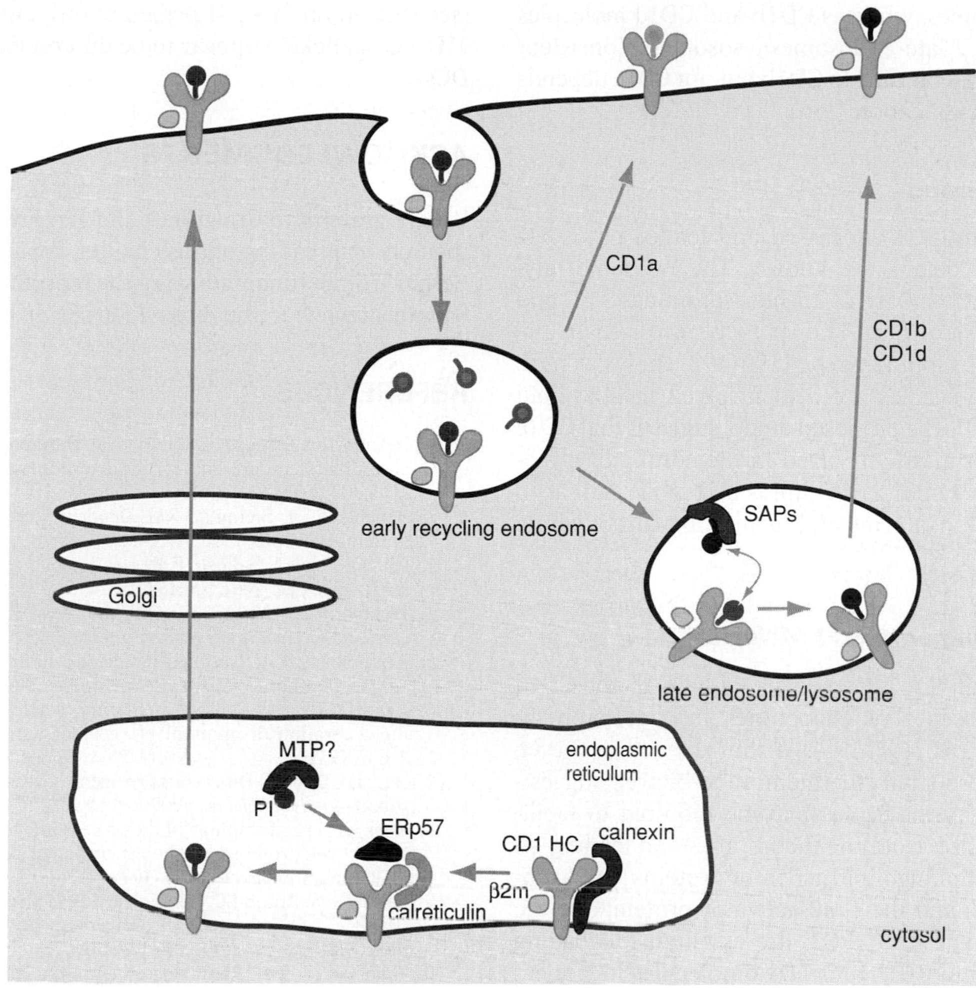

FIGURE 20.4 Overview of the CD1 pathway. CD1 molecules are major histocompatibility complex (MHC)–like proteins that bind lipid antigens from endogenous and exogenous origin. The newly synthesized CD1 heavy chain (HC) assembles with β_2-microglobulin (β_2m) in a process analogous to MHC I and requires the chaperones calnexin, calreticulin, and ERp57 in the endoplasmic reticulum (ER). The CD1b and CD1d molecules, and probably the other CD1 isoforms, then associate with the self-antigen phosphatidylinositol (PI) in the ER, possibly with the help of the microsomal triglyceride transfer protein (MTP). The antigen-loaded CD1 complexes then leave the ER and are transported to the cell surface via the Golgi apparatus. From the plasma membrane, CD1 isoforms traffic to different endocytic compartments, where they bind lipid antigens (CD1a molecules traffic to early endosomes, whereas CD1b and CD1d are targeted to the late endosomes/lysosomes). In lysosomes, sphingolipid activator proteins (SAPs) facilitate lipid extraction from the membranes and loading onto CD1 molecules. The lipid-loaded CD1 molecules are then transported to the cell surface for presentation to T cells.

of the CD1 presentation pathway may be regulated during DC maturation without affecting CD1 distribution. For example, it is unknown whether immature and mature DCs present a similar repertoire of lipid antigens. Of interest, CD1e molecules relocalize from the Golgi apparatus to the lysosomes, where they are cleaved into a stable soluble form upon DC maturation (171). CD1e molecules have been shown to be involved in the generation of glycolipid antigens presented by CD1b molecules (190). Thus, by regulating the intracellular distribution of CD1e molecules, DCs might regulate the processing of glycolipid antigens and their presentation by CD1 molecules.

Antigen Processing and Loading on CD1 Molecules

Lipid ligand selection is probably controlled by the intracellular distribution and the binding groove specificities of the CD1 isoforms. According to their intracellular localization, it is likely that CD1a molecules bind lipid antigens in the early endosomes, whereas CD1b and CD1d molecules are loaded in the late endosomes/lysosomes. Consistent with this idea, lipid binding to CD1b but not CD1a depends on endosomal acidification (186).

Antigen Processing

How are lipid antigens processed and loaded onto CD1 molecules? Few details are known. The lysosomal glycosidases α-galactosidase A, β-hexosaminidase β, and α-mannosidase have been shown to be involved in the trimming of glycolipid antigens (190–192). In lysosomes, soluble CD1e molecules are also involved in glycolipid degradation (190). The proposed model suggests that CD1e molecules are primarily involved in the editing of glycolipid antigens by binding glycolipids in a mode similar to that of other CD1 isoforms and facilitating carbohydrate degradation.

Antigen Loading onto CD1 Molecules

In vitro, lipids can directly associate with CD1b and CD1d molecules in absence of chaperones in a reaction favored by acidic pH (193–195). Within the cell, however, lipids tend to insert into the membrane bilayer, suggesting that accessory molecules may be required to facilitate lipid extraction from the membranes and loading on CD1 molecules. Sphingolipid activator proteins (SAPs), including saposins and the GM2-activator protein, and the Niemann-Pick type C2 (NPC2) are essential for loading lipid antigens onto CD1b and CD1d molecules in late endosomes/lysosomes (196–200). SAPs are believed to have multiples functions: (a) they extract lipids from the lysosomal membrane, making them available for processing by lysosomal enzymes or direct loading onto CD1 molecules and (b) they interact with CD1 molecules and exchange the lipids bound to CD1 molecules. By analogy with the chaperones, tapasin in the MHC pathway, and DM in the MHC II pathway, SAPs may serve an editing function by binding to and removing antigens that are weakly bound to CD1 molecules.

Cathepsin L–deficient mice exhibit a defect in CD1d presentation (201), although the underlying mechanism remains to be elucidated. Cathepsin L may be required for the conversion of the saponin precursor, or other unknown enzymes involved in the CD1 pathway, into mature active forms. Alternatively, cathepsin L may be directly involved in the processing of antigens that bind CD1d molecules.

The newly lipid-loaded CD1 molecules are then transported to the cell surface, where they present lipid antigens to T cells. CD1a molecules loaded in early endosomes reach the plasma membrane via the recycling endosomal pathway. How CD1b and CD1b molecules escape the late endosomes/lysosomes has not been characterized. One possibility is that they use the same pathway as MHC II molecules (see section on MHC II presentation), although CD1 and MHC II trafficking appear to be differentially regulated in DCs.

ACKNOWLEDGMENTS

We are grateful to Craig Platt and Jan Fredrik Simons for their critical reading of this chapter. We are indebted to E. Sergio Trombetta for allowing the reproduction of a figure from his review in the *Annual Review of Immunology* (4).

REFERENCES

1. Delamarre L, Pack M, Chang H, et al. Differential lysosomal proteolysis in antigen presenting cells determines antigen fate. *Science.* 2005;307:1630.
2. Banchereau J, Steinman RM. Dendritic cells and the control of immunity. *Nature.* 1998;392:245.
3. Lanzavecchia A, Sallusto F. Regulation of T cell immunity by dendritic cells. *Cell.* 2001;106:263.
4. Trombetta ES, Mellman I. Cell biology of antigen processing *in vitro* and *in vivo*. *Annu Rev Immunol.* 2005;23:975.
5. Reis e Sousa C. Activation of dendritic cells: translating innate into adaptive immunity. *Curr Opin Immunol.* 2004;16:21.
6. Heath WR, et al. Cross-presentation, dendritic cell subsets, and the generation of immunity to cellular antigens. *Immunol Rev.* 2004;199:26.
7. Dudziak D, et al. Differential antigen processing by dendritic cell subsets *in vivo*. *Science.* 2007;315:107.
8. Rock KL, et al. Inhibitors of the proteasome block the degradation of most cell proteins and the generation of peptides presented on MHC class I molecules. *Cell.* 1994;78:761.
9. Yewdell JW, Anton LC, Bennink JR. Defective ribosomal products (DRiPs): a major source of antigenic peptides for MHC class I molecules? *J Immunol.* 1996;157:1823.
10. Schubert U, et al. Rapid degradation of a large fraction of newly synthesized proteins by proteasomes. *Nature.* 2000;404:770.
11. Reits EA, Vos JC, Gromme M, et al. The major substrates for TAP *in vivo* are derived from newly synthesized proteins. *Nature.* 2000;404:774.
12. Lelouard H, et al. Transient aggregation of ubiquitinated proteins during dendritic cell maturation. *Nature.* 2002;417:177.
13. Shastri N, Schwab S, Serwold T. Producing nature's gene-chips: the generation of peptides for display by MHC class I molecules. *Annu Rev Immunol.* 2002;20:463.
14. Schwab SR, Li KC, Kang C, et al. Constitutive display of cryptic translation products by MHC class I molecules. *Science.* 2003;301:1367.
15. Rock KL, York IA, Saric T, et al. Protein degradation and the generation of MHC class I-presented peptides. *Adv Immunol.* 2002;80:1.
16. Kisselev AF, Akopian TN, Woo KM, et al. The sizes of peptides generated from protein by mammalian 26 and 20 S proteasomes. Implications for understanding the degradative mechanism and antigen presentation. *J Biol Chem.* 1999;274:3363.
17. Toes RE, et al. Discrete cleavage motifs of constitutive and immunoproteasomes revealed by quantitative analysis of cleavage products. *J Exp Med.* 2001;194:1.
18. Wilkinson KD. Ubiquitination and deubiquitination: targeting of proteins for degradation by the proteasome. *Semin Cell Dev Biol.* 2000;11:141.
19. Kuhlbrodt K, Mouysset J, Hoppe T. Orchestra for assembly and fate of polyubiquitin chains. *Essays Biochem.* 2005;41:1.
20. Kunisawa J, Shastri N. Hsp90alpha chaperones large C-terminally extended proteolytic intermediates in the MHC class I antigen processing pathway. *Immunity.* 2006;24:523.
21. Voges D, Zwickl P, Baumeister W. The 26S proteasome: a molecular machine designed for controlled proteolysis. *Ann Rev Biochem.* 1999;68:1015.

22. Strehl B, et al. Interferon-gamma, the functional plasticity of the ubiquitin-proteasome system, and MHC class I antigen processing. *Immunol Rev.* 2005;207:19.
23. Van Kaer L, et al. Altered peptidase and viral-specific T cell response in LMP2 mutant mice. *Immunity.* 1994;1:533.
24. Sijts AJ, et al. Efficient generation of a hepatitis B virus cytotoxic T lymphocyte epitope requires the structural features of immunoproteasomes. *J Exp Med.* 2000;191:503.
25. Morel S, et al. Processing of some antigens by the standard proteasome but not by the immunoproteasome results in poor presentation by dendritic cells. *Immunity.* 2000;12,:107.
26. Cascio P, Hilton C, Kisselev AF, et al. 26S proteasomes and immunoproteasomes produce mainly N-extended versions of an antigenic peptide. *EMBO J.* 2001:20:2357.
27. Ma CP, Slaughter, CA, DeMartino GN. Identification, purification, and characterization of a protein activator (PA28) of the 20 S proteasome (macropain). *J Biol Chem.* 1992;267:10515.
28. Cascio P, Call M, Petre BM, et al. Properties of the hybrid form of the 26S proteasome containing both 19S and PA28 complexes. *EMBO J.* 2002;21:2636.
29. Murata S, et al. Immunoproteasome assembly and antigen presentation in mice lacking both PA28alpha and PA28beta. *EMBO J.* 2001;20:5898.
30. Rock KL, York IA, Goldberg AL. Post-proteasomal antigen processing for major histocompatibility complex class I presentation. *Nat Immunol.* 2004;5:670.
31. Craiu A, Akopian T, Goldberg A, et al. Two distinct proteolytic processes in the generation of a major histocompatibility complex class I-presented peptide. *Proc Natl Acad Sci U S A.* 1997;94:10850.
32. Stoltze L, et al. Generation of the vesicular stomatitis virus nucleoprotein cytotoxic T lymphocyte epitope requires proteasome-dependent and -independent proteolytic activities. *Eur J Immunol.* 1998;28:4029.
33. Mo XY, Cascio P, Lemerise K, et al. Distinct proteolytic processes generate the C and N termini of MHC class I-binding peptides. *J Immunol.* 1999;163:5851.
34. Beninga J, Rock KL, Goldberg AL. Interferon-gamma can stimulate post-proteasomal trimming of the N terminus of an antigenic peptide by inducing leucine aminopeptidase. *J Biol Chem.* 1998;273:18734.
35. Stoltze L, et al. Two new proteases in the MHC class I processing pathway. *Nat Immunol.* 2000;1:413.
36. Reits E, et al. A major role for TPPII in trimming proteasomal degradation products for MHC class I antigen presentation. *Immunity.* 2004;20:495.
37. York IA, Bhutani N, Zendzian S, et al. Tripeptidyl Peptidase II Is the major peptidase needed to trim long antigenic precursors, but is not required for most MHC class I antigen presentation. *J Immunol.* 2006;177:1434.
37a. Saric 2001.
38. Serwold T, Gonzalez F, Kim J, et al. ERAAP customizes peptides for MHC class I molecules in the endoplasmic reticulum. *Nature.* 2002;419:480.
39. Saric T, et al. An IFN-gamma-induced aminopeptidase in the ER, ERAP1, trims precursors to MHC class I-presented peptides. *Nat Immunol.* 2002;3:1169.
40. Yan J, et al. *In vivo* role of ER-associated peptidase activity in tailoring peptides for presentation by MHC class Ia and class Ib molecules. *J Exp Med.* 2006;203:647.
41. Hammer GE, Gonzalez F, Champsaur M, et al. The aminopeptidase ERAAP shapes the peptide repertoire displayed by major histocompatibility complex class I molecules. *Nat Immunol.* 2006;7:103.
42. Hammer GE, Gonzalez F, James E, et al. In the absence of aminopeptidase ERAAP, MHC class I molecules present many unstable and highly immunogenic peptides. *Nat Immunol.* 2007;8:101.
43. Reits E, et al. Peptide diffusion, protection, and degradation in nuclear and cytoplasmic compartments before antigen presentation by MHC class I. *Immunity.* 2003;18:97.
44. York IA, et al. The ER aminopeptidase ERAP1 enhances or limits antigen presentation by trimming epitopes to 8-9 residues. *Nat Immunol.* 2002;3:1177.
45. Wei ML, Cresswell P. HLA-A2 molecules in an antigen-processing mutant cell contain signal sequence-derived peptides. *Nature.* 1992;356:443.
46. Abele R, Tampe R. The ABCs of immunology: structure and function of TAP, the transporter associated with antigen processing. *Physiology* (Bethesda). 2004;19:216.
47. Borst P, Elferink RO. Mammalian ABC transporters in health and disease. *Annu Rev Biochem.* 2002;71:537.
48. Powis SJ, et al. Restoration of antigen presentation to the mutant cell line RMA-S by an MHC-linked transporter. *Nature.* 1991;354:528.
49. Spies T, DeMars R. Restored expression of major histocompatibility class I molecules by gene transfer of a putative peptide transporter. *Nature.* 1991;351:323.
50. Uebel S, et al. Recognition principle of the TAP transporter disclosed by combinatorial peptide libraries. *Proc Natl Acad Sci U S A.* 1997;94:8976.
51. Peters B, Bulik S, Tampe R, et al. Identifying MHC class I epitopes by predicting the TAP transport efficiency of epitope precursors. *J Immunol.* 2003;171:1741.
52. Fruci D, et al. Quantifying recruitment of cytosolic peptides for HLA class I presentation: impact of TAP transport. *J Immunol.* 2003;170:2977.
53. Wright CA, Kozik P, Zacharias M, et al. Tapasin and other chaperones: models of the MHC class I loading complex. *Biol Chem.* 2004;385:763.
54. Garbi N, Tanaka S, van den Broek M, et al. Accessory molecules in the assembly of major histocompatibility complex class I/peptide complexes: how essential are they for CD8(+) T-cell immune responses? *Immunol Rev.* 2005:207:77.
55. Cresswell P, Ackerman AL, Giodini A, et al. Mechanisms of MHC class I-restricted antigen processing and cross-presentation. *Immunol Rev.* 2005;207:145.
56. Degen E, Cohen-Doyle MF, Williams DB. Efficient dissociation of the p88 chaperone from major histocompatibility complex class I molecules requires both beta 2-microglobulin and peptide. *J Exp Med.* 1992;175;1653.
57. Nossner E, Parham P. Species-specific differences in chaperone interaction of human and mouse major histocompatibility complex class I molecules. *J Exp Med.* 1995;181:327.
58. Farmery MR, Allen S, Allen AJ, et al. The role of ERp57 in disulfide bond formation during the assembly of major histocompatibility complex class I in a synchronized semipermeabilized cell translation system. *J Biol Chem.* 2000;275:14933.
59. Sadasivan B, Lehner PJ, Ortmann B, et al. Roles for calreticulin and a novel glycoprotein, tapasin, in the interaction of MHC class I molecules with TAP. *Immunity.* 1996;5:103.
60. Lindquist JA, Jensen ON, Mann M, et al. ER-60, a chaperone with thiol-dependent reductase activity involved in MHC class I assembly. *EMBO J.* 1998;17:2186.
61. Hughes EA, Cresswell P. The thiol oxidoreductase ERp57 is a component of the MHC class I peptide-loading complex. *Curr Biol.* 1998;8:709.
62. Park B, et al. Redox regulation facilitates optimal peptide selection by MHC class I during antigen processing. *Cell.* 2006;127:369.
63. Ortmann B, Androlewicz MJ, Cresswell P. MHC class I/beta 2-microglobulin complexes associate with TAP transporters before peptide binding. *Nature.* 1994;368:864.
64. Suh WK, et al. Interaction of MHC class I molecules with the transporter associated with antigen processing. *Science.* 1994;264:1322.
65. Ortmann B, et al. A critical role for tapasin in the assembly and function of multimeric MHC class I-TAP complexes. *Science.* 1997;277:1306.
66. Grandea AG 3rd, et al. Impaired assembly yet normal trafficking of MHC class I molecules in Tapasin mutant mice. *Immunity.* 2000;13:213.
67. Garbi N, et al. Impaired immune responses and altered peptide repertoire in tapasin-deficient mice. *Nat Immunol.* 2000;1:234.
68. Gao B, et al. Assembly and antigen-presenting function of MHC class I molecules in cells lacking the ER chaperone calreticulin. *Immunity.* 2002;16:99.
69. Garbi N, Tanaka S, Momburg F, et al. Impaired assembly of the major histocompatibility complex class I peptide-loading complex

in mice deficient in the oxidoreductase ERp57. *Nat Immunol.* 2006;7:93.
70. Lehner PJ, Surman MJ, Cresswell P. Soluble tapasin restores MHC class I expression and function in the tapasin-negative cell line .220. *Immunity.* 1998;8:221.
71. Garbi N, Tiwari N, Momburg F, et al. A major role for tapasin as a stabilizer of the TAP peptide transporter and consequences for MHC class I expression. *Eur J Immunol.* 2003;33:264.
72. Williams AP, Peh CA, Purcell AW, et al. Optimization of the MHC class I peptide cargo is dependent on tapasin. *Immunity.* 2002;16:509.
73. Zarling AL, et al. Tapasin is a facilitator, not an editor, of class I MHC peptide binding. *J Immunol.* 2003;171:5287.
74. Groothuis TA, Neefjes J. The many roads to cross-presentation. *J Exp Med.* 2005;202:1313.
75. Shen L, Rock KL. Priming of T cells by exogenous antigen cross-presented on MHC class I molecules. *Curr Opin Immunol.* 2006;18:85.
76. Norbury CC, Chambers BJ, Prescott AR, et al. Constitutive macropinocytosis allows TAP-dependent major histocompatibility complex class I presentation of exogenous soluble antigen by bone marrow-derived dendritic cells. *Eur J Immunol.* 1997; 27:280.
76a. Heit 2004.
76b. Tobian 2005.
77. Jung S, et al. *In vivo* depletion of CD11c(+) dendritic cells abrogates priming of CD8(+) T cells by exogenous cell-associated antigens. *Immunity.* 2002;17:211.
78. Neijssen J, et al. Cross-presentation by intercellular peptide transfer through gap junctions. *Nature.* 2005;434:83.
79. Norbury CC, et al. CD8+ T cell cross-priming via transfer of proteasome substrates. *Science.* 2004;304:1318.
80. Shen L, Rock KL. Cellular protein is the source of cross-priming antigen *in vivo*. *Proc Natl Acad Sci U S A.* 2004;101:3035.
81. Wolkers MC, Brouwenstijn N, Bakker AH, et al. Antigen bias in T cell cross-priming. *Science.* 2004;304:1314.
82. Blachère NE, Darnell RB, Albert ML. Apoptotic cells deliver processed antigen to dendritic cells for cross-presentation. *PLoS Biol.* 2005;3(6):e185.
83. Guermonprez P, Amigorena S. Pathways for antigen cross presentation. *Springer Semin Immunopathol.* 2005;26:257.
84. Shen L, Sigal LJ, Boes M, et al. Important role of cathepsin S in generating peptides for TAP-independent MHC class I crosspresentation *in vivo*. *Immunity.* 2004;21:155.
85. Lizee G, et al. Control of dendritic cell cross-presentation by the major histocompatibility complex class I cytoplasmic domain. *Nat Immunol.* 2003;4:1065.
86. Moore MW, Carbone FR, Bevan MJ. Introduction of soluble protein into the class I pathway of antigen processing and presentation. *Cell.* 1988;54:777.
87. Rodriguez A, Regnault A, Kleijmeer M, et al. Selective transport of internalized antigens to the cytosol for MHC class I presentation in dendritic cells. *Nat Cell Biol.* 1999;1:362.
88. Ackerman AL, Kyritsis C, Tampe R, et al. Early phagosomes in dendritic cells form a cellular compartment sufficient for cross presentation of exogenous antigens. *Proc Natl Acad Sci U S A.* 2003;100:12889.
89. Guermonprez P, et al. ER-phagosome fusion defines an MHC class I cross-presentation compartment in dendritic cells. *Nature.* 2003;425:397.
90. Houde M, et al. Phagosomes are competent organelles for antigen cross-presentation. *Nature.* 2003;425:402.
91. Ackerman AL, Kyritsis C, Tampe R, et al. Access of soluble antigens to the endoplasmic reticulum can explain cross-presentation by dendritic cells. *Nat Immunol.* 2005;6:107.
92. Ackerman, A. L, Giodini, A. Cresswell, P. A role for the endoplasmic reticulum protein retrotranslocation machinery during crosspresentation by dendritic cells. *Immunity.* 2006;25:607.
93. Touret N, et al. Quantitative and dynamic assessment of the contribution of the ER to phagosome formation. *Cell.* 2005;123:157.
94. Pelkmans L, Helenius A. Endocytosis via caveolae. *Traffic.* 2002; 3:311.
95. Accapezzato D, Visco V, Francavilla V, et al. Chloroquine enhances human CD8+ T cell responses against soluble antigens *in vivo*. *J Exp Med.* 2005:202:817.
96. Savina A, et al. NOX2 controls phagosomal pH to regulate antigen processing during crosspresentation by dendritic cells. *Cell.* 2006;126:205.
97. Burgdorf S, Kautz A, Bohnert V, et al. Distinct pathways of antigen uptake and intracellular routing in CD4 and CD8 T cell activation. *Science.* 2007;316:612.
98. Rescigno M, et al. Bacteria-induced neo-biosynthesis, stabilization, and surface expression of functional class I molecules in mouse dendritic cells. *Proc Natl Acad Sci U S A.* 1998;95:5229.
99. Cella M, et al. Maturation, activation, and protection of dendritic cells induced by double-stranded RNA. *J Exp Med.* 1999;189:821.
100. Delamarre L, Holcombe H, Mellman, I. Presentation of exogenous antigens on major histocompatibility complex (MHC) class I and MHC class II molecules is differentially regulated during dendritic cell maturation. *J Exp Med.* 2003;198:111.
101. den Haan JM, Bevan MJ. Constitutive versus activation-dependent cross-presentation of immune complexes by CD8(+) and CD8(−) dendritic cells *in vivo*. *J Exp Med.* 2002;196:817.
102. Gil-Torregrosa BC, et al. Control of cross-presentation during dendritic cell maturation. *Eur J Immunol.* 2004;34:398.
103. Miettinen HM, Rose J K, Mellman I. Fc receptor isoforms exhibit distinct abilities for coated pit localization as a result of cytoplasmic domain heterogeneity. *Cell.* 1989;58:317.
104. Amigorena S, et al. Cytoplasmic domain heterogeneity and functions of IgG Fc receptors in B lymphocytes. *Science.* 1992;256:1808. 105. Watts C, Amigorena S. Antigen traffic pathways in dendritic cells. *Traffic.* 2000;1:312.
106. Mellman, I. Endocytosis and molecular sorting. *Annu Rev Cell Dev Biol.* 1996;12:575.
107. Conner SD, Schmid SL. Regulated portals of entry into the cell. *Nature.* 2003;422;37.
107a. Underhill 2002.
108. Sallusto F, Cella M, Danieli C, et al. Dendritic cells use macropinocytosis and the mannose receptor to concentrate macromolecules in the major histocompatibility complex class II compartment: downregulation by cytokines and bacterial products. *J Exp Med.* 1995;182:389.
109. Garrett WS, et al. Developmental control of endocytosis in dendritic cells by Cdc42. *Cell.* 2000;102:325.
110. West MA, Prescott AR, Eskelinen EL, et al. Rac is required for constitutive macropinocytosis by dendritic cells but does not control its downregulation. *Curr Biol.* 2000;10:839.
111. West MA, et al. Enhanced dendritic cell antigen capture via Toll-like receptor–induced actin remodeling. *Science.* 2004;305:1153.
112. Munz C. Autophagy and antigen presentation. *Cell Microbiol.* 2006;8:891.
113. Paludan C, et al. Endogenous MHC class II processing of a viral nuclear antigen after autophagy. *Science.* 2005;307:593.
114. Schmid D, Pypaert M, Munz C. Antigen-loading compartments for major histocompatibility complex class II molecules continuously receive input from autophagosomes. *Immunity.* 2007;26:79.
115. Zhou D, et al. Lamp-2a facilitates MHC class II presentation of cytoplasmic antigens. *Immunity.* 2005;22:571.
116. Roche PA, Marks MS, Cresswell P. Formation of a nine-subunit complex by HLA class II glycoproteins and the invariant chain. *Nature.* 1991;354:392.
117. Hsing LC, Rudensky AY. The lysosomal cysteine proteases in MHC class II antigen presentation. *Immunol Rev.* 2005;207:229.
118. Lotteau V, et al. Intracellular transport of class II MHC molecules directed by invariant chain. *Nature.* 1990;348:600.
119. Marks MS, Blum JS, Cresswell P. Invariant chain trimers are sequestered in the rough endoplasmic reticulum in the absence of association with HLA class II antigens. *J Cell Biol.* 1990;111:839.
120. Roche PA, Cresswell P. Invariant chain association with HLA-DR molecules inhibits immunogenic peptide binding. *Nature.* 1990;345:615.
121. Teyton L, et al. Invariant chain distinguishes between the exogenous and endogenous antigen presentation pathways. *Nature.* 1990;348:39.

122. Bakke O, Dobberstein B. MHC class II–associated invariant chain contains a sorting signal for endosomal compartments. *Cell.* 1990;63:707.
123. Pieters J, Bakke O, Dobberstein B. The MHC class II–associated invariant chain contains two endosomal targeting signals within its cytoplasmic tail. *J Cell Sci.* 1993;106(Pt 3):831.
124. Odorizzi CG, et al. Sorting signals in the MHC class II invariant chain cytoplasmic tail and transmembrane region determine trafficking to an endocytic processing compartment. *J Cell Biol.* 1994;126:317.
125. Chow AY, Mellman I. Old lysosomes, new tricks: MHC II dynamics in DCs. *Trends Immunol.* 2005;26:72.
126. Driessen C, et al. Cathepsin S controls the trafficking and maturation of MHC class II molecules in dendritic cells. *J Cell Biol.* 1999;147:775.
127. Nakagawa TY, et al. Impaired invariant chain degradation and antigen presentation and diminished collagen-induced arthritis in cathepsin S null mice. *Immunity.* 1999;10:207.
128. Shi GP, et al. Cathepsin S required for normal MHC class II peptide loading and germinal center development. *Immunity.* 1999;10:197.
129. Morris P, et al. An essential role for HLA-DM in antigen presentation by class II major histocompatibility molecules. *Nature.* 1994;368:551.
130. Kropshofer H, Hammerling GJ, Vogt AB. How HLA-DM edits the MHC class II peptide repertoire: survival of the fittest? *Immunol Today.* 1997;18:77.
131. Alfonso C, Karlsson L. Nonclassical MHC class II molecules. *Annu Rev Immunol.* 2000;18:113.
132. Sloan VS, et al. Mediation by HLA-DM of dissociation of peptides from HLA-DR. *Nature.* 1995;375:802.
133. Kropshofer H, et al. Editing of the HLA-DR-peptide repertoire by HLA-DM. *EMBO J.* 1996;15:6144.
134. Weber DA, Evavold BD, Jensen PE. Enhanced dissociation of HLA-DR-bound peptides in the presence of HLA-DM. *Science.* 1996;274:618.
135. Denzin LK, Fallas JL, Prendes M, et al. Right place, right time, right peptide: DO keeps DM focused. *Immunol Rev.* 2005;207:279.
136. Glazier KS, et al. Germinal center B cells regulate their capability to present antigen by modulation of HLA-DO. *J Exp Med.* 2002;195:1063.
137. Watts C. The exogenous pathway for antigen presentation on major histocompatibility complex class II and CD1 molecules. *Nat Immunol.* 2004;5:685.
138. Maric M, et al. Defective antigen processing in GILT-free mice. *Science.* 2001;294:1361.
139. Manoury B, et al. An asparaginyl endopeptidase processes a microbial antigen for class II MHC presentation. *Nature.* 1998; 396:695.
140. Manoury B, et al. Destructive processing by asparagine endopeptidase limits presentation of a dominant T cell epitope in MBP. *Nat Immunol.* 2002;3:169.
141. Hsieh CS, deRoos P, Honey K, et al. A role for cathepsin L and cathepsin S in peptide generation for MHC class II presentation. *J Immunol.* 2002;168:2618.
142. Sercarz EE, Maverakis E. MHC-guided processing: binding of large antigen fragments. *Nat Rev Immunol.* 2003;3:621.
143. Donermeyer DL, Allen PM. Binding to Ia protects an immunogenic peptide from proteolytic degradation. *J Immunol.* 1989;142:1063.
144. Sette A, Adorini L, Colon SM, et al. Capacity of intact proteins to bind to MHC class II molecules. *J Immunol.* 1989;143:1265.
145. Davidson HW, Reid PA, Lanzavecchia A, et al. Processed antigen binds to newly synthesized MHC class II molecules in antigen-specific B lymphocytes. *Cell.* 1991;67:105.
146. Lindner R, Unanue ER. Distinct antigen MHC class II complexes generated by separate processing pathways. *EMBO J.* 1996;15:6910.
147. Castellino F, Zappacosta F, Coligan JE, et al. Large protein fragments as substrates for endocytic antigen capture by MHC class II molecules. *J Immunol.* 1998;161:4048.
148. Villadangos JA, Driessen C, Shi GP, et al. Early endosomal maturation of MHC class II molecules independently of cysteine proteases and H-2DM. *EMBO J.* 2000;19:882.
149. Moss CX, Tree TI, Watts C. Reconstruction of a pathway of antigen processing and class II MHC peptide capture. *EMBO J.* 2007;26:2137.
150. Pierre P, Mellman I. Developmental regulation of invariant chain proteolysis controls MHC class II trafficking in mouse dendritic cells. *Cell.* 1998;93:1135.
151. Beers C, Honey K, Fink S, et al. Differential regulation of cathepsin S and cathepsin L in interferon gamma–treated macrophages. *J Exp Med.* 2003;197:169.
152. Delamarre L, Couture R, Mellman I, et al. Enhancing immunogenicity by limiting susceptibility to lysosomal proteolysis. *J Exp Med.* 2006;203:2049.
153. Mellman I, Steinman RM. Dendritic cells: specialized and regulated antigen processing machines. *Cell.* 2001;106:255.
154. Villadangos JA, Schnorrer P, Wilson NS. Control of MHC class II antigen presentation in dendritic cells: a balance between creative and destructive forces. *Immunol Rev.* 2005;207:191.
155. Inaba K, et al. The formation of immunogenic major histocompatibility complex class II– peptide ligands in lysosomal compartments of dendritic cells is regulated by inflammatory stimuli. *J Exp Med.* 2000;191:927.
156. Turley SJ, et al. Transport of peptide–MHC class II complexes in developing dendritic cells. *Science.* 2000;288:522.
157. Li DN, Matthews SP, Antoniou AN, et al. Multistep autoactivation of asparaginyl endopeptidase *in vitro* and *in vivo*. *J Biol Chem.* 2003;278:38980.
158. Trombetta ES, Ebersold M, Garrett W, et al. Activation of lysosomal function during dendritic cell maturation. *Science.* 2003;299:1400.
159. Fiebiger E, et al. Cytokines regulate proteolysis in major histocompatibility complex class II–dependent antigen presentation by dendritic cells. *J Exp Med.* 2001;193:881.
160. Cella M, Engering A, Pinet V, et al. Inflammatory stimuli induce accumulation of MHC class II complexes on dendritic cells. *Nature.* 1997;388:782.
161. Pierre P, et al. Developmental regulation of MHC class II transport in mouse dendritic cells. *Nature.* 1997;388:787.
162. Ohmura-Hoshino M, et al. Inhibition of MHC class II expression and immune responses by c-MIR. *J Immunol.* 2006;177:341.
163. Shin JS, et al. Surface expression of MHC class II in dendritic cells is controlled by regulated ubiquitination. *Nature.* 2006;444: 115.
164. van Niel G, et al. Dendritic cells regulate exposure of MHC class II at their plasma membrane by oligoubiquitination. *Immunity.* 2006;25:885.
165. Kleijmeer M, et al. Reorganization of multivesicular bodies regulates MHC class II antigen presentation by dendritic cells. *J Cell Biol.* 2001;155:53.
166. Boes M, et al. T-cell engagement of dendritic cells rapidly rearranges MHC class II transport. *Nature.* 2002;418:983.
167. Chow A, Toomre D, Garrett W, et al. Dendritic cell maturation triggers retrograde MHC class II transport from lysosomes to the plasma membrane. *Nature.* 2002;418:988.
168. Unternaehrer JJ, Chow A, Pypaert M, et al. The tetraspanin CD9 mediates lateral association of MHC class II molecules on the dendritic cell surface. *Proc Natl Acad Sci U S A.* 2007;104:234.
169. Brigl M, Brenner MB. CD1: antigen presentation and T cell function. *Annu Rev Immunol* 2004;22:817.
170. Hava DL, et al. CD1 assembly and the formation of CD1-antigen complexes. *Curr Opin Immunol.* 2005;17:88.
171. Angenieux C, et al. The cellular pathway of CD1e in immature and maturing dendritic cells. *Traffic.* 2005;6:286.
172. Gumperz JE, et al. Murine CD1d-restricted T cell recognition of cellular lipids. *Immunity.* 2000;12:211.
173. Moody DB, et al. T cell activation by lipopeptide antigens. *Science.* 2004;303:527.
174. Moody DB, Zajonc DM, Wilson IA. Anatomy of CD1-lipid antigen complexes. *Nat Rev Immunol.* 2005;5:387.
175. van den Elzen P, et al. Apolipoprotein-mediated pathways of lipid antigen presentation. *Nature.* 2005;437:906.
176. Kang SJ, Cresswell P. Calnexin, calreticulin, and ERp57 cooperate in disulfide bond formation in human CD1d heavy chain. *J Biol Chem.* 2002;277:44838.

177. Park JJ, et al. Lipid–protein interactions: biosynthetic assembly of CD1 with lipids in the endoplasmic reticulum is evolutionarily conserved. *Proc Natl Acad Sci U S A.* 2004:101:1022.
178. Dougan SK, et al. Microsomal triglyceride transfer protein lipidation and control of CD1d on antigen-presenting cells. *J Exp Med.* 2005;202:529.
179. Brozovic, S, et al. CD1d function is regulated by microsomal triglyceride transfer protein. *Nat Med.* 2004;10:535.
180. SagivY, et al. A distal effect of microsomal triglyceride transfer protein deficiency on the lysosomal recycling of CD1d. *J Exp Med.* 2007;204:921.
181. Jayawardena-Wolf J, Benlagha K, Chiu YH, et al. CD1d endosomal trafficking is independently regulated by an intrinsic CD1d-encoded tyrosine motif and by the invariant chain. *Immunity.* 2001;15:897.
182. Kang SJ, Cresswell P. Regulation of intracellular trafficking of human CD1d by association with MHC class II molecules. *EMBO J.* 2002;21:1650.
183. Chiu YH, et al. Multiple defects in antigen presentation and T cell development by mice expressing cytoplasmic tail truncated CD1d. *Nat Immunol.* 2002;3:55.
184. Sugita M, et al. Cytoplasmic tail-dependent localization of CD1b antigen-presenting molecules to MIICs. *Science.* 1996;273:349.
185. Jackman RM, et al. The tyrosine-containing cytoplasmic tail of CD1b is essential for its efficient presentation of bacterial lipid antigens. *Immunity.* 1998;8:341.
186. Sugita M, et al. Separate pathways for antigen presentation by CD1 molecules. *Immunity.* 1999;11:743.
187. Briken V, Jackman RM, Dasgupta S, et al. Intracellular trafficking pathway of newly synthesized CD1b molecules. *EMBO J.* 2002;21:825.
188. Lawton AP, et al. The mouse CD1d cytoplasmic tail mediates CD1d trafficking and antigen presentation by adaptor protein 3-dependent and -independent mechanisms. *J Immunol.* 2005;174:3179.
189. van der Wel NN, et al. CD1 and major histocompatibility complex II molecules follow a different course during dendritic cell maturation. *Mol Biol Cell.* 2003;14:3378.
190. de la Salle H, et al. Assistance of microbial glycolipid antigen processing by CD1e. *Science.* 2005;310:1321.
191. Prigozy TI, et al. Glycolipid antigen processing for presentation by CD1d molecules. *Science.* 2001;291:664.
192. Zhou D, et al. Lysosomal glycosphingolipid recognition by NKT cells. *Science.* 2004;306:1786.
193. Ernst WA, et al. Molecular interaction of CD1b with lipoglycan antigens. *Immunity.* 1998;8:331.
194. Naidenko OV, et al. Binding and antigen presentation of ceramide-containing glycolipids by soluble mouse and human CD1d molecules. *J Exp Med.* 1999;190:1069.
195. Cheng TY, et al. Role of lipid trimming and CD1 groove size in cellular antigen presentation. *EMBO J.* 2006;25:2989.
196. Kang SJ, Cresswell P. Saposins facilitate CD1d-restricted presentation of an exogenous lipid antigen to T cells. *Nat Immunol.* 2004;5:175.
197. Winau F, et al. Saposin C is required for lipid presentation by human CD1b. *Nat Immunol.* 2004;5.
198. Zhou D, et al. Editing of CD1d-bound lipid antigens by endosomal lipid transfer proteins. *Science.* 2004;303:523.
199. Schrantz N, et al. The Niemann-Pick type C2 protein loads isoglobotrihexosylceramide onto CD1d molecules and contributes to the thymic selection of NKT cells. *J Exp Med.* 2007;204:841.
200. Yuan W, et al. Saposin B is the dominant saposin that facilitates lipid binding to human CD1d molecules. *Proc Natl Acad Sci U S A.* 2007;104:5551.
201. Honey K, et al. Thymocyte expression of cathepsin L is essential for NKT cell development. *Nat Immunol.* 2002;3:1069.

SECTION VI

Regulation and Effector Functions of the Immune Response

Chapter 21

Immunogenicity and Antigen Structure

Jay A. Berzofsky and Ira J. Berkower

THE NATURE OF ANTIGENIC DETERMINANTS RECOGNIZED BY ANTIBODIES

Haptens

In the antigen–antibody-binding reaction, the antibody-binding site is often unable to accommodate the entire antigen. The part of the antigen that is the target of antibody binding is called an *antigenic determinant*, and there may be one or more antigenic determinants per molecule. To study antibody specificity, we need to have antibodies against single antigenic determinants. Small functional groups that correspond to a single antigenic determinant are called *haptens*. For example, these may be organic compounds, such as trinitrophenyl or benzene arsonate, a mono- or oligosaccharide such as glucose or lactose, or an oligopeptide such as pentalysine. Although these haptens can bind to antibody, immunization with them usually will not provoke an antibody response (for exceptions, see online ref. *1*). Immunogenicity often can be achieved by covalently attaching haptens to a larger molecule, called the *carrier*. The carrier is immunogenic in its own right, and immunization with the hapten–carrier conjugate elicits an antibody response to both hapten and carrier. However, the antibodies specific for hapten can be studied by equilibrium dialysis using pure hapten (without carrier) or by immunoprecipitation using hapten coupled to a different (and non–cross-reacting) carrier, or by inhibition of precipitation with free hapten.

This technique was pioneered by Landsteiner *(2)* and helped to elucidate the exquisite specificity of antibodies for antigenic determinants. For instance, the relative binding affinity of antibodies prepared against succinic acid–serum protein conjugates shows marked specificity for the maleic acid analog, which is in the *cis* configuration, as compared to the fumaric acid (*trans*) form *(3)*. Presumably, the immunogenic form of succinic acid corresponds to the *cis* form *(3)*. This ability of antibodies to distinguish *cis* from *trans* configurations was re-emphasized in later studies measuring relative affinities of antibodies to maleic and fumaric acid conjugates *(4)* (Table 21.1A). Table 21.1B shows the specificity of antibodies prepared against *p*-azobenzene arsonate coupled to bovine gamma globulin *(5)*. Since the hapten is coupled through the *p*-azo group to aromatic amino acids of the carrier, haptens containing bulky substitutions in the para position would most resemble the immunizing antigen. In fact, *p*-methyl-substituted benzene arsonate has a higher binding affinity than unsubstituted benzene arsonate. However, methyl substitution elsewhere in the benzene ring reduces affinity, presumably because of interference with the way hapten fits into the antibody-binding site. Thus, methyl substitutions can have positive or negative effects on binding energy, depending on where the substitution occurs. Table 21.1C shows the specificity of antilactose antibodies for lactose versus cellobiose *(6)*. These disaccharides differ only by the orientation of the hydroxyl attached to C4 of the first sugar either above or below the hexose ring. The three examples in this table, as well as many others *(1)*, show the marked specificity of antibodies for *cis–trans*, *ortho–meta-para*, and stereoisomeric forms of the antigenic determinant.

Comparative binding studies of haptens have been able to demonstrate antibody specificity despite the marked heterogeneity of antibodies. Unlike the antibodies against a multideterminant antigen, the population of antibodies specific for a single hapten determinant is a relatively restricted population, because of the shared structural constraints necessary for hapten to fit within the antibody-combining site. However, the specificity of an antiserum depends on the collective specificities of the entire population of antibodies, which are determined by the structures of the various antibody-binding sites. When studying the cross-reactions of hapten analogs, some haptens bind all antibodies, but with reduced K_A. Other hapten analogs reach a plateau of binding because they fit some antibody-combining sites quite well but not others (see discussion of cross-reactivity in Chapter 5). Antibodies raised in different animals may show different cross-reactivities with related haptens. Even within a single animal, antibody affinity and specificity are known to increase over time following immunization under certain conditions *(7)*. Thus, any statements about the cross-reactivity of two haptens reflect both structural differences between the haptens that affect antigen–antibody fit and the diversity of antibody-binding sites present in a given antiserum.

Carbohydrate Antigens

The antigenic determinants of a number of biologically important substances consist of carbohydrates. These often occur as glycolipids or glycoproteins. Examples of the former include bacterial cell wall antigens and the major blood group antigens, whereas the latter group includes "minor" blood group antigens such as Rh. In addition, the capsular polysaccharides of bacteria are important for virulence and are often targeted by protective antibodies.

TABLE 21.1 Exquisite Specificity of Antihapten Antibodies

Hapten	*Structure*	*K_{rel} of Antibody Specific for*	
A.		Maleic (cis)	Fumarlc (trans)
Maleanilate		1.0	<0.01
Fumaranilate		<0.01	1.0
B.		Parasubstituted benzene arsonate	
Benzene arsonate		1.0	
o-Methyl benzene arsonate		0.2	
m-Methyl benzene arsonate		0.8	
p-Methyl benzene arsonate		1.9	
C.		Lactose	
Lactose	β gal (1→4) glu	1.00	
Cellobiose	β glu (1→4) glu	0.0025	

Part A from ref. 4; part B from ref. 5; and part C from ref. 6, with permission.

A number of spontaneously arising myeloma proteins have been found to show carbohydrate specificity, possibly reflecting the fact that carbohydrates are common environmental antigens. In the days prior to hybridoma technology, these carbohydrate-specific myeloma proteins provided an important model for studying the reaction of antigen with a monoclonal antibody.

Empirically, the predominant antigenic determinants of polysaccharides often consist of short oligosaccharides (one to five sugars long) at the nonreducing end of the polymer chain *(8)*. This situation is analogous to a hapten consisting of several sugar residues linked to a large nonantigenic polysaccharide backbone. The remainder of the polysaccharide is important for immunogenicity, just as the carrier molecule was important for haptens. In addition, branch points in the polysaccharide structure allow for multiple antigenic determinants to be attached to the same macromolecule. This is important for immunoprecipitation by lattice formation, as discussed in Chapter 5. Several examples illustrating structural studies of oligosaccharide antigens are given later.

The technique used most widely to analyze the antigenic determinants of polysaccharides is called *hapten inhibition (8)*. In this method, the precipitation reaction between antigen and antibody is inhibited by adding short oligosaccharides. These oligosaccharides are large enough to bind with the same affinity and specificity as the polysaccharide, but because they are monomeric, no precipitate forms. As more inhibitor is added, fewer antibody combining sites remain available for precipitation. Using antiserum specific for a single antigenic determinant, it is often possible to block precipitation completely with a short oligosaccharide corresponding to the nonreducing end of the polysaccharide chain. Besides showing the "immunodominance" of the nonreducing end of the chain, this result also shows that the structure of the antigenic determinant of polysaccharides depends on the sequence of carbohydrates and their linkage, rather than their conformation. For inhibition by hapten to be complete, the antigen–antibody system studied must be made specific for a single antigenic determinant. For optimal sensitivity, the equivalence point of antigen and antibody should be used.

We illustrate the types of carbohydrate antigens encountered by examining three classic examples in more detail: the salmonella O antigens, the blood group antigens, and dextrans that bind to myeloma proteins.

Immunochemistry of Salmonella O Antigens

The antigenic diversity among numerous salmonella species resides in the structural differences of the lipopolysaccharide (LPS) component of the outer membrane *(9)*. These molecules are the main target for antisalmonella antibodies. The polysaccharide moiety contains the antigenic determinant, whereas the lipid moiety is responsible for endotoxin effects. The chemical structure of LPS can be divided into three regions (Figure 21.1). Region I contains the antigenic O-specific polysaccharide, usually made up of repeated oligosaccharide units, which vary widely among different strains. Region II contains an oligosaccharide "common core" shared among many different strains. Failure to synthesize region II oligosaccharide or to couple completed region I polysaccharide to the growing region II core results in R (rough) mutants, which have "rough" colony morphology and lack the O antigen. Region III is the lipid part, called *lipid A*, which is shared among all salmonellae and serves to anchor LPS on the outer membrane. Early immunologic attempts to classify the O antigens of different salmonellae revealed a large number of cross-reactions between different strains. These were detected by preparing antiserum to one strain of salmonella and using it to agglutinate bacteria of a second strain. Each cross-reacting determinant was assigned a number, and each strain was characterized by a series of O antigen determinants (in aggregate, the "serotype" of the strain) based on its pattern of cross-reactivity. Each strain was classified within a group, based on sharing a strong O determinant. For example, group A strains share determinant 2, whereas group B strains share determinant 4 (Table 21.2). However, within a group, each strain possesses additional O determinants, which serve to differentiate it from other members of that group. Thus, determinant 2 coexists with determinants 1 and 12 on *Salmonella paratyphi A*.

This problem of cross-reactivity based on sharing of a subset of antigenic determinants is commonly encountered in complex antigen–antibody systems. The problem may be simplified by making antibodies monospecific for individual antigenic determinants. To do this, antibodies are absorbed to remove irrelevant specificities, or cross-reactive strains are chosen that share only a single determinant with the immunizing strain. The reaction of each determinant with its specific antibody can be thought of as an antigen–antibody system. Thus, for the strains shown in Table 21.2, antiserum to *Salmonella typhi* (containing anti-9 and anti-12 antibodies) may be absorbed with *S. paratyphi A* to remove anti-12, leaving a reagent specific for antigen 9 (21.2). Alternatively, the unabsorbed antiserum may be used to study the system antigen 12–anti-12 by allowing it to agglutinate *Salmonella paratyphi B*, which shares only antigen 12 with the immunogen. Because the other determinants on *S. paratyphi B* were absent from the immunizing strain, the antiserum contains no antibodies to them.

Once the antigen–antibody reaction is made specific for a single determinant, a variety of oligosaccharides can be added to test for hapten inhibition. Because the O antigens contain repeating oligosaccharide units, it is often possible to obtain model oligosaccharides by mild chemical or enzymatic degradation of the LPS polysaccharide itself. Once the most inhibitory oligosaccharide is found,

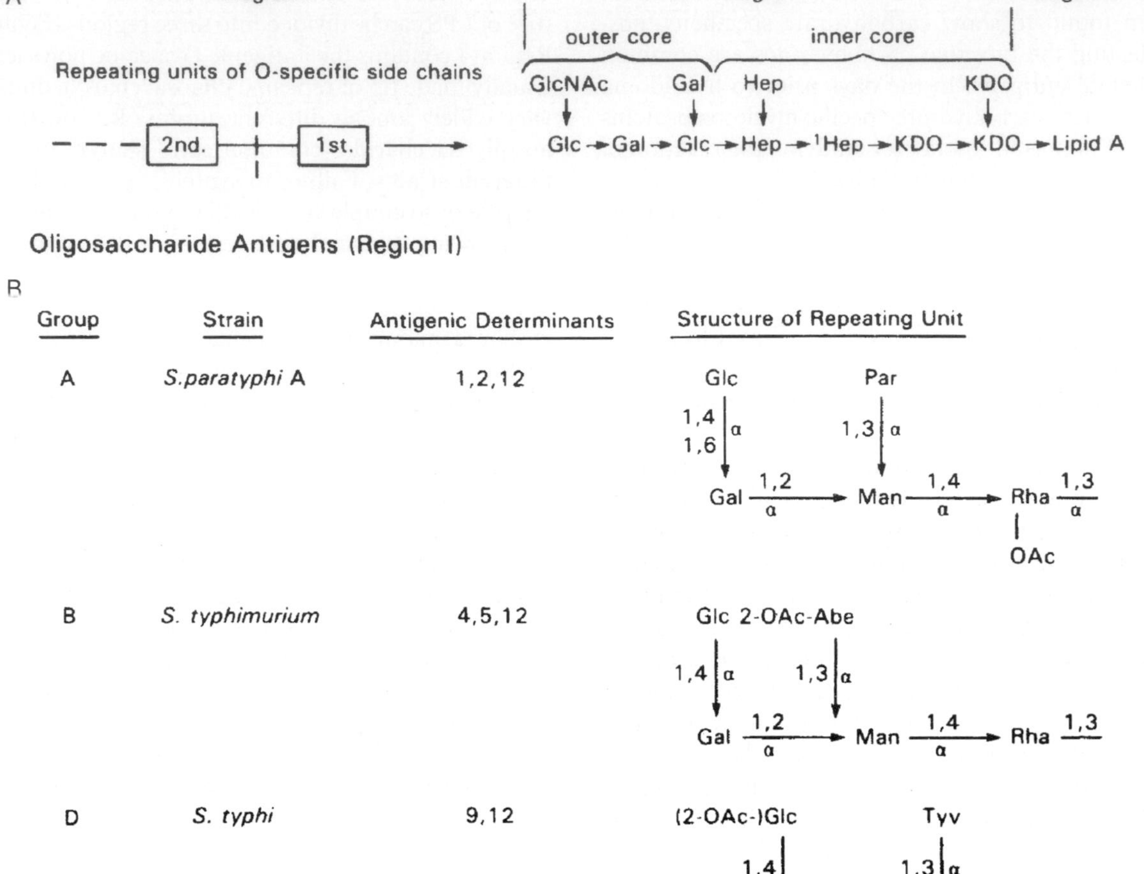

FIGURE 21.1 Structure of *Salmonella (S.)* lipopolysaccharide. Region I contains the unique O-antigen determinants, which consist of repeating units of oligosaccharides. These are attached to lipid moiety through the core polysaccharide. Three examples of oligosaccharide units are shown (9). (Part A adapted from ref. *8*, with permission; part B based on ref. *9*.)

its chemical structure is determined. Alternatively, a variety of synthetic mono-, di-, tri-, and oligosaccharides are tested for hapten inhibition of precipitation. For example, as shown in Table 21.3, antigen 1–anti-1 antibody precipitation is inhibited by methyl-αD-glucoside. Therefore, various disaccharides incorporating this structure were tested, of which αD-Glu(1→6)D-Gal was the most inhibitory. Then various trisaccharides incorporating this sequence were tested. The results indicate the sequence and size of the determinant recognized by anti-1 antibodies to be a disaccharide with the structure shown here. The test sequences can be guessed by analyzing the oligosaccharide

TABLE 21.2 *Salmonella* O Antigen Serotyping

Salmonella *Strain*	*Serogroup*	*O Antigenic Determinants*
S. paratyphi A	A	1, 2, 12
S. paratyphi B	B	1, 4, 5, 12
S. typhi	D	9, 12

Antiserum	*Absorbed*	*Tested on*	*Single Determinant Measured*
Anti–*S. typhi*		*S. paratyphi* B	12
Anti–*S. typhi*	*S. paratyphi* A	*S. typhi*	9

Reprinted with permission from ref. *8*.

TABLE 21.3 Analysis of *Salmonella* O-Antigen Structure by Hapten Inhibition

	Antigen System	
Maximum Inhibition by Hapten (%)	*1: anti-1*	*19: anti-19*
D-Glu	—	0
Me-α-D-Glu	35	10
α-D-Glu(1 → 6)-D-Gal	80	25
Glu.Gal.Man	80	70
Gtu.Gal.Man.L-Rham	>70	>70
Deduced structure	α-D-Glu(1→6)-D-Gal	D-Glu-D-Gal-D-Man-L-Rham

Reprinted with permission from ref. *8*.

breakdown products of the lipopolysaccharide, which include tetramers of D-Glu-D-Gal-D-Man-L-Rham.

The results in Table 21.3 also suggest that the difference between determinants 1 and 19 is the length of oligosaccharide recognized by antibodies specific for each determinant. This hypothesis is supported by the observation that determinant 1 is found in some strains with, and in other strains without, determinant 19; whereas determinant 19 is always found with determinant 1. As shown in the table, determinant 19 requires the full tetrasaccharide for maximal hapten inhibition, including the sequence coding for determinant 1. Besides identifying the antigenic structures, these results indicate that there is variation in the size of different antigenic determinants of polysaccharides.

Blood Group Antigens

The major blood group antigens A and B were originally detected by the ability of serum from individuals lacking either determinant to agglutinate red blood cells bearing them (for reviews, see refs. *8* and *10–12*). In addition, group O individuals have an H antigenic determinant that is distinct from A or B types, and individuals in all three groups may have additional determinants such as the Lewis (Le) antigens. Although the ABH and Le antigenic determinants are found on a carbohydrate moiety, the carbohydrate may occur in a variety of biochemical forms. On cell surfaces, they are either glycolipids that are synthesized within the cell (AB and H antigens) or glycoproteins taken up from serum (Le antigens). In mucinous secretions, such as saliva, they occur as glycoproteins. Milk, ovarian cyst fluid, and gastric mucosa contain soluble oligosaccharides containing blood group reactivity. In addition, these antigens occur frequently in other species, including about half of the bacteria in the normal flora of the gut *(10)*. This widespread occurrence may account for the ubiquitous anti-AB reactivity of human sera, even in people never previously exposed to human blood group substances through transfusion or pregnancy.

The immunochemistry of these antigens was simplified greatly by the use of oligosaccharides in hapten inhibition studies. Group A oligosaccharides, for example, would inhibit the agglutination of group A red blood cells by anti-A antibodies. They could also inhibit the immunoprecipitation of group A-bearing glycoproteins by anti-A antibodies. Because the oligosaccharides are monomeric, their reaction with antibody does not form a precipitate but does block an antibody-combining site.

The inhibitory oligosaccharides from cyst fluid were purified and found to contain D-galactose, L-fucose, *N*-acetyl galactosamine, and *N*-acetylglucosamine. The most inhibitory oligosaccharides for each antigen are indicated in Figure 21.2. As can be seen in the figure, the ABH and Le antigens all share a common oligosaccharide core sequence, and the antigens appear to differ from each other by the sequential addition of individual sugars at the end or at branch points. Besides hapten inhibition, other biochemical data support this relationship among the different determinants. Enzymatic digestion of A, B, or H antigens yields a common core oligosaccharide from each. This product cross-reacts with antiserum specific for pneumococcal polysaccharide type XIV, which contains structural elements shared with blood group determinants, as shown at the bottom of Figure 21.2. In addition, this structure, known as *precursor substance*, has been isolated from ovarian cyst fluid.

Starting from precursor substance, the H determinant results from the addition of L-fucose to galactose, whereas Lewis^a antigen (Le^a) determinant results from the addition of L-fucose to *N*-acetylglucosamine, and Le^b from the addition of L-fucose to both sugars. Addition of *N*-acetylgalactosamine to H substance produces the A determinant, whereas addition of galactose produces the B determinant, in each case blocking reactivity of the H determinant.

The genetics of ABH and Le antigens is explained by this sequential addition of sugars via glycosyltransferases. The allelic nature of the AB antigens is explained by the addition of *N*-acetylgalactosamine, galactose, or nothing to the H antigen. The rare inherited trait of inability to synthesize the H determinants from precursor substance (Bombay phenotype) also blocks the expression of A and B antigens, because the A and B transferases lack an

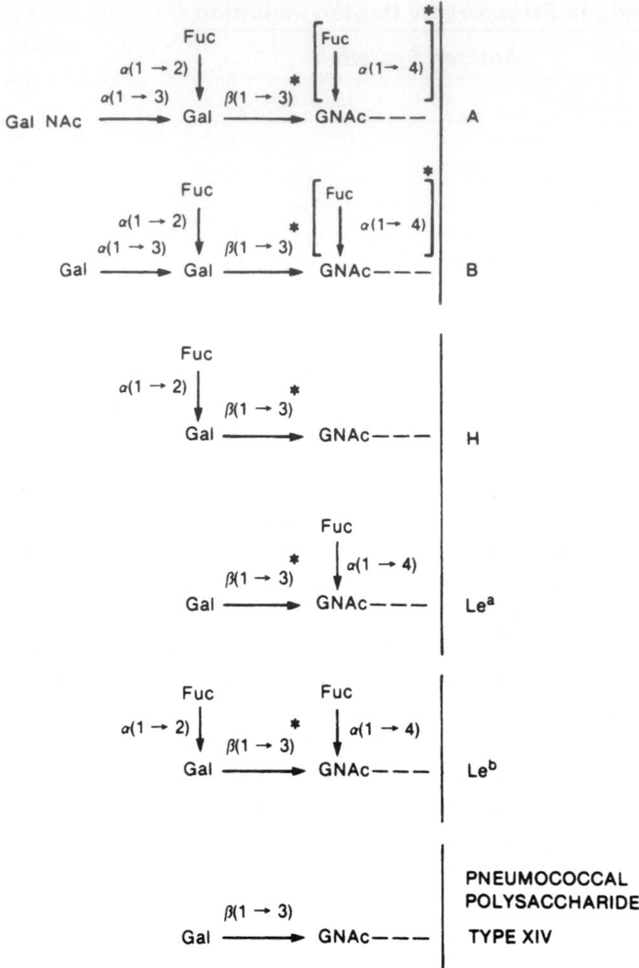

FIGURE 21.2 Oligosaccharide chain specificity. Structure of the ABH and Lewis (Le) blood group antigens, as determined by hapten inhibition studies *(8,11)*. There are two variants of each of these determinants. In type 1, the Gal-GNAc linkage is $\beta(1 \rightarrow 3)$, whereas in type 2, the Gal-GNAc linkage is $\beta(1 \rightarrow 4)$. In addition, there is heterogeneity in the A and B antigens with respect to the presence of the Le fucose attached to the GNAc. In the molecules that contain the extra fucose, when the Gal-GNAc linkage is $\beta(1 \rightarrow 3)$ (type 1), the fucose must be linked $\alpha(1 \rightarrow 4)$, whereas the type 2 molecules, with the $\beta(1 \rightarrow 4)$ Gal-GNAc linkage, contain $\alpha(1 \rightarrow 3)$-linked fucose. The *asterisks* indicate the sites of this variability in linkage.

acceptor substrate. However, the appearance of the Le^a on red cells is independent of H antigen synthesis. Its structure, shown in Figure 21.2, can be derived directly from precursor substance without going through an H antigen intermediate. Comparing different individuals, the appearance of Le^a antigen on red blood cells correlates with its presence in saliva, because the Le^a antigen is not an intrinsic membrane component but must be absorbed from serum glycoproteins, which, in turn, depend on secretion. In addition to the independent synthetic pathway, the secretion of Le^a antigen is also independent of the secretory process for ABH antigens. Therefore salivary nonsecretors of ABH antigens (which occur in 20% of individuals) may still secrete Le^a antigen if they have the fucosyl transferase encoded by the Le gene. In contrast, salivary secretion of ABH is required for red blood cells to express Le^b.

Dextran-Binding Myeloma Proteins

Because polysaccharides are common environmental antigens, it is not surprising that randomly induced myeloma proteins were frequently found to have carbohydrate specificities. Careful studies of these monoclonal antibodies support the clonal expansion model of antibody diversity: heterogeneous antisera behave as the sum of many individual clones of antibody with respect to affinity and specificity. In the case of the IgAκ myeloma proteins W3129 and W3434, both antibodies were found to be specific for dextrans containing α-glu (1→6)glu bonds *(12)*. Hapten inhibition with a series of mono- or oligosaccharides of increasing chain length indicated that the percentage of binding energy derived from the reaction with one glucose was 75%, two glucoses 95%, three 95% to 98%, and four 100%. This suggests that most binding energy between antidextran antibodies and dextran derives from the terminal monosaccharide, and that oligosaccharides of chain length 4 to 6 commonly fill the antibody-combining site. Human antidextran antisera behaved similarly, with tetrasaccharides contributing 95% of the binding energy. These experiments provided the first measure of the size of an antigenic determinant, 4 to 6 residues *(13,14)*. In addition, as was observed for antisera, binding affinity of myeloma proteins was highly sensitive to modifications of the terminal sugar and highly specific for $\alpha(1 \rightarrow 6)$ versus $\alpha(1 \rightarrow 3)$ glycosidic bonds. However, modification of the third or fourth sugar of an oligosaccharide had relatively less effect on hapten inhibition of either myeloma protein or of antisera reacting with dextran.

Studies with additional dextran-binding myeloma proteins *(15)* revealed that not all antipolysaccharide monoclonal antibodies are specific for the nonreducing end, as exemplified by QUPC 52. Competitive inhibition with mono- and oligosaccharides revealed that less than 5% of binding energy derived from mono- or disaccharides, 72% from trisaccharides, 88% from tetrasaccharides, and 100% from hexasaccharides, in marked contrast to other myeloma proteins. A second distinctive property of myeloma protein QUPC 52 was its ability to precipitate unbranched dextran of chain length 200. Because the unbranched dextran has only one nonreducing end, and because the myeloma protein has only one specificity, lattice formation due to cross-linking between the nonreducing ends is impossible, and precipitation must be explained by binding some other determinant. Therefore, QUPC 52 appears to be specific for internal oligosaccharide units of 3 to 7 chain length. W3129 is specific for end determinants and will not precipitate unbranched dextran chains.

Antibodies precipitating linear dextran were also detected in six antidextran human sera, comprising 48% to 90% of the total antibodies to branched chain dextran. Thus antidextrans can be divided into those specific for terminal oligosaccharides and those specific for internal oligosaccharides; monoclonal examples of both types are available, and both types are present in human immune serum. Cisar et al. *(15)* speculated as to the different topology of the binding sites of W3129 or QUPC 52 necessary for terminal or internal oligosaccharide specificity. Both terminal and internal oligosaccharides have nearly identical chemical structures, differing at a single C–OH or glycoside bond. Perhaps the terminal oligosaccharide specificity of W3129 is due to the shape of the antibody-combining site—a cavity into which only the end can fit; whereas the internal oligosaccharide-binding site of QUPC 52 could be a surface groove in the antibody, which would allow the rest of the polymer to protrude out at both ends. A more definitive answer depends on x-ray crystallographic studies of the combining sites of monoclonal antibodies with precisely defined specificity, performed with antigen occupying the binding site (see below).

With the advent of hybridoma technology, it became possible to produce monoclonal antibodies of any desired specificity. Immunizing mice with nearly linear dextran (the preferred antigen of QUPC 52), followed by fusion and screening (with linear dextran) for dextran-binding antibodies, yielded 12 hybridomas *(16)*, all with specificity similar to QUPC 52. Oligosaccharide inhibition of all 12 monoclonals showed considerable increments in affinity up to hexasaccharides, with little affinity for disaccharides and only 49% to 77% of binding energy derived from trisaccharides *(17)*. Second, all 12 monoclonals had internal $\alpha(1\rightarrow6)$ dextran specificity because they could all precipitate linear dextran. Third, 9 of 11 BALB/c monoclonals shared a cross-reactive idiotype with QUPC 52, whereas none shared idiotype with W3129 *(18)*. These data support the hypothesis that different antibodies with similar specificity and similar groove-type sites may be derived from the same family of germline V_H genes bearing the QUPC 52 idiotype *(18)*.

The large number of environmental carbohydrate antigens and the high degree of specificity of antibodies elicited in response to each carbohydrate antigen suggest that a tremendous diversity of antibody molecules must be available, from which some antibodies can be selected for every possible antigenic structure. Studies of a series of 17 monoclonal anti-$\alpha(1\rightarrow6)$ dextran hybridomas *(19,20)* have investigated whether the binding sites of closely related antibodies were derived from a small number of variable region genes, for both heavy and light chains, or whether antibodies of the same specificity could derive from variable region genes with highly divergent sequences. Each monoclonal had a groove-type site that could hold six or seven sugar residues (with one exception), based on inhibition of immunoprecipitation by different-length oligosaccharides. Thus, unlike monoclonals to haptenated proteins, the precise epitope could be well characterized and was generally quite similar among the entire series.

Studies of the V_κ sequences revealed that only three V_κ groups were used in these hybridomas. Use of each V_κ group correlated with the particular antigen used to immunize the animals, whether linear dextran or short oligosaccharides, so that 10 of the monoclonals from mice immunized the same way all used the same V_κ.

In contrast, the 17 V_H chains were derived from at least five different germline genes from three different V_H gene families *(21)*. The two most frequently used germline V_H genes were found in seven and five monoclonals, respectively, with minor variations explainable by somatic mutations. The remarkable finding is that very different V_H chains (about 50% homologous) can combine with the same V_κ to produce antibody-binding sites with nearly the same size, shape, antigen specificity, and affinity. Even when different V_H sequences combine with different V_κ sequences, they can produce antibodies with very similar properties. Dextran binding depends on the antigen fitting into the groove and interacting favorably with the residues forming the sides and bottom of the groove. The results indicate that divergent variable region sequences, both in and out of the complementarity-determining regions, can be folded to form similar binding site contours, which result in similar immunochemical characteristics. Similar results have been reported in other antigen–antibody systems, such as phenyloxazolone *(22)*.

Additional studies of carbohydrate binding monoclonal antibodies have revealed significant information about how the antibody variable regions can bind a carbohydrate structure with high affinity and specificity. Several examples are now available of crystal structures of carbohydrates bound to antibodies.

For example, monoclonal antibody Se155-4 is specific for the group B determinant of the Salmonella O antigen, which consists of the sugars Gal- Abequose- Man (23,24). The crystal structure of antibody bound to the polysaccharide shows that one hexose, abequose, fits into the binding pocket, while the rest of the interactions occur along the surface of the antibody, similar to the groove-type sites previously described. Binding energy depends on hydrogen bonds formed between the protein residues and the hydroxyl groups of the carbohydrate. The protein residues include aromatic amines, such as His 32, Trp91, and Trp 96 of the light chain, as well as His 97 and His 35 of the heavy chain. In addition, one of the sugars is hydrogen bonded via a water molecule bridge to the amide bonds of the protein backbone. About three fourths of all sugar hydroxyl groups are involved in hydrogen bonds with the protein. Although each H bond is relatively weak by itself, the combined effect of eight hydrogen bonds results in high affinity binding. Antibody specificity derives from the fact that the carbohydrate fits into a binding pocket, where H bond formation depends on precise interactions with amino acid residues that are oriented about the pocket. Surprisingly, most of these bonds are formed between sugar hydroxyls and aromatic amino acids that are neither charged nor very polar at neutral pH.

Similarly, monoclonal antibody BR96 and the humanized monoclonal hu3S193 are specific for the Lewis Y antigen, which resembles the Le b antigen described in Figure 21.2, except that the Fucose-*N* Acetyl Glucosamine bond is beta 1→3 instead of beta 1→4. The Le Y antigen is commonly expressed on tumor cells of epithelial origin. The crystal structures have revealed the sources of the binding energy that results in affinity and specificity for this carbohydrate antigen (25,26). These two monoclonals bind Le Y antigen in a large, deep pocket, which accommodates all four hexoses and corresponds to the cavity-type binding site predicted by Kabat (*15*). The terminal Fucose goes in first, while the other three sugars are hydrogen-bonded to amino acid side chains lining the pocket, including Tyr 33, Tyr 35, and Gln 52 of the heavy chain, and His 27 of the light chain. Once again, hydrogen bonds between hydroxyl groups of the sugars and aromatic amines (Trp and Tyr) of the protein play a dominant role in determining affinity and specificity of binding. A smaller number of H bonds depend on amide groups of the protein backbone.

A third example is provided by human monoclonal 2G12, which has neutralizing activity against a broad spectrum of HIV isolates. This antibody binds the mannose-rich oligosaccharide side chains that form a protective surface, called a *glycoshield*, on the envelope glycoprotein gp120. The crystal structure shows that the two terminal mannose sugars of each oligosaccharide bind end-on into a deep pocket of the antibody, in a cavity-type site (27,28). Twelve hydrogen bonds form between the two terminal mannose residues and the protein, depending mainly on the amide groups of the protein backbone. Additional hydrogen bonds form between the third mannose residue and the side chain of Asp 100 of the heavy chain and between the fourth mannose residue and Tyr 94 of the light chain and Tyr 56 of the heavy chain. A unique feature of this antibody is the cross over of variable regions between heavy and light chains, so that each binding site is made up of the V_H from one HL pair combining with the V_L chain of the opposite pair. This arrangement allows the antibody to bind one branch of an oligosaccharide and the opposite branch of a nearby oligosaccharide and makes it ideally suited for cross-linking the densely clustered oligosaccharides of gp120.

Immunogenicity of Polysaccharides

Capsular polysaccharides are the main target of protective antibodies against bacterial infection, and, as such, are important vaccine antigens. In adults, the chain length of the polysaccharide is an important determinant of immunogenicity, and the polysaccharides induce a T-independent response that cannot be boosted on repeat exposure. In young children, whose maternal antibodies wane by 6 months of age and who most need immunity to pathogens such as *Haemophilus influenzae* type b and *Streptococcus pneumoniae* of multiple serotypes, the T-independent response to these polysaccharides is weak, regardless of chain length. To immunize children, the polysaccharides were coupled to a protein carrier to create a new T-dependent antigen that gained immunogenicity from T-cell help and boosted antibody titers with each successive dose. This strategy has produced highly successful conjugate vaccines against *H. influenzae* type b *(29)* resulting in a markedly reduced incidence of meningitis caused by this agent in immunized children (30,31) and evidence of herd immunity even among unimmunized children. The same strategy has produced an effective vaccine against invasive disease (32) and otitis media (33) caused by the most prevalent serotypes of *Strep. pneumonia*.

Protein and Polypeptide Antigenic Determinants

Like the proteins themselves, the antigen determinants of proteins consist of amino acid residues in a particular three-dimensional array. The residues that make contact with complementary residues in the antibody-combining site are called *contact residues*. To make contact, of course, these residues must be exposed on the surface of the protein, not buried in the hydrophobic core. Because the complementarity-determining residues in the hypervariable regions of antibodies have been found to span as much as 30 to 40 Å × 15 to 20 Å × 10 Å (D. R. Davies, personal communication, 1982), these contact residues comprising the antigenic determinant may cover a significant area of protein surface, as measured by x-ray crystallography of antibody–protein antigen complexes (*34–36*,37). The size of the combining sites has also been estimated using simple synthetic oligopeptides of increasing length, such as oligolysine. In this case, a series of elegant studies *(38–40)* suggested that the maximum length of chain a combining site could accommodate was six to eight residues, corresponding closely to that found earlier for oligosaccharides *(13,14)*, discussed previously.

Several types of interactions contribute to the binding energy. Many of the amino acid residues exposed to solvent on the surface of a protein antigen will be hydrophilic. These are likely to interact with antibody contact residues via polar interactions. For instance, an anionic glutamic acid carboxyl group may bind to a complementary cationic lysine amino group on the antibody, or vice versa; or a glutamine amide side chain may form a hydrogen bond with the antibody. However, hydrophobic interactions can also play a major role. Proteins cannot exist in aqueous solution as stable monomers with too many hydrophobic residues on their surface. Those hydrophobic residues that are on the surface can contribute to binding to antibody for exactly the same reason. When a hydrophobic residue in a protein antigenic determinant or, similarly, in a carbohydrate determinant *(8)*, interacts with a corresponding hydrophobic residue in the antibody-combining site, the water molecules previously in contact with each of them are excluded. The result is a significant stabilization of the interaction. A thorough review of these aspects of the chemistry of antigen–antibody binding is in reference 41.

Mapping Epitopes: Conformation versus Sequence

The other component that defines a protein antigenic determinant, besides the amino acid residues involved, is the way these residues are arrayed in three dimensions. Because the residues are on the surface of a protein, we can also think of this component as the topography of the antigenic determinant. Sela *(42)* divided protein antigenic determinants into two categories, sequential and conformational, depending on whether the primary sequence or the three-dimensional conformation appeared to contribute the most to binding. On the other hand, because the antibody-combining site has a preferred topography in the native antibody, it would seem *a priori* that some conformations of a particular polypeptide sequence would produce a better fit than others and therefore would be energetically favored in binding. Thus, conformation or topography must always play some role in the structure of an antigenic determinant.

Moreover, when one looks at the surface of a protein in a space-filling model, one cannot ascertain the direction of the backbone or the positions of the helices (contrast Figs. 21.3A, B) *(43–47)*. It is hard to recognize whether two residues that are side by side on the surface are adjacent on the polypeptide backbone or whether they come from different parts of the sequence and are brought together by the folding of the molecule. If a protein maintains its native conformation when an antibody binds, then it must similarly be hard for the antibody to discriminate between residues that are covalently connected directly and those connected only through a great deal of intervening polypeptide. Thus, the probability that an antigenic determinant on a native globular protein consists of only a consecutive sequence of amino acids in the primary structure is likely to be rather small. Even if most of the determinant were a continuous sequence, other nearby residues would probably play a role as well. Only if the protein were cleaved into fragments before the antibodies were made would there be any reason to favor connected sequences.

This concept was analyzed and confirmed quantitatively by Barlow et al. *(48)*, who examined the atoms lying within spheres of different radii from a given surface atom on a protein. As the radius increases, the probability that all the atoms within the sphere will be from the same continuous segment of protein sequence decreases rapidly. Correspondingly, the fraction of surface atoms that would be located at the center of a sphere containing only residues from the same continuous segment falls dramatically as the radius of the sphere increases. For instance, for lysozyme, with a radius of 8 Å, fewer than 10% of the surface residues would lie in such a "continuous patch" of surface. These are primarily in regions that protrude from the surface. With a radius of 10 Å, almost none of the surface residues fall in the center of a continuous patch. Thus, for a contact area of about 20 Å × 25 Å, as found for a lysozyme–antibody complex studied by x-ray crystallography, none of the antigenic sites could be completely continuous segmental sites (see following discussion and Fig. 21.4).

Antigenic sites consisting of amino acid residues that are widely separated in the primary protein sequence but brought together on the surface of the protein by the way it folds in its native conformation have been called *assembled topographic* sites *(49,50)* because they are assembled from different parts of the sequence and exist only in the surface topography of the native molecule. By contrast, the sites that consist of only a single continuous segment of protein sequence have been called *segmental* antigenic sites *(49,50)*.

In contrast to T-cell recognition of "processed" fragments retaining only primary and secondary structures, the evidence is overwhelming that most antibodies are made against the native conformation when the native protein is used as immunogen. For instance, antibodies to native staphylococcal nuclease were found to have about a 5,000-fold higher affinity for the native protein than for the corresponding polypeptide on which they were isolated (by binding to the peptide attached to Sepharose) *(51)*. An even more dramatic example is that demonstrated by Crumpton *(52)* for antibodies to native myoglobin or to apomyoglobin. Antibodies to native ferric myoglobin produced a brown precipitate with myoglobin, but did not bind well to apomyoglobin, which, without the heme, has a slightly altered conformation. On the other hand, antibodies to the apomyoglobin, when mixed with native (brown) myoglobin, produced a white precipitate. These antibodies so strongly favored the conformation of apomyoglobin, from which the heme was excluded, that they trapped those molecules that vibrated toward that conformation and pulled the equilibrium state over to the apo form. One could almost say, figuratively, that the antibodies squeezed the heme out of the myoglobin. Looked at thermodynamically, it is clear that the conformational preference of the antibody for the apo versus native forms, in terms of free energy, had to be greater than the free energy of binding of the heme to myoglobin. Thus, in general, antibodies are made that are very specific for the conformation of the protein used as immunogen.

Synthetic peptides corresponding to segments of the protein antigen sequence can be used to identify the structures bound by antibodies specific for segmental antigenic sites. To identify assembled topographic sites, more complex approaches have been necessary. The earliest was the use of natural variants of the protein antigen with known amino acid substitutions, where such evolutionary variants exist *(49)*. Thus, substitution of different amino acids in proteins in the native conformation can be examined. The use of this method, which is illustrated later, is limited to studying the function of amino acids that vary among homologous proteins, that is, those that are polymorphic. It may now be extended to other residues by use of site-directed mutagenesis. A second method is to use the antibody that binds to the native protein to protect the antigenic site from modification *(53)* or proteolytic degradation *(54)*. A related but less sensitive approach makes use of competition with other antibodies *(55–57)*. A third approach, taking advantage of the capability of producing thousands of peptides on a solid-phase surface for direct binding assays *(58)*, is to study binding of a monoclonal antibody to every possible combination of six amino acids *(58)*. If the assembled topographic site can be mimicked by a combination of six amino acids not corresponding to any continuous segment of the protein sequence but structurally resembling a part of the surface, then one can produce a "mimotope" defining the specificity of that antibody *(58)*.

Myoglobin also serves as a good model protein antigen for studying the range of variation of antigenic determinants from those that are more sequential in nature to those that do not even exist without the native conformation of the protein (Fig. 21.3). A good example of the first, more segmental type of determinant, is that consisting of residues 15 to 22 in the amino terminal portion of the molecule. Crumpton and Wilkinson *(59)* first discovered that the chymotryptic cleavage fragment consisting of residues 15 to 29 had antigenic activity for antibodies raised to either native or apomyoglobin. Two other groups *(44,60)* then found that synthetic peptides corresponding to residues 15 to 22 bind antibodies made to native sperm whale myoglobin, even though the synthetic peptides were only 7 to 8 residues long. Peptides of this length do not spend much time (in solution) in a conformation corresponding to that of the native protein. On the other hand, these synthetic peptides had a several hundred-fold lower affinity for the antibodies than did the native protein. Thus, even if most of the determinant was included in the consecutive sequence 15 to 22, the antibodies were still much more specific for the native conformation of this sequence than for the random conformation peptide. Moreover, there was no evidence to exclude the participation of other residues, nearby on the surface of myoglobin but not in this sequence, in the antigenic determinant[1] *(61–64)*.

A good example of the importance of secondary structure is the case of the loop peptide (residues 64 to 80) of hen egg-white lysozyme *(65)*. This loop in the protein sequence is created by the disulfide linkage between cysteine residues 64 and 80 and has been shown to be a major antigenic determinant for antibodies to lysozyme *(65)*. The isolated peptide 60 to 83, containing the loop, binds antibodies with high affinity, but opening of the loop by cleavage of the disulfide bond destroys most of the antigenic activity for antilysozyme antibodies *(65)*.

At the other end of the range of conformational requirements are those determinants involving residues far apart in the primary sequences that are brought close together on the surface of the native molecule by its folding in three dimensions, called *assembled topographic determinants (49,50)*. Of six monoclonal antibodies to sperm whale myoglobin studied by Berzofsky et al. *(43,66)*, none bound to any of the three cyanogen bromide cleavage fragments of myoglobin that together span the whole sequence of the molecule. Therefore, these monoclonal antibodies (all with affinities between 2×10^8 and 2×10^9 M^{-1}) were all highly specific for the native conformation. These were studied by comparing the relative affinities for a series of native myoglobins from different species with known amino acid sequences. This approach allowed the definition of some of the residues involved in binding to three of these antibodies. Two of these three monoclonal antibodies were found to recognize topographic determinants, as defined previously. One recognized a determinant including Glu 4 and Lys 79, which come within about 2 Å of each other to form a salt bridge in the native molecule (Fig. 21.3A,B). The other antibody recognized a determinant involving Glu 83, Ala 144, and Lys 145 (Fig. 21.3A). Again, these are far apart in the primary sequence but are brought within 12 Å of each other by the folding of the molecule in its native conformation. Similar examples have been reported for monoclonal antibodies to human myoglobin *(67)* and to lysozyme (37,55).

Other examples of such conformation-dependent antigenic determinants have been suggested using conventional antisera to such proteins as insulin *(68)*, hemoglobin *(69)*, tobacco mosaic virus *(70)*, and cytochrome c *(71)*. Moreover, the crystallographic structures of

[1] This is the only segmental antigenic determinant of myoglobin that has clearly been confirmed by more than one independent group of investigators. Crumpton and Wilkinson *(59)* did measure antigenic activity for a chymotryptic fragment 147-153 that overlaps one of the other reported sequential determinants *(61)*. However, two of the other reported sequential determinants *(61)*, corresponding to residues 56 to 62 and 94 to 100, have not been reproducible when tested with other antisera, even raised in the same species *(62)*. For related studies, see refs. *63* and *64*.

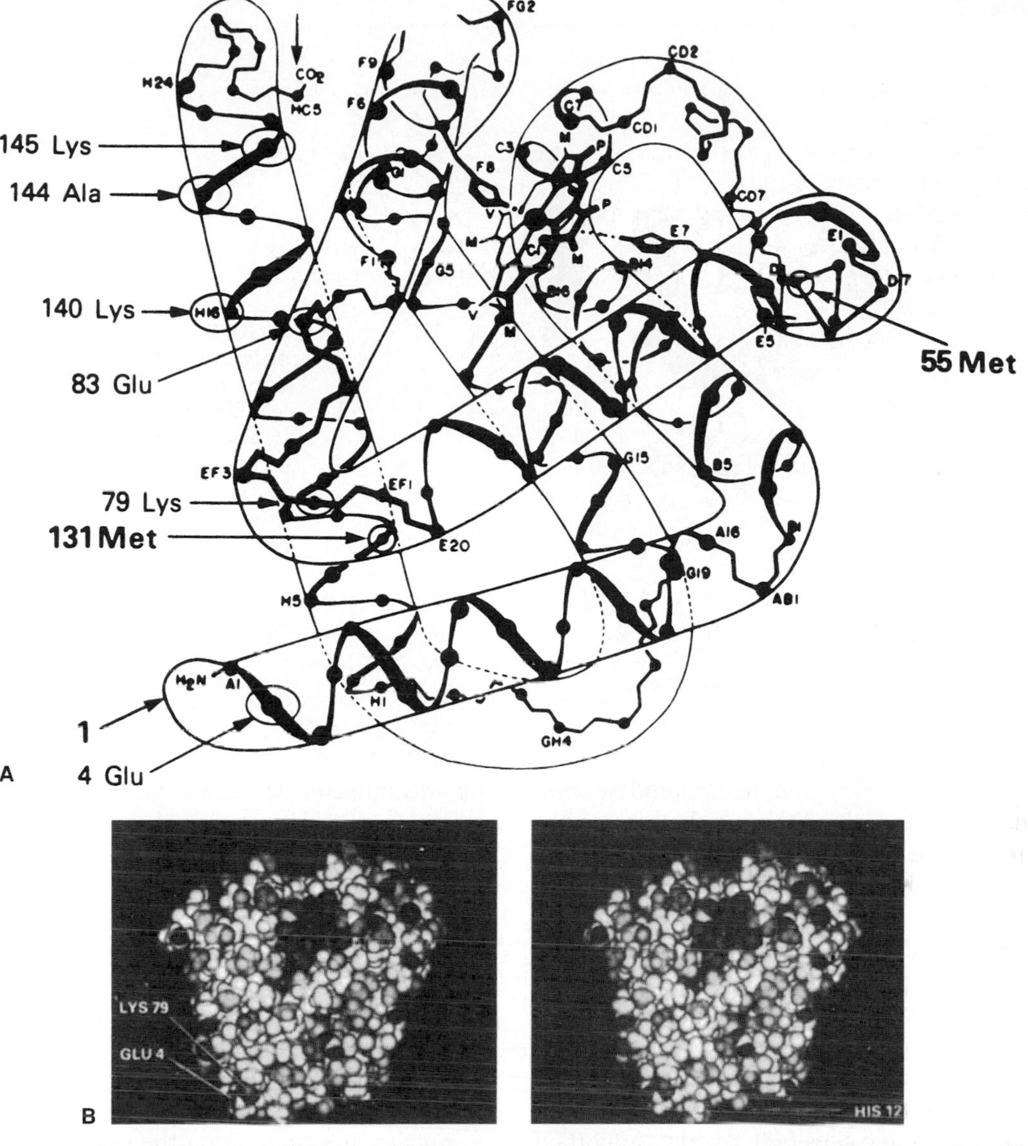

FIGURE 21.3 **A:** Artist's representation of the polypeptide backbone of sperm whale myoglobin in its native three dimensional conformation. The α helices are labeled A through H from the amino terminal to the carboxyl terminal. Side chains are omitted, except for the two histidine rings (F8 and E7) involved with the heme iron. Methionines at positions 55 and 131 are the sites of cleavage by cyanogen bromide (CNBr), allowing myoglobin to be cleaved into three fragments. Most of the helicity and other features of the native conformation are lost when the molecule is cleaved. A less-drastic change in conformation is produced by removal of the heme to form apomyoglobin, because the heme interacts with several helices and stabilizes their positions relative to one another. The other labeled residues (4 Glu, 79 Lys, 83 Glu, 140 Lys, 144 Ala, and 145 Lys) are residues that have been found to be involved in antigenic determinants recognized by monoclonal antibodies (*43*). Note that cleavage by CNBr separates Lys 79 from Glu 4 and separates Glu 83 from Ala 144 and Lys 145. The "sequential" determinant of Koketsu and Atassi (*44*) (residues 15 to 22) is located at the elbow, lower right, from the end of the A helix to the beginning of the B helix. (Adapted from ref. *45*, with permission.) **B:** Stereoscopic views of a computer-generated space-filling molecular model of sperm whale myoglobin, based on the Takano (*46*) x-ray diffraction coordinates. This orientation, which corresponds to that in Panel A, is arbitrarily designated the *front view*. The computer method was described by Feldmann et al. (*47*). The heme and aromatic carbons are shaded darkest, followed by carboxyl oxygens, then other oxygens, then primary amino groups, then other nitrogens, and finally side chains of aliphatic residues. The backbone and the side chains of nonaliphatic residues, except for the functional groups, are shown in white. Note that the direction of the helices is not apparent on the surface, in contrast to the backbone drawing in Panel A. The residues Glu 4, Lys 79, and His 12 are believed to be part of a topographic antigenic determinant recognized by a monoclonal antibody to myoglobin (*43*). This stereo pair can be viewed in three dimensions using an inexpensive stereoviewer such as the "stereoscopes" sold by Abrams Instrument Corp., Lansing, MI, or Hubbard Scientific Co., Northbrook, IL. (Adapted from ref. *43*, with permission.)

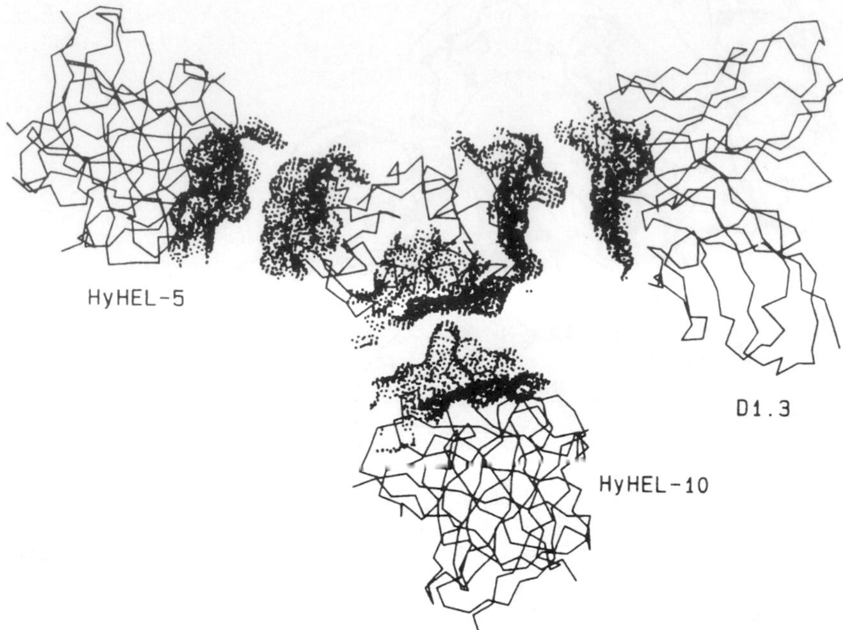

FIGURE 21.4 Assembled topographic sites of lysozyme illustrated by the footprints of three nonoverlapping monoclonal antibodies. Shown are the α carbon backbones of lysozyme in the center and the Fv portions of three antilysozyme monoclonal antibodies D1.3, HyHEL-5, and HyHEL-10. The footprints of the antibodies on lysozyme and lysozyme on the antibodies (i.e., their interacting surfaces) are shown by a dotted representation. Note that the three antibodies each contact more than one continuous loop of lysozyme and so define assembled topographic sites. (Reproduced from ref. *37*, with permission.)

lysozyme–antibody (*34,36*,37) and neuraminidase–antibody *(35)* complexes show clearly that, in both cases, the epitope bound is an assembled topographic site. In the case of the three monoclonal antibodies binding to nonoverlapping sites of lysozyme (Fig. 21.4), it is clear that the footprints of all three antibody-combining sites cover more than one loop of polypeptide chain and thus each encompasses an assembled topographic site (37). This result beautifully illustrates the concept that the majority of antibody-combining sites must interact with more than a continuous loop of polypeptide chain and thus must define assembled topographic sites *(48)*. Another important example is represented by neutralizing antibodies to the HIV envelope protein that similarly bind assembled topographic sites (72,73); see also the discussion at the end of this section.

How frequently are antibodies specific for topographic determinants compared with those that bind consecutive sequences when conventional antisera are examined? This question was studied by Lando et al. *(74)*, who passed goat, sheep, and rabbit antisera to sperm whale myoglobin over columns of myoglobin fragments, together spanning the whole sequence. After removal of all antibodies binding to the fragments, 30% to 40% of the antibodies remained that still bound to the native myoglobin molecule with high affinity but did not bind to any of the fragments in solution by radioimmunoassay. Thus, in four of four antimyoglobin sera tested, 60% to 70% of the antibodies could bind peptides and 30% to 40% could bind only native-conformation intact protein.

On the basis of studies such as these, it has been suggested that much of the surface of a protein molecule may be antigenic *(49,75)* but that the surface can be divided up into antigenic domains *(43,63,64,67)*. Each of these domains consists of many overlapping determinants recognized by different antibodies.

An additional interesting point is that in three published crystal structures of protein antigen–antibody complexes, the contact surfaces were broad, with local complementary pairs of concave and convex regions in both directions (*34–36*,37). Thus, the concept of an antigen binding in the groove or pocket of an antibody may be oversimplified, and antibodies may sometimes bind by extending into pockets on an antigen.

Further information on the subjects discussed in this section is available in the reviews by Sela *(42)*, Crumpton *(52)*, Reichlin *(76)*, Kabat *(77)*, Benjamin et al. *(49)*, Berzofsky *(50)*, Getzoff et al. *(41)*, and Davies et al. (37).

Conformational Equilibria of Protein and Peptide Antigenic Determinants

There are several possible mechanisms to explain why an antibody specific for a native protein will bind a peptide fragment in random conformation with lower affinity. Of course, the peptide may not contain all the contact residues of the antigenic determinant, so that the binding energy would be lower. However, for cases in which all the residues in the determinant are present in the peptide, several mechanisms still remain. First, the affinity may be lower because the topography of the residues in the peptide may not produce as complementary a fit in the antibody-combining site as the native conformation would. Second, the apparent affinity may be reduced because only a small fraction of the peptide molecules are in a nativelike conformation at any time, assuming that the antibody binds only to the native conformation. Because the concentration of peptide molecules in native conformation is lower than the total peptide concentration by a factor that corresponds to the conformational equilibrium constant of the peptide, the apparent affinity is also lower by this factor. This model is analogous to an allosteric model. A third, intermediate hypothesis would suggest that initial binding of the peptide in a nonnative conformation occurs with submaximal complementarity and is followed by an intramolecular conformational change in the peptide to achieve energy minimization by assuming a nativelike conformation. This third hypothesis corresponds to an induced-fit model. The loss of affinity is due to the energy required to change the conformation of the peptide, which in turn corresponds to the conformational equilibrium constant in the second hypothesis. To some extent these models could be distinguished kinetically because the first hypothesis predicts a faster "on" rate and a faster "off" rate than does the second hypothesis *(78)*.

Although not the only way to explain the data, the second hypothesis is useful because it provides a method to estimate the conformational equilibria of proteins and peptides (*51–71*,72,73,*74–79*). The method assumes the second hypothesis, which can be expressed as follows:

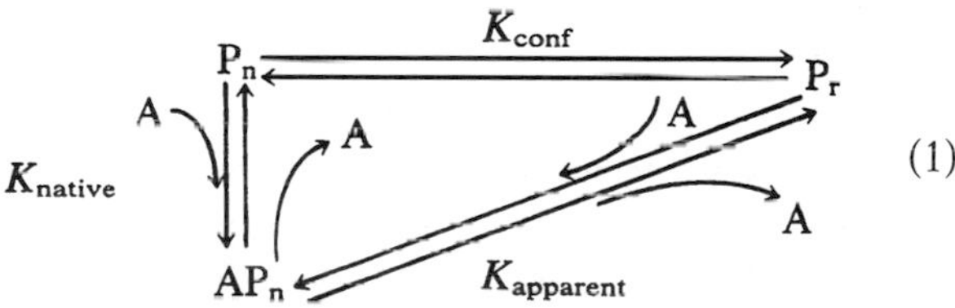

(1)

where A is antibody, P_n is native peptide, and P_r is random conformation peptide, so that

$$K_{apparent} = K_{conf}\,K_{native} \qquad (2)$$

Thus, the ratio of the apparent association constant for peptide to the measured association constant for the native molecule should give the conformational equilibrium constant of the peptide. Note the implicit assumption that the total peptide concentration can be approximated by $[P_r]$. This will generally be true because most peptide fragments of proteins demonstrate little native conformation; that is, $K_{conf} = [P_n]/[P_r]$ is much less than 1. Also note that if the first hypothesis (or third) occurs to some extent, this method will overestimate K_{conf}. On the other hand, if the affinity for the peptide is lower because it lacks some of the contact residues of the determinant, this method will underestimate K_{conf} (by assuming that all the affinity difference is due to conformation). To some extent, the two errors may partially cancel out. When this method was used to determine the K_{conf} for a peptide staphylococcal nuclease, a value of 2×10^{-4} (unitless because it is a ratio of two concentrations) was obtained *(51)*. Similarly, when antibodies raised to a peptide fragment were used, it was possible to estimate the fraction of time the native nuclease spends in nonnative conformations *(79)*. In this case, the K_{conf} was found to be about 3,000-fold in favor of the native conformation.

Antipeptide Antibodies that Bind to Native Proteins at a Specific Site

In light of the conformational differences between native proteins and peptides and the observed K_{conf} effects shown by antibodies to native proteins when tested on the corresponding peptides, it was somewhat surprising to find that antibodies to synthetic peptides show extensive cross-reactions with native proteins *(80,81)*. These two types of cross-reactions can be thought of as working in opposite directions: the binding of antiprotein antibodies to the peptide is inefficient, while the binding of antipeptide antibodies to the protein is quite efficient and commonly observed. This finding is quite useful because automated solid-phase peptide synthesis has become readily available. This has been particularly useful in three areas: exploitation of protein sequences deduced by recombinant DNA methods, preparation of site-specific antibodies, and the attempt to focus the immune response on a single protein site that is biologically important but may not be particularly immunogenic. This section focuses on the explanation of the cross-reaction, uses of the cross-reaction, and the potential limitations with regard to immunogenicity.

The basic assumption is that antibodies raised against peptides in an unfolded structure will bind the corresponding site on proteins folded into the native structure *(81)*. This is not immediately obvious because antibody binding to antigen is the direct result of the antigen fitting into the binding site. Affinity is the direct consequence of "goodness of fit" between antibody and antigen, while antibody specificity is the result of the inability of other antigens to occupy the same site. How then can the antipeptide antibodies overcome the effect of K_{conf} and still bind native proteins with good affinity and specificity? The whole process depends on the antibody-binding site forming a three-dimensional space and the antigen filling it in an energetically favorable way.

Because the peptides are randomly folded, they rarely occupy the native conformation, so they are not likely to elicit antibodies against a conformation they do not maintain. If the antibodies are specific for a denatured structure, then, like the myoglobin molecules that were denatured to apomyoglobin by antibody binding *(52)*, the cross-reaction may depend on the native protein's ability to assume different conformational states. If the native protein is quite rigid, then the possibility of its assuming a random conformation is quite small; but if it is a flexible three-dimensional spring, then local unfolding and refolding may occur all the time. Local unfolding of protein segments may permit the immunologic cross-reaction with antipeptide antibodies because a flexible segment could assume many of the same conformations as the randomly folded peptide *(81)*.

In contrast, the proteins' ability to crystallize (a feature that allows the study of their structure by x-ray crystallography) has long been taken as evidence of protein rigidity *(82)*. In addition, the existence of discrete functional states of allosteric enzymes *(83)* provides additional evidence of stable structural states of a protein. Finally, the fact that antibodies can distinguish native from denatured forms of intact proteins is well known for proteins such as myoglobin *(52)*.

However, protein crystals are a somewhat artificial situation because the formation of the crystal lattice imposes order on the components, each of which occupies a local energy minimum at the expense of considerable loss of randomness (entropy). Thus, the crystal structure may have artificial rigidity that exceeds the actual rigidity of protein molecules in solution. On the contrary, we may attribute some of the considerable difficulty in crystallizing proteins to disorder within the native conformation. Second, allosterism may be explained by two distinct conformations that are discrete without being particularly rigid. Finally, the ability to generate antiprotein antibodies that are conformation-specific does not rule out the existence of antipeptide antibodies that are not. All antibodies are probably specific for some conformation of the antigen, but this need not be the crystallographic native conformation in order to achieve a significant affinity for those proteins or protein segments that have a "loose" native conformation.

Antipeptide antibodies have proved to be very powerful reagents when combined with recombinant DNA methods of gene sequencing *(81,84)*. From the DNA sequence, the protein sequence is predicted. A synthetic peptide is constructed, coupled to a suitable carrier molecule, and used to immunize animals. The resulting polyclonal antibodies can be detected with a peptide-coated enzyme-linked immunosorbent assay plate (see Chapter 5). They are used to immunoprecipitate the native protein from a ^{35}S-labeled cell lysate and thus confirm expression of the gene product in these cells. The antipeptide antibodies can also be used to isolate the previously unidentified gene product of a new gene. The site-specific antibodies are also useful in detecting posttranslational processing, because they bind all precursors and products that contain the site. In addition, because the antibodies bind only to the site corresponding to the peptide, they are useful in probing structure–function relationships. They can be used to block the binding of a substrate to an enzyme or the binding of a virus to its cellular receptor.

Immunogenicity of Proteins and Peptides

Up to this point, we have considered the ability of antibodies to react with proteins or peptides as antigens. However, immunogenicity refers to the ability of these compounds to elicit antibodies following immunization. Several factors limit the immunogenicity of different regions of proteins, and these have been divided into those that are intrinsic to protein structure itself versus those extrinsic to the antigen that are related to the responder and vary from one animal or species to another *(50)*. In addition, we consider the special case of peptide immunogenicity as it applies to vaccine development. The features of protein structure that have been suggested to explain the results include surface accessibility of the site, hydrophilicity, flexibility, and proximity to a site recognized by helper T cells.

When the x-ray crystallographic structure and antigenic structure are known for the same protein, it is not surprising to find that a series of monoclonal antibodies binding to a molecule such as influenza neuraminidase choose an overlapping pattern of sites at the exposed head of the protein *(85)*. The stalk of neuraminidase was not immunogenic, apparently because it was almost entirely covered by carbohydrate.

Beyond such things as carbohydrate, which may sterically interfere with antibody binding to protein, accessibility on the surface is clearly a sine qua non for an antigenic determinant to be bound by an antibody specific for the native conformation, without any requirement for unfolding of the structure *(50)*. Several measures of such accessibility have been suggested. All these require knowledge of the x-ray crystallographic three-dimensional structure. Some have measured accessibility to solvent by rolling a sphere with the radius of a water molecule over the surface of a protein *(86,87)*. Others have suggested that accessibility to water is not the best measure of accessibility to antibody and have demonstrated a better correlation by rolling a sphere with the radius of an antibody-combining domain *(88)*. Another approach to predicting antigenic sites on the basis of accessibility is to examine the degree of protrusion from the surface of the protein *(89)*. This was done by modeling the body of the protein as an ellipsoid and examining which amino acid residues remain outside ellipsoids of increasing dimensions. The most protruding residues were found to be part of antigenic sites bound by antibodies, but usually these sites had been identified by using short synthetic peptides and so were segmental in nature. As previously noted, for an antigenic site to be contained completely within a single continuous segment of protein sequence, the site is likely to have to protrude from the surface, as otherwise residues from other parts of the sequence would fall within the area contacting the antibody *(48)*.

Because the three-dimensional structure of most proteins is not known, other ways of predicting surface exposure have been proposed for most antigens. For example, hydrophilic sites tend to be found on the water-exposed surface of proteins. Thus, hydrophilicity has been proposed as a second indication of immunogenicity *(90–92)*.

This model has been used to analyze 12 proteins with known antigenic sites: the most hydrophilic site of each protein was indeed one of the antigenic sites. However, among the limitations are the facts that a significant fraction of surface residues can be nonpolar *(86,87)* and that several important examples of hydrophobic and aromatic amino acids involved in the antigenic sites are known *(42,70,93,94)*. Specificity of antibody binding likely depends on the complementarity of surfaces for hydrogen bonding and polar bonding as well as van der Waals contacts *(95)*, while hydrophobic interactions and the exclusion of water from the interacting surfaces of proteins may contribute a large but nonspecific component to the energy of binding *(95)*.

A third factor suggested to play a role in immunogenicity of protein epitopes is mobility. Measurement of mobility in the native protein is largely dependent on the availability of a high-resolution crystal structure, so its applicability is limited to only a small subset of proteins. Furthermore, it has been studied only for antibodies specific for segmental antigenic sites; therefore, it may not apply to the large fraction of antibodies to assembled topographic sites. Studies of mobility have taken two directions. The case of antipeptide antibodies has already been discussed, in which antibodies made to peptides corresponding to more mobile segments of the native protein were more likely to bind to the native protein *(81,96)*. This is not considered just a consequence of the fact that more mobile segments are likely to be those on the surface and therefore more exposed, because in the case of myohemerythrin (which was used as a model), two regions of the native protein that were equally exposed but less mobile did not bind nearly as well to the corresponding antipeptide antibodies *(97)*. However, as is clear from the earlier discussion, this result applies to antibodies made against short peptides and therefore is not directly relevant to immunogenicity of parts of the native protein. Rather, it concerns the cross-reactivity of antipeptide antibodies with the native protein and therefore is of considerable practical importance for the purposes outlined in the section on antipeptide antibodies.

Studies in the other direction—that is, of antibodies raised against native proteins—would be by definition more relevant to the question of immunogenicity of parts of the native protein. Westhof et al. *(98)* used a series of hexapeptides to determine the specificity of antibodies raised against native tobacco mosaic virus protein and found that six of the seven peptides that bound antibodies to native protein corresponded to peaks of high mobility in the native protein. The correlation was better than could be accounted for just by accessibility because three peptides that corresponded to exposed regions of only average mobility did not bind antibodies to the native protein. However, when longer peptides—on the order of 20 amino acid residues—were used as probes, it was found that antibodies were present in the same antisera that bound to less mobile regions of the protein *(99)*. They simply had not been detected with the short hexapeptides with less conformational stability. Thus, it was not that the more mobile regions were necessarily more immunogenic but rather that antibodies to these were more easily detected with short peptides as probes. A similar good correlation of antigenic sites with mobile regions of the native protein in the case of myoglobin *(98)* may also be attributed to the fact that seven of the nine sites were defined with short peptides of six to eight residues *(61)*. Again, this result becomes a statement about cross-reactivity between peptides and native protein rather than about the immunogenicity of the native protein. (For reviews, see Van Regenmortel *[100]* and Getzoff et al. *[41]*).

To address the role of mobility in immunogenicity, an attempt was made to quantitate the relative fraction of antibodies specific for different sites on the antigen myohemerythrin *(101)*. The premise was that, although the entire surface of the protein may be immunogenic, certain regions may elicit significantly more antibodies than others and therefore may be considered immunodominant or at least more immunogenic. Because this study was done with short synthetic peptides from 6 to 14 residues long based on the protein sequence, it was limited to the subset of antibodies specific for segmental antigenic sites. Among these, it was clear that the most immunogenic sites were in regions of the surface that were most mobile, convex in shape, and often of negative electrostatic potential. The role of these parameters has been reviewed *(41)*.

These results have important practical and theoretical implications. First, to use peptides to fractionate antiprotein antisera by affinity chromatography, peptides corresponding to more mobile segments of the native protein should be chosen when possible. If the crystal structure is not known, it may be possible to use peptides from amino or carboxyl termini or from exon–intron boundaries, as these are more likely to be mobile *(96)*. Second, these results may explain how a large but finite repertoire of antibody-producing B cells can respond to any antigen in nature or even artificial antigens never encountered in nature. Protein segments that are more flexible may be able to bind by induced fit in an antibody-combining site that is not perfectly complementary to the average native structure *(41,50)*. Indeed, evidence from the crystal structure of antigen–antibody complexes (*102–103*,104) suggests that mobility in the antibody-combining site as well as in the antigen may allow both reactants to adopt more complementary conformations on binding to each other, that is, a two-way induced fit. A very nice example comes from the study of antibodies to myohemerythrin *(103)*, in which the data suggested that initial binding of exposed side chains of the antigen to the antibody promoted local displacements that allowed exposure and binding of other, previously buried residues that served as contact residues. The only way this could occur would be for such residues to become exposed during the course of an induced-fit conformational change in the antigen *(41,103)*. In a second very clear example of induced fit, the contribution of antibody mobility to peptide binding was demonstrated for a monoclonal antibody to peptide 75-110 of influenza hemagglutinin, which was crystallized with or without peptide in the binding site and analyzed by x-ray crystallography for evidence of an induced fit (104). Despite flexibility of the peptide, the antibody binding site probably could not accommodate the peptide without a conformational change in the third complementarity determining region (CDR3) of the heavy chain, in which an asparagine residue of the antibody was rotated out of the way to allow a tyrosine residue of the peptide to fit in the binding pocket of the antibody (104).

With regard to host-limited factors, immunogenicity is certainly limited by self-tolerance. Thus, the repertoire of potential antigenic sites on mammalian protein antigens such as myoglobin or cytochrome c can be thought of as greatly simplified by the sharing of numerous amino acids with the endogenous host protein. For mouse, guanaco, or horse cytochrome c injected into rabbits, each of the differences between the immunogen and rabbit cytochrome c is seen as an immunogenic site on a background of immunologically silent residues *(49,71,105)*. In another example, rabbit and dog antibodies to beef myoglobin bound almost equally well to beef or sheep myoglobin *(106)*. However, sheep antibodies bound beef but not sheep myoglobin, even though these two myoglobins differ by just six amino acids. Thus, the sheep immune system was able to screen out those clones that would be autoreactive with sheep myoglobin.

Ir genes of the host also play an important role in regulating the ability of an individual to make antibodies to a specific antigen *(107)*. These antigen-specific immune response genes are among the *MHC* genes that code for transplantation antigens. Structural mutations, gene transfer experiments, and biochemical studies *(107)* all indicate that *Ir* genes are actually the structural genes for major histocompatibility complex (MHC) antigens. The mechanism of action of the MHC antigens works through their effect on helper T cells (described later). There appear to be constraints on which B cells a T cell of a given specificity can help *(108,109)*, a process called *T–B reciprocity (110)*. Thus, if *Ir* genes control helper T-cell specificity, they will in turn limit which B cells are activated and thus which antibodies are made.

The immunogenicity of peptide antigens is also limited by intrinsic and extrinsic factors. With less structure to go on, each small peptide must presumably contain some nonself structural feature in order to overcome self-tolerance. In addition, the same peptide must contain antigenic sites that can be recognized by helper T cells as well as by B cells. When no T-cell site is present, three approaches may be helpful: graft on a T-cell site; couple the peptide to a carrier protein; or overcome T-cell nonresponsiveness to the available structure with various immunologic agents, such as interleukin (IL-2).

An example of a biologically relevant but poorly immunogenic peptide is the asparagine–alanine–asparagine–proline (NANP) repeat unit of the circumsporozoite (CS) protein of malaria sporozoites. A monoclonal antibody to the repeat unit of the CS protein can protect against murine malaria *(111)*. Thus, it would be desirable to make a malaria vaccine of the repeat unit of *Plasmodium falciparum* $(NANP)_n$. However, only mice of one MHC type (H-2^b) of all mouse strains tested were able to respond to $(NANP)_n$ *(112,113)*. One approach to overcome this limitation is to couple $(NANP)_n$ to a site recognizable by T cells, perhaps a carrier protein such as tetanus toxoid *(114)*. In human trials, this conjugate was weakly immunogenic and only partially protective. Moreover, as helper T cells produced by this approach are specific for the unrelated carrier, a secondary or memory response would not be expected to be elicited by the pathogen itself.

Another choice might be to identify a T-cell site on the CS protein itself and couple the two synthetic peptides together to make one complete immunogen. The result with one such site, called *Th2R*, was to increase the range of responding mouse MHC types by one, to include H-2^k as well as H-2^b *(115)*. This approach has the potential advantage of inducing a state of immunity that could be boosted by natural exposure to the sporozoite antigen. Because CS-specific T and B cells are both elicited by the vaccine, natural exposure to the antigen could help maintain the level of immunity during the entire period of exposure.

Another strategy to improve the immunogenicity of peptide vaccines is to stimulate the T- and B-cell responses artificially by adding IL-2 to the vaccine. Results with myoglobin indicate that genetic nonresponsiveness can be overcome by appropriate doses of IL-2 *(116)*. The same effect was found for peptides derived from malaria proteins (*117*; K. Akaji, D. T. Liu, and I. J. Berkower, unpublished results).

One of the most important possible uses of peptide antigens is as synthetic vaccines. However, even though it is possible to elicit with synthetic peptides anti-influenza antibodies to nearly every part of the influenza hemagglutinin *(80)*, antibodies that neutralize viral infectivity have not been elicited by immunization with synthetic peptides. This may reflect the fact that antibody binding by itself often does not result in virus inactivation. Viral inactivation occurs only when antibody interferes with one of the steps in the life cycle of the virus, including binding to its cell surface receptor, internalization, and virus uncoating within the cell. Apparently, antibodies can bind to most of the exposed surface of the virus without affecting these functions. Only those antibodies that bind to certain "neutralizing" sites can inactivate the virus. In addition, as in the case of the VP1 coat protein of poliovirus, certain neutralizing sites are found only on the native protein and not on the heat-denatured protein *(118)*. Thus, not only the site but also the conformation that is bound by the antibodies may be important for the antibody to inactivate the virus. These sites may often be assembled topographic sites not mimicked by peptide segments of the sequence. Perhaps binding of an antibody to such an assembled site can alter the relative positions of the component subsites so as to induce an allosteric neutralizing effect. Alternatively, antibodies to such an assembled site may prevent a conformational change necessary for activity of the viral protein.

One method of mapping neutralizing sites is based on the use of neutralizing monoclonal antibodies. The virus is grown in the presence of neutralizing concentrations of the monoclonal antibody, and virus mutants are selected for the ability to overcome antibody inhibition. These are sequenced, revealing the mutation that permits "escape" by altering the antigenic site for that antibody. This method has been used to map the neutralizing sites of influenza hemagglutinin *(119)* as well as poliovirus capsid protein VP1 *(120)*. The influenza escaping mutations are clustered to form an assembled topographic site, with mutations distant from each other in the primary sequence of hemagglutinin but brought together by the three-dimensional folding of the native protein. At first, it was thought that neutralization was the result of steric hindrance of the hemagglutinin binding site for the cell surface receptor of the virus *(121)*. However, similar work with poliovirus reveals that neutralizing antibodies that bind to assembled topographic sites may inactivate the virus at less than stoichiometric amounts, when at least half of the sites are unbound by antibody *(122)*. The neutralizing antibodies all cause a conformational change in the virus, which is reflected in a change in the isoelectric point of the particles from pH 7 to pH 4 *(120,123)*. Antibodies that bind without neutralizing do not cause this shift. Thus, an alternative explanation for the mechanism of antibody-mediated neutralization is the triggering of the virus to self-destruct. Perhaps the reason that neutralizing sites are clustered near receptor-binding sites is that occupation of such sites by antibody mimics events normally caused by binding to the cellular receptor, causing the virus to prematurely trigger its cell entry mechanisms. However, in order to transmit a physiologic signal, the antibody may need to bind viral capsid proteins in the native conformation (especially assembled topographic sites), which antipeptide antibodies may fail to do. Antibodies of this specificity are similar to the viral receptors on the cell surface, some of which have been cloned and expressed without their transmembrane sequences as soluble proteins. The soluble recombinant receptors for poliovirus (124) and HIV-1 *(125–127)* exhibit high-affinity binding to the virus and potent neutralizing activity *in vitro*. The HIV-1 receptor, CD4, has been combined with the human immunoglobulin heavy chain in a hybrid protein CD4–Ig *(128)*, which spontaneously assembles into dimers and resembles a monoclonal antibody, in which the binding site is the same as the receptor-binding site for HIV-1. In these recombinant constructs, high-affinity binding depends on the native conformation of the viral envelope glycoprotein gp120.

For HIV-1, two types of neutralizing antibodies have been identified. The first type binds a continuous or segmental determinant, such as the "V3 loop" sequence between amino acids 296 and 331 of gp120 *(129–131)*. Antipeptide antibodies against this site can neutralize the virus *(129)*. However, because this site is located in a highly variable region of the envelope, these antibodies tend to neutralize a narrow range of viral variants with nearly the same sequence as the immunogen. Even for this highly variable site, more broadly neutralizing antibodies can be obtained that recognize conserved conformations (132–134). The second type of neutralizing antibody binds conserved sites on the native structure of gp120, allowing them to neutralize a broad spectrum of HIV-1 isolates. These antibodies are commonly found in the sera of infected patients *(135)*, and a panel of neutralizing monoclonals derived from these subjects has been analyzed.

These monoclonals can be divided into three types. One group, possibly the most common ones in human polyclonal sera, bind at or near the CD4 receptor-binding site of gp120 (136–140). A second type of monoclonal, called *2G12*, binds a conformational site on gp120 that also depends on glycosylation, but has no direct effect on CD4 binding (141). A third type, quite rare in human sera, is represented by monoclonal antibody 2F5 (142) and binds a conserved site on the transmembrane protein gp41. Although this site is contained on a linear peptide ELDKWA, antibodies like 2F5 cannot be elicited by immunizing with the peptide, again suggesting the conformational aspect of this site (143,144).

These monoclonals neutralize fresh isolates, as well as laboratory-adapted strains, and they neutralize viruses tropic for T cells or macrophages (145), regardless of the use of CXCR4 or CCR5 as second receptor. These monoclonals, which target different sites, act synergistically. A cocktail combining all three types of monoclonals can protect monkeys against IV challenge or vaginal challenge with an SIV/HIV hybrid virus, indicating the potential for antibodies alone to prevent HIV infection (146,147). Because each of the three conserved neutralizing determinants depends on the native conformation of the protein (148), a prospective gp120 vaccine (or gp160 vaccine) would need to be in the native conformation to be able to elicit these antibodies.

ANTIGENIC DETERMINANTS RECOGNIZED BY T CELLS

Studies of T-cell specificity for antigen were motivated by the fact that the immune response to protein antigens is regulated at the T-cell level. A hapten, not immunogenic by itself, will elicit antibodies only when coupled to a protein that elicits a T-cell response in that animal. This ability of the protein component of the conjugate to confer immunogenicity on the hapten has been termed the *carrier effect*. Recognition of the carrier by specific helper T cells induces the B cells to make antibodies. Thus, the factors contributing to a good T-cell response appear to control the B-cell response as well.

"Nonresponder" animals display an antigen-specific failure to respond to a protein antigen, both for T cells and antibody responses. The "high responder" phenotype for each antigen is a genetically inheritable, usually dominant trait. Using inbred strains of mice, the genes controlling the immune response were found to be tightly linked to the MHC genes (*107*,149). MHC-linked immune responsiveness has been shown to depend on the T-cell recognition of antigen bound within a groove of MHC antigens of the antigen-presenting cell (APC) (discussed later; see also Chapters 19 and 20). The recognition of antigen in association with MHC molecules of the B cell is necessary for carrier-specific T cells to expand and provide helper signals to B cells.

In contrast to the range of antigens recognized by antibodies, the repertoire recognized by helper and cytotoxic T cells appears to be limited largely to protein and peptide antigens, although exceptions such as the small molecule tyrosine–azobenzene arsonate *(150)* exist. Once the antigenic determinants on proteins recognized by T cells are identified, it may be possible to better understand immunogenicity and perhaps even to manipulate the antibody response to biologically relevant antigens by altering the helper T cell response to the antigen.

Defining Antigenic Structures

Polyclonal T-Cell Response

Significant progress in understanding T-cell specificity was made possible by focusing on T-cell proliferation *in vitro*, mimicking the clonal expansion of antigen specific clones *in vivo*. The proliferative response depends on only two cells: the antigen-specific T cell and an APC, usually a macrophage, dendritic cell, or B cell. The growth of T cells in culture is measured as the incorporation of [^{3}H]thymidine into newly formed DNA. Under appropriate conditions, thymidine incorporation increases with antigen concentration. This assay permits the substitution of different APCs and is highly useful in defining the MHC and antigen-processing requirements of the APCs.

Using primarily this assay, several different approaches have been taken to mapping T-cell epitopes. First, T cells immunized to one protein have been tested for a proliferative response *in vitro* to the identical protein or to a series of naturally occurring variants. By comparing the sequences of stimulatory and nonstimulatory variants, it was possible to identify potential epitopes recognized by T cells. For example, the T-cell response to myoglobin was analyzed by immunizing mice with sperm whale or horse myoglobin and testing the resulting T cells for proliferation in response to a series of myoglobins from different species with known amino acid substitutions *(151)*. Reciprocal patterns were observed in T cells from mice immunized with sperm whale or horse myoglobin. The response to the cross-stimulatory myoglobins was as strong as to the myoglobin used to immunize the mice. This suggested that a few shared amino acid residues formed an immunodominant epitope and that most substitutions had no effect on the dominant epitope. A comparison of the sequences revealed that substitutions at a single residue could explain the pattern observed. All myoglobins that cross-stimulated sperm-whale-immune T cells had Glu at position 109, while all that cross-stimulated horse-immune T cells had Asp at 109. No member of one group could stimulate T cells from donors immunized with a myoglobin of the other group. This suggested that an immunodominant epitope recognized by T cells was centered on position 109, regardless of which amino acid was substituted. Usually, this approach has led to correct localization of the antigenic site in the protein *(151–153)*, but the possibility of long-range effects on antigen processing must be kept in mind (see "Antigen Processing"). Also, this approach using natural variants is limited in that it can focus on the correct region of the molecule but cannot define the boundaries of the site. Site-directed mutagenesis may therefore expand the capabilities of this approach.

A second approach is to use short peptide segments of the protein sequence, taking advantage of the fact that T cells specific for soluble protein antigens appear to see only segmental antigenic sites, not assembled topographic ones *(107,154–158)*. These may be produced by chemical or enzymatic cleavage of the natural protein (*156–163*,164), solid-phase peptide synthesis *(163,165–168)*, or recombinant DNA expression of cloned genes or gene fragments *(169)*. In the case of class I MHC molecule-restricted cytotoxic T cells, viral gene deletion mutants expressing only part of the gene product have also been used (*170,171*,172).

In the case of myoglobin-specific T cells, mapping of an epitope to residue Glu 109 was confirmed by use of a synthetic peptide 102–118, which stimulated the T cells *(167,173)*. The T cells elicited by a myoglobin with either Glu or Asp 109 could readily distinguish between synthetic peptides containing Glu or Asp at this position. Similar results were obtained with cytochrome c, where the predominant site recognized by T cells was localized with sequence variants to the region around residue 100 at the carboxyl end of cytochrome *(152)*. Furthermore, the response to cytochrome c peptide 81 to 104 was as great as the response to the whole molecule. This indicated that a 24-amino acid peptide contained an entire antigenic site recognized by T cells. The T cells could distinguish between synthetic peptides with Lys or Gln at position 99, although both were immunogenic with the same MHC molecule *(174–176)*. This residue determined T-cell memory and specificity and so presumably was interacting with the T-cell receptor. A similar conclusion could be drawn for residue 109 of myoglobin. However, this type of analysis must be used with caution. When multiple substitutions at position 109 were examined for T-cell recognition and MHC binding, residue 109 was found to affect both functions (177). The ultimate use of synthetic peptides to analyze the segmental sites of a protein that are recognized by T cells was to synthesize a complete set of peptides, each staggered by just one amino acid from the previous peptide, corresponding to the entire sequence of hen egg lysozyme, HEL (178). Around each immunodominant site, a cluster of several stimulatory peptides was found. The minimum "core" sequence consisted of just those residues shared by all antigenic peptides within a cluster, while the full extent of sequences spanning all stimulatory peptides within the same cluster defined the "determinant envelope." These two ways of defining an antigenic site differ, and one interpretation is that each core sequence corresponds to an MHC binding site, while the determinant envelope includes the many ways for T cells to recognize the same peptide bound to the MHC.

In each case, the polyclonal T-cell response could be mapped to a single predominant antigenic site. These results are consistent with the idea that each protein antigen has a limited number of immunodominant sites (possibly one) recognized by T cells in association with MHC molecules of the high responder type. If none of the antigenic sites could associate with MHC molecules on the APCs, then the strain would be a low responder, and the antigen would have little or no immunogenicity.

Monoclonal T Cells

Further progress in mapping T-cell sites depended on the analysis of cloned T-cell lines. These were either antigen-specific T-cell lines made by the method of Kimoto and Fathman *(179)* or T-cell hybridomas made by the method of Kappler et al. *(180)*. In the former method, T cells are allowed to proliferate in response to antigen and antigen-presenting cells, rested, and then restimulated again. After stimulation, the blasts can be cloned by limiting dilution and grown from a single cell in the presence of IL-2. In the second method, enriched populations of antigen-specific T cells are fused with a drug-sensitive T-cell tumor, and the fused cells are selected for their ability to grow in the presence of the drug. Then the antigen specificity of each fused cell line must be determined. The key to determining this in a tumor line is that antigen-specific stimulation of a T-cell hybridoma results in release of IL-2 even though proliferation is constitutive. T cells produced by either method are useful in defining epitopes, measuring their MHC associations, and studying antigen-processing requirements.

Monoclonal T cells may be useful in identifying which of the many proteins from a pathogen are important for T-cell responses. For instance, Young and Lamb *(181)* have developed a way to screen proteins separated by SDS–polyacrylamide gel electrophoresis and blotted onto nitrocellulose for stimulation of T-cell clones and have used this to identify antigens of *Mycobacterium tuberculosis (182)*. Mustafa et al. *(183)* have even used T-cell clones to screen recombinant DNA expression libraries to identify relevant antigens of *Mycobacterium leprae*. Use of T cells to map epitopes has also been important in defining tumor antigens (*184*,185–189).

Precise mapping of antigenic sites recognized by T cells was made possible by the fact that T cells would respond to peptide fragments of the antigen when they contain a complete antigenic determinant. A series of overlapping peptides can be used to walk along the protein sequence and find the antigenic site. Then, by truncating the peptide at either end, the minimum antigenic peptide can be determined. For example, in the case of myoglobin, a critical amino acid residue, such as Glu 109 or Lys 140, was found by comparing the sequences of stimulatory and nonstimulatory myoglobin variants and large CNBr cleavage fragments *(190)* as previously discussed, and then a series of truncated peptides containing the critical residue was synthesized with different overlapping lengths at either end *(163,167)*. Because solid-phase peptide synthesis starts from a fixed carboxyl end and proceeds toward the amino end, it can be stopped at various positions to produce a nested series of peptides that vary in length at the amino end. In this way, it was found that two of the Glu 109-specific T-cell clones responded to synthetic peptides 102 to 118 and 106 to 118 but not to peptide 109 to 118 *(167)*. One clone responded to peptide 108 to 118, and the other did not. Thus, the amino end of the peptide recognized by one clone was Ser 108, and the other clone required Phe 106 and/or Ile 107. Similar fine specificity differences have been observed with T-cell clones specific for the peptides 52 to 61 and 74 to 96 of hen egg lysozyme *(160,191,192)*, the peptide 323 to 339 of chicken ovalbumin *(161)*, and the peptide 81 to 104 of pigeon cytochrome c *(166)*: the epitopes recognized by several T-cell clones overlap but are distinct. In addition, nine T-cell clones recognized a second T-cell determinant in myoglobin located around Lys 140, and each one responded to the cyanogen bromide cleavage fragment 132 to 153 *(193)*. Further studies with a nested series of synthetic peptides showed that the stimulatory sequence is contained in peptide 136 to 145 *(163)*.

These findings can be generalized to characterize a large number of epitopes recognized by T cells from a number of protein antigens (Table 21.4) *(190–205)*. What these studies and others demonstrated about epitopes recognized by

TABLE 21.4 Examples of Immunodominant T-Cell Epitopes Recognized in Association with Class II MHC Molecules

Protein	T-Cell Antigenic Sites (ref.)	Amphipathic Segments
Sperm whale myoglobin	69–78 (148)	64–78
	102–118 (*159*)	99–117
	132–145 (*155*)	128–145
Pigeon cytochrome c	93–104 (158)	92–103
Beef cytochrome c	11–25 (*192*)	9–29
	66–80 (*193*)	58–78
Influenza	109–119 (186)	97–120
Hemagglutinin	130–140 (187)	—
A/PR/8/34	302–313 (187,188)	291–314
Pork Insulin	D 5–10 (*157*)	4–16
	A 4–14 (189)	1–21
Chicken lysozyme	46–61 (185)	—
	74–86 (*184*)	72–86
	81–96 (*175*)	86–102
	109–119 (145)	—
Chicken ovalbumin	323–339 (*153*)	329–346
Foot and mouth virus VP1	141–160 (*191*)	148–165
Hepatitis B virus		
Pre-S	120–132 (*190*)	121–135
Major surface antigen	38–52 (*194*)	36–49
	95–109 (*194*)	—
	140–154 (*194*)	—
λ Repressor protein CI	12–26 (*195*)	8–25
Rabies virus–spike glycoprotein precursor	32–44 (*196*)	29–46

MHC, major histocompatibility complex.
Adapted with permission from ref. 188.

T cells is that in each case, the entire site is contained on a short peptide. MHC class I-restricted antigens also follow this rule *(206)*, even when the protein antigen is normally expressed on the surface of infected cells. This applies to viral glycoproteins, such as influenza hemagglutinin, that are recognized by cytolytic T cells after antigen processing *(207)* (see "Antigen Processing"). These peptides consist of no more than about 12 to 17 amino acid residues for class II MHC or 8 to 10 residues for class I. Within this size, they must contain all the information necessary to survive processing within the APC, associate with the MHC antigen, and bind to the T-cell receptor, as discussed in the next sections.

Sequential Steps that Focus the T-Cell Response on Immunodominant Determinants

In contrast to antibodies that bind all over the surface of a native protein *(49)* (see "Protein and Polypeptide Antigenic Determinants"), it has been observed that T cells elicited by immunization with the native protein tend to be focused on one or a few immunodominant sites (*208,209*–210). This is true whether one deals with model mammalian or avian proteins such as cytochrome c *(157)*, myoglobin *(156,158)*, lysozyme *(160,192,211,212)*, insulin *(165,197)*, and ovalbumin *(161)*, or with bacterial, viral, and parasitic proteins from pathogens, such as influenza hemagglutinin *(195)* or nucleoprotein *(206)*, staphylococcal nuclease *(213)*, or malarial circumsporozoite protein *(115,214)*. Because the latter category of proteins shares no obvious homology to mammalian proteins, the immunodominance of a few sites cannot be attributed simply to tolerance for the rest of the protein because of homologous host proteins. Moreover, immunodominance is not simply the pre-emption of the response by a single clone of predominant T cells, because it has been observed that immunodominant sites tend to be the focus for a polyclonal response of a number of distinct T-cell clones recognizing overlapping subsites within the antigenic site or having different sensitivities to substitutions of amino acids within the site (*160,161,166,167*,178,*191,192*,215).

Immunodominant antigenic sites appear to be qualitatively different from other sites. For example, in the case of myoglobin, when the number of clones responding to different epitopes after immunization with native protein was quantitated by limiting dilution, it was observed that the bulk of the response to the whole protein in association with the high-responder class II MHC molecules was focused on a single site within residues 102 to 118 *(173)* (Fig. 21.5). When T cells in the (high × low responder) F1 hybrid restricted to each MHC haplotype were compared, there was little difference in the responses to nondominant epitopes, and all the overall difference in magnitude of response restricted by the high versus low responder MHC could be attributed to the high response to the immunodominant determinant in the former and the complete absence of this response in the latter (Fig. 21.5). Similar results were found for two different high-responder and two different low-responder MHC haplotypes *(173)*. Why did not the response to the other sites compensate for the lack of response to the immunodominant site in the low responders? The greater frequency of T cells specific for the immunodominant site may in part be attributed to the large number of ways this site can be recognized by different T-cell clones, as mentioned previously, but this only pushes the problem back one level. Why is an immunodominant site the focus for so many different T-cell clones? Because the answer cannot depend on any particular T cell, it must depend on other factors, primarily involved in the steps in antigen processing and presentation by MHC molecules.

It has also been observed that some peptides may be immunogenic themselves, but the T-cell response they elicit is specific only for the peptide and does not cross-react with the native protein, nor do T cells specific for the native protein recognize this site (*216,217*,218). These are called

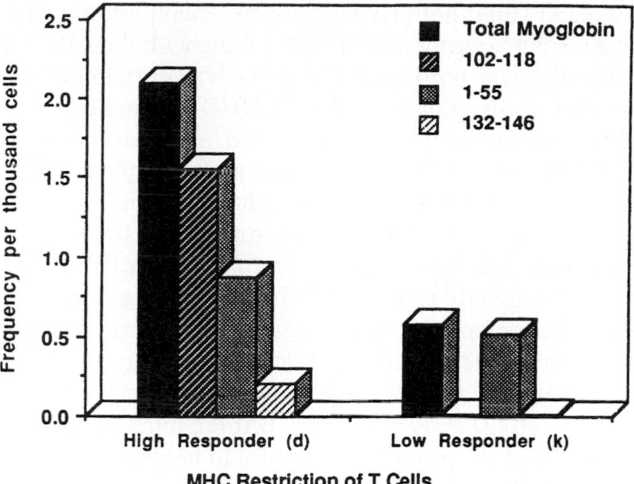

FIGURE 21.5 Frequency of high- and low-responder major histocompatibility complex (MHC)-restricted T cells in F1 hybrid. High responsiveness may be accounted for by the response to a single immunodominant epitope. Lymph node T cells from [low-responder (H-2^k) × high-responder (H-2^d)]F1 hybrid mice immunized with whole myoglobin were plated at different limiting dilutions in microtiter wells with either high- or low-responder presenting cells and myoglobin as antigen. The cells growing in each well were tested for responsiveness to whole myoglobin and to various peptide epitopes of myoglobin. The frequency of T cells of each specificity and MHC restriction was calculated from Poisson statistics and is plotted on the ordinate. Most of the difference in T-cell frequency between high- and low-responder restriction types (*solid bars*) can be accounted for by the presence of T cells responding to the immunodominant site at residues 102 to 118, accounting for more than two thirds of the high-responder myoglobin-specific T cells, in contrast to the absence of such T cells restricted to the low-responder MHC type. (Based on the data in ref. *173*.)

cryptic determinants (218). The reasons for these differences may involve the way the native protein is processed to produce fragments distinct from but including or overlapping the synthetic peptides used in experiments, and also the competition among sites within the protein for binding to the same MHC molecules, as discussed further in a later section. To understand these factors that determine dominance or crypticity, one must understand the steps through which an antigen must go before it can stimulate a T-cell response.

Unlike B cells, T-cell recognition of antigen depends on the function of another cell, the APC *(219)*. Antigen must pass through a number of intracellular compartments and survive processing and transport steps before it can be effectively presented to T cells. Following antigen synthesis in the cell (as in a virally infected cell) or antigen uptake via phagocytosis, pinocytosis, or, in some cases, receptor-mediated endocytosis, the subsequent steps include (a) partial degradation ("processing") into discrete antigenic fragments that can be recognized by T cells, (b) transport of these fragments into a cellular compartment where MHC binding can occur, (c) MHC binding and assembly of a stable peptide-MHC complex, and (d) recognition of that peptide-MHC complex by the expressed T-cell repertoire. At each step, a potential antigenic determinant runs the risk of being lost from the process, for example, by excessive degradation or failure to meet the binding requirements needed for transport to the next step. Only those peptides that surmount the four selective hurdles will prove to be antigenic for T cells. We will now consider each step in detail, for its contribution to the strength and specificity of the T-cell response to protein antigens.

A. Antigen Processing

Influence of Antigen Processing on the Expressed T-Cell Repertoire

Several lines of evidence indicate that antigen processing plays a critical role in determining which potential antigenic sites are recognized and therefore what part of the potential T-cell repertoire is expressed on immunization with a protein antigen. Because the T cell does not see the native antigen but only the products of antigen processing, it is not unreasonable that the nature of these products would at least partly determine which potential epitopes could be recognized by T cells.

One line of evidence that processing plays a major role in T-cell repertoire expression came from comparisons that were made of the immunogenicity of peptide versus native molecule in the cases of myoglobin *(216)* or lysozyme *(217)*. In the case of myoglobin, a site of equine myoglobin (residues 102 to 118) that did not elicit a response when H-2^k mice were immunized with native myoglobin nevertheless was found to be immunogenic when such mice were immunized with the peptide (*216*). Thus, the low responsiveness to this site in mice immunized with the native myoglobin was not due to either of the classical mechanisms of Ir gene defects—namely, a hole in the T-cell repertoire or a failure of the site to interact with MHC molecules of that strain. However, the peptide-immune T cells responded only poorly to native equine myoglobin *in vitro*. Thus, the peptide and the native molecule did not cross-react well in either direction. The problem was not simply a failure to process the native molecule to produce this epitope, because (H-2^k × H-2^s)F1-presenting cells could present this epitope to H-2^s T cells when given native myoglobin but could not present it to H-2^k T cells. Also, because the same results applied to individual T-cell clones, the failure to respond to the native molecule was apparently not due to suppressor cells induced by the native molecule.

Similar observations were made for the response to the peptide 74 to 96 of hen lysozyme in B10.A mice *(217)*. The peptide, not the native molecule, induced T cells specific for this site, and these T cells did not cross-react with the native molecule. With these alternative mechanisms excluded, we are left with the conclusion that an appropriate peptide was produced but it differed from the synthetic peptide in such a way that a hindering site outside the minimal antigenic site interfered with presentation by presenting cells of certain MHC types. Further evidence consistent with this mechanism came from the work of Shastri et al. *(220)*, who found that different epitopes within the 74 to 96 region of lysozyme were immunodominant in H-2^b mice when different forms of the immunogen were used.

Another line of evidence came from fine specificity studies of individual T-cell clones. Shastri et al. *(221)* observed that H-2^b T-cell clones specific for hen lysozymes were about 100-fold more sensitive to ring-necked pheasant lysozyme than to hen lysozyme. Nevertheless, they were equally sensitive to the cyanogen bromide cleavage fragments containing the antigenic sites from both lysozymes. Thus, regions outside the minimal antigenic site removable by cyanogen bromide cleavage presumably interfered with processing, presentation, or recognition of the corresponding site in hen lysozyme. Similarly, it was observed that a T-cell clone specific for sperm whale myoglobin, not equine myoglobin, responded equally well to the minimal epitope synthetic peptides from the two species *(216)*. Here too, residues outside the actual site must be distinguishing equine from sperm whale myoglobin. Experiments using F1-presenting cells that can clearly produce this epitope for presentation to other T cells proved that the problem was not a failure to produce the appropriate fragment from hen lysozyme *(217)* or equine myoglobin *(216)*. Thus, these cases provide evidence that a structure outside the minimal site can hinder presentation in association with a particular MHC molecule.

Such a hindering structure was elegantly identified in a study by Grewal et al. (222) comparing hen egg lysozyme peptides presented by strains C57BL/6 and C3H.SW that share H-2^b but differ in non-MHC genes. After immunization with whole lysozyme, a strong T-cell response was seen to peptide 46-61 in C3H.SW mice but not at all in C57BL/6 mice. Because the F1 hybrids of these two strains responded, the lack of response in one strain was not due to a hole in the T-cell repertoire produced by self-tolerance. It was found that peptide 46-60 bound directly to the I-A^b class II MHC molecule, whereas 46-61 did not, indicating that the C-terminal Arg at position 61 hindered binding. Evidently, a non-MHC–linked difference in antigen processing allowed this Arg to be cleaved off the 46-61 peptide in C3H.SW mice, in which the peptide was dominant, but not in C57Bl/6 mice, in which the peptide was cryptic.

Even a small peptide that does not need processing may nevertheless be processed, and that processing may affect its interaction with MHC molecules. Fox et al. *(223)* found that substitution of a tyrosine for isoleucine at position 95 of cytochrome c peptide 93 to 103 enhanced presentation with $E\beta^b$ but diminished presentation with $E\beta^k$ when live APCs were used but not when the APCs were fixed and could not process antigen. Therefore, the tyrosine residue was not directly interacting with the different MHC molecule but was affecting the way the peptide was processed, which in turn affected MHC interaction.

Besides the mechanisms suggested here, Gammon et al. *(217)* and Sercarz et al. *(224)* have proposed the possibility of competition between different MHC-binding structures ("agretopes") within the same processed fragment. If a partially unfolded fragment first binds to MHC by one such site already exposed, further processing may stop, and other potential binding sites for MHC may never become accessible for binding. Such competition could also occur between different MHC molecules on the same presenting cell *(217)*. For instance, BALB/c mice, expressing both A^d and E^d, produce a response to hen lysozyme specific for 108 to 120, not for 13 to 35 *(217)*, and this response is restricted to E^d. However, B10.GD mice that express only A^d respond well to 13 to 35 when immunized with lysozyme. BALB/c mice clearly express an A^d molecule, so the failure to present this 13 to 35 epitope may be due to competition from E^d, which may preempt by binding the 108 to 120 site with higher affinity and preventing the 13 to 35 site from binding to A^d. Competition between different peptides binding to the same MHC molecule could also occur.

All these results, taken together, indicate that antigen processing not only facilitates interaction of the antigenic site with the MHC molecule and/or the T-cell receptor but also influences the specificity of these interactions and in turn the specificity of the elicited T-cell repertoire. The molecular mechanisms behind such effects are just now being elucidated, as described in the next sections.

Processing of Antigen for T Cells Restricted to Class II MHC Molecules

It has long been known that T-cell responses such as delayed hypersensitivity *in vivo* or T-cell proliferation *in vitro* to exogenous proteins can be stimulated not only by the native protein but also by denatured protein *(154)* and fragments of native protein *(197)*. Indeed, this feature, along with the requirement for recognition in association with class II MHC molecules, distinguishes T- from B-cell responses. In a number of cases, the site recognized by cloned T cells has been located to a discrete synthetic peptide corresponding to a segment of the primary sequence of the protein. Examples include insulin *(165,197)*, cytochrome c *(166)*, lysozyme *(160,191)*, and myoglobin *(156,163,167)*. In each case, the stimulatory peptide must contain all the information required for antigen presentation and T-cell stimulation. The lack of conformational specificity does not indicate a lack of T-cell receptor specificity. Rather, it results from antigen processing into peptide fragments that destroys conformational differences prior to binding the T-cell receptor. One way to accomplish this is via antigen processing, which involves the partial

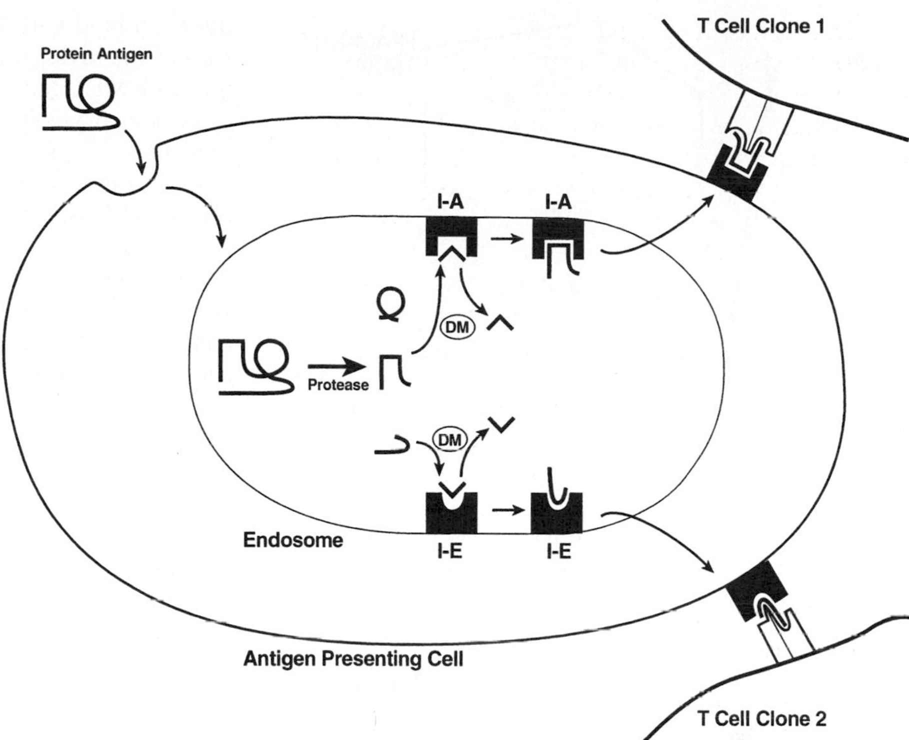

FIGURE 21.6 Steps in antigen presentation by class II major histocompatibility complex (MHC) molecules. Soluble antigen enters the presenting cell by phagocytosis, pinocytosis, or receptor-mediated endocytosis. It is partially degraded to peptide fragments by acid-dependent proteases in endosomes. Antigenic peptides associate with MHC class II molecules (I-A or I-E in the mouse) to form an antigenic complex that is transported to the cell surface. Before an MHC class II molecule can bind the peptide, it must release the class II-associated invariant chain peptide fragment of invariant chain from the binding groove, which is catalyzed by HLA-DM. Binding of T-cell receptors to the peptide/MHC complex triggers T-cell proliferation, resulting in clonal expansion of antigen-specific T cells.

degradation of a protein antigen into peptide fragments (Fig. 21.6).

Evidence of processing came from the fact that a single protein antigen could stimulate T cells to different epitopes, each specific for a different MHC antigen. For example, when a series of myoglobin-specific T-cell clones were tested for both antigen specificity and MHC restriction, six clones were specific for a site centering on amino acid Glu 109, and all six recognized the antigen in association with I-A^d. Nine additional T-cell clones were specific for a second epitope centered on Lys 140 and were restricted to a different MHC antigen, I-E^d. Thus, the antigen behaved as if it was split up into distinct epitopes, each with its own ability to bind MHC *(193)*.

That T cells recognize processed antigen was demonstrated by the fact that inhibitors of processing can block antigen presentation. Early experiments by Ziegler and Unanue *(225)* showed that processing depends on intracellular degradative endosomes because drugs like chloroquine and NH_4Cl, which raise endosomal pH and inhibit acid-dependent proteases, could block the process. However, prior degradation of proteins into peptide fragments allows them to trigger T cells even in the presence of these inhibitors of processing *(226)*. For example, T-cell clone 14.5 recognizes the Lys 140 site of myoglobin equally well on the antigenic peptide (residues 132 to 153) as on the native protein (Fig. 21.7). The difference between these two forms of antigen is brought out by the presence of processing inhibitors. Leupeptin, for example, inhibits lysosomal proteases and blocks the T-cell responses to native myoglobin but not to peptide 132 to 153. Thus, native myoglobin cannot stimulate T cells without further processing, whereas the peptide requires little or no additional processing *(227)*.

Why is antigen processing necessary? For class II MHC molecules, experiments suggest that antigen processing may uncover functional sites that are buried in the native protein structure. For example, a form of intact myoglobin that has been partially unfolded through chemical modification can behave like a myoglobin peptide and can be presented by APC even in the presence of enough protease inhibitor or chloroquine to completely block the presentation of native myoglobin *(227)*. Denatured lysozyme could also be presented without processing to one T-cell clone *(162)*. This result suggests that the requirement for processing may simply be a steric requirement, that is, to uncover the two sites needed to form the trimolecular complex between antigen and MHC and between antigen and T-cell receptor. Thus, unfolding may be sufficient without proteolysis, and proteolysis may simply accomplish an unfolding analogous to Alexander's approach to the Gordian knot.

The importance of antigen unfolding for T-cell recognition and the ability of unfolding to bypass the need for antigen processing apply to a range of polypeptide sizes from small peptides to extremely large proteins. At one extreme, Lee et al. *(228)* found that even fibrinogen, of Mr 340,000, does not need to be processed if the epitope recognized is on the carboxy terminal portion of the α chain, which is naturally unfolded in the native molecule. At the other

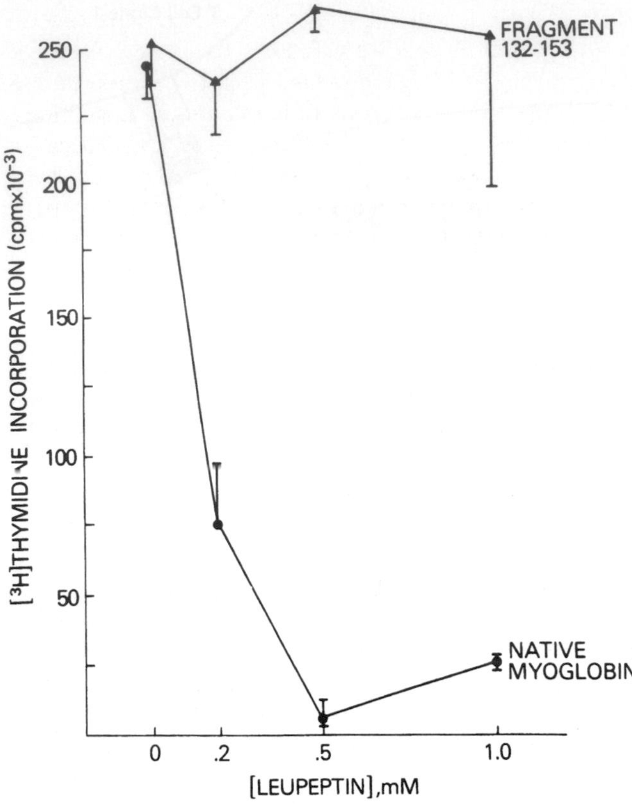

FIGURE 21.7 Inhibition of antigen presentation by the protease inhibitor leupeptin: differential effect on presentation of the same epitope of native myoglobin or peptide 132 to 153 to the same monoclonal T-cell population. Splenic cells from nonimmunized B10.D2 mice, as a source of antigen-presenting cells, were incubated with leupeptin at the concentration indicated for 15 minutes prior to and during exposure to 2-μM native myoglobin or 1-μM peptide fragment, washed, irradiated, and cultured at 400,000 cells/well with 10,000 T cells of clone 14.5; thymidine incorporation was measured after 4 days of culture. (See ref. *227*.)

extreme, even a small peptide of only 18 amino acid residues, apamin, requires processing unless the two disulfide bonds that hold it in the native conformation are cleaved artificially to allow unfolding *(229)*. Therefore, large size does not mandate processing, and small size does not necessarily obviate the need for processing, at least for class II presentation. The common feature throughout the size range seems to be the need for unfolding. This evidence, taken together with the earlier data on unfolding of myoglobin and lysozyme, strongly supports the conclusion that unfolding, rather than size reduction, is the primary goal of antigen processing and that either antigen presentation by MHC molecules or T-cell receptor recognition frequently requires exposure of residues not normally exposed on the surface of the native protein. This conclusion is supported by recent studies of peptides eluted from class II MHC molecules, and the crystal structures of class II MHC-peptide complexes, which show that longer peptides can bind with both ends extending beyond the two ends of the MHC groove (230–232) (see "Antigen Interaction with MHC Molecules").

Besides proteolysis, unfolding may require the reduction of disulfide bonds between or within protein antigens. A gamma interferon-inducible lysosomal thiol reductase, called *GILT*, is expressed in antigen-presenting cells and localizes to the late endosomal and lysosomal compartments where MHC class II peptide loading occurs (233). Unlike thioredoxin, this enzyme works at the acid pH of endosomes and uses Cys but not glutathione as a reducing agent. Antigen-presenting cells from GILT knockout mice were tested for the ability to present hen egg lysozyme to HEL-specific T-cell lines (234). For two epitopes, the T-cell response was insensitive to the GILT defect, even though they involved a disulfide bond in the native protein. But for one epitope, located between disulfide bonds, the T-cell response was completely inhibited when the antigen-presenting cells lacked GILT reductase. In this case, reduction of disulfide bonds was an essential step for antigen presentation, presumably needed to generate free peptides for MHC class II binding.

Processing of Antigen for T Cells Restricted to Class I MHC Molecules

Early studies on class I-restricted T cells, such as cytolytic T cells (CTLs) specific for virus-infected cells, assumed that they responded mainly to unprocessed viral glycoproteins expressed on the surface of infected cells. However, since the mid-1980s, it has been clear that CTLs, like other T cells, recognize processed antigens. For example, influenza nucleoprotein (NP) was a major target antigen for influenza-specific CTLs, even though NP remains in the nucleus of infected cells and none is detectable on the cell surface *(235)*. Further support came from the finding that target cells that take up synthetic NP peptide 366 to 379 were lysed by NP-specific CTLs *(206)*. This constitutes evidence that antigen presented in association with class I molecules requires processing into antigenic fragments. Also, the demonstration that synthetic peptides could sensitize targets for CTLs introduced a powerful tool for mapping and studying CTL epitopes.

Even for influenza hemagglutinin, which is expressed on the surface of infected cells, surface expression was not required for antigenicity, implying that it is the processed antigen that stimulates a T-cell response. Target cells expressing leader-negative hemagglutinin, which is not transported to the cell surface but remains in the cytosol, were lysed equally well as those with surface hemagglutinin *(207)*. Similar conclusions were drawn from anchor-negative mutants *(236)*. Indeed, studies of HIV-1 gp160 genes with or without a leader sequence suggest that removal of the leader sequence can increase the amount of protein that is retained in the cytosol and is available for processing and presentation through the class I MHC processing pathway (237). The explanation may be that the signal peptide results in cotranslational translocation of the growing peptide chain into the endoplasmic reticulum, whereas proteins without a signal peptide remain in the cytosol, where they are accessible to the processing machinery of the class I pathway (see later discussion). This cytosolic protein-processing machinery consists primarily of the 26S proteasomes (238,239). The specificity of such proteasomes to cleave at certain positions in a protein sequence thus provides the first hurdle that a potential epitope must surmount to be presented by class I MHC molecules, to be cut out correctly but not destroyed by the proteasome.

In the standard proteasome, 14 distinct subunits assemble to form a high-molecular-weight complex of about 580 kD with three distinct protease activities, located on different subunits. The proteasome is a barrel-shaped structure, with the protease activities arrayed on the inner surface, and unfolded proteins are believed to enter the barrel at one end, leaving as peptides at the other end. The different proteases cut preferentially after aromatic or branched chain amino acids (chymotrypticlike activity of the $\beta 5$ subunit), basic amino acids (trypsinlike activity of the $\beta 2$ subunit), or acidic residues (glutamate preferring activity of the $\beta 1$ subunit) (240,241). Protease activity is increased against misfolded proteins, such as senescent proteins, which are tagged with ubiquitin and directed to the proteasome. In addition, viral proteins produced during infection and proteins synthesized with artificial amino acids are particularly susceptible to degradation by proteasomes. The products of protease digestion are peptides ranging from to 3 to 14 amino acids in length, including nine-mers, of just the right size for MHC binding. The chymotryptic- and trypsinlike activities may be particularly important for antigenic peptides because many peptides that naturally bind MHC end in hydrophobic or basic residues (242).

The proteasome is the major processing machinery of the nonendosomal processing pathway. This is shown by the effect of proteasome inhibitors on MHC class I assembly and antigen presentation and by the effect of LMP-2 and LMP-7 mutations on antigen processing. A family of proteasome inhibitors have been described (240,241,243) which consist of short peptides, three to four amino acids in length, ending in an aldehyde, such as Ac-Leu Leu norLeu-al, carbobenzoxy-Leu Leu norVal-al (241), or nonpeptides such as lactacystin (244). Although the peptides appear to be directed primarily at the chymotrypsinlike protease activity, as false substrates, in fact they inhibit all three types of protease activity.

By inhibiting antigen processing, these inhibitors induce a phenotype of reduced expression of MHC class I and inability to present antigen to class I-restricted CTL (241). The MHC class I heavy chains remain in the endoplasmic reticulum (ER), as shown by failure to become resistant to endoglycosidase H (245), which occurs in the Golgi. They are also unable to form stable complexes with β_2-microglobulin because of a lack of peptides. These effects are specific for the protease function because the inhibitors do not block presentation of synthetic peptides, which also rescue MHC class I expression, and because inhibition is reversible when inhibitor is removed. These results suggest that proteasomes are the primary supplier of antigenic peptides for class I because other pathways are unable to compensate. However, it is also possible that the inhibitors could block other potential processing enzymes as well. An alternative processing pathway that bypasses the proteasome is provided by signal peptidase. As signal peptides are cleaved from proteins entering the endoplasmic reticulum, these hydrophobic peptides can bind MHC class I (246). Particularly for MHC molecules like HLA-A2, which prefer hydrophobic sequences, this peptidase can be an alternative source of antigenic peptides that are independent of proteasomes and TAP-1/2 transport (see "Transport") because they are formed inside the ER.

The proteins destined for proteasomal processing include some normally short-lived proteins with a half-life of about 10 minutes, which constitute about 25% of the proteins in the cell. The rest arise from long-lived proteins, with a half-life of about 1 day, which may be synthesized incorrectly. These defective ribosomal products, or DRiPs, are ubiquitinated and marked for rapid degradation in proteasomes (247,248). In a normal cell, these can arise from errors in RNA transcription, protein translation, assembly, folding, or targeting. But in a virally infected cell, misfolded viral proteins provide a ready supply of antigenic peptides for antigen presentation and T-cell recognition almost as soon as the virus starts to produce new viral proteins. Similarly, incorporation of amino acid analogues, such as canavanine in place of arginine, creates misfolded proteins that are rapidly processed and more efficiently presented via the proteasomal pathway (249).

Interestingly, the MHC itself encodes, near the class II region, three proteins, known as LMP-2 and LMP-7 for "low-molecular-weight protein," and MECL1, for "multicatalytic endopeptidase complexlike 1," that contribute to the proteasome structure. The LMP-2, MECL-1, and LMP-7 subunits are upregulated by interferon-γ, and substitute for the subunits $\beta 1$, $\beta 2$, and $\beta 5$, respectively, forming what has been dubbed an *immunoproteasome*, present in professional antigen-presenting cells. All complexes with LMPs contain proteasome proteins, but only 5% to 10% of proteasomes contain LMP-2 and LMP-7. The ones without LMPs are called *constitutive proteasomes*.

These MHC-encoded subunits of the immunoproteasome shift the preference of proteasomes for cleaving after certain sequences, resulting in the production of different peptide fragments (250–252). Proteasomes lacking LMP-2 through mutation or gene knockout have the same affinity, but decreased cleavage rate, for sequences ending in hydrophobic or basic amino acids. The effect is specific for these proteolytic sites because the activity against sequences containing acidic amino acids actually increased (251). Despite the shift in specific peptides released, the overall level of MHC class I expression was reduced only slightly in LMP-7 knockouts (252) and not at all in the LMP-2 knockouts. However, presentation of specific epitopes of the male H-Y antigen or of influenza nucleoprotein was reduced by three- to fivefold in these knockouts. Toes et al. (253) quantitatively compared the cleavage fragments produced by standard proteasomes and immunoproteasomes, and defined the prevalence of different amino acids on each side of the cleavage site. Consistent with the earlier studies, there is a strong preference for both to cleave after leucine, and also to a lesser extent after other hydrophobic residues, both aliphatic and aromatic. However, the immunoproteasomes have a stronger tendency to cleave after such hydrophobic residues and a much reduced cleavage frequency after acidic residues, Asp and Glu, than standard or constitutive proteaseomes. This shift in specificity is concordant with the observation that class I MHC molecules tend to bind peptides with C-terminal hydrophobic or basic residues, not acidic ones. Thus, the immunoproteasomes in professional antigen-presenting cells may be more effective at generating antigenic peptides that can be presented by MHC molecules (250,253). Protein degradation by proteasomes is processive, so the peptides released after 5% digestion are the same as the fragments released after 90% digestion. This suggests that intact proteins may enter the barrel, but they are not released at the other end until processing is complete.

Immunoproteasomes were shown to be essential for production of a hepatitis B virus core antigenic epitope (254), and to increase production of epitopes from adenovirus (255) and lymphocytic choriomeningitis virus (256). Similarly, certain epitopes of latent membrane protein 2 of Epstein-Barr virus depended on immunoproteasomes (257). In that case, the requirement for immunoproteasomes depended on the context of the peptide within the native protein. Incomplete protein synthesis due to puromycin, or expression of the epitope surrounded by protein fragments with fewer membrane-spanning domains, allowed epitope generation by constitutive proteasomes.

On the other hand, some epitopes are generated more effectively by the constitutive proteasome than the immunoproteasome (253,258). When the repertoire of seven defined class I MHC-restricted epitopes was compared in an elegant quantitative study in LMP2-deficient or wild-type C57BL/6 mice, it was found that responses to the two epitopes that are immunodominant in wild-type mice were greatly reduced in the LMP2-deficient mice, that lack immunoproteasomes, and two normally subdominant epitopes became dominant (259). However, from adoptive transfer experiments in both directions, it was found that the reduced response to one normally dominant epitope was due to decreased production without immunoproteasomes, but that to the other was due to an altered T-cell repertoire in the LMP2-deficient mice, presumably from alterations in the peptides presented in the thymus. Further, the increased response to one of the subdominant determinants was related to increased production of this peptide by the constitutive proteasomes compared to the immunoproteasomes. Thus, the immunoproteasome specificity plays a significant role in determining the repertoire of epitopes presented, and in selecting those that are immunodominant, as well as regulating the $CD8^+$ T-cell repertoire generated in the thymus.

Another protein associated with proteasomes is the proteasome activator PA28, which assembles into 11s structures (260). Like LMP-2 and 7 (250), PA28 is inducible by interferon-γ, and its induction causes a shift in proteasome function that may lead to the production of greater amounts of and different repertoires of antigenic peptides. For example, synthetic substrates were designed to test the ability of proteasomes to generate authentic MHC binding peptides. These substrates contained the MHC-binding ligand flanked by the natural sequence as found in the original protein.

To generate the MHC-binding ligand, the proteasome would have to cleave the substrate twice (261). By itself, the 20s proteasome was able to produce singly cleaved fragments, but with added PA28, doubly cut peptides were generated preferentially. Thus, PA28 favored the production of antigenic peptides, possibly by keeping the peptide in the proteasome until processing was complete. Alternatively, PA28 may coordinate the proteolytic activity of two adjacent sites to generate doubly cut peptides of just the right length (8 to 9-mers) to fit in the MHC groove. The distance between these nearby sites would determine the size of the peptides produced. PA28 has been shown to increase generation of a dominant lymphocytic choriomeningitis virus epitope independently of the presence of the other interferon-γ–inducible components LMP2, LMP7, and MECL-1 (262).

The specificity of this proteasomal processing system determines the first step in winnowing the number of protein segments that can become CTL epitopes, by selectively producing some peptide fragments in abundance and destroying others. Thus, it is probably not just coincidental that the C-terminal residues produced by proteasomal cleavage often serve as anchor residues for binding class I MHC molecules, or that the lengths of peptides produced are optimal for class I MHC binding (250,263). Better understanding of the specificity of proteasomes will contribute to the new methods to predict dominant $CD8^+$ T cell epitopes (210).

Additional downstream processing steps, after the proteasome, are known to be important for generation of antigenic peptides. One of these occurs in the cytoplasm, prior to TAP transport, and others occur after transport into the ER. The proteasome creates a first draft of the peptides, which are then selected and trimmed to produce the final pool of antigenic peptides of optimal size and sequence for MHC binding, while protecting the nascent peptides from degradation before they can bind MHC.

Recent studies have revealed that most peptides are released from the proteasome when they still need further processing to become antigenic peptides (264,265). In the cytoplasm, the major proteolytic activity comes from an enzyme called *tripeptidyl amino peptidase II*, or TPPII, which is located on a large particle. It has amino peptidase activity, which can remove one to three amino acids at a time, and is useful for peptides of 15 amino acids or less. It also has endopeptidase activity that can cut in the middle of peptides larger than 15 amino acids, with the release of fragments of at least 9 amino acids. These are a significant source of 9-mers with new carboxyl ends, and this may be the only way to generate carboxyl ends other than the proteasome itself.

The importance of TPPII activity for antigen processing is shown by the fact that a specific inhibitor, butabindide, can prevent peptide loading of MHC, resulting in reduced surface expression. The most likely path for most protein antigens is to enter the proteasome and emerge as peptides of 15 amino acids or larger. These are then trimmed by TPPII, resulting in peptides ready for TAP transport. Longer peptides are trimmed internally by TPPII endoprotease, which may generate carboxyl ends needed for TAP binding. The resulting peptides are then transported by TAP into the ER, where they may be trimmed further to prepare them for MHC binding. An additional role of TPPII is shown by the generation of unique epitopes that are not produced by proteasomes. For example, an important T-cell epitope of the Nef protein of HIV requires TPPII processing. Proteasomal inhibitors have no effect on it, but butabindide prevents its processing and presentation to HLA-A3 or A11 restricted T cells (266). This pathway seems particularly important for generating epitopes ending in lysine groups, which bind these two MHC types but are rarely generated by proteasomes alone. TPPII can act in parallel with proteasomes or in tandem with them to release this epitope from intact protein or its partially degraded fragments.

B. Transport into a Cellular Compartment where MHC Binding Can Occur

The second hurdle a potential epitope must surmount is to be transported into the cellular compartment for loading onto MHC molecules. These compartments are different for class I and class II molecules, as noted earlier.

Transport Pathways Leading to MHC Class I Presentation

The second hurdle for peptide presentation by class I MHC molecules is to get from the cytosol, where the peptides are produced, to the ER, where the newly synthesized class I MHC molecules are assembled and loaded with peptide. The discovery of a specific active transporter suggested that specificity of transport could further restrict the repertoire of peptides available to load onto class I MHC molecules. Genetic analysis of mutant cell lines that failed to load endogenous peptides onto class I molecules revealed homozygous deletions of part of the MHC class II region near the DR locus. Molecular cloning of DNA from this region revealed at least 12 new genes, of which two, called *TAP-1* and *TAP-2*, for "transporter associated with antigen processing," showed a typical sequence for ABC transporter proteins (267–269). Their function is to transport processed peptides from the cytosol to the ER. Once in this compartment, peptides are handed off by TAP to newly formed MHC class I molecules and stabilize a trimolecular complex with β_2-microglobulin. This complex is then transported to the cell surface, where antigen presentation occurs. Without the peptide transporters, empty dimers of MHC class I with β_2-microglobulin form, but these are unstable. Excess free peptide would rescue MHC class I by stabilizing the few short-lived empty complexes that reach the surface, as shown by Townsend et al. *(270)* and Schumacher et al. (271). Thus MHC-linked genes coding for proteolysis, peptide transport, and presentation at the cell surface have been identified. In effect, the MHC now appears to encode a complex system of multiple elements devoted to the rapid display of foreign protein determinants on the surface of an infected cell. By continuously sampling the output of the protein-synthesizing machinery, this system permits rapid identification and destruction of infected cells by CTL before infectious virus can be released.

In an infected cell, as soon as viral proteins are made, peptide fragments generated by the proteasome become available to the TAP-1 and TAP-2 transporter proteins (Fig. 21.8). These transport the peptide fragments into the ER for association with newly formed MHC class I molecules, which would carry them to the cell surface for antigen presentation, all within 30 minutes. Indeed, the finding of a physical association between TAP and the nascent class I heavy chain/β_2-microglobulin complex suggests that the peptide may be directly handed off from TAP to the new MHC molecule without being free in solution (272,273). If TAP transport is highly selective, then some cytosolic peptides may fail to enter the ER for presentation with class I, but if it is promiscuous, then some peptides may be transported that were better off not presented, such as those leading to autoimmunity.

The idea that other proteins may control accessibility of MHC class I binding sites for peptides originally came from the observation that two rat strains with the same MHC type (RT1.A^a) were nevertheless not histocompatible, and CTL could recognize the difference between them *(274)*. The difference, called a *cim* effect, for class I modification, occurred because different peptides were binding the same MHC in the two strains (275,276). The

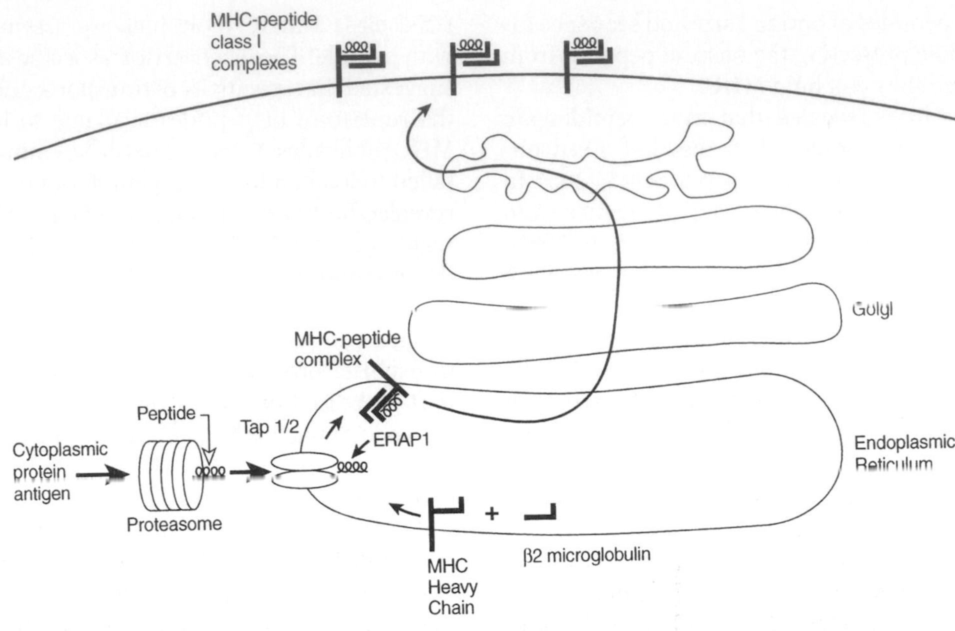

FIGURE 21.8 Cytoplasmic antigen-processing pathway leading to major histocompatibility complex (MHC) class I presentation. Cytoplasmic antigen is degraded in the proteasome to fragments, which are transported into the endoplasmic reticulum (ER) by the transporter associated with antigen processing (TAP). Peptide supplied by TAP forms a stable complex with MHC class I heavy chains and β_2-microglobulin, and the complex is transported through the Golgi, where it achieves mature glycosylation, and out to the cell surface for presentation to class I-restricted T cells. Additional processing options by tripeptidyl amino peptidase II in the cytoplasm and endoplasmic reticulum aminopeptidase I (ERAP 1) in the ER, before and after TAP transport, allow greater flexibility in meeting the requirements of binding both TAP and MHC molecules.

rat has two alleles for a peptide transporter supplying peptides to MHC. The one called TAP2A has peptide specificity matching that of RT1.A^a and delivers a broad set of peptides for MHC binding. The other transporter allele, called TAP2B, supplies a different set of peptides that are discordant with RT1.A^a, so fewer types of peptides are bound. Although RT1.A^a would prefer to bind peptides with Arg at position 9, it has to settle for peptides with hydrophobic termini as provided by TAP2B (277), thereby accounting for the apparent histocompatibility difference. Thus, the specificity of TAP transport was shown to provide a selective step in narrowing the potential repertoire of CTL epitopes.

To measure TAP specificity in other species, a transportable peptide bearing an N-linked glycosylation site was added to cells permeabilized by treatment with streptolysin. If the peptide was transported by TAP, it would enter the ER and *cis*-Golgi, where it would be glycosylated (278–280). The extent of glycosylation served as a measure of TAP function. When competitor peptides were added as well, TAP-mediated transport of the reporter peptide decreased, indicating saturation of peptide binding sites. In this way, a series of related peptides could be tested for the ability to compete for TAP binding and transport in order to identify the requirements for TAP binding and transport.

TAP binding and transport depended strongly on peptide length (280,281). Mouse TAP was shown to have a strong preference for peptides of nine residues or longer (281). For human TAP, peptides shorter than seven amino acids long were not transported, regardless of sequence (280). Peptides 8 to 11 amino acids long were almost all transported, with some variation in binding affinities depending on sequence. Peptides 14 to 21 amino acids in length were transported selectively, while those longer than 24 amino acids were almost never transported intact. Thus, human TAP transport selected against peptides less than 7 or more than 24 amino acids in length, regardless of sequence. Unlike the rat, human and mouse TAP do not show allelic differences in peptide transport.

Although TAP can and must transport a wide variety of peptides, it may still have preferences for which peptides are transported most efficiently and which MHC types are provided with the peptides they need. For example, a self-peptide that naturally binds HLA B27 was modified slightly to produce an N-linked glycosylation site, resulting in the sequence RRYQNSTEL (280). Using the glycosylation of this peptide to measure transport, saturation of TAP by homologous peptides occurred with a 50% inhibitory concentration of less than 1 μM. Other peptides with unrelated sequences also inhibited, often with equally high affinity.

Not only did natural HLA-binding peptides compete, but so did peptide variants lacking the MHC binding motif at positions 2 and 9 (see later discussion). Clearly, peptides binding different MHC types were transported by the same TAP protein, and even peptides that bound mouse MHC were transported by human TAP. In another example, using rat TAP proteins, peptides with Pro at position 2, 6, or 9 were found to be poor competitors for transport of a reference peptide (279).

In a different approach, using a baculovirus system overexpressing TAP proteins in microsomes, the affinity of TAP binding was determined for a wide variety of synthetic peptides, allowing mapping of the important residues (282,283). Binding, rather than transport, appears to be the major step determining TAP peptide selectivity (284). Indeed, artificial neural networks have been developed to predict peptide binding to human TAP (285). Using this scheme, it was found that peptides eluted from three different human class I molecules had higher predicted affinities for TAP than a control set of peptides with equal binding to those class I MHC molecules, supporting the hypothesis that TAP specificity contributes to the selection of the subset of peptides able to bind a class I molecule that actually binds *in vivo* (285). Unlike MHC class I, there were no anchor positions at which a specific amino acid was required. However, there were several positions where substituting the wrong amino acid caused a marked reduction in TAP binding. In a typical MHC class I binding 9-mer, the strongest substitution effects were observed at position 9 (P9), followed by substitutions at P2 and P3, followed by P1. At the carboxy terminal P9 position, the preferred residues were Tyr and Phe (as well as Arg and Lys), while Glu was worst, causing a 3 log reduction in binding. Similarly, substituting Pro at P2 caused a 1.5 to 2 log reduction in binding, as compared with preferred residues Arg, Val, and Ile. TAP preferences such as these would selectively transport some peptides more than others from cytoplasm to ER. Use of combinatorial peptide libraries independently confirmed that the critical residues influencing TAP transport were the first three N-terminal residues and the last C-terminal residue (286).

Interestingly, these preferred residues are many of the same ones forming the MHC class I binding motifs (P2 and P9). However, because the MHC binding motifs differ from each other, it is not possible for TAP preferences to match them all. For example, the TAP preference for Arg at P2 and Phe, Tyr, Leu, Arg, or Lys at P9 overlaps with the binding motif of HLA-B27 and may favor the transport of peptide ligands for this MHC type. Remarkably, the variant B2709, which does not prefer Tyr or Phe at P9, is not associated with autoimmune disease as in the more common form of HLA-B27. In contrast, HLA-B7 requires a Pro at P2, which greatly decreases TAP binding. Similarly, some peptides binding HLA-A2 have hydrophobic residues unfavorable for TAP binding, suggesting suboptimal compatibility between TAP and the most common HLA class I allele. Measurements with a series of naturally presented peptides from HLA-A2 and B27 indicated a mean 300-fold higher affinity of TAP for the B27 peptides than for those from A2, and some of the A2 peptides did not bind TAP at all (285). How are these low-affinity peptides delivered to MHC? One suggestion is that peptide ligands for HLA-A2 and B7 may be transported as a larger precursor peptide containing the correct amino acids, which are then trimmed off to fit the MHC groove.

A series of studies support this mechanism, showing that longer peptide precursors are trimmed at the N-terminus by aminopeptidases in the ER to form HLA-binding peptides (287). The ability to transport larger peptides, followed by trimming, could increase the range of permissible antigenic peptides, by facilitating transport of nonantigenic peptides, followed by trimming to the size and specificity needed for MHC binding. For example, following hepatitis B virus infection, certain peptide epitopes that are frequently recognized by CTL are nevertheless not bound or transported by TAP. By extending these peptides by one or two amino acids of the natural sequence at the amino end, their TAP binding was greatly enhanced, but at the expense of reduced MHC binding. When tested on permeabilized cells, the overall effect of the extended peptides was to increase MHC binding. Apparently, by improving TAP transport, these peptides were able to increase peptide delivery into the ER, where they were trimmed to produce peptides compatible with MHC binding (288).

Similarly, it is known that peptides with a Pro at position 2, needed to bind to certain MHC molecules but poorly transported, are produced from longer precursors that are transported by N-terminal trimming in the ER by aminopeptidases (289). In fact, the inability of the aminopeptidase to cleave beyond a residue preceding a Pro naturally leads to trimming of peptides to produce ones with a Pro at position 2. Alternatively, some of these peptides may derive from signal peptides and enter the ER in a TAP-independent manner. The ER trimming enzyme has been identified as endoplasmic reticulum aminopeptidase I (ERAP I) (290–292). This enzyme is a 106-kD zinc metalloproteinase, and it is the major ER protease with broad specificity. It is inducible by interferon-γ and inhibited by the aminopeptidase inhibitor leucinethiol. Down-regulation of ERAP I with siRNA results in decreased expression of MHC class I, indicating that ERAP I contributes to the supply of peptides. ERAP I prefers peptides of 9 or 10 amino acids or longer and ignores peptides of 8 amino acids or fewer, which may allow it to generate antigenic peptides for MHC binding without degrading them beyond recognition. The aminopeptidase provides a way to relax the requirement for proteasomes to generate ends that can simultaneously bind TAP and MHC. In contrast, the fact that a comparable carboxypeptidase has not been identified suggests that carboxyl ends generated by proteasomal processing must be suitable for TAP transport and compatible with MHC binding. This requirement is quite stringent because the carboxyl terminal residue is the most important for TAP binding, and it is frequently an anchor residue for MHC as well.

The significance of selective peptide transport may be to limit immunity to self-peptides. If the match between HLA-B27 and TAP specificity is too good, it may contribute to the increased incidence of autoimmune disease associated with HLA- B27 (282). An effect of human TAP specificity in loading of peptides in viral infection has confirmed the biological significance of TAP specificity (288). TAP binding specificity also limited the repertoire of alloantigenic peptides presented by HLA-B27 (293).

By combining the selectivity of proteasomal processing, TAP transport, and MHC binding, it has been possible to generate models that correlate with known antigenic peptides (294,295). These can be used to analyze the sequence of any given protein and to predict epitopes that may be recognized by T cells restricted to MHC class I. These may be important for analyzing the T-cell response to viral or neoplastic antigens and for generating synthetic vaccines capable of eliciting a T-cell response to these antigens.

The importance of TAP proteins to antiviral immunity is shown by the fact that herpesviruses have targeted TAP-1 function as a way to interfere with antigen presentation to $CD8^+$ CTL. A herpes simplex virus (HSV-1) immediate early viral protein called ICP47 binds to TAP and inhibits its function, causing reduced expression of new MHC class I molecules on the cell surface and inability to present viral or other antigens with MHC class I (296–298). As a way to evade immune surveillance, this strategy could contribute to viral persistence in chronic infection and viral activation in recurrent disease, as frequently occurs with HSV-1 and -2. These findings also raise the possibility of making a live attenuated ICP47-defective HSV vaccine that would be more immunogenic than natural infection.

Transport Pathways Leading to MHC Class II Presentation

Unlike the class I pathway, which delivers peptides to MHC, the MHC class II pathway transports MHC molecules to the endosomal compartment, where antigenic peptides are produced. During transport, the peptide binding groove must be kept free of endogenous peptides. The cell uses one protein, called *invariant chain* (and its processed fragment CLIP), to block the binding site until needed, and another protein, HLA-DM, to facilitate release of CLIP peptides and their exchange for antigenic peptides as they become available.

MHC class II molecules assemble in the ER, where alpha and beta chains form a complex with invariant chain (*299*–301). Invariant chain binds MHC and blocks the peptide-binding groove, so endogenous peptides transported into the ER, for example by TAP, cannot bind (300,*302*,303–307). The complex of alpha, beta, and invariant chains, consisting of nine polypeptide chains in all (308), is transported via the Golgi and directed by signals on invariant chain into endosome/lysosomelike vesicles called MHC class II compartments. The compartments contain acid-activated proteases capable of digesting foreign proteins into antigenic peptides. In addition, they degrade invariant chain to a fragment called *CLIP*, corresponding to amino acids 80–103. As long as CLIP remains in the binding groove, antigenic peptides cannot bind, so the rate of CLIP release limits the capacity of MHC to take up antigenic peptides.

Peptide loading can be measured by its effect on MHC structure. When an MHC class II molecule binds a peptide, it changes conformation, and certain monoclonal antibodies are specific for the peptide-bound conformation (309). Also, the alpha-beta complex becomes more stable after peptide binding, which can be detected by running the MHC on an SDS gel without boiling. The peptide bound form runs on gels as a large alpha-beta dimer, while MHC without peptides (but still bound to CLIP) is unstable under these conditions and falls apart to give alpha and beta chain monomers on SDS gels (310).

Mutant cell lines have been generated with a deletion between *HLA-DP* and *HLA-DQ* genes on chromosome 6 (309,311–313). These cells express normal levels of MHC class II structural proteins, HLA-DQ and DR, but fail to present protein antigens (313). Some of their class II MHC proteins appear on the cell surface, but more are retained in the MHC class II compartments. Biochemically, they still contain CLIP peptides (314), rather than peptide antigens, and they have not achieved the conformation (309) or SDS stability of peptide-binding MHC class II complexes (315). The defect was discovered to be due to loss of either of the two chains of a class II molecule, HLA-DM, and the phenotype can be corrected by adding back the missing gene (316). In the presence of normal HLA-DM, MHC releases CLIP and binds antigenic peptides for presentation to T cells.

The importance of HLA-DM function for T-cell help *in vivo* was studied in H2-DM knockout mice (317). These mice have reduced numbers of T cells, their class II MHC molecules reach the cell surface bearing high levels of CLIP peptide, and their B cells are unable to present certain antigens, such as ovalbumin, to T cells. When H2-DM knockout mice were immunized with 4-hydroxy 5-nitrophenyl acetyl ovalbumin, specific IgG antibodies were reduced 20-fold, as compared with wild type. Germinal center formation and class switching were greatly reduced, and affinity maturation was not observed. The phenotype was more pronounced for some MHC types, such as I-A^b, than for others, such as I-A^k. Because of tighter binding of CLIP peptides, these MHC types may be more dependent on H2-DM to

TABLE 21.5 Effect of HLA-DM on Peptide on Rates and Off Rates for Binding to HLA-DR1

Peptide	*HLA-DM*	*Half-Life for Binding*	*Half-Life for Release*
CLIP (80–103)	−	60 min	11 hr
	+	9 min	0.3 hr
MBP (90–102)	−	62 min	86 hr
	+	9 min	1 hr
HA (307–319)	−	67 min	144 hr
	+	10 min	144 hr

CLIP, class II-associated invariant chain peptide; HA, hemagglutinin; HLA, human leukocyte antigen; MBP, myelin basic protein.
The on (association) and off (dissociation) rates of biotinylated peptide from purified soluble HLA-DR1 were measured by fluorescence assay, in the presence or absence of HLA-DM. The on rates of all three peptides are increased similarly in the presence of HLA-DM and probably reflect the rate-limiting dissociation of the bound CLIP fragment of the invariant chain. In contrast, once the peptides are bound, the off rates differ as a result of differences in affinity. Thus, HLA-DM catalyzes release of more weakly binding peptides and allows stable binding of higher affinity peptides. In effect, this is an editing function of HLA-DM.
Adapted from the data of Sloan et al. (298).

maintain empty class II molecules in a peptide receptive state.

In vitro studies with purified MHC class II molecules and biotin-labeled peptides have shown that HLA-DM can accelerate loading of exogenous peptides into HLA-DR binding sites (318,319). For example, loading of myelin basic protein fragment 90–102 was accomplished in 9 minutes with HLA-DM versus 60 minutes without it (Table 21.5). Other peptides were also loaded at the same rate, suggesting that the rate-limiting step was the same for each: removal of CLIP peptides to expose the peptide binding sites on HLA-DR. The kinetic effect was optimal between pH 4.5 and 5.8, which is typical of the endosomal/lysosomal compartment where HLA-DM operates. HLA-DM did not affect the affinity, as measured by half-maximal binding, but it had a marked effect on the kinetics of binding.

Conversely, when biotinylated peptides were allowed to saturate HLA-DR binding sites overnight, and then free peptides were removed, the off rate could be measured over time (318,319). As shown in Table 21.5 (adapted from ref. 318), the off rate for different peptides could be compared in the absence or presence of HLA-DM. The half-life for CLIP peptides was reduced from 11 hours to 20 minutes by adding HLA-DM. This could explain the enhanced loading of all other peptides because they must wait for CLIP to come off. In the case of antigenic peptides, myelin basic protein 90–112 was released 80-fold faster in the presence of DM than in its absence. However, another peptide, influenza hemagglutinin 307–319, was not affected at all. The differential effect on these antigenic peptides suggests that HLA-DM can serve a potential role in editing which peptides stay on MHC long enough to be presented and which are removed (318). By releasing MBP preferentially and not the HA peptide, HLA-DM would favor the stable MHC binding and presentation of HA peptides over MBP peptides. The affinity of each peptide is determined by the fit between peptide and MHC groove, not by HLA-DM. However, DM can amplify the impact of the difference in affinity (i.e., signal-to-noise ratio), by facilitating release of low-affinity peptides and allowing the high-affinity ones to remain. This editing function could have an important effect on which peptides get presented and elicit a T-cell response, and which do not. HLA-DM could contribute to immunodominance of a peptide binding MHC with high affinity by releasing its lower affinity competitors. Alternatively, HLA-DM could contribute to self-tolerance by releasing self-peptides of low affinity before they could stimulate self-reactive T cells.

C. MHC Binding and Assembly of a Stable Peptide-MHC Complex

Antigen Interaction with MHC Molecules

Perhaps the most selective step a potential antigenic site must pass is to bind with sufficiently high affinity to an appropriate MHC molecule.

The response of T cells to antigens on APCs or target cells provided a number of hints that antigen interacts directly with MHC molecules of the APCs. First, genes coding for immune responsiveness to a specific antigen are tightly linked to genes for MHC-encoded cell surface molecules (*107*,149). Second, it became apparent that T-cell recognition of antigen is the step at which MHC restriction occurs *(107,157,197,320)*. For example, *in vitro* T-cell responses to small protein and polypeptide antigens were found to parallel *in vivo* responses controlled by *Ir* genes, and T cells were exquisitely sensitive to differences in MHC antigens of the APC in all their antigen recognition functions. This observation *in vitro* made it possible to separate the MHC of the T cell from that of the APC. The T-cell response to antigenic determinants on each chain of insulin depended on the MHC antigens of the APC. This was particularly apparent when T cells from an (A × B)F1 animal responded to antigen presented by APCs of either the A or B parental MHC type *(197,321)*. Neither parental APC stimulated an allogeneic response from (A × B)F1 T cells, and the response to antigen was now limited by the MHC of the APC. This ability of the APC to limit what could be presented to the T cells was termed *determinant selection (197,321)*. It became obvious that even in a single (A × B)F1 animal, distinct sets of antigen-specific T cells exist that respond to each antigenic determinant only in association with MHC type A or type B *(322)*.

Experiments on the fine specificity of antigen-specific T cell clones suggested that the MHC of the APC could influence the T-cell response in more subtle ways than just allowing or inhibiting it. Determinant selection implied that a given processed peptide should contain both a site for MHC interaction and a distinct functional site for T-cell receptor binding. Thus, a protein with multiple determinants could be processed into different peptides, each with a different MHC restriction, consistent with the independent *Ir* gene control of the response to each antigenic determinant on the same protein *(159)*. For example, T-cell clones specific for myoglobin responded to different antigenic determinants on different peptide fragments of myoglobin *(193)*: those specific for one of the epitopes were always restricted to I-A, while those specific for the other were always restricted to I-E. The simplest interpretation was that each antigenic peptide contained an MHC association site for interacting with I-A or I-E. At the level of *Ir* genes, mouse strains lacking a functional I-E molecule could respond to one of the sites only, and those with neither I-A nor I-E molecules capable of binding to any myoglobin peptide would be low responders to myoglobin.

Evidence for a discrete MHC association site on peptide antigens came from studies with pigeon cytochrome c. The murine T-cell response to pigeon cytochrome c and its carboxy terminal peptide (*81–103*,104) depends on the I-E molecules of the APCs *(157)*. However, distinct structural sites on the synthetic peptide antigen appear to constitute two functional sites: an epitope site for binding to the T-cell receptor and an "agretope" (for "antigen-restriction-tope") site for interacting with the MHC molecule of the APC *(157,174–176)*. Amino acid substitutions for Lys at position 99 on the peptide destroyed the ability to stimulate T-cell clones specific for the peptide, while the difference between Ala and a deletion at position 103 determined T-cell stimulation in association with some MHC antigens but not others, independent of the T-cell fine specificity. In addition, immunizing with the peptides substituted at position 99 elicited new T-cell clones that responded to the substituted peptide but not the original and showed the same pattern of genetic restriction, correlated with the residue at position 103, as the clones specific for the original peptide. These results implied that the substitutions at position 99 had not affected the MHC association site but independently altered the epitope site that interacts directly with the T-cell receptor. In contrast, position 103 was a likely subsite for MHC interaction, without altering the T-cell receptor binding site.

It remained to be shown that MHC molecules without any other cell surface protein were sufficient for presentation of processed peptide antigens. This was demonstrated by Watts et al. *(323)*, who showed that glass slides coated with lipid containing purified I-A molecules could present an ovalbumin peptide to an ovalbumin-specific T-cell hybridoma. This result meant that no other special steps were required other than antigen processing and MHC association. Likewise, Walden et al. *(324)* specifically stimulated T-cell hybridomas with liposomes containing nothing but antigen and MHC molecules. Second, Norcross et al. *(325)* transformed mouse L cells with the genes for the I-A α and β chains and converted the fibroblasts (which do not express their own class II molecules) into I-A-expressing cells. These cells were able to present several antigens to I-A-restricted T-cell clones and hybridomas *(325)*, and similar I-E transfectants presented to I-E–restricted T cells *(193)*. Thus, whatever processing enzymes are required are already present in fibroblasts, and the only additional requirement for antigen-presenting function is the expression of I-A or I-E antigens.

The planar membrane technique has been applied to determine the minimum number of MHC–antigen complexes per antigen-presenting cell necessary to induce T-cell activation (326). After pulsing the presenting cells with antigen, the cells were studied for antigen-presenting activity, and some of the cells were lysed to produce a purified fraction containing MHC charged with antigenic peptides. These MHC–peptide complexes were used to reconstitute planar membranes, and their potency was compared with a reference MHC preparation pulsed with a high peptide concentration *in vitro* and presumed to be fully loaded. In this way, the relative peptide occupancy of MHC binding sites corresponding to any level of antigen presentation could be determined. For B cells and macrophages, the threshold of antigen loading necessary for triggering T cells was 0.2% of I-E^d molecules occupied by peptide, corresponding to about 200 MHC–peptide complexes per presenting cell. For artificial presenting cells, such as L cells transfected with I-E^d, the threshold was 23 times greater, or 4.6% of MHC occupied by peptide. Similarly, when MHC–peptide binding was measured directly, using radiolabeled peptide to determine the minimum level of MHC–peptide complexes required for T-cell triggering, B cells were capable of presenting antigen with as few as 200 to 300 MHC–peptide complexes per cell (327). A similar number of peptide–MHC class I molecule complexes was reported to be required on a cell for recognition by CD8$^+$ cytotoxic T cells (328). These results explain how newly generated peptide antigens can bind enough MHC molecules to stimulate a T-cell response, even in the presence of competing cellular antigens, because a low level of MHC occupancy is sufficient. In addition, this threshold of presentation may explain how multivalent protein antigens, such as viral particles, with 100 to 200 protein copies each, can be more than 10^3-fold more immunogenic than the same weight of protein monomers (*329*,330,331). Studies of the number of T-cell receptors needed for triggering, based on titrating peptide and recombinant soluble class I MHC molecules on plastic, suggested that interaction of three to five T-cell receptors with peptide-MHC complexes was sufficient, consistent with several T cells interacting with one APC (332,333).

Biochemical evidence for the direct association between processed peptide and MHC molecules was demonstrated by competition between peptides for antigen presentation *(203,334–337)* and then more directly by equilibrium dialysis *(338)*, molecular sieve chromatography *(339)*, or affinity labeling *(340)*. Equilibrium dialysis was performed by incubating detergent-solubilized class II molecules with fluoresceinated or radioactive antigenic peptides, followed by dialysis against a large volume of buffer. Peptide can pass in or out of the dialysis bag, but the class II molecules are trapped inside. In the absence of binding by class II molecules, the labeled peptide would distribute itself equally between the inside and outside of the dialysis chamber. However, when the appropriate class II molecules were added to the chamber, extra peptide molecules were retained inside it due to formation of a complex with MHC class II. In this way, direct binding of antigen and MHC was shown, and an affinity constant was determined *(338,339)*.

A second approach was to form the antigen–MHC complex over 48 hours, followed by rapid passage over a Sephadex G50 sizing column. The bound peptide came off the column early because it is the size of class II molecules (about 58 kD), while free peptide was usually included in the column and eluted later because it is only approximately 2 kD *(339)*. Peptide bound to specific and saturable sites on MHC. Competitive binding showed that different peptide antigens with the same MHC restriction bind to the same site on the MHC class II molecule *(341,342)*. For example, Table 21.6 shows the results with peptide antigens that are known to be presented with I-A or I-E antigens of the d or k haplotype. We observe that Ova peptide 323 to 339, which is presented with I-A^d, also binds well to purified I-A^d, while nonradioactive peptide competes for the peptide binding sites of the I-A^d molecule. Similarly, the other I-A^d-restricted peptide, myoglobin 106–118, competes with Ova 323–339 for the same site. However, myoglobin 132–153, which is not restricted to I-A^d, does not compete for it but does compete for its own restriction element, I-E^d. Similarly, pigeon cytochrome c competes best for its restriction element I-E^k rather than I-A^k or I-E^d, which do not present cytochrome. Conversely, recombinant Eβ genes have been used to map separate sites on a class II MHC molecule for binding to peptide antigen and to the T-cell receptor *(343)*.

Using these two biochemical methods, it has been possible to explain major losses of peptide antigenicity resulting from amino acid substitutions in terms of their adverse effect on epitope or agretope function. For example, the response of each of two ovalbumin-specific T-cell clones was mapped to peptide 325 to 335 by using a nested set of synthetic peptides. Five substitutions were made for each amino acid in the peptide, and the resulting 55 different peptides were each tested for the ability to stimulate the clone *(344)*. Presumably, those peptides that failed to stimulate could be defective at an epitope or an agretope functional site. In fact, only two amino acids (Val 327 and Ala 332) were essential for MHC interaction, and changes at either of these resulted in a loss of antigenicity for the clone. Seven other amino acids were critical for T-cell stimulation but did not affect MHC binding. Thus, these must be part of the functional epitope. Interestingly, certain substitutions for His 328, Ala 330, and Glu 333 had effects on MHC binding, while others had effects on T-cell stimulation without affecting MHC binding. These amino acids might participate in both agretope and epitope functional sites, or, alternatively, the substitutions may affect the conformation of the peptide as it binds, thus indirectly affecting T-cell recognition (345) (see later discussion). The fact that substitutions at 9 of 11 amino acids could be tolerated without affecting MHC binding is consistent with the determinant selection hypothesis in that multiple antigenic peptides are capable of interacting with the same antigen binding site on the MHC molecule.

Similarly, by using a T-cell clone specific for peptide 52–61 of hen egg lysozyme, substitutions at each amino acid were analyzed for the ability to bind to I-A^k and stimulate the clone *(346)*. Four of 11 amino acid residues were silent, while substitutions at three positions resulted in reduced binding to I-A^k. Substitutions at the remaining three positions resulted in decreased T-cell stimulation without affecting MHC association. The epitope was very sensitive to substitutions, even conservative ones such as changing Leu 56 to Ile, norLeu, or Val. The results in both of these studies confirmed by competitive binding that the MHC molecule contains a single saturable site for peptide

TABLE 21.6 Correlation between MHC Restriction and Binding to MHC Molecules

Competitor Peptide		Ova + A^d	Myo + E^d	HEL + A^k	Cyto + E^k
Ova	323–339	++++	–	++	+
Myo	106–118	++++	–	++	+/–
Myo	132–153	–	++++	–	++
HEL	46–61	+	+	++++	+
Cytochrome c	88–104	++	+/–	++	++++

MHC, major histocompatibility complex.
Data from ref. *322*.

binding. This site must be capable of binding a broad range of antigenic peptides. In binding the MHC groove, antigenic peptides assume the extended conformation that exposes the epitope for recognition by the T-cell receptor.

Although a full set of general principles explaining the specificity of antigen presentation and T-cell recognition has not yet emerged, it is studies such as these, combined with complementary structural studies characterizing the antigen-interacting portions of MHC molecules (*192*,231,232,*343*,*347–349*,350–352,353,354) (see Chapters 19 and 20) and of T-cell receptors (*355–358*,359–361) (see Chapter 10) that will ultimately lead to an understanding of these principles.

One observation that came out of this type of structure–function study was that a single peptide can bind to a class II MHC molecule in more than one way, and thus be seen by different T cells in different orientations or conformations (345,*362*) The same conclusion can be reached from an entirely different type of study, in which mutations are introduced into the MHC molecule. Mutations in the floor of the peptide-binding groove, which cannot directly interact with the T-cell receptor, can differentially affect recognition of a peptide by one clone and not another (*363*,*364*,365). In a particularly thoroughly studied case, it was clear that the quantitative level of peptide binding was not affected by the mutation, but rather the change in the floor of the groove imposed an altered conformation on the peptide that differentially affected recognition by different T cells (365). If indeed the T-cell receptor cannot detect the mutation in the MHC molecule except indirectly by its effect on the peptide conformation, then one is forced to conclude that different T cells have preferences for different conformations of the same peptide bound to (what appears to the T cell as) the same MHC molecule.

Another general observation to come from this type of study is that substitution of amino acids often affects presentation by MHC and recognition by T cells through introduction of dominant negative interactions or interfering groups, whereas only a few residues are actually essential for peptide binding (366). Both for class II binding (366,*367*,368,*369*) and for class I MHC binding (370), most residues can be replaced with Ala or sometimes Pro without losing MHC binding, as long as a few critical residues are retained. Of course, T-cell recognition may require retention of other residues. If many of the amino acid side chains are not necessary for binding to the MHC molecule, then one might expect side chains of noncritical amino acids to occasionally interfere with binding, either directly or through an effect on conformation. That is exactly what was observed for a helper epitope from the HIV-1 envelope protein when a heteroclitic peptide—that is, one that stimulated the T cells at much lower concentrations than did the wild-type peptide—was obtained by replacing a negatively charged Glu with Ala or with Gln, which has the same size but no charge (366). An Asp, negatively charged but smaller, behaved like the Glu. Thus, this residue was not necessary for binding to the class II MHC molecule, but a negatively charged side chain interfered with binding to the MHC molecule as measured by competition studies. Information about residues that interfere with binding has allowed the refinement of sequence motifs for peptides binding to MHC molecules to permit more reliable prediction of binding (371) (see later discussion).

This observation also provides a novel approach to make more potent vaccines by "epitope enhancement," the process of modifying the internal sequence of epitopes to make them more potent, for example, by increasing affinity for an MHC molecule or T-cell receptor (TCR), or able to induce more broadly cross-reactive T cells specific for multiple strains of a virus (372–375). Proof of principle that this approach can make more potent peptide vaccines has recently been obtained (375). The modified "enhanced" helper T-cell epitope from the HIV-1 envelope protein described previously (366), with Ala substituted for Glu, was shown to be immunogenic at 10- to 100-fold lower doses for *in vivo* immunization than the wild-type HIV-1 peptide to induce a T-cell proliferative response specific for the wild-type peptide. Further, when a peptide vaccine construct using this helper epitope coupled to a CTL epitope (376,377) was modified with the same Glu-to-Ala substitution, it was more potent at inducing $CD8^+$ CTL specific for the CTL epitope than was the original vaccine construct, even though the CTL epitope was unchanged (Fig. 21.9) (375). The increased potency of the vaccine construct was shown to be due to improved class II MHC-restricted help by genetic mapping using congenic strains of mice expressing the same class I MHC molecule to present the CTL epitope and the same background genes, but differing in class II MHC molecules (375). Thus, class II-restricted help makes an enormous difference in induction of class I-restricted CTL, and epitope enhancement can allow construction of more potent vaccines, providing greater protection against viral infection (378). Further, the improved help was found to be qualitatively, not just quantitatively, different, skewed more toward Th1 cytokines (378). The mechanism was found to involve greater induction of CD40-ligand on the helper T cells, resulting in greater IL-12 production by the antigen-presenting dendritic cells, which in turn polarized the helper cells toward Th1 phenotype (378). The dendritic cells conditioned with the helper T cells and the higher affinity peptide and then purified were also more effective at activating $CD8^+$ CTL precursors in the absence of helper cells, supporting a mechanism of help mediated through activation of dendritic cells (379–381). This study showed also that such help was mediated primarily through up-regulation of IL-12 production and CD80 and CD86 expression on the dendritic cell (378). Understanding this mechanism of epitope enhancement may contribute to the design of improved vaccines.

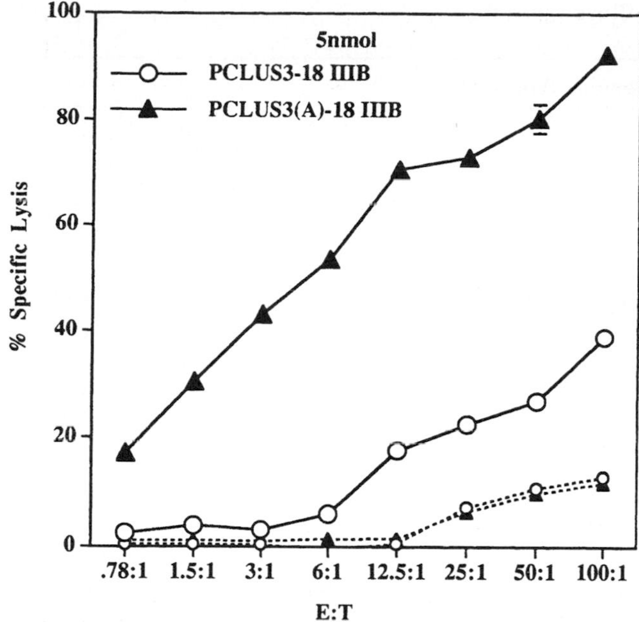

FIGURE 21.9 Enhancement of immunogenicity of a peptide vaccine for induction of class I major histocompatibility complex (MHC)-restricted cytotoxic T lymphocytes by modification of the class II MHC-binding portion to increase CD4$^+$ T-cell help. Peptide vaccine PCLUS3-18 IIIB contains a class II MHC binding helper region, consisting of a cluster of overlapping determinants from the human immunodeficiency virus (HIV)-1 envelope protein gp160, and a class I MHC-binding cytotoxic T-cell (CTL) epitope, P18 IIIB. Modification of the helper epitope to remove an adverse negative charge by replacement of a Glu with an Ala residue was shown to increase binding to the class II MHC molecule (366). Here, introduction of the same modification of the helper epitope, to produce PCLUS3(A)-18IIIB, is shown to greatly increase immunogenicity *in vivo* for induction of CTL to the class I-binding P18IIIB portion. Immunization of A.AL mice with 5 nmol of either vaccine construct subcutaneously in montanide ISA 51 adjuvant, and stimulation of resulting spleen cells with P18IIIB for 1 week in culture, resulted in 33-fold more lytic units for lysing targets coated with P18IIIB when mice were immunized with the modified second-generation vaccine than when they were immunized with the original construct with the natural sequence. Thus, class II-restricted CD4$^+$ T-cell help has a major impact on induction of class I-restricted CTL, and this process of "epitope enhancement" can be used to make vaccines more potent than the natural viral antigens. Targets: BALB/c 3T3 fibroblasts with P18IIIB (*solid lines*) or no peptide (*dashed lines*). (Modified from ref. 375 with permission.)

Similar epitope enhancement has been carried out for class I MHC-binding viral or tumor peptides as well (382,*383*,384), and in one case has been found to result in greater clinical efficacy of a melanoma vaccine used for human immunotherapy (385). These results emphasize the importance of affinity for MHC molecules vaccine efficacy (386), and suggest that rational design of vaccines with higher affinity epitopes may produce more effective second-generation vaccines (387,388). To that end, the discovery of sequence motifs predicting MHC molecule binding, and the development of bioinformatics strategies to predict peptide affinity, have proven a great impetus to the field (389).

In the case of class I MHC molecules, results defining sequence-binding motifs generalize the conclusion that only a few critical "anchor" residues determine the specificity of binding to the MHC molecule (Table 21.7) (242,370,390–394). These motifs were defined by a detailed study of one peptide–MHC system (392), by sequencing the mixture of natural peptides eluted from a class I MHC molecule and finding that at certain positions in the sequence a single residue predominated within the pool of peptides (390), and by separating and sequencing individual natural peptides eluted from a class I molecule and finding a conserved residue at certain positions (391). The latter two studies also made the important observation that the natural peptides eluted from class I MHC molecules were all about the same length, eight or nine residues, and this was confirmed for a much larger collection of peptides eluted from HLA-A2 and analyzed by tandem mass spectrometry (393). This finding was consistent with other studies demonstrating that a minimal nonapeptide was many orders of magnitude more potent than longer peptides in presentation by class I molecules to T cells (395,396). This conservation of length was critical to the success of the approach of sequencing mixtures of peptides eluted from a class I molecule (390), because such a method requires that the conserved anchor residues all be at the same distance from the N terminus. The fact that Falk et al. (390) could find a single amino acid at certain positions, such as a Tyr at position 2 in peptides eluted from K^d, implies not only that most or all of the peptides bound to K^d had a Tyr that could be aligned, but also that the peptides were already aligned as bound to the MHC molecule, with each one having just one residue N terminal to the Tyr. This result implies that the position of the N-terminal residue is fixed in the MHC molecule. It is this fact that has made the identification of motifs for binding to class I molecules much more straightforward than finding motifs for binding class II molecules.

This conclusion has not only been confirmed but also explained by the x-ray crystallographic data on class I peptide–MHC complexes (350–352). It appears that both the N-terminal α amino group and the C-terminal carboxyl group are fixed in pockets at either end of the MHC groove, independent of what amino acids are occupying those positions, and that the rest of the peptide spans these fixed points in a more or less extended conformation. The minimum length that can span the distance between these pockets is 8 residues, but 9 or 10 residues can be accommodated with a slight bulge or β turn in the middle of the peptide, explaining the narrow restriction on length. Between these ends, one or two pockets in the groove can accommodate the side chain of an amino acid, usually either at position 2 binding in the B pocket, or at position 5 binding in

TABLE 21.7 Examples of Motifs for Peptides Binding to Class I and II MHC Molecules

	Residue Number								
MHC Molecule	*1*	*2*	*3*	*4*	*5*	*6*	*7*	*8*	*9*
Class I									
H-2K^d		Y							I, L, V
H-2D^b					N				M, I
H-2K^b					F, Y			L, M	
H-2L^d		P			(hydrophilic K, R)				M, L, F
H-2D^d		G	P		K, R				L
H-2K^k		E						I	
HLA-A2.1		L, M							V
HLA-A3		L	(F)						Y, K
HLA-B27	K, R O	R	I, Y, F, W						K, R
Class II									
DRB1*0101	Y, V, L, F, I, A			L, A		A, G			L, A
DRB1*0301	L, I F, M V			D		K, R E, Q			Y, L F
DRB1*0401 (DR4Dw4)	F, Y W			no R, K		N, S T, Q Aliphatic	Polar Charged		Polar Aliphatic K
DRB1*0402 (DR4Dw10)	V, I, L, M		no	D, E		N, Q, S, T K	R, K H, N Q, P		Polar Aliphatic H
DRB1*1501 (DR2b)	L, V, I			F, Y I			I, L V, M F		
DQA1*0501 DQB1*0301	F, Y, I, M L, V				V, L I, M Y		Y, F M, L, V, I		

MHC, major histocompatibility complex.
Data from refs. 234, 350, and 370–374.

the C pocket, depending on the particular MHC molecule. Additionally the side chain of the C-terminal residue serves as an anchor in the F pocket at the end of the groove. These residues that fit into pockets correspond exactly to the "anchor" residues, at positions 2 or 5, and 8, 9, or 10, defined by the sequence motifs, and appear to be the primary determinants of specificity for peptide binding because the rest of the interactions are largely with peptide backbone atoms, including the α amino and carboxyl groups, and therefore do not contribute to sequence specificity. This finding can explain both the breadth of peptides that can bind to a single MHC molecule because most of the binding involves only backbone atoms common to all peptides, and also the exquisite specificity of binding is determined by the anchor residues that account for the *Ir* gene control of responsiveness.

In contrast, when natural self-peptides were eluted from class II MHC molecules (230,397), the lengths were much more variable, ranging from 13 to 18 residues, and several variants of the same peptide were found with different lengths of extra sequence at one end or the other ("ragged ends"). This finding suggested that both ends of the peptide-binding groove of class II MHC molecules are open, in contrast to class I, so that additional lengths of peptide can hang out either side, and trimming does not have to be precise. However, a corollary is that the peptides eluted from class II molecules would not be aligned in a motif starting from the exact amino terminus, and that was indeed what was found. Although a moderately conserved motif was found in some of the peptides eluted from the murine class II molecule I-A^d, consistent with the motif defined based on known antigenic peptides binding to I-A^d *(398)*, the motif was neither so clearly defined nor so highly conserved as in the class I case, and required aligning of sequences to identify a core motif of about 9 amino acid residues (397). Subsequently, a number of motifs for peptides binding to human class II MHC molecules have been defined (242,399–404). Unlike peptides eluted from

MHC class I grooves, these class II binding peptides may locate the core binding motif at various distances from the amino or carboxyl end of the peptide.

The crystal structure of a peptide bound to a human class II MHC molecule, DR1, revealed that indeed the ends of the groove are open and the peptide can extend beyond the groove in either direction (232,405). In addition, the more broadly defined class II motifs in Table 21.7 can be explained by less stringent requirements for amino acid side chains to interact with binding pockets in class II. In general, the MHC class II binding pockets are shallower than for class I, and a selected peptide derives less binding energy from each pocket. In fact, they form fewer H-bonds with the peptide side chains, and more H-bonds are directed at the peptide backbone, allowing a variety of different peptides to bind. Rather than requiring a specific amino acid at each position, the shallow binding pockets of MHC class II tend to exclude peptides based on unfavorable interactions, such as side chains too large to fit the binding pocket. Even one amino acid side chain that binds strongly to an MHC pocket is sufficient to anchor the peptide to MHC class II and set the frame for the interaction of the rest of the peptide with the MHC groove.

For example, binding of three peptides to the class II molecules I-A in mice or HLA-DQ in humans are shown in Figure 21.10. The first residue of the peptide motif is designated P1, the next is P2, and so on. The alpha-helical walls and beta-sheet floor of the MHC class II groove (Chapter 19) are peeled away to reveal the peptide backbone and side chains in relation to MHC binding pockets. For the ovalbumin peptide $Ova_{323-329}$ binding to $I\text{-}A^d$, residues P1, P4, and P9 all point down into the binding pockets (406). The best fit is between Val 327 and the P4 pocket, which creates mainly hydrophobic interactions with MHC, and serves as the anchor residue. Residues P5 (His 328) and P8 (His 331) project upward for binding to the TCR. The shallow P4 pocket can tolerate only small hydrophobic side chains, such as Val, so it dictates which peptides can bind here. The other MHC pockets, P1 and P9, accommodate many different residues, so they have little effect on which peptides can be presented by $I\text{-}A^d$.

For hen egg lysozyme peptide HEL_{50-62} binding to $I\text{-}A^k$, interactions with MHC are observed for P1, P4, P6, and P9 (407). The P1 interaction is very different from $I\text{-}A^d$ because the P1 pocket is a perfect fit for Asp and has an arginine at the end of the tunnel to neutralize charge. This structure explains why nearly all peptides presented by $I\text{-}A^k$ must have Asp at this position. In contrast, the P4 and P9 pockets are partially filled and will tolerate a number of different side chains at these positions. The P6 pocket requires a Glu or Gln here, even though the MHC residues deep in the pocket are acidic. It is presumed that one of the Glu residues must be protonated to allow Glu binding at this position. This arrangement of the peptide leaves P2, P5, and P8 exposed to solvent in the crystal structure and to the TCR during antigen presentation.

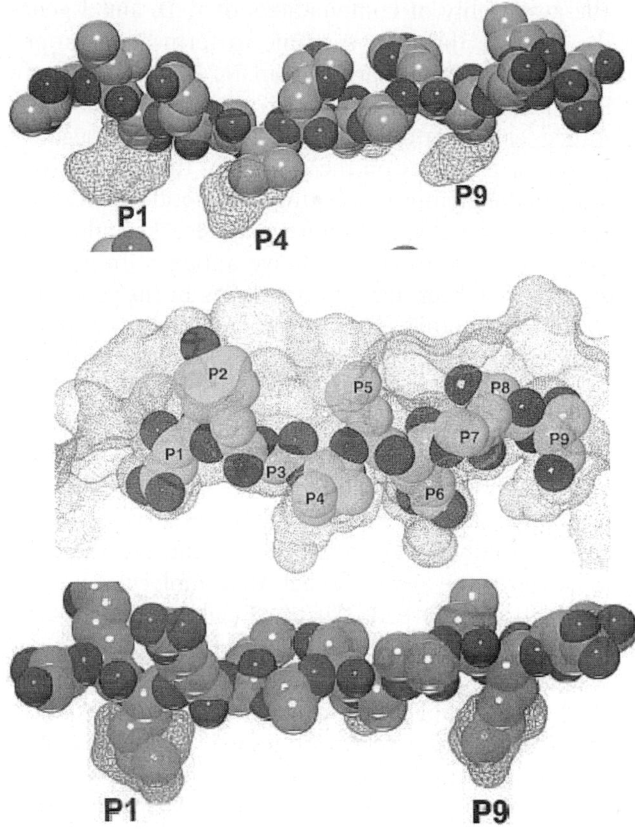

FIGURE 21.10 Interaction of peptides with the binding groove of major histocompatibility complex (MHC) class II, as determined by x-ray crystallography. Anchor residue side chains fill binding pockets to a greater or lesser extent, supplemented by H-bonds to the peptide backbone. Examples include: $I\text{-}A^d$ with ovalbumin peptide 323-334 (**top**) (406), $I\text{-}A^k$ with hen egg lysozyme 52-60 (**middle**) (407), and HLA-DR3 with class II-associated invariant chain peptide (**bottom**) (408).

For the CLIP peptide binding to HLA-DR3, deep pockets at P1 and P9 are more fully occupied by the peptide side chains (408). pH-dependent binding is important because CLIP must be stable at neutral pH and unstable at acid pH in the presence of HLA-DM in order to perform its function.

Based on affinity for MHC, these interactions explain the peptide-binding motifs for MHC class II that select which peptides can be presented to T cells. In addition, these interactions orient the peptide in the MHC groove and determine which residues are accessible for recognition by the TCR.

D. T-Cell Receptor Recognition

The last hurdle that a potential antigenic determinant must surmount is recognition by a TCR within the repertoire of the individual responding. This repertoire may be limited by the availability of combinations of V, D, and J genes in the genome that can combine to form an appropriate receptor, given the lack of somatic hypermutation in TCRs in contrast to antibodies *(357,409)*, and then by self-tolerance, as mediated by thymic or peripheral negative selection, or by limits on the repertoire that is positively selected in the thymus on existing self-peptide–MHC complexes. The available repertoire may also be influenced by prior exposure to cross-reactive antigens. In general, however, it has been hard to find holes in the repertoire *(410)*. Indeed, studies examining large panels of peptides binding to particular class I molecules for correlations between peptide affinity for MHC and T-cell responses have failed to find high-affinity peptides for which no T-cell response can be raised, whereas not all lower affinity peptides elicit a response (411,412). These results suggest that if the peptide can bind well enough to the MHC molecule, there is virtually always a T cell that can see the complex. However, the array of other MHC molecules present can influence the breadth of the T-cell repertoire (413). Furthermore, when TCR repertoires of mice and humans were compared for peptides presented by HLA-A2.1, they seemed to be capable of seeing the same spectrum of peptides (414). Eleven peptides from HCV proteins, each of which had a motif for binding to HLA-A2.1, were tested for recognition by CTL from HLA-A2.1 transgenic mice and human HLA-A2.1–positive patients infected with HCV. The same four peptides that were recognized by the T cells from the mice were the ones recognized by the human T cells, whereas the others were not recognized well by either murine or human T cells. The selection of which peptides were recognized seemed to be determined by binding to the HLA-A2.1 molecule, rather than by the availability of T cells. Thus, despite the differences in *TCR* genes in mice and humans, the repertoires are plastic enough that if a peptide passes the other three hurdles of processing, transport, and binding to MHC molecules, T cells can be elicited to respond to it in either species (414). Likewise, no hole in the helper T-cell repertoire could be found to explain low responders to the recombinant hepatitis B vaccine (415).

On the other hand, evidence exists that MHC binding is not the whole story. Schaeffer et al. *(416)* examined 14 overlapping peptides covering the sequence of staphylococcal nuclease with different class II MHC molecules, constituting 54 different peptide-MHC combinations. Clearly, MHC binding plays a major role because 12/13 immunogenic peptides were high or intermediate binders to MHC molecules, whereas only one of 37 poor binders were immunogenic. Of high-affinity binders, 5/5 peptides were immunogenic. However, for intermediate-affinity MHC-binding peptides, only 7/12 were immunogenic. Similar results were found for the class I MHC molecule HLA-B0702, in which it was found that 7/7 high-affinity binders but only 9/12 intermediate affinity binders were immunogenic (412). Thus, MHC binding alone is not sufficient to ensure immunogenicity. The T-cell repertoire was one factor suggested that might limit the spectrum of immunogenic peptides.

Indeed, examples for selection at the level of the TCR repertoire exist. A particularly elegant example described by Moudgil et al. (417) is one in which a peptide *(46–61)* of mouse lysozyme presented by I-A^k is recognized T cells from CBA/J and B10.A mice, expressing I-A^k and I-E^k, but not by T cells from B10.A(4R) mice expressing only I-A^k, even though the APC from B10.A(4R) mice can present the peptide to T cells from the other strains. T cells from the B10.A(4R) mice can respond to variant 46–61 peptides in which the C-terminal Arg is replaced by Ala, Leu, Phe, Asn, or Lys, indicating that the C-terminal Arg is hindering recognition, but not binding by I-A^k, and in this case, not processing because the B10.A(4R) APC can present the peptide. It appears that the hindrance interferes with recognition by TCRs available in B10.A(4R) mice, but not TCRs available in B10.A or CBA/J mice, or in (B10.A[4R] × CBA/J)F1 mice. Because the B10.A mice are congenic with the B10.A(4R) mice, the difference is not one of non–MHC-linked genes such as TCR structural genes or non-MHC self-antigens producing self-tolerance. Further, because the F1 mice respond, the difference is not due to a hole in the repertoire produced by a self-antigen of the B10.A(4R) mice. It was concluded that the CBA/J and B10.A mice contain an additional repertoire, positively selected on I-E^k or possibly an H-2D/L class I molecule, in which these strains differ, that can recognize the 46–61 peptide despite the hindering Arg at the C-terminus.

An alternative related explanation is that strains that express I-E^k or D^k or D^d/L^d have an additional repertoire of TCRs positively selected on I-A^k presenting self-peptides from processing of these other MHC molecules in the thymus. This example illustrates a case in point that subtle differences in TCR, presumably caused in this case by positive selection, can lead to responsiveness or nonresponsiveness to a determinant that has already passed all of the three earlier hurdles: processing, transport, and MHC binding. Of course, there are some holes related to self-tolerance, primarily related to the loss of response to dominant determinants (418) and especially loss of high-avidity T cells (419–422). Interestingly, not only is there no loss of response to cryptic determinants, but also T cells recognizing cryptic determinants of mouse lysozyme can be positively selected on other nonmouse lysozyme self-ligands in a lysozyme knockout mouse (418). The selective loss of high-avidity T cells to immunodominant determinants has suggested a strategy to apply epitope enhancement to modify subdominant lower affinity tumor antigen peptides to increase their affinity for MHC molecules and thereby make them more immunogenic in order to take advantage of a repertoire not already crippled by loss of the high-avidity clones (423).

Another elegant example of T-cell repertoire limitations on immunodominance comes from a study of mice deficient in LMP2, and so unable to make immunoproteasomes. Reduced response to one normally immunodominant influenza epitope was found by T-cell adoptive transfer studies to be due to an alteration in the T-cell repertoire, presumably because of altered processing of self-peptides in the thymus (259).

A recent study found another mechanism by which the T-cell repertoire contributes to immunodominance. It was found that the relative immunodominance of a dominant determinant of the HIV envelope protein among different strains of H-2^d mice all presenting the same peptide–H-2D^d complex correlated with the avidity of the T cells responding in those strains (423a). The mechanism found was that high-avidity T cells proliferate faster than low-avidity ones when exposed to antigen, and therefore dominate the response. This mechanism differs from those at earlier steps that progressively constrain the response and thereby narrow the repertoire to dominant epitopes, whereas this mechanism selectively expands the dominant repertoire. This mechanism may also explain other recent findings such as the higher affinity of dominant compared with subdominant TCRs specific for human cytomegalovirus (424). Because high avidity T cells are better able to clear virus infection (425,426), a recent study even suggests that the driving force for MHC polymorphism is to create a large enough repertoire to select for high-avidity T cells (427).

As more is understood about the molecular basis of TCR recognition, with crystallographic data now available (360,361,428), it becomes possible to apply epitope enhancement in a rational way to the affinity of the peptide-MHC complex to the TCR, as was previously described for the peptide affinity for MHC molecules. Sequence modifications in the peptide that increase the affinity for the TCR were shown to be more effective at expanding *in vivo* the T cells specific for tumor antigens (429–431). Most of these modifications were found empirically, but a systematic study of substitutions throughout a number of peptides revealed a pattern in which peptides with conservative substitutions at positions 3, 5, or 7 were most likely to yield increased TCR affinity, narrowing the candidate list of peptides that require empirical screening (432). This strategy provides a second type of epitope enhancement, derived from basic immunologic principles, to produce more effective vaccines.

Defining the Role of Individual Amino Acids and Effects of Altered Peptide Ligands

Once an antigenic peptide is identified, the next step is to map key amino acid residues by making a series of variant peptides, each of which differs from the native sequence by a single amino acid substitution, as described in section C. One approach, called an *alanine scan*, substitutes Ala for the natural amino acid at each position in the peptide, or uses Ser or Gly to replace naturally occurring Ala. Ala is used because the side chain is only a methyl group, so it replaces whatever functional side chain is present with the smallest one other than that of Gly, which is not used because of its effects on conformation. Thus, one can ask whether loss of the naturally occurring side chain affects function, without the introduction of a new side chain that might itself affect function. Generally, each peptide will have several amino acids wherein Ala substitution destroys antigenicity. Some of these correspond to contact residues for the TCR, while others are contact residues for MHC. In many cases, the MHC binding residues can be determined by testing the substituted peptides in a competitive MHC binding assay (previously discussed). The amino acid substitutions that knock out T-cell proliferation but not MHC binding are presumed to be in the epitope recognized by the TCR directly, and these can be studied with additional substitutions. For example, this technique was used to compare the residues interacting with the MHC molecule or TCR when the same HIV-1 V3 loop peptide P18 (residues 308–322) was presented by three different MHC molecules, a human class I molecule, a mouse class I molecule, and a mouse class II molecule (Fig. 21.11) (433,434). Interestingly, there was a striking concordance of function of several of the residues as presented by all three MHC molecules (Fig. 21.11). For example, Pro and Phe interacted with the MHC in all three cases, and the same Val interacted with the TCR in all three cases. Also, the same Arg in the middle of the peptide interacted with both the mouse class I and the mouse class II molecules, and the C-terminal Ile was an anchor residue for both human and murine class I molecules (433,434).

In the case of autoimmune T cells, these techniques have been used to study the number and variety of epitopes recognized by self-reactive T cells. In the diabetic NOD mouse, the B chain of insulin is a major target of T cells recovered from pancreatic islets (435). Alanine scanning of B chain peptide 9 to 23 revealed two patterns of T-cell recognition for the same peptide. Some T cells recognize peptide 9–16, and others respond to peptide 13–23. Each epitope appears to have distinct sites for MHC and TCR binding, even though they come from the same peptide chain. Similarly, in systemic lupus erythematosus, human T cells specific for the Sm antigen are narrowly restricted to a few epitopes that are found on a small group of proteins (436). On the Sm-B antigen, three epitopes were recognized. On Sm-D antigen, there were two. In each case, alanine scans showed that the same epitopes were recognized by distinct T-cell clones. These results are consistent with the hypotheses that the autoimmune response to insulin or to Sm antigen may be induced by abnormal exposure of a very few cryptic epitopes, or they may depend on

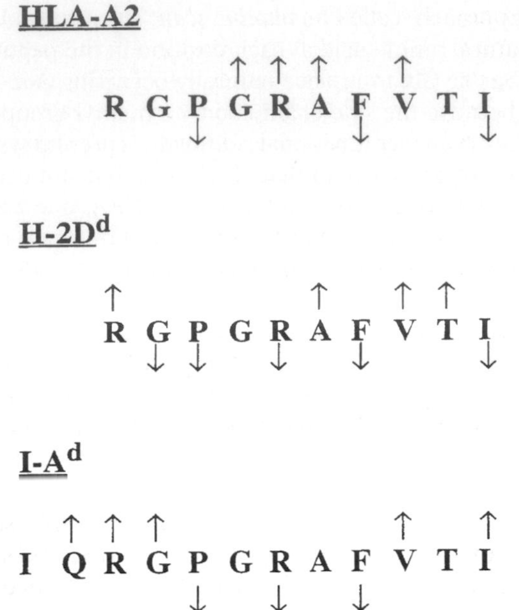

FIGURE 21.11 Comparison of the major histocompatibility complex (MHC)-interacting ("agretopic") and T-cell receptor interacting ("epitopic") residues of the same human immunodeficiency virus (HIV)-1 envelope V3 loop peptide as it is presented by human class I, murine class I, and murine class II MHC molecules to $CD8^+$ cytotoxic T cell (CTL) and $CD4^+$ helper T cells. Shown is the sequence of the optimal binding portion of peptide P18 IIIB from the HIV-1 envelope protein V3 loop for each MHC molecule, in single-letter amino acid code. *Arrows pointing up* indicate residues determined to interact with the T-cell receptor, and *arrows pointing down* indicate residues determined to interact with the MHC molecule. Mapping of residue function for binding to the human class I MHC molecule HLA-A2.1 was described in ref. 434, and binding to the murine class I molecule H-$2D^d$ and the murine class II molecule I-A^d was described in ref. 433. Note the common use of the Pro and Phe for binding all three MHC molecules, and the use of the key Val residue for binding all the T-cell receptors. Also, the murine MHC molecules both use the central Arg residue as a contact residue, whereas both class I molecules use the C-terminal Ile residue as an anchor residue. Thus, there is a surprising degree of concordance.

selective loss of tolerance for a limited number of epitopes shared by a small subset of self-proteins.

TCRs may distinguish different chemical classes of amino acid side chains. An example of structural differences between amino acid side chains recognized by the TCR comes from an analysis of non–cross-reactive CTL that distinguish homologous peptides from the V3 loop of different strains of HIV-1 envelope protein. The residue at position 8 in the minimal determinant was identified as a key "epitopic" TCR contact residue in both strain IIIB, which has a Val at this position, and strain MN, which has a Tyr at this position (433,437,*438*). CTL specific for strain IIIB do not recognize the MN sequence, but will recognize peptides identical to MN except for the substitution of any aliphatic amino acid at that position, such as Val, Leu, or Ile (374). In contrast, CTL specific for the MN strain do not recognize the IIIB sequence, but will recognize the IIIB peptide if the Val at this position is replaced by a Tyr (437). Moreover, they will see any MN variant in which the Tyr is replaced by another aromatic amino acid, such as Phe, Trp, or His (374). Thus, the two non–cross-reactive TCRs see similar peptides but discriminate strongly between peptides with amino acids with aliphatic versus aromatic side chains. On the other hand, they do not distinguish strongly among different aliphatic residues or among different aromatic residues. Interestingly, however, in each category, the least active is the bulkiest member of the category, Ile and Trp, respectively, suggesting that these residues must fit into a pocket of limited size in the TCR.

However, many T cell receptors can distinguish even conservative substitutions. The interaction of peptide ligand with TCR can be studied by introducing single substitutions of conservative amino acids at these contact residues, such as Glu for Asp, Ser for Thr, or Gln for Asn. The TCR readily distinguishes among peptides with these minor differences at a single residue, and the results have been revealing. Depending on affinity for the TCR, closely related (altered) peptides can elicit very different responses in T cells. Thus, although a substituted peptide may be very weak or nonstimulatory by itself, it may still act as a partial agonist, or even a strong antagonist of an ongoing T-cell response. Antagonistic peptides can be demonstrated by pulsing antigen-presenting cells with native peptide antigen first, so that one is not measuring competition for binding to MHC molecules, followed by pulsing with a 10-fold or greater excess of the antagonist, before adding T cells. In the case of influenza hemagglutinin peptide 307-319 presented with HLA-DR1, peptide analogues such as Gln substituted for Asn 313 inhibited the proliferation of a human T-cell clone, even though they did not stimulate the clone. Anergy was not induced, and the antagonist peptide had to be present throughout the culture to inhibit the response (439,440). Thus, lack of antagonist activity is another feature of the interaction between peptide (in complex with MHC molecule) and TCR that is required for the peptide to be a stimulatory antigenic determinant.

Partial agonists were first demonstrated using T-cell clones specific for an allelic form of mouse hemoglobin. These T cells were from CE/J mice, which express the Hb^s allele of mouse hemoglobin, after immunization with the Hb^d allele. The minimum antigenic peptide corresponds to amino acids 67-76 of the Hb^d sequence and differs from Hb^s at positions 72, 73, and 76 *(441)*. Peptides substituted at each residue from amino acid 69 to 76 were tested for T-cell proliferation and cytokine release. Some substitutions, such as Gln for Asn at position 72, blocked T-cell stimulation completely in both assays. Other substituted peptides, such as Asp for Glu at position 73, lost T-cell proliferation, but still stimulated IL-4 release, and these are considered

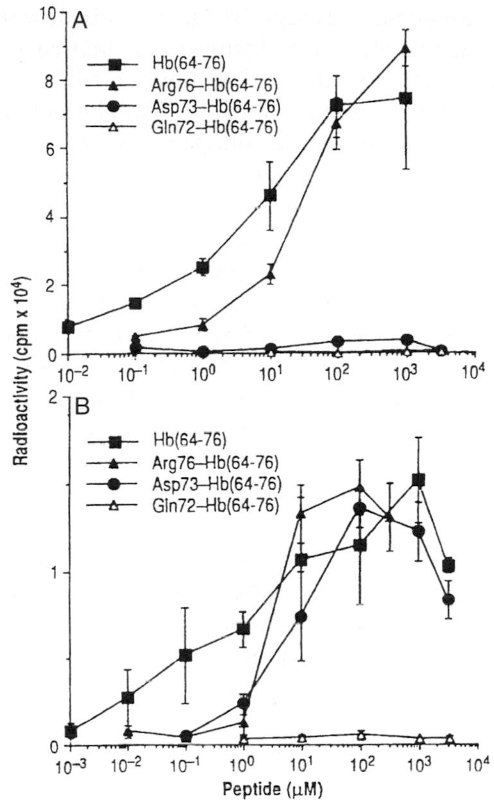

FIGURE 21.12 Differential effect of altered peptide ligands on the response to peptide 64 to 76 from hemoglobin. **A:** Proliferative response of a T-cell line incubated with antigen-presenting cells and the natural Hb (64-76) peptide or with peptides substituted at positions 72, 73, or 76. **B:** Interleukin 4 (IL-4) release by the T-cell line under the same conditions. The peptide substituted with Asp for Glu at position 73 is unable to induce T-cell proliferation, but it can still induce production of IL-4, so it is a partial agonist. In contrast, substitution of Gln for Asn at position 72 knocks out both responses equally. (Modified from ref. 442, with permission.)

partial agonists (Fig. 21.12) (442). Lack of stimulation was not due to failure to bind MHC because both substituted peptides gave reasonable binding in a competitive binding assay (443). Similar alteration of cytokine profile by altering the peptide ligand can be seen in other systems (440,444,445).

For one of the Hb 64-76–specific T-cell clones, PL.17, substitutions at amino acids 70, 72, 73, or 76 reduced antigenic potency by 1,000-fold or more, even though conservative amino acids were substituted. Although substitution of Ser for Ala 70 prevented T-cell stimulation in both assays, there was clearly some response to this peptide because it induced expression of the IL-2 receptor (446). In addition, once T cells were exposed to the Ser 70 peptide, they became unresponsive to subsequent exposure to the natural Hb^d peptide. This phenomenon closely resembled T-cell anergy and persisted for a week or more. The Ser 70 substitution alters a contact residue of the peptide for the TCR of clone PL.17 and affects its affinity. Other T-cell clones, however, can respond to this peptide presented on the same MHC molecule (I-E^k). Other Hb^d peptides substituted at this position, such as Met and Gly 70, also induced anergy but not proliferation, while nonconservative substitutions such as Phe, Asn, Asp, and His 70 induced neither (447)

Another well-studied example is influenza hemagglutinin peptide 306-318 as presented on human HLA-DR1. Based on the known crystal structure of the peptide-MHC complex (231) amino acid substitutions could be targeted to contact residues for the TCR, at positions 307, 309, 310, 312, 315, and 318 (448). At each position, nonconservative substitutions often rendered the peptide inactive, while conservative substitutions at several sites either gave full antigenicity, or gave progressively lower stimulatory activity, down to 1,000-fold less than native peptide, while retaining the ability to induce anergy. For example, substituting His or Gly for Lys 307 gave 1,000-fold reduced stimulation of T-cell proliferation, but full ability to induce tolerance. Similarly, substituting His for Lys 315 gave complete loss of stimulation, but nearly full anergy-inducing activity. As before, induction of the IL-2 receptor (CD25) was a sign of T-cell activation by these altered peptide ligands, even when they did not induce proliferation. Unlike these peptides, the antagonists do not induce interleukin receptors or secretion, and they do not cause long lasting tolerance. Overall, a number of altered peptide ligands have now been identified that, in appropriate complexes with MHC molecules, induce anergy or act as antagonists of the TCR and block activation by agonist ligands by delivering an abortive signal (440).

Several methods have been found to anergize T cells to a specific antigen for up to a week, and all have the common theme of delivering a partial signal via the TCR, resulting in tolerance rather than stimulation. The first method was to expose the T cells to peptide plus antigen-presenting cells treated with the carbodiimide cross-linker ECDI *(449)*. This treatment may prevent accessory molecules on the presenting cell from interacting with the TCR complex, or costimulatory signals from contributing to T-cell activation. The second method was to present peptide on presenting cells with mutated I-E molecules (450,451). The third method was to use altered peptide ligands that act as TCR antagonists as previously described (440,447,448). The final method was to block CD4 function with a monoclonal antibody, which would delay the recruitment of CD4 to the engaged TCR (452). Because generation of a complete stimulatory signal requires the interaction of TCR and accessory molecules, modifications that affect either component can block signaling. An altered peptide ligand, with decreased affinity for the TCR, may form an unstable complex, which cannot stay together long enough to recruit accessory molecules and generate a complete signal (452,453). Altered peptide ligands with low affinity for the TCR can also act as partial agonists that can compete with optimal agonists and reduce T-cell stimulation based on a similar mechanism (short dwell time of peptide-MHC complex on the TCR) (177).

Abnormal TCR signaling can be demonstrated by following the activity of protein kinases. Normal signaling produces phosphorylation of TCR subunits, such as ζ chain, as well as phosphorylation and activation of receptor-associated tyrosine kinases, such as ZAP-70. These kinases generate the downstream signal needed for T-cell activation. However, in each case studied, partial antigen signaling resulted in ζ chain phosphorylation without phosphorylation or activation of ZAP-70 (447,451,452), so downstream activation did not occur. This abnormal pattern occurred regardless of the method of anergy induction.

Partial signaling may be important for T-cell survival during negative selection in the thymus or in maintaining peripheral tolerance. By responding to self-antigens as if they were altered ligands presented in the thymus, T cells could use anergy induction as a successful strategy for avoiding clonal deletion. Similarly, peripheral tolerance may be an important mechanism for preventing autoimmune disease. Immunotherapy with altered peptide ligands could be envisioned as a way to block an ongoing response or induce tolerance to a specific antigen, such as the synovium in arthritis, or foreign MHC antigens in allograft rejection. However, a potential pitfall is that different T cells recognize the same peptide differently, so a peptide that is seen as an altered peptide ligand by some T-cell clones may be seen as a complete antigen by others. In addition, the choice of peptide would vary with MHC type. To be effective, an altered peptide ligand should antagonize or anergize polyclonal T cells and should work with each patient's MHC type.

A similar mechanism may be invoked to explain the generally weak immunogenicity of tumor antigens. According to this hypothesis, the only T cells capable of responding to self-antigens on tumors may have low-affinity receptors for them. In effect, the natural sequence is the altered ligand that induces tolerance. In some cases, this anergy can be overcome with modified peptides that have greater affinity for the TCR and induce a full stimulatory signal, resulting in an effective immune response to the tumor antigens (429), as described previously.

Prediction of T-Cell Epitopes

The fact that T cells recognize processed fragments of antigens presented by MHC molecules leads to the ironic situation that T-cell recognition of antigen, which is more complex than antibody recognition because of the ternary complex needed between TCR, antigen, and MHC molecule, may actually be focused on simpler structures of the antigen than those seen by most antibodies specific for native protein antigens. In contrast to the assembled topographic antigenic sites seen by many antibodies *(49,50)*, T cells specific for processed antigens are limited to seeing short segments of continuous sequence *(155,211)*. Therefore the tertiary structure of the protein plays little if any role in the structure of the epitope recognized by T cells, except as it may influence processing. However, the structure of the T-cell antigenic site itself must be limited to primary (sequence) and secondary structure, the latter depending only on local rather than long-range interactions. This limitation greatly simplifies the problem of identifying structural properties important to T-cell recognition because one can deal with sequence information, which can now be obtained from DNA without having a purified protein, and with the secondary structure implicit therein without having to obtain an x-ray crystallographic three-dimensional structure of the native protein, a much more difficult task.

Because the key feature necessary for a peptide to be recognized by T cells is its ability to bind to an MHC molecule, most approaches for predicting T-cell epitopes are based on predicting binding to MHC molecules. These approaches, which have been reviewed (389,454), can be divided into those that focus on specific individual MHC molecules one at a time, such as motif-based methods, and those that look for general structural properties of peptide sequences. We shall discuss first the methods based on general properties, and then those directed to individual MHC molecules.

The first structural feature of amino acid sequences found associated with T-cell epitopes that remains in use today is helical amphipathicity *(205,455–458)* which is statistically significant independent of the tendency to form a helix per se *(456)*. Because the x-ray crystallographic structures of both MHC class I (350–352,459) and class II molecules (231,408) have consistently shown peptides to be bound in extended, not alpha helical conformation, helicity per se has been abandoned as an associated structural feature of T-cell epitopes. However, as discussed later, other explanations of amphipathic structures have been discovered that do not require the peptide to be bound to the MHC molecule as an alpha helix. Amphipathicity is the property of having hydrophobic and hydrophilic regions separated in space. It was observed that the immunodominant T-cell epitopes of myoglobin and cytochrome c corresponded to amphipathic helices *(163,167,460)*. DeLisi and Berzofsky *(455)* developed an algorithm to search for segments of protein sequence that could fold as amphipathic helices, based on the idea that the hydrophobicity of the amino acids in the sequence must oscillate as one goes around an amphipathic helix. For the hydrophobic residues to line up on one side and the hydrophilic residues on the other, the periodicity of this oscillation must be approximately the same as the structural periodicity of the helix, about 100 degrees per residue (360 degrees per 3.6 residues per turn) (Fig. 21.13).

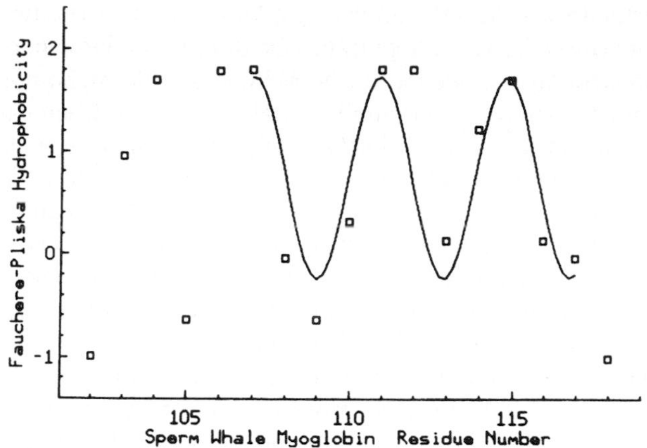

FIGURE 21.13 Plot of hydrophobicity of each amino acid in sperm whale myoglobin 102 to 118, according to the scale of Fauchère and Pliska (*529*), as a function of amino acid sequence, showing least-squares fit of a sinusoidal function to the sequence of hydrophobicities from 107 to 117. (From ref. *158*, with permission.)

A microcomputer program implementing this analysis was published *(458)*. Margalit et al. *(205)* optimized the original approach *(455)*, correctly identifying 18 of the 23 immunodominant helper T-cell antigenic sites from the 12 proteins in an expanded database ($p < .001$) *(205)* (Table 21.4). Indeed, when the database was expanded to twice and then 4 times its original size, the correlation remained highly significant, and the fraction of sites predicted remained relatively stable (34/48 sites = 71%, $p < .003$; 61/92 sites = 66%, $p < .001$) (*461*,462). A similar correlation was found for 65% of peptides presented by class I MHC molecules (462). A primary sequence pattern found in a substantial number of T-cell epitopes by Rothbard and Taylor *(463)* was consistent with one turn of an amphipathic helix. Also, another approach, called the *strip-of-the-helix* algorithm, that searches for helices with a hydrophobic strip down one face, found a correlation between amphipathic helices and determinants presented by both class II and class I MHC molecules *(457,464)*.

Newer data suggest at least two explanations, not mutually exclusive, for this correlation in the absence of helical structure found in the peptides bound to MHC molecules (465). First, crystal structures of peptides bound to class II MHC molecules have found that the peptides are bound in an extended conformation, but with a −130-degree twist like that of a type II polyproline helix (231,408), and can be quite amphipathic because of this twist (231). Although the -130-degree twist is distinct from that of an alpha helix, it gives a periodicity similar enough to be detected. Second, it was observed that spacing of the anchor residues in the motifs for peptides binding to class I and II MHC molecules was consistent with the spacing of turns of an alpha helix, for example, at positions 2 and 9 (7 residues apart like two turns of a helix) or at positions 5 and 9 (spaced like one turn of a helix) (465). Because the anchor residues are most often hydrophobic, this pattern resulted in an amphipathic periodicity pattern like that of an amphipathic alpha helix for just the anchor residues alone, seen in the majority of motifs (465). Thus, if the other residues have a random pattern, the anchor residue spacing alone, which is enforced by the spacing of the pockets in the MHC molecules that bind these anchor residues, will produce the amphipathic helical signal, even though the peptide is bound in an extended conformation. This amphipathic helical periodicity has held up as a correlate for peptides defined as T-cell epitopes (465), and has continued to be a useful predictive tool for identifying potential epitopes, successful in a number of studies, when one does not want to focus on individual MHC alleles or wants to find regions of high epitope density.

Other approaches to predicting T-cell epitopes are generally based on sequences found to bind to specific MHC molecules (389,454). The simplest approach is to apply standard sequence search algorithms to known protein sequences to locate motifs for peptides binding to particular MHC molecules, using collections of motifs identified in the literature (242). This approach showed early success for epitopes in proteins from *Listeria monocytogenes* (466) and malaria (467), but it also became apparent that only about 30% of sequences bearing motifs actually bound to the corresponding MHC molecules (466,468,469). This discrepancy may relate to adverse interactions created by nonanchor residues (366,371,470), and could be overcome to some extent by generating extended motifs taking into account the role of each residue in the sequence (371,470).

To determine whether one could locate regions of proteins with high densities of motifs for binding multiple MHC molecules, Meister et al. (471) developed the algorithm Epimer, which determined the density of motifs per length of sequence. A surprising result was that the motifs were not uniformly distributed, but clustered. This clustering may reflect the fact that many motifs are related, and that the same anchor residues are shared by several motifs, perhaps because MHC molecules are also related and their variable segments that define some of the binding pockets are sometimes exchanged by gene-conversion events *(472)*. This hypothesis has now been confirmed and extended by studies showing that each anchor pocket can be grouped into families of MHC molecules sharing similar pockets and therefore anchor residues, but the families for the B, C, and F pockets do not coincide, so there is a reassortment between pockets (473,474). These observations allow prediction of motifs for additional MHC molecules. In the case of HIV, the densities of motifs for class I MHC binding were anomalous at both the low and high ends of the spectrum (475). Clustering at the high end may be due to anchor sharing, and showed no correlation with conserved or variable regions of the sequence. However, at the low end, long stretches with low motif density occurred preferentially in variable regions, suggesting that the virus was mutating to escape the CTL immune system (475). This clustering may be useful in vaccine development, because identification of sequences containing overlapping motifs for multiple MHC molecules may define promiscuously presented peptides that would elicit responses in a broad segment of the population (471).

Another type of MHC allele-specific approach is the use of matrices defining the positive or negative contribution of each amino acid possible at each position in the sequence toward binding to an MHC molecule. A positive or negative value is assigned to each of the 20 possible amino acids that can occur at each position in a peptide sequence, and these are summed to give the estimated potential of that peptide for binding. The values in the matrix are derived from either experimental binding studies using peptide panels with single positions substituted with each possible amino acid (404,476–478), or from comparisons of peptides known to bind in a compilation of the literature, if the number known is sufficiently large (454,479). Davenport et al. (480,481) also developed a motif method based on Edman degradation sequencing of pooled peptides eluted from MHC molecules. All of these methods have had some success in predicting peptides binding to particular MHC molecules (454), but they all require the assumption that each position in a peptide must be acting independently of its neighbors, which is a reasonable first approximation, but exceptions are known (482). The more experimental data that go into generating the matrix, the more reliable the predictions. Therefore, the predictive success may be greater for some of the more common HLA molecules for which more data exists. This matrix approach has been used for both class I and class II MHC molecules. Current predictive matrix algorithms, compared with experimental screening, have been found to detect most $CD8^+$ T-cell epitopes detected experimentally, for example, in vaccinia virus, in which the top-ranked 300 peptides using 4 different algorithms predicted 40/49 epitopes found (483).

A potentially very useful observation is the finding that HLA class I molecules can be grouped into families (HLA supertypes) that share similar binding motifs (403,476,484,485). The broader motifs that encompass several MHC molecules have been called *supermotifs*. For example, HLA-A0301, A1101, A3101, A3401, A6601, A6801, and A7401 all fall into the HLA-A3 superfamily (484). A peptide that carried this supermotif should be active in a broader range of individuals than one that was presented by a single HLA molecule. Moreover, because several HLA supertypes have been defined, it should be possible to design a vaccine effective in a large fraction of the population with only a limited number of well-selected antigenic determinants (486).

Another approach for predicting peptides that bind to MHC molecules is based on free energy calculations of peptides docked into the groove of a known MHC structure, for which the crystallographic coordinates are known, or on structural modeling of the MHC molecule by homologous extension from another MHC molecule, when the crystal structure is not known, followed by peptide docking calculations (487,488) It is important to use free energy rather than energy because the latter alone cannot find the most stable orientation of a side chain and cannot correctly rank order different side chains at the same position. This approach correctly predicts the structure of several known peptide–MHC complexes when starting with the crystal structure of a different complex, in each case to within 1.2 to 1.6 Å all-atom root-mean square deviation (488). Using this structural modeling can allow one to extend motifs to nonanchor positions for cases in which only anchor residue motifs are known, and can allow one to predict new motifs for MHC molecules whose motifs have not yet been determined.

Another approach to predicting MHC binding sequences uses a technique called *threading* that has been developed for predicting peptide secondary structure, based on threading a sequence through a series of known secondary structures, and calculating the energies of each structure. Altuvia et al. (489,490) showed that threading could be applied to peptides in the groove of MHC molecules, because when several peptides that bind to the same MHC molecule are compared crystallographically, the conformation of the peptides is fairly similar, as for example in several peptides crystallized bound to HLA-A2.1 (459). In testing the threading approach, Altuvia et al. (489,490) showed that known antigenic peptides are highly ranked among all peptides in a given protein sequence, and the rank order of peptides in competitive binding studies could be correctly predicted. The advantage of this approach is that it is independent of known binding motifs, and can identify peptides that bind despite lack of the common motif for the MHC molecule in question. It can also be used to rank a set of peptides all containing a known motif.

Finally, artificial neural networks (ANN) can be trained on a set of peptides that bind to a given MHC molecule to recognize patterns present in binding peptides (491). When the predictions of the ANN are tested, the results can be used to further train the ANN to improve the predictive capability in an iterative fashion.

Recently, predictive algorithms for proteasomal cleavage sites (492) and TAP-transported peptides (294) have been developed. Combining these into approaches to predict epitopes based on all the steps a peptide must pass through, cleavage, transport, and MHC binding, (except for TCR binding), has led to the most recent comprehensive algorithms for epitope prediction, which can achieve up to 62% sensitivity (295,493–497).

As all these methods are further developed and refined, they promise to allow accurate prediction of peptides that will bind to different MHC molecules and thus allow the design of vaccines without empirical binding studies until the end of the process. Further, localization of clusters of adjacent or overlapping binding sequences in a short segment of protein sequence can also be useful for selecting sequences that will be broadly recognized.

RELATIONSHIP BETWEEN HELPER T-CELL EPITOPES AND B-CELL EPITOPES ON A COMPLEX PROTEIN ANTIGEN

As we have seen, the factors that determine the location of antigenic sites for T cells and for B cells, with the possible exception of self-tolerance, are largely different. Indeed, if B cells (with their surface antibody) bind sites that tend to be especially exposed or protruding—sites that are also more accessible and susceptible to proteolytic enzymes—then there is reason to think that T cells may have a lower probability of being able to recognize these same sites, which may be more likely to be destroyed during processing. Certainly, assembled topographic sites will be destroyed during processing. On the other hand, there are examples in which T cells and antibodies seem to see the same, or very closely overlapping, sites on a protein *(43,163,193,498–500)*, although fine specificity analysis usually indicates that the antibody and T-cell fine specificities are not identical. The question dealt with here is whether there are any functional or regulatory factors in T cell–B cell cooperation that would produce a relationship between helper T-cell specificity and B-cell specificity for the same protein antigen.

Early evidence that helper T cells might influence the specificity of the antibodies produced came from a number of studies showing that *Ir* genes, which appeared to act through effects of T-cell help, could influence the specificity of antibodies produced to a given antigen *(159,501–508)*. It was hard to imagine how MHC-encoded *Ir* genes could determine which epitopes of a protein elicit antibodies, when such antibodies are generally not MHC-restricted. One explanation suggested was that the *Ir* genes first select which helper T cells are activated, and these in turn influence which B cells, specific for particular epitopes, could be activated *(110)*. Because, for cognate help, the B cell has to present the antigen in association with an MHC molecule to the helper T cell, the *Ir* gene control of antibody specificity must operate at least partly at this step by selecting which helper T cell can be activated by and help a given B cell. Conversely, if the helper T cell selects a subset of B cells to be activated on the basis of their antibody specificity, then there is a reciprocal interaction between T and B cells influencing each other's specificity. Therefore, this hypothesis was called *T–B reciprocity (110)*. Steric constraints on the epitopes that could be used by helper T cells to help a B cell specific for another particular epitope of the same protein were also proposed by Sercarz et al. *(509)*.

The concept was first tested by limiting the fine specificity of helper T cells to one or a few epitopes and then determining the effect on the specificities of antibodies produced in response to the whole molecule. This was accomplished by inducing T-cell tolerance to certain epitopes *(510)* or using T cells from animals immune to peptide fragments of the protein *(108,511,512)*. In each case, the limitation on the helper T-cell specificity repertoire influenced the repertoire of antibodies produced.

One purpose of the B-cell surface immunoglobulin is to take up the specific antigen with high affinity, which is then internalized by receptor-mediated endocytosis and processed like any other antigen *(513–520)*. Therefore, the explanation was proposed that the surface immunoglobulin, which acts as the receptor to mediate endocytosis, sterically influences the rate at which different parts of the antigen are processed, because what the B cell is processing is not free antigen but a monoclonal antibody–antigen immune complex *(110)*. This concept presupposes that many antibody–antigen complexes are stable near pH 6 in the endosome and that what matters is the kinetics of production of large fragments, rather than the products of complete digestion, when both the antigen and the antibody may be degraded to single amino acids. Such protection from proteolysis of antigen epitopes by bound antibody can be demonstrated at least *in vitro (54)*. The effect of antigen-specific B-cell surface immunoglobulin on the fragments produced by proteolytic processing of antigen was elegantly demonstrated by Davidson and Watts *(521)*. They demonstrated that the pattern of fragmentation of tetanus toxoid, as measured by SDS–polyacrylamide gel electrophoresis, produced during processing by B lymphoblastoid clones specific for tetanus toxoid, varied among B-cell clones depending on their specificity for different epitopes within the antigen. Binding to the antibody may also influence which fragments are shuttled to the surface and which are shunted into true lysosomes for total degradation. Thus different B cells bearing different surface immunoglobulin would preferentially process the antigen differently to put more of some potential fragments than others on their surface, in contrast to nonspecific-presenting cells that would process the antigen indifferently. By this mechanism, it is proposed that B-cell specificity leads to selective antigen presentation to helper T cells and therefore to selective help from T cells specific for some epitopes more than from T cells specific for others *(110)*.

To test this hypothesis, Ozaki and Berzofsky *(109)* made populations of B cells effectively monoclonal for purposes of antigen presentation by coating polyclonal B cells with a conjugate of monoclonal antimyoglobin coupled to anti-IgM antibodies. B cells coated with one such conjugate presented myoglobin less well to one myoglobin-specific

T-cell clone than to others. B cells coated with other conjugates presented myoglobin to this clone equally well as to other clones. Therefore, the limitation on myoglobin presentation by this B cell to this T-cell clone depended on the specificity of both the monoclonal antibody coating the B cell and the receptor of the T-cell clone. It happened in this case that both the monoclonal antibody and the T-cell clone were specific for the same or closely overlapping epitopes. Therefore, it appears that the site bound by the B-cell surface immunoglobulin is less well presented to T cells. This finding is also consistent with a study of chimeric proteins in which one or more copies of an ovalbumin helper T-cell determinant were inserted in different positions (522). Although the position of the ovalbumin determinants did not affect the antibody response to one epitope, the position did matter for antibody production to an epitope of the chimeric protein derived from insulinlike growth factor I. An ovalbumin determinant inserted distal to this epitope was much more effective in providing help than one inserted adjacent to the same epitope, when both constructs were used as immunogens, even though both constructs elicited similar levels of ovalbumin-specific T-cell proliferation in the presence of nonspecific presenting cells *in vitro*, as a control for nonspecific effects of flanking residues on processing and presentation of the helper T-cell determinants. However, circumstantial evidence from the *Ir* gene studies mentioned previously suggests that T cells may preferentially help B cells that bind with some degree of proximity to the T-cell epitope, as there was a correlation between T cell and antibody specificity for large fragments of protein antigens under *Ir* gene control *(107,110,159,504,505,508)*. Therefore, antibodies may have both positive and negative selective effects on processing.

Further studies on presentation of β-galactosidase–monoclonal antibody complexes by nonspecific APCs suggest similar conclusions (*523*,524). Presumably, the conjugates are taken up via immunoglobulin fragment c (Fc) receptors on the presenting cells and processed differentially according to the site bound by the antibody, so that they are presented differentially to different T-cell clones. Thus, non–B-presenting cells can be made to mimic specific B-presenting cells. This also suggests that circulating antibody may have a role in the selection of which T cells are activated in a subsequent exposure to antigen.

The issue of whether bound antibody enhanced or suppressed presentation of specific determinants to T cells was explored further by Watts and Lanzavecchia (525) and their coworkers (Simitsek et al. [526]). They first found that a particular tetanus-toxoid–specific Epstein-Barr virus-transformed human B-cell clone 11.3 failed to present the tetanus-toxoid epitope 1174-1189 to specific T cells, whereas it presented another epitope as well as did other B cells, and another B-cell clone presented the 1174-1189 epitope well. Moreover, the free 11.3 antibody also inhibited presentation of this epitope to T cells at the same time that it enhanced presentation of other epitopes by Fc receptor facilitated uptake (525). They subsequently found that the same 11.3 B cell and antibody actually enhanced presentation of another epitope of tetanus toxoid, 1273-1284, by about 10-fold, even though both epitopes were within the footprint of the antibody, as determined by protection from proteolytic digestion (526). The enhancement could be mediated also by free antibody as well as Fab fragments thereof, indicating that the mechanism did not involve Fc receptor-facilitated uptake. Further, the 11.3 antibody had no effect on presentation of another determinant in the same tetanus toxoid C fragment, 947-967, that was not within the footprint of the antibody, and another antibody to the C fragment did not enhance presentation of 1273-1284. The authors conclude that the same antibody or surface immunoglobulin can protect two determinants from proteolysis, but sterically hinder the binding of one to class II MHC molecules while facilitating the binding of the other (526). The facilitation may involve protection from degradation. This antibody-mediated enhancement of presentation of selected epitopes to helper T cells can greatly lower the threshold for induction of a T-cell response, and may thereby elicit responses to otherwise subdominant epitopes. It can also contribute to epitope spreading, for example, in autoimmune disease, in which an initial response to one dominant determinant leads to a subsequent response to other subdominant determinants, perhaps by helping for antibody production, which in turn facilitates presentation of the other determinants.

Taken together, these results support the concept of T–B reciprocity in which helper T cells and B cells each influence the specificity of the other's expressed repertoire *(110)*. This mechanism may also provide an explanation for some of the cases in which *Ir* genes have been found to control antibody idiotype *(527,528)*. These relationships probably play a significant role in regulating the fine specificity of immune response of both arms of the immune system. Therefore, they will also be of importance in the design of synthetic or recombinant fragment vaccines that incorporate both T- and B-cell epitopes to elicit an antibody response.

CONCLUSION

Overall, antibodies and T cells recognize different structural features in different contexts or environments, and thus complement each other to detect the spectrum of foreign (or self) antigens encountered. Antibodies recognize three-dimensional structures on the exposed surface of molecules either in solution or on a cell surface. Therefore, they are very dependent on the conformation of the antigen and can recognize structures that are assembled on the surface of the antigen molecule by the way it folds but that are not contiguous in the primary sequence. However, they do not generally recognize structures buried within protein molecules or inside cells. In contrast, T cells are designed to recognize short segments of primary amino acid sequence of protein antigens, and thus are not dependent on the conformation of the original protein, unless it affects processing. Furthermore, T cells particularly provide internal surveillance of proteins inside cells, recognizing peptide fragments of these presented by MHC molecules that carry these fragments to the cell surface.

This surveillance of intracellular proteins requires a number of hurdles including proteolytic processing of the antigen into fragments, transport of these into the compartments where they are loaded onto MHC molecules, binding with appropriate specificity to the combining site of specific MHC molecules, and then finally recognition by an appropriate T-cell receptor. These hurdles limit the number of amino acid sequences that can be recognized and account in part for immunodominance. Furthermore, the two major subsets of T cells also complement each other by recognizing exogenous and endogenous proteins processed and transported through different pathways and presented by difference classes of MHC molecules. Thus, the two major classes of T cells complement the types of structures and the locales surveyed by antibodies. For example, in the case of viruses, antibodies can detect intact virions and shed viral proteins in solution as well as viral proteins expressed on the surface of infected cells, $CD4^+$ T cells can recognize viral proteins taken up by antigen-presenting cells and processed in an endosomal pathway, and $CD8^+$ T cells can detect proteins synthesized within the infected cell, whether or not they are ever expressed intact on the cell surface or secreted. Together, they provide the immune system with a strategy to detect all forms of foreign invaders as well as to protect the host through different effector mechanisms.

REFERENCES

23. Cygler M, Rose DR, Bundle DR. Recognition of a cell-surface oligosaccharide of pathogenic Salmonella by an antibody Fab fragment. *Science*. 1991;253:442–445.
24. Bundle DR, Eichler E, Gidney MA, et al. Molecular recognition of a Salmonella trisaccharide epitope by monoclonal antibody Se155-154. *Biochemistry*. 1994;33:5172–5182.
25. Jeffrey PD, Bajorath J, Chang CY, et al. The x-ray structure of an anti-tumour antibody in complex with antigen. *Nat Struct Biol*. 1995;2:466–471.
26. Ramsland PA, Farrugia W, Bradford TM, et al. Structural convergence of antibody binding of carbohydrate determinants in Lewis Y tumor antigens. *J Mol Biol*. 2004;340:809–818.
27. Calarese DA, Scanlan CN, Zwick MB, et al. Antibody domain exchange is an immunological solution to carbohydrate cluster recognition. *Science*. 2003;300:2065–2071.
28. Calarese DA, Lee HK, Huang CY, et al. Dissection of the carbohydrate specificity of the broadly neutralizing anti-HIV-1 antibody 2G12. *Proc Natl Acad Sci U S A*. 2005;102:13372–13377.
30. Robbins JB, Schneerson R, Anderson P, et al. The 1996 Albert Lasker Medical Research Awards. Prevention of systemic infections, especially meningitis, caused by *Haemophilus influenzae type b*. Impact on public health and implications for other polysaccharide-based vaccines. *JAMA*. 1996;276:1181–1185.
31. Murphy TV, White KE, Pastor P, et al. Declining incidence of Haemophilus influenzae type b disease since introduction of vaccination. *JAMA*. 1993;269:246–248.
32. Black S, Shinefield H, Fireman B, et al. Efficacy, safety and immunogenicity of heptavalent pneumococcal conjugate vaccine in children. Northern California Kaiser Permanente Vaccine Study Center Group. *Pediatr Infect Dis J*. 2000;19:187–195.
33. Eskola J, Kilpi T, Palmu A, et al. Efficacy of a pneumococcal conjugate vaccine against acute otitis media. *N Engl J Med*. 2001;344:403–409.
37. Davies DR, Padlan EA. Antibody-antigen complexes. *Annu Rev Biochem*. 1990;59:439–473.
72. Kwong PD, Wyatt R, Robinson J, et al. Structure of an HIV gp120 envelope glycoprotein in complex with the CD4 receptor and a neutralizing human antibody. *Nature*. 1998;393:648–659.
73. Wyatt R, Kwong PD, Desjardins E, et al. The antigenic structure of the HIV gp120 envelope glycoprotein. *Nature*. 1998;393:705–711.
104. Rini JM, Schulze-Gahmen U, Wilson IA. Structural evidence for induced fit as a mechanism for antibody-antigen recognition. *Science*. 1992;255:959–965.
124. Kaplan G, Freistadt MS, Racaniello VR. Neutralization of poliovirus by cell receptors expressed in insect cells. *J Virol*. 1990;64:4697–4702.
132. Gorny MK, VanCott TC, Hioe C, et al. Human monoclonal antibodies to the V3 loop of HIV-1 with intra- and interclade cross-reactivity. *J Immunol*. 1997;159:5114–5122.
133. Gorny MK, Williams C, Volsky B, et al. Human monoclonal antibodies specific for conformation-sensitive epitopes of V3 neutralize human immunodeficiency virus type 1 primary isolates from various clades. *J Virol*. 2002;76:9035–9045.
134. Sharon M, Kessler N, Levy R, et al. Alternative Conformations of HIV-1 V3 Loops Mimic beta Hairpins in Chemokines, Suggesting a Mechanism for Coreceptor Selectivity. *Structure (Camb)*. 2003;11:225–236.
136. Kang C-Y, Nara P, Chamat S, et al. Evidence for non-V3-specific neutralizing antibodies that interfere with gp120/CD4 binding in human immunodeficiency virus 1-infected humans. *Proc Natl Acad Sci U S A*. 1991;88:6171–6175.
137. Berkower I, Murphy D, Smith CC, et al. A predominant group-specific neutralizing epitope of human immunodeficiency virus type 1 maps to residues 342 to 511 of the envelope glycoprotein gp120. *J Virol*. 1991;65:5983–5990.
138. Thali M, Olshevsky U, Furman C, et al. Characterization of a discontinuous human immunodeficiency virus type 1 gp120 epitope recognized by a broadly reactive neutralizing human monoclonal antibody. *J Virol*. 1991;65:6188–6193.
139. Tilley SA, Honnen WJ, Racho ME, et al. A human monoclonal antibody against the CD4-binding site of HIV1 gp120 exhibits potent, broadly neutralizing activity. *Res Virol*. 1991;142:247–259.
140. Kessler JA, 2nd, McKenna PM, Emini EA, et al. Recombinant human monoclonal antibody IgG1b12 neutralizes diverse human immunodeficiency virus type 1 primary isolates. *AIDS Res Hum Retroviruses*. 1997;13:575–582.
141. Trkola A, Purtscher M, Muster T, et al. Human monoclonal antibody 2G12 defines a distinctive neutralization epitope on the gp120 glycoprotein of human immunodeficiency virus type 1. *J Virol*. 1996;70:1100–1108.
142. Muster T, Steindl F, Purtscher M, et al. A conserved neutralizing epitope on gp41 of human immunodeficiency virus type 1. *J Virol*. 1993;67:6642–6647.
143. Eckhart L, Raffelsberger W, Ferko B, et al. Immunogenic presentation of a conserved gp41 epitope of human immunodeficiency virus type 1 on recombinant surface antigen of hepatitis B virus. *J Gen Virol*. 1996;77:2001–2008.
144. Burton DR. A vaccine for HIV type 1: the antibody perspective. *Proc Natl Acad Sci U S A*. 1997;94:10018–10023.
145. Trkola A, Ketas T, Kewalramani VN, et al. Neutralization sensitivity of human immunodeficiency virus type 1 primary isolates to antibodies and CD4-based reagents is independent of coreceptor usage. *J Virol*. 1998;72:1876–1885.

146. Baba TW, Liska V, Hofmann-Lehmann R, et al. Human neutralizing monoclonal antibodies of the IgG1 subtype protect against mucosal simian-human immunodeficiency virus infection. *Nat Med.* 2000;6:200–206.
147. Mascola JR, Stiegler G, VanCott TC, et al. Protection of macaques against vaginal transmission of a pathogenic HIV-1/SIV chimeric virus by passive infusion of neutralizing antibodies. *Nat Med.* 2000;6:207–210.
148. Steimer KS, Scandella CJ, Skiles PV, et al. Neutralization of divergent HIV-1 isolates by conformation-dependent human antibodies to Gp120. *Science.* 1991;254:105–108.
149. Benacerraf B, McDevitt HO. Histocompatibility-linked immune response genes. *Science.* 1972;175:273–279.
164. Kurokohchi K, Akatsuka T, Pendleton CD, et al. Use of recombinant protein to identify a motif-negative human CTL epitope presented by HLA-A2 in the hepatitis C virus NS3 region. *J Virol.* 1996;70:232–240.
172. Hosmalin A, Clerici M, Houghten R, et al. An epitope in HIV-1 reverse transcriptase recognized by both mouse and human CTL. *Proc Natl Acad Sci U S A.* 1990;87:2344–2348.
177. England RE, Kullberg MC, Cornette JL, et al. Molecular analysis of a heteroclitic T-cell response to the immunodominant epitope of sperm whale myoglobin: implications for peptide partial agonists. *J Immunol.* 1995;155:4295–4306.
178. Gammon G, Geysen HM, Apple RJ, et al. T cell determinant structure: Cores and determinant envelopes in three mouse major histocompatibility complex haplotypes. *J Exp Med.* 1991;173:609–617.
185. Van der Bruggen P, Traversari C, Chomez P, et al. A gene encoding an antigen recognized by cytolytic T lymphocytes on a human melanoma. *Science.* 1991;254:1643–1647.
186. Guilloux Y, Lucas S, Brichard VG, et al. A peptide recognized by human cytolytic T lymphocytes on HLA-A2 melanomas is encoded by an intron sequence of the N-Acetylglucosaminyltransferase B gene. *J Exp Med.* 1996;183:1173–1183.
187. Kawakami Y, Eliyahu S, Delgado CH, et al. Cloning of the gene coding for a shared human melanoma antigen recognized by autologous T cells infiltrating into tumor. *Proc Natl Acad Sci U S A.* 1994;91:3515–3519.
188. Robbins PF, El-Gamil M, Li YF, et al. A mutated b-catenin gene encodes a melanoma-specific antigen recognized by tumor infiltrating lymphocytes. *J Exp Med.* 1996;183:1185–1192.
189. Wang R-F, Parkhurst MR, Kawakami Y, et al. Utilization of an alternative open reading frame of a normal gene in generating a novel human cancer antigen. *J Exp Med.* 1996;183:1131–1140.
210. Yewdell JW, Bennink JR. Immunodominance in major histocompatibility complex class I-restricted T lymphocyte responses. *Annu Rev Immunol.* 1999;17:51–88.
215. Nanda NK, Arzoo KK, Geysen HM, et al. Recognition of mutiple peptide cores by a single T cell receptor. *J Exp Med.* 1995;182:531–539.
218. Sercarz EE, Lehmann PV, Ametani A, et al. Dominance and crypticity of T cell antigenic determinants. *Annu Rev Immunol.* 1993;11:729–766.
222. Grewal IS, Moudgil KD, Sercarz EE. Hindrance of binding to class II major histocompatibility complex molecules by a single amino acid residue contiguous to a determinant leads to crypticity of the determinant as well as lack of response to the protein antigen. *Proc Natl Acad Sci U S A.* 1995;92:1779–1783.
230. Rudensky AY, Preston-Hurlburt P, Hong S-C, et al. Sequence analysis of peptides bound to MHC class II molecules. *Nature.* 1991;353:622–627.
231. Stern LJ, Brown JH, Jardetzky TS, et al. Crystal structure of the human class II MHC protein HLA-DR1 complexed with an influenza virus peptide. *Nature.* 1994;368:215–221.
232. Stern LJ, Wiley DC. Antigenic peptide binding by class I and class II histocompatibility proteins. *Structure.* 1994;2:245–251.
233. Arunachalam B, Phan UT, Geuze HJ, et al. Enzymatic reduction of disulfide bonds in lysosomes: characterization of a gamma-interferon-inducible lysosomal thiol reductase (GILT). *Proc Natl Acad Sci U S A.* 2000;97:745–50.
234. Maric M, Arunachalam B, Phan UT, et al. Defective Antigen Processing in GILT-Free Mice. *Science.* 2001;294:1361–1365.
237. Tobery T, Siliciano RF. Targeting of HIV-1 antigens for rapid intracellular degradation enhances cytotoxic T lymphocytes (CTL) recognition and the induction of De Novo CTL responses in vivo after immunization. *J Exp Med.* 1997;185:909–920.
238. York IA, Goldberg AL, Mo XY, et al. Proteolysis and class I major histocompatibility complex antigen presentation. *Immunol Rev.* 1999;172:49–66.
239. Yewdell JW, Bennink JR. Cut and trim: generating MHC class I peptide ligands. *Curr Opin Immunol.* 2001;13:13–18.
240. Vinitsky A, Antón LC, Snyder HL, et al. The generation of MHC class I-associated peptides is only partially inhibited by proteasome inhibitors Involvement of nonproteasomal cytosolic proteases in antigen processing? *J Immunol.* 1997;159:554–564.
241. Rock KL, Gramm C, Rothstein L, et al. Inhibitors of the proteasome block the degradation of most cell proteins and the generation of peptides presented on MHC class I molecules. *Cell.* 1994;78:761–771.
242. Rammensee H-G, Friede T, Stevanovíc S. MHC ligands and peptide motifs: first listing. *Immunogenetics.* 1995;41:178–228.
243. Vinitsky A, Cardozo C, Sepp-Lorenzino L, et al. Inhibition of the proteolytic activity of the multicatalytic proteinase complex (proteasome) by substrate-related peptidyl aldehydes. *J Biol Chem.* 1994;269:29860–29866.
244. Fenteany G, Standaert RF, Lane WS, et al. Inhibition of proteasome activities and subunit-specific amino-terminal threonine modification by lactacystin. *Science.* 1995;268:726–731.
245. Hughes EA, Ortmann B, Surman M, et al. The protease inhibitor, N-Acetyl-L-Leucyl-L-Leucyl-L-Norleucinal, decreases the pool of major histocompatibility complex class I-binding peptides and inhibits peptide trimming in the endoplasmic reticulum. *J Exp Med.* 1996;183:1569–1578.
246. Henderson RA, Michel H, Sakaguchi K, et al. HLA-A2.1-associated peptides from a mutant cell line: a second pathway of antigen presentation. *Science.* 1992;255:1264–1266.
247. Yewdell J. To DRiP or not to DRiP: generating peptide ligands for MHC class I molecules from biosynthesized proteins. *Mol Immunol.* 2002;39:139–146.
248. Princiotta MF, Finzi D, Qian SB, et al. Quantitating protein synthesis, degradation, and endogenous antigen processing. *Immunity.* 2003;18:343–354.
249. Qian SB, Reits E, Neefjes J, et al. Tight linkage between translation and MHC class I peptide ligand generation implies specialized antigen processing for defective ribosomal products. *J Immunol.* 2006;177:227–233.
250. Gaczynska M, Rock KL, Goldberg AL. g-Interferon and expression of MHC genes regulate peptide hydrolysis by proteasomes. *Nature.* 1993;365:264–267.
251. Van Kaer L, Ashton-Rickardt PG, Eichelberger M, et al. Altered peptidase and viral-specific T cell response in LMP2 mutant mice. *Immunity.* 1994;1:533–541.
252. Fehling HJ, Swat W, Laplace C, et al. MHC class I expression in mice lacking the proteasome subunit LMP-7. *Science.* 1994;265:1234–1237.
253. Toes RE, Nussbaum AK, Degermann S, et al. Discrete cleavage motifs of constitutive and immunoproteasomes revealed by quantitative analysis of cleavage products. *J Exp Med.* 2001;194:1–12.
254. Sijts AJ, Ruppert T, Rehermann B, et al. Efficient generation of a hepatitis B virus cytotoxic T lymphocyte epitope requires the structural features of immunoproteasomes. *J Exp Med.* 2000;191:503–514.
255. Sijts AJ, Standera S, Toes RE, et al. MHC class I antigen processing of an adenovirus CTL epitope is linked to the levels of immunoproteasomes in infected cells. *J Immunol.* 2000;164:4500–4506.
256. Schwarz K, van Den Broek M, Kostka S, et al. Overexpression of the proteasome subunits LMP2, LMP7, and MECL-1, but not PA28 alpha/beta, enhances the presentation of an immunodominant lymphocytic choriomeningitis virus T cell epitope. *J Immunol.* 2000;165:768–778.
257. Ito Y, Kondo E, Demachi-Okamura A, et al. Three immunoproteasome-associated subunits cooperatively generate a cytotoxic T-lymphocyte epitope of Epstein-Barr virus LMP2A by overcoming specific structures resistant to epitope liberation. *J Virol.* 2006; 80:883–890.

258. Morel S, Levy F, Burlet-Schiltz O, et al. Processing of some antigens by the standard proteasome but not by the immunoproteasome results in poor presentation by dendritic cells. *Immunity*. 2000;12:107–117.
259. Chen W, Norbury CC, Cho Y, et al. Immunoproteasomes shape immunodominance hierarchies of antiviral CD8(+) T cells at the levels of T cell repertoire and presentation of viral antigens. *J Exp Med*. 2001;193:1319–1326.
260. Dubiel W, Pratt G, Ferrell K, et al. Purification of an 11 S regulator of the multicatalytic protease. *J Biol Chem*. 1992;267:22369–22377.
261. Dick TP, Ruppert T, Groettrup M, et al. Coordinated dual cleavages induced by the proteasome regulator PA28 lead to dominant MHC ligands. *Cell*. 1996;86:253–262.
262. van Hall T, Sijts A, Camps M, et al. Differential influence on cytotoxic T lymphocyte epitope presentation by controlled expression of either proteasome immunosubunits or PA28. *J Exp Med*. 2000;192:483–494.
263. Goldberg AL, Rock KL. Proteolysis, proteasomes and antigen presentation. *Nature*. 1992;357:375–379.
264. Reits E, Neijssen J, Herberts C, et al. A major role for TPPII in trimming proteasomal degradation products for MHC class I antigen presentation. *Immunity*. 2004;20:495–506.
265. Kloetzel PM. Generation of major histocompatibility complex class I antigens: functional interplay between proteasomes and TPPII. *Nat Immunol*. 2004;5:661–669.
266. Seifert U, Maranon C, Shmueli A, et al. An essential role for tripeptidyl peptidase in the generation of an MHC class I epitope. *Nat Immunol*. 2003;4:375–379.
267. Monaco JJ, Cho S, Attaya M. Transport protein genes in the murine MHC: possible implications for antigen processing. *Science*. 1990;250:1723–1726.
268. Deverson EV, Gow IR, Coadwell WJ, et al. MHC class II region encoding proteins related to the multidrug resistance family of transmembrane transporters. *Nature*. 1990;348:738–741.
269. Trowsdale J, Hanson I, Mockridge I, et al. Sequences encoded in the class II region of the MHC related to the "ABC" superfamily of transporters. *Nature*. 1990;348:741–743.
271. Schumacher TNM, Heemels M-T, Neefjes JJ, et al. Direct binding of peptide to empty MHC class I molecules on intact cells and in vitro. *Cell*. 1990;62:563–567.
272. Ortmann B, Androlewicz MJ, Cresswell P. MHC class I/b2-microglobulin complexes associate with TAP transporters before peptide binding. *Nature*. 1994;368:864–867.
273. Suh W-K, Cohen-Doyle MF, Fruh K, et al. Interaction of MHC class I molecules with the transporter associated with antigen processing. *Science*. 1994;264:1322–1326.
275. Livingstone AM, Powis SJ, Günther E, et al. Cim: An MHC class II-linked allelism affecting the antigenicity of a classical class I molecule for T lymphocytes. *Immunogenetics*. 1991;34:157–163.
276. Powis SJ, Deverson EV, Coadwell WJ, et al. Effect of polymorphism of an MHC-linked transporter on the peptides assembled in a class I molecule. *Nature*. 1992;357:211–215.
277. Powis SJ, Young LL, Joly E, et al. The rat cim effect: TAP allele-dependent changes in a class I MHC anchor motif and evidence against C-terminal trimming of peptides in the ER. *Immunity*. 1996;4:159–165.
278. Neefjes JJ, Momburg F, Hämmerling GJ. Selective and ATP-dependent translocation of peptides by the MHC-encoded transporter. *Science*. 1993;261:769–771.
279. Neefjes J, Gottfried E, Roelse J, et al. Analysis of the fine specificity of rat, mouse and human TAP peptide transporters. *Eur J Immunol*. 1995;25:1133–1136.
280. Androlewicz MJ, Cresswell P. Human transporters associated with antigen processing possess a promiscuous peptide-binding site. *Immunity*. 1994;1:7–14.
281. Schumacher TNM, Kantesaria DV, Heemels M-T, et al. Peptide length and sequence specificity of the mouse TAP1/TAP2 translocator. *J Exp Med*. 1994;179:533–540.
282. van Endert PM, Riganelli D, Greco G, et al. The peptide-binding motif for the human transporter associated with antigen processing. *J Exp Med*. 1995;182:1883–1895.
283. van Endert PM. Peptide selection for presentation by HLA class I: A role for the human transporter associated with antigen processing? *Immunol Res*. 1996;15:265–279.
284. Gubler B, Daniel S, Armandola EA, et al. Substrate selection by transporters associated with antigen processing occurs during peptide binding to TAP. *Mol Immunol*. 1998;35:427–433.
285. Daniel S, Brusic V, Caillat-Zucman S, et al. Relationship between peptide selectivities of human transporters associated with antigen processing and HLA class I molecules. *J Immunol*. 1998;161:617–624.
286. Uebel S, Kraas W, Kienle S, et al. Recognition principle of the TAP transporter disclosed by combinatorial peptide libraries. *Proc Natl Acad Sci U S A*. 1997;94:8976–8981.
287. Fruci D, Niedermann G, Butler RH, et al. Efficient MHC class I-independent amino-terminal trimming of epitope precursor peptides in the endoplasmic reticulum. *Immunity*. 2001;15:467–476.
288. Lauvau G, Kakimi K, Niedermann G, et al. Human transporters associated with antigen processing (TAPs) select epitope precursor peptides for processing in the endoplasmic reticulum and presentation to T cells. *J Exp Med*. 1999;190:1227–1240.
289. Serwold T, Gaw S, Shastri N. ER aminopeptidases generate a unique pool of peptides for MHC class I molecules. *Nat Immunol*. 2001;2:644–651.
290. Serwold T, Gonzalez F, Kim J, et al. ERAAP customizes peptides for MHC class I molecules in the endoplasmic reticulum. *Nature*. 2002;419:480–483.
291. York IA, Chang SC, Saric T, et al. The ER aminopeptidase ERAP1 enhances or limits antigen presentation by trimming epitopes to 8–9 residues. *Nat Immunol*. 2002;3:1177–1184.
292. Saric T, Chang SC, Hattori A, et al. An IFN-gamma-induced aminopeptidase in the ER, ERAP1, trims precursors to MHC class I-presented peptides. *Nat Immunol*. 2002;3:1169–1176.
293. Paradela A, Alvarez I, Garcia-Peydro M, et al. Limited diversity of peptides related to an alloreactive T cell epitope in the HLA-B27-bound peptide repertoire results from restrictions at multiple steps along the processing-loading pathway. *J Immunol*. 2000;164:329–337.
294. Peters B, Bulik S, Tampe R, et al. Identifying MHC class I epitopes by predicting the TAP transport efficiency of epitope precursors. *J Immunol*. 2003;171:1741–1749.
295. Tenzer S, Peters B, Bulik S, et al. Modeling the MHC class I pathway by combining predictions of proteasomal cleavage, TAP transport and MHC class I binding. *Cell Mol Life Sci*. 2005;62:1025–1037.
296. York IA, Roop C, Andrews DW, et al. A cytosolic herpes simplex virus protein inhibits antigen presentation to CD8+ T lymphocytes. *Cell*. 1994;77:525–535.
297. Früh K, Ahn K, Djaballah H, et al. A viral inhibitor of peptide transporters for antigen presentation. *Nature*. 1995;375:415–418.
298. Hill A, Jugovic P, York I, et al. Herpes simplex virus turns off the TAP to evade host immunity. *Nature*. 1995;375:411–415.
300. Brodsky FM, Guagliardi LE. The cell biology of antigen processing and presentation. *Annu Rev Immunol*. 1991;9:707–744.
301. Germain RN, Margulies DH. The biochemistry and cell biology of antigen processing and presentation. *Annu Rev Immunol*. 1993;11:403–450.
303. Roche PA, Cresswell P. Invariant chain association with HLA-DR molecules inhibits immunogenic peptide binding. *Nature*. 1990;345:615–618.
304. Teyton L, O'Sullivan D, Dickson PW, et al. Invariant chain distinguishes between the exogenous and endogenous antigen presentation pathways. *Nature*. 1990;348:39–44.
305. Roche PA, Cresswell P. Proteolysis of the class II-associated invariant chain generates a peptide binding site in intracellular HLA-DR molecules. *Proc Natl Acad Sci U S A*. 1991;88:3150–3154.
306. Bodmer H, Viville S, Benoist C, et al. Diversity of endogenous epitopes bound to MHC class II molecules limited by invariant chain. *Science*. 1994;263:1284–1286.
307. Long EO, LaVaute T, Pinet V, et al. Invariant chain prevents the HLA-DR-restricted presentation of a cytosolic peptide. *J Immunol*. 1994;153:1487–1494.
308. Roche PA, Marks MS, Cresswell P. Formation of a nine-subunit complex by HLA class II glycoproteins and the invariant chain. *Nature*. 1991;354:392–394.

309. Fling SP, Arp B, Pious D. HLA-DMA and -DMB genes are both required for MHC class II/peptide complex formation in antigen-presenting cells. *Nature*. 1994;368:554–558.
310. Sadegh-Nasseri S, Stern LJ, Wiley DC, et al. MHC class II function preserved by low-affinity peptide interactions preceding stable binding. *Nature*. 1994;370:647–650.
311. Mellins E, Kempin S, Smith L, et al. A gene required for class II-restricted antigen presentation maps to the major histocompatibility complex. *J Exp Med*. 1991;174:1607–1615.
312. Riberdy JM, Newcomb JR, Surman MJ, et al. HLA-DR molecules from an antigen-processing mutant cell line are associated with invariant chain peptides. *Nature*. 1992;360:474–477.
313. Morris P, Shaman J, Attaya M, et al. An essential role for HLA-DM in antigen presentation by class II major histocompatibility molecules. *Nature*. 1994;368:551–554.
314. Sette A, Ceman S, Kubo RT, et al. Invariant chain of peptides in most HLA-DR molecules of an antigen-processing mutant. *Science*. 1992;258:1801–1804.
315. Denzin LK, Cresswell P. HLA-DM induces CLIP dissociation from MHC class II ab dimers and facilitates peptide loading. *Cell*. 1995;82:155–165.
316. Denzin LK, Robbins NF, Carboy-Newcome C, et al. Assembly and intracellular transport of HLA-DM and correction of the class II antigen-processing defect in T2 cells. *Immunity*. 1994;1: 595–606.
317. Alfonso C, Han JO, Williams GS, et al. The impact of H2-DM on humoral immune responses. *J Immunol*. 2001;167:6348–6355.
318. Sloan VS, Cameron P, Porter G, et al. Mediation by HLA-DM of dissociation of peptides from HLA-DR. *Nature*. 1995;375:802–806.
319. Sherman MA, Weber DA, Jensen PE. DM enhances peptide binding to class II MHC by release of invariant chain-derived peptide. *Immunity*. 1995;3:197–205.
326. Demotz S, Grey HM, Sette A. The minimal number of class II MHC-antigen complexes needed for T cell activation. *Science*. 1990;249:1028–1030.
327. Harding CV, Unanue ER. Quantitation of antigen-presenting cell MHC class II/peptide complexes necessary for T-cell stimulation. *Nature*. 1990;346:574–576.
328. Christinck ER, Luscher MA, Barber BH, et al. Peptide binding to class I MHC on living cells and quantitation of complexes required for CTL lysis. *Nature*. 1991;352:67–70.
330. Kirnbauer R, Booy F, Cheng N, et al. Papillomavirus L1 major capsid protein self-assembles into virus-like particles that are highly immunogenic. *Proc Natl Acad Sci U S A*. 1992;89:12180–12184.
331. Stoute JA, Slaoui M, Heppner G, et al. A preliminary evaluation of a recombinant circumsporozoite protein vaccine against plasmodium falciparum malaria. *New Engl J Med*. 1997;336:86–91.
332. Takeshita T, Kozlowski S, England RD, et al. Role of conserved regions of class I MHC molecules in the activation of CD8+ CTL by peptide and purified cell-free class I molecules. *Int Immunol*. 1993;5:1129–1138.
333. Brower RC, England R, Takeshita T, et al. Minimal requirements for peptide mediated activation of CD8+ CTL. *Molec Immunol*. 1994;31:1285–1293.
345. Kurata A, Berzofsky JA. Analysis of peptide residues interacting with MHC molecule or T-cell receptor: can a peptide bind in more than one way to the same MHC molecule? *J Immunol*. 1990;144: 4526–4535.
350. Madden DR, Gorga JC, Strominger JL, et al. The structure of HLA-B27 reveals nonamer self-peptides bound in an extended conformation. *Nature*. 1991;353:321–325.
351. Matsumura M, Fremont DH, Peterson PA, et al. Emerging principles for the recognition of peptide antigens by MHC class I molecules. *Science*. 1992;257:927–934.
352. Fremont DH, Matsumura M, Stura EA, et al. Crystal structures of two viral peptides in complex with murine MHC class I H-2Kb. *Science*. 1992;257:919–927.
359. Vasmatzis G, Cornette J, Sezerman U, et al. TcR recognition of the MHC-peptide dimer: Structural properties of a ternary complex. *J Mol Biol*. 1996;261:72–89.
360. Garcia KC, Degano M, Stanfield RL, et al. An ab T cell receptor structure at 2.5Å and its orientation in the TCR-MHC complex. *Science*. 1996;274:209–219.
361. Garboczi DN, Ghosh P, Utz U, et al. Structure of the complex between human T-cell receptor, viral peptide and HLA-A2. *Nature*. 1996;384:134–141.
365. Racioppi L, Ronchese F, Schwartz RH, et al. The molecular basis of class II MHC allelic control of T cell responses. *J Immunol*. 1991; 147:3718–3727.
366. Boehncke W-H, Takeshita T, Pendleton CD, et al. The importance of dominant negative effects of amino acids side chain substitution in peptide-MHC molecule interactions and T cell recognition. *J Immunol*. 1993;150:331–341.
368. Jardetzky TS, Gorga JC, Busch R, et al. Peptide binding to HLA-DR1: a peptide with most residues substituted to alanine retains MHC binding. *EMBO J*. 1990;9:1797–1803.
370. Maryanski JL, Verdini AS, Weber PC, et al. Competitor analogs for defined T cell antigens: peptides incorporating a putative binding motif and polyproline or polyglycine spacers. *Cell*. 1990;60: 63–72.
371. Ruppert J, Sidney J, Celis E, et al. Prominent role of secondary anchor residues in peptide binding to HLA-A2.1 molecules. *Cell*. 1993;74:929–937.
372. Berzofsky JA. Epitope selection and design of synthetic vaccines: molecular approaches to enhancing immunogenicity and crossreactivity of engineered vaccines. *Ann NY Acad Sci*. 1993;690:256–264.
373. Berzofsky JA. Designing peptide vaccines to broaden recognition and enhance potency. *Ann NY Acad Sci*. 1995;754:161–168.
374. Takahashi H, Nakagawa Y, Pendleton CD, et al. Induction of broadly cross-reactive cytotoxic T cells recognizing an HIV-1 envelope determinant. *Science*. 1992;255:333–336.
375. Ahlers JD, Takeshita T, Pendleton CD, et al. Enhanced immunogenicity of HIV-1 vaccine construct by modification of the native peptide sequence. *Proc Natl Acad Sci U S A*. 1997;94:10856–10861.
376. Shirai M, Pendleton CD, Ahlers J, et al. Helper-CTL determinant linkage required for priming of anti-HIV CD8+ CTL in vivo with peptide vaccine constructs. *J Immunol*. 1994;152:549–556.
377. Ahlers JD, Dunlop N, Alling DW, et al. Cytokine-in-adjuvant steering of the immune response phenotype to HIV-1 vaccine constructs: GM-CSF and TNFa synergize with IL-12 to enhance induction of CTL. *J Immunol*. 1997;158:3947–3958.
378. Ahlers JD, Belyakov IM, Thomas EK, et al. High affinity T-helper epitope induces complementary helper and APC polarization, increased CTL and protection against viral infection. *J Clin Invest*. 2001;108:1677–1685.
379. Ridge JP, Di Rosa F, Matzinger P. A conditioned dendritic cell can be a temporal bridge between a CD4+ T-helper and a T-killer cell. *Nature*. 1998;393:474–478.
380. Bennett SRM, Carbone FR, Karamalis F, et al. Help for cytotoxic-T-cell responses is mediated by CD40 signalling. *Nature*. 1998;393: 478–480.
381. Schoenberger SP, Toes REM, van der Voort EIH, et al. T-cell help for cytotoxic T lymphocytes is mediated by CD40-CD40L interactions. *Nature*. 1998;393:480–483.
382. Pogue RR, Eron J, Frelinger JA, et al. Amino-terminal alteration of the HLA-A0201-restricted human immunodeficiency virus pol peptide increases complex stability and in vitro immunogenicity. *Proc Natl Acad Sci U S A*. 1995;92:8166–8170.
384. Sarobe P, Pendleton CD, Akatsuka T, et al. Enhanced in vitro potency and in vivo immunogenicity of a CTL epitope from hepatitis C virus core protein following amino acid replacement at secondary HLA-A2.1 binding positions. *J Clin Invest*. 1998;102:1239–1248.
385. Rosenberg SA, Yang JC, Schwartzentruber DJ, et al. Immunologic and therapeutic evaluation of a synthetic peptide vaccine for the treatment of patients with metastatic melanoma. *Nature Medicine*. 1998;4:321–327.
386. Sette A, Vitiello A, Reherman B, et al. The relationship between class I binding affinity and immunogenicity of potential cytotoxic T cell epitopes. *J Immunol*. 1994;153:5586–5592.
387. Berzofsky JA, Ahlers JD, Derby MA, et al. Approaches to improve engineered vaccines for human immunodeficiency virus (HIV) and other viruses that cause chronic infections. *Immunol Rev*. 1999;170:151–172.

388. Berzofsky JA, Ahlers JD, Belyakov IM. Strategies for designing and optimizing new generation vaccines. *Nat Rev Immunol.* 2001;1:209–219.
389. DeGroot AS, Meister GE, Cornette JL, et al. Computer prediction of T-cell epitopes. In: Levine MM, Woodrow GC, Kaper JB, Cobon GS, eds. *New Generation Vaccines*. New York: Marcel Dekker, Inc., 1997: 127–138.
390. Falk K, Rötzschke O, Stevanovic S, et al. Allele specific motifs revealed by sequencing of self peptides eluted from MHC molecules. *Nature*. 1991;351:290–296.
391. Jardetzky TS, Lane WS, Robinson RA, et al. Identification of self peptides bound to purified HLA-B27. *Nature*. 1991;353:326–329.
392. Romero P, Corradin G, Luescher IF, et al. H-2Kd-restricted antigenic peptides share a simple binding motif. *J Exp Med.* 1991;174:603–612.
393. Hunt DF, Henderson RA, Shabanowitz J, et al. Characterization of peptides bound to the class I MHC molecule HLA-A2.1 by mass spectrometry. *Science*. 1992;255:1261–1263.
394. Corr M, Boyd LF, Padlan EA, et al. H-2Dd exploits a four residue peptide binding motif. *J Exp Med.* 1993;178:1877–1892.
395. Schumacher TNM, De Bruijn MLH, Vernie LN, et al. Peptide selection by MHC class I molecules. *Nature*. 1991;350:703–706.
396. Tsomides TJ, Walker BD, Eisen HN. An optimal viral peptide recognized by CD8+ T cells binds very tightly to the restricting class I major histocompatibility complex protein on intact cells but not to the purified class I protein. *Proc Natl Acad Sci U S A.* 1991;88:11276–11280.
397. Hunt DF, Michel H, Dickinson TA, et al. Peptides presented to the immune system by the murine class II major histocompatibility complex molecule I-Ad. *Science*. 1992;256:1817–1820.
399. Chicz RM, Urban RG, Gorga JC, et al. Specificity and promiscuity among naturally processed peptides bound to HLA-DR alleles. *J Exp Med.* 1993;178:27–47.
400. Chicz RM, Urban RG, Lane WS, et al. Predominant naturally processed peptides bound to HLA-DR1 are derived from MHC-related molecules and are heterogeneous in size. *Nature*. 1992;358:764–768.
401. Hammer J, Takacs B, Sinigaglia F. Identification of a motif for HLA-DR1 binding peptides using M13 display libraries. *J Exp Med.* 1992;176:1007–1013.
402. Hammer J, Valsasnini P, Tolba K, et al. Promiscuous and allele-specific anchors in HLA-DR binding peptides. *Cell.* 1993;74:197–203.
403. Sinigaglia F, Hammer J. Motifs and supermotifs for MHC class II binding peptides. *J Exp Med.* 1995;181:449–451.
404. Marshall KW, Wilson KJ, Liang J, et al. Prediction of peptide affinity to HLA DRB10401. *J Immunol.* 1995;154:5927–5933.
405. Jardetzky TS, Brown JH, Gorga JC, et al. Three-dimensional structure of a human class II histocompatibility molecule complexed with superantigen. *Nature*. 1994;368:711–718.
406. Scott CA, Peterson PA, Teyton L, et al. Crystal structures of two I-A(d)-peptide complexes reveal that high affinity can be achieved without large anchor residues. *Immunity*. 1998;8:319–329.
407. Fremont DH, Monnaie D, Nelson CA, et al. Crystal structure of I-A(k) in complex with a dominant epitope of lysozyme. *Immunity*. 1998;8:305–317.
408. Ghosh P, Amaya M, Mellins E, et al. The structure of an intermediate in class II MHC maturation: CLIP bound to HLA-DR3. *Nature*. 1995;378:457–462.
411. Alexander J, Snoke K, Ruppert J, et al. Functional consequences of engagement of the T cell receptor by low affinity ligands. *J Immunol.* 1993;150:1–7.
412. Alexander J, Oseroff C, Sidney J, et al. Derivation of HLA-B0702 transgenic mice: functional CTL repertoire and recognition of human B0702-restricted CTL epitopes. *Hum Immunol* 2003;64: 211–223.
413. Firat H, Cochet M, Rohrlich PS, et al. Comparative analysis of the CD8(+) T cell repertoires of H-2 class I wild-type/HLA-A2.1 and H-2 class I knockout/HLA-A2.1 transgenic mice. *Int Immunol* 2002;14:925–934.
414. Shirai M, Arichi T, Nishioka M, et al. CTL responses of HLA-A2.1-transgenic mice specific for hepatitis C viral peptides predict epitopes for CTL of humans carrying HLA-A2.1. *J Immunol.* 1995;154:2733–2742.
415. Soroosh P, Shokri F, Azizi M, et al. Analysis of T-cell receptor beta chain variable gene segment usage in healthy adult responders and nonresponders to recombinant hepatitis B vaccine. *Scand J Immunol.* 2003;57:423–431.
417. Moudgil KD, Grewal IS, Jensen PE, et al. Unresponsiveness to a self-peptide of mouse lysozyme owing to hindrance of T cell receptor-major histocompatibility complex/peptide interaction caused by flanking epitopic residues. *J Exp Med.* 1996;183:535–546.
418. Sinha P, Chi HH, Kim HR, et al. Mouse lysozyme-M knockout mice reveal how the self-determinant hierarchy shapes the T cell repertoire against this circulating self antigen in wild-type mice. *J Immunol.* 2004;173:1763–1771.
419. Hernandez J, Lee PP, Davis MM, et al. The use of HLA A2.1/p53 peptide tetramers to visualize the impact of self tolerance on the TCR repertoire. *J Immunol.* 2000;164:596–602.
420. Theobald M, Biggs J, Hernández J, et al. Tolerance to p53 by A2.1-restricted cytotoxic T lymphocytes. *J Exp Med.* 1997;185:833–841.
421. Sandberg JK, Franksson L, Sundback J, et al. T cell tolerance based on avidity thresholds rather than complete deletion allows maintenance of maximal repertoire diversity. *J Immunol.* 2000;165:25–33.
422. Slifka MK, Blattman JN, Sourdive DJ, et al. Preferential escape of subdominant CD8+ T cells during negative selection results in an altered antiviral T cell hierarchy. *J Immunol.* 2003;170:1231–1239.
423. Gross DA, Graff-Dubois S, Opolon P, et al. High vaccination efficiency of low-affinity epitopes in antitumor immunotherapy. *J Clin Invest.* 2004;113:425–433.
423a. Dzutsev AH, Belyakov IM, Isakov DV, et al. Avidity of CD8 T cells sharpens immunodominance. *Int Immunol.* 2007;19:497–507.
424. Trautmann L, Rimbert M, Echasserieau K, et al. Selection of T cell clones expressing high-affinity public TCRs within Human cytomegalovirus-specific CD8 T cell responses. *J Immunol.* 2005;175:6123–6132.
425. Alexander-Miller MA, Leggatt GR, Berzofsky JA. Selective expansion of high or low avidity cytotoxic T lymphocytes and efficacy for adoptive immunotherapy. *Proc Natl Acad Sci U S A.* 1996;93:4102–4107.
426. Gallimore A, Dumrese T, Hengartner H, et al. Protective immunity does not correlate with the hierarchy of virus-specific cytotoxic T cell responses to naturally processed peptides. *J Exp Med.* 1998;187:1647–1657.
427. Messaoudi I, Patino JA, Dyall R, et al. Direct link between MHC polymorphism, T cell avidity, and diversity in immune defense. *Science*. 2002;298:1797–1800.
428. Ding YH, Smith KJ, Garboczi DN, et al. Two human T cell receptors bind in a similar diagonal mode to the HLA-A2/Tax peptide complex using different TCR amino acids. *Immunity*. 1998;8:403–411.
429. Slansky JE, Rattis FM, Boyd LF, et al. Enhanced Antigen-Specific Antitumor Immunity with Altered Peptide Ligands that Stabilize the MHC-Peptide-TCR Complex. *Immunity*. 2000;13:529–538.
430. Zaremba S, Barzaga E, Zhu M, et al. Identification of an enhancer agonist cytotoxic T lymphocyte peptide from human carcinoembryonic antigen. *Cancer Res.* 1997;57:4570–4577.
431. Fong L, Hou Y, Rivas A, et al. Altered peptide ligand vaccination with Flt3 ligand expanded dendritic cells for tumor immunotherapy. *Proc Natl Acad Sci U S A.* 2001;98:8809–8814.
432. Tangri S, Ishioka GY, Huang X, et al. Structural features of peptide analogs of human histocompatibility leukocyte antigen class I epitopes that are more potent and immunogenic than wild-type peptide. *J Exp Med.* 2001;194:833–846.
433. Takeshita T, Takahashi H, Kozlowski S, et al. Molecular analysis of the same HIV peptide functionally binding to both a class I and a class II MHC molecule. *J Immunol.* 1995;154:1973–1986.
434. Alexander-Miller MA, Parker KC, Tsukui T, et al. Molecular analysis of presentation by HLA-A2.1 of a promiscuously binding V3 loop peptide from the HIV-1 envelope protein to human CTL. *Int Immunol.* 1996;8:641–649.
435. Abiru N, Wegmann D, Kawasaki E, et al. Dual overlapping peptides recognized by insulin peptide B:9–23 T cell receptor AV13S3 T cell clones of the NOD mouse. *J Autoimmun.* 2000;14:231–237.

436. Talken BL, Schafermeyer KR, Bailey CW, et al. T cell epitope mapping of the Smith antigen reveals that highly conserved Smith antigen motifs are the dominant target of T cell immunity in systemic lupus erythematosus. *J Immunol*. 2001;167:562–568.
437. Takahashi H, Merli S, Putney SD, et al. A single amino acid interchange yields reciprocal CTL specificities for HIV gp160. *Science*. 1989;246:118–121.
439. De Magistris MT, Alexander J, Coggeshall M, et al. Antigen analog-major histocompatibility complexes act as antagonists of the T cell receptor. *Cell*. 1992;68:625–634.
440. Sette A, Alexander J, Ruppert J, et al. Antigen analogs/MHC complexes as specific T cell receptor antagonists. *Annu Rev Immunol*. 1994;12:413–431.
442. Evavold BD, Allen PM. Separation of IL-4 production from Th cell proliferation by an altered T cell receptor ligand. *Science*. 1991;252:1308–1310.
443. Evavold BD, Williams SG, Hsu BL, et al. Complete dissection of the Hb(64–76) determinant using Th1, Th2 clones and T cell hybridomas. *J Immunol*. 1992;148:347–353.
444. Pfeiffer C, Stein J, Southwood S, et al. Altered peptide ligands can control CD4 T lymphocyte differentiation in vivo. *J Exp Med*. 1995;181:1569–1574.
445. Chaturvedi P, Yu Q, Southwood S, et al. Peptide analogs with different affinities for MHC alter the cytokine profile of T helper cells. *Int Immunol*. 1996;8:745–755.
446. Sloan-Lancaster J, Evavold BD, Allen PM. Induction of T-cell anergy by altered T-cell-receptor ligand on live antigen-presenting cells. *Nature*. 1993;363:156–159.
447. Sloan-Lancaster J, Shaw AS, Rothbard JB, et al. Partial T cell signaling: altered phospho-z and lack of Zap70 recruitment in APL-induced T cell anergy. *Cell*. 1994;79:913–922.
448. Tsitoura DC, Holter W, Cerwenka A, et al. Induction of anergy in human T helper 0 cells by stimulation with altered T cell antigen receptor ligands. *J Immunol*. 1996;156:2801–2808.
450. Racioppi L, Ronchese F, Matis LA, et al. Peptide-major histocompatibility complex class II complexes with mixed agonist/antagonist properties provide evidence for ligand-related differences in T cell receptor-dependent intracellular signaling. *J Exp Med*. 1993;177:1047–1060.
451. Madrenas J, Wange RL, Wang JL, et al. z phosphorylation without ZAP-70 activation induced by TCR antagonists or partial agonists. *Science*. 1995;267:515–518.
452. Madrenas J, Chau LA, Smith J, et al. The efficiency of CD4 recruitment to ligand-engaged TCR controls the agonist/partial agonist properties of peptide-MHC molecule ligands. *J Exp Med*. 1997;185:219–229.
453. McKeithan TW. Kinetic proofreading in T-cell receptor signal transduction. *Proc Nat Acad Sci U S A*. 1995;92:5042–5046.
454. DeGroot AS, Jesdale BM, Berzofsky JA. Prediction and determination of MHC ligands and T cell epitopes. In: Kaufmann SHE, Kabelitz D, eds. *Immunology of Infection*. London: Academic Press, 1998:79–108.
459. Madden DR, Garboczi DN, Wiley DC. The antigenic identity of peptide-MHC complexes: a comparison of the conformations of five viral peptides presented by HLA-A2. *Cell*. 1993;75:693–708.
462. Cornette JL, Margalit H, DeLisi C, et al. The amphipathic Helix as a structural feature involved in T-cell recognition. In: Epand RM, ed. *The Amphipathic Helix*. Boca Raton: CRC Press, 1993:333–346.
465. Cornette JL, Margalit H, Berzofsky JA, et al. Periodic variation in side-chain polarities of T-cell antigenic peptides correlates with their structure and activity. *Proc Nat Acad Sci U S A*. 1995;92:8368–8372.
466. Pamer EG, Harty JT, Bevan MJ. Precise prediction of a dominant class I MHC-restricted epitope of Listeria monocytogenes. *Nature*. 1991;353:852–855.
467. Hill AVS, Elvin J, Willis AC, et al. Molecular analysis of the association of HLA-B53 and resistance to severe malaria. *Nature*. 1992;360:434–439.
468. Lipford GB, Hoffman M, Wagner H, et al. Primary in vivo responses to ovalbumin: probing the predictive value of the Kb binding motif. *J Immunol*. 1993;150:1212–1222.
469. Nijman HW, Houbiers JGA, Vierboom MPM, et al. Identification of peptide sequences that potentially trigger HLA-A2.1-restricted cytotoxic T lymphocytes. *Eur J Immunol*. 1993;23:1215–1219.
470. Altuvia Y, Berzofsky JA, Rosenfeld R, et al. Sequence features that correlate with MHC restriction. *Molec Immunol*. 1994;31:1–19.
471. Meister GE, Roberts CGP, Berzofsky JA, et al. Two novel T cell epitope prediction algorithms based on MHC-binding motifs; comparison of predicted and published epitopes from Mycobacterium tuberculosis and HIV protein sequences. *Vaccine*. 1995;13:581–591.
473. Zhang C, Anderson A, DeLisi C. Structural principles that govern the peptide-binding motifs of class I MHC molecules. *J Mol Biol*. 1998;281:929–947.
474. Sturniolo T, Bono E, Ding J, et al. Generation of tissue-specific and promiscuous HLA ligand databases using DNA microarrays and virtual HLA class II matrices. *Nat Biotechnol*. 1999;17:555–561.
475. Zhang C, Cornette JL, Berzofsky JA, et al. The organization of human leukocyte antigen class I epitopes in HIV genome products: Implications for HIV evolution and vaccine design. *Vaccine*. 1997;15:1291–1302.
476. Hammer J, Bono E, Gallazzi F, et al. Precise prediction of major histocompatibility complex class II-peptide interaction based on peptide side chain scanning. *J Exp Med*. 1994;180:2353–2358.
477. Parker KC, Bednarek MA, Coligan JE. Scheme for ranking potential HLA-A2 binding peptides based on independent binding of individual peptide side-chains. *J Immunol*. 1994;152:163–175.
478. Fleckenstein B, Kalbacher H, Muller CP, et al. New ligands binding to the human leukocyte antigen class II molecule DRB10101 based on the activity pattern of an undecapeptide library. *Eur J Biochem*. 1996;240:71–77.
479. Jesdale BM, Mullen L, Meisell J, et al. Epimatrix and epimer, tools for HIV research. *Vaccines*: Cold Spring Harbor Laboratory Press, Cold Spring Harbor, NY; 1997:57–64.
480. Davenport MP, Ho Shon IAP, Hill AVS. An empirical method for the prediction of T-cell epitopes. *Immunogenetics*. 1995;42:392–397.
481. Davenport MP, Godkin A, Friede T, et al. A distinctive peptide binding motif for HLA-DRB10407, an HLA-DR4 subtype not associated with rheumatoid arthritis. *Immunogenetics*. 1997;45:229–232.
482. Leggatt GR, Hosmalin A, Pendleton CD, et al. The importance of pairwise interactions between peptide residues in the delineation of T cell receptor specificity. *J Immunol*. 1998;161:4728–4735.
483. Moutaftsi M, Peters B, Pasquetto V, et al. A consensus epitope prediction approach identifies the breadth of murine T(CD8+)-cell responses to vaccinia virus. *Nat Biotechnol*. 2006;24:817–819.
484. Sidney J, Grey HM, Southwood S, et al. Definition of an HLA-A3-like supermotif demonstrates the overlapping peptide-binding repertoires of common HLA molecules. *Hum Immunol*. 1996;45:79–93.
485. Kropshofer H, Max H, Halder T, et al. Self-peptides from four HLA-DR alleles share hydrophobic anchor residues near the NH2-terminal including proline as a stop signal for trimming. *J Immunol*. 1993;151:4732–4742.
486. Sette A, Sidney J. Nine major HLA class I supertypes account for the vast preponderance of HLA-A and -B polymorphism. *Immunogenetics*. 1999;50:201–212.
487. Vajda S, Weng Z, Rosenfeld R, et al. Effect of conformational flexibility and solvation on receptor-ligand binding free energies. *Biochem*. 1994;33:13977–13988.
488. Sezerman U, Vajda S, DeLisi C. Free energy mapping of class I MHC molecules and structural determination of bound peptides. *Protein Science*. 1996;5:1272–1281.
489. Altuvia Y, Schueler O, Margalit H. Ranking potential binding peptides to MHC molecules by a computational threading approach. *J Mol Biol*. 1995;249:244–250.
490. Altuvia Y, Margalit H. A structure-based approach for prediction of MHC-binding peptides. *Methods*. 2004;34:454–459.
491. Brusic V, Rudy G, Harrison LC. Prediction of MHC binding peptides using artificial neural networks. In: Stonier RJ, Yu XH, eds. *Complex systems mechanism of adaptation*. Amsterdam: IOS Press, 1994:253–260.
492. Altuvia Y, Margalit H. Sequence signals for generation of antigenic peptides by the proteasome: implications for proteasomal cleavage mechanism. *J Mol Biol*. 2000;295:879–890.

493. Donnes P, Kohlbacher O. Integrated modeling of the major events in the MHC class I antigen processing pathway. *Protein Sci.* 2005;14:2132–2140.
494. Peters B, Sette A. Generating quantitative models describing the sequence specificity of biological processes with the stabilized matrix method. *BMC Bioinformatics*. 2005;6:132.
495. Larsen MV, Lundegaard C, Lamberth K, et al. An integrative approach to CTL epitope prediction: a combined algorithm integrating MHC class I binding, TAP transport efficiency, and proteasomal cleavage predictions. *Eur J Immunol.* 2005;35:2295–2303.
496. Doytchinova IA, Flower DR. Class I T-cell epitope prediction: improvements using a combination of proteasome cleavage, TAP affinity, and MHC binding. *Mol Immunol.* 2006;43:2037–2044.
497. Doytchinova IA, Guan P, Flower DR. EpiJen: a server for multistep T cell epitope prediction. *BMC Bioinformatics*. 2006;7:131.
522. Löwenadler B, Lycke N, Svanholm C, et al. T and B cell responses to chimeric proteins containing heterologous T helper epitopes inserted at different positions. *Molec Immunol.* 1992;29:1185–1190.
524. Manca F, Fenoglio D, Li Pira G, et al. Effect of antigen/antibody ratio on macrophage uptake, processing, and presentation to T cells of antigen complexed with polyclonal antibodies. *J Exp Med.* 1991;173:37–48.
525. Watts C, Lanzavecchia A. Suppressive effect of antibody on processing of T cell epitopes. *J Exp Med.* 1993;178:1459–1463.
526. Simitsek PD, Campbell DG, Lanzavecchia A, et al. Modulation of antigen processing by bound antibodies can boost or suppress class II major histocompatibility complex presentation of different T cell determinants. *J Exp Med.* 1995;181:1957–1963.

Chapter 22

Fc Receptors and Their Role in Immune Regulation and Inflammation

Jeffrey V. Ravetch and Falk Nimmerjahn

HISTORICAL BACKGROUND

Cellular receptors for immunoglobulins were anticipated by the description of cytophilic antibodies of the immunoglobulin (Ig) G class, identified by Boyden and Sorkin in 1960 (1). These antibodies conferred on normal cells, like macrophages, the capacity to specifically absorb antigen. Using sheep red blood cells (RBCs) as the antigen resulted in rosette formation between the cytophilic anti–sheep RBC antibodies and macrophages and provided a convenient means of visualization of the binding of cytophilic antibodies with normal cells. Subsequent studies by Berken and Benacerraf (2) suggested that the crystallized fragment (Fc) of the cytophilic antibody interacted with a cell surface receptor on macrophages. Similar studies on B lymphocytes extended the generality of these receptors and led to the term *Fc receptor* (FcR) to denote the surface molecules on lymphoid and myeloid cells that are capable of interacting with the Fc of immunoglobulin molecules (3). Studies on IgE, IgM, and IgA also demonstrated the existence of distinct receptors for those isotypes various immune cell types. Detailed biochemical characterization of Fc receptors was inaugurated by the studies of Kulczycki et al. (4) on the high-affinity IgE FcR of mast cells, revealing a heterooligomeric $\alpha\beta\gamma_2$ subunit structure. A distinction between FcRs for the IgE and IgG isotypes emerged with the observation of the very high (10^{10} M^{-1}) binding affinity of IgE for its receptor in comparison with the low binding (10^6 M^{-1}) of IgG1 to its receptor. This distinction led to the realization that the functional IgG1 ligand was exclusively in the form of an immune complex, whereas IgE binding occurred through monomer interaction with its receptor. This difference in binding affinity had significant functional implications for the structures of these receptors and mechanisms by which each isotype activated its target cell. Determination of the structure of these receptors was facilitated by their molecular cloning, beginning with the IgG FcRs (5,6) and followed by the IgE FcR (7). Two distinct types of IgG receptors differing in their transmembrane and cytoplasmic sequences, were identified, which thus offered a molecular explanation for the apparent contradictory activation and inhibitory activities attributed to IgG FcRs. The primary structure of the subunits of the high-affinity IgE FcR revealed homology in the ligand-binding α subunit to its IgG counterparts. However, the extent of similarity between these receptors became apparent with the observation that the γ-chain subunit was common to both IgG and IgE FcRs, providing both assembly and signaling functions to these activation receptors (8,9). This common structure suggested a functional link between immune complex diseases and allergic reactions, a prediction that was confirmed through mouse knockout studies of IgG FcRs (10,11). The FcRs, through their dependence on the immunoreceptor tyrosine-based activation motif (ITAM) pathway of cellular activation, belonged to the family of immunoreceptors that included the antigen receptors on B cells and T cells. Three-dimensional crystal structures have been solved for the low-affinity IgG FcRs (12,13) and the high-affinity IgE FcR (14) alone and in complex with their immunoglobulin ligands (15,16), further establishing the close structural link between these immunoglobulin receptors.

The functional roles of IgG FcRs were suggested by the distribution of these receptors on both lymphoid and myeloid cells (17). On myeloid cells, they were presumed to mediate effector cell activation, resulting in phagocytosis, antibody-dependent cellular cytotoxicity (ADCC), and release of inflammatory mediators. However, the well-known ability of the classic pathway of complement to generate activated fragments in response to immune complexes capable of inducing inflammatory responses by myeloid cells complicated the interpretation of the physiologic role of IgG FcRs. Thus, the contribution of IgG FcRs to the mechanism of immune complex–mediated inflammation, as distinct from the role of complement, remained uncertain. Insight into this distinction was gained through the generation of mouse strains specifically deficient or blocked in either FcRs (10,18–20) or components of the classic complement pathway (21). Studies on immune complex–mediated inflammatory responses in these animals, such as the Arthus reaction, led to the realization that IgG FcRs and not the classic pathway of complement activation were the functional mediators of inflammatory responses triggered by immune complexes (20,22,23). The situation for IgE was less confounding, and the identification and characterization of a high-affinity receptor for this isotype on mast cells offered a plausible explanation for many of the inflammatory features of allergic reactions (24), validated later by mouse knockouts of this receptor. IgG immune complexes had also been observed to mediate suppression of B cell responses; thus, the presence of an IgG FcR activity on B cells provided a possible but uncharacterized mechanism for this inhibitory activity. Molecular characterization of this inhibitory activity for the B cell FcR, FcRIIB, resulted in the first detailed description of an inhibitory motif, now termed the immunoreceptor tyrosine-based inhibitory motif (ITIM) (25,26), and the signaling pathway by which it abrogates ITAM-triggered activation. The ITIM mechanism is now recognized as ubiquitous and has resulted in the recognition of a large family of inhibitory receptors on immune cells that function to maintain proper thresholds for activation and abrogate activation responses to terminate an immune reaction (27).

FcRs are now recognized as central mediators of antibody-triggered responses, coupling the innate and adaptive immune responses in effector cell activation (28). In addition to these specialized roles, the IgG FcRs have served as an example of the emerging class of balanced immunoreceptors, in which activation and inhibition are tightly coupled in response to ligand binding. Perturbations in either arm of the response have been shown to lead to pathologic consequences and have been taken as a paradigm of how these systems are likely to work for those paired immunoreceptors with unknown ligand-binding functions. The newly described roles for FcRs in maintaining peripheral tolerance, shaping the antibody repertoire, regulating antigen-presenting cell (APC) maturation, and promoting mast cell survival indicate the diversity of functions that these receptors possess and their central role in modulating both afferent and efferent responses in the immune response.

This chapter focuses primarily on the IgG and IgE FcRs, for which substantial data are available on their structure, function, regulation, and role in a variety of physiologic and pathologic conditions. The similarity in structure and signaling between those receptors and other members of this family, such as the IgA FcR, is also discussed. In addition, a brief overview of the recently discovered and rapidly expanding family of FcR homologous proteins is given. Other immunoglobulin receptors with specialized functions in the transport of immunoglobulins, such as the FcRn (29) and the poly-Ig FcR (30), are discussed elsewhere in this volume.

STRUCTURE AND EXPRESSION

Molecular Genetics

Two general classes of FcRs are now recognized: the activation receptors, characterized by the presence of a cytoplasmic ITAM sequence associated with the receptor, and the inhibitory receptor, characterized by the presence of an ITIM sequence. These two classes of receptors function in concert and are usually found coexpressed on the cell surface. Thus, coengagement of both signaling pathways is the rule, setting thresholds for and ultimately determining the physiologic outcome of effector cell responses. Among the factors that determine this threshold level are the actual affinities of the individual activating and inhibitory receptors for a specific IgG ligand and the expression level of the receptor pairs on immune effector cells. It is important to note that the affinity of different antibody isotypes and subclasses for their respective activating and inhibitory FcRs varies significantly, which explains the differential activity of antibody isotypes *in vivo* (20,31,32). In addition, alleles of specific FcRs have been described that alter their affinity for individual subclasses, thus accounting for the variable responses seen in a population to an antibody (see later discussion).

Subunit Composition

FcRs are typically type I integral membrane glycoproteins consisting of, at the least, a ligand recognition α subunit that confers isotype specificity for the receptor. The α subunits for IgG, IgE, and IgA have been described (17,33). These subunits typically consist of two extracellular domains of the immunoglobulin V type superfamily: a single transmembrane domain and a relatively short intracytoplasmic domain. In activation FcRs, a signaling subunit of the γ family is often found, resulting in an $\alpha\gamma_2$ complex. The inhibitory FcRIIB molecule, in contrast, is expressed as a single-chain receptor. The α subunits have apparent molecular weights of between 40 and 75 kDa and share significant amino acid sequence homology in their extracellular domains. Alternatively spliced forms of FcγRIIB modify the intracytoplasmic domain of this molecule. For example, the B2 form lacks sequences that inhibit internalization and thus demonstrates enhanced internalization of immune complexes in comparison with RIIB1. However, all the splice variants contain the ITIM motif, a necessary and sufficient domain for mediating inhibitory signaling. The conservation of this sequence in mice and humans, its presence in all splice variants, and the hyperresponsive phenotypes generated in mice deficient in this receptor all support inhibition as the central function of RIIB. The specific structures of the α subunits are shown in Figure 22.1. The notable exceptions to the general structure just outlined are seen for the high-affinity FcγRIα subunit, which has three extracellular domains; the activation FcγRIIAα subunit, which does not require additional subunits for assembly or signaling; and the glycosyl-phosphatidylinositol (GPI)–linked FcγRIIIB, which attaches to the cell surface through a GPI linkage rather than through a transmembrane domain.

The γ subunit is found associated with activation of IgG, IgE, and IgA FcRs, as well as with non-FcR molecules, such as paired immunoglobulin-like receptor A (PIR-A) and natural killer (NK) cell cytotoxicity receptors (34–36). It is required for assembly of the α subunits of these receptors by protecting them from degradation in the endoplasmic reticulum. The γ chain is found as a disulfide-linked homodimer with a short extracellular domain containing the cysteine involved in dimerization, a transmembrane domain, and an intracytoplasmic domain containing the ITAM. An aspartic acid residue found in the transmembrane domain is often associated with a basic amino acid residue in the transmembrane domain of the α subunit. The γ subunit belongs to a gene family that includes the T cell receptor–associated ζ chain and the NK receptor DAP-10– and DAP-12–associated molecules (37). FcγRIIIA can associate with the ζ chain, resulting in the $\alpha\zeta_2$ complex found in human NK cells.

A third subunit is found associated with the activation of FcRs, FcεRI, and FcγRIII, the β subunit. This 33-kDa subunit has four transmembrane-spanning domains and amino and carboxy intracytoplasmic domains, belonging to the CD20 family of tetraspan molecules (24). An ITAM sequence is found in the intracytoplasmic carboxy domain. In mast cells and basophils, the β chain assembles into an $\alpha\beta\gamma_2$ complex, with the α chain belonging to either FcγRIII or FcεRI. Its presence is required for assembly of FcεRI in rodents. In humans, however, $\alpha\gamma_2$ complexes of FcεRI are found in monocytes, Langerhans cells, and dendritic cells, in addition to the $\alpha\beta\gamma_2$ complexes found in mast cells and basophils. The ITAM motif found in the β subunit is not an autonomous activation sequence but functions as a signaling amplifier of the ITAM found in the γ subunits (38).

Gene Organization, Linkage, and Polymorphisms

All α subunits share a common gene organization, which indicates that the evolution of this family of receptors resulted from gene duplication from a common ancestor (39). Sequence divergence then resulted in the acquisition of distinctive specificities for these related sequences. Most of the genes belonging to the FcR family, including the recently identified group of FcR-homologous or -like (FCRL) proteins, are found on the long arm of chromosome 1, including the γ chain and the α chains of FcγRI, FcγRII, FcγRIII, and FcεRI (Figure 22.2) (40–42). This region is syntenic with a comparable region on mouse chromosome 1; however, FcγRIα and several FCRLs are found on mouse chromosome 3. In humans, the α subunit of the IgA receptor is found on chromosome 19, and the β subunit is on chromosome 11. The FcγRII–FcγRIII locus on chromosome 1 is further linked to a variety of lupus susceptibility genes found in that region, including the *Sle1* cluster (43). A locus linked to atopy has been identified at 11q12–13 and further delineated polymorphisms of the β chain (I181V and V183L) that are associated with a heightened risk of atopy. However, a direct functional association of these polymorphisms with the known biological activities of the β chain has not been found (44).

Polymorphisms in the α chains of the FcγRs have been described, most notably in FcγRIIA and FcγRIII; these polymorphisms result in differences in binding affinity to specific IgG subclasses (45). For example, a histidine at

	FcγRI CD64	FcγRIIA CD32	FcγRIIB CD32	FcγRIIIA CD16		FcγRIIIB CD16	FcεRI		FcαRI CD89
Structure Subunit composition	γ_2 α	α	ITIM α	γ_2 α β	γ_2 α	α-GPI	γ_2 α β	γ_2 α	γ_2 α
Ka	10^8 M^{-1}	2x10^6 M^{-1}	2x10^6 M^{-1}	5x10^5 M^{-1}	5x10^5 M^{-1}	2x10^5 M^{-1}	10^{10} M^{-1}	10^{10} M^{-1}	5x10^7 M^{-1}
Binding Specificity	1. IgG1=IgG3 2. IgG4 3. IgG2	1. IgG1 2. IgG2=IgG3 3. IgG4	1. IgG1 2. IgG2=IgG3 3. IgG4	1. IgG1=IgG3	1. IgG1=IgG3	1. IgG1=IgG3	IgE	IgE	IgA_1=IgA_2
Expression	Macrophages Neutrophils Eosinophils Dendritic Cells	Macrophages Neutrophils Mast cells Eosinophils Platelets Dendritic Cells	Macrophages Neutrophils Mast cells Eosinophils Dendritic Cells FDC B cells	Mast cells Basophils	Macrophages Mast cells Basophils NK cells Dendritic Cells	Neutrophilsa	Mast cells Basophils	Mast cells Basophils Eosinophils Platelets Dendritic Cells	Macrophages Neutrophils Eosinophils
Class	Activation	Activation	Inhibition	Activation		Decoy	Activation	Activation	Activation
Function	-Inducible by inflammatory cytokines -Enhance effector responses at inflammatory sites -IC capturing by DC	-Effector cell activation by IC's, cytotoxic Ab	-Set threshold for effector cell activation by Fc -B cell repression -Maintain tolerance	-Dominant pathway for effector activation by IgG -In vivo ADCC -Arthus reaction -IC capture by DC -IC mediated DC maturation		-Sink for IC -Focus IC to PMN -Synergize with FcγRIIA	-Degranulation -Allergic reactions (Type I)	-Degranulation -Allergy -Antigen caption by DC	-IgA binding -IgA activation of effector cells

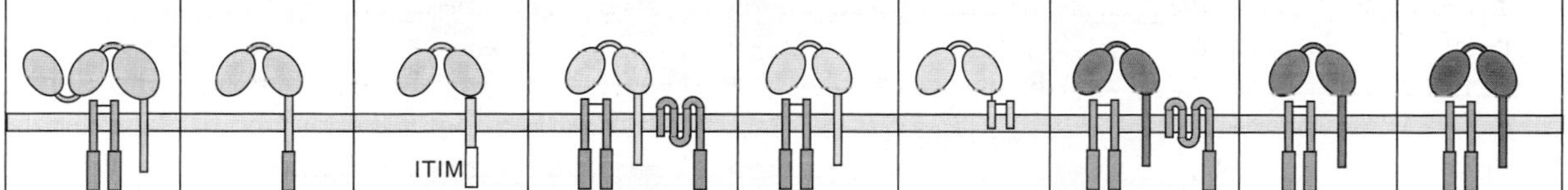

FIGURE 22.1 Summary of FcR structures, expression patterns, and *in vivo* functions. The immunoreceptor tyrosine-based activation motif (ITAM) signaling motif is indicated by the green rectangle; the immunoreceptor tyrosine based inhibitor motif (ITIM) is indicated as a red rectangle. Alleles of FcRIIA and FcRIIIB and their binding properties are discussed in the text. ADCC, antibody-dependent cellular cytotoxicity; DC, dendritic cells; FDC, follicular dendritic cells; GPI, glycosyl phosphatidylinositol; IC, immune complex; Ig, immunoglobulin; NK, natural killer; PMN, polymorphonuclear neutrophils.

position 131 in FcγRIIA results in higher-affinity binding to IgG2 and IgG3 than does an arginine at that position. Similarly, FcγRIIIA with valine at position 158 of the α chain has a higher binding affinity for IgG1 and 3 than does the polymorphic form with phenylalanine at that position. This polymorphism translates into a more robust ADCC response for the val/val haplotype *in vitro* and has been positively correlated with the degree of an *in vivo* response to a B cell–depleting, anti-CD20 antibody (46). Four amino acids are polymorphic for FcγRIIIB at positions 18, 47, 64, and 88, which contributes to the neutrophil antigen polymorphisms for this receptor. Several studies have attempted to link specific FcR polymorphisms to autoimmune diseases, specifically to systemic lupus erythematosus (SLE). Recent studies have reported associations in susceptibility to SLE in both murine and human populations with levels of RIIB expression or alleles of RIIB (47). Reduced expression of RIIB on activated B cells, such as memory cells, has been seen in lupus populations and is associated with a promoter polymorphism. In mouse strains that develop a spontaneous, lupus-like disease, restoring the level of RIIB expression on their B cells to a wild-type level reverses disease (48). A higher incidence of an allele of RIIB has been reported in several populations with autoimmune disease. This allele, found in the transmembrane domain of the receptor, is suggested to result in a hypomorphic phenotype, similar to the reduced expression observed.

Species Comparisons

Detailed comparisons between FcRs in mice and humans have revealed several notable differences in both structure and expression of these molecules (Figures 22.1 to 22.3). Whereas IgG and IgE FcRs are conserved in these species, IgA FcRs are not. A murine homolog for the IgA

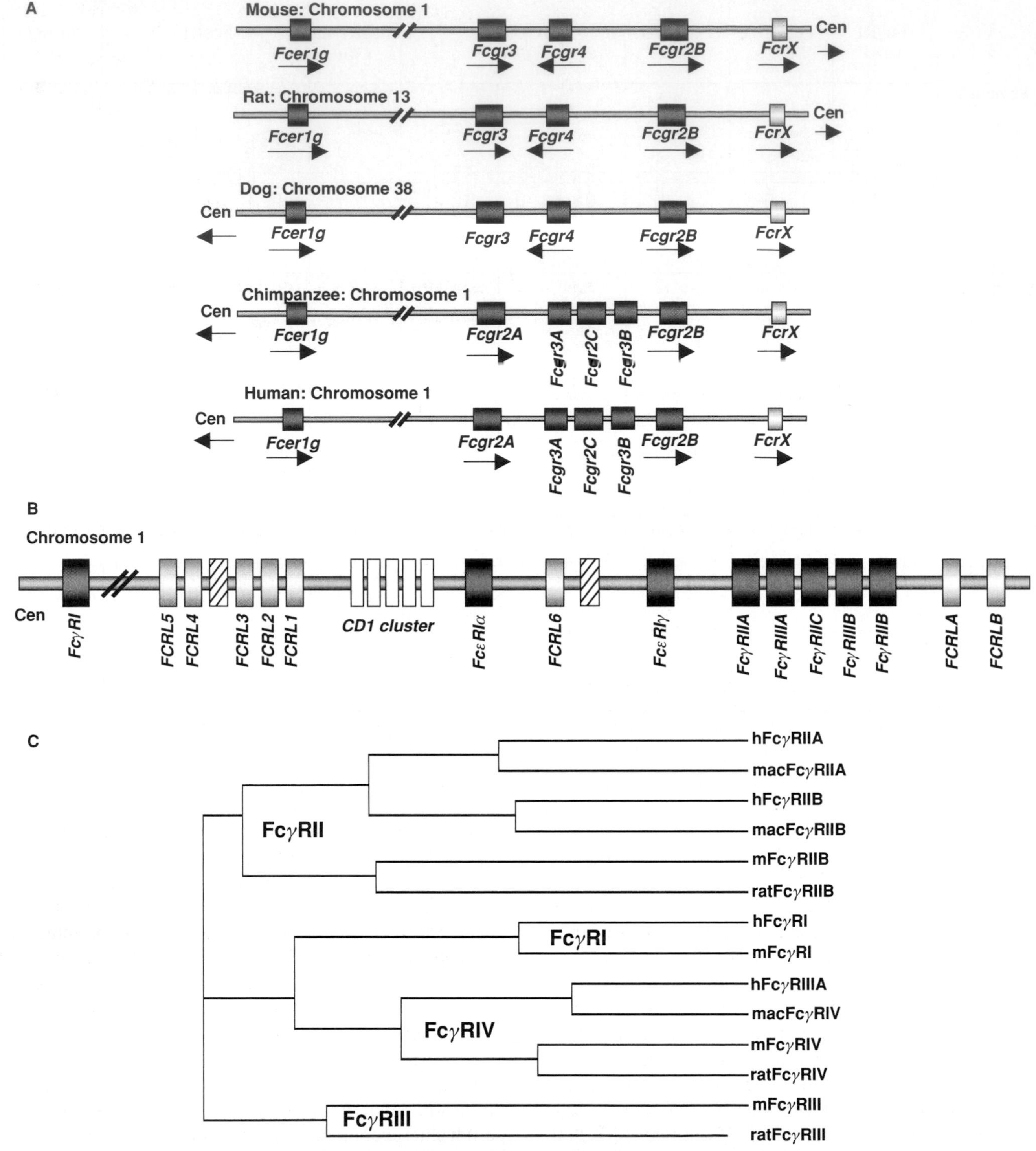

FIGURE 22.2 Chromosomal organization of FcR and FCRL genes. **A:** Localization of FcR genes in different species. **B:** The human FcR locus on chromosome 1. Classic FcR genes are shown in dark gray, FCRL genes as light gray, and the CD1 gene cluster on chromosome 1 as white boxes. Pseudogenes are indicated as hatched boxes. (Adapted from Davis RS, Dennis G Jr, Odom MR, et al. Fc receptor homologs: newest members of a remarkably diverse Fc receptor gene family. *Immunol Rev*. 2002;190:123, with permission.) **C:** The cladogram shows the alignment of selective classic FcRs of humans (h), macaques (mac), mice (m), and rats.

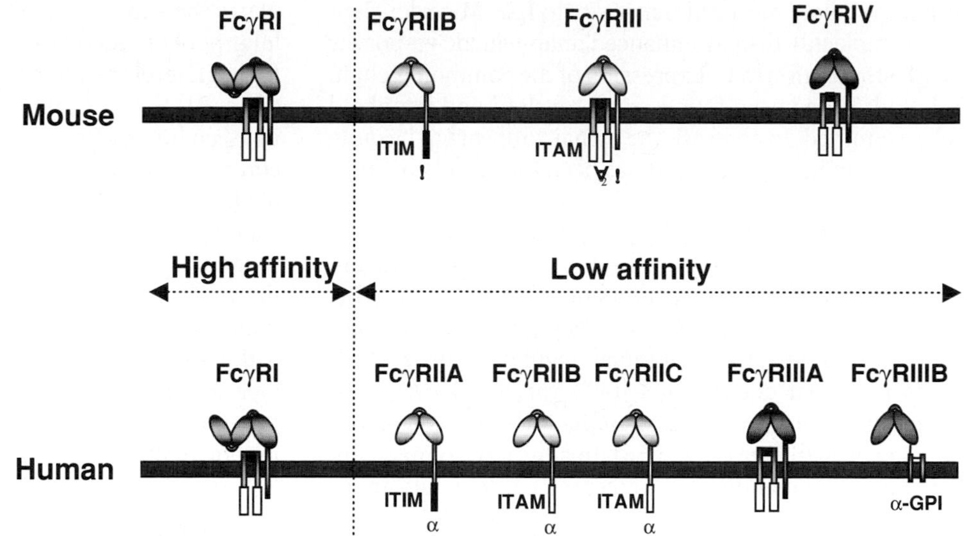

FIGURE 22.3 Comparison of the human and mouse Fcγ-receptor protein family. In both species FcγRs can be distinguished by their affinity for the antibody Fc portion (high or low affinity) and by the signaling pathways they trigger (activating versus inhibitory).

FcR has not been identified. In general, murine and human IgG FcRs display comparable degrees of heterogeneity and complexity (39,49). Specific differences, however, have been noted. For example, FcγRI is encoded by a single gene in the mouse and three genes in the human (41). Two genes for activation FcRs, FcγRIIA and C, are found in humans and not rodents, which is notable because of their unusual single-chain activation structure (50). Both mice and humans encode a gene referred to as FcγRIIIA, although recent studies have identified a novel mouse FcR with higher homology to the human FcγRIIIA called FcγRIV (31,49,51). As mentioned previously, FcγRIIIB is unique among FcRs in being expressed as a GPI-anchored protein. Its expression is limited to human neutrophils, in contrast with FcγRIIIA, which is expressed widely on cells of the myeloid lineage, such as macrophages, NK cells, mast cells, and dendritic cells. Finally, both mice and humans have only a single gene encoding the inhibitory FcγRIIB molecule.

The genes for the IgE FcR are conserved in mice and humans. The difference that is observed relates to the requirement for the β chain to achieve surface expression in mice, precluding the expression of the $\alpha\gamma_2$ complex (24). In humans, this form of the receptor is widely expressed on monocytes, Langerhans cells, and dendritic cells and is likely to be found on mast cells and basophils as well. This difference in FcεRI subunit composition is likely to result in functional differences as well. Although these specific interspecies differences are important, the fundamental organization of the FcR system, with activation and inhibitory signaling through a shared ligand specificity coupled to opposing signaling pathways, is well conserved. Thus, conclusions regarding the function of this system in immunity by the analysis of murine models are relevant to an understanding of the role of these receptors to human immunity as well.

Expression

FcRs are expressed widely on cells of the myeloid lineage, including monocytes, macrophages, dendritic cells, mast cells, basophils, neutrophils, eosinophils, and NK cells (17,33). In addition, B cells and follicular dendritic cells (FDCs) express the inhibitory FcRIIB receptor, whereas T cells are generally negative for FcR expression. Of interest, the majority of FCRL proteins are expressed during varying stages of B cell development. Despite their homology to the classic FcRs, however, the FCRL proteins seem not to bind to immunoglobulins, rendering FcγRIIB the only IgG-binding FcR on B cells. The specific expression pattern for each Fc-receptor varies; these patterns are summarized in Figure 22.1. Because FcRs represent a balanced system of activation and inhibition, the general rule of coexpression of FcRs of these classes is maintained. B cells use the B cell antigen receptor as the activation coreceptor for FcRIIB, whereas NK cells appear to use NK inhibitory receptors to modulate FcγRIIIA activation. The decoy FcγR, FcγRIIIB, is expressed exclusively on human neutrophils, on which it functions to concentrate and focus immune complexes without directly triggering cell activation, perhaps also playing a role in neutrophil recruitment (52). The FcγRIIA–FcγRIIB pair functions on neutrophils to modulate immune complex activation. FcεRI can be modulated by FcγRIIB, as demonstrated both *in vitro* and *in vivo*; mice deficient in FcγRIIB display enhanced IgE-triggered anaphylaxis (53) by virtue of the ability of IgE to bind with high affinity to FcεRI and with low affinity to FcγRIIB. Other mast cell inhibitory receptors, such as glycoprotein

49B1, modulate mast cell sensitivity to IgE: Mice deficient in this molecule display enhanced anaphylactic responses to IgE stimulation (54). Expression of the common γ chain is broad: It has been found on all myeloid and lymphoid cells examined. In contrast, the β chain appears to be quite restricted in its expression: It has been found only on mast cells and basophils.

Regulation of FcR expression can occur at several levels. In general, cytokines involved in activation of inflammatory responses induce expression of activation FcγRs, whereas inhibitory cytokines downregulate these activation receptors. Transcriptional regulation of α chain levels has been documented for a variety of cytokines, including interferon-γ, interleukin-4 (IL-4), and transforming growth factor-β (55,56). In addition, complement component C5a binding to its receptor, C5aR, results in the induction of expression of activation FcγRs (57). Induction of FcγRI, FcγRIIA, and FcγRIIIA α and γ chains in myeloid cells occurs on interferon-γ treatment: IL-4 generally inhibits expression of these activation receptors but induces expression of the inhibitory FcγRIIB. Administration of intravenous γ-globulin, a widely used treatment for inflammatory diseases, has been shown to induce expression of the inhibitory FcγRIIB on effector macrophages (58–60). This induction is not direct but is likely mediated through another, noncanonical Fc receptor pathway (60). The situation in B cells is likely to be more complex, whereby regulation of FcγRIIB is critical for the maintenance of peripheral tolerance. Germinal center B cells downregulate FcγRIIB, perhaps in response to IL-4 production by T cells. Regulation of FcR expression has also been documented to occur on binding of ligand. IgE regulates the expression of FcεRI by stabilizing the intracellular pool of receptor on receptor engagement (61). Thus, high IgE levels result in the induction of surface expression of FcεRI. However, this same mechanism of regulation is not seen for FcγRs: Mice deficient in IgG have FcγR levels comparable with those of wild-type animals. Competition for limiting subunits also contributes to regulation of receptor expression. In mast cells, it appears that the level of γ chain is limiting. Competition between α chains for the limiting concentration of γ chain has been documented in mouse knockouts, whereby levels of one receptor increase if the α chain of the other receptor is reduced (62). This type of reciprocal regulation is likely to be significant in the cross-regulation of FcRs by different isotypes of immunoglobulin.

Three-Dimensional Structure

The crystal structures of FcγRIIA, FcγRIIB, FcγRIIIA, and FcεRI have been solved, along with the cocrystals of FcγRIIIA–IgG1 Fc and FcεRI–IgE Fc (63) (Figure 22.4). These studies demonstrate that the receptors have a common structure in which the two extracellular immunoglobulin domains fold in a strongly bent overall structure arranged into a heart-shaped domain structure. A 1:1 stoichiometry between the receptor and ligand is observed, with the receptor inserted into the cleft formed by the two chains of the Fc fragment (Cγ2 or Cε3). The binding region of the FcR to Fc fragments consists mainly of rather flexible loops that rearrange on complex formation. Only domain 2 and the linker region connecting domains 1 and 2 interact in the complex with different regions of both

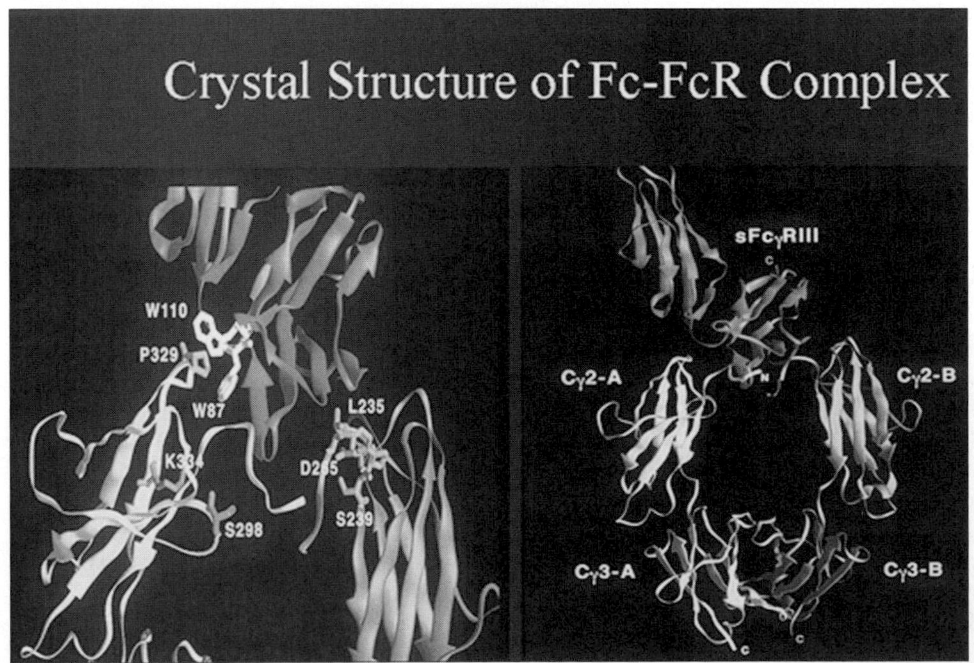

FIGURE 22.4 Ribbon diagram of crystallizable fragment (Fc) receptor III–immunoglobulin G1 (IgG1) Fc structure. The carbohydrate moiety has been removed from the IgG1 Fc fragment in this visualization, although it is present in the crystal structure. The extracellular domains of Fc receptor III are shown, together with the Fc fragment of IgG1. Some of the contact residues are shown for the binding interface. See text for details. (Adapted from Sondermann P, Huber R, Oosthuizen V, et al. The 3.2-A crystal structure of the human IgG1 Fc fragment-Fc gammaRIII complex. *Nature*. 2000;406(6793):267, with permission.)

chains of the Fc. Conserved tryptophans located on the FcRs interact with proline to form a "proline sandwich." A solvent-exposed hydrophobic residue at position 155 is conserved among all FcRs and represents a binding site for the important IgG1 residue Leu 235 (not found in IgE). Specificity is generated among the receptor–ligand pairs in a variable region connecting the two extracellular domains that is in contact with the lower hinge region of the Fc fragment (residues 234 to 238), a region not conserved among the IgGs and IgE. The binding region of FcRs to their immunoglobulin ligands does not overlap with other Fc-binding molecules such as protein A, protein G, and FcRn.

The structure of the FcR bound to their ligand reveal that the antigen-binding fragment (Fab) arms are quite sharply bent and may adopt a perpendicular orientation toward the Fc. This arrangement would give the Fab arms maximal flexibility to bind antigen when the Fc fragment is oriented parallel to the membrane of the FcR-expressing cell. The asymmetric interaction of the two Fc chains with a single FcR prevents a single antibody molecule from triggering dimerization of receptors and initiating signaling. Instead, dimerization is initiated by the interaction of antigen with the Fab arms, thus linking adaptive responses to effector cell triggering.

IN VITRO ACTIVITY

Binding Properties

As outlined in Figures 22.1 and 22.3, immunoglobulin binding to FcRs falls into either a high- or a low-affinity binding class. The high-affinity binding class is typified by FcεRI, with a binding affinity of 10^{10} M^{-1} for IgE, which ensures a monomeric interaction between IgE and its receptor. FcγRI binds with relatively high affinity for IgG1 and IgG3 (human) and IgG2a (mouse), with an affinity constant of 10^8 M^{-1}. In contrast to these high-affinity FcRs, the low-affinity receptors, such as the human FcγRIIA, FcγRIIB, FcγRIIIA, FcγRIIIB, and FcαRI and the mouse FcγRIIB, FcγRIII, and FcγRIV bind with affinities ranging from 5×10^5 M^{-1} (FcγRIII) to 2×10^7 M^{-1}. This low-affinity binding ensures that these receptors interact with immune complexes and not monomeric ligands. As described later, this dependence on high-avidity and low-affinity interactions ensures that these receptors are activated only by physiologically relevant immune complexes and not by circulating monomeric immunoglobulin, thus avoiding inappropriate activation of effector responses. In general, low-affinity FcγRs bind IgG1 and IgG3 preferentially; binding to IgG2 and IgG4 is observed at even lower affinities. As mentioned previously, polymorphisms in FcγRIIA and FcγRIIIA affect binding to IgG2 and IgG1, respectively, which may have significance *in vivo* in predicting responses to specific cytotoxic antibodies (Table 22.1). The isolated consideration of the affinity of antibody isotopes to their activating FcRs is not sufficient, however, to explain the differences in *in vivo* activity. More important, the ratio of the affinity of an antibody isotype to the activating FcRs compared to its affinity to the inhibitory FcγRIIB (the A/I ratio) predicts antibody activity more consistently (20,49). Thus, antibody isotypes with a high A/I ratio, such as mouse IgG2a and IgG2b, show a greater activity than counterparts with a lower ratio (Table 22.1). Binding has been observed between aglycosyl FcRs and immunoglobulin, with K_a values similar to those observed for the glycosylated forms. In contrast, the sugar moiety of the antibody Fc portion is essential for FcR binding, and the presence or absence of certain sugar residues can significantly affect antibody–FcR binding (20,64–66). The absence of fucose, for example, will selectively increase the affinity of human IgG1 or mouse IgG2b to FcγRIIIa or mouse FcγRIV, respectively. In contrast, the presence of terminal sialic acid on the N-linked Fc glycan reduces affinities for FcRs by an order of magnitude with a concomitant reduction in *in vivo* activity (66). Subunit interactions have also been reported to influence affinity for ligand, as demonstrated for the common γ chain associating with FcγRIIIA (67). Its affinity for IgG1 is higher than the GPI-anchored form of this receptor, FcγRIIIB.

The crystal structures of IgG1-FcγRIIIA and IgE-FcεRI reveal similarities in the binding properties of these two complexes. Of significance is the 1:1 stoichiometry of the complexes, which ensures that a single receptor binds to a single immunoglobulin molecule (15,16). This property in turn ensures that activation occurs on cross-linking of receptor complexes by multivalent ligands. Two binding sites on the receptor interact asymmetrically with two sites on the Fc molecule. The FcR inserts into the cleft formed by the two chains of the Fc molecule, burying a binding surface of 895 Å for each binding site. Alterations in the Fc structure that reduce the cleft, such as deglycosylation of IgG, inhibit FcR binding. Four distinct regions have been defined in the Fc domains involved in FcR interactions. For IgE, this includes residues 334 to 336, 362 to 365, 393 to 396, and 424. The homologous regions for IgG are residues 234 to 239, 265 to 269, 297 to 299, and 327 to 332, respectively. Interactions of these residues occur with the carboxy-terminal domain 2 of the respective FcRs. In view of the similarities of these complexes and the homologies among the receptors and their ligands, an obvious question that arises concerns the molecular basis for specificity. Attempts to resolve that question have relied on mutagenesis studies of the ligands and domain exchanges between receptors. For example, exchange of the FG loop in domain 2 of Fcε to Fcγ receptors confers detectable IgE binding; similarly, variation in this loop in FcγRs may provide interactions that determine IgG specificity for these receptors. Mutagenesis of IgG1 revealed that a common set of

TABLE 22.1 Affinity of Antibody Fc-Receptor Interactions

	Mouse Soluble FcγR (K_a, M^{-1})					Human Soluble FcγR (K_a, M^{-1})						
	FcγRI	FcγRIIB	FcγRIII	FcγRIV	A/I	FcγRI	FcγRIIA^{131R}	FcγRIIA^{131H}	FcγRIIB	FcγRIIIA^{158F}	FcγRIIIA^{158V}	A/I
mIgG1	n.b.	3.3×10^6	3.1×10^5	n.b.	0.1	n.d.	2.5×10^5	0.4×10^5	1×10^5	$<10^4$+	n.d.	
mIG2a	1.8×10^8	0.42×10^6	6.8×10^5	2.9×10^7	69	n.d.	3.2×10^5	1.7×10^5	1.6×10^5	1.0×10^5	n.d.	
mIgG2b	n.b.	2.2×10^6	6.4×10^5	1.7×10^7	7	n.d.	9.1×10^4	1.2×10^5	1.2×10^5	0.1×10^5	n.d.	
mIgG3	n.b.	n.b.	n.b.	n.b.	—	n.d.	$<10^4$+	$<10^4$+	$<10^4$–	$<10^4$+	n.d.	
hIgG1	3.8×10^6	2×10^5	3.5×10^4	2.2×10^6		9.1×10^8[a]	2.7×10^5	3.8×10^5	$1–3.8 \times 10^5$[b]	4.3×10^5	$1.9–4.8 \times 10^6$[b]	1/13[c]
hIgG2	n.b.	$<10^4$+	$<10^4$+	n.b.		n.b.	2.1×10^4	1.2×10^5	$<10^4$+	$<10^4$+	n.d.	(2/12)[d]
hIgG3	1.2×10^6	8.3×10^4	n.b.	$<10^4$+		n.d.	2.4×10^5	1.2×10^5	7.0×10^4	1.8×10^5	n.d.	3
hIgG4	7.2×10^4	$<10^4$+	$<10^4$+	$<10^4$+		n.d.	$<10^4$+	$<10^4$+	4.8×10^4	n.b.	n.d.	<<1

A/I, ratio of activating to inhibitory binding; h, human; Ig, immunoglobulin; m, mouse.
Binding constants were obtained by surface plasmon resonance (SPR) analysis with immobilized antibodies (fluorescein isothiocyanate–isotype switch variants) and soluble FcRs produced by transient transfection in 293T cells.
n.b., No detectable binding, or binding that is too low to be evaluated.
n.d., No SPR or other quantitative data are available.
+, Detectable but very low binding that did not allow determination of exact binding constants by SPR.
[a]Paetz et al. (137).
[b]Okazaki et al. (138), Maenaka et al. (139).
[c]The two numbers indicate the A/I ratios for the low- and high-affinity alleles of FcγRIIIA, respectively.
[d]Due to the low affinity of IgG2 to FcγRIIB, the values are approximate.

residues is involved in binding to all FcγRs, but FcγRII and FcγRIII also use distinct residues (68). Several IgG1 residues not found at the IgG–FcR interface by crystallographic determination had a profound effect on binding, which indicates the greater complexity of these interactions in solution.

The implications of these structural studies are that the Fc domain of IgG may be selectively mutated to direct its binding to specific FcγRs. Fc mutants that selectively engage activation FcRs (IIIA and IIA) while minimally interacting with inhibitory and decoy FcRs (IIB and IIIB) would confer optimal cytotoxic potential for tumoricidal applications. Indications that such Fc engineering is possible are suggested by IgG mutants with selective binding to FcRIII or FcRII.

Effector Cell Activation

The critical step in triggering effector cell response by FcRs is mediated by the cross-linking of these receptors by immunoglobulin. This can occur either by interactions of low-affinity, high-avidity IgG immune complexes or of IgG opsonized cells with activation FcγRs or by the cross-linking of monomeric IgG or IgE bound to FcγRI or FcεR, respectively, by multivalent antigens binding to the Fab of the antibody. Cross-linking of ITAM-bearing FcRs results in common cellular responses, determined by the cell type, rather than the FcR. Thus, for example, FcεRI or FcγRIII cross-linking of mast cells results in degranulation of these cells, whereas cross-linking of macrophage-expressed FcαRI or FcγRIII by opsonized cells triggers phagocytosis. These functions underlie the functional similarity of activation FcRs in which cross-linking mediates cellular responses by ITAM-mediated tyrosine kinase cascades. In addition to degranulation and phagocytosis, activation FcR cross-linking has been demonstrated to induce ADCC, the oxidative burst, and the release of cytokines and other inflammatory cell mediators. A sustained calcium influx is associated with these functions, as is transcription of genes associated with the activated state.

Cellular activation initiated by ITAM-bearing activation FcRs can be enhanced by coengagement with integrin and complement receptors. Although the ability of these receptors to mediate phagocytosis, for example, is modest, synergistic interactions with FcRs result in sustained activation and enhancement. Synergistic interactions between activation FcRs and Toll receptors, mannose receptors, and other pattern-recognition molecules have also been reported *in vitro* and suggest that interplay between the innate and adaptive effector mechanisms of an immune response are involved in mediating efficient protection from microbial pathogens.

In contrast to the activation of effector cell responses triggered by cross-linking of ITAM-bearing FcRs *in vitro*, cross-linking of an ITIM-bearing inhibitory receptor to an ITAM-bearing receptor results in the arrest of these effector responses. Homoaggregation of FcRIIB by its cross-linking on effector cells by immune complexes does not result in cellular responses; rather, it is the coengagement of ITAM- and ITIM-bearing receptors that results in the functional generation of an inhibitory signal. *In vitro,* it is possible to ligate any ITAM-bearing receptor to any ITIM-bearing receptor with a resulting inhibitory response. This activity is used functionally to define putative ITIMs and has proved to be a useful device in dissecting the signaling pathways induced by ITAM–ITIM coligation.

B Lymphocyte Suppression

B cell stimulation through the B cell antigen receptor can be arrested by the coligation of FcγRIIB to the B cell receptor (BCR). This occurs naturally when immune complexes retained on FDCs in the germinal center interact with both the BCR and FcγRIIB during the affinity maturation of an antibody response. *In vitro* suppression of B cell activation has been demonstrated by coligation of BCR and FcγRIIB, resulting in arrest of calcium influx and proliferative responses triggered by the BCR (25,69), the result of recruitment of the SH2-containing inositol 5′-phosphatase (SHIP)–1 (70). Calcium release from the endoplasmic reticulum is not affected, and there is thus an initial rise in intracellular calcium; however, this calcium flux is not sustained because SHIP recruitment blocks calcium influx by uncoupling of the capacitance channel. Homoaggregation of FcγRIIB by immune complexes can trigger apoptosis in B cells, as demonstrated in the DT40 B cell line and in murine splenocyte preparations (71). This activity is retained in ITIM mutants and depends on the transmembrane sequence of FcγRIIB. The *in vivo* relevance of this activity remains to be determined.

SIGNALING

Immunoreceptor Tyrosine-Based Activation Motif Pathways

The general features of signal transduction through ITAM receptors are conserved among all members of this family, including T cell receptors, BCRs, and various FcRs. The 19–amino acid–conserved ITAM is necessary and sufficient to generate an activation response, as demonstrated by the analysis of chimeric receptors. With a single exception, FcRs associate with accessory subunits that contain these signaling motifs. As described previously, the common γ chain contains an ITAM and is associated with FcεRI, FcγRI, FcγRIII, FcγRIV, and FcαRI. In addition, both FcεRI and FcγRIII may associate with the β subunit in mast cells. The ITAM found in the β chain does not function as an autonomous activation cassette, as has

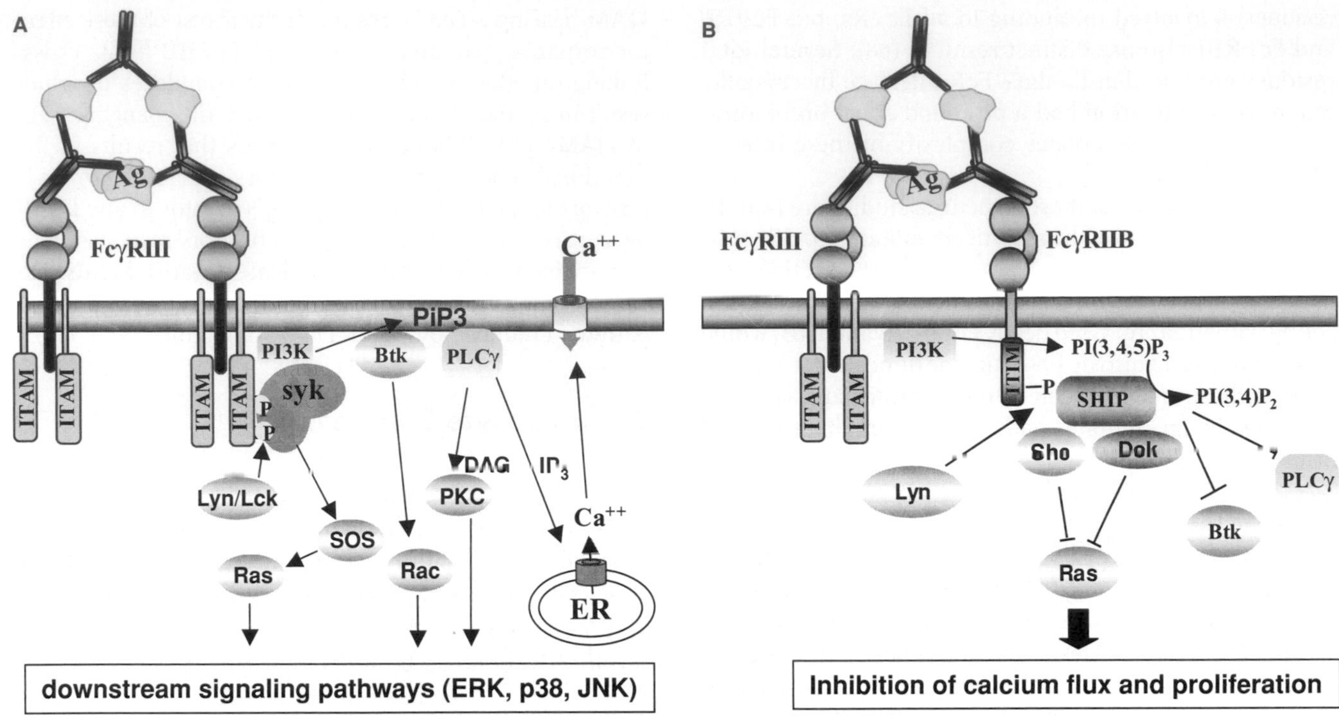

FIGURE 22.5 Signaling by activation and inhibitory FcRs. **A:** FcRIII signaling in natural killer cells is shown as an example of the activation class of FcRs. Cross-linking by an immune complex initiates the signaling cascade. The specific Src family kinase varies, depending on the cell type. **B:** FcR signaling in macrophages is shown as an example of simultaneous triggering of activation and inhibitory Fc receptors.

been found for most other ITAMs. Instead, it functions to amplify the activation response generated by the γ chain ITAM by increasing the local concentration of Lyn available for activation on aggregation of the receptor (38). FcγRIIA contains an ITAM in the cytoplasmic domain of its ligand recognition α subunit and is thus able to activate in the absence of any associated subunit.

On sustained receptor aggregation, Src-family kinases that may be associated with the receptor in an inactive form become activated and rapidly tyrosine-phosphorylate the ITAM sequences, creating SH2 sites for the docking and subsequent activation of Syk kinases. Ligands that become rapidly dissociated from the receptors result in nonproductive signaling complexes that fail to couple to downstream events and behave as antagonistic ligands (72). The specific Src kinase involved for each FcR depends on the receptor and cell type in which it is studied. Thus, Lyn is associated with the FcεRI pathway in mast cells, Lck is associated with FcγRIIIA in NK cells, and both of these kinases as well as Hck are associated with FcγRI and FcγRIIA in macrophages. After activation of the Src kinase, tyrosine phosphorylation of the ITAM motif rapidly ensues, leading to the recruitment and activation of Syk kinases. This two-step process is absolutely necessary to transduce the aggregation signal to a sustainable intracellular response.

Once activated, Syk kinases lead to the phosphorylation or recruitment of a variety of intracellular substrates, including PI3K, Btk and other Tec family kinases, phospholipase C-γ (PLCγ), and adaptor proteins such as SLP-76 and BLNK. The Ras pathway is also activated through Sos bound to Grb2 that is recruited on phosphorylation of Shc. Ras phosphorylates Raf, which in turn leads to MEK kinase and MAP kinase activation. A summary of these intracellular pathways is shown in Figure 22.5A. A crucial step in this sequential activation cascade occurs with the activation of PI3K by Syk. By generating phosphatidylinositol polyphosphates such as PIP_3, PI3K leads to the recruitment of pleckstrin homology (PH) domain–expressing proteins such as Btk and PLCγ, which in turn leads to the generation of inositol triphosphate (IP3) and diacylglycerol (DAG), intermediates crucial to the mobilization of intracellular calcium and activation of protein kinase C (PKC), respectively.

Immunoreceptor Tyrosine-Based Inhibitory Motif Pathways

The inhibitory motif, embedded in the cytoplasmic domain of the single-chain FcγRIIB molecule, was defined as a 13–amino acid sequence AENTITYSLLKHP, shown to be both necessary and sufficient to mediate the inhibition of BCR-generated calcium mobilization and cellular proliferation (25,26). Of significance, phosphorylation of the tyrosine of this motif was shown to occur on BCR coligation and was required for its inhibitory activity. This modification generated an SH2 recognition domain that is the binding site for the inhibitory signaling molecule SHIP (70,73). In addition to its expression on B cells, where it is the only IgG FcR, FcγRIIB is widely expressed on macrophages, neutrophils, mast cells, dendritic cells, and FDCs, absent only from T and NK cells. Studies on FcγRIIB provided the impetus to identify similar sequences in other surface molecules that mediated cellular inhibition and resulted in the description of the ITIM, a general feature of inhibitory receptors.

FcγRIIB displays multiple inhibitory activities. Coengagement of FcγRIIB to an ITAM-containing receptor leads to tyrosine phosphorylation of the ITIM by the Lyn kinase, recruitment of SHIP, and the inhibition of ITAM-triggered calcium mobilization and cellular proliferation (Figure 22.5B) (70,74,75). These two activities result from different signaling pathways; calcium inhibition requires the phosphatase activity of SHIP to hydrolyze PIP_3 and the ensuing dissociation of PH domain–containing proteins such as Btk and PLCγ (76). The net effect is to block calcium influx and prevent sustained calcium signaling. Calcium-dependent processes such as degranulation, phagocytosis, ADCC, cytokine release, and proinflammatory activation are all blocked. Arrest of proliferation in B cells also depends on the ITIM pathway, through the activation of the adaptor protein Dok and subsequent inactivation of MAP kinases (77,78). The role of SHIP in this process has not been fully defined, inasmuch as it can affect proliferation in several ways. SHIP, through its catalytic phosphatase domain, can prevent activation of the PH domain survival factor Akt by hydrolysis of PIP_3 (79,80). SHIP also contains PTB domains that could act to recruit Dok to the membrane and provide access to the Lyn kinase that is involved in its activation. Dok-deficient B cells are unable to mediate FcγRIIB-triggered arrest of BCR-induced proliferation while retaining their ability to inhibit a calcium influx, which demonstrates the dissociation of these two ITIM-dependent pathways.

Another inhibitory activity displayed by FcγRIIB is independent of the ITIM sequence and is displayed on homoaggregation of the receptor. Under these conditions of FcγRIIB clustering, a proapoptotic signal is generated through the transmembrane sequence. This proapoptotic signal is blocked by recruitment of SHIP, which occurs on coligation of FcγRIIB to the BCR because of the Btk requirement for this apoptotic pathway (71). This novel activity has been reported only in B cells and has been proposed to act as a means of maintaining peripheral tolerance for B cells that have undergone somatic hypermutation. The *in vivo* relevance of this pathway remains to be proven.

IN VIVO FUNCTIONS

Fcγ Receptors in the Afferent Response

The ability of IgG immune complexes to influence the afferent response has been known since the 1950s and can be either enhancing or suppressive, depending on the precise combination of antibody and antigen and the mode of administration (81). Investigators have attempted to define the molecular mechanisms behind these activities with the availability of defined mouse strains with mutations in activation or inhibitory FcRs and through the use of specific blocking antibodies to individual receptors. Direct effects on B cells stem from the ability of the inhibitory FcγRIIB molecule to influence the state of B cell activation and survival Because antigen is retained in the form of immune complexes on FDCs, it can interact with B cells by coengaging FcγRIIB with BCR, modulating the activation state of the cell. Mice deficient in this inhibitory receptor develop anti-DNA and anti-chromatin antibodies and die of a fatal, autoimmune glomerulonephritis at 8 months of age. The phenotype is strain dependent and is not seen in BALB/c or 129 strains of mice (82). Combining FcγRIIB deficiency with defects in other inhibitory receptor pathways, such as PD-1, results in autoantibodies with different specificities and distinct pathologic presentation. Thus, PD-1–deficient BALB/c mice develop cardiomyopathy resulting from anti–cardiac myosin antibodies. PD-1/RIIB double-deficient BALB/c mice develop antiuroepithelial antibodies and hydronephrosis (83). FcγRIIB thus acts as a modifier of autoimmune disease, a conclusion further supported by studies that determined the contribution of the C57B6 background to the spontaneous lupuslike disease observed in those mice. The B6 background, by virtue of an incomplete light chain editing pathway, provides a source of autoreactive B cells in the periphery, which, when combined with defects in the inhibitory RIIB pathway, lead to the accumulation of autoantibodies, pathogenic immune complexes, and disease (84). Further support for this conclusion is provided by the observations that autoimmune disease–prone strains of mice, such as New Zealand black (NZB), BXSB, SB/Le, MRL, and nonobese diabetic (NOD) strains, have reduced surface expression of FcγRIIB on activated B cells, attributed to DNA polymorphisms in the promoter region of the gene encoding this receptor (85,86). This reduced expression of FcγRIIB is thus suggested to contribute to the increased susceptibility of these animals to the development of autoantibodies and autoimmune disease. Direct evidence that this is indeed the case comes from studies in which FcγRIIB expression levels have been restored by retrovirus-mediated gene transfer in

BXSB, NZM, and FcγRIIB knockout animals. These mice had dramatically reduced levels of autoreactive antibodies and were protected from the development of fatal autoimmune disease (48).

Moreover, if FcγRIIB indeed functions *in vivo* to maintain peripheral tolerance, then its loss should allow for the emergence of autoantibodies when otherwise resistant animals are challenged with potentially cross-reactive antigens. This hypothesis has been validated in models of collagen-induced arthritis and Goodpasture's syndrome. FcγRIIB-deficient mice, with the nonpermissive H-2^b haplotype, develop arthritis when immunized with bovine type II collagen (87). The loss of FcγRIIB thus bypasses the requirement for the specific H-2^q and H-2^r alleles previously demonstrated to be necessary in this model by allowing FcγRIIB-deficient autoreactive B cell clones to expand and produce pathogenic autoantibodies. When the permissive DBA/1 strain (H-2^q) is made deficient in FcγRIIB, autoantibody development is augmented and disease is greatly enhanced. In a similar manner, immunization of H-2^b mice deficient in FcγRIIB with bovine type IV collagen results in cross-reactive autoantibodies to murine type IV collagen, with dramatic pathogenic effects (87,88). These mice develop hemorrhagic lung disease and glomerulonephritis with a "ribbon deposition" pattern of immune complexes in the glomeruli. These characteristics are indicative of Goodpasture's syndrome, a human disease not previously modeled in an animal species.

Expression of the inhibitory FcγRIIB on B cells thus provides a mechanism for the suppressive effects of immune complexes on antibody production. Although FcγRIIB is expressed throughout peripheral B cell development, recent data suggest that it represents a late checkpoint controlling the expansion of autoreactive IgG-positive plasma cells. In contrast, deficiency of the inhibitory receptor did not affect the generation of autoreactive IgM antibodies (84). Given the considerably higher pathogenic potential of IgG compared to IgM antibodies, this late stage of FcγRIIB-mediated regulation seems to be sufficient to prevent severe autoreactive processes.

The enhancing property of immune complexes on the afferent response is likely to arise from the expression of FcRs on APCs, such as dendritic cells (89–91). Dendritic cells express all three classes of IgG FcRs as well as FcεRI. Although *in vitro* studies have suggested that triggering of activation FcRs can induce dendritic cell maturation, the *in vivo* significance of this pathway has not been established (92). The ability of FcRs, particularly FcγRI, to internalize immune complexes could provide a mechanism for enhanced presentation and augmented antibody responses, whereas the presence of the inhibitory FcγRIIB molecule appears to reduce the enhancing effect. Mice deficient in FcγRIIB display enhanced antibody responses to soluble antibody–antigen complexes, in some cases dramatically so, which is likely to result from enhanced presentation (93,94). In addition, *in vitro* studies suggest that internalization through specific FcRs on APCs may influence the epitopes presented and T cell response generated as a result. A growing body of data suggests that FcRs are indeed involved in enhancement of the afferent response by influencing antigen presentation and cognate T cell interactions. FcγRIIB-deficient dendritic cells pulsed *ex vivo* with antigen in the form of immune complexes (ICs) induce a strong and protective cytotoxic immune response after transfer into naïve mice (95). In contrast, wild-type DCs induce a much smaller and nonprotective response, indicating that the threshold set by co-cross-linking of the inhibitory and activating Fc receptors prevents complete DC maturation. Moreover, blocking of IC binding to FcγRIIB on human DCs with an FcγRIIB-specific antibody resulted in spontaneous maturation of the cells by ICs present in low amounts in human serum (96,97). Taken together these data indicate that the inhibitory receptor is an important regulator of DC activation. Because the DC maturation state will determine whether an activating or a tolerogenic signal will be delivered to T cells, FcRs might be important factors for the maintenance of peripheral tolerance in the cellular immune system. Transiently blocking FcγRIIB activity with monoclonal antibodies *in vivo* might thus be an interesting strategy for optimizing immunotherapeutic and vaccination approaches. Further defining the precise role of each FcR expressed on APCs will require conditional knockouts of these molecules on specific dendritic cell populations to resolve the contribution of these systems to the generation of an appropriate antibody response.

Fcγ Receptors in the Efferent Response

The first FcR knockout to be described was for the common activation subunit, the γ chain, which resulted in the loss of surface assembly and signaling of FcγRI, FcγRIII, and FcγRIV as well as FcεRI (10). Mice deficient in the common γ chain were systematically studied in diverse models of inflammation and found to be unable to mediate IgG-triggered inflammatory responses for cytotoxic or immune complex reaction; attributed to low-affinity activation receptors, the high-affinity FcγRI played a minimal role in the *in vivo* inflammatory response triggered by IgG (22,98–100). The results were further confirmed by comparisons of mice deficient or blocked for FcγRI, FcγRIII, or FcγRIV (19,20,32,101). The loss of FcεRI ablated IgE-mediated anaphylaxis; this was demonstrated independently by gene disruption in the α subunit of that receptor (11). Subsequent studies on mice deficient in the inhibitory FcγRIIB molecule established the opposing action of this receptor, in which mice deficient in that receptor displayed enhanced B cell responses, autoimmunity, and augmented IgG-mediated inflammation in a subclass- and effector cell–dependent manner (18,20,32,100,102).

The general finding, which is discussed in detail later, illustrates that IgGs initiate their effector responses *in vivo* through coengagement of activating and inhibitory FcRs. The physiologic response is thus the net of the opposing activation and inhibitory signaling pathways that each receptor triggers and is determined by the level of expression of each receptor and the selective avidity of the IgG ligand (Table 22.1). This also explains the longstanding observation that different IgG isotypes have a differential activity *in vivo* (Figure 22.6A). The absence of a murine homolog for FcαRI has precluded similar studies for that receptor. Studies on mice bearing a human transgene of FcαRI suggest that this receptor is involved in IgA nephropathy (Berger's disease) (103).

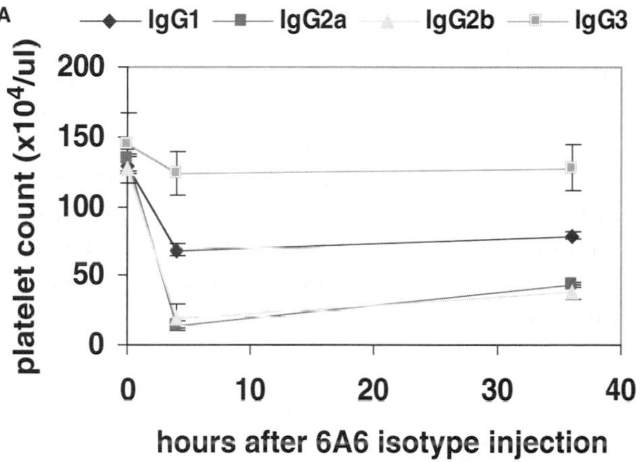

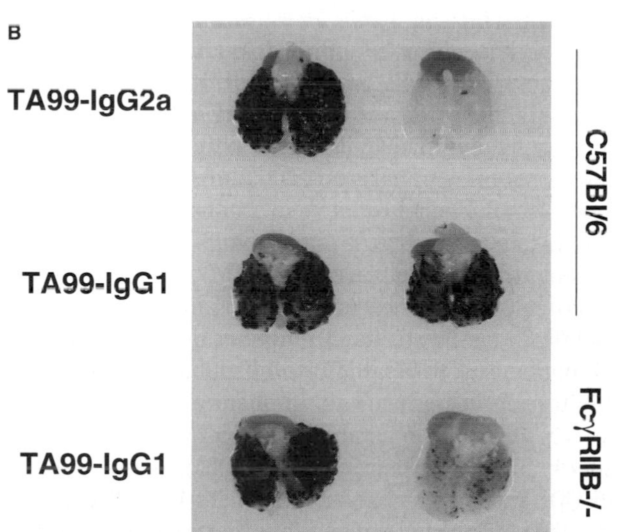

FIGURE 22.6 Antibody activity is determined by activating and inhibitory FcRs. **A:** Mice were injected with the same amount of different 6A6 antibody isotypes, which recognize an integrin on mouse platelets and lead to FcR-dependent clearance of platelets from the blood as observed by the drop in platelet count after antibody injection. **B:** Wild-type or FcγRIIB knockout mice were injected intravenously with B16 melanoma cells on day 0 and with IgG1 and IgG2a isotype switch variants of the monoclonal antibody TA99 on alternate days. Lungs were harvested on day 14. (Adapted from Nimmerjahn F, Ravetch JV. Divergent immunoglobulin g subclass activity through selective Fc receptor binding. *Science*. 2005;310(5753):1510, with permission.)

Type I: Immediate Hypersensitivity

Both cutaneous and systemic models of passive anaphylaxis induced by IgE were studied in FcRγ chain–deficient mice and were found to be absent, a finding fully consistent with the observations obtained in FcεRI-deficient mice and confirming the role of the high-affinity IgE receptor in mediating IgE-induced anaphylactic responses (10,11,38,104). FcγRIIB-deficient mice challenged in this model displayed an unexpected enhancement of IgE-mediated anaphylaxis, which suggests a physiologic interaction between this inhibitory receptor and FcεRI (53). The molecular basis for this modulation of FcεRI signaling by FcγRIIB has not been determined, although previous studies indicated that IgE can bind with low affinity to FcγRII/FcγIII, which suggests that there exists a mechanism for coengagement of these receptors. Deletion of the mast cell inhibitory receptor glycoprotein 49B1 also results in enhanced IgE-induced anaphylaxis (54). In addition to FcεRI, mast cells also express the IgG FcRIIB and FcRIII but not FcγRIV. Passive systemic anaphylaxis induced by IgG was attenuated in FcRγ chain–deficient and FcγRIII-deficient mice, which indicates the capacity of IgG and FcγRIII to mediate mast cell activation *in vivo*. FcγRIIB-deficient mice displayed enhanced IgG-induced anaphylaxis. Active anaphylaxis, induced by immunization with antigen in alum, was enhanced in FcεRI-, FcγRIIB-, and glycoprotein 49B1–deficient mice and attenuated in FcRγ- and FcγRIII-deficient mice. All of these animals displayed antigen-specific antibodies for IgE and IgGs, which indicates that the active anaphylaxis seen was attributed primarily to IgG antibodies. The reason for the enhancement of anaphylactic responses in FcεRI-deficient animals resulted from the increased expression of FcγRIII on mast cells in these mice, normally limited by competition of α chains for the available pool of the common γ chain (62). In the absence of FcεRI α chain, FcRγ chain is available to associate with FcγRIII α chain and assemble on the cell surface as a functional signaling receptor. These studies indicated the importance of the γ chain in regulating the level of surface expression of FcεRI and FcγRIII. Because γ chain is also associated with other members of the activation/inhibition paired receptors expressed on mast cells, such as PIR-A/PIR-B, the intracellular competition between these diverse α subunits and the common γ chain determines the level of surface expression of individual receptors and thus their ability to respond to specific biological stimuli. The absolute level of surface expression of FcRs on mast cells is clearly of therapeutic significance in both IgE- and IgG-mediated inflammatory responses; modulation of γ chain expression could thus represent a new therapeutic avenue for intervention in diseases such as anaphylaxis and asthma.

Type II Inflammation: Cytotoxic Immunoglobulin G

Cytotoxic IgGs are found in a variety of autoimmune disorders and have been developed for therapeutic indications in the treatment of infectious and neoplastic diseases. The mechanisms by which these antibodies trigger cytotoxicity *in vivo* have been investigated in FcR knockout mice. Anti-RBC antibodies trigger erythrophagocytosis of IgG-opsonized RBCs in an FcR-dependent manner; γ chain–deficient mice were protected from the pathogenic effect of these antibodies, whereas complement C3–deficient mice were indistinguishable from wild-type animals in their ability to clear the targeted RBCs (105,106). FcγRIII plays the exclusive role in this process for the mouse IgG1 isotype. Murine IgG2a anti-RBC antibodies use primarily the FcγRIV receptor pathway despite the singular ability of murine IgG2a antibodies to bind as monomers to FcγRI. These and other studies suggest that the role of the high-affinity FcγRI in IgG-mediated inflammation is likely to be restricted to augmenting the effector response (determined by FcγRIII and IV) in situations that involve high concentrations of murine IgG2a antibodies that are found at localized inflammatory sites where FcγRI expression is induced on recruited macrophages.

Experimental models of immune thrombocytopenic purpura (ITP) in which murine IgG1 antiplatelet antibodies trigger thrombocytopenia yielded results similar to those of the anti-RBC studies cited previously. The specific FcγR involved depended on the subclass of antibody used. IgG1 antibodies mediated their activity exclusively through FcγRIII, whereas IgG2a and 2b were RIV dependent. In contrast, FcγRI- or C3-deficient mice were fully susceptible to antibody-induced thrombocytopenia (20,31). FcγRIIB-deficient mice showed an isotype-specific enhancement of antibody-mediated platelet depletion, with the strongest impact on IgG1 and much smaller increases for IgG2a and IgG2b isotypes. This is consistent with the affinities of these isotypes for their specific activating and the inhibitory receptor, which will determine antibody activity *in vivo* (Table 22.1). In a passive protection model of *Cryptococcus neoformans*–induced disease, passive immunization with mouse IgG1, IgG2a, and IgG2b antibodies resulted in protection in wild-type animals but not in FcRγ chain–deficient animals (107).

IgG antibodies raised to murine glomerular basement membrane preparations induce acute glomerulonephritis in a model of Goodpasture's disease in wild-type but not FcRγ- or FcγRIV-deficient animals (59,108,109). FcγRIIB-deficient animals displayed enhanced disease in this model, which indicates that the effector cells involved were constitutively expressing significant levels of FcγRIIB. Similar results were obtained when DBA/1 animals were immunized with bovine type II collagen to induce arthritis. Deficiency of FcRγ chain protected these mice from the pathogenic effects of the anticollagen antibodies that were generated (110). As mentioned previously, deficiency of FcγRIIB in the DBA/1 collagen-induced arthritis model resulted in enhanced disease through increased autoantibody production and elevated effector responses.

A dramatic example of the importance of these pathways in determining the *in vivo* activity of cytotoxic antibodies was obtained in models of antitumor antibody response. In a syngenic murine model of metastatic melanoma, a murine IgG2a antimelanocyte antibody was able to reduce tumor metastasis in wild-type animals but was ineffective in FcRγ- or FcγRIV-deficient mice (20,111). In the absence of FcγRIIB, the activity of an IgG1 antibody, matched in its antigen-binding domain, was enhanced, which indicates that the *in vivo* cytotoxic activity of the antibody was the net of activation and inhibitory receptor engagement (20,102) (Figure 22.6B). These studies, together with similar studies performed with antiplatelet antibodies or defucosylated antibodies, demonstrated that the *in vivo* activity of a cytotoxic antibody could be predicted by a simple equilibrium binding model in which the ratio of the monomeric affinity constants for the activation and inhibitory Fc receptors (A/I ratio) are the dominant parameters, as demonstrated for TCR–MHC interactions (112). Xenograft models of human tumors transplanted into nude mice demonstrated, for a variety of tumors and cytotoxic antibodies, the requirement for FcR effector activity. For example, human breast carcinoma or lymphoma lines transplanted into nude mice and treated with either the humanized IgG1 or chimerized IgG1 antibodies trastuzumab (Herceptin) and rituximab (Rituxan), respectively, revealed that the ability of these antibodies to modulate tumor growth was abrogated in FcRγ chain–deficient mice. A point mutation that eliminated FcR binding of the anti-Her2/neu murine IgG1 antibody 4D5 abolished the *in vivo* cytotoxic activity of the antibody against a human xenograft but did not affect the *in vitro* growth-inhibitory activity; this again illustrates the difference between *in vivo* and *in vitro* mechanisms. Similar results were obtained for T cell lymphoma xenograft models and anti-CD2 antibodies, among others (113,114). The general conclusions that can be drawn from these studies support a dominant role for the low-affinity activating FcγRs in mediating cytotoxicity by IgG antibodies. FcγRIIB restricts the effector response for those antibodies with low A/I ratios and in situations in which the effector cell expresses this inhibitory molecule.

The relevance of these murine *in vivo* studies to the treatment of human populations with antitumor cytotoxic antibodies has been demonstrated in two studies that investigated the differential responses of patients treated with anti-CD20 (Rituximab) for lymphoma (115,116). Both studies demonstrated a highly significant correlation between patient response, as measured by the time to relapse, and alleles of FcγRIIIA. In patients with an allele of this low-affinity activation receptor (158V) that confers higher binding affinity for human IgG1 Fc, improved outcome was observed as compared to those with a lower-binding allele of this receptor (158F). In addition, lymphoma patients with the high-affinity allele showed a significantly better clinical response after receiving antiidiotype vaccination (117).

Type III Responses: Immune Complex–mediated Inflammation

The classic example of this reaction, the Arthus reaction, has been studied in a variety of FcR- and complement-deficient animals. The initial studies were performed by using the cutaneous reverse passive Arthus reaction in which antibody was injected intradermally and antigen was given intravenously. An inflammatory response, characterized by edema, hemorrhage, and neutrophil infiltration, developed within 2 hours. This reaction was elicited in a variety of complement- and FcR-deficient animals. The results from several independent studies confirmed the initial observations: IgG immune complexes triggered cutaneous inflammatory reactions even in the absence of complement but displayed an absolute requirement for FcγR activation (22). FcγRIIB modulated the magnitude of the response, with enhanced Arthus reactions observed in FcγRIIB-deficient strains (18). The effector cell in the cutaneous reaction was determined to be the mast cell, as demonstrated by the use of mast cell–deficient strains and by mast cell reconstitution studies (104). The generality of this result was demonstrated in similar reactions performed in the lung, illustrating the FcR dependence and relative complement independence of this response (88). Thus, all studies have demonstrated an absolute dependence on FcR expression in the Arthus reaction. One model for immune complex–induced arthritis, the KRN/NOD model, in which IgG1 anti-GPI antibodies are responsible for IC deposition in the synovium (118), has been shown to depend on both FcRIII and C3 but not on components of the classic pathway, such as C1q and C4; transfer of serum to animals deleted for FcRIII or C3 prevented the development of disease (119,120). Deficiency in the late components of complement, such as C5a or its receptor, have also been reported to result in a partial reduction in the magnitude of the response in immune complex–induced lung inflammation (121) and a result in a complete block in the KRN/NOD arthritis model. The likely mechanism by which C5a exerts its effects is through upregulation of activating FcγRs, resulting in an amplification loop (57). C5a is generated in this system as a result of FcR activation of effector cells and is independent of the classic, alternative and MBP pathways. Binding of C5a to the C5aR results in upregulation of activation receptors on these effector macrophages, thus augmenting the inflammatory response triggered by FcRs. These studies have led to a revision of the hypotheses about the mechanism of immune complex–mediated inflammation, typified by the Arthus reaction, in which there is an absolute requirement for activating FcγRs in initiating mast cell activation by immune complexes. FcγR activation is, in turn, modulated by the inhibitory receptor FcγRIIB. The A/I value of a specific IgG antibody and the densities of these opposing signaling receptors determine the concentration threshold for immune complex activation and the magnitude of the effector response that can be obtained. The classic pathway of complement activation is not required; however, C5a activation, through the FcγR pathway, may enhance the response under some circumstances through an amplifying loop. These release of inflammatory mediators such as vasoactive amines, chemokines, and cytokines leads to the hallmarks of this reaction: edema, hemorrhage, and neutrophil infiltration at the site of immune complex deposition.

The significance of the FcR pathway in initiating immune complex inflammation in autoimmune disease was further established by investigating a spontaneous murine model of lupus, the B/W F1 mouse. The Arthus reaction results predicted the absolute requirement of activation FcγR in initiating inflammation and tissue damage in immune complex diseases such as lupus. The FcRγ chain deletion was backcrossed onto the NZB and New Zealand white strains for eight generations, and the intercrossed progeny were segregated into B/W FcR$\gamma^{-/-}$ and FcR$\gamma^{+/-}$. Anti-DNA antibodies and circulating immune complexes developed in all animals; immune complex and complement C3 deposition was similarly observed in all animals. However, mice deficient in the common γ chain showed no evidence of glomerulonephritis and had normal life expectancy, despite comparable levels of circulating immune complexes and glomerular deposition of these complexes along with complement C3. Mice heterozygous for the γ chain mutation were indistinguishable from B/W F1 animals with wild-type γ chains in developing glomerulonephritis and displaying reduced viability (99). This spontaneous model supports the conclusions stated previously about the absolute requirement for FcRIII in the activation of inflammatory disease by immune complexes: In the absence of this receptor, deposited immune complexes and C3 are not sufficient to trigger effector cell activation, which indicates that it is possible to uncouple pathogenic immune complexes from inflammatory disease by removing activating FcR engagement. Similar conclusions were reached in a murine model of Goodpasture's disease in which immune complex deposition, composed of mouse IgG2b antibodies, resulted in a fulminant glomerulonephritis (59). Blocking the relevant activation FcR, FcRIV, with a monoclonal antibody protected the animals from fatal disease. These results further indicate that intervention in the effector stage of immune complex diseases, such as lupus and rheumatoid arthritis, would be accomplished by blocking activation FcγRs to prevent initiation of effector cell responses.

Fc Receptor Homologs

The family of FcR-homolog or FcR-like (FCRL) proteins was initially discovered by database searches based on a conserved motif in the Fc-binding region of classic FcRs. In humans the FCRL family consists of eight family members, termed FCRL1 to 6 and FCRLA, B (122). All the FCRL genes are located in close proximity to the classic FcRs on chromosome 1q21-23 (Figure 22.2B). A similar, although smaller family of FCRL proteins exists in mice also closely linked to classic FcRs on chromosomes 1 and 3 (42,123). In addition, the mouse has a unique FcR-like protein, called FCRLS, with a C-terminal type B scavenger receptor cysteine-rich domain. The majority of FCRL proteins consist of an extracellular domain of variable size, a transmembrane domain, and an intracellular portion that contains ITIM or ITAM motifs. The only exceptions are FCRLA, B, which lack a transmembrane domain and therefore represent intracellular or secreted proteins (122,123). The FCRL proteins do not depend on the common signaling γ chain, which is the crucial signaling adaptor for classic FcRs. Moreover, the FCRLs are predominantly expressed on B cells, with significant variation during B cell development and activation state. The ITAM-containing receptor FCRL1, for example, is widely expressed throughout B cell development starting from the pre-B cell stage (123,124). On activation, however, it is downregulated, and expression is restored on differentiation into memory but not into plasma cells. In contrast, FCRL4, which contains two ITIM motifs in its cytosolic domain, shows a more restricted expression pattern on a subpopulation of memory B cells (125). Co-cross-linking of FCRL4 with the BCR has been shown to dampen activating signals triggered by the BCR via recruitment of SHP-1 and SHP-2 (126). A functional variant of FCRL3 has recently been linked to rheumatoid arthritis and other autoimmune disorders in a group of Japanese patients (127). Despite significant sequence homology in some of the extracellular domains of FCRL proteins to classic FcRs, however, attempts to show binding to antibody Fc-portions have failed. Thus, the ligands of this interesting new family of proteins remain to be identified. More important, this renders the inhibitory FcγRIIB the only bona fide Fc receptor on B cells.

DISEASE ASSOCIATIONS

Autoimmunity and Tolerance

In view of their functional capacity to link autoantibodies to effector cells, FcRs have naturally been considered to have a pathogenic role in the development of autoimmune diseases. Several studies have attempted to correlate specific polymorphisms in FcRIIA, FcRIIIA, or FcRIIIB with incidence or severity of lupus or rheumatoid arthritis (128). In view of the heterogeneity of these diseases, it is perhaps not surprising that inconsistent results have been obtained. Alleles that increase the ability of FcRIIA to bind IgG2 or FcRIIIA to bind IgG1 might be expected to correlate with disease severity in some populations. Indeed, these types of associations have been reported in some studies but not in others. These variable results have often been explained as an indication that other genes may be in linkage disequilibrium with the FcR alleles under investigation. This is a plausible explanation when viewed in light of the autoimmunity susceptibility genes mapping in or near the region of the FcR genes, chromosome 1q21-24 (129). This region of chromosome 1 has been implicated in a variety of human and murine linkage studies. For example, the *Sle1* alleles derived from NZB flank the FcRIIB gene and form a linkage group with the ability to break tolerance to nuclear antigens, resulting in production of antichromatin antibodies. Epistatic interactions between FcRIIB and lupus susceptibility genes have been demonstrated in the murine lupus model of B6.RIIB. Crossing the *yaa* gene to this strain accelerates the development of disease; 50% survival is decreased from 8 months to 4 months, with 100% fatality by 8 months. This increase in severity correlates with a change in the specificity of the autoantibodies, from diffuse antinuclear antibodies to antibodies that stain with a punctate, nucleolar pattern on antinuclear antibody staining. Recently, it has been shown that the *yaa* susceptibility locus contains a duplication of the Toll-like receptor 7 (TLR7) gene in the pseudoautosomal region of the Y chromosome (130). Moreover, TLR7 and TLR9, with their ability to recognize potential self antigens such as RNA or DNA, respectively, were shown to be important components in the generation of pathogenic autoreactive antibodies (131,132).

Recent studies have identified two types of polymorphisms in the FcRIIB gene that are associated with SLE. Promoter polymorphisms have been described resulting in reduced expression of RIIB on activated B cells in both mouse and human SLE populations (85,133). In addition, a polymorphism in the transmembrane domain of FcRIIB has been identified that is associated with susceptibility to SLE in Japanese populations. This polymorphism results in an RIIB protein with reduced ability to enter lipid rafts and thus behaves as a hypomorphic allele for inhibitory function.

Together, these studies point to FcRIIB as a susceptibility factor in the development of autoimmunity, with the ability to interact with other susceptibility factors to modify both the afferent and efferent limbs of the autoimmune response

Inflammation

Antibody-mediated inflammatory diseases have been clearly demonstrated to involve the coupling of pathogenic autoantibodies or immune complexes to cellular FcRs.

Therapeutics targeted to disrupt these interactions are in development, beginning with a monoclonal antibody to human IgE that functions to reduce IgE binding to its high-affinity receptor and thereby prevent allergic and anaphylactic reactions (134). Because IgE is required for the survival of mast cells as well as in the regulation of FcεRI expression, reduction in IgE has synergistic effects on the ligand, receptor, and effector cell. The success of this approach will undoubtedly lead to other approaches that target the receptor or its signaling pathway. Blocking FcγRIIIA or IIA is expected to mimic the phenotype of FcRγ-deficient animals in models of IgG-induced disease. Early attempts to use this approach in ITP were promising but limited by the cross-reactivity to receptors on neutrophils, which led to neutropenia and the development of immune response to the murine antibody (135). Development of second-generation anti-FcRIIIA antibodies with greater specificity and reduced toxicity now appears to be a viable approach for the treatment of autoimmune diseases.

An alternative approach to limiting the activation of FcRs is to use the endogenous inhibitory pathway to abrogate IgE or IgG activation of their cognate receptors through coligation to FcγRIIB. This mechanism has been proposed to explain the ability to induce desensitization for the treatment of allergic diseases (33,136). Inducing production of IgG antibodies to an allergen may facilitate cross-linking of FcγRIIB to FcεRI. The ability to exploit the inhibitory pathway to reduce the activity of activation FcγRs has been demonstrated to account for some of the anti-inflammatory activity associated with high-dose intravenous γ-globulin (IVIG), which consists of the pooled IgG fraction of serum from thousands of donors (58). The use of IVIG for the treatment of ITP and other autoimmune diseases is well established, although the mechanism of action has been elusive. In murine models of ITP, arthritis, and nephritis, it has been demonstrated that protection by IVIG depends on the presence of FcRIIB; deletion of FcRIIB or blocking FcRIIB by a monoclonal antibody eliminates the ability of IVIG to protect the animal against an inflammatory response (58,60,66). IVIG was demonstrated to lead to the *in vivo* induction of FcRIIB on splenic effector macrophages, which would raise the threshold required for platelet clearance by FcRIII on these cells (60). Recently it has become clear that the sialic acid–rich fraction of IgG antibodies in the IVIG preparation is responsible for the antiinflammatory activity and FcγRIIB upregulation (66). Together with previous data on the dependence of FcRIIB upregulation on effector macrophages on CSF-1–dependent, so-called sensor macrophages, this suggests a two-cell model for the mechanism of IVIG activity (Figure 22.7). In this model, sialic acid–rich IVIG binds to a receptor on sensor macrophages, which in turn induces upregulation of FcRIIB on effector macrophages, thereby raising the threshold for activation. In addition, inducing expression of FcRIIB might be a clinically feasible approach and could be effective at modulating pathogenic autoantibodies from activation effector cell responses through activating FcRs.

Studies on the FcαRI receptor have demonstrated a role for this molecule in the pathogenesis of IgA nephropathy, in which circulating macromolecular complexes are deposited in the mesangium, resulting in hematuria and eventually leading to renal failure. Soluble FcαRI is found in the circulating IgA complexes, which suggests a role for the receptor in the formation of these pathogenic complexes. A transgenic mouse expressing FcαRI spontaneously develops IgA nephropathy resulting from the interaction of polymeric mouse IgA and the human FcαRI receptor to release soluble receptor–IgA complexes, which leads to deposition in the mesangium and the sequelae of IgA neuropathy.

SUMMARY AND CONCLUSIONS

Receptors for the Fc of immunoglobulins provide an essential link between the humoral and adaptive response, translating the specificity of antibody diversity into cellular responses. These receptors mediate their biological responses through the coupling of Fc recognition to ITAM/ITIM-based signaling motifs. A diverse array of biological responses depends on the FcR system, influencing both the afferent and efferent limbs of the immune response. Detailed biochemical, structural, and molecular biological data have provided a thorough understanding of how these receptors are regulated, are assembled, bind their ligand, and transduce specific cellular signals. FcRs play a significant role *in vivo* in maintaining peripheral tolerance by limiting the accumulation of autoreactive B cells that escape central tolerance checkpoints, such as light-chain editing, or that potentially arise during somatic hypermutation in germinal centers, in modulating T-cell responses by regulating both antigen presentation and maturation by dendritic cells, and in mediating the coupling of antigen recognition to effector cell activation. They are the primary pathways by which pathogenic IgG and IgE antibodies trigger inflammatory responses *in vivo*. Allergic reactions, cytotoxic IgG responses, and immune complex–mediated inflammation are all critically dependent on FcR cross-linking and have resulted in a fundamental revision of the mechanisms underlying such classic immunologic responses as the Arthus reaction. Blocking of these receptors uncouples the pathogenic potential of autoantibodies and represents an important new therapeutic target for the development of anti-inflammatory therapeutic agents. Central to the correct functioning of these responses is the balance that is maintained through the pairing of

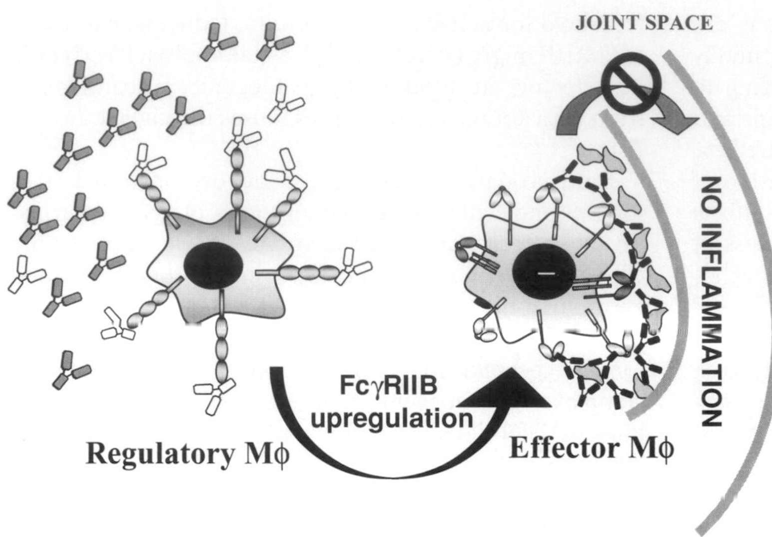

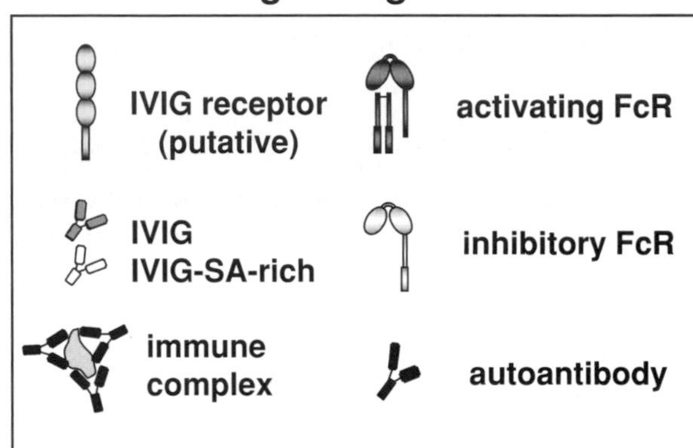

FIGURE 22.7 Two-cell model for the antiinflammatory activity of intravenous γ-globulin (IVIG). Sialic acid–rich antibodies in the IVIG preparation bind to an as-yet-unknown cell surface receptor on CSF-1–dependent sensor macrophages. This leads to the upregulation of the inhibitory FcγRIIB on effector macrophages, which results in a higher threshold for cell activation and thus inhibits the release of inflammatory mediators and tissue destruction. Falk Nimmerjahn is supported by grants from the DFG and Baygene.

activation and inhibitory receptors that coengage the IgG ligand; perturbations in either component can result in pathologic responses. The study of FcRs defined the ubiquitous inhibitory motif, the ITIM, and provided a paradigm for how these pathways modulate ITAM-based activation responses. Studies in mice deficient in individual FcRs have provided the necessary insights for defining comparable activities in human autoimmune diseases and suggest ways in which manipulation of the IgG–FcR interaction may lead to new classes of therapeutics for the treatment of these diseases. Modulation of the inhibitory response, a novel activity associated with IVIG to account for some of its anti-inflammatory activity *in vivo,* represents a novel approach to the regulation of immunoglobulin-mediated inflammation and suggests that therapeutic agents based on those pathways are likely to be effective. Conversely, engineering of therapeutic antibodies targeted to eliminate infectious or neoplastic disease will probably benefit from optimization of their Fc domains for interaction with specific FcRs.

ACKNOWLEDGMENTS

The Laboratory of Molecular Genetics and Immunology at the Rockefeller University is supported by grants from the National Institutes of Health, the Dana Foundation, the Juvenile Diabetes Research Foundation, the Cancer Research Institute, and Theresa and Eugene Lang.

REFERENCES

1. Boyden SV, Sorkin E. The adsorption of antigen by spleen cells previously treated with antiserum *in vitro*. *Immunology*. 1960;3:272.
2. Berken A, Benacerraf B. Properties of antibodies cytophilic for macrophages. *J Exp Med*. 1966;123(1):119.
3. Paraskevas F, Lee ST, Orr KB, et al. A receptor for Fc on mouse B lymphocytes. *J Immunol*. 1972;108(5):1319.
4. Kulczycki A Jr, Isersky C, Metzger H. The interaction of IgE with rat basophilic leukemia cells. I. Evidence for specific binding of IgE. *J Exp Med*. 1974;139(3):600.
5. Lewis VA, Koch T, Plutner H, et al. A complementary DNA clone for a macrophage-lymphocyte Fc receptor. *Nature*. 1986;324(6095):372.

6. Ravetch JV, Luster AD, Weinshank R, et al. Structural heterogeneity and functional domains of murine immunoglobulin G Fc receptors. *Science*. 1986;234(4777):718.
7. Kinet JP, Metzger H, Hakimi J, et al. A cDNA presumptively coding for the alpha subunit of the receptor with high affinity for immunoglobulin E. *Biochemistry*. 1987;26(15):4605.
8. Ra C, Jouvin MH, Blank U, et al. A macrophage Fc gamma receptor and the mast cell receptor for IgE share an identical subunit. *Nature*. 1989;341(6244):752.
9. Kurosaki T, Ravetch JV. A single amino acid in the glycosyl phosphatidylinositol attachment domain determines the membrane topology of Fc gamma RIII. *Nature*. 1989;342(6251):805.
10. Takai T, Li M, Sylvestre D, et al. FcR gamma chain deletion results in pleiotrophic effector cell defects. *Cell*. 1994;76(3):519.
11. Dombrowicz D, Flamand V, Brigman KK, et al. Abolition of anaphylaxis by targeted disruption of the high affinity immunoglobulin E receptor alpha chain gene. *Cell*. 1993;75(5):969.
12. Maxwell KF, Powell MS, Hulett MD, et al. Crystal structure of the human leukocyte Fc receptor, Fc gammaRIIa. *Nat Struct Biol*. 1999;6(5):437.
13. Sondermann P, Huber R, Jacob U. Crystal structure of the soluble form of the human fcgamma-receptor IIb: a new member of the immunoglobulin superfamily at 1.7 A resolution. *EMBO J*. 1999;18(5):1095.
14. Garman SC, Kinet JP, Jardetzky TS. Crystal structure of the human high affinity IgE receptor. *Cell*. 1998;95(7):951.
15. Garman SC, Wurzburg BA, Tarchevskaya SS, et al. Structure of the Fc fragment of human IgE bound to its high-affinity receptor Fc epsilonRI alpha. *Nature*. 2000;406(6793):259.
16. Sondermann P, Huber R, Oosthuizen V, et al. The 3.2-A crystal structure of the human IgG1 Fc fragment-Fc gammaRIII complex. *Nature*. 2000;406(6793):267.
17. Ravetch JV, Kinet JP. Fc receptors. *Annu Rev Immunol*. 1991;9:457.
18. Takai T, Ono M, Hikida M, et al. Augmented humoral and anaphylactic responses in Fc gamma RII-deficient mice. *Nature*. 1996;379(6563):346.
19. Hazenbos WL, Gessner JE, Hofhuis FM, et al. Impaired IgG-dependent anaphylaxis and Arthus reaction in Fc gamma RIII (CD16) deficient mice. *Immunity*. 1996;5(2):181.
20. Nimmerjahn F, Ravetch JV. Divergent immunoglobulin g subclass activity through selective Fc receptor binding. *Science*. 2005;310(5753):1510.
21. Carroll MC. The role of complement and complement receptors in induction and regulation of immunity. *Annu Rev Immunol*. 1998;16:545.
22. Sylvestre DL, Ravetch JV. Fc receptors initiate the Arthus reaction: redefining the inflammatory cascade. *Science*. 1994;265(5175):1095.
23. Ravetch JV, Clynes RA. Divergent roles for Fc receptors and complement *in vivo*. *Annu Rev Immunol*. 1998;16:421.
24. Kinet JP. The high-affinity IgE receptor (Fc epsilon RI): from physiology to pathology. *Annu Rev Immunol*. 1999;17:931.
25. Muta T, Kurosaki T, Misulovin Z, et al. A 13-amino-acid motif in the cytoplasmic domain of Fc gamma RIIB modulates B cell receptor signalling. *Nature*. 1994;368(6466):70.
26. Amigorena S, Bonnerot C, Drake JR, et al. Cytoplasmic domain heterogeneity and functions of IgG Fc receptors in B lymphocytes. *Science*. 1992;256(5065):1808.
27. Ravetch JV, Lanier LL. Immune inhibitory receptors. *Science*. 2000;290(5489):84.
28. Ravetch JV, Bolland S. IgG Fc receptors. *Annu Rev Immunol*. 2001;19:275.
29. Ghetie V, Ward ES. Multiple roles for the major histocompatibility complex class I–related receptor FcRn. *Annu Rev Immunol*. 2000;18:739.
30. Mostov KE. Transepithelial transport of immunoglobulins. *Annu Rev Immunol*. 1994;12:63.
31. Nimmerjahn F, Bruhns P, Horiuchi K, et al. FcgammaRIV: a novel FcR with distinct IgG subclass specificity. *Immunity*. 2005;23(1):41.
32. Hamaguchi Y, Xiu Y, Komura K, et al. Antibody isotype-specific engagement of Fcgamma receptors regulates B lymphocyte depletion during CD20 immunotherapy. *J Exp Med*. 2006;203(3):743.
33. Daeron M. Fc receptor biology. *Annu Rev Immunol*. 1997;15:203.
34. Kubagawa H, Chen CC, Ho LH, et al. Biochemical nature and cellular distribution of the paired immunoglobulin-like receptors, PIR-A and PIR-B. *J Exp Med*. 1999;189(2):309.
35. Maeda A, Kurosaki M, Kurosaki T. Paired immunoglobulin-like receptor (PIR)-A is involved in activating mast cells through its association with Fc receptor gamma chain. *J Exp Med*. 1998;188(5):991.
36. Moretta A, Bottino C, Vitale M, et al. Activating receptors and coreceptors involved in human natural killer cell–mediated cytolysis. *Annu Rev Immunol*. 2001;19:197.
37. Lanier LL. Face off—the interplay between activating and inhibitory immune receptors. *Curr Opin Immunol*. 2001;13(3):326.
38. Dombrowicz D, Lin S, Flamand V, et al. Allergy-associated FcRbeta is a molecular amplifier of IgE- and IgG-mediated *in vivo* responses. *Immunity*. 1998;8(4):517.
39. Qiu WQ, de Bruin D, Brownstein BH, et al. Organization of the human and mouse low-affinity Fc gamma R genes: duplication and recombination. *Science*. 1990;248(4956):732.
40. Su Y, Brooks DG, Li L, et al. Myelin protein zero gene mutated in Charcot-Marie-tooth type 1B patients. *Proc Natl Acad Sci U S A*. 1993;90(22):10856.
41. Maresco DL, Chang E, Theil KS, et al. The three genes of the human FCGR1 gene family encoding Fc gamma RI flank the centromere of chromosome 1 at 1p12 and 1q21. *Cytogenet Cell Genet*. 1996;73(3):157.
42. Davis RS, Dennis G Jr, Odom MR, et al. Fc receptor homologs: newest members of a remarkably diverse Fc receptor gene family. *Immunol Rev*. 2002;190:123.
43. Morel L, Blenman KR, Croker BP, et al. The major murine systemic lupus erythematosus susceptibility locus, Sle1, is a cluster of functionally related genes. *Proc Natl Acad Sci U S A*. 2001;98(4):1787.
44. Sandford AJ, Moffatt MF, Daniels SE, et al. A genetic map of chromosome 11q, including the atopy locus. *Eur J Hum Genet*. 1995;3(3):188.
45. van der Pol W, van de Winkel JG. IgG receptor polymorphisms: risk factors for disease. *Immunogenetics*. 1998;48(3):222.
46. Houghton AN, Scheinberg DA. Monoclonal antibody therapies—a 'constant' threat to cancer. *Nat Med*. 2000;6(4):373.
47. Floto RA, Clatworthy MR, Heilbronn KR, et al. Loss of function of a lupus-associated FcgammaRIIb polymorphism through exclusion from lipid rafts. *Nat Med*. 2005;11(10):1056.
48. McGaha TL, Sorrentino B, Ravetch JV. Restoration of tolerance in lupus by targeted inhibitory receptor expression. *Science*. 2005;307(5709):590.
49. Nimmerjahn F, Ravetch JV. Fcgamma receptors: old friends and new family members. *Immunity*. 2006;24(1):19.
50. Brooks DG, Qiu WQ, Luster AD, et al. Structure and expression of human IgG FcRII (CD32). Functional heterogeneity is encoded by the alternatively spliced products of multiple genes. *J Exp Med*. 1989;170(4):1369.
51. Ravetch JV, Perussia B. Alternative membrane forms of Fc gamma RIII (CD16) on human natural killer cells and neutrophils. Cell type–specific expression of two genes that differ in single nucleotide substitutions. *J Exp Med*. 1989;170(2):481.
52. Coxon A, Cullere X, Knight S, et al. Fc gamma RIII mediates neutrophil recruitment to immune complexes. A mechanism for neutrophil accumulation in immune-mediated inflammation. *Immunity*. 2001;14(6):693.
53. Ujike A, Ishikawa Y, Ono M, et al. Modulation of immunoglobulin (Ig)E-mediated systemic anaphylaxis by low-affinity Fc receptors for IgG. *J Exp Med*. 1999;189(10):1573.
54. Daheshia M, Friend DS, Grusby MJ, et al. Increased severity of local and systemic anaphylactic reactions in gp49B1-deficient mice. *J Exp Med*. 2001;194(2):227.
55. de Andres B, Mueller AL, Verbeek S, et al. A regulatory role for Fcgamma receptors CD16 and CD32 in the development of murine B cells. *Blood*. 1998;92(8):2823.
56. Pricop L, Redecha P, Teillaud JL, et al. Differential modulation of stimulatory and inhibitory Fc gamma receptors on human monocytes by Th1 and Th2 cytokines. *J Immunol*. 2001;166(1):531.
57. Schmidt RE, Gessner JE. Fc receptors and their interaction with complement in autoimmunity. *Immunol Lett*. 2005;100(1):56.

58. Samuelsson A, Towers TL, Ravetch JV. Anti-inflammatory activity of IVIG mediated through the inhibitory Fc receptor. *Science*. 2001;291(5503):484.
59. Kaneko Y, Nimmerjahn F, Madaio MP, et al. Pathology and protection in nephrotoxic nephritis is determined by selective engagement of specific Fc receptors. *J Exp Med*. 2006;203(3):789.
60. Bruhns P, Samuelsson A, Pollard JW, et al. Colony-stimulating factor-1–dependent macrophages are responsible for IVIG protection in antibody-induced autoimmune disease. *Immunity*. 2003;18(4):573.
61. Yamaguchi M, Lantz CS, Oettgen HC, et al. IgE enhances mouse mast cell Fc(epsilon)RI expression *in vitro* and *in vivo*: evidence for a novel amplification mechanism in IgE-dependent reactions. *J Exp Med*. 1997;185(4):663.
62. Dombrowicz D, Flamand V, Miyajima I, et al. Absence of Fc epsilonRI alpha chain results in upregulation of Fc gammaRIII-dependent mast cell degranulation and anaphylaxis. Evidence of competition between Fc epsilonRI and Fc gammaRIII for limiting amounts of FcR beta and gamma chains. *J Clin Invest*. 1997;99(5):915.
63. Sondermann P, Kaiser J, Jacob U. Molecular basis for immune complex recognition: a comparison of Fc-receptor structures. *J Mol Biol*. 2001;309(3):737.
64. Shinkawa T, Nakamura K, Yamane N, et al. The absence of fucose but not the presence of galactose or bisecting N-acetylglucosamine of human IgG1 complex-type oligosaccharides shows the critical role of enhancing antibody-dependent cellular cytotoxicity. *J Biol Chem*. 2003;278(5):3466.
65. Shields RL, Lai J, Keck R, et al. Lack of fucose on human IgG1 N-linked oligosaccharide improves binding to human Fcgamma RIII and antibody-dependent cellular toxicity. *J Biol Chem*. 2002;277(30):26733.
66. Kaneko Y, Nimmerjahn F, Ravetch JV. Anti-inflammatory activity of immunoglobulin G resulting from Fc sialylation. *Science*. 2006;313(5787):670.
67. Miller KL, Duchemin AM, Anderson CL. A novel role for the Fc receptor gamma subunit: enhancement of Fc gamma R ligand affinity. *J Exp Med*. 1996;183(5):2227.
68. Shields RL, Namenuk AK, Hong K, et al. High resolution mapping of the binding site on human IgG1 for Fc gamma RI, Fc gamma RII, Fc gamma RIII, and FcRn and design of IgG1 variants with improved binding to the Fc gamma R. *J Biol Chem*. 2001;276(9):6591.
69. Choquet D, Partiseti M, Amigorena S, et al. Cross-linking of IgG receptors inhibits membrane immunoglobulin-stimulated calcium influx in B lymphocytes. *J Cell Biol*. 1993;121(2):355.
70. Ono M, Bolland S, Tempst P, et al. Role of the inositol phosphatase SHIP in negative regulation of the immune system by the receptor Fc(gamma)RIIB. *Nature*. 1996;383(6597):263.
71. Pearse RN, Kawabe T, Bolland S, et al. SHIP recruitment attenuates Fc gamma RIIB-induced B cell apoptosis. *Immunity*. 1999;10(6):753.
72. Torigoe C, Inman JK, Metzger H. An unusual mechanism for ligand antagonism. *Science*. 1998;281(5376):568.
73. Tridandapani S, Pradhan M, LaDine JR, et al. Protein interactions of Src homology 2 (SH2) domain-containing inositol phosphatase (SHIP): association with Shc displaces SHIP from FcgammaRIIb in B cells. *J Immunol*. 1999;162(3):1408.
74. Daeron M, Latour S, Malbec O, et al. The same tyrosine-based inhibition motif, in the intracytoplasmic domain of Fc gamma RIIB, regulates negatively BCR-, TCR-, and FcR-dependent cell activation. *Immunity*. 1995;3(5):635.
75. Malbec O, Fong DC, Turner M, et al. Fc epsilon receptor I-associated lyn-dependent phosphorylation of Fc gamma receptor IIB during negative regulation of mast cell activation. *J Immunol*. 1998;160(4):1647.
76. Bolland S, Pearse RN, Kurosaki T, et al. SHIP modulates immune receptor responses by regulating membrane association of Btk. *Immunity*. 1998;8(4):509.
77. Tamir I, Stolpa JC, Helgason CD, et al. The RasGAP-binding protein p62dok is a mediator of inhibitory FcgammaRIIB signals in B cells. *Immunity*. 2000;12(3):347.
78. Yamanashi Y, Tamura T, Kanamori T, et al. Role of the rasGAP-associated docking protein p62(dok) in negative regulation of B cell receptor–mediated signaling. *Genes Dev*. 2000;14(1):11.
79. Aman MJ, Lamkin TD, Okada H, et al. The inositol phosphatase SHIP inhibits Akt/PKB activation in B cells. *J Biol Chem*. 1998;273(51):33922.
80. Liu Q, Sasaki T, Kozieradzki I, et al. SHIP is a negative regulator of growth factor receptor-mediated PKB/Akt activation and myeloid cell survival. *Genes Dev*. 1999;13(7):786.
81. Heyman B. Regulation of antibody responses via antibodies, complement, and Fc receptors. *Annu Rev Immunol*. 2000;18:709.
82. Bolland S, Ravetch JV. Spontaneous autoimmune disease in Fc(gamma)RIIB-deficient mice results from strain-specific epistasis. *Immunity*. 2000;13(2):277.
83. Okazaki T, Otaka Y, Wang J, et al. Hydronephrosis associated with antiurothelial and antinuclear autoantibodies in BALB/c-Fcgr2b−/−Pdcd1−/− mice. *J Exp Med*. 2005;202(12):1643.
84. Fukuyama H, Nimmerjahn F, Ravetch JV. The inhibitory Fcgamma receptor modulates autoimmunity by limiting the accumulation of immunoglobulin G+ anti-DNA plasma cells. *Nat Immunol*. 2005;6(1):99.
85. Jiang Y, Hirose S, Abe M, et al. Polymorphisms in IgG Fc receptor IIB regulatory regions associated with autoimmune susceptibility. *Immunogenetics*. 2000;51(6):429.
86. Pritchard NR, Cutler AJ, Uribe S, et al. Autoimmune-prone mice share a promoter haplotype associated with reduced expression and function of the Fc receptor FcgammaRII. *Curr Biol*. 2000;10(4):227.
87. Yuasa T, Kubo S, Yoshino T, et al. Deletion of fcgamma receptor IIB renders H-2(b) mice susceptible to collagen-induced arthritis. *J Exp Med*. 1999;189(1):187.
88. Nakamura A, Yuasa T, Ujike A, et al. Fcgamma receptor IIB-deficient mice develop Goodpasture's syndrome upon immunization with type IV collagen: a novel murine model for autoimmune glomerular basement membrane disease. *J Exp Med*. 2000;191(5):899.
89. Banchereau J, Steinman RM. Dendritic cells and the control of immunity. *Nature*. 1998;392(6673):245.
90. Amigorena S, Bonnerot C. Fc receptors for IgG and antigen presentation on MHC class I and class II molecules. *Semin Immunol*. 1999;11(6):385.
91. Hamano Y, Arase H, Saisho H, et al. Immune complex and Fc receptor-mediated augmentation of antigen presentation for *in vivo* Th cell responses. *J Immunol*. 2000;164(12):6113.
92. Regnault A, Lankar D, Lacabanne V, et al. Fcgamma receptor-mediated induction of dendritic cell maturation and major histocompatibility complex class I–restricted antigen presentation after immune complex internalization. *J Exp Med*. 1999;189(2):371.
93. Wernersson S, Karlsson MC, Dahlstrom J, et al. IgG-mediated enhancement of antibody responses is low in Fc receptor gamma chain-deficient mice and increased in Fc gamma RII-deficient mice. *J Immunol*. 1999;163(2):618.
94. Baiu DC, Prechl J, Tchorbanov A, et al. Modulation of the humoral immune response by antibody-mediated antigen targeting to complement receptors and Fc receptors. *J Immunol*. 1999;162(6):3125.
95. Kalergis AM, Ravetch JV. Inducing tumor immunity through the selective engagement of activating Fcgamma receptors on dendritic cells. *J Exp Med*. 2002;195(12):1653.
96. Dhodapkar KM, Kaufman JL, Ehlers M, et al. Selective blockade of inhibitory Fcgamma receptor enables human dendritic cell maturation with IL-12p70 production and immunity to antibody-coated tumor cells. *Proc Natl Acad Sci U S A*. 2005;102(8):2910.
97. Boruchov AM, Heller G, Veri MC, et al. Activating and inhibitory IgG Fc receptors on human DCs mediate opposing functions. *J Clin Invest*. 2005;15:15.
98. Clynes R, Ravetch JV. Cytotoxic antibodies trigger inflammation through Fc receptors. *Immunity*. 1995;3(1):21.
99. Clynes R, Dumitru C, Ravetch JV. Uncoupling of immune complex formation and kidney damage in autoimmune glomerulonephritis. *Science*. 1998;279(5353):1052.
100. Clynes R, Maizes JS, Guinamard R, et al. Modulation of immune complex–induced inflammation *in vivo* by the coordinate expression of activation and inhibitory Fc receptors. *J Exp Med*. 1999;189(1):179.

101. Hazenbos WL, Heijnen IA, Meyer D, et al. Murine IgG1 complexes trigger immune effector functions predominantly via Fc gamma RIII (CD16). *J Immunol.* 1998;161(6):3026.
102. Clynes RA, Towers TL, Presta LG, et al. Inhibitory Fc receptors modulate *in vivo* cytoxicity against tumor targets. *Nat Med.* 2000; 6(4):443.
103. Launay P, Grossetete B, Arcos-Fajardo M, et al. Fcalpha receptor (CD89) mediates the development of immunoglobulin A (IgA) nephropathy (Berger's disease). Evidence for pathogenic soluble receptor-Iga complexes in patients and CD89 transgenic mice. *J Exp Med.* 2000;191(11):1999.
104. Miyajima I, Dombrowicz D, Martin TR, et al. Systemic anaphylaxis in the mouse can be mediated largely through IgG1 and Fc gammaRIII. Assessment of the cardiopulmonary changes, mast cell degranulation, and death associated with active or IgE- or IgG1-dependent passive anaphylaxis. *J Clin Invest.* 1997;99(5):901.
105. Sylvestre D, Clynes R, Ma M, et al. Immunoglobulin G–mediated inflammatory responses develop normally in complement-deficient mice. *J Exp Med.* 1996;184(6):2385.
106. Fossati-Jimack L, Ioan-Facsinay A, Reininger L, et al. Markedly different pathogenicity of four immunoglobulin G isotype-switch variants of an antierythrocyte autoantibody is based on their capacity to interact *in vivo* with the low-affinity Fcgamma receptor III. *J Exp Med.* 2000;191(8):1293.
107. Yuan R, Clynes R, Oh J, et al. Antibody-mediated modulation of *Cryptococcus neoformans* infection is dependent on distinct Fc receptor functions and IgG subclasses. *J Exp Med.* 1998;187(4):641.
108. Suzuki Y, Shirato I, Okumura K, et al. Distinct contribution of Fc receptors and angiotensin II–dependent pathways in anti-GBM glomerulonephritis. *Kidney Int.* 1998;54(4):1166.
109. Park SY, Ueda S, Ohno H, et al. Resistance of Fc receptor–deficient mice to fatal glomerulonephritis. *J Clin Invest.* 1998;102(6):1229.
110. Kleinau S, Martinsson P, Heyman B. Induction and suppression of collagen-induced arthritis is dependent on distinct fcgamma receptors. *J Exp Med.* 2000;191(9):1611.
111. Clynes R, Takechi Y, Moroi Y, et al. Fc receptors are required in passive and active immunity to melanoma. *Proc Natl Acad Sci U S A.* 1998;95(2):652.
112. Stone JD, Cochran JR, Stern LJ. T-cell activation by soluble MHC oligomers can be described by a two-parameter binding model. *Biophys J.* 2001;81(5):2547.
113. Zhang Z, Zhang M, Ravetch JV, et al. Effective therapy for a murine model of adult T-cell leukemia with the humanized anti-CD2 monoclonal antibody, MEDI-507. *Blood.* 2003;102(1):284.
114. Zhang M, Zhang Z, Garmestani K, et al. Activating Fc receptors are required for antitumor efficacy of the antibodies directed toward CD25 in a murine model of adult t-cell leukemia. *Cancer Res.* 2004;64(16):5825.
115. Weng WK, Levy R. Two immunoglobulin G fragment C receptor polymorphisms independently predict response to rituximab in patients with follicular lymphoma. *J Clin Oncol.* 2003;21(21):3940.
116. Cartron G, Dacheux L, Salles G, et al. Therapeutic activity of humanized anti-CD20 monoclonal antibody and polymorphism in IgG Fc receptor FcgammaRIIIa gene. *Blood.* 2002;99(3):754.
117. Weng WK, Czerwinski D, Timmerman J, et al. Clinical outcome of lymphoma patients after idiotype vaccination is correlated with humoral immune response and immunoglobulin G Fc receptor genotype. *J Clin Oncol.* 2004;22(23):4717.
118. Ji H, Ohmura K, Mahmood U, et al. Arthritis critically dependent on innate immune system players. *Immunity.* 2002;16(2):157.
119. Korganow AS, Ji H, Mangialaio S, et al. From systemic T cell self-reactivity to organ-specific autoimmune disease via immunoglobulins. *Immunity.* 1999;10(4):451.
120. Matsumoto I, Staub A, Benoist C, et al. Arthritis provoked by linked T and B cell recognition of a glycolytic enzyme. *Science.* 1999;286(5445):1732.
121. Baumann U, Kohl J, Tschernig T, et al. A codominant role of Fc gamma RI/III and C5aR in the reverse Arthus reaction. *J Immunol.* 2000;164(2):1065.
122. Maltais LJ, Lovering RC, Taranin AV, et al. New nomenclature for Fc receptor-like molecules. *Nat Immunol.* 2006;7(5):431.
123. Davis RS, Ehrhardt GR, Leu CM, et al. An extended family of Fc receptor relatives. *Eur J Immunol.* 2005;35(3):674.
124. Leu CM, Davis RS, Gartland LA, et al. FcRH1: an activation coreceptor on human B cells. *Blood.* 2005;105(3):1121.
125. Davis RS, Stephan RP, Chen CC, et al. Differential B cell expression of mouse Fc receptor homologs. *Int Immunol.* 2004;16(9):1343.
126. Ehrhardt GR, Davis RS, Hsu JT, et al. The inhibitory potential of Fc receptor homolog 4 on memory B cells. *Proc Natl Acad Sci U S A.* 2003;100(23):13489.
127. Kochi Y, Yamada R, Suzuki A, et al. A functional variant in FCRL3, encoding Fc receptor–like 3, is associated with rheumatoid arthritis and several autoimmunities. *Nat Genet.* 2005;37(5):478.
128. Dijstelbloem HM, van de Winkel JG, Kallenberg CG. Inflammation in autoimmunity: receptors for IgG revisited. *Trends Immunol.* 2001;22(9):510.
129. Wakeland EK, Liu K, Graham RR, et al. Delineating the genetic basis of systemic lupus erythematosus. *Immunity.* 2001; 15(3):397.
130. Pisitkun P, Deane JA, Difilippantonio MJ, et al. Autoreactive B cell responses to RNA-related antigens due to TLR7 gene duplication. *Science.* 2006;312(5780):1669.
131. Pasare C, Medzhitov R. Control of B cell responses by Toll-like receptors. *Nature.* 2005;438(7066):364.
132. Ehlers M, Fukuyama H, McGaha TL, et al. TLR9/MyD88 signaling is required for class switching to pathogenic IgG2a and 2b autoantibodies in SLE. *J Exp Med.* 2006;203(3):553.
133. Blank MC, Stefanescu RN, Masuda E, et al. Decreased transcription of the human FCGR2B gene mediated by the 343 G/C promoter polymorphism and association with systemic lupus erythematosus. *Hum Genet.* 2005;117(2–3):220.
134. Heusser C, Jardieu P. Therapeutic potential of anti-IgE antibodies. *Curr Opin Immunol.* 1997;9(6):805.
135. Bussel JB. Fc receptor blockade and immune thrombocytopenic purpura. *Semin Hematol.* 2000;37(3):261.
136. Strait RT, Morris SC, Finkelman FD. IgG-blocking antibodies inhibit IgE-mediated anaphylaxis *in vivo* through both antigen interception and Fc gamma RIIb cross-linking. *J Clin Invest.* 2006;116(3): 833.
137. Paetz A, Sack M, Thepen T, et al. Recombinant soluble human Fcgamma receptor I with picomolar affinity for immunoglobulin G. *Biochem Biophys Res Commun.* 2005;338(4):1811.
138. Okazaki A, Shoji-Hosaka E, Nakamura K, et al. Fucose depletion from human IgG1 oligosaccharide enhances binding enthalpy and association rate between IgG1 and FcgammaRIIIa. *J Mol Biol.* 2004;336(5):1239.
139. Maenaka K, van der Merwe PA, Stuart DI, J et al. The human low affinity Fcgamma receptors IIa, IIb, and III bind IgG with fast kinetics and distinct thermodynamic properties. *J Biol Chem.* 2001;276(48):44898.

Chapter 23

Type I Cytokines and Interferons and Their Receptors

Warren J. Leonard

OVERVIEW AND ISSUES OF NOMENCLATURE

Cytokines are proteins that are secreted by cells and exert actions on either the cytokine-producing cell (autocrine actions) or on other target cells (paracrine actions) by binding to and transducing signals through specific cell surface receptors. From this operational type of description, it is clear that the distinction among cytokines, growth factors, and hormones is imprecise, even though all are secreted proteins. As a generalizaiton, cytokines and growth factors are similar, except that the term *cytokine* typically refers to a molecule involved in host defense that has actions on white blood cells (leukocytes), whereas the term *growth factor* more often refers to molecules acting on other somatic cell types. Cytokines generally act locally. For example, in the interaction between a T cell and an antigen-presenting cell, cytokines are produced and usually exert potent actions locally, with rather limited biologic half-lives in the circulation. In contrast, hormones are released and then disseminated via the bloodstream throughout the body, with actions on many distal target organs. Nevertheless, this distinction between cytokines and hormones is not absolute, with certain cytokines acting at longer distances as well.

In the immune system, terms such as *monokines* and *lymphokines* were originally devised to identify the cellular source for cytokines (1). Specifically, monokines included molecules such as interleukin-1 (IL-1), which was first recognized as being produced by monocytes, and lymphokines included molecules such as IL-2, which was first described as a T-cell growth factor produced by T lymphocytes. The monokine/lymphokine nomenclature has obvious limitation when a cytokine is synthesized by more than one type of cell. This resulted in the adoption of the term *cytokine,* as proposed by Stanley Cohen in 1974 (2,*3*). The term *cytokine* refers to a protein made by a cell ("cyto") that acts on target cells. Cytokines can have very broad ranges of actions, including effects on cell growth, cell differentiation, cytolytic activity of effector cells, apoptosis, and chemotaxis.

Many cytokines are referred to as *interleukins,* a term that refers to molecules that are produced by one leukocyte and act on another (4). Analogous to the inadequacy of the terms *monokine* and *lymphokine,* however, some interleukins (e.g, IL-1 and IL-6) are additionally produced by cells other than leukocytes and/or can exert actions on other cell types extending beyond the immune system. IL-7 is not ideally named, as it is a cytokine that is produced by stromal/epithelial cells rather than by typical leukocytes. Furthermore, nomenclature has also been inconsistent. For example, IL-7 is highly related to another cytokine that is denoted as thymic stromal lymphopoietin (TSLP) rather than as an interleukin (both are discussed later). Indeed, both are stromal factors that share a receptor component and have overlapping actions on T and B cells, but their very different types of names obscures these facts. The more descriptive name TSLP correctly describes its production by thymic stroma but obcures its production by skin epithelial cells and that major target cells include dendritic cells and CD4$^+$ T cells.

Among the many different cytokines, the "type I" cytokines share a similar four–α-helical–bundle structure, as detailed later, and correspondingly, their receptors also share characteristic features that have led to their description as the cytokine receptor superfamily, or type I cytokine receptors (5,6,7,*8*). Although many interleukins are type I cytokines, this is not true for all. For example, two of the major "proinflammatory cytokines," IL-1 and IL-6, are interleukins, but IL-6 is a type I cytokine whereas IL-1 is not (IL-1 is discussed in Chapter 24). TUF (see Chapter 25) is yet another very different type of proinflammatory cytokine. One interleukin, IL-8, is a CXC-family chemokine (see Chapter 26), an entirely different type of molecule involved in chemotaxis. Moreover, as discussed later, IL-10, IL-19, IL-20, IL-22, IL-24, IL-26, IL-28, and IL-29 are more similar to interferons and are denoted as type II cytokines.

In summary, the term inter*leuk*in indicates a relationship to *leuk*ocytes, whereas the identification of a cytokine as a type I or type II cytokine indicates general properties of the three-dimensional structure of the cytokine. Knowing that a molecule is a type I cytokine is instructive, as it indicates a likely general structure for the cytokine receptor as well as the mechanism of signal transduction. In contrast, the identification of a molecule as an interleukin provides little information other than that it typically, but not always, is a type I or type II cytokine of immunologic interest.

In addition to molecules that are primarily of immunologic interest, other extremely important proteins, such as growth hormone, prolactin, erythropoietin (Epo), thrombopoietin (Tpo), and leptin, are also type I cytokines and their receptors are type I cytokine receptors. Despite having major actions outside the immune system, these cytokines nevertheless share important signal transduction pathways with type I cytokines whose actions are primarily of immunologic interest. By focusing on type I cytokines and their receptors, this chapter necessarily focuses on cytokines that are evolutionarily related and that share common signaling pathways, instead of focusing on common functions per se. For example, although IL-6 has overlapping actions with IL-1 and TNF-α, these latter proinflammatory cytokines are discussed elsewhere because they are not type I cytokines, and the signaling pathways they use are distinct from those used by IL-6. This illustrates the important concept that similar end functions can be mediated via more than one type of signaling pathway. This is not to minimize the observation that many type I cytokines in fact do have similar/overlapping functions, as detailed later, in the section on cytokine redundancy.

The field of interferon (IFN) research is older than the cytokine field, but both fields more recently have developed in parallel. In fact, one should perhaps simply consider the IFNs to be the first cytokines that were identified. IFN was originally discovered as an antiviral activity in 1957. This turned out to be type I IFN (IFN-α/β). Type II IFN (IFN-γ) was discovered in 1965. Over time, it was recognized that type I cytokines and IFNs/type II cytokines share a number of common features. It is noteworthy that a number of years ago, the International Interferon Society changed its name to the International Society of Interferon and Cytokine Research and that the International Cytokine Society focuses on the IFNs as well as cytokines, underscoring the common features, both in basic science and clinically, of IFNs and cytokines.

TYPE I CYTOKINES AND THEIR RECEPTORS

Type I Cytokines—Structural Considerations

Type I cytokines typically share only limited amino acid sequence identity, but strikingly, all type I cytokines whose structures have been solved by nuclear magnetic resonance (NMR) and/or x-ray crystallographic methods are known to achieve similar three-dimensional structures

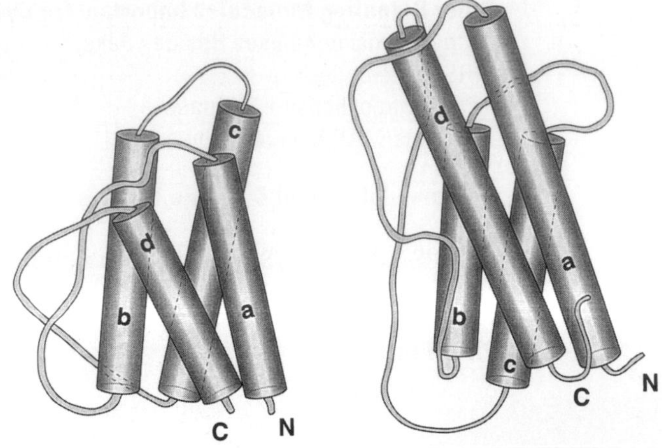

FIGURE 23.1 Schematic of four-α-helical-bundle cytokines. Schematic drawing showing typical short-chain and long-chain four-helical-bundle cytokines. Although these both exhibit an "up-up-down-down" topology to their four α helices, note that in the short-chain cytokines, the AB loop is behind the CD loop, whereas in the long-chain cytokines the situation is reversed. See text. The figure was provided by Dr. Alex Wlodawer, National Cancer Institute.

(5,6,7,*8*). Moreover, type I cytokines whose structures have not yet been solved also appear, based on modeling and comparison to the solved structures, to achieve similar three-dimensional structures (5,6,7,*8*). Type I cytokines contain four α helices and thus are designated as four-α-helical-bundle cytokines (Figure 23.1). Within their structures, the first two and last two α helices are each connected by long-overhand loops. This results in these cytokines achieving an "up-up-down-down" topologic structure, as the first two helices (A and B) can be oriented in an "up" orientation and the last two helices (C and D) can be oriented in a "down" orientation, as viewed from the NH_2- to COOH-terminal direction. As shown in Figure 23.1, the N and C termini of the cytokines are positioned on the same part of the molecule.

Type I cytokines fall into two groups, known as "short-chain" and "long-chain" four-α-helical-bundle cytokines, based on the lengths of the α helices *(8)*. Some of the short-chain cytokines include IL-2, IL-3, IL-4, IL-5, GM-CSF, IL-7, IL-9, IL-13, IL-15, IL-21, M-CSF, SCF, and TSLP, whereas long-chain cytokines include growth hormone, prolactin, erythropoietin, thrombopoietin, leptin, IL-6, IL-11, leukemia-inhibitory factor (LIF), oncostatin M (OSM), ciliary neurotrophic factor (CNTF), cardiotrophin-1 (CT-1), novel neurotrophin-1/B cell-stimulating factor-3/ cardiotrophinlike factor (NNT-1/BSF-3/CLC), and G-CSF (Table 23.1) *(8,9)*. The α helices are approximately 15 amino acids long in short-chain helical cytokines and 25 amino acids long in long-chain cytokines. Aditional differences include differences in the angles between the pairs of helices, and the AB loop is "under" the CD loop in the short cytokines, but "over" the CD loop in the long cytokines

TABLE 23.1 Four-Helical-Bundle Cytokines

Short-Chain Cytokines	*Long-Chain Cytokines*
IL-2	IL-6
IL-4	IL-11
IL-7	Oncostatin M
IL-9	Leukemia-inhibitory factor
IL-13	CNTF
IL-15	Cardiotropin-1
IL-21	NNT-1/BSF-3
TSLP	
IL-3	Growth hormone
IL-5[a]	Prolactin
GM-CSF	Erythropoietin
	Thrombopoietin
M-CSF[a,b]	Leptin
SCF[b]	G-CSF

[a]Dimers.
[b]Different from the other four-helical-bundle cytokines in that the M-CSF and SCF receptors (CSF-1R and c-kit, respectively) have intrinsic tyrosine kinase activity and are not type I cytokine receptors.

(Figure 23.1) (7,8,10). Moreover, short-chain cytokines have β structures in the AB and CD loops, whereas long-chain cytokines do not.

The division of type I cytokines into short-chain and long-chain cytokines has evolutionary considerations and also correlates with grouping of receptor chains for these two subfamilies of type I cytokines. An analysis of short-chain cytokines has revealed that 61 residues comprise the family framework, including most of the 31 residues that contribute to the buried inner core. The similarities and differences in the structures of IL-2, IL-4, and GM-CSF have been carefully analyzed (5). Among these cytokines, there is considerable variation in the intrachain disulfide bonds that stabilize the structures. For example, IL-4 has three intrachain disulfide bonds, GM-CSF has two, and IL-2 has only one. In IL-4, the first disulfide bond (between Cys 24 and Cys 65) connects loop AB to BC, the second disulfide bond (between Cys 46 and Cys 99) connects helix B and loop CD, and the third disulfide bond (between Cys 3 and Cys 127) connects the residue preceding helix B with helix D. In GM-CSF, the N terminus of helix B and the N terminus of β-strand CD are connected by one disulfide bond, whereas the other disulfide bond connects the C terminus of helix C and a strand following helix D. In IL-2, a single essential disulfide bond between Cys 58 and Cys 105 connects helix B to strand CD. Thus, each cytokine has evolved distinctive disulfide bonds to stabilize its structure, although it is typical that helix B is connected to the loop between helices C and D. The structures formed by helices A and D are more rigorously conserved than those formed by helices B and C, primarily because of the interhelical angles; helix D and the connecting region are the most highly conserved elements among the three cytokines (5).

This is of particular interest because the regions of type I cytokines that are most important for cytokine receptor interactions (based on analogy to the growth-hormone receptor structure, see later), include helices A and D and residues in the AB and CD loops, whereas helices B and C do not form direct contacts (5).

Certain variations on these typical four-α-helical-bundle structures can occur. For example, IL-5 is unusual in that it is a dimer positioned in a fashion so that the ends containing the N and C termini are juxtaposed *(11)*. Helix D is "exchanged" between the two covalently attached monomers so that helix D of each molecule actually forms part of the four-helix bundle of the other *(11)*. M-CSF is also a dimer, but no exchange of helix D occurs (10).

The interferons form related albeit distinctive structures from type I cytokines and are designated as type II cytokines *(8)*. IFN-β has an extra helix that is positioned in place of the CD strand *(12)*. IFN-γ is a dimer, each of which consists of six α helices *(13)*, as can be seen in Figure 23.2. Two of these helices are interchanged, including one from each four-α-helical bundle (10,*13*). IL-10, which is closely related to IFN-γ, has a similar structure *(14)*, and it can be predicted that more recently identified IL-10–like molecules, including IL-19, IL-20, IL-22, IL-24, IL-26, IL-28, and IL-29, have similar structures. Interestingly, although not universally the case, the majority of four α-helical cytokines have four exons, with helix A in exon 1, helices B and C in exon 3, and helix D in exon 4 *(7)*. A related organization is found for IFN-γ, as well as for the long-chain helical cytokines, growth hormone and G-CSF. However, there are exceptions; for example, IL-15 is divided into nine exons, whereas the IFN α and IFN β are encoded by single exons.

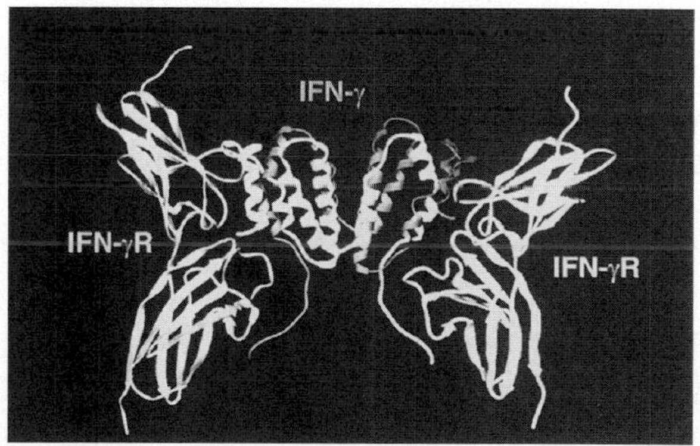

FIGURE 23.2 Structure of the IFN-γ receptor. Shown are ribbon diagrams of the structures of the IFN-γ/IFN-γ receptor complex as an example of a type II cytokine/cytokine receptor. In the IFN-γ receptor, only IFNGR-1 complexed to the IFN-γ dimer is shown, as the full structure with IFNGR-2 is not available. See text for discussion of the structure. The IFN-γ-IFNGR-1 structure is from (287). The figure was provided by Dr. Alex Wlodawer, National Cancer Institute.

Receptors for Type I Cytokines

The first report suggesting that type I cytokines interacted with receptors with similar features identified similarities in the sequences of the erythropoietin receptor and the IL-2 receptor β chain *(15)*, and subsequent analysis of a large number of type I cytokine receptors much more clearly established the existence of these receptors as a superfamily (16). Type I cytokine receptors are generally type I membrane-spanning glycoproteins (N terminus extracellular, C terminus intracellular). The only exceptions are proteins such as the CNTF receptor α chain (see later), which lacks a cytoplasmic domain and instead has a GPI anchor; however, the orientation of this protein is otherwise similar to that of a type I membrane protein. In their extracellular domains, a number of conserved features have been noted (Table 23.2). These include four conserved cysteine residues that are involved in intrachain disulfide bonding, and a tryptophan residue, located two amino acids C-terminal to the second conserved cysteine. In addition, a membrane-proximal region WSXWS (Trp-Ser-X-Trp-Ser) motif is generally conserved, although again exceptions exist: for example, in the growth hormone receptor, the motif is a substantially different YGEFS (Tyr-Gly-Glu-Phe-Ser) sequence, and in the IL-23R, it is a more similar WQPWS (Trp-Gln-Pro-Trp-Ser) motif. In some cases, such as the common cytokine receptor β chain, β_c, shared by the IL-3, IL-5, and GM-CSF receptors (see later), the extracellular domain is extended, with a duplication of the domains containing the four conserved cysteines and the WSXWS motif. Another shared feature of type I cytokine receptors is the presence of fibronectin type III domains.

The two pairs of conserved cysteine residues are typically encoded in two adjacent exons, and the exon containing the WSXWS motif is typically just 5′ to the exon encoding the transmembrane domain. Although serines can be encoded by six different codons (i.e, sixfold degeneracy in codon usage), only two of these (AGC and AGT) dominate as the codons used for the serines in WSXWS. All of these features indicate a common ancestral type I cytokine receptor.

TABLE 23.2 Features Common to Type I Cytokine Receptors

Extracellular domain

1. Four conserved cysteine residues, involved in intrachain disulfide bonds
2. WSXWS motif
3. Fibronectin type III modules

Cytoplasmic Domain

1. Box 1/Box 2 regions—The Box 1 region is a proline-rich region that is involved in the interaction of Janus family tyrosine kinases.

Overall, analogous to limited sequence identity between type I cytokines, there is only limited sequence identity among type I receptor molecules. Nevertheless, they appear to form similar structures, based on the known structures for the receptors for growth hormone, prolactin, erythropoietin, IL-4, and IL-2 (17,*18–20*,21), and the modeling of other cytokine receptor molecules based on the known structures. The cytokines and their receptors have presumably coevolved, with the differences in amino acid sequences between different cytokines allowing for their distinctive interactions with their cognate receptor chains. Despite amino acid differences, there are several sets of cytokines that coevolved to interact with shared receptor chains, thus forming type I cytokine and cytokine receptor subfamilies *(8)*.

In addition to the above-noted similarities in the extracellular domains, there are sequence similarities that are conserved in the cytoplasmic domain of cytokine receptors. In particular, membrane-proximal "Box 1/Box 2" regions are conserved (Table 23.2), with the proline-rich Box 1 region being the most conserved *(22)*. This will be discussed in greater detail later, related to its role in the binding of Jak kinases.

Type I Cytokine Receptors Are Homodimers, Heterodimers, or Higher-order Receptor Oligomers

The first cytokine receptor structure solved was that for growth hormone (Figure 23.3) (17). Prior to the x-ray crystallographic analysis, it was believed that growth hormone bound to its receptor with a stoichiometry of 1:1. Remarkably, however, the x-ray crystal solution structure revealed that a single growth hormone molecule interacted with a

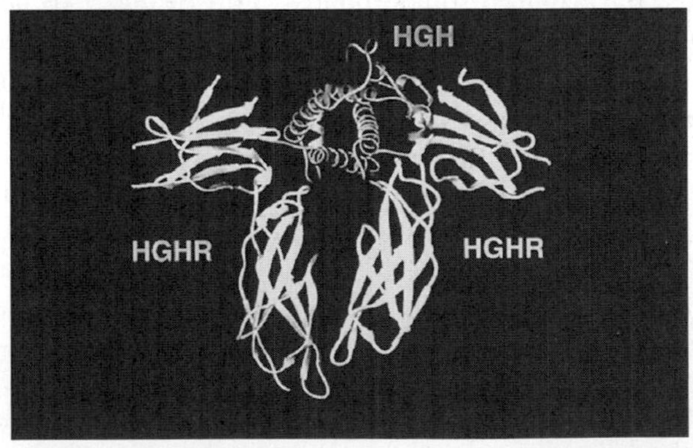

FIGURE 23.3 Structure of the growth hormone receptor. Shown are ribbon diagrams of the structure of the growth hormone receptor as an example of a type I cytokine receptor. For growth hormone, both growth hormone receptor monomers are shown. See text for discussion of the structures. The growth hormone/growth hormone receptor structure is from (17). The figure was provided by Dr. Alex Wlodawer, National Cancer Institute.

dimer of the growth hormone receptor, in which each receptor monomer contributes a total of seven β strands. Perhaps the most striking finding was that totally different parts of the growth hormone molecule interacted with the same general region of each receptor monomer. The three-dimensional x-ray crystal structure for the growth hormone/growth hormone receptor complex is shown in Figure 23.3. Solving the structure also clarified the basis for the assembly of the growth hormone receptor complex (17). Growth hormone appears first to interact with one receptor monomer via a relatively large and high-affinity interaction surface (site I), spanning approximately 1,230 Å^2. A second receptor monomer then interacts with the growth hormone/growth hormone receptor complex via two contact points—one on growth hormone (spanning approximately 900 Å^2) (site II), and the other on the first receptor monomer (spanning approximately 500 Å^2) (site III), located much more proximal to the cell membrane. Thus, a total of three extracellular interactions are responsible for the formation and stabilization of the growth hormone/growth hormone receptor complex. Mutations in critical residues in site I should prevent growth hormone binding to its receptor, whereas inactivating mutations in site II can be predicted to prevent dimerization and signal transduction. These considerations indicate a basis by which different classes of antagonists might be identified.

The growth hormone/growth hormone receptor structure revealed that the growth hormone receptor extracellular domain is composed of two fibronectin type III modules, each of which is approximately 100 amino acids long and contains seven β strands, resulting in the formation of an immunoglobulinlike structure. The contact surface between ligand and receptor occurs in the hinge region that separates these two fibronectin type III modules. Analysis of a growth hormone/prolactin receptor complex revealed the anticipated similar structure for the prolactin receptor *(18)*.

The growth hormone/growth hormone receptor structure was not only of great importance for the growth hormone field, it also served as a paradigm for the structures of other type I cytokine receptors. As a receptor homodimer, it immediately served as a model for other homodimers, such as the erythropoietin receptor, whose structure was solved *(19)* using a small protein mimetic (20-amino acid–long peptide) of erythropoietin *(23)*. The erythropoietin receptor structure is similar to that of the growth hormone receptor, although the "site III" stem region interaction surface in the erythropoietin receptor is much smaller than that in the growth hormone receptor, comprising only 75 Å^2 *(19)*.

In addition to the structural similarities for the growth hormone and erythropoietin receptors and perhaps other homodimeric type I cytokine receptors, a similar structure was achieved by the heterodimeric growth hormone/growth hormone receptor/prolactin receptor structure *(18)*, in which one of the growth hormone receptor monomers is replaced by a prolactin receptor molecule. Thus, the growth hormone/growth hormone receptor system is one in which two surfaces of growth hormone interact either with two identical monomers of growth hormone or with two nonidentical monomers in the case of the growth hormone receptor/prolactin receptor heterodimer.

It can be hypothesized that cytokine receptor systems with a homodimeric receptor are evolutionarily older than those with heterodimeric receptors, and that the coordination of two different receptor chains in heterodimeric receptors would have evolved in order to allow higher levels of specialization. In this regard, it is interesting that growth hormone and erythropoietin, whose actions are vital for growth and erythropoiesis, bind to receptors that are both homodimers, whereas the heterodimeric structures that typify the immune system are perhaps more "specialized" functions that arose later in evolution.

Interestingly, all type I cytokines known to interact with homodimers (growth hormone, prolactin, erythropoietin, and G-CSF) are long-chain helical cytokines, although other long-chain helical cytokines (e.g, the cytokines whose receptors contain gp130; see later) interact with heteromeric receptors. The short-chain cytokines that signal through homodimers are stem cell factor (SCF) and M-CSF, but in these cases the receptors (c-kit and CSF-1R, respectively) are different from type I cytokine receptors in that they contain intrinsic tyrosine kinase domains. Thus, SCF and M-CSF are not typical type I cytokines, and all other short-chain cytokines signal through heterodimers or more complex receptor structures (e.g, IL-2 and IL-15 receptors have three components).

Heterodimeric receptors are involved when site II on a cytokine has evolved to a point at which it interacts with a different receptor molecule than site I. This latter situation is the case for many cytokines, including all short-chain type I cytokines except for SCF and M-CSF. Overall, several sets of type I cytokines fall into distinct groups, wherein each group shares at least one common receptor component. This phenomenon is observed for certain sets of both short-chain and long-chain four–α-helical–bundle cytokines, and depending on the set of cytokines, the shared chain interacts either with site I or with site II.

The structures of the low- and high-affinity forms of the IL-2 receptor have now been solved (21,24). These are valuable structures in that they include the first complete structure for a short-chain cytokine/receptor complex (25). Moreover, they are of added interest in that the low-affinity receptor involves the interaction of IL-2 with IL-2Rα, which is not a type I cytokine receptor protein but instead is a distinctive sushi domain–containing protein, whereas the high-affinity receptor includes not only IL-2Rα but also IL-2Rβ and γ_c, which are both type I cytokine receptor proteins that are shared either with

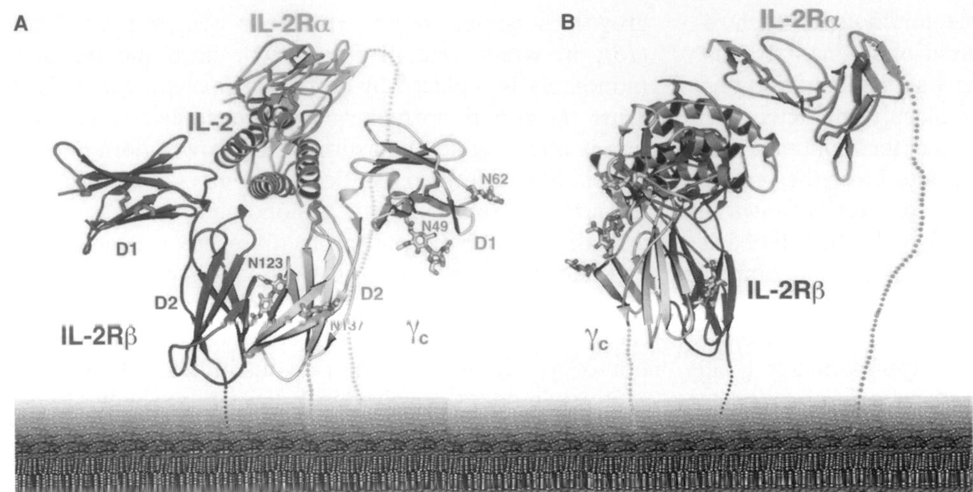

FIGURE 23.4 Structure of the high-affinity IL-2 receptor. This is the first structure for a short-chain type I cytokine complexed to its complete receptor. It is particularly interesting in that it includes the sushi domain containing the IL-2Rα chain as well. Reprinted from (21) with permission of Dr. Garcia and *Science* magazine.

IL-15 (IL-2Rβ) or with IL-4, IL-7, IL-9, IL-15, and IL-21(γ_c) (26), as discussed later. In the structure of IL-2 bound to its high-affinity receptor (Figure 23.4), there is a long peptide connecting the IL-2Rα globular head and transmembrane segment, allowing the binding site on this protein to extend relatively far from the cell surface in order to bind the dorsal surface of IL-2. Both the IL-2/IL-2Rα and IL-2/IL-2Rβ contacts are independent, and IL-2Rα does not appear to contact either IL-2Rβ or γ_c; however, IL-2 and IL-2Rβ together form a composite surface with γ_c, somewhat analogous to the composite surface formed by growth hormone and one growth hormone receptor monomer for binding to a second monomer. As anticipated, the surface interaction between IL-2 and γ_c is smaller than that between IL-2 and either of the other chains.

TYPE I CYTOKINE RECEPTOR FAMILIES AND THEIR RELATIONS

Cytokines That Share the Common Cytokine Receptor γ Chain (IL-2, IL-4, IL-7, IL-9, IL-15, and IL-21)

The receptors for six different immunologically important cytokines, IL-2, IL-4, IL-7, IL-9, IL-15, and IL-21, share the common cytokine receptor γ chain, γ_c (CD132) (27–29, *30*,*31*,32,*33*,34,*35*; reviewed in 26,*36*). These cytokines are all short-chain four–α-helical–bundle cytokines; basic features of these cytokines are summarized in Table 23.3. In the following, the properties of these cytokines and their unique receptor chains are summarized, followed by a discussion of the discovery that they share a common receptor component and the implications thereof.

Mature IL-2 is a 133-amino acid–long peptide that is produced by activated CD4$^+$ T lymphocytes and is the major T-cell growth factor, in keeping with its original discovery as a T-cell growth factor (TCGF) (37). IL-2 has other important actions as well (Table 23.3) (25). For example, it can increase immunoglobulin synthesis and J-chain transcription in B cells *(38–40)*, potently augment the cytolytic activity of natural killer (NK) cells (41,42,*43*) and induce the cytolytic activity of lymphokine-activated killer (LAK) cells, promote the elimination of auto-reactive cells in a process known as antigen-induced (or activation-induced) cell death (AICD; see Chapter 27) (25,*40*,44), promote the differentiation of regulatory T cells (T_{reg} cells) (45) (see Chapter 30), cells that suppress inappropriate responses and are important for immunologic tolerance (see Chapter 29), and it is important for proper T-helper cell differentiation. Interestingly, IL-2 can also prime CD8$^+$ T cells during a primary response to undergo enhanced proliferation in vivo during a secondary response *(46,47)*.

IL-2 is particularly important historically, as it is the first type I cytokine that was cloned (48), the first type I cytokine for which a receptor component was cloned (49,*50*), and was the first short-chain type I cytokine whose receptor structure was solved (21). Many general principles have been derived from studies of this cytokine, including its being the first cytokine demonstrated to act in a growth factor–like fashion through specific high-affinity receptors, analogous to the growth factors being studied by endocrinologists and biochemists *(40,51)*.

Although IL-2 is not produced by resting T cells, its production is rapidly and potently induced following antigen encounter with resting T cells. As a result, transcription and synthesis of IL-2 are often used as indicators of successful T-cell receptor–mediated cellular activation. Although the antigen determines the specificity of the T-cell immune response, the interaction of IL-2 with high-affinity IL-2 receptors regulates the magnitude and duration of the subsequent response, based on the amount of IL-2 produced, the levels of high-affinity receptors expressed, and the duration of IL-2 production and receptor expression. IL-2 can act in either an autocrine or paracrine fashion, depending on whether the producing cell is also the

TABLE 23.3 Features of Cytokines Whose Receptors Share γ_c

Cytokine	Major Source	Size[a]	Actions	Chromo. Location (h/m)	Genomic Org
IL-2	Activated T cells (Th1 cells)	h153 aa/20aa m169aa/20aa 15.5 kDa	T-cell growth factor B-cell growth, Ig production, J-chain expression Induce LAK activity Induce tumor-infiltrating lymphocyte activity Augment NK activity Critical role in antigen-induced cell death (AICD) Stimulate macrophage/monocyte antitumor effects	4q26-27/3	4 exons
IL-4	Activated T cells (Th2 cells) $CD4^+NK1.1^+$ natural T cells	h153/24 aa m140 aa/20 aa 18 kDa	B-cell proliferation Ig class switch—IgG1, IgE production Augment MHC II, Fcε receptors IL-4Rα and IL-2Rβ expression Th2 cell differentiation Antitumor effects	5q31.1/11	4 exons
IL-7	Stromal cells	h177 aa/25aa m154aa/25aa 17–25 kDa	Thymocyte growth T-cell growth Pre-B cell growth in mice but not humans Survival and growth of peripheral T cells	8q12-13/3	6 exons
IL-9	Activated helper T cells	h144aa/18aa m144aa/18aa 14 kDa	Th-helper clones Erythroid progenitors B cells Mast cells Fetal thymocytes	5q31-35/13	5 exons
IL-15	Monocytes and many cells outside the immune system[b]	h162aa/48aa m162aa/48aa 14–15 kDa	Mast-cell growth NK-cell development and activity T-cell proliferation	4q31/8	9 exons
IL-21	Activated $CD4^+$ T cells T_{FH} cells NKT cells Th17 cells	h162aa/31 aa m146aa/24 aa	Comitogen for T-cell proliferation Inhibits B cell proliferation to anti-IgM + IL-4 Augments B-cell proliferation to anti-CD40 Conflicting reports related to NK cells Cooperates with IL-7 and IL-15 to expand CD8 cells Antitumor effects Drives terminal B-cell differentiation to plasma cells Proapoptotic for B and NK cells	4q67-27	

[a] h and m refer to human and murine, respectively. The number of amino acids refers to the length of the open reading frame/length of signal peptide. The number of amino acids in the mature protein is therefore the difference between these numbers. Note that for IL-15, residues 1–29 have been identified as a signal peptide and residues 30–48 as a propeptide.

[b] More IL-15 mRNA is produced in skeletal muscle, kidney, placenta, and lung than in thymus or spleen. It is important to note, however, that IL-15 mRNA is widely expressed without concomitant production of IL-15 protein, so the source of biologically meaningful IL15 may be more limited.

responding cell or whether the responding cell is a nonproducing cell. The gene encoding IL-2 is located on chromosome 4 *(52)*, and, like many other helical cytokines, its gene consists of four exons *(7)*.

IL-2 binds to three different classes of receptors. These are formed by different combinations of three different chains, IL-2Rα (49,*50*,*53*), IL-2Rβ (54,55,*56*,57), and a protein initially called IL-2Rγ *(27)* but now known as the common cytokine receptor γ chain, γ_c (26,28). The different classes of IL-2 receptors are discussed in the following.

Like IL-2, IL-4 is produced primarily by activated $CD4^+$ T cells (58). IL-4 is also produced by $CD4^+NK1.1^+$

"natural" T cells, denoted as NKT cells *(59)*, and by mast cells and basophils (58). IL-4 is the major B-cell growth factor, and it promotes immunoglobulin class switch, enhancing the production and secretion of mouse IgG1 (human IgG4) and being essential for the production of IgE (58). IL-4 is involved in the physiologic response to parasites, including helminths, and for allergen sensitization. IL-4 induces expression of class II major histocompatibility complex (MHC) molecules and increases cell surface expression of the CD23 (the low-affinity IgE receptor) on B cells. In addition to its actions on B cells, IL-4 can also act as a T-cell growth factor, inducing proliferation in both human and murine T cells, and is critical for normal differentiation of Th2 cells (discussed later). When combined with PMA, IL-4 is also a potent comitogen for thymocytes. Importantly, IL-4 can inhibit certain responses of cells to IL-2 *(60)*. Moreover, IL-4 can exert actions on macrophages, hematopoietic precursor cells, stromal cells, and fibroblasts *(61)*. The gene encoding IL-4 is located on human chromosome 5 (5q23.3-31.2) and mouse chromosome 11 *(61,62)*, in the same region as IL-3, IL-5, IL-13, and GM-CSF. The type I IL-4 receptor expressed on T cells and other hematopoietic cells consists of the 140-kDa IL-4Rα protein (58,*63–65*) and γ_c (29,*30*). Expression of IL-4Rα tends to be quite low, and cells that respond potently to IL-4 often express only a few hundred receptors per cell. In addition to the type I IL-4 receptor, an alternate form of the receptor, containing IL-4Rα and IL-13Rα (now denoted IL-13Rα1), although it is not expressed on mature T cells, is expressed on many other cell types and can transduce IL-4 signals into these cells. For example, IL-13Rα1 is expressed on neonatal Th1 cells, and the type II IL-4R has been implicated as mediating apoptosis of these cells *(66)*.

IL-7 is not a lymphokine (i.e, it is not produced by lymphocytes) but instead is a 152-amino acid–long cytokine that is produced by stromal cells (67,*68*). Its major role is to enhance thymocyte survival, growth, and differentiation (*69,70*,71–73), as well as low-affinity peptide-induced proliferation, and thus it promotes homeostatic proliferation of naïve and memory CD8$^+$ T cells (73,*74*,75). Additionally, IL-7 can regulate homeostasis of CD4$^+$ memory T cells (76,77) and also can stimulate the growth of mature T cells (26,73,*78*,*79*). It is vital for the growth of murine pre-B cells (*65*,67,71,72,79), and transient IL-7 signaling can inhibit immunoglobulin heavy-chain gene rearrangements *(80)*. In contrast to the mouse situation as underscored by the normal B-cell development in patients with defective IL-7 signaling (patients with X-linked severe combined immunodeficiency [SCID], Jak3-deficient SCID, and IL-7Rα-deficient SCID, see later), human B cells can develop normally in the absence of IL-7 responsiveness, demonstrating that in humans, IL-7 is not vital for the growth of human pre-B cells (26,*81*), and it remains unknown whether IL-7 plays any important role for B-cell biology in humans. The gene encoding IL-7 is located on human chromosome 8q12-13 *(82)* and mouse chromosome 3. The functional IL-7 receptor contains the 75-kDa IL-7Rα *(83)* and γ_c (28,*31*). Based on chemical cross-linking experiments and Scatchard analyses, there is a suggestion, however, that the receptor may contain a still-unidentified third component as well (28).

IL-9 was originally described as a murine T-cell growth factor (84) that is produced by activated T cells and can support the growth of T-helper clones but not of cytolytic clones *(85)*. In contrast to IL-2, its production is delayed, suggesting its involvement in later, perhaps secondary signals. In the mouse, IL-9 can exert proliferative effects on erythroid progenitors, B cells, B1 cells, mast cells, and fetal thymocytes. IL-9 is identical to mast cell growth-enhancing activity (MEA), a factor present in conditioned medium from splenocytes *(86)*, and synergizes with IL-3 for maximal mast cell proliferation. The action of IL-9 on thymocytes in vitro is interesting in view of the development of thymomas in IL-9 transgenic mice coupled to the observation that IL-9 is a major antiapoptotic factor for thymic lymphomas (87). Nevertheless, IL-9 knockout mice do not have a defect in T-cell development (88). Instead, they exhibit a defect in pulmonary goblet cell hyperplasia and mastocytosis following challenge with *Schistoma manoni* eggs, a synchronous pulmonary granuloma formation model; however, there was no defect in eosinophilia or granuloma formation (88). Mice in which an IL-9 transgene is expressed in the lung exhibit airway inflammation and bronchial hyperresponsiveness; nevertheless, IL-9$^{-/-}$ mice exhibit normal eosinophilia and airway hyperreactivity in an ovalbumin-induced inflammatory model (*89,90*,91). Thus, although IL-9 can contribute to allergic/pulmonary responses, there are compensatory cytokines that substitute for IL-9 in at least certain settings. Although murine IL-9 is active on human cells, human IL-9 is not biologically active on murine cells (the opposite situation from that for IL-2). Human IL-9 is located on chromosome 5 in the 5q31-35 region *(92)*, which is also the location of the genes encoding IL-3, IL-4, IL-5, IL-13, and GM-CSF. In contrast, mouse IL-9 is "isolated" on chromosome 13, while IL-3, IL-4, IL-5, IL-13, and GM-CSF are clustered on chromosome 11. IL-9 binds to the 64-kDa IL-9Rα–binding protein, which is similar in size to γ_c *(93)*, and the functional IL-9 receptor consists of IL-9Rα plus γ_c (26,32,33).

IL-15 was identified as a novel T-cell growth factor that also unexpectedly was expressed in the supernatants of an HTLV-I–transformed T-cell line (94,95). Although IL-15 mRNA is produced by a range of nonlymphocytic cell types, it is difficult to detect physiologic levels of IL-15 protein (96). Its main site of synthesis appears to be dendritic cells and monocytes, and unlike IL-2, it is not produced by activated T cells (97). IL-15 receptors are widely expressed, but IL-15 is most important for the development of NK cells (98,99,*100*) and CD8$^+$ memory T cells (99,*100*). Interestingly, it also regulates the T-cell receptor repertoire of $\gamma\delta$ intraepithelial lymphocytes (101) and cross-talk between different types of dendritic cells (102). The receptor for IL-15 on T cells contains IL-2Rβ (34,96,*103*), γ_c (34) and one unique protein, IL-15Rα. IL-15Rα shares a number of structural similarities with IL-2Rα, including that it is a sushi domain–containing protein (IL-2Rα has two sushi domains, whereas IL-15Rα has one) *(104)*, and the *IL2RA* and *IL15RA* genes are closely positioned on human chromosome 10p14 *(105)*. What is distinctive about IL-15 signaling is that it signals substantially by a process called *trans presentation,* wherein IL-15Rα on the surface of dendritic cells or monocytes will trans-present IL-15 to responding cells such as CD8$^+$ T cells or NK cells that express IL-2Rβ + γ_c (97,106). The very high affinity of IL-15Rα for IL-15 is explained by a large number of ionic interactions mediated by the sushi domain *(107)*. Note that these responding cells can also express IL-15Rα. In contrast to IL-2, which is a growth factor as well as a mediator of AICD and promoter of T_{reg} differentiation, the role of IL-15 appears to be more focused on growth of CD8$^+$ T cells *(108)*, maintaining long-lasting, high-avidity T-cell responses to foreign pathogens (i.e, CD8$^+$ T-cell memory) (97,109). This ability has suggested that it could have potential as a vaccine adjuvant *(110)*.

IL-21 is the most recently identified member of the IL-2 family of cytokines (reviewed in 110a). IL-21 can bind to specific receptors and exert actions on T, B, asnd NK cells. It augments T-cell proliferation as a comitogen (111), can cooperate with IL-7 or IL-15 to drive the expansion of freshly isolated murine CD8$^+$ T cells, and can augment the antitumor activity of CD8$^+$ T cells (112). Its actions on B cells are particularly complex. It augments B-cell proliferation when combined with anti-CD40 or lipopolysaccharide (LPS) but inhibits proliferation in response to anti-IgM + IL-4 (111), but this inhibition is reversed if anti-CD40 is additionally provided. It induces apoptosis of incompletely activated B cells but drives terminal differentiation to plasma cells of more fully activated cells. Strikingly, IL-21 can drive plasma cell differentiation of both peripheral memory B cells and cord-blood B cells, at least in part explained by its ability to induce expression of Blimp1 (113,*114*). In IL-21R knockout mice, following immunization, IgG1 is diminished related to a role for IL-21 in class switching to IgG1 and IgG3, whereas IgE is elevated, related to the ability of IL-21 to inhibit Cε transcription (115). IL-21R/IL-4 double-knockout mice have revealed that IL-21 cooperates with IL-4 to globally regulate immunoglobulin production in that it causes a pan-hypogammaglobulinemia, mimicking the T-cell phenotype in humans with XSCID (116). IL-21 can also cooperate with IL-15 and Flt-3 ligand to increase development of NK cells (111), and augment antitumor activity (117), but yet it was also reported to oppose the actions of IL-15 (118) and it can also direct NK cell apoptosis. Interestingly, elevated IL-21 levels have been reported in the BXSB-*Yaa* mouse model of systemic lupus erythematosus (SLE) (113) and, moreover, elevated IL-21 levels have been found in a subset of humans with SLE (P. Lipsky, personal communication). Moreover, elevated IL-21 has also been associated with other autoimmune processes, including in the NOD mouse (reviewed in 115). More recently, IL-21 has been shown to be vital for the differentiation of Th17 cells (115a, 115b, 115c) and to be able to prime cells in vitro for antitumor effects in vivo following adoptive transfer in a melanoma tumor model (115d). The receptor for IL-21 consists of IL-21R plus γ_c (*35*; reviewed in 26). IL-21R is most related to IL-2Rβ, and like IL-2Rβ, its expression is induced following cellular stimulation with anti-CD3 or phytohemagglutinin, and in addition, its expression is augmented in T cells following transformation with HTLV-I (119). Both human and murine IL-21 can act on cells of the other species. IL-21 is on human chromosome 4q26-27, while its receptor is on chromosome 16p11, immediately downstream of the *IL4R* gene.

Thus, IL-2, IL-4, IL-7, IL-9, IL-15, and IL-21 collectively exhibit partially overlapping roles related to T cells, NK cells, B cells, and mast cells, and together would be expected to play vital roles for normal development and/or function of these cellular lineages. The fact that these six cytokines share γ_c is of particular interest given that the gene encoding this protein is mutated in the most common form of severe combined immunodeficiency in humans.

X-Linked Severe Combined Immunodeficiency Disease (XSCID) Results from Mutations in γ_c

The γ chain was originally identified as a third component of the IL-2 receptor (27), after it became clear that IL-2 receptor α and β chains alone were not sufficient to transduce an IL-2 signal. The hypothesis that the γ chain was a shared component of receptors in addition to the IL-2 receptor was motivated from a comparison of the clinical phenotypes in humans that result from defective expression of IL-2 versus the γ chain. In 1993, it was reported that the γ chain was defective in patients with X-linked severe combined immunodeficiency (XSCID; the disease is formally designated as SCIDX1) (26,120) (see also Chapter 46). XSCID is characterized by profoundly diminished numbers of T cells and NK cells (26,*36*,120,*121*,*122*,123,124), (Table 23.4). Although

TABLE 23.4 Features of XSCID

1. Absent or profoundly diminished numbers of T cells and mitogen responses.
2. Absence of NK cells
3. Normal numbers of B cells, but defective B-cell responses.
4. IgM can be normal, but greatly diminished immunoglobulins of other classes.
5. XSCID carrier females exhibit nonrandom X-inactivation patterns in their T cells and NK cells; the X-inactivation pattern is random in surface IgM-positive B cells but nonrandom in more terminally differentiated B cells

the B cells are normal in number, they are nonfunctional, apparently because of a lack of T-cell help as well as an intrinsic B-cell defect (*36*,123,*125*). In contrast to the profoundly decreased number of T cells in patients with XSCID, IL-2–deficient patients *(126,127)* and mice *(128)* have normal numbers of T cells (the phenotypes of mice deficient in type I and type II cytokines and their receptor, Jak kinases, and STAT proteins are summarized later, in Table 23.15). This observation minimized the possibility that a component of the IL-2 receptor was defective in XSCID, making the finding that the γ chain was mutated in XSCID all the more unexpected. Thus, the conundrum was why a defect in a component of a receptor would be more severe than a defect in the corresponding cytokine. This led to the hypothesis that the γ chain was part of other immunologically important cytokine receptors as well (120). In this model, defective IL-2 signaling either did not contribute to the defects in XSCID or these defects were explained by the simultaneous inactivation of multiple signaling pathways, rather than from a selective IL-2 signaling defect (*36*,120). Initially, it was shown that the γ chain was also an essential functional component of both the IL-4 and IL-7 receptors on T cells (28,29,*30,31*), leading to it being renamed as the common cytokine receptor γ chain, γ_c (28,29). IL-9, IL-15, and IL-21 were subsequently also shown to share γ_c (26) (Figure 23.5).

The sharing of γ_c by six different cytokine receptors revealed XSCID to be a disease of defective cytokine signaling. The major deficiencies in XSCID can be attributed

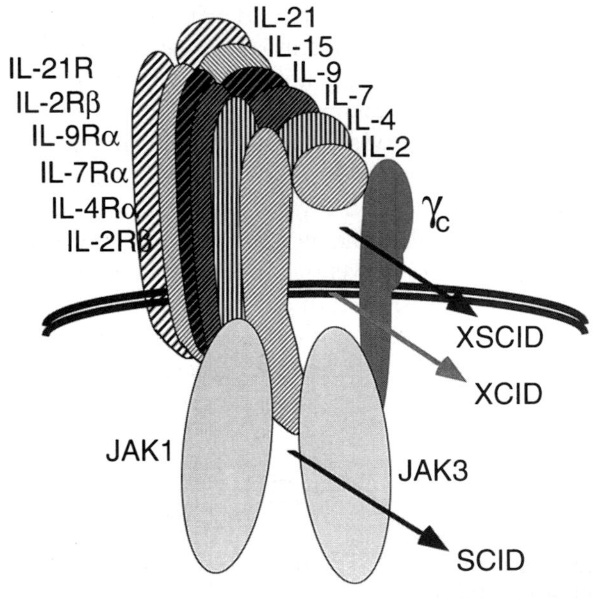

FIGURE 23.5 Schematic of the receptors for IL-2, IL-4, IL-7, IL-9, IL-15, and IL-21, showing interactions with Jak1 and Jak3. The cartoon shows that IL-2, IL-4, IL-7, IL-9, IL-15, and IL-21 all share γ_c. IL-2Rα and IL-15Rα are not shown. Whereas the distinctive chains associate with Jak1, γ_c associates with Jak3. Mutations in γ_c cause XSCID or more moderate forms of X-linked immunodeficiency (XCID). Mutations in Jak3 cause an autosomal recessive form of SCID (see text).

to defects related to different cytokines. Based on the dramatically diminished T-cell development not only in IL-7–deficient (72) or IL-7Rα–deficient mice (71), but also in *IL7R*-deficient humans with T$^-$B$^+$NK$^+$ SCID (129,*130*), yet normal T-cell development in mice deficient in either IL-2 *(128)*, IL-4 *(131,132)*, both IL-2 and IL-4 *(133)*, IL-9 (88), IL-15 *(100)*, IL-15Rα (99), and IL-21R (116,118), most if not all of the defect in T-cell development in patients with XSCID can be attributed to defective IL-7 signaling (26). In addition to profoundly diminished numbers of T cells, humans with XSCID lack NK cells. As discussed previously, NK-cell development is defective in IL-15– and IL-15Rα–deficient mice, indicating that it is defective IL-15 signaling that is responsible for the defective NK-cell development in XSCID (26).

In contrast to the greatly diminished number of T cells and absent NK cells in XSCID patients, B-cell numbers are normal. This is in marked contrast to the greatly diminished numbers of B cells in γ_c-deficient mice (134,135) and mice deficient in either IL-7 or IL-7Rα, indicating that IL-7 is not required for pre–B-cell development in humans and underscoring a major difference for IL-7 in human versus mouse biology. Indeed, *IL7R*-deficient SCID patients have a T$^-$B$^+$NK$^+$ form of SCID (129,*130*). Although B cells develop in XSCID patients, they are nonfunctional. This is due in part to a lack of T-cell help (given the near absence of T cells in XSCID), but a variety of data have suggested an intrinsic B-cell defect as well (26). As discussed earlier, analysis of IL-4/IL-21R double-knockout mice indicated that defective signaling by IL-4 and IL-21 appear to explain the intrinsic B-cell defect in XSCID.

Rationale for the Sharing of γ_c

Why should there have been evolutionary pressure to maintain the sharing of γ_c, given the obvious increased risk associated with sharing a receptor component when it is mutated? There are at least two different types of models *(36,136)*. First, given that IL-2, IL-4, IL-7, IL-9, IL-15, and IL-21 can each act as T-cell growth factors, at least in vitro, it is possible that γ_c might couple to signal-transducing molecule(s) that promote T-cell growth. The second type of model is diametrically different, and suggests that the sharing of γ_c is a means by which one cytokine using γ_c can modulate the signals of the others. To understand this model, it is important to emphasize that, in contrast to antigen receptor complexes, cytokine receptor components are targeted individually to the cell surface, and the formation/stability of receptor complexes is dependent on ligand binding. This was suggested earlier in the discussion of the growth hormone receptor, wherein the second receptor monomer recognizes the combined surface of growth hormone and the first growth hormone receptor monomer (17) or for the IL-2 receptor where γ_c "sees" a combined IL-2/IL-2Rβ surface (21), consistent with γ_c originally having been identified in coprecipitates with IL-2Rβ in the presence but not in the absence of IL-2 *(137)*, and dimerization of IL-2Rβ and γ_c is known to be required for efficient signaling (138,139). Thus, receptor heterodimerization at a minimum is stabilized by the cytokine and physiologically may be absolutely dependent on the presence of the cytokine. In the absence of stable preformed cytokine receptor complexes between γ_c and the other receptor chains, one can envision that γ_c might be differentially recruited to different receptors based on the relative amount of a cytokine or its binding efficiency. In a situation where γ_c is limiting, a cytokine might then not only induce its own action but could also simultaneously inhibit the action of another cytokine that was less efficient at recruiting γ_c to its cognate receptor complex.

An analysis of mice deficient in IL-2 *(128)*, IL-2Rα (140), IL-2Rβ (141), and γ_c (134, 135) provides the interesting observation that although the mice lacking γ_c have defective signaling in six different cytokine pathways, mice deficient in IL-2, IL-2Rα, and IL-2Rβ appear to be less healthy than the γ_c knockout mice with activated T cells and autoimmunity that is not evident in γ_c-deficient mice. This perhaps is explained by the fact that IL-2–deficient mice lack regulatory T cells and thus develop autoimmune disease, whereas γ_c-deficient mice lack T cells as a result of defective IL-7 signaling and thus lack effector T cells. These and other data indicate that γ_c plays a major role in regulating lymphoid homeostasis as originally indicated *(142)*.

Cytokines Whose Receptors Share the Common β Chain, β_c (IL-3, IL-5, and GM-CSF)

The hematopoietic cytokines, IL-3, IL-5, and GM-CSF (Table 23.5) are all synthesized by T cells and exert effects on cells of hematopoietic lineage (*143*,144,145). These cytokines are vital for proliferation as well as differentiation of myeloid precursor cells. Of these three cytokines, IL-3 is the most pluripotent (144) and historically was also called multi-CSF, reflecting the large number of lineages on which it can act. It can act to promote proliferation, survival, and development of multipotent hematopoietic progenitor cells and of cells that have become dedicated to a range of different lineages, including granulocyte, macrophage, eosinophil, mast cell, basophil, megakaryocyte, and erythroid lineages. IL-3 also can exert end-function effects, such as enhancing phagocytosis and cytotoxicity. GM-CSF is mainly restricted to the granulocyte and monocyte/macrophage lineages, but its actions are nevertheless still quite broad *(143)*. It is both a growth and a survival factor. In addition, it can expand the number of antigen-presenting cells, such as dendritic cells, and thereby may greatly expand the ability of the host to respond to antigen. Whereas IL-3 and GM-CSF can act on eosinophils, they act at much earlier stages than IL-5, presumably expanding the number of eosinophil-committed precursors cells. IL-5 stimulates the eosinophilic lineage and eosinophil release from the bone marrow and is essential for expanding eosinophils after helminth infections *(146,147)*, and it can mediate the killing of *Schistosoma mansoni*. IL-5 can also induce immunoglobulin production in B cells activated by contact with activated Th cells in murine systems, and IL-5 and IL-5Rα knockout mice have diminished $CD5^+$ B1 cells and decreased thymocytes until approximately 6 weeks of age *(146,147)*.

On cells that express receptors for more than one of these cytokines, such as eosinophilic progenitors that express receptors for IL-3, IL-5, and GM-CSF, or on murine pre-B cells, which express receptors for IL-3 and IL-5, the signals induced are indistinguishable (144,145). Thus, the different lineage specificities of these cytokines are determined by the cellular distribution of their receptors rather than by fundamental differences in the signals that are induced by each cytokine. These observations are explained by studies demonstrating that each of these three cytokines has its own unique 60- to 80-kDa α chain (i.e, IL-3Rα, IL-5Rα, and GM-CSFRα) (148,*149–154*), but that they share a common 120- to 130-kDa β chain, β_c (145,*155,156*,157). The α chains are the principal binding proteins for the cytokines, whereas the shared β_c subunit augments binding affinity but does not exhibit binding activity in the absence of the proper α chain. The α chains have relatively short cytoplasmic domains

TABLE 23.5 Features of Cytokines Whose Receptors Share β_c

Cytokine	Major Source	Size	Cellular Targets	Chr. Loc. (h/m)	Exons
IL-3	T cells	h152/19aa m166/26 aa 22–34 kDa	Multiple lineages	5q31.1/11	5
IL-5	T cells	h139/22aa m133/21 45-kDa dimer	Eosinophils B cells (?)	5 q31.1/11	4
GM-CSF	T cells	h144/17aa m141/17aa 23 kDa	Granulocytes Macrophages	5q31.1/11	4

(approximately 55 amino acids long for IL-3Rα, IL-5Rα, and GM-CSFRα) and are not believed to play major roles in signaling function, whereas β_c, with its cytoplasmic domain of 432 amino acids, is the primary determinant of the signal. As a result, there is a relative compartmentalization of binding and signaling function for these cytokines, although the cytoplasmic domains of the GM-CSFRα and IL-5Rα chains (and, by analogy, perhaps the IL-3Rα chain), as well as β_c, appear to be capable of at least modulating the growth signals in transfected cells (145,*158–160*). In any case, the sharing of β_c helps to explain why the signals induced by IL-3, IL-5, and GM-CSF are similar on cells that can respond to more than one of these cytokines. The situation for the β_c family of cytokines is therefore quite different from the receptors for γ_c family cytokines, wherein the chains with the largest cytoplasmic domains (IL-2Rβ, IL-4Rα, IL-7Rα, IL-9Rα, and IL-21R) not only contribute most to signaling specificity, but also are the proteins principally involved in ligand binding (note that in the case of IL-2 and IL-15, IL-2Rα and IL-15Rα serve important roles as well). The shared chain, γ_c, serves a vital accessory function (hence the development of XSCID when the *IL2RG* gene is mutated), but it contributes less to cytokine binding and does not provide an obvious basis for signaling specificity (see following).

An interesting feature of the β_c family of hematopoietic cytokines is that there appears to be considerable redundancy of function, so that knockout mice that lack the ability to respond to all three cytokines (GM-CSF, IL-3, and IL-5) as a result of deletion of β_c as well as the murine IL-3–specific β_c-like protein (discussed in the following) nevertheless exhibit relatively normal hematopoiesis. These observations do not minimize the potency of these particular cytokines, but instead underscore a substantial redundancy for a particularly important set of functions (144,145,*161*). It is also noteworthy that β_c-deficient mice exhibit defective host responses to infectious challenge, suggesting that these hematopoietic cytokines play a vital role in promoting immune function.

Cytokines Receptors That Share gp130 (IL-6, IL-11, Oncostatin M [OSM], Ciliary Neurotropic Factor [CNTF], Leukemia-Inhibitory Factor [LIF], Cardiotrophin-1 [CT-1], NNT/BSF-3/CLC, and IL-27)

There are now eight cytokines that are known to utilize gp130 as a signal-transducing molecule (162,*163–171*,172,173). Some of the properties of these cytokines are summarized in Table 23.6. This family is often referred to as the IL-6 family of cytokines and includes IL-6, IL-11, oncostatin M (OSM), leukemia-inhibitory factor (LIF), ciliary neurotrophic factor (CNTF), cardiotrophin-1 (CT-1), NNT/BSF-3/CLC, and IL-27. This group of cytokines comprises molecules with a diverse range of actions, ranging beyond the hematopoietic and immune systems to the central nervous and

TABLE 23.6 Cytokines Whose Receptors Share gp130[a]

Cytokine	Chr. Loc. *(h/m)*
IL-6	7p21/5
IL-11	19q13.3-13.4/7
LIF	22q12.1-12.2/11
OSM	22q12.1-12.2/11
CNTF	11q12.2/19
CT-1	16p11.1-11.2/7
NNT-1/BSF-3/CLC	11q13/
IL-27	

Overlapping actions of several gp130 cytokines

	IL-6	*IL-11*	*LIF*	*OSM*	*CNTF*	*CT-1*
Growth of myeloma cells	+	–	+	+	+	?
Maintenance of ES-cell pluripotency	–	–	+	+	+	+
Induction of hepatic acute-phase proteins	+	+	+	+	+	+
Induction of cardiac hypertrophy	–	+	+	+	+/–	+
Induction of osteoclast formation	–	+	+	+	?	?
Enhanced neuronal survival/differentiaion	+	+	+	+	+	+
Inhibit adipogenesis	?	+	+	?	?	?

[a]Most of the data in this table are derived from *(166)*.
Note that NNT-1 can support survival of chicken embryonic and sympathetic neurons, can induce amyloid A and analogous to IL-6 can induce B-cell hyperplasia.

cardiovascular systems, making them even more "multifunctional" than the γ_c and β_c families of cytokines, which appear to exert actions largely restricted to the lymphoid and hematopoietic systems.

IL-6 was originally identified and then cloned as a B-cell differentiation factor that stimulated terminal differentiation/maturation of B cells into antibody-producing plasma cells (*174*,175). However, IL-6 also can exert effects for T-cell growth and differentiation (and thus is a thymocyte "comitogen"), induce myeloid differentiation into macrophages, induce acute-phase protein synthesis of hepatocytes, and exert actions on keratinocytes, mesangial cells, hematopoietic stem cells, the development of osteoclasts, and neural differentiation of PC12 cells (168). IL-6 is also a mediator of amplified lymphocyte trafficking during febrile inflammatory responses, which is dependent on IL-6–mediated activation of L-selectin *(176)*. IL-6 binds to an 80-kDa IL-6–binding protein, denoted IL-6Rα, which has a comparatively short 82-amino acid–long cytoplasmic domain (175,*177*) This IL-6-IL-6Rα complex then interacts with and recruits the 130-kDa signal transducing molecule, gp130, which together with IL-6Rα can form a functional IL-6 receptor (168). From a structural perspective, gp130 contains a total of six fibronectin type III modules, with the four conserved cysteine residues and the WSXWS motif being located in the second and third of these modules, starting from the N terminus. As such, these regions are topologically positioned a greater distance external to the cell membrane than is the case for the other type I cytokine receptors discussed previously.

The IL-6 system illustrates a novel twist related to the properties of their principal binding proteins: the cytoplasmic domain of IL-6Rα is superfluous for signaling; a soluble form of the IL-6Rα extracellular domain is in fact sufficient for ligand binding and coordination with gp130, a process termed IL-6 trans signaling *(178)*. Thus, in the presence of soluble IL-6Rα and IL-6, many cell types that express gp130 but not IL-6Rα are capable of signaling in response to IL-6. It was observed that IL-6 signaling requires the dimerization of gp130 and that the overall complex contains two molecules each of IL-6, IL-6Rα, and gp130 (a dimer of a trimer or a hexamer) (*179–181*,183), providing a possible paradigm for the stoichiometry of subunits for other members of the IL-6 family of cytokines.

IL-11 was identified as a factor produced by a stromal cell line in response to stimulation with IL-1 *(184,185)*. It was noted to exert a number of effects on hematopoiesis, particularly in combination with IL-3 and stem cell factor. Because IL-11 exhibited "IL-6–like activities," a cDNA was isolated based on the presence of IL-6–like activity in the presence of antibodies to IL-6 *(186)*. Other actions of IL-11 include the ability to stimulate the proliferation of lymphoid and hematopoietic progenitor cells, stimulate megakaryocytic progenitors and megakaryocyte maturation, and stimulate erythroid progenitors (an action not shared by IL-6) *(184,185)*. Like IL-6, IL-11 can induce acute-phase proteins and augment antigen-specific B-cell responses, but it does not stimulate human myeloma cells *(184–187)*. Subsequently, adipogenesis-inhibitory factor was cloned and found to be identical to IL-11 *(188)*, revealing another action of IL-11. IL-11 is also produced in the lung eosinophils and various structural cells in the lung, and is expressed in patients with modest to severe asthma (189). IL-11 signals via a receptor complex containing both IL-11Rα *(190)* and gp130 (162). Interestingly, IL-11Rα mRNA can be alternatively spliced to yield a form lacking the cytoplasmic domain, and, like IL-6Rα, a soluble form of IL-11Rα can coordinate with IL-11 to trans-signal in cells expressing gp130 *(191)*. Studies on the stoichiometry of the IL-11 receptor complex failed to reveal dimerization of gp130 to itself or LIFRβ. Thus, assuming that it forms a hexameric receptor complex, only five members are known—two molecules of IL-11 and IL-11Rα, and one of gp130—suggesting that another component may still be found *(192)*.

Leukemia-inhibitory factor (LIF) is another multifunctional cytokine originally cloned based on the activity associated with its name *(193)*. LIF can suppress the differentiation of pluripotent embryonic stem cells, inhibit adipogenesis (like IL-11), and induce monocyte differentiation of the M1 murine leukemia cell line, thus mimicking a number of the actions of IL-6 *(194)*. In addition, it exerts a number of actions in the central nervous system, and LIF was shown to be identical to cholinergic neural differentiation factor (CDF) *(195)*. CDF can induce acetylcholine synthesis while simultaneously suppressing catecholamine production, thereby inducing cholinergic function while suppressing noradrenergic function *(195)*. LIF has been shown to be essential for embryo implantations *(196)*. LIF binds to a receptor (LIFRβ) that is structurally related to gp130 *(197)*, but the functional LIF receptor requires the heterodimerization of LIFRβ and gp130 as well *(164)*.

Ciliary neurotrophic factor was discovered based on its ability to promote neuronal survival (198,*199*). CNTF signals through a receptor comprising LIFRβ and gp130, but additionally requires a specific binding protein (200,201), now denoted CNTFRα. Interestingly, CNTFRα lacks transmembrane and cytoplasmic domains and instead is a glycosyl-phosphatidylinositol (GPI)–linked receptor molecule. CNTFRα appears to provide a receptor–cytokine surface with which gp130 and LIFRβ can interact. Thus, CNTF is like IL-6 in that each requires initial binding to a receptor component (CNTFRα or IL-6Rα) that does not require its own cytoplasmic domain for signaling. Whereas IL-6 signaling involves homodimerization of gp130, CNTF signaling involves the heterodimerization of LIFRβ and gp130. In fact, the functional CNTF receptor appears to be a hexameric structure containing two molecules of CNTF, two of CNTFRα, and one each of gp130 and LIFRβ

(202). The receptor is expressed largely within the nervous system and in skeletal muscle, accounting for largely restricted actions of CNTF (200).

Oncostatin M (OSM) is a growth regulator that was originally identified based on its ability to inhibit the growth of A375 human melanoma cells (203,204). OSM is a potent growth factor for Kaposi sarcoma in patients with acquired immunodeficiency syndrome (AIDS) (205,206). OSM can bind directly to gp130 and signals through a receptor combination of gp130 and LIFRβ (164), but it also has an alternative receptor comprising a specific OSM receptor subunit (OSMRβ) and gp130 (207). These are now known as the type I and type II OSM receptors, respectively. OSM is now known to enhance the development of both endothelial cells and hematopoietic cells, possibly by increasing hamangioblasts, a common precursor for endothelial and hematopoietic cells (169).

Cardiotrophin-1 (CT-1) was initially isolated based on its actions on cardiac muscle cells (208). However, it is now clear that it is a multifunctional cytokine with hematopoietic, neuronal, and developmental effects, in additional to its effects on cardiac development and hypertrophy (209,210). Like OSM and LIF, CT-1 can also signal through a heterodimer of LIFRβ and gp130 (167). Interestingly, the CT-1 receptor on motor neurons may involve a third receptor component, possibly GPI-linked (211,212).

Novel neurotrophin-1/B-cell stimulatory factor-3 (NNT-1/BSF-3), like CNTF, can also support the survival of chicken embryonic sympathetic and motor neurons (171). Interestingly, in mice, NNT-1/BSF-3 can augment the effects of IL-1 and IL-6 and is a B-cell–stimulating factor (hence the term BSF-3). The NNT-1 receptor contains LIFRβ and gp130 (171). NNT-1 is also known as cardiotrophinlike cytokine (CLC), and this forms a complex with a soluble receptor protein known as cytokinelike factor-1 (CLF-1). Together this complex is a second ligand for CNTFR (213). It appears that CLC can also interact directly with soluble CNTFR to form a related cytokine (172).

IL-27 is an IL-6–related cytokine (214) that represents a dimer of the p28 protein and EB13 (Epstein–Barr virus-induced gene 3), which can induce proliferation of naïve CD4^{+} T cells. p28 was also denoted as IL-30 but by itself has no known biologic action. Together with IL-12, IL-23, CLC/CLF-1, and CLC/soluble CNTFR, this is one of five cytokines that represent dimers comprising a type I cytokine and a soluble receptorlike protein. IL-27 signals via the WSX-1/TCCR receptor (214); discussed later in the section on diseases of cytokine receptors and related molecules) and gp130. IL-27 has pro- and anti-inflammatory effects. Although it was suggested to promote Th1 responses, it is clear that it can also antagonize such responses, and IL-27 can promote effector responses of both CD4^{+} and CD8^{+} T cells, of NK cells, and it additionally stimulates mast cells. The anti-inflammatory effects of IL-27 are indicated by the phenotype observed in the absence of WSX-1, which includes in increased mast cell and macrophage responses (215,216).

TABLE 23.7 Composition of Receptors for the IL-6 Family of Cytokines

Cytokines whose receptors do not contain LIFR β	
IL-6	IL-6Rα + gp130
IL-11	IL-11Rα + gp130
OSM	OSMRβ + gp130
Cytokines whose receptors contain LIFR β	
LIF	LIFRβ + gp130
OSM	LIFRβ + gp130
CNTF	CNTFRα + LIFRβ + gp130
CT-1	LIFRβ + gp130 + ?CT1Rα
NNT-1/BSF-3/CLC + CLF-1	CNTFRα + LIFRβ + gp130
CLC + soluble CNTFRα	LIFRβ + gp130
Cytokines whose receptors contain OSMR β	
OSM	OSMRβ + gp130
IL-31	IL-31R + OSMRβ

Note that the sharing of CNTFRα by CNTF and the dimeric NNT-1/BSF-3/CLC–CLF-1 ligand helps to explain why the phenotype in CNTF$^{-/-}$ mice is less severe than that found in CNTFR$\alpha^{-/-}$ mice.

Thus, eight cytokines (IL-6, IL-11, LIF, CNTF, OSM, CT-1, NNT-1/BSF-3, and IL-27) all have receptors that are dependent on gp130 (reviewed in 217). These can be divided into two sets of cytokines: those known to not require LIFRβ, namely, IL-6, IL-11, and IL-27; and those that use both gp130 and LIFRβ (LIF, CT-1, OSM, CNTF, and NNT-1/BSF-3) (see Table 23.7), with OSM having two forms of receptors, each of which contains gp130 but only one of which contains LIFRβ. When cytokines share essentially the same receptor, one can hypothesize that two cytokines might exert identical actions on cells that can respond to both cytokines. It is clear that the presence of IL-6Rα, IL-11Rα, and CNTFRα (either on the cell surface or as a soluble receptor form, discussed in the following) determines whether a cell can respond to IL-6, IL-11, and CNTF. This raises the interesting question of whether functional homologs of these proteins also exist for LIF, OSM, CT-1, NNT-1/BSF-3, and IL-27. As noted previously, a third, possibly GPI-linked component of the CT-1 receptor indeed may exist.

Significance of the Sharing of Receptor Chains

Interestingly, γ_c, β_c, and gp130 all contribute to signaling, but none of these shared cytokine receptor proteins has primary binding activity for any known cytokine. Instead, they each increase binding affinity in the context of the primary binding protein for each cytokine. Consequently, the capacity of a cell to respond to a given cytokine is determined by the unique binding chain, but signaling pathways can be shared.

Other Receptors with Similarities to gp130 (G-CSFR, OB-R, IL-12Rβ1, IL-12Rβ2, and IL-31R)

As noted earlier, LIFRβ and OSMRβ bear some similarities to gp130 (207). In addition, the G-CSFR, the leptin receptor (also denoted OBR, for obesity receptor), IL-12/IL-23 receptor components, and IL-31R all resemble gp130. The amino acid identity among these different receptors, compared pairwise, ranges from 18% to 32%, with LIFRβ and OSMRβ being the most similar.

Leptin

Leptin is the product of the obesity (ob) gene, an adipose tissue–derived cytokine that plays a role in body-weight homeostasis (*218,219*,220). Additionally, leptin affects thymic homeostasisis, increasing thymocyte number and having antiapoptotic effects in the thymus and periphery. It is proinflammatory, promoting Th1 differentiation, and augmenting the production of TNF-α, IL-1, and IL-6 by monocytes/macrophages (220). The leptin receptor, OB-R, was cloned and found to be most closely related to the gp130 signal transducer, G-CSFR, and LIFRβ *(221)*. Interestingly, this receptor is encoded by the "diabetes gene," which is mutated in db/db mice (222).

IL-12 and IL-23

IL-12 is primarily produced by phagocytic cells in response to bacterial and intracellular parasites, such as *Toxoplasma gondii*, but it is also produced by other antigen-presenting cells, such as B cells *(223)*. IL-12 potently induces the production of IFN-γ by NK cells and T cells and is also a growth factor for preactivated but not resting NK and T cells. IL-12 was originally discovered as natural killer cell-stimulatory factor (NKSF) *(224)*. IL-12 also is a unique inducer of Th1 cell differentiation (see below). IL-12 can also induce the production of IL-2, IL-3, GM-CSF, IL-9, TNF-α, and M-CSF, although inducing IFN-γ is its most important known action (*223*,225). As is discussed later, in the section on immunodeficiency diseases, IL-12 is essential for the proper clearing of mycobacterial infections.

IL-12 can be thought of as having vital roles in both innate immunity and acquired immune responses. It is rapidly produced by NK cells and then T cells in response to antigens or foreign pathogens. This rapid response facilitates the activation of first-line defense against infections. In addition, however, IL-12 is also required for the subsequent differentiation of specialized T-cell populations, including the priming of Th1 cells for optimal production of IFN-γ and IL-2. IL-12 can act synergistically with hematopoietic growth factors, such as IL-3 and stem cell factor, to support the proliferation and survival of hematpoietic stem cells *(223)*. Structurally, IL-12 is a covalently linked dimer of 35- and 40-kDa peptides *(223)*; thus successful production of IL-12 requires that a cell transcribe both the p35 and p40 genes *(226)*. Interestingly, whereas p35 bears sequence similarity to IL-6 and G-CSF, p40 is homologous to the extracellular domains of IL-6Rα, CNTFRα, and G-CSFR and bears some of the features typical of type I receptors, including four conserved cysteines, a conserved tryptophan, and a WSEWAS motif, which has similarity to the typical WSXWS motif *(223)*. Moreover, as both IL-12 receptor (IL-12Rβ1 and IL-12Rβ2) chains bear some similarity to gp130 *(224,226,227)*, one can think of p40 as a functional homolog of the soluble p80 IL-6Rα chain. Thus, for this cytokine, part of the "receptor" has become part of the cytokine. Interestingly, all cells that produce IL-12 synthesize much more p40 than p35, suggesting that the careful control of signaling is at the level of the "primordial" p35 cytokine part of IL-12. p40 is on human chromosome 5q31-33, whereas p35 is on 3p12-13.2 *(223)*.

IL-23 is similar to IL-12 in that it also contains p40 *(228)*. However, rather than also containing p35, IL-23 is a dimer of a p40 and p19. IL-23 signals via a receptor that contains IL-12Rβ1 but not IL-12Rβ2 (229). Instead, another receptor chain, denoted IL-23R, is the second component of the IL-23 receptor *(230)*; both IL-12Rβ2 and IL-23R are located on chromosome 1 within 150 kilobases (kb) of each other *(230)*. Both IL-12 and IL-23 activate Jak2 and Tyk2. IL-12 and IL-23 can activate Stat1, Stat3, Stat4, and Stat5. Stat4 is the dominant STAT protein activated by IL-12 *(230)*. Interestingly, as compared to human IL-23R, murine IL-23R contains a 20-amino acid–duplicated region that spans the WQPWS motif. IL-23 appears to play a vital role in the maintenance, rather than in the initial differentiation, of Th17 cells (IL-17–producing cells), and IL-23 is essential for resistance to certain diseases, such as experimental autoimmune encephalomyelitis (EAE), that were originally believed to be Th1-mediated diseases. In the CD40-mediated model of inflammatory bowel disease, IL-12 p35 secretion controlled wasting disease and serum cytokine production but did not affect mucosal pathology, which instead was associated with IL-23/p19 (231). IL-27 is a related cytokine (discussed earlier), but it can act as an inhibitor of Th1 responses associated with intracellular infections such as *Toxoplasma gondii*. Whereas host defense to *T. gondii* is dependent on IL-12 and IFN-γ, IL-27–deficient mice control the parasite replication but develop a lethal inflammatory disease that is dependent on $CD4^+$ T cells. Additionally, IL-27 can inhibit Th2 actions (216).

IL-31

IL-31 is a four–α-helical–bundle cytokine that fits into the greater IL-6 extended family in that its receptor consists of IL-31RA and the OSMRβ (232). IL-31R is a gp130-like type 1 receptor, with four splice variants. IL-31 is produced primarily by activated T cells, and when overexpressed results in pruritis, alopecia, and skin lesions, indicating a potential role in dermatitis.

Other Examples of Shared Receptor Molecules

IL-7 and Thymic Stromal Lymphopoietin (TSLP) Share IL-7Rα

In addition to IL-7, a second stromal factor, TSLP (originally called thymic stromal–derived lymphopoietin and now thymic stromal lymphopoietin) has been identified that shares at least some actions with IL-7 (233,234), and whose receptor is a heterodimer of TSLPR and IL-7Rα (235,236). Interestingly, TSLPR is a remarkable 24% identical to γ_c, making it the cytokine receptor most like γ_c (235). Human and murine TSLP share only 43% amino acid identity, and human and murine TSLPR share only 39% identity *(237)*. This is extremely low for human and murine orthologous cytokine receptors; for example, human and murine γ_c are 70% identical *(238)*. In addition to their wide sequence divergence, murine and human TSLP were originally suggested to differ substantially in their actions. The major actions of murine TSLP were first reported to be as a B-cell differentiation factor that is important for the development of IgM$^+$-immature B cells from pre-B cells and as a weak thymic comitogen. In contrast, human TSLP appeared not to exert effects on these lineages but was found to be an epithelial-derived cytokine that potently activated dendritic cells related to Th2 allergic responses, an action not known to be shared by murine TSLP (239,*240*,241). However, the differences are in fact not so dramatic, as it is now clear that mouse TSLP can also activate dendritic cells, it plays a critical role in both atopic disease and asthma in mouse models, and these murine effects of TSLP are mediated via actions on both dendritic cells and CD4$^+$ T cells (242–245). Interestingly, human TSLP is expressed by Hassall corpuscles *(246)*, and it appears to promote selection of T_{reg} cells in human thymus, thus contributing to central tolerance (247). It is interesting, however, that mice that lack TSLPR have normal numbers of T_{reg} cells, indicating that TSLP is not absolutely essential for this function and that other molecules can at least substitute for TSLP.

Two Types of IL-4 Receptors, One of Which Also Responds to IL-13

As detailed previously, on T cells, IL-4 acts through a receptor comprising IL-4Rα and γ_c (the type I IL-4 receptor) (29,*30*). However, IL-4 can also signal through type II IL-4 receptors that do not express γ_c (248). IL-13 is another cytokine that shares some actions with IL-4 and was originally described as a T-cell–derived cytokine capable of inhibiting inflammation (249), although it is now clear that other cells such as NK cells and mast cells can also produce IL-13. IL-13 can induce identical signals to IL-4 on non-T cells that respond to IL-4, but lacks effects on mature T cells, as these cells do not bind IL-13 *(250,251)*. The shared actions of IL-4 and IL-13 include the ability to (a) decrease expression of inflammatory cytokines, (b) induce MHC class II expression, (c) induce CD23 expression and IgE production by B cells in humans, (d) inhibit IL-2–induced proliferation of chronic lymphocytic leukemia cells of B-cell origin, and (e) costimulate with anti-CD40 antibodies. This is explained by the observation that the type II IL-4 receptor consists of IL-4Rα plus IL-13Rα1 (252,*253*), with both IL-4 and IL-13 inducing indistinguishable signals on cells expressing this receptor. Interestingly, IL-4 binds primarily to IL-4Rα and IL-13 binds primarily to IL-13Rα1. This situation may be analogous to the situation for LIF, CT-1, and OSM, which can all act through receptors containing LIFRβ and gp130 but differ in their abilities to interact directly with each of these receptor proteins. An additional IL-13–binding protein, IL-13Rα2, has much higher binding affinity for IL-13 than does IL-13Rα1 (254). IL-13Rα2 is nonfunctional in terms of signaling and instead acts as a "decoy" receptor.

Although IL-13 was originally believed to be redundant with IL-4, it clearly has important distinctive actions as well. IL-13 may be vital in asthma, as blocking IL-13 can inhibit pathophysiologic changes of asthma (*255*,256). It also is clear that IL-13 regulates eosinophilic infiltration, airway hyperresponsiveness, and mucus secretion, and that it is a potent mediator of fibrosis (249). The phenotype of IL-13 knockout mice suggested a role for IL-13 in the ability to expel helminths *(257)* and it is clear that IL-13 can specifically modulate resistance to intracellular organisms, including *Leishmania major* and *Listeria monocytogenes* (249). IL-13 has also been identified as a factor that is secreted by and can stimulate the growth of Hodgkin and Reed–Sternberg cells (258).

An Example of Multiple Affinities of Binding for a Single Cytokine: Three Classes of IL-2 Receptors

Although cytokines typically signal via a single class of high-affinity cell surface receptor, more complex situations exist. The IL-2 system provides the very interesting illustration of a system with three classes of affinities of receptors (Table 23.8). In addition to the high-affinity receptor (IL-2Rα + IL-2Rβ + γ_c, $K_d \approx 10^{-11}$ M), there are both low-affinity (IL-2Rα alone, $K_d \approx 10^{-8}$ M) and intermediate-affinity (IL-2Rβ + γ_c, $K_d \approx 10^{-9}$ M) receptors (reviewed in (25,*40*). Low- and high-affinity receptors are expressed on activated lymphocytes, whereas intermediate-affinity receptors are found on resting lymphocytes, particularly on natural killer cells. Both intermediate- and high-affinity

TABLE 23.8 Classes of IL-2 Receptors

Affinity	K_d	*Where Expressed*	*Composition*	*Functional*
Low	10^{-8} M	Activated cells	IL-2Rα	No
Intermediate	10^{-9} M	Resting cells	IL-2Rβ and γ_c	Yes
High	10^{-11} M	Activated cells	IL-2Rα, IL-2Rβ, and γ_c	Yes

receptors can signal, thus suggesting that IL-2Rβ and γ_c are necessary and sufficient for signaling, in keeping with the theme of dimerization indicated earlier. Given that the intermediate-affinity form is functional, what, then, is the rationale for having a high-affinity IL-2 receptor that also contains IL-2Rα? This is a particularly relevant question in view of the fact that IL-2Rα has an extremely short cytoplasmic domain that does not appear to play a role in signaling. The importance of IL-2Rα is clearly demonstrated by the severely abnormal phenotype of IL-2Rα–deficient mice, which exhibit autoimmunity, inflammatory bowel disease, and premature death (140), and by the recognition that IL-2Rα mutations can cause an autoimmune syndrome in humans as well (259). A clue to the importance of IL-2Rα comes from the kinetics of association of IL-2 with each chain. Although the IL-2Rα appears to lack a direct signaling function, it has a very fast "on" rate for IL-2 binding *(260)*. Thus, the combination of this rapid "on" rate with the slow "off" rate from IL-2Rβ/γ_c dimers results in high-affinity binding that is vital for responding to the very low concentrations of IL-2 that are physiologically present in vivo. Moreover, as activated T cells express approximately 10 times as many low-affinity as high-affinity receptors, IL-2Rα may serve as an efficient means of recruitment and concentration of IL-2 on the cell surface, allowing more efficient formation of IL-2/IL-2Rβ/γ_c signaling complexes.

As mentioned earlier, IL-2Rα is not a type I cytokine receptor. In the mid-1980s, it was noted to have homology to the recognition domain of complement factor B *(261)*. Subsequently, however, the IL-15 receptor α chain was shown to also have a similar structure *(104)*, with both IL-2Rα and IL-15Rα having what are called "sushi" domains, which contribute to ligand binding. The fact that IL-2 and IL-15 both have related α chains is consistent with the close relationship between IL-2 and IL-15 and the fact that the receptors for both IL-2 and IL-15 contain both IL-2Rβ and γ_c.

As IL-2Rα cannot transduce a signal by itself, the detection of IL-2Rα on the cell surface does not necessarily reflect IL-2 responsiveness. Because IL-2Rα was discovered before IL-2Rβ and γ_c, many early papers in the literature evaluated IL-2 receptor expression based on IL-2Rα expression alone, and, for example, the presence of this protein on a subpopulation of double-negative thymocytes is a useful phenotypic marker corresponding to a stage of development, but it does not by itself reflect IL-2 responsiveness. Each of the components of the IL-2 receptor is located on a different chromosome: Human IL-2Rα is located on chromosome 10p14-15 *(262)*; IL-2Rβ is at 22q *(263,264)*, and γ_c is at Xq13.1 (120), while the murine homologs are located at chromosomes 2, 15, and X.

Erythropoietin, Thrombopoietin, and Stem Cell Factor

Erythropoietin is vital for erythropoiesis and thrombopoietin for thrombopoiesis. These cytokines each bind to receptors that are homodimers *(19,265)*. Interestingly, erythropoietin signaling may depend in part on the functional cooperation of the erythropoietin receptor and c-kit, the receptor for stem cell factor *(266)*. This latter receptor has intrinsic tyrosine kinase activity and is not a type I cytokine receptor.

CYTOKINE AND CYTOKINE RECEPTOR PLEIOTROPY AND REDUNDANCY

It is well recognized that many cytokines exhibit the phenomena of cytokine "pleiotropy" and "redundancy" (217). Cytokine pleiotropy refers to the ability of a cytokine to exert many different types of responses, often on different cell types, whereas cytokine redundancy refers to the fact that many different cytokines can induce similar actions. One set of cytokines that exhibits cytokine pleiotropy is the γ_c family of cytokines. For example, IL-2 can induce T-cell growth, augment B-cell immunoglobulin synthesis, increase the cytolytic activity of lymphokine-activated killer and natural killer cells, and play an essential role in mediating activation-induced cell death; IL-4 can induce B-cell growth and immunoglobulin class switch; and IL-7 plays a major role in thymocyte development, but also can stimulate mature T cells, and at least in the mouse, can act as a pre–B-cell growth factor. The gp130 family cytokines also exhibit broad actions. For example, IL-6 exerts effects ranging from that of a comitogen for thymocyte activation to that of a mediator of the acute-phase response in liver. Regarding cytokine redundancy, it has already been highlighted that IL-2, IL-4, IL-7, IL-15, and IL-21 whose receptors contain γ_c, can act as T-cell growth factors, and that IL-3 has actions that overlap with IL-5 and GM-CSF.

The recognition that cytokines not only have overlapping actions but also share receptor components led to the concepts of "cytokine receptor pleiotropy" and "cytokine receptor redundancy" (reviewed in 217). The first of these terms can be defined by the ability of a single cytokine receptor subunit to function in more than one receptor. Thus, examples include the sharing of γ_c, β_c, gp130, IL-4Rα, LIFRβ, and OSMRβ, as summarized earlier, as well as the sharing of IL-2Rβ by IL-2 and IL-15 receptors, the sharing of IL4Rα and IL-13Rα in type II IL-4 receptors and IL-13 receptors, and the sharing of IL-7Rα by the IL-7 and TSLP receptors. Another way of viewing receptor pleiotropy is that certain receptor chains are useful "modules" that function in more than one context.

The final term, cytokine receptor subunit redundancy, is the one with fewest examples. There is one well-documented example in mice, but not humans. IL-3 signals through IL-3Rα plus either β_c or an alternative unique IL-3Rβ that shares 91% amino acid identity with β_c and appears to be a completely functionally redundant protein for IL-3 signaling, but IL-3Rβ cannot substitute for β_c in the context of IL-5 or GM-CSF signaling (157). Other potential examples exist. For example, in type I and type II IL-4 receptors, IL-4Rα coordinates with either γ_c or IL-13Rα, respectively, and there are two types of OSM receptors, both of which contain gp130, but one of which contains a specific OSMR while the other contains LIFRβ. What remains unknown, however, is whether the signals mediated by these different types of receptors are truly identical so that there is redundancy, or whether there are distinctive features to the signals that IL-4 and OSM induce via the different receptors.

In addition to the preceding examples related to type I cytokines, the IL-10 subfamily of type II cytokines is interesting in that IL-10Rβ, IL-20Rα, IL-20Rβ, and IL-22Rα are each shared components, collectively affecting signaling in response to IL-10, IL-19, IL-20, IL-22, and IL-24 (reviewed in 217 and references below related to the IL-10 family of cytokines). Specifically, IL-10 signals via a receptor containing IL-10Rα and IL-10Rβ, IL-19 signals via a receptor containing IL-20Rα and IL-20Rβ, IL-20 signals via receptors containing IL-20Rβ and either IL-20Rα or IL-22Rα, IL-22 signals via receptors containing IL-10Rβ and IL-22Rα, and IL-24 signals through receptors containing IL-20Rβ plus either IL-20Rα or IL-22Rα. Two other IL-10 family members, IL-28 and IL-29, both signal via IL-28R + IL-10Rβ (267).

SOLUBLE RECEPTORS

Soluble forms of many cytokine receptors have been identified, including those for IL-1, IL-2, IL-4, IL-5, IL-6, IL-7, IL-13Rα2, GM-CSF, type I and type II IFNs, IL-22, and TNF *(268–270)*. As is clear from this list of cytokines, soluble receptors are not restricted to receptors that are type I cytokine receptors, and in the case of IL-2, the principal soluble receptor protein is IL-2Rα, which is not a type I cytokine receptor. Soluble receptors can be created by alternative splicing that truncates the protein N-terminal to the transmembrane domain, resulting in a secreted protein rather than a membrane-anchored membrane in the case of IL-4Rα, IL-5Rα, IL-6Rα, IL-7Rα, IFNAR-2, and GM-CSFRα. Alternatively, they can be created by proteolytic cleavage of the membrane receptor, as is found for the receptors for IL-2Rα and TNFRI and TNFRII (reviewed in *269*) (Table 23.9). Although it is theoretically possible that a distinct gene might encode the soluble forms of a receptor, no such examples have been reported. In the cases in which proteolytic cleavage occurs, the identity of the proteases has not been identified. The major questions related to these soluble receptors are these: (a) Do they have physiologic or pathophysiologic functions? (b) How do their affinities compare to those of the corresponding cell surface receptor? (c) Do they have diagnostic, prognostic, and therapeutic applications?

TABLE 23.9 Soluble Cytokine Receptors

Generated by Alternative Splicing	*Generated by Proteolytic Cleavage of Mature Receptor*
sIL-4Rα	sIL-2Rα
sIL-5Rα	sTNFR
sIL-6Rα	
sIL-7Rα	
sGM-CSFRα	
sIFNAR-2	

Unfortunately, there is little information available on the in vivo role of soluble receptors. In general, in in vitro studies, soluble receptors can compete with their corresponding cell surface receptors, thereby serving negative regulatory roles. For example, this appears to be the case for the IL-22–soluble receptor. However, soluble IL-6Rα exerts an agonistic role because, as summarized earlier, IL-6 signaling occurs equally well via gp130 when the soluble rather than the transmembrane form of IL-6Rα interacts with IL-6. Nevertheless, a mutated form of IL-6Rα that cannot interact with gp130 but still binds IL-6 can effectively inhibit the actions of IL-6 *(271)*. In the case of IL-2Rα, there is no reported physiologic function for soluble IL-2Rα, as the affinity of the released receptor is, as expected, similar to that of the low-affinity receptor ($K_d \approx 10^{-8}$ M), making it unlikely to effectively compete with the high-affinity cell surface receptor ($K_d \approx 10^{-11}$ M). However, this and other soluble receptors could serve as cytokine carrier proteins and potentially could increase stability of a cytokine by protecting it from proteolysis *(269)*. Moreover, there are potential diagnostic and prognostic uses for measuring the level of shed receptors (Table 23.10).

TABLE 23.10 Soluble IL-2 Receptors in Human Disease

Malignancies
Hematologic
- Adult T-cell leukemia (ATL)
- Hairy-cell leukemia
- Acute lymphocytic leukemia
- Chronic lymphocytic leukemia (B-cell) (CLL)
- Acute myelogenous leukemia (AML)
- Chronic myelogenous leukemia (CML), especially in blast crisis
- Malignant lymphomas
  - Hodgkin's disease
  - Non-Hodgkin's lymphomas

Nonhematologic
- Adenocarcinoma of lung, breast, pancreas
- Small-cell bronchogenic carcinoma
- Ovarian, cervical, and endometrial cancers
- Nasopharyngeal carcinoma
- Melanoma

Infections
- HIV
- Tuberculosis
- Rubeola
- Infectious mononucleosis

Other Diseases
- End-stage renal disease
- Rheumatoid arthritis
- Systemic lupus erythematosis
- Scleroderma
- Sarcoidosis

After transplantation
After IL-2 administration

In adults, the mean sIL-2Rα levels are 280 ± 161 U/mL (levels tend to be higher in pediatric populations). The situations where the levels exceed 5,000 U/mL are ATL, hairy-cell leukemia, CML, and after IL-2 administration. The situations where levels are between 1,000 and 5,000 units/ml include AML, CLL, non Hodgkin's lymphomas, AIDS associated with Kaposi sarcoma, tuberculosis, rubeola, and end-stage renal disease. Data are from *(268,269)*.

INTERFERONS (TYPE II CYTOKINES) AND THEIR RECEPTORS

Interferons (IFNs) represent an evolutionarily conserved family (Table 23.11) of cytokines that are related to the IL-10 family of type II cytokines. IFNs were discovered in 1957 on the basis of their antiviral activity and were the first cytokines that were discovered (272). IFNs are known as either type I or type II IFNs (*273–277,*278–282), where type I interferons include IFN-α (originally known as leukocyte IFN) and IFN-β (originally known as fibroblast IFN), and IFN-ε, IFN-κ, IFN-ω, IFN-δ, and IFN-τ. IFN-δ and IFN-τ are absent in humans. IFN-ω is closely related to the IFN-α and was formerly designated as an IFN-α. There are multiple (at least 12) IFN-α in mice and humans. In contrast, the other type I IFNs, IFN-β and IFN-ω, are each encoded by single human and murine genes near the IFN-α cluster, and in addition there are multiple pseudogenes most closely related to IFN-α and IFN-ω. The type I IFNs are clustered on human chromosome 9 and murine chromosome 4. Type II interferon is IFN-γ, which is encoded by a single gene on human chromosome 12 and murine chromosome 10. IFN-α/β is produced after viral infection in many cell types, although plasmacytoid dendritic cells appear to be the largest producers of IFN-α/β. These type I IFNs inhibit viral replication and induce the apoptosis of virally infected cells. In addition, IFN-α/β mediate the activation of macrophages and NK cells, and they additionally affect the proliferation and survival of $CD8^+$ T cells.

TABLE 23.11 Type II Cytokines

		Chromosomal Location (h/m)
Type I interferons		
IFNα	Many genes	9p22/4
IFNβ	Single gene	9p21/4
IFNω	Single gene	9p21/4
IFNτ	Many genes	
Type II interferon		
IFNγ	Single gene	12q14/10
IL-10 family cytokines		
IL-10	Single gene	1q31-32/1
IL-19	Single gene	1q32/1
IL-20	Single gene	1q32/1
IL-22	Single gene	12q14-15/10
IL-24	Single gene	1q32/1
IL-26	Single gene	12q14-15/
IL-28	Single gene	19q13/7
IL-29	Single gene	19q13

The grouping of the IFN-α and IFN-β together as type I IFNs is logical not only because of the similar amino acid sequences and structures of these IFNs, but also based on the fact that they share the same receptor and induce essentially the same signals *(283,284)*; although DNA array analysis does show some differences in the genes induced by IFN-α and IFN-β, the basis for these differences is unclear *(285)*. These signals include antiproliferative and antiviral activities, but also the ability to stimulate cytolytic activity in lymphoyctes, natural killer cells, and macrophages. In contrast, IFN-γ has a distinct receptor. Type I and type II IFN receptors share a sufficient degree of similarity to each other so as to form a family *(286)*. The structure of the IFN-γ receptor (287) is shown in Figure 23.2. IFN receptors are referred to as type II cytokine receptors to reflect the substantial differences between these receptors and the type I cytokine receptors *(8)*. Because both type I and type II IFNs bind to type II cytokine receptors, IFNs are occasionally referred to as type II cytokines, but more generally are referred to as IFNs. Based on the similarity of the IL-10 receptor to the IFN-γ receptors *(8)*,

IL-10 was designated as a type II cytokine, and indeed, when its x-ray crystal was determined, IL-10 was found to be topologically related to IFN-γ *(14)*. As noted earlier, more recently a series of IL-10–related cytokines has been identified, including IL-19, IL-20, IL-22, IL-24, IL-26, IL-28, and IL-29, and these are also designated as type II cytokines. Among type II cytokines, IFN-γ has helices similar to those of the type I short-chain helical cytokines, but its short helices that occupy the AB and CD loops positions exhibit the long-chain cytokinelike AB-over-CD topology. IL-10 and IFN-α/β have long-chain structures *(8)*. Thus, the theme of short-chain and long-chain type I cytokines also extends to the interferons and the IL-10 family of type II cytokines.

Type I IFNs signal through a receptor known as the type I IFN receptor (*274*,278,280,282,*283*), The receptor consists of at least two chains *(288–291)*. In contrast to the α- and β-chain nomenclature typical for type I cytokine receptors, IFN receptor chains are officially denoted as IFNAR-1 (previously also denoted IFN-αR1, IFNAR1, and IFN-Rα) and IFNAR-2 (previously also known as IFN-α/β receptor [IFN-α/βR], IFN-αR2, IFNAR2, and IFN-Rβ) *(292)*. IFNAR-2 has both short and long forms as well as a soluble form *(293)*. The long form has a much larger cytoplasmic domain and serves a more important role in signal transduction. Whereas IFNAR-1 cannot bind IFN-α, IFNAR-2 binds with low affinity, and the combination of both chains results in high-affinity binding *(293)* and function. As detailed later, IFNAR-1 binds the Janus family tyrosine kinase Tyk2, whereas IFNAR-2 binds Jak1. In addition to these cellular receptors, it is interesting that vaccinia virus and other orthopoxviruses encode a soluble form of type I IFN receptor that is related to the IL-1 receptors and that is capable of binding IFN-α, IFN-β, and IFN-ω (294,295). This form of IFN receptor is therefore not a member of the type II cytokine family but instead is an immunoglobulin superfamily protein. The IFN-α are typically species-specific, although IFN-α8 is a human type I IFN that can bind to the mouse receptor. IFNAR-1 confers species specificity of binding.

IFN-γ was first recognized more than 40 years ago, in 1965, as immune IFN, named as IFN-γ in 1980, cloned in 1982, and then confirmed to be the same as primary macrophage-activating factor (MAF) (*274,283, 296,297*,298). Although IFN-γ clearly possesses antiviral activity, it also has a range of actions on proinflammatory and anti-inflammatory host responses (279) For example, IFN-γ can prime macrophages to manifest antimicrobial and antitumor effects. Moreover, following IL-12–mediated differentiation of Th1 cells, IFN-γ is a major secreted product. This production is critical for host response to a range of infectious pathogens, including, for example, *Toxoplasma gondii*. IFN-γ inhibits the generation of Th2 cells as well as Th17 cells. IFN-γ is produced by a range of cells, including T_{reg} cells, and in this context appears to result in apoptosis of naïve cells and Th2 effector T cells. It is produced by NK cells and can mediate NK-dependent lysis of tumor cells, augment IgG2a isotype switching of B cells, and activate dendritic cells. Moreover, IFN-γ can either contribute to disease protection or can be protective, depending on the context (298). Finally, IFN-γ– or anti-IFN-γ– based therapies are being tried for a range of conditions.

IFN-γ is encoded by four exons on chromosome 12. IFN-γ forms a functional homodimer with an apparent molecular weight of 34 kDa, whereas little of the monomeric form can be detected and it is not biologically active. Each IFN-γ monomer has six α helices, four of which resemble the short-chain helical cytokines, and there is no β-sheet structure. The subunits interact in an antiparallel fashion. In contrast to the ability of many different cells to produce IFN-α, IFN-γ is more restricted, with it being produced primarily by NK cells, $CD8^+$ T cells, and the Th1 subclass of $CD4^+$ T cells (reviewed in *274*). Many signals, including antigen stimulation, IL-12, and IL-18, can induce the production of IFN-γ. IFN-γ exerts its effects through specific receptors that are expressed on all types of cells except erythrocytes. Interestingly, even platelets express IFN-γ receptors, raising the possibility that they can serve a function in transporting IFN-γ in the circulation *(274)*. The functional human receptor consists of two chains *(299)*: IFNGR-1, formerly also denoted IFNγR1 or IFNγRα *(292,300)*, a 90-kDa protein whose gene is located on human chromosome 6q16-22 and murine chromosome 10 *(297)*; and IFNGR-2, also denoted as IFNγRβ *(301,302)*, located on human chromosome 21q22.1 and murine chromosome 16 *(297)*. IFNGR-1 is required for ligand binding, whereas IFNGR-2 plays a role in signaling. Jak1 associates with the Leu–Pro–Lys–Ser sequence in the membrane-proximal region of the cytoplasmic domain of IFNGR-1 *(303)*, whereas Jak2 binds to IFNGR-2 *(304)*. The fact that IFN-γ is a homodimer explains how its binding induces the homodimerization of IFNGR-1, which then allows the recruitment of IFNGR-2. Thus, the functional IFN-γ receptor is believed to contain two molecules each of IFNGR-1 and IFNGR-2. Normal IFN-γ production is dependent on IL-12, and defective IFN-γ signaling is associated with failure to appropriately clear mycobacterial and other infections (discussed later).

Interleukin-10, a Type II Cytokine, and the Related Cytokines IL-19, IL-20, IL-22, IL-24, IL-26, IL-28, and IL-29

IL-10 is a type II cytokine that is produced by activated T cells, B cells, monocytes, NK cells, keratinocytes, and dendritic cells (305). The IL-10 gene contains five exons and is located on chromosome 1 in both mice and humans (305). IL-10 has an open reading frame of 178 amino acids, including the signal peptide, and the mature protein is 18 kDa. Human IL-10 receptor maps to 11q23.3. IL-10 can inhibit the production of a number of cytokines, including IL-2, IL-3, IFN-γ, GM-CSF, and TNF-α, and falls in the category of a Th2 cytokine (305) (see later). IL-10 originally was identified as cytokine synthesis-inhibitory factor (CSIF) (267,*306*), produced by Th2 cells. However, it is also clear that B cells and dendritic cells also produce IL-10. IL-10 inhibits monocyte/macrophage/dendritic cell-dependent T-cell proliferation, in part by markedly decreasing synthesis of a variety of cytokines, expression of costimulatory molecules, and chemokines, to name just some of its inhibitory effects (267). Nevertheless, in addition to these indirect effects on T cells, IL-10 appears to exert direct stimulatory effects on thymocytes and T cells in vitro and to promote the development of B1 cells and activity of NK cells. IL-10–deficient mice develop a form of inflammatory bowel disease that is similar to Crohn's disease (305,*307*). Interestingly, the BCRF1 protein that is encoded by Epstein–Barr virus is very similar to IL-10 and shares many of its biologic properties as a macrophage "deactivating" factor, and as a costimulator of proliferation of B cells *(308)*. The EBV IL-10 homolog is a selective agonist, although its binding to the IL-10 receptor is somewhat impaired *(308)*. IL-10 is a major inhibitor of Th1 functions (305). Although it was suggested that IL-10 might also favor Th2 development, IL-4 is established as the major mediator of Th2 cell development. IL-10 instead plays a major role in limiting and terminating inflammatory responses (305).

The IL-10 receptor is most closely related to IFN receptors, making it a type II cytokine receptor *(309,310)*, thus corresponding to the close structural relationship of IL-10 to IFN-γ. The receptor for IL-10 consists of an IL-10Rα chain and IL-10Rβ (305); this latter protein is the same as CRF2-4, which was first identified as an "orphan" IFN receptor family member that is located on chromosome 21 within 35 kb of IFNGR-2 *(311,312)*.

A series of IL-10-related cytokines has been been identified, including IL-19, IL-20, IL-22, IL-24, IL-26, IL-28, and IL-29 (313,*314–317*). Data on biologic roles of some of these proteins is still limited. IL-19 was discovered as a gene that was induced in LPS-stimulated monocytes. Analogous to IL-20, IL-19 has been suggested to potentially be involved in the pathogenesis of chronic inflammatory diseases, such as psoriasis. IL-20 was found in epidermal cells, with overexpression resulting in aberrant epidermal differentiation; it was suggested to have a role in psoriasis. IL-22 was found as an IL-9–induced cytokine that can in turn induce acute-phase reactant production by hepatocytes and accordingly that it might be involved in inflammatory responses. It is produced mainly by activated Th1 cells, but its target cells are primarily in the digestive and respiratory systems, as well as keratinocytes, and it appears to promote innate immunity *(318)*. IL-22 is also produced by Th17 cells (318a). IL-24 was originally discovered as melanoma differentiation-associated antigen 7 (Mda-7). IL-24 is induced in peripheral blood mononuclear cells (PBMC) with mitogens. Overexpression of IL-24 can induce apoptosis in a wide range of tumor cells, including, for example, melanoma and malignant gliomas, and infection with adenoviral-driven Mda7 can sensitize tumors to ionizing radiation (267). IL-26 was originally discovered as AK155. Very little is known regarding the function of IL-26. IL-28 (which exists in two isoforms, IL-28A and IL-28B, originally also called IFN-λ1 and IFN-λ2) and IL-29 (originally also called IFN-λ3) are induced in plasmacytoid dendritic cells by viral infection and exhibit antiviral activity, analogous to type I IFNs; nevertheless, they bind to a receptor consisting of IL-10Rβ and IL-28Rα *(319)*. Interestingly, the genes encoding IL-10, IL-19, IL-20, and IL-24 collocalize at human chromosome 1q32, whereas those encoding IL-22 and IL-26 are at 12q14-15 near the *IFNG* gene, and IL-28 and IL-29 are at 19q13 (267,*320*). Thus, these type II cytokines can be subdivided into three different groups based at least in part on chromosome localization.

SPECIES SPECIFICITY OF CYTOKINES

There are no general rules for the species specificity of human and murine cytokines and how the cytokines and their receptor chains have coevolved. To provide illustrative examples of each situation, human IL-2 can stimulate both human and murine cells, whereas murine IL-2 exhibits little action on human cells *(39)*. Conversely, human IL-12 does not work on murine cells, whereas murine IL-12 is biologically active on both murine and human cells *(223)*. This selective property of IL-12 is dependent on the species origin of p35. Finally, IL-4 exhibits rather strict specificity, so that human and murine IL-4 only induce responses on human and murine cells, respectively *(61,62)*. As noted previously, the IFN-α are generally specifies-specific, although IFN-α8 is not. In addition to these examples, varying degrees of relative species specificity have been demonstrated, depending on the cytokine; in other words, at times a cytokine from one species will work on another species, but with attenuated potency. Thus, virtually any combination of species specificities has been observed.

SIGNALING THROUGH INTERFERON AND CYTOKINE RECEPTORS

Our understanding of signaling through interferon and cytokine receptors has increased tremendously in the past few years. Multiple signaling pathways/molecules have been observed for various cytokines. Collectively, these include the Jak-STAT pathway, IRF family proteins, Ras-MAP kinase pathway, Src and Zap70 and related proteins, phosphatidyl inositol 3-kinase (PI 3-kinase), IRS-1 and IRS-2, and phosphatases. Each of these pathways will be discussed in turn. The Jak-STAT pathways are very important for both type I and IFNs/type II cytokines, whereas the IRF proteins play central functions, more so for the IFNs than type I cytokines.

OVERVIEW OF JAKS AND STATS

The Jak-STAT pathway (26,*283*,321,322,*323*,324), serves as a rapid mechanism by which signals can be transduced from the membrane to the nucleus. Jak kinases are known as Janus family tyrosine kinases, and the acronym STAT denotes "signal transducer and activator of transcription." STAT proteins are substrates for Jak kinases. A tremendous amount of information is now available on Jaks and STATs that demonstrates their importance related to development, differentiation, proliferation, cellular transformation, and tumorigenesis.

Jaks

The Jak kinases are 116 to 140 kDa and comprise approximately 1 150 amino acids (*283*,322). The seven regions of conserved sequences in Jak kinases, denoted JH1 to JH7, are depicted in Figure 23.6. One of the hallmark features of these kinases is that, in addition to the presence of a catalytic tyrosine kinase domain (JH1), there is also a pseudokinase region (JH2). The name Janus kinase reflects the two faces of the mythological Roman god, with one face representing the true kinase and the other the pseudokinase. Although the JH nomenclature was used historically, it has obvious limitations in that, except for the JH1 catalytic domain and JH2 pseudokinase domain, it remains unclear whether the other JH regions correspond to discrete domains. Modeling has indicated five important regions, including an N-terminal domain, a FERM (4.1, ezrin, radixin, moesin) domain, SH2, kinaselike (which spans two of the JH domains), and kinase domains *(325)*.

TABLE 23.12 Features of Janus Family Kinases

Kinase	*Inducible vs. Constitutive*	*Size*	*Chromo. Loc. (h/m)*
Jak1	Constitutive	135 kDa	1p31.3/4
Jak2	Constitutive	130 kDa	9p23-24/19
Jak3	Inducible	116 kDa	19p13/8
Tyk2	Constitutive	140 kDa	19p13.2/9

There are four mammalian Jak kinases, Jak1 *(326)*, Jak2 *(327)*, Jak3 *(328,329)*, and Tyk2 *(330)*, each of which was identified as part of a study intended to identify new kinases (322). At least one Jak kinase is activated by every IFN and cytokine, and some cytokines activate two or three Jak kinases (*283*,321,322,*323*). Table 23.12 lists a number of features of each Jak kinase, whereas Table 23.13 summarizes the Jak kinases that are activated by a variety of cytokines.

Because Jak1, Jak2, and Tyk2 are expressed ubiquitously, each cell type expresses either three or in some cases all four Jak kinases (e.g, lymphoid cells that also express Jak3). The Jak kinases that are activated by a specific cytokine are those that can bind to its receptor's cytoplasmic domain. Jak kinases physically bind to the membrane proximal Box 1/Box 2 region of the cytoplasmic domains *(329–332*,333,*334)* and the N-terminal region of the Jaks is required for this function (*335,336*,337). In cytokine receptors, the Box 1 region is proline-rich *(22)*, suggesting that Jak kinases may have SH3-like domains in their N-terminal regions to mediate these interactions. As each cytokine or IFN receptor is a homodimer, heterodimer, or higher-order oligomer, it is reasonable to assume that at least two Jak molecules (either two molecules of one Jak or one molecule each of two different Jaks) typically will be activated, as one Jak will be associated with each

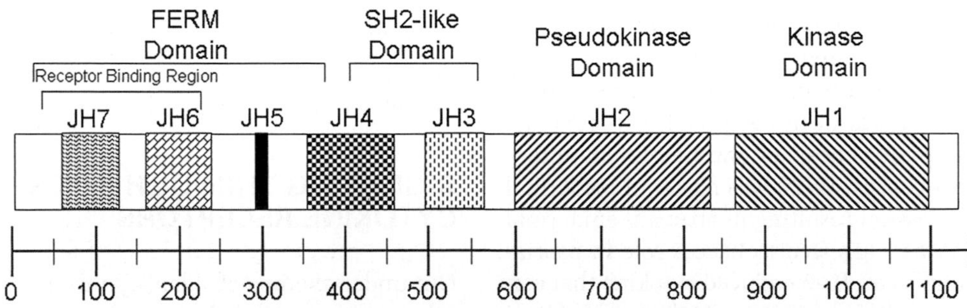

FIGURE 23.6 Schematic of Jak kinases. Shown are the locations of the seven JH domains. JH1 is the catalytic domain. JH2 is the pseudokinase domain, the presence of which prompted the naming of this family as Janus family tyrosine kinases. As noted in the text, the JH nomenclature has limitations and in fact masks the presence of an SH2 domain that spans parts of the JH4 and JH3 domains. Also shown is the conserved tyrosine (Y1007 in Jak2), whose phosphorylation is required for maximal catalytic activity.

TABLE 23.13 Cytokines and the Jaks They Activate

Cytokine	*Jak Kinase(s) Activated*
IFNα/β	Jak1, Tyk2
IFNγ	Jak1, Jak2
Growth hormone	Jak2
Prolactin	Jak2
Erythopoietin	Jak2
Thrombopoietin	Jak2
IL-10	Jak1, Tyk2
IL-12, IL-23	Jak2, Tyk2
G-CSF	Jak1, Jak2
γ_c family	
IL-2, IL-4*, IL-7, IL-9, IL-15, IL-21	Jak1, Jak3
β_c family	
IL-3, IL-5, GM-CSF	Jak2, ?Jak1
gp130 family	
IL-6, IL-11, CNTF, LIF, OSM, CT-1	Jak1, Jak2, Tyk2
TSLP	Instead of Jaks, TSLP was suggested to activate a Tec family kinase *(575)*

Note that IL-4 activates Jak1 and Jak3 when it acts through the type I IL-4 receptor (IL-4Rα + γ_c, found for example on T cells). However, Jak3 is not activated when IL-4 signals through the type II IL-4 receptors (IL-4Rα + IL13Rα1, a form of receptor that is expressed on a number of non-T cells, including fibroblasts).

receptor chain. In accord with their ubiquitous expression, Jak1, Jak2, and Tyk2 are activated by a variety of different sets of cytokines (Tables 23.12 and 23.13). For example, Jak1 is activated not only by type I and type II IFNs, but also by the γ_c family of cytokines (e.g, IL-2, IL-4, IL-7, IL-9, IL-15, and IL-21), whereas Jak2 is activated not only by IFN-γ but also by growth hormone, erythropoietin, prolactin, and the hematopoietic cytokines, IL-3, IL-5, and GM-CSF (321,322). Tyk2 is somewhat more restricted in that it is activated by IFN-α/β and IL-12/IL-23; the significance of its activation by gp130 family cytokines is less clear. Interestingly, Jak1, Jak2, and Tyk2 are recruited by each of the cytokine receptors that share gp130 as a signal-transducing molecule, raising the question of whether these cytokines require all three Jak kinases for optimal function or whether any one or two is/are sufficient. At least for IL-6, Jak1 is absolutely vital (338,*339*), whereas the importance of Jak2 and Tyk2 is less clear.

Jak3 is different from the other Jak kinases in that it is much more inducible. Moreover, Jak3 is activated only by the cytokines whose receptors contain γ_c (26,*36*). It is interesting that each cytokine whose receptor contains γ_c activates not only Jak3 but also Jak1. The basis for the activation of both Jak1 and Jak3 by IL-2, IL-4, IL-7, IL-9, IL-15, and IL-21 is that Jak1 associates with each of the unique signaling chains (IL-2Rβ, IL-4Rα, IL-7Rα, IL-9Rα, and IL-21R), whereas Jak3 associates with γ_c (26,*36*). Although this could be a coincidental result of coevolution of these cytokine systems, these observations raise the possibility that Jak1 is the Jak kinase that can most efficiently functionally cooperate with Jak3.

Given the wide range of cytokines that activate any particular Jak kinase and that in some cases multiple cytokines can activate the same set of Jaks, it is clear that the Jak kinases by themselves do not determine signaling specificity. For example, IL-2, IL-4, IL-7, IL-9, IL-15, and IL-21 all activate Jak1 and Jak3, but induce a range of actions. Moreover, Jak2 is the only Jak kinase that is activated by growth hormone and erythropoietin, cytokines with different target cells and biologic functions. Interestingly, Jak2 is the Jak that interacts with all cytokine receptors that form homodimers. Given that homodimeric receptors are most likely the oldest cytokine receptors in evolution, this suggests that Jak2 might be the "primordial" Jak kinase from which others evolved.

Importance of Jak Kinases in Signaling

In addition to the activation of Jak kinases by multiples cytokines and interferons, a variety of other data indicate their importance for signaling. One of the vital series of experiments that led to the establishment of the critical role of Jak kinases in IFN signaling involved a group of mutant cell lines that were defective for interferon signaling, but wherein signaling could be rescued by genetic complementation (reviewed in 283). Defective signaling in response to IFN-α and IFN-β was found in a mutant fibroblast cell line (U1 cells) lacking Tyk2; defective signaling in response to IFN-α, IFN-β, and IFN-γ was found in a mutant cell line lacking Jak1 (U4 cells), and defective IFN-γ signaling was found in cells lacking Jak2 *(283)*. A variety of other data have indicated the importance of Jak kinases for other cytokine pathways. First, dominant negative Jak2 inhibits signaling by erythropoietin and growth hormone *(340,341)*, whereas a dominant negative Jak3 inhibits signaling in response to IL-2 *(342)*, and, as noted earlier, Jak1 is vital for IL-6 signaling. Second, humans (343,344) and mice (345,346,*347*) that are deficient in Jak3 exhibit developmental and signaling defects consistent with defective signaling. Third, humans with an activating mutation in Jak2 develop polycythemia vera *(348)*, and a Jak2 inhibitor inhibited the growth of acute lymphoblastic leukemia cells in vitro *(349)*. Fourth, a patient with mutation in Tyk2 developed a form of immunodeficiency (350). Fifth, in *Drosophila*, the *hopscotch* gene encodes a Jak kinase wherein loss-of-function alleles result in lethality and decreased proliferation, whereas a gain-of-function allele, *hopscotch*$^{Tumorous\text{-}lethal}$ results in melanotic tumors and hypertrophy of the hematopoietic organs (351,*352*). Sixth, in zebrafish, Jak1 is vital for normal cell migration and anterior specification *(353)*.

Seventh, as discussed later, Jak kinases are constitutively activated in many cell lines infected with a number of viruses, including HTLV-I, v-Abl, spleen focus forming virus, and with v-src (354,*356*,357). These data together underscore the vital roles of Jaks in cytokine signaling. Depending on the function of the particular cytokine (e.g, development, differentiation, or proliferation), the particular Jak kinases potentially may be involved in a variety of processes, and when dysregulated, in at least certain settings, they appear to contribute to cellular transformation.

Jak3 Mutations Result in an Autosomal Recessive Form of Severe Combined Immunodeficiency (SCID) That is Indistinguishable from XSCID

A very large number of different mutations in γ_c have been observed in XSCID. As might be expected, in cases in which it has been examined, amino acid substitutions in the extracellular domain result in defective cytokine binding. In contrast, mutations or truncations in the γ_c cytoplasmic domain result in defective signaling. Analysis of a family in which a number of males exhibit a moderate form of X-linked combined immunodeficiency (XCID) revealed that this disease also resulted from a mutation in γ_c (32), (Leu 271 → Gln), that resulted in a decrease, but not total loss, of Jak3 association, in contrast to the loss of Jak3 interaction seen with mutations in the γ_c cytoplasmic domain that cause XSCID. Thus, the severity of the immunodeficiency correlated inversely with the degree of Jak3 activation (26,*36*). Moreover, it was predicted that Jak3 was required for T-cell and NK-cell development and that mutations in Jak3 might result in a clinical phenotype indistinguishable from that in XSCID (32). Indeed, this is the case in humans (343,344). As one would hypothesize, many mutations in Jak3 have been identified (322). Presumably, any mutation that interferes with its ability to interact with γ_c, with its catalytic activity, or with recruitment of substrates could result in clinical disease, ranging from moderate to severe immunodeficiency.

Analogous to the similarity of XSCID and Jak3-deficient SCID, mice deficient in either γ_c or Jak3 also have indistinguishable phenotypes (134,135,345,346,*347*). These in vivo data underscore the vital role of Jak3 in mediating γ_c-dependent functions and suggested that Jak3 is essential for most if not all γ_c functions. Some in vitro data indicate that γ_c may do more than recruit Jak3 *(342,358)*, and interestingly γ_c can interact with calpain *(359)*, but the recruitment of Jak3 is clearly essential and the defects in T-cell and NK-cell development associated with γ_c or Jak3 deficiency are indistinguishable. Because Jak3 deficiency is not clincially or phenotypically more severe than γ_c deficiency in humans and mice, it seems likely that γ_c is the major, if not only, protein with which Jak3 associates. Although Jak3 was suggested to associate with CD40 *(360)*, a functional role for Jak3 in CD40 signaling has been questioned *(361)*. The phenotypes of mice lacking each of the four Jak kinases are summarized in Table 23.14.

Jak2 Mutations and Translocations

The Jak2V617F mutations has now been identified in the vast majority of patients with polycythemia vera (*348*,362), some of whom had homozygous and some had heterozygous mutations. The homozygous patients had duplications of the mutated allele. This mutation results in a constitutively activated kinase and presumably confers factor-independent growth, something that has been demonstrated in transfected cell lines. Moreover, polycythemia patients exhibit erythropoietin-independent BFU-E. Furthermore, the *JAK2* locus is involved in a chromosomal translocation to create the TEL-JAK2 protein that is causally related to a human leukemia (363), further underscoring the relationship of Jak2 to the growth of hematopoietic cells.

Tyk2 Mutations and Human Immunodeficiency

A mutation in Tyk2 has now been identified in a patient with primary immunodeficiency (350). The patient had clinical defects more severe than anticipated from Tyk-deficient mice, with increased susceptibility to viral infections and atypical mycobacterial infections and defective signaling in response to IL-23, IL-6, and IL-10. Additionally, the patient had hyper IgE production, which perhaps corresponds to enhanced Th2 cell-mediated allergic inflammation in Tyk2$^{-/-}$ mice (364). Because this was a single patient, it remains to be determined if other individuals with Tyk2 deficiency will have this full range of clinical problems.

ACTIVATION OF JAKS AND THE JAK-STAT PARADIGM

The paradigm of Jak-STAT activation is shown in Figure 23.7, which also shows activation of other pathways, such as the Ras-MAP kinase and PI 3-kinase/Akt/p70 S6 kinase pathways. Following interferon or cytokine engagement, dimerization or higher-order oligomerization of receptor complexes is induced. This in turn allows the juxtapositioning of Jak kinases, facilitating transphosphorylation and activation. In receptors with only two chains, the direct transphosphorylation of one Jak by the other seems likely to occur. In more complex receptors, such as the IFN-γ system, because the receptor is a heterotetramer with two IFNGR-1 chains that each bind Jak1 and two IFNGR-2 chains that each bind Jak2, it is not clear if Jak1 and Jak2 transactivate each other or if one of the

TABLE 23.14 Phenotypes of Mice Deficient in Type I and Type II Cytokines, Their Receptors, STATs, and Jaks

Type I cytokines and their receptors	
γ_c Family	
IL-2 (*128,576*,577)	Normal thymic and peripheral T-cell development. Decreased polyclonal T-cell responses in vitro, but more normal in vivo responses to pathogenic challenges. Autoimmunity with marked changes in levels of serum immunoglobulin isotypes. Ulcerative colitis–like inflammatory bowel disease.
IL-4 *(131,132)*	Defective Th2 cytokine responses and class switch; detective IgG1 and IgE production.
IL-2/IL-4 *(133)*	Some features of both IL-2 and IL-4 knockout mice. No gross abnormalities of T-cell development.
IL-7 (72)	Greatly diminished thymic and peripheral T-cell development and B lymphopoiesis, resulting in profound lymphopenia.
IL-9 (88,*90*)	No T-cell defect. Defect in pulmonary goblet cell hyperplasia and mastocytosis following challenge with *Schistoma mansoni* eggs. No defect in eosinophilia or granuloma formation.
IL-15 *(100)*	Defective NK-cell development. Defect in CD8 memory T-cell homeostasis.
IL-2Rα (140)	Normal initial lymphoid development, but massive enlargement of peripheral lymphoid organs, polyclonal T- and B-cell expansions, and activated T cells, with impaired activation-induced cell death. Autoimmunity with increasing age, including hemolytic anemia and inflammatory bowel disease.
IL-2Rβ (141)	Severe autoimmunity including autoimmune hemolytic anemia. Die within approximately 3 mo. Deregulated T-cell activation. Dysregulated B-cell differentiation and altered immunoglobulin profile.
γc (134,135)	Greatly diminished thymic development but double negatives, double positives, and single positives all represented. Age-dependent accumulation of peripheral $CD4^+$ T cells with an activated memory phenotype. Greatly diminished numbers of conventional B cells, although B1 cells are present. No NK cells or $\gamma\delta$ cells. Absent gut-associated lymphoid tissue, including Peyer patches.
IL-4Rα *(578)*	Like IL-$4^{-/-}$ mice, they have defective Th2 cytokine responses and class switch; defective IgG1 and IgE production. In addition, they cannot expel *Nippostrongylus brasiliensis,* presumably because of defective IL-13 signaling.
IL-7Rα (71)	Greatly diminished thymic and peripheral T-cell development and B lymphopoiesis, resulting in profound lymphopenia.
IL-15Rα (99)	Defective NK-cell development. Defect in CD8 memory T cell homeostasis.
IL-21 (115a)	Normal development, defective Th17 development.
IL-21R (116,118,115c)	Normal development, diminished IgGl and elevated IgE, particularly after immunization. Defective Th17 development.
IL-4Rα/IL-21R (116)	Panhypogammaglobulinemia, with absent IgE production. Defective germinal center development with diminished or absent tingible body macrophages.
IL-13 *(257)*	Defective Th2-cell development and the ability to expel helminths.
β_c Family	
IL-5 *(146)*	Decreased basal level of eosinophils and defective induction of eosinophils following infectious challenge. Developmental defect in $CD5^+$ B1 cells. Normal antibody and cytotoxic T-cell responses.
GM CSF *(579,580)*	Normal basal hematopoiesis. Unexpected abnormalities of the lung; abnormal pulmonary homeostasis.
IL 3Rβ (581)	No defects (due to redundant function of β_c).
β_c (*161*,581)	Defective responses to IL-5 and GM-CSF, but normal responses to IL-3 (because of redundant function of IL-3Rβ). Diminished eosinophils—both basal levels and in responses to infectious challenge. Unexpected abnormalities of the lung characterized by pulmonary proteinosis and reduced phagocytosis by alveolar macrophages. In other words, the defects are a combination of those found in the IL-5– and GM-CSF–deficient mice.
IL-3Rβ + β_c double knockout (581)	Same phenotype as β_c-deficient mice, except that they cannot respond to IL-3.
gp130 Family	
IL-6 *(582)*	Impaired acute-phase responses following infection or tissue damage. Decreased numbers of hematopoietic progenitor cells.
gp130 (583,584)	Embryonic lethal. Extreme hypoplastic development of the myocardium; although the ventricular wall was very thin, traveculation within the ventricle chamber was normal. Hematologic abnormalities characterized by greatly reduced CFU-S and somewhat reduced CFU-Gm and BFU-E. Markedly diminished size of thymus and numbers of thymocytes. Reduced primordial germ cells in embryonic gonads. Diminished size of placenta.
LIF *(585–587)*	Decreased hematopoietic progenitor cells. Normal sympathetic neurons but deficient neurotransmitter switch in vitro. Defective blastocyst implantation.
LIFRβ *(588,589)*	Postnatal lethality. Normal hematopoietic and germ-cell compartments, but multiple neurologic, skeletal, placental, and metabolic defects. The greater severity than found in LIF-deficient mice reflects that LIFRβ is shared by several cytokines, including CNTF, LIF, OSM, and CT1.
CNTF *(590)*	Progressive atrophy and loss of motor neurons.
CNTFRα *(591)*	Severe motor neuron–deficient, resulting in perinatal mortality. The more severe phenotype than in CNTF-deficient mice was unexpected and suggests that another cytokine may utilize CNTFRα.
IL-11Rα *(592)*	Blastocysts can implant but decidulaization cannot occur, associated with failure of pregnancy. Fetal lethal phenotype.
IL-12 p40 *(593)*	Impaired but not completely lacking in ability to produce IFNγ and to mount a Th1 response in vivo. Elevated secretion of IL-4, normal production of IL-2 and IL-10. Substantially decreased CTL responses. Resistant to infection with intracellular pathogens.
IL-12Rβ 1 *(594)*	Defective IL-12 signaling. IL-2 but not IL-12 could augment NK activity. Defective IFNγ production in response to ConA or anti-CD3. Severe defect in Th1 differentiation.

(*continued*)

TABLE 23.14 Phenotypes of Mice Deficient in Type I and Type II Cytokines, Their Receptors, STATs, and Jaks (Continued)

IL-12 p35 (553,*595*)	Selective loss of IL-12 function without loss of IL-23. Less resistant to infection than p40 and IL-12Rβ 1 knockouts.
IL-12Rβ2 *(596)*	Selective loss of IL-12 function without loss of IL-23. Less resistant to infection than p40 and IL-12Rβ 1 knockouts.
IL-23 p19 (553,*597*)	Complete resistance to EAE, defective DTH response.
Epo, Tpo, G-CSF, and M-CSF	
Epo *(598)*	Embryonic lethal. Complete block of fetal liver erythropoiesis, resulting in severe anemia, yet normal development of BFI-E and CFU-E progenitor cells.
EpoR *(599)*	Same as Epo-deficient mice.
TpoR *(600)*	Decreased megakaryocytes and platelets, but other hematopoietic cells are present in normal numbers.
G-CSF *(601)*	Neutropenia and impaired neutrophil mobility. Diminished granulocytes, and macrophage precursors.
M-CSF *(602,603)*	Osteopetrosis, absence of teeth. Females are infertile, suggesting an unexpected role for M-CSF.
M-CSF + GM-CSF *(603)*	A combination of defects of both M-CSF and GM-CSF, with osteopetrosis and alveolar proteinosis. Die early of pneumonia.
Type II cytokines and their receptors	
IFNAR-1 *(604–606)*	Normal development. Defective immune defense against most viral infections tested, including lymphocytic choriomeningitis virus, Semliki Forest virus, Theiler virus, vesicular stomatitis virus. Normal resistance to *Listeria monocytogenes, Lesihmania major, Mycobacterium bovis* and *avium.*
IFNγ *(607–609)*	Normal lymphoid development. Impaired resistance to *Listeria monocytogenes, Lesihmania major, Mycobacterium bovis* and *avium.* Can mount curative responses to a number of viruses. CD4$^+$ effector cells default to the Th2 pathway after infection with *Leishmania.* Succumb to infection with *Toxoplasmosis gondii.*
IFNGR-1 *(605,606,610)*	Normal lymphoid development. Impaired resistance to *Listeria monocytogenes, Lesihmania major, Mycobacterium bovis* and *avium.* Can mount curative responses to a number of viruses.
IL-10 (305,*307*)	Normal lymphocyte development and antibody responses. Chronic entercolitis, anemia, and growth retardation. Augmented inflammatory responses.
STATs and Jaks	
Stat1 (*426*,427)	Defective responses to both type I and type II IFNs. Defective response to certain viruses and bacterial antigens.
Stat2 *(428)*	Defective signaling in response to type I IFNs; interestingly, the defect is not as severe in Stat2-deficient macrophages as it is in Stat2-deficient fibroblasts.
Stat3 *(429–433)*	Embryonic lethal. Embryos implant but cannot grow. The fact that this phenotype is even more severe than that seen with gp130 suggests a role for Stat3 via a gp130-independent cytokine. By Cre-lox methodology, Stat3 was also selectively targeted in T cells, which exhibit defective IL-2–induced proliferation that correlates with a defect in IL-2–induced IL-2Rα expression; as expected, T cells also exhibit defective signaling in response to IL-6. Stat3-deficient neutrophils and macrophages show defective IL-10 signaling. Stat3 is also essential for normal involution of the mammary epithelium, for wound healing, and for normal hair-cycle processes. Stat3-deficient DC exhibit defective Flt3L-dependent expansion of DC.
Stat4 (435,436)	Defective Th1 development. Essentially the same phenotype as in IL-12–deficient mice, including defective IL-12–mediated boosting of NK-cell cytolytic activity.
Stat5a (385,*440*)	Defective lobuloalveolar development in the mammary gland, a syndrome resulting from defective prolactin signaling. Defective IL-2–induced IL-2Rα expression and associated defects in IL-2–induced T-cell proliferation. Defective superantigen-induced expansion of Vβ 8 T cells. Defective antigen-induced recruitment of eosinophils into the lung as well as antigen-induced IgG1 production.
Stat5b (386,*441*)	Defective growth analogous to Laron dwarfism, a disease of defective growth-hormone signaling. Defective IL-2–induced IL-2Rα expression. More severe defects in IL-2–induced T-cell proliferation and NK-cell proliferation. Defective antigen-induced recruitment of eosinophils into the lung as well as antigen-induced IgG1 production. Defective NK cytolytic activity.
Partial Stat5a/Stat5b *(387,388)*	Defective signaling in response to prolactin and growth hormone. Absent NK-cell development. Major defect in T-cell proliferation and TCR signaling. Anemia.
Complete Stat5a/Stat5b (442)	Fetal lethality, absent T-cell development.
Stat6 (437,*438,439*)	Defective Th2 development, essentially the same phenotype as IL-4–deficient mice. Defective B-cell proliferation.
Jak1 (338)	Perinatal lethality, with defective signaling by gp130-dependent cytokines (IL-6, IL-11, CNTF, OSM LIF CT-1, and NNT-1/BSF-3). Defective signaling by γ_c-dependent cytokines (IL-2, IL-4, IL-7, IL-9, IL-15, IL-21; of these, IL-2 and IL-7 were formally evaluated).
Jak2 (611,*612*)	Fetal lethality with profound anemia due to defective signaling in response to erythropoietin.
Jak3 (345,346,*347*)	Very similar and possibly identical to γ_c-deficient mice. Defective signaling in response to γ_c-dependent cytokines (IL-2, IL-4, IL-7, IL-9, IL-15, IL-21). Greatly diminished T cells in thymus and spleen, but then age-dependent peripheral expansion of CD4$^+$ T cells. Unlike humans with JAK3 mutations, Jak3-deficient mice have greatly diminished B-cell numbers as well.
Tyk2 (613,*614*,615)	Mice lacking Tyk2 exhibit diminished signaling in response to IFNα/β and IL-12, but it is not abrogated. Primarily, Stat3 activation is diminished, even though Stat1/Stat2 and Stat4, respectively, are the STAT proteins that are primarily activated by IFNα/β and IL-12. Additionally, there are diminished responses to IFNγ and IL-18.

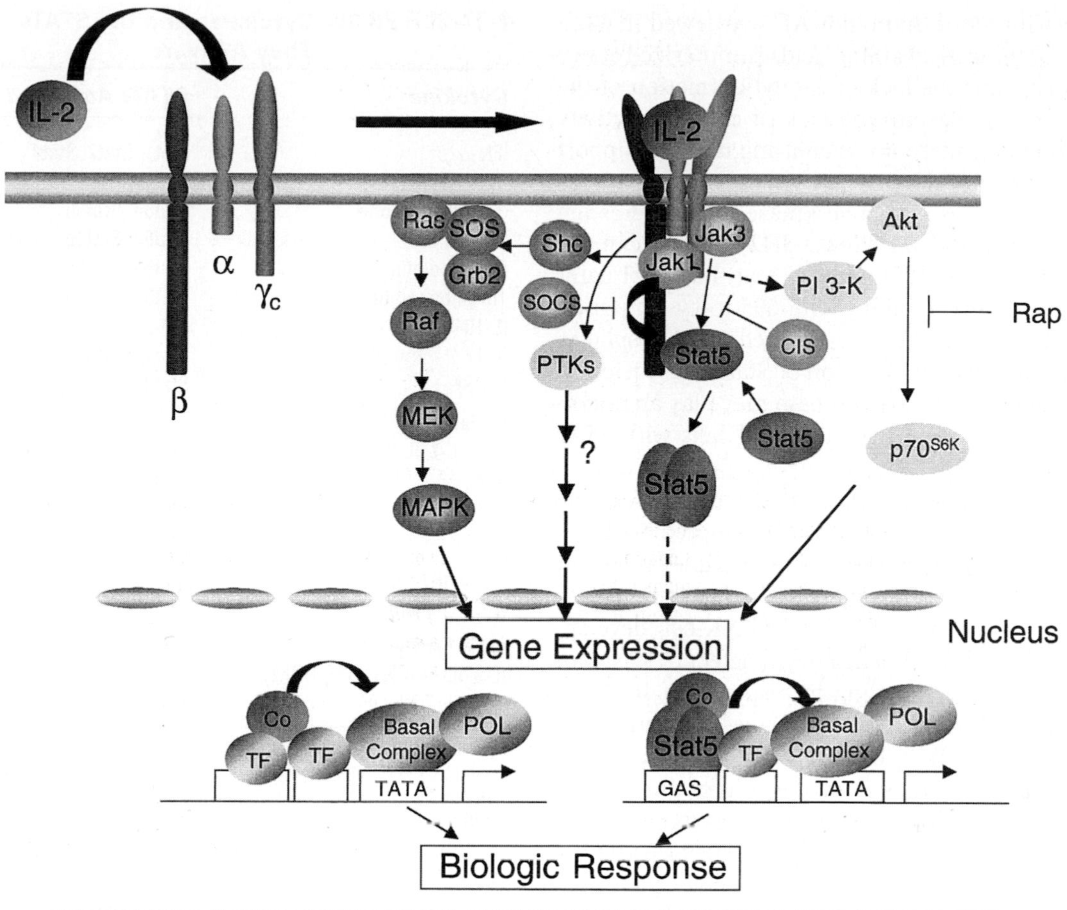

FIGURE 23.7 Schematic of cytokine signaling showing multiple signaling pathways activated by IL-2. Shown is the association of Jak1 and Jak3 with different chains of the receptor. Activation of Jak kinases results in tyrosine phosphorylation of IL-2Rβ. This allows the docking of Stat5 proteins via their SH2 domain. The STATs themselves are tyrosine-phosphorylated, dimerize, and translocate to the nucleus, where they modulate expression of target genes. The schematic also indicates that another phosphotyrosine mediates recruitment of Shc, which then can couple to the Ras/Raf/MEK/MAP kinase pathway. Also shown is the important PI 3-kinase pathway. These and other pathways are activated by many type I cytokines.

Jak kinases plays a dominant role. Indeed, one study suggests that Jak2 may phosphorylate both itself and Jak1, thereby increasing the catalytic activities of both kinases *(365)*. Jak1 in turn then phosphorylates IFNGR-1, allowing the recruitment of Stat1. In this model, it is additionally suggested that Jak2 phosphorylates Stat1 *(365)*. Interestingly, a kinase-dead mutant of Jak1 was able to mediate the induction of certain IFN-γ–induced genes, indicating a potential "structural" role for Jak1, but catalytically active Jak1 was essential for the establishment of the antiviral state *(365)*, emphasizing the essential role of both Jak1 and Jak2 for normal IFN-γ function.

The preceding discussion assumes that transphosphorylation of Jak kinases is a mechanism for the amplification of catalytic activity. Unless other kinases are involved, however, implicit to this idea is that the Jak kinases themselves must exhibit some basal activity that is amplified to a higher level by auto- or transphosphorylation. It is reasonable to speculate that both models may be operative, depending on the system. Consistent with Jak kinases being activated by phosphorylation, mutagenesis of a critical tyrosine in Tyk2 *(366)* or Jak2 *(367)* (e.g, tyrosine 1007 in the case of Jak2) in the activation loop of the kinase domain inhibits activity. It is also conceivable that phosphorylation of other tyrosines on the Jaks may create appropriate motifs for the recruitment of additional signaling molecules.

The function of the pseudokinase domain remains unclear. No other metazoan protein tyrosine kinases contain such a domain. The JH2 lacks the third glycine in the critical Gly–X–Gly–X–X–Gly motif, is missing an aspartic acid that serves as the proton acceptor that is typically conserved in the catalytic loop of both tyrosine and serine kinases, and is missing the conserved phenylalanine in the Asp–Phe–Glu motif that binds ATP (reviewed in 322). The absence of the critical amino acids summarized above presumably explains the lack of catalytic function of the JH2 domain *(327)*. Despite the lack of catalytic activity of the JH2 domain, there are increasing data in support of vital functions for this region. Although the kinase domain alone can act as an active kinase, it is interesting that a mutation in the Jak kinase JH2 domain can hyperactivate the *Drosophila* (*hop*$^{Tum-l}$/D-stat) Jak-STAT pathway and that the corresponding Glu 695-to-Lys mutation in murine Jak2 also resulted in increased autophosphorylation of Jak2 and phosphorylation of Stat5 in transfected cells *(368)*. Moreover, the JH2 domain may play an important role in mediating the interaction of Jaks with STAT proteins *(369)*.

Given that Jak kinases are associated with a wide range of IFN and cytokine receptors, it was to be predicted that Jaks would mediate signals involved in multiple processes. Indeed, these include important roles in development (as demonstrated by the lack of T-cell and NK-cell development associated with Jak3 deficiency, a defect at least partially due to defective signaling in response to IL-7 and IL-15), signaling in response to cytokines that are mitogenic growth factors (IL-2, IL-3, etc.), and in the antiviral response (IFNs). The analysis of the role of Jak1 in zebrafish not only revealed a role for Jak1 in early vertebrate development, it also demonstrated that during early development Jak1 kinase was exclusively of maternal origin *(353)*. These developmental roles for Jak1 in zebrafish are consistent with the importance of a Jak kinase in early *Drosophila* development as well *(370)*.

STAT PROTEINS ARE SUBSTRATES FOR JAKS THAT AT LEAST IN PART HELP DETERMINE SPECIFICITY

Given that there are only four Jak kinases and scores of cytokines, it is clear that Jaks by themselves cannot fully determine specificity. Indeed, different cytokines with different actions activate the same Jaks. One level of specificity comes from the same Jaks having different substrates, depending on the receptor. The best-characterized substrates for Jaks are the signal transducer and activator of transcription (STAT) proteins (321,322,*323*), and these appear to provide some but not all of the specificity, particularly given that there are only seven STAT proteins. Among the mutant cell lines with defects in IFN signaling, in addition to the ones with defects in Jaks that were noted previously, others were defective in STAT proteins, providing perhaps the earliest data proving a vital role for STAT proteins in signaling in response to IFNs.

STAT proteins are classically considered to be latent transcription factors that initially exist in the cytosol but then must be activated by phosphorylation, with subsequent translocation to the nucleus. STATs were first discovered as factors that bound to the promoters of interferon-inducible genes. The seven mammalian STAT proteins are Stat1 (371), Stat2 *(372)*, Stat3 *(373,374)*, Stat4 *(375,376)*, Stat5a (377,378,*379–381*), Stat5b *(379–382)*, and Stat6 *(383)*. Table 23.15 summarizes the cytokines that activate each of the STATs. Additionally, some STATs (e.g, Stat3) are known to have more than one isoform with distinct functions *(384)*. Although the STATs conserve a reasonable level of homology, Stat5a and Stat5b are unusually closely related, being 91% identical at the amino acid level *(379–382)*. It is interesting that murine and human Stat5a are more related than Stat5a and Stat5b within a single species. The same is true for murine and human Stat5b, suggesting that there has been evolutionary pressure to maintain the difference between Stat5a and Stat5b and that these two proteins might have certain distinctive functions. In this regard, Stat5a and Stat5b knockout mice exhibit both similarities as well as some differences in their phenotypes (385,386,*387,388*); however, given different levels of each Stat5 protein in certain tissues, it remains to be determined if the different phenotypes result from different intrinsic actions of Stat5a and Stat5b versus differences in the total level of Stat5.

Because active STAT proteins exist as dimers, the ability of at least some STATs to form heterodimers (e.g, Stat1

TABLE 23.15 Cytokines and the STATs They Activate

Cytokine	*STATs Activated*
IFN-α/β	Stat1, Stat2. Stat4
IFN-γ	Stat1
Growth hormone	Stat5a, Stat5b
Prolactin	Stat5a, Stat5b
Erythopoietin	Stat5a, Stat5b
Thrombopoietin	Stat5a, Stat5b
IL-10	Stat3
IL-12	Stat4, Stat3
G-CSF	Stat3
γ_c Family	
IL-2, IL-7, IL-9, IL-15, IL-21	Stat5a, Stat5b, Stat3, Stat1
IL-4	Stat6
IL-13	Stat6
TSLP	Stat5a, Stat5b
β_c Family	
IL-3, IL-5, GM-CSF	Stat5a, Stat5b
gp130 Family	
IL-6, IL-11, CNTF, LIF, OSM, CT-1	Stat3
Leptin	Stat3

Note that for IL-2, IL-7, IL-9, and IL-15, Stat5a and Stat5b appear to be the major STATs that are activated, although Stat3 in particular and Stat1 to a lesser degree can also be activated. For IL-21, Stat3 is the dominant STAT protein activated, followed by Stat1 and Stat5a/Stat5b *(35,454)*.

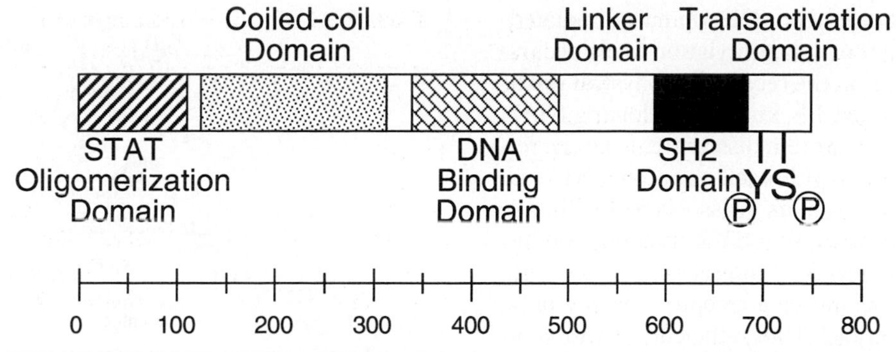

FIGURE 23.8 Architecture of a typical STAT protein. Shown are the locations of the following important regions: (a) the N-terminal region is shown to mediate the interaction of STAT dimers bound to adjacent GAS sites (known to be important for Stat1, but presumably true for all STATs); (b) the DNA-binding domain; (c) the SH2 domain that mediates STAT docking on receptors and STAT homodimerization/heterodimerization following tyrosine phosphorylation; and (d) the location of the conserved tyrosine whose phosphorylation allows the SH2-mediated dimerization. At least in Stat1 and Stat3, Serine 727, which is C-terminal to the conserved tyrosine, is an important site for phosphorylation. In the case of Stat1, p48 interacts downstream of the STAT dimerization domain. CBP/p300 interacts with two sites—at both the N terminus and the C terminus. Although it has been suggested that the region between the DNA-binding domains and the SH2 domain is an SH3 domain, this remains unproven and no interactions with proline-rich regions have been reported; as a result, I have omitted the labeling of this region as an SH3 domain. Note that this structure is typical of that for Stat1, Stat3, Stat4, Stat5a, and Stat5b. The main features are conserved in Stat2 and Stat6, but these are approximately 50 to 100 amino acids longer.

with Stat2 or Stat3 [reviewed in *323*]) increases the number of different complexes that can form. In addition, further complexity can be generated by the ability of at least some of the STATs to exist in alternatively spliced forms *(382,389)*. Some of these forms are inactive, and if alternative splicing of certain forms were regulated, it would allow for negative regulation.

A schematic of STAT proteins is shown in Figure 23.8. The STATs can be divided into two basic groups: those that are longer (Stat2 and Stat6, approximately 850 amino acids) and those that are shorter (Stat1, Stat3, Stat4, Stat5a, and Stat5b, between 750 and 800 amino acids). The STAT genes cluster in three locations. Murine Stat2 and Stat6 are both located on chromosome 10, Stat1 and Stat4 are located on chromosome 1, and Stat3, Stat5a, and Stat5b are located on chromosome 11 *(390)*. Correspondingly, human, Stat1 and Stat4 are on chromosome 2q32.2–2q32.3, Stat2 and Stat6 are on chromosome 12q13.2, and Stat 3, Stat5a, and Stat5b are closely positioned on chromosome 17q *(382)*.

The classic model is that in order for STATs to be "activated" and to be able to function as transcriptional activators, a number of cellular events must occur. They first bind to phosphorylated tyrosines on cytokine receptors, are tyrosine-phosphorylated, dissociate, dimerize, translocate from the cytosol to the nucleus, bind to target DNA sequences, and activate gene expression. A number of conserved structural features common to all STATs helps to explain these functions. These include an SH2 domain, a conserved tyrosine residue, a DNA-binding domain, a C-terminal transactivation domain, and an N-terminal STAT tetramerization region. Other regions as well contribute important functions. These special features of STATs are discussed in the following. In addition, however, there is now evidence for the biologic function of nuclear STATs that are not phosphorylated, as discussed in the following.

Docking of STATs on Receptors or Other Molecules, Tyrosine Phosphorylation of STATs, and STAT Dimerization

Each STAT protein has an SH2 domain that plays two important roles: (a) for receptor docking, as has been shown, for example, for Stat1 docking on IFNGR-1 *(391)*, Stat2 docking on IFNAR-1 *(392)*, Stat3 docking on gp130 (393), Stat5a and Stat5b docking on IL-2Rβ and IL-7Rα (248,*394*), and Stat6 docking on IL-4Rα (395); and (b) for STAT dimerization wherein dimerization is mediated by the SH2 of one STAT interacting with the conserved phosphorylated tyrosine of another STAT protein. In the case of the IFN-α receptor, no Stat1 docking site on IFNAR-1 or IFNAR-2 has been identified, and it is believed that Stat1 may interact with Stat2 after Stat2 is itself tyrosine-phosphorylated (322). It is also possible that STATs can dock on Jaks, given the ability to coprecipitate Jaks and STATs directly (355,*369*). After docking has occurred, a conserved tyrosine (tyrosine 701 in Stat1, tyrosine 694 in Stat5a, etc.) can be phosphorylated. This phosphorylation is required for SH2 domain–mediated STAT dimerization, and the phosphorylation likely occurs while the STAT is docked on the receptor in physical proximity to receptor-associated Jak kinases. Following STAT phosphorylation, the STAT protein dissociates from the receptor, and its dimerization with itself or another STAT is presumably then favored over its reassociation with the cytokine receptor chain, given that STAT dimerization involves two phosphotyrosine–SH2 interactions (a bivalent interaction), whereas docking on a receptor involves only one (monovalent interaction). Thus, efficient activation of STATs requires the presence in STATs of a conserved SH2 domain and a critical tyrosine.

Whereas some receptor proteins, such as IFNGR-1 *(391)* and IL-7Rα (248), have a single STAT docking site (for Stat1 and Stat5, respectively), a number of receptor molecules, including IL-2Rβ (248,*394*), IL-4Rα (395), gp130 (393), EPOR *(396)*, and IL-10Rα *(397)*, have more than one docking site for their respective STATs. The presence of more than one site provides functional redundancy, but also potentially could allow the simultaneous activation of two STAT molecules, providing a high local concentration of phosphorylated STATs, which called facilitate their dimerization.

STAT Nuclear Translocation and DNA Binding

Following dimerization, the STATs translocate into the nucleus, where they can bind to DNA as transcription factors. The mechanism for nuclear translocation was originally mysterious, given the absence of an obvious nuclear localization signal (398). However, it was shown that tyrosine-phosphorylated Stat1 dimers can interact directly with importin-α5, allowing internalization. This suggested that there indeed is a nuclear localization signal that is normally masked, and mutation of Leu 407 does not interfere with tyrosine phosphorylation, dimerization, or DNA binding, but prevents nuclear localization (398). Following its dephosphorylation, nuclear Stat1 is exported to the cytosol by a process that is dependent on the chromosome region maintenance 1 (CRM1) export reporter *(399)*. Thus, both import and export of Stat1 appear to be regulated processes. These findings also generalize to Stat3, Stat5a, and Stat5b (399a).

Whereas the majority of STAT dimers bind DNA directly, in the case of IFN-α/β, Stat1-Stat2 heterodimers are formed, and these bind DNA in conjunction with a 48-kDa DNA binding protein known as interferon regulatory factor 9 (IRF9); the Stat1-Stat2-IRF9 complex is known as ISGF3 (reviewed in *323*). In the case of other STAT dimers, accessory proteins are not required for DNA binding. The motif recognized by ISGF3 complexes is AGTTTNCNTTTCC (known as an ISRE, for interferon-stimulated response element), whereas the other STAT complexes bind more semi-

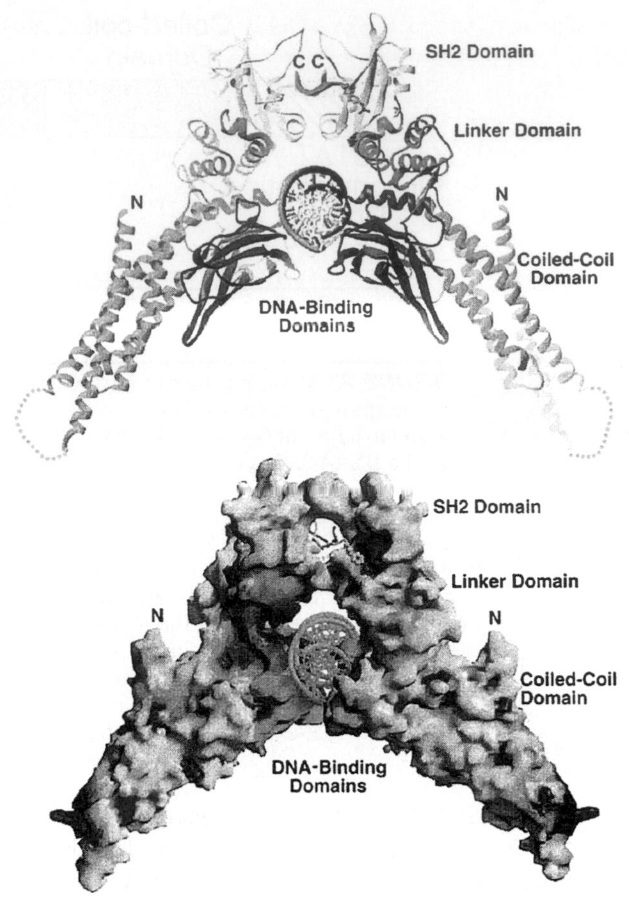

FIGURE 23.9 Three-dimensional structure of a Stat1 dimer bound to DNA. Reproduced from (400,401) with permission of Dr. Kuryian and Cell Press.

palindromic TTCN$_m$GAA motifs that are generally denoted as GAS motifs, for γ-interferon–activated sequences, reflecting their original discovery in the context of IFN-γ (*283*,321,322).

A series of chimeric STAT proteins were used to delineate a DNA-binding domain of approximately 180 amino acids, with two conserved subdomains. Although multiple STATs bind to the same motifs, their relative efficiencies vary, indicating fine specificities conferred by the different DNA-binding domains. For example, whereas Stat1 homodimers favor a TTCN$_3$GAA motif, Stat6 prefers a TTCN$_4$GAA motif (395). These differences partially explain why different STATs modulate the expression of nonidentical sets of target genes. The structures of Stat1 and Stat3β bound to DNA (400,401) (Figure 23.9) almost resemble that of a vertebral column, wherein the DNA represents the spinal cord. The N-terminal and coiled-coil domains are spatially the farthest from the DNA, whereas the DNA-binding domain, linker, and SH2 domain surround the DNA, with the stability apparently being provided by the SH2–phosphotyrosine interaction between the STAT monomers as well as each STAT monomer with interacting

DNA, presumably via a "half-GAS site" (402), as discussed under STAT tetramerization.

N-terminal regions mediate cooperative DNA binding of STAT proteins when multiple STAT binding sites occur in close proximity (*403*,404)—for example, in the IFN-γ gene (*403*). In the IL-2Rα gene, IL-2 response elements have been described in both the 5′-regulatory region and the first intron, each of which has tandem GAS motifs that cooperate functionally to mediate IL-2–induced IL-2Rα transcription (*405–407*,408).

STAT proteins were the first transcription factors that were identified as targets for tyrosine phosphorylation. Previously, tyrosine phosphorylation was associated primarily with membrane-proximal events, but the tyrosine phosphorylation of STATs is associated with a membrane-proximal event, as the STATs dock on cell surface receptors. This phosphorylation then allows the rapid dimerization that facilitates nuclear localization and DNA binding. STATs can interact directly with Jak kinases (first shown for Stat5 and Jak3) (355), suggesting that STATs may at times dock on Jaks rather than on receptors.

Nonphosphorylated STATs Can Be Nuclear

In addition to the classical tyrosine-phosphorylation–mediated dimerization and nuclear translocation, it is now clear that STAT proteins can exist in the nucleus even without being tyrosine-phosphorylated, and in that context can modulate gene expression (*409,410*,411). Moreover, nonphosphorylaed STATs (e.g, Stat4) can form N-domain–mediated dimers (412).

Optimal Binding Sites for STATs

The optimal binding motifs for several STAT proteins have been determined. For Stat1, Stat3, and Stat4, a TTCCSGGAA motif was defined (*323,403*), whereas Stat5a and Stat5b optimally bind a TTCYNRGAA motif (402) and Stat6 binds a TTCNTNGGAA motif (where Y is C or T and R is G or A) (395,402). Unexpectedly, purified Stat5a expressed in a baculoviral expression system binds efficiently as either a dimer or a tetramer, whereas similarly prepared Stat5b binds primarily as a dimer, suggesting a greater efficiency for homotetramerization of Stat5a than for Stat5b (402). Whereas dimeric STAT protein binding strongly preferred canonical motifs, the range of sequences recognized by Stat5a tetramers is broad, often occurring to two imperfect motifs or with one canonical motif with an associated "TTC" or "GAA" half-GAS motif. The optimal inter-GAS motif spacing is 5 to 7, although some naturally occurring sites, such as that in the PRRIII element of the IL-2Rα gene, has a spacing of 11 (402). The presence of suboptimal GAS motifs spaced at appropriate distances to allow tetrameric binding may allow greater specificity via cooperative binding of STAT oligomers. Interestingly, a number of STAT-regulated genes, such as Bcl-x and Pim-1, have "half-GAS motifs" located near full GAS motifs, suggesting that tetrameric binding is involved in the regulation of these genes (402).

Transcriptional Activation by STATs

In addition to tyrosine phosphorylation, some STATs can be phosphorylated on serine, and Stat1 and Stat3 phosphorylation at Ser 727 in the C-terminal transactivation domain is required for full activity (*413–415*). The Ser 727 region resembles a MAP kinase recognition site, and MAP kinase activity was reported to be required for IFN-α/β–induced gene expression (*416*). Ser 727 mediates the interaction of Stat1 with MCM5, a member of the minichromosome maintenance family of proteins; this interaction presumably is important for maximal transcriptional activation (417). In contrast, Stat2 is not serine-phosphorylated (*323*), and although Stat5a and Stat5b are serine-phosphorylated, the biologic role, if any, of this phosphorylation is unclear.

In addition to this regulated modification of the STAT proteins, STATs can also interact with other factors. For example, as noted earlier, Stat1-Stat2 heterodimers bind DNA only after interacting with IRF9 to form ISGF3 (*323*). Stat1 interacts with and synergizes with Sp1 for transcriptional activation in the ICAM-1 gene (*418*) and with TRADD to influence IFN-γ signaling (*419*). An alternatively spliced shorter form of Stat3, denoted Stat3β, associates with c-Jun to enhance transcriptional activity (420). Moreover, certain STATs can interact with the potent transcriptional coactivators CBP/p300 (*421–423*). In the case of Stat1, this is mediated by interactions involving both the N-terminal and C-terminal regions of Stat1 and the CREB and E1A-binding regions of CBP, respectively (*422*). Stat5a has been shown to associate with the glucocorticoid receptor (*424*). Additionally, the IL-2-response element in the IL-2Rα gene requires not only Stat5 binding but also the binding of Elf-1, an Ets family transcription factor, to a nearby site (*405*). Thus, active STAT complexes appear to involve the coordination of STAT proteins with other factors. The corepressor SMRT (silencing mediator for retinoic acid receptor and thyroid hormone receptor) was identified as a potential Stat5-binding partner that binds to both Stat5a and Stat5b, and potentially plays a negative regulatory role (*425*).

Specificity of STATs

Analogous to the Jaks, the same STATs are activated by multiple cytokines. The phenotypes of mice that lack expression of each of the seven STAT proteins are known, and these knockout models have helped to clarify which cytokines depend critically on a given STAT protein. Stat1 knockout mice exhibit defects that are very selective for the actions of type I and type II IFNs (*426*,427), suggesting that Stat1 is vital only for the actions of IFNs, even though a variety of other cytokines have been reported to activate Stat1. Although it is possible that Stat1 plays an important but redundant role for at least some of these other cytokines, the phenotype of Stat1-deficient mice indicates a need for caution in the interpretation of in vitro experiments that use high concentrations of cytokines or cell lines. Stat2-deficient mice exhibit defects consistent with selective inactivation of IFN-α/β signaling *(428)*. Stat3-deficient mice exhibit fetal lethality; the embryos implant, but they exhibit defective development and growth *(429)*. Deletion of Stat3 within specific lineages has revealed that mice that lack Stat3 in T cells *(430)* have normal lymphoid development but exhibit a defect in IL-2–induced IL-2Rα expression, somewhat analogous to what is seen in Stat5a- and Stat5b-deficient mice (see below). Neutrophils and macrophages that lack Stat3 exhibit defective signaling to IL-10, and it is known that Stat3 is important for the normal involution of the mammary epithelium, for wound healing, and for the normal hair cycle *(431,432)*. Dendritic cells that lack Stat3 exhibit a defect in Flt3L-dependent differentiation *(433)*, and APCs that are deficient in Stat3 exhibit disruption of priming of antigen-specific CD4$^+$ T cells *(434)*. Stat4-deficient mice exhibit a phenotype similar to that of IL-12–deficient mice (i.e, defective Th1 development), consistent with the observation that Stat4 is activated by IL-12 (435,436). Analogously, Stat6-deficient mice exhibit a phenotype similar to that of IL-4-deficient mice (i.e, defective Th2 development) (437,*438*,*439*), in keeping with the observation that Stat6 is activated only by IL-4 and the closely related cytokine, IL-13. Interestingly, mice that lack Stat5a exhibit a defect in prolactin-mediated effects, including defective lobuloalveloar proliferation *(440)*, whereas mice that lack Stat5b have defective growth similar to that found in Larons dwarfism *(441)*. Thus, although Stat5a and Stat5b appear to always be induced coordinately, each of these STATs is important in vivo. In addition to these defects, both Stat5a-deficient and Stat5b-deficient mice have defects in T-cell development and signaling (385,386). Stat5a-deficient mice have diminished numbers of splenocytes and exhibit a defect in IL-2–induced IL-2Rα expression (385). Stat5b-deficient mice have similar defects, but also have diminished thymocytes (386). Most dramatically, these mice have a major defect in the proliferation of freshly isolated splenocytes (386), and defective NK-cell development (386). Mice that lack both Stat5a and Stat5b in lymphoid cells exhibit a dramatic defect in T-cell development (442), and even hypomorphic expression of both Stat5a and Stat5b is sufficient to result in a lack of NK-cell development *(387)*. Presumably, the lack of T-cell development relates to defective IL-7 signaling, whereas the lack of NK-cell development relates to defective IL-15–dependent Stat5 activation. Stat5a/Stat5b double-knockout mice exhibit lethality associated with severe anemia that develops in these mice (443).

STATs Are Evolutionarily Old

Just as *Drosophila* has a Jak kinase, there is a *Drosophila* STAT, denoted as either DSTAT or STAT92E (444,*445*). The existence of Jak kinases and STAT proteins in lower organisms suggests that the system is evolutionarily old. A STAT has been identified in *Dictyostelium* that recognizes the sequence TTGA *(446)*, has highest sequence similarity to Stat5b, and can bind mammalian ISREs *(446)*. Interestingly, *Saccharomyces cerevisiae* do not appear to have STATs, as no SH2 domains have been identified in the entire *S. cerevisiae* genome.

What Types of Functions Are Mediated by STATs?

First and foremost, STAT proteins can translocate to the nucleus and bind to regulatory regions of target genes and influence transcription. Although STATs are generally activators of transcription, at least in the case of the *c-myc* gene, Stat1 can function as a transcriptional repressor *(447)*.

STAT proteins were discovered based on the study of IFN-inducible genes as part of studies intended to understand the cellular differentiation events that lead to development of the antiviral state. In addition to roles in differentiation, STAT proteins can contribute, directly or indirectly, to survival and/or mitogenic/proliferative responses that typify hematopoietic and immunologic cytokines, such as IL-3, IL-5, GM-CSF, IL-2, and IL-4 (322): First, a number of in vitro systems have demonstrated that viruses or viral oncogenes are associated with activated Jak-STAT pathways, suggesting a role for STATs in cellular transformation. Indeed, Stat3 and Stat5 have been implicated as oncogenes, with compelling data for transformation capability of Stat3 in cell lines, persistently tyrosine-phosphorylated STATs in several types of leukemia and lymphoma, and the development of T-lymphoblastic lymphomas in Stat5 transgenic mice (448). The role of Stat3 in the tumor microenvironment makes it an attractive target for cancer immunotherapy *(449)*. Second, there is diminished proliferation in a number of the STAT knockout mice that have been analyzed. For example, Stat4-deficient cells exhibit diminished cellular proliferation to IL-12 (435,436), whereas Stat6-deficient mice exhibit diminished proliferation to IL-4 (437,*438*), and Stat5-deficient mice have diminished T-cell proliferation to IL-2 (385,386). Some of these effects are indirect, based on modulation of receptor expression. For example, Stat6-deficient mice exhibit decreased IL-4Rα expression. Similarly, the absence of Stat5 results in decreased IL-2–induced IL-2Rα expression as well as decreased proliferation (385,386). Thus, in at least some cases, decreased proliferation results at least in part from decreased expression of receptor components. Stat5a and Stat5b appear to regulate Bcl-XL induction, indicating their ability to affect cell survival (443). Finally, it is interesting that Stat1 has been linked to cell growth arrest and induction of the cdk inhibitor $p21^{WAF1/CIP1}$ *(450)*, and that activation of Stat1 occurs in thanatrophoric dysplasia type II dwarfism as the result of a mutant fibroblast growth factor receptor (FGFR3) (451). In this chondrodysplasia, the mutant FGFR3 induces nuclear translocation of Stat1, expression of $p21^{WAF1/CIP1}$, and growth arrest, suggesting a possible relationship to the disease. Thus, different STATs may potentially mediate either growth expansion or growth arrest. Moreover, STATs may potentially play other types of roles, as well. For example, Stat3 has been reported to serve as an adapter to couple PI 3-kinase to the IFNAR-1 component of type I IFN receptors *(452)*.

A more complete understanding of the actions of the different STAT proteins may be facilitated with a compilation of the genes that are regulated by each STAT. Progress in this area has been made for a number of cytokines, but particularly for the IFNs *(285)*. It is also important to recognize that not all cytokine signals are dependent on STATs, as illustrated, for example, by Stat1-independent IFN signals *(453)*, Stat5-independent IL-2 signals *(394)*, and Stat1/Stat3-independent IL-21 signals *(454)*.

Do Other Proteins Bind to GAS Motifs?

At least one non-STAT protein can bind to GAS motifs. The *BCL6* gene is often mutated or has undergone translocations in diffuse large-cell B-cell lymphomas. Interestingly, Bcl-6 binds to GAS motifs capable of binding Stat6 and specifically can inhibit IL-4 action (455). Mice that lack Bcl-6 expression exhibit defective germinal-center formation, suggesting that formation of germinal centers may be at least partially dependent on Bcl-6–regulated (presumably negative) control of certain STAT-responsive genes (455).

OTHER LATENT TRANSCRIPTION FACTORS AS EXAMPLES OF CYTOPLASMIC-TO-NUCLEAR SIGNALING (NF-κB, NF-AT, AND SMADs)

An exciting feature of STAT proteins is that they exist in an inactive form in the cytosol and then are rapidly translocated to the nucleus. The rapid activation within minutes of signals from cell membrane to nuclear DNA binding makes the STAT acronym very apt, analogous to the urgency associated with "STAT" emergency physician orders in clinical medicine. The rapid activation of STAT proteins is somewhat analogous to several other transcription factors *(456)*. NF-κB also undergoes rapid nuclear translocation, but by a completely different mechanism from STATs. In contrast to STAT proteins, for which the tyrosine phosphorylation of the STATs is an initiator of nuclear translocation, for NF-κB it is the serine phosphorylation and/or uquitination of IκB that results in its dissociation and/or destruction, allowing the release and translocation of NF-κB. There is the classical NF-κB pathway used by many cytokines, which involves the IKKα/IKKβ/IKKγ-dependent phosphorylation of IκB, resulting in the activation of NFκB1 (p50)/Rel-A (p65) heterodimers as well as the alternative pathway in which a homodimer of IKKα mediates the activation of NFκB2 (p52)/Rel-B heterodimers *(457–459,*460). A third example of cytosolic to nuclear translocation occurs with NF-AT (nuclear factor of activated T-cell) family proteins *(461,*462), which are vital for regulating transcription of a number of cytokines, including, for example IL-2, IL-4, and GM-CSF. NF-AT is translocated to the nucleus, where it associates with AP-1 family proteins to form a functional complex. It is the activation of calcineurin and dephosphorylation of NF-AT that allows its nuclear translocation. A fourth example of cytosolic to nuclear translocation occurs with the SMAD proteins that mediate TGF-β signaling, which contributes to Th17 differentiation (discussed later). For SMADs, the phosphorylation is on serine and the kinase is intrinsic to the receptor, but like STATs, activation of these latent transcription factors is rapid and initiated by the binding of a growth factor. Thus, several mechanisms, each involving phosphorylation or dephosphorylation, have evolved to allow cytoplasmic to nuclear translocation of latent transcription factors.

OTHER SUBSTRATES FOR JAKS

Because Jaks are potent cytosolic tyrosine kinases, it is evident that the Jaks may do more than just phosphorylate tyrosine residues on receptors where STAT proteins dock as well as phosphorylating the STATs. In vitro data indicate that Jak kinases also can phosphorylate receptor tyrosines other than the docking sites for STATs. For example, in the case of IL-2Rβ, Jak1 can phosphorylate not only tyrosines 392 and 510, which are STAT docking sites, but also tyrosine 338, which is a docking site for Shc *(394)*, all of which are required for maximal proliferation. Jak kinases are known to autophosphorylate themselves or transphosphorylate other Jaks. Other molecules are potentially phosphorylated by Jak kinases, including the STAM adapter molecule *(463)* and the p85 subunit of PI 3-kinase *(464)*.

IRF Family Proteins

Interferon-regulatory factors form a family of nine proteins that are regulated by type 1 IFNs (281). They each have a well-conserved N-terminal DNA-binding domain that forms a helix–loop–helix structure as well as a C-terminal interaction domain. IRFs are critical for a number of actions, including type I IFN-dependent gene transcription (281). Select IRFs play critical roles in TLR-mediated IFN induction. IFRs can have negative as well as positive effects. For example, IFN-γ–mediated repression of IL-4 is mediated by IRF protein(s) *(465)*.

OTHER SIGNALING MOLECULES IMPORTANT FOR CYTOKINES

Other Tyrosine Kinases besides JAKS

In addition to their activation of Jak kinases, a number of cytokines can activate Src family kinases. For example, IL-2 can activate $p56^{lck}$ *(466,467)* in T cells and $p59^{fyn}$ and $p53/p56^{lyn}$ in B-cell lines *(468,469)*. The activation of some of these kinases has been reported to be mediated by associating with the "A" region of IL-2Rβ. Another tyrosine kinase, Syk, has been reported to associate with the S region of IL-2Rβ *(470)*. However, the significance of these interactions is less clear than that for Jak kinases. First, cells that lack Lck can proliferate vigorously in response to IL-2 *(471,472)*. Second, when the A region is deleted, proliferation still occurs, albeit at a lower level than seen with wild-type IL-2Rβ *(473)*. However, Y338, which is required for the recruitment of Shc, is in the A region and is required for normal proliferation *(394)*. Thus, it is possible that the decrease in proliferation associated with deletion of the A region relates more to the loss of Y338 than it does to the loss of association of Lck. Moreover, in $Il2rb^{-/-}$ mice reconstituted with an IL-2Rβ A–region mutant, proliferation is increased rather than decreased *(474)*. Additional investigation is required to clarify the role of activation of Src family kinases by IL-2 and other cytokines. The significance of the Syk interaction also remains unclear. As Syk and Jak1 both associate with the S region of IL-2Rβ, mutations that delete the S region simultaneous prevent both associations, making it hard to determine the specific role of Syk. Syk-deficient mice exhibit normal IL-2 proliferation *(475)*, further suggesting that Syk may not play an important role in IL-2–induced proliferation. The G-CSF receptor also can form a complex with Lyn and Syk *(476)*, but again, Syk-deficient mice do not exhibit a defect in G-CSF signaling *(475)*. β_c has also been reported to interact with Src family kinases *(477)*; gp130 has been reported to associate with a number of other kinases, including Btk, Tec, and Fes *(478–480)*; and IL-4Rα has been shown to interact with Fes *(481)*. However, relatively little is known about the significance of tyrosine kinases other than Jaks in cytokine signaling. Additionally, PI 3-kinase, p38, ERK, and JNK can each become activated, leading to activation of many downstream transcription factors, including NF-κB, AP1, PU.1, IRF1, IRF4, and IRF8, to mediate a program of gene expression.

IRS Proteins

IRS-1 was discovered as a tyrosine-phosphorylated substrate of the insulin receptor *(482)*. IRS proteins have a large number of phosphotyrosine docking sites, particularly for the p85 subunit of PI 3-kinase, and they presumably serve to recruit important accessory molecules. Interestingly, both insulin and IL-4 could induce tyrosine phosphorylation of an IRS-1–like molecule in hematopoietic cells, and 32D myeloid progenitor cells lack IRS-1 and could only signal in response to insulin or IL-4 when they were transfected with IRS-1 *(483)*. Both the insulin receptor and IL-4Rα proteins contain NPXY sequences that are important for IRS-1 or IRS-2 binding; in IL-4Rα, this is contained within a sequence denoted as the I4R motif *(484)*.

Other cytokines have subsequently been shown to activate IRS-1 and/or IRS-2. For example, growth hormone can induce phosphorylation of IRS-1 *(485)* and IRS-2 *(486)*, IFN-γ and LIF induce phosphorylation of IRS-2 *(486)*, and the γ_c-dependent cytokines, IL-2, IL-7, and IL-15, can induce tyrosine phosphorylation of IRS-1 and IRS-2 in T cells *(487)*. The significance of these findings remains unclear, as 32D cells reconstituted with a complete IL-2 receptor can proliferative vigorously in response to IL-2 *(471)*, whereas, as noted, in these same cells IL-4 responsiveness requires coexpression of both IL-4Rα and IRS-1, indicating different roles for IRS proteins for different cytokines.

Phosphatidylinositol 3-Kinase

PI 3-kinase is a lipid kinase that consists of an 85-kDa regulatory subunit and a 110-kDa catalytic subunit *(488)*. PI 3-K phosphorylation and activation can be induced by a number of cytokines *(489–492)*, and the use of inhibitors, such a wortmannin or LY294002, has demonstrated its importance in signaling for at least certain cytokines. IRS-1 has multiple docking sites for PI 3-kinase (YXXM motifs) and thus for some cytokines, such as IL-4, the association of IRS-1 might be the mechanism by which PI 3-K can be recruited.

The Ras/MAP Kinase Pathway

Another major signaling pathway for a number of cytokines is the Ras/MAP kinase pathway (493). This pathway presumably is used by cytokines whose receptors recruit the Shc adaptor molecule, which in turn mediates the recruitment of Grb2 and Sos, leading eventually to the activation of Ras. In turn, Ras couples to the MAP kinase pathway through a well-defined signaling cascade. Certain cytokines, such as IL-2 and IL-3, appear to use this pathway, whereas others, such as IL-4, do not, indicating that this pathway is differentially important depending on the cytokine that is being used.

DOWNMODULATION OF CYTOKINE SIGNALS

Much of the preceding discussion has centered on the mechanisms by which cytokines induce signals. However, the mechanisms by which cytokine signals can be terminated are also extremely important. There are multiple levels at which negative regulation can occur. These include (a) regulating a balance between the production (transcriptional and translational control) of the cytokine, its receptor, and/or downstream signaling molecules and the degradation of these same molecules; and (b) regulation of the activation state of the receptor and downstream signaling molecules. For example, these can be mediated by transcriptional repressors or molecules that either inhibit cytokine signaling (e.g, SOCS proteins) or reverse-activated states (e.g, phosphatases).

Transcriptional control of cytokine production is a widely used mechanism. Many T-cell–derived cytokines, such as IL-2, IL-3, and IL-4, are produced only by activated T cells, and their production is lost with the loss of activation. IL-15 provides an example in which translation of the protein is carefully regulated, in part, by the existence of multiple upstream ATGs (96). Most cytokine receptor chains are constitutively expressed, but some, such as IL-21R and IL-2Rβ, are regulated in part by signals that act through the T-cell receptor. The most regulated receptor chain may be IL-2Rα, whose expression is absent on resting lymphocytes but strongly induced following stimulation with antigens, mitogens, and certain cytokines; however, the transcriptional/translational control of most cytokine receptors is poorly studied.

Because phosphorylation events are vital for the creation of phosphotyrosine docking sites, dephosphorylation is an obvious mechanism of control. Indeed, two tyrosine phosphatases, Shp-1 (formerly also known as SHP, HCP, SH-PTP1, and PTP1C) and Shp-2 (formerly also known as Syp and PTP1D) have been shown to play roles related to cytokine signaling (*494*,495). Shp-1 mutations cause the motheaten (*me*) and viable motheaten (*me*^{v}) phenotypes in mice *(496,497)*. The viable motheaten mouse has a less severe phenotype that is associated with increased numbers of erythroid progenitor cells and hyperresponsiveness to Epo *(498)*, suggesting that Shp-1 might normally diminish responsiveness to Epo. Indeed, it was demonstrated that Shp-1 binds directly to the EpoR when Y429 is phosphorylated *(499)*. This tyrosine is located in a "negative" regulatory region of the EpoR, and when mutated, Epo-responsive cells can grow in lower concentrations of Epo. Following Shp-1 binding to Y429, dephosphorylation and inactivation of Jak2 is facilitated *(499)*. Thus, the negative regulation of Epo signaling appears to be at the level of a receptor-dependent inactivation of a Jak kinase. Shp-1 has also been shown to interact with β_c and to mediate diminished IL-3–induced signaling *(500)*, and to be able to associate with both Tyk-2 *(501)* and Jak2 *(502)*.

Shp-2 has generally been considered primarily an "activating" phosphatase; it is therefore interesting that it can also interact with Jak1, Jak2, and Tyk2 *(503)*. In addition to the presumed dephosphorylation of Jak kinases by phosphatases, STAT proteins also appear to be regulated at the level of tyrosine dephosphorylation *(504)*, and interestingly, it has been shown that dephosphorylation of phosphotyrosine on Stat1 dimers requires extensive spatial reorientation of the two monomers within the dimer, something that is facilitated by the N-terminal domain that is involved in tetramerization (505). Finally, another type of phosphatase, namely, the lipid phosphatases, known as SHIP and SHIP2, can act as negative regulators of cytokine signals *(506)*.

In addition to Shp1 and Shp2, CD45, PTP1B, and T-cell PTP (TCPTP) have been reported to regulate Jak kinases. CD45 appears to play roles related to erythropoietin and IFN signaling. PTP1B has been reported to dephosphorylate Jak2 and TYk2, and TCPTP has been reported to dephosphorylate Jak1 and Jak3 (324). In the cytosol, Shp2 and PTP1B have also been reported to dephosphorylate cytosolic Stat5 and nuclear Stat1 and Stat3, whereas TCPTP has been reported to dephosphorylate Stat1 and Stat3 in both cytosol and nucleus, but additional work is needed to determine whether these events are occurring physiologically in vivo (324).

In addition to tyrosine phosphatases,dual specificity phosphatases with specificity for both tyrosine and serine/threonine exist and multiple members can negatively regulate MAP kinases (508a). Some of these are relatively lineage-restricted and can regulate signaling by type I cytokines (508b).

In addition to dephosphorylation, another mode of negative regulation is by degradation. In addition to the degradation of receptor molecules, Stat1 itself is a target of the ubiquitin-proteasome pathway *(507)*. Finally, it is possible that regulation also can occur at the level of alternative splicing. In this regard, alternatively spliced versions of some of the STATs *(323,382,389)* have been reported.

THE CIS/SOCS/JAB/SSI FAMILY OF INHIBITORY ADAPTER PROTEINS

In 1995, the protoype molecule for an interesting class of proteins was discovered. The prototype molecule was named CIS, for cytokine-inducible, SH2-containing protein, and it was shown to negatively regulate the actions of a set of cytokines (508,*509*). CIS is rapidly induced by a variety of cytokines, including IL-2, IL-3, GM-CSF, and erythropoietin, to associate physically with both the β_c and erythropoietin receptors (508,*509*). Subsequently, a related protein, variably denoted SOCS-1 (suppressor of cytokine signaling-1), JAB (Jak-binding protein), and SSI-1 (STAT-induced STAT inhibitor-1), was identified that could negatively regulate the activity of other cytokines, including IL-6 (*510*,511,*512*) and IL-2, among others. Interestingly, this protein could associate with Jak family kinases, whereas this function has not been reported for CIS. A total of eight CIS/SOCS/JAB/SSI family members have been identified that collectively regulate signals in response to multiple cytokines (*513,514*,,515,*516*). These proteins are now generally known as SOCS proteins and share a central SH2 domain and a C-terminal region known as a SOCS box. Additional SOCS box–containing proteins lack SH2 domains and include proteins known as ASBs (ankyrin repeat-containing proteins with a SOCS box), SSBs (SPRY domain-containing proteins with a SOCS box), and WSBs (WD40 repeat-containing proteins with a SOCS box). SOCS proteins tend to be expressed at very low levels in nonactivated cells and to be induced by cytokines and pathogens. Following their induction, they negatively influence cytokine signaling, serving as negative feedback regulators. Their actions can extend beyond type I cytokines; for example, SOCS-1 can negatively regulate LPS responses *(517)*.

Knockout mice for a number of the SOCS proteins have been prepared, alone and in combination. CIS KO mice are relatively normal, but CIS transgenic mice exhibit low body weight, failure of lactation, and diminished numbers of NK and NKT cells as well as altered TCR-mediated responses, presumably related to its ability to inhibit Stat5-dependent responses including those related to growth hormone, prolactin, IL-15, and IL-2, as well as others. SOCS1 knockouts exhibit multiorgan inflammation and neonatal lethality as the result of augmented responsiveness to IFN-γ, and this lethality can be prevented if the mice are crossed to IFN-γ-deficient mice. Interestingly, Socs1$^{-/-}$ mice also indicate an essential role for SOCS1 in thymocyte differentiation, and there are diminished numbers of maturing B cells. Deletion of SOCS1 within thymocytes/T cells/NK T cells results in multiple lymphoid abnormalites with increased CD8^{+} T cells as a result of increased sensitivity to γ_c-dependent cytokines including IL-7 *(518)*. SOCS2 knockout mice exhibit gigantism, ostensibly due to dysregulated growth hormone signaling. SOCS3 knockout mice exhibit embryonic lethality as a result of placental insufficiency and dysregulated responses to LIF and IL-6, as well as hematopoietic defects. Conditional SOCS3 knockout mice have revealed a physiologic role for SOCS3 in regulating G-CSF signaling in myeloid cells and for "emergency" granulopoiesis (519) as well as for IL-6/gp130 signaling (520,*521*). SOCS6 knockous have mild growth retardation (324,515,*522*). Additional SOCS knockout mice and various combinations continue to be generated, adding additional information to this important area of negative regulation of STAT-dependent signaling.

PIAS PROTEINS

Protein inhibitors of activated STAT (PIAS) proteins are other negative regulators of cytokine actions (324,*523–527*), with PIAS-1 being an inhibitor of Stat1-binding activity and PIAS-3 being a similar inhibitor of Stat3-binding activity. These PIAS proteins block the DNA-binding activity of STAT dimers. Two other members, PIASx (which has both α and β splice variants) and PIASy, have also been described, with PIASx inhibiting Stat4 and PIASY inhibiting Stat1. They appear to act at least in part as transcriptional corepressors by recruiting other proteins such as histone deacetylase. In addition, PIASx and PIASy have added actions, not restricted to the context of STAT inhibition. For example, PIASy is a nuclear matrix–associated SUMO E3 ligase (a ubiquitin-related protein) that can repress the activity of the Wnt-responsive transcription factor, LEF1 *(526)*. PIASy coexpression results in the covalent modification of LEF1 by SUMO. Thus, as a class, PIAS proteins have more than one type of action (324).

THE T-HELPER PARADIGM: Th1, Th2, AND Th17

T-helper 1 (Th1) and Th2 cells were originally described based on the patterns of cytokine production by murine T cells (528), but the paradigm was extended to human cells as well (*529,530*,531–533). Th1 cells secrete IL-2, TNF, IFN-γ, and lymphotoxin, whereas Th2 cells produce IL-4, IL-5, IL-6, IL-9, IL-10, and IL-13. The cytokines produced by Th1 and Th2 cells are sometimes referred to as type 1 and type 2 cytokines (for Th1 and Th2 cytokines); unfortunately, this results in potential confusion as IL-4 is a type I (four-α-helical–bundle) cytokine that is functionally a type 2 cytokine (in that it is produced by Th2 cells).

In humans, the Th1 and Th2 patterns of cytokine production are similar, but not all the cytokines are as tightly restricted (*529,530*,531–533). IFN-γ is the cytokine most reliably produced by Th1 cells, whereas IL-4, IL-5, and IL-9 are produced by Th2 cells. In both species, certain cytokines, including IL-3 and GM-CSF, are produced by both Th1 and Th2 cells. The Th1/Th2 division of T-helper cells has proved useful in correlating the function of Th1 cells with cell-mediated immunity (inflammatory responses, delayed-type hypersensitivity, and cytotoxicity) and Th2 cells with humoral immunity. Of the Th2 cytokines, IL-4 is particularly important in driving IgE responses. As the division of Th1 and Th2 cells is not always perfect, when cells produce both Th1 and Th2 cytokines, they are called Th0 cells, whereas Th3 cells refer to cells that produce high levels of TGFβ.

A number of murine and human physiologic and disease states correspond to Th1 or Th2 responses/patterns (reviewed in 529–533). In general, among infectious diseases, resistance to intracellular bacteria, fungi, and protozoa is linked to mounting a successful Th1 response. Th1 responses can also be linked to pathology, such as arthritis, colitis, and other inflammatory states. Effective protection against extracellular pathogens, such as helminths, requires a Th2 response, and the enhanced humoral immunity may result in successful neutralization of pathogens by the production of specific antibodies. In humans, Th1 and Th2 cytokines are each dominant in the different types of lesions found in leprosy, with Th1 cytokines dominating in tuberculoid lesions and Th2 cytokines dominating in lepromatous lesions. In HIV infection, a simple Th1/Th2 pattern does not exist. The situation has been complicated by the fact that IL-4 expression is relatively transient, whereas IL-10 expression is more sustained. This has led to the current thought that IL-10 and IL-12 may be the most important cytokines controlling disease progression in AIDS *(529)*. Interestingly, Th0 and Th2 cells seem to be more susceptible to HIV than Th1 cells, potentially explaining why the virus can persist even in the absence of Th1 cells. Overall, human diseases that are characterized primarily by Th1 responses include Hashimoto thyroiditis, Graves ophthalmopathy, multiple sclerosis, type 1 diabetes mellitus, Crohn disease, rheumatoid arthritis, lyme arthritis, reactive arthritis, acute allograft rejection, unexplained recurrent abortions, *Helicobacter pylori*-induced peptide ulcer, and sarcoidosis (533). In contrast, diseases characterized primarily by Th2 responses include Omenn syndrome, vernal conjunctivitis, atopic disorders, progressive systemic sclerosis, crytptogenic fibrosing alveolitis, chronic periodontititis, progression to AIDS in HIV infection, and tumor progression (533).

It is believed that Th1 and Th2 cells are derived from a common precursor (Thp cells). IL-12 is the major driving force to induce Th1 differentiation, whereas IL-4 induces Th2 differentiation, although IL-2 and Stat5 are required for optimal Th2 differentiation (*534,*535). Corresponding to these findings, as discussed earlier in this chapter, Stat4-deficient mice are defective in IL-12 signaling and exhibit a defect in Th1 development. Lineage commitment to Th1 and Th2 is now better understood in terms of transcription factors, where T-bet, Stat4, HLX, and EOMES are transcription factors influencing Th1 commitment and Stat6, c-Maf, JunB, NFATc1, and GATA-3 are more specific for Th2 cells (536,*537,*538). The process by which the differentiated Th cells produce cytokines is one in which the genetic loci need to become competent for efficient transcription. One can think of this process as involving an initiation phase dependent on STAT proteins, a commitment phase mediated by factors such as T-bet and GATA3, and a final stabilization phase in which transcription is maintained without further stimulation *(539)*. Part of this process involves chromatin remodeling, a process that involves histone-modifying enzymes as well as specific transcription factors (540), to allow transcription, for example, of the IL-4/IL-13 locus *(539)*, with Th2 lineage commitment involving demethylation of the IL-4 gene (*541,*542), and Th1 commitment involving demethylation of the IFN-γ gene (298,543).

In addition to the major differences between Th1 and Th2 cells in the production of IFN-γ, it was observed that Th subsets differed markedly in their abilities to respond to IFN-γ, where the proliferation of Th2 clones was inhibited and that of Th1 clones was not *(544)*. Interestingly, the unresponsiveness of Th1 clones resulted from the absence of IFNGR-2, whereas Th2 cells express IFNGR-2 *(545,546)*. Thus, Th1 cells produce IFN-γ and can thereby inhibit the proliferation of Th2 cells. As noted earlier, IL-12 is the major inducer of Th1 cells. It is therefore interesting that Th2 cells do not respond to IL-12, and it is now clear that this extinction of IL-12 signaling results from their loss of expression of the IL-12Rβ2 subunit of the IL-12 receptor *(547)*. Apparently, IL-4 inhibits IL-12Rβ2 expression, whereas IFN-γ overcomes this inhibition *(547)*. The abilities of mice to survive infections is critically linked to the Th patterns of cytokines. For example, the ability to survive toxoplasmosis depends strictly on IFN-γ/IL-12 production (a Th1 pattern) (532).

In the past couple of years, another lineage of Th cells has been identified, known as Th17 cells *(548)*, which produce IL-17 in a manner dependent on IL-23 (549,*550*) and ROR-γ *(551)*. Interestingly, polarization of Th17 cells is dependent on TCR stimulation, TGFβ, and IL-6, but is independent of IL-23, which instead may be required for maintaining/expanding these cells (552,553,*554,555*). TGFβ may be less important for Th17 differentiation in the human (555a,555b). In a number of mouse autoimmune diseases that were believed to be caused by Th1 cells, the elimination of such cells paradoxically augmented the severity of disease, and it has become clear that Th17 cells are responsible, rather than Th1 cells. For example, EAE is exacerbated when IL-12/IFN-γ are eliminated. In contrast, the elimination of IL-23 (by eliminating either the p40 subunit shared by IL-12 and IL-23 or by eliminating p19) confers resistance to EAE (553,556). Whereas IL-23 promotes Th17 cell numbers, IL-27 can negatively regulate their development (556). It is now clear that IL-21/IL-21R play a critical role in Th17 differentiation (115a,115b,115c). Some specialized effector CD4$^+$ T cells have suppressor activity and are known as regulatory T cells (Treg cells) (discussed in Chapter 30).

DISEASES OF CYTOKINE RECEPTORS AND RELATED MOLECULES

A Range of Cytokine-Related Causes of SCID

As detailed earlier, mutations in the γ_c cause XSCID, and mutations in Jak3 cause a similar T$^-$B$^+$NK$^-$ SCID. Given that γ_c-dependent cytokines activate primarily Stat5a and Stat5b as signaling molecules downstream of the Jaks, it remains an open question as to whether mutations in these STAT proteins also cause human disease. Although one might hypothesize that mutations in either Stat5a or Stat5b alone might not cause a phenotype, because of potential redundancy, mice that lack Stat5a or Stat5b exhibit defects in T- and NK-cell numbers as well as T-cell proliferation and NK cytolytic activity (385,386), and mice that lack both Stat5a and Stat5b have an even more profound defect, with absent T-cell (442) and NK-cell development *(387)*. Given that Stat5a and Stat5b are tandem genes, perhaps a deletion of the Stat5a/Stat5b region of chromosome 17 would result in a new form of SCID, although it is likely that such a deletion could result in fetal lethality resulting from defective erythropoiesis, given the importance of Stat5a and Stat5b for Epo signaling.

It can be predicted that human immunodeficiencies might also result from mutations in some of the cytokines whose receptors contain γ_c, or from mutations in other components of the receptors for these cytokines. Indeed, as noted earlier, patients with IL-2 deficiency exhibit a SCID-like syndrome, due to inadequate function of their T cells, and recently an unusual immunodeficiency has been found to result from a mutation in IL-2Rα (259). One patient with defective IL-2Rβ expression also had an immunodeficient syndrome characterized by autoimmunity *(557)*, somewhat analogous to IL-2Rβ–deficient mice. Given that mutations in IL-7Rα in humans cause $T^-B^+NK^+$ SCID (129), mutations in IL-7 might be predicted to cause a similar syndrome. The one major difference might be that IL-7–deficient humans might not be capable of receiving a successful bone marrow transplant if stromal IL-7 is required for the graft. Such patients have not yet been identified. Given the defective NK-cell development and $CD8^+$ memory T-cell development in IL-15– and IL-15Rα–deficient mice, it is likely that these types of defects would also occur in humans lacking either of these proteins. However, again, such patients have not yet been identified. Although IL-9 transgenic mice develop lymphomas *(558)*, IL-9–deficient mice exhibit defects related to mast cells and mucous production rather than lymphoid defects. Thus, defects related to the IL-9 system seem unlikely as causes of SCID. At present, defective expression of IL-2, IL-2Rα, IL-2Rβ, IL-7Rα, γ_c, and Jak3 are the only cytokine-related mutations that have been found to cause SCID, with Tyk2 being implicated in another form of immunodeficiency. More time will be required to determine whether mutations in other cytokines, cytokine receptors, Jaks, or STATs can also cause SCID.

Defects in the Ability to Clear Mycobacterial Infections

A number of immunodeficiencies have been characterized in which affected individuals cannot properly clear mycobacterial infections. These have also turned out to be diseases of defective cytokine signaling. Mutations have been found in the components of either IL-12 itself or in the IFN or IL-12/IL-23 receptors, with mutations having been found in either the gene encoding the p40 subunit of IL-12 (which, as noted earlier, is also a component of IL-23) *(559)*, in IL-12Rβ1 (a component of both the IL-12 and IL-23 receptors) *(560)*, or in either the IFNGR-1 or IFNGR-2 components of IFN-γ receptors *(561,562)*. The critical role of IL-12 for Th1 cell-mediated differentiation and production of IFN-γ provides the explanation for finding similar clinical syndromes in humans lacking the p40, IL-12Rβ1, IFNGR1, or IFNGR-2. Moreover, one patient with a mutation in the STAT1 gene was also identified with a similar clinical syndrome (563), indicating that, as anticipated, Stat1 is a critical mediator of the IFN-γ signal. Interestingly, this patient had a mutation on only one STAT1 allele, but the mutation was a dominant negative mutation that selectively inhibited the formation of Stat1 dimers (hence abrogating IFN-γ signaling) but yet had at most only a modest effect on the ability to form ISGF3, hence leaving signaling in response to IFN-α/β relatively intact.

Mutations in the WSX-1/TCCR Type I Receptor

Interestingly, there is a type I cytokine receptor denoted as TCCR or WSX-1 that is related to IL-12β2, and its mutation results in defective Th1-related responses and diminished IFN-γ production, resulting in susceptibility to Leishmania major and *Listeria* monocytogenes (172,564,*565*). TCCR/WSX-1 is an essential component of the receptor for IL-27 (214) and also has been found to be required for resistance to *Trypanosoma cruzi* (566,*567*).

Other Diseases Associated with Cytokine Receptors

A number of other diseases have been reported that are related to cytokine receptors. First, mutations in the growth hormone receptor have been found in a form of dwarfism (Laron dwarfism) *(568)* in which target cells cannot respond to growth hormone. Interestingly, some aspects of Stat5b deficiency are related to this syndrome. Second, a single patient with a form of congenital neutropenia (Kostmann syndrome) has been found to have a mutation in one of his G-CSF receptor alleles *(569)*. Third, a kindred of patients with familial erythrocytosis has truncation in the erythropoietin receptor, resulting in hypersensitivity to erythropoietin *(570)*. Finally, an altered virally encoded form (v-mpl) of the thrombopoietin receptor (c-mpl) was originally identified as the oncogene of the myeloproliferative leukemia virus (MPLV) *(571)*.

Modulation of Cytokines and the Clinic

Certain diseases are associated with increased levels of cytokines or other situations in which treatment with an anti-cytokine receptor antibody is a rationale therapy. One example is Castleman disease, which is associated with overproduction of IL-6 by lymph node cells, leading to the successful treatment of this disease with IL-6 receptor blockade (175,572). Anti-IL-6R–based therapy also has utility for rheumatoid arthritis and possibly for Crohn's disease (175,573). Blocking the IL-2 receptor has been used in the treatment of patients with adult T-cell leukemia and other neoplasias, and the use of humanized and conjugated antibodies has produced responses in a number of individuals. Humanized anti-Tac monoclonal antibody, marketed under the name Daclizumab, has shown very strong efficacy in the treatment of allograft rejection as well as in T-cell–mediated autoimmune disorders including multiple sclerosis, uveitis, and tropical spastic paraparesis. Conjugated antibodies to both IL-2Rα and IL-2Rβ are also being tested for use in a variety of malignant disorders wherein the malignant cells express these proteins. Thus, there is the possibility of therapy, either based on blocking the cytokine or based on eliminating the responding cells (574).

CONCLUSION

Type I cytokines and IFNs are involved in the regulation of an enormous number of immunologic and nonimmunologic processes. There has been a progressive transition from viewing these as discrete molecules with special actions to sets of molecules that can be grouped according to shared receptor components and common signaling pathways. Signaling is one area in which our understanding has greatly expanded; the pathways that are activated are similar for many cytokines, even when the biologic functions they induce are dramatically different. Although some of the differences can be explained by "compartmentalization," according to which cells produce the cytokine and which cells express receptors that allow them to respond to the cytokine, a tremendous amount still needs to be learned about how distinctive signals are triggered, as well as more regarding the sets of genes that are induced by each cytokine. These will provide vital information important to the quest to completely understand the mechanisms by which type I cytokines and IFNs can effect their actions. At the same time, the generation of knockout mice for most cytokines and their receptors, as well as many signaling molecules, has provided in vivo clues as to vital functions served by these cytokines. Caution is clearly needed, however, in generalizing from these findings to human biology, given some apparently major differences in roles served, such as the essential role played by IL-7 in both humans and mice for T-cell development, whereas IL-7 is also essential for B-cell development in mice but not in humans. The identification of so many human disorders associated with cytokines and cytokine receptors has tremendously helped to teach us more about human biology as well.

REFERENCES

1. Dumonde DC, Wolstencroft RA, Panayi GS, et al. "Lymphokines": non-antibody mediators of cellular immunity generated by lymphocyte activation. *Nature*. 1969;224:38–42.
2. Cohen S, Bigazzi PE, Yoshida T. Commentary. Similarities of T cell function in cell-mediated immunity and antibody production. *Cell Immunol*. 1974;12:150–159.
4. Oppenheim JJ, Gery I. From lymphodrek to interleukin 1 (IL-1). *Immunol Today*. 1993;14:232–234.
5. Wlodawer A, Pavlovsky A, Gustchina A. Hematopoietic cytokines: similarities and differences in the structures, with implications for receptor binding. *Protein Sci*. 1993;2:1373–1382.
6. Bazan JF. Neuropoietic cytokines in the hematopoietic fold. *Neuron*. 1991;7:197–208.
10. Davies DR, Wlodawer A. Cytokines and their receptor complexes. *FASEB J*. 1995;9:50–56.
16. Bazan JF. Structural design and molecular evolution of a cytokine receptor superfamily. *Proc Natl Acad Sci U S A*. 1990;87:6934–6938.
17. de Vos AM, Ultsch M, Kossiakoff AA. Human growth hormone and extracellular domain of its receptor: crystal structure of the complex. *Science*. 1992;255:306–312.
21. Wang X, Rickert M, Garcia KC. Structure of the quaternary complex of interleukin-2 with its alpha, beta, and gammac receptors. *Science*. 2005;310:1159–1163.
25. Kim HP, Imbert J, Leonard WJ. Both integrated and differential regulation of components of the IL-2/IL-2 receptor system. *Cytokine Growth Factor Rev*. 2006;17:349–366.
26. Leonard WJ. Cytokines and immunodeficiency diseases. *Nat Rev Immunol*. 2001;1:200–208.
27. Takeshita T, Asao H, Ohtani K, et al. Cloning of the gamma chain of the human IL-2 receptor. *Science*. 1992;257:379–382.
28. Noguchi M, Nakamura Y, Russell SM, et al. Interleukin-2 receptor gamma chain: a functional component of the interleukin-7 receptor. *Science*. 1993;262:1877–1880.
29. Russell SM, Keegan AD, Harada N, et al. Interleukin-2 receptor gamma chain: a functional component of the interleukin-4 receptor. *Science*. 1993;262:1880–1883.
32. Russell SM, Johnston JA, Noguchi M, et al. Interaction of IL-2R beta and gamma c chains with Jak1 and Jak3: implications for XSCID and XCID. *Science*. 1994;266:1042–1045.
34. Giri JG, Ahdieh M, Eisenman J, et al. Utilization of the beta and gamma chains of the IL-2 receptor by the novel cytokine IL-15. *EMBO J*. 1994;13:2822–2830.
37. Morgan DA, Ruscetti FW, Gallo R. Selective in vitro growth of T lymphocytes from normal human bone marrows. *Science*. 1976;193:1007–1008.
41. Siegel JP, Sharon M, Smith PL, et al. The IL-2 receptor beta chain (p70): role in mediating signals for LAK, NK, and proliferative activities. *Science*. 1987;238:75–78.
42. Lanier LL, Phillips JH. Natural killer cells. *Curr Opin Immunol*. 1992;4:38–42.
44. Lenardo M, Chan KM, Hornung F, et al. Mature T lymphocyte apoptosis–immune regulation in a dynamic and unpredictable antigenic environment. *Annu Rev Immunol*. 1999;17:221–253.
45. Malek TR, Yu A, Vincek V, et al. CD4 regulatory T cells prevent lethal autoimmunity in IL-2Rbeta-deficient mice. Implications for the nonredundant function of IL-2. *Immunity*. 2002;17:167–178.
48. Taniguchi T, Matsui H, Fujita T, et al. Structure and expression of a cloned cDNA for human interleukin-2. *Nature*. 1983;302:305–310.
49. Leonard WJ, Depper JM, Crabtree GR, et al. Molecular cloning and expression of cDNAs for the human interleukin-2 receptor. *Nature*. 1984;311:626–631.
54. Sharon M, Klausner RD, Cullen BR, et al. Novel interleukin-2 receptor subunit detected by cross-linking under high-affinity conditions. *Science*. 1986;234:859–863.
55. Tsudo M, Kozak RW, Goldman CK, et al. Demonstration of a non-Tac peptide that binds interleukin 2: a potential participant in a multichain interleukin 2 receptor complex. *Proc Natl Acad Sci U S A*. 1986;83:9694–9698.
57. Hatakeyama M, Tsudo M, Minamoto S, et al. Interleukin-2 receptor beta chain gene: generation of three receptor forms by cloned human alpha and beta chain cDNA's. *Science*. 1989;244:551–556.

58. Nelms K, Keegan AD, Zamorano J, et al. The IL-4 receptor: signaling mechanisms and biologic functions. *Annu Rev Immunol.* 1999;17:701–738.
67. Namen AE, Lupton S, Hjerrild K, et al. Stimulation of B-cell progenitors by cloned murine interleukin-7. *Nature.* 1988;333:571–573.
71. Peschon JJ, Morrissey PJ, Grabstein KH, et al. Early lymphocyte expansion is severely impaired in interleukin 7 receptor-deficient mice. *J Exp Med.* 1994;180:1955–1960.
72. von Freeden-Jeffry U, Vieira P, Lucian LA, et al. Lymphopenia in interleukin (IL)-7 gene-deleted mice identifies IL-7 as a nonredundant cytokine. *J Exp Med.* 1995;181:1519–1526.
73. Fry TJ, Mackall CL. Interleukin-7: from bench to clinic. *Blood.* 2002;99:3892–3904.
76. Schluns KS, Lefrancois L. Cytokine control of memory T-cell development and survival. *Nat Rev Immunol.* 2003;3:269–279.
77. Seddon B, Tomlinson P, Zamoyska R. Interleukin 7 and T cell receptor signals regulate homeostasis of CD4 memory cells. *Nat Immunol.* 2003;4:680–686.
84. Van Snick J, Goethals A, Renauld JC, et al. Cloning and characterization of a cDNA for a new mouse T cell growth factor (P40). *J Exp Med.* 1989;169:363–368.
87. Renauld JC, Vink A, Louahed J, et al. Interleukin-9 is a major anti-apoptotic factor for thymic lymphomas. *Blood.* 1995;85:1300–1305.
88. Townsend JM, Fallon GP, Matthews JD, et al. IL-9-deficient mice establish fundamental roles for IL-9 in pulmonary mastocytosis and goblet cell hyperplasia but not T cell development. *Immunity.* 2000;13:573–583.
91. Renauld JC. New insights into the role of cytokines in asthma. *J Clin Pathol.* 2001;54:577–589.
94. Grabstein KH, Eisenman J, Shanebeck K, et al. Cloning of a T cell growth factor that interacts with the beta chain of the interleukin-2 receptor. *Science.* 1994;264:965–968.
96. Waldmann TA, Tagaya Y. The multifaceted regulation of interleukin-15 expression and the role of this cytokine in NK cell differentiation and host response to intracellular pathogens. *Annu Rev Immunol.* 1999;17:19–49.
97. Waldmann TA. The biology of interleukin-2 and interleukin-15: implications for cancer therapy and vaccine design. *Nat Rev Immunol.* 2006;6:595–601.
99. Lodolce JP, Boone DL, Chai S, et al. IL-15 receptor maintains lymphoid homeostasis by supporting lymphocyte homing and proliferation. *Immunity.* 1998;9:669–676.
101. Zhao H, Nguyen H, Kang J. Interleukin 15 controls the generation of the restricted T cell receptor repertoire of gamma delta intestinal intraepithelial lymphocytes. *Nat Immunol.* 2005;6:1263–1271.
102. Kuwajima S, Sato T, Ishida K, et al. Interleukin 15-dependent crosstalk between conventional and plasmacytoid dendritic cells is essential for CpG-induced immune activation. *Nat Immunol.* 2006;7:740–746.
106. Dubois S, Mariner J, Waldmann TA, et al. IL-15Ralpha recycles and presents IL-15 In trans to neighboring cells. *Immunity.* 2002;17:537–547.
109. Ma A, Koka R, Burkett P. Diverse functions of IL-2, IL-15, and IL-7 in lymphoid homeostasis. *Annu Rev Immunol.* 2006;24:657–679.
110a. Spolski R, Leonard WJ. Interleukin-21: Basic Biology and Implications for Cancer and Autoimmunity. *Annu Rev Immunol.* 2008;26:57–59.
111. Parrish-Novak J, Dillon SR, Nelson A, et al. Interleukin 21 and its receptor are involved in NK cell expansion and regulation of lymphocyte function. *Nature.* 2000;408:57–63.
112. Zeng R, Spolski R, Finkelstein SE, et al. Synergy of IL-21 and IL-15 in regulating CD8+ T cell expansion and function. *J Exp Med.* 2005;201:139–148.
113. Ozaki K, Spolski R, Ettinger R, et al. Regulation of B cell differentiation and plasma cell generation by IL-21, a novel inducer of Blimp-1 and Bcl-6. *J Immunol.* 2004;173:5361–5371.
115. Leonard WJ, Spolski R. Interleukin-21: a modulator of lymphoid proliferation, apoptosis and differentiation. *Nat Rev Immunol.* 2005;5:688–698.
115a. Nurieva R, Yang XO, Martinez G, et al. Essential autocrine regulation by IL-21 in the generation of inflammatory T cells. *Nature.* 2007;448:480–483.
115b. Korn T, Bettelli E. Gao W, et al. IL-21 initiates an alternative pathway to induce proinflammatory T(H)] 17 cells, *Nature.* 2007:448:484–487.
115c. Zhou L, Ivanov I I, Spolski R, et al. IL-6 programs T_H-17 cell differentiation by promoting sequential engagement of the IL-21 and IL-23 pathways. *Nature Immunol.* 2007;8:967–974.
115d. Hinrichs C, Spolski R, Paulos CM, et al. IL-2 and IL-21 confer opposing differentiation programs to $CD8^-$ T cells for adoptive immunotherapy. *Blood.* 2008, in press.
116. Ozaki K, Spolski R, Feng CG, et al. A critical role for IL-21 in regulating immunoglobulin production. *Science.* 2002;298:1630–1634.
117. Wang G, Tschoi M, Spolski R, et al. In vivo antitumor activity of interleukin 21 mediated by natural killer cells. *Cancer Res.* 2003;63:9016–9022.
118. Kasaian MT, Whitters MJ, Carter LL, et al. IL-21 limits NK cell responses and promotes antigen-specific T cell activation: a mediator of the transition from innate to adaptive immunity. *Immunity.* 2002;16:559–569.
119. Ozaki K, Kikly K, Michalovich D, et al. Cloning of a type I cytokine receptor most related to the IL-2 receptor beta chain. *Proc Natl Acad Sci U S A.* 2000;97:11439–11444.
120. Noguchi M, Yi H, Rosenblatt HM, et al. Interleukin-2 receptor gamma chain mutation results in X-linked severe combined immunodeficiency in humans. *Cell.* 1993;73:147–157.
123. Buckley RH. Primary immunodeficiency diseases due to defects in lymphocytes. *N Engl J Med.* 2000;343:1313–1324.
124. Cunningham-Rundles C, Ponda PP. Molecular defects in T- and B-cell primary immunodeficiency diseases. *Nat Rev Immunol.* 2005;5:880–892.
129. Puel A, Ziegler SF, Buckley RH, et al. Defective IL7R expression in T(-)B(+)NK(+) severe combined immunodeficiency. *Nat Genet.* 1998;20:394–397.
134. DiSanto JP, Muller W, Guy-Grand D, et al. Lymphoid development in mice with a targeted deletion of the interleukin 2 receptor gamma chain. *Proc Natl Acad Sci U S A.* 1995;92:377–381.
135. Cao X, Shores EW, Hu-Li J, et al. Defective lymphoid development in mice lacking expression of the common cytokine receptor gamma chain. *Immunity.* 1995;2:223–238.
138. Nakamura Y, Russell SM, Mess SA, et al. Heterodimerization of the IL-2 receptor beta- and gamma-chain cytoplasmic domains is required for signalling. *Nature.* 1994;369:330–333.
139. Nelson BH, Lord, JD. Greenberg PD. Cytoplasmic domains of the interleukin-2 receptor beta and gamma chains mediate the signal for T-cell proliferation. *Nature.* 1994;369:333–336.
140. Willerford DM, Chen J, Ferry JA, et al. Interleukin-2 receptor alpha chain regulates the size and content of the peripheral lymphoid compartment. *Immunity.* 1995;3:521–530.
141. Suzuki H, Kundig TM, Furlonger C, et al. Deregulated T cell activation and autoimmunity in mice lacking interleukin-2 receptor beta. *Science.* 1995;268:1472–1476.
144. Hara T, Miyajima A. Function and signal transduction mediated by the interleukin 3 receptor system in hematopoiesis. *Stem Cells.* 1996;14:605–618.
145. Geijsen N, Koenderman L, Coffer PJ. Specificity in cytokine signal transduction: lessons learned from the IL-3/IL-5/GM-CSF receptor family. *Cytokine Growth Factor Rev.* 2001;12:19–25.
148. Itoh N, Yonehara S, Schreurs J, et al. Cloning of an interleukin-3 receptor gene: a member of a distinct receptor gene family. *Science.* 1990;247:324–327.
157. Miyajima A, Kitamura T, Harada N, et al. Cytokine receptors and signal transduction. *Annu Rev Immunol.* 1992;10:295–331.
162. Hilton DJ, Hilton AA, Raicevic A, et al. Cloning of a murine IL-11 receptor alpha-chain; requirement for gp130 for high affinity binding and signal transduction. *EMBO J.* 1994;13:4765–4775.
168. Taga T, Kishimoto T. Gp130 and the interleukin-6 family of cytokines. *Annu Rev Immunol.* 1997;15:797–819.
172. Trinchieri G, Pflanz S, Kastelein RA. The IL-12 family of heterodimeric cytokines: new players in the regulation of T cell responses. *Immunity.* 2003;19:641–644.

173. Pflanz S, Hibbert L, Mattson J, et al. WSX-1 and glycoprotein 130 constitute a signal-transducing receptor for IL-27. *J Immunol.* 2004;172:2225–2231.
175. Kishimoto T. Interleukin-6: from basic science to medicine—40 years in immunology. *Annu Rev Immunol.* 2005;23:1–21.
182. Skiniotis G, Boulanger MJ, Garcia KC, et al. Signaling conformations of the tall cytokine receptor gp130 when in complex with IL-6 and IL-6 receptor. *Nat Struct Mol Biol.* 2005;12:545–551.
183. Boulanger MJ, Chow DC, Brevnova EE, et al. Hexameric structure and assembly of the interleukin-6/IL-6 alpha-receptor/gp130 complex. *Science.* 2003;300:2101–2104.
189. Zheng T, Zhu Z, Wang J, et al. IL-11: insights in asthma from overexpression transgenic modeling. *J Allergy Clin Immunol.* 2001;108:489–496.
198. Lin LF, Mismer D, Lile JD, et al. Purification, cloning, and expression of ciliary neurotrophic factor (CNTF). *Science.* 1989;246:1023–1025.
200. Davis S, Aldrich TH, Valenzuela DM, et al. The receptor for ciliary neurotrophic factor. *Science.* 1991;253:59–63.
201. Davis S, Aldrich TH, Stahl N, et al. LIFR beta and gp130 as heterodimerizing signal transducers of the tripartite CNTF receptor. *Science.* 1993;260:1805–1808.
207. Mosley B, De Imus C, Friend D, et al. Dual oncostatin M (OSM) receptors. Cloning and characterization of an alternative signaling subunit conferring OSM-specific receptor activation. *J Biol Chem.* 1996;271:32635–32643.
209. Pennica D, Wood WI, Chien KR. Cardiotrophin-1: a multifunctional cytokine that signals via LIF receptor-gp 130 dependent pathways. *Cytokine Growth Factor Rev.* 1996;7:81–91.
214. Pflanz S, Timans JC, Cheung J, et al. IL-27, a heterodimeric cytokine composed of EBI3 and p28 protein, induces proliferation of naive CD4(+) T cells. *Immunity.* 2002;16:779–790.
215. Hunter CA. New IL-12-family members: IL-23 and IL-27, cytokines with divergent functions. *Nat Rev Immunol.* 2005;5:521–531.
216. Kastelein RA, Hunter CA, Cua DJ. Discovery and biology of IL-23 and IL-27: related but functionally distinct regulators of inflammation. *Annu Rev Immunol.* 2007;25:221–242.
217. Ozaki K, Leonard WJ. Cytokine and cytokine receptor pleiotropy and redundancy. *J Biol Chem.* 2002;277:29355–29358.
220. La Cava A, Matarese G. The weight of leptin in immunity. *Nat Rev Immunol.* 2004;4:371–379.
222. Chen H, Charlat O, Tartaglia LA, et al. Evidence that the diabetes gene encodes the leptin receptor: identification of a mutation in the leptin receptor gene in db/db mice. *Cell.* 1996;84:491–495.
225. Trinchier G. Interleukin-12 and the regulation of innate resistance and adaptive immunity. *Nat Rev Immunol.* 2003;3:133–146.
229. Oppmann B, Lesley R, Blom B, et al. Novel p19 protein engages IL-12p40 to form a cytokine, IL 23, with biological activities similar as well as distinct from IL-12. *Immunity.* 2000;13:715–725.
231. Uhlig HH, McKenzie BS, Hue S, et al. Differential activity of IL-12 and IL-23 in mucosal and systemic innate immune pathology. *Immunity.* 2006;25:309–318.
232. Dillon SR, Sprecher C, Hammond A, et al. Interleukin 31, a cytokine produced by activated T cells, induces dermatitis in mice. *Nat Immunol.* 2004;5:752–760.
233. Friend SL, Hosier S, Nelson A, et al. A thymic stromal cell line supports in vitro development of surface IgM+ B cells and produces a novel growth factor affecting B and T lineage cells. *Exp Hematol.* 1994;22:321–328.
234. Sims JE, Williams DE, Morrissey PJ, et al. Molecular cloning and biological characterization of a novel murine lymphoid growth factor. *J Exp Med.* 2000;192:671–680.
235. Pandey A, Ozaki K, Baumann H, et al. Cloning of a receptor subunit required for signaling by thymic stromal lymphopoietin. *Nat Immunol.* 2000;1:59–64.
236. Park LS, Martin U, Garka K, et al. Cloning of the murine thymic stromal lymphopoietin (TSLP) receptor: formation of a functional heteromeric complex requires interleukin 7 receptor. *J Exp Med.* 2000;192:659–670.
239. Soumelis V, Reche PA, Kanzler H, et al. Human epithelial cells trigger dendritic cell mediated allergic inflammation by producing TSLP. *Nat Immunol.* 2002;3:673–680.
241. Liu YJ, Soumelis V, Watanabe N, et al. TSLP: An epithelial cell cytokine that regulates T cell differentiation by conditioning dendritic cell maturation. *Annu Rev Immunol.* 2007;25:193–219.
242. Al-Shami A, Spolski R, Kelly J, et al. A role for thymic stromal lymphopoietin in CD4(+) T cell development. *J Exp Med.* 2004;200:159–168.
243. Al-Shami A, Spolski R, Kelly J, et al. A role for TSLP in the development of inflammation in an asthma model. *J Exp Med.* 2005;202:829–839.
244. Yoo J, Omori M, Gyarmati D, et al. Spontaneous atopic dermatitis in mice expressing an inducible thymic stromal lymphopoietin transgene specifically in the skin. *J Exp Med.* 2005;202:541–549.
245. Zhou B, Comeau MR, De Smedt T, et al. Thymic stromal lymphopoietin as a key initiator of allergic airway inflammation in mice. *Nat Immunol.* 2005;6:1047–1053.
247. Liu YJ. IPC: professional type 1 interferon-producing cells and plasmacytoid dendritic cell precursors. *Annu Rev Immunol.* 2005;23:275–306.
248. Lin JX, Migone TS, Tsang M, et al. The role of shared receptor motifs and common Stat proteins in the generation of cytokine pleiotropy and redundancy by IL-2, IL-4, IL-7, IL-13, and IL-15. *Immunity.* 1995;2:331–339.
249. Wynn TA. IL-13 effector functions. *Annu Rev Immunol.* 2003;21:425–456.
252. Hilton DJ, Zhang JG, Metcalf D, et al. Cloning and characterization of a binding subunit of the interleukin 13 receptor that is also a component of the interleukin 4 receptor. *Proc Natl Acad Sci U S A.* 1996;93:497–501.
254. Caput D, Laurent P, Kaghad M, et al. Cloning and characterization of a specific interleukin (IL)-13 binding protein structurally related to the IL-5 receptor alpha chain. *J Biol Chem.* 1996;271:16921–16926.
256. Wills-Karp M, Luyimbazi J, Xu X, et al. Interleukin-13: central mediator of allergic asthma. *Science.* 1998;282:2258–2261.
258. Kapp U, Yeh WC, Patterson B, et al. Interleukin 13 is secreted by and stimulates the growth of Hodgkin and Reed-Sternberg cells. *J Exp Med.* 1999;189:1939–1946.
259. Sharfe N, Dadi HK, Shahar M, Roifman CM. Human immune disorder arising from mutation of the alpha chain of the interleukin-2 receptor. *Proc Natl Acad Sci U S A.* 1997;94:3168–3171.
267. Pestka S, Krause CD, Sarkar D, et al. Interleukin-10 and related cytokines and receptors. *Annu Rev Immunol.* 2004;22:929–979.
272. Isaacs A, Lindenmann J. Virus interference. I. The interferon. *Proc R Soc Lond B Biol Sci.* 1957;147:258–267.
278. Taniguchi T, Takaoka A. The interferon-alpha/beta system in antiviral responses: a multimodal machinery of gene regulation by the IRF family of transcription factors. *Curr Opin Immunol.* 2002;14:111–116.
279. Dunn GP, Koebel CM, Schreiber RD. Interferons, immunity and cancer immunoediting. *Nat Rev Immunol.* 2006;6:836–848.
280. van Boxel-Dezaire AH, Rani MR, Stark GR. Complex modulation of cell type-specific signaling in response to type I interferons. *Immunity.* 2006;25:361–372.
281. Honda K, Takaoka A, Taniguchi T. Type I interferon [corrected] gene induction by the interferon regulatory factor family of transcription factors. *Immunity.* 2006;25:349–360.
282. Vilcek J. Fifty years of interferon research: aiming at a moving target. *Immunity.* 2006;25:343–348.
287. Walter MR, Windsor WT, Nagabhushan TL, et al. Crystal structure of a complex between interferon-gamma and its soluble high-affinity receptor. *Nature.* 1995;376:230–235.
294. Symons JA, Alcami A, Smith GL. Vaccinia virus encodes a soluble type I interferon receptor of novel structure and broad species specificity. *Cell.* 1995;81:551–560.
298. Young HA, Romero-Weaver AL, Savan R, et al. Class II Cytokines. Trivandrum, Kerala, India: Research Signpost; 2007.
305. Moore KW, de Waal Malefyt R, Coffman RL, et al. Interleukin-10 and the interleukin-10 receptor. *Annu Rev Immunol.* 2001;19:683–765.
313. Xie MH, Aggarwal S, Ho WH, et al. Interleukin (IL)-22, a novel human cytokine that signals through the interferon receptor-related proteins CRF2-4 and IL-22R. *J Biol Chem.* 2000;275:31335–31339.

318a. Liang SC, Tan XY, Luxenberg DP, et al. Interleukin (IL)-22 and IL-17 are coexpressed by Th17 cells and cooperatively enhance expression of antimicrobial peptides. *J Exp Med*. 2006;203:2271–2279.
321. Darnell JE Jr, Kerr IM, Stark GR. Jak-STAT pathways and transcriptional activation in response to IFNs and other extracellular signaling proteins. *Science*. 1994;264:1415–1421.
322. Leonard WJ, O'Shea JJ. Jaks and STATs: biological implications. *Annu Rev Immunol*. 1998;16:293–322.
324. Shuai K, Liu B. Regulation of JAK-STAT signalling in the immune system. *Nat Rev Immunol*. 2003;3:900–911.
333. Witthuhn BA, Quelle FW, Silvennoinen O, et al. JAK2 associates with the erythropoietin receptor and is tyrosine phosphorylated and activated following stimulation with erythropoietin. *Cell*. 1993;74:227–236.
337. Chen M, Cheng A, Chen YQ, et al. The amino terminus of JAK3 is necessary and sufficient for binding to the common gamma chain and confers the ability to transmit interleukin 2-mediated signals. *Proc Natl Acad Sci U S A*. 1997;94:6910–6915.
338. Rodig SJ, Meraz MA, White JM, et al. Disruption of the Jak1 gene demonstrates obligatory and nonredundant roles of the Jaks in cytokine-induced biologic responses. *Cell*. 1998;93:373–383.
343. Russell SM, Tayebi N, Nakajima H, et al. Mutation of Jak3 in a patient with SCID: essential role of Jak3 in lymphoid development. *Science*. 1995;270:797–800.
344. Macchi P, Villa A, Giliani S, et al. Mutations of Jak-3 gene in patients with autosomal severe combined immune deficiency (SCID). *Nature*. 1995;377:65–68.
345. Nosaka T, van Deursen JM, Tripp RA, et al. Defective lymphoid development in mice lacking Jak3. *Science*. 1995;270:800–802.
346. Thomis DC, Gurniak CB, Tivol E, et al. Defects in B lymphocyte maturation and T lymphocyte activation in mice lacking Jak3. *Science*. 1995;270:794–797.
350. Minegishi Y, Saito M, Morio T, et al. Human tyrosine kinase 2 deficiency reveals its requisite roles in multiple cytokine signals involved in innate and acquired immunity. *Immunity*. 2006;25:745–755.
351. Harrison DA, Binari R, Nahreini TS, et al. Activation of a Drosophila Janus kinase (JAK) causes hematopoietic neoplasia and developmental defects. *EMBO J*. 1995;14:2857–2865.
354. Danial NN, Pernis A, Rothman PB. Jak-STAT signaling induced by the v-abl oncogene. *Science*. 1995;269:1875–877.
355. Migone TS, Lin JX, Cereseto A, et al. Constitutively activated Jak-STAT pathway in T cells transformed with HTLV-I. *Science*. 1995;269:79–81.
357. Yu CL, Meyer DJ, Campbell GS, et al. Enhanced DNA-binding activity of a Stat3-related protein in cells transformed by the Src oncoprotein. *Science*. 1995;269:81–83.
362. Levine RL, Gilliland DG. JAK-2 mutations and their relevance to myeloproliferative disease. *Curr Opin Hematol*. 2007;14:43–47.
363. Lacronique V, Boureux A, Valle VD, et al. A TEL-JAK2 fusion protein with constitutive kinase activity in human leukemia. *Science*. 1997;278:1309–1312.
364. Seto Y, Nakajima H, Suto A, et al. Enhanced Th2 cell-mediated allergic inflammation in Tyk2-deficient mice. *J Immunol*. 2003;170:1077–1083.
371. Fu XY. A transcription factor with SH2 and SH3 domains is directly activated by an interferon alpha-induced cytoplasmic protein tyrosine kinase(s). *Cell*. 1992;70:323–335.
377. Hou J, Schindler U, Henzel WJ, et al. Identification and purification of human Stat proteins activated in response to interleukin-2. *Immunity*. 1995;2:321–329.
378. Wakao H, Gouilleux F, Groner B. Mammary gland factor (MGF) is a novel member of the cytokine regulated transcription factor gene family and confers the prolactin response. *EMBO J*. 1994;13:2182–2191.
385. Nakajima H, Liu XW, Wynshaw-Boris A, et al. An indirect effect of Stat5a in IL-2-induced proliferation: a critical role for Stat5a in IL-2-mediated IL-2 receptor alpha chain induction. *Immunity*. 1997;7:691–701.
386. Imada K, Bloom ET, Nakajima H, et al. Stat5b is essential for natural killer cell-mediated proliferation and cytolytic activity. *J Exp Med*. 1998;188:2067–2074.
393. Stahl N, Farruggella TJ, Boulton TG, et al. Choice of STATs and other substrates specified by modular tyrosine-based motifs in cytokine receptors. *Science*. 1995;267:1349–1353.
395. Schindler U, Wu P, Rothe M, et al. Components of a Stat recognition code: evidence for two layers of molecular selectivity. *Immunity*. 1995;2:689–697.
398. McBride KM, Banninger G, McDonald C, et al. Regulated nuclear import of the STAT1 transcription factor by direct binding of importin-alpha. *EMBO J*. 2002;21:1754–763.
399a. Reich NC, Liu L. Tracking STAT nuclear traffic. *Nature Rev Immunol*. 2006;6:602–612.
400. Chen X, Vinkemeier U, Zhao Y, et al. Crystal structure of a tyrosine phosphorylated STAT-1 dimer bound to DNA. *Cell*. 1998;93:827–839.
401. Becker S, Groner B, Muller CW. Three-dimensional structure of the Stat3beta homodimer bound to DNA. *Nature*. 1998;394:145–151.
402. Soldaini E, John S, Moro S, et al. DNA binding site selection of dimeric and tetrameric Stat5 proteins reveals a large repertoire of divergent tetrameric Stat5a binding sites. *Mol Cell Biol*. 2000;20:389–401.
404. Vinkemeier U, Cohen SL, Moarefi I, et al. DNA binding of in vitro activated Stat1 alpha, Stat1 beta and truncated Stat1: interaction between NH2-terminal domains stabilizes binding of two dimers to tandem DNA sites. *EMBO J*. 1996;15:5616–5626.
408. Kim HP, Kelly J, Leonard WJ. The basis for IL-2-induced IL-2 receptor alpha chain gene regulation: importance of two widely separated IL-2 response elements. *Immunity*. 2001;15:159–172.
411. Yang J, Chatterjee-Kishore M, Staugaitis SM, et al. Novel roles of unphosphorylated STAT3 in oncogenesis and transcriptional regulation. *Cancer Res*. 2005;65:939–947.
412. Ota N, Brett TJ, Murphy TL, et al. N-domain-dependent nonphosphorylated STAT4 dimers required for cytokine-driven activation. *Nat Immunol*. 2004;5:208–215.
417. Zhang JJ, Zhao Y, Chait BT, et al. Ser727-dependent recruitment of MCM5 by Stat1alpha in IFN-gamma-induced transcriptional activation. *EMBO J*. 1998; 17:6963–6971.
420. Schaefer TS, Sanders LK, Nathans D. Cooperative transcriptional activity of Jun and Stat3 beta, a short form of Stat3. *Proc Natl Acad Sci U S A*. 1995;92:9097–9101.
427. Meraz MA, White JM, Sheehan KC, et al. Targeted disruption of the Stat1 gene in mice reveals unexpected physiologic specificity in the JAK-STAT signaling pathway. *Cell*. 1996;84:431–442.
435. Kaplan MH, Sun YL, Hoey T, et al. Impaired IL-12 responses and enhanced development of Th2 cells in Stat4-deficient mice. *Nature*. 1996;382:174–177.
436. Thierfelder WE, van Deursen JM, Yamamoto K, et al. Requirement for Stat4 in interleukin-12-mediated responses of natural killer and T cells. *Nature*. 1996;382:171–174.
437. Takeda K, Tanaka T, Shi W, et al. Essential role of Stat6 in IL-4 signalling. *Nature*. 1996;380:627–630.
442. Yao Z, Cui Y, Watford WT, et al. Stat5a/b are essential for normal lymphoid development and differentiation. *Proc Natl Acad Sci U S A*. 2006;103:1000–1005.
443. Socolovsky M, Fallon AE, Wang S, et al. Fetal anemia and apoptosis of red cell progenitors in Stat5a−/−5b−/− mice: a direct role for Stat5 in Bcl-X(L) induction. *Cell*. 1999;98:181–191.
444. Yan R, Small S, Desplan C, et al. Identification of a Stat gene that functions in Drosophila development. *Cell*. 1996;84:421–430.
448. Darnell JE Jr. Transcription factors as targets for cancer therapy. *Nat Rev Cancer*. 2002;2:740–749.
451. Su WC, Kitagawa M, Xue N, et al. Activation of Stat1 by mutant fibroblast growth-factor receptor in thanatophoric dysplasia type II dwarfism. *Nature*. 1997;386:288–292.
455. Dent AL, Shaffer AL, Yu X, et al. Control of inflammation, cytokine expression, and germinal center formation by BCL-6. *Science*. 1997;276:589–592.
460. Karin M, Greten FR. NF-kappaB: linking inflammation and immunity to cancer development and progression. *Nat Rev Immunol*. 2005;5:749–759.
462. Crabtree GR, Olson EN. NFAT signaling: choreographing the social lives of cells. *Cell*. 2002;109(suppl):S67–S79.
493. Dong C, Davis RJ, Flavell RA. MAP kinases in the immune response. *Annu Rev Immunol*. 2002;20:55–72.

495. Li L, Dixon JE. Form, function, and regulation of protein tyrosine phosphatases and their involvement in human diseases. *Semin Immunol.* 2000;12:75–84.
505. Mertens C, Zhong M, Krishnaraj R, et al. Dephosphorylation of phosphotyrosine on STAT1 dimers requires extensive spatial reorientation of the monomers facilitated by the N-terminal domain. *Genes Dev.* 2006;20:3372–3381.
508. Yoshimura A, Ohkubo T, Kiguchi T, et al. A novel cytokine-inducible gene CIS encodes an SH2-containing protein that binds to tyrosine-phosphorylated interleukin 3 and erythropoietin receptors. *EMBO J.* 1995;14:2816–2826.
508a. Jeffrey KL, Camps M, Rommel C, et al. Targeting dual-specificity phosphatases: manipulating MAP kinase signalling and immune responses. *Nat Rev Drug Discov.* 2007;6:391–403.
508b. Kovanen PE, Rosenwald A, Fu J, et al. Analysis of gamma c-family cytokine target genes. Identification of dual-specificity phosphatase 5 (DUSP5) as a regulator of mitogen-activated protein kinase activity in interleukin-2 signaling. *J Biol Chem.* 2003;278:5205–5213.
511. Starr R, Willson TA, Viney EM, et al. A family of cytokine-inducible inhibitors of signalling. *Nature.* 1997;387:917–921.
515. Alexander WS, Hilton DJ. The role of suppressors of cytokine signaling (SOCS) proteins in regulation of the immune response. *Annu Rev Immunol.* 2004;22:503–29.
519. Croker BA, Metcalf D, Robb L, et al. SOCS3 is a critical physiological negative regulator of G-CSF signaling and emergency granulopoiesis. *Immunity.* 2004;20:153–165.
520. Croker BA, Krebs DL, Zhang JG, et al. SOCS3 negatively regulates IL-6 signaling in vivo. *Nat Immunol.* 2003;4:540–545.
528. Mosmann TR, Cherwinski H, Bond MW, et al. Two types of murine helper T cell clone. I. Definition according to profiles of lymphokine activities and secreted proteins. *J Immunol.* 1986;136:2348–2357.
531. Mosmann TR, Sad S. The expanding universe of T-cell subsets: Th1, Th2 and more. *Immunol Today.* 1996;17:138–146.
532. Jankovic D, Sher A, Yap G. Th1/Th2 effector choice in parasitic infection: decision making by committee. *Curr Opin Immunol.* 2001;13:403–409.
533. Romagnani S. Cytokine Reference. Academic Press; San Diego, CA (J.J Oppenheim and M. Feledmann, editors) 2001:99–112.
535. Zhu J, Guo L, Min B, et al. Th1/Th2 Interleukins. In: Growth factor independent-1 induced by IL-4 regulates Th2 cell proliferation. *Immunity.* 2002;16:733–744.
536. Okamura H, Rao A. Transcriptional regulation in lymphocytes. *Curr Opin Cell Biol.* 2001;13:239 243.
538. Dong C. Diversification of T-helper-cell lineages: finding the family root of IL-17-producing cells. *Nat Rev Immunol.* 2006;6:329–333.
540. Lee GR, Kim ST, Spilianakis CG, et al. T helper cell differentiation: regulation by cis elements and epigenetics. *Immunity.* 2006;24:369–379.
542. Ansel KM, Djuretic I, Tanasa B, et al. Regulation of Th2 differentiation and Il4 locus accessibility. *Annu Rev Immunol.* 2006;24:607–656.
543. Szabo SJ, Sullivan BM, Peng SL, et al. Molecular mechanisms regulating Th1 immune responses. *Annu Rev Immunol.* 2003;21:713–758.
549. Harrington LE, Hatton RD, Mangan PR, et al. Interleukin 17-producing CD4+ effector T cells develop via a lineage distinct from the T helper type 1 and 2 lineages. *Nat Immunol.* 2005;6:1123–1132.
552. Weaver CT, Harrington LE, Mangan PR, et al. Th17: an effector CD4 T cell lineage with regulatory T cell ties. *Immunity.* 2006;24:677–688.
553. Cua DJ, Sherlock J, Chen Y, et al. Interleukin-23 rather than interleukin-12 is the critical cytokine for autoimmune inflammation of the brain. *Nature.* 2003;421:744–748.
555a. Acosta-Rodriguez EV, Napolitani G, Lanzavecchia A, et al. Interleukins 1 beta and 6 but not transforming growth factor-beta are essential for the differentiation of interleukin 17-producing human T helper cells. *Nat Immunol.* 2007;8:942–949.
555b. Wilson NJ, Boniface K, Chan JR, et al. Development, cytokine profile and function of human interleukin 17-producing helper T cells. *Nat Immunol.* 2007;8:950–957.
556. Stumhofer JS, Laurence A, Wilson EH, et al. Interleukin 27 negatively regulates the development of interleukin 17-producing T helper cells during chronic inflammation of the central nervous system. *Nat Immunol.* 2006;7:937–945.
563. Dupuis S, Dargemont C, Fieschi C, et al. Impairment of mycobacterial but not viral immunity by a germline human STAT1 mutation. *Science.* 2001;293:300–303.
564. Yoshida H, Hamano S, Senaldi G, et al. WSX-1 is required for the initiation of Th1 responses and resistance to L. major infection. *Immunity.* 2001;15:569–578.
566. Hamano S, Himeno K, Miyazaki Y, et al. WSX-1 is required for resistance to Trypanosoma cruzi infection by regulation of proinflammatory cytokine production. *Immunity.* 2003;19:657–667.
573. Ding C, Jones G. Technology evaluation: MRA, Chugai. *Curr Opin Mol Ther.* 2003;5:64–69.
574. Waldmann TA. The meandering 45-year odyssey of a clinical immunologist. *Annu Rev Immunol.* 2003;21:1–27.
577. Sadlack B, Merz H, Schorle H, et al. Ulcerative colitis-like disease in mice with a disrupted interleukin-2 gene. *Cell.* 1993;75:253–261.
581. Nishinakamura R, Nakayama N, Hirabayashi Y, et al. Mice deficient for the IL-3/GM-CSF/IL-5 beta c receptor exhibit lung pathology and impaired immune response, while beta IL3 receptor-deficient mice are normal. *Immunity.* 1995;2:211–222.
583. Yoshida K, Taga T, Saito M, et al. Targeted disruption of gp130, a common signal transducer for the interleukin 6 family of cytokines, leads to myocardial and hematological disorders. *Proc Natl Acad Sci U S A.* 1996;93:407–411.
584. Akira S, Yoshida K, Tanaka T, et al. Targeted disruption of the IL-6 related genes: gp130 and NF-IL-6. *Immunol Rev.* 1995;148:221–253.
611. Parganas E, Wang D, Stravopodis D, et al. Jak2 is essential for signaling through a variety of cytokine receptors. *Cell.* 1998;93:385–395.
613. Karaghiosoff M, Neubauer H, Lassnig C, et al. Partial impairment of cytokine responses in Tyk2-deficient mice. *Immunity.* 2000;13:549–560.

Chapter 24

Interleukin-1 Family of Ligands and Receptors

Charles A. Dinarello

HISTORICAL BACKGROUND

The history of interleukin-1 (IL-1) begins in the period 1943 to 1948 with studies by Menkin and Beeson on the pathogenesis of fever and the properties of the fever-producing protein called endogenous or leukocytic pyrogen. Many investigators primarily interested in the links connecting fever, infection, and inflammation studied leukocytic pyrogen. In 1972, Waksman and Gery reported that soluble factors from macrophages augmented lymphocyte proliferation in response to mitogenic stimuli. Kampschmidt contributed to the discovery phase of IL-1 by characterizing soluble factors that induced the synthesis of acute-phase proteins. In the field of rheumatoid arthritis, Krane and Dayer demonstrated that IL-1 induced prostaglandins and collagenases in synovial fibroblasts, and Saklatvala described IL-1 in the context of its ability to destroy cartilage. Others provided data that IL-1 was a colony-stimulating factor and induced neutrophilia. The term "interleukin" was established to streamline the description of the growing number of biological properties attributed to soluble factors from macrophages and lymphocytes. IL-1 was the name given to the macrophage product, and IL-2 was used for the lymphocyte product. At the time of the "interleukin" assignments, the amino acid sequences of IL-1 and IL-2 were unknown. Despite studies on highly purified preparations, the large number of diverse biological activities attributed to IL-1 as a single molecule engendered considerable skepticism. With the cloning of IL-1 in 1984 (1,2), however, study of the recombinant molecule established that IL-1 was indeed a pleiotropic cytokine that induced inflammation as well as augmented immunologic responses. In fact, humans injected with recombinant IL-1 manifested each of the biological properties that had been previously reported in animals using IL-1 purified from human blood monocytes. With the use of agents that specifically block IL-1 activity, it has been possible to define the role of this first interleukin in human disease, which has resulted in reduction of severity in some diseases.

OVERVIEW OF THE IL-1 FAMILY IN INFLAMMATION

Of the 11 members of the IL-1 family (IL-1F) of ligands, four gene products (IL-1α, IL-1β, IL-1 receptor antagonist, and IL-18) have been thoroughly studied *in vitro* and in animal models of disease. In the case of humans, the blocking of IL-1 activity has entered clinical medicine. The IL-1 receptor antagonist (IL-1Ra) is approved in several countries for treating the signs and symptoms, including joint destruction, of rheumatoid arthritis. It is estimated that more than 100,000 patients with rheumatoid arthritis and related diseases have been treated with IL-1Ra, some for more than 10 years. IL-1Ra has also been used in patients with type 2 diabetes, arresting the loss of the insulin-producing pancreatic beta cells in the islets of Langerhans (3). In addition to IL-1α, IL-1β, IL-1Ra, and IL-18, other members of the IL-1 family are found in various human tissues. The most recent addition to the IL-1 family is IL-1F11 (IL-33), the ligand for the former orphan receptor ST2. IL-33 plays a role in mast cell functions and the Th2 response.

The IL-1 Family as Proinflammatory Cytokines

Unlike IL-2 and other cytokines that affect lymphocyte function, differentiation, and expansion, most members of the IL-1 family of ligands primarily affect inflammation. Within the IL-1 family, several possess proinflammatory properties, whereas others possess antiinflammatory activities. The family of IL-1 receptors also transduce proinflammatory as well as antiinflammatory signals. What is meant by "proinflammatory"? The proinflammatory members of the IL-1 family stimulate the expression of genes associated with acute inflammation as well as chronic inflammation. The best example of an IL-1 family member in the context of inflammation is IL-1β. The ability of IL-1β to induce gene expression and synthesis of cyclooxygenase type 2 (COX-2), type 2 phospholipase A, and inducible nitric oxide synthase (iNOS) accounts for prostaglandin

E_2 (PGE_2), platelet-activating factor, and nitric oxide (NO) production. The results are fever, lowered pain threshold, vasodilation, and hypotension.

Another important proinflammatory property of IL-1β is its ability to increase the expression of adhesion molecules such as intercellular adhesion molecule-1 on mesenchymal cells and vascular-cell adhesion molecule–1 on endothelial cells. Together with the induction of chemokines, these properties of IL-1β promote the infiltration of inflammatory and immunocompetent cells from the circulation into the extravascular space and then into tissues, where tissue remodeling is the end result of chronic IL-1–induced inflammation. IL-1β is also an angiogenic factor and plays a role in tumor metastasis and blood vessel formation. In mice deficient in IL-1β, vascular endothelial cell growth factor (VEGF) cannot stimulate formation of blood vessels, and malignant melanoma cells do not spread. IL-1β also acts on bone marrow stem cells for differentiation of the myeloid series of progenitor cells. In humans injected intravenously with low doses of IL-1β, 1 to 10 ng/kg, fever is observed, as well as increased levels of adrenocorticotropic hormone, blood neutrophils, nitric oxide, acute-phase proteins, and several cytokines and chemokines. Humans are particularly sensitive to IL-1β, and a dose of 50 ng/kg results is frank hemodynamic shock.

Blocking IL-1 Activity

Specific blockade of IL-1 activity in humans has defined the role for this cytokine in several diseases. IL-1Ra is the specific receptor antagonist for IL-1α and IL-1β but not for any other member of the IL-1 family. When IL-1Ra occupies the IL-1 receptor type I (IL-1RI), bona fide IL-1 cannot bind to the receptor and there is no biological response to IL-1. The existence of this highly specific, naturally occurring receptor antagonist in cytokine biology appears to be unique to the IL-1 family. In addition to IL-1Ra, the administration of neutralizing monoclonal antibodies to IL-1β or the IL-1 Trap (4) has been used to treat patients with rheumatoid arthritis. Although each of the IL-1–blocking therapies reduces the severity of rheumatoid arthritis, other treatments are also used to treat this disease. For example, anti–tumor necrosis factor-α (TNFα), anti-CD20 monoclonal antibody, and CTLA4-Ig are also effective therapies for rheumatoid arthritis. There are, however, other inflammatory diseases that rapidly remit with IL-1–blocking therapies but are not responsive to blocking TNFα. Those diseases in which IL-1 blockade is highly effective are termed "autoinflammatory" diseases to distinguish them from "autoimmune" diseases.

IL-1 and the Autoinflammatory Diseases

One important criterion for characterizing a disease as "autoinflammatory" is that on the blocking of IL-1 activity, patients experience a rapid and sustained cessation of symptoms, as well as reductions in biochemical and hematologic markers of the disease. The clinical manifestations of the autoinflammatory syndromes are recurrent fevers, neutrophilic leukocytosis, rashes, painful and deforming arthritis, and high serum levels of acute-phase reactants. Progressive deafness, leptomeningitis, and amyloidosis may also be present in some patients. The adult and juvenile forms of Still's disease fall into the "autoinflammatory" group. Since the use of the IL-1 Trap and the use of monoclonal anti–IL-1β antibodies are equally effective in treating autoinflammatory diseases, the culprit in these diseases is IL-1β and not IL-1α. Another criterion for classification of an autoinflammatory disease is a reduction in disease severity with the use of caspase-1 inhibition, which, as discussed later, targets the processing and secretion of IL-1β.

The biological basis for "autoinflammatory" diseases appears to be an increase in the spontaneous as well as inducible secretion of active IL-1β from blood monocytes. Increased release of IL-1β from primary blood monocytes has been documented in many of these patients compared to healthy controls. Most autoinflammatory diseases are syndromes. They include neonatal-onset multi-inflammatory disease, the Muckle-Wells syndrome, familial cold-induced autoinflammatory syndrome, hyper–immunoglobulin D (IgD) syndrome, familial Mediterranean fever, and urate crystal arthritis (gout). Although these syndromes are rare, the clinical manifestations are common to many inflammatory and infectious diseases.

The Inflammasome

The "inflammasome" plays an important role in processing inactive IL-1β, IL-18, and IL-33 precursors into active cytokines. The inflammasome is an assembly of intracellular proteins that activates caspase-1. Caspase-1 is an intracellular cysteine protease that cuts the N-terminal amino acids at the aspartic acid residue in the P1 position. In the case of IL-1β, caspase-1 cleaves the N-terminal 116 amino acids from the IL-1β precursor, thereby converting the precursor into an active cytokine. As shown in Figure 24.1, there are several steps in the processing and secretion of mature IL-1β. Cryopyrin is one of the essential proteins that comprise the inflammasome. Some patients with an autoinflammatory disease have mutations in cryopyrin, resulting in a loss in the control of IL-1β processing by caspase-1. There are also patients who have the clinical and hematologic characteristics of autoinflammatory syndromes but not mutations in cryopyrin. Nevertheless, spontaneous and inducible secretion of IL-1β from blood monocytes is elevated in these patients. The increase is modest (three- to fourfold compared to monocytes from healthy subjects), but these patients are debilitated from the chronic inflammatory process of their disease.

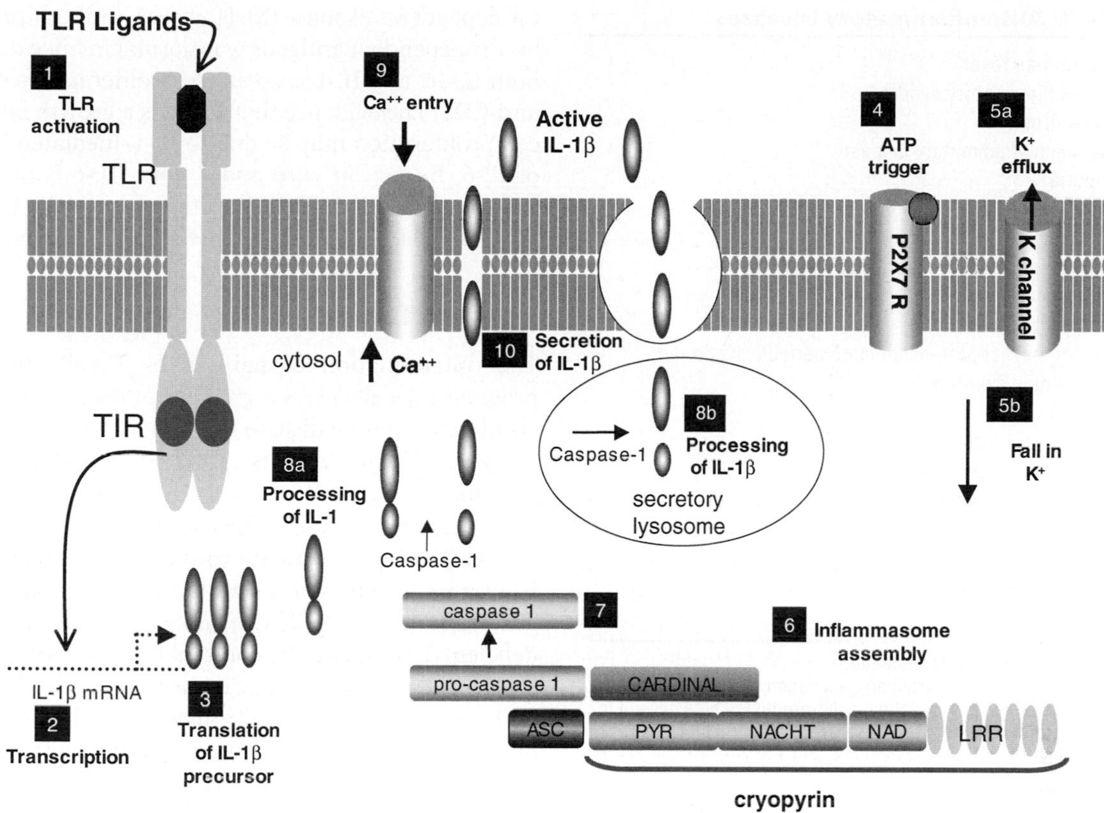

FIGURE 24.1 Steps in the activation of the caspase-1 inflammasome, processing of the interleukin-1β (IL-1β) precursor, and secretion of IL-1β. Primary blood monocytes from healthy human subjects are first activated by Toll-like receptor (TLR) ligands, for example, endotoxin binding to TLR-4 (1). The transcription (2) and translation into the IL-1β precursor (3) take place in the cytosol, not the endoplasmic reticulum (34). On activation of the P2X7 receptor by ATP (4), there is a rapid efflux of potassium from the cell (5a), resulting in fall in intracellular levels of potassium (5b). The fall in intracellular potassium levels triggers the assembly of the components of the caspase-1 inflammasome (6) with cryopyrin, ASC, and Cardinal. The assembled components of the inflammasome initiate the processing of pro-caspase-1, resulting in the formation of the active caspase-1 (7). Active casapse-1 cleaves the IL-1β precursor in the cytosol (8a) or in the secretory lysosome (8b), resulting in the carboxy-terminal mature IL-1β. An influx of calcium into the cell (9) with an increase in intracellular calcium levels (153,154) provides a mechanism by which mature IL-1β is released from the cell (10). The rise in intracellular calcium activates phosphatidylcholine-specific phospholipase C and calcium-dependent phospholipase A (2), which facilitate the secretion of IL-1β with exocytosis of the lysosomal contents (154). TIR, Toll-IL-1-receptor.

Table 24.1 lists examples of syndromes that fall into the "autoinflammatory" class and are treated by reducing the activity of IL-1β.

OVERVIEW OF THE IL-1 FAMILY IN IMMUNE RESPONSES

IL-1 as a Costimulator of T Cells

IL-1 (IL-1α or IL-1β) functions as a costimulator of T cell functions, primarily together with an antigen or a mitogen. For example, IL-1 is a costimulator for T cell proliferation, in that the combination of IL-1 plus a mitogen such as phytohemagglutinin (PHA) or concanavalin A (ConA) results in a greater production of IL-2 than either PHA or ConA alone. Alone, IL-1 does not induce IL-2. In fact, in the absence of a coactivator, IL-1 has no effect on T cells. The widely used bioassay for the immunologic activity of IL-1 for T cell proliferation is costimulation with a mitogen on murine thymocytes. Human thymic epithelium produces constitutive levels of IL-1α, which can function as a growth factor. However, it is unlikely that IL-1 plays a significant role in thymic growth and function because mice deficient in IL-1α or IL-1β or the IL-1RI have normal thymic development. Similar to IL-1α, IL-18 is strongly expressed

TABLE 24.1 Autoinflammatory Diseases[a]

Familial Mediterranean fever
Familial cold autoinflammatory syndrome
Muckle-Wells syndrome
Neonatal-onset multiinflammatory disease
Mevalonic aciduria
Hyper–immunoglobulin D syndrome
Adult-onset Still's disease
Systemic-onset juvenile idiopathic arthritis
Schnitzler's syndrome
Antisynthetase syndrome
Tumor necrosis factor receptor–associated periodic syndrome
Macrophage activation syndrome[b]
Behçet's syndrome
Normocomplementemic urticarial vasculitis
Pericarditis in adult Still's disease
PAPA syndrome (pyogenic arthritis, pyoderma gangrenosum, and acne)
Blau's syndrome
Sweet's syndrome
Urate crystal arthritis (Gout)
Type 2 diabetes[c]

[a]Responsive to interleukin-1 (IL-1) blockade.
[b]IL-18 likely contributes to the macrophage activation syndrome (152).
[c]IL-1 blockade with IL-1Ra protected the insulin-producing beta cells of the islets but did not affect peripheral insulin resistance. Hyperglycemia stimulates IL-1β secretion from the beta cell and accounts for the loss of the beta cell mass in type 2 diabetes (67).

in thymic epithelial cells. IL-18 induced CD11b-positive dendritic cells from thymocytes, and these IL-18–inducible dendritic cells were highly efficient at presenting antigen to CD4- and CD8-positive T cells.

IL-1 and Th2 Immune Responses

For the most part, IL-1 as a Th2 cytokine is derived from models of murine asthma. After airway sensitization to various antigens or haptens, the mice are challenged by inhalation of the antigen. The responses to antigen challenge are increased airway responsiveness to bronchoconstricting agents, infiltration of the lungs by eosinophils, and increased expression of IL-4. However, in mice deficient in IL-1RI or treated with neutralizing anti–IL-1β antibodies, the response to inhaled antigen is markedly reduced (5). By the use of airway sensitization with ovalbumin, eosinophil and neutrophil infiltration after inhalation antigen challenge was prevented in mice expressing IL-1Ra adenovirus (6). Suppression of IL-5 was also observed.

IL-1 and B Cell Functions

In 1983, a neutralizing antibody to human IL-1β was shown to inhibit pokeweed mitogen–stimulated human B cell proliferation and the generation of Ig-secreting cells (7). Since then, a role for IL-1β in antibody production has been repeatedly reported. For example, mice deficient in IL-1β do not produce anti–sheep red blood cell antibodies, a T-dependent response (8). However, antibody production by T-independent antigens was normal in mice deficient in both IL-1α and IL-1, as was the proliferative response to anti-CD3. The evidence that IL-1β is a growth factor for B cell proliferation may be due to IL-1–mediated induction of IL-6. In fact, *in vitro* and *in vivo*, IL-6 is often under the control of IL-1. Therefore the effect of IL-1 on B cell functions may reflect the ability of IL-1 to induce IL-6.

IL-1 and Th17

The differentiation of naive CD4 T cells into IL-17–producing T cells plays a greater pathogenic role in models of autoimmune disease than do Th1 T cells producing IFNγ. IL-17 production is sustained by IL-23, and several autoimmune and inflammatory diseases do not develop in mice deficient in IL-23. The place of IL-1 in the generation of Th17 responses appears essential because T cells from mice deficient in IL-1RI fail to induce IL-17 on antigen challenge (9). IL-23 does not sustain IL-17 in IL-1RI–deficient T cells, and the combination of IL-23 plus either IL-1α or IL-1β is synergistic in the induction of IL-17. Even TNFα enhancement of IL-23–induced IL-17 is IL-1 dependent. Although the combination of IL-6 plus TGFβ induces IL-17, IL-6 production is often under the control of IL-1, particularly IL-1β. Therefore, one interpretation of one role of IL-1 in one generation of Th17 responses is the dependency of IL-6 production on IL-1 activity.

These studies are consistent with results on mice deficient in IL-1Ra. These mice develop a spontaneous rheumatoid arthritis–like disease. However, the disease does not develop in mice deficient in IL-17 (10). Furthermore, IL-1 activation of the cosignaling receptor OX40 induces IL-17. Taken together, these findings indicate that IL-1 appears to be upstream of IL-6 and OX40 activation and thus IL-17 production. The findings are also consistent with the observation that mice deficient in both IL-1α and IL-1β do not develop experimental autoimmune encephalomyelitis (EAE) (11). Several studies show that IL-1 and IL-17 act synergistically on the induction of nitric oxide, PGE, and cartilage breakdown, which is not unexpected, because IL-1 induces IL-17,and IL-17 in turn stimulates the production and release of IL-1β from primary human blood monocytes. In general, proinflammatory cytokines induce each other.

IL-18 Induces Th1 and Th2 Cytokines

Because IL-18 participates with IL-12 and IL-15 in the production of IFNγ, IL-18 is considered a classic Th1-inducing cytokine; however, there is a well-described role for IL-18 in the Th2 response (12). For example, IL-18 induces IL-4 and the number of IL-4–positive cells from activated natural killer (NK) T cells in the absence of IL-12. In general, the presence of IL-12 shifts the activity of IL-18 toward IFNγ and the Th1 response, whereas IL-18 in the absence of IL-12 drives the Th2 response. Combined overexpression of IL-18 and caspase-1 results in the development of spontaneous atopic dermatitis with increased expression of Th2 cytokines and IgE (13). In transgenic mice overexpressing IL-18, serum levels of IgE, IgG1, IL-4, and IFNγ were significantly increased (14). Therefore, high IL-18 production can polarize toward both Th1 and Th2 responses.

CASPASE-1 AND THE PROCESSING OF IL-1 FAMILY MEMBER PRECURSORS

With the exception of IL-1Ra, each member of the IL-1 family is initially synthesized as an inactive precursor molecule without a signal peptide. After processing by the removal of N-terminal amino acids by the specific intracellular cysteine protease called caspase-1, the resulting molecules are called "mature" forms. Caspase-1 is the first member of a large family of intracellular cysteine proteases with important roles in programmed cell death. However, there is little evidence that caspase-1 participates in programmed cell death. Instead, caspase-1 seems to be primarily used by the cell to cleave the IL-1β and IL-18 precursors. IL-33 also uses caspase-1 for cleavage (15). As shown in Figure 24.1, caspase-1 cleaves IL-1β, but the same steps are likely involved for the cleavage of IL-18 and IL-33. In the word "caspase" the "asp" refers to the aspartic acid in the P1 position. The aspartic acid in the P1 position is the recognition amino acid for all caspases. After cleavage, the mature form of IL-1β is generated as a 17.5-kDa molecule. Figure 24.2 depicts the caspase-1 cleavage sites of IL-1β, IL-18, and IL-33. Although caspase-1 is primarily responsible for cleavage of the precursor intracellularly, other proteases such as proteinase-3 can process the IL-1β precursor extracellularly into an active cytokine (16). Proteinase-3 may also contribute to the processing of IL-18 (17).

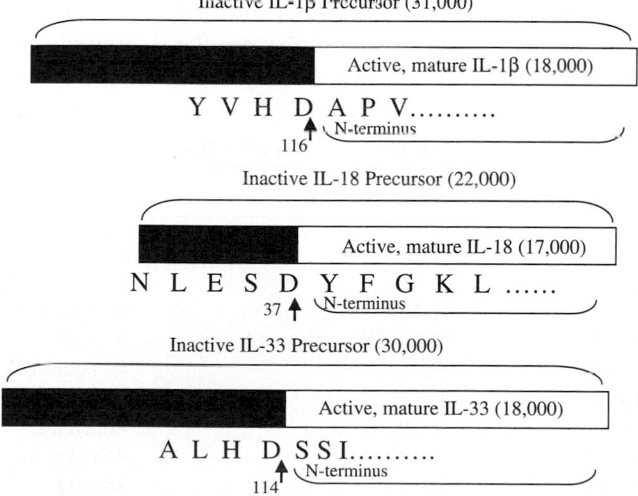

FIGURE 24.2 Three substrates for caspase-1. Caspase-1 cleaves the IL-1β, IL-18, and IL-33 precursors at the aspartic acid (D) in P1 position. Shown are the amino acids lengths of the mature cytokines.

DEFICIENCY IN IL-1 FAMILY MEMBERS

Mice deficient in IL-1RI, IL-1 receptor accessory protein (IL-1RAcP), IL-1α, or IL-1β or doubly deficient in IL-1α and IL-1β exhibit a phenotype no different from that of wild-type mice of the same strain. Thus, mice without IL-1 activity live in routine animal facilities. From these observations, one can conclude that IL-1α and IL-1β, which play important roles in disease, are not essential for normal embryonic development, postnatal growth, homeostasis, reproduction, or resistance to routine microbial flora. These mice also do not exhibit evidence of spontaneous carcinogenesis, and their life span appears to be normal. Lymphoid organ architecture is also normal. Each of these observations has been made regardless of background mouse strain. Nevertheless, in the context of an inducible disease, infection, or inflammatory challenge, a deficiency in IL-1 has a demonstrable effect on outcomes. In contrast, mice deficient in IL-1Ra do not exhibit normal reproduction, have stunted growth, and in selected strains develop spontaneous diseases such as rheumatoid arthritis–like polyarthropathy and a fatal arteritis (18,19).

In general, young mice deficient in IL-18 exhibit reduced responses in several models of disease. For example, IL-18–deficient mice are resistant to endotoxin lethality, collagen-induced arthritis, Fas ligand–mediated hepatitis, graft versus host disease, ConA-induced hepatitis, and allograft rejection. In contrast, a deficiency in the IL-18 receptor α chain results in a hyperresponsive phenotype to inflammatory challenges and greater production of TNFα, IFNγ, and chemokines (20). In a model of EAE, mice deficient in IL-18 exhibited the opposite in terms of disease severity to mice deficient in the IL-18 receptor (21). These findings challenge the underlying assumption that the IL-18 receptor is unique to IL-18. The conclusion from these findings is that an unknown ligand binds to the IL-18 receptor and delivers a negative signal, suppressing cytokine production and inflammation. As discussed later, the IL-1 family member IL-1F7 binds to the IL-18 receptor and may deliver an inhibitory signal.

PRODUCTION OF IL-1 FAMILY MEMBERS

Transcriptional Regulation of IL-1β

The primary sources of IL-1β are blood monocytes, tissue macrophages, and dendritic cells. B lymphocytes and NK cells also produce IL-1β. Fibroblasts and epithelial cells, however, generally do not produce the cytokine. In health, circulating human blood monocytes or bone marrow aspirate do not constitutively express IL-1β. Constitutive expression of IL-1β in the human hypothalamus has been described (22). Several malignant tumors express IL-1β as part of their neoplastic nature, particularly acute myelogenous leukemia, multiple myeloma, and juvenile myelogenous leukemia, each of which exhibits constitutive expression of IL-1β. In general, production of IL-1β in tumors contributes to their ability to spread and to induce neovascularization (23–25).

Nearly all microbial products induce IL-1β via the various ligands of the Toll-like receptors (TLRs). TLR–4 is used by lipopolysaccharide (LPS) to induce several cytokines, and the induction of IL-1β is particularly sensitive to low (1 to 10 pg/mL) concentrations of LPS. A LPS–IL-1 response element has been described in which a complex of STAT-1, tyrosine phosphorylated interferon response factor 8, and Spi/PU.1 is required (26). IL-1β mRNA levels rise rapidly within 15 minutes but begin to decline after 4 hours. This decrease is likely due to the synthesis of a transcriptional repressor and/or a decrease in mRNA half–life or the action of micro RNA. However, when IL-1 is used as a stimulant of its own gene expression, IL-1β mRNA levels are sustained for more than 24 hours compared to microbial stimulants. Raising intracellular cAMP levels with histamine enhances IL-1α–induced IL-1β gene expression and protein synthesis (27). Inhibition of translation by cycloheximide results in enhanced splicing of exons, excision of introns, and increased levels of mature mRNA (superinduction) by two orders of magnitude. Thus, synthesis of mature IL-1β mRNA requires an activation step to overcome an apparently intrinsic inhibition to process precursor mRNA.

Unlike the promoter of IL-1α, the promoter region for IL-1β contains a TATA box. Unlike most cytokine promoters, IL-1β regulatory regions are distributed over several thousand base pairs upstream and a few base pairs downstream from the transcriptional start site. The topic of IL-1β gene regulation has been reviewed in detail (26). In addition to a cAMP response element, there is an NFκB-like site. Activating protein-1 (AP-1) sites also participate in LPS-induced IL-1β gene expression.

There is no constitutive gene expression for IL-1β in freshly obtained human peripheral blood mononuclear cells (PBMCs) from healthy donors using more than 40 polymerase chain reaction cycles (28,29); however, the same PBMCs express constitutive mRNA for IL-18 (29). In Western blot analysis from the same PBMCs, the precursor for IL-18 was present but not the IL-1β precursor. Constitutive IL-18 gene expression and the precursor IL-18 protein were also observed in freshly obtained murine splenocytes (29). In these splenocytes, there was no constitutive expression of the IL-1β gene or protein. Other than to distinguish differences between IL-1β and IL-18 in the same cells, the clinical significance of constitutive gene and protein expression for IL-18 in health places IL-18 and the caspase-1 inflammasome in a unique situation.

Dissociation Between Transcription and Translation

Non-TLR ligands such as the complement component C5a, hypoxia, adherence to surfaces, or clotting of blood induce the synthesis of large amounts of IL-1β mRNA in monocytic cells without significant translation into the IL-1β protein (30). This dissociation between transcription and translation is characteristic of IL-1β but not most cytokines. It appears that these endogenous stimuli are sufficient to provide vigorous signal for transcription but not for translation. The IL-1β mRNA assembles into large polyribosomes without significant elongation of the peptide (31). Without translation, most of the IL-1β mRNA is degraded. However, adding TLR ligands or IL-1 itself to monocytes with high levels of IL-1β mRNA results in augmented translation in somewhat the same manner as the removal of cycloheximide after superinduction. One explanation is that stabilization of the AU-rich 3′ untranslated region takes place in cells stimulated with LPS. The stabilization of mRNA by microbial products may explain why low concentrations of LPS or a few bacteria or *Borrelia* organisms per cell induce the translation of large amounts of IL-1β (32). It is also possible that IL-1β mRNA is degraded by micro RNAs.

FUNCTIONS OF THE IL-1 FAMILY

Table 24.2 lists the members of the IL-1 family and their primary function. This chapter keeps the terms IL-1α, IL-1β, and IL-18, as well as IL-1Ra. The most recent addition to the IL-1 family, IL-1F11, is also termed IL-33, which is used in this chapter. Most members of the IL-1 family are

TABLE 24.2 Interleukin-1 Family Members

New Name	*Other Name*	*Property*
IL-1F1	IL-1α	Agonist
IL-1F2	IL-1β	Agonist
IL-1F3	IL-1Ra	Antagonist
IL-1F4	IL-18; IFNγ-inducing factor	Agonist
IL-1F5	FIL-1δ	Antagonist (?)
IL-1F6	FIL-1ε	Agonist
IL-1F7	IL-1H4, IL-1ζ	Antagonist
IL-1F8	IL-1H2	Agonist
IL-1F9	IL-1ε	Agonist
IL-1F10	IL-1Hy2	Antagonist
IL-1F11	IL-33	Agonist

IFNγ, interferon-γ; IL, interleukin.

located on the long arm of chromosome 2. All IL-1 family members are closely related to the primary amino acid sequences of IL-1β,L–1Ra, and IL-18. From the intron-exon organization, some members represent gene duplications. In the case of IL-1F5 and IL-1F10, the duplication of the IL-1Ra gene has taken place (33). IL-1F9 is also related to IL 1Ra; it does not function as a receptor antagonist, however, but rather as an agonist. IL-33 (IL-1F11) is closely related to IL-18. However, as described later, the activity of IL-1 family members is not determined by its structure but instead by its ability to transmit a signal or act as a receptor antagonist.

IL-1F1 (IL-1α)

The intron-exon organization of the IL-1 genes suggests duplications of a common gene 350 million years ago. Before this common IL-1 gene, there may have been another ancestral gene from which fibroblast growth factors (FGFs) also evolved because IL-1 and FGFs share significant amino acid homologies. Like FGFs, IL-1α is synthesized as a precursor molecule without a signal peptide; unlike IL-1β, the IL-1α precursor is biologically active. Most proteins are translated by the endoplasmic reticulum, but the 31-kDa IL-1α precursor is synthesized in association with cytoskeletal structures (microtubules and microfilaments). Immunohistochemical studies of IL-1α in LPS-stimulated human blood monocytes revealed a diffuse staining pattern. By comparison, in the same cell, IL-1Ra, which has a signal peptide, is localized to the Golgi complex (34). Even under conditions of cell stimulation, human blood monocytes do not process or readily secrete mature IL-1α. In contrast to IL-1β, IL-1α is not commonly found in the circulation or in body fluids except during severe disease, in which case the cytokine may be released from dying cells (36). Calpain, a calcium-activated cysteine protease associated with the plasma membrane, is responsible for cleavage of the IL-1α precursor into a mature molecule. It is unclear whether calpain cleavage of the IL-1α precursor is functional under physiologic conditions. The propiece of the IL-1α precursor is active intracellularly as a nuclear factor (35).

IL-1α as an Autocrine Growth Factor

The concept that IL-1α acts as an autocrine growth factor assumes that the intracellular IL-1α precursor regulates normal cellular differentiation, particularly in epithelial and ectodermal cells. In support of the concept, an antisense oligonucleotide to IL-1α reduces senescence in endothelial cells (37,38). In a murine Th2 cell line, IL-1α functions as an essential autocrine and paracrine growth factor, based on studies using an antisense IL-1α oligonucleotide or anti–IL-1α antibodies. Thymic epithelium also produces IL-1α constitutively, and a requirement for IL-1α has been demonstrated to regulate the expression of CD25 (IL-2 receptor α chain) and maturation of thymocytes. However, the concept that IL-1α acts as an autocrine growth factor for skin or thymic epithelial cells must be interpreted carefully because mice deficient in IL-1α show no demonstrable defects in growth and development, including skin, fur, epithelium, and gastrointestinal function (39).

Is there is a role for intracellular precursor IL-1α in normal cell function? The effect, if any, would arise from the presence of large amounts of the intracellular form of the IL-1Ra (icIL-1Ra) (40). This form of the IL-1Ra also binds to the IL-1RI and prevents signal transduction. In fact, icIL-1Ra is produced in the same cells that express the IL-1α precursor and are believed to compete with the intracellular pool of precursor IL-1α for nuclear binding sites. However, normal epithelial functions in the IL-1α–deficient mouse as well as the IL-1Ra–deficient mouse do not support the concept that there is a natural role for IL-1α in epithelial growth and differentiation.

Membrane IL-1α

Precursor IL-1α can be found on the surface of several cells, particularly on monocytes and B lymphocytes, in which case it is referred to as membrane IL-1α (41). Membrane IL-1α is biologically active; its biological activities are neutralized by antibodies to IL-1α but not to IL-1β. Membrane IL-1α is likely anchored to the cell membrane via a lectin interaction involving mannose residues. A mannose-like receptor appears to bind membrane IL-1α (42). Membrane IL-1α plays an important role in inflammation because mice deficient in IL-1α exhibit reduced inflammation in models in which cell death and the release of intracellular IL-1α does not take place (43).

Autoantibodies to IL-1α

Neutralizing autoantibodies directed against IL-1α may function as natural buffers for IL-1α. Autoantibodies to IL-1α have been detected in healthy subjects as well as in patients with various autoimmune diseases. Autoantibodies to IL-1α are neutralizing IgG antibodies that bind the IL-1α precursor as well as mature IL-1α (44). An inverse correlation has been observed between the levels of anti–IL-1α antibodies and clinical disease activity.

Biological Functions of Constitutive IL-1α

Primary cells contain constitutive levels of the IL-1α precursor and not IL-1β (45). Most cell lines, including tumor cell lines, contain constitutive levels of IL-1α (35,46,47). It is not surprising that, because the IL-1α precursor is biologically active and found in normal epithelial cells, including thymic epithelium, contents from necrotic cells contain biologically active IL-1α (36). It is well known that contents of necrotic cells are inflammatory, and hence their activity is due to IL-1α present in either the cytosol or the membrane fraction (35). Even if a cell contains the IL-1β precursor, any biological activities of its contents would be due to IL-1α because the IL-1β precursor is inactive (45). Furthermore, epithelial cells do not contain caspase-1, and therefore processing of the IL-1β or IL-18 precursor cannot yield the biologically active form of either cytokine. Therefore, using necrotic cells as a source of inflammation will favor IL-1α activity, not IL-1β or IL-18, because the IL-18 precursor is also inactive. Constitutively expressed IL-1α is critical for several IFNγ activities. In a study with the WISH epithelial cell line, what were considered to be intrinsic IFNγ activities depended largely on constitutively expressed IL-1α. IFNγ activities were inhibited by antibodies to IL-1α but not to IL-1β (47). It was also reported that antibodies to IL-1α and not to IL-1β prevent the biological activities of necrotic cells (36).

Studies in IL-1α–Deficient Mice

Mice deficient in IL-1α are born healthy and develop normally. After subcutaneous injection of turpentine, which induces a local inflammatory response, wild-type and IL-1α–deficient mice develop fever and acute-phase proteins, whereas IL-1β–deficient mice do not (39). In addition, although the induction of glucocorticoids after turpentine injection was suppressed in IL-1β–deficient mice, this suppression was not observed in IL-1α–deficient mice. However, expression of IL-1β mRNA in the brain decreased 1.5-fold in IL-1α–deficient mice, whereas expression of IL-1α mRNA decreased more than 30-fold in IL-1β–deficient mice. These data suggest that IL-1β exerts greater control over production of IL-1α than does IL-1α over the production of IL-1β. In caspase-1–deficient mice, IL-1α production is also reduced (48), suggesting that production of IL-1α is under the control of IL-1β.

The effects of IL-1 on atherogenesis caused by a high-cholesterol diet was evaluated in mice deficient in either IL-1α or IL-1β (43). Serum amyloid A protein, a marker of inflammation in atherogenesis, was markedly lower in IL-1α–deficient mice than in wild-type or IL-1β–deficient mice. IL-1α–deficient mice had significantly higher levels of non–high-density-lipoprotein cholesterol. The beneficial effect of IL-1α deficiency was due to bone marrow cells. Transplantation of bone marrow cells from IL-1α–deficient mice resulted in a reduction in aortic lesion size twice that observed in mice transplanted with IL-1β–deficient bone marrow cells. Therefore, IL-1α appears to play a greater role in the pathogenesis of lipid-mediated atherogenesis than IL-1β, and this may be due to an effect of membrane IL-1α. However, without IL-1α, the nuclear factor function of the IL-1α propiece is also absent.

IL-1F2 (IL-1β)

Processing and Secretion of IL-1β via the Caspase-1 Inflammasome

Inactive pro–caspase-1 is constitutively expressed in macrophagic cells as a primary transcript of 45 kDa requiring two internal cleavages before becoming an enzymatically active heterodimer comprised of a 10- and a 20-kDa chain. The active-site cysteine is located on the 20-kDa chain. Due to alternate RNA splicing, there are five isoforms of human caspase-1 (α, β, γ, δ, and ε); caspase-1α cleaves the caspase-1 precursor as well as the IL-1β precursor. It is presumed that caspase-1β and γ also process precursor caspase-1. In the presence of specific inhibitors of caspase-1, the generation and secretion of mature IL-1β is reduced, and precursor IL-1β accumulates mostly inside the cell. The precursor is also found outside the cell, supporting the concept that precursor IL-1β can be released from a cell independent of processing by caspase-1.

The rate-limiting step in the processing and secretion of active IL-1β takes place in the caspase-1 inflammasome. As shown in Figure 24.1, several intracellular proteins form a complex with cryopyrin, a large protein with a domain of leucine-rich repeats similar to those of TLR, to form the inflammasome. Cryopyrin was initially discovered in patients with familial cold autoinflammatory syndrome, a genetic disease characterized by hives, fevers, and elevated acute-phase proteins after exposure to cold (49). Assembly of the inflammasome components with inactive pro–caspase-1 takes place after a fall in intracellular potassium. ATP activation of the P2X7 receptor opens the potassium channel, and simultaneously, as potassium levels fall, caspase-1 is activated by the inflammasome. As shown in Figure 24.1, the cleavage of the IL-1β precursor by active caspase-1 can take place in the specialized secretory lysosomes or in the cytoplasm. An increase in intracellular calcium is also required for the mature IL-1β to exit the cell.

The function of caspase-1 inflammasome is primarily to convert inactive pro–caspase-1 into the active enzyme. This activation is triggered by the efflux of potassium and is rapidly followed by the appearance of mature IL-1β in the supernatant together with the processed caspase-1. However, a single amino acid mutation in cryopyrin results in activation of caspase-1 without a requirement for a sudden fall in the level of intracellular potassium to activate the inflammasome. Mutated cryopyrin allows for the assembly of the complex of interacting proteins in the presence of normal intracellular levels of potassium. Cells from patients with Muckle-Wells syndrome or neonatal-onset multiinflammatory disease secrete more IL-1β than do cells from healthy controls. Although studied using an exogenous stimulant such as endotoxin, monocyte secretion of IL-1β from these patients is stimulated by endogenous inflammation *in vivo*; in fact, the most likely endogenous stimulant is IL-1β itself.

Any disease process that includes an increase in the steady-state levels of caspase-1, components of the inflammasome, or the IL-1β precursor carries the potential to be an "autoinflammatory" disease. Blocking IL-1β in patients with mutations in cryopyrin is associated with an *in vitro* reduction in the secretion of IL-1β from monocytes when compared to secretion before treatment (50). IL-1β stimulates both its own gene expression and translation of the mRNA into the precursor (51,52).

Effects in Mice Deficient in IL-1β

The IL-1β–deficient mouse has shown no abnormal findings after 10 years of continuous breeding. However, on challenge, IL-1β–deficient mice exhibit specific differences from their wild-type controls. The most dramatic difference is in the response to local inflammation followed by a subcutaneous injection of turpentine. Within the first 24 hours, IL-1β–deficient mice injected with turpentine do not manifest an acute-phase response, do not develop anorexia, have no circulating IL-6, and have no fever (53,54). These findings are consistent with those reported in the same model using anti–IL-1R type I antibodies in wild-type mice (53). IL-1β–deficient mice also have reduced inflammation after zymosan-induced peritonitis (55). Additional studies have also found that IL-1β–deficient mice have elevated febrile responses to LPS, IL-1β, and IL-1α. In contrast, IL-1β–deficient mice have nearly the same responses to LPS as do wild-type mice (56), with some notable exceptions. IL-1β–deficient mice injected with LPS have little or no expression of leptin mRNA or protein (57).

As shown in Table 24.3, in the mouse, IL-1β is critical for local and systemic inflammation. Another characterization of IL-1β deficiency can be seen in relation to body temperature, activity, and feeding during live influenza virus infection. Body temperature and activity were lower in IL-1β–deficient mice (58). The anorexic effect of influenza infection was similar in both groups of mice. The mice deficient in IL-1β exhibited a higher mortality to influenza infection than the wild-type mice. In addition, mice deficient in IL-1α have a brisk inflammatory response to turpentine-induced inflammation, whereas IL-1β deficient mice have nearly no response.

TABLE 24.3 Effects in Interleukin-1β–Deficient Mice

Disease Model	*Effects*
LPS-induced fever	Fever similar to wild type or ↑ fever
LPS-induced leptin	↓ Circulating leptin
LPS-induced hypoglycemia	Normoglycemia
LPS-induced shock lung	No effect on neutrophil infiltration
LPS-induced coagulopathy	Plasminogen activator inhibitor unchanged
Disseminated *Canada albicans*	↓ Peritoneal neutrophils, ↓ superoxide production
Zymosan peritonitis	↓ Inflammation, ↓ mortality, and ↓ IL-6 and chemokines
Turpentine-induced inflammation	↓ Fever, ↓ IL-6; ↓ SAA ↓ cortisone, ↓ COX-2
C protein–induced myositis	↓ Disease severity
IL-1α–induced fever	↑ Fever, ↑ cytokines
B16 melanoma	↓ Hepatic metastasis, ↓ VCAM-1
Brain ischemia–reperfusion	↓ Neuronal death
Model of myasthenia gravis	↓ Disease development
Systemic lupus erythematosus	↓ Anti-dsDNA, ↓ disease severity
Collagen-induced arthritis	↓ Disease severity, ↓CD40 ligand, ↓OX40
Fas-expressing tumors	↓ Neutrophil infiltration
Turpentine-induced coagulopathy	↓ Plasminogen activator inhibitor
Contact hypersensitivity	↓ Langerhans cell activation
Steady-state levels p65 (NFκB)	↓ Levels and nuclear translocation
Delayed type hypersensitivity	↓ Sensitized CD4$^+$ T cells, ↓ proliferation to antigen
Airway hypersensitivity to antigen	↓ Bronchoconstriction, ↓ IgG1 and IgE
Carcinogen-induced tumors	↓ Tumors, ↓ neutrophil infiltration
Injury-induced astrogliosis	↓ Glial fibrillary acid protein
Meniscus model of osteoarthritis	↓ Damage to cartilage
VEGF-mediated neovascularization	↓ Hypoxia-inducible factor-1α, ↓ VEGF, ↓ VEGFR-2

COX-2, cyclooxygenase type 2; dsDNA, double-stranded DNA; Ig, immunoglobulin; IL, interleukin; LPS, lipopolysaccharide; SAA, serum amyloid A; VCAM-1, vascular cell adhesion molecule-1; VEGF, vascular endothelial cell growth factor; VEGFR-2, vascular endothelial cell growth factor receptor-2.

Differences in Carcinogenesis Between IL-1α– and IL-1β–Deficient Mice

Mice deficient in IL-1β were compared to mice deficient in IL-1α in the microenvironment after chemical carcinogenesis (25). In IL-1β–deficient mice, tumors developed more slowly or did not develop in some mice. A deficiency in IL-1α, on the other hand, did not impair tumor development compared to wild-type mice injected with the same carcinogen. In IL-1Ra–deficient mice, tumor development was the most rapid. A leukocyte infiltrate was found at the site of carcinogen injection. The neutrophilic infiltrate was almost absent in IL-1β–deficient mice, whereas in IL-1Ra–deficient mice, a dense neutrophilic infiltrate was observed. In wild-type mice, the leukocytic infiltrate was sparse, and the infiltrate that was observed in IL-1α–deficient mice was similar to that of control mice. These findings may reflect the fact that IL-1β is secreted into the microenvironment, resulting in the emigration of monocytes and neutrophils, whereas IL-1α, which remains cell associated, is less likely to affect the microenvironment. The relationship of neutrophil-derived oxygen radicals and carcinogenesis is known.

IL-1F3 (IL-1Ra)

The IL-1 receptor antagonist (IL-1Ra) was first termed the "IL-1 inhibitor." The "inhibitor" had been reported by several groups (59), but it was Phillipe Seckinger, working in the laboratory of Jean-Michel Dayer, who demonstrated that the inhibitor of IL-1 prevented IL-1 binding to cells. The IL-1 inhibitor was purified to homogeneity, and the amino acid sequence was used to clone the molecule from a monocyte cDNA library (60). The IL-1 inhibitor was renamed the IL-1 receptor antagonist (IL-1Ra), and the generic name anakinra is used for the recombinant form of IL-1Ra. The amino acid sequence of IL-1Ra is more homologous to that of IL-1β than to that of IL-1α. There is only one IL-1Ra gene, but several isoforms exist. Unlike IL-1β, IL-1Ra has a classic leader peptide and is readily secreted. Other forms of IL-1Ra, namely intracellular forms lacking a leader peptide but derived from the same gene, have been reported. When expressed as a mature recombinant molecule, intracellular IL-1Ra blocks IL-1 binding as well as does the secreted form.

The Structural Analysis of the IL-1RI/IL-1Ra Complex

X-ray crystallography reveals that IL-1β has two sites of binding to IL-1RI. IL-1Ra also has two binding sites, which are similar to those of IL-1β. However, one of the binding sites of IL-1Ra binds to IL-1RI with a high affinity such that the second binding site is not available to recruit the IL-1RAcP. After binding of IL-1Ra to IL-1RI–bearing cells, there was no phosphorylation of the epidermal growth factor receptor, a well-established and sensitive assessment of IL-1 signal transduction. Overwhelming evidence that IL-1Ra is a pure receptor antagonist comes from studies of intravenous injection of IL-1Ra into healthy humans. At doses 1 million–fold greater than that of IL-1α or IL-1β, IL-1Ra had no agonist activity in humans (61).

Studies Using IL-1Ra in Animals

Because IL-1Ra exhibits no species specificity, a large body of data exists revealing a role for IL-1 in animal models of disease. As shown in Figure 24.3, when IL-1Ra binds to IL-1RI, there is no formation of the heterodimer with the IL-1RAcP chain, and in the presence of IL-1β, there is no activity. IL-1β can also bind to the IL-1R type II (IL-1RII) either on the cell surface or in the extracellular space. Table 24.4 lists the effect of IL-1Ra in various animal models of disease.

IL-1Ra (Anakinra) Treatment in Humans with Rheumatoid Arthritis

The recombinant form of IL-1Ra is called by the generic name anakinra. There have been several randomized, placebo-controlled, double-blind trials with anakinra in

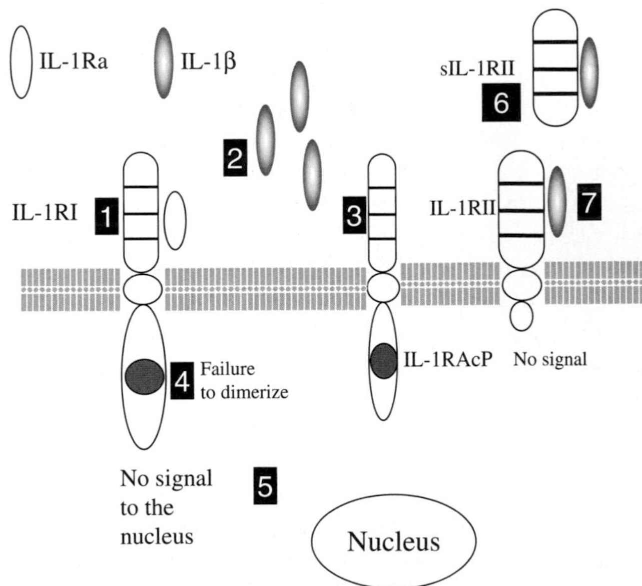

FIGURE 24.3 Events following the binding of IL-1Ra to IL-1RI. The IL-1RI binds IL-1Ra (1). The high-affinity binding of IL-1Ra to IL-1RI prevents the binding of IL-1β to the receptor (2). The complex of IL-1Ra with IL-1RI does not recruit the IL-1RAcP (3), and as a result there is failure for the receptor chains to dimerize (4). Without dimerization, there is no signal to the nucleus (5). In the extracellular compartment, IL-1β can bind to sIL-1RII (6) or cell surface IL-RII (7) and prevent active IL-1β from transmitting a signal.

TABLE 24.4 Effects of IL-1 Receptor Antagonist *in vivo*

Models of live infection
Improved survival, reductions in shock, nitric oxide production, intestinal inflammation and hypoglycemia. Decreased levels of circulating cytokines, insulin-like growth factor–1, thrombin, tissue plasminogen activator, plasminogen activator inhibitor, and elastase.
Models of local and systemic inflammation
Decreased accumulation of neutrophils. Reductions in loss of cartilage proteoglycan.
Decreased pancreatic and hepatic inflammation. Reduced myeloperoxidase levels and cytokines/chemokines.
Models of acute or chronic lung injury
Decreased neutrophil infiltration, eosinophil accumulation, capillary leak, and airway hyperactivity. Prevention of pulmonary fibrosis, hypoxia-induced pulmonary hypertension.
Models of central nervous system injury
Decreased lethality, stress-induced hypothalamic-pituitary axis, astrocytosis, edema, and infarct brain monoamine levels and number of necrotic neurons.
Models of metabolic dysfunction
Reduction in hepatocellular damage, muscle protein breakdown, hyperglycemia, weight loss, and bone loss.
Models of autoimmune diseases
Decreased in severity of experimental allergic encephalomyelitis, systemic lupus, graft versus host disease in mice, islet allograft rejection, contact hypersensitivity, adjuvant arthritis, and streptozotocin-induced diabetes.
Models of malignant disease
Increased survival. Reduction in subcutaneous and metastatic melanoma. Decreased tumor-mediated weight loss. Reduction in colony formation and cytokine production of human acute myelogenous leukemia cells *in vitro*. Reduced spontaneous interleukin-6 and prostaglandin E_2 production in multiple myeloma cells.
Models of angiogenesis
Decreased new blood vessel growth in tumors, reduced neovascularization by vascular endothelial cell growth factor.
Impairment of host responses

rheumatoid arthritis. A dose of 100 mg of anakinra administered subcutaneously daily has been approved in several countries. Due to a short serum half-life—less than 6 hours—daily dosing is effective when assessed by the number of swollen joints, activity, pain score, and C-reactive protein (CRP) levels. A total of 472 patients with severe rheumatoid arthritis were studied in a European multicenter trial (62). The rate of radiologic progression of joint destruction in the patients receiving anakinra was significantly less than in the placebo group at 24 weeks (63). An additional evaluation of these patients revealed a decrease in the rate of progression in erosion and joint space narrowing compared to placebo. These clinical findings are consistent with anakinra blocking the osteoclast-activating factor. Osteoclast activating factor, in fact, is IL-1β (64). In patients who received anakinra, synovial biopsies before and after 24 weeks of daily treatment revealed evidence of decreased cellular infiltration and expression of the adhesion molecules E-selectin and vascular cell adhesion molecule-1 using immunohistochemical techniques (65).

IL-1Ra (Anakinra) Treatment in Type 2 Diabetes

IL-1β was shown to be highly injurious to the insulin-producing pancreatic beta cell (66). High glucose concentrations induce IL-1β production from human beta cells, resulting in impaired insulin secretion, decreased cell proliferation, and beta cell death (67). In a placebo-controlled trial in patients with type 2 diabetes, anakinra treatment for 13 weeks resulted in a significantly lower levels of glycated hemoglobin level compared to the placebo group (3). The blockade of IL-1 was also associated with lower levels of CRP and IL-6.

IL-1Ra (Anakinra) Treatment of Autoinflammatory Diseases

Table 24.1 lists several autoinflammatory diseases that have been treated with anakinra. In most cases, the responses have been rapid and sustained with daily injections. However, because of the short half-life of anakinra, cessation of treatment results in a rapid return of disease activity (50,68). Nevertheless, on restarting treatment, disease activity is again controlled. As stated in the introductory remarks, autoinflammatory diseases are associated with increased secretion of IL-1β from blood monocytes (69–72).

Mice Deficient in IL-1Ra

Mice deficient in IL-1Ra have low litter numbers and exhibit growth retardation in adult life (73). These animals also have elevated basal concentrations of plasma IL-6 and exhibit higher levels of hepatic acute-phase proteins than wild-type control mice. Injection of LPS in

IL-1Ra–deficient mice results in increased lethality. The most dramatic phenotype has been observed in IL-1Ra–deficient mice crossed into a BALB/c background (18). In these mice, a chronic inflammatory polyarthropathy develops spontaneously. The joints show prominent synovial and periarticular infiltration of inflammatory cells, osteoclast activation, and bone erosion. The histologic pattern is similar to that of humans with rheumatoid arthritis. There are elevated levels of rheumatoid factor and anti–double-stranded DNA antibodies. Steady-state levels of COX-2, IL-1RI, IL-1β, IL-6, and TNFα mRNA in the affected joints are also increased. IL-17 is required for IL-1Ra–deficient mice to develop the arthritis (10). The onset of this autoimmune process also requires a genetic background favoring the Th2 response, which produces antibodies rather than cytotoxic T cells in response to antigens. The immunologic stimulus likely occurs when either an endogenous antigen or an antigen from the intestinal flora triggers a Th2 response, which, in the absence of endogenous IL-1Ra, results unopposed IL-1 activities.

IL-1Ra–deficient mice also develop a lethal arterial inflammation involving primary and secondary branch points of the aorta (19). These are stress points in the vessel wall due to blood flow and are also the same locations at which atherosclerotic plaques are commonly found. The lesions are characterized by transmural infiltration of neutrophils, macrophages, and CD4$^+$ T cells. Death is due to vessel wall collapse, stenosis, and organ infarction. Heterozygotes, which have reduced but detectable levels of endogenous IL-1Ra compared to wild-type controls, do not die from this severe arteritis but do develop small arterial lesions.

IL-1F4 (IL-18)

IL-18 is unquestionably a proinflammatory cytokine in the IL-1 family. The tertiary structure of the mature form of IL-18 closely resembles that of IL-1β (74). However, the biology of IL-18 is hardly the recapitulation of IL-1β. There are several unique and specific properties in the biology of IL-18. For example, in healthy human subjects and also in normal mice, gene expression for IL-1β in blood mononuclear cells and hematopoietic tissue is absent, and there is no evidence to suggest that the IL-1β precursor is constitutively present in cells (29). In contrast, in the same blood samples large amounts of the IL-18 precursor are present. Peritoneal macrophages and mouse spleen also contain the precursor in the absence of disease (29).

Together with IL-12, IL-18 participates the T helper-1 (Th1) paradigm. This property of IL-18 is due to its ability to induce IFNγ either with IL-12 or IL-15. Without IL-12 or IL-15, IL-18 does not induce IFNγ. IL-12 or IL-15 upregulates the IL-18 receptor β chain (IL-18Rβ), which is essential for IL-18 signal transduction. Without IL-12 or IL-15, IL-18 plays a role in Th2 diseases (12). The role of IL-18 in the Th17 responses is unclear, but, being an inducer of IFNγ, IL-18 likely contributes to the actions of Th17 cells. Several IL-18–linked diseases are associated with elevated levels of IFNγ. Indeed, the original description of IL-18 was "IFNγ inducing factor." Diseases such as systemic lupus erythematosus, macrophage activation syndrome, rheumatoid arthritis, type 1 diabetes, Crohn's disease, psoriasis, and graft versus host disease are believed to be mediated, in part, by IL-18.

Like IL-1β, IL-18 is initially synthesized as an inactive precursor (molecular weight 24,000) and requires caspase 1 cleavage for processing into a mature molecule of molecular weight 18,000 (Figure 24.2). After an injection of endotoxin, caspase 1–deficient mice do not have circulating IFNγ (75). IL-12–induced IFNγ is also caspase 1 dependent (76), again suggesting that microbial toxins (via TLR) require IL-18 for IFNγ production. In general, processing of the IL-18 precursor is caspase-1 dependent, but exceptions exist. For example, Fas ligand stimulation results in the release of biologically active IL-18 in caspase 1–deficient murine macrophages (77). Similar to IL-1β processing, proteinase–3 appears to activate processing to mature IL-18 (17).

IL-18–Binding Protein

The discovery of the IL-18–binding protein (IL-18BP) took place during the search for the soluble receptors for IL-18 in human urine (78). IL-18BP is a constitutively secreted protein with exceptional affinity to IL-18 (400 pM) (Figure 24.6). There is limited amino acid sequence homology between IL-18BP and cell-surface IL-18 receptors; IL-18BP lacks a transmembrane domain and contains only one Ig-like domain (79). Present in the serum of healthy humans at a 20-fold molar excess compared to IL-18 (80), IL-18BP may contribute to a default mechanism by which a Th1 response to foreign organisms is blunted to reduce triggering an autoimmune responses to a routine infection. IL-18BP is a naturally occurring, specific inhibitor of IL-18, neutralizing IL-18 activities. A clinical preparation of human IL-18BP has been shown to be safe in patients (81). Other options for reducing IL-18 activities include inhibitors of capsase-1, human monoclonal antibodies to IL-18, soluble IL-18 receptors, and anti–IL-18 receptor monoclonal antibodies.

Natural neutralization of human IL-18 by IL-18BP takes place during a common viral infection. In *Molluscum contagiosum*, characterized by raised but bland eruptions, there are large numbers of viral particles in the epithelial cells of the skin, but histologically there are few inflammatory or immunologically active cells in or near the lesions. Clearly, the virus fails to elicit an inflammatory or immunologic response. Amino acid similarity exists between human IL-18BP and a gene found in various members of the poxviruses, the greatest of which is found to be expressed in *Molluscum contagiosum* (82). The ability of viral IL-18BP to reduce the activity of mammalian IL-18 likely explains the lack of inflammatory and immune cells in the infected individual and provides further evidence for the natural ability of IL-18BP to interfere with IL-18 activity.

IL-18, Hyperphagia, and the Metabolic Syndrome

Starting at age 16 weeks, IL-18–deficient mice overeat, become obese, and exhibit lipid abnormalities, increased atherosclerosis, insulin resistance, and diabetes mellitus reminiscent of the metabolic syndrome (83). The higher body weight is attributed to enhanced food intake, which starts to diverge from those of wild-type animals at a relatively early age and reaches values of 30% to 40% higher than that of wild type mice. A striking finding was an increase of more than 100% in the percentage of adipose tissue in the IL-18–deficient animals, which was accompanied by fat deposition in the arterial walls. The insulin resistance was corrected by exogenous recombinant IL-18. Mice deficient in IL-18 respond normally to a challenge with exogenous leptin, suggesting that a unique mechanism is responsible for the higher food intake in the IL-18–deficient animals.

IL-1F5

IL-1F5 shares 47% amino acid identity with IL-1Ra and is expressed in human monocytes activated by LPS. From the gene sequence, the predicted amino acid sequence of IL-1F5 does not have a leader peptide for secretion, which is in sharp contrast to the IL-1Ra (IL-1F3). IL-1F5 failed to exhibit agonist activity using induction of IL-6 from fibroblasts, a well-described biological property of IL-1α and IL-1β (84). Furthermore, IL-1F5 did not block the IL-1α– or IL-1β–induced IL-6– or IL-18–induced production of IFNγ (84). Therefore, IL-1F5 possesses neither IL-1– or IL-18–like agonist activities nor the property to act as a receptor antagonist for IL-1, despite it close amino acid identity to IL-1Ra.

It appears, however, that IL-1F5 functions as an anti-inflammatory member of the IL-1 family. IL-1F5 induces IL-4, which can reduce IL-1 activity. The anti-inflammatory effects of IL-1F5 include downregulating the responses to IL-1β as well as LPS; in mice deficient in IL-4, IL-1F5 is less effective as an antiinflammatory cytokine (85). The ability of IL-1F5 to dampen inflammation is via its interaction with the single immunoglobulin IL-1–related receptor (SIGIRR), also known as Toll-IL-1-receptor-8 (TIR8). SIGIRR is an orphan member of the IL-1 family of receptors, and in mice deficient in SIGIRR, there is more inflammation than in wild-type control mice (85).

IL-1F6

IL-1F6 is a proinflammatory member of the IL-1 family. The cytokine binds to the IL-1R–related protein (IL-1Rrp2) as its ligand-binding chain and recruits the IL-1 receptor accessory protein (IL-1RAcP) to form the heterodimer. High levels of IL-1F6 are found in mouse embryonic tissues rich in epithelial cells (86). In humans, IL-1F6 is observed in keratinocytes but not fibroblasts, but it is believed to contribute to the inflammation of psoriasis. On forming the heterodimer with IL-1Rrp2 and IL-1RAcP, IL-1F6 activates NFκB, similar to IL-1β (87). In addition to NFκB activation, IL-1F6 also activates mitogen-activated protein kinase, c-Jun N-terminal kinase, and extracellular signal-related kinase (ERK) 1/2 (87).

IL-1F7

Although IL-1F7 (formerly IL-1H4) is structurally related to IL-1Ra (36%), this IL-1 family member binds to the IL-18 receptor α chain and therefore has attracted attention as being related to IL-18 (88). IL-1F7 has no leader peptide, and the recombinant form has been expressed with a N-terminus from a predicted caspase-1 site (89). There are two forms of IL-1F7: a full-length peptide and a splice variant with an internal 40–amino acid deletion (88). The binding of IL-1F7 to the soluble IL-18R α chain has also been observed. However, in contrast to IL-18, recombinant IL-1F7 does not induce IFNγ in whole human blood cultures, in PBMCs, or in various cell lines. Therefore, it is unlikely that IL-1F7 is a true agonist for the IL-18 receptor. In other studies, IL-1F7 bound to a recombinant form of the extracellular domains (soluble) of the IL-18 receptor α chain linked to the Fc of IgG but not to the extracellular domains (soluble) of the IL-1 type I receptor or ST2 (see later discussion) (90). Although IL-1F7 binds to the IL-18 receptor α chain, IL-1F7 is not a receptor antagonist for IL-18. When injected directly into murine tumors, adenovirus expressing IL-1F7 there was a significant reduction in tumor growth (91). The antitumor effects of IL-1F7 was diminished in mice deficient in IL-12, IFNγ, or Fas ligand (91).

IL-1F7 also binds to the IL-18–binding protein (IL-18BP) (92). This may be due to the similarities of IL-18BP to the third domain of the IL-18 receptor α chain. On formation of a complex with IL-18BP, there is decrease in IL-18 activity. In fact, there is increased inflammation in mice deficient in the IL-18 receptor α chain, whereas there is less inflammation in mice deficient in IL-18 itself (20). It is possible that IL-1F7 delivers a negative signal via the

IL-18 receptor α chain. In mice with experimental allergic encephalomyelitis, a deficiency in the IL-18 receptor α chain results in the opposite outcome to that in mice deficient in IL-18 (21). In the two studies, the investigators came to the conclusion that IL-18 receptor α chain binds another ligand in addition to IL-18 and that this ligand may be IL-1F7.

IL-1F8

The receptor for IL-1F8 is IL-1Rrp-2 (IL-1R6) and is expressed on human synovial fibroblasts and human articular chondrocytes. In response to stimulation by recombinant IL-1F8, there is increased production of proinflammatory mediators (93). Although IL-1F8 steady-state mRNA is constitutive in chondrocytes, the cytokine is inducible by IL-1β in synovial fibroblasts. Circulating levels of IL-1F8 patients with rheumatoid arthritis, osteoarthritis, or septic shock were similar to those in healthy subjects. It unclear what role extent IL-1F8 plays in joint disease, although constitutive expression in primary chondrocytes may indicate a role for the cytokine in osteoarthritis.

IL-1F9

IL-1F9 is constitutively expressed primarily in the placenta and the squamous epithelium of the esophagus. The three-dimensional folding of IL-1F9 is similar to that of IL-1Ra; nevertheless, IL-1F9 is a proinflammatory cytokine binding to IL-1Rrp2 and recruiting the IL-1RAcP. IL-1F9 triggers the same kinase cascade and NFκB as IL-1F6 (see previous discussion).

IL-1F10

IL-1F10 shares 37% amino acid identity with the IL-1Ra and a similar three-dimensional structure (94). This cytokine is secreted from cells and is expressed in human skin, spleen, and tonsil. Recombinant IL-1F10 has been shown to bind to the isolated extracellular domains IL-1 receptor type I, but it is unclear whether IL-1F10 binds to complete cell surface–bound IL-1 receptors. Although these data suggest that IL-1F10 is likely to be a receptor antagonist (95), compared to IL-1Ra, its role in health and disease is unclear.

IL-1F11

IL-1F11 is also known as IL-33. This new member of the IL-1 family requires caspase-1 processing and signals through the T1/ST2 receptor (15). ST2 is also termed the IL-33 receptor α chain (IL-33Rα). Activation of ST2, formerly an orphan member of the IL-1 receptor family for 16 years, drives T helper type 2 (Th2) responses. The new cytokine, IL-33, is the specific ligand for ST2. In 1994, the receptor termed ST2 was first reported as regulated by the estrogen-inducible transcription factor Fos (96). This receptor was very similar to the IL-1 receptor type I and the IL-18 receptor α chain in that ST2 also has three extracellular Ig domains and an intracellular Toll domain (Figure 24.3). Despite a search for its cognate ligand, there was never a convincingly specific candidate; it was always assumed, however, that the ligand for ST2 would be a member of the IL-1 family. IL-33 recapitulates much of the existing data that ST2 promotes Th2-type responses. IL-33 is identical to a nuclear factor primarily expressed in high endothelial venules (NF-HEV) (97), suggesting that, similar to IL-1α (35), IL-33 acts as a proinflammatory cytokine by binding to ST2 as well as a nuclear factor and regulates transcription (97).

There is no dearth of studies on ST2 tissue-specific localization, regulation of its expression, and its effects in transgenic mice overexpressing ST2, as well as on deletion, neutralization, and antibody cross-linking of ST2. Elevated levels of the soluble form of ST2 were present in the circulation of patients with various inflammatory diseases, and exogenous administration of pharmacologic doses of soluble ST2 neutralized the putative ligand and reduced inflammation (98). Furthermore, several studies suggested that whatever the ligand is for this orphan receptor, it plays a role in allergic-type diseases because activation of ST2 uniquely drives Th2 responses. Structurally, IL-33 is closest to IL-18 rather than IL-1β. The dominant property of IL-33 is the induction of IL-4, IL-5, and IL-13 in addition to properties anticipated for a Th2-type cytokine. Diseases believed to be due to increased immunoglobulin production may also be related to IL-33. IL-33 induces the production of IL-6, IL-1β, and PGE from mast cells.

Mice injected with human IL-33 exhibit impressive pathologic changes in the arterial walls, lungs, and intestinal tissues (15). Of particular relevance to the concept that IL-33 drives a Th2 response is that esosinophilic infiltration was a prominent finding in the lung. Although the interpretation of *in vivo* effects after the administration of an exogenous cytokine should be conservative, the findings are clearly consistent with IL-33 being a proinflammatory ligand of the IL-1 receptor family. Even before researchers had the ability to test IL-33–mediated activation, others had reported that neutralization of the putative ST2 ligand using soluble ST2 markedly reduced joint inflammation, synovial hyperplasia, and joint erosion when given in the therapeutic phase of collagen-induced arthritis in mice (98). Moreover, it appears that organs with high numbers of mast cells appear to undergo dramatic changes on injection of IL-33 into mice. Consistent with a role in allergic diseases, IL-33 induces the cytokines IL-5 and IL-13 *in vivo*, known contributors of allergic diseases. Mice deficient in ST2 do not develop a Th2 response to *Schistosoma* egg antigen.

It remains unclear how IL-33 favors the Th2 response. Similar to IL-1β, IL-33 induces IL-6, which is an adjuvant for antibody production. IL-33 signal transduction requires a coreceptor for biological activities, and similar to IL-1, IL-33 uses the IL-1 receptor accessory protein. IL-33 induction of IL-6 is prevented by a blocking antibody to IL-1RAcP (99). IL-33 initiates signal transduction via activation of NFκB, which is typical of IL-1α, IL-1β, and IL-18 (15), but other studies have shown that antibody cross-linking of ST2 does not result in activation of NFκB but instead that of AP-1. There are also studies that IL-33 has antiinflammatory properties by inhibiting angiotensin II–induced phosphorylation of IκB in cardiac fibroblasts (100). ST2 can sequester TLR adaptor molecules such as MyD88 and Mal (101).

The idea of IL-33 as a member of the IL-1 ligand family gains considerable legitimacy because processing of the IL-33 precursor is accomplished by caspase-1 (15), similar to IL-1β and IL-IL-18. It is possible that lack of processing IL-33 into an active cytokine may contribute to the protection afforded caspase-1–deficient mice. From the first report of the existence of ST2 (96), a high level of expression of this receptor on mast cells has been a prominent finding. The Th2 response favors antibody production, including IgE and IgG.

IL-1 RECEPTOR FAMILY

The IL-1 receptor family encodes 10 members, some of which are orphan receptors. As shown in Figure 24.3, most belong to the group containing three IgG-like segments for the extracellular domain of the receptor. In general, the extracellular domains of these receptors can be cleaved from the cell surface by proteases; they are then termed "soluble" receptors. Soluble receptors can serve two functions: By binding to the ligand, they can neutralize the activity of the ligand, but they can also act as ligand carriers. Although most soluble receptors are generated by proteolytic cleavage from the cell surface receptors, this is apparently not the mechanism for high levels of soluble IL-1RAcP (sIL-1RAcP) (102). sIL-1RAcP forms a complex with IL-1β and sIL-1RII and is an effective mechanism for neutralization of IL-1β activity (103). Constitutive secretion of sIL-1RAcP accounts for its high serum levels. Supporting this concept is the existence of a splice variant of the IL-1RAcP that lacks a transmembrane anchor. Once synthesized, sIL-1RAcP is released by the liver as an acute-phase protein, as is IL-1Ra (104). As shown in Figure 24.4, sIL-1RAcP forms a complex of IL-1β with sIL-1RII in the extracellular space. Thus, a large molar excess of sIL-1RAcP provides at least three mechanisms by which to neutralize secreted IL-1β.

Table 24.5 summarizes the IL-1 receptor family and their functions (105). IL-1R1, IL-1R2, and IL-1R3 are the bona fide receptors for IL-1α and IL-1β. IL-1R4, also known as ST2, is no longer an orphan receptor because IL-33 binds to this receptor (15). Before the identification of IL-33 as the ligand for ST2, a number of studies had examined the function, distribution, and gene regulation of this receptor, particularly on mast cells (106). IL-1R5 was formerly an orphan receptor termed IL-1R–related protein–1 (107), but it was subsequently discovered to be the ligand-binding (α) chain of the IL-18 receptor (108), now termed IL-18Rα.

The IL-1R–related protein–2 (IL-1R6) is the receptor for the agonists IL-1F6, IL-1F8, and IL-1F9, but is also the receptor for IL-1F5, which is the antagonist for IL-1F9 (86,105). IL-1R7, formerly the non–ligand-binding chain of the IL-18 receptor termed IL-1RAcPL (109), is now named IL-18Rβ chain. Similar to the IL-1R–AcP, the IL-18Rβ is essential for IL-18 signal transduction (109,110).

Two members of the IL-1 receptor family are particularly singular in that they are found on the X chromosome. These are IL-1R8 and IL-1R9, both homologous to IL-1RAcP and IL-18Rβ. IL-1R9 is highly homologous to IL-1R8. Both forms have no known ligands, and the receptors are found in the fetal brain. Nonoverlapping deletions and a nonsense mutation in the IL-1R8 gene were found in patients with cognitive impairment (111), in which expression in the adult hippocampal area may play a role in memory or learning. The cytoplasmic domains of IL-1R8 and IL-1R9 are longer than the other accessory chains. The IL-1R9 may function as a negative receptor. This was shown in cells overexpressing this receptor in addition to IL-1RI and IL-1RAcP, in which IL-1β signaling was blocked with a specific antibody to IL-1RAcP. In the presence of the antibody, IL-1β–induced luciferase was suppressed, suggesting that a possible complex of the type I receptor with IL-1β plus IL-1R9 results in a negative signal (112).

Single Ig IL-1 Related Receptor

Single Ig IL-1 related receptor (SIGIRR) is a negative regulator of both IL-1α and IL-1β activities and also of TLR agonists. Although there is only a single IgG domain for the extracellular segment, the cytoplasmic domain contains a Toll domain and has the longest cytoplasmic domain of all the members of the IL-1 receptor family (Figure 24.5). Initially, SIGIRR was thought to be expressed primarily in kidney, lung, and gastrointestinal tract, primarily in resting epithelial cells. However, SIGIRR is also expressed in human monocytes and mouse macrophages in response to the stresses associated with infection and transient hypoxia. Dendritic cells also express SIGIRR (113). In a study of patients resuscitated from cardiac arrest, the peripheral monocytes displayed increased steady-state levels of SIGIRR, which were associated with increased gene

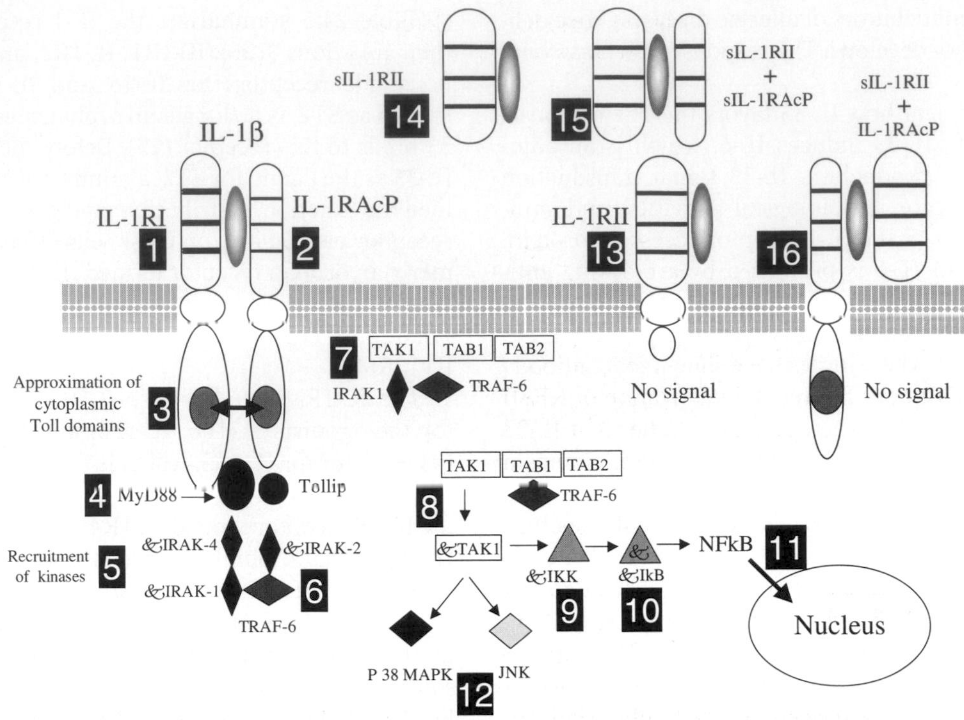

FIGURE 24.4 IL-1 signal transduction and decoy receptors. IL-1β binding to the IL-1RI (1) recruits the IL-1RAcP (2) to form a heterodimeric receptor (1 + 2). The cytoplasmic Toll domains on each receptor chain approximate (3). MyD88 and Tollip are recruited (4). MyD88 binding to the cytoplasmic domains triggers the phosphorylations of the IL-1–receptor associated kinases IRAK-4, IRAK-2, and IRAK-1 (5). TRAF-6 is recruited (6). Phosphorylated IRAK-1 and TRAF-6 migrate to the membrane and associate with TAK-1, TAB1, and TBA2 (7). The complex of TAK-1, TAB1, TAB 2, and TRAF-6 migrates to the cytosol, where TAK-1 is phosphorylated following the ubiquination of TRAF-6 (8). Phosphorylated TAK-1 activates IKKβ (9), and phosphorylated IKKβ phosphorylates IκB (10). Phosphorylated IκB degrades, releasing NFκB, which enters the nucleus (11). In addition to the phosphorylation of IKKβ, TAK-1 also activates MAPK p38 and JNK (12). On the surface of the cell, IL-1RII, a decoy receptor, may also bind IL-1β (13), but this complex does not recruit IL-1RAcP, and there is no signal. In the extracellular space, the extracellular domains (soluble or sIL-1RII) of the IL-1RII bind IL-1β and neutralize its activity (14). sIL-1RII can also bind IL-1β and form a complex with soluble IL-1RAcP (15) or cell-bound IL-1RAcP (16). In the latter two complexes, IL-1β is not available to bind to IL-1RI and therefore cannot transmit a signal.

expression for the antiinflammatory cytokine IL-10 and a decrease expression for TNFα. In microglia of mice infected with murine leukemia virus, a gene array of 14,000 genes revealed that only 3 genes were differentially expressed between the virulent and nonvirulent strains of the viruses, and one of these genes was SIGIRR (114).

With overexpression of SIGIRR in the form of a chimeric molecule with IL-1RAcP, suppression of

TABLE 24.5 The Interleukin-1 (IL-1) Receptor Family

Name	*Designation*	*Ligands*	*Coreceptor*
IL-1RI	IL-1R1	IL-1α, IL-1β, IL-1Ra	IL-1RAcP (IL-1R3)
IL-1RII	IL-1R2	IL-1β, IL-1β precursor	IL-1RAcP (IL-1R3)
ST2/Fit-1	IL-1 R4 (IL-33Rα)	IL-33	IL-1RAcP (IL-1R3)
IL-18Rα	IL-1R5	IL-18, IL-1F7	IL-18Rβ (IL-1R7)
IL-1Rrp-2	IL-1R6	IL-1F6, IL-1F8, IL-1F9	IL-1RAcP (IL-1R3)
TIGIRR-2/IL-1RAPL	IL-1R8	Unknown	Unknown
TIGIRR-1	IL-1R9	Unknown	Unknown
SIGIRR	TIR8	Unknown	Unknown

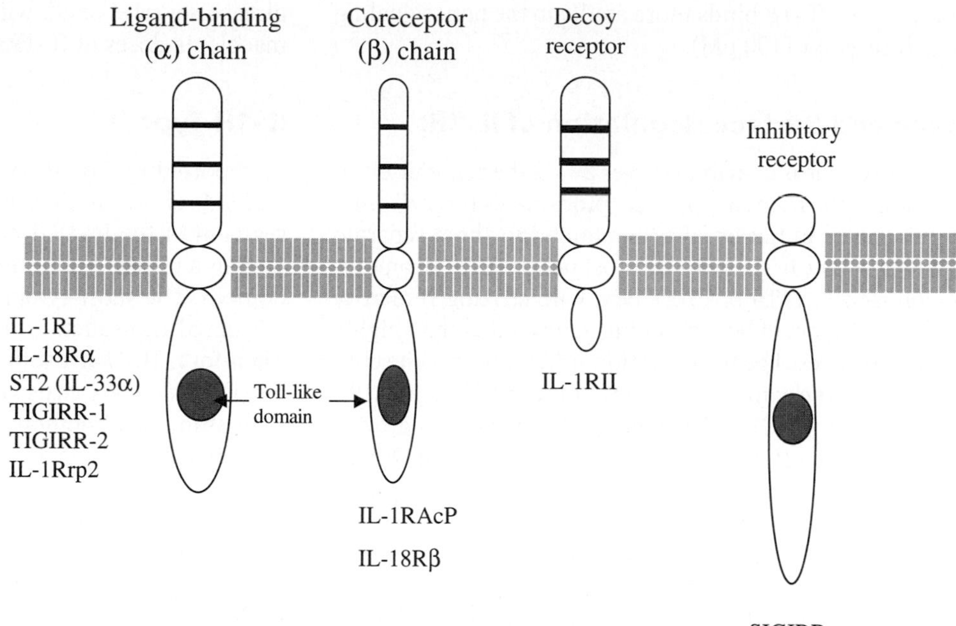

FIGURE 24.5 IL-1 family of receptors.

IL-1–driven NFκB was observed. SIGIRR inhibition of IL-1–driven NFκB does not require the presence of the extracellular domain of SIGIRR. The complex of IL-1 with IL 1RAcP activates NFkB, but in the presence of SIGIRR there is suppression of the response. In another study, inhibition of IL-1 activity required the extracellular single Ig domain of SIGIRR (115). The mechanism for suppression of the IL-1 responses in cells overexpressing SIGIRR is one of competitive inhibition of MyD88, such that there is no activation of IRAK or TRAF-6 (115). The inhibition of MyD88, IRAK, and TRAF-6 by SIGIRR is not due to the formation of complex with IL-1RAcP or IL-1RI. Overexpression of SIGIRR results in inhibition of LPS and IL-1 activities, whereas mice deficient in SIGIRR exhibit heightened inflammation. Mice deficient in SIGIRR develop a more severe disease in response to LPS or chronic colitis (113,116). Overexpression of SIGRR in 293 cells inhibits both IL-1– and IL-18–induced NFκB reporter activity but not IFNγ activity (116). Splenocytes from mice deficient in SIGRR produce severalfold greater levels of the mouse chemokines KC and MIP–2 and IFN-inducible protein 10 after LPS. In a model of live *Pseudomonas* keratitis, a blocking antibody to SIGIRR resulted in increased bacterial counts and increased steady-state mRNA levels of IL-1β, IL-18, and IL-18 (117). Overexpression of SIGIRR in macrophages resulted in decreased mRNA levels for IL-1RI, IFNγ, IL-12, and IL-IL-18. Thus SIGIRR downregulates the responses to IL-1 and TLR4.

IL-1 Receptor Type I

There is considerable amino acid homology between IL-1RI and IL-1RAcP in extracellular domains. IL-1RAcP does not bind IL-1 itself, but instead it "wraps around" the complex of IL-1:IL-1RI. As shown by X-ray crystallization studies, IL-1RI exhibits a conformational change when binding IL-1β, and apparently this shape change allows the IL-1RAcP to form the heterodimer (Figure 24.4). The cytoplasmic domain of IL-1RI is unique in that it contains homology to the *Drosophila* Toll protein. The area of homology is termed Toll-IL-1-receptor (TIR) domain. TIR domain is also found in the cytoplasmic domains of each TLR. The TIR domain of IL-1RI is necessary for signal transduction. The TIR domain of the coreceptor IL 1RAcP is also essential for IL-1 activity. Although most cells express IL-1RI constitutively, expression of IL-1RAcP is not constitutive in some cells.

In general, IL-1-responsiveness is more a reflection of receptor expression than ligand binding (118). The failure to show specific and saturable IL-1 binding to cells is often due to the low numbers of surface IL-1RI on primary cells. In cell lines, the number of IL-1RIs can reach 5,000 per cell, but primary cells usually express less than 200 receptors per cell. In some primary cells there are less than 50 per cell, and IL-1 signal transduction has been observed in cells expressing less than 10 type I receptors per cell.

Human IL-1α binds to cell surface and sIL-1RI with approximately the same affinity (100 to 300 pM) as does IL-1Ra. If one examines the binding of IL-1Ra, the affinity is even higher than that of IL-1α. IL-1Ra avidly binds to the surface type I receptor (50 to 100 pM). Of the three members of the IL-1 family (IL-1α, IL-1β, and IL-1Ra), IL-1β has the lowest affinity for the cell-bound form of IL-1RI (500 pM to 1 nM). The greatest binding affinity of the three IL-1 ligands for IL-1RI is IL-1Ra. In fact, the off-rate is slow, and binding of IL-1Ra to cell-bound IL-1RI is nearly irreversible. Compared to IL-1Ra, IL-1α binds to IL-1RI with affinities ranging from 100 to 300 pM. By comparison, IL-1β binds more avidly to the non–signaling type II receptor (100 pM).

Gene and Surface Regulation of IL-1RI

The entire gene is distributed over 29 kb; the genomic organization of the human type I receptor reveals three distinct transcription initiation sites contained in three separate segments of the first exon. The most proximal (5′) promoter region lacks a TATA or CAAT box, with striking similarity to the promoters of housekeeping genes rather than highly regulated genes. The transcription initiation start site contains nearly the same motif as that for the TdT gene (119). Phorbol esters, PGE_2, dexamethasone, epidermal growth factor, IL-2, and IL-4 increase surface expression of IL-1RI. In cells that synthesize PGE_2, IL-1 upregulates its own receptor via PGE_2; however, when PGE_2 synthesis is inhibited, IL-1 downregulates IL-1RI in the same cells. Part of the immunosuppressive properties of TGFβ may be due to downregulation of the IL-1RI on T cells. Despite the housekeeping nature of its promoters, IL-1RI is regulated in the context of inflammation and immune responses.

Studies in IL-1RI–Deficient Mice

Mice deficient in IL-1RI develop normally and exhibit no particular phenotype, similar to that observed in IL-1α– or IL-1β–deficient mice. When given a turpentine abscess, IL-1RI–deficient mice exhibited an attenuated inflammatory response compared with wild-type mice. Delayed-type hypersensitivity responses are reduced in IL-1RI–deficient mice. IL-1RI–deficient mice are susceptible to infection with *Listeria monocytogenes*. Lymphocytes from IL-1RI–deficient mice with major cutaneous leishmanial infection produced more IL-4 and IL-10 but less IFNγ than did those from wild-type mice. Although IL-1α is constitutively expressed in the skin, the barrier function of skin remains intact in mice deficient in IL-1RI (120). Cells deficient in IL-1RAcP have normal binding of IL-1α and IL-1Ra (binding to the IL-1RI being intact in these mice) but a 70% reduction in binding of IL-1β (121). In these cells, there is no biological response to IL-1α, despite binding of IL-1α to the type I receptor. The results suggest that IL-1RAcP and not IL-1RI is required for IL-1β binding and biological response to IL-1.

Mice injected with LPS have been studied. IL-1RI–deficient mice exhibit the same decrease in hepatic lipase as wild-type mice. Mice deficient in IL-1RI did not develop trabecular bone loss after ovariectomy compared to wild-type controls (122). Mice deficient in IL-1RI failed to develop inflammatory lesions of in the central nervous system or evidence of clinical EAE. Although cells from IL-1RAcP–deficient mice bound IL-1α, there was no activation of genes dependent on NFκB or activator protein-1 (121). In general, mice deficient in IL-1RI exhibit reduced disease severity, as do wild-type mice injected with pharmacologic doses of IL-1Ra.

IL-1R Type II

As reported by Colotta et al., IL-1RII is a decoy receptor (123). As shown in Figures 24.3 and 24.4, the extracellular segment of the IL-1RII has three typical Ig-like domains; there is a transmembrane segment but a short cytoplasmic domain. The short cytoplasmic domain is unable to initiate signal transduction because there is no TIR domain. Therefore, IL-1RII captures IL-1 without signaling. Vaccinia and cowpox virus genes encode for a protein with a high amino acid homology to the extracellular or soluble domains of sIL-1RII. The viral form of the sIL-1RII serves to reduce the inflammatory and immune response of the host to the virus. In humans, sIL-1RII is released from the cell surface by a protease; sIL-1RII has a particularly high affinity for mature IL-1β and therefore functions as a naturally occurring neutralization mechanism for IL-1β.

IL-1β binding to the sIL-1RII is nearly irreversible. The precursor form of IL-1β also preferentially binds to sIL-1RII. A more efficient function of the type II receptor is to form a trimeric complex of the IL-1β with sIL-1RII and the IL-1RAcP chain (124). This mechanism serves to deprive the cell of both IL-1β and a functional receptor accessory chain. As shown in Figure 24.4, the type II receptor participates in four different complexes to deprive the cell of a response to IL-1β.

Modulation of IL-1 Activity by IL-1RII

The type II receptor is selectively expressed on macrophages, B lymphocytes, and chondrocytes. For example, B lymphocytes express 20-fold more type II receptors than type I receptors, but in T lymphocytes, this ratio is only 5-fold. Relevant to IL-1–mediated cartilage breakdown and inhibition of proteoglycan synthesis, chondrocytes express an excess of type II receptors. As shown in Figure 24.4, sIL-1RAcP forms complexes on the cell surface of IL-1β bound to type II receptors and accounts for the ability of sIL-1RAcP to reduce B lymphocyte activation (125). sIL-1RAcP inhibits IL-1–induced NFκB activity in B cells but not T cells, whereas IL-1Ra inhibited IL-1 on both cell types (126). sIL-1RAcP inhibits IL-1 signaling on cells expressing either low levels of membrane IL-1RAcP or high levels of IL-1RII.

sIL-1RI

The administration of the extracellular domain of the type I receptor (sIL-1RI) has been used in models of inflammatory and autoimmune disease. Administration of murine sIL-1RI to mice increased the survival of heterotopic heart allografts, reduced the hyperplasic lymph node response to allogeneic cells, and inhibited responses to LPS, acute lung injury, and delayed-type hypersensitivity. In the accelerated model of autoimmune diabetes induced by cyclophosphamide in the nonobese diabetic mouse, repeated injections with sIL-1RI protected the mice from insulin-dependent diabetes mellitus in a dose- dependent fashion. sIL-1RI may act as ligand carrier. In mice, intravenous injection of sIL-1RI alone induced a rapid increase in circulating IL-1α but not of TNFα or IL-1β (127). This observation is consistent with the view that sIL-1RI acts as a carrier for IL-1α.

Effect of IL-1sRI in Humans

Recombinant human sIL-1RI has been administered intravenously to healthy humans without side effects or changes in physiologic, hematologic, or endocrinologic parameters. Thus, similar to infusions of IL-1Ra, administration of sIL-1RI reinforces the conclusion that IL-1 does not have a role in homeostasis in humans. sIL-1RI has also been injected into humans in an attempt to reduce the systemic responses to experimental endotoxin. There were no effects on fever or systemic symptoms (128). In contrast to sIL-1RI, pretreatment of subjects with IL-1Ra prior to intravenous endotoxin resulted in a statistically significant decrease (40%) in circulating neutrophils (129). High doses of sIL-1RI were associated with higher levels of circulating TNFα and IL-8 as well as cell-associated IL-1β (128). Although there was a decrease in the level of circulating IL-1β compared to placebo-treated subjects, there was also a 43-fold decrease in the level of circulating IL-1Ra ($p <$ 0.001) due to complexing of sIL-1RI with endogenous IL-1Ra. These results support the *in vitro* binding data showing that sIL-1RI binds IL-1Ra and reduces the biological effectiveness of this natural IL-1 receptor antagonist in inhibiting IL-1.

sIL-1RI was administered subcutaneously to patients with active rheumatoid arthritis in a randomized, double-blind study (130). Similar to the placebo-treated patients, lower doses of the soluble receptor did not result in improvement. Despite the lack of clinical improvement, cell surface monocyte IL-1α expression in patients receiving sIL-1RI was significantly reduced. Other parameters of altered immune function in common in patients with rheumatoid arthritis also showed reduction. One possible explanation for the lack of clinical response despite efficacy in suppressing immune responses could be the inhibition of endogenous IL-1Ra. A trial of sIL-1RI was conducted in patients with relapsed and refractory acute myeloid leukemia (131). Serum levels of IL-1β, IL-6, and TNFα did not change. The goal of any anti–IL-1 strategy is to prevent IL-1 binding to surface receptors. The disadvantage of sIL-sRI therapy is the possibility that these receptors will either prolong the clearance of IL-1 or bind the natural IL-1Ra.

The soluble form of IL-1RI and IL-1RII circulate in healthy humans at molar concentrations that are 10- to 50-fold greater than those of IL-1β measured in septic patients and 100–fold greater than the concentration of IL-1β after intravenous administration (132). Why do humans have a systemic response to an infusion of IL-1α (133) or IL-1β? One concludes that binding of IL-1 to the soluble forms of IL-1R types I and II exhibits a slow "on" rate compared to cell-bound IL-1RI.

IL-1 SIGNAL TRANSDUCTION

Binding of IL-1 to IL-1RI

This section examines signaling pathways following the binding of either IL-1α or IL-1β to IL-1RI; most of the structural analysis between IL-1 and IL-1RI is based on the binding of IL-1β. Once IL-1β binds to IL-1 RI, the distal first domain folds over IL-1β, and this exposes sites in the ligand that bind IL-1RAcP. Only after the formation of IL-1RI/IL-1β does IL-1RAcP join the complex and is high-affinity binding observed (Figure 24.4). Therefore, IL-1 binds to the IL-1RI with a low affinity, causing a structural change in the ligand followed by recognition by the IL-1RAcP. Antibodies to either IL-1RI or IL-1RAcP block IL-1 activity, supporting the concept that both chains, IL 1RI and IL-1RAcP, are needed for activity. Whereas most cells express surface IL-1RI, in IL-1-responsive cells, one assumes that there is also expression of IL-1RAcP.

Of special consideration to the study of IL-1 signal transduction is the unusual discrepancy between the low number of receptors (fewer than10 in some cells) and the low concentrations of IL-1 (10 pM) that induce a biological response. In primary cells, the number of IL-1RIs is low (fewer than 100 per cell), and a biological response occurs when only as few as 2% to 3% of IL-1RI receptors are occupied. An extensive "amplification" step(s) takes place following the initial post–receptor-binding event. The most likely mechanism for signal amplification is multiple and sequential phosphorylations (or dephosphorylations) of kinases.

Characteristics of the Cytoplasmic Domains of the IL-1RI and IL-1RacP

The cytoplasmic domains of the IL-1RI or IL-1RAcP do not contain a consensus sequence for intrinsic tyrosine phosphorylation, but deletion mutants of the receptor reveal specific functions of some domains. For example, there are four nuclear localization sequences, which share homology with the glucocorticoid receptor. Three amino acids (Arg-431, Lys-515, and Arg-518), also found in the Toll protein, are essential for IL–1-induced IL-2 production in mammalian cells (134). However, the significance of the nuclear localization sequences in IL-1RI is unknown.

Early Events in IL-1 Signaling

The earliest event after the formation of the IL-1 receptor heterodimer is the approximation of the cytoplasmic domains of each receptor chain (Figure 24.4). Within 1 minute, there is recruitment of the myeloid differentiation protein 88 (MyD88, a cytoplasmic adapter molecule), the Toll-interacting protein (Tollip), and the IL-1 receptor activating kinase (IRAK). There are four IRAKs. Deletion of specific amino acids in the IL-1RAcP TIR domain results in loss of IRAK association (135). It is the close proximity of the TIR domains of each chain that recruits MyD88. Limited sequence homology of the cytoplasmic domain of gp130 (the IL-6 family signaling receptors) with that of IL-1RI and IL-1RAcP suggests that complex formation of IL-1R/IL-1/IL-1RAcP transduces a signal similar to that observed with the dimerization of gp130. In fact, deletion of the gp130 shared sequences from the IL-1RI cytoplasmic domain results in a reduced response to IL-1. IL-1 shares several prominent biological properties with gp130 ligands; for example, fever, hematopoietic stem cell activation, and the stimulation of the hypothalamic-pituitary-adrenal axis are common to both IL-1 and IL-6.

Recruitment of MyD88 and IL-1 Receptor Activating Kinases

The small cytosolic protein MyD88 has many of the characteristics of cytoplasmic domains of receptors, but MyD88 lacks any known extracellular or transmembrane structure. Mice deficient in MyD88 do not respond to IL-1, IL-18, or most of the TLR ligands. It is unclear exactly how this protein functions because it does not have any known kinase activity. However, it may assist in the binding of the IRAKs to the complex and hence function as an adapter molecule. Of the four IRAKs (136), IRAK-2 associates with MyD88 and undergoes autophosphorylation (137). In mice with a deletion in IRAK-4, there is reduced LPS as well as IL-1 signaling (136). The binding of IRAK-1 and IRAK-2 to the IL-1R complex is an essential step in the activation of NFκB (138). In addition to MyD88, TNF receptor–associated factor-6 (TRAF-6) docks to the complex. TRAF-6 phosphorylates NFκB, inducing kinase (139), but some studies suggest that this kinase is not necessary for IL-1 signaling. However, in mice deficient in TRAF-6, there is no IL-1 signaling in thymocytes, and the phenotype exhibits severe osteopetrosis and defective formation of osteoclasts (140).

The IL-1 Signaling Cascade

Using immunoprecipitation and tandem mass spectrometry, a thorough analysis has been made of proteins that are rapidly phosphorylated after IL-1 binding. Within 15 seconds, the IL-1 signaling complex contains IL-1RI, IL-1RAcP, IL-1, and MyD88 (141). The complex appears to be stable with prolonged activation. In the stable complex, a 60-kD phosphorylated protein was identified as IRAK-4 (141). As in previous studies, only serine/threonine residues are phosphorylated in IL-1 signaling and not tyrosine. Although MyD88 is not phosphorylated, IRAK-1, 2, and 4 in the complex are phosphorylated. TRAF-6 also associates with IRAK–1. IRAK-1 is the only component of the IL-1 receptor complex that dissociates from the complex, and together with TRAF-6 it migrates to the membrane.

The Role of TGFβ-Activated Kinase-1 in IL-1 Signaling

TGFβ-activated kinase-1 (TAK-1), TAB1, and TAB2 form a membrane-associated complex to which IRAK-1–TRAF-6 binds (142). Polyubiquitination of TRAF-6 results in the phosphorylation of TAK-1, which then migrates to the cytoplasm (Figure 24.4). In the cytoplasm, phosphorylated TAK-1 activates several kinases. These are IκB kinases (IKK) (143), MAPK p38 (144), and JNK. Activated IKK degrades IκB, and NFκB is released to translocate to the nucleus and trigger gene expression.

Activation of MAP Kinases

Most consistently, IL-1 activates p38 MAP kinase, which phosphorylates serine and threonine residues on epidermal growth factor receptor, heat-shock protein p27, myelin basic protein, and serine 56 and 156 of casein. The p42/44 MAP kinase family is associated with signal transduction by growth factors including *ras-raf-1* signal pathways. In rat mesangial cells, IL-1 activates the p42/44 MAP kinase within 10 minutes and also increases *de novo* synthesis of p42 (145).

p38 MAP Kinase Activation

The p38 MAPK plays an important role in IL-1 activity. MAP kinases are highly conserved proteins homologous to the *HOG-1* stress gene in yeasts. In fact, when *HOG-1* is deleted, yeasts fail to grow in hyperosmotic conditions; however, the mammalian gene coding for the IL-1–inducible p38 MAP kinase (146) can reconstitute the ability of the yeast to grow in hyperosmotic conditions. In primary human monocytes stimulated with hyperosmolar NaCl, LPS, IL-1, or TNF, indistinguishable phosphorylation of the p38 MAP kinase takes place and results in IL-8, IL-1β, IL-1α, and TNFα gene expression, and synthesis takes place (28). Thus, the MAP p38 kinase pathways involved in IL-1, TNF, and LPS signal transductions share certain elements that are related to the primitive stress-induced pathway. The dependency of Rho members of the GTPase family (see later discussion) for IL-1–induced activation of p38 MAP kinases has been demonstrated (147).

This latter observation links the intrinsic GTPase domains of IL-1RI and IL-1R-AcP with activation of the p38 MAP kinase.

As discussed previously, signal transduction of IL-1 requires phosphorylation of TAK-1 for phosphorylation of MAPK. For the phosphorylation of TAK-1, polyubquitination of TRAF-6 is required. Ubquitination of TRAF-6 is dependent on E2 ubiquitin conjugating enzyme Ubc13. In cells conditionally deficient in Ubc13, IL-1–induced degradation of IκB was unaffected in mouse embryonic fibroblasts. However, IL-1–induced phosphorylation of p38 MAPK, JNK, and ERK was markedly reduced, whereas TNF-induced phosphorylation of MAPK was unaffected (148).

GTPases

Both a sequence and a structural comparison of the cytosolic segment of IL-1RI with the *ras* family of GTPases has been made. The known amino acid residues for GTP binding and hydrolysis by the GTPase family align with residues in the cytoplasmic domain of the IL-1RI. These finding are consistent with a model in which, with dimerization of the two IL-1 receptor chains, activation of the putative GTP-binding sites on the IL-1 receptor cytosolic domains takes place, followed by binding of small G proteins, hydrolysis of GTP, and activation of a phospholipase. In chondrocytes, IL-1 triggers an increase in intracellular calcium followed by the organization of filamentous actin in the cytoskeleton (149). IL-1 stimulation initiates a rise in the cellular level of calcium from intracellular stores, which is mediated by phospholipase C (150). The influx of calcium into the cell also takes place via activation of G protein–coupled receptors.

Some of the biochemical changes associated with signal transduction are likely cell specific. Within 2 minutes, hydrolysis of GTP, phosphatidylcholine, phosphatidylserine, or phosphatidylethanolamine and release of ceramide by neutral, not acidic, sphingomyelinase, have been reported. In general, multiple protein phosphorylations and activation of phosphatases can be observed with 5 minutes, and some are thought to be initiated by the release of lipid mediators. Phosphorylation of phospholipase A2–activating protein also occurs in the first few minutes, which leads to a rapid release of arachidonic acid.

IL-18 Signals Similarly to IL-1

MyD88-deficient mice do not respond to IL-18. Thus, MyD88 is an essential component in the signaling cascade that follows IL-1, TLR ligand, and IL-18 binding. The cascade of sequential recruitment of MyD88, IRAK-1, 2, 3, and 4 and TRAF-6 followed by the degradation of IκB and release of NFκB are nearly identical for IL-1 and for IL-18 (Figure 24.6). In IL-18–stimulated U1 macrophages, which already expresses the gene for IL-18Rα, there is translocation of NFκB and stimulation of human immunodeficiency virus type 1 production (151).

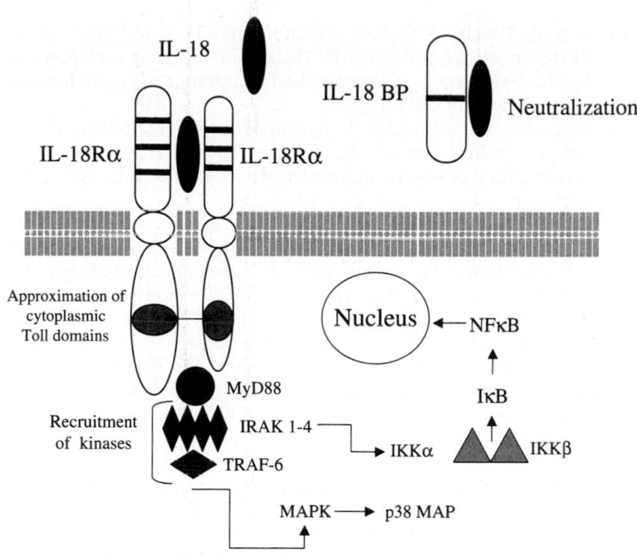

FIGURE 24.6 IL-18 signal transduction. The affinity of mature IL-18 for the IL-18Rα is low (K_d = 50 nM) but increases 100-fold with a complex of IL-18Rβ. Signal transduction in IL-18 involves MyD88 and IRAKs. TRAF-6 is also a part of IL-18 signaling. TRAF-6 is required for the phosphorylation of p38 MAP.

REFERENCES

1. Auron PE, Webb AC, Rosenwasser LJ, et al. Nucleotide sequence of human monocyte interleukin 1 precursor cDNA. *Proc Natl Acad Sci U S A.* 1984;81:7907.
2. Lomedico PT, Gubler R, Hellmann CP, et al. Cloning and expression of murine interleukin-1 cDNA in *Escherichia coli. Nature.* 1984;312:458.
3. Larsen CM, Faulenbach M, Vaag A, et al. Interleukin-1-receptor antagonist in type 2 diabetes mellitus. *N Engl J Med.* 2007;356:1517
4. Economides AN, Carpenter LR, Rudge JS, et al. Cytokine traps: multi-component, high-affinity blockers of cytokine action. *Nat Med.* 2003;9:47.
5. Johnson VJ, Yucesoy B, Luster MI. Prevention of IL-1 signaling attenuates airway hyperresponsiveness and inflammation in a murine model of toluene diisocyanate-induced asthma. *J Allergy Clin Immunol.* 2005;116:851.
6. Wang CC, Fu CL, Yang YH, et al. Adenovirus expressing interleukin-1 receptor antagonist alleviates allergic airway inflammation in a murine model of asthma. *Gene Ther.* 2006;13:1414.
7. Lipsky PE, Thompson PA, Rosenwasser LJ, et al. The role of interleukin 1 in human B cell activation: inhibition of B cell proliferation and the generation of immunoglobulin-secreting cells by an antibody against human leukocytic pyrogen. *J Immunol.* 1983;130:2708.
8. Nakae S, Asano M, Horai R, et al. Interleukin-1 beta, but not interleukin-1 alpha, is required for T cell-dependent antibody production. *Immunology.* 2001;104:402.
9. Sutton C, Brereton C, Keogh B, et al. A crucial role for interleukin (IL)-1 in the induction of IL-17-producing T cells that mediate autoimmune encephalomyelitis. *J Exp Med.* 2006;203:1685.
10. Nakae S, Saijo S, Horai R, et al. IL-17 production from activated T cells is required for the spontaneous development of destructive arthritis in mice deficient in IL-1 receptor antagonist. *Proc Natl Acad Sci U S A.* 2003;100:5986.

11. Matsuki T, Nakae S, Sudo K, et al. Abnormal T cell activation caused by the imbalance of the IL-1/IL-1R antagonist system is responsible for the development of experimental autoimmune encephalomyelitis. *Int Immunol.* 2006;18:399.
12. Nakanishi K, Yoshimoto T, Tsutsui H, et al. Interleukin-18 is a unique cytokine that stimulates both Th1 and Th2 responses depending on its cytokine milieu. *Cytokine Growth Factor Rev.* 2001; 12:53.
13. Konishi H, Tsutsui H, Murakami T, et al. IL-18 contributes to the spontaneous development of atopic dermatitis-like inflammatory skin lesion independently of IgE/stat6 under specific pathogen-free conditions. *Proc Natl Acad Sci U S A.* 2002;99:11340.
14. Hoshino T, Kawase Y, Okamoto M, et al. Cutting edge: IL-18-transgenic mice: in vivo evidence of a broad role for IL-18 in modulating immune function. *J Immunol.* 2001;166:7014.
15. Schmitz J, Owyang A, Oldham E, et al. IL-33, an interleukin-1-like cytokine that signals via the IL-1 receptor-related protein ST2 and induces T helper type 2-associated cytokines. *Immunity.* 2005; 23:479.
16. Coeshott C, Ohnemus C, Pilyavskaya A, et al. Converting enzyme-independent release of TNFα and IL-1β from a stimulated human monocytic cell line in the presence of activated neutrophils or purified proteinase-3. *Proc Natl Acad Sci U S A.* 1999;96:6261.
17. Sugawara S, Uehara A, Nochi T, et al. Neutrophil proteinase 3-mediated induction of bioactive IL-18 secretion by human oral epithelial cells. *J Immunol.* 2001;167:6568.
18. Horai R, Saijo S, Tanioka H, et al. Development of chronic inflammatory arthropathy resembling rheumatoid arthritis in interleukin 1 receptor antagonist-deficient mice. *J Exp Med.* 2000;191: 313.
19. Nicklin MJ, Hughes DE, Barton JL, et al. Arterial inflammation in mice lacking the interleukin 1 receptor antagonist gene. *J Exp Med.* 2000;191:303.
20. Lewis EC, Dinarello CA. Responses of IL-18- and IL-18 receptor-deficient pancreatic islets with convergence of positive and negative signals for the IL-18 receptor. *Proc Natl Acad Sci U S A.* 2006;103:16852.
21. Gutcher I, Urich E, Wolter K, et al. Interleukin 18-independent engagement of interleukin 18 receptor-alpha is required for autoimmune inflammation. *Nat Immunol.* 2006;7:946.
22. Breder CD, Dinarello CA, Saper CB. Interleukin-1 immunoreactive innervation of the human hypothalamus. *Science.* 1988;240: 321.
23. Voronov E, Shouval DS, Krelin Y, et al. IL-1 is required for tumor invasiveness and angiogenesis. *Proc Natl Acad Sci U S A.* 2003;100:2645.
24. Song X, Voronov E, Dvorkin T, et al. Differential effects of IL-1alpha and IL-1beta on tumorigenicity patterns and invasiveness. *J Immunol.* 2003;171:6448.
25. Krelin Y, Voronov E, Dotan S, et al. Interleukin-1beta-driven inflammation promotes the development and invasiveness of chemical carcinogen-induced tumors. *Cancer Res.* 2007;67:1062.
26. Unlu S, Kumar A, Waterman WR, et al. Phosphorylation of IRF8 in a pre-associated complex with Spi-1/PU.1 and non-phosphorylated Stat1 is critical for LPS induction of the IL1B gene. *Mol Immunol.* 2007;44:3364.
27. Vannier E, Dinarello CA. Histamine enhances interleukin (IL)-1-induced IL-1 gene expression and protein synthesis via H2 receptors in peripheral blood mononuclear cells: comparison with IL-1 receptor antagonist. *J Clin Invest.* 1993;92:281.
28. Shapiro L, Dinarello CA. Cytokine expression during osmotic stress. *Exp Cell Res.* 1997;231:354.
29. Puren AJ, Fantuzzi G, Dinarello CA. Gene expression, synthesis and secretion of IL-1β and IL-18 are differentially regulated in human blood mononuclear cells and mouse spleen cells. *Proc Natl Acad Sci U S A.* 1999;96:2256.
30. Schindler R, Clark BD, Dinarello CA. Dissociation between interleukin-1β mRNA and protein synthesis in human peripheral blood mononuclear cells. *J Biol Chem.* 1990;265:10232.
31. Kaspar RL, Gehrke L. Peripheral blood mononuclear cells stimulated with C5a or lipopolysaccharide to synthesize equivalent levels of IL-1β mRNA show unequal IL-1β protein accumulation but similar polyribosome profiles. *J Immunol.* 1994;153:277.
32. Miller LC, Isa S, Vannier E, et al. Live *Borrelia burgdorferi* preferentially activate IL-1β gene expression and protein synthesis over the interleukin-1 receptor antagonist. *J Clin Invest.* 1992;90:906.
33. Mulero JJ, Pace AM, Nelken ST, et al. IL1HY1: A novel interleukin-1 receptor antagonist gene. *Biochem Biophys Res Commun.* 1999; 263:702.
34. Andersson J, Björk L, Dinarello CA, et al. Lipopolysaccharide induces human interleukin-1 receptor antagonist and interleukin-1 production in the same cell. *Eur J Immunol.* 1992;22:2617.
35. Werman A, Werman-Venkert R, White R, et al. The precursor form of IL-1α is an intracrine proinflammatory activator of transcription. *Proc Natl Acad Sci U S A.* 2004;101:2434.
36. Chen C-J, Kono H, Golenbock D, et al. Identification of a key pathway required for the sterile inflammatory response triggered by dying cells. *Nature Med.* 2007;13:851.
37. Maier JAM, Voulalas P, Roeder D, et al. Extension of the life span of human endothelial cells by an interleukin-1α antisense oligomer. *Science.* 1990;249:1570.
38. Maier JAM, Statuto M, Ragnotti G. Endogenous interleukin-1 alpha must be transported to the nucleus to exert its activity in human endothelial cells. *Mol Cell Biol.* 1994;14:1845.
39. Horai R, Asano M, Sudo K, et al. Production of mice deficient in genes for interleukin (IL)-1α, IL- 1β, IL-1α/β, and IL-1 receptor antagonist shows that IL-1β is crucial in turpentine-induced fever development and glucocorticoid secretion. *J Exp Med.* 1998;187: 1463.
40. Hammerberg C, Arend WP, Fisher GJ, et al. Interleukin-1 receptor antagonist in normal and psoriatic epidermis. *J Clin Invest.* 1992;90:571.
41. Kurt-Jones EA, Beller DI, Mizel SB, et al. Identification of a membrane-associated interleukin-1 in macrophages. *Proc Natl Acad Sci U S A.* 1985;82:1204.
42. Brody DT, Durum SK. Membrane IL-1: IL-1α precursor binds to the plasma membrane via a lectin-like interaction. *J Immunol.* 1989;143:1183.
43. Kamari Y, Werman-Venkert R, Shaish A, et al. Differential role and tissue specificity of interleukin-1alpha gene expression in atherogenesis and lipid metabolism. *Atherosclerosis.* 2007;195(1):38.
44. Bendtzen K, Svenson M, Jonsson V, et al. Autoantibodies to cytokines—friends or foes? *Immunol Today.* 1990;11:167.
45. Hacham M, Argov S, White RM, et al. Different patterns of interleukin-1alpha and interleukin-1beta expression in organs of normal young and old mice. *Eur Cytokine Netw.* 2002;13:55.
46. Lonnemann G, Engler-Blum G, Müller GA, et al. Cytokines in human renal interstitial fibrosis. II. Intrinsic Interleukin (IL)-1 synthesis and IL-1-dependent production of IL-6 and IL-8 by cultured kidney fibroblasts. *Kidney Int.* 1995;47:845.
47. Hurgin V, Novick D, Werman A, et al. Antiviral and immunoregulatory activities of IFN-gamma depend on constitutively expressed IL-1alpha. *Proc Natl Acad Sci U S A.* 2007;104:5044.
48. Kuida K, Lippke JA, Ku G, et al. Altered cytokine export and apoptosis in mice deficient in interleukin-1β converting enzyme. *Science.* 1995;267:2000.
49. Hoffman HM, Mueller JL, Broide DH, et al. Mutation of a new gene encoding a putative pyrin-like protein causes familial cold autoinflammatory syndrome and Muckle-Wells syndrome. *Nat Genet.* 2001;29:301.
50. Goldbach-Mansky R, Dailey NJ, Canna SW, et al. Neonatal-onset multisystem inflammatory disease responsive to interleukin-1beta inhibition. *N Engl J Med.* 2006;355:581.
51. Dinarello CA, Ikejima T, Warner SJ, et al. Interleukin 1 induces interleukin 1. I. Induction of circulating interleukin 1 in rabbits in vivo and in human mononuclear cells in vitro. *J Immunol.* 1987;139:1902.
52. Warner SJC, Auger KR, Libby P. Interleukin-1 induces interleukin-1. II. Interleukin-1 induces production of interleukin-1 by adult human vascular endothelial cells in vitro. *J Immunol.* 1987;139:1911.
53. Zheng H, Fletcher D, Kozak W, et al. Resistance to fever induction and impaired acute-phase response in interleukin-1b deficient mice. *Immunity.* 1995;3:9.
54. Fantuzzi G, Ku G, Harding MW, et al. Response to local inflammation of IL-1β converting enzyme-deficient mice. *J Immunol.* 1997;158:1818.

55. Fantuzzi G, Sacco S, Ghezzi P, et al. Physiological and cytokine responses in interleukin-1β-deficient mice after zymosan-induced inflammation. *Am J Physiol.* 1997;273:R400.
56. Fantuzzi G, Zheng H, Faggioni R, et al. Effect of endotoxin in IL-1β-deficient mice. *J Immunol.* 1996;157:291.
57. Faggioni R, Fantuzzi G, Fuller J, et al. IL-1β mediates leptin induction during inflammation. *Am J Physiol.* 1998;274:R204.
58. Kozak W, Kluger MJ, Soszynski D, et al. IL-6 and IL-1 beta in fever. Studies using cytokine-deficient (knockout) mice. *Ann NY Acad Sci.* 1998;856:33.
59. Arend WP, Joslin FG, Massoni RJ. Effects of immune complexes on production by human monocytes of interleukin 1 or an interleukin 1 inhibitor. *J Immunol.* 1985;134:3868.
60. Eisenberg SP, Evans RJ, Arend WP, et al. Primary structure and functional expression from complementary DNA of a human interleukin-1 receptor antagonist. *Nature.* 1990;343:341.
61. Granowitz EV, Porat R, Mier JW, et al. Pharmacokinetics, safety, and immunomodulatory effects of human recombinant interleukin-1 receptor antagonist in healthy humans. *Cytokine.* 1992;4:353.
62. Bresnihan B, Alvaro-Gracia JM, Cobby M, et al. Treatment of rheumatoid arthritis with recombinant human interleukin-1 receptor antagonist. *Arthritis Rheum.* 1998;41:2196.
63. Genant HK, Bresnihan B, Ng E, et al. Treatment with anakinra reduces the rate of joint destruction and shows accelerated benefit in the second 6 months of treatment for patients with rheumatoid arthritis [abstract]. *Ann Rheum Dis.* 2001;40(Suppl 1):169.
64. Dewhirst FE, Stashenko PP, Mole JE, et al. Purification and partial sequence of human osteoclast-activating factor: identity with interleukin 1 beta. *J Immunol.* 1985;135:2562.
65. Cunnane G, Madigan A, Murphy E, et al. The effects of treatment with interleukin-1 receptor antagonist on the inflamed synovial membrane in rheumatoid arthritis. *Rheumatology (Oxford).* 2001;40:62.
66. Bendtzen K, Mandrup-Poulsen T, Nerup J, et al. Cytotoxicity of human pI 7 interleukin-1 for pancreatic islets of Langerhans. *Science.* 1986;232:1545.
67. Maedler K, Storling J, Sturis J, et al. Glucose- and interleukin-1beta-induced beta-cell apoptosis requires Ca2+ influx and extracellular signal-regulated kinase (ERK) 1/2 activation and is prevented by a sulfonylurea receptor 1/inwardly rectifying K+ channel 6.2 (SUR/Kir6.2) selective potassium channel opener in human islets. *Diabetes.* 2004;53:1706.
68. Fitzgerald AA, Leclercq SA, Yan A, et al. Rapid responses to anakinra in patients with refractory adult-onset Still's disease. *Arthritis Rheum.* 2005;52:1794.
69. Gattorno M, Tassi S, Carta S, et al. Pattern of interleukin-1beta secretion in response to lipopolysaccharide and ATP before and after interleukin-1 blockade in patients with CIAS1 mutations. *Arthritis Rheum.* 2007;56:3138.
70. Shoham NG, Centola M, Mansfield E, et al. Pyrin binds the PSTPIP1/CD2BP1 protein, defining familial Mediterranean fever and PAPA syndrome as disorders in the same pathway. *Proc Natl Acad Sci U S A.* 2003;100:13501.
71. Simon A, van der Meer JW. Pathogenesis of familial periodic fever syndromes or hereditary autoinflammatory syndromes. *Am J Physiol Regul Integr Comp Physiol.* 2007;292:R86.
72. Mandey SH, Kuijk LM, Frenkel J, et al. A role for geranylgeranylation in interleukin-1beta secretion. *Arthritis Rheum.* 2006;54:3690.
73. Hirsch E, Irikura VM, Paul SM, et al. Functions of interleukin 1 receptor antagonist in gene knockout and overproducing mice. *Proc Natl Acad Sci U S A.* 1996;93:11008.
74. Okamura H, Tsutsui H, Komatsu T, et al. Cloning of a new cytokine that induces interferon-γ. *Nature.* 1995;378:88.
75. Gu Y, Wu J, Faucheu C, et al. Interleukin-1β converting enzyme requires oligomerization for activity of processed forms in vivo. *EMBO J.* 1995;14:1923.
76. Fantuzzi G, Reed DA, Dinarello CA. IL-12-induced IFNγ is dependent on caspase-1 processing of the IL-18 precursor. *J Clin Invest.* 1999;104:761.
77. Tsutsui H, Kayagaki N, Kuida K, et al. Caspase-1-independent, Fas/Fas ligand-mediated IL-18 secretion from macrophages causes acute liver injury in mice. *Immunity.* 1999;11:359.
78. Novick D, Kim S-H, Fantuzzi G, et al. Interleukin-18 binding protein: a novel modulator of the Th1 cytokine response. *Immunity.* 1999;10:127.
79. Kim SH, Azam T, Novick D, et al. Identification of amino acid residues critical for biological activity in human interleukin-18. *J Biol Chem.* 2002;14:14.
80. Novick D, Schwartsburd B, Pinkus R, et al. A novel IL-18BP ELISA shows elevated serum il-18BP in sepsis and extensive decrease of free IL-18. *Cytokine.* 2001;14:334.
81. Tak PP, Bacchi M, Bertolino M. Pharmacokinetics of IL-18 binding protein in healthy volunteers and subjects with rheumatoid arthritis or plaque psoriasis. *Eur J Drug Metab Pharmacokinet.* 2006;31:109.
82. Xiang Y, Moss B. Correspondence of the functional epitopes of poxvirus and human interleukin-18-binding proteins. *J Virol.* 2001;75:9947.
83. Netea MG, Joosten LA, Lewis E, et al. Deficiency of interleukin-18 in mice leads to hyperphagia, obesity and insulin resistance. *Nat Med.* 2006;12:650.
84. Barton JL, Herbst R, Bosisio D, et al. A tissue specific IL-1 receptor antagonist homolog from the IL-1 cluster lacks IL-1, IL-1ra, IL-18 and IL-18 antagonist activities. *Eur J Immunol.* 2000;30:3299.
85. Costelloe C, Watson M, Murphy A, et al. IL-1F5 mediates anti-inflammatory activity in the brain through induction of IL-4 following interaction with SIGIRR/TIR8. *J Immunol.* 2007;in press.
86. Debets R, Timans JC, Homey B, et al. Two novel IL-1 family members, IL-1 delta and IL-1 epsilon, function as an antagonist and agonist of NF-kappa B activation through the orphan IL-1 receptor-related protein 2. *J Immunol.* 2001;167:1440.
87. Towne JE, Garka KE, Renshaw BR, et al. Interleukin (IL)-1F6, IL-1F8, and IL-1F9 signal through IL-1Rrp2 and IL-1RAcP to activate the pathway leading to NF-kappaB and MAPKs. *J Biol Chem.* 2004;279:13677.
88. Pan G, Risser P, Mao W, et al. IL-1H, an interleukin 1-related protein that binds IL-18 receptor/IL-1Rrp. *Cytokine.* 2001;13:1.
89. Kumar S, McDonnell PC, Lehr R, et al. Identification and initial characterization of four novel members of the interleukin-1 family. *J Biol Chem.* 2000;275:10308.
90. Kumar S, Hanning CR, Brigham-Burke MR, et al. Interleukin-1F7B (IL-1H4/IL-1F7) is processed by caspase-1 and mature IL-1F7B binds to the IL-18 receptor but does not induce IFN-gamma production. *Cytokine.* 2002;18:61.
91. Gao W, Kumar S, Lotze MT, et al. Innate immunity mediated by the cytokine IL-1 homologue 4 (IL-1H4/IL-1F7) induces IL-12-dependent adaptive and profound antitumor immunity. *J Immunol.* 2003;170:107.
92. Bufler P, Azam T, Gamboni-Robertson F, et al. A complex of the IL-1 homologue IL-1F7b and IL-18-binding protein reduces IL-18 activity. *Proc Natl Acad Sci U S A.* 2002;99:13723.
93. Magne D, Palmer G, Barton JL, et al. The new IL-1 family member IL-1F8 stimulates production of inflammatory mediators by synovial fibroblasts and articular chondrocytes. *Arthritis Res Ther.* 2006;8:R80.
94. Lin H, Ho AS, Haley-Vicente D, et al. Cloning and characterization of IL-1HY2, a novel interleukin-1 family member. *J Biol Chem.* 2001;276:20597.
95. Bensen JT, Dawson PA, Mychaleckyj JC, et al. Identification of a novel human cytokine gene in the interleukin gene cluster on chromosome 2q12-14. *J Interferon Cytokine Res.* 2001;21:899.
96. Bergers G, Reikerstorfer A, Braselmann S, et al. Alternative promoter usage of the Fos-responsive gene *Fit-1* generates mRNA isoforms coding for either secreted or membrane-bound proteins related to the IL-1 receptor. *EMBO J.* 1994;13:1176.
97. Carriere V, Roussel L, Ortega N, et al. IL-33, the IL-1-like cytokine ligand for ST2 receptor, is a chromatin-associated nuclear factor in vivo. *Proc Natl Acad Sci U S A.* 2007;104:282.
98. Leung BP, Xu D, Culshaw S, et al. A novel therapy of murine collagen-induced arthritis with soluble T1/ST2. *J Immunol.* 2004;173:145.
99. Ali S, Huber M, Kollewe C, et al. The interleukion-1 receptor accessory protein is essential for interleukin-33 induced activation of T cells and mast cells. *Proc Natl Acad Sci U S A.* 2007;in press.

100. Sanada S, Hakuno D, Higgins LJ, et al. IL-33 and ST2 comprise a critical biomechanically induced and cardioprotective signaling system. *J Clin Invest.* 2007;117:1538.
101. Gadina M, Jefferies CA. 2007. IL-33: a sheep in wolfs clothing? *Sci STKE.* 2007(12 June):pe31.
102. Smith DE, Hanna R, Della F, et al. The soluble form of IL-1 receptor accessory protein enhances the ability of soluble type II IL-1 receptor to inhibit IL-1 action. *Immunity.* 2003;18:87.
103. Dinarello CA. The many worlds of reducing interleukin-1. *Arthritis Rheum.* 2005;52:1960.
104. Gabay C, Smith MF, Eidlen D, et al. Interleukin 1 receptor antagonist (IL-1Ra) is an acute-phase protein. *J Clin Invest.* 1997;99:2930.
105. Boraschi D, Tagliabue A. The interleukin-1 receptor family. *Vitam Horm.* 200674:229.
106. Moritz D, Rodewald H-R, Gheyselinck J, et al. The IL-1 receptor-related T1 antigen is expressed on immature and mature mast cells an on fetal blood mast cell progenitors. *J Immunol.* 1998;161:4866.
107. Parnet P, Garka KE, Bonnert TP, et al. IL-1Rrp is a novel receptor-like molecule similar to the type I interleukin-1 receptor and its homologues T1/ST2 and IL-1R AcP. *J Biol Chem.* 1996;271:3967.
108. Torigoe K, Ushio S, Okura T, et al. Purification and characterization of the human interleukin-18 receptor. *J Biol Chem.* 1997;272:25737.
109. Born TL, Thomassen E, Bird TA, et al. Cloning of a novel receptor subunit, AcPL, required for interleukin-18 signaling. *J Biol Chem.* 1998;273:29445.
110. Kim SH, Reznikov LL, Stuyt RJ, et al. Functional reconstitution and regulation of IL-18 activity by the IL- 18R beta chain. *J Immunol.* 2001;166:148.
111. Carrie A, Jun L, Bienvenu T, et al. A new member of the IL-1 receptor family highly expressed in hippocampus and involved in X-linked mental retardation. *Nat Genet.* 1999;23:25.
112. Sana TR, Debets R, Timans JC, et al. Computational identification, cloning, and characterization of IL-1R9, a novel interleukin-1 receptor-like gene encoded over an unusually large interval of human chromosome Xq22.2-q22.3. *Genomics.* 2000;69:252.
113. Garlanda C, Riva F, Polentarutti N, et al. Intestinal inflammation in mice deficient in Tir8, an inhibitory member of the IL-1 receptor family. *Proc Natl Acad Sci U S A.* 2004;101:3522.
114. Dimcheff DE, Volkert LG, Li Y, et al. Gene expression profiling of microglia infected by a highly neurovirulent murine leukemia virus: implications for neuropathogenesis. *Retrovirology.* 2006;3:26.
115. Qin J, Qian Y, Yao J, et al. SIGIRR inhibits interleukin-1 receptor- and toll-like receptor 4-mediated signaling through different mechanisms. *J Biol Chem.* 2005;280:25233.
116. Wald D, Qin J, Zhao Z, et al. SIGIRR, a negative regulator of Toll-like receptor-interleukin 1 receptor signaling. *Nat Immunol.* 2003;4: 920.
117. Huang X, Hazlett LD, Du W, et al. SIGIRR promotes resistance against Pseudomonas aeruginosa keratitis by down-regulating type-1 immunity and IL-1R1 and TLR4 signaling. *J Immunol.* 2006;177:548.
118. Rosoff PM, Savage N, Dinarello CA. Interleukin-1 stimulates diacylglycerol production in T lymphocytes by a novel mechanism. *Cell.* 1988;54:73.
119. Ye K, Dinarello CA, Clark BD. Identification of the promoter region of the human interleukin 1 type I receptor gene: multiple initiation sites, high G+C content, and constitutive expression. *Proc Natl Acad Sci U S A.* 1993;90:2295.
120. Man MQ, Wood L, Elias PM, et al. Cutaneous barrier repair and pathophysiology following barrier disruption in IL-1 and TNF type I receptor deficient mice. *Exp Dermatol.* 1999;8:261.
121. Cullinan EB, Kwee L, Nunes P, et al. IL-1 receptor accessory protein is an essential component of the IL-1 receptor. *J Immunol.* 1998;161:5614.
122. Lorenzo JE, Naprta A, Rao Y, et al. Mice lacking the type I interleukin-1 receptor do not lose bone mass after ovariectomy. *Endocrinology.* 1998;139:3022.
123. Colotta F, Dower SK, Sims JE, et al. The type II "decoy" receptor: a novel regulatory pathway for interleukin-1. *Immunol Today.* 1994;15:562.
124. Neumann D, Kollewe C, Martin MU, et al. The membrane form of the type II IL-1 receptor accounts for inhibitory function. *J Immunol.* 2000;165:3350.
125. Malinowsky D, Lundkvist J, Laye S, et al. Interleukin-1 receptor accessory protein interacts with the type II interleukin-1 receptor. *FEBS Lett.* 1998;429:299.
126. Smeets RL, Joosten LA, Arntz OJ, et al. Soluble interleukin-1 receptor accessory protein ameliorates collagen-induced arthritis by a different mode of action from that of interleukin-1 receptor antagonist. *Arthritis Rheum.* 2005;52:2202.
127. Netea MG, Kullberg BJ, Boerman OC, et al. Soluble murine IL-1 receptor type I induces release of constitutive IL-1 alpha. *J Immunol.* 1999;162:4876.
128. Preas HL 2nd, Reda D, Tropea M, et al. Effects of recombinant soluble type I interleukin-1 receptor on human inflammatory responses to endotoxin. *Blood.* 1996;88:2465.
129. Granowitz EV, Porat R, Mier JW, et al. Hematological and immunomodulatory effects of an interleukin-1 receptor antagonist coinfusion during low-dose endotoxemia in healthy humans. *Blood.* 1993;82:2985.
130. Drevlow BE, Lovis R, Haag MA, et al. Recombinant human interleukin-1 receptor type I in the treatment of patients with active rheumatoid arthritis. *Arthritis Rheum.* 1996;39:257.
131. Bernstein SH, Fay J, Frankel S, et al. A phase I study of recombinant human soluble interleukin-1 receptor (rhu IL-1R) in patients with relapsed and refractory acute myeloid leukemia. *Cancer Chemother Pharmacol.* 1999;43:141.
132. Crown J, Jakubowski A, Kemeny N, et al. A phase I trial of recombinant human interleukin-1β alone and in combination with myelosuppressive doses of 5-fluoruracil in patients with gastrointestinal cancer. *Blood.* 1991;78:1420.
133. Smith JW, Longo D, Alford WG, et al. The effects of treatment with interleukin-1α on platelet recovery after high-dose carboplatin. *N Engl J Med.* 1993;328:756.
134. Heguy A, Baldari CT, Macchia G, et al. Amino acids conserved in interleukin-1 receptors and the *Drosophila* Toll protein are essential for IL-1R signal transduction. *J Biol Chem.* 1992;267:2605.
135. Wesche H, Korherr C, Kracht M, et al. The interleukin-1 receptor accessory protein is essential for IL-1-induced activation of interleukin-1 receptor-associated kinase (IRAK) and stress-activated protein kinases (SAP kinases). *J Biol Chem.* 1997;272:7727.
136. Suzuki N, Suzuki S, Duncan GS, et al. Severe impairment of interleukin-1 and Toll-like receptor signalling in mice lacking IRAK-4. *Nature.* 2002;416:750.
137. Boch JA, Yoshida Y, Koyama Y, et al. Characterization of a cascade of protein interactions initiated at the IL-1 receptor. *Biochem Biophys Res Commun.* 2003;303:525.
138. Croston GE, Cao Z, Goeddel DV. NFkB activation by interleukin-1 requires an IL-1 receptor-associated protein kinase activity. *J Biol Chem.* 1995;270:16514.
139. Malinin NL, Boldin MP, Kovalenko AV, et al. MAP3K-related kinase involved in NF-kappaB induction by TNF, CD95 and IL-1. *Nature.* 1997;385:540.
140. Lomaga MA, Yeh WC, Sarosi I, et al. TRAF6 deficiency results in osteopetrosis and defective interleukin-1, CD40, and LPS signaling. *Genes Dev.* 1999;13:1015.
141. Brikos C, Wait R, Begum S, et al. Mass spectrometric analysis of the endogenous IL-1RI signalling complex formed after IL-1 binding, identifies IL-1RAcP, MyD88 and IRAK-4 as the stable components. *Mol Cell Proteomics*. 2007;in press.
142. Holtmann H, Enninga J, Kalble S, et al. The MAPK kinase kinase TAK1 plays a central role in coupling the interleukin-1 receptor to both transcriptional and RNA-targeted mechanisms of gene regulation. *J Biol Chem.* 2001;276:3508.
143. Takaesu G, Surabhi RM, Park KJ, et al. TAK1 is critical for IkappaB kinase-mediated activation of the NF-kappaB pathway. *J Mol Biol.* 2003;326:105.
144. Kishimoto K, Matsumoto K, Ninomiya-Tsuji J. TAK1 mitogen-activated protein kinase kinase kinase is activated by autophosphorylation within its activation loop. *J Biol Chem.* 2000;275:7359.
145. Huwiler A, Pfeilschifter J. Interleukin-1 stimulates de novo synthesis of mitogen-activated protein kinase in glomerular mesangial cells. *FEBS Lett.* 1994;350:135.
146. Kracht M, Truong O, Totty NF, et al. Interleukin-1α activates two forms of p54α mitogen-activated protein kinase in rabbit liver. *J Exp Med.* 1994;180:2017.

147. Zhang S, Han J, Sells MA, et al. Rho family GTPases regulate p38 mitogen-activated protein kinase through the downstream mediator Pak1. *J Biol Chem.* 1995;270:23934.
148. Yamamoto M, Okamoto T, Takeda K, et al. Key function for the Ubc13 E2 ubiquitin-conjugating enzyme in immune receptor signaling. *Nat Immunol.* 2006;7:962.
149. Wang KZ, Wara-Aswapati N, Boch JA, et al. TRAF6 activation of PI 3-kinase-dependent cytoskeletal changes is cooperative with Ras and is mediated by an interaction with cytoplasmic Src. *J Cell Sci.* 2006;119:1579.
150. Pritchard S, Guilak F. Effects of interleukin-1 on calcium signaling and the increase of filamentous actin in isolated and in situ articular chondrocytes. *Arthritis Rheum.* 2006;54:2164.
151. Shapiro L, Puren AJ, Barton HA, et al. Interleukin-18 stimulates HIV type 1 in monocytic cells. *Proc Natl Acad Sci U S A.* 1998;95: 12550.
152. Mazodier K, Marin V, Novick D, et al. Severe imbalance of IL-18/IL-18BP in patients with secondary hemophagocytic syndrome. *Blood.* 2005;106:3483.
153. Kahlenberg JM, Dubyak GR. Mechanisms of caspase-1 activation by P2X7 receptor-mediated K+ release. *Am J Physiol Cell Physiol.* 2004;286:C1100.
154. Andrei C, Margiocco P, Poggi A, et al. 2004. Phospholipases C and A2 control lysosome-mediated IL-1 beta secretion: Implications for inflammatory processes. *Proc Natl Acad Sci U S A.* 2004;101: 9745.

Chapter 25

TNF-Related Cytokines in Immunity

Carl F. Ware

INTRODUCTION

Lymphocytes are highly mobile, transiting the vascular and lymphatic circulatory systems with limited stopovers in organized lymphoid tissues (lymph nodes, spleen, and Peyer's patches), in which they commune to initiate immune responses. Cytokines, both secreted and membrane-anchored proteins, serve as the communication media of the immune system. Cytokines in the tumor necrosis factor (TNF) superfamily help to orchestrate the development, homeostasis, and effector actions of cells in the immune system. The diversification of the TNF superfamily is evidenced by its roles in regulating cells of neuronal, skeletal, and ectodermal origin. This chapter focuses on members in the TNF superfamily that are primarily involved in regulating immunity.

The ligands belonging to the TNF superfamily initiate intercellular communication by binding specific receptors on the surface of the receiving cell. The TNF receptors (TNFRs) form a corresponding superfamily of cognate membrane proteins that initiate intracellular signaling pathways that influence growth, differentiation, and survival. The TNF-related ligands are membrane bound and require cell–cell contact to initiate signaling, although some ligands may be secreted in soluble form, influencing cellular responses at locations distant from the source of production. Each ligand–receptor pair forms a "system"; there are more than 40 distinct ligand–receptor systems. Many of the ligands and receptors engage more than one cognate, thereby forming "circuits" of signaling systems, which often function together as coordinated or integrated networks with other cytokines to regulate a specific cellular process. The signals delivered to the cytosol activate transcription factors such as NF-κB and AP1, which in turn initiate the expression of hundreds of genes that alter cellular differentiation. In addition, some TNFRs activate cell death pathways, both apoptotic and necrotic, terminating cellular life. Genetic mutations have revealed the importance of individual TNF superfamily members in human immune responses and development. Moreover, the beneficial effects of TNF antagonists in patients with certain autoimmune diseases have brought the need to understand the complexities of the TNF superfamily into sharp focus.

The nomenclature of the TNF superfamily is a bit of a morass for students new to the field, although introduction of a numerical system standardizing gene names (http://www.gene.ucl.ac.uk/nomenclature/) helps in accessing genomic databases. However, the use of more common, often colorful, acronyms continues. The name, rank, and genomic identification of each ligand (Table 25.1) and receptor (Table 25.2) are tabulated along with additional pertinent information for human and mouse genes.

TNF LIGAND FAMILY

The TNF-related cytokines are type II transmembrane proteins (intracellular N-terminus) with a short cytoplasmic tail (15 to 25 residues in length) and a larger extracellular region (approximately 150 amino acids) containing the signature TNF homology domain where the receptor-binding sites are located (Figure 25.1). The TNF homology domain assembles into trimers, the functional unit of the ligand. Atomic analysis of several members of the family (*1–5*) revealed that the ligands have a highly conserved tertiary structure folding into a β-sheet sandwich, and yet amino acid sequence conservation is limited to less than 35% among the family members. The conserved residues defining this superfamily are primarily located within the internal β strands that form the molecular scaffold, which promote assembly into trimers. Although most of the TNF ligands self-assemble into homotrimers, heterotrimers can also form between lymphotoxin-α (LTα) and LTβ (6), and between APRIL and BAFF (7). The stoichiometry of the LT heterotrimer is 1:2 (LT$\alpha\beta$2), which imparts its distinct receptor specificity from the LTα homotrimer. Of interest, complement component C1q and several related proteins are structurally related to the TNF family, containing a TNF homology domain, a rather surprising finding, given the apparent functional divergence between the complement and TNF systems (8). Alternate splicing can also generate distinct ligands, such as the splice form joining TWEAK and APRIL (TWE-PRIL) (9), the alternate ligands

TABLE 25.1 Tumor Necrosis Factor Superfamily Chromosomal Locations

	Chromosomal Location		*mRNA Accession Number*			
Gene Name/Alias	*Human*	*Mouse*	*Human*	*Mouse*	***Ligand Symbol***	***Human Unigene***
TNF	6p21.3	ch17 (19.06 cm)	NM_000594	NM_013693	TNF	Hs.241570
LTα	6p21.3	ch17 (19.06 cm)	NM_000595	NM_010735	LTA	Hs.36
LTβ	6p21.3	ch17 (19.06 cm)	NM_002341	NM_008518	LTB	Hs.890
OX40-L	lq25	ch1 (84.90 cM)	NM_003326	NM_009452	TNFSF4	Hs.181097
CD40-L, CD154	Xq26	chX (18.0 cM)	NM_000074	NM_011616	TNFSF5	Hs.652
Fas-L	1q23	ch1 (85.0 cM)	NM_000639	NM_010177	TNFSF6	Hs.2007
CD27-L, CD70	19p13	ch17 (20.0 cM)	NM_001252	NM_011617	TNFSF7	Hs.99899
CD30-L, CD153	9q33	ch4 (32.20 cM)	NM_001244	NM_009403	TNFSF8	Hs.1313
4-1BB-L	19p13	ch17 (20.0 cM)	NM_003811	NM_009404	TNFSF9	Hs.1524
TRAIL	3q26	ch3	NM_003810	NM_009425	TNFSF10	Hs.83429
RANK-L, TRANCE	13q14	ch14 (45.0 cM)	NM_003701	NM_011613	TNFSF11	Hs.115770
TWEAK	17p13	ch11	NM_003809	AF030100	TNFSF12	Hs.26401
APRIL/TALL2	17p13.1	ch13	NM_003808	NM_023517	TNFSF13	Hs.54673
BAFF, BLYS, TALL1	13q32-q34	ch8 (3 cM)	NM_006573	NM_033622	TNFSF13B	Hs.270737
LIGHT	19p13.3	ch7 (D-E1)	NM_003807	NM_019418	TNFSF14	Hs.129708
TL1A	9q33	ch4 (31.80 cM)	NM_005118	AF520786	TNFSF15	Hs.241382
GITRL, AITRL	1q23	ch 1 (84.95 cM)	NM_005092	NM_183391	TNFSF18	Hs.248197
EDA1	Xq12–q13.1	chX (37.0 cM)	NM_001399	NM_010099	EDA	Hs.105407
EDA2	Xq12–q13.1	chX (37.0 cM)	AF061189	AJ243657		Unknown

TABLE 25.2 Tumor Necrosis Factor Receptor Superfamily Chromosomal Locations

	Chromosomal Location		*mRNA Accession Number*				
Gene Name/Alias	*Human*	*Mouse*	*Human*	*Mouse*	***Gene Symbol***	***Human Unigene***	***Mouse Unigene***
TNFR-1, p55-60	12p13.2	ch6 (60.55cM)	NM_001065	NM_011609	TNFRSF1A	Hs.159	Mm.1258
TNFR2, p75-80	1p36.3-36.2	ch4 (75.5cM)	NM_001066	NM_011610	TNFRSF1B	Hs.256278	Mm.2666
LTβR	12p13	ch6 (60.4cM)	NM_002342	NM_010736	TNFRSF3	Hs.1116	Mm.3122
OX40	1p36	ch4 (79.4cM)	NM_003327	NM_011659	TNFRSF4	Hs.129780	Mm.13885
CD40	20q12–q13.2	ch2 (97.0cM)	NM_001250	NM_011611	TNFRSF5	Hs.25648	Mm.4966
FAS, CD95	10q24.1	ch19 (23.0cM)	NM_000043	NM_007987	TNFRSF6	Hs.82359	Mm.1626
DcR3	20q13	Unknown	NM_003823	Unknown	TNFRSF6B	Hs.348183	Unknown
CD27	12p13	ch6 (60.35)	NM_001242	L24495	TNFRSF7	Hs.355307	Mm.121
CD30	1p36	ch4 (75.5cM)	NM_001243	NM_009401	TNFRSF8	Hs.1314	Mm.12810
4-1BB	1p36	ch4 (75.5cM)	NM_001561	NM_011612	TNFRSF9	Hs.73895	Mm.198677
TRAILR-1, DR4	8p21	Unknown	NM_003844	Unknown	TNFRSF10A	Hs.249190	Unknown
TRAIL-R2, DR5	8p22-p21	ch14 (D1)	NM 003842	NM_020275	TNFRSF10B	Hs.51233	Mm.193430
TRAILR3, DcR1	8p22-p21	ch7 (69.6cM)	NM_003841	NM_024290	TNFRSF10C	Hs.119684	Mm.157724
TRAILR4, DcR2	8p21	ch7 (69.6cM)	NM_003840	NM_023680	TNFRSF10D	Hs.129844	Mm.156947
RANK, TRANCE-R	18q22.1	ch1	NM_003839	NM_009399	TNFRSF11A	Hs.114676	Mm.6251
OPG, TR1	8q24	ch15	NM_002546	NM_008764	TNFRSF11B	Hs.81791	Mm.15383
FN14	16p13.3	ch17	NM_016639	NM_013749	TNFRSF12A	Hs.355899	Mm.28518
TRAMP, DR3, LARD	1p36.3	ch4 (E1)	NM_003790	NM_033042	TNFRSF12	Hs.26401	Mm.101198
TACI	17p11.2	ch11	NM_012452	NM_021349	TNFRSF13B	Hs.158341	Mm.143787
BAFFR	22q13.1-q13.31	ch15	NM_052945	NM_028075	TNFRSF13C	Mm.131257	Mm.131257
HVEM, HveA, ATAR	1p36.3-p36.2	ch4	NM_003820	NM_178931	TNFRSF14	Hs.279899	Mm.215147
p75NTR, NGFR	17q12-q22	ch11 (55.6cM)	NM_002507	NM_033217	TNFRSF16	Hs.1827	Mm.103727
BCMA	16p13.1	ch16 (B3)	NM_001192	NM_011608	TNFRSF17	Hs.2556	Mm.12935
AITR, GITR	1p36.3	ch4 (E)	NM_004195	NM_009400	TNFRSF18	Hs.212680	Mm.3180
RELT	11q13.2	ch7	NM_152222	NM_177073	TNFRSF19L	Hs.79707	Mm.40336
TROY, TAJ	13q12.11-q12.3	ch14	NM_018647	NM_013869	TNFRSF19	Hs.283615	Mm.21526
EDAR	2q11–q13	ch10	NM_022336	NM_010100	EDAR	Hs.58346	Mm.89944
DR6	6P12.2-21.1	ch7	NM_014452	NM_052975	TNFRSF21	Hs.159651	Mm.200792
XEDAR	Xq11.1	chX	NM_021783	NM_175540	EDA2R	Hs.302017	Mm.189270
mTNFRH3	Unknown	ch7 (69.9cM)	Unknown	NM_175649	TNFRSF26	Unknown	Mm.247498

for ectodysplasin receptor (10), and a cytosolic form of LIGHT (11).

The genetic organization of TNF ligands is highly conserved, typically encoded in three or four exons, with the fourth exon encoding most of the extracellular TNF homology domain. The genes encoding TNF, LTβ, and LTα reside adjacent to each other in a compact locus in the class III region of the major histocompatibility gene complex (MHC) (in humans at chromosome 6p21) sandwiched between the antigenic-peptide-presenting MHC proteins encoded by MHC class I and II genes (6,*12*). Three other genetic clusters of TNF-related cytokines are found within the corresponding MHC paralogous regions, located on chromosomes 1, 9, and 19, with a remarkably conserved gene structure and transcriptional orientation and a function linked to regulating cellular immune responses (11). The evolutionary pressures retaining this genetic configuration of the MHC in general are encompassed in the paralogy theory of genome evolution (13). Conservation of gene structure of the TNF ligands outside of these MHC paralogs is limited. An evolutionarily conserved pathway in *Drosophila melanogaster*—the Eiger-Wengen system—is structurally and functionally related to the TNF superfamily (TNFSF)–related signaling pathway, although this system is predominantly expressed in the nervous system in invertebrates (*14*,15,*16*).

TNF RECEPTOR FAMILY

Members of the TNF receptor superfamily (TNFRSF) include proteins of vertebrate and viral origin. Most of the signaling receptors in the TNFRSF are type I transmembrane glycoproteins (N-terminus exterior to the cell). However, several TNFRSF members lack a membrane-anchor domain, are proteolytically cleaved from the surface, or are anchored via glycolipid linkage (e.g., TRAILR3). These soluble receptors, termed "decoy receptors," retain their

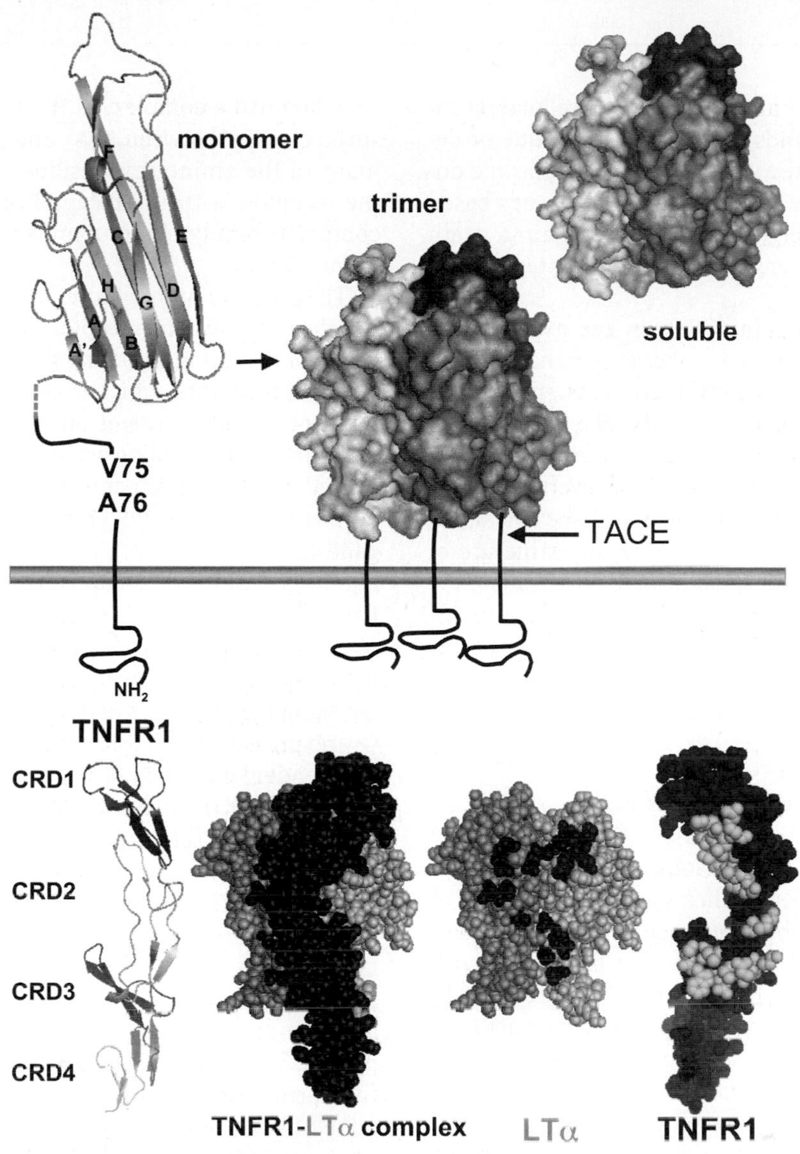

FIGURE 25.1 Structure of tumor necrosis factor (TNF) and TNF receptor (TNFR). **Top:** TNF. The β-sandwich of TNF monomer (1A8M.pdf) (shown as a ribbon diagram) contains two stacked β-pleated sheets each formed by five antiparallel β strands (wide ribbons given letter designations, A to G) that fold into a Greek key or "jelly-roll" topology (193). The inner β sheet (strands A, A′, H, C, and F) is involved in contacts between adjacent subunits, which promotes assembly into a trimer. The trimer is formed such that one edge of each subunit is packed against the inner sheet of its neighbor. The outer β sheet (strands B, B′, D, E, and G) is surface exposed. The trimeric structure is characteristic of all TNF-related ligands. The type II configuration of TNF (N-terminus inside the cell) anchors TNF to the membrane. The TNF trimer is approximately 60 Å in height with a relatively flat base residing close to the membrane, resembling a bell shape (shown as a surface representation with different shades of gray used for each subunit of the trimer). The surface-exposed loops between A-A′ and D-E strands are involved in receptor binding. TNF is cleaved by TNFα-converting enzyme (TACE), a member of the ADAM family of metalloproteinases (ADAM17) involved in processing of many cell surface proteins. TACE is a type I transmembrane protein that cleaves TNF between residues Val75 and Ala76; when all three sites are cleaved, TNF is released into a soluble form. **Bottom:** TNF receptor and ligand complex. The ectodomain of TNFR1 forms an elongated molecule with CRD1 proximal to the N-terminus (depicted as a ribbon diagram). The face of TNFR1 on the left engages LTα. In the ligand–receptor complex the elongated receptor (dark) lies along the cleft formed between adjacent subunits. Shown (space-filling) is a single TNFR1 in complex with two subunits of LTα (lighter shading); the receptor N-terminus points upward, closest to the base of the ligand (*trans* orientation). In the exploded view, TNFR1 is removed from in front of the ligand, revealing the contact residues in the ligand, which are primarily located in the D-E and the A′-A″ β strands (dark shading). TNFR1 is rotated 180 degrees, exposing the contact residues in the receptor (light shading). Structures from 1TRN.pdf (17) as visualized with MacPyMOL (http://www.pymol.org).

ligand-binding properties and compete with cellular receptors for the specific ligands, thus earning the title of decoy receptor. The structural motifs in the cytoplasmic domains further categorize the TNFR into two groups based on their signaling properties: those that contain a death domain and those that engage TNFR-associated factors (TRAFs).

The cysteine-rich domain (CRD) in the extracellular, ligand-binding region defines membership in the TNFRSF (Figure 25.1). Each CRD typically contains six cysteine residues forming three disulfide bonds. The CRD is pseudorepeated in different members, ranging from one to six. Based on the crystal structures solved for several TNFRSF members, the CRD confers an elongated shape and sidedness to the ectodomain (17,*18*). The crystal structure of the complex between TNFR1 and one of its ligands, the LTα homotrimer, revealed that residues in CRD2 and 3 of TNFR1 contact the ligand. Variation in binding interactions has been identified; for example, the receptors for BAFF have one functional CRD (*2*,19).

RECEPTOR–LIGAND COMPLEX

The binding specificity of the various members of the TNF ligand and receptor superfamilies show monotypic interaction, yet several members interact with multiple partners (20) (Figures 25.2 and 25.3). The binding interactions between TNF-related ligands and TNFR are typically of high affinity, with equilibrium binding constants measured in the high-picomolar to low-nanomolar range. The membrane position of the ligands further enhances the binding interaction with their receptors. In the membrane-anchored position the ligands and receptors must be in *trans* to form a complex. In the LTα-TNFR1 complex, the surface loops between A-A" and D-E β strands contain many of the amino acid residues that make contact with the receptor, with the receptor-binding site formed as a composite by adjoining subunits in the trimeric ligand (17) (Figure 25.1).

The trimeric architecture of the TNF ligands, containing three equivalent receptor-binding sites, provides the basis for initiating signaling through aggregation or clustering of receptors, which is supported by the finding that receptor-specific bivalent antibodies can act as agonists and mimic the signaling activity of the natural ligand *(21)*. Indeed, antibodies or peptides mimetic to TNFR can function as antagonists blocking the ability of the natural ligand to bind the receptor while simultaneously activating the receptor as an agonist (22). Some ligands, such as FasL, TRAIL, and BAFF, form higher-ordered oligomers of the basic trimer. These higher-ordered oligomers promote supraaggregation of receptors, enhancing or sustaining signaling pathways in the receptor-bearing cell (23,*24*). Overexpression of TNFR in cells can also lead to ligand-independent signaling, a feature bestowed in part by the propensity of the cytosolic tails to self-associate *(25)*. In the physiologic setting, the expression level and compartmentalization of these receptors are tightly controlled. A subregion in the first CRD of TNFR1, known as the preligand assembly domain (PLAD), may restrict the orientation of the unligated receptor to prevent spontaneous activation *(26)*. It is not known whether this mechanism applies to all members of the TNFRSF. Of interest, some patients with periodic fever syndrome have mutant TNFR1 that form abnormal disulfide-linked oligomers that are retained intracellullarly and provoke the misfolded protein response (27).

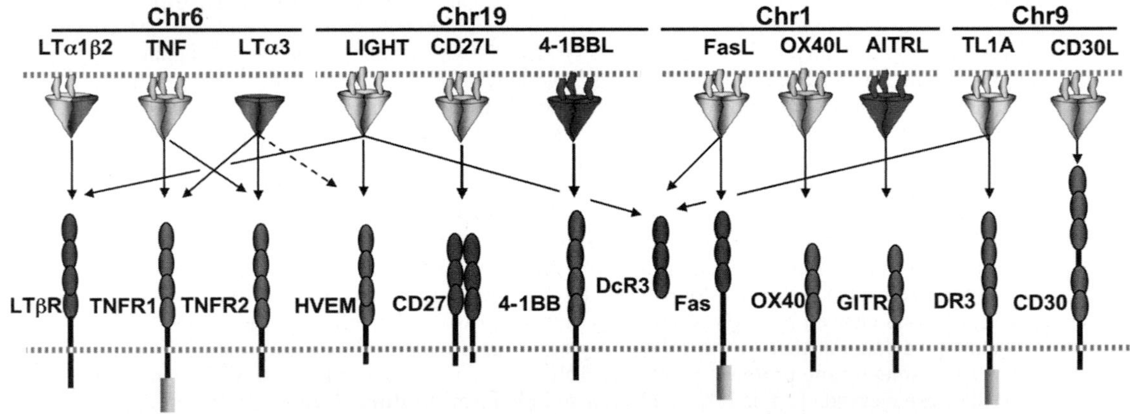

FIGURE 25.2 The tumor necrosis factor (TNF) superfamily major histocompatibility complex (MHC) paralogs. Members of the TNF ligand superfamily (above) and their corresponding receptors (below) are identified by connecting arrows. The ligands are grouped according to their chromosomal (Chr) locations in the MHC paralogous regions. The number of cysteine-rich domains is depicted for each TNF receptor (TFNR), and TNFRs containing a death domain are identified by cylinder in the cytoplasmic tail. (Modified from Ware CF. TNF superfamily. *Cytokine Growth Factors Rev*. 2003;14:181, with permission.)

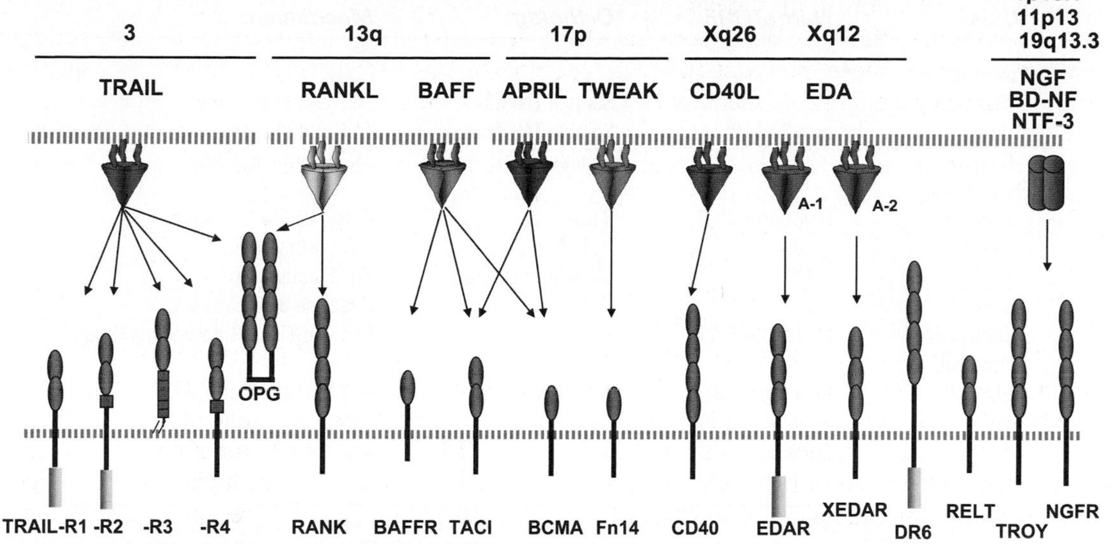

FIGURE 25.3 The tumor necrosis factor (TNF) superfamily, part 2. Members of the TNF ligand superfamily (above) and their corresponding receptors (below) are identified by connecting arrows. The ligands are grouped according to their chromosomal (Chr) locations. The number of cysteine-rich domains is depicted for each TNF receptor (TNFR), and TNFRs containing a death domain are identified by cylinder in the cytoplasmic tail. (Modified from Ware CF. TNF superfamily. *Cytokine and Growth Factors Rev*. 2003;14:181, with permission.)

Alternate Ligands

There is significant divergence in the ligands and the mechanisms of ligand binding by the TNFR family. A major branch point is exemplified by the ligands for p75 neurotrophin receptor (nerve growth factor and the other neurotrophins), which are structurally unrelated to the TNF ligand family. Molecular contacts between NGF and p75NTR occur through two spatially separated binding regions located at the first and second CRD and the junction between the CRD3 and CRD4 (28). The p75NTR functions in complex with two other proteins, Nogo66 and LINGO, and this complex engages myelin-associated inhibitory factors. TROY/Taj can supplant p75NTR in this complex (29). Like p75 NTR, DR6, RELT, and TROY/Taj do not bind any of the known TNF ligands. The pathways activated by p75NTR and TROY/Taj systems show both positive and inhibitory regulation of axonal regeneration (29,30).

The herpesvirus entry mediator (HVEM, TNFRSF14) provides an example of a TNFR system that binds an alternate ligand. Although HVEM binds two TNF-related ligands—LIGHT and LTα—it also engages a member of immunoglobulin superfamily—B and T lymphocyte attenuator (BTLA) (31). BTLA binding to HVEM occurs in CRD1, on the opposite face of where LIGHT/LTα binds CRD2 and 3. The BTLA-binding site in CRD1 of HVEM is a region also targeted by herpesviruses (32–34). The engagement of ligands distinct from TNFSF members implicates a higher level of integration with other signaling pathways.

Viral Orthologs

The TNFR-like proteins are found in several viral pathogens representing captured cellular genes imprisoned in the viral genome that evolved as part of that pathogen's immune evasion strategy (Table 25.3) (35). Poxvirus was the first pathogen identified harboring a version of a cellular TNFR (36). Poxvirus TNFR displays significant sequence conservation to TNFR2 and binds TNF and LTα. The rabbit poxvirus protein T2 is secreted by virally infected cells and contributes to the virulence of infection (37,38). Smallpoxvirus, the former scourge of mankind, also harbored viral versions of TNFR2 *(39)*.

SIGNALING PATHWAYS AND CELLULAR RESPONSES

Regulation

The cellular response activated by a TNF-related cytokine depends on several factors, including the temporal patterns of expression of the ligands and receptors in the interacting cells and the cellular context (the state of differentiation of the responding cell). Regulation is achieved at the level of transcriptional and translational controls and by modulating the availability of the ligand or receptors (Figure 25.4). For some ligands, transcriptional activation is a critical feature controlling the duration of mRNA expression. Some ligands exhibit inducible, transient

TABLE 25.3 Viral Orthologs and Modulators of the Tumor Necrosis Factor (TNF) Superfamily

Virus	Name/ORF	Ortholog[a]	Mechanism
Poxvirus:			
Myxoma	T2	Soluble TNFR2	TNF and LTα decoy
Virola	crm B (G2R)	Soluble TNFR2	TNF and LTα decoy
Coxpox	vCD30	Soluble CD30	CD30 ligand inhibitor
Herpesvirus:			
HSV1, 2	Glycoprotein D	BTLA	Entry; HVEM blockade
HCMV	UL144	HVEM	BTLA activation
EBV	LMP1	CD40 intracellular	TRAF activation
γHV	vFLIP	FLIP	Caspase 8 blockade
Adenovirus	E3-10.4,14.5,6.7	?	Fas and TRAILR downmodulation
Retrovirus:			
EIAV	Envelope gp90	?	HVEM entry factor
FIV	Envelope gp95	?	Ox40 entry factor
ASLV	Envelope gp85	?	TRAILR entry factor
Rabies virus	Envelope RVG	?	NTRp75 entry factor

ASLV, avian sarcosis and leucosis virus; BTLA, B and T lymphocyte attenuator; EBV, Epstein-Barr virus; EIAV, equine infectious anemia virus; FIV, feline immunodeficiency virus; FLIP, FLICE-inhibitory protein; γHV, equine gamma herpesvirus; HCMV, human cytomegalovirus; HEVM, herpesvirus entry mediator; HSV, herpes simplex virus; RVG, rabies virus glycoprotein, TRAF, TNF receptor–associated factor.

[a]Relationship determined by sequence or structural homology to the indicated TNF superfamily member; a question mark indicates that no homology is recognized.

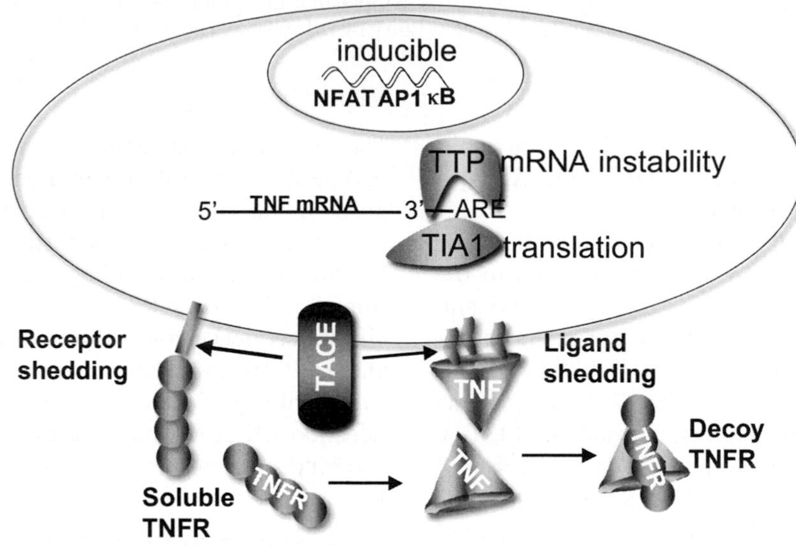

FIGURE 25.4 Regulation of tumor necrosis factor (TNF) bioavailability. The expression of TNF is regulated at the transcriptional and translational levels, and its bioavailability is affected by altering its physical location and cellular receptors. TNF transcription is regulated by the action of multiple transcription factors, including NFAT (nuclear factors of activated T cells), AP-1 (activated protein-1), and NF-κB (nuclear factor of the immunoglobulin κB locus). NFAT is a predominant transcription factor regulating TNF transcription in T and B lymphocytes, and NF-κB and AP-1 are important in myeloid lineage cells after activation via innate pattern recognition receptors, such as the Toll-like receptors. TNF mRNA stability is controlled by an AU-rich element (ARE) in the 3′ untranslated region present in many transiently expressed inflammatory genes (297). Stability of TNF mRNA is decreased by the action of tristetraprolin (TTP), and T cell intracellular antigen (TIA1) silences translation of TNF mRNA through the ARE (298). TACE proteolytically controls the TNF at the membrane, generating a soluble form of TNF. TACE also cleaves TNFR1 and 2 (299), downregulating cell surface receptors and releasing soluble receptors that retain TNF-binding activity. Soluble TNFRs can stabilize the TNF trimer at subsaturating concentrations, and at higher, saturating concentrations they act as decoys, competing for TNF binding to cellular receptors *(300)*.

expression of mRNA after antigen recognition or through innate receptor recognition systems. The half-life of mRNA levels may be controlled by an AU-rich element in the 3′ region (40), a feature very important in regulating TNF mRNA levels. Deletion of the AU-rich element in TNF mRNA in mice leads to a profound inflammatory disease (40,*41*). TNF mRNA is inducible in macrophages by multiple pathways, particularly innate activation pathways such as Toll-like receptor signaling, whereas other ligands, like 41BBL and Ox40L, are constitutively expressed in differentiated antigen-presenting dendritic cells. T and B lymphocytes require activation prior to expression of TNF. Signals via the antigen receptor using the NFAT transcription factor are needed for TNF inducibility. The inducible or constitutive patterns of expression are observed with the receptors as well.

Posttranslational regulation of signaling is achieved by proteolytic cleavage of the ligand or receptor from the cell's surface, which places the protein into the soluble phase, where its half-life may be dramatically shortened. TNF and Fas ligand, for example, are shed from the surface by membrane proteases. The enzyme processing TNF, ADAM17 (also known as TNFα converting enzyme [TACE]), into a soluble form is involved in cleaving multiple cell surface proteins, including transforming growth factor-α (TGFα), L-selectin, and TNFR1 and 2; the latter substrates may be important in regulating TNF bioavailability as decoy receptors (Figure 25.4).

Most of the TNF-related ligands are expressed by dendritic cells, activated lymphocytes, and myeloid cells, particularly macrophages, but they can also be produced by nonlymphoid cells. TNF is an example of a ligand expressed by many cell types, depending on the stimulus. In contrast, expression of TNFR is widespread. TNFR1 is expressed on most cells, although TNFR2 is limited to cells of hematopoietic origin and is expressed after activation of B or T cells. Macrophages are a primary source of TNF in response to TLR signaling, and T cells when activated by antigenic stimuli, but fibroblasts also produce TNF in response to virus infection, and nonlymphoid tumor cells may ectopically express TNF. FasL is another example of a ligand with varied cellular expression pattern. FasL is expressed by effector T cells and NK cells as a component of their cell lytic activity, yet FasL mRNA is detected in reproductive organs and epithelium of the eye, which may use this ligand to kill organ-infiltrating inflammatory cells, providing a mechanism to dampen inflammation.

Signal Transduction Pathways

TNF receptors initiate signaling pathways that alter gene expression patterns as well as apoptotic pathways terminating cellular life. The propagation of signals to enzymatically active proteins is mediated by two distinct types of signaling motifs in the cytosolic domain of the various TNFR: death domain (DD) receptors, such as Fas, TNFR1, and TRAILR1 and 2, and those that have a TRAF recruitment motif, including LTβR, CD40, and CD27, among others. Three basic schemes are used by TNF receptors to connect to enzymatically driven signaling pathways (Figure 25.5A). Adaptor molecules are required to establish the signaling connection. The DD connects TNFR to death effector domain (DED)–containing proteins, which in turn link to proteolytic active caspases (cysteine-based, aspartic acid–specific proteinases). Alternatively, the TRAF proteins connect to the cytosolic domain of the TNFR, linking to pathways that activate NF-κB and AP1 transcription factors. The third scheme involves an indirect link to TRAF adaptors via a DD adaptor, TRADD.

The apoptotic and NF-κB pathways activated by the TNFR family help to regulate cellular homeostasis by controlling cell death and survival. In the immune system, apoptosis is key to controlling homeostasis and eliminating antigen-bearing cells from the host. Many TNFRs can induce activation of survival or death pathways depending in part on the differentiated state of that cell. In all nucleated cells, the apoptotic pathway is the default, that is, all of the constituents are expressed and ready to be activated (Figure 25.6), whereas cellular survival requires transcriptional induction of genes that encode regulatory proteins that suppress progression of the apoptotic pathway. Ligation of TNFR promotes assembly of the death-inducing signaling complex (DISC), which promotes dimerization of pro-caspase 8, forming an active enzyme (42). Activated caspase 8 acts directly to cleave pro-caspase 3 and 7, which are known as the executioner caspases because they directly cleave critical cellular substrates leading to apoptotic death. Caspase 8 also cleaves BID, a crucial connection to the mitochondria-associated death mechanism, which greatly amplifies the apoptotic process. The inhibitors of apoptosis (IAP) are direct caspase inhibitors regulated at gene expression level by NF-κB. FLIP (FLICE/Fas-associated death domain [FADD] inhibitory protein) is an NF-κB–regulated gene, with a DED and pseudo caspase domain that attenuates the apoptotic pathway by blocking conversion of pro-caspase 8. As expected, many viruses have evolved different strategies to alter the proapoptotic pathways, and some use viral orthologs of IAP and FLIP (Figure 25.6).

Transcriptional activation by TNFR uses TRAF adaptors. After ligand binding, TRAFs are recruited to the activated receptor, but through different mechanisms. TRAF2, 3, and 5 bind directly to the receptor's cytosolic domain, whereas TRAF2 can also uses TRADD to couple to TNFR1. TRAF3 and TRAF6 appear to be preassociated with different protein kinases involved in multiple signaling pathways, including the pathogen recognition and interferon (IFN) pathways (43). TRAF adaptors link TNFR directly to protein kinase cascades, which in turn lead to activation of transcription factors, including NF-κB and AP1.

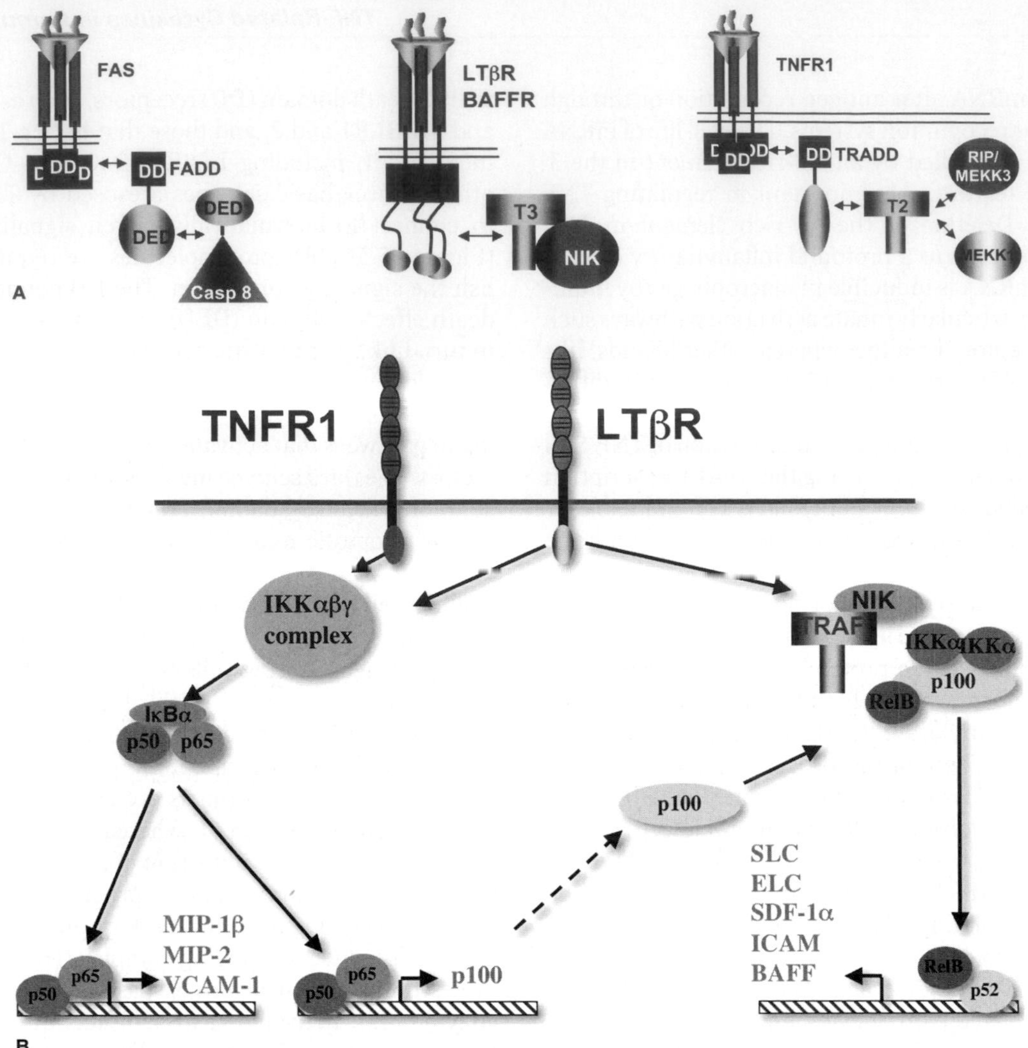

FIGURE 25.5 Signaling pathways and NF-κB. **A:** Adaptors link TNFR to proteinases and kinases. Three basic schemes link activated tumor necrosis factor receptors (TNFRs) to signaling pathways: The death-inducing signaling complex (DISC) formed with Fas is initiated by ligand clustering of Fas, promoting death domain (DD) interactions, which recruits FADD (heterotypic interaction). The death effector domain (DED) of Fas-associated death domain (FADD) links to the DED of pro-caspase (Casp) 8. The proximity of multiple pro-caspase 8 domains forms an active enzyme, which can process other caspase 8 molecules. By contrast, TNFRs bind TRAF adaptors (TNFR-associated factors) via short peptide motifs that release TRAF from associated kinases, such as NF-κB–inducing kinase (NIK). The third scheme is a combination of DD and TRAF recruitment. TNFR1 uses the DD protein TRADD to recruit RIP and TRAF2, promoting the activation of NF-κB. There are six TRAF members with distinct interaction patterns with the TNFR family. TRAF proteins may function as regulators of key kinases. TRAF3 and TRAF6 function as modulators of several different kinases involved in Toll-like receptor signaling, induction of type 1 interferon responses, and signaling by some TNFR family members. TRAF proteins contain an N-terminal RING finger motif, a coiled-coil domain (isoleucine zipper), and the receptor association (TRAF) domain. The TRAFs are trimers formed through their TRAF and coiled-coil domains. The TRAF domain can bind to several different TNFRs through a relatively short proline-anchored sequence that is responsible for binding directly to the mushroom head of various TRAF molecules (301). The zinc RING of TRAF6 functions together with Ubc13 and Uev1A as a ubiquitin ligase targeting proteins for proteasome degradation. (Modified from Ware CF. Tumor necrosis factors. In: Bertino JR, ed. *Encyclopedia of Cancer*, Vol. IV. San Diego, CA: Academic Press, 2002:475, with permission.) **B:** NF-κB activation. TNFR1 and LTβR induce distinct forms of the NF-κB family of transcription factors. TNFR1 signaling is a potent activator of RelA/p50 but does not activate the RelB pathway, whereas LTβR can activate both. The RelA and RelB forms of the κB family control transcription of distinct sets of genes; however, the two pathways are interrelated through the control of p100 expression by the RelA/p50 complex. (Modified from Dejardin E, Droin NM, Delhase M, et al. The lymphotoxin-beta receptor induces different patterns of gene expression via two NF-kappaB pathways. *Immunity*. 2002;17(4):525, with permission.)

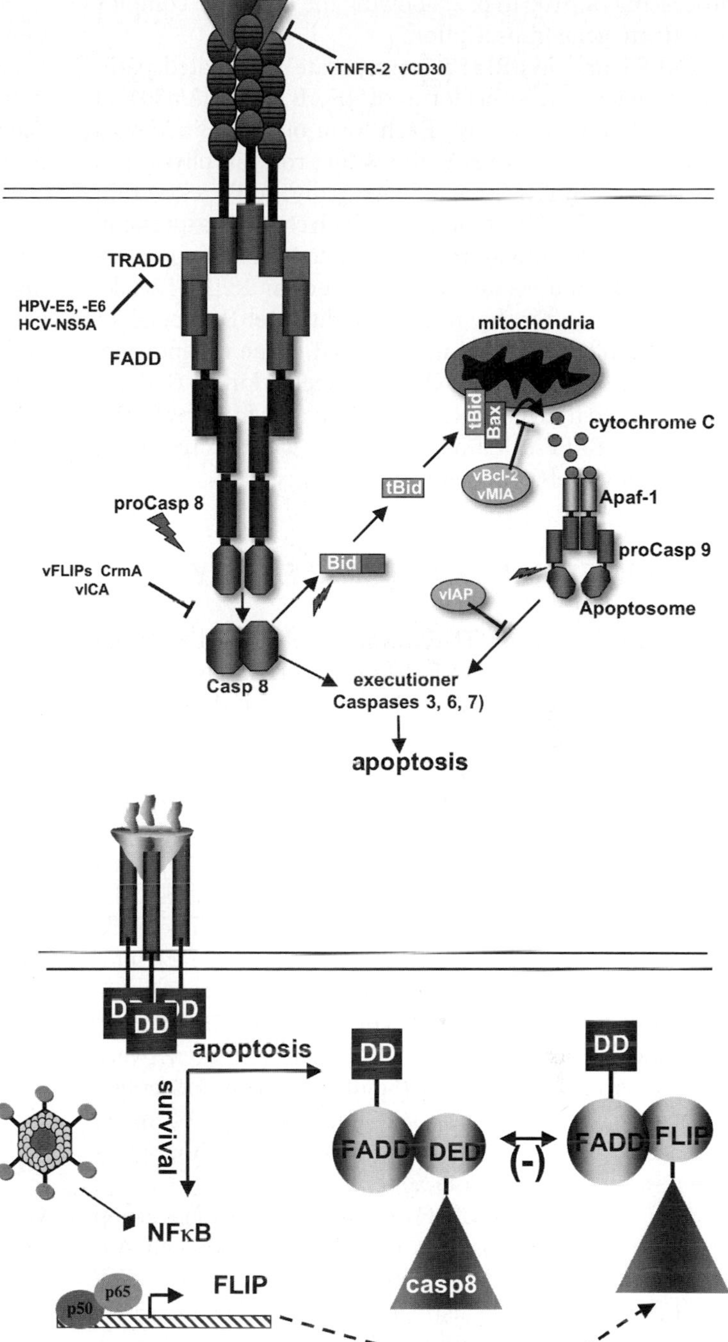

FIGURE 25.6 Apoptosis and survival signaling. **Top:** Ligation of TNFR1, Fas, or TRAILR1 and 2 activates apoptosis pathways. The nascent death-inducing signaling complex (DISC) can directly cleave the executioner caspases 3, 6, and 7. Caspase 8 also cleaves BID to truncated BID (tBID), activating the mitochondrial-regulated apoptotic pathway, dramatically accelerating cellular death. A number of viral proteins interfere with apoptosis induced through the tumor necrosis factor pathway, including human papilloma virus (HPV), hepatitis C virus (HCV), and herpesvirus FLICE-inhibitory proteins (vFLIPs) and virus orthologs of Bcl2 and vMIA that act on the mitochondria. (Adapted from Benedict CA, Banks TA, Ware CF. Death and survival: viral regulation of TNF signaling pathways. *Curr Opin Immunol.* 2003;15(1):59, with permission.) **Bottom:** The components of the apoptotic pathway are preformed in the cytosol, enabling the cell to respond rapidly to death signaling. In contrast, the key regulators of the apoptotic pathway, including Bcl2 and IAP (inhibitor of apoptosis) require new gene expression controlled by NF-κB. An important NF-κB–induced gene is cellular FLIP, which contains a pseudo caspase domain. The cFLIP protein interferes with caspase 8 activation, blocking the pro-death pathway. If the cell is transcriptionally inactive or unable to activate NF-κB, which often occurs in a pathogen-infected cell, then the proapoptotic pathway dominates the signals emanating from the TNFR1 signaling complex, leading to apoptosis and curtailing parasitism of the cell.

The NF-κB family of transcription factors controls expression of genes critical for cell survival, inflammatory, and immune responses. In mammalian cells, the NF-κB family consists of five members: RelA, RelB, c-Rel, p50/NF-κB B1, and p52/ NF-κB B2 (proteolytic processing of p105 and p100 yields the active forms p50 and p52, respectively) (*44*,45). Homo- and heterodimers of NF-κB family members are held inactive in the cytosol by inhibitors of κB (IκB), such as IκBα, masking nuclear localization motifs. The inhibitor of κB-kinase (IKK) complex is the common target of a variety of signals that control the activation of the RelA NF-κB transcription factor, which in turn regulates expression of several hundred genes within a signal-responsive cell. A distinct pathway regulates the activation of RelB NF-κB through a distinct complex comprised of NF-κB–inducing kinase (NIK)-IKKα kinases. Receptor ligation releases the active form of NIK that phosphorylates IKKα, which induces the proteasome-dependent processing of p100 to p52, allowing the RelB/p52 complex to activate gene transcription.

TNFR1 and LTβR activate separate yet related pathways that lead to distinct forms of NF-κB, the RelA/p50 and RelB/p52 complexes (46). Each form of NF-κB activates a large number of genes with distinct roles in physiology (Figure 25.5B). TNFR1 signaling rapidly mobilizes (within minutes) the RelA/p50 complex, which controls expression of many proinflammatory genes. By contrast, the processing of p100 and accumulation of nuclear RelB/p52 take several hours after the initial stimulus. Rel B–dependent genes are often involved in lymphoid tissue organogenesis and homeostasis. The NF-κB–inducing kinase (NIK) is also required for NF-κB RelB and RelA activation by CD27, CD40, and BAFF-R but not by TNFRI, which is restricted to activating RelA/p50 complex (47,48).

THE IMMEDIATE LT AND TNF FAMILY

Tumor necrosis factor (TNF, formerly TNFα, TNFSF2) and LTα (formerly TNFβ, TNFSF1) were originally pursued and characterized as inducers of tumor cell death, holding promise as antitumor therapeutics; however, the potent inflammatory action of TNF, particularly in the cardiovasculature, was quickly realized by observing the response of cancer patients injected with recombinant protein. We now recognize that TNF and LTα are two components of an interconnected network of "signaling circuits" that include LTβ and LIGHT (TNFSF14) and their specific receptors and regulatory proteins (Figure 25.2). Each individual pathway has unique and cooperative signaling activities with other members of this immediate family. The immunologic processes controlled by this cytokine network are extensive, ranging from the development and homeostasis of lymphoid organs to the mobilization of innate defense systems to cosignaling activity promoting adaptive immune responses (49,50,*51*).

TNF, LTα, LTβ, and LIGHT define the immediate group of TNF-related ligands that bind four cognate cell surface receptors with distinct but shared specificities. TNF and LTα both bind two distinct receptors, TNFR1 (p55-60, TNFR1A) and TNFR2 (p75-80, TNFR1B). The heteromeric LT$\alpha\beta$2 complex binds the LTβR, which also binds LIGHT (TNFSF14). LIGHT also engages the herpesvirus entry mediator (HVEM, TNFRSF14), which acts as a ligand for BTLA (31), an immunoglobulin (Ig) superfamily member. Two distinct human herpesviruses—herpes simplex virus and cytomegalovirus—target the HVEM-BTLA pathway using different mechanisms (34) (Figure 25.7).

TNF mediates a diverse range of cellular and physiologic responses linked to acute and chronic inflammatory processes. The diversity of responses is due in part to the broad expression of TNFR1 and the release of TNF as a soluble mediator, where it can act in a systemic fashion. TNF production is triggered by many of the innate recognition systems, such as the Toll-like receptors, and by T and B cells, whereby in chronic inflammation, TNF production can lead to tissue damage and organ failure. Genes expressed in response to TNF signaling coordinate the physiologic responses during inflammation (Table 25.4). The responses reflect the characteristic of the inflamed organ and the local or systemic source of TNF and the duration of TNF signaling. Acute inflammatory responses involve rapid changes in hemodynamics (plasma leakage and edema) and leukocyte adherence, extravasation, and organ infiltration induced by TNF. TNF production during chronic inflammation may contribute to systemic metabolic derangements and wasting (cachexia) or loss of organ structure and function (bone erosion in joints of patients with rheumatoid arthritis). In some models, TNF can promote an inflammatory environment that promotes tumor formation (52,53,*54*).

Elucidation of the functions associated with this TNF/LT signaling network has been aided by studies with genetically modified mice engineered with null or transgene expression of the cytokine or receptor (Table 25.5). Deficiency in TNF or TNFR1 but not TNFR2 leads to similar phenotypes with alterations in host defense to intracellular bacterial pathogens, like *Listeria monocytogenes* and *Mycobacterium tuberculosis*, but surprisingly modest susceptibility to some viral pathogens. These results demonstrated a role for TNF in acute-phase response of the host defense system. In contrast, LTα-deficient mice showed a failure in formation of peripheral lymphoid organs, a phenotype not observed in mice deficient in either TNFR or TNF, which implicated the LT$\alpha\beta$ complex signaling through the LTβR as a key developmental pathway for lymphoid organogenesis.

LT$\alpha\beta$-LTβR, a Mammalian Organ Development Pathway

Gene-deficient mice sharing a common phenotype of no lymph nodes revealed the framework of a signaling pathway involved in mammalian organ development. LTα-, LTβ-, or LTβR-deficient mice fail to develop secondary lymphoid tissues (55,*56*). Several other knockout mice, including transcriptional regulators Ikaros, ID2, and RORγt, also lack lymph nodes *(57–61)*, as do mice deficient in components of the NF-κB activation pathway, including TRAF6, NIK, IKKα, and Rel B and their gene targets. Deficiencies in target genes including CXCR5, the receptor for CXCL13, show defective lymphoid organ structure, as do CCR7$^{-/-}$ mice (receptor for CCL19/CCL21). The developmental program of secondary lymphoid organ formation initiates at 13 days postcoitus, progressing in an organized fashion from dorsal to lateral movement, with intestinal Peyer's patches forming during the first postnatal week *(62)*. The defect is irreversible, in that transferring

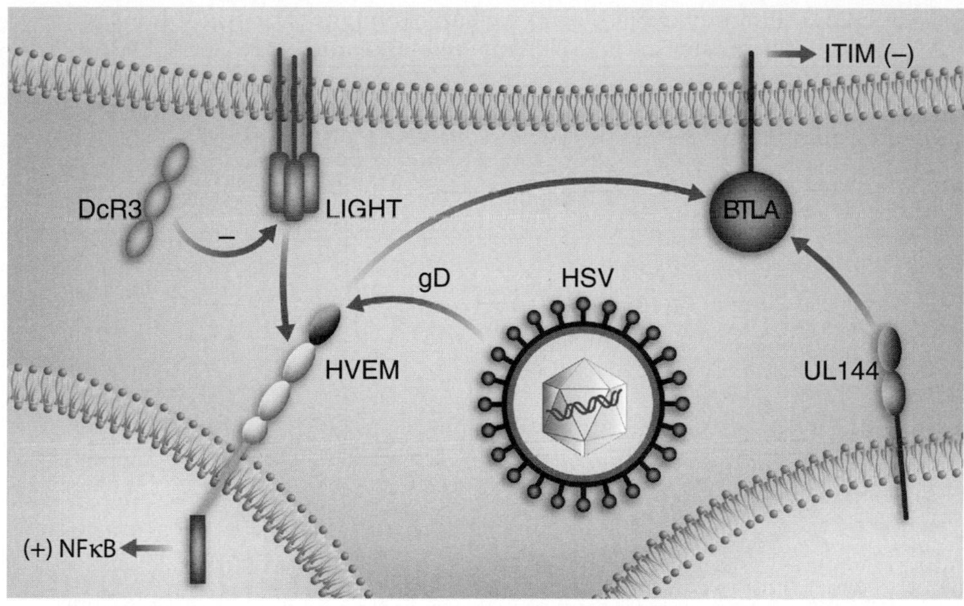

FIGURE 25.7 The herpesvirus entry mediator (HVEM)–B and T lymphocyte attenuator (BTLA) switch. The cartoon depicts the interactions involving HVEM that initiate positive cosignaling through LIGHT–HVEM interaction or inhibitory signaling through HVEM binding to BTLA. LIGHT bound to HVEM activates tumor necrosis factor receptor (TNFR)–associated factor–dependent activation of NF-κB, whereas HVEM-BTLA acts through an immuno tyrosine–based inhibitory motif (ITIM) of BTLA to recruit the phosphatase SHP2, attenuating kinases activated by TCR signaling. The herpes simplex virus (HSV) virion envelope protein gD attaches to HVEM, acting as an entry step for infection. The binding of glycoprotein D (gD) to HVEM can also competitively block BTLA binding and noncompetitively block the binding of LIGHT, inhibiting both intercellular communication pathways. UL144 of human cytomegalovirus binds BTLA but not LIGHT, selectively mimicking the inhibitory pathway of HVEM–BTLA. (From Kinkade A, Ware CF. The DARC conspiracy—virus invasion tactics. *Trends Immunol.* 2006;27:362, with permission.)

LT$\alpha\beta$-sufficient bone marrow into an adult LT-mutant mouse failed to induce lymph node formation. Accumulating studies indicate that the formation of lymphoid organs involves two distinct cell types: an embryonic, LTβR-expressing mesenchymal stromal cell that responds to LT$\alpha\beta$ expressed in a hematopoietically derived lineage, termed the lymphoid tissue inducer (LTi) cell. The LTi cell develops separately from lymphocytes and myeloid cells in a pathway dependent on ID2 and RORγt and different cytokines, including interleukin-7 (IL-7), RANK ligand (TRANCE, TNFSF11), and TNF. These cytokines induce surface LT$\alpha\beta$ in LTi cells that differentially engender formation of lymph nodes and Peyer's patches (63). Cells of the LTi lineage are maintained in the adult tissues at low levels (0.5%), presumably aiding in the homeostasis of lymphoid organs (*64*,65).

TABLE 25.4 Physiologic Correlates of Tumor Necrosis Factor–Mediated Gene Induction

Induced Gene	*Response*
iNOS	Vasodilation, edema
VCAM-1	Leukocyte margination and extravasation
IL-8	Leukocyte chemotaxis
MHC-1	Antigen presentation
Caspase 8 activation	Apoptosis
LPL	Cachexia

Caspase 8, cysteine-dependent aspartic acid specific proteinase-8; iNOS, inducible nitric oxide synthetase; IL-8, interleukin-8 (CXC chemokine); LPL, lipoprotein lipase; MHC-1, major histocompatibility complex-1; VCAM-1, vascular cell adhesion molecule-1.

The microarchitecture of the white pulp in the spleen (66) is disrupted in LT- and TNF-deficient mice *(67)*. Multiple features of the architecture, including missing macrophages in the marginal sinus and the loss of positional segregation of T and B cells into discrete zones, are observed in LT- and TNF-deficient mice. The segregation of T and B cells into discrete compartments depends on expression of the tissue-organizing chemokines, with CCL19 and CCL21 attracting T cells and CXC13L for B cells. CCL19 and CCL21 act through the chemokine receptor CCR7 expressed on T cells, and CXCR5 acting on B cells promotes localization in the follicles. An LT-chemokine

TABLE 25.5 Phenotypes in Mice Deficient in Lymphotoxin and Tumor Necrosis Factor (TNF) Immediate Family

	Phenotype					
Gene Deletion	***LN***[a]	***PP***[b]	***Architecture***[c]	***NK***[d]	***NK-T***[e]	***DC***[f]
LTα	–	–	Disrupted	Impaired	Impaired	CD8-DC
LTβ	–	–	Disrupted	Impaired	Impaired	CD8-DC
LIGHT	+	+	+	+	+	+
LTβ-B[g]	+	+	Disrupted	nr	nr	nr
LTβ-T[g]	+	+	+	nr	nr	nr
TNF[h]	+	+	+	+	+	Maturation
LTβR	–	–	Disrupted	–	–	CD8-DC
TNFR1	+	–	Disrupted MZ	+	+	Maturation
TNFR2	+	+	+	+	+	+

–, absent; +, normal; nr, not reported.

[a]Lymph nodes (LNs); LT$\beta^{-/-}$ mice have ~75% of mesenteric LNs; LIGHT/LT$\beta^{-/-}$ mice have fewer mesenteric nodes than LT$\beta^{-/-}$ mice (55,303,304).

[b]Peyer's patches (305,306).

[c]Architecture of the splenic white pulp includes T- and B-zone segregation; marginal zone (MZ); germinal center; follicular dendritic cell network.

[d]Natural killer (NK) cell deficiency includes reduced cell numbers and enhanced tumor susceptibility (307).

[e]NK-T cells, Vα14 subset (308).

[f]CD8[−] dendritic cell (DC) subsets in spleen are diminished from failure to proliferate (74).

[g]LTβ conditionally deleted in B cells or T cells (309). LTβ-B cells showed partial disruption in architecture; normal for LTβ-T, but combined knockout in both B and T cells was worse than LTβ-B.

[h]Normal architecture observed in TNF point mutant (305); abnormal architecture in TNFR1$^{-/-}$ mice (306).

Modified from Ware CF. Network communications: lymphotoxins, LIGHT, and TNF. *Annu Rev Immunol* 2005;23:787, with permission.

circuit is formed by migration of B cells to LTβR$^+$ stromal cells expressing CXCL13, which in turn induces expression of LTαβ on B cells (*68*,69,*70*). Circulating B cells lack surface LTαβ, but expression is regained on reentry into the CXCL13-rich microenvironment *(70)*. The formation of the splenic microarchitecture depends on B cell expression of LTαβ, which induces differentiation of specialized stromal cells (e.g., secretion of CCL20 and CXCL13 chemokines) in the spleen during postnatal maturation. Remodeling of the microarchitecture of the secondary lymphoid organs occurs during immune responses, which requires both TNF and LT pathways signaling on fibroblastic reticular cells (71). The viral pathogen cytomegalovirus can induce specific changes in the splenic microenvironment through modulation of CCL21 expression (72).

The LTβR and TNFR pathways facilitate lymphocyte entry into lymphoid tissues in part by modulating expression of adhesion molecules, such as peripheral node and mucosal addressins on high endothelial venules (73). LTβR signaling is necessary to maintain networks of follicular dendritic cells involved in capturing antigen and immune complexes that aid in activating B cells. These cellular interactions are further enhanced by LTβR signals that provides growth signal for some conventional myeloid dendritic cells (DCs) (CD8$^-$ subsets) within the lymphoid organ, whereas TNF plays a role in differentiation of DC progenitors in bone marrow (74).

T and B cells can communicate with stromal and myeloid cells via the LTαβ-LTβR pathway and thus during the course of an immune response modify their immediate microenvironment. Nonlymphoid tissues suffering from chronic inflammation associated with autoimmune disease, graft rejection, or microbial infection often contain organized accumulations of lymphocytes reminiscent of secondary lymphoid organs, called tertiary lymphoid organs. Activated T and B cells provide the source of LTαβ that helps to drive the process of forming these structures, but as antigen is cleared, immune responsiveness subsides and these structures resolve. A gradation of features may be found in the tertiary lymphoid organs, including presence of dendritic cells, expression of chemokines, high endothelial venules, segregated regions of T and B cells, and germinal centers, but they typically lack the permanence of a lymph node. TNF also contributes to formation of granuloma that assists in walling off bacteria (75). Thus, the LTαβ and TNF pathways operative in embryonic life also play critical roles in the adult in the formation of tertiary lymphoid structures.

Influence of the LTαβ Pathway on Lymphocyte Development

Mounting evidence indicates the LTαβ-LTβR pathway contributes to the ontogeny of unconventional T cells, including γδ T cells and invariant NK T cells, whereas conventional T cell subsets are normal in mice deficient in the TNF and LTβR pathways. The LTβR pathway seems to operate at distinct levels during thymic development (76).

Double-positive (DP) thymocytes regulate the differentiation of early thymocyte progenitors and $\gamma\delta$ T cells via the LTβR pathway *(77)*, yet the LTβR is not expressed in thymocytes, suggesting an indirect mechanism. In this regard, LTβR signaling is required for the proper formation and function of the thymic stroma, which influences T cell development *(78)*. The thymic medulla appears to control the export of iNKT cells from the thymus *(79,80)*. In addition, LTβR signaling in thymic stroma affects central tolerance to peripherally restricted antigens, which may be either dependent on or independent of the autoimmune regulator Aire *(81)*. Thymic differentiation depends on the LTβR pathway to mediate the cellular communication between lymphoid and stromal compartments.

Autoimmunity

Dysregulated expression of several members of the TNFSF leads to autoimmune-like diseases in humans and animal models. For example, enforced expression of TNF or LIGHT, which overrides the normal transient expression, causes severe autoimmune and inflammatory processes in mice (82–84). LTα or LT$\alpha\beta$ transgenic expression in the pancreas leads to insulitis and formation of tertiary lymphoid structures (85). These types of results have implicated members of the TNF superfamily as immune regulators and support the notion that LT$\alpha\beta$ and LIGHT pathways contribute to inflammation and tissue destructive processes.

Infectious Diseases

TNF is a major inflammatory cytokine required for the acute-phase response to bacterial infection. For instance, lipopolysaccharide (LPS) in gram-negative bacteria is a potent inducer of TNF secretion through the TLR4 innate recognition system, as are all the other TLRs. In mice, LPS induces a shock syndrome that is rapidly lethal owing to profound changes in blood circulation; however, mice survive LPS in the genetic absence of TNFR1 or if treated with a TNF-neutralizing antibody, indicating that host-derived TNF mediates pathogenesis (86,87,*88*). On the other hand, TNFR1 is essential for resistance to infection with a live organism, such as *L. monocytogenes*, through multiple processes including enhancement of phagocytosis and bacteriocidal destruction by macrophages. By contrast, T cell immunity is not overtly impaired in TNFR1$^{-/-}$ mice. Humans treated with TNF inhibitors show some increase in susceptibility to selective pathogens, particularly *M. tuberculosis*, reinforcing the role of TNF as a critical host defense system (89).

In contrast, LT-deficient mice showed significant variability in susceptibility to individual pathogens (Table 25.6). Increased susceptibility resulted from either

TABLE 25.6 Lymphotoxins in Host Defense: Mouse Models

Pathogen	*Mouse Model*[a]	*Susceptibility*	*Mechanism*	*Ref.*
Herpesvirus:				
MHV68	LT$\alpha^{-/-}$	Minimal	nd	*310*
HSV-1	LT$\alpha^{-/-}$	Increased	Decreased effector CD8$^+$ T cells	*311*
MCMV	LT$\alpha^{-/-}$	Increased	IFN response; adaptive immunity lost	*312, 313*
MCMV	LTβR-Fc Tg	Increased	Poor innate defenses	*312*
LCMV	LT$\beta^{-/-}$; LT$\alpha^{-/-}$	Increased	Defective architecture	*314–316*
LCMV	LTβR-Fc	Decreased	Decreased CD8$^+$/IFNγ	*317*
Theiler's virus	LT$\alpha^{-/-}$; LTβR-Fc	Increased	Defective architecture	*318*
Influenza	LT$\alpha^{-/-}$	Minimal	nd	*319*
Vesicular stomatitis virus	LT$\beta^{-/-}$	Increased	Defective architecture	*316*
Bacteria:				
Mycobacterium tuberculosis	LTβR$^{-/-}$	Increased	NO_2 synthase decreased	*320*
Mycobacterium tuberculosis	LT$\alpha^{-/-}$	Increased	No T cells in granuloma	*321*
Mycobacterium bovis	LTβR-Fc	Increased	Poor granuloma formation	*322*
Listeria monocytogenes	LTβR$^{-/-}$	Increased	nd	*320*
Leishmania major	LT$\beta^{-/-}$	Increased	Defective architecture	*323*
Toxoplasma gondii	LT$\alpha^{-/-}$	Increased	NO_2 synthase decreased	*324*
Plasmodium berghei	LT$\alpha^{-/-}$	Decreased	Decreased LTα-dependent inflammation	*325*

HSV1, herpes simplex virus (α-herpesvirus); IFN, interferon; LCMV, lymphocytic choriomenigitis virus; MCMV, mouse cytomegalovirus; MHV68, mouse γ-herpesvirus-68; nd, not determined.

[a]Studies conducted in gene-deficient mice ($^{-/-}$); LTβR-Fc Tg, mice expressing LTβR-Fc as a transgene; LTβR-Fc, mice injected protein.

Modified from Ware CF. Network communications: lymphotoxins, LIGHT, and TNF. *Annu Rev Immunol.* 2005;23:787, with permission.

developmentally controlled aspects of lymphoid organ structure (e.g., lymphocytic choriomenigitis virus, leishmania) or a requirement for LT$\alpha\beta$-LTβR pathway as an effector system in innate and adaptive immune systems (e.g., mouse cytomegalovirus). Viewed from an evolutionary perspective, this variation in the requirement for LT signaling may reflect specific contributions from the pathogen used to evade the broader TNF- and LT-dependent pathways (34,90).

TNF SUPERFAMILY AND T CELL COSIGNALING

Antigen recognition together with cooperative signaling or "cosignaling" systems determines the quality of the adaptive immune responses. Lymphocyte responses to antigen are dynamic processes that start with the activation of naive cells and transition through effector and memory phases. Cosignaling systems assist these phases by promoting more efficient engagement of antigen-binding T cell receptor (TCR) molecules to enhance initial cell activation and cell division (clonal expansion), augment cell survival (clonal contraction or memory cell differentiation), or induce effector functions such as cytokine secretion or killer function. Negative signals (inhibitory cosignaling) may also be delivered to T cells depending upon the particular system, which may prevent initial cellular activation or eliminate excess activated cells to dampen inflammation. Cosignaling can be quantitative, modifying thresholds of common signaling intermediates, or qualitative, involving signals distinct from other cosignaling systems or the TCR. Cosignaling receptors and ligands can be up- or downregulated at the transcriptional and protein levels depending on the stage of the T cell response and the inflammatory milieu. In the absence of cosignaling, T cells may become unresponsive (anergic) or die.

The TNF receptor superfamily is one of two major families of cosignaling regulators that modulate T cells. The other cosignaling systems belong to the immunoglobulin superfamily, such as CD28 *(91)*, CTLA-4 *(92)*, ICOS (93), PD1 (94), and BTLA (B-T lymphocyte attenuator) (95,96). TNF receptor superfamily members involved in cosignaling include Ox40, 41BB, DR3, CD27, CD30, and HVEM (97–99,*100*,101), whereas CD40 and BAFFR are more involved in cosignaling in B lymphocytes (102,103); however, considerable crossover of activities in both lymphocyte populations can be demonstrated. Death receptors such as Fas and TNFR1 are thought to be involved clonal contraction through apoptosis of activated effector cells, although TNF via TNFR2 also shows costimulatory action in naive T cells. In tissue culture models several of the TNF-related signaling pathways show costimulatory activities for T cells, which probably reflects the common induction of NF-κB–dependent survival genes, a common trait of TNFRSF members. However, analyses of physiologic models often reveal distinct roles for these molecules in the life of T cells. Cosignaling systems are emerging as important targets that enhance immune responses to tumors or attenuate autoimmune diseases (93,104,*105–107*,108).

Expression and Function of TNFRSF Cosignaling Molecules During Primary T Cell Responses

The TNFRs encoded on chromosome 1p36 share a common function as cosignaling systems for T cells (99,101). This region (human 1p36.33-1p36.21; syntenic with mouse 4E2-D3) contains the genes encoding GITR, Ox40, HVEM, DR3, 4-1BB, CD30, and TNFR2, representing an expansion of the region on chromosome12p13 where genes for TNFR1, LTβR, and CD27 reside. The TNF-related ligands for these receptors are linked in the MHC paralogs on chromosomes 1, 6, 9, and 19, reflecting a common functional link as costimulatory molecules modulating T cell differentiation (Figure 25.2).

Expression of TNFRSF members by T cells follows several distinct patterns during T cell activation: Expression on naive T cells in peripheral lymphoid tissues (e.g., CD27 and HVEM) that follow activation are upregulated or downregulated, respectively. Ox40, 4-1BB, TNFR2, and CD30 are only expressed by T cells after activation (99); TNFR2 is rapidly downmodulated after cleavage by TNFα-converting enzyme, generating soluble receptors that modulate TNF availability. The differing time course of expression of these molecules determines the phase at which they act in T cell differentiation.

Experimental activation of TNFRSF members can be achieved with agonist monoclonal antibodies. Antibodies specific for Ox40, 4-1BB, CD30, or CD27 all augment T cell clonal expansion and TCR-induced cytokine expression in tissue culture and mouse models. For example, CD27, which is expressed at very early stages of T cell activation, mediates initial cytokine production, cell division, and/or survival (*109*,110), whereas Ox40 and 4-1BB, which are expressed after cellular activation, promote T cell survival and proliferation during the later stages of the primary response (111,*112,113*). Although less is known regarding the exact timing and function of CD30 in T cell activation, CD30–CD30L interactions promote primary CD8$^+$ T cell expansion (114), suggesting functional parallels with other TNFRSF molecules. Coxpox virus encodes a specific CD30 mimic to block the action of CD30L as part of its immune evasion strategy (Table 25.3).

Death receptor-3 engages TL1A, promoting IFNγ expression by proinflammatory TH1 cells in mice (115) and humans (116), especially in intestinal tissues. The LIGHT-HVEM-LTβR pathway is also associated with T cell inflammatory processes in mucosal tissues (83,117). Similar cosignaling activities are reported for the glucocorticoid-induced TNF-related receptor (GITR) (118), with the potential of these systems to affect different subsets of T cells, such as GITR expression on T regulatory subsets. The role of these TNFRSFs in regulating different subsets is an active area of research. Deletion of genes for these members did not affect developmental pathways; however, immune deficiency is often revealed in response to infections.

By contrast, HVEM appears to play a role as an inhibitor of naive T cell activation though engagement of the Ig superfamily member BTLA (119). In this situation, HVEM acts as a ligand for BTLA, which, through a phosphatase recruitment domain (immuno tyrosine–based inhibitory motif [ITIM]) in its cytosolic tail limits signaling by antigen receptor–associated kinases (120). The BTLA-binding site on HVEM is distinct from the position occupied by LIGHT, yet membrane LIGHT can disrupt HVEM–BTLA binding, which suggests that HVEM acts as a regulatory switch between inhibitory and stimulatory cosignaling. The HVEM-BTLA pathway likely functions in maintaining inhibitory control over naive T cells. This pathway appears particularly effective in controlling CD4 T cell activation (121), but it is also important in regulating differentiating memory CD8 T cells (122). Together with the programmed death-1 cosignaling system (PD1), BTLA is needed to curtail antigen-induced lung inflammation (123).

T Cell Memory

Cosignaling through several TNFRSF members promotes the differentiation of memory T cells. Mice deficient in Ox40-Ox40L, CD27-CD70, or CD30-CD30L pathways all display defective memory responses to antigen (110,114,124–126). The Ox40 system is illustrative of the costimulatory signals provided to T cells by these TNFRs. Pharmacologic stimulation of Ox40 with an agonist antibody or ligand during a primary antigen-specific response in mice enhances the generation of memory CD4 T cells (*127*,128). The enhanced response of T cells includes increased accumulation of antigen-specific effector T cells at the site of inflammation producing effector cytokines such as IFNγ *(129)*. Moreover, blockade of Ox40-Ox40L interactions with monoclonal antibody specific to Ox40L during recall responses in models of collagen-induced arthritis (130) and experimental allergic lung inflammation (131) ameliorates inflammation. In Ox40-deficient mice, CD8 T cells expand normally; however, their accumulation and survival at later times in the primary response were significantly impaired, but the T cells also failed to fully differentiate as measured by loss of expression of effector cell surface markers, the synthesis of cytokines, and cytotoxic activity. In contrast, the formation of extrafollicular plasma cells, germinal centers, and antibody responses was independent of Ox40. Ox40 signaling induces transcription of survival genes such as Bcl2 and survivin in T cells, which may serve as the key targets that allow memory cell differentiation (*132*,133).

The discovery that HVEM can elicit inhibitory signaling in T cells through engagement of the Ig family member BTLA highlights the possibility that in certain situations TNFRSF molecules can counterregulate the stimulatory actions during T cell responses. Indeed, 4-1BB–deficient $CD4^+$ T cells in some models are hyperresponsive (134), and stimulation of 4-1BB can suppress immune responses in several models of autoimmune disease (*135–137*,138). Although activation of 4-1BB enhances the expansion of human antiviral memory $CD8^+$ T cells *in vitro* (139), several studies demonstrate that the absence of 4-1BB in mice leads to enhanced T cell responses (134,140), reminiscent of the phenotype associated with HVEM-deficient mice (141,142). Moreover, CD30 signals can, in some circumstances, suppress cytotoxic T lymphocyte activity (143). That TNFRSF molecules such as GITR or Ox40 are expressed on T regulatory cells suggests that costimulatory pathways may enhance the suppressive function of these cells during immune responses.

Mouse models of autoimmune diseases such as experimentally induced encephalomyelitis (EAE) and diabetes uncover critical roles for Ox40-Ox40L (*144*,145). Blockade of the CD27-CD70 pathway also ameliorates EAE through the suppression of TNF induction but not T cell priming (146). Furthermore, blockade of Ox40, 4-1BB, CD27, or CD30 costimulation can reduce transplant rejection and/or graft-versus-host disease (*147*,148,*149*,150).

Stimulation of these pathways may also be applicable for the treatment of diseases in which antigen-specific T cell responses are ineffective such as in cancer and infectious diseases. Stimulation of Ox40, 4-1BB, CD30, and CD27 with agonist antibodies augments T cell–mediated killing of a variety of tumors (reviewed in refs. 99,151). The critical roles of the cosignaling TNF-TNFRSF members are distinguished in immune responses to infectious pathogens. Similar to the immediate TNF family, the role of a specific cosignaling pathway in mediating protective T cell responses during infection depends on the pathogen (Table 25.7).

CD40L and the BAFF Systems

The CD40 and BAFF systems plays a major role in coordinating a range of costimulatory signals, including those important to B cell function, such as affinity maturation, isotype switching, immunoglobulin production, and clonal expansion (102,*152*,153–155). As are other TNF superfamily members, the CD40 system (Figure 25.3) is a key communication mechanism in host defense, autoimmunity, and cancer. Often these pathogenic processes are centered on the function of B cells. CD40 ligand maps to the X chromosome. Inducible CD40 ligand expression by

TABLE 25.7 Tumor Necrosis Factor Superfamily Cosignaling Pathways in Infectious Diseases

	Cosignaling Pathway			
Pathogen	*CD27-CD27L*	*Ox40-Ox40L*	*4-1BB-41BBL*	*CD30-CD30L*
Influenza	$CD4^+$, $CD8^+$ (110,*326*)	$CD4^+$ (126,*129,327*)	$CD8^+$ (124)	nd
LCMV	nd	$CD4^+$(*129*)	Normal $CD8^+$ (124)	nd
Leishmania major	No role	$CD4^+$ Th2 (*328*)	No role	No role
Helminths	nd	$CD4^+$ Th2 (*329*)	nd	nd
Cryptococcus neoformans	nd	Enhanced CD4 Th2 (*330*)	nd	nd
Mycobacterium avium	No role (*331*)	No role (*331*)	No role (*331*)	$CD4^+$, $CD8^+$ (*331*)
Listeria monocytogenes	$CD4^+$, $CD8^+$ (*332*)	nd	$CD8^+$ (*333*)	$CD8^+$ (*334*)

LCMV, lymphocytic choriomenigitis virus; nd, not done.
Unless indicated, the function of the T cells was impaired.
Adapted from Croft M. Co-stimulatory members of the TNFR family: keys to effective T-cell immunity? *Nat Rev Immunol.* 2003;3(8):609, with permission.

T helper cells promotes humoral immunity and is regulated by transcription factors NFAT, TFE3, and TFEB. CD40 ligand is also expressed on a variety of other cells, including activated B cells, endothelial cells, basophils, mast cells, and platelets. CD40 is expressed in many cells, prominently on B cells, using both TRAF3 and 6 to activate NF-κB and AP1 transcription factors, among other signaling pathways (156). Epstein-Barr virus, a B cell–transforming herpesvirus, mimics the CD40 pathway though its LMP1 protein, driving naive B cells into a memory state (*157*,158,*159*).

CD40 signaling is necessary for induction of activation-induced cytidine deaminase (AID), a key enzyme in class switching and somatic mutation of Ig genes. This process occurs in B cells in contact with T helper cells, which express CD40 ligand. The importance of the CD40 system in the activity of B cells was revealed in patients with hyper-IgM syndrome (HIGM). Several mutated genes underlie this syndrome, including CD40 ligand and CD40 *(160,161)*, the RelA NF-κB activating kinase subunit IKKγ (NEMO), and AID, among others (162). HIGM patients with mutated CD40L have elevated levels of IgM, often with no serum IgG, IgE, or IgA, and display increased susceptibility to bacterial and opportunistic infections. However, treatment of these patients with passive transfer of human immune IgG corrects infection by bacteria but not opportunistic pathogens such as *Pneumocystis carinii*. This latter result reflects the importance of CD40 system in T cell macrophage activation, which controls these opportunistic pathogens. In addition, the CD40 system can supplant T helper cell signals that allow DC and CD8 T cells to generate effector cells in the absence of CD4 T cells (*163*,164). In some patients, significant amounts of IgA and IgE are present in serum, even in the complete absence of CD40 ligand, a result indicating that another mechanism(s) can induce Ig class switching. Evidence has emerged for the BAFF/APRIL system in inducing Ig class switch independent of the CD40 system (165).

Since the discovery of B cell–activating factor of the TNF superfamily (BAFF, TNFSF13B, BLyS) and a proliferation-inducing ligand (APRIL, TNFSF13), much has been elucidated with regard to CD40 ligand-independent isotype switching and B cell development and survival in the periphery, as well as implications of BAFF-APRIL dysregulation in autoimmune disease and lymphomas (103,166). Although human BAFF maps to chromosome 13q34 and APRIL to 17p13.1, the proteins are strikingly more conserved (approximately 50% homology) than other TNF ligands. TWEAK (TNF-related ligand with weak apoptosis activity) maps adjacent to APRIL, part of a clade of genetically similar members that also includes ectodermal dysplasin (EDA1/EDA2). BAFF and APRIL form homo- and heterotrimers that interact with multiple receptors to form a complex signaling circuit (Figure 25.3). Membrane BAFF is shed via a furin protease at the cell surface, whereas APRIL is processed in the Golgi and secreted only in soluble form (167), although the receptor-binding domain of APRIL can be membrane anchored via an unusual splice variant with the TWEAK cytosolic and transmembrane domain (TWE-PRIL) (168). The significance of membrane-restricted local BAFF expression to systemic availability of soluble BAFF and APRIL remains to be established, although BAFF-APRIL heterotrimers are detected in serum from patients with systemic rheumatic diseases (7). BAFF and APRIL are inducibly expressed in monocytes, macrophages, dendritic cells, and T cells in the spleen and lymph nodes in response to certain cytokines such as type I and II IFN and IL-10; other TNF family members like CD40 and LTβR signaling also induce BAFF and APRIL. BAFF can be expressed in some B cell–derived chronic lymphocytic leukemia cells, and some epithelial-derived cancer cell lines and primary tumor tissues express APRIL. Stromal cell expression of BAFF maintains the major mature B cell pool, whereas inducible BAFF expression in myeloid cells aids in local B cell survival at sites of inflammation.

Three cognate receptors mediate the biological actions of BAFF. BAFFR (TNFRSF13C), TACI (transmembrane activator and calcium signal modulating cyclophilin ligand interactor, TNFRSF13B), and BCMA (B cell maturation antigen, TNFRSF17) are expressed on B cells and on other cell types. APRIL also engages matrix proteoglycans with weak binding, which may serve to enhance access to TACI and BCMA, or function as a distinct receptor–ligand interaction *(169)*. Signaling through BAFFR and BCMA are required for B cell survival and differentiation at different stages of B cell–mediated humoral response. BAFFR$^{-/-}$ mice display an almost complete loss of mature and marginal zone B cells acting at the late transitional phase of B cell maturation, whereas BCMA deficiency impaired the survival of long-lived bone marrow plasma cells (170,171).

By contrast, APRIL$^{-/-}$ mice develop normally but have altered class switching to IgA (172,*173*). TACI signaling may antagonize BAFFR and BCMA, because TACI$^{-/-}$ mice have elevated numbers of mature B cells (174). Both classical and alternative NF-κB pathways have been implicated in BAFFR and BCMA survival signals, with Bcl2 rescuing the B cell defect in BAFFR$^{-/-}$ mice. BAFFR and TACI engagement has also been shown to provide the necessary signals for CD40L-independent class switch recombination to IgG and IgE for BAFFR and IgG, IgE, and IgA for TACI in knockout mice, although IgA production seems specifically dependent on APRIL–TACI interaction (175). BAFFR is also connected to promoting the B cell coreceptor complex CD19/CD21/CD81, which binds to C3b-opsonized antigens to enhance rapid T-independent antibody response; however, overall impairment of T-independent antibody response appears to be greatest in TACI$^{-/-}$ mice and depends on APRIL–TACI interactions in B1 B cells. BAFFR, and not TACI, has also been proven to be important in T cell costimulation in *in vitro* and *in vivo* mouse models of allograft rejection response, where BAFFR$^{-/-}$ and BAFF$^{-/-}$ but not TACI$^{-/-}$ or BCMA$^{-/-}$ mouse recipients prolong graft survival due to weakened alloproliferative response (176).

Elevated levels of BAFF and APRIL have been detected in the serum, and especially the synovial fluid, of patients suffering from inflammatory autoimmune disorders such as systemic lupus erythematosus, rheumatoid arthritis, Sjörgen's syndrome, and multiple sclerosis (177). These levels tend to correlate with increasing amounts of autoreactive antibodies in serum, but soluble TACI-Ig treatment can lessen the severity of disease symptoms and progression in mouse models of lupus and collagen-induced arthritis (178). It is hypothesized that these excess quantities of BAFF and APRIL may contribute to the formation of autoreactive B lymphocytes and loss of tolerance during development and perpetuate their survival as plasmablasts. Emerging evidence connects the BAFF and APRIL systems to the pathology of B cell–derived cancers like B cell chronic lymphocytic leukemia, non-Hodgkin's lymphoma, and multiple myeloma. Malignant myeloma cells express high levels of BAFF and APRIL and receive ligand-induced survival signals, with upregulation of antiapoptotic Bcl-2 and Mcl-1 molecules (179). Therefore, BAFF and APRIL may bolster tumor survival via autocrine and paracrine signaling mechanisms.

TWEAK binds Fn14, a fibroblast growth factor (FGF)-2–inducible gene, limited to a monogamous interaction compared to its siblings (Figure 25.3). Fn14, a type I transmembrane protein with one CRD, binds TWEAK homotrimers in a manner similar to BAFF, APRIL, and their receptors (180,181). The biological functions of TWEAK-Fn14 system are broad, and perhaps paradoxical, promoting survival or inducing death; they are proinflammatory or immunorepressive. Due to these seemingly disparate observations, there is speculation that another, uncharacterized TWEAK receptor is involved, or that TWEAK acts in conjunction with other cosignaling systems that elicit different effects specific to its immunologic environment or context. TWEAK, like BAFF and APRIL, may be cleaved at its furin site to produce an active soluble form (180). Human and mouse TWEAK share 90% or greater sequence identity in the receptor-binding domain and manifest high-affinity cross-species interaction to respective Fn14 homologs (167). TWEAK has relatively wide organ mRNA expression, including heart, brain, spleen, lymph nodes, and human fibroblasts, although in some cells protein levels do not correlate with mRNA expression; it has also been detected in established cancer cell lines and primary tissue samples. TWEAK/Fn14 signaling induces apoptosis in some cancer lines (HT29, HSC3) and primary neurons (182,183,*184*). Other potential described capacities and proposed biological roles include induction of survival and growth in endothelial cells, migration and wound closure in endothelial monolayers, enhancement of proinflammatory cytokines (IL-6, IL-8), and angiogenesis (180,181). Very recent data connect TWEAK to regulation of the shift from innate to adaptive immune responsiveness by repressing innate inflammatory cytokines (IL-12, IFNγ) important in promoting TH1 immunity—a potential counterbalance to the proinflammatory actions of TNF (182). TWEAK may also have a potentiating influence in chronic tissue inflammation when dysregulated, such as its role in excessive demyelination and ultimate progression to excessive autoimmune encephalomyelitis *(185)*. In a mouse collagen-induced arthritis model, elevated levels of TWEAK in serum correspond to severe disease progression and enhanced arthritogenic mediator molecules (186). In obese patients with type 2 diabetes, TWEAK-Fn14 signaling augments proinflammatory cytokine release by adipocytes (187). TWEAK may prevent excessive luteinization after gonadotrophin-induced ovulation by controlling progesterone production in rats (188). This evidence suggests that the TWEAK-Fn14 system may provide important homeostatic functions to counteract inflammation in various tissues.

DEATH RECEPTORS AND LIGANDS

Fas Ligand and Fas System

The Fas (CD95, TNFRSF6)-Fas ligand (FasL, TNFSF6) system is an example of a direct signaling pathway to apoptotic cell death. The importance of the Fas-FasL system in immune regulation was revealed by the recognition that mice and humans with the autoimmune-like disorders lymphoproliferative (*lpr*) and generalized lymphoproliferative disorder (*gld*) harbored mutations in Fas and Fas ligand (*189,190,*191). Mice with the *lpr* or *gld* mutation display autoimmune phenotypes with high accumulation of activated T cells in the periphery and $CD4^-CD8^-$ T cells in the lymph nodes (lymphoadenopathy) and autoantibody production. The Fas-FasL system is involved in proinflammatory responses, tumor survival, and non–immune tissue homeostasis in osteoclastogenesis and angiogenesis (192). Activated lymphocytes are particularly sensitive to Fas-induced apoptosis, suggesting a role for Fas in the clonal contraction phase of the immune response. The finding that epithelial cells in the eye express FasL, suggest FasL may limit inflammation in organs sensitive to immune damage. FasL is believed to be one of several proapoptotic systems used as a killing mechanism by cytotoxic T cells and NK cells. Fas ligand binds Fas and, in primates, decoy receptor3 (DcR3), which also binds LIGHT and TL1A (193).

FasL can undergo cleavage by matrix metalloproteases to produce soluble FasL, which may induce markedly different events when it engages Fas compared to the membrane-bound form, such as loss in cytotoxicity (194). Other findings suggest that soluble FasL may counteract the proinflammatory properties of membrane-associated FasL as an immunosuppressive, particularly in the eye and tumor environments (195,196). Conversely, Fas has also been linked to lymphoproliferation and activation via NF-κB signaling pathways.

Essential biological roles of FasL-Fas include regulating lymphocyte homeostasis (via contraction of clonally expanded effector T and NK cells), directing cytotoxic T lymphocyte (CTL)–mediated apoptosis and lysis (immune surveillance), and establishing immune-privileged organs and sites. Fas is expressed in a wide variety of tissues such as the thymus, spleen, heart, and liver, whereas FasL can be found on activated T cells, NK cells tumor cells, immune-privileged sites, lung, and other tissues (192,197,198). In mature activated T and NK cells, Fas-FasL signaling plays a critical role in the induction of apoptosis during the latter stages of inflammation or activation-induced cell death and in shifting lymphocyte population numbers back to baseline (199). In certain organs like the liver, lung, and small intestines, FasL on stromal cells can be upregulated to control the overabundance of activated T cells after an inflammatory response and ultimately reduce tissue damage. Alternatively, dysregulation during hepatitis C infections can lead to death of hepatocytes and acute liver damage (200). The Fas system has also been implicated in curtailing autoantibody production by damping T cell helper–induced B cell activation and direct elimination of activated B cells, in which CD40 stimulation also upregulates Fas expression (192).

The Fas-FasL system, together with preforin and granzymes, is vital to CTL-mediated destruction and clearance of tumor and virally infected cells. Viruses have evolved multiple mechanisms of suppressing Fas signaling (90), including downmodulation of Fas (201) and blockade of caspase 8 activation (202). Tumor genome instability may lead to mutations that aid in escaping or resisting death pathways conducive to developing the metastatic phenotype (203). Uterine and breast cancer patients may have elevated levels of soluble FasL and Fas, which may aid in neutralizing CTL- and NK cell–induced lysis, or even killing Fas-expressing effector cells. HSV-1 infection *in vitro* of human neonatal neutrophils—critical effectors in innate and humoral immunity—upregulates Fas and FasL surface expression, leading to apoptosis, exemplifying a theme of pathogenic modulation of apoptotic signaling events to evade or attenuate immune responses (204). FasL is constitutively expressed in the eye, central nervous system (CNS), testis, fetal trophoblast, and placenta, where any lymphocyte infiltration could lead to unrestricted, irreversible bystander damage to these tissues (205). The implications of immune privilege have been applied to tissue transplantation rejection therapies; however, conflicting results on whether FasL expression reduces the likelihood of allograft rejection (*206*,207) or potentates effector responses (208,*209*) emphasize that induction of immune privilege by the Fas-FasL system is not that simple and is rather more complex. Fas-FasL interactions are at the core of graft-versus-host disease (GVHD), where contaminating donor effector T cells in an allograft expand to damage the recipient's tissues. In a mouse model for acute GVHD, p53-dependent upregulation of Fas on host stem cells leads to subsequent bone marrow depletion through FasL-mediated apoptosis (210). With regard to tissue homeostasis, FasL has been reported to enhance RANKL-mediated osteoclastogenesis and differentiation in mouse bone marrow–derived macrophages (211). Fas is also implicated in pulmonary inflammatory diseases resulting in fibrosis after acute lung injury (197).

TRAIL AND TRAIL-RECEPTOR SYSTEM

TRAIL (TNF-related apoptosis-inducing ligand, TNFSF10) is closely related based on sequence homology to FasL and TNF. Interest in TRAIL was spurred by its ability to selectively induce apoptosis in tumor cells (212).

TRAIL binds five different receptors: TRAILR1 (DR4, TNFRSF10A), TRAILR2 (DR5, TNFRSF10B), TRAILR3 (DcR1, TNFRSF10C), TRAILR4 (DcR2, TNFRSF10D), and osteoprotegerin (OPG, OCIF, TNFRSF11B) (Figure 25.3). TRAILR1, 2, and 4 are type I transmembrane proteins; all are membrane associated, with the exception of the more distantly related OPG, a dimeric, soluble decoy receptor, and the type III transmembrane protein TRAILR3 (213). TRAILR1 and 2 contain highly homologous DDs in their cytoplasmic tails that form the death-inducing signaling complex (214,215) responsible for apoptosis. TRAILR3 is anchored to the membrane via a glycophosphatidyl inositol tail, whereas TRAILR4 has a truncated, nonfunctional DD (193,216,*217*). How TRAILR3 and 4 antagonize TRAIL-induced apoptosis may not fully be explained by the "receptor decoy" paradigm of ligand competition. Nevertheless this does not preclude a "competition"-based mechanism for TRAILR3, especially if there is differential surface expression of death versus decoy receptors. Alternative splicing is a common feature among TRAIL and its receptors and is believed to regulate programmed cell death *(218)*. Two variants of human TRAIL, TRAILβ and TRAILγ, exhibit total loss of their proapoptotic potential due to incomplete receptor-binding domains. TRAILR2 has two forms, DR5A (short) and DR5B (long) *(219)*, and the TRAILR4-β variant lacks the first complete CRD1 of the ligand-binding site (220). The genetic organization of the TRAIL receptor loci in the mouse differs from that in humans. The mouse genome has TRAILR2, 3, and 4 homologs, but the TRAILR4 homolog does not bind TRAIL.

A major function of TRAIL-TRAILR signaling system is to induce apoptosis and to a lesser degree NF-κB activation. For example, the apoptotic function of TRAIL system is necessary for regulating the response of memory CD8$^+$ T cells to rechallenge with antigen. In the absence of CD4 T cell help, CD8 T cells undergo apoptosis mediated by TRAIL (221,222). In much the same way as Fas, TRAILR death domains are thought to recruit FADD and initiator caspases 8 and/or 10 into the DISC to activate downstream effector caspases in apoptosis. Caspase 8 contribution to this process is well defined, but caspase 10 involvement was less so until recent studies in autoimmune lymphoproliferative syndrome II patients and some carcinoma cell lines found that mutant caspase 10 ablates TRAIL-induced apoptosis (216). In some cell types, the extrinsic mitochondrial pathway is important in amplifying DISC signals in TRAIL-induced apoptosis, which is analogous to certain mechanisms for Fas-FasL signaling *(223)*. TRAIL is being intensely pursued as an anticancer therapeutic, and it has been found to be particularly potent in combination with chemotherapy because TRAILR2 expression can be increased in response to DNA damage (224).

TRAIL seems most involved in regulating immune homeostasis and immune surveillance and in clearing virally infected and cancerous cells. IFNγ treatment of tumor cells increases sensitization to TRAIL-induced death. This has been observed in melanoma and ovarian carcinoma cells (216) and is analogous to Fas-FasL apoptotic signaling in human colorectal carcinoma line HT-29. IFNα possesses powerful antiviral and antitumor properties as well and has been shown to upregulate TRAIL via JAK-STAT pathways in stimulated human multiple myeloma *in vitro*. TRAIL is also upregulated on NK cells in response to IFNγ, enhancing antitumor effector function (225).

TL1A-DR3 SYSTEM

TL1A (VEGI, TNFSF15) is a paralog of FasL, LIGHT, and LTβ, and its receptor, DR3, is a homolog of TNFR1 (APO3, TNFRSF25). TL1A also binds decoy receptor-3DcR3, potentially limiting any TL1A signaling mediated by DR3. Genetic deletion of TL1A or DR3 in mice revealed poor T cell responses to cosignaling but no overt developmental abnormalities (115,226,*227*,*228*). Specific mutations in the ligand-binding domain of DR3 are linked to rheumatoid arthritis, and, of interest, appear to be paralleled in other TNFRSF members and associated autoimmune pathologies (229).

ORPHAN RECEPTORS

The orphan death receptor-6 (DR6) has no known ligand related to the TNF superfamily. However, emerging evidence suggests that DR6 has a role in immune function. In a mouse EAE model, DR6 deficiency was shown to protect against CNS demyelination and leukocyte infiltration but also enhance overall CD4$^+$ T cell proliferation and Th2 differentiation, underscoring a role for DR6 in mediating Th1-specific immune responses in EAE progression (230).

Taj/TROY and RELT also do not bind any of the known TNF ligands; however, recent evidence indicates that Taj/TROY functions more like p75NTR, capable of binding myelin inhibitory factors (29,30). The role of Taj/TROY and RELT in immune function is unclear.

RANK LIGAND, RANK, AND OPG SYSTEM

Osteoprotegerin (OPG, TNFRSF11B) was initially identified as a key factor in the mechanism regulating bone density (231) (Figure 25.3). As a soluble receptor, OPG is a regulator of the RANK (receptor activator of NF-κB, TNFRSF11A) and RANK ligand (also known as TRANCE) signaling pathway involved in the differentiation of bone-resorptive osteoclasts from hematopoietic progenitors (osteoclastogenesis) (232–234). However, this system is also crucial for development of mammary glands *(235)*, lymph nodes, and DC–T cell interactions (*236*,237). Bone remodeling needed to sustain skeletal integrity and calcium homeostasis is regulated by a dynamic equilibrium between osteoblasts (bone forming) and osteoclasts (bone resorbing), which is regulated by the RANKL-RANK-OPG system. Dysregulation of the RANKL-RANK-OPG system has consequences in inflammatory, osteologic, and cancer pathophysiology, such as bone loss in inflammatory autoimmune diseases, preferential breast and prostate tumor metastasis to the bone, and gender bias in osteoporosis.

OPG functions as a decoy receptor that binds RANKL with high affinity, and it also binds TRAIL, albeit at low affinity in comparison to RANKL *(238,239)*. Despite such a weak binding, *in vitro* studies show that OPG can block TRAIL-mediated apoptosis, which suggests that the OPG-TRAIL system contributes to osteoclastogenesis. RANK interacts with TRAF2, 5, and 6. The membrane-proximal TRAF site is highly specific for TRAF6, and several studies have shown TRAF6 to be essential in RANKL-RANK signaling in osteoclastogenesis and lymph node genesis (240,*241*). Several "osteotropic" factors have been reported to regulate RANKL and OPG expression in osteoblast and osteoclast lineages, such as TGFβ, IL-1, TNF, estrogen, prostaglandin E_2, glucocorticoids, and vitamin D_3 (240,*242*). In a few cases, OPG and RANKL are differentially modulated by the same factor; parathyroid-related protein increases RANKL while decreasing OPG mRNA expression in osteoclast-like odontoclasts (243). The components in the RANK signaling triad are widely expressed. RANK is upregulated on CD40L-stimulated maturing DCs, whereas RANKL is upregulated during T cell activation and is constitutively expressed in some tumors and mammary gland epithelial cells.

TRAF6$^{-/-}$ and RANK$^{-/-}$ mice lack NF-κB activation in osteoclasts in response to RANKL and exhibit abnormally high bone density (osteopetrosis) (244,245). Osteoblasts and stromal cells stimulate differentiation via direct cell contact with osteoclast precursors. Macrophage colony stimulating factor (M-CSF) cooperates with RANKL-expressing osteoblasts to transmit positive signals through c-Fms and RANK expressed on precursors, promoting their differentiation (234), whereas OPG is a negative regulator by competitively binding RANKL, thus ablating all signals through RANK. RANK$^{-/-}$ and RANKL$^{-/-}$ mice phenocopy each other, displaying severe osteopetrosis due to absolute lack of osteoclasts (246). Complementing the observations in RANKL and RANK deficiencies is the finding that OPG blocks osteoclast differentiation in a dose-dependent manner. OPG overexpression in transgenic mice causes acute osteopetrosis, and OPG-deficient mice suffer from osteoporosis due to excessive osteoclastogenesis. In humans OPG and RANK mutations are linked to juvenile Paget's disease, familial expansile osteolysis, and other osteolytic disorders (233,240).

The RANKL-RANK system is proving to be an important enhancer of cell-mediated immune responses by promoting DC survival and naive T cell proliferation. RANKL stimulates DCs to produce proinflammatory cytokines such as IL-12 (247,*248*). The RANK pathway may serve to bolster CD40-CD40L interaction between DCs and T cells after TCR stimulation or prolong survival of activated DCs to ensure the establishment of T cell memory. For instance, in CD40L$^{-/-}$ mice, RANKL-RANK costimulation is protective against *Leishmania* infection by inducing IL-12 secretion and consequent Th1 immune response (249).

Bone loss in autoimmune and infectious models of inflammatory disease is mediated through slightly different mechanisms. In recent studies, activated, CD4$^+$RANKL$^+$ T cells have been shown to support osteoclastogenesis and mediate bone loss in humanized mouse models of *Actinobacillus*-specific periodontal disease, suggesting a role for Th1 immunity in inflammatory bone destruction (250,251). In HIV-positive patients, the virion envelope protein gp120 induces disease-related osteoporosis via induction of RANKL on CD4$^+$ T cells and augmentation of osteoclastogenesis (252).

In mouse models of tumor metastasis, high OPG and RANK levels are risk factors for metastasis to the bone and subsequent osteolysis, especially in breast tumors (253). OPG from human bone marrow stroma can protect prostate tumors from TRAIL-mediated apoptosis (254), and treatment with anti-TRAIL neutralizing antibodies reduces osteoclastogenesis in mixed lymphocyte–bone marrow cultures from patients with multiple myeloma, presumably by interfering with OPG-TRAIL complexes formed by activated T cells expressing TRAIL, OPG, and RANKL (255). The RANKL-RANK-OPG system has also been implicated in diabetes-associated osteopenia because serum levels of OPG are higher in patients with types 1 and 2 diabetes (256). Of interest, these patients are at greater risk for developing atherosclerotic plaques, perhaps reflected in the OPG-deficient mice, which suffer from arterial calcification (257), presumably from unrestricted bone resorption and Ca^{2+} release. Although elevated endogenous OPG levels are considered a risk factor in certain disease manifestations, the complexity of the cytokine networks that regulate RANKL-RANK-OPG interactions and vice versa render the clinical relevance difficult to interpret. Use of human anti-RANKL monoclonal antibody (denosumab) to disrupt RANKL-RANK signaling is being considered to reduce bone resorption in postmenopausal osteoporotic women and patients with multiple myeloma and osseous metastatic breast tumors (258).

TNF AND TNF INHIBITION IN THE THERAPY OF HUMAN DISEASE

TNF Inhibitors

The TNF superfamily is associated with a wide range of human diseases, as evidenced by genetic deficiencies or mutations in individual components of the TNF

TABLE 25.8 Human Genetic Diseases Associated with the Tumor Necrosis Factor (TNF) Superfamily

System	*Disease*	*Mutation*
TNFR1	Familial periodic fever	Mutation in first cysteine-rich domain
CD40 Ligand	Hyper–immunoglobulin syndrome	Multiple mutations affecting receptor binding and processing
EDA	X-linked hypohidrotic ectodermal dysplasia	Multiple mutations affecting receptor binding, trimerization, and secretion
RANK	Familial expansile osteolysis	Mutation in the signal peptide
Fas	Autoimmune lymphoproliferative syndrome	Multiple mutations/deletion in Fas

superfamily and in the therapeutic efficacy of TNF inhibitors in autoimmune diseases (Table 25.8). Although cancer therapy was the original motivation in developing TNF, the success of TNF inhibitors in autoimmune diseases such as rheumatoid arthritis, ankylosing spondilitis, psoriasis, and Crohn's disease provides significant motivation to explore therapeutics targeting other members of the TNF superfamily, and this is an active area of research.

In general, TNF inhibitors are designed along the properties of specific antibodies or soluble receptors (Figure 25.8). Both antibody- and receptor-based reagents block the capacity of the ligand to bind receptor, functioning as competitive antagonists. A partially humanized mouse monoclonal antibody to human TNF (infliximab) and fully human anti-TNF (adalimumab) are approved for use in humans. The ectodomain of the TNF receptor-2 genetically linked to the Fc region of human IgG1 (etanercept) was used to create a bivalent molecule that has higher avidity for TNF than naturally occurring soluble receptors. Soluble decoy receptors retain their ability to bind their native ligands, which in the case of TNFR2-Fc are TNF and LTα, whereas anti-TNF antibodies are specific for TNF and do not cross-react with LTα.

Bivalent antibodies directed to TNF receptors can function as agonists and mimic the ligand, but they are specific for a single receptor, a feature that may distinguish an antibody from a ligand, such as TRAIL, which has multiple receptors. Moreover, antibodies are inherently more stable than the native ligand and provide better pharmacodynamics (serum half-life and bioavailability). Agonist receptor antibodies (e.g., anti-TRAILR, anti-Ox40) are in preclinical studies and clinical trials. Although these drugs are classified as biologics (protein-based drugs) and are inherently safe, side effects like lymphoma and increased infections accompany TNF inhibition, as perhaps should be expected based on understanding the roles TNF plays in innate and adaptive immune responses.

Effect of TNF Blockade in Inflammatory Diseases

TNF inhibitors are approved for use in the treatment of rheumatoid arthritis (RA), psoriatic arthritis, ankylosing spondylitis, juvenile rheumatoid arthritis, Crohn's disease, and ulcerative colitis. Rheumatoid arthritis is a chronic autoimmune joint disease that occurs in genetically predisposed individuals. Treatment of RA is usually initiated with disease-modifying antirheumatic drugs (DMARDs), such as methotrexate or corticosteroids, to improve

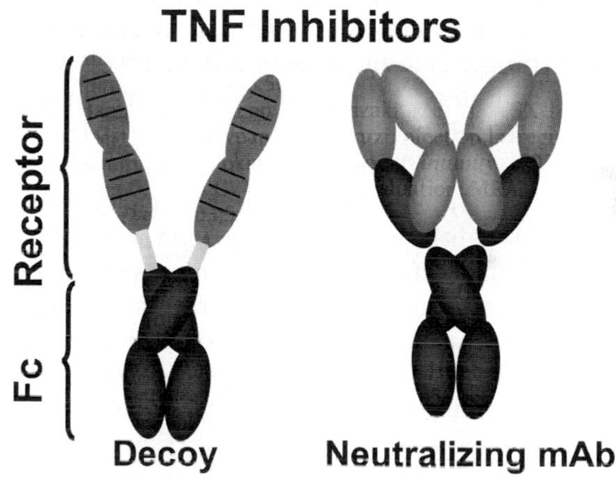

Inhibitor	Ligand	Disease
TNFR2-Fc (etanercept)	TNF, LTα	RA, psoriasis
IgG1κ (infliximab) (adalimumab)	TNF	RA, IBD

FIGURE 25.8 Tumor necrosis factor (TNF) inhibitors. The main structural features of TNF decoy receptor (etanercept) created as a genetic fusion protein of the ectodomain of TNFR2 with the Fc region of human immunoglobulin (Ig) G1, which forms a disulfide-linked dimer. Monoclonal antibody (mAb) specific for human TNF derived from mice and partially humanized (infliximab) or a fully human antibody (adalimumab) contain both H and L immunoglobulin chains. Both types of inhibitors are approved for use in treating autoimmune diseases: rheumatoid arthritis (RA), psoriasis, and inflammatory bowel diseases (IBD).

symptoms and reduce joint damage. The American College of Rheumatology uses clinical and laboratory measures to assess improvement in response to therapy in RA. A patient with a 70% or greater improvement according to these parameters is designated as having an ACR-70 response. TNF inhibitors in combination with methotrexate (the most widely used DMARD) produce ACR-70 responses in 33% to 40% of patients with early RA and in 10% to 27% percent of patients with established RA. In comparison to patients receiving methotrexate alone, the ACR-70 responses occurred in 19% to 21% of early RA patients and fewer than 5% of patients with established disease (259). In RA, joint damage begins early in the disease course as articular erosions when visualized by radiographic techniques in 40% of patients in the first year of disease and in 90% by the second year (260). TNF inhibitors slow radiographic progression in RA (261). Of interest, in a randomized, controlled trial of 428 patients with active RA, the combination of infliximab and methotrexate reduced the radiographic progression in patients that achieved ACR-20 responses as well as in those who did not meet these clinical criteria (262).

Inflammatory bowel disease, ulcerative colitis (limited to colon and bowel), and Crohn's disease (entire intestine) are chronic inflammatory conditions in which TNF is disproportionately expressed when the disease is active. Lamina propria mononuclear cells from patients with inflammatory bowel disease produce significantly higher levels of TNF after stimulation by lipopolysaccharide (263). The formation of fistulating inflammatory granulomas is a pathologic feature of Crohn's disease. Clinical trials demonstrated an initial response in 59% to 69% of patients and a dose-dependent clinical remission that ranged between 28% and 38% in nonfistulating Crohn's disease and between 64% and 97% of patients with complete fistula disease when categorized by location (264,*265*). In ulcerative colitis (UC), controlled trials (800 patients with active UC) showed an initial response at week 8 in 65% in patients treated with anti-TNF (infliximab) versus 35% in the placebo group, with remission achieved in 35% and 15% in infliximab- and placebo-treated patients, respectively (266). Anti-TNF of human origin (adalimumab) was efficacious in controlled trials in patients with moderate to severe Crohn's disease (264). By contrast, soluble TNFR2-Fc (etanercept) at doses known to be effective in rheumatoid arthritis failed to produce benefit in a controlled trial for Crohn's disease (267).

Erythrosquamous lesions containing infiltrating leukocytes and epidermal hypertrophy characterize psoriasis, a chronic inflammatory skin disease. Skin lesions of psoriatic patients contain elevated levels of TNF, and after treatment with TNF inhibitors, serum and skin levels of TNF decrease with clinical response (*268*,269). A significant subset of patients with psoriasis develops inflammatory, erosive arthritis (270). In clinical trials, both etanercept and infliximab significantly inhibited disease activity and improved the quality of life in patients with psoriatic arthritis (271–273,*274,275*).

Serious Adverse Effects

Side effects with the use of TNF inhibitors include lupus-like syndromes, aplastic anemia, hepatotoxicity, interstitial lung disease, optic neuritis, and exacerbations of quiescent multiple sclerosis. The rate of serious skin and soft tissue infections is also higher in treated patients, and there is also an increased risk of bacterial intracellular infections, primary tuberculosis and reactivation of latent *Mycobacterium tuberculosis* among patients treated with TNF inhibitors (276,277). Risk due to infection can be minimized and controlled (e.g., a tuberculosis skin test prior to treatment for patients that have not been previously vaccinated for *Mycobacterium*).

The contribution of anti-TNF therapy to increased risk of cancer is unclear. A systematic review of randomized clinical trials using infliximab and adalimumab found a dose-related increase of malignancies in RA patients (278). Some of the increased risk of malignancy (i.e., lymphoma) is difficult to dissect due to the increased association with RA (277).

TNF has been implicated in the pathogenesis of cardiac dysfunction, in part due to its negative ionotropic activities *in vitro* and *in vivo*; however, TNF blockade significantly increased the incidence of cardiac death. This observation led to the recommendation that TNF inhibitors be discontinued in patients with cardiac dysfunction (279,*280,281*).

Anti-CD40L

The interaction between CD40 and CD40L is involved in the pathogenesis of inflammatory diseases (102), and interference with this pathway induces amelioration of autoimmune disease and allograft rejection in animal models (282,283,*284–286*). Humanized anti-CD40L was tested in clinical trials of transplantation and autoimmunity including idiopathic thrombocytopenic purpura, psoriasis, Crohn's disease, and multiple sclerosis (287–289). However, controlled clinical trials using anti-CD40L for the treatment of proliferative lupus nephritis was halted because of thromboembolic events. A partial evaluation of the trial demonstrated decreased anti-dsDNA antibodies, increased serum complement levels, and reduced hematuria in some of the treated patients, consistent with the expected immunologic outcome (288). A phase II, double-blinded, placebo-controlled clinical trial in patients with mild to moderately active systemic lupus erythematosus using another anti-CD40L antibody was found to be safe but did not demonstrate efficacy when compared to placebo (287).

TNF in Cancer Chemotherapy

Tumor angiogenesis—the formation of vessels to support cancer growth—is a process essential for tumor growth. The ability of TNF to induce apoptosis of tumor-associated endothelial cells can result in the impairment of the tumor vasculature, leading to necrosis of the tumor. This mechanism involves perturbation of cell–cell adhesive junctions and inhibition of $\alpha v \beta 3$ integrin signaling in tumor-associated vessels (290). However, clinical phase I and II studies in cancer patients receiving recombinant TNF reported "septic shock–like syndrome," a dose-limiting toxicity, in quantities 10 times lower than the calculated antitumor dose extrapolated from animal studies (291,292). Animal studies also revealed the strong hemodynamic effects of TNF in the mediation of septic shock (293). Although anecdotal, reports of tumor regression after TNF administration *(294)* due to the induction of vasoplegia. TNF's use as an antitumor agent has been limited to treatment of locally advanced tumors by isolated limb perfusion, which limits systemic toxicity of TNF (295).

Preclinical and early clinical trials are in progress for many other members of the TNF superfamily. For example, antibodies to BAFF and LTβR-Fc decoy are in clinical trials for suppressing inflammation in autoimmune diseases and agonist antibodies to TRAILR for induction of cancer cell apoptosis. Modulation of immunity through the cosignaling members of the TNFR family such as Ox40, 41BB, LIGHT, and others is being considered for targeting to modify malignant diseases (108,151). Well-controlled studies are anticipated to help evaluate the efficacy of targeting these members of the TNF superfamily.

ACKNOWLEDGMENTS

I acknowledge the research assistance of April Kinkade, Rochelle Jean-Jacques, Ian Humphreys, and Pedro Ruiz, the graphic contributions of Grace Park, and support from the National Institutes of Health (R37AI33068).

REFERENCES

6. Browning JL, Ngam-ek A, Lawton P, et al. Lymphotoxin b, a novel member of the TNF family that forms a heteromeric complex with lymphotoxin on the cell surface. *Cell*. 1993;72:847.
7. Roschke V, Sosnovtseva S, Ward CD, et al. BLyS and APRIL form biologically active heterotrimers that are expressed in patients with systemic immune-based rheumatic diseases. *J Immunol*. 2002;169(8):4314.
8. Kishore U, Gaboriaud C, Waters P, et al. C1q and tumor necrosis factor superfamily: modularity and versatility. *Trends Immunol*. 2004;25(10):551.
9. Pradet-Balade B, Medema JP, Lopez-Fraga M, et al. An endogenous hybrid mRNA encodes TWE-PRIL, a functional cell surface TWEAK-APRIL fusion protein. *EMBO J*. 2002;21(21):5711.
10. Yan M, Wang LC, Hymowitz SG, et al. Two-amino acid molecular switch in an epithelial morphogen that regulates binding to two distinct receptors. *Science*. 2000:523.
11. Granger SW, Butrovich KD, Houshmand P, et al. Genomic characterization of LIGHT reveals linkage to an immune response locus on chromosome 19p13.3 and distinct isoforms generated by alternate splicing or proteolysis. *J Immunol*. 2001;167:5122.
13. Flajnik MF, Kasahara M. Comparative genomics of the MHC: glimpses into the evolution of the adaptive immune system. *Immunity*. 2001;15:351.
15. Kauppila S, Maaty WS, Chen P, et al. Eiger and its receptor, Wengen, comprise a TNF-like system in *Drosophila*. *Oncogene*. 2003;22(31):4860.
17. Banner DW, D'Arcy A, Janes W, et al. Crystal structure of the soluble human 55 kd TNF receptor-human TNF beta complex: implications for TNF receptor activation. *Cell*. 1993;73:431.
19. Hymowitz SG, Patel DR, Wallweber HJ, et al. Structures of APRIL-receptor complexes: like BCMA, TACI employs only a single cysteine-rich domain for high affinity ligand binding. *J Biol Chem*. 2005;280(8):7218.
20. Bossen C, Ingold K, Tardivel A, et al. Interactions of tumor necrosis factor (TNF) and TNF receptor family members in the mouse and human. *J Biol Chem*. 2006;281(20):13964.
22. Li B, Russell SJ, Compaan DM, et al. Activation of the proapoptotic death receptor DR5 by oligomeric peptide and antibody agonists. *J Mol Biol*. 2006;361(3):522.
23. Holler N, Tardivel A, Kovacsovics-Bankowski M, et al. Two adjacent trimeric Fas ligands are required for Fas signaling and formation of a death-inducing signaling complex. *Mol Cell Biol*. 2003;23(4): 1428.
27. Lobito AA, Kimberley FC, Muppidi JR, et al. Abnormal disulfide-linked oligomerization results in ER retention and altered signaling by TNFR1 mutants in TNFR1-associated periodic fever syndrome (TRAPS). *Blood*. 2006;108(4):1320.
28. He XL, Garcia KC. Structure of nerve growth factor complexed with the shared neurotrophin receptor p75. *Science*. 2004;304(5672): 870.
29. Shao Z, Browning JL, Lee X, et al. TAJ/TROY, an orphan TNF receptor family member, binds Nogo-66 receptor 1 and regulates axonal regeneration. *Neuron*. 2005;45(3):353.
30. Park JB, Yiu G, Kaneko S, et al. A TNF receptor family member, TROY, is a coreceptor with Nogo receptor in mediating the inhibitory activity of myelin inhibitors. *Neuron*. 2005;45(3):345.
31. Sedy JR, Gavrieli M, Potter KG, et al. B and T lymphocyte attenuator regulates T cell activation through interaction with herpesvirus entry mediator. *Nat Immunol*. 2005;6(1):90.
32. Montgomery RI, Warner MS, Lum B, et al. Herpes simplex virus 1 entry into cells mediated by a novel member of the TNF/NGF receptor family. *Cell*. 1996;87:427.
33. Compaan DM, Gonzalez LC, Tom I, et al. Attenuating lymphocyte activity: the crystal structure of the BTLA-HVEM complex. *J Biol Chem*. 2005;280(47):39553.
34. Cheung TC, Humphreys IR, Potter KG, et al. Evolutionarily divergent herpesviruses modulate T cell activation by targeting the herpesvirus entry mediator cosignaling pathway. *Proc Natl Acad Sci U S A*. 2005;102(37):13218.
35. Benedict CA. Viruses and the TNF-related cytokines, an evolving battle. *Cytokine Growth Factor Rev*. 2003;14(3–4):349.
36. Smith CA, Davis T, Anderson D, et al. A receptor for tumor necrosis factor defines an unusual family of cellular and viral proteins. *Science*. 1990;248:1019.
38. Rahman MM, McFadden G. Modulation of tumor necrosis factor by microbial pathogens. *PLoS Pathog*. 2006;2(2):e4.
40. Kontoyiannis D, Pasparakis M, Pizarro TT, et al. Impaired on/off regulation of TNF biosynthesis in mice lacking TNF AU-rich elements: implications for joint and gut-associated immunopathologies. *Immunity*. 1999;10(3):387.
42. Boatright KM, Salvesen GS. Mechanisms of caspase activation. *Curr Opin Cell Biol*. 2003;15(6):725.
43. Oganesyan G, Saha SK, Guo B, et al. Critical role of TRAF3 in the Toll-like receptor-dependent and -independent antiviral response. *Nature*. 2006;439(7073):208.
45. Karin M, Ben-Neriah Y. Phosphorylation meets ubiquitination: the control of NF-kappa.B activity. *Annu Rev Immunol*. 2000;18:621.
46. Pomerantz JL, Baltimore D. Two pathways to NF-kappaB. *Mol cell*. 2002;10(4):693.

47. Dejardin E, Droin NM, Delhase M, et al. The lymphotoxin-beta receptor induces different patterns of gene expression via two NF-kappaB pathways. *Immunity*. 2002;17(4):525.
48. Ramakrishnan P, Wang W, Wallach D. Receptor-specific signaling for both the alternative and the canonical NF-kappaB activation pathways by NF-kappaB-inducing kinase. *Immunity*. 2004;21(4): 477.
49. Kollias G. TNF pathophysiology in murine models of chronic inflammation and autoimmunity. *Semin Arthritis Rheum*. 2005;34(5 Suppl 1):3.
50. Ware CF. Network communications: lymphotoxins, LIGHT, and TNF. *Annu Rev Immunol*. 2005;23:787.
52. Kulbe H, Thompson R, Wilson JL, et al. The inflammatory cytokine tumor necrosis factor-alpha generates an autocrine tumor-promoting network in epithelial ovarian cancer cells. *Cancer Res*. 2007;67(2):585.
53. Balkwill F. TNF-alpha in promotion and progression of cancer. *Cancer Metastasis Rev*. 2006;25(3):409.
55. De Togni P, Goellner J, Ruddle NH, et al. Abnormal development of peripheral lymphoid organs in mice deficient in lymphotoxin. *Science*. 1994;264:703.
63. Nishikawa S, Honda K, Vieira P, et al. Organogenesis of peripheral lymphoid organs. *Immunol Rev*. 2003;195:72.
65. Eberl G. Inducible lymphoid tissues in the adult gut: recapitulation of a fetal developmental pathway? *Nat Rev Immunol*. 2005;5(5):413.
66. Mebius RE, Kraal G. Structure and function of the spleen. *Nat Rev Immunol*. 2005;5(8):606.
69. Luther SA, Bidgol A, Hargreaves DC, et al. Differing activities of homeostatic chemokines CCL19, CCL21, and CXCL12 in lymphocyte and dendritic cell recruitment and lymphoid neogenesis. *J Immunol*. 2002;169(1):424.
71. Katakai T, Hara T, Sugai M, et al. Lymph node fibroblastic reticular cells construct the stromal reticulum via contact with lymphocytes. *J Exp Med*. 2004;200(6):783.
72. Benedict CA, De Trez C, Schneider K, et al. Specific remodeling of splenic architecture by cytomegalovirus. *PLoS Pathog*. 2006;2(3):0164.
73. Drayton DL, Liao S, Mounzer RH, et al. Lymphoid organ development: from ontogeny to neogenesis. *Nat Immunol*. 2006;7(4):344.
74. Kabashima K, Banks TA, Ansel KM, et al. I ntrinsic lymphotoxin-beta receptor requirement for homeostasis of lymphoid tissue dendritic cells. *Immunity*. 2005;22(4):439.
75. Kindler V, Sappino AP, Grau GE, et al. The inducing role of tumor necrosis factor in the development of bactericidal granulomas during BCG infection. *Cell*. 1989;56(5):731.
76. Elewaut D, Ware CF. The unconventional role of LTalphabeta in T cell differentiation. *Trends Immunol*. 2007;28:169.
82. Keffer J, Probert L, Cazlaris H, et al. Transgenic mice expressing human tumour necrosis factor: a predictive genetic model of arthritis. *EMBO J*. 1991;10:4025.
83. Shaikh R, Santee S, Granger SW, et al. Constitutive expression of LIGHT on T cells leads to lymphocyte activation, inflammation and tissue destruction. *J Immunol*. 2001;167:6330.
84. Wang J, Chun T, Lo JC, et al. The critical role of LIGHT, a TNF family member, in T cell development. *J Immunol*. 2001;167:5099.
85. Drayton DL, Ying X, Lee J, et al. Ectopic LT alpha beta directs lymphoid organ neogenesis with concomitant expression of peripheral node addressin and a HEV-restricted sulfotransferase. *J Exp Med*. 2003;197(9):1153.
86. Beutler B, Cerami A. The biology of cachectin/TNF—a primary mediator of the host response. *Annu Rev Immunol*. 1989;7:625.
87. Pfeffer K, Matsuyama T, Kundig TM, et al. Mice deficient for the 55 kd tumor necrosis factor receptor are resistant to endotoxic shock, yet succumb to L. monocytogenes infection. *Cell*. 1993;73:457.
89. Wallis RS, Broder MS, Wong JY, et al. Granulomatous infectious diseases associated with tumor necrosis factor antagonists. *Clin Infect Dis*. 2004;38(9):1261.
90. Benedict CA, Banks TA, Ware CF. Death and survival: viral regulation of TNF signaling pathways. *Curr Opin Immunol*. 2003;15(1):59.
93. Riley JL, June CH. The CD28 family: a T-cell rheostat for therapeutic control of T-cell activation. *Blood*. 2005;105(1):13.
94. Greenwald RJ, Freeman GJ, Sharpe AH. The B7 Family Revisited. *Annu Rev Immunol*. 2005;23:515.
96. Han P, Goularte OD, Rufner K, et al. An inhibitory Ig superfamily protein expressed by lymphocytes and APCs is also an early marker of thymocyte positive selection. *J Immunol*. 2004;172(10):5931.
97. Granger SW, Ware CF. Commentary: turning on LIGHT. *J Clin Invest*. 2001;108:1741.
98. Locksley RM, Killeen N, Lenardo MJ. The TNF and TNF receptor superfamilies: Integrating mammalian biology. *Cell*. 2001;104:487.
99. Croft M. Co-stimulatory members of the TNFR family: keys to effective T-cell immunity? *Nat Rev Immunol*. 2003;3(8):609.
101. Watts TH. TNF/TNFR family members in costimulation of T cell responses. *Annu Rev Immunol*. 2005;23:23.
102. Toubi E, Shoenfeld Y. The role of CD40-CD154 interactions in autoimmunity and the benefit of disrupting this pathway. *Autoimmunity*. 2004;37(6–7):457.
103. Schneider P. The role of APRIL and BAFF in lymphocyte activation. *Curr Opin Immunol*. 2005;17(3):282.
104. Vonderheide RH, June CH. A translational bridge to cancer immunotherapy: exploiting costimulation and target antigens for active and passive T cell immunotherapy. *Immunol Res*. 2003;27(2–3):341.
108. Yu P, Lee Y, Liu W, et al. Priming of naive T cells inside tumors leads to eradication of established tumors. *Nat Immunol*. 2004;5(2):141.
110. Hendriks J, Gravestein LA, Tesselaar K, et al. CD27 is required for generation and long-term maintenance of T cell immunity. *Nat Immunol*. 2000;1(5):433.
111. Bansal-Pakala P, Halteman BS, Cheng MH, et al. Costimulation of CD8 T cell responses by OX40. *J Immunol*. 2004;172(8):4821.
114. Podack ER, Strbo N, Sotosec V, et al. CD30-governor of memory T cells? *Ann NY Acad Sci*. 2002;975:101.
115. Bamias G, Mishina M, Nyce M, et al. Role of TL1A and its receptor DR3 in two models of chronic murine ileitis. *Proc Natl Acad Sci U S A*. 2006;103(22):8441.
116. Papadakis KA, Prehn JL, Landers C, et al. TL1A synergizes with IL-12 and IL-18 to enhance IFN-gamma production in human T cells and NK cells. *J Immunol*. 2004;172(11):7002.
117. Wang J, Anders RA, Wang Y, et al. The critical role of LIGHT in promoting intestinal inflammation and Crohn's disease. *J Immunol*. 2005;174(12):8173.
118. Shimizu J, Yamazaki S, Takahashi T, et al. Stimulation of CD25+CD4+ regulatory T cells through GITR breaks immunological self-tolerance. *Nat Immunol*. 2002;3:135.
119. Gavrieli M, Sedy J, Nelson CA, et al. BTLA and HVEM cross talk regulates inhibition and costimulation. Advances in immunology. 2006;92:157–85.
120. Chemnitz JM, Lanfranco AR, Braunstein I, et al. B and T lymphocyte attenuator-mediated signal transduction provides a potent inhibitory signal to primary human CD4 T cells that can be initiated by multiple phosphotyrosine motifs. *J Immunol*. 2006;176(11): 6603.
121. Krieg C, Han P, Stone R, et al. Functional analysis of B and T lymphocyte attenuator engagement on CD4+ and CD8+ T cells. *J Immunol*. 2005;175(10):6420.
122. Krieg C, Boyman O, Fu YX, et al. B and T lymphocyte attenuator regulates CD8(+) T cell-intrinsic homeostasis and memory cell generation. *Nat Immunol*. 2007;8(2):162.
123. Deppong C, Juehne TI, Hurchla M, et al. Cutting edge: B and T lymphocyte attenuator and programmed death receptor-1 inhibitory receptors are required for termination of acute allergic airway inflammation. *J Immunol*. 2006;176(7):3909.
124. DeBenedette MA, Wen T, Bachmann MF, et al. Analysis of 4-1BB ligand (4-1BBL)-deficient mice and of mice lacking both 4-1BBL and CD28 reveals a role for 4-1BBL in skin allograft rejection and in the cytotoxic T cell response to influenza virus. *J Immunol*. 1999;163(9):4833.
125. Tan JT, Whitmire JK, Murali-Krishna K, et al. 4-1BB costimulation is required for protective anti-viral immunity after peptide vaccination. *J Immunol*. 2000;164(5):2320.
126. Dawicki W, Bertram EM, Sharpe AH, et al. 4-1BB and OX40 act independently to facilitate robust CD8 and CD4 recall responses. *J Immunol*. 2004;173(10):5944.
128. Gramaglia I, Jember A, Pippig SD, et al. The OX40 costimulatory receptor determines the development of CD4 memory by regulating primary clonal expansion. *J Immunol*. 2000;165:3043.

130. Yoshioka T, Nakajima A, Akiba H, et al. Contribution of OX40/OX40 ligand interaction to the pathogenesis of rheumatoid arthritis. *Eur J Immunol.* 2000;30(10):2815.
131. Salek-Ardakani S, Song J, Halteman BS, et al. OX40 (CD134) Controls memory T helper 2 cells that drive lung inflammation. *J Exp Med.* 2003;198(2):315.
133. Song J, So T, Cheng M, et al. Sustained survivin expression from OX40 costimulatory signals drives T cell clonal expansion. *Immunity.* 2005;22(5):621.
134. Lee SW, Vella AT, Kwon BS, et al. Enhanced CD4 T cell responsiveness in the absence of 4-1BB. *J Immunol.* 2005;174(11):6803.
138. Seo SK, Choi JH, Kim YH, et al. 4-1BB-mediated immunotherapy of rheumatoid arthritis. *Nat Med.* 2004;10(10):1088.
139. Serghides L, Bukczynski J, Wen T, et al. Evaluation of OX40 ligand as a costimulator of human antiviral memory CD8 T cell responses: comparison with B7.1 and 4-1BBL. *J Immunol.* 2005;175(10):6368.
140. Lee SW, Park Y, Song A, et al. Functional dichotomy between OX40 and 4-1BB in modulating effector CD8 T cell responses. *J Immunol.* 2006;177(7):4464.
141. Wang Y, Subudhi SK, Anders RA, et al. The role of herpesvirus entry mediator as a negative regulator of T cell-mediated responses. *J Clin Invest.* 2005;115(3):711.
142. Truong W, Hancock WW, Anderson CC, et al. Coinhibitory T-cell signaling in islet allograft rejection and tolerance. *Cell Transplant.* 2006;15(2):105.
143. Kurts C, Carbone FR, Krummel MF, et al. Signalling through CD30 protects against autoimmune diabetes mediated by CD8 T cells. *Nature.* 1999;398(6725):341.
145. Pakala SV, Bansal-Pakala P, Halteman BS, et al. Prevention of diabetes in NOD mice at a late stage by targeting OX40/OX40 ligand interactions. *Eur J Immunol.* 2004;34(11):3039.
146. Nakajima A, Oshima H, Nohara C, et al. Involvement of CD70-CD27 interactions in the induction of experimental autoimmune encephalomyelitis. *J Neuroimmunol.* 2000;109(2):188.
148. Tsukada N, Akiba H, Kobata T, et al. Blockade of CD134 (OX40)-CD134L interaction ameliorates lethal acute graft-versus-host disease in a murine model of allogeneic bone marrow transplantation. *Blood.* 2000;95(7):2434.
150. Blazar BR, Levy RB, Mak TW, et al. CD30/CD30 ligand (CD153) interaction regulates CD4+ T cell-mediated graft-versus-host disease. *J Immunol.* 2004;173(5):2933.
151. Weinberg AD. OX40: targeted immunotherapy—implications for tempering autoimmunity and enhancing vaccines. *Trends Immunol.* 2002;23(2):102.
153. Clark EA, Craxton A. A CD40 bridge between innate and adaptive immunity. *Immunity.* 2003;18(6):724.
154. Mackey MF, Barth RJ Jr, Noelle RJ. The role of CD40/CD154 interactions in the priming, differentiation, and effector function of helper and cytotoxic T cells. *J Leukoc Biol.* 1998;63:418.
155. Quezada SA, Jarvinen LZ, Lind EF, et al. CD40/CD154 interactions at the interface of tolerance and immunity. *Annu Rev Immunol.* 2004;22:307.
156. Craxton A, Otipoby KL, Jiang A, et al. Signal transduction pathways that regulate the fate of B lymphocytes. *Adv Immunol.* 1999;73:79.
158. Thorley-Lawson DA. Epstein-Barr virus: exploiting the immune system. *Nat Rev Immunol.* 2001;1(1):75.
162. Durandy A, Revy P, Fischer A. Human models of inherited immunoglobulin class switch recombination and somatic hypermutation defects (hyper-IgM syndromes). *Adv Immunol.* 2004;82:295.
164. Hernandez MG, Shen L, Rock KL. CD40-CD40 ligand interaction between dendritic cells and CD8+ T cells is needed to stimulate maximal T cell responses in the absence of CD4+ T cell help. *J Immunol.* 2007;178(5):2844.
165. Litinskiy MB, Nardelli B, Hilbert DM, et al. DCs induce CD40-independent immunoglobulin class switching through BLyS and APRIL. *Nat Immunol.* 2002;3(9):822.
166. Mackay F, Leung H. The role of the BAFF/APRIL system on T cell function. *Semin Immunol.* 2006 Oct;18(5):284–9.
167. Bossen C, Schneider P. BAFF, APRIL and their receptors: Structure, function and signaling. *Semin Immunol.* 2006;18(5):263.
168. Kolfschoten GM, Pradet-Balade B, Hahne M, et al. TWE-PRIL; a fusion protein of TWEAK and APRIL. *Biochem Pharmacol.* 2003;66(8):1427.
170. O'Connor BP, Raman VS, Erickson LD, et al. BCMA is essential for the survival of long-lived bone marrow plasma cells. *J Exp Med.* 2004;199(1):91.
171. Sasaki Y, Casola S, Kutok JL, et al. TNF family member B cell-activating factor (BAFF) receptor-dependent and -independent roles for BAFF in B cell physiology. *J Immunol.* 2004;173(4):2245.
172. Varfolomeev E, Kischkel F, Martin F, et al. APRIL-deficient mice have normal immune system development. *Mol Cell Biol.* 2004;24(3):997.
174. Yan M, Wang H, Chan B, et al. Activation and accumulation of B cells in TACI-deficient mice. *Nat Immunol.* 2001;2(7):638.
175. Castigli E, Wilson SA, Scott S, et al. TACI and BAFF-R mediate isotype switching in B cells. *J Exp Med.* 2005;201(1):35.
176. Ye Q, Wang L, Wells AD, et al. BAFF binding to T cell-expressed BAFF-R costimulates T cell proliferation and alloresponses. *Eur J Immunol.* 2004;34(10):2750.
177. Sutherland AP, Mackay F, Mackay CR. Targeting BAFF: immunomodulation for autoimmune diseases and lymphomas. *Pharmacol Ther.* 2006;112(3):774.
178. Dillon SR, Gross JA, Ansell SM, et al. An APRIL to remember: novel TNF ligands as therapeutic targets. *Nat Rev Drug Discov.* 2006;5(3):235.
179. Moreaux J, Legouffe E, Jourdan E, et al. BAFF and APRIL protect myeloma cells from apoptosis induced by interleukin 6 deprivation and dexamethasone. *Blood.* 2004;103(8):3148.
180. Wiley SR, Winkles JA. TWEAK, a member of the TNF superfamily, is a multifunctional cytokine that binds the TweakR/Fn14 receptor. *Cytokine Growth Factor Rev.* 2003;14(3–4):241.
181. Vince JE, Silke J. TWEAK shall inherit the earth. *Cell Death Differ.* 2006;13:1842.
182. Maecker H, Varfolomeev E, Kischkel F, et al. TWEAK attenuates the transition from innate to adaptive immunity. *Cell.* 2005;123(5):931.
183. Potrovita I, Zhang W, Burkly L, et al. Tumor necrosis factor-like weak inducer of apoptosis induced neurodegeneration. *J Neurosci.* 2004;24(38):8237.
186. Perper SJ, Browning B, Burkly LC, et al. TWEAK is a novel arthritogenic mediator. *J Immunol.* 2006;177(4):2610.
187. Chacon MR, Richart C, Gomez JM, et al. Expression of TWEAK and its receptor Fn14 in human subcutaneous adipose tissue. Relationship with other inflammatory cytokines in obesity. *Cytokine.* 2006;33(3):129.
188. De A, Park JI, Kawamura K, et al. Intraovarian tumor necrosis factor-related weak inducer of apoptosis/fibroblast growth factor-inducible-14 ligand-receptor system limits ovarian preovulatory follicles from excessive luteinization. *Mol Endocrinol.* 2006;20:2528–2538.
191. Fisher GH, Rosenberg FJ, Straus SE, et al. Dominant interfering Fas gene mutations impair apoptosis in a human autoimmune lymphoproliferative syndrome. *Cell.* 1995;81:935–946.
192. Lee HO, Ferguson TA. Biology of FasL. *Cytokine Growth Factor Rev.* 2003;14(3–4):325.
193. odmer JL, Schneider P, Tschopp J. The molecular architecture of the TNF superfamily. *Trends Biochem Sci.* 2002;27(1):19.
194. Schneider P, Holler N, Bodmer JL, et al. Conversion of membrane-bound Fas(CD95) ligand to its soluble form is associated with downregulation of its proapoptotic activity and loss of liver toxicity. *J Exp Med.* 1998;187(8):1205.
195. Gregory MS, Repp AC, Holhbaum AM, et al. Membrane Fas ligand activates innate immunity and terminates ocular immune privilege. *J Immunol.* 2002;169(5):2727.
196. Wajant H, Pfizenmaier K, Scheurich P. Non-apoptotic Fas signaling. *Cytokine Growth Factor Rev.* 2003;14(1):53.
197. Dosreis GA, Borges VM, Zin WA. The central role of Fas-ligand cell signaling in inflammatory lung diseases. *J Cell Mol Med.* 2004;8(3):285.
198. Houston A, O'Connell J. The Fas signalling pathway and its role in the pathogenesis of cancer. *Curr Opin Pharmacol.* 2004;4(4):321.
199. Green DR, Droin N, Pinkoski M. Activation-induced cell death in T cells. *Immunol Rev.* 2003;193:70.
200. Hayashi N, Mita E. Involvement of Fas system-mediated apoptosis in pathogenesis of viral hepatitis. *J Viral Hepatol* 1999;6(5):357.
201. Benedict CA, Norris PS, Prigozy TI, et al. Three adenovirus E3 proteins cooperate to evade apoptosis by tumor necrosis

factor-related apoptosis-inducing ligand receptor-1 and -2. *J Biol Chem*. 2001;276:3270.
202. Thome M, Schneider P, Hofmann K, et al. Viral FLICE-inhibitory proteins (FLIPs) prevent apoptosis induced by death receptors. *Nature*. 1997;386:517.
203. Kim R, Emi M, Tanabe K, et al. Tumor-driven evolution of immunosuppressive networks during malignant progression. *Cancer Res*. 2006;66(11):5527.
204. Ennaciri J, Menezes J, Proulx F, et al. Induction of apoptosis by herpes simplex virus-1 in neonatal, but not adult, neutrophils. *Pediatr Res*. 2006;59(1):7.
205. Niederkorn JY. See no evil, hear no evil, do no evil: the lessons of immune privilege. *Nat Immunol*. 2006;7(4):354.
207. Stuart PM, Yin X, Plambeck S, et al. The role of Fas ligand as an effector molecule in corneal graft rejection. *Eur J Immunol*. 2005;35(9):2591.
208. Turvey SE, Gonzalez-Nicolini V, Kingsley CI, et al. Fas ligand-transfected myoblasts and islet cell transplantation. *Transplantation*. 2000;69(9):1972.
210. Yada S, Takamura N, Inagaki-Ohara K, et al. The role of p53 and Fas in a model of acute murine graft-versus-host disease. *J Immunol*. 2005;174(3):1291.
211. Park H, Jung YK, Park OJ, et al. Interaction of Fas ligand and Fas expressed on osteoclast precursors increases osteoclastogenesis. *J Immunol*. 2005;175(11):7193.
212. Wiley SR, Schooley K, Smolak PJ, et al. Identification and characterization of a new member of the TNF family that induces apoptosis. *Immunity*. 1995;3:673.
213. Zauli G, Secchiero P. The role of the TRAIL/TRAIL receptors system in hematopoiesis and endothelial cell biology. *Cytokine Growth Factor Rev*. 2006;17(4):245.
214. Schneider P, Tschopp J. Apoptosis induced by death receptors. *Pharm Acta Helv*. 2000;74(2–3):281.
215. Kischkel FC, Lawrence DA, Chuntharapai A, et al. Apo2L/TRAIL-dependent recruitment of endogenous FADD and caspase-8 to death receptors 4 and 5. *Immunity*. 2000;12(6):611.
216. Almasan A, Ashkenazi A. Apo2L/TRAIL: apoptosis signaling, biology, and potential for cancer therapy. *Cytokine Growth Factor Rev*. 2003;14(3–4):337–48.
220. Krieg A, Schulte Am Esch J 2nd, Ramp U, et al. TRAIL-R4-beta: A new splice variant of TRAIL-receptor 4 lacking the cysteine rich domain 1. *Biochem Biophys Res Commun*. 2006;349(1):115.
221. Hamilton SE, Wolkers MC, Schoenberger SP, et al. The generation of protective memory-like CD8+ T cells during homeostatic proliferation requires CD4+ T cells. *Nat Immunol*. 2006;7(5):475.
222. Janssen EM, Droin NM, Lemmens EE, et al. CD4+ T-cell help controls CD8+ T-cell memory via TRAIL-mediated activation-induced cell death. *Nature*. 2005;434(7029):88.
224. Duiker EW, Mom CH, de Jong S, et al. The clinical trail of TRAIL. *Eur J Cancer*. 2006;42(14):2233.
225. Sato K, Hida S, Takayanagi H, et al. Antiviral response by natural killer cells through TRAIL gene induction by IFN-alpha/beta. *Eur J Immunol*. 2001;31:3138.
226. Papadakis KA, Zhu D, Prehn JL, et al. Dominant role for TL1A/DR3 pathway in IL-12 plus IL-18-induced IFN-gamma production by peripheral blood and mucosal CCR9+ T lymphocytes. *J Immunol*. 2005;174(8):4985.
229. Borysenko CW, Furey WF, Blair HC. Comparative modeling of TNFRSF25 (DR3) predicts receptor destabilization by a mutation linked to rheumatoid arthritis. *Biochem Biophys Res Commun*. 2005;328(3):794.
230. Schmidt CS, Zhao J, Chain J, et al. Resistance to myelin oligodendrocyte glycoprotein-induced experimental autoimmune encephalomyelitis by death receptor 6-deficient mice. *J Immunol*. 2005;175(4):2286.
231. Simonet WS, Lacey DL, Dunstan CR, et al. Osteoprotegerin: a novel secreted protein involved in the regulation of bone density. *Cell*. 1997;89(2):309.
232. Walsh MC, Kim N, Kadono Y, et al. Osteoimmunology: interplay between the immune system and bone metabolism. *Annu Rev Immunol*. 2006;24:33.
233. Tanaka S, Nakamura K, Takahasi N, et al. Role of RANKL in physiological and pathological bone resorption and therapeutics targeting the RANKL-RANK signaling system. *Immunol Rev*. 2005; 208:30.
234. Xing L, Schwarz EM, Boyce BF. Osteoclast precursors, RANKL/RANK, and immunology. *Immunol Rev*. 2005;208:19.
237. Fata JE, Kong YY, Li J, et al. The osteoclast differentiation factor osteoprotegerin-ligand is essential for mammary gland development. *Cell*. 2000;103(1):41.
240. Wada T, Nakashima T, Hiroshi N, et al. RANKL-RANK signaling in osteoclastogenesis and bone disease. *Trends Mol Med*. 2006; 12(1):17.
243. Fukushima H, Jimi E, Kajiya H, et al. Parathyroid-hormone-related protein induces expression of receptor activator of NF-kappaB ligand in human periodontal ligament cells via a cAMP/protein kinase A-independent pathway. *J Dent Res*. 2005;84(4):329.
244. Lomaga MA, Yeh WC, Sarosi I, et al. TRAF6 deficiency results in osteopetrosis and defective interleukin-1, CD40, and LPS signaling. *Genes Dev*. 1999;13(8):1015.
245. Naito A, Azuma S, Tanaka S, et al. Severe osteopetrosis, defective interleukin-1 signalling and lymph node organogenesis in TRAF6-deficient mice. *Genes Cells*. 1999;4(6):353.
246. Dougall WC, Glaccum M, Charrier K, et al. RANK is essential for osteoclast and lymph node development. *Genes Dev*. 1999;13(18):2412.
247. Josien R, Li HL, Ingulli E, et al. TRANCE, a tumor necrosis factor family member, enhances the longevity and adjuvant properties of dendritic cells *in vivo*. *J Exp Med*. 2000;191(3):495.
249. Padigel UM, Kim N, Choi Y, et al. TRANCE-RANK costimulation is required for IL-12 production and the initiation of a Th1-type response to *Leishmania* major infection in CD40L-deficient mice. *J Immunol*. 2003;171(10):5437.
250. Kotake S, Nanke Y, Mogi M, et al. IFN-gamma-producing human T cells directly induce osteoclastogenesis from human monocytes via the expression of RANKL. *Eur J Immunol*. 2005;35(11):3353.
251. Teng YT, Mahamed D, Singh B. Gamma interferon positively modulates *Actinobacillus actinomycetemcomitans*-specific RANKL+ CD4+ Th-cell-mediated alveolar bone destruction *in vivo*. *Infect Immun*. 2005;73(6):3453.
252. Fakruddin JM, Laurence J. HIV envelope gp120-mediated regulation of osteoclastogenesis via receptor activator of nuclear factor kappa B ligand (RANKL) secretion and its modulation by certain HIV protease inhibitors through interferon-gamma/RANKL cross-talk. *J Biol Chem*. 2003;278(48):48251.
253. Fisher JL, Thomas-Mudge RJ, Elliott J, et al. Osteoprotegerin overexpression by breast cancer cells enhances orthotopic and osseous tumor growth and contrasts with that delivered therapeutically. *Cancer Res*. 2006;66(7):3620.
254. Nyambo R, Cross N, Lippitt J, et al. Human bone marrow stromal cells protect prostate cancer cells from TRAIL-induced apoptosis. *J Bone Miner Res*. 2004;19(10):1712.
255. Colucci S, Brunetti G, Rizzi R, et al. T cells support osteoclastogenesis in an *in vitro* model derived from human multiple myeloma bone disease: the role of the OPG/TRAIL interaction. *Blood*. 2004; 104(12):3722.
256. Galluzzi F, Stagi S, Salti R, et al. Osteoprotegerin serum levels in children with type 1 diabetes: a potential modulating role in bone status. *Eur J Endocrinol*. 2005;153(6):879.
257. Bucay N, Sarosi I, Dunstan CR, et al. Osteoprotegerin-deficient mice develop early onset osteoporosis and arterial calcification. *Genes Dev*. 1998;12(9):1260.
258. Body JJ, Facon T, Coleman RE, et al. A study of the biological receptor activator of nuclear factor-kappaB ligand inhibitor, denosumab, in patients with multiple myeloma or bone metastases from breast cancer. *Clin Cancer Res*. 2006;12(4):1221.
259. Scott DL, Kingsley GH. Tumor necrosis factor inhibitors for rheumatoid arthritis. *N Engl J Med*. 2006;355(7):704.
260. van der Heijde DM, van Leeuwen MA, van Riel PL, et al. Biannual radiographic assessments of hands and feet in a three-year prospective followup of patients with early rheumatoid arthritis. *Arthritis Rheum*. 1992;35(1):26.
261. van der Heijde DM. Overview of radiologic efficacy of new treatments. *Rheum Dis Clin North Am*. 2004;30(2):285.
262. Lipsky PE, van der Heijde DM, St Clair EW, et al. Infliximab and methotrexate in the treatment of rheumatoid arthritis. Anti-Tumor

Necrosis Factor Trial in Rheumatoid Arthritis with Concomitant Therapy Study Group. *N Engl J Med*. 2000;343(22):1594.

263. Reinecker HC, Steffen M, Witthoeft T, et al. Enhanced secretion of tumour necrosis factor-alpha, IL-6, and IL-1 beta by isolated lamina propria mononuclear cells from patients with ulcerative colitis and Crohn's disease. *Clin Exp Immunol*. 1993;94(1):174.
264. Hanauer SB, Sandborn WJ, Rutgeerts P, et al. Human anti-tumor necrosis factor monoclonal antibody (adalimumab) in Crohn's disease: the CLASSIC-I trial. *Gastroenterology*. 2006; 130(2):323.
266. Rutgeerts P, Sandborn WJ, Feagan BG, et al. Infliximab for induction and maintenance therapy for ulcerative colitis. *N Engl J Med*. 2005;353(23):2462.
267. Sandborn WJ, Targan SR. Biologic therapy of inflammatory bowel disease. *Gastroenterology*. 2002;122(6):1592.
269. Schon MP, Boehncke WH. Psoriasis. *N Engl J Med*. 2005;352(18): 1899.
270. Mease PJ. Psoriatic arthritis therapy advances. *Curr Opin Rheumatol*. 2005;17(4):426.
271. Antoni CE, Kavanaugh A, Kirkham B, et al. Sustained benefits of infliximab therapy for dermatologic and articular manifestations of psoriatic arthritis: results from the infliximab multinational psoriatic arthritis controlled trial (IMPACT). *Arthritis Rheum*. 2005;52(4):1227.
272. Gordon KB, Langley RG, Leonardi C, et al. Clinical response to adalimumab treatment in patients with moderate to severe psoriasis: double-blind, randomized controlled trial and open-label extension study. *J Am Acad Dermatol*. 2006;55(4):598.
273. Leonardi CL, Powers JL, Matheson RT, et al. Etanercept as monotherapy in patients with psoriasis. *N Engl J Med*. 2003;349(21): 2014.
276. Dixon WG, Watson K, Lunt M, et al. Rates of serious infection, including site-specific and bacterial intracellular infection, in rheumatoid arthritis patients receiving anti-tumor necrosis factor therapy: results from the British Society for Rheumatology Biologics Register. *Arthritis Rheum*. 2006;54(8):2368.
277. Hochberg MC, Lebwohl MG, Plevy SE, et al. The benefit/risk profile of TNF-blocking agents: findings of a consensus panel. *Semin Arthritis Rheum*. 2005;34(6):819.
278. Bongartz T, Sutton AJ, Sweeting MJ, et al. Anti-TNF antibody therapy in rheumatoid arthritis and the risk of serious infections and malignancies: systematic review and meta-analysis of rare harmful effects in randomized controlled trials. *JAMA*. 2006;295(19):2275.
279. von Haehling S, Jankowska EA, Anker SD. Tumour necrosis factor-alpha and the failing heart—pathophysiology and therapeutic implications. *Basic Res Cardiol*. 2004;99(1):18.
282. Mohan C, Shi Y, Laman JD, et al. Interaction between CD40 and its ligand gp39 in the development of murine lupus nephritis. *J Immunol*. 1995;154(3):1470.
283. Kalled SL, Cutler AH, Datta SK, et al. Anti-CD40 ligand antibody treatment of SNF1 mice with established nephritis: preservation of kidney function. *J Immunol*. 1998;160(5):2158.
287. Kalunian KC, Davis JC Jr, Merrill JT, et al. Treatment of systemic lupus erythematosus by inhibition of T cell costimulation with anti-CD154: a randomized, double-blind, placebo-controlled trial. *Arthritis Rheum*. 2002;46(12):3251.
288. Boumpas DT, Furie R, Manzi S, et al. A short course of BG9588 (anti-CD40 ligand antibody) improves serologic activity and decreases hematuria in patients with proliferative lupus glomerulonephritis. *Arthritis Rheum*. 2003;48(3):719.
289. Bussel JB. Overview of idiopathic thrombocytopenic purpura: new approach to refractory patients. *Semin Oncol*. 2000;27(6 Suppl 12):91.
290. Ruegg C, Yilmaz A, Bieler G, et al. Evidence for the involvement of endothelial cell integrin alphaVbeta3 in the disruption of the tumor vasculature induced by TNF and IFN-gamma. *Nat Med*. 1998;4(4):408.
291. Taguchi T, Sohmura Y. Clinical studies with TNF. *Biotherapy*. 1991;3(2):177.
292. Skillings J, Wierzbicki R, Eisenhauer E, et al. A phase II study of recombinant tumor necrosis factor in renal cell carcinoma: a study of the National Cancer Institute of Canada Clinical Trials Group. *J Immunother*. 1992;11(1):67.
293. Tracey KJ, Lowry SF, Cerami A. The pathophysiologic role of cachectin/TNF in septic shock and cachexia. *Ann Inst Pasteur Immunol*. 1988;139(3):311.
295. Lejeune FJ, Lienard D, Matter M, et al. Efficiency of recombinant human TNF in human cancer therapy. *Cancer Immun*. 2006;6:6.
296. Ware CF. The TNF superfamily. *Cytokine Growth Factor Rev*. 2003;14(3–4):181.
297. Seko Y, Cole S, Kasprzak W, et al. The role of cytokine mRNA stability in the pathogenesis of autoimmune disease. *Autoimmunity Rev*. 2006;5(5):299.
298. Zhang T, Kruys V, Huez G, et al. AU-rich element-mediated translational control: complexity and multiple activities of trans-activating factors. *Biochem Soc Trans*. 2002;30(Pt 6):952.
299. Black RA, Doedens JR, Mahimkar R, et al. Substrate specificity and inducibility of TACE (tumour necrosis factor alpha-converting enzyme) revisited: the Ala-Val preference, and induced intrinsic activity. *Biochem Soc Symp*. 2003(70):39.
301. Li C, Norris PS, Ni CZ, et al. Structurally distinct recognition motifs in lymphotoxin-beta receptor and CD40 for tumor necrosis factor receptor-associated factor (TRAF)-mediated signaling. *J Biol Chem*. 2003;278(50):50523.
302. Kinkade A, Ware CF. The DARC conspiracy—virus invasion tactics. *Trends Immunol*. 2006;27(8):362.
305. Rutschmann S, Hoebe K, Zalevsky J, et al. PanR1, a dominant negative missense allele of the gene encoding TNF-alpha (Tnf), does not impair lymphoid development. *J Immunol*. 2006;176(12):7525.
306. Neumann B, Luz A, Pfeffer K, et al. Defective Peyer's patch organogenesis in mice lacking the 55-kD receptor for tumor necrosis factor. *J Exp Med*. 1996;184:259.
307. Iizuka K, Chaplin DD, Wang Y, et al. Requirement for membrane lymphotoxin in natural killer cell development. *Proc Natl Acad Sci U S A*. 1999;96(11):6336.
309. Tumanov AV, Grivennikov SI, Shakhov AN, et al. Dissecting the role of lymphotoxin in lymphoid organs by conditional targeting. *Immunol Rev*. 2003;195:106.

Chapter 26

Chemokines

Philip M. Murphy

INTRODUCTION

Chemokines (or chemotactic cytokines) are members of a family of extracellular immunoregulatory proteins defined by sequence homology and a common structural fold (1). Differentially expressed by most cell types, chemokines can be loosely divided into two main immunologic groups: homeostatic chemokines, which are expressed constitutively; and inflammatory chemokines, which are induced by infection and injury or in the setting of inappropriate inflammation (2–15). At the biochemical level, both types act by binding to one or more members of a large subfamily of seven-transmembrane-domain G-protein–coupled receptors, signaling mainly through G_{i2} (16,17). At the cellular level, chemokine action in the immune system is determined by differential expression of chemokine receptors on both lymphoid and myeloid cells, and classically results in directed cell migration (chemotaxis), although effects on activation, specific effector function, memory, proliferation, and apoptosis may also occur. At the biologic level, chemokines play critical roles in immunity and inflammation, acting at multiple levels, including immune system development (18), transendothelial migration (19,20), leukocyte positioning within microenvironments (21,22), and both phagocyte and lymphocyte activation (23–25). As a result, chemokines may function both beneficially, for example, in the setting of antimicrobial host defense and tissue repair, or harmfully, for example, in the setting of cancer, chronic inflammation, autoimmunity, and infectious disease. The discovery of pathogens that encode multispecific chemokine-binding proteins and chemokine receptor antagonists able to subvert chemokine action provides compelling evidence for the importance of chemokines in host defense and for the significance of their redundant functions (26–28). Some pathogens, most notably HIV and *Plasmodium vivax,* go further and actually co-opt and exploit parts of the host chemokine system as essential virulence factors (16,29,30). Some chemokines also have nonimmunologic functions, including regulation of organ development (31,32), angiogenesis (33), and cancer (34–36). Together these physiologic and pathologic properties have suggested potential chemokine-based therapeutic opportunities, both as drug targets (37,38) and as immunologic response modifiers, for example, as adjuvants in DNA vaccines (39,40). To date, >100 chemokines, chemokine receptors, and viral chemokine mimics have been discovered, each having its own interesting place in immunology. The goal of this chapter is to delineate the basic principles of how chemokines are organized as a system, and to illustrate classic and more recently discovered immunologic roles using well-established examples.

MOLECULAR ORGANIZATION OF THE CHEMOKINE SYSTEM

Chemokines

Chemokines are defined by structure, not by function, although almost all chemokines have strong chemotactic activity for at least one subtype of leukocyte. Most mature chemokines are 66 to 111 amino acids long, and all occupy a common sector of sequence space bounded loosely by ~20% identity for any pairwise comparison; tertiary structure is highly conserved, in part because of conservatively spaced disulfide-bonded cysteines (Figure 26.1) (41). Chemokines are subclassified based on variation in cysteine number and location; all have at least two cysteines, and all but two have at least four (Tables 26.1, 26.2). In the four-cysteine group, the first two are either adjacent (CC motif, $n = 24$) or separated by either one (CXC motif, $n = 16$) or three (CX3C motif, $n = 1$) nonconserved amino acids. The C chemokines ($n = 2$) have only two cysteines, corresponding to C-2 and C-4 in the other subgroups. Disulfide bonds link C-1 to C-3 and C-2 to C-4. The conserved chemokine fold contains three β sheets arranged in the shape of a Greek key, overlaid by a *C*-terminal α-helical domain and flanked by an N-terminal domain that lacks order. Sequence identity is <30% between members of different groups, but ranges from ~30% to 99% among members of the same group. The group motifs are used as roots, followed by the letter L for ligand and a number (e.g., CXCL1), in a systematic nomenclature that was established to resolve competing aliases (42).

CC and CXC chemokines can be subclassified by additional motifs that may have functional significance. The seven human CXC chemokines with Glu-Leu-Arg (ELR) N-terminal to C-1 are >40% identical, attract neutrophils, bind the same receptor CXCR2, and are angiogenic (Table 26.1) (43). Among CXC chemokines that lack ELR, only CXCL12 is angiogenic and attracts neutrophils, but by using a distinct receptor, CXCR4 (44); CXCL9–11 also are >40% identical and share a receptor (CXCR3), but are angiostatic, not angiogenic (45). The CC group has two large subgroups, the MCPs (monocyte chemoattractant protein) and the MIPs (macrophage inflammatory protein), whose members typically chemoattract monocytes/macrophages but not neutrophils, in addition to having differential cell targets (46). CXCL16 and CX3CL1 cross groups to form a unique multimodular subgroup (47,48). Each has a chemokine domain, a mucinlike stalk, a transmembrane domain, and a *C*-terminal cytoplasmic module and can exist as a membrane-bound or shed form, mediating direct

Structural Signature

Class	Structural Signature	Names	n
CX3C:	..........CXXXC.................. C.................C..............	CX3CL1	1
non-ELR CXC:	..........CX__C...................C.................C..............	CXCL#	9
ELR CXC:	...ELR...CX__C...................C.................C..............	CXCL#	7
4C CC:	..........C___C...................C.................C..............	CCL#	19
6C CC:	..........C___C..........C.........C.................C.....C........	CCL#	5
C:	.......................C...C..............	XCL#	2

FIGURE 26.1 Chemokine classification and nomenclature. Chemokine classes are defined by the number and arrangement of conserved cysteines, as shown. Brackets link cysteines that form disulfide bonds. ELR, Glu-Leu-Arg; X, an amino acid other than cysteine. The underscore is a spacer used to optimize the alignment. The N and C termini can vary considerably in length (not illustrated). For the molecules with four cysteines, there are approximately 24 amino acids between Cys-2 and Cys-3 and 15 amino acids between Cys-3 and Cys-4. At right are listed the nomenclature system and the number of human chemokines known in each class (n).

TABLE 26.1 The Human CXC, CX3C, and C Chemokine Families

ELR Motif	Chemokine	Common Aliases	Main Source	Main Immunologic Roles	Chromosomal Location
ELR+	CXCL1	GROα MGSA	Many tumors	Neutrophil trafficking	4q21.1
	CXCL2	GROβ			
	CXCL3	GROγ			
ELR−	CXCL4	PF-4	Preformed in platelets	Procoagulant	
	CXCL4L1		Preformed in platelets	ND	
ELR+	CXCL5	ENA-78	Induced in epithelial cells of gut & lung; N, Mo, Plts, EC	Neutrophil trafficking	
	CXCL6	GCP-2	Induced in lung microvascular EC; Mo; alveolar epithelial cells, mesothelial cells, EC & MΦ		
	CXCL7	NAP-2	Preformed in platelets		
	CXCL8	IL-8	Induced in most cell types		
ELR−	CXCL9	Mig	Induced in PMN, MΦ, T cells, astrocytes, microglial cells, hepatocytes, EC, fibroblasts, keratinocytes, thymic stromal cells	Th1 response	
	CXCL10	IP-10	Induced in ECs, Mo, keratinocytes, respiratory & intestinal epithelial cells, astrocytes, microglia, mesangial cells, smooth muscle cells		
	CXCL11	I-TAC	ECs, Mo,		
	CXCL12	SDF-1, PBSF	Constitutive in bone marrow stromal cells; most tissues	Myelopoiesis HPC, neutrophil homing to BM B lymphopoiesis	10q11.21
	CXCL13	BCA-1	Constitutive in follicular HEV of secondary lymphoid tissue	Naïve B- & T-cell homing to follicles B1-cell homing to peritoneum Natural Ab production	4q21.1
	CXCL14	BRAK	Constitutive in most tissues, breast and kidney tumors	Macrophage migration	5q31.1
ELR+	(CXCL15)	(mouse only)	Constitutive in lung epithelial cells	Neutrophil trafficking	NA
ELR−	CXCL16	Sexckine	Constitutive in spleen; DCs of the T zone	T-cell and DC homing to spleen	17p13
NA	CX3CL1	Fractalkine	EC, neurons, Mo, DC	NK, monocyte, MΦ,and Th1 cell migration; neuroprotection	16q13
	XCL1	Lymphotactin α	γδ epidermal T cells, NK, NK-T, activated $CD8^+$ and Th1 $CD4^+$ T cells	$CD62L^{low}$ T-effector cell migration	1q24.2
	XCL2	Lymphotactin β			

NA, not applicable; ND, not determined; Mo, monocyte; PMN, neutrophil; DC, dendritic cell; EC, endothelial cell; HEV, high-endothelial venule; MPC, myeloid progenitor cell; plt, platelet; MΦ, macrophage; GRO, growth-related oncogene; PF-4, platelet factor-4; GCP, granulocyte chemoattactant protein; ENA-78, 78-amino acid epithelial cell-derived neutrophil activator; NAP, neutrophil-activating protein; IL-8, interleukin-8; Mig, monokine induced by IFNγ; I-TAC; interferon-inducible T-cell α chemoattractant; SDF, stromal cell–derived factor; BCA, B-cell–activating chemokine; BRAK, breast- and kidney-associated chemokine.

cell–cell adhesion and chemotaxis, respectively. The discovery of "chemokine" DMC (human dendritic cell- and monocyte-attracting chemokinelike protein) by sequence threading techniques, not primary sequence homology (49), provides proof of principle that the boundaries of chemokine sequence space can expand substantially as protein structures are determined or modeled.

Chemokine monomer, dimer, and tetramer structures may occur, and complex quaternary structures bound to glycosaminoglycans (GAGs) on the surface of cells may be important for function in vivo (50). Location of the GAG-binding domains is variable and depends on the highly basic nature of these proteins. Chemokine heterodimers have been described, both CC/CC and CC/CXC (51,52),

TABLE 26.2 The Human CC Chemokine Family

Chromosomal Location	*Chemokine*	*Common Aliases*	*Sources*	*Main Immunologic Roles*
17q11-12	**CCL1**	I-309	Inducible in Mo & $CD4^+$ and $CD8^+$ $\alpha\beta$ and $CD4^-CD8^-$ $\gamma\delta$ T cells	Th2 response
	CCL2	MCP-1	Inducible in Mo, fibroblasts, keratinocytes, EC, PMN, synoviocytes, mesangial cells, astrocytes, lung epithelial cells & MΦ Constitutively made in splenic arteriolar lymphatic sheath and medullary region of lymph node, many tumors, & arterial plaque EC	Innate immunity Th2 response $CD4^+$ T-cell differentiation
	CCL3	MIP-1α LD78α MIP-1αS	Inducible in Mo/MΦ, $CD8^+$ T cells, B cells, plts, PMN, Eo, Ba, DC, NK, mast cells, keratinocytes, fibroblasts, mesangial cells, astrocytes, microglial cells, epith cells	Innate immunity Th1 response CD4 T-cell differentiation
	CCL3L1	LD78β MIP-1αP	Similar to CCL3	Probably similar to CCL3
	CCL4	MIP-1β	Similar to CCL3	Innate immunity Th1 response
	CCL5	RANTES	Inducible in EC, T cells, epithelial cells, Mo, fibroblasts, mesangial cells, NK cells Constitutively expressed and stored in plt and Eo granules	Innate immunity Th1 and Th2 response
NA	**(CCL6)**	Mouse only	Inducible in bone marrow and peritoneal-derived MΦ	ND
17q11-12	**CCL7**	MCP-3	Inducible in Mo, plts, fibroblasts, EC, skin, bronchial epithelial cells, astrocytes	Th2 response
	CCL8	MCP-2	Inducible in fibroblasts, PMN, astrocytes Constitutively expressed in colon, small intest, heart, lung, thymus, pancreas, spinal cord, ovary, placenta	Th2 response
NA	**(CCL9/10)**	Mouse only	Constitutively expressed in all mouse organs except brain; highest in lung, liver, & thymus Induced in heart & lung	ND
17q11	**CCL11**	Eotaxin	Epithelial cells, EC, smooth muscle, cardiac muscle, Eo, dermal fibroblasts, mast cells, MI, Reed–Sternberg cells	Th2 response Eosinophil trafficking Mast cell trafficking Basophil trafficking, degranulation
NA	**(CCL12)**	Mouse only	Inducible in lung alveolar MΦ & smooth muscle cells; spinal cord Constitutive expression in lymph node and thymic stromal cells	Allergic inflammation
17q11-12	**CCL13**	MCP-4	Inducible in nasal and bronchial epithelial cells; dermal fibroblasts; PBMCs; atherosclerotic plaque EC & MΦ Constitutively expressed in small intestine, colon, thymus, heart, & placenta	Th2 response
	CCL14a	HCC-1	Constitutively expressed in most organs; high plasma levels	ND
	CCL14b	HCC-3	Same as CCL14b except absent from skeletal muscle and pancreas	ND
	CCL15	HCC-2 Lkn-1	Inducible in Mo and DC Constitutive RNA expression in liver, gut, heart, & skeletal muscle, adrenal gland & lung leukocytes.	ND
	CCL16	HCC-4 LEC	Constitutively expressed in liver, possibly many other organs. Also, Mo, T cells, & NK cells express mRNA	DC maturation factor
16q13	**CCL17**	TARC	Constitutive in normal DC and Reed–Sternberg cells of Hodgkin's disease	Th2 response

(*continued*)

TABLE 26.2 The Human CC Chemokine Family (Continued)

Chromosomal Location	Chemokine	Common Aliases	Sources	Main Immunologic Roles
17q11.2	**CCL18**	DC-CK1 PARC	Constitutive in Mo/MΦ, germinal-center DC	DC attraction of naïve T cells Hematopoiesis
9p13.3	**CCL19**	ELC, MIP-3β	Constitutive on interdigitating DC in secondary lymphoid tissue	Naïve and memory T cell & DC homing to lymph node
2q36.3	**CCL20**	LARC MIP-3α	Constitutive in follicle-associated epithelium overlying GALT inductive sites (Peyer patches & isolated lymphoid follicles) Inducible in GALT, Th17 cells	GALT development B and DC homing to GALT IgA humoral response in gut Th17 response
9p13.3	**CCL21**	SLC 6Ckine	Constitutive in lymphatic EC, HEV, & interdigitating DC in T areas of 2° lymphoid tissue, thymic medullary epith cells, & EC	Naïve and memory T cell & DC homing to lymph node
16q13	**CCL22**	MDC	Constitutive in DC and MΦ Inducible in Mo, T & B cells	Th2 response
17q12	**CCL23**	MPIF-1	Constitutive in pancreas & skeletal muscle	ND
7q11.23	**CCL24**	Eotaxin-2	Inducible in Mo	Eosinophil migration
19p13.3	**CCL25**	TECK	Constitutive in thymic stromal cells & small intest	Thymocyte migration Homing of memory T cells to gut
7q11.23	**CCL26**	Eotaxin-3	Constitutive in heart & ovary Inducible on dermal fibroblasts & EC	Th2 response
9p13.3	**CCL27**	CTACK Eskine	Constitutive in placenta, keratinocytes, testis, & brain	Homing of memory and effector T cells to skin
5p12	**CCL28**	MEC	Constitutive in epith cells of gut, airway	Homing of T cells to mucosal surfaces

NA, not applicable. Mo, monocyte; PMN, neutrophil; DC, dendritic cell; EC, endothelial cell; HEV, high-endothelial venule; MPC, myeloid progenitor cell; plt, platelet; MΦ, macrophage MCP, monocyte chemoattractant protein; MIP, macrophage inflammatory protein; RANTES, regulated upon activation normal T cell expressed and secreted; MRP, MIP-related protein; HCC, hemofiltrate CC chemokine; TARC, thymus and activation-related chemokine; PARC, pulmonary and activation-related chemokine; ELC, Epstein–Barr virus–induced receptor ligand chemokine; LARC, liver and activation-related chemokine; SLC, secondary lymphoid tissue chemokine; MDC, macrophage-derived chemokine; MPIF, myeloid progenitor inhibitory factor; TECK, thymus-expressed chemokine; CTACK, cutaneous T-cell–associated chemokine; mucosal epithelium chemokine; MEC, mucosa-associated epithelial cell chemokine.

and some may form preferentially over homodimers in a GAG-dependent manner (53); native heterodimers have also been identified (54). It will be important to define the functional significance of this so-called interactome (55).

Chemokine Receptors

Chemokine receptors are defined as mediators that activate cellular responses upon binding chemokines. All 19 known human subtypes, together with receptors for the classical lipid and peptide chemoattractant receptors (16), are members of the rhodopsinlike 7TM superfamily of G-protein–coupled receptors (see www.gpcr.org/7tm for a Web site devoted to this superfamily). Apart from odorant receptors, this is the largest known subfamily of GPCRs, itself the largest protein family from *Caenorhabditis elegans* to human (16,17,56). Chemokine-binding, membrane-anchoring, and signaling domains are formed from a single polypeptide chain. Although homo- and heterodimers have been reported, the precise physiologic form has not been clearly delineated (57–59).

Usually the chemokine ligand–receptor relationship is promiscuous but chemokine subgroup–restricted (Table 26.3). A systematic nomenclature formula exploits this as follows: receptor name = ligand subgroup root + R (for "receptor") + number, in order of discovery. An exception is the C-chemokine receptor XCR1, where "X" distinguishes it from CR1, the previously assigned name for complement receptor 1. For consistency, the XCR1 ligands are named XCL1 and XCL2. Each chemokine has a unique receptor-specificity profile, and each receptor has a unique chemokine-specificity profile. Promiscuous ligands of a given receptor interact with the same receptor chain, which contrasts with other types of cytokines that share receptors. Almost all chemokines are chemotactic agonists, and a few are both agonists at one receptor and antagonists at another.

Atypical Chemokine System Components

Atypical chemokine system components have been known since 1993 and continue to be discovered in large numbers. Some have been shown to play important functional roles. Perhaps most intriguing are the functional chemokines and 7TM chemokine receptors encoded by poxviruses and herpesviruses, a clear result of "molecular piracy" of their hosts, and presumably of great importance in pathogenesis, although precise roles have not yet been well defined. A second category includes three human 7TM proteins (Duffy, D6, and CCX CKR) that bind chemokines promiscuously but do not signal (60,61). Several herpesviruses and poxviruses (26), as well as *Schistosoma mansoni* (62) and ectoparasitic ticks, also encode promiscuous chemokine-binding proteins, but they have unique non-7TM structures and are secreted. Duffy, also known as DARC (Duffy antigen receptor for chemokines), is expressed mainly on red cells and is an extreme exception to the ligand rule because it binds with high affinity many, but not all, CC and CXC chemokines. Expressed in placenta and on lymphatic endothelium, D6 is catalytic and not stoichiometrically restricted in its ability to scavenge inflammatory CC chemokines by a process of rapid internalization and recycling to plasma membrane. CCX CKR binds multiple CC chemokines (63). One theory is that nonsignaling chemokine-binding proteins function as anti-inflammatory chemokine buffers. Accordingly, they have been referred to as chemokine scavengers, interceptors, and silent or decoy receptors. Evidence from knockout mouse experiments with D6 and Duffy suggest that this may be the case in some but not all contexts.

Several endogenous nonchemokine ligands bind chemokine receptors, including aminoacyl tRNA synthetases, some of which function as autoantigens in autoimmune disorders (64); *β* defensin 2, which activates CCR6, possibly linking innate to adaptive immunity (65); chemokine-like factor 1, an agonist at CCR4 (66); and CD82 (KAI1), a tetraspanin expressed on leukocytes and cancer cells that binds to endothelial cell–expressed DARC, triggering senescence in tumor cells and suppression of metastasis (67). CCR5 acts as a dendritic cell pattern-recognition receptor for myHsp70, a heat-shock protein produced by *Mycobacterium tuberculosis*, promoting T-DC synapse formation and effector immune responses (68). Numerous chemokines bind scavenger-receptor ligands, such as oxidized LDL, through their receptor-binding domains (69). The prototype is CXCL16, which was originally called SR-PSOX (scavenger receptor for phosphatidyl serine and oxidized LDL). CXCL16 has also been shown to function as a transporter for CpG oligonucleotides across the plasma membrane for action at TLR9 (70), as well as to mediate bacterial phagocytosis by antigen-presenting cells (APCs) (71).

In contrast, a truncated form of CCL23, unlike full-length CCL23, has not been shown to activate any chemokine receptors yet is an agonist at FPRL1, a member of the classical chemoattractant fMet-Leu-Phe receptor subfamily (72). Perhaps the most surprising example of an alternative chemokine receptor agonist is the tripeptide Pro-Gly-Pro, a breakdown product of collagen from extracellular matrix that is found in bronchoalveolar lavage samples from patients with chronic obstructive pulmonary disease. This peptide shares structural homology with a domain in CXC chemokines (73), is a chemotactic agonist at CXCR2, and has been shown to recruit neutrophils via CXCR2 activation in a mouse model of lung inflammation. Examples of non-chemokine chemokine receptor ligands (agonists or antagonists) have been identified in numerous pathogens. For example, HIV Tat is an antagonist at CXCR4 (74), and *M. tuberculosis* heat-shock protein Hsp70, *Toxoplasma gondii* cyclophilin, and HIV gp120 are all agonists at CCR5.

Immunologic Classification of the Chemokine System

Chemokines and chemokine receptors have differential leukocyte specificities but together regulate the full spectrum of leukocytes. As such, they can be loosely divided into two main functional subsystems, *homeostatic* and *inflammatory* (Table 26.4). Homeostatic chemokines are differentially and constitutively expressed primarily in specific microenvironments of primary and secondary immune organs, and recruit hematopoietic precursor cells, mature dendritic cells (DCs), and naïve and central memory lymphocyte subsets via constitutively expressed receptors. Inflammatory chemokines are induced by noxious stimuli in diverse tissue cells and leukocytes. Inflammatory chemokine receptors are constitutively expressed on myeloid cells, natural killer (NK) cells, and effector but not naïve lymphocytes. Dynamic shifts in receptor expression occur during DC and NK cell maturation and during lymphocyte maturation, activation, and differentiation (75–78). This is not an absolute classification, because constitutive chemokines may be further induced, and chemokines that are highly inducible in some cell types may be constitutively expressed in others.

Evolution of the Chemokine System

Comparative whole-genome analysis has identified chemokine genes and chemokine receptor homologs in all vertebrates examined so far, including jawless fish, but not in any invertebrates including sea squirt and sea urchin, placing the system's origins between 564 and 650 million years ago. Forty-two human, 23 chicken (*Gallus galli*), 25 frog (*Xenopus tropicalis*), and, surprisingly, 63 zebrafish (*Danio rerio*) chemokine genes have been identified in the draft sequences for these organisms (79,80). Several human chemokines (e.g., CXCL8, CCL18) lack mouse counterparts and vice versa. CXCL12 and its receptors CXCR4 and RDC1/CXCR7 are all exceptionally highly conserved, and all three genes regulate both development and immunity and, at least in mouse, are essential for life (81). By

(text continues on page 813)

TABLE 26.3 Chemokine Specificities for Human 7TM Chemokine Receptors and Chemokine-Binding Proteins[a,b]

	CXCR1	CXCR2 (CD128)	CXCR3 (CD183)	CXCR4 (CD184)	CXCR5	CXCR6	CXCR7	CCR1	CCR2
CXCL1/Groα		+++							
CXCL2/Groβ		+++							
CXCL3/Groγ		+++							
CXCL4/PF-4			++						
CXCL4L1									
CXCL5/ENA-78	+	+++							
CXCL6/GCP-2	++	+++							
CXCL7/NAP-2		+++							
CXCL8/IL-8	+++	+++							
CXCL9/Mig			+++						
CXCL10/γIP-10			+++						
CXCL11/I-TAC			+++				++		
CXCL12/SDF-1				+++			+++		
CXCL13/BCA1			+		+++				
CXCL14/BRAK									
*CXCL15/lungkine									
CXCL16						+++			
CCL1/I-309									
CCL2/MCP-1								+	+++
CCL3/MIP-1α								+++	
CCL4/MIP-1β								Antag	
CCL5/RANTES								+++	
*CCL6/MRP-1									
CCL7/MCP-3								+++	+++
CCL8/MCP-2								++	+++
*CCL9/10/MRP-2								++	
CCL11/eotaxin			Antag						Antag
*CCL12/MCP-5									++
CCL13/MCP-4								+++	+++
CCL14a/HCC-1								+++	
CCL14b/HCC-3									
CCL15/HCC-2								+++	
CCL16/HCC-4								+	+
CCL17/TARC									
CCL18/PARC									
CCL19/ELC									
CCL20/LARC									
CCL21/SLC			+						
CCL22/MDC									
CCL23/MPIF-1								+++	
CCL24/eotaxin-2									
CCL25/TECK									
CCL26/eotaxin-3									
CCL27/CTACK									
CCL28/MEC									
XCL1/Lymphotactin α									
XCL2/ lymphotactin β									
CX3CL1/fractalkine									

[a]The standard name and most commonly used alias are listed for each chemokine.

[b]For each receptor, + indicates that the corresponding chemokine is an agonist, and "Antag" denotes an antagonist. For the 7TM chemokine-binding proteins CCX CKR, D6, and Duffy, the + signs indicate high-affinity binding without signaling.

*Denotes mouse chemokines that may not have human counterparts.

CCR3	CCR4	CCR5 (CD195)	CCR6	CCR7 (CD197)	CCR8	CCR9	CCR10	XCR1	CX_3CR1	CCX CKR	Duffy (CD234)	D6
											+++	
											++	
											++	
Antag												
Antag												
Antag												
					+++							
											++	++
		+++										
		+++			+							+++
++		+++									++	+++
++		Antag										+
++		+++										+++
+++		+										+
+++												++
		+++										+++
+++												
		+			+							
	+++				+							
				+++						+		
			+++									
				+++						+		
	+++											
+++												
						+++				+		
++												
							+++					
+							+++					
								+++				
								+++				
									+++			

TABLE 26.4 Specificities of Functional Human Chemokine Receptors for Human Leukocyte Subsets

	CXCR1	*CXCR2*	*CXCR3*	*CXCR4*	*CXCR5*	*CXCR6*	*CCR1*	*CCR2*	*CCR3*	*CCR4*	*CCR5*	*CCR6*	*CCR7*	*CCR7*	*CCR9*	*CCR10*	*XCR1*	*CX_3CR1*
$CD4^-CD8^-$ thymocytes				+														
$CD4^+CD8^+$ thymocytes				+											+			
$CD4^+CD8^-$ thymocytes				+						+			+					
$CD4^-CD8^+$ thymocytes				+					+	+			+					
$CD34^+$ HSC				+														
$CD56^{dim}$ $CD16^+$ NK	+		+	+	+	+	+			+	+	+			+			+
$CD56^{bright}$ $CD16^-$ NK	+		+	+	+	+	+				+	+	+		+			
CD4 NK-T			+	+				+		+	+							
CD8 NK-T			+	+		+	+	+			+	+						
$CD4^-CD8^-$ NK-T			+	+		+	+	+			+	+						
B cells			+	+	+		+	+				+	+					
Plasma cells				+		+			+							+		
IgA Ab-secreting cells				+											+	+		
Naïve T cells				+									+					
Follicular help T cells					+													
Central memory T cells			+							+		+	+					
Effector memory T cells							+		+		+							
Th1 Effector T cells			+	+		+		+			+		+					+
Th2 Effector T cells				+					+	+			+	+				
Th17 Effector T cells						+						+			+			
$\alpha4\beta7^+$ gut-homing memory T cells			+					+			+				+			
CLA^+ skin-homing memory T cells				+						+		−	+			+		
$CD4^+CD25^+Foxp3^+$ regulatory T cells										+	+	−		−				
Immature DC	+	+		+			+	+			+	+						
Mature DC				+								+	+					
$CD14^+$ monocytes	+	+		+			+	+										
$CD16^+$ monocytes				+														
Basophils		+		+			+		+		+							
Eosinophils			+	+			+		+									
Neutrophils	+	+		+			+	+										
Platelets	+			+			+		+	+								

Low
High

contrast, mice that lack CXCL14, the only other highly conserved chemokine, appear healthy and immunologically intact, and its putative receptor has not yet been identified (82). Orthologs for other chemokines among different vertebrate classes are difficult or impossible to assign. A model of chemokine system evolution has been proposed involving lineage-specific *en bloc* and tandem duplications. It has been speculated that the diverse roles of the chemokines were established early in their ontogeny, and that expansion accompanied the origin of recombination-activation gene (RAG)-based adaptive immunity (79).

Genes encoding inflammatory chemokines are found in two main clusters on human chromosomes 4q12-q21 (CXC) and 17q11-q21 (CC); CXCL16 is an exception, being located on chromosome 17 but on the other side of the centromere from the CC gene cluster. Genes for homeostatic chemokines are scattered alone or in small clusters on chromosomes 1, 2, 5, 7, 9, 10, and 16. Chemokine genes typically are ~4 kb long and usually have four exons in the case of CXC chemokines and three exons in the case of CC chemokines.

The 19 human chemokine receptor genes and three chemokine-binding-protein genes can be divided by chromosomal location into three groups: a large cluster on chromosome 3p21-23 including multiple CCRs, CX3CR1, XCR1, and CXCR6, plus D6 and CCX CKR ($n = 12$); CXCR1, CXCR2, and one receptor pseudogene clustered on 2q34-q35; and the rest unclustered. With the exception of CCR9, genes in the two clustered groups lack introns in the open reading frame (ORF) but have at least one and as many as 10 introns separating the promoter from the ORF. In contrast, an intron divides the N terminus of the majority of unclustered receptor genes (*CXCR3, 4,* and *5*; *CCR6,* and *10*). Several of these undergo alternative splicing creating isoforms with distinct N termini, and in the case of *CXCR3* this is functionally significant. CXCR3A and B both bind CXCL9, 10, and 11 with similar affinity, whereas only CXCR3B also binds the distantly related CXCL4. CXCR3A is selectively expressed on Th1 cells and mediates chemotactic responses in a G_i-dependent manner, whereas CXCR3B is expressed on microvascular endothelial cells and mediates the angiostatic effects of all four of its ligands through a distinct signaling mechanism (83).

With regard to horizontal evolution, variation in gene dosage among individuals has been observed for only a few chemokines. *CCL3* is an example in humans, and the *plt* locus (paucity of lymph node T cells) is an immunologically important example in mouse. In contrast, gene polymorphism is common among individuals for most chemokine and chemokine receptors, although the degree of polymorphism varies greatly among different genes. The most extreme and important example is the *CCR2-CCR5* locus, in which combinations of common dimorphic single-nucleotide polymorphisms (SNPs) in the CCR5 promoter with a SNP in the ORF of *CCR2* named *CCR2 V64I* and a 32-base pair (bp) deletion in the ORF of CCR5 named *CCR5Δ32* together form at least eight distinct haplotypes that may modulate susceptibility to and progression of various diseases, including HIV (84,85).

The Issue of Chemokine Redundancy

Two chemokines that bind to the same receptor may still have highly specific biologic roles, as a result of differential expression in time and space; activation of the same receptor via different signal transduction pathways or the same pathway with differential efficacy; or activation of additional differentially expressed receptors. A good example of differential expression is CXCL7 (NAP-2, neutrophil-activating protein-2) and CXCL8. Both are agonists for neutrophil CXCR2, but CXCL7 is stored in platelet α granules and released upon platelet activation, whereas CXCL8 is made by virtually all cell types upon gene induction by proinflammatory stimuli. There are few inflammatory processes in which only one chemokine is involved. They typically act cooperatively, on the same or separate cell types, but in a hierarchical manner through promiscuous receptors. The net result is that there may be enough functional redundancy in the whole system such that loss of a single inflammatory chemokine or chemokine receptor, for example, in a knockout mouse, does not cause altered susceptibility to naturally acquired infections or other diseases, yet there may not be sufficient redundancy to handle a stronger stress when one particularly important component is missing. In contrast, homeostatic chemokines act much less redundantly, with typically only one or two ligands per receptor, and their loss has been associated with major defects in development and basal leukocyte homing.

Chemokine Presentation Mechanisms

Chemokines typically act locally, and are thought to be concentrated for cell activation by tethering to endothelial cells via GAGs or transmembrane domains, or to matrix (22). GAG-dependent oligomerization has been shown to be important for in vivo activity of CCL5 and CXCL10 (86,87). The tethering cell may have produced the chemokine or else imported it by transcytosis from neighbors (88). The ligand-binding site includes the receptor N terminus and one or more extracellular loops, depending on the specific chemokine, which allow docking of the chemokine N-loop domain, and 7TM domains, which then accept the chemokine's N terminus and are critical for triggering. Tyrosine sulfation on the receptor N terminus has been shown to facilitate chemokine receptor binding to both chemokine and nonchemokine ligands (e.g., HIV gp120) (89).

LEUKOCYTE RESPONSES TO CHEMOKINES

Both homeostatic and inflammatory leukocyte trafficking require transendothelial migration, a multistep process involving an endothelium- and leukocyte-specific molecular code, in which chemokines regulate at least two steps (19,90). In an initial chemokine-independent step, leukocytes roll on inflamed endothelium in a selectin-dependent manner. Next, chemokines posted on endothelium stimulate rolling leukocytes to express activated $\beta 2$ integrins, which mediate shear-resistant adhesion via endothelial ICAMs. Leukocytes respond to chemokine gradients by changing their shape to produce a front and a back and by crawling toward the front (91,92). Motion is based on shear-dependent coordinated cytoskeletal remodeling, involving expansion of the front (lamellipodium), myosin based contraction at the back (uropod), release of the uropod from substrate, and membrane lipid movement. Navigation through tissue may require relays of chemokines and adhesion molecules. Fine navigation within tissue microenvironments has also been shown to be directed by specific chemokines up to the point of immunologic synapse formation (93,94), and there is now evidence that CCR5 and CXCR4 may accumulate in the immunologic synapse formed by $CD4^+$ T cells and dendritic cells *in vitro*, and that this may provide chemokine-dependent costimulatory signals (95,96).

Chemokines and their receptors have been increasingly implicated in other cell functions, including regulation of apoptosis (97–100), regulation of antigen sampling by immature DCs (e.g., CCR7 and CX3CR1), maturation of DCs (CCR7), and inhibition of mature DC endocytosis (CCR7) (101). Inflammatory chemokines may induce mediator release (e.g., defensins, proteases, perforins, histamine, eicosanoids), resulting in cytotoxic or vasomotor responses. Some chemokines even have direct antibacterial activity (102), which could explain why they may be found constitutively at high concentrations in body fluids such as sweat.

CHEMOKINE SIGNALING PATHWAYS

G_i-Dependent Effectors

Chemokines trigger chemokine receptors to act as guanine nucleotide exchange factors (GEFs), especially for G_{i2} (103). G-protein activation involves exchange of GDP for GTP by the α subunit, leading to dissociation of the trimer into α and $\beta\gamma$ subunits. The duration of G-protein signaling is regulated in part by intrinsic GTPase activity possessed by the α subunit, which can be markedly increased by GTPase-activating proteins (GAPs) known specifically as RGS proteins (regulators of G-protein signaling). Signaling appears to be mainly mediated by $\beta\gamma$, which activates diverse effectors, including phospholipases A2, C (subtypes $\beta 2$ and $\beta 3$) and D, phosphatidylinositol-3-kinase γ (PI3Kγ), protein tyrosine kinases (PTK) and phosphatases, low–molecular-weight GTPases, and mitogen-activated protein kinases (Figure 26.2). The requirements of these enzymes for chemotaxis are both chemoattractant- and cell-type dependent, and the complex mechanistic details underlying specificity remain to be elucidated.

PLC hydrolyzes PI(4,5) bisphosphate (PIP_2) to form 1,2-diacylglycerol (DAG) and inositol-1,4,5-trisphosphate (IP_3). IP_3 induces Ca^{2+} release from intracellular stores, which acts with DAG to activate protein kinase C (PKC). PI3Kγ phosphorylates PIP_2 to form PIP_3, which recruits proteins containing pleckstrin homology (PH) or Phox (PX) domains to lamellipodium, thereby converting shallow extracellular chemokine gradients to steep intracellular effector gradients (104,105). Four PH-domain–containing targets—Akt, and GEFs for Rac, Rho, and cdc42—modulate distinct phases of cell movement in various model systems. Rho regulates cell adhesion and chemotaxis, and myosin contraction. Rac and cdc42 control lamellipodia and filipodia formation, respectively. Downstream targets of Rac include PAK1, which also regulates myosin contraction. In neutrophils, signal amplification, gradient sensing, and cell orientation have been shown to be further amplified and reinforced by ATP release at the leading edge, which provides autocrine feedback signaling through P2Y2 nucleotide receptors. This is further amplified by conversion of ATP to extracellular adenosine, which signals through A3 receptors mobilized to the leading edge (106). Motility, phagocytosis, and immunologic synapse formation are all critically dependent on local polymerization of actin, coordinated by a large number of actin-binding proteins.

G_i-Independent Effectors

Many chemokine receptors couple to G proteins other than G_i *in vitro*; however, the role of these proteins *in vivo* is not well defined. There is *in vitro* evidence from studies of the fMet-Leu-Phe receptor that G12/13, through activation of Rho, may be important in formation of the uropod (107). Mice that lack both G12 and G13 selectively in B cells have reduced numbers of splenic marginal-zone B cells, resulting in a delay of antibody production in response to thymus-independent antigens. However, responsiveness of these cells to chemokines is normal. Instead, the phenotype may be a result of impaired sphingosine-1-phosphate signaling (108).

Chemokines may activate effectors such as MAP kinases and nonreceptor PTKs by a variety of G_i-independent mechanisms. A recent example is CXCR4, which has been shown to associate physically with TCR in a CXCL12-dependent manner, resulting in activation of ZAP-70 and

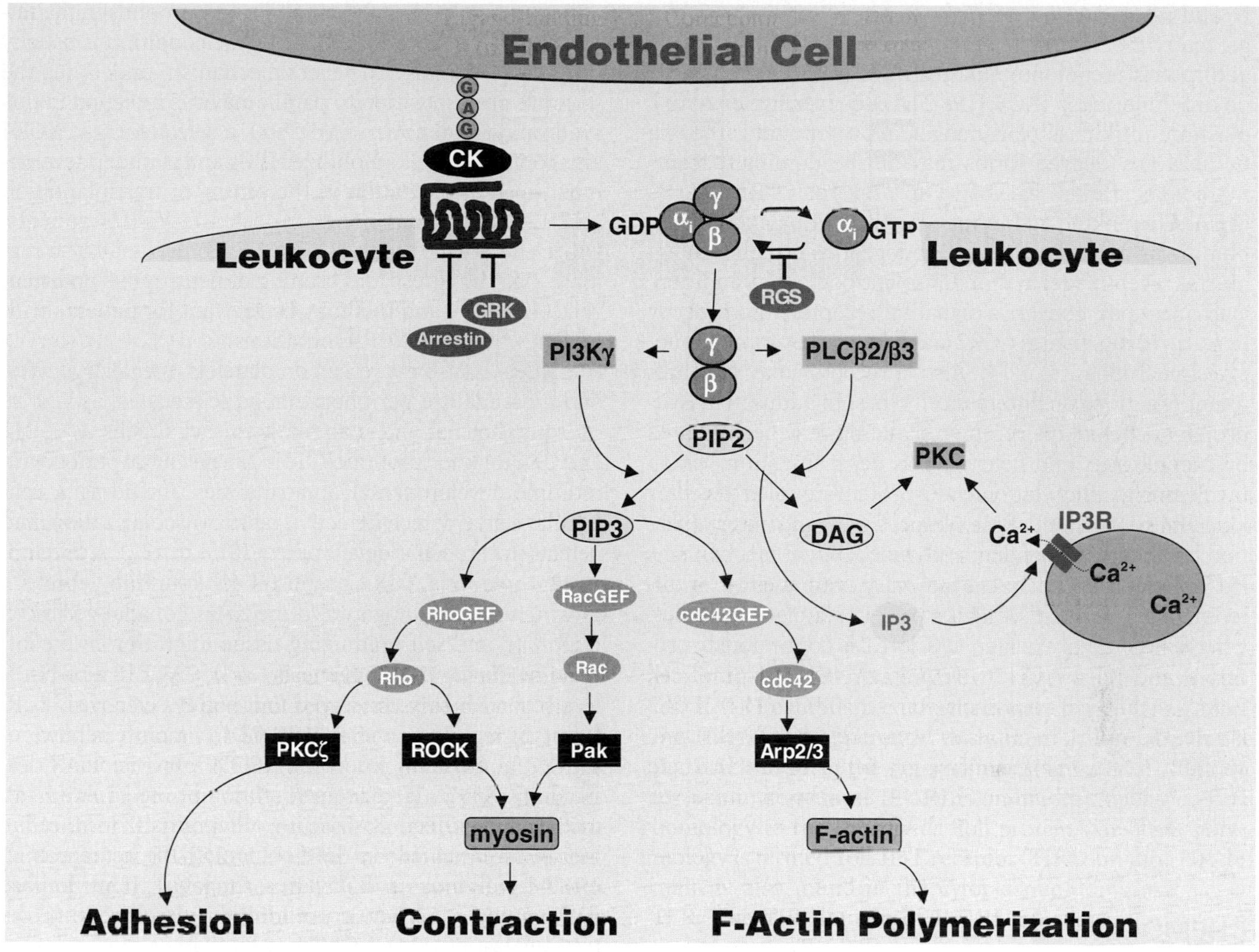

FIGURE 26.2 Chemokine signal transduction in chemotaxis. Depicted are key steps in two of the main pathways induced by most chemokines. The PI3Kγ pathway is particularly important for cell migration. Chemokines are able to activate other pathways as well, including non–G_i-type G proteins, protein tyrosine kinases, and MAP kinases, resulting in effects on cell proliferation and activation. Model is modified from the Alliance for Cell Signaling www.signaling-gateway.org). PLC, phospholipase C; PI3K, phosphatidylinositol 3-kinase; RGS, regulator of G-protein signaling; DAG, diacylglycerol; IP3, inositol trisphosphate; PIP, phosphatidylinsol phosphate; GAG, glycosaminoglycan; CK, chemokine; PKC, protein kinase C; GRK, G-protein–coupled receptor kinase; GEF, guanine nucleotide-exchange factor.

downstream effectors, including ERK, calcium flux, AP-1, and costimulation of cytokine secretion (96).

REGULATION OF CHEMOKINE ACTION

Chemokine and chemokine receptor expression may be positively or negatively regulated at the transcriptional level by diverse factors, including proinflammatory cytokines, hypoxia, viruses, bacterial products, cell adhesion, shear stress, antigen uptake, T-cell costimulation, and diverse transcription factors. Proinflammatory cytokines such as IL-1, TNF, and IL-15 induce expression of many of the inflammatory chemokines involved in innate immunity such as CXCL8, whereas immunoregulatory cytokines such as IFN-γ and IL-4 are more tightly focused on Th1 (e.g., CXCL9-11)- and Th2 (e.g., CCL11)-selective chemokines, respectively. Interferons, glucocorticoids, and anti-inflammatory cytokines (e.g., IL-10) may inhibit inflammatory chemokine gene expression. Chemokines may also be regulated at the level of mRNA stability and cell type–specific polyubiquitinylation and proteasomal degradation (109,110).

A chemokine gene may generate families of proteins that vary dramatically in activity and potency by alternative splicing and posttranslational modification, especially

N- and C-terminal proteolytic trimming. Proteases may target many chemokines (e.g., CD26 [dipeptidyl peptidase IV] and matrix metalloproteinases [MMP]) (111,112), or few or only one (e.g., TACE [the TNFα-converting enzyme], plasmin, urokinase plasminogen activator, and cathepsin G), and the cleaved forms may be the dominant forms in biologic fluids, as shown for several CCR1 ligands (113). Chemokine action may be blocked by chemokine-binding proteins (e.g., Duffy), endogenous receptor antagonists, receptor decoys, and autoantibodies. In addition, cytokines may convert a signaling receptor into a decoy (e.g., IL-10 inactivates CCR2 and other receptors on monocytes/macrophages) (114). Also, a receptor may have different functions on different cell types. In addition to RGS proteins, chemokine receptor signaling may be regulated by homologous and heterologous desensitization, which involves phosphorylation by G-protein–coupled receptor kinases or PKC and PKA, respectively, and internalization by clathrin-dependent and -independent mechanisms (115). Release mechanisms may vary dramatically for different chemokines. CXCL4 is stored in platelet α granules, whereas the highly related CXCL4L1 is continuously produced and released (116). CCL5 is released from T-cell granules that are preassociated with GAGs (117). CCL3 is released multidirectionally from activated T cells, presumably to create chemotactic gradients, unlike IL-2 and IFN-γ, which are secreted directly into the immunologic synapse (118).

CHEMOKINE REGULATION OF HEMATOPOIESIS

CXCL12 and CXCR4

Originally identified as a pre–B-cell-stimulatory factor from stromal cells that also enhanced HPC colony formation ex vivo, CXCL12 is the most abundant chemokine in bone marrow. Its production is under the control of G-CSF and adrenergic neurotransmission, among other factors (119). Mice that lack CXCL12 or its receptor CXCR4 have severe defects in bone marrow myelopoiesis and B-cell lymphopoiesis (81). The CXCL12/CXCR4 axis is also critical for mobilization of human peripheral blood progenitor cells and neutrophils from bone marrow in patients and for engraftment of human hematopoietic stem cells in SCID mice (120). Consistent with this, myelokathexis, or neutropenia without maturation arrest, is a defining phenotype of WHIM syndrome, a rare autosomal-dominant immunodeficiency disorder characterized by warts, hypogammaglobulinemia, infection, and myelokathexis, which has been linked to truncating mutations in the C tail of CXCR4 that prolong receptor signaling by delaying desensitization and blocking internalization (121). GM-CSF treatment overcomes this defect; moreover, patients can appropriately mobilize neutrophils in the setting of bacterial infection, so that the condition is usually not life-threatening. The exact mechanism underlying the selective predisposition to papillomavirus infection in this syndrome is unknown. AMD3100, a selective full CXCR4 antagonist, is able to mobilize HPCs and is under development for that indication in the setting of transplantation (122,123), but it has not been tested in WHIM patients. Other chemokines such as CXCR2 agonists may also regulate marrow egress and homing of neutrophils and stem cells (124,125), and this may be relevant for patients with WHIM who lack CXCR4 mutations.

CXCR4 is also expressed on platelets, megakaryocytes, and most mature peripheral blood leukocytes, as well as on some normal and malignant epithelial cells. CXCL12 and CXCR4 knockout mice die in the perinatal period with multiple developmental abnormalities, including a ventricular septal defect, defective gastric vascularization, and defects in cerebellar development (81,126,127). A developmental role for CXCR4 has also been found in zebrafish, in which the ortholog *cxcr4b* mediates gonadal germ-cell migration and self-organizing tissue migration in the lateral line during morphogenesis (128). CXCL12 also binds to a second highly conserved and highly selective GPCR, formerly known as the orphan RDC1, a close relative of the adrenomedullin receptor (129,130). Provisionally designated CXCR7, it appears to play a limited role in immunology (it affects positioning of marginal-zone B cells), but an essential role in development of the heart, particularly for all four cardiac valves. Curiously, mice that are deficient in CXCL12 do not exhibit this developmental defect, suggesting that CXCR7 may have other, more relevant ligands. Moreover, although CXCL12 binds to CXCR7 with high affinity, persuasive evidence of receptor triggering is lacking, thus the designation CXCR7 is provisional.

Consistent with a more general role in vascular biology, CXCR4 is expressed on vascular and cancer stem cells under the control of oxygen tension. These cells home to vascular niches under hypoxic conditions that occur during wound healing and in tumors. Hypoxia induces reduction of pVHL, which derepresses transcription factor HIF-1, a strong inducer of *CXCR4* expression (131–133).

Myelosuppressive Chemokines

When added to bone marrow culture systems ex vivo, many chemokines are able to suppress growth factor–dependent colony formation, apparently by acting directly on stem cells and early progenitors. The biologic significance of this remains unclear except for CXCR2. CXCR2$^{-/-}$ mice develop massive neutrophilia, splenomegaly, myeloid hyperplasia, and expansion of HPCs. CXCR2-dependent myelosuppression may be important for opposing overstimulation of hematopoiesis induced by environmental flora, because this phenotype is absent in mice derived in germ-free conditions. These mice also develop lymph node B-cell hyperplasia, which may occur by an indirect mechanism.

T Lymphopoiesis

During development, T cells must migrate from thymic cortex to medulla. Chemokines and chemokine receptors are differentially expressed in thymus and could coordinate migration, but precise roles have not been clearly delineated by phenotypes of gene-targeted mice or by other approaches. This is more likely to be a result of functional redundancy than lack of active chemokines in the thymus.

CCR9 and its ligand CCL25 may be important because competitive transplantation of CCR9$^{-/-}$ bone marrow is less efficient than normal marrow at repopulating the thymus of lethally irradiated Rag-1$^{-/-}$ mice (134). CCL25 is expressed by medullary dendritic cells and both cortical and medullary epithelial cells, and CCR9 is expressed on the majority of immature CD4^{+}CD8^{+} thymocytes, but is downregulated during transition to the CD4^{+} or CD8^{+} single-positive stage. Just before thymic egress, thymocytes become CCR9-negative and upregulate L-selectin. Transition from CD4^{+}CD8^{+} thymocytes in the cortex to CD4 or CD8 single-positive thymocytes in the medulla is also associated with upregulation of CCR4 and CCR7, receptors for CCL22, and CCL19 and CCL21, respectively, which are expressed on endothelial cells of medullary venules. Studies with knockout mice have suggested that CCR7-dependent cortex-to-medulla migration of positively selected thymocytes may be essential for establishing central tolerance but not for maturation or export of thymocytes in vivo (135).

Hematopoietic Cell Positioning in Peripheral Tissue

Recent work has begun to clarify chemokine-dependent mechanisms that control homeostatic positioning of leukocytes in peripheral tissues. The gut has been particularly well studied. CCL11 and its receptor CCR3 are important for migration of eosinophils to the gastrointestinal tract (and spleen) (136). CCL20 and its receptor CCR6 regulate positioning of immature myeloid CD11c^{+}CD11b^{+} DC in the subepithelial dome of Peyers patches (137,138), which may explain in part why humoral immune responses within the gut mucosa and defense against enteroinvasive pathogens are abnormal in CCR6$^{-/-}$ mice. CCR6 is also expressed on gut-homing B and T cells, which may become rapidly activated by CCR6^{+} DCs. CX3CR1 also regulates location of myeloid DCs in Peyers patches and may promote dendrite protrusion into the lumen as a method of antigen sampling. Consistent with this, CX3CR1 is important for controlling *Salmonella* infection after oral challenge (139). CCL25/CCR9 signaling regulates gut cryptopatch formation and subsequent positioning of intraepithelial lymphocytes (138).

CHEMOKINE REGULATION OF THE IMMUNE RESPONSE

Innate Immunity

Platelet-Derived Chemokines

Made primarily during platelet development, stored in platelet α granules, and rapidly released during platelet degranulation, CXCL4, CXCL4L1, and CXCL7 may be among the first chemokines to appear at sites of tissue injury and infection, particularly when there is hemorrhage and vascular damage, and may reach high concentrations (140). CXCL4 aggregates to form tetramers that are critical for binding to chondroitinsulfate proteoglycans and to CXCR3B on endothelial cells. In contrast, CXCL7 is activated by sequential proteolysis of its N terminus. The prepropeptide form, named platelet basic protein (92 amino acids [aa]), is trimmed during platelet maturation to produce the 85-aa major stored form, named connective tissue activating peptide-III (CTAP-III), which is inactive on neutrophils. CTAP-III is further processed during degranulation to 81-aa β-thromboglobulin, also inactive. This is then cleaved by a cell surface–bound, cathepsin G–like enzyme on neutrophils to form 70-aa CXCL7, which has high homology to CXCL4 (70% aa identity). Thus CXCL7 may function as an immediate-early mediator of neutrophil recruitment released from platelets at sites of inflammation. Although it is not a prominent leukocyte chemoattractant and does not induce degranulation of neutrophil lysosomal enzymes, CXCL4 is able to induce secondary granule exocytosis and release matrix-degrading enzymes, which may facilitate neutrophil penetration of infected or injured tissues. Both CXCL4 and CXCL4L1, the product of the highly homologous nonallelic variant gene of CXCL4, PF-4var1/PF-4alt, are strong angiostatic factors (141). In contrast, another platelet-derived chemokine, CXCL12, may be a major determinant of revascularization, as suggested by an ischemic hindlimb mouse model, in which its release could be regulated by Kit ligand and thrombopoietin and it functions to recruit CXCR4^{+} VEGFR^{+} hemangiocytes to the site of injury (142). The ultimate response in inflammation and revascularization may depend on the relative concentration and activities of these counterregulatory chemokines.

Neutrophil-Targeted Chemokines

All seven ELR^{+} CXC chemokines preferentially recruit neutrophils in vitro by binding to CXCR2. One of these, CXCL8, is also a potent agonist at CXCR1, which is coexpressed at similar levels on neutrophils (Figure 26.3) (143).

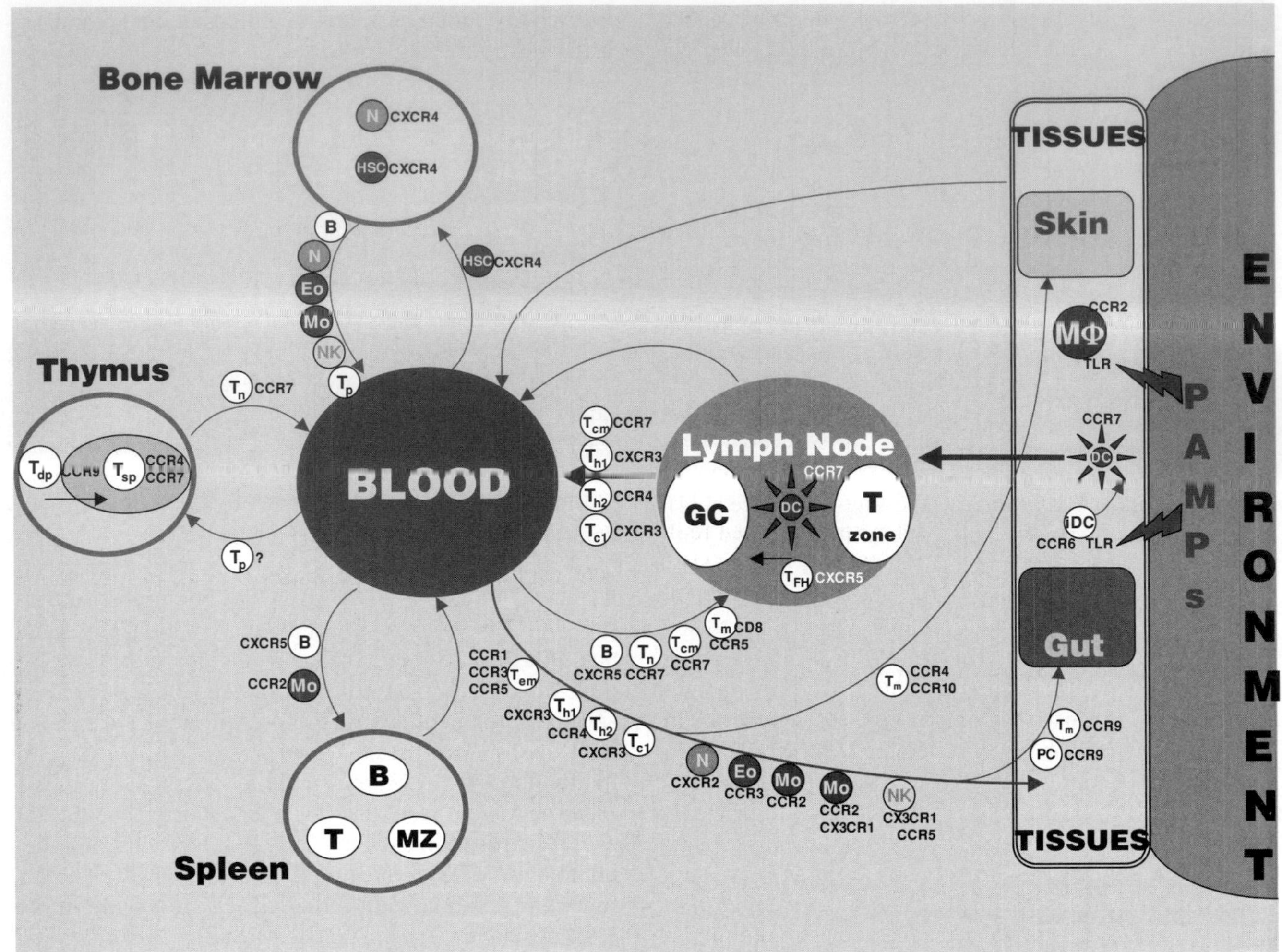

FIGURE 26.3 Chemokine receptor control of leukocyte trafficking. Shown are routes among primary and secondary immune organs and the periphery, leukocyte subtypes trafficking on those routes, and some of the chemokine receptors that appear to be most important in regulating each route. Tn, naïve T cells; Tp, precursor T cells; Tm, memory T cells; Tem, effector memory T cells; Tcm, central memory T cells; T_{FH}, follicular help T cells; iDC, immature dendritic cells; N, neutrophil; Eo, eosinophil; Mϕ, macrophage; Mo, monocyte; NK, natural-killer cell; PC, plasma cell; HSC, hematopoietic stem cell; GC, germinal center; Tdp, double positive T cells; Tsp, single positive T cells; MZ, marginal zone; TLR, Toll-like receptor; PAMP, pathogen-associated molecular patterns. Model is based primarily on studies in knockout mice.

These seven chemokines are rapidly inducible but may differ biologically as a result of temporal and spatial differences in expression, which may provide a mechanism for graded navigation of neutrophils through tissue. Blocking studies in multiple animal models have demonstrated the importance of CXCL8 and CXCR2 in neutrophil accumulation in response to infectious and noninfectious stimuli. The role of CXCR1 in vivo has not yet been defined and is difficult to analyze, because its major human agonist, CXCL8, is not found in the mouse; instead, the sole specific agonist identified for mouse CXCR1 is CXCL6 (GCP-2), which has relatively low potency in chemotactic assays in vitro. In a human blister model, endogenous CXCL8 peaks at ~24 hours, whereas C5a and leukotriene B4, which also recruit neutrophils, appear earlier. Thus the primary role of CXCL8 may be to amplify recruitment of neutrophils initiated by other chemoattractants.

Intradermal injection of CXCL8 in man causes rapid (<30 minutes) and selective accumulation of large numbers of neutrophils in perivascular regions of the skin without causing edema. Tissue-specific transgenic overexpression of the mouse CXCL8 paralogs KC and MIP-2 results in a similar picture, suggesting that in vivo these factors may recruit cells but not independently activate cytotoxic mechanisms. In vitro, the ability of CXC chemokines to activate neutrophil cytotoxic responses is modest. Instead, they may prolong survival of neutrophils in the setting of bacterial infection and paradoxically provide an intracellular niche in which at least some bacterial species such as *Staphylococcus aureus* may persist (144). Studies in mice have revealed that $\alpha\beta$ CD4$^+$ T cells are critical in providing CXC chemokines that foster abscess formation in several models of experimental *S. aureus* infection, and that the absence of these cells results paradoxically in smaller/fewer abscesses with reduced bacterial burden. In addition, pathogens such as *Streptococci* may actively interfere with the action of CXC chemokines by degrading them with specific proteases (145). Thus, although there is no question that neutrophils are critical in defense against bacterial and fungal pathogens and that CXCR2 agonists are critical for neutrophil trafficking in the setting of infectious disease, the ultimate outcome of infection may be determined by a balance between CXCR2-dependent neutrophil recruitment, niche development, and negative regulatory mechanisms.

CXCL1, -2, -3, -7, and -8 have also been reported to induce basophil chemotaxis and histamine release in vitro, which together with other factors such as complement-derived anaphylatoxins may promote vasodilatation during early stages of the innate immune response. CC chemokines can also activate human neutrophils, but this typically requires prestimulation of the cells with IFN-γ and other factors able to induce expression of appropriate receptors. Conversely, late apoptotic neutrophils can actively promote the resolution phase of acute inflammation by terminating chemokine signaling through scavenging by CCR5, which is expressed in a manner that depends on caspases and anti-inflammatory lipid mediators (146).

Monocyte/Macrophage-Targeted Chemokines

Circulating blood monocytes can be divided into two principal subsets with distinct migratory properties based on chemokine receptor expression (147). *Inflammatory* monocytes are short-lived CX3CR1^{low}CCR2$^+$Gr1$^+$ cells that are actively recruited to inflamed tissues in the mouse. These cells correspond to human CD14$^+$CD16$^-$ monocytes, which are CX3CR1^{low}. *Resident* monocytes are long-lived CX3CR1^{high}CCR2$^-$Gr1$^-$ cells in the mouse, characterized by CX3CR1-dependent engraftment and recruitment to noninflamed tissues. These cells correspond to human CD16$^+$ monocytes that are CX3CR1^{high} but do not express inflammatory chemokine receptors. Both subsets can differentiate in vivo into DCs that stimulate naïve T cells. There are numerous examples of the functional importance of these receptors in the monocyte/macrophage lineage in vivo. CX3CR1 is particularly important in microglial cell migration and function in the inflamed central nervous system (148), and has been linked to macular degeneration in aged mice and in human disease. Both receptors play a role in macrophage accumulation in atherosclerotic plaque (149). In a *Listeria* model, CCR2 was shown to be important for release of monocytes from the bone marrow to the circulation, but not for migration of circulating cells to the spleen (150).

Monocytes express additional inflammatory chemokine receptors including CCR1, CCR5, CXCR1, and CXCR2. Differentiation in vitro to macrophages is associated with downregulation of CCR2 and induction of CCR5 and CX3CR1. Polarized M1 and M2 subsets of macrophages have been described in keeping with the Th1/Th2 polarization paradigm for T cells. In this regard, the classic anti-inflammatory Th2 cytokine Il-10 is able to downregulate signaling by inflammatory chemokine receptors on macrophages (24). CCR4, which is a key receptor in Th2-mediated immune responses, has also been reported to play a dominant role in innate immunity in mouse models, including endotoxic shock and bacterial peritonitis, through effects on macrophage differentiation (151).

NK Cell–Targeted Chemokines

Human NK cell subsets express unique repertoires of chemokine receptors (77). The CD56^{dim}CD16$^+$ subset, which is associated with high cytotoxic capacity and low cytokine production, expresses primarily CXCR1 and CX3CR1, whereas the minor subset of CD56^{bright}CD16^{dim} cells, which produce large amounts of cytokines but have low killing capacity, preferentially express CCR7. The exact profile of chemokine receptor expression can be modulated by adherence and stimulation ex vivo with IL-2. Cognate chemokines chemoattract NK cells, and promote degranulation and killing. The importance of chemokines in NK cell function in vivo is well illustrated by mouse cytomegalovirus (MCMV) infection, a cause of hepatitis. MCMV induces CCL3 production in the liver that is required for recruitment of NK cells. NK cells are the major source of IFN-γ in this model, and IFN-γ induces CXCL9, which is required for protection. Thus a cytokine-to-chemokine-to-cytokine cascade is required for NK cell–mediated host defense against this pathogen (152).

Dendritic Cells and Transition to the Adaptive Immune Response

Transition from innate to adaptive phases of the immune response involves antigen uptake by antigen-presenting cells, especially dendritic cells, mediated by Fc and complement phagocytic receptors, as well as pattern-recognition receptors (PRRs), including DC-SIGN and Toll-like receptors (TLRs). Through specific PRR ligands, pathogens may shape the nature and magnitude of the immune response in a specific direction, in part by inducing production of specific sets of chemokines with distinct leukocyte specificities (153).

Chemokine receptor expression and function also depends on the nature of the inflammatory stimulus, but also on the type of DC. For example, blood-derived plasmacytoid and myeloid DCs express a similar repertoire of inflammatory chemoattractant receptors, but they are functional only on myeloid DCs. CCL3, CCL4, and CCL5 may be particularly important for recruiting additional mononuclear phagocytes and DCs to sites of infection. This can amplify the late stage of the innate immune response, and in the extreme may devolve into endotoxic shock. Consistent with this idea, genetic disruption of the CCL3/CCL4/CCL5 receptor CCR5 renders mice relatively resistant to LPS-induced endotoxemia. $CCR4^{-/-}$ mice are also resistant to endotoxic shock, and this is associated with reduced macrophage extravasation to the peritoneum and production of the CCR4 ligand CCL17, which can be produced by DCs (151).

Adaptive Immunity

Afferent Trafficking to Secondary Lymphoid Tissue

The homeostatic receptors CXCR4, CXCR5, and CCR7 and their ligands are major regulators of lymphoid development and the adaptive immune response (21,78,154–158). DC maturation in peripheral tissues is associated with downregulation of inflammatory receptors, which may be important for recruitment, migration, and retention in the periphery, and reciprocal upregulation of CCR7, which mediates mature DC migration via afferent lymphatics to draining lymph nodes in response to CCL21 expressed on lymphatic endothelial cells. Inflammatory receptors may also contribute, as demonstrated for CCR2 on Langerhans cells in a mouse model of *Leishmania* infection (159).

With regard to lymphocytes, CCR7, and to a lesser extent CXCR4, mediate both B- and T-cell entry from blood into lymph node. In lymph node and Peyers patch T zone, CCL21 is produced by HEV endothelial cells, whereas CCL19 (the second CCR7 ligand) and the CXCR4 ligand CXCL12 are produced by adjacent stromal cells. All three chemokines are displayed on the luminal and abluminal sides of the HEV, appropriately positioned to mediate transendothelial migration from the blood of naïve B and T lymphocytes, which both coexpress CCR7 and CXCR4 (160). CCR7 plays a dominant role in mediating B- and T-cell adhesion, but CXCR4 also contributes. $CCR7^{-/-}$ mice and the *plt* mouse, which is naturally deficient in CCL19 and the CCL21 isoform expressed in secondary lymphoid organs, have similar phenotypes: atrophic T-cell zones populated by a paucity of naïve T cells. This, plus the failure of activated DC to migrate to lymph node from the skin of these mice, explains why contact sensitivity, delayed-type hypersensitivity, and antibody production are severely impaired.

CXCR5 is expressed on all peripheral blood and tonsillar B cells, but on only a fraction of bone marrow B cells. Its ligand CXCL13, produced selectively by HEV endothelial cells and follicular stromal cells, is constitutively displayed on follicular HEV. CXCL13/CXCR5 supports ~50% of the signaling required for B-cell entry from blood to Peyers patch, although CXCR4 may also contribute (160,161). In $CXCR5^{-/-}$ mice, B cells do not migrate to lymph nodes, Peyers patches are abnormal, and inguinal lymph nodes are absent. CXCL13 is also required for B1-cell homing, natural antibody production, body cavity immunity, and lymphoneogenesis in the setting of autoimmunity. $CXCR5^{-/-}$ mice still can produce antibody, perhaps in part because B cells and follicular DC, by an unknown mechanism, are able to form ectopic germinal centers within T zones of the periarteriolar lymphocyte sheath of spleen. In Peyers patches, B-cell entry is also dependent on CCR7 and CXCR4.

CXCR5 and CCR7 are probably not the only chemokine receptors responsible for afferent trafficking of leukocytes to lymph node. CCL9 has been reported to mediate monocyte homing. In addition, inflamed peripheral tissues may exert "remote control" for monocyte homing to draining lymph nodes from the blood by "projecting" their local chemokine profile to HEVs of the draining lymph node (162). Migration of T cells to splenic red pulp may involve local production of CXCL16. NK-T cells and activated $CD4^+$ and $CD8^+$ T cells are found in this area and express the CXCL16 receptor CXCR6. CXCL16 is also made by DCs in the T zone, and CXCR6 is also found on intraepithelial lymphocytes. Thus, CXCL16 may function in T cell–DC interactions and in regulating movements of activated T cells in the splenic red pulp, and in peripheral tissues.

Migration within Lymph Node Microenvironments

CXCR5 and CCR7 also appear to be important for lymphocyte movement within the lymphoid microenvironment. So-called follicular helper T cells (T_{FH}), a $CD57^+$ subset, lack CCR7 but express CXCR5, which appears to facilitate migration from the T zone following activation to the follicles in response to CXCL13, where they provide help for B-cell maturation and antibody production. They do not produce Th1 or Th2 cytokines upon activation (163). Reciprocally, B cells activated by antigen in the follicles upregulate CCR7 and move toward the T zone in response to CCL21 (164). Thus B–T interaction may be facilitated by reciprocal movement of these cells, which may be determined in part by the balance of chemokines made in adjacent lymphoid zones.

CXCR4 signaling may also be important in naïve and memory B-cell trafficking to germinal centers. An active chemokine-dependent process has also been identified for $CD4^+$ T-cell–dependent activation of rare antigen-specific naïve $CD8^+$ T cells (94). After immunization in a TCR-transgenic mouse model, but before antigen recognition, naïve $CD8^+$ T cells in immunogen-draining lymph nodes upregulate CCR5, permitting the cells to home to sites of CD4$^+$ T cell–dendritic cell interaction in lymph nodes, where CCL3 and CCL4 are produced. Interference with this process inhibits antigen-specific memory CD8$^+$ T cell generation. There is also evidence that T-cell zone chemokines such as CCL21 are bound to the surface of lymph node DCs in vivo and function to capture and prime naïve T cells for activation by peptide-MHC. Thus T cells are costimulated "in trans" and sequentially after initial engagement with their chemokine-rich environment (165).

Efferent Trafficking

Critical determinants of lymphocyte egress from lymph node are sphingosine 1-phosphate and its receptor S1P (21). Naïve lymphocytes that do not encounter antigen continue to recirculate between the blood and secondary lymphoid tissue without acquiring any tissue-specific homing properties. In contrast, most antigen-stimulated T cells die by apoptosis. The survivors may be divided into functionally distinct subsets that preferentially express certain chemokine receptors. Within the CD4$^+$ subpopulation, three memory subsets and three primary effector subsets have been proposed. The memory subsets include T_{FH} cells, described previously, and effector memory (T_{EM}) and central memory cells (T_{CM}) (166). Memory cells classically express CD45RO. In addition to this, classic T_{CM} cells also express L-selectin (CD62L) and CCR7, which are thought to mediate homing of the cells from blood to secondary lymphoid organs across HEV; these cells are not polarized and lack immediate effector function. Instead, they are thought to interact with DCs in lymph node and differentiate into T_{EM} upon secondary stimulation. T_{EM} cells express L-selectin but lack CCR7, and were originally proposed to differentiate from T_{CM} and to traffic through peripheral tissues as immune surveillance cells, rapidly releasing cytokines in response to activation by recall antigens.

It is increasingly clear that the original T_{CM}/T_{EM} paradigm requires revision, in part because CCR7$^+$ effector memory cells have been detected in inflamed tissues and CCR7 facilitates their exit into lymphatics (167,168). Rather than a dualism with a single precursor–product relationship, analysis of freshly isolated human peripheral blood CD4$^+$ T cells has suggested that memory-cell differentiation may be a continuum with multiple branch points arising probabilistically, giving rise to many subpopulations that preferentially express certain chemokine receptors (169).

Upon activation, the classic polarized effector subsets, Th1 and Th2, downregulate CXCR5 and CCR7 and upregulate inflammatory chemokine receptors (170). This switch facilitates exit from lymph node via efferent lymphatics and homing to inflamed sites. In vivo, Th1 cells, which by the simplest definition secrete IFN-γ but not IL-4 and which control cellular and humoral immunity to intracellular pathogens, more frequently express CXCR3, CXCR6, CCR2, CCR5, and CX3CR1 than Th2 cells. The most highly differentiated CD4$^+$ memory T cells, so-called 'first responders,' express CCR2 and CCR5. In contrast, Th2 cells, which express IL-4 but not IFN-γ, and are associated with cellular and humoral immunity to extracellular pathogens and allergic inflammation, more frequently express CCR3, CCR4, and CCR8 than Th1 cells. CXCR3 expression is dependent on T-bet expression and has been most consistently associated with Th1 immune responses and Th1-associated disease. Consistent with this, its agonists CXCL9-11 are highly induced by IFN-γ but not by IL-4. Thus, in Th1 immunity there is the potential for a positive feedback loop in which IFN-γ induces production of CXCL9-11, which then recruit CXCR3$^+$ Th1 cells that produce IFN-γ. The "Th1 chemokines" may also help maintain Th1 dominance in part through their ability to block CCR3. Specific cytokines, microenvironments, and inflammatory stresses may differentially regulate CXCL9-11 expression, which may account for specialized biologic roles. For example, though all three chemokines are inducible by IFN-γ, CXCL10 and CXCL11 but not CXCL9 are also inducible by type I interferon. There is evidence that Th1 and Th2 cell recruitment into tissue is differentially regulated by Stat1 and Stat6, respectively, and that Stat1 controls recruitment of Th1 cells through the induction of CXCR3 ligands and CXCL16 (171).

Conversely, research on chemokine expression and targets has led to a model of Th2 immunity in which IL-4 and IL-13 made at inflamed sites in the periphery may induce production of CCL7, CCL11 and other CCR3 ligands, the CCR4 ligands CCL17 and CCL22, and the CCR8 ligand CCL1. CCR3 is expressed on a subset of Th2 T lymphocytes as well as on eosinophils and basophils, the three major cell types associated with Th2-type allergic inflammation, and Th2 cells are associated with CCR4 expression. Arrival of Th2 cells amplifies a positive feedback loop through secretion of additional IL-4. Moreover, CCL7 and CCL11 may block Th1 responses by antagonizing CCR2, CXCR3, and CCR5. Many chemokine receptors have been identified on CD4$^+$ regulatory T cells, including CCR4, CCR5, and CCR8. CCR5 has been shown to play an important role in homing of these cells to skin during *Leishmania major* infection, favoring pathogen persistence (172).

Recently, IL-17 producing T cells or Th17 cells, have emerged as an important third subset of CD4$^+$ effector cells, involved in autoimmunity and host defense. All Th17 cells express CCR6 (172a).

T-Cell Differentiation

Some chemokines appear to regulate not just trafficking but also T-cell polarization, at least in certain contexts. CCL2 and its receptor CCR2 have been most extensively studied in this regard, but the results are complex and appear at first glance contradictory because in vivo CCR2 is strongly associated with Th1 immune responses and CCL2 is associated with Th2 responses (173). CCL2 appears to promote Th2 polarization directly, by inhibiting IL-12 production in monocytes, and by enhancing IL-4 but not IFN-γ production in memory and activated T cells. Thus, CCL2 influences both innate immunity, through effects on monocyte trafficking, and adaptive immunity, through control of T-helper cell trafficking and potentially T-cell polarization. In the case of aerosol challenge with *M. tuberculosis* in CCR2$^{-/-}$- mice, DC migration to draining lymph node is markedly impaired, which preempts any direct effects of CCL2 on T cells. Why CCL2 and CCR2 have opposite effects on Th polarization is unclear but is most likely a result of ligand-receptor promiscuity.

Tissue-specific Lymphocyte Homing

CLA^{+} T lymphocytes, which home to skin, preferentially express CCR4 and CCR10. The CCR4 ligand CCL22 is made by resident dermal macrophages and DCs, whereas the CCR10 ligand CCL27 is made by keratinocytes. Blocking both of these pathways, but not either one alone, has been reported to inhibit lymphocyte recruitment to the skin in a DTH model, implying that in this model these two molecules act redundantly and independently of inflammatory chemokines (174).

Homing to small intestine is determined in part by T-lymphocyte expression of the integrin $\alpha_4\beta_7$ and CCR9. The $\alpha_4\beta_7$ ligand MAdCAM-1 and the CCR9 ligand CCL25 colocalize on normal and inflamed small intestinal endothelium, and most T cells in the intraepithelial and lamina propria zones of the small intestine express CCR9. These cells, which are mainly $\gamma\delta$ TCR (+) or CD8$\alpha\beta$(+)$\alpha\beta$TCR(+), are reduced in small intestine from CCR9$^{-/-}$ mice. CCL20 and its receptor CCR6 are also important in gut mucosal immune responses. CCL20 is constitutively expressed in follicle-associated epithelial cells (FAE) overlying GALT-inductive sites (Peyer patches and isolated lymphoid follicles), but can also be induced in GALT under inflammatory conditions. It is important for GALT development and for B and DC homing to GALT. CCR6^{+} DC recruited to the dome region of Peyer patches upon invasion of FAE by an enteric pathogen has been shown to mediate rapid activation of pathogen-specific T cells (175).

As B cells differentiate into plasma cells, they also downregulate CXCR5 and CCR7 and exit the lymph node. B immunoblasts expressing IgG coordinately upregulate CXCR4, which promotes homing to the bone marrow, whereas B immunoblasts expressing IgA migrate specifically to mucosal sites. Like gut-homing T cells, gut homing IgA-secreting B immunoblasts express $\alpha_4\beta_7$ integrin and CCR9 and respond to CCL25. Intestinal dendritic cells may help shape mucosal immunity by generating gut-homing IgA-secreting B cells through the synergistic action of several mediators, including retinoic acid, IL-5, and IL-6 (176–178). The chemokine requirements for trafficking to the colon and other mucosal sites have not been worked out yet.

CHEMOKINES AND DISEASE

There is a vast literature correlating the presence of chemokines with diverse human diseases, but strong evidence that they are actually involved in pathogenesis is available for only a small subset of these (Tables 26.5, 26.6). Many pathogenetic mechanisms have been proposed, including activation of innate immunity, activation of adaptive immunity, and cell trafficking. These mechanisms may cooperate so that, for example, nonspecific activation of innate immunity may markedly enhance susceptibility to destruction of a solid organ by adaptive immune mechanisms (179).

HIV

HIV infection requires fusion of the viral envelope to a target cell membrane, a process that is initiated by direct binding of the HIV envelope glycoprotein gp120 to both CD4 and a coreceptor on the target cell (30,180). Although many chemokine receptors and related GPCRs can function as coreceptors in vitro, CCR5 and CXCR4 appear to be the most relevant on primary cells. Their interaction with CD4 may be constitutive and stabilized by gp120. The usage of these receptors is so important that HIV strains are now functionally classified and named according to their specificity for CXCR4 (X4 strains), CCR5 (R5 strains), or both (R5X4 strains).

The importance of CCR5 in clinical HIV/AIDS was established by the seminal discovery that *CCR5Δ32*, a nonfunctional allele founded more than 5,000 years ago in Caucasians and now present in ~20% of North American Caucasians, is a strong AIDS-restriction factor, protecting homozygotes from initial infection and slowing the rate of progression to AIDS in infected heterozygotes (181). Additional genetic risk factors affecting the rate of HIV disease progression have been identified in the CCR5 signaling system, including SNPs in the promoters for *CCR5* and its ligand *CCL5*, and variation in the gene copy number of the CCR5 ligand CCL3L1, which cumulatively may account for ~9% of the risk of slow progression to AIDS (182–185). Genetic restriction factors have also been identified in some but not all studies for the CXCR4 ligand CXCL12 (*SDF1-3′A*) and the minor HIV coreceptors CCR2 (*CCR2-64I*) and CX3CR1 (*CX3CR1-M280*), but their biologic significance and mechanisms remain undefined. The pattern of genetic variation at *CCR5Δ32* is most consistent with neutral evolution (186). *CCR5Δ32* homozygotes appear healthy, as do unstressed CCR5 knockout mice. Drug development programs by several pharmaceutical companies targeting

TABLE 26.5 Some Phenotypes of Chemokine-Receptor Knockout Mice

	Phenotype		
Receptor	*Infectious Disease*	*Inflammation*	*Development*
CXCR2	*Increased susceptibility to:* *T. gondii* Brain abscess Onchocerca volvulus *E. coli* pyelonephritis	*Reduced:* Wound healing *A. fumigatus* AHR Urate crystal-induced synovitis	Expansion of neutrophils & B cells in blood, marrow, & lymphoid organs (not seen when derived in germ-free environment)
CXCR3	Increased susceptibility to MTb	Delayed cardiac allograft rejection	
CXCR4			Perinatal lethality *Defective:* Ventricular septum Bone marrow myelopoiesis B-cell lymphopoiesis Gastric vascularization Cerebellar granule cell migration
CXCR5			Few Peyer patches, no inguinal LN Defective germinal centers & B-cell homing to LN
CXCR7			Defective cardiac development
CCR1	*Increased susceptibility to:* *T gondii* Pneumonia virus of mice *A. fumigatus*	*Increased:* Th1 response and glomerular injury in nephrotoxic nephritis model Th2 response to SEA *Reduced:* Neutrophilic alveolitis in pancreatitis–ARDS model Airway remodeling and Th2 response in *A. fumigatus* model Th1 response & resistance to EAE Th1 response to PPD Delayed cardiac allograft rejection	NR
CCR2	*Increased susceptibility to:* *C. neoformans* *L. monocytogenes* *L. major* *M. tuberculosis* *Resistance to:* *L. donovani* Influenza A	*Decreased:* EAE DVT resolution Response to PPD Atherosclerosis Cardiac allograft rejection AHR to CRA Dextran sulfate–mediated colitis Thioglycollate-induced peritonitis FITC and bleomycin-induced pulmonary fibrosis MΦ recruited to injured nerve DTH Monocyte extravasation *Increased:* AHR to OVA AHR to *A. fumigatus* Glomerulonephritis in antiglomerular basement membrane antibody model	Enhanced myeloid progenitor cell cycling and apoptosis

(*continued*)

TABLE 26.5 Some Phenotypes of Chemokine-Receptor Knockout Mice (Continued)

	Phenotype		
Receptor	*Infectious Disease*	*Inflammation*	*Development*
		ip OVA sensitization → OVA challenge: Increased AHR & airway mast cells; decreased airway eos, trapped between elastic lamina and endothelial cells	
CCR3		*Epicutaneous OVA sensitization → OVA challenge:* Protection from allergic skin inflammation & AHR. Eos and mast cells not recruited to skin or lung Decreased IL-13–induced pulmonary eosinophilia & remodeling	
CCR4		Increased susceptibility to lps	
CCR5	*Increased susceptibility to:* *L. monocytogenes* *C. neoformans* *T. gondii* Influenza A *L. major* West Nile Virus *Resistance to:* *L. donovani*	Decreased: Dextran sulfate-mediated colitis Lps toxicity Mouse hepatitis virus-induced demyelination due to decreased MΦ recruitment to CNS Cardiac allograft rejection Increased: DTH Humoral response to T-dependent Ag	
CCR6	Impaired humoral immune response to orally administered antigen and to rotavirus	Defective CRA-induced allergic airway inflammation Increased contact hypersensitivity to 2,4-dinitrofluorobenzene Resistance to DTH to allogeneic splenocytes Decreased arthritis	Absent myeloid $CD11b^+$ $CD11c^+$ dendritic-cells in subepithelial dome of Peyer patches Increased T cells in intestinal mucosa
CCR7		Delayed humoral response Defective contact sensitivity Defective DTH Defective renal fibrosis & fibrocyte accumulation in unilateral ureteral obstruction	Defective lymphocyte and DC migration to LN Undeveloped T-cell zones Impaired trafficking of T cells and DC to LN
CCR8		Defective SEA-induced granuloma formation; decreased OVA- and CRA-induced allergic airway inflammation Decreased inflammation in IBD models	
CCR9			Decreased preproB cells, but nl T and B cells Decreased ratio of gut intraepithelial T-cell-to-epithelial cell ratio due to decreased $\gamma\delta$ T cells
CX3CR1	Increased susceptibility to *Salmonella* infection	Resistance to cardiac allograft rejection in cyclosporin A–treated animals	
Duffy		Increased or decreased neutrophil mobilization, depending on the model	
D6		Increased CFA- or TPA-induced psoriasiform dermatitis Reduced EAE	fetal loss

SEA, *Schistosoma mansoni*–soluble egg antigen; OVA, ovalbumin; CRA, cockroach antigen; AHR, airway hyperreactivity; LN, lymph node; DC, dendritic cell; DTH, delayed-type hypersensitivity; NR, not reported.

TABLE 26.6 Chemokine System and Human Disease[a]

WHIM syndrome (warts, hypogammaglobulinemia, infection, myelokathexis) and CXCR4
Plasmodium vivax malaria and Duffy
HIV/AIDS and CCR5
West Nile virus disease and CCR5
Kaposi sarcoma and human herpesvirus 8 vGPCR
Atherosclerotic cardiovascular disease and CX3CR1
Autoimmune heparin-induced thrombocytopenia and CXCL4
Chronic renal allograft rejection and CCR5
Rheumatoid arthritis and CCR5
Eosinophilic esophagitis and CCL26

[a]The list includes diseases for which there is consistent evidence for chemokine regulation of pathogenesis in humans. Chemokines have been implicated in many other human diseases by physical expression in disease sites, or by studies in animal models, but clear and consistent evidence for a functional role in human disease pathogenesis is not yet available, for example, from genetic studies or drug trials.

CCR5 have succeeded in identifying small-molecule antagonists, and Pfizer's Maraviroc has been approved by the FDA for the treatment of HIV/AIDS—the first approved drug targeting the chemokine system. Resistance to CCR5 antagonism has been documented for R5 HIV, but the mechanism involves usage of alternative drug-insensitive domains of CCR5, not conversion to CXCR4 tropism.

CCR5 is also important in the neuropathogenesis of West Nile virus (WNV) infection, in both humans and in a mouse model of disease, but unlike HIV, here it plays a protective role by facilitating antiviral leukocyte trafficking to the brain (187). CCR5-blocking agents could theoretically increase the risk of symptomatic WNV disease in infected patients, particularly in the setting of HIV/AIDS, in which the immune system is already compromised. Pathogenesis in the mouse model of WNV is also regulated by neuronal CXCL10 through recruitment of $CD8^+$ T cells to the brain (188). CXCL10 also controls pathogenesis in a mouse model of the related flavivirus Dengue virus, both by regulating T-cell recruitment through CXCR3 and by competitively inhibiting viral binding to cell-surface heparan sulfate (189).

X4 HIV strains typically do not transmit disease, but instead appear to evolve from R5 quasispecies in a minority of patients late in infection during the transition to clinical disease. Consistent with this, these strains appear more virulent than R5 strains in vitro. The reason is not fully defined, but it is important to note that the percentage of $CD4^+$ T cells expressing CXCR4 greatly exceeds that expressing CCR5. Moreover, the X4 envelope protein expressed on $CD4^+$ T cells has been shown to induce autophagic programmed cell death of uninfected bystander cells by binding to CXCR4 on the cell membrane, signaling in a non–G_i-, non–caspase 3-dependent manner (190). An unresolved question is why X4 strains do not readily transmit disease, given the broad expression of CXCR4 on macrophages and $CD4^+$ T cells.

Malaria

Analagous to CCR5 and HIV, Duffy, the 7TM promiscuous chemokine-binding protein, is required for infection of erythrocytes by *Plasmodium vivax*, a major cause of malaria. The parasite ligand, which is named the *Plasmodium vivax* Duffy-binding protein (PvDBP), is expressed in micronemes of merozoites and binds to the N-terminal domain of Duffy via a cysteine-rich domain (191). This interaction is required for junction formation during invasion, but not for initial binding or parasite orientation. Duffy deficiency, which is due mainly to an inherited single-nucleotide substitution named −46C at an erythroid-specific GATA-1 site in the Duffy promoter, is fixed in sub-Saharan Africa but not in other malaria-endemic regions of the world. Accordingly, *P. vivax* malaria is rare in sub-Saharan Africa but common in Central and South America, India, and Southeast Asia. Fixation of the mutation in Africa presumably occurred because of positive selective pressure from malaria. Together with *CCR5Δ32*, Duffy −46C is the strongest genetic resistance factor known for any infectious disease in humans. Duffy deficiency in humans and knockout mice is not associated with any known health problems under unstressed conditions. Chemokine control of *P. falciparum* malaria is less well studied, although in an intriguing development endothelial cell CX3CL1 was reported to bind parasite-infected erythrocytes in vitro (192), suggesting that the parasite expresses a mimic for the CX3CL1 receptor CX3CR1. Conversely, the G glycoprotein of respiratory syncytial virus has been reported to function as a CX3CL1 mimic, binding to CX3CR1 to induce chemotaxis and possibly promote viral entry (193), and human cytomegalovirus encodes US28, a chemokine receptor that is able to bind CX3CL1, possibly to mediate viral attachment to target cells. Together, these examples show the rich dialogue between hosts and pathogens using the chemokine system as a preferred method of communication.

Kaposi's Sarcoma

A full discussion of the many virally encoded chemokines and chemokine receptors is beyond the scope of this chapter (Table 26.7) but can be found in recent reviews (26,27). HHV8 ORF74 deserves special mention, however (194). HHV8 encodes three CC chemokines, vMIP-I, -II, and -III, as well as a constitutively active CC/CXC chemokine receptor named vGPCR, encoded by ORF74. All of these factors are angiogenic and may contribute to the pathogenesis of Kaposis sarcoma (KS), a highly vascular, multicentric, nonclonal tumor caused by HHV8, typically in a setting of immunosuppression such as in HIV/AIDS. Consistent

TABLE 26.7 The Viral Chemokine System[a]

Structural classification
Chemokines (e.g., HHV8 vMIP-I, -II, and -III; Molluscum contagiosum virus MC148-R)
7TM chemokine receptors: ligand-regulated and/or constitutively active (e.g., HCMV US28, HHV8 vGPCR)
Unique structure
Chemokine-binding proteins (e.g., γHV68 vCKBP-III)
Chemokine mimics (e.g., HIV gp120)
Functional classification
Cell entry factors (e.g., HIV gp120)
Leukocyte chemoattractants (e.g., HHV8 vMIP-II)
Immune evasion
Chemokine scavengers (e.g., γHV68 vCKBP-III)
Chemokine-receptor antagonists (e.g., Molluscum contagiosum virus MC148-R)
Angiogenic factors (e.g., HHV8 vGPCR)
Growth factors (e.g., HHV8 vGPCR)

[a]The role of chemokines in immunoregulation may be revealed by studying the viral chemokine system. Viral chemokine elements may also have applications as therapeutic agents.

with this, vGPCR induces KS-like tumors when expressed constitutively or inducibly in transgenic mice on endothelial cells. The mechanism may involve signaling through diverse pathways, including the nonconventional G protein Gq, and phosphorylation of tuberin, which promotes activation of mTOR, a rapamycin-sensitive target, through direct and paracrine mechanisms (195). The latter may include activation of NFκB and induction of angiogenic factors such as VEGF and proinflammatory chemokines and cytokines. Thus, this virus appears to have converted a hijacked receptor, probably CXCR2, into a regulator of gene expression. The model identifies rapamycin as a candidate therapeutic in Kaposi's sarcoma.

Atherosclerosis

There is now compelling genetic evidence from knockout mice and human disease cohorts that CX3CR1 is a significant proatherogenic factor. The mechanism remains unclear but may involve induction of CX3CL1 on vascular smooth muscle cells, and recruitment and retention of CX3CR1-positive monocytes to plaque through the dual chemotactic and adhesive functions of this ligand–receptor pair (196). The evidence in humans is based in part on consistent association of a defective receptor variant named CX3CR1 M280, with reduced risk of cardiovascular disease endpoints in multiple cohort studies (197). There is also extensive evidence in mouse models for a proatherogenic role for CCL2 and its receptor CCR2 (5).

Adoptive transfer studies of bone marrow from knockout mice have also revealed a role for CCR5 and CXCR2 in mouse models of atherosclerosis. CXCR2 may work by promoting monocyte adhesion to early atherosclerotic endothelium, through interaction with its mouse ligand KC and activation of the VLA-4/VCAM-1 adhesion system (198). Immunoneutralization experiments have revealed a role for CCR7 on foam cells in a mouse model of atheroregression (199). Surprisingly, CCR1 and CXCL16 deficiency appeared to increase inflammation in atherosclerosis models (200). CXCL10 has also been implicated in atherogenesis in a mouse model, possibly acting by recruitment of CXCR3^{+} Th1 cells. Lack of CXCL10 was also associated with a relative increase of regulatory T cells in plaque (201). Additional work will be needed to integrate these findings into a mechanistic model of how chemokines regulate atherosclerosis.

Autoimmunity

Two human diseases have been identified in which chemokines act as autoantigens for autoantibodies. The first, heparin-induced thrombocytopenia (HIT), is the only human autoimmune disease directly linked mechanistically to chemokines (202). An established risk factor for thromboembolic complications of heparin therapy, HIT occurs in 1% to 5% of patients treated with heparin and is the result of autoantibodies that bind specifically to CXCL4/heparin complexes in plasma. The second, autoimmune myositis, is associated with autoantibodies to histidyl tRNA synthetase, a protein synthesis factor that is also able to induce DC chemotaxis, apparently by acting as an agonist at CCR5 (64). Its exact importance in promoting inflammation in myositis has not been established. Several other autoantigens have also been shown to activate chemokine receptors in vitro.

In general, T-cell–dependent autoimmune diseases in humans such as psoriasis, multiple sclerosis (MS), rheumatoid arthritis (RA), and type 1 diabetes mellitus are associated with inflammatory chemokines and tissue infiltration by T lymphocytes and monocytes expressing inflammatory chemokine receptors. Rheumatoid arthritis has been consistently negatively associated with homozygous *CCR5Δ32*, suggesting that CCR5 is important in pathogenesis in humans (203). Consistent with this, Met-RANTES, a chemically modified variant of CCL5 that blocks CCR1, CCR3, and CCR5, was beneficial in a collagen-induced arthritis model in DBA/I mice.

Numerous chemokine receptors affect immunopathogenesis in mouse experimental allergic encephalomyelitis (EAE), a model of MS. In most cases, for example, CCL2, CCL3, and CCR2, gene disruption results in attenuation of disease. Neutralization of CCL3 and CCL2 with MAbs markedly reduced the early and relapsing phases of EAE, respectively. In contrast, CX3CR1$^{-/-}$ mice have increased mortality, nonremitting spastic paraplegia, and hemorrhagic inflammatory lesions in EAE. The phenotype is associated with a selective defect in migration of NK cells, which strongly express this receptor, to the central nervous system, suggesting that NK cells are negative immunoregulators in this context (204). Mice that lack D6, the chemokine scavenger, have decreased severity of EAE, because of decreased T-cell infiltration, which is opposite to prediction for a negative regulator, and opposite to what was observed for D6 knockouts in a psoriasis model (205). *CCR5Δ32* homozygotes have been reported who have MS, indicating that this receptor is not required for disease.

Paradoxically, in some cases, blocking chemokine receptors may lead to increased inflammation, as has been shown for CCR1 and CCR2 in nephrotoxic nephritis and glomerulonephritis mouse models. This is associated with increased renal recruitment of $CD4^+$ and $CD8^+$ T cells and macrophages and enhanced Th1 immune responses; however, the exact mechanism is not defined.

Acute Neutrophil-mediated Inflammatory Disorders

Many neutrophil-mediated human diseases have been associated with the presence of CXCL8, including psoriasis, gout, acute glomerulonephritis, acute respiratory distress syndrome (ARDS), rheumatoid arthritis, and ischemia-reperfusion injury. Systemic administration of neutralizing anti-CXCL8 antibodies is protective in diverse models of neutrophil-mediated acute inflammation in the rabbit (skin, airway, pleura, glomeruli), providing proof-of-concept that CXCL8 is a nonredundant mediator of innate immunity and acute pathologic inflammation in these settings. Moreover, CXCR2 knockout mice are less susceptible to acute urate crystal-induced gouty synovitis, and SB-265610, a nonpeptide small-molecule antagonist with exquisite selectivity for CXCR2, prevents neutrophil accumulation in the lungs of hyperoxia-exposed newborn rats. Together the results identify CXCL8 and its receptors as candidate drug targets for diseases mediated by acute neutrophilic inflammation. CXCR2 knockout mice also have delayed wound healing.

Transplant Rejection

An advantage of transplant rejection over other animal models of human disease is that in both the human and animal situations, the time of antigenic challenge is known precisely. The most extensive analysis of the role of chemokines in transplant rejection has been carried out in an MHC class I/II-mismatched cardiac allograft rejection model in the mouse, which is mediated by a Th1 immune response (206). Similar sets of inflammatory chemokines are found in the mouse model as in the human disease. ELR^+ CXC chemokines and CCL2 appear early, and are probably made by engrafted blood vessel endothelial cells. These are associated with neutrophil and mononuclear cell accumulation. On day 3 after engraftment, CCL2 is still present, and the three CXCR3 ligands CXCL9–11 and the CCR5 ligands CCL4 and CCL5 appear. Of the CXCR3 ligands, CXCL10 appears earliest and in largest amounts, probably in response to IFN-γ coming from NK cells. This phase is associated with transition to an adaptive immune response with accumulation of trafficking of recipient T cells, macrophages, and DCs to the graft, followed by acute and chronic rejection. Graft arteriosclerosis, which is distinct from the lipid-driven disease, may be driven in part by CXCL10 and IFN-γ. Analysis of knockout mice has demonstrated that while multiple chemokine receptors contribute to rejection in this model, there is a marked rank order: CXCR3 >> CCR5 > CCR1 = CX3CR1 = CCR2. Most impressively, rejection and graft arteriosclerosis do not occur if the recipient mouse, treated with a brief, subtherapeutic course of cyclosporin A, is $CXCR3^{-/-}$ or if the donor heart is $CXCL10^{-/-}$, identifying this axis as a potential drug target. Neutralization of CXCL9, a CXCR3 ligand that appears later than CXCL10, can also prolong cardiac allograft survival, and delay T-cell infiltration and acute rejection in class II MHC–disparate skin allografts. In rats, BX-471, a nonpeptide small-molecule antagonist of CCR1, was reported to be effective in heart transplant rejection. In humans, CCR5 may be important in chronic kidney allograft rejection, because individuals who are homozygous for *CCR5Δ32* are underrepresented among patients with this outcome in a large German kidney transplantation cohort (207).

Allergic Airway Disease

Chemokine receptors associated with asthma include CXCR2, CXCR4, CCR3, CCR4, and CCR8. CCR3 is present on eosinophils, basophils, mast cells, and some Th2 T cells, and CCR4 and CCR8 identify airway T cells of allergen-challenged atopic asthmatics. CCR8 knockout mice have reduced allergic airway inflammation in response to three different Th2-polarizing antigens: *Schistosoma mansoni* soluble egg antigen, ovalbumin, and cockroach antigen (208). The situation with the CCR4 axis is unsettled, because neutralization of the CCR4 ligand CCL22 was protective in a mouse model of airway hyperreactivity and eosinophilic inflammation, but CCR4 gene knockout was not. Because CCR4 is expressed on both Th2 effector cells and $CD4^+CD25^{high}Foxp3^+$ regulatory T cells, the relative functionality of other chemokine receptors on these cells would be expected to determine the overall effect of blocking CCR4 on allergic disease. A role for the CCR3 axis in asthma has been supported by CCL11 neutralization in guinea pig, and CCR3 gene knockout in mouse. Only one of three studies of CCL11 knockout mice found protection, ~40% reduction in airway eosinophils in ovalbumin-sensitized/challenged mice, possibly as a result of compensation by other CCR3 ligands. The net effect of CCR3 knockout was expected to be more profound, but the exact phenotype depends dramatically on the specific method of sensitization and challenge, because of complex and opposite effects on eosinophil and mast cell trafficking. Thus CCR3$^{-/-}$ mice sensitized IP have reduced eosinophil extravasation into the lung but an increase in mast cell homing to the trachea, with the net result being a paradoxical increase in airway responsiveness to cholinergic stimulation. Mast cell mobilization is not seen after epicutaneous sensitization, and these animals therefore have reduced airway eosinophilia on challenge and no increase in airway hyperresponsiveness (209,210). CCR3 and its ligands have also been clearly shown to play a critical role in an *Aspergillus*-induced chronic allergic airway disease mouse model, in part because of failure of eosinophils to traffic to the lung (211). CCR6 also appears to play a role, because CCR6$^{-/-}$ mice have decreased allergic airway inflammation in response to sensitization and challenge with cockroach antigen, which is consistent with the induction of its ligand CCL20 in this model. CXCL12/CXCR4 may be more than a homeostatic regulator, because neutralization of either ligand or receptor resulted in decreased lung eosinophilia and airway hyperreactivity in a mouse model of allergic airway disease (212).

Cancer

Many chemokines have been detected in situ in tumors, and cancer cells have been shown to produce chemokines and express chemokine receptors (34). However, the exact role played by endogenous tumor-associated chemokines in recruiting tumor-infiltrating lymphocytes and tumor-associated macrophages and in promoting an antitumor immune response has not been delineated. On the contrary, there are data from mouse models suggesting that the overall effect may be to promote tumorigenesis through additional effects on cell growth, angiogenesis, apoptosis, immune evasion, and metastasis (213). Controlling the balance of angiogenic and angiostatic chemokines may be particularly important (214). This has been shown in several instances, including human non-small-cell lung carcinoma (NSCLC), in which the ratio of ELR to non-ELR CXC chemokine expression is high, and where in a Scid mouse model neutralization of endogenous tumor-derived CXCL8 (angiogenic) could inhibit tumor growth and metastasis by about 50% through a decrease in tumor-derived vessel density, without directly affecting tumor-cell proliferation. Chemokine receptors on tumor cells have been shown to mediate chemokine-dependent proliferation directly, for example in the case of CXCL1 in melanoma, and metastasis, in the case of CXCR4 in a mouse model of breast cancer and glioblastoma. Moreover, chemokines may function in cancer by reprogramming cancer-associated stromal fibroblasts to a senescent pro-tumorigenic state, as shown recently in ovarian cancer for CXCL1 (215). It remains to be seen how general these effects are in other cancers.

THERAPEUTIC APPLICATIONS

Chemokines and Chemokine Receptors as Targets for Drug Development

Although chemokine-targeted drug development is still in the early stages and there are no approved drugs, there are already two accomplishments that deserve special mention: first, chemokine receptors are the first cytokine receptors for which potent, selective nonpeptide small-molecule antagonists have been identified that work in vivo, and second, targeting host determinants, as in the case of CCR5 and CXCR4 in HIV/AIDS, is a new approach in the development of antimicrobial agents. Other reasonable disease indications are Duffy in *P. vivax* malaria; CXCR2 in neutrophil-mediated inflammation such as chronic obstructive pulmonary disease; CXCR3 and CCR2 in Th1-driven disease; CCR2 and CX3CR1 in atherosclerosis; CCR3 and possibly CCR4 and CCR8 in Th2 diseases such as asthma; and CCR9 in inflammatory bowel disease.

As of early 2007, potent and selective nonpeptide small-molecule antagonists had been discovered for CXCR1-4 and CCR1-5, reported in ~250 patent applications, and tested in nine clinical trials (37). A nitrogen-rich core is a common structural feature for many of these molecules, which typically block ligand binding by acting at a conserved allosteric site analogous to the retinal-binding site in the transmembrane region of rhodopsin.

To date, Maraviroc is the only FDA-approved drug targeting the chemokine system, blocking CCCR5 in HIV/AIDS. AMD 3100 targeting CXCR4 has been shown to be as effective as GCSF in Phase 3 clinical trials for hematopoietic stem cell mobilization. Although small molecules taken as pills are the main goal, other blocking strategies are being actively pursued, including ribozymes, modified chemokines (e.g., amino-terminally modified versions of CCL5) and intrakines, which are modified forms of chemokines delivered by gene therapy that remain in the endoplasmic reticulum and block surface expression of newly synthesized receptors. Strategies to block chemokine/GAG binding are also under investigation (216).

Success in therapeutically targeting the chemokine system must overcome numerous potential and actual obstacles, including chemokine redundancy, the inability to treat in advance of most clinical illnesses, and the unreliability of many preclinical disease models.

Chemokines as Biologic Response Modifiers

Both inflammatory and homeostatic chemokines are being evaluated for therapeutic potential as biologic response modifiers, acting mainly as immunomodulators or as regulators of angiogenesis. Studies to date have not revealed major problems with toxicity, and efficacy has been observed in animal models of cancer, inflammation, and infection. To date, clinical trials in cancer and stem-cell protection have been disappointing. Chemokines are also being developed as vaccine adjuvants, delivered either as pure protein, as immunomodulatory plasmid, or as recombinant protein within antigen-pulsed DC. Chemokine gene administration has also been shown to induce neutralizing antibody against the encoded chemokine, and has successfully blocked immune responses and improved EAE and arthritis scores in rodent models.

Many chemokines, when delivered pharmacologically as recombinant proteins or by plasmid DNA or in transfected tumor cells, are able to induce immunologically mediated antitumor effects in mouse models and could be clinically useful. Mechanisms may differ depending on the model but may involve recruitment of monocytes, NK cells, and $CD8^+$ cytotoxic T cells to tumor. Chemokines may also function as adjuvants in tumor antigen vaccines. Chemokine–tumor antigen fusion proteins represent a novel twist on this approach that facilitate uptake of tumor antigens by APCs via the normal process of ligand-receptor internalization. Non-ELR CXC chemokines such as CXCL4 also exert antitumor effects through angiostatic mechanisms. Despite impressive antitumor effects in animal models, translating chemokines to patient therapy remains a major challenge.

CONCLUSION

The immune system, unlike all others, is a system in motion, and the study of chemokines has provided major new insights into how order is maintained as cells enter a tissue, traffic to a target, and in some cases leave and recirculate. In addition, chemokines are increasingly appreciated as multifunctional cytokines, playing large roles in some cases such as CXCL12 in development, and perhaps smaller or less well-appreciated ones in immune-activation processes. Most impressive is the degree to which pathogens and cancer cells have co-opted the chemokine system for harmful purposes. A major challenge for future research will be to attempt to target this misuse therapeutically, and great progress has been made in HIV toward this end.

ACKNOWLEDGMENTS

This review was supported with funding from the Division of Intramural Research, National Institute of Allergy and Infectious Disease.

REFERENCES

1. Lau EK, Allen S, Hsu AR, et al. Chemokine-receptor interactions: GPCRs, glycosaminoglycans and viral chemokine binding proteins. *Adv Protein Chem.* 2004;68:351–391.
2. Mantovani A. The chemokine system: redundancy for robust outputs. *Immunol Today.* 1999;20(6):254–257.
3. Luster AD. The role of chemokines in linking innate and adaptive immunity. *Curr Opin Immunol.* 2002;14(1):129–135.
4. Rollins BJ. Chemokines. *Blood.* 1997;90(3):909–928.
5. Charo IF, Ransohoff RM. The many roles of chemokines and chemokine receptors in inflammation. *N Engl J Med.* 2006;354(6):610–621.
6. Baggiolini M. Introduction to chemokines and chemokine antagonists. *Ernst Schering Res Found Workshop.* 2004(45):1–9.
7. Murphy PM, Baggiolini M, Charo IF, et al. International union of pharmacology. XXII. Nomenclature for chemokine receptors. *Pharmacol Rev.* 2000;52(1):145–176.
8. Oppenheim JJ, Zachariae CO, Mukaida N, et al. Properties of the novel proinflammatory supergene "intercrine" cytokine family. *Annu Rev Immunol.* 1991;9:617–648.
9. Premack BA, Schall TJ. Chemokine receptors: gateways to inflammation and infection. *Nat Med.* 1996;2(11):1174–1178.
10. Schall TJ. Biology of the RANTES/SIS cytokine family. *Cytokine.* 1991;3(3):165–183.
11. Baggiolini M, Dewald B, Moser B. Human chemokines: an update. *Annu Rev Immunol.* 1997;15:675–705.
12. Baggiolini M, Walz A, Kunkel SL. Neutrophil-activating peptide-1/interleukin 8, a novel cytokine that activates neutrophils. *J Clin Invest.* 1989;84(4):1045–1049.
13. Campbell DJ, Kim CH, Butcher EC. Chemokines in the systemic organization of immunity. *Immunol Rev.* 2003;195:58–71.
14. Yoshie O, Imai T, Nomiyama H. Chemokines in immunity. *Adv Immunol.* 2001;78:57–110.
15. Wolpe SD, Cerami A. Macrophage inflammatory proteins 1 and 2: members of a novel superfamily of cytokines. *FASEB J.* 1989;3(14):2565–2673.
16. Murphy PM. The molecular biology of leukocyte chemoattractant receptors. *Annu Rev Immunol.* 1994;12:593–633.
17. Murphy PM. International Union of Pharmacology. XXX. Update on chemokine receptor nomenclature. *Pharmacol Rev.* 2002;54(2):227–229.
18. Muller G, Hopken UE, Lipp M. The impact of CCR7 and CXCR5 on lymphoid organ development and systemic immunity. *Immunol Rev.* 2003;195:117–135.
19. Butcher EC, Picker LJ. Lymphocyte homing and homeostasis. *Science.* 1996;272(5258):60–66.
20. Laudanna C, Alon R. Right on the spot. Chemokine triggering of integrin-mediated arrest of rolling leukocytes. *Thromb Haemost.* 2006;95(1):5–11.
21. Cyster JG. Chemokines, sphingosine-1-phosphate, and cell migration in secondary lymphoid organs. *Annu Rev Immunol.* 2005;23:127–159.
22. Rot A, von Andrian UH. Chemokines in innate and adaptive host defense: basic chemokinese grammar for immune cells. *Annu Rev Immunol.* 2004;22:891–928.
23. Molon B, Gri G, Bettella M, et al. T cell costimulation by chemokine receptors. *Nat Immunol.* 2005;6(5):465–471.
24. Mantovani A, Sica A, Sozzani S, et al. The chemokine system in diverse forms of macrophage activation and polarization. *Trends Immunol.* 2004;25(12):677–686.
25. Bromley SK, Burack WR, Johnson KG, et al. The immunological synapse. *Annu Rev Immunol.* 2001;19:375–396.
26. Alcami A. Viral mimicry of cytokines, chemokines and their receptors. *Nat Rev Immunol.* 2003;3(1):36–50.
27. Murphy PM. Viral exploitation and subversion of the immune system through chemokine mimicry. *Nat Immunol.* 2001;2(2):116–122.
28. Lalani AS, McFadden G. Evasion and exploitation of chemokines by viruses. *Cytokine Growth Factor Rev.* 1999;10(3–4):219–233.
29. Berger EA, Murphy PM, Farber JM. Chemokine receptors as HIV-1 coreceptors: roles in viral entry, tropism, and disease. *Annu Rev Immunol.* 1999;17:657–700.
30. Lusso P. HIV and the chemokine system: 10 years later. *EMBO J.* 2006;25(3):447–456.
31. Raz E. Guidance of primordial germ cell migration. *Curr Opin Cell Biol.* 2004;16(2):169–173.

32. Murdoch C. CXCR4: chemokine receptor extraordinaire. *Immunol Rev.* 2000;177:175–184.
33. Strieter RM, Burdick MD, Gomperts BN, et al. CXC chemokines in angiogenesis. *Cytokine Growth Factor Rev.* 2005;16(6):593–609.
34. Balkwill F. Cancer and the chemokine network. *Nat Rev Cancer.* 2004;4(7):540–550.
35. Homey B, Muller A, Zlotnik A. Chemokines: agents for the immunotherapy of cancer? *Nat Rev Immunol.* 2002;2(3):175–184.
36. Zlotnik A. Chemokines and cancer. *Int J Cancer.* 2006;119(9):2026–2029.
37. Wells TN, Power CA, Shaw JP, et al. Chemokine blockers—therapeutics in the making? *Trends Pharmacol Sci.* 2006;27(1):41–47.
38. Ribeiro S, Horuk R. The clinical potential of chemokine receptor antagonists. *Pharmacol Ther.* 2005;107(1):44–58.
39. Kwak LW. Translational development of active immunotherapy for hematologic malignancies. *Int J Hematol.* 2002;76(suppl)1:320–321.
40. Scheerlinck JY. Genetic adjuvants for DNA vaccines. *Vaccine.* 2001;19(17–19):2647–2656.
41. Clore GM, Gronenborn AM. Three-dimensional structures of alpha and beta chemokines. *FASEB J.* 1995;9(1):57–62.
42. Zlotnik A, Yoshie O. Chemokines: a new classification system and their role in immunity. *Immunity*. 2000;12(2):121–127.
43. Clark-Lewis I, Kim KS, Rajarathnam K, et al. Structure-activity relationships of chemokines. *J Leuk Biol.* 1995;57(5):703–711.
44. Salcedo R, Oppenheim JJ. Role of chemokines in angiogenesis: CXCL12/SDF-1 and CXCR4 interaction, a key regulator of endothelial cell responses. *Microcirculation*. 2003;10(3–4):359–370.
45. Belperio JA, Keane MP, Arenberg DA, et al. CXC chemokines in angiogenesis. *J Leuk Biol.* 2000;68(1):1–8.
46. Van Coillie E, Van Damme J, Opdenakker G. The MCP/eotaxin subfamily of CC chemokines. *Cytokine Growth Factor Rev.* 1999;10(1):61–86.
47. Matloubian M, David A, Engel S, et al. A transmembrane CXC chemokine is a ligand for HIV-coreceptor Bonzo. *Nat Immunol.* 2000;1(4):298–304.
48. Bazan JF, Bacon KB, Hardiman G, et al. A new class of membrane-bound chemokine with a CX3C motif. *Nature.* 1997;385(6617):640–644.
49. Pisabarro MT, Leung B, Kwong M, et al. Cutting edge: novel human dendritic cell- and monocyte-attracting chemokine-like protein identified by fold recognition methods. *J Immunol.* 2006;176(4):2069–2073.
50. Handel TM, Johnson Z, Crown SE, et al. Regulation of protein function by glycosaminoglycans—as exemplified by chemokines. *Annu Rev Biochem.* 2005;74:385–410.
51. Dudek AZ, Nesmelova I, Mayo K, et al. Platelet factor 4 promotes adhesion of hematopoietic progenitor cells and binds IL-8: novel mechanisms for modulation of hematopoiesis. *Blood.* 2003;101(12):4687–4694.
52. Nesmelova IV, Sham Y, Dudek AZ, et al. Platelet factor 4 and interleukin-8 CXC chemokine heterodimer formation modulates function at the quaternary structural level. *J Biol Chem.* 2005;280(6):4948–4958.
53. Crown SE, Yu Y, Sweeney MD, et al. Heterodimerization of CCR2 chemokines and regulation by glycosaminoglycan binding. *J Biol Chem.* 2006;281(35):25438–25446.
54. Guan E, Wang J, Norcross MA. Identification of human macrophage inflammatory proteins 1alpha and 1beta as a native secreted heterodimer. *J Biol Chem.* 2001;276(15):12404–12409.
55. Weber C, Koenen RR. Fine-tuning leukocyte responses: towards a chemokine "interactome." *Trends Immunol.* 2006;27(6):268–273.
56. Zlotnik A, Yoshie O, Nomiyama H. The chemokine and chemokine receptor superfamilies and their molecular evolution. *Genome Biol.* 2006;7(12):243.
57. Mellado M, Rodriguez-Frade JM, Manes S, et al. Chemokine signaling and functional responses: the role of receptor dimerization and TK pathway activation. *Annu Rev Immunol.* 2001;19:397–421.
58. Springael JY, Urizar E, Parmentier M. Dimerization of chemokine receptors and its functional consequences. *Cytokine Growth Factor Rev.* 2005;16(6):611–623.
59. Babcock GJ, Farzan M, Sodroski J. Ligand-independent dimerization of CXCR4, a principal HIV-1 coreceptor. *J Biol Chem.* 2003;278(5):3378–3385.
60. Locati M, Torre YM, Galliera E, et al. Silent chemoattractant receptors: D6 as a decoy and scavenger receptor for inflammatory CC chemokines. *Cytokine Growth Factor Rev.* 2005;16(6):679–686.
61. Nibbs R, Graham G, Rot A. Chemokines on the move: control by the chemokine "interceptors" Duffy blood group antigen and D6. *Semin Immunol.* 2003;15(5):287–294.
62. Smith P, Fallon RE, Mangan NE, et al. Schistosoma mansoni secretes a chemokine binding protein with antiinflammatory activity. *J Exp Med.* 2005;202(10):1319–1325.
63. Gosling J, Dairaghi DJ, Wang Y, et al. Cutting edge: identification of a novel chemokine receptor that binds dendritic cell- and T cell-active chemokines including ELC, SLC, and TECK. *J Immunol.* 2000;164(6):2851–2856.
64. Howard OZ. Autoantigen signalling through chemokine receptors. *Curr Opin Rheumatol.* 2006;18(6):642–646.
65. Yang D, Chertov O, Oppenheim JJ. The role of mammalian antimicrobial peptides and proteins in awakening of innate host defenses and adaptive immunity. *Cell Mol Life Sci.* 2001;58(7):978–989.
66. Wang Y, Zhang Y, Yang X, et al. Chemokine-like factor 1 is a functional ligand for CC chemokine receptor 4 (CCR4). *Life Sci.* 2006;78(6):614–621.
67. Bandyopadhyay S, Zhan R, Chaudhuri A, et al. Interaction of KAI1 on tumor cells with DARC on vascular endothelium leads to metastasis suppression. *Nat Med.* 2006;12(8):933–938.
68. Floto RA, MacAry PA, Boname JM, et al. Dendritic cell stimulation by mycobacterial Hsp70 is mediated through CCR5. *Science.* 2006;314(5798):454–458.
69. Shimaoka T, Nakayama T, Hieshima K, et al. Chemokines generally exhibit scavenger receptor activity through their receptor-binding domain. *J Biol Chem.* 2004;279(26):26807–26810.
70. Gursel M, Gursel I, Mostowski HS, et al. CXCL16 influences the nature and specificity of CpG-induced immune activation. *J Immunol.* 2006;177(3):1575–1580.
71. Shimaoka T, Nakayama T, Kume N, et al. Cutting edge: SR-PSOX/CXC chemokine ligand 16 mediates bacterial phagocytosis by APCs through its chemokine domain. *J Immunol.* 2003;171(4):1647–1651.
72. Elagoz A, Henderson D, Babu PS, et al. A truncated form of CKbeta8-1 is a potent agonist for human formyl peptide-receptor-like 1 receptor. *Br J Pharmacol.* 2004;141(1):37–46.
73. Weathington NM, van Houwelingen AH, Noerager BD, et al. A novel peptide CXCR ligand derived from extracellular matrix degradation during airway inflammation. *Nat Med.* 2006;12(3):317–323.
74. Xiao H, Neuveut C, Tiffany HL, et al. Selective CXCR4 antagonism by Tat: implications for in vivo expansion of coreceptor use by HIV-1. *Proc Natl Acad Sci U S A.* 2000;97(21):11466–11471.
75. Allavena P, Sica A, Vecchi A, et al. The chemokine receptor switch paradigm and dendritic cell migration: its significance in tumor tissues. *Immunol Rev.* 2000;177:141–149.
76. Mantovani A, Allavena P, Vecchi A, et al. Chemokines and chemokine receptors during activation and deactivation of monocytes and dendritic cells and in amplification of Th1 versus Th2 responses. *Int J Clin Lab Res.* 1998;28(2):77–82.
77. Berahovich RD, Lai NL, Wei Z, et al. Evidence for NK cell subsets based on chemokine receptor expression. *J Immunol.* 2006;177(11):7833–7840.
78. Sallusto F, Mackay CR. Chemoattractants and their receptors in homeostasis and inflammation. *Curr Opin Immunol.* 2004;16(6):724–731.
79. DeVries ME, Kelvin AA, Xu L, et al. Defining the origins and evolution of the chemokine/chemokine receptor system. *J Immunol.* 2006;176(1):401–415.
80. Kaiser P, Poh TY, Rothwell L, et al. A genomic analysis of chicken cytokines and chemokines. *J Interferon Cytokine Res.* 2005;25(8):467–484.
81. Nagasawa T, Tachibana K, Kishimoto T. A novel CXC chemokine PBSF/SDF-1 and its receptor CXCR4: their functions in

development, hematopoiesis and HIV infection. *Semin Immunol.* 1998;10(3):179–185.

82. Meuter S, Schaerli P, Roos RS, et al. Murine CXCL14 is dispensable for dendritic cell function and localization within peripheral tissues. *Mol Cell Biol.* 2007;27(3):983–992.
83. Lazzeri E, Romagnani P. CXCR3-binding chemokines: novel multifunctional therapeutic targets. *Curr Drug Targets Immune Endocr Metabol Disord.* 2005;5(1):109–118.
84. Ioannidis JPA, Rosenberg PS, Goedert JJ, et al. Effects of CCR5-Delta 32, CCR2-641, and SDF-1 3′ A alleles on HIV-1 disease progression: an international meta-analysis of individual-patient data. *Ann Intern Med.* 2001;135(9):782–795.
85. O'Brien SJ, Moore JP. The effect of genetic variation in chemokines and their receptors on HIV transmission and progression to AIDS. *Immunol Rev.* 2000;177:99–111.
86. Proudfoot AE, Handel TM, Johnson Z, et al. Glycosaminoglycan binding and oligomerization are essential for the in vivo activity of certain chemokines. *Proc Natl Acad Sci U S A.* 2003;100(4):1885–1890.
87. Campanella GS, Grimm J, Manice LA, et al. Oligomerization of CXCL10 is necessary for endothelial cell presentation and in vivo activity. *J Immunol.* 2006;177(10):6991–6998.
88. Middleton J, Patterson AM, Gardner L, et al. Leukocyte extravasation: chemokine transport and presentation by the endothelium. *Blood.* 2002;100(12):3853–3860.
89. Kehoe JW, Bertozzi CR. Tyrosine sulfation: a modulator of extracellular protein-protein interactions. *Chem Biol.* 2000;7(3):R57–R61.
90. Springer TA. Traffic signals for lymphocyte recirculation and leukocyte emigration: the multistep paradigm. *Cell.* 1994;76(2): 301–314.
91. Manes S, Gomez-Mouton C, Lacalle RA, et al. Mastering time and space: immune cell polarization and chemotaxis. *Semin Immunol.* 2005;17(1):77–86.
92. Van Haastert PJ, Devreotes PN. Chemotaxis: signalling the way forward. *Nat Rev Mol Cell Biol.* 2004;5(8):626–634.
93. Castellino F, Germain RN. Chemokine-guided CD4+ T cell help enhances generation of IL-6RalphahighIL-7Ralpha high prememory CD8+ T cells. *J Immunol.* 2007;178(2):778–787.
94. Castellino F, Huang AY, Altan-Bonnet G, et al. Chemokines enhance immunity by guiding naive CD8+ T cells to sites of CD4+ T cell-dendritic cell interaction. *Nature.* 2006;440(7086):890–895.
95. Viola A, Contento RL, Molon B. T cells and their partners: The chemokine dating agency. *Trends Immunol.* 2006;27(9): 421–427.
96. Kumar A, Humphreys TD, Kremer KN, et al. CXCR4 physically associates with the T cell receptor to signal in T cells. *Immunity.* 2006;25(2):213–224.
97. Perfettini JL, Castedo M, Roumier T, et al. Mechanisms of apoptosis induction by the HIV-1 envelope. *Cell Death Differ.* 2005;12(suppl 1):916–923.
98. Boehme SA, Lio FM, Maciejewski-Lenoir D, et al. The chemokine fractalkine inhibits Fas-mediated cell death of brain microglia. *J Immunol.* 2000;165(1):397–403.
99. Sanchez-Sanchez N, Riol-Blanco L, de la Rosa G, et al. Chemokine receptor CCR7 induces intracellular signaling that inhibits apoptosis of mature dendritic cells. *Blood.* 2004;104(3):619–625.
100. Grayson MH, Holtzman MJ. Chemokine signaling regulates apoptosis as well as immune cell traffic in host defense. *Cell Cycle.* 2006;5(4):380–383.
101. Sanchez-Sanchez N, Riol-Blanco L, Rodriguez-Fernandez JL. The multiple personalities of the chemokine receptor CCR7 in dendritic cells. *J Immunol.* 2006;176(9):5153–5159.
102. Cole AM, Ganz T, Liese AM, et al. Cutting edge: IFN-inducible ELR-CXC chemokines display defensin-like antimicrobial activity. *J Immunol.* 2001;167(2):623–627.
103. Kehrl JH. Chemoattractant receptor signaling and the control of lymphocyte migration. *Immunol Res.* 2006;34(3):211–227.
104. Parent CA, Devreotes PN. A cell's sense of direction. *Science.* 1999;284(5415):765–770.
105. Wang F, Herzmark P, Weiner OD, et al. Lipid products of PI(3)Ks maintain persistent cell polarity and directed motility in neutrophils. *Nat Cell Biol.* 2002;4(7):513–518.
106. Chen Y, Corriden R, Inoue Y, et al. ATP release guides neutrophil chemotaxis via P2Y2 and A3 receptors. *Science.* 2006;314(5806): 1792–1795.
107. Xu J, Wang F, Van Keymeulen A, et al. Divergent signals and cytoskeletal assemblies regulate self-organizing polarity in neutrophils. *Cell.* 2003;114(2):201–214.
108. Rieken S, Sassmann A, Herroeder S, et al. G12/G13 family G proteins regulate marginal zone B cell maturation, migration, and polarization. *J Immunol.* 2006;177(5):2985–2993.
109. Peterson FC, Thorpe JA, Harder AG, et al. Structural determinants involved in the regulation of CXCL14/BRAK expression by the 26 S proteasome. *J Mol Biol.* 2006;363(4):813–822.
110. Kostyk AG, Dahl KM, Wynes MW, et al. Regulation of chemokine expression by NaCl occurs independently of cystic fibrosis transmembrane conductance regulator in macrophages. *Am J Pathol.* 2006;169(1):12–20.
111. Struyf S, Proost P, Van Damme J. Regulation of the immune response by the interaction of chemokines and proteases. *Adv Immunol.* 2003;81:1–44.
112. Overall CM, McQuibban GA, Clark-Lewis I. Discovery of chemokine substrates for matrix metalloproteinases by exosite scanning: a new tool for degradomics. *Biol Chem.* 2002;383(7–8):1059–1066.
113. Berahovich RD, Miao Z, Wang Y, et al. Proteolytic activation of alternative CCR1 ligands in inflammation. *J Immunol.* 2005;174(11): 7341–7351.
114. Mantovani A, Bonecchi R, Martinez FO, et al. Tuning of innate immunity and polarized responses by decoy receptors. *Int Arch Allergy Immunol.* 2003;132(2):109–115.
115. Neel NF, Schutyser E, Sai J, et al. Chemokine receptor internalization and intracellular trafficking. *Cytokine Growth Factor Rev.* 2005;16(6):637–658.
116. Lasagni L, Grepin R, Mazzinghi B, et al. PF-4/CXCL4 and CXCL4L1 exhibit distinct subcellular localization and a differentially regulated mechanism of secretion. *Blood.* 2007 Jan 11.
117. Wagner L, Yang OO, Garcia-Zepeda EA, et al. Beta-chemokines are released from HIV-1-specific cytolytic T-cell granules complexed to proteoglycans. *Nature.* 1998;391(6670):908–911.
118. Huse M, Lillemeier BF, Kuhns MS, et al. T cells use two directionally distinct pathways for cytokine secretion. *Nat Immunol.* 2006;7(3):247–255.
119. Katayama Y, Battista M, Kao WM, et al. Signals from the sympathetic nervous system regulate hematopoietic stem cell egress from bone marrow. *Cell.* 2006;124(2):407–421.
120. Dar A, Kollet O, Lapidot T. Mutual, reciprocal SDF-1/CXCR4 interactions between hematopoietic and bone marrow stromal cells regulate human stem cell migration and development in NOD/SCID chimeric mice. *Exp Hematol.* 2006;34(8):967–975.
121. Diaz GA. CXCR4 mutations in WHIM syndrome: a misguided immune system? *Immunol Rev.* 2005;203:235–243.
122. De Clercq E. The bicyclam AMD3100 story. *Nat Rev Drug Discov.* 2003;2(7):581–587.
123. Flomenberg N, DiPersio J, Calandra G. Role of CXCR4 chemokine receptor blockade using AMD3100 for mobilization of autologous hematopoietic progenitor cells. *Acta Haematol.* 2005;114(4):198–205.
124. Pelus LM, Fukuda S. Peripheral blood stem cell mobilization: the CXCR2 ligand GRObeta rapidly mobilizes hematopoietic stem cells with enhanced engraftment properties. *Exp Hematol.* 2006;34(8):1010–1020.
125. Martin C, Burdon PC, Bridger G, et al. Chemokines acting via CXCR2 and CXCR4 control the release of neutrophils from the bone marrow and their return following senescence. *Immunity.* 2003;19(4):583–593.
126. Tachibana K, Hirota S, Iizasa H, et al. The chemokine receptor CXCR4 is essential for vascularization of the gastrointestinal tract. *Nature.* 1998;393(6685):591–594.
127. Vilz TO, Moepps B, Engele J, et al. The SDF-1/CXCR4 pathway and the development of the cerebellar system. *Eur J Neurosci.* 2005;22(8):1831–1839.
128. Haas P, Gilmour D. Chemokine signaling mediates self-organizing tissue migration in the zebrafish lateral line. *Dev Cell.* 2006;10(5): 673–680.

129. Balabanian K, Lagane B, Infantino S, et al. The chemokine SDF-1/CXCL12 binds to and signals through the orphan receptor RDC1 in T lymphocytes. *J Biol Chem.* 2005;280(42):35760–35766.
130. Burns JM, Summers BC, Wang Y, et al. A novel chemokine receptor for SDF-1 and I-TAC involved in cell survival, cell adhesion, and tumor development. *J Exp Med.* 2006;203(9):2201–2213.
131. Ceradini DJ, Gurtner GC. Homing to hypoxia: HIF-1 as a mediator of progenitor cell recruitment to injured tissue. *Trends Cardiovasc Med.* 2005;15(2):57–63.
132. Zagzag D, Lukyanov Y, Lan L, et al. Hypoxia-inducible factor 1 and VEGF upregulate CXCR4 in glioblastoma: implications for angiogenesis and glioma cell invasion. *Lab Invest.* 2006;86(12):1221–1232.
133. Jin DK, Shido K, Kopp HG, et al. Cytokine-mediated deployment of SDF-1 induces revascularization through recruitment of CXCR4+ hemangiocytes. *Nat Med.* 2006;12(5):557–567.
134. Uehara S, Grinberg A, Farber JM, et al. A role for CCR9 in T lymphocyte development and migration. *J Immunol.* 2002;168(6):2811–2819.
135. Kurobe H, Liu C, Ueno T, et al. CCR7-dependent cortex-to-medulla migration of positively selected thymocytes is essential for establishing central tolerance. *Immunity.* 2006;24(2):165–177.
136. Rothenberg ME. Eotaxin. An essential mediator of eosinophil trafficking into mucosal tissues. *Am J Respir Cell Mol Biol.* 1999;21(3):291–295.
137. Rescigno M. CCR6(+) dendritic cells: the gut tactical-response unit. *Immunity.* 2006;24(5):508–510.
138. Onai N, Kitabatake M, Zhang YY, et al. Pivotal role of CCL25 (TECK)-CCR9 in the formation of gut cryptopatches and consequent appearance of intestinal intraepithelial T lymphocytes. *Int Immunol.* 2002;14(7):687–694.
139. Niess JH, Brand S, Gu X, et al. CX3CR1-mediated dendritic cell access to the intestinal lumen and bacterial clearance. *Science.* 2005;307(5707):254–258.
140. Gear AR, Camerini D. Platelet chemokines and chemokine receptors: linking hemostasis, inflammation, and host defense. *Microcirculation.* 2003;10(3–4):335–350.
141. Struyf S, Burdick MD, Proost P, et al. Platelets release CXCL4L1, a nonallelic variant of the chemokine platelet factor-4/CXCL4 and potent inhibitor of angiogenesis. *Circ Res.* 2004;95(9):855–857.
142. Massberg S, Konrad I, Schurzinger K, et al. Platelets secrete stromal cell-derived factor 1alpha and recruit bone marrow-derived progenitor cells to arterial thrombi in vivo. *J Exp Med.* 2006;203(5):1221–1233.
143. Bizzarri C, Beccari AR, Bertini R, et al. ELR+ CXC chemokines and their receptors (CXC chemokine receptor 1 and CXC chemokine receptor 2) as new therapeutic targets. *Pharmacol Ther.* 2006;112(1):139–149.
144. McLoughlin RM, Solinga RM, Rich J, et al. CD4+ T cells and CXC chemokines modulate the pathogenesis of Staphylococcus aureus wound infections. *Proc Natl Acad Sci U S A.* 2006;103(27):10408–10413.
145. Hidalgo-Grass C, Mishalian I, Dan-Goor M, et al. A streptococcal protease that degrades CXC chemokines and impairs bacterial clearance from infected tissues. *EMBO J.* 2006;25(19):4628–4637.
146. Ariel A, Fredman G, Sun YP, et al. Apoptotic neutrophils and T cells sequester chemokines during immune response resolution through modulation of CCR5 expression. *Nat Immunol.* 2006;7(11):1209–1216.
147. Geissmann F, Jung S, Littman DR. Blood monocytes consist of two principal subsets with distinct migratory properties. *Immunity.* 2003;19(1):71–82.
148. Rebenko-Moll NM, Liu L, Cardona A, et al. Chemokines, mononuclear cells and the nervous system: heaven (or hell) is in the details. *Curr Opin Immunol.* 2006;18(6):683–689.
149. Charo IF, Taubman MB. Chemokines in the pathogenesis of vascular disease. *Circ Res.* 2004;95(9):858–866.
150. Serbina NV, Pamer EG. Monocyte emigration from bone marrow during bacterial infection requires signals mediated by chemokine receptor CCR2. *Nat Immunol.* 2006;7(3):311–317.
151. Ness TL, Ewing JL, Hogaboam CM, et al. CCR4 is a key modulator of innate immune responses. *J Immunol.* 2006;177(11):7531–7539.
152. Salazar-Mather TP, Hamilton TA, Biron CA. A chemokine-to-cytokine-to-chemokine cascade critical in antiviral defense. *J Clin Invest.* 2000;105(7):985–993.
153. Coelho AL, Hogaboam CM, Kunkel SL. Chemokines provide the sustained inflammatory bridge between innate and acquired immunity. *Cytokine Growth Factor Rev.* 2005;16(6):553–560.
154. Lipp M, Muller G. Shaping up adaptive immunity: the impact of CCR7 and CXCR5 on lymphocyte trafficking. *Verh Dtsch Ges Pathol.* 2003;87:90–101.
155. Weninger W, von Andrian UH. Chemokine regulation of naive T cell traffic in health and disease. *Semin Immunol.* 2003;15(5):257–270.
156. Moser K, Tokoyoda K, Radbruch A, et al. Stromal niches, plasma cell differentiation and survival. *Curr Opin Immunol.* 2006;18(3):265–270.
157. Schaerli P, Moser B. Chemokines: control of primary and memory T-cell traffic. *Immunol Res.* 2005;31(1):57–74.
158. Randolph GJ, Sanchez-Schmitz G, Angeli V. Factors and signals that govern the migration of dendritic cells via lymphatics: recent advances. *Springer Semin Immunopathol.* 2005;26(3):273–287.
159. Sato N, Ahuja SK, Quinones M, et al. CC chemokine receptor (CCR)2 is required for langerhans cell migration and localization of T helper cell type 1 (Th1)-inducing dendritic cells. Absence of CCR2 shifts the *Leishmania major*-resistant phenotype to a susceptible state dominated by Th2 cytokines, b cell outgrowth, and sustained neutrophilic inflammation. *J Exp Med.* 2000;192(2):205–218.
160. Okada T, Ngo VN, Ekland EH, et al. Chemokine requirements for B cell entry to lymph nodes and Peyer's patches. *J Exp Med.* 2002;196(1):65–75.
161. Okada T, Miller MJ, Parker I, et al. Antigen-engaged B cells undergo chemotaxis toward the T zone and form motile conjugates with helper T cells. *PLoS Biol.* 2005;3(6):e150.
162. Palframan RT, Jung S, Cheng CY, et al. Inflammatory chemokine transport and presentation in HEV: A remote control mechanism for monocyte recruitment to lymph nodes in inflamed tissues. *J Exp Med.* 2001;194(9):1361–1373.
163. Moser B, Schaerli P, Loetscher P. CXCR5(+) T cells: follicular homing takes center stage in T-helper-cell responses. *Trends Immunol.* 2002;23(5):250–254.
164. Reif K, Ekland EH, Ohl L, et al. Balanced responsiveness to chemoattractants from adjacent zones determines B-cell position. *Nature.* 2002;416(6876):94–99.
165. Friedman RS, Jacobelli J, Krummel MF. Surface-bound chemokines capture and prime T cells for synapse formation. *Nat Immunol.* 2006;7(10):1101–1108.
166. Sallusto F, Lenig D, Forster R, et al. Two subsets of memory T lymphocytes with distinct homing potentials and effector functions. *Nature.* 1999;401(6754):708–712.
167. Debes GF, Arnold CN, Young AJ, et al. Chemokine receptor CCR7 required for T lymphocyte exit from peripheral tissues. *Nat Immunol.* 2005;6(9):889–894.
168. Bromley SK, Thomas SY, Luster AD. Chemokine receptor CCR7 guides T cell exit from peripheral tissues and entry into afferent lymphatics. *Nat Immunol.* 2005;6(9):895–901.
169. Song K, Rabin RL, Hill BJ, et al. Characterization of subsets of CD4+ memory T cells reveals early branched pathways of T cell differentiation in humans. *Proc Natl Acad Sci U S A.* 2005;102(22):7916–7921.
170. Sallusto F, Lenig D, Mackay CR, Lanzavecchia A. Flexible programs of chemokine receptor expression on human polarized T helper 1 and 2 lymphocytes. *J Exp Med.* 1998;187(6):875–883.
171. Mikhak Z, Fleming CM, Medoff BD, et al. STAT1 in peripheral tissue differentially regulates homing of antigen-specific Th1 and Th2 cells. *J Immunol.* 2006;176(8):4959–4967.
172. Yurchenko E, Tritt M, Hay V, et al. CCR5-dependent homing of naturally occurring CD4+ regulatory T cells to sites of Leishmania major infection favors pathogen persistence. *J Exp Med.* 2006;203(11):2451–2460.
172a. Singh SP, Zhang HH, Foley JF, et al. Human T cells that are able to produce IL-17 express the chemokine receptor CCR6. *J Immunol.* 2008;180(1):214–221.

173. Gerard C, Rollins BJ. Chemokines and disease. *Nat Immunol.* 2001;2(2):108–115.
174. Homey B, Alenius H, Muller A, et al. CCL27-CCR10 interactions regulate T cell-mediated skin inflammation. *Nat Med.* 2002;8(2):157–165.
175. Salazar-Gonzalez RM, Niess JH, Zammit DJ, et al. CCR6-mediated dendritic cell activation of pathogen-specific T cells in Peyer's patches. *Immunity.* 2006;24(5):623–632.
176. Mora JR, Bono MR, Manjunath N, et al. Selective imprinting of gut-homing T cells by Peyer's patch dendritic cells. *Nature.* 2003; 424(6944):88–93.
177. Mora JR, Iwata M, Eksteen B, et al. Generation of gut-homing IgA-secreting B cells by intestinal dendritic cells. *Science.* 2006; 314(5802):1157–1160.
178. Rodrigo Mora J, Von Andrian UH. Specificity and plasticity of memory lymphocyte migration. *Curr Top Microbiol Immunol.* 2006;308:83–116.
179. Lang KS, Georgiev P, Recher M, et al. Immunoprivileged status of the liver is controlled by Toll-like receptor 3 signaling. *J Clin Invest.* 2006;116(9):2456–2463.
180. Berger EA, Murphy PM, Farber JM. Chemokine receptors as HIV-1 coreceptors: roles in viral entry, tropism, and disease. *Annu Rev Immunol.* 1999;17:657–700.
181. Liu R, Paxton WA, Choe S, et al. Homozygous defect in HIV-1 coreceptor accounts for resistance of some multiply exposed individuals to HIV-1 infection. *Cell.* 1996;86(3):367–377.
182. Gonzalez E, Kulkarni H, Bolivar H, et al. The influence of CCL3L1 gene-containing segmental duplications on HIV-1/AIDS susceptibility. *Science.* 2005;307(5714):1434–1440.
183. O'Brien SJ, Moore JP. The effect of genetic variation in chemokines and their receptors on HIV transmission and progression to AIDS. *Immunol Rev.* 2000;177:99–111.
184. Arenzana-Seisdedos F, Parmentier M. Genetics of resistance to HIV infection: role of co-receptors and co-receptor ligands. *Semin Immunol.* 2006;18(6):387–403.
185. Nelson GW, O'Brien SJ. Using mutual information to measure the impact of multiple genetic factors on AIDS. *J Acquir Immune Defic Syndr.* 2006;42(3):347–354.
186. Sabeti PC, Walsh E, Schaffner SF, et al. The case for selection at CCR5-Delta32. *PLoS Biol.* 2005;3(11):e378.
187. Lim JK, Glass WG, McDermott DH, et al. CCR5: no longer a "good for nothing" gene—chemokine control of West Nile virus infection. *Trends Immunol.* 2006;27(7):308–312.
188. Klein RS, Lin E, Zhang B, et al. Neuronal CXCL10 directs CD8+ T-cell recruitment and control of West Nile virus encephalitis. *J Virol.* 2005;79(17):11457–11466.
189. Hsieh MF, Lai SL, Chen JP, et al. Both CXCR3 and CXCL10/IFN-inducible protein 10 are required for resistance to primary infection by dengue virus. *J Immunol.* 2006;177(3):1855–1863.
190. Levine B, Sodora DL. HIV and CXCR4 in a kiss of autophagic death. *J Clin Invest.* 2006;116(8):2078–2080.
191. Gaur D, Mayer DC, Miller LH. Parasite ligand-host receptor interactions during invasion of erythrocytes by *Plasmodium merozoites. Int J Parasitol.* 2004;34(13–14):1413–1429.
192. Hatabu T, Kawazu S, Aikawa M, et al. Binding of Plasmodium falciparum-infected erythrocytes to the membrane-bound form of Fractalkine/CX3CL1. *Proc Natl Acad Sci U S A.* 2003;100(26):15942–15946.
193. Tripp RA, Jones LP, Haynes LM, et al. CX3C chemokine mimicry by respiratory syncytial virus G glycoprotein. *Nat Immunol.* 2001;2(8):732–738.
194. Jensen KK, Lira SA. Chemokines and Kaposi's sarcoma. *Semin Cancer Biol.* 2004;14(3):187–194.
195. Sodhi A, Chaisuparat R, Hu J, et al. The TSC2/mTOR pathway drives endothelial cell transformation induced by the Kaposi's sarcoma-associated herpesvirus G protein-coupled receptor. *Cancer Cell.* 2006;10(2):133–143.
196. Barlic J, Zhang Y, Foley JF, et al. Oxidized lipid-driven chemokine receptor switch, CCR2 to CX3CR1, mediates adhesion of human macrophages to coronary artery smooth muscle cells through a peroxisome proliferator-activated receptor gamma-dependent pathway. *Circulation.* 2006;114(8):807–819.
197. McDermott DH, Fong AM, Yang Q, et al. Chemokine receptor mutant CX3CR1-M280 has impaired adhesive function and correlates with protection from cardiovascular disease in humans. *J Clin Invest.* 2003;111(8):1241–1250.
198. Smith DF, Galkina E, Ley K, et al. GRO family chemokines are specialized for monocyte arrest from flow. *Am J Physiol Heart Circ Physiol.* 2005;289(5):H1976–H1984.
199. Trogan E, Feig JE, Dogan S, et al. Gene expression changes in foam cells and the role of chemokine receptor CCR7 during atherosclerosis regression in ApoE-deficient mice. *Proc Natl Acad Sci U S A.* 2006;103(10):3781–3786.
200. Aslanian AM, Charo IF. Targeted disruption of the scavenger receptor and chemokine CXCL16 accelerates atherosclerosis. *Circulation.* 2006;114(6):583–590.
201. Heller EA, Liu E, Tager AM, et al. Chemokine CXCL10 promotes atherogenesis by modulating the local balance of effector and regulatory T cells. *Circulation.* 2006;113(19):2301–2312.
202. Aster RH. Drug-induced immune thrombocytopenia: an overview of pathogenesis. *Semin Hematol.* 1999;36(1 suppl 1):2–6.
203. Prahalad S. Negative association between the chemokine receptor CCR5-Delta32 polymorphism and rheumatoid arthritis: a meta-analysis. *Genes Immun.* 2006;7(3):264–268.
204. Huang D, Shi FD, Jung S, et al. The neuronal chemokine CX3CL1/fractalkine selectively recruits NK cells that modify experimental autoimmune encephalomyelitis within the central nervous system. *FASEB J.* 2006;20(7):896–905.
205. Liu L, Graham GJ, Damodaran A, et al. Cutting edge: the silent chemokine receptor D6 is required for generating T cell responses that mediate experimental autoimmune encephalomyelitis. *J Immunol.* 2006;177(1):17–21.
206. Hancock WW. Chemokine receptor-dependent alloresponses. *Immunol Rev.* 2003;196:37–50.
207. Fischereder M, Luckow B, Hocher B, et al. CC chemokine receptor 5 and renal-transplant survival. *Lancet.* 2001;357(9270):1758–1761.
208. Lukacs NW, Miller AL, Hogaboam CM. Chemokine receptors in asthma: searching for the correct immune targets. *J Immunol.* 2003;171(1):11–15.
209. Ma W, Bryce PJ, Humbles AA, et al. CCR3 is essential for skin eosinophilia and airway hyperresponsiveness in a murine model of allergic skin inflammation. *J Clin Invest.* 2002;109(5): 621–628.
210. Humbles AA, Lu B, Friend DS, et al. The murine CCR3 receptor regulates both the role of eosinophils and mast cells in allergen-induced airway inflammation and hyperresponsiveness. *Proc Natl Acad Sci U S A.* 2002;99(3):1479–1484.
211. Fulkerson PC, Fischetti CA, McBride ML, et al. A central regulatory role for eosinophils and the eotaxin/CCR3 axis in chronic experimental allergic airway inflammation. *Proc Natl Acad Sci U S A.* 2006;103(44):16418–16423.
212. Gonzalo JA, Lloyd CM, Peled A, et al. Critical involvement of the chemotactic axis CXCR4/stromal cell-derived factor-1 alpha in the inflammatory component of allergic airway disease. *J Immunol.* 2000;165(1):499–508.
213. Mantovani A, Allavena P, Sozzani S, et al. Chemokines in the recruitment and shaping of the leukocyte infiltrate of tumors. *Semin Cancer Biol.* 2004;14(3):155–160.
214. Strieter RM, Burdick MD, Mestas J, et al. Cancer CXC chemokine networks and tumour angiogenesis. *Eur J Cancer.* 2006;42(6):768–778.
215. Orimo A, Gupta PB, Sgroi DC, et al. Stromal fibroblasts present in invasive human breast carcinomas promote tumor growth and angiogenesis through elevated SDF-1/CXCL12 secretion. *Cell.* 2005;121(3):335–348.
216. Johnson Z, Proudfoot AE, Handel TM. Interaction of chemokines and glycosaminoglycans: a new twist in the regulation of chemokine function with opportunities for therapeutic intervention. *Cytokine Growth Factor Rev.* 2005;16(6):625–636.

Chapter 27

Programmed Cell Death

Nicolas Bidère, Helen C. Su, and Michael J. Lenardo

INTRODUCTION

Nontransformed cells have a finite lifespan. After a characteristic number of divisions, cells can undergo senescence, stop dividing, and subsequently die. Most of our cells will die long before we do, and evidence suggests that this is important for our health. However, adult vertebrates, as well as their internal organs, generally stay a constant size, so a form of homeostasis is implied (1). In certain organs, this involves a constantly fluctuating dynamic equilibrium. A prime example is the immune system, which employs cell renewal, expansion, and elimination in carrying out its function *(2,3,4,5)*. These changes can be systemic or localized to anatomic sites proximate to an antigen stimulus and may affect specific subsets of immune cells as dictated by the stimulus.

Programmed cell death (PCD) denotes a set of internal biochemical mechanisms that cause specific cells to die under defined conditions that are typically advantageous to the organism (6). Reasons for cell elimination include cell excess, improper cell differentiation, cell transformation, genetic damage to cells, and infection. In addition to this operational definition, considering a death event "programmed" usually means that one or more genes are required. This chapter has been organized so that we start with a broad overview of general immunoregulatory principles and then provide details on the molecules involved in PCD in specific sections at the end. Although there are conceptual antecedents from the 19th century, the selection of cells for survival or death by specific external stimuli was introduced by Levi-Montalcini for neural cells in the 1940s and later by Burnet for lymphocytes. Investigation into the molecular mechanism of PCD began in the mid-1980s and accelerated rapidly. DNA sequence databases permitted the rapid identification molecules involved in PCD *(7)*. Although PCD is a large and contentious area of cell biology research, molecular advances have established a firm and tractable theoretical foundation. Remarkably, much of what we will discuss was almost completely unknown two decades ago. Yet these pathways are at work every day in our bodies to control responses to infectious agents, establish cellular homeostasis, prevent autoimmunity, and avert lymphoid malignancies.

OVERVIEW: CELLULAR HOMEOSTASIS AND PCD IN MULTICELLULAR ORGANISMS

Internal programs of death are likely to exist in all mammalian cells. Martin Raff has suggested that these internal programs must be constantly and actively suppressed (8). For experimental investigation, it is thus important to discriminate between accidental cell death and that initiated or "programmed" by an internal biochemical mechanism. The term *apoptosis,* a Greek word meaning "falling off" as in leaves from a tree, was introduced in 1972 by Andrew Wyllie and coworkers to describe the normal, presumably programmed, attrition of cells (9). It was defined microscopically as cell shrinkage with nuclear and cytoplasmic condensation within an intact, but blebbed, cell membrane (10) (Figure 27.1B, C). This cell phenotype has long been associated with cell death *(11)*. Apoptosis is now mainly identified by the biochemical effects of the caspase family of proteases *(12)*. Caspases are important in two respects. First, they are a feature of most, if not all, apoptosis pathways. Second, once highly activated, they usually represent a commitment to apoptosis that is not reversible, although there are suggestions that low-level caspase activation may occur during lymphocyte activation *(13,14)*. For these reasons, caspases have been regarded as a final common pathway of apoptosis. In fact, the concept of PCD was significantly strengthened by the identification of caspases and other molecules that comprise dedicated internal biochemical death pathways. In general, the molecular components of the death mechanism are preassembled and available without new gene transcription or protein synthesis (6). For example, caspases are constitutively expressed in the cytoplasm of the cell as zymogens. Once proteolytically activated, caspases carry out specific protein cleavages leading to the morphological changes of apoptosis. The proteolytic substrates of caspases are highly selective because most proteins remain uncleaved. A panoply of molecular events entrained to caspases includes cleavage of chromosomal DNA, nuclear chromatin condensation, exposure of phosphatidylserine on the exterior of the cell membrane, proteolysis of specific proteins including other caspases, and mitochondrial changes. These processes are detectable by simple assays in tissue culture cells *in vitro* or, in some cases, *in vivo*. Protocols for these assays have been well described *(15,16)*.

Cells that die without the characteristics of apoptosis typically undergo what is usually called *necrosis*. While necrosis is often associated with accidental cell death, it may also result from programmed mechanisms. In certain cases, nonapoptotic mechanisms of cell death can be promoted by caspase inhibition (17). The appearance of a necrotic cell differs dramatically from apoptosis. Necrotic cells swell and lose the integrity of internal organelles and the cell membrane, giving an enlarged, "fractured" appearance under the microscope (Figure 27.1D). Recently, various research groups have begun to define molecular programs resulting in necrotic death (18). Several varieties of "programmed" necrosis that share the hallmarks of early loss of plasma membrane integrity and excessive reactive oxygen species (ROS) have been described. Programmed necrosis that involves the RIP serine/threonine kinase has been well documented in lymphocytes, especially under conditions of caspase inhibition (17,18). A closely related variant of this cell death program has been defined as necroptosis (19). Finally, the induction of autophagy has been genetically linked to a necrotic program of death (20). Autophagy is induced by starvation or other stimuli and involves internal membrane rearrangement leading to engulfment of portions of the cytoplasm, which are then degraded by fusion with lysosomes. Under death conditions, this mechanism leads to membrane damage and necrosis by ROS, which overaccumulate because of accelerated catalase degradation (21). The precise role of these necrosis programs, especially autophagic cell death, in immune function has not yet been worked out. However they are often provoked by the inhibition of caspase-dependent apoptosis.

Thus, it is important to distinguish between "programmed" necrosis and necrosis due to accidental causes, because these involve very different molecular events. It has been generally argued that apoptosis, which preserves membrane integrity, prevents inflammation from released cellular contents, whereas necrosis results in total cellular breakdown and content release which causes an inflammatory response *(22)*. There are contrasting views on whether remnants of apoptotic or necrotic cells are more immunogenic when engulfed by antigen presenting cells (APCs), though exposure to necrotic cells can cause dendritic cell (DC) maturation (*23,24,*25). The distinct immunological effects due to apoptosis and necrosis remain the subject of substantial experimental exploration.

As we will argue later in this chapter, the necessity of cellular homeostasis as well as the acute need to eliminate cells that are harmful or nonfunctional led to the early emergence of conserved cell death mechanisms during evolution *(11)*. Work by Horvitz and colleagues genetically identified several molecules essential for the death of specific cells during the development of the roundworm *C. elegans* that have subsequently been found to be homologues for mammalian PCD genes (26). It is clear from this

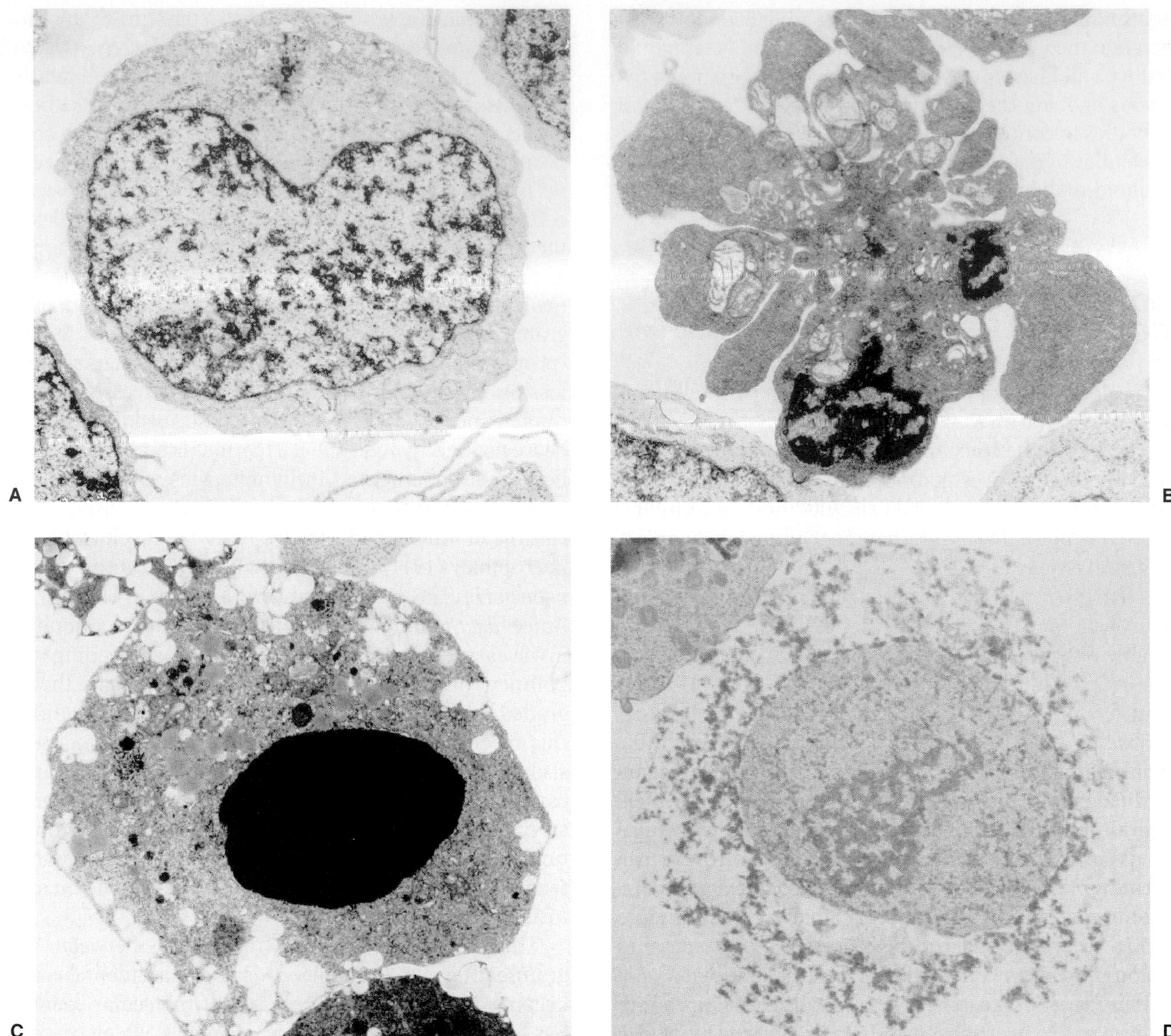

FIGURE 27.1 Electron microscopy elucidates the morphology of different forms of PCD. **A:** A normal, unstimulated Jurkat leukemia cell. **B:** Jurkat cell undergoing apoptosis in response to Fas receptor stimulation. Notice the condensed chromatin and the blebbing, but maintenance of plasma membrane integrity. **C:** Jurkat cell undergoing apoptosis in response to staurosporine treatment. Note the prominent nuclear condensation. **D:** Necrosis of human peripheral blood T lymphocyte infected with the human immunodeficiency virus. Notice the general loss of cellular integrity as well as the lack of chromatin condensation in the dying cell. (Figure courtesy of Diane Bolton and Jan Orenstein)

simplified system that the molecular logic of one form of cell death was likely established early in evolving multicellular organisms *(27)*. PCD mechanisms are now evident in most contemporary multicellular organisms from plants to humans, although it is not clear whether convergent evolution or conservation of function is responsible. However, the molecular pathways in worms and other simple organisms are rudimentary compared with the complexity found in mammalian PCD systems. To understand how these mechanisms contribute to immunity, we focus on mice and humans, which are the subjects of most immunological research.

PCD AND IMMUNE REGULATION

The fundamental unit of immune responsiveness is the cell. Lymphocytes, the major immune cells, are distinguished by expressing a unique clonotypic antigen receptor. A large number of lymphocytes with different receptor specificities are generated during ontogeny (e.g., the "immune repertoire"), and these cells can be programmed to expand or die throughout the life of the organism. Somatic hypermutation during B cell expansion in the germinal center can expand the repertoire. Although the level of antigen presentation, the degree of lymphocyte responsiveness (versus nonresponsiveness or anergy), and other factors also play important roles, the presence or absence of cells with specific recognition properties at any given time is a primary determinant of the quantitative response to any antigenic stimulus. The homeostasis of major lymphocyte populations is independently regulated such that deficits in B cells, T cells, or even major T cell subpopulations ($\alpha\beta$ versus $\gamma\delta$-, or CD4 versus CD8) may qualitatively alter but do not prevent the normal homeostasis of the remaining populations. During development, lymphocytes respond to the antigenic environment with either survival or death (28). Developmental PCD eliminates lymphocytes that cannot recognize antigen appropriately or have potentially dangerous self-reactivity (28,29). In the mature immune system, death is principally a negative feedback response that counterbalances proliferative responses to antigen (30). Although the clonal selection theory of F. M. Burnet encompassed clonal elimination during ontogeny, in the mature immune system, it allowed only selective expansion of antigen-stimulated lymphocytes. However, antigen-specific regulation of mature lymphocyte survival also powerfully controls immune responses and tolerance (4,30,31). Since the organism encounters an unpredictable universe of antigens in a lifetime, it is essential that there is feedback regulation of adaptive immune responses. Feedback is an essential element of any dynamic system in which final outcomes cannot be predicted from the starting conditions *(32)*. To achieve measured immune responses, proliferation and death are coordinated by feedback regulation to control the number of immunologically responsive cells. Moreover, during immune reactions, potentially harmful self-reactive cells may unexpectedly increase; because they continue to signal, these self-reactive cells are preferentially eliminated by feedback death mechanisms. Hence, homeostasis of both lymphocyte numbers and reactivities can be continuously maintained.

Thymic Deletion: Positive and Negative Selection

Thymic selection represents an intriguing example of apoptosis in which the same receptor—the clonotypic T cell receptor (TCR)—can lead to diametrically opposite outcomes depending on the level of stimulation (28,29). During development, when thymocytes express the TCR and both the CD4 and CD8 coreceptors (the "double-positive" stage), thymocytes will undergo apoptosis if they receive no TCR stimulation. This has been called *death by neglect (33)*. This process will eliminate thymocytes that have not productively rearranged the TCR genes or have no capacity to recognize antigen in the context of self–major histocompatibility complex (MHC). "Low-level" stimulation of the TCR antagonizes death by neglect. This protective event insures MHC-specific antigen recognition by T cells and is called *positive selection (34)*. While weak TCR signals can deliver an anti-apoptotic stimulus, strong TCR engagement of double-positive thymocytes delivers a pro-apoptotic signal. This event, termed *negative selection*, prevents the emergence of strongly autoreactive lymphocytes from the thymus *(33)*. This deletion step is a major mechanism of central tolerance and the prevention of autoimmunity *(35)*. These processes of selection employ caspase-dependent apoptosis and rapid phagocytosis of the dead thymocytes (*36*,37). Hence, thymocytes travel a narrow bridge of TCR avidity during development and will die if they deviate from it.

The differences between the neglect (or null), weak, and strong signals that result in life or death appear to be determined at early stages of TCR signaling (38,*39*). Death receptors (discussed later) appear not to be crucial; instead, there is a direct connection of the TCR signaling apparatus to mitochondrial death pathways (*40,41*,42,43). Although there is not complete certainty about how the TCR dictates life or death at specific antigen levels, the answer to this puzzle will almost certainly reside in the complex signal pathways emanating from this receptor. TCR engagement that causes transient induction of the Erk kinase is associated with positive selection, whereas slow but constant Erk activity is associated with negative selection (44–46). Other distinctions in TCR signaling have been identified. Signaling through phosphotidylinositol-3 kinase, the anti-apoptotic Akt kinase, and the retinoid orphan receptor (ROR)–gamma may promote thymocyte survival (reviewed in [38,47]). Gene knockouts in mice have revealed that several transcription factors, such as E2A, Id3, and IRF-1, can affect thymic cellularity, indicating that differential signaling may trigger transcriptional events that regulate cell survival (*48–50*,51). Finally, Andreas Strasser has emphasized that various forms of physiological cell death are likely to involve the subset of BH3-only proteins in the Bcl-2 family (52,53). The activation of proapoptotic BH3-only proteins, such as Bak, Bid, and especially Bim, by TCR signals initiates mitochondrial apoptosis during thymic selection processes. Thus, early TCR-induced signaling differences directly entrain transcriptional events that modulate BH3-only regulators of mitochondrial apoptosis. These distinct signals are tied to specific microenvironments within the thymus in which positive and negative selection occur (54). Hence, by intracellular communication with distinct apoptosis regulatory molecules, the TCR has a remarkable ability to signal life or death by the apparent strength of stimulus it receives.

PCD and the Homeostasis of Peripheral T Cells

Death of peripheral T cells differs markedly from thymocyte selection in that PCD of mature lymphocytes occurs mainly in cells that have proven usefulness (i.e., they have been already activated by antigen). This is because PCD of mature T cells is employed primarily to counter antigen-driven proliferation of activated T cells. In general, most naïve lymphocytes survive and circulate in the body in a resting state (G_0). The survival of such resting T cells is constitutively maintained by the presence of contact with MHC, the cytokine IL-7, and expression of the anti-apoptotic protein Bcl-2 (*35*,55,*56*,*57*). During an active immune response, T lymphocyte proliferation can involve as much as a 1,000-fold expansion within days. Such explosive proliferation is necessary to counter the extraordinarily rapid propagation of microbial pathogens. However, these activated and cycling T cells are potentially damaging due to toxic effector functions and potential cross-reactivity with self-antigens. Activated T cell expansion does not go unchecked and is subject to negative feedback in the form of cell death. However, because immune responses are directed at specific antigens, they must be independently regulated since some responses might expand while others contract. The immune system has developed propriocidal mechanisms to control independent populations of activated T cells. *Propriocidal regulation* refers to the various negative feedback death mechanisms that maintain homeostasis of mature peripheral T cells in an antigen-specific manner. These potently restrain antigen-activated T cells and tightly control lymphocyte numbers during and at the conclusion of immune responses.

Propriocidal regulation of T cells is triggered by remarkably simple attributes of T cell activation—the level of cell cycling and the level of antigen restimulation (30,55). These two features are ideally suited for triggering negative feedback death because they provide both a "sensing" mechanism for the level of active T cell proliferation and a negative response mechanism sensitive to the level of antigen stimulation. There are essentially two different mechanisms: 1) active or antigen-stimulated PCD, and 2) passive or lymphokine withdrawal PCD (Figure 27.2) (4,*58*,59,*60*). These have different roles and occur at

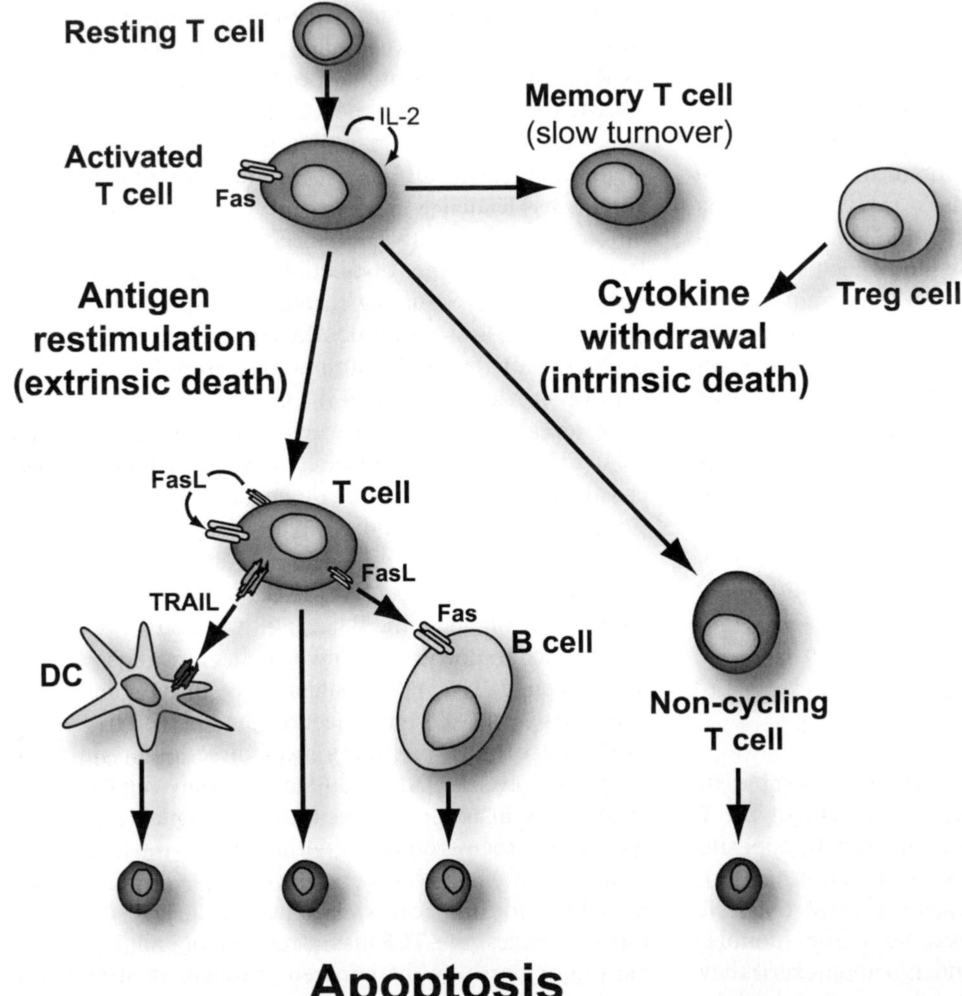

FIGURE 27.2 Propriocidal regulation of immune cells. Shown are the apoptosis pathways that govern T lymphocyte homeostasis by the antigen-restimulated (extrinsic death) and no antigen (cytokine withdrawal [intrinsic death]) pathways of apoptosis. Also shown are the regulation of B cells by FasL expressed by T cells, and DCs by TRAIL expressed by T cells.

different times, as will be described in detail later. In some respects, it is paradoxical that lymphocytes that respond well to foreign antigen and presumably could have protective value are actively eliminated. However, it is vital to constrain the number of activated T cells to prevent unhealthy effector or autoimmune reactions. During a strong immune response, lymphocytes that cross-react with self-antigens may proliferate. The propriocidal mechanisms that cause these cells to die upon encountering self-antigens could be an important mechanism of preserving self-tolerance. By this formulation, tolerance is a quantitative effect that is due to the low number of significantly self-reactive lymphocytes in the naïve organism. Clonal expansion during immune responses can unleash dormant or infrequent self-reactive clones, called *forbidden clones* by Burnet, creating an autoimmune diathesis. Propriocidal death reduces these clones and thereby promotes tolerance. Active antigen-induced propriocidal death, which is induced by high or repeated doses of antigen, is especially well suited for the elimination of self-reactive clones since self antigen is likely to be present in continuously high amounts (30,55).

Extrinsic or Antigen-stimulated T Lymphocyte Death

The extrinsic death mechanism involves apoptosis of mature T cells in response to antigen stimulation. This requires the T cells to be activated and cycling at the time that they undergo strong antigenic restimulation (30,55). The death is indirect in the sense that it requires the antigen-induced secretion of death ligands that engage specific apoptosis-inducing death receptors (DRs) in the tumor necrosis factor receptor (TNFR) and ligand superfamilies (Figure 27.2) (61,*62*). Current evidence suggests that Fas ligand (FasL) as well as TNF are the key death ligands that mediate this process in mature $CD4^+$ and $CD8^+$ T cells (4,*5*,63). Th2-differentiated CD4 cells are less sensitive than their Th1-differentiated counterparts to Fas-mediated killing (64). Instead, they preferentially die through a suicidal pathway that triggers internal release of granzyme B (65,*66*). Nagata originally observed that the lymphoproliferative and autoimmune phenotype of *lpr* mice was due to genetic alterations of Fas, and a similar disease in *gld* mice was due to a mutation in FasL (67,*68*). Defects in Fas (CD95) or FasL cause severe derangements of lymphocyte homeostasis and tolerance that will be detailed later in this chapter. In humans, defects in Fas and FasL cause the autoimmune lymphoproliferative syndrome (ALPS) types Ia and Ib, respectively (69). An alternative mechanism of propriocidal regulation is via perforin, which is a chief mediator of cytolytic T cell killing of target cells. Perforin defects in both mice and humans cause impaired clearance of activated $CD8^+$ T cells (*70*,71,*72*,73). Often these forms of death are called "activation-induced cell death" (AICD), but this is a misnomer *(74)*. AICD has been used to describe any form of death of activated T cells, thus causing confusion among investigators working on molecularly distinct death pathways (4,*75*). Activation *per se* does not directly cause cell death; instead, extrinsic death induction requires antigenic restimulation of activated T cells (i.e., TCR reengagement after the initial activation). For resting T cells, antigen encounter under costimulatory conditions leads to activation with very little cell death. Obviously, if the initial activation directly induced death, this would preclude immune responses. On the contrary, activated, cycling T cells do not spontaneously die by FasL or TNF unless they are strongly restimulated by antigen in the activated state, which causes up-regulation of the genes for these death cytokines and responsiveness to them (76).

Extrinsic death is a negative feedback mechanism, which explains why it is triggered by lymphokine-induced cell cycling (usually caused by IL-2) and reengagement of the TCR. IL-2-induced cell cycling indicates that there has been a productive antigen response and the T cells are multiplying. Because T cells can expand rapidly to great numbers, a large fraction of cycling T cells dictates a need to down-regulate the response to any further antigen exposure. The presence of repeated or continuously high amounts of antigen would be a powerful stimulus to greater proliferation. Under these conditions, the system programs a fraction of the restimulated cells to undergo apoptosis by death ligand production or perforin. Unchecked exponential T cell expansion is thereby prevented by a simple and specific feedback loop. Like most negative feedback systems, the propriocidal response directly reverses the ongoing process of proliferation by eliminating activated T cells. Antigen-induced death provides an explanation for many historical observations in the literature that show that reapplication or continuous presence of high concentrations of antigen can lead to suppression rather than augmentation of an immune response (reviewed in [55]).

Sensitivity to the extrinsic death mechanism is chiefly due to the effect of IL-2 in inducing cell cycle progression into late G1 or S phase, which confers susceptibility to death (77–79). The requirement for cell cycle progression has not been fully explained but appears to be necessary for apoptosis induced by TCR engagement or with direct Fas stimulation. Other cytokines that augment T cell cycling such as IL-4, IL-7, and IL-15 can also promote cell death to some degree but none with the potency of IL-2 (76). Hence, the theory of propriocidal regulation advanced the concept that IL-2 would have an important regulatory role in the elimination of activated T cells in addition to its previously known role in lymphocyte proliferation (55). This concept was later validated when genetic deficiencies of IL-2 and IL-2 receptor in mice were found to have defective apoptosis of activated T cells and autoimmunity

(80,*81,82*). Although the immunopathology in these animals has been also recently attributed to T regulatory cells, the latter may constitute another form of clonal deletion by cytokine competition. This surprising property of IL-2 is important to consider in the use of IL-2 as a therapeutic agent or vaccine adjuvant. It also underscores an important feature of feedback regulation—that to achieve a maximal response for, say, a vaccine, more stimulation is not necessarily better. In a variety of test situations, extrinsic antigen-induced death decreases the number of T cells, but does not completely eliminate the T cell immune response (30,31). In certain extraordinary conditions, such as high levels of a noncytopathic or chronic virus, essentially all responding T cells can be eliminated (83). FasL expressed on T cells also causes the death of B cells, which do not themselves express FasL (84). This causes a parallel regulation of B cell proliferation by Fas-induced death that can be antagonized by B cell receptor (BCR) engagement (Figure 27.2). Antigen-induced death therefore provides a mechanism to eliminate specific antigen-reactive lymphocytes under chronic stimulatory conditions when they might cause the host more harm than good.

Antigen-induced expression of death receptors and their ligands shunts a proportionate fraction of the antigen-specific activated cells, but not bystander cells, into the death pathway. The activated T cells still carry out their effector function when restimulated by antigen, but their ultimate fate is death instead of proliferation (76,83). Since the agents of cell death—Fas and other TNFRs—have no inherent antigen specificity, it is important to consider how the clonal specificity of antigen-induced apoptosis is achieved (30). For the death of activated T cells, the simple engagement of Fas by its ligand is insufficient (85,86). Efficient death induction also requires a "competency" signal from the TCR delivered at the same time FasL binds Fas (85,87). However, these signals do not require new protein synthesis and are delivered rapidly in a few hours or less (85,86). The requirement for simultaneous engagement of Fas and TCR plays a critical role in establishing the antigen-specificity of death. For example, it was shown that TCR stimulation of a specific subpopulation within a pool of Fas-expressing T cell blasts, such as with agonistic anti-Vβ8 antibody, leads only to the death of that subpopulation despite the apparent exposure of other subtypes of T cells to the Vβ8-expressing cells that have been induced to express FasL (30,85). Also, deletion *in vivo* is antigen-specific (88). The molecular nature of the competency signal is presently unknown.

Intrinsic Growth Factor Withdrawal T Cell Death

As important as it is to avert over-reaction during an immune response through extrinsic, TCR-induced death, it is equally important for the immune system to downmodulate the immune reaction after successful elimination of the pathogen. Lymphokine withdrawal death is a form of T cell apoptosis that occurs naturally at the end of an immune response when the accumulation of effector cells becomes unnecessary and potentially damaging *(89)*. When the trophic cytokine for activated T cells, typically IL-2, decreases because of reduced antigen stimulation, the excess T cells undergo apoptosis *(90)*. This form of negative feedback death may affect specific classes of T cells, for example, "effector" versus "memory" cells, though this distinction may be difficult to discern experimentally. Because most T cells in the expanded population are antigen-specific, this represents clonotype-specific T cell propriocidal regulation controlled by antigen and cell cycle progression. The activated cells can "sense" decreased antigen drive and decreased trophic cytokine, which programs them for apoptosis. The elimination of the expanded pool of activated cells, except for a small amount of memory cells, reestablishes homeostasis in T cell numbers. It has been shown that if IL-2 is exogenously delivered during a proliferative response to superantigen, the reactive T cells persist as long as lymphokine is provided (91). Therefore, the lack of IL-2 is a key element in the feedback regulation of the cellular response. Antigen and IL-2 therefore mediated propriocidal regulation in the midst of an immune response and at its conclusion downregulate T cell numbers.

Genetic studies reveal that the molecular mechanism of lymphokine withdrawal death is different than antigen-induced apoptosis (*58*,59). Although this event is often confused with extrinsic cell death mediated by Fas, DRs are not involved. Rather, cytokine withdrawal for 2 hours–4 hours commits the cell to a death pathway requiring new protein synthesis (92). Apoptosis is initiated through the mitochondrial pathway and is orchestrated by the Bcl-2 family of proteins. In fact, the ratio between the pro- and the anti-apoptotic Bcl-2 family members is believed to determine the fate of the cells. In the presence of growth factors, the anti-apoptotic Bcl-2, Bcl-X_L, and Mcl-1 proteins sequester the BH3-only activators Bim and Bid, thereby preventing the executioners Bax and Bak from permeabilizing the mitochondrial outer membrane (MOM) (see later discussion) *(93)*. Bim is an essential up-stream regulator of Bax and Bak during cytokine withdrawal-induced apoptosis in lymphocytes (for review, see [94]). Cytokine deprivation rapidly upregulates Bim mRNA levels through activation of the forkhead-like transcription factor FOXO3A. $CD4^+$ and $CD8^+$ T cells from mice homozygously deficient for Bim survived much longer than their wild-type counterparts following *in vitro* and *in vivo* activation with the superantigen *Staphylococcus aureus* enterotoxin B (95). Moreover, Bim is critical for both IL-2- and IL-7-withdrawal-induced cell death of T cells (52,95,96). PUMA, another BH3-only protein, functions synergistically with Bim downstream of FOXO3A in lymphoid cells and accounts for the Bim-independent death (97,98). When the trophic cytokine is present, the Ser/Thr kinase Akt phosphorylates key substrates and prevents mitochondrial collapse. For example, Akt suppresses FOXO3A activity. Akt also phosphorylates the pro-apoptotic Bad protein, which is then sequestered by the 14-3-3 scaffold protein (*99,*100). Another target inactivated by Akt is glycogen synthase kinase-3 (GSK-3), which phosphorylates Mcl-1 on residue S159 when cytokines are removed. The rapid degradation of phosphorylated Mcl-1 by the ubiquitin-proteasome pathway disrupts the fragile equilibrium between the pro- and the anti-apoptotic Bcl-2 family members and promotes cell death (101). Thus, Akt can preserve viability by targeting appropriate Bcl-2 family members.

T Regulatory Cells

An intriguing area of immune tolerance research is the emerging understanding of a subset of CD4 T cells, termed *T regulatory* or *Treg*. These cells express the forkhead box P3 (FoxP3) transcription factor and suppress the expression of many TCR-induced genes, including cytokines and cytokine receptors (*102,*103). Similar to other subsets of T cells in their "activated" state, Tregs require common gamma chain cytokines for survival. In particular, they characteristically express the IL-2 alpha chain receptor (CD25) and require IL-2 to persist in the periphery (104). IL-7 can also act as a survival factor for Treg cells (105). A postulated function of Treg cells has been an ability to "suppress" immune responses, although the mechanism by which this is achieved has been obscure (106). One line of evidence suggests that they may have the ability to cause death by a perforin or granzyme B mediated mechanism (107,108). Tregs have been proposed to use this mechanism to kill APCs, B cells, and T cells as a means to suppress immune responses (*109,*110). This possible death mechanism is still controversial but could involve clonal deletion *(110a)*.

T Cell Memory

T cells, once activated, can persist as "memory" cells. One view is that the process involves an escape from apoptosis (37,*111–113*). Hence, such cells would have to avoid elimination by the propriocidal mechanisms. Increasing evidence supports the concept that memory is due to the long-term survival of antigen-specific T cells even without further antigen exposure. Several means to achieve such survival are possible. To escape killing by Fas and other death receptors, T cells could express c-FLIP (cellular FLICE Inhibitory Protein), which is a homologue of caspase-8 and -10 that has no enzymatic function but can interpose itself into the death receptor complex and block caspase activation (114). This type of inhibition has been demonstrated in B cells by the ability of Ig stimulation, which upregulates c-FLIP (*115,*116), to block Fas killing *(117)*. Various "inhibitor of apoptosis proteins" (IAPs) might also interfere with DR killing (118,*119*). Further, the mitochondrial death pathway could be attenuated by upregulation of Bcl-2 and Bcl-X_L. These anti-apoptotic molecules, which are upregulated in CD8 and CD4 memory cells (*113,*120), have been shown to block lymphokine withdrawal apoptosis *(93)*. The necessity of these inhibitory molecules for the persistence of a memory population of T cells is unknown.

Another view is that long-term survival, in a nonproliferative "resting" state characteristic of "virgin" T cells, is never reestablished by memory cells. Recent work by Phillipa Marrack, Rafi Ahmed, and others reveal a surprisingly dynamic T cell memory pool. Their study proposes a constant, low-level proliferation of memory CD8$^+$ T cells that is antigen-dependent and maintained by IL-15 and to a lesser extent by IL-7 *(121,122)* (reviewed in [123]). Also, the fraction of memory cells remains constant over time, indicating that death is continuously maintaining a balance. Hence, the balance of slow proliferation and slow death ensures memory cell maintenance. As the molecular mechanism of the memory state is further elucidated, the differing views of "memory" are likely to be reconciled.

The mitochondrial pathway of death is likely to play a prominent role in the generation of memory cells. In addition to their proliferative effects, the cytokines IL-15 and IL-7 appear to promote survival of memory cells through their induction of anti-apoptotic molecules such as Bcl-2 *(124–126)*. This countervailing effect is consistent with a recently demonstrated Bim-dependent mechanism for limiting memory CD8 T cells (127). In addition, a Bim-independent mechanism for expunging memory T cells was shown (127), and this is likely to involve death receptors. For instance, CD4 T cell help is required for CD8 T cell memory. In the absence of CD4 help, TRAIL is expressed on and mediates apoptosis of CD8 cells upon antigen restimulation (128). TRAIL deficiency, however, only delayed the loss of CD8 memory cells, revealing that non-TRAIL mechanisms also contribute to the homeostasis of CD8 memory cells (129). Further studies are needed to dissect the PCD mechanisms contributing to T memory cell generation and homeostasis.

B Cell Homeostasis

We have focused most of our attention on T lymphocyte apoptosis thus far because it has received the greatest experimental examination and more details are known. However, PCD also governs B cell homeostasis and is regulated in ways that have similarities and differences with T cells. Both DR triggering and withdrawal of trophic stimuli contribute to B cell elimination. Similar to T cells, B cells developing in the bone marrow undergo a series of proliferative expansion and apoptotic contraction events to shape the final B cell repertoire *(130)*. Immunoglobulin (Ig) gene rearrangement starting at the pro-B stage generates the BCR. The cytokine IL-7, which promotes the survival of developing thymocytes (131,132), is crucial for sustaining survival at the pro-B/pre-B juncture (133,134). IL-7 induces transcription of the anti-apoptotic molecule Mcl-1, which selectively binds to and antagonizes the pro-apoptotic Bcl-2 family member Bim (*135*,136). Then selection for B cells occurs in two developmental steps with successive gene rearrangements at the heavy- and light chain Ig loci. B cells that fail to generate a productive BCR, due to abortive Ig gene rearrangements, are eliminated by PCD. At the other end of the spectrum, B cells that express BCRs directed against self-antigens are eliminated by apoptosis or undergo receptor editing to acquire new antigen specificity (137). The survival and antigen responsiveness of immature B cells can also be increased by lipopolysaccharide (LPS) exposure, presumably to enhance B cell production during infections *(138)*. Fas, TNFR-1 or perforin are not involved in the death of developing B cells (reviewed in [139]). Rather, death appears to be a consequence of a direct signaling event generated by the BCR (140).

In contrast to B cells in development, mature B cells rely heavily on TNFR family receptors such as CD40, Fas, and BAFF for regulating their survival and death. It is also clear that T cells control PCD of mature B cells. Christopher Goodnow and colleagues have illustrated the importance of CD40 and Fas in the balance of life and death in B cells using the hen egg lysozyme (HEL)–transgenic and HEL-specific TCR transgenic mice (141,142). Naïve, HEL-specific B cells undergo proliferation in the presence of HEL and HEL-specific CD4 T cell help. Hence, proper B cell activation requires triggering of the BCR as well as "help" in the form of CD40L expressed on activated T cells. The primary function of CD40L is to prevent death of the activated B cells. Survival allows further differentiation and function *(143)*. However, anergic HEL-specific B cells from HEL transgenic animals undergo apoptosis in the presence of the same HEL-specific CD4 T cell help. This antigen-specific B cell death is absent in Fas-deficient B cells (141), thus suggesting a role for Fas in causing the death of anergic antigen-specific B cells. Fas killing of mature B cells can also be abrogated by BCR engagement and IL-4, which promote antibody responses (144,*145*). An imbalance of CD40 and Fas signals might contribute to autoantibody production consequent to Fas and FasL mutations in both human and mouse. More recent studies using similar transgenic systems suggest that whereas Fas can mediate apoptosis of activated B cells by CD4 T cells, BCR-induced death of immature or resting mature B cells is primarily Fas-independent. Central to this Fas-independent pathway is up-regulation of the pro-apoptotic molecule Bim (*146*,147,148). Moreover, the recently discovered B cell survival and maturation factor BAFF serves as a survival factor for mature B cells by sustaining the MAPK Erk signals that in turn inhibit Bim accumulation (149).

The attenuation of B cell responses at the end of an immune reaction is likely to involve cytokine withdrawal death similar to that of T cells, but this phenomenon is less well characterized. Cytokines such as IL-7 and IL-15, which enhance cellular survival through the up-regulation of Bcl-2, Bcl-X_L, or Mcl-1, may be responsible (136,*150*). Lymphokine withdrawal death in B cells, like T cells, requires de novo RNA/protein synthesis *(151)*. An interesting observation is that a secreted lipocalin, identified through microarray analysis of an IL-3 dependent pro-B cell line, was implicated as a potential mediator for IL-3 withdrawal death (152). This protein appears to regulate intracellular iron levels, which may modulate Bim levels for apoptosis induction (153). However, it remains to be seen whether lipocalins or other similar molecules are involved in lymphokine withdrawal death in primary mature B or T cells. As we will discuss later in this chapter, survival genes such as Bcl-2 can protect cells against lymphokine withdrawal death and therefore play an important role in mature B cell homeostasis. Moreover, Bcl-2 can contribute to the survival of B lymphoma cells as revealed by the t(14:18) translocation of Bcl-2 to the Ig locus in follicular B cell lymphomas (154).

DC Homeostasis

Understanding the cell fate regulation of DCs is still in its infancy. However, emerging evidence suggests that these highly efficient APCs are also subject to homeostatic regulation by PCD. The natural turnover of DCs was demonstrated in the mouse by Jenkins and coworkers (155). Using elegant cell-labeling experiments, they showed that antigen-laden DCs stimulate the formation of a cluster of activated antigen-specific T cells and then disappear. This process was antigen- and T cell–dependent. Later, it was shown that the TNF homologue TRAIL (TNF-related apoptosis-inducing ligand), which is produced by activated T cells, could induce apoptosis in DCs and that this mechanism could be defective in patients harboring mutations in caspase-10 (156). Together these data introduced the concept that there is homeostatic regulation of DCs involving recruitment and differentiation followed by their active elimination by stimulated T cells. Early removal of DCs has the benefit of allowing the activation of T cells but avoiding T cell restimulation and propriocidal death too soon in the response to antigen. Recent work in mice genetically engineered to selectively express the p35 apoptosis inhibitory protein in DCs reveals that apoptotic removal of DCs is essential to preserve tolerance and prevent autoimmunity (157). Moreover, autoimmunity was accelerated when such mice were backcrossed onto the autoimmune-prone *MRL* strain. A similar acceleration in autoimmunity is observed when mice with T and B cell apoptosis defects are on an *MRL* genetic background. Thus, impaired DC apoptosis can collaborate with other genetic and environmental factors to powerfully predispose to autoimmunity.

PCD as an Immune Effector Mechanism

Although this topic will be covered authoritatively elsewhere in the book, it is important to recognize that the same pathways that participate in homeostatic cell death also are used as immune effector mechanisms. The Fas pathway is now recognized as the principal Ca^{2+}-independent pathway of cytotoxic T cell (CTL) killing (71). Fas ligand displayed by either $CD4^+$ or $CD8^+$ T cells can eliminate Fas-bearing cells that may be infected or malignant by inducing caspase-mediated apoptosis. Similarly, the Ca^{2+}-dependent CTL mechanism involving perforin and granzymes also can induce PCD in target cells. The two main proteases are granzyme A and granzyme B; this latter is the only serine protease capable of processing caspases *(158–162)*. When perforin breaches the target cell membrane, granzyme B gains access to the cytoplasm and proteolytically activates caspases leading to apoptosis. Although this cytoplasmic pathway of death does not emanate from the mitochondria, the latter may amplify the death signal by Bid cleavage (*163*,164,*165*,166,*167*). These parallels may provide an insight into why lymphocytes have evolved an indirect mechanism, involving the surface interaction of FasL and Fas or perforin/granzyme releases to homeostatically control their numbers by apoptosis. This mechanism permits the T cell to regulate itself, other immune cells, and expunge nonlymphoid cells that require immune elimination, such as those that are infected or malignant. Natural killer cells may also use PCD mechanisms for self-regulation and expunging infected or malignant cells (168,*169*). Hence, for mature T cells, the same molecules can subserve several death functions, perhaps even simultaneously. By contrast, a more direct connection of the TCR or BCR to death pathways is present in developing lymphocytes, which have no use for effector mechanisms or propriocidal regulation.

CELLULAR AND MOLECULAR MECHANISMS OF PCD

Apoptosis Initiation Mediated by Caspase Complexes: Two Principal Pathways

Caspases must be highly active within the cell cytoplasm to cause apoptosis. Like all proteases, these potentially destructive proteins are first produced as zymogens that are then proteolytically activated. In mammalian cells, the molecules and pathways regulating caspase activation are complex (Figure 27.3). Elucidating these complex pathways provides a window into the myriad of molecular abnormalities of apoptosis that contribute to immunological diseases and cancer. Fortunately, mammalian apoptosis can be understood with a few key concepts. Most importantly, the processing enzymes that activate caspases are caspases themselves. As explained later, activation and autoprocessing occur when caspase zymogens are brought into specific signaling complexes. In general there are two main forms of caspases. Those with long prodomains that have protein interaction domains capable of bringing them into activating platforms for autoprocessing are called *initiators,* upstream, or *apical caspases.* Those with short prodomains that must be cleaved by other proteases (caspases or granzyme B) are called *effectors,* downstream, or *executioner caspases.* This is achieved by various adapter molecules with domains that specifically recruit and assemble caspases into complexes: the death effector domains (DEDs) or the caspase recruitment domains (CARD) *(170,171)*. The DED and CARD are protein–protein interaction domains found in the caspase prodomains and other adapter molecules that generate the specific intermolecular assemblies. In contrast to executioner caspases, which require processing to become active, dimerization of initiator caspases drives their activation (172,*173*). When juxtaposed at the receptor complex, initiator caspases become proteolytically active and will cleave one another. This leads to the maturation of the enzyme through separation of the large and small enzymatic subunits. Autoprocessing also cleaves the enzymatic units from the prodomain, thereby liberating the highly active enzyme from the receptor complex. As discussed later in the chapter, structural studies suggest that active caspases are tetrameric species composed of two small and two large subunits. Hence, it is likely that activation and autoprocessing of caspases involves the cross-cleavage of at least two units of the unprocessed zymogen.

To initiate the caspase cascade, the enzyme must dock onto the appropriate adapter molecules. The adapter/caspase complex presumably provides a conformation that facilitates the initial autoprocessing step of the caspase zymogen. Adapter/caspase complexes originate from two principal sites in the cell: 1) the plasma membrane (through DRs), also known as extrinsic pathway, or 2) the mitochondrion, or intrinsic pathway (Figure 27.3). We will employ this primary dichotomy of intrinsic and extrinsic pathways since it recapitulates the two major forms of propriocidal apoptosis: antigen-induced and lymphokine withdrawal, respectively.

DR engagement by cognate ligand causes the formation of the death-inducing signaling complex (DISC), which comprises the cytoplasmic tail of the receptor, the FADD adapter protein, and caspase-8 or -10 (*174*,175). The recruitment of caspase-8 or -10 into the DISC triggers the processing of these proteases into their active form. An 80-amino acid death domain (DD) present in the Fas cytoplasmic tail and FADD causes their interaction. The DD

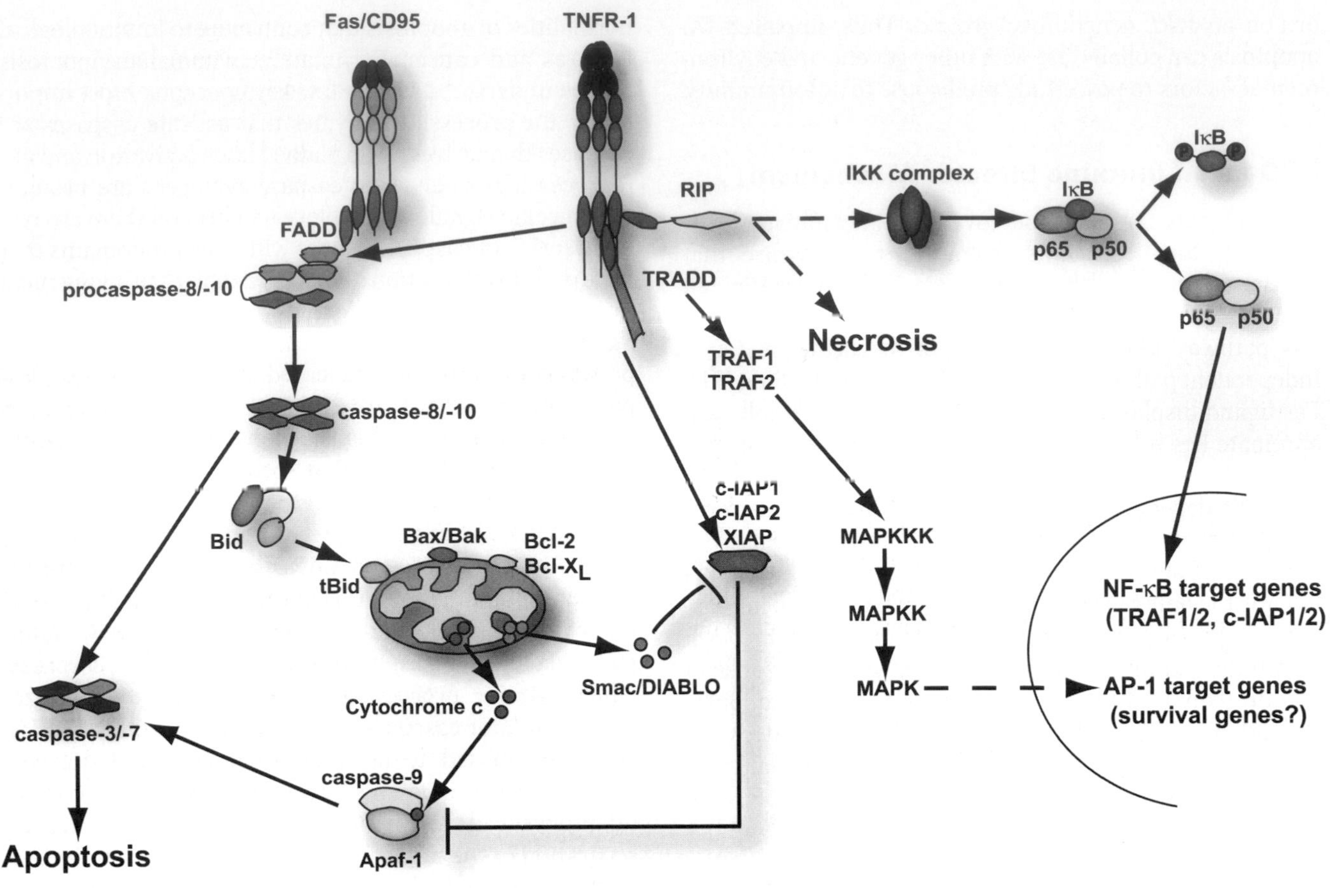

FIGURE 27.3 Signal transduction pathways of death receptors. Shown are the two principal apoptosis pathways associated with death receptors (Fas and TNFR-1) and that associated with the mitochondrial pathway of caspase-9 activation. The solid arrows indicate direct association of the steps involved, whereas the dashed arrows indicate that multiple steps are involved. Inhibitory interactions are shown by a barred line.

contains a "hexahelical bundle" that nucleates this complex, as described in greater detail later. There is an obligatory 3: 3 stoichiometry of the FADD adapter protein and the Fas receptor. FADD recruits caspase-8 or -10 by homotypic interaction between DEDs present in each of these molecules. The DED has a hexahelical bundle homologous but not identical to DDs. Sensitive energy transfer techniques showed that both caspases can enter the same receptor complex (176). FADD self-association at the receptor level also triggers the formation of microscopically visible clusters of Fas, termed *SPOTS* (signaling protein oligomerization transduction structures). These structures enhance caspase-8 recruitment and activation (177). Fas receptor capping and internalization in endosomal vesicles follow SPOTS formation and may promote the killing process *(178)*. The signal complex for TNFR-1 is different from Fas since it includes the DD-containing adapter TRADD in addition to FADD and caspase-8 and -10 (discussed later). Similar signaling complexes are likely formed with other DD-containing members of the TNFR superfamily including DR 3, TRAIL receptors (TR)-1 and -2 (also called DR-4 and -5, respectively), and DR 6 *(179–181)*. The physiological significance of apoptosis mediated by any of these receptors besides Fas and TNFR-1 in immune regulation is unknown, although DR6 has been implicated in Th2 cell differentiation *(182,183)*. It has been proposed that TR-1 and TR-2 may mediate the preferential killing of tumor cells (including lymphoid tumors) (184).

Activation of the mitochondrial pathway of apoptosis during lymphokine withdrawal or in response to developmental cues achieves the same end as DRs caspase activation. However, signal complex formation occurs in a different way. Intrinsic signals converge on the mitochondria, resulting in outer membrane permeabilization (MOMP) and the release of the pro-apoptotic molecules from the intermembrane space (IMS) into the cytosol. One key factor released is cytochrome c, a molecule also involved in the electron transport chain. Once liberated into the cytosol, cytochrome c binds and triggers the oligomerization of apoptotic protease-activating factor 1 (Apaf-1) in the presence of ATP/dATP, to form a heptameric complex often referred to as the *apoptosome* (*185*,186). The complex nucleates caspase-9 recruitment and activation (reviewed in [187,*188,189*]). There are specialized regulatory proteins for caspase-9 that provide additional levels of control: X-linked IAP (XIAP), which inhibits caspase-9, and Smac/Diablo, which counteracts XIAP (190,191). These mitochondrial events are tightly regulated since caspase-9 activation commits the cell to die.

The Central Role of the Mitochondrion

A special role for the mitochondrion in apoptosis was first suggested by the finding that Bcl-2 and related molecules were anchored predominantly in the outer mitochondrial membrane (OMM). The inner mitochondrial membrane (IMM) is devoted to energy conversion and ATP generation, but the OMM has emerged as a primary regulator of cell viability. A diversity of death inducers, including trophic factor withdrawal, drugs such as staurosporine or steroids, or DNA damage, can all generate signals that converge on the mitochondrion. Their principle effect is to increase OMM permeability to large proteins, leading to the release of apoptogenic factors into the cytosol. As described earlier, cytochrome c coalesces with Apaf-1 and caspase-9 into a lethal proteolytic complex soon after its release into the cytosol. The essential role of cytochrome c in apoptosis was elegantly demonstrated by generating "knock in" mice expressing a mutant cytochrome c (K72A) (192). This mutant version of cytochrome c retains its electron transfer function but lacks its ability to activate Apaf-1. The mutant mice display developmental abnormalities similar to Apaf-1 or caspase-9–deficient animals, and the surviving mice exhibit impaired lymphocyte homeostasis. In contrast to Apaf-1$^{-/-}$ cells, thymocytes from these mice were normally sensitive to intrinsic stimuli such as γ-irradiation, dexamethasone, and etoposide. This implies the existence of a cytochrome c- and apoptosome-independent but Apaf-1–dependent mechanism of caspase activation and cell death (192).

Interestingly, 85% of cytochrome c is sequestered inside the intra-cristae region formed by the convoluted folds of IMM, with a limited access to the IMS *(193)*. Therefore, the sudden "all-or-nothing" release of cytochrome c requires two steps: 1) a BH3-only–dependent (typically Bid) remodeling of the cristae structure allowing cytochrome c to access the IMS, and 2) the Bax- and Bak-dependent permeabilization of the OMM. The cristae structure was recently shown to be controlled by the IMM Presenilin-associated rhomboid-like protein (PARL) and by the IMS resident dynamin-related Optic Atrophy 1 (OPA1) (194,195). In yeast, homologues of these proteins, Rbd1 and Mgm1 respectively, regulate mitochondrial fusion, a process of mitochondrial metabolism. Mice deficient for PARL die between 8 weeks and 12 weeks of progressive cachexia, and their lymphocytes undergo massive apoptosis. Moreover, MEFs derived from these animals were significantly more sensitive to intrinsic stimuli, demonstrating the anti-apoptotic function of PARL. Normally, PARL cleaves OPA1, and both cleaved and uncleaved OPA1 form hetero-oligomers that maintain a tight bottleneck configuration of the cristae, keeping cytochrome c sequestered.

How the OMM releases its mortal poison is still unclear, and two models have been proposed. In one, the pro-apoptotic Bcl-2 family proteins Bax and Bak selectively permeabilize the OMM, without affecting the IMM. In the second model, a pore in the IMM known as the mitochondrial permeability transition complex (mPTC) opens and allows water and solutes up to 1.5 kDa to accumulate into the matrix. The matrix swells as water enters, and the OMM bursts *(196,197)*. Cells from mice lacking cyclophilin D, a critical component of the mPTC, remain sensitive to intrinsic death insults, favoring the first model. However, the mPTC appears to be essential for stimuli promoting necrosis such as calcium overload and ROS. Perhaps this accounts for the fact that the knockout mice were resistant to ischemia/reperfusion-induced cardiac injury (198,199). As detailed later in this chapter, MOMP appears to be regulated and coordinated by the large family of proteins related to Bcl-2.

In addition to cytochrome c, several other pro-apoptotic proteins from the IMS are released outside the mitochondria during apoptosis. The flavoprotein "apoptosis-inducing factor" (AIF) translocates from the mitochondria to the nucleus, causing DNA fragmentation and chromatin condensation in response to apoptotic stimuli (200,*201*). Genetic deficiency of this protein in mice inhibits the death of embryonic cells in response to serum starvation and leads to defects in embryonic morphogenesis and cavitation of the embryonic cell mass. The observation that these processes did not depend on caspase-3, caspase-9, or Apaf-1, suggests that unlike *C. elegans,* not all programmed death in mammalian cells is dependent on caspases (202). Further work with conditional genetic deficiencies of AIF in immune cell lineages will be needed to determine whether this mechanism has any role in immunity. Another mitochondrial protein important in apoptosis is endonuclease G (EndoG). EndoG is a resident mitochondrial nuclease that is released and translocates to the nucleus upon apoptotic stimulation. Once situated in the nucleus, EndoG cleaves DNA into nucleosomal sizes independent of caspases, thus distinguishing itself from the caspase-dependent activation of another apoptotic nuclease CAD (203) (see later discussion). Thus, the mitochondrion may participate in nuclear chromatin fragmentation, which is one of the chief effects of apoptosis. When released in the cytosol, Smac/DIABLO and Omi/HtrA2 neutralize the inhibitors of apoptosis proteins (IAPs), and thus promote caspase activation.

Studies on the mitochondrion have also focused on caspase-independent apoptosis. AIF, EndoG, and Omi/HtrA2 were proposed to mediate such a pathway. In general, this concept stemmed from examples of apoptosis that could not be blocked by small peptide caspase inhibitors such as zVAD (204,*205*). However, conclusions drawn from such experiments are limited by the short half-life of such inhibitors and the fact that they do not block all caspases. Also, kinetic experiments show that AIF release occurs slowly secondary to the fast simultaneous redistribution of cytochrome c, Smac/DIABLO, and Omi/HtrA2 (*206*,207). Finally, cells from double-knockout mice for the executioner caspases-3 and -7 exhibit a delayed translocation of cytochrome c and AIF, indicating that caspases act as an amplification loop necessary to fully permeabilize the mitochondria (208). Thus, it is uncertain if there is a truly caspase-independent form of apoptosis, although the possibility remains.

Programmed Necrosis

While PCD has generally been equated with apoptosis, recent evidence suggests that necrotic or alternative forms of death may also result from internal death programs (204,*205*,*209*,210). This is different from secondary necrosis that occurs in the late phase of apoptosis when membrane integrity is lost. Rather, PCD leading to a necrotic morphology without any intermediate stage of apoptosis or caspase activation is now well documented (18,202). For example, it has been found that DRs can trigger necrotic death rather than apoptotic death under certain circumstances (204,*205*,*209*). Although TNF stimulation through TNFR-1 can trigger caspase-dependent, classical apoptosis, necrosis may well be the dominant pathway for TNFR-1, at least in certain cell types (204,*209*). By contrast, Fas predominantly triggers apoptosis but can also induce necrosis (18). A shift from apoptosis to necrosis can be induced by tetrapeptide caspase inhibitors suggesting that a necrotic pathway may exist for cell elimination when apoptosis fails or is blocked *(205)*. Moreover, the recent identification and characterization of a small molecule that specifically inhibits necrosis but not apoptosis points to a distinct biochemical pathway for programmed necrosis (19). These observations have physiological relevance since propriocidal death of mature T cells is partly refractory to inhibition by caspase blockers and can manifest features of necrosis (18). For these reasons, we have chosen to introduce the name *programmed necrosis* to describe death by necrosis (or at least a clearly nonapoptotic phenotype) that results from a specific molecular pathway and appears to be advantageous to the host.

An interesting example of programmed necrosis has been investigated by Tschopp and coworkers. They have shown that necrosis can occur through strong Fas stimulation in a process that requires the receptor interacting protein (RIP) (18). Originally identified by a yeast two-hybrid interaction screen using the DD of Fas as bait *(211)*, RIP was later found to be an essential component of the TNFR-1 signaling complex that could induce the anti-apoptotic transcription factor NF-κB (211–213, *214*). Besides a carboxyl terminal DD that is required for homotypic binding to the receptor-signaling complex, RIP also contains an amino-terminal serine/threonine kinase domain that is dispensable to its apoptosis-inducing activity but is essential for its necrotic function. Both direct Fas engagement or TCR stimulation (which presumably indirectly triggers Fas by FasL induction) can stimulate necrosis *in vitro* (18). A similar form of RIP-dependent, caspase-independent necrosis has also been observed for TNFR-1 (17,215). Thus, RIP appears to be a bifunctional signaling molecule with stimulatory and necrosis-inducing effects. Paradoxically, RIP-deficient mice are severely runted and die shortly after birth, apparently due to increased TNF-induced death due impaired NF-κB induction (216). Because Fas-induced PCD has not been investigated extensively in the RIP-deficient animals, it remains to be seen whether RIP-dependent programmed necrosis has any role in normal physiology. Nevertheless, RIP appears to be the clearest talisman of a molecular pathway of programmed necrosis. The downstream signals in this pathway remain obscure, but in the case of TNF are distinct from the TRADD-dependent, caspase-dependent apoptotic pathway (215) and may partially involve oxidative stress (215,*217*). Cyclophilin D can regulate some forms of necrotic death induced by ROS and calcium but its role has not yet been studied in lymphocytes (198,199).

What is the potential role of DR-induced necrosis in immunity? Many viruses, particularly the poxviruses, encode inhibitors of caspases (17,*218*). Infection by poxviruses leads to blockade of caspase-dependent apoptosis. This sensitizes cells to TNF-induced necrosis *(219)*. Therefore, programmed necrosis may serve to counteract the effects of viral anti-apoptotic mechanisms by eliminating virally infected cells. From an immunological standpoint, necrotic cells may have a superior stimulatory activity than apoptotic cells for DC maturation *(23,24)*. During viral infection, TNF-induced necrosis may indirectly enhance the CTL response to the virus by promoting the maturation of DCs. Programmed necrosis may therefore have an immunostimulatory role in addition to directly eliminating virus-infected cells. Programmed necrosis could thereby serve as a "bridge" between the innate arm of immunity and the adaptive immune response.

Another important reason to further understand necrosis in the context of the immune system is that it may be responsible for the pathogenesis of viruses such as human immunodeficiency virus (HIV). Although many claims have been made that HIV causes apoptosis—of either directly infected or bystander T cells—most dying infected cells do not manifest hallmarks of apoptosis. Further, these cells actually appear necrotic when examined by electron microscopy (Figure 27.1) (220). Hence, apoptosis does not appear to be the major mode of death. HIV-induced necrosis is not impaired by the absence of RIP, thus distinguishing it from DR-induced necrosis. Further studies on identifying the molecules involved in virally induced necrosis are needed to determine whether it involves a specific molecular program or simply lethal cell injury.

FAMILIES OF MOLECULES PROVIDE PRECISE REGULATION OF PCD

Caspases

A key concept in understanding PCD is that it was apparently so vital to the successful evolution of multicellular organisms that a specific set of genes was dedicated to the task. Chief among these genes were those encoding caspases. Junying Yuan and H. Robert Horvitz in 1993 first observed that a gene crucial for PCD in *C. elegans*, ced-3, was related to a mammalian caspase, IL-1ß-converting enzyme (ICE), thus implicating specific proteolytic events in the death program (221). The "caspase" moniker is a rubric indicating that these enzymes contain an active site <u>C</u>ysteine, cleave substrates on the carboxyl side of **<u>ASP</u>**artate residues, and are prote**<u>ASES</u>**. Caspases have been called the "executioners" of apoptosis. Once activated, their cleavage of various cellular substrates, including other caspases, results in the morphological features of apoptotic cell death. Earnshaw et al. (222) authoritatively discuss the detailed biochemical features of caspases and their substrates, which are beyond the scope of this chapter. There are 15 caspases in mammals *(223)*. All appear to be involved in apoptosis except human caspase-1 (ICE) and caspase-4 (caspase-11 in the mouse), which serve to proteolytically process the precursors of cytokines such as IL-1ß into their mature forms. In addition to its pro-apoptotic role, caspase-12 was recently proposed to inhibit the proinflammatory functions of caspase-1. Indeed, caspase-12 functions as a FLIP and directly binds to caspase-1 to suppress its activity. Functionally, mice deficient in caspase-12 are resistant to sepsis and clear bacterial infection more efficiently. Further, humans with a caspase-12 polymorphism that results in an inactive truncated protein have increased LPS-stimulated cytokine production, as well as a correspondingly decreased risk for developing and dying from sepsis (224,225).

Much early work equated caspase enzymatic activity with processing. Although true for the so-called downstream "effector" caspases, recent studies have established that cleavage is neither necessary nor sufficient for activation of initiator caspases (172). Rather, oligomerization of procaspases-8 or -10 within the DISC, procaspase-9 within the apoptosome, or procaspase-2 within an Apaf-1–independent complex, is sufficient for activity *(226–229)*. The proximity-induced dimerization of the initiator caspases is due to their long N-terminal prodomains, which allow the caspases to enter into large activating multimeric complexes (as described later). Further processing of active procaspases may stabilize activity or allow for diffusion of active caspases intracellularly where they can access other protein substrates.

Because of the thermodynamic irreversibility of proteolysis, downstream caspase activation is a commitment to death that cannot be undone. Hence, caspases are tightly regulated. This regulation is achieved by three principle means: 1) Caspases are zymogens requiring proteolytic processing; 2) Certain caspases have long "prodomains" that allow them to enter complexes with adaptor molecules that promote autoprocessing; and 3) Specific inhibitors exist (6). How these mechanisms work is clear from the structures of caspases (Figure 27.4). Caspases have an NH_2-terminal "prodomain" that is removed in the active enzyme. The COOH-terminal protease domain comprises two catalytic subunits of the mature enzyme that are denoted by their processed molecular weights—for example, p20 and p10. The processing sites between these parts occur at short specific tetrapeptide sequences ending in aspartate residues that dictate that the major processing enzymes are caspases themselves (222). For caspases with short prodomains, namely caspases 3, 6, and 7, this event is believed to be the primary mode of regulation. Those with long prodomains harbor protein-interaction domains that allow them to enter activating complexes for specific death pathways as described earlier. Caspase-8 and -10 have DEDs and caspases-1, -2, -4/-11, -5, -9, -12, and -13 have CARD domains. How complex formation stimulates autoprocessing is not understood, but likely involves a stoichiometry in which multiple proenzymes come into close contact. Within such a complex, the proenzyme chains adopt a more active structure that may or may not resemble the final processed active structure. The liberated subunits form a heterotetramer of two large and two small enzyme subunits as reflected in the crystal structures of processed caspases (230,231,*232–234*). The consequences of subunit cleavage are dramatic: There is a 180° shift of the NH_2-terminus of the small subunit to bring it into apposition with the catalytic cleft (235). To begin autoprocessing, an active intermediate pseudoconformation could be stabilized by internal hydrophobic interactions or by the action of chaperones. After caspase zymogens are recruited to a trimeric DR complex, an enzyme pseudostructure formed by two precursors could process a third proenzyme molecule. Subsequent subunit rearrangements could then lead to processing of additional unprocessed chains. Once a processed heterotetramer is formed, it will be thermodynamically stable and move away from the activating complex. If the stoichiometry of the activating complexes requires three proenzymes, this would match the

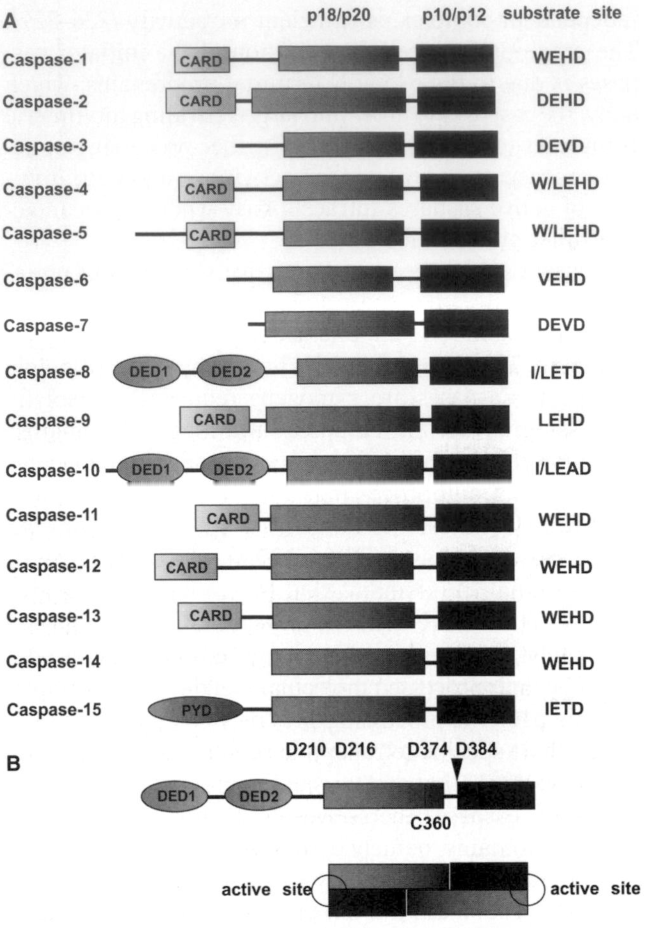

FIGURE 27.4 Mammalian caspases. **A:** The structures of the 15 known mammalian caspases are shown. Many of the caspases contain at their NH_2-terminal the CARD domain. Caspase-8 and caspase-10 contain a tandem copy of the DED at the NH_2-terminal end of the pro-enzyme, which is essential for recruitment to the DISC. Caspase-15 contains a pyrin (PYD) domain at the NH_2-terminus. The large (p18/p20) and small (p10/p12) subunits near the COOH-terminals are also shown. The optimal tetrapeptide substrate specificity of each caspase is shown on the right-hand column. Notice that the caspase-4 and caspase-11 are human and mouse homologues, respectively (asterisks). **B:** Proximity-induced oligomerization is crucial in activating initiator pro-enzymes, which also undergo autoproteolytic cleavage. Shown in the diagram by the arrows are the proteolytic cleavage sites of caspase-8 at aspartate residues 210, 216, 374, and 384, as well as the active site cysteine (C360) indicated by a bar. Two of each of the large and small subunits of the enzyme form the active enzyme in a head-to-tail conformation, resulting in a tetramer that contains two catalytic sites at the two ends of the molecule. The active sites of the enzyme, which are made up of residues from both the large and small subunits, are designated by the circles at the ends of the processed enzyme.

symmetry of DRs (see later discussion). Proteolytic activation is regulated by a variety of proteins. These inhibitors interact with the fully formed enzyme and remain bound as competitive inhibitors. Examples of such inhibitors are the CrmA protein, its homologs found in other viruses, and the IAP proteins *(218,236)*. Other viral proteins that harbor DEDs can enter the DR signaling complexes and inhibit cleavage of caspases-8 and -10 (114,*237*). Initially, it was thought that these inhibitors, termed *v-FLIPs* for *viral FLICE (caspase-8) inhibitory proteins,* inhibit apoptosis by competing with caspase-8 and -10 for entry into the DR complex. However, it is now clear that the inhibitor and the caspase enter the complex together. Resolution of the crystal structure of MC159, a v-FLIP from the pox virus Molluscum contagiosum virus, reveals that it cooperatively assembles with FADD and Fas through an extensive charge surface encompassing a conserved charge triad. This prevents FADD self-aggregation and disrupts higher order oligomerization necessary for activation of caspases-8 and -10 (238). Cellular FLIP, or *c-FLIP,* is structurally homologous to caspase-8 and -10 (indeed, it is encoded in the same locus on human chromosome 2 as these caspases) but has multiple mutations in the caspase domain that inactivate its protease function (116). It can also enter the Fas signaling complexes and prevent caspase recruitment and activation (238,239). However, c-FLIP can also induce apoptosis under certain conditions, which may be due to its ability to heterodimerize with and thus activate procaspase-8 *(240)*. The ability of antigen receptor stimulation to block Fas-induced death in B cells is regulated in part by c-FLIP *(117)*.

Another class of caspase regulators is the cellular IAPs (c-IAPs) that can directly inactivate mature caspases to avert the deleterious effects of inadvertent caspase activation (118,*119*). IAPs are characterized by the presence of up to three baculovirus IAP repeats (BIRs). Originally identified in baculovirus, the BIR domains are characterized by the presence of cysteine and histidine residues in defined spacing arrangements ($Cx_2Cx_6Wx_3Dx_5Hx_6C$) (for review, see [118]). The mechanisms of inhibition by IAPs on different caspases are quite distinct. For caspase-9, inhibition by XIAP depends on binding of the BIR3 domain with the tetrapeptide sequence ATPF at the NH_2-terminal of the p12 subunit that is exposed only in the mature enzyme. Hence, XIAP specifically inhibits active caspase-9, but not pro-caspase-9 (190). By contrast, XIAP inhibits caspase-7 and -3 by forming contacts in the catalytic groove with little involvement of the BIR domains (241). Interestingly, this mechanism of XIAP association is adopted by Smac/Diablo to inhibit the anti-apoptotic function of XIAP during the onset of mitochondrial PCD pathways (191). Smac/Diablo is a protein that resides in the intermembrane space of the mitochondria. It functions as an elongated dimer of α helices that adopts the shape of an arch. The NH_2-terminal amino acids AVPI generated from cleavage of the mitochondria targeting sequence are not well organized in the crystal structure. Nevertheless, they are critical for the inhibitory function of the protein. Mutation of alanine to methionine abolished the inhibitory activity of Smac/Diablo on XIAP (190,191).

This IAP-binding motif (IBM) is also shared by other IAP antagonists (Omi/HtrA2, and GSPT1/eRF3), and by caspase-9, suggesting that IAP antagonists and caspase-9 compete for binding to XIAP (190). The action of XIAP is flexible in order to carry out diverse functions. Instead of the BIR3 domain, XIAP uses the linker region between BIR1 and BIR2 to interact with and inhibit the function of caspases-3 and -7. In this case, the linker inserts into the catalytic groove of the caspase in reverse orientation to that of the tetrapeptide inhibitor DEVD-CHO. While BIR2 does not directly participate in the inhibitory activity, it may contribute to the stability of the association by making other contacts with caspase-3 (231,242,243).

The death-inducing effect of caspases is highly specific in that most proteins in the dying cell remain uncleaved. Lethality is therefore due to cleavage of a limited set of targets. Caspases have an absolute requirement for aspartate at the amino side of its cleavage sites (P1 site). Further specificity is dictated in part by the three amino acids preceding the obligatory aspartate in the substrate (P2-P4 positions) (222). Preferred tetrapeptides have been identified for each of the mammalian caspases so that, for example, caspase-3 is known to preferentially cleave at the sequence DEVD, whereas caspase-8 prefers IETD (*12,244,*245). Nicholson and coworkers have developed valuable tetrapeptide substrates and inhibitors based on these preferences, but they emphasize that these are not absolutely specific (*12,*222). In addition to primary amino acid sequence, additional secondary structural features of target proteins may be recognized. For example, many proteins harboring a DVED sequence may not be cleaved at that sequence by caspase-3 *(119)*. Thus, the tetrapeptide recognition sequences are required but not sufficient for apoptotic protein cleavage. Nevertheless, model caspase substrates and inhibitors based on short recognition peptides, such as zVAD- or DVED-fmk (fluoromethyl ketone), have been useful in assessing caspase function *in vitro* and *in vivo*.

Proteins known to be cleaved by caspases in the dying cells have been grouped according to apparent functional importance: a) cytoskeletal proteins such as actin, gelsolin, and α-fodrin, among others; b) nuclear structure proteins, especially lamins A and B; c) DNA metabolism and repair proteins such as poly (ADP-ribose) polymerase (PARP); d) protein kinases, such as various isoforms of PKC; e) signal transduction proteins such as STAT1, SREBP-1 and phospholipase C-γ1. A more extensive discussion of identified caspase substrates has been published (222). Since PCD typically involves the elimination of somatic cells, there may be little evolutionary constraint on random cleavage sites. Hence, it has been difficult to distinguish functional versus adventitious sites. Key caspase substrates that have unequivocal roles in apoptosis include caspases themselves, Bcl-2 and Bcl-X_L, the ICAD inhibitor (inhibitor of caspase activated deoxyribonuclease) of the DNase CAD, which is one enzyme causing apoptotic nuclear fragmentation, and the nuclear lamins *(246,247)*. Cleavage of the nuclear lamins was shown by Eileen White to be responsible for certain nuclear changes in apoptosis by experiments in which the aspartate cleavage sites were modified and the apoptotic changes were abrogated (248). This stringent test has been applied to very few proteins cleaved during apoptosis. In fact, evidence weighs against the role of many caspase substrates in apoptosis. The knockout of the PARP gene in mice revealed no abnormality of development, immunity, or apoptosis (249). Hence, further work is necessary to determine the importance of proteins cleaved during apoptosis.

Genetic analyses of human caspases have provided important information about their function. By contrast, homozygous deficiencies in mice have been associated with embryonic lethality or neurological defects but have not yielded specific immunological phenotypes (222). Inherited mutations of two caspases in humans cause prominent effects in the immune system. The first, an inherited mutation in caspase-10, was detected in the human disease ALPS, type II (156,250). Individuals with caspase-10 mutations exhibited defects in apoptosis triggered by multiple DRs affecting the homeostasis of T cells, B cells, and DCs. The abnormal accumulation of immune cells leads to the formation of a variety of autoantibodies that cause autoimmune conditions including hemolytic anemia, thrombocytopenia, and others. Individuals harboring mutations in caspase-8 have also been identified (251). These individuals also exhibit abnormal lymphocyte apoptosis and the accumulation of lymphocytes in secondary lymphoid tissues. However, unlike a caspase-10 mutant individual, the lack of caspase-8 leads to minimal autoimmunity. Rather, the affected individuals exhibit immunodeficiency manifested as recurrent sinopulmonary and viral infections. Biochemical analysis shows that caspase-8 is required for NF-κB induction by the TCR, BCR, and Fc receptor, which accounts for this T, B, and NK lymphocyte activation defects. These patients represent a novel clinical entity, termed *caspase-8 deficiency state* (CEDS) (252). The clinical differences between humans having caspase-10 or caspase-8 mutations may reflect differences in substrate specificities of these two closely related caspases (176,*253*).

TNF/TNFR Superfamily Members

The TNF/TNFR superfamily contains many key regulators of immunity (Figure 27.5). These receptors and their cognate ligands facilitate communication between immune cells in the orchestration of immune responses. They also comprise a major class of cellular sensors to external physiological cues that regulate PCD (254). The hallmark of these receptors is the presence of "cysteine-rich domains" (CRDs) in the extracellular region, which are required for receptor assembly and ligand binding. Each receptor

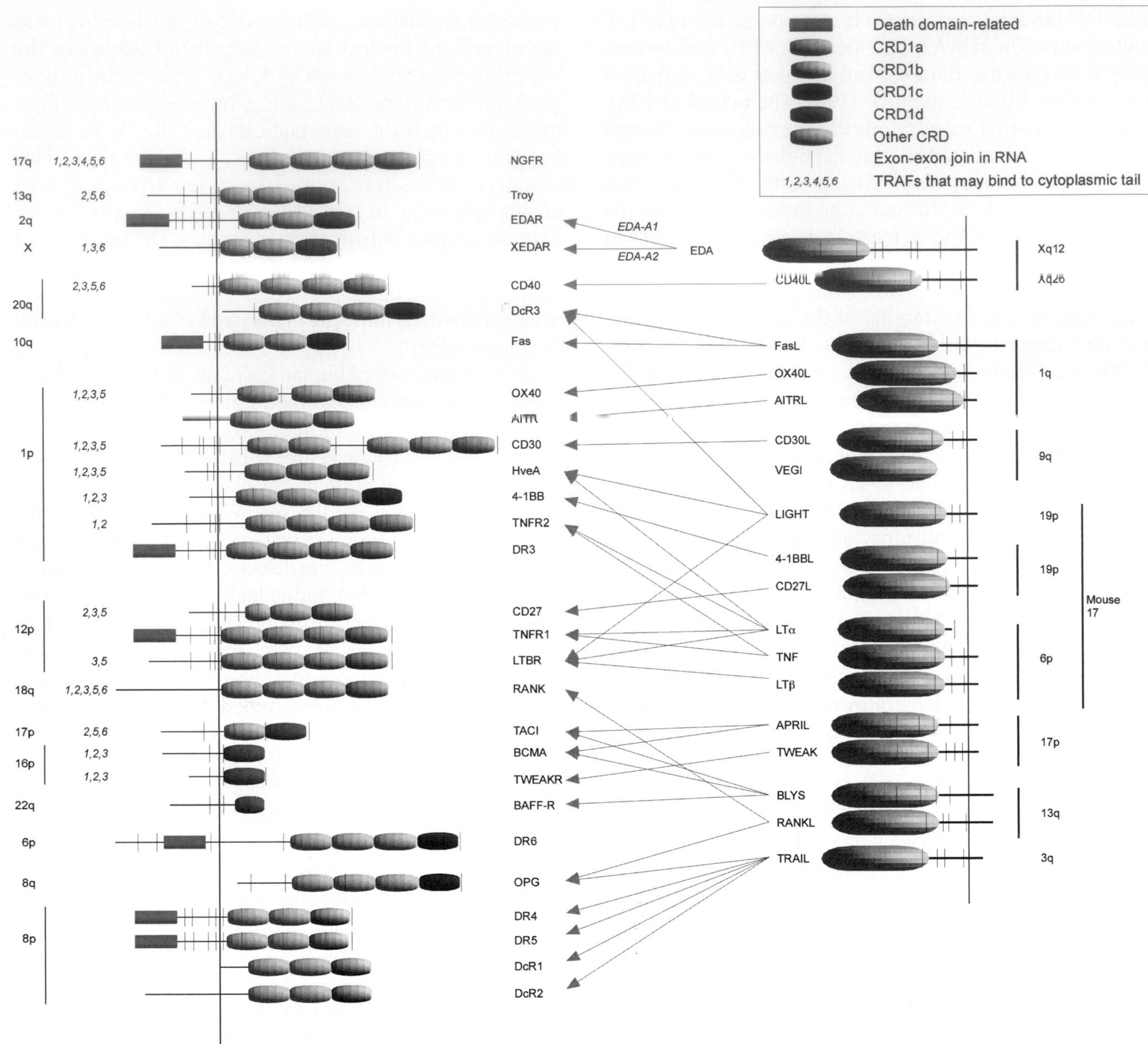

FIGURE 27.5 Interacting proteins of the TNF/TNFR superfamily. TNFR- and TNF-related proteins are shown at the left and right of the figure, respectively, with arrows connecting ligand-receptor pairs. CRDs are shown as small ovals. The NH_2-terminal CRDs (CRD1a,1b,1c,1d) are grouped on the basis of sequence similarity as indicated by the use of colors in the figure. Small vertical lines denote the locations of intron excision sites from the RNAs that encode the proteins (this information was not available for RANK, DcR1 and DcR2). Red boxes mark the locations of DD-related sequences in the cytoplasmic regions of the TNFR-related proteins. Numbers to the immediate left of the TNFR cytoplasmic regions denote known or inferred interactions with the indicated TRAFs. The locations of the human genes that encode the proteins are provided at the extreme left and right of the figure; the mouse cluster on chromosome 17 is also noted. (Figure adapted from [61] with permission from Cell Press by Nigel Killeen)

contains between one (BCMA and TWEAK-R) *(255,256)* to six (CD30) CRDs. The receptors can be further subdivided into two classes based on sequence homology within the cytoplasmic signaling domain. The DRs contain an 80-residue-long DD that is essential for death signaling *(174,*257). The majority of the receptors lack a DD, and therefore are not called DRs, but have a region that interacts with the TRAF (TNF receptor associated factors) proteins *(258)*. Interestingly, some of the DRs, including TNFR-1, can indirectly recruit TRAF proteins, which may explain cross-talk between certain DD-containing and DD-lacking receptors (259,260,*261*). Signals transduced by the non-DD-containing receptors are frequently pro-survival, while that of the DRs are typically pro-apoptotic. In all, more than 20 members of the TNF receptor family in humans have been identified (61). With a few exceptions (EDAR and XEDAR), essentially all TNFRs play important regulatory roles in the immune system.

Signaling by the TNFRs is initiated when the cognate ligands, which are obligate trimers, contacts the pre-formed receptor complex (reviewed in [*259*,262]). Down-stream signaling of DRs requires the recruitment of DD- or DED-containing proteins. For Fas, receptor engagement results in rapid recruitment of FADD and caspases-8 or -10 within the DISC, as detailed earlier (175). Other DRs such as TNFR-1 may require recruitment of an additional adaptor molecule like TRADD prior to the docking of FADD (263). These events rapidly culminate in caspase activation. The non-DD-containing receptors mediate NF-κB induction and the activation of c-Jun kinases through the recruitment of TRAF proteins, a property that is shared by some DRs such as TNFR-1. Recruitment of TRAF proteins by DRs may counter the pro-apoptotic response through their interactions with c-IAPs. "Knockout" analyses in mice reveal that many of these signaling intermediates, including TRAF2 (264), RIP (213), and components of the NF-κB activation pathway *(265–269)*, are essential for conferring protection against apoptosis induced by DR ligands. Deficiency of NF-κB tends to sensitize cells to TNF-induced death (270–272). Both TRAF2 and NF-κB induction through RIP may act in concert to promote survival in response to TNF (273). Interestingly, unlike the TNFR-1 and Fas-deficient mice, which are viable, knockout of the signaling components such as FADD or TRADD often results in embryonic lethality. The discordant results in knockout animals imply that TNFR signaling intermediates are involved in ontogenetic processes other than PCD. Alternatively, other TNFRs may mediate critical PCD events during development using the same set of signaling molecules. However, many other TNFR-deficient animals, including Fas-, DR6-, or multiply-deficient animals (TNFR1$^{-/-}$, TNFR2$^{-/-}$, and Fas$^{lpr/lpr}$ together) are viable, thus arguing against the latter hypothesis (*182,183*,274).

Bcl-2 Gene Family

Bcl-2 and Bcl-X$_L$ are the prototypes of a diverse family of apoptosis-regulatory proteins whose filial relationships are conferred by four impressively short homology regions, termed BH-1 to BH-4 (Figure 27.6) (275,*276*). Proteins in this family can be classified into three groups: 1) the "multidomain" anti-apoptotic proteins (Bcl-2, Bcl-X$_L$, Mcl-1, Bcl-w, A1, and BOO), which contain the four BH domains; 2) the "multidomain" pro-apoptotic Bax, Bak, and Bok that possess BH1–3 domains; and

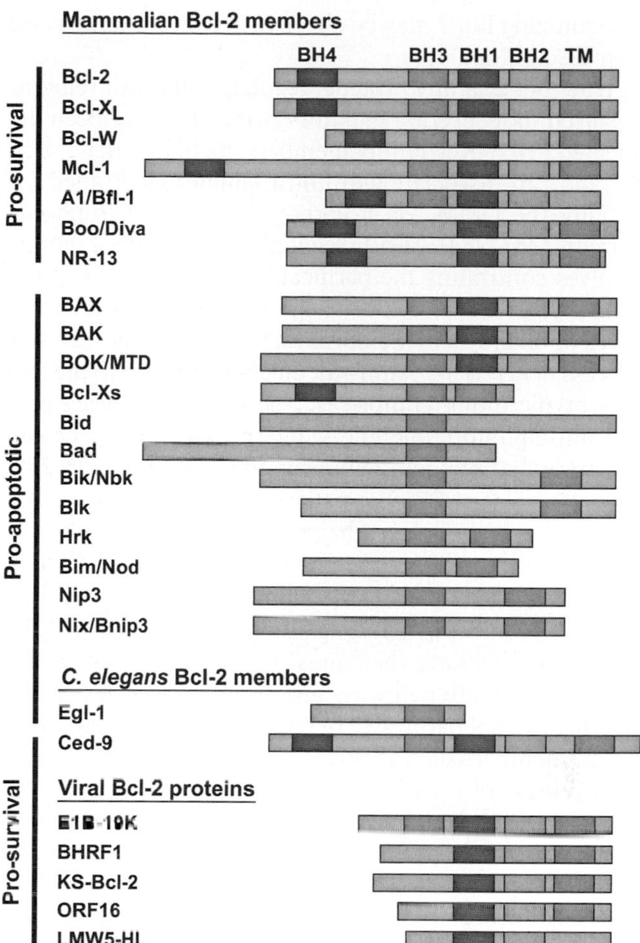

FIGURE 27.6 Schematic diagram of members of the Bcl-2 family. The dark blue, green, red, and orange boxes represent the different Bcl-2 homology (BH) domains and the gray boxes designate the hydrophobic transmembrane (TM) region that is required for insertion into the mitochondrial membrane.

3) the "BH3-only" proteins (Bid, Bad, Bim, Bik, Noxa, and Puma). Bcl-2 was identified at the chromosomal breakpoint of t(14;18)-bearing follicular B cell lymphomas. Vaux and Cory demonstrated that the oncogenic effect of Bcl-2 could be attributed to enhanced cell survival rather than proliferation (154,277). Consequently, Bcl-2 represented a new class of death-preventing oncogenes that collaborates with growth-promoting oncogenes, such as Myc (278). It is not uncommon to find abnormal overexpression of Bcl-2 in lymphoid and nonlymphoid malignancies *(279)*. Bcl-2 and Bcl-X$_L$ regulate various types of immune cell death caused by lymphokine withdrawal, γ-irradiation, and chemical death inducers such as glucocorticoids, phorbol esters, DNA-damaging agents, and ionomycin—all of which provoke mitochondrial apoptosis (reviewed in [280]). Apoptosis induction is one means by which cancer chemotherapeutics exert an anti-tumor effect. Thus, since apoptosis antagonism may be as important in transformation as mitogenesis, new therapeutic strategies aimed at

antagonizing Bcl-2 may be effective in cancer therapy (see later discussion).

How Bcl-2 family proteins regulate cell death remains unsolved, but several regulatory principles have been delineated (275). Key family members, including Bcl-2, Bcl-X_L, and Bax, associate with intracellular membranes, especially the OMM, via a carboxy-terminal hydrophobic domain *(281–284)*. Death regulation by the Bcl-2 family involves controlling the permeability and integrity of the OMM. Structural features suggest that Bcl-X_L may form pores or channels in membranes, which could govern this process *(171)*. Bcl-2 family members form homotypic and heterotypic dimer complexes. The balance between pro- and anti-apoptotic members determines cell fate probably through direct interactions with each other *(285–289*, 290). The precise stoichiometry of these associations that lead to survival or death have not been defined. Regulation by these proteins appears to be "upstream" of caspase activation, but they may also control caspase-independent forms of cell death, including autophagic cell death (202). These proteins have their most important effects on mitochondrial death pathways and comparatively less effect on DR-initiated pathways. In particular, the pro-apoptotic family members such as Bax and Bak can cause mitochondrial release of cytochrome c and activation of cytosolic caspases (291). Diverse pathways, such as transcriptional induction (Bim, Puma, Noxa, and Bcl-X_L), phosphorylation (Bad), processing (Bid), conformational changes (Bax and Bak), or organelle translocation (Bim, Bid, Bax), control the presence and biological activity of Bcl-2 family members (100,*292*). Each of these principles has reported exceptions, but they constitute the current basis for our understanding of the Bcl-2 family of proteins.

The biological function of Bcl-2 family members has been examined in genetically engineered mice and tissue culture cells (for a review see [94]). Bcl-X_L–deficient mice die around embryonic day 13 due to massive neuronal apoptosis (293). By contrast, Bcl-2–deficient mice survive a few weeks postnatally but then develop polycystic kidney disease, hypopigmentation due to decreased melanocyte survival, and, most important, massive apoptotic loss of all B and T lymphocytes (294). Thus, while Bcl-2 is not necessary for lymphocyte maturation, it is indispensable for the maintenance of mature lymphocytes. However, expression of Bcl-X_L is required for the survival of DP ($CD4^+CD8^+$) thymocytes, $B220^+$ bone marrow cells, and mature B cells (275). Mcl-1 deficiency results in peri-implantation lethality (295). A conditional knockout in the T cell compartment increases apoptosis at the double-negative 2 stage and arrests the development of both B and T lymphocytes. Mcl-1 is also essential for mature lymphocyte survival, and experimental elimination of this molecule triggers their rapid loss (136). Transgenic experiments in which Bcl-2 or Bcl-X_L were overexpressed suggest, however, that the two proteins can functionally substitute for one another and govern a final common death pathway (275). Selective transgenic overexpression of Bcl-2 in B or T cells leads to increased numbers of those cells and the late onset of lymphomas (296,297). Bcl-2 overexpression also blocks Apaf-1– and caspase-9–independent pathways of apoptosis, demonstrating the broad inhibitory effect of Bcl-2 (298). Further, Bcl-2 was recently shown to suppress Beclin 1 autophagic cell death, a novel form of nonapoptotic cell death (20,299). Deficiency of the pro-apoptotic Bax protein has a surprisingly mild phenotype in mice, causing only abnormalities in testis development and sterility (300). Deficiency of the pro-apoptotic Bak protein also causes very little effect in mice. However, a combined deficiency of Bax and Bak causes multiple organ abnormalities and perinatal death due to failed apoptosis (301). This includes an accumulation of lymphocytes and other hematopoietic cells, underscoring the importance of the Bax and Bak proteins for normal immune homeostasis.

Recent work has focused on the BH-3–only subset (Figure 27.6). Structural analysis has revealed that Bcl-2 family members interact through a hydrophobic pocket formed by the confluence of the BH-1, BH-2, and BH-3 helices. The interactions between Bcl-2 family members have a characteristic selectivity and hierarchy that may depend principally on binding to the BH-3 helix *(302)*. The BH-3–only proteins may selectively regulate the other family members through interactions at the hydrophobic pocket. Genetic ablation experiments have demonstrated the critical role of this family during developmentally programmed cell death as well as stress-induced death (94). So far, only one BH-3–only protein, called EGL-1 (egg laying defective 1), has been characterized in *C. elegans*. In mammals, the BH-3–only subset includes Bad, Bik, Bid, HRK, Bim, Noxa, Puma, Bmf, and perhaps others because the BH-3 motif is only a 9–16 amino acid long of alpha helix. Induction of cell death by BH-3–only proteins requires Bax and Bak, indicating that BH-3 proteins act upon or upstream of pro-apoptotic relatives *(303,304)*. The activity of BH-3–only proteins is governed transcriptionally and posttranscriptionally in a highly regulated fashion according to their function. Bid is cleaved by caspase-8, yielding a 15 kDa fragment that is myristoylated, which can insert into the mitochondrial membrane. This triggers the oligomerization of Bax and Bak thereby connecting the DRs to the mitochondrial pathway of death (*163,167*,291,305,*306*,307). Phosphorylation of Bad and Bim can control their association with 14-3-3 proteins or the microtubule-associated dynein motor complex, respectively (100). When released, Bad and Bim can induce apoptosis through the mitochondrial pathway. Interestingly, most of Bim is bound to Bcl-2 and Bcl-X_L at the mitochondria in both resting and activated T lymphocytes (308). Genetic deficiency of Bim protects against a variety of death inducers, such as cytokine deprivation, γ-radiation, glucocorticoids, ionomycin, DNA damage, etoposide, and Taxol but not FasL (52). Deficiency of Bim also significantly impairs TCR-induced thymocyte selection. These diverse forms of regulation provide a mechanism for a variety of different apoptosis inducers to converge on the mitochondrial pathway of death.

The mechanism by which the BH-3–only proteins control cell death is still an intense field of research. Studies carried out with peptides corresponding to the α-helical BH-3 domains distinguish two different subgroups of BH3–only proteins (*309,310*,311,*312*). The "activating BH-3" proteins (including Bim and Bid) can directly trigger death by Bax and Bak besides counteracting Bcl-2 and Bcl-X_L. The second group includes Bad and Bik and is called *derepressor BH3* or *sensitizing BH-3*. These molecules suppress the anti-apoptotic activity of Bcl-2 and Bcl-X_L but fail to activate the executioners Bax and Bak. They thus sensitize the mitochondria by increasing OMM permeability but require the intervention of an additional activator of Bax to induce apoptosis. The development of drugs mimicking sensitizing BH-3 protein associations represent an appealing therapeutic approach to modulate the anti-apoptotic Bcl-2 proteins during cancer treatment *(279)*. A small organic molecule (ABT-737) with mechanistic similarity to Bad was recently characterized as a potent inhibitor of the anti-apoptotic molecules Bcl-2, Bcl-X_L, and Bcl-w. Resembling a Bad-derived peptide, ABT-737 inhibits anti-apoptotic Bcl-2 proteins, but does not directly activate Bax and Bak. ABT 737 exhibits synergistic cytotoxicity with chemotherapeutics and radiation *in vitro* and *in vivo*. It displays single-agent activity against lymphoma, small-cell lung carcinoma, primary patient-derived cells, and promotes the regression of solid tumors (313).

Apaf Proteins

Mammalian Apaf-1 constitutes another class of proteins that is critical for the mitochondrial pathway of apoptosis. Apaf-1 is structurally and functionally homologous to the *C. elegans* Ced-4 protein (314). Both Apaf-1 and Ced-4 contain an NH_2-terminal CARD domain followed by a nucleotide-binding oligomerization domain (NOD). Ced-4 can complex with caspase-9 via CARD domains present in both molecules. The NOD domain is essential for binding ATP and homo-oligomerization. In addition, Apaf-1 also contains WD-40 repeats at the carboxy-terminal, which bind cytochrome c released from damaged mitochondria. Interestingly, *C. elegans* Ced-4 contains no carboxy-terminal WD-40 repeats and does not respond to mitochondrial insults *(315)*. Apaf-1, cytochrome c and ATP are all required to properly activate pro-caspase-9 (186,316). Genetic evidence from knockout animals revealed that Apaf-1 and caspase-9 are obligatory components of the apoptosis response through p53 to DNA damage and other mitochondrial death events (*317,318*,319).

Other proteins similar to Apaf-1/Ced-4 have been identified, most of which contain regions of homology to the NOD domain. Overexpression studies suggest that several of these (NOD1, NOD2, IPAF, and cryopyrin) may modulate apoptosis, but most evidence indicates they chiefly mediate proinflammatory responses. These proteins initiate intracellular responses to peptidoglycan or other bacterial antigens, through NF-κB induction or maturation of caspase-1 (320). One of these proteins, NOD2, has been mapped as a susceptibility gene for Crohn's disease (321,322). The CARD domain of NOD2 may allow it to be involved in apoptosis as well as inflammatory responses. Many members of the TNFR superfamily such as TNFR-1 and Fas have divergent effects (e.g., cellular activation versus apoptosis) that are apparent at different times and depend on the context of the immune response. Hence, combinations of protein interaction motifs like the CARD, NOD, and other signaling domains in single adapter proteins may allow bifurcation of biological responses from the same receptor.

STRUCTURAL REGULATION OF PCD

TNF/TNFR Structure

The recent determination of structures of components of the PCD pathways has led to a better physical sense of how these death programs work (Figure 27.7). In almost all cases, the formation of specific stoichiometric protein complexes is crucial for apoptosis signaling. Receptor-mediated apoptosis by DRs within the TNFR superfamily is triggered by receptor-specific ligands within the TNF superfamily (61). The defining structural motif of the TNFR superfamily, the CRD, is a 40 amino acid cluster of β strands folded back on themselves and pinned in place by three disulphide bonds formed by six cysteines in highly conserved positions (Figure 27.7A). Most of the TNFRs have multiple CRDs, which serve two primary functions depending on location. The membrane proximal or central CRDs mediate ligand binding. For example, in TNFR-1, the two central CRDs, CRD2 and 3, provide the key ligand-binding contacts. The membrane distal CRD mediates receptor pre-assembly on the cell surface (323,324). This membrane distal CRD along with adjacent amino-terminal sequences is called the *pre-ligand assembly domain* or PLAD. It promotes the oligomerization of like receptor chains prior to ligand engagement. Pre-assembly of receptor chains into trimers or perhaps other oligomeric complexes is obligatory for both ligand binding and signal transduction. The PLAD has been identified in both DRs such as Fas, TNFR-1, and TRAIL receptors, as well as in non-DD receptors, such as TNFR-2 (323,324). The orientation of the receptor chains is likely to change drastically between the unliganded and liganded complexes as reflected

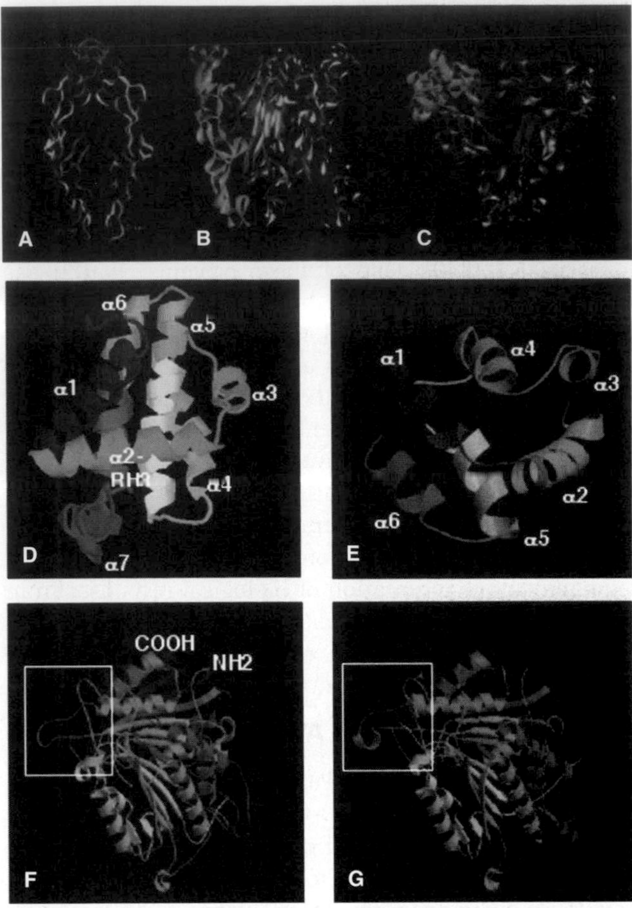

FIGURE 27.7 Structural biology of apoptosis. **A:** Structure of the unliganded TNFR-1. **B:** Side view of the TNFβ-bound TNFR-1 looking from plane of the membrane. Conserved disulphide bonds that are structurally essential are shown in red. **C:** Bird's eye view of the TNF/TNFR-1 structure looking down at the plane of the membrane. **D:** NMR structure of Bcl-X_L. The BH-3 (α2) domain runs perpendicularly across the molecule and the two central hydrophobic helices (α5 and α6) are buried in the middle portion of the molecule. **E:** Structure of the Fas DD, a prototypical hexahelical bundle. The bundle is composed of six helices, a structural scaffold that is also conserved in the DED and the CARD domain. The position of each of the helices is indicated. **F, G:** Structures of caspase-7 before (F) and after (G) proteolytic autoprocessing. Notice that the catalytic site (box) in the pro-enzyme is relatively "loose" (F). Processing of the pro-enzyme results in substantial "tightening" of the catalytic loops. The red-colored strand inside the boxed area in (G) denotes the position of the pseudosubstrate tetrapeptide DEVD.

in the extant crystal structures for unliganded and liganded TNFR-1 (see Figure 27.7A, B). The receptor chains are initially attached at the membrane distal CRD and then these interactions fall apart as the receptor admits the ligand between three receptor chains to interact with the CRDs closer to the membrane. The discovery of the PLAD overturned the prevailing model that TNFR family members signal by the ligand "cross-linking" solitary receptor chains into a trimeric complex. Instead, the ligand will bind to and change the configuration of pre-assembled receptor complexes. Hence, CRDs can regulate both intra- or intermolecular associations critical to receptor function.

The ligands for TNFRs are typically obligate homotrimers that adopt a compact "jelly-roll" conformation with a hydrophobic face where the individual subunits stably interact with each other (61,*325*). Certain exceptions, such as LTα and LTβ, can form heterotrimers. The ligand subunits are usually synthesized as type II transmembrane proteins and, following trimerization, may remain membrane bound or undergo metalloproteinase cleavage to a soluble form (326). Binding of the pre-assembled receptor complex with the trimeric ligand forms a symmetric three-to-three ligand-receptor complex that is evident in the crystal structures of the liganded TNFR1 and TRAIL receptors (241,327,328,*329,330*). Functionally, the ligand interaction appears to re-orient the receptor chains so that the intracellular domains adopt a specific juxtaposition favoring the binding of appropriate intracellular signaling proteins. The recently solved structure of the TRAIL trimer differs from the TNF structure in that it contains a loop insertion in the first β-strand that is critical for receptor association (241,327,328,*329,330*). In both the TNFR-1 and TRAIL-R2 crystals, ligand contacts appear to be restricted to the second and third CRDs. The extensive receptor–receptor interaction in the PLAD region found in the unliganded TNFR-1 receptor structure is absent in the ligand-bound receptor crystal structures (*331–333*,334). How the ligand initially contacts the pre-formed receptor complex and initiates chain rearrangement are important unresolved questions.

The fundamental three-fold symmetry of the TNF superfamily ligands and receptors appears to be conserved among the proximal signaling complexes. This includes the receptor–TRAF2 interaction (335,*336*), TRADD–TRAF2 interaction (337,*338*), and Fas–FADD interaction. The importance of the trifold symmetry in the receptor and signaling apparatus is highlighted by genetic mutations found in both human and mouse. For instance, heterozygous mutations in the cytoplasmic DD of Fas found in the *lpr*^{cg} (mouse) or Fas-defective form of ALPS resulted in a greater than 50% reduction in receptor signaling (339,*340*,341). This is likely due to the fact that inclusion of at least one bad subunit in the receptor trimer prevents the formation of a 3:3 Fas:FADD complex and thereby abrogates signaling (341).

The genetic effect by which a mutant allele encodes a protein that interferes with the same protein encoded by a wild-type allele is called *dominant interference*. Dominant interference is usually observed in proteins that function by forming multiprotein complexes, which is now known to be a common feature in PCD pathways. In the case of the trimeric Fas receptor, dominant interference may be potent due to the fact that with equal expression of a *wild-type* and mutant allele, $(1/2)^3$ or 1/8 would be expected to have solely *wild-type* subunits and 7/8 of the complexes would have at least one bad subunit by random reassortment of receptor chains (339,*340*,341). More generally, a dominant-interfering disease mechanism may be especially important in PCD disorders in outbred human populations, where most gene loci are heterozygous rather than homozygous. Thus, our understanding of the Fas receptor reveals that although higher order symmetric signaling complexes may provide rapid and selective signaling in immune regulation, they also create a vulnerability to genetic disease.

Bcl-2 Homology Structures

Bcl-X_L has the best-characterized structure, and it suggests interesting hypotheses regarding the function of Bcl-2 family members *(171)*. It contains a conserved nest of alpha helices including a backbone of two hydrophobic helices that are encircled by several amphipathic helices, including the BH4 helix, which is a key interaction site for members of the Bcl-2 family (Figure 27.7D). The structure has revealed a tantalizing similarity to pore-forming domains of bacterial toxins. This has stimulated a wealth of research into whether membrane pore formation is a key element of apoptosis modulation by Bcl-2 family proteins (342,*343*). It is interesting to consider that pore-forming toxins of bacteria have homology to regulatory proteins whose primary site of action is the mitochondria (which is believed to have evolved as a bacteria-like organism subsumed into eukaryotic cells). Structurally, Bcl-2 homology regions, BH1, BH2, and BH3 are widely spaced in the primary sequence but closely apposed in a hydrophobic pocket. Through this pocket, the pro- and anti-apoptotic members of the Bcl-2 family interact and cross-regulate one another. Proteins with only an amphipathic BH-3 helix can also interact with this pocket in the anti-apoptotic Bcl-2 family members and potentially nullify their protective function *(171)*. The specific amino acids contained in this pocket dictate a select hierarchy of interactions between various members of the Bcl-2 family. Hence, the structure reveals a possible functional interaction with the mitochondrial membrane and explains associations between members of the Bcl-2 family that determine survival or death.

The Hexahelical Bundle

The DD, DED, and CARD domains are critical protein–protein interaction motifs in DR-mediated PCD. Interestingly, all three domains adopt a similar structural scaffold of a compact bundle of six anti-parallel α-helices, which we will refer to as the "hexahelical bundle" (HHB) (Figure 27.7E). This structure is an ancient one that is related to the "ankyrin repeat," a protein interaction motif occuring in a plethora of proteins and conserved throughout phylogeny (61,*171*). Despite remarkable overall similarity, significant differences exist among the DD, DED, and CARD, which likely account for their binding specificities. They usually form homotypic associations. For example, the surfaces of Fas DD is made up of mostly charged residues (344), whereas the FADD DED contains hydrophobic patches that are important for binding to caspase-8 *(170)*. The six helices in CARD domain of RAIDD form an acidic surface on one side of the molecule and a basic region on the other side of the molecule, which may be important for binding of the corresponding CARD domain in caspase-2 (345). Structural and mutagenesis data corroborate the notion that helices 2 and 3 are critical contact regions for homophilic DD and DED interactions. In addition to $\alpha 2$ and $\alpha 3$, homophilic CARD–CARD interactions appear to involve electric dipole interactions between $\alpha 2$, $\alpha 3$, $\alpha 5$ on one molecule and $\alpha 1$, $\alpha 4$ on the partner. Examination of the CARD domain from Apaf-1 yields similar observations (346,*347*). Thus, specific molecular pathways are determined by defining residues in DD, DED, or CARDs presented on a common scaffold. It is also important to recognize that DDs, DEDs, and CARDs are primarily protein–protein interaction domains, and although they were initially discovered in apoptosis pathways, homologs of these motifs may be utilized by nature to associate proteins in pathways unrelated to apoptosis. In fact, a class of proteins containing the Pyrin domain also appears to use a HHB structural scaffold (*348*,*349*,350). The pyrin domain was originally identified in a protein mutated in patients with familial Mediterranean fever, thus providing a molecular link between apoptosis and inflammatory diseases.

An intriguing feature of HHBs is that they often occur in two tandem copies in proteins that promote or inhibit apoptosis. For example, the tandem DEDs in caspase-8 or -10 can augment apoptosis, whereas those in viral or cellular FLIPs inhibit apoptosis. The recent solution of the crystal structure of a viral FLIP, MC159, at 1.2 Angstroms resolution revealed a noncanonical fold of DEDs with a rigid dumbbell-shaped structure. Each DED played a unique role in the overall structure to generate an asymmetric interaction with DD proteins over an extensive surface (238). MC159 assembles into the DISC with Fas and FADD via a surface topology that differs from pro-apoptotic molecules. This blocks FADD self-association, which disrupts the higher-order oligomerization of the Fas receptors on the cell surface that is required for caspase activation.

Caspase Structure

The recruitment of DD-, DED-, or CARD-containing proteins eventually leads to the complex formation and activation of caspases. The structures of caspase-1, -3, -7, -8, and -9 have been determined (191,230,231,*233*,*234*,

235,242,243). Each caspase is composed of small and large subunits of approximately 10 kDa and 20 kDa (generally referred as p10 and -20, respectively). The catalytic subunits of all caspases are similarly composed of two p10/p20 heterodimers. Each p10/p20 heterodimer is folded into a compact cylindrical structure of six β strands and five α helices. The active site of the enzyme is formed by loops contributed by both the p10 and p20 subunits that come together at the top of the cylinder of β strands. The two heterodimers are aligned in an anti-parallel fashion where the β sheet forms the vertical axis of the tetrameric complex (Figures 27.6, 27.7F, G). Despite the overall structural similarity, distinct differences, especially in loops surrounding the catalytic active site, can explain the respective substrate preferences between different caspases.

Regulation of caspases by viral inhibitors has also been elucidated by structural studies. The baculovirus p35 is a potent inhibitor of many caspases that requires cleavage at its caspase recognition residue D87 to manifest inhibitory activity. Crystallographic studies reveal the formation of a thioester bond between the active site cysteine of caspase-8 (C360) and the aspartate of the amino-terminal cleavage product of p35 (351). Lu et al. showed that following caspase-8 processing, the buried p35 NH_2-terminus portion is liberated and undergoes a native chemical ligation reaction between residues D87 and C2. This mechanism, also used by self-splicing proteins, leads to the formation of a circular NH2-terminal p35 peptide, which is kept bound to the caspase-8 active site to ensure its long-lasting inhibitory effect (352).

PCD as Immune Therapy

Because of its exquisite antigen specificity, the possibility of using antigen-induced death, particularly of T lymphocytes, for the treatment of immunological diseases has been suggested *(353,354)*. In particular, the T cell components of graft rejection, autoimmune diseases, and allergic reactions could potentially be suppressed by antigen-induced elimination. This concept has been tested in both mice and monkeys with clearly beneficial effects on disease outcome. For example, it was found that the repetitive administration of a myelin basic protein antigen could suppress experimental allergic encephalomyelitis in mice by deleting the disease-causing T cells (88). This suggests that antigen-specific therapy is achievable if antigens relevant to the disease process are sufficiently well-defined and death of the culpable T cells can be triggered without exacerbation of symptoms (31).

Because these requirements have limited further evaluation of antigen-specific therapy in human clinical trials, other ways of triggering death have been explored. Fas or TNF agonist administration results in systemic toxicities limiting their potential utility (355,356). However, TRAIL agonists potentially induce death of neoplastic cells preferentially (184,357). Intracellular apoptosis signaling molecules targeted in preclinical or clinical trials include caspases, IAPs, Smac, and pro- or anti-apoptotic BCL2 family members (*253*,313,358,359). Many of these are rationally designed small molecules or peptidomimetics, which have demonstrated promising results, particularly against lymphoid and other malignancies.

PCD and Development of Lymphoid Malignancy

In this last section, we return to the question of why the mature immune system assiduously eliminates lymphocytes that have been activated by antigen and therefore have proven usefulness. Why can't the immune system adopt a laissez-faire economy of previously activated cells, which might have great value if the same pathogen is reencountered? Several lines of evidence strongly suggest that in addition to potential loss of tolerance and autoimmunity, lymphoid malignancy is also promoted by defective apoptosis. Hence, the accumulation of immune cells that have a propensity to proliferate and can undergo additional genetic changes may be deleterious to the organism. The association of translocations of the Bcl-2 gene with diffuse large cell lymphoma suggested that somatic aberrations in apoptosis pathways might be important in the transformation process. Since then, somatic changes in a variety of apoptosis molecules including Fas, caspases, and Bcl-2 family members have been documented in lymphoid tumors *(360)*. By contrast, the well-known inheritable apoptosis defect in p53 in the Li-Fraumeni syndrome seems to cause predominantly solid tumors but not lymphomas. Examination of large kindreds of patients with ALPS has revealed a 15-fold greater incidence of lymphomas. It is striking that these families have several different classes of lymphoma, suggesting that Fas protects against transformation not for a single cell type but generally for B and T lymphocytes (361). Moreover, Fas stimulation not only results in death induction, but also induction of signals for survival and proliferation such as NF-κB and MAPK activation; these dichotomous signals may have different thresholds, which can contribute to lymphomagenesis *(362)*. Thus, besides autoimmune manifestations, we can infer that protection against lymphoid malignancy demands strict control over the accumulation of activated lymphocytes.

CONCLUSION

The study of PCD has provided insights into many aspects of immune function, particularly in the establishment of central and peripheral tolerance and the numerical homeostasis of immune cells. PCD plays a vital part in the clonal composition, both qualitatively and quantitatively, of the immune repertoire. Immune cells utilize conserved mechanisms of apoptosis and necrosis that are common to perhaps all mammalian cells. Indeed, the immune system has been one of the most instructive model systems for understanding how these networks function. Finally, death is regulated by cues from the environment. For developing lymphocytes, the antigen environment determines cell survival and elimination. For mature cells, antigen and growth cytokines determine life or death. In this manner, the immune system can develop a wide repertoire of reactive cells, select the most useful members of the repertoire, and then expand and contract specific clonotypes as needed for specific immune responses. Such homeostatic control allows rapid cell proliferation in protective responses while preserving tolerance and avoiding autoimmunity and immune cell malignancies. There are still important challenges in this area of investigation. The molecular mechanisms of antigen receptor–induced apoptosis and necrosis are still not fully understood. In fact, fundamental questions such as what the crucial proteolytic substrates of caspases are for apoptosis remain unanswered. Also, the genetic or environmental influcences that cause autoimmunity in certain individuals with Fas defects but not others await definition. Also, the death effects by various lymphocytes subsets, particularly FoxP3$^+$ CD4$^+$ T cells, have not been fully explored. Finally, harnessing our understanding of PCD in the immune system for the diagnosis, prevention, and treatment of immunological diseases is an exciting frontier for the future.

ACKNOWLEDGMENTS

This manuscript was supported by the Intramural Research Program of the National Institute of Allergy and Infections Disease, National Institutes of Health. H.C.S. is a recipient of a Burroughs Wellcome Fund Career Award in the Biomedical Sciences. The views expressed in this chapter by the authors do not necessarily represent the views of the agency (Department of Health and Human Services, National Institutes of Health, National Institute of Allergy and Infections Diseases) or the U.S. government. The authors would like to thank Francis Ka-Ming Chan, Pushpa Pandiyan, and Jennifer Reed for thoughtful suggestions on the manuscript.

REFERENCES

1. Conlon I, Raff M. Size control in animal development. *Cell.* 1999;96(2):235–244.
4. Lenardo M, Chan KM, Hornung F, et al. Mature T lymphocyte apoptosis–immune regulation in a dynamic and unpredictable antigenic environment. *Annu Rev Immunol.* 1999;17:221–253.
6. Raff M. Cell suicide for beginners. *Nature.* 1998;396(6707):119–122.
8. Raff MC, Barres BA, Burne JF, et al. Programmed cell death and the control of cell survival. *Philos Trans R Soc Lond B Biol Sci.* 1994; 345(1313):265–268.
9. Kerr JF, Wyllie AH, Currie AR. Apoptosis: a basic biological phenomenon with wide-ranging implications in tissue kinetics. *Br J Cancer.* 1972;26(4):239–257.
10. Wyllie AH, Kerr JF, Currie AR. Cell death: the significance of apoptosis. *Int Rev Cytol.* 1980;68:251–306.
17. Chan FK, Shisler J, Bixby JG, et al. A role for tumor necrosis factor receptor-2 and receptor-interacting protein in programmed necrosis and antiviral responses. *J Biol Chem.* 2003;278(51):51613–51621.
18. Holler N, Zaru R, Micheau O, et al. Fas triggers an alternative, caspase-8-independent cell death pathway using the kinase RIP as effector molecule. *Nat Immunol.* 2000;1(6):489–495.
19. Degterev A, Huang Z, Boyce M, et al. Chemical inhibitor of non-apoptotic cell death with therapeutic potential for ischemic brain injury. *Nat Chem Biol.* 2005;1(2):112–119.
20. Yu L, Alva A, Su H, et al. Regulation of an ATG7-beclin 1 program of autophagic cell death by caspase-8. *Science.* 2004;304(5676):1500–1502.
21. Yu L, Wan F, Dutta S, et al. Autophagic programmed cell death by selective catalase degradation. *Proc Natl Acad Sci U S A.* 2006;103(13): 4952–4957.
25. Larsson M, Fonteneau JF, Bhardwaj N. Dendritic cells resurrect antigens from dead cells. *Trends Immunol.* 2001;22(3):141–148.
26. Metzstein MM, Stanfield GM, Horvitz HR. Genetics of programmed cell death in C. elegans: past, present and future. *Trends Genet.* 1998; 14(10):410–416.
28. Ashton-Rickardt PG, Tonegawa S. A differential-avidity model for T-cell selection. *Immunol Today.* 1994;15(8):362–366.
29. Ashton-Rickardt PG, Bandeira A, Delaney JR, et al. Evidence for a differential avidity model of T cell selection in the thymus [see comments]. *Cell.* 1994;76(4):651–63.
30. Lenardo MJ. Interleukin-2 programs mouse alpha beta T lymphocytes for apoptosis. *Nature.* 1991;353(6347):858–861.
31. Critchfield JM, Lenardo MJ. Antigen-induced programmed T cell death as a new approach to immune therapy. *Clin Immunol Immunopathol.* 1995;75(1):13–19.
37. Sprent J, Tough DF. T cell death and memory. *Science.* 2001; 293(5528):245–248.
38. Berg LJ, Kang J. Molecular determinants of TCR expression and selection. *Curr Opin Immunol.* 2001;13(2):232–241.
42. Page DM, Roberts EM, Peschon JJ, et al. TNF receptor-deficient mice reveal striking differences between several models of thymocyte negative selection. *J Immunol.* 1998;160(1):120–133.
43. Sidman CL, Marshall JD, Von Boehmer H. Transgenic T cell receptor interactions in the lymphoproliferative and autoimmune syndromes of lpr and gld mutant mice. *Eur J Immunol.* 1992;22(2): 499–504.
44. Alberola-Ila J, Forbush KA, Seger R, et al. Selective requirement for MAP kinase activation in thymocyte differentiation. *Nature.* 1995;373(6515):620–623.
45. Mariathasan S, Jones RG, Ohashi PS. Signals involved in thymocyte positive and negative selection. *Semin Immunol.* 1999;11(4):263–272.
46. Werlen G, Hausmann B, Palmer E. A motif in the alphabeta T-cell receptor controls positive selection by modulating ERK activity. *Nature.* 2000;406(6794):422–426.
47. Kruisbeek AM, Amsen D. Mechanisms underlying T-cell tolerance. *Curr Opin Immunol.* 1996;8(2):233–244.
51. Williams O, Brady HJ. The role of molecules that mediate apoptosis in T-cell selection. *Trends Immunol.* 2001;22(2):107–111.
52. Bouillet P, Metcalf D, Huang DC, et al. Proapoptotic Bcl-2 relative Bim required for certain apoptotic responses, leukocyte homeostasis, and to preclude autoimmunity. *Science.* 1999;286(5445):1735–1738.
53. Huang DC, Strasser A. BH3-Only proteins-essential initiators of apoptotic cell death. *Cell.* 2000;103(6):839–842.
54. Ladi E, Yin X, Chtanova T, et al. Thymic microenvironments for T cell differentiation and selection. *Nat Immunol.* 2006;7(4):338–343.
55. Critchfield JM, Boehme SA, Lenardo MJ. The Regulation of Antigen-Induced Apoptosis in Mature T Lymphocytes. In: *Apoptosis and the Immune Response.* Gregory CC, ed. New York: Wiley-Liss, Inc., 1995:55–114.

59. Strasser A, Harris AW, Huang DC, et al. Bcl-2 and Fas/APO-1 regulate distinct pathways to lymphocyte apoptosis. Embo J. 1995;14(24):6136-47.
61. Locksley RM, Killeen N, Lenardo MJ. The TNF and TNF receptor superfamilies: integrating mammalian biology. *Cell.* 2001;104(4):487–501.
63. Zheng L, Fisher G, Miller RE, et al. Induction of apoptosis in mature T cells by tumour necrosis factor. *Nature.* 1995;377(6547):348–351.
64. Oberg HH, Lengl-Janssen B, Kabelitz D, et al. Activation-induced T cell death: resistance or susceptibility correlate with cell surface fas ligand expression and T helper phenotype. *Cell Immunol.* 1997;181(1):93–100.
65. Devadas S, Das J, Liu C, et al. Granzyme B is critical for T cell receptor-induced cell death of type 2 helper T cells. *Immunity.* 2006;25(2):237–247. Epub 2006 Aug 10.
67. Watanabe-Fukunaga R, Brannan CI, Copeland NG, et al. Lymphoproliferation disorder in mice explained by defects in Fas antigen that mediates apoptosis. *Nature.* 1992;356(6367):314–317.
69. Straus SE, Sneller M, Lenardo MJ, et al. An inherited disorder of lymphocyte apoptosis: the autoimmune lymphoproliferative syndrome. *Ann Intern Med.* 1999;130(7):591–601.
71. Kagi D, Vignaux F, Ledermann B, et al. Fas and perforin pathways as major mechanisms of T cell-mediated cytotoxicity. *Science.* 1994;265(5171):528–530.
73. Stepp SE, Dufourcq-Lagelouse R, Le Deist F, et al. Perforin gene defects in familial hemophagocytic lymphohistiocytosis. *Science.* 1999;286(5446):1957–1959.
76. Zheng L, Trageser CL, Willerford DM, et al. T cell growth cytokines cause the superinduction of molecules mediating antigen-induced T lymphocyte death. *J Immunol.* 1998;160(2):763–769.
77. Boehme SA, Lenardo MJ. Propriocidal apoptosis of mature T lymphocytes occurs at S phase of the cell cycle. *Eur J Immunol.* 1993;23(7):1552–1560.
78. Li QS, Tanaka S, Kisenge RR, et al. Activation-induced T cell death occurs at G1A phase of the cell cycle. *Eur J Immunol.* 2000;30(11):3329–3337.
79. Lissy NA, Davis PK, Irwin M, et al. A common E2F-1 and p73 pathway mediates cell death induced by TCR activation. *Nature.* 2000;407(6804):642–645.
80. Hunig T, Schimpl A. Systemic autoimmune disease as a consequence of defective lymphocyte death. *Curr Opin Immunol.* 1997;9(6):826–830.
83. Moskophidis D, Lechner F, Pircher H, et al. Virus persistence in acutely infected immunocompetent mice by exhaustion of antiviral cytotoxic effector T cells. *Nature.* 1993;362(6422):758–761.
84. Rothstein TL, Wang JK, Panka DJ, et al. Protection against Fas-dependent Th1-mediated apoptosis by antigen receptor engagement in B cells. *Nature.* 1995;374(6518):163–165.
85. Hornung F, Zheng L, Lenardo MJ. Maintenance of clonotype specificity in CD95/Apo-1/Fas-mediated apoptosis of mature T lymphocytes. *J Immunol.* 1997;159(8):3816–3822.
86. Wong B, Arron J, Choi Y. T cell receptor signals enhance susceptibility to Fas-mediated apoptosis. *J Exp Med.* 1997;186(11):1939–1944.
87. Combadiere B, Reis e Sousa C, Trageser C, et al. Differential TCR signaling regulates apoptosis and immunopathology during antigen responses in vivo. *Immunity.* 1998;9(3):305–313.
88. Critchfield JM, Racke MK, Zuniga-Pflucker JC, et al. T cell deletion in high antigen dose therapy of autoimmune encephalomyelitis. *Science.* 1994;263(5150):1139–1143.
91. Kuroda K, Yagi J, Imanishi K, et al. Implantation of IL-2-containing osmotic pump prolongs the survival of superantigen-reactive T cells expanded in mice injected with bacterial superantigen. *J Immunol.* 1996;157(4):1422–1431.
92. Duke RC, Cohen JJ. IL-2 addiction: withdrawal of growth factor activates a suicide program in dependent T cells. *Lymphokine Res.* 1986;5(4):289–299.
94. Strasser A. The role of BH3-only proteins in the immune system. *Nat Rev Immunol.* 2005;5(3):189–200.
95. Hildeman DA, Zhu Y, Mitchell TC, et al. Activated T cell death in vivo mediated by proapoptotic bcl-2 family member bim. *Immunity.* 2002;16(6):759–767.
96. Pellegrini M, Belz G, Bouillet P, et al. Shutdown of an acute T cell immune response to viral infection is mediated by the proapoptotic Bcl-2 homology 3-only protein Bim. *Proc Natl Acad Sci U S A.* 2003;100(24):14175–14180.
98. You H, Pellegrini M, Tsuchihara K, et al. FOXO3a-dependent regulation of Puma in response to cytokine/growth factor withdrawal. *J Exp Med.* 2006;203(7):1657–1663.
100. Zha J, Harada H, Yang E, et al. Serine phosphorylation of death agonist BAD in response to survival factor results in binding to 14-3-3 not BCL-X(L). *Cell.* 1996;87(4):619–628.
101. Maurer U, Charvet C, Wagman AS, et al. Glycogen synthase kinase-3 regulates mitochondrial outer membrane permeabilization and apoptosis by destabilization of MCL-1. *Mol Cell.* 2006;21(6):749–760.
103. Wing K, Fehervari Z, Sakaguchi S. Emerging possibilities in the development and function of regulatory T cells. *Int Immunol.* 2006;18(7):991–1000.
104. Maloy KJ, Powrie F. Fueling regulation: IL-2 keeps CD4+ Treg cells fit. *Nat Immunol.* 2005;6(11):1071–1072.
105. Harnaha J, Machen J, Wright M, et al. Interleukin-7 is a survival factor for CD4+ CD25+ T-cells and is expressed by diabetes-suppressive dendritic cells. *Diabetes.* 2006;55(1):158 170.
106. Shevach EM. Regulatory T cells in autoimmmunity. *Annu Rev Immunol.* 2000;18:423–449.
107. Gondek DC, Lu LF, Quezada SA, et al. Cutting edge: contact-mediated suppression by CD4+CD25+ regulatory cells involves a granzyme B-dependent, perforin-independent mechanism. *J Immunol.* 2005;174(4):1783–1786.
108. Grossman WJ, Verbsky JW, Barchet W, et al. Human T regulatory cells can use the perforin pathway to cause autologous target cell death. *Immunity.* 2004;21(4):589–601.
110. Shevach EM, DiPaolo RA, Andersson J, et al. The lifestyle of naturally occurring CD4+ CD25+ Foxp3+ regulatory T cells. *Immunol Rev.* 2006;212:60–73.
114. Thome M, Schneider P, Hofmann K, et al. Viral FLICE-inhibitory proteins (FLIPs) prevent apoptosis induced by death receptors. *Nature.* 1997;386(6624):517–521.
116. Irmler M, Thome M, Hahne M, et al. Inhibition of death receptor signals by cellular FLIP. *Nature.* 1997;388(6638):190-5.
118. Deveraux QL, Reed JC. IAP family proteins–suppressors of apoptosis. *Genes Dev.* 1999;13(3):239–252.
120. Garcia S, DiSanto J, Stockinger B. Following the development of a CD4 T cell response in vivo: from activation to memory formation. *Immunity.* 1999;11(2):163–171.
123. Marrack P, Kappler J. Control of T cell viability. *Annu Rev Immunol.* 2004;22:765–787.
127. Wojciechowski S, Jordan MB, Zhu Y, et al. Bim mediates apoptosis of CD127(lo) effector T cells and limits T cell memory. *Eur J Immunol.* 2006;36(7):1694–1706.
128. Janssen EM, Droin NM, Lemmens EE, et al. CD4+ T-cell help controls CD8+ T-cell memory via TRAIL-mediated activation-induced cell death. *Nature.* 2005;434(7029):88–93.
129. Badovinac VP, Messingham KA, Griffith TS, et al. TRAIL deficiency delays, but does not prevent, erosion in the quality of "helpless" memory CD8 T cells. *J Immunol.* 2006;177(2):999–1006.
131. Akashi K, Kondo M, von Freeden-Jeffry U, et al. Bcl-2 rescues T lymphopoiesis in interleukin-7 receptor-deficient mice. *Cell.* 1997;89(7):1033–1041.
132. Maraskovsky E, O'Reilly LA, Teepe M, et al. Bcl-2 can rescue T lymphocyte development in interleukin-7 receptor-deficient mice but not in mutant rag-1-/- mice. *Cell.* 1997;89(7):1011–1019.
133. Grabstein KH, Waldschmidt TJ, Finkelman FD, et al. Inhibition of murine B and T lymphopoiesis in vivo by an anti-interleukin 7 monoclonal antibody. *J Exp Med.* 1993;178(1):257–264.
134. Namen AE, Lupton S, Hjerrild K, et al. Stimulation of B-cell progenitors by cloned murine interleukin-7. *Nature.* 1988;333(6173):571–573.
136. Opferman JT, Letai A, Beard C, et al. Development and maintenance of B and T lymphocytes requires antiapoptotic MCL-1. *Nature.* 2003;426(6967):671–676.
137. Sandel PC, Monroe JG. Negative selection of immature B cells by receptor editing or deletion is determined by site of antigen encounter. *Immunity.* 1999;10(3):289–299.
139. Hardy RR, Hayakawa K. B cell development pathways. *Annu Rev Immunol.* 2001;19:595–621.

140. King LB, Norvell A, Monroe JG. Antigen receptor-induced signal transduction imbalances associated with the negative selection of immature B cells. *J Immunol.* 1999;162(5):2655–62.
141. Rathmell JC, Cooke MP, Ho WY, et al. CD95 (Fas)-dependent elimination of self-reactive B cells upon interaction with CD4+ T cells. *Nature.* 1995;376(6536):181–184.
142. Rathmell JC, Townsend SE, Xu JC, et al. Expansion or elimination of B cells in vivo: dual roles for CD40- and Fas (CD95) ligands modulated by the B cell antigen receptor. *Cell.* 1996;87(2):319–329.
144. Foote LC, Marshak-Rothstein A, Rothstein TL. Tolerant B lymphocytes acquire resistance to Fas-mediated apoptosis after treatment with interleukin 4 but not after treatment with specific antigen unless a surface immunoglobulin threshold is exceeded. *J Exp Med.* 1998;187(6):847–853.
147. Enders A, Bouillet P, Puthalakath H, et al. Loss of the pro-apoptotic BH3-only Bcl-2 family member Bim inhibits BCR stimulation-induced apoptosis and deletion of autoreactive B cells. *J Exp Med.* 2003;198(7):1119–1126. Epub 2003 Sep 29.
148. Oliver PM, Vass T, Kappler J, et al. Loss of the proapoptotic protein, Bim, breaks B cell anergy. *J Exp Med.* 2006;203(3):731–741. Epub 2006 Mar 6.
149. Craxton A, Draves KE, Gruppi A, et al. BAFF regulates B cell survival by downregulating the BH3-only family member Bim via the ERK pathway. *J Exp Med.* 2005;202(10):1363–1374.
152. Devireddy LR, Teodoro JG, Richard FA, et al. Induction of apoptosis by a secreted lipocalin that is transcriptionally regulated by IL-3 deprivation. *Science.* 2001;293(5531):829–834.
153. Devireddy LR, Gazin C, Zhu X, et al. A cell-surface receptor for lipocalin 24p3 selectively mediates apoptosis and iron uptake. *Cell.* 2005;123(7):1293–1305.
154. Cleary ML, Smith SD, Sklar J. Cloning and structural analysis of cDNAs for bcl-2 and a hybrid bcl-2/immunoglobulin transcript resulting from the t(14;18) translocation. *Cell.* 1986;47(1):19–28.
155. Ingulli E, Mondino A, Khoruts A, et al. In vivo detection of dendritic cell antigen presentation to CD4(+) T cells. *J Exp Med.* 1997; 185(12):2133–2141.
156. Wang J, Zheng L, Lobito A, et al. Inherited human Caspase 10 mutations underlie defective lymphocyte and dendritic cell apoptosis in autoimmune lymphoproliferative syndrome type II. *Cell.* 1999;98(1):47–58.
157. Chen M, Wang YH, Wang Y, et al. Dendritic cell apoptosis in the maintenance of immune tolerance. *Science.* 2006;311(5764):1160–1164.
164. Heibein JA, Goping IS, Barry M, et al. Granzyme B-mediated cytochrome c release is regulated by the Bcl-2 family members bid and Bax. *J Exp Med.* 2000;192(10):1391–1402.
166. Sutton VR, Davis JE, Cancilla M, et al. Initiation of apoptosis by granzyme B requires direct cleavage of bid, but not direct granzyme B-mediated caspase activation. *J Exp Med.* 2000;192(10):1403–1414.
168. Ortaldo JR, Mason AT, O'Shea JJ. Receptor-induced death in human natural killer cells: involvement of CD16. *J Exp Med.* 1995;181(1):339–344.
172. Boatright KM, Salvesen GS. Mechanisms of caspase activation. *Curr Opin Cell Biol.* 2003;15(6):725–731.
175. Kischkel FC, Hellbardt S, Behrmann I, et al. Cytotoxicity-dependent APO-1 (Fas/CD95)-associated proteins form a death-inducing signaling complex (DISC) with the receptor. *Embo J.* 1995;14(22):5579–5588.
176. Wang J, Chun HJ, Wong W, et al. Caspase-10 is an initiator caspase in death receptor signaling. *Proc Natl Acad Sci U S A.* 2001;98(24): 13884–13888.
177. Siegel RM, Muppidi JR, Sarker M, et al. SPOTS: signaling protein oligomeric transduction structures are early mediators of death receptor-induced apoptosis at the plasma membrane. *J Cell Biol.* 2004;167(4):735–744.
184. Ashkenazi A, Dixit VM. Apoptosis control by death and decoy receptors. *Curr Opin Cell Biol.* 1999;11(2):255–260.
186. Zou H, Li Y, Liu X, et al. An APAF-1.cytochrome c multimeric complex is a functional apoptosome that activates procaspase-9. *J Biol Chem.* 1999;274(17):11549–11556.
187. Schafer ZT, Kornbluth S. The apoptosome: physiological, developmental, and pathological modes of regulation. *Dev Cell.* 2006;10(5): 549–561.
190. Srinivasula SM, Hegde R, Saleh A, et al. A conserved XIAP-interaction motif in caspase-9 and Smac/DIABLO regulates caspase activity and apoptosis. *Nature.* 2001;410(6824):112–116.
191. Wu G, Chai J, Suber TL, et al. Structural basis of IAP recognition by Smac/DIABLO. *Nature.* 2000;408(6815):1008–1012.
192. Hao Z, Duncan GS, Chang CC, et al. Specific ablation of the apoptotic functions of cytochrome C reveals a differential requirement for cytochrome C and Apaf-1 in apoptosis. *Cell.* 2005;121(4):579–591.
194. Cipolat S, Rudka T, Hartmann D, et al. Mitochondrial rhomboid PARL regulates cytochrome c release during apoptosis via OPA1-dependent cristae remodeling. *Cell.* 2006;126(1):163–175.
195. Frezza C, Cipolat S, Martins de Brito O, et al. OPA1 controls apoptotic cristae remodeling independently from mitochondrial fusion. *Cell.* 2006;126(1):177–189.
198. Baines CP, Kaiser RA, Purcell NH, et al. Loss of cyclophilin D reveals a critical role for mitochondrial permeability transition in cell death. *Nature.* 2005;434(7033):658–662.
199. Nakagawa T, Shimizu S, Watanabe T, et al. Cyclophilin D-dependent mitochondrial permeability transition regulates some necrotic but not apoptotic cell death. *Nature.* 2005;434(7033):652–658.
200. Susin SA, Lorenzo HK, Zamzami N, et al. Molecular characterization of mitochondrial apoptosis-inducing factor. *Nature.* 1999;397(6718):441–446.
202. Joza N, Susin SA, Daugas E, et al. Essential role of the mitochondrial apoptosis-inducing factor in programmed cell death. *Nature.* 2001;410(6828):549–554.
203. Li LY, Luo X, Wang X. Endonuclease G is an apoptotic DNase when released from mitochondria. *Nature.* 2001;412(6842):95–99.
204. Vercammen D, Beyaert R, Denecker G, et al. Inhibition of caspases increases the sensitivity of L929 cells to necrosis mediated by tumor necrosis factor. *J Exp Med.* 1998;187(9):1477–1485.
207. Munoz-Pinedo C, Guio-Carrion A, Goldstein JC, et al. Different mitochondrial intermembrane space proteins are released during apoptosis in a manner that is coordinately initiated but can vary in duration. *Proc Natl Acad Sci U S A.* 2006;103(31):11573–11578.
208. Lakhani SA, Masud A, Kuida K, et al. Caspases 3 and 7: key mediators of mitochondrial events of apoptosis. *Science.* 2006;311(5762): 847–851.
210. Wyllie AH, Golstein P. More than one way to go. *Proc Natl Acad Sci U S A.* 2001;98(1):11–13.
211. Stanger BZ, Leder P, Lee TH, et al. RIP: a novel protein containing a death domain that interacts with Fas/APO-1 (CD95) in yeast and causes cell death. *Cell.* 1995;81(4):513–523.
212. Hsu H, Huang J, Shu HB, et al. TNF-dependent recruitment of the protein kinase RIP to the TNF receptor-1 signaling complex. *Immunity.* 1996;4(4):387–396.
213. Kelliher MA, Grimm S, Ishida Y, et al. The death domain kinase RIP mediates the TNF-induced NF-kappaB signal. *Immunity.* 1998;8(3):297–303.
215. Zheng L, Bidere N, Staudt D, et al. Competitive control of independent programs of tumor necrosis factor receptor-induced cell death by TRADD and RIP1. *Mol Cell Biol.* 2006;26(9):3505–3513.
216. Lin Y, Devin A, Cook A, et al. The death domain kinase RIP is essential for TRAIL (Apo2L)-induced activation of IkappaB kinase and c-Jun N-terminal kinase. *Mol Cell Biol.* 2000;20(18):6638–6645.
220. Bolton DL, Hahn BI, Park EA, et al. Death of CD4(+) T-cell lines caused by human immunodeficiency virus type 1 does not depend on caspases or apoptosis. *J Virol.* 2002;76(10):5094–5107.
221. Yuan J, Shaham S, Ledoux S, et al. The C. elegans cell death gene ced-3 encodes a protein similar to mammalian interleukin-1 beta-converting enzyme. *Cell.* 1993;75(4):641–652.
222. Earnshaw WC, Martins LM, Kaufmann SH. Mammalian caspases: structure, activation, substrates, and functions during apoptosis. *Annu Rev Biochem.* 1999;68:383–424.
224. Saleh M, Mathison JC, Wolinski MK, et al. Enhanced bacterial clearance and sepsis resistance in caspase-12-deficient mice. *Nature.* 2006;440(7087):1064–1068.
225. Saleh M, Vaillancourt JP, Graham RK, et al. Differential modulation of endotoxin responsiveness by human caspase-12 polymorphisms. *Nature.* 2004;429(6987):75–79.

230. Blanchard H, Kodandapani L, Mittl PR, et al. The three-dimensional structure of caspase-8: an initiator enzyme in apoptosis. *Structure Fold Des.* 1999;7(9):1125–1133.
231. Riedl SJ, Renatus M, Schwarzenbacher R, et al. Structural basis for the inhibition of caspase-3 by XIAP. Cell. 2001;104(5):791–800.
235. Chai J, Wu Q, Shiozaki E, et al. Crystal structure of a procaspase-7 zymogen. Mechanisms of activation and substrate binding. *Cell.* 2001;107(3):399–407.
238. Yang JK, Wang L, Zheng L, et al. Crystal structure of MC159 reveals molecular mechanism of DISC assembly and FLIP inhibition. *Mol Cell.* 2005;20(6):939–949.
241. Cha SS, Sung BJ, Kim YA, et al. Crystal structure of TRAIL-DR5 complex identifies a critical role of the unique frame insertion in conferring recognition specificity. *J Biol Chem.* 2000;275(40):31171–31177.
242. Chai J, Shiozaki E, Srinivasula SM, et al. Structural basis of caspase-7 inhibition by XIAP. *Cell.* 2001;104(5):769–780.
243. Huang Y, Park YC, Rich RL, et al. Structural basis of caspase inhibition by XIAP: differential roles of the linker versus the BIR domain. *Cell.* 2001;104(5):781–790.
245. Thornberry NA, Rano TA, Peterson EP, et al. A combinatorial approach defines specificities of members of the caspase family and granzyme B. Functional relationships established for key mediators of apoptosis. *J Biol Chem.* 1997;272(29):17907–17911.
248. Rao L, Perez D, White E. Lamin proteolysis facilitates nuclear events during apoptosis. *J Cell Biol.* 1996;135(6 Pt 1):1441–1455.
249. Wang ZQ, Stingl L, Morrison C, et al. PARP is important for genomic stability but dispensable in apoptosis. *Genes Dev.* 1997;11(18):2347–2358.
250. Zhu S, Hsu AP, Vacek MM, et al. Genetic alterations in caspase-10 may be causative or protective in autoimmune lymphoproliferative syndrome. *Hum Genet.* 2006;119(3):284–294.
251. Chun HJ, Zheng L, Ahmad M, et al. Pleiotropic defects in lymphocyte activation caused by caspase-8 mutations lead to human immunodeficiency. *Nature.* 2002;419(6905):395–399.
252. Su H, Bidere N, Zheng L, et al. Requirement for caspase-8 in NF-kappaB activation by antigen receptor. *Science.* 2005;307(5714):1465–1468.
254. Wallach D, Varfolomeev EE, Malinin NL, et al. Tumor necrosis factor receptor and Fas signaling mechanisms. *Annu Rev Immunol.* 1999;17:331–367.
257. Tartaglia LA, Ayres TM, Wong GH, et al. A novel domain within the 55 kd TNF receptor signals cell death. *Cell.* 1993;74(5):845–853.
260. Rothe M, Wong SC, Henzel WJ, et al. A novel family of putative signal transducers associated with the cytoplasmic domain of the 75 kDa tumor necrosis factor receptor. *Cell.* 1994;78(4):681–692.
262. Siegel RM, Chan FK, Chun HJ, et al. The multifaceted role of Fas signaling in immune cell homeostasis and autoimmunity. *Nat Immunol.* 2000;1(6):469–474.
263. Hsu H, Xiong J, Goeddel DV. The TNF receptor 1-associated protein TRADD signals cell death and NF-kappa B activation. *Cell.* 1995;81(4):495–504.
264. Yeh WC, Shahinian A, Speiser D, et al. Early lethality, functional NF-kappaB activation, and increased sensitivity to TNF-induced cell death in TRAF2-deficient mice. *Immunity.* 1997;7(5):715–725.
270. Beg AA, Baltimore D. An essential role for NF-kappaB in preventing TNF-alpha-induced cell death [see comments]. *Science.* 1996;274(5288):782–784.
271. Van Antwerp DJ, Martin SJ, Kafri T, et al. Suppression of TNF-alpha-induced apoptosis by NF-kappaB [see comments]. Science. 1996;274(5288):787–9.
272. Wang CY, Mayo MW, Baldwin AS, Jr. TNF- and cancer therapy-induced apoptosis: potentiation by inhibition of NF-kappaB [see comments]. *Science.* 1996;274(5288):784–787.
273. Lee SY, Kaufman DR, Mora AL, et al. Stimulus-dependent synergism of the antiapoptotic tumor necrosis factor receptor-associated factor 2 (TRAF2) and nuclear factor kappaB pathways. *J Exp Med.* 1998;188(7):1381–1384.
274. Adachi M, Suematsu S, Suda T, et al. Enhanced and accelerated lymphoproliferation in Fas-null mice. *Proc Natl Acad Sci U S A.* 1996; 93(5):2131–2136.
275. Chao DT, Korsmeyer SJ. BCL-2 family: regulators of cell death. *Annu Rev Immunol.* 1998;16:395–419.
278. Vaux DL, Cory S, Adams JM. Bcl-2 gene promotes haemopoietic cell survival and cooperates with c-myc to immortalize pre-B cells. *Nature.* 1988;335(6189):440–442.
280. Opferman JT, Korsmeyer SJ. Apoptosis in the development and maintenance of the immune system. *Nat Immunol.* 2003;4(5):410–415.
290. Danial NN, Korsmeyer SJ. Cell death: critical control points. *Cell.* 2004;116(2):205–219.
291. Wei MC, Zong WX, Cheng EH, et al. Proapoptotic BAX and BAK: a requisite gateway to mitochondrial dysfunction and death. *Science.* 2001;292(5517):727–730.
293. Motoyama N, Wang F, Roth KA, et al. Massive cell death of immature hematopoietic cells and neurons in Bcl-x-deficient mice. *Science.* 1995;267(5203):1506–1510.
294. Veis DJ, Sorenson CM, Shutter JR, et al. Bcl-2-deficient mice demonstrate fulminant lymphoid apoptosis, polycystic kidneys, and hypopigmented hair. *Cell.* 1993;75(2):229–240.
295. Rinkenberger JL, Horning S, Klocke B, et al. Mcl-1 deficiency results in peri-implantation embryonic lethality. *Genes Dev.* 2000;14(1):23–27.
296. Linette GP, Hess JL, Sentman CL, et al. Peripheral T-cell lymphoma in lckpr-bcl-2 transgenic mice. *Blood.* 1995;86(4):1255–1260.
297. Strasser A, Harris AW, Cory S. E mu-bcl-2 transgene facilitates spontaneous transformation of early pre-B and immunoglobulin-secreting cells but not T cells. *Oncogene.* 1993;8(1):1–9.
298. Marsden VS, O'Connor L, O'Reilly LA, et al. Apoptosis initiated by Bcl-2-regulated caspase activation independently of the cytochrome c/Apaf-1/caspase-9 apoptosome. *Nature.* 2002;419(6907):634–637.
299. Pattingre S, Tassa A, Qu X, et al. Bcl-2 antiapoptotic proteins inhibit Beclin 1-dependent autophagy. *Cell.* 2005;122(6):927–939.
300. Knudson CM, Tung KS, Tourtellotte WG, et al. Bax-deficient mice with lymphoid hyperplasia and male germ cell death. *Science.* 1995;270(5233):96–99.
301. Lindsten T, Ross AJ, King A, et al. The combined functions of proapoptotic Bcl-2 family members bak and bax are essential for normal development of multiple tissues. *Mol Cell.* 2000;6(6):1389–1399.
305. Luo X, Budihardjo I, Zou H, et al. Bid, a Bcl2 interacting protein, mediates cytochrome c release from mitochondria in response to activation of cell surface death receptors. *Cell.* 1998;94(4):481–490.
307. Eskes R, Desagher S, Antonsson B, et al. Bid induces the oligomerization and insertion of Bax into the outer mitochondrial membrane. *Mol Cell Biol.* 2000;20(3):929–935.
308. Zhu Y, Swanson BJ, Wang M, et al. Constitutive association of the proapoptotic protein Bim with Bcl-2-related proteins on mitochondria in T cells. *Proc Natl Acad Sci U S A.* 2004;101(20):7681–7686.
311. Kuwana T, Bouchier-Hayes L, Chipuk JE, et al. BH3 domains of BH3-only proteins differentially regulate Bax-mediated mitochondrial membrane permeabilization both directly and indirectly. *Mol Cell.* 2005;17(4):525–535.
313. Oltersdorf T, Elmore SW, Shoemaker AR, et al. An inhibitor of Bcl-2 family proteins induces regression of solid tumours. *Nature.* 2005;435(7042):677–681.
314. Zou H, Henzel WJ, Liu X, et al. Apaf-1, a human protein homologous to C. elegans CED-4, participates in cytochrome c-dependent activation of caspase-3. *Cell.* 1997;90(3):405–413.
316. Li P, Nijhawan D, Budihardjo I, et al. Cytochrome c and dATP-dependent formation of Apaf-1/caspase-9 complex initiates an apoptotic protease cascade. *Cell.* 1997;91(4):479–489.
319. Soengas MS, Alarcon RM, Yoshida H, et al. Apaf-1 and caspase-9 in p53-dependent apoptosis and tumor inhibition. *Science.* 1999;284(5411):156–159.
320. Inohara N, Nunez G. NODs: intracellular proteins involved in inflammation and apoptosis. *Nat Rev Immunol.* 2003;3(5):371–382.
321. Hugot JP, Chamaillard M, Zouali H, et al. Association of NOD2 leucine-rich repeat variants with susceptibility to Crohn's disease. *Nature.* 2001;411(6837):599–603.

322. Ogura Y, Bonen DK, Inohara N, et al. A frameshift mutation in NOD2 associated with susceptibility to Crohn's disease. *Nature.* 2001;411(6837):603–606.
323. Chan FK, Chun HJ, Zheng L, et al. A domain in TNF receptors that mediates ligand-independent receptor assembly and signaling. *Science.* 2000;288(5475):2351–2354.
324. Siegel RM, Frederiksen JK, Zacharias DA, et al. Fas preassociation required for apoptosis signaling and dominant inhibition by pathogenic mutations. *Science.* 2000;288(5475):2354–2357.
326. McGeehan GM, Becherer JD, Bast RC, Jr., et al. Regulation of tumour necrosis factor-alpha processing by a metalloproteinase inhibitor. *Nature.* 1994;370(6490):558–561.
327. Banner DW, D'Arcy A, Janes W, et al. Crystal structure of the soluble human 55 kd TNF receptor-human TNF beta complex: implications for TNF receptor activation. *Cell.* 1993;73(3):431–445.
328. Cha SS, Kim MS, Choi YH, et al. 2.8 A resolution crystal structure of human TRAIL, a cytokine with selective antitumor activity. *Immunity.* 1999;11(2):253–261.
334. Naismith JH, Sprang SR. Modularity in the TNF-receptor family. *Trends Biochem Sci.* 1998;23(2):74–79.
335. Park YC, Burkitt V, Villa AR, et al. Structural basis for self-association and receptor recognition of human TRAF2. *Nature.* 1999;398(6727):533–538.
337. Park YC, Ye H, Hsia C, et al. A novel mechanism of TRAF signaling revealed by structural and functional analyses of the TRADD-TRAF2 interaction. *Cell.* 2000;101(7):777–787.
339. Fisher GH, Rosenberg FJ, Straus SE, et al. Dominant interfering Fas gene mutations impair apoptosis in a human autoimmune lymphoproliferative syndrome. *Cell.* 1995;81(6):935–946.
341. Martin DA, Zheng L, Siegel RM, et al. Defective CD95/APO-1/Fas signal complex formation in the human autoimmune lymphoproliferative syndrome, type Ia. *Proc Natl Acad Sci U S A.* 1999;96(8):4552–4557.
342. Minn AJ, Velez P, Schendel SL, et al. Bcl-x(L) forms an ion channel in synthetic lipid membranes. *Nature.* 1997;385(6614):353–357.
344. Huang B, Eberstadt M, Olejniczak ET, et al. NMR structure and mutagenesis of the Fas (APO-1/CD95) death domain. *Nature.* 1996;384(6610):638–641.
345. Chou JJ, Matsuo H, Duan H, et al. Solution structure of the RAIDD CARD and model for CARD/CARD interaction in caspase-2 and caspase-9 recruitment. *Cell.* 1998;94(2):171–180.
346. Qin H, Srinivasula SM, Wu G, et al. Structural basis of procaspase-9 recruitment by the apoptotic protease-activating factor 1. *Nature.* 1999;399(6736):549–557.
350. Martinon F, Hofmann K, Tschopp J. The pyrin domain: a possible member of the death domain-fold family implicated in apoptosis and inflammation. *Curr Biol.* 2001;11(4):R118–120.
351. Xu G, Cirilli M, Huang Y, et al. Covalent inhibition revealed by the crystal structure of the caspase-8/p35 complex. *Nature.* 2001;410(6827):494–497.
352. Lu M, Min T, Eliezer D, et al. Native chemical ligation in covalent caspase inhibition by p35. *Chem Biol.* 2006;13(2):117–122.
355. Ogasawara J, Watanabe-Fukunaga R, Adachi M, et al. Lethal effect of the anti-Fas antibody in mice. *Nature.* 1993;364(6440):806–809.
356. Tracey KJ, Beutler B, Lowry SF, et al. Shock and tissue injury induced by recombinant human cachectin. *Science.* 1986;234(4775):470–474.
357. Walczak H, Miller RE, Ariail K, et al. Tumoricidal activity of tumor necrosis factor-related apoptosis-inducing ligand in vivo. *Nat Med.* 1999;5(2):157–163.
358. Li L, Thomas RM, Suzuki H, et al. A small molecule Smac mimic potentiates TRAIL- and TNFalpha-mediated cell death. *Science.* 2004;305(5689):1471–1474.
359. Walensky LD, Kung AL, Escher I, et al. Activation of apoptosis in vivo by a hydrocarbon-stapled BH3 helix. *Science.* 2004;305(5689):1466–1470.
361. Straus SE, Jaffe ES, Puck JM, et al. The development of lymphomas in families with autoimmune lymphoproliferative syndrome with germline Fas mutations and defective lymphocyte apoptosis. *Blood.* 2001;98(1):194–200.

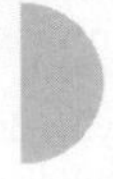

Immunologic Memory

Stephen P. Schoenberger and Shane Crotty

MEMORY AS A BIOLOGICAL CONCEPT

The Protected State

> *Yet it was with those who had recovered from the disease that the sick and the dying found most compassion. These knew what it was from experience, and had now no fear for themselves; for the same man was never attacked twice—never at least fatally. And such persons not only received the congratulations of others, but themselves also, in the elation of the moment, half entertained the vain hope that they were for the future safe from any disease whatsoever (1).*

The preceding quote comes from the Greek historian Thucydides (ca. 460 BCE to ca. 395 BCE) and describes his first-hand account of a plague that struck Athens during a protracted war with Sparta. Although the identity of the causative agent continues to be a matter of speculation (2), these words transcend the ages to vividly illustrate the concept of immune memory—the phenomenon in which prior exposure to an infectious pathogen endows an individual with immunity, a durable state of protection against reinfection with the same organism. Unknown to Thucydides and his fellow Greeks, the immunity observed in the survivors of this plague reflected changes in the operational status of their immune systems as a result of the first (primary) response to the infecting pathogen. In the act of responding to the initial infection, the immune system expands a diverse population of antigen-specific B and T lymphocyte clones possessing a range of affinities and effector capacities. Through a process that is just now beginning to be understood at the molecular level, a portion of this repertoire is retained within the memory pool in the form of cells that are able to persist for long periods of time at relatively stable numbers by maintaining a slow but steady rate of division that is roughly equivalent to their rate of loss (death). When faced with a renewed challenge from the same (or antigenically related) infectious agents, memory cells mount a strong and rapid effector response that is capable of stopping reinfection at its earliest stages. The functional units of immune memory, therefore, are the long-lived B and T cells that mount rapid secondary (recall) responses on reencounter with their cognate antigen. In the broader teleologic concept of memory, however, it is the antigen receptors that were shown to be "useful" in combating the initial infection that are selected and preserved at an increased frequency on clonal progeny that possess enhanced response kinetics and specialized functions. Whether generated through infection or vaccination, the value of the protected state that they confer to the individual is self-evident because preexisting immunity can prevent or limit the potential damage of an otherwise unrestrained infection. This can be of benefit from the earliest days of life, as seen in the example of maternal antibodies transmitted to the neonate in milk and serum that may serve to limit infections and transform them into "natural vaccinations" and thereby diminish the severity of childhood infections that will be encountered during the next 1 to 2 years (3,3a).

This chapter examines the phenomena and mechanisms of long-lasting protection that can develop following infection or vaccination and focuses on the factors that govern the establishment and maintenance of specialized subsets of lymphocytes generated from the naïve repertoire during the primary response to a given antigen. This concept stands in contrast to the "memory" associated with immune tolerance, through which the adaptive arm of the immune system can prevent inappropriate responses against ubiquitous self-antigens. Immune memory involves a stable increase in the number of antigen-experienced B and T lymphocytes that have acquired specialized functional properties allowing them to generate secondary responses that are more rapid and effective than those made by their clonal antecedents during the primary response. It is in the establishment, maintenance, and execution of memory responses that the adaptive immune system finds its greatest purpose for the preservation of both the individual and population. As shown in this chapter, immune memory depends on a remarkable degree of interaction and cooperation among many different cell types in an elegant division of labor aimed at preserving those T and B cell specificities that have proved useful in the battles fought and won against previously encountered pathogens. It is important in considering the concept of immune memory, however, that distinctions be drawn between the protected state, an operational definition that can vary with the nature and magnitude of the antigenic challenge used to test its integrity, and memory cells, the clonal elements of memory whose contribution to the protected state can only be inferred from their phenotypic and functional properties.

Lifelong Memory Can Be Induced Through Infection or Vaccination

Observations of acquired resistance to recurring diseases are recorded throughout the history of human epidemics. The careful observations of the Danish physician Ludwig Panum were among the first clearly to illustrate just how durable the protected state can be in an individual. Working on the remote Faroe Islands in the North Sea, Panum studied two separate measles epidemics that took place 65 years apart between the 18th and 19th centuries. In the apparent absence of outbreaks in the intervening period, he found that people who had contracted measles in the first epidemic were not affected during the second, whereas those of appropriate age who were infected during the second outbreak had not been affected during the first (4). Thus, Panum observed, a single infection was capable of endowing an individual with lifelong immunity through a process that did not require reexposure to the pathogen. Although immune reactivity can be boosted by repeated exposure to a given organism, the extent to which this determines the maintenance of immune memory remains a source of some controversy (5,507). A source of uncertainty in applying this concept to human immunology is the difficulty in determining whether a single exposure or multiple exposures have taken place before the memory state is assessed. With infrequently encountered life-threatening infections such measles, yellow fever, or polio it is relatively straightforward to infer that a single exposure can establish a state of protection for up to 75 years that appears to be mediated by antibodies (4,6,7). With less threatening ubiquitous agents such as those causing the childhood infections chicken pox (varicella zoster) and whooping cough (*Bordatella pertussis*), it is unclear whether immune memory may depend on occasional subclinical reinfection (8,507).

Given the long history of immunity in survivors of infectious disease, it is notable that even the most rudimentary understanding of how the protected state could be achieved was realized long after methods for its induction had been devised. Among the earliest practices was that of variolation, which had long been in practice in China and India as a means for enhancing protection against the deadly smallpox virus, which had been a major source of mortality in humans since recorded history (9). Variolation involves the intentional inoculation with dessicated material obtained from the open pustules of smallpox victims in the hope that exposed individual would develop a milder form of the disease and, on recovery, be immune to smallpox (variola virus). Although effective in many cases, the procedure was not without risk to the recipient, who risked contracting a more serious life-threatening form of the disease that could be spread to others. In 1796, Edward Jenner famously (and dramatically) overcame these obstacles by using material obtained from the pustules of milkmaids infected with cowpox (vaccinia virus), an antigenically related but less virulent type of poxvirus, to inoculate young James Phipps, who subsequently survived his exposure to infectious smallpox patients (10). In the 19th century, Louis Pasteur further developed the concept of using less-virulent or intentionally disabled forms of infectious organisms to confer immunity to bacterial diseases such as chicken cholera and anthrax and viral diseases such as rabies. Pasteur used the word "vaccine" as a generic term to describe antigenic preparations administered to produce immunity, in reference to Jenner's earlier work with cowpox (vaccinia) virus (*vacca* is Latin for "cow"). As described in more detail in the chapter on vaccines, current vaccines can be generated from organisms that are antigenically related to the one against which immunity is desired, from inactivated forms of the entire disease-causing organism, or from specific constituent portions of the infectious organism such as proteins, polysaccharides, or nucleic acids.

Despite their various compositions, all effective vaccines recapitulate several important aspects of the immune response leading to memory formation: they mimic the threat of an infectious pathogen through stimulation of innate immunity via Toll-like receptors (TLRs), and they contain distinct antigens that can become recognizable by cells of the adaptive immune system (11,12). The power of vaccination to induce long-lasting immune memory is best illustrated by the example of the smallpox vaccine (vaccinia). This once-devastating organism has been virtually eradicated since the late 1970s through a worldwide mass vaccination program that stands as one of the crowning achievements of the 20th century (13). The immunity induced by the smallpox vaccine is of remarkable durability, with both antibody and $CD4^+$ and $CD8^+$ T cell responses detectable 50 years after initial priming (14–16), and effectiveness, with a lifelong protection rate of 90% to 95% in vaccinated individuals and a fatality rate of only 2% in those vaccinated within a decade before exposure (17,18). With the advent of modern immunologic tools such as enzyme-linked immunosorbent assay (ELISA), intracellular cytokine staining (ICCS), and enzyme-linked immunospot (ELISPOT) assays for the detection of rare vaccinia-specific T and B cells, a more detailed longitudinal picture of the response to the smallpox vaccine has emerged. These studies suggest that humoral immunity is more durable than cellular immunity: Increased numbers of vaccinia-specific memory B cells remain stable for more than 50 years after vaccination, whereas $CD4^+$ and $CD8^+$ T cell responses continue to decline over time, with a half-life of 8 to 15 years (14,16). This indicates that memory B cell responses, and to a lesser extent memory T cell responses, are maintained by robust mechanisms. The reason for the apparent discrepancy between the longevity of memory B versus T cell responses is unknown, but it may involve the selective ability of mature B cells to perform more extensive DNA repair than T cells through their recombination and somatic hypermutation machinery (19).

Given the remarkable longevity of the immunity induced through either infection or vaccination, it is clear that the cells mediating the protected state must possess several key properties to preserve useful specificities generated in previous antigenic experiences; the study of memory T cells has revealed insights into a number of these features. First among these is that antigen-specific memory cells must be present in the immune repertoire in greater numbers than in the naïve repertoire as a result of their initial proliferation (20–25). Second, they must have undergone a program of differentiation involving alterations in chromatin structure and activation of specific transcription factors to allow the expression of key effector molecules such as perforin, granzyme B, and interferon-γ (IFNγ) to be constitutively expressed and to be available immediately on recognition of antigen-expressing target cells (26–32). Memory cells must be able to survive as a clonal population over time; that is, they must be able to replace cells lost to normal homeostatic turnover (reviewed in refs. 33, 34). Memory cells also must perform a sentinel function by occupying specific physiologic niches where naïve cells are not usually found and where antigen exposure will either occur or be detected such as the mucosa of the lung or gastrointestinal tract (reviewed in refs. 35, 36). Consistent with this sentinel function, memory cells are found to be capable of responding to lower concentrations of antigen than naïve cells through the selective expansion of high-affinity clones and the upregulation of adhesion molecules and reorganization of their T cell receptor (TCR) (37–40). Lastly, memory cells should be able to respond quickly to reencounter with their cognate antigen with the induction of rapid effector functions and renewed rounds of clonal expansion (41). Memory cells have developed a variety of mechanisms to achieve each of these specialized properties. In the following section, we examine how memory cells are generated during immune responses and how these key features are imparted during priming, maintained over long periods of time, and expressed when needed to confer rapid protection from reinfection.

THE GENERATION OF MEMORY T CELLS

Antigen-driven T cell responses can be broadly categorized as having two main components: a comparatively short-lived effector arm that comprises large numbers of cells that mediate direct functional response against target cells, and a smaller but longer-lived memory population that ensures the potential of rapid and potent recall responses against the inducing antigen. The memory component can be distinguished into two separate activities: one that resides mainly within lymph nodes, where it can respond to antigenic challenge by renewed clonal expansion and production of secondary effectors ("central memory" phenotype T cells [T_{CM}s]), and one that is largely disseminated throughout peripheral tissues, where the first contact with infectious pathogens is likely to occur ("effector memory" phenotype T cells [T_{EM}s]), and is capable of mediating immediate effector functions on antigen recognition (35,42). These subsets were first distinguished in humans based on their expression of the lymph node homing receptor CD62L and CCR7 and by their effector functions and proliferative capacity (41,43). The specific roles in immunity and the signals that may govern the development of these subsets are discussed in subsequent sections in this chapter. Although the effector and memory responses typically display notable quantitative, qualitative, and temporal differences in their function, it is generally accepted that both originate from the same primary response to antigen, with memory population being endowed with an enhanced capacity for self-renewal and recall responsiveness. It is the precise relationship between the effector and memory populations that has been the focus of intense experimental interest over the last 10 to 15 years, with distinct and often contradictory results emerging from different experimental systems. This is due in part to kinetic and functional differences in which effector and memory populations are detected, their shared expression of many surface markers, and the paucity of methods for reliably tracking both their emergence from naïve precursors and determining their lineage relationships over time.

There are several models for how both effector and memory populations could be concomitantly generated, either in parallel or sequentially (Figure 28.1). The first model suggests that memory cells are the clonal progeny of a distinct precursor population that follows a separate differentiation fate from that of the primary effectors and instead survive to execute these effector functions during the recall phase (separate precursor model). The second model posits that memory cells derive from the same precursor pool as the effectors but are descended from cells that have received qualitatively and/or quantitatively distinct signals at the time of their the initial priming or subsequent development (instructive model) (44). The inductive signals that can influence memory versus effector fates in this view include a range of antigen-specific and nonspecific stimuli, such as the strength and duration of TCR signals, the nature of costimulatory molecules and cytokines produced, or the type of antigen-presenting cell(s) (APCs) involved. An alternative model supports the notion that memory cells are generated in a stochastic manner via asymmetric cell division that occurs at a preprogrammed stage of antigen-driven clonal expansion (stochastic model) (45,46). This model envisions memory as a cellular fate governed by the same common biological strategy used during ontogeny and development to specify distinct functional properties in selected cells and their clonal progeny (47). Finally, memory T cells may constitute a functionally distinct population generated through progressive differentiation of the same precursors that give rise to short-lived effectors (progressive differentiation model) (48). Two mutually nonexclusive pathways have been suggested through which this can occur: linear and nonlinear differentiation. In the linear pathway, T cells proceed sequentially through distinct functional states, first as effectors, with a subset of these developing into the memory population (reviewed in refs. 49, 50). Alternatively, memory development may follow a nonlinear pathway in which environmental signals and an individual cell's stimulation history influence whether primary effectors develop into T_{EM} or T_{CM} subsets. Variations applicable to the latter three models have been proposed in which sequential encounters with antigen can decrease the potential of a given cell to differentiate fully into a memory cell (51,52). In each of these models, the initiating event leading to memory cell development is the primary activation of a naïve T cell in response to immunization or infection. We therefore begin our consideration of memory T cell generation with the illustrative example of the $CD8^+$ T cell response. Many of the concepts relevant for $CD8^+$ T cell priming are also applicable to the generation of $CD4^+$ T cell memory, whose unique characteristics are discussed in the following section.

The Generation of Memory $CD8^+$ T Cells

$CD8^+$ T cells are critical for the control of acute and chronic infections by a range of pathogens, including viruses, intracellular bacteria, and single- and multicellular parasites, and can mediate the destruction of tumor cells (53–60). Most of our understanding of how memory $CD8^+$ T cells are formed has emerged from studies on the response to acute infection in mice. This is partly due to the nature of the immunogens used to generate robust T cell responses in these models, such as lymphochoriomeningitis virus (LCMV), influenza A (flu), or *Listeria monocytogenes* (LM), which produce significant numbers of effector $CD8^+$ T cells specific for a subset of immunodominant class I major histocompatibility complex (MHC)–restricted antigens on infection of inbred mice (61–63). Another reason is the availability of superior tools for the detection and longitudinal tracking of antigen-specific $CD8^+$ T cells such as intracellular cytokine staining (ICS), which allows enumeration of cells secreting cytokines in response to their cognate peptide antigen, and the use of peptide/MHC tetramers, which are soluble forms of the ligand structure recognized by T cells and which allow the detection of cells recognizing a specific antigenic determinant (64,65). When combined with more traditional antibody-based immunophenotyping approaches used in flow cytometry, these techniques have revealed important features of the specificity, kinetics, magnitude, and functional differentiation of antigen-specific $CD8^+$ T cells following infection and have allowed new insights into the process of memory T cell development (66,67). Finally, the use of TCR-transgenic T cells in adoptive transfer experiments has allowed the fate of a monoclonal population of antigen-specific $CD8^+$ T cells to be followed throughout their development from naïve to memory cells. Such studies have established that the $CD8^+$ T cell response to infection can be divided into four main phases: priming, contraction, memory maintenance, and recall (Figure 28.2). As explained in this section, the first two phases involve a complex and carefully orchestrated series of cellular interactions to transport antigen from the site of inflammation or infection to the secondary lymphoid organs where the events leading to memory formation can take place. The

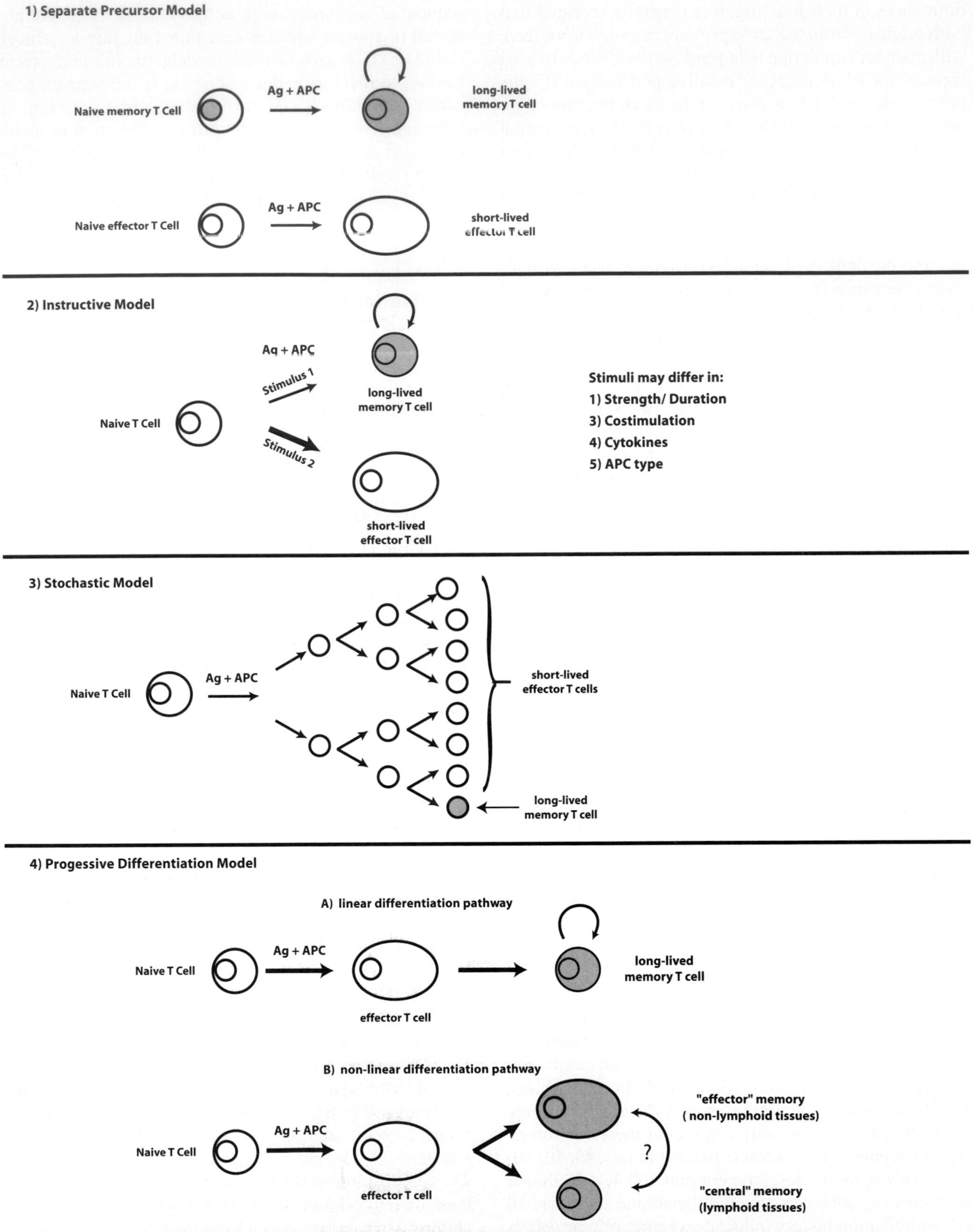

1) Separate Precursor Model
Naive memory T Cell
Ag + APC
long-lived
memory T cell
Naive effector T Cell
Ag + APC
short-lived
effector T cell
2) Instructive Model
Ag + APC
Stimulus 1
Stimulus 2
long-lived
memory T cell
Naive T Cell
short-lived
effector T cell
Stimuli may differ in:
1) Strength/ Duration
3) Costimulation
4) Cytokines
5) APC type
3) Stochastic Model
Naive T Cell
Ag + APC
short-lived
effector T cells
long-lived
memory T cell
4) Progessive Differentiation Model
A) linear differentiation pathway
Naive T Cell
Ag + APC
effector T cell
long-lived
memory T cell
B) non-linear differentiation pathway
Naive T Cell
Ag + APC
effector T cell
"effector" memory
(non-lymphoid tissues)
?
"central" memory
(lymphoid tissues)

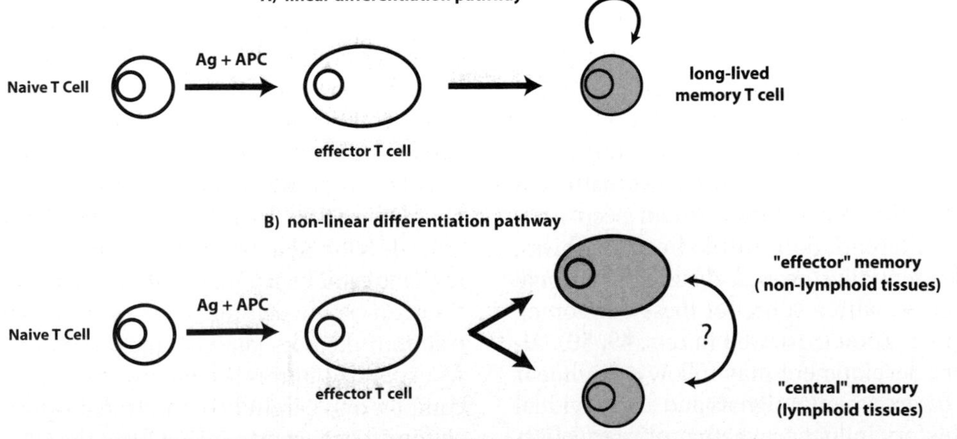

FIGURE 28.1 Models of memory T cell generation.

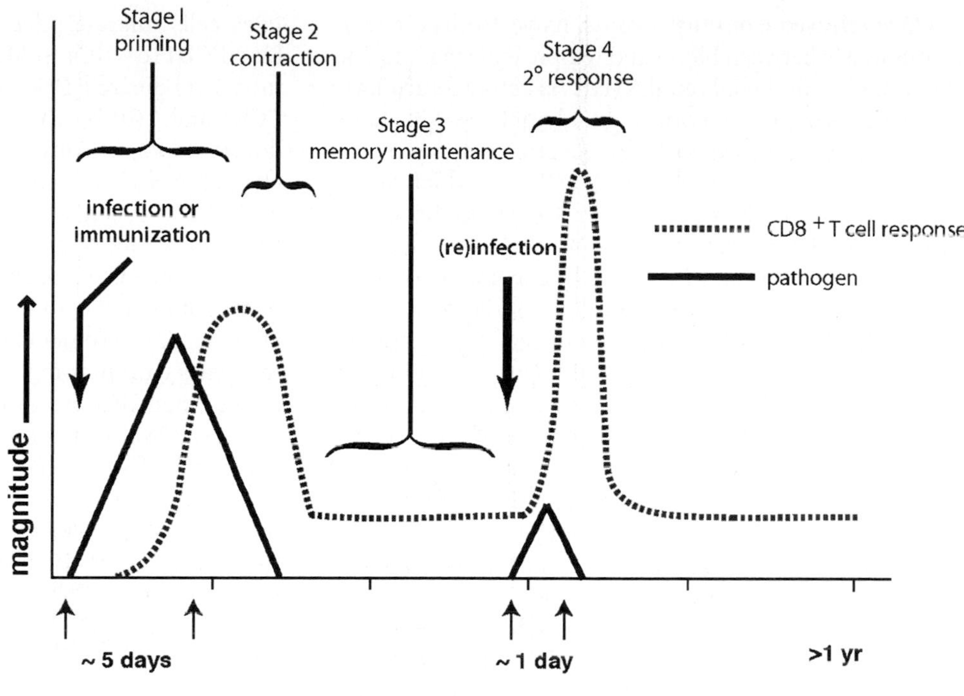

FIGURE 28.2 Stages of the T cell response to infection

next phases (maintenance and recall) of the CD8+ T cell response are considered in a subsequent section.

Phase I: Priming and Clonal Expansion

The process of generating T cell memory begins at priming, which is the initial activation of mature postthymic precursors by peripheral antigens. Before the priming phase can be initiated, however, antigen-specific naïve precursors must sample a network of professional antigen-presenting cells, usually dendritic cells (DCs), within the spleen and lymph nodes (LNs) and locate the rare few that present the specific surface class I MHC/peptide complex recognized by their TCR. This is not a simple task because CD8+ T cells recognizing any one single antigen are rare in the naïve repertoire, occurring with a frequency of perhaps 1 in 10^5 to 10^6 among the total population (68). The antigen-bearing APCs are also likely to be infrequent among the (tens of) millions of cells within a given LN or in the spleen because in most cases they must first obtain their antigenic cargo at peripheral sites of infection and then migrate via the lymphatics to LNs or via the bloodstream to the spleen (69). As will be described, the complex interaction of rare and migrating cell types necessary for the generation of immune responses is facilitated by highly regulated patterns of migration and by the structural features of the secondary lymphoid organs themselves.

Naïve T cells are produced at a modest rate by the thymus, with approximately 1–2 × 10^6 cells per day emerging into the bloodstream in young mice (70,71). These recent thymic emigrants (RTEs) are preferentially incorporated into the periphery regardless of the size of the existing pool (72). The homeostatic survival of naïve cells/RTE requires at least two types of extrinsic signals: (a) MHC molecules that are presumably occupied with low-affinity ligands (self or environmental peptides) and provide tonic TCR stimulation, and (b) a critical cytokine, interleukin-7 (IL-7) (73–79). IL-7 is a nonredundant member of the type I cytokine family that signals through a heterodimer comprised of the common cytokine signaling γ-chain (γc) and IL-7Rα (reviewed in ref. 80). Neither of these components is unique to IL-7; γc is shared with IL-2, IL-4, IL9, IL-15, and IL-21, and IL-7Rα is shared with thymic stromal lymphopoetin (TSLP). IL-7 is produced by nonhematopoietic stromal cells in multiple organs, including the thymus, where it promotes survival of developing T cells, and within peripheral lymphoid organs, intestine, and liver, among other sites. IL-7 has many roles in lymphopoiesis, promoting the survival, proliferation, and development of B cells, thymocytes, and mature T cells (81). Because γc is expressed widely among lymphocytes, IL-7 responsiveness is governed by surface levels of IL-Rα that are tightly regulated through thymopoiesis (high on double negative cells, absent on double positive cells, and high once again on thymocytes undergoing positive selection) and, as will be discussed, on naïve and memory T cells (82,83). Consequently, mice deficient in either IL-7 or IL-Rα have severely reduced numbers of peripheral T cells, and excess IL-7 provided exogenously or through transgenic expression leads to cycling and expansion of the naïve T cell pool (84–88).

Once released from the thymus, naïve T cells circulate continuously between blood and lymph, entering into LNs via the high endothelial venules (HEVs) before returning to the blood through the thoracic duct lymph (89–93). Naïve T cells express high levels of two receptors that are critical for this pattern of recirculation: (a) CD62L, which allows T cells to arrest at the site of expression of specific ligands expressed on HEV and initiate the process of translocation into the LN cortex, and (b) CCR7, a chemokine receptor that allows T cells to follow a gradient of the chemokines CCL19 (ELC) and CCL21 (SLC) produced by LN endothelial cells at the point of entry (94,95). Once inside the LN environment, naïve T cells are guided by a network of collagen fibers ensheathed in specialized stromal cells (called fibroblast reticular cells [FRCs]) toward specialized T cell compartments, where they encounter APCs that have arrived from peripheral sites via afferent lymph drainage and transport through pores in the subcapsular sinus (96–100). Thus the entry of naïve T cells into the LN is a highly regulated process that is facilitated by specific homing receptors, chemokines, and the structural features of the LN environment. Entry of naïve T cells into the spleen, by contrast, is nonspecific, with blood-borne precursors carried in by the splenic artery and deposited in the marginal zone between the red and white pulp before moving selectively to the white pulp, where they accumulate around central arterioles called periarteriolar lymphocyte sheaths (PALS). The movement of naïve T cells from the marginal zone to the PALS is guided by CCR7-mediated recognition of ligands expressed on stromal cells; activated CD8$^+$ T cells lacking this receptor are excluded from the white pulp and effector cells, with enforced expression of CCR7 localized almost exclusively to this compartment (101,102). Continuous migration of naïve T cells through the secondary lymphoid organs ensures their rapid exposure to antigens derived from pathogens. In the absence of antigenic stimulation, the blood-to-lymph process takes about 12 to 18 hours for circulation through LNs, whereas the average residence time of a naïve T cell in the spleen is 12 hours (103). To become stimulated (primed), naïve T cells must recognize antigens in the form of peptide fragments bound to MHC molecules on professional antigen-presenting cells such as DCs. Within the T cell areas of LN and spleen, DCs form a dense cellular network that is continuously sampled by recirculating T cells for the presence of antigenic peptides, that is, those peptides for which a TCR repertoire exists and which are presented in an immunogenic context by an activated APC.

In their response to microbial pathogens, immature DCs migrate to sites of infection and inflammation in response to a range of CC and CXC chemokines. For example, immature DCs respond to CCL3, CCL4, CCL5, and CCL20, which are inducible on inflammatory stimuli (104–107). Of note, each immature DC population displays a unique spectrum of chemokine responsiveness. Langerhans cells migrate selectively to CCL20 (via CCR6) and blood CD11c$^+$ DCs to MCP chemokines (via CCR2), and monocyte-derived DCs respond to CCL3 and CCL4 (via CCR1 and CCR5), whereas blood CD11c$^-$ DC precursors do not respond to any of these chemokines. Each of these chemokines is inducible on inflammatory stimuli, such as CCL20, which is only detected within inflamed epithelium, a site of antigen entry known to be infiltrated by immature DCs. Once at the site of infection, DCs acquire both soluble and particulate antigens through various phagocytic (pinocytosis, phagocytosis) and endocytic pathways (receptor-mediated endocytosis) that are highly active when DCs are in the immature state (reviewed in refs. 69, 108). As a consequence of antigen uptake at the site of an infection, these DCs will be exposed to a range of immunostimulatory adjuvants derived from the infectious microorganisms themselves, such as lipopolysaccharide (LPS), double-stranded RNA, or unmethylated CpG DNA that can be recognized by a family of highly conserved germline-encoded sensor molecules called Toll-like receptors (109–111). These receptors, expressed on the plasma membrane and within cells, signal through a set of intracellular adaptor molecules called TIR adaptor proteins because they share a common Toll-like/IL-1 receptor domain used for homophilic association with the TLRs (112). Four 4TIR proteins are identified that transduce TLR-mediated signals (MyD88, MAL/Tirap, TRIF/Ticam-1/Lps2, TRAM), and a fifth (SARM) appears to negatively regulate TRIF (113–120). Each of the TIR adaptor proteins associates with a specific set of TLRs (MyD88 with all TLRs, TRIF with TLR-3 and TLR4, etc.), and it is believed that differential use of these TIR domain–containing adaptors provides specificity to individual TLR-mediated signaling pathways (121,122). Ligation of different TLRs induces gene programs in DCs that lead not only to the robust production of general proinflammatory mediators and upregulation of costimulatory molecules, but also to the production of unique effectors, which provide pathogen-tailored immune responses. In addition to directly sensing the presence of infectious microbes, DCs can also react to the tissue damage caused by these microorganisms via endogenous "danger" signals such as heat-shock proteins, nucleotides, reactive oxygen intermediates, extracellular-matrix breakdown products, neuromediators that are released by stressed or damaged tissues, or those undergoing abnormal death (123). Damaged or infected cells can also produce alarm signals through the production of interferons, such as type I interferons (IFNα, IFNβ) that can lead to complex signaling events within DCs that synergize with those emanating from TLRs to promote a range of gene expression and functional changes in DCs (reviewed in refs. 124, 125).

After exposure to either endogenous or exogenous alarm signals, DCs undergo a transition from an immature to a mature state and begin to express new chemokine receptors that facilitate their migration away from sites of inflammation and toward the T cell areas of secondary lymphoid organs (126). The most important among these is CCR7, the same receptor used by naïve T cells for LN chemokinesis (reviewed in ref. 127). The CCL19-CCL21-CCR7 chemokine system, therefore, plays a critical role in orchestrating immune responses by guiding both naïve T cells and migrating DCs to high-traffic areas within the deep cortex of LNs, where they can interact and T cell priming can occur. Consistent with this, mice lacking either CCR7 or CCL19/CCL21 have profound defects in T cell and DC motility and mount substantially depressed antiviral T cell responses (128–132). In addition to altered migration characteristics, DCs undergoing maturation initiate a variety of other changes that enhance their capacity to present antigen in an immunogenic form. These include a marked cellular redistribution of major histocompatibility complex class II molecules (MHC II) from late endosomal and lysosomal compartments to the plasma membrane that is accompanied by downregulation of some forms of endocytosis (133–137). The result of this is the surface presentation of MHC class II molecules with a substantially increased half-life, thus preserving the "antigenic fingerprint" of the material (in the form of peptides bound to MHC molecules) ingested at the site of infection for subsequent presentation to T cells in the secondary lymphoid organs (138).

Another critical consequence of DC activation is the upregulated expression of numerous costimulatory molecules and cytokines that contribute to T cell priming by promoting cell division, survival, and differentiation (69,139–141). The primary activation of naïve T cells has traditionally been believed to require at least two signals: an antigen-specific "signal 1" that is transmitted on TCR-mediated recognition of its cognate peptide/MHC complex and an antigen nonspecific "signal 2" costimulus (142,143). This "two-signal" model predicted that engagement of the TCR in the absence of costimulation is insufficient for sustained clonal expansion and cytokine production, and cells instead become anergic and unresponsive to further stimulation (144). Although this outcome has been demonstrated in a number of studies, the number of ligand/receptor pairs capable of functioning as "signal(s) two" has grown considerably in the last decade. CD80 and CD86 are considered to be the prototypical costimulatory molecules expressed on APC capable of transmitting "signal 2" through their interaction with CD28 expressed on T cells. CD80/86-mediated ligation of CD28 produces signals in T cells that are distinct from that of the TCR and enhances clonal expansion, effector functions, and memory development (145–148). Although many $CD4^+$ and $CD8^+$ T cell responses depend on CD28, the requirement is not absolute because many types of T cell responses can occur in its absence *in vivo*, including allograft rejection, induction of allogeneic graft-versus-host and delayed-type hypersensitivity responses, and the generation of cytotoxic $CD8^+$ T cells (149–153). These observations suggest that additional pathways exist for costimulation of T cells other than CD28 (154). A number of these have emerged from the tumor necrosis factor receptor (TNFR) family [CD27/CD70, 4-1BB (CD137)/4-1BBL, OX40 (CD134)/OX40-L, HVEM-LIGHT, CD30/CD30-L, and GITR], each of which can provide costimulatory stimuli that synergize with TCR signals to sustain T cell activation after priming and have been shown to be important for the magnitude and longevity of $CD8^+$ T cell responses *in vivo* in studies of knockout mice lacking either ligand or receptor (reviewed in refs. 154–156). It should be pointed out that the influence of costimulatory interactions on the regulation of $CD8^+$ T cells responses is by no means limited to the priming event: Several receptor–ligand pairs, notably 4-1BB/4-1BBL, OX4O/OX40L, BTLA/HVEM, and PD-1/PDL1/PDL1, can act on the expanded population with either positive or negative effects on T cell function and survival (156–158).

In addition to contact-dependent costimulation, a number of inflammatory cytokines including IL-12, IFN$\alpha\beta$, and IFNγ, have been implicated in the transmission of a "signal 3" that is required for optimal development of $CD8^+$ T cells (reviewed in ref. 159). One of these is IL-12, produced by DCs after some infections and by CD40 stimulation; it helps to drive the development of Th1-polarized $CD4^+$ responses (reviewed in ref. 160). Addition of IL-12 to $CD8^+$ T cells primed by peptide/MHC and B7 or IL-2 substantially promotes their proliferation, survival, and cytotoxic potential (161–163). The effect appears to be directly on the $CD8^+$ T cells because IL-12 can support wild-type $CD8^+$ T cell responses in IL-12Rβ_1-deficient hosts (164). The evidence for IFN$\alpha\beta$ as a signal 3 for $CD8^+$ T cells is less clear and may be influenced by the nature of the immunogen. Studies on $CD8^+$ T cells primed *in vitro* with peptide/MHC and CD80 showed that optimal expansion and development of lytic functions required addition of IFNα (165). *In vivo* studies with IFN$\alpha\beta$R-deficient LCMV GP-specific $CD8^+$ T cells transferred to wild-type mice showed dramatic reductions in their ability to undergo clonal expansion and to generate a memory pool following infection with LCMV (166,167). When the LCMV GP was expressed from a recombinant vaccinia virus, however, only a modest defect in $CD8^+$ T cell expansion and survival was observed, suggesting that the IFN$\alpha\beta$ dependence of $CD8^+$ T cell memory is influenced not by the target antigen but rather by the immunogen (166). This idea has found support in a recent study showing that the response of IFN$\alpha\beta$R-deficient transgenic $CD8^+$ T cells to the same peptide-pulsed DC vaccine offered in the context of four different infections (LCMV, vaccinia virus, vesicular stomatitis virus, and *Listeria monocytogenes*) were most severely inhibited for LCMV infection (166a). IFNγ has also been shown to support optimal $CD8^+$ T cell expansion

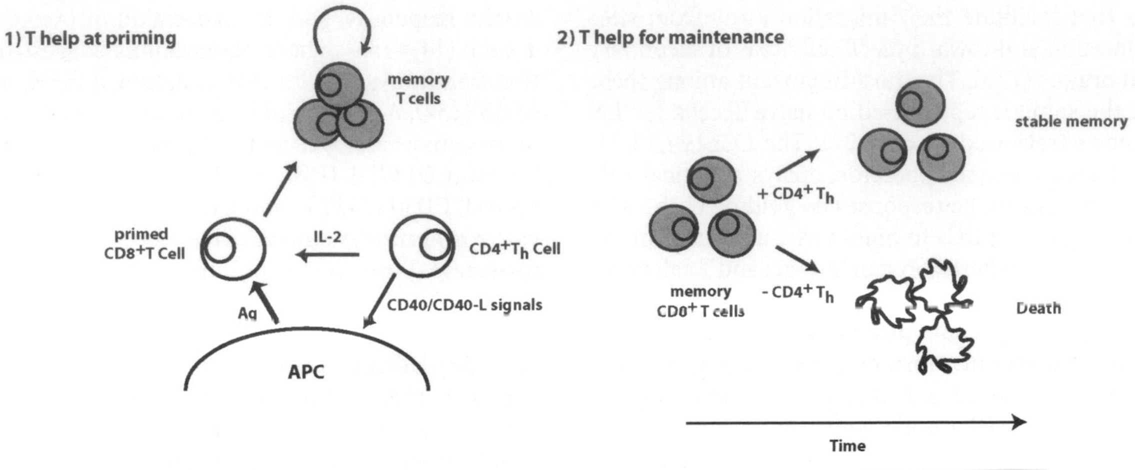

FIGURE 28.3 Models of CD4+ T cell help for CD8+ memory formation.

after LCMV infection or peptide vaccination, and transgenic CD8+ T cells lacking the IFNγR1 display reduced expansion compared to wild-type cells in the same host (168–170). It is unclear why a range of factors can serve as signal 3, but the answer may have something to do with pathogen-specific innate responses and the range of inflammatory cytokines (i.e., IFNαβ versus IL-12, etc.) that each produces (159). Alternatively, the kinetics with which the various signal 3 cytokines are produced could ensure that CD8+ T cell responses are exposed to at least one during the course of their priming.

Although DCs increase their immunogenicity in response to inflammatory stimuli delivered at peripheral sites of antigen uptake, their stimulatory capacity can be further enhanced within the LNs through the action of CD4+ "helper" cells (Th) that recognize peptide antigens bound to MHC class II molecules at the surface of the same APC presenting to the CD8+ T cell (171–173) (Figure 28.3). The contribution of Th cells to CD8+ priming had initially been thought to be conditional, that is, required for response to some immunogens but not others, and limited in mechanism to the production of paracrine IL-2 for the benefit of CD8+ T cells present in a "three-cell cluster" together with APCs (174–176). More recent evidence, however, has shown that CD4+ T cells make important contributions to the generation and maintenance of CD8+ T cell responses at a number of discrete steps (reviewed in refs. 172, 177). Several studies have shown that a key function of Th cells involves the engagement of CD40 on DCs, which leads to a number of immunostimulatory alterations, including high-level expression of costimulatory and adhesion molecules, including CD80, CD86, 4-1BB, OX40, and CD70, as well as high-level production of IL-12 (156,178–182). CD4+ T cells can also help to guide naïve CCR5-expressing CD8+ T cell precursors to relevant APCs within secondary lymph nodes by enhancing production of the chemokines CCL3 and CCL4 at the CD4+ T cell/DC interface (183,184). NKT cells are also able to provide CD40-dependent "help" for CD8+ T cell responses, likely through recognition of glycolipid ligands such as α-galactosyl ceramide that are presented by CD1 molecules at the surface of DCs (185–187). Finally, CD4+ T cells have been shown to be important for the maintenance of CD8+ T cells whether they were primed in the presence or absence of Th cells (188). The "help" under these conditions apparently need not be cognate (antigen specific) as it is in the case of help for priming, suggesting that its role may involve the direct or indirect provision of homeostatic survival factors (discussed in the next section) (34). The absence of Th cells can have different effects on the CD8+ T cell response depending on the immunogen and the functional parameter measured. In most cases, the primary response to immunization or acute infection is only modestly decreased. In acute infections using higher challenge doses and in chronic viral infections, however, CD8+ T cells responses wane over time, leading to either deletion or exhaustion, a state of persistence without effector function (189–195). An explanation for these findings may be based in the "helpless" or "lethargic" phenotype displayed by CD8+ T cells primed in the absence of Th cells in which they proliferate less, produce fewer cytokines during primary responses, and are defective in their ability to mount secondary proliferative responses, a hallmark of immune memory (196–200). In the case of recall responses to a cellular vaccine, the mechanism responsible involves the Th-mediated modification of the CD8+ T cell developmental program to avoid apoptosis on secondary stimulation by TRAIL (TNF-related apoptosis-inducing ligand) *(201)*. The role of TRAIL in this process may be limited in its duration because, although TRAIL appears to regulate the secondary expansion defect of "helpless" CD8+ T cells for at least 4 weeks after priming in the absence of Th cells, additional factors conferred by CD4+ T cells are required for their homeostatic survival in the months afterward *(202)*.

Once a naïve CD8+ T cell recognizes its cognate peptide/MHC ligand on an activated DC within the secondary lymphoid organs, the interactions of priming (i.e., the 'antigenic signal') can take place. The molecular details of this process involves the formation of immune synapses at the T/APC contact site that are composed of rapidly clustering TCR molecules binding peptide/MHC complexes on APCs plus the local accumulation of intracellular signaling molecules such PKC-θ, LAT, and LCK. The signaling events and downstream consequences for T cell activation are discussed in Chapters 11 and 13. To elucidate the cellular details of CD8+ T cell priming, several groups have used multiphoton and confocal microscopy to visualize the process within intact LNs. These studies have revealed that the lymph node environment is dynamic, with T cell migration at a velocity of approximately 12 mm/min in their search for antigen and DCs able to sample 500 T cells per hour and make contacts with 10 T cells at any given moment *(203–206)*. By applying these visualization techniques to LNs within living animals (intravital microscopy), the priming of naïve CD8+ T cells by DC was observed to occur in three distinct phases *(207)*. The first lasts several hours and is characterized by short interactions between T cells and DCs, with upregulation of activation markers such as CD44 and CD69.

Phase 2 of priming lasts for approximately 12 hours and features sustained (1 hour or longer) contacts between T cells and DCs as well as initiation of cytokine production. In the third phase, the T cells disengage from the DCs, proliferate, and return to their pattern of high motility. The rate of CD8+ T cell clonal expansion can be remarkable, with cells undergoing sequential divisions approximately every 6 to 8 hours during their initial rounds (32,*208–211*). The extent of CD8+ T cell division and magnitude of their numerical increase can be equally impressive, with cells undergoing 15 to 20 rounds of division and number of effector cells increasing more than 10^4-fold over their initial frequency in the naïve repertoire in the setting of acute infection with LCMV or *Listeria (212–215)*. The factors that govern the extent of CD8+ T cell division *in vivo* are unclear but may relate to the availability of antigen, as demonstrated in studies that have revealed a relationship between antigen load and the number of effector cells generated *(209,210,216–218)*. Coincident with their clonal expansion, the growing population of CD8+ T cells develop the key effector capacities that are important to their function as cytotoxic cells. The full differentiation of CD8+ T cells into cytotoxic effectors appears to be tightly linked to proliferation because the same stimulus provided to clonal precursors to induce their clonal expansion also results in the development of effector functions such as secretion of IFNγ and TNF and to kill target cells *(209–211)*. These observations suggest that at least for CD8+ T cells, the commitment to division and effector differentiation are elements of an instructional program of development that is established in clonal precursors by inductive signals transmitted during their primary activation. Because memory CD8+ T cells appear to originate from this same event, their development can also be seen as a resulting from instructional programs established during priming (44,*219*). Although many details remain to be elucidated, programming appears to involve the acquisition of specific functional capacities in response to discrete signals received during the priming phase. For example, the presence of CD4+ T cells during the priming of CD8+ T cell precursors endows their clonal progeny with the ability to undergo secondary proliferative responses on reencounter with antigen (198). More recently, a role for IL-2–mediated signals transmitted via CD25, the high-affinity subunit of the IL-2 receptor, to CD8+ T cells has been demonstrated in programming their capacity for secondary expansion *(220)*. These experiments used radiation bone marrow chimeras to control the expression of CD25 on CD8+ T cells and IL-2/anti–IL-2 immune complexes to provide IL-2 signals. They revealed that secondary expansion of memory CD8+ T cells detected at day 60 required that IL-2 signals were provided during the first week of priming by infection *(220)*. The IL-2 signal was not required for the primary expansion of the CD8+ T cells, and its source in this scenario is unknown, being either autocrine, from the CD8+ T cells themselves, or paracrine, from either CD4+ Th cells or activated DCs that have been shown to produce IL-2 in response to microbial stimuli *(221–224)*.

After commitment to clonal expansion and acquisition of effector functions, CD8+ T cells begin to express new surface patterns of chemokine, homing, and adhesion receptors that mediate their egress from LNs and facilitate their migration to peripheral sites. An initial event in this process is the downregulation of CD62L and CCR7, the receptors used by naïve precursors to enter the lymph node, and restoration of the chemotactic response to the lysophospholipid sphingosine-1-phosphate (S1P) through reexpression of its receptor (S1P-receptor-1), which promotes migration to blood and lymph by distinct sources of its ligand (35,*225–227*). After this, the migration of effector CD8+ T cells to nonlymphoid tissues is largely determined by homing receptors and chemokines *(228)*. These include chemokine receptors such as CCR2 and CCR5 that guide cells to inflammatory sites through recognition of a variety of ligands, as well as α1- and β1-integrins such as LFA-1 that allow activated T cells to bind to and penetrate the walls of small blood vessels and thereby gain access to extravascular spaces throughout the body. In some cases, and for reasons that are poorly understood, a subset of these cells reexpress CD62L and CCR7, thereby allowing their reentry into the LN, where they can function as central memory cells (T_{CM}s), the functional properties of which are described in the following section *(229)*. Others migrate to the spleen via the blood and take up residence in the red pulp and are largely excluded from the white pulp (101). The ultimate "address" to which the cell will migrate, however, can be influenced by the conditions under which it was activated. In response to systemic infection, for example, the migration of effector CD8$^+$ T cells can be relatively nonspecific and promiscuous, with cells able to access all nonlymphoid compartments (35,*230,231*). This has been confirmed in parabiosis studies (involving surgically conjoined animals) showing that effector cells primed in the infected parabiont equilibrate in essentially all tissues of its noninfected partner within 2 weeks *(232)*. In other cases, however, the migration of T cells can be tissue specific, reflecting the particular homing receptors they expressed. The homing of activated T cells to inflamed skin, for example, depends on binding to E- and P-selectins and tissue-specific chemokines, such as CCL17, expressed by skin vascular epithelium, and TACK, expressed on keratinocytes that are recognized by complimentary receptors on T cells, that is, E- and P-selectin ligands, CCR4, and CCR10 (for CCL17 and TACK, respectively) *(233,234)*.

In some instances, the pattern of homing receptors expressed by CD8$^+$ T cells can result from imprinting by the DCs responsible for their priming or reactivation. DCs from Peyer's patches—specialized secondary lymphoid organs within the intestine—have been shown to induce the selective expression of the integrin $\alpha4\beta7$ and the CCR9 chemokine receptor, both of which are essential for gut homing, in CD8$^+$ T cells *(235–238)*. The migration pattern of gut versus skin homing appears to be "reprogrammable," however, because restimulation of gut-tropic T cells by peripheral LN DCs can restore a skin-homing phenotype *(235–238)*. Thus, DCs not only can transmit information to naïve T cells regarding the presence of an infectious pathogen encountered at the site of inflammation through exogenous and endogenous danger signals, but they also can instruct T cells to express the appropriate homing receptors needed to enable their migration to the specific anatomic site where they are needed, that is, where ligands for these receptors are produced (36).

Contraction

After clonal expansion and effector differentiation, CD8$^+$ T cells migrate to the periphery, where they can engage the pathogen through direct killing of infected cells through use of death receptors (Fas, TNF, etc.), secretion of lytic granules (containing perforin, granzymes, etc.), or production of effector cytokines such as TNF or IFNγ that can act either directly or through activation of accessory cells such as macrophages and DCs *(239–241)*. Coincident with pathogen clearance at the end of the primary response, the majority of effector CD8$^+$ T cells within secondary lymphoid organs will be eliminated through a complex and poorly understood process that involves their orderly apoptosis (programmed cell death [PCD]) via interactions among various member of the TNF family of cell surface receptors and well as elements of the mitochondrial pathway of apoptosis (reviewed in refs. *242, 243*). Effector molecules such as perforin and IFNγ can play a role in contraction, in that mice deficient in either of these have increased numbers of CD8$^+$ T cells in both the expansion and contraction phases (168). The contraction phase leaves a small population of cells, perhaps 5% to 10% of the numbers present at the peak of the response, to survive as the memory subset at levels that remain stable for the life of the animal (reviewed in refs. *244, 245*). Although the disappearance of CD8$^+$ T cells has traditionally been considered as causally related to the elimination of the infectious pathogen and the disappearance of antigen, recent evidence suggests that contraction, like many other aspects of the CD8$^+$ T cell response, can be "programmed," that is, independent of the extent of clonal expansion, the dose and duration of infection, or the amount of antigen displayed *(246,247)*. The removal of effector cells achieves two important goals for the immune system, in that it prevents the T cell repertoire from being skewed to a focused population of cells that have outlived their usefulness, and it restores homeostasis to the available environmental niches for support of T cells so that new antigenic challenges can be met. The loss of CD8$^+$ T cells from secondary lymphoid organs at the end of immune responses is largely attributable to apoptotic death, although some portion of this is also due to the irreversible migration of cells into peripheral tissues such as the lung, intestine, and bone marrow, where activated cells are maintained more stably over long periods of time *(248–253)*.

The apoptotic death of T cells during the contraction phase can occur by two main pathways: (a) activation-induced cell death (AICD), also called antigen (Ag)-driven ("active") apoptosis, and (b) cell autonomous or activated T cell autonomous cell death (ACAD). AICD is believed to operate toward the end of the expansion phase following priming and can be triggered by TCR stimulation and signals transmitted via various surface-expressed members of the TNF receptor family such as Fas, Fas ligand, and TNF and the p55 and p75 TNF receptors (reviewed in ref. *254*). The degree to which CD8$^+$ T cells are eradicated through AICD *in vivo* depends on their subsequent encounter with antigen and death receptor ligands such as CD95-L (FasL), TNF, and TRAIL during or near the end of their clonal expansion phase and on the balance of proapoptotic (FADD, FLICE, etc.) and antiapoptotic (c-FLIP, Bcl-2, Bcl-XL, etc.) proteins they express *(255,256)*. The anatomic location of the T cell also plays a role, in that T cells in peripheral nonlymphoid tissues such as the lungs, fat pad, and peritoneal cavity are more resistant to apoptosis than those in secondary lymphoid organs *(253)*. It is not known whether this reflects intrinsic properties of the effector memory subset that occupy these nonlymphoid niches, or whether the local cellular environment (through cells and/or cytokines) controls T cell turnover in the periphery (33–35).

In contrast to the Ag-driven pathway, ACAD does not depend on death cytokines, receptors, or antigen but appears to involve the proapoptotic activities of the Bcl-2–related protein Bim and PUMA (p53-upregulated modulator of apoptosis), which are induced by a variety of cellular stressors, including the withdrawal of key survival cytokines such as IL-2, IL-7, and IL-15 *(243,257–263)*. BIM or PUMA can bind Bcl-2 or BCL-XL on the mitochondrial membrane and promote the release of cytochrome c and the induction of cell death *(264,265)*. During their expansion phase, T cells also decrease their expression levels of Bcl-XL and thereby allow for activation of the intrinsic ACAD pathway *(266)*. Both AICD and ACAD are believed to work through a final common pathway involving cysteinyl aspartate–specific proteases (caspases) that activate the apoptotic cascade *(245,267)*. ACAD, rather than AICD, is believed to be responsible for the contraction of $CD8^+$ T cells that follows the expansion phase. The extent of contraction within a given $CD8^+$ T cell response can be variable, with decreases of 95% of peak numbers observed in cases of acute systemic infections with virus or bacteria and more modest decreases seen when the infection is limited, for example, with antibiotics in the case of *Listeria* infection, although this may also limit the size of the memory pool generated (32,*213–215,268,269*).

Generation of $CD4^+$ T Cell Memory

Although a number of unique features characterize the generation of $CD4^+$ memory T cells, many of the basic processes described in the preceding section on $CD8^+$ memory T generation are also relevant for the initiation of $CD4^+$ T cell responses. Common features include the factors governing the ontogeny of naïve T cells, the role of extrinsic signals in their survival, and the range of homing receptors and migration patterns that guide them to the secondary lymphoid organs where priming occurs. In addition, the role APCs in the acquisition and transport of Ag and the role of inflammatory signals in determining the (co)stimulatory context in which it will ultimately be presented are also shared between $CD4^+$ and $CD8^+$ T cells. Other aspects of their biology related to priming and memory development are distinct from $CD8^+$ T cells and will be discussed in this section. These include their capacity develop into long-lived memory cells, key aspects of their functional specialization, and the extent of their clonal expansion and contraction. $CD4^+$ T cells contribute to immunity in a number of ways, including through activation of DC via CD40–CD40L interactions, the secretion of inflammatory cytokines such as IFNγ that activate the antimicrobial response of macrophages, and by providing help to both B cells for antibody responses and to $CD8^+$ T cells for their optimal development into memory cells (141,179,*270–273*). In addition, regulatory $CD4^+$ T cells (Treg) identified by expression of the transcription factor FoxP3 can profoundly suppress the development of immune responses directed against self and non-self antigens (reviewed in refs. *274–276*).

Less is known about memory development in $CD4^+$ than in $CD8^+$ T cells. This is due in part to the apparent reduced capacity of $CD4^+$ T cells to develop into long-term resting memory cells compared to $CD8^+$ T cells in the widely used murine models of infection such as vaccinia, LCMV, Sendai virus, and *L. monocytogenes (208,277–279)*. Likewise, adoptive transfer studies with $CD44^{high}$ memory phenotype $CD4^+$ T cells have shown that a nondividing subset disappears with a half-life similar to that of naïve cells *(280)*. A comparatively smaller number of studies have been undertaken using sensitive tools such as peptide/MHC tetramers and transgenic T cells that have facilitated memory $CD8^+$ T cells studies through the detection and phenotyping of responding populations at the single-cell level *(281,282)*. As with $CD8^+$ T cell responses, the generation of $CD4^+$ memory T cells is believed to occur during the same priming event that produces the effector cells. Once primed, however, $CD4^+$ and $CD8^+$ T cells display intrinsic differences in both their kinetics of activation and proliferative potential. For example, it has been observed that $CD8^+$ T cells require a comparatively shorter period of stimulation (2 to 4 hours) for commitment to clonal expansion and effector development than do $CD4^+$ T cells (approximately 20 hours) *(209,211,283,284)*. $CD8^+$ T cells also begin dividing earlier after priming than $CD4^+$ T cells and have a faster rate of division *(284–287)*. In addition, and in contrast to $CD8^+$ T cells, it has been observed that $CD4^+$ T cells require continued antigenic stimulation throughout their period of expansion to achieve full proliferative and effector potential *(288,289)*. Based on these and other findings, Lanzavecchia and Sallusto suggested that the optimal development of memory T cells will occur in cells that receive a specific level of antigenic stimulation during their priming and subsequent expansion that enables them to use and access survival signals in a process termed progressive differentiation (48,*283,290,291*).

Naïve $CD4^+$ T cells constitute a multipotent precursor population in which clonal precursors expressing a single antigenic specificity can be directed toward distinct differentiation fates by the actions of both the innate and adaptive arms of the immune system. A surprising variety of functional subsets of $CD4^+$ T cells can be generated through a complex process of differentiation involving the interactions of specific cytokines, cell-signaling proteins, and transcription factors that lead to stable and heritable changes in gene expression patterns that are established and maintained by chromatin remodeling (26,160,292). Th1 cells, for example, are generated by priming of $CD4^+$ T cells in the presence of IL-12 produced by APCs that are stimulated in response to TLR signals or CD40 signals (from activated CD4+ T cells or NKT cells) *(293,294)*. TCRs and cytokine signals then act together through signaling and transcription factors such as signal transducer and activator of transcription factor 4 (STAT4) and T-bet to induce functional differentiation into IFNγ-producing effector cells that promote development of cellular immune responses *(295,296)*. Similarly, Th2 cells are generated by priming of CD4+ T cells in the presence of IL-4, thereby activating STAT4 and GATA-3 to induce differentiation into effector cells that produce IL-4, IL-5, and IL-13 as "signature cytokines" and favor the development of humoral responses and those against certain parasites *(297–299)*. There is considerable evidence for cross-regulation of these two subsets through the cytokines they produce, with the development of Th1 cells being inhibited by Th2-produced IL-4 and the development of Th2 subset being inhibited by IFNγ-produced Th1 cells. Thus as each subset becomes polarized, its development into Th1 versus Th2 cells will be reinforced by its specific pattern of autocrine cytokine production. More recently, a new cytokine-polarized subset of the CD4+ T cell subset has been described that produces the cytokine IL-17 and is suspected of playing a central role in inflammatory responses and autoimmunity *(300–303)*. Although the exact details of Th17 development remain to be elucidated, the cytokines IL-6 and transforming growth factor-β (TGFβ) appear to play an instructive role in their differentiation through engagement of the IL-21 and IL-23 pathways, as well as the transcription factor STAT-3 and the nuclear orphan receptor RORg *(304–307)*. The development of Th17 cells may be a reciprocal fate to that of Tregs for naïve CD4+ T cells primed in the presence of a TGFβ cytokine milieu, with the vitamin A metabolite retinoic acid functioning as a key regulator of inflammatory signals that determine the developmental path chosen under these conditions *(308–310)*.

Once activated, the magnitude of clonal expansion is more modest for CD4+ T cells than for CD8+ T cells, although unusually vigorous clonal bursts have been reported for responses against the bacterium *Salmonella* (50,*208,311*). The activation of naïve CD4+ has been shown to involve distinct costimulatory requirements from those of CD8+ T cell priming. These studies have mostly been carried out through infection experiments performed in knockout mice lacking specific ligand or receptors for these pathways. Whereas LCMV-specific CD8+ T cells can efficiently be generated in mice lacking CD28, CD40L, or OX40, virus-specific CD4+ T cell responses are substantially reduced. The opposite situation is seen in mice lacking 4-1BB, which mount normal CD4+ but diminished CD8+ T cell responses to LCMV infection (reviewed in ref. *312*). CD4+ T cells also display quantitative and kinetic differences in their contraction compared to CD8+ T cells. For example, after initial viral clearance, LCMV-specific CD4+ T cells initially contract rapidly but then substantially reduce their rate of disappearance and take a full 6 months to reach stable numbers of memory cells, whereas the CD8+ T response in this study achieved a stable "set-point" of memory after approximately 30 days *(279)*. Similarly, the numbers of CD4+ Sendai virus–specific T cells in the lung declined during the first 3 months after pulmonary infection, whereas the CD8+ T cell response remained stable during this period *(277)*. These observations of decreased longevity and diminished secondary responsiveness in Th1 T cells may relate to their production of IFNγ gas an effector cytokine. IFNγ-deficient mice generate 30% to 50% more activated CD4+ T cells in murine models of mycobacterial infection and experimental autoimmune encephalitis *(313,314)*. The regulatory capacity of IFNγ in CD4+ T cells is further supported by the observation that their longevity within homogeneous populations can be extended if this cytokine is inhibited during activation *(315,316)*. The mechanism underlying the selective susceptibility of IFNγ-producing Th1 cells appears to involve the induction of apoptosis via a caspase 8–dependent pathway and is selective for this CD4+ T cell subset because Th2 cells display a greater propensity for memory formation *(317,318)*. There is little information on the ability of the Treg and Th17 subsets to form memory, although this will certainly change in the near future due to active experimentation in these fields. Finally, in contrast to CD8+ memory T cells, the majority of CD4+ memory T cells do not reexpress CD62L: Only 30% of polyclonal CD4+ T cells express this marker as compared with 90% of memory CD8+ T cells in some systems *(319,320)*. The absence of CD62L expression does not preclude access into lymph nodes, however, because these CD4+ T cells can access lymph nodes via the afferent lymph, as shown by the presence of memory phenotype CD4+ T cells found in the lymph nodes of CD62L$^{-/-}$ mice *(321)*.

Generation of Memory B Cells and Plasma Cells

Immunologic memory in the B cell compartment consists of two very different cell types: memory B cells and long-lived plasma cells. These two cell types perform two different functions. Long-lived plasma cells can be considered "active memory" because they continuously secrete voluminous quantities of antibodies that circulate in the blood. Memory B cells can be considered "quiescent memory" because these cells are resting, waiting for a second infection or reexposure to antigen to reactivate them. The proposed basic lineage relationship among naïve mature B cells, memory B cells, and plasma cells is shown in Figure 28.4. Different stages of B cell differentiation occur in histologically defined locations, as illustrated in Figure 28.5. In this basic model (Figures 28.4, 28.5), naïve mature B cells are activated by antigen (protein in adjuvant, viral infection, or autoantigen), and CD4 T cell help.

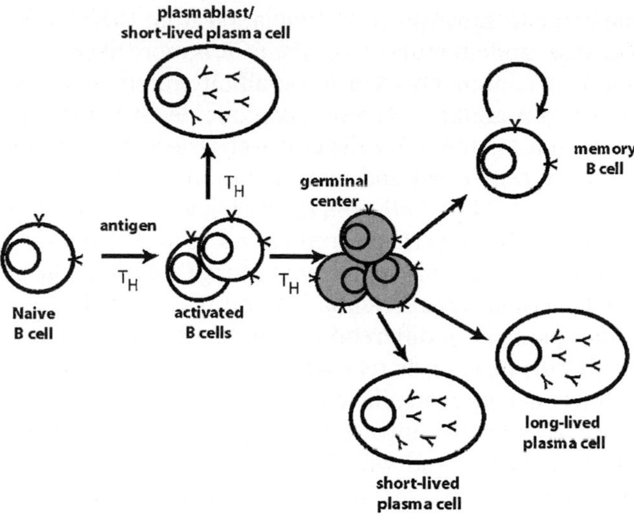

FIGURE 28.4 Development of B lineage immune response and memory. After antigenic stimulation, naïve B cells undergo clonal expansion and form clusters of activated B cells known as extrafollicular foci. These activated B cells can either differentiate into short-lived plasma cells or migrate back into the follicle and initiate a germinal center reaction. After proliferation and affinity maturation, germinal center B cells produce both long-lived plasma cells that produce high-affinity antibodies and memory B cells that have high-affinity B cell receptors. Memory B cells can self-renew by homeostatic proliferation. Memory B cells may also periodically differentiate, in an antigen-dependent or antigen-independent manner, into long-lived plasma cells to maintain long-term antibody production.

These initial interactions occur at the border between the T and B cell areas of the lymphoid organ (spleen or lymph node) *(322,323)*. The activated B cells undergo clonal expansion. During this initial phase of activation, B cells can class switch from immunoglobulin M (IgM) to IgG or other isotypes if stimulated strongly. B cells can initiate germinal centers in the follicle, or they can proliferate and differentiate into plasmablasts (intermediately differentiated antibody-secreting plasma cells) and plasma cells and migrate to the red pulp *(322)*, where they can be observed as extrafollicular foci, frequently residing adjacent to blood vessels *(322,324,325)*. Given the complexity of the biology involved, it is perhaps not surprising that there are clear examples of exceptions to the basic model of B cell memory generation outlined in Figures 28.4 and 28.5 where steps are bypassed or significantly altered *(326–329)*. Nevertheless, the model appears to hold true for most conditions *(273,330,331)*.

A second phase of clonal expansion and differentiation of activated B cells occurs within the specialized microenvironment of a germinal center (GC) *(325,332,333)*. Because antigen-specific memory B cells and long-lived plasma cells come from germinal centers, germinal centers are the critical sites for the development of long-term humoral immunity. The detailed mechanics of the germinal center reaction are unclear, but extensive research has been done into the processes of germinal center B cell selection and differentiation *(332)*. It is normally within the germinal centers that affinity maturation occurs. Affinity maturation is the process by which a B cell clone improves the affinity of its B cell receptor (BCR) for the cognate antigen through multiple rounds of somatic hypermutation and selection. It is known that germinal center B cells are the only mature cells in the body that undergo somatic hypermutation. This reflects both the importance of germinal centers in immunity and the difficulties inherent in trying to produce high-affinity antibodies to the universe of possible antigens. In the germinal center, an antigen-specific B cell will undergo somatic hypermutation in its BCR gene via the enzymatic activities of AID and other factors *(331)* (also see other chapters in this volume). The mutated BCR is then expressed on the surface of

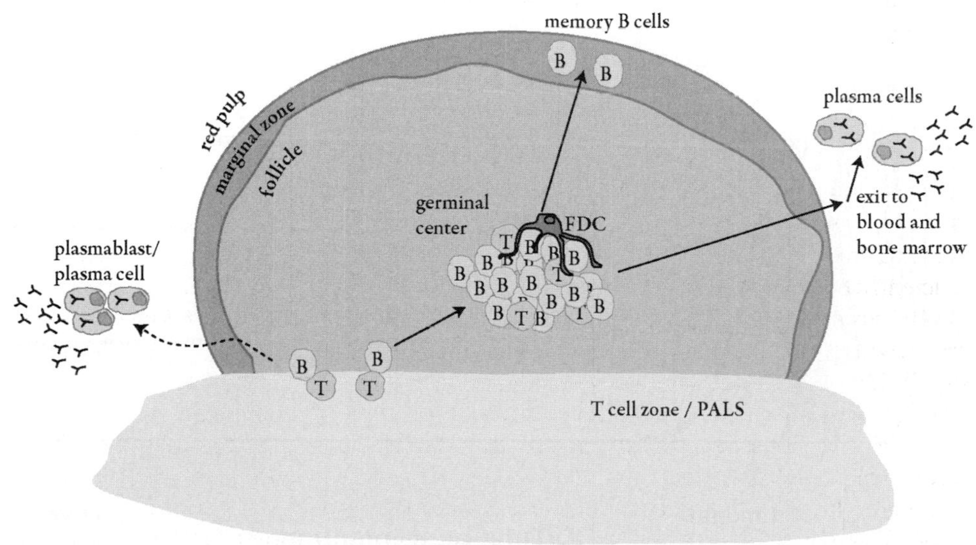

FIGURE 28.5 Anatomic features of effector and memory B cell differentiation. See text for details.

the B cell. If the mutant BCR is of higher affinity, the new clone more efficiently binds cognate antigen in the germinal center [tethered to follicular dendritic cells or otherwise present as an antigen depot *(328,335,336)*], processes and then presents peptides derived from the protein antigen in class II, and receives appropriate stimulatory signals from antigen-specific germinal center–resident CD4 T cells *(273,337)*. Germinal centers contain antigen-specific $CD4^+$ T cells, and both the generation and maintenance of germinal centers normally depend on antigen-specific CD4 T cells *(338–341)*. The germinal center CD4 T cells, often referred to as follicular helper CD4 T cells (T_{FH}s), provide stimulatory signals to germinal center B cells believed to consist of both T–B cell surface receptor–ligand interactions [e.g., CD40–CD40L *(338)*] and cytokines secreted by the CD4 T cells and bound by cytokine receptors expressed on the surface of the germinal center B cells [e.g., IL-21–IL21R *(342)*]. On receiving the appropriate stimulatory signals, the newly mutated, higher-affinity B cell proliferates and then repeats the cycle of somatic hypermutation, selection, and proliferation in the germinal center. Trafficking of B cells in germinal centers has recently been intensively examined *(343–346)*. Failure to bind cognate antigen and subsequently receive appropriate stimulatory signals from CD4 T cells or follicular dendritic cells (FDCs) results in apoptotic death. Given that these processes are acting on a population of antigen-specific B cells simultaneously, those B cells with the highest-affinity BCRs are expected to rapidly outcompete lower-affinity clones for antigen and subsequent costimulation from CD4 T cells. Because random mutation of the BCR is more likely to result in a nonfunctional or lower-affinity receptor instead of a higher-affinity receptor, apoptotic death is rampant in germinal centers. B cells positively selected within the germinal center exit and mature into memory B cells or plasma cells *(347–349)*. It is unclear how B cells are triggered to exit the germinal center and become memory B cells or plasma cells. It is known that CD40 ligation inhibits plasma cell differentiation and IL-10 and IL 21 enhance plasma cell differentiation of human germinal center B cells *(350)*. It is reasonable to propose that once B cell has undergone sufficient BCR affinity maturation to reach a certain affinity/avidity threshold, it will exit the germinal center and will differentiate into a memory B cell or plasma cell based on the combination of signals it receives from CD4 T cells immediately prior to exiting the germinal center. However, this is mostly a speculative model. Alternatively, both the exit from a germinal center and the memory B cell/plasma cell differentiation decision may be stochastic. On exit from a germinal center, memory B cells primarily reside in the marginal zones of the spleen, whereas the plasma cells exit into the blood.

A subset of plasma cells produced in the germinal centers migrates from blood to bone marrow, where they reside as long-lived plasma cells *(351–357)*. The kinetics and anatomic location of antibody production after an immunization (in this case an acute viral infection) in mice is shown in Figure 28.6. There are two phases of antibody

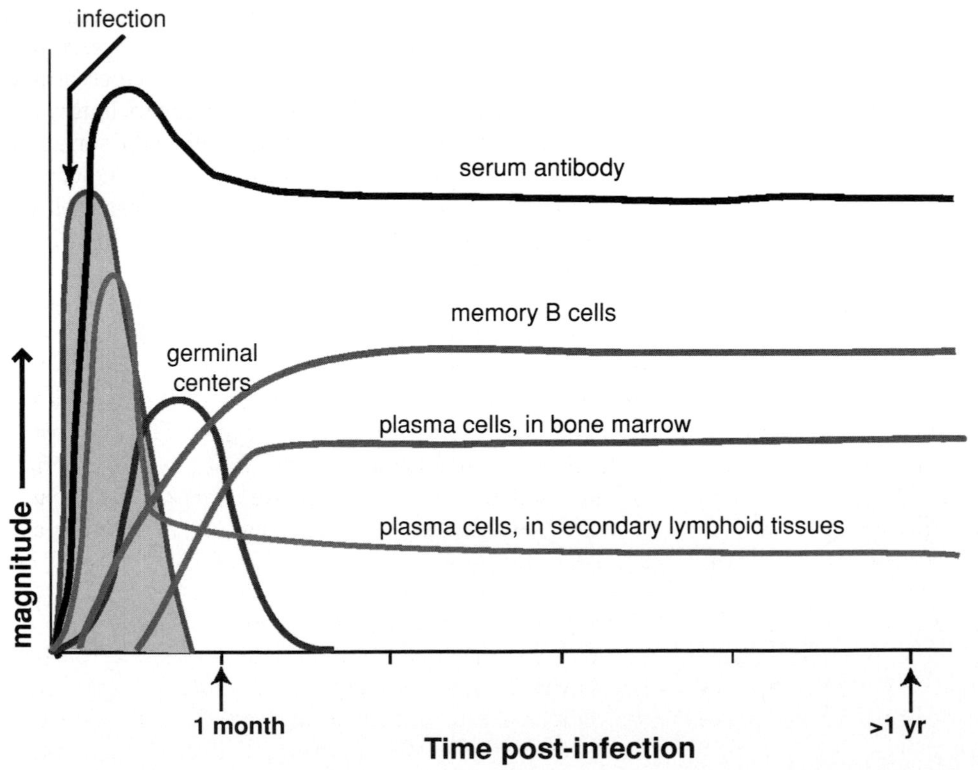

FIGURE 28.6 Kinetics of B cell responses after acute viral infection of mice. The plasma cell response in secondary lymphoid tissues peaks during the first 2 weeks and then declines within 2 to 4 weeks after infection (14,354). As splenic plasma cell populations decline, antigen-specific plasma cells begin to migrate to and/or accumulate in the bone marrow compartment (344,351,355,359). After the germinal center reaction subsides, the bone marrow becomes the predominant site of antibody production, with up to 90% of the host's plasma cells located in this compartment (14,354).

production: acute and long term. Because preexisting antibody provides the first line of defense against repeat infection by microbial pathogens, the importance of long-term antibody production by plasma cells in protective immunity cannot be overstated. There are at least two populations of plasma cells: the early antibody-secreting cells forming extrafollicular foci, which produce antibody only for a short period after antigen exposure, and long-lived plasma cells, which survive for extended periods (the half-life is 3 to 4 months in mice) (Figure 28.6) (14,*353,356,358*). Data indicate that plasmablasts and plasma cells generated from B cells in extrafollicular foci are short lived, with a half-life of less than 3 days *(359–361)*. The acute responding, extrafollicular population of antibody-secreting cells has various names in the literature—plasmablast, antibody-secreting cell, plasma cell, short-lived plasma cell—due to the different assays used to identify the cells and the uncertainty surrounding plasma cell differentiation states. Plasmablasts are antibody-secreting B cells that still have the ability to proliferate. Plasma cells are terminally differentiated nonproliferating cells with greater capacity for antibody secretion. Plasmablasts can develop from naïve B cells, germinal center B cells, or memory B cells, but it is unclear whether all plasmablasts have the capacity for complete differentiation into plasma cells and whether all plasma cells are competent to become long-lived plasma cells (Figures 28.1, 28.5). Naïve B cells specific for any given antigen are rare (10^{-5}-10^{-6}), and therefore only a small number of B cells are recruited into the initial response. Within this small set of B cells, it is likely that there exists a range of B cell receptor affinities for the antigen. The recruited B cells with the highest affinity for the target antigen appear preferentially to differentiate into plasmablasts/plasma cells and form extrafollicular foci. The recruited B cells with intermediate to lower affinities appear preferentially to initiate germinal centers *(362,363)*. At the molecular level, this indicates that stronger BCR signals drive proliferation and then plasma cell differentiation, and weaker BCR signals drive proliferation without plasma cell differentiation. This suggests that the B cell differentiation program has evolved under selective pressure to produce an early wave of high-affinity, antigen-specific secreted antibody as rapidly as possible, presumably reflecting the importance of rapid antibody responses in blunting viral or bacterial replication after infection; it is also important, however, to evolve high-affinity antibodies that are much more efficient at controlling and eliminating the pathogen, which is done by the antigen-specific B cells that initiate germinal centers. Long-lived plasma cells predominantly (or possibly exclusively) come from post–germinal center B cells, as evidenced by defects in long-lived plasma cell generation in mice with germinal center defects *(364)* and the observation that bone marrow plasma cells exhibit DNA and antibody affinity signatures of affinity maturation *(349,365)*.

MAINTENANCE AND FUNCTION OF MEMORY CELLS

Maintenance and Function of T Cell Memory

The small fraction of effector T cells that survive contraction initiates the memory pool that confers lifelong protection to the individual. Despite their extensive culling from peak numbers, antigen-specific cells in the postcontraction population are found at a far higher precursor frequency than in the naïve repertoire, a fact that undoubtedly affects the increased speed and intensity that is characteristic of secondary responses. Although they possess some features associated with memory, having arisen in response to an antigenic challenge and being able to persist after the majority of their fellow effectors have been eliminated, the postcontraction T cells nonetheless comprise a heterogeneous population whose maintenance in the memory pool is a dynamic process involving phenotypic changes that determine their function, distribution, and protective capacity over time (35,41,*366*). A central theme governing this process involves adaptation to the homeostatic control mechanisms that regulate the equilibrium of naïve versus memory T cells. These pathways appear to be distinct and under independent control because the mechanism regulating naïve T cell homeostasis that prevents overcrowding of the available niches by thymic emigrants cannot compensate for cell loss when production falls below a critical threshold, whereas the mechanism regulating the memory pool can both reequilibrate memory cell numbers after the increased input that results from normal immune responses and promote reexpansion to match the set threshold after physiologic loss of T cells, as often occurs during viral infections *(367–369)*. As will be described, the homeostatic mechanisms that regulate the naïve and memory T cell pools also differ in their requirement for extrinsic factors such as TCR stimulation by self-MHC molecules (presumably occupied with peptide derived from self or environmental antigens) and signals provided by the γ-chain (γc) cytokines IL-7 and IL-15.

Before discussing the factors responsible for the survival of memory T cells, it is important to understand the types of experimental approaches that have been used in their study and how these influence the various conclusions that can be drawn from the experimental data. In general, there have been two main experimental settings through which memory T cells have been studied *in vivo*. One involves enumeration of cells that express markers associated with prior antigen experience such as CD44^{high} or CD62L^{low} for activated cells in either immunized or unmanipulated normal mice. In the latter case, the cells in question are the spontaneously arising "memory phenotype" (MP) T cells of unknown derivation and specificity, which increase in frequency with age *(370,371)*. In the case of antigen (Ag)-specific T cells, these can be generated from either the endogenous polyclonal repertoire or adoptive transferred monoclonal transgenic T cells. A concern about immunization/infection studies is that antigens can persist for long periods of time in host animals, so that one may be studying continuous activation and not true memory. For this reason, a number of studies have monitored T cells that either arise spontaneously in normal mice (ostensibly in response to environmental antigens or self-MHC) or are specifically primed in one host and are transferred to a new, antigen-free host. This method has been used extensively for $CD8^+$ T cells, although the comparably modest expansion of activated $CD4^+$ T cells after priming has made their recovery in numbers sufficient for adoptive transfer a technical challenge. An additional concern for transfer of MP cells is that their antigenic specificity is unknown, precluding transfer to an antigen-free host. Lastly, many studies have involved transfer of naïve versus memory T cells to lymphopenic environments (irradiated or recombination activating gene [rag]–deficient mice). Under these conditions, the transferred T cells will expand to fill the available "space" (i.e., environmental niches), with the cell and molecular requirements for this type of proliferation termed "homeostatic expansion" to reflect the substantial increase in cell numbers it involves, being a topic of great interest in recent years *(372–376)*. This type of proliferation is clearly different in magnitude and, when applied to the various types of memory T cells described previously, perhaps in mechanism from the slower "basal" proliferation of T cells that maintains their numbers within intact mice *(377)*. Adding to the potential for confusion in the literature is the fact that different studies have used the term "homeostatic proliferation" to refer to the division of cells transferred to lymphopenic hosts as well as in normal T cell–replete hosts. For the purposes of this section, we refer to the slow turnover of T cells in a normal immunocompetent host as "basal homeostatic proliferation" and the faster, more extensive division of T cells within lymphopenic hosts as "homeostatic expansion."

As discussed earlier in this chapter, adoptive transfer studies have shown that the long-term survival of naïve T cells in lymphopenic hosts requires contact with self-MHC (73–78). Whereas initial studies in the 1990s suggested that both types of memory cells were maintained by occasional TCR contact with undetectable amounts of sequestered foreign or cross-reactive environmental antigens, more recent studies have shown that $CD8^+$ memory T cells can survive and remain functionally competent in the absence of either antigen or MHC molecules, arguing against any obligatory role for TCR stimulation in their maintenance (32,78,*378–381*). The situation for $CD4^+$ memory T cells is less clear, with studies on both antigen-specific and MP $CD4^+$ T cells revealing that maintenance of the pool size does not strictly depend on MHC or TCR (73,*382*). The rate of both basal homeostasis and homeostatic expansion of MP $CD4^+$ T cells, however, does appear to depend on the TCR–MHC interactions and declines significantly when these signals are extinguished, leaving the cells in one study critically dependent on IL-7 (73,*382–385*). These findings suggest a more prominent role for TCR than cytokines for the homeostatic survival of MP $CD4^+$ T cells. Supporting data for this notion comes from a study of Ag-specific transgenic $CD4^+$ memory T cells, which, on transfer to MHC-deficient hosts, display impaired responses to antigen reencounter *in vitro* and *in vivo (386)*. These observations indicate that $CD4^+$ and $CD8^+$ memory T cells differ in their requirement for TCR signals for maintenance and further suggest the non–mutually exclusive ideas that different mechanisms regulate the maintenance versus functional responsiveness of MP and antigen-specific memory $CD4^+$ T cells and that significant heterogeneity exists in the rates of homeostatic proliferation within the Ag-specific memory versus MP $CD4^+$ T cell populations, as demonstrated in several systems (71,*280,387,388*).

These findings of MHC-independent survival of memory T cells have brought cytokines into focus as the main extrinsic factors responsible for their maintenance, with particular emphasis on the common γc family members IL-7 and IL-15. One of the important initial observations linking cytokines with memory T cell survival came from studies in which agents capable of stimulating interferon production by cells of the innate immune system, such as LPS and Poly I:C, caused a transient burst of TCR-independent proliferation from the major $CD122^{high}$ $CD44^{high}$ subset of antigen-experienced $CD8^+$ T cells through the IFN-α/β-induced production of IL-15 *(389–394)*. Of note, the IFN-α/β-induced proliferative burst of $CD122^{high}$ $CD44^{high}$ $CD8^+$ T cells was not observed in IL-$15^{-/-}$ mice, and the *in vivo* administration of exogenous IL-15 was found to mimic the effect of IFNs in stimulating the bystander proliferation of the MP $CD8^+$ T cell subset *(390,395,396)*. The receptor for IL-15 is composed of three subunits: a unique α chain, a β chain (CD122) that is shared with the IL-2 receptor, and the common γc that is shared with IL-2, IL-4, IL-7, IL9, and IL-21 *(397–399)*. Although a soluble cytokine under *in vivo* conditions, IL-15 is presented in *trans* via cell-associated complexes bound to IL-15Rα that are preassembled in the cytoplasm of the (non-T) cells that make both molecules *(400–402)*. Paradoxically, $CD8^+$ T cells also express IL-15Rα, and although this is not essential for them to respond to IL-15 (which requires expression of only the β and γ chains), it may enable them to activate other cells types such as T cells or APC via *trans* presentation *(400,401,403,404)*. The expression of CD122 is selectively elevated on the MP ($CD44^{high}$) subset of $CD8^+$ T cells that undergo bystander proliferation in response to IL-15, whereas it is expressed at low but detectable levels on naïve $CD8^+$ cells *(394)*. IL-15 is nonetheless important for the survival for both subsets because IL-$15^{-/-}$ mice show a 50% reduction in the number of naïve $CD8^+$ T cells, and both IL-$15^{-/-}$ and IL-15R$\alpha^{-/-}$ mice contain significantly reduced numbers of $CD44^{high}$ $CD122^{high}$ MP $CD8^+$ T cells *(390,405–407)*. The effect of IL-15 on MP CD8$^+$ T cells may reflect its role in cell survival rather than development because these fail to proliferate and disappear rapidly on transfer to IL-15$^{-/-}$ recipients *(390)*. Consistent with this view, IL-15 transgenic mice were found to contain elevated numbers of MP CD8$^+$ T cells *(396,408)*. Taken together, these findings have led to the current view that the generation, survival, and basal homeostatic proliferation of MP CD8$^+$ T cells is mediated through contact with ambient IL-15 that is most likely produced by dendritic cells in the steady state, because these make both IL-15 and IL-15Rα, and by a variety of other cell types including skeletal muscle, kidney, placenta, and hematopoietic stromal cells under conditions of innate immune activation via the IFN pathway *(393,409,410)*. Studies of Ag-specific CD8$^+$ T cell responses have used MHC class I tetramers to follow the response to viral infection (LCMV or vesicular stomatitis virus) in IL-15$^{-/-}$ or IL-15R$\alpha^{-/-}$ mice, and have shown that, similar to MP CD8$^+$ T cells, IL-15 is also important for the maintenance of Ag-specific memory CD8$^+$ T cells *(377,411,412)*. These studies found that, although Ag-specific CD8$^+$ T cells were generated in the absence of IL-15 signals, they did not proliferate, and their numbers declined over time *(411,412)*. Taken together, these observations show that IL-15 mediates the homeostatic turnover of both MP and Ag-specific memory CD8$^+$ T cells. Although important for memory CD8$^+$ T cell homeostasis, IL-15 does not appear to be required for their function because LCMV-specific memory CD8$^+$ T cells are able to produce the effector cytokines IFNγ and TNF and are capable of responding to secondary infection *(411,412)*. The main effect of IL-15 on the homeostatic survival of CD8$^+$ T cells is likely mediated through upregulation of antiapoptotic factors such as BCL-2 and BCL-XL and avoidance of death via the mitochondrial pathway of apoptosis, a common mechanism of γc cytokines (79,*413–415*). The bone marrow may be the preferred site for homeostatic survival of memory CD8$^+$ T cells, as it contains a major pool of dividing memory cells and those that migrate there undergo division *(392)*.

In contrast to its clear role in the homeostatic survival of CD8$^+$ T cells, the requirement for IL-15 in memory CD4$^+$ T cell survival has been more difficult to define. This may have to do with the different survival requirements for the various types of memory cells used to study this phenomenon (MP, Ag-specific, and transgenic) and with the compensatory mechanisms that lymphocytes can develop in the absence of physiologic stimuli involved in their growth and development. For example, IL-15 has been considered to be irrelevant for the development and homeostasis of MP CD4$^+$ T cells because these express low levels of CD122 and can be found in normal numbers in IL-15$^{-/-}$ mice *(394,406)*. Given that the homeostasis of MP CD4$^+$ T cells appears to be governed more by TCR stimulation than by cytokines, as discussed previously, and that they are a homogeneous population containing a subset that undergoes a significantly faster rate of homeostatic expansion, it is possible that the MP CD4$^+$ T cells undergoing homeostatic proliferation in IL-15–deficient environment do so because they are chronically stimulated by foreign antigens, perhaps derived from commensal bacteria. In contrast to MP cells, the homeostasis of Ag-specific CD4$^+$ T cells appears to be exclusively under the control of cytokines because these cells can survive and undergo homeostatic expansion in lymphopenic hosts lacking MHC II molecules *(382,416)*. Studies with Ag-specific memory CD4$^+$ T cells generated in IL-15$^{-/-}$ hosts indicate that they too are independent of IL-15 for their maintenance *(387,406)*. It has been suggested, however, that the CD4$^+$ T cells arising in IL-15$^{-/-}$environment can become permanently conditioned to cope with IL-15 deficiency and may not represent the requirement of normal CD4$^+$ memory T cells formed in a T cell–replete environment (34,*417*). Similarly, the lymphopenic environment may also represent a nonphysiologic condition because the ambient levels of homeostatic cytokines can significantly increase in the absence of other T cells and NK cells that would normally compete for these resources *(418)*. In support of this idea, recent studies using transgenic and endogenous LCMV-specific CD4$^+$ memory T cells generated in normal mice and then transferred to lymphopenic versus normal nonlymphopenic hosts have shown that memory CD4$^+$ T cells depend on IL-15 for their basal homeostatic proliferation and long-term survival *(419)*. Consistent with this view, it has been shown that human and mouse CD4$^+$ T cells respond to exogenous IL-15, and IL-15-transgenic mice display enhanced CD4$^+$ T cell responses to infectious pathogens *(408,420)*. Taken together, these data indicate that both CD4$^+$ and CD8$^+$ memory T cells depend on IL-15 for their homeostatic survival.

The other cytokine known to affect the homeostatic survival of memory T cells is IL. As discussed previously, IL-7 is constitutively produced by nonhematopoietic cells, and perhaps some DC subsets, and is recognized by a heterodimeric receptor consisting of an α chain (shared with the receptor for TSLP) and γc *(421,422)*. Although memory CD8$^+$ T cells show a strong bias for IL-15, increasing the level of IL-7 *in vivo* through transgenic expression can overcome the requirement for IL-15 in promoting survival and homeostatic expansion of CD122^{high} memory CD8$^+$ T cells *(423)*. This finding is reminiscent of the apparent redundancy of IL-7 and IL-15 in promoting the homeostatic expansion of memory CD8$^+$ T cells, which has been shown to occur at a similar rate and magnitude in IL-15$^{-/-}$ hosts as in normal irradiated hosts *(377,388)*. Given the well-documented role of IL-15 as necessary for the survival of memory CD8$^+$ T cells, it would seem paradoxical that the lymphopenia, such as exists in both IL-15$^{-/-}$ and irradiated wild-type recipients, could alleviate this requirement. The reason turned out to be that IL-7, which in the absence of "consumers" such as naïve T cells and NK cells that normally compete for this key cytokine, is able to reach ambient higher levels in lymphopenic hosts that can compensate for the lack of IL-15. When both IL-7 and IL-15 are removed through gene knockouts and use of antireceptor antibodies, homeostatic static expansion ceases. These results indicate a degree of functional overlap between IL-7 and IL-15 in promoting the homeostatic expansion of memory T cells, but they suggest that this pathway is operates only when IL-7 reaches higher levels than normally exist in immunocompetent animals. Both naïve and memory $CD8^+$ T cells express high levels of IL-7Rα, with most effector cells sustaining the downregulation that occurs on activated cells during their primary expansion phase (75,85,*377,424,425*). The presence of elevated IL-7Rα expression on a subset of $CD8^+$ T cells detected early in the response to acute LCMV infection has been suggested specifically to identify precursors that are destined to develop into memory $CD8^+$ T cells *(424)*. This conclusion emerged from adoptive transfer experiments in which IL-7Rα^{high} and IL-7Rα^{low} populations of LCMV-specific $CD8^+$ effector T cells were transferred from infected mice into antigen-negative recipients, with the latter population displaying better long-term survival and recall responsiveness *(424)*. Subsequent experiments have indicated that this is more likely due to a survival advantage mediated by IL-7Rα expression in conferring enhanced sensitivity to ambient IL-7, and that $CD8^+$ memory T cells are not selected solely on the basis of IL-7/IL-7Rα interactions but result from a more complex series of differentiative events *(426–429)*.

The role of IL-7 in the maintenance of $CD4^+$ memory T cells has been a question of continuing interest, with conflicting results coming from different systems. Despite numerous reports that IL-7 is essential for the thymic development and homeostasis of naïve $CD4^+$ T cells, one study found that transgenic $CD4^+$ T cells from mice lacking γc expression, and therefore lacking the ability to transmit signals from either IL-7 or IL-15, display a short lifespan as naïve cells but survived efficiently after developing into memory cells *(417)*. Another study found that neither IL-7 nor IL-15 was required for the homeostatic expansion of MP $CD4^+$ T cells in lymphopenic hosts, despite the fact that memory $CD4^+$ T cells express high levels of IL-7Rα (388). Although these results would appear to support the idea that IL-7 is unimportant for the homeostasis of $CD4^+$ T cells, the development of the γc-independent $CD4^+$ T cells in the former case may have proceeded via an abnormal alternative pathway that obviates the normal role of IL-7, and the MP cells in the latter example were found to be the fast-dividing subset discussed previously that is thought to be under chronic TCR stimulation by endogenous ligands (77,*430*). Thus, these experimental systems may not accurately reflect the physiologic requirement for IL-7 in maintaining $CD4^+$ memory T cells, which itself is related to TCR signals and can apparently be masked by chronic TCR stimulation. In support of this, it has been found that when TCR signals are extinguished in MP $CD4^+$ T cells, they become acutely dependent on IL-7 for survival and homeostatic expansion in lymphopenic hosts *(385)*. Similarly, Ag-specific transgenic $CD4^+$ T cells that do not undergo homeostatic proliferation were found to depend on IL-7 for their survival under lymphopenic conditions *(431)*. More recently, it has been found that the survival and basal homeostatic proliferation of newly formed Ag-specific polyclonal memory $CD4^+$ T cells was substantially reduced after treatment with antibodies against IL-7R *(387,432)*. In addition, both MP and Ag-specific memory $CD4^+$ T cells lacking IL-7Rα were unable to survive in intact and lymphopenic hosts *(432)*. Together, these observations support the idea that IL-7 is essential to the maintenance and survival of $CD4^+$ memory T cells. The molecular mechanism through which this occurs is not entirely clear, although, as with IL-15, regulation of the balance of pro- and antiapoptotic members of the Bcl-2 family represents one potential explanation *(433)*. IL-7 protects T cells from death by inducing the antiapoptotic factors Bcl-2 and Mcl-1 and inhibiting the proapoptotic factors Bax, Bad, and Bim *(434–439)*. Furthermore, the T cell developmental defect in IL-7– or IL-Rα–deficient mice can be rescued by a bcl-2 transgene or deletion of Bax, and addition of anti-IL-7/anti-IL-7Rαa to memory cell cultures was found to reduce Bcl-2 expression *(431,434,440,441)*.

Function of T Cell Memory: The Secondary Response

From an operational perspective, it can be argued that the ultimate purpose for the long-term maintenance of memory T cells is found in the secondary response to previously encountered antigens, which comprises both direct effector functions and renewed proliferation. Although both aspects of the recall response can be readily demonstrated *in vitro*, under physiologic conditions this task requires that memory cells be present wherever invading pathogens enter the body and where they are first detected by the APC system. Accordingly, T_{EM} cells can be found in the blood and in a variety of peripheral tissues such as bone marrow, liver, gastrointestinal tract, lung parenchyma and fat pads, where they can mediate immediate effector functions, and T_{CM} cells are found mostly within the lymph nodes, where they are able to produce IL-2 (in addition to IFNγ) and mount proliferative responses to restimulation *(249–251,320)*. Although initial studies supported a clear division of labor between these subsets, it has become clear that some degree of overlap exists in their location, function, and phenotype. In the $CD8^+$ lineage, T_{EM}s can undergo substantial secondary expansion, and, conversely, T_{CM}s have been shown to migrate to and accumulate in the bone marrow and can display cytotoxic potential and production of effector cytokines equivalent to that of T_{EM} (131,*320,442,443*). The relative contribution of T_{EM} versus T_{CM} subsets to recall responses and effective immunity can depend on the nature of the antigenic challenge. For example, T_{CM} generated by immunization with virus-like particles (VLPs) are better able to protect from challenge with LCMV, a pathogen that replicates within lymphoid organs and is controlled perforin rather than $CD8^+$ T cell cytokines, whereas T_{EM} can be superior in mediating protection from vaccinia virus, which replicates in peripheral solid organs and is controlled by cytokines rather than by direct cytotoxicity *(444–448)*. Other studies, in contrast, have shown that T_{EM} are superior in mediating protection from viral challenge *(320)*. The timing of the challenge can also play a role because T_{EM} in the lung have been shown to be more effective at mediating protection against Sendai virus at early time points, whereas T_{CM} are superior at later time points *(449)*.

In addition to the increased frequencies of Ag-specific cells, the T cells that comprise the secondary response display a higher functional avidity and lower signaling thresholds than primary responders, and consequently they can mount faster and more effective responses to infection that the naïve repertoire (27,*450–453*). This "faster and better" response of memory T cells involves alterations in TCR signal transduction components that result in enhanced sensitivity to antigen, as well as epigenetic modification of key cytokine gene targets for TCR-mediated transcriptional activation, such as IFNγ and IL-2, resulting in more efficient and higher-level production (23,*451,452*). In the case of some effector molecules, including IL-4, and RANTES, memory T cells contain stored mRNA that is rapidly translated on TCR stimulation *(454–457)*. The enhanced functionality of the memory cells at the population level may reflect a mechanism in which Ag-driven clonal selection is controlled by affinity-based thresholds (40,*453,458*). In addition, a number of studies have shown that the secondary T cell response is prolonged compared to the primary response, with emerging evidence suggesting that renewed exposure to antigen can further improve the function of the available repertoire because secondary memory $CD8^+$ T cells have been shown to provide better per-cell protective immunity while retaining the capacity to undergo expansion in numbers similar to primary memory cells after reinfection (32,*246,249,268, 459–462*).

The structures and signals required to elaborate the secondary responses differ somewhat from those involved in the priming of naïve T cells. For many infections, the secondary response to antigenic challenge can proceed in the absence of encapsulated lymph nodes or spleen *(463,464)*. Mice deficient in lymphotoxin-α, which lack all secondary lymphoid organs, revealed the *de novo* generation of lymphoid organ–like structures within the airways called inducible bronchus-associated lymphoid tissue (iBALT) after pulmonary infection that were able to assume many of the T cell–activating functions of normal lymphoid organs *(463–465)*. The optimal secondary response to infection nonetheless appears to require DCs and, depending on the model, can require costimulation by molecules such as CD28 and 4-1BB *(466–468)*.

Maintenance and Function of B Cell Memory

How does B cell memory persist? The mechanisms involved in sustaining memory B cells can be divided into two categories: antigen dependent and antigen independent. There are three antigen-dependent mechanisms for maintaining B lineage memory: reinfection/immunization, latent infection, and antigen depot. Periodic reexposure to the pathogen is an effective way to maintain high levels of immunity and serves as a natural "booster" to the immune system. Frequently, such reinfections are mild or asymptomatic due to the preexisting immunity. When using vaccines, booster immunizations serve the same purpose of recalling preexisting memory. Latent or very low grade persistent infections can also serve as efficient antigen-dependent mechanisms for maintaining memory. It is believed that this occurs extensively for reactivating herpes virus infections and possibly other infectious diseases. A third antigen-dependent mechanism for maintaining B lineage memory is the presence of persisting nonreplicating antigen. This antigen can be present as an antigen depot or bound to the surface of follicular dendritic cells or possibly other professional antigen-presenting cells *(328,335,336,469)*. Distinguishing antigen-dependent from antigen-independent maintenance of B lineage memory and understanding their biological relevance and contributions are central problems in examining memory B cells and long-lived plasma cells because antigen-dependent and antigen-independent mechanisms may affect these memory cell types in different ways. These issues are a constant challenge for experimentalists studying B lineage memory. It is equally important to understand immune memory in the absence of reexposure to antigen to know how long immunity intrinsically lasts, particularly in the context of understanding human vaccines to understand how to maximize their success.

There are several classic examples that have clearly documented long-term protective immunity lasting up to 75 years in humans in the absence of reexposure to the pathogen (Table 28.1) (64,70,*471*). These observations have been crucial in shaping our ideas about immunologic memory because they showed that the immune system could remember an encounter that occurred many years ago. Because antibodies are the main protective mechanism for poliovirus, the case of measles immunity on the Faroe Islands mentioned at the beginning of this chapter suggested that B cell memory lasts at least 65 years after measles infection in the absence of reexposure to the virus. A similar situation was observed with polio outbreaks in a remote Eskimo village. Three serotypes of poliovirus exist, and antibodies against one serotype were observed only

TABLE 28.1 Long-Term Human Immunity in the Absence of Reexposure to the Pathogen

Infection	*Duration of Immunity (yr)*
Measles on the Faroe Islands (470)	65
Yellow fever virus in Norfolk, Virginia (471)	75
Polio in remote Eskimo villages (6)	40
Inactivated poliovirus vaccine in Sweden (472)	30+
Smallpox vaccine in United States, Israel, Italy (14–16,513,626)	30–60+

in Eskimos older than 40 years, and antibodies against a second serotype were observed only in individuals older than 20 years. Therefore, this epidemiologic observation indicated that production of antipoliovirus antibodies is long lived even in the absence of reexposure to the virus. A third example of long-term human immunity was an experiment. Yellow fever was an uncommon epidemic disease in the southeast United States during the 19th century. Seventy-five years after the last known outbreak in Norfolk, Virginia, serum samples were taken from individuals known to have been infected 75 years prior. The serum was transferred to primates, which were then challenged with yellow fever virus. Primates receiving the serum from immune humans were protected from disease, showing that individuals make anti–yellow fever virus antibodies for greater than 75 years after an infection. All of these examples are observations related to immunologic memory after acute viral infections. More recent studies have examined long-term immunologic memory in humans by quantifying antigen-specific serum antibody or memory B cell levels (14,16,*472*,*473*), as discussed later in the context of maintenance of memory.

Maintenance and Value of Memory B Cells: Quiescent Memory

The longevity of memory B cells in mice in the absence of antigen was controversial. Adoptive transfer studies of B cells into irradiated animals indicated that memory B cells have an extremely short lifespan in the absence of antigen (approximately 3 days) *(474)*. However, experiments done in intact animals suggested that the memory B cell numbers were stable, and a slow rate of memory B cell proliferation was observed (less than one division per month), indicating that the proliferation was homeostatic and not antigen driven *(475)*. Two additional studies observed a similar antigen-independent long lifespan of memory B cells with slow proliferation consistent with homeostatic cycling *(330,476)*. Studying antigen-independent maintenance of memory B cells in mice is extremely challenging because it has been shown that antigen can persist in mice at low levels for more than 18 months in some conditions *(477)*, which is effectively the full life of a mouse. A transgenic switch approach has largely settled the matter by circumventing the issue of possible antigen persistence *(478)*. Mice were engineered with a genetic switch, such that memory B cells expressing an NP-specific B cell receptor (BCR) could be changed *in vivo* to instead express a PE-specific BCR. By inducing the switch in memory B cells, PE-specific memory B cells that had never seen cognate antigen (PE) could be examined. The cells persisted in an antigen-independent manner just as well as other memory B cells *(478)*. These results were consistent with results obtained in intact mice *(330,475,476)*. It should be noted that naïve mature B cells, and presumably memory B cells, must constantly maintain BCR expression for survival *(479)*, and therefore it is possible that constant very low affinity self cross-reactive binding is an intrinsic component of B cell survival.

Immunologic memory is not necessarily maintained in the same way in mice and humans. There are classic reports of long-term immunity in humans in the absence of reexposure to a pathogen, as mentioned earlier (Table 28.1) (64,70,*471*). However, those studies have left many important questions unanswered. How stable is long-term immune memory in humans? Is the stability similar or different in the multiple compartments of the adaptive immune system (circulating antibodies, memory $CD8^+$ T cells, memory $CD4^+$ T cells, and memory B cells)? If immune memory is not stable, what is the kinetics of decline? What are the cellular and molecular processes involved in memory cell maintenance? These questions are generally difficult to answer in humans, both because the time frame of interest is decades and it is difficult to find situations in which reexposure to antigen/vaccine/pathogen can be excluded as a source of intermittent "booster immunizations" maintaining the immune memory. Many vaccines induce serum antibody responses that persist for decades *(480)*, but most reports of durable antibody responses in humans are plagued by questions about the potential of intermittent reexposure to the antigen (live measles/mumps/poliovirus vaccines given to nearby children, tetanus in the soil, etc.). Furthermore, memory B cell levels have only been directly examined in a few studies, and it is unclear what the relationship is between serum antibody titers and memory B cell levels. Immune memory after smallpox vaccination is a valuable benchmark for understanding the kinetics and longevity of memory B cells in the absence of reexposure to antigen because immunization against smallpox was standard in the United States and throughout the Western world but was stopped in the mid 1970s, and smallpox disease was declared eradicated worldwide in 1980 after the last known case was observed in eastern Africa in 1977 *(481)*. Because the smallpox vaccine is a live virus vaccine, it is also an excellent model of a well-defined acute infection. Smallpox vaccine–specific memory B cells can be detected for 60 years or more after vaccination (14). Of note, memory B cell levels appeared to be stable from 10 to 60 years postvaccination, indicating that antigen-specific memory B cells are maintained by robust mechanisms.

There are four models for how human memory B cells are maintained: (a) antigen dependent, (b) intermittent stimulation by cross-reactive antigens, (c) bystander activation, and (d) programmed homeostatic maintenance. These models are not mutually exclusive, and all are topics of active research to determine their importance in memory maintenance. The first model, antigen-dependent maintenance, was introduced earlier in the chapter. Reinfection or reimmunization is one clear mechanism for maintaining memory via recall. Microbial persistence is another clear mechanism for maintaining memory. A number of microbes (herpesviruses being the best-known examples) can persist at low levels in healthy individuals, and this chronicity can provide either a continuous or an intermittent antigenic stimulus to the immune system. This can be an effective mechanism of maintaining a higher frequency of antigen-specific T and B cells but requires a careful balance between pathogen levels and immune responses. This critical balance is necessary to avoid excessive immunopathology and also to avoid overstimulation of the antigen-specific T cells to such an extent that these cells get deleted or functionally exhausted (193,*482*). Antigen depots are an antigen-dependent mechanism for memory maintenance that does not depend on reinfection/exposure or microbial replication. The antigen depot model of memory maintenance relies on the ability of FDCs to trap antigen–antibody complexes on their cell surface and retain them for extended periods of time *(483,484)*. FDCs express Fc receptors on their cell surface, and antigen–antibody complexes can bind to these Fc receptors. It appears that FDCs do not internalize these antigen–antibody complexes but instead display them on their cell surface for long periods, thus promoting maintenance of germinal centers and continued affinity maturation of B cells *(335)*. It is well described that follicular dendritic cells bind antigen and present antigen to B cells in germinal centers. This antigen presentation is generally agreed to be a key component of the affinity maturation and selection process within the germinal center *(332,333,335,476,485)*, although this is debated *(328,336)*. It is generally agreed that antigen is required to maintain germinal center reactions to provide a substrate for positive selection and prevent apoptosis. Some studies have suggested that antigen can persist on FDCs for greater than 1 year, and it has been proposed that after the generation of memory B cells, the memory cells are maintained by periodic reencounter with antigen presented long term by follicular dendritic cells *(483)*. Data from the only study directly tracking antigen in germinal centers after a viral infection, using a mouse model, indicated that germinal centers are sustained by antigen on FDCs for approximately 30 days after clearance of the virus, after which there is a drop of greater than 90% in the number of germinal centers and a drop of greater than 90% in the amount of viral antigen bound by the FDCs *(484)*. This was corroborated by a second study with a nonreplicating antigen, indicating that FDCs were critical for maintenance of the germinal center reaction but were not involved in the maintenance of memory B cells after the subsidence of the germinal center reaction *(476)*. It is unlikely that viral particles or protein antigens *in vivo* can survive the wear and tear of antibody binding for long before being broken into pieces or destroyed. Essentially all proteins have a finite lifespan, with a half-life in the range of hours to weeks. Proteins and protein structures are damaged by environmental conditions, proteases, and interactions with other proteins, and presumably they would be consumed during memory B cell activation, antigen uptake, and presentation to CD4 T cells. Therefore, retention of biologically relevant levels of antigen by follicular dendritic cells may only be expected to occur for a period of weeks to months before exhaustion of the antigen depot *(476,484)*. Therefore, nonreplicating antigen is unlikely to maintain human memory B cells for greater than 50 years (14). Furthermore, murine memory B cells are maintained in the absence of antigen (discussed in detail previously), suggesting that human memory B cells are also likely to be maintained long term in the absence of antigen.

A second proposal is that memory is maintained by stimulation of memory B cells by cross-reactive environmental or self-antigens. B cells are stimulated by direct interaction of the B cell receptor with antigen, and the specificity of a B cell receptor is not absolute; cross-reactivity is observed. Therefore, it is possible that memory B cells are maintained long term by intermittent interaction with environmental antigens (i.e., allergens, food products, unrelated pathogens) or self-antigens. This hypothesis is exceptionally difficult to test. On a related topic, Rajewsky and colleagues showed that mature naïve B cells must constantly maintain BCR expression for survival *(479)*, presumably due to a need for tonic signaling through the BCR. Tonic signaling may or may not be dependent on low-affinity binding of the BCR to self-antigens. If the signaling is dependent on self-reactivity, memory B cell BCRs may also have a requirement for low-grade self cross-reactivity. On the other hand, memory B cells may have different requirements for BCR stimulation and may no longer require antigen for their survival or homeostatic proliferation. This would be similar to the differential requirements observed between naïve T cells and memory T cells for stimulation through the TCR *(486)*.

A third potential mechanism for the maintenance of memory B cells is bystander polyclonal activation. This model is based on the observation that memory B cells stimulated *in vitro* with TLR ligands or select polyclonal activators will undergo several rounds of proliferation and differentiate into plasma cells, whereas naïve B cells will not *(473,487)*. If this same process occurs *in vivo*, memory B cells would be likely to proliferate in response to irrelevant microbes containing TLR ligands or proliferate due to production of cytokines secreted by responding cells of the immune system *(473,488)*. Intermittent bystander activation in this manner would result in small-scale expansion of memory B cells, thereby maintaining the population by replacing any memory B cells dying over time. This model is mechanistically plausible but seems unlikely. Although one study observed bystander activation of human memory B cells *in vivo*, as measured by increased antigen-specific serum antibody titers *(473)*, two others human studies observed no bystander activation *in vivo (489,490)*. Bystander activation was not observed in a mouse model system *(491)*. Adoptive transfer experiments involving co-transfer of human cytomegalovirus (HCMV)– and tick-borne encephalitis virus (TBEV)–specific memory B cells into T cell–deficient hosts showed that a memory B cell recall response only occurred when the mice were challenged with the correct cognate antigen *(491)*. Like each of the memory B cell maintenance models discussed in this chapter, this bystander activation hypothesis requires further examination, particularly by directly measurement of antigen-specific memory B cell proliferation and maintenance *in vivo* before, during, and after a number of heterologous infections and/or immunizations.

A fourth potential mechanism for the maintenance of memory B cells is programmed homeostatic proliferation. This hypothesis draws from the known mechanisms of CD8 T cell memory maintenance in mice (52,*411*). As discussed elsewhere in the chapter, murine memory CD8 T cells accomplish prolonged maintenance by proliferation primarily via IL-15 signals. Memory CD8 T cells are believed to undergo homeostatic proliferation when they migrate through the bone marrow, where there are high concentrations of IL-15 and other proliferation and survival signals *(492,493)*. Therefore, antigen-specific memory B cells may maintain themselves by a similar programmed homeostatic maintenance involving intermittent proliferation triggered by certain autocrine/paracrine cytokines or other as-yet-unknown factors. Data from both mice and humans indicate that memory B cells undergo a slow rate of proliferation in the absence of rechallenge *(330,475, 476,494,495)*. This is consistent with slow homeostatic proliferation and does not require CD4 T cells *(496)*.

What is the value of long-term maintenance of memory B cells? Memory B cells have several features that indicate they are valuable for protection against infections. First, memory B cells are present in much greater numbers than naïve mature B cells of a given antigen specificity (14,*473,475,497,498*). Second, memory B cells respond to reactivation faster than naïve B cells *(473,499)*, differentiate into plasma cells faster *(499)*, and have a larger burst size, indicative of resistance to apoptosis *(500)*. Third, memory B cells have undergone affinity maturation and therefore produce antibodies after reactivation that have substantially higher affinity and/or avidity than antibody produced from naïve B cells. Each of these properties likely makes memory B cells highly valuable for protection against reinfection because the memory B cells are able to make a rapid recall response and produce high levels of high-affinity antibodies quickly to limit the spread of the infecting microbe and quell the infection. In situations in which antibodies are known to be protective but are not present at high enough levels for sterilizing immunity (i.e., able completely to block infection by the microbial exposure or inoculation), memory B cells are likely to contribute to the observed protection against disease. The hepatitis B virus (HBV) vaccine is a well-characterized example known for antibody titers that drop over several years *(501–503)*. Antibodies against HBsAg are the defined correlate of protection for the HBV vaccine, and the minimum protective level has been established as 10 mIU/mL *(480)*. When serum anti-HBsAg antibody levels drop below that level, booster immunization is recommended. However, many individuals with low or undetectable levels of HBsAg fail to obtain booster immunizations, and some fraction of that population subsequently becomes exposed to HBV. Of interest, nearly of those individuals are still protected from HBV infection *(504)*. Why? Memory B cells are an appealing explanation because HBV surface antigen–specific antibodies are the correlate of protection for the vaccines, and memory B cells will rapidly differentiate into anti-HBsAg antibody-secreting cells within 3 to 5 days of virus exposure *(501,504,505)*. This may also be observed with the anthrax vaccine *(506,507)* and other vaccines or infections when the levels of circulating antibody do not result in sterilizing immunity. In any situation in which antibodies contribute to protective immunity, reactivation of memory B cells is likely to contribute to protection as long as the infectious agent is not so virulent as to cause disease before the memory B cells have time to proliferate and differentiate into plasma cells.

Maintenance of Long-lived Plasma Cells: Active Memory

There are at least two populations of plasma cells: long-lived and short-lived. Long-lived plasma cells are a central part of immune memory because these cells are largely responsible for the long-term continuous secretion of antibody. In contrast to memory B cells, plasma cells are terminally differentiated and cannot be stimulated by antigen to either divide or increase their rate of antibody production. Because preexisting antibody provides the first line of defense against infection by microbial pathogens, the importance of plasma cells in protective immunity cannot be overstated.

The traditional view was that all plasma cells are short-lived cells with a half-life of approximately 3 to 14 days *(359)*, and therefore continuous antigenic stimulation of memory B cells was necessary to replenish the pool of rapidly dying plasma cells and thereby maintain antibody production. This view has been replaced by a model describing two major populations of plasma cells: short-lived plasma cells that produce antibody soon after antigen exposure, and long-lived plasma cells that survive for extended periods (the half-life is 3 to 4 months in mice) (Figure 28.1) (14,*353,357,476,508*). The majority of serum antibodies are produced by plasma cells residing in bone marrow *(354,509–511)*. The secondary lymphoid tissue plasma cell response to an immunization or acute infection peaks within 1 to 2 weeks and then declines within 2 to 4 weeks after infection *(349,354,361,364)*. As splenic plasma cell populations decline, antigen-specific plasma cells begin to migrate to and/or accumulate in the bone marrow compartment *(349,351,355,361)*. After the germinal center reaction subsides, the bone marrow becomes the predominant site of antibody production, with bone marrow plasma cells responsible for 80% to 95% of the host's antibody production (14,*354,509,512*).

Many human vaccines induce serum antibody responses that persist for decades *(480)*, but it is usually unclear whether there is a long-term decline in the antibody levels, and there are usually questions about the potential of intermittent reexposure to the antigen, as stated earlier. An impressive study of long-term antibody levels that avoided the reexposure issue was the large cross-sectional study of poliovirus immunity done in Sweden (Table 28.1) *(472)*. The Swedish population was almost ideal for such a study, for several reasons: (a) poliomyelitis had been eliminated in Sweden since 1962; (b) only inactivated poliovirus vaccine (IPV, the Salk vaccine) provided by a single supplier has ever been used in the Swedish population; (c) the final booster immunization was given at the young age of 5 years; (d) the enterovirus infection burden in Sweden has been extremely low, and there were very few opportunities for introduction of poliovirus from foreign sources; and (e) Sweden has excellent health care records and public health surveillance. Given those factors, it was striking to see that when the Swedish population was surveyed for poliovirus immunity in 1991, substantial antipoliovirus antibody titers were detected in all age groups *(472)*. Of interest, there was virtually no difference in serum antibody titers among the different age groups (all at greater than 10 years postvaccination), indicating that antipoliovirus antibody titers are stably maintained in the absence of additional immunizations or exposure to live virus *(472)*. Of interest, declining levels of antitetanus and antidiptheria antibody titers were observed in that same study, suggesting that not all immune memory is created equal *(472)*. In other human studies, antibody responses after smallpox immunization can be maintained for greater than 60 to 75 years (14,16,*513*). It is impressive that the serum levels of anti–vaccinia virus (VV) antibodies were stable from 1 to more than 60 years postimmunization (14,16). Immune memory after smallpox vaccination is a valuable benchmark for memory in the absence of antigen reexposure because immunization against smallpox was stopped in the mid-1970s and neither smallpox nor the smallpox vaccine virus exists in the wild. Total anti-VV antibody levels in vaccines correlated reasonably well with neutralizing anti-VV antibody levels, providing some indication that antibody responses of different specificities were maintained equally well (14,16). Data from yet another group of studies examining immunity to HBV in humans showed that anti-HBV serum antibody levels decline over time in vaccinated individuals *(501–503)*. Altogether these studies show than human antibodies can be maintained for greater than 60 years in the absence of reexposure to antigen, but long-term maintenance of antibody levels does not occur in all cases, indicating that not all memory is created or maintained equally.

How is the antibody production maintained for 60 or more years? Long-lived plasma cells are crucial for the maintenance of antibody levels. There are two main theories for how numbers of antigen-specific long-lived plasma cells are sustained for years after vaccination (Figure 28.7): (a) competitive/conditional longevity of long-lived plasma cells, and (b) replenishment of long-lived plasma cells from differentiating memory B cells. The first model proposes that long-lived plasma cells are long lived because of the survival niche they occupy in bone marrow or spleen (358). Once a long-lived plasma cell is produced and homes to specific sites such as the bone marrow, the plasma cell may survive for decades without requiring replenishment from the memory B cell pool. Plasma cells generated *in vitro* or isolated *ex vivo* die rapidly, but their survival *in vitro* can be extended somewhat by providing stimuli found in bone marrow *(514)*. The conditional survival model proposes that a plasma cell will survive for as long as it physically stays in a survival niche *(358)*. If the plasma cell leaves the survival niche or is dislodged from the survival niche, it will die. Because the number of bone marrow plasma cells in mice and humans is relatively stable over a lifetime, old plasma cells must somehow be eliminated to make room for new plasma cells. This model proposes that the generation of a new immune response somehow induces the loss of longer-lived plasma cells *(358)*. There is human data indicating that bone marrow plasma cells can be mobilized into the blood after an irrelevant immunization *(515)*. At least one murine model study has detected a loss of plasma cells after a new immunization with a second antigen, and the survival of the long-lived plasma cells was correlated with lack of FcγRII expression *(516)*. A caveat to this model is that long-lived plasma cells in mice have a measured half-life of 3 to 4 months *(353,476)*, suggesting that plasma cells may have an intrinsic lifespan.

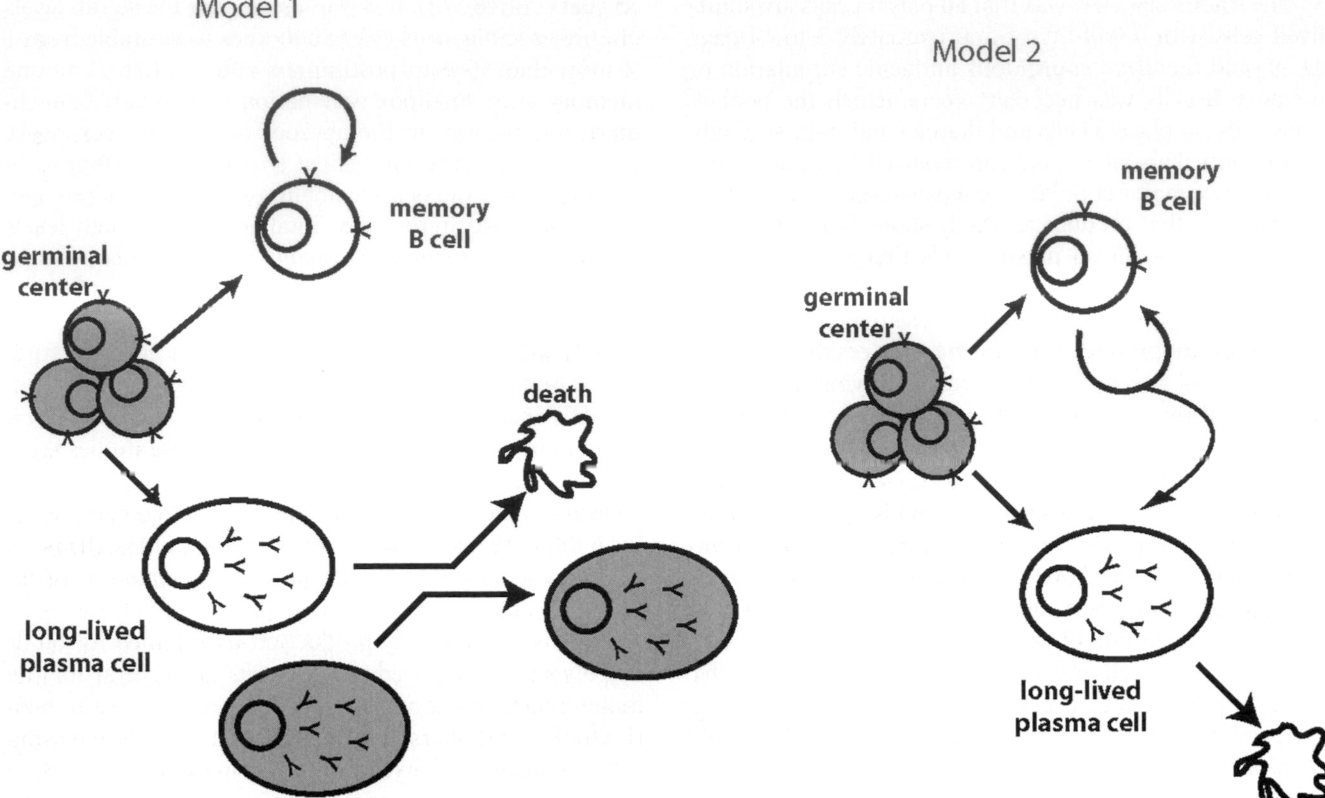

FIGURE 28.7 Two hypothetical models of antigen-independent long-term maintenance of antibody levels. Hypothetical model 1: Independent memory B cell and plasma cell populations are generated. If a plasma cell migrates to a survival niche (such as those present in bone marrow), the plasma cell becomes a long-lived plasma cell and will live indefinitely as long as it remains in the survival niche. New long-lived plasma cells can survive by occupying a survival niche vacated by an old, long-lived plasma cell. Hypothetical model 2: Memory B cell and long-lived plasma cell populations are generated. Plasma cells have a certain half-life, and die over time. Both memory B cell and long-lived plasma cell numbers are maintained or replenished by intermittent divisions by memory B cells coupled to differentiation of a plasma cell at the same time, such that one memory B cell effectively gives rise to one daughter memory B cell and one daughter plasma to maintain both the antigen-specific memory B cell and plasma cell compartments.

However, in a third study an indefinite half-life was observed *(512)*.

The second model is replenishment of long-lived plasma cells from memory B cells. Plasma cells are terminally differentiated and unable to proliferate. Therefore, repopulation of their numbers can be accomplished by proliferation and differentiation of memory B cells into antibody-secreting plasma cells. This replenishment is known to occur in an antigen-dependent manner after a booster immunization or reexposure to infection. It is proposed that there can be antigen-independent differentiation of memory B cells to long-lived plasma cells (Figure 28.2) *(488,507)*. There are models of long-term memory B cell maintenance that propose that antigen-specific memory B cells maintain themselves within the pool of total memory B cells either by intermittent bystander activation or by a programmed homeostatic maintenance proliferation, as described in the previous section. A corollary to those memory B cell maintenance models is that the antigen-independent proliferation of memory B cells to maintain their numbers may be coupled to differentiation of a plasma cell at the same time, such that one memory B cell effectively gives rise to one daughter memory B cell and one daughter plasma cell to maintain both the antigen-specific memory B cell and plasma cell compartments. If this model is accurate, there should be a correlation between memory B cell numbers and plasma cell numbers (or serum antibody levels). Two human studies have shown a positive correlation between antigen-specific memory B cell frequencies and serum antibody levels (14,473). In both cases the correlation was moderate, indicating that there may be multiple factors controlling the relationship between circulating memory B cell levels and circulating antibody levels. Two other human studies observed no correlation looking at other antigens *(498,505)*, again indicating that multiple factors may control the relationship between memory B cells and serum antibody levels.

Neither of these models fully accounts for the observation that some antibody responses appear to be more stable and long-lived than others, as discussed earlier. Resolution of these disparate models of memory B cell and antibody maintenance requires further study, particularly in humans, in whom the issues of longevity are amplified due to interest in understanding immunologic memory that lasts for a decade or longer. In addition, understanding the detailed physiologies of memory B cells and plasma cells in both mice and humans will help to illuminate the functions of these cell types and the relationships among memory B cells, long-lived plasma cells, and the maintenance of humoral immunity.

THE PHENOTYPIC HETEROGENEITY OF THE CELLS CLASSIFIED AS MEMORY CELLS

Identification of T Cell Memory

A number of key questions regarding the origin, maintenance, and function of immune memory would be informed by a marker or set of markers through which memory cells could be identified and distinguished from the naïve and effector subsets. Unfortunately, this goal has been difficult to realize for a number of reasons, including the fact that the many of the phenotypic changes that occur in activated lymphocytes are often transient and can revert back to their status as naïve cells over time and that many of the surface proteins expressed by long-lived Ag-experienced cells that would otherwise qualify them as memory markers are also expressed on recently activated effectors. Furthermore, T cells can be found to express markers of prior activation without having responded to antigen in the conventional sense, such as occurs in lymphopenic hosts or in the rapidly dividing subset of $CD4^+$ T cells described previously in this chapter that appears to be under chronic antigenic stimulation. Finally, there is substantial heterogeneity within the memory population with regard to phenotype, function, and anatomic location, both in $CD4^+$ and $CD8^+$ compartments. Immunologists have nonetheless tried to define the features that distinguish populations of T cells that are presumed never to have previously encountered antigens (i.e., those from umbilical cord blood or germ-free mice) with those that are known to have recently undergone primary or secondary stimulation, with most studies focusing on surface molecules expressed in the different populations. Such studies have revealed a surprising degree of heterogeneity in putative memory markers with respect to both temporal and anatomic aspects of the expression.

It has long been appreciated that memory T cells express surface markers that distinguish them from naïve cells *(517,518)* (Figure 28.8). Much early work was focused on the high– and low–molecular weight isoforms of the surface-expressed tyrosine phosphatase CD45, which can be generated through differential splicing of three extracellular exons, called A, B, and C, which are differentially expressed on naïve versus memory T cells *(519)*. In the human system, naïve T cells express the high–molecular weight form called CD45RA that contains all three of the spliced exons, whereas memory cells tend to more often express the low–molecular weight form called CD45RO, with the different phenotypes assigned based on reactivity with isoform-specific monoclonal antibodies *(520,521)*. There is significant heterogeneity in CD45 expression, however, with variation in surface levels of the low–molecular weight isoforms on memory T cells as a result of reexpression of CD45RA after its initial downregulation, which itself occurs at different rates on $CD4^+$ versus $CD8^+$ T cells (reviewed in ref. *522*). Furthermore, although murine T cells also express variant isoforms of CD45, this has also proven to be a less reliable marker of naïve versus memory cells *(523–525)*. A number of studies have attempted to correlate the upregulation of adhesion molecules on memory cells, including members of the $\beta 1$ (CD49d, CD40e, CD29) and $\beta 2$ (CD11a, CD11b, CD18) family of integrins, as well as CD2, CD44, CD54, and CD58 (reviewed in ref. *371*). Among these, however, most appear to reflect recent activation status of the T cells; only CD44 appears to be a stably expressed marker of memory cells that is expressed at high levels when T cells are transferred to antigen-free recipient mice *(379,486,526–528)*. However, high-level CD44 expression is also found on the memory phenotype T cells discussed in a previous section that are believed to be subject to chronic stimulation by ubiquitous environmental antigens, so that CD44 expression alone cannot serve as an informative marker for memory cells. When used in conjunction with other markers, however, CD44 can be used more specifically to distinguish memory from naïve T cells.

A number of other molecules can differentiate between naïve and antigen-experienced cells. These include both CD122, a component of both the IL-2 and IL-15 receptors, and Ly-6c, a small GPI-linked surface protein, although this involves increased rather than *de novo* expression on memory cells, and this only on $CD8^+$ and not $CD4^+$ T cells *(394,529–531)*. $CD8^+$ T cells have also been shown to undergo changes in their cell-surface glycosylation that can help to distinguish effectors from resting memory cells (reviewed in ref. *532*). After activation, $CD8^+$ T cells undergo an elimination of sialic acid from core 1 O-glycans and an induction of core 2 O-glycans

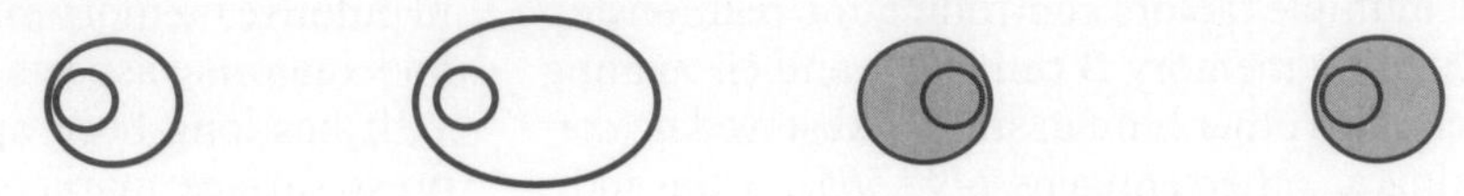

		Naive	1° effectors	T_{EM}	T_{CM}
Surface Markers					
Human		$CD45RA^+$ $CD62L^{hi}$ $CCR7^+$		$CD45RA^{+/-}$ $CD62L^{hi/lo}$ $CCR7^-$	$CD45RA^-$ $CD62L^{hi}$ $CCR7^-$
Mouse		$CD44^{lo}$ $CD62L^{hi}$ $CCR7^+$	$CD44^{hi}$ $CD62L^{lo}$ $CCR7^{+/-}$	$CD44^{hi}$ $CD62L^{lo}$ $CCR7^{+/-}$	$CD44^{hi}$ $CD62L^{hi}$ $CCR7^+$
Functional potential					
$CD4^+$					
T_H1	Proliferation	+++	+	++	++
	Effector Function (IFN-γ)	–	+++	+++	++
	Homing	2° L.O.	2° L.O. P.T.	P.T.	2° L.O.
T_H2	Proliferation	+++	+	?	++
	Effector Function (IL-4, IL-5, IL-13)	–	+++	+++	+/–
	Homing	2° L.O.	2° L.O.	P.T.	2° L.O.
$CD8^+$	Proliferation	++++	++	++	++++
	Effector Function (cytotoxicity, IFN-γ)	–	++++	+++	++
	Homing	2° L.O.	2° L.O. P.T.	P. T.	2° L.O.

2° L.O.: Seccondary Lymphoid Organs
P.T.: Peripheral Tissues

FIGURE 28.8 Phenotypic heterogeneity of memory T cells.

until they differentiate into memory cells *(533)*. This difference allows selective binding of the 1B11 antibody, which binds to CD43 only when modified by core 2 O-glycans *(534)*. Of interest, although core 2 O-glycan expression decreases after conversion of $CD8^+$ effectors into memory cells, peanut agglutinin staining (which reflects the expression of unsialylated core 1 O-glycans) is slightly higher on memory than on naïve T cells, and it has been proposed that this influences their reduced TCR signaling threshold *(534–536)*.

In addition to these phenotypic markers of memory T cells, efforts have been made to identify these cells based on their function, usually defined by the parameters of protection, proliferation, and persistence. The unambiguous assignment of a unique set of functional markers through which they can be identified has also been difficult because many of the capacities they possess are simply not unique to the memory subset. For example, naïve T cells, like memory T cells, are capable of self-renewal in response to homeostatic cytokines and can proliferate extensively in response to antigen. Similarly, effector cells, which differ from effector-competent memory cells only in their longevity, can mediate potent functional responses and, if present in sufficient numbers, protective immunity, depending on the nature of the challenge. The physiologic location of memory cells has been held to represent a defining feature because naïve T cells are not normally believed to occupy extralymphoid environments (90). Recent studies using S1P-receptor antagonists, however, have revealed that naïve cells may pass through peripheral tissues as part of their normal recirculation pattern (90,*537,538*).

Chemokine receptors represent another class of molecules used to functionally define different subsets of memory T cells, in this case based on their specific homing behavior *(539–541)*. Skin-homing memory T cells, for example, express high levels of $\beta 1$ and $\beta 2$ integrins and cutaneous lymphocyte antigen (CLA), a molecule involved in lymphocyte homing to the dermis, as well as a number of receptors for inflammatory chemokines, including CCR1, CCR3, and CCR5, but neither of the lymph node–homing receptors CCR7 or CD62L (41). $CCR7^+$ memory T cells, in contrast, express lower integrin levels and no CLA, but express chemokine receptors that will guide them to lymphoid tissues such as CCR4, CCR6, and CXCR3, as well as CD62L. Based on the distinct homing potential of these two subsets (e.g., $CCR7^+$ $CD62L^+$ and $CCR7^-$ $CD62L^-$), it was proposed that they represent two specialized types of memory T cells, each charged with a specific task in host defense (reviewed in ref. *542*). The $CCR7^-$ $CD62L^-$ effector memory subset (T_{EM}) resides in peripheral tissues, where pathogens are likely to first gain access to the body, and can mediate direct effector functions against infected cells. The $CCR7^+$ $CD62L^+$ central memory subset (T_{CM}) is found mostly within lymph nodes, where it responds to antigenic stimulation by renewed proliferation and the generation of secondary effectors. It should be pointed out that expression of both CD62L and CCR7 also defines naïve T cells, so that additional markers are required to distinguish T_{CM} such as high-level expression of CD44 in the mouse or the absence of CD45RA in the human. Although CD62L and CCR7 do not represent perfect sets of phenotypic markers with which to define memory subsets because significant heterogeneity exists in their respective expression patterns among memory T cells, the concept of a functional division of labor between T_{EM} and T_{CM} has been remarkably influential, with numerous studies dedicated to elucidating their lineage relationship and relative role in maintaining the protected state. Some of these have concluded that T_{EM} and T_{CM} arise sequentially through a linear pathway of differentiation, whereas others support the idea that they are separate populations that arise independently *(320,543–549)*. More recently, it has been suggested that the initial precursor frequency of antigen-specific T cells may influence the commitment of T cells to one or the other lineage, or that changing the anatomic location (e.g., from lymphoid to peripheral tissues) can cause the conversion from T_{CM} to T_{EM} phenotype *(546,550)*. Numerous laboratories are working on the elucidation of the origins and lineage relationships of T_{EM} and T_{CM} phenotypes, their relative roles in protective immunity, and their potential for interconversion.

Although much remains to be revealed about the phenotypic and functional characteristics by which memory T cells can be identified, a sufficient body of knowledge has been acquired so that an initial framework can be used to distinguish them from naïve and short-lived effector cells (Figure 28.8). As might be expected from the information discussed previously, memory T cells constitute a heterogeneous population with respect to surface phenotype, anatomic location, and functional capacity. Still, using a combination of markers for these parameters together with an understanding of the time that has elapsed since their initial priming, it is often possible positively to identify memory T cells.

Identification of B Cell Memory

Memory B cell and plasma cells markers differ in mice and humans. There is no widely accepted memory B cell marker in mice. CD27 expression does not selectively distinguish mouse memory B cells, in contrast to what is observed for human memory B cells (see later discussion). Mouse memory B cells are usually identified by flow cytometry as isotype-switched B cells (e.g., IgG^+ IgD^-) that are neither germinal center B cells (e.g., not PNA^+ $FashiCD38loGL7^+$) nor plasma cells (not $CD138^+$) *(363,551)*. This is problematic for the identification of IgM memory B cells, limiting our current understand of that compartment *(552,553)*. Antigen-specific memory B cells can be identified by their ability to bind fluorescently labeled antigen *(475,478,497,554)*, which is a rich source for experimental study, although it can be technically challenging *(331,555)*. Antigen-specific memory B cells can also be identified by *ex vivo* functional assays (14,*556*) or adoptive transfers *(557)*, although *ex vivo* reactivation assays are limited in their ability to provide single-cell-level analysis, and adoptive transfers can have unexpected complications *(491)*. Although some surface phenotypic markers have been proposed to be differentially expressed by mouse memory B cells ($CD38^{high}$, $CD11b^+$, Fasint) or

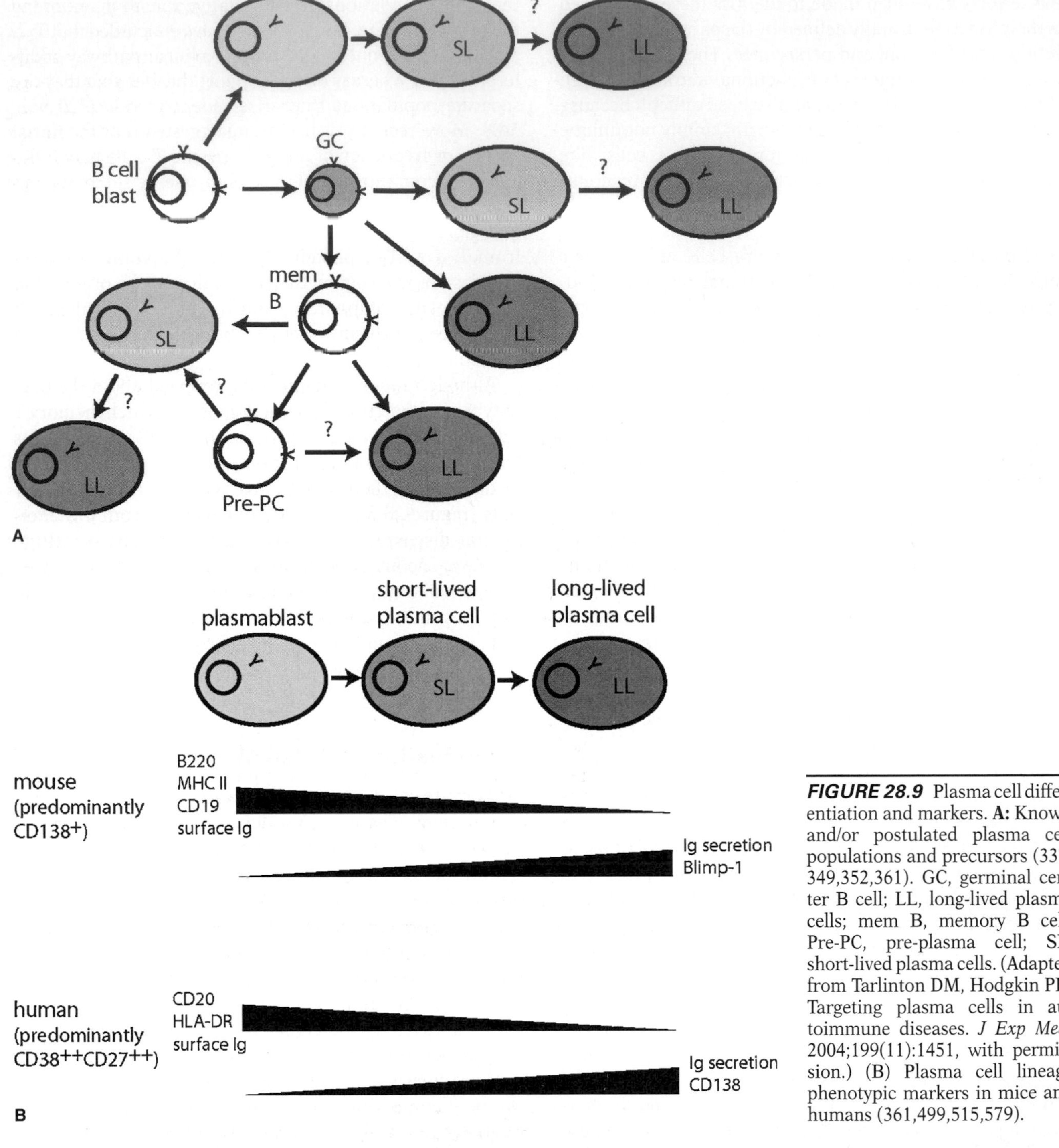

FIGURE 28.9 Plasma cell differentiation and markers. **A:** Known and/or postulated plasma cell populations and precursors (337, 349,352,361). GC, germinal center B cell; LL, long-lived plasma cells; mem B, memory B cell; Pre-PC, pre-plasma cell; SL, short-lived plasma cells. (Adapted from Tarlinton DM, Hodgkin PD. Targeting plasma cells in autoimmune diseases. *J Exp Med.* 2004;199(11):1451, with permission.) (B) Plasma cell lineage phenotypic markers in mice and humans (361,499,515,579).

subsets of memory cells (B220$^-$), there is debate about their utility, and none is widely adopted *(330,331,485,558)*. This suggests that memory B cells are either phenotypically heterogeneous or similar to naïve B cells in their cell surface protein expression profile *(330,331,485)*.

Plasma cells are identified histologically by their large size, eccentric nucleus, and high concentration of intracellular immunoglobulin. Plasma cells are identified functionally by their ability to secrete immunoglobulin *(477,559)*. Plasma cells are also identified by the surface phenotypic marker CD138 *(560)*. Fully differentiated murine plasma cells do not express CD19, B220, or MHC II *(512,561,562)*. Plasmablasts are larger than resting B cells and also have high concentrations of intracellular immunoglobulin *(562,563)*. Plasmablasts express CD138, but they still express intermediate levels of B220, CD19, and

MHC II *(352,561,562)*. It is unclear whether there are multiple distinct plasma cell differentiation pathways *in vivo* distinguishing short-lived from long-lived plasma cells and their precursors or there is one plasma cell differentiation pathway and the percentage of plasma cells with access to a long term survival niche acquire a distinct phenotype based on their location (Fig. 28.9) *(352)*.

Humans

Human memory B cells selective express CD27 *(564–566)*, a member of the TNF receptor superfamily *(567)*. Surface expression of CD27 is now widely used as a specific marker, in conjunction with lack of IgD expression, to discriminate human memory B cells from naïve B cells. CD27 was initially determined as a marker of human memory B cells in both peripheral blood and spleen by demonstrating that $CD27^+$ B cells express somatically mutated Ig V genes, whereas $CD27^-$ B cells do not *(565,566)*. This was also consistent with the observation that nearly all isotype-switched B cells in peripheral blood are $CD27^+$, and the majority of IgD^+ B cells are not *(564,565)*. Memory B cells in tonsillar tissue can be identified as IgD^- $CD38^-$ B cells as well as IgD^- $CD38^-$ $CD27^+$ *(568,569)*. Vaccine induced antigen-specific memory B cells have also been shown to be predominantly $CD27^+$ *(473,570)*. Human $CD27^+$ memory B cells in the spleen localize to the marginal zone *(566)*, comparable to what has been observed in rats and mice. There does exist a small population of $CD27^-$ human memory B cells, and it has been proposed that differential expression of ABC transporter B1 (ABCB1) can be used to distinguish those memory B cells from naïve B cells *(495)*. There has also been debate as to whether somatically mutated IgM^+ IgD^- $CD27^+$ B cells represent a true memory compartment, discussed in two recent reviews *(552,571)*.

Antigen-specific human memory B cells can be identified by fluorescent antigen binding and flow cytometry *(572,573)* or functional identification by *in vitro* reactivation *(473,570)*. Antigen-specific memory B cells are present at low frequencies [approximately 0.005% to 0.2% of total peripheral blood B cells (14,498)]. Using either approach, antigen-specific human memory B cells have been identified to the smallpox vaccine (14), the anthrax vaccine *(507)*, the tetanus vaccine *(473,489,498)*, measles *(473)*, malaria *(574)*, influenza (flu) *(575,576)*, rotavirus *(573,577)*, severe acute respiratory syndrome *(578)*, and wasp venom allergen *(498)*.

Human plasma cells express higher levels of CD27 than memory B cells and are conventionally distinguished in flow cytometry by their high level of CD38 expression and downregulation of CD20 expression *(515, 579,580)*. Human bone marrow plasma cells are similar to murine plasma cells, in that they express CD138, but this marker is not observed on tonsillar or splenic human plasma cells *(499,579)* or on *in vitro*–generated plasmablasts. Our understanding of human plasma cells is limited in large part due to the low frequency of plasma cells in peripheral blood (100 to 1,000 per million cells) and the very brief presence of antigen-specific cells in peripheral blood, making detailed analysis difficult. For studies of human antigen-specific plasma cells, serum antibody levels are classically used as a surrogate indicator.

THE MOLECULAR BASIS OF IMMUNE MEMORY

The Genetic Program of T Cell Memory

Although memory T cells share many features with short-lived effectors, their capacity for self-renewal and recall response suggests that they are guided by a distinct program of gene expression. The phenotypic distinction and functional specialization inherent within the T_{CM} and T_{EM} subsets give further evidence of this notion. Investigations into the molecular events that guide the generation and maintenance of memory T cells are at a relatively early stage in comparison to the phenotypic studies through which these phenomena have been defined. Nonetheless, a framework for understanding the genetic program of memory is beginning to emerge through the identification of genes and regulatory elements that control key functional parameters of T cell memory (30,*581*). Initial studies focused on performing genome-scale gene expression analysis in T cells using gene array hybridization techniques, first to resting versus-activated T cells and subsequently to T cells undergoing homeostatic proliferation (31,*582–584*). These studies revealed that the gene expression in T cells is a dynamic process that undergoes substantial alterations in response to TCR-mediated and environmental stimuli during the transition from resting to activated status. The phenotypic features of this process (e.g., proliferation, effector differentiation, survival) are matched in the global patterns of genes expressed (e.g., cyclins, effector molecules, anti-apoptotic factors, etc).

A key study on the transcriptional profile of memory T cells comes from Kaech et al., who performed genome-wide analyses of gene expression on naïve, effector, and memory transgenic $CD8^+$ T cells activated *in vivo* by LCMV (30). Among the findings emerging from a comparative analysis was that each phase of development was characterized by specific patterns of gene expression directly related to the development or function of the cells at that stage of differentiation; approximately 30% of the genes expressed by effector cells were also maintained in the memory cells, supporting the direct lineage relationship between these cell types (30). In some cases, the expression level of the genes was set at the peak of the effector response (d8), but in others the level of expression decreased as the gradual conversion to memory occurred, perhaps reflecting a global reduction in transcriptional activity in these cells. Whereas the distinction of T_{EM} and T_{CM} subsets has traditionally been defined by phenotypic markers, Willinger at al. used transcriptional profiling to analyze the molecular signature of these subsets in human CD8$^+$ T cells and found that the T_{CM} subset had a pattern of gene expression that was intermediate between naïve and T_{EM} and effector/T_{EM} phenotype cells *(585)*. It has long been appreciated that memory T cells share several notable features related to self-renewal with long-term hematopoietic stem cells (Lt-HSCs). Consistent with this, Hyatt et al. found that both memory T and B cells appear to share many elements of their transcriptional program with Lt-HSCs, with notable increases in the expression of prosurvival and antiapoptosis genes *(581)*.

In parallel with the genome-wide studies of gene expression at the population level in T cells, efforts have been made to define the genetic program of memory in single cells or with respect to specific transcription factors. The recent study of Peixoto et al. is notable in its study of gene expression patterns at the level of single cells at various stages during an immune response *(586)*. This study revealed surprisingly heterogeneous and dynamic patterns of gene expression from the earliest point in the response, with both proinflammatory and effector functionality revealed in discrete cells, followed by a more uniform pattern in secondary responders. It is unclear whether the reduction in heterogeneity at later time points reflects a selection process or a progressive development of the entire memory populations. A number of studies have analyzed the contribution of specific transcription factors to the enhanced longevity and function of memory T cells. These include T-bet and eomesodermin (Eomes), the transcription factors that coordinately regulate a number of genes related to lineage commitment and effector differentiation in both CD4$^+$ and CD8$^+$ T cells *(295,296,587–589)*. T-bet$^{-/-}$ Eomes$^{+/-}$ mice have a near-total loss of effector and memory T cells through a mechanism that is believed to involve their role in regulating the expression of CD122 and thereby responsiveness to IL-15 *(590)*. The roles of T-bet and Eomes in determining whether effector cells are selected for memory development may involve their reciprocal regulation in response to inflammatory signals via IL-12. In response to pathogen-induced IL-12, Eomes is repressed and T-bet levels are increased, which can lead to inhibition of IL-7Rα expression and decreased survival in short-lived effectors *(591,592)*. When IL-12 signals are reduced, Eomes levels rise, whereas T-bet levels decrease, favoring the development of long-lived memory cells *(592,593)*. Another transcription factor that is relevant for memory formation is inhibitor of DNA binding-2 (Id2), an antagonist of E protein transcription factors that is upregulated in CD8$^+$ T cells during infection and maintained on their conversion to memory cells. Although Id2-deficient naïve CD8$^+$ T cells recognized antigen and proliferate normally early after infection, the effector cells become highly susceptible to apoptosis and fail to accumulate. Id2-deficient CD8$^+$ T cells responding to infection show defective memory formation and have altered patterns of expression in genes that influence survival *(594)*.

In addition to the transcription factors described previously, several transcriptional repressors have emerged as regulators of T cell memory. Bcl-6, first described as a transcriptional repressor with pleiotropic functions in B cell differentiation, appears to play a role the generation of both CD4$^+$ and CD8$^+$ T cell memory because the survival of Bcl-6 deficient CD4$^+$ effector T cells was greatly diminished compared to wild-type controls after priming, and Bcl-6–deficient mice were found to lack memory phenotype CD8$^+$ T cells after immunization *(595,596)*. The Bcl-6 homolog Bcl-6b, known to repress IL-2–induced B cell differentiation, is expressed by a small subset of CD8$^+$ T cells and regulates their capacity for secondary expansion in response to antigenic challenge *(597)*. Another transcriptional repressor first described in B cells that influences T cell homeostasis is Blimp-1, which is required for terminal differentiation of B cells through coordinate regulation of hundreds of genes (reviewed in refs. *598,599*). Mice lacking Blimp-1 suffer from a variety of immune-mediated pathologies including colitis and multiorgan inflammatory diseases that are characterized by accumulation of effector and memory T cells *(600,601)*.

It is worth noting that in the case of both the transcriptional activators and repressors that have been implicated in T cell memory, very little is known about the downstream genes they control or the effect these have on the phenotypic and functional parameters through which memory T cells have traditionally been defined. An especially exciting prospect for the near future is that meaningful connections can be made among these transcriptional regulators, the myriad of genes that the array-based approaches have identified at each stage of memory T cell development, and the variety of phenotypic and functions displayed by memory T cells in the generation and maintenance of the protected state.

The Genetic Program of B Cell Memory

The genetic program of B cell memory can be considered to be made up of different genetic programs regulating four cell types: genes regulating germinal center B cells, genes regulating CD4 T cells, genes regulating memory B cells, and genes regulating plasma cells. For example, mice and humans with defects in SAP (SLAM-associated protein, the product of the *sh2d1a* gene) have severe memory B cell deficiencies *(364,602)*. This defect is due to the requirement for SAP expression in CD4 T cells to provide B cell help and generate germinal centers *(340,364,603)*. Genes that regulate CD4 T cell help to B cells affect memory

B cell generation. Additional prominent examples include CD40L, ICOS, CD28, and CXCR5 *(273)*. Human genetic deficiencies in CD40L and ICOS have been identified and are associated with severe germinal center B cell defects and overall reductions in memory B cell numbers *(604,605)*.

Memory B cells are generated in germinal centers, and therefore genes necessarily expressed in B cells for germinal center B cell differentiation and function control memory B cell development. Prominent examples of genes expressed in B cells that are important for differentiation into germinal center B cells or function (class switching and hypermutation) of germinal center B cells include BCL6, AID, CD40, ICOSL, and IL21R *(342,606–609)*. An exhaustive list is available elsewhere *(332)*, with several notable recent additions *(610–612)*. Human genetic deficiencies in CD40 and AID have been identified and are associated with severe B cell defects, including overall reductions in memory B cell numbers *(605)*. Genes that are required for fully functional mature peripheral B cells also generally affect subsequent germinal center formation after infection/immunization. Genes in this category include B cell development and/or survival regulators including CD19, OBF, and BAFF-R *(613–616)*. All of these genes are important in germinal center development and are therefore directly or indirectly important for the differentiation of memory B cells. Genes have not been identified that are specifically required for the maintenance of memory B cells in a cell-intrinsic manner. Because memory B cells are believed to maintain themselves via slow homeostatic proliferation *(475,494,495)*, comparable to what is observed for CD8 T cells (34,52,*411*), it is likely that genes involved in cell survival, homeostatic proliferation, and the stem cell–like property of self-renewal (which may include quiescence factors) are important for memory B cell maintenance.

Genes necessary for plasma cell differentiation in a cell-intrinsic manner are necessary for the development of long-lived plasma cells and the long-term maintenance of serum antibody levels. Blimp-1 and XBP-1 are two prominent examples of important regulators of plasma cell differentiation *(617–620)*. The selective effects of Blimp-1 on plasma cell differentiation are highly informative. Blimp-1 expression in B cells is tightly correlated with plasma cell differentiation *(361)*, and Blimp-1 deficiency in mice leads to normal (or enlarged) germinal center development and memory B cell development but results in a complete lack of plasma cells after immunization *(621)*. These observations demonstrate that the memory B cell and plasma cell lineages are distinct and are controlled by different genetic programs. Regarding long-lived plasma cell survival, CXCR4 is a chemokine receptor important for homing of long-lived plasma cells to the bone marrow and other locations of survival niches *(358)*, and constitutive expression of Blimp-1 is required for maintenance of long-lived plasma cells *(622)*.

A fourth category of genes that affect B cell memory comprises genes important for lymphoid organ architecture and organization. Genes encoding cytokines in the TNF superfamily, including LTα, LTβ, the LTβ receptor, and TNF and TNFR1, and are crucial for the development of appropriate lymphoid architecture *(623,624)*. In the absence of these genes, germinal center formation is severely disrupted. It is believed that this disruption of germinal center development is due to the combined factors of defective lymphoid architecture and defective follicular dendritic cell differentiation. B cell expression of LT$\alpha\beta$ is key for establishing gradients of chemokines, which are important molecules affecting germinal center development (and therefore B cell memory generation) by organizing the cellular compartments of lymphoid organs *(625)*.

CONCLUSION

The salient features related to the phenomenon of immune memory have been recognized for decades and can be easily replicated in both *in vitro* and *in vivo* experimental systems. Despite this, a detailed molecular understanding of just how memory cells are able to persist and protect has yet to be realized. Key steps towards this goal have been the development of standard definitions for what memory cells are and can do and an appreciation of the remarkable phenotypic and functional heterogeneity they possess. The next advances in our understanding of immune memory will come from the application of more holistic molecular approaches to the study of physiologic immune responses *in vivo*, which will allow activities of the immune system, as opposed to a specific immune cell, to be studied. Although this might seem a daunting task in terms of its complexity and sheer volume of information to be obtained, the results will be transformative in terms of our fundamental understanding of the immune system and our ability to manipulate it for the prevention of disease.

REFERENCES

1. Thucydides. *History of the Peloponnesian war*. New York: Dover, 2004.
2. Cunha BA. The cause of the plague of Athens: plague, typhoid, typhus, smallpox, or measles? *Infect Dis Clin North Am*. 2004;18(1): 29–43.
3. Zinkernagel RM. On natural and artificial vaccinations. *Annu Rev Immunol*. 2003;21:515–546.

3a. Ahmed R, Gray D. Immunological memory and protective immunity: understanding their relation. *Science*. 1996;272:54–60.

4. Panum PL. Beobachtungenuber das maserncontagium. *Virchows Arch*. 1847;1:492–512.
5. Zinkernagel RM. On differences between immunity and immunological memory. *Curr Opin Immunol*. 2002;14(4):523–536.
6. Paul JR, Riordan JT, Melnick JL. Antibodies to three different antigenic types of poliomyelitis virus in sera from North Alaskan Eskimos. *Am J Hygiene*. 1951;54(2):275–285.

7. Sawyer WA. The persistence of yellow fever. *Immunity J Prevent Med.* 1931;5:413–428.
8. Zinkernagel RM, Hengartner H. Protective 'immunity' by pre-existent neutralizing antibody titers and preactivated T cells but not by so-called "immunological memory." *Immunol Rev.* 2006;211:310–319.
9. Barquet N, Domingo P. Smallpox: the triumph over the most terrible of the ministers of death. *Ann Intern Med.* 1997;127(8 Pt 1):635–642.
10. Jenner E. *An inquiry into the causes and effects of the variolae vaccinae.* London: Samson Low, 1798.
11. Iwasaki A, Medzhitov R. Toll-like receptor control of the adaptive immune responses. *Nat Immunol.* 2004;5(10):987–995.
12. Pulendran B, Ahmed R. Translating innate immunity into immunological memory: implications for vaccine development. *Cell.* 2006;124(4):849–863.
13. Henderson DA. The eradication of smallpox. *Sci Am.* 1976;235(4): 25–33.
14. Crotty S, Felgner P, Davies H, et al. Cutting edge: long-term B cell memory in humans after smallpox vaccination. *J Immunol.* 2003;171(10):4969–4673.
15. Demkowicz WE Jr, Littaua RA, Wang J, et al. Human cytotoxic T-cell memory: long-lived responses to vaccinia virus. *J Virol.* 1996;70(4):2627–2631.
16. Hammarlund E, Lewis MW, Hansen SG, et al. Duration of antiviral immunity after smallpox vaccination. *Nat Med.* 2003;9(9):1131–1137.
17. Gayton W. T*he value of vacciniation as shown by an analysis of 10,403 cases of smallpox.* London: Gillet & Henty, 1885.
18. Mack TM. Smallpox in Europe, 1950–1971. *J Infect Dis.* 1972; 125(2):161–169.
19. Honjo T, Alt F, Neuberger M. *Molecular biology of B cells.* Amsterdam: Elsevier, 2004.
20. Bousso P, Levraud JP, Kourilsky P, et al. The composition of a primary T cell response is largely determined by the timing of recruitment of individual T cell clones. *J Exp Med.* 1999;189(10):1591–1600.
21. Busch DH, Pilip IM, Vijh S, et al. Coordinate regulation of complex T cell populations responding to bacterial infection. *Immunity.* 1998;8(3):353–362.
22. Hou S, Hyland L, Ryan KW, et al. Virus-specific CD8+ T-cell memory determined by clonal burst size. *Nature.* 1994;369(6482):652–654.
23. Northrop JK, Thomas RM, Wells AD, et al. Epigenetic remodeling of the IL-2 and IFN-gamma loci in memory CD8 T cells is influenced by CD4 T cells. *J Immunol.* 2006;177(2):1062–1069.
24. Varga SM, Welsh RM. High frequency of virus-specific interleukin-2-producing CD4(+) T cells and Th1 dominance during lymphocytic choriomeningitis virus infection. *J Virol.* 2000;74(9):4429–4432.
25. Whitmire JK, Asano MS, Murali-Krishna K, et al. Long-term CD4 Th1 and Th2 memory following acute lymphocytic choriomeningitis virus infection. *J Virol.* 1998;72(10):8281–8288.
26. Agarwal S, Rao A. Modulation of chromatin structure regulates cytokine gene expression during T cell differentiation. *Immunity.* 1998;9(6):765–775.
27. Bachmann MF, Barner M, Viola A, et al. Distinct kinetics of cytokine production and cytolysis in effector and memory T cells after viral infection. *Eur J Immunol.* 1999;29(1):291–299.
28. Grayson JM, Murali-Krishna K, Altman JD, et al. Gene expression in antigen-specific CD8+ T cells during viral infection. *J Immunol.* 2001;166(2):795–799.
29. Hathcock KS, Kaech SM, Ahmed R, et al. Induction of telomerase activity and maintenance of telomere length in virus-specific effector and memory CD8+ T cells. *J Immunol.* 2003;170(1): 147–152.
30. Kaech SM, Hemby S, Kersh E, et al. Molecular and functional profiling of memory CD8 T cell differentiation. *Cell.* 2002;111(6):837–851.
31. Teague TK, Hildeman D, Kedl RM, et al. Activation changes the spectrum but not the diversity of genes expressed by T cells. *Proc Natl Acad Sci U S A.* 1999;96(22):12691–12696.
32. Veiga-Fernandes H, Walter U, Bourgeois C, et al. Response of naïve and memory CD8+ T cells to antigen stimulation *in vivo*. *Nat Immunol.* 2000;1(1):47–53.
33. Schluns KS, Lefrancois L. Cytokine control of memory T-cell development and survival. *Nat Rev.* 2003;3(4):269–279.
34. Surh CD, Boyman O, Purton JF, et al. Homeostasis of memory T cells. *Immunol Rev.* 2006;211:154–163.
35. Lefrancois L. Development, trafficking, and function of memory T-cell subsets. *Immunol Rev.* 2006;211:93–103.
36. Rodrigo Mora J, Von Andrian UH. Specificity and plasticity of memory lymphocyte migration. *Curr Top Microbiol Immunol.* 2006;308:83–116.
37. Busch DH, Pamer EG. T cell affinity maturation by selective expansion during infection. *J Exp Med.* 1999;189(4):701–710.
38. Fahmy TM, Bieler JG, Edidin M, et al. Increased TCR avidity after T cell activation: a mechanism for sensing low-density antigen. *Immunity.* 2001;14(2):135–143.
39. Rees W, Bender J, Teague TK, et al. An inverse relationship between T cell receptor affinity and antigen dose during CD4(+) T cell responses *in vivo* and *in vitro*. *Proc Natl Acad Sci U S A.* 1999;96(17):9781–9786.
40. Savage PA, Boniface JJ, Davis MM. A kinetic basis for T cell receptor repertoire selection during an immune response. *Immunity.* 1999;10(4):485–492.
41. Sallusto F, Lenig D, Forster R, et al. Two subsets of memory T lymphocytes with distinct homing potentials and effector functions. *Nature.* 1999;401(6754):708–712.
42. Lanzavecchia A, Sallusto F. Understanding the generation and function of memory T cell subsets. *Curr Opin Immunol.* 2005;17(3):326–332.
43. Hamann D, Baars PA, Rep MH, et al. Phenotypic and functional separation of memory and effector human CD8+ T cells. *J Exp Med.* 1997;186(9):1407–1418.
44. Masopust D, Kaech SM, Wherry EJ, et al. The role of programming in memory T-cell development. *Curr Opin Immunol.* 2004;16(2):217–225.
45. Chang JT, Palanivel VR, Kinjyo I, et al. Asymmetric T lymphocyte division in the initiation of adaptive immune responses. *Science.* 2007;315(5819):1687–1691.
46. Reiner SL, Sallusto F, Lanzavecchia A. Division of labor with a workforce of one: challenges in specifying effector and memory T cell fate. *Science.* 2007;317(5838):622–625.
47. Roegiers F, Jan YN. Asymmetric cell division. *Curr Opin Cell Biol.* 2004;16(2):195–205.
48. Lanzavecchia A, Sallusto F. Progressive differentiation and selection of the fittest in the immune response. *Nat Rev.* 2002;2(12):982–987.
49. Carter LL, Swain SL. From naïve to memory. Development and regulation of CD4+ T cell responses. *Immunol Res.* 1998;18(1):1–13.
50. Seder RA, Ahmed R. Similarities and differences in CD4+ and CD8+ effector and memory T cell generation. *Nat Immunol.* 2003;4(9):835–842.
51. Kaech SM, Wherry EJ. Heterogeneity and cell-fate decisions in effector and memory CD8+ T cell differentiation during viral infection. *Immunity.* 2007(27):393–405.
52. Kaech SM, Wherry EJ, Ahmed R. Effector and memory T-cell differentiation: implications for vaccine development. *Nat Rev.* 2002;2(4):251–262.
53. Harari A, Dutoit V, Cellerai C, et al. Functional signatures of protective antiviral T-cell immunity in human virus infections. *Immunol Rev.* 2006;211:236–254.
54. Hikono H, Kohlmeier JE, Ely KH, et al. T-cell memory and recall responses to respiratory virus infections. *Immunol Rev.* 2006;211:119–132.
55. Hinrichs CS, Gattinoni L, Restifo NP. Programming CD8+ T cells for effective immunotherapy. *Curr Opin Immunol.* 2006;18(3):363–370.
56. Huster KM, Stemberger C, Busch DH. Protective immunity towards intracellular pathogens. *Curr Opin Immunol.* 2006;18(4): 458–464.

57. Martin D, Tarleton R. Generation, specificity, and function of CD8+ T cells in *Trypanosoma cruzi* infection. *Immunol Rev*. 2004;201:304–317.
58. Morrot A, Zavala F. Effector and memory CD8+ T cells as seen in immunity to malaria. *Immunol Rev*. 2004;201:291–303.
59. Williams MA, Holmes BJ, Sun JC, et al. Developing and maintaining protective CD8+ memory T cells. *Immunol Rev*. 2006;211:146–153.
60. Woodworth JS, Behar SM. *Mycobacterium tuberculosis*-specific CD8+ T cells and their role in immunity. *Crit Rev Immunol*. 2006;26(4):317–352.
61. Butz E, Bevan MJ. Dynamics of the CD8+ T cell response during acute LCMV infection. *Adv Exp Med Biol*. 1998;452:111–122.
62. Harty JT, Bevan MJ. Responses of CD8(+) T cells to intracellular bacteria. *Curr Opin Immunol*. 1999;11(1):89–93.
63. Kedzierska K, La Gruta NL, Turner SJ, et al. Establishment and recall of CD8+ T-cell memory in a model of localized transient infection. *Immunol Rev*. 2006;211:133–145.
64. Altman JD, Moss PA, Goulder PJ, et al. Phenotypic analysis of antigen-specific T lymphocytes. *Science*. 1996;274(5284):94–96.
65. Labalette-Houache M, Torpier G, Capron A, et al. Improved permeabilization procedure for flow cytometric detection of internal antigens. Analysis of interleukin-2 production. *J Immunol Meth*. 1991 Apr 25;138(2):143–153.
66. Appay V, Rowland-Jones SL. The assessment of antigen-specific CD8+ T cells through the combination of MHC class I tetramer and intracellular staining. *J Immunol Meth*. 2002;268(1):9–19.
67. Badovinac VP, Harty JT. Detection and analysis of antigen-specific CD8+ T cells. *Immunol Res*. 2001;24(3):325–332.
68. Blattman JN, Antia R, Sourdive DJ, et al. Estimating the precursor frequency of naïve antigen-specific CD8 T cells. *J Exp Med*. 2002;195(5):657–664.
69. Steinman RM. The dendritic cell system and its role in immunogenicity. *Annu Rev Immunol*. 1991;9:271–296.
70. Scollay RG, Butcher EC, Weissman IL. Thymus cell migration. Quantitative aspects of cellular traffic from the thymus to the periphery in mice. *Eur J Immunol*. 1980;10(3):210–218.
71. Tough DF, Sprent J. Turnover of naïve- and memory-phenotype T cells. *J Exp Med*. 1994;179(4):1127–1135.
72. Berzins SP, Uldrich AP, Sutherland JS, et al. Thymic regeneration: teaching an old immune system new tricks. *Trends Mol Med*. 2002;8(10):469–476.
73. Polic B, Kunkel D, Scheffold A, et al. How alpha beta T cells deal with induced TCR alpha ablation. *Proc Natl Acad Sci U S A*. 2001;98(15):8744–8749.
74. Rooke R, Waltzinger C, Benoist C, et al. Targeted complementation of MHC class II deficiency by intrathymic delivery of recombinant adenoviruses. *Immunity*. 1997;7(1):123–134.
75. Schluns KS, Kieper WC, Jameson SC, et al. Interleukin-7 mediates the homeostasis of naïve and memory CD8 T cells *in vivo*. *Nat Immunol*. 2000;1(5):426–432.
76. Takeda S, Rodewald HR, Arakawa H,. MHC class II molecules are not required for survival of newly generated CD4+ T cells, but affect their long-term life span. *Immunity*. 1996;5(3):217–228.
77. Tan JT, Dudl E, LeRoy E, et al. IL-7 is critical for homeostatic proliferation and survival of naïve T cells. *Proc Natl Acad Sci U S A*. 2001;98(15):8732–8737.
78. Tanchot C, Lemonnier FA, Perarnau B, et al. Differential requirements for survival and proliferation of CD8 naïve or memory T cells. *Science*. 1997;276(5321):2057–2062.
79. Marrack P, Kappler J. Control of T cell viability. *Annu Rev Immunol*. 2004;22:765–787.
80. Boyman O, Purton JF, Surh CD, et al. Cytokines and T-cell homeostasis. *Curr Opin Immunol*. 2007;19(3):320–326.
81. Hofmeister R, Khaled AR, Benbernou N, et al. Interleukin-7: physiological roles and mechanisms of action. *Cytokine Growth Factor Rev*. 1999;10(1):41–60.
82. Mazzucchelli R, Durum SK. Interleukin-7 receptor expression: intelligent design. *Nat Rev*. 2007;7(2):144–154.
83. Akashi K, Kondo M, Weissman IL. Role of interleukin-7 in T-cell development from hematopoietic stem cells. *Immunol Rev*. 1998;165:13–28.
84. Rathmell JC, Farkash EA, Gao W, et al. IL-7 enhances the survival and maintains the size of naïve T cells. *J Immunol*. 2001;167(12):6869–6876.
85. Vella A, Teague TK, Ihle J, et al. Interleukin 4 (IL-4) or IL–7 prevents the death of resting T cells: stat6 is probably not required for the effect of IL. *J Exp Med*. 1997;186(2):325–330.
86. Boise LH, Minn AJ, June CH, et al. Growth factors can enhance lymphocyte survival without committing the cell to undergo cell division. *Proc Natl Acad Sci U S A*. 1995;92(12):5491–5795.
87. von Freeden-Jeffry U, Vieira P, Lucian LA, et al. Lymphopenia in interleukin (IL)-7 gene-deleted mice identifies IL-7 as a nonredundant cytokine. *J Exp Med*. 1995;181(4):1519–1526.
88. Peschon JJ, Morrissey PJ, Grabstein KH, et al. Early lymphocyte expansion is severely impaired in interleukin 7 receptor-deficient mice. *J Exp Med*. 1994;180(5):1955–1960.
89. Gowans JL, Knight EJ. The route of re-circulation of lymphocytes in the rat. *Proc R Soc Lond B Biol*. 1964;159:257–282.
90. Mackay CR. Homing of naïve, memory and effector lymphocytes. *Curr Opin Immunol*. 1993;5(3):423–427.
91. Marchesi VT, Gowans JL. The migration of lymphocytes through the endothelium of venules in lymph nodes: an electron microscope study. *Proc R Soc Lond B Biol*. 1964;159:283–290.
92. Picker LJ, Butcher EC. Physiological and molecular mechanisms of lymphocyte homing. *Annu Rev Immunol*. 1992;10:561–591.
93. Sprent J. *Recirculating lymphocytes*. New York: Dekker, 1977.
94. Berg EL, Robinson MK, Warnock RA, et al. The human peripheral lymph node vascular addressin is a ligand for LECAM-1, the peripheral lymph node homing receptor. *J Cell Biol*. 1991;114(2):343–349.
95. Gunn MD, Tangemann K, Tam C, et al. A chemokine expressed in lymphoid high endothelial venules promotes the adhesion and chemotaxis of naïve T lymphocytes. *Proc Natl Acad Sci U S A*. 1998;95(1):258–263.
96. Bajenoff M, Egen JG, Koo LY, et al. Stromal cell networks regulate lymphocyte entry, migration, and territoriality in lymph nodes. *Immunity*. 2006;25(6):989.
97. Gretz JE, Anderson AO, Shaw S. Cords, channels, corridors and conduits: critical architectural elements facilitating cell interactions in the lymph node cortex. *Immunol Rev*. 1997;156:11–24.
98. Katakai T, Hara T, Lee JH, et al. A novel reticular stromal structure in lymph node cortex: an immuno-platform for interactions among dendritic cells, T cells and B cells. *Int Immunol*. 2004;16(8):1133–1142.
99. Katakai T, Hara T, Sugai M, et al. Lymph node fibroblastic reticular cells construct the stromal reticulum via contact with lymphocytes. *J Exp Med*. 2004;200(6):783–795.
100. Miller MJ, Wei SH, Cahalan MD, et al. Autonomous T cell trafficking examined *in vivo* with intravital two-photon microscopy. *Proc Natl Acad Sci U S A*. 2003;100(5):2604–2609.
101. Potsch C, Vohringer D, Pircher H. Distinct migration patterns of naïve and effector CD8 T cells in the spleen: correlation with CCR7 receptor expression and chemokine reactivity. *Eur J Immunol*. 1999;29(11):3562–3570.
102. Unsoeld H, Voehringer D, Krautwald S, et al. Constitutive expression of CCR7 directs effector CD8 T cells into the splenic white pulp and impairs functional activity. *J Immunol*. 2004;173(5):3013–3019.
103. Sprent J. Circulating T and B lymphocytes of the mouse. I. Migratory properties. *Cell Immunol*. 1973;7(1):10–39.
104. Caux C, Ait-Yahia S, Chemin K, et al. Dendritic cell biology and regulation of dendritic cell trafficking by chemokines. *Springer Semin Immunopathol*. 2000;22(4):345–369.
105. Caux C, Vanbervliet B, Massacrier C, et al. Regulation of dendritic cell recruitment by chemokines. *Transplantation*. 2002;73(1 suppl):S7–S11.
106. Sallusto F, Palermo B, Lenig D, et al. Distinct patterns and kinetics of chemokine production regulate dendritic cell function. *Eur J Immunol*. 1999;29(5):1617–1625.
107. Sozzani S, Mantovani A, Allavena P. Control of dendritic cell migration by chemokines. *Forum* (Genoa, Italy). 1999;9(4):325–338.
108. Banchereau J, Steinman RM. Dendritic cells and the control of immunity. *Nature*. 1998;392(6673):245–252.

109. Janeway CA Jr, Medzhitov R. Innate immune recognition. *Annu Rev Immunol*. 2002;20:197–216.
110. Medzhitov R, Preston-Hurlburt P, Janeway CA Jr. A human homologue of the *Drosophila* Toll protein signals activation of adaptive immunity. *Nature*. 1997;388(6640):394–397.
111. Takeda K, Kaisho T, Akira S. Toll-like receptors. *Annu Rev Immunol*. 2003;21:335–376.
112. Beutler B, Hoebe K, Georgel P, et al. Genetic analysis of innate immunity: identification and function of the TIR adapter proteins. *Adv Exp Med Biol*. 2005;560:29–39.
113. Bin LH, Xu LG, Shu HB. TIRP, a novel Toll/interleukin-1 receptor (TIR) domain-containing adapter protein involved in TIR signaling. *J Biol Chem*. 2003;278(27):24526–24532.
114. Fitzgerald KA, Palsson-McDermott EM, Bowie AG, et al. Mal (MyD88-adapter-like) is required for Toll-like receptor-4 signal transduction. *Nature*. 2001;413(6851):78–83.
115. Fitzgerald KA, Rowe DC, Barnes BJ, et al. LPS-TLR4 signaling to IRF-3/7 and NF-kappaB involves the toll adapters TRAM and TRIF. *J Exp Med*. 2003;198(7):1043–1055.
116. Hoebe K, Du X, Georgel P, et al. Identification of Lps2 as a key transducer of MyD88-independent TIR signalling. *Nature*. 2003; 424(6950):743–748.
117. Horng T, Barton GM, Medzhitov R. TIRAP: an adapter molecule in the Toll signaling pathway. *Nat Immunol*. 2001;2(9):835–841.
118. Muzio M, Ni J, Feng P, et al. IRAK (Pelle) family member IRAK-2 and MyD88 as proximal mediators of IL-1 signaling. *Science*. 1997;278(5343):1612–1615.
119. Oshiumi H, Sasai M, Shida K, et al. TIR-containing adapter molecule (TICAM)-2, a bridging adapter recruiting to Toll-like receptor 4 TICAM-1 that induces interferon-beta. *J Biol Chem*. 2003;278(50):49751–49762.
120. Yamamoto M, Sato S, Mori K, et al. Cutting edge: a novel Toll/IL-1 receptor domain-containing adapter that preferentially activates the IFN-beta promoter in the Toll-like receptor signaling. *J Immunol*. 2002;169(12):6668–6672.
121. Hoebe K, Beutler B. LPS, dsRNA and the interferon bridge to adaptive immune responses: Trif, Tram, and other TIR adaptor proteins. *J Endotoxin Res*. 2004;10(2):130–136.
122. O'Neill LA, Bowie AG. The family of five: TIR-domain-containing adaptors in Toll-like receptor signalling. *Nat Rev*. 2007;7(5):353–364.
123. Gallucci S, Matzinger P. Danger signals: SOS to the immune system. *Curr Opin Immunol*. 2001;13(1):114–119.
124. Honda K, Taniguchi T. IRFs: master regulators of signalling by Toll-like receptors and cytosolic pattern-recognition receptors. *Nat Rev*. 2006;6(9):644–658.
125. O'Neill LA. How Toll-like receptors signal: what we know and what we don't know. *Curr Opin Immunol*. 2006;18(1):3–9.
126. Sallusto F, Mackay CR, Lanzavecchia A. The role of chemokine receptors in primary, effector, and memory immune responses. *Annu Rev Immunol*. 2000;18:593–620.
127. von Andrian UH, Mempel TR. Homing and cellular traffic in lymph nodes. *Nat Rev*. 2003;3(11):867–878.
128. Forster R, Schubel A, Breitfeld D, et al. CCR7 coordinates the primary immune response by establishing functional microenvironments in secondary lymphoid organs. *Cell*. 1999;99(1):23–33.
129. Junt T, Scandella E, Forster R, et al. Impact of CCR7 on priming and distribution of antiviral effector and memory CTL. *J Immunol*. 2004;173(11):6684–6693.
130. Luther SA, Tang HL, Hyman PL, et al. Coexpression of the chemokines ELC and SLC by T zone stromal cells and deletion of the ELC gene in the plt/plt mouse. *Proc Natl Acad Sci U S A*. 2000;97(23):12694–12699.
131. Unsoeld H, Krautwald S, Voehringer D, et al. Cutting edge: CCR7+ and CCR7− memory T cells do not differ in immediate effector cell function. *J Immunol*. 2002;169(2):638–641.
132. Worbs T, Mempel TR, Bolter J, et al. CCR7 ligands stimulate the intranodal motility of T lymphocytes *in vivo*. *J Exp Med*. 2007; 204(3):489–495.
133. Chow A, Toomre D, Garrett W, et al. Dendritic cell maturation triggers retrograde MHC class II transport from lysosomes to the plasma membrane. *Nature*. 2002;418(6901):988–994.
134. Inaba K, Turley S, Iyoda T, et al. The formation of immunogenic major histocompatibility complex class II-peptide ligands in lysosomal compartments of dendritic cells is regulated by inflammatory stimuli. *J Exp Med*. 2000;191(6):927–936.
135. Shin JS, Ebersold M, Pypaert M, et al. Surface expression of MHC class II in dendritic cells is controlled by regulated ubiquitination. *Nature*. 2006;444(7115):115–118.
136. Turley SJ, Inaba K, Garrett WS, et al. Transport of peptide-MHC class II complexes in developing dendritic cells. *Science*. 2000;288(5465):522–527.
137. van Niel G, Wubbolts R, Ten Broeke T, et al. Dendritic cells regulate exposure of MHC class II at their plasma membrane by oligoubiquitination. *Immunity*. 2006;25(6):885–894.
138. Cella M, Engering A, Pinet V, et al. Inflammatory stimuli induce accumulation of MHC class II complexes on dendritic cells. *Nature*. 1997;388(6644):782–787.
139. Guermonprez P, Valladeau J, Zitvogel L, et al. Antigen presentation and T cell stimulation by dendritic cells. *Annu Rev Immunol*. 2002;20:621–667.
140. Lanzavecchia A, Sallusto F. Regulation of T cell immunity by dendritic cells. *Cell*. 2001;106(3):263–266.
141. Banchereau J, Briere F, Caux C, et al. Immunobiology of dendritic cells. *Annu Rev Immunol*. 2000;18:767–811.
142. Fuchs E. Two signal model of lymphocyte activation. *Immunol Today*. 1992;13(11):462.
143. Lafferty KJ, Warren HS, Woolnough JA, et al. Immunological induction of T lymphocytes: role of antigen and the lymphocyte costimulator. *Blood Cells*. 1978;4(3):395–406.
144. Chambers CA, Allison JP. Costimulatory regulation of T cell function. *Curr Opin Cell Biol*. 1999;11(2):203–210.
145. Slavik JM, Hutchcroft JE, Bierer BE. CD28/CTLA-4 and CD80/CD86 families: signaling and function. *Immunol Res*. 1999; 19(1):1–24.
146. Chambers CA. The expanding world of co-stimulation: the two-signal model revisited. *Trends Immunol*. 2001;22(4): 217–223.
147. Greenfield EA, Nguyen KA, Kuchroo VK. CD28/B7 costimulation: a review. *Crit Rev Immunol*. 1998;18(5):389–418.
148. Lenschow DJ, Walunas TL, Bluestone JA. CD28/B7 system of T cell costimulation. *Annu Rev Immunol*. 1996;14:233–258.
149. Shahinian A, Pfeffer K, Lee KP, et al. Differential T cell costimulatory requirements in CD28-deficient mice. *Science*. 1993;261(5121):609–612.
150. Kawai K, Shahinian A, Mak TW, et al. Skin allograft rejection in CD28-deficient mice. *Transplantation*. 1996;61(3): 352–355.
151. Speiser DE, Bachmann MF, Shahinian A, et al. Acute graft-versus-host disease without costimulation via CD28. *Transplantation*. 1997;63(7):1042–1044.
152. Wen T, Kono K, Shahinian A, et al. CD28 is not required for rejection of unmanipulated syngeneic and autologous tumors. *Eur J Immunol*. 1997;27(8):1988–1993.
153. Suresh M, Whitmire JK, Harrington LE, et al. Role of CD28-B7 interactions in generation and maintenance of CD8 T cell memory. *J Immunol*. 2001;167(10):5565–5573.
154. Watts TH, DeBenedette MA. T cell co-stimulatory molecules other than CD28. *Curr Opin Immunol*. 1999;11(3):286–293.
155. Croft M. Co-stimulatory members of the TNFR family: keys to effective T-cell immunity? *Nat Rev*. 2003;3(8):609–620.
156. Watts TH. TNF/TNFR family members in costimulation of T cell responses. *Annu Rev Immunol*. 2005;23:23–68.
157. Keir ME, Francisco LM, Sharpe AH. PD-1 and its ligands in T-cell immunity. *Curr Opin Immunol*. 2007;19(3):309–314.
158. Sharpe AH, Freeman GJ. The B7-CD28 superfamily. *Nat Rev*. 2002;2(2):116–126.
159. Haring JS, Badovinac VP, Harty JT. Inflaming the CD8+ T cell response. *Immunity*. 2006;25(1):19–29.
160. Murphy KM, Ouyang W, Farrar JD, et al. Signaling and transcription in T helper development. *Annu Rev Immunol*. 2000;18:451–494.
161. Curtsinger JM, Schmidt CS, Mondino A, et al. Inflammatory cytokines provide a third signal for activation of naïve CD4+ and CD8+ T cells. *J Immunol*. 1999;162(6):3256–3262.

162. Schmidt CS, Mescher MF. Adjuvant effect of IL-12: conversion of peptide antigen administration from tolerizing to immunizing for CD8+ T cells *in vivo*. *J Immunol*. 1999;163(5):2561–2567.
163. Valenzuela J, Schmidt C, Mescher M. The roles of IL-12 in providing a third signal for clonal expansion of naïve CD8 T cells. *J Immunol*. 2002;169(12):6842–6849.
164. Schmidt CS, Mescher MF. Peptide antigen priming of naïve, but not memory, CD8 T cells requires a third signal that can be provided by IL-12. *J Immunol*. 2002;168(11):5521–5529.
165. Curtsinger JM, Valenzuela JO, Agarwal P, et al. Type I IFNs provide a third signal to CD8 T cells to stimulate clonal expansion and differentiation. *J Immunol*. 2005;174(8):4465–4469.
166. Aichele P, Unsoeld H, Koschella M, et al. CD8 T cells specific for lymphocytic choriomeningitis virus require type I IFN receptor for clonal expansion. *J Immunol*. 2006;176(8):4525–4529.
166a. Thompson LJ, Kolumam GA, Thomas S, et al. Innate inflammatory signals induced by various pathogens differentially dictate the IFN-1 dependence of CD8 T cells for clonal expansion and memory formation. *J Immunol*. 2006;177:1746–1754.
167. Kolumam GA, Thomas S, Thompson LJ, et al. Type I interferons act directly on CD8 T cells to allow clonal expansion and memory formation in response to viral infection. *J Exp Med*. 2005;202(5): 637–650.
168. Badovinac VP, Tvinnereim AR, Harty JT. Regulation of antigen-specific CD8+ T cell homeostasis by perforin and interferon-gamma. *Science*. 2000;290(5495):1354–1358.
169. Sercan O, Hammerling GJ, Arnold B, et al. Innate immune cells contribute to the IFN-gamma-dependent regulation of antigen-specific CD8+ T cell homeostasis. *J Immunol*. 2006;176(2):735–739.
170. Whitmire JK, Benning N, Whitton JL. Cutting edge: early IFN-gamma signaling directly enhances primary antiviral CD4+ T cell responses. *J Immunol*. 2005;175(9):5624–5628.
171. Bennett SR, Carbone FR, Karamalis F, et al. Induction of a CD8+ cytotoxic T lymphocyte response by cross-priming requires cognate CD4+ T cell help. *J Exp Med*. 1997;186(1):65–70.
172. Castellino F, Germain RN. Cooperation between CD4+ and CD8+ T cells: when, where, and how. *Annu Rev Immunol*. 2006;24:519–540.
173. Smith CM, Wilson NS, Waithman J, et al. Cognate CD4(+) T cell licensing of dendritic cells in CD8(+) T cell immunity. *Nat Immunol*. 2004;5(11):1143–1148.
174. Bevan MJ. Immunology. Stimulating killer cells. *Nature*. 1989; 342(6249):478–479.
175. Keene JA, Forman J. Helper activity is required for the *in vivo* generation of cytotoxic T lymphocytes. *J Exp Med*. 1982;155(3):768–782.
176. Mitchison NA, O'Malley C. Three-cell-type clusters of T cells with antigen-presenting cells best explain the epitope linkage and noncognate requirements of the *in vivo* cytolytic response. *Eur J Immunol*. 1987;17(11):1579–1583.
177. Bevan MJ. Helping the CD8(+) T-cell response. *Nat Rev*. 2004;4(8): 595–602.
178. Bennett SR, Carbone FR, Karamalis F, et al. Help for cytotoxic-T-cell responses is mediated by CD40 signalling. *Nature*. 1998;393(6684):478–480.
179. Grewal IS, Flavell RA. The role of CD40 ligand in costimulation and T-cell activation. *Immunol Rev*. 1996;153:85–106.
180. Ridge JP, Di Rosa F, Matzinger P. A conditioned dendritic cell can be a temporal bridge between a CD4+ T-helper and a T-killer cell. *Nature*. 1998;393(6684):474–478.
181. Schoenberger SP, Toes RE, van der Voort EI, et al. T-cell help for cytotoxic T lymphocytes is mediated by CD40-CD40L interactions. *Nature*. 1998;393(6684):480–483.
182. Cella M, Scheidegger D, Palmer-Lehmann K, et al. Ligation of CD40 on dendritic cells triggers production of high levels of interleukin-12 and enhances T cell stimulatory capacity: T-T help via APC activation. *J Exp Med*. 1996;184(2):747–752.
183. Beuneu H, Garcia Z, Bousso P. Cutting edge: cognate CD4 help promotes recruitment of antigen-specific CD8 T cells around dendritic cells. *J Immunol*. 2006;177(3):1406–1410.
184. Castellino F, Huang AY, Altan-Bonnet G, et al. Chemokines enhance immunity by guiding naïve CD8+ T cells to sites of CD4+ T cell-dendritic cell interaction. *Nature*. 2006;440(7086):890–895.
185. Fujii S, Liu K, Smith C, et al. The linkage of innate to adaptive immunity via maturing dendritic cells *in vivo* requires CD40 ligation in addition to antigen presentation and CD80/86 costimulation. *J Exp Med*. 2004;199(12):1607–1618.
186. Fujii S, Shimizu K, Smith C, et al. Activation of natural killer T cells by alpha-galactosylceramide rapidly induces the full maturation of dendritic cells *in vivo* and thereby acts as an adjuvant for combined CD4 and CD8 T cell immunity to a coadministered protein. *J Exp Med*. 2003;198(2):267–279.
187. Stober D, Jomantaite I, Schirmbeck R, et al. NKT cells provide help for dendritic cell-dependent priming of MHC class I-restricted CD8+ T cells *in vivo*. *J Immunol*. 2003;170(5):2540–2548.
188. Sun JC, Williams MA, Bevan MJ. CD4+ T cells are required for the maintenance, not programming, of memory CD8+ T cells after acute infection. *Nat Immunol*. 2004;5(9):927–933.
189. Battegay M, Moskophidis D, Rahemtulla A, et al. Enhanced establishment of a virus carrier state in adult CD4+ T-cell-deficient mice. *J Virol*. 1994;68(7):4700–4704.
190. Belz GT, Wodarz D, Diaz G, et al. Compromised influenza virus-specific CD8(+)-T-cell memory in CD4(+)-T-cell-deficient mice. *J Virol*. 2002;76(23):12388–12393.
191. Cardin RD, Brooks JW, Sarawar SR, et al. Progressive loss of CD8+ T cell-mediated control of a gamma-herpesvirus in the absence of CD4+ T cells. *J Exp Med*. 1996;184(3):863–871.
192. Matloubian M, Concepcion RJ, Ahmed R. CD4+ T cells are required to sustain CD8+ cytotoxic T-cell responses during chronic viral infection. *J Virol*. 1994;68(12):8056–8063.
193. Moskophidis D, Lechner F, Pircher H, et al. Virus persistence in acutely infected immunocompetent mice by exhaustion of antiviral cytotoxic effector T cells. *Nature*. 1993;362(6422): 758–761.
194. von Herrath MG, Yokoyama M, Dockter J, et al. CD4-deficient mice have reduced levels of memory cytotoxic T lymphocytes after immunization and show diminished resistance to subsequent virus challenge. *J Virol*. 1996;70(2):1072–1079.
195. Zajac AJ, Blattman JN, Murali-Krishna K, et al. Viral immune evasion due to persistence of activated T cells without effector function. *J Exp Med*. 1998;188(12):2205–2213.
196. Bourgeois C, Rocha B, Tanchot C. A role for CD40 expression on CD8+ T cells in the generation of CD8+ T cell memory. *Science*. 2002;297(5589):2060–2063.
197. Bourgeois C, Veiga-Fernandes H, Joret AM, et al. CD8 lethargy in the absence of CD4 help. *Eur J Immunol*. 2002;32(8): 2199–2207.
198. Janssen EM, Lemmens EE, Wolfe T, et al. CD4+ T cells are required for secondary expansion and memory in CD8+ T lymphocytes. *Nature*. 2003;421(6925):852–856.
199. Shedlock DJ, Shen H. Requirement for CD4 T cell help in generating functional CD8 T cell memory. *Science*. 2003;300(5617): 337–339.
200. Sun JC, Bevan MJ. Defective CD8 T cell memory following acute infection without CD4 T cell help. *Science*. 2003;300(5617): 339–342.

Chapter 29

Immunologic Tolerance

Ronald H. Schwartz

In 1905, Ehrlich and Morgenroth *(1)* observed that goats injected with red blood cells (RBCs) from another goat always made hemolytic antibodies directed against the immunizing cells, but these antisera never reacted against the recipient's own RBCs. Furthermore, they deliberately immunized a goat with its own RBCs and also observed that no antibody response was elicited. They coined the Latin phrase *horror autotoxicus* to describe this situation. To them, the term meant that the animals avoided self-destructive responses, although it was often interpreted by others to mean a failure to make any immune responses against self-components. In fact, in a footnote in their article *(1)*, they made clear the distinction between autoreactivity and autoimmune disease when they discussed the experiments of Metalinikoff *(2)*, who found that guinea pigs injected with homologous sperm made cytotoxic antibodies against these cells. Because the antibodies did not kill the sperm *in vivo*, they deemed the antibodies not to be autotoxic.

In this chapter I retain the perspective of Ehrlich and Morgenroth. Hence, I define tolerance as a physiologic state in which the immune system does not react destructively against the components of the organism that harbors it or against antigens that are introduced into it.

Destructive responses are prevented by a variety of mechanisms that operate during development of the immune system *and* during the course of each immune response. Pharmacologic manipulations are not included. This broad view allows one to consider immunoregulation as part of the tolerance process. Finally, I will focus on the adaptive immune system only and not discuss the tolerance processes for either natural killer (NK) cells or the innate like NK T (NKT) cells, B-1 cells, and TCR$\gamma\delta$ cells.

TOLERANCE IS AN ADAPTIVE PROCESS

Why did the goats not make antibodies against their own RBCs? The first observations that shed light on this issue were made by Owen (3) on dizygotic bovine twins and Owen et al. *(4)* on quintuplets. They analyzed the surface antigens of RBCs from these cattle using alloantisera of the type raised by Ehrlich and Morgenroth *(1)* in goats, and showed that each offspring possessed all of the antigens found in the parents, even though some of these determinants were not expressed by both parents. In the quintuplets this seemed unlikely to result from codominant heterozygosity as the outbred parents would have had to be homozygous at multiple genetic loci. Instead, Owen and colleagues were able to show in cytotoxicity assays that the offspring were chimeric, that is, their blood contained a mixture of cells with different phenotypes. Based on the earlier work of Lillie *(5)*, who had suggested that dizygotic cattle could exchange products through anastomoses of the blood vessels in their two placentas, Owen and colleagues postulated that hemopoietic stem cells from each sibling migrated to the bone marrow of the other sibs to create a stable chimeric state that persisted after the sibs were separated at birth. Because the chimerism of the antigenically disparate cells was not disturbed by an immune response, Owen and colleagues described this state of peaceful coexistence as one of tolerance. The observations suggested that a foreign substance could be either reacted against or tolerated by an immune system depending on when the antigen was presented to it. The observations also suggested that there was no fundamental distinction between self-molecules (encoded by the host's genome) and foreign molecules (coming from the sibling's hematopoietic cells) in their ability to induce a tolerant state.

Burnet and Fenner *(6)* were strongly influenced by Owen's observations, as well as by those of Traub *(7)*, who demonstrated that a carrier state for the lymphocytic choriomeningitis virus (LCMV) could be induced in mice by natural exposure to this virus *in utero* or during the neonatal period. Their interpretation of both sets of results was that the developing immune system was malleable and that if a foreign substance were introduced early enough, it would induce tolerance rather than immunity. The first experimental data to support this hypothesis were generated by Billingham et al. (8,9). They injected cell suspensions from mixed tissues of mouse strain A into neonatal or fetal mice of strain B and showed that as adults, the strain B mice could accept skin grafts from a strain A mouse, although they would rapidly reject skin grafts from a third-party strain C mouse. The concept derived from this work, that tolerance was an acquired state, was confirmed by Hašek *(10)*, who experimentally reproduced the observations of Owen *(3,4)* by parabiosis of chick embryos. After separation at birth, the adult birds could not make an antibody response against their partner's RBCs (Ehrlich's experiment *(1)*) and could not reject each other's skin grafts (Medawar's experiment *(8,9)*). Burnet subsequently gave a theoretical framework to all of these results in his clonal selection theory, in which he postulated that clones of lymphocytes with receptors on their surface specific for molecules present during the development of the immune system would be selectively eliminated by a deletion process (11). Similar ideas were put forth by Talmage *(12)*.

Consistent with the idea that the immune system learns to be tolerant during its development was the subsequent experiment of Triplett (13). He removed the pituitary anlage from tree frog larvae and let them differentiate under the skin of other larvae. When the tadpoles went through metamorphosis, he gave back to the adult frogs their own pituitaries and found that the animals rejected the autografts. Partial hypophysectomized animals did not reject the grafts, arguing that the rejection was not caused by the acquisition of new antigens, through either abnormal differentiation or carryover of the temporary host's tissues. Thus, even for self-antigens, tolerance appeared to be an acquired state requiring the presence of the antigen to induce it.

The adaptive nature of tolerance is a fundamental property of the vertebrate immune system. Given the task of the system, which is to recognize and respond to unexpected molecules using the random structural diversity generated from rearranging T- and B-cell antigen-receptor genes, there is no way to genetically program it to know what molecules will lead to self-destructive responses. Instead, a series of steps must be undertaken somatically during which the environment is sampled and the system fine-tuned to avoid its own destruction. The nature of these steps in both the mature and developing immune system will be the principal focus of this chapter.

NEGATIVE SELECTION DURING B-CELL DEVELOPMENT

Receptor Editing and Clonal Deletion

Tolerance that occurs in the primary organs in which lymphocytes develop (bone marrow and thymus) is called *central tolerance* and the process for B cells is referred to as *negative selection*. The first direct demonstration of negative selection at the B-cell level was made by Nemazee and Bürki (14). They constructed a transgenic mouse expressing an IgM B-cell receptor (BCR) reactive with major histocompatibility complex (MHC^k) class I molecules. On a neutral MHC^d background, 25% to 50% of splenic B cells ($B220^+$, IgM^+) expressed this receptor and IgM antibodies with this specificity were found at significant levels in the serum. When crossed to an MHC^k mouse, however, both the splenic B cells and the antibody did not emerge. The site of tolerance induction appeared to be the bone marrow because IgM and transgene receptor levels on the cells there were low to undetectable, but $B220^{low}$ expression (indicative of Pro- and Pre-B cell development) was normal (see Chapter 7 for a review of B cell development). This suggested that the tolerance process involved the down-modulation (cross-linking, capping, and internalization) of the BCR following antigen encounter immediately after the receptor was expressed at the cell surface of the immature B cell. This idea was consistent with much earlier studies, which showed that treatment of bone marrow or fetal liver B cells with high concentrations of anti-IgM antibody for 48 hours caused the permanent disappearance of immunoglobulin from the surface of the B cell (15,*16*).

There is now uniform agreement that sufficient engagement of the BCR on immature B cells can lead to a state of maturational arrest (17,18,*19*). BCR transgenic bone marrow cells placed in culture with membrane bound antigen or anti-kappa antibody down-regulate their receptors. If the cells come from double transgenic animals expressing both the BCR and the relevant antigen, the arrested cells persist in culture in the presence of antigen for up to 3 days, but do not make an antibody response (17). Interestingly, the cells can come out of this unresponsive state if the antigen is removed; the cells then differentiate into more mature B cells ($B220^{high}$, IgM^{high} IgD^{low}) and can proliferate and secrete antibody in response to lipopolysaccharide (LPS). Thus, the maturational arrest is a reversible process. More recent studies suggest that if one purifies the immature B cells away from other cell types in the bone marrow, then treatment with anti-BCR leads rapidly to apoptosis *(20)*. The death can be prevented by adding back a special bone marrow cell ($Thy1^{low}$, $DX5^+$), which in bone sections was seen to be interacting with immature B cells in the marrow, presumably facilitating maturational arrest over BCR-induced apoptosis *(21)*.

What is the function of the maturational arrest? Early experiments using BCR transgenics uncovered evidence that the B cells could undergo a qualitative change in their IgM receptors during this period, a process termed *receptor editing* (18,22). BCR transgenic bone marrow cells arrested at the immature B-cell stage increased the level of their recombinant activating gene (RAG) enzymes and underwent further light chain gene rearrangements when stimulated with an anti-kappa chain antibody *(19)*. Secondary rearrangements at the kappa locus can occur by deletion or inversion of the intervening DNA (see Chapter 6). New kappa light chains that emerge (referred to as "editors") allow escape from negative selection (23). Some cells switch to the use of the lambda chain locus when deletion of both kappa constant region genes occurs following recombination to a conserved downstream element referred to as the recombination sequence (see Chapter 6). Immature B cells from normal mice also showed an increased percentage of lambda-bearing cells (without undergoing cell division) following stimulation with an anti-kappa antibody *(19)*. Similar results were observed in hybridomas derived from BCR transgenic mice specific for dsDNA *(24)*. The editing process requires the activity of the *RAG* genes as it is not observed in mice in which at least one of these genes have been disrupted. Thus, the immature B cell can modify its receptor by light chain exchange in order to escape silencing when it encounters self-antigens in the bone marrow.

What happens to the B cell if the light chain replacement fails to shift the cell's specificity sufficiently away from autoreactivity? There is a mechanism for heavy chain editing involving V_H gene and/or D element replacement by recombination with cryptic heptamer sequences embedded in the 3′ end of many (70%) V_H genes *(24,25)*. However, under inescapable conditions, such as stimulating immature B cells with anti-$C\mu$, the maturational arrest is eventually followed by cell death (15,*16*). Early *in vivo* experiments, in which anti-μ antibodies were given *in utero* to chickens or mice, led to the elimination of IgG antibody production by what appeared to be an apoptotic mechanism (26). In the BCR transgenic mice, exposure to the membrane-bound antigens during development also resulted in a depleted peripheral B-cell pool (17,18). Thus, the bone marrow compartment has two mechanisms for dealing with autoreactive cells: one is a receptor selection process that allows cell survival following encounter with self-antigens at an immature stage of development by exchange of light chains and/or V_H replacement; the second is a clonal deletion process by apoptosis, which ensues if the receptor is repeatedly occupied over a sufficient period of time without relief by receptor editing. Note that the latter is not really a simple direct clonal deletion process following receptor stimulation as originally envisioned by Burnet (11). It is instead a programmed bailout mechanism when all else fails, although it can be delayed experimentally by transgenic overexpression of the *Bcl-2* survival gene (17). Normal B-cell development, in contrast, involves a low level of basal (ligand independent) signaling from the assembled, unoccupied BCR. This positively selects the B cell for further maturation *(27)*.

Which of these two processes is the dominant mechanism for B-cell–negative selection? Early on it was thought that receptor editing was a rare rescue event, because membrane-antigen and BCR double-transgenic mice showed mostly a loss of BCR^+ cells in the peripheral spleen and lymph nodes. However, this outcome is mainly a consequence of integration of the transgene outside the immunoglobulin locus. In this case, secondary light chain rearrangements and V_H replacement cannot alter the original transgene. This allows for the continued expression of an autoreactive receptor, unless a breakdown in allelic exclusion leads to the production of a second heavy and/or light chain, which decreases the density of the autoreactive receptor on the cell membrane or physically interferes with the transgene protein expression (e.g., by preferential chain pairing). In contrast, when the transgenic technology advanced to the point of allowing the construction of knockin mice, wherein the rearranged BCR transgene could be inserted directly into the immunoglobulin locus (referred to as *site-directed transgenics*), then the results were completely the opposite *(24,28,29,*30). With this new model, receptor editing could now rescue 85% to 98% of the B cells in as little as a 2- to 6-hour period *(29,*31). Multiple rearrangements were often required, and if this was impaired, for example, by eliminating downstream J-kappa segments, then a component of deletion was also observed (23,31). The same conclusion was reached for normal B cells, in a transgenic mouse that produced a membrane-bound, single-chain antibody reactive against the kappa constant region *(28)*. Here, the numbers of $B220^+$ cells in the spleen were reduced by 40% and the 60% of edited cells expressed exclusively lambda light chains (at three- to fourfold increased number compared with controls). In other studies, the total extent of receptor editing in the mouse B-cell repertoire was estimated to be around 25% of the repertoire *(32)*. This is in line with estimates of more than 50% for the prevalence of self-reactive antibodies in the germ line repertoire *(33)*. Thus, the current consensus in the field is that receptor editing is the major central tolerance mechanism during B-cell development and that clonal deletion is only undertaken as a last resort after several days of trying to replace the receptor.

In the process of receptor editing, the up-regulation of the *RAG* genes that follows BCR engagement also allows for a primary rearrangement to occur at the light chain locus on the other chromosome. This process is known as *allelic inclusion* and produces B cells with two receptors, one of which is still autoreactive. It had been predicted on theoretical grounds that such cells would be deleted by signaling through the autoreactive receptor *(34)*. However, in one well-studied BCR transgenic case, it was discovered that a large fraction of the escape variants of this type were not deleted, but rather survived by chronically down-regulating the autoreactive receptor and degrading it in lysosomes *(35)*. These receptors could be re-expressed on the cell surface if the cell was removed from the antigen in its extracellular environment. The cells also could be signaled *in vitro* through their other receptor using anti-BCR antibodies, and in the mouse, after many months, autoantibodies secreted by these cells could be detected in the serum. Estimates on the percentage of such double cells in the normal mouse B cell population are as high as 10% *(32,36,37)*; but how many of them can go on to produce autoantibodies is currently unknown.

Signaling Aspects of B-Cell Negative Selection

Insights into what characteristics of self-reactive B cells and their autoantigens determine whether they will be negatively selected have been inferred from the early studies on B-cell tolerance induction to foreign antigens (38). With an *in vivo* limiting dilution splenic focus assay, it was demonstrated that if immunoglobulin-negative bone marrow cells were exposed for 24 hours to a hapten in the absence of T-cell help, they became unresponsive to subsequent stimulation by the hapten in the presence of T-cell help. In order to induce tolerance in this system, the antigen had to be multivalent. DNP_4-ovalbumin was tolerogenic for DNP-specific B cells, but DNP_1-papain was not. This observation suggests that signaling through the immunoglobulin receptor requires cross-linking in order to induce tolerance. In the BCR transgenic experiments of Nemazee and colleagues used to directly study B-cell central tolerance, the MHC^k class I antigen made an excellent tolerogen, presumably because it is a transmembrane glycoprotein and therefore displayed on cell surfaces in the bone marrow in a multimeric array *(39)*. In contrast, when the BCR transgenic mouse was crossed to a mouse strain expressing a soluble form of the $MHCK^k$ molecule, no deletion of the B cells was observed (40). A similar difference in outcome was noted in the hen egg lysozyme (HEL) transgenic model depending on whether the antigen was expressed as a membrane bound (maturational arrest and deletion) or a soluble form (nondeletional, peripheral tolerance) (17). The latter can become deletional, however, if the BCR transgenic is made deficient in signaling molecules, such as CD22, Lyn, or SHP-1, that normally negatively regulate B-cell activation *(41–43)*. In these cases the enhanced strength of signaling converts a low-avidity BCR occupancy event into a high-avidity outcome. In a third BCR transgenic, B cells specific for a RBC surface antigen were eliminated from the conventional (B-2) splenic follicular pool (although the receptor was expressed in B-1 cells in the peritoneal cavity) *(44)*. Interestingly, when the cytoplasmic domain of the membrane bound HEL molecule was altered to retain it in the endoplasmic reticulum, it no longer induced deletion of HEL-specific B cells *(45)*. Instead, the cells differentiated into B-1 cells capable of secreting IgM autoantibody.

Also consistent with the idea that surface-displayed antigens are good tolerogens while intracellular molecules are not, is the general finding that many of the natural autoreactive antibodies are specific for intracellular molecules (46,*47,48*); only a few have been identified that react with cell surface proteins *(49,50)*, and these also arise (as in the anti-RBC and anti-HEL transgenics) from the B-1 subset of B cells, which may have different signaling properties. Finally, immature B cells with receptors specific for ds-DNA are heavily negatively selected against in both normal mice *(51–53)* and BCR transgenics *(54–56)*. The structural reason for this is not fully clear, but may result from the stability of oligonucleosomes released from dying cells *(57)*, which could allow for multimeric display of the antigen.

The affinity of the BCR for antigen is another important variable. In the anti-MHC^k BCR transgenics, the receptor cross-reacts with several different MHC alleles, allowing an analysis of the tolerance process in the same model under different affinity conditions. The MHC K^{bm3} allele has a binding constant of only 2×10^4 M^{-1} and yet the phenotype of the negative selection was the same as that for other allelic MHC proteins with 10- or 100-fold higher affinity; this was observed with both conventional and site-directed BCR transgenics (31,*39*). This suggests a high degree of sensitivity for the immature BCR. Indeed, when compared with mature B cells in their ability to mobilize intracellular calcium using a K^k mimetic peptide, the immature B cells were found to respond at lower antigen concentrations, even though they had less surface IgM (58). This increased sensitivity was associated with enhanced tyrosine phosphorylation of Igα and Lyn and increased levels of the signaling intermediates SLP-65, Btk, and PLCγ2 (see Chapter 8). The activity of PLCγ2 was also prolonged, resulting in enhanced calcium mobilization, even though the size of the intracellular store of calcium was smaller. One suggested mechanism for this increased sensitivity has been a diminished content of free cholesterol in the plasma membrane resulting in predominant BCR signaling from outside of lipid rafts *(59,60)*.

In addition to an increase in sensitivity, the immature B cell also has a different program of response to BCR stimulation than the mature B cell. Although it will up-regulate transcription of the *RAG* genes at low receptor occupancy, the immature B cell fails to up-regulate CD69, CD86 (B7-2), or MHC class II molecules, even when stimulated with high concentrations of antigen *(61)*. In contrast, at high antigen concentrations, mature naive B cells up-regulate CD69, CD86, and MHC class II molecules, but not the *RAG* genes. Mature cells also enter the cell cycle and proliferate, whereas immature cells make cyclin D2, activate CDK4, and enter the G1 phase of the cell cycle, but do not go on to make cyclin E, activate CDK2, or enter S phase *(62)*. Instead, the cells undergo growth arrest or apoptosis, depending on their immediate environment (as discussed earlier). This difference from mature B cells may be mediated by the level of c-myc expression, which is only transiently up-regulated in immature B cells, but shows sustained elevation in mature B cells *(59)*. This is again related to the levels of cholesterol in the plasma membrane and can be reversed in immature B cells by the introduction of exogenous cholesterol into their membranes. Finally, mobilization to the nucleus of the transcription factor NFκB is thought to play a key role in the signaling of mature B cells to proliferate *(63)* as well as in the reactivation of receptor editing in immature B cells *(64)*. A contribution from the costimulatory receptor BAFF-R3 augments NFκB p52 levels in mature cells and facilitates cell survival by up-regulating the antiapoptotic kinase Pim2 (*65*,66). Differences in the activation of particular NFκB family members may contribute to unique phenotypic outcomes.

The increased signaling sensitivity of immature B cells, which can range more than 10,000-fold, is thought to provide a margin of safety in assuring that central tolerance eliminates as many potentially autoreactive B-cell clones as possible from the mature peripheral repertoire. In addition, by raising the threshold for activation during maturation of the remaining B cells, the chance of their being activated in the periphery by self-antigens should remain quite low. It is important to keep in mind, however, that even with this purging process, there will be B cells with receptors that can recognize self-antigens with low affinity *(67)*, which may become activated to secrete antibody if provided with adequate T-cell help and a sufficient quantity of antigen (68,*69–71*). These types of observations in the past led investigators to question whether central tolerance occurred at all in the B-cell repertoire. But careful studies of affinity measurements in such systems have generally shown that clones with high-affinity receptors for the antigen have been purged, leaving mostly clones that produce only low-affinity antibodies (72). Nonetheless, such clones, once activated, may undergo somatic hypermutation and potentially generate autoantibodies of higher affinity (73).

NEGATIVE SELECTION DURING T-CELL DEVELOPMENT

Clonal Deletion

The first demonstration of negative selection as a central tolerance mechanism operating during T-cell development was made by Kappler et al. (74). They used a monoclonal antibody against the variable region of a T-cell receptor (TCR) beta chain (anti-Vβ17a) to follow the fate of T cells expressing this receptor. In mice that did not express an I-E molecule encoded by MHC class II genes, Vβ17a-bearing cells in the T-cell population were present at a frequency of 10%. In contrast, mice expressing I-E molecules did not possess Vβ17a$^+$ cells in the spleen. When I-E$^+$ and I-E$^-$ strains were crossed, the F_1 offspring contained no Vβ17a$^+$ cells in the periphery. A dominant elimination process was then shown to take place in the thymus.

Cells expressing Vβ17a were found in only slightly reduced numbers in the immature CD4$^+$8$^+$ TCR-low population, but these cells were greatly depleted in the more mature, single positive (CD4$^+$8$^-$ and CD4$^-$8$^+$) thymocyte subset. The possibility that the cells had simply down-regulated their receptors was subsequently ruled out by showing that Vβ17a mRNA was also absent in mature T-cell populations (P. Marrack and J. Kappler, unpublished data). Similar observations were made by others for Vβ6$^+$ T cells *(75)*. In this model the deletion process was exactly pinpointed to the late double-positive stage when TCR expression becomes elevated and CD4 and CD8 coreceptors have begun to down-modulate *(76,77)*. Physical evidence that the process is in fact clonal deletion by an apoptotic mechanism was subsequently published (*78*,79).

The antigens involved in these Vβ-specific deletion processes are endogenous superantigens encoded by open reading frames (ORF) in the 3′ Long Terminal Repeats of mouse mammary tumor viruses (Mtvs) *(80)*. These proteins are capable of activating the T cell by interacting with both the Vβ and the I-E molecule at the same time. However, this activation mechanism is slightly different from that of peptide/MHC stimulation as it bypasses the need for the Src-family kinase, Lck *(81)*. Hence, it was important that Kisielow et al. (82) were able to extend the observations on clonal deletion to a more conventional antigen system, the male-specific antigen H-Y. They took advantage of the first alpha/beta T-cell receptor (TCR$\alpha\beta^+$) transgenic mouse—developed by Blüthmann et al. *(83)*—to follow the fate of a large cohort of T cells expressing the same anti-H-Y receptor, either in females, which do not express the antigen (controls), or in males, that do. The male mice had a thymus of greatly reduced size (less than 10% of normal) and a tremendous reduction in the percentage of double-positive thymocytes. Similar observations were made by others with TCR transgenic mice specific for an alloantigen (L^d) *(84)*. These mice deleted T cells bearing the receptor at the early double-positive (DP) stage when they were crossed to mice expressing the alloantigen. Thus, the basic model postulated by Burnet appears to be correct for the standard CD4$^+$ and CD8$^+$ TCR$\alpha\beta^+$ cells, that is, immature T cells encountering their antigen during development are clonally deleted instead of activated to make an immune response (11). This process is referred to as *negative selection*. An exception to this process involving the selection of regulatory T cells will be discussed later.

Stages of T-Cell Development at which Negative Selection Occurs

The experiments involving tolerance to the H-Y and L^d antigens suggested that clonal deletion takes place at the early DP stage, whereas the experiments involving tolerance to superantigens suggested that clonal deletion takes place at the transition from the DP to the SP stage. This dichotomy has been observed in a single transgenic mouse that carried a receptor specific for both a viral antigen and an Mtv-7 encoded superantigen (85). The T cells were deleted at the early DP stage if the mice were carriers of the virus, but deleted closer to the SP stage when the mice did not harbor virus, and instead were mated to animals expressing the Mtv-7 superantigen. Thus, it seemed likely that the nature of the recognition event—where and how the antigen and the receptor were expressed at the time of antigen presentation—would determine the stage at which the cells were deleted.

In the case of superantigens, the major cell type found to express these proteins is the B cell *(86)*. In the adult mouse thymus, these cells are mainly CD5$^+$ B1 cells located in the medulla, near the corticomedullary junction *(87,88)*. Interestingly, these B1 cells are not present in neonatal thymus, and Vβ6$^+$ T cells are not deleted by the Mtv-7 superantigen in the neonate *(88,89)*. In the case of the Mtv-6 superantigen, however, expression takes place in thymic dendritic cells (90) and deletion is completed earlier *(91)*. Vβ3$^+$ T cells are deleted in fetal thymic organ cultures (FTOCs), but not in reaggregated cultures that lack the dendritic cells. When compared with Mtv-1, which encodes an identical protein expressed in B cells, Mtv-6 mRNA expression is eightfold higher. This results in 50% deletion of DP thymocytes as well as all of the SP thymocytes, compared with one-half that effect in both compartments for Mtv-1. Thus, the amount and location of superantigen expression can determine the extent of clonal deletion that is observed.

In the case of the TCR transgenics, it now seems clear that the receptors are prematurely expressed at high levels at the double-negative (DN) stage of T-cell development when the TCR beta genes normally become active (DN2–DN3) *(92)*. If the antigen is sufficiently present in the environment at this time, then the TCR signaling induces a maturational arrest at the CD4$^-$,CD8$^-$ (DN) or CD4$^-$,CD8^{low} pre-T-cell stage, depending on the strength of signal and the exact timing of receptor expression (92,93,94). In the case of the H-Y transgenic mouse, this must be at the CD4$^-$,CD8^{low} stage because CD8 interaction with the MHC class I molecule is required for deletion *(95)*. Some of the cells, however, do manage to survive, either by differentiating toward other lineages ($\gamma\delta$ T cells or CD8$\alpha\alpha$-intraepithelial lymphocytes) or by rearranging their endogenous alpha chain genes, which in some instances can interfere with signaling through the transgenic receptor by preferential chain pairing or by decreasing the cell surface density of the transgenic receptor *(96,97)*. As a consequence, the periphery is usually populated with these surviving, dual receptor T cells and T cells of other lineages. Under normal circumstances, of course, the T cells would not express their full surface $\alpha\beta$ receptor until the DP stage, after the alpha chain gene rearrangement has been completed. When the H-Y-specific TCR was engineered to separately express the alpha chain gene under the control of a modified CD4 promotor, it emerged correctly at the DP stage and deletion in the male mice occurred later (98). In this case there was only a 50% decrease in the number of DP cells, while most of the SP cells were deleted.

But why did all the DP thymocytes not delete as soon as they expressed the H-Y–specific receptor? In contrast to the superantigens, whose expression is mostly restricted to the medulla, the H-Y antigens are ubiquitously expressed and in the thymic cortex could clearly produce substantial thymocyte deletion in the original TCR transgenic at the DN to DP transition. Indeed, a variety of experiments have demonstrated that if the antigen is introduced into the cortical environment at high concentrations, then all the DP thymocytes quickly die by apoptosis. This was first demonstrated by adding soluble superantigens or anti-CD3 antibody to FTOCs and observing apoptosis of DP cells in 18 hours *(78,99)*. This was subsequently confirmed in TCR transgenic mice by administration of soluble peptide *(100–104)*. The *in vitro* culture experiments were critical because *in vivo* administration of peptides can lead to peripheral activation of mature T cells and release of cytokines such as tumor necrosis factor (TNF), which kill DP thymocytes independent of negative selection *(105,106)*. Yet even some FTOC gave outcomes different from *in vivo* results. Isolated cortical epithelial cells from mice expressing the circulating complement protein C5 were able to present this antigen in reaggregation FTOC as efficiently as isolated thymic dendritic cells for the deletion of TCR transgenic DP thymocytes, suggesting an adequate amount of antigen loading and effectiveness (107). However, *in vivo*, the deletion of the TCR$^+$ cells did not occur until the DP to SP transition *(97)*. Thus, physiological levels of the processed C5 antigen on cortical epithelial cells were not adequate to induce clonal deletion of thymocytes *in vivo* at an early DP stage. However, this particular transgenic TCR may not delete early because it is expressed under the control of an hCD2 locus control region, which yields lower than normal TCR expression levels.

Recently it has been possible to examine clonal deletion in the thymus of normal B6 mice by two different methods. The first used a monoclonal antibody against a CD3ε conformational determinant that becomes exposed when the TCR receives a strong antigenic signal (108). By immunohistochemistry, this marker was greatly elevated in TCR transgenic mice undergoing negative selection and was associated with a marker of apoptosis occurring in the same cells. When this technique was applied to tissue sections of normal B6 thymus, only a small number of cells were positive, and these were mostly DP thymocytes located in the cortex and corticomedullary junction. The second approach looked at thymocytes that have up-regulated expression of the orphan steroid nuclear receptor Nur77 (109). This molecule is expressed within 1 hour after TCR stimulation, leading to cell death, and it is elevated in a small subset of thymocytes in both alloantigen-induced and superantigen-induced clonal deletion. In B6 mice, the 0.5% Nur77$^+$ cells were found in both the DP and CD4 SP subpopulations. All these cells expressed high levels of CD69 and the DP cells were TCR^{int} and low for both CD4 and CD8, suggesting that they had just been positively selected. The CD4 SP cells were TCR^{high} and CD24(HSA)^{high}, implying that they were semimature T cells normally found in the medulla (see later discussion). Thus, with this technique, normal negative selection appears to mainly occur at the late DP to SP transition.

Receptor Editing?

Why are the immature DP thymocytes not usually deleted *in vivo*? One possibility is that, similar to immature B cells (see previous discussion), the T cells undergo a receptor editing process instead. There are two intriguing experiments in the literature that suggest that this might be possible. A standard TCR transgenic mouse expressing its receptor under the control of an IgH enhancer assembled its receptor during the DN stage and deleted most of the TCR$^+$ cells as they matured to the DP stage, when the mice were crossed to another transgenic mouse expressing the antigen *(110)*. In contrast, if the rearranged Vα-Jα gene was knocked into the TCRα locus and then crossed to a separate TCRβ chain-only transgenic mouse to reconstitute the original receptor, the DP thymocytes in this hybrid mouse were *not* deleted when crossed to the antigen transgenic. Instead, most of the knocked in TCRα chains disappeared and seemed to be replaced by other alpha chains. That this might be a receptor editing process was suggested by experiments with another TCR transgenic mouse, which, when its DP thymocytes were exposed to antigen in the cortex, up-regulated expression of the *RAG* genes, enhanced gene rearrangement at the TCRα locus, and increased expression of receptors bearing endogenous TCRα chains *(111)*. In neither set of experiments, however, was it proven that the loss of transgene expression was the direct result of receptor driven rearrangement of the knock-in allele.

In contrast to this work, a second major attempt to examine TCR editing by knocking in a rearranged anti–H-Y Vα-Jα gene and expressing it on both chromosomes failed to produce any evidence for receptor editing *(112)*. All that was observed was clonal deletion. Although these mice might not have shown editing because the transgenic receptor was expressed too early (at the DN stage), the conclusion of "no editing" was subsequently substantiated by studies with a β chain-only transgenic mouse in which pairing with the normal Vα repertoire generated a variety of anti-H-Y-specific T cells at the DP stage (113). Examination of the effect of the presence of the male antigen on a particular subset of anti–H-Y-specific receptors demonstrated no molecular evidence for receptor editing in the form of excess T-cell excision circles bearing the rearranged Vα-Jα gene. In fact, what was observed was a decrease in the ratio of male-reactive T-cell excision circles, relative to out-of-frame sequences, in males compared with females. This result is more consistent with clonal deletion. Thus, in contrast to B cells, T cells mainly use clonal deletion as their mechanism for negative selection. The purpose of early receptor revision in T cells appears instead to be reserved for optimizing positive selection, in which the task is to generate as many receptors as possible that are capable of recognizing self MHC molecules *(114–116)*.

Antigen-presenting Cells for Negative Selection

If DP thymocytes do not undergo receptor editing in response to antigens presented by thymic epithelial cells, why do they not undergo clonal deletion more frequently? The dominant idea in the literature throughout the years has been that cortical epithelial cells are not very effective at presenting antigens for negative selection, either because they do not access and process the antigen adequately or because they are incapable of providing appropriate costimulatory signals. The earliest experiments giving rise to this concept involved various types of thymic and bone marrow MHC chimeras *(117)*. When (MHC-A × MHC-B)F_1 bone marrow cells were transferred into lethally irradiated strain B recipients, tolerance resulted for both strain A and strain B peptide MHC complexes as measured in a mixed leukocyte response (MLR) or a cytotoxic T lymphocyte (CTL) response (118). In superantigen models, this process involved deletion of thymocytes at the DP-to-SP transition stage, suggesting a role for hematopoietic cells, such as thymic dendritic and B cells, which repopulate an irradiated thymus quickly from bone marrow precursors *(119,120)*. In a more direct experiment (121), it was shown that allogeneic dendritic cells from the spleen introduced into a FTOC could induce tolerance to the alloantigens as measured in a CTL assay. Thus, a professional antigen-presenting cell (APC) capable of activating T cells in the periphery, tolerized thymocytes, again consistent with Burnet's original clonal deletion model (11). Other experiments with thymocyte suspensions from TCR transgenic mice showed directly that splenic APCs could induce deletion of $CD4^+CD8^+$ T cells *in vitro (122)*.

In contrast, the role of thymic stromal (nonhematopoietic) cells in negative selection has always been more controversial. Initial experiments with parental MHC-B bone marrow into (A × B)F_1 irradiated hosts revealed tolerance to strain B MHC molecules, but alloreactivity against strain A APC *(123)*. Similarly, deoxyguanosine-treated fetal thymuses (depleted of hematopoietic cells) when grafted into allogeneic nude mice, produced T cells that reacted in MLR *(124)* and CTL response *(125)* against the alloantigens of the thymus donor (126). The initial conclusion from these types of experiments was that thymic stromal cells could not induce negative selection at all. A careful examination of the data, however, reveals that some negative effects do take place. For example, alloreactivity in the MLRs was often quantitatively diminished and the nude mice did not reject their thymus grafts *(127)*. How then does one account for the failure to completely induce tolerance by thymic stromal cell antigen presentation? One possibility is that the tolerance induced is tissue-specific (128). Although alloantigens have the virtue of directly presenting their peptides without cell transfer, they can only tolerize for the subset of bound peptides that are expressed in the stromal cells. Hence, MLR and CTL assays, in which splenic dendritic cells do the presenting, will still be capable of stimulating T cells specific for hematopoietic cell-derived peptides not expressed by the thymic stromal cells. When a second whole thymus graft is given, only the hematopoietic cells, not the stromal cells, are rejected (128). For example, when the MHC class II gene I-A^b_β was targeted using a keratin-14 (K14) promoter for transgenic expression in the thymic cortical epithelium of MHC class II-deficient (I-$A_\beta^{b-/-}$) mice, the $CD4^+$ T cells from these animals were strongly responsive to "self" splenic dendritic cells in an MLR *(129)*. However, when given syngeneic thymus grafts, they accepted them because they were tolerant to peptide/MHC complexes expressed on the epithelial cells *(130)*. The MLR was due to dendritic cell peptide/MHC complexes that were not expressed on the thymic epithelium. The fate of other tissue grafts in this type of experiment depends on how much peptide overlap there is between the thymus and the grafts (128). Similar observations were made for $CD8^+$ T cells tolerized to MHC class I molecules that were targeted for expression in thymic cortical epithelial cells of a $\beta 2$-microglobulin ($\beta 2$m) knockout mouse with the K14 promoter driving expression of $\beta 2$m *(131)*.

The second possibility to explain the presence of alloreactivity in parent into F_1 chimeras is that only T cells with high-avidity receptors are deleted, leaving low-avidity clones to respond to strong dendritic cell presentation *(127)*. This explanation has the virtue of being able to explain the absence of clonal deletion in chimera experiments involving viral superantigens. For the most part, these molecules stimulate regardless of what peptides are bound to the MHC class II molecule. Although in some cases the failure to delete *in vivo* may be the result of the inaccessibility of the superantigens to the MHC molecules on thymic cortical epithelium, an *in vitro* experiment with deoxyguanosine-treated FTOC reconstituted with fresh T cells plus or minus dendritic cells, showed that an exogenous superantigen could only rapidly induce clonal deletion in the presence of dendritic cells, even though the superantigen was shown to bind to the MHC class II molecules on the epithelial cells *(132)*. Cultures lacking dendritic cells, however, did demonstrate deletion on prolonged exposure to superantigen, suggesting that the stromal cells are just inefficient at antigen presentation. For $CD8^+$ T cells, targeting of an MHC class I molecule to the thymic medullary epithelium with either a keratin IV promoter or an aberrantly expressed $E\mu$ promoter resulted in tolerance that was "spilt"; that is, the animals accepted skin grafts but manifested a CTL response *in vitro* in the presence of interleukin 2 (IL-2) *(133,134)*. Crossing this mouse to a $CD8^+$ TCR transgenic mouse specific for the MHC class I molecule deleted only T cells expressing high densities of the TCR, and not those with lower densities (135). The latter exist because of endogenous TCRα chain expression and are probably of lower avidity and thus less readily activated.

In contrast to experiments involving alloantigens, negative selection experiments using peptides from non-MHC antigens were more straightforward to interpret. Chimera experiments with TCR transgenic animals revealed strong evidence for thymic stromal cell-mediated deletion. For example, transfer of TCR-transgenic bone marrow cells from a mouse expressing a nondeleting MHC allele, into a virus-infected irradiated host expressing on its stromal cells the MHC molecule capable of viral peptide-specific presentation and deletion, led to massive elimination of the cells in the thymus at the early DP stage (either because of premature TCR expression or high levels of antigen expression) (94). In experiments with the H-Y antigen, the early deletion was less dramatic if the bone marrow-derived cells expressed an allo-MHC molecule that could not present the peptide (136). In this case, thymocyte yields in the male were 25% of what was observed in the female, showing that partial deletion was occurring from stromal cell antigen presentation. However, the surviving DP cells all had high TCR expression and many made it to the $CD8^+$ SP stage, suggesting that a significant fraction were not being deleted by the cortical epithelial cells. Similar results were observed in experiments using deoxyguanosine-treated, male thymic epithelial cell grafts into thymectomized females (136). In still other experiments, clonal deletion of the DP thymocytes was observed when the H-Y peptide was expressed as a transgene under the control of the K14 promoter, which limited expression to cortical thymic epithelial cells (93).

A particularly interesting result was obtained when a human papilloma virus protein (E7) was targeted to the cortical thymic epithelium with the K14 promoter *(137)*. This expression resulted in a reduction, following antigen priming, of the antiviral CTL response, but an enhanced T-cell proliferative response and normal B-cell help. This "split" result suggests that presentation by cortical epithelial cells of a particular peptide/MHC class I molecule can be more effective for tolerance induction than that of a particular peptide/MHC class II molecule derived from the same antigen. In another set of experiments with $CD4^+$ T cells, a transgenic TCR specific for pigeon cytochrome c deleted only SP T cells when crossed to a transgenic mouse expressing limited amounts of that antigen, but deleted at the DP stage when crossed to a second transgenic mouse that expressed three-to tenfold more antigen (138). Both antigen-transgenic mice expressed cytochrome mRNA in the cortex and medulla, but only the high antigen expressor induced observable apoptosis of thymocytes in the cortex. Interestingly, a second cytochrome c-specific TCR transgenic mouse expressing a receptor of lower affinity for the antigen, deleted only at the SP stage, even when crossed to the high antigen-expressing mouse. In contrast, cells with this same receptor were completely deleted at the DP stage when crossed to a strain very highly expressing an inducible form of the peptide embedded in an invariant chain transgene (108,*139*). Thus, the level of antigen expression and the affinity of the receptor for antigen determined whether deletion took place in the cortex at the DP stage of development.

What then are the differences that sometimes allow the same T cell to be deleted by thymic dendritic cells at the corticomedullary junction and not by epithelial cells in the cortex? One key factor on the T-cell side is that positive selection leads to a tenfold increase in TCR expression *(140,141)*. This allows TCR occupancy to be enhanced and could allow previously suboptimal signals to become adequate for negative selection. The second factor, on the APC side, is that thymic dendritic cells are in general more potent APCs. The ability of the two cell types to present antigens has been directly tested *in vitro*. Cortical epithelial cells were clearly inferior to thymic dendritic cells when asked to stimulate mature T cells to express CD69 or proliferate (107,*142*). Some of this inferiority may relate to a lack of expression of costimulatory molecules (such as B7), which have been shown in a number of different models to be required for clonal deletion in the thymus (*143–145*,146,*147*,148). Nonetheless, when tested in a direct assay for clonal deletion of thymocytes, cortical epithelial cells were found to be as potent as dendritic cells (107), perhaps because very few peptide/MHC complexes are required for clonal deletion *in vitro (149)*. *In vivo*, however, their weaker presentation capacity under nonsaturating conditions may normally hinder adequate stimulation of DP thymocytes for clonal deletion. Overall, the published results suggest that, although thymic epithelial cells are less efficient at antigen presentation, they can effectively induce DP T-cell clonal deletion in certain cases, depending on the affinity of the particular TCR, the density of the peptide/MHC complexes that are present, and the amount of costimulation available.

If one accepts that bone marrow-derived dendritic cells are the primary mediators of clonal deletion in the thymus, then it is possible to obtain a minimal estimate for the extent of clonal deletion that occurs during normal T-cell development by examining radiation chimeras in which the bone marrow is derived from MHC class II-deficient or MHC class I and II double-deficient mice. If the irradiated host is normal for MHC expression, then positive selection will be unaffected. In contrast, negative selection by thymic dendritic cells would be completely eliminated. When this experiment was performed (150), the percentage of single-positive $CD4^+$ T cells in the chimeric thymus increased 1.7-fold over control chimeras, suggesting that about 40% of the positively selected cells normally undergo clonal deletion induced by bone marrow-derived cells. This result is consistent with studies on positive selection of $CD4^+$ T cells in the presence of a single peptide/MHC ligand wherein 65% of the repertoire sampled (by generating T-cell hybridomas) was autoreactive against the same MHC molecule plus other peptides (151). An experiment in which both approaches were combined, confirmed a steady-state 1.7-fold increase in $CD4^+$ T cells when bone marrow-derived dendritic cells expressed only a single peptide/MHC ligand, and conversely a deletion of two thirds of the repertoire positively selected on the single peptide/MHC ligand when the bone marrow-derived dendritic cells expressed a normal complement of multiple peptide complexes with the same MHC molecule *(152)*. Thus, at least 40% to 70% of selected thymocytes undergo negative selection.

Clonal Deletion in the Thymic Medulla

Evidence that clonal deletion can still occur even after thymocytes have reached the single-positive stage in the medulla is very compelling. For T cells reactive with endogenous superantigens, the tolerance process often begins only after birth. Mtv-7 reactive $CD4^+CD8^-$ $V\beta6^+$ thymocytes disappear during the first week of life, when B1 cells expressing the viral ORF arrive in the thymic medulla *(89,153)*. *In vitro* culture of these $V\beta6^+$ cells demonstrated that the disappearance was not just a migration out of the thymus, but an active death process that could be inhibited by low temperature, cycloheximide, or actinomycin D. *In vivo* experiments have suggested that it is the earliest $CD24^{high}$ $CD4^+8^-$ cells that are being deleted (154). The mechanism includes costimulation, with both CD40L/CD40 and often CD28/B7 interactions being required for maximum effect (*145*,148). Involvement of other molecules such as ICAM, CD5, and CD43 has also been suggested (146,*147*). Thus, again, full activation leads to negative selection, indicating that even semimature thymocytes are tolerizable only.

These cells are also susceptible to glucocorticoid-induced cell death and are functionally immature like DP thymocytes *(155–157)*. Thus, this thymocyte subpopulation appears to be in transition from an immature to a mature T-cell stage. This is quite similar to the transitional stage in B-cell development, which occurs after the immature B cells migrate from the adult bone marrow to the spleen. In that stage, they are still highly susceptible to BCR-induced cell death (see later discussion). The thymic medulla can in some sense be regarded as a peripheral lymphoid organ, like the spleen, as it is readily accessible to circulating antigens and to recirculating activated lymphocytes such as the B1 cells and effector T cells *(88,158–160)*. Thus, in both lineages, these semimature cells are still preferentially susceptible to cell death following strong receptor stimulation. Other mechanisms of tolerance can also be induced at this stage and will be discussed in the sections on peripheral tolerance mechanisms. The importance of the medullary tolerance process has recently been shown in CCR7 and CCR7 L gene-targeted mice (161). Cortical cells in these mice leave the thymus after the DP-to-SP transition, instead of moving into the medulla under CCR7 chemokine direction. As a consequence, the mice are not fully tolerant, and develop autoimmune disease of the salivary and lacrimal glands. Presumably some of the T cells reactive against the autoantigens in these tissues are normally inactivated in the thymic medulla.

Signaling Aspects of T-Cell–Negative Selection

Burnet (11), Talmage *(162)*, and Lederberg *(163)* postulated early on that negative selection occurs by signaling through the antigen-specific receptor followed by cell death. Although histologic examination of the thymus does not reveal much evidence for ongoing cell death, kinetic labeling studies have demonstrated that about 95% of the cells generated in the thymus die there *(164)*. Experiments using a more sensitive TUNEL assay to detect DNA strand breaks showed that macrophages contain the debris of thymocytes that have died by apoptosis (79). In a TCR $V\beta5$ transgenic mouse expressing MHC class II I-E molecules and an endogenous $V\beta5$-reactive Mtv-9 ORF-superantigen, the medulla of the thymus was found to contain aggregates of apoptotic cells that were engulfed by $MAC3^+$ macrophages. This first visualization of apoptosis established that the final death process induced by superantigens was taking place in the thymic medulla. Others have since used this technique to visualize apoptosis in the cortex with TCR transgenic models (108,138).

Although a consensus now exists that thymocytes die by apoptosis during negative selection, the molecular pathways leading to this programmed cell death are not fully understood *(165)*. Negative selection is a process elicited by TCR stimulation and needs to be distinguished from the death by neglect that occurs at the DP stage, when thymocytes fail to have their TCR engaged for positive selection. A strong receptor occupancy signal leads to a conformational change in the cytoplasmic domain of the $CD3\varepsilon$ chain of the TCR, which is thought to reflect the initiation of signal transduction (108). An exposed proline-rich sequence then binds the SH3 domain of the Nck adaptor protein, which recruits the serine/threonine kinase MINK to activate the negative selection pathway *(166)*.

MINK-deficient mice display enhanced production of TCR^{high} DP and CD4 SP thymocytes, including $V\beta5^+$ T cells that are normally deleted by the Mtv-9 superantigen. MINK deficiency also completely prevents clonal deletion of DP thymocytes in the H-Y male transgenic model. MINK expression is greatly up-regulated at the DP stage of thymocyte development and then declines back down at the SP stage, suggesting that it might be a critical component of the signaling machinery that makes thymocytes tolerizable only.

In addition to MINK activation, the more conventional tyrosine kinase activation pathway is also critical for negative selection. A point mutation in the SH2 domain of Zap-70, which interferes with TCRζ binding and Zap-70 phosphorylation following anti-CD3 cross-linking, leads to impaired positive and negative selection in TCR transgenic models. Interestingly, these mice develop an autoimmune arthritis *(167)*. To achieve negative selection, Zap-70 must adequately phosphorylate LAT, which then recruits Grb2 and PLCγ1 to the plasma membrane. The adaptor protein Grb2 is involved in activation of Ras at the plasma membrane via the guanine nucleotide exchange factor mSOS. The lipase PLCγ1 generates diacylglycerol and inositol-tris-phosphate/calcium release and facilitates N-Ras activation via activation and recruitment of RasGRP1 to the plasma membrane or Golgi *(168,169)*. Ras activation at the plasma membrane is the critical event. This is followed by activation of the mitogen-activated protein (MAP) kinase family of enzymes *(170)*. All experiments support a role for sustained Jun N-terminal kinase (JNK) activity (171), and the Grb2-SOS pathway of Ras activation plays a key role in this process *(168)*. The p38 pathway is also activated via Zap-70 phosphorylation *(172)*. Data for involvement of the extracellular signal-regulated kinase (ERK) pathway has been conflicting; however, an early peak of ERK activation at the plasma membrane is now thought to be required (*169,173*,174,*175,176*). Interestingly, MINK-deficient DP thymocytes show an impairment in receptor-induced JNK phosphorylation, but not in ERK phosphorylation *(166)*, reinforcing the importance of JNK in clonal deletion. The involvement of the calcium/calcineurin pathway is also controversial, but most of the experiments using cyclosporin A, which inhibits calcineurin in this pathway, suggest that NF-AT activation does not play a key role in cases of strong deletion, although elevated intracellular calcium levels are critical *(104,177–179)*. Finally, experiments expressing a superinhibitory form of the NF-κB inhibitory protein in the T-cell lineage had no effect on the negative selection of two different CD8-restricted TCR transgenics *(180)*.

Further downstream there is good evidence for the induction of the proapoptotic transcription factor Nur77, an "orphan" steroid nuclear receptor (*178*,181). Transcription of this receptor is negatively controlled by HDAC7, a thymocyte-enriched histone deacetylase that normally resides in the nucleus *(182)*. On TCR engagement, activation of protein kinase delta1 leads to serine phosphorylation of HDAC7 and redistribution of the protein into the cytoplasm *(183,184)*. Within 1 hour this facilitates transcription and translation of Nur77. In the presence of adequate intracellular calcium, the protein activates transcription of downstream genes. Although the Nur77 knockout mouse shows normal clonal deletion *(185)*, a DN form of Nur77 inhibits negative selection in the F5 and H-Y transgenic mouse models, suggesting redundancy in the pathway, possibly mediated by other family members such as Nurr1 (181,*186*). Nur77 is also induced in mature T cells following TCR and CD28 signaling. Under these circumstances, however, the protein is hyperphosphorylated by continued signaling through the PI3 K/Akt and Erk/MAP kinase pathways (187). This inactivates its DNA binding domain, allowing the protein to be removed from the nucleus to the cytoplasm, where presumably it is inactive *(188)*. The difference in the response between immature thymocytes and mature T cells is not fully understood, but one observation is that immature thymocytes fail to strongly activate Akt kinase activity (187). Finally, gene knockout experiments have shown that the BH3-only Bcl-2 family member BimL is required for complete thymocyte negative selection *(189)*. This protein is up-regulated in thymocytes following TCR ligation and combines with $Bcl\text{-}X_L$ to inhibit its survival function (190). Transcription of BimL requires both protein kinase C (PKC) activation and an increase in intracellular calcium *(179)*. BimL up-regulation is attenuated in MINK-deficient cells *(166)* and its induction has been shown to require JNK activation in neurons *(191)*. In the autoimmune prone NOD mouse both Nur77 and BimL up-regulation are impaired *(192)*. BimL is a critical initiator of apoptosis in both DP and semimature CD4 SP thymocytes (193); however, the KO phenotype is fairly mild (only late B-cell–mediated immune complex glomerulonephritis) *(194)* and its effect in reversing deletion in the male H-Y transgenic model was only partial *(189)*. This suggests that other BH3-only family members, such as PUMA, may also play a role in negative selection *(195)*. Null mutations in death receptors and their ligands, such as TNF, TRAIL, and TNF-receptor, have no effect on thymic negative selection *(196,197)*, but the role of the Fas/FasL pair still remains controversial (193,*198,199*). Some experiments suggest that Fas-mediated deletion of semimature $CD4^+$ SP thymocytes can occur at high levels of receptor cross-linking *(199)*; other experiments do not (193).

Activation Versus Tolerance Thresholds

After T cells complete their maturation in the thymus, they are capable of responding to a foreign antigen when the concentration of peptide/MHC complexes derived from that antigen reach a certain critical density for activation. The relationship between this threshold and the concentration of intact antigen depends on processing and presentation requirements, in addition to the intrinsic affinity of the TCR for the peptide/MHC complex. An important question is the relationship between this threshold for peripheral activation and the one involved in negative selection. If a self-antigen presented in the thymus induces clonal deletion in only a subset of high-affinity T cells, what happens if that antigen is subsequently expressed or processed in peripheral tissues in increased amounts during tissue destruction in an inflammatory response? Will T-cell clones with slightly lower affinity for the self-peptide MHC complexes now become activated? This usually is not the case; that is, trauma rarely leads to autoimmunity. The question is, why?

Early observations on endogenous viral superantigens suggested that T cells bearing certain Vβs could be deleted *in vivo* if the mice carried the proper Mtv, but that these same cells could not be stimulated *in vitro* to give a T cell proliferative response with APCs expressing that Mtv *(200)*. This suggested that tolerance induction in the thymus was achieved at a lower threshold than peripheral T-cell activation. The use of thymic organ cultures and TCR transgenic mice allowed a more quantitative analysis of this comparison. Deletion of TCR^{high} V$\beta8^+$ cells by the superantigen SEB in thymic organ culture occurred at concentrations that were 30- to 100-fold lower than those required to activate mature CD4$^+$ cells to proliferate *(201)*. For T-cell help generated in FTOC, exposure to the liver F protein during *in vitro* culture induced tolerance at a tenfold lower concentration than that required for proliferation of mature T cells (202). Finally, for CD8 responses, variant lymphocytic choriomeningitis viruses were compared for their ability to elicit antiviral responses in TCR transgenic mice and for their ability to induce neonatal tolerance in these mice *(203)*. One viral variant could not activate a CTL response or be cleared by the animal over a 1000-fold range of viral challenge doses; yet it was capable of inducing a partial deletion (40%) of transgenic TCR CD8$^+$ T cells in the thymus after neonatal tolerization. Thus, all the experiments suggest that the concentration threshold required for tolerance induction of immature T cells is lower than the threshold required by the mature T cell for activation.

A direct estimate of the sensitivity of immature thymocytes to clonal deletion in FTOC established from a TCR transgenic showed that as few as three to four peptide/MHC complexes were sufficient to delete 50% of the cells *(149)*. This, however, was with the strong, high-affinity agonist peptide. More revealing results have emerged in experiments performed with partial (weak) agonist peptides. In some cases these peptides allowed development of TCR transgenic thymocytes that were no longer responsive to the partial agonist after maturation, suggesting that the T cells had somehow altered their threshold for activation during the selection process *(204)*. Another study, using a CD69 expression assay for the readout of a response, revealed the requirement for a 10- to 30-fold higher concentration of partial agonist to stimulate peripheral CD4$^+$ T cells compared with DP transgenic thymocytes (205). In contrast, there was little or no difference in the response of cells from the two tissues using a high-affinity peptide agonist. Thus, the adjustment in the responsiveness threshold has its critical impact only on low-avidity interacting ligands. Biochemical experiments showed that these functional observations were associated with decreases in proximal TCR signaling of the mature cells by the weak agonist peptides, affecting the level of tyrosine phosphorylation of TCRζ and ZAP 70. Similar observations have been made for CD8$^+$ T cells, where the weak agonist peptide could elicit both CD69 and a calcium response from DP thymocytes, but no detectable calcium response from mature CD8$^+$ T cells *(206)*. Recently, it was suggested that this difference might be due to increased sialylation of the T cell on maturation, which reduces the avidity of the CD8 coreceptor for MHC class I molecules *(207)*. The general conclusion from these studies is that T-cell maturation is accompanied by a raising of the activation threshold of the cell, which helps prevent the activation of low-affinity anti–self-clones in the periphery by small changes in the concentration of self-peptide/MHC complexes. A conceptually similar maturation phenomenon occurs for B cells, as discussed earlier.

In addition to this differentiation event for altering thymocyte activation thresholds, there also exists mechanisms for altering thresholds in response to environmental cues. This process has been referred to as *T-cell tuning (208)*. The best example involves the cell surface molecule CD5 *(209)*. The membrane levels of CD5 increase as thymocytes mature from DN to DP to SP cells. The final level achieved on a particular T cell depends on its TCR avidity and the strength of signal it transmits into the cell. Transgenic TCRs of higher avidity emerge as cells with higher levels of CD5, while TCRs with impaired signaling function, such as those with inactivated TCRζ ITAMS, emerge with lower levels of CD5 (210). T cells from CD5$^{-/-}$ mice display an enhanced responsiveness to antigen, suggesting that the molecule has a negative impact on TCR signaling. This involves ITAM and ITIM motifs in its cytoplasmic domain, but the exact biochemical mechanism of its negative signaling and the mechanism by which TCR strength of signal is converted to alterations in CD5 levels are not understood. Nonetheless, the consequences for thymocyte positive and negative selection are clear. In the case of a TCR with a high avidity for a positively selecting self-peptide/MHC ligand, gene targeting of CD5 can create an environment in which many of the cells are negatively selected *(209)*. In a TCR transgenic mouse with weak alloreactivity, introduction of the alloantigen leads to deletion of many of the cells, but those that exit the thymus have higher levels of CD5 (210). This "adjustment" occurs at the DP stage. In contrast, high constitutive expression of a CD5 transgene had the opposite effect. This

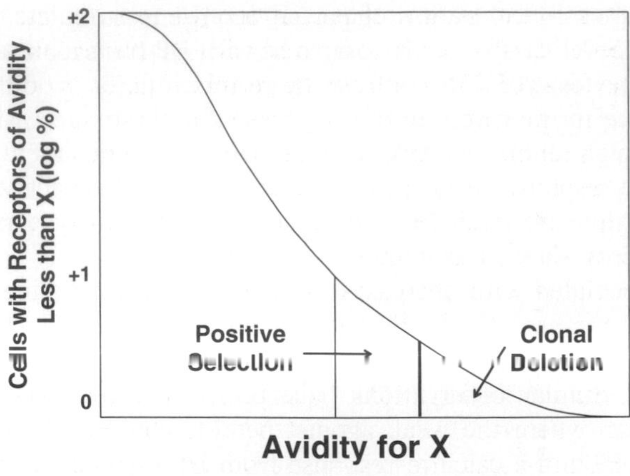

FIGURE 29.1 Selection of the T-cell repertoire as a consequence of T-cell receptor avidity for self-antigens expressed in the thymus. The 10% of cells whose receptors have an avidity greater than that indicated by the thin vertical bar on the left undergo positive selection. Of those, cells with receptors of the highest avidities (to the right of the thick vertical bar) undergo negative selection by clonal deletion.

prevented positive selection in both the female CD8$^+$ MHC class I-restricted H-Y TCR transgenic mouse and the CD4$^+$ MHC class II-restricted DO11.10 TCR transgenic mouse *(211)*. These results suggest that thymocytes use the regulation of CD5 expression to fine tune their TCR responsiveness during selection, and could explain some of the puzzling observations made with weak peptide agonists *(204)*. This adjustment would optimize the capture of cells by positive selection and minimize the loss of cells from negative selection at the DP stage.

Despite these mechanisms to fine tune the negative selection process to ensure the optimum deletion of self-reactive T cells, the cutoff inherently has an arbitrary aspect to its nature. If one thinks of the generated T-cell repertoire as having various degrees of affinity for a particular self-antigen (pedtide/MHC complex), then only a small fraction of TCRs will have a high enough avidity to be negatively selected (Figure 29.1). Another, presumably larger, cohort of cells of more modest affinity would be positively selected during thymic development. But where do you set the line that distinguishes between these two cohorts? Studies on a set of peptide analogs with differing avidities for a particular TCR showed that the distinction is quite sharply demarcated *(169)*. Most analogs are either only positively selected or negatively selected in FTOC, no matter what dose of antigen was added. However, a rare few could do both, positively selecting at low doses and negatively selecting at high doses. How the T-cell molecularly makes such a sharp distinction is not understood, but these rare peptides that can do both clearly present a potential challenge to self-tolerance if they are subsequently expressed at high levels in the periphery.

DOMINANT TOLERANCE: NATURAL T REGULATORY CELLS (NTREGs)

Perhaps because of this inherent leakiness of negative selection, the immune system seems to have evolved an additional mechanism to deal with the problem of autoreactivity at the T-cell level. This entails the selection of a subpopulation of CD4$^+$ T cells that expresses the transcription factor Foxp3 and low levels of the alpha chain of the IL-2R (CD25) *(212–214)*. Nishizuka and Sakakura (215) first showed that neonatal thymectomy of female mice at 3 days of age (but not at day 1 or 7) led to oophoritis and sterility. Subsequent studies showed that other organs could be affected such as the thyroid, stomach, prostate, and testis, and that the target tissue varied depending on the genetic background of the inbred mouse strain *(216,217)*. Disease could be prevented either by thymus grafting or by injection of normal day 7 or adult spleen cells. A transfer model into lymphopenic hosts eventually allowed the identification of the protecting cells as CD4$^+$ T cells *(218)* and then later as constitutively expressing CD25$^+$ (219) and the transcription factor Foxp3 (220,*221*,*222*). These cells are referred to as *natural T regulatory cells* (nTregs)

The presence of CD4$^+$CD25$^+$Foxp3$^+$ T cells in the thymus suggests that they develop there, although the possibility that the cells recirculate back from the periphery had to be considered. The first convincing evidence that nTregs arise in the thymus came from studies on embryonic epithelial grafts of thymic primordium (223,*224*). These experiments were initially done in a chicken/quail chimera model and then in the mouse using different strains. They showed that allogeneic grafts were tolerated because of a dominant suppressive mechanism directed against the epithelial cell alloantigens. Subsequently, a mouse expressing MHC class II molecules only in the thymic cortex was shown to support the development of CD4$^+$CD25$^+$ immunoregulatory T cells, while mice deficient in all MHC class II molecules did not *(225)*. Finally, nTregs develop in FTOC *(213,226)*, and a mouse in which an eGFP reporter protein was knocked into the Foxp3 locus revealed selection of T cells into this lineage at the transition from DP to SP thymocytes *(227)*, although recent work suggests that initial commitment might occur earlier at the DN2 stage *(228)*.

What antigens do nTregs recognize? Most TCR transgenic mice made with receptor genes from CD4$^+$ helper T-cell clones do not contain nTregs when expressed on a Rag-deficient background (so there are no other receptors expressed), suggesting that the repertoires of these two subsets do not overlap much. This has recently been confirmed by extensive sequencing of TCRs from both CD4 subsets selected under conditions of restricted TCR diversity (229). Not only was there little overlap, but the diversity was greater in the nTreg subpopulation. One TCR transgenic mouse has been described, however, which

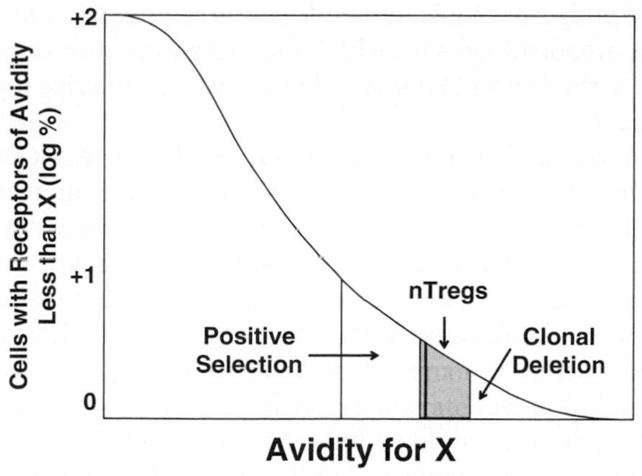

FIGURE 29.2 The same as Figure 29.1 except that the proposed repertoire for natural T regulatory cells (nTregs) is superimposed. They are mainly cells with receptors of high enough avidity to choose this alternative fate rather than die from negative selection by clonal deletion.

gives rise to a high frequency of both CD4$^+$CD25$^-$ helper T cells and nTregs; but the latter were only generated when the animal was also engineered to express the antigen to which the TCR is specific (230). Interestingly, a second TCR transgenic with a lower-affinity receptor for the same antigen did not generate nTregs under the same conditions. This observation suggests that a relatively high affinity for the selecting ligand is required to generate nTregs. This concept is supported by the observation that nTregs are generated in higher frequency in SHP-1 phosphatase-deficient mice (which signal more strongly through their TCR) *(226)*. The current working model for how this might happen is shown in Figure 29.2. Positive selection of CD4 thymocytes is favored when TCR signaling is relatively strong or sustained. If the avidity of this interaction is too high, however, the cell undergoes a different fate. This can be deletion by negative selection or alternatively a commitment to the nTreg lineage. Which fate is adopted may be influenced by exposure to the growth factor, thymic stromal lymphopoietin, which favors survival and differentiation *(231)*, or other *trans* signals delivered by DP thymocytes *(228)*. In either case, though, only a few of the T cells would have receptors with affinities in the usual positive selection only range. Hence, little overlap would exist in the repertoires between nTregs and conventional CD4$^+$ effector T cells.

The self-antigen recognition by nTregs can be organ-specific, at least in the way the cells prevent autoimmune disease. For example, in the day 3 thymectomy models for orchitis and prostatitis, CD4$^+$CD25$^+$ regulatory T cells from the spleens of normal male mice were tenfold more effective at preventing disease than spleen cells from either female mice or males that had been castrated at birth (and who therefore do not express antigens of the testes or the testes-dependent prostate) *(232)*. Tissue ablation experiments in adults suggest that peripheral antigen expression is needed to sustain prolonged survival and/or expansion of the CD4$^+$CD25$^+$ T cells in the periphery *(233)*. Whether the generation and continued presence of these cells in the thymus requires ectopic expression of peripheral antigens in epithelial cells of the thymic medulla (see later discussion), or cross-reaction with other self-antigens expressed only in the thymus, remains to be determined.

Peripheral and thymic CD4$^+$CD25$^+$ regulatory T cells have an activated phenotype. In addition to being CD25$^+$, they express high levels of CD44, CD5, and CD54 as well as low levels of CD45RB and the glucocorticoid-induced TNF-receptor family-related protein (GITR) *(234)*. They also express CTLA4, and there is some evidence that this molecule is involved in their *trans* suppressive function *(235–237)*. The molecule is not essential, however, because CTLA4$^{-/-}$ gene-targeted mice show normal nTreg development and function *(238)*. Interestingly, the resting CD4$^+$CD25$^+$ T cells appear to be in a clonal anergic state (see later discussion). They do not make IL-2 or proliferate when stimulated through their TCR *in vitro*. This is partly due to alterations in diacylglycerol kinase activity *(239)* and partly because Foxp3 competes with AP-1 for NF-AT binding to the IL-2 promoter, preventing transcription of this gene (240). The cells can proliferate if IL-2 is added to the cultures along with anti-CD3 *(241)* and this approach has been used to expand them *in vitro (242)*. *In vivo* their expansion and survival also seems to depend on IL-2 *(243)* because gene-targeted mice deficient in either IL-2 or its co-signaling receptors, CD28 and CD40L, have fewer numbers of CD4$^+$CD25$^+$ cells (*244*,245,*246*,*247*). IL-2 does not appear to be required for nTreg development *(248,249)*.

In vitro studies have shown that nTregs function either by suppressing the proliferative response of naive CD4$^+$ and CD8$^+$ T cells through blocking of their IL-2 production and arresting the cells in the G1 phase of the cell cycle *(250)* or by consuming IL-2 in the culture, leading to apoptosis of these cells by cytokine withdrawal *(250a)*.To accomplish these things the regulatory cells must be activated through their TCRs and come into close proximity with the naive T cells. Once Treg activation is initiated by antigen or anti-TCR antibodies, the suppression becomes completely antigen independent. There is some controversy about whether an APC is also involved in the process *in vitro (250–252)*, but recent evidence *in vivo* suggests they can play a critical role in the effector function of Tregs *(214,253)*. Another controversy is whether the mechanism of inhibition involves cytokines such as IL-10 and TGF-β *(254–256)*. The regulatory cells clearly make these cytokines when they are stimulated, and in some cases this is required for suppressive function (*257–259*,260). They also produce IL-9, which can recruit and activate mast cells to mediate immune suppression *(261)*. In any case, the antigen-nonspecific, bystander mechanism(s) of the suppression makes it hard to understand why these cells do not also suppress responses to foreign antigens *(262)*. Some experiments suggest that activation of the innate immune system might lead to an inactivation of nTregs while at the same time facilitating naive T-cell activation via up-regulation of costimulation by APCs *(263)*. TLR-mediated stimulation of IL-6 and IL-1 production has been shown to be critical in this regard *(264)*.

In addition to $CD4^+$ nTregs, recent experiments have suggested that there might also be populations of $CD8^+$ nTregs. Mice deficient in the CD122 IL-2R beta chain show enhanced granulopoiesis and severe anemia that is caused by the expansion of hyperactivated T cells *(265,266)*. This defect was corrected by the addition of $CD8^+CD122^{high}$ T cells *(267)*. In addition, $Rag2^{-/-}$ mice injected with normal $CD8^+CD122^{low}$ T cells die within 10 weeks of transfer, and this autoimmunity could also be prevented by the addition of $CD8^+CD122^{high}$ T cells *(267)*. *In vitro* experiments showed that the regulatory T cells suppressed both proliferation and interferon (IFN)-γ production by the $CD8^+CD122^{low}$ T cells via an IL-10-dependent mechanism (268). A very different population of nTregs that is $CD8^+CD25^+$ has been detected in MHC class II-deficient mice and it has almost all of the properties of $CD4^+CD25^+$ T cells *(269)*. It is $Foxp3^+GITR^+CTLA\text{-}4^+$, found in the thymus, and inhibits $CD25^-$ naive T-cell responses to anti-CD3 stimulation *in vitro*. However, it produces IFN-γ in addition to IL-10 on stimulation, and proliferates without the addition of IL-2. The exact functional role for either of these types of $CD8^+$ nTregs is still not clear.

TOLERANCE TO PERIPHERAL ANTIGENS

At the completion of development, T and B cells emerge from the primary lymphoid organs and enter the recirculating pool of peripheral lymphocytes. One of the first things these naive cells encounter in their fully mature state is antigens from various nonlymphoid organs that were thought to be restricted in their expression to a particular peripheral tissue. These antigens would be processed by dendritic cells in the tissues and brought to the draining lymph nodes for presentation to the naive lymphocytes. In this section is discussed whether these tissue-restricted antigens are recognized by the immune system, whether the antigens are only expressed in the peripheral tissues, and whether the immune system is tolerant to them.

Tissue-specific Antigens

When Medawar was asked if he could distinguish dizygotic from monozygotic bovine twins, he was certain this could be done by skin grafting; however, when his group attempted to test this, they found that most of the time (7/8) skin grafts exchanged between dizygotic twins were not rejected (270). This surprising result led them to conclude that skin does not contain any unique transplantation antigens, that is, none other than those found on the hematopoietic cells for which the twins were chimeric (3). Thus, the concept emerged that blood cells tolerize for all tissues.

The first challenge to this intellectual framework came from the studies of Billingham and Brent (271) on neonatal tolerance in mice. They found that B6 newborns injected with A spleen cells were not tolerant of A skin grafts. Boyse and colleagues *(272)* corroborated this finding in radiation-induced bone marrow chimeras [$(A \times B6)F_1 \rightarrow B6$], where they were able to show that the recipient contained $(A \times B6)F_1$ hematopoietic cells but still rejected A skin. Tolerance could be induced, however, if A strain epidermal cells were injected along with the F_1 bone marrow (273). They concluded that there must be a skin-specific transplantation antigen (Sk) expressed by A and not by B6 mice. Subsequent studies showed that two genes controlled the expression of this antigen(s) *(274)* and that Sk antigens could be identified in other strain combinations *(275)*. These studies thus appeared at odds with the original Medawar results (270). A resolution of the contradiction was achieved by Emery and McCullagh (276). They repeated the early experiments with a small technical modification. In the original study, skin grafts were prepared from the ears of the donor and placed on the back (whithers) of the recipient. Instead, Emery and McCullagh exchanged flank skin grafts. In this case, all dizygotic twins rejected their sib's graft. Repeating the technique of Anderson et al. (270), they confirmed that many animals did not reject under these conditions (in their hands, 50%). Thus, cattle also have skin-specific antigens.

The failure to elicit a rejection with ear skin grafts most likely relates to the "strength" of antigen presentation (e.g., the density of Langerhans cells), which has been shown to vary in different areas of mouse skin *(277)*. Although Medawar's group demonstrated that their ear skin grafts were antigenic across a complete MHC genetic disparity (i.e., outbred cattle), differences in skin-specific (minor histocompatibility) antigens between dizygotic twins is a situation in which the two immune systems are tolerant to all processed peptides derived from proteins of hematopoietic cells, but not to peptides derived from proteins unique to the skin. In the cases in which the gene encoding a skin protein exists in two allelic forms, the potential arises for peptides to be expressed by the graft tissue that are not present in the host's skin. To elicit an immune response such peptides have to be able to bind (one each) to the MHC class I and class II molecules, perhaps explaining why two genes "control" the expression of the Sk antigen. These three constraints could explain why not all mouse strain combinations reveal an immune response to skin-specific antigens: (a) requirement for allelic polymorphism, (b) requirement for peptide binding to MHC molecules (immune response [Ir] gene control), and (c) tolerance to minor histocompatibility antigens that are also expressed by hematopoietic cells. Outbred animals like cattle, however, should show this reactivity more frequently because of potentially greater diversity in the genes encoding their skin-specific proteins.

The concept of tissue-specific antigens is not unique to skin. The experiment of Triplett (13) demonstrating that immunologic tolerance is an acquired state showed that frog pituitary also expresses tissue-specific antigens. Because an attempt to confirm that study for pituitary, thyroid, and eye in other species of frog failed *(278)*, McCullagh (279) also readdressed this issue using the thyroid of fetal lambs. At 54 days of gestation, the lamb's immune system has not yet developed and the animal will accept allografts of adult skin. If the thyroid gland was removed at that time, implanted into a nude mouse (lacking T cells for rejection) for 5 to 9 weeks, and then reimplanted subcutaneously into the same lamb after birth, autoimmune thyroiditis developed. Partial thyroidectomized lambs did not get the disease, arguing that the immune response was specific for thyroid antigens and not any xenogeneic mouse tissue. These observations demonstrate that the immune system normally learns to become tolerant of other self-tissues and that it has mechanisms for dealing with the problem of tolerance to antigens that are predominantly synthesized in peripheral nonlymphoid tissues or that are expressed later in development (e.g., at puberty). These other mechanisms will be the topic of the rest of this chapter.

Ectopic Expression of Peripheral Antigens in the Thymus

The existence of tissue-specific antigens (TSAs) creates a problem for the immune system because the primary mechanism for induction of tolerance in the T-cell compartment is by clonal deletion or generation of nTregs, processes which both occur in the thymus. One possible solution to this problem is for these antigens to also be expressed in the thymus. The first hint that this might occur came from studies with transgenic mice expressing foreign antigens under the control of tissue-restricted promoters (*280*,281). In particular, the rat insulin promoter was found to sometimes express in the thymus in addition to the beta cells of the pancreas *(282–284)*. This expression was initially viewed as an artifact resulting from insertion of the transgene into regions of active chromatin *(285)*; however, the expression was observed in the thymus by several groups, a similar phenomenon was also seen when using other promoters, and importantly was not observed very often in other nontarget tissues *(286–288)*. In most cases the expression levels in the thymus were very low (e.g., for the rat insulin promoter 3,000 to 10,000 times less than in the pancreas) and could only be detected at the message level by reverse transcription polymerase chain reaction (RT-PCR) *(284)*; yet this expression had clear immunologic effects. For example, the LCMV glycoprotein expressed under the control of the rat insulin promoter produced two types of transgenic founders, one with detectable expression in the thymus, the other not *(283)*. The former showed only a slow onset of diabetes following LCMV infection, mediated by low-affinity CD8 T cells requiring CD4 help, while disease onset in the latter was rapid and independent of CD4 help. These observations suggested that the thymic expression had induced a partial state of tolerance. Convincing evidence that it is only the thymic expression that is responsible for the tolerance process was achieved in the insulin and other models (LCMV, lactalbumin, elastase, and C-reactive protein) in which the thymus from the transgenic mouse was transplanted to a normal recipient and found to induce the same tolerant state *(282,283,288,289,290)*.

Subsequent studies using RT-PCR on human and normal murine thymuses revealed expression of many peripheral antigens, including somatostatin, insulin, myelin basic protein, glutamic acid decarboxylase 67, glucagon, elastase, trypsin, astrocyte S100β, C-reactive protein, lactalbumin, and thyroglobulin, although a few proteins such as human glutamic acid decarboxylase 65 and mouse preproinsulin 1 were not detected (291). Again, the expression was mostly confined to the thymus and the amounts expressed were small. In some cases sensitive assays were used to detect protein expression *(292)*. Which cell types in the thymus express these proteins was initially controversial (281). All investigators agreed that they were rare cells, mostly in the medulla *(293)*, and bone marrow chimera experiments showed that the cells were radioresistant *(290)*. Subsequent experiments using cell isolation and RT-PCR found that almost all of the TSAs were expressed in purified populations of medullary epithelial cells (291). A few antigens such as elastase, trypsin, somatostatin, lens crystallin, and retinal S antigen were also expressed in cortical epithelial cells. Very few were expressed in dendritic cells and then only at low levels. Thus, the current model is that TSA expression is mostly confined to the epithelial lineage and the expression begins in the common precursor to cortical and medullary epithelial cells, but increases enormously in diversity at the fully differentiated medullary stage, peaking in the mature MHC class II$^+$ and CD80$^+$ cells of this lineage, which are capable of presenting the antigen to both CD4$^+$ and CD8$^+$ thymocytes (294). Interestingly, for any given TSA, only 1-3% of medullary cells seem to express it *(295)*. This explains why the mRNA levels are so low in the whole thymus, but creates the cellular problem of how the system screens all maturing thymocytes for potential autoreactivity. It is estimated that scanning 30,000 mTECs by 15 million medullary thymocytes would take about 4 days (294). BrdUrd-labeling studies, however, have shown that maturing thymocytes can spend from 9 to 14 days in the medullary compartment *(296,297)*. Furthermore, for some antigens, transfer and cross-presentation by dendritic cells has been shown to be required and achieved for negative selection *(298)*.

A critical question is whether the low levels of expression of TSAs play a role in the tolerance process. Detectable expression of TSAs in the thymus has been correlated with resistance to autoimmune disease induction among mouse and rat strains, for example, for interphotoreceptor retinoid-binding protein in experimental autoimmune uveoretinits *(299)* and for myelin basic protein in experimental autoimmune encephalomyelitis (EAE) *(300)*. For EAE caused by immunization with proteolipid protein, the dominant immunogenic epitope is encoded by an exon that is not present in the mRNA splice variant expressed in the thymus, suggesting that the T cells responsive to all other potential epitopes have been tolerized by the thymic expression *(301)*. This mechanism also influenced strain susceptibility to EAE as SJL mice could recognize an immunodominant peptide from this region, while B6 mice could not.

For insulin, an interesting correlation exists in the human population between a genetic susceptibility locus for diabetes (IDDM2) and proinsulin expression in the thymus. Two groups showed that variation in a minisatellite repeat element (VNTR) 0.5 kb upstream of the human insulin gene results in variation in proinsulin expression (*292*,302). The higher expressing alleles (three- to fourfold) show a dominant form of protection with a three- to fivefold reduction in the risk of developing Type 1 diabetes. Finally, impairment in the development of mature (UEA-1^+) mTECs occurs in TRAF6- and RelB-deficient mice *(303)*, and this is accompanied by multiorgan autoimmunity (304). Grafting thymuses from these knockouts into nude mice recapitulated the disease as did thymic grafts from NF-κB-inducing kinase mutants *(305)*. All three proteins are part of the NF-κB signaling pathway. The disruptions of this pathway in mTECs resulted in abnormal nTreg development and decreased expression of TSAs. Reconstitution of thymus-grafted mice with $CD4^+CD25^+$ T cells reduced the severity of the autoimmunity, but did not totally eliminate it, suggesting that the decreased TSA expression was also contributing to the disease process *(305)*. Overall, these results suggest an important tolerogenic role for the ectopic expression of TSAs in the thymus.

How do thymic medullary epithelial cells express proteins normally functioning in other tissues? Some insight into this mechanism has come from the characterization of mutations in a gene called *AIRE* (autoimmune regulator) (306). Such mutations were first identified as responsible for a human autosomal recessive disease called autoimmune polyendocrine syndrome type-1 (APS-1) *(307,308)*. When an *AIRE*-deficient mouse was created, it became clear that many TSAs were no longer expressed in the thymic medulla and this correlated with an increase in autoimmunity against the peripheral tissues expressing those antigens (306). In transgenic models, *AIRE*-deficient mice (in a gene dosage-dependent manner) lost the ability to delete high avidity $CD4^+$ T cells recognizing their antigen expressed under the control of the insulin or thyroglobulin promoter *(309)*. The molecular mechanism of action of the *AIRE* gene is still not clear, but it can transactivate in a GAL4 transcription assay and has been found associated with the general transcription regulatory protein CBP in nuclear bodies (*310*,311,*312*). Not all TSA genes require *AIRE* for expression *(313)*, but those that do tend to be clustered *(314)*. The imprinted genes Igf2, insulin2, and H19 all require *AIRE* for ectopic expression, but only Igf2 loses its imprinting in mTECs *(315)*. Thus, generalized DNA demethylation does not seem to be involved. Finally, *AIRE* has effects beyond just regulation of the expression of TSAs. The presence of *AIRE* is associated with increased expression of MHC class I and II genes as well as a cluster of chemokine genes *(314)*. Interestingly, isolated mTECs from *AIRE*-deficient mice were less efficient at presenting antigen to T cells *in vitro (316)*. Thus, *AIRE* might also help to facilitate tolerance induction by enhancing antigen presentation of TSAs by mTECs.

A role for TSAs in the selection of $CD4^+$ nTregs was initially postulated when both were first located to the thymic medulla. Subsequently, however, mice in which MHC class II molecules were limited to expression in the thymic cortex, using the K14 promoter, were found to develop normal numbers of functional nTregs *(225)*. In more recent experiments, *AIRE*-deficient mice (with normal nTreg numbers) and the Foxp3-scurfy mutant (deficient in nTregs) were crossed *(317)*. The offspring showed an additive effect of the two genetic alterations on the shortening of lifespan. Half the double-mutant mice died by 16 days of age from lymphocytic infiltration and severe inflammation of the lung and liver, whereas the parents lived well beyond 35 days of age and showed less severe pathology. It is still possible, however, that a subset of ectopically expressed, *AIRE*-dependent TSAs are involved in selecting a part of the nTreg repertoire.

Delivery of Peripheral Antigens to the Thymus

The presence of a mechanism for ectopic expression of TSAs in the thymus would now seem adequate to explain the original observations of Boyse et al. (272,273) described previously, wherein the irradiated host would lack A-type antigens in the thymus as well as the skin, thus preventing tolerance induction. In contrast, this mechanism cannot explain the observations of Triplett (13) or McCullagh (279) because removal of the peripheral organ (pituitary or thyroid) should not eliminate the central tolerance mechanism. It is possible that expression of some TSAs from these tissues is not *AIRE*-dependent, but then how would tolerance come about normally? Another plausible mechanism for achieving central tolerance to molecules that are not normally expressed in the thymus is to bring them there. Proteins and their fragments derived from peripheral tissues through secretion or cell necrosis could easily enter the thymic medulla through its arterial circulation *(318)*. Exogenous antigens injected intravenously can reach and be processed by thymic dendritic cells as well as presented on MHC class II molecules in a form that stimulates T-cell clones to proliferate *(158,319)*. Early experiments showed that direct injection of soluble proteins into the thymus could induce tolerance to them, as measured in antibody responses and prevention of EAE (*320*,321). More recently, in a double-transgenic model with a TCR specific for the human C-reactive protein (hCRP), central tolerance could be mediated by bone marrow-derived dendritic cells when the transgenic antigen was induced in the liver of females (289). This T-cell deletion occurred even if the thymus was replaced with a nontransgenic thymus graft so that ectopic expression of hCRP in mTECs could not take place. Experiments on the fifth component of complement also showed that circulating proteins could reach the thymus and induce central tolerance (97,107).

Another possible mechanism for antigens to be transported to the thymus is for dendritic cells to pick them up in the periphery and then migrate back to the medulla. Small numbers of DCs have been detected in thoracic duct lymph returning to the bloodstream *(322)*. The first convincing data for migration to the thymus came from parabiosis experiments in which DCs from one CD45-marked host were found in low levels in the thymus of the other host after the shared blood vessel circulation was created *(323,324)*. In addition, intravenous injection of labeled CD11c$^+$ DCs yielded a small fraction appearing in the corticomedullary region of the thymus next to endogenous DCs *(324)*. This immigration process required recognition of endothelial P-selectin, integrin VLA4/VCAM-1 interaction, and activation of a pertussis toxin sensitive chemokine receptor, a three-step process normally required for most hemopoietic cell transcytosis events. Only immature CD11c$^+$ DC could do this and their ability disappeared if they were preactivated with LPS (possibly in order to prevent the delivery of foreign antigens to the thymus). When injected into irradiated mice prior to reconstitution with bone marrow cells from a TCR transgenic mouse, the DCs induced clonal deletion, if they had been preloaded with the OVA peptide recognized by the TCR. Finally, OVA transgenic mice expressing antigen in cardiac myocytes were also shown to delete the TCR transgenic thymocytes, and this negative selection was prevented by treatment with an anti-VLA4 mAb, which presumably prevented peripheral DC from entering into the thymus *(324)*. The number of such DCs in the thymus is estimated from the parabiosis experiments to be about 14,000. Although these experiments demonstrate that peripheral DCs can deliver TSAs back to the thymus to mediate negative selection, it should be noted that this process has not been detected in several other experimental models *(301,325)*. Nonetheless, this tolerance mechanism is capable of explaining the Triplett (13) and McCullagh (279) experiments described earlier.

Despite the clear evidence for two ways that the immune system has for bringing TSAs into the thymus to mediate a central tolerance mechanism, the possibility that the antigens could also induce tolerance in the periphery was raised by experiments in which allogeneic MHC class I and II molecules were expressed in the periphery using tissue-restricted promoters. In contrast to soluble proteins, these MHC class I molecules must remain intact in order to present their tissue-specific peptides. In other words, if shed and processed by dendritic cells for presentation in the thymus, they would not tolerize T cells that are specific for the peptide/MHC complexes expressed in the original peripheral tissue.

The first transgenic model of this type expressed the MHC class II E molecule either in β cells of the pancreas under the control of the rat insulin promoter (326) or in acinar cells of the pancreas under the control of the elastase promotor *(327)*. These animals were tolerant of the E molecule in a MLR, and they failed to eliminate certain Vβ-expressing T cells that are normally deleted by endogenous superantigens when this E molecule is expressed in the thymus. Some of the cells expressing those Vβs were unresponsive when stimulated in culture with anti-Vβ antibodies immobilized on a plate *(328)*. This tolerance process is referred to as *anergy* and will be discussed further in a later section. The possibility that the tolerance was induced by low-level ectopic expression of the transgenic E molecule in the thymus was eliminated by introducing nontransgenic thymus grafts into adult thymectomized, lethally irradiated and bone marrow-reconstituted (AT $\times$ BM) transgenic mice. Under these conditions the T cells mature in a thymic environment that does not endogenously express the transgene. These mice were also tolerant, arguing in favor of a peripheral mechanism for the tolerance induction. However, the possibility that the tissue-specific peptide/MHC molecules were transferred intact (via episomal bodies) to pancreatic DCs, which then migrated to the thymus to induce central tolerance, has not been ruled out. A similar series of experiments was done with MHC class I molecules expressed in a variety of peripheral tissues and the outcome was the same *(329–331)*, although thymic transplant experiments were rarely performed to rule out ectopic expression. Interestingly, the tolerance mechanism(s) involved in these situations, similar to the I-E molecule example discussed, were often not deletional. In the next sections of this chapter such mechanisms will be examined in more detail.

PERIPHERAL TOLERANCE MECHANISMS

Transitional B Cells

Peripheral tolerance deals with events that take place once the lymphocyte has fully matured and entered the peripheral circulation. For the T cell, this process is completed in the thymic medulla, and naïve T cells that seed out into the spleen and lymph nodes are viewed as mature. B cells, however, must travel to the spleen to complete their maturation. Here they are called *transitional cells* (T1 to T3) and are defined by a series of cell surface markers (such as CD21 and CD23) that they acquire during final maturation (see Chapter 7 for a review of B-cell development). During this stage the B cell is still subject to negative selection and clonal deletion. In contrast to the bone marrow environment, BCR-stimulated transitional cells can no longer escape by receptor editing, but rather die by apoptosis if they encounter high-avidity multivalent antigen (*332*,333). Alternatively, the B cell can undergo a process of receptor desensitization and developmental arrest at the T1/T2 stage if it encounters persistent, soluble antigen of lower avidity and valency *(29,334)*. This process is known as *B-cell anergy* and will be discussed in detail later. In contrast, if the B cell also receives T cell help, it survives and both proliferates and differentiates into an antibody-forming cell (335). In early experiments, neonatal spleen cells were transferred at limiting dilution to keyhole limpet hemocyanin (KLH) carrier-primed irradiated recipients (38,*336*). As the naive B cells matured in splenic focus cultures *in vitro*, presentation of the DNP hapten coupled to KLH led to an IgM antibody response. In contrast, if the hapten was presented on another carrier (DNP-HGG), to which the T cells were not primed, then there was no antibody made to DNP. The antigen was recognized, however, because an initial 24-hour exposure to DNP-HGG prevented the antibody response to DNP-KLH. This showed that the developing immature B cells were tolerized to the hapten in the absence of T-cell help. Thus, the same B cells could be activated or tolerized depending on the presence of helper T cells.

In more recent studies, transitional B cells stimulated *in vitro* with anti-μ antibodies were shown to die by apoptosis; however, if IL-4 was also added to the cultures, the apoptosis was prevented and some of the B cells proliferated (333,*337*). IL-4 is one of the known cytokines to participate in T-cell help. At a molecular level, the anti-IgM–induced cyclin-dependent kinase (CDK)-4 and its regulatory subunit cyclin D2, which only allowed the cell to go from G0 into the G1 phase of the cell cycle. With the addition of IL-4, however, the expression of cyclin E and CDK2 was also induced, and this allowed some of the cells to transit into the S phase of the cell cycle. More complete help is provided by signaling through CD40 (333,*338*). These experiments support the idea that tolerizable immature B cells can be rescued by T-cell help.

These observations are not consistent with the clonal selection ideas proposed by Burnet (11), but fit nicely with the general model for B-cell activation originally proposed by Bretscher and Cohn (339). In an attempt to explain why immune responses require the recognition of two different determinants on the antigen and how the same antigen could both tolerize and immunize when given at different doses, these theoreticians first suggested that antibody-forming cells must be only tolerizable when stimulated through their antigen-specific receptor (this was referred to as signal one), but activated if they also received a second signal (referred to as signal two). This second signal was also postulated to be antigen-specific, and both antigenic determinants were required to be linked together on the same molecule. In the original model, the second signal was delivered by antibody from another B cell via an antigen bridge. With the subsequent discovery of T lymphocytes, the second signal became help from T cells specific for the same antigen. In today's way of thinking, the B cell binds the antigen via its BCR, which then transduces the first signal into the cell by activation of tyrosine kinases, such as Lyn and Syk. The receptor-antigen complex is then internalized, the antigen processed, and peptide/MHC complexes displayed on the B-cell surface. If T cells exist with receptors that can recognize these peptide/MHC complexes, then the ensuing T-cell/B-cell interaction provides the second signals in the form of a CD40 ligand/CD40 interaction and the release of stimulatory cytokines such as IL-4 and IL-5. In this framework then, antigen stimulation of B cells in the absence of T-cell help leads to peripheral tolerance, while stimulation in the presence of antigen-specific T-cell help leads to B-cell proliferation and differentiation. Based on the experiments described previously, it appears that these rules govern the response of transitional B cells to antigens.

Costimulation and the Two Signal Model for T-Cell Activation

The population of naive T cells that shows up in a lymph node on any given day is largely devoid of T cells with high-avidity receptors specific for self-antigens. Nonetheless, there are plenty of cells with low-avidity receptors and possibly a few with high-avidity receptors that have escaped central tolerance mechanisms. What happens if they encounter peptide/MHC complexes from a self-antigen that has been picked up in the tissues by DCs and brought to the draining lymph node? The immune system has a failsafe mechanism to thwart the stimulation of such high-avidity naive T cells, and that is the activation state of the APCs. Resting and immature DCs are not very effective in stimulating naive T cells, even when fully loaded with the proper peptide/MHC complexes (*340*,341).

Our understanding of this phenomenon traces back to the original dispute between Ehrlich and Morgenroth (1) and Metchnikov (2) discussed in the introduction section of this chapter. Immunizing with self-tissues often produces tissue-specific antibodies but these seldom caused any disease *(342)*. This changed in 1942 when Freund and McDermott introduced the use of an oil in water emulsion containing mycobacterial extracts as an adjuvant to enhance the magnitude of antibody responses *(343)*.

When Kabat et al. *(344)* used this complete Freund's adjuvant (CFA) to immunize monkeys with rabbit brain extracts, three of four animals developed a demyelinating encephalitis. When CFA was later tried by Freund et al. *(345)* with a guinea pig testis suspension (a variant of the Metchnikov experiment), all the guinea pigs developed aspermatogenesis. Thus, the animals appeared not to be tolerant to their own tissues if these were presented to the immune system in the presence of CFA.

Further insight into this phenomenon emerged from the work of Dresser *(346)*. He discovered that protein antigens could be tolerogenic when injected into adult mice, if the preparations were first spun in an ultracentrifuge to remove protein aggregates. Interestingly, this same preparation was immunogenic (produced an antibody response) if administered in CFA. Dresser concluded that paralysis (failure to produce an antibody response following prior exposure to antigen) ensued when lymphocytes recognized the deaggregated antigen alone. In contrast, if this was accompanied by a second component, which he termed *adjuvanticity*, then an antibody response was obtained. Claman (347) subsequently reproduced these observations and showed that an antigen-nonspecific, bacterial endotoxin (LPS) could work as an adjuvant. Frei et al. *(348)* then demonstrated that *in vivo* filtration of protein antigens in rabbits could remove the aggregated material and convert an immunogen into a tolerogen. They interpreted the role of the adjuvant to be the stimulation of antigen uptake by macrophages. The proper role for the APC, however, was subsequently elucidated by Lafferty and Woolnough *(349)*. In their studies of allogeneic reactions, they found that only hemopoietic cells could stimulate an MLR, because in addition to expressing the alloantigen (signal 1) they delivered a nonspecific "inductive stimulus" (signal two) that they called *costimulation* (350). This antigen-nonspecific signal could be eliminated by ultraviolet irradiation without affecting the presentation of specific alloantigens. Using a related approach, Jenkins and Schwartz (351) extended this work to the study of protein antigens. They showed that cloned $CD4^+$ T cells failed to produce IL-2 and proliferate when stimulated with chemically fixed, antigen-bearing APC. In addition, these cells entered a state of hyporesponsiveness in which they persisted in not responding even when rechallenged with antigen and normal APCs. Consistent with the loss of a nonspecific "costimulatory activity" following chemical treatment of the APCs, the addition of allogeneic APCs (which were not capable of presenting the antigenic peptide) promoted proliferation of the T cells and prevented development of the unresponsive state *(352)*. Similar observations were made with purified peptide/MHC complexes presented in planar lipid membranes, showing that signal one was indeed solely TCR occupancy *(353)*. Taken together, these *in vitro* studies provided the basis for our current thinking that APCs must provide both a stimulatory peptide/MHC complex as well as an antigen nonspecific costimulatory activity to promote T-cell clonal expansion and IL-2 production.

What then is the role of CFA in this two signal model? Note that this model is different from the one proposed by Bretscher and Cohn (339). In the latter, the second signal needs to be antigen-specific. In the Lafferty/Cunningham model the second signal is not antigen-specific (350). This requires one to rethink the importance of self-nonself discrimination in the induction of tolerance because the APC providing the nonspecific costimulation has no obvious direct way to tell whether it is presenting a self or a foreign antigen. The first person to confront this problem was Janeway (*354*,355), who suggested that costimulation (and not foreign antigen) was the switch that controlled whether the organism made an immune response. He proposed that the innate immune system first evolved to recognize and respond to pathogen-associated molecular patterns (PAMPS) that were common to infectious agents and absent from the host (see Chapter 14 on innate immunity). At a later time in evolution, the adaptive immune system emerged with the recognition of foreign determinants by antigen-specific receptors as a means to focus and sustain the immune response initiated by the detection of PAMPs. In his model, the PAMPS activate pattern recognition receptors (PRRs) on APCs and this leads to the up-regulation of costimulatory activities, which subsequently deliver the second signals required to activate naive T cells. Thus, the absence or presence of a PAMP signal becomes the critical determinant in peripheral self/nonself discrimination. The subsequent discovery by Medzhitov et al. *(356)*, as well as many others, of multiple NOD and Toll-like receptors (TLRs) in and on innate immune cells (which are capable of mediating the recognition of PAMPs and activating APCs) has provided considerable support for this model (357,358,*359*,360). These receptors recognize lipids, carbohydrates, or nucleic acids specifically produced by pathogens and then activate the APCs through the NF-κB signaling pathway. The mycobacterial extract in CFA is now known to contain several PAMPs that act on TLRs 2 and 9 *(361–363)* and the incomplete oil in water emulsion (IFA) alone has been shown to up-regulate TLR2 in the liver *(364)*.

Despite this elegant framework, PRRs cannot be the whole explanation for how adaptive immune responses are initiated. For example, graft rejection following transplantation usually does not involve exposure to infectious agents. The first person to conceptualize that there must be other mechanisms for activating APCs was Matzinger (365), who presented the idea that the immune system distinguished not between self and nonself, but between things that were dangerous and things that were not ("The Danger Model"). In this model, the response would be initiated by perturbations in the organism's internal environment and propagated by alarm or "danger" signals, which in turn would stimulate the ability of the APCs to deliver costimulation. In the case of transplantation, it would be the response to injury, initiated through necrotic cell death that would provide the inductive signal. The molecular stimuli are thought to come from heat-shock proteins released into the environment by the dying cells *(366)*. These molecules carry potentially immunogenic peptides that are first internalized by binding to CD91 receptors on the APCs *(367)* and then cross-presented by MHC molecules to T cells (368,*369,370*). Interestingly, the heat-shock proteins also interact with TLRs 2 and 4 *(371,372)* to activate expression of costimulatory molecules and proinflammatory cytokines such as TNF-α and IL-1-β through stimulation of the NF-κB signaling pathway *(366)*. However, the possibility of trace contamination with endotoxin to explain this result has been difficult to exclude (373). Such indirect pathways could also be triggered by pathogens, which might infect and kill host cells, or otherwise perturb the host's internal milieu in a manner that could be recognized by a family of molecular sensors. A conceptually similar model called the "guard hypothesis" was subsequently proposed to explain certain aspects of plant immunity (374). In a recently described new twist, it was discovered that mycobacterial HSP-70 molecules from infected immature DCs, can stimulate human T cells through their CCR5 chemokine receptor to cluster with the DCs and activate them to kill the bacteria *(375)*. In this case, a chemokine receptor involved in the normal physiology of the immune system has been co-opted to function as a PRR.

In general, tissue dendritic cells can be activated by a variety of endogenous alarm signals generated by stressed or necrotic peripheral tissues. Dead cells can serve as adjuvants when coinjected with foreign antigens *(376,377)*. Recent studies have shown that uric acid released from these dying cells can stimulate dendritic cell maturation (B7 expression) and act as an adjuvant for enhancing the cytotoxic response of CD8$^+$ T cells to 3T3 cells expressing HIV gp120 *(378,379)*. It is actually crystalline monosodium urate (MSU) that is the biologically active form and this phase change *in vivo* may be the critical initiating danger signal. Depletion of uric acid with a combination of allopurinol to block its synthesis and uricase to metabolize it inhibited the CTL response to gp120 by 80% (380). Another strong candidate for an endogenous danger signal is the high mobility group one protein (HMGB1) which normally bends gene-targeted DNA in the nucleus, but which can be released from necrotic (but not apoptotic) cells *(381)* and induce inflammation by binding to the RAGE receptor *(382)*. Freeze/thawed necrotic fibroblasts from Hmgb1$^{-/-}$ mice fail to elicit tumor necrosis factor (TNF)-α production from monocytes or bone marrow cells the way WT cells do *(381,383)* and antibodies to HMGB1 can attenuate endotoxin-induced lethality in mice (384). Activated macrophages can also secrete HMGB1 but only after overnight stimulation with LPS (*381*,384). The mechanism for release from dying cells is more rapid and does not depend on TLRs.

Such endogenous danger signals may in fact play the dominant role in the facilitating effects seen with adjuvants. Gene-targeted mice lacking both MyD88 and TRIF, the two critical intracellular signaling components required for all Toll receptor function, still showed normal augmentation of antibody responses to protein antigens by adjuvants such as CFA or alum *(385)*, although other PRRs such as NODs might be playing a role (360). Thus, it could be argued that danger signals were in fact the first form of defense involved in recognizing both tissue injury and infection. It is even possible that the PRRs evolved from the original receptors concerned with sensing danger during wound repair and the clearance of molecular waste *(386)*.

Costimulatory Molecules

Activated DCs up-regulate their level of MHC class II molecules *(387)* and express a number of costimulatory molecules that facilitate their ability to activate naive T cells (341). Two critical ones are the B7 family member CD86 *(388)*, and the TNF superfamily member CD40 *(389)*. B7 molecules engage the CD28 receptor on T cells and promote naive T-cell proliferation by lowering the threshold for cell activation in response to a given number of serial engagements by the TCR and its associated coreceptor CD4 or CD8 *(390)*. CD28 costimulation induces the movement of lipid- and kinase-rich membrane raft microdomains to the interface between the T cell and the APC *(391)*, leading to more effective and persistent tyrosine kinase activity, c-Jun N-terminal kinase activation, and NF-κB translocation to the nucleus *(392)*. As a consequence, CD28 costimulation has the capacity to enhance transcription of the *IL-2* gene and increase the stability of resulting *IL-2* transcripts, as well as induce Bcl-xL protein expression, leading to greater proliferation, differentiation to cytokine production, and improved T-cell survival (*393*,394,395).

CD154/CD40 interactions at the T cell/APC interface during antigen priming can also act to amplify costimulatory signaling within CD4$^+$ T cells *(396)*. In contrast to CD28, CD154 is not constitutively expressed on the naive T cell. Its expression requires TCR- and CD28 stimulation. Subsequently CD154 binds to CD40 molecules on the APC, which have been up-regulated following APC activation by PAMPS or danger signals. CD40 signaling then reinforces the priming of the T cells by, among other things, promoting higher levels of expression of the B7 molecules (397). In the absence of CD154, this positive feedback loop is disrupted and antigen-bearing APC remain only weak stimulators of CD4$^+$ T cell growth and helper cell differentiation. Similarly, mice treated with a neutralizing anti-CD154 mAb demonstrate only a suboptimal CD4$^+$ T cell clonal expansion following immunization in the presence of antigen and adjuvant.

Following CD40 stimulation of the APC, another important molecule that is up-regulated is OX40 ligand (OX40L) (*398*,399). This molecule interacts with CD134 (OX40), which is expressed on activated T cells 1 to 2 days after stimulation with antigen and adjuvant. This up-regulation is partially dependent on CD28 signaling and augmented by costimulation with proinflammatory cytokines such as IL-1. During the response to antigen, agonist anti-CD134 mAb prolongs T cell proliferation through a molecule called Survivin *(400)* and reduces apoptosis by augmenting *Bcl-xL* and *Bcl-2* expression *(401)*. This provides better help for antigen-specific IgG production and enhances the frequency of the memory T-cell population. Genetic deficiency of OX40L leads to defective contact hypersensitivity as a consequence of poor naive T-cell priming. Similarly, mice treated with a neutralizing anti-OX40L mAb show defective priming for T-cell proliferation and recall lymphokine production. Finally, treatment of mice with ongoing inflammatory bowel disease using a blocking CD134/Fc fusion protein reduces both the number of T cells infiltrating the lamina propria as well as the amount of proinflammatory cytokine gene expression. The effect on migration is likely a consequence of OX40L expression on vascular endothelial cells where it facilitates adhesion and migration into tissues by activated T cells.

These experiments illustrate that costimulation is a series of positive feedback loops required to sustain an immune response (399). The process involves multiple receptor/ligand interactions. In addition to CD28/B7, CD154/CD40, and CD134/OX40L, there are also CD137/4-1BBL, ICOS/ICOSL, LIGHT/HVEM, and CD27/CD70, which coordinately amplify T-cell proliferation, differentiation, and survival. In addition, proinflammatory cytokines such as IL-1 help to amplify the immune response by enhancing the expression of these receptors (CD134 and CD154) on T cells *(402)*. Thus, the original idea of costimulation as a simple second signal required to allow TCR occupancy to lead to an immune response (350,351) has now given way to the idea of a family of non antigen specific positive signals that help both initiate and sustain the immune response *(403)*.

APCs Favor Tolerance in the Absence of Activation

What happens in the opposite situation, when the naive T cell encounters DCs in the absence of PAMPs and danger signals? In the complete absence of costimulatory ligands, isolated $CD4^+$ TCR ligation by solid-phase high-affinity peptide/MHC complexes (immobilized on plastic culture plates, latex beads, or gluteraldehyde-fixed cells) elicits only a weak and transient proliferative response that is accompanied by suboptimal IL-2 secretion (351,*353,404,405*). In addition, the studies on $CD4^+$ T cell clones showed the induction of a peripheral tolerance process called *clonal anergy* (see later section). However, these $CD4^+$ T cells were already preactivated. The induction of this tolerance has been more difficult to show with naive T cells *in vitro* (406). It cannot be easily demonstrated with immature dendritic cells because these cells become activated in culture when they adhere to the plastic culture dish *(407)*. The best data have been generated using as APCs Drosophila cells transfected with MHC class II molecules and various additional costimulatory molecules *(408)*. It was assumed that the Drosophila cells did not express any other molecules that could play a role in a mammalian immune response. These experiments revealed that mouse peptide/MHC complexes alone could elicit little or no naive T cell response, while the addition of ICAM-1 for an LFA-1 interaction to improve cell adhesion resulted in the induction of anergy. Further addition of CD86 for the delivery of CD28 costimulation caused the cells to proliferate and differentiate into preactivated T cells. Thus, adequate TCR signaling in the absence of CD28 costimulation could induce a hyporesponsive state. By contrast, for $CD8^+$ T cells, experiments with high-avidity peptide Ag/MHC class I tetramers showed that single, isolated naive TCR transgenic T cells could be stimulated to proliferate *(409)*. Adding costimulation in the form of CD28 cross-linking did not enhance this response. In addition, populations of these cells produced IL-2 and differentiated into cytotoxic effector cells making IFN-γ. When the tetramers for the H-Y peptide were injected into female mice, they primed for a more rapid graft rejection of male skin *(410)*. Thus, under very strong TCR stimulating conditions it appears that the need for costimulation can initially be bypassed for $CD8^+$ T cells without inducing an unresponsive state (but see later discussion). Interestingly, however, multiple injections *in vivo* induced a partial tolerant state by a mechanism involving the generation of $CD8^{low}$ regulatory T cells *(411)*.

A more compelling case for what happens to naive T cells in vivo has emerged from experiments designed to target foreign protein/peptide antigens to DCs using mAbs directed against their cell surface molecules, such as 33D1 or DEC-205, that do not activate the dendritic cells (412). The first experiment looked at the mouse antibody response to rat IgG2b. Pretreatment with small amounts of a monoclonal rat IgG2b directed against the 33D1 molecule greatly reduced the subsequent antibody response to a stimulatory IgG2b Ab (413). This tolerant state also involved a reduction in T-cell cytokine production (both IL-4 and IFN-γ) and could be prevented by coinjection of the proinflammatory cytokine IL-1 along with the anti-33D1 mAb. In contrast, a mAb directed against the CD11c molecule was immunogenic. Later experiments looked directly at T cells using $CD4^+$ cells from a TCR transgenic mouse specific for lysozyme (HEL) *(414)*. In this case, the HEL peptide was engineered to be part of a mAb specific for the DEC-205 protein on DCs. Injection of the antibody stimulated CD4$^+$ T cell proliferation and IL-2, but not IFN-γ or IL-4 production. After four to seven rounds of division, most of the T cells disappeared and the remaining cells were anergic. This tolerance induction was prevented by simultaneous administration of an agonist anti-CD40 mAb, a potent stimulator of the NF-κB pathway and an activator of the APCs. Subsequent studies with OVA delivery to DCs *in vivo* showed a similar phenomenon for CD8$^+$ T cells *(415)* and studies with the MOG peptide in an EAE model showed some evidence for involvement of the CD5 molecule in the tolerance process *(416)*.

Are these abortive responses a consequence of partial activation of the APCs by the mAbs against 33D1 and DEC-205? Arguing against this is a series of experiments in which CFSE-labeled, naive TCR transgenic T cells were transferred into an unmanipulated host expressing native or transgenic antigen in a tissue-specific manner *(329,417,418,419)*. The CD4$^+$ or CD8$^+$ T cells that entered the draining lymph node of that tissue were observed to initially proliferate, and then they either died off or became anergic. It is thought by many that this abortive response represents the consequence of antigen-induced T-cell activation in the absence of costimulation, although this has not been rigorously demonstrated in most of these *in vivo* models. The general strategy is to show that addition of a costimulatory signal allows for a full response *(419)*, but seldom is the inverse experiment done to genetically remove the possibility of costimulation and show that this abortive response still takes place.

Another postulated reason for the failure to sustain an immune response has been attributed to the induction of molecules that exert negative feedback on TCR signaling. The two best-studied molecules are CTLA-4 (420) and PD-1 (421). Soon after activation, T cells express the CD28-homolog CTLA-4, and ligation of this receptor by B7 molecules on the APC promotes the activation of an associated SHP-2 tyrosine phosphatase, leading to reduced IL-2 production and inhibited progression through the cell cycle. *In vivo*, the cells stop interacting with the APCs *(422)*. This inhibition is in part responsible for the anergy induction that occurs *in vivo* under conditions wherein B7 levels have not been sufficiently up-regulated by infection or injury *(423,424)*, although not in all cases *(425,426)*. Because CTLA-4 has a higher affinity for the B7 molecules than does CD28, its negative signaling can be expected to dominate under conditions of weak APC activation and limiting B7 expression *(427)*. The PD-1/PD-L1/2 receptor/ligand pair also inhibits T-cell activation by recruitment of the SHP-2 phosphatase to this receptor *(428)*, although its exact molecular mechanism of inhibition seems to be different than that of CTLA-4 *(429)*. Both PD-ligands are inducible on APCs with IFN-γ, but PD-L1 is constitutively expressed on many peripheral tissues such as heart, lung, and kidney, and thus may be mostly involved in downregulation of T cells during their effector phase. Blocking PD-L1 in chronic LCMV infection allows the anergic effector CD8$^+$ T cells to become more active and greatly reduces the viral load in the mouse *(430)*. Deficiency for CTLA-4 leads to the development of a T-cell lymphoproliferative disorder with massive lymphocyte infiltration of many organs and early death of the mouse *(431)*. PD-1 deficiency is less severe and leads to selective autoimmune disease with different phenotypes depending on the genetic background of the animal *(432,433)*. Targeting of CTLA-4 has a much more rapid and profound effect than targeting PD-1, possibly because the former also plays an important role in nTreg function *(237)*. Therefore, it is likely that in the absence of serious infection or injury, ligation of CTLA-4 and/or PD-1 by their respective ligands on the APC limits T-cell responsiveness and favors the maintenance of a hyporesponsive state.

Despite the existence of these two negative-feedback mechanisms and the ability to bypass costimulation under strong TCR occupancy conditions that avoid tolerance induction, it is quite clear that B7 molecules (CD80 and CD86) do become more highly expressed on APC *in vivo* following exposure to agonist anti-CD40 mAb, PAMPS such as LPS, or danger signals (341). Thus, their presence or absence could still play a critical role in the induction decision between tolerance and immunity under suboptimal activation conditions. *In vivo* blocking experiments with soluble CTLA-4, especially those in which the receptor has been mutated to have a higher affinity for masking B7 molecules, have revealed modest, but clinically significant, disruption of immunity, mostly involving negative effects on antibody responses *(434–437)*. Similar partial effects were observed with CD28 knockout mice, but these are complicated by the continued presence of CTLA4 *(438)*. The most revealing experiments on this issue have been carried out with gene-targeted mice lacking both B7-1 and B7-2 (439). These mice fail to reject heart allografts *(440)*, do not get allergic pulmonary inflammation following sensitization to OVA *(441)* or experimental autoimmune encephalomyelitis following injection of myelin oligodendrocyte glycoprotein (MOG) in CFA *(442)*, although the last outcome is strain-dependent *(443)*. When crossed onto the MRL/Mp-*lpr/lpr* background, the mice failed to develop autoimmunity *(444)*. An analysis *in vitro* showed that B7-deficient APCs are impaired in stimulating IL-2 production and proliferation from both naive and primed CD4$^+$ T cells *(445)*. In addition, the differentiation of naive CD4$^+$ T cells into IL-4 producers was impaired, although IFN-γ production was not, resulting in a T-helper cell 1 (Th1) bias to the weak response *(445)*. CD8$^+$ T-cell–mediated contact sensitivity was impaired at low antigen doses, but not at high doses *(446)*. Thus, B7 molecules play a critical role in the tolerance/immunity decision *in vivo*; however, they do not represent the only molecules involved in the process of costimulation and their absence can be circumvented in some immune responses of either a Th1 or Th2 nature *(446,447)*.

In general, unperturbed dendritic cells appear to be maintained in a state that predisposes to tolerance rather than immunity. This is achieved by the steady-state phagocytosis of apoptotic cell products from their environment (*448*,449). Unlike necrotic cells that promote the maturation of dendritic cells and increase their expression of costimulatory activities, many apoptotic cell products inhibit the production of proinflammatory cytokines such as IL-1, IL-8, TNF-α, granulocyte macrophage-colony stimulating factor, leukotriene C_4, and thromboxane B2 *(448,450)* and down-regulate the activation phenotype of dendritic cells by decreasing MHCII and B7-2 expression *(451)*. They also actively inhibit the response of DCs to proinflammatory stimuli such as LPS and promote the production of anti-inflammatory substances such as TGF-β1, IL-10, prostaglandin-E_2 and platelet-activating factor *(448,450,452)*. This process can be prevented by coating the apoptotic cells with antibodies that signal the phagocytic cell through the Fc receptor *(450,453)*. The induction of the "anti-inflammatory" cell program occurs via the recognition and binding of apoptotic cell products to surface receptors such as the phosphatidyl serine receptors, CD36, thrombospondin, the $\alpha v\beta 3$ and $\alpha v\beta 5$ integrins, pentraxins including serum amyloid P and C-reactive protein, collectins such as the mannose binding lectin, and the complement component C1q *(452,454–458)*. Receptor tyrosine kinases of the Tyro3/Axl/Mer family and their ligands GAS6 and protein S have been shown to be necessary for the phagocytosis of these apoptotic cell products and these receptors act as intermediates in the production of the immunosuppressive activities (459). Notably, mice that are genetically deficient for one or more of these kinases are selectively impaired in their ability to phagocytose apoptotic cells *(460–462)*. They constitutively express high levels of costimulatory molecules and develop spontaneous systemic autoimmunity. Thus, the quiescent immune system normally acts as a buffer against immune responses to discarded self-components from peripheral tissues by efficiently removing these antigens without activating costimulation.

Finally, there is the question of what happens when a dendritic cell simultaneously ingests apoptotic cells and an infectious agent expressing PAMPs? Recent work suggests that each phagocytic vacuole is independent of the other, and that TLRs in the PAMP-containing vessicle can signal the NF-κB pathway without interference from the Mer signaling pathway (463). This allows strong enough danger signals to override the anti-inflammatory program and activate the APC.

Priming of CD8$^+$ Cytotoxic T Cells Requires Three Signals

Naive CD8$^+$ T cells can be directly activated to proliferate by antigen and APC or peptide/MHC tetramers *(409,464)*. Nevertheless, many normal cytotoxic responses depend on concomitant priming of CD4$^+$ T cells in order to be sustained. Furthermore, in the Qa1 CTL model of Keene and Forman *(465)*, it was shown that activation of the CD8$^+$ T cells in the absence of CD4$^+$ T cell help resulted in CD8$^+$ T cell tolerance *(466,467)*. The nature of the help in this model was initially viewed as a three-cell interaction in which a single APC presented the antigen to activate both T cells in close proximity; then the activated CD4$^+$ T cell produced IL-2, which helped the CD8$^+$ T cell to expand and differentiate *(465)*. Subsequent studies, however, demonstrated that the information actually flows through two sequential two-cell interactions (468,*469*). The need for CD4$^+$ T-cell help could be bypassed by antibodies to CD40, which made the APC competent to present the antigen to naive CD8$^+$ T cells. B7 molecules were essential for effective stimulation, but they were not sufficient, suggesting the need for another form of costimulation. *In vitro* studies from Mescher's laboratory with a microbead presentation system showed that IL-12 can synergize with antigen and either B7 or IL-2 to prime naive CD8$^+$ T cells for IFN-γ production and CTL activity as well as stimulating proliferative expansion and increased survival through a Bcl-3–mediated mechanism *(470,471)*. Several laboratories have also shown *in vivo* that IL-12 can act as well as CFA as an adjuvant to prime naive transgenic CD8$^+$ T cells *(470,472)*. Because CD40L stimulation of APCs through CD40 greatly increases APC expression of IL-12 *(473)*, this molecule would seem to be one good candidate for the third required signal induced by CD4$^+$ T-cell help. However, it is not the only one as CD8$^+$ T-cell priming can occur in IL-12 p40-deficient mice if they are stimulated with antigen in CFA (474). Recent experiments have demonstrated that type I IFNs can also subserve the third signal function by stimulation through a STAT4-dependent pathway *(475)*. Finally, once the CD8$^+$ T cells have been activated, they express CD137, which can interact with the 4-1BB ligand on the APC to sustain CD8$^+$ T-cell proliferation and prevent apoptosis in long-term culture *(476)*.

In the absence of a third signal, the naive CD8$^+$ T cells are tolerized even though the APCs express B7 (468). As shown by Albert et al. *(472)*, the T cells undergo a weak expansion and then many of them die, similar to what is observed *in vivo* during the cross-presentation of self-antigens *(325)*. They may also undergo activation-induced cell death through a TRAIL/DR5-dependent mechanism when restimulated with antigen and APCs (477). However, many of the remaining cells appear to be anergic, that is, they fail to produce IL-2 on restimulation *(470)*. In this regard, addition of IL-12 augments the amount of CD25 expression and proliferation, which helps prevent anergy induction. It also is required for granzyme B production *(478)*. The model can also explain why CD8$^+$ T-cell priming occurs in certain viral infections in the absence of CD4$^+$ T-cell help *(479,480)*. If the virus is capable of infecting the APC, the cell can turn on IFN-$\alpha\beta$ production and up-regulate B7 expression to provide the optimal costimulatory environment required for priming of CD8 $^{+}$ T cells.

TOLERANCE INDUCTION IN MATURE B CELLS

Receptor Blockade

The induction of tolerance to foreign antigens in adult animals has a long experimental history because of its importance for potentially treating autoimmune diseases and facilitating organ transplantation. One of the earliest bodies of work was performed by Felton and colleagues (*481*,482). They studied the immunogenicity of polysaccharides from *Pneumococcus pneumoniae* and found that a dose of 0.5 mg paralyzed the immune system such that subsequent infection with the bacterium often led to death of the animal. The major immunologic effect appeared to be an inhibition of the antibody response to an optimal dose (0.5 μg) of the polysaccharide. This paralysis was specific for the particular polysaccharide used, was induced in adult animals, and lasted for a long time, presumably because of the poor degradability of the molecules. Although Felton was sure that the effect was on antibody-forming cells, it was difficult at the time to rule out a masking of the antibody response by adsorption on the persisting antigen.

In the 1950 s, a number of investigators extended these observations to protein antigens by showing that high doses of protein would paralyze the immune system and prevent it from making an antibody response to a subsequent immunogenic dose of the antigen *(346,483)*. Subsequently, Katz and colleagues *(484–486)* extended the polysaccharide experiments of Felton by examining haptens coupled to poorly degradable synthetic D amino acid copolymers. They showed that guinea pig B cells were directly affected by these antigens, even if the cells had been primed. Initially, it was thought that the B-cell unresponsiveness induced in these models might be due to receptor blockade by poorly degradable antigens stuck to the B-cell surface. Diener and Paetkau *(487)* were the first to discover that antigen given to adult animals in tolerogenic doses could persist on the surface of lymphocytes. Such cells with bound antigen were also observed in the hapten IgG model of Aldo-Benson and Borel *(488,489)*. Only tolerogenic conjugates such as DNP_{12} IgG_1 produced these cells, not closely related nontolerogenic conjugates such as DNP_{52} IgG_3 (490). At high doses of tolerogen the cells persisted for weeks, as did the tolerance, and when the tolerance waned, the cell-bound antigen was no longer detected. Culturing the cells *in vitro* allowed the antigen to be shed and the tolerance to disappear on adoptive transfer.

Physical properties of the antigen, such as size *(491–493)* and hapten density *(494)*, were shown to be important variables in receptor blockade. In a rigorous series of experiments, Dintzis et al. (495,*496*) made linear polymers of acrylamide of various lengths, coupled with haptens at various densities, and found that large polymers with high hapten density were immunogenic, whereas small polymers with low hapten density were not. The latter, however, could block activation by the former. These results were interpreted as the need for B-cell receptors to be clustered into complexes of 10 to 15 receptors each in order to signal the cell. The small polymers with low hapten density could not achieve this configuration but they were able to tie up receptors in nonproductive complexes and therefore block activation by the larger polymers. This model provides one molecular mechanism for a receptor blockade, although the type of B cell being affected (B1 vs. B2) was never fully characterized.

Another mechanism emerged from the comparison of DNP_{12} IgG_1 and DNP_{52} IgG_3 by Waldschmidt et al. (490). The class of antibody turned out to be the critical variable in determining the outcome. TNP_{11} IgG_1 induced tolerance, while TNP_{11} IgG_3 was immunogenic. Furthermore, removal of the Fc portion of the antibody from human gamma globulin to make TNP_{10} $F(ab')_2$ created an immunogen out of a tolerogen. These results suggested that engagement of the Fc receptor on B cells might be responsible for the tolerance (*497*,498). More recent studies have shown that signaling through the BCR can be inhibited if Fc receptors are simultaneously engaged in the same complex, most typically brought about by the binding of antigen-antibody complexes *(499)*.

B-Cell Anergy

The early studies convincingly demonstrated that some forms of tolerance induction in adult B cells could be reversed by trypsinization of the cells to remove bound antigen and the receptors *(500)*. This was followed by receptor re-expression. Unresponsiveness in these cases was likely caused by receptor blockade without signaling. Tolerance induced by other antigens, however, could not be reversed by simply removing the surface molecules, indicating a requirement for active metabolic processes during induction *(501)*. For example, the D amino acid copolymers induced unresponsiveness at 37°C even if the B cells were subsequently trypsinized to clear the bound immunoglobulin receptors from the cell surface. In contrast, exposure of the cells to antigen at 4°C did not induce tolerance. The low temperature presumably prevented the necessary signaling to the cell required for the tolerance. In several other systems, stimulation with mitogens such as LPS was also required to reverse B-cell tolerance (*502*,503). These observations suggested that there might exist a stable but reversible unresponsive state for mature B cells in the short-term absence of antigen.

The introduction of fluorescein-tagged and radiolabeled antigens in the late 1960s allowed for the first time the quantitation of antigen-binding cells. Most of the cells detected were B cells as defined by the expression of surface immunoglobulin. When this technique was applied to tolerant animals, whether natural or acquired through injection of high doses of antigen, the surprising observation was made that the animals had antigen-binding cells specific for the tolerogen. For example, cells binding thyroglobulin were observed repeatedly in human peripheral blood, but cells specific for human serum albumin were not *(504)*. This suggested that self-tolerance did not always involve deletion of clones as postulated by Burnet (11). Similar observations were made for protein antigens administered to adult animals *(505)*. Because the total number of B cells capable of binding labeled antigen was not diminished in these models, the tolerant state was referred to by Nossal as clonal anergy rather than clonal deletion or abortion *(505)*. This was difficult to prove, however, because in a normal mouse only 1% to 3% of the antigen-binding cells (assayed at limiting dilution) were responsive to antigen or produced specific antibodies when stimulated with LPS. Thus, a small fraction of functionally important cells might have been deleted, but their absence would have been hard to detect amidst the mass of low-affinity antigen-binding cells. Subsequent limiting dilution experiments, with a more potent mitogenic mixture of dextran sulfate and LPS as a stimulant, revealed that at least some tolerized B cells could be stimulated to differentiate into antibody-forming cells when the BCR was bypassed (503). This reversal suggested that at least a portion of the cells had been rendered functionally unresponsive (anergized) rather than deleted.

A much clearer picture of the nature of B-cell anergy became possible with the introduction of BCR transgenic mice (*334*,506). A mouse model was created by Goodnow and colleagues that expressed on its B cells a high-affinity receptor (both IgM and IgD) specific for HEL (506). About 90% of the B cells in this mouse expressed the transgenic receptor. When this BCR transgenic mouse was crossed with a second transgenic mouse constitutively expressing the lysozyme antigen in a soluble form, the double-transgenic offspring still expressed large numbers of lysozyme-binding B cells in their spleens and lymph nodes. On immunization with lysozyme, however, these B cells failed to make an antibody- or plaque-forming cell response. Because the failure to respond could have been caused by tolerance at the level of the T cells, spleen cells from these animals were transferred to irradiated, nontransgenic recipients along with spleen cells from mice primed to horse or sheep RBCs as a source of T-cell help. The recipients were then boosted with lysozyme-RBC conjugates. Compared with control BCR transgenic mice, the B cells from double-transgenic mice made a 10- to 100-fold lower plaque-forming cell response. Thus, not only had the B cells not been deleted, but they also appeared to be functionally hyporesponsive. Such a lymphocyte intrinsic, functionally unresponsive state has become the general definition for anergy.

Why are the lysozyme-specific B cells not negatively selected in the bone marrow by a central tolerance mechanism? When the gene encoding the transgenic BCR light chain was inserted into the immunoglobulin kappa locus, receptor editing was observed *(507,508)*. If lysozyme was then introduced as a transgene expressed in a membrane-bound form, all of the developing B cells underwent editing; however, if lysozyme was introduced in a soluble form, only 50% of the B cells escaped by editing *(29)*. The other 50% were found in the spleen arrested between the immature T1 ($CD23^{low}$) and T2 ($CD23^{high}$) stages *(509)*. The cells still expressed the transgenic BCR and were in an anergic state. B-cell tolerance to secreted self-antigens is thus different from that to antigen presented in a membrane-bound form. From the early *in vitro* experiments of Metcalf and Klinman (38) it is clear that to induce B-cell tolerance a molecule must be presented in a multivalent form, be present at a high enough concentration, and react with the BCR with a high enough affinity. The affinity of the transgenic BCR for lysozyme is 2×10^9 M^{-1} *(334)*. The importance of antigen concentration was confirmed *in vivo* with a series of transgenic mice that expressed lysozyme at different circulating levels (510). When the serum concentration was greater than 10^{-10} M, the B cells were anergic and the animals were tolerant, even if they were immunized in Freund's complete adjuvant with lysozyme coupled to a foreign carrier to provide T-cell help. Below 10^{-10} M, the animals were still tolerant at the T-cell level, but they could make a normal high-affinity antibody response if given heterologous T-cell help. This model for natural tolerance is also consistent with the early mouse experiments of Chiller et al. (511) done with injection of the foreign antigen human gamma globulin, where the soluble antigen dose required to tolerize T cells was lower than that required to tolerize B cells. Both these experiments support the notion that available antigen concentrations can produce situations in which only the T-cell compartment is unresponsive. The absolute concentrations required to tolerize a particular B cell will obviously vary with the affinity of the receptor; but the valency of the antigen is also critical. Basten et al. *(512)* have suggested that the tolerogenic form of lysozyme is in fact molecules bound to a high-molecular-weight serum protein, a modification that presumably would make the lysozyme multivalent. However, why this form of antigen induces anergy while a membrane bound form induces central tolerance is still not clear.

The most striking characteristic of the anergic state is a 90% reduction of IgM on the surface of the B cells resulting from endocytosis and a block in IgM re-expression during transport from the endoplasmic reticulum to the Golgi *(513)*. IgD levels are normal, as are other surface markers such as B220 and CD24. Hence, the cells are still capable of binding lysozyme and the antigen was detected on the surface of B220$^+$ cells freshly isolated from both the bone marrow and the spleen. When the BCR transgenic was crossed to an inducible lysozyme transgenic, which expressed tenfold lower levels of circulating antigen, the B cells were not tolerant and no decrease in surface IgM was noted *(514)*. Interestingly, if these animals were then fed zinc in their drinking water, induction of the metallothionein promoter of the lysozyme transgene enhanced the circulating concentrations of lysozyme by 70-fold during a 4-day period. During this time membrane IgM gradually decreased on the surface of all the transgenic BCR-bearing B cells, eventually reaching the low levels found in the initial double-transgenic mice previously described. These mature cells appeared to have been tolerized as they failed to respond well to lysozyme-RBC conjugates when adoptively transferred into irradiated mice along with horse RBC-primed helper T cells. Similar results were observed when B cells from the BCR-transgenic mice were transferred into a lysozyme transgenic mouse expressing high levels of circulating antigen. Thus, the anergic state could be induced in mature adult B cells within 4 days.

The impairment in anergic B-cell activation appears to be at the level of BCR signaling because activation for proliferation through either CD40 or TLR-2/4 is unaffected in the absence of antigen *(515,516)*. Biochemically, the anergic block is at the earliest events in signal transduction, as tyrosine kinase activity is greatly reduced *(517)*. In the presence of antigen, the IgD receptor continuously recycles between the plasma membrane and endosomes, and a large fraction is always found intracellularly, in contrast to the BCR on nonanergic B cells (518). This results in diminished calcium oscillations and a failure to activate the transcription factor NF-κB, as well as the JNK MAP kinase pathway *(519)*. In contrast, activation of the NF-AT transcription factor and stimulation through the ERK pathway is normal. The former induces the negative regulator CD5, while the later inhibits plasma cell differentiation *(520,521)*. The BCR signaling block prevents the normal up-regulation of the B7 costimulatory molecules *(522,523)*. Finally, PKC-δ is required to achieve an anergic state as shown by the development of autoimmunity instead of anergy when a PKC-δ–deficient mouse was crossed onto the lysozyme double-transgenic background *(524)*. PKC-δ seems to be necessary for the IgD endocytosis (518).

The anergic state can be reversed in culture by stimulation with LPS *(515)*. Although the initial proliferative response is somewhat less than for normal B cells, the anergic B cells fully re-express surface IgM by 2 days and after 3 days their antibody production increases. If antigen was included in the culture along with LPS, however, the B cells' ability to secrete antibody remained inhibited, even though they proliferated just as well during the treatment. This suggests that BCR occupancy by antigen is the critical signal for maintaining the state as well as inducing it. In this sense anergy can be viewed as a BCR-desensitization process stemming from the constant signaling of the receptor.

The fate of anergic B cells *in vivo* was examined by bromodeoxyuridine-labeling studies to determine the turnover of the cells *(525)*. In contrast to normal mature B cells, which have a half-life of 4 to 5 weeks, anergic B cells were found to last for only 3 to 4 days, and they tended not to enter into lymphoid follicles during their migration *(526)*. The rate of emergence of B cells into the mature pool was similar for the two types of cells, suggesting that anergic B cells died more quickly in the periphery *(525)*. These events, however, occurred only in the presence of antigen. If the anergic B cells were adoptively transferred into irradiated, antigen-free recipients, the cells survived as long as normal B cells *(515,526)*. Interestingly, their IgM levels returned to normal after 5 to 10 days, but when challenged with antigen, they still did not respond well. Thus, decreased IgM serves as a marker for some anergic cells, but it is not the only component needed for the unresponsiveness.

Surprisingly, the fate of the anergic cells in response to antigen and T-cell help turned out to be cell death *(527)*. Nontolerant B cells from the BCR single-transgenic mice proliferated and made antibodies against lysozyme when stimulated with antigen in the presence of CD4$^+$ T cells from a lysozyme-specific TCR transgenic. In contrast, if the B cells came from a double-transgenic mouse, where they had been exposed continuously to soluble circulating lysozyme, the anergic B cells underwent cell death by apoptosis in response to the same stimulus. Death was prevented on a CD95-deficient (lpr) background, suggesting that the Fas/Fas ligand pathway was necessary for the killing. Subsequent studies demonstrated that the CD40 receptor also had to be engaged in order to obtain cell death, because signaling through CD40 was required to up-regulate Fas expression on anergic B cells (528). Normal transgenic B cells did not die under the same circumstances and in fact required both CD40 ligation and Fas expression for optimal clonal expansion and antibody production (528,*529*). If, however, BCR occupancy by antigen was bypassed, by pulsing the B cells with the peptide recognized by T cells, then even nontolerant B cells were killed (528). These results suggest that for mature B cells signal two alone (as might occur in certain bystander situations) can be tolerogenic. Thus, signaling through the BCR is critical for determining the outcome of helper T-cell/B-cell interactions, and, presumably, anergic B cells die because of their partial block in BCR signaling.

In contrast, two other groups were able to get the anergic B cells to make an antibody response in an *in vivo* adoptive transfer system by providing antigen-specific T-cell help *(516,529)*. In the lysozyme system they achieved this by immunizing with the antigen in CFA *(516)*. One interpretation of this result is that the PAMPS and danger signals provided by the adjuvant induced the up-regulation of antiapoptotic proteins (such as bcl-2), which counteract the elevated levels of Bim present in anergic B cells, and thus protect the cells from apoptosis (530). In a like manner, anergic B cells survive poorly when in the presence of other B cells because of competition for the costimulatory molecule BAFF, which maintains B-cell viability through enhancement of the levels of NF-κB p52 and the prosurvival kinase Pim2 (530). When on their own, however, a large fraction of the anergic B cells survive much longer as there is now sufficient BAFF available per cell to stimulate them adequately through the BAFF-R. Low levels of CD40 signaling from CD40L engagement can also help sustain these cells *(531)*.

Recently a number of investigators have examined BCR transgenics specific for autoantigens involved in systemic lupus erythematosus pathogenesis such as double-stranded (ds) and single-stranded (ss) DNA and the ribonucleoprotein Smith antigen (Sm) *(529,532)*. Several of these transgenes were placed on a Rag2$^{-/-}$ or a C$\kappa^{-/-}$ background to eliminate complications in the phenotype stemming from receptor editing. These studies have revealed a spectrum of tolerance states that the B cell can adopt to suppress antibody production against self-antigens. At one extreme is a high-affinity BCR for ds-DNA in which all of the cells in the transgenic mouse are deleted in the bone marrow *(533)*. In contrast, another transgenic with the same heavy chain and a different light chain showed modest deletion in the bone marrow and a significant cohort of cells surviving in the spleen (534). The latter manifested an unusual surface phenotype that was immature for B-cell maturation markers, for example, CD24^{int}, but showed the presence of activation markers such as CD44^{high}. Their IgM levels were decreased tenfold and the cells did not proliferate *in vitro* to either LPS or anti-IgM stimulation. They also did not differentiate into antibody-secreting cells. This anergic state could be partially overcome *in vitro* by stimulation with CD154 and IL-4, which restored IgM expression, tyrosine phosphorylation of Syk, up-regulation of B7, and proliferation. However, the cells did not differentiate into antibody-forming cells even if IL-5 was added to the cultures. *In vivo*, the anergic cells were found only at the T-B interface of splenic follicles; they did not secrete antibodies; and they had a very fast turnover rate, suggesting that they were dying quickly. However, if given strong T-cell help, the B cells lost their anergic phenotype and secreted autoantibody *(529)*. Interestingly, this secretion could be prevented if the anergy was reversed in the presence of CD4^{+}CD25^{+} Tregs.

At the other end of the spectrum are transgenic mice with BCRs specific for ss-DNA *(535)* and one with a low-avidity BCR for Sm *(532)*. In both cases, the B cells fully matured and had a normal follicular distribution and lifespan. IgM levels were normal or only slightly decreased and signaling for tyrosine phosphorylation of Syk and increases in intracellular calcium were intact. Nonetheless, the cells showed decreased antibody and proliferative responses to both LPS and anti-IgM stimulation *in vitro* and did not secret antibody *in vivo*. The proliferative block could be overcome by addition of CD154 and IL-4 to the anti-IgM, but antibody production was still impaired, most likely because of continued antigen stimulation of the ERK Map kinase pathway *(520)*. This maturational arrest occurs at an early CD138^{+} preplasma cell (Blimp-1–negative) stage and is followed by B-cell apoptosis (536). Overall, this anergic state appears to be less profound than that observed for B cells in the soluble lysozyme double-transgenic mouse, while the lysozyme BCR transgenic is less repressed than the state for ds-DNA. These experiments suggest that B-cell anergy (like T-cell anergy) can exist at different levels, consistent with the tuning idea of Grossman and Paul (537).

B-Cell Clonal Deletion

The first experiments to show peripheral clonal deletion with BCR transgenic mice were done by Russell et al. (538) using a receptor specific for the K^{b} MHC class I molecule. This mouse was crossed to an MHC transgenic mouse expressing K^{b} in the liver, pancreas, and kidney, under the control of a metallothionein promoter. The double-transgenic offspring had only a few transgene-receptor positive B cells in the spleen and lymph node, although there were large numbers in the bone marrow. Because the number of B220^{+} cells was also greatly reduced in the peripheral lymphoid tissues and because no mRNA encoding the transgenic receptor could be detected, it was concluded that the B cells had been deleted. Thus, B-cell recognition of K^{b} in certain peripheral tissues, even with low affinity in this particular case, resulted in a tolerant state. The mechanism of this tolerance is likely to be clonal deletion, but cells undergoing apoptosis were not detected. In contrast, expression in thyroid epithelium of a membrane-bound form of lysozyme under the control of a thyroglobulin promoter did not lead to either clonal elimination or functional inactivation of BCR-transgenic B cells specific for lysozyme *(539)*. The reason for the discrepancy between the two models is not known, but may relate to the accessibility of naive B cells to the antigen in the different target tissues.

In general, once a B cell has been activated by a foreign antigen and divides, many of its progeny terminally differentiate into antibody-forming cells and die. This process is retarded in *lpr* and *gld* mice because of genetic defects in the Fas or Fas ligand molecules required for cell death *(540)*. These mice get an antibody-mediated autoimmune disease similar to systemic lupus erythematosis in humans with the production of anti-ds DNA autoantibodies and the development of glomerulonephritis *(541)*. B-cell death is also impaired in bcl-2 transgenic mice, which express the antiapoptotic bcl-2 protein at high levels in the B-cell lineage *(542)*. These mice get B-cell lymphomas *(543)* as well as autoimmunity (544). Based on these indirect experiments it is assumed that apoptotic cell death is a normal part of the B-cell response to foreign antigens and that this is at least in part Fas/FasL-mediated. The observations also suggest that Fas-dependent death helps maintain self-tolerance by deleting peripheral B cells that have generated autoreactive receptors.

A substantial portion of the activated B cells also migrate to germinal centers where they undergo the process of somatic hypermutation *(545)*. These B cells first remove the BCR from their surface, undergo several rounds of division, and re-express mutated immunoglobulin receptors *(546)*. The cells then undergo a negative selection process similar to that of transitional B cells. The antigen is provided from antigen-antibody complexes on follicular dendritic cells *(547)*. Survival requires the receptor to be of high enough affinity to out-compete the already circulating antibody and allow B-cell uptake and processing of antigen for display of peptides to primed helper T cells, which have also moved into the germinal centers (545,548). If the B cell receives T-cell help it survives and is stimulated to undergo another round of expansion and differentiation. If T-cell help is not received, the B cells can become anergized or die by apoptosis. Apoptotic cell death was demonstrated by two groups by giving large amounts of soluble antigen at the time of optimal germinal center formation (549,*550*). The antigen was selected to either lack the critical T-cell determinant required for help or deaggregated by ultracentrifugation (in the manner of Dresser *[346]*) to reduce APC processing for T-cell activation. In each case, the high-affinity B cells, located in both the germinal centers and the nearby lymphoid zones rich in T cells, underwent apoptosis rather than the affinity maturation seen with T-cell help. Thus, just as for transitional B cells, signaling of primed B cells in the absence of T-cell help can result in deletional tolerance. In the opposite vein, if excess costimulation is provided by microbial infection, then even low-avidity T cells that have escaped central tolerance might migrate into germinal centers and provide help to low-avidity cross-reactive or somatically mutated autoreactive B cells. An ENU-induced mutation in an E3 ubiquitin ligase that normally down-regulates mRNA stability, resulted in an overexpression of CXCR5, ICOS and IL-21 in all its T cells *(551)*. This led to an excess of follicular T cells in an increased number of germinal centers, and resulted in high titers of autoantibodies and a lupus-like immunopathology.

TOLERANCE INDUCTION IN MATURE T CELLS

Activation-induced Cell Death and Homeostasis

The frequency of responding T cells in an MLR is quite high, ranging from 2% to 5% of the $CD4^+$ T-cell population *(552)*. Proliferation following priming does not increase this frequency, suggesting that many of the dividing cells must die *(553)*. Sprent *(554)* and Sprent and Miller *(555)* followed the fate of the reactive cells in this assay by isolating 4-day blasts from the thoracic duct of F_1 mice injected with parental cells, labeling the cells and transferring them back to syngeneic parental hosts. These cells homed to the spleen and intestine and then most of them disappeared, appearing to die *in situ* and be degraded by macrophages or be excreted into the lumen of the gut over a 2-week period. Only a few survived to become memory cells, which were capable of responding more rapidly.

Modern studies on the fate of T cells stimulated with superantigens have confirmed these early findings with alloreactive T cells. Injection of spleen cells expressing Mtv-7 into mice lacking Mtv-7 (556) or injection of staphylococcal enterotoxin B (SEB) *(557)* or A *(558)* into strains expressing Vβ8 and/or Vβ3 T cells, results in an initial expansion of the reactive T cells followed by extensive death via apoptosis. This is not simply a phenomenon observed with superantigens because transfer into male nude mice of spleen cells from a transgenic female mouse expressing the TCR$\alpha\beta$ anti-H-Y receptor resulted in a similar expansion and disappearance of $CD8^+$ T cells (559). The general pattern of response to all of these stimuli is shown in Figure 29.3.

The biochemical pathway responsible for signalling the cell to die is still not fully understood. *In vivo* studies have suggested that killing of $CD4^+$ T cells can be mediated by reactive oxygen species *(560)*. Also in an *in vitro* reactivation model it was shown that IFN-γ produced by activated $CD4^+$ cells could stimulate granulocytes to make NO and reactive oxygen intermediates, which in turn killed the activated $CD4^+$ cells *(561)*. For death receptor (e.g., Fas)-mediated killing, the activated T cell is initially resistant because the cells express a signaling antagonist called *c-Flip (562)* and because the costimulation accompanying T-cell stimulation increases the synthesis of antiapoptotic bcl-2 family members such as Bcl-2 and Bcl-X_L (190,420). When the latter decay, however, the proapoptotic BH3-only molecule Bim predominates and the cell becomes vulnerable to apoptotic cell death (563). If restimulated through the antigen-receptor, the surviving cells can now be killed by a rapid re-expression of Fas or TNF ligands (*564*,565) (see discussion of active death in Chapter 27). Other cells die simply when their growth factors are withdrawn (passive death) *(566)*. This last mechanism involves down-regulation of the glucose transporter, atrophy of the cell, and mitochondrial changes leading to cytochrome c release and apoptosis (567). These mechanisms are important for maintaining peripheral tolerance as shown by genetic mutations in their pathways (e.g., *lpr* [Fas] and *gld* [FasL]), which lead to autoimmune disease *(568)*.

Several experiments have demonstrated that the initial expansion phase of the T-cell response is started by the

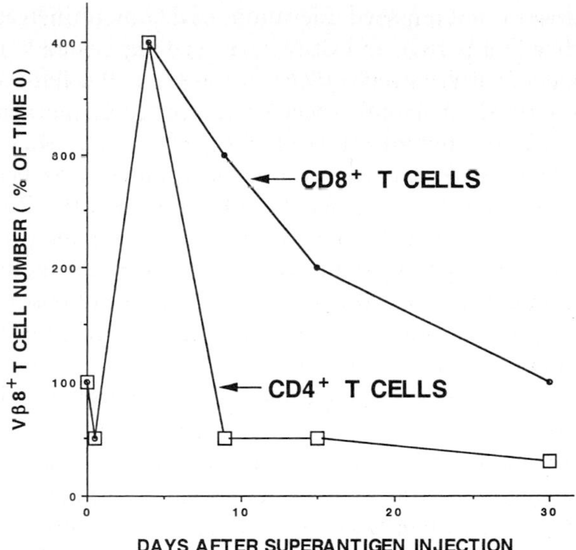

FIGURE 29.3 The general pattern of *in vivo* responses of CD4+ and CD8+ T cells to superantigen and antigen stimulation. The response of Vβ8+ T cells to staphylococcal enterotoxin B is shown as a model. The response occurs in four phases. During the first 12 hours, the massive release of cytokines from memory T cells can result in significant cell death in the stimulated cells. In the second phase, the remaining stimulated cells divide, increasing two- to eightfold over a period of 4 days. In the third phase, CD4+ T cells die off rapidly but leave a residue of cells that appear to be anergized. In the fourth phase, the anergized cells slowly disappear. CD8+ T cells, in contrast, slowly decrease in number from their peak expansion, returning to normal levels after 30 days. Whether these cells become anergic depends on the presence or absence of effective CD4+ T-cell help.

first encounter with antigen and that the cells are then programmed under optimum conditions to go through four to eight rounds of division without any restimulation (569,*570,571*). At the end of this period the cells stop proliferating and then must receive further instructions to determine their fate. Death is only one possible outcome and all the quantitative parameters that influence the cell's fate at this point are not understood. CD28 signaling does not protect against activation-induced cell death induced by superantigens or antigen (572). Only LPS or proinflammatory cytokines such as IL-1 and TNF-α prevented it (572,*573*). One way these molecules act is through up-regulation of the IκB family member Bcl-3, which in expression experiments was shown to have antiapoptotic effects *(574)*.

Interestingly, only the CD4+ T cells die rapidly at day 4 following SEB injection; CD8+ T cells do not (Figure 29.3). Thus, a completely different explanation for CD4+ T cell depletion has been proposed. Removal of CD8+ T cells from the mice prior to SEB injection, by treatment with anti-CD8 antibody, prevented the rapid loss of CD4+ T cells *(575)*. Similar results were observed with CD8 removal in an EAE resistance model following secondary immunization with myelin basic protein (576). The authors postulated that the activated CD8+ T cells kill off the activated CD4+ T cells by a perforin/granzyme-mediated cytotoxicity mechanism involving recognition of the Qa-1 molecule. Recent experiments with Qa-1–deficient mice have demonstrated that both antigen- and superantigen-mediated CD4+ T cell secondary expansion is greatly exaggerated in the knockout, which can lead to augmented autoimmune disease subsequent to decreased CD8+ T-cell–mediated inhibition (577). The molecular mechanism for initiating this inhibition is not known, but may involve a TAP-independent, Qa-1 presentation of hydrophobic peptides derived from the CD4+ TCR *(578–580)*.

One of the most interesting aspects of all these observations is that 90% of T cells responding to antigen or superantigen die. This is best understood in the context of homeostatic regulation of the immune system rather than antigen-specific tolerance per se. There is only so much space in the body for lymphocytes and room must be maintained for the influx of new naive cells from the thymus as well as the preservation of memory T cells for an extended period of time. Transfer of splenic T cells into nude mice showed that the cells could expand only until a critical cell number is reached (approximately 2×10^8 cells per mouse) *(581–583)*. Surprisingly, memory T cells and naive T cells were independently regulated, that is, each subpopulation did not influence the expansion of the other (584). Their half-lives were also controlled in different manners as many naive T cells were dependent on TCR recognition of self-MHC molecules for survival, whereas memory T cells were not *(585–587)*. The latter depended on cytokines such as IL-7 and IL-15 (*588*,589). In the immune response to a virus, Masopust et al. *(590)* have shown that the frequency of the responding antigen-specific cells increases dramatically over an 8-day period, up to a frequency of 80% or more of the total CD8+ T cells in the spleen. As these cells begin to effectively eliminate the virus, however, their frequency drops and in the memory phase of the response it becomes only 1/300 to 1/1000 of the total CD8+ pool *(591)*. Thus, homeostasis is maintained by allowing most of the newly generated cells to die by an apoptotic mechanism once the antigen is cleared *(592)*.

T-Cell Anergy

Anergy is a peripheral tolerance mechanism in which the lymphocyte intrinsically becomes functionally inactivated following an antigen encounter, but remains alive for an extended period of time as a hyporesponsive cell (406). The first description of a CD4+ T-cell anergic state was in human (593) and mouse (351) clones and is now referred to as T-cell clonal anergy (406). Activation of CD4+ Th1 clones to proliferate requires intact APCs. If the APCs are chemically treated with fixatives such as paraformaldehyde and then used to present peptide antigens, the T cells do not proliferate. Instead, by 6 to 18 hours they have entered a new state in which they fail to make IL-2 or proliferate when restimulated with normal APC and antigen (351). The T cells are still alive because they can proliferate in response to added IL-2, and in fact this response brings them out of the state (*594*,595). Without IL-2 the unresponsiveness can last for several weeks in the absence of any further antigen addition. Simultaneous studies using planar lipid membranes, composed of MHC class II molecules on a plastic surface and pulsed with peptide antigen, induced the same state *(353)*. This suggested that TCR occupancy was all that was required to induce clonal anergy. Subsequent reconstitution experiments supported this idea. Addition of untreated, allogeneic APC (which could not present the peptide), along with chemically fixed syngeneic APC and peptide, prevented the induction of the unresponsive state *(352)*. It also reconstituted the initial proliferative response. This suggested that the fixed cells were presenting antigen properly but that the fixation prevented other signals from being delivered by the APC. No soluble cytokines were effective in substituting for the allogeneic APC, and eventually the CD28 molecule was identified as the costimulatory receptor on the T cell required for the IL-2 production *(596)*. Agonist anti-CD28 antibodies were subsequently shown to prevent clonal anergy induction *(597)*. The ligand on the APC could be either B7-1 (CD80) or B7-2 (CD86). The biochemical block in clonal anergy was subsequently shown to be at the level of activation of the Ras/MAP kinase pathway by inhibiting the usual increase in GTP-$p21^{Ras}$ following TCR stimulation *(598,599)* Recent experiments suggest that this stems at least in part from an increased expression of the protein diacylglycerol kinase-α, which depletes the second messenger diacylglycerol by phosphorylating it; this prevents RasGRP1 from mobilizing to the plasma membrane and activating Raf (600,*601*). The block in MAP kinase activation prevents the induction of transcription factors such as AP-1, and this in turn prevents the production of IL-2 *(602)*.

In addition to induction by TCR occupancy in the absence of costimulation, clonal anergy has also been achieved by stimulation with low-affinity peptide ligands (partial agonists) in the presence of costimulation (603,*604*). This stimulus represents a suboptimal activation of the T cell that is inadequate to drive the cell into division, but adequate to induce the dominant biochemical feedback mechanism(s) that blocks subsequent proliferative responses to normal activating stimuli. Both types of clonal anergy induction require activation of the calcium/calcineurin pathway with mobilization of NF-AT to the nucleus and activation of genes not requiring AP-1, such as Egr2/3 (605,*606*). Induction can be partially mimicked by calcium ionophore stimulation (605,*607*), but the fully stable state also requires other signaling pathways such as PKC activation *(606)*. Activation of the MAP kinase pathway is not required. Elevations of E3 ubiquitin ligases such as Cbl-b, Itch, and Grail have been implicated in the induction process (608,*609,610*). A role for the cell-cycle inhibitor $p27^{kip1}$ has also been suggested for anergic states derived from costimulatory blockade *(611,612)*. CD28 costimulation prevents anergy induction indirectly by its enhancement of IL-2 production, and subsequent IL-2R signaling to activate the downstream kinase mTOR (613). Thus, the drug rapamycin, which blocks mTOR function, favors anergy induction even in the presence of costimulation. How activation of mTOR prevents or reverses the increase in the level of diacylglycerol kinase-α, which maintains the state of clonal anergy, is currently not understood.

Murine T cell clonal anergy is primarily a growth arrest state (406). The production of cytokines such as IL-2 and IL-3, which can augment T-cell proliferation, is strongly inhibited, while IL-4 production is unaffected (595). Instead, the proliferative response to IL-4 is blocked *(614)*. C-C chemokine production is also unaffected and there is only a small effect on IFN-γ production in Th1 clones *(615)*. This pattern, however, is not universal for all models of clonal anergy. In humans, antigen presentation by T cells to a $CD4^+$ T cell clone, even in the presence of costimulation, leads to an unresponsive state (593). In mice, overnight treatment of T-cell clones with just a calcium ionophore can induce a similar state (605). In these cases the anergic cells fail to produce IL-4 and IFN-γ in addition to IL-2. The cells also display a block in calcium signaling (605,*616*), which is not observed in other murine models *(617)*, and which could account for their more profound inhibition. There are also cases of deeper states of clonal anergy in other murine systems *(618,619)*. In several of these, CTLA-4 signaling has been shown to play a critical role in preventing certain of the T-cell responses and inducing anergy (*423,424*,620,*621*), but not in other models *(425,426)*.

$CD8^+$ murine T-cell clones can also be induced into a clonal anergic state by antigen/APC stimulation in the absence of costimulation *(622)*. The phenotype is again an inhibition of IL-2 production and proliferation with little effect on IFN-γ production or CTL activity. More recently, a form of clonal anergy has been described following $CD8^+$ T-cell stimulation called *activation-induced nonresponsiveness* (AINR) (474). This state ensues several days after optimal T-cell stimulation through the TCR, CD28, and the IL-12R. The $CD8^+$ T cells lose the capacity to proliferate in response to the continued presence of antigen *(623)*. They also lose their ability to make IL-2, but retain effector functions such as IFN-γ production and CTL activity. AINR biochemically resembles the clonal anergic state of $CD4^+$ T cells in that activation of all the MAP kinase pathways (ERK, JNK, and p38) is inhibited *(624)*. Also similar is the fact that AINR can be overcome if large enough quantities of IL-2 are provided either by $CD4^+$ T-cell help or by IL-2 added exogenously during the course of the immune response (625). The induction of AINR even in the presence of B7 costimulation and some division is presumably because the CD8$^+$ T cells cannot produce enough IL-2 on their own (usually 1/8 of what a CD4$^+$ T cell produces under optimal stimulation conditions *[626]*) to generate sufficient mTOR activation. This phenomenon helps to make long-term CD8$^+$ T cell expansion dependent on CD4$^+$ T-cell help *(627)*.

The first description of an anergic state *in vivo* was made in mice injected with superantigens (628). In animals given SEB or Mtv7$^+$ spleen cells, there remains a population of Vβ8$^+$ CD4$^+$ T cells that fails to proliferate or produce IL-2 on restimulation with the superantigens *in vitro* *(629–631)* (Figure 29.3). These cells stay in this functionally unresponsive state for weeks, especially if the animals have been thymectomized, but eventually the state reverses or the cells disappear (556,*558*). Similar phenomena were observed in radiation-induced bone marrow chimeras expressing MHC Class II E molecules and Mtv7 solely in cells of the irradiated host (632). The Vβ6$^+$ and Vβ17$^+$ T cells (CD4$^+$ and CD8$^+$) interacting with the Mtv superantigen were not deleted, although these cells (either mature thymocytes or peripheral lymph node cells) appeared to be functionally unresponsive in a MLR *in vitro* as well as in a graft-versus-host response following adoptive transfer *in vivo*. Furthermore, attempts to directly stimulate the cells to proliferate using anti-Vβ antibodies on a plate were unsuccessful. Addition of exogenous IL-2 gave only a partial recovery of the proliferative response, suggesting that both IL-2 production and responsiveness to IL-2 were blocked. Subsequent experiments showed that the unresponsive state could be reversed if the T cells were cultured in the absence of antigen (either *in vitro* or *in vivo*), thus proving that the cells had not been deleted *(633)*. This tolerance process most likely ensued in the thymic medulla, but it is not clear at which T-cell stage.

Such observations were extended to conventional antigens with TCR transgenic mice either by crossing them to a mouse expressing the antigen they recognized or by transferring their mature T cells directly into this second mouse (559,634,*635–637*). In the H-Y transgenic model described earlier (638), the CD8$^+$ T cells become unresponsive when the cells are put into an environment in which the male antigen they recognize is highly expressed and cannot be eliminated (e.g., following transfer into a male nude mouse). If the CD8$^+$ T cells are subsequently removed from this environment and placed in a female nude mouse, they recover their function *(639)*. Dependence of CD4$^+$ T cell unresponsiveness on the persistence of antigen has also been reported *(636)*. The unresponsiveness in these models has been called *adaptive tolerance* (406), and appears to be similar to anergic states seen following certain persistent viral and bacterial infections (*640*,641,*642*). Another possibly similar *in vivo* anergic state has been described when CD4$^+$ transgenic T cells are first transferred into a syngeneic host and then stimulated with soluble peptide ligand in the absence of a costimulatory signal such as LPS *(643)*.

The unresponsive state for both CD4$^+$ and CD8$^+$ T cells involves a failure to produce IL-2 on restimulation with the antigen and APC; however, the production of other cytokines varies with the model. In many cases, all cytokine production is inhibited *(636)*, while in others the cells were found to make IL-10 (634). Proliferation in most of these models is inhibited, and a few also show a failure to respond to IL-2. In all of them, the T cells regain responsiveness if they are transferred into an environment that is no longer expressing the antigen *(633,636,637,643)*. If transferred into a host expressing the antigen, the T cells can sometimes even go into a more profound unresponsive state *(636)*. Persistent antigen expression is the critical variable determining the fate of the T cells *(644)*, with repetitive low doses favoring deletion and high doses favoring anergy *(645)*. Even if the T cells are initially activated in the presence of strong costimulation (such as anti-CD40), their eventual fate is tolerance if the antigen persists *(637)*.

A number of biochemical studies have been done with the *in vivo* models involving TCR transgenics, because there is a large enough number of cells to study. It appears for many of them that the anergic state represents a block at the earliest steps of TCR-induced tyrosine phosphorylation *(631,646–648)*. Activation-induced ZAP-70 phosphorylation is generally reduced and the downstream phosphorylation of the LAT adaptor molecule is strongly inhibited *(648–650)*. This impairs PLC-γ1, Grb2-mSOS, and RasGRP1 activation, resulting in inhibition of both calcium mobilization and activation of the Ras/MAP kinase pathway. This pattern is different from some of the *in vitro* clonal anergy models *(648)*. In addition, the individual *in vivo* models show their own idiosyncrasies. For example, in the superantigen models, Cbl-b appears to play a critical role in maintaining the unresponsive state (608,*609*), as does an enhancement in the activity of the p38 pathway *(651)*. The former acts in preactivated T cells by ubiquitination and targeting of PLC-γ1 for degradation; the latter acts by inhibiting activation of the ERK pathway. Neither of these components, however, plays a critical role in adaptive tolerance. Similarly, a key role has been demonstrated for CTLA-4 signaling in the anergy induced by soluble peptide stimulation *(423)*, but it plays no role in the onset of adaptive tolerance *(426)*. Overall, these studies suggest that there may be multiple ways in which a T cell can exert negative feedback on its TCR signaling pathways. Thus, *in vivo* anergy models may have several different molecular mechanisms operating to ensure unresponsiveness.

What is the biological purpose of *in vivo* anergy? Because in many cases the state reverses when the antigen is removed, perhaps it represents an adaptation of the cell to the persistence of antigen in its environment, a form of TCR desensitization consistent with the Tunable Activation Threshold model of Grossman and Paul (537). In a

CD4 adaptive tolerance model, it was possible to show that the biochemical and functional response to the same dose of antigen of a TCR transgenic, anergic population varied depending on the level of chronic antigen exposure responsible for first inducing the state *(652)*. Thus, the function of the anergic state would be to retain a potentially useful cell in a harmless mode by raising its threshold for activation for a certain period of time until a decision can be made as to whether it is autoreactive or critical for host defense. The half-life of these cells in the absence of other T cells is long, but in the presence of normal T cells the anergic cells disappear more quickly by an unknown competitive or suppressive mechanism (653). In these transgenic models, the anergic T cells often retain partial effector functions and can eventually cause autoimmunity (653,654). In the case of chronic viral infections, however, the dampening of proliferative capacity is followed by the dampening of effector function: B-cell help for $CD4^+$ cells and TNF-α and IFN-γ production as well as CTL-activity for $CD8^+$ cells (641,*655*,656). In $CD8^+$ T cells the anergic state has been called *functional exhaustion*. It can be tuned to different levels of unresponsiveness, at least partly depending on signaling through the PD-1 receptor *(430)*. The anergic antiviral $CD4^+$ and $CD8^+$ cells persist for a long period of time even in the presence of normal T cells, possibly because the viral load continually fluctuates from replication or because the virus continues to elicit danger signals and costimulation. Premature entry into this anergic state can have deleterious effects, such as impairment of an effective immune response to a subsequent viral infection *(657)*. However, if appropriately timed with the clearance of the virus it can reduce immunopathology. When this state is induced in the thymus, it can also serve as a central tolerance mechanism in cases where the antigen is expressed both there and in the periphery *(658)*.

IMMUNOREGULATION

Once an immune response is underway, the nature of that response can feed back on the system in a number of ways to focus it on particular effector functions or to inhibit immunopathologic consequences. This section will briefly outline some of these mechanisms as they can formally be considered tolerance mechanisms when the immune system fails to reject the antigen because of them. A number of these topics, however, are covered in much greater detail in other sections of this book.

Immune Deviation (Th1 vs. Th2 and Th17 $CD4^+$ helpers)

The phenomenon of immune deviation was first described by Asherson and Stone (659). They injected guinea pigs with soluble or alum-precipitated antigens 2 weeks prior to challenge with the same antigen in Freund's complete adjuvant. The pretreatment prevented the usual delayed-type hypersensitivity (DTH) response measured as 24-hour skin reactions on rechallenge. In contrast, antibody production was normal, although the class of antibody was deviated from IgG2 toward IgG1 *(660)*. Parish and Liew (661) subsequently discovered a general reciprocal relationship between antibody production and DTH reactions as a function of antigen dose. When small doses of antigen were administered, the immune response was predominantly DTH. As the antigen dose was increased, an antibody response was observed, while the DTH response diminished. At very high doses of antigen, the antibody response also declined and in some cases the DTH response re-emerged. With the introduction of T-cell cloning technology, Mosmann et al. *(662)* discovered that fully differentiated mouse T-cell clones generally exhibit one of two discrete lymphokine production profiles *(662)*. Th1 cells make IL-2, IFN-γ, and TNF-β, while Th2 cells make IL-4, IL-5, and IL-13. This cellular dichotomy provided a potential explanation for immune deviation because these two cell types could cross-regulate each other. Lymphokines produced by Th1 cells turned out to be primarily mediators for stimulating macrophage activation via induction of IFN-γ and complement fixing IgG_{2a} antibodies, as well as CD8 T-cell activation for viral clearance, while those produced by Th2 cells were primarily activators of eosinophils and mediators of helper T-cell function for IgG_1 and IgE antibody production to aid in the clearance of parasites (663,664). The cross-regulation is also mediated by these lymphokines. Thus, IFN-γ produced by Th1 cells inhibits the proliferation of Th2 cells *(665)* by blocking costimulation by IL-1 *(666)*. A comparable antagonism occurs within the Th1 cell, where up-regulation of the transcription factor T-bet opposes the expression of the Th2 master regulator GATA-3 *(667)*. In a reciprocal manner, in Th2 cells GATA-3 expression inhibits STAT4 and the IL12Rβ2 protein preventing IL-12 augmentation of Th1 differentiation *(668)*. In naive cells IL-4 signaling also prevents colocalization of the IFN-γ receptor with the TCR at the immunologic synapse, which impairs Th1 development *(669)*. The initial discovery of IL-10 was as an inhibitory cytokine produced by Th2 cells *(670)*. It prevented the stimulation of Th1 cells by blocking APC function and by preventing lymphocyte production of IL-2 and TNF-α *(670,671)*. However, subsequent work showed that both cell types could produce IL-10 (672) and that it primarily facilitates the generation of T-regulatory 1 (Tr1) cells from naive $CD4^+$ T cells (673). It also can augment the effector function of both B cells *(674)* and $CD8^+$ T cells *(675)*. Thus, IL-10 is now generally thought of as immunosuppressive for both Th1 and Th2 cell differentiation.

The forces that operate to determine the dominance of Th1 versus Th2 cells in any given immune response are not completely understood. The dose of antigen is critical and the genetic constitution of the responding individual determines which particular doses are perceived as high and low. In the *Leishmania major* parasite model, BALB/c mice make predominantly a nonprotective Th2 response, whereas C3H and C57BL/6 mice make predominantly a protective Th1 response *(676)*. If, however, the BALB/c mice are inoculated with a minute number of parasites (less than 30), they become protected against a normal challenge dose because of immune deviation toward an IFN-γ response *(677)*. The antigen specificity of the response is also a critical variable. A single immunodominant determinant of the *Leishmania* is recognized in the early response of the BALB/c mouse *(678)*. If tolerance is induced to the protein containing this determinant, then the mouse mounts a protective Th1 immune response *(679)*. Another critical parameter is the cytokine milieu. High concentrations of IL-4 deviate the response toward Th2 (680), while high concentrations of IL-12 deviate the response toward Th1 *(681)*. Furthermore, the molecular form of the antigen is also influential, with particulate antigens favoring macrophage uptake and IL-12 production, which helps skew the response toward a Th1 phenotype *(681,682)*. CD8$^+$ T cells can similarly be affected by these parameters to give rise to Tc1 and Tc2 cells (683).

Recently another subset, Th17, has been described that augments recruitment of neutrophils to sites of inflammation to deal with extracellular bacterial pathogens (684). This subset is uniquely induced by the combined stimulation of naive T cells with IL-6 and TGF-β *(685–687)* through activation of the orphan nuclear receptor RORγt *(688)*, and is augmented in number and survival by subsequent stimulation with IL-23, once the IL-23R is induced *(689–691)*. The molecular details of how this subset is regulated have not yet been fully worked out, but it is already clear that Th1 and Th2 cells compete with it and that IFN-γ and IL-4 negatively regulate Th17 generation *(692,693)*. Thus, the principle of class regulation of the immune response by different T-cell subsets will most certainly be a generalizable phenomenon. A tolerance process could then be defined from this regulation as one that deviates the immune response toward a class of effector cells that does not cause immunopathology.

Induced CD4$^+$ T Regulatory Cells (Tr1 and iTreg)

Tr1 cells were first discovered in severe combined immunodeficient (SCID) patients who had received HLA-mismatched hemopoietic stem cells and appeared to be tolerant (*694*,695). The cells were CD4$^+$ and produced IL-10 on stimulation with host APC. They also made TGF-β, IL-5, and small amounts of IFN-γ, but not much IL-2 and no IL-4 *(696)*. They did not proliferate well when stimulated through their TCR and were described as anergic *(697)*. This clonal anergy also included a lack of IL-2R expression. Most interestingly, the cells were found to suppress the activation of other naive and memory CD4$^+$ and CD8$^+$ T cells by indirectly inhibiting APC function, through down-regulation of both MHC class II molecules and costimulatory molecules *(675)*, as well as by directly inhibiting T-cell cytokine production: IL-2, TNF-α, and IL-5 (*671*,698,699). Much of this suppression was of a bystander nature, mediated by the cytokines IL-10 *(700)* and TGF-β *(701)* released from the cells following antigen stimulation; however, in transwell experiments the suppression was only optimum if the two T cells were in contact, suggesting that there might also be cell-surface molecule(s) participating in the negative regulation (702). Tr1 cells can be differentiated from naive T cells in human by stimulating with antigen plus IL-10 and IFN-α *(703)*. In the mouse the cells emerge following antigen activation in the presence of vitamin D_3 and dexamethasone to suppress Th1 and Th2 responses *(704)*. They also can be induced by bone marrow-derived DC that had been previously exposed to IL-10 *(705)*. The major growth factor for Tr1 cells is IL-15 *(706)*. Naive CD8$^+$ T cells can also differentiate into Tr1-like cells in the presence of plasmacytoid DCs *(707)*.

The effector properties of Tr1 cells have many things in common with the CD4$^+$CD25$^+$Foxp3$^+$ nTreg population generated in the thymus (see earlier discussion). The possibility that such Tregs could also be induced in the periphery from CD4$^+$CD25$^-$ T cells was first raised for human T-cell populations *(708)*, and then more rigorously demonstrated in murine systems using low-dose antigen stimulation in thymectomized animals (709) and by transfer of monoclonal-naive TCR transgenic T cells into antigen-bearing hosts *(710)*. Subsequently it was discovered that such a switch could be greatly facilitated by stimulation with antigen/APC in the presence of TGF-β1 (711). Since then these so-called induced (or adaptive) T-regulatory cells (iTregs) have been generated under a variety of conditions including during transplantation tolerance *(712,713)* and chronic infectious diseases (*714*,715,*716*). They are distinguished from Tr1 cells in terms of their expression of CD25 and Foxp3 and in terms of the cytokines that generate them (TGF-β1 vs. IL-10) (673). In functional properties, however, they are very similar. In fact, under some conditions both types of cells can be found at the same site of inflammation *(714,717)*. Under other conditions, however, they can inhibit different aspects of the same immune response *(717)*.

Tr1 and iTreg cells negatively regulate many cells in the immune system, including APCs, B cells, and T cells. In mouse models they can suppress Th1-mediated inflammatory bowel disease (698,718) as well as Th-2–mediated immediate hypersensitivity responses *(719)*, the latter by blocking IgE production and Th2 cell priming. For CD8$^+$ targets, TGF-β1–induced inhibition of granule exocytosis (initiated by Tregs) can prevent CTL activity *(259)*. In humans, Tr1 cells have been observed in patients tolerant to kidney, liver, and bone marrow grafts, although a causal role in the tolerance process has not been established (673). Administration of alloreactive CD25$^+$ Tregs in bone marrow transplantation has been used to prevent acute graft-versus-host disease while sparing graft-versus-leukemia function *(720)*. In mice, pancreatic islet grafts have been facilitated by administration of IL-10 in addition to rapamycin *(721)*. In NOD mice these manipulations delayed disease onset by generating both Tr1 and iTregs. The former were found in the spleen and blocked proliferation and migration to the pancreas of effector T cells, while the latter were found in the islets of the pancreas and prevented diabetes *(717)*. In chronic infectious diseases caused by organisms such as the parasite *Leishmania major* (260) and the nematode *Onchocerca volvulus (722)*, the presence of Tr1 and/or Treg cells and their cytokine production (mostly IL-10) has been associated with persistence of the infection. Interestingly, the response can give rise to a state of concomitant immunity in which the host is resistant to rechallenge with the same parasite while still harboring the organism at a local site (260). This creates a state of equilibrium between host and parasite in which neither is completely destroyed by the other. In this regard a number of pathogenic viruses (Epstein-Barr virus, cytomegalovirus, and Pox) (723,*724,725*) have also taken advantage of the negative regulation of Tr1/iTreg cytokines such as IL-10 by evolutionarily capturing and modifying these genes for their own use in down-regulating host immune responses.

Mucosal Tolerance

The route of antigen introduction is a critical variable in determining the outcome of an immune response. Intravenous administration generally favors induction of tolerance *(726,727)*, whereas subcutaneous administration favors immunity (728). Intravenous injection might allow antigen presentation by costimulatory molecule-deficient naive B cells in the spleen *(729)*, whereas subcutaneous injection would favor uptake and presentation by Langerhans cells, which, following activation, are very effective at initiating immune responses in the draining lymph nodes *(730)*.

Oral and nasal administration of antigen have also been shown to favor tolerance induction (731,*732*). From the earliest studies of Wells *(733)* and Chase (734), it was clear that the oral route of administration induces some form of immunoregulation. Orally immunized animals usually make an initial systemic antibody response that subsequently diminishes (735). The tolerance state is often associated with large amounts of IgA production in the gut *(736)*. In other cases (e.g., for myelin basic protein), in which the antigen is administered in a form (peptides) preferentially recognized by T cells rather than B cells *(737)*, the immunoregulation has been reported to be mediated either by T cells that secrete TGF-β on antigen stimulation *(738)* or by induction of anergy and deletion *(739,740)*. The mechanism observed depends on the antigen dose, with high doses inducing direct inactivation of the antigen-specific T cells and low doses eliciting TGF-β–mediated immunoregulation *(741)*. These cells and cytokines precondition the environment of the gut so that APCs become educated to present antigen to naive T cells in a skewed fashion, propagating the induction of T cells producing IL-4, IL-10, and TGF-β *(742)*. Nasal administration of soluble proteins or peptides prevents or reduces ongoing Th1 IFN-γ responses by similar mechanisms. In this model, roles for $\gamma\delta$ T cells *(743)* and dendritic cells *(744)* secreting IL-10 have also been suggested.

The T cells in the gut, referred to as *Th-3 cells*, are unusual in that they can make substantial amounts of TGF-β following antigen stimulation *(745)*. This cytokine acts as a critical switch factor for B cells, favoring the production of IgA *(746)*. TGF-β, however, is also an anti-inflammatory cytokine that blocks T-cell proliferation by inhibiting IL-2 production and cell-cycle progression, although at the same time it also enhances T-cell survival *(747,748)*. TGF-β–deficient mice as well as mice harboring a dominant negative form of the receptor transgenically expressed in T cells develop inflammatory bowel disease, suggesting that this cytokine, like IL-10, is critical for anti-inflammatory immune regulation (749,750). After initial activation in the gut, Th-3 cells can leave and migrate to other sites in the body, where they can act as direct or indirect (bystander) suppressor cells, if they recognize their peptide/MHC ligand at that site and release TGF-β. In this sense oral tolerance is not really the absence of an immune response, but rather a form of immune regulation initiated in the gut to deal with the problem of the large number of commensal bacteria that colonize this tissue in a symbiotic fashion *(751,752)*. The relationship among Th-3, Tr1, and iTreg cells in the mucosa has not been clearly established. These cell types may represent a family of regulatory CD4$^+$ T cells whose members have differentiated in different places and times to produce (to varying degrees) the same set of inhibitory cytokines (IL-10 and TGF-β) required to provide negative feedback regulation on T-cell immune responses.

Indoleamine 2,3-Dioxygenase and Suppressive APC

A subset of plasmacytoid DCs (CD8α^+, CD19$^+$) can produce indoleamine 2,3-dioxygenase (IDO), an enzyme that catabolizes the essential amino acid tryptophan *(753)*. IDO expression is induced in these cells by either IFNs or LPS and TNF signaling (754,*755*). IDO can also be induced by cross-linking B7 molecules on the DC, which stimulates

IFN-α production and STAT1 and IRF1 signaling *(756)*. B7 cross-linking can be achieved experimentally with soluble CTLA4-Ig and it may be accomplished physiologically by CD4$^+$ regulatory T cells, which constitutively express CTLA4 on their surface (754). Mature DCs that express active IDO can inhibit T-cell expansion by depleting tryptophan in the environment *(757)*. This is sensed by the T cell as an increase in uncharged tRNA and leads to activation of the stress kinase GCN2, which inhibits entry into cell cycle *(758)*. Instead, the T cell enters an anergic state and can differentiate into iTregs in the presence of TGF-β *(758,759)*. Furthermore, toxic metabolites of tryptophan following its IDO breakdown to kynurenine (such as 3-hydroxy-anthranilic acid) can induce apoptosis in thymocytes and Th1 clones *in vitro (760,761)*. The role of IDO in immune responses *in vivo* has been explored by using the pharmacologic inhibitor 1-methyl-tryptophan to block the enzyme. This drug increased the severity of EAE *(762)* and inflammatory bowel disease *(763)* in mouse models and prevented CTLA4-Ig from facilitating islet transplantation *(756)*. When administered during pregnancy it resulted in rejection of allogeneic but not syngeneic fetuses *(764)*. In contrast, overexpression of IDO in tumors and lung tissue makes them resistant to rejection *(765–767)*. *In vitro*, IDO-expressing APC dominate, that is, they inhibit an MLR even when mixed with stimulatory APC not expressing IDO *(753,757,767)*. Although IDO has an inhibitory effect on the adaptive immune response, which favors the induction of tolerance, it can also function as an innate host defense because it inhibits the replication of pathogens that cannot synthesize their own tryptophan, such as *Toxoplasma gondii*, mycobacteria, and group B streptococci *(768–770)*. How the DCs maintain their own function and survival under these tryptophan-depleted conditions is still not understood.

CD8$^+$ iTregs and Anti-TCR Regulation

Studies on CD8$^+$ suppressor T cells in immunoregulation and tolerance were a dominant theme in cellular immunology in the 1970s. Looking back at those systems now, it is possible to classify some of them as forms of immune deviation. For example, CD8$^+$ T cells are particularly good at making IFN-γ *(771)*; thus, they should be capable of functioning as potent suppressors of Th2 and Th17 responses *(665,692)*. Furthermore, recent experiments have demonstrated that Th2-like CD8$^+$ T cells (Tc2) can be generated in the presence of IL-4 and these could function as suppressors in CD4$^+$ Th1 DTH responses (772,773). Thus, regulatory cytokines could provide a sufficient explanation for some of the old experiments.

One clear exception to this cytokine model, however, is the Qa1-restricted CD8$^+$ regulatory T-cell population discussed earlier (774). The original observation in the 1970s was that CD4$^+$ T cells were necessary to induce CD8$^+$ suppressor T cells and that this interaction required the presence of Qa-1 *(775)*. In rats, lines of these CD8$^+$ T cells could mediate resistance to EAE induction when transferred *in vivo (776)*. More recently the CD8 cells were shown to play a key role in the prevention of relapses in mouse EAE and to require Qa-1 for their generation (*575,576,577,777, 778*). Interestingly, these CD8 suppressor cells showed specificity for the Vβ^+ subset of CD4$^+$ T cells involved in the response *(575,777)*. How this specificity is generated is not completely clear. Standard T-cell activation involves recognition of antigenic peptides bound to MHC molecules. However, the generation of regulatory T cells that can suppress an immune response by recognizing the receptor on responding T cells requires the recognition of unique peptides derived from that TCR. Evidence that this can occur comes from the EAE studies of Vandenbark and colleagues (779,*780,781*). The CD4$^+$ T-cell response to myelin basic protein in Lewis rats is dominated by cells expressing Vβ8. Animals immunized with a synthetic peptide corresponding to the CDR2 region of this Vβ were protected against the demyelineating disease. Not all TCR peptides were effective, presumably because of the failure of some to bind to that animal's MHC molecules. Thus, a possible regulatory mechanism is that the Qa1/TCR peptide-specific CD8$^+$ T cells generated are cytotoxic for the activated CD4$^+$ T cells expressing the Vβ8 receptor *(782)*.

Another model of CD8$^+$ suppressor T cells has been described in humans *(783)*. These cells were generated by multiple rounds of antigen stimulation and inhibited either alloantigen or protein antigen proliferative and antibody responses in a specific manner. The cells were subsequently shown to lack expression of CD28 and to express all the markers of CD4$^+$Foxp3$^+$CD25$^+$ Tregs *(784)*. However, they did not produce IL-10 or TGF-β. Their mechanism of action was through alteration of the APC (785). When the CD8$^+$ iTregs were activated by peptide/MHC class I complexes on the APC, they induced the expression of a pair of KIR-like inhibitory receptors, ILT3 and ILT4, on the APC surface *(786)*. These two molecules could also be up-regulated on DCs by IL-10 and/or IFN-α stimulation *(787)*. ILT4 recognizes the α3 domain of HLA class I *(788)* and, like inhibitory NK cell receptors, recruits a phosphatase to prevent calcium signaling and NF-κB-mediated up-regulation of B7 costimulatory molecules on the APC (785,*789,790*). ILT3, in contrast, directly alters CD4$^+$ T cells. In response to antigen presentation in its presence, CD4$^+$ cells up-regulate Foxp3 and become anergic instead of differentiating into effector cells *(787,791)*. This same effect could be achieved with soluble recombinant ILT3-Fc and this form of the molecule could induce new CD8$^+$ iTregs in primary mixed leukocyte cultures *(792)*. Thus, the net result from the actions of ILT3 and ILT4 is to induce naive T cells into the Treg lineage. This represents another example of how a preconditioned APC can dictate the nature of the response by a naive T cell.

CD8$^+$ Veto Cells

A mechanism for directly tolerizing naive CD8$^+$ precytotoxic T cells has been described that involves negative immunoregulation by previously activated CD8$^+$ cells (T cells or NK cells) *(793,794)*. In the model system, a population of precultured MHC-incompatible CD8$^+$ T cells was recognized by unprimed allogeneic CD8$^+$ T cells and the former inactivated the latter. Hence, the name *veto cells*. These cells acted late in culture (after 20 hours), mediated their effects by cell-cell interaction (not secreted products), and did not compete for lysis of target cells in the CTL assay (as they could be eliminated prior to the assay with anti-MHC antibodies and complement without reversing the effect) *(795,796)*. The TCR specificity of the veto cell did not matter and engagement of its TCR was not required for its veto function *(797,798)*. Instead, it was the recognition of cell surface peptide/MHC class I antigens on the veto cell by the responding CD8$^+$ T cell that led to the latter's inactivation. Evidence that the veto phenomenon can also operate *in vivo* has come largely from the experiments of Rammensee, Fink, and Bevan (*796,799–800*,801). Injection of splenic CD8$^+$ T cells into mice differing at MHC class I loci resulted in inhibition of a subsequent *in vitro* CTL response by the recipient's T cells against donor class I molecules.

A molecular mechanism for vetoing has been described that involves signaling back through the MHC class I molecule following its interaction with CD8 on the veto cell (802). CD8-negative variants of clones otherwise capable of vetoing were found to lose their ability to veto. Furthermore, cell lines expressing the correct peptide/MHC complex, but which were not veto cells, became veto cells when transfected with a CD8 gene. Finally, a veto effect could be activated with peptide/MHC-positive, CD8-negative cells by adding a monoclonal antibody against the $\alpha 3$ domain of the MHC class I molecule (the molecular region for CD8 binding). Conversely, a CD8$^+$ veto cell could be prevented from killing by a monoclonal antibody against CD8, which blocked its interaction with the MHC molecule. These results suggest that the veto signal is initiated by the interaction of CD8 on the veto cell with the $\alpha 3$ domain of an MHC class I molecule on the target cell, but only when the latter cell simultaneously becomes activated through its TCR via recognition of a peptide/MHC molecule on the veto cell. The effect of this dual signaling by veto cells is to make the responding T cells susceptible to Fas/FasL-mediated apoptosis *(803,804)*. The function of this mechanism in self-tolerance is not clear, but it may play a role in eliminating autoreactive CD8$^+$ T cells specific for blast antigens expressed on activated CTLs. In a clinical setting CD8$^+$ veto cells raised against irrelevant third-party targets have been used to prevent graft rejection in allogeneic bone marrow transplantation using large doses of CD34$^+$ stem cells under minimal conditioning regimens such as treatment with rapamycin *(805–807)*.

Antibody-mediated Immunoregulation

Passive transfer of antibodies into a naive animal often prevents the priming of that animal with a subsequent injection of antigen (808). High-affinity antibodies are more effective than low-affinity ones *(809)*. Some of this effect is the result of formation and clearance of antigen-antibody complexes. The antibodies can also prevent the formation of particular peptides during antigen processing that are needed for T-cell recognition *(810,811)*. The antigen-antibody complexes are also likely to be responsible for the phenomenon known as *original antigenic sin* (*812*,813), in which memory B cells, generated during a prior exposure to a cross-reacting antigen, prevent or down-regulate the response to the unique new determinants on the antigen *(814)*. Memory B cells seem to have an advantage for rapid activation and this produces antibodies that feed back to inhibit the priming of naive B cells possessing receptors that are specific for unique determinants of the second immunogen. This feedback mechanism is most likely mediated through antigen-antibody complexes that interact with the FcγRIIb1 receptors on the naive B cells (815) and inhibit signal transduction through their IgM receptors by bringing the SHIP phosphatase into the receptor complex *(816,817)*. The sialylation state of the Fc core of the antibody is also critical for favoring its interaction with inhibitory Fcγ receptors *(818)*.

Anti-Idiotypic B-Cell Regulation

In 1974 Jerne *(819)* proposed that antibody production could be regulated by other antibodies that recognized unique idiotypic determinants in the V regions of the first antibody. He postulated that an increase in the production of the first antibody could negatively regulate the production of anti-idiotypic antibodies, and vice versa. Because of the interconnected pathways in such a network, perturbation of one segment would be dampened by the presence of other segments and thus the original steady state would be buffered.

In recent years, studies have focused on the analysis of IgM hybridomas from nonimmunized neonatal mice *(820)* or IgM antibodies derived from human cord blood Epstein-Barr virus–transformed B cells (46,*48,821,822*). Individual antibodies show the ability to react with several different self-ligands, many of which are intracellular proteins, such as cytoskeletal proteins *(47,48,821–825)*. In both species their major source appears to be B1 and marginal zone B cells *(49,50,826)*. The relation to immunologic networks is that these antibodies also interact with other members of the set *(820,827)*. Administration of such antibodies to neonatal mice perturbs the B-cell repertoire and affects the subsequent adult response to particular antigens (828,829). This effect is either positive or negative depending on the timing and the antibody. Whether the natural dominance of B cells expressing certain idiotypes is related to such network interactions *(826)* or is due to early exposure to commensal bacteria *(830)* remains controversial. However, clonally dominant idiotypes emerge in germ-free animals *(831,832)* and can be disrupted in their appearance by early antigen priming with heat-killed bacteria *(833)*. Interestingly, the non–idiotype-positive antibodies elicited by the premature priming proved *not* to be protective for subsequent challenge with virulent bacteria, suggesting that the natural network-derived antibodies played a crucial role in host defense (829).

IMMUNE PRIVILEGED SITES

Transplant surgeons have known for a long time that certain areas in the body are more favorable than others for grafting of tumors *(834)* and normal allogeneic tissues *(835)*. In particular, the brain, the anterior chamber of the eye, and the testis in rodents as well as the cheek pouch in hamsters seem to be privileged in their capacity to accept grafts readily *(836)*. The idea thus emerged that antigens contained in these tissues could not be seen by the immune system because they were sequestered in some way, for example, by the blood brain barrier or because the grafts failed to become vascularized (e.g., corneal transplants) (837). Subsequent studies, however, have shown that activated lymphocytes can migrate into most of these tissues *(838)*. Nonetheless, the tissues do have mechanisms for curtailing the initiation of an immune response. The nervous system has very few dendritic cells and little lymphatic drainage *(839)*. Instead, antigens end up via lymphatic links in the cerebrospinal fluid *(840)*. The hamster cheek pouch also has very few lymphatic vessels *(841)*. In fact, even the skin can be converted into a privileged site for primary grafts, if one surgically creates an alymphatic skin pedicle *(842)*. On the effector end, neurons express few if any MHC molecules, and, even in the presence of inflammatory cytokines, they only express low levels of MHC class I molecules for effector T cells to recognize *(843,844)*. Another mechanism by which a tissue may obtain privileged status, even if exposed to activated T cells, is by the expression of Fas ligand (845). This was first demonstrated for Sertoli cells of the testes *(846)*. In a transplantation model, testis grafts from normal mice survived indefinitely under the kidney capsule of allogeneic recipients while similar grafts from mice carrying a mutation in the Fas ligand gene (*gld*) were rejected. Similarly, in a tissue-destruction model, viral infection of the anterior chamber of the eye of *gld* mice caused massive tissue damage, whereas the same infection in normal mice resulted in Fas/FasL-dependent killing of the inflammatory lymphoid cells *(847)*. Fas ligand expression has been detected in both corneal epithelial and endothelial cells *(848)*.

Another mechanism that has been described to participate in the immune privilege of the eye is called *anterior chamber-associated immune deviation (849)*. Injections of exogenous antigens and allogeneic tissues into the anterior chamber results in a systemic impairment of the production of complement-fixing antibodies and DTH to that antigen, that is, Th1 responses are blocked *(850)*. The immune deviation appears to be an effect of inhibitory cytokines such as TGF-β secreted from the iris and ciliary body cells in the eye and IL-10 released from ocular APC *(851)*, as well as neuropeptides such as α MSH and vasoactive intestinal peptide released by corneal nerves *(852)*. These molecules alter the presentation properties of the F4/80$^+$ APCs in the eye. The APCs then migrate to the thymus *(853)* and spleen *(854)* where they induce NK T cells to make IL-10 *(855)*. The NK T cells, along with $\gamma\delta$ T cells *(856)* and B cells *(857)*, somehow induce Qa-1 class Ib–restricted CD8$^+$ regulatory T cells *(850,858)*. How these effector T cells suppress the CD4$^+$ DTH response in an antigen-specific manner has yet to be clearly elucidated (859,860). Finally, recent studies have demonstrated that some privileged sites can favor the induction of T-regulatory cells in response to tissue grafts *(861)*.

THE FETAL-MATERNAL RELATIONSHIP

A number of examples exist in the reproduction of vertebrates in which one organism successfully grafts itself onto another as a parabiont, completely circumventing rejection by the host's immune system (862). Perhaps the most interesting example of this natural tolerance induction is in viviparous mammals, where the fetus successfully implants itself in the uterus *(863)*. When any inbred mammalian strain A female is mated to a strain B male, the (A $\times$ B)F_1 fetus expresses histocompatibility antigens of the father to which the mother is not tolerant; yet the fetus is not rejected. This is also true for completely allogeneic fetuses that have been experimentally created by embryo transfer *(864,865)*.

The possibility that the fetal trophoblast represents a privileged immunologic tissue was first tested by transferring day 2 fertilized (A $\times$ B)F_1 ova or day 7.5 F_1 ectoplacental cones under the kidney capsule of strain A females *(866)*. These grafts were not rejected even if the recipient had been primed with strain B skin grafts. Witebski and Reich *(867)* were the first to suggest that this protection from immune attack might be because the placenta does not express histocompatibility antigens. Evidence to support this idea is very good in primates *(868,869)*.

Syncytiotrophoblasts of the human fetus do not express polymorphic MHC class Ia or class II molecules (with the exception of HLA-C) *(870)*. These cells are the closest in proximity to the maternal blood vessels in the villi of the placenta, and even when stimulated with IFN-γ, they do not express HLA-A and HLA-B class I molecules *(871)*. The remaining cells, cytotrophoblasts, express only the relatively nonpolymorphic class Ib MHC molecules, HLA-G and HLA-E *(872,873)*. Although early ideas suggested that the function of these molecules is to provide a ligand for the inhibitory receptor(s) on maternal NK cells and CD8$^+$ T cells, thus preventing them from killing fetal cells (874), more recent work has raised the possibility that instead they play a role in controlling vascularization of the maternal decidua (875).

One puzzling fact, however, is that rodent placental cells do express classical polymorphic MHC class Ia molecules, although at significantly lower levels in the fetus than in the adult *(876)*. Hence, other mechanisms must also play a role in preventing maternal immune attack. Of note is the fact that syncytiotrophoblasts synthesize the enzyme indoleamine 2,3-dioxygenase *(877)*, which, as discussed earlier, breaks down the essential amino acid tryptophan and has negative effects on T-cell activation. If a pharmacologic inhibitor of this enzyme is administered at the time of embryo implantation, it causes the loss of allogeneic fetuses in normal, but not Rag1-deficient, mice *(764)*. There was no effect on syngeneic litters. Conversely, feeding hamsters a high-tryptophan diet has been reported to cause fetal loss *(878)*. These observations suggest that control of tryptophan availability is a key mechanism by which trophoblasts maintain their immune privilege. However, it is not the only mechanism because IDO-deficient female mice produce normal litters when crossed to allogeneic IDO-deficient males *(877)*.

In the early experiments on multiparous rodents, allogeneic paternal skin grafts placed on mothers that had been mated several times to males of that allogeneic strain were rejected more slowly than the same grafts placed on mothers that had been mated to syngeneic males *(879–882)*. Also, the response of multiparous inbred females to the male-specific antigen H-Y is usually impaired *(883,884)* even though primed CD8$^+$ CTLs can be detected with tetramers (885). This suggests that there exists an immunosuppressive effect of the fetus on the mother's T-cell immune responses *(884)*. This was demonstrated clearly in TCR transgenic female mice whose CD8$^+$ T cells were specific for a paternal MHC class I molecule (K^b) (886). During pregnancy these cells were reduced in numbers and appeared to have down-regulated their receptor levels. They were also functionally impaired as the mother failed to reject Kb-bearing tumor grafts during this period. Following birth, the immune system returned to normal. Furthermore, these effects were antigen-specific as they were not observed in syngeneic or non-K^b allogeneic pregnancies. In another study, CD8$^+$ transgenic T cells specific for the male H-Y antigen were tolerized during pregnancy by mechanisms involving anergy and Fas-dependent deletion *(887)*. In a similar manner, a B-cell receptor transgenic mouse specific for K^k deleted about 80% of its idiotype$^+$ B cells starting at midpregnancy and then reverting to normal levels at birth *(888)*. Thus, pregnancy transiently can result in a state of specific tolerance to paternal alloantigens.

Several mechanisms have been proposed for this transient immunosuppressed state. One is expression of Fas ligand in the placenta, which, similar to its action in other privileged sites, would kill activated T cells entering the tissue *(889)*. In the human placenta, Fas ligand is expressed early on cytotrophoblasts as well as at term in syncytiotrophoblasts *(889,890)*. In the *gld* mouse, which lacks a functional Fas ligand, fetal resorption sites are common and litter sizes are small *(890)*. A second mechanism is the presence of suppressor T cells *(891)*. There is a generalized increase in the percentage of CD25$^+$Foxp3$^+$ Tregs that occurs during pregnancy (892). In the uterus about 30% of the CD4$^+$ T cells are Tregs by embryonic day 10.5, and this occurs in syngeneic as well as allogeneic matings. Depletion of CD25$^+$ cells prior to T-cell adoptive transfer into nude females led to gestational failure when these mice were bred to allogeneic males, but not if they were bred to syngeneic males. In the allogeneic combination fetal resorption was detected at embryonic day 10.5 and characterized by infiltration of CD3$^+$ T cells and hemorrhage at the maternal-fetal interface. Thus, the physiologic enhancement of Tregs during pregnancy may play a key role in preventing alloreactivity against paternal antigens. This enhancement may also be responsible for the amelioration of autoimmune diseases, such as rheumatoid arthritis, that often occurs with pregnancy *(893,894)*.

A third mechanism to explain systemic immunosuppression in pregnancy is the production of cytokines and hormones by the placenta, which would inactivate T cells or deviate them away from a cell-mediated immune response *(895)*. Progesterone, which is present in high concentrations in the placenta, has been shown to prolong allogeneic skin graft survival (*896*,897) and to favor the development of Th2 responses from antigen-specific T-cell lines and clones *(898)*. IL-4, IL-5, and IL-10 have been detected in the placenta, as has an immunosuppressive cytokine related to TGFβ2 *(895,899–901)*. The latter is made by trophoblasts rather than immune cells, as is much of the IL-10 produced in the placenta (902,*903*). A study of the effect of pregnancy on susceptibility to *Leishmania* infection in B6 mice, which normally resist the parasite with a vigorous Th1 response, showed an impaired clearance of the organism resulting from a general decrease in IFN-γ production (904). Reciprocally, infection with *Leishmania* enhanced both spontaneous abortion and failed implantation rates, as well as decreasing the production of IL-4 and IL-10 in the placenta *(905)*. In humans, spontaneous abortions are also associated with an increased capability of producing IL-2 and IFN-γ and a decrease in IL-4, IL-10, and leukemia inhibitory factor production *(906,907)*. Finally, the excess fetal loss observed in the CBA and DBA/2 mouse mating combination, which is mediated by activated NK cells and macrophages, is associated with decreased IL-4 and IL-10 production and can be reversed by administration of IL-10 or anti–IFN-γ antibody (*144*,902). Although not all Th-2 cytokines are necessary for a successful pregnancy *(908)*, the cytokine milieu of the placenta does appear to play an important role in the maternal acceptance of the fetus, and may provide another example of where immune deviation contributes to tolerance.

Often after multiple pregnancies the mother makes an antibody response to the father's histocompatibility antigens *(909,910)*. Occasionally, the antibodies formed are harmful to the fetus, as in Rh incompatibility causing erythrocyte destruction *(911)*, but for the most part the antibodies are not destructive. Several laboratories have demonstrated that many of these antibodies do not fix complement *(912)*. When they do fix complement, cells in the placenta are equipped with molecules such as decay-accelerating factor and membrane cofactor protein, which destroy or block the binding of complement (see Chapter 33). The importance of these protective mechanisms has been shown in a targeted mutation of a broadly distributed complement regulatory protein called *Crry*, a major complement inactivator in rodents (913). Homozygous knockout mice die *in utero* around embryonic day 10. The embryos at this time have C3 deposited in the placenta and the tissue is invaded with granulocytes. Crossing these mice to C3-deficient mice corrected the defect, demonstrating that the regulation of complement was an important variable in fetal survival.

SUMMARY

The immune system is often thought of as a protective device for responding to the dangers of pathogenic invaders and injury. However, one of the most serious threats to the organism is the immune system itself. Without the various phenomena referred to as tolerance, the organism would surely self-destruct. Hence, the mechanisms required to guard against this possibility are numerous and nonredundant (Table 29.1). First, in the central lymphoid organs, cells reactive to available endogenous antigens are

TABLE 29.1 Tolerance Mechanisms

Central Lymphoid Tissues	*Peripheral Lymphoid Tissues*
T cells in the thymus	**T cells in the spleen and lymph nodes**
1. Negative selection via clonal deletion by thymic dendritic cells presenting ubiquitous self-antigens	1. Programmed cell death following stimulation by antigen-bearing APCs. Usually mediated by growth factor withdrawal.
2. Deletion or anergy resulting from self-antigen presentation by thymic epithelial cells. This includes ectopically expressed tissue-specific antigens.	2. Clonal anergy due to TCR occupancy that is unaccompanied by sufficient costimulation
3. Deletion of thymocytes recognizing tissue-specific antigens by dendritic cells migrating to the thymus from the peripheral tissues	3. Receptor desensitization resulting from persistent antigen stimulation
4. Generation of CD4$^+$CD25$^+$Foxp3$^+$ regulatory T cells that act in the periphery to inhibit self-antigen reactivity	4. Th1/Th2/Th17 immune deviation via cytokine cross-regulatory effects
	5. Tr1, Th3 and iTreg cells acting via suppressive effects of IL-10 and TGF-β
	6. CD8$^+$ veto cells delete naive CD8$^+$ T cells by a Fas/FasL mechanism
	7. CD8$^+$ T cells delete activated CD4$^+$ T cells by recognition of TCR peptides presented on Qa1 molecules
	8. CD8$^+$ suppressor cells induce inhibitory receptors on APC
	9. Plasmacytoid DC inhibition of T-cell proliferation thru tryptophan depletion by indoleamine 2,3-dioxygenase
B cells in the bone marrow	**B cells in the spleen and lymph nodes**
1. Receptor editing as a consequence of growth arrest and immunoglobulin V-region substitution in response to polyvalent, high concentration self-antigens	1. Clonal anergy due to persistent antigen stimulation that leads to B-cell receptor desensitization and functional unresponsiveness
2. Clonal deletion following persistent stimulation of high-affinity clones by polyvalent, high concentration self-antigens leading to apoptosis	2. Clonal deletion by high concentration, high affinity, polyvalent antigens in the absence of T-cell help
3. Clonal anergy as a result of maturation arrest and subsequent loss of antigen-responsiveness to soluble self-antigens	3. Receptor blockade by smaller, soluble, low-valency antigens that tie up antigen receptors in nonfunctional clusters
4. Differentiation to B1 cells to allow survival of intermediate-affinity self-antigen reactive clones early in life	4. Antibody feedback inhibits naive B-cell activation via Fc receptors
	5. Anti-idiotypic IgM antibody network regulates levels of natural antibodies

APC, antigen-presenting cell; TCR, T-cell receptor; Th, T-helper cell; TGF-β, transforming growth factor-β; IgM, immunoglobulin M.

clonally deleted by an apoptotic process. In addition, editing allows B cells to replace their receptors in order to avoid autoimmunity. As the lymphocytes mature they next encounter peripheral antigens. Some of these are brought to the primary lymphoid organs by the bloodstream and migrating immature DCs. Other antigens are expressed ectopically in the medulla of the thymus. Here the cells are tolerized by a deletional or anergic process. In addition $CD4^{+}CD25^{+}Foxp3^{+}$ regulatory T cells are selected, which later can dampen immune responses against many peripheral self-antigens. Maturing transitional B cells can also be tolerized by an anergic or deletional process if they encounter antigen in the absence of T-cell help.

Once T cells have matured, their activation to antigen is still constrained by the requirement for two types of signaling, one antigen-specific and the other costimulatory. APCs are normally in a quiescent state and thus only present antigens in a tolerogenic fashion (signal one alone). The cells may respond to this stimulation and even divide, but the process is ultimately abortive and the cells either die or become anergic. B cells require T-cell help as their form of costimulation and antigen encounter without it leads to anergy or death. Finally, even following a strong immune response, the system can regulate itself by negative feedback mechanisms, which include various induced T-regulatory cells making IL-10 and TGF-β in response to antigen, cells killing effectors by recognizing idiotypic determinants or vetoing them, or by deviating the response toward a nonharmful state. B cells can be turned off by antibody signaling through Fc receptors.

Despite this plethora of mechanisms that exists to ensure that tolerance is enforced in the immune system, the safeguards can occasionally break down, resulting in autoimmune disease. When and how this occurs is the topic of Chapters 41 and 42 on systemic and organ-specific autoimmunity.

REFERENCES

3. Owen RD. Immunogenetic consequences of vascular anastomoses between bovine twins. *Science.* 1945;103:400.
8. Billingham RE, Brent L, Medawar PB. "Actively acquired tolerance" of foreign cells. *Nature.* 1953;172:603–607.
11. Burnet FM. A modification of Jerne's theory of antibody production using the concept of clonal selection. *Aust J Sci.* 1957;20:67–69.
13. Triplett EL. On the mechanism of immunologic self recognition. *J Immunol.* 1962;89:505–510.
14. Nemazee DA, Burki K. Clonal deletion of B lymphocytes in a transgenic mouse bearing anti-MHC class I antibody genes. *Nature.* 1989;337(6207):562–566.
15. Raff MC, Owen JJ, Cooper MD, et al. Differences in susceptibility of mature and immature mouse B lymphocytes to anti-immunoglobulin-induced immunoglobulin suppression in vitro. Possible implications for B-cell tolerance to self. *J Exp Med.* 1975;142(5):1052–1064.
17. Hartley SB, Cooke MP, Fulcher DA, et al. Elimination of self-reactive B lymphocytes proceeds in two stages: arrested development and cell death. *Cell.* 1993;72(3):325–335.
18. Tiegs SL, Russell DM, Nemazee D. Receptor editing in self-reactive bone marrow B cells. *J Exp Med.* 1993;177(4):1009–1020.
23. Li H, Jiang Y, Prak EL, et al. Editors and editing of anti-DNA receptors. *Immunity.* 2001;15(6):947–957.
26. Kincade PW, Lawton AR, Bockman DE, et al. Suppression of immunoglobulin G synthesis as a result of antibody-mediated suppression of immunoglobulin M synthesis in chickens. *Proc Natl Acad Sci U S A.* 1970;67(4):1918–1925.
30. Pelanda R, Schwers S, Sonoda E, et al. Receptor editing in a transgenic mouse model: site, efficiency, and role in B cell tolerance and antibody diversification. *Immunity.* 1997;7(6):765–775.
31. Halverson R, Torres RM, Pelanda R. Receptor editing is the main mechanism of B cell tolerance toward membrane antigens. *Nat Immunol.* 2004;5(6):645–650.
38. Metcalf ES, Klinman NR. In vitro tolerance induction of neonatal murine B cells. *J Exp Med.* 1976;143(6):1327–1340.
40. Nemazee D, Buerki K. Clonal deletion of autoreactive B lymphocytes in bone marrow chimeras. *Proc Natl Acad Sci U S A.* 1989; 86(20):8039–8043.
46. Guilbert B, Dighiero G, Avrameas S. Naturally occurring antibodies against nine common antigens in human sera. I. Detection, isolation and characterization. *J Immunol.* 1982;128(6):2779–2787.
58. Benschop RJ, Brandl E, Chan AC, et al. Unique signaling properties of B cell antigen receptor in mature and immature B cells: implications for tolerance and activation. *J Immunol.* 2001;167(8):4172–4179.
66. Lesley R, Xu Y, Kalled SL, et al. Reduced competitiveness of autoantigen-engaged B cells due to increased dependence on BAFF. *Immunity.* 2004;20(4):441–453.
68. Iverson GM, Lindenmann J. The role of a carrier-determinant and T cells in the induction of liver-specific autoantibodies in the mouse. *Eur J Immunol.* 1972;2(3):195–197.
72. Tsubata T, Nishikawa S, Katsura Y, et al. B cell repertoire for anti-DNA antibody in normal and lupus mice: differential expression of precursor cells for high and low affinity anti-DNA antibodies. *Clin Exp Immunol.* 1988;71(1):50–55.
73. Radic MZ, Weigert M. Genetic and structural evidence for antigen selection of anti-DNA antibodies. *Annu Rev Immunol.* 1994;12:487–520.
74. Kappler JW, Roehm N, Marrack P. T cell tolerance by clonal elimination in the thymus. *Cell.* 1987;49(2):273–280.
79. Surh CD, Sprent J. T-cell apoptosis detected in situ during positive and negative selection in the thymus. *Nature.* 1994;372(6501):100–103.
82. Kisielow P, Bluthmann H, Staerz UD, et al. Tolerance in T-cell-receptor transgenic mice involves deletion of nonmature CD4+8+ thymocytes. *Nature.* 1988;333(6175):742–746.
85. Pircher H, Burki K, Lang R, et al. Tolerance induction in double specific T-cell receptor transgenic mice varies with antigen. *Nature.* 1989;342(6249):559–561.
90. Moore NC, Anderson G, McLoughlin DE, et al. Differential expression of Mtv loci in MHC class II-positive thymic stromal cells. *J Immunol.* 1994;152(10):4826–4831.
93. Mayerova D, Hogquist KA. Central tolerance to self-antigen expressed by cortical epithelial cells. *J Immunol.* 2004;172(2):851–856.
94. Speiser DE, Pircher H, Ohashi PS, et al. Clonal deletion induced by either radioresistant thymic host cells or lymphohemopoietic donor cells at different stages of class I-restricted T cell ontogeny. *J Exp Med.* 1992;175(5):1277–1283.
98. Baldwin TA, Sandau MM, Jameson SC, et al. The timing of TCR alpha expression critically influences T cell development and selection. *J Exp Med.* 2005;202(1):111–121.
107. Volkmann A, Zal T, Stockinger B. Antigen-presenting cells in the thymus that can negatively select MHC class II-restricted T cells recognizing a circulating self antigen. *J Immunol.* 1997;158(2):693–706.
108. Risueno RM, van Santen HM, Alarcon B. A conformational change senses the strength of T cell receptor-ligand interaction during thymic selection. *Proc Natl Acad Sci U S A.* 2006;103(25):9625–9630.
109. Cho HJ, Edmondson SG, Miller AD, et al. Cutting edge: identification of the targets of clonal deletion in an unmanipulated thymus. *J Immunol.* 2003;170(1):10–13.

113. Holman PO, Walsh ER, Hogquist KA. The central tolerance response to male antigen in normal mice is deletion and not receptor editing. *J Immunol.* 2003;171(8):4048–4053.
118. Marrack P, Lo D, Brinster R, et al. The effect of thymus environment on T cell development and tolerance. *Cell.* 1988;53(4):627–634.
121. Matzinger P, Guerder S. Does T-cell tolerance require a dedicated antigen-presenting cell? *Nature.* 1989;338(6210):74–76.
126. Kindred B. Functional activity of T cells which differentiate from nude mouse precursors in a congenic or allogeneic thymus graft. *Immunol Rev.* 1978;42:60–75.
128. Bonomo A, Matzinger P. Thymus epithelium induces tissue-specific tolerance. *J Exp Med.* 1993;177(4):1153–1164.
135. Hoffmann MW, Heath WR, Ruschmeyer D, et al. Deletion of high-avidity T cells by thymic epithelium. *Proc Natl Acad Sci U S A.* 1995;92(21):9851–9855.
136. Carlow DA, Teh SJ, Teh HS. Altered thymocyte development resulting from expressing a deleting ligand on selecting thymic epithelium. *J Immunol.* 1992;148(10):2988–2995.
138. Oehen S, Feng L, Xia Y, et al. Antigen compartmentation and T helper cell tolerance induction. *J Exp Med.* 1996;183(6):2617–2626.
146. Kishimoto H, Sprent J. Several different cell surface molecules control negative selection of medullary thymocytes. *J Exp Med.* 1999;190(1):65–73.
148. Buhlmann JE, Elkin SK, Sharpe AH. A role for the B7-1/B7-2:CD28/CTLA-4 pathway during negative selection. *J Immunol.* 2003;170(11):5421–5428.
150. van Meerwijk JP, Marguerat S, Lees RK, et al. Quantitative impact of thymic clonal deletion on the T cell repertoire. *J Exp Med.* 1997;185(3):377–383.
151. Ignatowicz L, Kappler J, Marrack P. The repertoire of T cells shaped by a single MHC/peptide ligand. *Cell.* 1996;84(4):521–529.
154. Kishimoto H, Sprent J. Negative selection in the thymus includes semimature T cells. *J Exp Med.* 1997;185(2):263–271.
161. Kurobe H, Liu C, Ueno T, et al. CCR7-dependent cortex-to-medulla migration of positively selected thymocytes is essential for establishing central tolerance. *Immunity.* 2006;24(2):165–177.
171. Rincon M, Whitmarsh A, Yang DD, et al. The JNK pathway regulates the In vivo deletion of immature CD4(+)CD8(+) thymocytes. *J Exp Med.* 1998;188(10):1817–1830.
174. Mariathasan S, Ho SS, Zakarian A, et al. Degree of ERK activation influences both positive and negative thymocyte selection. *Eur J Immunol.* 2000;30(4):1060–1068.
181. Calnan BJ, Szychowski S, Chan FK, et al. A role for the orphan steroid receptor Nur77 in apoptosis accompanying antigen-induced negative selection. *Immunity.* 1995;3(3):273–282.
187. Cunningham NR, Artim SC, Fornadel CM, et al. Immature CD4+CD8+ thymocytes and mature T cells regulate Nur77 distinctly in response to TCR stimulation. *J Immunol.* 2006;177(10):6660–6666.
190. Marsden VS, Strasser A. Control of apoptosis in the immune system: Bcl-2, BH3-only proteins and more. *Annu Rev Immunol.* 2003;21:71–105.
193. Villunger A, Marsden VS, Zhan Y, et al. Negative selection of semimature CD4(+)8(−)HSA+ thymocytes requires the BH3-only protein Bim but is independent of death receptor signaling. *Proc Natl Acad Sci U S A.* 2004;101(18):7052–7057.
202. Robertson K, Simon K, Schneider S, et al. Tolerance of self induced in thymus organ culture. *Eur J Immunol.* 1992;22(1):207–211.
205. Lucas B, Stefanova I, Yasutomo K, et al. Divergent changes in the sensitivity of maturing T cells to structurally related ligands underlies formation of a useful T cell repertoire. *Immunity.* 1999;10(3):367–376.
210. Azzam HS, Grinberg A, Lui K, et al. CD5 expression is developmentally regulated by T cell receptor (TCR) signals and TCR avidity. *J Exp Med.* 1998;188(12):2301–2311.
215. Nishizuka Y, Sakakura T. Thymus and reproduction: sex-linked dysgenesia of the gonad after neonatal thymectomy in mice. *Science.* 1969;166(906):753–755.
219. Sakaguchi S, Sakaguchi N, Asano M, et al. Immunologic self-tolerance maintained by activated T cells expressing IL-2 receptor alpha-chains (CD25). Breakdown of a single mechanism of self-tolerance causes various autoimmune diseases. *J Immunol.* 1995;155(3):1151–1164.
220. Hori S, Nomura T, Sakaguchi S. Control of regulatory T cell development by the transcription factor Foxp3. *Science.* 2003;299(5609):1057–1061.
223. Ohki H, Martin C, Corbel C, et al. Tolerance induced by thymic epithelial grafts in birds. *Science.* 1987;237(4818):1032–1035.
229. Pacholczyk R, Ignatowicz H, Kraj P, et al. Origin and T cell receptor diversity of Foxp3+CD4+CD25+ T cells. *Immunity.* 2006;25(2):249–259.
230. Jordan MS, Boesteanu A, Reed AJ, et al. Thymic selection of CD4+CD25+ regulatory T cells induced by an agonist self-peptide. *Nat Immunol.* 2001;2(4):301–306.
240. Wu Y, Borde M, Heissmeyer V, et al. FOXP3 controls regulatory T cell function through cooperation with NFAT. *Cell.* 2006;126(2):375–387.
245. Furtado GC, Curotto de Lafaille MA, Kutchukhidze N, et al. Interleukin 2 signaling is required for CD4(+) regulatory T cell function. *J Exp Med.* 2002;196(6):851–857.
260. Belkaid Y, Piccirillo CA, Mendez S, et al. CD4+CD25+ regulatory T cells control Leishmania major persistence and immunity. *Nature.* 2002;420(6915):502–507.
268. Endharti AT, Rifa'i M, Shi Z, et al. Cutting edge: CD8+CD122+ regulatory T cells produce IL-10 to suppress IFN-gamma production and proliferation of CD8+ T cells. *J Immunol.* 2005;175(11):7093–7097.
270. Anderson D, Billingham RE, Lampkin GH, et al. The use of skin grafting to distinguish between monozygotic and dizygotic twins in cattle. *Heredity.* 1951;5:379–397.
271. Billingham RE, Brent L. Quantitative studies on tissue transplantation immunity. IV. Induction of tolerance in newborn mice and studies on the phenomenon of runt disease. *Proc R Soc Lond B Biol Sci.* 1959;242:439–477.
273. Boyse EA, Carswell EA, Scheid MP, et al. Tolerance of Sk-incompatible skin grafts. *Nature.* 1973;244(5416):441–442.
276. Emery D, McCullagh P. Immunological reactivity between chimeric cattle twins. I. Homograft reaction. *Transplantation.* 1980;29(1):4–9.
279. McCullagh P. Interception of the development of self tolerance in fetal lambs. *Eur J Immunol.* 1989;19(8):1387–1392.
281. Hanahan D. Peripheral-antigen-expressing cells in thymic medulla: factors in self-tolerance and autoimmunity. *Curr Opin Immunol.* 1998;10(6):656–662.
289. Klein L, Klein T, Ruther U, et al. CD4 T cell tolerance to human C-reactive protein, an inducible serum protein, is mediated by medullary thymic epithelium. *J Exp Med.* 1998;188(1):5–16.
291. Derbinski J, Schulte A, Kyewski B, et al. Promiscuous gene expression in medullary thymic epithelial cells mirrors the peripheral self. *Nat Immunol.* 2001;2(11):1032–1039.
294. Kyewski B, Klein L. A central role for central tolerance. *Annu Rev Immunol.* 2006;24:571–606.
302. Pugliese A, Zeller M, Fernandez A, Jr., et al. The insulin gene is transcribed in the human thymus and transcription levels correlated with allelic variation at the INS VNTR-IDDM2 susceptibility locus for type 1 diabetes. *Nat Genet.* 1997;15(3):293–297.
304. Akiyama T, Maeda S, Yamane S, et al. Dependence of self-tolerance on TRAF6-directed development of thymic stroma. *Science.* 2005;308(5719):248–251.
306. Anderson MS, Venanzi ES, Klein L, et al. Projection of an immunological self shadow within the thymus by the aire protein. *Science.* 2002;298(5597):1395–1401.
311. Pitkanen J, Rebane A, Rowell J, et al. Cooperative activation of transcription by autoimmune regulator AIRE and CBP. *Biochem Biophys Res Commun.* 2005;333(3):944–953.
321. Ellison GW, Waksman BH. Role of the thymus in tolerance. IX. Inhibition of experimental autoallergic encephalomyelitis by intrathymic injection of encephalitogen. *J Immunol.* 1970;105(2):322–326.
326. Lo D, Burkly LC, Widera G, et al. Diabetes and tolerance in transgenic mice expressing class II MHC molecules in pancreatic beta cells. *Cell.* 1988;53(1):159–168.
333. Sater RA, Sandel PC, Monroe JG. B cell receptor-induced apoptosis in primary transitional murine B cells: signaling requirements and modulation by T cell help. *Int Immunol.* 1998;10(11):1673–1682.
335. Nossal GJ. Choices following antigen entry: antibody formation or immunologic tolerance? *Annu Rev Immunol.* 1995;13:1–27.

339. Bretscher P, Cohn M. A theory of self-nonself discrimination. *Science.* 1970;169(950):1042–1049.
341. Gallucci S, Matzinger P. Danger signals: SOS to the immune system. *Curr Opin Immunol.* 2001;13(1):114–119.
347. Claman HN. Tolerance to a protein antigen in adult mice and the effect of nonspecific factors. *J Immunol.* 1963;91:833–839.
350. Lafferty KJ, Cunningham AJ. A new analysis of allogeneic interactions. *Aust J Exp Biol Med Sci.* 1975;53(1):27–42.
351. Jenkins MK, Schwartz RH. Antigen presentation by chemically modified splenocytes induces antigen-specific T cell unresponsiveness in vitro and in vivo. *J Exp Med.* 1987;165(2):302–319.
355. Janeway CA, Jr. The immune system evolved to discriminate infectious nonself from noninfectious self. *Immunol Today.* 1992;13(1): 11–16.
357. Janeway CA, Jr., Medzhitov R. Innate immune recognition. *Annu Rev Immunol.* 2002;20:197–216.
358. Takeda K, Kaisho T, Akira S. Toll-like receptors. *Annu Rev Immunol.* 2003;21:335–376.
360. Martinon F, Tschopp J. NLRs join TLRs as innate sensors of pathogens. *Trends Immunol.* 2005;26(8):447–454.
365. Matzinger P. Tolerance, danger, and the extended family. *Annu Rev Immunol.* 1994;12:991–1045.
368. Binder RJ, Srivastava PK. Essential role of CD91 in re-presentation of gp96-chaperoned peptides. *Proc Natl Acad Sci U S A.* 2004; 101(16):6128–6133.
373. Bausinger H, Lipsker D, Ziylan U, et al. Endotoxin-free heat-shock protein 70 fails to induce APC activation. *Eur J Immunol.* 2002; 32(12):3708–3713.
374. Dangl JL, Jones JD. Plant pathogens and integrated defence responses to infection. *Nature.* 2001;411(6839):826–833.
380. Shi Y, Galusha SA, Rock KL. Cutting edge: elimination of an endogenous adjuvant reduces the activation of CD8 T lymphocytes to transplanted cells and in an autoimmune diabetes model. *J Immunol.* 2006;176(7):3905–3908.
384. Wang H, Bloom O, Zhang M, et al. HMG-1 as a late mediator of endotoxin lethality in mice. *Science.* 1999;285(5425):248–251.
394. Lenschow DJ, Walunas TL, Bluestone JA. CD28/B7 system of T cell costimulation. *Annu Rev Immunol.* 1996;14:233–258.
395. McAdam AJ, Schweitzer AN, Sharpe AH. The role of B7 co-stimulation in activation and differentiation of CD4+ and CD8+ T cells. *Immunol Rev.* 1998;165:231–247.
397. Quezada SA, Jarvinen LZ, Lind EF, et al. CD40/CD154 interactions at the interface of tolerance and immunity. *Annu Rev Immunol.* 2004;22:307–328.
399. Watts TH. TNF/TNFR family members in costimulation of T cell responses. *Annu Rev Immunol.* 2005;23:23–68.
406. Schwartz RH. T cell anergy. *Annu Rev Immunol.* 2003;21:305–334.
412. Steinman RM, Hawiger D, Nussenzweig MC. Tolerogenic dendritic cells. *Annu Rev Immunol.* 2003;21:685–711.
413. Finkelman FD, Lees A, Birnbaum R, et al. Dendritic cells can present antigen in vivo in a tolerogenic or immunogenic fashion. *J Immunol.* 1996;157(4):1406–1414.
417. Morgan DJ, Kreuwel HT, Sherman LA. Antigen concentration and precursor frequency determine the rate of CD8+ T cell tolerance to peripherally expressed antigens. *J Immunol.* 1999;163(2):723–727.
420. Alegre ML, Frauwirth KA, Thompson CB. T-cell regulation by CD28 and CTLA-4. *Nat Rev Immunol.* 2001;1(3):220–228.
421. Okazaki T, Honjo T. The PD-1-PD-L pathway in immunological tolerance. Trends Immunol 2006;27(4):195–201.
439. Sharpe AH, Freeman GJ. The B7-CD28 superfamily. *Nat Rev Immunol.* 2002;2(2):116–126.
449. Savill J, Dransfield I, Gregory C, et al. A blast from the past: clearance of apoptotic cells regulates immune responses. *Nat Rev Immunol.* 2002;2(12):965–975.
459. Lemke G, Lu Q. Macrophage regulation by Tyro 3 family receptors. *Curr Opin Immunol.* 2003;15(1):31–36.
463. Blander JM, Medzhitov R. Toll-dependent selection of microbial antigens for presentation by dendritic cells. *Nature.* 2006;440(7085): 808–812.
468. Ridge JP, Di Rosa F., Matzinger P. A conditioned dendritic cell can be a temporal bridge between a CD4+ T-helper and a T-killer cell. *Nature.* 1998;393(6684):474–478.
474. Mescher MF, Curtsinger JM, Agarwal P, et al. Signals required for programming effector and memory development by CD8+ T cells. *Immunol Rev.* 2006;211:81–92.
477. Janssen EM, Droin NM, Lemmens EE, et al. CD4+ T-cell help controls CD8+ T-cell memory via TRAIL-mediated activation-induced cell death. *Nature.* 2005;434(7029):88–93.
482. Felton LD, Prescott B, Kauffmann G, et al. Pneumococcal antigenic polysaccharide substances from animal tissues. *J Immunol.* 1955;74(3):205–213.
490. Waldschmidt TJ, Borel Y, Vitetta ES. The use of haptenated immunoglobulins to induce B cell tolerance in vitro. The roles of hapten density and the Fc portion of the immunoglobulin carrier. *J Immunol.* 1983;131(5):2204–2209.
495. Dintzis HM, Dintzis RZ, Vogelstein B. Molecular determinants of immunogenicity: the immunon model of immune response. *Proc Natl Acad Sci U S A.* 1976;73(10):3671–3675.
498. Sinclair NR, Chan PL. Relationship between antibody-mediated immunosuppression and tolerance induction. *Nature.* 1971;234(5324): 104–105.
503. Pike BL, Abrams J, Nossal GJ. Clonal anergy: inhibition of antigen-driven proliferation among single B lymphocytes from tolerant animals, and partial breakage of anergy by mitogens. *Eur J Immunol.* 1983;13(3):214–220.
506. Goodnow CC. Transgenic mice and analysis of B-cell tolerance. *Annu Rev Immunol.* 1992;10:489–518.
510. Adelstein S, Pritchard-Briscoe H, Anderson TA, et al. Induction of self-tolerance in T cells but not B cells of transgenic mice expressing little self antigen. *Science.* 1991;251(4998):1223–1225.
511. Chiller JM, Habicht GS, Weigle WO. Kinetic differences in unresponsiveness of thymus and bone marrow cells. *Science.* 1971; 171(973):813–815.
518. Blery M, Tze L, Miosge LA, et al. Essential role of membrane cholesterol in accelerated BCR internalization and uncoupling from NF-kappa B in B cell clonal anergy. *J Exp Med.* 2006;203(7):1773–1783.
528. Rathmell JC, Townsend SE, Xu JC, et al. Expansion or elimination of B cells in vivo: dual roles for CD40- and Fas (CD95)-ligands modulated by the B cell antigen receptor. *Cell.* 1996;87(2):319–329.
530. Lesley R, Xu Y, Kalled SL, et al. Reduced competitiveness of autoantigen-engaged B cells due to increased dependence on BAFF. *Immunity.* 2004;20(4):441–453.
534. Roark JH, Bui A, Nguyen KA, et al. Persistence of functionally compromised anti-double-stranded DNA B cells in the periphery of non-autoimmune mice. *Int Immunol.* 1997;9(11):1615–1626.
536. Culton DA, O'Conner BP, Conway KL, et al. Early preplasma cells define a tolerance checkpoint for autoreactive B cells. *J Immunol.* 2006;176(2):790–802.
537. Grossman Z, Paul WE. Adaptive cellular interactions in the immune system: the tunable activation threshold and the significance of subthreshold responses. *Proc Natl Acad Sci U S A.* 1992;89(21):10365–10369.
538. Russell DM, Dembic Z, Morahan G, et al. Peripheral deletion of self-reactive B cells. *Nature.* 1991;354(6351):308–311.
544. Strasser A, Whittingham S, Vaux DL, et al. Enforced BCL2 expression in B-lymphoid cells prolongs antibody responses and elicits autoimmune disease. *Proc Natl Acad Sci U S A.* 1991;88(19):8661–8665.
548. Kearney ER, Pape KA, Loh DY, et al. Visualization of peptide-specific T cell immunity and peripheral tolerance induction in vivo. *Immunity.* 1994;1(4):327–339.
549. Shokat KM, Goodnow CC. Antigen-induced B-cell death and elimination during germinal-centre immune responses. *Nature.* 1995;375(6529):334–338.
556. Webb S, Morris C, Sprent J. Extrathymic tolerance of mature T cells: clonal elimination as a consequence of immunity. *Cell.* 1990;63(6):1249–1256.
559. Rocha B, von Boehmer H. Peripheral selection of the T cell repertoire. *Science.* 1991;251(4998):1225–1228.
563. Hildeman DA, Zhu Y, Mitchell TC, et al. Activated T cell death in vivo mediated by proapoptotic bcl-2 family member bim. *Immunity.* 2002;16(6):759–767.
565. Zheng L, Fisher G, Miller RE, et al. Induction of apoptosis in mature T cells by tumour necrosis factor. *Nature.* 1995;377(6547):348–351.

567. Lum JJ, Bauer DE, Kong M, et al. Growth factor regulation of autophagy and cell survival in the absence of apoptosis. *Cell.* 2005;120(2):237–248.
569. van Stipdonk MJ, Lemmens EE, Schoenberger SP. Naive CTLs require a single brief period of antigenic stimulation for clonal expansion and differentiation. *Nat Immunol.* 2001;2(5):423–429.
572. Vella AT, McCormack JE, Linsley PS, et al. Lipopolysaccharide interferes with the induction of peripheral T cell death. *Immunity.* 1995;2(3):261–270.
576. Jiang H, Zhang SI, Pernis B. Role of CD8+ T cells in murine experimental allergic encephalomyelitis. *Science.* 1992;256(5060):1213–1215.
577. Hu D, Ikizawa K, Lu L, et al. Analysis of regulatory CD8 T cells in Qa-1-deficient mice. *Nat Immunol.* 2004;5(5):516–523.
584. Tanchot C, Rocha B. The peripheral T cell repertoire: independent homeostatic regulation of virgin and activated CD8+ T cell pools. *Eur J Immunol.* 1995;25(8):2127–2136.
589. Surh CD, Sprent J. Regulation of mature T cell homeostasis. *Semin Immunol.* 2005;17(3):183–191.
593. Lamb JR, Skidmore BJ, Green N, et al. Induction of tolerance in influenza virus-immune T lymphocyte clones with synthetic peptides of influenza hemagglutinin. *J Exp Med.* 1983;157(5):1434–1447.
595. Beverly B, Kang SM, Lenardo MJ, et al. Reversal of in vitro T cell clonal anergy by IL-2 stimulation. *Int Immunol.* 1992;4(6):661–671.
600. Zha Y, Marks R, Ho AW, et al. T cell anergy is reversed by active Ras and is regulated by diacylglycerol kinase-alpha. *Nat Immunol.* 2006;7(11):1166–1173.
603. Sloan-Lancaster J, Evavold BD, Allen PM. Induction of T-cell anergy by altered T-cell-receptor ligand on live antigen-presenting cells. *Nature.* 1993;363(6425):156–159.
605. Macian F, Garcia-Cozar F, Im SH, et al. Transcriptional mechanisms underlying lymphocyte tolerance. *Cell.* 2002;109(6):719–731.
608. Heissmeyer V, Macian F, Im SH, et al. Calcineurin imposes T cell unresponsiveness through targeted proteolysis of signaling proteins. *Nat Immunol.* 2004;5(3):255–265.
613. Powell JD, Lerner CG, Schwartz RH. Inhibition of cell cycle progression by rapamycin induces T cell clonal anergy even in the presence of costimulation. *J Immunol.* 1999;162(5):2775–2784.
620. Wells AD, Walsh MC, Bluestone JA, et al. Signaling through CD28 and CTLA-4 controls two distinct forms of T cell anergy. *J Clin Invest.* 2001;108(6):895–903.
625. Tham EL, Shrikant P, Mescher MF. Activation-induced nonresponsiveness: a Th-dependent regulatory checkpoint in the CTL response. *J Immunol.* 2002;168(3):1190–1197.
628. Rammensee HG, Kroschewski R, Frangoulis B. Clonal anergy induced in mature V beta 6+ T lymphocytes on immunizing Mls-1b mice with Mls-1 a expressing cells. *Nature.* 1989;339(6225):541–544.
632. Ramsdell F, Lantz T, Fowlkes BJ. A nondeletional mechanism of thymic self tolerance. *Science.* 1989;246(4933):1038–1041.
634. Lanoue A, Bona C, von Boehmer H, et al. Conditions that induce tolerance in mature CD4+ T cells. *J Exp Med.* 1997;185(3):405–414.
638. Rocha B, Grandien A, Freitas AA. Anergy and exhaustion are independent mechanisms of peripheral T cell tolerance. *J Exp Med.* 1995;181(3):993–1003.
641. Oxenius A, Zinkernagel RM, Hengartner H. Comparison of activation versus induction of unresponsiveness of virus-specific CD4+ and CD8+ T cells upon acute versus persistent viral infection. *Immunity.* 1998;9(4):449–457.
653. Singh NJ, Chen C, Schwartz RH. The impact of T cell intrinsic antigen adaptation on peripheral immune tolerance. *PLoS Biol.* 2006;4(11):e340.
656. Wherry EJ, Blattman JN, Murali-Krishna K, et al. Viral persistence alters CD8 T-cell immunodominance and tissue distribution and results in distinct stages of functional impairment. *J Virol.* 2003;77(8):4911–4927.
659. Asherson GL, Stone SH. Selective and specific inhibition of 24 hour skin reactions in the guinea-pig. I. Immune deviation: description of the phenomenon and the effect of splenectomy. *Immunology.* 1965;9(3):205–217.
661. Parish CR, Liew FY. Immune response to chemically modified flagellin. 3. Enhanced cell-mediated immunity during high and low zone antibody tolerance to flagellin. *J Exp Med.* 1972;135(2):298–311.
663. Mosmann TR, Coffman RL. TH1 and TH2 cells: different patterns of lymphokine secretion lead to different functional properties. *Annu Rev Immunol.* 1989;7:145–173.
672. Pestka S, Krause CD, Sarkar D, et al. Interleukin-10 and related cytokines and receptors. *Annu Rev Immunol.* 2004;22:929–979.
673. Roncarolo MG, Gregori S, Battaglia M, et al. Interleukin-10-secreting type 1 regulatory T cells in rodents and humans. *Immunol Rev.* 2006;212:28–50.
680. Seder RA, Paul WE, Davis MM, et al. The presence of interleukin 4 during in vitro priming determines the lymphokine-producing potential of CD4+ T cells from T cell receptor transgenic mice. *J Exp Med.* 1992;176(4):1091–1098.
683. Li L, Sad S, Kagi D, et al. CD8Tc1 and Tc2 cells secrete distinct cytokine patterns in vitro and in vivo but induce similar inflammatory reactions. *J Immunol.* 1997;158(9):4152–4161.
684. Weaver CT, Harrington LE, Mangan PR, et al. Th17: an effector CD4 T cell lineage with regulatory T cell ties. *Immunity.* 2006;24(6):677–688.
695. Bacchetta R, Bigler M, Touraine JL, et al. High levels of interleukin 10 production in vivo are associated with tolerance in SCID patients transplanted with HLA mismatched hematopoietic stem cells. *J Exp Med.* 1994;179(2):493–502.
698. Groux H, O'Garra A, Bigler M, et al. A CD4+ T-cell subset inhibits antigen-specific T-cell responses and prevents colitis. *Nature.* 1997;389(6652):737–742.
702. Roncarolo MG, Bacchetta R, Bordignon C, et al. Type 1 T regulatory cells. *Immunol Rev.* 2001;182:68–79.
709. Apostolou I, von Boehmer H. In vivo instruction of suppressor commitment in naive T cells. *J Exp Med.* 2004;199(10):1401–1408.
711. Chen W, Jin W, Hardegen N, et al. Conversion of peripheral CD4+CD25- naive T cells to CD4+CD25+ regulatory T cells by TGF-beta induction of transcription factor Foxp3. *J Exp Med.* 2003;198(12):1875–1886.
715. Belkaid Y, Rouse BT. Natural regulatory T cells in infectious disease *Nat Immunol.* 2005;6(4):353–360.
718. Coombes JL, Robinson NJ, Maloy KJ, et al. Regulatory T cells and intestinal homeostasis. *Immunol Rev.* 2005;204:184–194.
723. Moore KW, Vieira P, Fiorentino DF, et al. Homology of cytokine synthesis inhibitory factor (IL-10) to the Epstein-Barr virus gene BCRFI. *Science.* 1990;248(4960):1230–1234.
728. Ptak W, Rozycka D, Askenase PW, et al. Role of antigen-presenting cells in the development and persistence of contact hypersensitivity. *J Exp Med.* 1980;151(2):362–375.
731. Faria AM, Weiner HL. Oral tolerance. *Immunol Rev.* 2005;206:232–259.
734. Chase M. Inhibition of experimental drug allergy by prior feeding of the sensitizing agent. *Proc Soc Exp Biol Med.* 1946;61:257–259.
735. Asherson GL, Zembala M, Perera MA, et al. Production of immunity and unresponsiveness in the mouse by feeding contact sensitizing agents and the role of suppressor cells in the peyer's patches, mesenteric lymph nodes and other lymphoid tissues. *Cell Immunol.* 1977;33(1):145–155.
749. Letterio JJ, Geiser AG, Kulkarni AB, et al. Autoimmunity associated with TGF-beta1-deficiency in mice is dependent on MHC class II antigen expression. *J Clin Invest.* 1996;98(9):2109–2119.
750. Gorelik L, Flavell RA. Abrogation of TGFbeta signaling in T cells leads to spontaneous T cell differentiation and autoimmune disease. *Immunity.* 2000;12(2):171–181.
754. Mellor AL, Munn DH. IDO expression by dendritic cells: tolerance and tryptophan catabolism. *Nat Rev Immunol.* 2004;4(10):762–774.
772. Bloom BR, Salgame P, Diamond B. Revisiting and revising suppressor T cells. *Immunol Today.* 1992;13(4):131–136.
774. Chess L, Jiang H. Resurrecting CD8+ suppressor T cells. *Nat Immunol.* 2004;5(5):469–471.
779. Vandenbark AA, Hashim G, Offner H. Immunization with a synthetic T-cell receptor V-region peptide protects against experimental autoimmune encephalomyelitis. *Nature.* 1989;341(6242):541–544.
785. Chang CC, Ciubotariu R, Manavalan JS, et al. Tolerization of dendritic cells by T(S) cells: the crucial role of inhibitory receptors ILT3 and ILT4. *Nat Immunol.* 2002;3(3):237–243.

801. Fink PJ, Shimonkevitz RP, Bevan MJ. Veto cells. *Annu Rev Immunol.* 1988;6:115–137.
802. Sambhara SR, Miller RG. Programmed cell death of T cells signaled by the T cell receptor and the alpha 3 domain of class I MHC. *Science.* 1991;252(5011):1424–1427.
808. Uhr JW, Moller G. Regulatory effect of antibody on the immune response. *Adv Immunol.* 1968;8:81–127.
813. Fazekas de SG, Webster RG. Disquisitions on Original Antigenic Sin. II. Proof in lower creatures. *J Exp Med.* 1966;124(3):347–361.
815. Ravetch JV, Bolland S. IgG Fc receptors. *Annu Rev Immunol.* 2001;19:275–290.
828. Lundkvist I, Coutinho A, Varela F, et al. Evidence for a functional idiotypic network among natural antibodies in normal mice. *Proc Natl Acad Sci U S A.* 1989;86(13):5074–5078.
829. Briles DE, Nahm M, Schroer K, et al. Antiphosphocholine antibodies found in normal mouse serum are protective against intravenous infection with type 3 streptococcus pneumoniae. *J Exp Med.* 1981;153(3):694–705.
837. Simpson E. A historical perspective on immunological privilege. *Immunol Rev.* 2006;213:12–22.
845. Green DR, Ferguson TA. The role of Fas ligand in immune privilege. *Nat Rev Mol Cell Biol.* 2001;2(12):917–924.
860. Niederkorn JY. The induction of anterior chamber-associated immune deviation. Chem Immunol Allergy 2007;92:27–35.
862. Beer AE, Billingham RE. Transplantation in nature. *Perspect Biol Med.* 1979;22(2 Pt 1):155–169.
874. Pazmany L, Mandelboim O, Vales-Gomez M, et al. Protection from natural killer cell-mediated lysis by HLA-G expression on target cells. *Science.* 1996;274(5288):792–795.
875. Parham P. NK cells and trophoblasts: partners in pregnancy. *J Exp Med.* 2004;200(8):951–955.
885. James E, Chai JG, Dewchand H, et al. Multiparity induces priming to male-specific minor histocompatibility antigen, HY, in mice and humans. *Blood.* 2003;102(1):388–393.
886. Tafuri A, Alferink J, Moller P, et al. T cell awareness of paternal alloantigens during pregnancy. *Science.* 1995;270(5236):630–633.
892. Aluvihare VR, Kallikourdis M, Betz AG. Regulatory T cells mediate maternal tolerance to the fetus. *Nat Immunol.* 2004;5(3):266–271.
897. Stites DP, Siiteri PK. Steroids as immunosuppressants in pregnancy. *Immunol Rev.* 1983;75:117–138.
902. Chaouat G, Assal MA, Martal J, et al. IL-10 prevents naturally occurring fetal loss in the CBA × DBA/2 mating combination, and local defect in IL-10 production in this abortion-prone combination is corrected by in vivo injection of IFN-tau. *J Immunol.* 1995;154(9):4261–4268.
901. Krishnan L, Guilbert LJ, Russell AS, et al. Pregnancy impairs resistance of C57 BL/6 mice to Leishmania major infection and causes decreased antigen-specific IFN-gamma response and increased production of T helper 2 cytokines. *J Immunol.* 1996;156(2):644–652.
913. Xu C, Mao D, Holers VM, et al. A critical role for murine complement regulator crry in fetomaternal tolerance. *Science.* 2000;287(5452):498–501.

Chapter 30

Regulatory/Suppressor T Cells

Ethan M. Shevach

INTRODUCTION

T cells are crucial in the immune response because they can function as both effector cells in cell-mediated responses and as helper cells in both humoral and cell-mediated responses. Most biologic systems are subject to complex regulatory controls, and the immune system is not an exception. In addition to T cells that upregulate (help), other populations that downregulate (suppress) the immune response must exist. Once a normal immune response is initiated by antigenic stimulation, mechanisms must be in place to control the magnitude of that response and to terminate it over time. Downregulation should contribute to the homeostatic control of all immune responses, serving to limit clonal expansion and effector-cell activity in response to any antigenic stimulus. An active mechanism of T-cell suppression is also needed to control potentially pathogenic autoreactive T cells. The primary mechanism that leads to tolerance to self-antigens is thymic deletion of autoreactive T cells, but some autoreactive T cells may escape thymic deletion or recognize antigens that are expressed only extrathymically. T-cell anergy *(1)* and T-cell ignorance/indifference *(2)* have been proposed as the primary mechanisms used to control autoreactive T cells

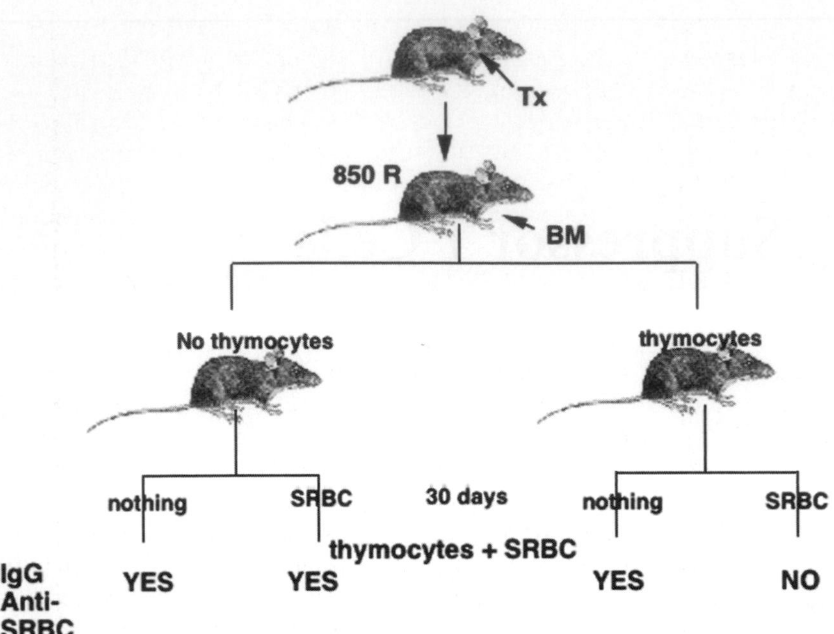

FIGURE 30.1 First demonstration of suppressor T cells. Adapted from Gershon RK, Kondo K. Cell interactions in the induction of tolerance: The role of thymic lymphocytes. *Immunology.* 1970;18:723–735.

in the periphery, although these "passive" mechanisms for self-tolerance may not be sufficient to control potentially pathogenic T cells.

It was proposed more than 30 years ago that a distinct subset of T cells is responsible for immune suppression (3). A suppressor T cell is functionally defined as a T cell that inhibits an immune response by influencing the activity of another cell type. Although a strong theoretical basis exists for T-cell–mediated suppression, this area of immunologic research has been plagued by controversy. The past decade has seen a resurgence of interest in the concept of T-cell suppression mediated by a distinct subset of T cells that are uniquely equipped to mediate suppressor activity.

HISTORICAL PERSPECTIVE

Suppressor T cells were first identified by Gershon and Kondo (3,4) during studies designed to understand the process of "high-zone" tolerance. Injection of supraoptimal doses of an antigen including sheep red blood cells (SRBC) resulted in specific tolerance or nonresponsiveness to subsequent challenge with that antigen. It was believed at that time that the antibody-producing B cell was rendered nonresponsive by exposure to the high concentration of antigen. To investigate whether B-cell tolerance was dependent on the presence of T cells, Gershon and Kondo injected high doses (2.5×10^{10}) of SRBC into thymectomized (Tx), irradiated, bone marrow–reconstituted mice and then assayed the functional status of B cells from these mice by a secondary challenge with SRBC in the presence of added thymocytes as a source of T-cell help. Surprisingly, nonresponsiveness as measured by deficient antibody production was only induced in the B cells of animals that had received thymocytes as well as bone marrow cells during the initial exposure to high-dose antigen, but not in mice that received bone marrow alone (Figure 30.1). This result fulfilled Gershon's prediction that under certain conditions antigen seen by T cells can induce not only helper and effector cells, but also cells that are able to suppress immune responses. Furthermore, when spleen cells from tolerized animals were transferred into secondary recipients together with normal thymocytes and bone marrow cells, they were capable of suppressing the otherwise competent response of these animals to SRBC. This suppression, or "infectious tolerance," as it was originally termed, was antigen-specific, as the immune response to an unrelated antigen, horse RBC, was not inhibited (4). T cells were necessary for the induction of B-cell tolerance, and these T-suppressor cells were assumed to be a distinct cell population with a fully differentiated gene program that allowed them to perform a very specialized function. Other studies (5,6,7) during the 1970s supported the existence of T-cell–mediated suppression.

Most of the early studies in these models demonstrated that the T cells mediating suppression were distinct from T cells mediating help because the former were $CD8^+$, whereas the latter were $CD8^-$. The finding that T-suppressor effector cells were $CD8^+$ distinguished them from helper cells, but did not allow them to be distinguished from cytotoxic cells, which are also $CD8^+$. It remained possible that suppressor T cells were actually cytotoxic cells that killed the helper or effector T cells. A cell surface marker that seemed to identify a suppressor-cell–specific antigen was discovered in 1976. It was found that an antiserum raised by immunizing the congenic strains

B10.A(3R) with cells from B10.A(5R) mice or vice versa gave rise to an antiserum that seemed to react exclusively with suppressor cells (8). CD8$^+$ suppressor cells were also shown to bind antigen in the absence of MHC molecules. These experiments suggested that the suppressor effector cells differed from other T cells in that they were capable of binding antigen directly, and did not recognize processed antigenic peptides in association with products of the major histocompatibility complex (MHC) on the surface of antigen-presenting cells (APC). Soon after the existence of T-cell–mediated suppression was appreciated, some studies suggested that interactions among multiple distinct T-cell subpopulations might be involved. A CD4$^+$ cell was described that appeared to induce CD8$^+$ suppressor cells and was called the suppressor inducer cell. Contrasuppressor T cells had no independent helper, suppressor, or cytotoxic activity on an immune response, but enhanced immune responses by preventing the downregulation mediated by suppressor cells.

Research in this area rapidly shifted from studies of the function of intact T cells to studies of their soluble products *(9)*. By the late 1970s, soluble factors from T-suppressor cells were described by several groups, and cloned T-cell hybridomas that produced such factors were generated. T-cell suppression was regarded as being mediated by numerous soluble antigen-specific and nonspecific factors that comprised a functionally unique network (10,*11,12*). The cascade involved antigen-specific, I-J–restricted CD4$^+$ suppressor inducer cells (Ts1 cells), CD8$^+$ anti-idiotype–specific cells (Ts2 cells), followed by CD8$^+$ antigen-specific effector cells (Ts3 cells), whose suppressor function was not restricted by the MHC. Some of these cells were capable of binding directly to immobilized antigen in the absence of MHC molecules. Connectivity in this cellular cascade was mediated by a series of soluble factors: TsF1 was idiotypic, antigen-specific, and immunoglobulin heavy-chain variable (V_H) region restricted. TsF2 was anti-idiotypic and required delivery by a macrophage. TsF3 acted totally nonspecifically. TsF1 and TsF2 required antigen-presenting cells, but TsF3 did not. Most of these factors were composed of two polypeptide chains, one of which was capable of binding native antigen and the other of which bore a determinant recognized by anti-I-J antibodies.

These elaborate, highly convoluted suppressor cell pathways and circuits fell out of favor in the mid-1980s for a number of important reasons. The existence of I-J was called into question by the finding that the region of the MHC complex to which I-J mapped did not contain a gene that could encode a unique I-J polypeptide *(13)*. When the genes encoding the T-cell receptor were isolated, they were completely unrelated to the genes encoding Ig heavy chains, thereby calling into question the existence of T-cell factors that expressed Ig V region products. Many of the suppressor T-cell hybridomas that produced antigen-specific suppressor factors were found either to have unrearranged genes for the α or β-chains of the TCR or to have deleted genes for TCR β chain (14). No studies were ever performed that convincingly characterized at the molecular level any of the suppressor T-cell factors. These studies, together with the inability to identify a marker specific for suppressor T cells and the inability to purify suppressor T cells, raised considerable doubts about the existence of a distinct functional lineage of suppressor T cells.

Two completely different approaches to the demonstration of the importance of regulatory or suppressor T cells in the prevention of organ-specific autoimmunity were also developed in the 1970s. In one, mice that were Tx on the third day of life (d3Tx) were shown to develop organ-specific autoimmune diseases (Figure 30.2). The specific disease that developed varied with the strain of mouse under study; more than one organ could be involved in a given mouse. Most important, autoimmunity was not seen if the mouse was Tx on day 1 or day 7 of life, and disease could be completely prevented if the d3Tx mouse received a thymus transplant between days 10 and 15 of life (15). These observations led to the hypothesis that autoreactive T cells were exported from the thymus during the first 3 days of life and that somewhat later in ontogeny a population of suppressor cells emigrated from the thymus that controlled

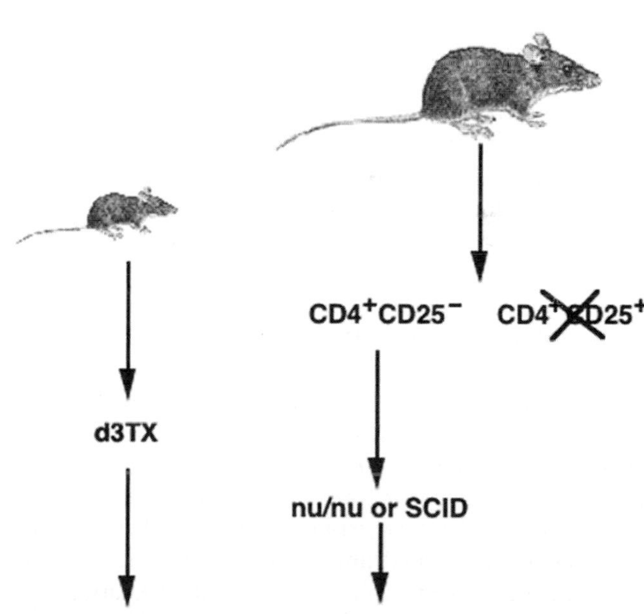

FIGURE 30.2 Depletion of CD4$^+$CD25$^+$ T cells results in organ-specific autoimmunity. Adapted from Nishizuka Y, Sakakura T. Thymus and reproduction: sex-linked dysgenesia of the gonad after neonatal thymectomy in mice. *Science.* 1969;166:753–755; and Sakaguchi S, Sakaguchi N, Asano M, et al. Immunologic self-tolerance maintained by activated T cells expressing IL-2 receptor α-chains (CD25). *J Immunol.* 1995;155:1151–1164.

TABLE 30.1 Organ-specific Autoimmune Disease and Lymphopenia

- 3dTx
- Neonatal administration of cyclosporine
- Thymectomy + repeated low-dose irradiation
- High-dose fractionated total lymphoid irradiation
- Adult thymectomy + cyclophosphamide
- Single TCR α-chain mice
- Transfer of T cells to T-cell–deficient mice

Adapted from Sakaguchi S, Sakaguchi N. Thymus, T cells, and autoimmunity: various causes but a common mechanism of autoimmune disease. In: Coutinho A, Kazatchkine MD, Eds. *Autoimmunity: Physiology and Disease.* Wiley-Liss; 1994:203–227.

the autoreactive T cells. Removal of the thymus before the suppressor cells reached the periphery resulted in autoimmune disease. A number of other protocols (Table 30.1) that induced a lymphopenic state also resulted in the development of organ-specific autoimmunity. It was believed that these procedures resulted in a selective depletion of suppressor T cells, while leaving the autoreactive effector populations intact. Subsequent studies demonstrated that the effector cells in this model were CD4$^+$ T cells. The suppressor T cells were also CD4$^+$ cells, and the development of autoimmune disease could be prevented by reconstitution of the d3Tx animals with peripheral CD4$^+$ T cells from normal adult mice *(16)*.

A second approach to define the role of T-regulatory cells (Treg) in the control of autoimmunity was described by Penhale and coworkers in the 1970s (17,*18*). They devised a procedure to deplete Treg from adult animals, while leaving the helper population responsible for autoantibody production intact. The disease model was autoimmune thyroiditis, because circulating antibody to thyroglobulin was believed to play an important pathogenic role. Spontaneous thyroiditis and circulating IgG autoantibodies developed in 60% of rats following the selective depletion of T cells by adult Tx followed by irradiation. Tx was performed between 3 and 5 weeks of age, and the rats were then given four to five repeated doses of 200 rad at 14-day intervals (Figure 30.3). No evidence of thyroiditis was seen in rats that received only local irradiation to the thyroid region, indicating that irradiation itself did not induce pathologic changes. The conclusion drawn from these studies was that in the normal animal, B cells that recognized thyroid antigens were prohibited from differentiating into autoantibody-producing cells by an active controlling T-cell mechanism. It was assumed that the suppressor T-cell population was mediating its functions by acting directly on the B cell and not by regulating other T cells. The active role of T cells in preventing the development of autoimmunity in this model was confirmed by reconstituting, shortly after the final dose of irradiation, the Tx-irradiated mice with lymphoid cells from normal donors. Penhale and colleagues (*19*) also demonstrated that autoimmune diabetes

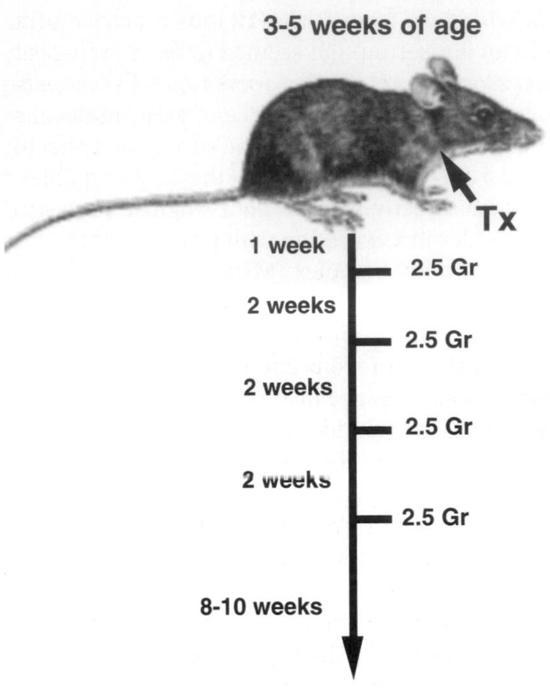

FIGURE 30.3 Induction of organ-specific autoimmunity in rats by adult thymectomy and irradiation. Adapted from Penhale WJ, Farmer A, Irvine WJ. Thyroiditis in T cell-depleted rats: influence of strain, radiation dose, adjuvants and antilymphocyte serum. *Clin Exp Immunol.* 1975:21:362–375.

would develop following the Tx-irradiation protocol in a strain of rats that was normally not susceptible to this disease. Taken together, the d3Tx model in the mouse and the Tx-irradiation model in the rat demonstrated that normally autoreactive helper and suppressor cells may coexist and that certain autoimmune responses are held in check by the equilibrium favoring suppressor activity.

IDENTIFICATION OF CD4$^+$CD25$^+$Foxp3$^+$ Treg

An important extension of this hypothesis was that inhibition of autoreactive T cells by suppressor T cells was not a phenomenon unique to the neonate, but that in the normal adult animal, autoreactive T cells are also under the constant control of the suppressor T cells. If the suppressor lineage was deleted, damaged, or compromised in the adult animal, autoimmune disease might develop. Although a number of studies suggested that the regulatory T cells in the normal adult animal might be identified by the expression of certain membrane antigens, for example, high levels of CD5 *(20)*, a major advance in our understanding of the role of regulatory T cells was the demonstration by Sakaguchi et al. (21,*22*), that a minor population of CD4+ T cells (10%) that coexpressed the CD25 antigen (the IL-2R α chain) appeared to function as regulatory T cells in the normal adult. When CD25+ T cells were depleted from a population of normal adult CD4+ T cells and the remaining CD4+CD25− T cells transferred to an immunocompromised recipient such as a *nu/nu* mouse, the recipients developed a spectrum of autoimmune diseases that closely resembled those seen following d3Tx (Figure 30.2). Co-transfer of the CD25+ cells prevented the development of autoimmunity. Similarly, the induction of disease post-d3Tx could also be prevented by reconstitution of the animals with CD4+CD25+, but not CD4+CD25−, normal adult T cells before day 14 of life (23). CD8+CD25− T cells alone were not capable of inducing autoimmunity and enhanced the induction of disease induced by CD4+CD25− T cells. These studies solidified the role of the CD4+CD25+ T cells as a major subset of cells that plays a unique role in the regulation of the immune response. The autoimmune diseases induced by depletion of CD4+CD25+ T cells are uniformly accompanied by the development of organ-specific autoantibodies, suggesting that this mode of loss of T-cell tolerance results in the breakdown of B-cell tolerance as well. It is likely that the activated self-reactive T-helper cells provide signals to self-reactive B cells, rescue them from apoptosis, and stimulate autoantibody production.

Powrie and Mason (24) were the first to identify cell surface markers that distinguished between regulatory and effector T-cell populations in the rat. When athymic rats were reconstituted with small numbers of CD4+CD45RC^{high} T cells, they developed a severe wasting disease characterized by extensive mononuclear cell infiltration in the lungs, liver, thyroid, stomach, and pancreas 6 to 10 weeks later. No pathology developed in rats that received unseparated CD4+ T cells or CD45RC^{low} cells. It seemed likely from these studies that the CD45RC^{low} subset controlled the capacity of the RC^{high} subset to mediate the wasting disease. The suppressive effect of the RC^{low} subset was directly demonstrated by Fowell and Mason (25) using the Tx-irradiation model develped by Penhale. Transfer of RC^{low} CD4+ T cells completely inhibited the development of diabetes and insulitis. RC^{low} T cells from long-term Tx donors could protect as efficiently as cells from normal donors, demonstrating that the regulatory T cell is long-lived in the periphery. Subsequently, CD4+CD45RB^{low} subset in the mouse was shown to have regulatory properties similar to the CD4+CD45RC^{low} subset of the rat (26). Taken together, these studies in mouse and rat model systems demonstrated for the first time that two well-characterized cell surface antigens (CD25 and CD45RC^{low}/CD45RB^{low}) could be used to identify suppressor CD4+ T-cell subpopulations present in normal animals. More recent studies have shown that the majority of the suppressor activity of the CD4+CD45RB^{low} population is mediated by the CD25+ T cells within that population (27).

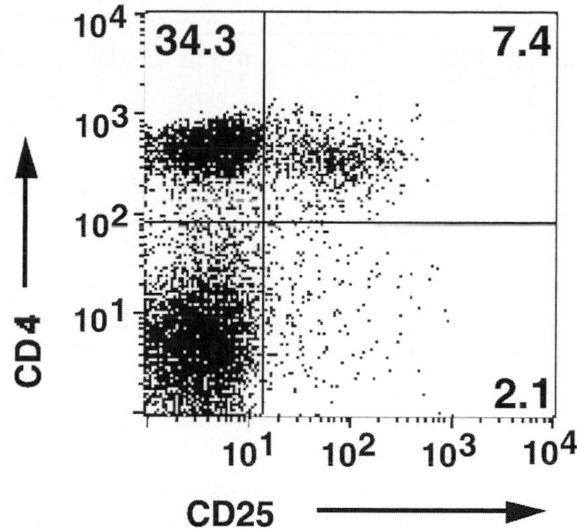

FIGURE 30.4 Identification of CD4+CD25+ T cells in normal mouse lymph node. Adapted from Thornton AM, Shevach EM. CD4+CD25+ immunoregulatory T cells suppress polyclonal T cell activation *in vitro* by inhibiting interleukin 2 production. *J Exp Med.* 1998;188:287–296.

CD4+CD25+ T cells typically represent 5% to 8% of the total population of T cells in the normal mouse lymph node (LN), or 10% to 15% of mouse CD4+ T cells (Figure 30.4). CD4+CD25+ T cells can also be found in the thymus, where they also represent about 5% to 10% of the mature CD4+CD8− population, or 0.5% of mouse thymocytes (21,*28*). A population with an identical phenotype has been identified in the rat, in human peripheral blood, and in human thymus (29,*30*,*31*,32,33,*34*,*35*,36). When compared directly to CD4+CD25− T cells, CD4+CD25+ T cells express slightly higher levels of CD5, have a slightly higher proportion of CD62L^{low} cells, and have a higher proportion of CD69+ cells. They express both intermediate and low levels of CD45RB, and are completely absent from the CD45RB^{high} population *(37)*. All of the CD4+CD25+ T cells express the TCR α/β receptor and are NK 1.1–negative. The distribution of expression of a given TCR Vα or Vβ specificity is similar on CD4+CD25+ and CD4+CD25− T cells *(28)*. One other unique property of CD25+ T cells in both mouse and human is that they are the only nonactivated T-cell population that expresses high levels of the CTLA-4 antigen intracellularly (27,38,39). The glucocorticoid-induced TNF-like receptor (GITR, TNFRSF18) has also been shown to be expressed on the majority of resting CD4+CD25+ T cells and to be expressed at very low levels on CD4+CD25− T cells (40,41). The GITR is upregulated on CD4+CD25− T cells following TCR-mediated activation.

A major advance in the study of Treg was derived from two related experiments of nature. Although CD4+CD25+ T cells were shown to display suppressive properties in multiple disease models, the value of CD25 has a marker is limited, as CD25 is highly expressed on both activated CD4

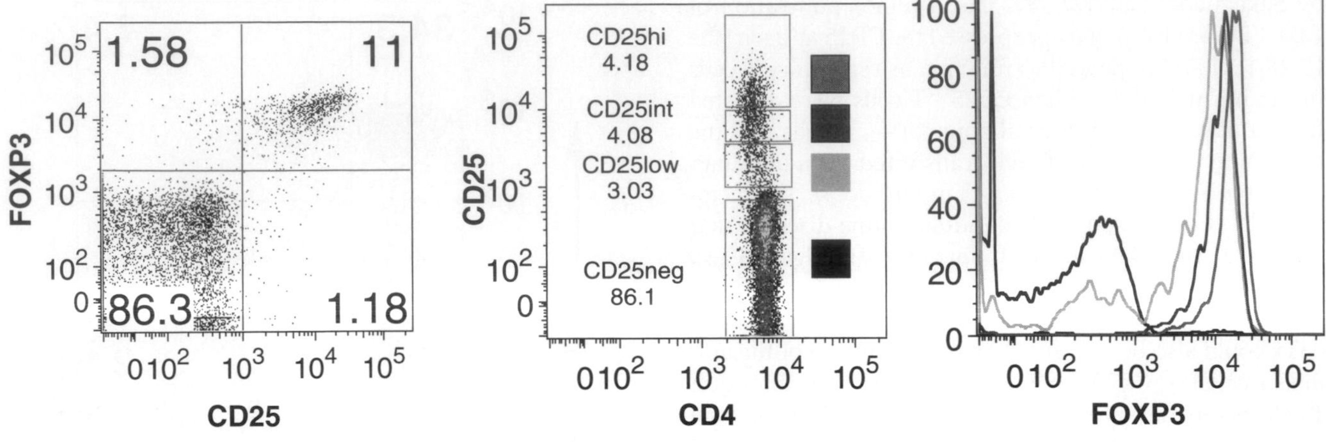

FIGURE 30.5 Correlation between CD25 expression and Foxp3 expression in mouse CD4+ cells.

and CD8 T cells, compromising its usefulness in studying Treg cells in settings of immune activation. Studies over the past 5 years have identified the X-chromosome–encoded forkhead transcription factor, Foxp3, as the key player in the biology of CD4+CD25+ Treg (*42*,43–45). Young males with the IPEX syndrome (immune dysregulation, polyendocrinopathy, enteropathy, X-linked) or a mutant mouse strain, scurfy, both succumb to similar autoimmune and inflammatory diseases as a result of uncontrolled activation and expansion of CD4+ T cells. Both IPEX patients and scurfy mice have mutations in a common gene, *Foxp3*, which encodes a forkhead-winged-helix transcription factor. There is an excellent correlation between expression of Foxp3 and CD25, but a minor population (~10%) of Foxp3+ cells is CD25− and about 10% of CD25+ cells are Foxp3− (Figure 30.5). It is likely that the latter represent activated effector cells. Expression of Foxp3 only in the thymus using a proximal lck-driven transgene does not prevent disease in scurfy mice. Foxp3 expression in peripheral T cells is thus required for maintenance of Treg function. Retroviral-mediated transduction of Foxp3 expression in naïve T cells can convert these cells to a regulatory phenotype functioning *in vitro* in a manner similar to CD4+CD25+ Treg. Furthermore, Foxp3-transduced naïve CD25− T cells also manifest suppressor activity *in vivo* and can inhibit the weight loss, diarrhea, and histologic development of colitis induced by transfer of CD25−CD45RB^{high} cells as effectively as Treg.

Fontenot et al. (46) generated Foxp3-deficient ($^{-/-}$) mice and demonstrated that Foxp3 is specifically required for the thymic development of Treg. Mixed bone marrow chimeras using wild-type (WT) and Foxp3$^{-/-}$ bone marrow demonstrated that Foxp3$^{-/-}$ T cells behaved normally in the presence of wild-type Foxp3+ Treg. Thus, the lethal autoimmune syndrome in Foxp3$^{-/-}$ mice results from a deficiency of Treg and not from a cell-intrinsic defect of CD4+CD25− T cells. Further study of the role of Foxp3 in Treg function has been greatly facilitated by the development of strains of mice in which a fluorescent protein such as GFP has been "knocked in" to the Foxp3 locus, permitting ready identification and isolation of Foxp3+ Treg by cell sorting (47). Studies of Treg development in the thymus of the Foxp3^{gfp} mice demonstrated that less than 0.1% of the CD4+CD8− thymocytes expressed Foxp3 within 12 hours after birth, and that the percentage of Foxp3+ CD4 SP thymocytes increased slowly over the following days and reached a plateau of ~4% at ~21 days after birth. The largest single-day change in the percentage of Foxp3 expressing SP occurred between days 3 and 4. Eighty percent of the Foxp3+ T cells on day 1 were CD4+CD8− SP cells. No DP-to-SP developmental progression was observed. This result correlates with the early studies on the d3Tx mice that suggested that the generation of Treg cells is delayed relative to generation of nonregulatory CD4+ T cells. Foxp3 was not expressed in nonhematopoietic tissues. Foxp3 expression in peripheral TCR $\alpha\beta$+ T cells regardless of CD25 expression correlates with suppressor activity.

Direct proof that Foxp3+ T cells maintain control of autoreactive T cells in the periphery has been shown by using a targeting construct encoding the human diptheria toxin receptor fused to sequences encoding GFP and equipped with an internal ribosome entry site into the 3′-untranslated region of Foxp3 (48). Complete elimination of Foxp3+ cells was achieved after 7 days of treatment with diptheria toxin. Foxp3 elimination at birth led to a syndrome very similar to that seen in Foxp3$^{-/-}$ mice. Treg cell elimination in adult nonlymphopenic mice resulted in an even more rapid development of terminal autoimmune disease than in neonates. This study demonstrates that self-reactive T cells, in the peripheral T-cell compartment of normal mice, must be controlled by Foxp3+ Treg cells to prevent the development of autoimmunity. Furthermore, Foxp3-independent recessive and dominant tolerance mechanisms established in adult mice are not sufficient

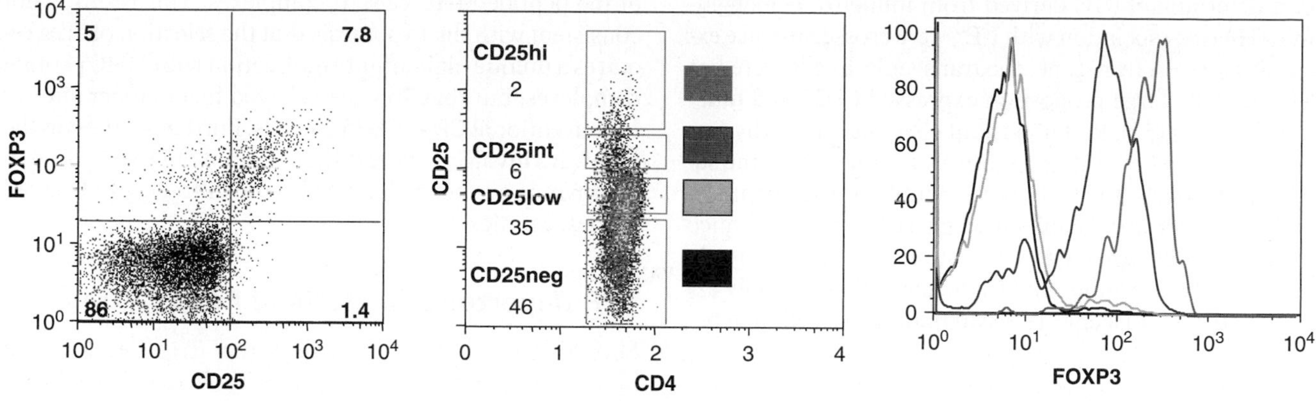

FIGURE 30.6 Correlation between CD25 expression and Foxp3 expression in human CD4+ cells.

to protect mice from fatal autoimmunity after elimination of Treg.

Isolation of human Treg continues to be a problematic, as one must rely on expression of cell surface antigens. It was reported that among T cells, only the highest expressors of CD25 (~2% of CD4+ T cells) exerted significant suppressive effects *in vitro (29)*. This observation was substantiated by a comparison of Foxp3 expression with CD25 expression on human CD4+ T cells. Almost all human CD4+CD25^{high} cells are Foxp3+, but a variable percentage of CD25^{int} cells express lower, but substantial, amounts of Foxp3 (Figure 30.6). Flow cytometric isolation of the CD25^{high} cells does allow one to obtain a population that is almost uniformly Foxp3+, but a substantial subset of Foxp3+ cells present in the CD25^{int} population will be lost. It has been proposed that almost all of human Foxp3+ T cells can be identified as expressing low levels of the IL-7 receptor (CD127), and that CD127^{low} expression can be used to isolate human Treg (48). However, CD127 is downregulated early in the course of T-cell activation, so the CD127^{low} phenotype is also unlikely to be Treg-specific during an ongoing immune or inflammatory response. In addition, only about 40% of the CD127^{low} population is Foxp3+, and even purified CD4+CD127^{low}CD25+ cells were only 85% to 90% Foxp3+. The utility of using the differential expression of CD127 for the isolation of human Treg requires further study.

Because the number of CD4+CD25+Foxp3+ T cells is remarkably constant in normal animals in the absence of perturbation of the immune system, they have been frequently referred to as thymic-derived, "naturally occurring" Treg (49). This nomenclature is not accurate, as biologically active Foxp3+ Treg can also be generated extrathymically in peripheral lymphoid tissues as well as *in vitro*. Many of the studies described in this chapter characterizing CD4+CD25+ T cells were performed prior to the availability of antibodies that recognized Foxp3. We will therefore use the terminology, Treg, to refer all T cells with regulatory properties, and we will attempt to further define the population where appropriate.

BIOLOGIC PROPERTIES OF CD4+CD25+ Foxp3+ Treg

Thymic Origin of Treg

The potential role of the thymus in the generation of regulatory T cells was first described several years ago *(50)*. Most studies strongly support the view that the Foxp3+ Treg population is produced in the thymus as a functionally mature, distinct T-cell subpopulation. Thymic Foxp3+ Treg is not derived from peripheral cells that have recirculated from the periphery to the thymus, because Treg developed *in vitro* in organ cultures of fetal thymus. CD4+CD25+ thymocytes are nonresponsive and suppress T-cell activation *in vitro* in a manner similar to Treg derived from the periphery *(28)*. The capacity of CD25+ T cells to migrate from the thymus to the periphery was documented by injection of FITC intrathymically. The percentage of CD4+CD25+ T cells within migrants and resident T cells was identical, suggesting that CD25+ T cells in the periphery can originate in the thymus *(51)*. Thymectomy at 4 to 5 weeks of age did not modify the number of CD25+ T cells in the periphery even when tested 19 months later.

It is widely accepted that conventional CD4+ and CD8+ T cells develop in the thymus by a process of positive and negative selection. Positive selection is mediated by interaction of developing T cells with MHC antigens on thymic cortical epithelium. Negative selection is mediated both by DC and thymic medullary epithelium. It is not known if a similar process is used for selection of Foxp3+ Treg. A number of studies have suggested that Treg undergoes a unique developmental process during its generation in the thymus. When TCR transgenic mice bearing a TCR specific for a determinant (S1) derived from influenza hemagglutinin (HA) in association with I-E^d were crossed to mice expressing the HA transgene, the transgenic T cells were not deleted and a large proportion expressed CD25 and functioned as Treg (52). Radioresistant elements of the thymus were shown to be both necessary and sufficient for the selection of CD25$^+$ T cells in these doubly transgenic mice. Similar results were obtained when TCR transgenic mice on a RAG$^{-/-}$ background were mated to the HA transgenic mice, clearly indicating that thymocytes that can only express a single transgenic TCR can undergo selection to become Treg.

A second TCR transgenic mouse was generated that expressed a variant determinant of HA, but that recognized the S1 determinant with 100-fold less affinity. When these mice were bred to the HA transgenic mouse (S1), they did not have an increased frequency of CD25$^+$ T cells. Thus, thymocytes with a low intrinsic affinity for the S1 peptide did not develop into CD25$^+$ thymocytes in response to HA. These data are consistent with a model in which selection of Treg that expresses a transgenic TCR depends on a high-affinity interaction of the TCR with its ligand. It could not be determined from these studies whether this selection process occurs on cortical or medullary epithelial cells. It is also not clear why only 50% rather than 100% of the exported thymocytes express CD25.

Although the affinity-based model of selection of Treg in the thymus is attractive and supported by some experiments, an alternative model for the differentiation of Treg in the thymus has been proposed by van Santen et al. (53). Most of the studies that demonstrated that MHC class II–restricted TCR transgenic thymocytes differentiated into Treg when they encountered their peptide/MHC ligand in the thymus demonstrated an increase in the relative percentage of Treg in the thymus and periphery, but failed to demonstrate an absolute increase in the numbers of Treg. If Treg in the thymus are more resistant than their non-Treg counterparts to clonal deletion, then conventional CD4$^+$ T cells will be deleted when they recognize their ligand in the thymus, and an increase in the proportion, but not the absolute numbers, of Foxp3$^+$ Treg will be observed. As a significant component of the repertoire of Treg is normally self-reactive, the repertoire of Treg cells molded by resistance to clonal deletion will be enriched in self-reactive specificities. The conventional CD4$^+$ repertoire will be decreased in self-reactive cells, as most will be removed by clonal deletion.

Other approaches (54) have suggested that the process of selection of CD4$^+$CD25$^+$ T cells is precisely the same as that involved in positive/negative selection of CD4$^+$CD25$^-$ T cells. Studies comparing the differentiation of Treg in mice expressing a single or many different peptides coupled to MHC class II demonstrate that the proportion of CD25$^+$ T cells in the CD4$^+$CD8$^-$ T-cell pool remains constant and that their total number reflects the complexity of the peptide/MHC class II complexes. This result is not consistent with the hypothesis that the selection of Treg requires a unique high-affinity interaction with MHC peptide complexes, but that Treg are selected in a manner similar to conventional CD4$^+$CD25$^-$ T cells. Further studies on the pathways involved in the differentiation of Foxp3$^+$ Treg in the thymus are needed to resolve the differences observed in these studies.

TCR Repertoire Analysis of Foxp3$^+$ Treg

Several lines of evidence suggest that Treg development hinges on a particular TCR specificity. Foxp3$^+$ Treg do not develop in TCR transgenic mice that lack RAG genes, suggesting that only cells with certain TCR specificities can develop into Treg. Very few studies have addressed in detail either the TCR repertoire of Foxp3$^+$ Treg or their antigen specificity. Hsieh et al. (55) have directly compared the sequences of the CDR3 region on Treg and conventional T cells and found that they are only partially overlapping. When immunodeficient mice were reconstituted with T cells expressing diverse Vα2 TCR α chains from Treg or conventional T cells paired with a single Vβ chain, some of the Treg TCR-reconstituted T cells were self-reactive, as they induced wasting disease in lymphopenic hosts but not in conventional recipients. Although 40% of the TCR were strongly self-reactive *in vivo*, others were only intermittently and moderately self-reactive or nonreactive as measured by T-cell expansion in lymphopenic hosts.

TCR repertoire analysis has also been used to determine the relationship between Foxp3$^+$ Treg cells generated in the thymus and Foxp3$^+$ Treg generated in the periphery. When thymic and peripheral Foxp3$^-$ and Foxp3$^+$ T-cell clones in mice that express a controllable set of TCR encoded by a transgenic TCR α-chain minilocus, the TCR from Foxp3$^+$CD4$^+$ peripheral T cells resembled those of thymic precursors and differed from TCR expressed by Foxp3$^-$CD4$^+$ T cells; in addition, the diversity of Foxp3$^+$ TCR was greater than TCR on Foxp3$^-$CD4$^+$ naïve T cells (56). These studies support the view that the great majority of peripheral Foxp3$^+$ Treg derive from thymic precursors and that peripheral conversion from Foxp3$^-$ to Foxp3$^+$ is rare. Nevertheless, the intrathymic pathway of Treg maturation is still unclear. They may separate from conventional T cells during thymic selection of CD4$^+$CD8$^+$ thymocytes in the cortex or differentiate later from more mature CD4$^+$ thymocytes in the medulla. Although some studies have raised the possibility that Treg are generated in the thymic cortex (57), others favor the view that the thymic medulla is the site where Treg precursors mature after contacts with tissue-specific peptides presented by thymic medullary epithelial cells (58) or DC. However, Treg maturation is normal in AIRE$^{-/-}$ mice that have impaired presentation of either tissue-specific antigens and in CCR7$^{-/-}$ mice that have defects in thymocyte trafficking, raising the possibility that the cortex and not the medulla is required for Foxp3 induction.

TCR repertoire analysis has also been applied to autoreactive T cells in mice deficient in Foxp3 (59). These mice did not exhibit a defect in negative selection. Activated, but not naïve, T cells in Foxp3$^{-/-}$ mice often used TCR found in the Foxp3^{+} Treg TCR repertoire of normal mice, suggesting that T cells expressing these self-reactive TCR are not eliminated, but instead contribute to the pathology associated with Foxp3 deficiency. Thus, thymocytes expressing Treg cell TCR survive thymic deletion in Foxp3$^{-/-}$ mice, complete thymic development as non-Treg expressing self-reactive Treg TCR, and enhance the severity of disease in Foxp3$^{-/-}$ mice. It is also possible that WT mice have a population of self-reactive non-Treg that express the Treg self-reactive TCR repertoire that are not subject to negative selection, but potentially can induce autoimmune disease.

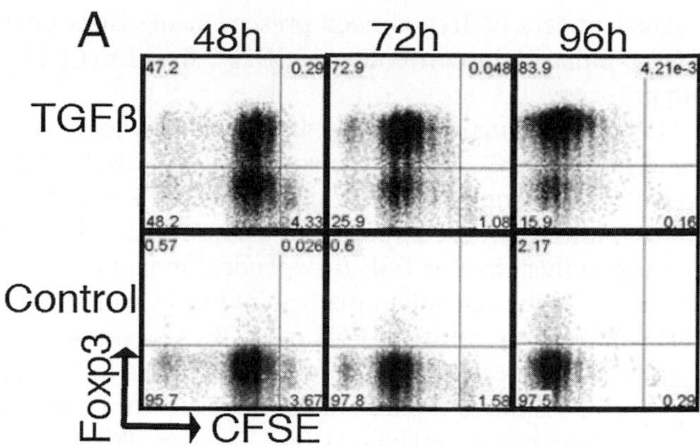

FIGURE 30.7 Naïve Foxp3^{-} T cells were cultured and stimulated in the presence of TGF-β. Foxp3 expression was determined by intracellular staining at the indicated times. Adapted from Davidson T, DiPaolo RJ, Andersson J, Shevach EM. Cutting Edge: IL-2 is essential for TGF-β-mediated induction of Foxp3^{+} regulatory cells. *J Immunol.* 2007;178:4027–4032.

Extrathymic Origin of Foxp3^{+} Treg

One important question that must be addressed is whether the thymus is the only site for the generation of Foxp3^{+} Treg. A number of studies performed both *in vivo* and *in vitro* have demonstrated that under certain conditions Foxp3^{+} Treg can be generated extrathymically and that TGF-β is a key component in this process. Administration of peptide antigen to TCR transgenic mice bred onto the RAG background, which lack Treg, resulted in prolonged expression of CD25 only when the antigen was administered under tolerogenic conditions *(60)*. The CD25^{+} cells had some Treg properties. Similarly, when Apostolou et al. (61) transferred splenic CD4^{+}CD25^{-} T cells specific for HA from RAG$^{-/-}$ mice to sublethally irradiated recipients that express HA under control of the Ig promoter, 5% of the injected T cells were CD25^{+}, while 95% of the cells were CD25^{-}. Both populations were anergic and were able to suppress the response of naïve T cells expressing the transgenic TCR. The mechanism of suppression used by these induced Treg was not explored. One highly effective method for the induction Treg with antigen was to expose TCR transgenic T cells on a RAG$^{-/-}$ background *in vivo* to a continuous supply of subimmunogenic doses of agonist peptides delivered via a mini-osmotic pump. Many of the T cells became Foxp3^{+} and resembled thymic-derived Treg in all their phenotypic and functional properties (62). It was postulated from these studies that low doses of peptide presented over relatively long periods of time on nonactivated DC represented a important mechanism by which Treg could be generated in the periphery particularly to self-components that do not lead to tolerance in the thymus. Further evidence in support of this hypothesis was obtained from studies in which peptide agonist ligands were targeted to DC in minute doses by coupling them to antibodies directed to DC under conditions of suboptimal DC activation (63). Treg induced with subimmunogenic conditions could subsequently be expanded by delivery of antigen in immunogenic conditions.

A number of groups (64–67) have presented studies that demonstrate a pivotal role for TGF-β in the generation of Foxp3^{+} Treg *in vitro*. TCR activation in the presence of TGF-β converted naïve T cells into Foxp3^{+} (Figure 30.7) cells with an anergic/suppressor phenotype. IL-2 plays a nonredundant role in TGF-β–mediated induction of Foxp3 expression in mouse CD4^{+} T cells. Once induced, Foxp3 expression was maintained both *in vitro* and *in vivo* in the absence of IL-2. Other cytokines utilizing the common γ chain as part of their receptors were unable to induced Foxp3 expression in IL-2$^{-/-}$ cells. The converted cells not only exhibit unresponsiveness to TCR stimulation, they also suppress normal CD4^{+} T-cell activation and Th1 and Th2 cytokine production *in vitro*. The induction of Foxp3 results in downregulation of Smad7 and renders T cells highly susceptible to the regulatory effects of TGF-β signaling via Smad3/4 (65). Foxp3^{+} T cells induced *in vitro* can suppress antigen-specific proliferation of CD4^{+} T cells *in vivo* and prevent house dust mite–induced mouse asthma. The ability of TGF-β to induce Foxp3 expression and endow the cell with a suppressive phenotype suggests a potential therapeutic intervention whereby antigen-specific, autoaggressive effector T cells could be transformed ex vivo into antigen-specific suppressors. Some studies suggest that TGF-β may also be capable of inducing Foxp3 expression *in vivo*. Peng et al. (68) used an inducible system for the transient induction of TGFβ in the pancreatic islets during the priming phase of diabetes. Approximately 40% to 50% of intraislet CD4^{+} T cells expressed CD25 and other characteristics of Treg. However, it is not clear if high levels of TGF-β resulted in the in situ expansion of the small numbers of Treg already present in the islets or if TGF-β induced the conversion of $CD25^-$ T cells to $CD25^+$ suppressors.

It thus remains unresolved whether and under what conditions $Foxp3^-$ T cells are converted to $Foxp3^+$ Treg *in vivo*. It is unknown whether any of the $Foxp3^+$ T cells in normal mice or, more important, in humans, are derived in the periphery by this TGF-β–dependent induction pathway. It is likely that inflammatory infiltrates would contain sufficient quantities of IL-2 and TGF-β, so this induction pathway should be operative *in vivo*. Thus far, it has not been possible to induce stable expression of Foxp3 in naïve human peripheral blood $CD4^+$ T cells by TCR stimulation in the presence of TGF-β. One additional major unresolved issue in humans relates to the origin of $Foxp3^+$ Treg in adults. Whereas mice live for 2 to 5 years, humans can live for eight decades, well beyond thymic involution early in life. It is far from clear whether the full complement of $Foxp3^+$ Treg is generated early in life and then persists for decades or if Treg might be generated from antigen-specific $CD4^+$ T cells that are approaching end-stage differentiation. A subpopulation of human Treg was highly proliferative *in vivo* with a doubling time of 8 days (69). However, these cells were also susceptible to apoptosis and had critically short telomeres and low telomerase activity, raising the possibility that they must be produced from another population source. Heteroduplex analysis of TCR from memory T cells and Treg suggested that they are closely clonally related, raising the possibility that some human Treg are not thymus-derived, but are generated from rapidly dividing, highly differentiated, memory $CD4^+$ T cells.

Cytokine Requirements for the Generation and Maintenance of Treg

It was initially observed that $CD4^+CD25^+$ T cells were absent from the periphery and from the $CD4^+CD8^-$ thymocyte population of IL-$2^{-/-}$ mice (51). Partial or more profound defects both in the number and function of $CD4^+CD25^+$ T cells have been reported in mice deficient for CD28 *(38)*, CD80/CD86, CD40 *(70)*, CD40L (71), CD122 (IL-2Rβ, (72)), and Stat5a (73). The one common factor that characterizes these mice is that the products of all the deficient genes have important roles in the production or responsiveness to IL-2. Treatment of mice with anti–IL-2 or with CTLA-4Ig to inhibit co-stimulatory signals also leads to a rapid decline in the number of $CD4^+CD25^+$ T cells (38). As $CD25^+$ T cells do not produce IL-2, this deficiency may be secondary to the capacity of $CD25^-$ T cells to produce IL-2, or to some intrinsic defect in the $CD25^+$ T cells in their capacity to respond to IL-2. Many, but not all, of these strains develop an autoimmune syndrome associated with lymphoproliferation. NOD mice have also been reported to have a defect in the numbers of $CD25^+$ T cells, but these cells appear to function normally (38). Blockade of the TRANCE-RANK pathway also has been shown to inhibit the generation and/or function of $CD4^+CD25^+$ T cells in a model of autoimmune diabetes (74).

IL-2 could be required for the generation of $CD4^+CD25^+$ T cells in the thymus and/or for their maintenance and survival in the periphery. One study (72) that suggests that IL-2 plays a nonredundant role in the differentiation of $CD4^+CD25^+$ T cells in the thymus was performed in mice deficient for the CD122. $CD122^{-/-}$ mice rapidly develop a lethal autoimmune syndrome. Transgenic expression of CD122 exclusively in the thymus prevents the development of autoimmunity and prolongs the lifespan of these mice from 8 to 12 weeks up to 12 to 16 months. $CD4^+CD25^+$ T cells are barely detectable in the thymus and absent from the periphery of $CD122^{-/-}$ mice. In contrast, $CD122^{-/-}$ mice with thymic-only expression of CD122 had twofold higher numbers of $CD4^+CD25^+$ T cells in the thymus and lymph nodes than WT mice. The $CD4^+CD25^+$ T cells from these mice were also fully capable of suppressing proliferative responses of T cells from WT mice. As cells from the peripheral lymphoid tissues of these mice are completely unresponsive to IL-2, these results suggest that IL-2 may only be required for the growth or survival of $CD4^+CD25^+$ T cells in the thymus, not in the periphery. It remains possible that other cytokines (e. g., IL-4) may in some circumstances be able to maintain $CD4^+CD25^+$ T cells in the periphery or that a higher output of $CD4^+CD25^+$ in the mice that express CD122 exclusively in the thymus may compensate for a lack of IL-2 in the periphery.

Other studies have proposed that in the absence of IL-2, Treg cannot survive or expand their numbers in the thymus or in the periphery (75), while other functional studies have suggested that IL-2 is directly required for Treg cell function and that in its absence Treg cells fail to suppress T-cell proliferation (76). One major problem with all these experiments is that they have relied on CD25 as a Treg cell marker. As CD25 expression is directly linked to IL-2 signaling, it has been impossible to detect and isolate Treg from mice with impaired IL-2 signaling based on CD25 expression. Fontenot et al. (77) analyzed mice expressing $Foxp3^{gfp}$ knock-in allele that were genetically deficient in either IL-2 or CD25. They found that IL-2 signaling was not required for the induction of Foxp3 expression in developing thymocytes, as Foxp3 was induced in a subset of developing thymocytes and $Foxp3^+$ Treg cells were present in substantial numbers, though reduced by one half compared to WT mice. BrdU incorporation of cells in the thymus differentiating into the Treg lineage was not substantially affected by the absence of IL-2. Thus, IL-2 signaling is not required for the development of $Foxp3^+$ Treg cells in the thymus. Both IL-$2^{-/-}$ and $CD25^{-/-}$ Treg cells were able to suppress T-cell proliferation *in vitro*. However, the numbers of Foxp3+ Treg cells in the periphery of IL-$2^{-/-}$, IL-2Rα, and IL-2R$\beta^{-/-}$ mice were substantially decreased or almost absent (78) and Foxp3+ IL-2R$\alpha^{-/-}$ T cells in mixed bone marrow chimeras had a substantially decreased competitive fitness compared to wild-type Foxp3+ Treg. The conclusion drawn from these studies was that IL-2 is an essential Treg cell growth factor *in vivo* and that in the absence of IL-2, Treg cells exhibit impaired metabolic fitness. IL-2 may be important in the maintenance of Foxp3 expression, as Foxp3 is increased in both wild-type and IL-$2^{-/-}$ mice after overnight treatment with exogenous IL-2. It appears that Foxp3 expression in Treg establishes a gene expression program that renders Treg critically dependent on paracrine IL-2 signaling, resulting in repression of IL-2 production and the induction of high IL-2Rα. No Foxp3-expressing thymic and peripheral CD4+ T cells can be detected in IL-2R$\gamma^{-/-}$ mice, indicating that other cytokines that utilize the common γ chain as part of their receptor complex may compensate for the absence of IL-2.

Analysis of Gene Expression by Foxp3+ Treg

Both DNA microarray technology and serial analysis of gene expression (SAGE) technology have been used to compare patterns of gene expression among different cell types (40,79,80). These technologies have also been applied to compare the patterns of gene expression in Treg with CD4+CD25− T cells and other cell types with regulatory functions. One major goal of this approach is to determine whether Treg simply represent a population of previously activated T cells, or whether they display a unique pattern of gene expression that is correlated with their functional properties. Most of the results are consistent with the latter possibility. Some genes are differentially expressed between the resting CD25− T cells and Treg, whereas others are differentially expressed following activation. A comparison of a number of these studies has permitted the identification of groups of genes that are relatively Treg-specific and allow one to begin to define a distinct Treg molecular signature (Table 30.2). Many of these identify activation antigens expressed on activated conventional T cells, including CTLA-4, GITR, and other members of the TNF-receptor superfamily that are expressed by activated effector cells. Some, including neuropilin, GITR, CD38, and CD5, appear to be shared with Foxp3−-anergic T cells that do not exert suppressive functions (81). Although some of the data from the SAGE analysis (80) suggested that Treg may be related to the subpopulation of T cells that secrete Th2 cytokines, on balance the studies on global gene expression indicate that Treg express a unique pattern of gene expression that may contribute to their survival and anergic state.

A Foxp3 chromatin immunoprecipitation method has been used to analyze the direct targets of Foxp3 (82,83). About 700 to 1,000 genes contain Foxp3-binding regions, and many of these genes are up- or downregulated in Foxp3+ T cells confirming that Foxp3 can function as both a transcriptional activator and a repressor. However, Foxp3 target genes comprise only a small portion of Foxp3-dependent gene expression, suggesting that Foxp3 regulates a large part of its transcriptional program by acting on other transcription factors (Table 30.3). It is likely that some genes encoding molecules that could potentially mediate suppressor function (e. g., IL-10, Granzyme B) are secondary Foxp3 targets, as they are not found in the group of genes that are direct Foxp3 targets.

One novel approach to understand the role of Foxp3 in directing Treg function is to engineer a mouse expressing the coding sequence of GFP knocked into the *Foxp3* locus together with disruption of Foxp3 protein expression (84,85). Surprisingly, the GFP+Foxp3− T cells in these mice shared many phenotypic features with their GFP+Foxp3+ counterparts. The former are what might be termed Treg "wannabees," as they develop in normal mice and respond to signals required to induce Foxp3 expression. The GFP+Foxp3− cells were unable to produce IL-2, effector cytokines, expressed elevated levels of CD25, were relatively nonresponsive to TCR stimulation, but lacked suppressor activity. Therefore, it is likely that Foxp3 does not function as the master inducer of the Treg lineage, but rather to stabilizes or enhances certain Treg characteristics. Suppression is exclusively dependent on Foxp3.

TABLE 30.2 *Genes* Selectively Activated in *CD4+ CD25+* T Cells

- *Signaling: COS, SOCS-1, SOCS-2, SLAP-130*
- *Secreted* molecules: *IL-10, IL-17,* enkephalin, *ETA-1, ECM-1, MIP-1α, MIP-1β*
- *Cell* surface molecules: *CD2, OX40, CD25, CD122, GPCR83, GITR, Ly-6, Galectin-1, Thy-1*

Adapted from McHugh RS, Whitters MJ, Piccirillo CA, et al. CD4+CD25+ immunoregulatory T cells: gene expression analysis reveals a functional role for the glucocorticoid-induced TNF receptor. *Immunity.* 2002;16:311–323.

TABLE 30.3 Transcription Factors Bound and Regulated by Foxp3

Prdm1
Irf6
CREM
Helios

Adapted from Zheng Y, Josefowicz SZ, Kas A, et al. Genome-wide analysis of Foxp3 target genes in developing and mature regulatory T cells. *Nature.* 2007;445:936–940; and Marson A, Kretchmer K, Frampton GM, et al. Foxp3 occupancy and regulation of key target genes during T-cell stimulation. *Nature.* 2007;445:931–935.

SUPPRESSOR MECHANISMS UTILIZED BY Foxp3$^+$ Treg

In vitro Studies

An *in vitro* model system has been established for the analysis of CD4$^+$CD25$^+$ Treg cell function that allows rapid assays and that may offer some insights to the mechanism of action of Treg function *in vivo* (37,86,87,88). This approach also allows a comparison of the requirements for activation (co-stimulation, antigen concentration) of CD25$^+$ T cells compared to CD25$^-$ T cells. Purified CD25$^+$ T cells were completely unresponsive to high concentrations of IL-2 alone, to stimulation with plate-bound or soluble anti-CD3, or to the combination of anti-CD3 and anti-CD28. They could be induced to proliferate when stimulated with the combination of anti-CD3 and IL-2, but not by stimulation of endogenous IL-2 production with anti-CD28. The most striking property of the CD25$^+$ T cells is their ability to suppress proliferative responses of both CD4$^+$ and CD8$^+$CD25$^-$ T cells (Figure 30.8). The CD25$^+$ T cells must be activated via their TCR to suppress. No suppression was seen when CD25$^+$ T cells were separated by semipermeable membrane from the CD25$^-$ T cells. This demonstrates that cell contact between CD25$^+$ and CD25$^-$ T cells is required. Neutralization of the suppressor cytokines IL-4, IL-10, and TGF-β individually or in combination also had no effect on the CD25-mediated suppression. Similarly, CD25$^+$ T cells from mice deficient in IL-4, IL-10, or TGF-β were fully competent suppressors. Indo-1–loaded CD25$^+$ T cells did not flux calcium in response to TCR stimulation (79), suggesting that they have a block in proximal signaling similar to that seen in T cells rendered anergic *in vitro*.

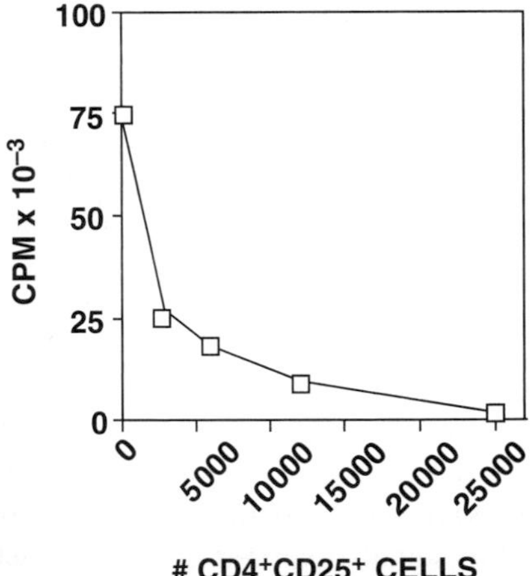

FIGURE 30.8 CD4$^+$CD25$^+$ T cells suppress the proliferative response of CD4$^+$CD25$^-$ T cells. Graded numbers of CD4$^+$CD25$^+$ T cells were mixed with 5 × 104 CD4$^+$CD25$^-$ T cells, T-depleted spleen cells, and soluble anti-CD3. Proliferation was measured after 72 hours. Adapted from Thornton AM, Shevach EM. CD4$^+$CD25$^+$ immunoregulatory T cells suppress polyclonal T cell activation *in vitro* by inhibiting interleukin 2 production. *J Exp Med.* 1998;188:287–296.

CD25$^+$ T cells mediate suppression by inhibiting the induction of IL-2 mRNA in the responder CD25$^-$ T cells. Thus, the trivial explanation for their suppressive properties that they bind IL-2 and function as IL-2 "sinks" *(89)* is completely ruled out, as no IL-2 is produced in the co-cultures. Suppression can be abrogated by the addition of IL-2, thereby circumventing the block. Although IL-2 gene transcription was inhibited in the presence or absence of exogenous IL-2, the addition of anti-CD28 overcomes suppression by potently stimulating the production of endogenous IL-2 and overriding the suppressive effects of the CD25$^+$ cells. Surprisingly, transcription of IL-2 mRNA was also restored in the co-cultures in the presence of anti-IL-2. These results suggest that Treg do not suppress the initial activation of CD4$^+$CD25$^-$ T cells, but mediate their suppressive effects following production of IL-2 by the responder cells, resulting in both the expansion of the Treg and induction/enhancement of their suppressor functions (76). CD25$^+$ T cells do not directly mediate the death of the responders, but induce a cell-cycle arrest at the G_1-S phase of the cell cycle. Such a cell-cycle arrest is often followed by cell death, and it is difficult to recover significant numbers of viable cells when the suppressors and responders are co-cultured for periods longer than 48 hours. Suppression of T-cell proliferation is the exclusive property of CD25$^+$ T cells isolated from normal animals. The induction of CD25 expression by stimulating CD25$^-$ T cells via the TCR, in the absence of TGF-β, does not render the stimulated cells suppressive. In this regard, it is important to emphasize that expression of CD25 does not indicate that a cell is likely to have suppressive properties.

CD25$^+$ T cells can be easily propagated *in vitro* for 3 to 14 days by stimulation initially with anti-CD3 and IL-2 and then expansion in IL-2 alone (88). It has also been possible to clone murine CD25$^+$ T cells by repeated stimulation with anti-CD3 and IL-2 (41). Following 7 to 14 days of activation and culture in IL-2, activated CD25$^+$ T cells remain nonresponsive and cannot be induced to proliferate when restimulated via their TCR in the absence of IL-2. The activated CD25$^+$ T cells have more potent suppressor activity on a per-cell basis (three- to fourfold) than freshly explanted CD25$^+$ T cells. CD25$^+$ T cells that appear to be antigen-specific can be identified in mice that express a transgenic TCR. In general, the percentage of CD25$^+$ cells is reduced in TCR transgenic mice (3% to 5%, compared to 10% in normal animals). The expression of the transgenic TCR α chain is a convenient tool that allows activation of the CD25$^+$ T cells with peptide/MHC rather than with anti-CD3 (88). When T cells from TCR transgenic mice are activated with their peptide/MHC ligand and then expanded *in vitro* in IL-2, the activated suppressors are subsequently capable of suppressing the

TABLE 30.4 The Suppressor Effector Function of Activated CD4$^+$CD25$^+$ T Cells Is Completely Nonspecific

First Culture		*Second Culture (TCR Tg CD4$^+$ CD25$^-$ T Cells for Specific for)*	*Percent Suppression*
CD4$^+$CD25$^+$ from HA		I-A^d + $HA_{126-138}$	99
TCR Tg stimulated with	→	I-E^d + $HA_{110-119}$	99
$HA_{126-138}$ + IL-2		I-E^k + PCC_{88-104}	95
3–7 days		I-A^u + MBP_{Ac1-11}	91

CD$^+$CD25$^+$ T cells from mice expressing a TCR transgene specific for $HA_{126-138}$ were cultured with peptide, T-depleted spleen cells, and IL-2. They were then washed and mixed with CD4$^+$CD25$^-$ T cells from mice expressing the same or different TCR transgenes and then stimulated with the appropriate peptide.
Adapted from Thornton AM, Shevach EM. Suppressor effector function of CD4$^+$CD25$^+$ immunoregulatory T cells is antigen nonspecific. *J Immunol.* 2000;164:183–190.

proliferative responses of fresh CD4$^+$CD25$^-$ T cells from mice that express a different transgenic TCR. There is no MHC restriction in the interaction of the activated suppressors and the CD25$^-$ responders. Therefore, the suppressor effector function of activated CD25$^-$ T cells is completely nonspecific (Table 30.4).

CD25-mediated suppression is highly sensitive to antigenic stimulation. For example, when CD25$^+$ and CD25$^-$ T cells are prepared from the same TCR transgenic mouse and stimulated with a specific peptide, the antigen concentration required to stimulate the CD25$^+$ T cells to suppress is 10- to 100-fold lower than that required for triggering the proliferation of the CD25$^-$ T-cell population (86). The partially activated phenotype of CD25$^+$ T-cell population, combined with their enhanced sensitivity to antigen stimulation, suggests that they are highly differentiated in their function and are ready to mediate their suppressive functions immediately upon encounter with their target antigens. Their capacity to rapidly suppress responses *in vitro* suggests that they have been continuously stimulated by self-antigens in the normal physiologic state and continuously exert some degree of suppression *in vivo*.

CD25$^+$ T cells suppress the proliferative responses of CD8$^+$ T cells in a manner similar to that seen with CD4$^+$ CD25$^-$ responders (90). Marked suppression of the effector cytokine IFN-γ, is also seen in the presence of CD25$^+$ T cells. Whereas suppression of the proliferation of CD4$^+$ responders by CD25$^+$ T cells can be completely reversed by the addition of IL-2 or anti-CD28, the suppression of CD8$^+$ T-cell responses is not reversed by the addition of IL-2 or anti-CD28. The failure of IL-2 to abrogate suppression is secondary to a failure of full upregulation of the expression of CD25 on the responder CD8$^+$ T cells. CD4$^+$CD25$^+$ T cells thereby prevent responses mediated by CD8$^+$ T cells both by inhibiting their ability to produce IL-2 and by inhibiting their ability to respond to IL-2, thus disrupting CD4$^+$ T cell help for CD8$^+$ T cells.

Recent studies have attempted to define the biochemical and molecular pathways that mediate the anergic or nonresponsive state of Foxp3$^+$ Treg (91,92). A number of studies have shown that Treg exhibit diminished responses of both proximal and distal signaling pathways both in absolute amplitude and in duration when compared to the responses of CD25$^-$ T cells. Treg have reduced phosphorylation of the TCR ζ chain, reduced recruitment of ZAP-70, and reduced phosphorylation of SLP-76. Defects were seen in the activity of PLC-γ1 and in signals downstream of this enzyme, including calcium mobilization, NFAT, NF-κB, and Ras-ERK-AP-1 activation. The diminished activity of PLC-γ1 in Treg is likely to contribute not only to the delay and reduced appearance of NFAT in the nucleus, but also to the attenuated activation of the PKC and Ras-ERK–directed pathways as well. Other studies (93) have suggested that the proximal promoter of the IL-2 gene fails to undergo chromatin remodeling and remains in a closed chromatin configuration.

Foxp3$^+$ Treg constitutively express all three chains (α, β, and γ) of the high-affinity IL-2 receptor. Despite the widely recognized importance of IL-2 in Treg homeostasis, very little is known about the intracellular mechanisms that regulate IL-2R signaling in Treg. Indeed, a defining characteristic of Treg is their inability to expand *in vitro* upon stimulation with IL-2 alone, despite expression of all three chains of the high-affinity IL-2 receptor. It has been shown that JAK/STAT-dependent signaling is intact in Treg stimulated with IL-2, but that downstream mediators of PI3 K are not activated (94). The nonresponsiveness of Treg is associated with elevated levels of PTEN, a phosphoinositol 3,4,5-triphosphatase, which catalyzes the reverse reaction of PI3 K, negatively regulating the activation of downstream signaling pathways. In conventional T cells, the level of PTEN is downregulated after T-cell activation, but PTEN remains highly expressed in Treg. A critical role of PTEN in the nonresponsiveness of Treg to IL-2 was established by studying PTEN$^{-/-}$ mice (95). PTEN$^{-/-}$ Treg proliferated readily after stimulation with IL-2 alone *in vitro* and exhibited enhanced peripheral turnover *in vivo*. They retained their ability to suppress effector T-cell responses both *in vitro* and *in vivo*. Forced expression of PTEN in recently activated non-Treg inhibited their ability to expand in response to IL-2, confirming the ability of this lipid phosphatase to negatively regulate IL-2–dependent proliferation.

Until very recently, little was known about the direct involvement of Foxp3 in controlling the activation of Treg. Bettelli et al. (96) have shown that forced expression of Foxp3 dramatically suppressed endogenous cytokine expression driven by NFAT and NF-κB. Foxp3 was shown to associate physically with the REL-domain proteins NFAT and NF-κB and to suppress their transcriptional activity. Many of the genes regulated by Foxp3 are also target genes for NFAT. The IL-2 and IL-4 genes are activated by NFAT and repressed by Foxp3, whereas the CD25 and CTLA-4 genes are upregulated by both NFAT and Foxp3. It is possible that Foxp3 represses IL-2 expression by competing with NFAT for binding to DNA. Alternatively, based on the finding of Bettelli et al. that NFAT and Foxp3 interact physically in cell lysates, Foxp3 might repress NFAT-driven cytokine transcription by sequestering NFAT away from DNA. Examination of the crystal structure of an NFAT:FOXP2:DNA complex revealed an extensive protein–protein interaction interface between NFAT and Foxp2 (97). Structure-guided mutations of Foxp3, predicted to disrupt its interaction with NFAT, interfere in a graded manner with the ability of Foxp3 to repress expression of IL-2 and upregulate Treg markers CTLA-4 and CD25. Thus, NFAT can switch its transcription partner from AP-1, which drives T-cell activation, to Foxp3, which programs Treg function. Foxp3 also has been shown to interact with the transcription factor AML1/Runx1, which is required for normal hematopoiesis, as well as activation of IL-2 and IFN-γ gene expression (98).

Much less is known about the molecular/biochemical signals generated in the responder cell following interaction with Foxp3$^+$ Treg. Detailed time-course studies *in vitro* have shown that suppression is established after 6 to 12 hours of contact with Treg, and that responders are refractory to suppression after 12 hours of activation. As suggested by the requirements for IL-2 to activate suppressor function (76), the IL-2 response of the responders is normal for the first 6 hours of the co-culture and then abruptly terminates. Co-stimulation with anti-CD28 generated resistance to suppression by stabilizing IL-2 transcripts, enabling the responder T cells to counterbalance transcriptional downregulation by Treg (99). Treg do not inhibit the induction of CD69 or CD25 early, and viability of responder cells was excellent at 36 hours. Gene expression analysis in responder T cells using a microarray approach has shown that one set of genes was expressed after culture with Treg and this set of genes was distinct from genes induced in anergized T cells, T cells deprived of IL-2, or T cells treated with TGFβ_1 (100). Hopefully, further detailed studies of these genes will elucidate the specific pathways involved in Treg-mediated inhibition.

Cellular Targets for Suppression *in vitro*

In general, murine Treg failed to inhibit responses induced by plate-bound anti-CD3, but readily inhibited responses induced by soluble anti-CD3 (37). This finding raised the possibility that the cellular target of the Treg was the APC rather than the responder T cell, as responses to plate-bound anti-CD3 are relatively APC-independent. It was originally proposed that the Treg target APC by inhibiting the induction of the expression of costimulatory molecules, or perhaps by competition for costimulatory signals. In cocultures of CD4$^+$CD25$^+$ T cells, CD4$^+$CD25$^-$ T cells, and T-depleted spleen cells as APC, the induction of expression of CD80, CD86, CD54, and CD40 on the APC (primarily B cells) appeared to be normal. Treg were also potent suppressors of T-cell proliferation when LPS-activated APC were used, suggesting that they did not inhibit the expression of an unknown costimulatory molecule. Suppression was also observed when the LPS-activated APC were fixed with paraformaldehyde. Lastly, suppression could not be overcome by adding an excess of LPS-activated APC to the cocultures (88).

These studies strongly suggested that the APC was not the target of Treg-mediated suppression. To prove that the Treg were capable of acting directly on the responder T-cell population, the effects of the Treg on the responses of CD8$^+$ T cells to activation by soluble MHC tetramers in a completely APC-independent cell culture system were studied (90). Both T-cell proliferation and IFN-γ production were markedly inhibited by activated CD25$^+$ T cells in the complete absence of APC. This result is most consistent with the view that CD25$^+$ T cells mediate suppression *in vitro* via a T–T cell interaction and that the APC is not directly required for delivery of the suppressive signal. Similar conclusions were drawn in other studies in which CD25$^+$ T cells were shown to suppress responses of either mouse *(101)* or human (33) CD25$^-$ T cells induced by anti-CD3 coupled to beads in the absence of APC.

In contrast to these studies that support the concept that Treg function by directly suppressing responder T cells, a number of studies have shown that Treg can suppress the maturation of DC. In short-term cultures, Treg cells downregulated the expression of markers on immature bone marrow–derived DC and inhibited their ability to elicit antigen-specific CD8$^+$ T cell responses *in vitro*. Activation of immature DC with CpG DNA or LPS abrogated the ability of the Treg to downregulate DC activation markers or to inhibit T-cell activation. Similarly, systemic activation of DC with CpG DNA or an agonistic anti-CD40 antibody completely inhibited the antidiabetogenic activity of Treg cells in NOD mice (102). Although these results suggest that Treg exert their suppressive effects by keeping DC in an immature state and that mature DC are resistant to the effects of Treg, other studies have shown that Treg are capable of inactivating CD40L-prestimulated human DC (103) and that Treg can dampen immune responses induced by fully mature DC *in vivo*. Some of the differences in these studies may be secondary to Treg modulation of cytokine production by the DC. For example, although Treg were unable to prevent DC maturation or induction of IL-6 transcription in the presence of strong inflammatory stimuli, they were still able to modulate mature DC responses by enhancing transcription of the anti-inflammatory cytokine IL-10 (104). Treg-mediated enhancement of IL-10 production by fully mature DC may result in inhibition of T-cell activation and is one mechanism by which Treg can modulate the function of mature DC.

Although the preceding studies focused on the inhibition of DC-induced effector cell activation by Treg, a number of studies have suggested that certain subpopulations of DC can modulate the function of the Treg. Treg will proliferate when stimulated with mature bone marrow DC in the absence of IL-2 in an antigen-specific manner *in vitro* and *in vivo* for several days at a rate that is comparable to that of $CD25^-$ T cells (105). The expanded T cells, after several cycles of cell division, retain their suppressor phenotype and function. Cell contact is essential and CD80/CD86 on the DC is required. Because DC induce proliferation of both $CD25^+$ and $CD25^-$ T cells in cocultures, it is impossible to assay the suppressive functions of $CD25^+$ T cells in proliferation assays. However, when IL-2 production was measured using an IL-2 secretion assay, Treg still suppressed IL-2 secretion by $CD25^-$ T cells without inhibiting their proliferation (106). These results suggest that DC can induce the expansion of Treg cells while simultaneously activating their ability to suppress cytokine secretion by effector cells. Because mature DC are likely to represent the major population of APC during inflammatory states and are also likely to be activated by TLR ligands, one must therefore question the relevance of the anergic/suppressor phenotype of Treg when they are stimulated with a heterogeneous population of splenic APC.

In the d3Tx model of organ-specific autoimmune disease, Treg cells suppressed the activation of autoantigen-specific T cells and inhibited the production of autoantibodies to the target organ. As B cells and autoantibody production are prominent mediators of pathology in many autoimmune diseases, it is critical to understand the potential for Treg to control autoantibody production. Although it is clear that Treg can suppress antibody production by blocking T-helper functions, a number of other studies have suggested that Treg can exert a direct effect on certain B-cell functions. Bystry et al. *(107)* were the first to suggest that Treg cells could inhibit LPS-mediated B-cell activation. Lim et al. (108) demonstrated that human Treg cells can suppress B-cell–dependent immunoglobulin production and class switch recombination by a cell contact–dependent mechanism in the absence of T-helper cells. $Foxp3^+$ Treg cells were identified in T–B area borders and within germinal centers of human lymphoid tissues (109). Treg cells were also able to suppress the expression of AID, a key enzyme involved in class-switch recombination and affinity maturation. The biochemical mechanisms for the suppression of B-cell function in these studies remain unclear.

Zhao et al. (110) demonstrated that Treg cells, that had been activated/expanded in the presence of TCR stimulation and IL-2 inhibited the proliferative responses of B cells to polyclonal B-cell activators. Suppression of proliferation was a result of increased cell death caused by the Treg cells in a cell contact–dependent manner. The induction of B-cell death was not mediated by Fas-Fas ligand pathway, but depended on the upregulation of perforin and granzymes in the Treg. One of the most interesting findings in this study was that activated Treg cells selectively killed activated antigen-presenting B cells and not bystander B cells in the cocultures (Figure 30.9). This result raised the possibility that one site of action of regulatory T cells in mediating suppression *in vivo* is the APC. If activated Treg cells are also lytic for activated DC, lysis of DC by activated Treg cells may be an important mechanism whereby they produce suppression of T-cell activation *in vivo*.

Although a role for Treg in modulating the function of NK cells was suggested in some of the early experiments describing enhancement of NK function following

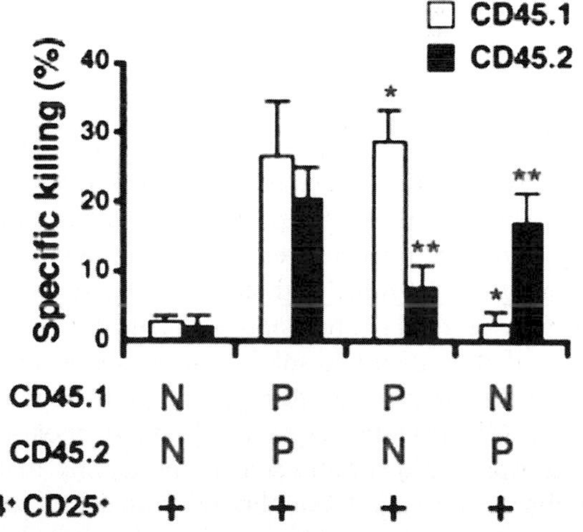

FIGURE 30.9 Activated OVA-specific Treg were mixed with activated B cells that were pulsed (P) or unpulsed (N) with OVA-peptide. Cell death was determined after 6 hours of culture. Adapted from Zhao D-M, Thornton AM, DiPaolo RJ, Shevach EM. Activated $CD4^+CD25^+$ regulatory T cells selectively kill B lymphocytes. *Blood.* 2006;107:3925–3932.

depletion of Treg (111), Treg–NK cell interactions have not been widely studied. Treg were shown to inhibit NKG2D-mediated cytolysis *in vitro* largely by a TGF-β–dependent, IL-10–independent mechanism. Similarly, Treg directly inhibited NKG2D-mediated NK-cell cytotoxicity *in vivo*, resulting in suppression of NK-cell–mediated tumor rejection (112). Other studies have shown that human Treg could also directly inhibit NK cell effector functions by a TGF-β–dependent mechanism with a concomitant down-regulation of NKG2D receptors on the NK-cell surface (113). NK-cell cytotoxicity was restored in the presence of Treg when the cocultures were performed in the presence of cytokines known to activate NK cells, such as IL-2, IL-4, IL-7, and IL-12. Curiously, in both of these studies, Treg cells did not induce a global inhibition of NK-activating receptors, but only an inhibition of NKG2D. In other experiments, depletion of Treg resulted in enhanced proliferation of NK cells as well as their cytotoxic potential. Treg may normally control NK-cell functions, but any imbalance in the frequency of Treg may affect NK-cell homeostasis. One explanation for the susceptibility of NK cells to Treg control is that uninhibited NK cells might be a danger to the host in autoimmune diseases. Future studies need to carefully examine Treg–NK interactions in situations that involve activation of the innate immune response, particularly during the course of an infectious challenge. The role of Treg in the regulation of NK-cell function has also been studied in a bone marrow graft rejection model (114). Following depletion of Treg *in vivo*, graft rejection was increased in both fully allogeneic and hybrid resistance situations. Rejection was dependent on host NK cells, because it was significantly impaired in NKcell–depleted recipients. TGF-β also appeared to play a role in this, as injection of anti-TGF-β before grafting significantly increased rejection.

Role of TGF-β

Although TGF-β has been clearly shown to play a critical role in the induction of Foxp$^+$ Treg *in vitro*, its role as a suppressor effector molecule remains controversial. Although the majority of studies with either human or mouse Treg that have studied suppression of T-cell activation *in vitro* have failed to identify a soluble suppressor cytokine, it is very difficult to rule out the involvement of a cytokine that acts over short distances or a cell-bound cytokine. Nakamura et al. (115) have raised the possibility that TGF-β produced by Treg and then bound to their cell surface by an as yet uncharacterized receptor might mediate suppression in a cell contact–dependent fashion. In their studies, TGF-β was detected on the surface of resting and activated CD25$^+$ T cells, and suppression could be reversed by high concentrations of anti-TGF-β mAbs. They postulated that latent (inactive) TGF-β, bound to the cell surface of activated Treg is delivered directly to responder CD25$^-$ T cells and is then locally converted to its active form. In contrast to these studies, Piccirillo et al. (116) were unable to show a requirement for either the production of TGF-β or responsiveness to TGF-β in Treg-mediated suppression. CD25$^-$ T cells from *Smad3*$^{-/-}$ and from mice expressing a dominant negative form of the TGF-β receptor II (TGFβRII), which are completely resistant to the immunosuppressive effects of TGF-β, were readily suppressed by Treg cells from WT mice (Table 30.5). Treg from TGF-β$^{-/-}$ mice were as efficient as Treg from WT mice in mediating suppression of WT CD25$^-$ T cells. High concentrations of anti-TGF-β did not reverse suppression, nor did anti-TGF-β or a soluble form of the TGF-βPII inhibit suppression mediated by activated CD25$^+$ T cells.

TABLE 30.5 ***CD4$^+$CD25$^+$* Suppressor Function Occurs Independently *of TGF-β***

CD4$^+$ CD25$^+$	*CD4$^+$ CD25$^-$*	*Suppression*
Wild type	Wild type	Yes
Wild type	Wild type + anti-TGF-β	Yes
Wild type	*SMAD3*$^{-/-}$	Yes
SMAD3$^{-/-}$	Wild type	Yes
Wild type	DNTGFβRII	Yes

CD4$^+$CD25$^+$ T cells were mixed with CD4$^+$CD25$^-$ T cells in the presence of T-depleted spleen cells and soluble anti-CD3. Proliferation was measured at 72 hours.

Adapted from Piccirillo CA, Letterio JJ, Thornton AM, et al. CD4$^+$CD25$^+$ regulatory T cells can mediate suppressor function in the absence of transforming growth factor β1 production and responsiveness. *J Exp Med.* 2002;196:1–10.

A number of *in vivo* experiments have also demonstrated that autocrine TGF-β1 expression is not essential for Treg suppression *in vivo*. Transfer of TGF-β1$^{-/-}$ splenocytes to RAG-2$^{-/-}$ mice induced disease with features similar to those of the TGF-β1$^{-/-}$ mice, and disease transfer was accelerated by the depletion of TGF-β$^{-/-}$ CD25$^+$ T cells. Importantly, cotransfer of TGF-β1$^{-/-}$ Treg clearly attenuated disease in RAG2$^{-/-}$ recipients of CD25-depleted spleen and lymph nodes, but suppression was incomplete when compared to WT Treg (117). Although TGF-β appears to play a nonredundant role in control of intestinal inflammation, Treg from TGF-β1$^{-/-}$ mice were capable of inhibiting IBD induced by CD45RB^{high} (118) or CD4$^+$CD25$^-$ T cells (119) *in vivo*. Furthermore, Treg from mice expressing a dominant negative form of the TGF-βRII are also capable of inhibiting colitis, suggesting that TGF-β is not required for the development or peripheral function of thymic-derived Treg. Importantly, the function of TGF-β$^{-/-}$ Treg cells was abrogated by anti-TGF-β, indicating that TGF-β is absolutely required for protection from IBD in this model, but can be provided by a non-Treg cell source. The requirement for non-Treg–produced TGF-β was confirmed by demonstrating that CD4$^+$CD45RB^{high} cells from the mice expressing the dominant negative receptor escaped control by Treg cells *in vivo*. It is possible that Treg induce TGF-β production by other hematopoietic cells or that production of TGF-β is independent of Treg and produced by healing gut epithelial cells.

These studies argue strongly against a role for secreted or cell surface–associated TGF-β as a major mediator of the *in vitro* or *in vivo* suppressive functions of Treg. An alternative possibility is that TGF-β plays a role in the enhancement or maintenance of Foxp3$^+$ Treg-suppressor activity. Indeed, Marie et al. (120) have demonstrated that peripheral TGF-$\beta1^{-/-}$ Treg expressed diminished levels of Foxp3. These studies suggested that TGF-β is required for maintenance of Foxp3 expression in peripheral Treg, that the source of the TGF-β is not the Treg, and that paracrine production of TGF-β by APC is needed for optimal Treg survival and suppressor function. Further evidence for the role of TGF-β in the maintenance of Treg was derived from studies of mice with T cell–specific deletion of TGF-βRII (121). In these mice, TGF-β was not required for induction of Foxp3 expression in the thymus and for the thymic development of Treg cells. In fact, TGF-βRII$^{-/-}$ mice have an increase in the percentage and number of Foxp3$^+$ T cells in the thymus and increased BrdU uptake, suggesting that TGF-β normally inhibits the proliferation of thymic Treg. Increased Treg proliferation was also seen in the periphery of TGF-βRII$^{-/-}$ mice, but these mice have a decrease in the percentage of Foxp3$^+$ Treg in the periphery, consistent with the possibility that TGF-β is essential for their survival in the periphery. When mixed bone marrow chimeras between TGF-βRII$^{-/-}$ and WT mice were generated, the knockout CD25$^-$ T cells demonstrated complete resistance to suppression by WT Treg. Although one interpretation of this experiment is that Treg-derived TGF-β mediates suppression, preliminary studies using TGF-$\beta^{-/-}$ and Foxp3$^{-/-}$ bone marrow chimeras show that TGF-$\beta^{-/-}$ Treg cells are fully capable of preventing systemic lymphoproliferation associated with Foxp3 deficiency. This result suggests that there is a defect in a cell intrinsic mechanism of TGF-β–mediated control of T-cell reactivity in the TGF-βRII$^{-/-}$ T cells.

Role of CTLA-4

Considerable controversy exists regarding the significance of the expression of CTLA-4 on Treg and its potential involvement in their suppressor function. Takahashi et al. (39) have shown that the addition of the Fab fragment of anti-CTLA reverses suppression in cocultures of Treg and CD4$^+$CD25$^-$ T cells. This finding, together with the observation of Read et al. (27) that treatment of mice with anti–CTLA-4 abrogates suppression of inflammatory bowel disease (IBD) mediated by Treg T cells, has been interpreted as indicating that a costimulatory signal mediated by interaction of CTLA-4 with its ligands, CD80/CD86, is required for activation of Treg to mediate their suppressive effects. Reversal of suppression by anti–CTLA-4 or its Fab fragment *in vitro* has not been seen in all studies (*31*,32,33,*34*,*35*,36,37). In studies (101) in which Treg suppress the activation of CD25$^-$ T cells in the absence of APC, the addition of anti-CTLA-4 or anti-CD80/CD86 did not reverse suppression, suggesting that engagement of CTLA-4 is not required for suppressor function. Treg from CTLA-4$^{-/-}$ mice are as efficient as WT Treg in mediating suppressor function *in vitro*, but, in contrast to WT Treg, their suppressive effects were partially dependent on TGF-β (122). One possible functional role for CTLA-4 on Treg would be to ligate CD80/CD86 on DC. Some (123) but not all studies (124) have claimed that CD80/CD86$^{-/-}$ CD25$^-$ T cells are refractory to Treg suppression *in vivo* and *in vitro*, and that interaction of CD80/CD86 on CD25$^-$ T cells with a molecule on Treg, most likely CTLA-4, is needed for suppression to be manifest.

Other Potential Suppressor Mechanisms

Overall, studies over the past 10 years have failed to identify a single molecular species that is responsible for Treg-mediated suppression *in vitro*. It remains possible that other well-characterized suppressor mechanisms may contribute, in part, to the suppressor function of Treg. The interaction of CTLA-4 on Treg with CD80 or CD86 on DC results in the activation of indoleamine 2,3 dioxygenase (IDO). IDO is responsible for the metabolism of the essential amino acid tryptophan. Reduced amounts of tryptophan after induction of IDO are associated with decreased activation of T cells. Induction of IDO production would represent an APC-dependent mechanism of *in vitro* suppression (125), but suppression by Treg can readily be observed in APC-free cultures.

One other potential mechanism for Treg-mediated suppression would be cytolysis of target cells. Human CD4$^+$CD25$^+$Foxp3$^+$ Treg can be activated by a combination of antibodies to CD3 and CD46 to express granzyme A and kill activated CD4$^+$ and CD8$^+$ T cells and other cell types in a perforin-dependent, Fas-FasL–independent manner (126). Significant cell death occurred at very low effector-to-target cell ratios (1:1), indicating potent cytotoxicity by the activated Treg. Activation of mouse Treg also results in upregulation of granzyme B expression, and one report has claimed that suppression of T-cell activation by Treg was mediated by a perforin-independent, granzyme B–dependent mechanism (127). These findings could not be confirmed in a second study that demonstrated that highly activated Treg could kill antigen-presenting but not bystander B cells or T cells (110). Nevertheless, these studies suggest that one should re-evaluate the concept of "cytotoxic/suppressor cell," because it appears at least *in vitro* that Treg can mediate both of these functions. It remains to be determined whether Treg can develop into cytotoxic cells *in vivo*.

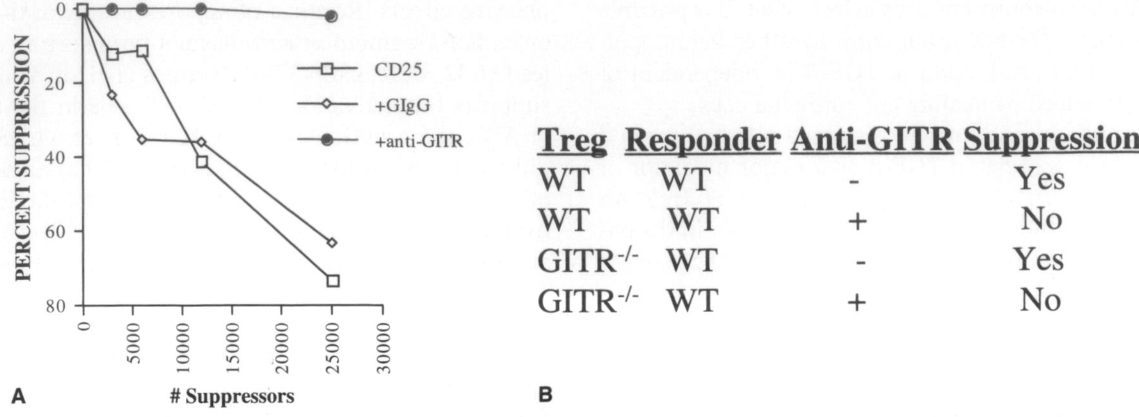

FIGURE 30.10 Anti-GITR reverses suppression by inducing resistance to suppression in responder $CD4^+CD25^-$ T cells. **A:** $CD4^+CD25^+$ T cells were cultured with $CD4^+CD25^-$ T cells in the presence of T-depleted spleen cells and soluble anti-CD3. Normal goat IgG or polyclonal goat-anti-mouse GITR were added as indicated. Proliferation was measured at 72 hours. **B:** $CD4^+CD25^+$ T cells from WT or $GITR^{-/-}$ mice were cocultured with $CD4^+CD25^-$ T cells in the presence or absence of anti-GITR. Adapted from McHugh RS, Whitters MJ, Piccirillo CA, et al. $CD4^+CD25^+$ immunoregulatory T cells: gene expression analysis reveals a functional role for the glucocorticoid-induced TNF receptor. *Immunity.* 2002;16:311–323; and Stephens GL, McHugh RS, Whitters MJ, et al. Engagement of glucocorticoid-induced TNFR family related receptor on effector T cells by its ligand mediates resistance to suppression by $CD4^+CD25^+$ T cells. *J Immunol.* 2004;173:5008–5020.

Resistance to Suppression

Although the mechanism of Treg-mediated cell contact–dependent inhibition of T-cell activation remains unknown, one approach to determining potential cell surface antigens involved in this process has been to reverse suppression with antibodies to candidate antigens. One member of the TNFRSF, the GITR (TNFRSF18), has been shown to play an important role in regulation of T-cell suppressor activity. Both a polyclonal antiserum and an mAb to the GITR appeared to be able to reverse suppression (Figure 30.10A), mediated by freshly isolated $CD25^+$ T cells (40,41). However, the GITR is expressed on two populations of cells (resting Treg and activated $CD4^+CD25^-$ cells) that do not manifest suppressor activity. It is therefore very unlikely that the GITR is the molecule responsible for mediating suppressor effector function. Surprisingly, culturing $CD25^+$ T cells with the anti-GITR in the presence of IL-2, but in the absence of anti-CD3, resulted in a vigorous proliferative response and breaking the nonresponsive state of the Treg to stimulation with IL-2.

Although these studies were originally interpreted as indicating that anti-GITR functioned as an agonist for the GITR, resulting in a signal that instructs the Treg not to mediate their suppressive functions, more recent studies have suggested an alternative explanation. As both $CD25^-$ and Treg can express the GITR, it was impossible to conclude that the anti-GITR mediated its effects by acting solely on the Treg. When combinations of WT and $GITR^{-/-}$ $CD4^+CD25^-$ and Treg were used in coculture experiments (Figure 30.10B), ligation of the GITR on the $CD25^-$ responders, not the Treg, was required to abrogate suppression (128). These results suggest that interactions of the GITR with its ligand, the GITR-L, provided a signal that renders effector T cells resistant to the inhibitory effects of Treg. Similar conclusions were drawn from studies in which the costimulatory effects of anti-GITR *in vivo* were maintained following depletion of Treg (129). The GITR-L was shown to be expressed on a number of different resting APC populations, including DC, macrophages, and B cells, and to be downregulated upon activation. Thus, engagement of the GITR on effector cells by its ligand on APC early during the course of an immune response may render the responder cells resistant to suppression by Treg. This model is also compatible with the observations of Pasare and Medzhitov (130) that soluble factors released by activated DC can act directly on effector, but not Treg, to render them resistant to suppression.

In addition to the role of APC-derived signals in rendering responder cells resistant to suppression, a number of mutations in TCR signaling and costimulatory pathways also appear to render responder cells completely resistant to the inhibitory signals delivered by Treg. One of the best examples of a defect in resistance to regulation is the cbl-$b^{-/-}$ mouse. Cbl-b is an E3 ubiquitin ligase that negatively regulates the CD28 costimulatory pathway and downregulates the PI3 K/Akt pathway. In the absence of cbl-b, mice develop CD28-independent hyperactive

TABLE 30.6 Genetically Deficient Mice That Are Resistant to Treg Suppression

$Cbl\text{-}b^{-/-}$
$TGF\text{-}\beta\text{-}RII^{-/-}$
$TRAF6^{-/-}$ T-cell–specific
$NFATc2^{-/-}/NFATc3^{-/-}$

Adapted from Marie JC, Liggitt D, Rudensky AY. Cellular mechanisms of fatal early-onset autoimmunity in mice with the T cell-specifc targeting of transforming growth factor-β receptor. *Immunity.* 2006;25:441–454; and Wohlfert EA, Gorelik L, Mittler R, et al. Cutting Edge: Deficiency in the E3 ubiquitin ligase cbl-b results in a multifunctional defect in T cells TGF-β sensitivity *in vitro* and *in vivo*. *J Immunol.* 2006;176:1316–1320

responses and autoimmunity. Treg from cbl-$b^{-/-}$ mice function normally *in vitro*, but $CD25^{-}$ T cells from cbl-$b^{-/-}$ mice are resistant to suppression *in vitro* and *in vivo* by wild-type Treg (131). Effector T cells from a number of other mutant mouse strains exhibit a resistance to suppression similar to that seen with cbl-$b^{-/-}$ effectors (Table 30.6). Many of these strains have in common a hyperactivated PI3 K/Akt pathway that may be a direct or indirect target for Treg-mediated suppression.

Suppression *in vivo*

As has been summarized, a clear understanding of the molecular mechanism(s) for Treg-mediated inhibition of T-cell activation *in vitro* has remained elusive. Analysis of the potential pathways of Treg suppression *in vivo* is even more complex. The Treg must able to localize to various parts of the body such that close contact with most effector T cells with a given antigen specificity, either directly or through an APC intermediate, becomes possible. Unlike the culture situation, there is ample space for T cells to evade suppression *in vivo* unless Treg can localize with them in response to antigenic stimulation that begins in antigen-draining lymph nodes. There are also a number of major differences between the properties of Treg *in vivo* compared to *in vitro*. First, although Treg are nonresponsive or anergic to stimulation via the TCR *in vitro*, Treg expand following engagement of their TCR by cognate antigen in a manner indistinguishable from conventional $CD4^{+}$ T cells *in vivo* (132). Second, most studies of Treg suppression *in vitro* have failed to define a role for suppressor cytokines, whereas multiple studies have shown that secretion of suppressor cytokines by Treg constitutes an important component of their suppressive effects *in vivo*. Lastly, the major effect of Treg on T-cell activation *in vitro* is to inhibit IL-2 production and effector-cell expansion. The role of IL-2 in the antigen-driven expansion of $CD4^{+}$ T cells *in vivo* is not clear, as antigen-specific T cells from IL-$2^{-/-}$ mice expand normally following stimulation by antigen *in vivo*.

Some studies have suggested that the primary effect of Treg *in vivo* is to inhibit the differentiation, but not the expansion, of T effector cells *in vivo*. Klein et al. (133) cotransferred into normal mice equal numbers of effectors and Treg, expressing the same transgene, followed by immunization with the antigen in incomplete adjuvant. For the first 4 days after transfer, both populations expanded in an equivalent manner. However, 6 to 8 days after transfer, the expansion of the Treg continued, but additional accumulation of effectors was suppressed. In contrast to the studies demonstrating inhibition of T effector differentiation, the remaining effector cells appeared to be fully competent to produce either IL-2 or IFN-γ. One problem with the interpretation of this study is that the studies can be conducted only for short periods of time, as the transferred cells migrate out of the draining lymph nodes.

Very little is known about the cell surface antigens that might play a role in Treg-mediated inhibition *in vivo*. Anti-CTLA-4 has been shown to abrogate suppression of IBD *in vivo* by Treg. In order to distinguish whether the effects of anti-CTLA-4 on reversal of Treg suppression of IBD are mediated indirectly by hyperactivation of effector T cells or directly via their effects on Treg, Treg were derived from CTLA-$4^{-/-}$ mice on a CD80/$CD86^{-/-}$ background that do not develop an autoimmune syndrome (134). When combinations of genetically deficient mice and WT T cells were used, it could be shown that anti-CTLA-4 or its Fab fragment disrupts Treg activity by targeting Treg and not the effector T cells. Anti-CTLA-4 did not overcome the regulatory activity of CTLA-$4^{-/-}$ Treg, showing that ligation of CTLA-4 on the effector population had limited impact on the induction of colitis in this system. The effects of anti-CTLA-4 were not mediated by depletion of CTLA-4^{+} Treg. Although anti-CTLA-4 Fab may block the interaction of CTLA-4 with its ligands, it is also possible that the interaction of CLTA-4 with antibody, or even Fab fragments, may modulate the expression of CTLA-4 on the cell surface or inhibit its recycling and thereby block the TCR-mediated signals required for induction of suppressor activity.

Many of the *in vitro* studies of Treg function have concluded that the target for suppression is the responder T cell. In contrast, recent studies suggest that the suppressive effects of Treg *in vivo* might also be mediated by the reduction of the stimulatory capacity of DC or other types of APC. Intravital two-photon laser scanning microscopy has been used to visualize the behavior of autoantigen-specific T cells in the presence or absence of Treg in intact lymph nodes (135,136). In the absence of Treg cells, the locomotion of autoantigen-specific T cells inside lymph nodes is decreased, and the contact between effector T cells and antigen-loaded DC are prolonged, while contacts between T cells and antigen-presenting DC are of shorter duration in the presence of Treg cells. Thus, Treg attenuate the establishment of stable contacts during priming of naïve T cells by DC and thereby may decrease the magnitude of TCR activation. Importantly, no stable interactions between the Treg cells and effector T cells were observed in these studies. These observations are most consistent with the concept that Treg cells can inactivate DC directly or that DC-activated Treg cells produce soluble mediators that prevent T effector–DC interactions.

Foxp3⁻ Treg

Thymic-derived Foxp3+ Treg or Foxp3+ Treg induced in peripheral sites represent the major population of Treg that have been characterized in both normal physiologic studies and in disease models. A number of other Treg populations have been described in both mouse and human, and many of these also appear to exert potent Treg functions in certain defined situations. One important distinction between these induced populations of Treg and the Foxp3+ Treg is that the former are very frequently specific for known antigens, whereas the antigen specificity of the latter remains to be defined.

Th3 Cells

One of the first approaches used for the induction of Treg was the administration of antigen via the oral route. Oral tolerance takes advantage of the normal physiologic process that is needed to prevent systemic immune responses to ingested proteins. Oral administration of antigen at low doses induces populations of Treg that secrete suppressor cytokines, whereas higher antigen doses result in deletion or clonal anergy of autoreactive precursors. Pretreatment with orally administered antigen induced suppressor populations that suppressed pathology in a number of different animal models of autoimmunity, including experimental allergic encephalomyelitis (EAE), collagen-induced arthritis (CIA), and uveitis (137). Bulk T cells from orally tolerized animals can suppress active immune responses to other antigens in the microenvironment, a phenomenon called antigen-driven bystander suppression. The suppressor cells from orally tolerant mice have been termed Th3 cells and mediate their suppressive effects primarily by secreting TGF-β. A major advance in our understanding of the function of regulatory cells following oral tolerance was a study by Chen et al. (138), which successfully isolated T-cell clones from the mesenteric lymph nodes of SJL mice that had been orally tolerized to MBP. These clones produced large amounts of TGF-β and varying amounts of IL-4 and IL-10. Most important, upon adoptive transfer to normal recipients, they suppressed EAE induced with either myelin basic protein (MBP) or proteolipid protein (PLP). Their *in vivo* suppressive activity could be neutralized with anti-TGF-β. The selective induction of Treg via the oral route is thought to be secondary to certain poorly characterized properties of the gut mucosal microenvironment, most likely the type of resident APC (139,*140*).

Although the oral administration of antigen represents a potentially easy way to induce Treg, progress in this area has been slow because it has been difficult to determine the antigen concentration that is capable of inducing Treg but that does not induce deletion. It has also been very difficult to isolate the types of clones described earlier in the EAE model in other systems or to identify Treg cells that exclusively produce TGF-β in other models. The therapeutic utility of orally administered antigens in autoimmunity has primarily been demonstrated in pretreatment protocols, and oral administration of antigen has been ineffective in treating animals once disease has been initiated.

T Regulatory 1 (Tr1) Cells

One important lesson that can be derived from the experiments on oral tolerance is that the milieu in which T cells are primed is critically important in determining whether regulatory rather than effector T cells will be generated. Decreased expression of costimulatory molecules on APC or the presence of suppressor cytokines such as IL-10 and TGF-β may generate suppressor T cells rather than effector T cells. The production of these suppressor cytokines by Treg may lead to the generation or expansion of additional regulatory cells via a positive feedback loop (Figure 30.11).

One of the first studies demonstrating the potential importance of IL-10 in the generation of Treg was derived from an analysis *(141)* of patients with severe combined immunodeficiency who received transplants of HLA-mismatched hematopoietic stem cells. Complete immunologic reconstitution was achieved in the absence of graft-versus-host disease. CD4+ T-cell clones reactive with host MHC antigens from these patients produced IL-10, but not IL-2, after antigen-specific stimulation *in vitro*. It therefore seemed likely that endogenous IL-10 production in the transplanted patients was responsible for maintaining tolerance *in vivo*. The IL-10 may prevent the activation

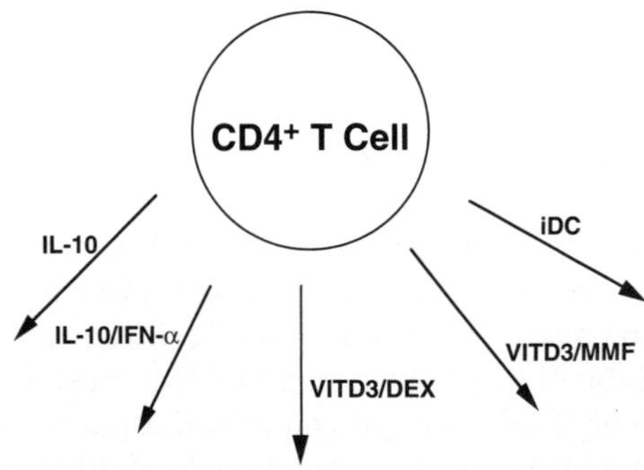

FIGURE 30.11 Multiple factors can induce the differentiation of IL-10–producing T cells.

of host reactive T cells or suppress APC function and cytokine production by host APC. The high IL-10 production *in vivo* may reflect a chronic activation of donor T cells and host monocytes.

IL-10 is a cytokine produced by numerous cell types, including activated T cells, B cells, mast cells, and macrophages, and acts primarily by inhibiting the maturation and function of APC. The activation of $CD4^+$ human T cells in the presence of IL-10 renders them nonresponsive or anergic (142). Activation of human $CD8^+$ T cells with allogeneic APC and IL-10 also results in reduced proliferation and cytotoxicity. T cells rendered anergic by the addition of exogenous IL-10 in an MLR become unable to respond to a rechallenge with the same antigen. IL-10–induced anergy is strictly antigen-specific, because treated T cells retain normal proliferative and cytotoxic responses toward other protein antigens and third-party alloantigens.

Collectively, these studies suggested that IL-10 itself is a major factor for the induction of suppressive IL-10–producing T cells. Culture of mouse or human $CD4^+$ T cells with antigen or alloantigen in the presence of IL-10 results in the generation of IL-10–producing T-cell clones. Most of these T-cell clones produce high levels of IL-10 and TGF-β, moderate amounts of IFN-γ and IL-5, but not IL-2 or IL-4. $CD4^+$ T cells generated in this manner have been termed T regulatory 1 (Tr1) cells (143). Tr1 cells proliferate poorly following polyclonal TCR-mediated or antigen specific activation and do not expand significantly under standard T-cell culture conditions. This low proliferative capacity is a result in part to autocrine production of IL-10, because anti–IL-10 mAbs partially restore proliferative responses. The intrinsic low proliferative capacity of Tr1 cells has been a major limitation and has hindered their detailed characterization. The ability to generate human Tr1 cells is enhanced by the addition of IFN-α *(144)*. Tr1 cells can be generated from human cord blood with IFN-α alone, as cord blood T cells have the intrinsic ability to produce IL-10. IFN-α and IL-10 do not act as general antiproliferative agents, but rather as factors that induce the differentiation of Tr1 cells and inhibit the growth of non-Tr1 cells in the culture. TGF-β played no role in the induction of Tr1 cells in this model. A global suppression of all cytokine production was seen when TGF-β was added to the cultures.

Tr1 cells do not express Foxp3 and can be generated in the absence of $Foxp3^+$ Treg. Both human and mouse Tr1 clones suppress immune responses *in vitro*. Antigen-induced proliferation of naïve $CD4^+$ T cells was dramatically reduced following coculture with activated Tr1 clones that were separated from the responding cells by a transwell insert. The capacity of either human or mouse Tr1 clones to suppress $CD4^+$ T cells proliferation was reversed by the addition of anti-TGF-β and IL-10 mAbs (143). Some IL-10–producing Tr1 cells suppress the proliferation of naïve $CD4^+$ T cells by an IL-10–independent, cell contact–dependent mechanism (145). Human Tr1 cell clones also suppress the production of immunoglobulin by B cells, as well as the antigen-presenting capacity of monocytes and DC. Most important, it could be shown (143) that mouse Tr1 clones have regulatory effects *in vivo* and suppress Th1-mediated colitis induced by transfer of $CD45RB^{high}$ cells into SCID mice. Suppression was seen only if the Tr1 clones were activated by antigen-specific stimulation via their TCR. Because the function of Tr1 cells is mediated by IL-10 and TGF-β, these studies imply that Tr1 clones can suppress active immune responses to unknown antigens in the microenvironment by an antigen-driven bystander suppression mechanism similar to the mechanism proposed for Th3 cells in oral tolerance. Although IL-10 was originally described as a product of mouse Th2 cells, Tr1 clones are also capable of regulating Th2 responses, including antigen-specific IgE production (146). Anti-IL-10R antibodies reversed this inhibitory effect.

An alternative approach to the generation of Tr1 cells *in vitro* has involved pharmacologic manipulation of the microenvironment during T-cell priming (147). The immunosuppressive drug 1, 25(OH)2-vitamin D3 (VitD3), acts on APC and activated T cells. VitD3 inhibits antigen-induced T-cell proliferation, cytokine production, and the maturation of human DC, leading to inhibition of the expression of CD40/CD80/CD86. Similarly, the glucocorticoid dexamethasone inhibits key transcription factors involved in the regulation of a number of inflammatory cytokine genes. When naïve $CD4^+$ T cells were stimulated through their TCR in the presence of the combination of VitD3 and dexamethasone, the primed T cells produced IL-10, but not IFN-γ, IL-4, or IL-5 (79). The IL-10–producing cells developed independently of Th1 (IL-12, IFN-γ) and Th2 (IL-4) polarizing cytokines, and addition of these cytokines inhibited the development of the IL-10–producing cells. Although the induction of these Treg could not be induced by IL-10, endogenous IL-10 production was required, because addition of anti-IL-10R antibodies substantially reduced the number of IL-10–producing T cells. These cytokines have the potential to mediate inflammatory pathologies. The development of the IL-10–producing T cells occurred under conditions in which the expression and/or activation of key transcription factors involved in Th1 (T-bet) and Th2 (GATA3) differentiation was minimal, suggesting that the IL-10 producers were completely unrelated to conventional Th1 or Th2 cells. VitD3/dexamethasone-induced Tr1 cells are also capable of inhibiting the induction of Th1-mediated autoimmune disease *in vivo*.

One common theme to emerge from the studies on the *in vitro* induction of Tr1 cells, by the addition of either IL-10 or pharmacologic agents, is that both of these modalities are likely to inhibit the maturation and activation of DC and to generate what has been termed "tolerogenic DC." Treg have been generated by culturing human $CD4^+$ cord-blood lymphocytes with allogeneic immature DC (iDC). Stimulation with mature DC resulted in expansion of alloreactive T cells of the Th1 phenotype, but stimulation in the presence of iDC resulted in the induction of poorly growing IL-10–producing T cells (148). These T cells suppressed the alloantigen-driven proliferation of syngeneic Th1 cells in cocultures in a cell contact–dependent manner. The suppressor effector function was nonspecific and was not mediated by IL-10 or TGF-β, but suppression could be partially be overcome by addition of IL-2. The suppressor population generated by stimulation with iDC in many respects resembles naturally occurring $CD25^+$ cells. It is not known if these iDC-induced Treg express Foxp3.

$CD8^+$ Treg

Most of the early studies on T-suppressor cells in the mouse demonstrated that they were confined to the $CD8^+$ subset. Although almost all of the recent studies on suppressor/regulatory T cells in mouse or human have focused on $CD4^+$ T cells, a number of recent studies have suggested that potent $CD8^+$ suppressor cells may also exist. Repeated stimulation of human T cells in the MLR resulted in a progressive decrease of the capacity of $CD4^+$ T cells to proliferate when rechallenged with the APC used for priming. The relative nonresponsiveness of the stimulated $CD4^+$ T cells could be restored by depletion of $CD8^+CD28^-$, but not $CD8^+CD28^+$, T cells from these cultures. The stimulated $CD8^+CD28^-$ T cell population was devoid of cytotoxic activity for either $CD4^+$ T cells or the APC used for priming. When the $CD8^+CD28^-$ T cells were added to mixtures of CD4 cells and APC, they inhibited proliferation (149), but suppression was observed only when the stimulatory APC shared at least one HLA class I allele with the original stimulator population. The regulatory effect of the $CD8^+$ suppressors was not restricted either by class I or class II MHC antigens expressed by the responder $CD4^+$ T cells. Suppression mediated by $CD8^+CD28^-$ T cells required cell–cell contact and was not reversed by antisuppressor cytokine antibodies. Coincubation of the $CD8^+$ suppressors with $CD4^+$ responders had no effect, whereas coincubation of the $CD8^+$ T cells with the APC rendered the APC unable to stimulate $CD4^+$ proliferation. Phenotypic analysis indicated that the $CD8^+$ suppressors blocked the upregulation of costimulatory molecules such as CD80/CD86, CD54, and CD58 on the APC *(150)*. The mechanism by which the $CD8^+$ suppressors deactivate APC functions has been shown to involve upregulation of the genes encoding immunoglobulinlike transcript 3 (ILT3) and ILT4 (151). These inhibitory receptors are structurally and functionally related to killer cell–inhibitory receptors (KIR). Thus far, the biologic activity of these $CD8^+CD28^-$ suppressor populations has only been studied *in vitro*. Their potential roles in mediating immunosuppression *in vivo* as well as their relationship to $CD4^+$ suppressor cells remain to be explored. It has been proposed that antigen-specific MHC class I–restricted $CD8^+CD28^-$ Treg first induce ILT-expressing tolerogenic DC, which in turn generate $CD4^+$ Treg (152).

Regulatory $CD8^+$ T cells have also been generated *in vitro* by stimulation with unique subpopulations of DC *(153)*. When naïve $CD8^+$ T cells were stimulated *in vitro* with CD40L-activated, monocyte-derived DC (DC1), the primed $CD8^+$ T cells proliferated when restimulated with allogeneic targets, secreted large amounts of IFN-γ and had potent cytotoxic activity. In contrast, when naïve $CD8^+$ T cells were stimulated with CD40L-activated plasmacytoid DC (DC2), the primed $CD8^+$ T cells proliferated poorly, displayed weak cytotoxic activity, and secreted primarily IL-10. DC2-primed $CD8^+$ T cells inhibited the ability of naïve $CD8^+$ T cells to proliferate to allogeneic monocytes, iDC, or mature DC. Both the generation of $CD8^+$ suppressor cells and their suppressor function could be markedly inhibited by anti-IL-10, but not by anti-TGF-β. Dhodapkar et al. *(154)* have measured the ability of iDC1 cells to modulate the immune response *in vivo* in humans. Injection of iDC pulsed with influenza matrix peptide resulted in an expansion of antigen-specific, tetramer-binding $CD8^+$ T cells. These $CD8^+$ cells were capable of proliferating when stimulated with antigen *in vitro*, but were defective in IFN-γ secretion and lacked cytotoxic function. These findings indicate that iDC can dampen pre-existing antigen-specific effector function in humans. The potential suppressive function of the $CD8^+$ T cells that responded to the iDC was not studied. The relationship of these $CD8^+$ T cells to those induced *in vitro* with DC2 cells is unknown. Wei et al. (155) have isolated plasmacytoid DC from malignant ascites of patients with ovarian cancer. These DC, upon CD40L activation, could induce antigen-specific $CD8^+$ IL-10, producing Treg that suppressed the responses of tumor antigen-specific $CD4^+$ T cells.

$CD8^+CD122^+$ Treg

A unique subpopulation of $CD8^+$ T cells that expresses high levels of the IL-2R β chain (CD122) has been shown to have immunoregulatory activity (156). The percentage of $CD8^+CD122^+$ T cells is high in young mice (~50%), but decreases to ~10% at 7 to 10 weeks of age. $CD122^{-/-}$ mice develop an autoimmune syndrome that can be prevented when neonates are injected with $CD8^+CD122^+$ T cells. Importantly, $RAG^{-/-}$ mice reconstituted with $CD8^+CD122^-$ T cells develop an autoimmune syndrome that can be prevented by cotransfer of $CD8^+CD122^+$ T cells, but not $CD4^+Foxp3^+$ T cells. $CD8^+CD122^-$ are $Foxp3^-$ and inhibit the activation of both $CD8^+$ and $CD4^+$ T cells *in vitro* by an IL-10–dependent mechanism, as $CD8^+CD122^+$ T cells from $IL\text{-}10^{-/-}$ could not suppress T-cell activation *in vitro*, but may exert some suppressive effects *in vivo* (157).

Qa-1 Restricted CD8$^+$ Treg

Mice that are genetically deficient or depleted of CD8$^+$ T cells have demonstrated a clear role for CD8$^+$ T cells in regulating EAE. CD8$^+$ T cells from mice that had recovered from EAE downregulated or killed some CD4$^+$ neuroantigen-specific T-cell clones. Inhibition was blocked by antibodies to the MHC class Ib molecule Qa-1, but not by anti-MHC class Ia molecules (158). It has been proposed that Qa-1 self-peptide complexes expressed by activated CD4$^+$ T cells trigger the TCR on CD8$^+$ cells. These CD8$^+$ T cells then differentiate into suppressor cells that in turn suppress the CD4$^+$ T cells that express the same Qa-1 self-peptide complex. Other studies suggest that a peptide from the conserved region of the TCR is targeted by the CD8$^+$ Treg population (159). The mechanism of suppression has not been fully defined, although it may involve cytotoxicity or the secretion of suppressor cytokines. Human CD8$^+$ T cells restricted by HLA-E, the human homolog of mouse Qa-1, may have similar functions (160).

Double-Negative (DN) Treg

The majority of T cells in normal mice and humans that express the TCR $\alpha\beta$ chains also express either the CD4 or CD8 co-receptor molecules. However, 1% to 5% of the peripheral TCR $\alpha\beta$ population expresses CD3, but not CD4 or CD8. DN T cells can be divided into NKT cells and NK-marker-negative DN Treg. DN Treg do not develop from CD8$^+$ precursors, nor is CD8 expression required for their development *in vivo* (161). Functional DN Treg develop outside of the thymus and may mature from a previously uncharacterized lineage of T cells. DN T cells have been shown to have immunoregulatory activity both *in vivo* and *in vitro* in both mouse and human (162). These DN populations were derived following administration of donor antigens to induce tolerance to allografts, and are presumably derived from precursors present in normal peripheral lymphoid populations (163). DN suppressors generated in this way kill alloreactive CD4$^+$ and CD8$^+$ T responders that express functional Fas by a mechanism involving Fas/Fas-L interactions. These activated DN cells were only able to kill syngeneic targets activated by the same alloantigenic stimulus.

Treg-Induced Treg

One possible mechanism to increase the efficiency of Treg is that Treg induce anergy or suppressor activity in the CD25$^-$ responders as a form of infectious immunologic tolerance. It has been shown that human CD4$^+$CD25$^+$ T cells induce CD4$^+$CD25$^-$ T cells to become Treg that are capable suppressing by producing IL-10 *(164)* or TGF-β (165) and thereby mediating suppression of naïve CD4$^+$ T cells. Similar studies in the mouse demonstrated that coculture of Treg with Foxp3$^-$ responder cells resulted in the induction of both TCR and IL-2 unresponsiveness in the responder population (166). The responder cells remained Foxp3$^-$ and exerted suppressor activity in a cell contact–dependent manner that was partially abrogated by anti-TGF-β.

CONTROL OF AUTOIMMUNE DISEASE BY Treg

Autoimmune Gastritis (AIG)

The role of Treg in the prevention of organ-specific autoimmune diseases has been studied in a number of different animal models. One of the best-studied models is autoimmune gastritis (AIG) that develops when BABL/c mice are subjected to d3Tx or when *nu/nu* mice on a BALB/c background are reconstituted with CD4$^+$CD25$^-$ T cells. A large body of evidence had implicated the major protein pump of the gastric parietal cell, the H/K ATPase, as the target antigen for the CD4$^+$ T cells that are responsible for inducing this disease *(167,168)*. To evaluate whether Treg could prevent disease induced by primed, fully differentiated effector-cell populations, two H/K ATPase-reactive T-cell lines were derived from d3Tx animals *(23)*. Both of these lines were CD4$^+$, I-A^d–restricted and recognized distinct peptides derived from the H/K ATPase α chain. One of the cell lines secreted Th1 cytokines and the other Th2, but both were equally pathogenic in inducing gastritis when transferred to immunocompromised, but not normal, recipients. The capacity of both of these clones to transfer disease to *nu/nu* recipients could be inhibited by cotransfer of CD4$^+$CD25$^+$ Treg from normal BALB/c mice. Thus, Treg are able to inhibit not only the initiation of disease after d3Tx, but also the function of fully activated effector cells. To address the possible involvement of cytokines in suppression of AIG, Treg from a number of different cytokine deficient mice were utilized to prevent induction of disease either after d3Tx or in *nu/nu* recipients of CD25$^-$ T cells. Treg from both IL-4 and IL-10$^{-/-}$ mice were as efficient as wild-type Treg in preventing the induction of disease (169,*170*). Furthermore, the protective capacity of Treg from wild-type mice was not reduced when the reconstituted mice were treated with an antibody to TGF-β (116).

It remains unknown whether Treg prevent autoimmune disease by inhibiting the priming and expansion of effector cells, by acting on APC, by preventing migration from the draining LN into the target organ, or by preventing the differentiation of naïve precursors into pathogenic effector cells. One important tool in furthering our understanding of the mechanism of action of Treg-mediated inhibition of AIG was the development of a line of TCR transgenic mice whose receptors recognize a defined peptide of the H/K

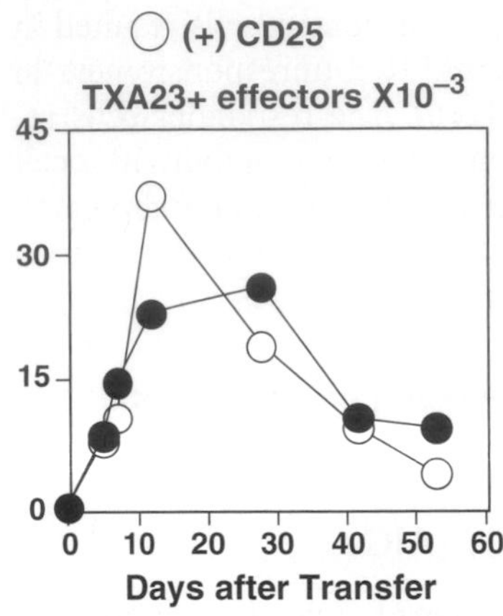

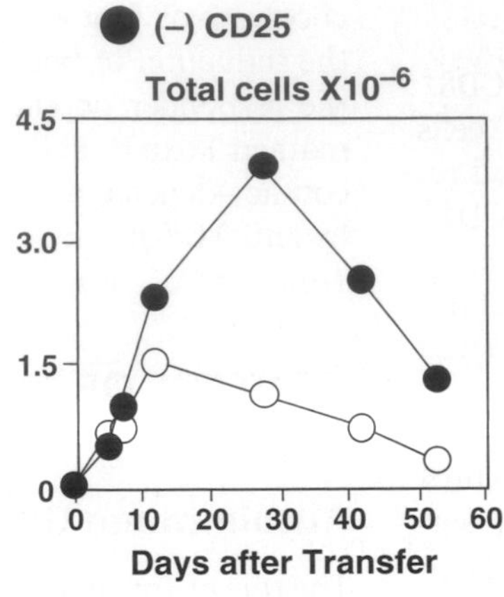

FIGURE 30.12 Treg do not block the expansion of effector T cells in the gastric lymph node, but they do inhibit the total number of cells. Adapted from DiPaolo RJ, Glass DD, Bijwaard KE, Shevach EM. CD4$^+$CD25$^+$ T cells prevent the development of organ-sepcifc autoimmune disease by inhibiting the differentiation of autoreactive effector cells. *J Immunol.* 2005;175:7135–7142.

ATPase and that spontaneously develop AIG (171). Small numbers of CD4$^+$CD25$^-$ thymocytes from this transgenic line can transfer AIG, home to the gastric lymph node, and be activated by DC that have acquired the H/K ATPase from parietal cells in the gastric mucosa. Cotransfer of polyclonal Treg with a small number of naïve auto-antigen–specific T cells under conditions in which lymphopenia-induced proliferation was partially controlled, was quite effective in inhibiting the development of AIG, demonstrated by suppression of parietal cell destruction and lack of autoantibody production. Treg failed to inhibit the migration of autoreactive T cells into the gastric lymph or into the target organ and did not inhibit the antigen-driven expansion of autoreactive T cells in the gastric lymph node (Figure 30.12). The primary effect of the Treg appeared to be inhibition of the differentiation of the self-specific T cells to Th1 effector cells, as reflected by a decrease in antigen-stimulated IFN-γ production and reduction in Tbet expression. A decrease in the total cellularity of the gastric lymph node was also seen in recipients of the Treg and likely reflects decreased cytokine/chemokine production by the effector T cells secondary to the suppressive effects of Treg.

It is widely assumed that Treg must be activated via the TCR to exert their suppressive effects *in vitro* and *in vivo*. The source of the TCR signal during *in vivo* activation of polyclonal populations of Treg is not known. In the AIG model, suppression of the antigen-specific induction of IFN-γ production could be observed as early as 7 days after transfer. It seems highly unlikely that this suppression is secondary to the activation and expansion of the limited number of gastric antigen-specific Treg within the polyclonal population. An alternative possibility is that Treg are able to control various responses because they are continuously recognizing and being partially activated by ubiquitous self-peptides.

To evaluate whether organ or antigen-specific Treg are more efficient at preventing autoimmunity than a polyclonal population of Treg with diverse antigen specificities, antigen-specific Foxp3$^+$ Treg were generated from naïve H/K ATPase-specific T cells following *in vitro* activation in the presence of TGF-β. After transfer, they maintained Foxp3 expression and inhibited the development of AIG. The mechanism of action of the antigen-specific-induced Treg was different from that of the polyclonal Treg, as they suppressed disease by preventing the initial activation and expansion of the autoreactive effector cells. The major effect of the induced Treg was to inhibit the priming of autoreactive T cells within the gastric lymph node. A 40-fold reduction in the number of autoreactive effectors was observed within the first 5 days. DC that had been in the presence of the induced Treg had a reduced capacity to present endogenous antigen compared to those from noninjected mice or mice injected only with effector cells. Thus, one mechanism by which induced Treg exert their function *in vivo* is by reducing the ability of DC to prime autoreactive T cells, hence stopping the autoimmune reaction before it even starts. The data from the AIG studies are most consistent with a model in which the Treg exert their negative effect by decreasing the stimulatory capacity of DC, rather than by competing with the effectors for antigen or by acting directly with the effectors to prevent their interaction with DC.

Inflammatory Bowel Disease (IBD)

The differential expression of the CD45RB isoforms initially used to define effector and regulatory T cells in the rat was extended to the mouse. Transfer of CD4$^+$CD45RB^{high} cells to SCID mouse recipients resulted in the development of a wasting disease and colitis 6 to 8 weeks after T-cell transfer. This disease was characterized pathologically by epithelial cell hyperplasia, goblet cell depletion, and transmural inflammation (172). There was a 20- to 30-fold accumulation of Th1 cells in the intestine compared to normal mice. Treatment of recipients with anti-IFN-γ, anti-TNF-α, or anti-IL-12 inhibited the induction of disease. Transfer of CD45RB^{low} cells did not induce colitis, and cotransfer of RB^{high} and RB^{low} cells prevented the development of colitis. A ratio of 1:8 RB^{low} to RB^{high} was able

TABLE 30.7 Role of Cytokines in the Pathogenesis and Treatment of Inflammatory Bowel Disease

Treatment	*Effect on Disease*
Anti-IFN-γ (d 1 + 4)	Substantial protection
Anti-TNF-5α (d 1 + 4)	No protection
Anti-TNF (weekly)	Protection during treatment only
IL-10	Protection during treatment only
IL-4	No protection
CD4$^+$CD25$^+$ T cells	Complete protection
CD4$^+$CD25$^+$ T cells + anti-IL-4	Complete protection
CD4$^+$CD25$^+$ T cells + anti-IL-10R	Protection with naïve CD45RB^{high}
CD4$^+$CD25$^+$ T cells + anti-IL-10R	No protection with naïve CD45RB^{low}
CD4$^+$CD25$^+$ T cells + anti-TGF-β	No protection

Adapted from Powrie F, Leach MW, Mauze S, et al. Inhibition of TH1 responses prevents inflammatory bowel-disease in SCID mice reconstituted with CD45RB^{high} T cells. *Immunity.* 1994;1:553–562; Asseman C, Read S, Powrie F. Colitogenic Th1 cells are present in the antigen-experienced T cell pool in normal mice: Control by CD4$^+$ regulatory T cells and IL-10. *J Immunol.* 2003;171:971–978; and Powrie F, Carlino J, Leach MW, et al. A critical role for transforming factor-β but not interleukin 4 in the suppression of T helper 1-mediated colitis by CD45RB^{low}CD4$^+$ T cells. *J Exp Med.* 1996;183:2669–2674.

to prevent disease. When CD45RB^{low} cells were fractionated into CD25$^+$ and CD25$^-$ fractions, control of intestinal inflammation was mediated primarily by the CD25$^+$ fraction (27). CD45RB^{low} CD25$^-$ cells did exert some suppressive function when transferred at high cell concentrations.

Treatment of recipients of RB^{high} cells with IL-10 inhibited the development of colitis (Table 30.7). This treatment inhibited the accumulation of Th1 cells in the intestine, but did not induce Treg, because colitis developed when IL-10 administration ceased. Treg isolated from IL-10$^{-/-}$ mice are able to inhibit colitis induced by CD4$^+$CD45RB^{high} cells, indicating that IL-10 secretion by Treg themselves is not required. However, control of colitis induced with CD25$^-$CD45RB^{low} cells was found to be highly dependent on IL-10 (173). The ability of Treg to inhibit colitis did not involve IL-4, but was dependent on TGF-β, because administration of anti-TGF-β abrogated the protective effect of these cells (174). It should be emphasized that Treg-mediated suppression of AIG involves a cell contact–dependent mechanism of suppression, and IL-10 and TGF-β are not involved, whereas Treg-mediated suppression of IBD is abrogated by anti-IL-10 and/or anti-TGF-β. One reason for this difference is that the pathogenesis of AIG and IBD are quite distinct. Bacteria play a required role in IBD, whereas AIG can be induced by d3Tx of germ-free mice. It remains possible that suppression of IBD involves both the cell contact–dependent and the cytokine-mediated pathways of suppression. IL-10 and TGF-β are required to first dampen the inflammatory response induced by intestinal bacteria. Once this response is reduced, cell contact–mediated suppression can become operative.

Mice with colitis have an accumulation of activated CD4$^+$ T cells in the mesenteric LN and colon. This T-cell infiltrate is accompanied by an accumulation of DC that in the mesenteric LN, but not the colon, express CD134L (OX-40L). Binding of CD134L to CD134 on T cells provides a costimulatory signal for T-cell activation. Administration of anti-CD134L prevented the development of colitis (175). Blockade of CD134/CD134L interactions does not inhibit signals involved in the early activation of pathogenic T cells, but may inhibit amplification of the response. DC may pick up intestinal antigens in the colon and transport them to the mesenteric lymph node, where they activate T-effector cells. In the absence of Treg, CD134$^+$ DC may magnify this response leading to colitis. Treg may inhibit the migration of DC to the lymph node or inhibit macrophage activation in the colon.

One advantage of the IBD model is that CD4$^+$CD25$^+$ CD45RB^{low}, but not CD4$^+$CD25$^-$CD45RB^{low}, T cells can cure ongoing colitis 4 weeks after transfer of CD4$^+$ CD45RB^{high} T cells *(176)*. Treg proliferate and accumulate in the mesenteric LN and also in the colonic lamina propria. At both sites, the progeny of the Treg are in direct contact with CD11c$^+$ DC as well as effector T cells. These findings suggest that regulation of an active immune response by Treg occurs in the draining LN as well as at the site of inflammation. During the cure of intestinal inflammation, the majority of the Foxp3$^+$ T cells are IL-10–secreting cells. Whereas Foxp3$^+$ cells are present in similar frequencies in both the secondary lymphoid organs and lamina propria of colitic animals, the IL-10–producing cells are selectively enriched in the colonic lamina propria. The gut environment may condition the Treg to differentiate into IL-10–producing Treg in the colon. Alternatively, the accumulation of Treg in the colon may be attributed to the preferential expansion of a minor subset of IL-10 producers contained in the transferred population. Treg from IL-10$^{-/-}$ mice, although less potent than wild-type Treg, are able to cure colitis. It is also likely that other cell types, possibly under the instruction of Treg, can make a significant amount of IL-10 and contribute to the cure of disease. Cure of colitis was not dependent on a reduction the proportion of IFN-γ–secreting cells among the effector cells, but the total number of CD4$^+$ T cells was greatly reduced.

Autoimmune Thyroiditis

In studies using the adult Tx-irradiation model for the induction of autoimmune thyroiditis, Seddon and Mason *(176)* demonstrated that disease could be prevented by the injection of CD4$^+$CD45RC^{low} peripheral T cells or by CD4$^+$CD8$^-$ thymocytes. In fact, the thymocytes were 10 times more potent that the Treg derived from the periphery. Suppression of thyroiditis mediated by both cell populations could be reversed by treatment of the recipients with either anti-IL-4 or anti-TGF-β. These studies strongly suggest that the mature $CD4^+CD8^-$ thymocyte population contains a high frequency of Treg or Treg precursors with the potential to differentiate in the periphery into Treg that prevent organ-specific autoimmunity. Detailed studies of Foxp3 expression by $CD25^+$ and $CD25^-$ T cells in this rat model have not as yet been performed.

Insulin-Dependent Diabetes Mellitus (IDDM)

The nonobese diabetic mouse (NOD) represents the best experimental model for autoimmune diabetes. It is widely accepted that $CD4^+$ Treg play a critical role in the regulation of disease in this animal model *(177)*. The islets of Langerhans become rapidly infiltrated with immune cells several weeks before the onset of diabetes. Diabetes progression may relate to a subsequent failure in the maintenance of Treg function. Because diabetes could only be transferred from sick mice to normal syngeneic recipients if the recipients were less than 5 weeks of age (female) or 3 weeks of age (male), it was assumed that Treg was deficient in young mice. Cyclophosphamide treatment, which may preferentially deplete Treg, accelerated the development of disease in young NOD mice. $CD4^+$ T cells from nondiabetic NOD mice could prevent the transfer of diabetes from overtly diabetic mice into sublethally irradiated NOD recipients. The protective cell population was not present in the spleen until 3 weeks of age and reached its highest activity at 8 weeks of age; suppressor cells were present in the thymus of neonates, which may explain why thymectomy at weaning accelerated disease. Diabetes could also be efficiently transferred to nonirradiated adult NOD recipients, if they were Tx and depleted of $CD4^+$ T cells. Depletion of T cells alone was not sufficient for disease transfer, suggesting that Tx was needed to limit emergence of newly generated $CD4^+$ Treg from the thymus. Islet infiltrating T cells from young nondiabetic mice could transfer diabetes to NOD/SCID mice, but cotransfer of $CD4^+CD45RB^{low}$ T cells from spleen of the same mouse delayed the onset of disease. Some studies demonstrated that the Treg could also be distinguished from the effector T cells by differential expression of CD62L.

Chatenoud et al. (178) have examined whether $CD4^+$ $CD25^+$ Treg play a protective role in the NOD mouse. Young NOD/SCID recipients were injected IV with mixtures of splenocytes from diabetic NOD mice, and Treg and $CD25^-$ T cells from the spleens of prediabetic NOD mice. Treg from young (6-week-old) prediabetic mice significantly protected against diabetes in this model. Protection could be reversed by treatment of the recipient mice with anti-TGF-β, but not anti-IL-4 or anti-IL-10. Interestingly, anti-TGF-β did not reverse protection mediated by Treg derived from the thymus. $CD4^+CD25^-$ T cells from young NOD mice could also exert some degree of protection in adoptive transfer studies. Analysis of Treg function in the NOD mouse is difficult because not all animals will develop disease and it takes a long time for disease to develop. Green et al. (74) have developed a model of IDDM in which a regulatable TNF gene is expressed in the pancreatic islets. When these mice were crossed to mice expressing CD80 in their islets and TNF was expressed for 25 days from birth, diabetes was delayed. In contrast, if TNF expression was allowed to continue for 28 days, the regulatory mechanisms were overcome and the animals rapidly developed diabetes. The autoreactive effector cells in this model are exclusively $CD8^+$ T cells. Treg could be isolated from the islets and draining pancreatic node, but not from other nodes or spleen, and they could suppress the development of disease in animals in which TNF was expressed for 28 days. These regulatory cells were extremely potent, and protection could be transferred with as few as 2×10^3 Treg. This site-specific accumulation of regulatory cells may be the result of localized production of chemokines that specifically recruit Treg to the site of inflammation. Alternatively, the Treg in the draining node may be antigen-specific and generated in situ by stimulation by islet-derived antigens.

Antigen-specific Treg from the TCR transgenic BDC2.5 mice that recognize an islet-derived antigen have been expanded with co-immobilized anti-CD3/anti-CD28 in the presence of IL-2 (179). These expanded Treg prevented the development of diabetes in NOD mice, survived long-term *in vivo*, but required antigen exposure for functional activity. Islet autoantigen-specific BDC2.5 Treg were significantly more effective than polyclonal Treg in regulating autoimmune responses *in vivo*. Importantly, expanded BDC2.5 Treg were able to reverse diabetes when transferred into NOD mice that had been diabetic for 2 weeks in conjunction with 500 syngeneic NOD islets. The expanded Treg were also capable of inhibiting diabetes in newly diagnosed NOD mice.

These results raise the possibility that Treg might be isolated from patients during remission or soon after disease onset, expanded, and used to treat patients at the time of maximal disease activity to moderate the inflammatory response. Indeed, Masteller et al. (180) were able to expand Treg with the BDC2.5 specificity by stimulating NOD Treg with beads coated with a mimitope peptide complexed to MHC class II (I-Ag^7) that is recognized by the BDC2.5 TCR. The expanded Treg were more efficient than polyclonal Treg in suppressing autoimmune diabetes. Thus, small numbers of autoantigen-specific Treg may be clinically efficacious because they can suppress polyclonal pathogenic T-cell responses either by bystander cytokine production or by recruitment of endogenous Treg, while avoiding pan-immune suppression that might be induced by polyclonal Treg. As many organ-specific antigens have been identified, it may be possible to use human MHC multimer reagents to expand organ-specific Treg from peripheral blood for effective treatment of human autoimmune disease.

Several studies have explored the site of action and mechanisms of action of Treg in autoimmune diabetes models (181). Treg had little or no effect on the activation of effector cells but suppressed IFN-γ production by the effectors in the pancreatic LN and seemed to slow the migration of effector cells into the islets, perhaps through a reduction in CXCR3 in the pancreatic LN. One problem with studies of Treg-mediated protection from autoimmune disease is that they frequently involve transfer into lymphopenic hosts, where interpretation of the results may be difficult secondary to stimulation of the effector population that is seen in response to lymphopenia. Foxp3$^{-/-}$ NOD mice have been used to analyze where and how Treg cells exert their control on diabetes under experimental conditions not influenced by homeostatic expansion of effector populations (182). Treg did not delay or hinder the activation and expansion of anti-islet T cells in the pancreatic LN nor the timing of their infiltration into the islets, but primarily prevented locally damaging consequences of autoimmune infiltration in the islets. It appears the Treg primarily impinge on autoimmune diabetes by suppressing destructive T cells inside the islets, more than during the initial activation in the draining LN. Further studies are clearly needed to resolve these conflicting findings, as a detailed understanding of the site and mechanism of suppression of experimental autoimmune disease will facilitate translation of the therapeutic use of Treg for treatment of autoimmune disease in humans.

Experimental Autoimmune Encephalomyelitis (EAE)

EAE is the major animal model for the study of multiple sclerosis, and Treg have been shown to play a role in this model. When the Treg population of naïve C57 BL/6 mice was supplemented with CD4$^+$CD25$^+$ Treg from a normal donor before the active induction of EAE by immunization with an encephalitogenic peptide from myelin oligodendrocyte glycoprotein (MOG), the Treg conferred significant protection. Protection was associated with the presence of Th2 cytokines and a marked decreased CD4$^+$ T-cell and APC infiltrates in the central nervous system (CNS) (183). These studies suggested that Treg might inhibit the homing of pathogenic T cells to the CNS. McGeachy et al. (184) demonstrated that that the accumulation of CD25$^+$Foxp3$^+$ cells in the CNS correlated with the recovery phase of EAE. As few as 10^4 CNS-derived CD25$^+$ cells significantly reduced disease severity in recipients, whereas the same number of naïve CD25$^+$ T cells had no effect. Although the mechanism of action of the Treg in protection from EAE was not completely elucidated, CD25$^+$ T cells were the major source of IL-10 in the CNS and IL-10 production was crucial for full recovery from EAE.

Antigenic Specificity of Treg in Autoimmunity

Very little progress has been made in the identification of the target antigen recognized by polyclonal Treg. They could recognize ubiquitously expressed self-peptides or a target antigen derived from the organ that is under autoimmune attack. A number of studies have shown that when the developing immune system is prevented from gaining access to a tissue-specific antigen, tissue specific tolerance fails to develop. For example, when fetal rat thyroid glands were destroyed by exposure to radioactive iodine and syngeneic thyroid tissue was then implanted into the athyroid rats as adults, autoimmune thyroiditis developed in the grafted tissue *(185)*. The development of thyroiditis in such rats could be prevented by parabiosis to normal syngeneic partners. Parabiosis was protective only if it was instituted at the time of thyroid grafting, but not 1 to 2 weeks after graft implantation. This approach was extended by Seddon and Mason (186) to demonstrate that peripheral CD45RC^{low} T cells from rats rendered athyroid were unable to prevent thyroid-specific autoimmunity induced by the adult-Tx irradiation protocol. The loss of Treg was specific for the extirpated organ, as T cells from the athyroid rats could prevent the development of diabetes. CD4$^+$CD8$^-$ thymocytes from the same athyroid donors were effective at preventing thyroiditis. It appears that regulatory T cells were normally generated in the thymus in the absence of the target organ, but the target organ was needed for their survival and/or expansion in the periphery.

Spleen cells from normal adult male mice were much more effective suppressors of autoimmune orchitis induced post-d3Tx than were spleen cells from female mice or male mice that had undergone a neonatal orchiectomy (187). In contrast, spleen cells from male and female mice exerted equivalent potency in protecting against gastritis. Taguchi et al. *(188)* have shown that the suppressor-cell population that was capable of inhibiting the induction of prostatitis was organ-specific, because cells from males, but not females, or males orchiectomized at birth, inhibited disease post-d3Tx. Other studies in autoimmune prostatitis suggested that the differences were relative rather than absolute, because protection could be achieved with 4×10^6 cells from normal males, but only with 4×10^7 spleen cells from females. Moreover, normal male, normal female, and spleen cells from females that were oophorectomized at birth were found to suppress d3Tx-induced oophoritis with comparable efficiency *(189)*.

Important insights into determining the antigenic specificity of regulatory T cells have also been derived from studies of the requirements for induction of organ-specific autoreactive effector cells (190). When susceptible strains of mice are immunized with the ovary-specific antigen, pZP3, 100-fold more pZP3 in CFA was required to elicit the same pathogenic response in female mice compared to male mice that had been grafted with an ovary. This differential responsiveness to stimulation by the autoantigen indicates that female mice have a certain level of tolerance to pZP3 that is dependent on the presence of physiologically expressed ZP3 antigen. Neonatal oophorectomy converts the female response to that of a male. Oophorectomy between the ages of 1 and 6 weeks also leads to conversion of the female to a male responsiveness profile when the ovaries are removed for more than 7 days, but not 3 days, before challenge with pZP3 in CFA. It remains to be determined whether tolerance in the female is mediated by Treg and whether continued expression of the endogenous antigen is required for the maintenance/survival of the Treg in the periphery. More recent studies (191) have demonstrated that Treg from lymph nodes draining the target organ were 15 to 50 times more efficient than Treg from the nondraining lymph node in suppressing oophoritis, prostatitis, and dacryoadenitis that developed post-d3Tx. It was concluded from these studies that the accumulation of Treg is not random and that organ-specific Treg are increased in frequency where they are needed to protect against autoimmunity that might develop in their target organ in response to infection or inflammation.

Treg and Th2-Mediated Diseases

Several early studies suggested that CD4$^+$CD25$^+$ Treg cells bias the differentiation of CD4$^+$ T cells toward Th2 cells and might express a subset of Th2 genes, indicating that Treg might promote Th2 development. However, more recent studies have reported that the depletion of CD25$^+$ Treg cells *in vivo* led to an in increased development of Th2 cells. It has also been shown that Treg suppress the differentiation and function of Th1 and Th2 cells *in vitro* and *in vivo* (192,193). Other studies (194) have shown that freshly isolated Treg inhibited the IL-4–induced development of Th2 cells, but had no influence on established Th2 cells. In contrast, preactivated Treg inhibited cytokine production and proliferation of established Th2 cells.

CD4$^+$Foxp3$^+$ Treg modulate the development of experimentally induced asthma in mice genetically predisposed or comparatively resistant to the development of AHR. *In vivo* depletion of Treg in resistant animals before initial antigen contact increased airway hypersensitivity reaction (AHR), airway eosinophilia, and IgE synthesis, and was associated with Th2 cytokine production, whereas Treg cell depletion had no effect on allergen-driven AHR in susceptible mice (195). Enhancement of allergic phenotype in resistant mice was associated with stimulation of DC function, suggesting that the Treg do not act on effector T cells, but act indirectly via the DC. Similarly, Th2 polarized CD4$^+$ T cells depleted of CD25$^+$ cells induce increased airway eosinophilia after adoptive transfer (196). Allergen-specific CD4$^+$CD25$^+$ T cells from TCR transgenic mice inhibited the classical pathology associated with allergic asthma, including AHR, lung eosinophilia, and Th2 cytokine production in immunocompetent mice. Their effects were dependent on IL-10, but Treg cells exerted their suppressive effects *in vivo* independently of their capacity to produce IL-10, by inducing IL-10 production from recipient CD4$^+$ T cells (197).

Mice with an established helminth infection are less prone to allergic airway inflammation as measured by inflammatory infiltrate in bronchial lavage fluid or peribronchial and perivascular inflammation. Helminth infection with *Helicobacter polygyrus* protects from allergic airway responses by acting downstream from allergen sensitization, and protection can be transferred from infected mice to uninfected presensitized animals by CD25$^+$ T cells. Th2 effector cytokines (IL-5 and IL-13) were diminished, but allergen-specific IgE responses were not changed. Thus, chronic parasite infection may maintain a high level of activation in Treg, so that they primarily target the effector mechanisms resulting in decreased inflammation in a previously sensitized allergy-prone host (198).

Lymphocyte Homeostasis and Autoimmunity

Lymphocyte numbers in a normal adult animal remain stable throughout life. A homeostatic equilibrium exists among the numbers of newly produced cells, self-renewal of peripheral T cells, and the numbers of dying cells. The mechanism that controls the number of peripheral lymphocytes is unknown. The regulation of the numbers of naïve and memory CD4$^+$ and CD8$^+$ T cells is independently controlled. Most studies of the effects of Treg *in vivo* in the suppression of autoimmune disease involve the transfer of the effector populations to a T-cell–deficient mouse. T lymphocytes undergo a rapid, vigorous proliferative response when transferred to an immunodeficient recipient. We assume that some of the inhibitory effects of Treg in autoimmunity are related to their ability to be specifically activated by autoantigens. An alternative possibility is that a major component of Treg function is to nonspecifically inhibit lymphopenia-induced proliferation (199) and thereby prevent the development of autoimmune disease. CD4$^+$Foxp3$^+$ T cells might be potent inhibitors of lymphopenia-induced proliferation, but any T-cell population with an activated effector/memory phenotype might also be capable of mediating inhibition (200).

Surprisingly, both CD4$^+$CD25$^-$ (including RB^{high} cells) T cells and CD4$^+$CD25$^+$ T cells were capable of proliferating in a lymphopenic host, with proliferation beginning on day 3 or 4 posttransfer, and reaching as many as eight divisions by days 21 to 28 after transfer. CD4$^+$CD25$^+$ T cells did

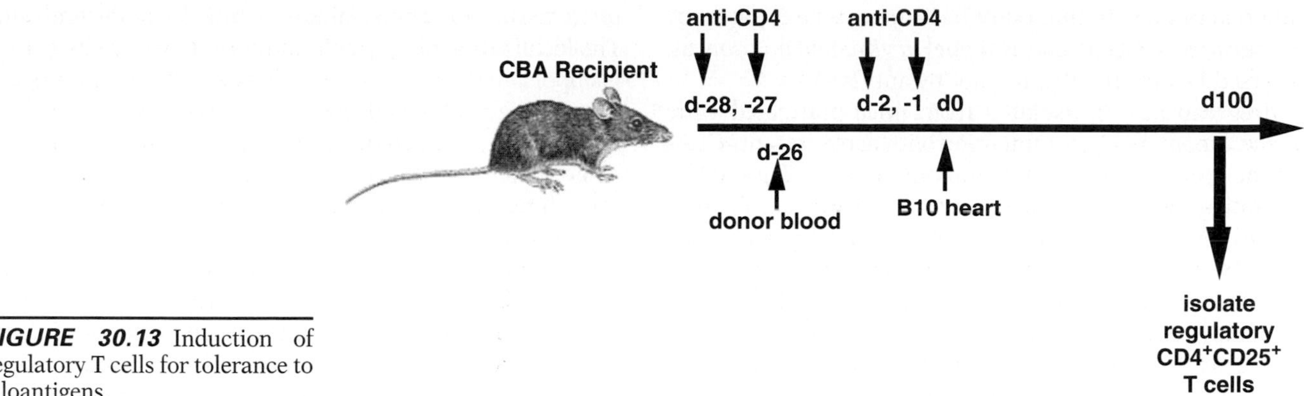

FIGURE 30.13 Induction of regulatory T cells for tolerance to alloantigens.

not inhibit this early phase of "homeostatic proliferation" of CD4$^+$CD25$^-$ T cells *(201)*. Although CD4$^+$CD25$^+$ T cells have been shown to inhibit the accumulation of CD25$^-$ T cells 2 to 6 months after transfer to a RAG$^{-/-}$ recipient by an IL-10–dependent mechanism, this result must be interpreted with caution (202). The fact that CD25$^-$ T cells almost always induce some form of organ-specific autoimmune disease demonstrates that CD25$^-$ T cells have undergone some form of autoantigen-specific proliferation in addition to the lymphopenia-induced proliferation. As described previously, CD4$^+$Foxp3$^+$ T cells are highly efficient inhibitors of the induction of these autoimmune diseases. It should be noted that transfer of CD25$^+$Foxp3$^+$ T cells to immunodeficient mice results in loss of expression of CD25 by a majority of the transferred cells (79). The significance of this finding is unknown, as the recovered CD25$^-$ T cells retain the ability to suppress T-cell activation *in vitro*.

Although the role of Treg cells in controlling lymphopenia-induced proliferation remains unresolved, one major factor that has only recently been considered is the avidity of the TCR for self-ligands. When monoclonal or polyclonal T cells with low avidity for self, as determined by expression of low levels of CD5, were transferred to lymphopenic recipients, their proliferation was substantially inhibited by CD4$^+$CD25$^+$ Treg. In contrast, T cells with high avidity for self-antigens that expressed high levels of CD5 entered the cell cycle in the presence of Treg, but failed to differentiate from naïve to memory phenotype (203).

CONTROL OF ALLOGRAFT REJECTION AND GRAFT-VERSUS-HOST DISEASE (GVHD) BY Treg

A considerable body of data exists that regulatory/suppressor T cells exist in patients and animals with long-term surviving allografts *(204)*. Analysis of the properties of these cells *in vitro* has been hampered because bulk populations of T cells from tolerant recipients proliferate normally when cultured *in vitro* with donor alloantigens and frequently secrete a proinflammatory Th1 pattern of cytokines. It appears that the Treg are masked by the presence of naïve T cells responding to alloantigens. In animal models, a number of protocols have been used to induce tolerance to allografts (Figure 30.13). Tolerance to cardiac allografts in mice can be induced by pretreatment with a donor-specific blood transfusion combined with depleting or nondepleting anti-CD4 antibody. It is likely that the protective effects of this protocol were mediated by the induction of CD4$^+$ Treg, because complete depletion of CD4$^+$ T cells fails to induce tolerance. Pretreated mice accepted cardiac grafts, and cells from these mice could transfer tolerance to naïve recipients. CD4$^+$ T cells were responsible for both the induction and maintenance of tolerance.

In studies of allograft rejection across a full H-2 difference, the differential expression of CD45RB has facilitated separation of nontolerant naïve T cells from the induced regulatory T cells *(204)*. RB^{high} cells from tolerant mice responded normally to challenge with alloantigen *in vitro* and were able to reject allogeneic skin grafts when transferred alone to T-cell–deficient mice. In contrast, CD45RB^{low} cells failed to mount a proliferative response, to secrete cytokines in response to alloantigen *in vitro*, and to induce allograft rejection *in vivo*. The addition of CD45RB^{low} cells to an MLR with CD45RB^{high} cells as responders resulted in inhibition of proliferation. CD45RB^{low} T cells from long-term-tolerant mice were able to suppress responses to alloantigen *in vitro* only when the donor alloantigens were presented by the indirect pathway of allorecognition by the APC present in the culture. One explanation for this result is that it is potentially advantageous for the Treg to respond to alloantigens via the indirect pathway because Treg may require constant stimulation to maintain their function. Passenger leukocytes rapidly migrate out of the graft, and the graft tissues lack costimulatory molecules. Donor-derived allopeptides must be presented by recipient APC for stimulation of the Treg *in vivo* and for the detection of functional activity of these cells *in vitro*. All of the suppressive activity of the CD45RB^{low} cells was mediated by the CD4$^+$CD25$^+$ T-cell subset contained in that pool. The suppressive capacity of the regulatory T cells in this model *in vitro* and *in vivo* was reversed by anti-IL-10R, but not by anti-IL-4.

Treg can also be isolated from mice pretreated with donor alloantigen in combination with depleting anti-CD4, but not transplanted with an allograft (205). These cells are fully competent in prolongation of cardiac graft survival when transferred to naïve recipients. Treg can be isolated 28 days after pretreatment, and regulation is antigen-specific. Both treatments are required, and $CD25^+$ T cells from naïve donors do not prolong graft rejection. It is possible that the precursor frequency of alloantigen-specific regulatory $CD25^+$ T cells from naïve animals is too low to observe suppression at the cell doses used, and that the pretreatment regimen serves to increase their frequency. No major increase in the percentage of $CD25^+$ cells is observed in the pretreated animals, and it remains to be proven that the $CD25^+$ T cells isolated from the pretreated animals are derived from the Treg pool and not generated from $CD25^-$ T cells. In either case, it is likely that the pretreatment protocol maximizes the conditions for activation of Treg.

In studies examining induction of tolerance to minor histocompatibility antigens on allografts following protocols similar to those used above, both $CD4^+CD25^+$ and $CD4^+CD25^-$ T cells from tolerant mice could mediate suppression, but suppression required 10 times more $CD4^+CD25^-$ T cells (206). Both populations may have a significant role in maintaining transplantation tolerance, as the number of $CD25^-$ T cells is 10 times higher than the number of $CD25^+$ T cells in the tolerant mouse. It is possible that some of the $CD25^+$ T cells have lost expression of CD25 during the tolerance-induction protocol, that effector cell death in the $CD25^-$ T-cell pool unmasked the presence of Treg, or that some of the $CD25^-$ T cells express Foxp3. In contrast to the results with a major MHC difference, $CD4^+CD25^+$ T cells from naïve mice could also prevent naïve T cells from rejecting skin grafts, although five times more cells were required than from tolerant donors. The enhanced potency of $CD25^+$ T cells from tolerant mice may be secondary to expansion of an alloantigen-specific population. The capacity of T cells from tolerant donors or $CD25^+$ T cells from normal mice to mediate their suppressive function could not be neutralized by anti-CTLA-4, anti-IL-10, or anti-IL-4 (205).

A short treatment of mice with saturating amounts of nondepleting anti-CD4 can induce tolerance to foreign protein antigens and enables long-term survival of minor antigen–mismatched skin or MHC-mismatched cardiac grafts. The addition of anti-CD40L can extend this effect to full donor-specific tolerance, such that second donor grafts are accepted at any later time, while third-party grafts are rapidly rejected. The maintenance of tolerance is dependent on $CD4^+$ Treg that can suppress both $CD4^+$ and $CD8^+$ naïve T cells after transfer into secondary recipients. Treg cells are found not only in recipient lymphoid tissue after transplantation, but also at the graft site. The localization of Treg cells at more than one site *in vivo* is important if Treg are to control aggressive immune reactivity to the graft effectively. In lymphoid tissues, Treg cells might be effective at blocking the initiation of an aggressive response against the graft, whereas at the graft site, they can inhibit the effector activity of aggressive cells that have escaped regulation and migrated to the graft.

Regulation observed in therapeutic tolerance probably is maintained both by pre-existing Treg together with induced Treg. In the continued presence of donor antigen, $CD4^+$ Treg are able to convert naïve, potentially aggressive $CD4^+$ T cells into Treg, a process termed infectious tolerance. Little is known about the molecular mechanisms involved in the conversion, whether they act systemically or within the graft, and how they relate to $Foxp3^+$ Treg. In one model, antigen stimulation in the presence of a nondepleting anti-CD4 has been shown to convert $CD4^+Foxp3^-$ T cells into $Foxp3^+$ Treg in a TGF-β–dependent manner *in vivo*, and this correlates with life-long acceptance of the graft (207). Treg cells that recognize donor MHC molecules through the indirect pathway of allorecognition have been shown to be responsible for the phenomenon of linked unresponsiveness (208). Linked suppression *in vivo* seems to correlate with the *in vitro* finding that once Treg are activated, they can suppress the activation of other T cells responding to antigen presented by the same APC in an antigen-nonspecific manner.

The inability of T-cell populations containing large numbers of $CD25^+$ T cells to mediate GVHD strongly raised the possibility that $CD25^+$ T cells might actually be capable of inhibiting $CD25^-$ effectors in cotransfer studies. Freshly isolated $CD25^+$ T cells only modestly inhibited GVHD when mixed with $CD25^-$ T cells in equal numbers, while alloantigen-stimulated, cultured $CD25^+$ T cells profoundly inhibited the capacity of $CD25^-$ T cells to inhibit rapidly lethal GVHD *(209)*. In murine models, transplantation of bone marrow into a lethally irradiated host does not cause GVHD, and cotransfer of naïve donor T cells ($CD4^+$, $CD8^+$, or both) is required to induce GVHD. The onset and course of GVHD depends on the degree of major and minor MHC disparity and the T-cell dose. Depletion of Treg from the donor graft accelerated the course of GVHD and increased lethality. These findings provided evidence for the role of Treg in suppressing GVHD. Transfer of Treg with naïve T cells from the donor protected lethally irradiated recipients from GVHD morbidity and decreased GVHD-related mortality (210) across minor and major MHC class I and/or class II barriers in various mouse strain combinations. The mechanisms by which Treg suppress GVHD is not well understood. The effect of Treg on GVHD is likely to be early and to affect the maturation and expansion of effector cells. $CD62L^{high}$ Tregs are more potent suppressors of GVHD, presumably because of their ability to migrate to secondary lymph nodes, where they are primed and activated *(211)*. Because host APC are necessary to trigger acute GVHD, it is possible that the activated Treg function by downregulating costimulatory molecules and thereby prevent the activation of effector T cells. Hoffman et al. showed decreased protection from GVHD with Treg derived from IL-$10^{-/-}$ animals (212).

The most analogous model to the murine models of GVHD induction is the administration of donor lymphocyte infusions to humans with relapsed leukemia after allogeneic hematopoietic cell transplantation (HCT) so as to obtain a graft-versus-tumor effect. The development of GVHD after donor lymphocyte infusion is associated with tumor clearance. However, Treg controlling GVHD may also cause suppression of tumor immunity. Edinger and coworkers (213) found that adoptive transfer of donor Treg effectively decreased the incidence and severity of GVHD without abrogating the graft-versus-tumor response. In this model, cotransfer of Treg markedly decreased the proliferation of alloreactive effector cells in secondary lymphoid organs by >90% at day 7, but did not inhibit the activation of the effectors as judged by activation-marker expression and cytokine production. One possibility is that the decrease in the proliferation and expansion of the alloreactive T-effector cells was sufficient to control acute GVHD, but this decrease was not complete, and the remaining donor T-effector cells were sufficient to mount an effective graft-versus-tumor effect.

Treg also play a facilitating role in bone marrow engraftment. Joffre et al. (214) found that Treg provided allospecific protection of transplanted bone marrow from host rejection. Enhanced engraftment with Treg also increased long-term donor chimerism in animals that received Treg compared to those that received bone marrow transplants only. Recipients of Treg demonstrated tolerance to host and donor antigens, but mounted responses to third-party antigens (215). Encouraging preclinical data have set the stage for the potential therapeutic application of Treg in patients. Patients undergoing haploidentical transplantation are at high risk for severe GVHD and therefore are the ideal candidates for adoptive transfer of donor Treg.

REGULATORY T CELLS AND TUMOR IMMUNITY

Studies by R. North and associates in the early 1980s (216) demonstrated the role of suppressor T cells in the prevention of tumor immunity. In their studies, primed antitumor T cells were incapable of causing regression of a tumor when passively transferred into a normal host. If the tumor recipient was rendered T-cell–deficient by Tx and lethal irradiation, followed by bone marrow reconstitution combined with sublethal irradiation, or treated with cyclophosphamide, the transferred cells could induce tumor regression. Cotransfer of T cells from tumor-bearing recipients prevented T-cell–mediated tumor regression. T cells taken on day 6 after tumor implantation were capable of transferring protection to T-cell–depleted recipients. By day 9 of tumor growth, the antitumor T cells were lost, and transfer of cells from the tumor-bearing animals suppressed antitumor immune effectors. Immediately after tumor implantation, mice developed concomitant immunity and would reject a challenge implant of cells of the same tumor given at another site. Later in the course of tumor development, concomitant immunity decayed.

The suppressor T cells in the experiments of North and coworkers were shown to be $CD4^+CD8^-$, but were not characterized further *(217)*. Their susceptibility to sublethal irradiation and cyclophosphamide is similar to that of $CD4^+CD25^+$ T cells. As most tumor antigens are normal self-antigens, it is likely that those mechanisms that maintain immunologic tolerance to self-antigens may impede the generation of effective tumor immunity against autologous tumor cells. In many cases, successful immunotherapy of cancer often leads to the appearance of autoimmunity because of cross-reactions between antigens expressed on tumors and normal tissue antigens. Onizuki et al. (218) were the first to suggest that $CD4^+CD25^+$ T cells played an important role in inhibiting tumor immunity. They first depleted $CD4^+CD25^+$ T cells by injecting a depleting anti-CD25 mAb and noted that this led to regression of a number of tumors that grew progressively in non depleted mice. The depletion had to be performed not later than day 2 after injection of the tumor. Coadministration of anti-CD8 inhibited the tumor regression induced by anti-CD25 depletion, suggesting that CD8 T cells were responsible for tumor regression. Similar conclusions were drawn by Shimizu et al. (111), who transferred CD25-depleted or CD25-containing spleen cells to *nu/nu* recipients and then challenged them with normally nonimmunogenic tumors. In the recipients of CD25-depleted cells, tumors grew, but regressed; in contrast, all recipients of spleen cells containing $CD25^+$ T cells died from rapidly growing tumors. Long-lasting tumor immunity to rechallenge could also be demonstrated in the recipients of the CD25-depleted spleen cells.

Taken together, the studies on depletion of $CD4^+CD25^+$ T cells and the transfer of $CD4^+CD25^-$ T cells suggest strongly that the effectiveness of a tumor vaccine would be greatly enhanced by removal of $CD4^+CD25^+$ T-cell suppressor activity. Indeed, Sutmuller et al. (219) were able to demonstrate that antibody-mediated depletion of $CD25^+$ T cells followed by vaccination with a GM-CSF–transfected melanoma cell line resulted in enhanced tumor rejection. Tumor rejection was accompanied by skin depigmentation, suggesting that autoreactive immune responses are involved in this process. Depletion of $CD25^+$ T cells followed by anti-CTLA-4 treatment and vaccination resulted in the most potent antitumor response (Table 30.8). Thus, CD25 depletion and anti-CTLA-4 treatment increase the

TABLE 30.8 Depletion of CD4+CD25+ T Cells Augments the Immune Response to a Tumor Vaccine

Treatment	*Percent Surviving at d 90*
None	0
Anti-CD25 (d −4)	20
GM-CSF vaccine (d 0, 3, 6) + Anti-CD25 (d −4)	50
GM-CSF vaccine (d 0, 3, 6) + Anti-CTLA-4 (d 0, 3, 6)	50
GM-CSF vaccine (d 0, 3, 6) + Anti-CD25 (d −4) + Anti-CTLA-4 (d 0, 3, 6)	100

Adapted from Sutmuller RPM, van Duivenvoorde LM, van Elsas A, et al. Synergism of cytotoxic T lymphocyte-associated antigen 4 blockade and depletion of $CD25^+$ regulatory T cells in antitumor therapy reveals alternative pathways for suppression of autoreactive cytotoxic T lymphocyte responses. *J Exp Med.* 2001;194:823–832.

immunogenicity of a tumor vaccine by distinct mechanisms that involve nonredundant pathways. CTLA-4 blockade enhances the induction of antitumor effector cells by removing the normal inhibitory signals generated by CD80/CD86 interactions with CTLA-4.

Experiments with adoptively, transferred mouse Treg cells provided a direct link between Treg cells and reduced tumor immunity. Tumor-specific $CD8^+$ T cells were transferred with either Treg cells or conventional T cells into mice bearing B16 melanoma. In mice that received Treg cells, but not in mice that received $CD25^-$ T cells, $CD8^+$ T-cell–mediated immunity was abolished. Treg cells may mediate their suppressive effect by inhibiting T-cell priming in lymphoid organs or by reducing the effector function of tumor antigen-specific cells. Antony et al. (220) have shown that transfer of Treg cells reduced the therapeutic efficiency of adoptively transferred tumor antigen-specific effector T cells in a mouse melanoma model. Depletion of intratumoral Treg cells induced potent T-cell tumor immunity and resulted in regression of large established tumors. Administration of anti-GITR antibody protected mice from B16 tumor challenge and induced tumor regression in mice bearing carcinogen-induced sarcomas and colon carcinomas (221). The anti-GITR likely costimulates T-effector functions to make the effector cells resistant to Treg-mediated suppression.

Although the preceding studies in well-characterized animals models demonstrate the role of $CD4^+CD25^+$ T cells in inhibiting tumor rejection, it is often difficult to extrapolate from tumor immunity studies in rodents to humans. Woo et al. (222) have shown that $CD4^+CD25^+$ T cells exist in high proportions (~33%) in the tumor-infiltrating lymphocytes of patients with non-small-cell lung cancer. It is not known if these tumor-infiltrating $CD4^+CD25^+$ T cells arise from the naturally occurring $CD4^+CD25^+$ population or are generated from $CD4^+CD25^-$ T cells. Nevertheless, these findings suggest that one component of the immune response to tumors in humans is the generation of tumor-specific suppressor T cells. A high frequency of Treg cells has been noted in many other human cancers. Treg cell have been extensively studied in human ovarian cancer (223). Treg cells within the ovarian tumor microenvironment expressed Foxp3, inhibited tumor antigen-specific $CD8^+$ T-cell cytotoxicity, and contributed to tumor growth *in vivo* in a human–SCID mouse chimeric model. An accumulation of Treg cells in the tumor predicted a striking reduction in survival.

A number of mechanisms have been proposed for Treg-mediated suppression of tumor immunity. Because Treg express CTLA-4, one possible model is that engagement of CD80/CD86 on tumor APC may induce production of the immunosuppressive molecule, IDO. IDO-expressing APC are found in human tumors and within draining lymph nodes. Alternatively, ovarian tumor-associated macrophages, but not normal macrophages, express B7-H4, a negative regulator of T-cell responses. B7-$H4^+$ macrophages isolated from tumors inhibited tumor antigen-specific responses, and suppression could be reversed by anti-B7-H4 (224). Treg, but not normal, T cells induced B7-H4 on monocytes, macrophages, and myeloid DC and rendered them immunosuppressive through B7-H4.

The spectrum of tumor-specific antigens recognized by Treg has not yet been defined. In one case, cloned Treg from a melanoma recognized LAGE-1, a cancer- and testis-specific antigen, and suppressed LAGE-1-specific T-cell activation (225). It is important to identify the ligands for Treg cells to compare them to the ligands for tumor-specific effector cells and to determine whether there are ligands that are exclusively recognized by Treg cells and whether Treg cells recognize mutated tumor antigens. A major concern that remains to be addressed is whether vaccination with certain tumor antigens might promote Treg cell clonal expansion.

The concept of reversing immunosuppression in cancer has merit as a therapeutic approach. CTLA-4 blockade improves tumor immunity but also resulted in severe manageable autoimmune responses in patients (226). The mechanistic link between the effects of treatment with anti-CTLA and Treg function remain to be determined. Depletion of Treg should be beneficial for cancer patients. Denileukin diftitox (Ontak), a ligand-toxin fusion protein, consists of full-length IL-2 fused to the enzymatically active and translocating domains of diptheria toxin. It has been hypothesized that this agent will lead to depletion of Treg *in vivo*, but it also might deplete $CD25^+$ effector cells. In one trial, patients received a single does of Ontak followed by vaccination with DC transfected with total tumor RNA (227). Treg cells were eliminated in a dose-dependent manner, and Ontak-treated vaccinated patients had an improved tumor-specific effector T-cell response. In other studies, Ontak had variable effects on Foxp3 mRNA expression in CD4+ T cells in patients with melanoma, and no significant clinical efficacy was observed (228). Further clinical trials are needed to link Treg depletion with improved immunity and an objective clinical response. An alternative strategy would be to selectively block Treg trafficking into tumors.

Although the majority of studies indicate that Treg cells suppress tumor immunity, other models raise the possibility that Treg may have a beneficial effect in preventing tumorigenesis. A widely used model for human colorectal carcinogenesis is the multiple intestinal neoplasia mouse, which has a germline mutation in the *Apc* tumor suppressor gene (229). Transfer of CD4+CD25+ Treg cells reduced the multiplicity of epithelial adenomas in these mice by an IL-10–dependent mechanism. Recipients of Treg showed increased apoptosis and downregulation of cyclo-oxygenase-2 within tumors, coinciding with tumor regression. In this model, aspirin and cyclo-oxygenase inhibitors also decrease the risk for colon cancer by inhibiting cyclo-oxygenase-2. Because Treg can suppress bacterially triggered inflammatory responses in the bowel of mice, the ability of Treg to traffic and suppress inflammation likely explains their therapeutic efficacy in this model. As inflammatory mediators drive tumor development, Treg and anti-inflammatory drugs exert their effect by modulating the levels of these molecules.

Treg CONTROL OF IMMUNITY TO INFECTIOUS AGENTS

Most of the studies of Treg have focused on their role in the suppression of the immune response to autoantigens, tumor antigens, or alloantigens. One of the most important roles of Treg may, in fact, involve modulation of the immune response to infectious agents to prevent the lethal consequences of an overwhelming inflammatory response during the course of a productive immune response to an invading microorganism. Treg and effector cells must maintain equilibrium between no immunity at all and immunopathology. This critical role of Treg is well illustrated by the immune response of mice to infection with *Pneumocystis carinii* (PC). When SCID mice chronically infected with PC are reconstituted with CD4+CD25− T cells, they develop a severe inflammatory response in their lungs that is ultimately fatal. Animals injected with CD25+ T cells alone did not become moribund and only manifested transient weight loss. Cotransfer of CD25+ T cells prevented the development of the PC-driven fatal pulmonary inflammation induced by CD25− T cells, but also suppressed the elimination of PC mediated by the CD25− T cells. Protective CD25+ T cells are needed to inhibit the lethal immunopathologic response mediated by the PC-specific CD4+CD25− T cells, but they also inhibited complete clearing of the organism (230). PC-associated immunopathology is often seen in lymphopenic animals/humans, and this may reflect a relative deficiency in regulatory T cells. Although Treg may target CD4+ and CD8+ T cells responding to an infectious challenge, Treg have also been shown to act on the innate immune system in the response to *Helicobacter hepaticus* (231).

The role of CD4+CD25+ T cells in the immune response to infection includes more than suppression of inflammation (232). CD4+CD25+ T cells also maintain persistence of infection and promote chronicity. The persistence of pathogens following clinical cure is a hallmark of certain viral, bacterial, and parasitic infections. In clinical and experimental forms of leishmaniasis, small numbers of viable organisms persist within lymphoid tissue and within the site of former skin lesions following self-cure or successful chemotherapy. Because low numbers of parasites persisting in the dermis can be efficiently transmitted back to their vector sandflies, the expansion and/or recruitment of regulatory T cells to the site of *L. major* infection might reflect a parasite adaptive strategy to maintain its transmission cycle in nature. Despite the absence of sterilizing immunity, these individuals maintain strong life-long immunity to reinfection, a status similar to the concomitant immunity described in tumor models *(233)*.

In healed C57 BL/6 mice, CD4+CD25+ regulatory T cells accumulate in sites of *L. major* infection in the skin (Figure 30.14) (234). These cells are derived exclusively from CD25+ T cells and not from activated CD25− T cells. They suppress the expansion of and killing mediated by *L. major*–specific effector cells. Although IL-10 produced by CD25+ T cells is essential to the establishment of persistent infection, early in the infectious process CD25+

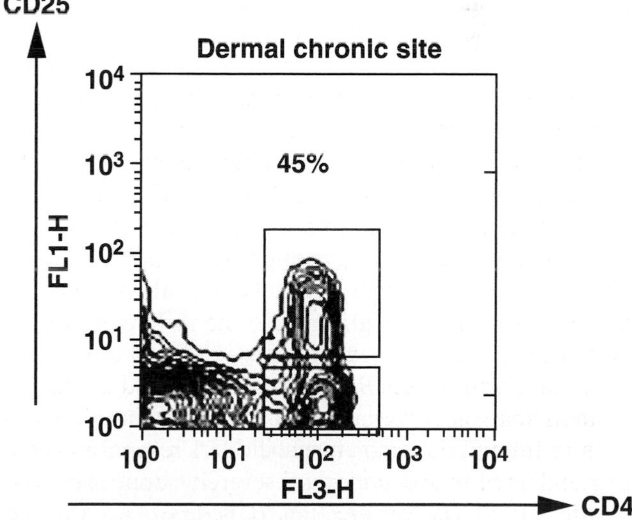

FIGURE 30.14 CD4+CD25+ T cells comprise ~50% of the CD4+ T cells in chronic *L. major* infection. Adapted from Belkaid Y, Piccirillo CA, Mendez S, et al. CD4+CD25+ immunoregulatory T lymphocytes control *Leishmania major* persistence and the development of concomitant immunity. *Nature.* 2002;420:502–507.

T cells can promote parasite survival and growth in an IL-10–independent manner. Later in the course of infection, IL-10 is absolutely required for development of the chronic lesion, Because recipients of $CD25^+$ T cells from IL-$10^{-/-}$ mice ultimately healed and completely cleared the parasite from the site. IL-10 produced by Treg contributes directly to parasite persistence by either modulating APC function, inhibiting cytokine production by Th1 cells, or rendering macrophages refractory to IFN-γ, which is needed for intracellular killing.

Although one consequence of this regulation is parasite persistence and the potential for disease reactivation, parasite persistence itself is a major benefit to the host that is needed for life-long immunity to reinfection. When rechallenge studies were performed in IL-$10^{-/-}$ mice or in WT mice that were treated during the chronic stage of their primary infection with anti-IL-10R, conditions that result in complete clearance of parasites from the skin and draining lymph node, reinfection at a site distant from the initial infection resulted in parasite loads that were comparable to those following primary infection in naïve mice. Healed mice treated with control antibody maintained strong immunity to reinfection, so the maintenance of a residual source of infection, secondary to IL-10 production by $CD25^+$ T cells at the lesion site is required for preservation of acquired immunity to *L. major*. One important question that must be addressed is whether the regulatory function of $Foxp3^+$ Treg cells is associated with their capacity to recognize foreign antigens or is the result of bystander activation through self-antigen recognition. Treg cell lines isolated from chronic *L. major* are able to respond to parasite-infected DC by proliferating and producing IL-10 (235). The cells that have undergone proliferation express and maintain Foxp3 expression. It appears that the parasite has specifically evolved to manipulate DC in a manner that favors and sustains Treg proliferation. Most important, the *L. major*–specific cell lines maintain their suppressive functions *in vivo*, as transfer of the lines to chronically infected mice results in massive disease reactivation and dissemination.

Certain pathogen-derived molecules such as bacterial DNA containing CpG motifs are powerful inducers of the differentiation of Th1 effector cells, but other pathogen-derived components might induce the differentiation of Treg. Although Th1 effector cells are induced during the course of infection with *Bordetella pertussis* and ultimately play a critical role in the clearance of bacteria from the respiratory tract (236), antigen-specific Th1 responses in the lung and local lymph nodes are severely suppressed during the acute phase of infection. *B. pertussis* has evolved a number of strategies to circumvent protective immune responses. One bacterial component, filamentous hemagglutinin (FHA), is capable of inhibiting LPS-driven IL-12 production by macrophages and DC and stimulating IL-10 production. FHA may contribute to the suppressed Th1 responses during acute infection with *B. pertussis* by the induction of T cells with regulatory activity as a result of its interactions with cells of the innate immune system. Repeated stimulation of T cells from the lungs of mice acutely infected with *B. pertussis* resulted in the generation of Tr1 clones that were specific for FHA. Tr1 cells could only be generated from the lungs of infected animals, and not from spleen. These Tr1 cells secreted high levels of IL-10 and inhibited protective immune responses against *B. pertussis in vivo* and *in vitro*. Suppression was substantially reversed by anti-IL-10 *in vivo*. The capacity to induce Tr1 cells is thereby exploited by a respiratory pathogen to evade protective immunity and suppress protective Th1 responses at local sites of infection.

Analysis of cytokine production by T cells from patients with chronic hepatitis C virus (HCV) infection identified antigen-specific regulatory T cells that secreted IL-10 in addition to IFN-γ circulating Th1 cells (237); no IL-4 producing T cells were identified. IL-10–producing cells were detected in a higher proportion of patients with chronic infection than in those who had cleared the virus. Taken together with the studies on *L. major* and *B. pertussis*, these studies on HCV strongly support the general concept that many infectious agents have evolved mechanisms for selective activation of either naturally occurring $CD25^+$ T cells or the generation of IL-10–producing Tr1 cells from $CD25^-$ T cells. The ultimate result is perpetuation of the chronic infectious state, with incomplete clearing of the infection. Depending on the extent of suppression of effector T cells in the host, the consequences of the chronic state may be protective immunity (*L. major*) or continued pathogen-mediated organ destruction (HCV).

Many viruses, such as herpesviruses, hepatitis viruses, and retroviruses, evade immunologic destruction during acute infection and establish chronic persistent infections that may culminate in life-threatening diseases. Friend virus (FV) infection in mice has been used as an experimental model to study retrovirus-induced immunosuppression and may offer insights into our understanding of immunosuppression associated with HIV. Mice that are chronically infected with FV are unable to reject both FV-induced and unrelated immunogenic tumors. $CD8^+$ T cells from acutely infected mice produced perforin, granzyme A, and granzyme B and display recent evidence of degranulation and *in vivo* cytotoxicity. Activated T cells from chronically infected mice were deficient in cytolytic molecules and showed little evidence of recent degranulation and *in vivo* cytotoxicity. These results demonstrate a broad impairment of cytotoxic $CD8^+$ T-cell effector function during chronic retroviral infection and explain the inability of virus-specific $CD8^+$ T cells to eliminate persistent virus. $CD4^+$, but not $CD8^+$, T cells from infected mice can transfer suppression to normal mice and can inhibit the generation of CTL in culture (238). Suppression could be substantially reversed by the addition of anti-CTLA-4, but not anti-IL-10R, to the cultures. FV-induced Treg suppress $CD8^+$ T cells *in vitro* regardless of the TCR specificity of the $CD8^+$ T cells (239). It is unknown whether the Treg in chronically infected mice are specific for any viral proteins or whether they are derived from $Foxp3^+$ Treg. Nevertheless, it appears that an important component of the generalized immunosuppression seen in retroviral infections involves the induction of suppressor T cells.

As HIV infection in humans in many respects mimics the animal models of chronic retroviral infections, several studies have begun to examine Treg function as different stages of HIV infection. Kinter et al. (240) found that in a majority of HIV-infected, but still healthy, individuals, $CD25^{high}$ Treg cells significantly suppressed cellular proliferation and cytokine production by $CD4^+$ and $CD8^+$ T cells in response to HIV antigens *in vitro*. Suppression was cell contact–dependent and IL-10– and TGF-β–independent. Patients with strong HIV-specific suppression *in vitro* had lower levels of viremia and higher CD4/CD8 T-cell ratios than patients who did not have Treg activity. These data suggest that the suppression of $CD4^+$ T-cell activation by Treg may make HIV replication less favorable, as the virus must replicate within the $CD4^+$ T cell itself. Thus, in this chronic infection model, the suppressive functions of Treg may actually be beneficial to the patient.

The role of Treg has been most clearly shown in responses to chronic infections. Much less is known about the role of Treg in modulating acute viral infections. In the murine model of herpetic stromal keratitis, depletion of Treg before infection resulted in lesions of greater severity and permitted the induction of disease with lower infecting doses of virus (241). Cotransfer of Treg with $CD25^-$ T cells reduced lesion severity and diminished the Ag-specific cytokine response of splenic $CD4^+$ T cells. The mechanism of action of Treg in this model is not fully elucidated. Treg inhibit the induction of virus-specific $CD4^+$ T-cell induction but may also modify the expression of homing molecules involved in T-cell migration to the ocular inflammatory site or the extra-lymphoid inflammatory sites of pathogenic T cells. Treg can also control the intensity of secondary responses to HSV and may also influence the magnitude of immunologic memory.

Treg FUNCTION IN HUMAN DISEASE

In this chapter a number of distinct Treg populations have been described, and their potential role in the regulation of the immune response in animal models of disease has been reviewed. A large body of data supports the existence of $CD4^+CD25^+Foxp3^+$ T cells in humans (29,*30*,*31*,32,33,*34*,*35*,36), and the *in vitro* characterization of human $CD4^+CD25^+Foxp3^+$ cells suggests that they are identical to their murine counterpart. Tr1 cells have been readily induced in cultures of human T cells, and a number of studies have supported the existence of cell populations with Tr1-like properties in humans. The finding that autoreactive T cells found in patients with autoimmune disease are more easily activated compared to those from normal subjects suggests that Treg are either reduced in number or have reduced suppressor effector function. More important, Danke et al. (242) have shown that deletion of Treg *in vitro* allows marked clonal expansion of autoreactive T cells *in vitro*.

TABLE 30.9 Human Diseases with Abnormal Treg Function

Disease	*Reference*
Multiple sclerosis	243
Myasthenia gravis	244
Rheumatoid arthritis	*245*
Autoimmune polyglandular II	*246*
Lupus erythematosis	*247*
Psoriasis	*248*
Type 1 diabetes	*249*
HIV/AIDS	*250*

A number of studies in a wide variety of autoimmune diseases have demonstrated a defect in the function of Treg, raising the issue of whether this may be a common denominator in the cause of human autoimmune disease (Table 30.9). In many of these studies, it was definitively shown that the decrease in Treg function was due to defect in Treg subset rather than secondary to responder T cells that were refractory to suppression. One possibility is that Treg may have migrated into the target tissue, so that blood Treg function is depressed but Treg function from the target tissue may actually be enhanced. For example, the frequency of $CD25^{high}$ T cells was much greater in synovial fluid compared to peripheral blood in adult patients with rheumatoid arthritis, and synovial fluid Treg demonstrated normal suppressive activity *in vitro (251)*.

Appropriate caution should be exercised in interpretation of these studies. As discussed previously, identification of human $Foxp3^+$ Treg is difficult, and many of the studies published thus far have only utilized high levels of CD25 expression to identify human Treg and did not validate the isolated populations for Foxp3 expression by intracellular staining. An additional issue is whether Foxp3 expression is a bona-fide marker of human Treg, as some studies have suggested that Foxp3 can be induced in activated effector cells, but such cells do not adopt a regulatory phenotype (252,253). Thus, human $CD25^{high}Foxp3^+$ T cells from inflammatory sites may not be true Treg.

Enhancement of either the numbers or the function of Treg represents a goal for the treatment of autoimmune and allergic diseases as well as for inhibition of allograft rejection. One might expand either $CD4^+CD25^+$ T cells or Tr1 T cells to generate sufficient numbers of cells for infusion back into patients (254). If Foxp3$^+$ Treg recognize organ-specific antigens, and if these antigens can be identified, it may be possible to generate lines or clones of antigen-specific suppressor T cells *in vitro* that could be used therapeutically. Such an approach will probably need to be combined with attempts to delete or anergize the effector cells. Organ-specific Treg would home to their target, be activated by their target autoantigen, but mediate bystander suppression, because their effector function would be nonspecific. Alternatively, as a number of factors (e. g., IL-6 or the GITR-L) can render effector cells resist to the suppressor function of Treg, blocking or neutralizing these factors may enhance Treg function. Ultimately, further studies of the molecular basis of Treg-mediated suppression should allow the development of mAbs or small molecules that could enhance their suppressor effector function.

A second issue related to the therapeutic modulation of Treg function in humans is the development of approaches to decrease the numbers or function of Treg either to augment tumor immunity or increase the immunogenicity of weak vaccines. Depletion of CD4$^+$CD25$^+$ T cells with a depleting anti-CD25 mAb has resulted in potent antitumor immune responses in mouse models. Humanized anti-CD25 mAb approved for human use are nondepleting and block the binding of IL-2 to CD25. Even in the mouse, the mechanism of action and the extent of depletion of CD4$^+$CD25$^+$ T cells remain controversial (255). Depletion of CD25$^+$ T cells would also not affect the Foxp3$^+$CD25$^-$ Treg compartment. Caution should also be used to develop better approaches to deplete Treg, as Treg play an important role in the modulation of the acute inflammatory response that is an integral part of the response to any infectious agent. In the absence of Treg, the consequences of this exuberant response can be deleterious. If future studies successfully define the cell surface molecules on Treg cells that deliver the suppressive signal to the responder cell, then an antibody to this molecule(s) might be the ideal reagent to transiently inhibit suppressor cell activity, facilitating immune responses to tumor antigens. An alternative approach to the downmodulation of suppressor T-cell function might be to increase the resistance of the responder cells to Treg-mediated suppression by using an agonistic anti-GITR mAb or soluble GITR-L or by administering anti-CTLA-4 (226).

REFERENCES

3. Gershon RK, Kondo K. Cell interactions in the induction of tolerance: the role of thymic lymphocytes. *Immunology.* 1970;18:723–735.
4. Gershon RK, Kondo K. Infectious immunological tolerance. *Immunology.* 1971;21:903–914.
6. Tada T, Taniguchi M, Okumura K. Regulation of homocytotropic antibody response in the rat. II. Effect of X-irradiation. *J Immunol.* 1971;106:1012–1018.
7. Okumura K, Tada T. Regulation of homocytotrophic antibody in the rat. VI. Inhibitory effect of thymocyte on homocytotrophic antibody response. *J Immunol.* 1971;107:1682–1689.
10. Germain RN, Benacerraf B. A single major pathway of T-lymphocyte interactions in antigen-specifc immune suppression. *Scand J Immunol.* 1981;13:1–10.
15. Nishizuka Y, Sakakura T. Thymus and reproduction: sex-linked dysgenesia of the gonad after neonatal thymectomy in mice. *Science.* 1969;166:753–755.
17. Penhale WJ, Farmer A, Irvine WJ. Thyroiditis in T cell-depleted rats: influence of strain, radiation dose, adjuvants and antilymphocyte serum. *Clin Exp Immunol.* 1975:21:362–375.
21. Sakaguchi S, Sakaguchi N, Asano M, et al. Immunologic self-tolerance maintained by activated T cells expressing IL-2 receptor α-chains (CD25). *J Immunol.* 1995;155:1151–1164.
23. Suri-Payer E, Amar AZ, Thornton AM, et al. CD4$^+$CD25$^+$ T cells inhibit both the induction and effector function of autoreactive T cells and represent a unique lineage of immunoregulatory cells. *J Immunol.* 1998;160:1212–1218.
24. Powrie F, Mason D. OX-22^{high}CD4$^+$ T cells induce wasting disease with multiple organ pathology: prevention by the OX-22^{low} subset. *J Exp Med.* 1990;172:1701–1708.
25. Fowell D, Mason D. Evidence that the T cell repertoire of normal rats contains cells with the potential to cause diabetes. Characterization of the CD4$^+$ T cell subset that inhibits this autoimmune potential. *J Exp Med.* 1993;177:627–636.
26. Powrie F, Leach MW, Mauze S, et al. Phenotypically distinct subsets of CD4$^+$ T cells induce or protect from chronic intestinal inflammation in C.B-17 scid mice. *Int Immunol.* 1993;5:1461–1471.
27. Read S, Malmstrom V, Powrie F. Cytotoxic T lymphocyte-associated antigen 4 plays an essential role in the function of CD25$^+$CD4$^+$ regulatory cells that control intestinal inflammation. *J Exp Med.* 2000;192:295–302.
29. Baecher-Allan C, Brown JA, Freeman GJ, Hafler DA. CD4$^+$CD25^{high} regulatory cells in human peripheral blood. *J Immunol.* 2001;167: 1245–1253.
32. Jonuleit H, Schmitt E, Stassen M, et al. Identification and functional characterization of human CD4$^+$CD25$^+$ T cells with regulatory properties isolated from peripheral blood. *J Exp Med.* 2001;193: 1285–1294.
33. Dieckmann D, Plottner H, Berchtold S, et al. Ex vivo isolation and characterization of CD4$^+$CD25$^+$ T cells with regulatory properties from human blood. *J Exp Med.* 2002;193:1303–1310.
36. Stephens LA, Mason D. CD25 is a marker for CD4$^+$ thymocytes that prevent autoimmune diabetes in rats, but peripheral T cells with this function are found in both CD25$^+$ and CD25- subpopulations. *J Immunol.* 2001;165:3105–3110.
37. Thornton AM, Shevach EM. CD4$^+$CD25$^+$ immunoregulatory T cells suppress polyclonal T cell activation *in vitro* by inhibiting interleukin 2 production. *J Exp Med.* 1998;188:287–296.
38. Salomon B, Lenschow DJ, Rhee L, et al. B7/CD28 costimulation is essential for the homeostasis of the CD4$^+$CD25$^+$ immunoregulatory T cells that control autoimmune diabetes. *Immunity.* 2000;12:431–440.
39. Takahashi T, Tagami T, Yamazaki S, et al. Immunologic self-tolerance maintained by CD25$^+$CD4$^+$ regulatory T cells constitutively expressing cytotoxic T lymphcyte-associated antigen 4. *J Exp Med.* 2000;192:303–309.
40. McHugh RS, Whitters MJ, Piccirillo CA, et al. CD4$^+$CD25$^+$ immunoregulatory T cells: gene expression analysis reveals a functional role for the glucocorticoid-induced TNF receptor. *Immunity.* 2002;16:311–323.
41. Shimizu J, Yamazaki S, Takahashi T, et al. Stimulation of CD25$^+$ CD4$^+$ regulatory T cells through GITR breaks immunological self-tolerance. *Nat Immunol.* 2002;3:135–142.
43. Fontenot JD, Gavin MA, Rudensky AY. Foxp3 programs the development and function of CD4$^+$CD25$^+$ regulatory T cells. *Nat Immunol.* 2003;4:330–336.
44. Hori S, Nomura T, Sakaguchi S. Control of regulatory T cell development by the transcription factor *Foxp3*. *Science.* 2003;299:1057–1061.
45. Khattri R, Cox T, Yasayko S-A, et al. An essential role for scurfin in CD4$^+$CD25$^+$ T regulatory cells. *Nat Immunol.* 2003;4:337–342.

46. Fontenot JD, Rasmussen JP, Williams LM, et al. Regulatory T cell lineage spcification by the Forkhead Transcription Factor Foxp3. *Immunity.* 2005;22:329–341.
47. Fontenot JD, Dooley JL, Farr AG, et al. Development regulation of Foxp3 expression during ontogeny. *J Exp Med.* 2005;202:901–906.
48. Kim JM, Rasmussen JP, Rudensky AY. Regulatory T cells prevent catastrophic autoimmunity throughout the lifespan of mice. *Nat Immunol.* 2007;8:191–197.
52. Jordan MS, Boesteanu A, Reed AJ, et al. Thymic selection of $CD4^+CD25^+$ regulatory T cells induced by an agonist self-peptide. *Nat Immunol.* 2001;2:301–306.
53. Van Santen H-M, Benoist C, Mathis D. Number of T reg that differentiate does not increase upon encounter of agonist ligand on thymic epithelial cells. *J Exp Med.* 2004;200:1221–1230.
54. Pacholczyk P, Kraj P, Ignatowicz L. Peptide specificity of thymic selection of $CD4^+CD25^+$ T cells. *J Immunol.* 2002:168:613–620.
55. Hsieh C-S, Liang, Y, Tyznik AJ, et al. Recognition of peripheral self by naturally arising $CD25^+CD4^+$ T cell receptors. *Immunity.* 2004;21:267–277.
56. Pacholczyk R, Ignatowicz H, Kraj P, et al. Origin and T cell receptor diversity of $Foxp3^+CD4^+CD25^+$ T cells. *Immunity.* 2006;25:249–259.
57. Bensinger SJ, Bandeira A, Jordan MS, et al. Major histocompatibility complex class II-positive cortical epithelium mediates the selection of $CD4^+25^+$ immunoregulatory T cells. *J Exp Med.* 2001;194:427–438.
58. Aschenbrenner K, D'Cruz LM, Vollman EH, et al. Selection of $Foxp3^+$ regulatory T cells specific for self-antigen expressed and presented by $Aire^+$ medullary thymic epithelial cells. *Nat Immunol.* 2007;8:351–358.
59. Hsieh C-S, Zheng, Y, Liang Y, et al. An intersection between self-reactive regulatory and nonregulatory T cell receptor repertoires. *Nat Immunol.* 2006;7:401–410.
61. Apostolou I, Sarukhan A, Klein L, et al. Origin of regulatory T cells with known specificity for antigen. *Nat Immunol.* 2002:3:756–763.
62. Apostoulou I, von Boehmer H. *In vivo* instruction of suppressor commitment in naïve T cells. *J Exp Med.* 2004;199:1401–1408.
63. Kretschmer K, Apostolou I, Hawiger D, et al. Inducing and expanding regulatory T cell populations by foreign antigen. *Nat Immunol.* 2005;6:1219–1227.
64. Chen WJ, Jin W, Hardegen N, et al. Conversion of peripheral $CD4^+CD25^-$ naïve T cells to $CD4^+CD25^+$ regulatory T cells by TGF-β induction of transcription factor Foxp3. *J Exp Med.* 2003;198: 1875–1886.
65. Fantini MC, Becker C, Monteleone G, et al. Cutting Edge: TGF-β induces a regulatory phenotype in $CD4^+CD25^-$ T cells through Foxp3 induction and down-regulation of Smad7. *J Immunol.* 2004;172:5149–5153.
66. Horwitz DA, Zheng SG, Gray JD, et al. Regulatory T cells generated ex vivo as an approach for the therapy of autoimmune disease. *Semin Immunol.* 2004;16:135–143.
67. Davidson T, DiPaolo RJ, Andersson J, et al. Cutting Edge: IL-2 is essential for TGF-β-mediated induction of $Foxp3^+$ regulatory cells. *J Immunol.* 2007;178:4027–4032.
68. Peng Y, Laouar Y, Li MO, et al. TGF-β regulates *in vivo* expansion of Foxp3-expressing $CD4^+CD25^+$ regulatory T cells responsible for protection against diabetes. *Proc Natl Acad Sci U S A.* 2004;101: 4572–4577.
69. Vukmanovic-Stejic M, Zhang Y, Cook JE, et al. Human $CD4^+$ $CD25^{high}Foxp3^+$ regulatory T cells are derived by rapid turnover of memory populations *in vivo*. *J Clin Invest.* 2006;116:2423–2433.
71. Singh B, Read S, Asseman C, et al. Control of inflammation by regulatory T cells. *Immunol Rev.* 2001;182:190–200.
72. Malek TR, Yu A, Vincek V, et al. CD4 regulatory T cells prevent lethal autoimmunity in IL-2Rβ-deficient mice: implications for the nonredundant function of IL-2. *Immunity.* 2002;17:167–178.
73. Kagami S-I, Nakajima H, Suto A, et al. Stat5 a regulates T helper cell differentiation by several distinct mechanisms. *Blood.* 2001;97: 2358–2365.
74. Green EA, Choi Y, Flavell RA. Pancreatic lymph node-derived $CD4^+$ $CD25^+$ treg cells: highly potent regulators of diabetes that require TRANCE-RANK signals. *Immunity.* 2002;16:183–191.
75. Furtado GC, Curotto de Lafaille MA, Kutchukhidze N, et al. Interleukin 2 signaling is required for $CD4^+$ regulatory T cell function. *J Exp Med.* 2002;196:851–857.
76. Thornton AM, Donovan EE, Piccirillo CA, et al. Cutting Edge: IL-2 is critically required for the *in vitro* activation of $CD4^+CD25^+$ T cell suppressor function. *J Immunol.* 2004;172:6519–6523.
77. Fontenot JD, Rasmussen JP, Gavin MA, et al. A function for interleukin 2 in Foxp3-expressing regulatory T cells. *Nat Immunol.* 2005;6:1142–1151.
78. D'Cruz LM, Klein L. Development and function of agonist-induced $CD24^+Foxp3^+$ regulatory T cells in the absence of interleukin 2 signaling. *Nat Immunol.* 2005;6:1152–1159.
79. Gavin MA, Clarke SR, Negrou E, et al. Homeostasis and anergy of $CD4^+CD25^+$ suppressor T cells *in vivo*. *Nat Immunol.* 2002;3:33–41.
80. Zelenika D, Adams E, Humm S, et al. Regulatory T cells overexpress a subset of Th2 gene transcripts. *J Immunol.* 2002;168:1069–1079.
81. Knoechel B, Lohr J, Zhu S, et al. Functional and molecular comparison of anergic and regulatory T lymphocytes. *J Immunol.* 2006;176:6473–6483.
82. Zheng Y, Josefowicz SZ, Kas A, et al. Genome-wide analysis of Foxp3 target genes in developing and mature regulatory T cells. *Nature.* 2007;445:936–940.
83. Marson A, Kretchmer K, Frampton GM, et al. Foxp3 occupancy and regulation of key target genes during T-cell stimulation. *Nature.* 2007;445:931–935.
84. Gavin MA, Rasmussen JP, Fontenot JD, et al. Foxp3-dependent programme of regulatory T cell differentiation. *Nature.* 2007;445:771–775.
85. Lin W, Haribhai D, Relland LM, et al. Regulatory T cell development in the absence of functional Foxp3. *Nat Immunol.* 2007;8:359–368.
86. Takahashi T, Kuniyasu Y, Toda M, et al. Immunologic self-tolerance maintained by $CD25^+CD4^+$ naturally anergic and autoimmune disease by breaking their anergic/suppressive state. *Int Immunol.* 1998;10:1969–1980.
88. Thornton AM, Shevach EM. Suppressor effector function of $CD4^+CD25^+$ immunoregulatory T cells is antigen nonspecific. *J Immunol.* 2000;164:183–190.
90. Piccirillo CA, Shevach EM. Cutting Edge: Control of $CD8^+$ T cell activation by $CD4^+CD25^+$ immunoregulatory cells. *J Immunol.* 2000;167:1137–1140.
91. Hickman SP, Yang J, Thomas RM, et al. Defective activation of protein kinase C and Ras-ERK pathways limits IL-2 production and proliferation by $CD4^+CD25^+$ regulatory T cells. *J Immunol.* 2006;177:2186–2194.
92. Tsang JY-S, Camara NOS, Eren E, et al. Altered proximal T cell receptor signaling in human $CD4^+CD25^+$ regulatory T cells. *J Leuk Biol.* 2006;80:145–151.
93. Su L, Creusot RJ, Gallo EM, et al. Murine $CD4^+CD25^+$ regulatory T cells fail to undergo chromatin remodeling across the proximal promoter region of the IL-2 gene. *J Immunol.* 2004;173:4994–5001.
94. Bensinger SJ, Walsh PT, Zhang J, et al. Distinct IL-2 receptor signaling pattern in $CD4^+CD25^+$ regulatory T cells. *J Immunol.* 2004;172: 5287–5296.
95. Walsh PT, Buckler JL, Zhang J, et al. PTEN inhibits IL-2 receptor-mediated expansion of $CD4^+CD25^+$ Tregs. *J Clin Invest.* 2006;116: 2521–2531.
96. Bettelli E, Dastrange M, Oukka M. Foxp3 interacts with nuclear factor of activated T cells and NF-κB to repress cytokine gene expression and effector functions of T helper cells. *Proc Natl Acad Sci U S A.* 2005;102:5138–5143.
97. Wu Y, Borde M, Heissmeyer V, et al. FOXP3 controls regulatory T cell function through cooperation with NFAT. *Cell.* 2006;126:375–387.
98. Ono M, Yaguchi H, Ohkura N, et al. Foxp3 controls regulatory T-cell function by interacting with AML1/Runx1. *Nature.* 2007;446:685–689.
99. Sojka DK, Hughson A, Sukiennicki TL, et al. Early kinetic window of target T cell susceptibility to $CD25^+$ regulatory T cell activity. *J Immunol.* 2005;175:7274–7280.
100. Sukiennicki TL, Fowell DJ. Distinct molecular program imposed on $CD4^+$ T cell targets by $CD4^+CD25^+$ regulatory T cells. *J Immunol.* 2006;177:6952–6961.
102. Serra P, Amrani A, Yamanouchi J, et al. CD40 ligation releases

immature dendritic cells from the control of Regulatory CD4+CD25+ T cells. *Immunity.* 2003;19:877–889.
103. Misra N, Bayry J, Lacroix-Desmazes S, et al. Cutting Edge: Human CD4+CD25+ T cells restrain the maturation and antigen-presenting function of dendritic cells. *J Immunol.* 2004;172:4676–4680.
104. Veldhoen M, Moncrieffe H, Hocking RJ, et al. Modulation of dendritic cell function by naïve and regulatory CD4+ T cells. *J Immunol.* 2006;176:6202–6210.
105. Yamazaki S, Iyoda T, Tarbell K, et al. Direct expansion of functional CD25+CD4+ regulatory T cells by antigen-processing dendritic cells. *J Exp Med.* 2003;198:235–247.
106. Brinster C, Shevach EM. Bone marrow-derived dendritic cells reverse the anergic state of CD4+CD25+ regulatory T cells without reversing their suppressive function. *J Immunol.* 2005;175:7332–7340.
108. Lim HW, Hillsamer P, Banham AH, et al. Cutting Edge: Direct suppression of B cells by CD4+CD25+ regulatory T cells. *J Immunol.* 2005;175:4180–4183.
109. Lim HW, Hillsamer P, Kim CH. Regulatory T cells can migrate to follicles upon T cell activation and suppress GC-Th and GC-Th cell driven B cell responses. *J Clin Invest.* 2002;114:1640–1649.
110. Zhao D-M, Thornton AM, DiPaolo RJ, et al. Activated CD4+CD25+ regulatory T cells selectively kill B lymphocytes. *Blood.* 2006;107: 3925–3932.
111. Shimizu J, Yamazaki S, Sakaguchi S. Induction of tumor immunity by removing CD25+CD4+ T cells: a common basis between tumor immunity and autoimmunity. *J Immunol.* 1999;163:5211–5218.
112. Smyth MJ, Teng MWL, Swann J, et al. CD4+CD25+ T regulatory cells suppress NK cell-mediated immunotherapy of cancer. *J Immunol.* 2006;176:1582–1587.
113. Ghiringhelli, F, Menard C, Terme M, et al. CD4+CD25+ regulatory T cells inhibit natural killer cell functions in a transforming growth-factor-β-dependent manner. *J Exp Med.* 2005;202:1075–1085.
114. Barao I, Hanash AM, Hallett W, et al. Suppression of natural killer cell-meidated bone marrow cell rejection by CD4+CD25+ regulatory T cells. *Proc Natl Acad Sci U S A.* 2006;103:5460–5465.
115. Nakamura K, Kitani A, Strober W. Cell contact-dependent immunosuppression by CD4+CD25+ regulatory T cells is mediated by cell surface-bound transforming growth factor β. *J Exp Med.* 2001;194:629–644.
116. Piccirillo CA, Letterio JJ, Thornton AM, et al. CD4+CD25+ regulatory T cells can mediate suppressor function in the absence of transforming growth factor β1 production and responsiveness. *J Exp Med.* 2002;196:1–10.
117. Mamura M, Lee W, Sullivan TJ, et al. CD28 disruption exacerbates inflammation in *TGF-β1*$^{-/-}$ mice: *in vivo* suppression by CD4+CD25+regulatory T cells independent of autocrine TGF-□1. *Blood.* 2002;103:4594–4601.
118. Fahlen L, Read S, Gorelik L, et al. T cells that cannot respond to TGF-β escape control by CD4+CD25+ regulatory T cells. *J Exp Med.* 2005;201:737–746.
119. Kullberg MC, Hay V, Cheever AW, et al. TGF-β1 production by CD4+CD25+ regulatory T cells is not essential for suppression of intestinal inflammation. *Eur J Immunol.* 2005;35:2886–2895.
120. Marie JC, Letterio JJ, Gavin M, et al. TGF-β1 maintains suppressor function and Foxp3 expression in CD4+CD25+ regulatory T cells. *J Exp Med.* 2005;201:1061–1067.
121. Marie JC, Liggitt D, Rudensky AY. Cellular mechanisms of fatal early-onset autoimmunity in mice with the T cell-specifc targeting of transforming growth factor-β receptor. *Immunity.* 2006;25:441–454.
122. Tang Q, Boden EK, Henriksen KJ, et al. Distinct roles of CTLA-4 and TGF-β in CD4+CD25+ regulatory cell function. *Eur J Immunol.* 2004;34:2996–3005.
123. Paust S, Cantor H. Regulatory T cells and autoimmune disease. *Immunol Rev.* 2005;204:195–207.
124. May KF, Chang X, Zhang HM, et al. B7-deficient autoreactive T cells are highly susceptible to suppression by CD4+CD25+ regulatory T cells. *J Immunol.* 2007;178:1542–1552.
125. Grohmann U, Fallarino F, Puccetti P. Tolerance DCs and tryptophan: much ado about IDO. *Trends Immunol.* 2003;24:242–248.
126. Grossman, WJ, Verbsky JW, Barchet W, et al. Human regulatory T cells can use the perforin pathway to cause autologous target cell death. *Immunity.* 2004;21:589–601.
127. Gondek DC, Lu L-F, Quezada SA. Cutting Edge: Contact-mediated suppression by CD4+CD25+ regulatory cells involves a granzyme B-dependent, perforin-independent mechanism. *J Immunol.* 2005;174:1783–1786.
128. Stephens GL, McHugh RS, Whitters MJ, et al. Engagement of glucocorticoid-induced TNFR family related receptor on effector T cells by its ligand mediates resistance to suppression by CD4+CD25+ T cells. *J Immunol.* 2004;173:5008–5020.
129. Kohm AP, Williams JS, Miller SD. Cutting Edge: Ligation of the glucocorticoid-induced TNF receptor enhances autoreactive CD4+ T cell activation and experimental autoimmune encephalomyelitis. *J Immunol.* 2004;172:4686–4690.
130. Pasare C, Medzhitov R. Toll pathway-dependent blockade of CD4+CD25+ T cell-mediated suppression by dendritic cells. *Science.* 2003;299:1033–1036.
131. Wohlfert EA, Gorelik L, Mittler R, et al. Cutting Edge: Deficiency in the E3 ubiquitin ligase cbl-β results in a multifunctional defect in T cells TGF-β sensitivity *in vitro* and *in vivo*. *J Immunol.* 2006;176:1316–1320.
132. Walker LSK, Chodos A, Eggene M, et al. Antigen-dependent proliferation of CD4+CD25+ regulatory T cells *in vivo*. *J Exp Med.* 2003;198:249–258.
133. Klein L, Khazaie K, von Boehmer H. *In vivo* dynamics of antigen-specific regulatory T cells not predicted from behavior *in vitro*. *Proc Natl Acad Sci U S A.* 2003;100:8886–8891.
134. Read S, Greenwald R, Izcue A, et al. Blockade of CTLA-4 on CD4+CD25+ regulatory T cells abrogates their function *in vivo*. *J Immunol.* 2006;177:4376–4383.
135. Tang Q, Adams JY, Tooley AJ, et al. Visualizing regulatory T cell control of autoimmune responses in nonobese diabetic mice. *Nat Immunol.* 2006;7:83–92.
136. Tadokoro CE, Shakhar G, Shen S, et al. Regulatory T cells inhibit stable contacts between CD4+ T cells and dendritic cells *in vivo*. *J Exp Med.* 2006;203:505–511.
137. Weiner HL, Friedman A, Miller A, et al. Oral tolerance—immunological mechanisms and treatment of animal and human organ-specific autoimmune-diseases by oral-administration of autoantigens. *Annu Rev Immunol.* 1994;12:809–837.
138. Chen Y, Kuchroo VK, Inobe J-I, et al. Regulatory T cell clones induced by oral tolerance: suppression of autoimmune encephalomyelitis. *Science.* 1994:265:1237–1240.
139. Weiner HL. The mucosal milieu creates tolerogenic dendritic cells and T_R1 and T_H3 regulatory cells. *Nat Immunol.* 2001;2:671–672.
142. Roncarolo MG, Bacchetta R, Bordignon C, et al. Type 1 regulatory cells. *Immunol Rev.* 2001;182:68–79.
143. Groux H, O'Garra A, Bigler M, et al. A CD4+ T-cell subset inhibits antigen-specific T-cell responses and prevents colitis. *Nature.* 1997;389:737–742.
145. Viera PL, Christensen JR, Minaee S, et al. IL-10 secreting T cells do not express Foxp3 but have comparable regulatory functions to naturally occurring CD4+CD25+ regulatory T cells. *J Immunol.* 2004;172:5986–5993.
146. Cottrez F, Hurst SD, Coffman RL, et al. T regulatory cells 1 inhibit a TH2-specific response *in vivo*. *J Immunol.* 2000;165:4848–4853.
147. Barrat FJ, Cua DJ, Boonstra A, et al. *In vitro* generation of interleukin 10-producing regulatory CD4+ T cells is induced by immunosuppressive drugs and inhibited by T helper type 1 (Th1)- and Th2-inducing cytokines. *J Exp Med.* 2002;195:603–616.
148. Jonuleit H, Schmitt E, Schuler G, et al. Induction of interleukin 10-producing, nonproliferating CD4+ T cells with regulatory properties by repetitive stimulation with allogeneic immature human dendritic cells. *J Exp Med.* 2000;192:1213–1222.
149. Liu Z, Tugulea S, Cortesini R, et al. Specific suppression of T helper alloreactivity by all-MHC class I-restricted CD8+CD28- T cells. *Int Immunol.* 1998;10:775–783.
151. Chang CC, Ciubotariu R, Manavalan JS, et al. Tolerization of dendritic cells by Ts cells: the crucial role of inhibitory receptors ILT3 and ILT4. *Nat Immunol.* 2002;3:237–243.
152. Vlad G, Cortesini R, Suciu-Foca N. License to heal: bidirectional interaction of antigen-specific regulatory T cells and tolerogenic APC. *J Immunol.* 2005;174:5907–5914.

155. Wei S, Kryczek I, Zou L, et al. Plasmacytoid dendritic cells induce $CD8^+$ regulatory T cells in human ovarian carcinoma. *Cancer Res.* 2005;65:5020–5026.
156. Rifa'I M, Kawamoto Y, Nakashima I, et al. Essential roles of $CD8^+CD122^+$ regulatory T cells in the maintenance of T cell homeostasis. *J Exp Med.* 2004;200:1123–1134.
157. Endharti AT, Rifa'I, Shi Z, et al. Cutting Edge: $CD8^+CD122^+$ regulatory T cells produce IL-10 to suppress IFN-β production and proliferation of $CD8^+$ T cells. *J Immunol.* 2005;175:7093–7097.
158. Jiang H, Chess L. The specific regulation of immune responses by $CD8^+$ T cells restricted by the MHC class IB molecule, Qa-1. *Annu Rev Immunol.* 2000;18:185–216.
159. Tang X, Maricic I, Purohit N, et al. Regulation of immunity by a novel population of Qa-1-restricted $CD8\alpha\alpha^+$ $TCR\alpha\beta^+$ T cells. *J Immunol.* 2006;177:7645–7655.
160. Li J, Goldstein I, Glickman-Nir, et al. Induction of TCR Vbeta-specific $CD8^+$ CTLs by TCR Vbeta-derived peptides bound to HLA-E. *J Immunol.* 2001;167:3800–3808.
161. Ford MS, Zhang Z-X, Chen W, et al. Double-negative T regulatory cells can develop outside the thymus and do not mature from $CD8^+$ T cell precursors. *J Immunol.* 2006;177:2803–2809.
162. Fischer K, Voekl S, Heymann J, et al. Isolation and characterization of human antigen-specific $TCR\alpha\beta^+$ $CD4^-CD8^-$double-negative regulatory T cells. *Blood.* 2005;105:2826–2835.
163. Zhang Z-X, Yang L, Young KJ, et al. Identification of a previously unknown antigen-specific regulatory T cells and its mechanism of suppression. *Nat Med.* 2000;6:782–789.
165. Jonuleit H, Schmitt E, Kakirman H, et al.. Infectious tolerance: Human $CD25^+$ regulatory T cells convey suppressor activity to conventional $CD4^+$ T helper T cells. *J Exp Med.* 2002;196:255–260.
166. Qiao M, Thornton AM, Shevach EM. $CD4^+CD25^+$ T cells render naïve $CD4^+$CD25- T cells anergic and suppressive. *Immunology.* 2007;120:447–455.
169. McHugh RS, Shevach EM, Thornton AM. Control of organ-specific autoimmunity by immunoregulatory $CD4^+CD25^+$ T cells. *Microbes Infect.* 2001;3:919–927.
171. DiPaolo RJ, Glass DD, Bijwaard KE, et al. $CD4^+CD25^+$ T cells prevent the development of organ-sepcifc autoimmune disease by inhibiting the differentiation of autoreactive effector cells. *J Immunol.* 2005;175:7135–7142.
172. Powrie F, Leach MW, Mauze S, et al. Inhibition of TH1 responses prevents inflammatory bowel-disease in SCID mice reconstituted with $CD45RB^{high}$ T cells. *Immunity.* 1994;1:553–562.
173. Asseman C, Read S, Fowrie F. Colitogenic Th1 cells are present in the antigen-experienced T cell pool in normal mice: Control by $CD4^+$ regulatory T cells and IL-10. *J Immunol.* 2003;171:971–978.
174. Powrie F, Carlino J, Leach MW, et al. A critical role for transforming factor-β but not interleukin 4 in the suppression of T helper 1-mediated colitis by $CD45RB^{low}CD4^+$ T cells. *J Exp Med.* 1996;183:2669–2674.
175. Malmstrom V, Shipton D, Singh B, et al. CD134L expression on dendritic cells in the mesenteric lymph nodes drives colitis in T cell restored SCID mice. *J Immunol.* 2001;166:6972–6981.
178. Chatenoud L, Salomon B, Bluestone JA. Suppressor T cells—they're back and critical for regulation of autoimmunity. *Immunol Rev.* 2001;182:149–163.
179. Tang Q, Henriksen KJ, Bi M, et al. *In vitro*-expanded antigen-specific regulatory T cells suppress autoimmune diabetes. *J Exp Med.* 2004;199:1455–1465.
180. Masteller EL, Warner MR, Tang Q, et al. Expansion of functional endogenous antigen-specific $CD4^+CD25^+$ regulatory T cells from nonobese diabetic mice. *J Immunol.* 2005;175:3053–3059.
181. Sarween N, Chodos A, Raykundalia C, et al. $CD4^+CD25^+$ cells controlling a pathogenic CD4 response inhibit cytokine differentiation, CXCR-3 expression, and tissue invasion. *J Immunol.* 2004;173:2942–2951.
182. Chen Z, Herman AE, Matos M, et al. Where $CD4^+CD25^+$ T reg cells impinge on autoimmune diabetes. *J Exp Med.* 2005;202:1387–1397.
183. Kohm AP, Carpentier PA, Anger HA, et al. Cutting Edge: $CD4^+$ $CD25^+$ regulatory T cells suppress antigen-specific autoreactive immune responses and central nervous system inflammation during active experimental autoimmune encephalomyelitis. *J Immunol.* 2002;169:4712–4716.
184. McGeachy MJ, Stephens LA, Anderton SM. Natural recovery and protection from autoimmune encephalomyelitis: contribution of $CD4^+CD25^+$ regulatory cells within the central nervous system. *J Immunol.* 2005;175:3025–3032.
186. Seddon B. Mason D. Peripheral autoantigen induces regulatory T cells that prevent autoimmunity. *J Exp Med.* 1999;189:877–881.
187. Taguchi O, Nishizuka Y. Self-tolerance and localized autoimmunity. Mouse models of autoimmune disease that suggest tissue-specific suppressor T cells are involved in self-tolerance. *J Exp Med.* 1987;165:146–156.
190. Tung KSK, Agersborg SS, Alard P, et al. Regulatory T cell, endogenous antigen and neonatal environment in the prevention and induction of autoimmune disease. *Immunol Rev.* 2001;182:135–148.
191. Samy ET, Parker LA, Sharp CP, et al. Continuous control of autoimmune disease by antigen-dependent polyclonal $CD4^+CD25^+$ regulatory T cells in the regional lymph node. *J Exp Med.* 2005;202: 771–782.
192. Asefa A, Gumy A, Launois P, et al. The early IL-4 response to *Leishmania major* and the resulting Th2 cell maturation steering progressive disease in BALB/c mice are subject to the control of regulatory $CD4^+CD25^+$ T cells. *J Immunol.* 2002;169:3232–3241.
193. Xu D, Lin H, Koami-Koma M, et al. $CD4^+CD25^+$ regulatory T cells suppress differentiation and functions of Th1 and Th2 cells, Leishmania infection, and colitis in mice. *J Immunol.* 2003;170:394–399.
194. Stassen M, Jonuleit H, Muller C, et al. Differential regulatory capacity of $CD25^+$ T regulatory cells and preactivated $CD25^+$ T regulatory cells on development, functional activation, and proliferation of Th2 cells. *J Immunol.* 2004;173:267–274.
195. Lewkowich IP, Herman NS, Schliefer KW, et al. $CD4^+CD25^+$ T cells protect against experimentally induced asthma and alter pulmonary dendritic cell phenotype and function. *J Exp Med.* 2005;202:1549–1561.
196. Jaffar S, Sivakuru T, Roberts K. $CD4^+CD25^+$ T cells regulate airway eosinophilic inflammation by modulating Th2 cell phenotype. *J Immunol.* 2004;172:3842–3849.
197. Veldhoen M, Moncrieffe H, Hocking RJ, et al. Modulation of dendritic cell regulatory $CD4^+$ T cells. *J Immunol.* 2006;176:6202–6210.
198. Wilson MS, Taylor MD, Balic A, et al. Suppression of allergic airway inflammation by helminth-induced regulatory T cells. *J Exp Med.* 2005;202:1199–1212.
199. Stockinger B, Barthlott T, Kassiotis G. T cell regulation: a special job or everyone's responsibility. *Nat Immunol.* 2001;2:757–759.
200. Bourgeoios C, Stockinger B. $CD25^+CD4^+$ regulatory T cells and memory T cells prevent lymphopenia-induced proliferation of naïve T cells in transient state of lymphopenia. *J Immunol.* 2006;177: 4558–4566.
202. Annacker O, Pimenta-Araujo R, Burlen-Defranoux O, et al. $CD25^+CD4^+$ T cells regulate the expansion of peripheral CD4 T cells through the production of IL-10. *J Immunol.* 2001;166:3008–3018.
203. Shin S, Ding Y, Tadokoro, CD, et al. Control of homeostatic proliferation by regulatory T cells. *J Clin Invetst.* 2005;115: 3517–3526.
205. Hara M, Kingsley CI, Niimi M, et al. IL-10 is required for regulatory T cells to mediate tolerance to alloantigens *in vivo*. *J Immunol.* 2001;166:3789–3796.
206. Graca L, Thompson S, Lin C-Y, et al. Both $CD4^+CD25^+$ and $CD4^+$CD25- regulatory cells mediate dominant transplantation tolerance. *J Immunol.* 2002;168:5558–5567.
207. Cobbold SP, Castejon R, Adams E, et al. Induction of *foxp3*$^+$ regulatory T cells in the periphery of T cell receptor transgenic mice tolerized to transplants. *J Immunol.* 2004;172;6003–6010.
208. Karim M, Feng G, Wood KJ, et al. $CD25^+CD4^+$ regulatory T cells generated by exposure to a model protein antigen prevent allograft rejection: antigen-specific reactivation *in vivo* is critical for bystander regulation. *Blood.* 2005;105:4871–4877.
210. Cohen JL, Trenado A. Vasey D, et al. $CD4^+CD25^+$ immunoregulatory T cells: new therapeutics for graft-versus-host disease. *J Exp Med.* 2002;196:401–406.
212. Hoffman P, Ermann J, Edinger M, et al. Donor-type $CD4^+CD25^+$ regulatory T cells suppress lethal acute graft-versus-host disease after allogeneic bone marrow transplantation. *J Exp Med.* 2002;196: 389–399.

213. Edinger M, Hoffman P, Ermann J, et al. CD4+CD25+ regulatory T cells preserve graft-versus-tumor activity while inhibiting graft-versus-host disease after bone marrow transplantation. *Nat Med.* 2003;9:1144–1150.
214. Joffre O, Gorsse N, Romagnoli P, et al. Induction of antigen-specific tolerance to bone marrow allografts with CD4+CD25+ T lymphocytes. *Blood.* 2004;103:4216–4221.
215. Hanash AM, Levy RB. Donor CD4+CD25+ T cells promote engraftment and tolerance following MHC-mismatched hematopoietic cell transplantation. *Blood.* 2005;105:1828–1836.
216. North, RJ, Bursuker I. Generation and decay of the immune response to a progressive fibrosarcoma. I. Ly-1+2- suppressor T cells down-regulate the generation of Ly-1-2+ effector T cells. *J Exp Med.* 1984;159:1295–1311.
218. Onizuka S, Tawara I, Shimizu J, et al. Tumor rejection by *in vivo* administration of anti-CD25 (interleukin-2 receptor α) monoclonal antibody. *Cancer Res* 1999;59:3128–3133.
219. Sutmuller RPM, van Duivenvoorde LM, van Elsas A, et al. Synergism of cytotoxic T lymphocyte-associated antigen 4 blockade and depletion of CD25+ regulatory T cells in antitumor therapy reveals alternative pathways for suppression of autoreactive cytotoxic T lymphocyte responses. *J Exp Med.* 2001;194:823–832.
220. Antony PA, Piccirillo CA, Akpinarli A, et al. CD8+ T cell immunity against a tumor/self-antigen is augmented by CD4+ T helper cells and hindered by naturally occurring T regulatory cells. *J Immunol.* 2005;174:2591–2601.
221. Turk MJ, Guevara-Patino JA, Rizzuto GA, et al. Concomitant tumor immunity to a poorly immunogenic melanoma is prevented by regulatory T cells. *J Exp Med.* 2004;200:771–782.
222. Woo, EY, Yeh H, Chu CS, et al. Cutting Edge: regulatory T cells from lung cancer patients directly inhibit autologous T cell proliferation. *J Immunol.,* 2002;168:4272–4276.
223. Curiel TJ, Cooukos G, Zou LH, et al. Specific recruitment of regulatory T cells in ovarian carcinoma fosters immune privilege and predicts reduced survival. *Nat Med.* 2004;10:942–949.
224. Kryczek I, Wei S, Zou LH, et al. Cutting Edge: Induction of B7-H4 on APCs through IL-10: novel suppressive mode for regulatory T cells. *J Immunol.* 2006;177:40–44.
225. Wang HY, Lee DA, Peng GY, et al. Tumor-specific human CD4+ regulatory T cells and their ligands: implications for immunotherapy. *Immunity.* 2004;20:107–118.
226. Phan GQ, Yang JC, Sherry RM, et al. Cancer regression and autoimmunity induced by cytotoxic T lymphocyte-associated antigen 4 blockade in patients with metastatic melanoma. *Proc Natl Acad Sci U S A.* 2003;100:8372–8377.
227. Dannull J, Su Z, Rizzieri D, et al. Enhancement of vaccine-mediated antitumor immunity in cancer patients after depletion of regulatory T cells. *J Clin Invest.* 2005;115:3623–3633.
228. Attia P, Maker AV, Haworth LR, et al. Inability of a fusion protein of IL-2 and diptheria toxin (Denileukin Diftitox, DAB(389) IL-2, ONTAK) to eliminate regulatory T lymphocytes in patients with melanoma. *J Immunother.* 2005;28:582–592.
229. Erdman SE, Sohn JJ, Rao VP, et al. CD4+CD25+ regulatory lymphocytes induce regression of intestinal tumors in $APC^{Min/+}$ mice. *Cancer Res.* 2005;65:3998–4004.
230. Hori S, Carvalho TL, Demengeot J. CD25+CD4+ regulatory T cells suppress CD4+ T cell-mediated pulmonary hyperinflammation driven by Pneumocystis carinii in immunodeficient mice. *Eur J Immunol.* 2002;32:1282–1291.
231. Maloy KJ, Salaun L, Cahill R, et al. CD4+CD25+ T-R cells suppress innate immune pathology through cytokine-dependent mechanisms. *J Exp Med.* 2003;197:111–119.
232. Belkaid Y, Rouse BT. Natural regulatory T cells in infectious disease. *Nat Immunol.* 2005;6:353–360.
234. Belkaid Y, Piccirillo CA, Mendez S, et al. CD4+CD25+ immunoregulatory T lymphocytes control *Leishmania major* persistence and the development of concomitant immunity. *Nature.* 2002;420:502–507.
235. Suffia IJ, Reckling SK, Piccirillo CA, et al. Infected site-restricted Foxp3+ natural regulatory T cells are specific for microbial antigens. *J Exp Med.* 2006;203:777–788.
236. McGuirk P, McCann C, Mills KHG. Pathogen-specific T regulatory 1 cells induced in the respiratory tract by a bacterial molecule that stimulates interleukin 10 production by dendritic cells: a novel strategy for evation of protective T helper type 1 responses by Bordetella pertussis. *J Exp Med.* 2002;195:221–231.
237. MacDonald AJ, Duffy M, Brady MT, et al. CD4 T helper type 1 and regulatory T cells induced against the same epitopes on the core protein in hepatitis C virus-infected persons. *J Infect Dis.* 2002;185:720–707.
238. Iwashiro M, Messer RJ, Peterson KE, et al. Immunosuppression by CD4+ regulatory T cells induced by chronic retroviral infection. *Proc Natl Acad Sci U S A.* 2001;98:9226–9230.
239. Robertson SJ, Messer RJ, Carmody AB, et al. *In vitro* suppression of CD8+ T cell function by Friend virus-induced regulatory T cells. *J Immunol.* 2006;176:3342–3349.
240. Kinter AL, Hennessey M, Bell A, et al. CD25+CD4+ regulatory T cells from the peripheral blood of asymptomatic HIV-infected individuals regulate CD4+ and CD8+ HIV-specific T cell immune responses *in vitro* and are associated with favorable clinical markers of disease status. *J Exp Med.* 2004;200:331–343.
241. Suvas S, Azkur AK, Kim BS, et al. CD4+CD25+ regulatory T cells control the severity of viral neuroinflammatory lesions. *J Exp Med.* 2004;172:4123–4132.
242. Danke NA, Koelle DM, Yee C, et al. Autoreactive T cells in healthy individuals. *J Immunol.* 2004;172:5967–5972.
243. Viglietta V, Baecher-Allan C, Weiner HL, Hafler DA. Loss of functional suppression by CD4+CD25+ regulatory T cells in patients with multiple sclerosis. *J Exp Med.* 2004;199:971–979.
244. Baladina A, Lecart S, Dartevelle P, et al. Functional defect of regulatory CD4+CD25+ T cells in the thymus of patients with autoimmune myasthenia gravis. *Blood.* 2005;105:735–741.
252. Allen SE, Crome SQ, Crellin NK, et al. Activation-induced FOXP3 in human T effector cells does not suppress proliferation or cytokine production. *Int Immunol.* 2007;190:345354.
253. Wang J, Ioan-Facsinay A, van der Voort AEIH, et al. Transient expression of FOXP3 in human activated nonregulatory CD4+ T cells. *Eur J Immunol.* 2007;37:129–138.
254. Tang QZ, Bluestone JA. Regulatory T-cell physiology and application to treat autoimmunity. *Immunol Rev.* 2006;212:217–237.
255. Kohm AP, McMahon JS, Podojil JR, et al. Cutting Edge: Anti-CD25 monoclonal antibody injection results in the functional inactivation, not depletion, of CD4+CD25+ T regulatory cells. *J Immunol.* 2006;176:3301–3305.

Chapter 31

The Mucosal Immune System

Hiroshi Kiyono, Jun Kunisawa, Jerry R. McGhee, and Jiri Mestecky

INTRODUCTION

The most important source of stimulation of the entire immune system is the external environment comprising the indigenous mucosal microbiota, potential pathogenic microorganisms, abundant food antigens (Ags), and allergens, all of which are encountered mainly at the vast surface areas of mucosal membranes. This enormous and highly variable antigenic load has resulted in a strategic distribution of cells involved in the uptake, processing and presentation of Ags, production of antibodies (Abs), secretion of cytokines, and cell-mediated immune (CMI) defenses at the front line of defense—mucosal tissues and associated secretory glands. Quantitative data concerning the distribution of phagocytic cells, T and B lymphocytes, and Ab-producing cells illustrate the point: mucosal tissues, particularly those of the intestinal tracts, contain more macrophages (MΦ), plasma cells (PCs), and T cells than any other lymphoid tissue in the entire immune system.

Notwithstanding the global importance of systemically acquired infections such as malaria and neonatal tetanus, the majority of infectious diseases worldwide either directly afflicts or is acquired through mucosal surfaces of the gastrointestinal (GI), respiratory, and genital tracts. Consequently, innate and adoptive immune mechanisms operational at mucosal surfaces are of great importance to the protection and survival in a hostile environment. The induction of preventive and protective immune responses to mucosal infectious agents, and to ingested food Ags and environmental allergens that would limit their absorption, is usually the most emphasized functional aspect of the mucosal immune system. Yet, recently revived interest in the induction of systemic unresponsiveness to Ags applied first by the mucosal route, so called *oral* or *nasal* (mucosal) *tolerance,* has directed the attention of immunologists working in the field of autoimmunity, transplantation, and hypersensitivity to the exploitation of this fundamental principle. Although there are limited numbers of clinical successes, the phenomenon of mucosal tolerance is an essential feature and critical functional component that efficiently prevents and suppresses otherwise unavoidable overstimulation of the entire immune system by the most common environmental Ags primarily of food and indigenous bacterial origins. The enhancement of protective mucosal immune responses to infectious agents sought by vaccinologists, and the desired suppression of systemic immune responses to autoAgs and transplantation Ags, may seem paradoxical. Yet, such outcomes are not mutually exclusive due to the hierarchy in the quality of immune responses induced by mucosal Ag delivery: Mucosal immunity manifested by the appearance of secretory Abs and systemic tolerance evaluated by diminished CMI-responses may be concomitantly induced. Thus, the fundamental objectives of the mucosal immune system—containment of the vast onslaught of environmental Ags without compromised integrity of mucosal barriers and prevention of overstimulation of the systemic compartment—are achieved by concerted interactions of lymphoid and nonlymphoid cells, epithelial cells (ECs) in particular, and their respective products as a mucosal internet of communication. Thus, an orchestrated mucosal immune system consisting of innate immunity as well as acquired immunity including secretory IgA (S-IgA) Abs and mucosal cytotoxic T lymphocytes (CTLs), add additional layers of host defense.

INNATE MUCOSAL IMMUNE SYSTEM

Epithelial Cells

Physical Barrier Function of ECs

The epithelium of the mucosa-associated lymphoid tissues (MALTs) of the lung, gut and genitourinary tracts, and, others have been clearly shown to play an active role in both innate and adaptive types of mucosal immunity. Given the physical proximity of the ECs to the external milieu and, therefore, the primary site of initial Ag exposure, ECs may be a central cell type in both defining the Ags with which the mucosal immune system is confronted and regulating the ultimate responses to these antigenic exposures. Initially, prevention of luminal Ag transport is through a thick layer of mucus. Mucin 2 (MUC2) is a dominant intestinal mucus-formation molecule that is abundantly produced by goblet cells located at the intestinal villous epithelium (1). Mucus not only provides a physical and biological protective barrier, but also ensures maintenance of an appropriate concentration of Abs at the mucosal surface by preventing Ag-specific S-IgA Abs from being physically carried away. Additionally, paracellular transport of luminal Ag is prevented by the juncture between adjacent ECs that is mediated by physical structures associated with the epithelium including the tight junctions (TJs) and the subjacent desmosomes and adherence junctions (2). The TJs are composed of a number of interacting cellular proteins, which include claudin, occuludin, ZO-1, ZO-2, and cingulin, among others. Under normal circumstances, the TJs exclude Ags greater than 6 to 12 Å (> 500 to 900 Daltons) in molecular diameter.

In addition to these physical barrier functions of ECs, the epithelium of the MALTs of the lung, gut and genitourinary tracts, have been clearly shown to play an active role in both innate and adaptive types of mucosal immunity by collaboration with adjunct neighboring ECs as well as subjacent parenchymal cells (fibroblasts and mesenchymal cells and their connective tissue substances) and hematopoietic cells [MΦ, dendritic cells (DCs), polymorphonuclear cells (PMN) and lymphocytes] and likely microbial components in the lumen (3).

Antimicrobial Peptides

The epithelium also secretes a variety of antimicrobial peptides (defensins, cathelicidins, cryptdin-related sequence [CRS] peptides) and bacteriolytic enzymes (lysozyme, secretory phospholipase-A2 [PLA2], peroxidase, and lactoferrin), and others (Figure 31.1). In the intestinal epithelium, ECs, Paneth cells, and PMNs mainly produce these molecules (4,5). Paneth cells reside at the base of the crypt regions of the small intestine, but not the stomach or colon. They produce α-defensins constitutively. In contrast, β-defensins are produced by ECs of the whole intestine, which requires microbial stimulation (4,5). Both defensins are cationic small peptides with a characteristic β-sheet–rich fold and a framework of six disulphide-linked cysteines and exhibit antimicrobial activity by damaging and permeabilizing the bacterial cell membrane by pore formation. Defensins also inhibit viral infection (e.g., human immunodeficiency virus [HIV], herpes simplex virus [HSV], vesicular stomatitis virus, and influenza virus) by interupting their invasion at an early step, such as receptor binding (4,5). In addition to the antimicrobial properties, defensins have chemotactic activities for monocytes, T cells, and B cells, implying that defensins may bridge between mucosal innate and acquired immunity via the augmentation of T and B cell interactions (6). The cathelicidin is also a cationic small peptide containing a cathelin-like domain produced by ECs, PMNs, and keratinocytes (4,5). The expression of cathelicidin by ECs is regulated by butyrate and other short-chain fatty acids produced by fermenting bacteria. The CRS peptide is produced by Paneth cells and shows antimicrobial activity through its cationic feature (4,5).

Antimicrobial enzymes are other molecules showing antimicrobial activities (Figure 31.1). PLA2 is a small

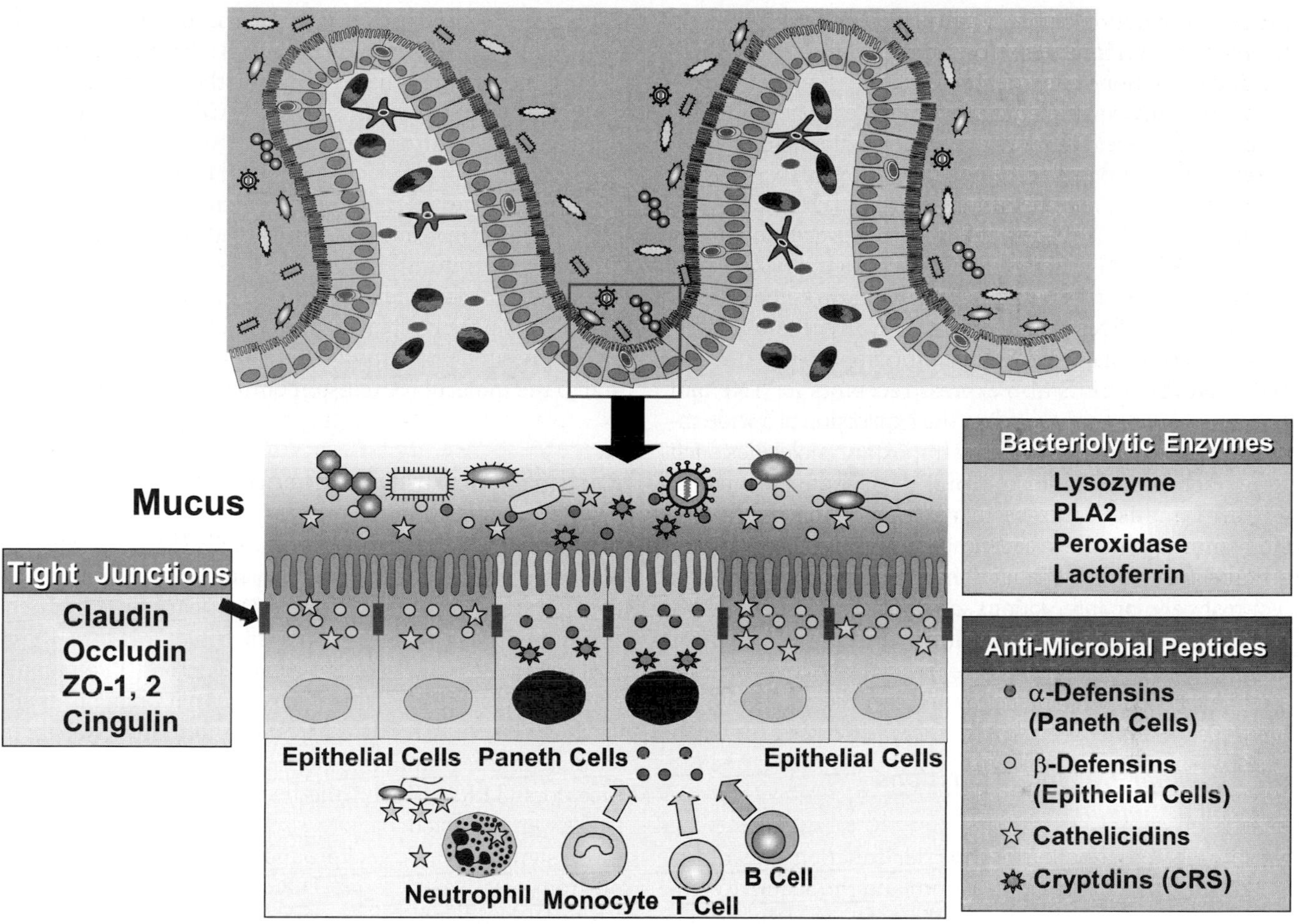

FIGURE 31.1 Various types of antimicrobial molecules protect mucosal surfaces against invading microbes. Epithelial cells (ECs) and Paneth cells secrete bacteriolytic enzymes (lysozyme, PLA2, peroxidase, and lactoferrin) and antimicrobial peptides (defensins, cathelicidins and cryptdin related sequence [CRS]) in mucosal sites. Neutrophils also produce antimicrobial molecules. Defensins have been shown to possess the capability to recruit immunocompetent cells for the initiation of innate and adaptive immune responses.

enzyme produced by Paneth cells and PMNs, which degrades bacterial phospholipids and subsequently disrupts bacterial integrity (4,5). Lysozyme is another bactericidal component produced by Paneth cells, PMNs, and ECs. Lysozyme is a muramidase cleaving the glycosidic linkage between *N*-acetylglucosamine and *N*-acetyl muramic acid of peptidoglycan, and thus it is preferentially effective against gram-positive bacteria (4,5). Surfactant proteins A-D (SPs) are highly hydrophobic proteins in the lung produced by alveolar type II cells. Several lines of evidence revealed that SPs are actively involved in lung innate immunity following bacterial penetration into the lower airways (7). SPs bind to LPS and the interaction between SPs and CD14 may explain their ability to affect some LPS responses.

Antimicrobial molecules are also produced by PMNs induced following infection by pathogens. It is well established that PMNs take up invading microorganisms through a complement lysis-dependent phagocytosis and kill them by antimicrobial tools such as toxic oxygen radicals, cationic peptides, and lytic enzymes in the phagocytic vacuoles. In addition, PMNs produce extracellular fibers containing DNA, histones, and granule proteins after stimulation by bacterial endotoxins (8). These fibers are known as *neutrophil extracellular traps* (NETs). NETs bind to both gram-negative and -positive bacteria, and kill them by their esterase and antimicrobial peptides and enzymes.

Cytokines and Cytokine Receptors

ECs are able to secrete both constitutively and inducibly a large number of inflammatory and regulatory cytokines. Using EC lines, it has been shown that the epithelium can constitutively express proinflammatory cytokines such as IL-1-α, IL-1-β, IL-15, TNF-α, and IL-6 and anti-inflammatory and barrier-promoting cytokines such as TGF-β and IL-10, whose levels may be further increased by interactions with pathogens and their toxic products

(3). The production of these cytokines by the epithelium is likely to play an important role in both promoting intestinal inflammation (e.g., IL-1 and TNF-α), regulating the activation and expansion of mucosal T cells within the epithelium (e.g., stem cell factor [SCF], IL-5, IL-7, and IL-15), regulating local B cell production of Igs (e.g., TGF-β, IL-5, IL-6, and IL-10), and, finally, regulating barrier function, *per se* (IL-10, IL-15, and TGF-β). With regards to barrier function, ECs also express a large number of cytokine receptors (3). Intestinal EC (IEC) lines and freshly isolated IECs express mRNA for the common IL-2 receptor γ-chain and specific α-chains of the receptors for IL-2, IL-4, IL-7, IL-9, and IL-15. IECs also express receptors for TNF and IFN-γ, which not only regulate the expression of a wide variety of other immunologically important molecules such as the polymeric Ig receptor (pIgR), for example, but also tend to diminish epithelial barrier function. The expression of these cytokines and cytokine receptors thus further emphasize the integration of the epithelium into the network of cellular interactions associated with the MALTs. In this regard, bacterial infection can influence the interactions of the EC-mediated mucosal internet with mucosal T and B cells via IL-7/IL-7R and IL-15/IL-15R.

Transcellular Transport Functions of the Epithelium

Another aspect of epithelial barrier function that represents a link between the epithelium and the adaptive components of the MALT is the ability of the epithelium to transport macromolecules, especially Igs, transcellularly in a process termed *transcytosis,* which reflects the polarized nature of the epithelium. Two receptors for Ig have been shown to have such properties. The pIgR, whose itinerary is now well defined, transports polymeric forms of IgA (pIgA) and IgM (pIgM) from the basal to apical direction with unloading of its cargo in association with an extracellular proteolytic fragment of the pIgR receptor (secretory component, SC) (9). This pathway is not only able to deliver large quantities of secretory Ig onto the mucosal surfaces, but it is also able to exclude Ags that have entered the secretory pathway either apically or basally (discussed later). This type of defense, which takes advantage of a component of the adaptive immune response, is likely to be important in resistance against pathogenic viral infections.

In a related but distinct manner, the epithelium also expresses the neonatal Fc receptor for IgG (FcRn) (10). Recent evidence indicates that this molecule is expressed by adult human epithelium and MΦ of the intestine (and, likely, other surfaces) and thus is not strictly limited to neonatal life as predicted by earlier studies in rodents wherein the FcRn was responsible for the passive acquisition of IgG neonatally (10). In the context of expression postnatally in adult humans, FcRn may therefore be in a position to provide luminal immunosurveillance against pathogenic exposure. FcRn binds IgG, its cargo, in a pH-dependent process (pH 6 on, pH 7.4 off) due to critical histidine residues in the Fc-region of the IgG molecule. In contrast to the itinerary associated with pIgR-associated transport, the transport pathway associated with FcRn is bidirectional; both apical to basal and basal to apical (10). In addition, the FcRn is not associated with proteolytic cleavage allowing for reiterative rounds of transport. It is predicted, therefore, that the FcRn is at least in part responsible for the steady state distribution of IgG on either side of an epithelial barrier given the unlikely possibility that paracellular transport of this macromolecule occurs due to the molecular exclusion of the TJs.

Pattern Recognition Receptors

Toll-like Receptors

The extrinsic barrier functions of the epithelium associated with innate immunity are at least partially mediated by the interaction with luminal microbiota. It is well established that pattern recognition receptors (PRRs) play an important role in the recognition of microbial products (Figure 31.2) (11,12). Most prominent among PRRs that regulate innate immune responses are an array of Toll-like receptors (TLRs). ECs in the respiratory, genital, and GI tracts were reported to express several types of TLRs binding to signature microbial products such as peptidoglycan of gram-positive bacteria (TLR2), viral double-stranded RNA (dsRNA) (TLR3), bacterial LPS of gram-negative bacteria (TLR4), bacterial flagellin (TLR5), and microbial CpG motifs of DNA (TLR9) (13,14). Pathogens have more than one TLR ligand so multiple TLRs are co-ordinately regulated. These molecules were initially characterized as the pathogen-associated molecular patterns (PAMPs), but these are produced by both pathogenic and commensal microorganisms. Although TLR signaling induces an inflammatory cascade in the sterile circumstance of the systemic immune compartment, mucosal TLRs should take a different strategy to distinguish pathogenic microorganisms from commensal microorganisms for the immunosurveillance in the mucosal tissues directly and continuously exposed to the large numbers of commensal as well as occasional pathogenic microorganisms.

Evidence has been emerging that underlying molecular pathways exist to achieve the discrimination of pathogenic from commensal microorganisms in the innate mucosal system (Figure 31.2). First, it has been proposed that decreased surface expression of TLRs and coreceptors leads to the down-regulation of TLR signaling (13,14). Notably, peptidoglycan and LPS are abundantly produced by the commensal microflora, and thus their receptors (TLR2 and TLR4) should have an immune quiescent system against these commensal-derived PAMPs. Along these lines, TLR2 and TLR4 are expressed on the surface of ECs but

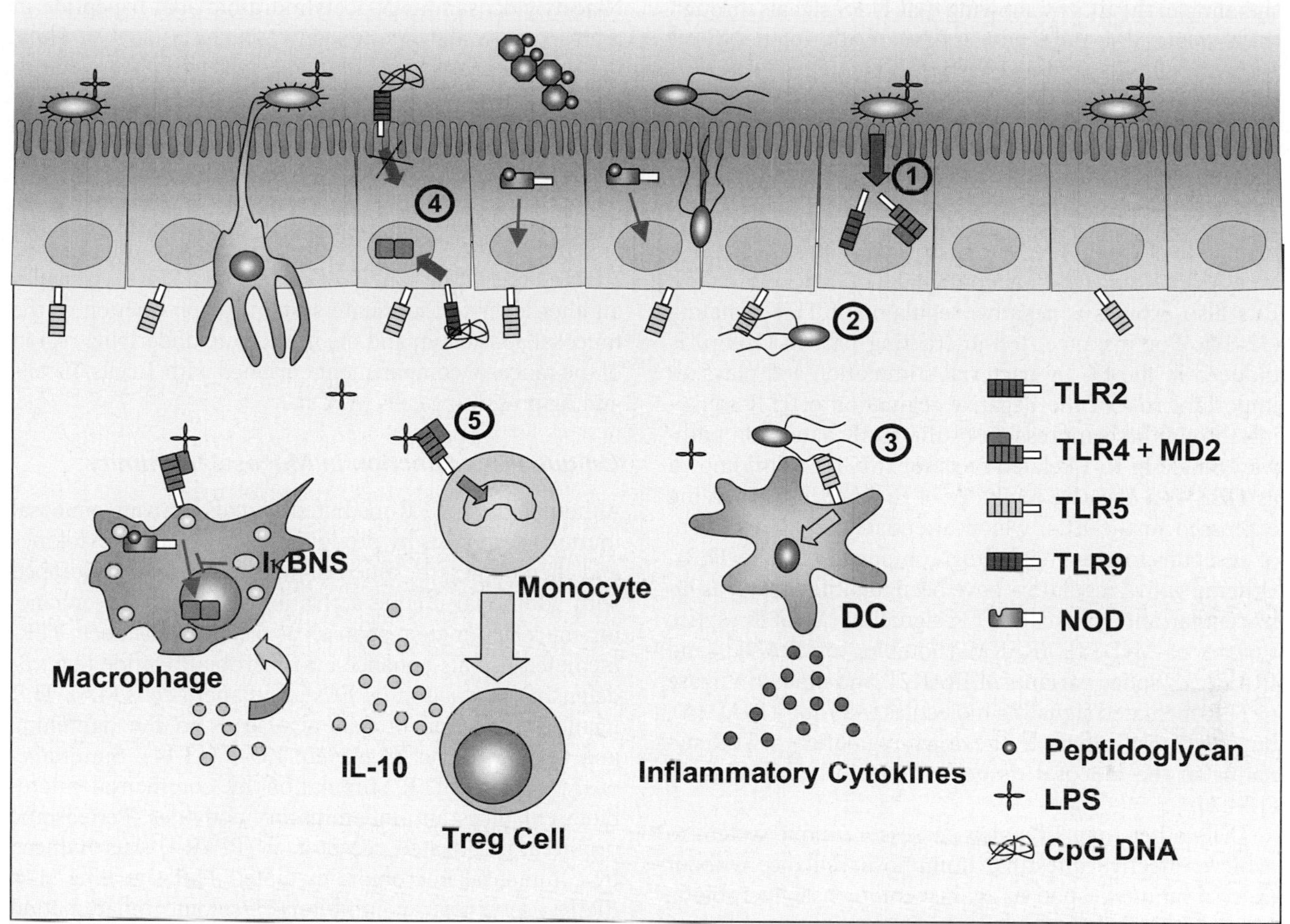

FIGURE 31.2 Uniqueness of recognition and discrimination of microbes. Toll-like receptors and nucleotide-binding oligomerisation domains (NODs) recognize bacterial products (peptidoglycan [PG], lipopolysaccharide [LPS] and CpG DNA). The host mucosal immune system employs various mechanisms to distinguish pathogenic from commensal bacteria: 1, continuous bacterial stimulation leads to down-regulation of TLR expression; 2, TLR5 is preferentially expressed on the basolateral side of ECs; 3, pathogenic bacteria are recognized by LP DCs which express TLR5; 4, TLR9 signals through the basolateral side induces the activation of the NF-κB pathway while apical TLR9 stimulation prevents NF-κB activation; 5, LPS from commensal bacteria induces regulatory T cell differentiation.

prolonged stimulation with their ligands resulted in their down-regulation. Thus, TLR2 and TLR4 are expressed on fetal ECs and adult crypt ECs, but their expression was lost on mature ECs (15). In addition to ligand stimulation, down-regulation of TLR expression is induced by TGF-β, a regulatory cytokine predominantly produced in the intestine (12). In the case of TLR4, LPS recognition is coupled to CD14 binding of LPS, wherein LPS bound to CD14 interacts with a TLR4/MD-2 protein heterodimer. The absence or reduction of CD14 and MD-2 expression on ECs was reported, which presumably was associated with a lack of reactivity with LPS (14).

Secondly, the reduced reactivity of ECs to PAMPs is explained by the unique distribution of TLRs. For example, it has been shown that the LPS-induced reduction of TLR2 and TLR4 was mediated by the alteration of their distribution from the apical site to intracellular compartments (13). It is interesting to note that intracellular TLR4 maintains its activity to detect intracellular bacteria. This unique intracellular distribution of TLR4 but not outer cell membrane allows the EC to discriminate pathogenic cells invading the ECs and commensal cells generally attaching on their cell surface. Another example of this was shown by TLR5, which recognizes bacterial flagellin. TLR5 is exclusively expressed on the basolateral site of ECs, allowing them to sense bacteria when they invade into the lamina propria (LP) regions (14). A recent study has provided an additional example of polarity-mediated regulation of TLR signaling in the ECs by showing that TLR9 signals through the basolateral site and induces the activation of the NF-κB pathway, while apical TLR9 stimulation prevents NF-κB activation (16).

As the third mechanism, several negative regulatory pathways for TLR expression have been identified. It was reported that the loss of postnatal LPS responsiveness of ECs was associated with a post-transcriptional down-regulation of the IL-1 receptor-associated kinase 1 (IRAK1), an essential molecule for epithelial TLR4 signaling (15). ECs also express a negative regulator of TLR signaling (12–14). For instance, toll-interacting protein (Tollip) is induced in the EC by bacterial stimulation and plays an important role in the negative regulation of TLR signaling through its suppression of the IRAK activation pathway. Single Ig IL-1-related receptor (SIGIRR, also known as TIR8) is a negative regulator of IL-1 and TLR signaling expressed in the ECs, which attenuates the recruitment of receptor-proximal signaling components to the TLRs. Other negative regulators have been identified, such as intracellular antagonists of TLR signaling (MyD88s [splice variant of MyD88], IRAKM [homolog of IRAK1], and IRAK2c/d [splice variants of IRAK2]) and ubiquitin ligase of TLR-mediated signaling molecules (A20 and TRIAD3A), but their involvement in the down-regulation of TLR signaling in the mucosal tissues remain to be investigated (12–14).

Cells other than ECs also possess a unique system to achieve effective intestinal immunosurveillance without excess immune responses against commensal microbiota. Like the ECs, LP MΦ lack reactivity to LPS due to failure to express CD14 (17). It is interesting to note that the unresponsiveness of intestinal MΦ to LPS was intrinsic but that of EC was acquired immediately after birth by exposure to exogenous LPS, as mentioned earlier (15). Additionally, LP MΦ selectively express IκBNS, an inhibitor of NFκB activation (18). In the case of mucosal DCs, a unique pathogen recognition system is achieved by the distinct expression of TLR4 and TLR5. Unlike conventional DCs in systemic immune compartments (e.g., spleen), intestinal LP DCs predominantly express TLR5, but not TLR4 (19). Thus, the LP DCs can detect pathogenic bacteria in a TLR5-dependent manner when luminal pathogens break the epithelial barrier and become exposed to LP DCs. However, these DCs do not secrete pro-inflammatory cytokines after exposure to commensal bacteria.

Cytoplasmic PAMPs Receptors

Besides the TLRs, other receptors for detecting cytoplasmic PAMPs have been identified (Figure 31.2). Nucleotide-binding oligomerization domain 1 (NOD1) and NOD2 are well-characterized cytoplasmic PRRs expressed by both ECs and MΦ, which recognize a peptidoglycan motif containing a diaminopimelate-containing N-acetylglucosamine-N-acetylmuramic acid tripeptide in gram-positive and gram-negative bacteria (11,12). Thus, the NOD family plays a crucial role in distinguishing invading pathogens and commensal bacteria. For the detection of invading viruses, retinoic acid inducible gene-I (RIG-I) and melanoma differentiation-associated gene 5 (MDA5) have been identified. Both recognize dsRNA generated during viral replication and trigger the activation of NF-κB and IRF3/7 with subsequent production of antiviral type I IFN (11,12). The family of intracellular PRRs provides another layer to the innate system for production of the mucosal epithelium and the immediate underlying region of the mucosal compartment enriched with T cells, B cells and Ag presenting cells (APCs).

Unique PRRs Function in Mucosal Immunity

Although these PRR-mediated signals activate mucosal immune responses by producing inflammatory cytokines and chemokines, the mucosal immune system is equipped with additional unique activation pathways for enhancing mucosal innate responses as well. For instance, TLR-mediated signals enhance antimicrobial peptide (e.g., β-defensin) production by ECs and Paneth cells (4,5). TLR ligand stimulation of ECs also leads to the tightening and sealing of the TJ protein ZO-1 (13,14). Simultaneously, mucosal TLR stimulation by commensal microbiota enhances anti-inflammatory activities. Peroxisome proliferator-activated receptor γ (PPARγ) was induced by commensal microbiota-mediated TLR signaling (14). PPARγ serves as an inhibitor of colonic inflammation through its ability to inhibit NF-κB activation. Additionally, LPS from the commensal microbiota, but not from pathogenic bacteria, induces the development of regulatory T (Treg) cells producing an inhibitory cytokine, IL-10 (12). In the lungs, TLR stimulation induces the production of indoleamine 2,3-dioxygenase (IDO) in the parenchyma. The lung-specific production of IDO leads to the inhibition of T cell–mediated lung inflammation and airway hyperreactivity by inhibiting T cell migration into the lung and by killing T cells (20).

An Involvement of PRRs in the Development of Mucosal Inflammation and Allergy

As one may envision, a dysregulated mucosal innate system leads to inflammatory responses in mucosal tissues. For instance, TLR2 and TLR4 expression is upregulated during inflammatory bowel disease (IBD) development, and polymorphisms in TLR4 have been shown to be linked to IBD development (13). Similarly, mutation of NOD2 contributes to IBD pathogenesis (21). Additionally, mutation or down-regulation of negative regulators for TLR signaling (e.g., IκBNS) resulted in IBD development (18). It is interesting to note that MyD88-deficient mice showed a higher mortality than wild-type mice when exposed to dextran sulfate sodium (DSS)-induced colitis (22). The disease susceptibility was at least partially attributable to an impaired epithelial proliferation caused by the TLR-mediated signaling. Commensal bacteria and TLRs are also involved in the development of food allergy, another serious mucosal disease. It has been shown that commensal biota-derived signaling through TLR provides a protective function against food allergy (14).

In addition to intestinal inflammation, PRRs are involved in airway inflammatory diseases such as asthma. It was previously reported that an insertion-deletion polymorphism of NOD was strongly associated with asthma (23). Additionally, a recent study suggests that TLR4-mediated signaling is involved in the development of allergic airway inflammation through a modification in mast cell function (24). These studies indicate that signaling through PRRs is also important for the creation and maintenance of a quiescent status in the immune environment of mucosal compartments. This includes intestinal homeostasis rather than induction of inflammatory responses since the destruction of the PRR system is associated with the development or acceleration of mucosa-associated diseases. Taken together, PRR-mediated signals play an important role in both immunosurveillance and immune homeostasis in mucosal tissues.

Intraepithelial T Lymphocytes

Close Communication between ECs and Intraepithelial Lymphocytes

The major interface between internal organs and the outside environment is the columnar intestinal epithelial cell (IEC) layer, which covers mucosal tissues. In addition to IECs, the columnar epithelium includes a population of lymphocytes commonly termed *intraepithelial lymphocytes* (IELs) (25). As their name implies, IELs reside between the basolateral surfaces of IECs. It has been estimated that 1 IEL occurs for every 4 to 10 IECs seen in the small intestine and for every 30 to 50 IECs found in the large intestine. This shows that large numbers of lymphocytes are situated in the surface regions of intestinal mucosal tissues. Thus, IELs have been shown to closely communicate with each other and with the IECs that surround them. Indeed, several interacting molecules were expressed between IECs and IELs. For example, CD103 (α_E integrin) expressed on IELs interacts with the E-cadherin expressed on IECs, playing an important role in the retention of IELs in the intestinal epithelium (26). Additionally, IEL retention may be mediated by expression of certain integrins (e.g., $\alpha_1\beta_1$, $\alpha_4\beta_1$, and β_2 integrins), the adhesion molecule, Ep-CAM and TJ molecules (e.g., ZO-1 and occludins) (25). These intimate biological interactions between IECs and IELs provide physiological barriers that act as a first line of innate defense in the intestine.

As mentioned earlier, IECs are in constant contact with the luminal microbiota. In addition, IECs become the target of microbial pathogen attachment and replication leading to the establishment of infection. Given the presence of immune and inflammatory cells within the epithelium and their obvious changes during infection or inflammation, it is worthwhile to consider the role of IECs and IELs in orchestrating these responses. It is logical to assume that these IELs are important lymphoid cells that participate in the mucosal innate response. Indeed, the majority of human and murine IELs are classified as T cells because they express the CD3 molecule in association with either of the two forms of T cell receptor (TCR), $\gamma\delta$ or $\alpha\beta$. Concerning the expression of CD4 and CD8 by IELs, it has been shown that approximately 80% of small intestinal IELs belong to the CD8 subset; however, a substantial number of IELs can be grouped as CD4-bearing cells including $CD4^+CD8^-$ and $CD4^+CD8^+$ subsets. The CD8 molecules expressed on IELs consist of either $\alpha\beta$ heterodimeric or $\alpha\alpha$ homodimeric chains. $CD8\alpha\beta^+$ IELs express Thy-1 and express the $\alpha\beta$ TCR. In contrast, $CD8\alpha\alpha^+$ IELs and $CD4^-CD8^-$ double-negative (DN) IELs contain both TCR$\gamma\delta$ and TCR$\alpha\beta$ fractions (25).

Innate Homeostatic and Protective Immune Function of $\gamma\delta$ IELs

Among IELs, those expressing the TCR$\gamma\delta$ ($\gamma\delta$ IELs) have been considered to be involved in mucosal innate defense because cell-transfer studies have indicated that the $\gamma\delta$ IELs have only minimal pathogen-specific activity (25,27). The less Ag-specificity of $\gamma\delta$ IELs is supported by the finding that $\gamma\delta$ IELs are present in mice deficient in the transporter associated either with antigen processing (TAP) or with the classical class I molecules ($K^{b-/-}D^{b-/-}$), while $\gamma\delta$ IELs were drastically reduced in numbers in β2-microglobulin–deficient mice (25,27), suggesting that $\gamma\delta$ IELs recognize a TAP-independent nonclassical MHC molecule (Figure 31.3). In humans, the TCR$\gamma\delta$ expressed by IELs predominantly use Vδ1. These human TCR$\gamma\delta$ recognize the MIC molecules MICA and MICB, members of the nonclassical MHC molecule family (27). MIC molecules on ECs are induced by stress such as heat shock and microbial infections and are not capable of presenting peptides, but instead act as ligands for $\gamma\delta$TCRs. In mice, $\gamma\delta$ IELs predominantly use the Vγ5 (also known as Vγ7) gene segment together with several Vδ genes. Although mice do not have a functional MIC gene ortholog, they express molecules that resemble MIC such as H60, members of the RAE class I–like family, and other nonclassical MHC class I molecules (e.g., T10/T22) (Figure 31.3) (27).

Upon TCR$\gamma\delta$-mediated stimulation by nonclassical MHC molecules, $\gamma\delta$ IELs synthesize an array of cytokines that includes IL-2, IL-3, IL-6, IFN-γ, TNF-α, and TGF-β

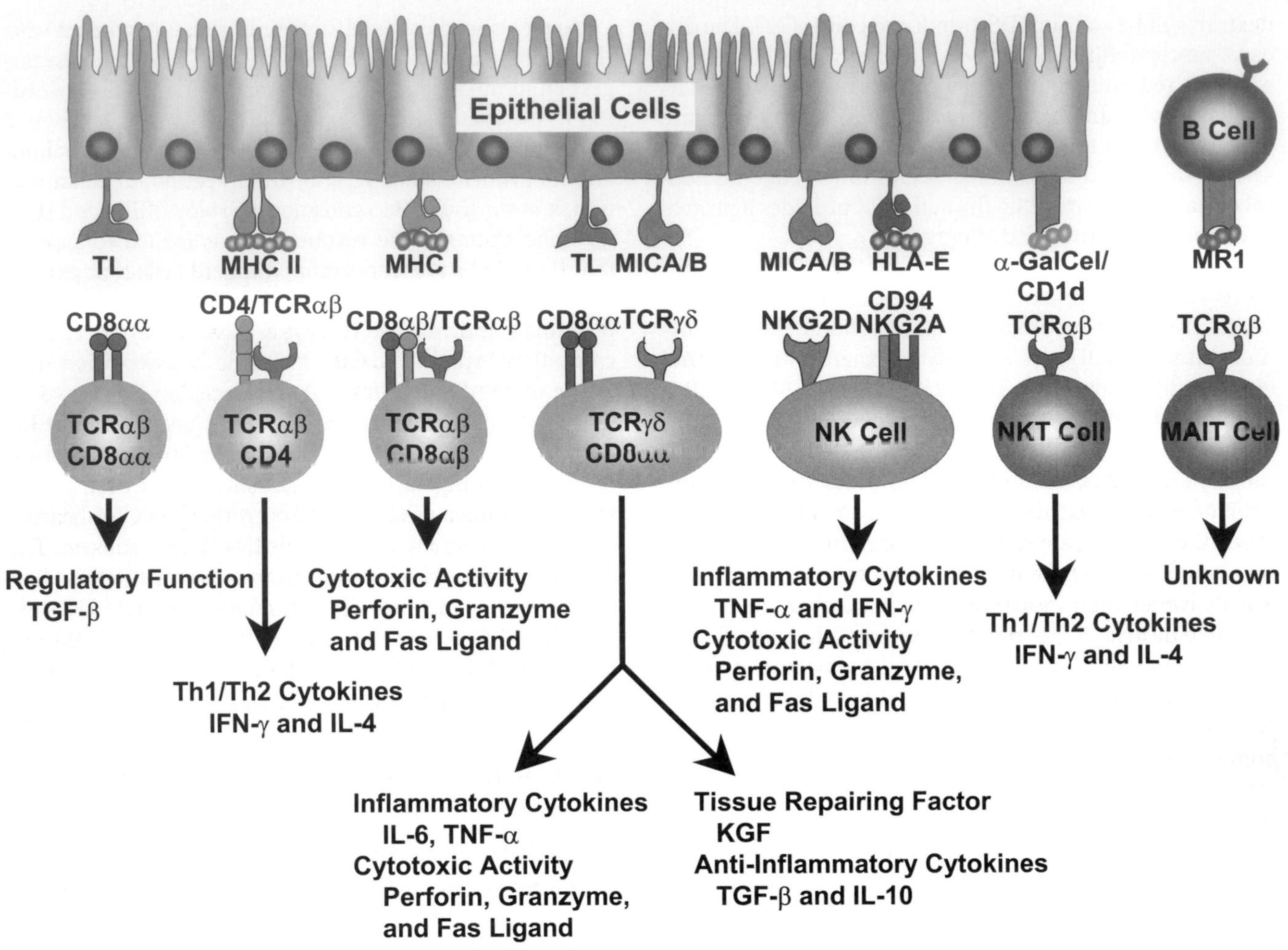

FIGURE 31.3 Molecular machinery for mucosal lymphocyte and EC interactions. Unique populations of mucosal lymphocytes are located in or underneath the intestinal epithelium. Immunological functions of these lymphocytes are regulated via molecular interactions between MHC family molecules and corresponding receptors. The ECs express MHC molecules including broad types of nonclassical MHC molecules interacting with specific receptors expressed on lymphocytes, which allow the establishment of induction of productive and quiescent immune responses in mucosal tissues.

(25,27). It was also shown that freshly isolated and activated $\gamma\delta$ IELs express high levels of mRNA specific for lymphotactin, a chemokine important for $CD8^+$ T cell chemotaxis (27). These results suggest that IELs actively produce cytokines and chemokines to provide specific immunologic functions in the mucosal compartment. In addition to cytokine production, $\gamma\delta$ IELs produces cytotoxic molecules such as perforin, granzyme, and Fas ligand, and show cytotoxic activity against stressed or microbial infected IECs (28).

Alternatively, because activated $\gamma\delta$ IELs can produce keratinocyte growth factor (KGF), which is important for epithelial growth and repair of damaged tissues, some $\gamma\delta$ IELs could be involved in repair of tissue damage elicited during inflammatory responses (27). In addition to KGF, $\gamma\delta$ IELs synthesize anti-inflammatory and regulatory cytokines such as TGF-β and IL-10. In agreement with production of these cytokines, TCRδ chain–deficient mice show an increased susceptibility to epithelial damage caused by dextran sulfate sodium (DSS)-induced colitis (27). Thus, $\gamma\delta$ IELs also play a critical role in the maintenance of mucosal homeostasis in epithelial regions. However, not all immune responses mediated by $\gamma\delta$ IELs are beneficial. For example, it was shown that dysregulated production of IL-15 and overexpression of MICA/MICB on IECs led to the aberrant activation of IELs in the case of celiac disease (29).

To prevent the disruption of the epithelium by activated IELs, it is essential that IELs produce cytokines without self-proliferation. To achieve this opposite regulation (cytokine production without proliferation), the mucosal immune system has evolved a unique interaction between IECs and IELs. Thymus leukemia antigen (TL) is a nonclassical MHC molecule expressed almost exclusively by IECs of the small intestine (Figure 31.3) (27). Like other nonclassical MHC molecules, TL does not present antigenic peptides but strongly interacts with CD8$\alpha\alpha$ on IELs. The interaction between CD8$\alpha\alpha$ and TL enhances cytokine production by IELs but inhibits self-proliferation and cytotoxic activity. By inhibiting proliferation, CD8$\alpha\alpha$-TL interactions prevent the disruption of a sheeted form of epithelium that results from attack by dividing IELs (27).

Recent studies show that a naïve population of IELs is made up of recent CD8$^+$ thymic emigrants (RTEs) (30). RTEs are distinguished by their ability to migrate into the small intestine without activation because of their expression of $\alpha_4\beta_7$ integrin, α_E integrin, and CCR9 in the thymus (30). After migrating directly into the intestinal epithelium from the thymus, these RTEs begin to proliferate in response to Ag exclusively present in the gut. These IELs show diverse TCR repertoires, which is important in their maintenance of TCR diversity in the intestine.

Unique Developmental Pathways for IELs

In addition to their immunological uniqueness, IELs also have a special development pathway, even though controversy remains as to what extent the IELs require thymic dependency (31,32). Like naïve lymphocytes circulating in systemic immune compartments, the major IEL populations in CD4 or CD8$\alpha\beta$ subsets expressing TCR$\alpha\beta$ originate from conventional single-positive (SP) thymocytes. In contrast, some populations of double-negative (DN) IELs and CD8$\alpha\alpha$ IELs expressing either TCR$\alpha\beta$ or TCR$\gamma\delta$ originate from unconventional thymocytes. Several lines of evidence have revealed that these IEL precursors in the DN thymocytes, including TCR$\alpha\beta^+$ DN thymocytes, TCR$\gamma\delta^+$ DN thymocytes, and TCR$\alpha\beta^-$ CD4$^-$ CD8$^-$ triple-negative (TN) thymocytes (31). TCR$\alpha\beta^+$ DN thymocytes are thought to be mature postselected DN thymocytes because they arose from the CD8$\alpha\alpha^+$ CD4$^+$ CD8$\alpha\beta^+$ triple-positive (TP) thymocytes after agonist selection and migration into the intestine where they further reinduce CD8$\alpha\alpha$ under the influence of IL-15 (31). In addition to the postselected DN thymocytes, some subsets among the TN thymocytes emigrated from the thymus during the CD44$^+$ CD25$^+$ TN2 or the CD44$^-$ CD25$^+$ TN3 stages and migrated into the intestinal epithelium where they characteristically expressed *c-kit* and IL-7 receptor (IL-7R) and subsequently expressed TCR$\alpha\beta$ or TCR$\gamma\delta$ (31). It was recently found that thymic IEL precursors could be divided into two groups based on the requirement of sphingosine 1-phosphate (S1P), a lipid mediator, in the regulation of trafficking of thymic IEL precursors into the intestine (33). CD4 or CD8$\alpha\beta$ naïve IELs originating from single-positive (SP) thymocytes express high levels of type 1 S1P receptor. In contrast, unconventional thymic IEL precursors, including RTEs and DN thymocytes expressing either TCR$\alpha\beta$ or TCR$\gamma\delta$, migrate into intestine in a S1P-independent manner (33).

In addition to the conventional and unconventional thymic IEL precursors, it has been proposed that certain populations of IEL subsets (e.g., TCR$\gamma\delta$ CD8$\alpha\alpha$ IELs) develop extrathymically (32,34). As a candidate lymphoid tissue for extrathymic IEL development, cryptopatches (CryPs) were identified (35). CryPs were shown to be lymphocyte clusters in the crypt LP of the murine small and large intestine. Cells within the CryPs are composed mostly of lymphoid progenitors expressing stem cell factor (SCF) receptor (c-kit), and IL-7Rα, but lacking the lineage markers (CD3, B220, Mac-1, Gr-1, and TER-119). They possess transcripts for germline TCR genes, mRNA for CD3ε, as well as proteins (i.e., *RAG*-2 and preTα) involved in TCR gene rearrangement and are able to generate CD8$\alpha\alpha$ $\alpha\beta$ as well as $\gamma\delta$ IELs, albeit with a strong bias toward the generation of $\gamma\delta$ T cells, in irradiated severe combined immune-deficient (SCID) mice. These findings demonstrated that c-kit$^+$ CryP cells are committed to the T cell lineage and are competent for the generation of IELs.

Natural Killer and NKT Cells

In addition to the T cells, the epithelium includes natural killer (NK) and NKT cells. For instance, the human nonclassical MHC molecules MICA and MICB predominantly expressed on damaged or transformed IECs act as ligands for the NK receptor, NKG2D (Figure 31.3) (27). Interestingly, as mentioned earlier, TCR$\gamma\delta$ recognizes the same MICA and MICB molecules (Figure 31.3), implying that the mucosal immune system can use both TCR$\gamma\delta$ and NKG2D to recognize damaged or stressed IECs through the nonclassical MHC molecules. Additionally, the expression of HLA-E on the epithelium is associated with ligation of killer inhibitory-related receptors (CD94/NKG2) on activated mucosal NK cells in humans (Figure 31.3) (29). It was previously shown that the cytotoxic effects of NK IELs were enhanced by IL-15 through the up-regulation of IFN-γ production and Fas ligand-mediated killing activity and simultaneous enhancement of MICA expression (29).

NKT cells also play an important role in mucosal innate immunity (Figure 31.3). NKT cells express invariant TCR. The TCRα chain comprises a Vα14 in the murine system, and TCR Vα24 is a homologue expressed on human NKT cells (36). In contrast to the invariant expression of TCRα, NKT cells possess a wide variety of TCRβ chains (36), which allows them to contribute to various immune responses including mucosal homeostasis. These NKT cells recognize lipid-derived Ag presented by the CD1d, one of the nonclassical MHC molecules (Figure 31.3). IECs and DCs in the intestinal compartments express the CD1d (37). However, several studies have identified lipid

Ags presented by CD1d, such as α-glucuronosylceramide and α-galacturonosylceramide from nonpathogenic sphingomonas bacteria and a diacylglycerol from pathogenic *Borrelia burgdorferi* (36). In addition, it has been proposed that infection with bacteria (e.g., *E. coli, Bacillus subtilis, S. aureus,* or *Mycobacterium bovis-Bacillus Calmette Guerín*) or their derived bacterial components such as LPS, lipoteichoic acid, or $Pam_3CysSerLys_4$ (P_3CSK_4) allows $CD1d^+$ cells to present endogenous glycosphingolipid, isoglobotrihexosylceramide, and stimulate NKT cells, which may contribute to initial sensing of pathogenic or infected cells (Figure 31.3) (36).

After stimulation via CD1d, NKT cells can secrete both Th1- and Th2-type cytokines (Figure 31.3). It is still unclear how the hierarchy between Th1- and Th2-biased NKT cells is determined, but this may account for the contribution of NKT cells to both protective and anti-inflammatory functions (36). Consistent with this, it was reported that CD1d-deficient mice were susceptible to infections (e.g., *Listeria* and *Pseudomonas aeruginosa*) at mucosal sites. NKT cells are also involved in the amelioration of DSS-induced colitis through their ability to produce regulatory cytokines such as IL-4 and IL-10. NKT cells are also thought to be involved in the suppression of allergen-induced airway hyperreactivity by the induction of a Th1 shift from an allergy-associated Th2 environment or the creation of anergy. These results generally suggest a critical role for NKT cells in the down-regulation of inflammatory responses; however, other studies demonstrated that NKT cells induced asthma. Although the NKT cell subset is a minor population of mucosal immune compartments, the cells are involved in the recognition of self- and exogenic-glycolipid Ags as a part of the mucosal innate defense system (36).

Mucosa-associated Invariant T Cells

A recent study has discovered MHC-related 1 (MR1)–restricted mucosal-associated invariant T cells (MAIT cells) as a novel subset of unconventional T cells abundantly present in the intestinal LP (Figure 31.3) (38). MAIT cells express invariant TCR α chain, TCR Vα7.2-Jα33 in humans and TCR Vα19-Jα33 in mice. Like conventional T and NKT cells, MAIT cells develop in the thymus, but their selection is independent of the TAP and invariant chain, suggesting that putative ligands presented by MR1 are different from those presented by conventional MHC class I and II molecules. In this context, several lines of evidence have revealed that MAIT cells can be activated by both peptide Ag and glycolipid Ags (e.g., α-GalCer and other α-mannosylceramides) (Figure 31.3). MAIT cells additionally require $MR1^+$ B cells for their development. It is interesting to note that MAIT cells are markedly decreased in germ-free mice, suggesting that some microbial stimulation is required for the selection, migration, and expansion of MAIT cells. MAIT cells have been suggested to be involved in the immunosurveillance and the establishment of immunological homeostasis in the intestine, because MAIT cells possess regulatory functions where the cells inhibit autoimmune responses (39).

ACQUIRED MUCOSAL IMMUNE SYSTEM

Mucosal Migration System for Acquired Immunity

In addition to the innate mucosal immune system, the mucosal immune system is equipped for well-organized and controlled acquired immunity. The mammalian host has evolved organized secondary lymphoid tissues in the upper respiratory and GI tract regions that facilitate Ag uptake, processing, and presentation for priming immunocompetent cells for subsequent induction of Ag-specific mucosal immune responses. Collectively, these tissues are termed mucosal inductive sites. The gut-associated lymphoid tissues (GALT) consist of several family members of inductive sites including the Peyers patches (PPs), colonic patches (CPs), the appendix, and isolated lymphoid follicles (ILFs) (34). The major inductive tissues for nasal/inhaled Ags in humans, and primates appear to be the palatine tonsils and adenoids (nasopharyngeal tonsils), which together form a physical barrier of lymphoid tissues termed the *Waldeyers ring,* as well as nasal-associated lymphoid tissues (NALT) for mice and rats (40). To summarize, then, NALT and GALT in humans and mice and possibly primates comprise a MALT network.

Through the interaction with APCs in MALTs, naïve B and T cells are primed by Ag and then emigrate from the inductive environment via lymphatic drainage, circulate through the bloodstream, and home to mucosal effector sites, especially the LP regions of the intestinal, respiratory, and reproductive tracts where they further differentiate into effector cells that protect mucosal surfaces (41,42). These mucosal networks are known as the common-mucosal immune system (CMIS) or recently suggested to be named as mucosal migration system (MMS) bridging between the inductive (e.g., MALTs) and effector sites (e.g., LP), a network that plays a key role in the induction of Ag-specific acquired immunity against mucosally encountered Ag.

Structure and Cellular Composition of Mucosal Inductive Sites

Among several MALTs, the most extensively studied mucosal inductive tissues are the PPs of the murine GI tract. PPs are large enough to be observed upon gross examination, and usually number 8 to 10 in murine small intestine. In humans, up to 200 PPs were detected. Like PPs in the small intestine, there are lymphoid organs in the

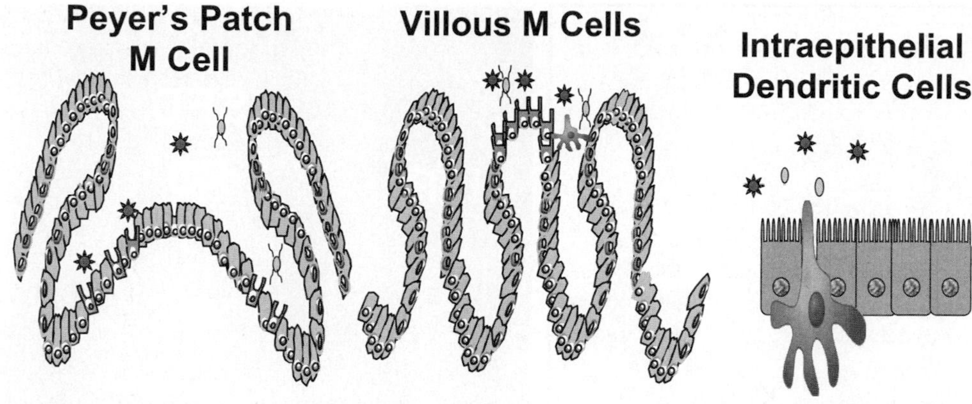

FIGURE 31.4 Multiple Ag uptake pathways for the induction of mucosal immune responses. At least three distinct Ag sampling sites have been reported. M cells were originally discovered in FAE of MALTs including PPs, ILFs, and NALT for sampling of orally administered Ags. In addition to MALT-associated M cells. M cells are also capable of developing at the tip region of villous epithelium from FAE of MALTs and have been termed villous M cells. Finally, DCs can extend their dendrites expressing the TJ molecule claudin between ECs and directly take up GI tract luminal Ags.

large intestine. These tissues are known as CPs, or rectal-associated lymphoid tissue (RALT), which are smaller in size than PPs (34). An additional lymphoid structure resembling PPs and CPs in composition and architecture has been identified as numbering at least 30,000 (in humans), and 100 to 200 (in mice) clusters on the antimesenteric wall of the murine small intestine, which are now known as solitary lymphoid follicles or ILFs (34). In the respiratory tract, NALT is found on both sides of the nasopharyngeal duct dorsal to the cartilaginous soft palate in rodents (40). In humans, there are unpaired nasopharyngeal tonsils (adenoids) and the paired palatine tonsils that play an important role for human airway immunity. The latter makes up most of Waldeyers ring in humans (40). Further, a NALT-like structure of lymphocyte aggregation with follicle formation was identified in human nasal mucosa, especially that of the middle concha in children less than 2 years old (43). In the bronchial tract, bronchus-associated lymphoid tissues (BALT) was classically defined as an aggregated lymphoid structure separated from the bronchial lumen by a specialized lymphoepithelium in several species, including rats, rabbits, and sheep, although the presence of murine and human BALT as an aggregated lymphoid follicle under normal conditions remains a subject of debate (40).

Although each MALT exists in different regions of the mucosal tissues, MALTs share several interesting features associated with their role as the major mucosal inductive tissue (41,42). First, MALTs are unique in that they contain efferent lymphatics but no afferent lymphatics, reducing the possibility that an Ag will be encountered via the afferent lymphatics. Instead, MALTs are covered with the specialized EC termed a *follicle-associated epithelium* (FAE). FAE contains a specialized cell type called a *microfold/membraneous cell* (*M cell*) that is closely associated with lymphoid cells (Figure 31.4) (44). M cells are noted in the MALTs of both humans and rodents (e.g., PPs, ILFs, CPs, and NALT). The M cells, which have short microvilli, small cytoplasmic vesicles, and few lysosomes, are adept at takeup and transport of luminal Ags, including proteins and particulates such as viruses, bacteria, small parasites, and microspheres, allowing the selective transport of these Ag into the MALTs. The human palatine and nasopharyngeal tonsils (adenoids) are largely covered by a squamous epithelium and are often not appreciated as mucosal inductive tissues. However, the palatine tonsils usually contain 10 to 20 crypts that increase their surface area where M cells locate in the deeper regions (44). Although this issue remains a subject of debate, several studies demonstrated that M cells could be differentiated from the absorptive ECs through interactions with B cells (45).

MALTs contain organized regions for the generation of IgA-committed B cells. Distinct B cell zones are located beneath the dome area of PPs and contain germinal centers (GCs) where significant B cell division is seen (Figure 31.5). These GCs contain the majority of surface IgA-positive (sIgA$^+$) B cells (46), but, unlike the spleen and secondary lymph nodes (LNs) in the systemic compartment, PC development does not effectively occur. In addition to the GCs, the underlying dome region of the PPs consist of sparse sIgA$^+$ cells that may provide a first line of IgA-mediated defense for the dome region of PPs. Since germ-free mice have PPs but lack GCs, it has been postulated that the continuous exposure of the PPs to the commensal bacteria or viruses from the outside environment induce the constant GC formation seen in PPs (47). In contrast to the PPs, GCs are absent in the NALT of normal mice (41,42). Thus, PPs contain a high frequency (10% to 15%)

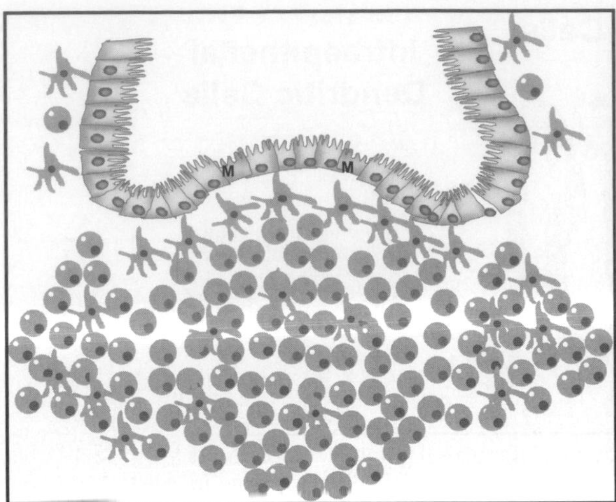

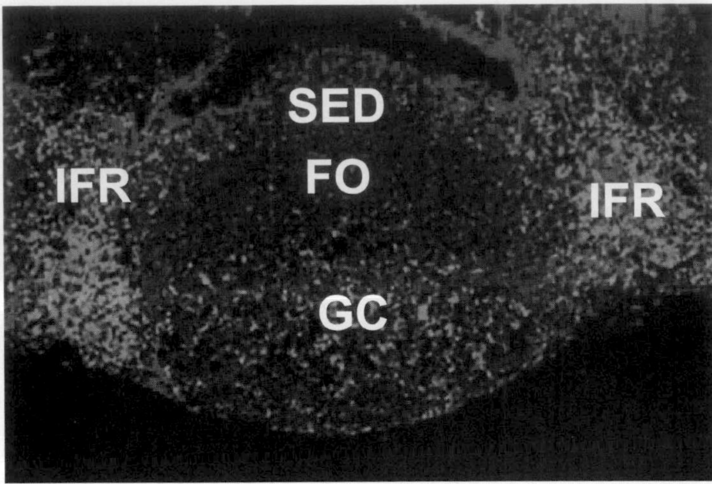

CD4 B220 CD11c

FIGURE 31.5 Segregated cell distribution in the PPs. CD4$^+$ T cells (green) are mainly present in the intrafollicular regions (IFRs) and B cells (red) are located in the subepithelial dome (SED) and follicle (FO) regions. DCs (blue) are distributed in the SED and IFRs. GCs are enriched in B cells with small numbers of T cells and DCs for the creation of a cellular environment for the efficient generation of IgA-committed B cells. (See color insert.)

of sIgA$^+$ B cells, while NALT was found to contain fewer IgA-committed B cells, even though nasal immunization induces higher numbers of sIgA$^+$ B cells in NALT (41,42). In human tonsils, approximately one half of cells are B lymphocytes, and they mainly occur in follicle-containing GCs (46). Most human tonsillar B cells are actually surface IgG-positive (sIgG$^+$); however, significant numbers of sIgM$^+$ and sIgA$^+$ B cells are also present. The human palatine tonsil also contains a distinct subepithelial B cell population, as is seen in the FAE region of PPs. This B cell subset differs from both GCs and follicular mantle B cells (46). These subepithelial B cells located in NALT and GALT may play a crucial role in immediate Ab production toward Ag taken up through M cells.

All major T cell subsets are found in the T cell–dependent areas adjacent to follicles, the interfollicular regions (IFRs) (Figure 31.5). The parafollicular T cells are mature and > 97 % of these T cells use the $\alpha\beta$ heterodimer form of TCR. Approximately two-thirds of TCR$\alpha\beta^+$ T cells in the PPs are CD4$^+$ and exhibit properties of Th cells, including support for IgA Ab responses (48). Approximately one-third of the TCR$\alpha\beta^+$ T cells in the PPs are CD8$^+$; this cell subset contains precursors of CTLs (28). These IFRs contain high endothelial venules (HEVs), a main entry site for lymphocytes into PPs. The HEVs express mucosal vascular addressin cell adhesion molecule 1 (MAdCAM-1), a ligand for the $\alpha_4\beta_7$ integrin, which determines a selective gut-tropism migration for lymphocytes (49,50). The T cell-rich IFRs overlap with the B cell follicles in some areas, providing an important place for initial T–B cell interactions.

Immunohistologic studies have revealed the unique distribution of DCs. In the PPs, DCs are divided into at least three distinct populations (51,52). First, myeloid-type DCs expressing CD11b are located in the subepitheliual dome (SED) region. The second DC population in the PPs is CD8α^+ lymphoid DCs residing in the T cell–rich IFRs. Additionally, PPs contain DCs expressing neither CD11b nor CD8α, which are called DN DCs. The DN DCs are exclusively found in both SED and IFRs. The distribution of different populations of DCs in the PPs is at least partially determined by chemokines and their receptors (51,52). CD11b$^+$ myeloid DCs express CCR6, which allow their migration toward CCL20 selectively expressed by FAE. Consistent with this, CD11b$^+$ DCs were markedly reduced in the SED of PPs in CCR6-deficient mice (53). In addition to the interaction between CCR6 and CCL20, the interaction between CCR1 and CCL9 plays a nonredundant role in the migration of CD11b$^+$ DCs into the FAE of PPs. Additionally, all DCs in the PPs expressed CCR7, allowing them to migrate into the IFRs toward cells producing CCL19 and CCL21. It has been demonstrated that DCs also play an important role in the respiratory immune system; however their distribution remains unclear.

Distinct Pathway for MALT Organogenesis

GALT Organogenesis

Although similar in terms of anatomy and histology, the MALTs of the respiratory and intestinal immune system differ in their organogenesis (34,41,42). The models

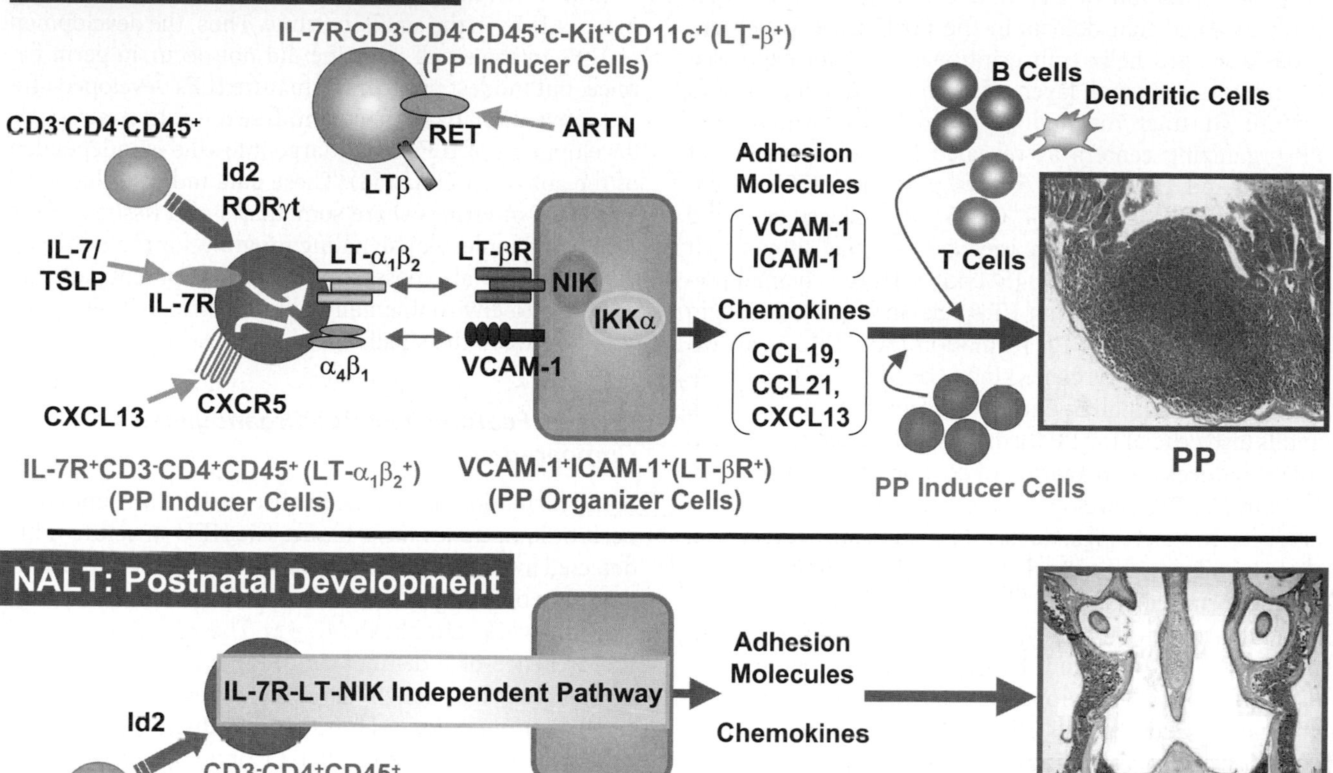

FIGURE 31.6 Distinctively orchestrated organogenesis of MALTs of PPs and NALT. Initial phase of the tissue genesis program of PPs operates during embryogenesis. The development of IL-7R$^+$CD3$^-$CD4$^+$CD45$^+$ PP inducer cells requires Id2 and RORγt genes. IL-7R$^+$CD3$^-$CD4$^+$CD45$^+$ PP inducer cells accumulate initially at the tissue anlagen and specifically interact with VCAM-1$^+$ PP organizer cells. This cell-to-cell interaction induces subsequent activation of LT-βR–associated molecules such as NIK and IKKα for the induction of adhesion molecules and chemokines by PP organizer cells, which leads to the further recruitment of T cells, B cells, and DCs. Recently, RET$^+$CD11c$^+$ cells expressing LT-β have been identified as a new member of inducer cells that contribute to the initiation phase prior to the appearance of IL-7R$^+$CD3$^-$CD4$^+$CD45$^+$ PP inducer cells. In comparison to the PP organogenesis program, NALT organogenesis is initiated in a postnatal manner and is totally independent of IL-7R-LT/LT-βR-NIK–mediated tissue genesis signaling pathway. For the development of NALT inducer cells, like PPs, Id2 is necessary for the differentiation of CD3$^-$CD4$^+$CD45$^+$ NALT inducer cells but does not require RORγt.

describing the development of PPs have been studied in some detail in mice. A cluster of mesenchymal-lineage VCAM-1$^+$/ICAM-1$^+$ cells occur in the upper small intestine beginning at embryonic day 15 to 16 (Figure 31.6). These cells are termed *PP organizers* and express lymphotoxin β receptor (LT-βR). Subsequently, lymphoid-lineage IL-7R$^+$CD3$^-$CD4$^+$CD45$^+$ PP inducer cells appear to be the anlagen of the PPs at embryonic day 17.5. Following stimulation signals provided through IL-7R, PP inducer cells express LT-$\alpha 1\beta 2$ to activate PP organizer cells through LT-βR, and then PP organizer cells produce chemokines such as CXCL13 and CCL19 to stimulate PP inducer cells through CXCR5 and CCR7 (Figure 31.6). The reciprocal interaction between inducer and organizer cells through the chemokine and cytokine receptors is essential for the initiation of PP formation, and the loss of any part of the signaling program is sufficient to disrupt PP development, as evidenced by the loss of PPs in LTβR$^{-/-}$ and IL-7R$\alpha^{-/-}$ mice and the partial reduction in the formation and number of PPs in CXCR5$^{-/-}$ mice (34,41,42). In addition, alymphoplasia (*aly/aly*) mice, with a mutation in the NF-κB-inducing kinase, which appears to act downstream of LT-$\alpha 1\beta 2$/LT-βR signaling, also fail to develop PPs (54). Further evidence in support of this model comes from studies showing that mice lacking the CD3$^-$CD4$^+$ CD45$^+$ IL-7R$^+$ inducer cells due to genetic deletion of the transcription regulators Id2 or RORγt also completely lack the formation of PPs and LNs (34,41,42). Another study revealed that defects in the Foxl1 gene, which encodes a winged helix transcriptional regulator expressed in the mesenchymal layer of both the developing and mature GI tract resulted in the delayed formation of PP organizing centers as revealed by the expression of VCAM1 and IL-7R at 17.5 days postcoitus (55). In addition to IL-7R$^+$CD3$^-$CD4$^+$CD45$^+$ PP inducer cells and stromal organizer cells, a recent study has shown that the IL-7R$^-$CD3$^-$CD4$^-$CD45$^+$c-kit$^+$CD11c$^+$ hematopoietic population expressing LT-β has an important role in the initiation stage of PP formation (56). These cells express the receptor tyrosine kinase (RET), which is essential for the mammalian enteric nervous system formation and is also crucial for PP formation. Thus, the RET ligand ARTN induces the formation of ectopic PP-like structures. In humans, PPs develop during prenatal life, a situation also seen in sheep, pigs, dogs, and horses, and it is thought that a similar tissue genesis program is involved.

The formation of ILFs also requires LT-β and LT-βR–dependent events (34,41,42). However, the LT-β and LT-βR–dependent events in ILF formation are chronologically different from PP development. ILF formation can occur postnatally and requires LT-β-expressing B lymphocytes (34). Consistent with this fact, treatment with LT-βR-Ig fusion protein during the postnatal period suppresses ILFs but not PPs (42). It was also demonstrated that immature ILFs with clusters of B220$^+$ cells are present in the intestine of germ-free mice, but exogenous stimuli including bacterial Ags/mitogens are required for the completion of the lymphoid organization of ILFs, including GC formation (34,41,42). In activation-induced cytidine deaminase (AID)-deficient mice, ILFs developed hyperplasia. A subsequent study demonstrated that the lack of hypermutated IgA production into the intestinal lumen resulted in the expansion of segmented filamentous bacteria in the small intestine of AID-deficient mice (57). Since antibiotic treatment of AID-deficient mice abolished the hyperplasia, it was proposed that anaerobic bacterial growth induced ILF hyperplasia. Taken together, these findings suggest that postnatal and physiological inflammatory signals are essential for the formulation of ILFs in the small intestine.

Like the PPs, inhibition of LT-β–mediated signaling during the embryonic stage leads to the inhibition of CP formation in the large intestine (34,41,42). In contrast, increased numbers and enlargement of CPs were noted in Foxl1-deficient mice, while the size and numbers of PPs were decreased (55). Additionally, ILFs in the large intestine showed a different requirement for LT-β signaling for their development. Normal ILFs were present in the small intestine of mice treated with LT-β-Ig fusion protein *in utero* (42). However, the same treatment resulted in the acceleration of ILF formation in the large intestine (58), suggesting that LT-mediated signaling behaves as a negative regulator for ILF formation in the large intestine during the gestational period. One study demonstrated a critical involvement of the GI tract flora for the development of ILFs in the small intestine. Thus, the development of ILFs in the small intestine did not occur in germ-free mice, but modest numbers of mature ILFs developed after the conventionalization of germ-free mice. In contrast, the development of ILFs in the large intestine is independent of the gut microbiota (58). These data indicate that small and large intestines share some parts of a tissue genesis-associated molecular signaling program for their development, but they also possess unique development pathways to adjust to environmentally different circumstances that occur between the small and large intestines.

Distinct Features of NALT Organogenesis Compared with PPs

NALT formation has not been observed during embryogenesis or in newborn nasal tissue. The HEV structure is first detected in bilateral nasal tissue 1 week after birth, and the complete bell-shaped NALT formation with lymphoid cells is seen 8 weeks after birth (40–42). These findings indicate the presence of a distinct tissue genesis program in the PPs and NALT, although these tissues have a similar structure and immunological function as inductive tissues (Figure 31.6). As mentioned earlier, PP organogenesis requires a cytokine-signaling cascade involving IL-7R and LT-βR, and these deficiencies resulted in the lack of PP formation. However, mice lacking PPs or both PPs and LNs due to a deficiency in the LT-βR–mediated inflammatory cytokine cascade, including LT-β–deficient, IL-7R–deficient, and *aly/aly* mice, and mice treated *in utero* with LT-β-Ig fusion protein have a normal NALT structure (40–42). These findings further support the idea that NALT genesis does not follow the "programmed physiological inflammation" model typical of PPs. In contrast, deletion of Id2, which is responsible for the induction of CD3$^-$CD4$^+$CD45$^+$ inducer cells, impaired the genesis of all secondary lymphoid tissues including both NALT and PPs (Figure 31.6) (40–42). However, the deletion of the gene encoding RORγt, the additional transcriptional regulator for the development of CD3$^-$CD4$^+$CD45$^+$ inducer cells, resulted in the suppression of PP organogenesis, while NALT development was normal (40–42). These findings suggest that although NALT and PPs development depends on inducer cells of the same phenotype, CD3$^-$CD4$^+$CD45$^+$, those inducer cells can be categorized as those either dependent on Id2 alone (for NALT) or dependent on both Id2 and RORγt (for PPs).

Antigen Sampling and Presentation in MALTs

As mentioned earlier, MALTs have unique epithelial regions or FAE containing specialized ECs, termed *M cells*, to achieve preferential transport of luminal Ag (Figure 31.4) (44). M cells are characterized by a pocket structure (M cell pocket) at the basolateral side harboring a wide variety of lymphoid cell subsets such as DCs, MΦ, and lymphocytes. Unique features of M cells include the fact that in spite of high uptake of luminal Ag via pinocytosis and endocytosis, they contain only a few lysosomes. In addition, IgA preferentially binds to the apical sides of M cells (44,59). Thus, it has been suggested that M cells contribute to the transport of luminal Ags to underlying APCs without any Ag digestion or processing.

In addition to serving as a means of transport for luminal Ags, the unique structural features of M cells (e.g., short microvilli and the thick glycocalx) and their predominant expression of receptors for some microorganisms also provide entry sites for pathogens (44,59). For instance, *Yersinia* adheres to M cells via the invasin and the $\beta 1$ integrin expressed on the *Yersinia* and M cells, respectively. *Salmonella* initiate murine infection by invading the M cells of the PPs. Reoviruses also initiate infection of the mouse through the M cell, an ability that has been associated with the reovirus sigma protein. It has also been suggested that M cells act as the entry site for Prions. Lung M cells were reported to be the site for entry of *Mycobacterium tuberculosis* into the host, with subsequent uptake in draining LNs (60). Thus, M cells act as a gateway to the outside environment, delivering antigenic substrate to the underlying immune-competent cells for the subsequent induction of Ag-specific immune responses.

Several lines of evidence demonstrated that DCs are present in the MALTs. Among them, detailed studies have been performed mainly using PPs and showed that there are several distinct types of DCs in the PPs, which are distinguished by the surface expression of CD11b, CD8, and B220, as described earlier (51,52). In the FAE regions, CD11b$^+$ DCs and CD11b$^-$ CD8$^-$ DN DCs are present, and some of them are associated with M cells, suggesting that they reside in the M cell pockets (44,52). Upon stimulation of CD11b$^+$ DCs and DN DCs through microbial infection or uptake of their products, CD11b$^+$ DCs and some populations of DN DCs begin to express CCR7, allowing them to migrate into the IFRs of PPs. Hence, it is likely that blood-derived CCR6$^+$ DCs migrate into FAE regions via interactions with CCL20, and their activation by microbial stimulation through M cells results in their migration into the IFRs. Here, they present Ag to T cells for priming and subsequent induction of the productive phase of the Ag-specific immune response. In the IFRs, additional types of DCs occur. These DC subsets express CD8, but not B220. The exclusive expression of CCR7 on CD8$^+$ DCs allows them to reside in the IFRs. A fourth population, the B220$^+$ plasmacytoid DCs (pDCs), are also present in the IFRs and FAE (51,52). The pDCs perhaps are involved in the generation of Treg cells for the establishment of a quiescent state of immune response (termed *tolerance*) in the harsh environment of mucosal tissues. These different types of DCs cooperatively regulate the activation or inhibition of immune responses induced via MALTs.

Priming of T Cells in Mucosal Inductive Sites

As CD4$^+$ Th cells mature in response to foreign Ags, they assume unique characteristics, such as production of distinct cytokine arrays. The naïve CD4$^+$ T cells have substantial plasticity for development of distinct effector or regulatory lineages (Figure 31.7). The environment and cytokine milieu greatly influences the differentiation of naïve T cells into Th1 (IFN-γ), Th2 (IL-4, IL-13), Th3 (TGF-β), Th17 (IL-17) T cells, or CD25$^+$ Foxp3$^+$ IL-10–producing Treg cells (48). For example, the differentiation of Th1 cells producing IFN-γ was induced by certain pathogens. These cells often develop following production of IL-12 by DCs. In this context, it was previously reported that both DN DCs and CD8$^+$ DCs secreted high levels of IL-12p70 following microbial stimulation, which led to the predominant Th1-type responses (51,52). However, CD11b$^+$ DCs predominantly exist in the FAE regions and produce high levels of IL-10 in response to microbial stimulation, but produce little IL-12, which leads to the induction of Ag-specific T cells secreting IL-4 and IL-10. Of note, IL-10–producing Treg cells are preferentially induced by CD11b$^+$ DCs, indicating that CD11b$^+$ DCs have a unique ability to induce Treg cells.

Recently, an IL-17–producing T cell subset, termed *Th17 cells*, has also been identified as a new subset of the intestinal T cell repertoire and considered to be responsible for pathologic inflammatory reactions (61). It is interesting to note that stimulation of naïve T cells with both TGF-β and IL-6 resulted in the induction of Th17 cells, while IL-6 inhibited the development of Treg cells in the presence of TGF-β (62,63). Taken together, the mucosal immune system has unique T cell–inducing and balancing mechanisms for matching CD4$^+$ T cell effector and regulatory lineage specification, and clearly DCs play a central role in the education of naïve T cells to be an immunosuppressive and active under normal conditions.

Other T cell families involved in mucosal immunity are CTLs. Most CTLs are CD8$^+$ TCR$\alpha\beta^+$ and recognize antigenic peptides through MHC class I–restricted presentation by infected cells. An obvious question is how a CTL immune response is initiated given that mucosal inductive sites, which harbor CTL precursors (pCTLs), are separate from effector sites, such as infected ECs where activated CD8$^+$ CTLs function. A partial answer is that the M cell has specific receptors for mucosal viruses, best exemplified by reovirus. As described earlier, using the sigma one protein, the reovirus enters the M cell in both NALT and GALT (44,59). It is likely, though less well documented that other enteric viruses, such as rotavirus and respiratory pathogens, such as influenza and respiratory syncytial virus (RSV), also enter the mucosal inductive pathway via M cells (44,59). Further, it was shown that administration of attenuated virus into the GI tract results in the induction of increased pCTL

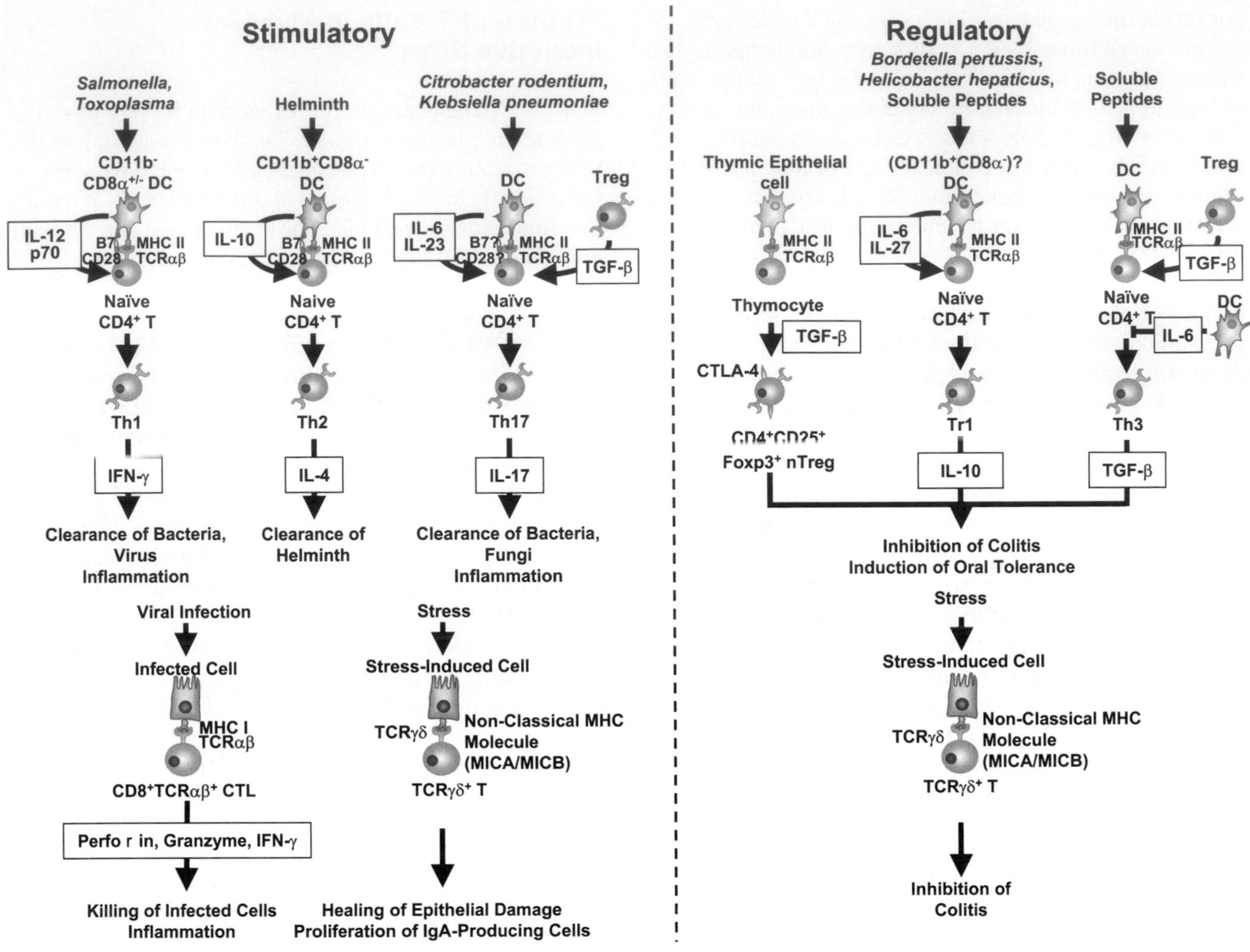

FIGURE 31.7 Various induction pathways for the generation of versatile mucosal T cells for the induction of productive and quiescent immune responses. Naïve T cells are primed and stimulated via a molecular network with the recognition of peptide Ag presented by MHC molecules, costimulatory molecules, and cytokines. After receiving stimulation, naïve T cells differentiate into immunologic (effector T cells) or tolerogenic (Treg cells) cell types for subsequent immunity.

frequencies in the PPs (64). Similarly, virus-specific CTLs were detected in NALT as well as in mediastinal, submandibular, and cervical LNs after nasal immunization with attenuated virus (65). These findings clearly demonstrate that PPs and NALT play a pivotal role in the induction of Ag-specific CTLs in addition to the generation of Ag-specific IgA-committed B cells; the molecular and cellular pathways underlying the CTL induction in the inductive tissues (e.g., involvement of DCs) remain obscure.

Immunoglobulin Isotype Switching in Mucosal Inductive Sites

T Cells for IgA Class Switching

The cross-talk among DCs, T cells, and B cells in mucosal inductive tissues promotes the IgA-commitment of B cells, which undergo μ to α isotype class swich recombination (CSR) (Figure 31.8) (66). This μ to α isotype CSR is likely dependent on Ag stimulation in GCs, where naïve B cells interact with local CD4$^+$ T cells and with follicular Ag-trapping DCs (FDCs) in the presence of specific cytokines. Hence, depletion of CD4$^+$ T cell subsets markedly affects mucosal immune responses, including diminished levels of sIgA$^+$ B cells (67). Consistent with this, clear evidence was presented that clones of T cells from murine GALT, when mixed with noncommitted sIgM$^+$ B cells, induced isotype switching to B cells expressing surface IgA (sIgA$^+$) (68). The initial studies with murine T switch (Tsw) cells used T cell clones derived by mitogen stimulation and IL-2 supported outgrowth, and when Tsw cells were added to sIgM$^+$ sIgA$^-$ B cell cultures resulted in marked increases in sIgA$^+$ cells (68). This result suggests that cognate interactions between Tsw and B cells are required for induction of the IgA class switch. Other studies have revealed that

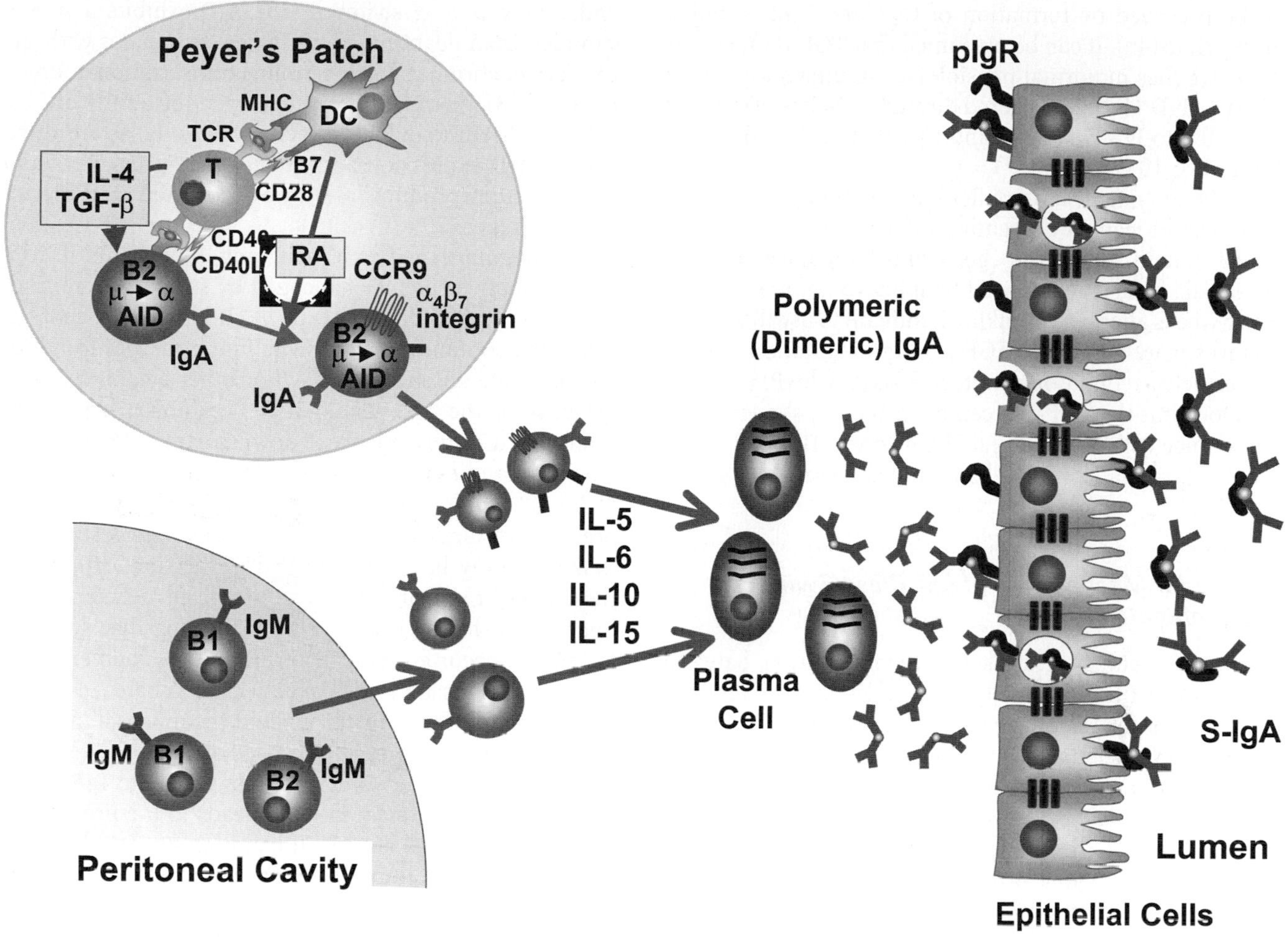

FIGURE 31.8 MALT-dependent and alternative pathways for the production of intestinal S-IgA Abs. In the MALT-dependent pathway (e.g., Peyer's patch), DCs take up luminal Ag via M cells, and then present the peptide to $CD4^+$ Th cells after intracellular processing of Ags in PPs. Ag-primed Th cells produce IL-4 and TGF-β, allowing B cells to undergo μ to α CSR. Simultaneously, retinoic acid (RA) produced by DCs increases gut homing receptors ($\alpha_4\beta_7$ integrin and CCR9) on Ag-primed IgA-committed B cells. In the LP, Th2 cell-derived IL-5 and IL-6 induce terminal differentiation of $sIgA^+$ B cells to become IgA-producing PCs secreting dimeric (or polymeric) forms of IgA. The dimeric IgA (dIgA) binds to the pIgR expressed on the basolateral surface of ECs and transports the dIgA into the lumen as S-IgA. In the alternative pathway, peritoneal B cells (mainly B1 cells) migrate into the LP, where they differentiate into IgA-producing PCs under the influence of IL-5 and IL-15.

T–B cell interactions support B cell switches and have postulated a major role for the CD40 receptor on GC B cells with CD40 L on activated T cells (66,69). Evidence for Tsw cells in human IgA responses has stemmed from an earlier study with T cell clones obtained from human appendix. These T cell clones and their derived culture supernatants exhibited preferential help for IgA synthesis (70).

Cytokines for IgA Class Switches

The most definitive studies to date suggest that several cytokines are involved in the B cell switching to IgA (66). The first studies showed that addition of TGF-β to LPS-triggered mouse splenic B cell cultures resulted in switching to IgA, and IgA synthesis was markedly enhanced by IL-2 (71) or IL-5 (72). It was also shown that TGF-β induced sterile Cα germline transcripts (72), an event that clearly precedes actual switching to IgA. Molecular pathways of TGF-β–induced Cα germline transcripts have been clarified (46). For example, transcriptional activation of the $C_H\alpha$ gene requires the TGF-β–mediated activation of Smad3/4 and the *de novo* synthesis of core-binding factor (CBF) α3 that binds to the Smad-binding elements (SBEs) and CBF sites on the intronic $C_H\alpha$ promoter region (46,66). Other studies showed that TGF-β induced human B cells to switch to either IgA1 or IgA2, an event clearly shown to be preceded by formation of Cα1 and Cα2 germline transcripts (46). It can be presumed that TGF-β induces μ to α switches in normal physiologic circumstances, since sIgM$^+$, sIgD$^+$ B cells triggered through CD40 were induced to switch to IgA by TGF-β and to secrete IgA in the presence of IL-10 (73,74).

Although one would predict that deletion of the TGF-β gene would lead to a negative influence on the IgA immune system, the TGF-β gene knockout mice unfortunately die from a generalized lymphoproliferative disease 3 to 5 weeks after birth, making it difficult to use this model to investigate the role of TGF-β in IgA regulation *in vivo*. Nevertheless, conditional mutagenesis (Cre/loxP) was used to knock out the TGF-β receptor in B cells, showing that these mice exhibited expanded peritoneal B1 cells and B cell hyperplasia in PPs and a complete absence of serum IgA (75).

Molecular Mechanisms of IgA Class Switch Recombination

Isotype switching involves the recombination between tandem repetitive DNA sequences (switch or S regions) located 5′ of the respective C_H genes. Switching is an irreversible DNA deletional event in which recombination between upstream and downstream S regions forms a DNA circle containing the deleted intervening C_H genes. Isotype switching can also be induced by cytokines in combination with activation signals provided by mitogens such as LPS or through the more physiological T cell CD40 L and B cell CD40 interactions as discussed earlier (46,66). Several tangible events, including demethylation of 5′ flanking region DNA, DNAse hypersensitivity, and transcription of unrearranged H chain genes, precede cytokine-induced switching. Germline transcription initiates 5′ of the targeted C_H gene upstream of so-called *I region exons* that contain stop codons in all translational reading frames, thus the resulting transcripts are "sterile." I exons have been identified for all isotypes and subclasses, and in general their deletion, for example, in I exon-knockout mice, results in impaired switching to that isotype or subclass (76). An apparent exception has been observed for IgA switching, where replacement of the Iα exon with an irrelevant human gene construct in the gene transcriptional orientation did not impair B cell switching to IgA (77). These studies rule out a direct role for the I exon in controlling switch recombination. However, transcription of the Cα locus was found to be constitutive in the Iα-targeted mice, in contrast to other I region KO mice. It seems likely that cytokine-induced germline transcripts themselves direct cytokine-regulated isotype switching (46,66).

A dramatic breakthrough in our understanding of CSR came with the discovery of the AID gene, initially identified in GC B cells and subsequently cloned from B lymphoma cells stimulated with CD40 L, IL-4, and TGF-β, which were undergoing μ to α switches (78). AID exhibits a single-stranded DNA deaminase activity and associates with the CSR target chromatin in a germline transcription-coupled manner (78). As may be expected given the ability of PPs, ILFs, and NALT to induce the generation of IgA-committed B cells, AID expression and Iα-Cμ circle transcripts and their reaction products are always detected in these inductive tissues (79).

The dogma that μ to α switching only occurs in mucosal inductive sites is challenged by several recent findings. Overexpression of AID in μ^+ B lymphoma cells resulted in spontaneous class switching from IgM to IgA in the complete absence of TGF-β or other cytokines. Mice defective in the AID gene (AID$^{-/-}$) exhibit a hyper IgM syndrome with no evidence of downstream switching (78). However, studies revealed that AID$^{-/-}$ mice have a subset of B220$^+$ sIgA$^+$ B cells in LP (an effector site) and the presence of circles of "looped out" DNA suggest that μ to α switching had just occurred in this site (80). Along these lines, it was also revealed that B cell–deficient μMT mice also exhibit LP IgA$^+$ PCs, suggesting that switches to IgA can occur even during preB cell development (81). Although this issue is still a subject of debate, μ to α B cell switches may occur throughout the mucosal immune system and in the complete absence of GCs.

In contrast to the dominant class switch to IgA in the PPs, B cell development in NALT leads to the production of both IgA and IgG (41,42). It had been previously established that the development of IgA-committed cells in the presence of TGF-β was characterized by sequential CSR from Cμ to Cα via a Cγ pathway-mediated by CD40 engagement (82). It is also interesting to note that human tonsils have been shown to contain a high frequency of IgG B cells in addition to IgA (83). These findings may explain the equal commitment of B cells to IgG and to IgA in NALT, but further analysis will be required to reveal the molecular mechanism involved in the generation of mucosal B cells with those two different isotypes.

Trafficking and Homing from Mucosal Inductive into Effector Sites

Following T cell priming and CSR to IgA-committed B cells through their interaction with DCs, both B and T cells emigrate from the inductive tissue (e.g., PPs and NALT), circulate through the bloodstream, and home to distant mucosal effector compartments, especially the LP regions of the GI, respiratory and reproductive tracts (Figure 31.8).

Several early studies demonstrated that lymphocytes circulated from blood to LNs and that thoracic duct lymphocytes were retained primarily in the intestine (50). A direct route for B cell migration between PPs and distant LP was revealed by the finding that rabbit GALT B cells repopulated the gut with IgA PCs (84). Further, the mesenteric lymph nodes (MLNs) of orally immunized animals were found to contain Ag-specific precursors of IgA PCs that repopulated the LP of gut and mammary, lacrymal, and salivary glands (50). Studies of the origin, migration, and homing of lymphoid cells from mucosal inductive to effector tissues were of basic importance for parallel attempts to induce Ag-specific immune responses. Consequently, specific Abs in glandular secretions could be induced in human and animal experiments by oral or bronchial immunization. These studies served as the basis for demonstrating the existence of a CMIS. This may explain the phenomena that immunization via one mucosal site often activates other, remote mucosal sites. However, immunization via certain mucosal inductive tissues can lead to the preferential induction of humoral immune responses in the same mucosal site, which is basically determined by site-specific combination of adhesion molecules and chemokines.

Recently, a lipid mediator, S1P has been identified as a key regulator of lymphocyte emigration from the organized lymphoid structures including the thymus and secondary lymphoid organs (85). Lymphocytes increase the S1P receptor, especially type 1 S1P receptor, when they emigrate from the secondary lymphoid organs, allowing them to emigrate from the lymphoid tissues to the blood where S1P is present in high concentrations (100 nM to 300 nM) (85). Several studies have now suggested that the S1P-mediated pathway is involved in the regulation of T cell emigration from mucosal inductive tissues (e.g., PPs) (85). In addition to T cells, it was recently found that B cell trafficking, especially IgA$^+$ plasmablasts, is selectively regulated by S1P in the emigration of B cells from the PPs and their entry into the macosal migration pathway for the final destination of LP (85a).

Lymphocyte Homing in the GI Tract

Lymphocytes enter mucosal or systemic lymphoid tissues from the blood through specialized HEVs, which consist of cuboidal endothelial cells. In GALT, HEVs are present in the interfollicular zones rich in T cells (41,42,50). The endothelial venules in effector sites such as the LP of the GI tract are less pronounced and tend to occur near villus crypt regions. Mucosal addressin cell adhesion molecule-1 (MAdCAM-1) is the most important addressin expressed by HEVs in the PPs and LP (Figure 31.9) (50). Likewise, peripheral lymph node addressin (PNAd) and vascular cell adhesion molecule (VCAM)-1 are the principal addressins expressed by peripheral lymph node (PLN) and skin HEVs, respectively. The major homing receptors expressed by lymphocytes are the integrins, a large class of molecules characterized by a heterodimeric structure of α and β chains. In general, the type of homing receptor is determined by the integrin expressed with the α_4 chain; the β_1 integrin characterizes the homing receptor for the skin and the β_7 integrin that for the GI tract. Thus, the pairing of α_4 with β_7 represents the major integrin molecule responsible for lymphocyte binding to MAdCAM-1 expressed on HEVs in the PPs and LP (Figure 31.9) (49). In addition to $\alpha_4\beta_7$ integrin, the C-type lectin family of selectins that includes L-, E-, and P-selectins, also serve as homing receptors. L-selectin has a high affinity for carbohydrate-containing PNAd, and this lectin addressin is of central importance in PLN homing of B and T cells (41,42,50). Despite this homing pair, L-selectin can also bind to carbohydrate-rich MAdCAM-1 and is an important initial receptor for homing into GALT HEVs. Interestingly, naïve B and T cells destined for GALT express L-selectin; moderate levels of $\alpha_4\beta_7$ ($\alpha_4\beta_7{}^+$) and memory lymphocytes destined for LP express higher levels of $\alpha_4\beta_7$ ($\alpha_4\beta_7^{\text{high}}$) and lack L-selectin (Figure 31.9). Similarly, human tissues revealed naïve T and B cells in HEVs, which expressed both L-selectin and $\alpha_4\beta_7$ integrin, while memory T and B cells in efferent lymphatics expressed $\alpha_4\beta_7$ integrin but not L-selectin (86). These data indicate that naïve and memory lymphocytes utilize a different regulation pathway for their migration into the GI tract.

In addition to the integrin-mediated regulation, chemokines have been directly involved in lymphocyte homing, and different chemokine-receptor pairs control migration into different lymphoid tissues (Figure 31.9) (50,85). For example, loss of secondary lymphoid tissue chemokine (SLC/CCL21) results in lack of naïve T cell or DC migration into PPs or spleen. Further, the chemokine receptor CCR4, which responds to the thymus activation-regulated chemokine (TARC/CCL17) and MΦ-derived chemokine (MDC/CCL22), mediates arrest of skin-homing T cells but does not affect $\alpha_4\beta_7^{\text{high}}$ T cell migration in the GI tract. However, gut-tropism, especially into the small intestine, is determined by the CCR9, selectively expressed on IgA-, but not IgM- or IgG-committed B cells (Figure 31.9) (50,85). The ligand of CCR9 is CCL25, also known as thymus-expressed chemokine TECK, which is produced dominantly by the small intestinal epithelium, determining the selective homing of sIgA$^+$ B cells into the small intestinal LP (50,85). Although the detailed mechanism remains to be investigated, it has been reported that the migration of sIgA$^+$ B cells to the large intestine may be due to the expression of MEC/CCL28 (50). Similarly, human memory T cell migration into the LP of the GI tract is mediated by the TECK/CCL25 expressed on intestinal epithelium, and gut-homing $\alpha_4\beta_7^{\text{high}}$ T cells specifically express CCR9 (50). In addition to the LP T cells, $\alpha_E\beta_7^+$ and $\alpha_4\beta_7^{\text{high}}$ IELs also expressed CCR9 in human and mouse, suggesting that TECK-CCR9 is also involved in lymphocyte homing and arrest of IEL in the small intestinal epithelium (50).

Several lines of evidence have suggested that GALT DCs play a crucial role in determining the gut tropism of T and B cells (Figure 31.8) (87). $\alpha_4\beta_7$ integrin and CCR9 were induced on Ag-primed T cells by GALT DCs, but not

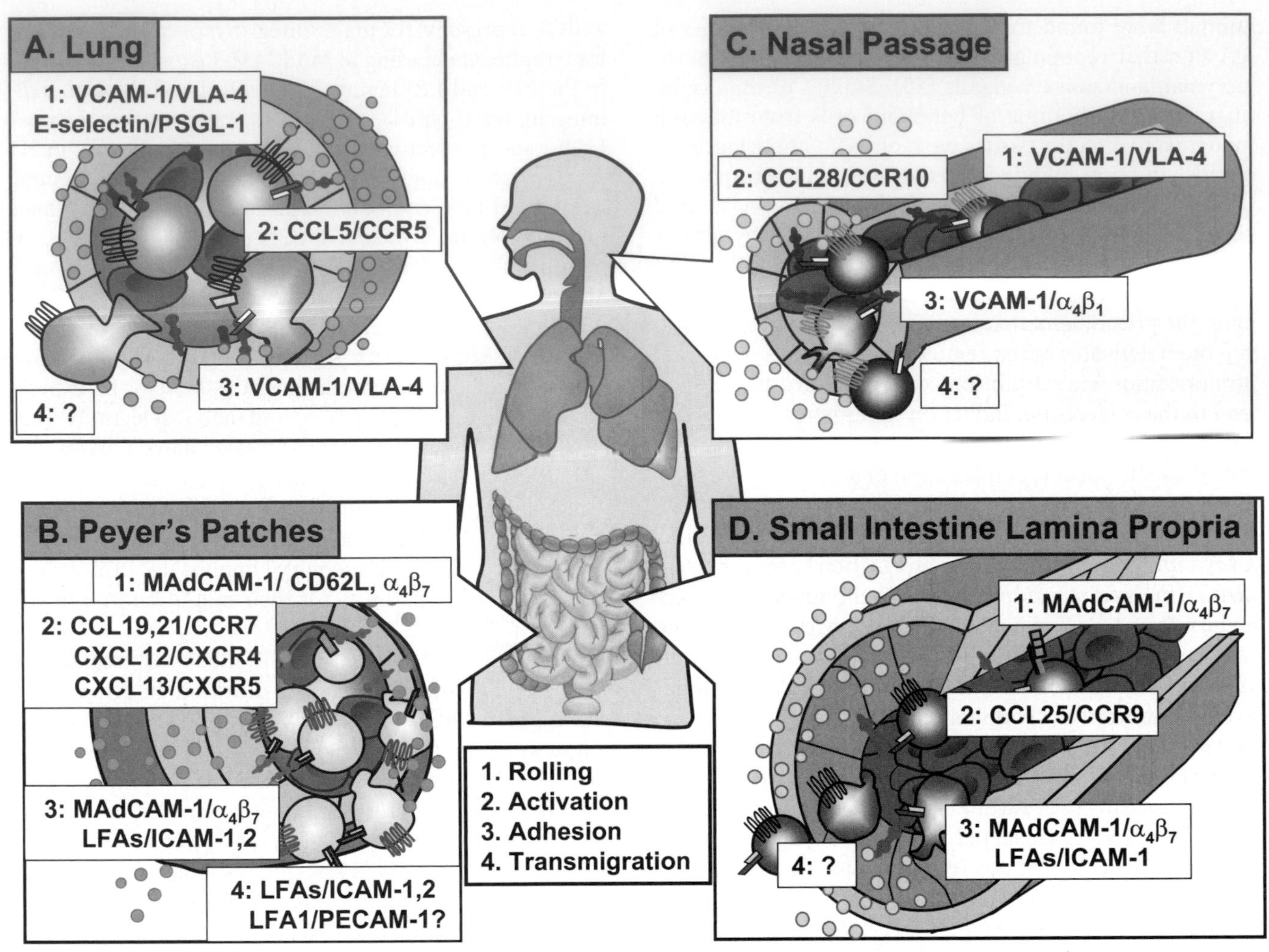

FIGURE 31.9 Mucosal lymphocyte migration-adhesion pathway. Lymphocyte migration is consistent with 1) rolling, 2) activation, 3) adhesion, and 4) transmigration or diapedesis. Effector/activated lymphocytes migrate to the mucosal effector sites, such as pulmonary tissue via the pulmonary vasculature (**A**), nasal passages (**C**), and intestinal LP (**D**) via endothelial venules. Naïve lymphocytes migrate into the PPs with interaction of lymphocytes and HEVs (MadCAM-1/$\alpha_4\beta_7$ integrin) in a chemokine-dependent pathway (e.g., CCL19, 21/CCR7 (T cells), CXCL12/CXCR4, CXCL13/CXCR5 (B cells) (**B**).

other DCs, respectively interacting with the MAdCAM-1 expressed by HEVs in the intestinal LP and the TECK/CCL25 produced by small IECs. Recent work has revealed that retinoic acid (RA) produced by GALT DCs is involved in the imprinting of T and B cells for gut homing (88,89). RA is a metabolite of vitamin A, and GALT DCs express RA-producing enzymes (alcohol dehydrogenases). Thus, significantly decreased numbers of gut T and B cells were noted in vitamin A–deficient mice (88,89).

Although $CD8^+$ CTLs utilize similar migration pathways into mucosal immune compartments, $CD8^+$ CTLs additionally migrate into the epithelium. This is reasonable because ECs are the primary cells infected with many viruses and bacteria and should be recognized by $CD8^+$ CTLs. Although mucosal effector tissues such as the intestinal epithelium contain high numbers of $\gamma\delta$ T cells as key players in innate immunity as mentioned earlier (25), virus-specific CTLs in IELs greatly contribute to the acquired phase of immunosurveillance in the epithelium itself. The homing of IELs into the epithelium is also determined by the adhesion molecules and chemokines (25). Like migration of other T cells into the intestinal compartment, CCR9 play an important role in the determination of IEL trafficking into the epithelium. In addition, the various chemokine receptors expressed on IELs, such as CCR3, CCR4, CCR5, and CXCR3, may play pivotal roles in the alternative pathway of IEL trafficking (Figure 31.9) (25). The $\alpha_4\beta_7$ integrin also contributes to the regulation of IEL trafficking. Thus, β_7 integrin-deficient mice showed critically reduced numbers of IELs in the intestine (49). Integrin-mediated interactions between IECs and IELs play a pivotal role not only in the migration of the IELs into the intestine, but also in the retention of IELs at the epithelium. CD103 (α_E integrin) is exclusively expressed on IELs; it interacts with E-cadherin expressed on ECs (Figure 31.9) (26). It was previously reported that TGF-β induced down-regulation of $\alpha_4\beta_7$ integrin and simultaneously up-regulated CD103. Thus, $\alpha_4\beta_7$ integrin expression was reduced following IEL entry into the small intestinal epithelium, a reduction that coincided with an increase in CD103 expression (87). In addition to the TGF-β–mediated pathway, a recent study proposed that CCR9-mediated signaling promoted the induction of CD103, a retention molecule of IELs in the epithelium (87).

Lymphocyte Homing in NALT and Lung-associated Tissues

Unlike PP HEVs, which are found in T cell zones, murine NALT HEVs are found in B cell zones and express PNAd either alone or associated with MAdCAM-1 (Figure 31.9) (41,42). Further, anti-L-selectin but not anti-MAdCAM-1 Abs blocked the binding of naïve lymphocytes to NALT HEVs, suggesting predominant roles for both L-selectin and PNAd. Consistent with this, the failure of human tonsillar cells to demonstrate selective $\alpha_4\beta_7$ expression and the lack of MAdCAM-1 expression on tonsil or adenoid HEVs make it likely that gut-homing does not extend to human NALT and associated LNs. However, nasal immunization induces up-regulation of $\alpha_4\beta_1$ integrin and CCR10, allowing selective trafficking of B cells to nasal passage epithelium expressing their ligands, VCAM-1 and CCL28, respectively (Figure 31.9) (41,42). It is interesting to note that the same molecules are involved in the trafficking to the genitourinary tract (41,42), which may explain why high levels of Ag-specific immune responses are induced in the genital tract after nasal immunization (Figure 31.9).

Early induction of VCAM-1, E-selectin, and P-selectin in the pulmonary vasculature was reported during pulmonary immune responses with an initially increased expression of P-selectin ligand by peripheral blood CD4$^+$ and CD8$^+$ T cells (50). The number of cells expressing P-selectin ligand then declined in the blood as they accumulated in the bronchoalveolar lavage fluid. The very late antigen (VLA-4) could be an important adhesion molecule involved in the migration of activated T cells into the lung since migration of VLA-4$^+$ cells into bronchoalveolar fluid is impaired following treatment with anti-α_4 Ab. Other investigators have shown that Ag-specific L-selectin^{low} CTL effectors rapidly accumulate in the lung following adoptive transfer to naïve mice with reduced pulmonary viral titers early during infection.

An interesting approach used to address the homing of human cells in the NALT was the analysis of tissue-specific adhesion molecules after systemic, enteric, or nasal immunization (90). This study showed that following systemic immunization, most effector B cells expressed L-selectin, with only few cells expressing $\alpha_4\beta_7$, while after enteric (oral or rectal) immunization the opposite held true. Interestingly, effector B cells induced by nasal immunization displayed a more promiscuous pattern of adhesion molecules with a large majority of these cells expressing both L-selectin and $\alpha_4\beta_7$ integrin.

S-IgA Formation and Transport

Distribution of Ig Isotypes

Measurement of combined synthesis of Ig of all isotypes indicates that in a 70 kg individual, around 8 g of Ig are produced every day (Table 31.1) (91). Divided by individual isotypes, humans produce ~5 g IgA, ~2.5 g IgG, ~0.6 g IgM, and trace amounts of IgD and IgE per day. Approximately one half of IgA is internally catabolized mainly in the liver, and the remainder is actively and passively transported into external secretions (91). It is estimated that ~50% to 70% of total IgA is selectively transported into external secretions; daily, over 3 g of IgA are deposited on a large surface area of mucosal membranes. Studies that addressed the tissue origin of S-IgA demonstrated that ~99% is produced locally in mucosal tissues and glands. Extensive studies of the distribution of Ig-producing cells in various mucosal tissues and glands by the immunofluorescence technique and ELISPOT convincingly

TABLE 31.1 Levels of Immunoglobulins in Human External Secretions (μg/ml)[a]

	IgA	IgG	IgM
Tears	80–400	trace-16	0–18
Nasal fluid	70–846	8–304	0
Parotid saliva[b]	15–319	0.4–5	0.4
Whole saliva	194–206	42	64
Bronchoalveolar fluid	3	13	0.1
Colostrum and milk	470–12,340	40–168	50–610
Hepatic bile	58–77	88–140	6–18
Gallbladder bile	92	12	46
Duodenal fluid	313	104	207
Jejunal fluid	32–276	4–340	2
Colonic fluid	240–827	1	trace-860
Intestinal fluid[c]	166	4	8
Urine	0.1–1.0	0.06–0.56	
Ejaculate	11–23	16–33	0–8
Cervical fluid	3–133	1–285	5–118
Vaginal fluid	35	52	

[a] High variability in Ig levels is due to the method of collection, dilution of specimens by lavage fluids, methods of measurements, including the use of appropriate standards (S-IgA versus monomeric IgA) flow rates and stimulation of secretions, hormonal states, and the health status of the individual.
[b] Unstimulated or stimulated.
[c] Whole gut lavage.

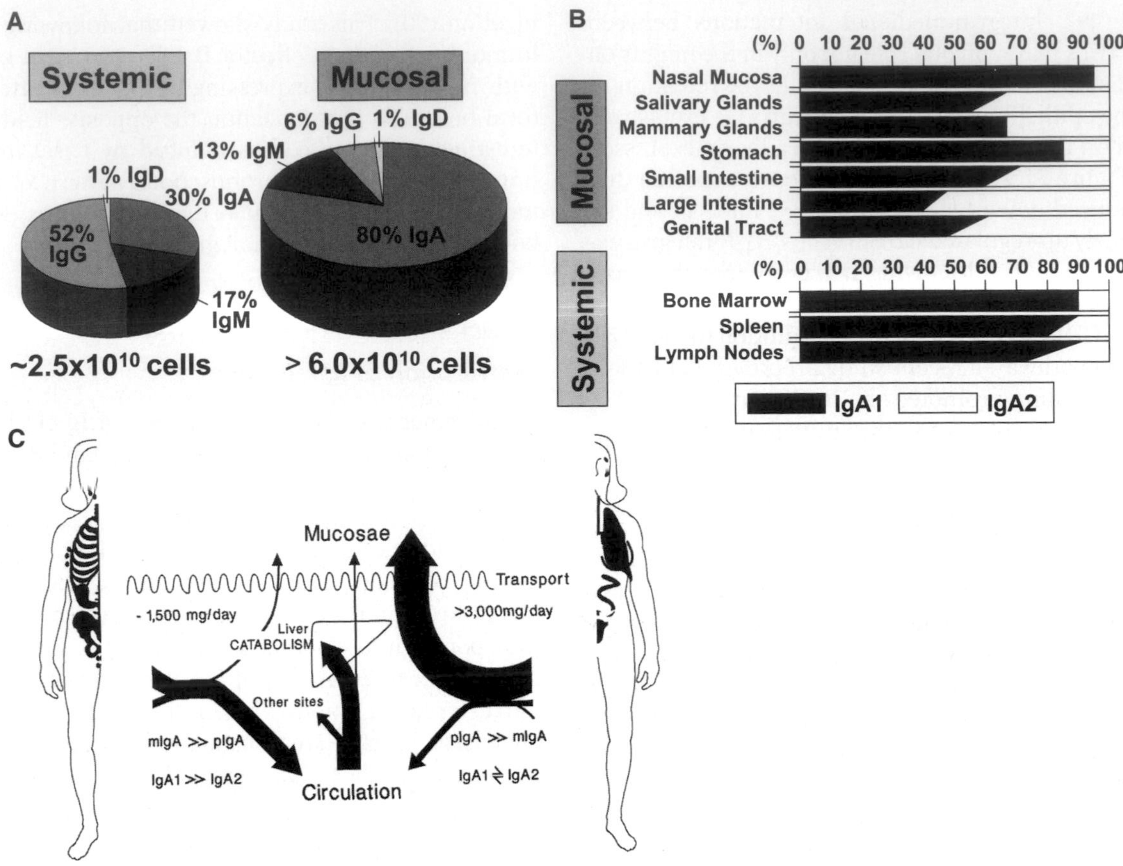

FIGURE 31.10 Comparative distribution of human B cells in systemic and mucosal compartments. **A:** Quantitative distribution and Ig isotypes. **B:** Distribution of IgA subclasses. **C:** Distribution and properties of IgA produced in the systemic and mucosal compartments.

demonstrated a remarkable preponderance of IgA-producing cells in all such tissues (Figure 31.10A) (46). The only exception is the uterine cervix, where the numbers of IgG-producing cells are equal or slightly exceed IgA-producing cells (91). However, there are tissue-specific differences in the proportions of IgA-, IgG-, IgM-, and IgD-positive PCs. For example, nasal mucosa contains on average 69% IgA-, 17% IgG-, 6% IgD-, and 6% IgM-positive cells, while in the large intestine 90% of cells are positive for IgA, 6% for IgM, and 4% for IgG (46). Moreover, cells producing IgA1 or IgA2 also display a characteristic tissue distribution (Figure 31.10B) (46,91). Systemic lymphoid tissues (e.g., spleen, tonsils, LNs, and bone marrow), as well as most of the mucosal tissues (nasal, gastric, and small intestinal mucosa and to a lesser degree glandular tissues) contain more IgA1- than IgA2-producing cells, while in the large intestine and the female genital tract tissues, IgA2-producing cells are more frequent than IgA1 cells (Figure 31.10B). Although direct experimental evidence is not available, it has been speculated that this tissue-specific distribution of IgA1- or IgA2-producing cells is related to the differences in the origin of IgA1 and IgA2 precursors and perhaps their distinct homing patterns. Alternatively, Ag-driven clonal expansion in various mucosal tissues may also be involved. For example, most of the naturally occurring S-IgA Abs to bacterial endotoxin is associated with the IgA2 isotype (91). Thus, it is likely that endotoxin abundantly present in the large intestine induces clonal expansion of IgA2-producing cells in this locale.

Distribution of Polymeric or Monomeric IgA-Producing Cells

Analyses of molecular forms of IgA in supernatants of cells and tissue explants obtained from systemic and mucosal compartments, tissue perfusates, and immunohistochemical studies of such tissue demonstrated that the separate populations of pIgA- and monomeric IgA (mIgA)-secreting cells display a characteristic tissue distribution (46,91). Typically, almost all IgA-producing cells in the normal bone marrow produce mIgA (Figure 31.10C). The admixture of peripheral blood in the bone marrow specimens grossly influences the results because peripheral blood lymphocytes secrete, especially after stimulation, predominantly pIgA and little mIgA (92). Supernatants collected from *in vitro* cultured human LNs and spleen contained both forms, usually with the preponderance of mIgA. In contrast, such supernatants or perfusates of mucosal tissues, especially in the GI tract, contain pIgA as the dominant form (Figure 31.10C).

Structure of Secretory IgA (S-IgA)

When compared to its serum counterpart, IgA in external secretions (called S-IgA) displays unique structural features with respect to its molecular form, chain composition, and IgA subclass distribution (91). Examinations of sera and mucosal secretions, culture supernatants, and cell lysates, and immunohistochemical studies of systemic and mucosal lymphoid tissues indicated that pIgA contains joining (J) chain as a typical component and that J chain–containing pIgA is capable of binding to pIgR and its extracellular region, SC (9). Consequently, the presence of intracellular J chain and the ability to bind SC have been taken as markers for pIgA- or IgM-producing cells. In humans, almost all serum IgA is present in a monomeric form (sedimentation constant 7S) and contains two heavy (α) and two light (either κ or λ) chains, and ~85% belongs to the IgA1 and ~15% to the IgA2 subclass. Only a small but variable fraction (1% to 10%) of serum IgA is found in a polymeric form and contains an additional polypeptide-joining (J) chain. In contrast, ~90% of S-IgA occurs in a polymeric form (dimers and tetramers with sedimentation constants 11S and 15.5S, respectively) and is associated with J chain acquired during the transepithelial transport via the pIgR. The structure of a typical dimeric IgA molecule is shown in Figure 31.11. Two mIgA molecules are mutually linked by disulfide bridges through their Fc regions; J chain is bound to the penultimate Cys residues of α chains. Although SC interacts noncovalently with the Fc regions of both monomers, it is attached by disulfide bridges to only one of them, and there are no covalent bonds formed between J chain and SC.

Mammalian α chains with molecular mass ~50 kDa contain one variable and three constant region domains. There are high numbers of Cys residues involved in the formation of intrachain and interchain disulfide bridges with another α chain, L and J chains, and SC (91). In addition, α chains can form complexes with a number of plasma and secretory proteins including albumin, amylase, lactoferrin, glycosyltransferases, and proteolytic enzymes. An unusual hinge region is present in the middle of the α chain of IgA1, between Cα1 and Cα2 domains (46,91). This 13 amino acid–long hinge region is reminiscent of mucin (high content of Pro, Ser, and Thr residues) and carries 3-5 *O*-linked oligosaccharide side chains (Figure 31.11). Although IgA is quite resistant to common proteolytic enzymes, the hinge region contains peptide bonds susceptible to the cleavage by highly substrate-specific IgA1 proteases of bacterial origin (e.g., *Streptococcus pneumoniae, Neisseria meningitidis, N. gonorrhoeae, Haemophilus influenzae,* and several other species of bacteria) (93). Comparative structural and genetic studies of IgA molecules from many species indicate that molecules of the IgA2 subclass represent phylogenetically older forms and that the IgA1 subclass arose in hominoid primates by insertion of a gene segment encoding the hinge region (91). The Fcα region, particularly its C terminus, displays a high degree of sequence homology to the μ chain of IgM, including the characteristic C terminae "tail" (an ~18 amino acid extension over the C terminus of γ, δ, and ε chains of corresponding Ig isotypes) involved in the polymerization and ability of α and μ chains to bind J chain. Both IgA1 and IgA2 contain 6% to 8% of glycans associated in the form of ~2 to 5 *N*-linked side chains within the Fc region; as described earlier, the hinge region of IgA1 also contains *O*-linked glycans (91).

J chain is a chacteristic polypeptide chain present in pIgA and IgM (94). It has a molecular mass of 15 kDa

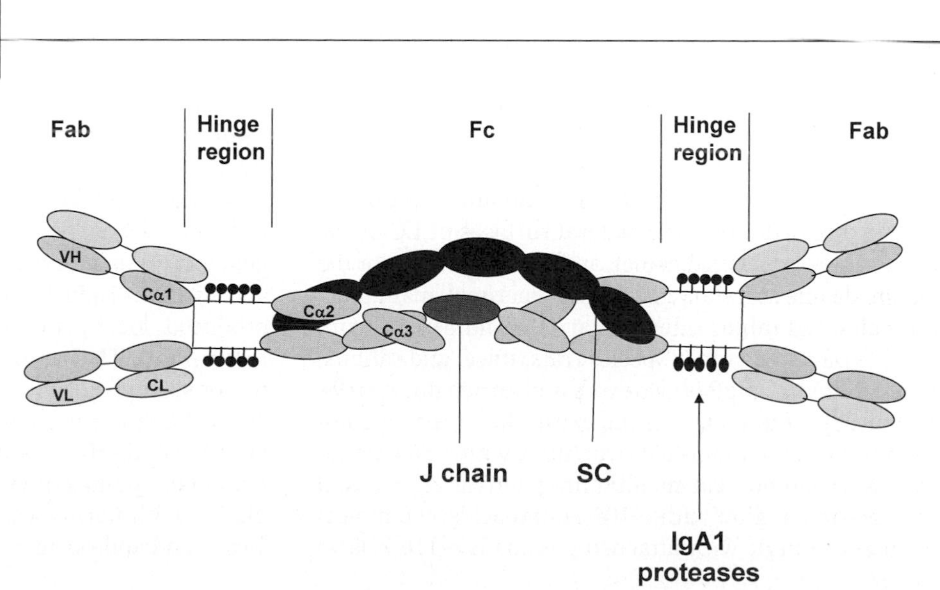

FIGURE 31.11 Molecular dimensions, proteolytic fragments, and domain structure of the human dimeric S-IgA1 molecule. Dimeric or polymeric IgA was formed by joining each IgA by J chain. The dimeric or polymeric forms of IgA are associated with SC, an extracellular domain of pIgR. Hinge region between Fab and Fc is a target site of IgA1 proteases.

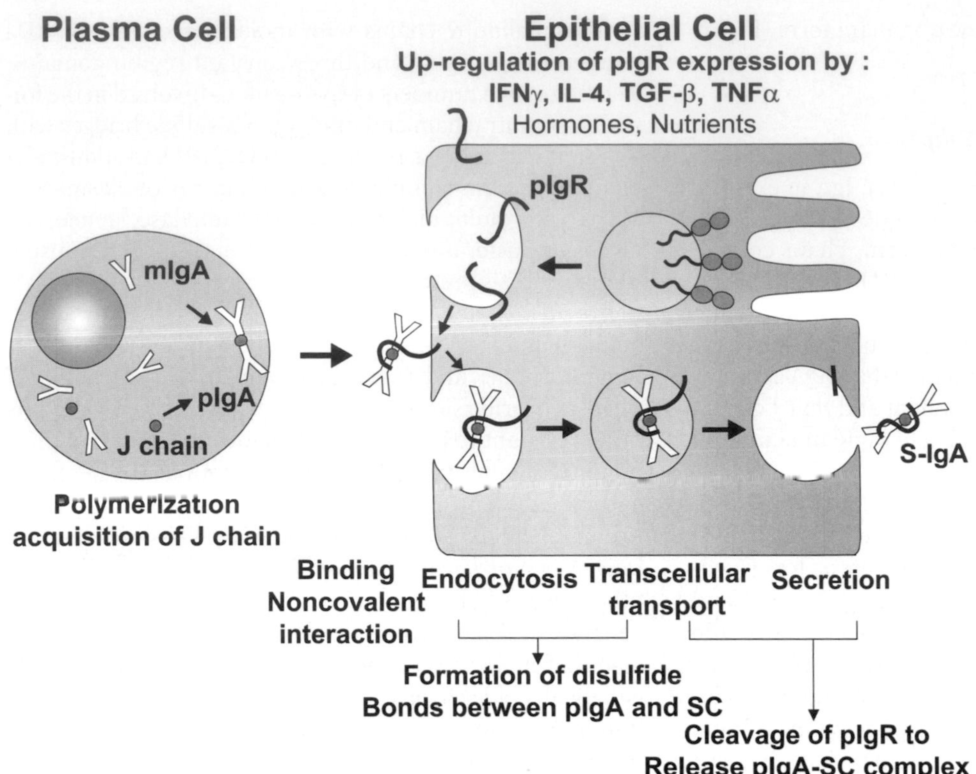

FIGURE 31.12 12 Transcellular transport of pIgA (or dIgA) by the pIgR-mediated mechanism and regulation of pIgR expression. Subepithelial PCs produce J chain–associated pIgA that interacts with the epithelial pIgR, and the pIgA-pIgR complex is transcytosed through the epithelial cells and released, after the proteolytic clevage of pIgR, as S-IgA.

and a single *N*-linked glycan chain and displays an Ig domain folding pattern. Of eight Cys residues, six are involved in three intrachain disulfide bridges, and two participate in linkages to the penultimate Cys residues of α and μ chains. A very high degree of homology exists in the primary structures and antigenic cross-reactivities of mammalian and avian J chains, indicating that the basic properties have remained conserved throughout evolution (91). PCs in mucosal effector tissues and glands assemble pIgA intracellularly from mIgA and J chain as a last step before its externalization (Figure 31.12). Although the incorporation of J chain is not absolutely required for polymerization, the ability of pIgA and IgM to interact with pIgR expressed on ECs or SC depends on the presence of J chain as demonstrated in J chain knockout mice (95).

The pIgR specific for the J chain-containing pIgA and IgM is expressed on the basolateral surfaces of EC of the GI tract and endocervix, acinar, and ductal epithelia of the small and large secretory glands (e.g., lacrimal, mammary, and major and minor salivary glands) in humans (Figure 31.12) (9). In some other species (rats, mice, and rabbits, but not humans), pIgR is also expressed on hepatocytes (9). Structurally, pIgR comprises an extracellular region composed of five Ig domain-like structures, with ~560 amino acids, a 23 amino acid membrane-spanning region, and a cytoplasmic region with ~103 amino acids; the molecular mass of pIgR with attached glycans is ~110 kDa to 120 kDa. The similarity of the general structural features of pIgR from a number of mammalian species indicates that this receptor and its ability to interact with pIg are conserved in phylogeny.

The N-terminal domain of pIgR interacts with Cα domains (9). The pIgA-pIgR complex is internalized, transcytosed, and finally released at the apical end of the ECs with the entire process taking ~30 minutes (Figure 31.12). Signals for basolateral targeting of pIgR, its endocytosis, and its transcytosis are encoded in the cytoplasmic region of pIgR as revealed by deletion mutants. In the final steps, pIgR is proteolytically cleaved, thus releasing the pIgA-SC complex; the intracellular and transmembrane regions are endocytosed and degraded or released from the apex. Unlike several other receptors, pIgR does not recycle; instead, it remains permanently associated with the ligand as bound SC (9). Therefore, the transport of pIgA and IgM is directly dependent on the availability of pIgR on EC (or hepatocyte) membranes. A number of substances of local and distant origin influence pIgR expression. Cytokines produced locally in mucosal tissues and glands (e.g., IFN-γ, IL-4, TNF-α, and TGF-β) up-regulate in an additive or synergistic pattern the expression of pIgR on established EC lines, usually of intestinal or endometrial origin (9). Similarly, ECs from the female genital tract and mammary gland express pIgR as a consequence of stimulation with hormones, particularly with estrogens, prolactin, and androgens.

Other IgA Receptors

The Fc region of IgA can interact with other receptors expressed on structurally and functionally diverse cell populations including monocytes/MΦ/mesangial cells, PMNs, granulocytes, ECs, hepatocytes, B and T cells, and PCs (96). Some of these receptors have been structurally defined and specific reagents are now available for their detection.

The best-characterized receptor expressed on monocytes, neutrophils, and eosinophils recognizes Fcα regions of both IgA1 and IgA2 with a certain degree of preference for pIgA, probably due to the presence of multiple binding sites on pIgA. This Fcα receptor, designated as FcαRI (CD89) and detectable by monoclonal Abs, occurs in several isoforms and is heavily glycosylated (96). Another study indicates that CD89 is present in minute quantities also in the circulation in complexes with high molecular mass IgA (96). Additionally, eosinophils, but not PMNs, express a receptor for SC, suggesting that S-IgA has the potential to stimulate eosinophils through an interaction with SC. Detailed analysis of the molecular properties of such complexes revealed that FcαRI and IgA were covalently linked, but the high molecular mass IgA complexes lacked J chain; it can be speculated that the soluble FcαRI is linked to the binding site occupied in pIgA by J chain.

Binding studies indicate that the sites of interactions include the first extracellular domain of FcαRI and the boundary between the Cα2 and Cα3 domains of IgA heavy chains (96). Cross-linking of FcαRI on cell surfaces triggers phagocytosis, superoxide generation, and release of inflammatory mediators from PMNs, eosinophils, and MΦ (Table 31.2). A receptor specific for the Fc regions of IgA and IgM has been described and designated as Fcα/μR (97). However, the biological function of the receptor remains to be elucidated.

It has been previously reported that the transferrin receptor (CD71) is surprisingly effective in binding IgA1 molecules, especially in their monomeric form (98). Because the binding of IgA1 is inhibitable by transferrin, it appears that this novel receptor binds two structurally highly dissimilar ligands—transferrin as well as IgA1. Although the function of this receptor remains to be determined, its expression on intestinal ECs suggests it may be involved in the appearance of mIgA in GI tract secretions.

TABLE 31.2 Functions/Biological Properties of IgA

Protective Functions in External Secretions
Prevention of Ag absorption from mucosal surfaces due to the formation of Ag-IgA complexes
Mucus trapping (IgA-mucin complexes entrap microorganisms)
Virus neutralization (in some experiments nonneutralizing Abs may also be protective)
Enzyme and toxin neutralization
Enhancement of antimicrobial activities of innate factors (e.g., lysozyme, lactoperoxidase, and lactoferrin)
Biological Activities in Tissues
Inhibition of C activation in some experiments (polymeric IgA or glycan-altered IgA may activate complement by the alternative or lectin pathways)
Enhancement (opsonization) or inhibition of phagocytosis
Inhibition of type I and II hypersensitivity reactions (e.g., anaphylaxis and Arthus reaction)
Degranulation of eosinophils
Intracellular virus neutralization
Elimination of Ag-IgA immune complexes by ECs and hepatocytes expressing IgA receptors
Ab-dependent cell-mediated cytotoxicity
Inhibition of NK cell activity
Regulation of the release of inflammatory cytokines

T Cell Help for IgA Production

Earlier studies revealed that addition of culture supernatants from DC-T cell clusters, T cell clones, or T cell hybridomas to cultures of PP or splenic B cells resulted in enhanced secretion of IgA (99). One factor responsible for this activity was subsequently shown to be IL-5 (Figure 31.8) (66,72). Removal of sIgA$^+$ B cells from PP B cell cultures abrogated IgA synthesis, demonstrating that this cytokine affected postswitched IgA-committed B cells (100). If splenic B cells were used, these cells required stimulation with LPS before increased IgA secretion occurred. Taken together, these results suggest that IL-5 induces sIgA$^+$ B cells that are in cell cycle (blasts) to differentiate into IgA-producing cells. Human IL-5 is thought to act mainly as an eosinophil differentiation factor and thus may have little effect on B cell isotype switching and differentiation. It has been reported, however, that human B cells, when stimulated with the bacterium *Moraxella (Branhamella) catarrhalis,* could be induced by IL-5 to secrete IgA, and also to possibly undergo isotype switching to IgA (99). This effect could not be demonstrated using other more conventional B cell mitogens, a finding that demonstrates the importance of the primary *in vitro* activation signal for B cell switching.

IL-6, when added to PP B cells in the absence of any *in vitro* stimulus, causes a marked increase in IgA secretion with little effect on either IgM or IgG synthesis (46,66). IL-6–induced two- to three-fold more IgA secretion than IL-5 (101). The removal of sIgA$^+$ B cells abolished the effect of IL-6, demonstrating that like IL-5, this cytokine also acted on postswitched B cells. In IL-6$^{-/-}$ mice, the numbers of IgA$^+$ B cells in the LP were markedly reduced, and Ab responses following mucosal challenge with OVA or vaccinia virus were greatly diminished (102). It was shown that human appendix sIgA$^+$ B cells express IL-6 receptors, while other B cell subsets do not. Further, appendix B cells were induced by IL-6 to secrete both IgA1 and IgA2 in the absence of any *in vitro* activation (103). This effect was also shown in IgA-committed B cells, again demonstrating the importance of IL-6 for inducing the terminal differentiation of $sIgA^+$ B cells into IgA-producing PCs (Figure 31.8).

An additional Th2 cytokine, IL-10, has also been shown to play an important role in the induction of IgA synthesis in humans (46,66). Stimulation of human B cells with anti-CD40 and *Staphylococcus aureus* Cowan (SAC) resulted in B cell differentiation for IgM and IgG synthesis in patients with IgA deficiency. Further, naïve $sIgD^+$ B cells could be induced to produce IgA after co-culture with IL-10 in the presence of TGF-β and anti-CD40 (74). Taken together, these findings demonstrate that Th2 cytokines such as IL-5, IL-6, and IL-10 all play major roles in the induction of IgA responses by the generation of IgA-producing cells (Figure 31.8).

Since IL-2 has been shown to enhance IgA synthesis in LPS-stimulated B cell cultures, it would be too simplistic to conclude that Th2-type cells and their derived cytokines are the only elements important in the generation of IgA responses. IL-2 also synergistically augmented IgA synthesis in B cell cultures in the presence of LPS and TGF-β (46,66). Although IFN-γ is not directly involved in the enhancement of IgA B cell responses, this cytokine has been shown to enhance the expression of pIgR, an essential molecule for the transport of S-IgA (9). In summary, an optimal relationship between Th1- and Th2-derived cytokines is essential for the induction, regulation and maintenance of appropriate IgA responses in mucosa-associated tissues.

Further, a helper function of IELs has been proposed for support of IgA synthesis (104). Thus, IELs may be actively involved in the induction and regulation of S-IgA Ab responses at mucosal surfaces. It was shown that the numbers of IgA-producing cells in mucosa-associated tissues, such as the intestinal LP of $TCR\gamma\delta^{-/-}$ mice, was significantly lower than that observed in control ($TCR\gamma\delta^{+/+}$) mice of the same genetic background (104). In contrast, identical numbers of IgM- and IgG-producing cells were found in systemic compartments of $TCR\gamma\delta^{-/-}$ and $TCR\gamma\delta^{+/+}$ mice. Further, when $TCR\gamma\delta^{-/-}$ mice were orally immunized with tetanus toxoid (TT) plus cholera toxin (CT) as mucosal adjuvant, significantly lower IgA anti-TT Ab responses were induced in PPs and LP when compared with identically treated $TCR\gamma\delta^{+/+}$ mice. These findings indicate that $\gamma\delta$ T cells are involved in the induction and regulation of Ag-specific IgA Ab responses in both mucosal and systemic compartments.

ALTERNATIVE INDUCTION PATHWAY FOR MUCOSAL IMMUNITY

Although the MALT (e.g., PP and NALT)-mediated pathway is a major mechanism for the induction of Ag-specific mucosal immune responses, an alternative way (or MALT-independent pathway) exists for the induction of appropriate productive immunity at mucosa-associated tissues. This is supported by the fact that Ag-specific immune responses have been induced in PP- and/or ILF-null mice following oral immunization (41,42). Indeed, a number of those pathways have been identified, especially in the GI tract at the levels of Ag sampling and S-IgA Ab production.

Other Ag Sampling Systems in the Intestinal Epithelium

In the MALT-independent acquired immune system, the epithelium is also likely to play an important role as alternative Ag-sampling routes. At least three different scenarios have been offered regarding the alternative Ag-sampling routes in the epithelium. First, M cells were identified on the intestinal villous epithelium (villous M cells), not in proximity to PPs (Figure 31.4) (105). Villous M cells developed in various PP/ILF-null mice and are capable of taking up bacteria, such as *Salmonella*, *Yersinia*, and invasin-expressing *Escherichia coli* (105). A recent study has suggested that villous M cells locate closer to the upper half of the villus and are preferentially observed in the terminal ileum when compared with other parts of the small intestine, suggesting that the microbiota influences villous M cell development (106). In addition, villous M cells are present in mice lacking both B and T cells, indicating that villous M cell differentiation and maintenance does not require lymphocytes (106).

A second route for Ag uptake is the EC itself. As mentioned earlier, ECs are involved in innate immunity by expressing nonclassical MHC molecules that can be sensed by $\gamma\delta$ IEL and NK cells (25,27,37). In addition, there is evidence to suggest that ECs could process and then present Ags to T cells via MHC class I as well as class II molecules in humans and rodents (37). The presentation by MHC class II exhibits polarity with uptake of Ag primarily apical and presentation basal under normal noninflammatory conditions and in inflammatory conditions when MHC class II expression is enhanced through the action of the MHC class II transactivator, CIITA (37). Under normal circumstances, ECs do not express classical costimulatory molecules such as CD80 and CD86 but may do so, at least in the case of CD86, in the context of intestinal inflammation (37). However, intestinal ECs express a number of potential costimulatory molecules, which, in certain circumstances, are functional. For example, LFA-3 or CD58 is constitutively expressed on ECs *in vivo* and *in vitro*, is upregulated in response to inflammation, and may provide crucial costimulatory signals to mucosal T cells through its ligand, CD2, which is constitutively expressed on mucosal T cells (107).

Recent studies identified various DC populations in the unorganized intestine (Figure 31.4). Among them are DCs located between intestinal ECs. These intraepithelial

DCs are frequent in the terminal ileum and express TJ-associated proteins (e.g., occuludin, claudin 1, and *zona occuludens* 1), and thus are capable of extending their dendritic arms into the lumen via the TJ between ECs (108). A previous study had already demonstrated that CD18-expressing phagocytes were involved in an M cell–independent pathway for bacterial invasion (109). A recent study has revealed that these intraepithelial DCs are characterized by the expression of CX_3CR1 and that the interaction between CX_3CR1 and its ligand fractalkine/CX_3CL1 is required for extension of transepithelial dendrites into the epithelium (110). Once intraepithelial DCs take up luminal Ags, it is likely that they leave the epithelium and migrate into the LP or draining LNs for the presentation of Ag to T cells.

A recent study has demonstrated that Ag/IgG complexes from the intestinal lumen can be taken up into the LP across intestinal ECs through FcRn *in vivo* (10,37). These transported Ag/IgG complexes may be captured by LP DCs because they express FcRn (10). In addition to sampling a wide variety of foreign Ags, the mucosal immune system must contend with the high number of apoptotic ECs that result from the frequency with which the epithelium is replaced. Although most of these apoptotic ECs are shed by the epithelium to the lumen, some of these apoptotic ECs have been shown to be potentially immunogenic and transportable to T cell areas of MLNs by mucosal DCs (111).

Contribution of B1 Cells for Mucosal IgA Responses

In addition to conventional B cells (or B2 cells) located in MALTs (e.g., PPs), peritoneal B1 cells have been considered to be a precursor of intestinal IgA PCs (112,113). B1 and B2 cells can be distinguished by their cell surface molecules (*e.g.*, B220, IgM, IgD, CD5, and Mac-1), origins, and growth properties (112). Further, B1 cells exhibit different V_H repertoires and Ig specificities, and they are thought to be specialized in responding to T cell–independent Ag conserved on common pathogens like DNA and phosphatidylcholine, while B2 cells recognize most T-dependent protein Ags (112). Consistent with this notion, IgA production from B1 cells was noted in MHC class II–deficient mice as well as TCR β and δ chain–deficient mice (114,115). Of note, about 65% of fecal bacteria were reactive with B1 cell–derived IgA, and 30% of bacteria were bound with B2 cell-derived IgA, indicating that S-IgA derived from B1 cells recognized a large population of commensal bacteria as well as pathogenic bacteria (112).

B1 and B2 cell responses have distinct IgA-associated cytokine requirements. It was shown that IL-5, a well-known IgA-enhancing cytokine, and IL-15 are also involved in the proliferation and differentiation of B1 but not of B2 cells into IgA-producing cells (113). Thus, mucosal EC-derived IL-15 promoted the proliferation and differentiation of B1 cells into IgA-producing cells. Based upon these findings, it appears that intestinal B1 cells migrate presumably from the peritoneal cavity into mucosal effector sites, where they further differentiate into IgA-producing PCs under the influence of IL-5 and IL-15 for IgA production against T-independent Ags and commensal microbiota-associated Ags.

Although precisely where CSR might occur for B1 cells is an unresolved issue, several lines of evidence have demonstrated B1 cell migration into intestinal LP. Using *aly/aly* mice that carried a point mutation in the NIK, there was a complete absence of B cell populations in the intestinal LP, but elevated B cell levels were seen in the peritoneal cavity (54). In this context, another report proposed that the migratory pathway of B1 cells to the peritoneal cavity depended upon the BCL/CXCL13 produced by peritoneal MΦ (85). These results imply that the NFKB-inducing kinase (NIK)-mediated pathway is involved in the B1 cell mucosal migration, which may be dependent on specific but not yet identified chemokine receptor(s). Additionally, a recent study showed that peritoneal B cells express comparable levels of the receptor for S1P, a lipid mediator, and that S1P plays an important role in the regulation of peritoneal B cell trafficking into the intestine (116). It was also previously reported that B1 cells existed in nasal passages (113), but the actual molecular machinery for B1 cell migration into nasal passages remains an open question. These findings suggested the presence of a unique migration mechanism for the continuous supply of B1 cells as a part of a MALT-independent mucosal immunity.

MICROBIAL MUCOSAL IMMUNE SYSTEM

Protection

Mucosal Igs

Large amounts of Ig are delivered onto mucosal surfaces as a result of receptor-mediated transepithelial transport and passive transudation of plasma-derived Igs. Depending upon the species as well as type of external secretion, IgA, IgM, and IgG are present in variable proportions (Table 31.1). Igs of all of these isotypes provide, by different mechanisms, protection against pathogenic microorganisms, interact with commensal microbiota, and interfere with the absorption of undigested food Ags from the large surface area of the digestive tract.

The dominant presence of S-IgA has several important functional advantages that render Abs of this isotype and molecular form particularly suitable for functioning in the mucosal environment (Table 31.2) (117). Dimeric and tetrameric S-IgA and pentameric S-IgM display 4 to 10 Ag binding sites. Although of lower affinity than, for example, IgG Abs of the same specificity, this multivalency of pIg enhances their effectiveness over mIg by at least an order of magnitude. The presence of such low-affinity IgA Abs that are also "polyreactive" and thus are capable of binding to a variety of bacterial Ags, and autoAgs have been shown in human external secretions. Further, the intrinsic resistance of pIgA to proteolysis, enhanced by association with SC, is of functional advantage in secretions, particularly those of the GI tract rich in proteolytic enzymes. Finally, due to the inability to activate complement (C) and thus generate C3 and C5 fragments, IgA displays strong anti-inflammatory properties (Table 31.2). This fact is of special importance in the GI tract in which the external milieu rich in microbial and food Ags, and the internal milieu are separated by only a single layer of ECs.

As demonstrated in a number of studies, mucosal Ig inhibits the absorption of soluble and particulate Ags from mucosal surfaces by forming large immune complexes. Further, endogenous commensal microorganisms are coated *in vivo* with corresponding Abs that, in turn, prevent their adherence to epithelial receptors. In this respect, mucosal Abs and especially IgA may function by two independent mechanisms. Specific Abs interact with corresponding Ags through the Ag binding site. In addition, glycans that are abundant on the Fc region of IgA can aggregate bacteria based upon the interaction of bacterial glycan-binding lectins, with glycan side chains present on IgA molecules (117). Consequently, such IgA-coated bacteria are prevented from adhering to ECs expressing analogous mannose-rich glycans on their luminal surfaces without the need for Ag-specific Abs.

Biologically active Ags such as viruses, enzymes, and toxins can be effectively neutralized by mucosal Abs (117). The neutralization activity that is operational in a fluid phase may also extend to the intracellular compartment. In addition, it was demonstrated that virus-specific pIgA also exhibit their neutralization activity intracellularly (117). Apparently, the transcytosis route of pIgA intercepts the pathways involved in virus assembly, resulting in intracellular neutralization. Further, elimination of immune complexes composed of noninfectious Ags, absorbed by ECs and corresponding internalized pIgA Abs, has been demonstrated *in vitro*. Small circulating immune complexes containing soluble Ags and pIgA can be eliminated from the circulation into the bile by binding to hepatocytes that in some species (e.g., rats, mice, and rabbits) express pIgR (117). It appears that this mechanism of disposal of immune complexes is primarily restricted to species whose plasma IgA is dominated by pIgA, which in humans represent normally only a minor component (117). However, it is possible that immune complexes containing locally produced pIgA and absorbed Ags that may be formed within mucosal tissues are eliminated by this mechanism.

The noninflammatory nature of IgA is probably of considerable importance for the maintenance of the structural and functional integrity of mucosal tissues (117). The concept that IgA Abs are anti-inflammatory is exemplified by studies in which intact, native, and fully glycosylated human IgA Abs failed to activate C when complexed with Ags; actually in competition experiments, IgA effectively inhibited C activation by IgM and IgG Abs (Table 31.2) (117). Close examination of the frequently cited ability to activate C reveals that this may be largely due to artificial aggregation and conformational alterations caused by purification procedures and binding to hydrophobic surfaces in C activation assays and aberrancies in glycosylation frequently seen in IgA proteins. Indeed, specific IgA Abs with modified glycan moieties have been shown to activate the alternative and perhaps the lectin pathways of C activation.

Although phagocytic cells including monocytes/MΦ, PMNs, and eosinophils express receptors for the Fc region of IgA (96), the ability of IgA alone to effectively promote phagocytosis of bacteria remains controversial and depends upon the experimental system used in such studies. However, the binding of IgA and IgA-containing immune complexes to such receptors may provide transducing signals for cell activation, proliferation, and oxidative metabolism and prompt degranulation of eosinophils with local inflammatory consequences and extensive tissue damage (96).

The function of mucosal S-IgA also depends on the subclass distribution of specific Abs (46,91,117). Naturally occurring and immunization-induced Abs to protein and glycoprotein Ags are predominantly present in the IgA1 subclass, while Abs to polysaccharide Ags, LPS, and lipoteichoic acid are mainly of the IgA2 subclass. Because of its unique hinge region, IgA1 is susceptible to the cleavage by bacterial IgA1 proteases that are considered as one of the virulence factors produced by *S. pneumoniae, H. influenzae, N. gonorrhoeae, N. meningitidis,* and other microorganisms (93). It was also shown that bacteria coated with Fabα are refractory to IgM- and IgG-mediated and C-dependent killing action due to blocking. The antibacterial activity of IgA may be further potentiated by cooperation with innate factors of immunity including the peroxidase system, mucin, lactoferrin, and lysozyme (Table 31.2) (117).

Although S-IgA is the dominant isotype in most external secretions, the protective effects of Abs of IgM and IgG isotypes are evident from many studies. In external secretions of some IgA-deficient individuals, S-IgM and IgG may functionally compensate for the absence of S-IgA (118). Further, systemic immunization, particularly with conjugated polysaccharide-protein vaccines induces, vigorous and long-lasting IgG immune responses that protect children from infections with upper respiratory tract pathogens causing otitis media and meningitis (*H. influenzae, N. meningitides*) (119). In animal species (e.g., horses, cows, and pigs) in which prenatal transplacental active transport of IgG is not operational, consumption of milk rich in IgG is of life-saving importance. Abs of this isotype are absorbed during the first 7 to 14 days of life from the gut into the circulation presumably by the action of FcRn (10).

Mucosal CTLs

In the mucosal setting, natural infection of the epithelium by enteric (rotavirus or reovirus) or by respiratory viral pathogens (influenza or RSV) leads to endogenous viral peptide processing that induces pCTLs to become effector (activated) and memory CTLs. Most virus-specific CTLs are CD8$^+$ TCR$\alpha\beta^+$, and recognition of viral peptides is associated with MHC class I presentation by infected cells. In this regard, high numbers of CD8$^+$ T cells reside in the mucosal epithelium as a subpopulation of IELs (25). These CD8$^+$ IELs are thought to represent an important cytotoxic effector population that can eliminate virus-infected ECs. When freshly isolated IELs were examined using a redirected cytotoxicity assay, these T lymphocytes were found to constitutively possess lytic activity (28).

Significant progress is being made in areas related to the roles of APCs for induction of pCTLs and for mechanisms of perforin-mediated or Fas-Fas ligand-associated killing of target cells (28). It should be noted that the same processes occur during host responses to intracellular bacteria, to tumor-associated antigens, and in certain mucosal parasite infections. Although this focus is on CD8$^+$ CTLs, cell- and Ab-mediated cytotoxicity and NK cell activity are major responses associated with IELs (28).

An obvious question is how a CTL immune response is initiated given that mucosal inductive sites, which harbor pCTLs, are separate from effector sites, such as infected ECs where activated CD8$^+$ CTLs function. A partial answer is that the M cell has specific receptors for mucosal viruses, best exemplified by reovirus. As described earlier, the sigma protein of the reovirus enters the M cell in both NALT and GALT (59). It is likely, though less well documented, that other enteric viruses, such as rotavirus and respiratory pathogens, such as influenza and RSV, also enter the mucosal inductive pathway via M cells (59). Further, it now established that administration of virus into the GI tract results in the induction of increased pCTL frequencies in PPs (28). These findings suggest that, after enteric infection or immunization, Ag-stimulated CTLs are disseminated from PPs into MLNs via the lymphatic drainage. Further, virus-specific CTLs were also found among LP lymphocytes, IELs, and spleen cells of mice mucosally immunized with reovirus or rotavirus (28). Although mucosal effector tissues such as intestinal epithelium contain high numbers of $\gamma\delta$ T cells in addition to $\alpha\beta$ T cells, virus-specific CTLs in IELs were associated with the latter T cell subset (25,28). These studies suggest that oral immunization with live virus can induce Ag-specific CTLs in both mucosal inductive and effector tissues and in systemic lymphoid tissues.

Detailed studies of immune responses after nasal infection with influenza virus have also revealed that both humoral and cellular pathways are involved in virus clearance (120). However, it was shown that using mice lacking CD8$^+$ T cells (β2-microglobulin knockout mice) or treating with anti-CD8 mAbs did not alter clearance of influenza (121). These results support the presence of multiple pathways for immunity and suggest that CD4$^+$ Th cell pathways are important for mucosal Ab responses and CD8$^+$ CTLs for respiratory tract immunity. Several studies have also established that effector CTLs protect mice from RSV infection. The murine RSV model was used to determine the relative importance of CD4$^+$ T cells, including Th1 and Th2 subsets, which resulted in inflammation versus immunity. These studies clearly suggest that CD4$^+$ IFN-γ-producing Th1 cells as well as CD8$^+$ T cells are associated with recovery, while CD4$^+$ Th2-type pathways are not (122). Interestingly, priming with inactivated RSV or F glycoprotein induced CD4$^+$ Th2 cells while live RSV elicited the Th1-type pathway. When one considers mucosal vaccine development for virus infections, these findings suggest that the outcome of Th1- (including induction of CTLs) and Th2-type immune responses could be regulated by the nature and form of viral Ag used for immunization.

CTLs also play an important role in the inhibition of HIV infection. It was shown that CTLs recognized Ags derived from gp120, p27, nef, gag, tat, and pol proteins (123,124). Thus, infection of rhesus macaques with simian immunodeficient virus (SIV) resulted in the induction of CTL responses in the vaginal mucosa, which played a crucial role in the control of viral replication in the acute phase of viral infection. CTLs killed HIV-infected cells in a granzyme, perforin, or FasL-dependent manner. It is interesting to note that chemokines (e.g., CCL3, 4, and 5, and CXCL12) were produced by CTLs, which prevented HIV infection by blocking CCR5 and CXCR4, which are specific receptors for HIV infection.

Symbiotic Interactions with the Mucosal Microbiota

Mucosal surfaces of the oral cavity; the GI, genital, and respiratory tracts; and conjunctiva are populated by a large number of bacteria of more than 200 species with a characteristic distribution (Figure 31.13) (125). The mucosal microbiota comprises some 10^{14} bacteria present mostly in the large intestine. Considering the relative numbers of host's eukaryotic cells and prokaryotic bacteria, it is estimated that the mucosal microbiota outnumbers mammalian host cells by a factor of at least 10. Mutually beneficial coexistence of the mucosal microbiota with the effective mucosal immune system is one of the most

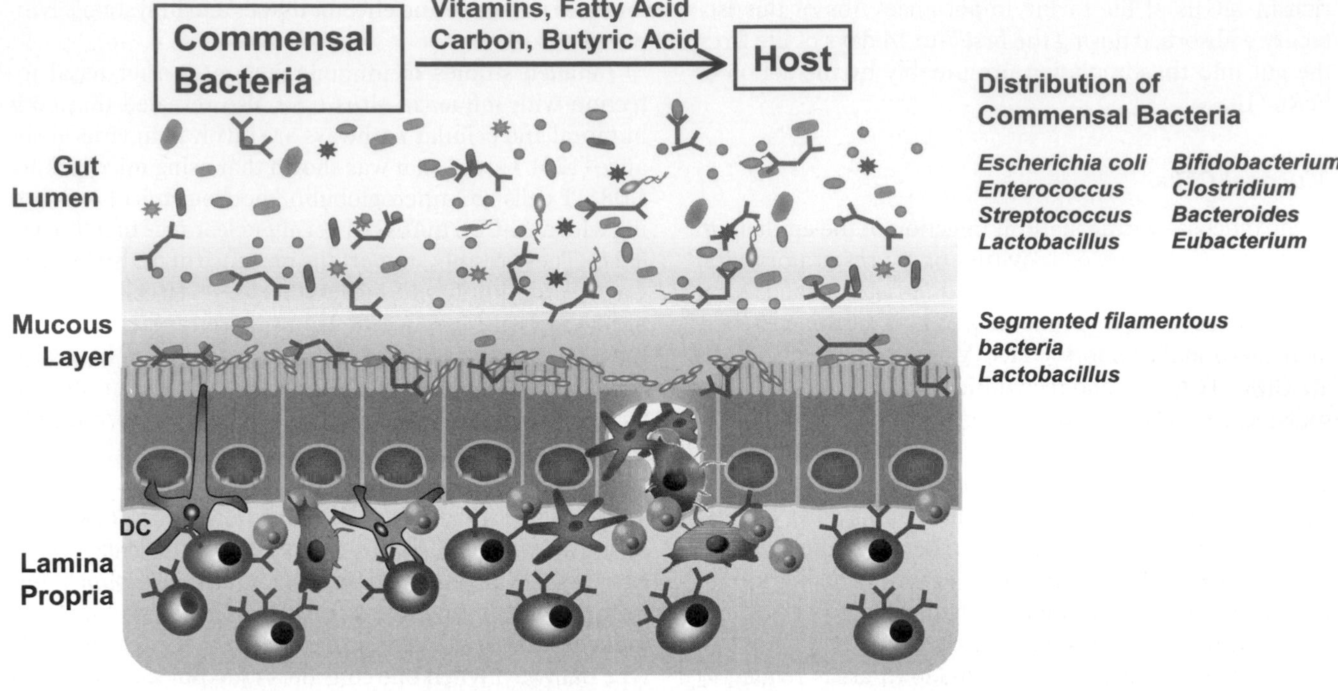

FIGURE 31.13 Symbiotic interactions between the mucosal immune system and commensal microbiota. Most microorganisms are present in the lumen and some preferably reside in the mucous layer. The host mucosal immune system regulates the diversity and quantity of intestinal microbiota by secreting S-IgA Abs into the lumen. In mice, these Abs have been suggested to originate from B1 cells. These Abs may limit the adherence of commensal bacteria to ECs for an appropriate cohabitation environment and thus their ability to continuously produce beneficial bioactive molecules such as vitamins, fatty acids, carbon, and butyric acid for the host.

interesting problems in mucosal immunology. Although the innate and specific immune factors present in the mucosal secretions and tissues may limit the adherence of bacteria to mucosal ECs and prevent penetration of such bacteria into the mucosal tissues with subsequent systemic dissemination, the mucosal microbiota continues to survive with remarkable tenacity in the presence of an immune response manifested by corresponding Abs (47). As a matter of fact, oral, intestinal, and probably other mucosal bacteria are coated *in vivo* with Abs, particularly of the IgA isotype, that may prevent their adherence to the epithelial receptors but do not significantly interfere with their elimination and metabolism (112). Therefore, products generated as a result of fermentation by mucosal bacteria such as butyric acid, fatty acids and vitamins can be important sources of energy and carbon for the human host, thus further stressing the immunological and physiological interdependence of the host on the mucosal microbiota (Figure 31.13) (125).

Quantitative and Qualitative Aspects of the Mucosal Microbiota

Quantitative data concerning the distribution of the indigenous microbiota on mucosal surfaces of the oral cavity, conjunctiva, and genital, GI, and respiratory tracts indicate that of approximately 10^{14} of bacteria, 99.9% are present in the large intestine (125). In this locale, bacteria are found free in the lumen and in feces, bound to the desquamated ECs, entrapped in the mucus layer, and deep in intestinal crypts (Figure 31.13). Despite the inherent difficulties with representative sampling, culture conditions, identification of cultured bacteria, as well as obvious host variables (e.g., hormonal status, diet, use of antibiotics, etc.), hundreds of species in 40 to 50 bacterial genera have been identified and described. These studies revealed that gram-negative and gram-positive, spore- and non–spore-forming, and aerobic as well as strictly anaerobic bacteria are present and are characteristically distributed in specific mucosal compartments. Although it is beyond the scope of this chapter to provide detailed information concerning the specific species distribution of indigenous microbiota in individual mucosal compartments, a brief summary of the colonic microbiota may illustrate the most important points. The intestinal microbiota is acquired shortly after birth and its composition is greatly influenced by the route of delivery (vaginal versus Cesarean section), the environment, and most profoundly by the diet (breastfeeding versus bottled formula and addition of solid food). Colonic microbiota changes from the dominant bifidobacteria at the initial stage to other species, particularly *Bacteroides* and anaerobic cocci with a significant presence of coliforms, streptococci and clostridia. Quantitative representation of bacteria in feces from adults indicates the dominance of bacteria of the genera *Bacteroides, Clostridium, Eubacterium, Lactobacillus, Streptococcus,* and *Bifidobacterium*; *E. coli* constitutes only a minor contribution (~ 1 %) of the colonic microbiota.

Regulation of Mucosal Immune Development and Immunological Homeostasis by Commensal Microbiota

The presence of the mucosal microbiota has a profound influence on the evolution and functionality of the immune system (47,126,127). As evidenced by a large number of studies performed on gnotobiotic (germ-free) animals, the development of both mucosal and systemic lymphoid tissues and the hosts' ensuing ability to respond to environmental Ags is, to a large extent, dependent on the previous exposure to a mucosal microbiota. Specifically, when compared to conventionally reared animals, lymphoid tissues of germ-free animals are hypotrophic, lack well-developed GCs, display minute numbers of mucosal PCs, and respond poorly to mitogens and polyclonal stimulants. Upon colonization with even a few representative species of mucosal microbiota, a prompt development of lymphoid tissues and restoration of responsiveness to a plethora of Ags and other stimuli ensues. Importantly, the development and responsiveness of both humoral and cell-mediated compartments of the immune system are profoundly affected by the mucosal microbiota as documented by the presence and numbers of B cells and ultimately AFC or PCs in mucosal and nonmucosal tissues, levels of mucosal and plasma Abs, and T cells of various phenotypes in the IEL and LP compartments of mucosal tissues, as well as in the systemic secondary lymphoid tissues (47,126,127).

The presence of the mucosal microbiota in the intestinal lumen induces S-IgA Ab synthesis. It was shown that induction of polyreactive S-IgA Ab responses to commensal bacteria is mainly derived from T cell–independent B1 cells (112). The T cell–independent IgA Abs originating from B1 cells possessed reactivity to conserved bacterial products (e.g., phosphorylcholine), which resulted in the nondiscriminating blockade of commensal bacterial attachment to mucosal surfaces. In this B1 cell Ab production pathway, IL-15 may be involved in IgA production facilitated by the intestinal microbiota, since it was previously reported that B1 cells proliferated in the LP when reacted with IL-15, an event induced by TLR-mediated signaling (113).

Another study revealed a unique pathway for specific Ab production against commensal microbiota in the intestine. It was shown that intestinal MΦ rapidly kill commensal bacteria, while intestinal DCs retain small numbers of live commensal bacteria and migrate only into MLNs but do not penetrate beyond MLNs (128). This function ensures a commensal bacteria-specific IgA Ab response that is specifically produced at the gut mucosa, but not in systemic immune compartments.

Mucosal microbiota-mediated innate immunity (e.g., TLR-mediated signaling) also plays an important role in the maintenance of mucosal homeostasis (47,126,127). For instance, the TLR-mediated cross-talk between the mucosal microbiota and IECs is biologically significant in the maintenance of epithelial homeostasis. EC cycles such as renewal, differentiation, and mitosis are significantly changed in germ-free or MyD88-deficient mice (22). In this regard, it was shown that TLR-mediated signals from the intestinal microbiota regulated the production of tissue protective factors such as IL-6, KC-1, and heat shock proteins (22). In addition to ECs, it was shown that TLRs were selectively expressed on $CD25^+$ $CD4^+$ Treg cells, which have been considered to be involved in the induction of oral tolerance, as discussed later in this chapter (129). Thus, bacterial products such as LPS directly enhance their survival and proliferation. These products and host responses may explain why C3H/HeJ mice lacking TLR4-mediated signaling and germ-free mice show less sensitivity to oral tolerance induction (130).

Additional examples of molecules in the microbiota-dependent intestinal homeostasis are bacterial DNA. Bacterial DNA contains unmethylated CpG motifs within consensus sequences and is the ligand for TLR9 (11). Several lines of evidence have demonstrated that CpG targets DCs to induce the inhibitory environment (131), and it has been considered that some types of DCs are involved in these inhibitory immune responses (51,52); it appears that the intestinal microbiota stimulates intestinal DCs through the interactions between CpG and TLR9 for the maintenance of intestinal homeostasis. These inhibitory effects of bacterial DNA have led to the development of probiotics-mediated anti-inflammatory therapy, as discussed later in this chapter (131).

MUCOSAL TOLERANCE

Basic Concepts

In addition to the protective function of Ag-specific S-IgA and serum IgG Ab responses after mucosal immunization, the mucosal route of Ag delivery can also induce systemic unresponsiveness (132). Oral administration of a single high dose or repeated oral delivery of low doses of proteins has been shown to induce systemic unresponsiveness. Additional studies have shown that the nasal administration of proteins also induces systemic unresponsiveness and has led to the more general term mucosal tolerance to include nasal or oral Ag induction of unresponsiveness (132). The inhibition of Ag-specific immune responses in systemic compartments by mucosal Ag delivery is important for the prevention of overstimulation of responses and frequently encountered and hypersensitivity responses to food proteins and allergens. Further, this system could potentially be applied to the prevention and possibly treatment of autoimmune diseases by feeding relevant Ags.

Role of PPs in Oral Tolerance

The precise site of Ag uptake in the GI tract during oral tolerance induction has not been firmly established. One possible route is that Ags may enter the GALT via M cells and lead to APC–T cell interactions that down-regulate T and B cell responses. Some investigators have suggested that organized lymphoid tissue in the GI tract was not required for oral tolerance to OVA, since B cell defective mice, which contain poorly developed PPs, were fully tolerized at the level of T cells (133). The availability of mice without PPs has allowed reinvestigation of the notion that GALT may be involved in oral tolerance. In one study, it was shown that mice that lack GALT but retain MLNs could be orally tolerized to OVA (134). However, others found that mice that lack PPs but retain MLNs were resistant to oral tolerance to protein (135); however, these mice showed normal mucosal S-IgA Ab responses to oral protein given with CT as adjuvant (41,42). Although one cannot yet conclude whether GALT is a strict requirement for oral tolerance to proteins, it is plausible to suggest that the nature of the Ag itself may influence the site of entry into the host.

CD4$^+$ T Cells in Oral Tolerance

The $\alpha\beta$ T cells appear to be the major players in down-regulation of systemic immune responses to orally administered Ags. It is generally agreed that the status of oral tolerance can be explained by: 1) clonal anergy or deletion of T cells, or 2) by active suppression by regulatory-type T cells through the secretion of inhibitory cytokines (132). Low doses of oral Ag tend to favor the latter form of inhibition, while higher doses of feeding induce clonal anergy of immunocompetent T cells. These two forms of oral tolerance are not mutually exclusive and may occur simultaneously following oral administration of Ags.

Anergy is defined as a state of T cell unresponsiveness characterized by the lack of proliferation and IL-2 synthesis and diminished IL-2R expression, a condition reversed by pre-culturing T cells with IL-2 (132). It was shown that Th1-type cells appear to be more sensitive to the induction of tolerance *in vitro* than Th2-type cells; *in vivo* evidence has demonstrated that Th1 cells are likely to be anergized in oral tolerance. This may be an oversimplification since it has been shown that oral tolerance can be induced in mice defective in Th1 (STAT4$^{-/-}$) or Th2 (STAT6$^{-/-}$) cells (136). Further, to identify which lymphocyte compartment (e.g., CD4$^+$ versus CD8$^+$ T cells) preferentially mediates the induction of oral tolerance, cell transfer experiments were performed using SCID and *nu/nu* mice, demonstrating that oral tolerance was induced by anergized CD4$^+$ but not CD8$^+$ T cells (137).

Clonal deletion has been considered as another pathway for the induction of oral tolerance. Clonal deletion of Ag-specific CD4$^+$ T cells was detected after oral feeding of high doses of Ag (132). Accumulating evidence has revealed that the clonal deletion induced by feeding high doses of Ag was due to an increase in the susceptibility of lymphocyte apoptosis via increased expression of caspase.

Mucosal Regulatory T Cell Networks

Regulatory- and suppressor type T cells are crucial players in the induction of peripheral tolerance to self and foreign Ags. It is now accepted that several populations of T cells expressing CD4 or CD8 show regulatory or suppressive functions to other T cell-mediated mucosal immune responses. They can be classified as: 1) naïve, or those which have not yet encountered Ag; 2) activated (effector); and 3) memory, where both effector and memory T cells have engaged in the regulation of immune responses (48,132). CD4$^+$ T cells including CD4$^+$CD25$^+$Foxp3$^+$ Treg cells, Th3 cells (secreting TGF-β), and Tr1 cells (secreting IL-10) and CD8$^+$ T cells were shown to be key players for the creation of a mucosal regulatory T cell network in the establishment of quiescent immunity (or mucosal tolerance) (Figures 31.7, 31.14).

CD25$^+$ CD4$^+$ Treg Cells

Recent evidence has revealed that naturally arising CD25$^+$ CD4$^+$ Treg cells play a pivotal role in the negative control of a variety of physiological and pathological immune responses (138). Naturally arising Treg cells specifically express a forkhead winged-helix transcription factor family member (Foxp3) for the process of Treg cell lineage commitment. Thus, Foxp3 deficiency results in early onset, fatal, systemic autoimmune disease. The Foxp3$^+$ CD25$^+$ CD4$^+$ Treg cells are present in the PPs, suggesting that Foxp3$^+$ CD25$^+$ CD4$^+$ Treg cells are involved in the maintenance of intestinal homeostasis.

In addition to inhibitory cytokines, such as IL-10 and TGF-β, several inhibitory molecules have been shown to be expressed on CD25$^+$ CD4$^+$ Treg cells (138). Although naïve T cells express CTLA-4 (or CD152) after activation, which competes with the cellular interaction between CD28 on effector T cells and CD80/CD86 on APCs, CD25$^+$ CD4$^+$ Treg cells constitutively express CTLA-4 (Figures 31.7, 31.14). The CTLA-4 on Treg cells plays a pivotal role in the maintenance of mucosal homeostasis (139). Thus, anti-CTLA-4 mAb treatment inhibited the regulatory function of CD25$^+$ CD4$^+$ Treg cells and subsequently led to the development of IBD. Several mechanisms have been proposed for the

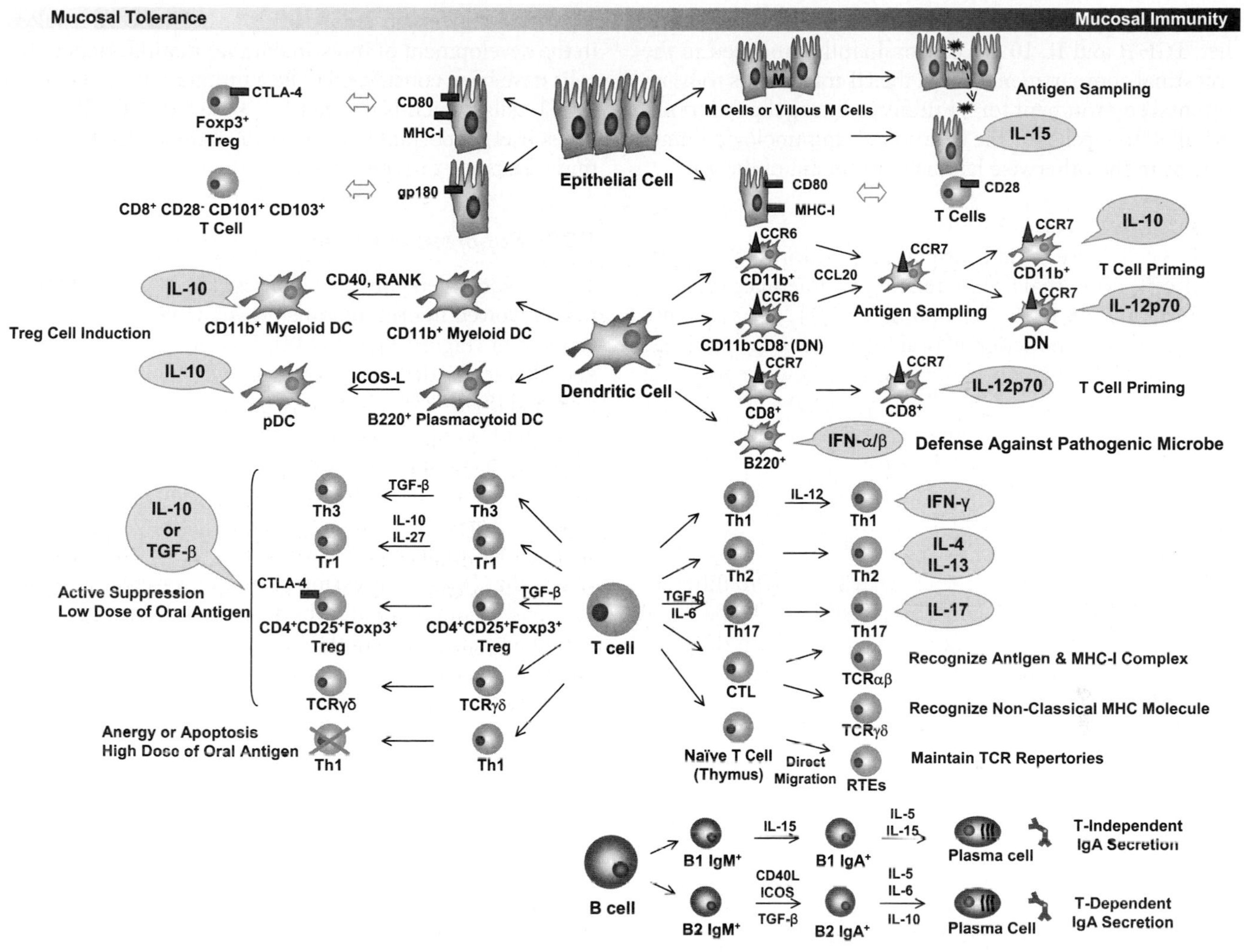

FIGURE 31.14 Cellular and molecular mechanisms for the induction and regulation of mucosal immunity and tolerance. A unique aspect of the mucosal immune system is the simultaneous presence of active (e.g., effector T cells and S-IgA Abs) and quiescent (e.g., Treg cells and mucosal tolerance) immunity. To smoothly operate two opposite types of immunity, ECs, DCs, and T cells play central roles by providing appropriate inflammatory and anti-inflammatory cytokine networks together with costimulatory and chemokine molecular families.

inhibitory function of CTLA-4 on Treg cells, including the enhancement of Treg cell activity through the interaction with CD80/CD86 on APCs (138). Since ECs also express CD80 as mentioned earlier (37), it is possible that Treg cells recognize CD80 on the ECs in order to exhibit their immunosuppressive function. Another possible mechanism is the induction of the inhibitory molecule, IDO (140). As mentioned earlier, IDO exhibits immunosuppressive effects by catalyzing the catabolism of tryptophan, an essential amino acid for T cell proliferation (20). In addition to CTLA-4, Treg cells also express high levels of glucocorticoid-induced TNF-like receptor (GITR), another important suppressive function-associated molecule, that contributes to the maintenance of a quiescent condition in mucosal immune compartments (138). Thus, transfer of GITR^{high} Treg cell–depleted spleen cells to athymic nude mice resulted in the development of autoimmune diseases including gastritis (141). GITR-mediated signaling triggers Treg cell proliferation, which has been considered to be one molecular mechanism for GITR-mediated suppressive function of Treg cells in the presence of IL-2, but detailed mechanisms remain unclear.

Although naturally arising CD25^{+} CD4^{+} Treg cells develop in the thymus and their survival in the periphery is dependent on IL-2 (138), accumulating evidence has demonstrated that Foxp3^{+} Treg cells can be induced from Foxp3^{-} precursors and, like naturally arising CD25^{+} CD4^{+} Treg cells, the induced Treg cells express CD25 and CTLA-4, and also produce IL-10 and TGF-β (142). It is interesting to note that cytokines such as TGF-β and IL-10 contribute to the differentiation of Treg cells (142). As mentioned earlier, TGF-β and IL-10 are predominantly produced in the intestinal compartments; thus, the GI tract seems to be an optimal environment for naturally inducing the differentiation of Treg cells for the creation of immunologic homeostasis in the otherwise harsh environment of the gut.

Th3 Cells

Th3 cells were initially discovered as a form of suppressor T cell subset that accounted for oral tolerance (Figures 31.7, 31.14) (48,132). The finding of CD4$^+$ T cell clones generated after induction of oral tolerance to myelin basic protein (MBP), led to the description of a new phenotype of regulatory or suppressor T cell. Clones of CD4$^+$ T cells were MBP-specific, and of 48 clones assessed, 42 produced the active form of TGF-β, which is also an essential cytokine to induce Th3 cells (143). Th3 cells have different cytokine requirements for their growth from CD25$^+$ CD4$^+$ Treg cells. As mentioned earlier, the survival of CD25$^+$ CD4$^+$ Treg cells is dependent upon IL-2 (138), while *in vitro* differentiation of Th3 cells is enhanced by TGF-β, IL-4, and IL-10 (48). These findings suggest that Th3 cells are a different linage from naturally arising CD25$^+$ CD4$^+$ Treg cells, but it is still unclear whether Th3 cells are the same as induced Treg cells because of the lack of a specific marker for Th3 cells. It was previously shown that TGF-β was produced by intestinal DCs (51,52), which has been considered to be the source of cytokines for the induction of Th3 cells in the intestine. Additionally, since TGF-β production was induced by CTLA-4, which is constitutively expressed on naturally arising Treg cells (142), it is possible that TGF-β production from Treg cells through CTLA-4–mediated signaling may stimulate the differentiation of both induced Treg cells and Th3 cells.

Tr1 Cells

Another regulatory type of T cell is one that secretes IL-10 and TGF-β and has been termed a Tr1 cell (Figures 31.7, 31.14) (144). Similar to IL-10–secreting induced-type Treg cells, Tr1 cells are induced by Ag stimulation in the presence of IL-10, which is abundantly produced by DCs in GALT and in pulmonary tissues, as mentioned earlier (51,52). The function of Tr1 cells is to suppress Ag-specific effector T cell responses in a cytokine-dependent manner. Ag-specific activation of TCR is required for the Tr1 suppressive function, but Tr1 cells can also mediate bystander suppressive activity against other Ags once they are activated. Although the migratory capacity of Tr1 cells has not been elucidated yet, it is interesting to note that Tr1 cells in the blood circulation express the GI tract migration chemokine receptor, CCR9, suggesting that these cells intrinsically home to the intestine (145). Consistent with this idea, previous studies reported an important role for Tr1 cells in IBD and celiac diseases (144,146). Although Tr1 cells do not express Foxp3 the lack of Tr1 cells resulted in the development of intestinal inflammation. Hence, Tr1 cells have been considered to be a unique subset of regulatory T cells, which is distinct from the CD4$^+$ CD25$^+$ Treg cell subset, important in the control of undesired hyperimmune responses in the intestine.

CD8$^+$ Suppressor T Cells

The first identified population of regulatory T cells thought to be involved in oral tolerance was a CD8$^+$ suppressor T cell subset (Figure 31.14) (147). However, their functions and characteristics have not been clearly defined. It was reported that CD8$^+$ CD28$^-$ suppressor T cells induced the up-regulation of Ig-like transcript 3 (ILT3) and ILT4 expressed on human monocytes and DCs, rendering these APCs tolerogenic by inducing Ag-specific unresponsiveness of CD4$^+$ T cells through reduced expression of costimulatory molecules (148). Subsequent study has revealed that ILT3/4 expression in human vascular endothelial cells was up-regulated by IL-10 (149). Since IL-10 is abundantly produced in the intestinal compartments, it is plausible that IL-10 produced in the intestinal compartments may regulate ILT3/4-mediated suppressive function as suppressor T cell–mediated maintenance of intestinal homeostasis. In addition, it was suggested that CD8$^+$ CD122$^+$ (IL-2/IL-15 receptor β chain) T cells behave like naturally occurring regulatory T cells, where the depletion of the CD8$^+$ T cells resulted in the high incidence of pulmonary inflammation (150). Although CD8$^+$ CD122$^+$ T cells are also involved in the intestinal immune system, the finding further suggested the existence of multiple layers of a mucosal regulatory network for the creation and maintenance of the quiescent status of the immune environment in the mucosal compartments of both the GI and respiratory tracts.

Factors in Determining the Type of Regulatory T Cells

Recent studies have identified several factors determining whether T cells differentiate into pathogenic or regulatory T cells. For instance, as mentioned earlier, TGF-β is known to be an essential molecule for the induction of Treg cells and Th17 cells; however, Th17 cells additionally require IL-6 for their development. Therefore, in the presence of IL-6 plus TGF-β, only Th17 cells developed (62,63). A recent separate study shows that stimulation with TGF-β and IL-6 triggers initial lineage commitment of Th17, but IL-23 is required for the full differentiation of Th17 cells (151). In contrast to the effects of IL-23 for the full differentiation of IL-6– and TGF-β-treated T cells into Th17 cells, IL-27 plus IL-6 and TGF-β–induced T cells producing IL-10, which resembled Tr1 cells (152,153). Thus, it seems that IL-23 and IL-27 both play important roles in the fate decision of IL-6– and TGF-β–exposed T cells either become pathogenic Th17 cells or regulatory Tr1 cells. Several separate studies have revealed that mucosal DC–derived retinoic acid, a key molecule for the induction of gut-homing $\alpha 4\beta 7$ integrin and CCR9, as mentioned earlier (88,89), also enhanced conversion of TGF-β–treated T cells to Treg cells and simultaneously suppressed the differentiation to Th17 cells (154–157). These data suggest the presence of versatile pathways for regulating T cell fate.

Role of IELs in Mucosal Tolerance

Since the intestinal epithelium is directly and continuously exposed to gut environmental Ags, it was logical to consider that IELs and IECs contribute to the mucosal regulatory network for the induction of mucosal tolerance (25,132). Interestingly, it has been shown that depletion of TCR$\gamma\delta$ cells resulted in the failure to induce the systemic unresponsiveness after oral administration of Ags (158). Another study demonstrated that when either TCR$\delta^{-/-}$ or TCR$\delta^{+/+}$ mice were immunized orally with a high dose of OVA prior to parenteral challenge, systemic IgG and IgE Ab responses were markedly reduced in both types of mice (159). Reduced T cell proliferative responses and delayed-type hypersensitivity were seen in both TCR$\delta^{-/-}$ and TCR$\delta^{+/+}$ mice given high-doses of OVA. In contrast, while oral tolerance associated with increased levels of IL-10 synthesis was induced by low-dose OVA in TCR$\delta^{+/+}$ mice, TCR$\delta^{-/-}$ mice were not tolerized and failed to produce IL-10 (159). These findings indicate that $\gamma\delta$ T cells play an important role in IL-10–mediated, low-dose oral tolerance induction, but are not essential participants in the induction of systemic tolerance induced by oral administration of large doses of Ag. It has been suggested that oral tolerance induced by repeated administration of small doses of Ag is mediated by T cells involved in the generation of active suppression, while systemic unresponsiveness induced by large doses of Ag is caused by clonal anergy or clonal deletion (132). Thus, it is likely that $\gamma\delta$ T cells play regulatory roles for the induction of active suppression, although they are not involved in the induction of clonal anergy or deletion.

DCs and IECs in Oral Tolerance

It has been demonstrated that intestinal DCs contribute to the induction of tolerance. The initial evidence of DC involvement in the induction of oral tolerance was provided by the demonstration that Flt3 ligand-mediated expansion of DCs led to enhanced oral tolerance (160). Among several kinds of DCs in the intestinal compartments, two subsets of DCs have gained attention. As mentioned earlier, CD11b^{+} myeloid DCs in the PPs have the unique feature of producing predominantly IL-10 in response to CD40 ligation or receptor activator of NF-κB (RANK)/RANK ligand interactions (51,52). A second DC population involved in the induction of oral tolerance is pDCs. One study described that CD11c^{low} DCs displayed a plasmacytoid morphology and a stable immature phenotype and secreted IL-10 for the induction of IL-10–secreting Tr1 cells, and a recent study has revealed that inducible costimulator ligand (ICOS-L) plays an important role in pDC-mediated Tr1 induction (161). High levels of ICOS-L expression on pDCs allow them to induce the differentiation of naïve CD4 T cells to IL-10 but not the other Th2 cytokines (161). In addition to Tr1 cells, pDCs induced IL-10–producing CD8^{+} regulatory T cells (162). Taken together, IL-10 produced by DCs is a key factor in the differentiation of regulatory-type T cells.

ECs are also thought to contribute to the induction of oral tolerance by capturing and presenting luminal Ag by MHC molecules with low expression of costimulatory molecules (37). As an additional pathway of IEC-mediated oral tolerance, it was demonstrated that gp180, an associated molecule with cold, mediated interaction between IECs and CD8^{+} CD28^{-} CD101^{+} CD103^{+} cells, causing the CD8^{+} CD28^{-} CD101^{+} CD103^{+} cells to develop into regulatory cells (37,163). IECs also mediated suppression of CD4^{+} T cell activation in a cell contact-dependent and TGF-β–independent manner (164). A recent study has demonstrated that IEC-primed T cells secreted lower amounts of IFN-γ and IL-2 and exhibited an increased expression of IL-10 and Foxp3, providing direct evidence that IECs induced IL-10–producing Foxp3^{+} T cells (165). Thus, IECs can be involved in the creation of a mucosal regulatory network in two phases including Ag-presentation and priming of regulatory-type T cells.

Nasal Tolerance

The initial dogma that mucosal tolerance requires intestinal processing of the Ag was challenged by the observation that systemic unresponsiveness could be achieved by administration of the Ag via the nasal or aerosol routes (132). These routes were found to require lower doses of Ags than did oral administration, a discrepancy that can be explained by the dilution effect, as well as the potential degradation of the Ag in the GI tract. Although the precise mechanism behind nasally induced tolerance is not yet known, several studies have demonstrated a similar pathway for the induction of both nasal tolerance and oral tolerance. For example, the membrane-bound form of TGF-β–expressing CD4^{+} Foxp3^{+} T cells are involved in tolerance induction to inhaled Ag (166). It was also shown that airway pDCs suppressed the generation of effector T cells primed by myeloid DCs via the induction of IL-10–producing Treg cells (167).

Mucosal Tolerance in Humans

Increasing attention is being paid to oral tolerance and the role it could play in the prevention or treatment of autoimmune diseases, including multiple sclerosis, rheumatoid arthritis, uveitis, as well as type I diabetes and contact hypersensitivity (132). Indeed, humans immunized with the neoantigen keyhole limpet hemocyanin (KLH) either by the oral or nasal route developed systemic unresponsiveness evaluated by delayed type hypersensitivity (DTH) and T cell proliferative responses. However, B cell responses were primed in both systemic and mucosal sites. In other studies, humans naturally ingesting the dietary Ags bovine gamma globulin, OVA, and soybean protein developed a T cell tolerance characterized by anergy (132). Antigen-specific Th3 cells secreting TGF-β have been observed in the blood of multiple sclerosis patients orally treated with a bovine myelin preparation, demonstrating that oral administration of autoantigen can induce antigen-specific TGF-β–secreting cells in a human autoimmune disease.

Pilot clinical trials of oral tolerance have been conducted in patients with autoimmune diseases, and promising clinical benefits have been reported (132). Despite encouraging initial results regarding oral delivery of autoantigens for the treatment of human autoimmune diseases, a followup study did not demonstrate statistically significant beneficial effects. Further, oral feeding of autoantigen in mice resulted in the generation of antigen-specific $CD8^+$ CTL responses that could lead to the aggravation of autoimmune disease (132). Thus, one must also keep in mind that oral administration of autoantigen may induce undesirable $CD8^+$ CTLs that may worsen the disease instead of preventing the development of autoimmunity.

A description of extensive experiments and clinical studies based on the exploitation of principles of mucosal tolerance in the prevention and treatment of T and B cell–mediated hypersensitivity diseases (e.g., contact dermatitis and inhalation allergies), other autoimmune diseases (e.g., uveoretinitis, glomerulonephritis, and diabetes), and prolonged survival of allografts are beyond the scope of this review. However, these efforts have not yet reached fruition. Thus, the experience of most investigators is that once antigen-specific systemic immune response has been induced, it is difficult to achieve a reversal through mucosal tolerance.

MUCOSAL IMMUNE SYSTEM FOR HOST DEFENSE

Mucosal Vaccines

Mucosal surfaces are also the most frequent portals of entry of common viral, bacterial, fungal, and parasitic agents causing both local and systemic infectious diseases. The fascinating characteristics of the mucosal immune system in the prevention of infections by pathogens has led to much attention for the development of mucosal (e.g., oral and nasal) vaccines (6). Mucosal vaccines offer numerous advantages over traditional injection-type parenteral vaccines, including needleless and easy administration. Most important, mucosal vaccines can induce both mucosal and systemic immune responses, while parenteral immunization yields only systemic immune responses. Hence, traditional parenteral immunization does not induce mucosal immunity, which would inhibit the initial attachment of pathogens, while mucosal vaccines can establish a first line of immunological defense at mucosal sites as well as provide a systemic immune surveillance to detect and destroy invading pathogens. Therefore, numerous studies have been conducted to harness the enormous potential of the mucosal immune system to induce protective immune responses at the site of entry of infectious agents.

However, due to the difficulties with dosing of relevant Ags, their limited absorption, proteolytic degradation, low pH, and detergent activity by bile salts, unique Ag delivery systems and mucosal adjuvants have been explored to avoid such problems (6). At a minimum, these systems should protect the Ag from physical and biological elimination. In addition, a major research focus has been aimed at molecular and cellular elucidation of key immunological mechanisms for the simultaneous induction and regulation of active (e.g., S-IgA) and silent (e.g., mucosal tolerance) immune responses.

Administration Route of Mucosal Vaccines

Stimulation of local and generalized mucosal immune responses can be achieved by ingestion of Ags or their introduction by the rectal route. The former route exploits the inductive potential of lymphoepithelial tissues distributed in the small intestine, while the latter route primarily stimulates cells accumulated in structures termed *rectal tonsils* (6). Immune responses induced by infections or immunization through the nasal mucosa and oropharyngeal lymphoid tissues (Waldeyers ring or NALT) have been evaluated with particular emphasis on local respiratory tract pathogens such as influenza, parainfluenza, and RSV (120). Individuals naturally infected or locally immunized with attenuated viruses responded by formation of S-IgA and IgG Abs in nasal secretions and when examined also in saliva (120). In general, nasal immunization in contrast to intestinal administration, induces prominent systemic immune responses manifested by the presence of AFCs in peripheral blood with mucosal as well as systemic homing receptors, and plasma Ab responses. Examination of other external secretions of nasally immunized humans and animals revealed another significant feature: the female genital tract secretions contained high levels of antimicrobial Abs of IgA and IgG isotypes, which, in some experiments, were higher than those induced by local, oral, rectal, or systemic immunizations (168). Thus, it appears that nasal exposure with Ags is the route of choice for the induction of female genital tract responses.

The mucosal immune system of the female and male genital tracts displays several features distinct from other mucosal sites, such as the absence of lymphoepithelial structures analogous to intestinal PPs, and a dominance of IgG-AFCs in tissues and IgG in cervical mucus, vaginal washes, and serum (168,169). Although repeated administration of Ags with adjuvants, or infection with live viruses generated local immune responses, Abs were absent or present in low levels in secretions of remote glands, probably due to the lack of organized inductive sites, equivalent to PPs, in the genital tract. However, systemic immunization followed by local mucosal booster or targeted immunization in the vicinity of local LNs enhanced genital tract responses (168,169). Further, sequential combination of several immunization routes (systemic, oral, rectal, vaginal, tracheal, or nasal) generates better results than repeated immunization at a single site.

Enterotoxin-based Mucosal Adjuvants

Two bacterial enterotoxins, CT and the closely related heat labile toxin (LT), are the most well-studied mucosal adjuvants, which are derived from *Vibrio cholerae* and *Escherichia coli*, respectively (6,170,171). They are not only potent immunogens, but also adjuvants that enhance both mucosal and systemic immune responses against mucosally coadministered Ags. CT and LT are structurally similar (83% homology at the amino acid level) hexameric toxins consisting of two structurally and functionally separate A (CT-A or LT-A) and B (CT-B_5 or LT-B_5) subunits (6,170,171). The A subunit possesses ADP-ribosyltransferase activity, and the B subunit participates in the binding to host cells. Different binding activities between CT-B and LT-B have been reported. The CT-B binds to GM1-ganglioside, whereas the LT-B binds to GM1-ganglioside as well as asialo GM1 and GM2. The binding of B subunits to their receptors on ECs allows the A subunit to reach the cytosol of target cells, where it binds to nicotinamide adenosyl diphosphate (NADP) and catalyzes the ADP ribosylation of Gsα. The latter GTP-binding protein activates adenyl cyclase with subsequent elevation of cAMP in ECs, followed by secretion of water and chloride ions into the intestinal lumen. Although both CT and LT have strong adjuvant activities, the clinical use of CT and LT has been hampered by the fact that both enterotoxins induce severe diarrhea after oral administration or from natural infection. Both enterotoxins also have undesirable side effects involving their entry into the central nervous system when given by the nasal route (6,170,171).

To circumvent toxicity linked to these enterotoxins, several groups have attempted to generate mutants of CT (mCT) and LT (mLT) devoid of their toxic activity or replacement of the toxic A subunit (6,170,171). The first approach involves the introduction of single amino acid substitutions in the active site (i.e., the site responsible for the ADP-ribosylation activity) of the A subunit of CT or LT or in the protease sensitive loop of LT. mCTs constructed by substitution of serine by phenylalanine at position 61 (CT-S61F) and glutamate by lysine at position 112 (CT-E112K) in the ADP-ribosyltransferase activity center of the CT gene from *V. cholerae* 01 strain GP14 display no ADP-ribosyltransferase activity or enterotoxicity (6,170,171). The levels of Ag-specific serum IgG and S-IgA Abs induced by the mutants are comparable to those induced by wild-type CT. Further, the mutant CT-E112K, like native CT, induces Th2-type responses through a preferential inhibition of Th1-type $CD4^+$ T cells. Subsequent studies demonstrated that the mutant forms of CT were effective for the induction of immune responses against tetanus toxin, *S. pneumoniae*, influenza virus, diphtheria toxin, HIV, and botulinum neurotoxin (6,170,171). Mutations in other sites of the CT molecule were reported to induce nontoxic derivatives, but the adjuvant activity was also affected. Similarly, mLTs have also been successfully developed as safe mucosal adjuvants and used with vaccines against measles virus, tetanus toxin, *Helicobacter pylori*, and influenza among many others, and some of them have been examined clinically (6,170,171).

Another strategy that exploits the binding potential of CT and CT-B to gangliosides on mucosal cells involves the genetic construction of recombinant chimeric proteins. The toxic subunit A of CT consists of two segments, A1 (carrier of toxicity) and A2, that interact with the B subunit. Genetic replacement of the A1 segment with DNA encoding a desired Ag (e.g., Ag I/II of *Streptococcus mutans*) results in the assembly of a molecule composed of CT-B/A2-Ag (6,170,171). When given intragastrically and especially nasally, potent Ag-specific humoral immune responses were generated in mice.

In addition to CT and LT, several toxins have been shown to exhibit mucosal adjuvant activity. For instance, Shiga toxin 1 (STX1) and the mutant form of STX1 have been shown to exhibit mucosal adjuvanticity. A genetically engineered pertussis toxin (PTX) developed by removal of its ADP-ribosylating activity was an effective adjuvant for enhancing mucosal immune responses (6). The PTX recognizes glycoprotein with a branched mannose core and an N-acetyl glucosamine expressed on various types of mammalian cells. Nasal immunization with tetanus toxoid and PTX augmented parenteral and mucosal Ab responses. *Zonula occludens* toxin (Zot) is a single polypeptide encoded by the filamentous bacteriophage infecting toxigenic strain of *V. cholerae*. Nasal or rectal immunization with Zot resulted in the induction of plasma IgG and mucosal S-IgA Ab responses against coadministered Ag mediated by both Th1- and Th2-type cells (6). CTA1-DD is composed of an enzymatically active CT-A and a dimer of an Ig-binding element of *S. aureus* protein A. Thus, it targets to B cells (172). When CTA1-DD was applied nasally, it enhanced Ag-specific immune responses in both mucosal and systemic sites without causing inflammation. A subsequent study indicated that the adjuvanticity of CTA1-DD was at least mediated by promoting GC formation (172). Surprisingly, CTA1-DD is nontoxic although it contains the intact form of holotoxin.

It should be noted that, except for a few results, almost all mutant forms of adjuvants derived from the bacterial toxin retained full adjuvant activity at least after nasal and parenteral immunization, but possess less adjuvant activity when they were given orally. The reasons for different adjuvant activities after nasal versus oral delivery remains an open question, and further experiments are necessary for effective oral delivery use of toxin-based mutant adjuvants.

Mucosal Cytokines, Chemokines, and Innate Factors as Adjuvants

Mucosal delivery of cytokines allowed the use of these molecules that primarily interact with their corresponding receptors without the important adverse effects that are often associated with the large and repeated parenteral cytokine doses generally required for the effective targeting of tissues/organs. Considerable numbers of cytokines such as type I IFNs, IL-1, IL-2, IL-12, IL-15, and IL-18 have been shown to have mucosal adjuvant activity (6). Although these cytokines showed adjuvant activities after a single use, previous reports have provided evidence for synergistic effects of cytokines. For instance, the adjuvant activity for induction of mucosal S-IgA and systemic IgG Abs after simultaneous administration of IL-1, IL-12, and IL-18 was much stronger than those induced by the treatment with each cytokine alone or a combination of IL-12 plus IL-18. In contrast to the synergistic effects of IL-1, IL-12, and IL-18, coexpression of IL-15 with IL-12 did not enhance adjuvanticity. These findings suggest that the adjuvant mechanism mediated by cytokines is complex and should be carefully examined for the suitability of a particular cytokine for use in the development of effective mucosal vaccines.

In addition to cytokines, chemokines have been shown to act as innate-type mucosal adjuvants (6). For instance, nasal administration of XCL1/lymphotactin with Ag resulted in the marked enhancement of Ag-specific S-IgA Abs in various mucosal secretions (e.g., feces, saliva, vaginal, and nasal washes) and plasma IgG Ab responses. Similarly, nasal coadministration of RANTES with Ag induced high levels of S-IgA, plasma IgG, and preferential Th1-type responses. MIP-1 is another CC chemokine that was analyzed for its ability to act as a mucosal adjuvant. MIP-1 contains two homologous subtypes, MIP-1α and MIP-1β. It was demonstrated that nasal administration of MIP-1α enhanced Ag-specific Ab responses to coadministered Ag in systemic but not in mucosal sites. In contrast, MIP-1β promoted mucosal S-IgA Ab responses with less efficient induction of systemic immune responses, although they both share the same ligand (CCR5).

Defensins belong to a family of antimicrobial peptides produced by Paneth cells, as mentioned earlier (4,5). Defensins also possess chemotactic activity against T cells and exert adjuvant activity (6). It is interesting to note that no mucosal S-IgA Ab responses were induced after nasal immunization with defensins, although they promoted systemic IgG Ab responses associated with IFN-γ, IL-5, IL-6, and IL-10 production. Thus, defensins are unique adjuvants that enhance systemic immune responses without induction of mucosal S-IgA Ab production.

PRR-Targeted Mucosal Adjuvants

Innate immunity plays a pivotal role in host defense against invading microbial pathogens at early stages of infection through recognition by PRRs (11). The PRR-mediated signals induce cytokine production like type I IFN, IL-1 and IL-12, as well as antimicrobial peptides like defensins that are all known to have adjuvant activity, as discussed earlier. As one may expect from the fact that cytokines that function as mucosal adjuvants, PAMPs, also act as mucosal adjuvants. For example, monophosphoryl lipid A (MLA) that has already been shown to be a systemic adjuvant pre-clinically and clinically effectively works as a mucosal adjuvant (6). Until now, the target cells of TLR agonists remained obscure but were presumably DCs, since TLR4 expression is very low or absent on ECs, as mentioned earlier. TLR2 is also a target of a specific mucosal adjuvant. Muramyl dipeptide (MDP) is derived from the cell wall of mycobacteria and has been shown to be one of the ligands for TLR2. Before identification of TLR2, MDP was shown to stimulate PP cells for the enhancement of IgA Ab responses (6). Recent studies have demonstrated that mycoplasma-derived MΦ-activating 2 kDa lipopeptide (MALP-2) promoted Th2-type responses, plasma IgG, and mucosal S-IgA Ab responses against coadministered Ags such as β-galactosidase and HIV-1 Tat protein through TLR2 (173).

The discovery that gene-associated molecules (e.g., DNA and RNA) had immune-stimulating activities allowed us to extend this system for development of mucosal adjuvants. Bacterial, but not eukaryotic, DNA generally contains nonmethylated "CpG motifs" and acts as a ligand for TLR9, thus, initiating innate and adaptive immunity (11). Thus, plasmid DNA for gene vaccination can be functionally divided into two distinct units: a transcription unit and an adjuvant/mitogen unit (131). The latter unit contains immunostimulatory sequences consisting of short palindromic nucleotides centered on a CpG dinucleotide core. It is now clear that CpG motifs can induce B cell proliferation and Ig synthesis as well as cytokine secretion (i.e., IL-6, IFN-α, IFN-β, IFN-γ, IL-12, and IL-18) by a variety of immune cells (131). Numerous studies have shown that mucosal administration of Ag with CpG promoted mucosal S-IgA, plasma IgG, and T cell responses, including CD8$^+$ CTLs and CD4$^+$ Th1 cells accompanied with type I IFN production by DCs, which induced protective immunity against various types of infections, such as *S. pneumoniae,* HIV, HSV-2, and *Helicobacter pylori* (131).

Mucosal Ag Delivery Systems

The mucosal delivery of Ag is another important subject in the area of mucosal vaccine development. Various approaches toward the development of an ideal mucosal Ag delivery system have been developed using inert particles, including biodegradable polymer-based particles (microspheres and nanospheres) as well as lipid-based particles such as liposomes and ISCOMs (6,174). Incorporation of Ags into these particles usually protects them from proteolytic degradation by mucosal enzymes and acids; however particles by themselves are nonimmunogenic. Further, variation in microsphere chemical composition allows generation of particles with fast or slow degradation to stimulate long-lasting responses. Several different Ags can be incorporated into a single preparation, and other substances such as cytokines can be co-incorporated with Ags to show ensuing immune responses (6). These obvious attractive features are, however, counterbalanced by serious disadvantages. Specifically, the disappointingly low uptake from mucosal surfaces (<1%), low rate of incorporation, and the use of organic solvents that may denature Ags are negative features.

To overcome this limitation, several modifications have been attempted to deliver the Ag selectively to M cells, the major targets for delivery of encapsulated Ag. Lectins have been widely exploited to gain or to enhance access to M cells. It has been considered that *Ulex europaeus agglutinin* 1 (UEA-1), a lectin specific for α-L-fucose residues, binds almost exclusively to the apical surface of M cells of murine PPs and NALT (44). The unique reactivity of UEA-1 to M cells allowed the selective and effective delivery of microspheres or liposomes to M cells after oral administration, which led to the significant enhancement of Ag-specific Ab responses (175). Recent advances in biomedical technology have been utilized to identify organic molecules or peptides that mimic the functional activity of UEA-1 using mixture-based positional scanning of synthetic combinatorial libraries or of phage peptide libraries. The former study revealed that a digalloyl D-Lysine amide construct and a tetragalloyl D-Lysine amide construct bound effectively to M cells, and the coating of particles with these compounds resulted in the selective delivery of the particles to M cells with high efficacy (176). The latter study demonstrated that specific peptide (YQCSYTMPHPPV) selectively bound to the M cell–rich subepithelial dome region of the PPs and enhanced the delivery of microspheres to M cells (177). In addition to these molecules, an M cell–specific monoclonal antibody (mAb) (NKM16-2-4) was recently developed, which can be used for the M cell–targeted delivery of vaccine antigen (178). This mAb recognized carbohydrate-modified molecules selectively expressed on M cells and thus, effectively delivered the conjugated vaccine Ag to M cells for the induction of mucosal and systemic Ag-specific immune responses (178).

Microbial adhesins have been applied to the targeted delivery of synthetic particles to M cells. As expected given the selectivity of ligands, enhanced Ag uptake was achieved by coating polystyrene nanospheres with *Yersinia*-derived invasin, a ligand for β1 integrins on the apical side of M cells (44,59). Similarly, reoviruses are known to invade through M cells using a 45-kDa viral haemagglutinin σ1 protein (44,59). Subsequent studies demonstrated that mucosal immune responses were significantly increased by mucosal immunization by coupling a reovirus-derived σ1 protein (179). As another approach, hybrid Ag delivery vehicles have been developed (180). These vehicles are composed of a synthetic liposome and virus, such as influenza and Sendai viruses (6). Using fusion activity that originates from the virus, the virus-mimicked liposomes could effectively deliver the encapsulated Ag to MALTs and induce high levels of Ag-specific immune responses.

Attenuated live microorganisms have been developed as vaccines, and some of them have already been used as mucosal vaccines (e.g., poliovirus, *S. typhi* Ty21a, and *V. cholerae*) (6,181,182) since the attenuation may not affect the natural abilities of bacteria to survive in the hostile environment of the intestinal and respiratory tracts and to bind to M cells to promote vaccine uptake for the effective induction of mucosal and systemic immune responses. Recent progress in genetic technology has allowed the creation of a new application of attenuated vaccines for Ag delivery, namely recombinant attenuated vaccines carrying DNA encoding heterologous Ag (6,181,182). In the attenuated recombinant vaccines, several genes determining pathogenicity have been mutated or disrupted, and a gene encoding a heterologous Ag has been inserted, which ensures both safety and effectiveness. Vectors that have been tested include various species of attenuated bacteria such as *S. typhi*, *Shigella flexneri*, and *Listeria monocytogenes*, *V. cholerae*, *Lactobacillus*, and *Y. enterocolitica* (181). Similarly, recombinant viruses have been established as vehicles for mucosal vaccine delivery (182). Since CTL responses appear to be pivotal in chronic viral infections, these efforts have been aimed at developing mucosal vaccines that induce both mucosal S-IgA and CTL responses to prevent initial contact of pathogens with host cells in mucosal sites and for surveillance of virus-infected cells, respectively. Several types of viruses have the advantage of their natural transmission via mucosal sites. These include poxvirus, adenovirus, HSV, adeno-associated virus, alphavirus (e.g., Semliki Forest virus and Sindbis virus), vesicular stomatitis virus, and poliovirus (182).

Novel molecular methods have allowed the production of subunit vaccines in transgenic plants (183). Plant-based vaccines offer some advantages over other systems, including: 1) the ability to carry out posttranslational modifications similar to eukaryotes; 2) ease of production of large quantities at reduced costs; 3) no requirement to use a human pathogen. Assemblies of one or more Ags that retain both T and B cell epitopes have been expressed in genetically modified plants (GM plants) and are now being tested for their potential use as human or animal vaccines. To date, many plant species have been employed for vaccine usage. Early studies used tobacco and potato plants, but now tomato, banana, corn, lupine, lettuce, wheat, rice, and other plants are being used for this purpose (183). To circumvent potential denaturation of Ag during cooking, recombinant plants such as tomatoes, lettuce, and bananas have been developed. To overcome the "cold chain" problem, grain (e.g., corn, wheat, and rice) are suitable because they can be stored at ambient temperature for a long time. Along these lines, a rice-based vaccine technology was introduced. In mice orally immunized with rice expressing CT-B kept over 18 monthes under normal temperature condition (or without any refergiration), CT-B–specific intestinal S-IgA Ab responses were elicited, which enabled them to protect against CT-induced diarrhea (183a). Like this one example, considerable progress has been achieved to show that protective immune responses are induced in animal model studies and, more recently, in completing application trials for target animals for veterinary vaccines (183). Thus, although many problems need to be overcome for use of this technology clinically, including low yields and inconsistent product quality for GM plant standards, there is no doubt that plant-based vaccines are still considered to be a most promising mucosal vaccine system.

MUCOSAL DISEASES AND IMMUNOTHERAPY

IgA Deficiency

Deficiency of IgA is the most common primary immunodeficiency disease in humans (184). Serological data indicate that in Western Europe and the United States, one out of 400 to 700 individuals are affected; in Japan, the disease is less frequent (~1:18,000). Deficiency of IgA frequently escapes detection, because a large percentage of afflicted individuals have no clinical symptoms. In an absolute majority of cases, both serum IgA1 and IgA2 are either deficient or are present in low levels (<50 mg/100 ml). Although rare, selective deficiencies of IgA1 or IgA2 subclasses, due to the deletion of Cα1 or Cα2 genes, have been described (184). It is well recognized that the majority of IgA-deficient individuals are asymptomatic presumably due to alternative compensatory presence of S-IgM in external secretions that functionally substitutes for the deficient S-IgA. However, it appears that in comparison to normal individuals, patients with IgA deficiency have a higher incidence of recurrent infections, especially in the upper respiratory tract, allergic diseases, autoimmune disorders, and malignancies, particularly intestinal adenocarcinomas (184). Absence or low levels of S-IgA Abs to microbial and food Ags may result in higher rates of absorption of such Ags from mucosal surfaces, induction of higher levels of corresponding Abs in plasma, and formation of circulating immune complexes. Although S-IgM may replace S-IgA in deficient patients, it appears that S-IgM does not fully substitute for the IgA-associated functions. This may be partly ascribed to the anti-inflammatory nature of IgA manifested by its inability to activate C with potential inflammatory consequences. In contrast, both IgM and IgG are potent C activators, and it has been demonstrated that the formation of immune complexes composed of protein Ags and IgM or IgG within mucosal tissues leads to local damage and increased absorption of bystander Ags. Diminished functional substitution of S-IgA with S-IgM is also apparent in frequency of viral and bacterial infections, and responses to vaccines (184).

HIV-1 Infection and the Mucosal Immune System

Mucosal tissues of the genital and intestinal tracts are the most important portals of entry of HIV (124). Epidemiological studies indicate that worldwide ~80%–90% of HIV infections are acquired by mucosal routes through heterosexual and homosexual intercourse and the vertical transmission route *in utero*, during delivery or by breast feeding (124). Further, application of SIV on the surfaces of vagina, penile urethra, or nasopharyngeal lymphoid tissues was sufficient to infect rhesus monkeys (123).

Several mucosal cell types may be involved in the initial uptake of HIV and SIV (123,124). In animal models, specialized M cells found in the intestinal PPs, in analogous lymphoepithelial structures of the rectum, and also in tonsils are capable of internalization of HIV/SIV and presumably passing the virus to adjacent infectable cells including T cells, MΦ and DCs (123,124). Human intestinal and oral EC lines and primary IECs internalize HIV and are infectable *in vitro* due to the expression of HIV receptors/coreceptors (CD4, galactosyl-ceramide, and CC-chemokine receptors, mainly CCR5 and to a lesser extent CXCR4) on their surfaces (185). However, direct *in vivo* evidence for the presence of HIV in enterocytes is not available. In rhesus macaques vaginally exposed to cell-free

SIV, Langerhans cells dispersed in the stratified squamous vaginal epithelium were the first cells that were infected (185). Previous studies indicate that SIV and HIV primarily targets and destroys mucosal CD4$^+$ cells perhaps due to the selective expression of chemokine receptors (123,124). Isolated mucosal MΦ are less permissive for HIV infection than phenotypically distinct blood monocytes probably due to the reduced expression of HIV coreceptors (123,124). In addition to the initial HIV infection sites, mucosal tissues, especially gastrointestinal sites, are involved in the chronic activation of the systemic immune system, a hallmark of progressive HIV infection. A recent study demonstrated that chronically HIV-infected individuals and rhesus macaques infected with SIV showed increased amounts of LPS in the blood, which was presumably derived from commensal microbiota in the GI tracts (186). It was also shown that the microbial translocation from gastrointestinal mucosa to systemic compartments correlated with chronic activation through both innate and acquired immune systems, providing evidence for chronic systemic immune activation in HIV infection mediated by the GI mucosa.

HIV-1–specific Abs become detectable in sera shortly after infection. In all seropositive individuals, these Abs are of the IgG isotype; IgA Abs are present less frequently and occur at much lower levels. Extensive studies of external secretions, including tears, saliva, nasal, intestinal, and vaginal washes; semen; cervical mucus; milk; fecal extracts; and urine yielded often controversial results with respect to the presence and isotypes of HIV-1–specific Abs (123,124). Differences in the collection procedures, processing of samples, dilutions of some secretions by washing fluids, and methodologies used for Ab detection may account for some of these discrepancies. Surprisingly, HIV-1–specific Abs of the IgG isotype are dominant in all secretions despite the overwhelming levels of total IgA and route of infection (systemic or mucosal) (123,124). For example, in human milk, intestinal fluid, and saliva, in which IgA represents ~98% to 99% and IgG only ~1% of total Igs, HIV-1–specific Abs are present mainly in the IgG isotype. In external secretions of individuals with HIV-1–specific IgA Abs, there is a pronounced restriction to the IgA1 subclass (187). Absence or presence of levels of HIV-1–specific IgA Abs in external secretions is not due to a defect in the production of total IgA or unresponsiveness to viral Ags: IgA Abs to, for example, influenza virus are readily detectable in secretions of HIV-1–infected individuals (188). The mechanisms involved in this diminished responsiveness to HIV-1 but not the influenza virus in the S-IgA isotype have not been clarified. The site of original infection and the presence of effective mucosal inductive sites in the upper respiratory tract but not in the genital tract may play a role. Initial reports (188) of the selective occurrence of HIV-1–specific Abs in secretions of HIV-1–exposed but seronegative individuals have not been confirmed in other studies. Studies concerning the presence of CTLs in mucosal tissues of HIV-infected individuals are rather limited mainly due to the unavailability of tissues to perform extensive analyses. The progressive decline of immune functions in long-term HIV-1–infected and untreated individuals also compromise the mucosal immune system. An increased incidence of infections with mucosal opportunistic pathogens, including viruses, bacteria, fungi and protozoa, and of mucosal neoplasms has been observed.

IBD

IBD represents a chronic, relapsing, and remitting inflammatory condition of the GI tract that is manifest as one of the two, usually distinct but significantly overlapping, clinical entities, ulcerative colitis (UC) and Crohn's disease (CD). Increasing evidence suggests that IBD is a dysregulated mucosal immune response to components of the normal commensal luminal microbiota in a genetically susceptible host that is further modified by a variety of environmental factors. The majority of these insights have come through a variety of animal models of IBD, including those that occur spontaneously and those that are induced by administration of exogenous agents, gene targeting through knockout or transgenic approaches, or transfer of cells into immunodeficient animals (189,190).

The incidence of IBD is reduced when bacterial colonization is eliminated through germ-free conditions or reduced such as through antibiotic administration, suggesting that the intestinal microflora is involved in the development of IBD (189,190). However, not all bacteria are equal in this regard. For example, some groups of organisms are known to trigger colitis in genetically susceptible animal strains, such as the ability of *Bacteroides vulgatus* to stimulate colitis in HLA-B27 transgenic rats (191). However, some groups of organisms are able to prevent colitis such as *Lactobacillus sp.*, which are considered to be probiotics and are known to prevent colitis in genetically susceptible hosts such as IL-10 knockout mice (192). Consistent with the protective role of MyD88 signaling in the intestine as mentioned earlier (22), it is now clear that probiotics mediate their anti-inflammatory effects at least partially through TLR9-mediated CpG signaling (131). Thus, TLR9$^{-/-}$ mice showed impaired inhibitory function of probiotics or CpG against experimental colitis. Further, methylated probiotic DNA, calf thymus DNA, and DNase-treated probiotics had no effect on the inhibition of colitis (131).

In addition, colitis in mouse models appears to be triggered by a subset of protein Ags that largely activate effector T cells as manifested by the evidence of private and, to a lesser extent, public TCR motifs in bacterially driven disease models such as the CD45RB^{high} transfer model in *scid/scid* mice consistent with observations in humans (189,190). Interestingly, the response in the involved IBD intestine is associated with T cell activation and production of Th1 (IFN-γ), Th2 (IL-4), Th17 (ZL-17) and regulatory cytokines (IL-10 and TGF-β). This is consistent with the concept that the final common pathway of excessive Th1, Th2 or Th17 cytokine production that underlies the pathogenesis of these IBDs is achieved by either excessive Th1 or Th2 effector T cells or ineffective counterbalance of effector T cells by regulatory subsets of cells that secrete anti-inflammatory cytokines such as IL-10 and TGF-β. This has placed significant emphasis on defining the regulatory subsets of cells involved in blocking disease pathogenesis and has allowed for drawing significant similarities between and insights from mechanisms previously related to the study of oral tolerance. Indeed, oral tolerance has been shown to be effective in the prevention of IBD through production of these regulatory cytokines in animal models (132). Additionally, a recent study reveals evidence of a genetic defect in oral tolerance in IBD patients (193). As such, the role of Treg cells in intestinal homeostasis has been gained from studies using the T cell transfer colitis model. In this model, cotransfer of CD4$^+$ CD45RB^{low} T cells together with CD4$^+$ CD45RB^{high} T cells prevents the pathology due to the IL-10– and TGF-β–dependent activity of Treg cells (139). In addition to Treg cells, the iNKT cell type has also been shown to inhibit IBD (194). Thus, an amelioration of IBD symptoms was noted in mice treated with αGalCer, but not αManCer, via the IL-10 production by iNKT cells.

Mucosal Allergies

The majority of allergic immunologic diseases are of mucosal origin, and their clinical manifestations are locally expressed. The diseases tend to mainly affect the upper respiratory and GI tracts. Numerous anti-allergic drugs have been developed, but these drugs do not achieve a permanent cure for the allergic diseases. There is a general belief that this increase is due to "cleanliness" in our environment so that exposure to allergens can more often result in hypersensitivity and not classical immunity to infections like tuberculosis, measles, or hepatitis A (195). Asthma is the most common of the severe atopic diseases, which also include allergic rhinitis. The three hallmarks of asthma include: 1) variable airflow obstruction, 2) airway hyperresponsiveness (AHR), and 3) airway inflammation (196). However, hypersensitivity in the GI tract emanates from ingestion of large amounts of food Ags, including cow's milk proteins, eggs, and peanuts (197). It is generally agreed that Th2-type responses, characterized by the enhanced production of IL-4, IL-5, IL-9, and IL-13, and IgE-mediated Ab responses to common inhaled and fed allergens are major factors in the development of both asthma and food allergy (196,197). Therefore, inhibition of allergen-specific Th2 cells and blocking Th2 differentiation among new responses are reasonable goals for disease manipulation. The former is achieved, for example, by treatment with anti-IL-4 or IL-13 mAbs or soluble cytokine receptors, and the latter was mediated by blocking the interaction between CD28 and CD80/CD86, inhibiting ICOS function, or IL-12 expression (197). In addition, new drugs targeting Th2 effector molecules include PPAR agonists (e.g., cyclopentenone, prostaglandins, and thiazolidinediones) (198). The treatment with PPAR agonists inhibited GATA-3, a Th2-specific transcription factor, and decreased Th2-driven IgE production and inhibited asthma. Further, a Th1-dominant environment is also achieved by TLR-mediated stimulation because these triggers tend to induce Th1 responses as mentioned above. Thus, some TLR ligands (e.g., CpG oligodeoxynucleotides) have been established as agents effective against mucosal allergy in animal models, and clinical trials have been initiated (131). Similarly, blocking IgE activity resulted in the inhibition of allergic responses by suppression of inflammatory cell (e.g., mast cells and basophils) migration and degranulation (199).

Induction of tolerance is another strategy against mucosal allergy (132). Induction of tolerance by repeated subcutaneous injection of allergen has been used in clinical practice for nearly 100 years and is successful in selected allergic patients sensitive to a limited number of allergens. In addition to subcutaneous injection, oral or nasal administration has been employed to induce tolerance in animal models and clinical trials against various allergens such as pollen and house dust (132). In this context, a rice-based vaccine system expressing multiple T cell epitopes has been developed to induce oral tolerance and inhibit allergy (200). In addition to allergy, mucosal tolerance has been applied to other diseases, including EAE, arthritis, diabetes, myasthenia gravis, transplantation, and others (132).

As mentioned earlier, Treg cells play an important role in the induction of mucosal tolerance (132,139). The relationship between Treg cells and mucosal allergy was implicated by reports that the ratio of allergen-specific effector Th2 cells and Treg cells may be linked to the pathogenesis of food allergy (201). Among several types of Treg cells (e.g., naturally arising Treg cells, Tr1, and Th3), allergen-specific IL-10–producing Treg cells display strong immunosuppressive potential (201). Consistent with this, several studies suggested that IL-10 levels were inversely correlated with the severity of human allergic disease (201). However, recent studies revealed a novel pathway mediated by naturally arising Treg cells to inhibit asthma via an IL-10–independent pathway (202), suggesting that mucosal allergies can be treated by the versatile Treg cell system.

The recruitment of effector cells at the sites of allergen exposure is a target for treating mucosal allergy (197). This could be achieved by interfering selectively with the system of adhesion molecules regulating the trafficking of Th2 cells and inflammatory cells (e.g., eosinophils, basophils, and mast cells). For example, blocking the adhesion molecule LFA-1 has been shown to be effective in the inhibition of airway inflammation in animals and in allergic patients (197). Chemokines are other target molecules in preventing allergic inflammation (197). A recent study demonstrated that Th17 cells reduced AHR by down-regulation of CCL11/eotaxin and CCL17/TARC production in the lungs (203). In addition, several other chemokines (e.g., CCL17, CCL1, and CXCL12) have been considered to facilitate preferentially the development of Th2 inflammation (204). Using a food allergy model, it was recently reported that S1P, a lipid mediator, contributes to the regulation of migration of pathogenic CD4 T and mast cells from the systemic immune compartment into the large intestine and inhibition of S1P-mediated pathway results in the inhibition of development of allergic diarrhea (205).

Celiac Disease

Celiac disease is another related disorder of mucosal immunity, which is characterized by small-intestinal mucosal injury in response to the dietary ingestion of gluten (29). Gluten is a proline- and glutamine-rich protein that is found in wheat, rye, and barley. Pathologic features of celiac disease include increased numbers of IELs and less extensive villous atrophy and crypt hypertrophy (29). IELs from patients with celiac disease preferentially include NK-like cells, which recognize stress-induced MICA molecules expressed on IECs (29). This process has been considered to be mediated by IL-15. IL-15 induces increased expression of MICA and subsequent interaction between MICA and its receptor, NKG2D, and up-regulates gluten-specific CTL activity in the small intestine (206). Gluten-free diet currently is the only accepted therapy for celiac disease, and various immunological approaches such as blocking IL-15 and treatment with IL-10 have been examined (29). However, in terms of quality of life, it is doubtful that this treatment will be effective with so many potential side effects. Thus, it is essential to identify the gluten-specific pathogenic immunocompetent cell population for the development of novel strategies to selectively delete the specific pathogenic populations.

ACKNOWLEDGMENTS

We thank all members of our laboratories for their assistance with the preparation of this chapter. The experimental results included in this chapter were supported by U.S. Public Health grant U19 AI 28147; MSM 0021620812 from the Czech Republic; Core Research for Evolutional Science and Technology (CREST) of the Japan Science and Technology Corporation (JST), the Ministry of Education, Science, Sports, and Culture, and the Ministry of Health and Welfare in Japan.

REFERENCES

1. Cone RA. Mucus. *Mucosal Immunology*, 3rd ed. Mestecky J, Lamm ME, Strober W, Bienenstock J, McGhee JR, Mayer L, eds. San Diego: Academic Press. 2005;35–48.
2. Furuse M, Tsukita S. Claudins in occluding junctions of humans and flies. *Trends Cell Biol*. 2006;16:181–188.
3. Vijay-Kumar M, Gewirtz AT. Role of epithelium in mucosal immunity. *Mucosal Immunology*, 3rd ed. Mestecky J, Lamm ME, Strober W, Bienenstock J, McGhee JR, Mayer L, eds. San Diego: Academic Press. 2005;423–434.
4. Lehrer RI, Bevins CL, Ganz T. Defensins and other antimicrobial peptides and proteins. *Mucosal Immunology*, 3rd ed. Mestecky J, Lamm ME, Strober W, et al., eds. San Diego: Academic Press. 2005;73–94.
5. Russell MW, Bobek LA, Brock JH, et al. Innate humoral defense factors. *Mucosal Immunology*, 3rd ed. Mestecky J, Lamm ME, Strober W, et al., eds. San Diego: Academic Press. 2005;73–94.
6. Kunisawa J, McGhee J, Kiyono H. Mucosal S-IgA enhancement: development of safe and effective mucosal adjuvants and mucosal antigen delivery vehicles. In: *Mucosal Immune Defense: Immunoglobulin A*. Kaetzel C, ed. New York: Kluwer Academic/Plenum Publishers. 2007;346–389.
7. Chaby R, Garcia-Verdugo I, Espinassous Q, et al. Interactions between LPS and lung surfactant proteins. *J Endotoxin Res*. 2005;11: 181–185.
8. Brinkmann V, Reichard U, Goosmann C, et al. Neutrophil extracellular traps kill bacteria. *Science*. 2004;303:1532–1535.
9. Kaetzel CS. The polymeric immunoglobulin receptor: bridging innate and adaptive immune responses at mucosal surfaces. *Immunol Rev*. 2005;206:83–99.
10. Lencer WI, Blumberg RS. A passionate kiss, then run: exocytosis and recycling of IgG by FcRn. *Trends Cell Biol*. 2005;15:5–9.
11. Akira S, Uematsu S, Takeuchi O. Pathogen recognition and innate immunity. *Cell*. 2006;124:783–801.
12. Lee MS, Kim YJ. Signaling pathways downstream of pattern-recognition receptors and their cross talk. *Annu Rev Biochem*. 2007;76:447–480.
13. Cario E, Podolsky DK. Toll-like receptor signaling and its relevance to intestinal inflammation. *Ann NY Acad Sci*. 2006;1072:332–338.
14. Kelly D, Conway S, Aminov R. Commensal gut bacteria: mechanisms of immune modulation. *Trends Immunol*. 2005; 26:326–333.
15. Lotz M, Gutle D, Walther S, et al. Postnatal acquisition of endotoxin tolerance in intestinal epithelial cells. *J Exp Med*. 2006; 203:973–984.
16. Lee J, Mo JH, Katakura K, et al. Maintenance of colonic homeostasis by distinctive apical TLR9 signalling in intestinal epithelial cells. *Nat Cell Biol*. 2006;8:1327–1336.
17. Schenk M, Mueller C. Adaptations of intestinal macrophages to an antigen-rich environment. *Semin Immunol*. 2007;19:84–93.
18. Kuwata H, Matsumoto M, Atarashi K, et al. IκBNS inhibits induction of a subset of Toll-like receptor-dependent genes and limits inflammation. *Immunity*. 2006;24:41–51.
19. Uematsu S, Jang MH, Chevrier N, et al. Detection of pathogenic intestinal bacteria by Toll-like receptor 5 on intestinal CD11c$^+$ lamina propria cells. *Nat Immunol*. 2006;7:868–874.
20. Munn DH, Sharma MD, Lee JR, et al. Potential regulatory function of human dendritic cells expressing indoleamine 2,3-dioxygenase. *Science*. 2002;297:1867–1870.
21. Watanabe T, Kitani A, Murray PJ, et al. Nucleotide binding oligomerization domain 2 deficiency leads to dysregulated TLR2

signaling and induction of antigen-specific colitis. *Immunity.* 2006;25:473–485.

22. Rakoff-Nahoum S, Paglino J, Eslami-Varzaneh F, et al. Recognition of commensal microflora by toll-like receptors is required for intestinal homeostasis. *Cell*. 2004;118:229–241.
23. Hysi P, Kabesch M, Moffatt MF, et al. NOD1 variation, immunoglobulin E and asthma. *Hum Mol Genet.* 2005;14:935–941.
24. Nigo YI, Yamashita M, Hirahara K, et al. Regulation of allergic airway inflammation through Toll-like receptor 4-mediated modification of mast cell function. *Proc Natl Acad Sci U S A.* 2006;103:2286–2291.
25. Kunisawa J, Takahashi I, Kiyono H. Intraepithelial lymphocytes: their shared and divergent immunological behaviors in the small and large intestine. *Immunol Rev*. 2007;215:136–153.
26. Cepek KL, Shaw SK, Parker CM, et al. Adhesion between epithelial cells and T lymphocytes mediated by E-cadherin and the $\alpha E\beta 7$ integrin. *Nature*. 1994;372:190–193.
27. Cheroutre H. Starting at the beginning: new perspectives on the biology of mucosal T cells. *Annu Rev Immunol.* 2004;22:217–246.
28. Lefrancois L. Cytotoxic T cells of the mucosal immune system. In: *Mucosal Immunology*, 3rd ed. Mestecky J, Lamm ME, Strober W, Bienenstock J, McGhee JR, Mayer L. eds. San Diego: Academic Press. 2005;559–564.
29. Kagnoff MF. Celiac disease: pathogenesis of a model immunogenetic disease. *J Clin Invest.* 2007;117:41–49.
30. Staton TL, Habtezion A, Winslow MM, et al. $CD8^{+}$ recent thymic emigrants home to and efficiently repopulate the small intestine epithelium. *Nat Immunol.* 2006;7:482–488.
31. Lambolez F, Kronenberg M, Cheroutre H. Thymic differentiation of $TCR\alpha\beta^{+}$ $CD8\alpha\alpha^{+}$ IELs. *Immunol Rev*. 2007;215:178–188.
32. Ishikawa H, Naito T, Iwanaga T, et al. *Curriculum vitae* of intestinal intraepithelial T cells: their developmental and behavioral characteristics. *Immunol Rev*. 2007;215:154–165.
33. Kunisawa J, Kurashima Y, Higuchi M, et al. Sphingosine 1-phosphate dependence in the regulation of lymphocyte trafficking to the gut epithelium. *J Exp Med*. 2007;204:2335–2348.
34. Ishikawa H, Kanamori Y, Hamada H, et al. Development and function of organized gut-associated lymphoid tissues. In: *Mucosal Immunology*, 3rd ed. Mestecky J, Lamm ME, Strober W, et al., eds. San Diego: Academic Press. 2005;385–406.
35. Saito H, Kanamori Y, Takemori T, et al. Generation of intestinal T cells from progenitors residing in gut cryptopatches. *Science*. 1998; 280:275–278.
36. Bendelac A, Savage PB, Teyton L. The biology of NKT cells. *Annu Rev Immunol.* 2007;25:297–336.
37. Mayer L Blumberg RS. Role of epithelial cells in mucosal antigen presentation. In: *Mucosal Immunology*, 3rd ed. Mestecky J, Lamm ME, Strober W, et al., eds. San Diego: Academic Press. 2005;435–450.
38. Treiner E, Duban L, Bahram S, et al. Selection of evolutionarily conserved mucosal-associated invariant T cells by MR1. *Nature.* 2003;422:164–169.
39. Croxford JL, Miyake S, Huang YY, et al. Invariant $V\alpha 19i$ T cells regulate autoimmune inflammation. *Nat Immunol.* 2006;7:987–994.
40. Bienenstock J, McDermott MR. Bronchus- and nasal-associated lymphoid tissues. *Immunol Rev*. 2005;206:22–31.
41. Kiyono H, Fukuyama S. NALT- versus Peyers-patch-mediated mucosal immunity. *Nat Rev Immunol.* 2004;4:699–710.
42. Kunisawa J, Fukuyama S, Kiyono H. Mucosa-associated lymphoid tissues in aerodigestive tract: their shared and divergent traits and their importance to the orchestration of mucosal immune system. *Curr Mol Med.* 2005;5:557–572.
43. Debertin AS, Tschernig T, Tonjes H, et al. Nasal-associated lymphoid tissue (NALT): frequency and localization in young children. *Clin Exp Immunol.* 2003;134:503–507.
44. Neutra MR Kraehenbuhl J. Cellular and molecular basis for antigen transport across epithelial barriers. In: *Mucosal Immunology*, 3rd ed. Mestecky J, Lamm ME, Strober W, et al., eds. San Diego: Academic Press. 2005;111–132.
45. Kerneis S, Bogdanova A, Kraehenbuhl JP, et al. Conversion by Peyers patch lymphocytes of human enterocytes into M cells that transport bacteria. *Science.* 1997;277:949–952.
46. Brandtzaeg P Johansen FE. Mucosal B cells: phenotypic characteristics, transcriptional regulation, and homing properties. *Immunol Rev.* 2005;206:32–63.
47. Cebra JJ, Jiang HQ, Boiko NV, et al. The role of mucosal microbiota in the development, maintenance, and pathologies of the mucosal immune system. In: *Mucosal Immunology*, 3rd ed. Mestecky J, Lamm ME, Strober W, et al., eds. San Diego: Academic Press. 2005;335–368.
48. Fujihashi K McGhee J. Th1/Th2/Th3 cells for regulation of mucosal immunity, tolerance, and inflammation. In: *Mucosal Immunology*, 3rd ed. Mestecky J, Lamm ME, Strober W, et al., eds. San Diego: Academic Press. 2005;539–558.
49. Wagner N, Lohler J, Kunkel EJ, et al. Critical role for $\beta 7$ integrins in formation of the gut-associated lymphoid tissue. *Nature.* 1996;382:366–370.
50. Youngman K, Lazarus N, Butcher EC. Lymphocyte homing: chemokines and adhesion molecules in T call and IgA plasma cell. In: *Mucosal Immunology*, 3rd ed. Mestecky J, Lamm ME, Strober W, et al., eds. San Diego: Academic Press. 2005;667–380.
51. Johansson C, Kelsall BL. Phenotype and function of intestinal dendritic cells. *Semin Immunol.* 2005;17:284–294.
52. Iwasaki A. Mucosal dendritic cells. *Annu Rev Immunol*. 2007;25: 381–418.
53. Cook DN, Prosser DM, Forster R, et al. CCR6 mediates dendritic cell localization, lymphocyte homeostasis, and immune responses in mucosal tissue. *Immunity*. 2000;12:495–503.
54. Fagarasan S, Shinkura R, Kamata T, et al. Alymphoplasia (aly)-type nuclear factor kappaB-inducing kinase (NIK) causes defects in secondary lymphoid tissue chemokine receptor signaling and homing of peritoneal cells to the gut-associated lymphatic tissue system. *J Exp Med*. 2000;191:1477–1486.
55. Fukuda K, Yoshida H, Sato T, et al. Mesenchymal expression of Foxl1, a winged helix transcriptional factor, regulates generation and maintenance of gut-associated lymphoid organs. *Dev Biol.* 2003;255:278–289.
56. Veiga-Fernandes H, Coles MC, Foster KE, et al. Tyrosine kinase receptor RET is a key regulator of Peyers patch organogenesis. *Nature*. 2007;446:547–551.
57. Fagarasan S, Muramatsu M, Suzuki K, et al. Critical roles of activation-induced cytidine deaminase in the homeostasis of gut flora. *Science.* 2002;298:1424–1427.
58. Kweon MN, Yamamoto M, Rennert PD, et al. Prenatal blockage of lymphotoxin beta receptor and TNF receptor p55 signaling cascade resulted in the acceleration of tissue genesis for isolated lymphoid follicles in the large intestine. *J Immunol*. 2005;174:4365–4372.
59. Brayden DJ, Jepson MA, Baird AW. Keynote review: intestinal Peyers patch M cells and oral vaccine targeting. *Drug Discov Today.* 2005;10:1145–1157.
60. Teitelbaum R, Schubert W, Gunther L, et al. The M cell as a portal of entry to the lung for the bacterial pathogen *Mycobacterium tuberculosis*. *Immunity*. 1999;10:641–650.
61. Weaver CT, Harrington LE, Mangan PR, et al. Th17: an effector CD4 T cell lineage with regulatory T cell ties. *Immunity.* 2006;24:677–688.
62. Mangan PR, Harrington LE, O'Quinn DB, et al. Transforming growth factor-β induces development of the T(H)17 lineage. *Nature*. 2006;441:231–234.
63. Bettelli E, Carrier Y, Gao W, et al. Reciprocal developmental pathways for the generation of pathogenic effector TH17 and regulatory T cells. *Nature.* 2006;441:235–238.
64. Ward RL, Greenberg HB, Estes MK. Viral gastroenteritis vaccines. In: *Mucosal Immunology*, 3rd ed. Mestecky J, Lamm ME, Strober W, et al., eds. San Diego: Academic Press. 2005;887–904.
65. Schmid DS, Rouse BT. Respiratory viral vaccines. In: *Mucosal Immunology*, 3rd ed. Mestecky J, Lamm ME, Strober W, et al., eds. San Diego: Academic Press. 2005;923–936.
66. Strober W, Fagarasan S, Lycke N. IgA B cell development. In: *Mucosal Immunology*, 3rd ed. Mestecky J, Lamm ME, Strober W, et al., eds. San Diego: Academic Press. 2005;583–616.
67. Mega J, Bruce MG, Beagley KW, et al. Regulation of mucosal responses by $CD4^{+}$ T lymphocytes: effects of anti-L3T4 treatment on the gastrointestinal immune system. *Int Immunol*. 1991;3:793–805.

68. Kawanishi H, Ozato K, Strober W. The proliferative response of cloned Peyers patch switch T cells to syngeneic and allogeneic stimuli. *J Immunol.* 1985;134:3586–3591.
69. Zan H, Cerutti A, Dramitinos P, et al. CD40 engagement triggers switching to IgA1 and IgA2 in human B cells through induction of endogenous TGF-β: evidence for TGF-β but not IL-10-dependent direct Sμ->Sα and sequential Sμ->Sγ, Sγ->Sα DNA recombination. *J Immunol.* 1998;161:5217–5225.
70. Benson EB, Strober W. Regulation of IgA secretion by T cell clones derived from the human gastrointestinal tract. *J Immunol.* 1988;140:1874–1882.
71. Lebman DA, Lee FD, Coffman RL. Mechanism for transforming growth factor β and IL-2 enhancement of IgA expression in lipopolysaccharide-stimulated B cell cultures. *J Immunol.* 1990;144:952–959.
72. Sonoda E, Matsumoto R, Hitoshi Y, et al. Transforming growth factor β induces IgA production and acts additively with interleukin 5 for IgA production. *J Exp Med.* 1989;170:1415–1420.
73. Rousset F, Garcia E, Banchereau J. Cytokine-induced proliferation and immunoglobulin production of human B lymphocytes triggered through their CD40 antigen. *J Exp Med.* 1991;173:705–710.
74. Defrance T, Vanbervliet B, Briere F, et al. Interleukin 10 and transforming growth factor β cooperate to induce anti-CD40-activated naive human B cells to secrete immunoglobulin A. *J Exp Med.* 1992;175:671–682.
75. Cazac BB Roes J. TGF-β receptor controls B cell responsiveness and induction of IgA *in vivo*. *Immunity.* 2000;13:443–451.
76. Jung S, Rajewsky K, Radbruch A. Shutdown of class switch recombination by deletion of a switch region control element. *Science.* 1993;259:984–987.
77. Harriman GR, Bradley A, Das S, et al. IgA class switch in I α exon-deficient mice. Role of germline transcription in class switch recombination. *J Clin Invest.* 1996;97:477–485.
78. Honjo T, Nagaoka H, Shinkura R, et al. AID to overcome the limitations of genomic information. *Nat Immunol.* 2005;6:655–661.
79. Shikina T, Hiroi T, Iwatani K, et al. IgA class switch occurs in the organized nasopharynx- gut-associated lymphoid tissue, but not in the diffuse lamina propria of airways and gut. *J Immunol.* 2004;172:6259–6264.
80. Fagarasan S, Kinoshita K, Muramatsu M, et al. *In situ* class switching and differentiation to IgA-producing cells in the gut lamina propria. *Nature.* 2001;413:639–643.
81. Macpherson AJ, Lamarre A, McCoy K, et al. IgA production without μ or δ chain expression in developing B cells. *Nat Immunol.* 2001;2:625–631.
82. Iwasato T, Arakawa H, Shimizu A, et al. Biased distribution of recombination sites within S regions upon immunoglobulin class switch recombination induced by transforming growth factor β and lipopolysaccharide. *J Exp Med.* 1992;175:1539–1546.
83. Brandtzaeg P, Surjan L, Jr., Berdal P. Immunoglobulin-producing cells in clinically normal, hyperplastic and inflamed human palatine tonsils. *Acta Otolaryngol Suppl.* 1979;360:211–215.
84. Craig SW, Cebra JJ. Peyers patches: an enriched source of precursors for IgA-producing immunocytes in the rabbit. *J Exp Med.* 1971;134:188–200.
85. Cyster JG. Chemokines, sphingosine-1-phosphate, and cell migration in secondary lymphoid organs. *Annu Rev Immunol.* 2005;23:127–159.
85a. Gohda M, Kunisawa J, Kurashima Y, et al. Sphingosine 1-phosphate regulates the egress of IgA plasmablasts from Peyers patches for intestinal IgA responses. *J Immunol.* 2008 (in press).
86. Farstad IN, Halstensen TS, Kvale D, et al. Topographic distribution of homing receptors on B and T cells in human gut-associated lymphoid tissue: relation of L-selectin and integrin $\alpha 4\beta 7$ to naive and memory phenotypes. *Am J Pathol.* 1997;150:187–199.
87. Agace WW. Tissue-tropic effector T cells: generation and targeting opportunities. *Nat Rev Immunol.* 2006;6:682–692.
88. Iwata M, Hirakiyama A, Eshima Y, et al. Retinoic acid imprints gut-homing specificity on T cells. *Immunity.* 2004;21:527–538.
89. Mora JR, Iwata M, Eksteen B, et al. Generation of gut-homing IgA-secreting B cells by intestinal dendritic cells. *Science.* 2006; 314:1157–1160.
90. Quiding-Jarbrink M, Nordstrom I, Granstrom G, et al. Differential expression of tissue-specific adhesion molecules on human circulating antibody-forming cells after systemic, enteric, and nasal immunizations. A molecular basis for the compartmentalization of effector B cell responses. *J Clin Invest.* 1997;99:1281–1286.
91. Mestecky J, Moro I, Kerr MA, et al. Mucosal Immunoglobulins. In: *Mucosal Immunology*, 3rd ed. Mestecky J, Lamm ME, Strober W, Bienenstock J, McGhee JR, Mayer L, eds. San Diego: Academic Press. 2005;153–182.
92. Kutteh WH, Koopman WJ, Conley ME, et al. Production of predominantly polymeric IgA by human peripheral blood lymphocytes stimulated in vitro with mitogens. *J Exp Med.* 1980;152:1424–1429.
93. Kilian M, Russell MW. Microbial evasion of IgA function. In: *Mucosal Immunology*, 3rd ed. Mestecky J, Lamm ME, Strober W, Bienenstock J, McGhee JR, Mayer L, eds. San Diego: Academic Press. 2005;291–303.
94. Halpern MS, Koshland ME. Novel subunit in secretory IgA. *Nature.* 1970;228:1276–1278.
95. Sorensen V, Sundvold V, Michaelsen TE, et al. Polymerization of IgA and IgM: roles of Cys309/Cys414 and the secretory tailpiece. *J Immunol.* 1999;162:3448–3455.
96. Monteiro RC, Van De Winkel JG. IgA Fc receptors. *Annu Rev Immunol.* 2003;21:177–204.
97. Shibuya A, Honda S. Molecular and functional characteristics of the Fcα/μR, a novel Fc receptor for IgM and IgA. *Springer Semin Immunopathol.* 2006;28:377–382.
98. Moura IC, Centelles MN, Arcos-Fajardo M, et al. Identification of the transferrin receptor as a novel immunoglobulin (Ig)A1 receptor and its enhanced expression on mesangial cells in IgA nephropathy. *J Exp Med.* 2001;194:417–425.
99. McGhee JR, Mestecky J, Elson CO, et al. Regulation of IgA synthesis and immune response by T cells and interleukins. *J Clin Immunol.* 1989;9:175–199.
100. Murray PD, McKenzie DT, Swain SL, et al. Interleukin 5 and interleukin 4 produced by Peyers patch T cells selectively enhance immunoglobulin A expression. *J Immunol.* 1987;139:2669–2674.
101. Beagley KW, Eldridge JH, Lee F, et al. Interleukins and IgA synthesis. Human and murine interleukin 6 induce high rate IgA secretion in IgA-committed B cells. *J Exp Med.* 1989;169:2133–2148.
102. Ramsay AJ, Husband AJ, Ramshaw IA, et al. The role of interleukin-6 in mucosal IgA antibody responses in vivo. *Science.* 1994;264:561–563.
103. Fujihashi K, McGhee JR, Lue C, et al. Human appendix B cells naturally express receptors for and respond to interleukin 6 with selective IgA1 and IgA2 synthesis. *J Clin Invest.* 1991;88:248–252.
104. Fujihashi K, Taguchi T, Aicher WK, et al. Immunoregulatory functions for murine intraepithelial lymphocytes: gamma/delta T cell receptor-positive (TCR$^+$) T cells abrogate oral tolerance, while α/β TCR$^+$ T cells provide B cell help. *J Exp Med.* 1992;175:695–707.
105. Jang MH, Kweon MN, Iwatani K, et al. Intestinal villous M cells: an antigen entry site in the mucosal epithelium. *Proc Natl Acad Sci U S A.* 2004;101:6110–6115.
106. Mach J, Hshieh T, Hsieh D, et al. Development of intestinal M cells. *Immunol Rev.* 2005;206:177–189.
107. Ebert EC. Proliferative responses of human intraepithelial lymphocytes to various T-cell stimuli. *Gastroenterology.* 1989;97:1372–1381.
108. Rescigno M, Urbano M, Valzasina B, et al. Dendritic cells express tight junction proteins and penetrate gut epithelial monolayers to sample bacteria. *Nat Immunol.* 2001;2:361–367.
109. Vazquez-Torres A, Jones-Carson J, Baumler AJ, et al. Extraintestinal dissemination of *Salmonella* by CD18-expressing phagocytes. *Nature.* 1999;401:804–808.
110. Niess JH, Br S, Gu X, et al. CX3CR1-mediated dendritic cell access to the intestinal lumen and bacterial clearance. *Science.* 2005;307:254–258.
111. Huang FP, Platt N, Wykes M, et al. A discrete subpopulation of dendritic cells transports apoptotic intestinal epithelial cells to T cell areas of mesenteric lymph nodes. *J Exp Med.* 2000;191:435–444.

112. Bos NA, Kroese FG, Cebra JJ. B-1 cells and the mucosal immune system. In: *Mucosal Immunology*, 3rd ed. Mestecky J, Lamm ME, Strober W, et al., eds. San Diego: Academic Press. 2005;655–666.
113. Kunisawa J, Kiyono H. A marvel of mucosal T cells and secretory antibodies for the creation of first lines of defense. *Cell Mol Life Sci*. 2005;62:1308–1321.
114. Snider DP, Liang H, Switzer I, et al. IgA production in MHC class II-deficient mice is primarily a function of B-1 a cells. *Int Immunol*. 1999;11:191–198.
115. Macpherson AJ, Gatto D, Sainsbury E, et al. A primitive T cell-independent mechanism of intestinal mucosal IgA responses to commensal bacteria. *Science*. 2000;288:2222–2226.
116. Kunisawa J, Kurashima Y, Gohda M, et al. Sphingosine 1-phosphate regulates peritoneal B-cell trafficking for subsequent intestinal IgA production. *Blood*. 2007;109:3749–3756.
117. Russell MW, Kilian M. Biological activities of IgA. In: *Mucosal Immunology*, 3rd ed. Mestecky J, Lamm ME, Strober W, et al., eds. San Diego: Academic Press. 2005;267–289.
118. Gunninghan-Rundles C. Immunodeficiency and mucosal immunity. In: *Mucosal Immunology*, 3rd ed. Mestecky J, Lamm ME, Strober W, et al., eds. San Diego: Academic Press. 2005;1145–1158.
119. Underdown BJ. Passive immunization: systemic and mucosal. In: *Mucosal Immunology*, 3rd ed. Mestecky J, Lamm ME, Strober W, et al., eds. San Diego: Academic Press. 2005;841–851.
120. Murphy BR. Mucosal immunity to viruses. In: *Mucosal Immunology*, 3rd ed. Mestecky J, Lamm ME, Strober W, et al., eds. San Diego: Academic Press. 2005;799–814.
121. Eichelberger M, Allan W, Zijlstra M, et al. Clearance of influenza virus respiratory infection in mice lacking class I major histocompatibility complex-restricted CD8$^+$ T cells. *J Exp Med*. 1991;174:875–880.
122. Graham BS, Bunton LA, Wright PF, et al. Role of T lymphocyte subsets in the pathogenesis of primary infection and rechallenge with respiratory syncytial virus in mice. *J Clin Invest*. 1991; 88:1026–1033.
123. Lehner T, Bergmeier LA. Mucosal infection and immune responses to simian immunodeficiency virus. In: *Mucosal Immunology*, 3rd ed. Mestecky J, Lamm ME, Strober W, et al., eds. San Diego: Academic Press. 2005;1179–1197.
124. Smith PD, Wahl SM. Immunobiology of mucosal HIV-1 infection. In: *Mucosal Immunology*, 3rd ed. Mestecky J, Lamm ME, Strober W, et al., eds. San Diego: Academic Press. 2005;1999–1211.
125. Savage DC. Mucosal Microbiota. In: *Mucosal Immunology*, 3rd ed. Mestecky J, Lamm ME, Strober W, et al., eds. San Diego: Academic Press. 2005;19–33.
126. Macpherson AJ, Geuking MB, McCoy KD. Immune responses that adapt the intestinal mucosa to commensal intestinal bacteria. *Immunology*. 2005;115:153–162.
127. Hooper LV, Gordon JI. Commensal host-bacterial relationships in the gut. *Science*. 2001;292:1115–1118.
128. Macpherson AJ. Uhr T. Induction of protective IgA by intestinal dendritic cells carrying commensal bacteria. *Science*. 2004; 303:1662–1665.
129. Caramalho I, Lopes-Carvalho T, Ostler D, et al. Regulatory T cells selectively express toll-like receptors and are activated by lipopolysaccharide. *J Exp Med*. 2003;197:403–411.
130. Kiyono H, McGhee JR, Wannemuehler MJ, et al. Lack of oral tolerance in C3H/HeJ mice. *J Exp Med*. 1982;155:605–610.
131. Krieg AM. Therapeutic potential of Toll-like receptor 9 activation. *Nat Rev Drug Discov*. 2006;5:471–484.
132. Mowat AM, Faria AM, Weiner HL. Oral tolerance: physical basis and clinical applications. In: *Mucosal Immunology*, 3rd ed. Mestecky J, Lamm ME, Strober W, et al., eds. San Diego: Academic Press. 2005;487–538.
133. Alpan O, Rudomen G, Matzinger P The role of dendritic cells, B cells, and M cells in gut-oriented immune responses. *J Immunol*. 2001;166:4843–4852.
134. Spahn TW, Fontana A, Faria AM, et al. Induction of oral tolerance to cellular immune responses in the absence of Peyers patches. *Eur J Immunol*. 2001;31:1278–1287.
135. Fujihashi K, Dohi T, Rennert PD, et al. Peyers patches are required for oral tolerance to proteins. *Proc Natl Acad Sci U S A*. 2001;98:3310–3315.
136. Shi HN, Grusby MJ, Nagler-Anderson C. Orally induced peripheral nonresponsiveness is maintained in the absence of functional Th1 or Th2 cells. *J Immunol*. 1999;162:5143–5148.
137. Hirahara K, Hisatsune T, Nishijima K, et al. CD4$^+$ T cells anergized by high dose feeding establish oral tolerance to antibody responses when transferred in SCID and nude mice. *J Immunol*. 1995;154:6238–6245.
138. Sakaguchi S, Ono M, Setoguchi R, et al. Foxp3$^+$ CD25$^+$ CD4$^+$ natural regulatory T cells in dominant self-tolerance and autoimmune disease. *Immunol Rev*. 2006;212:8–27.
139. Izcue A, Coombes JL, Powrie F. Regulatory T cells suppress systemic and mucosal immune activation to control intestinal inflammation. *Immunol Rev*. 2006;212:256–271.
140. Grohmann U, Orabona C, Fallarino F, et al. CTLA-4-Ig regulates tryptophan catabolism *in vivo*. *Nat Immunol*. 2002;3:1097–1101.
141. Ono M, Shimizu J, Miyachi Y, et al. Control of autoimmune myocarditis and multiorgan inflammation by glucocorticoid-induced TNF receptor family-related protein^{high}, Foxp3$^-$expressing CD25$^+$ and CD25$^-$ regulatory T cells. *J Immunol*. 2006;176:4748–4756.
142. Chen W, Jin W, Hardegen N, et al. Conversion of peripheral CD4$^+$CD25$^-$ naive T cells to CD4$^+$CD25$^+$ regulatory T cells by TGF-β induction of transcription factor Foxp3. *J Exp Med*. 2003;198:1875–1886.
143. Chen Y, Kuchroo VK, Inobe J, et al. Regulatory T cell clones induced by oral tolerance: suppression of autoimmune encephalomyelitis. *Science*, 1994; 265:1237–1240.
144. Roncarolo MG, Gregori S, Battaglia M, et al. Interleukin-10-secreting type 1 regulatory T cells in rodents and humans. *Immunol Rev*. 2006; 212:28–50.
145. Papadakis KA, Landers C, Prehn J, et al. CC chemokine receptor 9 expression defines a subset of peripheral blood lymphocytes with mucosal T cell phenotype and Th1 or T-regulatory 1 cytokine profile. *J Immunol*. 2003;171:159–165.
146. Gianfrani C, Levings MK, Sartirana C, et al. Gliadin-specific type 1 regulatory T cells from the intestinal mucosa of treated celiac patients inhibit pathogenic T cells. *J Immunol*. 2006;177:4178–4186.
147. Mowat AM, Lamont AG, Bruce MG. A genetically determined lack of oral tolerance to ovalbumin is due to failure of the immune system to respond to intestinally derived tolerogen. *Eur J Immunol*. 1987;17:1673–1676.
148. Chang CC, Ciubotariu R, Manavalan JS, et al. Tolerization of dendritic cells by T(S) cells: the crucial role of inhibitory receptors ILT3 and ILT4. *Nat Immunol*. 2002;3:237–243.
149. Gleissner CA, Zastrow A, Klingenberg R, et al. IL-10 inhibits endothelium-dependent T cell costimulation by up-regulation of ILT3/4 in human vascular endothelial cells. *Eur J Immunol*. 2007; 37:177–192.
150. Rifa'i M, Kawamoto Y, Nakashima I, et al. Essential roles of CD8$^+$CD122$^+$ regulatory T cells in the maintenance of T cell homeostasis. *J Exp Med*. 2004;200:1123–1134.
151. McGeachy MJ, Bak-Jensen KS, Chen Y, et al. TGF-β and IL-6 drive the production of IL-17 and IL-10 by T cells and restrain T(H)-17 cell-mediated pathology. *Nat Immunol*. 2007;8:1390–1397.
152. Awasthi A, Carrier Y, Peron JP, et al. A dominant function for interleukin 27 in generating interleukin 10-producing anti-inflammatory T cells. *Nat Immunol*. 2007;8:1380–1389.
153. Stumhofer JS, Silver JS, Laurence A, et al. Interleukins 27 and 6 induce STAT3-mediated T cell production of interleukin 10. *Nat Immunol*. 2007;8:1363–1371.
154. Coombes JL, Siddiqui KR, Arancibia-Carcamo CV, et al. A functionally specialized population of mucosal CD103$^+$ DCs induces Foxp3$^+$ regulatory T cells via a TGF-β and retinoic acid-dependent mechanism. *J Exp Med*. 2007;204:1757–1764.
155. Sun CM, Hall JA, Blank RB, et al. Small intestine lamina propria dendritic cells promote de novo generation of Foxp3 Treg cells via retinoic acid. *J Exp Med*. 2007;204:1775–1785.
156. Benson MJ, Pino-Lagos K, Rosemblatt M, et al. All-trans retinoic acid mediates enhanced T reg cell growth, differentiation, and gut homing in the face of high levels of co-stimulation. *J Exp Med*. 2007;204:1765–1774.
157. Mucida D, Park Y, Kim G, et al. Reciprocal Th17 and regulatory T cell differentiation mediated by retinoic acid. *Science*. 2007;317:256–260.

158. Ke Y, Pearce K, Lake JP, et al. $\gamma\delta$ T lymphocytes regulate the induction and maintenance of oral tolerance. *J Immunol.* 1997;158:3610–3618.
159. Fujihashi K, Dohi T, Kweon MN, et al. $\gamma\delta$ T cells regulate mucosally induced tolerance in a dose-dependent fashion. *Int Immunol.* 1999;11:1907–1916.
160. Viney JL, Mowat AM, O'Malley JM, et al. Expanding dendritic cells *in vivo* enhances the induction of oral tolerance. *J Immunol.* 1998;160:5815–5825.
161. Ito T, Yang M, Wang YH, et al. Plasmacytoid dendritic cells prime IL-10-producing T regulatory cells by inducible costimulator ligand. *J Exp Med.* 2007;204:105–115.
162. Gilliet M, Liu YJ. Generation of human CD8 T regulatory cells by CD40 ligand-activated plasmacytoid dendritic cells. *J Exp Med.* 2002;195:695–704.
163. Allez M, Brimnes J, Dotan I, et al. Expansion of $CD8^+$ T cells with regulatory function after interaction with intestinal epithelial cells. *Gastroenterology*. 2002;123:1516–1526.
164. Cruickshank SM, McVay LD, Baumgart DC, et al. Colonic epithelial cell mediated suppression of CD4 T cell activation. *Gut.* 2004;53:678–684.
165. Westendorf AM, Bruder D, Hansen W, et al. Intestinal epithelial antigen induces $CD4^+$ T cells with regulatory phenotype in a transgenic autoimmune mouse model. *Ann NY Acad Sci.* 2006;1072:401–406.
166. Ostroukhova M, Seguin-Devaux C, Oriss TB, et al. Tolerance induced by inhaled antigen involves $CD4^+$ T cells expressing membrane-bound TGF-β and FOXP3. *J Clin Invest.* 2004;114: 28–38.
167. Oriss TB, Ostroukhova M, Seguin-Devaux C, et al. Dynamics of dendritic cell phenotype and interactions with $CD4^+$ T cells in airway inflammation and tolerance. *J Immunol.* 2005;174:854–863.
168. Kutteh WH, Mestecky J, Wira CR. Mucosal immunity in the human female reproductive tract. In: *Mucosal Immunology*, 3rd ed. Mestecky J, Lamm ME, Strober W, et al., eds. San Diego: Academic Press. 2005;1631–1646.
169. Anderson DF, Pudney J. Human male genital tract immunity and experimental models. In: *Mucosal Immunology*, 3rd ed. Mestecky J, Lamm ME, Strober W, et al., eds. San Diego: Academic Press. 2005;1647–1660.
170. Peppoloni S, Ruggiero P, Contorni M, et al. Mutants of the *Escherichia coli* heat-labile enterotoxin as safe and strong adjuvants for intranasal delivery of vaccines. *Expert Rev Vaccines.* 2003;2:285–293.
171. Elson CO, Dertzbaugh MT. Mucosal Adjuvants. In: *Mucosal Immunology*, 3rd ed. Mestecky J, Lamm ME, Strober W, et al., eds. San Diego: Academic Press. 2005;967–986.
172. Lycke N. Targeted vaccine adjuvants based on modified cholera toxin. *Curr Mol Med.* 2005;5:591–597.
173. Borsutzky S, Kretschmer K, Becker PD, et al. The mucosal adjuvant macrophage-activating lipopeptide-2 directly stimulates B lymphocytes via the TLR2 without the need of accessory cells. *J Immunol.* 2005;174:6308–6313.
174. Michalek SM, O'Hagan D, Childers NK, et al. Antigen delivery systems I: Nonliving microparticles, liposomes, and immune stimulating complexes (ISCOMs). In: *Mucosal Immunology*, 3rd ed. Mestecky J, Lamm ME, Strober W, et al., eds. San Diego: Academic Press. 2005;987–1008.
175. Jepson MA, Clark MA, Hirst BH. M cell targeting by lectins: a strategy for mucosal vaccination and drug delivery. *Adv Drug Deliv Rev.* 2004;56:511–525.
176. Lambkin I, Pinilla C, Hamashin C, et al. Toward targeted oral vaccine delivery systems: selection of lectin mimetics from combinatorial libraries. *Pharm Res.* 2003;20:1258–1266.
177. Higgins LM, Lambkin I, Donnelly G, et al. In vivo phage display to identify M cell-targeting ligands. *Pharm Res.* 2004;21:695–705.
178. Nochi T, Yuki Y, Matsumura A, et al. A novel M cell specific carbohydrate-targeted mucosal vaccine effectively induces antigen-specific immune responses. *J Exp Med.* 2007;2004:2789–2796.
179. Wu Y, Wang X, Csencsits KL, et al. M cell-targeted DNA vaccination. *Proc Natl Acad Sci U S A.* 2001;98:9318–9323.
180. Kunisawa J, Nakagawa S, Mayumi T. Pharmacotherapy by intracellular delivery of drugs using fusogenic liposomes: application to vaccine development. *Adv Drug Deliv Rev.* 2001; 52:177–186.
181. Curtiss R 3rd. Antigen delivery system II: development of live recombinant attenuated bacterial antigen and DNA vaccine delivery vector vaccines. In: *Mucosal Immunology*, 3rd ed. Mestecky J, Lamm ME, Strober W, Bienenstock J, McGhee JR, Mayer L, eds. San Diego: Academic Press. 2005;1009–1038.
182. Rosenthal KL. Recombinant live viral vectors as vaccines for mucosal immunity. In: *Mucosal Immunology*, 3rd ed. Mestecky J, Lamm ME, Strober W, Bienenstock J, McGhee JR, Mayer L, eds. San Diego: Academic Press. 2005;1039–1052.
183. Mason HS, Chikwamba R, Santi L, et al. Transgenic plants for mucosal vaccines. In: *Mucosal Immunology*, 3rd ed. Mestecky J, Lamm ME, Strober W, Bienenstock J, McGhee JR, Mayer L, eds. San Diego: Academic Press. 2005;1053–1060.
183a. Nochi T, Takagih H, Yuki Y, et al. Rice-based mucosal vaccine as a global strategy for cold-chain- and needle-free vaccination. *Proc Natl Acad Sci U S A.* 2007;104:10986–10991.
184. Cunningham-Rundles C. Immunodeficiency and mucosal immunity. In: *Mucosal Immunology*, 3rd ed. Mestecky J, Lamm ME, Strober W, Bienenstock J, McGhee JR, Mayer L, eds. San Diego: Academic Press. 2005;1145–1158.
185. Meng G, Wei X, Wu X, et al. Primary intestinal epithelial cells selectively transfer R5 HIV-1 to $CCR5^+$ cells. *Nat Med.* 2002; 8:150–156.
186. Brenchley JM, Price DA, Schacker TW, et al. Microbial translocation is a cause of systemic immune activation in chronic HIV infection. *Nat Med.* 2006;12:1365–1371.
187. Kozlowski PA, Jackson S. Serum IgA subclasses and molecular forms in HIV infection: selective increases in monomer and apparent restriction of the antibody response to IgA1 antibodies mainly directed at env glycoproteins. *AIDS Res Hum Retroviruses.* 1992;8:1773–1780.
188. Kaul R, Trabattoni D, Bwayo JJ, et al. HIV-1-specific mucosal IgA in a cohort of HIV-1-resistant Kenyan sex workers. *AIDS.* 1999;13: 23–29.
189. Elson CO, Cong Y, McCracken VJ, et al. Experimental models of inflammatory bowel disease reveal innate, adaptive, and regulatory mechanisms of host dialogue with the microbiota. *Immunol Rev.* 2005;206:260–276.
190. Powrie F, Uhlig H. Animal models of intestinal inflammation: clues to the pathogenesis of inflammatory bowel disease. *Novartis Found Symp.* 2004;263:164–174; discussion 174–168, 211–168.
191. Rath HC, Wilson KH, Sartor RB. Differential induction of colitis and gastritis in HLA-B27 transgenic rats selectively colonized with *Bacteroides vulgatus* or *Escherichia coli. Infect Immun.* 1999;67:2969–2974.
192. Gionchetti P, Rizzello F, Lammers KM, et al. Antibiotics and probiotics in treatment of inflammatory bowel disease. *World J Gastroenterol.* 2006;12:3306–3313.
193. Kraus TA, Cheifetz A, Toy L, et al. Evidence for a genetic defect in oral tolerance induction in inflammatory bowel disease. *Inflamm Bowel Dis.* 2006;12:82–88.
194. Kaser A, Nieuwenhuis EE, Strober W, et al. Natural killer T cells in mucosal homeostasis. *Ann NY Acad Sci.* 2004;1029:154–168.
195. Vercelli D. Mechanisms of the hygiene hypothesis—molecular and otherwise. *Curr Opin Immunol.* 2006;18:733–737.
196. Cohn L, Elias JA, Chupp GL. Asthma: mechanisms of disease persistence and progression. *Annu Rev Immunol.* 2004; 22:789–815.
197. Kweon M Kiyono H. Allergic diseases in the gastrointestinal tract. In: *Mucosal Immunology*, 3rd ed. Mestecky J, Lamm ME, Strober W, Bienenstock J, McGhee JR, Mayer L, eds. San Diego: Academic Press. 2005;1351–1360.
198. Popescu FD. New asthma drugs acting on gene expression. *J Cell Mol Med.* 2003;7:475–486.
199. Brownell J, Casale TB. Anti-IgE therapy. *Immunol Allergy Clin North Am.* 2004;24:551–568, v.
200. Takagi H, Hiroi T, Yang L, et al. A rice-based edible vaccine expressing multiple T cell epitopes induces oral tolerance for inhibition of Th2-mediated IgE responses. *Proc Natl Acad Sci U S A.* 2005; 102:17525–17530.

201. Hawrylowicz CM. Regulatory T cells and IL-10 in allergic inflammation. *J Exp Med*. 2005;202:1459–1463.
202. Lewkowich IP, Herman NS, Schleifer KW, et al. $CD4^{+}CD25^{+}$ T cells protect against experimentally induced asthma and alter pulmonary dendritic cell phenotype and function. *J Exp Med*. 2005;202:1549–1561.
203. Schnyder-Candrian S, Togbe D, Couillin I, et al. Interleukin-17 is a negative regulator of established allergic asthma. *J Exp Med*. 2006;203:2715–2725.
204. Bisset LR, Schmid-Grendelmeier P. Chemokines and their receptors in the pathogenesis of allergic asthma: progress and perspective. *Curr Opin Pulm Med*. 2005;11:35–42.
205. Kurashima Y, Kunisawa J, Higuchi M, et al. Sphingosine 1-phosphate-mediated trafficking of pathogenic Th2 and mast cells for the control of food allergy. *J Immunol*. 2007;179:1577–1585.
206. Hue S, Mention JJ, Monteiro RC, et al. A direct role for NKG2D/MICA interaction in villous atrophy during celiac disease. *Immunity*. 2004; 21:367–377.

Chapter 32

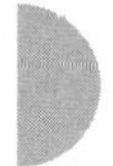

Neural Immune Interactions

Jeanette I. Webster Marketon and Esther M. Sternberg

INTRODUCTION

A bidirectional communication exists between the central nervous system (CNS) and the immune system whereby neurotransmitters and neurohormones regulate immunity and, in turn, immune molecules signal the central nervous system to activate these extra–immune system regulatory pathways in a negative feedback loop that maintains homeostasis. Perturbation of this balance in either direction results in disease. Overregulation of the immune system results in an ineffective immune response and increased susceptibility to infections, whereas underregulation results in an unchecked immune response and the development of autoimmune/inflammatory disease. This chapter focuses on these routes of communication, with particular emphasis on the hypothalamic-pituitary-adrenal (HPA) axis and resultant glucocorticoid release. Dysregulation of the HPA axis and glucocorticoid signaling is discussed.

EFFECTS OF IMMUNE FACTORS ON THE CNS

Immune factors, including immune cells and cytokines, affect the CNS at molecular, cellular, and whole-organ levels. These factors have different effects on the CNS depending on whether they are expressed within the CNS or produced at peripheral sites.

Effects of Immune Factors Within the CNS

Cells of the brain, such as glia, neurons, and macrophages, are able to produce cytokines locally, which have been shown to be involved in neuronal cell death (*1*,*2*,3,*4*) and survival (*5*,*6*). Cytokine-mediated neuronal cell death is believed to play an important role in several neurodegenerative diseases, such as neuroAIDS, Alzheimer's disease, multiple sclerosis, stroke, and nerve trauma (7,*8*–*10*).

Effects of Peripheral Immune Factors on the CNS

Cytokines produced at peripheral sites during inflammation are able to signal the brain and change brain function and in this sense act like hormones. In addition to inducing fever, cytokines induce a set of symptoms called "sickness behavior." The symptoms include decreased locomotion, depressed cognition, memory, and mood, decreased appetite, and decreased interest in social interactions and sexual behavior (11,*12*,13). Peripherally produced cytokines can access and stimulate the CNS by several routes. They can cross the blood–brain barrier (BBB) at "leaky points" such as at the organum vasculosum lamina terminalis (OVLT) or median eminence, and they can also be actively transported in small amounts across the BBB (14). In addition, they can activate the vagus nerve to signal the CNS rapidly by binding to receptors on paraganglia cells adjacent to vagal ganglia (15,16,*17*). Finally, they can activate second messengers, such as nitric oxide and prostaglandins, by binding to receptors on brain endothelial cells (15,*18–20*). For further reading the reviews by Masek et al. (21) and Sternberg (22) are recommended.

CNS REGULATION OF THE IMMUNE SYSTEM

The CNS is able to communicate with the immune system through both neural pathways and hormonal pathways. In general, neural routes innervate immune organs and regulate immunity at regional and local levels, and hormonal routes regulate immunity systemically.

Neural Pathways That Regulate Immune Function

Neural pathways that participate in CNS regulation of the immune system include the sympathetic nervous system (SNS), the parasympathetic nervous system, and the peripheral nervous system (PNS).

Sympathetic Nervous System

The SNS regulates the immune system at a regional level, through innervation of immune organs. Norepinephrine and neuropeptide Y, synthesized and secreted together from nerve endings (23), regulate the immune system regionally. In contrast, when these neuropeptides are released into the bloodstream from the adrenal medulla they regulate the immune system at a systemic level. Extensive studies indicate that norepinephrine affects adaptive immunity and antibody production (24). The effects on innate immunity have not been as well studied and are reviewed by Sternberg (22) and Maestroni (25). Norepinephrine and neuropeptide Y together inhibit interleukin-6 (IL-6) secretion from macrophages (*26*,27). Recent comprehensive reviews are available of the regulation of the immune system by the sympathetic nervous system (25,28).

Parasympathetic Nervous System

The parasympathetic nervous system regulates immune responses regionally through the vagus nerve. The primary parasympathetic neurotransmitter is acetylcholine, which binds to nicotinic and muscarinic cholinergic receptors (22). During inflammation, IL-1 is released by activated immune cells; this then activates the afferent fibers of the vagus nerve, which rapidly activate the parasympathetic brainstem regions through IL-1 receptors on the parasympathetic ganglia (29). This is the first step in the "inflammatory reflex" that leads to acetylcholine release from efferent vagus nerve fibers as a negative feedback control of inflammation (30). Cutting the vagus nerve prevents immune signaling to brain and activation of parasympathetic brainstem regions and, in turn, prevents vagal control of inflammation and toxic shock (29,30,*31*).

Peripheral Nervous System

At sites of inflammation, the PNS releases neurotransmitters from sensory peripheral nerves that are generally proinflammatory and increase local inflammatory responses. These neuropeptides include corticotrophin-releasing hormone (CRH), substance P, and calcitonin gene–regulated peptide (CGRP) (*32*,33,*34*). Vasoactive intestinal peptide (VIP) is released by peripheral nerves and microglia (35) and inhibits inflammation through G protein–coupled receptors VPAC1 and VPAC2 (36).

Neuropeptides released centrally from the CNS or pituitary gland have different effects and tend to be antiinflammatory. For example α-melanocyte-stimulating hormone (α-MSH), a 13–amino acid peptide, has antiinflammatory actions (*37*,38). It is released from the pituitary, the neurons of the arcuate nucleus and paraventricular nucleus of the hypothalamus, and the peripheral nerves (*39*,40). Opioids, synthetic (morphine) and endogenous (endorphins and enkephalins), are also antiinflammatory molecules released by pituitary (41). These can also stimulate HPA axis and glucocorticoid release (42).

Hormonal Pathways That Regulate Immune Function

In addition to neural control of inflammation, hormones are also released in response to stimuli of brain regions that control the immune system. Prolactin secreted by the pituitary gland binds to the prolactin receptor on immune cells and enhances immune function. Hyperprolactinemia has been described in some autoimmune diseases (43,*44*). Growth hormone, another pituitary hormone also produced by lymphoid organs such as the thymus, spleen, and peripheral blood, also plays a role in enhancing immune function, stimulating T and B cell proliferation and antibody production (45). Ghrelin is predominantly produced in the stomach after stimulation through the gut–brain axis and has been shown to have antiinflammatory actions (46,47). Leptin, also part of the gut–brain axis, has been shown to act as a proinflammatory hormone (48,*49*) and signals the hypothalamus from adipose tissue, forming a negative feedback loop (47).

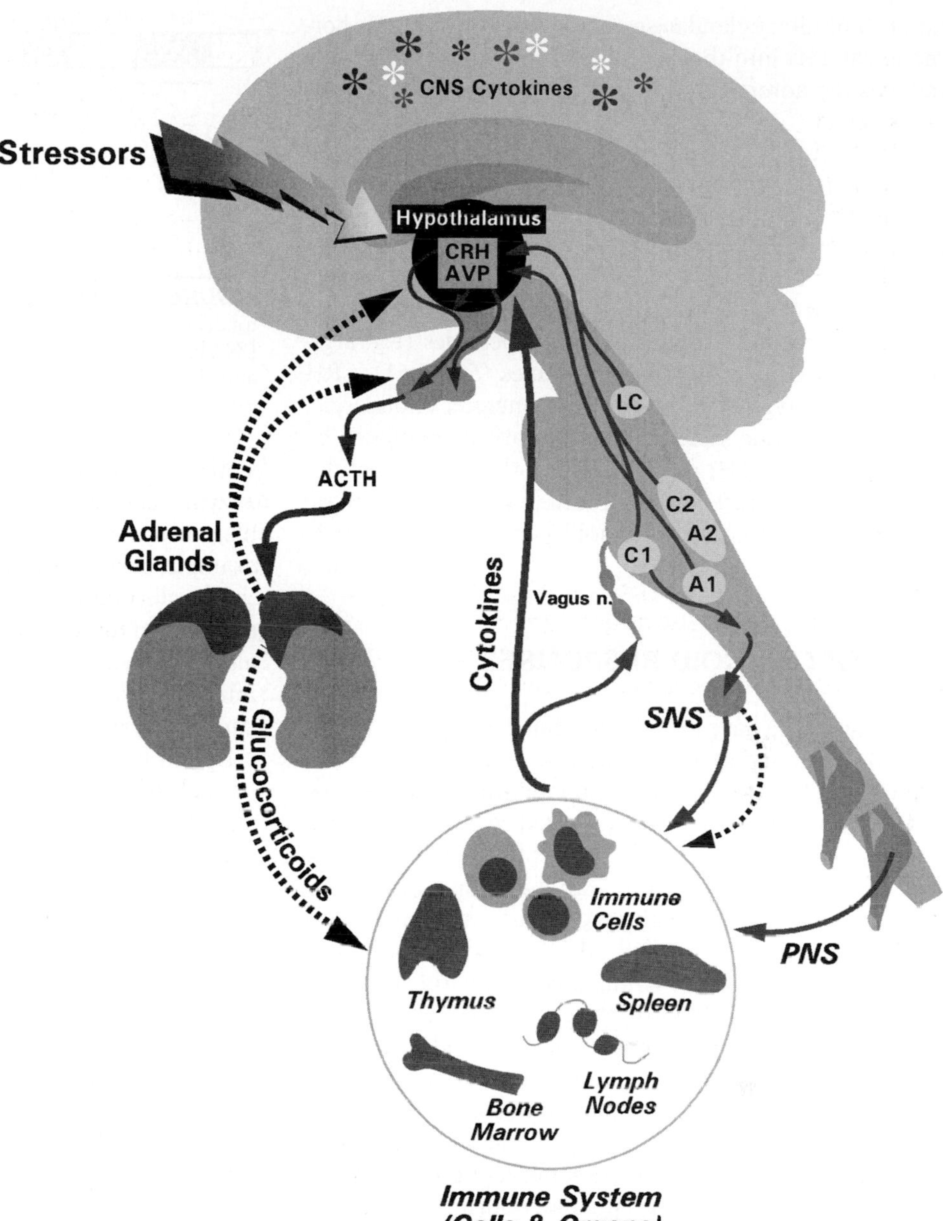

FIGURE 32.1 Two-way communication between the immune and nervous systems. The immune system and the central nervous system (CNS) communicate with and regulate each other. Cytokines made in the periphery signal the CNS by several routes, including passage across the blood–brain barrier and via the vagus nerve. Peripheral cytokines affect many aspects of CNS function, including activation of the neuroendocrine stress response, or hypothalamic-pituitary-adrenal (HPA) axis. When activated, the hypothalamus releases corticotrophin-releasing hormone (CRH) and arginine vasopressin (AVP), which together stimulate the pituitary grand to release adrenocorticotrophin (ACTH). This in turn stimulates the adrenal cortex to release glucocorticoids. These hormones suppress immunity at a molecular, cellular, and organ level. Other routes by which the CNS regulates immunity are through the sympathetic nervous system (SNS) and peripheral nervous system (PNS). Stress both activates the HPA axis to release these immunosuppressive hormones and activates the SNS. The HPA axis and SNS communicate through brainstem routes that involve noradrenergic nuclei, including the locus ceruleus, C1, C2, A1, and A2. Cytokines are also expressed within the CNS, and in this compartment they play a role in neuronal cell death and survival.

The Hypothalamic-Pituitary-Gonadal Axis

The hypothalamic-pituitary-gonadal (HPG) axis is also involved in regulation of immune responses (50,*51*). Estrogen is generally immunoenhancing at lower concentrations (*52–54*,55,*56*), whereas testosterone and progesterone are generally immunosuppressive (55,56). Increases in estrogens relative to androgens have been shown in rheumatoid arthritis and lupus (57). The differences in immune regulation by the sex hormones may, at least in part, explain the well-recognized phenomenon that females of all species are more susceptible to autoimmune and inflammatory diseases than males, expressing a 2- 10-fold higher incidence or severity of autoimmune diseases compared to males (52,55).

The Hypothalamic-Pituitary-Adrenal Axis

The HPA axis is a major regulator of the immune system via the production of adrenal glucocorticoids (Figure 32.1). The HPA axis consists of the paraventricular nucleus (PVN) of the hypothalamus, the anterior pituitary gland located at the base of the brain, and the adrenal glands. CRH is secreted on stimulation from the PVN into the hypophyseal portal blood supply. This subsequently stimulates the anterior pituitary gland to secrete adrenocorticotropic hormone (ACTH) into the systemic circulation. In turn, this induces the adrenal glands to synthesize and release glucocorticoids.

The HPA axis is regulated by both factors within the central nervous system and from the periphery. Glucocorticoids, the end product of the HPA axis, negatively regulate the axis at the level of the hypothalamic and pituitary. The HPA axis is also regulated by other factors, such as neurotransmitters and neuropeptides of the sympathetic nervous system, other neuropeptides (e.g. arginine vasopressin [AVP]), and cytokines (*58–60*,61). CRH is positively regulated by the serotonergic, cholinergic, and histaminergic systems but is negatively regulated by itself and by ACTH, as well as by other neuropeptides and neurotransmitters in the brain (e.g., γ-aminobutyric acid–benzodiazepines and opioid peptide systems) (*62–64*,65,*66*,*67*).

GLUCOCORTICOID RESPONSES

Glucocorticoids have been known for many years to influence the immune system and because of this have been used in the treatment of inflammatory diseases since the 1940s. The Nobel prize was awarded to Kendall, Reichstein, and Hench for the discovery of this effect in 1950 (68). Since then, extensive research has investigated the pharmacologic effects of glucocorticoids on many aspects of immune cell function (69–70,*71*). However, only relatively recently has the essential physiologic role of glucocorticoids in the regulation of the immune system in health and disease been fully appreciated. To understand the pathogenesis of inflammatory/autoimmune disease and ultimately to develop effective therapies for such diseases, one needs a better understanding of the mechanisms involved in glucocorticoid secretion/production and regulation of the immune system both under normal and disease conditions.

The Glucocorticoid Receptor

Glucocorticoids function through a cellular receptor to modulate gene transcription. Two receptors are activated by glucocorticoids: the higher-affinity type I receptor, the mineralocorticoid receptor (MR); and the lower-affinity type II receptor, the glucocorticoid receptor (GR). Glucocorticoids bind preferentially to MR at low concentrations, and only at high stress levels do they bind to GR (72). It has been suggested that MR functions in a proactive capacity in the maintenance of homeostasis in the brain, whereas GR functions in a reactive role in the recovery from disturbance (73). However, GR is the primary receptor for glucocorticoids in immune cells. Other factors can regulate the availability of glucocorticoids, such as the expression of 11β hydroxysteroid dehydrogenase (11β-HSD), an enzyme that converts the active form of steroids, for example, cortisol and corticosterone, into the inactive form, for example, cortisone and 11-dehydrocortisone (74,75,*76*).

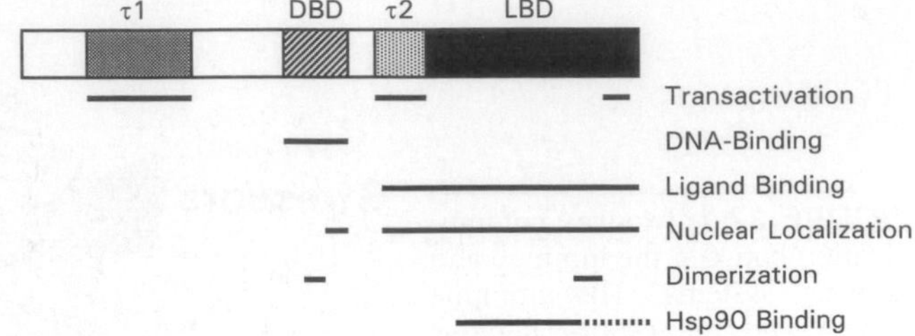

FIGURE 32.2 Molecular structure of the glucocorticoid receptor. The areas associated with the functions of transactivation, DNA binding, ligand binding, nuclear localization, dimerization, and Hsp90 binding are shown.

The glucocorticoid receptor (NR3C1) is a member of the steroid and thyroid hormone receptor superfamily, which also includes the receptors for progesterone, estrogen, mineralocorticoid, and thyroid hormones. These receptors can essentially be thought of as ligand-dependent transcription factors that mediate the endpoint tissue effects of such hormones (77). The nuclear hormone receptors all share a common three-domain structure (Figure 32.2) consisting of an N-terminal transactivation domain, a central DNA-binding domain (DBD), and a C-terminal ligand-binding domain (LDB) (78,79).

Circulating glucocorticoids are bound to cortisol-binding globulin (CBG) or albumin in the peripheral blood stream. Glucocorticoids are small hydrophobic molecules that can enter the cell mainly by passive diffusion, although evidence exists for some active transport processes *(80)*. GR is located in the cytoplasm and held in a conformation accessible to the ligand by a multiprotein complex containing Hsp90 and immunophilins. On activation by ligand binding, GR dissociates from the Hsp complex, dimerizes, and translocates to the nucleus, where it binds as a homodimer to a specific DNA sequence—hormone response element (HRE) or glucocorticoid response element (GRE). GR can modulate gene expression, either upregulating or downregulating target genes, by interacting with many coactivators or corepressors (Figure 32.3) (78,*81*,82). Repression of target genes by GR can occur via a negative glucocorticoid response element (nGRE), for example, the bovine prolactin gene and the POMC gene (83,*84*,*85*), but primarily occurs by interaction with other transcription factors, such as activator protein-1 (AP-1) and nuclear factor-kappa B (NF-κB) (82,86,87,*88*,89). Similarly GR activity can be repressed by AP-1 and NF-κB (*90*,91).

The presence of other receptors that also bind glucocorticoids would affect glucocorticoid responses. Such receptors include the mineralocorticoid receptor and an inactive splice variant of the glucocorticoid receptor, GRβ, which

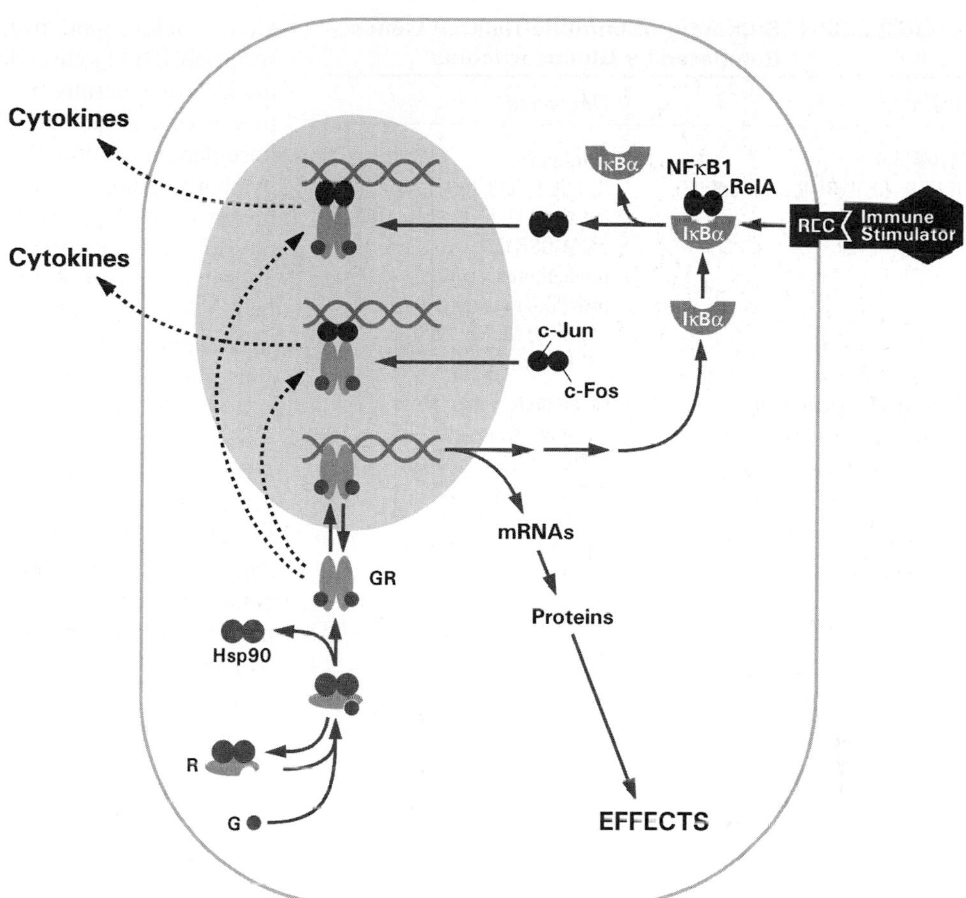

FIGURE 32.3 Molecular mechanisms of glucocorticoid effects on immune cell function. Schematic diagram of the mechanism of action of the glucocorticoid receptor, including interactions with the NF-κB and AP-1 pathways. Dotted lines represent repressive pathways.

differs in the C-terminal LBD (92). Like GR, GRβ is also found in the cytoplasm complexed to hsp90, but, in addition, it is also located in the nucleus regardless of ligand status. Due to a unique 15–amino acid C-terminus, GRβ is unable to bind ligand or activate gene transcription. It has been suggested that GRβ forms transcriptionally inactive heterodimers with GRα, thereby acting as a dominant negative receptor or, effectively, as a GR antagonist *in vitro* (*93–98*,99). However, this mechanism is still under dispute because other studies have shown no effect of GRβ on GRα-mediated transactivation or transrepression (100,*101*,102,*103*). Monocytes and T cells exhibit differential GR sensitivity, and this has been suggested to be due to the differential expression of GRβ (104). GRβ has also been shown to repress MR (105).

Effects of Glucocorticoids on Immune Responses

Pharmacologic and physiologic doses or forms of glucocorticoids exhibit very different responses. Physiologic doses of glucocorticoids modulate transcription of inflammatory genes, whereas pharmacologic doses totally suppress the inflammatory response (106). In addition, different immune responses are elicited by synthetic glucocorticoids, such as dexamethasone, compared to natural glucocorticoids, such as hydrocortisone. For example, dexamethasone exerts a greater suppression on IL-12 than does hydrocortisone, consistent with the greater affinity of dexamethasone than hydrocortisone for GR (107). Physiologic doses of the natural glucocorticoid corticosterone have been shown to have immunoenhancing effects in skin delayed-type hypersensitivity (DTH) in rats. However, if the dose of corticosterone is increased to pharmacologic concentrations or the pharmacologic glucocorticoid dexamethasone is used, immunosuppressive effects are observed (108). This suggests that acute administration of a natural glucocorticoid is immunoenhancing, whereas chronic administration of a natural glucocorticoid or administration of a pharmacologic glucocorticoid is immunosuppressive. This is in agreement with the observation that acute stress can be beneficial, for example, in enhancement of immune function, whereas chronic stress is detrimental to health, for example, in enhancing susceptibility to infections and impaired wound healing (109,*110–114*,115,*116–118*).

A wide variety of immune genes and immune cell functions are regulated by glucocorticoids through GR and the molecular mechanisms described earlier. For example, glucocorticoids modulate gene expression of cytokines,

TABLE 32.1 Summary of Immune-Related Genes Regulated by Glucocorticoids

Increase	*Decrease*
Cytokines	**Cytokines**
IL-4, IL-10, IL-RI, IL-1 receptor antagonist	IL-1, IL-2, IL-3, IL-4, IL-5, IL-6, IL-8, IL-11, IL-12, IL-13, TNFα, GM-CSF, IFNγ
	Chemokines
	RANTES, eotaxin, MIPα, MCP-1, MCP-2, MCP-3, CINC/gro
Inflammatory mediators	**Inflammatory mediators**
Lipocortin-1 (annexin-1), SLPI, MKP-1	Prostaglandins, NO, NOS II, iNOS, COX-2, cPLA$_2$
	Adhesion molecules
	ICAM-1, ELAM-1, VCAM-1, E-selectin, L-selectin
Receptors	**Receptors**
β_2-Adrenoceptor	IL-2R, NK$_1$R, NK$_2$R, IL-4Rα
IκBα	

CINC, cytokine-induced neutrophil chemoattractant; COX-2, cyclooxygenase type 2; cPLA$_2$, cytosolic phospholipase A$_2$; ELAM-1, endothelial-leukocyte adhesion molecule-1; GM-CSF, granulocyte-macrophage colony-stimulating factor; ICAM-1, intracellular adhesion molecule-1; INFγ, interferon-γ; iNOS, inducible nitric oxide synthase; IL, interleukin; NO, nitric oxide; NOS II, nitric oxide synthase II; MCP, monocyte chemoattractant protein; MKP-1, mitogen-activated protein kinase phosphatase-1; SLPI, secretory leukocyte protease inhibitor; TNFα, tissue necrosis factor-α; VCAM-1; vascular adhesion molecule-1.

adhesion molecules, chemoattractants, inflammatory mediators, and other inflammatory molecules (Table 32.1); for a comprehensive review see Webster et al. (119).

Cytokines

In general, proinflammatory cytokine gene expression is repressed by glucocorticoids, for example, IL-1 (*120,121*, 122), IL-2 (123), IL-5 (124,*125*,126,*127*), IL-6 (*128,129*,130, 131), IL-8 (131,132,*133,134*), IL-11 (135), IL-12 (*136,137*, 138,139), tumor necrosis factor-α (TNFα) (*140,141*,142), interferon-γ (IFNγ) (123,143) and granulocyte-macrophage colony-stimulating factor (GM-CSF) (131,*144*,145), whereas antiinflammatory cytokine expression is upregulated, for example, IL-4 (*125,146*,147) and IL-10 (143,148).

Regulation of cytokine expression by glucocorticoids can also be achieved by modulation of mRNA stabilization, for example, IL-1β (*120,121*,122), IL-5 (124), IL-8 (132), and IL-11 (135); modulation of receptors and decoy receptor expression, for example, IL-1R II (*149,150*,151,*152*), IL-1 receptor antagonist (153),and IL-12R (*136,137*,138); regulation of translation, for example, TNFα (*140*,142); or modulation of cytokine signaling pathways, for example, dexamethasone inhibition of IL-2 signaling via the Janus kinase (Jak)–signal transducers and activators of transcription (STAT) cascade (154). As mentioned, glucocorticoids are generally thought to upregulate antiinflammatory cytokines; however, there are some specific cell- and dose-dependent effects. For example, IL-10 is upregulated by pharmacologic doses of glucocorticoids, whereas physiologic doses suppress IL-10 (143,148). IL-4 is induced by physiologic concentrations of glucocorticoids in the lymph nodes and spleen of mice (*155*,156) but is downregulated in T cells by high stress levels of dexamethasone (123).

Modulation of cytokine expression by glucocorticoids causes a shift from a T helper (Th) 1 (cellular immunity) to a Th2 (humoral immunity) pattern of immunity. This is evident in some autoimmune diseases, such as rheumatoid arthritis, multiple sclerosis (MS), and type 1 diabetes mellitus, where a shift toward Th1 immunity has been observed, however, in systemic lupus erythematosus (SLE) there is a shift toward Th2 immunity (*136*,157,158). In cases of excessive glucocorticoid production, for example, in animal models with a hyperactive HPA axis (F344/N rats) or in women in the third trimester of pregnancy, a relative resistance to Th1-associated autoimmune diseases has been described (158). However, in cases of low glucocorticoid production, for example, animals lacking glucocorticoids or exhibiting a hypoactive HPA axis (LEW/N rats), susceptibility to Th1-associated autoimmune diseases has been described (*159*,160).

Cell Adhesion Molecules and Chemoattractants

The proteins involved in the attraction and adhesion of leukocytes to areas of inflammation are also downregulated by glucocorticoids. These include intracellular adhesion molecule-1 (ICAM-1) (91,*161,162*,163,164,*165*), endothelial-leukocyte adhesion molecule-1 (ELAM-1) (164), vascular adhesion molecule-1 (VCAM-1) (*165,166*, 167), E-selectin (168,*169*), L-selectin (*170*,171), cytokine-induced neutrophil chemoattractant (CINC)/gro (172), eotaxin (*173*,174), RANTES (regulated on activation normal T cell expressed and secreted) (175), and monocyte chemoattractant protein-1 (MCP-1), MCP-2, and MCP-3 (176,*177–179*).

Inflammatory Mediators

Glucocorticoids also suppress the production of inflammatory mediators, such as prostaglandins and nitric oxide (NO). Glucocorticoids inhibit prostaglandin synthesis at multiple stages; they repress expression of the key enzymes cytosolic phospholipase A$_2$ (PLA$_2$) and cyclooxygenase type 2 (COX-2) (180,*181,182*) and induce lipocortin-1 (or annexin-1), an inhibitor of arachadonic acid release (*183*,184,*185*). NO is suppressed by glucocorticoids by repression of cytokine induction of nitric oxide synthase II (NOS II) (186) and inhibition of inducible nitric oxide

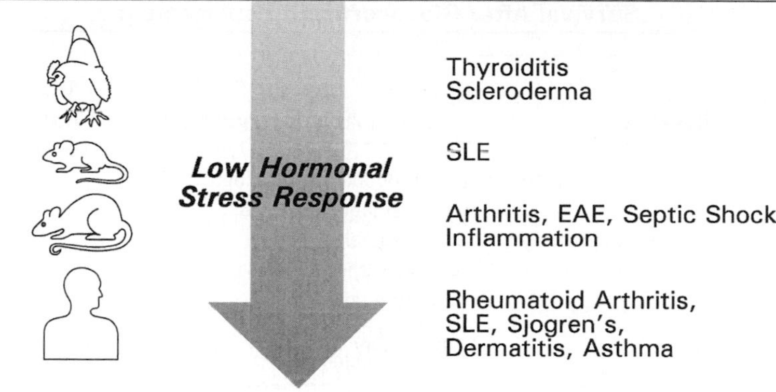

FIGURE 32.4 Blunted hypothalamic-pituitary-adrenal (HPA) axis associated with autoimmune/inflammatory disease. The diagram shows animal models and human studies in which a blunted HPA axis has been found to be associated with autoimmune/inflammatory disease.

synthase (iNOS) gene transcription (*187,188*,189). In addition, secretory leukocyte protease inhibitor (SLPI), an inflammatory gene, is enhanced by GR (82,190), and mitogen-activated protein kinase (MAPK) phosphatase-1 (MKP-1), an inhibitor of the MAPK pathways that induce inflammatory genes, is induced by GR (*191*,192,*193–196*).

Other Inflammatory Response Factors

Glucocorticoids also regulate several receptors involved in the regulation of the immune system. For example, glucocorticoids upregulate the β_2-adrenergic receptor, which is involved in the adrenergic control of the immune system (197,*198,199*), and downregulate the NK_1 receptor, the receptor for substance P (200), and the NK_2 receptor (201).

DYSREGULATION OF HPA AXIS IN THE PATHOGENESIS OF IMMUNE-RELATED DISEASES

Fluctuations in glucocorticoid levels, such as during exercise and with circadian rhythm, have been shown to be associated with changes in cytokine levels and production by leukocytes (202,*203–205*), suggesting a role of physiologic glucocorticoids in the regulation of the immune system. However, animal models have provided the strongest evidence that endogenous glucocorticoids are essential physiologic regulators of the immune response and that disruption of this regulation plays a role in inflammatory/autoimmune disease.

Blunted HPA Axis Associated with Immune Disease: Animal Models

Blunted HPA axis responses have been shown in a number of animal models that are predisposed to autoimmune disease, such as the obese strain (OS) chicken (a model for autoimmune thyroiditis) (206); certain mouse SLE models (MRL strain but not NZB/NZW) (*207*,208); and the inbred Lewis rat strain (LEW/N) (160) (Figure 32.4). For a review of animal models of inflammatory diseases see Jafarian-Tehrani and Sternberg (209) and Tonelli et al. (160).

Two histocompatible inbred rat strains—LEW/N and Fischer (F344/N) rats—that exhibit differential HPA axis responsiveness and differential susceptibility and resistance to autoimmune/inflammatory disease have been extensively used to examine this relationship between HPA axis responses and autoimmune/inflammatory disease. LEW/N rats exhibit a blunted HPA response on stimulation and are highly susceptible to development of a wide range of autoimmune/inflammatory diseases in response to a variety of antigenic or proinflammatory stimuli, whereas F344/N rats have a hyperactive HPA axis and are relatively resistant to such disease on exposure to the same stimuli (210–213,*214*). For example, LEW/N rats, but not F344/N rats, develop experimental allergic encephalomyelitis (EAE) on immunization with myelin basic protein (215) and develop arthritis in response to heat-killed *Mycobacterium tuberculosis* in adjuvant or streptococcal cell walls and inflammation in response to carrageenan (212,213,216,*217*). The molecules involved in the HPA axis regulation and glucocorticoid action have been shown to be different in these two rat strains, for example, hypothalamic CRH (213), pro-opiomelanocortin (POMC) (211), CBG (210), and GR expression and activation (210,218,219).

In a model for Hashimoto's thyroiditis, OS chickens, which have a blunted HPA axis, spontaneous develop thyroiditis (206). These chickens also have increased CBG, which results in decreased free corticosterone levels (220). In a model for human scleroderma, UCD-200 chickens exhibit an ACTH-hyporesponsive adrenal gland (221). Blunted HPA axis responses have also been shown in MRP lupus-prone mice (*207*,208) but not other strains, such as NZB. These associations between a blunted HPA axis and susceptibility to inflammatory/autoimmune disease do not prove cause and effect. Intervention studies, such as those described later, must be performed to do this.

TABLE 32.2 Increased Mortality Rates After Intervention of Hypothalamic-Pituitary-Adrenal (HPA) Axis and Subsequent Survival After Glucocorticoid Replacement

Infection/Disease	*HPA Axis Intervention*	*Mortality Rate (%)*	*Mortality Rate After Corticosterone Replacement (%)*	*Reference*
Streptococcal cell wall–induced arthritis	Glucocorticoid receptor antagonist RU486	100	13	212
Myelin basic protein–induced EAE	Adrenalectomy	80	22	229
Salmonella	Hypophysectomy	100	5	227
MCMV	Adrenalectomy	100	20	228
Shiga toxin 2	Adrenalectomy	100	N/A	230
Anthrax LeTx	Adrenalectomy	90	N/A	231

EAE, experimental allergic encephalomyelitis; LeTx, lethal toxin; MCMV, murine cytomegalovirus; N/A, not available.

It must be emphasized that HPA axis responsiveness is just one variable among many factors that contribute to overall susceptibility and resistance to such complex autoimmune diseases. Genetic linkage studies in rat models have identified genes in more than 20 regions on 15 chromosomes involved in susceptibility and resistance to inflammatory arthritis (*222*,223,*224*,225). These include many genes that are related to immunity and some neuroendocrine genes but also many that are unknown. Similarly, in humans there are likely to be many factors that contribute to susceptibility/resistance to autoimmune/inflammatory disease.

Interruption of the HPA axis, either surgically or pharmacologically, can alter the course and enhance the severity of inducible autoimmune/inflammatory disease in rodents. This link between the requirement of an intact HPA axis for survival from exposure to proinflammatory stimuli is further enforced by the demonstration that the inflammatory disease is attenuated and mortality rates deceased in these animal models by reconstitution of the HPA axis, pharmacologically with glucocorticoids, or surgically by intracerebral fetal hypothalamic tissue transplantation. Administration of the glucocorticoid receptor antagonist RU486 together streptococcal cell walls in otherwise inflammatory resistant F344/N rats results in severe arthritis and high mortality rates that can be reversed by low-dose dexamethasone treatment (212) or prevented by intracerebroventricular transplantation of F344/N hypothalamic tissue (226). Increased mortality rates after *Salmonella typhimurium* infection were also observed in hypophysectomized rats compared to nonhypophysectomized animals (227). Similarly, adrenalectomy resulted in increased mortality following murine cytomegalovirus (MCMV) virus infection, which could be reversed by glucocorticoid treatment (228), and in myelin basic protein (MBP)–induced experimental allergic EAE in LEW/N rats (229). Increased mortality rates in response to Shiga toxin (230) and *Bacillus anthracis* lethal toxin (231) have also been observed in adrenalectomized animals (Table 32.2). These animal models provide evidence for the critical importance of an intact HPA axis and glucocorticoids in protection against septic shock after exposure to a wide range of antigenic, proinflammatory or infectious stimuli.

Blunted HPA Axis Associated with Immune Disease: Human Disease

A blunted HPA axis with resultant low glucocorticoid levels or low glucocorticoid responses has been associated with a number of inflammatory diseases in humans. For example, dysregulation of HPA axis and glucocorticoid responses have been shown in rheumatoid arthritis (*232*,*233*,234,*235–237*,238), SLE (234,*239*), Sjogren's syndrome (234,*240*,*241*), allergic asthma and atopic skin disease (*242*,243,*244*), chronic fatigue syndrome (CFS) (245,*246*,*247*,248,*249*), fibromyalgia (234,*246*,250), multiple sclerosis (251,*252*,253,*254*), and inflammatory and irritable bowel syndrome (255,*256*) (Table 32.3).

Conversely, excessive stimulation of the HPA axis and chronically elevated glucocorticoid levels that result from chronic stress situations, such as those experienced by caregivers of Alzheimer's patients, students taking exams,

TABLE 32.3 Human Diseases That Exhibit a Blunted Hypothalamic-Pituitary-Adrenal Axis

Human Disease	*Reference*
Rheumatoid arthritis	*232*,*233*,234,*235–237*,238
Systemic lupus erythematosus	234,*239*
Sjogren's syndrome	234,*240*,*241*
Allergic asthma	*242*,243,*244*
Atopic skin disease	*242*,243,*244*
Chronic fatigue syndrome	245,*246*,*247*,248,*249*
Fibromyalgia	234,*246*,250
Multiple sclerosis	251,*252*,253,*254*
Inflammatory and irritable bowel syndrome	255,*256*

couples during marital conflict, and Army Rangers undergoing extreme exercise, have been associated with enhanced susceptibility to viral infection, prolonged wound healing, or decreased antibody production after vaccination (*114*,115,*116*,257,*258*,*259*,260).

HPA axis responses can be measured in patients by stimulation of the HPA axis using, for example, exogenous hormones (ovine CRH, AVP, ACTH) (*247*,253), physical stress (exercise) (*203*,248), psychosocial stress (the Trier Social Stress Test [TSST], which involves public speaking and mental arithmetic) (*242*,*244*,248), or insulin hypoglycemia (*239*,248).

Glucocorticoid Resistance in Immune Disease

Glucocorticoid resistance is a phenomenon exhibited in many autoimmune/inflammatory diseases. This resistance can be hereditary or acquired. The molecular mechanisms by which glucocorticoid resistance can occur are described in the following.

Glucocorticoid Receptor

Several mutations and polymorphisms have been found in the glucocorticoid receptor associated with defective glucocorticoid signaling and glucocorticoid resistance. Familial glucocorticoid resistance, a hereditary disease, results from mutations of GR that may result in decreased number, stability, nuclear translocation, or ligand binding of GR. Three different point mutations in the LBD of GR—one in the hinge region—and a deletion in the LBD have been identified in families with familial glucocorticoid resistance [for a review see Charmandari et al. (261)]. Some GR mutations and polymorphisms have been found in other diseases and glucocorticoid resistance states. For example, a phase shift mutation in GR has been described in patients with lupus nephritis (262), and a mutation in the LBD has been found in patients with lupus (263). A mutant GR (amino acid 559 Ile-Asn) that cannot translocate to the nucleus and therefore prevents translocation of wild-type GR was found in a heterozygotic patient with severe glucocorticoid resistance (264). The majority of GR mutations found in glucocorticoid resistance patients affect ligand binding; however, other mutations in GR could affect GR function. A mutation in the DBD of GR has been described in a patient with primary cortisol resistance (*265*,266). Recently, a novel C-terminal mutation that interferes with GR–p160 coactivator interactions was found in a French family with familial glucocorticoid resistance (267). Another mutant has been described that prevented GR–glucocorticoid receptor interacting protein-1 (GRIP1) binding (268). However, not all GR polymorphisms result in glucocorticoid resistance. For example, a polymorphism in GR (codon 363) has been associated with increased sensitivity to glucocorticoids (269), but five polymorphisms in GR (including the one at codon 363) have been described in a normal population (270).

In some patients with glucocorticoid resistance no mutation in GR has been detected, and it is plausible that in these patients there is a defect in another aspect of GR function (271). Defects in other aspects of GR signaling may also result in glucocorticoid resistance without a mutation in the receptor. Decreased glucocorticoid receptor numbers may play a role in glucocorticoid resistance, as is seen in pulmonary fibrosis (272). Decreased ligand affinity has been described in Cushing's syndrome (273). Defective GR transactivation and reduced stability of the receptor can be the result of a mutation in the phosphorylation sites on GR (274). Although no such mutation has yet been identified, phosphorylation of GR has been implicated in a group of steroid-resistant asthma patients. In this case, IL-2 and IL-4 have been suggested to activate p38 MAPK phosphorylation of GR, resulting in reduced nuclear GR activity and glucocorticoid resistance in these patients (275). A defect in GR nuclear translocation has been described in a group of glucocorticoid resistance patients (276). In another group, nuclear translocation was normal but there was a defect in histone acetylation (276).

Glucocorticoid resistance can occur without a mutation in wild-type GR by differences in the expression of the splice variant and proposed dominant repressor GRβ. This could potentially contribute to enhanced inflammatory susceptibility in these subjects through relative antagonism of the GR and resultant relative glucocorticoid resistance. However, the physiologic significance of GRβ as an endogenous GR antagonist is not clear; *in vivo* GRβ exists in a very low ratio compared to the fully active GRα (277). Nonetheless, supporting the physiologic relevance of GRβ abnormalities in disease is the finding of increased expression of GRβ relative to GRα, which has been described in other diseases, including rheumatoid arthritis (*278*,279,280), asthma (*281*,*282*,283,*284*–*288*,289), Cushing's syndrome (290), Crohn's disease (291), ulcerative colitis (*292*,293), inflammatory bowel disease (294), chronic lymphocytic leukemia (295), septic shock (280), ankylosing spondylitis (296), and nasal polyposis disease (*297*,298). Another splice variant, GRγ, has an insertion of three bases in the DBD of GR. This insertion decreases the transactivation activity of GR (299). However, it has been suggested that it does not play a role in glucocorticoid sensitivity (300).

Cortisol-binding Globulin

CBG limits the amount of free cortisol available in the blood. Therefore, theoretically, changes in the expression of this protein or in its binding capacity can also affect the availability of cortisol and glucocorticoid responses. Changes in CBG have not been overly implicated in patients with glucocorticoid resistance. However, increased expression of CBG has been suggested to be responsible for the partial or complete resistance to steroids described in some patients with long-standing Crohn's disease (301). In chronic fatigue syndrome patients, a similar increase in CBG levels has also been described (250).

11β-Hydroxysteroid Dehydrogenase

Glucocorticoid availability can also be regulated by other factors, such as the expression of 11β-HSD, an enzyme that converts the active form of steroids, for example, cortisol and corticosterone, into the inactive form, for example, cortisone and 11-dehydrocortisone (74,75). Changes in the levels of this enzyme could, therefore, cause differences in circulating or tissue glucocorticoid concentrations and glucocorticoid resistance (302). For example, decreased plasma cortisol levels were noted in obese men as a result of type I 11β-HSB impairment (303), and decreased 11β-HSD mRNA was shown in ulcerative colitis (304).

Cofactors

GR is able to influence gene transcription by interacting with the basal transcription machinery through many cofactors, coactivators, or corepressors. Thus, defects in these cofactors could also affect GR function. However, no mutations in cofactors have been found associated with glucocorticoid resistance. However, one interesting recent study showed that a viral protein acting as a cofactor can alter GR responses. The human immunodeficiency virus (HIV-1) accessory protein virion-associated protein (Vpr) binds directly to GR and p300/cAMP-response element binding protein (CREB)–binding protein (CBP) cofactors, thereby functioning as an adapter protein between these components and enhancing GR-mediated gene transaction. This explains the observed glucocorticoid-hypersensitive state associated with HIV-1 infection (*305*,306). Vpr has been shown to enhance the endogenous glucocorticoid suppression of IL-12 but not IL-10 in human peripheral blood monocytes (307). There is one example in which a cofactor defect is thought to be involved in glucocorticoid resistance in two sisters with resistance to multiple steroids (*308*,309). Smoking has been shown to cause oxidative stress, and this can reduce the expression of histone deacetylases (HDACs). There is a decrease in HDAC2 in chronic obstructive pulmonary disease, a glucocorticoid-resistant disease (310,*311*).

Transport Proteins

Intracellular ligand concentration is yet another factor that if altered could affect GR function. Although glucocorticoids are believed passively to diffuse into cells, evidence for an active transport process out of cells exists. Multidrug resistance (MDR) proteins, members of the ATP binding cassette (ABC) family of transporters (312), have been shown to transport glucocorticoids out of cells (*313*,314,315,*316*,317), and their involvement in glucocorticoid-unresponsive disease states has begun to be investigated. Increased expression of the human MDR1 (ABCB1) has been shown in patients with inflammatory bowel disease who have failed medical therapy (318,*319*,*320*,321,322) and also in patients with rheumatoid arthritis (323), Crohn's disease *(320)*, and SLE (324). The novel orphan receptor pregnane X receptor (PXR) (also known as steroid and xenobiotic receptor [SXR]) or PXR ligands have been shown to be regulated by these transporter proteins (325–328). This receptor is activated by many ligands, including glucocorticoids (329), suggesting a possible mechanism by which acquired glucocorticoid resistance during long-term therapy might develop.

EFFECTS OF INFECTION ON HPA AXIS AND GR FUNCTION

Another possible mechanism by which glucocorticoid resistance may occur is through bacterial or viral infections. As one might expect, such infections activate the HPA axis, but, as will be discussed, some bacterial and viral proteins are known directly to interfere with GR signaling. We have recently shown that the anthrax lethal toxin is also able to repress GR signaling, as will be described.

Effect of Infection as a Stimulus to the HPA Axis

Many bacterial and viral infections result in an activation of the HPA axis and increased glucocorticoid release. These include endotoxins, such as lipopolysaccharides, *Mycoplasma fermentans*, *Clostridium difficile* toxin A, Shiga toxin 2, tetanus toxoid, bacterial superantigens, MCMV, lymphocytic choriomeningitis virus (LCMV), herpes simplex virus type 1 (HSV-1), the Sindbis virus, Newcastle disease virus (NDV), influenza virus, and HIV. This activation of the HPA axis is probably the result of the action of inflammatory mediators such as cytokines. In some cases the inflammatory mediators have been identified. Activation of the HPA axis will not be further discussed here; we recently reviewed it elsewhere (330) (Table 32.4).

Direct Effects of Infection on GR Signaling

Several bacterial infections/proteins have been shown to influence GR signaling. These include endotoxin (*331*,332–336), *Chlamydia pneumoniae* (337), bacterial superantigens (338), Shiga toxin 2 (230), and the anthrax lethal toxin (231,*339*,240,341) (Table 32.5). In addition, some viral proteins also interfere with GR signaling. The best studied is

TABLE 32.4 Bacterial and Viral Infections That Activate the Hypothalamic-Pituitary-Adrenal Axis

Bacterial	*Viral*
Lipopolysaccharide	Murine cytomegalovirus
Endotoxin	Lymphocytic choriomeningitis virus
Mycoplasma fermentans	Poly(I:C)
Clostridium difficile toxin A	HIV
Shiga toxin 2	Herpes simplex virus type 1
Tetanus toxoid	Sindbis virus
Staphylococcal enterotoxin A	Newcastle disease virus
Staphylococcal enterotoxin B	Influenza virus

TABLE 32.6 Viruses That Interact with the Glucocorticoid Receptor (GR)

Virus/Viral Product	*Effect*	*Ref.*
HIV (Vpr)	Enhances GR activity (acts as cofactor)	*305*,306,307
Poxvirus MC protein MC013L	Inhibits GR activity	342
Influenza virus	Increases GR activity	343
HSV-1	Increases GR number and activity	344
Epstein-Barr virus	Increases GR number	*345*,346
Murine cytomegalovirus	Decreases GR binding in spleen	347

the HIV protein Vpr, which we have previously described. Others include the poxvirus MC protein MC013L (342), influenza virus (343), HSV-1 (344), Epstein-Barr virus (EBV) (*345*,346), and MCMV (347) (Table 32.6). For a comprehensive review of these interactions see our recent review article (330).

Effect of Anthrax Lethal Toxin on GR

We recently showed that a bacterial toxin—the anthrax lethal toxin (LeTx)—represses the glucocorticoid receptor and other members of the nuclear hormone receptor superfamily, such as the progesterone receptor. LeTx is a noncompetitive inhibitor that does not affect GR numbers or interfere with ligand binding or nuclear translocation. It does prevent GR binding to DNA in the context of a native gene. We have suggested that LeTx interferes with one of the many cofactors involved in GR signaling (340,341). Adrenalectomy has been shown to convert a LeTx-resistant animal into one that is susceptible to lethality from LeTx, suggesting the importance of an intact HPA axis response and glucocorticoids in protection from the lethal effects of LeTx (231). Further studies are underway further to understand these effects and to determine the generalizability of this phenomenon to other bacterial toxins and its role in contributing to shock.

TABLE 32.5 Bacteria That Interact with the Glucocorticoid Receptor (GR)

Bacteria/Bacterial Product	*Effect*	*Ref.*
Endotoxin	GR downregulation	*331*,332
	Downregulation of leukocyte GR number	333
	Inhibition of dexamethasone binding (rat liver nuclei)	334
	Inhibition of dexamethasone binding (peritoneal macrophages)	335
	Increased GR number, reduced affinity (bronchial epithelial cells)	336
Chlamydia pneumoniae	Activation of GR	337
Superantigen SEB	Induction of GRβ	338
Shiga toxin 2	Increased GR expression	230
Anthrax lethal toxin	Repression of GR activity	231,*339*, 340,341

CONCLUSION

A bidirectional regulation occurs between the CNS and immune system. Perturbations of this balance result in disease. An intact HPA axis and glucocorticoid signaling are essential for survival from a number of proinflammatory insults. Dysregulation of this HPA axis has been shown in many autoimmune/inflammatory diseases, and defects in all aspects of GR signaling can result in glucocorticoid resistance. In addition, bacterial or viral infections can also affect GR signaling. Thus, all aspects of this bidirectional communication should be considered when assessing risk factors for immune-mediated diseases.

REFERENCES

3. Gibson RM, Rothwell NJ, Le Feuvre RA. CNS injury: the role of the cytokine IL-1. *Vet J.* 2004;168:230.
6. Strle K, Zhou JH, Shen WH, et al. Interleukin-10 in the brain. *Crit Rev Immunol.* 2001;21:427.
7. Rosenberg PB. Clinical aspects of inflammation in Alzheimer's disease. *Int Rev Psychiatry.* 2005;17:503.
11. Watkins LR, Maier SF, Goehler LE. Immune activation: The role of pro-inflammatory cytokines in inflammation, illness responses and pathological pain states. *Pain.* 1995;63:289.
13. Dantzer R. Cytokine-induced sickness behaviour: a neuroimmune response to activation of innate immunity. *Eur J Pharmacol.* 2004;500:399.
14. Banks WA, Kastin AJ, Broadwell RD. Passage of cytokines across the blood-brain barrier. *Neuroimmunomodulation.* 1995;2:241.

15. Dantzer R, Konsman JP, Bluthe RM, et al. Neural and humoral pathways of communication from the immune system to the brain: parallel or convergent? *Auton Neurosci.* 2000;85:60.
16. Goehler LE, Gaykema RP, Hansen MK, et al. Vagal immune-to-brain communication: A visceral chemosensory pathway. *Auton Neurosci.* 2000;85:49.
21. Masek K, Slansky J, Petrovicky P, et al. Neuroendocrine immune interactions in health and disease. *Int Immunopharmacol.* 2003;3:1235.
22. Sternberg EM. Neural regulation of innate immunity: a coordinated nonspecific host response to pathogens. *Nat Rev Immunol.* 2006;6:318.
23. Schwarz H, Villiger PM, von Kempis J, et al. Neuropeptide Y is an inducible gene in the human immune system. *J Neuroimmunol.* 1994;51:53.
24. Sanders VM. Interdisciplinary research: noradrenergic regulation of adaptive immunity. *Brain Behav Immun.* 2006;20:1.
25. Maestroni GJ. Sympathetic nervous system influence on the innate immune response. *Ann NY Acad Sci.* 2006;1069:195.
27. Straub RH, Schaller T, Miller LE, et al. Neuropeptide Y cotransmission with norepinephrine in the sympathetic nerve-macrophage interplay. *J Neurochem.* 2000;75:2464.
28. Kin NW, Sanders VM. It takes nerve to tell T and B cells what to do. *J Leukoc Biol.* 2006;79:1093.
29. Watkins LR, Maier SF. Implications of immune-to-brain communication for sickness and pain. *Proc Natl Acad Sci U S A.* 1999;96:7710.
30. Tracey KJ. The inflammatory reflex. *Nature.* 2002;420:853.
33. Cuesta MC, Quintero L, Pons H, et al. Substance P and calcitonin gene-related peptide increase IL-1 beta, IL-6 and TNF alpha secretion from human peripheral blood mononuclear cells. *Neurochem Int.* 2002;40:301.
35. Blondel O, Collin C, McCarran WJ, et al. A glia-derived signal regulating neuronal differentiation. *J Neurosci.* 2000;20:8012.
36. Delgado M, Pozo D, Ganea D. The significance of vasoactive intestinal peptide in immunomodulation. *Pharmacol Rev.* 2004;56:249.
38. Taylor AW. The immunomodulating neuropeptide alpha-melanocyte-stimulating hormone (alpha-MSH) suppresses LPS-stimulated TLR4 with IRAK-M in macrophages. *J Neuroimmunol.* 2005;162:43.
40. Roselli-Rehfuss L, Mountjoy KG, Robbins LS, et al. Identification of a receptor for gamma melanotropin and other proopiomelanocortin peptides in the hypothalamus and limbic system. *Proc Natl Acad Sci U S A.* 1993;90:8856.
41. Grimm MC, Ben-Baruch A, Taub DD, et al. Opiate inhibition of chemokine-induced chemotaxis. *Ann NY Acad Sci.* 1998;840:9.
42. Mellon RD, Bayer BM. The effects of morphine, nicotine and epibatidine on lymphocyte activity and hypothalamic-pituitary-adrenal axis responses. *J Pharmacol Exp Ther.* 1999;288:635.
43. De Bellis A, Bizzarro A, Pivonello R, et al. Prolactin and autoimmunity. *Pituitary.* 2005;8:25.
45. Meazza C, Pagani S, Travaglino P, et al. Effect of growth hormone (GH) on the immune system. *Pediatr Endocrinol Rev.* 2004;1(Suppl 3):490.
46. Dixit VD, Taub DD. Ghrelin and immunity: a young player in an old field. *Exp Gerontol.* 2005;40:900.
47. Popovic V, Duntas LH. Brain somatic cross-talk: ghrelin, leptin and ultimate challengers of obesity. *Nutr Neurosci.* 2005;8:1.
48. Otero M, Lago R, Gomez R, et al. Leptin: a metabolic hormone that functions like a proinflammatory adipokine. *Drug News Perspect.* 2006;19:21.
50. Cutolo M, Sulli A, Pizzorni C, et al. Hypothalamic-pituitary-adrenocortical and gonadal functions in rheumatoid arthritis. *Ann NY Acad Sci.* 2003;992:107.
55. Bouman A, Heineman MJ, Faas MM. Sex hormones and the immune response in humans. *Hum Reprod Update.* 2005;11:411.
57. Cutolo M, Sulli A, Capellino S, et al. Sex hormones influence on the immune system: Basic and clinical aspects in autoimmunity. *Lupus.* 2004;13:635.
61. Volpi S, Rabadan-Diehl C, Aguilera G. Vasopressinergic regulation of the hypothalamic pituitary adrenal axis and stress adaptation. *Stress.* 2004;7:75.
65. Giordano R, Pellegrino M, Picu A, et al. Neuroregulation of the hypothalamus-pituitary-adrenal (HPA) axis in humans: effects of GABA-, mineralocorticoid-, and GH-secretagogue-receptor modulation. *Sci World J.* 2006;6:1.
68. Hench P. Effects of cortisone in the rheumatic diseases. *Lancet.* 1950;2:483.
69. Adcock IM. Glucocorticoids: new mechanisms and future agents. *Curr Allergy Asthma Rep.* 2003;3:249.
70. Barnes PJ. Anti-inflammatory actions of glucocorticoids: molecular mechanisms. *Clin Sci.* 1998;94:557.
72. Funder JW. Glucocorticoid receptors. *J Steroid Biochem Mol Biol.* 1992;43:389.
73. De Kloet ER. Hormones and the stressed brain. *Ann NY Acad Sci.* 2004;1018:1.
74. Draper N, Stewart PM. 11beta-hydroxysteroid dehydrogenase and the pre-receptor regulation of corticosteroid hormone action. *J Endocrinol.* 2005;186:251.
75. Seckl JR. 11beta-hydroxysteroid dehydrogenases: changing glucocorticoid action. *Curr Opin Pharmacol.* 2004;4:597.
77. Nuclear Receptor Nomenclature Committee. A unified nomenclature system for the nuclear receptor superfamily. *Cell.* 1999;97:161.
78. Aranda A, Pascual A. Nuclear hormone receptors and gene expression. *Physiol Rev.* 2001;81:1269.
82. Hayashi R, Wada H, Ito K, et al. Effects of glucocorticoids on gene transcription. *Eur J Pharmacol.* 2004;500:51.
83. Dostert A, Heinzel T. Negative glucocorticoid receptor response elements and their role in glucocorticoid action. *Curr Pharm Des.* 2004;10:2807.
86. Smoak KA, Cidlowski JA. Mechanisms of glucocorticoid receptor signaling during inflammation. *Mech Ageing Dev.* 2004;125:697.
87. Adcock IM, Caramori G. Cross-talk between pro-inflammatory transcription factors and glucocorticoids. *Immunol Cell Biol.* 2001;79:376.
89. Karin M, Chang L. AP-1-glucocorticoid receptor crosstalk taken to a higher level. *J Endocrinol.* 2001;169:447.
91. Caldenhoven E, Liden J, Wissink S, et al. Negative cross-talk between RelA and the glucocorticoid receptor: a possible mechanism for the antiinflammatory action of glucocorticoids. *Mol Endocrinol.* 1995;9:401.
92. Encio IJ, Detera-Wadleigh SD. The genomic structure of the human glucocorticoid receptor. *J Biol Chem.* 1991;266:7182.
99. Lewis-Tuffin LJ, Cidlowski JA. The physiology of human glucocorticoid receptor beta (hGRbeta) and glucocorticoid resistance. *Ann NY Acad Sci.* 2006;1069:1.
100. de Lange P, Koper JW, Brinkmann AO, et al. Natural variants of the beta isoform of the human glucocorticoid receptor do not alter sensitivity to glucocorticoids. *Mol Cell Endocrinol.* 1999;153:163.
102. Carlstedt-Duke J. Glucocorticoid receptor beta: view II. *Trends Endocrinol Metab.* 1999;10:339.
104. Li LB, Leung DY, Hall CF, et al. Divergent expression and function of glucocorticoid receptor beta in human monocytes and T cells. *J Leukoc Biol.* 2006;79:818.
105. Bamberger CM, Bamberger AM, Wald M, et al. Inhibition of mineralocorticoid activity by the beta-isoform of the human glucocorticoid receptor. *J Steroid Biochem Mol Biol.* 1997;60:43.
106. Munck A, Guyre PM, Holbrook NJ. Physiological functions of glucocorticoids in stress and their relation to pharmacological actions. *Endocr Rev.* 1984;5:25.
107. Visser J, van Boxel-Dezaire A, Methorst D, et al. Differential regulation of interleukin-10 (IL-10) and IL-12 by glucocorticoids *in vitro*. *Blood.* 1998;91:4255.
108. Dhabhar FS, McEwen BS. Enhancing versus suppressive effects of stress hormones on skin immune function. *Proc Natl Acad Sci U S A.* 1999;96:1059.
109. Cohen S, Williamson GM. Stress and infectious disease in humans. *Psychol Bull.* 1991;109:5.
115. Glaser R, Kiecolt-Glaser JK. Stress-induced immune dysfunction: implications for health. *Nat Rev Immunol.* 2005;5:243.
119. Webster JI, Tonelli L, Sternberg EM. Neuroendocrine regulation of immunity. *Annu Rev Immunol.* 2002;20:125.
122. Schmidt M, Pauels HG, Lugering N, et al. Glucocorticoids induce apoptosis in human monocytes: Potential role of IL-1 beta. *J Immunol.* 1999;163:3484.
123. Moynihan JA, Callahan TA, Kelley SP, et al. Adrenal hormone modulation of type 1 and type 2 cytokine production by spleen cells:

dexamethasone and dehydroepiandrosterone suppress interleukin-2, interleukin-4, and interferon-gamma production *in vitro*. *Cell Immunol*. 1998;184:58.
124. Staples KJ, Bergmann MW, Barnes PJ, et al. Evidence for post-transcriptional regulation of interleukin-5 by dexamethasone. *Immunology*. 2003;109:527.
126. Mordvinov VA, Kok CC, Arthaningtyas E, et al. Dexamethasone suppresses human interleukin-5 gene promoter. *Bull Exp Biol Med*. 2005;140:80.
130. Vanden Berghe W, Vermeulen L, De Wilde G, et al. Signal transduction by tumor necrosis factor and gene regulation of the inflammatory cytokine interleukin-6. *Biochem Pharmacol*. 2000;60:1185.
131. Tobler A, Meier R, Seitz M, et al. Glucocorticoids downregulate gene expression of GM-CSF, NAP-1/IL-8, and IL-6, but not of M-CSF in human fibroblasts. *Blood*. 1992;79:45.
132. Chang MM, Juarez M, Hyde DM, et al. Mechanism of dexamethasone-mediated interleukin-8 gene suppression in cultured airway epithelial cells. *Am J Physiol Lung Cell Mol Physiol*. 2001;280:L107.
135. Wang J, Zhu Z, Nolfo R, et al. Dexamethasone regulation of lung epithelial cell and fibroblast interleukin-11 production. *Am J Physiol*. 1999;276:L175.
138. Wu CY, Wang K, McDyer JF, et al. Prostaglandin E2 and dexamethasone inhibit IL-12 receptor expression and IL-12 responsiveness. *J Immunol*. 1998;161:2723.
139. Ma W, Gee K, Lim W, Chambers K, et al. Dexamethasone inhibits IL-12p40 production in lipopolysaccharide-stimulated human monocytic cells by down-regulating the activity of c-Jun N-terminal kinase, the activation protein-1, and NF-kappa B transcription factors. *J Immunol*. 2004;172:318.
142. Joyce DA, Gimblett G, Steer JH. Targets of glucocorticoid action on TNF-alpha release by macrophages. *Inflamm Res*. 2001;50:337.
143. Verhoef CM, van Roon JA, Vianen ME, et al. The immune suppressive effect of dexamethasone in rheumatoid arthritis is accompanied by upregulation of interleukin 10 and by differential changes in interferon gamma and interleukin 4 production. *Ann Rheum Dis*. 1999;58:49.
145. Smith PJ, Cousins DJ, Jee YK, et al. Suppression of granulocyte-macrophage colony-stimulating factor expression by glucocorticoids involves inhibition of enhancer function by the glucocorticoid receptor binding to composite NF-AT/activator protein-1 elements. *J Immunol*. 2001;167:2502.
147. Yoshikawa H, Nakajima Y, Tasaka K. Glucocorticoid suppresses autocrine survival of mast cells by inhibiting IL-4 production and ICAM-1 expression. *J Immunol*. 1999;162:6162.
148. Hodge S, Hodge G, Flower R, et al. Methyl-prednisolone up-regulates monocyte interleukin-10 production in stimulated whole blood. *Scand J Immunol*. 1999;49:548.
151. Pousset F, Cremona S, Dantzer R, et al. Dexamethasone up-regulates type II IL-1 receptor in mouse primary activated astrocytes. *J Neurochem*. 2001;76:901.
153. Levine SJ, Benfield T, Shelhamer JH. Corticosteroids induce intracellular interleukin-1 receptor antagonist type I expression by a human airway epithelial cell line. *Am J Respir Cell Mol Biol*. 1996;15:245.
154. Bianchi M, Meng C, Ivashkiv LB. Inhibition of IL-2-induced Jak-STAT signaling by glucocorticoids. *Proc Natl Acad Sci U S A*. 2000;97:9573.
156. Daynes RA, Araneo BA, Dowell TA, et al. Regulation of murine lymphokine production *in vivo*. III. The lymphoid tissue microenvironment exerts regulatory influences over T helper cell function. *J Exp Med*. 1990;171:979.
157. Crane IJ, Forrester JV. Th1 and Th2 lymphocytes in autoimmune disease. *Crit Rev Immunol*. 2005;25:75.
158. Elenkov IJ. Glucocorticoids and the Th1/Th2 balance. *Ann NY Acad Sci*. 2004;1024:138.
160. Tonelli L, Webster JI, Rapp KL, et al. Neuroendocrine responses regulating susceptibility and resistance to autoimmune/inflammatory disease in inbred rat strains. *Immunol Rev*. 2001;184:203.
163. Shirasaki H, Watanabe K, Kanaizumi E, et al. Effect of glucocorticosteroids on tumour necrosis factor-alpha-induced intercellular adhesion molecule-1 expression in cultured primary human nasal epithelial cells. *Clin Exp Allergy*. 2004;34:945.
164. Cronstein BN, Kimmel SC, Levin RI, et al. A mechanism for the anti-inflammatory effects of corticosteroids: the glucocorticoid receptor regulates leukocyte adhesion to endothelial cells and expression of endothelial-leukocyte adhesion molecule 1 and intercellular adhesion molecule 1. *Proc Natl Acad Sci U S A*. 1992;89:9991.
167. Kang H, Wei EQ, Yang XH, et al. VCAM-1 expression, eosinophil infiltration, and pharmacological modulation in rat allergic airway inflammation. *Acta Pharmacol Sin*. 2002;23:157.
168. Ray KP, Farrow S, Daly M, et al. Induction of the E-selectin promoter by interleukin 1 and tumour necrosis factor alpha, and inhibition by glucocorticoids. *Biochem J*. 1997;328(2):707.
171. Weber PS, Toelboell T, Chang LC, T et al. Mechanisms of glucocorticoid-induced down-regulation of neutrophil L-selectin in cattle: evidence for effects at the gene-expression level and primarily on blood neutrophils. *J Leukoc Biol*. 2004;75:815.
172. Ohtsuka T, Kubota A, Hirano T, et al. Glucocorticoid-mediated gene suppression of rat cytokine-induced neutrophil chemoattractant CINC/gro, a member of the interleukin-8 family, through impairment of NF-kappa B activation. *J Biol Chem*. 1996;271:1651.
174. Matsukura S, Kokubu F, Kurokawa M, et al. Molecular mechanisms of repression of eotaxin expression with fluticasone propionate in airway epithelial cells. *Int Arch Allergy Immunol*. 2004;134(Suppl 1):12.
175. Wingett D, Forcier K, Nielson CP. Glucocorticoid-mediated inhibition of RANTES expression in human T lymphocytes. *FEBS Lett*. 1996;398:308.
176. Matsuo H, Tamura M, Kabashima N, et al. Prednisolone inhibits hyperosmolarity-induced expression of MCP-1 via NF-kappaB in peritoneal mesothelial cells. *Kidney Int*. 2006;69:736.
180. Dolan-O'keefe M, Nick HS. Inhibition of cytoplasmic phospholipase A2 expression by glucocorticoids in rat intestinal epithelial cells. *Gastroenterology*. 1999;116:855.
184. Buckingham JC, Flower RJ. Lipocortin 1: a second messenger of glucocorticoid action in the hypothalamo-pituitary-adrenocortical axis. *Mol Med Today*. 1997;3:296.
186. Kleinert H, Euchenhofer C, Ihrig-Biedert I, et al. Glucocorticoids inhibit the induction of nitric oxide synthase II by down-regulating cytokine-induced activity of transcription factor nuclear factor-kappa B. *Mol Pharmacol*. 1996;49:15.
189. Shinoda J, McLaughlin KE, Bell HS, et al. Molecular mechanisms underlying dexamethasone inhibition of iNOS expression and activity in C6 glioma cells. *Glia*. 2003;42:68.
190. Abbinante-Nissen JM, Simpson LG, Leikauf GD. Corticosteroids increase secretory leukocyte protease inhibitor transcript levels in airway epithelial cells. *Am J Physiol*. 1995;268:L601.
192. Abraham SM, Lawrence T, Kleiman A, et al. Antiinflammatory effects of dexamethasone are partly dependent on induction of dual specificity phosphatase 1. *J Exp Med*. 2006;203:1883.
197. Mak JC, Nishikawa M, Barnes PJ. Glucocorticosteroids increase beta 2-adrenergic receptor transcription in human lung. *Am J Physiol*. 1995;268:L41.
200. Ihara H, Nakanishi S. Selective inhibition of expression of the substance P receptor mRNA in pancreatic acinar AR42J cells by glucocorticoids. *J Biol Chem*. 1990;265:22441.
201. Katsunuma T, Mak JC, Barnes PJ. Glucocorticoids reduce tachykinin NK2 receptor expression in bovine tracheal smooth muscle. *Eur J Pharmacol*. 1998;344:99.
202. DeRijk R, Michelson D, Karp B, et al. Exercise and circadian rhythm-induced variations in plasma cortisol differentially regulate interleukin-1 beta (IL-1 beta), IL-6, and tumor necrosis factor-alpha (TNF alpha) production in humans: high sensitivity of TNF alpha and resistance of IL-6. *J Clin Endocrinol Metab*. 1997;82:2182.
206. Wick G, Sgonc R, Lechner O. Neuroendocrine-immune disturbances in animal models with spontaneous autoimmune diseases. *Ann NY Acad Sci*. 1998;840:591–598.
208. Lechner O, Hu Y, Jafarian-Tehrani M, et al. Disturbed immunoendocrine communication via the hypothalamo-pituitary-adrenal axis in murine lupus. *Brain Behav Immun*. 1996;10:337.
209. Jafarian-Tehrani M, Sternberg EM. Animal models of neuroimmune interactions in inflammatory diseases. *J Neuroimmunol*. 1999;100:13.
210. Dhabhar FS, McEwen BS, Spencer RL. Stress response, adrenal steroid receptor levels and corticosteroid-binding globulin levels-a

comparison between Sprague-Dawley, Fischer 344 and Lewis rats. *Brain Res*. 1993;616:89.
211. Moncek F, Kvetnansky R, Jezova D. Differential responses to stress stimuli of Lewis and Fischer rats at the pituitary and adrenocortical level. *Endocr Regul*. 2001;35:35.
212. Sternberg EM, Hill JM, Chrousos GP, et al. Inflammatory mediator-induced hypothalamic-pituitary-adrenal axis activation is defective in streptococcal cell wall arthritis-susceptible Lewis rats. *Proc Natl Acad Sci U S A*. 1989;86:2374.
213. Sternberg EM, Young WS, Bernardini R, et al. A central nervous system defect in biosynthesis of corticotropin-releasing hormone is associated with susceptibility to streptococcal cell wall-induced arthritis in Lewis rats. *Proc Natl Acad Sci U S A*. 1989;86:4771.
215. Stefferl A, Linington C, Holsboer F, et al. Susceptibility and resistance to experimental allergic encephalomyelitis: relationship with hypothalamic-pituitary-adrenocortical axis responsiveness in the rat. *Endocrinology*. 1999;140:4932.
216. Aksentijevich S, Whitfield HJ, Young WS, et al. Arthritis-susceptible Lewis rats fail to emerge from the stress hyporesponsive period. *Brain Res Dev Brain Res*. 1992;65:115.
218. Dhabhar FS, Miller AH, McEwen BS, et al. Differential activation of adrenal steroid receptors in neural and immune tissues of Sprague Dawley, Fischer 344, and Lewis rats. *J Neuroimmunol*. 1995; 56:77.
219. Smith CC, Omeljaniuk RJ, Whitfield HJ, et al. Differential mineralocorticoid (type 1) and glucocorticoid (type 2) receptor expression in Lewis and Fischer rats. *Neuroimmunomodulation*. 1994;1:66.
220. Wick G, Hu Y, Schwarz S, et al. Immunoendocrine communication via the hypothalamo-pituitary-adrenal axis in autoimmune diseases. *Endocr Rev*. 1993;14:539.
221. Brezinschek HP, Gruschwitz M, Sgonc R, et al. Effects of cytokine application on glucocorticoid secretion in an animal model for systemic scleroderma. *J Autoimmun*. 1993;6:719.
223. Listwak S, Barrientos RM, Koike G, et al. Identification of a novel inflammation-protective locus in the Fischer rat. *Mamm Genome*. 1999;10:362.
225. Wilder RL, Griffiths MM, Cannon GW, et al. Genetic factors involved in central nervous system/immune interactions. *Adv Exp Med Biol*. 2001;493:59.
226. Misiewicz B, Poltorak M, Raybourne RB, et al. Intracerebroventricular transplantation of embryonic neuronal tissue from inflammatory resistant into inflammatory susceptible rats suppresses specific components of inflammation. *Exp Neurol*. 1997;146:305.
227. Edwards CK, Yunger LM, Lorence RM, et al. The pituitary gland is required for protection against lethal effects of Salmonella typhimurium. *Proc Natl Acad Sci U S A*. 1991;88:2274.
228. Ruzek MC, Pearce BD, Miller AH, et al. Endogenous glucocorticoids protect against cytokine-mediated lethality during viral infection. *J Immunol*. 1999;162:3527.
229. MacPhee IA, Antoni FA, Mason DW. Spontaneous recovery of rats from experimental allergic encephalomyelitis is dependent on regulation of the immune system by endogenous adrenal corticosteroids. *J Exp Med*. 1989;169:431.
230. Gomez SA, Fernandez GC, Vanzulli S, et al. Endogenous glucocorticoids attenuate Shiga toxin-2-induced toxicity in a mouse model of haemolytic uraemic syndrome. *Clin Exp Immunol*. 2003;131: 217.
231. Moayeri M, Webster JI, Wiggins JF, et al. Endocrine perturbation increases susceptibility of mice to anthrax lethal toxin. *Infect Immun*. 2005;73:4238.
234. Crofford LJ. The hypothalamic-pituitary-adrenal axis in the pathogenesis of rheumatic diseases. *Endocrinol Metab Clin North Am*. 2002;31:1.
238. Neeck G, Kluter A, Dotzlaw H, et al. Involvement of the glucocorticoid receptor in the pathogenesis of rheumatoid arthritis. *Ann NY Acad Sci*. 2002;966:491.
243. Buske-Kirschbaum A, Hellhammer DH. Endocrine and immune responses to stress in chronic inflammatory skin disorders. *Ann NY Acad Sci*. 2003;992:231.
245. Cleare AJ. The neuroendocrinology of chronic fatigue syndrome. *Endocr Rev*. 2003;24:236.
248. Gaab J, Huster D, Peisen R, et al. Hypothalamic-pituitary-adrenal axis reactivity in chronic fatigue syndrome and health under psychological, physiological, and pharmacological stimulation. *Psychosom Med*. 2002;64:951.
250. Demitrack MA, Crofford LJ. Evidence for and pathophysiologic implications of hypothalamic-pituitary-adrenal axis dysregulation in fibromyalgia and chronic fatigue syndrome. *Ann NY Acad Sci*. 1998;840:684.
251. Gold SM, Mohr DC, Huitinga I, et al. The role of stress-response systems for the pathogenesis and progression of MS. *Trends Immunol*. 2005;26:644.
253. Michelson D, Stone L, Galliven E, et al. Multiple sclerosis is associated with alterations in hypothalamic-pituitary-adrenal axis function. *J Clin Endocrinol Metab*. 1994;79:848.
255. Niess JH, Monnikes H, Dignass AU, et al. Review on the influence of stress on immune mediators, neuropeptides and hormones with relevance for inflammatory bowel disease. *Digestion*. 2002;65: 131.
257. Friedl KE, Moore RJ, Hoyt RW, et al. Endocrine markers of semistarvation in healthy lean men in a multistressor environment. *J Appl Physiol*. 2000;88:1820.
260. Vedhara K, Cox NK, Wilcock GK, et al. Chronic stress in elderly carers of dementia patients and antibody response to influenza vaccination. *Lancet*. 1999;353:627.
261. Charmandari E, Kino T, Chrousos GP. Familial/sporadic glucocorticoid resistance: clinical phenotype and molecular mechanisms. *Ann NY Acad Sci*. 2004;1024:168.
262. Jiang T, Liu S, Tan M, et al. The phase-shift mutation in the glucocorticoid receptor gene: Potential etiologic significance of neuroendocrine mechanisms in lupus nephritis. *Clin Chim Acta*. 2001;313:113.
263. Lee YM, Fujiwara J, Munakata Y, et al. A mutation of the glucocorticoid receptor gene in patients with systemic lupus erythematosus. *Tohoku J Exp Med*. 2004;203:69.
264. Kino T, Stauber RH, Resau JH, et al. Pathologic human GR mutant has a transdominant negative effect on the wild-type GR by inhibiting its translocation into the nucleus: importance of the ligand-binding domain for intracellular GR trafficking. *J Clin Endocrinol Metab*. 2001;86:5600.
266. Charmandari E, Kino T, Ichijo T, et al. Functional characterization of the natural human glucocorticoid receptor (hGR) mutants hGRalphaR477H and hGRalphaG679S associated with generalized glucocorticoid resistance. *J Clin Endocrinol Metab*. 2006;91:1535.
267. Vottero A, Kino T, Combe H, et al. A novel, C-terminal dominant negative mutation of the GR causes familial glucocorticoid resistance through abnormal interactions with p160 steroid receptor coactivators. *J Clin Endocrinol Metab*. 2002;87:2658.
268. Kunz S, Sandoval R, Carlsson P, et al. Identification of a novel glucocorticoid receptor mutation in budesonide-resistant human bronchial epithelial cells. *Mol Endocrinol*. 2003;17:2566.
269. Huizenga NA, Koper JW, De Lange P, et al. A polymorphism in the glucocorticoid receptor gene may be associated with and increased sensitivity to glucocorticoids *in vivo*. *J Clin Endocrinol Metab*. 1998;83:144.
270. Koper JW, Stolk RP, de Lange P, et al. Lack of association between five polymorphisms in the human glucocorticoid receptor gene and glucocorticoid resistance. *Hum Genet*. 1997;99:663.
271. Huizenga NA, de Lange P, Koper JW, et al. Five patients with biochemical and/or clinical generalized glucocorticoid resistance without alterations in the glucocorticoid receptor gene. *J Clin Endocrinol Metab*. 2000;85:2076.
272. Pujols L, Xaubet A, Ramirez J, et al. Expression of glucocorticoid receptors alpha and beta in steroid sensitive and steroid insensitive interstitial lung diseases. *Thorax*. 2004;59:687.
273. Huizenga NA, De Herder WW, Koper JW, et al. Decreased ligand affinity rather than glucocorticoid receptor down-regulation in patients with endogenous Cushing's syndrome. *Eur J Endocrinol*. 2000;142:472.
274. Webster JC, Jewell CM, Bodwell JE, et al. Mouse glucocorticoid receptor phosphorylation status influences multiple functions of the receptor protein. *J Biol Chem*. 1997;272:9287.
275. Irusen E, Matthews JG, Takahashi A, et al. p38 Mitogen-activated protein kinase-induced glucocorticoid receptor phosphorylation reduces its activity: role in steroid-insensitive asthma. *J Allergy Clin Immunol*. 2002;109:649.

276. Matthews JG, Ito K, Barnes PJ, et al. Defective glucocorticoid receptor nuclear translocation and altered histone acetylation patterns in glucocorticoid-resistant patients. *J Allergy Clin Immunol.* 2004;113:1100.
277. Pujols L, Mullol J, Roca-Ferrer J, et al. Expression of glucocorticoid receptor alpha- and beta-isoforms in human cells and tissues. *Am J Physiol Cell Physiol.* 2002;283:C1324.
279. Derijk RH, Schaaf MJ, Turner G, et al. A human glucocorticoid receptor gene variant that increases the stability of the glucocorticoid receptor beta-isoform mRNA is associated with rheumatoid arthritis. *J Rheumatol.* 2001;28:2383.
280. Goecke A, Guerrero J. Glucocorticoid receptor beta in acute and chronic inflammatory conditions: clinical implications. *Immunobiology.* 2006;211:85.
283. Goleva E, Li LB, Eves PT, et al. Increased glucocorticoid receptor beta alters steroid response in glucocorticoid-insensitive asthma. *Am J Respir Crit Care Med.* 2006;173:607.
289. Tliba O, Cidlowski JA, Amrani Y. CD38 expression is insensitive to steroid action in cells treated with tumor necrosis factor-alpha and interferon-gamma by a mechanism involving the up-regulation of the glucocorticoid receptor beta isoform. *Mol Pharmacol.* 2006;69:588.
290. Hagendorf A, Koper JW, de Jong FH, et al. Expression of the human glucocorticoid receptor splice variants alpha, beta, and P in peripheral blood mononuclear leukocytes in healthy controls and in patients with hyper- and hypocortisolism. *J Clin Endocrinol Metab.* 2005;90:6237.
291. Towers R, Naftali T, Gabay G, et al. High levels of glucocorticoid receptors in patients with active Crohn's disease may predict steroid resistance. *Clin Exp Immunol.* 2005;141:357.
293. Zhang H, Ouyang Q, Wen ZH, et al. Significance of glucocorticoid receptor expression in colonic mucosal cells of patients with ulcerative colitis. *World J Gastroenterol.* 2005;11:1775.
294. Orii F, Ashida T, Nomura M, et al. Quantitative analysis for human glucocorticoid receptor alpha/beta mRNA in IBD. *Biochem Biophys Res Commun.* 2002;296:1286.
295. Shahidi H, Vottero A, Stratakis CA, et al. Imbalanced expression of the glucocorticoid receptor isoforms in cultured lymphocytes from a patient with systemic glucocorticoid resistance and chronic lymphocytic leukemia. *Biochem Biophys Res Commun.* 1999;254:559.
296. Lee CK, Lee EY, Cho YS, et al. Increased expression of glucocorticoid receptor beta messenger RNA in patients with ankylosing spondylitis. *Korean J Intern Med.* 2005;20:146.
298. Pujols L, Mullol J, Benitez P, et al. Expression of the glucocorticoid receptor alpha and beta isoforms in human nasal mucosa and polyp epithelial cells. *Respir Med.* 2003;97:90.
299. Rivers C, Levy A, Hancock J, et al. Insertion of an amino acid in the DNA-binding domain of the glucocorticoid receptor as a result of alternative splicing. *J Clin Endocrinol Metab.* 1999;84:4283.
300. Stevens A, Donn R, Ray D. Regulation of glucocorticoid receptor gamma (GRgamma) by glucocorticoid receptor haplotype and glucocorticoid. *Clin Endocrinol.* 2004;61:327.
301. Mingrone G, DeGaetano A, Pugeat M, et al. The steroid resistance of Crohn's disease. *J Invest Med.* 1999;47:319.
302. Pretorius E, Wallner B, Marx J. Cortisol resistance in conditions such as asthma and the involvement of 11beta-HSD-2: a hypothesis. *Horm Metab Res.* 2006;38:368.
303. Rask E, Olsson T, Soderberg S, et al. Tissue-specific dysregulation of cortisol metabolism in human obesity. *J Clin Endocrinol Metab.* 2001;86:1418.
304. Takahashi KI, Fukushima K, Sasano H, et al. Type II 11beta-hydroxysteroid dehydrogenase expression in human colonic epithelial cells of inflammatory bowel disease. *Dig Dis Sci.* 1999;44:2516.
306. Kino T, Gragerov A, Slobodskaya O, et al. Human immunodeficiency virus type 1 (HIV-1) accessory protein Vpr induces transcription of the HIV-1 and glucocorticoid-responsive promoters by binding directly to p300/CBP coactivators. *J Virol.* 2002;76:9724.
307. Mirani M, Elenkov I, Volpi S, et al. HIV-1 protein Vpr suppresses IL-12 production from human monocytes by enhancing glucocorticoid action: potential implications of Vpr coactivator activity for the innate and cellular immunity deficits observed in HIV-1 infection. *J Immunol.* 2002;169:6361.
309. New MI, Nimkarn S, Brandon DD, et al. Resistance to multiple steroids in two sisters. *J Steroid Biochem Mol Biol.* 2001;76:161.
310. Barnes PJ. How corticosteroids control inflammation: Quintiles Prize Lecture. 2005. *Br J Pharmacol.* 2006;148:245.
312. Borst P, Elferink RO. Mammalian ABC transporters in health and disease. *Annu Rev Biochem.* 2002;71:537.
314. Medh RD, Lay RH, Schmidt TJ. Agonist-specific modulation of glucocorticoid receptor-mediated transcription by immunosuppressants. *Mol Cell Endocrinol.* 1998;138:11.
315. Meijer OC, de Lange EC, Breimer DD, et al. Penetration of dexamethasone into brain glucocorticoid targets is enhanced in mdr1A P-glycoprotein knockout mice. *Endocrinology.* 1998;139:1789.
317. Webster JI, Carlstedt-Duke J. Involvement of multidrug resistance proteins (MDR) in the modulation of glucocorticoid response. *J Steroid Biochem Mol Biol.* 2002;82:277.
318. Farrell RJ, Murphy A, Long A, et al. High multidrug resistance (P-glycoprotein 170) expression in inflammatory bowel disease patients who fail medical therapy. *Gastroenterology.* 2000;118:279.
321. Hirano T, Onda K, Toma T, et al. MDR1 mRNA expressions in peripheral blood mononuclear cells of patients with ulcerative colitis in relation to glucocorticoid administration. *J Clin Pharmacol.* 2004;44:481.
322. Farrell RJ, Kelleher D. Glucocorticoid resistance in inflammatory bowel disease. *J Endocrinol.* 2003;178:339.
323. Llorente L, Richaud-Patin Y, Diaz-Borjon A, et al. Multidrug resistance-1 (MDR-1) in rheumatic autoimmune disorders. Part I: Increased P-glycoprotein activity in lymphocytes from rheumatoid arthritis patients might influence disease outcome. *Joint Bone Spine.* 2000;67:30.
324. Diaz-Borjon A, Richaud-Patin Y, Alvarado de la Barrera C, et al. Multidrug resistance-1 (MDR-1) in rheumatic autoimmune disorders. Part II: Increased P-glycoprotein activity in lymphocytes from systemic lupus erythematosus patients might affect steroid requirements for disease control. *Joint Bone Spine.* 2000;67:40.
325. Geick A, Eichelbaum M, Burk O. Nuclear receptor response elements mediate induction of intestinal MDR1 by rifampin. *J Biol Chem.* 2001;276:14581.
326. Kast HR, Goodwin B, Tarr PT, et al. Regulation of multidrug resistance-associated protein 2 (ABCC2) by the nuclear receptors pregnane X receptor, farnesoid X-activated receptor, and constitutive androstane receptor. *J Biol Chem.* 2002;277:2908.
327. Kauffmann HM, Pfannschmidt S, Zoller H, et al. Influence of redox-active compounds and PXR-activators on human MRP1 and MRP2 gene expression. *Toxicology.* 2002;171:137.
328. Johnson DR, Klaassen CD. Regulation of rat multidrug resistance protein 2 by classes of prototypical microsomal enzyme inducers that activate distinct transcription pathways. *Toxicol Sci.* 2002;67:182.
329. Moore LB, Parks DJ, Jones SA, et al. Orphan nuclear receptors constitutive androstane receptor and pregnane X receptor share xenobiotic and steroid ligands. *J Biol Chem.* 2000;275:15122.
330. Webster JI, Sternberg EM. Role of the hypothalamic-pituitary-adrenal axis, glucocorticoids and glucocorticoid receptors in toxic sequelae of exposure to bacterial and viral products. *J Endocrinol.* 2004;181:207.
332. Stith RD, McCallum RE. Down regulation of hepatic glucocorticoid receptors after endotoxin treatment. *Infect Immun.* 1983;40:613.
333. Li F, Xu RB. Changes in canine leukocyte glucocorticoid receptors during endotoxin shock. *Circ Shock.* 1988;26:99.
334. Vaptzarova KI, Baramova EN, Popov PG. Endotoxin inhibition of glucocorticoid enzyme induction and *in vivo* 3H-dexamethasone labelling of rat liver nuclei. *Int J Biochem.* 1989;21:701.
335. Jiayi D, Chen YZ. LPS-induced decrease of specific binding of 3H-dexamethasone to peritoneal macrophages of C57BL/6 mice. *J Recept Res.* 1992;12:451.
336. Verheggen MM, van Hal PT, Adriaansen-Soeting PW, et al. Modulation of glucocorticoid receptor expression in human bronchial epithelial cell lines by IL-1 beta, TNF-alpha and LPS. *Eur Respir J.* 1996;9:2036.

337. Gencay MM, Tamm M, Glanville A, et al. *Chlamydia pneumoniae* activates epithelial cell proliferation via NF-kappaB and the glucocorticoid receptor. *Infect Immun*. 2003;71:5814.
338. Hauk PJ, Hamid QA, Chrousos GP, et al. Induction of corticosteroid insensitivity in human PBMCs by microbial superantigens. *J Allergy Clin Immunol*. 2000;105:782.
340. Webster JI, Sternberg EM. Anthrax lethal toxin represses glucocorticoid receptor (GR) transactivation by inhibiting GR-DNA binding *in vivo*. *Mol Cell Endocrinol*. 2005;241:21.
341. Webster JI, Tonelli LH, Moayeri M, et al. Anthrax lethal factor represses glucocorticoid and progesterone receptor activity. *Proc Natl Acad Sci U S A*. 2003;100:5706.
342. Chen N, Baudino T, MacDonald PN, et al. Selective inhibition of nuclear steroid receptor function by a protein from a human tumorigenic poxvirus. *Virology*. 2000;274:17.
343. Ghoshal K, Majumder S, Zhu Q, et al. Influenza virus infection induces metallothionein gene expression in the mouse liver and lung by overlapping but distinct molecular mechanisms. *Mol Cell Biol*. 2001;21:8301.
344. Erlandsson AC, Bladh LG, Stierna P, et al. Herpes simplex virus type 1 infection and glucocorticoid treatment regulate viral yield, glucocorticoid receptor and NF-kappaB levels. *J Endocrinol*. 2002;175:165.
346. Sinclair AJ, Jacquemin MG, Brooks L, et al. Reduced signal transduction through glucocorticoid receptor in Burkitt's lymphoma cell lines. *Virology*. 1994;199:339.
347. Miller AH, Spencer RL, Pearce BD, et al. 1996 Curt P. Richter Award. Effects of viral infection on corticosterone secretion and glucocorticoid receptor binding in immune tissues. *Psychoneuroendocrinology*. 1997;22:455.

Chapter 33

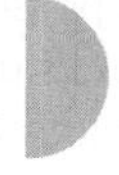

Complement

Cornelia Speth, Wolfgang M. Prodinger, Reinhard Würzner, Heribert Stoiber, and Manfred P. Dierich

OVERVIEW

Complement as a Functional System

Complement, with its more than 35 plasma or membrane proteins (Table 33.1), serves as an auxiliary system in immunity and antimicrobial defense. Its activation is due predominantly to a cascade of proteolytic steps, performed by serine protease domains in some of the components. Three different pathways of activation are distinguished (Figure 33.1), triggered by either target-bound antibody (the classical pathway), by microbial repetitive polysaccharide structures (the lectin pathway), or by recognition of other "foreign" surface structures (the alternative pathway). The alternative pathway also amplifies C3 activation triggered by the other pathways. All three merge in the pivotal activation of C3 and, subsequently, of C5 by highly specific enzymatic complexes, so-called convertases. In the common terminal pathway, downstream of C5 further complement components are activated in a nonproteolytic manner and assembled into the membrane attack complex (MAC). The entire powerful activation machinery is controlled redundantly by >10 negative regulators.

Complement can be activated by a variety of stimuli, such as immune complexes, appearance of apoptotic cells, presence of non–self-tissue (e.g., after transplantation) and microbial surface patterns directly (Figure 33.2). The broad spectrum of effector functions includes clearance of immune complexes or apoptotic cells, enhancement of inflammation (e.g., by the anaphylatoxins C3a and C5a), and cooperation with other host defense mechanisms as well as direct antimicrobial attack with subsequent opsonization and/or lysis.

Historical Roots

In the second half of the nineteenth century a first concept of complement emerged with the distinction of "alexin," a heat-labile fraction in normal serum that, in addition to antibody, is necessary for killing of bacteria. The term *complement* was introduced by Paul Ehrlich in 1899. In the 1950s, Louis Pillemer advanced the concept of complement, which at that time comprised primarily the classical pathway, by postulating an antibody-independent mechanism of activation (1) that is now referred to as the alternative pathway. As in archeological excavations, however, the oldest layer is often discovered last: The third and phylogenetically old lectin pathway was discovered a little more than 10 years ago and, despite recent cloning of several new components, remains incompletely understood.

Phylogenetic Aspects

It is difficult to define exactly when the complement system emerged in evolution, because the precise consensus definition of early precursor molecules may be ambiguous. At the preceding stage of complement evolution, between emergence of metazoa and emergence of deuterostomes, the individual domains used by mammalian complement components were created. Being absent from plants or yeast, primitive protostomes such as *Limulus* or the dipterans *Drosophila* and *Anopheles* possess proteins of the C3/α_2-macroglobulin superfamily of thioester proteins that are either homologues of α_2-macroglobulin (and thus unspecific protease inhibitors) or opsonins (and, as such, upregulated during infectious challenges). Between the emergence of deuterostomes and the emergence of jawed vertebrates, the unique combination of complex domain structure and proteolytic cleavage/activation sites in complement factors C3, C4, and C5 evolved, suggesting that basic functions of these complement components were established at this stage. The lectin and alternative pathways can be seen as descendants of a primordial surveillance system for microbes. At the modern stage, after emergence of jawed vertebrates and evolution of the adaptive immunity, the classical pathway was "added" and developed into a major effector mechanism for the powerful humoral immune system. This immunologic extension with the classical pathway involved gene duplication events with subsequent modification and functional divergence leading to pairs of related genes in the old (lectin or alternative) and new (classical) pathways, e.g., factor B and C2 (2).

Nomenclature

Classical and terminal pathway components were early designated C1 through C9. Notably, the (later-determined) activation sequence of the cascade is C1–C4–C2–C3–C5–C6–C7–C8–C9. Alternative pathway components are called *factors* and are distinguished by letters (factors B, D, H, I, P). Proteolytic activation of C2 through C5 produces smaller fragments and larger ones remaining in a complex required for the next activation step. The small, liberated fragments are denoted by the letter *a* (e.g., for C4, C4a), the larger ones by *b* (e.g., C4b), the notable exception being C2 (i.e., C2a is the large active fragment). Inactivation of C3b or C4b yields even smaller fragments (C4c, C4d, etc.). These must not be confused with the chains of C3 and C4 (e.g., C4α, C4β, C4γ) or isotypic proteins (e.g., C4A and C4B derived from two genetic C4 loci).

BIOSYNTHESIS OF COMPLEMENT: LOCATION AND REGULATION

The majority of plasma complement components are synthesized in the liver (3), which therefore represents the major site of complement protein synthesis. Exceptions are C1 (produced in the intestinal epithelium) and factor D (produced in adipose tissue). C7, of hepatic origin, was found to contribute less than 60% to plasma C7, with bone

TABLE 33.1 Complement Components

Component	Molecular Weight (in kDa) of Intact Protein (Subunits)	Plasma Concentration (μg/mL)	Chromosomal Assignment
Classical pathway			
C1q	460 (6 subunits each of 3 chains: A, 26; B, 26; C, 24)	150	1p34-1p36: 3 genes for A, B, C
C1r	85	50	12p13
C1s	85	50	12p13
C4	205 (α, 97; β, 75; γ, 33)	300–600	6p21: 2 loci (*C4A*, *C4B*), MHC-III region
C2	102	20	6p21: MHC-III region
C3	185 (α, 110; β, 75)	1,200–1,300	19p13
Alternative pathway:			
Factor B	93	200	6p21: MHC-III region
Factor D	24	2	19
Properdin	Oligomers of 110, 165, 200 (monomer: 55)	25	Xp11
Lectin pathway			
MBL	200–600, i.e., 2–6 subunits (1 subunit = 3 chains, each 32)	0.05–5	10q22
M-ficolin (ficolin-1)	Oligomer (monomer: 35)	n.d.	9q34: tail to tail with L-ficolin
L-ficolin (ficolin-2, ficolin/p35)	Oligomer: up to 320 (monomer: 35)	3	9q34: tail to tail with M-ficolin
H-ficolin (ficolin-3, Hakata antigen)	Oligomer: up to 650 (monomer: 34)	18	1p35.3
MASP-1	90	2–12	3q27-3q28: splice variant of MASP-1/3 gene
MASP-2	74	0.4	1p36: splice variant of MASP-2/sMAP gene
MASP-3	94	3	3q27-3q28: splice variant of MASP-1/3 gene
sMAP/MAp19	19	n.d.	1p36: splice variant of MASP-2/sMAP gene
Terminal pathway			
C5	190 (α,115; β, 75)	80	9q33
C6	110	45	5p14-5p12: MAC gene cluster
C7	100	90	5p14-5p12: MAC gene cluster
C8	150 (α, 64; β, 64; γ, 22)	55	1p22: genes for α, β 9q22-9q32: gene for γ
C9	70	60	5p14-5p12: MAC gene cluster
Control proteins (in plasma)			
Factor I	88	35	4q25
C1-INH	105	240	11q12-11q13
Factor H	150	300–450	1q32
FHL-1	42	5–20	1q32: splice variant of Factor H/ FHL-1 gene, *RCA* gene cluster
C4bp	550 (7 α chains each 70, 1 β-chain, 45)	250	1q32: *RCA* gene cluster
S protein (vitronectin)	84	500	17q11
Clusterin (SP-40,40)	70 (2 × 35)	50	8p21-8p12
Carboxypeptidase N	280 (2 × 83 and 2 × 50)	35	8p23-8p22: 83-kDa subunit 10: 50-kDa subunit
Membrane-bound complement control proteins			
CR1 (CD35)	190–280 (due to isoforms)	—	1q32: *RCA* gene cluster
DAF (CD55)	70	—	1q32: *RCA* gene cluster
MCP (CD46)	45–70 (due to glycosylation)	—	1q32: *RCA* gene cluster
CD59	18–20	—	11p13

(*continued*)

TABLE 33.1 Complement Components (Continued)

Component	Molecular Weight (in kDa) of Intact Protein (Subunits)	Plasma Concentration (μg/mL)	Chromosomal Assignment
Complement proteins with unclear function			
FHR-1	39 and 42 (due to glycosylation)	60	1q32: *RCA* gene cluster
FHR-2	24 and 29 (due to glycosylation)	40	1q32: *RCA* gene cluster
FHR-3	55	n.d.	1q32: *RCA* gene cluster
FHR-4A	86	n.d.	1q32: splice variant of FHR4 gene, *RCA* gene cluster
FHR4B	42	n.d.	1q32: splice variant of FHR4 gene, *RCA* gene cluster
FHR-5	80	5	1q22-1q23

MBL, mannan-binding lectin; MHC, major histocompatibility complex; MASP, MBL-associated serine protease; sMAP/MAp19, small MBL-associated protein or MBL-associated protein of 19 kDa; MAC, membrane attack complex; n.d., not determined; C1-INH, C1 inhibitor; RCA, regulator of complement activation; FHL, factor H like protein; C4bp, C4 binding protein; CR, complement receptor; DAF, decay-accelerating factor; MCP, membrane cofactor protein; FHR, factor H–related protein.

marrow–derived cells, in particular granulocytes, representing a major alternative source (4). The local contribution of C7 may exert an even stronger modulating effect than the concentration of complement inhibitors (5).

In addition to the liver, complement components are synthesized in many cell types, such as epithelial and endothelial cells, lymphocytes, and in reproductive organs. Recently, synthesis of complement components has been demonstrated in the retina (6). Notably, production of virtually all components has been observed not only in monocytes/macrophages, but also in dendritic cells (7) and astrocytes (8). Extrahepatic complement production appears to be important: Like astrocytes or other glial cells, it is the only source for complement behind an intact blood–brain barrier. At sites of infection, effective upregulation of local complement synthesis may contribute to host defense (9). Local complement production also plays a somewhat neglected role in transplantation, promoting allograft rejection (10).

The production of plasma complement components is augmented in the acute-phase response. The main common transcriptional inducer of complement genes is IFN-γ, others being IL-1- and IL-6–type cytokines (i.e., IL-1α, IL-1β, IL-6, IL-11, and others) (11). Cell surface–bound complement regulators are expressed on a variety of tissues (3).

COMPLEMENT COMPONENTS: A NETWORK OF PROTEIN FAMILIES

Complement C3/α_2-Macroglobulin Superfamily

C3, C4, and C5 (Figures 33.1, 33.3) are derived from one ancestral protein that supposedly has served as a multispecific protease inhibitor. Detailed structural insights of C3 have been provided recently (12). A pivotal feature is an internal thioester formed during biosynthesis in C3, C4, and α_2-macroglobulin, which allows the activation-dependent formation of covalent bonds. This thioester is formed between a cysteine and a glutamine residue three positions apart (Figure 33.3) (13). In C5, no thioester is formed. C3, C4, and C5 are activated by proteolytic cleavage at a conserved peptide bond that induces a gross conformational change and new epitopes being exposed, e.g., the then-protected thioester in C3 or C4. This leads to the formation of a reactive intermediate that enables the glutamyl residue to form a covalent ester or amide bond with water or with NH_2 or OH residues of surrounding molecules. C3 and the C4B isotype of C4 possess a histidine positioned in close proximity to the thioester, which acts as the catalyst for the formation of ester bonds. In contrast, the C4A isotype lacks this histidine and preferentially forms amide bonds (14).

Proteins with Short Consensus Repeat Units

Short consensus repeats (SCRs) or, synonymously, complement control proteins (CCP) modules, are individually folding domains of about 60 amino acids displaying a β-barrel structure (15) and distinct conserved residues, e.g., tryptophane, prolines and—most important—four cysteines, which form two disulfide bonds (Cys_1 to Cys_3 and Cys_2 to Cys_4) (16). Although SCRs can be found in various noncomplement proteins (e.g., in the selectins), proteins that consist predominantly of SCRs are encoded by genes in the *R*egulator of *C*omplement *A*ctivation (*RCA*) gene cluster. The *RCA* comprises the genes for factor H and the factor H-family proteins, for C4bp, DAF, CR2, CR1, and MCP (17). The number of SCRs in these proteins ranges from 4 to 34, and some proteins possess

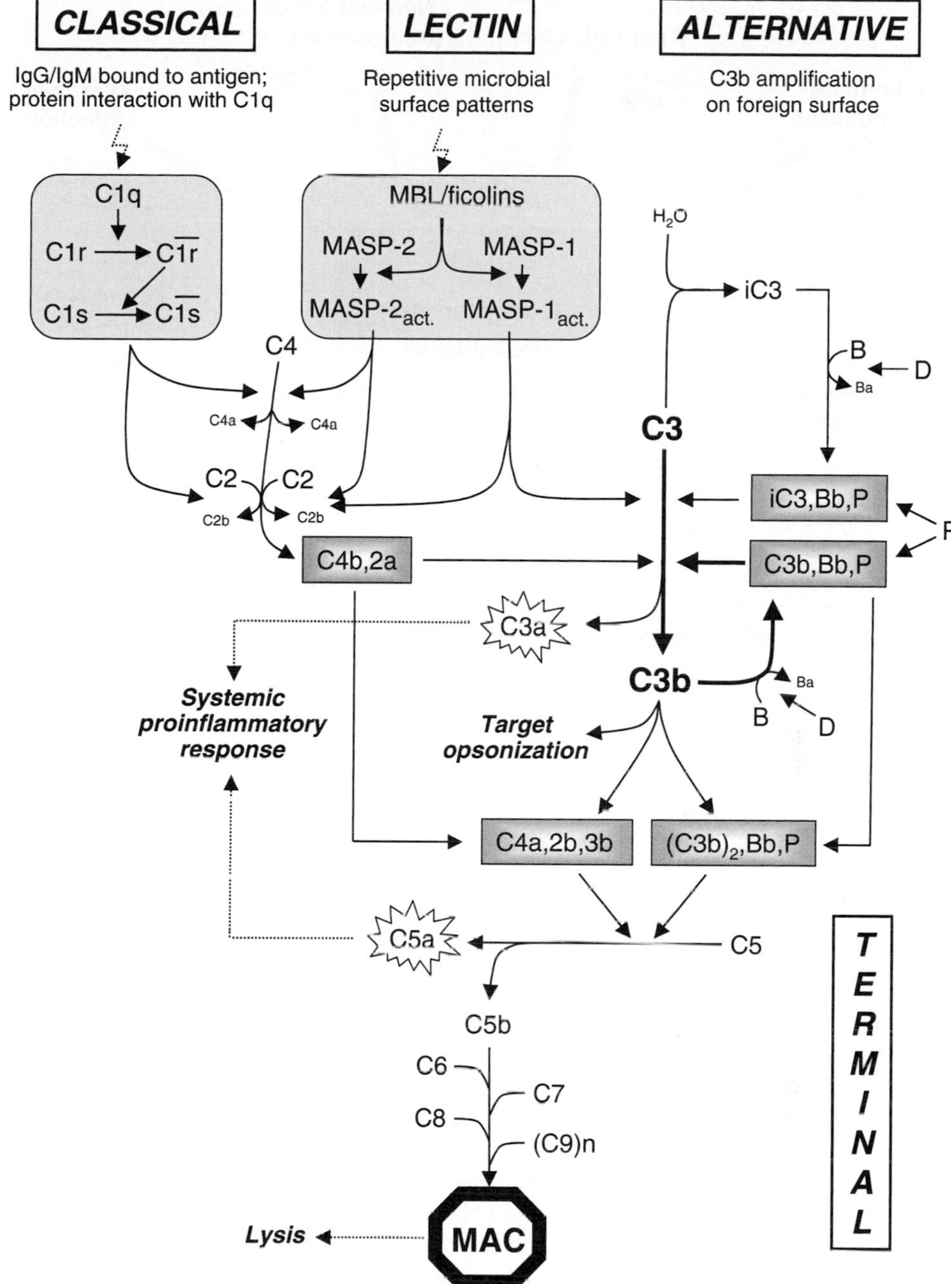

FIGURE 33.1 Overview of complement activation pathways (detailed explanation in the text). The C3 and C5 convertases of the pathways are boxed. The alternative-pathway amplification loop of C3b generation is indicated by bold line arrows. Note the systemic action of the anaphylatoxins in contrast to the effect of opsonization or lysis via membrane-attack complex, which occur on the target surface.

transmembrane and short intracytoplasmic parts (CR1, CR2, MCP) or glycosylphosphatidylinositol (GPI) anchors (DAF, CD59). RCA proteins are elongated in shape: e.g., CR1 extends 90 nm from the cell membrane.

The *RCA* is thought to have evolved from one ancestral prototypic SCR by duplication and gene conversion events as a family of genes for proteins controlling C3 and C4 activation. Nevertheless, the binding of activated C3 or C4 can be attributed to distinct, often adjacent, SCRs in each member. Few SCRs are present in mosaic proteins like factor B, C2, the members of the MASP-like family (C1r, C1s, MASP-1, MASP-2, MASP-3), C6, and C7, all of which interact with thioester proteins.

Proteins with a Serine Protease Module

Proteins with serine protease activity are crucially involved in the early, amplifying steps of complement activation. Serine protease domains are present in the two homologous proteins C2 and factor B, and, furthermore, in factor I, factor D, and in the members of the MASP-like family. The latter proteins contain a serine protease domain

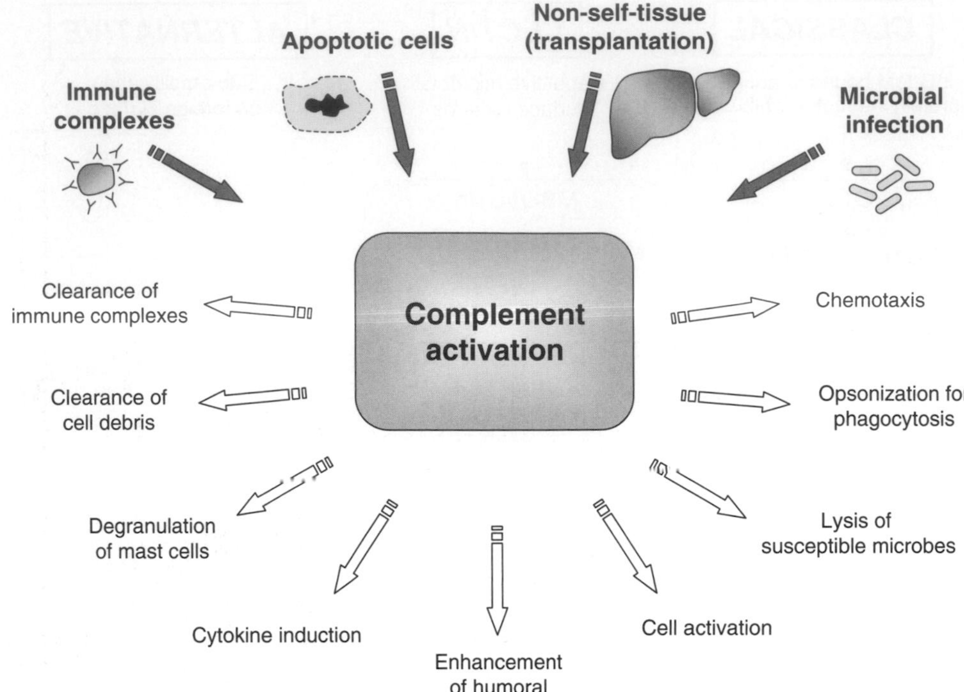

FIGURE 33.2 Overview: Induction of complement activation and effector functions.

together with two CUB domains,[1] an epidermal growth factor–like (EGF-like) domain, and two SCRs.

Protein Motifs Found in Terminal Pathway Components

C6 through C9 have an amphiphilic character that allows them to act in plasma and on lipid membranes, an important feature for MAC formation. As true mosaic proteins, they assemble a variety of modules in a characteristic sequence: thrombospondin type 1 repeats (TSRs), also found in the extracellular matrix protein thrombospondin and in properdin; a low-density lipoprotein receptor (LDLR) domain; a conserved cysteine-poor region (18) also found in perforin; an EGF module; SCRs; and factor I modules (FIMs). Functional activity is preserved even in the absence of the latter, at least for C6 (19).

ACTIVATION OF C3: THE CRUCIAL STEP

The three aforementioned pathways lead to activation of C3 (Figure 33.1). The physiologically relevant activators of C3 are the C3 convertases, although proteases such as plasmin can activate C3 *in vitro*. Four distinct protein entities act on C3 or C3b:

1. *The C3- convertases.* C3b,Bb and C4b,2a consist of proteins with an activated serine protease domain in complex with C3b and C4b, respectively; each cleaves C3 into C3a and C3b.
2. *Factor I.* A plasma serine protease specific only for C3b and C4b, factor I inactivates C3b and C4b by cleaving them into iC3b and iC4b, respectively. Factor I requires a cofactor.
3. *RCA family proteins composed of SCRs.* These negatively regulate C3 and C4 activation by disintegrating the C3 convertases and serving as cofactors for factor I.
4. *The receptors for fragments of C3.* this heterogeneous group comprises integrins, seven-transmembrane receptors, and RCA-family members: They use C3-activation products to mediate induction of phagocytosis or chemotaxis.

The native C3 molecule becomes cleaved at a conserved arginine residue in the α chain into C3a and C3b. The peptide C3a (77 amino acids) is a potent anaphylatoxin. The large "nascent" C3b has a half-life of 60 microseconds, during which it changes its conformation, exposes the internal thioester bond, and binds through the now highly reactive thioester to nearby nucleophils, e.g., OH groups of any surrounding molecule, including H_2O.

ACTIVATION VIA THE CLASSICAL PATHWAY

C1, C4, C2, and C3 (in this order) represent the activation cascade of the classical pathway. C1-INH, C4bp, CR1,

[1] CUB domains are widespread protein modules and are found (among others) in complement C1r/C1s, sea urchin EGF (Uegf), and bone morphogenetic protein-1.

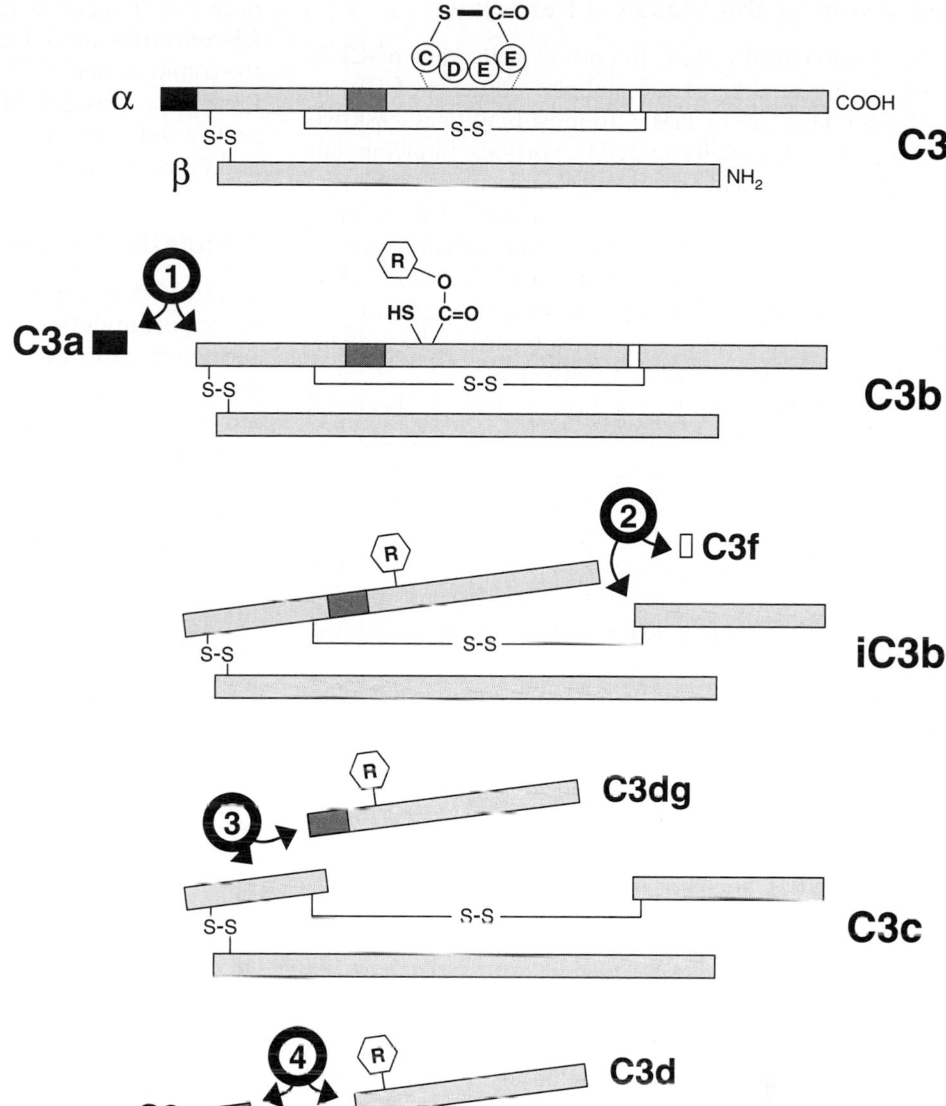

FIGURE 33.3 Activation and inactivation of C3. The thioester bond (bold line) formed between Cys and Glu is shown for native C3 (amino acids of the thioester region are in circles). (*1*) Activation of native C3 by C3-convertases yields C3a and C3b bound to an acceptor R (here via ester linkage). (*2*) C3b inactivation by factor I and a cofactor. (*3*) iC3b is further degraded by factor I and CR1. (*4*) Acceptor-bound C3dg is trimmed by unspecific plasma proteases to C3d.

factor I, DAF, and MCP function as control proteins. C1 consists of one C1q molecule bound noncovalently to two C1r and two C1s molecules (Figure 33.4). Calcium ions are required for formation of the stable C1 complex. About 70% of the C1 components in plasma are present in C1 complexes at a given time. One C1q protein is assembled from six identical subunits. In turn, each subunit consists of three homologous chains (A, B, and C) that form a globular domain at the C terminus, followed by the "neck" and a coiled coil in the "stalk." The six subunits are held together by the collagenous stalk parts (a "bunch of six tulips" appearance under the electron microscope). The stalks also interact with the $C1r_2C1s_2$ tetramer assembled in a linear chain (20). Each C1s and C1r possesses a serine protease domain (catalytic domain) and a contact domain. Before activation, all four catalytic domains remain inside the cone-shaped stalk of C1q (21) (Figure 33.4).

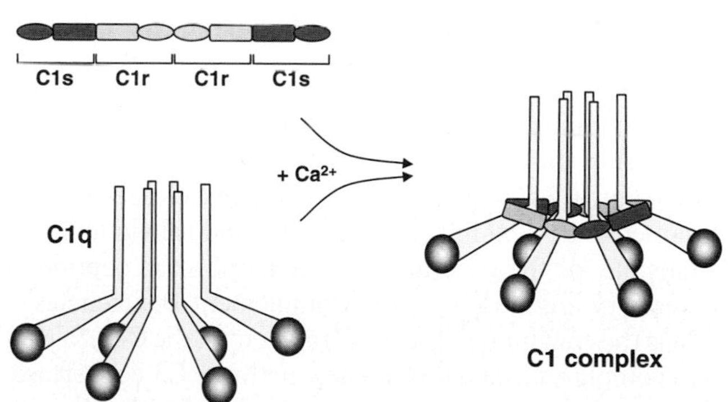

FIGURE 33.4 Assembly of the C1 complex. The model for the C1 complex proposes that the folding of the rodlike $C1r_2$-$C1s_2$ tetramer around the arms of C1q causes the catalytic domains of C1s to contact the catalytic domains of C1r. Inactivation of C1 occurs by covalent binding of C1r and C1s to C1 inhibitor.

Initiation of the Classical Pathway

The physiologically most important activation of C1 is initiated by binding of the globular domains of C1q to antigen-bound IgG or IgM. C1q must bind to at least two of the conformationally altered Fc portions, implying that one single IgM, but at least two IgG molecules in sufficient proximity (i.e., <40 nm apart) are required. This restricts C1 activation by IgG to substrates with a critical density of bound antibody. The C1q-binding potential of human IgG subclasses is highest with IgG3 (followed by IgG1, IgG2, and IgG4), which is important with regard to the humanization of murine monoclonal antibodies.[2]

Other triggers of C1 activation include bacterial lipopolysaccharide, polyanionic compounds, myelin, C-reactive protein (CRP), and viral envelopes (e.g., of HIV-1). C1q binding followed by classical pathway activation also plays a role in the clearance of apoptotic cells through phagocytosis by macrophages (22). This mechanism may explain the strong association of systemic lupus erythematosus with complete deficiencies of classical pathway components, especially C1q (23).

The binding of C1q to its substrate induces a conformational change in C1q and subsequently a change in position of the two C1r serine esterase domains relative to each other. This allows for reciprocal cleavage of the C1r molecules. Such activated C1r in turn cleaves and activates C1s, which is the enzyme to activate C4 and C2. Cleavage of C1r and C1s does not liberate proteolytic fragments. Altogether, one active C1 molecule can produce about 35 C4b molecules, as a result of its low K_m value and the high plasma concentration of C4 (24).

C4 is cleaved into the small C4a and the large C4b fragment (termed nascent C4b), which undergoes a gross conformational change. The internal thioester in C4b becomes exposed and able to form covalent bonds with surrounding molecules. These reactions take place within microseconds (13), and most nascent C4b are "lost" by reacting with water. About 5% of the C4b become covalently attached to the surface, clustered around the activating Ig–C1 complex.

C2 activation proceeds more slowly than C4 activation, because of the lower plasma concentration of C2 (25). C2 forms a complex with C4b in a Mg^{2+}-dependent manner and within this complex becomes accessible for cleavage by C1s into C2a (*larger* fragment) and C2b (released *smaller* fragment). C2b exhibits kinin activity and is held to be responsible for the generation of the pathogenic peptide in hereditary angioedema (see "Complement Deficiencies"). C2a is the enzymatically active fragment in the C4b,2a protein complex, termed the classical pathway C3-convertase. C2a is active only as long as it is associated with C4b and, once it is dissociated, cannot bind to C4b again. With the C3-convertase formation, the classical pathway leads into the common step of C3 activation (see below). Recently, a C1r-like protease (C1r-LP) has been identified that represents a different way to generate a classical-pathway C3- and C5-convertase (26).

[2] Some mouse IgG subclasses (e.g., IgG2a, but not IgG1) can also activate human complement that is exploited for selective *in vitro* killing of human cells by monoclonal antibodies.

Regulation of the Classical Pathway

C1s and C1r are tightly controlled by C1-INH, a member of the *serpin* family (*ser*ine *p*rotease *in*hibitors) and inactivate serine proteases by a suicide substrate mechanism, i.e., forming a covalent bond with the active serine of the substrate protease domain. C1-INH is already associated with native C1, which tends toward autoactivation. Activated C1r and C1s are rapidly bound by C1-INH in a stoichiometric relation, yielding two C1rC1s(C1-INH)$_2$ molecules per C1. Notably, C1-INH, unlike other complement inhibitors, is not abundant in plasma. It may become a limiting factor, e.g., in septic shock, where extensive complement activation control is required. Inhibitors downstream of C1 are C4bp, DAF, and CR1 (Table 33.2). C4b,2a disassembles spontaneously, but its decay is accelerated by CR1 or DAF, and C4b is inactivated through factor I (Table 33.2).

ACTIVATION VIA THE LECTIN PATHWAY

The concept of the lectin pathway of complement activation has emerged relatively recently and therefore not all details are yet fully understood. Its main constituent is the plasma protein mannan-binding lectin or mannose-binding lectin, MBL (27). MBL is a member of the *collectins,* proteins with *coll*agenlike stalk parts and *lectin* domains (28). It is made up of subunits that consist of three polypeptide chains, each with an N-terminal cross-linking region followed by a collagenlike region, a neck par,t and a globular carbohydrate recognition domain (CRD). The three collagenous parts form a coiled-coil structure, and this subunit structure is stabilized by interchain disulfide bonds and hydrophobic interactions. Two to six subunits (i.e., 6 to 18 CRDs), held together by disulfide bonds in the crosslinking region, form an MBL oligomer with a multipronged appearance. Plasma MBL is a mixture of these oligomers, but the complement-activating potential is associated only with the higher oligomeric forms in which multiple CRDs facilitate multivalent ligand binding. The two major MBL forms present in human serum are MBL-I and MBL-II, which contain 9 and 12 disulfide-linked chains, respectively, and therefore are trimers and tetramers of the structural unit (27).

The broad variation of MBL plasma levels among presumably normal individuals (up to 1,000-fold) is largely influenced by the alleles of the *MBL* gene. Different point mutations in exon 1 result in altered collagenous domains

TABLE 33.2 Mode of Action of Complement Control Proteins

Regulator	Site of Action	Mode of Action			
Early activation steps, anaphylatoxins					
C1-INH	Plasma	Covalent binding to active C1s, C1r, MASPs			
Carboxypeptidase N	Plasma	Cleavage of carboxy-terminal arginine from C3a, C5a			
Convertases					
		Decay Acceleration of		**Cofactor for Cleavage of**	
		C3b,Bb	*C4b,2a*	*C3b*	*C4b*
Factor H	Plasma, nonactivator surface	+	−/+[a]	+	−
C4bp	Plasma	−	+	−	+
CR1 (CD35)	(Homologous) cell membrane[b]	+	+	+	+
MCP (CD46)	(Homologous) cell membrane[b]	−	−	+	+
DAF (CD55)	(Homologous) cell membrane[b]	+	+	−	−
Terminal pathway					
S protein; clusterin	Plasma	Binding to soluble C5b-7, blocking of integration into membranes			
CD59	(Homologous) cell membrane[b]	Inhibition of binding and polymerization of C9			

[a]Decays acceleration of classical pathway C5 convertase, but not of classical pathway C3 convertase.

[b]CR1 has a narrow tissue distribution, in contrast to DAF, MCP, and CD59.

and, as a consequence, interfere with the formation of high-order oligomers. This impairment of polymerization for the three variant *MBL* alleles (B, C, D variants) is associated with low MBL plasma levels compared to the wild type *MBL* allele (termed A variant) (28). Additionally, promoter polymorphisms influence MBL plasma levels. Nevertheless, there is still considerable variation in MBL plasma levels even among individuals with the same genotype.

Many studies underline that MBL plasma levels and allotypes influence the predisposition to infections (29). MBL-deficiency is not considered a major risk factor, but may coexist with other common deficiencies in the immune system. A population-based prospective study showed twice as many acute respiratory infections in infants with MBL deficiency, although that risk is largely confined to a "window of vulnerability" at the age of 6 to 18 months, when maternal antibodies disappear (30). On the other hand, a positive correlation between the presence of low-producer MBL alleles and a low incidence of both HIV infection and active tuberculosis has been discussed (31).

MBL in plasma is found in complexes with the proenzymes *MBL-a*ssociated *s*erine *p*roteases, MASP-1, MASP-2, and MASP-3 (Table 33.1). A large proportion of the MASPs in circulation, however, are not complexed with MBL. MBL can also form complexes with MAp19 or sMAP (small MBL-associated protein), a truncated version of MASP-2 without serine protease domain that is generated by alternative splicing. The role of the nonenzymatic sMAP is not clear.

In addition to MBL, the ficolins also form aggregates with MASPs. *Ficolins* are lectins with a *fi*brinogenlike and a *col*lagenlike domain. Three types of ficolins have been identified in humans, L-ficolin, H-ficolin, and M-ficolin. The two serum lectins L-ficolin and H-ficolin associate with MASPs, and both activate the lectin pathway (32). Recent reports describe similar results for M-ficolin, which is detected on the surface of monocytes, but also in secretory granules of neutrophils, monocytes, and lung epithelial cells. Forming complexes with MASP-1 and MASP-2, it functions as a pattern-recognition molecule and activates complement (33).

Initiation of the Lectin Pathway

The CRDs of MBL function as C-type lectins, as they recognize a range of carbohydrates such as D-mannose, N-acetyl-glucosamine, N-acetyl-mannosamine, glucose, and L-fucose. The affinity of a single CRD to these ligands is low ($K_d = 10^{-3}$M), so multiple CRDs have to interact for avid binding, which is best achieved with repetitive carbohydrate structures found as common constituents of bacterial, viral, fungal, and parasitic surfaces. MBL is also involved in the recognition of self-targets, such as apoptotic and necrotic cells, thus being a prototypic pattern-recognition molecule of the innate immune system (34).

Carbohydrate binding is also performed by ficolins via their fibrinogenlike domains. The sugar specificity is still unclear but might include N-acetyl-glucosamine for L-ficolin and N-acetyl-glucosamine, N-acetyl-galactosamine and fucose for H-ficolin (35), and acetyl groups for M-ficolin (36). Similar to MBL, H-ficolin and L-ficolin also recognize apoptotic cells and subsequently activate complement.

Upon ligand binding by CRD (MBL) or fibrinogenlike domains (ficolins), MASPs are auto-activated from a single-chain zymogen precursor by proteolytic cleavage

(37). Activated MASP-2 seems to be the main mediator of complement activation because it cleaves and activates the complement proteins C2 and C4, thereby generating the C3 convertase C4b,2a in a C1-independent manner (38). MASP-1 cleaves C2 almost as efficiently as MASP-2 does, but it does not cleave C4 (39). In addition, MASP-1 cleaves C3, although much less efficiently than the convertases, and this mechanism has been hypothesized to provide an initial source for amplification of surface-deposited C3b by alternative pathway activation (27). Compared to MASP-1 and MASP-2, MASP-3 has distinct substrate specificity and inhibitor profile, and its role in complement activation is unclear (40).

Regulation of the Lectin Pathway

Control of the lectin pathway seems to be exerted mainly through covalent binding of C1-INH to active MASPs and to be very similar to control of the classical pathway in general, although the different effects of synthetic inhibitors suggest that differences do exist (41). Furthermore, altered mammalian cell membranes can trigger lectin pathway activation via MBL in situations such as ischemia followed by reoxygenation (42). Complement activation does not appear to be the only contribution of MBL to host defense. An MBL receptor or collectin receptor has long been postulated, but not identified unequivocally. An MBL receptor is thought to mediate a C3b-independent opsonic effect on phagocytes that may also attribute a new role to the noncomplement-activating forms of MBL.

ACTIVATION VIA THE ALTERNATIVE PATHWAY

Alternative pathway activation requires C3 and C3b, factors B, D, and properdin. Alternative pathway activation is a positive feedback mechanism to augment C3b generation (C3b-amplification loop). The starting C3b is generated through either of the other two pathways. The alternative pathway may also be triggered directly via iC3.

The C3b-Amplification Loop

Whether a given structure (e.g., a cell membrane, viral envelope, bacterial polymer) will allow alternative pathway activation depends on the affinity of factor H for C3b deposited on that structure and on the presence of other regulators (Figures 33.5, 33.6). Surface structures that allow alternative pathway activation are called activator

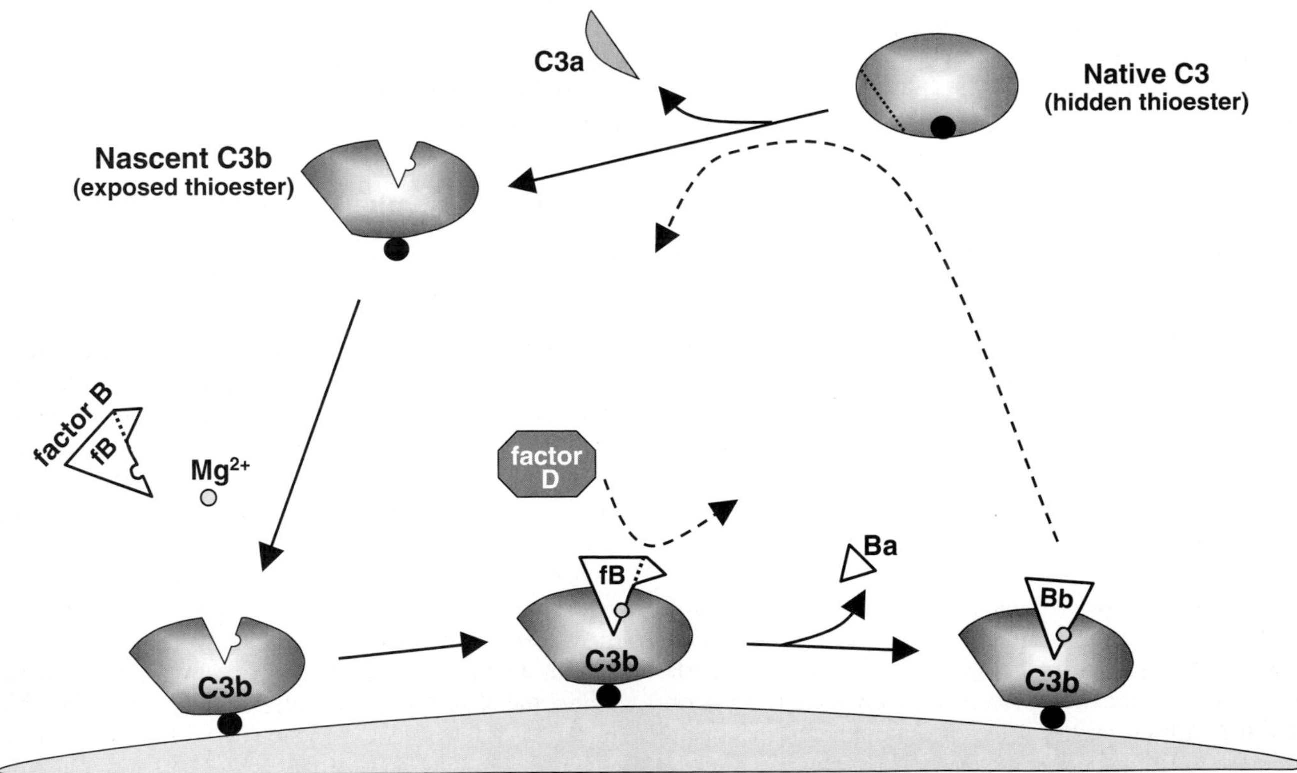

FIGURE 33.5 Generation of the alternative-pathway C3 convertase. Upon cleavage of C3 to C3b, the reactive thioester (full black circle) is exposed and forms covalent bonds to activator surface molecules. C3b associates with factor B in the presence of Mg^{2+}, which is then cleaved by factor D. Bb bound to C3b is the proteolytically active part of the convertase C3b,Bb. Dashed-lined arrows represent enzymatic action, dotted lines within molecules indicate cleavage sites for enzymes.

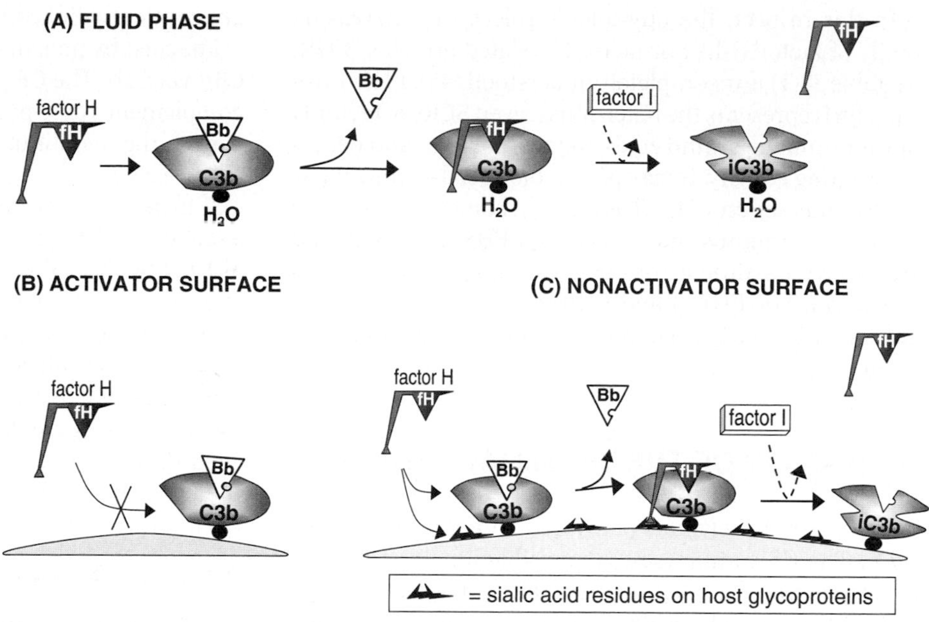

FIGURE 33.6 Control of C3b amplification by factor H depends on its binding affinity to the respective C3b target. **Upper part:** In the fluid phase, C3b,Bb is rapidly disassembled through factor H binding. C3b cleavage through factor I generates iC3b, which has no complement-activating potential. **Lower part:** Factor H binding to C3b is low on activator surfaces such as microbial cell walls, and C3b,Bb remains active. On nonactivator surfaces, e.g., host cells with sialic acid residues, factor H has a higher affinity to C3b, and binding is followed by convertase dissociation and C3b inactivation.

surfaces, whereas those that effectively limit activation are termed nonactivators. When a first C3b molecule becomes covalently attached to an activator surface, factor B subsequently associates with this C3b in the presence of Mg^{2+}. In this complex, the zymogen factor B is accessible to cleavage by factor D, a serine protease present in plasma in minute amounts. Factor D is brought into its active conformation through recognition of its substrates, C3b,B or iC3,B, and returns to its "inactive" state after the cleaved Ba fragment is released from B (43). The enzymatically active Bb fragment remains attached to C3b, forming the C3 convertase of the alternative pathway, C3b,Bb (Figure 33.5). Surface-attached C3b,Bb activates further C3 molecules, and more nascent C3b will attach to the same surface. C3b,Bb remains active as long as Bb remains bound to C3b (half-life 90 seconds). Properdin stabilizes the convertase against decay. A microbe may thus rapidly become covered with C3b, which is slowly (i.e., relatively inefficiently compared to C3b on nonactivators) turned into iC3b. Recently, it has been postulated that rapid alternative pathway activation is facilitated by binding properdin first, followed by C3b attachment (44).

Initiation of the Alternative Pathway via iC3

A long-standing conceptual problem was to explain the generation of the initial C3b and thus whether the alternative pathway can be triggered on its own. The concept of "C3 tickover" provided such an explanation (25). Plasma C3 is constantly transformed at a low rate into inactive C3 (iC3 or "C3b-like" C3) through spontaneous reaction of the C3 internal thioester bond with H_2O. iC3 can be described as uncleaved C3 in a C3b-like conformation and accounts for 0.5% of total plasma C3. Like C3b, iC3 can associate with factor B in a Mg^{2+}-dependent reaction, thus forming iC3,Bb. It is thought that this initial C3 convertase of the alternative pathway is formed constantly but is rapidly inactivated in plasma. Nevertheless, by this mechanism nascent C3b molecules randomly attach onto nearby microbes and trigger the amplification loop.

The concept of C3 tickover preceded the discovery of the MBL pathway. The targeted generation of C3b via MBL/MASP-1 provides an alternative explanation of initial C3b generation. Even to date, the relative contributions of both mechanisms are not fully understood.

Inactivation and Degradation of C3b and Regulation of the Alternative Pathway

Because of its self-amplifying capacity, C3b circulating in plasma is subject to tight control (Table 33.2). The spontaneous decay of C3-convertases (approximate half-life, 2 minutes) is accelerated by CR1, factor H, or DAF, an activity termed decay acceleration. Considerable redundancy in control proteins exists for these steps, although CR1 can actually substitute for all other regulatory RCA proteins in this respect. Cleavage of C3b and thus its inactivation relies on factor I and its cofactors. Becaue of the high plasma concentration of factor H, virtually all C3b or iC3 present in plasma will quickly bind to H. The low K_m of factor I for C3b,H permits efficient cleavage of C3b into iC3b, which is then split into the biologically inert C3c and the smaller C3dg fragment that remains bound to the target (see Figure 33.3). Thus, C3b degradation eliminates the complement-activating C3b, but produces fragments with other biologic functions. Notably, control proteins of other species normally have no effect on human complement components.

In this respect, the physiologic role of the increasing family of factor H-like or factor H–related proteins (FHR; see Table 33.1) is incompletely understood (45). FHL-1 (reconectin) represents the N-terminal seven SCRs of factor H plus four unique amino acids and has cofactor and decay-accelerating activity. It may play a role in cell–extracellular matrix interaction. All FHRs share homology with the factor-H C terminus that binds C3b. FHR-1, FHR-2, and FHR-4 are constituents of lipoproteins, and FHR-3 binds to heparin. For FHR-3 and FHR-4, interaction with C3b and thus a potential role in C3b regulation has been proposed (45).

ACTIVATION OF THE TERMINAL PATHWAY

Activation of the terminal pathway is initiated by cleavage of C5. The C5 convertases, responsible for this cleavage, are composed of a C3 convertase with an additional C3b molecule deposited covalently in the immediate vicinity: C3b,Bb,C3b or C4b,2a,3b. The (second) C3b acts like an anvil for C5: It interacts with C5 and presents C5 in the correct conformation for cleavage by the C2a or Bb enzyme. Cleavage of C5 in the α chain generates the 11-kDs C5a peptide, whereas C5b starts the membrane-attack-complex formation. It should be noted that the classical C3 convertase together with another C4b was shown to cleave C5 directly to some extent (46). However, C5 may be activated directly by different enzymes (47), in particular thrombin (48).

After cleavage of C5, the terminal complement components C6, C7, C8, and C9 are sequentially, but nonenzymatically, activated, resulting in the formation of the terminal complement complex, TCC (49). On a cellular target membrane, TCC can be generated as the potentially membranolytic membrane attack complex (MAC), or in extracellular fluids as nonlytic SC5b-9 in the presence of S protein (vitronectin). Both forms consist of C5b and the complement proteins C6, C7, C8, and C9. After cleavage of C5, C5b undergoes conformational changes and exposes a binding site for C6. The ability of C5b, staying near the C5 convertase on the target surface, to bind C6 decays rapidly, but once it is bound, C5b6 forms a stable bimolecular complex. C5b6 binds C7, resulting in the exposure of membrane-binding sites and incorporation into target membranes. If C7 concentrations near the site of complement activation are limiting, the stable bimolecular C5b6 complex dissociates from the C5-activating complex and accumulates in solution. In the presence of C7 fluid phase C5b-7 is formed that will not necessarily stay soluble, as it has a transient ability to attach to membranes, bind C8 and C9, and initiate lysis, a process called *reactive lysis* (50). Both the membrane-bound C5b-7 complex as well as the fluid-phase C5b-7 complex can bind C8. C8 consists of three nonidentical polypeptide chains: the α and γ chains are covalently linked by a disulfide bond, and the β chain is attached by noncovalent forces. Nascent C5b-7 binds to C8β via C5b. The C8 γ chain has no apparent function in complement lysis, probably because it does not lie adjacent to the membrane but faces the extracellular plasma (Figure 33.7).

Efficient lysis is dependent on an interaction of the C8 α-moiety with C9, although some lytic activity is expressed already by the C5b-8 complex alone. C5b-8 acts as a polymerizing agent for C9. The first C9 bound to C5b-8 undergoes major structural changes enabling formation of an elongated molecule and allows binding of further C9 molecules and insertion of C9 cylinders into the target membrane (Figure 33.7). Whereas only one molecule of each C5b, C6, C7, and C8 is involved in TCC formation, the number of C9 molecules varies from one to three in the fluid phase and from one to 12 in the membrane-bound form, although polymers containing up to 15 C9 molecules are also possible.

Two mutually nonexclusive hypotheses have been proposed to explain the precise mechanism of terminal complement-mediated cytotoxicity after insertion of C9. According to one model, the polar domains of inserted complement proteins, particularly C9, cause local distortion of the phospholipid bilayer, resulting in "leaky patches" (51). The other theory postulates that the terminal complement proteins form a hydrophilic channel ("pore") through the membrane, with consequent disruption of the cell (52).

Regulation of the Terminal Pathway

Control is executed before the integration of the assembling MAC into the membrane and at the stage of pore formation, i.e., association of C8 and polymerization of C9 (Table 33.2) A number of different membrane and plasma molecules are involved in modulating TCC assembly, of which C8 is probably the most important. It represents not only an essential component of the lytic complex but, paradoxically, also prevents membrane damage by binding to the nascent C5b-7 complex in the fluid phase, thereby precluding its firm insertion into the membrane (53).

Not only C8 but also the abundant S protein, clusterin, lipoproteins, antithrombin III, proteoglycans such as heparin, and protamine are able to bind to nascent C5b-7 and to prevent its membrane insertion. The final step of MAC assembly, subsequent to C5b-7 insertion, when the MAC becomes more firmly inserted into the lipid bilayer, is safeguarded by a well-characterized 18- to 20-kDa glycolipid-anchored membrane molecule (CD59), which protects against complement-mediated lysis by interfering with polymerization of C9.

Membrane perforation by complement is not a unique feature. Damage to mammalian cells by proteins that destroy target membranes can be also caused by perforin,

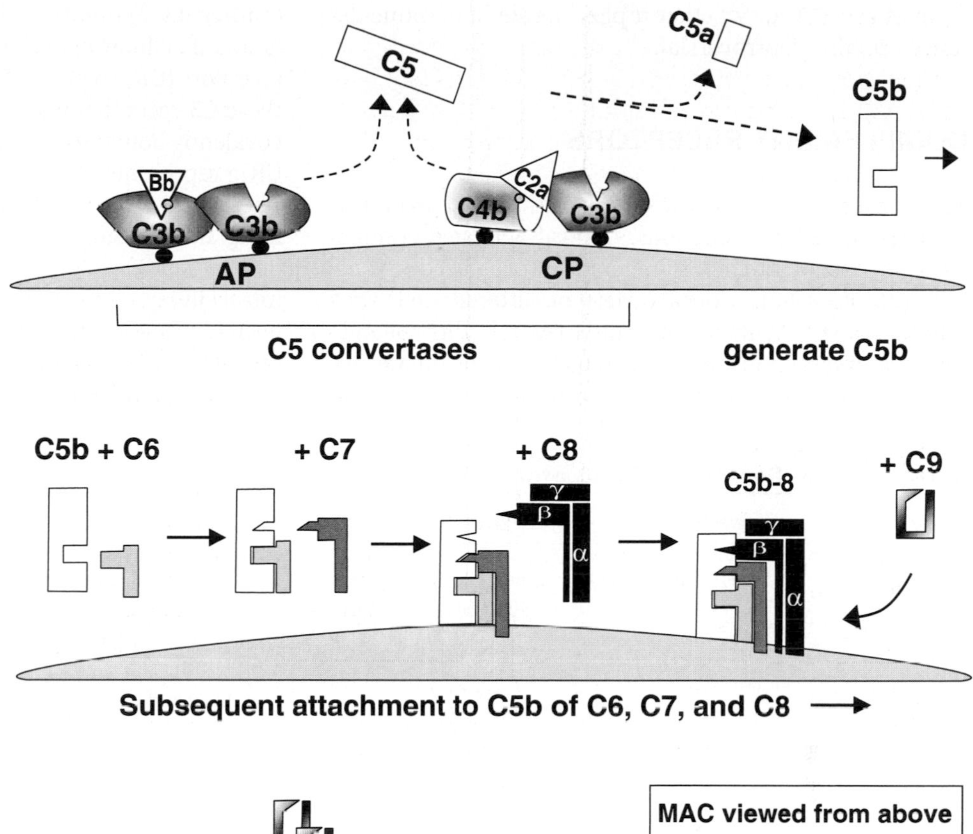

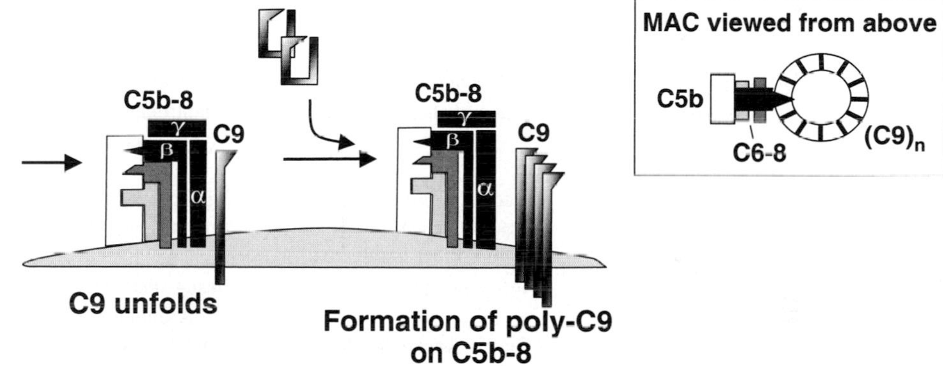

FIGURE 33.7 Activation of C5 and terminal complement pathway. C5 is activated by C5 convertases of the classical (CP) or alternative (AP) pathway. Nascent C5b interacts sequentially with C6, C7, and C8, and attaches to lipid membranes. C9 polymerization on C5b-8 completes the membrane attack complex (MAC).

which is contained in the cytoplasmic granules of cytotoxic T lymphocytes and natural killer cells (see Chapters 16 and 34) and actually shows a strong homology with C9 (54).

Biologic Properties of the Terminal Complement Complex

The MAC deposited on cells may either exert lytic properties that are important in host defense (see "Complement Defense against Infection") or may induce so-called sublytic effects on nucleated cells that are not unequivocally identified as "non-self" (55). The term *sublytic* refers to the fact that nucleated cells can withstand single (and erroneous) attacks, unlike erythrocytes. Furthermore, previous sublytic effects may even protect these cells from further, otherwise lytic effects, favoring the host cells that are constantly in contact with complement (56). Sublytic attack also stimulates protein synthesis and arachidonic acid metabolism and activates attacked polymorphonuclear leukocytes. In particular, sublytic TCC on nucleated cells transiently increases intracellular Ca^{2+}, activates protein kinase C and G proteins, induces procoagulant and proinflammatory activities, and activates cell-cycle activation and transcription (57). Therefore, the presence of TCC on the surface of viable immune cells suggests a modulating role in the physiology of cells to which it attaches (58). In autoimmune demyelination and multiple sclerosis, terminal complement activation exerts a dual role: C5b-9 not only promotes demyelination of oligodendrocytes, it also, in sublytic concentrations, protects them from apoptosis (59). Whether SC5b-9 represents simply the inactivated form of the TCC or whether it plays a role in immune defence remains controversial.

COMPLEMENT RECEPTORS

The consequences of complement activation encompass changes in cellular functions. Central activated complement proteins or their fragments are recognized by specific receptors found on a variety of different cell types (Table 33.3). Primary consequences of this ligand–receptor interaction are the enhancement of innate immune responses to increase removal of foreign material (pathogens, apoptotic cells, immune complexes) or modulation of cellular responses. The best-studied complement receptors (CR) so far are CR1 to CR4. A common feature of these C3 receptors is the recognition of the C3 fragments covalently bound to surfaces upon complement activation. CRIg represents a further receptor for C3 fragments (60). The anaphylatoxin receptors C3aR, C5aR, and C5L2 bind as ligands the anaphylatoxins C3a and C5a as well as their derivatives $C3a^{desArg}$ and $C5a^{desArg}$. A growing number of intracellular and cellular surface receptors for C1q have been identified, which are discussed as modulators of cell responses after ligand binding (Table 33.3). This group of receptors includes cloned proteins such as $C1qR_p$, gC1qbp,

TABLE 33.3 Complement Receptors

Type	*Ligand*	*Structure, MW*	*Distribution*	*Function*
CR1 (CD35)	C3b > C4b > iC3b	Single-chain glycoprotein, 160–250 kDa; allotypes A through D with 30, 37, 23, or 44 SCRs	Monocytes, macrophages, neutrophils, eosinophils, erythrocytes, B and T cells, FDC, mesangium cells in glomeruli	Immune complex clearance, immune complex localization to germinal centers, regulator of C3 and C5 activation
CR2 (CD21)	C3dg/C3d, iC3b, EBV, CD23, IFN-α	Single-chain glycoprotein, 140–145 kDa; two isoforms: CD21S or CD21L (15 or 16 SCRs)	B cells, activated T cells, epithelial cells, FDC (CD21L)	B cell activation, immune complex localization to germinal centers, rescue of germinal center cells from apoptosis
CR3 (CD11b/CD18)	iC3b, ICAM-1, LPS, fibrinogen, clotting factor X, carbohydrates	Heterodimeric glycoprotein, $\alpha + \beta$ chain: 165 + 95 kDa	Monocytes, macrophages, neutrophils, NK cells, FDC, T cells, mast cells	Phagocytosis, cell adhesion, signal transduction, oxidative burst
CR4 (CD11c/CD18)	iC3b, fibrinogen	Heterodimeric glycoprotein, $\alpha + \beta$ chain: 165 + 95 kDa	Monocytes, macrophages, neutrophils, NK cells, T cells, mast cells	Phagocytosis, cell adhesion
CRIg	C3b, iC3b	IgG superfamily	Tissue-resident and sinusoid macrophage	Phagocytosis of circulating pathogens
C3aR	C3a	Single chain of 48 kDa, G-protein–linked receptor	Mast cells, basophils, smooth muscle cells, lymphocytes	Increases vascular permeability, triggers serosal type mast cells
C5aR (CD88)	C5a, $C5a_{desArg}$	Single chain of 43 kDa, G-protein–linked receptor	Mast cells, basophils, neutrophils, monocytes, macrophages, endothelial cells, smooth muscle cells, lymphocytes	Increases vascular permeability, triggers serosal type mast cells, promotes chemotaxis
C5L2	C5a, $C5a_{desArg}$ C3a, $C3a_{desArg}$	Single chain of 37 kDa, G-protein–linked receptor	Neutrophils, immature DCs, preadipocytes, adipocytes	Stimulates triglyceride synthesis Limits pro-inflammatory response
$C1qR_p$	C1q (collagenous part), MBL, SP-A	Single chain of 126 kDa, highly glycosylated	Monocytes, macrophages, neutrophils, endothelial cells, microglia	Phagocytosis
cC1qR "collectin-receptor"	C1q (collagenous part), MBL, SP-A, CL-43	Single chain of 60 kDa, acidic glycoprotein	B cells, monocytes, macrophages, platelets, endothelial cells, fibroblasts	Phagocytosis, localization of immune complexes; enhances ADCC, oxidative metabolism
gC1qR	C1q (globular heads)	Tetramer of 33-kDa subunits, acidic protein	B cells, monocytes, macrophages, platelets, endothelial cells, neutrophils	Inhibits complement activation, phagocytosis

cC1qR (also termed calreticulin or collectin receptor), and a putative $C1qR_{O2}^{-}$ (61).

C3 Receptors

Antigen–antibody complexes or pathogens with C3 fragments linked covalently to their surface are immunologic tags for phagocytes and other immunocompetent cells. Uptake of such opsonized particles and subsequent activation of intracellular pathways are the main functions of C3 receptors (i.e., CR1 through CR4 and CRIg).

Complement Receptor Type 1 (CR1, C3b/C4b Receptor, CD35)

Human CR1 is a multifunctional glycoprotein that belongs to the family of complement regulator proteins (62). A common feature of these proteins is repeats of tandemly arranged modules of about 60 amino acids, referred to as short consensus repeats (SCRs). Within the CR1, larger structural elements are formed, called long homologous repeats (LHRs), each consisting of seven SCRs. The four known polymorphic forms of human CR1 differ in the number of SCRs (up to 34) or LHRs. The ligand-binding sites for C3b and C4b are localized in LHR B (SCR 8–10) and LHR C (SCR 15–17). LHR A harbors an additional C4b-binding region and decay-accelerating activity for both C3 convertases (62). This modular arrangement provides the basis for multivalent CR1–C3b/C4b interactions. In addition to C3b and C4b, CR1 also binds iC3b, although with low affinity. The tissue distribution of CR1 covers a broad spectrum of peripheral blood cells, and it is also found on follicular dendritic cells (FDCs). Because of the numerical predominance of erythrocytes, about 90% of CR1 is found on this cell type.

A main function of CR1 on erythrocytes is a result of its ability to serve as an immune adherence receptor for transport of C3b/C4b opsonized immune complexes (IC), which, after binding, are transported to the liver and spleen. In these organs, IC are transferred to phagocytic cells for removal. On activated phagocytes such as neutrophils or macrophages, CR1 mediates phagocytosis of opsonized pathogens, whereas on nonactivated cells, CR1 cooperates with FcR or CR3 to bind and ingest foreign material. The possible C1q-mediated binding of IC to CR1 for clearing of IC seems to be of minor physiologic importance, because patients who lack complement components downstream of C1q are unable to clear IC via CR1-C1q interactions (63). On B cells, CR1 is suggested to participate in B-cell proliferation and differentiation. In germinal centers of the lymphoid follicles, CR1 expressed on FDC may be of importance in the induction of immunologic memory. CR1 has decay-accelerating activity for the C3 and C5 convertases and cofactor activity for factor I—mediated cleavage of C3b and iC3b. This broad regulatory activity is the basis for the anticomplement therapeutic strategies that use recombinant CR1 (see "Complement in Therapy").

Complement Receptor Type 2 (CR2, C3d Receptor, CD21)

CR2 consists of 15 or 16 SCRs, termed CD21S and CD21L, respectively. CD21L contains an additional exon, which codes for the additional SCR 10a (64). CD21L seems to be selectively expressed on FDC, while CD21S is found mainly on B cells but is also expressed to a small extent on activated T cells and epithelial cells. CR2 interacts with C3d, C3dg, and iC3b, and is the receptor for the Epstein–Barr virus (EBV), facilitating viral entry into B cells and epithelial cells. The binding site for EBV envelope protein gp350/220 within the first two SCRs overlaps with, but is not identical to, the C3d site that has been assigned to SCR 2 (65). CR2 has been reported to interact with CD23, the low-affinity receptor for IgE, which is thought to be involved in regulation of IgE production (66).

The most important role of CR2 is bridging parts of innate and adaptive immunity (67), because it is involved in antibody maturation and induction of B-cell memory. On the surface of human B cells, CD21 is associated with CD19 and CD81, forming a trimolecular coreceptor complex (68). Through C3d-opsonized antigens, the CR2/CD19/CD81 complex is cross-linked with the B-cell–receptor complex (BCR), a process that is stabilized in lipid rafts. As shown in detail in Chapter 8, BCR-associated kinases can phosphorylate cytoplasmic tyrosines of CD19, thus allowing activation of downstream kinases (69). Altogether, cross-linking of the CD19/CR2/CD81 and the BCR complexes lowers the threshold for B-cell activation by the specific antigen by two orders of magnitude compared to antigen alone (68).

Complement Receptor Type 3 (CR3, Mac-1, Mo-1, $\alpha_M\beta_2$, CD11b/CD18)

Together with LFA-1 (CD11a/CD18) and CR 4 (CD11c/CD18), CR3 belongs to the family of β_2 integrins (70). The heterodimeric CR3 consists of a 165-kDa α chain (CD11b) and a 95-kDa β chain (CD18). A remarkable feature of CR3 is its promiscuous interaction with numerous ligands, including the C3 fragment iC3b, ICAM-1 and -2, proteins of the clotting system, or molecules of microbial origin, e.g., from *Leishmania, Klebsiella pneumoniae, Mycobacterium tuberculosis, Candida albicans* (70), and probably HIV (71).

Most ligands investigated so far bind to a specialized region in the α chain, referred to as the I (for "inserted") domain, in a Ca^{2+}-dependent manner (72). In addition, a C-terminal extracellular domain of CD11b has been identified as a high-affinity interaction site for β-glucans, which may interact with carbohydrate structures of different pathogens (73). CR3 is found on mononuclear phagocytes, neutrophils, mast and NK cells, FDC, and T-cell subsets and contributes considerably to leukocyte adherence and migration. The crucial role of CD11b/CD18 as complement receptor in phagocytosis has been recognized in patients with reduced or absent expression of β_2 integrins, known as leukocyte adhesion deficiency (74). Evidence is provided that interaction of CR3 with iC3b is not sufficient to induce phagocytosis and requires additional coligation of the CR3 lectin site with microbial surface polysaccharides (73); alternatively, CR3 can cooperate with other phagocytic receptors such as FcγRIII, FcαRI, or CD14. CR3 is associated on the cell surface with these GPI-anchored surface proteins and may be used as adaptor for their intracellular signalling (75).

Complement Receptor Type 4 (CR4, p150/95, $\alpha_X\beta_2$, CD11c/CD18)

CR4 belongs to the same β_2-integrin subfamily as CR3 (Table 33.3). Ligand specificities of CR4 tested so far seem to be similar to CR3. Also, the tissue distribution of CD11c is comparable to that of CR3, although CR4 seems to be more prominent on distinct dendritic cell subsets (76).

Complement Receptor CRIg

CRIg, a very recently characterized member of the IgG superfamily, is recognized by C3b and iC3b (60). Expression on Kupffer cells is required for the interaction and internalization of C3-opsonized particles even in the presence of CR3. The absence of CRIg, at least in the mouse, significantly increases the infection and mortality rates of the host for bacterial pathogens. Thus, CRIg seem to play a pivotal role in the clearance of opsonized pathogens (60). In addition, evidence is provided that CRIg acts as an inhibitor of the alternative pathway of complement (77).

Anaphylatoxin Receptors C3aR, C5aR (CD88), and C5L2

As discussed previously, cleavage of C3, C4, and C5 results in generation of the small fragments C3a, C4a, and C5a, with a C-terminal arginine residue, which are termed anaphylatoxins (AT). Although C4a is thought to be inactive, C3a and C5a exert various effects when they are bound to their specific receptors C3aR, C5aR (CD88), and C5L2, respectively (78). C3aR, C5aR, and C5L2 are seven-transmembrane receptors of the rhodopsin superfamily. Expression of C3Ra and C5aR was thought to be restricted to cells of myeloid origin, until recent studies demonstrated the presence of C5aR on epithelial, endothelial, and parenchymal cells as well as on B and T lymphocytes. C5L2 is localized on immature dendritic cells (DCs), neutrophils, and in adipocytes and preadipocytes in human subcutaneous and omental adipose tissue (78).

C5a is the best-characterized AT. It is a potent proinflammatory mediator that, via binding to C5aR, induces chemotactic migration and the release of various inflammatory mediators such as histamine or cytokines, enhances cell adhesion, and stimulates the oxidative burst (77). Although the C5a concentration in the blood is 10-fold lower than that of C3a, C3a is believed to be less potent. By binding to C3aR C3a is spasmogenic, stimulates the release of PEG_2 from macrophages, induces degranulation and chemotaxis of eosinophils, attracts mast cells, and exhibits proinflammatory characteristics that overlap with C5a-induced responses (79). Phosphorylation of AT receptors is a key event that regulates their biologic function. Because excessive inflammation may result in tissue damage, the biologic activities of C3a and C5a are tightly controlled. Carboxypeptidase N, a plasma enzyme, rapidly removes the C-terminal arginine residue from C3a and C5a, thereby converting the AT into the desArg form. In contrast to C5aR, the third AT receptor, C5L2, binds both C5a and $C5a^{desArg}$ with high affinity. Becaue C5L2 couples only weakly to signaling G proteins, because of the lack of the exact interaction motifs, it seems likely that C5L2 serves as a nonsignaling decoy receptor and thus limits proinflammatory effects of the anaphylatoxin (80). The binding of C3a and $C3a^{desArg}$ to C5L2 is still controversial (81).

C1q Receptors

Several reports indicate that C1q binds to a variety of different cell types, presumably via distinct receptors, and mediates, e.g., enhanced phagocytosis or oxidative-burst metabolism (82). The best-characterized C1q receptor is $C1qR_p$. Monoclonal antibodies against $C1qR_p$ block C1q-mediated enhancement of phagocytosis in human monocytes and macrophages. The receptor has also been localized on human endothelial cells. The collagenlike tail of C1q also interacts with cC1qR, CR1, or a putative $C1qR_{O2}$, whereas the globular region of C1q interacts with gC1qR (83) (Table 33.3). Ligands of cC1qR besides C1q appear to be the collectins MBL and the surfactant protein SpA. Therefore, cC1qR is also referred to as collectin receptor. cC1qR is identical with calreticulin, a chaperone and Ca^{2+}-dependent signaling molecule that is most abundant in the endoplasmic reticulum. It is unclear how calreticulin may become associated with the cell surface, but together with CD91, surface calreticulin is involved in uptake and removal of cell remnants (84) when it is opsonized with C1q.

COMPLEMENT AS PART OF THE IMMUNE NETWORK

The complete understanding of an immune response requires an integrated view of how immunologic entities work together to achieve the range of physiologic and pathologic characteristics of immune function. The immune network encompasses all of the connections and regulatory associations in the antimicrobial defence armamentarium. Different arms of the innate immunity are activated in parallel by local or systemic infections and closely interact and supplement each other to discriminate between nonself and self and to provide critical danger signals instructing adaptive immune responses. Therefore complement factors maintain a variety of connections to other pathways and elements of innate and adaptive immunity.

Complement, Pentraxins, and Toll-like Receptors

One complement-interacting innate immune molecular family are the pentraxins, a superfamily of conserved acute-phase proteins with characteristic cyclic multimeric structure. Classical short pentraxins are C-reactive protein (CRP) and serum amyloid P (SAP); a prototypic long pentraxin is pentraxin 3 (PTX3). The pentraxins show striking functional parallels to C1q in immune defence to microbes and in scavenging cellular debris.

The major acute-phase protein CRP readily complexes to substances with exposed phosphocholine groups, such as apoptotic cells and C-polysaccharides of the bacterial cell wall (85). Complexed CRP ignites the classical complement pathway by recognition of and interaction with the globular head region of C1q (86). However, CRP-mediated activation of complement proceeds only "halfway," generating C3 convertase but no effective C5 convertase or membrane attack complex (87). The reason for that ineffectual CRP-induced complement flow might be based in the interaction of CRP with factor H and C4bp (88). The collaboration between CRP and complement may nevertheless be functional, resulting in the opsonization of phosphocholine structures by C3 fragments with subsequent phagocytosis. On the other hand, CRP may limit excessive complement activation by directing C4bp and factor H to the targets and thus protecting the host from inflammation-induced tissue damage (88).

A similar Janus-faced role is established for PTX3, which binds to C1q with high affinity and specificity (89). PTX3 enhances C1q binding and complement activation on apoptotic cells but blocks its interaction with immunoglobulins in fluid phase, with subsequent inhibition of complement activation (34).

Toll-like receptors (TLRs) represent another class of pattern-recognition receptors that act as primary sensors of invading pathogens. Both TLRs and complement are activated by invading pathogens, and their cross-talk affects the outcome of infections. Interaction of lipopolysaccharides from gram-negative bacteria with TLR4 induces production of the cytokine IL-12, a key mediator of cell-mediated immunity and a critical link between innate resistance and adaptive immunity (90). Complement factors via binding to their receptors C3aR, C5aR, and CR3 control TLR4-mediated IL-12 release and thus limit the pathogen-induced inflammatory response (90).

Complement and the T-Cell Response

There is increasing evidence for an important role of complement for the induction and promotion of T-cell immunity. Upon infection of mice deficient in C3 ($C^{-/-}$) with influenza virus, the priming of CD4 helper cells and virus-specific CTLs is strongly impaired, resulting in delayed clearance of the infection and increased viral titers (91). Similarly, the induction and expansion of CD8 T cells during infection with lymphocytic choriomeningitis virus relies on C3 (92).

It is likely that macrophages and/or DCs are involved in the C3-mediated T-cell priming. Macrophages derived from $C3^{-/-}$ mice have impaired ability to trigger a robust alloreactive T-cell response. The synthesis of C3 by DCs is thought to be necessary for an alloreactive T-cell activation of a Th1 phenotype in a transplantation model (93). C3 may also play a role in both Th1 and Th2 responses to antigens upon epicutaneous sensitization or intraperitoneal immunization (94).

In addition to C3, membrane-anchored RCAs (CD46, CD55, CD59) modulate the T-cell response. Cross-linking of CD46 with TCR induces regulatory T cells (Treg) (95). CD55 modulates the induction of T cells by controlling T-cell–APC-induced alternative complement activation during cognate interaction (96). A further negative regulator of T-cell activation is CD59. Engagement of CD59 on T cells during APC–T-cell interactions downmodulates T-cell activity in a complement-independent manner (97).

Complement and the B-Cell Response

On mature B lymphocytes, the binding of C3d(g)-opsonized antigens to the CR2/CD19/CD81 complex enables coclustering with the B-cell antigen receptor (BCR). This, in turn, drastically lowers the threshold for B-cell activation by antigens and enhances immunoglobulin production by several orders of magnitude (68). Because this effect is dependent on the amount of C3d molecules interacting with the complex, model vaccines have been designed that include C3d sequences as adjuvant (see: "Complement in Therapy").

The expression of CR2 on FDC in germinal centers (GC) seems to play a profound role in development of antibody response and B-cell memory, too. As soon as low-affinity antibodies are produced during a primary immune response, opsonized immune complexes are trapped on FDC via complement and Fc receptors. C3d-opsonized antigen retained on FDCs via interaction with CR2 provide a survival signal for centroblasts in the GC and thus inhibit their apoptosis (68). The subsequent exposure of trapped antigen to B cells is critical for induction of B-cell maturation and humoral immune response.

Based on results obtained with mice deficient for C4 or CD21/CD35, respectively, CR2 may also be involved in maintenance of B-cell tolerance (98). Normally, self-reactive B cells are either deleted or become anergic. In mice that are deficient for both C4 and CD21/CD35, self-antigens are not efficiently localized in the bone marrow or in GC, which keeps B cells reactive against soluble self-antigens.

Thus, the C3d–CR2 interaction provides an important link between adaptive and innate immunity by contributing to the induction and maturation of the humoral immune response and the maintenance of self-tolerance (99).

COMPLEMENT AS A PATHOGENIC FACTOR IN DISEASE

By "complementing" the destructive action of antibodies via an activation of the whole cascade system, complement may become a pathogenic factor in disease, either alone or, more often, together with other cofactors. In addition, complement may contribute to diseases, e.g., by improper clearance and disposal of complement-coated immune complexes from the circulation (100); the fixation of C4 and C3 fragments into the antigen–antibody lattice significantly reduces the size of the single immune complex, giving rise to a larger number of small complexes ("detergent-like" effect of complement). Furthermore, the presence of C4b and C3b on the immune complexes facilitates efficient fixation of these smaller immune complexes to complement receptors, predominantly erythrocyte-CR1, and ensures transportation and sequestration into the liver and spleen, where antigenic material can be removed by reticulohistiocytic cells, followed by degradation of the antigen. Consequently, pathophysiologically detrimental effects of complement become apparent when a failure in this clearance system occurs, leading to an uptake of these immune complexes by endothelial cells and their sequestration into various organs or tissues ("trapping"), giving rise to further inflammation and immune complex formation with concomitant destruction of surrounding tissue. These pathological conditions include:

1. Inherited, often complete, classical pathway complement deficiency ($C1q^-$, $C4^-$ deficiency)
2. Acquired complement consumption resulting from constant activation on continuously generated immune complexes, as in autoimmune diseases or chronic bacteremia
3. Inherited or acquired low CR1-per-erythrocyte ratio, as in lupus, or low red cell count
4. Extensive liver or spleen disease, impairing the removal of the antigen

Because immune complexes are in particular trapped in small capillaries of the skin or the renal glomeruli, clearance disorders manifest predominantly in the skin and the kidney.

Complement also contributes to inflammation and tissue damage in neurodegenerative and autoimmune diseases, and also in ischemia and reperfusion injury or in shock (Table 33.4). Recently, defects in complement

TABLE 33.4 Human Diseases with a Contribution of Complement to Pathogenesis and/or to Perpetuation

Biocompatibility/Shock	***Neurologic***	***Rheumatologic***
Postbypass syndrome	Myasthenia gravis	Rheumatoid arthritis
Acute respiratory distress syndrome	Multiple sclerosis	Systemic lupus erythematosus
Anaphylaxis	Cerebral lupus erythematosus	Behcet syndrome
Tissue incompatibility/transplantation	Guillain–Barré syndrome	Juvenile rheumatoid arthritis
Pre-eclampsia	Alzheimer's disease	Sjogren syndrome
Biomaterial-induced inflammation	Stroke	
	Pick disease	
	Parkinson's disease	
	Transmissible spongiform encephalopathies	
Dermatologic	***Renal***	***Other Diseases***
Pemphigus vulgaris/pemphigoid	Lupus nephritis	Liver fibrosis, cirrhosis
Phototoxic reactions	Dense deposit disease	Atheroma
Vasculitis	Membranous nephritis	Thyreoiditis
Chronic urticaria	Atypical hemolytic uremic syndrome	Infertility
		Age-related macular degeneration
		Infectious diseases, sepsis
		Tumorigenesis

inhibitors have been implicated in age-related macular degeneration (AMD) (101), because, e.g., avidity of factor H binding to retinal epithelial cells is dependent on tyrosine at position 402 (102). Such a mutated factor H may not be employable by pathogens (see "Evasion Strategies of Micro-organisms"), so AMD in old age may be the prize to pay for protection from infectious disease in youth.

Complement in Renal Disease

Because complement action takes place not only locally, within tissues, but also in circulation, it is somewhat predictable that the kidney as a major filter organ will be affected in case of complement malfunctions. Indeed, preformed immune complexes are often trapped in the kidneys in case of a clearance disorder and the characteristic hypocomplementemia is usually a result of systemic complement activation in the circulation. Intraglomerular complement activation has only a minimal, if any, effect on serum complement levels. C3 and TCC, however, are frequently found in glomerular deposits. These are usually accompanied by local production of cytokines, prostaglandins, proteolytic enzymes, and reactive oxygen metabolites, which create, together with leukocytes, an extended area of inflammation. The crucial role of complement for this inflammation has long been known from animal studies showing that complement-deficient or -depleted animals do not develop induced nephritis (103).

A second important role of complement in renal disease with increased complement-related inflammation is a result of so called nephritic factors (NeF), circulating IgG autoantibodies that bind and stabilize the alternative pathway C3 convertase (103), slowing down its physiologic decay by more than 10-fold. The respective clinical conditions are partial lipodystrophy, an acute condition characterized by loss of fat from the face and upper body as a result of adipocyte lysis via the alternative pathway (104), and MPGN type II (also termed dense deposit disease, DDD) (105).

DDD may also be caused by complement control protein deficiency. However, whereas homozygous deficiency preferably leads to DDD, heterozygous deficiency of these proteins often leads to atypical (because of the lack of preceding diarrhea) hemolytic uremic syndrome (HUS) (106). Interestingly for the latter, heterozygous factor H mutations do not cluster in the N-terminal part of factor H that is involved in complement regulatory functions, but particularly in the C-terminal part of the molecule, which targets factor H action to the surface of the host cell. Factor H heterozygosity (107) or certain allotypes (not necessarily deficiency mutations) (108) predispose to disease, and it may be that it is not the absence of 50% of functionally active molecules that predisposes to HUS, but rather the presence of dysfunctional molecules, attaching to but not protecting the host cells and also preventing attachment of the active molecules (109). Antihuman C5 antibodies (see "Complement as Target in Drug Therapy") may represent an interesting therapy option for patients suffering from renal diseases caused by unrestricted complement activation.

Complement in Neurologic Disease

The human brain is immunologically sheltered from the peripheral immune system by the tight and selective blood–brain barrier. Additional immunologic barriers are manifested by limited antigen presentation and expression of immunosuppressive cytokines (110). To adjust this restricted immunosurveillance, astrocytes, microglia, neurons, and oligodendrocytes produce at least some complement proteins, including soluble factors, regulators, and receptors (111). Of these cell types, astrocytes, the most abundant glial cells, are the major source of complement in the brain, thereby providing immune defense against invading pathogens.

However, a harmful role for complement is implicated for tissue destruction and cell damage in some pathologic conditions such as Alzheimer's disease (AD), Huntington disease, Pick disease, multiple sclerosis (MS), and stroke. Complement is also thought to participate in neurodegeneration induced by cerebral infections.

AD, the most common cause of dementia, is characterized by neuronal loss, neuritic dystrophy, and the accumulation of senile plaques in the brain. Activation of the complement system has been widely investigated as a potential mechanism for these processes. Complement components of classical and terminal pathway are highly upregulated in AD brains, especially in the senile plaques (112). The main component of these plaques, the β-amyloid peptide, can activate complement by binding specifically to the collagenlike domain of C1q (113). Consecutive complement-dependent processes likely contribute to neuronal injury in the proximity of these plaques, especially because neurons are extremely sensitive to complement-induced bystander lysis, because of the low or even absent expression of complement inhibitors on their surface.

MS is an inflammatory autoimmune disease characterized by demyelination of axons, failure of remyelination, and loss of oligodendrocytes. Demyelination results not only from an autoimmune response against myelin components and subsequent activation of the classical pathway, but also from direct binding of complement factors to myelin. Myelin oligodendrocyte glycoprotein (MOG) harbors a protein domain similar to the C1q-binding sequence of IgG antibodies (114). Complement activation results in lysis of oligodendrocytes and chemoattraction of phagocytes, which accumulate at the site of inflammation and degrade the myelin sheath. These processes are mediated by complement receptor CR3 on the phagocyte surface and induce production of inflammatory substances such as TNF-α and nitric oxide (115).

Complement is also hypothesized to contribute to pathogen-induced neural damage. The human immunodeficiency virus HIV-1 is detected in >80% of brains from individuals with AIDS and causes meningitis, neuropathies, and a subcortical dementia that manifests in cognitive, motor, and behavioral dysfunctions. Atrophy, appearance of multinucleated giant cells, reactive astrogliosis, microgliosis, loss of neurons, and inflammation are visible. The discrepancy between the small number of HIV-infected brain cells and the severity of neurologic impairment suggests the existence of detrimental mediator molecules rather than direct virus-induced cell damage. Several hints imply a role of complement in this virus-induced neurologic damage. The expression of different complement factors and receptors is upregulated in HIV-infected astrocytes as well as *in vivo* in the brains of HIV-infected patients (116). Complement activation products such as C3a, C5a, and MAC exert a variety of proinflammatory biologic effects on brain cells. Furthermore, the HIV-1 transmembrane protein gp41 downmodulates the expression of CD59 in human neuronal and astroglial cell lines, thus enhancing the susceptibility of neurons toward complement-dependent bystander cell lysis (110).

COMPLEMENT IN DEFENSE AGAINST INFECTION

The dominant role of complement in the innate immune system, as important first-line defence of higher vertebrates against invading microorganisms, is displayed twofold. First, complement recognizes "nonself" immediately after infection as a primitive surveillance system independent of antibodies or immune cells; and second, it serves as an executor of antibody-mediated immunity.

Nonself structures activate the alternative and lectin pathways (triggered by the surface composition of the invader, e.g., lipopolysaccharides, sialic acids, glycoproteins, and peptidoglycans) or the classical pathway, mainly via C1q-binding moieties. Stimulation of phagocytic cells, by generated anaphylatoxins, attract them to the site of infection (chemotaxis). Generation of C3 fragments, mainly C3b and iC3b (opsonization), on the microbial surface and their recognition via complement receptors on phagocytic cells, mainly CR1 and CR3 (see "Complement Receptors"), followed by phagocytosis or lysis of the microbe, then mostly lead to a control of the infection. Intracellular processing in phagolysosomes and presentation of phagocytosed material on the cell surface by professional antigen-presenting cells will initiate adaptive immune responses and trigger production of specific antibodies, thereby linking innate immunity to adaptive response.

Whereas lysis is effective against some viruses and gram-negative bacteria, chemotaxis followed by opsonophagocytosis represents probably the main mechanism for destruction of most viruses, bacteria, and fungi that cannot be lysed by complement.

Not only the number of C3-fragment molecules deposited on the invader, but also the amount of C5b-9 inserted into the target membrane, are decisive for host defense. The particularly frequent occurrence of terminal complement deficiencies in patients with meningococcal infections suggests that the cytolytic activity of complement is especially important in resistance to gram-negative bacteria (117). Lysis is accomplished via induction of injurious processes or by terminal complement components via the outer membrane attack leaks (118).

Evasion Strategies of Micro-organisms

Highly pathogenic microorganisms are attacked by complement, but in turn may evade appropriate recognition or constrain suitable attack and destruction (119) (Figure 33.8). To achieve these goals a range of strategies has been developed during evolution to (a) avoid or minimize complement activation by displaying special surface moieties, (b) resist C3-dependent opsonophagocytosis, or (c) prevent complement-mediated cytolytic damage (119). The two latter are, e.g., facilitated by displaying proteins antigenically and/or functionally mimicking C3, which can bind to complement receptors. This can mediate uptake in a complement-independent manner, i.e., even when the invader has not been opsonized before. Proteolytic degradation of complement proteins by micro-organisms may also protect them from opsonization and/or lysis (119). Cleavage of C1-INH by proteases, e.g., leads to constant activation (and also consumption) of C1. Micro-organisms that evade complement by consuming it must ensure that this occurs at a secure distance from their cellular membranes.

Another mechanism is the use of complement proteins provided by the host. When HIV-1 buds from an infected cell, it is encoated with a lipid bilayer obtained from the host-cell membrane and as a consequence carries, in addition to viral, also host-cell membrane proteins. Of the latter, especially DAF and CD59 are of particular importance, as they protect HIV-1 from complement lysis (120). Attachment of factor H to C3b on the virus and to several sites on the external portion of gp41 and to one site on gp120 confers an additional protective effect against efficient destruction (121). Because of this acquisition of complement regulators, HIV accumulates in the plasma of infected hosts and spreads with the aid of erythrocytes that interact via their CR1 with the C3b deposited on the viral surface. Furthermore, the dynamic processing of virus-coating C3b into iC3b allows the interactions with CR3-positive cells (Figure 33.9). As a consequence, CR-positive cells contribute to the spread of HIV within an infected host. Acquisition of host-derived fluid-phase complement regulatory proteins, in particular factor H and C4bp, is also executed by bacteria in order to evade complement (122).

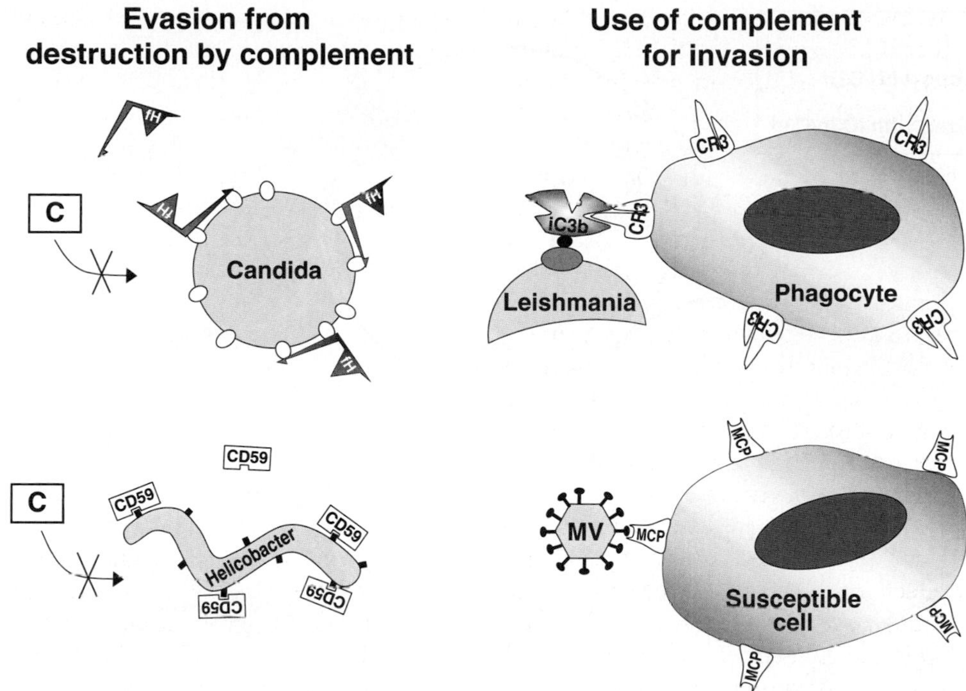

FIGURE 33.8 Micro-organisms display surface moieties that bind to complement proteins. By employing inhibitors from the fluid phase, microorganisms can evade destruction by complement (C) (defensive manner, *left*). Via binding of factor H or CD59, *Candida (upper left)* or *Helicobacter (lower left)* restrict complement activation or membrane-attack complex assembly, respectively. By allowing complement activation and use of complement receptors or via direct binding, they can invade host cells (aggressive manner, *right*). *Leishmania* induces complement activation by displaying complement-activating structures on its surface, followed by opsonization with iC3b, phagocytic CR3-based recognition, and phagocytosis of the parasite; a small but significant portion of the pathogens will survive this procedure *(upper right)*. Measles virus (MV) uses CD46 (MCP) as cellular receptor directly—previous complement activation does not appear to be necessary here *(lower right)*.

Acquisition of the respective gene during evolution is another sophisticated way of evasion. Vaccinia virus complement control protein (VCP), a functionally CR1-like and structurally C4bp-like protein, has evolved after uptake to retain only the most essential domains; any further manipulation of the small viral protein results in loss of function, indicating that the gene has achieved maximum efficiency (123). In other pathogens, molecular mimicry may represent the conservation of ancestral molecular recognition motifs. Many are related to mammalian CR1, DAF, MCP, or C4bp, confirming the importance of C3- and C4-fragment–binding molecules.

The trematode *Schistosoma mansoni* has a highly elaborated anticomplement arsenal: First, it can modify its surface sialic acids, thus modulating activation; second, it can acquire DAF to accelerate decay of surface bound C3; third, it can bind and cleave C4 and C3, mimicking in part CR1; fourth, it can cleave C9, preventing MAC assembly; and fifth, but probably not last, it encodes a protein that mimics CD59, inhibiting membrane attack (124).

The yeast *Candida albicans* possesses an integrin/CR3-like molecule on its surface (125) that is involved in inducing morphology changes. Furthermore, it facilitates cellular adherence like other human integrins and is not only functionally (125) but also antigenically and structurally related to human CR3. There is strong evidence that HIV-1 is able to bind to *Candida* directly, possibly via C3-like regions on gp41 and the CR3-like molecule on *Candida* (126). This interaction enhances fungal proteinase release and suppresses phagocytosis by PMNs (127). Thus, the concerted mimicry of both pathogens may contribute to the virulence of both *Candida* and HIV (126).

COMPLEMENT GENETICS

Many decades of complement genetics research has led to the conclusion that usually only homozygous deficient subjects (or animals) show a significant phenotype, whereas specific allotypes do not normally predispose to disease. However, more and more exceptions are being reported, and interestingly, these are often not related to the typical complement-related functions. The donor C3 allotype has been reported to determine late renal transplantation

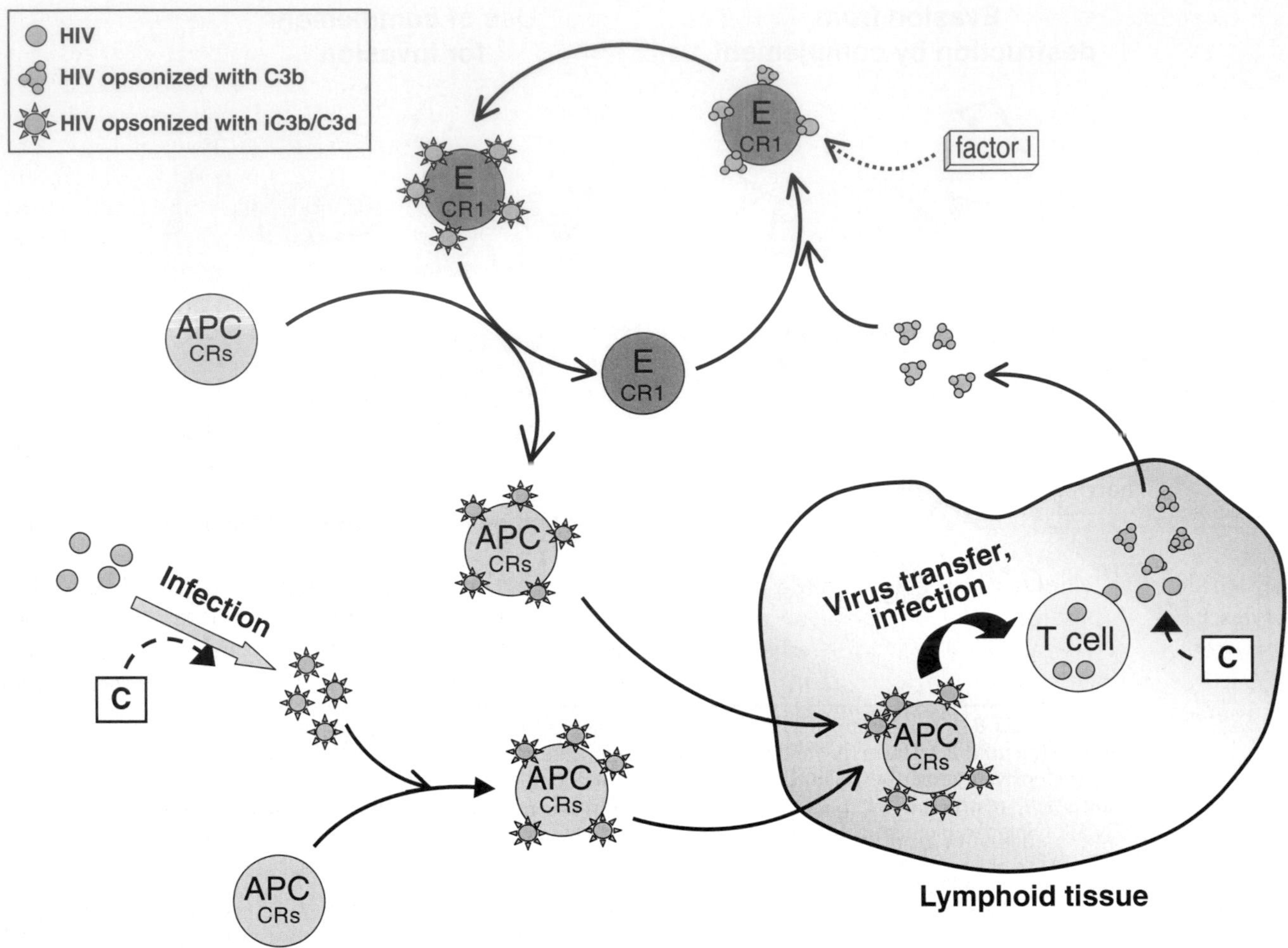

FIGURE 33.9 Complement-mediated enhancement of viral dissemination in early stages of HIV infection. Complement on mucosal surfaces and in seminal fluid opsonizes HIV even in the absence of virus-specific antibodies. Thus, upon crossing the mucosal barrier and entering the host, opsonized HIV is subsequently trapped by antigen-presenting cells (APC), mainly dendritic cells, via complement receptors (CRs). The APC are thought to transport the viral particles into the lymphoid tissue, where the virus is transferred to T cells. Progenitor viruses produced by the infected T cells are subsequently opsonized with C3b and bind to CR1 on erythrocytes (E). Factor I together with CR1 promotes the cleavage of C3b into iC3b. The low affinity of CR1 to iC3b favors the transfer of iC3b-covered virions to CR3 on APC. APC loaded with HIV migrate into lymphoid tissues again, where further T cells are infected.

outcome (128); the pattern of breast cancer metastasis correlates with a single-nucleotide C1q polymorphism (129); the factor H allotype Y402H is associated with a significantly higher likelihood of developing macular degeneration (see "Complement in Renal Disease") (101); and a common fH polymorphism, with an increased risk of myocardial infarction (130).

Furthermore, complement genetics has also been a valuable tool with which to investigate plasma protein genetics in general and their evolution. The chromosomal locations of the complement protein genes are given in Table 33.1. These are not scattered around the chromosomes, but form linkage groups of structurally homologous components, confirming previous assumptions based on homology studies on the protein level that the majority of complement proteins has evolved by duplication and diversion events from only a small number of precursor genes (131).

Because complement receptors and certain regulatory proteins are expressed on erythrocytes, they also represent blood-group antigens; e.g., the Knops, McCoy, Swain-Langley, and York antigens are on CR1. Variations in the DAF antigen are responsible for the Cromer blood-group system, with the rare Inab phenotype lacking DAF altogether. Chido and Rogers blood-group antigens are associated with C4 (131). In this respect, complement genetics has been widely applied to anthropologic investigations and forensic medicine.

Progress in DNA work has facilitated the characterization of complement allotypes on the molecular level. Both phenotypic assessments of protein variants (phenotyping, e.g., by isoelectric focusing or monoclonal antibodies) and characterizations of genomic DNA (genotyping, e.g., by RFLP or PCR) are currently used (132). Phenotyping has the advantage that the presence and even the functional activity of a protein can be ascertained. Genotyping does not allow identification of silent or null alleles as such, however, once a mutation is known, a defective gene may be traced in family studies, providing a basis for genetic counseling.

COMPLEMENT DEFICIENCIES

Inherited deficiencies, either complete or subtotal, have been described for most complement components and regulatory proteins. These abnormalities are relatively rare and usually inherited in an autosomal recessive manner, which means that only homozygous subjects are readily detected and susceptible to disease. One important exception is the autosomal dominant inherited hereditary angioedema (see below). Another, only recently discovered heterozygous deficiency is that of factor H and other complement-regulatory proteins (see "Complement in Renal Disease").

Complement defects can be ascertained by the traditional total hemolytic complement assays (CH_{50}, $APCH_{50}$) followed by radial immunodiffusion (Mancini), electroimmunodiffusion (rocket electrophoresis, Laurell), or enzyme immunoassays (ELISA) (133). The latter are of particular importance as so-called subtotal deficiencies, in which residual functionally active amounts can only be detected by sensitive ELISA, and may have a different clinical picture and prognosis (134). Low concentrations of terminal components, for example, may be sufficient for preventing meningococcal disease and can be tested for their ability to incorporate into the TCC by ELISA based on neoepitope-specific anti-C9 monoclonal antibodies (135). None of these quantitative assays allows, although widely practiced, the assumption that approximately half-normal concentrations indicate heterozygous deficiency. Heterozygous subjects may present with almost normal concentrations of the component in question. A very sophisticated assay in ELISA format has recently been elaborated by a European consortium, which can be used as a screening assay for detecting complement deficiencies (136).

Complement-deficient subjects are usually detected because of their increased propensity to infection or, especially for deficiencies of the early classical pathway components, in association with systemic lupus erythematosus (SLE) (Table 33.5). As only *C4* and *C2* are encoded on the same chromosome (within the MHC-III region; see Table 33.1), the possibility that these deficiencies are all linked to a disease-susceptibility gene can be excluded. In contrast, it is the absent "detergentlike" effect of complement (see "Complement as Pathogenic Factor in Disease") that leads to impaired clearance of immune complexes and to their sequestration at peripheral sites, giving rise to further inflammation and immune complex formation.

It is not surprising that deficiency of mannan-binding lectin (MBL), a major plasma protein of the innate immune

TABLE 33.5 Complement-Deficiency States

Component	*No. of Reported Patients*	*Functional Defect*	*Disease Associations*[a]
C1	50–100	Impaired immune-complex handling	SLE, bacterial infections
C4	20–50	Impaired immune-complex handling	SLE, bacterial infections
C2	>1,000	Impaired immune-complex handling	SLE, bacterial infections
C3	20–50	Impaired opsonization	Bacterial infections
C1-INH	>>10,000	Excessive C2 and kinin activation	HAE
B	None		Not incompatible with life in mouse
D	<5	Impaired alternative-pathway activation	Bacterial infections?
P	>100	Impaired alternative-pathway activation	Meningococcal infections
H	>100	Excessive alternative-pathway activation	Meningococcal infections, glomerulonephritis
I	20–50	Excessive alternative pathway activation	Bacterial infections
Carboxy-peptidase N	<5	Absent inhibition of C5a and C3a	Angioedema, chronic urticaria
C5	20–50	Impaired chemotaxis, absent lytic activity	Meningococcal infections
C6; C7; C8	>100 each (independent)	Absent lytic activity	Meningococcal infections
C9	>1,000	Impaired lytic activity	Meningococcal infections

[a] Only established and typical disease associations are listed (i.e., >50% of deficient subjects suffering from disease).

system with the ability to initiate antimicrobial and inflammatory actions, results in a higher susceptibility to infection. MBL deficiency is common, as more than 10% of the general population may, depending on definition, be classified as MBL-deficient (137).

In individuals with homozygous C3 deficiency, pyogenic infections with encapsulated bacteria are severe, recurrent, and life-threatening, usually starting in early childhood. Deficiencies of factor I or factor H are associated with the inability to degrade C3b, leading to uncontrolled amplification of cleavage of C3 by C3b,Bb and resulting in a state of acquired, severe C3 deficiency (138).

Whereas deficiencies of properdin predispose to (usually singular) meningococcal infections, deficiencies of a terminal complement component lead to recurrent infections by gram-negative bacteria as a result of an inability to generate a bactericidal membrane attack complex. Recurrent infection or infection with uncommon serogroups should alert the clinician in nonendemic regions, whereas recurrent disease is the important indicator in endemic areas (134). Associations of terminal complement deficiencies with susceptibility to autoimmune diseases, such as SLE, are likely the result of ascertainment artefacts (134).

Hereditary angioedema (HAE), the clinically most relevant, by far most acute, and, if untreated, potentially lethal, complement deficiency, is the clinical manifestation of an inherited or acquired C1-inhibitor deficiency (139). An absent, depleted (also via autoantibodies), or dysfunctional C1 inhibitor will allow unrestricted activation of the classical pathway, as there is no sufficient backup for the C1 inhibitor. The C2b fragment generated also exhibits kinin activity and is thus responsible for the classical symptoms of HAE; affected patients suffer intermittently from multiple edemas, predominantly in the skin, the gastrointestinal tract, or the oropharynx, usually when the patient experiences minor trauma or infection that triggers unrestricted complement activation. Edemas in the larynx may be life-threatening (i.e., danger of suffocation). Although laryngeal edema in HAE usually develops within hours, and not within minutes as does allergic laryngeal edema, HAE is, even today, associated with a high mortality rate. The frequent association with abdominal colic may also delay the correct diagnosis. The acute treatment of HAE consists of replacement of C1 inhibitor in purified form or, if unavailable, infusion of fresh frozen plasma. Testosterone derivatives (e.g., Danazol) have been used successfully for the long-term prevention of attacks.

A particular deficiency, which is primarily not a complement deficiency, is paroxysmal nocturnal hemoglobinuria (PNH). Mutations in the *PIG-A* gene affect the synthesis of a competent glycosylphosphatidylinositol (GPI) anchor, which leads to failure of expression of all molecules attached to the membrane via this anchor, including CD55 and CD59. The lack of these two complement-control proteins is responsible for the extreme susceptibility of PNH erythrocytes to lysis by complement that is either activated by the alternative pathway or via acidic generation of C56, i.e., the activation of C6 without cleaving off C5a, especially at the physiologically lower blood pH at night (140).

COMPLEMENT IN THERAPY: TARGET AND TOOL

The cloning of the complement components, the determination of their functional domains, and increasing knowledge of immunologic relationships have made it feasible to design therapeutic approaches that (a) interfere with excess complement activation in pathophysiologic settings or in therapeutic approaches; (b) stimulate complement attack on tumor cells; or (c) take advantage of complement to optimize therapeutic or prophylactic tools (Table 33.6).

Interference with Complement Activation

Dysregulated complement activation exerts detrimental effects on organs and cells, and is involved in the pathogenesis of a broad variety of diseases. Furthermore, the unintentional activation of the complement cascade can limit therapeutic interventions, such as (xeno)transplantation, gene therapy via viral vectors, or use of biomaterials (hemodialysers, catheters, prostheses, stents, etc.) (141). This situation creates a strong need for controlled and adequate interference with complement activation.

Different mechanistic concepts for the inhibition of complement activation include (a) native or modified complement regulators, (b) transfer of genes encoding complement regulators, (c) monoclonal antibodies recognizing complement factors or fragments derived thereof, or (d) peptides that block complement factors or its receptors (Table 33.6).

Native regulatory proteins generally have the advantage of being perfectly specific and having a low antigenic potential. Plasma-derived C1-INH is used for standard substitution therapy in hereditary or acquired angioedema (142), but also favorably influences the outcome in life-threatening conditions associated with a relative deficiency of functional C1-INH (143). C1-INH substitution has been used with success in animal models or open, uncontrolled clinical trials in septic shock, capillary leak syndrome, or ischemia/reperfusion injury.

Recombinant soluble CR1, designated TP10, is a truncated derivate of the cell surface CR1. Clinical studies showed that TP10 improves the outcome of lung transplant recipients and inhibited complement activation in patients undergoing cardiac surgery on cardiopulmonary bypass (144). However, this was not associated with a reduced morbidity and mortality. New complement-inhibitor substances are often modified to prolong the bioavailability

TABLE 33.6 Complement in Therapeutic Approaches

Target/Mechanism	*Potential and Established Indication*	*References*
I. Inhibition of complement activation		
Application of soluble CR1 or fragments thereof (e.g., TP10, APT070, TP20) Inhibition of C3/C5 convertases and cofactor activity for factor I	Rheumatoid arthritis Systemic lupus erythematosus Ischemia-reperfusion injury Cardiac surgery Transplantation Acute respiratory distress syndrome ABO incompatibility in blood transfusion	179, 146, 179, 180, 181, 182, 183, 184
Application of C1-INH protein: Inactivation of C1r, C1s, MASP2	Hereditary or acquired angioedema Brain/liver ischemia Septic shock, burn (capillary leakage syndrome) Antiphospholipid syndrome in pregnant women Myocardial infarction, myocardial surgery Transplantation	143, 185, 186, 187, 188, 189, 190
Application of modified soluble CD59 (e.g., sCD59-APT542)	Rheumatoid arthritis Paroxysmal nocturnal hemoglubinuria	145, 190
CD55-transgenic animals, vector-mediated transfer of CD55 Inhibition of C3/C5 convertases	(Xeno)transplantation	147, 149
Incorporation of CD55 into viral vectors Inhibition of C3/C5 convertases	Protection of viral vectors in gene therapy	150, 151
Antibodies to C5 (pexelizumab, eculizumab) Inhibition of C5 cleavage by convertases	Myocardial infarction Stroke Coronary artery bypass, aortic valve replacement Membraneous nephritis Rheumatoid arthritis Paroxysmal nocturnal hemoglobinuria Dermatomyositis	152, 153, 154, 192, 193
Antibodies to C5a Prevention of anaphylatoxin activity	Septic shock Pulmonary edema	194
Antibodies to Factor D Inhibition of factor B cleavage/activation from alternative pathway	Myocardial injury, surgery	155
Synthetic peptides binding to C3 (e.g., compstatin) Inhibition of C3 cleavage by convertases	Hyperacute rejection in transplantation Organ preservation ex vivo	156
Antagonists to C3a receptor (e.g., SB290157) Blocking the anaphylatoxin receptor	Inflammation, e.g., after surgery Allergic asthma Arthritis	157, 195
Antagonists to C5a receptor (e.g., PMX53, PMX205) Blocking the anaphylatoxin receptor	Inflammation after injury or surgery Septic shock Rheumatoid arthritis Ischemia-reperfusion injury Inflammatory bowel disease Abdominal aortic aneurysm Liver fibrosis Neurodegeneration	158, 159, 196
II. Stimulation of complement activation		
Optimization of therapeutic monoclonal antibodies for complement stimulation Complement-dependent lysis of tumor cells	Several forms of tumors	161, 162, 163, 165, 197, 198, 199
Antibodies to CD55 Reduced inhibition of C3/C5 convertases	Several forms of tumors	166
Monoclonal antibody that mimics CD55 Induction of immune response to CD55	Several forms of tumors	166, 167, 168
Small interfering RNA (siRNA) to CD55 Reduced inhibition of C3/C5 convertases	Several forms of tumors	169

(*continued*)

TABLE 33.6 Complement in Therapeutic Approaches (Continued)

Target/Mechanism	*Potential and Established Indication*	*References*
III. Exploitation of complement molecules for therapy and vaccination		
CD46 as measles virus receptor	Several forms of tumors	171, 172, 173
Measles virus–induced lysis of tumor cells		
CD46 as receptor for adenovirus subgroup B	Several forms of tumors	174, 175, 176
Adenovirus-induced lysis of tumor cells	Vaccination	
Adenovirus as antigen carrier to CD46-bearing APC	Gene therapy	
Adenovirus as vehicle for therapeutic genes		
CD55 as coxsackievirus receptor	Several forms of tumors	171
Coxsackie virus–induced lysis of tumor cells		
C3d-enhanced DNA vaccination	Vaccination	177, 178, 200
Increase of humoral immune response		

and to retain them after local administration at the inflammatory site(s) of interest. Soluble CR1 or CD59 were chemically coupled to a short synthetic address tag that confers membrane-binding activity. These modified complement regulators are therapeutically effective in animal models of rheumatoid arthritis or paroxysmal nocturnal hemoglobinuria (145,146). In another tagging approach, sCR1 was expressed with high amounts of the sialyl Lewis^x carbohydrate, the ligand for E-selectin. The resulting compound, TP20, is targeted to E-selectin, which is upregulated on inflamed endothelium, and thus blocks the attachment of neutrophils. TP20 showed benefits over the unmodified TP10 in a murine model of stroke and in a rat-lung transplantation model, but has not been studied further (147).

Gene transfer is suggested or under development for complement inhibition in xenotransplantation and protection of viral vectors for gene therapy. In xenotransplantation, hyperacute rejection is due primarily to the attachment of preformed xenoreactive antibodies to the donor vascular endothelium, which results in hyperactivation of the complement system. Organs from donor pigs transgenic for human CD55 showed less parenchymal injury and decreased sequestration of platelets when perfused with human blood, thus representing an interesting organ pool for transplantation (148). Expression of CD55 can also be achieved by adenoviral transduction and results in reduced sensitivity to complement-mediated lysis (149). Incorporation of genes for complement inhibitors protects lentiviral or baculovirus-derived vectors from inactivation by human complement and thereby enables the development of more potent delivery stems for gene therapy (150)

Monoclonal antibodies (mAbs) represent a third strategy to interfere with complement activation. Anti-C5 antibodies (151) are the best-studied representatives of that class. Both pexelizumab and eculizumab are humanized mAbs that bind to C5 with high affinity and prevent C5 cleavage, C5a generation, and MAC formation, but allow C3 activation and deposition. Pexelizumab is currently being tested in a Phase III clinical trial in patients undergoing coronary artery bypass graft surgery, and has significantly reduced mortality and myocardial infarction (152,153). Eculizumab was shown in an open-label extension trial to be well tolerated and to reduce hemolysis in patients with paroxysmal nocturnal hemoglobinuria (154). Surprisingly, data presented with an anti-factor D antibody showed effective complement inhibition, neutrophil activation, and IL-6 production in a baboon model of cardiopulmonary bypass, obviously a result of the selective inactivation of the alternative pathway (155).

Small synthetic molecules inhibit complement activation by binding to complement factors or its receptors. Compstatin is a synthetic 13-residue cyclic peptide that binds to the β chain of C3 and inhibits its cleavage by C3-convertases, presumably by an induced conformational change of C3 (156). Compstatin has been successfully tested in animal models of hyperacute rejection in kidney xenotransplatation and of extracorporeal circulation, where it inhibits the activation of C3 and downstream pathways.

The role of C3a and C5a in anaphylaxis, sepsis, adverse reactions in extracorporeal circulation, or dialysis, has led to the generation of receptor antagonists. The C3a receptor antagonist SB 290157 blocked C3a-triggered effects of the C3aR and showed anti-inflammatory activity in animal models for allergic asthma and intestinal ischemia-reperfusion injury. Recent results, however, implied that SB290157 can also have an unwanted agonist activity, which urgently warrants further studies before any therapeutic use (157). The cyclic hexapeptide PMX53 and its more lipophilic derivative PMX205 competitively inhibit the interaction between C5a and its receptor (158). The substances were tested successfully in animal models of e.g., ischemia-reperfusion injury, rheumatoid arthritis, and neurodegeneration, where they reduced morbidity and mortality, as well as neutrophil infiltration, apoptosis, and synthesis of inflammatory cytokines (159).

Stimulation of Complement Activation

Immunotherapy using mAbs holds great promise to improve therapy of malignancies, because of its ability to specifically target malignant cells while ignoring surrounding normal tissue. However, only seven mAbs are currently approved for clinical use. To improve antibody tools, it is therefore a priority to optimize their triggering of the complement attack against tumor cells. Complement initiates two mechanisms that are effective against mAb-coated tumor cells: direct killing by MAC (complement-depending cytotoxicity; CDC) and CR3-dependent enhancement of antibody-dependent cytotoxicity (ADCC), in which CR3 binds to iC3b, thus enhancing FcγR-mediated effector-cell binding. A third mechanism, the priming of CR3 by β-glucans, which, in concert with target-associated iC3b, elicit phagocytosis, is usually activated only by microorganisms but not by tumors (160). However, strategies to support this third way, the CR3-dependent cellular cytotoxicity (CR3-DCC), are under investigation.

Many anticancer antibodies (e.g., rituximab against CD20 on B-lymphoma cells) depend strictly on complement activation in their therapeutic activity (161). Subclass IgG1 is especially effective at directing CDC via the classical pathway; novel human mAbs against tumor antigens may be genetically converted to IgG1 to optimize CDC and ADCC activities (162). To fine-tune the immunologic activity of a given IgG1, novel strategies may include the engineering of its hinge region in order to increase C1q binding (163).

Another putative approach to amplify complement-dependent killing of tumor cells by mAbs is the addition of β-glucans, which bind to CR3 and prime it for binding to iC3b. Thus, β-glucans promote killing of the cancer cells by phagocytes in concert with iC3b opsonization of tumor cells, engendered by administration of antitumor antibodies (164). Other ways to increase complement activation include amplification of the amount of mAb deposited on tumor cells by use of a second mAb directed against the iC3b bound on the tumor cell after binding of the therapeutic antibody. Injection of an anti-iC3b mAb following rituximab treatment in a monkey lymphoma model resulted in enhanced complement activation, iC3b deposition, and killing of $CD20^+$ lymphoma cells (165).

Because complement-regulatory proteins are often upregulated on malignant cells and thus provide relative resistance against complement attack, it is desirable to undermine this evasion mechanism. Besides CD46 and CD59, CD55 has been detected in a variety of different malignancies and is regarded as a requisite for cancer development and progression (reviewed in: 166). To restore tumor sensitivity to complement, several studies applying anti-CD55 mAbs or vaccinating against CD55 have been started recently, and first promising results reveal a significant regression of tumor mass. These strategies to block CD55 on the tumor cells are associated with comparatively low toxicity in humans (166).

Anti-CD55 vaccination can be achieved with monoclonal antibodies mimicking CD55. The following immune response directed against CD55 makes the tumor more susceptible against complement attack. The best-known example is the anti-idiotypic antibody 105AD7, which mimics the first two SCR domains of CD55. 105AD7 stimulated strong CD4 and CD8 responses in initial clinical trials in patients with osteosarcoma or colorectal cancer and was surprisingly well tolerated (167,168). The resistance of lymphoma to complement-dependent cytotoxicity may also be overcome by RNA interference. Small interfering RNA (siRNA) designed for CD55 potently decreased CD55 expression and resistance to CDC in breast cancer cells and lymphoma cells (169).

Exploitation of Complement Molecules for Therapy and Vaccination

New strategies to treat cancer include virotherapy with replication-competent viral vectors obtaining oncolytic properties. The selective upregulation of complement regulators on the tumor cell surface makes complement inhibitor–binding viruses attractive tools and permits targeting virus-mediated destruction of malignant cells within nonmalignant tissue. CD55 is the attachment site of a common cold virus, Coxsackievirus A21 (CAV21). CAV21 rapidly destroys human melanoma cells in a mouse model, highlighting its putative application as an effective oncolytic agent (170).

The attenuated measles virus (MV) vaccine strain Edmonston B (MV-Edm) elicits extensive cell-to-cell fusion and ultimately cell death. Tumor cells—e.g., from breast cancer—that normally express high levels of the MV-Edm receptor CD46 are preferentially targeted by the virus (171). The first clinical trials in patients with cutaneous T-cell lymphomas revealed that MV-Edm therapy was well tolerated, with local viral activity in the tumor and increased immune parameters (172). The tumor selectivity of MV-Edm may be enhanced by making the virus dependent from matrix metalloproteinases; by introduction of a specific sequence into the viral fusion protein F, the proteolytic activation of F can be performed exclusively by these proteolytic enzymes that are secreted in high amounts by cancer cells (173).

CD46 is also the receptor for most B-group adenoviruses (Ad). Recombinant Ad-based vectors with B-group fibers target tumors that express CD46 at high levels and revealed oncolytic effects in animal models (174). CD46-binding adenoviruses can also deliver therapeutic genes to cancer cells, because the CD46 expression on tumor cells was elevated (175). CD46-binding adenoviruses could also be valuable tools for vaccination. B-group adenoviruses encoding test antigens efficiently target CD46^{+} dendritic cells and antigen-presenting cells in a monkey model, thus enabling an efficient immune response (176).

Complement provides another interesting tool to support vaccination strategies (177). The C3-fragment C3d, when covalently bound to antigen, serves as a molecular adjuvant in immunization by targeting this antigen to CD21 on B cells and follicular dendritic cells. Complement tagging of antigens may thus help to raise an effective immune response against poorly immunogenic but protective antigens (178). It influences the magnitude of humoral immune response, as it may determine the valence of the constructs; polyvalent CR2-ligands have an immunostimulatory effect, whereas monovalent CR2 ligands are immunosuppressive. Recombinantly or chemically attached C3d as a "natural adjuvant" has been shown to elicit enhanced immune response against prominent pathogens such as measles virus, influenza virus, pneumococci, or HIV.

CONCLUSION

Complement comprises plasma proteins (i.e., substrates and regulators of the activation cascades) and cell membrane proteins (i.e., receptors and cell-protecting regulators). Complement activation, triggered by bound antibody or microbial patterns directly, proceeds in three intertwined pathways (classical, lectin, and alternative) and either leads directly to destruction of foreign structures through insertion of a lytic pore or contributes to their elimination, e.g., through promotion of phagocytosis and antibody formation.

Recent findings have advanced our understanding of complement, especially of the ways it can be dealt with in clinical therapy. The genotype of *MBL*, standing for the activity of the lectin pathway, was shown to correlate widely with disposition to infection. The three-dimensional structures of core components (e.g., C3) have been solved. Finally, several specific complement inhibitors (chimeric constructs derived from natural regulators, monoclonal antibodies, or small molecules found by combinatorial approaches) are in the stage of advanced clinical trials. Ischemic and inflammatory diseases, including ischemia-reperfusion injury in surgery and transplantation, are particularly interesting for therapeutic complement inhibition.

ACKNOWLEDGMENTS

The authors would like to acknowledge the European Community, the Austrian Science Fund (FWF), the Austrian National Bank, and the Ludwig-Boltzmann-Society for support of their research.

REFERENCES

1. Pillemer L, Blum L, Lepow IH. The properdin system and immunity. I. Demonstration and isolation of a new serum protein, properdin, and its role in immune phenomena. *Science.* 1954;120:279–285.
2. Fujita T, Matsushita M, Endo Y. The lectin-complement pathway—its role in innate immunity and evolution. *Immunol Rev.* 2004;198:185–202.
3. Morgan BP, Gasque P. Extrahepatic complement biosynthesis: where, when and why? *Clin Exp Immunol.* 1997;107:1–7.
4. Würzner R, Joysey VC, Lachmann PJ. Complement component C7. Assessment of *in vitro* synthesis after liver transplantation reveals that hepatocytes do not synthesize the majority of the C7. *J Immunol.* 1994;152:4624–4629.
5. Würzner R. Modulation of complement membrane attack by local C7 synthesis. *Clin Exp Immunol.* 2000;121:8–10.
6. Kuehn MH, Kim CY, Ostojic J, et al. Retinal synthesis and deposition of complement components induced by ocular hypertension. *Exp Eye Res.* 2006;83:620–628.
7. Reis ES, Barbuto JA, Isaac L. Human monocyte-derived dendritic cells are a source of several complement proteins. *Inflamm Res.* 2006;55:179–184.
8. Morgan BP, Gasque P. Expression of complement in the brain: role in health and disease. *Immunol Today.* 1996;17:461–466.
9. Bruder C, Hagleitner M, Darlington G, et al. HIV-1 induces complement factor C3 synthesis in astrocytes and neurons by modulation of promoter activity. *Mol Immunol.* 2004;403:949–961.
10. Sacks SH, Zhou W. Allograft rejection: effect of local synthesis of complement. *Springer Semin Immunopathol.* 2005;27:332–344.
11. Volanakis JE. Transcriptional regulation of complement genes. *Annu Rev Immunol.* 1995;13:277–305.
12. Janssen BJ, Huizinga EG, Raaijmakers HC, et al. Structures of complement component C3 provide insights into the function and evolution of immunity. *Nature.* 2005;437:505–511.
13. Law SKA, Dodds AW. The internal thioester and the covalent binding properties of the complement proteins C3 and C4. *Protein Sci.* 1997;6:263–274.
14. Carroll MC, Fathallah DM, Bergamaschini L, et al. Substitution of a single amino acid (aspartic acid for histidine) converts the functional activity of human complement C4B to C4A. *Proc Natl Acad Sci U S A.* 1990;87:6868–6872.
15. Barlow PN, Steinkasserer A, Norman DG, et al. Solution structure of a pair of complement modules by nuclear magnetic resonance. *J Mol Biol.* 1993;232:268–284.
16. Janatova J, Reid KB, Willis AC. Disulfide bonds are localized within the short consensus repeat units of complement regulator proteins: C4b-binding protein. *Biochemistry.* 1989;28:4754–4761.
17. Heine-Suner D, Diaz-Guillen MA, Pardo F, et al. A high resolution map of the regulator of the complement activation gene cluster on 1q32 that integrates new genes and markers. *Immunogenetics.* 1997;45:422–427.
18. Hobart MJ, Fernie BA, DiScipio RG. Structure of the human C7 gene and comparison with the C6, C8A, C8B, and C9 genes. *J Immunol.* 1995;154:5188–5194.
19. Würzner R, Hobart MJ, Fernie BA, et al. Molecular basis of subtotal complement C6 deficiency. A carboxy-terminally truncated but functionally active C6. *J Clin Invest.* 1995;95:1877–1883.
20. Tschopp J, Villiger W, Fuchs H, et al. Assembly of subcomponents C1r and C1s of the first component of complement: Electron microscopic and ultracentrifugal studies. *Proc Natl Acad Sci U S A.* 1980;77:7014–7018.
21. Arlaud GJ, Rossi V, Thielens NM, et al. Structural and functional studies on C1r and C1s: new insights into the mechanisms involved in C1 activity and assembly. *Immunobiology.* 1998;199:303–316.
22. Taylor PR, Carugati A, Fadok VA, et al. A hierarchical role for classical pathway complement proteins in the clearance of apoptotic cells *in vivo*. *J Exp Med.* 2000;192:359–366.

23. Navratil JS, Korb LC, Ahearn JM. Systemic lupus erythematosus and complement deficiency: clues to a novel role for the classical complement pathway in the maintenance of immune tolerance. *Immunopharmacology.* 1999;42:47–52.
24. Ziccardi R. Activation of the early components of the classical complement pathway under physiologic conditions. *J Immunol.* 1981;126:1769–1773.
25. Müller-Eberhard HJ. Molecular organization and function of the complement system. *Annu Rev Biochem.* 1988;57:321–347.
26. Ligoudistianou C, Xu Y, Garnier G, et al. A novel human complement-related protein, C1r-like protease (C1r-LP), specifically cleaves pro-C1s. *Biochem J.* 2005;387:165–173.
27. Petersen SV, Thiel S, Jensenius JC. The mannan-binding lectin pathway of complement activation: biology and disease association. *Mol Immunol.* 2001;38:133–149.
28. Madsen HO, Garred P, Kurtzhals JA, et al. A new frequent allele is the missing link in the structural polymorphism of the human mannan-binding protein. *Immunogenetics.* 1994;40:37–44.
29. Turner MW, Hamvas RM. Mannose-binding lectin: structure, function, genetics and disease associations. *Rev Immunogenet.* 2000;2:305–322.
30. Koch A, Melbye M, Sorensen P, et al. Acute respiratory tract infections and mannose-binding lectin insufficiency during early childhood. *JAMA.* 2001;285:1316–1321.
31. Garcia-Laorden MI, Pena MJ, Caminero JA, et al. Influence of mannose-binding lectin on HIV infection and tuberculosis in a Western-European population. *Mol Immunol.* 2006;43:2143–2150.
32. Matsushita M, Fujita T. Ficolins and the lectin complement pathway. *Immunol Rev.* 2001;180:78–85.
33. Liu Y, Endo Y, Iwaki D, et al. Human M-ficolin is a secretory protein that activates the lectin complement pathway. *J Immunol.* 2005;175:3150–3156.
34. Nauta AJ, Raaschou-Jensen N, Roos A, et al. Mannose-binding lectin engagement with late apoptotic and necrotic cells. *Eur J Immunol.* 2003;33:2853–2863.
35. Holmskov U, Thiel S, Jensenius JC. Collectins and ficolins: humoral lectins of the innate immune defense. *Annu Rev Immunol.* 2003;21:547–578.
36. Frederiksen PD, Thiel S, Larsen CB, et al. M-ficolin, an innate immune defence molecule, binds patterns of acetyl groups and activates complement. *Scand J Immunol.* 2005;62:462–473.
37. Gal P, Harmat V, Kocsis A, et al. A true autoactivating enzyme. Structural insight into mannose-binding lectin-associated serine protease-2 activations. *J Biol Chem.* 2005;280:33435–33444.
38. Thiel S, Vorup-Jensen T, Stover CM, et al. A second serine protease associated with mannan-binding lectin that activates complement. *Nature.* 1997;386:506–510.
39. Chen CB, Wallis R. Two mechanisms for mannose-binding protein modulation of the activity of its associated serine proteases. *J Biol Chem.* 2004;279:26058–26065.
40. Cortesio CL, Jiang W. Mannan-binding lectin-associated serine protease 3 cleaves synthetic peptides and insulin-like growth factor-binding protein 5. *Arch Biochem Biophys.* 2006;449:164–170.
41. Petersen SV, Thiel S, Jensen L, et al. Control of the classical and the MBL pathway of complement activation. *Mol Immunol.* 2000;37:803–811.
42. Collard CD, Vakeva A, Morrissey MA, et al. Complement activation after oxidative stress: role of the lectin complement pathway. *Am J Pathol.* 2000;156:1549–1556.
43. Volanakis JE, Narayana SVL. Complement factor D, a novel serine protease. *Protein Sci.* 1996;5:553–564.
44. Hourcade DE. The role of properdin in the assembly of the alternative pathway C3 convertases of complement. *J Biol Chem.* 2006;281:2128–2132.
45. Zipfel PF, Jokiranta TS, Hellwage J, et al. The factor H protein family. *Immunopharmacology.* 1999;42:53–60.
46. Masaki T, Matsumoto M, Yasuda R, et al. A covalent dimer of complement C4b serves as a subunit of a novel C5 convertase that involves no C3 derivatives. *J Immunol.* 1991;147:927–932.
47. Vogt W. Cleavage of the fifth component of complement and generation of a functionally active C5b6-like complex by human leukocyte elastase. *Immunobiology.* 2000;201:470–477.
48. Huber-Lang M, Sarma JV, Zetoune FS, et al. Generation of C5a in the absence of C3: a new complement activation pathway. *Nat Med.* 2006;12:682–687.
49. Müller-Eberhard HJ. The membrane attack complex of complement. *Annu Rev Immunol.* 1986;4:503–528.
50. Thompson RA, Lachmann PJ. Reactive lysis: the complement-mediated lysis of unsensitized cells. I. The characterization of the indicator factor and its identification as C7. *J Exp Med.* 1970;131:629–641.
51. Esser AF. Big MAC attack: complement proteins cause leaky patches. *Immunol Today.* 1991;12:316–318.
52. Bhakdi S, Tranum Jensen J. Complement lysis: a hole is a hole. *Immunol Today.* 1991;12:318–320.
53. Nemerow GR, Yamamoto KI, Lint TF. Restriction of complement-mediated membrane damage by the eighth component of complement: a dual role for C8 in the complement attack sequence. *J Immunol.* 1979;123:1245–1252.
54. Peitsch MC, Amiguet P, Guy R, et al. Localization and molecular modelling of the membrane-inserted domain of the ninth component of human complement and perforin. *Mol Immunol.* 1990;27:589–602.
55. Morgan BP. Complement membrane attack on nucleated cells: resistance, recovery and non-lethal effects. *Biochem J.* 1989;264:1–14.
56. Reiter Y, Ciobotariu A, Fishelson Z. Sublytic complement attack protects tumor cells from lytic doses of antibody and complement. *Eur J Immunol.* 1992;22:1207–1213.
57. Fosbrink M, Niculescu F, Rus H. The role of C5b-9 terminal complement complex in activation of the cell cycle and transcription. *Immunol Res.* 2005;31:37–46.
58. Würzner R, Xu H, Franzke A, et al. Blood dendritic cells carry terminal complement complexes on their cell surface as detected by newly developed neoepitope-specific monoclonal antibodies. *Immunology.* 1991;74:132–138.
59. Rus H, Cudrici C, Niculescu F. C5b-9 complement complex in autoimmune demyelination and multiple sclerosis: dual role in neuroinflammation and neuroprotection. *Ann Med.* 2005;37:97–104.
60. Helmy KY, Katschke KJ, Gorgani NN, et al. CRIg: a macrophage complement receptor required for phagocytosis of circulating pathogens. *Cell.* 2006;124:915–927.
61. Ghebrehiwet B, Lim BL, Kumar R, et al. gC1q-R/p33, a member of a new class of multifunctional and multicompartmental cellular proteins, is involved in inflammation and infection. *Immunol Rev.* 2001;180:65–77.
62. Krych-Goldberg M, Atkinson JP. Structure-function relationships of complement receptor type 1. *Immunol Rev.* 2001;180:112–122.
63. Eggleton P, Tenner AJ, Reid KB. C1q receptors. *Clin Exp Immunol.* 2000;120:406–412.
64. Liu YJ, Xu JC, de Bouteiller O, et al. Follicular dendritic cells specifically express the long CR2/CD21 isoform. *J Exp Med.* 1997;185:165–170.
65. Szakonyi G, Guthridge JM, Li D, et al. Structure of complement receptor 2 in complex with its C3d ligand. *Science.* 2001;292:1725–1728.
66. Aubry JP, Pochon S, Graber P, et al. CD21 is a ligand for CD23 and regulates IgE production. *Nature.* 1992;358:505–507.
67. Chen Z, Koralov SB, Kelsoe G. Regulation of the humoral immune responses by CD21/CD35. *Immunol Rev.* 2000;176:194–204.
68. Fearon DT, Carroll MC. Regulation of B lymphocyte responses to foreign and self-antigens by the CD19/CD21 complex. *Annu Rev Immunol.* 2000;18:393–422.
69. Tedder TF, Inaoki M, Sato S. The CD19-CD21 complex regulates signal transduction thresholds governing humoral immunity and autoimmunity. *Immunity.* 1997;6:107–118.
70. Ehlers MR. CR3: a general purpose adhesion-recognition receptor essential for innate immunity. *Microbes Infect.* 2000;2:289–294.
71. Stoiber H, Frank I, Spruth M, et al. Inhibition of HIV-1 infection *in vitro* by monoclonal antibodies to the complement receptor type 3 (CR3): an accessory role for CR3 during virus entry? *Mol Immunol.* 1997;34:855–863.
72. Diamond MS, Garcia-Aguilar J, Bickford JK, et al. The I domain is a major recognition site on the leukocyte integrin Mac-1 (CD11b/CD18) for four distinct adhesion ligands. *J Cell Biol.* 1993;120:1031–1043.

73. Thornton BP, Vetvicka V, Pitman M, et al. Analysis of the sugar specificity and molecular location of the beta-glucan-binding lectin site of complement receptor type 3 (CD11b/CD18). *J Immunol.* 1996;156:1235–1246.
74. Hogg N, Stewart MP, Scarth SL, et al. A novel leukocyte adhesion deficiency caused by expressed but nonfunctional beta2 integrins Mac-1 and LFA-1. *J Clin Invest.* 1999;103:97–106.
75. Stockinger H. Interaction of GPI-anchored cell surface proteins and complement receptor type 3. *Exp Clin Immunogenet.* 1997;14:5–10.
76. Bilsland CA, Diamond MS, Springer TA. The leukocyte integrin p150,95 (CD11c/CD18) as a receptor for iC3b. Activation by a heterologous beta subunit and localization of a ligand recognition site to the I domain. *J Immunol.* 1994;152:4582–4589.
77. Wiesmann C, Katschke KJ, Yin JP, et al. Structure of C3b in complex with CRIg gives insights into regulation of complement activation. *Nature.* 2006;444:217–220.
78. Guo RF, Ward PA. Role of C5a in inflammatory responses. *Annu Rev Immunol.* 2005;23:821–852.
79. Hugli TE. Structure and function of C3a anaphylatoxin. *Curr Top Microbiol Immunol.* 1990;153:181–208.
80. Gerard NP, Lu B, Lui P, et al. An anti-inflammatory function for the complement anaphylatoxin C5a-binding protein, C5L2. *J Biol Chem.* 2005;280:39677–39680.
81. Johswich K, Martin M, Thalmann J, et al. Ligand specificity of the anaphylatoxin C5L2 receptor and its regulation on myeloid and epithelial cell-lines. *J Biol Chem.* 2006;281:39088–39095.
82. Eggleton P, Reid KB, Tenner AJ. C1q—how many functions? How many receptors? *Trends Cell Biol.* 1998;8:428–431.
83. Ghebrehiwet B, Lim BL, Kumar R, et al. gC1q-R/p33, a member of a new class of multifunctional and multicompartmental cellular proteins, is involved in inflammation and infection. *Immunol Rev.* 2001;180:65–77.
84. Henson PM, Bratton DL, Fadok VA. The phosphatidylserine receptor: a crucial molecular switch? *Nat Rev Mol Cell Biol.* 2001;2:627–633.
85. Agrawal A. CRP after 2004. *Mol Immunol.* 2005;42:927–930.
86. McGrath FD, Brouwer MC, Arlaud GJ, et al. Evidence that complement protein C1q interacts with C-reactive protein through its globular head region. *J Immunol.* 2006;176:2950–2957.
87. Berman S, Gewurz H, Mold C. Binding of C-reactive protein to nucleated cells leads to complement activation without cytolysis. *J Immunol.* 1986;136:1354–1359.
88. Sjoberg AP, Trouw LA, McGrath FD, et al. Regulation of complement activation by C-reactive protein: targeting of the inhibitory activity of C4b-binding protein. *J Immunol.* 2006;176:7612–7620.
89. Roumenina LT, Ruseva MM, Zlatarova A, et al. Interaction of C1q with IgG1, C-reactive protein and pentraxin 3: mutational studies using recombinant globular head modules of human C1q A, B, and C chains. *Biochemistry.* 2006;45:4093–4104.
90. Hawlisch H, Kohl J. Complement and Toll-like receptors: key regulators of adaptive immune responses. *Mol Immunol.* 2006;43:13–21.
91. Kopf M, Abel B, Gallimore A, et al. Complement component C3 promotes T-cell priming and lung migration to control acute influenza virus infection. *Nat Med.* 2002;8:373–378.
92. Suresh M, Molina H, Salvato MS, et al. Complement component 3 is required for optimal expansion of CD8 T cells during a systemic viral infection. *J Immunol.* 2003;170:788–794.
93. Peng Q, Li K, Patel H, et al. Dendritic cell synthesis of C3 is required for full T cell activation and development of a Th1 phenotype. *J Immunol.* 2006;176:3330–3341.
94. Yalcindag A, He R, Laouini D, et al. The complement component C3 plays a critical role in both Th1 and Th2 responses to antigen. *J Allergy Clin Immunol.* 2006;117:1455–1461.
95. Kemper C, Chan AC, Green JM, et al. Activation of human CD4+ cells with CD3 and CD46 induces a T-regulatory cell 1 phenotype. *Nature.* 2003;421:388–392.
96. Heeger PS, Lalli PN, Lin F, et al. Decay-accelerating factor modulates induction of T cell immunity. *J Exp Med.* 2005;201:1523–1530.
97. Longhi MP, Sivasankar B, Omidvar N, et al. Cutting edge: murine CD59a modulates antiviral CD4+ T cell activity in a complement-independent manner. *J Immunol.* 2005;175:7098–7102.
98. Prodeus AP, Goerg S, Shen LM, et al. A critical role for complement in maintenance of self-tolerance. *Immunity.* 1998;9:721–731.
99. Cherukuri A, Cheng PC, Pierce SK. The role of the CD19/CD21 complex in B cell processing and presentation of complement-tagged antigens. *J Immunol.* 2001;167:163–172.
100. Lachmann PJ. Complement. In: McGee JOD, Isaacson PG, Wright NA, eds. *Oxford Textbook of Pathology.* Oxford, UK: Oxford University Press; 1992:259–266.
101. Hageman GS, Anderson DH, Johnson LV, et al. A common haplotype in the complement regulatory gene factor H (HF1/CFH) predisposes individuals to age-related macular degeneration. *Proc Natl Acad Sci U S A.* 2005;102:7227–7232.
102. Zipfel PF, Skerka C. Complement dysfunction in hemolytic uremic syndrome. *Curr Opin Rheumatol.* 2006;18:548–555.
103. West C. Complement and glomerular disease. In: Volanakis JE, Frank MM, eds. *The Human Complement System in Health and Disease.* New York: Marcel Dekker; 1998:571–596.
104. Mathieson PW, Würzner R, Oliveria DB, et al. Complement-mediated adipocyte lysis by nephritic factor sera. *J Exp Med.* 1993;177;1827–1831.
105. Appel G, Cook TH, Hageman G, et al. Disease of the month: membranoproliferative glomerulonephritis type II (dense deposit disease): An update. *J Am Soc Nephrol.* 2005;16:1392–1403.
106. Goodship TH. Factor H genotype-phenotype correlations: lessons from aHUS, MPGN II, and AMD. *Kidney Int.* 2006;70:12–13.
107. Dragon-Durey MA, Fremeaux-Bacchi V, Loirat C, et al. Heterozygous and homozygous factor H deficiencies associated with hemolytic uremic syndrome or membranoproliferative glomerulonephritis: report and genetic analysis of 16 cases. *J Am Soc Nephrol.* 2004;15:787–795.
108. Esparza-Gordillo J, Goicoechea de Jorge E, Buil A, et al. Predisposition to atypical hemolytic uremic syndrome involves the concurrence of different susceptibility alleles in the regulators of complement activation gene cluster in 1q32. *Hum Mol Genet.* 2005;14:703–712.
109. Würzner R, Zimmerhackl LB. Therapeutic strategies for atypical and recurrent hemolytic uremic syndromes (HUS). In: Zipfel PF, ed. *Complement and Kidney Disease.* Basel: Birkhäuser; 2006:149–163.
110. Speth C, Dierich MP, Gasque P. Neuroinvasion by pathogens: a key role of the complement system. *Mol Immunol.* 2002;38:669–679.
111. Gasque P, Dean YD, McGreal EP, et al. Complement components of the innate immune system in health and disease in the CNS. *Immunopharmacology.* 2000;49:171–186.
112. Bonifati DM, Kishore U. Role of complement in neurodegeneration and neuroinflammation. *Mol Immunol.* 2007;44:999–1010.
113. Jiang H, Burdick D, Glabe CG, et al. Beta-amyloid activates complement by binding to a specific region of the collagen-like domain of the C1q A chain. *J Immunol.* 1994;152:5050–5059.
114. Johns TG, Bernard CC. Binding of complement component Clq to myelin oligodendrocyte glycoprotein: a novel mechanism for regulating CNS inflammation. *Mol Immunol.* 1997;34:33–38.
115. van der Laan LJ, Ruuls SR, Weber KS, et al. Macrophage phagocytosis of myelin *in vitro* determined by flow cytometry: phagocytosis is mediated by CR3 and induces production of tumor necrosis factor-alpha and nitric oxide. *J Neuroimmunol.* 1996;70:145–152.
116. Speth C, Dierich MP, Sopper S. HIV-infection of the central nervous system: the tightrope walk of innate immunity. *Mol Immunol.* 2005;42:213–228.
117. Figueroa JE, Densen P. Infectious diseases associated with complement deficiencies. *Clin Microbiol Rev.* 1991;4:359–395.
118. Taylor PW. Complement-mediated killing of susceptible gram-negative bacteria: an elusive mechanism. *Exp Clin Immunogenet.* 1992;9:48–56.
119. Würzner R. Evasion of pathogens by avoiding recognition or eradication by complement, in part via molecular mimicry. *Mol Immunol.* 1999;36:249–260.
120. Marschang P, Sodroski J, Würzner R, et al. Decay-accelerating factor (CD55) protects human immunodeficiency virus type I from inactivation by human complement. *Eur J Immunol.* 1995;25:285–290.
121. Stoiber H, Pinter C, Siccardi AG, et al. Efficient destruction of human immunodeficiency virus in human serum by inhibiting the protective action of complement factor H. *J Exp Med.* 1996;183:307–310.

122. Kraiczy P, Würzner R. Complement escape of human pathogenic bacteria by acquisition of complement regulators. *Mol Immunol.* 2006;43:31–44.
123. Jha P, Kotwal GJ. Vaccinia complement control protein: multifunctional protein and a potential wonder drug. *J Biosci.* 2003;28: 265–271.
124. Fishelson Z. Complement evasion by parasites: search for "Achilles' heel." *Clin Exp Immunol.* 1991;86(suppl 1):47–52.
125. Heidenreich F, Dierich MP. *Candida albicans* and *Candida stellatoidea,* in contrast to other *Candida* species, bind iC3b and C3d but not C3b. *Infect Immun.* 1985;50:598–600.
126. Würzner R, Gruber A, Stoiber H, et al. Human immunodeficiency virus type I gp41 binds to *Candida albicans* via complement C3-like regions. *J Infect Dis.* 1997;176:492–498.
127. Gruber A, Lukasser-Vogl E, Borg-von Zepelin M, et al. Human immunodeficiency virus type 1 gp160/gp41 binding to *Candida albicans* enhances candidal virulence *in vitro*. *J Infect Dis.* 1998;177:1057–1063.
128. Brown KM, Kondeatis E, Vaughan RW, et al. Influence of donor C3 allotype on late renal-transplantation outcome. *N Engl J Med.* 2006;354:2014–2023.
129. Racila E, Racila DM, Ritchie JM, et al. The pattern of clinical breast cancer metastasis correlates with a single nucleotide polymorphism in the C1qA component of complement. *Immunogenetics.* 2006;58:1–8.
130. Kardys I, Klaver CC, Despriet DD, et al. A common polymorphism in the complement factor H gene is associated with increased risk of myocardial infarction: the Rotterdam Study. *J Am Coll Cardiol.* 2006;47:1568–1575.
131. Schneider PM, Rittner C. Complement genetics. In: Dodds A, Sim RB, eds. *Complement—A Practical Approach.* Oxford, UK: Oxford University Press; 1997.165–198.
132. Mauff G, Würzner R. Complement Genetics. In: Herzenberg LA, Weir DM, Blackwell C, eds. *Weir's Handbook of Experimental Immunology.* Malden, MA: Blackwell Science; 1997:77.1–77.11.
133. Kirschfink M. The clinical laboratory: testing the complement system. In: Rother K, Till GO, Hansch GM, eds. *The Complement System.* Berlin, Heidelberg, New York: Springer-Verlag; 1998:522–547.
134. Würzner R, Orren A, Lachmann PJ. Inherited deficiencies of the terminal components of human complement. *Immunodefic Rev.* 1992;3:123–147.
135. Würzner R, Mollnes TE, Morgan BP. Immunochemical assays for complement components. In: Johnstone AP, Turner MW, eds. *Immunochemistry 2: A Practical Approach.* Oxford, UK: Oxford University Press; 1997:197–223.
136. Seelen MA, Roos A, Wieslander J, et al. Functional analysis of the classical, alternative, and MBL pathways of the complement system: standardization and validation of a simple ELISA. *J Immunol Methods.* 2005;296:187–198.
137. Thiel S, Frederiksen PD, Jensenius JC. Clinical manifestations of mannan-binding lectin deficiency. *Mol Immunol.* 2006;43:86–96.
138. Morgan BP, Walport MJ. Complement deficiency and disease. *Immunol Today.* 1991;12:301–306.
139. Carugati A, Pappalardo E, Zingale LC, et al. C1-inhibitor deficiency and angioedema. *Mol Immunol.* 2001;38:161–173.
140. Bessler M, Schaefer A, Keller P. Paroxysmal nocturnal hemoglobinuria: insights from recent advances in molecular biology. *Transfus Med Rev.* 2001;15:255–267.
141. Nilsson B, Ekdahl KN, Mollnes TE, et al. The role of complement in biomaterial-induced inflammation. *Mol Immunol.* 2007;44:82–94.
142. Frank MM. Hereditary angioedema. *Curr Opin Pediatr.* 2005;17:686–689.
143. Caliezi C, Wuillemin WA, Zeerleder S, et al. C1-Esterase inhibitor: an anti-inflammatory agent and its potential use in the treatment of diseases other than hereditary angioedema. *Pharmacol Rev.* 2000;52:91–112.
144. Lazar HL, Bokesch PM, van Lenta F, et al. Soluble human complement receptor 1 limits ischemic damage in cardiac surgery patients at high risk requiring cardiopulmonary bypass. *Circulation.* 2004;110(suppl 1):II274–II279.
145. Fraser DA, Harris CL, Williams AS, et al. Generation of a recombinant, membrane-targeted form of the complement regulator CD59: activity *in vitro* and *in vivo*. *J Biol Chem.* 2003;278:48921–48927.
146. Linton SM, Williams AS, Dodd I, et al. Therapeutic efficacy of a novel membrane-targeted complement regulator in antigen-induced arthritis in the rat. *Arthritis Rheum.* 2000;43:2590–2597.
147. Schmid RA, Hillinger S, Hamacher J, et al. TP20 is superior to TP10 in reducing ischemia/reperfusion injury in rat lung grafts. *Transplant Proc.* 2001;33:948–949.
148. Poling J, Oezkur M, Kogge K. Hyperacute rejection in ex vivo-perfused porcine lungs transgenic for human complement regulatory proteins. *Transplant Int.* 2006;19:225–232.
149. Schmidt P, Goto M, Le Mauff B, et al. Adenovirus-mediated expression of human CD55 or CD59 protects adult porcine islets from complement-mediated cell lysis by human serum. *Transplantation.* 2003;75:697–702.
150. Schauber-Plewa C, Simmons A, Tuerk MJ, et al. Complement regulatory proteins are incorporated into lentiviral vectors and protect particles against complement inactivation. *Gene Ther.* 2005;12:238–245.
151. Würzner R, Schulze M, Happe L, et al. Inhibition of terminal complement complex formation and cell lysis by monoclonal antibodies. *Complement Inflamm.* 191;8:328–340.
152. Smith PK, Carrier M, Chen JC, et al. Effect of pexelizumab in coronary artery bypass graft surgery with extended aortic cross-clamp time. *Ann Thorac Surg.* 2006;82:781–788.
153. Mahaffey KW, Van de Werf F, Shernan SK, et al. Effect of pexelizumab on mortality in patients with acute myocardial infarction or undergoing coronary artery bypass surgery: a systematic overview. *Am Heart J.* 2006;152:291–296.
154. Hill A. Eculizumab for the treatment of paroxysmal nocturnal hemoglobinuria. *Clin Adv Hematol Oncol.* 2005;3:849–850.
155. Undar A, Eichstaedt HC, Clubb FJ, et al. Novel anti-factor D monoclonal antibody inhibits complement and leukocyte activation in a baboon model of cardiopulmonary bypass. *Ann Thorac Surg.* 2002;74:355–362.
156. Soulika AM, Holland MC, Sfyroera G, et al. Compstatin inhibits complement activation by binding to the beta-chain of complement factor 3. *Mol Immunol.* 2006;43:2023–2039.
157. Baelder R, Fuchs B, Bautsch W, et al. Pharmacological targeting of anaphylatoxin receptors during the effector phase of allergic asthma suppresses airway hyperresponsiveness and airway inflammation. *J Immunol.* 2005;174:783–789.
158. Woodruff TM, Arumugam TV, Shiels IA, et al. A potent human C5a receptor antagonist protects against disease pathology in a rat model of inflammatory bowel disease. *J Immunol.* 2003;171:5514–5520.
159. Proctor LM, Woodruff TM, Sharma P, et al. Transdermal pharmacology of small molecule cyclic C5a antagonists. *Adv Exp Med Biol.* 2006;586:329–345.
160. Gelderman KA, Tomlinson S, Ross GD, et al. Complement function in mAb-mediated cancer immunotherapy. *Trends Immunol.* 2004;25:158–164.
161. Golay J, Cittera E, Di Gaetano N, et al. The role of complement in the therapeutic activity of rituximab in a murine B lymphoma model homing in lymph nodes. *Haematologica.* 2006;91:176–183.
162. Huang J, Shibaguchi H, Zhao J, et al. IgG isotype conversion of a novel human anti-carcinoembryonic antigen antibody to increase its biological activity. *Anticancer Res.* 2006;26:1057–1063.
163. Dall'Acqua WF, Cook KE, Damschroder MM, et al. Modulation of the effector functions of a human IgG1 through engineering of its hinge region. *J Immunol.* 2006;177:1129–1138.
164. Li B, Allendorf DJ, Hansen R, et al. Yeast beta-glucan amplifies phagocyte killing of iC3b-opsonized tumor cells via complement receptor 3-Syk-phosphatidylinositol 3-kinase pathway. *J Immunol.* 2006;177:1661–1669.
165. Kennedy AD, Solga MD, Schuman TA, et al. An anti-C3b(i) mAb enhances complement activation, C3b(i) deposition, and killing of CD20+ cells by rituximab. *Blood.* 2003;101:1071–1079.
166. Mikesch JH, Buerger H, Simon R, et al. Decay-accelerating factor (CD55): a versatile acting molecule in human malignancies. *Biochim Biophys Acta.* 2006;1766:42–52.
167. Pritchard-Jones K, Spendlove I, Wilton C, et al. Immune responses to the 105AD7 human anti-idiotypic vaccine after intensive chemotherapy, for osteosarcoma. *Br J Cancer.* 2005;92:1358–1365.

168. Maxwell-Armstrong C. Studies using the anti-idiotypic monoclonal antibody 105AD7 in patients with primary and advanced colorectal cancer. *Ann R Coll Surg Engl.* 2002;84:314–318.
169. Terui Y, Sakurai T, Mishima Y, et al. Blockade of bulky lymphoma-associated CD55 expression by RNA interference overcomes resistance to complement-dependent cytotoxicity with rituximab. *Cancer Sci.* 2006;97:72–79.
170. Shafren DR, Au GG, Nguyen T, et al. Systemic therapy of malignant human melanoma tumors by a common cold-producing enterovirus, coxsackievirus a21. *Clin Cancer Res.* 2004;10:53–60.
171. Ong HT, Timm MM, Greipp PR, et al. Oncolytic measles virus targets high CD46 expression on multiple myeloma cells. *Exp Hematol.* 2006;34:713–720.
172. Heinzerling L, Kunzi V, Oberholzer PA, et al. Oncolytic measles virus in cutaneous T-cell lymphomas mounts antitumor immune responses *in vivo* and targets interferon-resistant tumor cells. *Blood.* 2005;106:2287–2294.
173. Springfeld C, von Messling V, Frenzke M, et al. Oncolytic efficacy and enhanced safety of measles virus activated by tumor-secreted matrix metalloproteinases. *Cancer Res.* 2006;66:7694–7700.
174. Ni S, Gaggar A, DiPaolo N, et al. Evaluation of adenovirus vectors containing serotype 35 fibers for tumor targeting. *Cancer Gene Ther.* 2006;13:1072–1081.
175. Suominen E, Toivonen R, Grenman R, et al. Head and neck cancer cells are efficiently infected by Ad5/35 hybrid virus. *J Gene Med.* 2006;8:1223–1231.
176. DiPaolo N, Ni S, Gaggar A, et al. Evaluation of adenovirus vectors containing serotype 35 fibers for vaccination. *Mol Ther.* 2006;13:756–765.
177. Fearon DT. Innate immunity—beginning to fulfill its promise? *Nat Immunol.* 2000;1:102–103.
178. Bergmann-Leitner ES, Leitner WW, Tsokos GC. Complement 3d: from molecular adjuvant to target of immune escape mechanisms. *Clin Immunol.* 2006;121:177–185.
179. Quigg RJ. Use of complement inhibitors in tissue injury. *Trends Mol Med.* 2002;8:430–436.
180. Stammberger U, Hamacher J, Hillinger S, Schmid RA. sCR1sLe ameliorates ischemia/reperfusion injury in experimental lung transplantation. *J Thorac Cardiovasc Surg.* 2000;120:1078–1084.
181. Rioux P. TP-10 (AVANT Immunotherapeutics). *Curr Opin Investig Drugs.* 2001;2:364–371
182. Manzi L, Montano R, Abad MJ, et al. Expression of human soluble complement receptor 1 by a pig endothelial cell line inhibits lysis by human serum. *Xenotransplantation.* 2006;13:75–79
183. Szebeni J, Fontana JL, Wassef NM, et al. Hemodynamic changes induced by liposomes and liposome-encapsulated hemoglobin in pigs: a model for pseudoallergic cardiopulmonary reactions to liposomes. *Circulation.* 1999;99:2302–2309.
184. Yazdanbakhsh K. Complement receptor 1 therapeutics for prevention of immune hemolysis. *Immunohematology.* 2005;21:109–118.
185. Frank MM. Hereditary angioedema. *Curr Opin Pediatr.* 2005;17:686–689.
186. Heijnen BH, Straatsburg IH, Padilla ND, et al. Inhibition of classical complement activation attenuates liver ischaemia and reperfusion injury in a rat model. *Clin Exp Immunol.* 2006;143:15–23.
187. Radke A, Mottaghy K, Goldmann C, et al. C1 inhibitor prevents capillary leakage after thermal trauma. *Crit Care Med.* 2000;28:3224–3232.
188. Benson EM. Immunologic manipulation for the threatened fetus. *Thromb Res.* 2004;114:427–434.
189. Thielmann M, Marggraf G, Neuhauser M, et al. Administration of C1-esterase inhibitor during emergency coronary artery bypass surgery in acute ST-elevation myocardial infarction. *Eur J Cardiothorac Surg.* 2006;30:285–293.
190. Kirschfink M. C1-inhibitor and transplantation. *Immunobiology* 2002;205:534–541.
191. Hill A, Ridley SH, Esser D, et al. Protection of erythrocytes from human complement-mediated lysis by membrane-targeted recombinant soluble CD59: a new approach to PNH therapy. *Blood.* 2006;107:2131–2137
192. Kaplan M. Eculizumab (Alexion). *Curr Opin Investig Drugs.* 2002;3:1017–1023.
193. Carrier M, Menasche P, Levy JH, et al. Inhibition of complement activation by pexelizumab reduces death in patients undergoing combined aortic valve replacement and coronary artery bypass surgery. *J Thorac Cardiovasc Surg.* 2006;131:352–356.
194. Hangen DH, Stevens JH, Satoh PS, et al. Complement levels in septic primates treated with anti-C5a antibodies. *J Surg Res.* 1989;46:195–199.
195. Ames RS, Lee D, Foley JJ et al. Identification of a selective non-peptide antagonist of the anaphylatoxin C3a receptor that demonstrates antiinflammatory activity in animal models. *J Immunol.* 2001;166:6341–6348.
196. Woodruff TM, Crane JW, Proctor LM et al. Therapeutic activity of C5a receptor antagonists in a rat model of neurodegeneration. *FASEB J.* 2006;20:1407–1417.
197. Taylor RP. Of mice and mechanisms: identifying the role of complement in monoclonal antibody-based immunotherapy. *Haematologica.* 2006;91:146a.
198. Takami A, Hayashi T, Kita D, et al. Treatment of primary central nervous system lymphoma with induction of complement-dependent cytotoxicity by intraventricular administration of autologous-serum-supplemented rituximab. *Cancer Sci.* 2006;97:80–83.
199. Adams GP, Weiner LM. Monoclonal antibody therapy of cancer. *Nat Biotechnol.* 2005;23:1147–1157.
200. Tong T, Fan H, Tan Y, et al. C3d enhanced DNA vaccination induced humoral immune response to glycoprotein C of pseudorabies virus. *Biochem Biophys Res Commun.* 2006;347:845–851.

Chapter 34

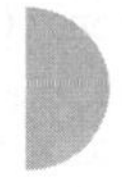

Cytotoxic T Lymphocytes

R. Chris Bleackley

The cell-mediated immune system serves to defend organisms against intracellular pathogens through the action of cytolytic effector cells. These effectors can destroy targets infected by a virus or harboring microbes and are also believed to be involved in the eradication of tumors, the rejection of transplants, and the pathogenesis of a number of autoimmune diseases. In vertebrates, defense occurs through two distinct mechanisms: the innate and the adaptive responses. During innate immunity pathogens are destroyed when macrophages and monocytes perform phagocytosis and when granulocytic cells, such as eosinophils, release cytotoxic substances. Natural killer (NK) cells are also considered part of innate immunity. These responses are extremely important for the successful removal of many pathogens and are also involved in the body's ability to inhibit tumorigenesis. However, the innate immune response is unable to adapt to changing pathogens that may be encountered during the host's lifetime. This is achieved via the adaptive immune response, which is specifically activated by, and targeted against, the antigens expressed by the invading organism. Although this type of response requires a few days to develop, it is able to eliminate the pathogen with minimum damage to noninfected tissues. An adaptive response is also able to retain memory of antigen exposure and thus is able to mount a quicker and more powerful response when again presented with the same antigens. The adaptive immune response therefore possesses two main advantages of specificity and memory that contributes to the success of pathogen removal.

The adaptive effectors are T lymphocytes (both CD8$^+$ and CD4$^+$ cells). It was originally believed that CD4 cells were exclusively regulators and CD8 the major effectors of cell mediated immune responses. This is still a convenient way of thinking, but it is now clear that there is some overlap in functions. For the sake of simplicity most of the discussion in this chapter will deal primarily with CD8 cells, but it should be realized that CD4 killers can use similar molecules to destroy targets. In addition, T and NK cells are very similar in their mechanisms of killing, although the ways in which they recognize targets are different. NK cells are discussed in detail in Chapter 16.

BASIC BIOLOGY/HISTORY OF CTL-MEDIATED KILLING

The first experimental models of killing were developed in the 1960s with *in vivo* sensitized effectors acting *ex vivo* to destroy targets (1). Early progress was rather slow because there was no easy way to measure lysis other than by direct observation. However, a major breakthrough came with the development of an assay to monitor and quantify lytic activity based on the release of radioactive chromium (Cr^{51}) from targets undergoing lysis (2). Healthy cells will take up the isotope in the form of chromate, and the reduced chromium becomes stably complexed with intracellular proteins. When the cell lyses the chromium is released and can be quantified as a measure of lytic activity. Using this assay, a series of insightful experiments were performed during the next decade that provided the fundamental description of the biology of cytotoxic T lymphocyte (CTL)–mediated killing (3,4). Indeed, this measurement of lysis by chromium release was used by Zinkernagel and Doherty to establish the basis of MHC restriction (5).

Target cell lysis was observed to be quite rapid and was not blocked by inhibitors of protein synthesis (6), suggesting that preformed mediators of cell death were carried by activated CTL. The lytic reaction required cell–cell contact, was unidirectional, and the effector came away uninjured to kill multiple targets (7). In addition, neighboring cells that were not recognized by the effectors were spared which led to the concept of a directed, local mechanism of cytolysis (2).

During these early days, the discovery of interleukin (IL)-2 and its use to generate functional clones of CTL was particularly significant (8). This allowed investigators to generate large numbers of functional cells and thus pursue the biochemical and genetic analyses of CTL-killing mechanisms. The model of killing that was developed divided the process into three stages: CTL-target binding; programming the target for lysis; and finally, target cell death. The initial contact between the cells was independent of antigen and mediated by the interactions of LFA-1 (lymphocyte function-associated antigen 1) and CD2 on the T cell with ICAM-1 and LFA-3 on the target. This early adhesion step required a few minutes and was dependent on magnesium. The importance of these initial interactions was underscored by transfection experiments showing that antigen-specific lysis does not occur unless the nonspecific binding occurs (9). Indeed, recent data provide evidence that LFA-1 delivers a signal that is essential for the degranulation process discussed later (10). Specific interactions then occur between TCR and antigen/MHC, and without this critical step the cells move apart. Finally, CD8 strengthens the interaction by binding directly to MHC.

The end result of these signal transduction events is a dramatic reorganization of the CTL and the polarized exocytosis of cytoplasmic granules discussed in detail later. After delivery of the kiss of death, it takes a couple of hours to see significant lysis as measured by the chromium release assay. However, recent studies that monitor events, such as mitochondria depolarization and DNA fragmentation, demonstrate that the target is on the road to death much sooner. Interestingly, the killer cell is no longer needed and can detach to go in search of its next target.

CTL DIFFERENTIATION AND FORMATION OF GRANULES

$CD8^+$ T cells are stimulated through recognition of antigen bound to major histocompatibility complex (MHC) class I protein through the T cell receptor (TCR) and CD8 coreceptor. The initial activation involves three cellular players. First, antigen is presented by professional APCs, such as macrophages, which secrete IL-1. This acts on helper T cells to stimulate proliferation and production of IL-2, which stimulate the differentiation of precursor CTL into active killers.

Several intracellular events are triggered by this intimate contact between CTL and antigen presenting cells (APC). The signal transduction pathway involves the TCR-associated CD3 complex and kinases, such as lymphocyte cell kinase ($p56^{lck}$) and protein kinase C. At the same time, inositol triphosphate, produced by the action of phospholipase C on phosphatidyl bisphosphate, induces the release of calcium from intracellular stores. This is accompanied by an influx of extracellular calcium, and a net result is an increase in intracellular calcium. This lymphocyte activation can be duplicated *in vitro* with factors such as CD3 antibodies (αCD3) and concanavalin A (con A) in the presence of the cytokine IL-2.

Early events in effector differentiation have been studied extensively in $CD4^+$ T cells and to a lesser extent in $CD8^+$ T cells. Downstream signaling pathways are initiated almost immediately after TCR stimulation and within hours induce the transcription of hallmarks of early T cell activation such as the IL-2 gene. Effector CTL differentiation occurs 3 to 5 days after activation and a number of CTL effector-specific genes, including the granzymes, granulysin, perforin, and RANTES are up-regulated at this

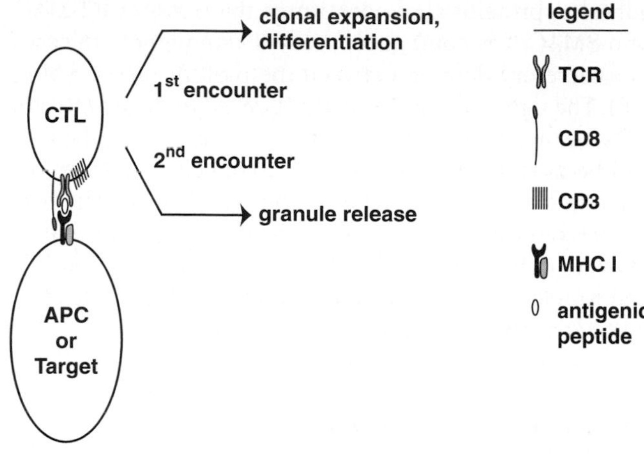

FIGURE 34.1 CTL binds to an antigen expressing cell. The CTL binds to an APC during the initial activation events. This results in clonal expression, differentiation, and expression of cytotoxicity-related proteins. When the activated CTL then binds to a target, the granules polarize and are released towards the target.

time. For example, granzyme B gene transcription, an important granule constituent of the CTL, begins after 48 hours of *in vitro* activation of primary murine CD8$^+$ T cells, and peaks after 5 days have passed (11). Little is known about the processes inducing transcription of these late genes, many of which are important for the establishment of CTL cytotoxicity and are essential components of the granules that develop in the CTL.

When CD8$^+$ T cells differentiate into effector CTLs, a number of proteins are expressed that allow the CTL to perform their effector functions. Naïve CD8$^+$ T lymphocytes are unable to kill and do not contain cytotoxic granules. During the period of effector differentiation, many effector proteins unique to CTLs are transcribed and translated. These nascent proteins are then packaged within the new cytoplasmic granules. However, MHC class I molecules are not restricted to so-called *professional APCs,* but are expressed by every cell in the body. Therefore, CD8$^+$ T cells can recognize when a cell of the body displays an altered self-protein via the MHC class I receptor. Thus, although the signal transduction events are similar, there is a fundamental difference between a naïve T cell being stimulated and an armed killer that encounters an antigen-positive target (Figure 34.1). In the latter case, the interaction now results in the polarization of granules and delivery of the kiss of death.

CYTOTOXIC GRANULES AND EXOCYTOSIS

Cytotoxic granules are also known as *secretory lysosomes.* They have a dense core of proteins required for granule-mediated target cell death, surrounded by a multilamellar region similar to lysosomes. They first appear as multivesicular structures that slowly acquire dense cores as newly translated secretory proteins accumulate within the organelles (12). The targeting of some of the granule-proteins (e.g., granzymes, discussed later) is directed to the organelle via a mannose-6-phosphate signal, while others (e.g., perforin) must use a different mechanism (13). The organelles are acidic, with a pH around 5, and act in the CTL both as a lysosomal organelle, and as a secretory granule (14).

The secretory lysosome differs from normal lysosomes in that it can fuse with the plasma membrane in a regulated fashion in response to activation of the TCR by a virus-infected or tumor cell. TCR engagement initiates tyrosine kinase signaling cascades and calcium influx that causes a dramatic reorganization of the CTL. Shortly after contact, the microtubule organizing center (MTOC) and Golgi apparatus reorient toward the point of contact with the target, and the nucleus moves away (15). This suggested that a polarized secretory mechanism was involved in the killing process. At around the same time, it was demonstrated that cytoplasmic granules isolated from NK and CTL were cytolytic (16,17). The observations that the granules polarize and contained lytic effectors led to the formulation of the granule exocytosis model of CTL function (18). A simplified view of the process is depicted in Figure 34.2.

Henkart suggested that CTL produce potent lytic molecules and store them in cytoplasmic granules. Upon target cell recognition, the granules move toward the point of contact and the contents are exocytosed to deliver the lethal hit. Immunofluorescent staining revealed that the actin and tubulin in the CTL were also polarized toward the target. These provide the tracks for the movement of granules toward the target. This view was substantiated by direct visualization of cell conjugates using high-resolution Nomarski optics cinematography (19). The

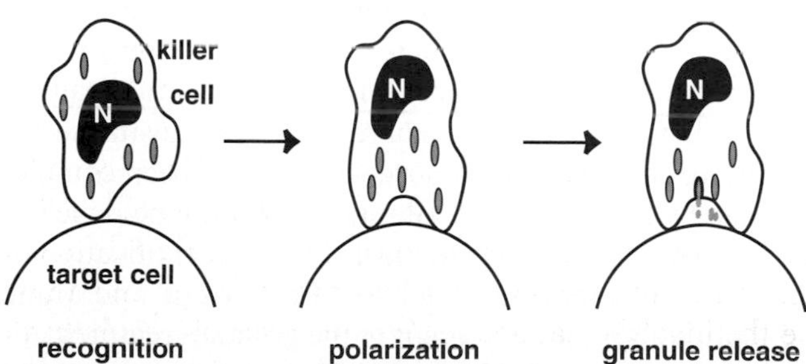

FIGURE 34.2 The steps during CTL-mediated killing. The target is recognized by the CTL via nonspecific adhesion, then specific interaction with the TCR. This latter tight binding results in the polarization of the microtubule organizing center; the Golgi and the granules move toward the target. The nucleus appears to move to the side, and the granules fuse with the CTL membrane in the region of contact with the target. This results in the release of the granule contents including perforin and granzymes.

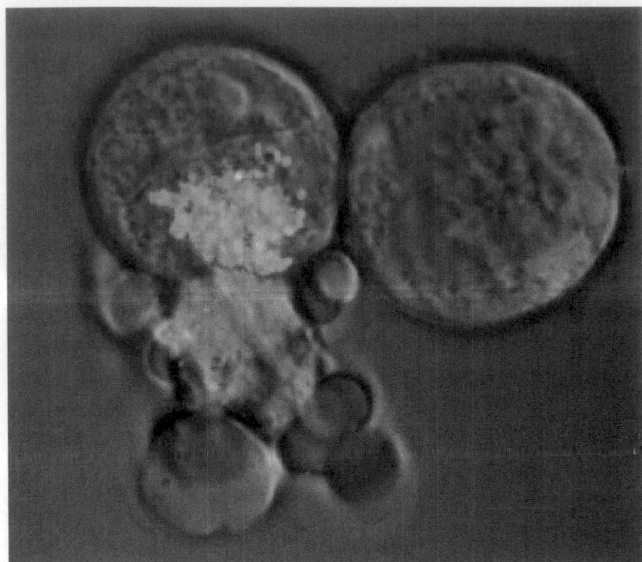

FIGURE 34.3 Killing in action. This cytotoxic cell appears to contact two targets (red); however, the granules (green) are polarized to the left-hand target. The cell exhibits the characteristic blebbing of apoptosis. The other target seems unaffected. Figure provided by Dr. I.S. Goping, University of Alberta. (See color insert.)

nucleus was seen to be displaced and the granules migrated toward the contact site. Importantly, microtubule-disrupting drugs inhibited target cell lysis (20), suggesting that the polarization of granules toward the target was critically important. Figure 34.3 shows, quite dramatically, a cytolytic cell in action. The granules are polarized toward one cell and the nucleus is shifted aside. Clearly, the target involved in degranulation is dying (the blebbing is characteristic of apoptosis, and this will be discussed later), while the other target appears unaffected.

The movement of the granules has been shown in an *in vitro* assay to be dependent on kinesin (21), but the components of the molecular machinery that control granule exocytosis are only now coming to light. Interestingly, a number of candidates were identified through the analysis of coat color mutant strains of mice when it was realized that melanocytes and CTL share the same unusual secretory lysosome (22). The mouse studies have been complemented by the analysis of albinism and immune deficiencies in patients (23), which has led to the identification of regulators of exocytosis, such as AP3, Rab27a, and Munc 13-4. Although the movement of the granules requires microtubules it appears that the final step of delivery to the plasma membrane is dependent on polarization of the centrosome (24).

After CTL-target conjugation there is also a redistribution of adhesion and signalling molecules to the region of contact (25). The central area, called the *central supramolecular activation complex* (c-SMAC), contains the TCR and CD8 molecules and is surrounded by a ring of adhesion proteins that constitutes the peripheral-SMAC, or p-SMAC. The contents of the lytic granules are released in a secretory domain between the p-SMAC and c-SMAC (26). The tight synapse formed between target and effector cells ensures that the lytic proteins released from the CTL will be quickly taken up to the target cell, and therefore avoid damage to other neighboring cells. This mechanism of targeted exocytosis of granules allows the CTL killing machinery to be directed very specifically to the target cell and to release the contents of the cytotoxic granules in a very concentrated manner.

GRANULE CONTENTS

The most abundant proteins found in granules are perforin and granzymes. However, proteoglycans, some Fas ligand protein, and a few cytokines are also present. Other proteins that are contained in granules, but not exclusively found in CTLs, are calreticulin, and lysosomal proteins.

Perforin

Perforin was first identified as a lytic molecule found in cytotoxic granules (27,28). The protein, also known as *cytolysin* in the early days, is a 65 kDa polypeptide that can bind to lipids. The gene was cloned (29,30) and the amino acid sequence predicted a region of strong homology to the pore-forming C9 protein of complement (31). Perforin was consequently shown to polymerise and form pores in the membranes of red blood cells (32). It is sorted into lytic granules by a mannose phosphate–independent, unknown mechanism. Once inside the granules perforin is proteolytically activated into a mature form (33). It is inactive in the acidic environment of the cytotoxic granule, but forms pores when released into the neutral environment of the intermembrane space in the presence of Ca^{2+}. This led to the proposition that CTLs caused death by releasing perforin to disrupt the plasma membrane of the target cell through pore formation. However, CTL-induced apoptosis does not only result in cell lysis and membrane damage, but includes DNA fragmentation, suggesting additional factors besides perforin were involved in CTL-mediated cell death (34). These factors were later identified as a family of serine proteases, now called *granzymes,* which will be discussed in the next section.

The generation of perforin knockout mice showed the critical role of perforin for granule-mediated cytotoxicity of the CTL (35), and to allow the delivery of granzymes into the cytoplasm of target cells. This delivery was originally visualized with granzymes simply entering into target cells through perforin pores formed in the plasma membrane. However, addition of sublytic concentrations of perforin that do not form pores in the plasma membrane is still sufficient to enable granzyme entry into target cells.

Surprisingly, granzymes have also been shown to enter into target cells independently of perforin, but the proteases remain harmlessly confined to endocytic vesicles until perforin, or another permeabilizing agent, releases them (36). Granzyme B entry into target cells will be discussed in more detail later.

The structure function analysis of perforin has not been well studied because of the inability to express the recombinant protein. Recently, a baculovirus system has been developed and used to confirm that the carboxyl C2 motif is responsible for membrane binding and to define the residues important for lysis (37). In addition, the functional analysis of a number of the mutant forms of perforin present in patients have been carried out (38).

Granzymes

The granzymes are a family of serine proteinases that colocalize with perforin in the granules. Only granzymes A (grA) and B (grB) are found in any abundance in CTL, and they will be a major focus of discussion in this chapter. Both are synthesized as preproenzymes with the hydrophobic leader sequence removed upon entry into the endoplasmic reticulum. The proenzyme is activated by the removal of the aminoterminal dipeptide by the enzyme cathepsin C as the granzymes are packaged into granules (39). All family members are highly basic, which likely contributes to their interaction with proteoglycans.

The genes for granzymes A and B were first cloned (40,41), and then the proteins isolated (42). Granzyme B was predicted to have unusual substrate specificity for cleavage at aspartate (43), and this was confirmed biochemically (44). No other eukaryotic serine protease cleaves at an aspartic acid, and this specificity allows granzyme B to act like an initiator caspase to activate apoptosis, as will be discussed later. Granzyme A resembles trypsin as it cleaves after argine and lysine residues and can conveniently be detected using benzoyl lysine thioester as a substrate (45). Both granzymes are targeted to granules by the mannose-6-phosphate receptor (46).

Proteoglycan

Serglycin is the proteoglycan that is found in CTL granules. It is believed to be involved in the packing of lytic compounds within the organelles. The protein consists of serine-glycine repeats to which sulphated glycosaminoglycan chains are linked. Overall, the molecule is very negatively charged, which likely contributes to its ability to bind to the basic granule components. In isolated granules, there are stable interactions between the serglycin and granzyme A (47), granzyme B (48), and perforin (49). The interaction appears to be ionic since high salt disrupts the complexes. Knocking out the serglycin gene leads to impaired ability to produce dense granules and a reduction in granule protease activity (50). The complexes of serglycin with granzymes and perforin are maintained after exocytosis. Interestingly, these complexes can still mediate killing (48,51).

Other Cytotoxic Granule Proteins

Fas ligand was first thought to be present exclusively on the surface of CTLs, but it has also been shown to be stored in cytotoxic granules (52). The protein activates cell death at the plasma membrane, and the stored FasL translocates in a polarized manner to the plasma membrane, where the synapse with the target cell has formed. This allows FasL-induced apoptosis to occur in a directed manner to the target cell and avoids nonspecific bystander killing. The nascent protein is delivered to the granules from the trans-Golgi network following a distinct sorting mechanism (52).

Chemokines, such as RANTES and macrophage inflammatory protein (MIP-1α), have also been found in cytotoxic granules and are important in lysis of virion-producing cells in HIV-1 infection (53). Another protein present is granulysin (54), a member of the saposin-like protein family (55). This novel cationic protein is active against a broad range of gram-positive and -negative bacteria, fungi, and parasites (56). It has been also suggested that granulysin may play a role in CTL action on tumors and act as a chemoattractant and pro-inflammatory mediator (57). Rather surprisingly, no mouse homologue has been described.

Calreticulin (CRT) is a calcium storage protein and chaperone normally found in the endoplasmic reticulum, but has also been found in the cytotoxic granules of CTLs (58). CRT expression is up-regulated upon CTL activation and is found to interact with perforin to inhibit its lytic activity (59). The exact role for CRT in lytic granules is not fully understood, as CTLs derived from knockout mice possess functional lytic machinery. The effectors from the deficient mice did, however, show a compromised level of killing that correlated with reduced conjugate formation and defects in calcium signalling (60,61).

Lysosomal hydrolases, such as cathepsin B, C, D, and cathepsin A-like protective protein, acid phosphatase, arylsulphatase, and α-glucosidase, are found in the periphery of the cytolytic granules. Also present is cathepsin C, which is responsible for the proteolytic maturation of the enzymes granzyme A and B (39). Lysosomal membrane proteins, such as Lamp-1, Lamp-2, and CD63, are also present on the membrane surface of cytotoxic granules.

GRANULE-INDEPENDENT MECHANISMS OF TARGET CELL LYSIS

Although the granule-mediated mechanism became the accepted paradigm for target cell death, it soon became clear that this was not the complete story. CTL lines were described that would kill targets in the absence of calcium, did not express perforin or granzymes, and were lytic without exocytosis (62,63). This alternate form of death was found to be mediated by Fas ligand on the surface of the CTL, which binds Fas expressed by the target (64). These mechanisms are not mutually exclusive and often may act in concert. Most short-term assays are dominated by granule exocytosis, and Fas is only revealed if this is blocked pharmacologically by, for example, concanamycin A (65) or in perforin knock out CTL (66). For long-term assays, the Fas pathway becomes more important, and death induced by TNF is also apparent (67).

APOPTOSIS AND NECROSIS

The observation that CTL-mediated death was accompanied by fragmentation of the target cell DNA led to the hypothesis that apoptosis was being activated. This, indeed, proved to be the case, but it is now clear that the targets can also die by necrosis, particularly if apoptosis is inhibited. Clearly, the *in vitro* death induced by perforin resembles necrotic death. Necrosis was originally thought to be a passive process resulting from extreme environmental pressure, such as heat or a noxious chemical. The process begins in the cell with organelle swelling and is accompanied by early disruption of the cell membrane resulting in the release of cellular contents that leads to inflammation of surrounding tissues. Apoptosis, in contrast, is a quiet form of cell death where cellular contents remain neatly packaged in membrane-enclosed apoptotic bodies that are rapidly engulfed by phagocytic cells.

Cells undergoing apoptosis can be recognized by a variety of distinct morphological and biochemical changes. There is characteristic blebbing of the plasma membrane, and condensation and fragmentation of the chromatin. The cell breaks up into small apoptotic bodies that are phagocytosed efficiently by macrophages (68). The apoptotic cells are phagocytosed so efficiently because of the appearance of novel molecules on the surface that can be recognized by phagocytes. One such example is the movement of phosphatidyl serine (PS) from the inner to the outer membrane. PS exposure is an "eat me" signal for phagocytic cells like macrophages and dendritic cells (69), allowing apoptotic cells to be removed with minimal inflammation (70). It is rather surprising to realize that the membrane rupture that is revealed by the chromium release assay likely never occurs *in vivo* when a target under attack by a CTL dies by apoptosis. Long before membrane rupture, the doomed cell is removed by the extremely efficient phagocytic process.

The most striking biochemical change during CTL-mediated apoptosis is the characteristic internucleosomal degradation of chromosomal DNA. This creates a "ladder" of oligonucleosomal fragments when apoptotic DNA is visualised by agarose gel electrophoresis (71). Degradation occurs when caspase-activated DNAse, or CAD, is activated in the apoptotic process. The active caspase actually cleaves the inhibitor of CAD (ICAD). The freed nuclease then translocates to the nucleus and induces double-strand breaks between the nucleosomes (hence the ladder). These caspases are at the very heart of apoptosis and, as we will see, are very much involved in granzyme B and Fas-mediated death.

Caspases

Caspases (cysteinyl aspartate-specific proteinases) are proteases that have a cysteine residue in the active site and cleave substrates on the carboxyl side of aspartate residues (72). These proteins are present in every cell as inactive pro-enzymes that contain an inhibitory domain at their amino-terminal and a small and large subunit. The enzyme is activated when the pro-domain is cleaved from the rest of the protein. Upstream or initiator caspases are activated at the beginning of apoptotic cascades, generally after recruitment to a receptor as during Fas-mediated cell death. Downstream or effector caspases are directly or indirectly activated by upstream caspases and can also be cleaved by the CTL protein granzyme B. Effector caspases, such as caspase-3, act as the executioners and cleave substrates throughout the cell.

One of the key substrates is ICAD, or inhibitor of caspase-activated DNAse. This inhibitory protein is normally bound to CAD (caspase-activated DNAse) in the cytoplasm of a healthy cell. When cleaved by an effector caspase, ICAD no longer inhibits the CAD enzyme, which translocates to the nucleus and is responsible for the internucleosomal degradation of the chromosomal DNA (73). Caspases also cleave a number of structural proteins, such as lamins, actin, and fodrin, leading to cell shrinkage and cytoskeletal rearrangements. The loss of mitochondrial potential and leakage of mitochondrial proteins can also be caused by caspase activity during apoptosis. All of these features are seen in CTL-mediated death. As seen in Figure 34.3, the dying target cell shows the classic apoptotic blebbing.

FAS-MEDIATED CELL DEATH

Death receptors of the tumor-necrosis factor receptor (TNFR) family, including the FasL protein, are expressed on the surface of effector CTLs. The FasL protein has been found to induce Ca^{2+}-independent apoptosis in target cells expressing the Fas receptor, also known as CD95 (64). This receptor-ligand binding causes clustering of the receptor molecules and recruitment of signaling molecules to form a multiprotein complex called the DISC, or death-inducing signalling complex (74). The DISC consists of a docking protein FADD (Fas-associated death domain) and pro-caspase-8. The clustering of the Fas protein causes FADD proteins to bind to the intracellular tail of the Fas receptors via the presence of homologous death domain protein motifs in both FADD and Fas (75). This protein scaffold then recruits pro-caspase-8 molecules by binding of homologous death effector domains (DEDs) present in both FADD and the pro-domain of caspase-8. The close association of a number of pro-caspase-8 proteins allows the slight activity of the pro-enzyme to trans-activate other caspase-8 molecules in close proximity (76).

The consequences of caspase-8 activation are shown in Figure 34.4. Activated caspase-8 initiates apoptosis in one of two ways, depending on the cell type (77). In type I cells, the effector caspase-3 is activated directly by caspase-8, while in type II cells, caspase-8 cleaves Bid, a pro-apoptotic member of the Bcl family of proteins, to create a truncated form, or tBid (78). This protein will move to the mitochondria to initiate the mitochondrial pathway of apoptosis. As a result of cytochrome c release from the mitochondria, caspase-9 is activated in the apoptosome (79). The activated caspase-9 then acts with caspase-8 to amplify cleavage of the executioner caspase-3. This is really the point of no return, as the activated caspase-3 then cleaves a variety of substrates, including ICAD, leading to DNA fragmentation.

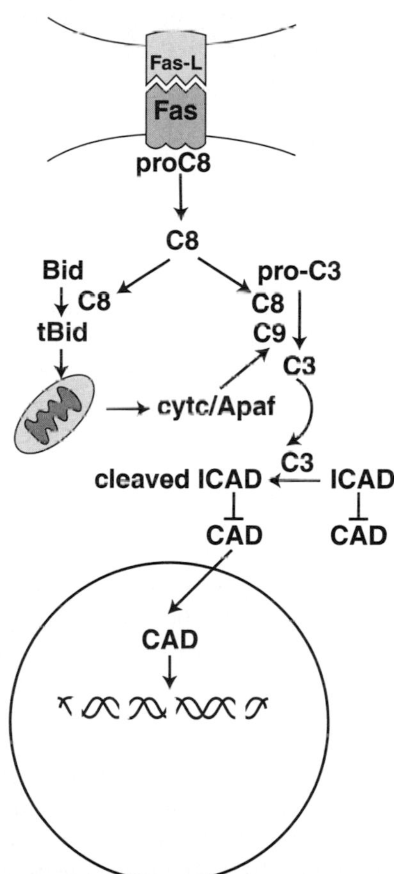

FIGURE 34.4 The pathway activated by Fas. Ligation of Fas on the target by Fas-ligand on the CTL results in activation of caspase-8 (C8). This protease can cleave and activate caspase-3 (C3). It also cleaves Bid, which then translocates to the mitochondria. Cytochrome c (cytc) is released and activates caspase-9 (C9) in the apoptosome. The caspase-9 then amplifies the amount of active caspase-3, which acts on ICAD. The released CAD translocates to the nucleus and generates double-stranded breaks.

GRANULE-MEDIATED CELL DEATH

Granule exocytosis has become well established as the major mechanism of CTL-induced cell death. This pathway begins with the targeted secretion of granules that releases the granule contents into a target cell to induce both caspase-dependent and caspase-independent cell death. The purification and characterization of perforin was critical for our current understanding of CTL-induced death. However, it was soon realized that other components were needed to duplicate all of the features of killing by intact CTL. In particular, perforin could not induce the DNA fragmentation observed in a cell–cell killing assay. Three lines of experimentation came together to conclude that granzyme B was critical for the DNA fragmentation activity. First, a classic biochemical approach to purify the "fragmentin" activity identified the factor as granzyme B (80,81). The second was a more molecular/cell biology investigation in which noncytotoxic RBL mast cell tumors had to be transfected with both perforin and granzyme B cDNAs in order to mediate both membrane damage and DNA fragmentation. Importantly, transfection with just perforin endowed the cell with only membranolytic activity (82,83). The final approach took advantage of knockout technology to develop mice with no functional granzyme B. CTL from the deficient animals could still cause chromium release in targets, but were severely compromised in early DNA fragmentation (84). Although knocking out granzyme A alone had little effect, the combination of removing both A and B reduced DNA fragmentation still further. Cytolytic effectors from these double knockout mice could still mediate membrane damage (85), but their effectiveness *in vivo* was severely compromised (86). Collectively, these results suggest that perforin facilitates entry of granzymes into targets that then actually provide the lethal hit. This results in the activation of the pre-programmed suicide signal within the target and death by apoptosis.

Granzyme Entry into Target Cells

In the presence of high concentrations of perforin, target cells are rapidly lysed. Early EM studies also provided evidence for a putative perforin channel in the membrane of cells under attack by cytolytic effectors (87). These and other studies led to the hypothesis that perforin polymerized in the target cell membrane to create a channel through which granzymes could pass. However, evidence for a channel large enough to accommodate a 30 kDa protein is lacking (88).

Granzyme B was also found to bind to the cell surface in a saturable manner and to be internalized independently of perforin (36). These results suggested the existence of a cell surface receptor for granzyme B, and a candidate was identified as the cation-independent mannose-6-phosphate receptor (CI-MPR) (89). It was postulated that granzyme B binding occurs through its posttranslational modifications, namely mannose-6-phosphorylation, and the protease entered the target cell through receptor-mediated endocytosis. Although this study showed granzyme B entry into target cells as dependent on MPR expression, other work has suggested that the CI-MPR pathway can be circumvented in cells lacking MPR expression (90,91). Recent evidence suggests that granzyme B is complexed with proteoglycans, specifically serglycin (SG), and this large macromolecule (greater than 250 kDa) is the native form of granzyme B *in vivo* (92,93). This could suggest that granzyme B would not be able to bind directly to a receptor, but also adds a caveat to uptake studies using purified granzyme B. It is entirely possible that there are multiple routes of entry of granzymes into cells depending on the nature of the target. A specific receptor could mediate one mechanism of uptake, but it is also likely that less specific ionic interactions facilitate binding followed by entry via repair-mediated endocytosis induced after perforin damage (94).

Recent results suggest that cell surface heparin sulphate may be important for this nonspecific binding of granzyme B (95,96). The interaction with heparin sulphate could mediate receptor independent uptake, but may also facilitate granzyme B internalization via receptor-mediated endocytosis (51). Indeed, heparin sulfate is an important cofactor in other receptor binding mechanisms (97,98). Whatever the mechanism of internalization, it is believed that once inside the cell, the proteolytic activity of granzymes serves to activate cell death through the cleavage and activation of specific substrates.

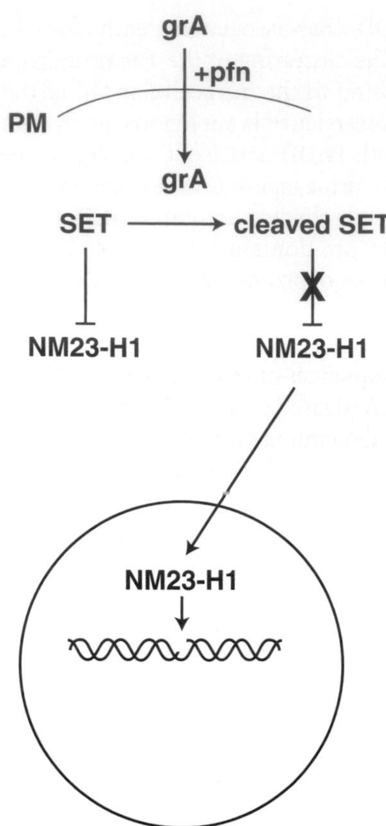

FIGURE 34.5 The granzyme A pathway. Perforin (pfn) facilitates the entry of granzyme A (grA) into the cytoplasm of the target. The protease cleaves a number of targets, including SET protein, which is an inhibitor of the nuclease NM23-H1. The released nuclease translocates to the nucleus and generates single-stranded DNA breaks.

Granzyme A Substrates

Granzyme A is the most abundant of the granzymes in the granules of CTLs (45). This protease induces caspase-independent apoptosis by inducing DNA damage by single-stranded nicks (99) and disrupting the mitochondrial membrane potential without the release of cytochrome c (100). Granzyme A cleaves proteins after arginine or lysine and targets proteins found in the SET complex (101–103). This SET complex contains proteins involved with repairing DNA, modulating chromatin, and regulating transcription and is also thought to help repair DNA in response to oxidative damage (103). As depicted in Figure 34.5, the cleavage of the SET protein by granzyme A releases the NM23-H1, a nuclease responsible for the single-stranded nicking of the DNA in association with TREX1 (104). The granzyme A–dependent cleavage of Ape1, a SET protein involved in DNA repair, also contributes to DNA damage. Ku70, another key double-stranded repair protein is also a substrate (105), and its inactivation has been shown to facilitate granzyme A–mediated death. Granzyme A also induces nuclear destruction by cleaving nuclear structural proteins lamins (106) and histones, resulting in chromatin unfolding (107). The mechanism of granzyme A–dependent mitochondrial disruption has not yet been elucidated.

Granzyme B Substrates

The discovery of a key substrate for granzyme B came from two rather unrelated observations. First, it had been shown that granzyme B has an unusual ability to cleave following asparate residues (43,44). Secondly, a mutation in nematodes was described that resulted in defective cell death (108). The gene involved, named ced3, was a caspase essential for apoptosis and required activation at an aspartate. The mammalian equivalent of ced3 was discovered as CPP32 and later named caspase-3 (109). It was, therefore, hypothesized that granzyme B could act to initiate apoptosis through the cleavage of caspase-3. Indeed, granzyme B was shown to cleave directly caspase-3 both *in vitro* and *in vivo* (110). The activation itself was a two-step process in which granzyme B acts to cleave the protein, and this is followed by self-catalytic activation by caspase-3 (111).

A single substrate did not explain all aspects of lysis since granzyme B was also shown to initiate cell death independent of caspases (112). It was also observed that granzyme B–induced cell death still proceeded, in the presence of caspase inhibitors, with a loss of mitochondrial membrane potential and the release of cytochrome c from the intermembrane space (113). However, these were blocked by transfection of the targets with the antiapoptotic gene Bcl2, thus suggesting the existence of a granzyme B substrate upstream of mitochondria. Studies showed that granzyme B–induced mitochondrial damage was the result of granzyme B cleavage of the pro-apoptotic protein Bid to form granzyme B–truncated Bid (gtBid) (114). Another Bcl2 family member, Mcl-1, has also been shown to be a substrate for granzyme B (115). This can interfere with mitochondria via interaction with Bim. The importance of the mitochondrial pathway will be discussed later.

Granzyme B has also been shown to cleave and activate other members of the caspase family, but *in vivo* caspase-3 appears to be the initiating event (116). A number of clinically important auto antigens are also cleaved by granzyme B, and these may be important in autoimmunity (117). Proteomic approaches have also been employed to discover novel granzyme B substrates, but it remains to be seen how many actually play a role in the mode of action of the protease (118). More detailed analyses on some of these other substrates have been conducted, such as α-tubulin (119,120), Hsp-70 (121), and Hop (Hsp-70/Hsp-90 organizing protein), an anti-apoptotic chaperone of Hsp70/Hsp-90 (122). The presence of multiple granzyme B substrates within a cell may enhance apoptosis, but more importantly may provide alternate pathways of cell death in the event of immune evasion of a virally infected or tumor cell.

A Key Role for Mitochondria in Killing

Once granzyme B is released into the cytoplasm, it acts to cleave and activate key substrates to induce apoptosis. It was rather surprising to find that this pathway was blocked by the overexpression of Bcl2. The Bcl2 family is intimately linked to the mitochondria and can either negatively or positively regulate the process of cell death. The anti-apoptotic family member Bcl2 is a membrane protein anchored to the mitochondria. Once in the membrane, Bcl2 and the related protein bcl-x_L associate with the mitochondrial permeability transition pore (PTP), a large multiprotein complex localized to the mitochondrial membrane contact sites. During apoptosis, the PTP has been reported to open, allowing loss of ψ_m along with release of apoptogenic factors such as cytochrome c. Inhibitors of PTP opening, such as cyclosporine A, are unable to inhibit mitochondrial disruption by granzyme B, indicating that the PTP is not the only site of action for Bcl2 in the mitochondria (123). Overexpression of Bcl2 attenuates granzyme B–mediated cell death, revealing a functional requirement for mitochondria in granzyme B–mediated apoptosis. This implied that the mitochondrial apoptotic machinery was activated in cells destined to die due to exposure to granzyme B. Most important, both the loss of ψ_m (123,124) and cytochrome c efflux following granzyme B treatment (125,126) occurred in a caspase-independent fashion, which suggested that granzyme B substrates other than the caspases were involved.

Granzyme B can cleave the pro-apoptotic member of the Bcl2 family, bid. In fact, granzyme B catalyzes bid cleavage more efficiently than caspases 3 or 8 (127). This gr-truncated bid (gtbid) is produced by hydrolysis at D75 and thus has a different amino terminus than the D59-caspase-8 cleaved form (tbid) (128). Nevertheless, both forms of cleaved bid translocate to the mitochondria resulting in the release of cytochrome c. The requirement of bid for cytochrome c release was demonstrated in a cell-free system in which cytosolic extracts immuno-depleted of bid were no longer able to promote granzyme B–induced cytochrome c release from purified mitochondria (114). Importantly, transfection of targets with a noncleavable mutant bid also interfered with apoptosis (129). The cleaved bid was required for the translocation of bax to the mitochondria, and this regulated import of bax was abolished in granzyme B–treated Bcl2-overexpressing cells. Bax, and the related protein bak, have been implicated in pore formation in the mitochondrial outer membrane and may provide the link between granzyme B and cytochrome c release. Indeed, bax/bak null cells do not release cytochrome c after incubation with granzyme B (130).

As described earlier for Fas killing, factors released from mitochondria include cytochrome c, which causes the formation of an oligomeric complex of APAF1 and caspase-9 known as the *apoptosome*. The recruitment of caspase-9 allows its autoactivation, and this, in turn, activates effector caspases. It was therefore possible that the granzyme B death pathway was dependent on this branch of the pathway. Using dominant-negative caspase-9–expressing cells as targets, it was demonstrated that the requirement for caspase-9 activity can be bypassed (131). This was not the case with Fas where the interference with caspase-9 activity efficiently blocked death. This suggested that in the granzyme B–mediated mechanism some other pathway was involved downstream of mitochondria.

Two other caspase activators have been shown to be released from mitochondria, SMAC/DIABLO (second mitochondrial activator of caspases/direct IAP binding protein with low pI) (132) and HtrA2/Omi. These share a short (~5 amino acids) motif at the N-terminus, which is revealed upon removal of the mitochondrial import signal. This peptide acts as a binding site for the inhibitor of apoptosis proteins (IAPs), which are natural inhibitors of activated caspases. Both SMAC/DIABLO and HtrA2/Omi function by binding IAPs and displace activated caspases associated with the IAP allowing the apoptotic program to proceed. Granzyme B–treated cells released SMAC/DIABLO from the mitochondria and thus relieve the inhibition of caspase-3 by XIAP (131,133). These experiments suggest that although granzyme B is capable of directly cleaving pro-caspase-3, SMAC/DIABLO release is required to allow full caspase-3 enzymatic activity and ultimately, cell death.

This mechanism (outlined in Figure 34.6) has been referred to as the *safety brake model* (134): granzyme B is delivered to the cytosol where it cleaves caspase 3. The foot is on the gas pedal, but the safety brake (IAP) is on. The brake is removed via cleavage of bid and release of SMAC. Now the cell speeds down the road to death. A detailed knowledge of the mechanism of death provides the tools to analyze how it might be defective, for example in tumors, or can be manipulated therapeutically. The clinical relevance has been recently highlighted by a drug designed on the basis of the model, which sensitizes Hodgkin's lymphoma to CTL (135).

Although the major focus of this discussion has been on the control of apoptosis, it should be noted that mitochondria function is also compromised. Mitochondria are also affected by granzyme A. These organelles are the powerhouses of the cell and supply energy in the form of ATP. Thus, by halting energy production the survival of the cell is compromised and, in time, would die by necrosis. This might be quite relevant in cells infected with a virus that encodes anti-apoptotic proteins. Surprisingly, overexpression of Bcl2 has little if any effect on CTL-mediated killing (136). CTLs are, therefore, able to bypass or inactivate Bcl2 in target cells. The mechanism for this is, as yet, unknown.

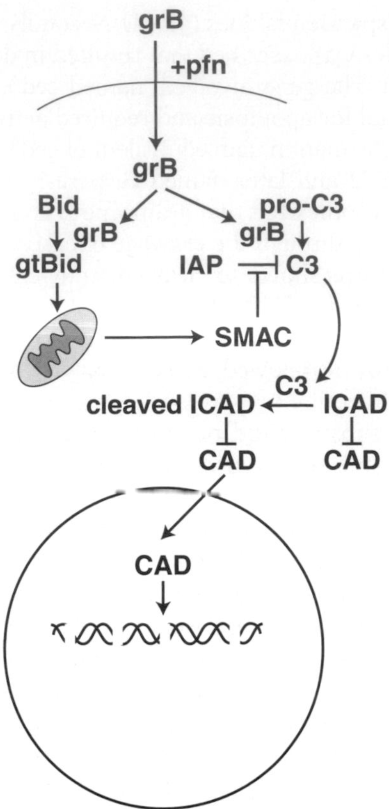

FIGURE 34.6 The granzyme B pathway. Perforin (pfn) facilitates the entry of granzyme B (grB) into the cytoplasm of the target. The protease cleaves caspase-3 (C3), but the enzymatic activity is inhibited by an IAP. The granzyme B also cleaves Bid and the truncated Bid (gtBid) translocates to the mitochondria. This results in leakage of mitochondrial proteins into the cytosol. One of these, SMAC, binds tightly to IAP and thus relieves the caspase-3 inhibition. The active caspase-3 then acts on ICAD to free CAD. The active nuclease then translocates to the nucleus and generates double-stranded breaks.

Extracellular Substrates

The majority of studies on granzyme substrates have focused on proteins within the target cell. It is becoming increasingly clear, however, that significant levels of extracellular granzyme can be detected and that extracellular substrates can be important targets. Indeed, elevated granzyme levels have been measured in numerous diseases ranging from viral and bacterial infections to inflammatory disorders (137). The exact mechanism of release is not clear, but it may be due to loss of granzyme from the synapse during CTL attack. Alternatively, granzyme may be released through constitutive secretion independent of granules after stimulation of the TCR or by cytokines. Finally, granzyme release has been shown to occur by the presence of bacteria through a cytokine-dependent mechanism (138).

Both granzyme A and granzyme B have been shown to cleave extracellular matrix proteins. This could influence migration of lymphocytes, but may also lead to perforin-independent death due to disruption of cell–cell interactions (139). Granzyme A has been proposed to cleave cell surface receptors, such as the thrombin receptor, that may lead to a cellular response (140). The neuronal glutamate receptor has also been shown to be cleaved by granzyme B (141). Interestingly, this activity was found to be influenced by glycosylation, which was thought to change accessibility of the cleavage site. Degradation of some of the extracellular matrix (ECM) substrates was also affected by conformation, but this does not seem to be the case for granzyme A (142).

DISTINGUISHING CELL DEATH MECHANISMS

Historically, the two main features of cell death that are convenient to measure are membrane damage (chromium or lactate dehydrogenase (LDH) release) and DNA fragmentation. Although apoptosis is characterized by DNA fragmentation, this is also seen in necrotic death. The key difference in the DNA fragmentation pattern is only revealed by gel electrophoresis. In apoptotic cell death, there is a laddering of the DNA, while in necrosis the stained DNA is just a smear. Typically, the early DNA fragmentation seen with granzyme B is apoptotic, while the late nucleolytic activity induced by granzyme A is necrotic, or at least is a caspase-independent form of death with only single-strand breaks (99). In addition, it should be appreciated that some lines respond preferentially to granzymes. In the mouse lymphoma L1210.3, for example, DNA damage is mediated exclusively by granzyme B, whereas in another lymphoma, EL4.F15, both granzymes contributed (143).

There are now numerous convenient ways to monitor death, but they must be used judiciously (144). For example, exposure of PS on the surface of an apoptotic cell can be monitored by binding of annexin V (145). However, at late stages of necrosis when the membrane is permeable, the annexin can enter the cell and bind to the internal PS. Thus, it is of paramount importance that this assay must be combined with propidium iodide exclusion to monitor membrane integrity. Loss of membrane potential of mitochondria is easily measured by release of fluorescent dyes, such as tetramethyl rhodamine ethyl ester (TMRE) (146). However, apoptosis is not the only way in which mitochondrial dysfunction can occur. Probably the most common method used to measure apoptosis is DNA fragmentation detected by terminal deoxynucleotidyl transferase mediated dUTP-linked nick end labeling (TUNEL) (147). However, this assay will detect any kind of nicking in DNA, not just apoptosis. More recently, reagents that detect caspase activation using either substrates or antibodies to neoepitopes have become available and are very useful (148,149). Probably the bottom line is that the researcher should never restrict analysis to one measure of death.

In the specific case of distinguishing between granzyme- and Fas-mediated killing, there is considerable confusion. The common dogma is that granzyme-mediated killing is dependent on calcium, whereas Fas-induced death is not. Consequently, many investigators distinguish the two on the basis of sensitivity to EGTA. However, as some Fas-ligand has now been shown to be in granules, it will also be inhibited by chelation of calcium. A better method is to use an antibody directed against the Fas receptor that blocks, rather than activates, Fas killing.

PROTECTION OF CTL FROM LYSIS

The granule exocytosis model provides an explanation for the directed lysis of a bound target, but it does not explain why the CTL remains alive. Indeed, if there is enough granzyme and perforin in the synapse, why does the CTL not die? Many explanations have been put forward, but this is still an open question. Originally, it was hypothesized that CTLs were inherently resistant to their own lytic machinery. Indeed, it has been shown that they do express a granzyme B inhibitor (150). However, even though they are more resistant than the typical hemopoietic target cell used in routine assays, they can be killed by other CTLs (151). Protective membrane proteins that bind perforin have also been proposed, but have remained fairly elusive. It is more likely that the process of degranulation may provide the CTL with a transient resistance. As the degranulation is so local, it is possible that the inside of the granule becomes the only region of the CTL that is exposed to the granzyme/perforin. One candidate for such a mechanism is membrane-bound cathepsin B, which is known to be within the granule. According to the model, it was hypothesized that the enzyme would cleave and inactivate perforin (152). Recent experiments with cathepsin B knockout mice, however, have not shown any evidence of death in CTLs after killing (153). Hence, this cannot be the only mechanism for the protection observed.

T CELL HOMEOSTASIS

In addition to a role in target cell lysis, there is increasing evidence that perforin may play a role in lymphocyte homeostasis. Perforin-deficient mice have an increased expansion and persistence of CTL after stimulation. Similar observations were made with alloreactive clones with cells from perforin knockout mice. Taken together, these results suggest a role for perforin in activation induced cell death (154,155). Recently, evidence has been provided for a similar role for granzyme B in TH2 cells (156).

Perforin deficiency has also been documented in children who suffer from familial haemophagocytic lymphohistiocytosis (FHL) (157). This rare disease is characterized by overproduction of T cells and inflammatory cytokines. The activated cells infiltrate various organs, including spleen, lymph nodes, and the central nervous system, leading to a variety of pathologies. Patients with this disorder generally have been found to carry mutations in the perforin gene. This is not always the case, however, and a mutation in a protein involved in granule fusion has also been shown to give rise to the same clinical phenotype

(158). Lymphocytes from the patients have no cytolytic activity, and perforin is absent from the granules.

EXPRESSION OF GRANZYME/PERFORIN IN TREGS

Although most of the chapter has discussed the role of CTLs, there has been considerable excitement generated by the discovery that granzymes and perforin are in a subset of $CD4^+$ regulatory T cells (159). Both adaptive and activated natural Tregs appear to express perforin and granzymes. These Tregs seem to be able to kill APCs and activated T cells through a granule-dependent mechanism, thus suggesting one pathway by which these cells can regulate immune responses (160). The cytotoxicity is dependent on adhesive interactions, but surprisingly not on MHC/TCR. They do not appear to act through a Fas/Fas-ligand pathway.

EFFECTOR MOLECULES IN DISEASE

Virus Infection

The importance of perforin in mediating protection against viruses, such as lymphocytic choriomeningitis virus and ectromelia, has been firmly established using knockout mice (161,162). The results with granzyme-deficient mice have been less clear-cut, but this is likely due to the functional redundancy of the granzyme family. Although mice deficient in granzyme A and all granzymes in the B cluster are susceptible to ectromelia, they do seem to be able to mount an effective response to other viruses (162). The interpretation of *in vivo* experiments can also be difficult, as it is known that interferon-gamma (IFN^{γ}), produced by CTL, can up-regulate Fas on targets (163). Even more confounding, it has also been demonstrated that the granule-mediated mechanism of killing may actually promote immunopathology associated with acute viral infections (164). In humans, we do not generally have knockouts for experimental analyses; rather, results are limited to correlating expression with diseases. It is believed that $CD8^+$ T cells play a pivotal role in the control of viral infections and expression of key effector molecules is thought to be important. In particular, studies with HIV patients have revealed an interesting reduction in perforin expression in CTL (165). This may not be confined to HIV and might be a general feature of chronic infection (166).

Cancer

The situation with tumor immunosurveillance is also suggestive of a critical role for perforin, particularly in eradication of spontaneous tumors. However, the role for granzyme is not so obvious. It is clear that many tumors are infiltrated by perforin and granzyme-positive CTLs, but often they are ineffective *in vivo*. An interesting speculation is that their cytolytic potential is kept in check by Treg cells (167), so perhaps tumor destruction has to be mediated by other mechanisms. However, if the Treg-mediated block could be reversed perhaps the granule-mediated effector mechanism could be unmasked. *In vivo* experiments with perforin-deficient mice have confirmed an important role for perforin in destruction of tumors (168). In addition, there is an increased incidence of spontaneous malignancy in these knockout mice (169). Whether this is due to the direct involvement of perforin with the lytic machinery or due to its immunoregulatory properties is unclear.

The innate immune response seems to be particularly important in protection against nonlymphoid tumors. Again, this seems, in part, to be due to perforin, but Fas can also be up-regulated on targets leading to death receptor–mediated death (170). Although the evidence for involvement of CTLs is not clear, it should be noted that in states of immunosuppression—for example, HIV—increased cases of malignancy are often seen. Further, with vaccines that stimulate CTLs or with adoptive therapy of tumor-infiltrating lymphocytes, there is clear evidence of protection (171,172).

Autoimmunity

CTLs have long been implicated in the destruction of ß cells during type 1 diabetes. A number of transgenic models of autoimmune diabetes have shown $CD8^+$ T cells can efficiently kill beta cells (173,174). Perforin-deficient nonobese diabetic (NOD) mice are protected from diabetes (175) and isolated islets are susceptible to granzyme/perforin-induced death (176). However, *in vitro* studies suggest that in the absence of perforin, the Fas pathway is operative (177). In another modal of autoimmune disorder, experimental autoimmune encephalomyelitis (EAE), Fas-mediated killing was required for the pathogic events in perforin-deficient mice (178). However, recent evidence has suggested that granzyme B may be an important mediator of the neuronal injury (179).

Transplant Rejection

Organ allograft rejection is strongly associated with CTLs, and the presence of granzyme and perforin closely correlate with rejection. However, allografts transplanted into hosts with disrupted genes for perforin and granzymes A and B showed no decrease in tubulitis and were still rejected (180). Fas-ligand is also up-regulated in rejecting allografts, but it is not required for graft rejection (181). Thus, despite the striking expression of these potential lytic effectors in the grafts, their activities do not seem to be required for rejection. The effector mechanisms and, indeed, the cells responsible for rejection remain unclear. In bone marrow transplantation, donor T cells play a key role in preventing graft rejection by the attacking recipient T cells. This can occur by both perforin- and Fas-mediated mechanisms (182,183).

VISUALIZATION OF CTL *in vivo*

One possible reason that the role of effector molecules in disease still remains unclear is that the *in vitro* assays used previously do not truly reflect what occurs *in vivo*. To remedy this, it will be necessary to develop techniques to visualize CTL and immune responses *in vivo*. This is now becoming possible through the generation of transgenic mice that express green fluorescent protein in specific subsets of T cells, and the utilization of two-photon microscopy. Indeed, using this kind of technology, CTLs have now been observed in the act of killing a tumor target (167).

CONCLUSION

This chapter describes the biological features and molecular mechanisms used by CTL to destroy antigen bearing target cells. *In vitro* studies suggest that there are primarily two major pathways used to induce cell death. The first is mediated by effector molecules contained within granules that are vectorally exocytosed upon target cell recognition. The other occurs via ligation of Fas on the surface of the target by Fas-ligand carried by the killer. A detailed knowledge of the mechanisms that lead to the death of the target cell mediated by granyzmes A and B, as well as Fas, have now been elucidated. These involve induction of both apoptotic and necrotic death pathways, depend on the proteolytic activities of the granzymes and caspases, and involve target organelles, such as mitochondria. Such knowledge can now be used to design drugs that may modulate CTL activities.

The genes for a number of effector molecules involved in killing have been knocked out, which has allowed investigation of their roles in disease pathogenesis. These studies implicate the effectors in a number of responses *in vivo*, but the results are not definitive. Part of the problem centers on the redundancy of the killing mechanisms used, and when one is inactivated another appears to substitute. However, it is certainly suggested by this line of investigation that alternate killing mechanisms may exist in *in vivo* situations.

It has also become clear that effector molecules, such as perforin and granzymes, may be involved in homeostasis of T lymphocytes. There is also an increasing appreciation that granzymes may act on substrates outside the target and this may play a role in disease pathogenesis. Finally, the effectors may play a role in regulation of immune responses via their expression in regulatory T cells. All of these new functions suggest very exciting possibilities for the future development of novel immunomodulatory strategies.

REFERENCES

1. Govaerts A. Cellular antibodies in kidney homotransplantation. *J Immunol.* 1960;85:516–522.
2. Cerottini JC, Nordin AA, Brunner KT. Specific *in vitro* cytotoxicity of thymus-derived lymphocytes sensitized to alloantigens. *Nature.* 1970;228(5278):1308–1309.
3. Berke G. Cytotoxic T-lymphocytes. How do they function? *Immunol Rev.* 1983;72:5–42.
4. Nabholz M, MacDonald HR. Cytolytic T lymphocytes. *Annu Rev Immunol.* 1983;1:273–306.
5. Zinkernagel RM, Doherty PC. Restriction of *in vitro* T cell-mediated cytotoxicity in lymphocytic choriomeningitis within a syngeneic or semiallogeneic system. *Nature.* 1974;248(450):701–702.
6. Thorn RM, Henney CS. Studies on the mechanism of lymphocyte-mediated cytolysis. VI. A reappraisal of the requirement for protein synthesis during T cell-mediated lysis. *J Immunol.* 1976;116(1): 146–9.
7. Zagury D, Bernard J, Dufer J, et al. The biology of isolated immunocytes. I. Isolation into a closed liquid microchamber: application to PFC. *Ann Immunol (Paris).* 1975;126(1):23–30.
8. Gillis S, Smith KA. Long term culture of tumour-specific cytotoxic T cells. *Nature.* 1977;268(5616):154–156.
9. Spits H, van Schooten W, Keizer H, et al. Alloantigen recognition is preceded by nonspecific adhesion of cytotoxic T cells and target cells. *Science.* 1986;232(4748):403–405.
10. Anikeeva N, Somersalo K, Sims TN, et al. Distinct role of lymphocyte function-associated antigen-1 in mediating effective cytolytic activity by cytotoxic T lymphocytes. *Proc Natl Acad Sci U S A.* 2005; 102(18):6437–6442.
11. Kelso A, Costelloe EO, Johnson BJ, et al. The genes for perforin, granzymes A-C and IFN-gamma are differentially expressed in single CD8+ T cells during primary activation. *Int Immunol.* 2002;14(6):605–613.
12. Stinchcombe JC, Page LJ, Griffiths GM. Secretory Lysosome Biogenesis in Cytotoxic T Lymphocytes from Normal and Chediak Higashi Syndrome Patients. *Traffic.* 2000;1(5):435–444.
13. Griffiths GM. Protein sorting and secretion during CTL killing. *Semin Immunol.* 1997;9(2):109–115.
14. Clark R, Griffiths GM. Lytic granules, secretory lysosomes and disease. *Curr Opin Immunol.* 2003;15(5):516–521.
15. Kupfer A, Dennert G, Singer SJ. The reorientation of the Golgi apparatus and the microtubule-organizing center in the cytotoxic effector cell is a prerequisite in the lysis of bound target cells. *J Mol Cell Immunol.* 1985;2(1):37–49.
16. Podack ER, Konigsberg PJ. Cytolytic T cell granules. Isolation, structural, biochemical, and functional characterization. *J Exp Med.* 1984;160(3):695–710.
17. Henkart PA, Millard PJ, Reynolds CW, et al. Cytolytic activity of purified cytoplasmic granules from cytotoxic rat large granular lymphocyte tumors. *J Exp Med.* 1984;160(1):75–93.
18. Henkart PA. Mechanism of lymphocyte-mediated cytotoxicity. *Annu Rev Immunol.* 1985;3:31–58.
19. Yannelli JR, Sullivan JA, Mandell GL, et al. Reorientation and fusion of cytotoxic T lymphocyte granules after interaction with target cells as determined by high resolution cinemicrography. *J Immunol.* 1986;136(2):377–382.
20. Kupfer A, Dennert G, Singer SJ. Polarization of the Golgi Apparatus and the Microtubule-Organizing Center within Cloned Natural Killer Cells Bound to Their Targets. *PNAS.* 1983;80(23):7224–7228.
21. Burkhardt JK, McIlvain JM, Jr., Sheetz MP, et al. Lytic granules from cytotoxic T cells exhibit kinesin-dependent motility on microtubules *in vitro*. *J Cell Sci.* 1993;104 (Pt 1):151–162.
22. Stinchcombe J, Bossi G, Griffiths GM. Linking albinism and immunity: the secrets of secretory lysosomes. *Science.* 2004;305(5680): 55–9.

23. Bossi G, Booth S, Clark R, et al. Normal lytic granule secretion by cytotoxic T lymphocytes deficient in BLOC-1, -2 and -3 and myosins Va, VIIa and XV. *Traffic*. 2005;6(3):243–51.
24. Stinchcombe JC, Majorovits E, Bossi G, et al. Centrosome polarization delivers secretory granules to the immunological synapse. *Nature*. 2006;443(7110):462–465.
25. Lin J, Miller MJ, Shaw AS. The c-SMAC: sorting it all out (or in). *J Cell Biol.* 2005;170(2):177–182.
26. Stinchcombe JC, Bossi G, Booth S, et al. The Immunological Synapse of CTL Contains a Secretory Domain and Membrane Bridges. *Immunity.* 2001;15(5):751–761.
27. Millard PJ, Henkart MP, Reynolds CW, et al. Purification and properties of cytoplasmic granules from cytotoxic rat LGL tumors. *J Immunol.* 1984;132(6):3197–3204.
28. Podack ER, Young JD-E, Cohn ZA. Isolation and Biochemical and Functional Characterization of Perforin 1 from Cytolytic T-Cell Granules. *PNAS.* 1985;82(24):8629–8633.
29. Lowrey DM, Aebischer T, Olsen K, et al. Cloning, analysis, and expression of murine perforin 1 cDNA, a component of cytolytic T-cell granules with homology to complement component C9. *Proc Natl Acad Sci U S A.* 1989;86(1):247–251.
30. Shinkai Y, Takio K, Okumura K. Homology of perforin to the ninth component of complement (C9). *Nature.* 1988;334(6182):525–527.
31. Tschopp J, Masson D, Stanley KK. Structural/functional similarity between proteins involved in complement- and cytotoxic T-lymphocyte-mediated cytolysis. *Nature.* 1986;322(6082):831–834.
32. Sauer H, Pratsch L, Tschopp J, et al. Functional size of complement and perforin pores compared by confocal laser scanning microscopy and fluorescence microphotolysis. *Biochimica et Biophysica Acta (BBA) - Biomembranes.* 1991;1063(1):137–146.
33. Uellner R, Zvelebil M, Hopkins J, et al. Perforin is activated by a proteolytic cleavage during biosynthesis which reveals a phospholipid-binding C2 domain. *EMBO J.* 1997;16(24):7287–7296.
34. Duke RC, Chervenak R, Cohen JJ. Endogenous Endonuclease-Induced DNA Fragmentation: An Early Event in Cell–Mediated Cytolysis. *PNAS.* 1983;80(20):6361–6365.
35. Kagi D, Ledermann B, Burki K, et al. Molecular Mechanisms of Lymphocyte-Mediated Cytotoxicity and Their Role in Immunological Protection and Pathogenesis *In Vivo*. *Annu Rev Immunol.* 1996;14(1):207–232.
36. Froelich CJ, Orth K, Turbov J, et al. New Paradigm for Lymphocyte Granule–mediated Cytotoxicity. Target Cells Bind and Internalize Granzyme B, but an Endosomolytic Agent Is Necessary for Cytosolic Delivery and Subsequent Apoptosis. *J Biol Chem.* 1996;271(46): 29073–39079.
37. Voskoboinik I, Thia MC, Fletcher J, et al. Calcium-dependent plasma membrane binding and cell lysis by perforin are mediated through its C2 domain: A critical role for aspartate residues 429, 435, 483, and 485 but not 491. *J Biol Chem.* 2005;280(9):8426–8434.
38. Voskoboinik I, Trapani JA. Addressing the mysteries of perforin function. *Immunology and cell biology.* 2006;84(1):66–71.
39. Pham CTN, Ley TJ. Dipeptidyl peptidase I is required for the processing and activation of granzymes A and B *in vivo*. *PNAS.* 1999;96(15):8627–8632.
40. Lobe CG, Finlay BB, Paranchych W, et al. Novel Serine Proteases Encoded by Two Cytotoxic T Lymphocyte-specific Genes. *Science.* 1986;232(4752):858–861.
41. Gershenfeld HK, Weissman IL. Cloning of a cDNA for a T cell-specific serine protease from a cytotoxic T lymphocyte. *Science.* 1986;232(4752):854–858.
42. Masson D, Tschopp J. A family of serine esterases in lytic granules of cytolytic T lymphocytes. *Cell.* 1987;49(5):679–685.
43. Murphy ME, Moult J, Bleackley RC, et al. Comparative molecular model building of two serine proteinases from cytotoxic T lymphocytes. *Proteins.* 1988;4(3):190–204.
44. Odake S, Kam CM, Narasimhan L, et al. Human and murine cytotoxic T lymphocyte serine proteases: subsite mapping with peptide thioester substrates and inhibition of enzyme activity and cytolysis by isocoumarins. *Biochemistry.* 1991;30(8):2217–2227.
45. Pasternack MS, Eisen HN. A novel serine esterase expressed by cytotoxic T lymphocytes. *Nature.* 1985;314(6013):743–745.
46. Griffiths GM, Isaaz S. Granzymes A and B are targeted to the lytic granules of lymphocytes by the mannose-6-phosphate receptor. *J Cell Biol.* 1993;120(4):885–896.
47. Stevens RL, Kamada MM, Serafin WE. Structure and function of the family of proteoglycans that reside in the secretory granules of natural killer cells and other effector cells of the immune response. *Current topics in microbiology and immunology.* 1989;140:93–108.
48. Metkar SS, Wang B, Aguilar-Santelises M, et al. Cytotoxic cell granule–mediated apoptosis: perforin delivers granzyme B-serglycin complexes into target cells without plasma membrane pore formation. *Immunity.* 2002;16(3):417–428.
49. Masson D, Peters PJ, Geuze HJ, et al. Interaction of chondroitin sulfate with perforin and granzymes of cytolytic T-cells is dependent on pH. *Biochemistry.* 1990;29(51):11229–11235.
50. Grujic M, Braga T, Lukinius A, et al. Serglycin-deficient Cytotoxic T Lymphocytes Display Defective Secretory Granule Maturation and Granzyme B Storage. *J Biol Chem.* 2005;280(39):33411–8.
51. Veugelers K, Motyka B, Goping IS, et al. Granule-mediated Killing by Granzyme B and Perforin Requires a Mannose 6-Phosphate Receptor and Is Augmented by Cell Surface Heparan Sulfate. *Mol Biol Cell.* 2006;17(2):623–633.
52. Bossi G, Griffiths GM. Degranulation plays an essential part in regulating cell surface expression of Fas ligand in T cells and natural killer cells. *Nat Med.* 1999;5(1):90–96.
53. Wagner L, Yang OO, Garcia-Zepeda EA, et al. beta.-Chemokines are released from HIV-1-specific cytolytic T-cell granules complexed to proteoglycans. *Nature.* 1998;391(6670):908–911.
54. Clayberger C, Krensky AM. Granulysin. *Curr Opin Immunol.* 2003;15(5):560–565.
55. Munford RS, Sheppard PO, O'Hara PJ. Saposin-like proteins (SAPLIP) carry out diverse functions on a common backbone structure. *J Lipid Res.* 1995;36(8):1653–1663.
56. Gamen S, Hanson DA, Kaspar A, et al. Granulysin-Induced Apoptosis. I. Involvement of at Least Two Distinct Pathways. *J Immunol.* 1998;161(4):1758–1764.
57. Deng A, Chen S, Li Q, et al. Granulysin, a cytolytic molecule, is also a chemoattractant and proinflammatory activator. *J Immunol.* 2005;174(9):5243–5248.
58. Dupuis M, Schaerer E, Krause KH, et al. The calcium-binding protein calreticulin is a major constituent of lytic granules in cytolytic T lymphocytes. *J Exp Med.* 1993;177(1):1–7.
59. Andrin C, Pinkoski MJ, Burns K, et al. Interaction between a $Ca2^{+}$-binding protein calreticulin and perforin, a component of the cytotoxic T-cell granules. *Biochemistry.* 1998;37(29):10386–10394.
60. Sipione S, Ewen C, Shostak I, et al. Impaired Cytolytic Activity in Calreticulin-Deficient CTLs. *J Immunol.* 2005;174(6):3212–3219.
61. Porcellini S, Traggiai E, Schenk U, et al. Regulation of peripheral T cell activation by calreticulin. *J Exp Med.* 2006;203(2):461–471.
62. Ostergaard HL, Kane KP, Mescher MF, et al. Cytotoxic T lymphocyte mediated lysis without release of serine esterase. *Nature.* 1987;330(6143):71–72.
63. Berke G, Rosen D. Highly lytic *in vivo* primed cytolytic T lymphocytes devoid of lytic granules and BLT-esterase activity acquire these constituents in the presence of T cell growth factors upon blast transformation *in vitro*. *J Immunol.* 1988;141(5):1429–1436.
64. Rouvier E, Luciani MF, Golstein P. Fas involvement in $Ca(2^{+})$-independent T cell-mediated cytotoxicity. *J Exp Med.* 1993;177(1): 195–200.
65. Kataoka T, Shinohara N, Takayama H, et al. Concanamycin A, a powerful tool for characterization and estimation of contribution of perforin- and Fas-based lytic pathways in cell-mediated cytotoxicity. *J Immunol.* 1996;156(10):3678–86.
66. Kagi D, Vignaux F, Ledermann B, et al. Fas and perforin pathways as major mechanisms of T cell-mediated cytotoxicity. *Science.* 1994;265(5171):528–530.
67. Lee RK, Spielman J, Zhao DY, et al. Perforin, Fas ligand, and tumor necrosis factor are the major cytotoxic molecules used by lymphokine-activated killer cells. *J Immunol.* 1996;157(5):1919–1925.
68. Kerr JFR, Wyllie AH, Currie AR. Apoptosis: a basic biological phenomenon with wide-ranging implications in tissue kinetics. *Br J Cancer.* 1972;26(4):239–257.

69. Fadok VA, Savill JS, Haslett C, et al. Different populations of macrophages use either the vitronectin receptor or the phosphatidylserine receptor to recognize and remove apoptotic cells. *J Immunol.* 1992;149(12):4029–4035.
70. Fadok VA, Bratton DL, Konowal A, et al. Macrophages That Have Ingested Apoptotic Cells *In Vitro* Inhibit Proinflammatory Cytokine Production Through Autocrine/Paracrine Mechanisms Involving TGF-beta, PGE2, and PAF. *J Clin Invest.* 1998;101(4):890–898.
71. Skalka M, Matyasova J, Cejkova M. Dna in chromatin of irradiated lymphoid tissues degrades *in vivo* into regular fragments. *FEBS Lett.* 1976;72(2):271–274.
72. Stennicke HR, Salvesen GS. Catalytic properties of the caspases. *Cell Death Differ.* 1999;6(11):1054–1059.
73. Liu X, Zou H, Slaughter C, et al. DFF, a Heterodimeric Protein That Functions Downstream of Caspase-3 to Trigger DNA Fragmentation during Apoptosis. *Cell.* 1997;89(2):175–184.
74. Kischkel FC, Hellbardt S, Behrmann I, et al. Cytotoxicity-dependent APO-1 (Fas/CD95)-associated proteins form a death-inducing signaling complex (DISC) with the receptor. *Embo J.* 1995;14(22):5579–5588.
75. Chinnaiyan AM, O'Rourke K, Tewari M, et al. FADD, a novel death domain-containing protein, interacts with the death domain of fas and initiates apoptosis. *Cell.* 1995;81(4):505–512.
76. Muzio M, Stockwell BR, Stennicke HR, et al. An Induced Proximity Model for Caspase-8 Activation. *J Biol Chem.* 1998;273(5):2926–2930.
77. Scaffidi C, Fulda S, Srinivasan A, et al. Two CD95 (APO-1/Fas) signaling pathways. *EMBO J.* 1998;17(6):1675–1687.
78. Luo X, Budihardjo I, Zou H, et al. Bid, a Bcl2 interacting protein, mediates cytochrome c release from mitochondria in response to activation of cell surface death receptors. *Cell.* 1998;94(4):481–490.
79. Boatright KM, Salvesen GS. Mechanisms of caspase activation. *Curr Opin Cell Biol.* 2003;15(6):725–731.
80. Shi L, Kam CM, Powers JC, et al. Purification of three cytotoxic lymphocyte granule serine proteases that induce apoptosis through distinct substrate and target cell interactions. *J Exp Med.* 1992;176(6):1521–1529.
81. Shi L, Kraut RP, Aebersold R, et al. A natural killer cell granule protein that induces DNA fragmentation and apoptosis. *J Exp Med.* 1992;175(2):553–566.
82. Nakajima H, Park HL, Henkart PA. Synergistic roles of granzymes A and B in mediating target cell death by rat basophilic leukemia mast cell tumors also expressing cytolysin/perforin. *J Exp Med.* 1995;181(3):1037–1046.
83. Shiver JW, Su L, Henkart PA. Cytotoxicity with target DNA breakdown by rat basophilic leukemia cells expressing both cytolysin and granzyme A. *Cell.* 1992;71(2):315–322.
84. Heusel JW, Wesselschmidt RL, Shresta S, et al. Cytotoxic lymphocytes require granzyme B for the rapid induction of DNA fragmentation and apoptosis in allogeneic target cells. *Cell.* 1994;76(6):977–987.
85. Simon MM, Hausmann M, Tran T, et al. *In Vitro*- and ex vivo-derived cytolytic leukocytes from granzyme A × B double knockout mice are defective in granule-mediated apoptosis but not lysis of target cells. *J Exp Med.* 1997;186(10):1781–1786.
86. Shresta S, Graubert TA, Thomas DA, et al. Granzyme A initiates an alternative pathway for granule-mediated apoptosis. *Immunity.* 1999;10(5):595–605.
87. Dourmashkin RR, Deteix P, Simone CB, et al. Electron microscopic demonstration of lesions in target cell membranes associated with antibody-dependent cellular cytotoxicity. *Clin Exp Immunol.* 1980;42(3):554–560.
88. Browne KA, Blink E, Sutton VR, et al. Cytosolic delivery of granzyme B by bacterial toxins: evidence that endosomal disruption, in addition to transmembrane pore formation, is an important function of perforin. *Mol Cell Biol.* 1999;19(12):8604–8615.
89. Motyka B, Korbutt G, Pinkoski MJ, et al. Mannose 6-Phosphate/Insulin-like Growth Factor II Receptor Is a Death Receptor for Granzyme B during Cytotoxic T Cell-Induced Apoptosis. *Cell.* 2000;103(3):491–500.
90. Trapani JA, Sutton VR, Thia KYT, et al. A clathrin/dynamin- and mannose-6-phosphate receptor-independent pathway for granzyme B-induced cell death. *J Cell Biol.* 2003;160(2):223–233.
91. Dressel R, Raja SM, Honing S, et al. Granzyme-mediated Cytotoxicity Does Not Involve the Mannose 6-Phosphate Receptors on Target Cells. *J Biol Chem.* 2004;279(19):20200–20210.
92. Metkar SS, Wang B, Aguilar-Santelises M, et al. Cytotoxic Cell Granule-Mediated Apoptosis: Perforin Delivers Granzyme B-Serglycin Complexes into Target Cells without Plasma Membrane Pore Formation. *Immunity.* 2002;16(3):417–428.
93. Raja SM, Wang B, Dantuluri M, et al. Cytotoxic Cell Granule-mediated Apoptosis. Characterization of the Macromolecular Complex of Granzyme B with Serglycin. *J Biol Chem.* 2002;277(51):49523–49530.
94. Keefe D, Shi L, Feske S, et al. Perforin Triggers a Plasma Membrane-Repair Response that Facilitates CTL Induction of Apoptosis. *Immunity.* 2005;23(3):249–262.
95. Bird CH, Sun J, Ung K, et al. Cationic Sites on Granzyme B Contribute to Cytotoxicity by Promoting Its Uptake into Target Cells. *Mol Cell Biol.* 2005;25(17):7854–7867.
96. Shi L, Keefe D, Durand E, et al. Granzyme B Binds to Target Cells Mostly by Charge and Must Be Added at the Same Time as Perforin to Trigger Apoptosis. *J Immunol.* 2005;174(9):5456–5461.
97. Yayon A, Klagsbrun M, Esko JD, et al. Cell surface, heparin-like molecules are required for binding of basic fibroblast growth factor to its high affinity receptor. *Cell.* 1991;64(4):841–848.
98. Zioncheck TF, Richardson L, Liu J, et al. Sulfated Oligosaccharides Promote Hepatocyte Growth Factor Association and Govern Its Mitogenic Activity. *J Biol Chem.* 1995;270(28):16871–16878.
99. Beresford PJ, Xia Z, Greenberg AH, et al. Granzyme A loading induces rapid cytolysis and a novel form of DNA damage independently of caspase activation. *Immunity.* 1999;10(5):585–594.
100. Lieberman J, Fan Z. Nuclear war: the granzyme A-bomb. *Curr Opin Immunol.* 2003;15(5):553–559.
101. Beresford PJ, Zhang D, Oh DY, et al. Granzyme A Activates an Endoplasmic Reticulum-associated Caspase-independent Nuclease to Induce Single-stranded DNA Nicks. *J Biol Chem.* 2001;276(46):43285–43293.
102. Fan Z, Beresford PJ, Zhang D, et al. HMG2 Interacts with the Nucleosome Assembly Protein SET and Is a Target of the Cytotoxic T-Lymphocyte Protease Granzyme A. *Mol Cell Biol.* 2002;22(8):2810–2820.
103. Fan Z, Beresford PJ, Zhang D, et al. Cleaving the oxidative repair protein Ape1 enhances cell death mediated by granzyme A. *Nat Immunol.* 2003;4(2):145–153.
104. Chowdhury D, Beresford PJ, Zhu P, et al. The exonuclease TREX1 is in the SET complex and acts in concert with NM23-H1 to degrade DNA during granzyme A-mediated cell death. *Mol Cell Biol.* 2006;23:133–142.
105. Zhu P, Zhang D, Chowdhury D, et al. Granzyme A. which causes single-stranded DNA damage, targets the double-strand break repair protein Ku70. *EMBO.* 2006;7:431–437.
106. Zhang D, Beresford PJ, Greenberg AH, et al. Granzymes A and B directly cleave lamins and disrupt the nuclear lamina during granule-mediated cytolysis. *PNAS.* 2001;98(10):5746–5751.
107. Zhang D, Pasternack MS, Beresford PJ, et al. Induction of Rapid Histone Degradation by the Cytotoxic T Lymphocyte Protease Granzyme A. *J Biol Chem.* 2001;276(5):3683–3690.
108. Avery L, Horvitz HR. A cell that dies during wild-type C. elegans development can function as a neuron in a ced-3 mutant. *Cell.* 1987;51(6):1071–1078.
109. Nicholson DW, Ali A, Thornberry NA, et al. Identification and inhibition of the ICE/CED-3 protease necessary for mammalian apoptosis. *Nature.* 1995;376(6535):37–43.
110. Darmon AJ, Nicholson DW, Bleackley RC. Activation of the apoptotic protease CPP32 by cytotoxic T-cell-derived granzyme B. *Nature.* 1995;377(6548):446–448.
111. Martin SJ, Amarante-Mendes GP, Shi L, et al. The cytotoxic cell protease granzyme B initiates apoptosis in a cell-free system by proteolytic processing and activation of the ICE/CED-3 family protease, CPP32, via a novel two-step mechanism. *Embo J.* 1996;15(10):2407–2416.

112. Sarin A, Williams MS, Alexander-Miller MA, et al. Target Cell Lysis by CTL Granule Exocytosis Is Independent of ICE/Ced-3 Family Proteases. *Immunity*. 1997;6(2):209–215.
113. Heibein JA, Barry M, Motyka B, et al. Granzyme B-Induced Loss of Mitochondrial Inner Membrane Potential ({Delta}{Psi}m) and Cytochrome c Release Are Caspase Independent. *J Immunol.* 1999;163(9):4683–4693.
114. Heibein JA, Goping IS, Barry M, et al. Granzyme B-mediated Cytochrome c Release Is Regulated by the Bcl-2 Family Members Bid and Bax. *J Exp Med.* 2000;192(10):1391–1402.
115. Han J, Goldstein LA, Gastman BR, et al. Degradation of Mcl-1 by granzyme B: implications for Bim-mediated mitochondrial apoptotic events. *J Biol Chem*. 2004;279(21):22020–22029.
116. Yang X, Stennicke HR, Wang B, et al. Granzyme B mimics apical caspases. Description of a unified pathway for trans-activation of executioner caspase-3 and -7. *J Biol Chem*. 1998;273(51):34278–34283.
117. Casciola-Rosen L, Andrade F, Ulanet D, et al. Cleavage by granzyme B is strongly predictive of autoantigen status: implications for initiation of autoimmunity. *J Exp Med*. 1999;190(6):815–826.
118. Bredemeyer AJ, Lewis RM, Malone JP, et al. A proteomic approach for the discovery of protease substrates. *PNAS*. 2004;101(32):11785–11790.
119. Goping IS, Sawchuk T, Underhill DA, et al. Identification of alpha-tubulin as a granzyme B substrate during CTL-mediated apoptosis. *J Cell Sci*. 2006;119(5):858–865.
120. Adrain C, Duriez PJ, Brumatti G, et al. The cytotoxic lymphocyte protease, granzyme B, targets the cytoskeleton and perturbs microtubule polymerization dynamics. *J Biol Chem*. 2006;281(12):8118–8125.
121. Loeb CRK, Harris JL, Craik CS. Granzyme B proteolyzes receptors important to proliferation and survival, tipping the balance towards apoptosis. *J Biol Chem*. 2006;281(38):28326–28335.
122. Bredemeyer AJ, Carrigan PE, Fehniger TA, et al. Hop cleavage and function in granzyme B-induced apoptosis. *J Biol Chem*. 2006;281(48):37130–37141.
123. Heibein JA, Barry M, Motyka B, et al. Granzyme B-induced loss of mitochondrial inner membrane potential (Delta Psi m) and cytochrome c release are caspase independent. *J Immunol.* 1999; 163(9):4683–4693.
124. MacDonald G, Shi L, Vande Velde C, et al. Mitochondria-dependent and -independent regulation of Granzyme B-induced apoptosis. *J Exp Med.* 1999;189(1):131–144.
125. Heibein JA, Goping IS, Barry M, et al. Granzyme B-mediated cytochrome c release is regulated by the Bcl-2 family members bid and Bax. *J Exp Med.* 2000;192(10):1391–1402.
126. Alimonti JB, Shi L, Baijal PK, et al. Granzyme B Induces BID-mediated Cytochrome c Release and Mitochondrial Permeability Transition. *J Biol Chem*. 2001;276(10):6974–6982.
127. Pinkoski MJ, Waterhouse NJ, Heibein JA, et al. Granzyme B-mediated Apoptosis Proceeds Predominantly through a Bcl-2-inhibitable Mitochondrial Pathway. *J Biol Chem.* 2001;276(15): 12060–12067.
128. Li H, Zhu H, Xu CJ, et al. Cleavage of BID by caspase 8 mediates the mitochondrial damage in the Fas pathway of apoptosis. *Cell.* 1998;94(4):491–501.
129. Sutton VR, Davis JE, Cancilla M, et al. Initiation of apoptosis by granzyme B requires direct cleavage of bid, but not direct granzyme B-mediated caspase activation. *J Exp Med*. 2000;192(10):1403–1414.
130. Thomas DA, Scorrano L, Putcha GV, et al. Granzyme B can cause mitochondrial depolarization and cell death in the absence of BID, BAX, and BAK. *Proc Natl Acad Sci U S A*. 2001;98(26):14985–14990.
131. Goping IS, Barry M, Liston P, et al. Granzyme B-induced apoptosis requires both direct caspase activation and relief of caspase inhibition. *Immunity.* 2003;18(3):355–365.
132. Verhagen AM, Ekert PG, Pakusch M, et al. Identification of DIABLO, a Mammalian Protein that Promotes Apoptosis by Binding to and Antagonizing IAP Proteins. *Cell.* 2000;102:43–53.
133. Sutton VR, Wowk ME, Cancilla M, et al. Caspase activation by granzyme B is indirect, and caspase autoprocessing requires the release of proapoptotic mitochondrial factors. *Immunity.* 2003;18(3):319–329.
134. Bleackley RC. A molecular view of cytotoxic T lymphocyte induced killing. *Biochem Cell Biol.* 2005;83:747–751.
135. Kashkar H, Seeger JM, Hombach A, et al. XIAP targeting sensitizes Hodgkins Lymphoma cells for cytolytic T cell attack. *Blood.* 2006;108(10):3434–3440.
136. Sutton V, Vaux D, Trapani J. Bcl-2 prevents apoptosis induced by perforin and granzyme B, but not that mediated by whole cytotoxic lymphocytes. *J Immunol.* 1997;158(12):5783–5790.
137. Buzza MS, Bird PI. Extracellular granzymes. *Curr Perspectives Bio Chem*. 2006;387(7):827–837.
138. Lauw FN, Simpson AJ, Hack CE, et al. Soluble granzymes are released during human endotoxemia and in patients with severe infection due to gram-negative bacteria. *J Infect Dis*. 2000;182(1): 206–213.
139. Choy JC, Hung VH, Hunter AL, et al. Granzyme B induces smooth muscle cell apoptosis in the absence of perforin: involvement of extracellular matrix degradation. *Arterioscler Thromb Vasc Biol.* 2004;24(12):2245–2250.
140. Suidan HS, Bouvier J, Schaerer E, et al. Granzyme A released upon stimulation of cytotoxic T lymphocytes activates the thrombin receptor on neuronal cells and astrocytes. *Proc Natl Acad Sci U S A.* 1994;91(17):8112–8116.
141. Gahring L, Carlson NG, Meyer EL, et al. Granzyme B proteolysis of a neuronal glutamate receptor generates an autoantigen and is modulated by glycosylation. *J Immunol.* 2001;166(3):1433–1438.
142. Buzza MS, Zamurs L, Sun J, et al. Extracellular Matrix Remodeling by Human Granzyme B via Cleavage of Vitronectin, Fibronectin, and Laminin. *J Biol Chem.* 2005;280(25):23549–23558.
143. Pardo J, Balkow S, Anel A, et al. The differential contribution of granzyme A and granzyme B in cytotoxic T lymphocyte-mediated apoptosis is determined by the quality of target cells. *Eur J Immunol.* 2002;32(7):1980–1985.
144. Barry M, Heibein J, Pinkoski M, et al. Quantitative measurement of apoptosis induced by cytotoxic T lymphocytes. *Methods Enzymol.* 2000;322:40–46.
145. Koopman G, Reutelingsperger CP, Kuijten GA, et al. Annexin V for flow cytometric detection of phosphatidylserine expression on B cells undergoing apoptosis. *Blood*. 1994;84(5):1415–1420.
146. Farkas DL, Wei MD, Febbroriello P, et al. Simultaneous imaging of cell and mitochondrial membrane potentials. *Biophysical Journal.* 1989;56(6):1053–1069.
147. Gavrieli Y, Sherman Y, Ben-Sasson SA. Identification of programmed cell death in situ via specific labeling of nuclear DNA fragmentation. *J Cell Biol.* 1992;119(3):493–501.
148. Komoriya A, Packard BZ, Brown MJ, et al. Assessment of caspase activities in intact apoptotic thymocytes using cell-permeable fluorogenic caspase substrates. *J Exp Med.* 2000;191(11):1819–1828.
149. Leers MP, Kolgen W, Bjorklund V, et al. Immunocytochemical detection and mapping of a cytokeratin 18 neo-epitope exposed during early apoptosis. *J Pathology*. 1999;187(5):567–572.
150. Sun J, Bird CH, Sutton V, et al. A cytosolic granzyme B inhibitor related to the viral apoptotic regulator cytokine response modifier A is present in cytotoxic lymphocytes. *J Bio Chem*. 1996;271(44):27802–27809.
151. Walden PR, Eisen HN. Cognate peptides induce self-destruction of CD8+ cytolytic T lymphocytes. *Proc Natl Acad Sci U S A.* 1990; 87(22):9015–9019.
152. Balaji KN, Schaschke N, Machleidt W, et al. Surface cathepsin B protects cytotoxic lymphocytes from self-destruction after degranulation. *J Exp Med*. 2002;196(4):493–503.
153. Baran K, Ciccone A, Peters C, et al. Cytotoxic T lymphocytes from cathepsin B-deficient mice survive normally *in vitro* and *in vivo* after encountering and killing target cells. *J Bio Chem*. 2006;281(41): 30485–30491.
154. Spaner D, Raju K, Rabinovich B, et al. A role for perforin in activation-induced T cell death *in vivo*: increased expansion of allogeneic perforin-deficient T cells in SCID mice. *J Immunol.* 1999;162(2):1192–1199.
155. Kagi D, Odermatt B, Mak TW. Homeostatic regulation of $CD8^+$ T cells by perforin. *Eur J Immunol.* 1999;29(10):3262–3272.
156. Shi X, Leng L, Wang T, et al. CD44 Is the Signaling Component of the Macrophage Migration Inhibitory Factor-CD74 Receptor Complex. *Immunity.* 2006;25(4):595–606.

157. Stepp SE, Dufourcq-Lagelouse R, Le Deist F, et al. Perforin gene defects in familial hemophagocytic lymphohistiocytosis. *Science.* 1999;286(5446):1957–1959.
158. Feldmann J, Callebaut I, Raposo G, et al. Munc13-4 is essential for cytolytic granules fusion and is mutated in a form of familial hemophagocytic lymphohistiocytosis (FHL3). *Cell.* 2003;115(4): 461–473.
159. Grossman WJ, Verbsky JW, Tollefsen BL, et al. Differential expression of granzymes A and B in human cytotoxic lymphocyte subsets and T regulatory cells. *Blood.* 2004;104(9):2840–2848.
160. Grossman WJ, Verbsky JW, Barchet W, et al. Human T regulatory cells can use the perforin pathway to cause autologous target cell death. *Immunity.* 2004;21(4):589–601.
161. Kagi D, Ledermann B, Burki K, et al. Cytotoxicity mediated by T cells and natural killer cells is greatly impaired in perforin-deficient mice. *Nature.* 1994;369(6475):31–37.
162. Mullbacher A, Hla RT, Museteanu C, et al. Perforin is essential for control of ectromelia virus but not related poxviruses in mice. *J Virol.* 1999;73(2):1665–1667.
163. Mullbacher A, Lobigs M, Hla RT, et al. Antigen-dependent release of IFN-gamma by cytotoxic T cells up-regulates Fas on target cells and facilitates exocytosis-independent specific target cell lysis. *J Immunol.* 2002;169(1):145–150.
164. Alsharifi M, Lobigs M, Simon MM, et al. NK cell-mediated immunopathology during an acute viral infection of the CNS. *Eur J Immunol.* 2006;36(4):887–896.
165. Appay V, Nixon DF, Donahoe SM, et al. HIV-specific CD8(+) T cells produce antiviral cytokines but are impaired in cytolytic function. *J Exp Med.* 2000;192(1):63–75.
166. Zhang D, Shankar P, Xu Z, et al. Most antiviral CD8 T cells during chronic viral infection do not express high levels of perforin and are not directly cytotoxic. *Blood.* 2003;101(1):226–235.
167. Mempel TR, Pittet MJ, Khazaie K, et al. Regulatory T cells reversibly suppress cytotoxic T cell function independent of effector differentiation. *Immunity.* 2006;25:129–141.
168. Smyth MJ, Thia KY, Cretney E, et al. Perforin is a major contributor to NK cell control of tumor metastasis. *J Immunol.* 1999;162(11):6658–6662.
169. Smyth MJ, Thia KY, Street SE, et al. Perforin-mediated cytotoxicity is critical for surveillance of spontaneous lymphoma. *J Exp Med.* 2000;192(5):755–760.
170. Screpanti V, Wallin RP, Ljunggren HG, et al. A central role for death receptor-mediated apoptosis in the rejection of tumors by NK cells. *J Immunol.* 2001;167(4):2068–2073.
171. Morgan RA, Dudley ME, Wunderlich JR, et al. Cancer regression in patients after transfer of genetically engineered lymphocytes. *Science.* 2006;314(5796):126–129.
172. van Elsas A, Sutmuller RP, Hurwitz AA, et al. Elucidating the autoimmune and antitumor effector mechanisms of a treatment based on cytotoxic T lymphocyte antigen-4 blockade in combination with a B16 melanoma vaccine: comparison of prophylaxis and therapy. *J Exp Med.* 2001;194(4):481–489.
173. Ohashi PS, Oehen S, Buerki K, et al. Ablation of "tolerance" and induction of diabetes by virus infection in viral antigen transgenic mice. *Cell.* 1991;65(2):305–317.
174. Morgan DJ, Liblau R, Scott B, et al. CD8(+) T cell-mediated spontaneous diabetes in neonatal mice. *J Immunol.* 1996;157(3):978–983.
175. Kagi D, Odermatt B, Seiler P, et al. Reduced incidence and delayed onset of diabetes in perforin-deficient nonobese diabetic mice. *J Exp Med.* 1997;186(7):989–997.
176. Estella E, McKenzie MD, Catterall T, et al. Granzyme B-mediated death of pancreatic beta-cells requires the proapoptotic BH3-only molecule bid. *Diabetes.* 2006;55(8):2212–2219.
177. McKenzie MD, Dudek NL, Mariana L, et al. Perforin and Fas induced by IFNgamma and TNFalpha mediate beta cell death by OT-I CTL. *International Immunol.* 2006;18(6):837–846.
178. Malipiero U, Frei K, Spanaus KS, et al. Myelin oligodendrocyte glycoprotein-induced autoimmune encephalomyelitis is chronic/relapsing in perforin knockout mice, but monophasic in Fas- and Fas ligand-deficient lpr and gld mice. *Eur J Immunol.* 1997;27(12): 3151–3160.
179. Wang T, Allie R, Conant K, et al. Granzyme B mediates neurotoxicity through a G-protein-coupled receptor. *Faseb J.* 2006;20(8):1209–1211.
180. Halloran PF, Urmson J, Ramassar V, et al. Lesions of T-cell-mediated kidney allograft rejection in mice do not require perforin or granzymes A and B. *Am J Transplant.* 2004;4(5):705–712.
181. Larsen CP, Alexander DZ, Hendrix R, et al. Fas-mediated cytotoxicity. An immunoeffector or immunoregulatory pathway in T cell-mediated immune responses? *Transplantation.* 1995;60(3):221–224.
182. Martin PJ, Akatsuka Y, Hahne M, et al. Involvement of donor T-cell cytotoxic effector mechanisms in preventing allogeneic marrow graft rejection. *Blood.* 1998;92(6):2177–2181.
183. Graubert TA, DiPersio JF, Russell JH, et al. Perforin/granzyme-dependent and independent mechanisms are both important for the development of graft-versus-host disease after murine bone marrow transplantation. *J Clin Invest.* 1997;100(4):904–911.

SECTION VII

Immunity to Infectious Agents

Chapter 35

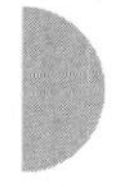

The Immune Response to Parasites

David L. Sacks, Alan Sher, Eleanor M. Riley, and Thomas A. Wynn

PARASITES AND THE IMMUNE SYSTEM

Distinct Features and Global Health Importance of Parasitic Pathogens

The term "parasite" is formally used as a designation for eukaryotic protozoan and metazoan pathogens residing within or on their hosts. The exact origin of this usage is not clear, but almost certainly it relates to the common historical period and tropical disease context in which many of these agents were identified. Indeed, parasites are the most phylogenetically diverse of pathogens, and at the lower end of their evolutionary tree they are often difficult to distinguish from fungi and protista in both their morphology and genomic organization.

Although the taxonomic basis of their classification into a single group is under question, parasites as infectious agents do share many biological characteristics. They frequently (although not always) display complex life cycles consisting of morphologically and antigenically distinct stages and produce long-lived chronic infections to ensure transmission between their hosts. The induction of severe morbidity or mortality is an atypical outcome. However, in the tropical and subtropical regions where transmission is high, the low frequency of disease translates into a major global health and economic problem because of the sheer number of people exposed and because of the confounding issues of malnutrition and coinfection. As illustrated by outbreaks in the last decade of disease caused by the protozoa *Giardia*, *Cryptosporidia*, *Cyclospora*, and *Toxoplasma*, parasites also represent a continuing threat to populations in wealthier countries. Indeed, all of the major food and water-borne protozoa have been classified as Category B bioterrorism pathogens because of their potential to cause acute epidemic illness. The AIDS epidemic has also increased the impact of parasitic disease in both developed and developing regions because immunocompromised hosts become highly susceptible to some normally tolerated parasites such as *Cryptosporidia*, *Toxoplasma gondii*, and *Leishmania*. Finally, parasitic disease remains an important problem in livestock, causing annual economic losses in the billions of dollars and, in the case of trypanosomiasis, limiting the agricultural development of huge areas of potential grazing lands on the African continent.

The immune system plays a central role in determining the outcome of parasitic infection, establishing a critical balance meant to ensure both host and pathogen survival. As with other infectious agents, disease emerges when the scales tip toward either a deficient or excessive immune response. Manipulation of that response by means of vaccination or immunotherapy remains a key approach for global intervention in parasitic disease. A list of the most important parasitic infections of humans, along with estimates of their prevalence, annual mortality, health impact (measured in disability-adjusted life years), and current control methods, is presented in Table 35.1. The data testify to the continued enormity of the problem, reflected in the numbers of people annually infected and dying of diseases such as malaria, schistosomiasis, and trypanosomiasis, as well as the high level of morbidity in those surviving. A striking situation reflected in the data is the complete absence of effective vaccines for protecting human populations. In the case of malaria, the need for a global immunization strategy has become particularly acute as drug resistance spreads worldwide.

Clearly, the development of vaccines to prevent parasitic diseases remains one of the major unachieved goals of modern immunology and one of its greatest and most difficult challenges. The scientific challenge lies with the extraordinary complexity of parasites as immunologic targets and their remarkable adaptability to immunologic pressure. The field of immunoparasitology is focused on developing a basic understanding of this important host–pathogen interface for the ultimate purpose of intervention. At the same time, the work in this area—particularly in recent years—has provided immunology with a series

TABLE 35.1 Global Impact of Parasitic Disease and Current Control Measures

	Estimated Prevalence (Millions)	Disease Burden (DALYs, Thousands)[a]	Annual Deaths (Thousands)	Control Method Used
Malaria	515	42,279	1,124	Vector control, chemotherapy
Schistosomiasis[c]	187	4,500	155–280	Chemotherapy, hygiene
Soil-transmitted helminths[b]	2,000	38,900	139	Chemotherapy, hygiene
African trypanosomiasis	0.3	1,332	50–100	Vector control
Leishmaniasis	12	1,757	51	Vector control, chemotherapy
Chagas' disease	10	586	13	Vector control
Lymphatic filariasis	120	4,600	0	Vector control, chemotherapy
Onchocerciasis	37	2,000	0	Vector control, chemotherapy

Data compiled from World Health Organization, *Disease control priorities in developing countries*, 2nd ed., 2006, available at http://www.dcp2.org/pubs/DCP, and from ref. 336.

[a]Disability-adjusted life years, a measure of the time lived with a disability, combined with the time lost due to premature mortality *(337)*.

[b]Hookworm, ascariasis, and trichuriasis. The data are combined values for all three infections.

[c]Currently being revised upward.

of major insights concerning effector and regulatory responses as they occur *in vivo*. Indeed, because of their years of close encounter with and adaptation to the vertebrate immune system, parasites can be thought of as the "ultimate immunologists," and there is much to be learned from them about the fundamental nature of immune responses.

Some Hallmarks of the Immune Response to Parasites

The interaction of parasites with the immune system has several distinguishing features that are of special interest to fundamental immunologists. Most parasitic pathogens are able to survive the initial host response and produce long-lasting chronic infections designed to promote transmission. In the case of many protozoa (e.g., *Toxoplasma, Leishmania*), *chronicity* is characterized by a state of *latency* in which replication of the parasite is minimal and infection cryptic. The development of chronicity depends not only on the ability of the parasite to escape protective immune responses (*immune evasion*), but also on the generation of finely tuned mechanisms of *immunoregulation* that serve both to prevent parasite elimination and suppress host immunopathology. As discussed in detail later in this chapter, the study of these immunomodulatory pathways in both human and experimental parasitic infections has yielded important insights concerning the mechanisms by which regulatory T cells and cytokines control immune effector functions *in vivo*.

An additional prominent feature of the immune response to parasites is *Th1/Th2 polarization*. For reasons that are not entirely clear, parasitic infections often induce $CD4^+$ T cell responses that are highly polarized in terms of their Th1/Th2 lymphokine profiles. This phenomenon is particularly striking in the case of helminths, which, in contrast to nearly all other pathogens, routinely trigger strong Th2 responses leading to high immunoglobulin E (IgE) levels, eosinophilia, and mastocytosis. At the opposite pole, many intracellular protozoa (in common with their bacterial counterparts) induce $CD4^+$ T cell responses with Th1-dominated lymphokine secretion patterns. This striking difference presents a beautiful example of immunologic class selection. Of interest, in murine *Leishmania major* infection, $CD4^+$ cells polarize to either Th1 or Th2, depending on the strain of mouse infected, and the association of these responses with healing or exacerbation provided the first demonstration of a functional role for this dichotomy (1,2). Parasite models have also been used to reveal new effector functions, such as the ability of eosinophils to kill pathogens, and, as discussed later, they are now being used extensively to study microbial innate recognition and immune response initiation. This ability to uncover and investigate basic immune and immunopathogenic mechanisms while studying the host response to a group of phylogenetically unique pathogens of global importance is perhaps the most engaging and rewarding aspect of research in immunoparasitology.

INNATE RECOGNITION AND HOST DEFENSE

Innate recognition plays an important role in determining the outcome of the host–parasite encounter by both providing an initial barrier to infection and influencing the magnitude and class of the subsequent adaptive immune response. At the same time, from the parasite's point of view, innate immune defenses must be subverted for infection to be established, and it is clear that many parasitic pathogens have evolved specific mechanisms for evading them. Moreover, in some cases parasites appear actually to hijack the process of innate recognition to redirect adaptive immunity to promote their own persistence.

Humoral Mechanisms

Innate resistance against parasitic infection is mediated in part by preexisting soluble factors that recognize and destroy invading developmental stages or target them for killing by effector cells. The alternative pathway of complement activation provides a first line of defense against extracellular parasites. Invading forms of many of these pathogens lack the complement regulatory factors that normally promote the degradation of C3b on the surface of host cells. The resulting activation of the complement cascade leads to formation of the potentially lytic membrane attack complex (MAC), as well as opsonic recognition by C3 receptors on phagocytes. In addition, other products of complement activation are chemotactic and attract immune cells to the site of infection. There is also a lectin-mediated pathway in which recognition of mannose residues on parasite surfaces by a mannan-binding protein triggers the complement cascade.

Because the complement system represents such an important first line of defense in resistance to pathogens, the infectious stages of parasitic protozoa and helminths have developed a variety of strategies to subvert complement-mediated attack. In some instances blood and tissue parasites have evolved redundant mechanisms to ensure their survival during serum exposure. For example, infective metacyclic and bloodstream trypomastigotes of *Trypanosoma cruzi* express multiple stage-specific surface glycoproteins, such as gp160 and the 87- to 93-kDa trypomastigote decay accelerating factor (T-DAF), which are actively released by the parasite and are functional homologs of human DAF, which interferes with assembly of C3 convertases by binding to C3b (3). Another trypomastigote glycoprotein, gp58/68, inhibits alternative pathway C3 convertase assembly by binding to factor B. *T. cruzi* trypomastigotes have also been found continuously to shed acceptor molecules with covalently bound C3 fragments, believed to be due to an endogenous phospholipase that cleaves glycosylphosphatidylinositol (GPI)–anchored membrane proteins. *T. cruzi* amastigotes have been shown to resist complement lysis by preventing membrane insertion of the MAC C5b-9. An identical mechanism of resistance has been observed for the infective-stage, metacyclic promastigotes of *Leishmania*, which expresses an elongated form of the abundant surface lipophosphoglyan, such that it behaves as an effective barrier to membrane insertion and pore formation by MAC (4). Metacyclics also increase expression of the surface metalloproteinase gp63 *(5)*, which can cleave C3b to the inactive iC3b form, thus preventing deposition of MAC *(6)*. Both C3b and iC3b effectively opsonize the complement-resistant forms for uptake by macrophages, its host cell of choice. Tissue-invasive strains of *Entamoeba histolytica* also activate alternative complement pathway but are resistant to lysis due to the action of a Gal/GalNAc lectin, which mediates adherence of trophozoites to host cells and binds to C8 and C9 terminal components (7). Of interest, the lectin shares sequence similarities with CD59, a membrane inhibitor of MAC in human blood cells.

Another set of soluble mediators providing a barrier to parasitic infection comprises the primate-specific trypanosome lysis factors (TLFs) that contribute to the innate resistance of humans to *Trypanosoma brucei* infection. Biochemical analysis of the activity present in human serum revealed that high-density lipoproteins (HDLs) are part of the substance that mediates cytolysis of the parasite, and initial studies demonstrated that this complex, TLF, is composed of several common apolipoproteins, as well as a haptoglobin-related protein (Hpr) and apolipoprotein L-1 (ApoL-1) (8–10). Both Hpr and ApoL-1 are cytotoxic to *T. b. brucei* and act synergistically to provide enhanced trypanosome killing when assembled into the same HDL particle. To mediate cytotoxicity, TLF has to undergo receptor-mediated uptake and enter an intracellular acidic compartment. Hpr and ApoL-1 have different proposed activities; ApoL-1 is able to form ion pores in lysosomal membranes, whereas Hpr is able to accelerate lysosomal membrane peroxidation. A combination of these two activities may be needed for the complete protection TLF affords against *T. b. brucei* infection. Whereas TLF is capable of killing *T. brucei*—the species that infect humans—both *T. b. gambiense* and *T. b. rhodesiense* are refractory to TLF-mediated cytolysis. This resistance has been correlated with the expression of a serum resistance associated (SRA) gene that is homologous to the variant surface glycoprotein. Of note, transfection of SRA from *T. b. rhodesiense* into *T. brucei* confers resistance to lysis by human serum, suggesting that its expression may have been a critical step in the adaptation of the former parasite for infection of primates *(11)*.

The damage caused to worms as a consequence of alternative pathway activation is due primarily to the bound C3 activation products that act as ligands for cellular adherence and killing by eosinophils, neutrophils, and macrophages. Unlike the examples of parasitic protozoa cited earlier, worms may not rely on synthesizing their own complement regulatory proteins to subdue the activation cascade, but rely instead on acquisition of these proteins from the host. In the case of *Schistosoma mansoni*, DAF molecules are acquired from the host and incorporated into the worm tegument (12). The infective L3 stage larvae of *Onchocerca volvulus*, the causative agent of river blindness, were shown to bind the main fluid-phase regulator—human factor H—and to promote C3b inactivation *(13)*. By contrast, the infective stage L3 larvae of the mouse nematode *Nippostrongylus brasiliensis* are extremely vulnerable to complement-dependent attack by eosinophils, but by 24 hours the lung-stage L4 larvae no longer fix complement and are no longer susceptible (14). Whether the lung-stage larvae acquire complement-regulatory proteins from the host or secrete/excrete complement-inhibitory proteins, as has been shown for nematode larvae of *Toxocara canis (15)*, has not been determined.

Cellular Mechanisms

Phagocytosis by macrophages represents an innate first line of defense against protozoan pathogens. Macrophages possess primary defense mechanisms, including activation of macrophage oxidative metabolism, that are induced by the attachment and engulfment of microbial agents. The major source of reactive oxygen species (ROSs) in macrophages is the multimeric enzyme complex NADPH oxidase. Early studies suggested that *Leishmania* parasites avoid triggering the oxidative burst by actively inhibiting the macrophage protein kinase C (PKC) activation (16) that is required for phosphorylation of several sites on the cytosolic oxidase subunit p47phox. Inhibition of PKC-mediated protein phosphorylation and suppression of respiratory burst induction was observed using purified lipophosphoglycan (LPG), which is rapidly transferred from the parasite to the inner leaflet of the phagosomal membrane *(17)*. Insertion of the glycolipid has been shown to alter the physical properties of the bilayer to inhibit PKC membrane translocation, and might similarly inhibit translocation of the cytosolic components of the NADPH oxidase. Because some LPG-deficient *Leishmania* strains still manage to survive in macrophages, redundant mechanisms exist for the parasite to avoid macrophage triggering, including opsonic ingestion through receptors that are uncoupled from the activation of NADPH oxidase. A number of "silent" entry receptors have been described that are variably used by different species and developmental stages of *Leishmania*, including complement and mannose receptors *(18)*, galectin-3 *(19)*, and receptors for apoptotic cells (20,*21*). In contrast to *Leishmania*, *Toxoplasma* enters all nucleated cells, including macrophages, by an active invasion mechanism that excludes most host cell proteins, including membrane components of the NADPH oxidase, from the parasitophorous vacuole (22). Malaria parasites are also sensitive to oxidative stress, in this case generated primarily as a result of the degradation of host hemoglobin within parasitized red blood cells (RBCs) *(23)*. The detoxification of ROS is achieved with a range of low-molecular weight antioxidants, including the tripeptide glutathione, and a number of host- and parasite-encoded enzymes *(24)*.

The development of phagosomes into digestive organelles represents the heart of the defensive machinery of macrophages, and intracellular parasites have evolved diverse strategies to avoid, escape from, or withstand the acidified, hydrolytic environment of phagolysosomes. For *Toxoplasma*, the integral membrane proteins that are excluded from the nascent vacuole include those involved in acidification and fusion with the endosomal network (25). If instead the parasite is forced to enter the cell by a phagocytic pathway, as a consequence of, for example, antibody opsonization, it is targeted through the normal phagolysosomal system and is killed (26). For *T. cruzi*, which trigger a wound repair pathway involving lysosome exocytosis to enter into cells, the early vacuole is acidified and potentially fusogenic. Intracellular survival of *T. cruzi* depends on its ability to escape from the vacuole, a process facilitated by its expression of a homolog of C9 that can disrupt the phagosome membrane and allow egress of the parasite into the cytoplasm (27). *Leishmania* promastigotes, again via transfer of their surface LPG, transiently inhibit normal phagosome maturation (28). LPG was found to increase the periphagosomal accumulation of F-actin and to disrupt phagosome microdomains, which in each case will impair normal endocytic trafficking and fusion. The delay in phagosome maturation may be necessary to allow sufficient time for metacyclic promastigotes to differentiate into more-acidophilic, hydrolase-resistant amastigotes. The various strategies employed by parasitic protozoa to evade the innate defenses of host cell macrophages are depicted in Figure 35.1.

Unlike protozoa, helminths are too big to be engulfed by phagocytes and can only be killed by these cells when the latter have been activated by products of the adaptive immune response. Instead, eosinophils, which frequently accumulate in tissues soon after worm invasion, may mediate innate cellular defense against helminth larvae by the discharge of the major basic protein and cationic proteins present in the granules of these cells (29,30).

In contrast to intracellular killing by phagocytes and extracellular killing by eosinophils, other innate cellular defenses do not eliminate parasites directly but instead trigger other effector cells to do so. Perhaps the best-studied example of this form of innate immunity is the natural killer (NK) cell pathway of interferon-γ (IFNγ) and tissue necrosis factor-α (TNFα) production. NK cell numbers and nonspecific lytic activity are increased as a consequence of a variety of parasitic infections, and *Leishmania* promastigotes, *Plasmodium falciparum*–infected red blood cells, components of *T. gondii, T. cruzi, E. histolytica,* and *Cryptosporidium parvum* (reviewed in ref. 31), and excretory-secretory (ES) proteins of the hookworm *Necator americanus (32)* all activate human peripheral blood NK cells to produce IFNγ. These findings suggest that NK cells may provide a T lymphocyte–independent pathway for cytokine-mediated defense and as such serve to prevent parasites from overwhelming the host prior to the development of adaptive responses. For the majority of pathogens, NK cell IFNγ is triggered by monokines, critically interleukin-12 (IL-12) *(33)*, produced by macrophages and dendritic cells (DCs) in response to microbial products. Trafficking of NK cells to parasite-infected tissues is critically dependent on chemokines binding to CCR5 *(34)*. Both IL-10 and transforming growth factor-β (TGFβ) have been shown to serve as negative regulators of NK cell IFNγ production by means of their suppression of monokine and B7 expression by antigen-presenting cells (APCs) or, in the case of TGFβ, by directly affecting NK cell function (35). Such suppression may be important in protecting the host against the tissue-damaging effects of excessive NK-derived IFNγ and TNFα. NK cell responses are further regulated by calibration of signals from activating and inhibitory receptors for major histocompatibility class (MHC) molecules; moderation of NK responses to malaria-infected red blood cells by inhibitory receptors such as NKG2A/CD94 and polymorphic killer-cell immunoglobulin-like receptors (KIRs) has been proposed (36). Although NK cell–derived IFNγ can limit the initial phase of protozoal replication (37) and may a play a role in the polarization and expansion of Th1 cells, in some situations adaptive T cell immunity is sufficient to control infection even in the absence of this early NK response (38,39). The role of NK cell cytotoxicity in resistance to protozoan infection is less well understood; for murine malaria it is not required for NK-mediated resistance to blood stages (38), but cytotoxic NK killing of malaria-infected liver cells has been reported *(40)*.

Two other cell populations that may function to provide a rapid cytokine response to invading parasites are $\gamma\delta$ lymphocytes and NK T cells. These "unconventional T lymphocytes" express T cell receptor chains of limited diversity, which may be designed for innate recognition of microbial structures or self-components revealed by infection of host cells. Although the function of NK T cells in innate resistance to parasites is under debate, there is considerable evidence supporting a protective role for $\gamma\delta$ T cells. $\gamma\delta$ T cells can respond to heat shock proteins (HSPs), and because invasion and intracellular replication by different parasites results in increased expression of HSPs, this may provide a mechanism that allows $\gamma\delta$ T cells to nonspecifically restrict infection either by direct host cell

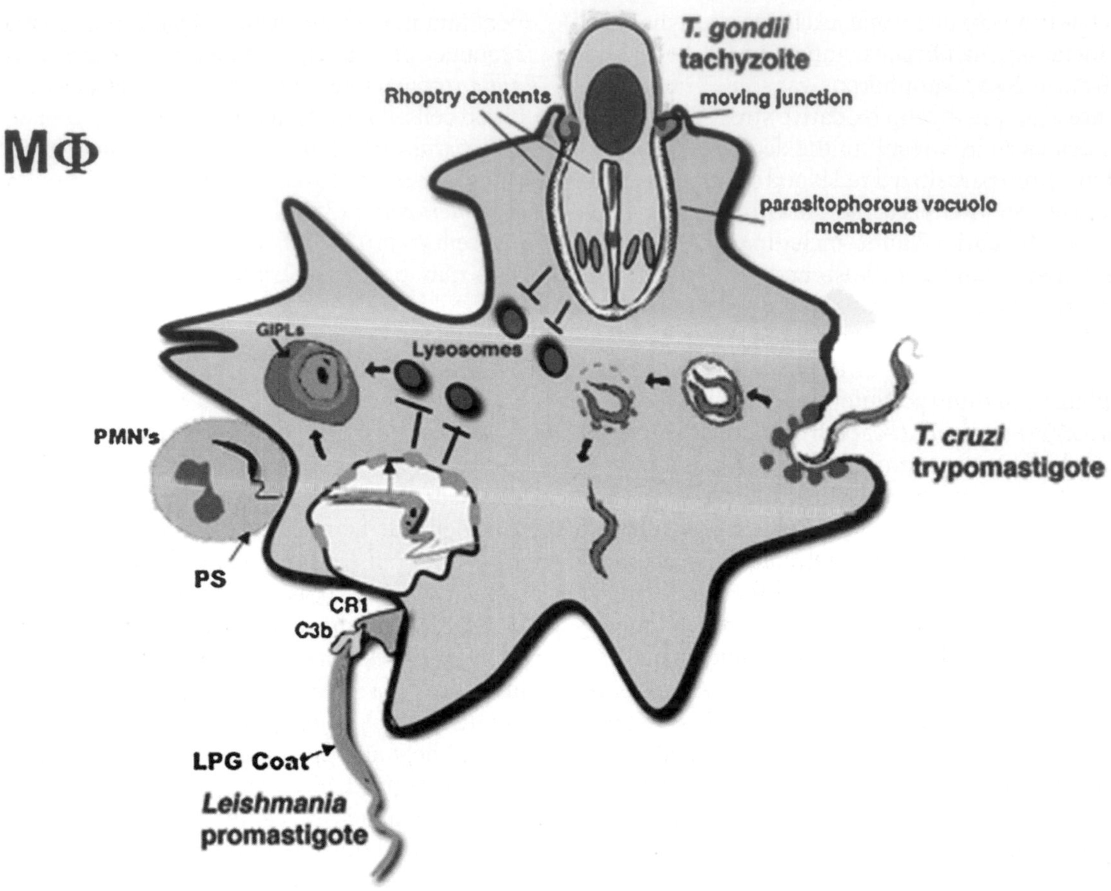

FIGURE 35.1 Evasion of innate immune mechanisms in infected macrophages by parasitic protozoa. Macrophages possess potent antimicrobial functions that are initiated by uptake of pathogens. Opsonization of *Leishmania* with C3 cleavage fragments C3b and C3bi results in uptake by CR1 and CR3 receptors that are unlinked from the signaling pathways involved in induction of reactive oxygen intermediates or proinflammatory cytokines. Silent uptake using receptors for apoptotic, phosphatidyl serine (PS)–positive neutrophils delivering viable promastigotes has also been described. In addition, the transfer of surface lipophosphoglycan (LPG) to the phagosome membrane results in delayed fusion with lysosomes. After transformation to amastigotes, which are more hydrolase resistant due to an abundance of surface glycoinositolphopsholipids (GIPLs), phagosome maturation proceeds. *Toxoplasma* actively invades by rapid discharge of adhesive proteins from secretory organelles called rhoptries, then by inserting and squeezing past a moving junction in the plasma membrane that acts as a molecular sieve, excluding from its vacuole host proteins required for acidification and fusion with the endosomal network. *Trypanosoma cruzi* trypomastigotes enter the macrophage by inducing the recruitment of lysosomes to the plasma membrane; they only transiently reside in the vacuole before escaping into the cytoplasm via secretion of a pore-forming molecule.

lysis or, more likely, by the production of IFNγ and other effector lymphokines. Although $\gamma\delta$ T cells represent a small percentage of lymphocytes in the periphery, they are abundant in epithelial and mucosal tissues, the sites of initial host invasion by many parasites. Moreover, their numbers increase in peripheral blood in response to a number of protozoan infections *(41)*, in which they appear to play a protective role (42,*43*). Nevertheless, rather than being essential for host resistance, it is likely that $\gamma\delta$ T lymphocytes (in common with NK cells) provide an adjunct to conventional $\alpha\beta$ CD4 and CD8 cells, restricting parasite growth during the vulnerable period when the adaptive responses mediated by these effectors are emerging.

Role of Pattern Recognition Receptors in Innate Recognition of Parasites

The innate immune system, in addition to providing a natural barrier that limits infection, also plays a critical role in the initial recognition of parasites and the triggering of adaptive immunity. Invading parasites, like other pathogens, are sensed by host pattern recognition receptors (PRRs) that recognize microbe-associated molecular patterns (MAMPs) shared by different groups of organisms. These PRRs are highly expressed on both epithelial and antigen-presenting cells and when ligated trigger cytokine and costimulatory signals that initiate both innate and adaptive cellular responses. Until quite recently little was known about pattern recognition of parasites, which, in contrast to bacteria and viruses, are eukaryotes. The last few years have seen an enormous expansion of research on this topic, in part driven by the need to better understand how specific effector responses against parasitic pathogens are initiated.

Toll-like receptors (TLRs) are the major group of PRRs known to be triggered by parasites (Table 35.2), although the role of non-TLR PRRs (e.g., NOD-like receptors, c-type lectins) has yet to be carefully examined. The study of TLR involvement in parasitic infection began with the identification of parasite ligands that stimulate cytokine production from macrophages and DCs. In the case of protozoa, an important class of such molecular structures is made up of the GPI lipid anchors present on many parasite surface proteins and membrane-associated but nonanchored glycoinositolphospholipids (GIPLs). Thus, GPIs from *T. brucei*, *Leishmania*, and *P. falciparum* can stimulate macrophages to upregulate inducible nitric oxide synthase (iNOS) expression and produce TNF and IL-1. Similarly, the GPI anchor fraction of mucin-like molecules from *T. cruzi* trypomastigotes triggers macrophage production of IL-12 and TNF. GIPLS from *T. cruzi*, *T. brucei*, and *P. falciparum* possess similar agonist activities (reviewed in ref. 44). Studies using reporter cell lines transfected with specific TLR molecules or TLR-specific knockouts have demonstrated that the responses induced by these parasite glycolipids are due to stimulation of TLR2 and to a lesser extent TLR4 (preferentially triggered by GIPLS in the case of *T. cruzi*). Both of the two TLR2 heterodimers have been implicated, with GPIs from *T. cruzi* and *P. falciparum* selectively triggering the TLR2–TLR6 and TLR2–TLR1 complexes, respectively.

A chemically different class of TLR ligands is made up of the profilin proteins expressed by apicomplexan protozoa. These molecules are unique to eukaryotes and are typically associated with intracellular actin. Profilins from *T. gondii*, *Eimeria*, and *Cryptosporidium parvum* potently trigger IL-12 production from murine DCs as well as systemically following *in vivo* inoculation *(45)*. Studies in the murine *T. gondii* model established that this response is due to the stimulation of TLR11, a TLR that, although present in mice and other lower animals, is not functionally expressed in primates. Finally, genomic DNAs from several protozoan species have been shown to stimulate host proinflammatory cytokine production, presumably through the recognition of unmethylated CpG motifs by TLR9, although this interaction has been directly

TABLE 35.2 Parasite Molecular Patterns (MAMPs) Recognized by Toll-Like Receptors (TLRs)

MAMPs	*Parasite*	*Structure*	*TLR Stimulated*	*Ref.*
GPI anchors	*Leishmania* ssp.	LPG	TLR2	44
	Trypanosoma cruzi	GPI anchors containing unsaturated alkylacylglycerol	TLR2	
		GIPLs containing ceramide	TLR4	
	Trypanosoma brucei	GPI anchors of VSG	Undefined	
	Plasmodium falciparum	GPI anchors of merozoite surface proteins	TLR2 TLR4	*338*
	Toxoplasma gondii	GIPLs and GPI anchors	TLR2 TLR4	
Genomic DNA	*T. brucei*	Contain unmethylated CpG motifs	TLR9	*47*
	T. cruzi	Contain unmethylated CpG motifs	TLR9	46,344
Hemazoin	*P. falciparum*	Polymerized heme from degradation of hemoglobin	TLR9	48,345
Protein	*T. gondii* (and related apicomplexa)	Profilin molecules	TLR11	*45*
Phospholipid	*Schistosom mansoni*	Lysophosphatidylserine in tegument	TLR2	51
Phosphorylcholine	Filarial nematodes	Phosphorylcholine-containing glycoconjugates on ES-62 glycoprotein	TLR4	50
RNA	*Schistosoma mansoni*	Double-stranded RNA in parasite ova	TLR3	52

ES-62, filarial excretory-secretory antigen; GIPL, glycoinositolphospholipid; GPI, glycosylphosphatidylinositol; LPG, lipophosphoglycan; VSG, variant surface glycoproteins.
Adapted from Gazzinelli RT, Denkers EY. Protozoan encounters with Toll-like receptor signalling pathways: implications for host parasitism. *Nat Rev Immunol.* 2006;6(12):895, with permission.

demonstrated only with *T. brucei* and *T. cruzi* DNAs (*46,47*). In the case of *P. falciparum*, hemazoin, a product of malaria-induced hemoglobin degradation, is a TLR9 agonist *(48)*, although there is controversy as to whether this results from contamination with immunostimulatory DNA fragments of parasite origin.

Helminth parasites also appear to express TLR ligands, although, as discussed later, their role in immune response has been harder to define than those characterized in protozoa. Moreover, in many studies the possibility of contamination by bacterial or viral TLR ligands from symbionts has not been systematically ruled out. Indeed, *Wolbachia* symbionts confer strong TLR4 and TLR2 agonist activity on filarial parasites due to endotoxin-like components present in these bacteria (49). Well-studied examples of helminth TLR MAMPs include the phosphorylcholine-containing moieties of the filarial glycoprotein ES-62 (50) and the lysophosphatidylserine components of schistosome membranes (51), which trigger TLR4 and TLR2, respectively. In addition, schistosome eggs possess double-stranded RNA molecules that stimulate TLR3 in DCs (52).

The role played by TLR in the host response to parasites is complex and not fully delineated in any of the host–parasite models studied. The main evidence for TLR involvement comes from experiments in mice deficient in MyD88, a major adaptor protein required for signaling by most TLR/IL-R receptors. These animals exhibit a loss in resistance to *T. gondii, T. cruzi, L. major,* and *T. brucei* and, in the case of *Plasmodium berghei,* decreased immunopathology (44), reflecting the role of TLR signaling in the initiation and maintenance of Th1 responses. Of significance, no major alterations in helminth-induced immune responses have been reported in MyD88-deficient hosts on susceptible genetic backgrounds, arguing against a major role for the TLR signaling in Th2-dependent host resistance and pathology against worm infections.

In contrast to the dramatically increased susceptibility often observed in MyD88$^{-/-}$ mice after protozoan infection, mice deficient in a single TLR exposed to the same parasites rarely show pronounced changes in resistance even when such animals display major immune response impairments. For example, whereas TLR11$^{-/-}$ mice infected with *T. gondii* develop severely blunted IL-12 responses both *in vitro* and *in vivo*, they nevertheless survive the acute-phase infection and show only a minor increase in parasite load in comparison to fully susceptible IL-12–deficient animals *(45)*. Such findings may reflect redundant functions for different TLRs or a requirement for multiple MyD880-dependent TLR (or IL-1/IL-18) signals in host resistance. Indeed, mice doubly deficient in TLR2 and TLR9 show greater susceptibility to *T. cruzi* infection than either of the single knockouts *(46)*. Additional synergy in TLR function is seen in mice engineered to be deficient in both MyD88$^{-/-}$ and TRIF (an adaptor used by TLR3 and TLR4 in triggering type I IFN production). These double knockouts are even more susceptible to *T. cruzi* than MyD88$^{-/-}$ mice, an effect attributed to defective IFNβ production (53). An additional complexity is that mice deficient in a single TLR may show unaltered (or even enhanced) resistance because the TLR in question controls an immunopathologic response or downregulates host effector functions (54). A major challenge of research in this area is to decipher such positive and negative parasite-induced TLR signals and to elucidate their interactions with other PRRs both within and without the TLR family.

DCs play a major role in linking parasite pattern-recognition signals to the induction of both NK-mediated innate responses and T cell–dependent adaptive immunity *(33)*. As discussed previously, in the case of many protozoa, DC-produced IL-12 provides a major stimulus for the initiation of both host defense pathways. The critical role of DCs is underscored by the impaired IL-12 production as well as control of protozoan *(T. gondii)* infection (55) seen in mice in which CD11c^{+} DC populations have been genetically depleted. Such DC-depleted mice are also unable to generate CD8^{+} CTL responses against *Plasmodium yoelii* sporozoites (56). The requirement for protozoan invasion in DC activation is complex and depends on the parasite species and DC subset in question. Indeed, as discussed later, infection of DCs can result in suppressed responsiveness to activation stimuli. Nevertheless, live infection of DCs with, for example, *Leishmania (57)* or *T. gondii (58)* appears to be important for efficient priming of CD8^{+} T cells despite the sequestration of many of the protozoa in question within parasitophorous vacuoles physically removed from the class I MHC antigen presentation machinery of the host cell. In addition, it appears that under certain situations [e.g., immunization with irradiated sporozoites *(59)*] infected apoptotic host cells are taken up by DCs as a mechanism of CD8^{+} T cell priming.

Downregulation of Proinflammatory Signaling Pathways in Macrophages and DCs

In addition to upregulating APC function, parasite products can also dampen their activity either as a mechanism of immune evasion or for the purpose of protecting the host against an uncontrolled immune response. *Leishmania*, *T. cruzi*, and *Toxoplasma* have in common their ability to inhibit proinflammatory and IFNγ-inducible responses in infected macrophages, such that the parasites might not only prevent or delay the induction of Th1 responses, but also render infected macrophages unresponsive to activation signals during the effector phase of the immune response. For *Leishmania*, the inhibition is due in part to activation of host cell tyrosine phosphatases, including SHP-1, which inactivates JAK2 and ERK1/2 MAP kinases involved in the IFNγ-inducible phosphorylation cascade (60). The major *Leishmania* GPI-anchored glycolipids LPG and GIPLS have been shown to inhibit signaling pathways in macrophages, resulting in impaired production of IL-12 *(61)*, essential for the development of protective immunity. By contrast with *Leishmania*, the ability of GPI anchors derived from *T. cruzi* trypomastigotes to trigger macrophages to produce proinflammatory cytokines is, as already discussed, well described (44). The GPI-mucin-like glycoprotein signals through TLR2, and it functions similarly to lipopolysaccharide (LPS) in inducing a state of tolerance in macrophages, such that subsequent responses to itself and even other TLR agonists are suppressed (62). Both LPS and the trypanosome GPI-mucin induce host cell phosphatase activities that are associated with defective MAPK activation and IκB degradation. The GPI anchor substituents associated with the shed variant surface glycoprotein (VSG) of African trypanosomes also potentiate the proinflammatory cytokine response in macrophages exposed simultaneously to IFNγ (63). If, however, the macrophages are preexposed to released VSG, the subsequent IFNγ-induced response, including Stat-1 phosphorylation, is markedly reduced. Infection with *T. gondii* is also characterized by the strong production of proinflammatory cytokines, such as IL-12 and TNFα required for host resistance; however, nuclear translocation of both NF-κB and Stat1 is blocked in infected cells, despite the fact that both transcription factors undergo phosphorylation-dependent activation in infected cells (64). Thus, although both *T. cruzi* and *T. gondii* initiate strong proinflammatory responses in host macrophages, these signaling pathways appear to be subsequently impaired to avoid reaching pathologic levels that may be lethal to the host and/or lethal to the parasite during the adaptive phase of the immune response.

In addition to their suppressive effects on macrophages, parasite products can also negatively regulate dendritic cell function. For example, CCR5-dependent IL-12 production by splenic DCs is rapidly suppressed after initial *in vivo* stimulation with *T. gondii* (STAg) and cannot be restimulated for approximately 1 week thereafter. This inhibition appears to result from the induction by parasite products of lipoxin A4, an arachadonic acid metabolite that downregulates both CCR5 expression on DCs and IL-12 production by the same cells (65). Similarly, in murine malaria infections, the initial burst of inflammatory cytokine production is downregulated as DCs become refractory to further TLR signalling (66). A similar phenomenon is observed with human DCs exposed to *P. falciparum*, in which case it appears to be mediated by direct binding of infected red blood cells to the scavenger receptor CD36 on the DCs (67). Human DCs exposed to *T. cruzi* trypomastigotes also become unresponsive to subsequent LPS-induced activation, a refractory state that can be achieved by the ceramide portion of the parasite-derived GIPL *(68)*. Studies with *Leishmania* suggest a more passive strategy for avoidance or delayed initiation of immune control mechanisms. In the case of *L. major*, the metacyclic promastigotes that are deposited in the skin by vector sand flies are poorly taken up by DCs, whereas the efficient uptake of amastigotes by DCs *in vitro* and *in vivo* was found to depend on parasite-reactive IgG and involved FcgRI and FcgRIII that primed them for efficient production of IL-12 *(69)*. Furthermore, the initial encounter of other *Leishmania* species associated with more chronic infections fail to activate DCs on their own or to prime them for further maturation and IL-12 p70 secretion in response to endogenous agonists such as IFNγ and CD40L (70). Similarly, DCs exposed to helminths show only minor signs of maturation, and in the case of DCs exposed to schistosome egg antigens (SEA) or to microfilaria, their Th1-inducing capacity in response to TLR ligands or CD40L/IFNγ became severely impaired (71–73).

Mechanisms Underlying Th1/Th2 Response Selection

Because parasites often stimulate CD4$^+$ T cell responses that are highly polarized in either the Th1 or Th2 direction, parasitic infection models have become important tools for studying the cellular basis of Th1/Th2 subset selection. As discussed previously, DCs are believed to be an important source of the signals that determine CD4$^+$ T cell effector choice, and their role is best understood for Th1 responses. *T. gondii, T. cruzi, Plasmodium,* and to a lesser extent *Leishmania* have been shown to activate DCs, resulting in upregulated expression of IL-12 and costimulatory molecules. One of the costimulatory molecules induced on such DCs is CD40. Of interest, when upregulated CD40 on DCs interacts with CD40L on T cells, IL-12 p70 synthesis is enhanced, which in the case of *Leishmania* provides an essential positive feedback loop for Th1 activation and immunity *(74)*. In addition to its role in initiating Th1 differentiation, an unexpected requirement for continuous IL-12 signaling was observed for the maintenance of host resistance to *T. gondii* and *Leishmania* infections even in the chronic state (75,76). Also contrary to accepted dogma, there is the evidence that IL-12 signaling is not obligatory for initial Th1 subset selection. Thus, in studies in which parasite-induced CD4$^+$ T lymphocyte responses were analyzed at a single-cell level, wild-type and IL-12–knockout mice exposed to *T. gondii* developed comparable frequencies of splenic IFNγ^+ CD4$^+$ T cells, despite different levels of IFNγ being detected in the culture supernatants, suggesting that IL-12 may be more important for Th1 effector competence than for Th1 cell priming per se *(77)*. It is likely that in addition to IL-12 there are signals delivered by other cytokines, including IL-18, IFNα, and IL-1, that may be provided by protozoan-conditioned DCs to bias CD4$^+$ T cell priming toward a proinflammatory Th1$^-$ cell fate. For example, intrinsic differences were observed in high versus low production of IL-1α by DCs from BALB/c susceptible versus resistant strains, respectively, after uptake of *Leishmania* amastigotes, and injection of IL-1α around the time of *L. major* challenge enhanced protective immunity in BALB/c mice *(78)*.

As noted, the first direct demonstrations of the relevance of the Th1/Th2 balance to the regulation of disease outcome *in vivo* were made in studies on the *Leishmania major*/mouse model. The mechanisms controlling the polarized Th2 response in susceptible BALB/c mice have been of enormous interest. A key finding is that much of the early IL-4 derives from an oligoclonal population of CD4 cells with the Vβ4 Vα8 TCR that recognize the *Leishmania* antigen LACK (79). It was initially believed that these cells might represent a unique lineage in BALB/c mice that are precommitted to releasing large amounts of IL-4. Subsequent studies have revealed, however, that the Th2 response in BALB/c mice may reflect an intrinsic defect in their ability to mount or sustain a parasite-driven Th1 response. BALB/c mice appear to have an intrinsically poor Th1-differentiating capacity, because even in the absence of IL-4 or IL-4 receptor signaling, IFNγ responses remain relatively weak *(80,81)*. Of likely relevance is the observation that under conditions of neutral priming, IL-12Rβ2 expression is not maintained during Th development in BALB/c mice *(82)*.

Additional differences in the factors controlling Th1 differentiation that are intrinsic not to CD4$^+$ T cells but to components of the innate response were noted earlier with respect to IL-1 production by DCs after uptake of amastigotes. An additional strain difference that may influence Th-subset development relates to the finding that the dissemination of parasites from the site of inoculation to the draining lymph nodes and spleen occurs early in BALB/c mice, whereas early parasite containment is observed in resistant mice *(83)*. These differences in parasite dissemination raise the possibility that distinct populations of DCs with the capacity to induce preferential priming for either Th1 or Th2 cells become activated in resistant versus susceptible mice. Such populations might not represent distinct APC lineages, but instead they may reflect modulation of APC function by specific tissue environments. That the site of antigen delivery can influence T cell priming has been clearly demonstrated in the *L. major* model; parasites delivered intravenously, intranasally, or even to different skin environments can elicit Th2 responses and nonhealing infections in normally resistant mice *(84,85)*.

Whereas *L. major* infection in BALB/c mice remains an extraordinary tool for investigating the factors controlling Th2 response selection *in vivo*, the fact that the model reflects an aberrant response arising, at least in part, from inherent Th1 developmental defects suggests that these defects might not reflect the mechanisms underlying the Th2 polarization that is a hallmark of helminth infections in virtually all mammalian hosts. Furthermore, whereas the Th2 immune deviation is clearly an inappropriate host response to an intracellular pathogen like *Leishmania*, it is an evolutionarily driven, integral aspect of acquired resistance to parasitic worms. The role of DC in Th2 response selection in helminth infection seems clear because DCs conditioned by exposure to helminth products (*Brugia* or *Schistosoma*) have been shown to polarize naive T cells toward a Th2 phenotype (86,87). In this case, however, activation of DCs as judged by the upregulation of prototypic MHC and costimulatory markers appears to be minimal, as is production of IL-12 or IL-4. Furthermore, Th2 polarization is MyD88 independent, whereas Th1 differentiation is in most instances MyD88 dependent. These observations are consistent with a model of Th2 induction by DCs that occurs via a default pathway, in the absence of Th1 priming signals, especially IL-12. However, such defaulting to Th2 is not observed when IL-12–deficient mice are infected with either *T. gondii* or *Leishmania* (see earlier discussion). Furthermore, in the case of DCs exposed to schistosoma antigens, there is a requirement for expression of signaling (NF-κB) and costimulatory (CD40 and OX40L) molecules for the induction of Th2 responses (88). Notch signaling, initiated by upregulated expression of the Notch ligand Jagged 1 on APCs, has also been implicated in Th2 differentiation, and mice that lacked signaling from all four Notch receptors failed to develop a protective Th2 cell response against the gastrointestinal helminth *Trichuris muris* (89). Therefore, it is more likely that helminth-conditioned DCs, rather than initiating a default differentiation pathway in naive T cells, provide a set of positive signals that result in Th2 priming.

The concept that IL-4 provides an essential instructive signal for Th2 differentiation is also under scrutiny. As noted earlier, helminth-conditioned DCs will polarize a Th2 response *in vitro* in the absence of IL-4, and mice deficient in IL-4, IL-4R, or the Th2-promoting transcription factor STAT-6, when infected with the helminth parasite *Nippostrongylus brasiliensis* or *Schistosoma mansoni*, develop diminished but still physiologically significant Th2 responses. In the case of IL-4–deficient mice, such residual Th2 cytokine secretion was shown to mediate, through the action of IL-13, protective or immunopathologic effects against *N. braziliensis* or *S. mansoni*, respectively (90,91). Although these findings argue that whereas IL-4R/STAT-6 signaling is not essential for priming of IL-4$^+$ CD4$^+$ T lymphocytes, it is clear that IL-4 plays a critical role in the maturation and stabilization of Th2 cells once their phenotype has been decided. For example, STAT-6–deficient animals exposed to a helminth stimulus display not only diminished numbers of Th2, cells but also an expanded population of Th1 cells that appears to be IL-12 independent (92). This observation supports data from other studies arguing that an important function of the IL-4R/STAT-6 pathway may be to silence IFNγ gene expression, a mechanism that would indirectly lead to elevated Th2 frequencies. Finally, Th2 cells need not be the only source of IL-4 for maturation of the Th2 response; basophils committed to express IL-4 are recruited to the liver and lungs of mice infected with the migrating intestinal helminth *N. brasiliensis* (93,94).

EFFECTOR MECHANISMS OF HOST RESISTANCE

Once parasites have successfully evaded innate host defenses and had their antigens processed by APCs, adaptive cellular and humoral immune responses are invariably induced, usually against a wide array of antigenic constituents of each pathogen. The problem is that because of the nature of the host–parasite adaptation, these responses are rarely orchestrated in a manner that will completely eliminate the parasite or restrict its growth. The design of successful immune intervention strategies depends on the identification of relevant target antigens but even more importantly on an understanding of the type of immune response and protective mechanism that must be induced. These effector mechanisms can be broadly classified based on the type of parasite (intracellular or extracellular) against which they are directed.

Intracellular Parasites

Because of their primary habitat within host cells, intracellular parasites are believed to be susceptible mainly to cell-mediated immune effector mechanisms, often involving a mixture or succession of $CD4^+$ and $CD8^+$ T cell responses. The extent of CD8 involvement appears to be partially related to the degree of class II versus class I MHC expression on the host cells infected. $CD8^+$ T cells are especially critical effector cells for the control of *T. cruzi* or *T. gondii* infections because these parasites can infect many nucleated cell types that express only MHC class I molecules. Nevertheless, even in *Leishmania* infection, in which parasites reside almost exclusively in macrophages, $CD8^+$ T cells can be highly protective against both primary infection and challenge exposure (95,96). In addition to their contribution of IFNγ to the effector response, $CD8^+$ T cells might also control intracellular parasitic infection through the lysis of host cells. This would be of particular benefit to the host if the target cells from which viable parasites are released are themselves defective in intracellular killing (e.g., fibroblasts, DCs) and if the parasites are subsequently made available for uptake by cells that are more responsive to activation signals (e.g., macrophages). In every protozoan infection analyzed, however, including *T. gondii (97)*, malaria (98), and *T. cruzi* (99), mice deficient in the lytic molecules perforin or granzyme B show no or minimal loss of host resistance. The foregoing observations suggest that, as already noted for NK cells (see earlier discussion), the protective functions of $CD4^+$ and $CD8^+$ T cells against intracellular parasites are mediated primarily through lymphokine production rather than target cell lysis.

IFNγ is the key lymphokine involved in control of intracellular protozoan parasites, as demonstrated by the extreme susceptibility of IFNγ-deficient mouse strains to infections with *Leishmania* (100), *T. cruzi* (101), *T. gondii* (102), *Plasmodium (103)*, and even *Cryptosporidium parvum (104)*, which dwells in epithelial cells inside the gut. Its mechanism of action is perhaps clearest in the case of *Leishmania*, which replicate primarily, if not exclusively, in macrophages—a cell type readily activated by this cytokine. The major function of IFNγ in restricting parasite growth appears to be the induction of inducible nitrogen oxide synthase (iNOS) and the subsequent generation of toxic reactive nitrogen intermediates (RNIs) within infected macrophages. Thus, disruption of the iNOS gene in a normally resistant strain leads to a susceptible phenotype, and macrophages from the same knockout strain show defective IFNγ-induced control of parasite growth (105). In addition to IFNγ, optimal production of RNI depends on costimulation with TNF or triggering by alternative signals such as IFNα/β or by CD40L and LFA-1 produced by parasite-induced $CD4^+$ T cells *(106)*. The production of RNI by IFNγ-activated macrophages is inhibited by IL-4, IL-10, IL-13, and TGFβ (107), and this is likely to be a major but not the sole mechanism by which the Th2 response prevents healing in leishmaniasis.

In contrast to *Leishmania*, most intracellular protozoa, including *T. cruzi*, *T. gondii*, *Cryptosporidium*, *Eimeria*, and *Plasmodium* spp., preferentially invade cells not traditionally believed to possess microbicidal mechanisms that can be activated by IFNγ. In the case of these pathogens, the role of RNIs or respiratory oxygen intermediates (ROIs) in IFNγ-mediated control of parasite growth is more tissue restricted. A good example is the role of IFNγ in immunity against the exoerythrocytic stages of malaria. IFNγ produced primarily by $CD8^+$ T cells in response to vaccination induces RNIs within hepatocytes invaded early after sporozoite challenge and restricts further pathogen development (108). However, when malaria parasites escape the liver they take up residence in erythrocytes, which, in contrast to hepatocytes, are unable to produce RNIs.

Lymphokine-mediated intracellular control of *T. gondii* infection involves a more complicated mechanism than induction of RNIs. The immunity induced cannot be attributed solely to activated macrophages as originally believed because the parasite infects multiple host cell types and host resistance requires IFNγ signaling in cells of both hemapoietic and nonhemapoietic origin *(109)*. Accordingly, the role of RNIs in resistance has been shown to be limited, functioning predominantly in the chronic stage of infection. An important clue concerning the mechanism controlling acute infection came from studies in mice deficient for members of the p47GTPase family. These proteins are induced by IFNγ in a variety of hemapoietic as well as nonhemapoietic cell types. Mice deficient in either interferon induced GTPase (IGTP) or a second family member, LRG-47, were found to be highly susceptible to infection with *T. gondii* although they developed a normal IFNγ response (110). On IFNγ stimulation of *T. gondii*–infected cells, IGTP has been shown to traffic from the endoplasmic reticulum to the parasitophorous vacuole, where it participates in a process involving disruption of the vacuole, stripping of the tachyzoite membrane, and autophagic elimination of the parasites in the host cell cytosol (111,*112*). Although LRG-47 is similarly required for effective IFNγ-dependent control of *T. gondii*, it is not recruited to the parasitophorous vacuole and thus must serve a different function. Of interest, LRG-47 also plays a major role in IFNγ-dependent host resistance to *T. cruzi* and, in addition to regulating intracellular killing of the parasite, is required for a normal hematopoietic response to the infection. Thus, *T. cruzi*-infected LRG47$^{-/-}$ mice, although they develop a higher parasitemia, also undergo profound bone marrow failure that is likely to be the direct cause of their early mortality (113). Another IFNγ-dependent mechanism of intracellular parasite killing that limits *T. gondii* replication in human but not mouse nonhemapoietic cells is the induction of indolamine 2,3-dioxygenase, an enzyme that catabolizes tryptophan, an essential amino acid for growth of this protozoan (114). The foregoing examples underscore the complexity of the effector pathways triggered by IFNγ that act against different parasites in different host cells.

Although resistance to the erythrocytic stages of malaria is believed to be mediated primarily by humoral mechanisms, blood-stage immunity develops after infection in B cell–deficient mice and can be transferred with defined CD4$^+$ T cell lines and clones, suggesting that cell-mediated effector mechanisms also exist (115). Direct killing of infected red blood cells by lymphocytes is believed to be unlikely; instead, parasite clearance seems to depend on activation of phagocytosis by Th-1–type cytokines (of which IFNγ is absolutely crucial). Although it is possible to augment this mechanism by vaccination, experimental vaccines relying exclusively on T cell–mediated effector mechanisms have been associated with high mortality. For example, 60% of mice receiving a vaccine designed to induce CD4$^+$ Th1 responses to an immunodominant blood-stage antigen of *P. yoelii* died despite being able very effectively to eliminate infected erythrocytes (116). Even when the role of antibody is clear, as with the passive transfer of immune serum, the extent of protection is reduced by prior splenectomy or T cell depletion. The relevant pathways seem to function through cytokine (e.g., IFNγ, TNFα) activation of macrophages that phagocytose and destroy infected RBCs in spleen. This process is augmented when infected RBCs are opsonized by FcR-binding antibodies, providing an excellent example of cooperation between cellular and humoral arms of the immune response. In support of this concept, resistance to human malaria has been correlated with T cell production of IFNγ (117) and generation of NO (118) *in vitro* and with FcR-binding antibody subclasses (119).

Intracellular protozoa live briefly in the extracellular milieu during initial host infection and when they invade new cells during their *in vivo* multiplication. During this period they are vulnerable to attack by antibody (Ab). In addition, although they do not directly kill free parasites, Abs can block their invasion of new cells, thereby suppressing infection. These forms of humoral immunity are of special interest in vaccine development. After repeated infection, humans living in areas endemic for *P. falciparum* gradually develop immunity to asexual blood stages, preventing high-density parasitemia and thereby preventing clinical disease. The contribution of Abs to this resistance was demonstrated in experiments in which serum from highly immune adults was transferred to acutely infected children, resulting in a temporary but highly significant reduction in parasitemia (120). The generally accepted explanation for slow acquisition of immunity to malaria is that it is strain specific and that an individual becomes immune only after being exposed to the strains circulating in his or her community. Furthermore, humoral immunity to malaria is likely to depend on an array of Abs of differing antigen specificities and functions, including agglutination of sporozoites, merozoites, or parasitized RBCs, inhibition of parasitized RBC cytoadherence to small blood vessels, and/or blocking of hepatocyte or red cell invasion by sporozoites or free merozoites, respectively (115). For the latter mechanism, the antigenic fine specificity of the Ab is crucial because some Ab specificities are able to block merozoite invasion into erythrocytes, whereas others, with distinct but overlapping specificities, either have no effect or, in the worst case, impede the activity of invasion inhibitory specificities (121). Although many of these mechanisms operate independently of FcR binding, an additional *in vitro* mechanism has been described, Ab-dependent cellular inhibition (ADCI), in which IgG1 and IgG3 in donor serum interact with monocytes or granulocytes via FcR, triggering them to produce TNFα, which is proposed to be inhibitory for parasite development *(122)*.

A well-studied example is the antibody response against the circumsporozoite (CS) protein present on preerythrocytic stages of malaria (123). Monoclonal Abs (mAbs) directed against CS protein prevent the invasion and development of sporozoites in cultured hepatocytes and *in vivo*, in passive transfer studies, confer protective immunity against *Plasmodium berghei, P. yoelii, P. vivax*, or *P. knowlesi* sporozoite challenge *(124)*. With the advent of intravital imaging techniques, it has become apparent that sporozoites are initially inoculated into dermal connective tissues, where they may take up to 30 minutes to locate and invade a blood vessel. In immunized animals or those that have been passively transfused with anti-CS antibodies, sporozoites become immobilized within minutes and fail to invade blood vessels [see Vanderberg and Frevert (125) for excellent video imaging showing these effects]. Although incomplete sporozoite neutralization or inhibition of hepatocyte invasion allows the development of forms that can infect red cells, reducing the number of developing hepatic schizonts can significantly reduce the size of the blood inoculum and delay the onset of patent parasitemia and may allow the host more time to develop effective anti–blood stage immunity. Sporozoite antigens may therefore prove to be very valuable components of a multivalent vaccine.

Extracellular Parasites

The extracellular parasites are a highly diverse group of pathogens, which include nematoda (round worms), platyhelminthes (flat worms), and a few extracellular protozoa. Because they exhibit variability in size, tissue tropism, and mechanism of immune evasion, it is not surprising that immunity against many of these pathogens often requires more than one immune effector mechanism to mediate resistance. A variety of immune cells and mediators are activated during infection, including T cells, eosinophils, mast cells, basophils, macrophages, and antibodies. Immunity is achieved through a variety of direct and indirect mechanisms that include ADCC, increased mucus production, alterations in gut physiology, and exposure to toxic mediators produced by activated macrophages and eosinophils, which ultimately cooperate to facilitate worm expulsion. Such complex mechanisms are needed against helminths in particular because they live in the gut, blood, lymphatics, and a variety of other host tissues.

Helminth parasites induce highly polarized Th2 responses that contribute to the mast cell, eosinophil, giant cell, IgE/IgA, and mucosal responses that are typically associated with these infections. For the intestinal helminths, it is clear that elements of the type 2-response are crucial for resistance to infection. Several worms have been studied in detail in this regard: *Trichuris muris*, a natural parasite of the mouse and closely related to human whipworm, *Heligomosoides polygyrus*, *Litomosoides sigmodontis*, *Trichinella spiralis*, *Nippostrongylus brasiliensis* (the rat hookworm), and *Strongyloides stercoralis*. Although Th2 cytokines are clearly involved in resistance to many of the intestinal nematodes, the importance of Th2 immunity is less certain with many of the filarial (*Brugia malayi*, *Wuchereria bancrofti*, *Litomosoides sigmodontis*) (126–128) and schistosome species *(129)*, as discussed in detail later.

T. muris and *H. polygyrus* are both transmitted by the oral-fecal route independent of an intermediate host, and, in some strains of mice, they can establish chronic infections. In the case of *T. muris*, immunity is strictly dependent on the genetic background of the host, with resistant animals rejecting the parasite soon after exposure and susceptible animals developing long-lived chronic infections *(130)*. In this model, resistant mice develop type 2 responses, whereas susceptible mice mount type 1 responses, with a variety of immunoregulatory cytokines and mediators influencing this decision. For example, in normally susceptible strains, IFNγ, IL-12, MyD88, and Toll-like receptor-4 deficiencies (*130*,131) can promote the expansion of type 2 responses and effective clearance of the parasites.

For both *H. polygyrus* and *T. muris*, primary immunity depends on the development of a parasite-specific CD4$^+$ T cell response *(132)*. Most mouse strains are susceptible to primary *H. polygyrus* infections, but after drug clearance the animals develop strong type 2 responses and are highly resistant to secondary infection. The maintenance of immunity during recall infections is crucially dependent on the presence of memory CD4$^+$ Th2 cells at the site of infection (133). The memory Th2 response also triggers the development of alternatively activated macrophages, which help to clear secondary *H. polygyrus* infections (134). Exogenous IL-4 can cure primary *T. muris* and *H. polygyrus* infections, whereas anti-IL-4R mAb treatment suppresses immunity to both. Of interest, however, the individual roles of IL-4 and IL-13 in these infections appear to depend on the genetic background of the host because C57BL/6 IL-4 knockout mice are susceptible to *T. muris* infection, whereas BALB/c IL-4 knockouts are completely resistant *(135,136)*. These latter studies were the first to suggest an IL-4–independent role for IL-13 in resistance, which was confirmed by treating BALB/c IL-4–deficient mice with a soluble IL-13 inhibitor. IL-13–deficient mice also generate chronic infections despite developing relatively normal IL-4 responses, further emphasizing the important contribution of IL-13 to the mechanism of resistance *(135)*.

Other cytokines, chemokines, and signaling pathways, including TNF, IL-18, IL-1, IL-25, IL-10, IL-27R (WSX-1), CCL2, Notch, and the NF-κB, family were also identified as important regulators of protective IL-13 responses during *T. muris* infection. For example, mice treated with neutralizing antibodies to TNF develop relatively normal Th2 responses after infection with *T. muris*, yet they fail to expel their parasites, illustrating a critical downstream role for TNF in the mechanism of IL-13–mediated immunity *(137)*. IL-1α and IL-1β are also protective, although, unlike TNF deficiency, which does not affect the Th2 response, IL-1 deficiency has a profound inhibitory effect on Th2 cytokine production, thus identifying a unique role for IL-1 signaling in the development of immunity *(138)*. Chronic *T. muris* infections are also established in IL-10 and IL-10/IL-4 double-deficient mice, with IL-10 enhancing type 2–dependent immunity by downregulating the type 1 response (139,140). IL-10–deficient mice also display marked morbidity and mortality after *T. muris* infection, suggesting a particularly critical role for IL-10 in the development of either immunity or pathology. Mortality is reduced if the animals are treated with a broad-spectrum antibiotic, suggesting that an outgrowth of opportunistic bacteria in the gut contributes to the uncontrolled inflammation and high morbidity of IL-$10^{-/-}$ animals (140). IL-25 was also identified as an important regulator of Th2 responses *(141)*. Studies conducted with IL-$25^{-/-}$ mice showed that IL-25 is required for the rapid development of type 2 immunity during both *T. muris* and *N. brasiliensis* infection (142,143). Like IL-10, IL-25 also limited the development of pathogenic inflammation in the gut. Thus, multiple pathways are involved in the generation of protective IL-4/IL-13 responses during *T. muris* infection.

The normal development of immunity in *N. brasiliensis* infection appears to be almost entirely IL-4 independent, as demonstrated in experiments with IL-$4^{-/-}$ and anti–IL-4 mAb–treated mice (144). The IL-4–independent mechanism is, however, dependent on the IL-4 receptor and Stat6 signaling, suggesting a critical contribution of IL-13, which was confirmed in IL-13 blocking studies. IL-13- and IL-4/IL-13–deficient mice are also more susceptible to *N. brasiliensis* than IL-$4^{-/-}$ mice, further illustrating the critical role of IL-13 in the development of immunity (145). Immunity to *T. spiralis* also requires STAT6 *(146)* and IL-4R signaling but not IL-4 (126), again suggesting a dominant role for IL-13 in the development of antihelminth immunity. The fact that IL-4 and IL-13 are capable of stimulating immunity in immunodeficient hosts suggests that a non–bone marrow–derived cell expressing the IL-4R is being targeted in the gut, which was recently confirmed in elegant experiments using bone marrow chimeras *(147)*.

Notwithstanding the clear results in mice, the relative contribution of type 2 cytokines to the development of immunity in humans is uncertain. The most straightforward hypothesis, and one predicted for many years, that IgE is protective against intestinal helminths, has either been refuted following intensive investigation using mouse models or at least received little direct confirmation (148,*149*). The possibility exists, however, that there are host species differences in this regard because in rats the rapid expulsion of a secondary *T. spiralis* infection is easily transferred to naive animals with IgE *(150)*. IgE$^{-/-}$ mice can expel adult worms but at a slower pace, and they develop nearly twice as many muscle larvae as IgE$^{-/-}$ mice (151). Although type 2 cytokines promote IgE class switching in B cells, the exact mechanism by which IL-4 and IL-13 mediate worm expulsion in the gut is undefined. Nevertheless, many important advances have been made in this area over the last few years. For example, IL-4, IL-13, and *H. polygyrus* infection all have dramatic effects on intestinal physiology, causing decreased peristalsis, increased mucosal permeability, reduced sodium-linked glucose absorption, and decreased chloride secretion in response to 5-hydroxytryptamine and acetylcholine (152,*153*), which together may facilitate expulsion of enteric nematodes from the gut. Smooth muscle hypercontractility and goblet cell hyperplasia are also induced by type 2 cytokines and inhibited by IL-12 and the IL-13 decoy receptor (140,*154*,155). Intestinal permeability and smooth muscle contractility are also regulated by the actions of mast cell–derived proteases and protease-activated receptors, which are expressed throughout the small intestine. The net effect of these processes is to trap parasites in mucus within the gut lumen, increase intestinal fluid content, and peristalsis, which presumably leads to the expulsion of luminal dwelling parasites. More recently, a Th2-induced protein made by goblet cells (RELMbeta/FIZZ2) was found to inhibit *T. muris* chemotaxis by interacting with the parasite's chemosensory apparatus, suggesting an additional role for Th2-induced effector molecules in resistance to gastrointestinal nematode infection (156).

Eosinophils are also frequently associated with helminth infections. Surprisingly, they do not appear to play a significant role in protective immunity to *T. muris*, *H. polygyrus*, or *N. brasiliensis (149)*. Nevertheless, there is evidence from experiments with anti–IL-5 mAb–treated, IL-5 transgenic, and IL-5Rα-chain knockout mice that eosinophils play a significant role in immunity against tissue-invasive larval forms of *Strongyloides* spp. and *Angiostrongylus cantonensis* (*157*,*158*,159). Immunity against primary *T. spiralis* infection is also impaired in IL-5–deficient mice and is associated with decreased muscle hypercontractility *(160)*. Because eosinophils can produce significant quantities of IL-4 and/or IL-13 (161,*162*), one of their key functions may be to amplify the effector mechanisms that are controlled by type 2 cytokines (163). There is a large body of literature, primarily from studies in rats and humans, that suggests that eosinophils play a role in protection against (non–gut dwelling) schistosomes (164,165), although anti-IL–5 treated and eosinophil-deficient animals display no changes in susceptibility to these parasites, again suggesting host-species differences (161,164). Overall, despite the prevailing dogma, the majority of studies have failed to support a critical role for eosinophils in immunity to the intestinal helminths.

Mast cells, which have been linked with IL-4–induced changes in intestinal physiology, appear to play an important role in immunity to *T. spiralis*; mice treated with mAbs against stem cell factor (SCF, a non–T cell–derived cytokine) or c-kit (both of which play a central role in mast cell development) are unable to expel their parasites *(166)*. In these experiments, there was no inhibitory effect on the CD4 response, and when the mAb treatment was stopped, the parasites were quickly expelled. These data suggest that the CD4 T cell–dependent response cooperates with SCF to promote the mast cell response, which ultimately facilitates parasite expulsion. Several cytokines made by CD4 cells, including IL-3, IL-4, IL-9, IL-10, and IL-18, have been implicated in the protective mast cell responses (91,139,*167*). The contribution of IL-9 seems especially convincing because high concentrations of IL-9 accelerate the clearance of *T. spiralis (168)* and *T. muris (169)*, whereas anti–IL-9 mAb treatment inhibits immunity to *T. muris (170)*. IL-9–producing dendritic cells have been used as adjuvants to generate the protective CD4$^+$ Th2 responses (171), raising the possibility that IL-4 derived from mast cells is feeding back to enhance Th2 cell differentiation *(169)*. A similar Th2-promoting mechanism was proposed for tissue basophils, which have been identified as an important source of IL-4 in schistosome, filarial, and *N. brasiliensis* infections (93,*172*,173). In filariasis patients, the presence of antigen-specific IgE appears to be critical for basophil IL-4 production (173). Thus, CD4$^+$ Th2 cells, eosinophils, mast cells, and basophils may all contribute to the protective type 2 responses that are induced after infection with helminth parasites.

In addition to playing roles in immunity to gastrointestinal helminths, there is growing epidemiologic evidence that type 2 responses, particularly in the form of antigen-specific IgE, mediate the resistance that develops with age in endemic areas. Although the exact mechanism by which IgE Ab mediates protection is unclear, it is possible that parasite-specific IgE cooperates with eosinophils or macrophages in an ADCC type mechanism (174). Consistent with this hypothesis, carriage of the HLA-DRB1*13 class II allele is associated with increased posttreatment IgE levels against *S. mansoni* antigens and lower long-term reinfection levels (175), whereas field studies in Brazil suggested that resistance is controlled by a major gene that localizes to a region of chromosome 5, which encodes the type 2 cytokines *(176)*. IgE-primed basophils may also enhance immunity by producing Th2 cytokines (93,*172*,173).

Both type 1 and type 2 associated effector mechanisms may be needed for the efficient clearance of lymphatic filariasis *(177)* because the primary immune response to live filarial parasites is dominated by both Th2 cytokines and several proinflammatory mediators, including IFNγ, TNFα, granulocyte-macrophage colony-stimulating factor, IL-1α, and IL-8. In the *Brugia* mouse model of filariasis, B cells are required for the development of immunity (178), with IgM antibodies participating in the clearance of both primary and secondary infections and IgE assisting with primary but not secondary infections (179). Eosinophils are also required for resistance to primary *Brugia pahangi* infection *(180)*, suggesting that an ADCC-type effector mechanism facilitates parasite clearance. In the *L. sigmodontis* model of filariasis, IL-4 blocks nematode development in resistant hosts but not in susceptible strains of mice, suggesting that additional immune effector molecules are required in some hosts *(181)*. Related studies have suggested important synergy between IFNγ and IL-5 in the development of antifilarial immunity (182), although the role of IFNγ is unclear.

As with many of the extracellular parasites, resistance to protozoan trypanosomes appears to require elements of both cell-mediated and humoral immunity. The African trypanosomes are tsetse-transmitted parasites that inhabit the extracellular compartment of their host's blood and avoid detection by the humoral immune system by switching among antigenically distinct variant surface glycoproteins (VSGs) (see later discussion). Trypanosome-infected hosts typically do not produce antibodies that destroy the parasite other than those that are VSG specific. Parasitemias manifest as recurring waves, with each wave of parasites expressing a different VSG, and are cleared after development of VSG-specific Ab. Before an effective antibody response can be generated, however, the host can develop quite high parasitemias, severe trypanosomiasis-associated pathology, generalized immunosuppression, and, in some circumstances, debilitating secondary infections *(183)*. It is clear that overproduction of IFNγ and nitric oxide appears to be the root cause of these deleterious side effects *(184)* while also contributing to host resistance, because parasite control within the extravascular tissue compartment has been shown to involve a parasite antigen-specific Th1 response, associated with IFNγ-dependent activation of macrophages (*185*,186).

Another important extracellular protozoan, *Giardia*, is a flagellated intestinal parasite that causes both acute and chronic diarrheal disease. Despite its intestinal habitat, *Giardia* appears to be controlled by mechanisms distinct from those mediating resistance to most gastrointestinal nematodes, although recent studies suggest that mast cell–derived IL-6 may be important for the rapid elimination of *Giardia* in mice (187,*188*). Although a T cell–dependent mechanism is also clearly essential for resistance to acute infections, numerous studies have suggested that antibodies, particularly of the IgA isotype, are required to control chronic *G. lamblia* infections (reviewed in ref. *189*). More recently, it was suggested that neuronal NOS (NOS1) might facilitate clearance of *Giardia* from the gut by increasing gastrointestinal motility and parasite-induced diarrhea (190).

The foregoing examples stress that whereas intracellular and extracellular parasites often stimulate distinct immune response profiles, their immune control may involve overlapping immunologic effector arms.

MECHANISMS OF IMMUNE EVASION

Pathogens that rely on an invertebrate vector to complete their life cycle or are only sporadically transmitted from one host to another are under strong evolutionary pressure to prolong their survival within the mammalian host.

Because the adaptive immune response is the principal barrier to the persistence of pathogens in the mammalian host, parasites have evolved diverse strategies to evade immune control mechanisms, either by evading immune recognition or by suppressing the immune response. The former strategy refers to the ability of some parasites to sequester within sites that are inaccessible to immune attack, to mask themselves with host antigens, to shed their own target antigens, or, most notably, to undergo antigenic variation. The later strategy refers to the active suppression of established, ongoing immune responses that may contribute to the state of equilibrium that is established between host and parasite in sites of chronic infection.

Evasion of Immune Recognition

The asexual, blood stage of malaria would seem the most obvious example of a well-hidden parasite. Its ability to invade mature erythrocytes, which lack both class I and class II histocompatibility molecules, in theory at least should protect it from recognition by antibodies or effector T cells. However, because parasitized erythrocytes are efficiently cleared by the spleen, additional immune evasion strategies, that is, antigenic variation, are required (described later). Other intracellular protozoa appear to hide within immunologically privileged sites. The persistence of *T. cruzi* within heart or skeletal muscle, which is believed to underlie the pathogenesis of Chagas' disease, occurs despite the fact that parasites are cleared from most other tissue (191). Infected muscle cells may be only poorly recognized as targets for cytotoxic T lymphocytes (CTLs) or poorly accessible to their homing, or they may have intrinsic defects in immune-mediated killing mechanisms. A similar form of sequestration has been proposed to explain the long-term persistence of *Leishmania* within fibroblasts and dendritic cells following their efficient killing by activated macrophages during the acute stage of infection (192). Although persistent low-level infection of host cells has been proposed as an explanation for latency in *T. gondii* infection, the major parasite reservoir during chronic infection is undoubtedly provided by the tissue cyst, essentially a modified host cell carrying a specialized dormant parasite stage, the bradyzoite. Helminths (with the exception of *Trichinella*) do not invade host cells and therefore cannot use this strategy for evading immune recognition. Furthermore, because most multicellular helminth parasites do not replicate themselves within their mammalian hosts, they are not equipped to evade immune recognition by undergoing antigenic variation. Instead, they employ alternative mechanisms such as disguising their surfaces with host molecules and rapidly shedding membrane (tegument)-bound immune complexes (193). In addition, helminths have evolved a series of elaborate processes for inactivating antibody, complement, and cellular effector elements that threaten the parasite surface (194). Of interest, recent data suggest that helminths may take advantage of host T lymphocyte and cytokine signals as developmental triggers, and if these signals are in low abundance or lacking *in vivo* parasite growth may be aborted or severely attenuated (195–197). In the case of schistosome parasites, development of female parasites is not directly influenced by the adaptive immune system, whereas male development is *(198)*. In this sequential model, adaptive immune signals trigger development of mature males, which subsequently stimulate development of mature females. Thus, in this example, chronic infection is achieved only when specific features of the host adaptive immune system are successfully exploited.

Antigenic variation is an important mechanism of immune evasion shared by diverse classes of pathogenic protozoa, including African trypanosomes, *Giardia*, and malaria. In each case, the antigens involved are highly immunogenic but poorly cross-reactive and are encoded by large families of nonallelic genes. The best-studied example of antigenic variation in parasites is that of African trypanosomes, the etiologic agents of sleeping sickness (reviewed in ref. 199). As mentioned, these organisms, such as *T. brucei*, produce waves of parasitemia by generating subpopulations that express antigenically different forms of the major surface variant-specific glycoprotein (VSG). This switching occurs independent of antibody and at relatively high frequency. An internal subregion of the VSG appears to be the major epitope driving the Th1 response, and this region is also highly variable.

In the case of *Giardia lamblia*, surface antigenic variation occurs within a family of variant-specific, cysteine-rich, zinc finger proteins (VSPs). After inoculation into mice of a single *G. lamblia* clone, the original VSP is expressed for approximately 2 weeks and then is gradually replaced by other VSPs, coincident with the appearance of variant-specific antibodies (reviewed in ref. 200). Mice that are unable to make antibodies, however, are still able to control acute *G. lamblia* infection, and, even in immunodeficient mice or gerbils, certain clones of *G. lamblia* are selected for or against, depending on the parasite clone and the host species *(201)*. Thus, in addition to immune evasion, antigenic variation may be involved in other aspects of biological selection, such as diversifying the host range of the parasite.

Although the need for antigenic variation might be obvious for extracellular protozoa such as trypanosomes and *Giardia*, it is less obvious why malaria parasites—hiding inside red blood cells—should have evolved a similar strategy of immune evasion (reviewed in ref. 202). The most plausible explanation is as follows. Developing schizonts cause erythrocyte distortion, loss of flexibility, and abnormal surface exposure of various membrane components, all of which make infected erythrocytes vulnerable to clearance from the circulation during passage through the spleen in a manner very similar to that by which normally aged red cells are removed and destroyed. To avoid passage through the spleen, the parasite exports to the red cell surface a range of molecular anchors—of which the best characterized is *P. falciparum* erythrocyte membrane protein-1 (PfEMP-1)—which bind to endothelial receptors, allowing the parasite to sequester in peripheral tissues. Parasite sequestration contributes to malaria pathology, clogging blood vessels and triggering focal inflammation, giving rise to cerebral, respiratory, and renal symptoms; sequestration in the placenta gives rise to pregnancy-associated malaria. Because these molecular anchors are parasite derived, they are recognized by the immune system; antibodies bind to them, prevent endothelial sequestration (and disease), and allow parasitized RBCs to be cleared in the spleen. Thus, for the parasite to establish a chronic infection, a system of clonal antigenic variation is required. The importance of these molecular anchors as a parasite survival strategy is demonstrated by the fact that there are upward of 50 copies of the gene for PfEMP-1 (*var* genes) per parasite, more than 200 copies of other clonally variant surface protein genes *(203)*, and innumerable allelic variants of each gene in the global parasite population.

Evasion by Immune Suppression

Generalized immunodepression, which is a feature of many chronic parasitic infections, including malaria, African trypanosomiasis, and visceral leishmaniasis, appears in most instances to be secondary to other immune evasion strategies, and results from the need to downregulate inflammation to prevent immune pathology (see next section) or from a variety of immune dysfunctions that high systemic parasite burdens can produce. These dysfunctions include disruption of normal lymphoid architecture, such as occurs in the mouse spleen during chronic infection with *Leishmania donovani,* in which excess TNF production leads to destruction of stromal cells in the periarteriolar lymphoid sheath and the loss of the chemokines that these cells would normally produce to recruit naive T cells and mature DCs (204). The accumulation of parasite-derived metabolic products can also be directly inhibitory to lymphocyte function. Metabolic products of *S. mansoni* adult worms, for example, have also been shown to strongly inhibit lymphocyte proliferation, including primary and secondary Th2 responses (205,*206*).

There is evidence from *in vitro* studies that clonally variant or polymorphic antigens of parasitic protozoa may also promote parasite survival by modulating the immune response. The simultaneous presence of variant CS T cell epitopes (also referred to as altered peptide ligands), as might occur in African children infected with multiple allelic variants of malaria, was found to deliver an altered signal to the responding T cells that induced nonresponsiveness to its target agonist epitope *(207)*. In the case of *T. cruzi,* which can express and secrete multiple members of the highly polymorphic surface sialidase superfamily at one time, epitope-specific T cell responses are suppressed either by altered peptide ligand inhibition or because immune recognition is impeded by a flood of competing targets *(208)*. Some variants of PfEMP-1 appear to mediate binding of malaria-infected erythrocytes to dendritic cells and inhibit their maturation (209), whereas erythrocytes infected with nonbinding parasite lines failed to adhere to dendritic cells or to affect their function. However, whether these phenomena are of any functional immunologic consequence in the infected host is not known. Similarly, lymphocyte polyclonal activation, which can result in depression of antigen-specific responses, is a feature of many parasitic protozoan infections, including blood and tissue trypanosomes, *L. donovani*, *T. gondii*, and rodent malarias, but again, a causal link between polyclonal activation and immune evasion has not been established. The original hypothesis—that these organisms possess mitogenic or superantigenic moieties (210)—has been substantiated in the case of *T. cruzi*, in which the B cell mitogen has been cloned and characterized as a eukaryotic proline racemase *(211)*. For malaria there is evidence that some domains of PfEMP-1 may be mitogenic for human B cells *(212)*.

Regulatory T Cells and Parasite Persistence

The modulation of ongoing immune responses in sites of chronic infection, such as the gut or the skin, may in many instances reflect not only parasite survival strategies, but also normal mechanisms of immune homeostasis that operate to control immunopathology associated with antimicrobial effector mechanisms. Accumulating evidence has implicated a crucial role for regulatory T cells in the dynamic equilibrium that is established between parasites and their hosts. Regulatory T cells is the name given generally to the subsets of $CD4^+$ T cells, and more recently $CD8^+$ T cells, that negatively regulate multiple immune functions. Among the different subsets of $CD4^+$ regulatory T cells that have been described, the best characterized are the so-called naturally occurring $CD4^+$ $CD25^+$ T cells that are present in naive animals. These cells also express CTLA-4 and the transcription factor Foxp3, which are actively involved in their development and suppressive function. T cells with regulatory activity can also be induced from conventional naive cells after encounter with antigen in the periphery (Tr1, Th3, and $CD8^+$ Treg cells). In addition to the critical role that Treg play in suppressing potentially pathogenic T cell responses directed against self-antigens or gut flora, they may also suppress potentially beneficial immune responses, such as those directed against infectious pathogens and tumors. Both natural and inducible Treg can produce downmodulatory cytokines (IL-10 and TGFβ) that switch off inflammatory and protective immune responses and can interfere with effector T cell activation in a contact-dependent manner. The evidence that natural Treg contribute to pathogen persistence was initially demonstrated in the *L. major* mouse model, in which IL-10 produced by $CD4^+$ $CD25^+$ T cells was required for the persistence of amastigotes in the skin following clinical cure in resistant mice (213). These cells, at least some of which are *Leishmania* specific, were found to accumulate in the dermal lesion and to suppress the frequency of Th1 cells and their ability to mediate parasite killing in the site. Similarly, in a model of mouse malaria characterized by extremely rapid parasite growth (*P. yoelii* YM or 17XL), very early induction of TGFβ and IL-10 appears to inhibit the development of responses that are required for parasite clearance. Neutralization of IL-10 and TGFβ (214)—or, in some studies, depletion of natural regulatory T cells (215)—at the onset of infection allows parasite replication to be contained, and mice are able to resolve their infections and survive. A similar scenario has been observed in experimental human infections within the context of malaria vaccine trials (216).

The ability of natural Treg to suppress Th2 responses has also been demonstrated, such that *L. major*–infected BALB/c mice treated with anti-CD25 antibody developed even more severe disease *(217)*. The persistence of filarial worms as a consequence of Treg-mediated suppression of Th2 responses was shown for *Litomosoides sigmodontis* infection of mice, although in this case the effects were independent of IL-10 (218). The isolation of T cells with regulatory characteristics from humans infected with filarial nematodes and the observation that CTLA-4$^+$ T cells contribute to their suppressed production of IL-5 indicate that regulatory T cells may be involved in suppression of protective immune responses in patients with onchocerciasis or lymphatic filariasis (219,220). The role of natural Treg in modulating immunopathology associated with helminth infections is discussed later.

The role of IL-10 in parasite persistence is especially striking in the case of *Leishmania*, although in some cases this powerful deactivating cytokine was found to be produced by cells other than natural Treg. Of interest, the inability to heal infection with a substrain of *L. major* that induces a polarized Th1 response in C57Bl/6 mice was associated with IL-10 production by CD4$^+$ CD25$^-$ Foxp3$^-$ T cells that also produced IFNγ (221). A similar phenotype is associated with control of Th1-driven immune pathology associated with *T. gondii* infection in mice (discussed later). The data suggest that in sites of strong inflammation, IL-10–producing Th1 cells may be activated as an especially powerful mechanism of feedback control. The *L. major* mouse model has also revealed a potential role for suppression mediated by IL-10 and TGFβ produced by macrophage after uptake of Ig-opsonized parasites (222,*223*). Thus redundant mechanisms of homeostatic control, including innate cells and natural and adaptive Treg, may be activated to control immune pathology associated with antimicrobial immune responses in tissues that are especially susceptible to injury, for example, the skin and mucosa. The regulatory T cell subsets that have been described in parasitic infections are summarized in Table 35.3.

IMMUNOPATHOLOGIC MECHANISMS AND THEIR REGULATION

If the appropriate adaptive immune mechanisms fail to develop or if they are not able fully to eradicate the infection, then persistent inflammation and other nonspecific responses may be the only way of limiting the infection. This is the situation for many parasitic diseases, and it carries an inevitable risk of pathologic side effects. This does not mean that all infections with the same parasite species lead to the same immune pathology. One of the most striking features of human parasitic disease is the great variability in clinical outcome, ranging from asymptomatic infection to fatal disease. Esophageal disease due to *T. cruzi*, liver fibrosis and portal hypertension due to *S. mansoni,* and cerebral malaria due to *P. falciparum* are a few examples of the many immunopathologic complications that may occur in some individuals but not others. Part of this variability is determined by host genetics, whereas other potential determinants include parasite virulence factors, infection intensity, and the prior level of immunity. The picture may be further complicated by coinfection with other infectious agents: For example, the severity of *P. falciparum* malaria is increased by concomitant bacteremia but reduced by concomitant *P. vivax* infection (224). HIV antiretroviral drugs also impair CD36-mediated cytoadherence and nonopsonic phagocytosis of parasitized erythrocytes by human macrophages, which may lead to altered malaria disease outcomes in treated coinfected individuals (225). The pathology associated with chronic *S. mansoni* infections reduces the CD4$^+$ T cell count, which can exacerbate the effects of HIV-1 in coinfected individuals (226). *S. mansoni* infection has also been shown to increase susceptibility to AIDS virus infection, transmission, and replication in nonhuman primates *(227)*, and similar observations have been made in malaria-infected HIV patients (228). Concomitant exposure to malaria affects the regression of hepatosplenomegaly after treatment for *S. mansoni* infection *(229)*. Coinfections of *T. gondii* and *S. mansoni* are also more lethal *(230)*. Finally, even more surprising was the finding that endosymbiotic *Wolbachia* LPS is the principal cause of river blindness in filariasis (231).

It is impossible to do justice to the remarkably broad range of immunologic mechanisms that contribute to the pathology of parasitic disease. Twenty years ago, much of the research in this field concerned the role of immune complexes, complement, and anaphylaxis. These areas remain important, but the focus has shifted to the molecular basis of cellular processes such as inflammation, granuloma formation, and tissue remodeling. An important issue is how the host maintains the fine balance between a protective immune response and one that is liable to cause pathologic complications. It is becoming increasingly clear that this is one of the most critical determinants

TABLE 35.3 Regulatory T Cells and Parasitic Infections

Parasite	Host	Treg Phenotype	Cytokine Secreted	Suppressive Function	Ref.
Leishmania					
L. major	C57Bl/6	$CD4^+CD25^+Foxp3^+$	IL-10	Suppress Th1 responses and sterile cure in healed mice	213
L. major	BALB/c	$CD4^+CD25^+$	nd	Suppress Th2 responses, moderate lesion progression	*217*
L. major	C57Bl/6	$CD4^+IFN\gamma^+CD25^-Foxp3^-$	IL-10	Suppress Th1 responses and healing	221
L. brasiliensis	Human	$CD4^+CD25^+CTLA^+$ $Foxp3^+$	IL-10/TGFβ	Treg from lesion suppress proliferative responses *in vitro*	*339*
Malaria					
Plasmodium yoelii	BALB/c	$CD4^+CD25^+$	nd	Suppress CD4 response and resistance to lethal infection	215
P. yoelii	C57Bl/6	$CD8^+$	IL-10/ TGFβ	Suppress type 1 cytokine response; inhibit parasite clearance	214
P. chabaudi	C57Bl/6	nd	IL-10/ TGFβ	Suppress immunopathology in nonlethal infection	*245, 246*
P. falciparum	Human	$CD4^+CD25^+Foxp3^+$	TGFβ	Suppress systemic type 1 response; facilitate parasite growth	216
P. falciparum	Human	$CD4^+CD25^+$	L-10	Suppress antigen-specific IFNγ from cord blood lymphocytes	*340*
Toxoplasma	Mouse	$CD4^+IFN\gamma^+CD25^-Foxp3^-$	IL-10	Suppress Th1-mediated pathology	238
Filaria					
Onchocerca volvulus	Human	Tr1	IL-10	Antigen specific IL-10, suppressive activity not shown	219
Litomosoides sigmodontis	Mouse	$CD4^+CD25^+CTLA^+$	IL-10 indep	Suppress Th2 response and resistance	218
Brugia malayi	Human	$CD4^+CD25^+CTLA^+$	TGFβ	Suppress antigen-specific Th1/Th2 responses *in vitro*	220
Schistosoma					
S. mansoni	Mouse	$CD4^+CD25^+$	IL-10	Suppress immunopathology and lethality of infection	264
		$CD4^+CD25^+$	IL-10	Suppress Th1 response and polarize Th2 response	*341*
		$CD4^+CD25^+Foxp3^+$	IL-10 indep	Natural Tregs limit egg-induced cytokine response	*342*
		$CD4^+CD25^+Foxp3^+$	IL-10 indep	Inhibit Th1 and suppress Th2 response	*265*

IFNγ, interferon-γ; IL, interleukin; indep, independent; nd, not determined; TGFβ, transforming growth factor-β.

of a successful host–parasite relationship, and, as such, it is of considerable importance for vaccinologists. Of interest, in many parasitic infections this balance appears to be regulated by the coordinated actions of a growing list of important immunoregulatory mechanisms.

Achieving Balance Between the Antiinfective Immune Response and Host Pathology

Whereas a proinflammatory Th1 response is usually required to control intracellular infections, there is also a need to balance the response. The potentially harmful effector molecules induced by Th1 responses include NO, ROIs, and TNF, which often operate in a synergistic fashion. IL-10, TGFβ, and to a lesser extent IL-4 produced by distinct subsets of regulatory cells including Tregs, Th2, Th3, and Tr1 cells appear to be important in preventing the Th1 responses from overshooting during intracellular infections. There are also several examples in which Th2 responses appear to be detrimental. Strong antibody responses may lead to the formation of antigen–antibody complexes or complement activation resulting in bystander lysis *(232)*. Eosinophils, typically associated with the Th2 response, are involved in hypersensitivity reactions to the filarial worm *O. volvulus* and can contribute to fibrotic tissue remodeling (161). Th2 responses appear to be the primary cause of hepatic fibrosis and chronic morbidity in *S. mansoni*–infected mice *(233)*. The data suggest that a variety of mediators, including IFNγ, IL-12, IL-10, Tregs, and decoy receptors cooperate to keep Th2 responses in check. Finally, a new subset of T helper cells designated Th17 was recently described, which have replaced Th1 cells as the critical pathogenic cells in several autoimmune diseases *(234)*. Although they provide adaptive immunity tailored to specific classes of pathogens, most notably extracellular bacteria, it is unclear whether Th17 cells regulate immunity or immunopathology during parasitic infection (235). In summary, a successful resolution to infection typically requires precise titration of T helper cell responses appropriate to the type of pathogen (Figure 35.2). This is not just in terms of amount, but also of where, when, and for how long polarized responses persist.

Pathogenesis of Chronic Th1 Responses

As discussed, control of intracellular pathogens such as *Leishmania* spp., *T. gondii*, and *T. cruzi* requires the coordinated activation of both antigen-specific cells (T lymphocytes) and less specific responses (NK cells, neutrophils, and macrophages), with IFNγ and TNF playing critical roles by upregulating macrophage activation and nitric oxide production. Of interest, IL-10–deficient mice inoculated with a normally avirulent *T. gondii* strain or with a virulent strain of *T. cruzi* succumb to infection within the first 2 weeks of infection (236,237). In both of these infections, animals lacking IL-10 show increased suppression of parasite growth, and, in the case of *T. cruzi*, inflammation and necrosis within the endocardium and interstitium of the myocardium is reduced. The increase in mortality appears to be caused by high systemic levels of IL-12, IFNγ, and TNF produced in large part by activated CD4$^+$ lymphocytes and macrophages. The livers of both *T. gondii*– and *T. cruzi*–infected mice show numerous and prominent necrotic foci together with dramatically increased mononuclear cell infiltration. Similarly, macrophages from the mutant mice activated *in vitro* or *in vivo* with *T. gondii* secrete higher levels of TNF, IL-12, and inducible NO than macrophages from IL-10–sufficient animals. The combined clinical manifestations suggest that the IL-10 knockout mice die in response to an overwhelming systemic immune response, resembling that observed during septic shock. In support of this conclusion, administration of anti-CD4, anti-IL-12, or anti-TNF Abs reduces mortality in IL-10 knockout mice (236,237). Thus in these

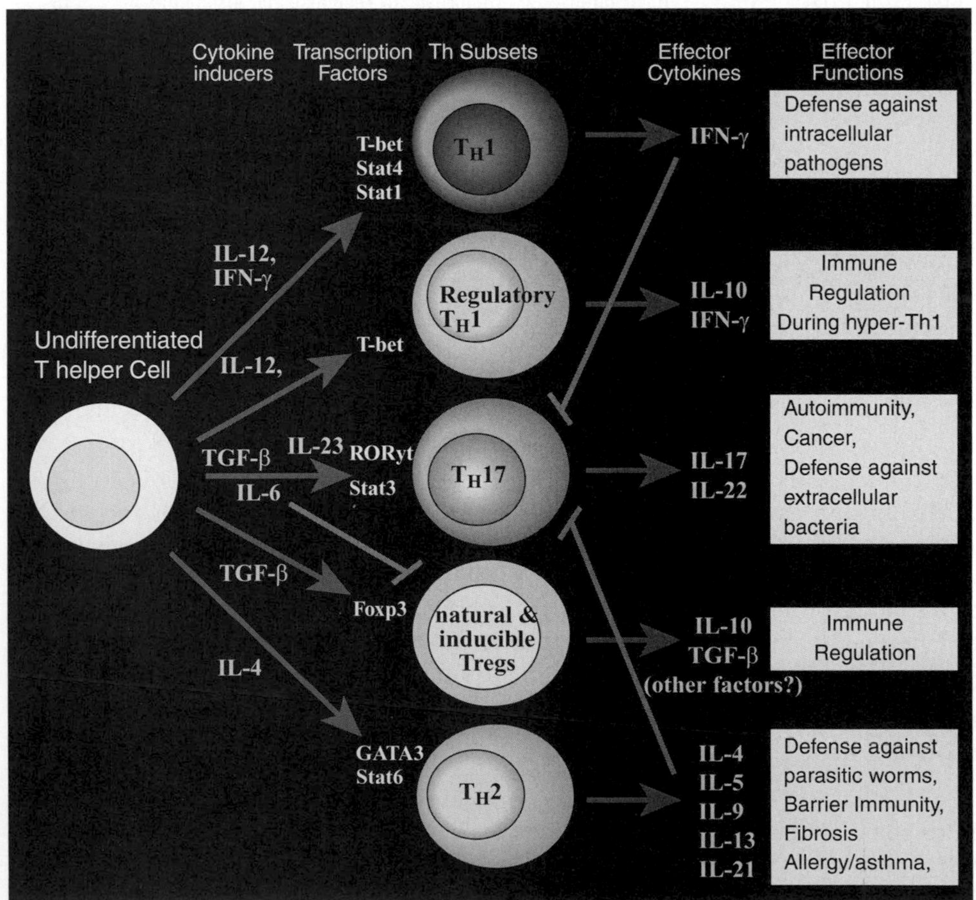

FIGURE 35.2 Effector and regulatory CD4$^+$ T cell subsets involved in achieving the balance between the antiinfective immune response and host pathology.

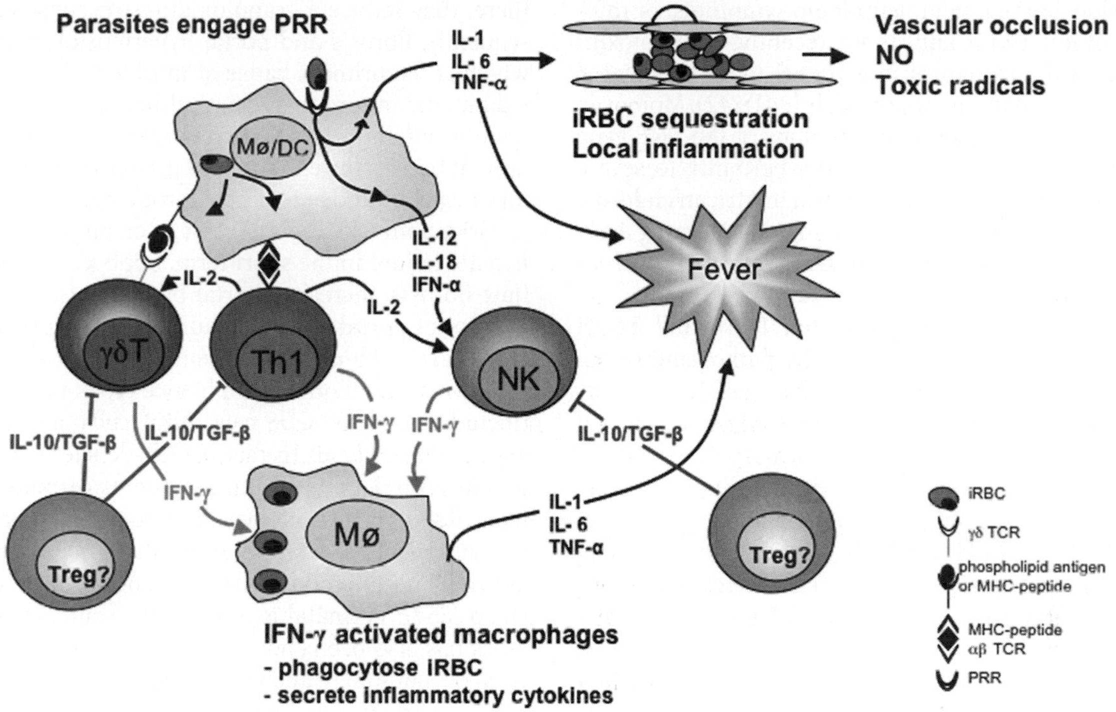

FIGURE 35.3 Immunopathogenesis of malaria. Infected red blood cells (iRBCs) and parasite products bind to pattern recognition receptors (PRRs, e.g., TLR2 and TLR9) on monocytes and dendritic cells (DCs) and induce a cascade of proinflammatory cytokines (most importantly interleukin-12 [IL-12], interferon-γ [IFNγ], and tumor necrosis factor-α [TNFα]). These inflammatory signals initiate numerous pathologic processes. They cause upregulation of adhesion molecule expression on vascular endothelium, promoting vascular sequestration of iRBCs, which clogs the vessels, reduces blood flow, and simultaneously raises intracranial pressure. iRBC products also bind to PRRs in tissue, initiating local inflammatory loops that amplify iRBC sequestration. Vascular occlusion and subsequent tissue damage contribute to cerebral malaria, respiratory distress, and multiorgan failure. Other cytokines such as IL-1, TNFα, and IL-6 induce the fever response, which includes elevated temperature, nausea, headache, prostration, and muscle pain. The actions of inflammatory cytokines are antagonized by antiinflammatory cytokines, principally IL-10 and TGFβ, which inhibit both production of, and cellular responses to, inflammatory signals.

models, IL-10 plays a major role in protecting the host against an excessive and lethal type 1 cytokine response.

Recent studies in the murine *T. gondii* model have demonstrated that CD4$^+$ T lymphocytes are the major source of the host-protective IL-10 (238). Of interest, CD25$^-$, Foxp3$^-$-producing Th1 cells are the principal CD4$^+$ subpopulation producing the cytokine, and these same cells can trigger macrophages to control the parasite through their simultaneous synthesis of IFNγ. These and other findings suggest that IL-10 is triggered in parasite-induced IFNγ-producing Th1 cells as means of suppressing IL-12 synthesis in APCs and downregulating further Th1 expansion.

Much has been written about the protective versus pathologic consequences of proinflammatory cytokine production in malaria (Figure 35.3) (reviewed in ref. 239). During the preerythrocytic stage in the liver, when parasite burden is relatively low and the infection is clinically asymptomatic, there is evidence that IL-12, IFNγ, and NO each plays an important role in preventing the infection from progressing further *(240)*. Once the parasites invade erythrocytes and grow to large numbers, the risk–benefit equation is less clear. Although TNF, IL-12, and IFNγ can inhibit blood-stage parasites and thereby exert a protective function, at this stage the cytokine response is systemic, and some pathologic side effects are inevitable. The most common clinical consequence in humans is fever, whereas life-threatening complications such as profound anemia and cerebral malaria occur in a proportion of infections due to *P. falciparum* but not other species. Mice with malaria do not develop fever (instead, systemic inflammation leads to a decrease in core temperature), but, depending on the specific host–parasite combination, they may develop anemia, fatal neurologic symptoms, or multiorgan failure; TNFα and, more recently, lymphotoxin-α have been the cytokines most consistently associated with severe pathology in these models (241,*242*). Moreover, polymorphisms of the promoter regions of the TNF gene (243) have been associated with susceptibility to severe complications of *P. falciparum* malaria in African children. One interpretation of these findings is that a strong early proinflammatory cytokine response is protective, whereas a strong late response is pathologic (244).

Experimental studies suggest that IL-10 and TGFβ cooperate to downregulate potentially pathogenic proinflammatory cytokine responses in malaria *(245)*. IL-10–deficient mice infected with *P. chabaudi chabaudi* showed increased mortality compared with normal wild-type littermates, although peak parasitemias did not differ markedly *(246)*. Instead, acute infection was characterized by an enhanced TNF response, which directly contributed to pathology; neutralization of TGFβ in *P. chabaudi*–infected IL-10–deficient mice was rapidly and universally fatal (247). Thus, susceptibility of IL-10–deficient mice to an otherwise nonlethal infection results not from fulminant parasitemia but from a sustained and enhanced proinflammatory cytokine response. Similarly, treatment of infected mice with a neutralizing antibody to TGFβ exacerbated the virulence of *P. berghei* and caused *P. c. chabaudi* infection, which normally resolves spontaneously, to become lethal; it was concluded that the protective effects of this cytokine are also due to downregulation of inflammatory responses (244). However, as described previously, very early induction of TGFβ and IL-10 can inhibit the effector response that is required for parasite clearance (214,215); thus, the outcome of malaria infections is determined, in part at least, by the sequence and timing of proinflammatory and antiinflammatory (immune regulatory) responses.

Pathogenesis of Chronic Th2 Responses

With many of the nematode infections, the protective Th2 response can cause significant pathologic changes in the gut (inflammation, excess mucus, damage to epithelium, and diarrhea). However, these effects are often transient and quickly resolve after parasite expulsion. If the parasites are not expelled quickly, the immune response typically shifts to a more Th1-polarized reaction (248). Thus, there are only a few examples in which persistent Th2 reactions are established as a result of chronic infection. Perhaps the most widely studied in this regard are the schistosome parasites, which are extremely successful at establishing long-term infections in their definitive hosts. On infection, adult parasites of *S. mansoni* migrate to the mesenteric veins, where they live up to 10 years or more, laying hundreds of eggs per day. Some of the eggs become entrapped in the microvasculature of the liver, and once there, they induce a granulomatous response (249). Subsequently, fibrosis and portal hypertension may develop, which is the primary cause of morbidity in infected individuals and in some cases may ultimately be lethal. Consequently, much of the symptomatology of schistosomiasis is attributed to the egg-induced granulomatous inflammatory response and associated fibrotic pathology (250).

Granulomas are pathogenic, not because they cause hepatic failure in the short term, but because they precipitate fibrosis, increased portal blood pressure, and development of portal systemic shunts that are prone to bleed *(251)*. CD4$^+$ Th cells are essential for granuloma formation, whereas all other lymphocyte types examined so far (including B cells, CD8 cells, NKT cells, and $\gamma\delta$ T cells) appear less critical. In fact, B cell–deficient (μMT) mice mount an exacerbated granulomatous response, and unlike wild-type animals, they fail to downmodulate pathology late in infection, suggesting that B cells play an important immunomodulatory role, perhaps by producing IL-10 *(252)*. Perinatal exposure to specific anti-SEA idiotypes has also been shown to induce long-term effects on survival, pathology, and immune response patterns in mice subsequently infected with *S. mansoni (253)*. These cross-reactive regulatory idiotypes can also predict clinical outcomes of chronic disease (254).

The critical role of Th2 cells in granulomatous inflammation and fibrosis was confirmed in experiments in which mice vaccinated with egg antigen plus IL-12 to induce an egg-specific Th1 response on subsequent infection developed smaller granulomas and less severe fibrosis than did nonvaccinated infected controls (255). Decreased fibrosis was associated with a diminished Th2 response and increased Th1 cytokine production. Anti–IL-4 mAbs were also shown to reduce granuloma size and fibrosis in infected mice, although the effects of IL-4 deficiency varies in different strains of IL-4$^{-/-}$ mice *(256)*.

Although egg-induced granulomas are widely believed to be detrimental to the infected host, it is clear that the lesions also serve an important host-protective function, particularly in *S. mansoni* infections. In chronically infected hosts, schistosome eggs provide a continuous antigenic stimulus for the immune response. If these antigens are not sequestered or neutralized effectively, they may damage the affected tissues, with the liver being particularly sensitive. Indeed, T-cell–deprived, nude, severe combined immune deficiency (SCID), and egg-tolerized mice infected with *S. mansoni* all die earlier than comparably infected immunologically intact control mice because they are unable to mount a normal granuloma response *(257)*. Widespread microvesicular hepatic damage induced by toxic egg products contributes to the poorer survival of infected immunosuppressed mice. Granuloma formation therefore seems to be a compromise solution to allow the host to live with the infection.

During granuloma development, the primary CD4$^+$ T cell response switches from a Th1 response of short duration to a persistent Th2 response, which dominates soon after the acute stage of infection. The development of the Th2 response was thought to be highly dependent on IL-4; therefore, it was hypothesized that depleting IL-4 might slow the development of severe hepatosplenic disease. Nevertheless, studies conducted with IL-4–deficient mice demonstrated that IL-4 plays an essential host-protective role during infection with *S. mansoni (256,258)*. Unlike wild-type mice, that develop chronic infections without significant complications, infected IL-4–deficient mice suffer from an acute inflammatory disease, which is characterized by cachexia and significant mortality. Of interest, IL-4R-signaling is required for the efficient passage of eggs through the intestine into the lumen *(257)*. Consequently, the eggs are trapped in the intestinal wall, which causes localized inflammation and ultimately increased systemic exposure to bacterial toxins such as LPS. This, combined with the decreased Th2- and enhanced Th1-type response, results in increased proinflammatory cytokine production that contributes to the weight loss and death of the IL-4–deficient animals.

IL-10 appears to also play a role in inhibiting inflammation during both murine and human *S. mansoni* infections *(233,259)*. In mouse studies, marked increases in IFNγ, TNF, and iNOS expression were detected in infected IL-10–deficient animals, and this correlated with the development of morbidity and mortality. Even more striking effects were observed in mice that are deficient in both IL-4 and IL-10 (DKO mice), which developed the most highly polarized Th1-type response and in which 100% mortality was seen by week 9 postinfection *(233)*. The mice had elevated serum aspartate transaminase levels, suggesting that mortality was likely attributable to uncontrolled proinflammatory cytokine production and acute hepatotoxicity. Other studies suggest that IL-4 and perhaps IL-10 protect the host by downregulating the generation of reactive oxygen and nitrogen intermediates that can damage the liver *(260)*. Regardless of the exact mechanisms involved, IL-4 and IL-10 are both required to prevent the Th1 responses from overshooting and becoming pathogenic. IL-10 has also been implicated in the control of the Th2-driven granulomatous response, the failure of which is thought to be responsible for the development of hepatosplenic disease in some chronically infected individuals. Roles for IL-10 in immune downmodulation have also been documented in *Schistosoma mansoni*– and *S. haematobium*–infected humans (*261,262*,263). Recent studies in mice have focused on defining the cellular sources of IL-10, and although a role for Treg-derived IL-10 has been reported, it is clear that IL-10 derived from a variety of sources, including Th2 cells, macrophages, dendritic cells, and B cells, can help to regulate type 2 responses and perhaps, development of hepatosplenic disease (88,*252*,264,*265*).

Because fibrosis is driven by the Th2 response, many of the complications associated with chronic infection (portal hypertension, collateral vessel formation, bleeding from esophageal and gastric varices) likely result from the persistent production of type 2 cytokines (266). Although it is clear that intact IL-4 receptor signaling is critical for the development of granulomas and fibrosis, IL-13 was identified as the dominant profibrotic mediator in schistosomiasis (90). Infected IL-13–deficient mice also survive longer than wild-type animals, further highlighting the pathogenic role of IL-13 in chronic infections *(267)*. Thus, IL-4 appears to play a host-protective role, whereas IL-13 is pathogenic during chronic schistosome infections. A valid approach toward immunoprophylaxis of schistosomiasis may be to design a vaccine that minimizes IL-13 activity and egg-induced pathology. In mice, the progression of hepatic fibrosis correlates with the intensity of the type 2 cytokine response, and immunologic interventions that block IL-4 and IL-13 were found to reduce collagen deposition significantly (*268*,269) (Figure 35.4). Fibrosis can also be slowed or prevented in mice that are sensitized with egg antigens and IL-12 or CpG oligonucleotides before infection (255,*270*). Thus, an antipathology vaccine that is based on "immune deviation" could be envisioned for schistosomiasis, and novel immunodominant eggs antigens are being identified with this goal in mind.

Over the last several years, immune deviation has been used extensively as a research tool to study the mechanisms of granuloma formation and fibrosis in detail. Several mediators and cell types that characterize type 1 cytokine responses were shown to inhibit fibrosis, including TNFα, IL-12, and NO *(271,272)*. Because macrophages and dendritic cells are important sources of these mediators, a significant effort has been made to elucidate their roles in the pathogenesis of schistosomiasis. In the case of NO, the protective antifibrotic effects of type 2–to–type 1 immune deviation are completely inhibited in the absence of nitric oxide synthase-2 (NOS-2). Activated macrophages are capable of expressing two cytokine inducible enzymes, NOS-2 and arginase, which share L-arginine as a substrate, and type 1 and type 2 cytokines were shown to induce NOS-2 and arginase-1 (Arg-1) expression, respectively *(273)*. The Th1-associated cytokines IFNγ and TNFα induced NOS-2 in macrophages designated "classically activated," whereas the type 2 cytokines induced Arg-1 activity in cells termed "alternatively activated" (274). Studies conducted in the schistosomiasis model identified IL-13 as the major arginase inducer *(275)*, and arginase activity correlated consistently with the size of granulomas and the severity of fibrosis. In contrast, NOS-2 dominated in Th1-polarized mice, and these animals developed small granulomas with little fibrosis. These data served as a first

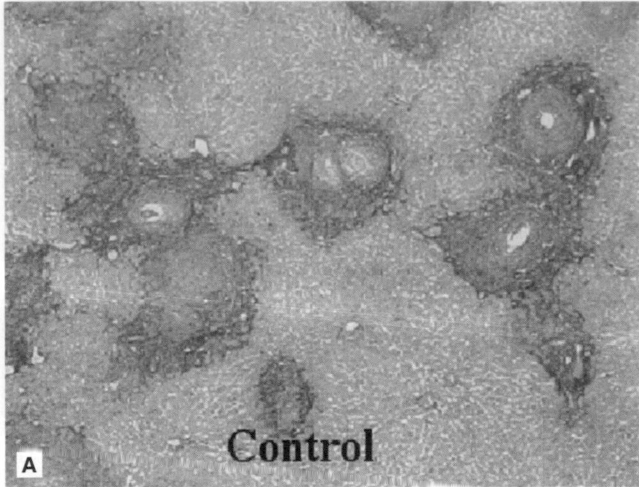

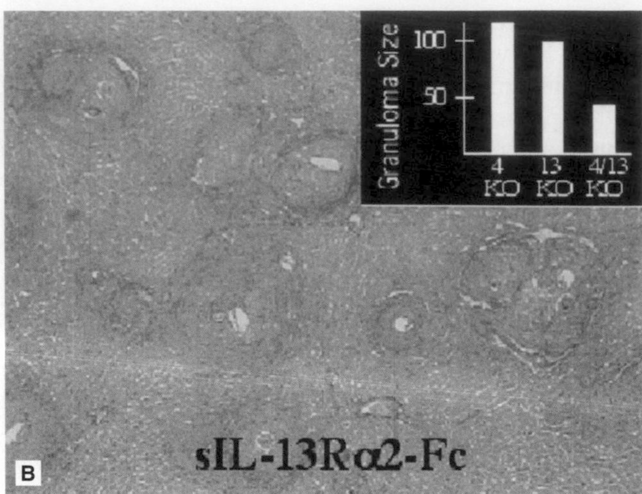

FIGURE 35.4 Pivotal role of interleukin-13 (IL-13) in schistosome egg–induced hepatic fibrosis. C57BL/6 mice were infected with *Schistosoma mansoni* cercariae and treated with sIL-13Rα2-Fc or control immunoglobulin (Ig) on weeks 6 through 12 postinfection. Mice were sacrificed, and liver sections were stained with picrosirius red (dark-staining areas around granulomas) to identify collagen and examined at 25× magnification. Note the presence of granulomas in the liver of sIL-13Rα2–treated mice, yet the absence of significant collagen staining. The inset in the second panel shows the relative change in granuloma size in animals deficient in IL-4 or IL-13 or simultaneously deficient in IL-4 and IL-13, relative to wild-type (WT) mice. Note that granuloma size decreases only in mice deficient in both cytokines.

example of the differential regulation of NOS-2/Arg-1 by type 1/type 2 cytokines *in vivo*. More importantly, they clarified how CD4$^+$ Th2 cells and "alternatively activated" cells (macrophages/DCs/fibroblasts) might cooperate to control disease progression in schistosomiasis.

PARASITE VACCINE STRATEGIES

There is no safe, uniformly effective vaccine against any human parasitic infection. The lack of progress in this field is due to many factors, including the low priority that has historically been given to development of vaccines against diseases confined mainly to the developing world. By contrast, the perceived economic benefit to the agricultural industry of vaccines against livestock parasites has led to the licensing of several anthelminthic vaccines for veterinary use (276). The greater impediments, however, may be related to the nature of parasitic infections themselves. In contrast to those bacterial and viral infections for which highly effective vaccines exist and for which there is complete immunity induced by primary infection, most antiparasite vaccines will need to outperform the immune response to natural infection. Furthermore, virtually all bacterial or viral vaccines that are in use mediate their protection by inducing a strong, long-lived humoral response that inhibits attachment or invasion, promotes clearance, or neutralizes released toxins. By contrast, there are no vaccines that are uniformly effective against diseases caused by intracellular pathogens that require cellular immunity to mediate protection. Thus, the manner in which potentially protective antigens can be administered to generate and maintain appropriate T cell responses has yet to be proven in a clinical setting. Consequently, for the development of vaccines against intracellular protozoa, for example, malaria, *Leishmania*, *T. cruzi*, and *Toxoplasma*, it will not be sufficient simply to identify target antigens; novel and rational approaches to vaccine design and delivery will need to be explored. In fact, from the examples discussed later, it is clear that ample numbers of potentially protective antigens have been identified and cloned from most of the major human parasitic disease agents, and the completion of their genomic sequences has already led to the identification of additional vaccine candidates based on their predicted developmental stage specificity, surface expression, secretion, or virulence associations (277–279). The vaccination strategies that are being explored to meet the challenge of both antigen selection and delivery will be considered in the general context of B and T cell antiparasite vaccines. Note that the examples provided are by no means exhaustive but reflect general principles of vaccination against extracellular and intracellular targets.

B Cell Vaccines

Vaccination Against Intestinal Protozoa

Parasitic protozoa that have an exclusive extracellular lifestyle in their mammalian hosts and are sensitive to antibody-mediated control include the intestinal pathogens

Entamoeba histolytica and *Giardia lamblia*. Most deaths from *E. histolytica* arise from amebic liver abscess, the major extraintestinal manifestation of disease. Clinical studies suggest that the presence of mucosal antibodies to the surface Gal/GalNAc lectin of *E. histolytica* capable of blocking amebic adherence to intestinal epithelial cells correlates with reduced risk of recolonization *(280)*. A recent vaccine study provides direct evidence that vaccination with the Gal/GalNAc lectin can produce IgA antilectin antibodies and provide protection against intestinal amebiasis in a mouse model of disease *(281)*. An amebic serine-rich protein (SREHP) is a highly immunogenic surface antigen of *E. histolytica* containing multiple tandem octapeptide and dodecapeptide repeats. Passive immunization with antibodies to SREHP protects SCID mice from amebic liver abscess. Parenteral immunization with recombinant SREHP or with a SREHP-based DNA vaccine was highly effective in protecting gerbils against amebic liver abscess (282). Specific serum and mucosal antibodies targeting surface antigens are also known to be important in elimination of *Giardia* from the host intestine. *Giardia* vaccines containing whole-trophozoite preparations protected animals even when challenged with heterologous strains (283). Thus an immune response to variant surface antigens that are known to be targets of cytotoxic antibodies appears not to be essential for control of acute infection, and this supports an alternative role for antigenic variation in, for example, diversifying the host range of the parasite *(201)*. The cloning and expression of *Giardia* antigen genes for vaccine testing is in its infancy. Genes coding for cyst wall proteins (CWPs), which could be used for developing a transmission-blocking vaccine, have been cloned, and a recombinant protein induced IgA antibodies such that immunized mice shed fewer cysts after challenge with live cysts *(284)*.

Vaccines Targeting Extracellular Stages of Malaria

Because both preerythrocytic- and erythrocytic-stage malaria parasites are at least transiently exposed to humoral antibody, vaccine strategies based on eliciting high-titered antibodies that can inhibit their invasion of red blood cells or hepatocytes have long been favored (Figure 35.5). As discussed, antibodies to sporozoite surface proteins can immobilize invading parasites, preventing them from reaching or invading hepatocytes; such antibodies can be protective, and the dominant antibody epitope is represented by the CS central repeat sequences (NANP*n* in *P. falciparum*). These observations have made the CS protein the most extensively studied of all the malaria vaccine candidates (reviewed in ref. *285*). The latest version of the vaccine—RTS,S—comprises a recombinant CS polypeptide fused to the surface protein of hepatitis B virus and administered together with an adjuvant containing lipopolysaccharide (monophosphoryl lipid A) and a water-soluble glycoside obtained from tree bark (*Quillaja saponaria*) *(286)*. The vaccine has been designed to induce both antibodies and T cell–mediated effector mechanisms, and it is not clear which of these mechanisms is most important in conferring immunity. This vaccine is discussed in more detail later.

Antibodies that inhibit the invasion of erythrocytes by the extracellular merozoite stage of malaria *in vitro* are found in many but not all individuals living in malaria-endemic regions. Although the significance of these inhibitory antibodies to naturally acquired resistance is unclear, their target antigens nonetheless remain prime candidates for asexual malaria vaccines (reviewed in ref. *287*) (Figure 35.5). One of the targets of invasion-inhibitory antibodies is merozoite surface protein (MSP-1), which was the first purified malaria protein to be used as a vaccine *(288)*. The 19-kDa C-terminal fragment of MSP-1 is the only part of the larger molecule to be taken into the red cell during invasion. Although MSP-1 proteins from different isolates of *P. falciparum* show considerable allelic polymorphism, the regions corresponding to the 19-kDa fragment are relatively conserved, and antibodies raised to one version of the protein cross-react with antibodies raised to other variants *(289)*. Native and recombinant forms of *P. falciparum* MSP-1_{19} and a longer fragment, MSP-1_{42}, can protect *Aotus* monkeys *(290)*. MSP-1_{42} is in clinical trials *(291)*. Apical membrane antigen-1 (AMA-1) is also the target of efficient invasion inhibitory antibodies and is being developed as a potential vaccine *(292)*, but problems may lie ahead because the target epitopes of invasion inhibitory antibodies appear to be highly polymorphic.

Despite their extreme polymorphism, the variant surface antigens present on infected erythrocytes that mediate adhesion to endothelial cells are potential vaccine candidates. Epidemiologic data suggest that the risk of severe manifestations of the disease is reduced after only a very few clinical episodes *(293)* and that parasites causing severe disease tend to express a subset of variant surface antigens *(294)*. Thus, a finite number of variant antigens might be sufficient to elicit broad immunity against severe disease. Two structural domains, termed DBLα and CIDR1α, which are present in the semiconserved head structure of all PfEMP-1 molecules sequenced to date (295), are attractive candidates for inclusion in such a vaccine. Similarly, relatively few PfEMP-1 variants appear to mediate parasite sequestration in placenta, and a pregnancy malaria vaccine might work by targeting the DBLγ domain that binds to chondroitin sulfate, the major placental ligand for parasitized RBC sequestration (296).

Antimalarial transmission-blocking immunity works primarily by antibody-mediated, complement-dependent lysis of extracellular sexual stages of the parasite within the midgut of a blood-feeding mosquito (reviewed in ref. 297). Transmission-blocking immunity has been induced *in vivo*

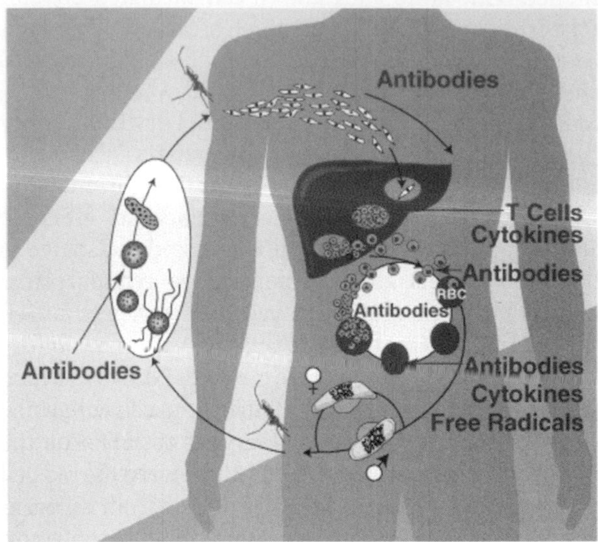

STAGES	ANTIGENS [a]	MECHANISM
Sporozoite	**CSP, TRAP/SSP2,** STARP, SALSA	**Anti-infection vaccine.** Antibody binds surface antigens to inhibit hepatocyte invasion
Hepatocyte	**CSP, TRAP/SSP2,** LSA1, EXP1, LSA3, STARP, SALSA	**Anti-infection vaccine.** T-cell recognition of infected hepatocytes; cytokine-mediated inhibition of growth, schizogony
Merozoite	**MSP1,** MSP2, MSP3, MSP4, PfEBA175, PvDABP, **AMA1,** SERA, GLURP, Pf155/RESA, RAP1, RAP2	**Anti-morbidity/mortality vaccine.** Antibody binds to parasite antigens to block erythrocyte invasion
Erythrocyte (asexual)	PfEMP1, rifins, Pf332	**Anti-morbidity/mortality vaccine.** Antibody binds to antigens on infected erythrocyte to inhibit sequestration
	Glycosylphosphatidyl-inositol (GPI) anchors	Antibody binds to GPI to inhibit inflammation and pathology
Mosquito	**Pfs25,** Pfs28, Pfs48/45, Pfs230	**Transmission-blocking vaccine** Antibody binds to parasite antigens to inhibit fertilization, oogenesis

[a] Antigens in **bold type** represent those currently in major clinical trials

FIGURE 35.5 Stage-specific vaccine targets in malaria parasites. **Left:** The life cycle of malaria and the immune effector mechanisms that target the different developmental forms of the parasite. (From Malaria Vaccine Initiative, *What is malaria?*, available at http://www.malariavaccine.org/mal-what_is_malaria.htm, with permission). **Right:** The major candidate vaccine antigens identified on these stages and the proposed mechanism by which immunization would act against each target. (Adapted from Richie TL, Saul A. Progress and challenges for malaria vaccines. *Nature.* 2002;415[6872]:694, with permission.)

by immunization with gametes of avian, rodent, and monkey malarias. Several potential transmission-blocking vaccine candidates have been identified, and the genes encoding these surface proteins have been isolated and sequenced, but their production as recombinant proteins is hampered by failure to recreate the highly complex tertiary structures that are the targets of inhibitory antibodies. Furthermore, for those antigens expressed only by invertebrate stages of the parasite, lack of natural boosting may prevent maintenance of sufficiently high antibody titers.

Clearly, an optimal vaccine against malaria would need to target multiple antigens and induce immunity against all stages. However, by targeting certain antigens confined to asexual blood stages, the induction of an adult-like immune status among high-risk infants in sub-Saharan Africa could greatly diminish severe disease and death caused by *P. falciparum.*

T Cell Vaccines

Vaccination Against Leishmaniasis

Vaccines against intracellular parasites will need to induce long-lived cellular immune responses. As already discussed, for diseases such as malaria, leishmaniasis, Chagas' disease, and toxoplasmosis, Th1 and/or $CD8^+$ T cell responses are the effector mechanisms required for protective immunity. An inherent problem with most nonliving vaccines is their relative inefficiency in generating these sorts of cellular responses. A major advance in T cell vaccine development was the demonstration that proteins derived from *L. major* could elicit a powerful Th1 response and protective immunity if given with recombinant IL-12 as adjuvant (298). IL-12, or IL-12–inducing adjuvants such as bacillus Calmette-Guérin (BCG), CpG-oligodinucleotides (CpG-ODN), or CD40L have since been used extensively in animal models to potentiate the efficacy of whole-cell killed vaccines or a diversity of recombinant protein *Leishmania* vaccines (reviewed in ref. 299). A polyprotein containing several *Leishmania* antigens (TSA, LmSTI1, and LeIF), formulated with the TLR4 agonist MPL, a detoxified derivative of 4′-monophosphoryl lipid A of LPS *(300)*, is the only defined, subunit vaccine against leishmaniasis in human trials.

The shortcomings of nonliving vaccines with respect to their potency and durability have been revealed in experimental studies. When mice were challenged with *L. major* 3 months as opposed to 2 weeks after immunization, a protein plus rIL-12 vaccine was no longer effective *(301)*. In contrast, a DNA vaccine encoding the same antigen remained effective, presumably due to more sustained expression of the antigen. Immunization with plasmid DNA is thus an attractive approach because it mimics the persistent antigenic stimulation of subclinical infection, and a large number of DNA vaccines encoding a diversity of *Leishmania* antigens have demonstrated some efficacy in mouse models of cutaneous and visceral leishmaniasis (302). The gold standard of the protection that can be achieved by vaccination protocols, and the only vaccination strategy against leishmaniasis that has worked in humans, is "leishmanization," which is based on the lifelong convalescent immunity that is acquired after induction of a lesion at a selected site with small doses of a cutaneous strain. The requirement for antigen persistence in this live "vaccine" is indicated by the mouse studies in which immunity to rechallenge infection was lost following manipulations that completely cleared the persisting parasites (213,*303*). Thus, whereas nonpersisting antigens delivered with appropriate adjuvants may contribute to vaccine efficacy by generating Th1 central memory cells, the presence at the time of challenge exposure of a population of antigen-dependent, effector memory cells that are tissue seeking and readily secrete cytokine on encounter with antigen in the periphery appears to be critical for the full expression of acquired immunity in the challenge site (304). Such loss of effector memory T cells after antigen clearance might well explain the failures of a whole-cell killed *L. major* vaccine plus BCG significantly to reduce the incidence of cutaneous leishmaniasis in individuals living in areas of relatively low transmission, where natural boosting is unlikely to have occurred *(305)*. The requirement for persistent antigens reinforces the rationale for live, attenuated vaccines. The generation of safe, live attenuated vaccines demonstrating some efficacy in mice has been accomplished by targeted deletion of genes involved in parasite survival or virulence, including mutants lacking dihydrofolate reductase *(306)*, cysteine proteinases *(307)*, or LPG-related molecules *(308)*. However, because live parasite vaccines will be extremely difficult to standardize and to deliver in field settings, there has been considerable interest in developing DNA vaccination, particularly as a component of herterologous prime/boost strategies involving viral vectors, capable of eliciting longer-lived cellular immune responses *in vivo*.

Another advantage of DNA vaccines is their ability to elicit specific $CD8^+$ T cells. Although $CD8^+$ T cells contribute to *Leishmania* resistance, they are especially important to the control of infections involving *T. cruzi* and *T. gondii*, which require effector $CD8^+$ T cells to kill parasites within cells lacking MHC class II molecules. Furthermore, because *T. cruzi* escapes from the parasitophorous vacuole and becomes cytoplasmic, many of its released antigens have access to the class I processing pathway. Immunization using plasmid DNA or viral vectors expressing the trans-sialidase surface antigen (TSSA) can induce $CD8^+$ T cell–mediated protective immunity against lethal *T. cruzi* infection in mice (309,*310*). Protection was also achieved using DNA encoding the KMP11-HSP70 fusion protein *(311)* and the *T. cruzi* complement regulatory protein *(312)*. Recombinant proteins, including cruzipain, the cysteinyl proteinase of *T. cruzi*, and purified paraflagellar rod proteins derived from the flagellum of *T. cruzi* trypomastigotes and mixed with either CpG-ODN or IL-12 have been used to elicit cellular immune responses in mice and enhanced survival against *T. cruzi* challenge infection *(313,314)*. It is important to note that in no case have these experimental vaccines been capable of achieving sterile immunity, and protection against the chronic phase of Chagas' disease involving myocardial dysfunctions was not evaluated in these models.

Vaccination Against Malaria Liver Stages

Because malaria parasites infect and replicate in hepatocytes, which express MHC class I, infected hepatocytes are potential targets of $CD8^+$ T cell responses. Irradiated *Plasmodium* sporozoites, which can infect hepatocytes but do not progress to a blood-stage infection, have been shown to protect rodents, monkeys, and humans against malaria by inducing IFNγ-producing $CD8^+$ T cells specific for preerythrocytic antigen (reviewed in ref. 315). Overirradiation of sporozoites negates their ability to immunize, suggesting that the targets of protective mechanisms are novel antigens expressed only if sporozoites undergo partial differentiation within hepatocytes. On the other hand, killed sporozoites can efficiently prime long-lived memory T cells, which, although they do not protect against immediate challenge with viable parasites, can protect against secondary infection (316). These observations suggest that live and dead parasites differentially prime T cell responses, although the molecular basis of this has not yet been elucidated. Similar to that described following sterile cure in leishmaniasis, immunity using irradiated sporozoites was lost in rats that were treated with a drug that eliminated parasites in the liver before rechallenge (317).

Efforts to mimic the protection generated by irradiated sporozoites using nonliving protein- and DNA-based vaccines have yielded encouraging results. A synthetic peptide representing the 102–amino acid–long C-terminal region of the *P. falciparum* CS protein and fused to hepatitis B surface antigen elicited strong $CD8^+$ and $CD4^+$ T cells responses, as well as antisporozoite antibodies, in human volunteers, particularly when given with the water-in-oil adjuvant Montanide ISA-720. The vaccine 'RTS,S' induced strong antibody and T cell responses in adults already primed to CS by preexposure to malaria. Most significantly, in this trial, vaccine efficacy during the first 9 weeks of follow-up was 71%, but it decreased to 0% over the next 6 weeks (318). In another trial, despite the apparently short-lived nature of protection, vaccinated children were less likely than those receiving the placebo to develop clinical malaria in a second year of follow-up (319), raising hopes that 'RTS,S' may be the first malaria vaccine to be licensed for use in humans. Nevertheless, the vaccine does not confer sterilizing immunity, and the level of protection is much lower than has been obtained with irradiated sporozoites *(320)*.

Despite initial enthusiasm that DNA vaccination strategies might improve the durability and potency of the cellular response, clinical trials have been disappointing, and the use of sequential immunizations using various heterologous prime/boost protocols is being tested to enhance the effectiveness of preerythrocytic vaccines (reviewed in ref. 123). Priming with plasmid DNA encoding CS and various liver stage–specific proteins and boosting with recombinant adenovirus or pox virus, such as modified vaccinia virus Ankara (MVA) or fowlpox, has induced complete protection and very high levels of IFNγ-secreting $CD8^+$ T cells in mice. Although protection in human trials has been less convincing, delays in time to emergence of blood-stage parasites have been consistently obtained, suggesting that the vaccination substantially reduces, but does not eliminate, liver-stage parasites.

Vaccination to Prevent Pathology

In many parasitic infections, disease is a consequence of the host immune response. Because these pathogens are so well adapted to their hosts, it may therefore be easier and more efficient to design immune interventions that prevent parasite-induced immunopathology rather than eliminate the infection itself. Although this approach will not lead to eradication of the parasite, it would likely reduce or alleviate the health consequences of infection. The feasibility of antipathology vaccines was demonstrated in a murine model of schistosomiasis (255). Because disease in schistosomiasis is largely due to the granulomatous pathology that develops around parasite eggs trapped in target host tissues, a valid approach toward immunoprophylaxis for schistosomiasis is to vaccinate to minimize granulomatous pathology. In wild-type mice, granuloma size and collagen deposition are correlated with the intensity of the type 2 response, and immunologic interventions, such as the administration of IL-4 and IL-13 antagonists, reduces both the size of granulomas and magnitude of fibrosis (discussed earlier) (269,*321*). In extensions of these studies, mice immunized with parasite egg antigens plus IL-12 *(322)* or CpG oligonucleotides *(270)* to induce an egg-antigen–specific type 1 response, on subsequent infection exhibited far less severe egg-associated liver disease than did infected, nonimmunized controls. Of importance, several immunodominant egg antigens have been described in recent studies *(323,324)*, and thus it may be possible to design recombinant antipathology vaccines that duplicate the promising results produced with these crude parasite extracts.

Parasite-derived GPI has been implicated in much of the pathology of malaria (325), binding to TLRs on dendritic cells and macrophages and inducing release of TNFα and other proinflammatory cytokines. As a proof of principle that GPI might serve as a target of an antidisease vaccine, mice immunized with synthetic GPI were protected against the acute immune pathology associated with *P. berghei* infection; however, because the mice were not immune to the parasite itself, they were unable to control parasite replication and eventually died of overwhelming parasitemia *(326)*. These observations suggest that whereas vaccines that prevent immune pathology might reduce some aspects of morbidity, they are unlikely to be deployed in the absence of vaccine components that also limit parasite burden.

Vaccines Against Helminths

Infection with helminthic parasites remains a significant health problem in many tropical countries. Although control measures are available in some areas, in most cases, patients living in endemic regions are quickly reinfected. Therefore, vaccines that reduce parasite and/or egg burdens would be a valuable tool to complement existing disease-prevention programs and could represent a less costly and more practical approach than repeated chemotherapy. Nevertheless, although many subunit vaccines have been described and tested in various animal models, suboptimal levels of protection have hindered the development of all but a few of these candidate vaccines *(327)*. Significant advances in vaccination technology over the last decade have made it possible to engineer vaccines that elicit strong cellular and humoral immunity. Novel DNA vectors, improved delivery systems, new adjuvants, and immunomodulatory cytokines allow significant augmentation of the immune response to vaccines and preferential induction of specific effector mechanisms, including antibody isotypes, T helper cell subsets, and cytotoxic T cells. However, to effectively harness and implement these advances, it will be necessary first to better elucidate the immune mechanisms responsible for killing helminth parasites.

The best examples of successful immunization against helminths are provided by vaccine models using radiation-attenuated larval parasites. With the irradiated schistosome vaccine, although complete sterilizing immunity appears to be an unachievable goal, immunity approaching 60% to 80% is clearly possible and has served as the gold standard for schistosome vaccine development *(328)*. The cumulative evidence from vaccine studies conducted in numerous gene knockout mice suggests that irradiated parasites can induce protection via both Th1- and Th2-dependent pathways *(129)* and that humoral and cellular mechanisms are both required for the generation of optimal immunity *(329,330)*.

Although there has been extensive research on defined vaccines against helminth infection [reviewed recently by Maizels et al. (331)], none of the candidate antigens has been shown to be protective in humans. Based on antibody responses in schistosome-vaccinated mice, several vaccine candidate antigens have been put forward for phase I trials, and at least one of the antigens (GST) has completed phase I and is entering phase II trial. These antigens include glutathione-*S*-transferase (P28/GST); paramyosin (Sm97); IrV5 (myosin-like 62-kDa protein); triose phosphate isomerase (TPI); Sm23 and tetraspanin-2, both integral membrane proteins; and Sm14, a fatty acid–binding protein *(332,333)*. With the recent advances in schistosome genomics and proteomics, a new panel of potential vaccine antigens is being identified, and these warrant further investigation (334). A number of filarial vaccine candidates have also been described and are being tested, including chitinase, tropomyosin, paramyosin, and several larval antigens called the "abundant larval transcript family" (ALT) (331). Finally, a novel recombinant larval protein antihookworm vaccine is in clinical trial (335). Although these accomplishments represent a significant advance for the field of helminthology, it is important to note that all of the candidate antischistosome vaccine antigens have, at best, provided only partial immunity, with few consistently reaching a required threshold of 40% protection. It is hoped, however, that ongoing improvements in vaccination technology, combined with greater knowledge of the mechanisms controlling resistance, will allow development of more-efficacious and better-defined vaccines for these complex organisms.

CONCLUSION

The last 4 to 5 years have seen a rapid expansion in research dealing with innate determinants of the immune response to parasites and in innate effector functions. This work has important implications not only for understanding the basis of Th-subset selection by parasites, but also for providing insights useful in the design of new adjuvants and immunomodulators. The studies on helminth infections will in addition provide a unique opportunity to decipher the innate determinants of the Th2 response and should represent an exciting research area in the coming years. The study of immunoregulatory mechanisms in parasitic infection has also seen important progress in recent years, with much of this work testifying to the multilayered complexity and tightly balanced interaction of antiparasitic immune responses. This work has forced us to rethink many of the paradigms concerning polarized effector functions and their regulation in parasitic infection. Thus, it is becoming increasingly evident that rather than being the product of a single arm of the immune response, effective control of parasites involves the coordination of both humoral and cellular elements dependent on both Th1 and Th2 cytokines. Moreover, the simplified notion that Th2 immune polarization underlies susceptibility to intracellular pathogens such as *Leishmania* has had to contend with accumulating evidence in mice and humans that regulatory cells and cytokines (e.g., IL-10 and TGFβ) modulating concurrent Th1 immunity better explain nonhealing and persistent infections. Targeting regulatory T cells or their cytokines, especially in conjunction with antiparasitic drugs, offers the potential for more efficient or even sterile cures.

The last 4 or 5 years has also seen remarkable progress in molecular parasitology that should affect immunologic approaches to disease control. For instance, the ability to target virulence genes for deletion in *Leishmania* and *Toxoplasma* has led to the generation of safe, live attenuated vaccines that promote more durable immunity than nonliving vaccines. The completion of the *L. major, T. cruzi, T. brucei, and P. falciparum* genomes should foster further discoveries of virulence molecules for deletion or drug targeting and identify additional protective antigens for vaccine development. The genomic sequence of an important helminth parasite, *B. malayi*, was recently completed *(343)* although transgenesis for helminths is still in its infancy. Given the overlapping pathways of immune regulatory and effector mechanisms in chronic parasitic infections and the dynamic nature of host responses during different phases of infection and in different tissues, there is clearly a danger in confining immune analyses to selected cells obtained from a fixed place and time. A systems biology approach that employs host–parasite genomic databases along with computer algorithms may be needed to reveal control points in immune networks that are associated with parasite killing, persistence, or pathology. Perhaps the most compelling need is for more human immunology to determine the clinical relevance of the mouse models and as an adjunct to clinical development of particular vaccines or immune-based therapies.

During the period since the publication of the last version of this chapter in the previous edition of this book, public recognition of the importance of malaria as one of three major global infectious diseases (along with AIDS and tuberculosis) has resulted in the expansion of government- and private foundation–supported vaccine programs, in some instances with industrial partners, aimed primarily at moving candidate immunogens into clinical trials. It is to be hoped that the initial encouraging results of the phase II 'RTS,S' vaccine trial in reducing the incidence of clinical malaria and severe disease in Mozambican children will be sustained and will provide a road map as to how public/private partnerships supporting translational research can achieve genuine progress in the control of these significant neglected diseases.

REFERENCES

1. Scott P, Natovitz P, Coffman RL, et al. Immunoregulation of cutaneous leishmaniasis. T cell lines that transfer protective immunity or exacerbation belong to different T helper subsets and respond to distinct parasite antigens. *J Exp Med.* 1988;168:1675–1684.
2. Heinzel FP, Sadick MD, Holaday BJ, et al. Reciprocal expression of interferon gamma or interleukin 4 during the resolution or progression of murine leishmaniasis. Evidence for expansion of distinct helper T cell subsets. *J Exp Med.* 1989;169(1):59–72.
3. Norris KA, Bradt B, Cooper NR, et al. Characterization of a *Trypanosoma cruzi* C3 binding protein with functional and genetic similarities to the human complement regulatory protein, decay-accelerating factor. *J Immunol.* 1991;147(7):2240–2247.
4. Puentes SM, Da Silva RP, Sacks DL, et al. Serum resistance of metacyclic stage *Leishmania major* promastigotes is due to release of C5b-9. *J Immunol.* 1990;145(12):4311–4316.
7. Braga LL, Ninomiya H, McCoy JJ, et al. Inhibition of the complement membrane attack complex by the galactose-specific adhesion of *Entamoeba histolytica*. *J Clin Invest.* 1992;90(3):1131–1137.
8. Raper J, Fung R, Ghiso J, et al. Characterization of a novel trypanosome lytic factor from human serum. *Infect Immun.* 1999; 67(4):1910–1916.
9. Smith AB, Esko JD, Hajduk SL. Killing of trypanosomes by the human haptoglobin-related protein. *Science.* 1995;268(5208):284–286.
10. Vanhamme L, Paturiaux-Hanocq F, Poelvoorde P, et al. Apolipoprotein L-I is the trypanosome lytic factor of human serum. *Nature.* 2003;422(6927):83–87.
12. Pearce EJ, Hall BF, Sher A. Host-specific evasion of the alternative complement pathway by schistosomes correlates with the presence of a phospholipase C-sensitive surface molecule resembling human decay accelerating factor. *J Immunol.* 1990;144(7):2751–2756.
14. Giacomin PR, Wang H, Gordon DL, et al. Loss of complement activation and leukocyte adherence as *Nippostrongylus brasiliensis* develops within the murine host. *Infect Immun.* 2005;73(11):7442–7449.
16. Olivier M, Brownsey RW, Reiner NE. Defective stimulus-response coupling in human monocytes infected with *Leishmania* donovani is associated with altered activation and translocation of protein kinase C. *Proc Natl Acad Sci U S A.* 1992;89(16):7481–7485.
20. van Zandbergen G, Bollinger A, Wenzel A, et al. *Leishmania* disease development depends on the presence of apoptotic promastigotes in the virulent inoculum. *Proc Natl Acad Sci U S A.* 2006;103(37):13837–13842.
22. Mordue DG, Hakansson S, Niesman I, et al. *Toxoplasma gondii* resides in a vacuole that avoids fusion with host cell endocytic and exocytic vesicular trafficking pathways. *Exp Parasitol.* 1999;92(2): 87–99.
25. Sibley LD, Weidner E, Krahenbuhl JL. Phagosome acidification blocked by intracellular *Toxoplasma gondii*. *Nature.* 1985;315(6018): 416–419.
26. Joiner KA, Fuhrman SA, Miettinen HM, et al. *Toxoplasma gondii*: fusion competence of parasitophorous vacuoles in Fc receptor-transfected fibroblasts. *Science.* 1990;249(4969):641–646.
27. Andrews NW. The acid-active hemolysin of *Trypanosoma cruzi*. *Exp Parasitol.* 1990;71(2):241–244.
28. Lodge R, Descoteaux A. Modulation of phagolysosome biogenesis by the lipophosphoglycan of *Leishmania*. *Clin Immunol.* 2005;114(3):256–265.
29. Galioto AM, Hess JA, Nolan TJ, et al. Role of eosinophils and neutrophils in innate and adaptive protective immunity to larval *Strongyloides stercoralis* in mice. *Infect Immun.* 2006;74(10):5730–5738.
30. Klion AD, Nutman TB. The role of eosinophils in host defense against helminth parasites. *J Allergy Clin Immunol.* 2004;113(1): 30–37.
31. Korbel DS, Finney OC, Riley EM. Natural killer cells and innate immunity to protozoan pathogens. *Int J Parasitol.* 2004;34(13–14): 1517–1528.
35. Hunter CA, Bermudez L, Beernink H, et al. Transforming growth factor-beta inhibits interleukin-12-induced production of interferon-gamma by natural killer cells: a role for transforming growth factor-beta in the regulation of T cell-independent resistance to *Toxoplasma gondii*. *Eur J Immunol.* 1995;25(4):994–1000.
36. Artavanis-Tsakonas K, Eleme K, McQueen K, et al. Activation of a subset of human natural killer cells upon contact with *Plasmodium falciparum*–infected erythrocytes. *J Immunol.* 2003;171:5396–5405.
37. Stevenson MM, Riley EM. Innate immunity to malaria. *Nat Rev Immunol.* 2004;4:169–180.
38. Mohan K, Moulin P, Stevenson MM. Natural killer cell cytokine production, not cytotoxicity, contributes to resistance against blood-stage *Plasmodium chabaudi AS* infection. *J Immunol* 1997;159: 4990–4998.
39. Satoskar AR, Stamm LM, Zhang X, et al. Mice lacking NK cells develop an efficient Th1 response and control cutaneous *Leishmania major* infection. *J Immunol.* 1999;162(11):6747–6754.
42. Tsuji M, Mombaerts P, Lefrancois L, et al. Gamma delta T cells contribute to immunity against the liver stages of malaria in alpha beta T-cell-deficient mice. *Proc Natl Acad Sci U S A.* 1994;91(1):345–349.
44. Gazzinelli RT, Denkers EY. Protozoan encounters with Toll-like receptor signalling pathways: implications for host parasitism. *Nat Rev Immunol.* 2006;6(12):895–906. Epub 2006 Nov 17.
49. Brattig NW, Bazzocchi C, Kirschning CJ, et al. The major surface protein of *Wolbachia* endosymbionts in filarial nematodes elicits immune responses through TLR2 and TLR4. *J Immunol.* 2004; 173(1):437–445.
50. Goodridge HS, Marshall FA, Else KJ, et al. Immunomodulation via novel use of TLR4 by the filarial nematode phosphorylcholine-containing secreted product, ES-62. *J Immunol.* 2005;174(1):284–293.
51. van der Kleij D, Latz E, Brouwers JF, et al. A novel host-parasite lipid cross-talk. Schistosomal lyso-phosphatidylserine activates toll-like receptor 2 and affects immune polarization. *J Biol Chem.* 2002;277(50):48122–48129.
52. Aksoy E, Zouain CS, Vanhoutte F, et al. Double-stranded RNAs from the helminth parasite *Schistosoma* activate TLR3 in dendritic cells. *J Biol Chem.* 2005;280(1):277–283.
53. Koga R, Hamano S, Kuwata H, et al. TLR-dependent induction of IFNbeta mediates host defense against *Trypanosoma cruzi*. *J Immunol.* 2006;177(10):7059–7066.
54. Akira S, Uematsu S, Takeuchi O. Pathogen recognition and innate immunity. *Cell.* 2006;124(4):783–801.
55. Liu CH, Fan YT, Dias A, et al. Cutting edge: dendritic cells are essential for *in vivo* IL-12 production and development of resistance against *Toxoplasma gondii* infection in mice. *J Immunol.* 2006; 177(1):31–35.
56. Jung S, Unutmaz D, Wong P, et al. *In vivo* depletion of CD11c(+) dendritic cells abrogates priming of CD8(+) T cells by exogenous cell-associated antigens. *Immunity.* 2002;17(2):211–220.

60. Olivier M, Gregory DJ, Forget G. Subversion mechanisms by which *Leishmania* parasites can escape the host immune response: a signaling point of view. *Clin Microbiol Rev*. 2005;18(2):293–305.
62. Ropert C, Gazzinelli RT. Signaling of immune system cells by glycosylphosphatidylinositol (GPI) anchor and related structures derived from parasitic protozoa. *Curr Opin Microbiol* 2000;3(4):395–403.
63. Coller SP, Mansfield JM, Paulnock DM. Glycosylinositolphosphate soluble variant surface glycoprotein inhibits IFNgamma-induced nitric oxide production via reduction in STAT1 phosphorylation in African trypanosomiasis. *J Immunol*. 2003;171(3):1466–1472.
64. Denkers EY, Butcher BA. Sabotage and exploitation in macrophages parasitized by intracellular protozoans. *Trends Parasitol*. 2005;21(1):35–41.
65. Aliberti J, Hieny S, Sousa CR, et al. Lipoxin-medited inhibition of IL-12 production by DCs: a mechanism for the regulation of microbial immunity. *Nat Immunol*. 2002;3(1):76–82.
66. Perry JA, Olver CS, Burnett RC, et al. Cutting edge: the acquisition of TLR tolerance during malaria infection impacts T cell activation. *J Immunol*. 2005;174(10):5921–5925.
67. Urban B, Willcox N, Roberts D. A role for CD36 in the regulation of dendritic cell function. *Proc Natl Acad Sci U S A*. 2001;98:8750–8755.
70. McDowell MA, Marovich M, Lira R, et al. *Leishmania* priming of human dendritic cells for CD40 ligand-induced interleukin-12p70 secretion is strain and species dependent. *Infect Immun*. 2002;70(8):3994–4001.
71. Jankovic D, Kullberg MC, Caspar P, et al. Parasite-induced Th2 polarization is associated with down-regulated dendritic cell responsiveness to Th1 stimuli and a transient delay in T lymphocyte cycling. *J Immunol*. 2004;173(4):2419–2427.
72. Kane CM, Cervi L, Sun J, et al. Helminth antigens modulate TLR-initiated dendritic cell activation. *J Immunol*. 2004;173(12):7454–7461.
73. Semnani RT, Liu AY, Sabzevari H, et al. *Brugia malayi* microfilariae induce cell death in human dendritic cells, inhibit their ability to make IL-12 and IL-10, and reduce their capacity to activate CD4+ T cells. *J Immunol*. 2003;171(4):1950–1960.
75. Park AY, Hondowicz BD, Scott P. IL-12 is required to maintain a Th1 response during *Leishmania major* infection. *J Immunol*. 2000;165(2):896–902.
76. Yap G, Pesin M, Sher A. Cutting edge: IL-12 is required for the maintenance of IFNgamma production in T cells mediating chronic resistance to the intracellular pathogen, *Toxoplasma gondii*. *J Immunol*. 2000;165(2):628–631.
79. Launois P, Maillard I, Pingel S, et al. IL-4 rapidly produced by V beta 4 V alpha 8 CD4+ T cells instructs Th2 development and susceptibility to *Leishmania major* in BALB/c mice. *Immunity*. 1997;6(5):541–549.
86. MacDonald AS, Straw AD, Bauman B, et al. CD8- dendritic cell activation status plays an integral role in influencing Th2 response development. *J Immunol*. 2001;167(4):1982–1988.
87. Whelan M, Harnett MM, Houston KM, et al. A filarial nematode-secreted product signals dendritic cells to acquire a phenotype that drives development of Th2 cells. *J Immunol*. 2000;164(12):6453–6460.
88. Perona-Wright G, Jenkins SJ, MacDonald AS. Dendritic cell activation and function in response to *Schistosoma mansoni*. *Int J Parasitol*. 2006;36(6):711–721.
89. Tu L, Fang TC, Artis D, et al. Notch signaling is an important regulator of type 2 immunity. *J Exp Med*. 2005;202(8):1037–1042.
90. Chiaramonte MG, Schopf LR, Neben TY, et al. IL-13 is a key regulatory cytokine for T helper 2 cell-mediated pulmonary granuloma formation and IgE responses induced by *Schistosoma mansoni* eggs. *J Immunol*. 1999;162:920–930.
91. Finkelman FD, Urban JF Jr. The other side of the coin: the protective role of the TH2 cytokines. *J Allergy Clin Immunol*. 2001;107(5):772–780.
92. Jankovic D, Kullberg MC, Noben-Trauth N, et al. Single cell analysis reveals that IL-4 receptor/Stat6 signaling is not required for the *in vivo* or *in vitro* development of CD4+ lymphocytes with a Th2 cytokine profile. *J Immunol*. 2000;164(6):3047–3055.
93. Min B, Prout M, Hu-Li J, et al. Basophils produce IL-4 and accumulate in tissues after infection with a Th2-inducing parasite. *J Exp Med*. 2004;200(4):507–517.
94. Voehringer D, Shinkai K, Locksley RM. Type 2 immunity reflects orchestrated recruitment of cells committed to IL-4 production. *Immunity*. 2004;20(3):267–277.
95. Belkaid Y, Von Stebut E, Mendez S, et al. CD8+ T cells are required for primary immunity in C57BL/6 mice following low-dose, intradermal challenge with *Leishmania major*. *J Immunol*. 2002;168(8):3992–4000.
98. Doolan DL, Hoffman SL. The complexity of protective immunity against liver-stage malaria. *J Immunol*. 2000;165(3):1453–1462.
99. Kumar S, Tarleton RL. The relative contribution of antibody production and CD8+ T cell function to immune control of *Trypanosoma cruzi*. *Parasite Immunol*. 1998;20(5):207–216.
100. Belosevic M, Finbloom DS, Van Der Meide PH, et al. Administration of monoclonal anti-IFNgamma antibodies *in vivo* abrogates natural resistance of C3H/HeN mice to infection with *Leishmania major*. *J Immunol*. 1989;143(1):266–274.
101. Torrico F, Heremans H, Rivera MT, et al. Endogenous IFNgamma is required for resistance to acute *Trypanosoma cruzi* infection in mice. *J Immunol*. 1991;146(10):3626–3632.
102. Scharton-Kersten TM, Wynn TA, Denkers EY, et al. In the absence of endogenous IFNgamma, mice develop unimpaired IL-12 responses to *Toxoplasma gondii* while failing to control acute infection. *J Immunol*. 1996;157(9):4045–4054.
105. Wei XQ, Charles IG, Smith A, et al. Altered immune responses in mice lacking inducible nitric oxide synthase. *Nature*. 1995;375(6530):408–411.
107. Bogdan C, Rollinghoff M, Diefenbach A. Reactive oxygen and reactive nitrogen intermediates in innate and specific immunity. *Curr Opin Immunol*. 2000;12(1):64–76.
108. Good MF, Doolan DL. Immune effector mechanisms in malaria. *Curr Opin Immunol*. 1999;11(4):412–419.
110. Taylor GA, Feng CG, Sher A. p47 GTPases: regulators of immunity to intracellular pathogens. *Nat Rev Immunol*. 2004;4(2):100–109.
111. Ling YM, Shaw MH, Ayala C, et al. Vacuolar and plasma membrane stripping and autophagic elimination of *Toxoplasma gondii* in primed effector macrophages. *J Exp Med*. 2006;203(9):2063–2071.
113. Santiago HC, Feng CG, Bafica A, et al. Mice deficient in LRG-47 display enhanced susceptibility to *Trypanosoma cruzi* infection associated with defective hemopoiesis and intracellular control of parasite growth. *J Immunol*. 2005;175(12):8165–8172.
114. Pfefferkorn ER. Interferon gamma blocks the growth of *Toxoplasma gondii* in human fibroblasts by inducing the host cells to degrade tryptophan. *Proc Natl Acad Sci U S A*. 1984;81(3):908–912.
115. Good MF. Towards a blood-stage vaccine for malaria: are we following all the leads? *Nat Rev Immunol*. 2001;1(1):117–125.
116. Makobongo MO, Riding G, Xu H, et al. The purine salvage enzyme hypoxanthine guanine xanthine phosphoribosyl transferase is a major target antigen for cell-mediated immunity to malaria. *Proc Natl Acad Sci U S A*. 2003;100(5):2628–2633.
117. Luty AJ, Lell B, Schmidt-Ott R, et al. Interferon-gamma responses are associated with resistance to reinfection with *Plasmodium falciparum* in young African children. *J Infect Dis*. 1999;179(4):980–988.
118. Anstey NM, Weinberg JB, Hassanali MY, et al. Nitric oxide in Tanzanian children with malaria: inverse relationship between malaria severity and nitric oxide production/nitric oxide synthase type 2 expression. *J Exp Med*. 1996;184(2):557–567.
119. Bouharoun-Tayoun H, Attanath P, Sabchareon A. Antibodies that protect humans against *Plasmodium falciparum* blood stages do not on their own inhibit parasite growth and invasion *in vitro* but act in co-operation with monocytes. *J Exp Med*. 1990;172:1633–1641.
120. Cohen S, McGregor IA, Carrington S. Gamma globulin and acquired immunity to malaria. *Nature*. 1961;192:733–737.
121. Uthaipibull C, Aufiero B, Syed S, et al. Inhibitory and blocking monoclonal antibody epitopes on merozoite surface protein 1 of the malaria parasite *Plasmodium falciparum*. *J Mol Biol* 2001;307:1381–1394.
123. Hill AV. Pre-erythrocytic malaria vaccines: towards greater efficacy. *Nat Rev Immunol*. 2006;6(1):21–32.
125. Vanderberg JP, Frevert U. Intravital microscopy demonstrating antibody-mediated immobilisation of *Plasmodium berghei* sporozoites injected into skin by mosquitoes. *Int J Parasitol*. 2004;34(9):991–996.

126. Finkelman FD, Wynn TA, Donaldson DD, et al. The role of IL-13 in helminth-induced inflammation and protective immunity against nematode infections. *Curr Opin Immunol*. 1999;11(4):420–426.
127. Maizels RM, Balic A, Gomez-Escobar N, et al. Helminth parasites—masters of regulation. *Immunol Rev*. 2004;201:89–116.
128. Nutman TB, Kumaraswami V. Regulation of the immune response in lymphatic filariasis: perspectives on acute and chronic infection with *Wuchereria bancrofti* in South India. *Parasite Immunol*. 2001;23(7):389–399.
131. Helmby H, Grencis RK. Essential role for TLR4 and MyD88 in the development of chronic intestinal nematode infection. *Eur J Immunol*. 2003;33(11):2974–2979.
133. Mohrs K, Harris DP, Lund FE, et al. Systemic dissemination and persistence of Th2 and type 2 cells in response to infection with a strictly enteric nematode parasite. *J Immunol*. 2005;175(8):5306–5313.
134. Anthony RM, Urban JF Jr, Alem F, et al. Memory T(H)2 cells induce alternatively activated macrophages to mediate protection against nematode parasites. *Nat Med*. 2006;12(8):955–960.
139. Helmby H, Grencis RK. Contrasting roles for IL-10 in protective immunity to different life cycle stages of intestinal nematode parasites. *Eur J Immunol*. 2003;33(9):2382–2390.
140. Schopf LR, Hoffmann KF, Cheever AW, et al. IL-10 is critical for host resistance and survival during gastrointestinal helminth infection. *J Immunol*. 2002;168:2383.
142. Fallon PG, Ballantyne SJ, Mangan NE, et al. Identification of an interleukin (IL)-25-dependent cell population that provides IL-4, IL-5, and IL-13 at the onset of helminth expulsion. *J Exp Med*. 2006; 203(4):1105–1116.
143. Owyang AM, Zaph C, Wilson EH, et al. Interleukin 25 regulates type 2 cytokine-dependent immunity and limits chronic inflammation in the gastrointestinal tract. *J Exp Med*. 2006;203(4):843–849.
144. Urban JF Jr, Noben-Trauth N, Donaldson DD, et al. IL-13, IL-4Ralpha, and Stat6 are required for the expulsion of the gastrointestinal nematode parasite *Nippostrongylus brasiliensis*. *Immunity*. 1998;8(2):255–264.
145. McKenzie GJ, Fallon PG, Emson CL, et al. IL-10 is critical for host resistance. Simultaneous disruption of interleukin (IL)-4 and IL-13 defines individual roles in T helper cell type 2-mediated responses. *J Exp Med*. 1999;189(10):1565–1572.
148. Faulkner H, Turner J, Kamgno J, et al. Age- and infection intensity-dependent cytokine and antibody production in human trichuriasis: the importance of IgE. *J Infect Dis*. 2002;185(5):665–672.
151. Gurish MF, Bryce PJ, Tao H, et al. IgE enhances parasite clearance and regulates mast cell responses in mice infected with *Trichinella spiralis*. *J Immunol*. 2004;172(2):1139–1145.
152. Madden KB, Yeung KA, Zhao A, et al. Enteric nematodes induce stereotypic STAT6-dependent alterations in intestinal epithelial cell function. *J Immunol*. 2004;172(9):5616–5621.
155. Zhao A, McDermott J, Urban JF Jr, et al. Dependence of IL-4, IL-13, and nematode-induced alterations in murine small intestinal smooth muscle contractility on Stat6 and enteric nerves. *J Immunol*. 2003;171(2):948–954.
156. Artis D, Wang ML, Keilbaugh SA, et al. RELMbeta/FIZZ2 is a goblet cell-specific immune-effector molecule in the gastrointestinal tract. *Proc Natl Acad Sci U S A*. 2004;101(37):13596–13600.
159. Yoshida T, Ikuta K, Sugaya H, et al. Defective B-1 cell development and impaired immunity against *Angiostrongylus cantonensis* in IL-5R alpha-deficient mice. *Immunity*. 1996;4(5):483–494.
161. Reiman RM, Thompson RW, Feng CG, et al. Interleukin-5 (IL-5) augments the progression of liver fibrosis by regulating IL-13 activity. *Infect Immun*. 2006;74(3):1471–1479.
163. Padigel UM, Lee JJ, Nolan TJ, et al. Eosinophils can function as antigen-presenting cells to induce primary and secondary immune responses to *Strongyloides stercoralis*. *Infect Immun*. 2006;74(6): 3232–3238.
164. Ganley-Leal LM, Mwinzi PN, Cetre-Sossah CB, et al. Correlation between eosinophils and protection against reinfection with *Schistosoma mansoni* and the effect of human immunodeficiency virus type 1 coinfection in humans. *Infect Immun*. 2006;74(4):2169–2176.
165. Reimert CM, Fitzsimmons CM, Joseph S, et al. Eosinophil activity in *Schistosoma mansoni* infections *in vivo* and *in vitro* in relation to plasma cytokine profile pre- and posttreatment with praziquantel. *Clin Vaccine Immunol*. 2006;13(5):584–593.
171. Leech MD, Grencis RK. Induction of enhanced immunity to intestinal nematodes using IL-9–producing dendritic cells. *J Immunol*. 2006;176(4):2505–2511.
173. Mitre E, Taylor RT, Kubofcik J, et al. Parasite antigen-driven basophils are a major source of IL-4 in human filarial infections. *J Immunol*. 2004;172(4):2439–2445.
174. Dombrowicz D, Capron M. Eosinophils, allergy and parasites. *Curr Opin Immunol*. 2001;13(6):716–720.
175. Booth M, Shaw MA, Carpenter D, et al. Carriage of DRB1*13 is associated with increased posttreatment IgE levels against *Schistosoma mansoni* antigens and lower long-term reinfection levels. *J Immunol*. 2006;176(11):7112–7118.
178. Paciorkowski N, Shultz LD, Rajan TV. Primed peritoneal B lymphocytes are sufficient to transfer protection against *Brugia pahangi* infection in mice. *Infect Immun*. 2003;71(3):1370–1378.
179. Spencer LA, Porte P, Zetoff C, et al. Mice genetically deficient in immunoglobulin E are more permissive hosts than wild-type mice to a primary, but not secondary, infection with the filarial nematode *Brugia malayi*. *Infect Immun*. 2003;71(5):2462–2467.
182. Saeftel M, Arndt M, Specht S, et al. Synergism of gamma interferon and interleukin-5 in the control of murine filariasis. *Infect Immun*. 2003;71(12):6978–6985.
186. Magez S, Radwanska M, Drennan M, et al. Interferon-gamma and nitric oxide in combination with antibodies are key protective host immune factors during *Trypanosoma congolense* Tc13 Infections. *J Infect Dis*. 2006;193(11):1575–1583.
187. Li E, Zhou P, Petrin Z, et al. Mast cell-dependent control of *Giardia lamblia* infections in mice. *Infect Immun*. 2004;72(11):6642–6649.
190. Li E, Zhou P, Singer SM. Neuronal nitric oxide synthase is necessary for elimination of *Giardia lamblia* infections in mice. *J Immunol*. 2006;176(1):516–521.
191. Tarleton RL, Zhang L. Chagas disease etiology: autoimmunity or parasite persistence? *Parasitol Today*. 1999;15(3):94–99.
192. Bogdan C, Gessner A, Solbach W, et al. Invasion, control and persistence of *Leishmania* parasites. *Curr Opin Immunol*. 1996;8(4):517–525.
193. Pearce EJ, Sher A. Mechanisms of immune evasion in schistosomiasis. *Contrib Microbiol Immunol*. 1987;8:219–232.
194. Maizels RM, Bundy DA, Selkirk ME, et al. Immunological modulation and evasion by helminth parasites in human populations. *Nature*. 1993;365(6449):797–805.
195. Davies SJ, Grogan JL, Blank RB, et al. Modulation of blood fluke development in the liver by hepatic CD4+ lymphocytes. *Science*. 2001;294(5545):1358–1361.
196. Osman A, Niles EG, Verjovski-Almeida S, et al. *Schistosoma mansoni* TGFbeta receptor II: role in host ligand-induced regulation of a schistosome target gene. *PLoS Pathog*. 2006(Jun);2(6):e54.
197. Wolowczuk I, Nutten S, Roye O, et al. Infection of mice lacking interleukin-7 (IL-7) reveals an unexpected role for IL-7 in the development of the parasite *Schistosoma mansoni*. *Infect Immun*. 1999;67(8):4183–4190.
199. Pays E, Vanhamme L, Perez-Morga D. Antigenic variation in *Trypanosoma brucei*: facts, challenges and mysteries. *Curr Opin Microbiol*. 2004;7(4):369–374.
200. Nash TE. Surface antigenic variation in *Giardia lamblia*. *Mol Microbiol*. 2002;45(3):585–590.
202. Dzikowski R, Templeton TJ, Deitsch K. Variant antigen gene expression in malaria. *Cell Microbiol*. 2006;8(9):1371–1381.
204. Kaye PM, Svensson M, Ato M, et al. The immunopathology of experimental visceral leishmaniasis. *Immunol Rev* 2004;201:239–253.
205. Gomez-Escobar N, Bennett C, Prieto-Lafuente L, et al. Heterologous expression of the filarial nematode alt gene products reveals their potential to inhibit immune function. *BMC Biol*. 2005;3:8.
209. Urban BC, Ferguson DJ, Pain A, et al. *Plasmodium falciparum*–infected erythrocytes modulate the maturation of dendritic cells. *Nature*. 1999;400(6739):73–77.
210. Greenwood BM. Possible role of a B-cell mitogen in hypergammaglobulinaemia in malaria and trypanosomiasis. *Lancet*. 1974;1(7855):435–436.

213. Belkaid Y, Piccirillo CA, Mendez S, et al. CD4+ CD25+ regulatory T cells control *Leishmania major* persistence and immunity. *Nature*. 2002;420(6915):502–507.
214. Omer FM, de Souza JB, Riley EM. Differential induction of TGFbeta regulates proinflammatory cytokine production and determines the outcome of lethal and nonlethal *Plasmodium yoelii* infections. *J Immunol*. 2003;171(10):5430–5436.
215. Hisaeda H, Maekawa Y, Iwakawa D, et al. Escape of malaria parasites from host immunity requires CD4(+)CD25(+) regulatory T cells. *Nat Med*. 2004;10(1):29–30.
216. Walther M, Tongren JE, Andrews L, et al. Upregulation of TGF-beta, FOXP3, and CD4+ CD25+ regulatory T cells correlates with more rapid parasite growth in human malaria infection. *Immunity*. 2005;23(3):287–296.
218. Taylor MD, LeGoff L, Harris A, et al. Removal of regulatory T cell activity reverses hyporesponsiveness and leads to filarial parasite clearance *in vivo*. *J Immunol*. 2005;174(8):4924–4933.
219. Satoguina J, Mempel M, Larbi J, et al. Antigen-specific T regulatory-1 cells are associated with immunosuppression in a chronic helminth infection (onchocerciasis). *Microbes Infect*. 2002;4(13):1291–1300.
220. Steel C, Nutman TB. CTLA-4 in filarial infections: implications for a role in diminished T cell reactivity. *J Immunol*. 2003;170(4):1930–1938.
221. Anderson CF, Oukka M, Kuchroo VJ, et al. CD4+CD25-Foxp3- Th1 cells are the source of IL-10 mediated immune suppression in chronic cutaneous leishmaniasis. *J Exp Med*. 2007;204:285.
222. Miles SA, Conrad SM, Alves RG, et al. A role for IgG immune complexes during infection with the intracellular pathogen *Leishmania*. *J Exp Med*. 2005;201(5):747–754.
224. Wynn TA, Kwiatkowski D. Pathology and pathogenesis of parasitic disease. In: Kaufmann S, Sher A, Ahmed R, eds. Immunology of infectious diseases. Washington DC: ASM Press,. 2001:293–306.
225. Nathoo S, Serghides L, Kain KC. Effect of HIV-1 antiretroviral drugs on cytoadherence and phagocytic clearance of *Plasmodium falciparum*–parasitised erythrocytes. *Lancet*. 2003;362(9389):1039–1041.
226. Mwinzi PN, Karanja DM, Kareko I, et al. Short report: Evaluation of hepatic fibrosis in persons co-infected with *Schistosoma mansoni* and human immunodeficiency virus 1. *Am J Trop Med Hyg*. 2004;71(6):783–786.
228. Kublin JG, Steketee RW. HIV infection and malaria—understanding the interactions. *J Infect Dis*. 2006;193(1):1–3.
231. Andre AvS, Blackwell NM, Hall LR, et al. The role of endosymbiotic *Wolbachia* bacteria in the pathogenesis of river blindness. *Science*. 2002;295(5561):1892–1895.
235. Rutitzky LI, Lopes da Rosa JR, Stadecker MJ. Severe CD4 T cell-mediated immunopathology in murine schistosomiasis is dependent on IL-12p40 and correlates with high levels of IL-17. *J Immunol*. 2005;175(6):3920–3926.
236. Gazzinelli RT, Wysocka M, Hieny S, et al. In the absence of endogenous IL-10, mice acutely infected with *Toxoplasma gondii* succumb to a lethal immune response dependent on CD4+ T cells and accompanied by overproduction of IL-12, IFNgamma and TNF alpha. *J Immunol*. 1996;157(2):798–805.
237. Holscher C, Mohrs M, Dai WJ, et al. Tumor necrosis factor alpha-mediated toxic shock in *Trypanosoma cruzi*-infected interleukin 10-deficient mice. *Infect Immun*. 2000;68(7):4075–4083.
238. Jankovic D, Kullberg MC, Feng C, et al. Conventional T-bet Foxp3 Th1 cells are the major source of regulatory IL-10 during intracellular protozoan infection. *J Exp Med*. 2007;204(2):273.
239. Schofield L, Grau GE. Immunological processes in malaria pathogenesis. *Nat Rev Immunol*. 2005;5(9):722–735.
241. Engwerda C, Mynott T, Sawhney S, et al. Locally up-regulated lymphotoxin alpha, not systemic tumor necrosis factor alpha, is the principle mediator of murine cerebral malaria. *J Exp Med*. 2002; 195:1371–1377.
243. Knight JC, Udalova I, Hill AV, et al. A polymorphism that affects OCT-1 binding to the TNF promoter region is associated with severe malaria. *Nat Genet*. 1999;22(2):145–150.
244. Omer FM, Kurtzhals JA, Riley EM. Maintaining the immunological balance in parasitic infections: a role for TGFbeta? *Parasitol Today*. 2000;16(1):18–23.
247. Li C, Sanni LA, Omer FM, et al. Pathology and mortality of *Plasmodium chabaudi chabaudi* infection in IL-10-deficient mice is ameliorated by anti-TNFa and exacerbated by anti-TGFb antibodies. *Infect Immun*. 2003;71:4850.
248. Cliffe LJ, Grencis RK. The *Trichuris muris* system: a paradigm of resistance and susceptibility to intestinal nematode infection. *Adv Parasitol*. 2004;57:255–307.
249. Pearce EJ, MacDonald AS. The immunobiology of schistosomiasis. *Nat Rev Immunol*. 2002;2(7):499–511.
250. Wynn TA, Thompson RW, Cheever AW, et al. Immunopathogenesis of schistosomiasis. *Immunol Rev*. 2004;201:156–167.
254. Montesano MA, Colley DG, Willard MT, et al. Idiotypes expressed early in experimental *Schistosoma mansoni* infections predict clinical outcomes of chronic disease. *J Exp Med*. 2002;195(9):1223–1228.
255. Wynn TA, Cheever AW, Jankovic D, et al. An IL-12-based vaccination method for preventing fibrosis induced by schistosome infection. *Nature*. 1995;376(6541):594–596.
263. Wamachi AN, Mayadev JS, Mungai PL, et al. Increased ratio of tumor necrosis factor-alpha to interleukin-10 production is associated with *Schistosoma haematobium*–induced urinary-tract morbidity. *J Infect Dis*. 2004;190(11):2020–2030.
264. Hesse M, Piccirillo CA, Belkaid Y, et al. The pathogenesis of schistosomiasis is controlled by cooperating IL-10–producing innate effector and regulatory T cells. *J Immunol*. 2004;172:3157.
266. Wynn TA. Fibrotic disease and the T(H)1/T(H)2 paradigm. *Nat Rev Immunol*. 2004;4(8):583–594.
269. Chiaramonte MG, Donaldson DD, Cheever AW, et al. An IL-13 inhibitor blocks the development of hepatic fibrosis during a T-helper type 2-dominated inflammatory response. *J Clin Invest*. 1999;104(6):777–785.
274. Gordon S. Alternative activation of macrophages. *Nat Rev Immunol*. 2003;3(1):23–35.
276. Vercruysse J, Knox DP, Schetters TP, et al. Veterinary parasitic vaccines: pitfalls and future directions. *Trends Parasitol*. 2004;20(10): 488–492.
277. Bhatia V, Sinha M, Luxon B, et al. Utility of the *Trypanosoma cruzi* sequence database for identification of potential vaccine candidates by *in silico* and *in vitro* screening. *Infect Immun*. 2004;72(11):6245–6254.
278. Stober CB, Lange UG, Roberts MT, et al. From genome to vaccines for leishmaniasis: screening 100 novel vaccine candidates against murine *Leishmania major* infection. *Vaccine*. 2006;24(14):2602–2616.
279. Tongren JE, Zavala F, Roos DS, et al. Malaria vaccines: if at first you don't succeed. *Trends Parasitol*. 2004;20(12):604–610.
282. Snow MJ, Stanley SL Jr. Recent progress in vaccines for amebiasis. *Arch Med Res*. 2006;37(2):280–287.
283. Olson ME, Ceri H, Morck DW. *Giardia* vaccination. *Parasitol Today*. 2000;16(5):213–217.
295. Duffy PE, Craig AG, Baruch DI. Variant proteins on the surface of malaria-infected erythrocytes—developing vaccines. *Trends Parasitol*. 2001;17(8):354–356.
296. Duffy PE. Maternal immunization and malaria in pregnancy. *Vaccine*. 2003;21(24):3358–3361.
297. Stowers A, Carter R. Current developments in malaria transmission-blocking vaccines. *Expert Opin Biol Ther*. 2001;1(4): 619–628.
298. Afonso LCC, Scharton TM, Vieira LQ, et al. The adjuvant effect of interleukin 12 in a vaccine against *Leishmania major*. *Science*. 1993;263:235–237.
299. Coler RN, Reed SG. Second-generation vaccines against leishmaniasis. *Trends Parasitol*. 2005;21(5):244–249.
302. Handman E. Leishmaniasis: current status of vaccine development. *Clin Microbiol Rev*. 2001;14(2):229–243.
304. Zaph C, Uzonna J, Beverley SM, et al. Central memory T cells mediate long-term immunity to *Leishmania major* in the absence of persistent parasites. *Nat Med*. 2004;10(10):1104–1110.
309. Miyahira Y, Takashima Y, Kobayashi S, et al. Immune responses against a single CD8+ -T-cell epitope induced by virus vector vaccination can successfully control *Trypanosoma cruzi* infection. *Infect Immun*. 2005;73(11):7356–7365.

315. Hoffman SL, Doolan DL. Malaria vaccines—targeting infected hepatocytes. *Nat Med*. 2000;6(11):1218–1219.
316. Hafalla JC, Rai U, Morrot A, et al. Priming of CD8+ T cell responses following immunization with heat-killed *Plasmodium* sporozoites. *Eur J Immunol*. 2006;36(5):1179–1186.
317. Scheller LF, Azad AF. Maintenance of protective immunity against malaria by persistent hepatic parasites derived from irradiated sporozoites. *Proc Natl Acad Sci U S A*. 1995;92(9):4066–4068.
318. Bojang KA, Milligan PJ, Pinder M, et al. Efficacy of RTS,S/AS02 malaria vaccine against *Plasmodium falciparum* infection in semi-immune adult men in the Gambia: a randomised trial. *Lancet*. 2001;358(9297):1927–1934.
319. Alonso PL, Sacarlal J, Aponte JJ, et al. Duration of protection with RTS,S/AS02A malaria vaccine in prevention of *Plasmodium falciparum* disease in Mozambican children: single-blind extended follow-up of a randomised controlled trial. *Lancet*. 2005;366(9502):2012–2018.
325. Schofield L, Mueller I. Clinical immunity to malaria. *Curr Mol Med*. 2006;6(2):205–221.
331. Maizels RM, Holland MJ, Falcone FH, et al. Vaccination against helminth parasites—the ultimate challenge for vaccinologists? *Immunol Rev*. 1999;171:125–147.
334. Dalton JP, Brindley PJ, Knox DP, et al. Helminth vaccines: from mining genomic information for vaccine targets to systems used for protein expression. *Int J Parasitol*. 2003;33(5–6):621–640.
335. Loukas A, Bethony J, Brooker S, et al. Hookworm vaccines: past, present, and future. *Lancet Infect Dis* 2006;6(11):733–741.
336. Mascie-Taylor CG, Karim E. The burden of chronic disease. *Science*. 2003;302(5652):1921–1922.

Immunity to Viruses

Hildegund Ertl

INTRODUCTION

Viruses are the simplest of all life forms. They can be viewed as selfish genes with the single-minded purpose to replicate. Viruses are parasites, and their replication depends strictly on the machinery of cellular organisms. They have developed vehicles that allow for efficient transfer of their genes into host cells, supporting their replication. Replication of viruses is rarely subtle; instead it commonly results in damage or even death of the invaded cells. Hosts have in turn developed defense mechanisms against this invasion. Mechanisms used directly by the attacked cells to block virus entry or virus replication have evolved to protect individual cells and are employed by both primitive monocellular organisms such as bacteria and sophisticated mammalian hosts alike. More complex organisms have also developed specific organs and cells to form an immune system to ward off invading pathogens. In turn, viruses, which are much more flexible than their hosts because of their rapid replication allowing for genetic modifications, are constantly mutating to dodge the defense mechanisms of their unwilling production facilities.

Altogether, >400 viruses cause disease in their human hosts. More than 100 of those belong to the *Rhinovirus* genus. Considering the multitude of viruses that are pathogenic in humans, it is not surprising that in spite of advances in modern medicine, viral infections remain one of the leading causes of human morbidity and mortality worldwide. Constant evolution allows more efficient replication of viruses, in part through an increase in host range from animals to humans. Therefore, although not long ago governments of some developed countries declared infectious diseases a problem of the past, the fight against infectious diseases became one of the main topics of the last G-8 summit, the meeting of eight of the world's leading industrialized nations.

One major current threat is a new influenza A virus pandemic of potentially catastrophic outcome. Three influenza A virus pandemics struck in the last century. The influenza pandemic of 1918 killed more young Americans than all of the wars of the twentieth century combined and claimed an estimated 20 to 50 million human lives globally. Additional pandemics occurred in 1957, which caused approximately 2 million human deaths, and in 1968, which resulted in approximately 1 million human deaths. The currently evolving H5N1 virus, which could be the precursor for the next pandemic, has disturbing similarities to the highly virulent virus of 1918, which was reconstructed through reverse genetics with the help of bits and pieces of viral genome isolated from a human cadaver that had been preserved in the arctic permafrost. H5N1 virus was first detected in Asian poultry in 1997. By July 2006, 229 human cases of H5N1 virus infection had been reported, mainly from Asia, but also from Africa and Europe. These cases resulted in 131 fatalities, which is far in excess of previously observed mortality rates of influenza A virus infections. So far the virus has been transmitted by human contact with infected birds, and only a few isolated cases suggest direct human-to-human transmission. Further mutations of H5N1 virus, either in the form of adaptive point mutations, that is, antigenic drift, or through reassortment in humans concomitantly infected with a different influenza A virus, called antigenic shift, could eventually allow for sustained and efficient human-to-human transmission.

The human immunodeficiency virus (HIV)-1 was first identified in 1981. It evolved from a simian immunodeficiency virus that infects chimpanzees and crossed the species barrier less than 100 years ago. Since then it has gained an irreversible foothold in the human population.

A corona virus that had spilled over for years into humans from a yet-to-be-identified animal reservoir failed to cause serious symptoms, but then suddenly began to result in life-threatening acute respiratory infections in 2003. This change in virulence was the result of a deletion mutation within the viral genome.

Vaccines are currently available for only a fraction of the identified human viral pathogens. Vaccines to viruses that only infect humans, that is, without an animal reservoir, can eradicate a virus, as was shown for smallpoxvirus, which was eliminated through global vaccination campaigns by 1977. Other human viruses for which vaccines are available, such as poliovirus, measles virus, or hepatitis B virus, could potentially be eliminated by global mass vaccination as well.

SOME BASICS IN VIROLOGY

Virus Classification

The International Committee on Taxonomy of Viruses has approved 3 orders, 56 families, 9 subfamilies, 233 genera, and 1,550 virus species. The three orders include DNA viruses, DNA and RNA reverse transcribing viruses, and RNA viruses. DNA viruses are divided into double-stranded (ds) DNA viruses (e.g., poxviruses, herpes viruses, adenoviruses, and papilloma viruses) and single-stranded (ss) DNA viruses (e.g., parvoviruses). RNA viruses are divided into dsRNA viruses (e.g., reoviruses), negative-sense ssRNA viruses (e.g., influenza virus and rabies virus), and positive-sense ssRNA viruses (e.g., poliovirus and yellow fever virus). The genome can be linear (e.g., poxvirus), circular (e.g., papillomaviruses), or segmented (e.g., influenza virus) and can range in size from 375 kp (poxvirus) to 4 to 6 kb (adeno-associated viruses). Viruses are further classified into enveloped or naked, that is, nonenveloped viruses. Viruses can also be divided according to their morphology, which can be polymorphic or structured. To given an example of the taxonomic division of viruses, measles virus belongs to the genus *Morbillivirus*, the subfamily Paramyxovirinea, and the family Paramyxoviridae. In this chapter, examples of viruses are used to clarify antiviral immunity. A list of these viruses, their classifications, abbreviations, and antigens that are mentioned throughout the text is given in Table 36.1.

Virus Transmission

Viruses are transmitted either through the mucosal surfaces of the airways, the intestinal or genital tract, or the eye, abrasions of the skin, or by directly gaining access to the bloodstream. Mucosal entry is most common. Viruses, such as influenza viruses, parainfluenza viruses, certain types of adenoviruses, or rhinoviruses spread through the airways and are transmitted by droplets that are formed during coughing or sneezing of an infected individual. Such viruses can be extraordinarily contagious, as attested by influenza viruses, which cause periodic pandemics that spread around the globe within less than half a year. Aquatic birds serve as influenza A virus reservoirs. The virus mutates rapidly, and antigenic variations of the two surface proteins, the hemaglutinin (HA) and the neuraminidase (NA), allow for the development of antigenic drift strains that can evade protective humoral immune responses induced by previous infections. Most annual epidemics are caused by antigenic drift variants. Rearrangements of the HA or NA encoding gene segments between viral strains circulating in humans with those endemic in animals result in more dramatic changes, also called antigenic shifts, and the pandemics of 1957 with H2N2 and 1968 with H3N2 were caused by such new strains of influenza virus. Influenza A virus can also gain human-to-human transmissibility through adaptive mutations. This was the case with the H1N1 virus that caused the pandemic of 1918. During this and subsequent pandemics, some countries prohibited public coughing or sneezing, a control measure that was shown to be ineffective. Control measures such as quarantine of infected individuals to stop transmission can be effective, as was shown during the severe acute respiratory symptom (SARS) outbreak caused by a corona virus in 2003–2004, but they will not stop an influenza virus pandemic.

TABLE 36.1

Family	Genus	Virus	Abbreviation	Proteins
Poxviridae	Orthopoxvirus	Vaccinia virus	—	B18R, B13R, GIF, C10L, NIL, A46R, A52R, B8R, M104L, E3L, K3L, MT1, T2, crmA-D, VCP
		Ectromelia virus	—	p28
	Leporipoxvirus	Shope fibroma virus	—	N1R
		Myxoma virus		M57, M135R, F2, SEPP-2, M-T2, M-T4, M-T5
	Mulluscipox	Molluscum contagiosum virus	MCV	MC159, MC160, MC066. M11L, MC148
Herpesviridae	Herpesvirus	Human cytomegalovirus	HCMV	US11, US2, UL33, UL78, US27, US28, UL146, UL145, UL147, UL111A, UL144, UL16, US10, US3, US6, US11, UL40, UL35, UL36, UL18
		Mouse cytomegalovirus	MCMV	m157, m144, m152, m6/gp48, m144
		Karposi sarcoma–associated herpesviruses (human herpesvirus-8)	KSHV (HHV-8)	K3, K4, K5, N5, mκ3
		Herpesvirus samiri	—	CCPH
		Epstein–Barr virus	EBV	BHRF1
		Herpes simplex virus	HSV	ICP47, gc
Adenoviridae	Adenovirus	Human serotype adenoviruses	—	E1B/19K, E1B/55K, E3/10.4K, E3/14.5K, E3/19K
Polyomaviridae	Papillomavirus	Human papillomavirus	HPV	E6, E7
Flaviviridae	Hepacivirus	Hepatitis C virus	HCV	NS3/4, NS5A, E2
Filoviridae	Ebolavirus	—	—	Vp35
Orthomyxoviridae	Influenza virus A	—	—	NS1

Intestinal transmission is caused by virus shedding in feces, from where viruses gain access to oral ingestion. Orally transmitted pathogens are in general remarkable stable. They can pass through the acidic environment of the stomach or survive in water for prolonged times. Infection of aquatic birds with influenza viruses, which are transmitted orally in birds, is linked to contamination of lake water. Outbreaks of rotaviruses have been caused by contaminated water. Poliovirus, which prior to worldwide immunization programs caused devastating infection of children worldwide, was commonly transmitted in public swimming pools. Hepatitis A virus can be transmitted by ingestion of raw oysters that have become infected by viruses in water.

Genital transmission by sexual contact maintains the pandemic of acquired immunodeficiency (AIDS), which is caused by human immunodeficiency virus (HIV). AIDS is by now the leading cause of death in humans aged 18 to 59 worldwide. Between 1981 and 2003, an estimated 20 million humans died of AIDS. By 2005, 40.3 million people were infected with HIV-1. In 2005, it was estimated that an additional 3.1 million humans had died of AIDS, while 4.9 million people became newly infected with HIV-1. Sub-Saharan Africa has by far the highest incidence rates of HIV-1 infections, and in some sub-Saharan nations, such as in Botswana, a staggering 37.3% of the adult population is infected. HIV-1 is starting to spread in other regions, including highly populated countries of Asia such as India and China. India has a population of 1 billion with an estimated infection rate of 0.9%, China has a population of 1.2 billion with an estimated infection rate of 0.1%, and both countries are at risk for an explosive increase in HIV-1 infection rates. Women are at a higher risk than men to become infected by heterosexual contact, and currently 60% of all HIV-1 infected individuals are women. Infected women in turn can transmit virus to their offspring during pregnancy, birth, or breastfeeding, and it is estimated that more than 2.2 million infants have become infected from their mothers.

Certain types of human papillomaviruses (HPV), such as types 16 and 18, are sexually transmitted. Although these viruses cause benign infections in most men and in the majority of women, who can clear virus-infected cells through adaptive immune responses, oncogenic types of papillomaviruses can persist and cause cervical cancer. Cervical cancer is currently the second most common cause of cancer death in women worldwide, claiming approximately 300,000 to 400,000 lives each year. In the United States, approximately 4,800 women die each year from cervical cancer. Worldwide, cervical cancer affects about 1% of all women and is the most common cause of cancer death in women under the age of 50. A vaccine to HPV-16 and HPV-18 was licensed recently, and it is expected that this vaccine will reduce the incidence of cervical cancer induced by these two types of HPV. Notwithstanding, over 50 types of HPV are known, and some others besides types 16 and 18 are oncogenic.

A number of viruses can only infect humans if they gain direct access to the bloodstream. These viruses rely on intermediate hosts, which commonly include blood-feeding insects such as mosquitoes, ticks, or flies. Rabies virus can only infect warm-blooded mammals. It causes a fatal encephalitis, and one of the symptoms in rabies virus–infected animals is increased aggressiveness resulting in unprovoked attacks, which in turn allows rabies virus to spread from the saliva of the infected animal into the bite wound of its victim.

Virus Cell Entry

Many viruses enter cells through the use of specific cell surface receptors, which in turn influences the tropism of the virus. Examples of viral receptors include sialic acid for influenza viruses, the coxsackie adenovirus receptor (CAR) for coxsackie virus and most types of adenoviruses (1,2), CD46, a complement component, for adenoviruses of subfamily B2, measles virus, or human herpes virus 6 (3–5), CD4 for HIV-1, CD54, an intercellular adhesion molecule used by 78 of the more than 100 rhinovirus types (6), CD155 used by poliovirus (7), the herpes virus entry mediator (HVEM), a member of the TNF family used by herpes simplex virus (8), or heparan sulfate protoglycan used by some strains of adeno-associated virus (AAV) (9). Many viruses, in addition to their primary binding receptor, use coreceptors for cell entry. For example, the envelope protein of HIV-1, upon binding to CD4, changes its structure and then binds to CCR5 to gain access into the cells. Adenoviruses gain entry into cells after binding of the fiber knob to CAR, followed by interactions between the viral penton and cell surface–expressed integrins. Once viruses bind to cell membranes, they employ a variety of pathways to gain access into the cell. Naked virus particles can cross the cell membrane directly, or they can form a pore within the membrane and inject their genome into the cytoplasm. Other nonenveloped viruses, such as adenoviruses or AAVs, sink into clathrin-coated pits upon binding to cell surface receptors, which invaginate and close off, forming clathrin-coated vesicles within the cytoplasm. There the clathrin dissociates into triskelions, which leave the vesicles. The resulting uncoated vesicles transport the virions to endosomes, from where virus can be released.

Enveloped viruses such as influenza virus enter cells by receptor-mediated endocytosis. The membrane of some enveloped viruses can fuse with cell and the release virus components such as its protein-covered genome into the cytoplasm. Parainfluenza viruses such as Sendai virus or HIV-1 enter cells through direct fusion between the viral and cell membrane, allowing the viral contents access into the cytoplasm. Most but not all viruses replicate in the nucleus. Poxviruses, which are the largest of all viruses and encode several hundred proteins, can transcribe their DNA in the cytoplasm, and the viruses carry the enzymes needed for transcription of the early viral genes. Other viruses have to transport their genome into the nucleus. Some viruses, such as adenoviruses, travel through the cytoplasm to the nuclear pore complex, taking advantage of cellular transport systems such as microtubules. Once the virus reaches the nuclear pores, it uncoates, and the genome, still complexed with some of the viral proteins such as factor VII for adenoviruses, is injected into the nucleus. HIV, an RNA virus, carries a reverse transcriptase that in the cytoplasm converts viral RNA into DNA. The DNA in turn moves into the nucleus through nuclear pores.

Cells have evolved mechanisms to recognize viruses at these early stages while viruses gain access to the host cell replication machinery. Pathogen-recognition receptors such as Toll-like receptors are located at the cell surface or within cells. They recognize patterns, rather than specific sequences, that are not present in normal healthy cells but are associated with pathogens. Such patterns include motifs on viral proteins, DNA, or RNA. Viral RNA can also be sensed by RNA helicases such as RIG-1, resulting in the induction of interferon responses. Within the nucleus, incoming viral DNA can be complexed into so-called nuclear dots, and there is circumstantial evidence that binding of viral genomes to such nuclear dots inhibits their replication and is thus part of the cellular defense machinery.

Virus Replication

Once the virus gains access to the nucleus, virus propagation is initiated. Transcription of the more complex DNA viruses occurs in two stages and starts with transcription of the so-called early genes, which encode proteins needed for transcription and nuclear export of viral RNA, followed by replication of the genome and then transcription of the late genes, which encode the structural proteins.

This process can be exemplified by transcription of the adenovirus genome, a double-stranded DNA virus with a genome of 30 to 35 kb in length that is read in both directions and increases its repertoire of polypeptides through further splicing (10). The E1A proteins are produced first. They modulate the cellular metabolism to make the cell more susceptible to virus replication, primarily by interfering with NF-κB and p53 pathways. The E1B gene products prolong cell survival by inhibiting cell apoptosis. The E2 gene products provide the machinery for replication of virus DNA and, together with cellular factors, promote transcription of late genes. The E3 gene products, which are not essential for adenovirus replication, provide a compendium of proteins that subverts the host defense mechanisms. The E4 gene products facilitate virus messenger RNA metabolism and provide functions to promote virus DNA replication and shutoff of host protein synthesis. They also prevent viral DNA concatemer formation. Adenoviruses also transcribe a set of hairloop-structured RNAs that are not translated, termed virus-associated (VA)-RNAs, and these play a role in combating cellular defense mechanisms. DNA replication begins from both DNA termini, followed by transcription of the late genes that encode the structural proteins. The encapsidation process of the viral DNA is governed by the presence of a packaging signal at the conventional left end of the virus DNA, which consists of a series of AT-rich sequences. These events are accompanied by major changes in the nuclear infrastructure and the permeabilization of the nuclear membrane of the host cells. This facilitates the egress of the virus into the cytoplasm and is followed by the disintegration of the plasma membrane and the release of infectious virus.

Some RNA viruses, such as influenza A viruses, carry enzymes that are needed to initiate viral transcription. The influenza A virus genome is composed of eight segments of linear negative-sense single-stranded RNA. The genome sequence has terminal repeated sequences at both ends that are 12 to 13 nucleotides long. The viral endonuclease (PB2) cuts terminal nucleotides from the RNA, which are then used as primers for the transcription of the genes. Once the initial proteins have been synthesized, eight complementary positive-sense RNA strands are made from the eight negative-sense RNA segments. From this cRNA, a negative-sense RNA is produced. Assembly of virus particles takes place in the cytoplasm at the plasma membrane.

Upon replication, some viruses exit their host cells by budding through the plasma membrane, in a process of reverse endocytosis. Other viruses are released upon the death of the infected cells. Still other viruses pass from one cell into adjacent cells without exposure to the extracellular environment.

ANTIVIRAL IMMUNE RESPONSES

Immune responses are essential to protect their host from pathogens. Humans with severe immnodeficiencies, whether due to inheritance, infection with HIV-1, or immuno-ablating medical interventions, commonly die as a result of overwhelming viral infections.

Viruses come in different flavors, and the immune system has evolved to respond accordingly. Although all viruses have the ultimate goal of replicating, their approach differs and can roughly be divided into "hit and run" or "hit and hide" varieties. The hit-and-run variety infects an individual, replicates rapidly, and then spreads to the next victim. Such viruses can cause fulminate and fatal infections, because survival of the host is not essential for their continued existence once they have spread to the next organism. Many of the small viruses, but also some of the more complex DNA viruses, take this hit-and-run approach. A typical example is influenza virus, which causes an acute infection and then spreads to the next host. The host either dies or completely clears the infection. The success of influenza virus is linked to its ease of transmission, so there is no reason for this virus to rely on continued infection of a given host.

Another example is rabies virus. This virus in interesting because its incubation time varies tremendously; patients can develop symptoms within 2 to 3 weeks, or the infection can stay asymptomatic for decades and then suddenly flare up. It is unknown where the virus hides during this time, and it is also unknown why rabies virus suddenly starts to replicate in the central nervous system years later, causing disease. Humans or animals that develop symptoms of rabies nearly always die, and the very few humans who have survived have severe neurologic deficits. The virus is by no means as contagious as influenza virus but instead requires direct and fairly intimate contact between an infected host's saliva and its next victim. Notwithstanding, the virus is very successful, for it has a broad host range and ensures that infected individuals who become contagious at the end stage of their disease exhibit the aggressive behavior that is needed for rabies virus to spread.

To ward off hit-and-run viruses requires a rapid and robust immune response to blunt viral spread within an individual without causing undue damage to the infected host. Hit-and-hide viruses are usually more complex, because much of their genome is devoted to combating immune responses. These viruses replicate upon infection, but they do not focus on seeking a new host; rather, they focus on extending their survival within an infected host. Examples are herpes viruses, which, upon an acute and lytic cycle, become latent and persist for the lifetime of an infected host. Another example is HIV-1, which initially replicates to high titers, causing influenzalike symptoms. An adaptive immune response is triggered and reduces viral load. Nevertheless, the virus cannot be cleared and persists until the host eventually succumbs to virus-associated complications. HIV-1 is far less contagious than influenza virus and does not have the luxury of the broad host range of rabies virus. Chronic infections thus allow the survival of viruses that are less easily transmitted. Chronic or persistent infections pose different demands on the immune system than transient and acute infections, because viral loads need to be controlled for long periods of time.

VIRUSES AND THE INNATE IMMUNE SYSTEM

The innate immune system has two roles: It provides an early defense system against pathogens; and it alerts and assists in activating the adaptive immune system.

Pathogen Recognition Receptors

The innate immune system lacks the exquisite specificity of the adaptive immune system. Specificity for recognition of foreign antigens is provided by receptors called pattern recognition receptors (PRRs), which recognize pathogen-associated molecular patterns (PAMP) (11). Toll-like receptors (TLR) serve as PRRs, and 12 TLRs have been identified to date in mammals (12). Of those, TLR-3, -7, -8, and -9 recognize viral genomes (13); TLR-3 recognizes dsRNA, TLR-7 and -8 recognize G/U-rich ssRNA, and TLR-9 recognizes unmethylated CpG motifs on dsDNA present in bacteria or large DNA viruses such as herpes viruses. TLR-2 and TLR-4 recognize mainly bacterial products but can also be activated by viral proteins, such as the hemagglutinin of measles virus (TLR-2) (14) or the fusion protein of respiratory syncytial virus (TLR-4) (15). TLRs that recognize viral genomes are in the endosome, whereas those that bind proteins are on the cell surface. Expression of TLRs in the endosomes ensures access to viral genomes while preventing interaction with host cell–derived RNA. Most of the TLRs use MyD88 as an adaptor molecule (16), which upon binding to TIRAP activates IRAK and TRAF6 and then NF-κB and IRF-3. TLR-3 signals through TRIF (17), which binds to TRAF6 and RIP1, which activate NF-κB. Alternatively, TRIF can bind to TBK1, which activates IRF3 and IRF7. The latter pathway can also be used by TLR-4. Activation of NF-κB followed by its translocation to the nucleus results in production of proinflammatory cytokines such as IL-6, TNF-α, and IL-12; activation of IRF-3 or -7 causes production of type I interferons (IFN).

DsRNA is further recognized by two kinases, protein kinase R (PKR) (18) and RNAseL (19). Upon activation, PKR phosphorylates the eukaryotic initiation factor 2 (eIF-2) α subunit. This inhibits translation in virus-infected cells. PKR thus functions to protect cells against synthesis of viral proteins once the kinase is activated by dsRNA, a common by-product of viral propagation. Activation of PKR furthermore induces production of type I interferons (20). RNAseL affects degradation of RNA and thus also inhibits protein synthesis.

DsRNA can activate two cytoplasmic IFN-inducible DExD/H box RNA helicases termed retinoic acid–inducible protein 1 (RIG-1) and melanoma differentiation–associated gene 5 (mda-5) (21,22). In addition to helicase domains, these proteins contain a tandem caspase recruitment domain, which results in signal transduction cascades that activate NF-κB and IRF-3. The specificity of the helicases is comparable to that of TLR-3, and it is currently unclear how their roles in antiviral defense differ. TLR-3 is localized in intracellular vesicles and may encounter viral RNA upon phagocytosis of viral particles. The helicases as well as PKR are located in the cytoplasm and are likely to react to dsRNA produced during viral replication. TLR-3 is expressed on NK cells and may play an important role in their activation. Binding of West Nile virus to TLR-3 was shown to initiate an inflammatory response that increases the permeability of the blood–brain barrier, thus allowing the virus to enter the brain (23). Overall, TLR3 is the most abundantly expressed TLR in the central nervous system (24), indicating that this TLR may have a specific and yet-to-be-identified role in the brain.

Early Antiviral Cytokines

Stimulation of NF-κB or the interferon pathways by viral PAMPs results in production of a series of proinflammatory cytokines and chemokines. Some of the cytokines, such as interferons, have direct antiviral activity. Interferons are subdivided into type I interferons (IFN-1), which in humans include one type of IFN-β, IFN-ε, IFN-κ, IFN-ω, and at least 13 variants of IFN-α, type II interferon, also called immune interferon or IFN-γ, and type III interferon, also called IFN-λ or IL-28/29 (25).

All nucleated cells can produce type I IFNs, although during a primary infection most of it originates from dendritic cells (DCs), especially plasmacytoid DCs (pDCs). IFN-γ is produced mainly by T and NK cells. Type III IFN can be produced by a number of cells, including DCs. Both IFN-α and IFN-β use the same receptor and have interchangeable functions. The receptor for type I IFNs consists of two subunits, IFNAR-1 and IFNAR-2. Binding of type I IFN to its receptor leads to phosphorylation of the tyrosine kinase (Tyk)-2 and Janus kinase (Jak)-1 (26). This in turn causes tyrosine phosphorylation of Stat1 and 2 proteins, which upon translocation into the nucleus form a complex with other proteins, leading to activation of interferon-inducible genes (27). Type I IFN acts mainly through Stat1 and Stat2 but can also activate Stat3, Stat4, and Stat5.

Mainly NK cells produce IFN-γ in response to PAMPS or other cytokines such as IL-12 or IL-18. Binding of IFN-γ to its receptor, which contains two chains called IFNGR-1 and IFNGR-2, leads to the phosphorylation of Stat1 via Jak-1 (28,29).

Type III IFN acts through a receptor complex composed of the IL-28 receptor (R) α chain and the IL-10Rβ chain. Binding of IFN-λ to its receptor activates Stat1 and 2 but, similar to type I IFN, can act through Stat3, 4, or 5. Type III IFN can signal through non-Jak-Stat pathways either through the kinase AKT or mitogen-activated kinases (MAPK) JNK and ERK1/2. Although type I IFN can use some of these alternative pathways as well, its action through JNK has not yet been reported. Type I and type III IFNs are commonly produced by the same cells in response to virus infections (25). However, in one study, expression of IFN-λ but not type I IFNs was demonstrated from liver biopsy samples of patients infected with hepatitis C virus (HCV), indicating differential regulation of their expression (25,30).

Type I IFNs are in general 10 to 100 times more potent as antiviral agents compared to IFN-γ. All types of IFNs affect viral multiplication at several levels. They can inhibit entry of the viruses into host cells by reducing expression of the viral receptors. IFN-1 induces production of the Mx protein that inhibits transcription of influenza viruses through a still ill-defined pathway (31). IFNs downregulate viral promoters. They trigger expression of 2′5′-oligoadenylsynthase and double-stranded RNA kinase, which inhibits production of viral progeny. For some viruses, IFN-γ can promote transcription. For example, the long terminal repeat of HIV-1 is activated by IFN-γ (32). IFN-γ induces nitric oxide synthases, which converts L-arginine to L-citrulline and NO. The latter has direct effects on poxviruses and herpes viruses by inhibiting DNA replication, synthesis of late viral proteins, and viral assembly (33).

In addition to their antiviral activity, IFNs play a dominant role in other host defense mechanisms. They activate macrophages and NK cells. They promote Th1-type immune responses. They drive maturation of DCs, induce or augment expression of MHC class I and II determinants, costimulatory molecules of the B7 family, and proteins involved in antigen processing. They enhance cross-priming. IFN or IFN-receptor knockout mice show increased susceptibility to some viral infections. IFN-α has been licensed for treatment of chronic infections with hepatitis B (34) and C virus (35) and for treatment of human papilloma virus-associated genital warts (*Condyloma acuminata*) (36).

Activation of Cells of the Innate Immune System

Chemokine-mediated Recruitment of Leukocytes

Most viruses cause an inflammatory reaction through chemokine-mediated recruitment of leukocytes to the site of infection. At least 50 different chemokines have been identified in humans to date (37,38). Most of them can be divided into CXC or CC chemokines, depending on the positioning of their cystein residues. Chemokines are either constitutively expressed to maintain normal trafficking of leukocytes, or they are induced under conditions of inflammation to recruit a cellular infiltrate. The chemokine system is redundant, and receptors and their ligands involved in inflammatory reactions are commonly promiscuous. Chemokines as well as cytokines are induced in response to interactions between PAMPs and PRRs. This affects a local increase of the expression of adherent molecules on blood vessel walls, which causes leukocytes to slow down and to start rolling. This is followed either by detachment of the rolling cells as a result of the shearing forces of the blood flow or by firm adhesion and then extravasation from the blood into the tissue, where leukocytes migrate to the site of infection. The latter two events are controlled by chemokines. Neutrophils are attracted first through CXC chemokines such as CXCL8, CXCL5, and CXCL1. Monocytes and other mononuclear cells that express CCR2, CCR3, or CCR5 are recruited later through CCL2, CCL3, and CCL5 chemokines. The role of chemokines that recruit different NK cell subsets remains controversial. Resting NK cells express CXCR4, whereas activated NK cells upregulate CCR2, CCR4, CCR7, and CCR8, indicating that they migrate in response to the corresponding chemokines.

Activity of Natural Killer (NK) Cells

NK cells are activated by viruses either directly, upon recognition of viral sequences by TLRs such as TLR-3, or indirectly through IL-12. NK cells contribute to early viral control through direct lysis of virus-infected cells and through the production of IFN-γ (39,40). NK cells carry a multitude of activating as well as inhibitory receptors to ensure selective lysis of infected cells (41,42). The overall balance of signals through both types of receptors determines NK-cell activity. Some of the NK-cell receptors belong to the killer immunoglobulinlike receptors (KIR), which can be activating or inhibitory and which differ in their specificity to HLA. Inhibitory KIRs contain immunotyrosine-based inhibitory motifs in their cytoplasmic tail. Some of the inhibitory KIR receptors recognize MHC class I determinants, and loss of MHC class I molecules upon virus infections activates NK cells, provided that an activating receptor is engaged by a host cell ligand or a pathogen-derived sequence. Some activating KIRs are sensitive not only to modulation of MHC class I expression, but also to peptides displayed by class I molecules. This specificity for viral peptides displayed by MHC class I is not as exclusive as that of T-cell receptors but rather resembles that of PRRs. The inhibitory KIR receptors include KIR2DL1 specific for HLA-C/C2, KIR2DL2/3 specific for HLA C/C1, KIR3DL1 specific for HLA-B Bw4, and KIR3DL2 specific for HLA-a/A3/A11. The corresponding activating receptors KIR2DS1, KIR2DS2, and KIR3DS1 have the same specificity, whereas KIR2DL4 appears to recognize HLA-G. Of the two lectinlike receptors, CD94/NKG2A is inhibitory whereas CD94/NKG2C is activating. Both recognize HLA-E, which binds the leader sequence of HLA-A, -B, and -C molecules as well as the leader sequence of nonclassical MHC molecules, and thus signals global changes in MHC expression. Additional activating receptors are NKG2D, NKp46, and NKp30, which are constitutively expressed on NK cells, whereas NKp44 is induced upon activation of NK cells. These receptors are termed cytotoxicity receptors because their ligation causes release of perforin or granzyme, which kills the target cells through pore formation in the cell membrane. NKG2D recognizes the stress-induced MHC class I–related MICA and MICB proteins, whereas NKp46 and NKp44 recognize viral hemagglutinins (43). NK cells also express TLRs involved in viral sensing, although the role of such TLRs remains to be established. IL-12 and type I interferon also provide potent activating signals to NK cells. NK cells are linked to the adaptive immune system through their interactions with immature DCs. Activated NK cells can lyse immature DCs upon ligation of the NKp30 receptor. Upon maturation, DCs upregulate MHC class I molecules and become resistant to NK-cell lysis. NK cells can drive maturation of DCs through production of proinflammatory cytokines such as TNF-α. In turn, mature DCs can activate the CD56^{high} subset of NK cells through IL-12. NK cells are pivotal in providing early control of virus infection, as was shown in animal models, in which lack of NK cells resulted in enhanced susceptibility to infections with a number of different viruses such as sendai virus, influenza virus, or cytomegalovirus, a finding that was confirmed in human patients with NK deficiency (44).

Dendritic Cells

DCs provide a crucial connection between the innate and the adaptive immune system. Two main subsets of DCs have been identified to date, called myeloid DCs (mDCs) (45) and plasmacytoid DCs (pDCs) (46), which differ in morphology, surface marker expression, and function. A third subset, called lymphoid DCs, has also been described (47). mDCs have a typical dendroid morphology. They are CD11b$^+$ and CD11c$^+$. pDCs have a plasma cell-like morphology. They are CD11c^{low} and CD11b$^-$. Human pDCs express CD123, whereas mouse pDCs express Ly6c. Both mDCs and pDCs are bone marrow–derived. They show distinct migration patterns; immature mDCs migrate to peripheral tissues, whereas immature pDCs, which are CD62L^{high}, migrate to lymphatic tissues, where they enter the T-cell zones. Immature mDCs constantly monitor their environment by phagocytosing particles including viruses, but are unsuited to present antigen to naive T cells until they differentiate into mature DCs. Such differentiation signals are provided by cytokines such as TNF-α or type I IFNs and by activation of PRRs such as the TLRs. Interestingly, mDCs express many of the TLRs that recognize bacterial products such as TLR-2, -4, and -5. They also express TLR-3. In contrast, pDCs express TLRs that recognize viral genomes such as TLR-7, -8 (expressed only by mouse pDC, not by human pDCs), and -9, indicating a pivotal role of pDCs in antiviral defense (48). Upon receiving an activation signal, mDCs initially increase phagocytosis and start secreting chemokines that attract an additional inflammatory infiltrate, which includes cells of the innate and adaptive immune system and additional immature mDCs and pDCs. Activated mDCs then cease to take up antigen, rearrange their actin cables, and upregulate CCR7 expression, which drives their migration to draining lymph nodes. Activated DCs furthermore upregulate their antigen-processing machinery as well as expression of MHC class I molecules, and translocate MHC class II determinants from intracellular vesicles to the cell surface. At this stage, MHC molecules are loaded with antigen-derived peptides. In addition, mature DCs start to express or upregulate positive costimulatory molecules of the B7 family such as CD80 and CD86 as well as CD40, and secrete cytokines such as IL-12 and type I IFNs. Once mature mDCs reach the lymph nodes, they migrate to the T-cell zones and commence activation of naïve T cells. In contrast, upon activation, pDCs produce type I IFN at levels that are 10 to 100 times higher on a per-cell basis than those produced by mature mDCs. In mDCs, stimulation through a PAMP, through cytokines, or through CD40 ligation activates IRF-3, which leads initially to the production of low amounts of type I IFN. Upon binding to its receptor, type I IFN then increases its own production through a positive feedback mechanism, which requires upregulation of IRF-7. pDCs constitutively express IRF-7, which renders these cells independent of positive feedback, and they can therefore produce large amounts of type I IFN immediately upon activation (49). pDCs can present antigen to naïve T cells; they upregulate MHC determinant and costimulatory molecules upon differentiation into mature pDCs. Nevertheless, levels of these crucial cell surface molecules are lower than those on mature mDCs. Furthermore, pDCs do not phagocytose antigen and are thus poorly suited to present antigen (50). It is unclear whether pDCs indeed present antigen *in vivo* to cells of the adaptive immune system or if their primary role is to produce type I IFNs and to assist maturation of mDCs.

Antigen presentation by DCs can influence the homing behavior of activated T cells. Mucosal surfaces are particularly vulnerable to pathogen invasion. Especially the intestinal mucosal membrane is constantly bombarded with bacteria and food-derived antigens and has thus evolved a distinct immune system. DCs within the intestine have been shown to activate T cells that preferentially home to gut-associated lymphoid tissues. Such homing is mediated by expression of CCR9 and $\alpha 4\beta 7$ on T cells. Lamina propria–derived DCs, unlike DCs in the spleen or in central lymph nodes, express the integrin chain of CD103, which induces T cells with gut-homing preference (51).

DCs not only activate adaptive immune responses, they also have important regulatory functions. Immature DCs fail to activate T-cell responses but instead cause T-cell anergy once a T cell encounters its cognate antigen on DCs, which lack expression of costimulatory signals. In addition, immature or "semimature" DCs are thought to induce regulatory T cells, which suppress adaptive immune responses (52,53). Mature DCs can also downregulate T-cell activation through the expression of negative costimulatory molecules. CD28 expressed on T cells can bind to CD80 and CD86, which provide positive costimulation. CD80 and CD86 bind with higher affinity to CTLA-4, which is expressed later on activated T cells and delivers a negative signal (54). The ICOS:ICOS ligand pathway has overlapping functions with CD28 and appears to be particularly important for stimulating cytokine production by effector T cells (55). However, ICOS also has a negative regulatory role, influencing the function of IL-10 production by regulatory T cells (56). Functional studies support both stimulatory and inhibitory roles for B7-H3 (57). The newest member of the B7 family, B7-H4, has a negative regulatory function (58). PD-1 is an inhibitory receptor expressed on T cells and B cells, and it induces cell cycle arrest (59). PD-1 interacts with two receptors, PD-L1 and PD-L2, which exhibit distinct patterns of expression. PD-L1 is expressed more broadly than PD-L2; PD-L1 is expressed on T cells, B cells, macrophages, DCs, endothelium, syncytiotrophoblasts, and other cell types, whereas PD-L2 expression is restricted to macrophages and DCs. Chronic viral infection seems to cause activation of the PD1-PDL1/L2 pathways, potentially resulting in an impairment of T-cell functions (60). The B- and T-lymphocyte attenuator (BTLA) (34) provides inhibitory signals upon binding to the herpes virus entry mediator (HVEM) (61), which is expressed on DCs, and also interacts with gD of herpes virus and with a distinct region with two TNF family members, LIGHT and lymphotoxin-A.

ANTIGEN-SPECIFIC IMMUNE RESPONSES

Activation of the innate immune system is followed by stimulation of adaptive immune responses to viral pathogens. Cells of the adaptive immune system have exquisite specificity to their respective antigen through clonally expressed receptors that maintain a complex repertoire through genetic rearrangement and, in the case of B-cell receptors, through additional somatic hypermutations. To maintain the large repertoire that is needed to mount a response against the multitude of pathogens, cells with a given receptor specificity are present at very low numbers. Upon activation, B and T cells need to undergo extensive proliferation to reach more effective numbers. T and B cells replicate very rapidly, with an approximate doubling time of 6 hours. Notwithstanding, viruses can multiply 1,000 fold during the same period. The 4- to 5-day delay between viral infection and onset of adaptive immunity caused by the initial proliferation of T and B cells with the appropriate receptor specificities leaves the host susceptible to capacious virus replication, which at this stage is controlled mainly by cells and factors of the innate immune system.

The adaptive immune system is composed of B and T cells; T cells are divided into CD4$^+$ and CD8$^+$ T cells. T cells are stimulated by peptides derived from foreign antigens that are displayed by MHC molecules on the surface of mature DCs. CD4$^+$ T cells, which have immunoregulatory functions, are activated by peptides derived from exogenous antigen displayed by MHC class II molecules, whereas CD8$^+$ T cells, which have effector functions and can lyse virus-infected cells directly, are activated by peptides that are in general derived from de novo–synthesized antigens, and that are displayed on MHC class I molecules. B cells are activated by native antigen. Effector T cells have the task of eliminating virus-infected cells preferentially by killing them before new viral progeny have been assembled. Restricting their receptor specificity to virus-derived peptides that are bound to transplantation antigens prevents them from being sidetracked by free virus.

CD8$^+$ T Cells

During a primary virus infection, viral control is achieved predominantly by specific CD8$^+$ T cells that can eliminate virus-infected cells through direct lysis of MHC class I–expressing infected cells, and that can further reduce virus replication through the release of cytokines such as IFN-γ.

Antigen Processing and Presentation for CD8$^+$ T-Cell Activation

CD8$^+$ T cells respond to peptides that are 8 to 10 amino acids long and displayed by MHC class I determinants (62). Such peptides are commonly derived from early viral proteins and allow for early destruction of the infected cells (63). Naïve CD8$^+$ T cells are activated by MHC class I/peptide complexes displayed on mature DCs. Other cells, such as B cells, macrophages, or tissue cells, cannot activate naïve CD8$^+$ T cells (64), although they can trigger a recall response. Minute amounts of MHC class I/peptide complexes suffice to trigger activation of CD8$^+$ T cells, though immunogenic levels most likely vary and depend in part on the affinity between the MHC peptide complex and the T-cell receptor, as well as on the duration of antigen presentation.

Peptide loading of MHC complexes in most cases occurs in the endoplasmic reticulum (ER) although, at least *in vitro*, empty cell surface–expressed MHC class I molecules can bind exogenous peptides. Because empty cell surface–expressed MHC class I molecules are unstable, this process may not play a role *in vivo*. The most common pathway for peptide/MHC class I complex formation involves productive infection of cells followed by synthesis of viral antigens. Proteins that are not translated faithfully or that are folded incorrectly are degraded in the cytoplasm into peptides by proteolytic enzymes that form the proteosome complex (65). Synthesis and posttranslational modifications of this complex are increased by IFN-γ (66). Peptides that are derived upon enzymatic cleavage of proteins are transported into the ER through transporter associated with antigen presentation (TAP) (67,68). TAP shows preference for peptides that are 8 to 13 amino acids in length and, depending on the species of the host cell, for peptides with certain motifs such as hydrophobic carboxy termini (69).

Newly synthesized MHC class I heavy chains are also transported into the ER, where they bind to calnexin, which promotes appropriate folding of the protein. The folded heavy chain then binds $\beta 2$ microglobulin. The correct folding of the MHC class I heavy chain is further facilitated by calreticulin. The resulting complex binds to tapasin, providing a link to TAP (70). Upon TAP-facilitated transport into the ER, peptides with the appropriate anchoring residues bind to the groove that is displayed on top of the MHC class I heavy-chain/$\beta 2$ microglobulin complexes. If necessary, peptides are further clipped by peptidase present in the ER until they reach a size that is optimal for binding to MHC. Some peptides contain signal sequences that allow for TAP-independent transport into the ER. Binding of peptides to MHC class I molecules causes release of calreticulin and tapasin and is followed by transport of the MHC/peptide complex through the Golgi apparatus to the cell surface.

Not all viruses infect DCs directly, so alternative pathways exist to ensure that their antigens are presented to CD8$^+$ T cells. DCs present exogenous antigen in the context of MHC class I determinant through a process called cross-presentation or cross-priming (71). This process is enhanced by type I IFNs. Cross-priming involves direct uptake of viruses or viral proteins by DCs through phagocytosis or pinocytosis into lysosomes, from where they are transported to early endosomes. Here some of the viral proteins are degraded by enzymes present in these compartments. Viruses and viral degradation products can egress the endosomes and reach the cytoplasm for further degradation by proteasome complexes and TAP-dependent transport of peptides into the ER. Alternatively, phagosomes (the endosomal vehicles that contain material that is phagocytosed by DCs) can fuse directly with the ER, generating compartments that have been dubbed ergosomes (72). Loading of peptides onto MHC class I molecules within ergosomes was shown to be TAP-dependent, suggesting that viruses, proteins, or peptides first have to leave the ergosome and then re-enter the ergosomes with the help of TAP, most likely upon further degradation. Upon association with MHC class I molecules, the peptide/MHC class I complexes within the ergosomes are transported to the cell surface through a process that is not completely inhibited by the drug brefeldin, which blocks transport through the Golgi complex, suggesting that ergosomes can fuse directly with the outer cell membrane like endosomes (73).

A second mechanism of cross-priming has been suggested in which preformed MHC class I/peptide complexes are transferred from cells that are productively infected with a virus to DCs. Direct proof that this pathway is used *in vivo* is missing. A third and related pathway has been suggested in which peptides formed in infected cells are transported by chaperone proteins to DCs (74). Again, proof that this pathway is used *in vivo* is missing, and current evidence suggests that the chaperone model of cross-presentations is likely to be an *in vitro* artifact, as the efficiency of cross-priming was shown to correlate directly with the stability of the antigen. The model of cross-presentation through chaperones would predict that unstable proteins that are readily degraded into peptides would be more efficiently presented by cross-presentation than antigens that are relatively resistant to proteolysis, but, in contrast, cross-presentation of unstable proteins can be increased through proteasome inhibitors.

Once MHC/peptide complexes reach the cell surface, they are remarkably stable. It has been estimated that each MHC class I molecule has the potential to bind any of 10,000 different peptides. Nevertheless, upon virus infection, CD8$^+$ T-cell populations that recognize one or two epitopes of a virus commonly dominate the response. This in turn allows viruses to escape immunosurveillance by CD8$^+$ T cells through mutation of such epitopes (75).

Nonclassical MHC class I molecules such as CD1 (76) can also present antigen, in part nonpeptide antigens such as lipids, to the immune system. The role of these alternative pathways for antiviral defense is not yet understood.

Primary CD8$^+$ T-Cell Responses

Activation of primary CD8$^+$ T-cell responses occurs in lymphatic tissues and requires antigen presentation by DCs. Activation occurs rapidly, within hours after peptide-loaded mature DCs reach the T-cell–rich zones of lymphatic tissues. DCs migrate primarily to lymph nodes draining the site of infection, and T cells are stimulated primarily within these draining nodes. Viruses that cause systemic infections are presented in multiple lymph nodes as well as in the spleen. Upon receiving activation signals, CD8$^+$ T cells proliferate extensively in a 6- to 8-hour cycle. For example, during an experimental infection of mice with lymphocytic choriomeningitis virus (LCMV), 10^2 naive CD8$^+$ T cells can expand within a few days to 10^7 effector cells. Activation of CD8$^+$ T cells to some viruses is dependent on help from CD4$^+$ T cells, whereas other viruses induce CD8$^+$ T cells in the absence of CD4$^+$ T cells. It has been suggested that CD4$^+$ T cells provide additional differentiation signals to DCs, enabling them to prime CD8$^+$ T cells (77). Some viruses can apparently induce a similar differentiation pathway of DCs, allowing for activation of CD8$^+$ T cells in the absence of T help. CD8$^+$ T cells that are deprived of CD4$^+$ T-cell help are commonly short-lived and fail to establish functional memory (78).

During activation, CD8$^+$ T cells undergo a number of phenotypic changes (79). They reduce expression of CD62L and CCR7, which allows their egress from lymphatic tissues. Early during activation, they transiently upregulate expression of CD69 and CD25. The latter is the receptor for IL-2 and may be required for IL-2–driven T-cell proliferation. Upon activation, $CD8^+$ T cells upregulate expression of CD27 and CD44. A subset of $CD8^+$ effector T cells augments expression of the IL-7 receptor αchain (CD127). $CD8^+$ effector T cells express granzyme and perforin, and they produce cytokines and chemokines upon encounter with their cognate antigens, including IFN-γ, TNF-α, IL-2, and MIP-1α/β. A number of parameters during antigen presentation, such as costimulatory signals, type of T-cell help, strength of T-cell–receptor engagement, and duration of presentation, are likely to influence the breadth of $CD8^+$ T-cell functions, which in turn determines their effectiveness in limiting viral spread (80). Once they are fully activated, $CD8^+$ T cells leave the lymph nodes and migrate to sites of infection. Activated T cells express different chemokine receptors and a higher density of certain types of adhesion molecules (LFA-1 or integrin $\alpha 4$) than naïve T cells, which allows them to leave the blood vessels and enter sites of inflammation (81). Once activated T cells reach an area of inflammation, their adhesion molecules interact with P- and E-selectins, ICAM, VCAM, and CD34, which are expressed at increased levels on vascular endothelial cells in the presence of cytokines such as IL-1 or TNF-α. This interaction initially causes a loose attachment of the lymphocytes, followed by their rolling along the vessel walls (82). Chemokines secreted at the site of inflammation carry heparin-binding sites that cause them to be retained in the extracellular matrix close to their site of origin. Once the lymphocytes reach an area that is rich in chemokines corresponding to their receptors, they bind firmly to the vascular endothelial cells and eventually emigrate out of the vessels into the tissue. Recruitment of activated T cells is thus driven by chemokines and not by the antigen specificity of the T-cell receptors (83). Once $CD8^+$ T cells reach infected tissue and re-encounter their antigen on MHC class I–positive cells, they commence effector functions by releasing cytokines and mediating lysis of virus-infected cells. IFN-γ, which is released by most activated antiviral $CD8^+$ T cells, upregulates the antigen-processing machinery and MHC class I expression, thus facilitating interactions between infected cells and activated $CD8^+$ T cells. $CD8^+$ T cells predominantly lyse their target cells through the release of granzyme and perforin, which form pores in target-cell membranes and cause apoptotic cell death. Another lytic pathway involves interactions between Fas ligand (CD95) expressed by activated T cells and Fas expressed by some types of target cells. Interactions between CD95 and Fas trigger activation of caspases and apoptotic cell death of the target cells (84). Although each $CD8^+$ T cell can lyse several target cells, direct lysis appears to be rather inefficient, because it requires direct interactions between $CD8^+$ T cells and each infected cell. Nevertheless, it is crucial for viral clearance. Mice that lack perforin were shown to have an increased susceptibility to a number of viral infections.

$CD8^+$ T-Cell Memory and Recall Responses

Once virus-infected T cells have been eliminated during an acute viral infection, approximately 90% of the activated $CD8^+$ T cells undergo activation-induced cell death. Effector T cells that express high levels of CD127 preferentially survive the contraction phase and differentiate into memory cells (85). During this process they undergo a number of functional and phenotypic changes. At least two types of memory $CD8^+$ T cells have been identified to date, so-called central memory $CD8^+$ T cells (T_{CM}) and effector memory $CD8^+$ T cells (T_{EM}) (86,87). T_{CM} T cells express CD62L and CCR7 and home to lymphatic tissues, whereas effector memory T cells lack expression of CCR7 and CD62L and remain in peripheral tissues. It was initially argued that upon re-encounter of antigen, T_{EM} can immediately commence effector function such as secretion of cytokines or target cell lysis, whereas T_{CM} initially need to proliferate and hence assume effector functions with a delay (88). Accordingly, it was argued that T_{EM} provide a crucial first barrier against virus infections. Subsequent studies showed that T_{CM} can release cytokines as rapidly as T_{EM} and that they also assume lytic activity quite rapidly, although not as instantaneously as T_{EM}. In addition, it was shown that in some virus infections, such as with LCMV, T_{CM} provide superior protection to T_{EM} (89). This may in part reflect that, although both memory $CD8^+$ T cells can proliferate upon re-encounter of their antigen, T_{CM} have a higher proliferative capacity than T_{EM}, allowing for a more robust recall response. In other virus infections, such as pulmonary infection with influenza A virus or with sendai virus, T_{EM} rather than T_{CM} were shown to protect from virus-associated disease (90). One would assume that the type of virus and the site of infection in part dictate which subset is needed for efficient early viral clearance, and that in most cases both subsets are beneficial. T_{EM} have the advantage of location, T_{CM} have the advantage of numbers.

Whether T_{EM} and T_{CM} reflect distinct T-cell subsets or rather distinct stages of differentiation remains debated. Overall, numbers of $CD8^+$ memory T cells are maintained at remarkably stable levels during the lifetime of a creature. Each individual memory $CD8^+$ T cell has a finite lifespan of about 2 months and requires IL-7 as a survival factor. At the population level, constant numbers are maintained through homeostatic proliferation, which is dependent on IL-15 and takes place primarily in the bone marrow (91). In the absence of antigen, numbers of T_{EM} gradually decline while numbers of T_{CM} increase. As demonstrated in the LCMV system, this is caused by differentiation of T_{EM} into T_{CM}, suggesting a linear relation between these two T-cell populations (92).

Upon repeated re-exposure to antigen, the overall ratio of T_{EM} to T_{CM} increases, with more of the memory $CD8^+$ T cells retaining an activated phenotype (93). $CD8^+$ T cells induced by repeated immunization have a reduced proliferative capacity and accumulate preferentially in nonlymphatic tissues.

Effect of Chronic or Persistent Infections on CD8+ T Cells

During chronic viral infections, $CD8^+$ T cells can become exhausted (94). In mice persistently infected with LCMV, specific $CD8^+$ T cells gradually lose the ability to mediate target cell lysis, secrete TNF-α or IFN-γ. Exhausted $CD8^+$ T cells lose the ability to proliferate to antigen. Exhausted T cells express high levels of PD-1, an inhibitory receptor of the CD28 family. Blockage of PD-1/PD-L1 interaction by monoclonal antibodies was shown to restore T-cell functions and their proliferative capacity (95). Impairments of $CD8^+$ T cells were also observed in humans chronically infected with HIV-1, hepatitis B virus (HBV), or HCV. In HIV-infected patients, $CD8^+$ T-cell functionality rather than frequencies was shown to correlate with progression; compared to patients with HIV-1–specific $CD8^+$ T cells showing a broad range of functions, patients with $CD8^+$ T cells showing limited function progress faster to disease, reflected by increased viral loads, loss of CD4 T cells, and opportunistic infections (80).

Other persistent infections are characterized by periodic virus replication rather than perpetually high levels of replication. For example, certain types of herpes viruses, such as herpes simplex virus (HSV) or cytomegalovirus (CMV), persist in a latent form during which viral protein synthesis is virtually shut off. Upon reactivation of the virus as a result of certain stress factors, viral replication is reinitiated and, in response, specific memory $CD8^+$ T cells expand and in healthy individuals rapidly control the infection. The repeated recall responses result in very high frequencies of specific memory $CD8^+$ T cells over time. In the elderly, who have commonly impaired immune responses, frequencies of $CD8^+$ T cells with a naïve phenotype decline while those with a memory phenotype increase, suggesting exhausting of the repertoire as a result of chronic exposure to antigens. It is not uncommon that in elderly humans up to 30% of peripheral $CD8^+$ T cells show specificity to antigens of herpes viruses. It has been suggested that aging is infectious, as morbidity and mortality of the elderly is linked to the functionality of their immune system (96).

Mucosal CD8+ T Cells

The immune system can be roughly subdivided into two separate, albeit interactive, entities: a central immune system localized in the spleen and lymph nodes, which patrols the inner tissues and organs; and a mucosal immune system, which in humans covers a total surface area of approximately 400 m^2 of mucosa of the airways, the intestines, and the urogenital tract, which are the most common ports of entry for pathogens. Mucosal surfaces, such as those of the intestinal tract or the airways, are constantly bombarded with "harmless" antigens that are best ignored. The inner tissues and organs, on the other hand, are in a sterile environment, warranting more stringent control against foreign antigens. The two immune systems that control the central and the mucosal surfaces are faced by different challenges and in consequence have distinct characteristics. The central immune system has been exceedingly well characterized over the last 30 years. Less is known about the mucosal immune system, which provides the first line of defense against most viral infections.

The mucosal immune system consists anatomically of local inductive sites, called organized mucosa-associated lymphoid tissue (O-MALT), such as tonsils, Peyer patches, and the appendix, and effector sites that are present directly in the mucosa, called diffuse mucosa-associated lymphoid tissue (97). In the intestine, T cells can be found within the lamina propria (LP), and these T cells are phenotypically similar to those found in the central immune system. T cells can also be found within the epithelium. The intraepithelial lymphocytes (IELs) are distinct from those that reside in the LP. The epithelium that covers the mucosal surfaces differs depending on the anatomic location; for example, the intestine is covered by a single epithelial layer, whereas the vagina is covered by a multilayered squamous epithelium that varies in thickness with the menstrual cycle. Transport of antigen from the mucosal surface to the O-MALT system or the local lymph nodes is accomplished by M cells in the intestine and the airways, whereas mucosal surfaces covered by a squamous epithelium rely on local DCs for transport of antigen to the inductive sites. Mucosal DCs may differ functionally from those in the central immune system (98). For example, they express CD103, which induces $\alpha 4\beta 7$ expression of $CD8^+$ T cells. This in turn promotes their homing to mucosal sites (31). The best-studied mucosal T-cell populations are the intraepithelial lymphocytes (IELs) of the intestine. They appear relatively late in development (about 2 to 4 weeks after birth in mice) (99) and are initially composed mainly of T cells that express the γ/δ receptor (100). These γ/δ^+ cells are eventually joined by T cells that carry the α/β receptor (100). A portion of α/β T cells is double-positive for CD4 and CD8, in contrast to T cells found in the spleen or lymph nodes. The majority of these double-positive T cells carry homodimers of the CD8α chain. T cells that carry the γ/δ T-cell receptor (TcR) and are single-positive for CD8 also lack CD8β-chain expression (101). A portion of the intraepithelial T cells (both α/β and γ/δ TcR^+) develop within the mucosal immune system independent of the thymus (102).

Antigen recognition by double-positive CD8α/β and TcRγ/δ T cells is different from that of single-positive and α/β TcR-expressing T cells. The latter subsets, which are present in the central and the mucosal immune system, recognize antigenic peptides in association with classical MHC class I or II determinants. The double-positive CD8α/βT cells of the mucosal immune system fail to respond to activation with anti-TcR antibodies and furthermore express potentially autoreactive antigen receptors (103). T cells that express the γ/δ receptor have been shown to have effector functions; they conduct antimicrobial activity (104–107) and promote the development of IgA-secreting B cells (108). Many of the γ/δ^+ T cells seem to recognize antigen directly, including nonprotein structures, without the need for presentation by classical MHC determinants (109). T cells that express either the α/β or γ/δ receptor are present in vaginal epithelium. The vaginal γ/δ T cells have a distinctive phenotype that resembles those in the skin: They are CD4$^-$CD8$^-$, CD45$^+$ and express an invariant TcR (110).

Mucosal T cells show an activated phenotype. They can be primed locally within Peyer patches by viruses that target the intestine, such as rotavirus or reovirus. In some instances, CD8$^+$ T cells induced in lymphatic tissues of the central immune system migrate to mucosal sites. This migration is facilitated by expression of $\alpha 4\beta 7$ (111) and certain chemokine receptors such as CCR9 (112). Mucosal homing of effector CD8$^+$ T cells has been observed upon systemic infection of mice with LCMV virus. Other systemic infections fail to trigger CD8$^+$ T cells that migrate efficiently to the mucosa, suggesting that the quality and strength of the activation signal may influence mucosal homing of CD8$^+$ T cells. Mucosal CD8$^+$ T cells have lytic activity and secrete cytokines such as IFN-γ in response to antigen. Memory CD8$^+$ T cells can also be detected at mucosal sites (113). Memory CD8$^+$ T cells within the LP differ from those within the intestinal epithelium, and the presence of such cells in the LP is not indicative of the presence of such cells within the epithelium. Memory CD8$^+$ T cells within the LP resemble T_{EM} cells within other tissues, whereas the phenotype of memory CD8$^+$ T cells within the epithelium differs. Memory CD8$^+$ T cells within the epithelium express granzyme. They express high levels of CD69, CD103, and the integrin chain $\beta 7$. They express only low levels of CD27, CD122, or Ly6C. Levels of CD127 are intermediate. They can proliferate upon re-exposure to antigen, albeit less efficiently than CD8$^+$ T_{CM}. They produce IFN-γ and TNF-α but no IL-2. Overall, this phenotype suggests that memory CD8$^+$ T cells within the intestinal epithelium are highly activated. Lack of expression of receptors for memory CD8$^+$ T-cell survival and proliferation factors indicate that either they will decline over time, that homeostatic proliferation within the mucosa is driven by other cytokines than those that operate to maintain central memory CD8$^+$ T cells, or that the mucosal memory CD8$^+$ T cells are constantly being replaced from the pools of memory CD8$^+$ T cells within the central immune system.

Role of CD8$^+$ T Cells in Viral Infections

CD8$^+$ T cells are crucial to control acute viral infections caused by cytopathic viruses that kill the infected cells. Accordingly cytopathic viruses are either cleared successfully by the immune system or they result in the death of the infected individual. Examples of cytopathic viruses include orthomyxoviruses (influenza virus), paramyxoviruses (mumps virus, measles virus, respiratory syncytial virus), reoviruses (rotavirus), picornaviruses (poliovirus, hepatitis A virus, rhinoviruses), Ebola virus, or poxviruses. In mice, clearance of infections with influenza virus, Theiler virus, HSV-1, Ebola virus (114), and Friends retrovirus depends on CD8$^+$ T cell–derived perforin or granzyme rather than IFN-γ. Clearance of neuronal infections such as measles also requires CD8$^+$ T cells, although within the central nervous system IFN-γ production by CD8$^+$ T cells rather than release of toxic granules is needed to resolve viral infections (115). Neurons lack expression of MHC class I determinants, although such molecules are induced by IFN-γ. Neurons have limited capacity for self-renewal, and it is tempting to speculate that viral inhibition by antiviral cytokines is more beneficial to the host than killing irreplaceable neutrons. The relative paucity of MHC class I determinants on neurons may favor cytokine release over directly lytic mechanisms.

Noncytopathic viruses can establish very long-lasting infections and successfully evade complete destruction by immune effector mechanisms. CD8$^+$ T cells are instrumental in controlling such infections. A role for CD8$^+$ T cells in controlling infections with retroviruses was documented in nonhuman primates infected with a chimeric simian/human immunodeficiency virus, which, like HIV-1, infects CD4$^+$ cells and causes their eventual loss (116). Similarly, in human HIV-1 patients, protection against CD4$^+$ T-cell loss and control of viral load is correlated with the functionality of virus-specific CD8$^+$ T cells.

HPVs can cause persistent infections upon integration into the host cells' genome. Most types of HPV cause harmless proliferation of keratinocytes in the skin or the genital mucosa. Skin warts, which are common in children, often regress spontaneously, presumably upon activation of an immune response. Genital warts that are highly infectious can be treated either surgically or by topic application of interferon. Genital infections with oncogenic types of HPV, most notably 16 and 18, are cleared by most patients rapidly as a result of cellular immune responses to the early viral proteins. Some patients develop persistent infections, which after years of latency can lead to cervical cancer. Immunosuppressed women have a significantly higher incidence of cervical cancer, indicating that viral clearance is mediated by cellular immune responses.

HCV, a flavivirus, and HBV, a hepadnavirus, can establish persistent hepatic infections that cause chronic inflammatory liver disease and liver failure or hepatocellular carcinoma. It is currently not clear why a fraction of patients develop persistent infections whereas others clear the viruses completely during the acute infection. Patients chronically infected with HBV have relatively weak $CD8^+$ T-cell responses to this virus, which may contribute to the lack of complete eradication of virus-infected cells. In contrast, carriers of HCV have vigorous $CD8^+$ T-cell responses to multiple viral antigens. HCV mutates more rapidly than HBV, and the resulting viral variants may continuously escape immune-mediated destruction. During chronic infections, $CD8^+$ T cells control the viral load and at the same time contribute to liver injury. Patients with chronic hepatitis virus infections are currently treated with type I IFN, which in some but not all patients results in clearance of the virus-infected cells.

Some strains of LCMV can cause chronic infections in mice. In these mice, LCMV-specific $CD8^+$ T cells become exhausted and cease to function. Exhausted T cells express PD-1, and elegant studies by the Ahmed group showed that treatment of mice with monoclonal antibodies that block PD-1/PD-L1 interactions can restore $CD8^+$ T-cell functions, which in turn results in a reduction of virus titers in infected tissue, again proving that $CD8^+$ T cells are required to control chronic infections.

Persistent infections, which are characterized by periodic production of low levels of virus such as seen with most types of herpes virus, do not appear to impair T-cell functions, although they may take a toll on the overall capacity of the immune system as a result of very high frequencies of $CD8^+$ T cells activating over time, thus reducing the number of T cells available for other infections. Chronic infections during which large numbers of virus particles are produced each day, on the other hand, do impair T-cell functions over time, which in the extreme can lead to $CD8^+$ T-cell exhaustion. Attempts to improve the outcome of chronic viral infections through vaccination should take this into account, as immunization with additional antigen without signals that readjust the impairment of the $CD8^+$ T cell responses are unlikely to be of benefit to the host.

The role of memory $CD8^+$ T cells in protecting against reinfection remains debated. Once an individual has cleared an infection, the ensuing immune response in general provides life-long protection against the same virus. This was already appreciated in ancient history. In China, during smallpoxvirus epidemics, patients were inoculated with scab material from infected individuals because it was known that this would provide long-term resistance to a natural infection. Needless to say, this practice killed many and was eventually abandoned. In 1781, a measles epidemic struck the isolated islands of Faeroe off the coast of Scandinavia. Once the epidemic ran its natural course, Faeroe did not re-encounter this pathogen until 65 years later, when a new epidemic infected nearly every one of its inhabitants except for the elderly population that had been infected more than six decades earlier. Immunologic memory is long-lived and provides protection against some pathogens for life without further encounter of the antigen.

What is not clear is whether and to what degree different adaptive immune mechanisms contribute to this long-lasting protection in humans. In many viral infections, $CD8^+$ T cells do not appear to prevent reinfection, and resistance is linked to virus-neutralizing antibodies. For example, different strains of influenza A viruses show heterogeneity of their surface antigens, which bind neutralizing antibodies. Their internal proteins, which carry T-cell epitopes, are relatively conserved. Humans infected with a given strain of influenza virus are rendered resistant to reinfection with the same virus, but remain susceptible to infection with a serologically distinct influenza A virus even if this virus shares T-cell epitopes with the initially infecting strain. The same applies for infections with adenoviruses. Fifty-six serotypes of adenovirus have been identified in humans to date. They cause a variety of symptoms ranging from mild to deadly respiratory infections, gastroenteritis, or conjunctivitis. Adenoviruses are grouped into six families, and members of each family show extensive sequence homology (>90%). Most of the sequence variability is seen in the viral hexon, which binds neutralizing antibodies. Humans infected with one serotype of adenovirus are rendered resistant to reinfection with the same serotype but remain fully susceptible to infection with a different serotype even if this serotype belongs to the same subfamily. Both of these findings suggest that $CD8^+$ T cells are inefficient to protect against a second infection, although there is some evidence that humans with high frequencies of circulating $CD8^+$ T cells to influenza A virus develop relatively milder forms of disease following infections with a serologically different influenza virus strain (117). Both influenza A viruses and adenoviruses cause infections that are limited to the respiratory tract, the intestinal tract, or the eye. Although this remains to be confirmed experimentally, one could postulate that $CD8^+$ T_{EM} cells that home to these compartments are required for solid protection, and that this subset of T cells is relatively short-lived and differentiates over time into T_{CM}, which home to lymph nodes. In other viral infections, when viruses are spread throughout the organism or infect lymphatic tissues, long-lived T_{CM} may provide better protection against infection-associated disease. In one of his articles, Rolf Zinkernagel compared memory $CD8^+$ T cells to an urban police force that tries to protect taxpayers from thieves (118). The police cars mainly cruise on highways, so thieves who target houses in little alleys (the equivalent of tissues) get away, for by the time the victim calls the police and they actually arrive, the deed is done. Police may happen to cruise by a robbery of a store next to a major highway (the equivalent of viremia, i.e., virus in the bloodstream), notice that something is amiss, and apprehend the culprits. Thieves that are dumb enough to rob the police station (the lymphatic tissues) would most likely be stopped instantly unless the police are totally incompetent (impaired immune system).

Answers to the question of whether and to what degree antigen-specific memory CD8$^+$ T cells can prevent viral infections are needed in order to develop effective vaccines to viral pathogens that continue to take a major toll on human lives. One example is HIV-1. Currently available vaccines to many other viral agents provide protective immunity mainly through the induction of circulating virus-neutralizing antibodies. Passive transfer studies have indicated that neutralizing antibodies to HIV-1 can protect nonhuman primates from an experimental mucosal infection with a pathogenic chimeric simian/human immunodeficiency virus (119). Unfortunately, attempts to generate vaccines that express the HIV-1 envelope protein in a form able to induce protective titers of broadly cross-reactive HIV-1–neutralizing antibodies have failed thus far (120), and current vaccine efforts are focused mainly on inducing protection through T cells directed against more conserved epitopes of HIV-1 (121). Unfortunately, it is unknown if vaccine-induced T cells can indeed prevent infections, or at least reduce viral setpoint loads and thus lessen progression to disease and further spread of the virus.

Vaccines against influenza A virus used annually against the prevailing human strains are available. They induce protective immunity through the induction of subtype-specific neutralizing antibodies. The most commonly used vaccines are based on whole, subunit, or surface (HA + NA) formulations of influenza virus grown in embryonated chicken eggs. Vaccines are usually trivalent, containing two strains of influenza A and one strain of influenza B virus. As influenza vaccines induce protection through strain-specific neutralizing antibodies, vaccine composition is reviewed annually and updated to incorporate antigenic drift or shift strains. It takes approximately 6 months to develop sufficient stockpiles of an influenza virus vaccine, so new vaccine compositions are designed in spring to have the annual vaccines available to prevent the seasonal influenza virus outbreaks that typically occur in winter.

Influenza virus pandemics are caused by newly evolved strains of influenza A virus. Advanced stockpiling of a pandemic influenza virus vaccine is unrealistic, as the vaccine's antigen composition, especially that of HA and NA, must closely resemble the pandemic strain. Once such a strain has evolved, it is expected to spread throughout the world within less than 6 months, overwhelming production capacity of vaccine manufacturers. Rather that relying on rapid production of traditional vaccines to induce protection through stimulation of type-specific neutralizing antibodies, and for which precise knowledge of the molecular composition of the coming pandemic influenza A virus strain is a prerequisite, one could develop and stockpile vaccine compositions that induce CD8$^+$ T cell–mediated cross-reactive protection against heterotypic strains of influenza A virus. Such vaccines provide resistance to heterotypic strains of influenza virus in experimental animals, but it is unknown whether and to what degree such T-cell–inducing vaccines would protect humans against influenza A virus–associated disease.

CD4$^+$ T Cells

CD4$^+$ T cells have regulatory functions; CD4$^+$ T-helper cells promote activation of B and CD8$^+$ T cells, while CD4$^+$ regulatory T cells inhibit the induction or the effector functions of such responses.

Antigen Processing and Presentation for CD4$^+$ T-Cell Activation

CD4$^+$ T cells recognize peptides displayed by MHC class II molecules (122). Although MHC class I and II molecules are closely related structurally, their peptide-binding grooves are distinct. The MHC class I groove is closed at both ends, which limits access to peptides of 8 to 10 amino acids in length, whereas the MHC class II groove is open at both ends, permitting association with peptides of varied lengths. Unlike MHC class I molecules, which are displayed on nearly all nucleated cells, MHC class II expression is restricted to a small subset of cells such as macrophages, B cells, and DCs. Upon synthesis of the α and β subunits, MHC class II molecules assemble in the ER into a nonameric complex composed of three α chains, three β chains, and three invariant chains. Binding of the invariant chain stabilizes the overall structure of the complex. The invariant chain contains a peptide sequence termed CLIP (Class II–associated invariant peptide) that binds promiscuously to the groove of MHC class II dimmers, thus preventing binding of other peptides within the ER. The MHC class II–invariant chain complexes are translocated to endosomes/lysosomes, where proteins taken up from the extracellular domain are broken down by disulfide reduction and enzymatic proteolysis. Within the endosomes the invariant chain, which blocks access of peptides to the MHC class II groove, is degraded by cathepsin S. Upon dissociation of the invariant chain, an accessory protein termed DM associates with the N-terminal part of the peptide-binding groove. DM is then replaced with an antigenic polypeptide. These polypeptides can be short and fit readily into the groove, or they can be quite large, with long chains extending beyond the groove at either end. The portions of the polypeptides that fit into the groove are protected from proteolysis, while the overhanging parts are removed by cleavage. The MHC class II peptides complexes are then transported to the cell surface. In immature DCs, most MHC class II molecules are stored within the endosome and are released to the cell surface once DCs receive a maturation signal. Although immature DCs constantly synthesize MHC class II molecules to replace those that are degraded in the endosomes/lysosomes, mature DCs shut off synthesis of MHC class II molecules and rely on the long (>10 hours) half-life of cell surface–expressed and recycled MHC class II molecules to present antigen to CD4$^+$ T cells.

CD4$^+$ T-Cell Responses

Activation of naïve CD4$^+$ T cells requires presentation of antigen by MHC class II molecules in context of the costimulatory molecules CD80 and CD86 and the adhesion molecule CD54 (123). Upon antigen recognition, CD4$^+$ T cells proliferate in response to autocrine IL-2. Proliferation of CD4$^+$ T cells is not as extensive as that of CD8$^+$ T cells, and during most infections the frequencies of specific CD8$^+$ effector T cells exceed those of CD4$^+$ T cells. It has been estimated that CD4$^+$ T cells undergo approximately 8 to 10 cycles, whereas CD8$^+$ T cells can cycle 20 times or more, depending on the scope of the infection. Activation and proliferation of CD4$^+$ T cells is augmented by proinflammatory cytokines such as IL-1, IL-6, and TNF-α, which are produced by cells of the innate immune system in response to viral infections. The type of activation determines CD4$^+$ T-helper cell polarization into Th1- or Th2-type cells; Th1 cells are induced in the presence of IFN-γ and IL-12 or agents that block IL-4, whereas Th2 cells develop in the presence of IL-4. Once T cells commit to either pathway, epigenitic imprinting of the chromatin ensures the stability of this phenotype.

Virus infections induce both Th1 and Th2 cells. Th1 cells secrete IL-2, IFN-γ, and TNF-α; Th2 cells produce IL-4, IL-5, IL-10, and IL-13. Some viruses, such as measles virus, induce a non-antigen–specific global shift toward Th2, resulting in transient suppression of Th1-linked immune responses (124). Once CD4$^+$ T cells are activated in the T-cell–rich zones of the lymph nodes, they are ready to commence effector functions. Within the lymph nodes, CD4$^+$ T cells are needed for formation of germinal centers at which CD4$^+$ T cells interact with B cells through CD40–CD40 ligand interactions. CD4$^+$ T-cell–derived cytokines are instrumental for isotype switching of B cells. In mice, Th1-cell–derived IFN-γ promotes switching to IgG2a, whereas Th2-derived IL-4 preferentially induces IgG1 switching. CD4$^+$ T-cell–derived cytokines also drive proliferation of B cells and their differentiation into long-lived antibody-secreting plasma cells. As mentioned previously, some of the cytopathic viruses, such as LCMV, sendai virus, influenza virus, or ectromelia virus (a mouse poxvirus), can induce CD8$^+$ effector T cells without CD4$^+$ T help, although the help is required for efficient memory CD8$^+$ T-cell formation. Other viruses, such as mouse hepatitis virus, HSV, or adenoviruses, only elicit a CD8$^+$ T-cell response in the presence of functional CD4$^+$ T cells. CD4$^+$ T cells help differentiation of naïve CD8$^+$ T cells into effector cells by providing activation signals to DCs and by secretion of growth factors, most notably IL-2, which promotes CD8$^+$ T-cell proliferation and under certain circumstances CD8$^+$ T-cell survival.

Once they are activated, CD4$^+$ T cells downregulate CCR7 and CD62L, which allows their migration to peripheral tissues. In the periphery, CD4$^+$ T cells can contribute to viral clearance either indirectly, through the release of antiviral cytokines produced in response to viral peptides displayed on MHC class II–positive cells, which are dispersed throughout most tissues and accumulate at sites of inflammation, or directly, by killing infected MHC class II molecule–expressing cells. MHC class II antigens are constitutively expressed on some cells such as B cells, and it has been shown that CD4$^+$ T cells can kill Epstein–Barr virus (EBV)–infected B cells (125). In other cell types that normally fail to express MHC class II, expression can be induced by cytokines such as IFN-γ. Following the effector phase, CD4$^+$ T-cell responses contract, and about 10% of the cells survive to form the memory CD4$^+$ T-cell pool (126). Whereas contraction of CD8$^+$ T cells occurs very rapidly, within a few days, CD4$^+$ T cells undergo activation-induced cell death over a period of several weeks. Similarly to CD8$^+$ T cells, memory CD4$^+$ cells can be grouped into T_{EM} and T_{CM} memory cells, which can be differentiated based on expression levels of CD62L and CCR7. Memory CD4$^+$ T cells are maintained at constant levels through IL-7–regulated homeostatic proliferation. Nevertheless, the longevity of CD4$^+$ T-cell memory and its dependence on antigen remains debated. Upon re-encounter of antigen, memory CD4$^+$ T cells proliferate and differentiate into effector T cells. Memory CD4$^+$ T cells assume effector functions more rapidly than naïve T cells, in part through storage of RNA for key cytokines and chemokines, which are available for immediate translation once the T-cell receptor has been engaged. Reactivation of memory CD4$^+$ T cells is relatively independent of costimulation, allowing for reactivation by antigen-presenting B cells or macrophages. Notwithstanding, costimulation affects the quality of the recall response; CD4$^+$ T cells activated in the absence of costimulation proliferate and produce IL-2 but fail to produce IFN-γ and are poorly suited to assist reactivation of CD8$^+$ T cells.

Role of CD4$^+$ T Cells in Protection against Viral Infections

In adoptive transfer studies in which naïve mice were injected with T-helper cells generated *in vitro*, CD4$^+$ T cells have been shown to protect against a subsequent pulmonary challenge with a lethal dose of influenza A virus. Protection was in part mediated by perforin, suggesting that the T-helper cells eliminated infected cells by direct killing. Protection was also linked to an accelerated antibody response (127). Earlier studies showed that selective presence of CD4$^+$ T cells in the absence of CD8$^+$ T cells or neutralizing antibodies increases influenza virus–associated immunopathology and thus mouse mortality following infection (128). In other mouse models of viral infections, CD4$^+$ T cells were also shown to contribute to protection, commonly acting in concert with CD8$^+$ T cells. One would expect that because of their restricted recognition of cells that express MHC class II, CD4$^+$ T cells would be poorly suited to single-handedly control virus infections unless such infections are limited to MHC class II–positive cells. Their primary role is indirect; they facilitate stimulation of naive CD8$^+$ T cells, assist in memory CD8$^+$ T-cell development, and promote antibody responses.

Regulatory CD4$^+$ T Cells

The notion of T cells that suppress activation of adaptive T cells was first proposed in the 1970s (129). These cells were supposed to act through complicated idiotypic–anti-idiotypic receptor interactions in which antigen-specific (that is, idiotypic) receptors on effector T cells induced T cells with corresponding anti-idiotypic receptors that then released suppressor factors. The suppressor T cells could never be isolated, and the experimental evidence for their existence was circumstantial. Experiments that were conducted to prove the existence of suppressor T cells were so complex that artifacts were probable. By the late 1970s the majority of immunologists concluded that suppressor T cells were a product of fantasy and poor experimentation, and for two decades manuscripts that described suppressor T cells or grant applications that proposed to study such T cells were viewed with scorn. In the mid-1990s, suppressor T cells were finally isolated. To avoid public ridicule, they were termed regulatory T cells (129,130). A number of cell subsets can have immunomodulatory functions, including NK cells and CD8$^+$ T cells. By far the best-studied populations of regulatory cells are two subsets of CD4$^+$ T cells; one subset is constitutively present and is termed natural Treg, while the other is induced by antigen and is called Tr.

Natural Treg are CD4$^+$CD25$^+$CTLA-4$^+$GITR$^+$ and express the transcription factor forkhead box (Fox)p3 (131,132). They comprise approximately 5% to 10% of the circulating pool of CD4$^+$ T cells. Natural Treg respond to self-antigens and are crucial to maintain tolerance. They play a role in infectious diseases by reducing the magnitude of primary immune responses, by limiting effector T-cell functions, and by reducing secondary immune responses. Treg recognize antigen through polyclonal T-cell receptors, and it is assumed that their receptors that respond primarily to self-antigens cross-react with antigens expressed by pathogens. They control adaptive immune responses through secretion of anti-inflammatory cytokines such as IL-10 or TGF-β, through modulation of DCs, and through direct cell-to-cell contact. Treg express TLRs including TLR-7 and -8 and are activated by infectious agents. After activation, they migrate to the sites of infection. Mice that lack Treg are better able to control viral infections, but they are also prone to more damaging immune responses, indicating that Treg activity reduces immunopathology, which in turn can allow for more extensive and prolonged survival of infectious agents and for the development of persisting infections. This has been documented for a number of bacterial infections and for HCV, for which the degree of liver inflammation in humans correlates inversely with frequencies of circulating Treg. During ocular infections with HSV, CD4$^+$ T cells cause severe blinding infections of the eye in the absence of Treg. That Treg reduce the adaptive immune system's ability to eliminate infected cells and consequently promotes persistence of the pathogen was also shown in mice chronically infected with Friend leukemia virus, in which depletion of Treg restored CD8$^+$ T-cell functions, resulting in a reduction of viral loads.

Antigen-induced suppressor T cells are commonly referred to as Th3 or Tr cells (133). They appear to be triggered preferentially upon mucosal immunization, presumably to prevent induction of immune responses against antigens present in food or inhaled air. Tr cells are induced by DCs and preferentially by mucosal DCs that are not fully matured and secrete IL-10. This immunosuppressive cytokine appears also to favor Tr induction if it is derived from other cell types. For example, nonstructural proteins of HCV induce monocytes to produce IL-10, which in turn promotes Tr activation. Other cytokines, such as IL-4, IL-6, and TGF-β, have been implicated to sponsor Tr differentiation. The role of Tr cells during viral infections appears to be similar to that of CD4$^+$CD25$^+$ Treg. Tr cells inhibit T-cell responses and thus infection-associated immunopathology, which in turn promotes viral persistence.

B Cells

B cells recognize viral antigens through cell surface–expressed receptors, which are membrane-anchored immunoglobulin molecules. Upon virus infection, antigen is translocated by DCs to the T-cell zones of lymph nodes draining the sites of infection. Here they induce antigen-specific CD4$^+$ T cells, which, once activated, migrate to the T/B interphase of the primary B-cell follicles. Naïve B cells can pick up their antigen through specific cell surface–expressed IgM. The antigen is internalized and degraded within the lysosomes/endosomes into peptides that, provided they have suitable anchoring residues, associate with MHC class II molecules. The peptide/MHC complexes are transported back to the cell surface. Once B cells receive activation signals through PAMPs, they move to the T/B border of the follicles, where they interact with

CD4$^+$ T cells that recognize the MHC/peptide complex on the B cells' surface. T-cell help requires direct interactions between T and B cells in which CD40 expressed on B cells binds to CD40 ligands expressed by T-helper cells. A number of other surface molecules on B cells and their corresponding ligands on T cells participate in forming the synapsis between activated T cells and naive B cells. Cytokines secreted by activated CD4$^+$, such as IL-4 and IL-6, are also required for B-cell proliferation and differentiation. Once B cells are primed, they migrate to the T-cell zones and develop into short-lived plasma cells, or they return to the B-cell zones, where they initiate formation of germinal centers. In either case, isotype switching occurs through genetic rearrangement of the immunoglobulin genes. Hypermutation, on the other hand, happens only in B cells that differentiate into long-lived plasma cells. Short-lived plasma cells start to secrete antibodies within 3 to 5 days but then die rapidly. B cells that return to the B-cell zones undergo more massive proliferation, creating regions that are called secondary follicles, which eventually form the germinal centers. Formation of germinal centers requires T-cell help. Within the germinal centers, B cells undergo affinity maturation through hypermutation of their immunoglobulin (Ig) variable-region genes. B cells with deleterious Ig mutation die by apoptosis, while those that produce antibodies with increased affinity to the antigen continue to proliferate. T-helper cells are present in the germinal center and are thought to deliver signals to promote B-cell memory formation.

Two other B-cell subsets have been described in addition to the B cells that home to the B-cell–rich areas of lymphatic tissues. One subset, which is commonly found in the peritoneal cavity, carries an activated phenotype, presumably due to interactions with self-peptides. These B cells secrete IgM and IgG3 and are the source of naturally occurring antibodies that are found in naïve animals (134). Natural antibodies play a crucial role in inhibiting early viral dissemination. They are able to form complexes with a wide variety of viral pathogens. Such complexes are selectively retained in lymphoid tissues, facilitating induction of adaptive immune responses and reducing the spread of the pathogen to other vital organs. An additional B-cell subset is found in the marginal zone of the spleen at the juncture of white and red pulp (135). This subset, called marginal-zone B cells, also has a preactivated phenotype and is able to respond very rapidly to viral pathogens by secretion of IgM antibodies. This response, which is independent of T-helper cells, peaks after 3 to 4 days and is then followed by antibodies originating from follicular B cells in lymph nodes and spleens. Once peritoneal-cavity B cells or marginal-zone B cells become activated, they terminally differentiate into plasma cells. They do not contribute to the memory response but instead undergo programmed cell death. B cells have thus evolved to respond very rapidly with "unedited" antibodies of low affinity to an incoming pathogen. These antibodies are secreted without further input from T-helper cells that are not yet fully activated at this early stage after an infection. A T-helper cell–independent B-cell response has an increased risk for cross-reactivity with self-antigen. To lessen the threat of permanent damage due to auto-antibodies, the B cells that provide early antibodies are not destined to become part of the memory B-cell pool.

B-cell effector functions are mediated by secreted antibodies. B cells can produce five different types of antibodies, IgA, IgD, IgE, IgG, and IgM, which can express the same antigen-binding site but differ in the composition of their constant regions. IgA, IgG, and IgM contribute to the control of viral infections. IgM is produced first and is then, over time, replaced by IgG upon isotype switching. IgGs are most commonly found in blood, and they are divided into four subtypes. All IgGs with the appropriate specificity can prevent infection of cells by neutralizing viruses. Antibodies can lyse virus particles directly, or they can activate the complement cascade to disrupt the viral membrane. Human IgG3 is particularly effective at activating complement. IgGs can also facilitate uptake of viruses by Fc receptor–positive phagocytes, which degrade the virus. IgA has similar functions to IgG but can be transported actively across epithelial surfaces, allowing for its secretion at mucosal surfaces. IgA is thus crucial for protection against pathogens that invade through the mucosal epithelium.

B cells terminally differentiate either into antibody-producing plasma cells or into memory B cells (136). Memory B cells are long-lived and persist for many years. It is unknown whether this survival involves homeostatic proliferation or whether individual cells have an extended lifespan. Survival of memory B cells requires expression of the B-cell receptor, which led to the notion that periodic receptor engagement is required through low-affinity interaction with cross-reactive self-proteins or through periodic exposure to antigen. Antigen can form very stable complexes with antibodies, and such complexes can be captured by Fc receptors expressed on follicular DCs within lymphatic tissues, from where they are released slowly over a long period of time. These small amounts of antigen may suffice to maintain memory B cells.

Antibodies have short half-lives. Nevertheless, after viral infections, specific antibodies can commonly be detected years later. This suggested that antibody-producing plasma cells are maintained for a very long time, either through longevity or by periodic activation of memory B cells through exposure to antigen. Plasma cells die rapidly in culture, and it was initially assumed that they were short-lived and that antibody titers were maintained through constant antigen-driven activation by memory B cells. Subsequent studies showed that plasma cells that home to bone marrow are long-lived. Their survival depends on IL-6 and on interactions with bone marrow stromal cells. An alternative pathway to maintain antibody-producing plasma cells has been proposed; during infections with unrelated pathogens that carry PAMPs, memory B cells receive signals through PRRs such as TLRs, which drives antigen-independent differentiations of memory B cells into antibody-producing plasma cells (137).

Antiviral antibodies play a role in primary infections. Pre-existing natural antibodies provide an immediate layer of defense, which is rapidly joined by antibodies secreted by marginal-zone B cells or B cells that reside outside lymphoid tissues. Peak production of affinity-matured antibodies takes up to 2 weeks, and such antibodies would not be expected to play a dominant role in primary infections, although they are crucial to ward off secondary infections. Most antiviral vaccines are based on the concept that circulating IgG antibodies or IgA antibodies secreted at mucosal surfaces prevent infections by immediately neutralizing viral pathogens. Under ideal conditions such neutralization leads to so-called sterilizing immunity, in which none of the virus particles are able to infect host cells. Protection by neutralizing antibodies has been documented for rabies virus, influenza A virus, poliovirus, human papillomavirus, and many others. Nonneutralizing antibodies also contribute to protection. For example, antibodies to the ectodomain of the matrix protein of influenza A virus lack neutralizing activity but can nevertheless prevent fatal infection with influenza A virus in animal models (138). Sexually transmitted viruses cross the epithelial cell layer of the genital tract by transcytosis. This can be blocked intracellularly by IgA antibodies, as was shown in experimental SIV infections of nonhuman primates (139).

Antibodies of the IgG isotype are transferred from females to their offspring through transport across the placenta. After birth, IgAs and IgGs are secreted in breast milk and are taken up by the infants' intestines, which are highly permeable shortly after birth. The immune system of newborns is relatively incompetent, and during the time needed for the neonatal immune system to mature, maternally transferred antibodies provide protection against common pathogens. R. Zinkernagel has argued that immunologic memory evolved solely to protect newborns through maternal antibodies (140). He argues that anyone who survives a first infection is likely to be of sufficient genetic fitness to survive a second infection with the same pathogen and that therefore immunologic memory does not offer a survival advantage to a species. One could counterargue that most common infections strike in childhood. Individuals who develop protective immunologic memory against common infectious agents have a far better chance to reproduce successfully once they are sexually mature than those who are constantly ill because of crippling infections with viruses, which not only affect the desire of the prospective parents to become parents but are also commonly transmitted across the placenta, causing abortion or malformations of the fetus.

Autoimmunity/Allergies and Viral Infections

Although epidemiologic data implicate pathogens as causative agents for autoimmune diseases, a direct infectious etiology has yet to be proven. Evidence implicating viruses or bacteria in triggering destructive responses against self-antigens remains circumstantial, at least in a clinical setting. Direct evidence has been gained in transgenic mouse models in which T-cell–receptor transgenic mice that express the corresponding antigen in selective tissues were shown to develop autoimmunity upon stimulation of the T cells by external addition of antigen (141).

Several mechanisms can be envisioned for viruses to cause autoimmune responses. Some viruses cause polyclonal activation of adaptive immune responses, which could lead to inadvertent activation of T and/or B cells with self-reactive receptors. Such polyclonal activation signals may be provided by so-called superantigens that are expressed by some bacteria or viruses (142). Superantigens can activate $CD4^+$ T-cell responses without processing and presentation by MHC class II molecules. They bind to MHC II molecules directly, outside the conventional peptide-binding groove, and then interact with the variable region of the β chain of the T-cell receptor. Each superantigen can bind to a number of different $V\beta$ chains and cause activation of the corresponding $CD4^+$ T cells independent of their antigen specificity. A superantigen can thus activate up to 25% of the entire $CD4^+$ T-cell repertoire, resulting in fulminate cytokine release, which can cause toxic shock and death. A number of viral antigens have superantigen activity, such as the nucleoprotein of rabies virus, nef of HIV-1, and a yet-to-be-identified component of EBV. The polyclonal activation of T cells by contact with superantigens is thought to lead to stimulation of self-reactive T cells that are otherwise kept in check through negative immunoregulatory mechanisms.

Antigenic mimicry, in which a viral antigen resembles a self-antigen, could also elicit autoimmune responses (143). Bioinformatic searches for sequence homology between viral proteins and self-proteins show that such homologies are quite common. For example, a sequence in Coxsackie B virus is homologous to one in glutamic acid decarboxylase (GAD), a protein expressed by insulin-producing pancreatic islet cells. Antibodies to GAD are linked to type I diabetes, and Coxsackie B virus has been shown to trigger loss of insulin production in animals. The polymerase of HBV mimics myelin basic protein, and immunization of rabbits with the shared peptide sequence induces pathology that resembles allergic encephalomyelitis. Nevertheless, in humans, neither multiple sclerosis (which is similar to allergic encephalomyelis) nor type I diabetes has been linked to specific infections, which may in part reflect the long latency between a certain infection and overt symptoms caused by either autoimmune disease.

Organ-specific autoimmunity may be caused by local viral infections in which the strong inflammatory response to viral antigens promotes presentation of self-antigens. For example, upon infection with Theiler virus, mice develop a virus-associated encephalomyelitis in which T cells respond to the antigens of the virus. This is replaced by T cells recognizing myelin basic protein or proteolipid protein, causing continued neurologic damage (144). Infection of mice with Coxsackie B3 viruses causes cardiomyopathy that develops in two stages: at first, virus-specific T cells develop and damage the infected cells; they are then replaced by an even more destructive autoimmune T-cell response (145). In either model, the damage caused by antigen-specific T cells is limited to clearance of infected cells, but the associated inflammation triggers self-reactive T cells, which prolong and exacerbate disease.

Viral and bacterial infections have not only been implicated in causing autoimmunity, they are also thought to protect against autoimmunity and allergy (146). In the last 30 years, developed countries have experienced a steady and alarming increase in autoimmune diseases and allergies. This epidemic is not seen in undeveloped countries, and it is more pronounced in colder countries than in warmer countries. Although these allergies and autoimmunity have opposing underlying mechanisms, with allergies being basically a misguided Th2 response while autoimmunity is associated with Th1 responses, epidemiologic evidence shows that their prevalence is linked to increased hygiene and decreased infections. One could postulate several mechanisms for this linkage. One could argue that adaptive immune responses against strong antigens of pathogens will outcompete the comparatively weaker immune responses to self-antigens or allergens. One could argue that immune responses to infectious agents increase negative regulatory responses that dampen adaptive immunity to strong antigens and abolish weaker responses to self-antigens or allergens.

IMMUNOEVASION BY VIRUSES

Viruses and their hosts coevolved through the millennia. While the hosts developed a more sophisticated immune system to limit damage inflicted by viral infections, viruses changed in tandem and acquired traits that allowed them to dodge destruction by their hosts' immune responses. RNA viruses, which have small genomes, primarily but not exclusively evade by rapid mutations caused by the infidelity of their replication machinery that lacks the proofreading capacity of mammalian polymerases. Although lack of faithful genome replication is costly in that many of the resulting viruses lack the fitness of the parent virus, in the end it serves the virus population, which produces thousands of new infectious viruses from each original virus and can thus afford to lose some to defective genomes. The larger, more complex DNA viruses have the space to devote a significant percentage of their genome to encode polypeptides that allow their evasion from the forces of the hosts' immune systems. Considering the size limitations of the genomes of even the larger viruses, the multitude of genes that serve to subvert immune responses must clearly provide them with an evolutionary advantage. Also, pathways that are targeted by viruses give insight to immunologists to what degree such pathways play a role in the immunologic defense against viruses.

Escape by Hiding

Viruses can hide by changing their molecular shape through mutations that modify sites targeted by antibodies, T-cell receptors, or antiviral cytokines. In the face of neutralizing antibodies, viral variants, also termed quasispecies, are selected for that have lost or modified the neutralizing antibodies' target sites, which are generally located on viral surface proteins (147). Selection of viral variants with mutated internal viral proteins is prompted by the activity of T cells (148). The latter is found during HIV-1 or HCV infections, in which, over time, virus particles are selected for that carry mutations in dominant $CD8^+$ T-cell epitopes. IFNs, which have potent antiviral activity, can drive outgrowth of viral mutants with increased resistance to its activity. This has been observed in chronic infections with HCV, in which lack of a response to IFN therapy can be associated with selection of therapy-resistant viral variants (149).

The central nervous system is an immunologically privileged site where viruses are relatively sheltered from the immune system. A number of viruses take advantage of this and establish neuronal infections. A typical example is rabies virus, which multiplies in neurons. Once the virus is ready to be transmitted to the next host, it spreads via axonal flow to the periphery to infect, for example, cells of the salivary gland. Although effector or memory T lymphocytes can cross the blood–brain barrier, the immune system lacks the needed signals in the periphery to efficiently activate rabies virus-specific T cells and is thus incapable of controlling the infection. Herpes viruses can shut off viral protein synthesis upon infection of cells and enter a state of latency. The immune system remains ignorant of latently infected cells that do not express viral antigens. This allows the virus to evade complete destruction during the height of an acute immune response. Once the immune system assumes a more relaxed stage of memory, the virus can reactivate and replicate unhindered for a few days, until T cells convert from memory cells back to effector cells. These short bursts of viral replication suffice to produce ample amounts of virus to allow its spread to other organisms.

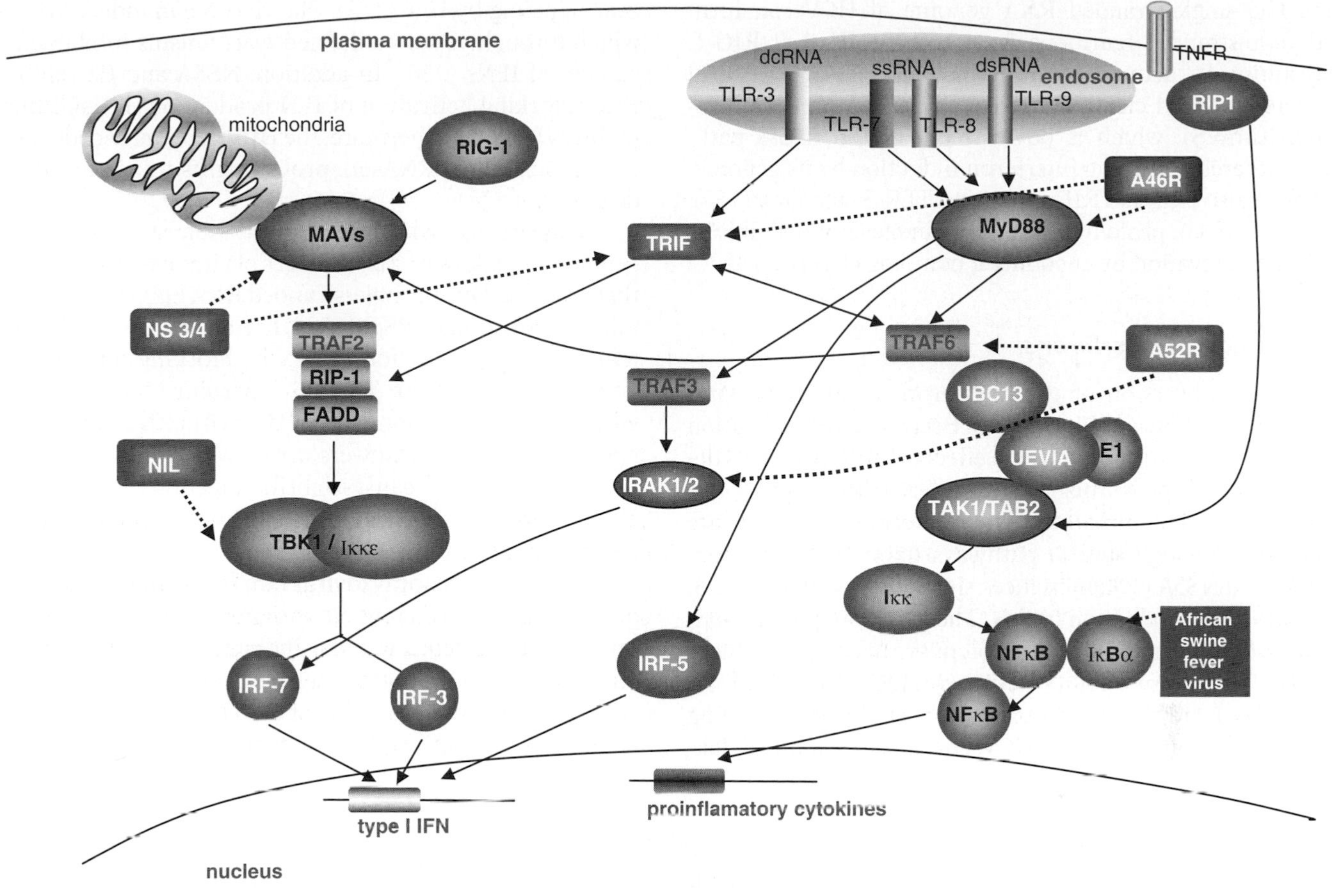

FIGURE 36.1 Activation of innate immune responses through viral PAMPs. FADD, Fas-associated protein with death domain; IKK, IκB kinase; IRAKs, IL-1R–associated kinases; IRF, interferon regulatory factor/interferon response factor; MAVS, mitochondrial antiviral signaling protein; MyD88, myeloid differentiation factor 88; NFκB, nuclear factor κB; RIG1, retinoid-inducible gene 1; RIP3, receptor-interacting protein 3; TAB1/TAB2, adaptor proteins that associate with TAK1; TAK1, TGFβ-activating kinase 1; TANK, TNFR-associated factor family member-associated NF-κB activator; TBK1, (TANK)-binding kinase; TLR, Toll-like receptors; TRAF, TNF receptor-associated factor; TRIF, Toll-IL-1 receptor domain-containing adapter-inducing IFN-β factor; Uev1A, Ubc, ubiquitination proteins—Uev1A, together with Ubc13, serves as an E2 in the ubiquitination of Tak1.

Escape by Destruction of Immune Cells

A number of viruses infect cells of the adaptive immune system, leading to their demise. The best example is HIV-1 virus, which infects and destroys $CD4^+$ T cells (150). This is probably mediated in part by the viral envelope protein, which forms spikes on the surface of the virions that can contribute to killing uninfected $CD4^+$ T cells, susceptible to being killed by cells that express Fas.

Escape from Early Innate Immune Responses

Inhibition of PRR Activation

Innate immune responses are rapidly initiated once a viral PAMP is recognized by a cellular PRR. A number of viruses, such as poxviruses, HCV, and adenoviruses, have evolved pathways to block activation of cellular inflammatory reactions to their PAMPs (Figure 36.1).

The poxvirus protein N1L interrupts TLR signaling to NF-κB by blocking the TANK-binding kinase (TBK)1, which is part of the TLR–NF-κB and TLR–TRF-3 activation pathways (151). The vaccinia virus A46R protein has a toll-like-interleukin-1 resistance (TIR) domain and inactivates MyD88, a crucial adapter molecule for TLR signaling. In addition, A46R interferes with the activity of TRIF, thus also shutting off MyD88-independent pathways used by TLR-4 and TLR-3. Vaccinia virus protein A52R blocks tumor necrosis–activated factor 6 (TRAF6) and interleukin 1-receptor–associated kinase 2 (IRAK2), inhibiting activation of NF-κB or IRF-3 upon TLR signaling (152).

The single-stranded RNA genome of HCV can form double-stranded hairloops that activate TRL-3 or RIG-1, resulting in activation of NF-κB and IRF-3. The viral protease NS3/4 cleaves the mitochondrial signaling protein (MAVS), which is downstream of the RIG-1 pathway, thereby blocking interferon induction by its genome. NS3/4 also cleaves TRIF, inhibiting TLR-3 signaling (153).

The A238L protein of African swine fever virus inhibits KF-κB activation by encoding a homolog of IκB (154).

Inhibition of Interferons

Immunosubversion of the interferon pathways by viral proteins is shown in Figure 36.2. Because HCV replication is very sensitive to the antiviral effects of IFNs, the virus developed multiple strategies to interfere with the induction of early proinflammatory cytokine responses, which are induced through several pathways upon HCV infection. The viral NS5A protein induces signaling to activate Stat3, resulting in production of IFN. The viral core protein activates PKR, which shuts off protein synthesis and induces IFN. The genomic PAMP activates TLR-3 and RIG-1. As described previously, the viral protease blocks signaling through either PRR. The HCV core protein inhibits Jak-Stat signaling by IL-6 (155). The viral NS5A induces IL-8, which through yet-to-be-defined mechanisms inhibits the activity of IFNs (156). In addition, NS5A and E2 inhibit PKR, blocking activation of IFN production through this pathway (157). Furthermore, the HCV genome encodes decoy sequences for RNAseL, protecting its transcript from degradation.

Adenoviruses, which carry a double-stranded DNA genome, encode one or two species of viral-associated RNA that are folded into double-stranded RNA hairloops, which inhibit activation of PKR (158). The ebolavirus VP35 protein prevents production of IFN by blocking phosphorylation of IRF-3 (159). The NS-1 protein of influenza A virus inhibits activation of NF-κB by viral RNA (160). The NSs protein of Bunyamwera virus, which is transmitted by mosquitoes and causes febrile infections in humans, also blocks induction of IFN production through yet-to-be-identified pathways (161).

Viruses of the paramyxovirus family, which is composed of a number of different viruses including sendai virus, human parainfluenza viruses, and mumps virus, have several strategies to abrogate interferon signaling. They can cause proteolytic degradation of Stat-1, thus inhibiting signaling through both type I and type II IFNs. They inhibit

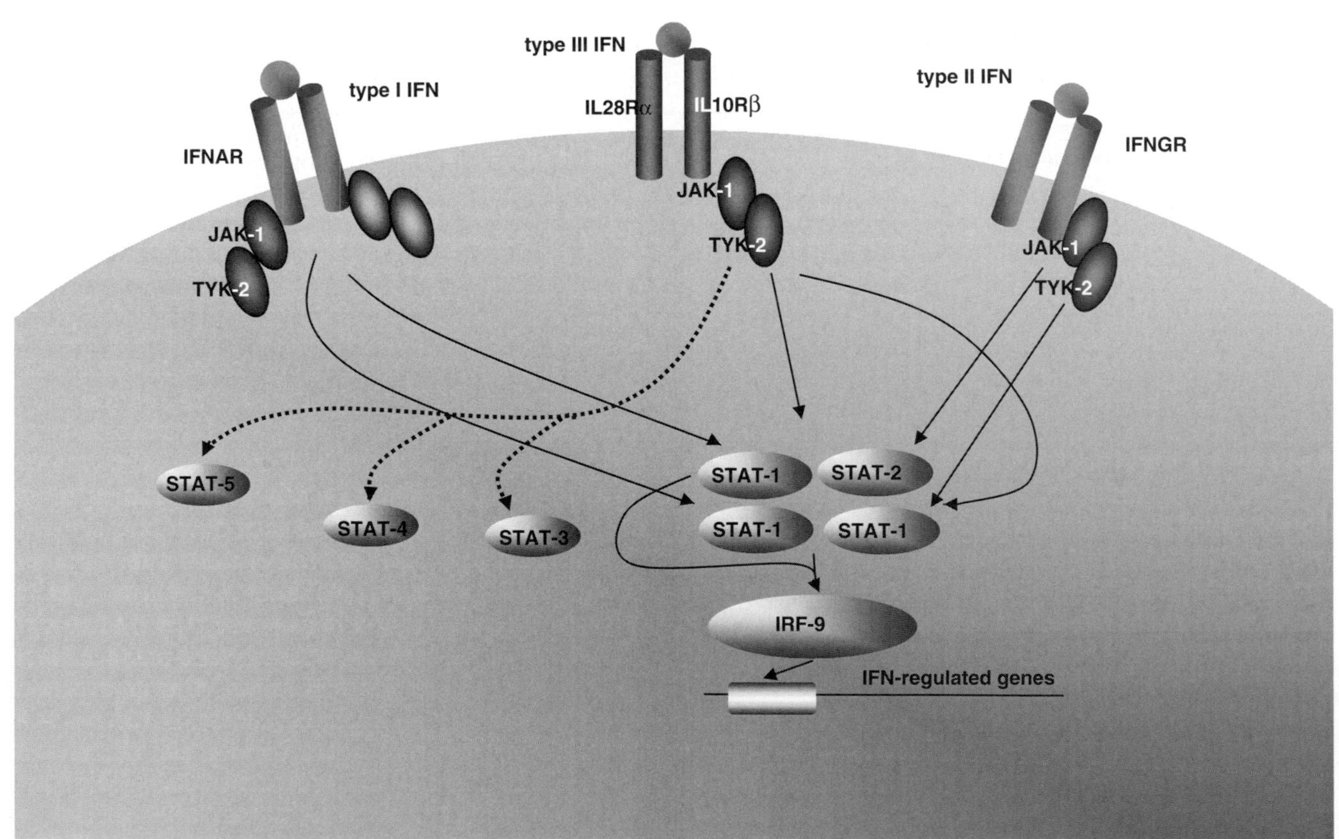

FIGURE 36.2 IFN-regulated genes. IFNAR, interferon α/β receptor; IFNGR, interferon γ receptor 1; IRF, interferon regulatory factor/interferon response factor; JAK, Janus kinase; STAT, signal transducers and activators of transcription; TYK, tyrosine kinase.

formation of transcription complexes essential for IFN signaling or they prevent phosphorylation of serine 727 on Stats, which is needed for their optimal transcriptional activity (162).

HPVs inhibit the activity of interferon through the early proteins E6 and E7 that interfere with cell-cycle regulation in oncogenic types of papillomavirus. The E6 protein binds and inactivates IRF-3 (230). The E7 protein binds to IRF-1 and histone deacetylase, thus silencing the activity of the transactivator on IFN-inducible promoters (163).

IL-18 is a cytokine that, like IL-12, induces IFN-γ production. Molluscum contagiosum virus (MCV) as well as orthopoxviruses secrete IL-18–binding proteins, which prevent the cytokine's interaction with its natural receptor. IL-18 is produced as a precursor molecule that is cleaved by caspase 1 into its active form. The crmA protein of vaccinia virus inhibits the activity of this caspase (164).

Other viral proteins act downstream on the activity of IFN-induced proteins. The M-T7 protein of myxoma virus and the B8R protein of vaccinia virus (both belonging to the poxvirus family) show sequence homology with the IFN-γ receptor (165). Both proteins bind to IFN-γ, inhibiting ligation to its receptor. Vaccinia virus also encodes a type I interferon inhibitor that shows sequence homology with the IFN-1 receptor.

The E3L protein of vaccinia virus inhibits activation of PKR. The K3L protein of vaccinia virus is a homolog of eIF-2, which serves as a decoy for activated PKR (166).

Interference with Other Cytokines/Chemokines

Collectively, herpes and poxviruses encode 40 members of the chemokine receptor family that serve as decoys for chemokines (167). Four proteins of human cytomegalovirus (HCMV), UL33, UL78, US27, and US28, show homology with the CCR1 receptor. UL146 and UL147 of HCMV encode CXC chemokine homologies; mouse CMV (MCMV) encodes a CC chemokine homolog, MC148 protein of Molluscipox virus shows similarity to the CCR8 chemokine receptor. Both leporipox (infectious for rodents) and orthopoxviruses encode secreted proteins (M-T1 and p35, respectively) that have functional homology to chemokine receptors. The M104L protein of poxvirus shows some similarity to MIG, an interferon-induced CXC chemokine. The effect that these different chemokine receptor mimetics have on the innate and adaptive immune responses to pox and herpes viruses remains under investigation. One would assume that sequestration of chemokines will affect leukocyte migration and thus reduce inflammatory reactions to the infections.

Herpes and poxviruses in addition produce proteins that bind or mimic cytokine receptors. The B8R protein of vaccinia virus binds to IFN-γ (168), whereas B18R binds to type I IFN (169). The poxvirus-encoded GIF binds to both GM-CSF and IL-2 (170). Poxviruses encode M135R (myxoma virus) and B18R (vaccinia virus), two proteins that bind and consequently inhibit IL-1β. The C10L protein of vaccinia virus encodes a protein that blocks the IL-1 receptor. IL-1β is synthesized as a precursor that requires cleavage by caspase 1 to gain functional activity. The same caspase also cleaves the precursor molecule of IL-18. Cowpoxvirus encodes a serine protease inhibitor called crmA that inhibits the function of caspase 1. The activity of crmA is not restricted to caspase 1 but also affects additional caspases involved in apoptosis (171).

Parapoxvirus, which infects sheep and goats, as well as CMV and EBV, encode an IL-10–like protein that inhibits synthesis of IL-12 and thus generation of Th1 immune responses. Similarly, the UL111A open reading frame of HCMV has sequence homology with IL-10 (172). UL146 and 147 of HCMV encode an IL-8–like molecule that may affect lymphocyte trafficking and IFN activity (173). IL-18 mimics are encoded by poxviruses such as molluscum contagiosum, ectromelia, cowpox, or vaccinia viruses (171). Kaposi sarcoma–associated herpes virus (KSHV), also called human herpes virus 8 (HHV-8), encodes an IL-6–like protein (174).

HCMV encodes UL144, which is a homolog of the TNF-receptor (TNFR) supergene family [222]. Its functions are currently unknown. Shope fibroma virus and myxoma virus encode a single TNFR homolog called T2 (223), whereas orthopoxviruses encode one to three different TNFR homologs called crmB, crmC, and crmD (224). T2, crmB, and crmD bind TNFI and lymphotoxin A, whereas crmC associates only with TNFα. T2, crmC, and crmD block TNFα–mediated cell lysis. The T2 protein in addition prevents apoptosis of $CD4^+$ T cells. This activity is independent of TNF-α (175).

Inhibition of NK Cell and Macrophage Activity

Cells infected with some viruses have reduced MHC class I surface expression and become susceptible to lysis by NK cells. In order to avoid this destruction by NK cells, some viruses either selectively spare downregulation of certain types of MHC, they encode MHC class I homologs, they directly inhibit the activating receptors on NK cells, they reduce recruitment of NK cells by interfering with chemokines as described earlier, or they affect NK cells directly (176) (Figure 36.3). MCMV and HCMV encode two proteins, m144 and UL18, which serve as MHC class I decoys. MCMV m157 interacts with inhibitory and activating NK receptors; in MCMV-resistant strains of mice, m157 is a ligand for the NK-activating Ly49H receptor, whereas in susceptible strains of mice it binds the inhibitory Ly491 receptor. HCMV proteins US2, US3, US6, and US11 downregulate the expression of most types of HLA molecules. They do not impair HLA-C and HLA-E expression, which are the dominant ligands for the inhibitory receptors of NK cells. Cell surface expression of HLA-E is generally

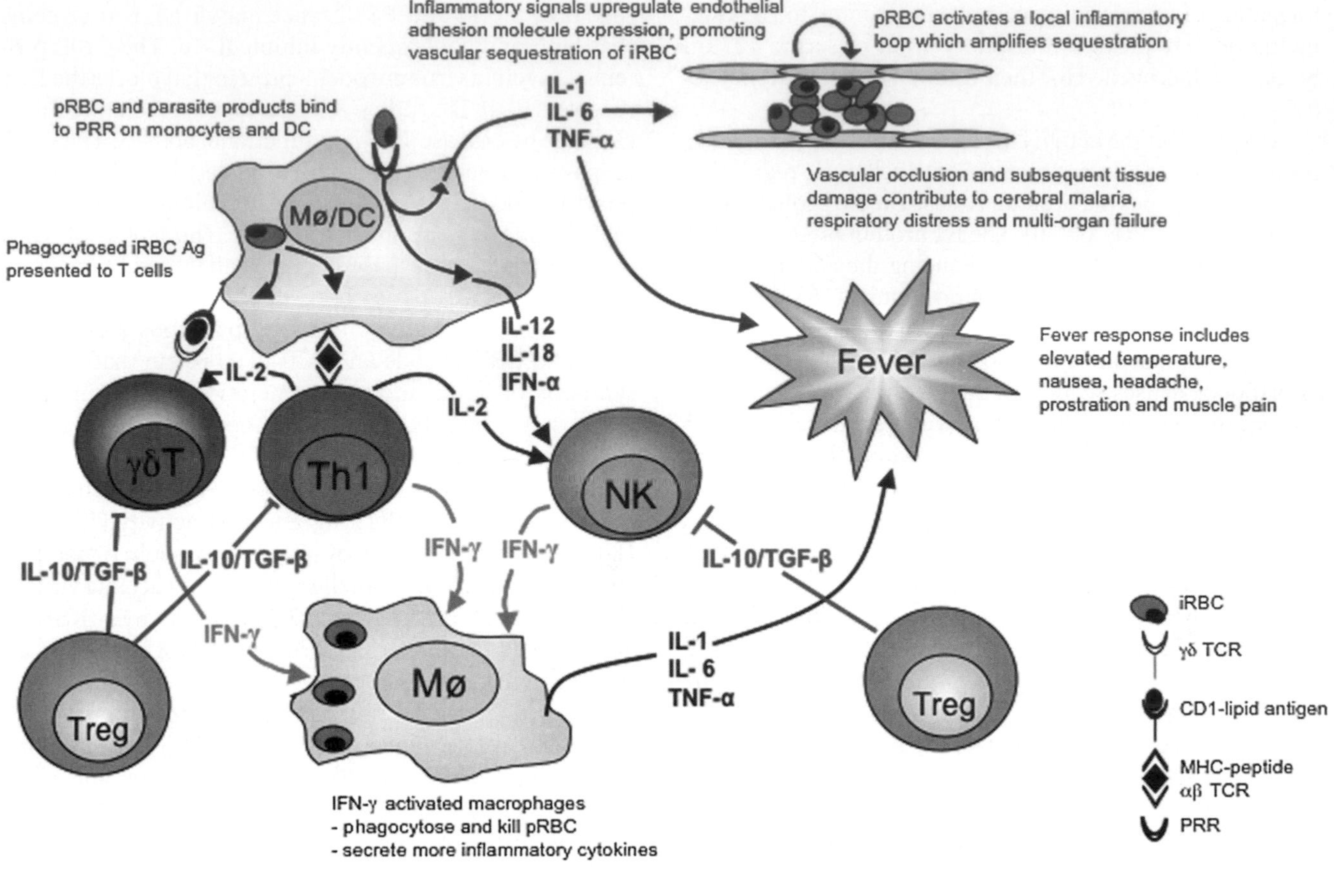

FIGURE 36.3 Immunopathogenesis of malaria.

TAP-dependent. In uninfected cells, HLA-E presents a peptide present in the signal sequence of HLA-C. Processing of this peptide, needed for its transport into the endoplasmic reticulum for binding to HLA-E, requires TAP, which is inhibited in HCMV-infected cells. The signal sequence of UL40, another HCMV-encoded protein, carries a sequence with a potential binding motif to HLA-E. It is possible that this peptide associates with HLA-E independently of TAP, thus allowing its translocation to the cell surface. KSHV encodes K3 and K5, which reduce MHC class I expression by causing their rapid endocytosis and degradation in lysosomes. Although K3 reduces expression of all of the HLA class I molecules, K5 selectively downregulates HLA-A and HLA-B but spares HLA-C and HLA-E. The *nef* gene of primate lentiviruses such as HIV-1 or SIV encodes a protein that acts in a similar way; it selectively downregulates expression of HLA-A and HLA-B but not of HLA-C or HLA-E.

Viruses not only increase the strength of inhibitory signals to NK cells but also interfere with activating receptors. HCMV downregulates expression of LFA-3, an adhesion molecule that binds to CD2 on NK cells. MCMV encodes a protein m152 that reduces expression of H60, a ligand for the NK-cell–activating receptor KG2D. N5 of KSHV reduces expression of ICAM-1 and CD86, which can both serve as ligands for activating NK receptors. NKG2D, one of the activating receptors of NK cells, binds to the UL16-binding protein (ULBP), which triggers the release of toxic granules. HCMV encodes UL16, which can bind ULBP and thus prevent its interaction with NKG2D. The tat protein of HIV binds to a calcium channel on NK cells, which blocks calcium influx and calcium-calmodulin kinase II, which is needed for NK-cell cytotoxicity.

Some viruses, such as HSV and HIV, can infect and kill NK cells directly. The major envelope protein E2 of hepatitis C virus binds to CD81, which in turn inhibits NK-cell activation and effector functions (177).

Activated phagocytes in particular macrophages produce inducible nitric oxide synthase (iNOS), which generates nitric oxide, a compound with antimicrobial functions. Production of iNOS is induced by type I IFNs, and viruses indirectly reduce iNOS production by interfering with the type I IFN pathways.

Inhibition of Complement Activation

Complement can directly lyse some viruses, promote phagocytosis, or kill virus-infected cells upon binding of antibodies to cell surface–expressed viral antigens. Viruses have thus evolved strategies to subvert activation of

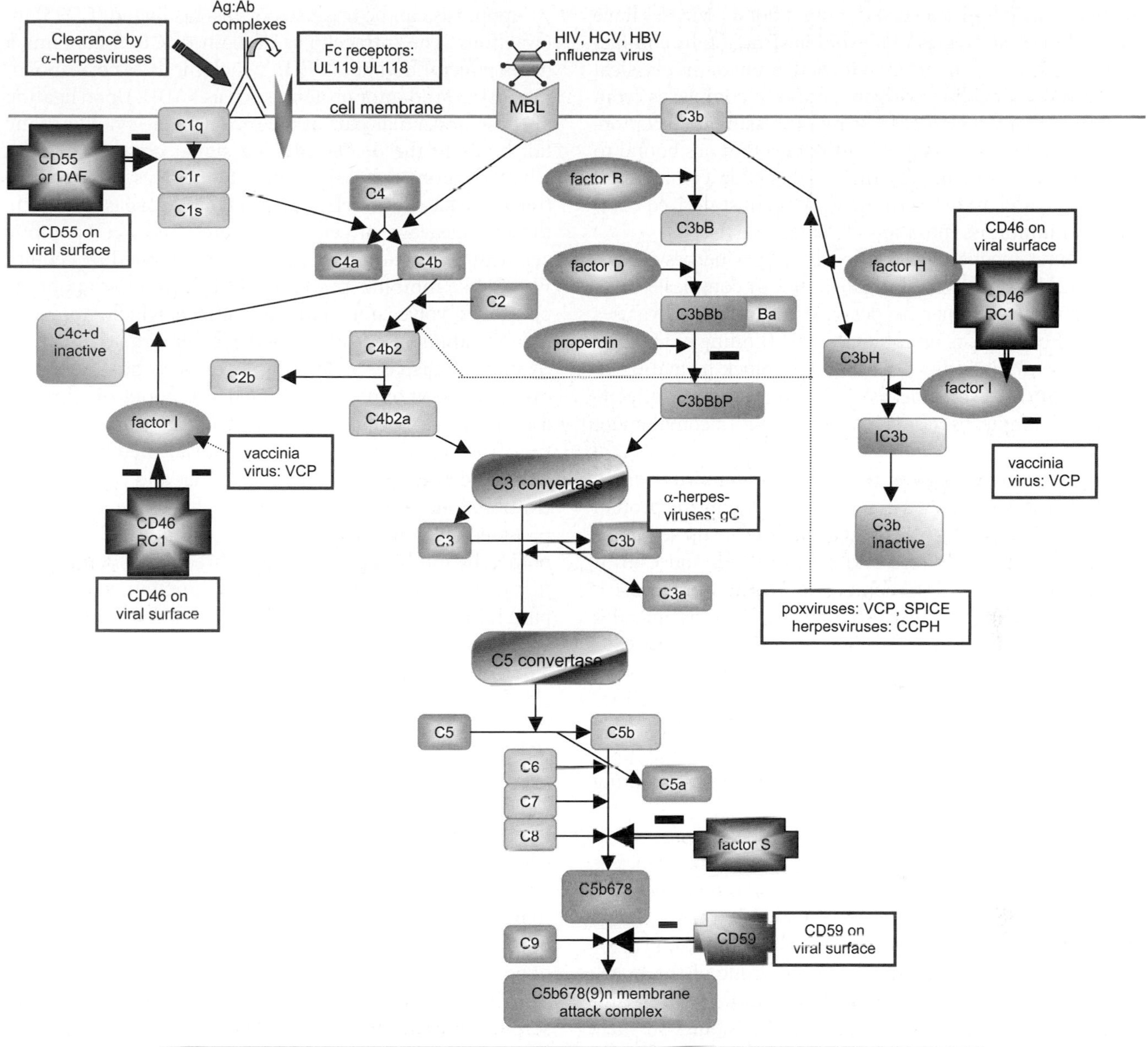

FIGURE 36.4 Interference of activation of the complement cascade pathways. CCPH, complement control protein homolog; CD, cluster of differentiation; HBV, hepatitis B virus; HCV, hepatitis C virus; HIV, human immunodeficiency virus; MBL, mannose-binding lectin; SPICE, smallpox inhibitor of complement enzymes; VCP, vaccinia virus complement control protein.

complement (178) (Figure 36.4). The complement system is composed of dozens of proteins that are sequentially activated through three distinct pathways called the classical, alternative, and lectin pathways. The classical pathway is activated once a virus, such as HIV or HCMV, or an antigen–antibody complex, binds to C1q, which forms a complex with C1r and C1s. Conformational changes of C1q enable the protein to activate C1r, which cleaves C1s into a protease, which in turn cleaves C4. Complement is activated through the alternative pathway as a direct consequence of C3b deposition on the surface of membranes. The mannose-binding lectin (MBL) pathway is induced through the binding of monosaccharides to MBL, which activates the attached protease and causes cleavage of C4. A number of viruses can bind MBL, such as HIV, HCV, HBV, and influenza virus. All three pathways converge after formation of the C3 complex, and after a few more steps, eventually form a complex that pokes holes into membranes, causing cell or viral death. Complement activation is tightly controlled through inhibitory molecules such as the C1 inhibitor, the decay-accelerating factor (DAF or CD55), the membrane cofactor protein (MCP or CD46), the C4-binding protein, CD59, and factor H. Many of these molecules contain a short 60-amino acid consensus sequence with four conserved cystein bonds. Viruses have evolved three strategies to a avoid destruction by complement: (a) They can interfere with activation of the classical pathway by shedding antigen–antibody complexes from the surface of infected cells or by expressing Fc receptor–like structures that complex antibodies that are bound to viral surface proteins; (b) they can encode complement inhibitors; and (c) they can incorporate host-derived complement inhibitors into their envelope.

The first mechanism is used by alpha herpesviruses, which rapidly eliminate antigen–antibody complexes from the cell surface. Other herpes viruses and coronaviruses express Fc receptors on infected cells. Binding of these Fc receptors to antibodies can sterically block formation of antigen–antibody complexes, or they may bind to antigen–antibody complexes in such a way as to block complement activation.

The second pathway is used by vaccinia virus, which encodes the vaccinia virus complement control protein (VCP). This protein has the typical consensus sequence of complement inhibitors and binds to C3b and C4b. It also acts as a cofactor to complement-regulating factor I. Variola virus, which causes smallpox in humans, encodes the smallpox inhibitor of complement enzymes (SPICE), which inactivates C3b. Herpes virus saimiri encodes a complement control protein homolog (CCPH), which resembles DAF and inhibits C3 convertase activity. Alpha herpesviruses produce glycoprotein gC, which can bind C3b. EBV can cleave serum C3 into an inactive form, preventing activation of the alternative pathway.

The third pathway is used by enveloped viruses. Budding of such viruses from the cell membrane takes place at lipid rafts that are rich in cholesterol and other lipids and also contain glycosyl phosphatidyl inositol anchored complement control proteins such as CD46, CD55, and CD59, which are incorporated into the membrane of the extracellular enveloped form of poxviruses, herpesviruses, and HIV. Alpha viruses pick up sialic acid residues on their surface during budding, inhibiting C3b deposition on the virus surface, which would initiate the alternative pathway of complement activation.

It should be noted that CD46, one of the inhibitors of complement activation, is used as a receptor by several viruses, such as adenoviruses of subfamily B2 and measles virus. To what degree this affects complement activation is unknown.

Inhibition of Apoptosis

The damage caused by virus infection can induce cells to undergo programmed cell death. Premature cell death is counterproductive for viruses if it occurs before they have successfully completed their replication cycle. Viruses, especially poxviruses, have developed a number of pathways to inhibit apoptosis (179,180) (Figure 36.5).

Apoptosis can be triggered by fas–fas ligand (CD95) interactions. The intracellular domain of CD95 contains a death effector domain (DED), which binds to corresponding DEDs on adaptor proteins such as FADD. Upon ligation of the extracellular part of the receptor, the cytoplasmatic tail binds to the death-inducing signal complex (DISC), which contains the caspase FLICE. This results in activation of caspase 8, which in turn activates caspase 3, which, through cleavage of cellular proteins, induces apoptotic cell death. Activation of caspase 8 is inhibited by cellular FLICE-like inhibitor proteins (cFLIP). Another apoptotic pathway involves mitochondial damage, which, upon permeabilization of the mitrochondrial membrane, causes activation of caspase 9. Apoptosis can also be induced by overexpression of p53, which mediates apoptosis through a pathway involving activation of Bax and its translocation from the cytosol to mitochondrial membranes, cytochrome c release from mitochondria, and caspase 9 activation, followed by the activation of caspase 3, 6, and 7. p53-Mediated apoptosis can be blocked at multiple checkpoints, by inhibiting p53 activity directly, by Bcl-2 family members regulating mitochondrial function, and by caspase inhibitors.

Poxviruses inhibit apoptosis of infected cells through a number of pathways. Molluscum contagiosum virus (MCV) prevents caspase 8 activation through two viral proteins called MC159 and MC160, which bind to FADD and procaspase 8, inhibiting activation of caspase 8. Some poxviruses produce a serine protease inhibitor–like molecule called crmA or SPI-2. CrmA inhibits the activity of caspases such as ICE (IL-1β–converting enzyme) and caspase 8, which are part of the death pathway. In addition, both proteins bind to granzyme B, a serine protease that is part of the lytic granules secreted by cytolytic T cells upon recognition of their target antigen. The SPI-2 family of poxvirus serpins, such as B13R from vaccinia virus, can inhibit fas- or TNF-mediated apoptosis. SERP-2, another serpin expressed by myxoma virus, inhibits caspase 1 and granzyme B protein. PKR not only inhibits translation of proteins, it may also activate caspase 8.

Intracellular reactive oxygen intermediates trigger apoptotic cell death. H_2O_2 can be reduced by cellular enzymes such as glutathione peroxidase, which is a selenocysteine-containing protein. The MC066 of MCV shows 74% sequence homology to this enzyme and was shown to protect cells from death due to reactive oxygen intermediates. MC066 does not interfere with apoptosis induced through fas.

The p28 of ectromeliavirus (mousepox) and the N1R of Shope fibroma virus have a RING finger motif that inhibits apoptosis induced by UV light. Inhibition is upstream of caspase 3. The M11L protein of myxoma virus localizes to mitochondrial membranes and prevents their permeabilization upon cell damage, thus inhibiting activation of caspase 3. The M-T4, M-T2, and M-T5 of

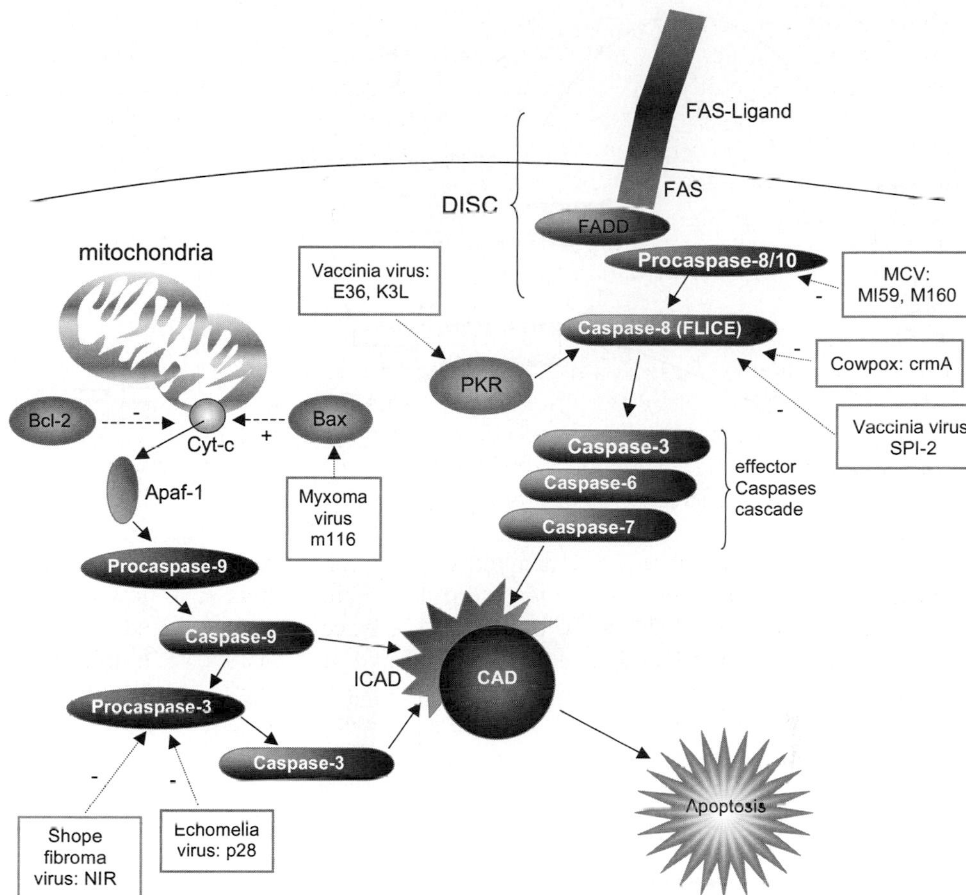

FIGURE 36.5 The pathway to viral apoptosis. Apaf-1, apoptosis protease activating factor-1; Bax, Bcl-2–associated X protein; Bcl-2, B-cell lymphoma 2; CAD, caspase-activated DNase; Cyt-c, cytochrome c; DISC, death-inducing signaling complex; FADD, Fas-associated death-domain protein; FAS, fatty acid synthase; FLICE, Fadd-like ICE (caspace 8); ICAD, inhibitor of CAD; PKR, dsRNA-dependent protein kinase.

myxomaviruses also inhibit apoptosis through as-yet-undefined pathways.

HCMV encodes at least two proteins that interfere directly with pathways that cause programmed cell death. UL35 protein is an inhibitor of caspase 8–induced apoptosis. UL36 binds to pro-caspase 8 and blocks its recruitment to the death-inducing signaling complex (DISC), a step preceding caspase 8 activation. vMIA binds and sequesters Bax at mitochondria, and interferes with BH3-only-death-factor/Bax-complex-mediated permeabilization of mitochondria.

A number of viruses encode antiapoptotic proteins with Bcl2-like activity. Examples include the E1B 19K polypeptide of adenoviruses, BHRF1 of EBV, and A179 of African swine fever. The E1B/55K protein of adenovirus, furthermore, inhibits p53-mediated apoptosis, whereas E3/10.4K and 14.5K proteins accelerate degradation of Fas and TRAIL receptors from the cell surface.

Escape by Subverting Antigen Processing and Antigen Presentation

A number of viruses have devised strategies to impair presentation of their antigens by the MHC class I pathway, thus reducing activation and effector functions of antigen-specific $CD8^+$ T cells, again stressing the importance of this cell subset for antiviral defense (181,182). Nearly every step of the MHC class I presentation pathway can be interfered with, and some viruses encode multiple proteins that act at different levels of the MHC class I processing pathway. Interference of MHC class II processing is less common but has also been described (Figure 36.6).

Viruses can escape detection T cells by inhibiting synthesis of MHC molecules. For example, tat of HIV-1 represses the MHC class I promoter. Human cytomegalovirus (HCMV) can impair MHC class II expression through two pathways. MHC class II molecules are expressed on only a subset of cells, and their transcription is tightly regulated, mainly through the class II transcactivator (CIITA), a non-DNA–binding protein that interacts with transcription factors that associate with the MHC class II promoter. CIITA is the rate-limiting factor of MHC class II production and thus determines the expression pattern of these molecules. CIITA production is regulated by four promoters, two of which sponsor constitutive expression of CIITA in antigen-presenting cells. One is activated by IFN-γ and causes increased MHC class II expression in the presence of this cytokine. Upon binding of IFN-γ to its receptor, Jak1 and Jak2 thyrosine-phosphorylate the intracellular domain of the receptor, which then recruits Stat1.

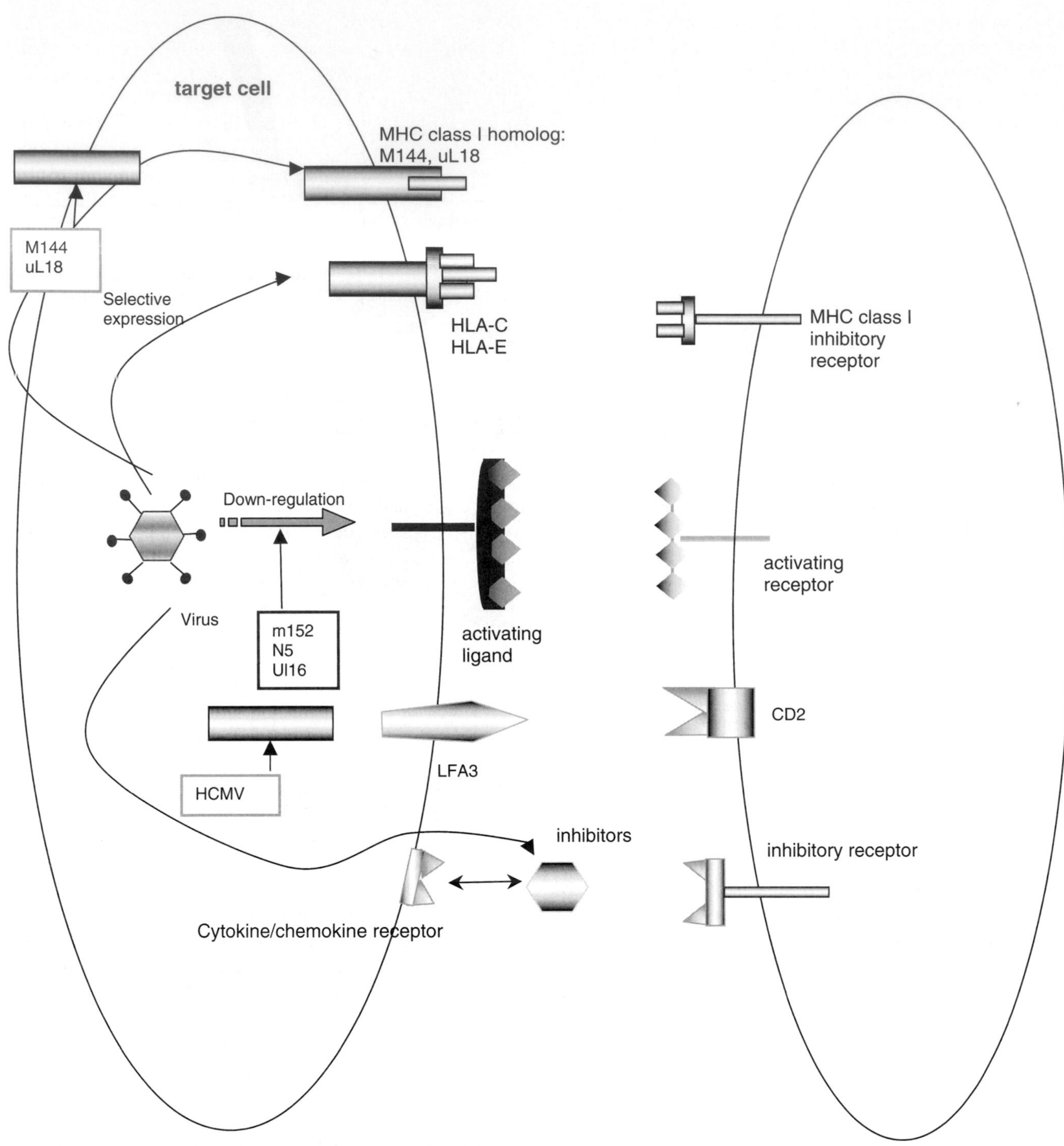

FIGURE 36.6 MHC class II processing. CD2, cluster of differentiation 2; HCMV, human cytomegalovirus; HLA, human leukocyte antigen; LFA-3, lymphocyte function–associated antigen type 3; MHC, major histocompatibility complex.

Stat1 phosphorylated by Jak1 and Jak2 forms a homodimer that is translocated to the nucleus. The Stat1 homodimers bind to the IFN-γ activation sequence GAS present in promoters of IFN-γ–inducible genes. This causes production of IRF-1 (interferon regulatory factor-1), a transcription factor that, together with Stat-1 homodimers and the ubiquitously expressed upstream factor-1 (USF-1), activate the inducible promoter of CIITA. Proteins of HCMV can increase degradation of Jak1 kinase and can further decrease CIITA activity in a Stat1-independent way.

Transport of MHC molecules to the cell membranes requires their binding to peptides, which for loading of MHC class I molecules depends on active transport of peptides from the cytoplasm to the ER with the help of TAP. The E7 of HPV-18 and the E1A protein of adenovirus human serotype 12 inhibit the promoter controlling TAP production. The mK3 protein of mouse gamma herpesviruses such as HHV-8 binds to TAP and tapasin, resulting in their ubiquination and degradation. The 19K polypeptide encoded by the E3 domain of adenoviruses binds to TAP and prevents association between TAP and tapasin. Other herpesviruses, such as HSV and HCMV, encode proteins that inhibit TAP-mediated peptide transport. US6, a protein encoded by HCMV, binds to TAP and prevents binding of ATP, which is needed for peptide transport. The ICP47 polypeptide from herpes simplex virus (HSV) inhibits TAP by blocking its peptide-binding site, thus preventing its association with other peptides. EBV encodes a protein that weakly binds the IL-10 receptor. Similar to cellular IL-10, the EBV protein reduces expression of TAP.

CD10 and CD13 serve aminopeptidases to trim peptides to a size that allows their binding to the groove of MHC class I or II molecules. Yet-to-be-identified proteins of HCMV block the activity of CD10 and CD13. Although CD10 expression is apparently blocked at the transcriptional or translational level, CD13 seems to be retained within the ER.

Once MHC class I molecules have bound peptides, they are transported to the cell surface to present the peptides to $CD8^+$ T cells. A number of viral products interfere with this transport, by retaining MHC class I molecules within the ER, by affecting their export into the cytoplasm, or by interfering with passage through the Golgi apparatus. The cytosolic tail of the 19K gene product of the E3 domain of adenovirus contains a dilysine motif that inhibits MHC class I trafficking by acting as an ER retrieval motif. The US3 and US10 proteins of HCMV also prevent the exit of MHC class I from the ER through pathways that are still poorly understood. The m152 of murine cytomegalovirus (MCMV), which encodes a 40-kDa glycoprotein, affects retention of peptide-loaded MHC class I molecules in a pre-Golgi compartment.

US11 and US2 of HCMV dislocate the MHC class I molecules from the ER to the cytoplasm, where they are rapidly degraded. In the presence of US2, the intracellular half-life of MHC class I is reduced from about 6 hours to less than 2 minutes, demonstrating that this pathway of MHC class I destruction is highly efficient. US2 binds to MHC class I molecules in the ER while the protein is being glycosylated, causing its incorrect folding. The complex is then transported through Sec61 pores back into the cytoplasm, where, upon deglycosylation, both proteins—i.e., the MHC class I molecule and the viral protein—are degraded. US11 has a similar mode of action, but unlike US2, it does not become demolished upon translocation into the cytoplasm. The m6/gp48 protein of MCMV binds to MHC class I/β2-microglobulin complexes in the ER. During transport of the complex to the cell surface, the m6/gp48 protein, whose cytoplasmic tail has a dileucin motif, targets the complex to lysosomes where they are proteolytically digested.

The K3 and K4 proteins of HHV8 lower expression of cell surface MHC class I molecules by enhancing their endocytosis into clathrin-coated pits. In addition, K5 downregulates cell surface expression of the costimulatory molecule CD86. Nef of HIV-1 reduces cell surface expression of MHC class I by redirecting the molecules from the trans-Golgi network to the endosomes. In addition, nef reduces expression of costimulatory molecules of the B7 family.

USE OF VIRAL VECTORS FOR GENE TRANSFER

The ease with which viruses move their genes into mammalian host cells has led scientists to explore their use for gene replacement therapy to correct missing or faulty genes. Needless to say, after millions of years of evolution that empowered complex organisms to fight virus infections, 20 years of viral gene replacement therapy research has thus far met with very little success in humans.

To allow for their use in gene replacement therapy, viruses are typically rendered replication-defective, and part or all of their genome is replaced with the gene that produces the therapeutic protein under the control of regulatory elements. Numerous types of viruses have been explored or are currently under scrutiny. Two of those, replication-defective adenovirus vectors and adeno-associated virus (AAV) vectors, well attest to the vows of viral gene therapy.

Twenty years ago, E1-deleted adenovirus vectors, most commonly based on the human serotype 5, were heralded as the potential solution to all genetic diseases (183). E1-deleted adenovirus vectors, or subsequent second-, third-, and fourth-generation vectors in which more and more of the viral genome had been removed, indeed succeeded in transferring genes into experimental animals (184). In animals that were immunoincompetent, such as SCID mice, expression of the transferred genes was sustained. In immunocompetent animals the transgene product and the antigens of the vector stimulated, as one would expect, potent B- and T-cell responses; $CD8^+$ T cells rapidly eliminated the transduced cells, while neutralizing antibodies to the hexon protein of adenovirus prevented successful reapplication of the vectors. In spite of limited success in experimental animals, human trials were initiated, in which the potent innate immune responses to the adenovirus vectors caused significant morbidity and resulted in the death of one patient (185).

AAVs vectored for use in gene replacement therapy are so-called dependo-viruses of the parvovirinae subfamily that in nature infect concomitantly with a helper virus such as adenovirus or herpes virus. Helper viruses are needed for multiple steps in the replicative cycle of AAV. So far, six distinct serotypes have been identified in humans, termed AAV-1 through -6. Of those, AAV-2–based vectors have been used most commonly for gene therapy. The AAV-2 genome is composed of a 4.7-kb single-stranded DNA flanked by inverted terminal repeats (ITRs). ITRs initiate DNA replication and are required for encapsidation of the genome. The genome contains two open reading frames (ORFs), one encoding proteins needed for DNA replication and for integration, the other encoding the three capsid proteins, which are generated from a single ORF by alternative splicing and distinct translation-initiation sites. In AAVs used for gene transfer, the ORFs are removed and replaced with the gene of interest, including regulatory elements flanked by the ITRs (186). The resulting vector can be grown in cells that provide the proteins encoded by AAV in trans and that furthermore provide helper virus functions commonly provided through gene products of adenovirus. Humans are naturally exposed to AAV, which they acquire together with a helper virus. The gene therapy literature shows that AAV vectors, depending on the dose, the amount of vector, the type of the transgene product, and the host's genetic makeup, can be poorly immunogenic, allowing for long-term expression of the transferred gene in mice, canines, and nonhuman primates (187). In particular, AAVs appear to escape detection by the innate immune system and thus fail to elicit the inflammatory reactions (188) that are needed to induce adaptive immunity. Nevertheless, in spite of very promising preclinical data, in a clinical trial in which AAV-2 expressing factor IX was transferred to the liver for correction of hemophilia B, patients eliminated the transduced hepatocytes, most likely through $CD8^+$ T cells directed against the capsid proteins of AAV-2 (189). It is likely that in humans during natural infections with AAV together with a helper virus, the innate immune response to the helper virus promotes adaptive immune responses including $CD8^+$ T cells against antigens of AAV. Upon AAV-mediated gene transfer, even if AAV by itself fails to cause a strong inflammatory reaction, pre-existing memory $CD8^+$ T cells would be expected to be reactivated and do what they are supposed to do—eliminate the AAV vector-transduced cells.

It is of interest to note that both E1-deleted adenovirus vectors and AAV vectors that remain favored tools of gene therapists are currently in clinical trials as vaccine carriers (190,191).

CONCLUSION

Our immune system is in constant battle with viruses, which in spite of their puny sizes are formidable opponents. Viruses continue to take a tremendous toll on human lives, outpacing wars and natural disasters combined. Although vaccines and antiviral drugs have lessened the impact of some viral infections, new viruses that can cause disease and death in humans are constantly evolving, raising havoc in human societies. Our best defense against viruses remains our immune system, which in most cases can rapidly control acute infections. Adaptive immunity appears to be less suited to eliminate viruses that have mastered the art to establish chronic infections. This results in part from defense mechanisms of those viruses, but it also results from a shortcoming in adaptive immunity, which has to eliminate pathogens without causing undue damage to its own host. During chronic infection, negative immunoregulatory mechanisms hamper the effectiveness of adaptive immune responses. A full understanding of the delicate balance between immunity and persistent viruses is still evolving, and further knowledge may help to devise treatments that lessen the burden of chronic viral infection.

REFERENCES

1. Bergelson JM, Cunningham JA, Droguett G, et al. Isolation of a common receptor for Coxsackie B viruses and adenoviruses 2 and 5. *Science.* 1997;275:1320–1323.
2. Roelvink PW, Lizonova A, Lee JG, et al. The coxsackievirus-adenovirus receptor protein can function as a cellular attachment protein for adenovirus serotypes from subgroups A, C, D, E, and F. *J Virol.* 1998;72:7909–7915.
3. Gaggar A, Shayakhmetov DM, Liszewski MK, et al. Localization of regions in CD46 that interact with adenovirus. *J Virol.* 2005;79:7503–7513.
4. Naniche D, Varior-Krishnan G, Cervoni F, et al. Human membrane cofactor protein (CD46) acts as a cellular receptor for measles virus. *J Virol.* 1993;67:6025–6032.
5. Santoro F, Kennedy PE, Locatelli G, et al. CD46 is a cellular receptor for human herpesvirus 6. *Cell.* 1999;99:817–827.
6. Giranda VL, Chapman MS, Rossmann MG. Modeling of the human intercellular adhesion molecule-1, the human rhinovirus major group receptor. *Proteins.* 1990;7:227–233.
7. Lopez M, Aoubala M, Jordier F, et al. The human poliovirus receptor related 2 protein is a new hematopoietic/endothelial homophilic adhesion molecule. *Blood.* 1998;92:4602–4611.
8. Montgomery RI, Warner MS, Lum BJ, et al. Herpes simplex virus-1 entry into cells mediated by a novel member of the TNF/NGF receptor family. *Cell.* 1996;87:427–436.
9. Summerford C, Samulski RJ. Membrane-associated heparan sulfate proteoglycan is a receptor for adeno-associated virus type 2 virions. *J Virol.* 1998;72:1438–1445.
10. Liu H, Naismith JH, Hay RT. Adenovirus DNA replication. *Curr Top Microbiol Immunol.* 2003;272:131–164.
11. Janeway CA Jr, Medzhitov R. Innate immune recognition. *Annu Rev Immunol.* 2002;20:197–216.
12. Takeda K, Akira S. Toll-like receptors in innate immunity. *Int Immunol.* 2005;17:1–14.
13. Schroder M, Bowie AG. TLR3 in antiviral immunity: key player or bystander? *Trends Immunol.* 2005;26:462–468.
14. Bieback K, Lien E, Klagge IM, et al. Hemagglutinin protein of wild-type measles virus activates toll-like receptor 2 signaling. *J Virol.* 2002;76:8729–8736.
15. Kurt-Jones EA, Popova L, Kwinn L, et al. Pattern recognition receptors TLR4 and CD14 mediate response to respiratory syncytial virus. *Nat Immunol.* 2000;1:398–401.
16. Akira S. Toll-like receptors: lessons from knockout mice. *Biochem Soc Trans.* 2000;28:551–556.

17. Yamamoto M, Takeda K, Akira S. TIR domain-containing adaptors define the specificity of TLR signaling. *Mol Immunol.* 2004;40:861–868.
18. Samuel CE, Kuhen KL, George CX, et al. The PKR protein kinase—an interferon-inducible regulator of cell growth and differentiation. *Int J Hematol.* 1997;65:227–237.
19. Samuel CE. Antiviral actions of interferons. *Clin Microbiol Rev.* 2001;14:778–809.
20. Diebold SS, Montoya M, Unger H, et al. Viral infection switches non-plasmacytoid dendritic cells into high interferon producers. *Nature.* 2003;424:324–328.
21. Meylan E, Tschopp J. Toll-like receptors and RNA helicases: two parallel ways to trigger antiviral responses. *Mol Cell.* 2006;22:561–569.
22. Werts C, Girardin SE, Philpott DJ. TIR, CARD and PYRIN: three domains for an antimicrobial triad. *Cell Death Differ.* 2006;13:798–815.
23. Wang T, Town T, Alexopoulou L, et al. Toll-like receptor 3 mediates West Nile virus entry into the brain causing lethal encephalitis. *Nat Med.* 2004;10:1366–1373.
24. McKimmie CS, Johnson N, Fooks AR, et al. Viruses selectively up-regulate Toll-like receptors in the central nervous system. *Biochem Biophys Res Commun.* 2005;336:925–933.
25. Ank N, West H, Paludan SR. IFN-lambda: novel antiviral cytokines. *J Interferon Cytokine Res.* 2006;26:373–379.
26. Honda K, Yanai H, Takaoka A, et al. Regulation of the type I IFN induction: a current view. *Int Immunol.* 2005;17:1367–1378.
27. Taniguchi T, Ogasawara K, Takaoka A, et al. IRF family of transcription factors as regulators of host defense. *Annu Rev Immunol.* 2001;19:623–655.
28. Platanias LC. Mechanisms of type-I- and type-II-interferon-mediated signalling. *Nat Rev Immunol.* 2005;5:375–386.
29. Darnell JE Jr. Studies of IFN-induced transcriptional activation uncover the Jak-Stat pathway. *J Interferon Cytokine Res.* 1998;18:549–554.
30. Mihm S, Frese M, Meier V, et al. Interferon type I gene expression in chronic hepatitis C. *Lab Invest.* 2004;84:1148–1159.
31. Zurcher T, Pavlovic J, Staeheli P. Mechanism of human MxA protein action: variants with changed antiviral properties. *EMBO J.* 1992;11:1657–1661.
32. Warfel AH, Belsito DV, Thorbecke GJ. Activation of an HIV-LTR-CAT transgene in murine macrophages by interferon-gamma in synergism with other cytokines or endotoxin. *Adv Exp Med Biol.* 1995;378:489–492.
33. Karupiah G, Xie QW, Buller RM, et al. Inhibition of viral replication by interferon-gamma-induced nitric oxide synthase. *Science.* 1993;261:1445–1448.
34. Malik AH, Lee WM. Chronic hepatitis B virus infection: treatment strategies for the next millennium. *Ann Intern Med.* 2000;132:723–731.
35. Lauer GM, Walker BD. Hepatitis C virus infection. *N Engl J Med.* 2001;345:41–52.
36. Gross G. Therapy of human papillomavirus infection and associated epithelial tumors. *Intervirology.* 1997;40:368–377.
37. Nelson PJ, Krensky AM. Chemokines, lymphocytes and viruses: what goes around, comes around. *Curr Opin Immunol.* 1998;10:265–270.
38. Salazar-Mather TP, Hokeness KL. Calling in the troops: regulation of inflammatory cell trafficking through innate cytokine/chemokine networks. *Viral Immunol.* 2003;16:291–306.
39. Hamerman JA, Ogasawara K, Lanier LL. NK cells in innate immunity. *Curr Opin Immunol.* 2005;17:29–35.
40. Bottino C, Moretta L, Pende D. Learning how to discriminate between friends and enemies, a lesson from Natural Killer cells. *Mol Immunol.* 2004;41:569–575.
41. Yokoyama WM, Plougastel BF. Immune functions encoded by the natural killer gene complex. *Nat Rev Immunol.* 2003;3:304–316.
42. Tomasello E, Blery M, Vely F, et al. Signaling pathways engaged by NK cell receptors: double concerto for activating receptors, inhibitory receptors and NK cells. *Semin Immunol.* 2000;12:139–147.
43. Mandelboim O, Porgador A. NKp46. *Int J Biochem Cell Biol.* 2001;33:1147–1150.
44. Eidenschenk C, Dunne J, Jouanguy E, et al. A novel primary immunodeficiency with specific natural-killer cell deficiency maps to the centromeric region of chromosome 8. *Am J Hum Genet.* 2006;78:721–727.
45. Leon B, Lopez-Bravo M, Ardavin C. Monocyte-derived dendritic cells. *Semin Immunol.* 2005;17:313–338.
46. Barchet W, Cella M, Colonna M. Plasmacytoid dendritic cells—virus experts of innate immunity. *Semin Immunol.* 2005;17:253–261.
47. McLellan AD, Kampgen E. Functions of myeloid and lymphoid dendritic cells. *Immunol Lett.* 2000;72:101–105.
48. Barchet W, Cella M, Colonna M. Plasmacytoid dendritic cells—virus experts of innate immunity. *Semin Immunol.* 2005;17:253–261.
49. Honda K, Ohba Y, Yanai H, et al. Spatiotemporal regulation of MyD88-IRF-7 signalling for robust type-I interferon induction. *Nature.* 2005 21;434:1035–1040.
50. Haeryfar SM. The importance of being a pDC in antiviral immunity: the IFN mission versus Ag presentation? *Trends Immunol.* 2005;26:311–317.
51. Johansson-Lindbom B, Svensson M, Pabst O, et al. Functional specialization of gut CD103+ dendritic cells in the regulation of tissue-selective T cell homing. *J Exp Med.* 2005;202:1063–1073.
52. Bacchetta R, Gregori S, Roncarolo MG. CD4+ regulatory T cells: mechanisms of induction and effector function. *Autoimmun Rev.* 2005;4:491–496.
53. Mahnke K, Enk AH. Dendritic cells: key cells for the induction of regulatory T cells? *Curr Top Microbiol Immunol.* 2005;293:133–150.
54. Linsley PS, Ledbetter JA. The role of the CD28 receptor during T cell responses to antigen. *Annu Rev Immunol.* 1993;11:191–212.
55. Wassink L, Vieira PL, Smits HH, et al. ICOS expression by activated human Th cells is enhanced by IL-12 and IL-23: increased ICOS expression enhances the effector function of both Th1 and Th2 cells. *J Immunol.* 2004;173:1779–1786.
56. Herman AE, Freeman GJ, Mathis D, et al. CD4+CD25+ T regulatory cells dependent on ICOS promote regulation of effector cells in the prediabetic lesion. *J Exp Med.* 2004;199:1479–1489.
57. Loke P, Allison JP. Emerging mechanisms of immune regulation: the extended B7 family and regulatory T cells. *Arthritis Res Ther.* 2004;6:208–214.
58. Kryczek I, Wei S, Zou L, et al. Cutting Edge: Induction of B7-H4 on APCs through IL-10: novel suppressive mode for regulatory T cells. *J Immunol.* 2006;177:40–44.
59. Greenwald RJ, Latchman YE, Sharpe AH. Negative co-receptors on lymphocytes. *Curr Opin Immunol.* 2002;14:391–396.
60. Barber DL, Wherry EJ, Masopust D, et al. Restoring function in exhausted CD8 T cells during chronic viral infection. *Nature.* 2006;439:682–687.
61. Croft M. The evolving crosstalk between co-stimulatory and co-inhibitory receptors: HVEM-BTLA. *Trends Immunol.* 2005;26:292–294.
62. Yewdell J, Anton LC, Bacik I, et al. Generating MHC class I ligands from viral gene products. *Immunol Rev.* 1999;172:97–108.
63. Koszinowski U, Ertl H. Role of early viral surface antigens in cellular immune response to vaccinia virus. *Eur J Immunol.* 1976;6:679–683.
64. Larsson M, Messmer D, Somersan S, et al. Requirement of mature dendritic cells for efficient activation of influenza A-specific memory CD8+ T cells. *J Immunol.* 2000;165:1182–1190.
65. York IA, Goldberg AL, Mo XY, et al. Proteolysis and class I major histocompatibility complex antigen presentation. *Immunol Rev.* 1999;172:49–66.
66. Pamer E, Cresswell P. Mechanisms of MHC class I–restricted antigen processing. *Annu Rev Immunol.* 1998;16:323–358.
67. Elliott T. How does TAP associate with MHC class I molecules? *Immunol Today.* 1997;18:375–379.
68. McCluskey J, Rossjohn J, Purcell AW. TAP genes and immunity. *Curr Opin Immunol.* 2004;16:651–659.
69. Latron F, Pazmany L, Morrison J, et al. A critical role for conserved residues in the cleft of HLA-A2 in presentation of a nonapeptide to T cells. *Science.* 1992;257:964–967.
70. Cresswell P, Bangia N, Dick T, et al. The nature of the MHC class I peptide loading complex. *Immunol Rev.* 1999;172:21–28.
71. Heath WR, Carbone FR. Cytotoxic T lymphocyte activation by cross-priming. *Curr Opin Immunol.* 1999;11:314–318.

72. Gagnon E, Duclos S, Rondeau C, et al. Endoplasmic reticulum-mediated phagocytosis is a mechanism of entry into macrophages. *Cell.* 2002;110:119–131.
73. Yewdell JW, Haeryfar SM. Understanding presentation of viral antigens to CD8+ T cells *in vivo*: the key to rational vaccine design. *Annu Rev Immunol.* 2005;23:651–682.
74. Srivastava P. Interaction of heat shock proteins with peptides and antigen presenting cells: chaperoning of the innate and adaptive immune responses. *Annu Rev Immunol.* 2002;20:395–425.
75. Lichterfeld M, Yu XG, Le Gall S, et al. Immunodominance of HIV-1-specific CD8(+) T-cell responses in acute HIV-1 infection: at the crossroads of viral and host genetics. *Trends Immunol.* 2005;26: 166–171.
76. Brossay L, Burdin N, Tangri S, et al. Antigen-presenting function of mouse CD1: one molecule with two different kinds of antigenic ligands. *Immunol Rev.* 1998;163:139–150.
77. Ridge JP, Di Rosa F, Matzinger P. A conditioned dendritic cell can be a temporal bridge between a CD4+ T-helper and a T-killer cell. *Nature.* 1998;393:474–478.
78. Shedlock DJ, Shen H. Requirement for CD4 T cell help in generating functional CD8 T cell memory. *Science.* 2003;300:337–339.
79. Henkart PA, Catalfamo M. CD8+ effector cells. *Adv Immunol.* 2004; 83:233–252.
80. Betts MR, Exley B, Price DA, et al. Characterization of functional and phenotypic changes in anti-Gag vaccine-induced T cell responses and their role in protection after HIV-1 infection. *Proc Natl Acad Sci U S A.* 2005;102:4512–4517.
81. LFA-1/ICAM-1 in the binding and transendothelial migration of T lymphocytes and T lymphoblasts across high endothelial venules. *Int Immunol.* 2000;12:241–251.
82. Li X, Abdi K, Rawn J, et al. LFA-1 and L-selectin regulation of recirculating lymphocyte tethering and rolling on lung microvascular endothelium. *Am J Respir Cell Mol Biol.* 1996;14: 398–406.
83. Kowalczyk DW, Wlazlo AP, Blaszczyk-Thurin M, et al. A method that allows easy characterization of tumor-infiltrating lymphocytes. *J Immunol Methods.* 2001;253:163–175.
84. Podack ER. Execution and suicide: cytotoxic lymphocytes enforce Draconian laws through separate molecular pathways. *Curr Opin Immunol.* 1995;7:11–16.
85. Kaech SM, Tan JT, Wherry EJ, et al. Selective expression of the interleukin 7 receptor identifies effector CD8 T cells that give rise to long-lived memory cells. *Nat Immunol.* 2003;4:1191–1198.
86. Lefrancois L. Development, trafficking, and function of memory T-cell subsets. *Immunol Rev.* 2006;211:93–103.
87. Wherry EJ, Ahmed R. Memory CD8 T-cell differentiation during viral infection. *J Virol.* 2004;78:5535–5545.
88. Masopust D, Vezys V, Marzo AL, et al. Preferential localization of effector memory cells in nonlymphoid tissue. *Science.* 2001;291:2413–2417.
89. Wherry EJ, Teichgraber V, Becker TC, et al. Lineage relationship and protective immunity of memory CD8 T cell subsets. *Nat Immunol.* 2003;4:225–234.
90. Cerwenka A, Morgan TM, Dutton RW. Naive, effector, and memory CD8 T cells in protection against pulmonary influenza virus infection: homing properties rather than initial frequencies are crucial. *J Immunol.* 1999;163:5535–5543.
91. Surh CD, Sprent J. Regulation of mature T cell homeostasis. *Semin Immunol.* 2005;17:183–191.
92. Wherry EJ, Teichgraber V, Becker TC, et al. Lineage relationship and protective immunity of memory CD8 T cell subsets. *Nat Immunol.* 2003;4:225–234.
93. Masopust D, Ha SJ, Vezys V, et al. Stimulation history dictates memory CD8 T cell phenotype: implications for prime-boost vaccination. *J Immunol.* 2006;177:831–839.
94. Wherry EJ, Blattman JN, Murali-Krishna K, et al. Viral persistence alters CD8 T-cell immunodominance and tissue distribution and results in distinct stages of functional impairment. *J Virol.* 2003;77:4911–4927.
95. Barber DL, Wherry EJ, Masopust D, et al. Restoring function in exhausted CD8 T cells during chronic viral infection. *Nature.* 2006;439:682–687.
96. Pawelec G, Koch S, Franceschi C, et al. Human immunosenescence: does it have an infectious component? *Ann NY Acad Sci.* 2006;1067:56–65.
97. Neutra M, Pringault E, Kraehenbuhl JP. Antigen sampling across epithelial barriers and induction of mucosal immune responses. *Annu Rev Immunol.* 1996;14: 275–300.
98. Holt PG, Stumbles PA, McWilliam AS. Functional studies on dendritic cells in the respiratory tract and related mucosal tissues. *J Leukoc Biol.* 1999;66:272–275.
99. Ferguson A, Parrott DVM. The effect of antigen deprivation on thymus-dependent and thymus-independent lymphocytes in the small intestine of the mouse. *Clin Exp Immunol.* 1972;12: 477–488.
100. Yoshikai Y, Ishida A, Murosaki S, et al. Sequential appearance of T-cell receptor $\gamma\delta$- and $\alpha\beta$-bearing intestinal intra-epithelial lymphocytes in mice after irradiation. *Immunology.* 1991;74: 583–588.
101. Poussier P, Julius M. Thymus independent T cell development and selection in the intestinal epithelium. *Annu Rev Immunol.* 1994;12:521–553.
102. Bandiera A, Itohara S, Bonneville M, et al. Extrathymic origin of intestinal epithelial lymphocytes bearing T-cell antigen receptor $\gamma\delta$. *Proc Natl Acad Sci U S A.* 1991;88:43–47.
103. Poussier P, Edouard P, Lee C, et al. Thymus-independent development and negative selection of T cells expressing T cell receptor α/β in the intestinal epithelial: evidence for distinct circulation patterns of gut- and thymus derived T lymphocytes. *J Exp Med.* 1992;176:187–199.
104. Beagley KW, Husband AJ. Intraepithelial lymphocytes: origins, distribution, and function. *Crit Rev Immunol.* 1998;18:237–254.
105. Hiromatsu K, Yoshikai Y, Matsuzaki G, et al. A protective role of $\gamma\delta$ T-cells in primary infection with *Listeria monocytogenes* in mice. *J Exp Med.* 1992;175:49–56.
106. Rosat J, MacDonald H, Louis J. A role for $\gamma\delta$+ T-cells during experimental infection of mice with *Leishmania major*. *J Immunol.* 1993;150:550–555.
107. Beagley K, Fujihashi K, Black C, et al. The *Mycobacterium tuberculosis* 71-kDa heat-shock protein induces proliferation and cytokine secretion by murine gut intraepithelial lymphocytes. *Eur J Immunol.* 1993;23:2049–2052.
108. Horner A, Jabara H, Ramesh N, et al. γ-δ T lymphocytes express CD40 ligands and induce isotype-switching in B lymphocytes. *J Exp Med.* 1995;181:1239–1244.
109. Chien Y, Jores R, Crowley MP. Recognition by γ/δ T cells. *Annu Rev Immunol.* 1996;14:511–532.
110. Nandi D, Allison JP. Phenotypic analysis and γ/Δ T cell receptor repertoire of murine T cells associated with the vaginal epithelium. *J Immunol.* 1991;147:1773–1778.
111. Shaw SK, Brenner MB. The beta 7 integrins in mucosal homing and retention. *Semin Immunol.* 1995;7:335–342.
112. Williams IR. Chemokine receptors and leukocyte trafficking in the mucosal immune system. *Immunol Res.* 2004;29:283–292.
113. Cheroutre H, Madakamutil L. Mucosal effector memory T cells: the other side of the coin. *Cell Mol Life Sci.* 2005;62:2853–2866.
114. Gupta M, Greer P, Mahanty S, et al. CD8-mediated protection against Ebola virus infection is perforin dependent. *J Immunol.* 2005;174:4198–4202.
115. Patterson CE, Lawrence DM, Echols LA, et al. Immune-mediated protection from measles virus-induced central nervous system disease is noncytolytic and gamma interferon dependent. *J Virol.* 2002;76:4497–4506.
116. Miller CJ, Abel K. Immune mechanisms associated with protection from vaginal SIV challenge in rhesus monkeys infected with virulence-attenuated SHIV 89.6. *J Med Primatol.* 2005;34:271–281.
117. Rhodes CJ, Anderson RM. A scaling analysis of measles epidemics in a small population. *Phil Trans R Soc Lond B Biol Sci.* 1996;351:1679–1688.
118. Epstein SL. Prior H1N1 influenza infection and susceptibility of Cleveland Family Study participants during the H2N2 pandemic of 1957: an experiment of nature. *J Infect Dis.* 2006;193:49–53.
119. Zinkernagel RM. On natural and artificial vaccinations. *Annu Rev Immunol.* 2003;21:515–546.
120. Ferrantelli F, Rasmussen RA, Buckley KA, et al. Complete protection of neonatal rhesus macaques against oral exposure to pathogenic simian-human immunodeficiency virus by human anti-HIV monoclonal antibodies. *J Infect Dis.* 2004;189:2167–2173.

121. McMichael AJ, Hanke T. HIV vaccines 1983–2003. *Nat Med.* 2003;9:874–880.
122. Castellino F, Zhong G, Germain RN. Antigen presentation by MHC class II molecules: invariant chain function, protein trafficking, and the molecular basis of diverse determinant capture. *Hum Immunol.* 1997;54:159–169.
123. Swain SL. CD4 T cell development and cytokine polarization: an overview. *J Leukoc Biol.* 1995;57:795–798.
124. Ward BJ, Griffin DE. Changes in cytokine production after measles virus vaccination: predominant production of IL-4 suggests induction of a Th2 response. *Clin Immunol Immunopathol.* 1993;67:171–177.
125. Nikiforow S, Bottomly K, Miller G, et al. Cytolytic CD4(+)-T-cell clones reactive to EBNA1 inhibit Epstein-Barr virus-induced B-cell proliferation. *J Virol.* 2003;77:12088–12104.
126. Swain SL, Agrewala JN, Brown DM, et al. CD4+ T-cell memory: generation and multi-faceted roles for CD4+ T cells in protective immunity to influenza. *Immunol Rev.* 2006;211:8–22.
127. Brown DM, Roman E, Swain SL. CD4 T cell responses to influenza infection. *Semin Immunol.* 2004;16:171–177.
128. Leung KN, Ada GL. Cells mediating delayed-type hypersensitivity in the lungs of mice infected with an influenza A virus. *Scand J Immunol.* 1980;12:393–400.
129. Bach BA, Greene MI, Benacerraf B, et al. Mechanisms of regulation of cell-mediated immunity. IV. Azobenzenearsonate-specific suppressor factor(s) bear cross-reactive idiotypic determinants the expression of which is linked to the heavy-chain allotype linkage group of genes. *J Exp Med.* 1979;149:1084–1098.
130. Sugihara S, Maruo S, Tsujimura T, et al. Autoimmune thyroiditis induced in mice depleted of particular T cell subsets. III. Analysis of regulatory cells suppressing the induction of thyroiditis. *Int Immunol.* 1990;2:343–351.
131. Suvas S, Rouse BT. Treg control of antimicrobial T cell responses. *Curr Opin Immunol.* 2006;18:344–348.
132. Belkaid Y, Rouse BT. Natural regulatory T cells in infectious disease. *Nat Immunol.* 2005;6:353–360.
133. Veldman C, Nagel A, Hertl M. Type I regulatory T cells in autoimmunity and inflammatory diseases. *Int Arch Allergy Immunol.* 2006;140:174–183.
134. Boes M. Role of natural and immune IgM antibodies in immune responses. *Mol Immunol.* 2000;37:1141–1149.
135. Zandvoort A, Timens W. The dual function of the splenic marginal zone: essential for initiation of anti-TI-2 responses but also vital in the general first-line defense against blood-borne antigens. *Clin Exp Immunol.* 2002;130:4–11.
136. McHeyzer-Williams MG, Ahmed R. B cell memory and the long-lived plasma cell. *Curr Opin Immunol.* 1999;11:172–179.
137. Lanzavecchia A, Bernasconi N, Traggiai E, et al. Understanding and making use of human memory B cells. *Immunol Rev.* 2006;211:303–309.
138. Mozdzanowska K, Feng J, Eid M, et al. Induction of influenza type A virus-specific resistance by immunization of mice with a synthetic multiple antigenic peptide vaccine that contains ectodomains of matrix protein 2. *Vaccine.* 2003;21:2616–2626.
139. Schwartz-Cornil I, Benureau Y, Greenberg H, et al. Heterologous protection induced by the inner capsid proteins of rotavirus requires transcytosis of mucosal immunoglobulins. *J Virol.* 2002;76:8110–8117.
140. Zinkernagel RM. On natural and artificial vaccinations. *Annu Rev Immunol.* 2003;21:515–546.
141. Yang Y, Santamaria P. T-cell receptor-transgenic NOD mice: a reductionist approach to understand autoimmune diabetes. *J Autoimmun.* 2004;22:121–129.
142. Samarkos M, Vaiopoulos G. The role of infections in the pathogenesis of autoimmune diseases. *Curr Drug Targets Inflamm Allergy.* 2005;4:99–103.
143. Fujinami RS, von Herrath MG, Christen U. Molecular mimicry, bystander activation, or viral persistence: infections and autoimmune disease. *Clin Microbiol Rev.* 2006;19:80–94.
144. Miller SD, Katz-Levy Y, Neville KL, et al. Virus-induced autoimmunity: epitope spreading to myelin autoepitopes in Theiler's virus infection of the central nervous system. *Adv Virus Res.* 2001;56:199–217.
145. Maier R, Krebs P, Ludewig B. Immunopathological basis of virus-induced myocarditis. *Clin Dev Immunol.* 2004;11:1–5.
146. Christen U, von Herrath MG. Infections and autoimmunity—good or bad? *J Immunol.* 2005;174:7481–7486.
147. Burns DP, Desrosiers RC. Envelope sequence variation, neutralizing antibodies, and primate lentivirus persistence. *Curr Top Microbiol Immunol.* 1994;188:185–219.
148. Sanchez-Merino V, Nie S, Luzuriaga K. HIV-1-specific CD8+ T cell responses and viral evolution in women and infants. *J Immunol.* 2005;175:6976–6986.
149. Pavio N, Lai MM. The hepatitis C virus persistence: how to evade the immune system? *J Biosci.* 2003;28:287–304.
150. Perfettini JL, Castedo M, Roumier T, et al. Mechanisms of apoptosis induction by the HIV-1 envelope. *Cell Death Differ.* 2005;12:916–923.
151. DiPerna G, Stack J, Bowie AG, et al. Poxvirus protein N1L targets the I-kappaB kinase complex, inhibits signaling to NF-kappaB by the tumor necrosis factor superfamily of receptors, and inhibits NF-kappaB and IRF3 signaling by toll-like receptors. *J Biol Chem.* 2004;279:36570–36578.
152. Bowie A, Kiss-Toth E, Symons JA, et al. A46R and A52R from vaccinia virus are antagonists of host IL-1 and toll-like receptor signaling. *Proc Natl Acad Sci U S A.* 2000;97:10162–10167.
153. Breiman A, Grandvaux N, Lin R, et al. Inhibition of RIG-I-dependent signaling to the interferon pathway during hepatitis C virus expression and restoration of signaling by IKKepsilon. *J Virol.* 2005;79:3969–3978.
154. Dixon LK, Abrams CC, Bowick G, et al. African swine fever virus proteins involved in evading host defence systems. *Vet Immunol Immunopathol.* 2004;100:117–134.
155. Hosui A, Ohkawa K, Ishida H, et al. Hepatitis C virus core protein differently regulates the JAK-STAT signaling pathway under interleukin-6 and interferon-gamma stimuli. *J Biol Chem.* 2003;278:28562–28571.
156. Polyak SJ, Khabar KS, Paschal DM, et al. Hepatitis C virus nonstructural 5A protein induces interleukin-8, leading to partial inhibition of the interferon-induced antiviral response. *J Virol.* 2001;75:6095–6106.
157. Reyes GR. The nonstructural NS5A protein of hepatitis C virus: an expanding, multifunctional role in enhancing hepatitis C virus pathogenesis. *J Biomed Sci.* 2002;9:187–197.
158. Burgert HG, Ruzsics Z, Obermeier S, et al. Subversion of host defense mechanisms by adenoviruses. *Curr Top Microbiol Immunol.* 2002;269:273–318.
159. Hartman AL, Towner JS, Nichol ST. A C-terminal basic amino acid motif of Zaire ebolavirus VP35 is essential for type I interferon antagonism and displays high identity with the RNA-binding domain of another interferon antagonist, the NS1 protein of influenza A virus. *Virology.* 2004;328:177–184.
160. Wang X, Li M, Zheng H, et al. Influenza A virus NS1 protein prevents activation of NF-kappaB and induction of alpha/beta interferon. *J Virol.* 2000;74:11566–11573.
161. Weber F, Bridgen A, Fazakerley JK, et al. Bunyamwera bunyavirus nonstructural protein NSs counteracts the induction of alpha/beta interferon. *J Virol.* 2002;76:7949–7955.
162. Young DF, Didcock L, Goodbourn S, et al. Paramyxoviridae use distinct virus-specific mechanisms to circumvent the interferon response. *Virology.* 2000;269:383–390.
163. Nees M, Geoghegan JM, Hyman T, et al. Papillomavirus type 16 oncogenes downregulate expression of interferon-responsive genes and upregulate proliferation-associated and NF-kappaB-responsive genes in cervical keratinocytes. *J Virol.* 2001;75:4283–4296.
164. Xiang Y, Moss B. IL-18 binding and inhibition of interferon gamma induction by human poxvirus-encoded proteins. *Proc Natl Acad Sci U S A.* 1999;96:11537–11542.
165. Mossman K, Upton C, McFadden G. The myxoma virus-soluble interferon-gamma receptor homolog, M-T7, inhibits interferon-gamma in a species-specific manner. *J Biol Chem.* 1995;270:3031–3038.
166. Langland JO, Jacobs BL. The role of the PKR-inhibitory genes, E3L and K3L, in determining vaccinia virus host range. *Virology.* 2002;299:133–141.
167. Seet BT, McFadden G. Viral chemokine-binding proteins. *J Leukoc Biol.* 2002;72:24–34.

168. Symons JA, Tscharke DC, Price N, et al. A study of the vaccinia virus interferon-gamma receptor and its contribution to virus virulence. *J Gen Virol.* 2002;83:1953–1964.
169. Alcami A, Symons JA, Smith GL. The vaccinia virus soluble alpha/beta interferon (IFN) receptor binds to the cell surface and protects cells from the antiviral effects of IFN. *J Virol.* 2000;74:11230–11239.
170. Deane D, McInnes CJ, Percival A, et al. Orf virus encodes a novel secreted protein inhibitor of granulocyte-macrophage colony-stimulating factor and interleukin-2. *J Virol.* 2000;74:1313–1320.
171. Moss B, Shisler JL. Immunology 101 at poxvirus U: immune evasion genes. *Semin Immunol.* 2001;13:59–66.
172. Redpath S, Ghazal P, Gascoigne NR. Hijacking and exploitation of IL-10 by intracellular pathogens. *Trends Microbiol.* 2001;9:86–92.
173. Beisser PS, Goh CS, Cohen FE, et al. Viral chemokine receptors and chemokines in human cytomegalovirus trafficking and interaction with the immune system. CMV chemokine receptors. *Curr Top Microbiol Immunol.* 2002;269:203–34.
174. Klouche M, Carruba G, Castagnetta L, et al. Virokines in the pathogenesis of cancer: focus on human herpesvirus 8. *Ann NY Acad Sci.* 2004;1028:329–339.
175. McFadden G, Murphy PM. Host-related immunomodulators encoded by poxviruses and herpesviruses. *Curr Opin Microbiol.* 2000;3:371–378.
176. Braud VM, Tomasec P, Wilkinson GW. Viral evasion of natural killer cells during human cytomegalovirus infection. *Curr Top Microbiol Immunol.* 2002;269:117–129.
177. Agrati C, Nisii C, Oliva A, et al. Lymphocyte distribution and intrahepatic compartmentalization during HCV infection: a main role for MHC-unrestricted T cells. *Arch Immunol Ther Exp.* 2002;50:307–316.
178. Favoreel HW, Van de Walle GR, Nauwynck HJ, et al. Virus complement evasion strategies. *J Gen Virol.* 2003;84:1–15.
179. Aubert M, Jerome KR. Apoptosis prevention as a mechanism of immune evasion. *Int Rev Immunol.* 2003;22:361–371.
180. Cuff S, Ruby J. Evasion of apoptosis by DNA viruses. *Immunol Cell Biol.* 1996;74:527–537.
181. Hewitt EW. The MHC class I antigen presentation pathway: strategies for viral immune evasion. *Immunology.* 2003;110:163–169.
182. Yewdell JW, Bennink JR. Mechanisms of viral interference with MHC class I antigen processing and presentation. *Annu Rev Cell Dev Biol.* 1999;15:579–606.
183. Kozarsky KF, Wilson JM. Gene therapy: adenovirus vectors. *Curr Opin Genet Dev.* 1993;3:499–503.
184. Cao H, Koehler DR, Hu J. Adenoviral vectors for gene replacement therapy. *Viral Immunol.* 2004;17:327–333.
185. Marshall E. Gene therapy death prompts review of adenovirus vector. *Science.* 1999;286:2244–2245.
186. Grieger JC, Samulski RJ. Adeno-associated virus as a gene therapy vector: vector development, production and clinical applications. *Adv Biochem Eng Biotechnol.* 2005;99:119–45.
187. High KA. Gene therapy: a 2001 perspective. *Haemophilia.* 2001;7.23–27.
188. Bessis N, GarciaCozar FJ, Boissier MC. Immune responses to gene therapy vectors: influence on vector function and effector mechanisms. *Gene Ther.* 2004;11:S10–S17.
189. Manno CS, Pierce GF, Arruda VR, et al. Successful transduction of liver in hemophilia by AAV-Factor IX and limitations imposed by the host immune response. *Nat Med.* 2006;12:342–347.
190. Clinical trials yield promising results from two adenovirus-based vaccines. *IAVI Rep.* 2005;9:24.
191. Use of AAV vectors in AIDS vaccine. *Expert Rev Vaccines.* 2002;1:7.

Chapter 37

Immune Responses to Intracellular Bacteria

Eric Pamer

INTRODUCTION

Despite the development of new antibiotics and vaccines, bacterial pathogens remain a major cause of human infection. Bacteria are diverse prokaryotic organisms that can be classified according to morphology (rod vs. coccus), staining characteristics (gram-positive vs. gram-negative), oxygen tolerance (anaerobe vs. aerobe), and growth rates (slow vs. rapid grower). Bacterial pathogens—i.e., those organisms that can cause disease in higher forms of life—can also be divided into those that infect the host and remain extracellular and those that invade host cells and become intracellular. Invasion of eukaryotic cells and intracellular survival and replication represent the strategy that a subset of pathogenic bacteria, the intracellular bacteria, have developed in order to survive and replicate within a mammalian host. Intracellular bacteria express factors that circumvent or inactivate microbicidal effector mechanisms that eukaryotic cells have evolved to eliminate invading pathogens. These bacterially expressed factors are referred to as *virulence factors* because they enable intracellular bacteria to cause disease by invading cells and promoting bacterial survival, replication, and spread. Pathogenic intracellular bacteria that lose these virulence factors, for example, by mutation or loss of a virulence factor-encoding plasmid, generally become avirulent, that is, incapable of causing disease.

In contrast to intracellular bacteria, extracellular bacterial pathogens survive and replicate outside of mammalian cells and have evolved a variety of mechanisms to avoid complement-mediated killing or phagocytic uptake by inflammatory cells. Although extracellular pathogens do not replicate within mammalian cells, some, such as *Staphylococcus aureus,* are capable of surviving within phagocytic cells (1) and others, such as *Neisseria meningitidis,* transiently invade cells to traverse epithelial barriers (2). Some extracellular pathogens, such as *Pseudomonas aerigunosa,* cause disease by injecting microbial proteins into the cytosol of adjacent epithelial cells (3), and in this fashion manipulate host cells using virulence mechanisms that are shared by some intracellular bacteria (4). Thus, the dividing line between intra- and extracellular pathogens is not completely distinct, and the immune mechanisms that are activated in defense against intracellular and extracellular bacteria share many features. Nevertheless, the components of the immune system that provide protection against intracellular and extracellular bacterial pathogens are only partially overlapping. With respect to protection against intracellular bacterial infection, macrophages, T cells and cytokines and accessory cells that facilitate antigen-specific T-cell responses are especially important for immune defense. On the other hand, neutrophils and humoral immunity play a more important role in defense against extracellular bacterial pathogens.

INTERACTIONS BETWEEN INTRACELLULAR BACTERIA AND THE IMMUNE SYSTEM

Intracellular bacterial pathogens differ from one another in a variety of ways that affect the innate and adaptive immune responses induced in the mammalian host. In the following sections, some of the key characteristics of different intracellular bacterial pathogens are described. and their implications for the host immune response are discussed.

Effect of Cell Wall Composition

The bacterial cell wall and outer membrane represent one of the major ligands for innate immune receptors and trigger signals that shape the inflammatory responses. The signal transduction pathways and inflammatory responses triggered by different innate immune receptors and bacterial ligands are diverse. Thus, the composition of the bacterial cell wall and membrane has a direct effect on the innate immune response and indirectly influences adaptive immune responses. A classical method to distinguish different bacterial pathogens, first described in 1884 by the Danish microbiologist Hans Christian Gram, is the Gram stain: Organisms that retain crystal violet dye are termed gram-positive, whereas those that do not are gram-negative. *Listeria monocytogenes,* a rod-shaped bacterium that infects macrophages, hepatocytes, and intestinal epithelial cells, is gram-positive and thus is enveloped by a thick layer of peptidoglycan, lacks lipopolysaccharide (LPS), and expresses lipoteichoic acid (LTA) on its surface (5). Other intracellular bacterial pathogens, such as *Salmonella enterica,* are gram-negative rods and have a cell wall consisting of a relatively thin layer of peptidoglycan surrounded by lipopolysaccharide (4). The distinct cell wall composition of *S. enterica* and *L. monocytogenes* has implications for the inflammatory response induced within the mammalian host. A third group of intracellular bacterial pathogens, which includes *Mycobacterium tuberculosis,* contains yet a different outer surface that consists of a complex array of glycolipids that include mycolic acids and lipoarabinomannans (6). These components induce inflammatory responses that are distinct from those elicited by peptidoglycan, LPS, and LTA. It is interesting that apparently minor modifications in surface molecules of microbial pathogens can affect the inflammatory responses induced in the infected host. For example, lipid chains of mycolic acids are modified by specific cyclopropane synthetases, which are encoded by a family of *M. tuberculosis* genes. Each cyclopropane synthetase generates a specific cyclopropane ring that structurally modifies the mycolic acid side chain, thereby altering the virulence and pathogenicity of *M. tuberculosis* (7,8). Thus, *M. tuberculosis* has evolved a mechanism to subtly modify the surface lipids that interface with the mammalian host (9,10). These modifications modify the host's innate inflammatory response and thus alter *in vivo* mycobacterial growth and survival.

Effect of Bacterial Growth Rate

In addition to the molecular composition of intracellular bacterial pathogens, other microbial characteristics also influence immune responses. The rate of bacterial replication is a factor that has significant consequences for innate and adaptive immune responses. Some intracellular bacteria, such as *Salmonella enterica* or *Listeria monocytogenes,* can divide every 30 to 40 minutes in the mammalian host. In this setting, the tempo of the disease can be very rapid and the amount of antigen can be quite large. In contrast, *Mycobacterium tuberculosis,* even under optimal growth conditions, divides only once every 24 hours. In this setting, particularly when the inoculum of a slow-growing pathogen is small, the threshold for activating the adaptive immune response may not be met for many weeks following infection. Thus, the *in vivo* kinetics of microbial growth, the production of ligands for innate immune receptors, and the generation of antigens that can be detected by T lymphocytes are quite variable following infection with different intracellular bacterial pathogens. Rapid bacterial growth, with resultant production of microbial products that trigger innate immune receptors and the production of large amounts of antigen, can increase the tempo and magnitude of innate inflammatory and adaptive immune responses. On the other hand, slow *in vivo* bacterial growth with attenuated innate inflammatory responses and potentially subthreshold levels of antigen may result in suboptimal immune responses that are incapable of clearing the pathogen.

Targeting Different Host Cells

Although a range of mammalian cells can be infected by intracellular bacterial pathogens, most intracellular bacteria are only capable of infecting and replicating within a limited subset of cell types. For example, *Mycobacterium tuberculosis* and *Salmonella enterica* survive and replicate predominantly within macrophages (11,12), whereas *Listeria monocytogenes* infects macrophages and hepatocytes (13,14). The type of cell that bacteria infect has implications for the immune response. Epithelial cells, for example, are not efficient at presenting antigens via the MHC class II pathway and have a limited capacity to kill intracellular bacteria. Macrophages, on the other hand, are efficient antigen-presenting cells and, upon activation, are highly effective at bacterial killing. Natural infections with *Salmonella enterica* and *Listeria monocytogenes* are acquired by oral ingestion, and thus, both of these pathogens encounter, invade, and traverse intestinal epithelial cells before gaining access to macrophages.

Traversing Epithelial Barriers

Intestinal epithelial cells form a defensive barrier against microbes, and pathogens that are acquired by the intestinal route infect intestinal epithelial cells in order to establish systemic infections in the mammalian host. In the case of *Listeria monocytogenes,* E-cadherin is postulated to be a receptor for the bacterial surface protein internalin-A and mediates bacterial entry into the intestinal epithelial cell (15). *Salmonella enterica,* on the other hand, traverses the intestinal epithelial barrier by entering M cells, which overlay Peyer patches in the gut (16). *Salmonella enterica* can also traverse the intestinal epithelial barrier by invading CD18-expressing phagocytes (17).

Bacterial entry into epithelial cells is a complex process because, unlike macrophages, epithelial cells are not phagocytic. Thus, in order to enter intestinal epithelial cells, intracellular bacterial pathogens have evolved complex pathogenesis strategies to induce their uptake (4). *Salmonella enterica,* for example, upon contacting the surface of intestinal epithelial cells, induces membrane ruffling at the site of contact that results from actin polymerization and other cytoskeletal changes (18). This process, which is essential for *S. enterica* virulence following oral ingestion, involves a multicomponent virulence complex referred to as the type III secretion system (TTSS) (19). TTSSs enable gram-negative bacteria to secrete proteins across their membranes and cell wall and into the cytosol of adjacent mammalian cells. This remarkable feat is accomplished by the highly organized assembly of a bacterially encoded multicomponent needle complex, which, by spanning all bacterial and eukaryotic membrane and cell wall barriers, provides a narrow channel that connects the bacterial cytosol with the cytosol of the mammalian cell. The *S. enterica* chromosome contains two "pathogenicity islands" that encode two distinct TTSSs on its chromosome, SPI-1 and SPI-2, which each contain roughly 20 genes that confer bacterial virulence (4). Inactivation of SPI-1 results in bacteria that are unable to infect intestinal epithelial cells, rendering the pathogen incapable of causing infection following oral ingestion (19). SPI-1 encodes the structural components of the needle complex and also effector proteins that are injected into the epithelial cell. Three *S. enterica* proteins, SopE, SopE2, and SopB, interact with CDC42 and Rac1 of the epithelial cell to induce actin polymerization that ultimately leads to the internalization of the bacterium (20). Other proteins, such as SptP, are secreted by the TTSS into the epithelial cell cytosol in order to revert the cytoskeletal changes induced by invasion (21). Expression of virulence factors is highly regulated, and different factors are secreted at distinct times and in different locations during cellular infection. For example, the SPI-2-encoded TTSS is not expressed by *S. enterica* until the bacteria have entered a host cell (22,23). Proteins secreted by the SPI-2–encoded complex appear to be essential for the modification of the macrophage phagosome, specifically, evasion of phagocyte NADPH oxidase–mediated killing (24).

Effect of Subcellular Localization

Different intracellular bacterial pathogens inhabit distinct compartments within mammalian host cells (Table 37.1). Most intracellular bacteria remain within vacuoles and thus are separated from the cytosol by a host cell–derived membrane. *Salmonella typhimurium, Mycobacterium tuberculosis,* and *Legionella pneumophila,* the cause of Legionaire's disease, reside and replicate within macrophage vacuoles or phagosomes. The nature of the vacuole varies with the pathogen, with some intracellular bacteria, such as *Legionella pneumophila,* residing within vacuoles that resemble the endoplasmic reticulum (25,26) while others, such as *Mycobacterium tuberculosis,* reside within vacuoles with endosomal characteristics (27). *M. tuberculosis*

TABLE 37.1 Intracellular Bacteria

Bacterial Species	Cell Type Infected	Subcellular Localization
Anaplasma phagocytophilum	Neutrophil	Vacuole
Brucella abortus	Macrophage	Vacuole
Bartonella bacilliformis	Erythrocyte/endothelial cell	Vacuole
Burkholderia pseudomallei	Macrophage	Vacuole
Calymmatobacterium granulomatosis	Monocyte	Vacuole
Chlamydia trachomatis	Mucosal epithelial cell	Vacuole
Chlamydia psittaci	Macrophage	Vacuole
Coxiella burnettii	Macrophage	Vacuole
Ehrlichia canis	Neutrophil/monocyte	Vacuole
Franciscella tularensis	Macrophage	Vacuole
Legionella pneumophila	Macrophage	Vacuole
Listeria monocytogenes	Macrophages/hepatocyte	Cytoplasm
Mycobacterium tuberculosis	Macrophage	Vacuole
Mycobacterium leprae	Macrophage/Schwann cell	Vacuole
Rickettsia rickettsii	Endothelial cell	Cytoplasm/nucleus
Rickettsia prowazekii	Endothelial cell	Cytoplasm
Salmonella enterica	Intestinal epithelial cell/macrophage	Vacuole
Shigella flexneri	Epithelial cell	Cytoplasm

impairs vacuolar acidification and the acquisition of lysosomal hydrolases and thus, to prevent destruction, arrests endosomal maturation (28). The MHC class II antigen–processing pathway intersects with endosomal compartments to present antigens to CD4 T cells and some pathogens, such as *Mycobacterium tuberculosis,* segregate their vacuoles from the MHC class II molecules (29).

In contrast to bacteria that remain within phagosomes, some intracellular bacterial pathogens escape vacuoles and enter the cytosol of infected cells. *Listeria monocytogenes* accomplishes this feat by secreting a membranolytic protein, listeriolysin, which ruptures the phagocytic membrane and enables bacterial entry into the cytosol (30). *L. monocytogenes* replicates rapidly in the host cell cytosol and moves by polymerizing actin on one pole, a process that pushes bacteria throughout the infected host cell and also into neighboring cells (31). Upon invading the neighboring cell, *L. monocytogenes* again produces listeriolysin, which lyses the phagosome, thus allowing bacteria to enter the next cell without an intervening extracellular phase. Vacuolar escape is essential for the virulence of *L. monocytogenes,* and deletion of listeriolysin O renders bacteria completely avirulent (32).

Several other intracellular bacterial pathogens also escape the vacuole, such as *Shigella flexneri* and *Rickettsia rickettsiae*. In the case of *Shigella flexneri* infections, although bacteria escape the vacuole and enter the host-cell cytoplasm in cell culture (33), it is unclear whether this process is a component of *in vivo* virulence. Entry into the host-cell cytoplasm and nucleus is also a feature of infections with *Rickettsia rickettsii,* a tick borne pathogen that infects endothelial cells and vascular smooth muscle cells and causes Rocky Mountain spotted fever (34).

As might be expected, cytosolic localization has important implications for both the innate and adaptive immune response to intracellular bacterial pathogens. For one, antigens secreted by cytosolic bacteria have direct access to the MHC class I antigen–processing pathway and thus prime CD8 T-cell populations that often play a substantial role in bacterial clearance and long-term protective immunity. On another level, innate immune receptors that associate with microbial molecules are present in the cytosol and result in the activation of inflammatory processes (35).

ROUTE OF ACQUISITION: IMPLICATIONS FOR SYSTEMIC AND MUCOSAL IMMUNITY

Intracellular bacterial pathogens can be acquired by inhalation, oral ingestion, or through the epidermis. Some bacterial pathogens, such as *Mycobacterium tuberculosis* and *Legionella pneumophila,* are acquired by the respiratory route and thus their initial interactions are with phagocytic cells of the lungs, most likely alveolar macrophages and dendritic cells. Other intracellular bacterial pathogens, such as *Salmonella typhimurium* and *Listeria monocytogenes,* enter the mammalian host via the intestinal tract and thus their initial encounters are with intestinal epithelial cells and M cells of the gut and also CX3CR1-expressing dendritic cells that extend dendrites into the gut lumen (36,37). Other intracellular bacterial pathogens, such as the *Rickettsia rickettsii* or *Anaplasma phagocytophilum,* are transmitted to the mammalian host by bites of the lone star tick or the deer tick, respectively (34,38). In these circumstances, the pathogens bypass the mammalian epidermis and enter the bloodstream, presumably after interacting with phagocytic cells in subcutaneous tissues. The lung, gut, and skin have associated lymphoid tissues that are distinct in terms of cellular composition, chemokine and integrin expression, and cytokine production. In the lung, macrophages and dendritic cells deliver microbes, such as the respiratory intracellular bacterial pathogens *M. tuberculosis* and *Legionella pneumophila,* to draining lymph nodes in the peribronchial and mediastinal region. During inflammation, lymphoid tissues can develop in the lungs and serve as auxiliary sites for T-cell priming (39). Gut-associated lymphoid tissues, which initiate immune responses against enteric intracellular pathogens such as *Salmonella enterica* and *Listeria monocytogenes,* are also complex. Peyer patches, which occur in the small intestine, consist of B cells and dendritic cells and lie beneath a layer of M cells, which transport antigens, including bacteria, from the intestinal lumen to the underlying lymphoid tissues. The intestinal epithelium also contains a variety of T cells, referred to as intraepithelial lymphocytes (IELs), which express either the $\alpha\beta$ or $\gamma\delta$ T-cell receptor (40). The lamina propria of the gut contains a large number of T cells that are predominantly of the memory phenotype (41,42). Although these immune cells very likely play a key role in immunity to intestinal intracellular bacterial pathogens, very little is known about their precise contributions to antimicrobial defense.

INNATE IMMUNE RESPONSES TO INTRACELLULAR BACTERIA

Mammalian cells express a range of innate immune receptors that bind to different microbial molecules and transmit signals that activate antimicrobial defense mechanisms (43). Innate immune receptors are present on the cell surface, within the vacuolar compartments of mammalian cells, and also in the cytoplasm. These receptors contain sequences that associate with microbial molecules and either contain domains that directly signal or that associate with adaptor molecules that initiate a signaling cascade that culminates in the expression of genes that provide antimicrobial defense. The following sections outline the recently defined innate immune signaling pathways that are involved in the recognition of intracellular bacterial pathogens. Many of these pathways are also involved in defense against extracellular bacterial pathogens and pathogenic viruses, fungi, and protozoa.

Toll-like Receptors (TLRs) in Defense against Intracellular Bacteria

The most completely characterized interactions between microbial molecules and innate immune receptors involve the members of the Toll-like receptor (TLR) family (44). Mammalian genomes contain up to 12 distinct TLR genes that encode transmembrane proteins that bind distinct microbial molecules, such as LPS (TLR-4), CpG (TLR-9), LTA (TLR-2), and flagellin (TLR-5 and TLR-11). MyD88 is an intracellular adaptor protein that mediates many, but not all, TLR signals, and mice that lack MyD88 are highly susceptible to infection with *Listeria monocytogenes* and *Mycobacterium tuberculosis* (45–47). MyD88-deficient macrophages are less effective at killing *Salmonella enterica* because of decreased phagocyte oxidase activation (48). Although the absence of MyD88 markedly increases susceptibility to a number of bacterial infections, the absence of individual TLR genes often does not noticeably affect susceptibility to infections, most likely reflecting the redundancy of these innate immune receptors. Thus, although TLR-2 recognizes and signals in response to components of *L. monocytogenes,* mice that lack this receptor have normal resistance to infection (46). Remarkably, although TLR-5 is expressed on lamina propria dendritic cells and responds to flagellin derived from *Salmonella enterica,* TLR-5–deficient mice are more resistant to infection with *S. enterica,* presumably because of diminished transport of bacteria from the lamina propria to mesenteric lymph nodes (49).

In contrast to the proposed detrimental effect of TLR-5 on murine *Salmonella* infections, in humans TLR-5 appears to play a protective role in defense against *Legionella pneumophila* infection. Genetic analysis of humans that became infected at a tulip festival in the Netherlands revealed a greater incidence of a TLR-5 mutation that results in a nonfunctional receptor in infected patients than in uninfected controls (50). Because TLR-5 is stimulated by bacterial flagellins, this result suggests that detection of *L. pneumophila* flagellin contributes to defense against infection.

Expression of TLRs is regulated and cell type-specific and thus, different cell types express different combinations of TLRs. TLRs are also targeted to different cellular compartments, with some TLRs residing on the plasma membrane (TLR-2 and TLR-4) and others residing within membrane-bound compartments of the cell (TLR-3, -7, and -9) (51). Thus, in the setting of intracellular bacterial infection, TLR signaling differs depending on the compartment occupied by the microbial pathogen and the TLR ligands that are available for association with their respective receptor. Parallel innate immune signaling pathways mediated by the ITAM-containing DAP12 adaptor molecule appear to inhibit TLR signaling, and mice that lack DAP12 are more resistant to *L. monocytogenes* infection (52).

Nod Signaling in Defense against Intracellular Bacterial Infection

Innate immune recognition of microbial molecules also occurs in the cytosol of mammalian cells. The most completely characterized cytoplasmic innate immune receptors are the Nod proteins, Nod1 and Nod2, which contain leucine-rich CARD and nucleotide-binding domains (53). These proteins recognize fragments of peptidoglycan in the cytosol and induce NFκB signaling and innate immune activation via the adaptor molecule RIP2. Mice that lack RIP2 are more susceptible to *Listeria monocytogenes* infection (54), and mice that lack Nod2 are defective in clearing *L. monocytogenes* upon enteric challenge (55). Thus, the Nod recognition pathway contributes to defense against infection with this gram-positive intracellular pathogen. Although CpG motifs within bacterial DNA are detected by TLR-9, bacterial DNA is also detected in the cytosol by non–Toll-like receptors, and triggers innate immune activation and secretion of type I interferons. These signaling pathways play a role in defense against *L. monocytogenes* and *L. pneumophila* infections (56).

Inflammasome-mediated Defense against Intracellular Bacteria

Recognition of microbial molecules in the cytosol of mammalian cells is mediated in part by the inflammasome, a roughly 700-kDa complex of proteins that includes apoptosis-associated specklike protein (ASC), Ipaf, and cryopyrin (also known as Nalp-3), which, upon stimulation, result in the activation of caspase-1 and the secretion of IL-1 and IL-18 (57). Inflammasome components are also involved in bacterially induced apoptosis of infected macrophages, a process that contributes to pathogenesis by some intracellular bacterial pathogens, including *S. enterica*. Genetic deletion of individual inflammasome components in mice has revealed their contribution to defense against a number of intracellular bacterial infections. Caspase-1–deficient mice, for example, are more susceptible to infection by *L. monocytogenes* (58) and *Salmonella enterica* (59). Macrophages derived from mice with a genetic deletion of ASC do not activate caspase-1 and are resistant to bacterially induced apoptosis (60), suggesting that macrophage apoptosis may enhance *in vivo* bacterial clearance. ASC-deficient macrophages also produce diminished amounts of IL-1 and IL-18 upon cytosolic invasion by *L. monocytogenes* (61). Along similar lines, macrophages that lack Ipaf, another component of inflammasomes, do not activate caspase-1 in response to intracellular infection with *Salmonella enterica* (60), and cells that lack Ipaf are resistant to *S. enterica*–induced apoptosis. On the other hand, macrophages that lack cryopyrin, a component of inflammasomes also referred to as NALP-3, produce IL-1 and IL-18 in response to *S. enterica* infection but do not undergo bacterially induced apoptosis (62,63). In contrast to *S. enterica* infection, NALP-3–deficient macrophages infected with *L. monocytogenes* do not produce IL-1β or IL-18. These studies indicate that inflammasomes interact with different intracellular bacterial pathogens distinctly. Although most studies have characterized the response of inflammasome-deficient macrophages to bacterial infection, characterization of the *in vivo* response of deficient mice to infection are fewer but demonstrate that mice that lack caspase-1 are more susceptible to infection with *Salmonella typhimurium*, whereas mice that lack Ipaf, ASC, or NALP-3 are not (59).

In the case of *Legionella pneumophila* infection of macrophages, bacterial flagellin plays a particularly important role in the induction of innate immune responses. Studies of human populations indicate that TLR-5 plays a role in defense against *L. pneumophila* by recognizing bacterial flagellin (50), but experiments with mouse macrophages have identified another receptor that detects *L. pneumophila* flagellin. Although most commonly used laboratory mouse strains are innately resistant to *L. pneumophila* infection, the A/J mouse strain is highly susceptible to infection with *L. pneumophila*. The susceptibility of A/J mice was traced to mutations within a gene encoding Naip-5 or Birc1e (64,65). Naip-5 is structurally similar to Nod proteins, containing a nucleotide-binding domain and a leucine-rich region. Naip-5 activation in *L. pneumophila*–infected macrophages results in caspase-1–mediated apoptosis and IL-1β production. *L. pneumophila* that lack the Dot/Icm type IV secretion system do not activate macrophage apoptosis, are less virulent, and do not activate Naip-5. Caspase-1–deficient mice are similar to mice with deficient Naip-5, indicating that caspase-1 is the mediator of the Naip-5 effect. Naip-5 also interacts with inflammasome components. For example, Ipaf-deficient macrophages, similar to caspase-1– or Naip-5–deficient cells, do not restrict *L. pneumophila* growth (66). In contrast, ASC-deficient macrophages do not produce IL-1β but effectively restrict *L. pneumophila* growth (67). Thus, IL-1β production, in response to Naip-5/caspase-1 activation, does not play a role in restricting *L. pneumophila* growth, but other caspase-1– and Ipaf-dependent processes restrict of bacterial growth (67).

Mutants of *L. pneumophila* that lack flagellin do not induce caspase-1 activation, do not induce macrophage apoptosis, and escape macrophage-mediated innate immune defense (68). Thus, innate immune defenses mediated by Naip-5 (also called Birc1e) respond to bacterial flagellin in a process that is independent of TLR-5 and MyD88. Flagellar assembly or motility are not required for innate immune activation, and introduction of purified fagellin into the cytosol induces caspase-1 activation and macrophage apoptosis (69).

NEUTROPHILS AND DEFENSE AGAINST INTRACELLULAR BACTERIA

From the perspective of a bacterial pathogen, one of the major benefits of intercellular survival is avoiding contact with neutrophils. Nevertheless, neutrophils can play an important role in defense against intracellular pathogens.

In the case of *S. enterica* infections, neutrophils play a particularly important role in the gut and a less important role in systemic sites of infection (70). In the mouse model of *L. monocytogenes* infection, antibody-mediated depletion of neutrophils greatly exacerbates infection, implicating neutrophils in the *in vivo* clearance of bacteria (71). How neutrophils detect and kill bacteria that are within hepatocytes, for example, remains unclear (72). It is likely, however, that neutrophils are recruited to sites of bacterial infection by the localized induction of the CXC-chemokines Mip-2 and KC (in humans, IL-8). Release of formyl-methionine–containing peptide, which can bind to formyl-peptide receptors on neutrophils and induce chemotaxis and degranulation, may also contribute to neutrophil recruitment and clearance of intracellular bacteria. Although neutrophils are highly bacteriocidal, one pathogen, *Anaplasma phagocytophylum,* infects and survives within granulocytes by preventing fusion with cytochrome b_{558}–containing vesicles and by diminishing transcription of gp91^{phox} (38).

MONOCYTE-MEDIATED DEFENSE AGAINST INTRACELLULAR BACTERIA

Mammalian monocytes can differentiate into tissue macrophages and dendritic cells and mediate immune defense against a broad range of pathogens, including intracellular bacteria. Monocytes derive from progenitors in the bone marrow and enter the bloodstream and then peripheral tissues. In the setting of *L. monocytogenes* infection, monocytes enter infected tissues such as the liver in a CD11b-mediated fashion, and blocking CD11b with a specific antibody results in uncontrolled bacterial growth in infected organs and death (14). CCR2 is a chemokine receptor that is expressed on a subset of monocytes that contributes to inflammatory responses, and mice with genetic deletions of CCR2 have increased susceptibility to infection with several intracellular bacterial pathogens (73). For example, CCR2-deficient mice succumb to infection with small doses of *L. monocytogenes* because monocytes are not recruited to bacterially infected tissues (73,74). MCP-1, a CC-chemokine that is a ligand for CCR2, is induced by *L. monocytogenes* infection and promotes the recruitment of monocytes (75). The first step in monocyte recruitment is emigration from the bone marrow into the bloodstream, and this step is mediated by MCP-1 and requires CCR-2–mediated signals (76). Thus, in mice that lack either CCR2 or MCP-1, inflammatory monocytes are retained in the bone marrow upon infection with *L. monocytogenes*. CCR2-mediated recruitment of monocytes is also required for effective control of pulmonary infection with *Mycobacterium tuberculosis* (77).

TNF and iNOS are essential for the efficient clearance of *L. monocytogenes* from infected mice (78,79), and monocytes are the major source of these proteins in infected tissues. Thus, in spleens of CCR2-deficient mice infected with *L. monocytogenes,* TNF and iNOS levels are markedly reduced (74). Although recruitment of monocytes does not require TLR-mediated signals, induction of TNF at the sites of infection is TLR-driven (75).

CYTOKINES MEDIATING DEFENSE AGAINST INTRACELLULAR BACTERIAL INFECTION

IFN-γ plays a central role in defense against intracellular bacterial pathogens (80). Genetic analysis of humans with an increased incidence of mycobacterial and *Salmonella* infections uncovered mutations in the IFN-γ receptor (IFNGR1) that in some cases abolished and in other cases diminished transduction of IFN-γ–mediated signals (81–83). Additional individuals with increased susceptibility to mycobacterial and *Salmonella* infections were identified with mutations in the genes that encode IL-12 p40, a subunit shared by IL-12 and IL-23 (84). These individuals, as well as individuals with mutations in the IL-12-receptor, produced less IFN-γ in response to stimulation with mycobacterial extracts. Mutations in the gene that encodes STAT-1, which in the homodimeric form mediates IFN-γ signaling, also predispose individuals to mycobacterial and *Salmonella* infections, again demonstrating the importance of IFN-γ in defense against these pathogens (85). An X-linked form of increased susceptibility to mycobacterial infections has been attributed to mutations in the gene that encodes NF-κB essential modulator (NEMO) (86). In these individuals, monocytes produce less IL-12 in response to stimulation with activated T cells, a result of decreased responsiveness to CD40 triggering (86).

Studies performed in mice with genetic deletions of IFN-γ also demonstrate the important role of this cytokine in defense against infections with intracellular bacteria. IFN-γ–deficient mice are highly susceptible to infection with *Mycobacterium tuberculosis* (87,88), *Listeria monocytogenes* (89), and also attenuated strains of *Salmonella typhimurium* (90). In the murine model of *M. tuberculosis* infection, IFN-γ promotes the expression of inducible nitric oxide synthase, an enzyme that produces NO, an essential participant in *in vivo* mycobacterial killing (91). As in humans, murine deficiency of IL-12 p40 is also associated with increased susceptibility to *M. tuberculosis* infection. Comparison of mice that lack p40 (common to IL-12 and IL-23), p30 (IL-12), and p19 (IL-23) revealed that IL-12 is essential for optimal IFN-γ–mediated immune defense against *M. tuberculosis*, whereas an effect of IL-23 on antimycobacterial defense was detectable only if IL-12 was concurrently absent (92). IL-12 probably makes its most important contribution to antimicrobial immune defense by enhancing the induction of Th1 CD4 T-cell–mediated immunity, but IL-12–mediated signals also enhance the migration of pulmonary dendritic cells from the lung to draining lymph nodes following intrapulmonary challenge with *M. tuberculosis* (93).

Tumor necrosis factor (TNF) is a pleuripotent cytokine that contributes to monocyte and granulocyte activation, enhances inflammatory cell migration, induces the production of other inflammatory cytokines, and increases the permeability of endothelial cells. Monoclonal antibodies or soluble receptors that block TNF receptor–mediated signaling are used clinically to ameliorate autoimmune inflammatory diseases such as rheumatoid arthritis and are very effective. Blocking TNF signaling, however, also increases susceptibility to a range of infectious pathogens, most prominently intracellular bacterial pathogens such as *M. tuberculosis* (94) and *L. monocytogenes* (95). The increased incidence of infections caused by these pathogens was not entirely surprising, because studies in mice, using either TNF- or TNF receptor–deficient mice, demonstrated their marked susceptibility to infection with these pathogens (79,96). TNF is synthesized as a membrane-bound protein that is cleaved from the cell surface by a metalloprotease, TNF-α–converting enzyme (TACE). Mice that lack this enzyme or that lack the metalloprotease cleavage site produce only membrane-bound TNF but are resistant to low-dose *L. monocytogenes* infection, suggesting that soluble TNF is not required for T-cell–mediated antimicrobial defense (97). Instead, it is likely that the TNF-mediated signals that are essential for microbial clearance are mediated by direct cell–cell contact. The nature of this interaction and the cellular participants remain incompletely defined.

In contrast to TNF and IFN-γ, type I interferons (IFN-α and IFN-β) are principally involved in defense against viral infections. Infection with some bacterial pathogens, however, also induces type I interferon production. *L. monocytogenes* infection of macrophages induces IFN-β, for example, in a process that requires bacterial invasion of the cytosol (98). However, in contrast to TNF and IFN-γ, type I interferons play a detrimental role in defense against *L. monocytogenes* infection. Mice that lack the receptor for type I interferons are more resistant to *L. monocytogenes,* with decreased numbers of bacteria in the spleen and liver after intravenous inoculation of bacteria (99–101). Some studies indicate that the recruitment and survival of monocytes is enhanced in the absence of type I interferon signaling, but another, potentially more important, mechanism may involve the effect of type I interferon on T-cell survival. *L. monocytogenes* infection, specifically LLO production by virulent bacteria, induces T-cell apoptosis, but this process is markedly attenuated in mice that lack the type I interferon receptor (102). The immunosuppressive effect of bacterially induced, type I interferon–mediated T-cell apoptosis is most clearly demonstrated by the finding that $Rag^{-/-}$ mice, which lack T cells, are remarkably resistant to *L. monocytogenes* at early time points following infection. Reconstitution of $Rag^{-/-}$ mice with wild-type T cells, but not with T cells lacking the type I interferon receptor, renders them more susceptible to *L. monocytogenes* infection (102). The immunosuppression induced by T-cell apoptosis in this setting is partially the result of IL-10 production by phagocytic cells internalizing apoptotic cells.

T-CELL RESPONSES TO INTRACELLULAR BACTERIA

In contrast to extracellular bacterial pathogens, which are eliminated by antibody-, complement-, and phagocyte-mediated mechanisms, clearance of intracellular bacterial pathogens is generally dependent on the activation and expansion of pathogen-specific T lymphocytes. The T-cell subsets that are involved and the mechanisms of microbial clearance differ for different bacterial pathogens, to a large extent reflecting the subcellular localization of the bacterium within the host cell. To activate CD4 and CD8 T cells, bacterial antigens must intersect the MHC class II and MHC class I antigen-processing pathways, respectively. Dendritic cells, although not a major reservoir of infection with intracellular bacterial pathogens, play a predominant role in priming naïve T cells. In some cases, dendritic cells are infected with bacteria directly, in others dendritic cells acquire apoptotic fragments of infected cells and cross-present antigens to naïve T cells (103).

Interactions of Intracellular Bacteria with Dendritic Cells

A subset of intracellular bacterial pathogens causes disease by traversing the intestinal epithelium and disseminating throughout the body. *Salmonella enterica* is one such organism, and its interaction with the intestinal epithelium has been well characterized. *S. enterica* contains several virulence regions in its genome that enable invasion and intracellular survival. The SP1 locus, which encodes the components of the type III secretion system, enables *S. typhimurium* to invade the intestinal epithelium via M cells in follicle-associated epithelial areas and to enter Peyer patches. Dendritic cells in Peyer patches respond to bacterial infection in a CCR6-dependent manner and rapidly prime CD4 T cells specific for *S. typhimurium* (104). Invasion via M cells, however, appears to be only one of several ways that *S. typhimurium* can dive below the intestinal epithelial surface. SP1-deficient *S. typhimurium* can disseminate from the gut without traversing M cells and are taken up by CD18-expressing cells (17), which carry them to the spleen. Remarkably, dendritic cells in the lamina propria of the gut extend dendrites into the gut lumen by disrupting tight junctions between intestinal epithelial cells and, in this process, capture luminal bacteria and transport them to mesenteric lymph nodes (36). Indeed, the lamina propria has an extensive network of dendritic cells that depends on the expression of CX3CR1 to enable dendrite extension into the gut lumen (37).

Intracellular bacteria also interact with dendritic cells following systemic infection, an interaction that is essential for effective priming of T lymphocytes. Experiments using a mouse strain in which dendritic cells can be selectively deleted by administration of a toxin demonstrated that CD8 T-cell priming following *L. monocytogenes* infection is entirely dependent on the presence of dendritic cells (105). Dendritic cells in spleen are directly infected by *L. monocytogenes* following intravenous inoculation, and toxin-mediated depletion of dendritic cells diminishes the number of bacteria that localize to the spleen (106).

CD4 T-Cell Responses to Intracellular Bacteria

T lymphocytes play a key role in the immune response to intracellular bacterial pathogens. In the case of bacteria residing in phagosomes, MHC class II–restricted CD4 T cells play a particularly important role in immune defense. Mice that lack MHC class II molecules, and consequently that also lack CD4 T cells, have markedly enhanced susceptibility to infection with *Mycobacterium tuberculosis* and *Salmonella enterica* (107,108). Along similar lines, patients infected with the human immunodeficiency virus (HIV) who have low CD4 counts are also more susceptible to infection with *M. tuberculosis*, *M. avium complex,* and several species of *Salmonella* (109). It is believed that IFN-γ production by pathogen-specific CD4 T cells is essential for activation of macrophages that harbor intracellular bacteria. IFN-γ induces the expression of iNOS by macrophages and thus contributes to bacterial killing.

In the setting of *M. tuberculosis* infection, clinical findings in patients and experimental results using murine models indicate that CD4 T cells, though essential for preventing progressive disease, fail to mediate complete bacterial clearance (110). Immunocompetent individuals can harbor viable *M. tuberculosis* for decades after initial exposure, and despite detectable CD4 T-cell responses, the pathogen persists, presumably in a latent state within macrophages. In mouse models of *M. tuberculosis* infection, vaccines that prime *M. tuberculosis*–specific CD4 T cells enhance resistance to challenge infection, diminishing *in vivo* mycobacterial growth in the immunized host by a factor of 10 to 100. No vaccine, however, has been able to prevent infection upon challenge with live, virulent *M. tuberculosis* (111). Along similar lines, immunization with *Mycobacterium bovis* BCG, a TB-preventive vaccine that has been administered extensively outside the United States, also provides only partial protection against infection (111).

The kinetics and differentiation of *M. tuberculosis*–specific CD4 T cells has been investigated in the mouse model. In mice, ESAT-6 is an immunodominant *M. tuberculosis* antigen detected by CD4 T cells, and the magnitude of the immune response to this antigen can be measured by intracellular staining of IFN-γ. Kinetic analysis of the CD4 T-cell response demonstrated that, in contrast to viral infections, such as influenza virus infection of the lung where CD4 T-cell responses are maximal 6 to 8 days following viral inoculation, CD4 T-cell responses to inhaled *M. tuberculosis* are delayed and do not peak until 21 to 28 days after exposure (112). This expansion of IFN-γ–producing CD4 T cells coincides with the inhibition of further increases in the number of viable bacteria in the lungs of infected mice.

CD4 T cell responses to *Salmonella enterica* have been investigated using T-cell receptor transgenic mice specific for an epitope derived from the bacterial flagellin. Following intestinal infection, flagellin-specific T cells are primed within 3 hours and undergo extensive proliferation in Peyer patches and mesenteric lymph nodes (113). In this system, the inoculum of *S. enterica* must be quite high to obtain T-cell priming, and at lower inocula, flagellin-specific CD4 T cells do not undergo proliferation (114). T-bet expression is required for Th1 differentiation of *S. enterica*–specific CD4 T cells (115).

Listeria monocytogenes infection of mice also induces CD4 T-cell responses, with peak responses occurring about 1 week after bacterial inoculation (116). The tissue distribution of pathogen-specific CD4 T cells differs, depending on the route of initial infection, with greater numbers of memory CD4 T cells in liver and intestinal epithelium following oral infection (116). CD4 T cells primed by *L. monocytogenes* infection produce IFN-γ and can mediate protective immunity. In contrast to CD8 T cells (see below), *L. monocytogenes*–specific CD4 T cells must produce IFN-γ in order to mediate protective immunity and thus, it is believed that CD4 T cells activate and enhance the bacteriocidal capacity of macrophages harboring intracellular bacteria (117). In contrast to *Salmonella* infections, T-bet is not required for IFN-γ production following *L. monocytogenes* infection (118). In addition to mediating bacterial clearance, *L. monocytogenes*–specific CD4 T cells have also been implicated in the generation of long-term CD8 T-cell memory against this pathogen (119,120). This role for CD4 T cells will be discussed in greater detail in the following section.

T-Regulatory Cells in Defense against Intracellular Bacteria

T-regulatory cells prevent the development of autoimmunity and also temper adaptive T-cell responses to microbial pathogens. Depletion of T-regulatory cells therefore enhances T-cell responses to *L. monocytogenes* (121) and also increases the immunigencity of killed bacterial pathogens (122), which usually do not induce substantial CD8 T-cell populations (123). In protozoal infections, such as that caused by *Leishmania,* T-regulatory cells prevent the complete clearance of the pathogen from the site of infection and thereby enhance the maintenance of long-term CD4 T-cell–mediated memory (124). It is likely that T-regulatory cells also influence the clearance and persistence of intracellular bacterial pathogens.

MHC Class I–Restricted T-Cell Responses

The MHC class I antigen-processing pathway and CD8 T lymphocytes are primarily involved in the recognition and eradication of viral infections. Viral antigens are synthesized in the host cytosol and thus have direct access to the MHC class I antigen-processing pathway. Many intracellular bacteria, however, also introduce protein antigens into the host-cell cytosol, either by invading the cytosol directly or by injecting proteins across plasma or vacuolar membranes into the cytosol.

Listeria monocytogenes has been used extensively to characterize CD8 T-cell responses to bacterial infection (35). Early studies of T-cell responses to this pathogen revealed that CD8 T cells are primed and that adoptive transfer of *L. monocytogenes*–specific CD8 T cells into naïve mice conferred protective immunity (125). As noted previously, *L. monocytogenes* escape killing in the macrophage vacuole by secreting listeriolysin O, a pore-forming toxin that perforates the vacuolar membrane and enables bacterial access to the cytosol (32). In the cytosol, *L. monocytogenes* secretes a number of proteins that are rapidly degraded by cytosolic proteasomes (126), in a manner that conforms to the N-end rule of protein degradation (127), and peptide fragments are transported into the ER and bound by newly synthesized MHC class I molecules. Studies in cell cultures demonstrated that the efficiency of epitope production is quite high, with one bound epitope requiring the degradation of 10 to 35 whole protein molecules (126,128). As might be expected, the quantities of different bacterially derived epitopes varied, with those derived from highly secreted proteins being more prevalent and those derived from scarce proteins being less prevalent. Quantitation of CD8 T-cell responses to these different epitopes, however, revealed little correlation between the frequency of epitopes and the magnitude of the CD8 T-cell responses (129,130). Indeed, the dominant response, which is specific for a peptide derived from listeriolysin O, recognizes a peptide that is presented in only small amounts on the cell surface. Comparison of CD8 T-cell responses to different MHC class Ia–restricted epitopes demonstrated similar expansion and contraction kinetics, suggesting that the duration of T-cell proliferation is not determined by the amount of antigen that is presented (130). Interestingly, inhibiting bacterial growth by administering antibiotics to infected mice has little effect on T-cell expansion or contraction but does limit CD8 memory T-cell development (131,132). Studies characterizing the duration of *in vivo* T-cell priming demonstrated that T-cell priming is restricted to a relatively narrow period of time during the first 72 hours of infection, suggesting that a negative feedback mechanism downregulates T-cell priming at later time points (133).

Adoptive transfer of *L. monocytogenes*–specific CD8 T cells into naïve mice protects these mice from bacterial challenge (134). How CD8 T cells mediate protection against *L. monocytogenes* infection remains incompletely understood, however. Surprisingly, CD8 T cells that lack IFN-γ, TNF, or perforin can still mediate protective immunity upon transfer into recipient mice (89,135,136). CD8 T-cell effector functions likely make distinct contributions to bacterial clearance in different tissues, as indicated by the finding that CD8 T cells lacking perforin and TNF can mediate protection in the liver but not the spleen of *L. monocytogenes*–infected mice (136).

As noted in the previous section, *L. monocytogenes* infection also induces CD4 T-cell responses that can mediate protective immunity (134). In addition to cytokine-mediated effects of CD4 T cells on bacterial clearance, CD4 T cells also provide stimuli that enhance the long-term survival of *L. monocytogenes*–specific memory CD8 T cells (119,120). Initial studies of *L. monocytogenes* infection of mice lacking CD4 T cells demonstrated normal primary CD8 T-cell responses, but careful, longer-term follow-up studies demonstrated that the frequency of memory CD8 T cells gradually diminished in the absence of CD4 T cells. This gradual loss of CD8 T-cell memory results from events that occur during the priming of CD8 T cells and can be attributed, at least in part, to the production of IL-2 by responding CD4 T cells (137).

Oral infection with *L. monocytogenes* induces robust antigen-specific CD8 T-cell responses in the intestinal lamina propria and in the intestinal epithelial layer (41,42). CD8 T cells in the gut undergo expansion with kinetics that are similar to those in the spleen and liver, but their frequency remains higher following clearance of the pathogen. It remains unclear whether intestinal CD8 T cells play a role in protection from subsequent reexposure to *L. monocytogenes*.

In contrast to *L. monocytogenes*, which enters and secretes proteins into the cytosol, *S. enterica* remains within a vacuole. Nevertheless, in order for *S. enterica* to survive within the host cell, it injects bacterial proteins into the cytosol of the infected cells using the type III secretion system, an essential process for *S. enterica* virulence. Experimental studies have demonstrated that recombinant *S. enterica* engineered to secrete known antigens into the cytosol of infected cells via the type III secretion system can prime antigen-specific CD8 T-cell responses (138), albeit with delayed kinetics compared to responses induced by either viral or *L. monocytogenes* infection (139). Recombinant *S. enterica* expressing viral antigens are being investigated as potential vaccine candidates (140,141).

CD8 T cells are also postulated to contribute to defense against *M. tuberculosis* infection. Initial studies demonstrated that mice lacking β2-microglobulin are more susceptible to *M. tuberculosis* infection, suggesting that CD8 T cells promote mycobacterial clearance (142). Analysis of T cells in lungs of mice cured of *M. tuberculosis* and then reinfected demonstrated the activation and expansion of memory CD8 T cells (143). Other studies, however, using mice lacking CD8α or mice depleted of CD8 T cells by antibody administration, suggest that expression of MHC class I molecules may contribute more to mycobacterial clearance than CD8 T cells, leading to the hypothesis that other MHC class I–binding receptors, such as the NK receptors, may contribute to the control of mycobacterial infections (144). Thus, the precise contribution of MHC class I molecules and CD8 T cells in defense against *M. tuberculosis* infection remains incompletely defined.

MHC Class Ib–Restricted T-Cell Responses

Conventional MHC molecules, also referred to as MHC class Ia molecules, are highly polymorphic and are responsible for allogeneic graft rejection and graft-versus-host disease. In addition to MHC class Ia molecules, the major histocompatibility complex of mice and humans encodes additional MHC class I molecules that are far less polymorphic. These molecules, referred to as MHC class Ib molecules, are structurally very similar to MHC class Ia molecules in terms of containing peptide-binding grooves and associating with β2-microglobulin. Two MHC class Ib molecules, murine H2-M3 and human HLA-E, have been implicated in defense against intracellular bacterial infections.

H2-M3 is an MHC class Ib molecule that binds endogenous peptide of mitochondrial origin, specifically selecting peptides that contain the N-formylated amino terminus of mitochondrially encoded proteins (145). Structural analysis of the H2-M3 protein revealed that H2-M3 contains a peptide-binding groove with a binding pocket specific for N-formyl-methionine (146). Because bacterial and mitochondrial ribosomes initiate protein synthesis with N-formyl methionine, while eukaryotic ribosomes do not, H2-M3 was suspected to play a role in defense against bacterial infection (147). Characterization of the CD8 T cell response to *L. monocytogenes* infection revealed that a substantial fraction of responding T cells were restricted by H2-M3 and specific for bacterially secreted N-formyl methionine containing peptides (148,149). Mice with genetic deletion of H2-M3 are more susceptible to *L. monocytogenes* infection, clearly establishing the role of H2-M3–restricted CD8 T cells in antimicrobial defense (150). N-formyl methionine–containing peptides from *M. tuberculosis* (151) and *S. enterica* (152) are also presented by H2-M3 to CD8 T cells following murine infection with these pathogens. In the case of murine *S. enterica* infection, Qa-1, another MHC class Ib molecule, has also been implicated in peptide presentation and CD8 T-cell activation (153).

Although CD8 T cells restricted by H2-M3 and MHC class Ia molecules following *L. monocytogenes* infection are phenotypically similar, their relative expansion kinetics following primary and secondary infection are distinct. H2-M3–restricted T cells expand more rapidly during primary infection than MHC class Ia–restricted T cells, and, in marked contrast to "conventionally" restricted T cells, H2-M3–restricted T cells undergo little expansion after secondary exposure to *L. monocytogenes* (154,155). Although the mechanisms responsible for this disparity remain undefined, these findings suggest that MHC class Ib–restricted T-cell responses may play a more prominent role during primary infection while making only minor contributions to memory responses.

HLA-E is a human MHC class Ib molecule that contains a binding groove that binds peptides derived from signal sequences of MHC class Ia molecules. Consistent with other MHC class Ib molecules, HLA-E is highly conserved between different individuals, that is, it lacks the polymorphism typical of MHC class Ia molecules. Characterization of T lymphocytes from individuals with a history of exposure to tuberculosis revealed that many CD8 T-cell clones that are specific for *M. tuberculosis* are restricted by HLA-E (156). Along similar lines, a subset of CD8 T cells specific for *Salmonella typhi* following immunization with the Ty21a typhoid vaccine were also found to be HLA-E–restricted (157). Although the contribution of HLA-E–restricted CD8 T cells to antimicrobial defense remains unclear, HLA-E–presented antigens are exciting vaccine candidates because they, unlike MHC class Ia–presented antigens, are likely to be immunogenic in HLA-disparate individuals.

CD1 MOLECULES AND PRESENTATION OF MYCOBACTERIAL LIPIDS

CD1 molecules are structurally similar to MHC class I molecules, associate with β2-microglobulin, and present antigens to T lymphocytes (158). In contrast to conventional MHC class I molecules, CD1 molecules have a deeper groove that, instead of binding peptides, accommodates hydrocarbon chains of lipids. Humans express four different CD1 molecules, CD1a, CD1b, CD1c, and CD1d, which differ in terms of intracellular trafficking, antigen presentation, and the T-cell populations that they stimulate (158).

CD1d molecules, for example, present lipid antigens to NK T cells in humans and mice. Mice do not express CD1a, CD1b, or CD1c, but in humans these molecules have been shown to present lipids derived from mycobacteria to T-cell populations. Mycolic acid, one of the major components of the mycobacterial outer surface, is a microbial antigen that is presented by CD1b (159). Subsequent studies demonstrated that lipoarabinomannan, phosphatidyl inositol mannoside, glucose monomycolate, and isoprenoid glycolipids are also bound by CD1 molecules and presented to T cells (160,161). The mechanism by which these highly hydrophobic hydrocarbons are inserted into the groove of the CD1 molecule remains unclear, but saposins, lysosomal lipid-binding proteins, have been implicated in lipid loading of CD1 molecules (162,163). Because CD1-restricted T cells can produce IFN-γ upon stimulation with mycobacterial lipids presented by CD1-expressing antigen-presenting cells, CD1-restricted T cells are believed to play a role in immune defense against *M. tuberculosis*. A particularly interesting feature of antigen presentation by CD1 molecules is their distinct subcellular localization, which allows them to present antigens from different endosomal compartments (158). Thus, CD1a traffics to early endosomes, CD11c to intermediate endosomes, and CD1d and CD1b traffic and derive antigens from late endosomes, lysosomes, and MHC class II compartments of antigen-presenting cells (158).

KILLING OF INTRACELLULAR BACTERIAL PATHOGENS

Although microbial killing is arguably the most important outcome of immune activation during infection, the molecular mechanisms that result in killing of intracellular bacterial pathogens are only partially understood. Killing of *S. enterica* in macrophages is mediated by NADPH phagocyte oxidase and inducible nitric oxide synthase. The oxidative burst, mediated by NADPH oxidase, kills bacteria in the first few hours following cellular infection, and nitric oxide–derived products synergize with oxidative products, in the form of superoxide anion, hydrogen peroxide, and peroxynitrite, to enhance early killing (164). At later time points following cellular infection, NO-mediated inhibition of bacterial growth predominates (164). Cytokines such as IFN-γ enhance NO-mediated bacterial killing by inducing nitric oxide synthase, while TNF enhances collocalization of NADPH phagocyte oxidase–containing vesicles with *Salmonella*-containing vacuoles (165). At another level, MyD88-dependent TLR-mediated signals activates p38 MAPK, which phosphorylates $p47^{phox}$, thereby enhancing NADPH oxidase assembly (48).

In addition to enhancing NADPH oxidase– and iNOS-mediated intracellular bacterial killing, IFN-γ also induces LRG-47, a 47-kDa GTPase that associates with vacuolar membranes. Mice that lack LRG-47 are markedly more susceptible to infection with *M. tuberculosis*, *S. enterica*, and *L. monocytogenes* (166). In fact, mice that lack LRG-47 are essentially comparable to IFN-γ–deficient mice in terms of susceptibility to infection by these intracellular bacterial pathogens. Initial studies indicated that LRG-47–deficient, *M. tuberculosis*–containing vacuoles did not acidify normally, thereby enhancing intracellular mycobacterial growth (167). More recent experiments demonstrate that autophagy is a major mechanism by which IFN-γ induces macrophage-mediated killing of *M. tuberculosis* (168,169) and that LRG-47 is essential for this process. Although *L. monocytogenes*, in contrast to *M. tuberculosis*, does not reside in a vacuole, LRG-47 is also essential for *in vivo* control of *L. monocytogenes* infection (170). Although autophagic elimination of intracellular bacteria may also play a role in this setting, it remains unclear how LRG-47 enhances killing of intracellular *L. monocytogenes*.

Although IFN-γ plays an essential role in defense against *M. tuberculosis* infection, the long-term persistence of mycobacteria in humans indicates that IFN-γ–mediated immune defense is not completely effective. Studies in murine and human macrophages demonstrated that *M. tuberculosis* infection reduces their responsiveness to IFN-γ (171). Inhibited responsiveness to IFN-γ is not general but specific for a subset of IFN-γ–induced effects, such as activation of the class II transactivator, but iNOS induction is maintained (172). Inhibition of INF-γ signaling is not the result from interference with STAT-1 phosphorylation or targeting to promoters and has both MyD88/TLR2-dependent and -independent components (173). Inhibition of IFN-γ signaling in part results from IL-6 production by *M. tuberculosis*–infected macrophages. Although the mechanism by which *M. tuberculosis* infection impairs macrophage responsiveness to IFN-γ remains incompletely defined, incomplete cytokine-mediated macrophage activation provides a plausible explanation for the inability of infected macrophages to eliminate *M. tuberculosis*.

T lymphocytes, by virtue of their MHC restriction, interact principally with other mammalian cells and do not recognize or respond to microbes directly. Microbial killing, therefore, is largely the purview of inflammatory cells such as macrophages, monocytes, dendritic cells, and neutrophils, which take their cues either directly or indirectly from T lymphocytes. Human T lymphocytes, however, release a protein, granulysin, which can directly kill microbes such as *L. monocytogenes* and *M. tuberculosis* (174). In patients with leprosy, caused by *Mycobacterium leprae*, higher frequencies of CD4 T cells expressing granulysin in infected cutaneous tissues correlated with fewer mycobacteria, suggesting that granulysin mediates microbial killing *in vivo* (175). Granulysin kills bacteria by altering their membrane permeability (176).

BACTERIAL MECHANISMS TO SUBVERT HOST IMMUNE RESPONSES

Intracellular bacteria have evolved complex strategies to invade cells, localize to distinct intracellular compartments, and spread to other cells. Mammalian cells, on the other hand, have evolved complex mechanisms to detect intracellular bacteria and activate antimicrobial effector processes. Some microbial pathogenesis strategies, in addition to enabling intracellular survival, also can be viewed as subverting immune recognition by the host. For example, *M. tuberculosis*, by avoiding intracellular compartments containing MHC class II molecules, may limit detection by pathogen-specific CD4 T cells (29). Along similar lines, by preventing the acidification of phagosomes, *M. tuberculosis* may inhibit the proteolytic generation of peptides that can associate with MHC class II molecules (177).

At the level of cytokine-mediated immune defenses, infection with *L. monocytogenes* induces IL-10 production, which attenuates both innate and adaptive immune responses. IL-10–deficient mice clear *L. monocytogenes* infections more rapidly (178). As described previously, virulent *L. monocytogenes* also induces type I interferon production, and mice that lack the receptor for type I interferon clear *L. monocytogenes* infections more rapidly (99–101). It has been postulated that *L. monocytogenes* induces type I interferon production in order to enhance its *in vivo* survival, a notion that remains speculative at this time.

CONCLUSION

Intracellular bacteria remain a major cause of human disease, and the generation of effective vaccines has been frustratingly difficult. The last decade has seen remarkable progress in defining the mechanisms that important pathogens such as *Mycobacterium tuberculosis, Salmonella enterica, Listeria monocytogenes,* and *Legionella pneumophila* use to invade cells and survive. Mechanisms by which host cells recognize intracellular bacteria are increasingly being identified and characterized and, importantly, their effects on adaptive immunity and their potential for enhancing long-term T-cell–mediated immunity determined.

REFERENCES

1. Fournier B, Philpott DJ. Recognition of *Staphylococcus aureus* by the innate immune system. *Clin Microbiol Rev.* 2005;18:521–540.
2. Merz AJ, So M. Interactions of pathogenic neisseriae with epithelial cell membranes. *Annu Rev Cell Dev Biol.* 2000;16:423–457.
3. Coburn J, Frank DW. Macrophages and epithelial cells respond differently to the *Pseudomonas aeruginosa* type III secretion system. *Infect Immun.* 1999;67:3151–3154.
4. Galan JE. Salmonella interactions with host cells: type III secretion at work. *Annu Rev Cell Dev Biol.* 2001;17:53–86.
5. Dussurget O, Pizarro-Cerda J, Cossart P. Molecular determinants of *Listeria monocytogenes* virulence. *Annu Rev Microbiol.* 2004;58:587–610.
6. Glickman MS, Jacobs WR Jr. Microbial pathogenesis of *Mycobacterium tuberculosis:* dawn of a discipline. *Cell.* 2001;104:477–485.
7. Glickman MS. The mmaA2 gene of *Mycobacterium tuberculosis* encodes the distal cyclopropane synthase of the alpha-mycolic acid. *J Biol Chem.* 2003;278:7844–7849.
8. Makinoshima H, Glickman MS. Regulation of *Mycobacterium tuberculosis* cell envelope composition and virulence by intramembrane proteolysis. *Nature.* 2005;436:406–409.
9. Rao V, Fujiwara N, Porcelli SA, et al. *Mycobacterium tuberculosis* controls host innate immune activation through cyclopropane modification of a glycolipid effector molecule. *J Exp Med.* 2005;201:535–543.
10. Rao V, Gao F, Chen B, et al. Trans-cyclopropanation of mycolic acids on trehalose dimycolate suppresses *Mycobacterium tuberculosis*-induced inflammation and virulence. *J Clin Invest.* 2006;116:1660–1667.
11. Mackaness GB. Relationship between host cell and parasite in tuberculosis. *Br Med Bull.* 1954;10:100–104.
12. Blanden RV, Mackaness GB, Collins FM. Mechanisms of acquired resistance in mouse typhoid. *J Exp Med.* 1966;124:585–600.
13. Mackaness GB. Cellular resistance to infection. *J Exp Med.* 1962;116:381–406.
14. Rosen H, Gordon S, North RJ. Exacerbation of murine listeriosis by a monoclonal antibody specific for the type 3 complement receptor of myelomonocytic cells. Absence of monocytes at infective foci allows *Listeria* to multiply in nonphagocytic cells. *J Exp Med.* 1989;170:27–37.
15. Mengaud J, Ohayon H, Gounon P, et al. E-cadherin is the receptor for internalin, a surface protein required for entry of *L. monocytogenes* into epithelial cells. *Cell.* 1996;84:923–932.
16. Vazquez-Torres A, Fang FC. Cellular routes of invasion by enteropathogens. *Curr Opin Microbiol.* 2000;3:54–59.
17. Vazquez-Torres A, Jones-Carson J, Baumler AJ, et al. Extraintestinal dissemination of *Salmonella* by CD18-expressing phagocytes. *Nature.* 1999;401:804–808.
18. Francis CL, Ryan TA, Jones BD, et al. Ruffles induced by *Salmonella* and other stimuli direct macropinocytosis of bacteria. *Nature.* 1993;364:639–642.
19. Galan JE, Collmer A. Type III secretion machines: bacterial devices for protein delivery into host cells. *Science.* 1999;284:1322–1328.
20. Chen LM, Hobbie S, Galan JE. Requirement of CDC42 for *Salmonella*-induced cytoskeletal and nuclear responses. *Science.* 1996;274:2115–2118.
21. Murli S, Watson RO, Galan JE. Role of tyrosine kinases and the tyrosine phosphatase SptP in the interaction of *Salmonella* with host cells. *Cell Microbiol.* 2001;3:795–810.
22. Cirillo DM, Valdivia RH, Monack DM, et al. Macrophage-dependent induction of the *Salmonella* pathogenicity island 2 type III secretion system and its role in intracellular survival. *Mol Microbiol.* 1998;30:175–188.
23. Pfeifer CG, Marcus SL, Steele-Mortimer O, et al. *Salmonella typhimurium* virulence genes are induced upon bacterial invasion into phagocytic and nonphagocytic cells. *Infect Immun.* 1999;67:5690–5698.
24. Vazquez-Torres A, Xu Y, Jones-Carson J, et al. *Salmonella* pathogenicity island 2-dependent evasion of the phagocyte NADPH oxidase. *Science.* 2000;287:1655–1658.
25. Horwitz MA. Formation of a novel phagosome by the Legionnaires' disease bacterium *(Legionella pneumophila)* in human monocytes. *J Exp Med.* 1983;158:1319–1331.
26. Tilney LG, Harb OS, Connelly PS, et al. How the parasitic bacterium *Legionella pneumophila* modifies its phagosome and transforms it into rough ER: implications for conversion of plasma membrane to the ER membrane. *J Cell Sci.* 2001;114:4637–4650.
27. Vergne I, Chua J, Singh SB, et al. Cell biology of *Mycobacterium tuberculosis* phagosome. *Annu Rev Cell Dev Biol.* 2004;20:367–394.
28. Russell DG, Mwandumba HC, Rhoades EE. *Mycobacterium* and the coat of many lipids. *J Cell Biol.* 2002;158:421–426.

29. Clemens DL, Horwitz MA. Characterization of the *Mycobacterium tuberculosis* phagosome and evidence that phagosomal maturation is inhibited. *J Exp Med.* 1995;181:257–270.
30. Tilney LG, Portnoy DA. Actin filaments and the growth, movement, and spread of the intracellular bacterial parasite, *Listeria monocytogenes*. *J Cell Biol.* 1989;109:1597–1608.
31. Kocks C, Gouin E, Tabouret M, et al. *L. monocytogenes*-induced actin assembly requires the actA gene product, a surface protein. *Cell.* 1992;68:521–531.
32. Gaillard JL, Berche P, Sansonetti P. Transposon mutagenesis as a tool to study the role of hemolysin in the virulence of *Listeria monocytogenes*. *Infect Immun.* 1986;52:50–55.
33. Sansonetti PJ, Ryter A, Clerc P, et al. Multiplication of *Shigella flexneri* within HeLa cells: lysis of the phagocytic vacuole and plasmid-mediated contact hemolysis. *Infect Immun.* 1986;51:461–469.
34. Walker DH, Valbuena GA, Olano JP. Pathogenic mechanisms of diseases caused by Rickettsia. *Ann NY Acad Sci.* 2003;990:1–11.
35. Pamer EG. Immune responses to *Listeria monocytogenes*. *Nat Rev Immunol.* 2004;4:812–823.
36. Rescigno M, Urbano M, Valzasina B, et al. Dendritic cells express tight junction proteins and penetrate gut epithelial monolayers to sample bacteria. *Nat Immunol.* 2001;2:361–367.
37. Niess JH, Brand S, Gu X, et al. CX3CR1-mediated dendritic cell access to the intestinal lumen and bacterial clearance. *Science.* 2005;307:254–258.
38. Carlyon JA, Fikrig E. Mechanisms of evasion of neutrophil killing by *Anaplasma phagocytophilum*. *Curr Opin Hematol.* 2006;13: 28–33.
39. Moyron-Quiroz JE, Rangel-Moreno J, Kusser K, et al. Role of inducible bronchus associated lymphoid tissue (iBALT) in respiratory immunity. *Nat Med.* 2004;10:927–934.
40. Lefrancois L. Phenotypic complexity of intraepithelial lymphocytes of the small intestine. *J Immunol.* 1991;147:1746–1751.
41. Pope C, Kim SK, Marzo A, et al. Organ-specific regulation of the CD8 T cell response to *Listeria monocytogenes* infection. *J Immunol.* 2001;166:3402–3409.
42. Huleatt JW, Pilip I, Kerksiek K, et al. Intestinal and splenic T cell responses to enteric *Listeria monocytogenes* infection: distinct repertoires of responding CD8 T lymphocytes. *J Immunol.* 2001;166: 4065–4073.
43. Akira S, Uematsu S, Takeuchi O. Pathogen recognition and innate immunity. *Cell.* 2006;124:783–801.
44. Medzhitov R. Toll-like receptors and innate immunity. *Nat Rev Immunol.* 2001;1:135–145.
45. Seki E, Tsutsui H, Tsuji NM, et al. Critical roles of myeloid differentiation factor 88-dependent proinflammatory cytokine release in early phase clearance of *Listeria monocytogenes* in mice. *J Immunol.* 2002;169:3863–3868.
46. Edelson BT, Unanue ER. MyD88-dependent but Toll-like receptor 2-independent innate immunity to *Listeria:* no role for either in macrophage listericidal activity. *J Immunol.* 2002;169:3869–3875.
47. Scanga CA, Bafica A, Feng CG, et al. MyD88-deficient mice display a profound loss in resistance to *Mycobacterium tuberculosis* associated with partially impaired Th1 cytokine and nitric oxide synthase 2 expression. *Infect Immun.* 2004;72:2400–2404.
48. Laroux FS, Romero X, Wetzler L, et al. Cutting Edge: MyD88 controls phagocyte NADPH oxidase function and killing of gram-negative bacteria. *J Immunol.* 2005;175:5596–5600.
49. Uematsu S, Jang MH, Chevrier N, et al. Detection of pathogenic intestinal bacteria by Toll-like receptor 5 on intestinal CD11c+ lamina propria cells. *Nat Immunol.* 2006;7:868–874.
50. Hawn TR, Verbon A, Lettinga KD, et al. A common dominant TLR5 stop codon polymorphism abolishes flagellin signaling and is associated with susceptibility to legionnaires' disease. *J Exp Med.* 2003;198:1563–1572.
51. Barton GM, Kagan JC, Medzhitov R. Intracellular localization of Toll-like receptor 9 prevents recognition of self DNA but facilitates access to viral DNA. *Nat Immunol.* 2006;7:49–56.
52. Hamerman JA, Tchao NK, Lowell CA, et al. Enhanced Toll-like receptor responses in the absence of signaling adaptor DAP12. *Nat Immunol.* 2005;6:579–586.
53. Inohara N, Chamaillard M, McDonald C, et al. NOD-LRR proteins: role in host-microbial interactions and inflammatory disease. *Annu Rev Biochem.* 2005;74:355–383.
54. Chin AI, Dempsey PW, Bruhn K, et al. Involvement of receptor-interacting protein 2 in innate and adaptive immune responses. *Nature.* 2002;416:190–194.
55. Kobayashi KS, Chamaillard M, Ogura Y, et al. Nod2-dependent regulation of innate and adaptive immunity in the intestinal tract. *Science.* 2005;307:731–734.
56. Stetson DB, Medzhitov R. Recognition of cytosolic DNA activates an IRF3-dependent innate immune response. *Immunity.* 2006;24:93–103.
57. Petrilli V, Papin S, Tschopp J. The inflammasome. *Curr Biol.* 2005; 15:R581.
58. Tsuji NM, Tsutsui H, Seki E, et al. Roles of caspase-1 in *Listeria* infection in mice. *Int Immunol.* 2004;16:335–343.
59. Lara-Tejero M, Sutterwala FS, Ogura Y, et al. Role of the caspase-1 inflammasome in *Salmonella typhimurium* pathogenesis. *J Exp Med.* 2006;203:1407–1412.
60. Mariathasan S, Newton K, Monack DM, et al. Differential activation of the inflammasome by caspase-1 adaptors ASC and Ipaf. *Nature.* 2004;430:213–218.
61. Ozoren N, Masumoto J, Franchi L, et al. Distinct roles of TLR2 and the adaptor ASC in IL-1beta/IL-18 secretion in response to *Listeria monocytogenes*. *J Immunol.* 2006;176:4337–4342.
62. Mariathasan S, Weiss DS, Newton K, et al. Cryopyrin activates the inflammasome in response to toxins and ATP. *Nature.* 2006;440:228–232.
63. Sutterwala FS, Ogura Y, Szczepanik M, et al. Critical role for NALP3/CIAS1/Cryopyrin in innate and adaptive immunity through its regulation of caspase-1. *Immunity* 2006;24:317–327.
64. Diez E, Lee SH, Gauthier S, et al. Birc1e is the gene within the Lgn1 locus associated with resistance to *Legionella pneumophila*. *Nat Genet.* 2003;33:55–60.
65. Wright EK, Goodart SA, Growney JD, et al. Naip5 affects host susceptibility to the intracellular pathogen *Legionella pneumophila*. *Curr Biol.* 2003;13:27–36.
66. Amer A, Franchi L, Kanneganti TD, et al. Regulation of *Legionella* phagosome maturation and infection through flagellin and host Ipaf. *J Biol Chem.* 2006;281:35217–35223.
67. Zamboni DS, Kobayashi KS, Kohlsdorf T, et al. The Birc1e cytosolic pattern-recognition receptor contributes to the detection and control of *Legionella pneumophila* infection. *Nat Immunol.* 2006;7:318–325.
68. Ren T, Zamboni DS, Roy CR, et al. Flagellin-deficient *Legionella* mutants evade caspase-1- and Naip5-mediated macrophage immunity. PLoS Pathog. 2006;2:e18.
69. Molofsky AB, Byrne BG, Whitfield NN, et al. Cytosolic recognition of flagellin by mouse macrophages restricts *Legionella pneumophila* infection. *J Exp Med.* 2006;203:1093–1104.
70. Cheminay C, Chakravortty D, Hensel M. Role of neutrophils in murine salmonellosis. *Infect Immun.* 2004;72:468–477.
71. Rogers HW, Unanue ER. Neutrophils are involved in acute, nonspecific resistance to *Listeria monocytogenes* in mice. *Infect Immun.* 1993.61:5090–5096.
72. Conlan JW, Dunn PL, North RJ. Leukocyte-mediated lysis of infected hepatocytes during listeriosis occurs in mice depleted of NK cells or CD4+ CD8+ Thy1.2+ T cells. *Infect Immun.* 1993;61:2703–2707.
73. Kurihara T, Warr G, Loy J, et al. Defects in macrophage recruitment and host defense in mice lacking the CCR2 chemokine receptor. *J Exp Med.* 1997;186:1757–1762.
74. Serbina NV, Salazar-Mather TP, Biron CA, et al. TNF/iNOS-producing dendritic cells mediate innate immune defense against bacterial infection. *Immunity.* 2003;19:59–70.
75. Serbina NV, Kuziel W, Flavell R, et al. Sequential MyD88-independent and -dependent activation of innate immune responses to intracellular bacterial infection. *Immunity.* 2003;19:891–901.
76. Serbina NV, Pamer EG. Monocyte emigration from bone marrow during bacterial infection requires signals mediated by chemokine receptor CCR2. *Nat Immunol.* 2006;7:311–317.
77. Peters W, Cyster JG, Mack M, et al. CCR2-dependent trafficking of F4/80dim macrophages and CD11cdim/intermediate dendritic cells

is crucial for T cell recruitment to lungs infected with *Mycobacterium tuberculosis*. *J Immunol.* 2004;172:7647–7653.

78. MacMicking JD, Nathan C, Hom G, et al. Altered responses to bacterial infection and endotoxic shock in mice lacking inducible nitric oxide synthase. *Cell.* 1995;81:641–650.
79. Pfeffer K, Matsuyama T, Kundig TM, et al. Mice deficient for the 55 kD tumor necrosis factor receptor are resistant to endotoxic shock, yet succumb to *L. monocytogenes* infection. *Cell.* 1993; 73:457–467.
80. Casanova JL, Abel L. Genetic dissection of immunity to mycobacteria: the human model. *Annu Rev Immunol.* 2002;20:581–620.
81. Newport MJ, Huxley CM, Huston S, et al. A mutation in the interferon-gamma-receptor gene and susceptibility to mycobacterial infection. *N Engl J Med.* 1996;335:1941–1949.
82. Jouanguy E, Altare F, Lamhamedi S, et al. Interferon-gamma-receptor deficiency in an infant with fatal bacille Calmette-Guerin infection. *N Engl J Med.* 1996;335:1956–1961.
83. Jouanguy E, Lamhamedi-Cherradi S, Altare F, et al. Partial interferon-gamma receptor 1 deficiency in a child with tuberculoid bacillus Calmette-Guerin infection and a sibling with clinical tuberculosis. *J Clin Invest.* 1997;100:2658–2664.
84. Altare F, Lammas D, Revy P, et al. Inherited interleukin 12 deficiency in a child with bacille Calmette-Guerin and *Salmonella enteritidis* disseminated infection. *J Clin Invest.* 1998;102:2035–2040.
85. Dupuis S, Dargemont C, Fieschi C, et al. Impairment of mycobacterial but not viral immunity by a germline human STAT1 mutation. *Science.* 2001;293:300–303.
86. Filipe-Santos O, Bustamante J, Haverkamp MH, et al. X-linked susceptibility to mycobacteria is caused by mutations in NEMO impairing CD40-dependent IL-12 production. *J Exp Med.* 2006;203:1745–1759.
87. Cooper AM, Dalton DK, Stewart TA, et al. Disseminated tuberculosis in interferon gamma gene-disrupted mice. *J Exp Med.* 1993;178:2243–2247.
88. Flynn JL, Chan J, Triebold KJ, et al. An essential role for interferon gamma in resistance to *Mycobacterium tuberculosis* infection. *J Exp Med.* 1993;178:2249–2254.
89. Harty JT, Bevan MJ. Specific immunity to *Listeria monocytogenes* in the absence of IFN gamma. *Immunity.* 1995;3:109–117.
90. Raupach B, Kurth N, Pfeffer K, et al. *Salmonella typhimurium* strains carrying independent mutations display similar virulence phenotypes yet are controlled by distinct host defense mechanisms. *J Immunol.* 2003;170:6133–6140.
91. MacMicking J, Xie QW, Nathan C. Nitric oxide and macrophage function. *Annu Rev Immunol.* 1997;15:323–350.
92. Khader SA, Pearl JE, Sakamoto K, et al. IL-23 compensates for the absence of IL-12p70 and is essential for the IL-17 response during tuberculosis but is dispensable for protection and antigen-specific IFN-gamma responses if IL-12p70 is available. *J Immunol.* 2005;175:788–795.
93. Khader SA, Partida-Sanchez S, Bell G, et al. Interleukin 12p40 is required for dendritic cell migration and T cell priming after *Mycobacterium tuberculosis* infection. *J Exp Med.* 2006;203:1805–1815.
94. Keane J, Gershon S, Wise RP, et al. Tuberculosis associated with infliximab, a tumor necrosis factor alpha-neutralizing agent. *N Engl J Med.* 2001;345:1098–1104.
95. Slifman NR, Gershon SK, Lee JH, et al. *Listeria monocytogenes* infection as a complication of treatment with tumor necrosis factor alpha-neutralizing agents. *Arthritis Rheum.* 2003;48:319–324.
96. Flynn JL, Goldstein MM, Chan J, et al. Tumor necrosis factor-alpha is required in the protective immune response against *Mycobacterium tuberculosis* in mice. *Immunity.* 1995;2:561–572.
97. Musicki K, Briscoe H, Tran S, et al. Differential requirements for soluble and transmembrane tumor necrosis factor in the immunological control of primary and secondary *Listeria monocytogenes* infection. *Infect Immun.* 2006;74:3180–3189.
98. O'Riordan M, Yi CH, Gonzales R, et al. Innate recognition of bacteria by a macrophage cytosolic surveillance pathway. *Proc Natl Acad Sci U S A.* 2002;99:13861–13866.
99. Auerbuch V, Brockstedt DG, Meyer-Morse N, et al. Mice lacking the type I interferon receptor are resistant to *Listeria monocytogenes*. *J Exp Med.* 2004;200:527–533.
100. Carrero JA, Calderon B, Unanue ER. Type I interferon sensitizes lymphocytes to apoptosis and reduces resistance to *Listeria* infection. *J Exp Med.* 2004;200:535–540.
101. O'Connell, RM, Saha SK, Vaidya SA, et al. Type I interferon production enhances susceptibility to *Listeria monocytogenes* infection. *J Exp Med.* 2004;200:437–445.
102. Carrero JA, Calderon B, Unanue ER. Lymphocytes are detrimental during the early innate immune response against *Listeria monocytogenes*. *J Exp Med.* 2006;203:933–940.
103. Winau F, Weber S, Sad S, et al. Apoptotic vesicles crossprime CD8 T cells and protect against tuberculosis. *Immunity.* 2006;24:105–117.
104. Salazar-Gonzalez RM, Niess JH, Zammit DJ, et al. CCR6-mediated dendritic cell activation of pathogen-specific T cells in Peyer's patches. *Immunity.* 2006;24:623–632.
105. Jung S, Unutmaz D, Wong P, et al. In vivo depletion of CD11c(+) dendritic cells abrogates priming of CD8(+) T cells by exogenous cell-associated antigens. *Immunity.* 2002;17:211–220.
106. Neuenhahn M, Kerksiek KM, Nauerth M, et al. CD8alpha+ dendritic cells are required for efficient entry of *Listeria monocytogenes* into the spleen. *Immunity.* 2006;25:619–630.
107. Hess J, Ladel C, Miko D, et al. *Salmonella typhimurium* aroA– infection in gene-targeted immunodeficient mice: major role of CD4+ TCR-alpha beta cells and IFN-gamma in bacterial clearance independent of intracellular location. *J Immunol.* 1996;156:3321–3326.
108. Caruso AM, Serbina N, Klein E, et al. Mice deficient in CD4 T cells have only transiently diminished levels of IFN-gamma, yet succumb to tuberculosis. *J Immunol.* 1999;162:5407–5416.
109. Sepkowitz KA. Opportunistic infections in patients with and patients without acquired immunodeficiency syndrome. *Clin Infect Dis.* 2002;34:1098–1107.
110. North RJ, Jung YJ. Immunity to tuberculosis. *Annu Rev Immunol.* 2004;22:599–623.
111. Kaufmann SH, McMichael AJ. Annulling a dangerous liaison: vaccination strategies against AIDS and tuberculosis. *Nat Med.* 2005;11:S33–S44.
112. Winslow GM, Roberts AD, Blackman MA, et al. Persistence and turnover of antigen-specific CD4 T cells during chronic tuberculosis infection in the mouse. *J Immunol.* 2003;170:2046–2052.
113. McSorley SJ, Asch S, Costalonga M, et al. Tracking salmonella-specific CD4 T cells *in vivo* reveals a local mucosal response to a disseminated infection. *Immunity.* 2002;16:365–377.
114. Srinivasan A, Foley J, Ravindran R, et al. Low-dose *Salmonella* infection evades activation of flagellin-specific CD4 T cells. *J Immunol.* 2004;173:4091–4099.
115. Ravindran R, Foley J, Stoklasek T, et al. Expression of T-bet by CD4 T cells is essential for resistance to *Salmonella* infection. *J Immunol.* 2005;175:4603–4610.
116. Kursar M, Bonhagen K, Kohler A, et al. Organ-specific CD4+ T cell response during *Listeria monocytogenes* infection. *J Immunol.* 2002;168:6382–6387.
117. Kaufmann SH. Immunity to intracellular bacteria. *Annu Rev Immunol.* 1993;11:129–163.
118. Way SS, Wilson CB. Cutting Edge: Immunity and IFN-gamma production during *Listeria monocytogenes* infection in the absence of T-bet. *J Immunol.* 2004;173:5918–5922.
119. Sun JC, Bevan MJ. Defective CD8 T cell memory following acute infection without CD4 T cell help. *Science.* 2003;300:339–342.
120. Shedlock DJ, Shen H. Requirement for CD4 T cell help in generating functional CD8 T cell memory. *Science.* 2003;300:337–339.
121. Kursar M, Bonhagen K, Fensterle J, et al. Regulatory CD4+CD25+ T cells restrict memory CD8+ T cell responses. *J Exp Med.* 2002;196:1585–1592.
122. Kursar M, Kohler A, Kaufmann SH, et al. Depletion of CD4+ T cells during immunization with nonviable *Listeria monocytogenes* causes enhanced CD8+ T cell-mediated protection against listeriosis. *J Immunol.* 2004;172:3167–3172.
123. Lauvau G, Vijh S, Kong P, et al. Priming of memory but not effector CD8 T cells by a killed bacterial vaccine. *Science.* 2001;294:1735–1739.
124. Belkaid Y, Piccirillo CA, Mendez S, et al. CD4+CD25+ regulatory T cells control *Leishmania major* persistence and immunity. *Nature.* 2002;420:502–507.

125. De Libero G, Kaufmann SH. Antigen-specific Lyt-2+ cytolytic T lymphocytes from mice infected with the intracellular bacterium *Listeria monocytogenes*. *J Immunol.* 1986;137:2688–2694.
126. Villanueva MS, Sijts AJ, Pamer EG. Listeriolysin is processed efficiently into an MHC class I-associated epitope in *Listeria monocytogenes*-infected cells. *J Immunol.* 1995;155:5227–5233.
127. Sijts AJ, Pilip I, Pamer EG. The *Listeria monocytogenes*-secreted p60 protein is an N-end rule substrate in the cytosol of infected cells. Implications for major histocompatibility complex class I antigen processing of bacterial proteins. *J Biol Chem.* 1997;272: 19261–19268.
128. Villanueva MS, Fischer P, Feen K, et al. Efficiency of MHC class I antigen processing: a quantitative analysis. *Immunity.* 1994.1:479–489.
129. Vijh S, Pamer EG. Immunodominant and subdominant CTL responses to *Listeria monocytogenes* infection. *J Immunol.* 1997;158: 3366–3371.
130. Busch DH, Pilip IM, Vijh S, et al. Coordinate regulation of complex T cell populations responding to bacterial infection. *Immunity.* 1998;8:353–362.
131. Mercado R, Vijh S, Allen SE, et al. Early programming of T cell populations responding to bacterial infection. *J Immunol.* 2000;165:6833–6839.
132. Williams MA, Bevan MJ. Shortening the infectious period does not alter expansion of CD8 T cells but diminishes their capacity to differentiate into memory cells. *J Immunol.* 2004;173:6694–6702.
133. Wong P, Pamer EG. Feedback regulation of pathogen-specific T cell priming. *Immunity.* 2003;18:499–511.
134. Harty JT, Schreiber RD, Bevan MJ. CD8 T cells can protect against an intracellular bacterium in an interferon gamma-independent fashion. *Proc Natl Acad Sci U S A.* 1992;89:11612–11616.
135. White DW, Harty JT. Perforin-deficient CD8+ T cells provide immunity to *Listeria monocytogenes* by a mechanism that is independent of CD95 and IFN-gamma but requires TNF-alpha. *J Immunol.* 1998;160:898–905.
136. White DW, Badovinac VP, Kollias G, et al. Cutting Edge: Antilisterial activity of CD8+ T cells derived from TNF-deficient and TNF/perforin double-deficient mice. *J Immunol.* 2000;165:5–9.
137. Williams MA, Tyznik AJ, Bevan MJ. Interleukin-2 signals during priming are required for secondary expansion of CD8+ memory T cells. *Nature.* 2006;441:890–893.
138. Russmann H, Shams H, Poblete F, et al. Delivery of epitopes by the *Salmonella* type III secretion system for vaccine development. *Science.* 1998;281:565–568.
139. Luu RA, Gurnani K, Dudani R, et al. Delayed expansion and contraction of CD8+ T cell response during infection with virulent *Salmonella typhimurium*. *J Immunol.* 2006;177:1516–1525.
140. Shams H, Poblete F, Russmann H, et al. Induction of specific CD8+ memory T cells and long lasting protection following immunization with *Salmonella typhimurium* expressing a lymphocytic choriomeningitis MHC class I-restricted epitope. *Vaccine.* 2001;20:577–585.
141. Kotton CN, Lankowski AJ, Scott N, et al. Safety and immunogenicity of attenuated *Salmonella enterica* serovar Typhimurium delivering an HIV-1 Gag antigen via the *Salmonella* Type III secretion system. *Vaccine.* 2006;24:6216–6224.
142. Flynn JL, Goldstein MM, Triebold KJ, et al. Major histocompatibility complex class I-restricted T cells are required for resistance to *Mycobacterium tuberculosis* infection. *Proc Natl Acad Sci U S A.* 1992;89:12013–12017.
143. Serbina NV, Flynn JL. CD8(+) T cells participate in the memory immune response to *Mycobacterium tuberculosis*. *Infect Immun.* 2001;69:4320–4328.
144. Urdahl KB, Liggitt D, Bevan MJ. CD8+ T cells accumulate in the lungs of *Mycobacterium tuberculosis*-infected Kb–/– *Db* –/– mice, but provide minimal protection. *J Immunol.* 2003;170:1987–1994.
145. Lindahl KF, Dabhi VM, Hovik R, et al. Presentation of N-formylated peptides by H2-M3. *Biochem Soc Trans.* 1995;23:669–674.
146. Wang CR, Castano AR, Peterson PA, et al. Nonclassical binding of formylated peptide in crystal structure of the MHC class Ib molecule H2-M3. *Cell.* 1995;82:655–664.
147. Vyas JM, Shawar SM, Rodgers JR, et al. Biochemical specificity of H-2M3a. Stereospecificity and space-filling requirements at position 1 maintain N-formyl peptide binding. *J Immunol.* 1992;149: 3605–3611.
148. Kurlander RJ, Shawar SM, Brown ML, et al. Specialized role for a murine class I-b MHC molecule in prokaryotic host defenses. *Science.* 1992;257:678–679.
149. Pamer EG, Wang CR, Flaherty L, et al. H-2M3 presents a *Listeria monocytogenes* peptide to cytotoxic T lymphocytes. *Cell.* 1992;70:215–223.
150. Xu H, Chun T, Choi HJ, et al. Impaired response to *Listeria* in H2-M3-deficient mice reveals a nonredundant role of MHC class Ib-specific T cells in host defense. *J Exp Med.* 2006;203:449–459.
151. Chun T, Serbina NV, Nolt D, et al. Induction of M3-restricted cytotoxic T lymphocyte responses by N-formylated peptides derived from *Mycobacterium tuberculosis*. *J Exp Med.* 2001;193:1213–1220.
152. Ugrinovic S, Brooks CG, Robson J, et al. H2-M3 major histocompatibility complex class Ib-restricted CD8 T cells induced by *Salmonella enterica* serovar Typhimurium infection recognize proteins released by *Salmonella* serovar Typhimurium. *Infect Immun.* 2005;73:8002–8008.
153. Lo WF, Woods AS, DeCloux A, et al. Molecular mimicry mediated by MHC class Ib molecules after infection with gram-negative pathogens. *Nat Med.* 2000;6:215–218.
154. Kerksiek KM, Busch DH, Pilip IM, et al. H2-M3-restricted T cells in bacterial infection: rapid primary but diminished memory responses. *J Exp Med.* 1999;190:195–204.
155. Seaman MS, Wang CR, Forman J. MHC class Ib-restricted CTL provide protection against primary and secondary *Listeria monocytogenes* infection. *J Immunol.* 2000;165:5192–5201.
156. Heinzel AS, Grotzke JE, Lines RA, et al. HLA-E-dependent presentation of Mtb-derived antigen to human CD8+ T cells. *J Exp Med.* 2002;196:1473–1481.
157. Salerno-Goncalves R, Fernandez-Vina M, Lewinsohn DM, Sztein MB. Identification of a human HLA-E-restricted CD8+ T cell subset in volunteers immunized with *Salmonella enterica* serovar Typhi strain Ty21a typhoid vaccine. *J Immunol.* 2004;173:5852–5862.
158. Moody DB, Porcelli SA. Intracellular pathways of CD1 antigen presentation. *Nat Rev Immunol.* 2003;3:11–22.
159. Beckman EM, Porcelli SA, Morita CT, et al. Recognition of a lipid antigen by CD1-restricted alpha beta+ T cells. *Nature.* 1994;372:691–694.
160. Moody DB, Reinhold BB, Guy MR, et al. Structural requirements for glycolipid antigen recognition by CD1b-restricted T cells. *Science.* 1997;278:283–286.
161. Moody DB, Ulrichs T, Muhlecker W, et al. CD1c-mediated T-cell recognition of isoprenoid glycolipids in *Mycobacterium tuberculosis* infection. *Nature.* 2000;404:884–888.
162. Kang SJ, Cresswell P. Saposins facilitate CD1d-restricted presentation of an exogenous lipid antigen to T cells. *Nat Immunol.* 2004;5:175–181.
163. Winau F, Schwierzeck V, Hurwitz R, et al. Saposin C is required for lipid presentation by human CD1b. *Nat Immunol.* 2004;5:169–174.
164. Vazquez-Torres A, Jones-Carson J, Mastroeni P, et al. Antimicrobial actions of the NADPH phagocyte oxidase and inducible nitric oxide synthase in experimental salmonellosis. I. Effects on microbial killing by activated peritoneal macrophages *in vitro*. *J Exp Med.* 2000;192:227–236.
165. Vazquez-Torres A, Fantuzzi G, Edwards CK 3rd, et al. Defective localization of the NADPH phagocyte oxidase to *Salmonella*-containing phagosomes in tumor necrosis factor p55 receptor-deficient macrophages. *Proc Natl Acad Sci U S A.* 2001;98:2561–2565.
166. Taylor GA, Feng CG, Sher A. p47 GTPases: regulators of immunity to intracellular pathogens. *Nat Rev Immunol.* 2004;4:100–109.
167. MacMicking JD, Taylor GA, McKinney JD. Immune control of tuberculosis by IFN-gamma-inducible LRG-47. *Science.* 2003;302:654–659.
168. Gutierrez MG, Master SS, Singh SB, et al. Autophagy is a defense mechanism inhibiting BCG and *Mycobacterium tuberculosis* survival in infected macrophages. *Cell.* 2004;119:753–766.
169. Singh SB, Davis AS, Taylor GA, et al. Human IRGM induces autophagy to eliminate intracellular mycobacteria. *Science.* 2006;313: 1438–1441.

170. Collazo CM, Yap GS, Sempowski GD, et al. Inactivation of LRG-47 and IRG-47 reveals a family of interferon gamma-inducible genes with essential, pathogen-specific roles in resistance to infection. *J Exp Med.* 2001;194:181–188.
171. Ting LM, Kim AC, Cattamanchi A, et al. *Mycobacterium tuberculosis* inhibits IFN-gamma transcriptional responses without inhibiting activation of STAT1. *J Immunol.* 1999;163:3898–3906.
172. Kincaid EZ, Ernst JD. *Mycobacterium tuberculosis* exerts gene-selective inhibition of transcriptional responses to IFN-gamma without inhibiting STAT1 function. *J Immunol.* 2003;171:2042–2049.
173. Fortune SM, Solache A, Jaeger A, et al. *Mycobacterium tuberculosis* inhibits macrophage responses to IFN-gamma through myeloid differentiation factor 88-dependent and -independent mechanisms. *J Immunol.* 2004;172:6272–6280.
174. Stenger S, Hanson DA, Teitelbaum R, et al. An antimicrobial activity of cytolytic T cells mediated by granulysin. *Science.* 1998;282:121–125.
175. Ochoa MT, Stenger S, Sieling PA, et al. T-cell release of granulysin contributes to host defense in leprosy. *Nat Med.* 2001;7:174–179.
176. Ernst WA, Thoma-Uszynski S, Teitelbaum R, et al. Granulysin, a T cell product, kills bacteria by altering membrane permeability. *J Immunol.* 2000;165:7102–7108.
177. Sturgill-Koszycki S, Schlesinger PH, Chakraborty P, et al. Lack of acidification in *Mycobacterium* phagosomes produced by exclusion of the vesicular proton-ATPase. *Science.* 1994;263:678–681.
178. Dai WJ, Kohler G, Brombacher F. Both innate and acquired immunity to *Listeria monocytogenes* infection are increased in IL-10-deficient mice. *J Immunol.* 1997;158:2259–2267.

Chapter 38

Immunity to Extracellular Bacteria

Jeffrey N. Weiser and Moon H. Nahm

INTRODUCTION

Human interactions with bacteria are complex. A consortial relationship has developed between humans and microbes. We are composed of 10^{12} human cells and are inhabited by 10^{14} bacteria composed of innumerable species (1). More than 500 distinct species are estimated to reside in the human oropharynx alone (2). Relatively few of these bacteria are harmful to us in any way. We know little about the innate or acquired immune mechanisms that maintain this equilibrium. In large part, many diseases caused by bacteria are mistakes in which this consortial relationship breaks down and lines are crossed. The innate and adaptive responses to these transgressions can in themselves lead to dire consequences. In *Lives of the Cell*, Lewis Thomas points out

> The microorganisms that seem to have it in for us in the worst way—the ones that really appear to wish us ill—turn out on close examination to be rather more like bystanders, strays, strangers in from the cold. They will invade and replicate if they get the chance, and some of them will get into our deepest tissues and set forth in the blood, but it is our response to their presence that makes the disease. Our arsenals for fighting off bacteria are so powerful, and involve so many different defense mechanisms, that we are in more danger from them than from the invaders. We live in the midst of explosive devices; we are mined (3).

Although certain bacterial species are classified as pathogens, they can live in harmony on our surfaces for long periods and never cause disease. The bacteria that can cause human disease are quite diverse. Based on the pathogenesis of infection and the resulting immune response, these bacteria can be categorized into two general types: those causing intracellular infections and those causing extracellular infections. Most bacteria causing intracellular infections avoid being killed after phagocytosis by either interfering with phagosome-lysosome fusion or escaping from the phagosome and into the cytoplasm. Cellular immunity is critical against bacteria that reside mainly within an intracellular milieu, as is described in Chapter 37. In contrast, the bacteria causing extracellular infections survive in the host by avoiding engulfment by professional phagocytic cells such as neutrophils and macrophages. They do this by presenting a surface that minimizes the opsonic and lytic effects of antibody and complement. Although extracellular bacteria have the ability to enter and pass through cells as a means of moving from one *in vivo* environment to another, they are readily killed once captured by phagocytes. Accordingly, the host defense against extracellular bacteria is critically dependent on humoral immunity complement and the production of specific antibody. Table 38.1 lists many of the important bacteria that can cause extracellular infections in humans, together with the diseases they cause and some of their major virulence factors. In this chapter, we describe the surface structures of many of these bacteria and provide examples of how they are able to infect their hosts and cause disease. We also describe the salient aspects of the innate immunity and antigen-induced immunity important in the host's defense against these bacteria.

SURFACE STRUCTURE OF GRAM-POSITIVE AND GRAM-NEGATIVE BACTERIA

Differences among bacteria contribute to their specific adaptation to either a particular host species or to microenvironments within their host. In general, our current understanding of the limitations of nutrients and the specificity of enzymes and bacterial adhesins, or host receptors, that account for these highly specific microbial tropisms is limited. The diversity of bacterial structures encountered by the host offers a major challenge to immune detection of potential pathogens. There are no structural features that reliably differentiate pathogens from nonpathogens. Moreover, many important extracellular pathogens exist mainly as commensals, only causing damage when the balance between host and microbe is perturbed (opportunistic pathogens). Thus, their diversity requires that initial recognition through innate immunity be focused on the more conserved structural features or "molecular patterns" of bacteria. These molecular patterns are, in general, structures such as peptidoglycan, lipoteichoic acid (LTA), and lipopolysaccharide (LPS) that are also essential for bacterial viability and are thus unlikely to be modified so as to evade innate immunity. A further consideration is that these structural differences among types of bacteria may dictate differences in host responses and contribute to distinct patterns of disease. That said, different types of bacteria may also give rise to remarkably similar host responses. The syndrome of sepsis, for instance, looks very similar regardless of whether it is caused by a gram-positive or a gram-negative organism, although there may be little overlap in the specific bacterial mediators involved.

Most extracellular, as well as intracellular, pathogenic bacteria can be divided into two major groups (gram-negative and gram-positive) based on their response to staining with Gram's stain. To illustrate the surface of the bacteria in the two groups, the surface structures of *Streptococcus pneumoniae* and *Neisseria meningitidis* are shown in Figure 38.1A and B, respectively. Three layers are commonly recognized: cytoplasmic membrane, cell wall, and outer layer. Although these layers are described later in detail, it is important to note that these definitions are operational and that, in reality, the layers are not entirely distinct. For instance, molecules anchored in the cytoplasmic membrane or cell wall may extend into or through other layers. It is also important to note that the capsule, O antigens, and cell wall are not contiguous shields; rather, they are permeable enough to allow through secreted products and nutrients, as well as some immunologic factors (e.g., antibodies and complement).

All bacteria have a cytoplasmic membrane, a non-sterol-containing phospholipid bilayer. This membrane is an osmotic barrier and also forms a barrier for most molecules. The cytoplasmic membrane encompasses various proteins, many of which function in transport. Some of these proteins, referred to as lipoproteins (e.g., pneumococcal surface adhesion A [PsaA], which is a manganese permease in *S. pneumoniae*), are noncovalently anchored to the membrane through lipid modifications and are especially common among some bacteria (e.g., *Borrelia burgdorferi* and *Mycobacterium tuberculosis*). Proteins not exposed on the surface generally display a greater degree of structural and functional conservation compared with those exposed to the selective pressure of host immunity.

A cell wall is found in all of the pathogenic bacteria of both groups, with the exception of mollicutes (which include the genus *Mycoplasma*). The cell wall surrounds the cytoplasmic membrane and is made of peptidoglycan, which is a polymer of alternating sugars *N*-acetyl glucosamine and muramic acid, the latter being connected to a stem peptide. The stem peptides include four to five D- and L-amino acids that are extensively cross-linked by bridges that provide rigidity to the cell wall and protect it from environmental extremes (especially differences in osmolarity). These cell wall peptides include atypical amino acids and are highly conserved within a species and relatively conserved across gram-negative species. Peptidoglycan polymerization is carried out by enzymes, many of which are the target of β-lactam antibiotics and are referred to as penicillin-binding proteins. Compared with gram-negative bacteria, gram-positive organisms may have different stem peptides and cross-linking, as well as a thicker (20 to 30 nm compared with 2 to 4 nm) cell wall layer that can retain the Gram's stain better. The thick cell wall of the gram-positive bacteria may be responsible for their greater resistance to complement-mediated lysis. Other features of the cell wall, such as O-acetylation of muramic acid found in some species, mediate resistance to lysozyme, an enzyme that lyses bacteria by cleavage of the peptidoglycan backbone (4).

In addition to peptidoglycan, many gram-positive bacteria have polysaccharide (PS) associated with their cell walls, with this cell wall PS often extending into the outer layer. The structure of the cell wall PS of gram-positive bacteria varies among species but is relatively invariant within

TABLE 38.1 Extracellular Bacteria Commonly Associated with Diseases

Species	Disease	Important Virulence Structures/Molecules	Special Adaptations Critical to Host Infection
Neisseria gonorrhoeae	Urethritis, cervicitis, salpingitis, endometritis, prostatitis, arthritis, proctitis, pharyngitis	Lipopolysaccharide, fimbria, peptidoglycan, Opa protein adhesin, IgA1 protease	Phase and antigenic variation, molecular mimicry of human antigens
Neisseria meningitidis	Bacteremia, meningitis, septic arthritis	Capsule, lipopolysaccharide, fimbria, IgA1 protease	Phase and antigenic variation, molecular mimicry of human antigens, asymptomatic carriage common
Haemophilus influenzae	Otitis media bronchitis, pneumonia, sepsis, meningitis (encapsulated strains)	Lipopolysaccharide with phosphorylcholine, fimbria, high–molecular weight adhesions, IgA1 protease	Phase and antigenic variation, molecular mimicry of human antigens
Bordetella pertussis	Whooping cough in children, chronic cough syndrome in adults	Pertussis toxin, pertactin, filamentous hemagglutinin, fimbria	Coordinate regulation of multiple virulence factors upon exposure to the host onvironment
Pseudomonas aeruginosa	Infections in compromised hosts, pneumonia, sepsis	Lipopolysaccharide, proteases, lipases, lecithinases, exotoxin A, elastase, flagella	Relatively large genomic size (~6 megabases) allows considerable adaptability to changes in environmental conditions, biofilms
Escherichia coli	Urinary tract infection, sepsis, traveler's diarrhea, dysentery, neonatal meningitis, hemolytic-uremic syndrome	Capsular polysaccharide, lipopolysaccharide, fimbria, toxins, siderophores	Antigenic heterogeneity of capsule and lipopolysaccharide
Vibrio cholerae	Diarrhea	Cholera toxin, fimbria	Bacterial dispersal via cholera toxin, which induces copious watery diarrhea
Helicobacter pylori	Peptic ulcer disease	Urease, flagella, CagA	Ability to survive at low pH provides a niche lacking bacterial competition or efficient immune surveillance
Streptococcus pneumoniae	Pneumonia, otitis media, meningitis, sinusitis	Capsule, PspA and C, pneumolysin, neuraminidase, hyaluronidase, teichoic acids with phosphorylcholine, IgA1 protease	Asymptomatic colonization, genetic transformation permitting continual generation of new genotypes
Streptococcus pyogenes (group A *Streptococcus*)	Acute pharyngitis, scarlet fever, necrotizing fasciitis, streptococcal toxic shock syndrome, rheumatic fever, glomerulonephritis	Hyaluronic acid capsule, M protein, streptococcal pyrogenic exotoxins, streptolysin O, streptolysin S, NAD-glycohydrolase, C5a peptidase	Molecular mimicry of human antigens, high diversity of M proteins
Streptococcus agalactiae (group B *Streptococcus*)	Bacteremia, neonatal pneumonia and meningitis	Capsule, β-hemolysin, hyaluronidase, C5a peptidase	Asymptomatic colonization, acquisition by infants during parturition
Staphylococcus aureus	Impetigo, folliculitis, boils, cellulitis, wound infections, toxic shock, osteomyelitis, endocarditis, bacteremia, pneumonia, food poisoning	Tissue-degrading enzymes, alpha toxin and other membrane-damaging toxins, epidermolytic toxins, enterotoxins, capsule, protein A, TSST1, pigment	Resistant to dehydration, asymptomatic colonization
Bacillus anthracis	Cutaneous infection, inhalation anthrax	Capsule, lethal and edema factors	Opportunistic infection by a spore-forming soil organism
Corynebacterium diphtheria	Diphtheria (pharyngitis/tonsillitis)	Diphtheria toxin	Toxin gene contained in temperate phage and expression regulated by iron concentration
Clostridium tetani	Tetanus (spastic paralysis)	Tetanus toxin (blocks inhibitory neurotransmitters)	Opportunistic infection by a spore-forming soil anaerobe
Clostridium perfringens	Gas gangrene, anaerobic cellulitis, endometritis, food poisoning	More than 10 exotoxins	Opportunistic infection of wounds
Clostridium botulinum	Flaccid paralysis: cutaneous, infant, ingestion forms	Botulism toxin blocks acetylcholine release at synapses	Opportunistic infection by a spore-forming anaerobe

Ig, immunoglobulin; TSST1, toxic shock syndrome toxin-1.

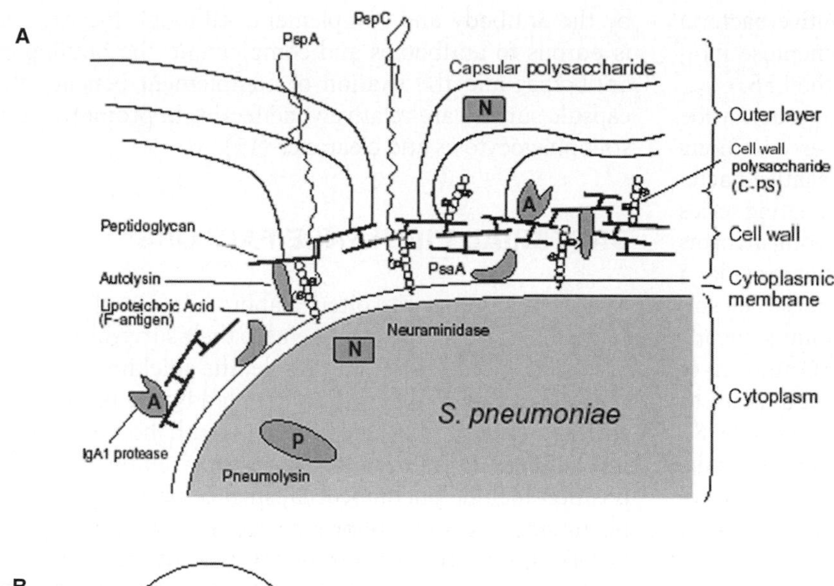

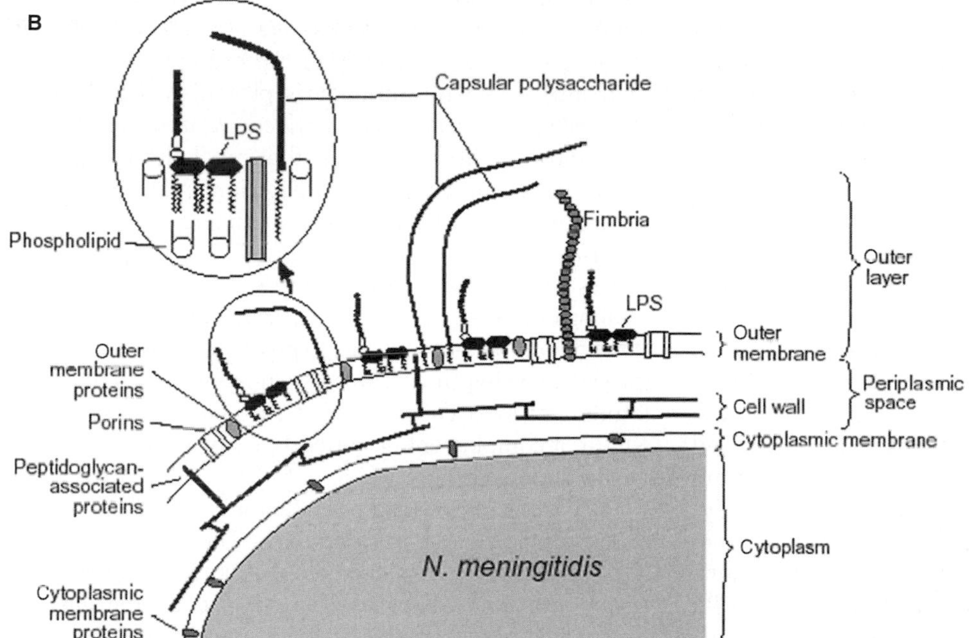

FIGURE 38.1 Schematic representation of the surfaces of **(A)** *Streptococcus pneumoniae* and **(B)** *Neisseria meningitidis* as examples of gram-positive and gram-negative bacteria, respectively. The cell wall polysaccharide of *S. pneumoniae* is often called C-polysaccharide (C-PS). The inset in panel B shows lipopolysaccharide (LPS) anchored to the outer leaflet of the outer membrane.

a species. Differences in the antigenicity of the cell wall PS have been used to distinguish species (e.g., separate streptococci into groups A, B, C, etc.) (5). Cell wall PS often has phosphate group(s) in repeating units of glycerol or ribitol in a structure known as teichoic acid. Teichoic acid may also be linked to lipid molecules, when it is then called lipoteichoic acid (LTA), which is anchored to the cytoplasmic membrane and extends out through the cell wall (6). In pneumococci, the overall PS structures of LTA and cell wall teichoic acid (also referred to as C-polysaccharide) are very similar, with the difference being their mode of attachment to the bacterial surface (7).

Another major difference in surface structure between gram-negative and gram-positive bacteria is the presence of an outer membrane on gram-negative bacteria. The outer membrane is an asymmetric bilayer. The inner leaflet is comprised primarily of phospholipids, whereas the outer leaflet contains lipid A, the hydrophobic component of LPS. LPS, also called endotoxin, is an amphipathic glycolipid with four distinct regions: lipid A, the inner core, the outer core, and, in some species, the O antigen. Lipid A is composed of a dihexosamine backbone to which between four and seven saturated (12- to 16-carbon) fatty acids are attached through amide and ester linkages. Lipid A is the principal "toxin" associated with most gram-negative bacteria, although it is now clear that lipid A is not a true toxin. Instead, its ability to induce cytokines accounts for its potentially detrimental effects. The carbohydrate portion of the LPS, which makes a minimal contribution to its endotoxin activity, is attached to lipid

A through a molecule unique to gram-negative bacteria called keto-deoxyoctanoate. Together with heptose moieties, this molecule forms the inner core of the LPS.

The outer core is composed of 7 to 10 monosaccharide units whose arrangement is relatively conserved among gram-negative species (8). In many gram-negative bacteria, the outer core of LPS is connected to a repeating series of carbohydrates called the O antigen. The O antigen forms a hydrophilic shield around the bacterium that provides a barrier to complement deposition on the bacterial cell surface. The O antigen is variable in length, is antigenically diverse, and confers serotypic specificity. The O antigens of *Escherichia coli*, *Klebsiella*, and *Salmonella* have as many as 30 repeating units composed of four to six sugars each (8). Members of the genera *Neisseria* and *Haemophilus*, on the other hand, lack O antigens, and the size of their carbohydrate regions, also called lipooligosaccharides (LOSs), does not exceed 7,000 daltons. Proteins, including channel-forming porins, are also found in their outer membrane.

For many pathogenic extracellular bacteria, PS components dominate the outer layer. In addition to the PS on LPS (gram-negative) and teichoic acid (gram-positive), there is often another thick layer of carbohydrate referred to as "capsule" that may account for more than half of the bacterial mass. An exception to this general rule is *Bacillus anthracis*, whose capsule is made of poly-D-glutamic acid rather than a polysaccharide (9). *S. pneumoniae* has capsular PS that is covalently attached to the cell wall in most (but not all) serotypes (10). In contrast, the capsule PS is anchored to the outer membrane by acyl chains in *N. meningitidis* (11) and *Haemophilus influenzae* type b (12). Capsular PSs may be highly diverse both within and between species. In the case of *S. pneumoniae*, each strain expresses a single type of capsular PS, with members of this species being capable of synthesizing at least 90 structurally distinct types (13). This diversity limits immune recognition until antibody is generated to the capsular PS of the infecting strain (antigenic variation).

The outer layer is well developed in bacteria that cause extracellular infections and has many features that help the bacteria circumvent the host immune system. First, the outer layer has properties that reduce the attachment of extracellular bacteria to eukaryotic surfaces, including those of phagocytes. Generally, the PS capsules render the bacteria hydrophilic and negatively charged like eukaryotic cell surfaces, which are rich in sialic acid. The negatively charged surface makes the bacteria partly resistant to the deposition of complement by the alternative pathway by enhancing the degradation of C3b (14) (Chapter 33). Second, in some cases, elicitation of antibody is minimized because the capsular PS or LPS mimics host antigens, as is more fully described later in this chapter (page 1193). Third, the outer layer can physically mask most of the other bacterial surface components and thus minimize the number of exposed epitopes that can be recognized by the antibody and complement. Although the capsule is porous to antibodies and complement, the binding of antibodies and the fixation of complement beneath the capsule surface are relatively ineffective in promoting opsonophagocytosis and clearance (15).

BACTERIAL VIRULENCE FACTORS

Extracellular bacteria often elaborate molecules called "virulence factors" that are useful to their survival and proliferation in the host. For example, the shielding function of the outer layer is further augmented by the presence of surface proteins that can interfere with host clearance mechanisms. Proteins inhibiting effective complement deposition include pneumococcal surface protein A (PspA); pneumococcal surface protein C (PspC), alternatively called choline-binding protein A (CbpA); and the C3-binding protein in *S. pneumoniae* (16,17) or M protein in *Streptococcus pyogenes* (18). An example of a protein that interferes with antibody is protein A, which is expressed on the surface of *Staphylococcus aureus* and binds immunoglobulin in a manner that precludes recognition of its target antigen (19). In addition, many successful mucosal pathogens, including members of the *Neisseria*, *Haemophilus*, and *Streptococcus* genera, express proteases with specificity for the hinge region of human immunoglobulin A1 (IgA1) (20). These IgA1 proteases remove the Fc_{α} component required to promote the inflammatory process, leaving the organisms' antigens obscured by the binding of inert Fab_{α} fragments. By inhibiting the deposition of complement or antibody, many of these proteins act to diminish phagocytosis.

The best-known virulence factors are toxins, which interrupt specific host functions. These proteinaceous molecules (also referred to as exotoxins to differentiate them from endotoxin) can be grouped on the basis of their molecular structure and their mechanism of action (21). The largest group is called A-B toxins, which are comprised of two subunits, each with a different function. The A subunit has enzymatic activity, and the B subunit targets the A subunit to the host cells. This group includes diphtheria toxin, cholera toxin, pertussis toxin, and two anthrax toxins (lethal factor and edema factor). For instance, lethal factor of *B. anthracis* behaves as the A subunit and requires a B subunit protein named "protective antigen" to enter into target cells. In some cases, the toxin alone is sufficient to account for the detrimental symptoms of its respective infection. Cholera toxin causes ADP ribosylation of G proteins, which stimulates adenylate cyclase and increases cAMP in cells lining the gut. This results in secretion of electrolytes and is responsible for a severe diarrhea, promoting transmission but often causing dehydration that, if not treated, may be fatal. Uptake of botulism toxin by nerve endings leads to retrograde transport that interrupts synaptic transmission and causes a flaccid paralysis (22). Staphylococcal enterotoxin A (a toxin that acts from the gut lumen), which is one of five membrane-damaging toxins produced by staphylococci, is the primary cause of staphylococcal food poisoning and plays a major role in invasive infections (23). Some strains of *Escherichia coli* produce a protein-synthesis-inhibiting verotoxin, which may damage the microvasculature of the kidney and cause hemolytic uremic syndrome (24). Another group of proteins secreted by *S. aureus* and *S. pyogenes* have toxin-like effects but lack any enzymatic activity. These "superantigens" cause a nonclonal stimulation of T cells by bridging major histocompatibility complex (MHC) class II molecules (outside the antigen-binding site) on antigen-presenting cells and the Vβ region of the T cell receptor on T cells. The ensuing massive release of cytokines by localized release of a superantigen, such as the toxic shock syndrome toxin-1 (TSST1) expressed by some strains of *S. aureus*, results in systemic symptoms that are collectively known as toxic shock syndrome (25).

Another class of virulence factors neutralizes host defenses. Pneumolysin from *S. pneumoniae* is a member of a large class of cholesterol-dependent cytotoxins that oligomerize to form large pores, which interfere with a number of host cell functions or induce cell death when present at higher concentrations (26). Pneumolysin also depletes complement at a distance from the pneumococci and interferes with both the function of phagocytes and the development of protective immunity (27). *S. pyogenes* and group B streptococci produce a C5a peptidase that inhibits the chemotaxic effects (recruitment of host phagocytes to the sites of infections) of C5a, a product of complement activation (28). *Helicobacter pylori* produces urease, which can generate ammonia that can neutralize acid in the stomach and thereby promotes its survival. *S. aureus* produces a pigment that makes the bacterium more resistant to oxidative stress and killing by neutrophils (29).

Whereas evasion of professional phagocytes is critical for extracellular pathogens, the ability to attach to other cell types, including both mucosal and nonmucosal surfaces, is important for their persistence. Many bacterial surface proteins have an adhesive function that confers a high affinity for binding to specific host cell receptors. Nasopharyngeal carriage of pneumococci is mediated largely by adherence to the host molecule *N*-acetyl-D-glucosamine $\beta1\rightarrow3$ galactose or *N*-acetyl-D-glucosamine $\beta1\rightarrow4$ galactose (30). Bacteria often mimic host ligands to coopt their receptors for their own purposes. Many pathogens of the airway express phosphorylcholine (phosphocholine [PC]) on their surfaces (31). This molecule, which is otherwise unusual in bacteria, is found on platelet-activating factor and allows bacterial binding to its receptor (rPAF) (32). To facilitate their attachment to host cells, many bacteria use a pilus (fimbria)—a long filamentous structure extending from the organism. The Pap pilus of *E. coli* binds the Gal$\alpha1\rightarrow4$Gal unit of cell surface globoside in urethral epithelial cells (33). The *Vibrio cholerae* pilus allows the bacterium to attach to the enterocyte for more efficient toxin delivery (34,35). *Bordetella pertussis* has three adherence factors—a filamentous hemagglutinin, pertactin, and a pilus—which allow it to attach to ciliated respiratory epithelial cells in the trachea and bronchi and thus resist the cleansing action of mucus flow (36,37).

Another group of virulence factors helps bacteria acquire essential nutrients. Motile bacteria (e.g., *Pseudomonas aeruginosa*) express flagellin, a complex motor apparatus that allows the bacterial cell to transit along a concentration gradient of nutrients (38). Although in some cases the host and microbe provide nutrients for one another, for some nutrients there is fierce competition. Mucosal fluid and blood are low in free ferric iron due to the presence of iron-binding proteins such as lactoferrin and transferrin. To successfully compete with the host for this vital metabolite, *N. meningitidis*, *Neisseria gonorrhoeae*, and *H. influenzae* have complex surface transport systems that can obtain iron from human transferrin, lactoferrin, and hemoglobin (39). Other bacteria, such as *E. coli* and *Salmonella*, use a different mechanism to acquire iron; they secrete small, high-affinity iron chelators called siderophores that remove iron from human proteins in the environment surrounding the bacteria. The iron–siderophore complex is then taken up by the bacterium, and the siderophore is degraded so that the iron can be freed for use (40).

Production of virulence factors is often highly regulated by bacteria to accommodate changes in environmental stimuli. In staphylococci, it has been shown that the amount of capsule is regulated in response to environmental stimuli (41). One of the best studied of such regulatory systems is the BvgAS, a two-component regulatory system in *B. pertussis* (42). This system, which regulates the expression of adhesins, toxins, and other virulence factors, is controlled by external signals including Mg^{2+}, temperature, and nicotinic acid. Two proteins are involved in this regulatory system, BvgS and BvgA. BvgS, the sensor, is a kinase and is able to autophosphorylate itself in response to the environmental signal. BvgA, the response regulator, is in turn phosphorylated by BvgS. Phosphorylated BvgA is able to activate transcription of virulence genes through a change in its interaction with a 70-bp consensus sequence repeated in Bvg-regulated promoters (42). Analogous two-component regulatory systems in other pathogens are frequently used to regulate the expression of genes associated with virulence (43).

A common theme among extracellular bacteria is the ability rapidly to modify their cell surfaces to adapt to different host environments, such as the natural environment outside of a host, the mucosa of a host, or more invasive sites within a host. For some pathogens, these modifications occur through sensing signals in their environment followed by programmed alterations in gene expression as described for the *Bordetella*.

Another strategy used by extracellular pathogens depends on selection among a heterogeneous population for those members with permissive characteristics. This heterogeneity in a population is commonly generated through genomic rearrangements, such as recombinational events or slip-stranded mispairing in highly repetitive DNA sequences (44). This latter mechanism allows for reversible on–off switching (phase variation) and is especially prevalent in genes encoding cell surface structures subject to immune pressure. For instance, the capsular PS on *N. meningitidis* is needed to protect the organism during invasive infection but inhibits adherence on the mucosal surface, where complement is less abundant. Phase variation of a gene required for capsule synthesis allows for selection of organisms without capsule (phase-off) (45). This change facilitates the bacterial adhesion to the epithelial cells, perhaps by exposing the bacterial adhesins. Alternatively, by decreasing capsule production, the bacteria become less hydrophilic and less negatively charged. This change facilitates their entry into the epithelial cells and their subsequent invasion into deeper tissues. On the emergence of the bacteria from the epithelial cells in the submucosa, capsule synthesis is restored (phase-on) because of the selective pressure of complement-mediated clearance and the requirement for the capsule to survive where the concentration of complement is higher. The flexibility to express different surface properties helps bacteria successfully evade the host immune system and survive in many niches within the host.

Bacteria-to-bacteria signaling is another important mechanism for the control of virulence factors. This phenomenon, called "quorum sensing" (46), has been shown to be operative in a large number of gram-negative and gram-positive species. The signal transmitted between the bacteria can be an acylated lipid (e.g., homoserine lactone) in gram-negative bacteria (e.g., vibrios) or a peptide in gram-positive bacteria (e.g., *S. aureus*). Quorum sensing has been shown to be important in biofilm formation in a number of bacterial species, in the expression of "competence" for the uptake and incorporation of exogenous DNA (transformation), and for the regulation of a number of virulence factors (47). Biofilms are communities of one or multiple bacterial species that adhere both to each other and to a target surface. These extensive aggregates are particularly resistant to many host clearance mechanisms and to antibiotics that are effective against free-living (planktonic) bacteria. Biofilms, therefore, are often a contributing factor in more-chronic bacterial infections such as those involving foreign bodies.

An important characteristic of virulence factors is their structural polymorphism. For instance, there are at least 100 different serologic types of M proteins of *S. pyogenes* (48). Similarly, pneumococci have 90 serologically distinct capsular PSs (13). The polymorphism in the structure of many virulence factors allows the bacteria making them to avoid antigen-specific host immunity. For example, antibodies to the immunodominant region on one serotype of M protein do not cross-react with M proteins of other serotypes and thus do not provide protection against strains expressing other serotypes. Similarly, newly acquired pneumococci can escape recognition by anticapsular antibodies produced in response to previous pneumococcal infections with other serotypes.

The polymorphism in virulence factors is achieved by various genetic mechanisms. Variation in M proteins is the result of sequence differences in the N-terminal (but not C-terminal) half of M proteins (49). *S. pneumoniae* has the genes for synthesizing capsular PS as a "genetic cassette" that can be exchanged among different strains (50) and may result in the shift in the serotype distribution after the use of vaccines designed to elicit serotype-specific protection (13). *Neisseria* has genetic machinery for rapid gene rearrangement (51) through gene conversion using the multiple "silent" pili genes with different sequences. This process, similar to gene rearrangements that generate specific immunoglobulins, permits an individual bacterium quickly to produce progeny expressing pili with different characteristics. The number of potential pilus–antigen variants within the progeny of a single organism is estimated to be greater than 100,000 (52). In addition, *Neisseria* contain large numbers of genes with tandem repeats that undergo phase variation through slip-stranded mispairing of these sequences. Based on predictions from whole-genome sequencing, through this mechanism alone the organism may be able to generate more than 2^{65} different phenotypic variants (53).

Sequencing of the entire genomes of bacteria has shown that the genes for virulence factors have generally originated from other organisms and exist as a part of large blocks of DNA containing multiple genes. These DNA blocks are called "pathogenicity islands" (PAIs). For instance, strains of "enteropathogenic" *E. coli* (EPEC) contain a PAI encompassing about 41 genes encoding a surface ligand required for intimate association of the bacterial and host cell and a bacterial secretion apparatus (54). This system (type IV secretion system) allows for delivery of the receptor for its own adhesin, encoded on the same PAI, into host cells. Elaborate secretion mechanisms (types III and IV) and pore-forming toxins are mechanisms whereby extracellular organisms gain access to the host cell cytoplasm to modify its activity to suit the needs of the extracellular pathogen. Another example is *H. pylori*, which injects cytotoxin-associated gene A (CagA) molecules directly into host cells using a syringe-like type IV secretory apparatus. CagA is then phosphorylated by the host cells, and the phosphorylated CagA alters host cell function, with the *H. pylori* strains producing the CagA molecules being more likely to cause ulcers (55). In the case of *S. pyogenes*, its pore-forming toxin, streptolysin O, allows for translocation of an enzyme (NAD-glycohydrolase) that is capable of producing the potent cytoplasmic second messenger cyclic ADP-ribose (56).

BACTERIAL INVASION OF THE HOST

Both keratinized skin and mucosal surfaces have inherent nonimmune defense mechanisms that modulate bacterial growth and minimize the risk of invasion. Healthy human skin is an effective physical barrier to infection by most human extracellular and intracellular pathogens. The keratinization of fully differentiated skin epithelium results in a relatively impermeable surface. In addition, lysozymes, toxic lipids, and hydrogen ions secreted by cutaneous glands offer bacteriostatic protection for cutaneous pores and hair follicles. Occasionally, this defense can be breached by extracellular bacteria such as *S. pyogenes* or *S. aureus,* causing cellulitis and abscess. More commonly, bacterial invasion through intact skin requires physical damage, such as abrasions, burns, or other trauma. For instance, cutaneous anthrax develops when *B. anthracis* enters the body through a break in the skin. *Staphylococcus epidermidis*, a member of the commensal skin flora, can infect indwelling catheters by spreading through the puncture site in the skin and may lead to bacteremia or colonization of prosthetic devices, including artificial heart valves and shunts. A major factor allowing these bacteria to cause disease is their ability to elaborate within the bacterial population a biofilm (see prior discussion) that facilitates their adhesion, is antiphagocytic, and acts as a barrier to antibiotic penetration (57).

Unlike the skin, the mucosal epithelium is not keratinized. Instead, mucosal areas, such as the gastrointestinal tract, nasopharynx, upper airway, and vagina, are moist and nutritionally rich. Thus, it is not surprising that mucosal areas contain a large number of bacteria. In oral secretions and gastrointestinal products, 10^8 and 10^{11} bacteria/mL may be found, respectively. To ensure their survival in the mucosal environment, extracellular bacteria elaborate many virulence factors required for the acquisition of essential nutrients or for their adherence to the host cells. In some cases, bacteria may subvert the host inflammatory response. *Salmonella* species can block the activation of NF-κB and the subsequent activation of the inflammatory response. They achieve this by preventing the degradation of IκB, which is essential for the translocation of NF-κB from the cytoplasm to the nucleus (58). In some cases, pathogens locate in a less well-protected microenvironment within the mucosal areas. *H. pylori* survives in the very acidic stomach by burying itself in the mucus, which protects it from direct exposure to the acid and from phagocytes. There are also few other species for *H. pylori* to compete with in this more hostile environment.

Mucosal sites have an especially diverse array of bacterial species. Most of the bacteria species found at the mucosal sites are harmless. In addition, polymerase chain reaction analysis of 16S ribosomal RNA sequences suggests the presence of many additional unidentified (and so far unculturable) bacterial species on the mucosal surface (59). Many potentially pathogenic bacterial strains are also often found in the mucosal areas of healthy individuals without causing symptoms. *S. pneumoniae, N. meningitidis, H. influenzae*, and *S. aureus* are examples of pathogenic extracellular bacteria that are frequently carried in the nasopharynx of healthy individuals. The carriage rate of pathogenic bacteria can be relatively high, as shown by the fact that 50% to 60% of healthy young children may carry *S. pneumoniae* in their throats (60). Maintenance of species diversity is dynamic. In some situations, collaboration among bacteria is essential for their successful colonization, as seen among the complex hierarchical communities adhering to tooth surfaces. In other situations, bacterial species compete and regulate diversity among themselves (31). Many bacterial species produce molecules that suppress the growth of other bacterial species. These molecules may include bacteriocins, small molecules that target members of the same or different species that do not express its cognate immunity protein (61). Some species can take advantage of host responses to which they are resistant to outcompete another member of the same niche that is less resistant (31). The host may also control the diversity of colonizing bacteria by modifying the pH or other environmental conditions in the mucosal area. Interference with these homeostatic mechanisms as occurs with antibiotic therapy may alter the flora and predispose the host to disease. As noted, stomach acid is an effective barrier to reaching the nutrient-rich environment of the gut. When stomach acid is pharmacologically reduced, the inoculum of organisms like *V. cholerae* required to infect the intestines is greatly diminished.

Several explanations have been advanced to explain why many pathogens do not cause disease when resident at mucosal sites during colonization. One explanation is that the maintenance of diverse bacterial population is responsible for the prevention of the disease. For instance, the destruction of the normal gastrointestinal bacterial flora with some antibiotics can be associated with a selective expansion of *Clostridium difficile* and the development of pseudomembranous colitis (62). Another explanation may be that the pathogenic bacteria carried in healthy persons are different from those isolated in the setting of disease. For instance, during nonepidemic periods, approximately 5% to 10% of the population carries *N. meningitidis,* which are mostly nonencapsulated (63). During epidemics, 30% to 60% of the population may carry meningococci, which are mostly encapsulated, and the majority of which are of the same capsular type as the case strain causing the epidemic (64). A third explanation is that the pathogenic bacteria are effectively confined to the mucosal surface, where they do not cause damage or induce inflammation. Group B streptococci are carried asymptomatically in the lower intestine and the female genital tract. In the same host, in the setting of parturition, group B streptococci may access the bloodstream and cause septic infection. A fourth explanation is centered on the differences among hosts. Group B streptococci that colonize the mother may cause life-threatening infection when the same strain is passed to the neonate at or before birth (65).

Although pathogenic extracellular bacteria can exist asymptomatically in the mucosa, they can passively enter into less defended sites and cause focal infections. For instance, *E. coli*, which is normally present in the gut, may enter the normally sterile urogenital tract and cause urinary tract infections. *S. pneumoniae* and *H. influenzae* are often carried in the nasopharyngeal space, but they can invade nearby, normally sterile cavities (e.g., lungs, sinuses, and middle ear) and cause focal infections. Aspiration of bacteria from the nasopharynx into the lung most likely occurs frequently with no ill effects; however, aspiration may lead to an infection when there is damage to the epithelial surface, particularly when the protective effects of mucociliary activity are lost, as often occurs in a smoker or during recent viral infection (respiratory syncytial virus or influenza) (5). Some bacteria produce enzymes such as hyaluronidase (66), which may aid in their passage though tissue barriers.

Bacteria can actively invade deeper tissues by multiple pathways. They can enter through specialized cells. *Shigella*, for example, can breach the gut mucosa by transcytosing through the M cells in the gut (67). Alternatively, extracellular bacteria can breach a cellular barrier (epithelium or endothelium) by going through (transcytosis) or between (paracellular pathway) the cells (67). *Porphyromonas gingivalis*, an organism associated with adult periodontitis, may breach the epithelial layer by the paracellular pathway through the production of enzymes useful in digesting the tight junction (68). Two different mechanisms of transcytosis have been described for pneumococci. In one, pneumococci may cross the bronchial epithelial cells by binding the polymeric Ig receptor of the epithelial cells and traveling in a retrograde manner by the IgA secretory pathway (69). In the other, pneumococci may use PC to bind to rPAF, which is abundant on activated endothelial cells, epithelial cells, or pneumocytes (30,70). In many cases, bacterial adhesion triggers changes in the host cell function, and these changes can assist transcytosis. For instance, nontypeable *H. influenzae* with LPS glycoform-containing PC can bind to rPAF on endothelial cells and initiate signaling through this receptor (71).

ANTIGEN-NONSPECIFIC HOST DEFENSE RESPONSE

To protect from infections caused by highly adaptable bacteria, the host uses a multilayered defense. This includes the mechanical barriers and iron sequestration described previously, as well as phagocytes, complement fixation, lysozyme, and (cytokine-induced) local inflammation. In addition, the host is protected with antigen-specific antibody (see later discussion) and T cell–mediated cellular immunity. Antigen-specific immunity, although exquisitely protective, takes from several days to weeks to develop after exposure to a pathogen. Because many extracellular pathogens are capable of causing overwhelming infection in periods of hours to days, other, more rapidly acting forms of protection are needed. Consequently, the primary defense against bacteria during the early phase of infection remains antigen-nonspecific host immunity. The importance and significance of nonspecific immunity is readily demonstrated by the relative ease with which colonies of severe combined immunodeficiency (SCID) mice, which lack antigen-specific immunity, can be maintained (72). This section describes several antigen-nonspecific host defense mechanisms; for additional information, see the chapter on innate immunity (Chapter 14).

Mucosal Defense

Although mucosal areas are rich with nutrients for bacteria, uncontrolled local proliferation of bacteria is held in check by mechanical cleansing actions and the lack of available iron. In the gastrointestinal tract, normal peristaltic motility, the secretion of mucus, and the detergent action of bile limit the number of bacteria. The normally sterile lower respiratory tract is protected by the movement of mucus by cilia lining the airway, which continually remove aspirated bacteria. Normal epithelial and tissue architecture is essential for drainage and expulsion of bacteria, and disruption of this mechanism by smoking, viral infections (e.g., influenza), or bacterial infection (e.g., pertussis) makes the host markedly susceptible to infection by bacteria that otherwise only exist as commensals of the upper airway. The increased frequency of lower respiratory tract infections in the elderly is due, in large part, to the loss of function of the mucociliary elevator and the increased aspiration from the upper respiratory tract of secretions containing bacteria (73,74).

In addition to the removal of bacteria by mucus flow, mucosal fluid contains many antibacterial products such as lactoferrin, lactoperoxidase, mucin, lysozyme, and defensins (75). Lactoferrin, which is found in various body fluids such as milk, saliva, and tears, binds iron and lowers the level of available iron (especially in areas with a low pH) (76). Mucin traps microbes and facilitates their removal. IgA antibodies in mucosal fluid may inhibit colonization by interfering with microbial adherence or by inactivating toxins (77). In addition, the polymeric structure of secretory IgA promotes agglutination, which in turn facilitates removal by mucus. Lysozyme reduces the bacterial load by cleaving the 1→4 linkage of *N*-acetylmuramic acid in the bacterial peptidoglycan. A number of antimicrobial peptides, including defensins, disrupt bacterial membranes (78). In the intestine, Paneth cells at the base of intestinal crypts produce defensins that are important in defense against intestinal infections (79). In the lung, collectin-like surfactant proteins, such as SP-A and SP-D, may be important in host defense by opsonizing bacteria for alveolar macrophages (80). SP-A–deficient mice, for example, are more susceptible to group B streptococcal infection of the lung (81). Epithelial cells that interface with the microbial world must exist in a quiescent state in response to colonizing organisms. If not, chronic inflammation may result in a disease (e.g., chronic inflammatory bowel disease). When the epithelial barrier is breached, these cells are able to elaborate cytokines and chemokine as an early trigger to the inflammatory response.

Local Response to Bacterial Invasion (Acute Inflammation)

On entry into the host, many bacterial products initiate local inflammatory processes. The list of the bacterial products initiating these processes includes peptidoglycan, LPS, lipoteichoic acid, exotoxins, lipoproteins, and glycolipids (82). Antibiotics used for treatment may make bacteria produce additional inflammatory products. Most of these molecules (pathogen-associated molecular patterns [PAMPs]) trigger responses through interaction with pathogen pattern recognition molecules, including Toll-like receptors (TLRs) (see Chapter 14). Of the 13 described TLRs, those anchored on the cell surface and recognizing bacterial PAMPs appear to be most important in responses to extracellular bacteria, although, in some cases, direct binding of the PAMPs has yet to be demonstrated. Cellular amounts of TLRs may also be an important factor in controlling inflammatory responses because TLRs are generally most abundant on inflammatory cells but are in lower levels in the epithelial barrier continuously exposed to microbial products (83). Lipoproteins and lipoteichoic acid are detected by TLR2. TLR2 requires a binding partner (TLR1 or 6) to transmit signals leading to cytokine production (84). Mice lacking the TLR2 gene are more susceptible to mucosal and systemic infection with staphylococci and streptococci (85,86). Although LPS binds to CD14 and lipid-binding proteins, it requires binding to TLR4 for cell signaling, because mice without functional TLR4 are unresponsive to LPS. Bacterial flagellin signals through TLR5 (87). Bacterial DNA, rich in unmethylated CpG motif, is a potent inducer of inflammation through its binding to TLR9. However, the importance of TLR9, an intracellular signaling receptor, in bacterial infection is unclear.

There are a number of TLR-independent mechanisms for the recognition of bacterial products. Many components of bacteria (e.g., peptidoglycan) can enhance the inflammatory process by activating complement through the alternative pathway (88) via the generation of chemoattractant fragments (e.g., C5a). The Nod family of cytosolic molecules transmits proinflammatory signals in response to peptidoglycan fragments and may contribute to the response of phagocytes to typical extracellular pathogens (89). In addition, several mechanisms have been described whereby penetration of the cytoplasmic membrane by extracellular bacteria allows access to the Nod proteins in nonphagoctic cells (90). Protein A on *S. aureus* binds to the tissue necrosis factor-α (TNFα) receptor (TNFR1), and this interaction reproduces the inflammatory effects of its natural ligand (91). Bacteria produce formylmethionyl peptides (e.g., f-Met-Ile-Leu-Phe), which are potent chemoattractants for neutrophils and macrophages (92).

During the initial phase of inflammation after a bacterial invasion, many cell types residing in the mucosa or skin (e.g., keratinocytes) may produce molecules important in controlling infections. Several studies revealed that mast cells are among the important resident host cells. Mast cells, classically known for their stores of histamine and serotonin (93), are abundant along the bronchial tree and epidermis of the skin. They are now known to contain preformed TNFα as well as to be a major source of various cytokines. Mast cells account for 90% of IL-4– and IL-6–producing cells in the nasal cavity (94). On exposure to various bacterial products (e.g., LPS), mast cells release these cytokines, which are essential for the recruitment of neutrophils to the site of inflammation. The absence of mast cells can increase the susceptibility of animals to bacterial infections in the peritoneum or the lung; their absence can be partially compensated for by administration of TNFα (95).

As the inflammatory process persists, additional cell types come to the site of inflammation. In the case of experimental pneumococcal pneumonia, neutrophils come to the lung in 12 to 24 hours, followed by the appearance of monocytes and macrophages in 48 hours (96). Few lymphocytes are observed in the lung during this time period. Neutrophils and macrophages become activated by the bacterial products (e.g., LPS) and chemokines (e.g., IL-8) on their arrival at the site of infection. Neutrophils and macrophages can rapidly phagocytize and kill the bacteria. (See Chapter 18 for a detailed description of phagocytosis.) Phagocytosis can occur when phagocytic cells recognize certain native molecular structures of the bacteria such as lectins, PS, and peptides (RGD sequence) (97) or, aided by their CR3 and Fc receptors, recognize the host opsonins on the bacterial surface.

Inflammatory processes trigger the cascade of chemokine and cytokine release at the site of inflammation. Sequential appearance of chemokines has been noted in the pneumonia model (96). The peak levels of chemokines macrophage inflammatory protein-2 (MIP-2) and KC are achieved in the lung less than 6 hours after infection. The peak levels of MIP-1α and monocyte chemotactic protein-1 (MCP-1) are observed in 12 to 24 hours. Neutralizing MIP-1α and MCP-1 along with RANTES (regulated on activation, normal T cell expressed and secreted) reduces macrophage recruitment. The cytokines produced during acute inflammation can be divided into two groups: proinflammatory cytokines (e.g., IL-1 and TNFα) and antiinflammatory cytokines (e.g., IL-4). The molecules produced during inflammation can induce the expression of endothelial leukocyte adhesion molecule (ELAM), intercellular adhesion molecule (ICAM), and vascular cell adhesion molecule (VCAM) on endothelial cells and selectins and integrins on leukocytes, thereby modifying the properties of the cells at the site of inflammation (cell adhesion, vascular permeability, etc.).

Systemic Response to Bacterial Invasion

Once extracellular bacteria enter the systemic circulation, they are rapidly removed by the spleen or the liver (15,92). Persons lacking splenic function (due to sickle cell disease or splenectomy) are at an increased risk of overwhelming sepsis from encapsulated pathogens (e.g., *S. pneumoniae*) (98). Clearance of bacteria from the blood by these organs is facilitated because phagocytes are abundant and blood circulates slowly in these organs, preexisting cross-reactive antibodies can fix complement (99), and the alternative pathway or mannose-binding lectin can fix complement nonspecifically. The bacteria release many inflammatory bacterial products into the systemic circulation and trigger many systemic changes, such as fever and accumulation of leukocytes at the sites of infection.

Cytokines (e.g., IL-6, IL-1) and glucocorticoids trigger the acute-phase response by stimulating hepatocytes to produce and secrete a variety of molecules that are termed acute-phase reactants, such as coagulation factors, serum amyloid A protein, C-reactive protein (CRP), TREM-1 (100), and collectins (101). Collectin molecules, which have a C-type lectin motif and a collagen-like motif, can bind to the surface of bacteria, activate complement along the classic pathway, and opsonize bacteria. For instance, mannose-binding lectin, a collectin, binds bacterial surface glycoproteins that contain mannose and *N*-acetyl glucosamine. Increased incidence of infection has been associated with low serum levels of mannose-binding lectin in individuals (102).

CRP, named for its ability to bind to pneumococcal C-polysaccharide, is found in highest concentrations in serum. Transgenic mice expressing human CRP are more resistant to systemic pneumococcal infection (98). After CRP binds to PC, which is expressed on many respiratory tract pathogens, it activates complement or functions like anti-PC antibody by engaging FcR. Indeed, CRP can kill PC-expressing *H. influenzae in vitro* in the presence of complement. Because many pathogens use phosphorylcholine to bind to the host cells via rPAF, CRP also blocks bacterial adhesion that involves this receptor (103).

One systemic response to infection is to lower the serum concentration of iron. This is achieved by an increase in the transferrin concentration in serum and by an increase in iron storage by tissues. Iron at the site of inflammation may be reduced by neutrophil-secreted lactoferrin. The reduction in the amount of iron available to bacteria can be a significant defensive measure (104). Moreover, even a moderate reduction in iron intake (105) and the use of an iron chelator have been shown to be beneficial against infections by extracellular bacteria. In contrast, an excess of iron may predispose an individual to infections (106).

In the past, the study of the role of molecules in host defense *in vivo* was limited by the availability of a few natural mutations (or alleles). With the widespread use of targeted gene-deletion and transgenic technology, many new molecules have now been investigated for their *in vivo* role. Some of these studies that are relevant to extracellular bacterial infections are listed in Table 38.2. Although the story is evolving, these studies have begun to show the complexity of the host defense in molecular detail. For instance, studies have revealed the unexpected relevance of some molecules to protection against bacterial infections. Lipoproteins are relevant to bacterial infections because lipoproteins can bind and neutralize LPS (107). Surfactant molecules are also important, and their mechanisms are under investigation. These studies further illustrate the differences in the protective mechanisms used against different groups of bacteria. C9 deficiency predisposes one to infection by gram-negative organisms such as *N. meningitidis* but not to infection by gram-positive bacteria. This information has supported our understanding that serum bactericidal activity is not the major protective mechanism for gram-positive bacteria.

Several additional mutations are found to affect predominantly the defense against gram-negative organisms (108). The *IL-1B* gene is allelic at various locations, but only the allelic homozygosity at position –511 of the IL-1B gene is associated with an increased fatal outcome to *N. meningitidis* infections in humans compared with heterozygosity at that position (109). The fact that heterozygous individuals are more protected than homozygotes also complicates the potential explanations. In addition, *in vivo* manifestations of the same genetic defect can be different in different genetic backgrounds. The effect of the *btk* mutation is largely limited to production of antibodies to PS antigens in mice (110), but the same mutation produces agammaglobulinemia in humans (111). Of

TABLE 38.2 Examples of Genes Associated with Changes in the Susceptibility to Extracellular Bacterial Infections

Gene	Susceptible	Reference
Low-density-lipoprotein receptor	Gram-negative bacteria (lipopolysaccharide)	241
C3	Group B streptococcus	242
C4	Group B streptococcus	242
C9	*Neisseria meningitidis*	243
SP-A	Group B streptococcus	81
TNFRI	*Streptococcus pneumoniae, Staphylococcus aureus*	244
TNFR1 and type1 IL-1R	*Escherichia coli*	245
IL-6	*E. coli*	246
IFNγ	*Brucella abortus*	247
IL-10	*E. coli* fewer bacteria but more damage	113
IL-23	*Citrobacter rodentium, Klebsiella pneumoniae*	221, 222
IL-17R	*K. pneumoniae*	221
bcl-3	*S. pneumoniae*	108
P50 unit of NF-κB	*S. pneumoniae, Listeria monocytogenes*	248
Nude mice	*Helicobacter pylori*	249
BTK	*S. pneumoniae*	164
TLR2	*S. pneumoniae*	85, 86
TLR4	*E. coli*	228
CXCL15	*K. pneumoniae*	250
CXCR2	*Pseudomonas aeruginosa*	251
IL-8R murine homolog	*E. coli*	252
LFA-1 CD11a/CD18	*S. pneumoniae*	253
Mac-1 CD11b/CD18	*S. pneumoniae*	253
Mrp-1	More resistant to *S. pneumoniae*	114
Nod1	*H. pylori*	90
IL-1 receptor associated kinase IRAK-4	*S. pneumoniae*	254

interest, an immunodeficient human patient with the inability to produce antibodies to PS (but not protein) antigens was found to have a mutation at *btk* (112), further emphasizing that background genes can have a profound effect on the *in vivo* role of one mutation. Finally, phenotypic changes are complex. IL-10 gene deletion results in fewer bacteria but more tissue damage after an infection (113). Mrp-1 gene deletion results in an increased resistance to pneumococcal infections (114). As additional information becomes available, a more comprehensive picture will emerge. This should help us to expand the use of immunoregulators (e.g., TNFα antagonist) for treating autoimmune diseases (115) without compromising the patient's ability to combat infections.

ANTIGEN-SPECIFIC HOST DEFENSE RESPONSE

Accompanying antigen-nonspecific responses, the host also mounts an adaptive, antigen-specific immune response. For protective responses to extracellular bacteria, B cell–mediated (but not T cell–mediated) immune responses are critical, as shown by clinical observations of patients with Bruton's agammaglobulinemia. These patients, who have relatively normal T cell function but lack B cells, suffer primarily from infections caused by extracellular bacteria, which can be very successfully treated with the passive administration of pooled γ-globulin (116). Consequently, protective B cell responses are described in detail in what follows.

Responses of the Host (B Cell) Immune System to Bacteria

After an asymptomatic exposure or an infection, the host develops antibodies to many different bacterial antigens. For instance, the level of antibodies to various pneumococcal antigens increases in young children as they age, even if they never have clinical infections (117). However, the antibody levels remain low in those young children without evidence of asymptomatic nasopharyngeal carriage of pneumococci. This finding suggests that asymptomatic carriage of pneumococci is sufficient to raise antibody levels (117).

When an infection occurs, it presents the host with a large load of free antigens released from bacteria such as capsular PSs and proteins (e.g., toxins). Bacterial proteins induce strong immune responses in a conventional

T cell–dependent manner; indeed, the antibody response induced by bacterial proteins has been used to diagnose infections (118). In addition, the released PSs that are readily detectable in the urine of many patients (119) are used to diagnose pneumococcal pneumonia (120). The released PSs may neutralize the anti-PS antibodies in the host. For example, vaccination with hemophilus vaccines may neutralize preexisting anti-PS antibody and briefly increase disease susceptibility immediately after the vaccination (121).

In contrast to proteins, bacterial PSs generally elicit antibody responses with minimal help from T cells (122). Because bacterial PSs usually have many repeating units and multiple epitopes, they can efficiently cross-link BCR and stimulate B cells. The PSs primarily stimulate two subsets of B cells: B1 B cells (123) and marginal zone (MZ) B cells (124,125). These two types of B cells along with follicular B cells are the three recognized subsets of mature B cells with preferential anatomic locations. B1 B cells are associated with the peritoneum, MZ B cells are found in the splenic marginal zone, and follicular B cells are in splenic follicles. In mice, the subsets can be distinguished by their surface phenotypes. Follicular B cells are IgM^{low}, IgD^{high}, $CD23^{+}$, $CD21^{int}$, and $CD1d^{low}$, whereas MZ B cells are IgM^{high}, IgD^{low}, $CD23^{low}$, $CD21^{high}$, and $CD1d^{high}$ (126). B1 B cells express CD11b and B220, with CD5 expression being used to divide them into B1a ($CD5^{+}$) and B1b ($CD5^{-}$) subsets (123). Furthermore, these subsets have distinct developmental requirements. MZ B cells require a proline-rich tyrosine kinase (Pyk-2) (124), Aiolos, and Notch2 (126). B1 B cell deficiency was noted in mice without the regulatory B1 subunit of calcineurin (127). B1a B cells are absent in CD19-deficient mice (128), and the development of B1 and follicular B cells requires BTK (129).

Several observations support the contention that the antibody response to PS antigens is largely independent of T cells. Athymic mice can produce antibodies to PS antigens. PS antigens do not bind class II molecules as protein antigens do (130) and may actually interfere with the presentation of protein antigens (131). In addition, they do not usually induce the formation of germinal centers (132), elicit poor immune memory (133), and easily tolerize B cells (134). Nonetheless, there have been past reports of T cell involvement in the antibody response to PS antigens (135), and recent studies suggest that CD40 is involved in this response (136). Because the PS antigens used for the studies may have had contaminants that affected their immune properties (137) and zwitterionic PSs may behave differently from other PSs (138), additional studies with pure PSs would be needed to define the role of non-B cells in the antibody response to PS antigens.

Polysaccharide antigens commonly elicit oligoclonal antibodies, which use a restricted number of V region genes (139,140) even among genetically unrelated humans (141). In addition, the antibodies to PS exhibit few somatic mutations (141,142) and generally have a low affinity to the antigen (143). However, because the capsular PS and LPS O antigens present repeating epitopes, even low-affinity antibodies can bind with enough avidity to fix complement and cause opsonization and/or bacteriolysis.

Capsular PSs have been used as vaccines because their antibodies are protective. Young children, however, do not produce antibodies to most PS antigens until they are several years old (144), and they are particularly susceptible to infections by encapsulated bacteria during their first few years of life (145). However, young children readily produce antibodies to PS when it is conjugated to a protein carrier. The clinical use of "conjugate" vaccines to induce antibodies to *H. influenzae* type b (Hib)-PS in young children has virtually eliminated Hib meningitis as well as oropharyngeal colonization by Hib (146). Similar "conjugate" vaccine approaches have been used to produce 7-valent pneumococcal and 4-valent meningococcal conjugate vaccines (147,148). The pneumococcal conjugate vaccine has been used for young children since 2000 and has markedly reduced the incidence of invasive pneumococcal infections in both young children and older adults (149).

The immunobiology of conjugate vaccines can differ based on the protein carriers used. Among hemophilus conjugate vaccines, Hib-PS conjugated to the meningococcal outer membrane protein complex (OMPC) can elicit antibody responses after only one immunization (150), presumably because, unlike other protein molecules used as carriers, OMPC stimulates TLR2 (151).

Not all bacterial antigens are presented to the host as free molecules, and some antigens remain associated with the bacteria. When the bacteria enter the blood circulation, they preferentially localize at the marginal zone of the spleen. The marginal zone has features useful in capturing particles in the blood: the zone is where the terminal arteriole ends and empties into sinuses and has several characteristic macrophages and dendritic cells (DCs) (126). After the localization of the bacteria at the marginal zone of the spleen, even without T cells, within 2 to 3 days MZ B cells can be activated and become plasma cells secreting antibodies to bacterial PSs (125). Marginal zone B cells have additional unique characteristics. They are rapidly stimulated by LPS (152), and their maturation may be facilitated by other bacterial molecules as well. MZ B cells may facilitate the activation of follicular B cells because they can capture IgM immune complex and transport it to follicular dendritic cells (153,154).

Although MZ B cells can mature and differentiate independent of T cells (125), other cells, including T cells, may help their maturation and antibody responses to various bacterial antigens. MZ B cells can present bacterial (protein) antigens to naive T cells (153). In addition to protein antigens, antibody responses to bacterial PSs require cofactors such as B7-2 (155) and CD40 (155,156) and can be reduced with simultaneous injection of anti-CD4 and CD8 antibodies (157,158). Indeed, studies have shown antibody responses to PSs attached to bacteria to be T cell dependent (159). MZ B cell response may depend on DCs as well. On taking up dead bacteria, CD11c^{low}, CD11b^{high} DCs in the blood locate to the spleen and may provide TACI ligand(s) helpful in MZ B cell survival (160). Adoptive transfer of live dendritic cells after an *in vitro* exposure to dead pneumococci can transfer antibody responses to pneumococcal proteins and PS antigens (161). NK T cells may be involved in MZ B cell maturation, because MZ B cells express CD1 and may activate NK T cells (153).

Preimmune animals have antibodies that cross-react with many structurally unrelated antigens. These antibodies are often labeled as "natural antibodies." The majority of these antibodies are of the IgM isotype, and they frequently bind autologous antigens. Anti-PC antibodies may be examples of natural antibodies. Recent studies suggest that these natural antibodies are important in the early phase of bacterial and viral infections (162). For instance, anti-PC antibodies react with a PC epitope found on *S. pneumoniae*, *H. influenzae*, and *Wuchereria bancrofti* (a tissue nematode) (163–165). Anti-PC antibodies can reduce the susceptibility of mice to pneumococcal infections (164). A recent study suggested that the natural antibodies are from B1a B cells. CD19-deficient mice lack B1a B cells and have a reduced number of MZ B cells. These mice also lack anti-PC antibodies and are susceptible to pneumococcal infections (128). In contrast, another mouse strain that exhibits both a reduced number of MZ B cells and a deficiency of B1b cells can produce anti-PC antibodies and is as resistant to pneumococcal infections as are normal mice (128).

In addition to natural antibodies, animals often have preexisting antibodies to a PS that cross-react with structurally similar PSs (166–168), probably because many PS molecules have very similar structures. Sometimes it is difficult to distinguish usual "anti-PS antibodies" from "natural antibodies." Cross-reactions may play an important role in protecting the host against its first exposure to a bacterial species. For instance, human adults carry detectable amounts of antibodies to the *H. influenzae* type b PS (Hib-PS)—even in the absence of vaccination—and are thus relatively resistant to *H. influenzae* infections (145). Although some of the antibodies may be the result of immunization by subclinical infections, the majority of human preimmune (but not postimmune) anti-Hib PS antibodies cross-react with *E. coli* K100, the PS capsule of which is an isopolymer of Hib PS (169). Experimental colonization of rats with *E. coli* K100 can protect them against Hib (170). About 1% of human IgG binds a carbohydrate epitope [gal(1→3)gal] (171), and this antibody can kill *Trypanosoma* and *Leishmania in vitro* (172). Cross-reactive antibodies binding the LPS core components are thought to be responsible for the protection from bacteremic dissemination of gonococci in nonimmune patients (99), although they cannot prevent infection of the genital tract (99).

Normal gut flora may be the antigenic stimulus for many of the cross-reactive anti-PS antibodies. About 1% of the human population carries *E. coli* K100 in its gut at any moment (173). Antibodies to gal(1→3)gal are found to bind many species of bacteria isolated from normal stool specimens (171). The gut flora may have additional interesting effects on the immune system. For example, in some transgenic mice, inflammatory bowel diseases develop in the presence of normal intestinal flora but not in the absence of gut flora. In addition, in some animals, such as chickens and rabbits, microbial colonization of the gut appears to be necessary for the normal development of antibody V region repertoires (174). Bacteria should therefore be considered as active participants in shaping the host immune system.

Protective Mechanisms of Antibodies

Antibodies to virulence factors may act by neutralizing the function of those factors. Antitoxin antibodies can protect a host by blocking the action of the toxins or by increasing the removal rate of the toxins (e.g., blocking the binding of the toxins to the host cell receptors). Antibodies to superantigens or tetanus toxin can inactivate them and thereby provide protection to the host. Antibodies to an *E. coli* adhesin can prevent experimental infections of *E. coli* (175). Antibodies to M protein neutralize its ability to interfere with complement and provide protection against *S. pyogenes* infections. Antibodies to LPS (176,177), or perhaps to LTA (178), can be protective. Antibodies to PspA, pneumolysin, autolysin, or PspC (CbpA) can protect animals from fatal pneumococcal sepsis. Although these antigens are being investigated as potential replacements for the expensive pneumococcal conjugate vaccines, the protective mechanisms that they use are unclear. The most recent hypothesis suggests that antibodies to PspA may alter the complement fixation on pneumococci (27,179). Antibodies to IgA1 protease or iron-transport systems (180,181) can also protect against bacterial infections, most likely by neutralizing the normal functions of the target antigens. Finally, in the presence of antibodies and complement, the ability of the liver to remove bacteria increases significantly (15). Thus, another protection mechanism provided by antibodies may be to facilitate the *in vivo* removal of bacteria from circulation by enhancing the ability of the reticuloendothelial system to clear bacteria.

Antibodies to capsule PS can provide protection by fixing complement on the surface of bacteria and by inducing bacteriolysis or opsonization. The bacteriolysis pathway can provide significant *in vivo* in protection against gram-negative bacteria, as is illustrated by the susceptibility to *N. meningitidis* infections of persons with deficiencies of C5-9 components (182). In contrast, antibodies and complement do not lyse gram-positive bacteria but opsonize them for phagocytic killing, as explained later (88). Host phagocytes cannot readily recognize and kill the intact encapsulated gram-positive bacteria. However, once they are coated with antibodies and complement fragments, the host phagocytes can readily recognize the bacteria with various recognition receptors and engulf the bacteria for intracellular killing. An Fc receptor (CD16b) and a complement receptor (CR3) are among the important recognition receptors. CR3, an integrin molecule, is a heterodimer of CD11b and CD18. Protection mediated by this antibody/complement-mediated opsonization is probably very important *in vivo*, because both complement deficiency and agammaglobulinemia predispose individuals to infections by many different extracellular bacteria (116,182). To be effective for opsonization, the epitope of the surface antigens must be exposed on the surface of the bacteria. Effective antibodies to the porins of *N. meningitidis* recognize the surface loop of the molecule (183). In most pneumococci, C-polysaccharide (C-PS) is mostly buried underneath the PS capsule. Although antibodies to the C-PS can fix complement (15), anti–C-PS antibodies were ineffective in protecting mice against most *S. pneumoniae*, unlike antibodies to capsular PS, which are protective (184). However, a recent study found that purified human anti–C-PS antibodies can opsonize pneumococci (185); thus, additional studies are needed.

Because antibody-mediated opsonization and bacteriolysis depend on the complement-fixing properties of the Fc region, the relative efficacies of antibodies of different immunoglobulin isotypes have been compared. IgM antibodies are produced early in the course of infections and should be important in the early phase of infections because they fix complement very efficiently and can opsonize bacteria. Selective deficiency of IgM antibodies was found to increase susceptibility to bacterial infections (186). Studies found that specific IgM antibodies agglutinate erythrocytes, fix complement, and lyse erythrocytes more readily than IgG antibodies (187), and IgM antibodies are more effective in complement-mediated bacteriolysis (188); however, IgG antibodies are more effective than IgM antibodies in preventing pneumococci infections of mice (189) or in opsonizing Hib *in vitro* (190). Moreover, antibodies to some IgG subclasses have been reported to be more protective against specific viral (191) and fungal (192) infections than antibodies to other subclasses. These results suggest that optimal opsonization requires not only complement receptors but also Fc receptors for IgG. In the absence of inflammation, IgM antibodies are confined to the intravascular space, whereas IgG antibodies can enter the extracellular space. However, inflammation can make the vessels at the infection site permeable, at which point antibodies of all isotypes may enter the infection site. Compared with IgM antibodies, IgG antibodies may be especially efficient at neutralizing toxins because they have a longer half-life, generally have a higher affinity, and are already present in extravascular spaces prior to infection (193).

IgG subclasses differ in their ability to fix complement and to bind Fc receptors (194,195). It was also reported that IgG1 mouse monoclonal antibody is protective against *Cryptococcus neoformans* but that IgG3 mouse antibody is not (192). Consequently, the fact that antibodies to bacterial PS are found to be largely restricted to a single IgG subclass (IgG2 in humans and IgG3 in mice) has led to many studies of the differences in the protective properties of antipolysaccharide antibodies of different isotypes. Mouse IgG3 antibodies (but not antibodies of other IgG subclasses) can associate with each other through their Fc regions (196). This feature may make the IgG3 antibodies with a low affinity to PS more effective in binding the antigen than antibodies of other isotypes of the same affinity. Although the foregoing observations provide a theoretical advantage for mouse IgG3 antibodies, this same aggregation phenomenon has not been observed for human IgG2 antibodies, even though some human IgG2 can form covalently joined dimers (197). The full significance of IgG3 aggregation is not clear, however, because antipolysaccharide antibodies of the IgG3 isotype have not been observed to be any more efficacious against pneumococcal infections than antibodies of other isotypes (198). IgG2 antibody levels can be significant, however. People expressing the Gm23$^-$ IgG2 allele have higher IgG2 antibody levels than people with the Gm23$^+$ allele. Among C2-deficient persons, Gm23$^-$ persons are more susceptible to bacterial infections than Gm23$^+$ individuals (199).

Moreover, in contrast to expectations, many studies found that human IgG1 antibodies are slightly more effective at opsonization and bacteriolysis than are human IgG2 antibodies (195,200). Neither of these isotypes appears to be essential, however, because individuals lacking IgG1 and IgG2 subclass genes are healthy (201). Furthermore, human IgG2 antibodies bind less strongly to CD16, CD32, and CD64 than do IgG1 or IgG3 antibodies (202) and may not be effective for neutrophil opsonization in individuals homozygous for a specific CD32 allele (200). These observations, taken together, strongly suggest that the human IgG2 (or mouse IgG3) subclass may not provide any unique advantage in defense against bacteria.

IgA is highly heterogeneous in structure: It can exist as a monomer, a polymer, or in secretory forms. However, its function is unclear. Although it has been reported that IgA can opsonize (203), fix complement (204), and facilitate the lysis of *N. meningitidis* (205), other studies have found that IgA does not fix complement *in vitro* (206) and may even inhibit the IgG-mediated complement-dependent killing (207). The ability of IgA to fix complement may also depend on its denaturation or its glycosylation status (208,209). Nevertheless, other studies indicate that IgA antibodies may fix complement by the mannose-binding lectin pathway (210) and that human IgA antibodies against pneumococcal capsular PS can opsonize pneumococci for killing by neutrophils (211).

Bacteria that commonly colonize or infect mucosal areas often produce IgA1 protease, and IgA antibody has been found to provide protection in at least some of these cases (212). These findings suggest that IgA may play an important role as a part of the complex mucosal immune defense. IgA antibodies may be important in reducing nasopharyngeal colonization by bacteria, inasmuch as the mice deficient in IgA or polymeric immunoglobulin receptor can carry pneumococci in the nasopharynx even after an immunization against pneumococci (213). IgA may function by aggregating the bacteria and facilitating their expulsion from mucosal areas. IgA may also block the invasion of bacteria through the mucosal epithelial cells, because endocytosed IgA has been found to block the transport of virus through epithelial cells (214). However, IgA-deficient persons or mice are relatively healthy, and IgA-deficient mice can elicit normal protective immunity to experimental infections with influenza virus. IgM antibodies may function as secretory antibodies in IgA-deficient individuals (215).

Responses by T Cell Immune System to the Extracellular Bacteria

Although immune responses to toxins from extracellular bacteria are T cell dependent, antibodies to the toxins mediate protection; therefore, the protective immunity against extracellular bacteria is clearly centered on the B cell responses. However, recent studies suggest additional roles for T cells in responses to extracellular bacteria and their products. PS associated with lipid can stimulate T cells in association with CD1 molecules (216). In addition, studies of abscess formation in response to *Bacteroides fragilis* infection showed that its zwitterionic capsular PS can be taken up by antigen-presenting cells, which can process the PS with a nitric oxide–dependent mechanism and present it in association with MHC class II molecules (138) to stimulate $CD4^+$ T cells to produce IL-17 (217). T cell stimulation also requires participation of cofactors CD86 and CD40L (218). IL-17 is an important part of the host response to *B. fragilis,* because antibody to IL-17 can block the *B. fragilis*–induced abscess formation (219). Recently, Th17 T cells were defined as a distinct $CD4^+$ T cell subset that secretes IL-17 and requires a novel set of cytokines for Th17 lineage commitment (TGFβ and IL-6) and stabilization (IL-23) (220). Although the role of Th17 T cells in immune responses to extracellular bacteria is being investigated, IL-17 receptor deficiency or deficiency of IL-23 has been associated with increased susceptibility to extracellular bacterial infections (221,222).

DELETERIOUS HOST RESPONSES

Inflammatory response by the host inevitably causes some tissue damage. In some bacterial infections such as pneumonia and meningitis, this damage plays a significant role in disease pathology and symptoms. For instance, animal models of meningitis have shown that inflammation associated with bacterial products (primarily cell walls) is the primary cause of neurologic damage. Treatment of animals with antibiotics alone can eradicate the bacteria, but it does not prevent neurologic damage. In contrast, when inflammation was controlled by steroids administered along with the antibiotics, the amount of neurologic damage was considerably reduced (223).

Antigen-nonspecific Deleterious Response

Uncontrolled inflammation at the systemic level can produce septic shock, which can be triggered by several factors, including exotoxins (e.g., staphylococcal enterotoxin B) of gram-positive bacteria, the combination of LTA and peptidoglycan from gram-positive bacteria (224), or LPS from gram-negative bacteria. The staphylococcal enterotoxin B superantigen binds the host's class II molecules of the MHC region and can stimulate large numbers of helper T cells to release cytokines. Septic shock can also be initiated when LPS from gram-negative bacteria binds CD14 and a TLR and stimulates macrophages or monocytes to secrete inflammatory cytokines. (See Chapter 14.) In addition to cytokines, the stimulation of host cells by bacterial products leads to the release of other mediators of inflammation, such as arachidonic acid metabolites; activation of the complement cascade; and activation of the coagulation cascade. Excess release of the mediators leads to the failure of the vascular system and, finally, the failure of multiple organ systems. Studies using transgenic mice with defective genes have identified several molecules critical in developing septic shock, such as TNFα, one of its receptors TNFRI, IL-1–converting enzyme, and ICAM-1 (225). This approach also showed that CD14 and TLR4 are critical for LPS-induced septic shock and that CD28, a T cell costimulation molecule, is necessary for superantigen-induced septic shock (225).

Anthrax infections provide another example of uncontrolled host response. "Lethal factor" binds the "protective antigen" immobilized on the macrophages and then stimulates the cells to secrete cytokines and reactive oxygen intermediates. These macrophage products are believed to kill the host, because the host dies even when the proliferation of the bacteria is controlled. When macrophage cells are removed from animals, the animals are resistant to anthrax toxins (226). This suggests that the macrophage response to the toxins is actually responsible for the death of the host.

Although inflammation is a significant cause of morbidity and mortality, it must also be regarded as the host's primary protection from bacterial infections. Evidence for this hypothesis comes from studies with TLR4-deficient mice, which, although they are nonreactive to LPS and are completely resistant to LPS shock, are more susceptible to infection with gram-negative bacteria than are normal mice (227,228). Perhaps LPS is "toxic" because the host has evolved to use this common bacterial component as a trigger for host responses.

Antigen-specific Deleterious Response

Many bacterial antigens express the epitopes cross-reactive with host antigens and thus have the potential to elicit antibodies during infections that cross-react with host tissue. For instance, the PS capsule of *N. meningitidis* group B mimics epitopes expressed in the central nervous system (229), such as the *N*-acetylneuramic acid epitope in the embryonic N-CAM (230). The LPS of many strains of *N. meningitidis*, *N. gonorrhoeae*, *H. influenzae*, and *H. ducreyi* expresses the epitope of blood group antigen pK (231). The LPS of *Campylobacter jejuni* and *Helicobacter pylori* expresses epitopes mimicking other host antigens, such as ganglioside and Lewis X, respectively (231). Epidemiologic studies associated *C. jejuni* infections with the development of an autoimmune disease—Guillain-Barré syndrome (232).

Although the association between the abovementioned examples of cross-reacting bacterial antigens and autoimmunity is unclear, *S. pyogenes* infection is associated with rheumatic fever and acute glomerulonephritis. Studies found that *S. pyogenes* can be divided into two classes with a monoclonal antibody to M protein (233) and that rheumatic fever develops only after an infection of *S. pyogenes* with class I strains (233). Class I and class II strains of *S. pyogenes* can also be readily distinguished by the linkage relationship of the M protein genes with the genes encoding related surface proteins (233,234). M proteins from some class I *S. pyogenes* express epitopes highly cross-reactive with epitopes of cardiac myosin, tropomyosin, vimentin, laminin, and keratin (235–237). An antibody molecule may bind to all of these protein molecules because a major portion of these proteins are coiled-coil α-helix (237). The polyreactive antibodies to M protein may directly damage myocardial and endothelial cells (238). In addition to antibodies, $CD4^+$ and $CD8^+$ T cells are found at rheumatic heart valves (239), and the T cells proliferate to M protein peptides and heart proteins (240). These observations suggest that the T cells with cross-reactivity between M protein and myosin may be involved in the pathogenesis of rheumatic fever as well.

CONCLUSION

Because extracellular bacteria can grow rapidly and produce toxins, some are potent pathogens. To combat these bacteria, higher organisms primarily depend on two arms of the immune system: innate immunity and adaptive immunity centered on antibody molecules. The two arms of the immune system comprise of multiple layers of protection. In the early stage of an infection, innate immunity involving pattern recognition receptors, complement, phagocytes, and natural antibodies cross-reacting with many antigens is important in host defense. During the late stage of an infection, pathogen-specific antibodies appear. These antibodies generally mediate the ultimate protection against extracellular bacteria by triggering the protective effects of complement and phagocytes. Nevertheless, innate and adaptive immune responses may cause damage instead of protection. A better understanding of how our immune system protects against each pathogen will aid in the development of more effective preventive and therapeutic measures against these pathogens.

REFERENCES

1. Hooper LV, Gordon J I. Commensal host-bacterial relationships in the gut. *Science.* 2001;292:1115.
2. Aas J, Paster B, Stokes L, et al. Defining the normal bacterial flora of the oral cavity. *J Clin Microbiol.* 2005;43:5721.
3. Thomas L. *The lives of a cell: notes of a biology watcher*. New York: Bantam Books, 1974.
4. Bera A, Biswas R, Herbert S, et al. The presence of peptidoglycan O-acetyltransferase in various staphylococcal species correlates with lysozyme resistance and pathogenicity. *Infect Immun.* 2006; 74:4598.
5. Gray BM. Streptococcal infection. In: Evans AS, Brachman PE, ed. *Bacterial infection*. New York: Plenum Press, 1998;673–711.
6. Fischer W. Lipoteichoic acid and lipoglycans. *New Compr Biochem.* 1994;27:199.
7. Fischer WT, Behr R, Hartmann J, et al. Teichoic acid and lipoteichoic acid of *Streptococcus pneumoniae* possess identical chain structures. A reinvestigation of teichoic acid (C-polysaccharide). *Eur J Biochem*. 1993;215:851.
8. Nikaido H. Outer membrane. In: Neidhardt FC., ed. *Escherichia coli and Salmonella: cellular and molecular biology*. Washington, DC: ASM Press, 1996:29.
9. Ezzell JW, Welkos SL. The capsule of *Bacillus anthracis*, a review. *J Appl Microbiol.* 1999;87:250.
10. Yother, J. Capsules. In: Tuomanen EI, Mitchell TJ, Morrison DA, et al., eds. *The Pneumococcus*. Washington DC: ASM Press, 2004:30.
11. Gotschlich, EC, Fraser BA, Nishimura O, et al. Lipid on capsular polysaccharides of gram-negative bacteria. *J Biol Chem.* 1981;256:8915.
12. Kuo JS-C, Doelling VW, Graveline JF, et al. Evidence for covalent attachment of phospholipid to the capsular polysaccharide of *Haemophilus influenzae* type b. *J Bacteriol.* 1985;163:769.
13. Bentley SD, Aanensen DM, Mavroidi A, et al. Genetic analysis of the capsular biosynthetic locus from all 90 pneumococcal serotypes. *PLoS Genet*. 2006;2:e31.
14. Kazatchkine MD, Fearon DT, Austen KF. Human alternative complement pathway: membrane-associated sialic acid regulates the competition between B and beta 1H for cell-bound C3b. *J Immunol.* 1979;122:75.
15. Brown EJ, Hosea SW, Hammer CH, et al. A quantitative analysis of the interactions of antipneumococcal antibody and complement in experimental pneumococcal bacteremia. *J Clin Invest*. 1982;69:85.

16. Tu AH, Fulgham RL, McCrory MA, et al. Pneumococcal surface protein A inhibits complement activation by *Streptococcus pneumoniae*. *Infect Immun*. 1999;67:4720.
17. Cheng Q, Finkel D, Hostetter MK. Novel purification scheme and functions for a C3-binding protein from *Streptococcus pneumoniae*. *Biochemistry*. 2000;39:5450.
18. Horstmann RD, Sievertsen HJ, Knobloch J, et al. Antiphagocytic activity of streptococcal M protein: selective binding of complement control protein factor H. *Proc Natl Acad Sci U S A*. 1988;85:1657.
19. Roben P, Salem A, Silverman G. VH3 family antibodies bind domain D of staphylococcal protein A. *J Immunol*. 1995;154:6437.
20. Kilian M, Reinholdt J. Immunoglobulin A1 proteases of pathogenic and commensal bacteria of the respiratory tract. In: Nataro JP, ed. *Colonization of mucosal surfaces*. Washington, DC: American Society for Microbiology Press, 2005:119.
21. Finlay B, Falkow BS. Common themes in microbial pathogenicity revisited. *Microbiol Mol Biol Rev*. 1997;61:136.
22. Salyers AA, Whitt DD. *Bacterial pathogenesis*. Washington DC: ASM Press, 1994:47.
23. Barg NL, Harris T. Toxin-mediated syndromes. In: Crossely KB, ed. *The staphylococci*. New York: Churchill Livingston, 1997:527.
24. Noel JM, Boedeker EC. Enterohemorrhagic *Escherichia coli*: a family of emerging pathogens. *Dig Dis*. 1997;15:67.
25. Krakauer T. Immune response to staphylococcal superantigens. *Immunol Res*. 1999;20(2):163.
26. Tweten R. Cholesterol-dependent cytolysins, a family of versatile pore-forming toxins. *Infect Immun*. 2005;73:6199.
27. Briles DE, Paton JC, Nahm MH, et al. Immunity to *Streptococcus pneumoniae*. In: Cunningham MW, Fujinami RS, eds. *Effects of microbes on the immune system*. Philadelphia: Lippincott-Raven, 1999:263.
28. Ji Y, Carlson B, Kondugunta A, et al. Intranasal immunization with C5a peptidase prevents nasopharyngeal colonization of mice by the group A streptococcus. *Infect Immun*. 1997;65:2080.
29. Liu GA, Essex J, Buchanan V, et al. *Staphylococcus aureus* golden pigment impairs neutrophil killing and promotes virulence through its antioxidant activity. *J Exp Med*. 2005:202:209.
30. McCullers JA, Tuomanen EI. Molecular pathogenesis of pneumococcal pneumonia. *Front Biosci*. 2001;6:D877.
31. Lysenko ES, Ratner AJ, Nelson AL, et al. The role of innate immune responses in the outcome of interspecies competition for colonization of mucosal surfaces. *PLoS Pathog*. 2005;1:e1.
32. Cundell DR, Gerard NP, Gerard C, et al. *Streptococcus pneumoniae* anchor to activated human cells by the receptor for platelet activating factor. *Nature*. 1995;377:435.
33. Striker R, Nilsson U, Stonecipher A, et al. Structural requirements for the glycolipid receptor of human uropathogenic *Escherichia coli*. *Mol Microbiol*. 1995;16:1021.
34. Sengupta TK, Sengupta DK, Ghose AC. A 20-kDa pilus protein with haemagglutination and intestinal adherence properties expressed by a clinical isolate of a non-01 *Vibrio cholerae*. *FEMS Microbiol Lett*. 1993;112:237.
35. Chiang SL, Taylor RK, Koomey M, et al. Single amino acid substitutions in the N-terminus of *Vibrio cholerae* TcpA affect colonization, autoagglutination, serum resistance. *Mol Microbiol*. 1995;17:1133.
36. Brennan MJ, Shahin RD. Pertussis antigens that abrogate bacterial adherence and elicit immunity. *Am J Respir Crit Care Med*. 1996;154:S145.
37. Geuijen CA, Willems RJ, Bongaerts M, et al. Role of the *Bordetella pertussis*; minor fimbrial subunit, FimD, in colonization of the mouse respiratory tract. *Infect Immun*. 1997;65:4222.
38. Prince A. Flagellar activation of epithelial signaling. *Am J Respir Cell Mol Biol*. 2006;34:548.
39. Otto B, Verweij-van Vught A, MacLaren D. Transferrins and heme-compounds as iron sources for pathogenic bacteria. *Crit Rev Microbiol*. 1992;18:217.
40. Earhart CF. Uptake and metabolism of iron and molybdenum. In: Neidhardt FC, ed. *Escherichia coli and Salmonella: Cellular and Molecular Biology*. Washington DC: ASM Press, 1996:1075.
41. Dassy B, Hogan T, Foster TJ, et al. Involvement of the accessory gene regulator (agr) in expression of type-5 capsular polysaccharide by *Staphylococcus aureus*. *J Gen Microbiol*. 1993;139:1301.
42. Uhl MA, Miller JF. Autophosphorylation and phosphotransfer in the *Bordetella pertussis* BvgAS signal transduction cascade. *Proc Nat Acad Sci U S A*. 1994;91:1163.
43. Hoch JA, Silhavy TJ. *Two-component signal transduction*. Washington DC: ASM Press, 1995:488.
44. Moxon E, Lenski R, Rainey P. Adaptive evolution of highly mutable loci in pathogenic bacteria. *Perspect Biol Med*. 1998;42:154.
45. Hammerschmidt SA, Muller H, Sillmann M, et al. Capsule phase variation in *Neisseria meningitidis* serogroup B by slipped-strand mispairing in the polysialyltransferase gene (siaD): correlation with bacterial invasion and the outbreak of meningococcal disease. *Mol Microbiol*. 1996;20:1211.
46. de Kievit TR, Iglewski BH. Bacterial quorum sensing in pathogenic relationships. *Infect Immun*. 2000;68:4839.
47. Withers H, Swift S, Williams P. Quorum sensing as an integral component of gene regulatory networks in gram-negative bacteria. *Curr Opin Microbiol*. 2001;4:186.
48. Fischetti VA. Streptococcal M protein: molecular design and biological behavior. *Clin Microbiol Rev*. 1989;2:286.
49. Fischetti VA, Bessen DE, Schneewind O, et al. Protection against streptococcal pharyngeal colonization with vaccines composed of M protein conserved regions. *Adv Exp Med Biol*. 1991;303:159.
50. Dillard JP, Vandersea MW, Yother J. Characterization of the cassette containing genes for type 3 capsular polysaccharide biosynthesis in *Streptococcus pneumoniae*. *J Exp Med*. 1995;181:973.
51. Zhang QY, DeRyckere D, Lauer P, et al. Gene conversion in *Neisseria gonorrhoeae*: evidence for its role in pilus antigenic variation. *Proc Natl Acad Sci U S A*. 1992;89:5366.
52. Seifert HS. Questions about gonococcal pilus phase- and antigenic variation. *Mol Microbiol*. 1997;21:433.
53. Saunders N, Jeffries A, Peden J, et al. Repeat-associated phase variable genes in the complete genome sequence of *Neisseria meningitidis* strain MC58. *Mol Microbiol*. 2000;37:207.
54. Nougayrede J, Fernandes P, Donnenberg M. Adhesion of enteropathogenic *Escherichia coli* to host cells. *Cell Microbiol*. 2003;5:359.
55. Covacci A, Rappuoli R. Tyrosine-phosphorylated bacterial proteins: Trojan horses for the host cell. *J Exp Med*. 2000;191:587.
56. Madden J, Ruiz N, Caparon M. Cytolysin-mediated translocation (CMT): a functional equivalent of type III secretion in gram-positive bacteria. *Cell*. 2001;104:143.
57. Rupp ME, Archer GL. Coagulase-negative staphylococci: pathogens associated with medical progress. *Clin Infect Dis*. 1994;19:231.
58. Neish AS, Gewirtz AT, Zeng H, et al. Prokaryotic regulation of epithelial responses by inhibition of IkappaB alpha ubiquitination. *Science*. 2000;289:1560.
59. Eckburg PE, Bik C, Bernstein E, et al. Diversity of the human intestinal microbial flora. *Science*. 2005;308:1635.
60. Mbelle N, Huebner RE, Wasas AD, et al. Immunogenicity and impact on nasopharyngeal carriage of a nonavalent pneumococcal conjugate vaccine. *J Infect Dis*. 1999;180:1171.
61. Riley M, Wertz J. Bacteriocins: evolution, ecology and application. *Annu Rev Microbiol*. 2002;56:117.
62. Bartlett JG, Chang TW, Taylor NS, et al. Colitis induced by *Clostridium difficile*. *Rev Infect Dis*. 1979;1:370.
63. Caugant DA, Hoiby EA, Magnus P, et al. Asymptomatic carriage of *Neisseria meningitidis* in a randomly sampled population. *J Clin Microbiol*. 1994;32:323.
64. Kuhns DM, Nelson CT, Feldman HA, et al. The prophylactic value of sulfadiazine in the control of meningococcic meningitis. *JAMA*. 1943:335.
65. Zangwill KM, Schuchat A, Wenger JD. Group B streptococcal disease in the United States, 1990: report from a multistate active surveillance system. *MMWR*. 1992;41:25.
66. Berry AM, Lock RA, Paton JC. Cloning and characterization of *nanB*, a second *Streptococcus pneumoniae* neuraminidase gene, purification of the NanB enzyme from recombinant *Escherichia coli*. *J Bacteriol*. 1996;178:4854.
67. Kazmierczak BI, Mostov K, Engel JN. Interaction of bacterial pathogens with polarized epithelium. *Annu Rev Microbiol*. 2001;55:407.
68. Katz J, Sambandam V, Wu J, et al. Characterization of *Porphyromonas gingivalis*-induced degradation of epithelial cell junctional complexes. *Infect Immun*. 2000;68:1441.

69. Zhang JR, Mostov KE, Lamm ME, et al. The polymeric immunoglobulin receptor translocates pneumococci across human nasopharyngeal epithelial cells. *Cell*. 2000;102:827.
70. Cundell DR, Weiser JN, Shen J, et al. Relationship between colonial morphology and adherence of *Streptococcus pneumoniae*. *Infect Immun*. 1995;63:757.
71. Swords WE, Ketterer MR, Shao J, et al. Binding of the non-typeable *Haemophilus influenzae* lipooligosaccharide to the PAF receptor initiates host cell signalling. *Cell Microbiol*. 2001;3:525.
72. Bancroft GJ, Kelly JP. Macrophage activation and innate resistance to infection in SCID mice. *Immunobiology*. 1994;191:424.
73. Musher DM. *Streptococcus pneumoniae*. In: *Principles and practice of infectious diseases*. New York: Churchill Livingstone, 1995: 1811.
74. Donowitz GR, Mandell GL. Acute pneumonia. In: Mandell GL, Bennett JE, Dolin R, eds. *Principles and practices of infectious diseases*. New York: Churchill Livingstone, 1995:619.
75. Pruitt KM, Rahemtulla F, Mansson-Rahemtulla B. Innate humoral factors. In: Ogra PL, ed. *Handbook of mucosal immunology*. New York: Academic Press, 1994:53.
76. Vorland LH. Lactoferrin: a multifunctional glycoprotein. *APMIS* 1999;107:971.
77. Mestecky J, McGhee J. Immunoglobulin A (IgA): molecular and cellular interactions involved in IgA biosynthesis and immune response. *Adv Immunol*. 1987;40:153.
78. Fellermann K, Stange EF. Defensins—innate immunity at the epithelial frontier. *Eur J Gastroenterol Hepatol*. 2001;13:771.
79. Bevins CL. Events at the host–microbial interface of the gastrointestinal tract. V. Paneth cell alpha-defensins in intestinal host defense. *Am J Physiol Gastrointest Liver Physiol*. 2005;289:G173.
80. Crouch E, Wright JR. Surfactant proteins a and d and pulmonary host defense. *Annu Rev Physiol*. 2001;63:521.
81. LeVine AM, Bruno MD, Huelsman KM, et al. Surfactant protein A–deficient mice are susceptible to group B streptococcal infection. *J Immunol*. 1997;158:4336.
82. Henderson B, Poole S, Wilson M. Bacterial modulins: a novel class of virulence factors which cause host tissue pathology by inducing cytokine synthesis. *Microbiol Rev*. 1996;60:316.
83. Melmed G, Thomas L, Lee N, et al. Human intestinal epithelial cells are broadly unresponsive to Toll-like receptor 2-dependent bacterial ligands: implications for host–microbial interactions in the gut. *J Immunol*. 2003;170:1406.
84. Kirschning C, Schumann R. TLR2: cellular sensor for microbial and endogenous molecular patterns. *Curr Top Microbiol Immunol*. 2002;270:121.
85. Echchannaoui H, Frei K, Schnell C, et al. Toll-like receptor 2-deficient mice are highly susceptible to *Streptococcus pneumoniae* meningitis because of reduced bacterial clearing and enhanced inflammation. *J Infect Dis*. 2002;186:798.
86. Takeuchi O, Hoshino K, Akira S. Cutting edge: TLR2-deficient and MyD88-deficient mice are highly susceptible to *Staphylococcus aureus* infection. *J Immunol*. 2000;165:5392.
87. Hayashi F, Smith KD, Ozinsky A, et al. The innate immune response to bacterial flagellin is mediated by Toll-like receptor 5. *Nature*. 2001;410:1099.
88. Frank MM, Fries LF. The role of complement in defense against bacterial disease. *Baillieres Clin Immunol Allergy*. 1988;2:335.
89. Worsaae N, Staehr Johansen K, et al. Impaired *in vitro* function of neutrophils in Crohn's disease. *Scand J Gastroenterol*. 1982; 17:91.
90. Viala J, Chaput C, Boneca I, et al. Nod1 responds to peptidoglycan delivered by the *Helicobacter pylori* cag pathogenicity island. *Nat Immunol*. 2004;5:1166.
91. Gomez M, Lee A, Reddy B, et al. *Staphylococcus aureus* protein A induces airway epithelial inflammatory responses by activating TNFR1. *Nat Med*. 2004;10:842.
92. Schiffmann E, Corcoran B, Wahl S. N-Formylmethionyl peptides as chemoattractants for leucocytes. *Proc Natl Acad Sci U S A*. 1975; 72:1059.
93. Galli SJ. New concepts about the mast cell. *N Engl J Med*. 1993;328:257.
94. Bradding P, Feather IH, Wilson S, et al. Immunolocalization of cytokines in the nasal mucosa of normal and perennial rhinitic subjects. The mast cell as a source of IL-4, IL-5, IL-6 in human allergic mucosal inflammation. *J Immunol*. 1993;151:3853.
95. Malaviya R, Ikeda T, Ross E, et al. Mast cell modulation of neutrophil influx and bacterial clearance at sites of infection through TNFa. *Nature*. 1996;381:77.
96. Fillion I, Ouellet N, Simard M, et al. Role of chemokines and formyl peptides in pneumococcal pneumonia–induced monocyte/macrophage recruitment. *J Immunol*. 2001;166:7353.
97. Ofek I, Goldhar J, Keisari Y, et al. Nonopsonic phagocytosis of microorganisms. *Annu Rev Microbiol*. 1995;49:239.
98. Szalai AJ, Briles DE, Volanakis JE. Human C-reactive protein is protective against fatal *Streptococcus pneumoniae* infection in transgenic mice. *J Immunol*. 1995;155:2557.
99. Apicella MA, Westerink MAJ, Morse SA, et al. Bactericidal antibody response of normal human serum to the lipooligosaccharide of *Neisseria gonorrhoeae*. *J Infect Dis*. 1986;153:520.
100. Gibot S, Cravoisy A, Levy B, et al. Soluble triggering receptor expressed on myeloid cells and the diagnosis of pneumonia. *N Engl J Med*. 2004;350:451.
101. Steel DM, Whitehead AS. The major acute phase reactants: C-reactive protein, serum amyloid P component and serum amyloid A protein. *Immunol Today*. 1994;15:81.
102. Turner MW. Mannose-binding lectin: the pluripotent molecule of the innate immune system. *Immunol Today*. 1996;17:532.
103. Gould JM, Weiser JN. The inhibitory effect of C-reactive protein on bacterial phosphorylcholine platelet-activating factor receptor-mediated adherence is blocked by surfactant. *J Infect Dis*. 2002;186:361.
104. Bullen JJ. *Iron and infection*. New York: Wiley, 1999.
105. Weinberg ED, Weinberg GA. The role of iron in infection. *Curr Opin Infect Dis*. 1997;8:164.
106. Patruta SI, Horl WH. Iron and infection. *Kidney Int Suppl*. 1999;69:S125.
107. Parker T, Levine D, Chang J, et al. Reconstituted high-density lipoprotein neutralizes gram-negative bacterial lipopolysaccharides in human whole blood. *Infect Immun*. 1995;63:253.
108. Schwarz EM, Krimpenfort P, Verma IM. Immunological defects in mice with a targeted disruption in Bcl-3. *Genes Dev*. 1997;11:187.
109. Read RC, Camp NJ, di Giovine FS, et al. An interleukin-1 genotype is associated with fatal outcome of meningococcal disease. *J Infect Dis*. 2000;182:1557.
110. Perlmutter RM, Nahm M, Stein KE, et al. Immunoglobulin subclass-specific immunodeficiency in mice with an X-linked B-lymphocyte defect. *J Exp Med*. 1979;149:993.
111. Kinnon C, Hinshelwood S, Levinsky RJ, et al. X-linked agammaglobulinemia—gene cloning and future prospects. *Immunol Today*. 1993;14:554.
112. Wood PM, Mayne A, Joyce H, et al. A mutation in Bruton's tyrosine kinase as a cause of selective anti-polysaccharide antibody deficiency. *J Pediatr*. 2001;139:148.
113. Sewnath ME, Olszyna DP, Birjmohun R, et al. IL-10–deficient mice demonstrate multiple organ failure and increased mortality during *Escherichia coli* peritonitis despite an accelerated bacterial clearance. *J Immunol*. 2001;166:6323.
114. Schultz MJ, Wijnholds J, Peppelenbosch MP, et al. Mice lacking the multidrug resistance protein 1 are resistant to *Streptococcus pneumoniae*–induced pneumonia. *J Immunol*. 2001;166:4059.
115. Firestein GS, Zvaifler NJ. Anticytokine therapy in rheumatoid arthritis. *N Engl J Med*. 1997;337:195.
116. Lederman HM, Winkelstein JA. X-linked agammaglobulinemia: an analysis of 96 patients. *Medicine*. 1985;64:145.
117. Rapola S, Jäntti V, Haikala R, et al. Natural development of antibodies to pneumococcal surface protein A, pneumococcal surface adhesion A, pneumolysin in relation to pneumococcal carriage and acute otitis media. *J Infect Dis*. 2000;182:1146.
118. Scott JA, Obiero J, Hall AJ, et al. Validation of immunoglobulin G enzyme-linked immunosorbent assay for antibodies to pneumococcal surface adhesin A in the diagnosis of pneumococcal pneumonia among adults in Kenya. *J Infect Dis*. 2002;186:220.
119. Scott JA, Hannington A, Marsh K, et al. Diagnosis of pneumococcal pneumonia in epidemiological studies: evaluation in Kenyan adults of a serotype-specific urine latex agglutination assay. *Clin Infect Dis*. 1999;28:764.

120. Smith MD, Derrington P, Evans R, et al. Rapid diagnosis of bacteremic pneumococcal infections in adults by using the Binax NOW *Streptococcus pneumoniae* urinary antigen test: a prospective, controlled clinical evaluation. *J Clin Microbiol*. 2003;41:2810.
121. Marchant CD, Band E, Froeschle JE, et al. Depression of anticapsular antibody after immunization with *Haemophilus influenzae* type b polysaccharide-diphtheria conjugate vaccine. *Pediatr Infect Dis J*. 1989;8:508.
122. Humphrey JH, Parrott DMV, East J. Studies of globulin and antibody production in mice thymectomized at birth. *Immunology*. 1964;7:419.
123. Herzenberg LA, Stall AM, Lalor PA, et al. The LY-1 B cell lineage. *Immunol Rev*. 1986;93:81.
124. Guinamard R, Okigaki M, Schlessinger J, et al. Absence of marginal zone B cells in Pyk-2–deficient mice defines their role in the humoral response. *Nat Immunol*. 2000;1:31.
125. Martin F, Oliver AM, Kearney JF. Marginal zone and B1 B cells unite in the early response against T-independent blood-borne particulate antigens. *Immunity*. 2001;14:617.
126. Pillai S, Cariappa A, Moran ST. Marginal zone B cells. *Annu Rev Immunol*. 2005;23:161.
127. Winslow MM, Gallo EM, Neilson JR, et al. The calcineurin phosphatase complex modulates immunogenic B cell responses. *Immunity*. 2006;24:141.
128. Haas KM, Poe JC, Steeber DA, et al. B-1a and B-1b cells exhibit distinct developmental requirements and have unique functional roles in innate and adaptive immunity to *S. pneumoniae*. *Immunity*. 2005;23:7.
129. Khan WN, Alt FW, Gerstein RM, et al. Defective B cell development and function in Btk-deficient mice. *Immunity*. 1995;3(3):283.
130. Harding CV, Roof RW, Allen PM, et al. Effects of pH and polysaccharides on peptide binding to class II major histocompatibility complex molecules. *Proc Natl Acad Sci U S A*. 1991;88:2740.
131. Leyva-Cobian F, Unanue ER. Intracellular interference with antigen presentation. *J Immunol*. 1988;141:1445.
132. Weissman IL, Gutman GA, Friedberg SH, et al. Lymphoid tissue architecture. III. Germinal centers, T cells, thymus dependent vs thymus-independent antigens. *Adv Exp Med Biol*. 1976;66:229.
133. Baker PJ, Stashak PW, Amsbaugh DF, et al. Characterization of the antibody response to type III pneumococcal polysaccharide at the cellular level. I. Dose-response studies and the effect of prior immunization on the magnitude of the antibody response. *Immunology*. 1971;20:469.
134. Klaus GGB, Humphrey JH. The immunological properties of haptens coupled to thymus-independent carrier molecules. I. The characteristics of the immune response to dinitrophenol-lysine-substituted pneumococcal polysaccharide (SIII) and levan. *Eur J Immunol*. 1974;4:370.
135. Baker PJ. Regulation of magnitude of antibody response to bacterial polysaccharide antigens by thymus-derived lymphocytes. *Infect Immun*. 1990;58:3465.
136. Jeurissen A, Billiau AD, Moens L, et al. CD4+ T lymphocytes expressing CD40 ligand help the IgM antibody response to soluble pneumococcal polysaccharides via an intermediate cell type. *J Immunol*. 2006;176:529.
137. Sen G, Khan AQ, Chen Q, et al. *In vivo* humoral immune responses to isolated pneumococcal polysaccharides are dependent on the presence of associated TLR ligands. *J Immunol*. 2005;175:3084.
138. Cobb BA, Kasper DL. Zwitterionic capsular polysaccharides: the new MHCII-dependent antigens. *Cell Microbiol*. 2005;7:1398.
139. Carroll WL, Adderson EE, Lucas AH, et al. Molecular basis of antibody diversity. In: Ellis RW, Granoff DM, eds. *Development and clinical uses of Haemophilus b conjugate vaccines*. New York: Marcel Dekker, 1994:207.
140. Claflin JL, Hudak S, Maddalena A. Anti-phosphocholine hybridoma antibodies. I. Direct evidence for three distinct families of antibodies in the murine response. *J Exp Med*. 1981;153:352.
141. Scott MG, Crimmins DL, McCourt DW, et al. Clonal characterization of the human IgG antibody repertoire to *Haemophilus influenzae* type b polysaccharide. III. A single VKII gene and one of several JK genes are joined by an invariant arginine to form the most common L chain V region. *J Immunol*. 1989;143:4110.
142. Gearhart PJ, Johnson ND, Douglas R, et al. IgG antibodies to phosphorylcholine exhibit more diversity than their IgM counterparts. *Nature*. 1981;291:29.
143. Hetherington SV. The intrinsic affinity constant (K) of anticapsular antibody to oligosaccharides of *Haemophilus influenzae* type b. *J Immunol*. 1988;140:3966.
144. Robbins JB, Austrian R, Lee CJ, et al. Considerations for formulating the second-generation pneumococcal capsular polysaccharide vaccine with emphasis on the cross-reactive types within groups. *J Infect Dis*. 1983;148:1136.
145. Fothergill LD, Wright J. Influenzal meningitis: the regulation of age incidence to the bactericidal power of blood against the causal organism. *J Immunol*. 1933;24:273.
146. Takala AK, Eskola J, Leinonen M, et al. Reduction of oropharyngeal carriage of *Haemophilus influenzae* type b (Hib) in children immunized with an Hib conjugate vaccine. *J Infect Dis*. 1991;164:982.
147. Girard MP, Preziosi MP, Aguado MT, et al. A review of vaccine research and development: meningococcal disease. *Vaccine*. 2006;24:4692.
148. Shinefield HR, Black S. Efficacy of pneumococcal conjugate vaccines in large scale field trials. *Pediatr Infect Dis J*. 2000;19:394.
149. Whitney CG, Farley MM, Hadler J, et al. Decline in invasive pneumococcal disease after the introduction of protein-polysaccharide conjugate vaccine. *N Engl J Med*. 2003;348:1737.
150. Donnelly JJ, Deck RR, Liu MA. Immunogenicity of a *Haemophilus influenzae* polysaccharide–*Neisseria meningitidis* outer membrane protein complex conjugate vaccine. *J Immunol*. 1990;145:3071.
151. Latz E, Franko J, Golenbock DT, et al. *Haemophilus influenzae* type b-outer membrane protein complex glycoconjugate vaccine induces cytokine production by engaging human toll-like receptor 2 (TLR2) and requires the presence of TLR2 for optimal immunogenicity. *J Immunol*. 2004;172:2431.
152. Oliver AM, Martin F, Gartland GL, et al. Marginal zone B cells exhibit unique activation, proliferative and immunoglobulin secretory responses. *Eur J Immunol*. 1997;27:2366.
153. Lopes-Carvalho T, Foote J, Kearney JF. Marginal zone B cells in lymphocyte activationandregulation. *Curr Opin Immunol*. 2005;17:244.
154. Ferguson AR, Youd ME, Corley RB. Marginal zone B cells transport and deposit IgM-containing immune complexes onto follicular dendritic cells. *Int Immunol*. 2004;16:1411.
155. Wu ZQ, Vos Q, Shen Y, et al. *In vivo* polysaccharide-specific IgG isotype responses to intact *Streptococcus pneumoniae* are T cell dependent and require CD40- and B7-ligand interactions. *J Immunol*. 1999;163:659.
156. Hwang Y, Nahm M, Briles D, et al. Acquired, but not innate, immune responses to *Streptococcus pneumoniae* are compromised by neutralization of CD40L. *Infect Immun*. 2000:68(2):511.
157. Wu ZQ, Khan AQ, Shen Y, et al. B7 Requirements for primary and secondary protein- and polysaccharide-specific Ig isotype responses to *Streptococcus pneumoniae*. *J Immunol*. 2001;165:6840.
158. Snapper CM, Shen Y, Khan AQ, et al. Distinct types of T-cell help for the induction of a humoral immune response to *Streptococcus pneumoniae*. *Trends Immunol*. 2001;22:308.
159. Briles DE, Nahm M, Marion TN, et al. Streptococcal group A carbohydrate has properties of both a thymus-independent (TI-2) and a thymus-dependent antigen. *J Immunol*. 1982;128:2032.
160. Balazs M, Martin F, Zhou T, et al. Blood dendritic cells interact with splenic marginal zone B cells to initiate T-independent immune responses. *Immunity*. 2002;17:341.
161. Colino J, Shen Y, Snapper CM. Dendritic cells pulsed with intact *Streptococcus pneumoniae* elicit both protein- and polysaccharide-specific immunoglobulin isotype responses *in vivo* through distinct mechanisms. *J Exp Med*. 2002;195:1.
162. Bouvet J, Dighiero G. From natural polyreactive autoantibodies to à la carte monoreactive antibodies to infectious agents: is it a small world after all? *Infect Immun*. 1998;66:1.
163. Lal RB, Paranjape RS, Briles DE, et al. Circulating parasite antigen(s) in lymphatic filariasis: Use of monoclonal antibodies to phosphocholine for immunodiagnosis. *J Immunol*. 1987;138:3454.
164. Briles DE, Nahm M, Schroer K, et al. Antiphosphocholine antibodies found in normal mouse serum are protective against intravenous infection with type 3 *Streptococcus pneumoniae*. *J Exp Med*. 1981;153:694.

165. Weiser JN, Shchepetov M, Chong ST. Decoration of lipopolysaccharide with phosphorylcholine: a phase-variable characteristic of *Haemophilus influenzae*. *Infect Immun*. 1997;65:943.
166. Heidelberger M, Rebers PA. Immunochemistry of the pneumococcal types II, V, VI. The relation of type VI to type II and other correlations between chemical constitution and precipitation in antisera to type VI. *J Bacteriol*. 1960;80:145.
167. MacPherson CFC, Heidelberger M, Alexander HE, et al. The specific polysaccharides of types A, B, C, D, F *Hemophilus influenzae*. *J Immunol*. 1946;52:207.
168. Heidelberger M, Bernheimer A. W. Cross-reactions of polysaccharides of fungi, molds, yeasts in anti-pneumococcal and other antisera. *Proc Natl Acad Sci U S A*. 1984;81:5247.
169. Lucas AH, Langley RJ, Granoff DM, et al. An idiotypic marker associated with a germ-line encoded kappa light chain variable region that predominates the vaccine-induced human antibody response to the *Haemophilus influenzae* b polysaccharide. *J Clin Invest*. 1991;88:1811.
170. Moxon ER, Anderson P. Meningitis caused by *Haemophilus influenzae* in infant rats: protective immunity and antibody priming by gastrointestinal colonization with *Escherichia coli*. *J Infect Dis*. 1979;140:471.
171. Galili U, Mandrell RE, Hamadeh RM, et al. Interaction between human natural anti-alpha-galactosyl immunoglobulin G and bacteria of the human flora. *Infect Immun*. 1988;56:1730.
172. Avila JL, Rojas M, Galili U. Immunogenic Gal-alpha-1–3Gal carbohydrate epitopes are present on pathogenic American *Trypanosoma* and *Leishmania*. *J Immunol*. 1989;142:2828.
173. Ginsburg CM, McCracken GH Jr, Schneerson R, et al. Association between cross-reacting *Escherichia coli* K100 and disease caused by *Haemophilus influenzae* type b. *Infect Immun*. 1978;22:339.
174. Knight KL, Crane MA. Generating the antibody repertoire in rabbit. *Adv Immunol*. 1994;56:179.
175. Langermann S, Palaszynski S, Barnhart M, et al. Prevention of mucosal *Escherichia coli* infection by FimH-adhesin-based systemic vaccination. *Science*. 1997;276:607.
176. Cross AS, Opal S, Cook P, et al. Development of an anti-core lipopolysaccharide vaccine for the prevention and treatment of sepsis. *Vaccine*. 2004;22:812.
177. Ziegler EJ, McCutchan JA, Fierer J, et al. Treatment of gram-negative bacteremia and shock with human antiserum to a mutant *Escherichia coli*. *N Engl J Med*. 1982;307:1225.
178. Theilacker C, Kaczynski Z, Kropec A, et al. Opsonic antibodies to *Enterococcus faecalis* strain 12030 are directed against lipoteichoic acid. *Infect Immun*. 2006;74:5703.
179. Ren B, McCrory MA, Pass C, et al. The virulence function of *Streptococcus pneumoniae* surface protein A involves inhibition of complement activation and impairment of complement receptor-mediated protection. *J Immunol*. 2004;173:7506.
180. Lewis LA, Gray E, Wang YP, et al. Molecular characterization of hpuAB, the haemoglobin-haptoglobin-utilization operon of *Neisseria meningitidis*. *Mol Microbiol*. 1997;23:737.
181. Pettersson A, Poolman JT, van der Ley P, et al. Response of *Neisseria meningitidis* to iron limitation. *Antonie Van Leeuwenhoek*. 1997;71:129.
182. Winkelstein JA. The complement system. In: Gorbach SL, Bartlett JG, Blacklow NR, eds. *Infectious Diseases*. Philadelphia: WB Saunders, 1992:37.
183. Van der Lay P, Heckels JE, Virji M, et al. Topology of outer membrane porins in pathogenic *Neisseria* spp. *Infect Immun*. 1991;59:2963.
184. Nielsen SV, Sorensen UBS, Henrichsen J. Antibodies against pneumococcal C-polysaccharide are not protective. *Microb Pathog*. 1993;14:299.
185. Goldenberg HB, McCool TL, Weiser JN. Cross-reactivity of human immunoglobulin G2 recognizing phosphorylcholine and evidence for protection against major bacterial pathogens of the human respiratory tract. *J Infect Dis*. 2004;190:1254.
186. Boes M, Prodeus AP, Schmidt T, et al. A critical role of natural immunoglobulin M in immediate defense against systemic bacterial infection. *J Exp Med*. 1998;188:2381.
187. Cooper NR. The classical complement pathway: activation and regulation of the first complement component. *Adv Immunol*. 1985;37:151.
188. Mostov KE. Transepithelial transport of immunoglobulins. *Annu Rev Immunol*. 1994;12:63.
189. McDaniel LS, Benjamin WH, Forman C, et al. Blood clearance by anti-phosphocholine antibodies as a mechanism of protection in experimental pneumococcal bacteremia. *J Immunol*. 1984;133:3308.
190. Schreiber JR, Barrus V, Cates KL, et al. Functional characterization of human IgG, IgM, IgA antibody directed to the capsule of *Haemophilus influenzae* type b. *J Infect Dis*. 1986;153:8.
191. Schlesinger JJ, Foltzer M, Chapman S. The Fc portion of antibody to yellow fever virus NS1 is a determinant of protection against YF encephalitis in mice. *Virology*. 1993;192:132.
192. Yuan R, Casadevall A, Spira G, et al. Isotype switching from IgG3 to IgG1 converts a nonprotective murine antibody to *Cryptococcus neoformans* into a protective antibody. *J Immunol*. 1995;154:1810.
193. Possee RD, Schild GC, Dimmock NJ. Studies on the mechanism of neutralization of influenza virus by antibody: evidence that neutralizing antibody inactivates influenza virus by inhibiting virion transcriptase activity. *J Gen Virol*. 1997;58:373.
194. Jefferis R, Pound J, Lund J, et al. Effector mechanisms activated by human IgG subclass antibodies: clinical and molecular aspects. *Ann Biol Clin*. 1994;52:57.
195. Burton DR, Woof JM. Human antibody effector function. *Adv Immunol*. 1992;51:1.
196. Cooper LJ, Shikhman AR, Glass DD, et al. Role of heavy chain constant domains in antibody-antigen interaction. Apparent specificity differences among streptococcal IgG antibodies expressing identical variable domains. *J Immunol*. 1993;150:2231.
197. Yoo EM, Wims LA, Chan LA, et al. Human IgG2 can form covalent dimers. *J Immunol*. 2003;170:3134.
198. Briles DE, Forman C, Hudak S, et al. The effects of subclass on the ability of anti-phosphocholine antibodies to protect mice from fatal infection with *Streptococcus pneumoniae*. *J Mol Cell Immunol*. 1984;1:305.
199. Jonsson G, Oxelius VA, Truedsson L, et al. Homozygosity for the IgG2 subclass allotype G2M(n) protects against severe infection in hereditary C2 deficiency. *J Immunol*. 2006;177:722.
200. Bredius RGM, de Vries CEE, Troelstra A, et al. Phagocytosis of *Staphylococcus aureus* and *Haemophilus influenzae* type b opsonized with polyclonal human IgG1 and IgG2 antibodies. *J Immunol*. 1993;151:1463.
201. Lefranc M, Lefranc G, Rabbitts TH. Inherited deletion of immunoglobulin heavy chain constant region genes in normal human individuals. *Nature*. 1982;300:760.
202. Ravetch JV, Kinet J. Fc Receptors. *Annu Rev Immunol*. 1991;9:457.
203. Gorter A, Hiemstra PS, Leijh PCJ, et al. IgA- and secretory IgA-opsonized *S. aureus* induce a respiratory burst and phagocytosis by polymorphonuclear leucocytes. *Immunology*. 1987;61:303.
204. Hiemstra PS, Gorter A, Stuurman ME, et al. Activation of alternative pathway of complement by human serum IgA. *Eur J Immunol*. 1987;17:321.
205. Jarvis GA, Griffiss JM. Human IgA1 initiates complement-mediated killing of *Neisseria meningitidis*. *J Immunol*. 1989;143:1703.
206. Imai H, Chen RJ, Wyatt RJ, et al. Lack of complement activation by human IgA immune complexes. *Clin Exp Immunol*. 1988;73:479.
207. Jarvis GA, Griffiss JM. Human IgA1 blockade of IgG-initiated lysis of *Neisseria meningitidis* is a function of antigen-binding fragment binding to the polysaccharide capsule. *J Immunol*. 1991;147:1962.
208. Nikolova EB, Tomana M, Russell MW. All forms of human IgA antibodies bound to antigen interfere with complement (C3) fixation induced by IgG or by antigen alone. *Scand J Immunol*. 1994;39:275.
209. Russell MW, Mansa B. Complement-fixing properties of human IgA antibodies. Alternative pathway complement activation by plastic-bound, but not specific antigen-bound, IgA. *Scand J Immunol*. 1989;30:175.
210. Roos A, Bouwman LH, van Gijlswijk-Janssen DJ, et al. Human IgA activates the complement system via the mannan-binding lectin pathway. *J Immunol*. 2001;167:2861.
211. Janoff EN, Fasching C, Orenstein JM, et al.. Killing of *Streptococcus pneumoniae* by capsular polysaccharide-specific polymeric IgA, complement, phagocytes. *J Clin Invest*. 1999;104:1139.
212. Michetti P, Mahan MJ, Slauch JM, et al. Monoclonal secretory immunoglobulin A protects mice against oral challenge with

the invasive pathogen Salmonella typhimurium. *Infect Immun.* 1992;60:1786.
213. Sun K, Johansen FE, Eckmann L, et al. An important role for polymeric Ig receptor-mediated transport of IgA in protection against *Streptococcus pneumoniae* nasopharyngeal carriage. *J Immunol.* 2004;173:4576.
214. Lamm ME. Interaction of antigens and antibodies at mucosal surfaces. *Annu Rev Microbiol.* 1997;51:311.
215. Brandtzaeg P, Fjellanger I, Gjeruldsen ST. Immunoglobulin M: local synthesis and selective secretion in patients with immunoglobulin A deficiency. *Science.* 1968;160:789.
216. Sieling PA, Chatterjee D, Porcelli SA, et al. CD1-restricted T cell recognition of microbial lipoglycan antigens. *Science.* 1995;269:227.
217. Tzianabos AO, Finberg RW, Wang Y, et al. T cells activated by zwitterionic molecules prevent abscesses induced by pathogenic bacteria. *J Biol Chem.* 2000;275:6733.
218. Stephen TL, Niemeyer M, Tzianabos AO, et al. Effect of B7-2 and CD40 signals from activated antigen-presenting cells on the ability of zwitterionic polysaccharides to induce T-cell stimulation. *Infect Immun.* 2005;73:2184.
219. Chung DR, Kasper DL, Panzo RJ, et al. CD4+ T cells mediate abscess formation in intra-abdominal sepsis by an IL-17-dependent mechanism. *J Immunol.* 2003;170:1958.
220. Weaver CT, Harrington LE, Mangan PR, et al. Th17: an effector CD4 T cell lineage with regulatory T cell ties. *Immunity.* 2006;24:677.
221. Happel KI, Dubin PJ, Zheng M, et al. Divergent roles of IL-23 and IL-12 in host defense against *Klebsiella pneumoniae*. *J Exp Med.* 2005;202:761.
222. Mangan PR, Harrington LE, O'Quinn DB, et al. Transforming growth factor-beta induces development of the T(H)17 lineage. *Nature.* 2006;441:231.
223. Bhatt SM, Cabellos C, Nadol JB, et al. The impact of dexamethasone on hearing loss in experimental pneumococcal meningitis. *Pediatr Infect Dis J.* 1995;14:93.
224. Kengatharan KM, De Kimpe S, Robson C, et al. Mechanism of gram-positive shock: identification of peptidoglycan and lipoteichoic acid moieties essential in the induction of nitric oxide synthase, shock, multiple organ failure. *J Exp Med.* 1998;188:305.
225. Gutierrez-Ramos JC, Bluethmann H. Molecules and mechanisms operating in septic shock: lessons from knockout mice. *Immunol Today.* 1997;18:329.
226. Hanna PC, Acosta D, Collier RJ. On the role of macrophages in anthrax. *Proc Natl Acad Sci U S A.* 1993;90:10198.
227. O'Brien AD, Rosenstreich DL, Scher I, et al. Genetic control of susceptibility to *Salmonella typhimurium* in mice: role of the Lps gene. *J Immunol.* 1980;124:20.
228. Hagberg L, Briles DE, Eden CS. Evidence for separate genetic defects in C3H/HeJ and C3HeB/FeJ mice that affect susceptibility to gram-negative infections. *J Immunol.* 1985;134:4118.
229. Finne J, Leinonen M, Makela PH. Antigenic similarities between brain components and bacteria causing meningitis. Implications for vaccine development and pathogenesis. *Lancet.* 1983;2:355.
230. Rougon G, Dubois C, Buckley N, et al. A monoclonal antibody against meningococcus group B polysaccharides distinguishes embryonic from adult N-CAM. *J Cell Biol.* 1986;103:2429.
231. Moran AP, Prendergast MM, Appelmelk BJ. Molecular mimicry of host structures by bacterial lipopolysaccharides and its contribution to disease. *FEMS Immunol Med Microbiol.* 1996;16:105.
232. Rees JH, Soudain SE, Gregson NA, et al. *Campylobacter jejuni* infection and Guillain-Barre syndrome. *N Eng J Med.* 1995;333:1374.
233. Bessen D, Jones KF, Fischetti VA. Evidence for two distinct classes of streptococcal M protein and their relationship to rheumatic fever. *J Exp Med.* 1989;169:269.
234. Hollingshead SK, Bessen DE. Evolution of the emm gene family: virulence gene clusters in group A streptococci. *Dev Biol Standard.* 1995;85:163.
235. Cunningham MW, McCormack JM, Fenderson PG, et al. Human and murine antibodies cross-reactive with streptococcal M protein and myosin recognize the sequence gln-lys-ser-lys-gln in M protein. *J Immunol.* 1989;143:2677.
236. Cunningham MW, Antone SM, Gulizia JM, et al. Alpha-helical coiled-coil molecules: A role in autoimmunity against the heart. *Clin Immunol Immunopathol.* 1993;68:118.
237. Cunningham MW. Streptococci and rheumatic fever. In: Friedman H, Rose NR, Bendinelli M, eds. *Microorganisms and autoimmune disease.* New York: Plenum Press, 1996:13.
238. Cunningham MW, Antone SM, Gulizia JM, et al. Cytotoxic and viral neutralizing antibodies crossreact with streptococcal M protein, enteroviruses and human cardiac myosin. *Proc Natl Acad Sci U S A.* 1992;89:1320.
239. Chow LH, Yuling Y, Linder J, et al. Phenotypic analysis of infiltrating cells in human myocarditis. An immunohistochemical study in paraffin-embedded tissue. *Arch Pathol Lab Med.* 1989;113:1357.
240. Guilherme L, Chuna-Neto E, Coelho V, et al. Human heart-infiltrating T cell clones from rheumatic heart disease patients recognize both streptococcal and cardiac proteins. *Circulation.* 1995;92:415.
241. Netea MG, Demacker PN, Kullberg BJ, et al. Low-density lipoprotein receptor-deficient mice are protected against lethal endotoxemia and severe gram-negative infections. *J Clin Invest.* 1996;97:1366.
242. Wessels MR, Butko P, Ma M, et al. Studies of group B streptococcal infection in mice deficient in complement component C3 or C4 demonstrate an essential role for complement in both innate and acquired immunity. *Proc Natl Acad Sci U S A.* 1995;92:11490.
243. Ross SC, Densen P. Complement deficiency states and infection: epidemiology, pathogenesis and consequences of neisserial and other infections in an immune deficiency. *Medicine* (Baltimore). 1984;63:243.
244. OBrien DP, Briles DE, Szalai A, et al. Tumor necrosis factor alpha receptor I is important for survival from *Streptococcus pneumoniae* infections. *Infect Immun.* 1999;67:595.
245. Mizgerd JP, Spieker MR, Doerschuk CM. Early response cytokines and innate immunity: essential roles for TNF receptor 1 and type I IL-1 receptor during *Escherichia coli* pneumonia in mice. *J Immunol.* 2001;166:4042.
246. Khalil A, Tullus K, Bartfai T, et al. Renal cytokine responses in acute *Escherichia coli* pyelonephritis in IL-6-deficient mice. *Clin Exp Immunol.* 2000;122:200.
247. Murphy EA, Sathiyaseelan J, Parent MA, et al. Interferon-gamma is crucial for surviving a *Brucella abortus* infection in both resistant C57BL/6 and susceptible BALB/c mice. *Immunology.* 2001;103:511.
248. Sha WC, Liou HC, Tuomanen EI, et al. Targeted disruption of the p50 subunit of NF-kappa B leads to multifocal defects in immune responses. *Cell.* 1995;80:321.
249. Engstrand, L. Potential animal models of *Helicobacter pylori* infection in immunological and vaccine research. *FEMS Immunol Med Microbiol.* 1995;10:265.
250. Chen SC, Mehrad B, Deng JC, et al. Impaired pulmonary host defense in mice lacking expression of the CXC chemokine lungkine. *J Immunol.* 2001;166:3362.
251. Tsai WC, Strieter RM, Mehrad B, et al. CXC chemokine receptor CXCR2 is essential for protective innate host response in murine *Pseudomonas aeruginosa* pneumonia. *Infect Immun.* 2000;68:4289.
252. Frendeus B, Godaly G, Hang L, et al. Interleukin 8 receptor deficiency confers susceptibility to acute experimental pyelonephritis and may have a human counterpart. *J Exp Med.* 2000;192:881.
253. Prince JE, Brayton CF, Fossett MC, et al. The differential roles of LFA-1 and Mac-1 in host defense against systemic infection with *Streptococcus pneumoniae*. *J Immunol.* 2001;166:7362.
254. Picard C, Puel A, Bonnet M, et al. Pyogenic bacterial infections in humans with IRAK-4 deficiency. *Science.* 2003;299:2076.

Chapter 39

Immunology of HIV Infection

Norman L. Letvin

INTRODUCTION

Acquired immunodeficiency syndrome (AIDS) has rapidly emerged as a devastating worldwide medical problem. Although the first cases of AIDS were described as recently as 1981 and its etiologic agent human immunodeficiency virus type 1 (HIV-1) was only isolated in 1983, the rapid pandemic spread of HIV-1/AIDS has changed the world in which we live. Five million new HIV-1 infections occur each year (1). HIV-1 has ravaged sub-Saharan Africa, where more than 25% of adults are infected by HIV-1 in such countries as Botswana and Zimbabwe (Figure 39.1). At the present time the virus is spreading most rapidly in India, Central Asia, and Eastern Europe. It continues to be a serious problem in the West, with more than 1 million HIV-1 infections diagnosed to date in the United States. Twenty million people have died from AIDS, and 40 million are currently living with HIV-1 infections.

Although antiretroviral drug treatment is available for infected individuals, these therapies are not curative. Moreover, antiretroviral drugs are prohibitively expensive for most people in the developing world. Thus, the consequences of this infection at both an individual and societal level make the development of strategies for the control of HIV-1 an absolute priority.

The immunopathogenesis of AIDS is unique among human viral diseases. Although humans mount a vigorous immune response against HIV-1, containment of replicating virus is incomplete. This incomplete immune control of the virus can be explained, at least in part, by the ability of the virus to persist in nonreplicating forms, by its propensity to mutate, and by its ability to destroy the cellular elements of the immune system. The immunobiology of the virus–host interactions of HIV-1 must be understood if we are to succeed in generating new drug therapies or in harnessing the immune response to create a vaccine to contain viral replication in infected individuals.

This chapter will provide an overview of our current understanding of the immunopathogenesis of AIDS. The overview will include a description of HIV-1 and other closely related primate lentiviruses. The mechanisms of HIV-1 spread from one infected individual to another will be examined. The immunologic dysfunction that occurs as a consequence of persistent HIV-1 infection will be

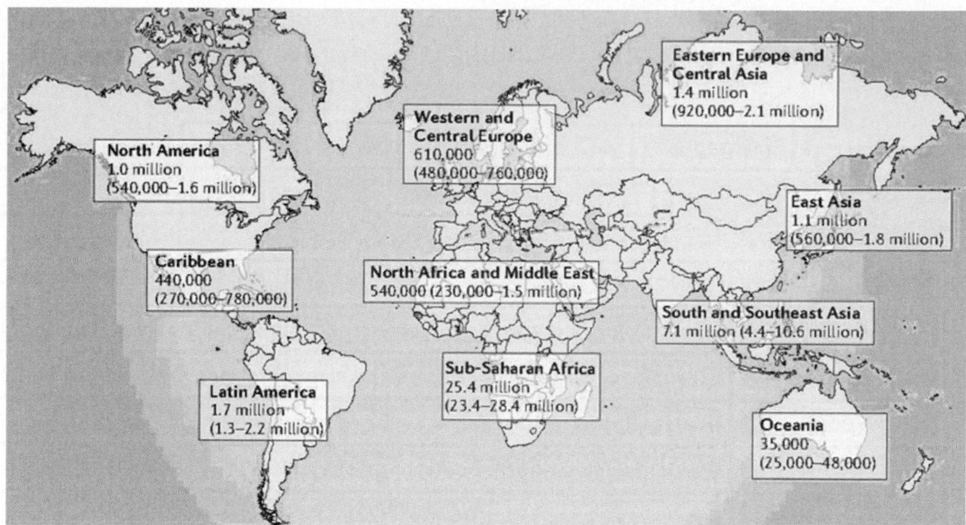

FIGURE 39.1 Prevalence of HIV-1 infections in different geographical regions worldwide. HIV-1 is a worldwide epidemic, and sub-Saharan Africa, the Indian subcontinent, and Southeast Asia are the areas most affected. Estimates of the number of infections are shown in the boxes. Adapted from (1) and (189).

detailed, and the factors that contribute to the extreme variability of the clinical course in infected individuals will be explored. The humoral and cellular immune responses induced by HIV-1 will be described, with an exploration of the ramifications of the incomplete immune control of the virus. Finally, we will examine the progress made to date and the obstacles we are still facing in the creation of an effective HIV-1 vaccine.

THE HIV-1 VIRUS

HIV-1 is a retrovirus and a member of a family of primate lentiviruses (2). An infectious HIV-1 virion contains two copies of a 9.2 kb single-stranded viral RNA genome (Figure 39.2). Once the virus enters the cell, the RNA is converted to double-stranded DNA by a virus-encoded enzyme, reverse transcriptase. This double-stranded DNA enters the cell nucleus and integrates into the host cell genome to generate a provirus using the virally encoded enzyme integrase. The integrated provirus becomes the primary template for the subsequent transcription of the virus' structural, regulatory, and accessory genes.

HIV-1 encodes three structural gene products (Figure 39.3). The *gag* gene encodes precursors for the virion capsid proteins (capsid, nucleocapsid, and matrix) that package genomic viral RNA into virions and participate in viral uncoating. The *pol* gene encodes precursors for several virion enzymes required for viral replication (protease, reverse transcriptase, RNase, and integrase). The *env* gene

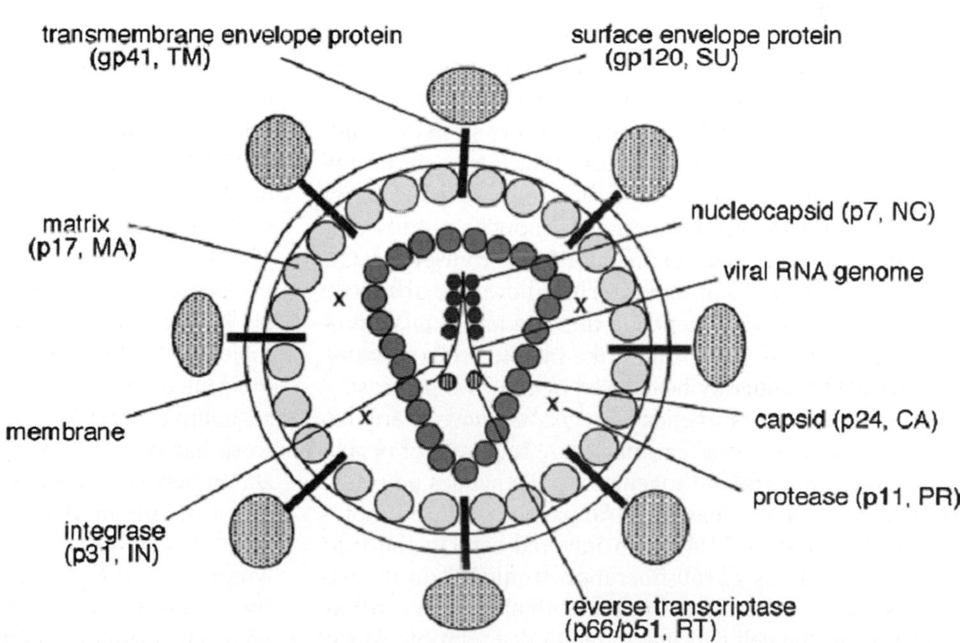

FIGURE 39.2 HIV-1 virion structure. Lentivirus particles are spherical and consist of a lipid bilayer surrounding a conical nucleocapsid. Adapted from (190).

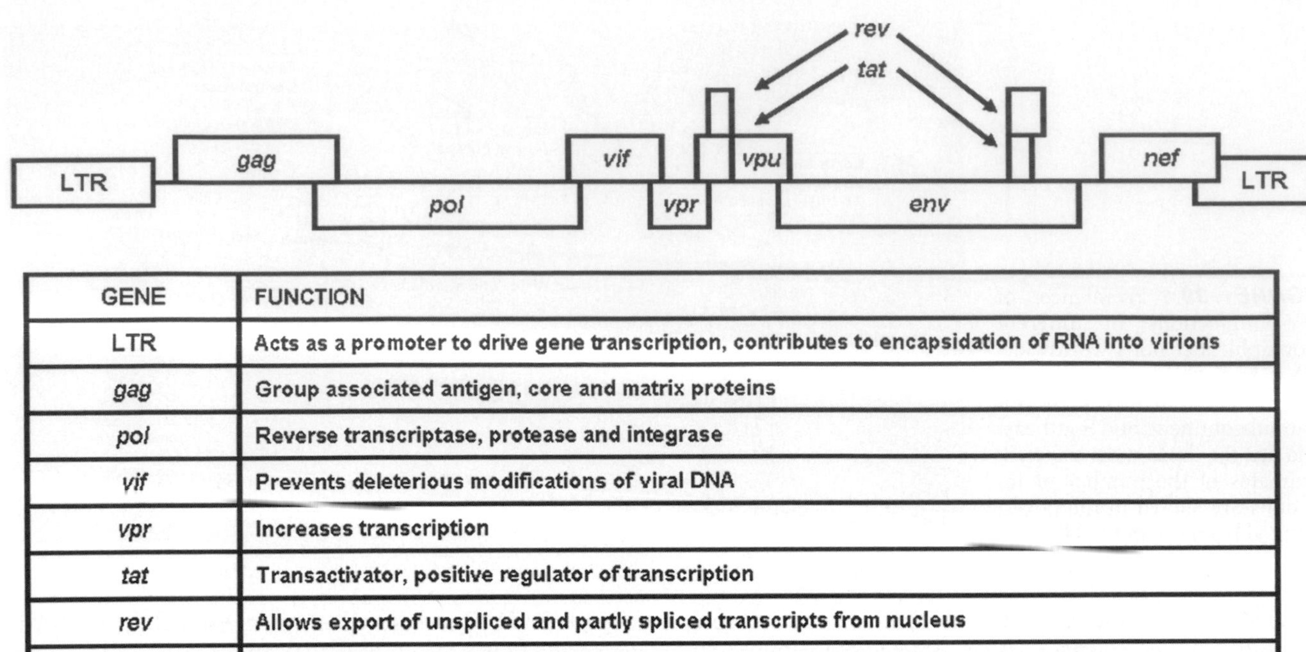

GENE	FUNCTION
LTR	Acts as a promoter to drive gene transcription, contributes to encapsidation of RNA into virions
gag	Group associated antigen, core and matrix proteins
pol	Reverse transcriptase, protease and integrase
vif	Prevents deleterious modifications of viral DNA
vpr	Increases transcription
tat	Transactivator, positive regulator of transcription
rev	Allows export of unspliced and partly spliced transcripts from nucleus
vpu	Promotes intracellular degradation of CD4 and enhances release of virus from membrane
env	Viral entry
nef	Downregulates host CD4

FIGURE 39.3 Genomic organization of HIV-1. The genomic organization of the linear double-stranded proviral DNA form of the virus is shown. The presumed function of each of the viral gene products is shown in the associated table.

encodes precursors for the envelope glycoproteins gp41 and gp120, which form the envelope protein gp160. The HIV envelope protein binds to CD4 and to chemokine receptors to facilitate entry into and infection of $CD4^+$ T cells or macrophages as will be discussed later.

The virus also encodes a series of small regulatory gene products, *tat* and *rev,* that are both essential for *in vitro* and *in vivo* virus replication. While the basal transcription of integrated HIV-1 is very low, the *tat* gene product dramatically augments this RNA synthesis. It does this by binding to an RNA stem-loop structure that is present on the 5′-terminus of viral mRNAs and thus acts to enhance transcriptional elongation. The *rev* gene product binds to a particular sequence present in unspliced viral transcripts, targeting them for nuclear export. This allows the unspliced viral transcripts, which encode the Gag and GagPol proteins, to enter the cytoplasm of the infected cell, be translated, and subsequently be cleaved by the viral protease.

The viral accessory genes *vpu, vpr, nef,* and *vif* are dispensible for *in vitro* replication but are required for *in vivo* replication and viral pathogenicity. *vpu* encodes a protein that enhances the release of viral particles and promotes the degradation of CD4 in an infected cell. In the host cell, vpu catalyzes gp160 liberation from CD4 in the endoplasmic reticulum, resulting in both an increase in Env transport to the cell surface and CD4 degradation via the ubiquitin/proteosome pathway. The functions of the *vpr* gene product include stimulation of gene expression from the HIV-1 LTR, induction of arrest in the G2 phase of the cell cycle in the host cell, and facilitation of transport of double-stranded viral DNA, produced by reverse transcription in the cytoplasm, to the nucleus in the infected cell. The functions associated with the *nef* gene product include down-regulation of both CD4 and major histocompatibility complex (MHC) class I on the surface of the infected cell, stimulation of virus infectivity, and modulation of cellular activation pathways. Finally, as described in more detail later, the *vif* gene product allows the virus to circumvent the potent antiviral activity of the host cell protein APOBEC3G.

Viral entry into cells usually requires an interaction of the envelope glycoprotein of the virus with the CD4 molecule (3) (Figure 39.4). Since CD4 is a cell signaling molecule and $CD4^+$ T lymphocyte dysfunction is a clinical hallmark of HIV-1 infection, considerable experimental work has been invested in determining whether an interaction between CD4 and gp120 is responsible for immune abnormalities in AIDS. While recombinant gp120 added to $CD4^+$ T lymphocytes *in vitro* has been shown to induce T lymphocyte abnormalities, there has never been conclusive evidence to suggest that viral gp120, either virion-associated or shed, can trigger T cell abnormalities *in vivo*.

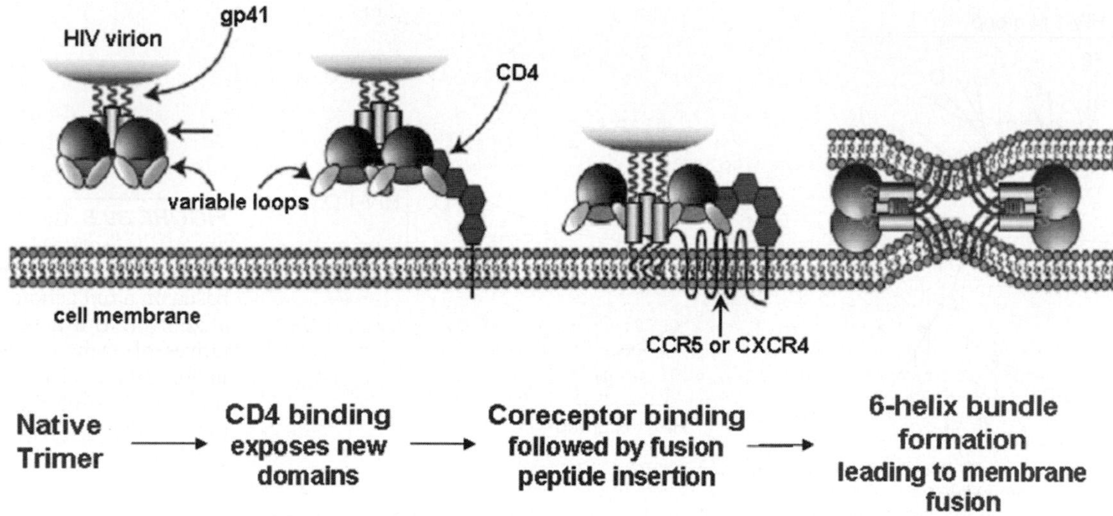

FIGURE 39.4 HIV-1 binding and entry into a cell. HIV-1 envelope binding to CD4 expressed on a cell surface results in conformational changes in the envelope that facilitate coreceptor binding. These events lead first to the insertion of the fusion peptide into the cell membrane and then membrane fusion. Adapted from (191).

It has also been demonstrated that HIV-1 makes use of other co-receptors for cell entry after binding to CD4 in a two-step binding mechanism (4–6). Those molecules are chemokine receptors and members of the seven transmembrane G-protein–coupled receptor family. The chemokine receptor used by a particular HIV-1 isolate has important ramifications for the cellular tropism of that isolate. It has been shown that infection of a transformed T cell line *in vitro* can only occur with viral isolates that employ the CXCR4 molecule as their second receptor. Infection of primary macrophage populations occurs with isolates that employ the CCR5 molecule as a second receptor. Entry of viruses into primary human T cells can occur through either the CXCR4 or the CCR5 receptor.

The demonstration that these seven transmembrane G-protein–coupled receptors are important for HIV-1 entry into cells provided an explanation for some previously puzzling biologic properties of HIV-1 isolates. This finding provided a rationale for how $CD4^{-}$ cells, such as endothelial cells, can be infected *in vivo* (7). It explained why HIV-1 replication in lymphocytes can be inhibited *in vitro* by a number of beta chemokines, including MIP-1α, MIP-1β, and RANTES, since these molecules are ligands for viral coreceptors (8).

This viral requirement for second receptors also explained some of the well-described idiosyncratic biologic events in the viral transmission process and in clinical progression to AIDS in those who are infected. It has been known for some time that only a subpopulation of HIV-1 isolates appears to be transmitted by sexual contact. Those viral isolates are almost universally macrophage-tropic (9). It is now clear that the isolates of HIV-1 that are most likely to be transmitted are macrophage-tropic because they are CCR5-tropic. It has also been known for some time that clinical conversion from an asymptomatic infection to AIDS in chronically infected individuals is associated with a phenotypic change in the infecting viral isolates (10). It is now appreciated that this phenotypic change is associated with a change of second receptor use by the virus from CCR5 to CXCR4. HIV-1 replication increases substantially in the infected individual as that individual progresses clinically to symptomatic AIDS. It is unclear whether the associated conversion from CCR5-tropic to CXCR4-tropic virus in these individuals results in a virus with particularly high replication potential, or rather that high levels of replicating virus select for CXCR4-tropic viruses.

An understanding of the immunobiology of AIDS must be built upon an appreciation that HIV-1 represents an extraordinarily diverse population of antigenically distinct viruses, both at a population level and at an individual level. This diversity is a result of a continuous process of mutation that occurs during HIV-1 replication. One of every 10,000 nucleotides of the replicating virus mutates because the HIV-1 reverse transcriptase lacks 3′ exonuclease proofreading activity.

The virus therefore rapidly becomes an antigenically heterogeneous swarm of viral quasispecies, even in a single infected individual. With more than 1 billion new viral particles created daily during the period of peak viral replication in an infected individual early after infection, there is reason to assume that virtually any mutation that the virus can tolerate will be generated. To contain HIV-1 replication, the immune system must therefore deal with a diverse population of viruses in an infected individual. The HIV-1 virus is also heterogenous at a population level. Analysis of viral sequences from HIV-1 has shown that the

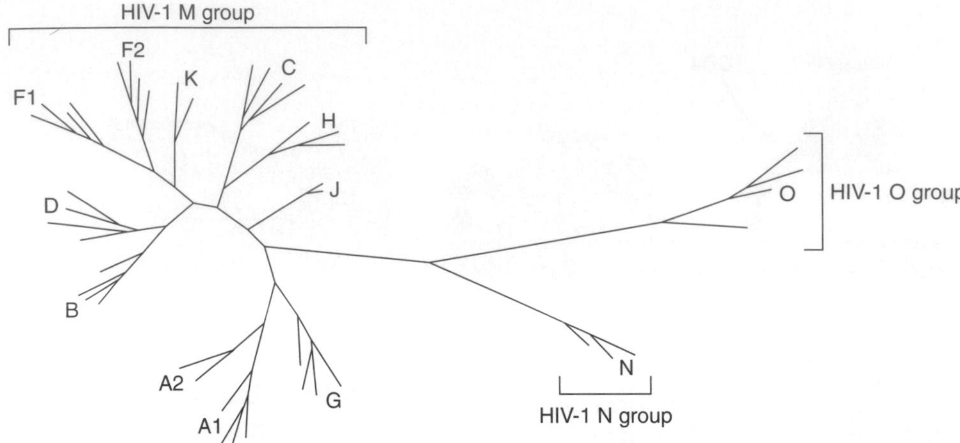

FIGURE 39.5 Genetic diversity of HIV-1 isolates. This figure depicts a neighbor-joining tree, based on a full genome sequence alignment with a few representatives of each of the M group major HIV-1 clades. The tree was drawn using the Treemaker tool at the Los Alamos HIV-1 database. Adapted from (189).

viruses cluster into distinct groups that are referred to as *subtypes* or *clades* (Figure 39.5). Most HIV-1 isolates that are found in the Western hemisphere and Europe are clade B viruses, whereas those in India are clade C viruses.

INTRINSIC MECHANISMS OF ANTIVIRAL DEFENSE

Recent work has defined a number of intracellular proteins that have anti–HIV-1 activity. The most intensively studied of these proteins is APOBEC3G (11). APOBEC3G is incorporated into budding HIV-1 virions and causes extensive deamination of dC to dU on the minus single-stranded viral DNA as it is being synthesized during reverse transcription in the target cell. This causes an accumulation of dG to dA mutations in the subsequently synthesized plus-strand DNA of the virus. This phenomenon is termed *hypermutation* because the deamination can occur in greater than 10% of all viral C residues, a level of mutation that is not tolerable to the virus. APOBEC3G is a member of a family of closely related cytidine deaminases that includes APOBEC1 and activation induced deaminase (AID), which deaminate the apolipoprotein B mRNA in gastrointestinal tissue and antibody genes in B cells, respectively.

The HIV-1 auxiliary protein Vif allows the virus to circumvent the potent antiviral activity of APOBEC3G through at least two complementing mechanisms. Vif recruits a ubiquitin ligase complex that mediates the polyubiquitylation of APOBEC3G, targeting this protein for destruction by the 26S proteasome. Moreover, Vif also impairs de novo APOBEC3G synthesis. Thus, Vif blocks the incorporation of APOBEC3G into HIV-1 virions.

Trim5α is another recently described intrinsic mediator of potent defense against primate lentiviruses (12). It is a member of the tripartite motif family of molecules and is composed of RING, B-box 2, and coiled-coil domains, as well as a C-terminal B30.2 (SPRY) domain. By directly recognizing the viral capsid of select primate lentiviruses, it accelerates uncoating of the capsid of viral particles following their entry into cells. By disrupting the ordered process of viral uncoating and reverse transcription, this protein acts to block cross-species transmission of certain immunodeficiency viruses.

In further studies to define genetic restriction factors for HIV-1, Murr1 has been shown to inhibit HIV-1 replication in unstimulated CD4$^+$ T lymphocytes (13). This gene product, previously implicated in copper regulation, appears to mediate this inhibition by stimulating basal and cytokine-mediated nuclear factor (NF)–κB activity. With considerable research activity ongoing at the present time in the area of host genetic restriction factors for HIV-1 replication, there is reason to believe that more of these molecules will be characterized in the near future.

ANIMAL MODELS OF AIDS

Animal models have proven of central importance in elucidating aspects of HIV-1 pathogenesis and evaluating AIDS vaccine strategies. Because HIV-1 is a member of a family of primate lentiviruses that are species-restricted in their ability to replicate, HIV-1 does not infect small laboratory animals. Mice therefore cannot be used to assess the immunobiology of HIV-1 infections. Nevertheless, several small laboratory animal models have been developed with the hope of applying them to studying HIV-1 biology. These models have relied on the tactic of reconstituting the immune systems of immune-incompetent mice with human lymphoid tissue. However, the use of these models has been limited because the complex biology associated with the dissemination of HIV-1 in humans is not reproduced in these mice.

Much of our current understanding of AIDS immunobiology has come from studies of nonhuman primates infected with primate immunodeficiency viruses. Many African nonhuman primate species are infected with lentivirus isolates that are closely related to HIV-1. These viruses are referred to as *simian immunodeficiency viruses*, or *SIVs*. It is, in fact, the transmission of selected SIVs across primate species barriers that led to the AIDS epidemic in human populations. HIV-2, the virus responsible for much of the AIDS in humans in West Central Africa, is indistinguishable at the genomic level from the SIV that endemically infects the West Central African monkey the sooty mangabey (14). Thus, a cross-species transmission of SIVsm from the sooty mangabey introduced this virus into humans.

Similarly, an SIV referred to as *SIVcpz* has been found endemically in chimpanzees living in the wild in West Central and East Africa. This virus arose as a result of cross-species transmissions and subsequent recombinations of two distinct SIVs that endemically infect nonhuman primate species on which chimpanzees prey. In fact, SIVcpz is so similar at the genomic level to HIV-1, it has been suggested that HIV-1 first entered humans in West Central Africa through blood–blood contact as humans were hunting SIVcpz-infected chimpanzees for food (15).

Interestingly, the various SIV isolates have dramatically different levels of pathogenicity in different primate species. The diverse SIVs that endemically infect various monkey species in Africa have little or no pathogenicity in their natural host species. SIVagm isolates that infect African Green monkeys replicate to only very low levels in this species and have not been reported to induce an AIDS-like illness. Studies of large numbers of sooty mangabeys that are naturally infected with their own SIVsm isolates have shown that this virus replicates at a very high level, comparable to the level of replication seen in HIV-1–infected humans. However, only a single case of AIDS has been reported in a sooty mangabey, and that occurred in a monkey infected for greater than 19 years.

The pathogenicity of the virus isolates that are responsible for AIDS in humans is quite variable. SIVsm/HIV-2, a virus that has very little pathogenic potential in its natural host species, causes AIDS in humans, although it appears to be less pathogenic in humans than SIVcpz/HIV-1. While the pathogenicity of SIVcpz in chimpanzees remains unknown, there is reason to think that the virus may have a low pathogenic potential in this species. This thinking derives from the observation that many HIV-1 isolates obtained from humans have been inoculated into chimpanzees, and only one of these isolates has been shown to induce AIDS in this species of great apes.

Importantly, selected SIV isolates induce an AIDS-like illness when inoculated under experimental conditions into certain Asian macaque species. The best studied of these is the infection of rhesus monkeys with SIVsm. SIVsm is also referred to in the literature as SIVmac because it was first isolated from macaques inadvertently infected with this sooty mangabey virus. Rhesus monkeys infected with SIVsm/SIVmac develop peak and set-point plasma virus RNA levels that are even higher than those observed in HIV-1–infected humans. The virus is R5-tropic and accordingly causes profound depletion of the CCR5-expressing memory CD4$^+$ T lymphocytes in rhesus monkeys. Infected monkeys develop wasting, and a spectrum of opportunistic infections and tumors indistinguishable from that seen in HIV-1–infected humans (16).

Chimeric viruses that express HIV-1 envelopes on an SIV backbone can be constructed in the laboratory. These viruses are known as *simian human immunodeficiency viruses* or *SHIVs*. A variety of HIV-1 envelopes have been incorporated into SHIVs, resulting in viruses with distinctive pathogenic profiles. SHIVs expressing R5-tropic envelopes have been able to replicate in macaques, but only to low levels, and have not proven consistently pathogenic. Selected SHIV isolates constructed with X4- or dual-tropic envelopes induce profound CD4$^+$ T lymphocyte loss, immunodeficiency, and an AIDS-like illness in macaques (17). However, this SHIV-induced clinical syndrome differs from HIV-1–induced disease in humans because the X4-tropic SHIVs selectively eliminate the naïve rather than the memory CD4$^+$ T lymphocyte populations targeted by the R5-tropic HIV-1 isolates in humans.

In spite of the distinct pathogenic profiles of these different primate immunodeficiency viruses in Asian monkeys, both the SIV- and SHIV-infected macaques have proven enormously powerful models for exploring mechanisms of AIDS immunopathogenesis and approaches to HIV-1 vaccination. They have been particularly useful in characterizing virologic and immunologic events that occur during the initial days following infection, a period of time during which HIV-1–infected humans are rarely recognized by clinical investigators. These models have also proven invaluable for evaluating a diversity of strategies for HIV-1 vaccination.

HIV-1 TRANSMISSION

HIV-1 is transmitted primarily by sexual exposure. It is also spread by needle sharing among intravenous drug users. Transfusion of virus-contaminated blood products occurred quite frequently before blood screening procedures were developed in the mid-1980s. However, with the introduction first of antibody testing and later of nucleic acid testing by blood banks, transfusion-associated transmission of HIV-1 has been nearly eliminated. Mother-to-infant spread of the virus also occurs and remains a serious problem worldwide (18). Testing for HIV-1 and treatment of infected women with a short course of antiretroviral drugs can reduce the frequency of intrapartem and peripartem transmission from as many as 30% to less than 2% of newborn infants. However, HIV-1 transmission from mother-to-infant during breastfeeding remains a major problem in the developing world.

Although we understand the epidemiology of HIV transmission in human populations, its transmission at the cellular level is not well defined. It is well established that

HIV is transmitted in genital secretions and blood products, with most transmission occurring across a mucosal surface during sexual contact (19). However, the extent to which HIV associates with cells during the process of transmission remains poorly understood. In infected individuals, viable virus exists both in a cell-free state and within cells. While viral transmission can presumably occur through exposure to either cell-free or cell-associated virus, the form in which the virus is usually transmitted during sexual contact remains unknown.

Studies in the SIV/macaque model of AIDS initially suggested that the first infected cell is of the dendritic or monocyte/macrophage lineage (20). That observation led to the hypothesis that virus in a dendritic cell (DC) or macrophage travels from the mucosal site of initial infection to local draining lymph nodes and then replicates in those lymph nodes (21). This scenario would explain why there appears to be selectivity for macrophage-tropic viruses at the time of viral transmission. While that paradigm is certainly intuitively attractive, recent studies in the SIV/macaque model have raised questions concerning its validity. In experiments in which SIV was applied to the tonsils or vaginal mucosa and local mucosal tissue was then evaluated, viral RNA was found only in T lymphocytes and not in DCs or macrophages (22,23). These studies suggest that viral infection might occur in T lymphocytes in addition to the previously defined DC/macrophage infection early after viral exposure.

HIV IMMUNOBIOLOGY AND CLINICAL CONSEQUENCES OF HIV-1 INFECTION

Following transmission across a mucosal barrier, HIV-1 is thought to begin replicating in subsets of T lymphocytes, monocyte/macrophages, and DCs that express CD4 and CCR5. Virus is presumed to spread from the mucosal area to local draining lymph nodes, and then disseminate rapidly via the blood stream to lymphatic tissue and other anatomic compartments throughout the body. Peak viral replication occurs 2 to 4 weeks after the transmission event, at a time before the virus-specific cellular and humoral immune responses are fully mobilized. Levels of virus in the blood can exceed 10^7 copies of viral RNA/mL plasma at this time.

Systemic viral replication, however, is quickly dampened in association with the emergence of virus-specific immune responses. Thus, by 9 to 12 weeks following initial infection, systemic viral loads usually reach a relatively consistent, low steady-state level. The steady-state level, referred to as *set-point,* is approximately 30,000 to 50,000 copies of viral RNA/mL plasma in untreated individuals. Clinical prognosis of HIV-1–infected individuals has been tied to the set-point viral load, with lower levels associated with better prognosis (24).

Because memory CD4$^+$ T cells express CCR5, the usual coreceptor for transmitted HIV-1, and activated cells are particularly susceptible to HIV-1 replication, there is a rapid and dramatic loss of activated, memory CD4$^+$ T cells during the first days following HIV infection (25). A very large number of lymphocytes are found in the gut-associated lymphatic tissue, including the majority of CCR5-expressing memory CD4$^+$ T cells. Therefore, the gastrointestinal tract is a site of extensive CD4$^+$ T lymphocyte loss in the early days following infection with HIV-1. Activated, memory CD4$^+$ T lymphocytes are, however, destroyed in all anatomic compartments of infected individuals.

The eventual pathogenic consequences of HIV-1 infection reflect the close association of viral replication and CD4$^+$ T lymphocyte destruction (Figure 39.6). Normal CD4$^+$ T lymphocyte counts are 800 to 1,050/mm^3, with a range (2 standard deviations) of 500 to 1,400/mm^3.

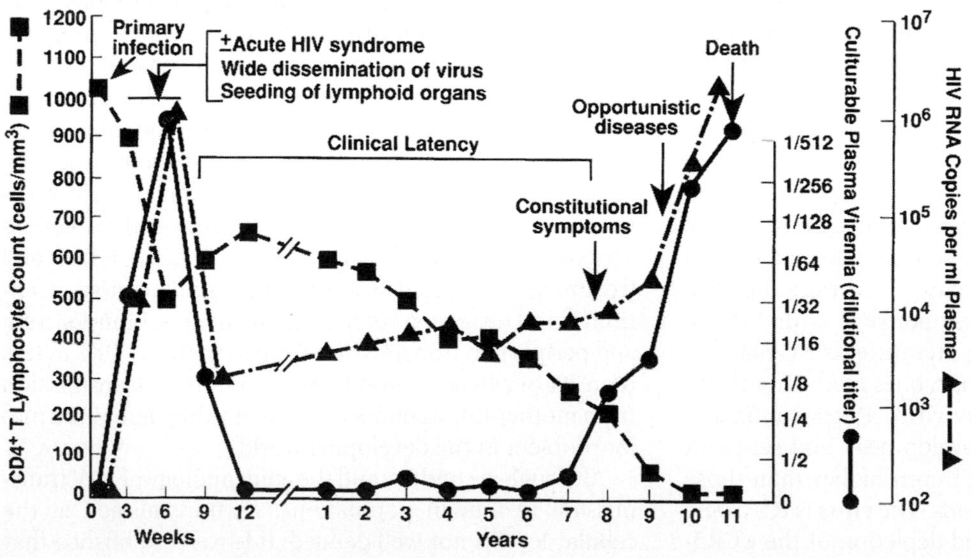

FIGURE 39.6 Usual clinical course of the untreated HIV-1–infected individual. A burst of viral replication with an associated loss of CD4$^+$ T lymphocytes occurs during the first weeks following viral infection. Partial control of the virus then occurs, with a slowing of CD4$^+$ T lymphocyte loss. When the CD4$^+$ T lymphocyte count eventually decreases to below 200 cells/mm^3, opportunistic diseases occur that lead to death. Adapted from (192).

T lymphocyte decline from this normal level is directly correlated with viral load. A CD4$^+$ T lymphocyte decline of approximately 4% per year occurs for every $\log_{10}$ HIV-1 RNA copies/mL plasma in an infected individual. The rate of CD4$^+$ T lymphocyte decline, in turn, is correlated with the rate of disease progression in the HIV-1–infected person.

A clinical condition referred to as an *acute retroviral syndrome* occurs in association with the intense viral replication during the first days following HIV-1 infection. This syndrome is characterized by the sudden onset of a fever with associated lymph node enlargement, sore throat, muscle pain, weight loss, and a skin rash. This self-limited syndrome is often not recognized by infected individuals. When it is recognized, the infected person often simply dismisses the condition as a "flu" because the symptoms are indistinguishable from those associated with many other acute viral infections. Evidence suggests that individuals with more severe symptoms during primary infection have a more rapid progression to clinical AIDS than those who are relatively asymptomatic.

Even without the introduction of therapy, the acute retroviral syndrome is followed by a prolonged asymptomatic period. During this time, on average a period of 8 years, the individual is most often unaware that he or she is infected with HIV-1. Nevertheless, ongoing viral replication during this asymptomatic period leads to inexorable CD4$^+$ T lymphocyte loss (26).

The diagnosis of AIDS is eventually made when the HIV-1–infected individual develops an opportunistic infection or tumor. Some of these medical complications, including tuberculosis, pneumococcal pneumonia, shingles, and thrush, can become manifest when the CD4$^+$ T lymphocyte count is $>200/mm^3$. However, most of the medical problems, referred to as *AIDS defining clinical events*, occur when the CD4$^+$ T lymphocyte count is $<200/mm^3$. The usual AIDS defining infections include *Pneumocystis carinii* pneumonia, toxoplasmosis, cryptococcal meningitis, *Candida* esophagitis, disseminated cytomegalovirus infection, and disseminated *Mycobacterium avium* infection. AIDS defining opportunistic tumors include Kaposi's sarcoma and non-Hodgkin's lymphoma.

The same pathogenic process underlies this diversity of clinical diseases. All are caused by microorganisms that commonly infect healthy individuals. In the setting of intact immune function, the spread of these microorganisms is held in check and they cause no disease. However, as the immune system is destroyed in the HIV-1–infected individual, these microorganisms are no longer contained and they cause diseases that can be fatal.

ANTIRETROVIRAL THERAPY

Without specific therapy, the average life expectancy following clinical recognition of an AIDS-defining opportunistic infection or tumor is 1.3 years. However, therapies to provide prophylaxis against the development of opportunistic infections and, more important, the use of antiretroviral drugs to contain HIV-1 replication have dramatically altered the natural history of HIV-1 infections (27). AZT, the first drug found to have activity against HIV-1, was introduced in 1987. This drug is a member of a family of drugs known as *nucleoside analogue reverse transcriptase inhibitors.* These nucleoside analogues are incorporated into viral RNA and lead to termination of the nucleotide chain being synthesized, blocking reverse transcriptase activity and the generation of proviral DNA. Other nucleoside analogue reverse transcriptase inhibitors have been introduced into clinical use since 1987. However, the use of these drugs as stand alone therapeutic agents was associated with only a modest prolongation of life in infected individuals.

A number of new classes of anti-HIV-1 drugs have been developed since the mid-1990s. The first of these new classes of drugs to be introduced into clinical use, the protease inhibitors, acts by inhibiting the activity of protease, the viral enzyme that cleaves developing viral proteins. The non–nucleoside analogue reverse transcriptase inhibitors, introduced soon after the protease inhibitors, affect the activity of the reverse transcriptase enzyme. Further, the first drug that acts by blocking the ability of the virus to fuse to a cell membrane was introduced as a clinical agent in 2003. Drugs that block the activity of the viral integrase or virus-CCR5 binding are currently undergoing clinical evaluation.

The use of representative drugs from these different classes in combination with one anther has revolutionized the care of the HIV-1–infected patient. A combination of these drugs has substantially more antiviral activity than a single drug used alone. Moreover, HIV-1 can rapidly develop mutations that allow the virus to escape from the activity of one of these drugs if that drug is used as a single therapeutic agent. The simultaneous use of combinations of drugs from these different classes of therapeutic agents dramatically slows the emergence of drug-resistant mutant viruses. By the late 1990s, there was a 60% to 80% decrease in mortality from HIV-1 infections in populations receiving these new combination therapies (28). These combination therapies are often referred to as *highly active antiretroviral therapy* (HAART).

In spite of these considerable advances in the treatment of HIV-1 infections, there is a growing realization that drug therapies will, in the end, not solve the problem posed by the worldwide AIDS epidemic. While these therapies clearly decrease viral replication, they do not eradicate HIV-1 from infected individuals. Antiretroviral drug treated patients who have undetectable plasma viral RNA levels still harbor replicating virus. This ongoing viral replication has been demonstrated in a number of ways. The virus in treated individuals continues to accumulate mutations, a phenomenon that can only occur in the setting of continuing viral replication (29). Moreover, interruption of antiretroviral therapy in individuals with undetectable plasma viral RNA can result in a dramatic rebound of viral replication (30). In fact, plasma viral RNA levels often reach pretreatment levels in these individuals.

A number of reservoirs of replicating or replication competent HIV-1 have been described in individuals who have been successfully treated with antiretroviral drugs (31). These sites include lymphoid tissue, where virus has been demonstrated in CD4^{+} T lymphocytes in the germinal centers of lymphoid tissue and trapped on follicular DCs. Other reservoirs of virus include resting CD4^{+} T lymphocytes in the peripheral blood, monocytes/macrophages, DCs, the central nervous system (CNS), and the reproductive tract.

Other factors also limit the impact of drugs on the AIDS epidemic. The antiretroviral therapies are often associated with toxicities that limit the ability of patients to use the drugs. The emergence of mutant HIV-1 isolates in treated individuals that are resistant to the activity of available drugs and the transmission of these mutant viruses to uninfected individuals may also limit the ultimate efficacy of these therapies. Finally, the populations in the developing world most severely affected by the AIDS epidemic cannot bear the economic burden of the costs of these therapies. Moreover, developing nations often do not have the medical infrastructure needed to use the therapies optimally.

VARIATION IN CLINICAL COURSE OF HIV INFECTION

Investigators have devoted considerable attention to studying infected individuals who are particularly successful in containing HIV-1 replication to help define the immunologic and virologic factors that may contribute to the control of HIV-1 spread in the infected individual. The rate of disease progression can vary dramatically among those infected with HIV-1. A small number of infected individuals, referred to as *long-term nonprogressors* (LTNP) or *elite controllers,* maintain relatively normal CD4^{+} T lymphocyte counts and have unmeasurable plasma viral RNA levels for years or even decades following infection, even without antiretroviral therapy (32,33). While some of these individuals have eventually developed progressive disease, a very small percentage of them have shown no evidence of replicating virus as determined by usual assays and have remained free of clinical disease. A number of immunologic, virologic, and host genetic factors have been implicated in this rare but potentially important cohort of HIV-1–infected individuals.

Most LTNPs demonstrate preserved immune function; however, it is not clear whether this accounts for control of HIV-1 replication or is a consequence of that control. These patients have been shown to have persisting neutralizing antibody responses, preserved lymphoid architecture, and preserved virus-specific T cells (34,35). The preserved antibody responses may, however, simply be a consequence of their preserved helper CD4^{+} T responses rather than the explanation for their benign clinical status. Similarly, while the usual HIV-1–infected individuals have dramatic lymphoid hyperplasia with destruction of the normal architecture of their lymph nodes, there is evidence of only mild follicular hyperplasia in the lymph nodes of these rare patients. This observation may, however, simply be a consequence of the low level of viral replication that occurs in these individuals rather than an etiologic explanation for the limited virus replication. Finally, reports indicate that HIV-1–specific CD8^{+} T lymphocyte populations are present at only very low frequencies in these individuals. This finding would be expected in the setting of low levels of viral replication where there is little viral antigen being produced to stimulate the expansion of effector lymphocytes. Thus, the immunologic correlates of the extraordinary virologic control in these patients may be consequences rather than causes of their effective viral containment.

Occasional individuals have a benign clinical course and are found to be infected with an HIV-1 isolate with a mutation that attenuates the pathogenicity of the virus. The most dramatic of these reported cases was a cluster of transfusion-associated infections in Australia where the mutant virus originated from a single blood donor (36). This virus contained deletions in the *nef* gene, the *nef*/U3 LTR overlap region and rearrangements of the NFκB/SP-1 sites in the viral LTR. Importantly, long-term follow-up of the clinical status of this cluster of infected individuals demonstrated that they went on to develop AIDS, albeit with a delayed time course (37). However, while infection with mutant viruses can certainly result in disease with a relatively benign or delayed clinical course, such cases constitute a very small percentage of the reported long-term nonprogressors.

Host genetic factors appear to account for the majority of cases of elite control of HIV-1 infection. One of the most intensively studied of these host factors is the relationship of particular MHC class I alleles with slow clinical progression (38). Heterozygosity at MHC class I loci is associated with slow clinical progression, while homozygosity at these loci is associated with more rapid progression (39). The presumptive explanation for this phenomenon is that heterozygosity facilitates CTL responses to a greater breadth of HIV-1 epitopes than is seen in individuals who are homozygous for particular MHC class I alleles. Broad CTL responses presumably mediate more effective control of HIV-1 replication than do more focused responses.

In addition to the impact of MHC class I heterozygosity, a number of particular MHC class I alleles have been associated with slow clinical progression in HIV-1–infected individuals. This relationship is most marked in infected individuals expressing HLA B57*01 or HLA B27 (40). Since MHC class I alleles play a central role in the CD8$^+$ T lymphocyte response to a virus and HLA B57*01-restricted CD8$^+$ T lymphocytes dominate the HIV-1–specific cytotoxic T lymphocyte (CTL) response in B57*01$^+$ infected individuals, it is likely that this MHC class I association with long-term nonprogression reflects a particularly effective B57*01-restricted CD8$^+$ T lymphocyte response to the virus. Other MHC class I alleles have also been associated with slow clinical progression, including HLA B14 and C8.

Interestingly, expression of the HLA Bw4–80I allele in association with the activating killer immunoglobulin-like receptor (KIR) allele KIR3DS1 has also been shown to be associated with slow clinical progression following HIV-1 infection (41). Since KIR molecules are expressed on the surface of natural killer (NK) cells, this provocative finding suggests a possible contribution of innate immunity to the control of HIV-1 replication.

Among genetic host factors involved in HIV-1 resistance, the allelic form of the CCR5 molecule expressed by the infected individual has been shown to contribute most profoundly. CCR5, the second receptor for most of the transmitted isolates of HIV-1, can exist in Caucasian populations either as an intact molecule or with a 32 base-pair deletion. The so-called *delta 32* form of CCR5 has a deletion in the portion of the gene that encodes the third extracellular domain of the molecule, resulting in a frame shift and premature stop codon in the fifth transmembrane domain of the molecule. Homozygosity for this delta 32 allelic form of CCR5, which occurs in 1% of Caucasians, confers almost absolute protection against acquisition of the virus (42). Thus, only a handful of CCR5-delta 32 homozygotes have been reported that are infected with HIV-1. This protection is evidence that the virus cannot infect cells that do not express an intact second receptor.

Importantly, while heterozygosity for the delta 32 form of the CCR5 molecule does not confer absolute protection against HIV-1 infection, it is associated with slower progression to AIDS and death in infected individuals (43). When compared to infected individuals expressing CCR5 alleles coding for full-length CCR5, HIV-1–infected CCR5 delta 32 heterozygotes have lower plasma viral RNA levels, slower rates of CD4$^+$ T lymphocyte decline, and a 2- to 4-year delay in time-to-death following seroconversion. These findings are likely a consequence of the fact that heterozygotes have a reduced expression of full-length CCR5 on the surface of their CD4$^+$ T lymphocytes, which likely decreases the efficiency of HIV-1 infection of those cells.

A number of other chemokine receptor allelic polymorphisms have also been associated with delayed progression to AIDS following HIV-1 infection. CCR2, a molecule with 82% sequence homology to CCR5, is only rarely a second receptor for *in vitro* HIV-1 infection. Nevertheless, homozygous or heterozygous expression of a CCR2 protein that contains a single valine to isoleucine substitution at position 64 of the first transmembrane domain CCR2-64I, is associated with a slowing by 2 years of progression to AIDS following infection (44). Finally, allelic forms of the ligands for various other chemokine receptors, including SDF and RANTES, have been assessed for their contributions to the rate of AIDS progression; some studies have suggested associations between particular allelic forms and progression while other studies have not shown such associations.

Polymorphisms in genes associated with molecules that participate in immune cell interactions have also been evaluated for their contribution to AIDS progression in HIV-1–infected individuals. Polymorphisms in the IL-10 promoter, a regulatory region associated with IL-4 production, the tumor necrosis factor (TNF) promoter, and the mannose-binding lectin promoter have all been implicated in influencing the rate of AIDS progression (45). This complex network of associations between allelic forms of molecules and the rate of AIDS clinical progression underscore the importance of both virus–cell interactions and immune activation in the pathogenesis of this disease.

An even more extreme of protection against HIV-1–induced disease has also been described. An extensive but controversial literature has appeared in recent years describing rare cohorts of individuals who are repeatedly exposed to HIV-1 but never convert to virus seropositivity (46). These subjects have been identified both in serodiscordant couples and also among commercial sex workers. Determining immune correlates of protection in such individuals could prove extremely valuable for developing novel strategies for HIV-1 vaccination. These individuals develop virus-specific peripheral blood CD4$^+$ and CD8$^+$ T lymphocyte responses. Mucosal virus-specific T lymphocytes and antibodies have also been described in exposed, uninfected subjects. However, studies have also been published suggesting that these claims of virus-specific immunity in the absence of detectable infection are based on experimental artifact rather than reliable data (47). Interesting studies have also been published suggesting that at least a subpopulation of multiply exposed but seronegative individuals harbor replicating virus at a level that cannot be detected with usual assays (48). Thus, levels of replicating virus in these individuals may be high enough to drive cellular and humoral immune responses, but too low to be detected by usual laboratory assays.

There remains considerable skepticism of these claims because of the low level and inconsistency of the measured immune responses in these exposed, uninfected subjects. Very low responses have been reported in these subjects, considerably lower than are seen in normally infected individuals. Moreover, these responses may be present at the time of one blood sampling and absent at the time of the next sampling. The ultimate importance of these cohorts of subjects for elucidating the basis of sterile protection remains to be determined.

CD4$^+$ T LYMPHOCYTE LOSS FOLLOWING HIV-1 INFECTION

While HIV-1 replication is controlled by the immune response in the early weeks following infection, the containment of the virus is not complete. The incomplete nature of containment of viral replication eventually results in viral destruction of the immune system. The immunologic hallmark of persistent replication of HIV-1 in humans is a gradual loss of CD4$^+$ T lymphocytes, most of which occurs during the period of clinical latency following primary infection.

The mechanism by which CD4$^+$ T lymphocytes are lost in the HIV-1–infected individual has remained an issue of considerable controversy. Early in the AIDS epidemic, at a time when the assays for measuring cell-associated virus were quite insensitive, it was assumed that only approximately 1 in 10^7 peripheral blood CD4$^+$ T cells were infected with HIV-1. Explanations were, therefore, sought to account for the occurrence of profound CD4$^+$ T cell loss in the absence of viral infection of CD4$^+$ T cells. The presumption that there were insufficient numbers of cells infected to account for CD4$^+$ T cell killing led to the suggestion that CD4$^+$ T cells were dying through a secondary apoptotic process (49). However, as assays for cell-associated virus improved in sensitivity, it became clear that large numbers of CD4$^+$ T cells harbored replicating virus in the infected individual. These observations led some to conclude that the CD4$^+$ T cell loss in HIV-1–infected individuals occurs solely as a result of virus replicating in and killing individual cells (50). Others have implicated CD8$^+$ T lymphocytes or general chronic immune activation in the killing of infected CD4$^+$ T helper cells. A number of studies have been done in recent years to characterize the mechanism and dynamics of CD4$^+$ T lymphocyte loss in AIDS and the interpretations of these studies have generated conflicting explanations for CD4$^+$ T cell decline.

With the advent of highly active antiretroviral therapy, it became clear that an early and rapid reconstitution of some of the lost peripheral blood CD4$^+$ T cell population occurred in HIV-1–infected individuals upon initiation of treatment (51–53). In fact, carefully observed clinical responses to HAART in HIV-1–infected subjects have been used to draw conclusions concerning AIDS immunopathogenesis. Thus, the rapid repopulation of CD4$^+$ T lymphocytes following the initiation of HAART has led to the proposal that there is a continuous, high rate of CD4$^+$ T cell turnover in HIV-1–infected individuals and that the decline in CD4$^+$ T cells in infected individuals occurs as a result of exhaustion of the capacity to replenish this rapidly turning-over CD4$^+$ T cell population. The data generated in these studies allowed a calculation of the life span of a CD4$^+$ T cell following infection with HIV-1: a $t_{1/2}$ of 1.6 days. While this explanation for CD4$^+$ T cell loss in HIV-1–infected individuals was attractive, further studies have not substantiated this model.

The first study to raise doubts about the validity of the exhaustion model previously discussed was an experiment done to assess telomere length in CD4$^+$ and CD8$^+$ T cells in HIV-1–infected subjects (54). Telomeres shorten in length as cells divide. Therefore, one can approximate the relative past proliferation of a lymphocyte by measuring the length of its telomeres. When peripheral blood T cells from HIV-1–infected individuals were assessed for their rate of turnover on the basis of telomere length, it was demonstrated that CD4$^+$ T lymphocytes turn over in these individuals at a rate no different than those in uninfected individuals. Interestingly, these studies showed that CD8$^+$ T cell populations in infected individuals have an increased rate of turnover. Studies were also done to assess the dynamics of CD4$^+$ T cell loss and repopulation in AIDS in the SIV/macaque model (55,56). BrdU labeling was employed to measure lymphocyte turnover in both infected and uninfected animals. These studies showed some increase in the rate of CD4$^+$ T cell turnover in infected as compared to uninfected monkeys. However, consistent with the studies of T lymphocyte telomere length, the rate of CD8$^+$ T cell turnover in these infected animals was greater than that of CD4$^+$ T cells. Finally, in studies performed using deuterium-labeled lymphocytes in humans, no evidence of an increased rate of CD4$^+$ T cell turnover could be documented in HIV-1–infected subjects (57). In fact, in those studies decreased numbers of circulating CD4$^+$ T cells in HIV-1–infected individuals appeared to be attributable to a decrease in the production of those lymphocytes.

The demonstration that HIV-1 infection can only occur in a subset of CD4$^+$ T lymphocytes has considerably clarified the longstanding puzzle of how CD4$^+$ T lymphocytes are destroyed. It is now apparent that HIV-1 infects the subset of CD4$^+$ T lymphocytes that express a chemokine receptor, usually CCR5, and that these cells support viral replication more readily if they are activated (25). The gastrointestinal tract is therefore an important site of CD4$^+$ T lymphocyte loss early following infection, since CCR5-expressing, activated CD4$^+$ T lymphocytes are found in large numbers in this anatomic compartment (58). Moreover, since CCR5 is selectively expressed on the memory subset of CD4$^+$ T lymphocytes, these important immune cells are preferentially lost following infection (59). These data suggest that immune cell loss in AIDS occurs in a subpopulation of CD4$^+$ T lymphocytes, and this cell loss occurs as a result of direct killing by replicating virus.

Other facets of the biology of CD4$^+$ T lymphocytes in HIV-1–infected individuals have also been explored. Attempts have been made to characterize the CD4$^+$

T lymphocytes that repopulate infected individuals after the initiation of highly active antiretroviral therapy (60). Early after the start of therapy, a rise in the memory ($CD45RO^+$) $CD4^+$ T cell pool is seen. Later, a reduction in the activation status of all T cells can be demonstrated. Finally, there is a rise in $CD4^+$ T lymphocytes with a naïve phenotype ($CD45RA^+CD62L^+$). The early rise in circulating memory $CD4^+$ T cells probably reflects the peripheral expansion of preexisting, mature T lymphocytes. The reduction of T cell activation likely occurs as a consequence of the sustained decrease in production of infecting virus in those individuals. Therefore, immune reactivity and the associated T cell activation is no longer being driven by the virus. Finally, the late increase in circulating naïve $CD4^+$ T cells probably reflects repopulation of the periphery with immature, uncommitted lymphocytes from bone marrow and thymus. These events suggest that some reconstitution of the pool of helper T lymphocytes can occur with the institution of HAART.

OTHER IMMUNOLOGIC DYSFUNCTION IN AIDS

While $CD4^+$ T lymphocyte loss is the best-studied immunologic abnormality seen in those infected with HIV-1, other evidence of immunologic dysfunction is clearly observed in these individuals. Perhaps the most striking of these abnormalities is the destruction of the lymphoid microenvironment (61). As HIV-1–induced disease progresses clinically, there is an inexorable destruction of lymph node germinal centers. Although the etiology of this germinal center destruction has not been fully explained, the loss of follicular DCs (FDCs) is prominently seen. FDCs do not express CD4, and there is no evidence that these cells themselves become infected with HIV-1 (62). FDCs trap viral particles in germinal centers during the course of infection. This contact with the virus, or local cytokine production that occurs as a consequence of infection, may contribute to the degeneration of these cells. $CD8^+$ T lymphocyte populations also migrate into the germinal centers of lymph nodes during the course of HIV-1 infection. These cell populations may secrete cytokines or lytic granules that mediate destruction of FDCs. Whatever the etiology of FDC loss proves to be, the destruction of the infrastructure upon which the germinal center is built contributes to germinal center dysfunction and eventual disintegration.

Chronic HIV-1 infection also destroys the thymus (63) (Figure 39.7). Thymic tissue loss is so marked that it can be demonstrated radiographically (64). The loss of thymic function in AIDS is also apparent at a molecular level. Genetic rearrangements of the antigen recognition domains of the T cell receptor (TCR) alpha and beta chains of maturing T lymphocytes occur in the thymus as T lymphocytes become committed to a single antigen recognition specificity. These rearrangements include a deletion of TCR delta genetic material, resulting in the generation of so-called *TCR excision circles* (TRECs) that can be detected in developing T lymphocyte populations. High levels of circulating T lymphocytes containing these excision circles is an indication of ongoing thymic maturation of T lymphocytes. As AIDS progresses clinically, the proportion of circulating T lymphocytes that contain these TRECs decreases (65). This suggests a waning of thymic function. The etiology of thymic loss and dysfunction in AIDS remains unclear. Importantly, however, both the radiographic evidence of thymus loss and molecular evidence of thymic dysfunction have been shown to reverse in HIV-1–infected individuals receiving antiretroviral therapy. These observations suggest that thymic dysfunction is

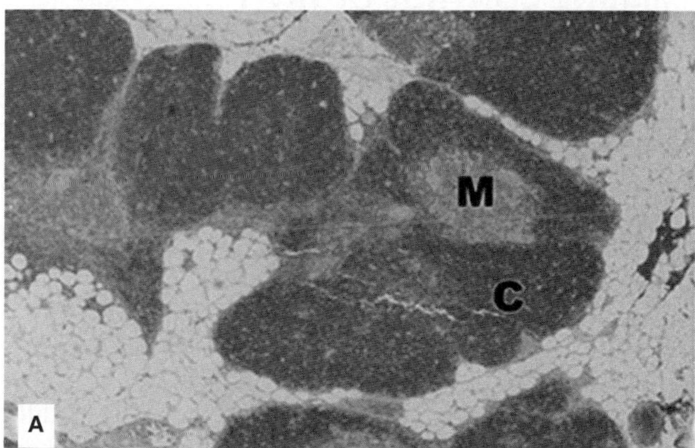

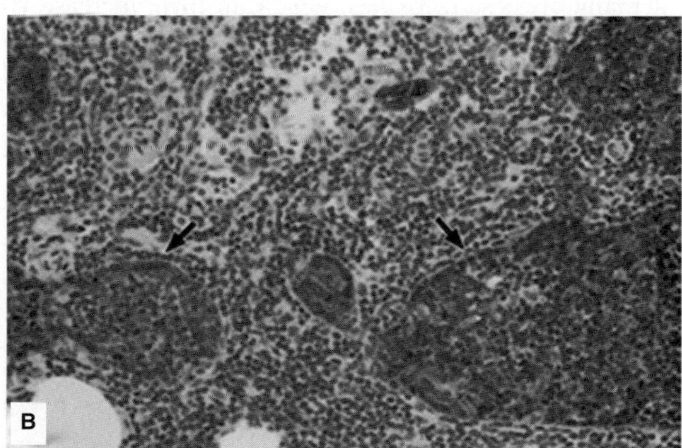

FIGURE 39.7 Immunohistochemical analysis of a thymus from an HIV-1–infected adult. Anti-CD1a staining of a thymus from a normal individual (**A**) is shown with the medulla (M) and cortex (C) noted. A similarly stained thymus from an HIV-1–infected adult (**B**) is also shown with arrows pointing to thymopoietic areas, consistent with persistent thymic function in chronically infected individuals. Adapted from (193).

indeed reversible in individuals who respond to antiviral therapy.

Evidence continues to accrue indicating that the bone marrow is also abnormal in HIV-1–infected individuals. It has been clear since the earliest clinical descriptions of AIDS that all bone marrow–derived cell populations are abnormal in infected individuals (66). Abnormalities are apparent in their number, morphology, and function (67). Anemia, thrombocytopenia, and neutropenia are quite commonly seen as clinical manifestations of AIDS. Assays of bone marrow progenitors that assess their potential to generate mature, functional cells invariably show diminished activity in infected subjects. Since the major constituent cell populations that comprise the immune system are generated in the bone marrow, there is reason to presume that these cell populations are not produced normally in HIV-1–infected individuals. In fact, studies suggest that at least a small component CD4$^+$ T cell loss in AIDS may be attributable to decreased production of these cells, presumably in the bone marrow (57). The etiology of this bone marrow dysfunction remains poorly understood. However, studies have shown that viral infection of bone marrow macrophage populations may contribute to an abnormal microenvironment that is responsible for at least some of this dysfunction (68).

HIV-1 infection also leads to profound cytokine dysregulation. Endogenous cytokines, including TNF alpha, GM-CSF, IL-6, and IFN gamma, have been shown to increase HIV-1 replication in various cell populations *in vitro* (69–71). The mechanisms by which this cytokine-induced up-regulation of viral replication occurs can differ and sometimes be complementary. For example, TNF alpha is a transcriptional activator of HIV-1 via NF kappa B, while IL-6 induces HIV-1 replication by a posttranscriptional mechanism. It is assumed that immune cells in the infected individual produce increased quantities of many of these cytokines, which, in turn, increase viral replication *in vivo*. It has, however, also been shown that other immunologically active cytokines, such as IFN alpha and IFN beta, can suppress HIV-1 replication *in vitro*. Therefore, the sum effect of cytokine dysregulation on HIV-1 replication *in vivo* is difficult to gauge.

Although B lymphocytes have never been shown to harbor replicating HIV-1 *in vivo* in infected individuals, B lymphocyte abnormalities have been described in individuals infected with HIV-1. An increase in circulating B lymphocytes has been described during primary HIV-1 infection as well as during primary infection of macaques with SIV (72). Cytokine production by B lymphocytes in infected individuals has also been shown to be abnormal, with increased levels of TNF alpha and IL-6 spontaneously produced by these cells (73,74). In fact, it has been suggested that these B lymphocyte-produced cytokines may actually upregulate HIV-1 replication in CD4$^+$ T lymphocytes and macrophages. It is likely that the B lymphocyte activation that occurs in HIV-1–infected individuals contributes to the striking incidence of AIDS-related B cell malignancies (75).

Finally, HIV-1 infects CD4-expressing antigen presenting cell populations, including monocytes, macrophages, and DCs. Very few circulating cells of these lineages are actually infected by the virus, and this infection does not appear to mediate the obligatory death of these cells. Rather, these infected cells are felt to represent an important reservoir of virus that will probably prove difficult to eradicate by antiviral therapies. Relevant to this postulated role as a reservoir, the infected DC has been shown to mediate an extremely efficient transfer of virus to normal T lymphocyte populations, at least under *in vitro* culture conditions (76). In fact, the DC-specific C-type lectin DC-SIGN has been shown to bind HIV-1 envelope, perhaps promoting capture of virus by DCs and facilitating infection of CD4$^+$ T lymphocytes (77). While very few infected monocyte/macrophages have been documented in the circulation, large numbers of resident macrophages have been shown to be infected in various organs, including the lungs and the brain.

In light of the infectability of cells of the monocyte/macrophage lineage, it is not surprising that these cells do not function normally in infected individuals. The abnormalities of these cells include problems with oxidative burst response, C3 receptor–mediated clearance, Fc receptor function, and chemotaxis (78). These cells in HIV-1–infected individuals also have been shown to have a decreased ability to mediate antibody-dependent cell-mediated cytotoxicity and microbicidal activity (79). Infection of resident brain macrophages probably initiates a cascade of cytokine abnormalities that change the milieu of the CNS, leading to neuronal damage and AIDS dementia (80).

IMMUNE CONTROL OF HIV-1

While the containment of HIV-1 spread is incomplete in the infected individual, the substantial damping of viral replication that occurs during primary infection in humans suggests that immune mechanisms are contributing to viral control. Considerable work has been done to define the contribution of innate, humoral, and cellular immune responses to this partial control of HIV-1 replication. These studies are reviewed later in this chapter.

Although there is circumstantial evidence to suggest that innate immune mechanisms contribute to early HIV-1 containment in infected individuals, it has proven difficult to demonstrate this unequivocally. An NK cell contribution to viral clearance is suggested by the genetic correlative data showing that the expression of the HLA Bw4-80I allele in association with the activating KIR allele KIR3DS1 is associated with slow clinical progression following HIV-1 infection (41). NK cells have been shown *in vitro* to mediate killing of HIV-1–infected cells (81). However, NK cell–mediated control of the virus has never been directly demonstrated. Studies in the SIV/macaque model in which cobra venom toxin was administered to monkeys prior to infection to eliminate the activity of specific limbs of the complement cascade failed to demonstrate a definitive role for complement in early viral control (82). Some have suggested that the resistance to HIV-1 infection in cohorts of exposed, uninfected individuals could be most readily explained by innate immune mechanisms. Yet, no such innate immune-mediated protection has been demonstrated to date.

ANTIBODY RESPONSE TO HIV-1

Since the immune control of many viruses depends on antibody-mediated virus neutralization, considerable effort has been invested in characterizing the mechanisms by which HIV-1 may be neutralized by antibody. Virus is neutralized when antibody binds to virions and blocks the ability of those virions to enter their target cells. HIV-1 engages both the CD4 molecule and the virus coreceptor, either CCR5 or CXCR4, on the cell surface. This engagement triggers HIV-1 fusion with its target cell mediated by a trimeric envelope complex that includes three molecules of gp160. A neutralizing antibody must therefore block the series of events that begins with HIV-1–coreceptor binding and ends with HIV-1 fusion.

Current models suggest that neutralizing antibodies block HIV-1 infection by binding to the mature trimer on the virion surface and blocking the events associated with initial receptor engagement or by binding after virion-target cell attachment and inhibiting the fusion process (83). Blocking of virion–cell engagement presumably occurs when a threshold number of envelope glycoprotein spikes are occupied by antibody. If the antibody blocks the fusion process that occurs after virion–cell engagement, the antibody presumably binds to domains of the virus that are exposed as a result of this process of engagement.

Progress in the elucidation of antibody-mediated neutralization of HIV-1 has been slowed by a lack of comparability of neutralization data generated in different laboratories. Until recently, HIV-1 neutralization assays were performed in different laboratories using different target cells, different techniques for detecting virus replication, and different types of indicator viruses. This has made it impossible to compare experimental results from different laboratories. However, recent technological advances have provided an approach that will finally allow standardization of these assays (84). Engineered cell lines can be generated that express high levels of the receptors for HIV-1, and neutralization can be assessed using these cells as targets. Moreover, pseudotyped viruses can be generated *in vitro* by cotransfecting cells with both an *env*-deficient HIV-1 and any selected *env* gene. The pseudovirions created by these cotransfections can initiate a single round infection that can be assessed by monitoring expression of a reporter gene carried either by the virus or the engineered cell line. By assessing an antibody's ability to block the single round infection of a panel of pseudovirions expressing different Envs, the potency and breadth of that antibody's neutralizing ability can be ascertained.

It was assumed at the outset of the AIDS epidemic that a neutralizing antibody response to HIV-1 would play a crucial role in containing the replication of this virus. However, a number of observations have raised doubts about that assumption. It has been clear for some time that the HIV-1 neutralizing antibody response in patient sera against primary patient isolates of HIV-1 is quite weak (85,86). Moreover, the burst of HIV-1 replication that occurs during the period of primary infection is contained well before the emergence of a neutralizing antibody response in infected individuals (87–89). Monkeys depleted of B lymphocytes by infusion of an anti-CD20 antibody and then infected with SIV show normal early virus clearance. Interestingly, recent evidence does suggest that immune pressure mediated by antibodies results in the selection of HIV-1 mutants that are not susceptible to antibody neutralization (90,91). Although this process of autologous neutralization escape by virus occurs, it does not appear to be associated with clinical deterioration in the infected individual. Hence, treatment of chronically infected humans with monoclonal antibodies that have *in vitro* HIV-1 neutralizing activity has very little impact on viral replication *in vivo*. These observations suggest that the antibody response may not be of central importance in controlling HIV-1 replication in the setting of infection.

In fact, a number of unique characteristics of HIV-1 appear to protect the virus from antibody-mediated neutralization (92). The envelope of HIV-1 is heavily glycosylated, and these sugars can shield the underlying viral protein structures from access by antibodies. Neutralization-sensitive domains of the envelope appear to be hidden from antibodies due to steric hindrance caused by this glycosylation, steric hindrance caused by adjacent protein domains, or the fact that these domains are only exposed upon ligand binding. While the loops of the virus envelope appear to be particularly good targets for neutralizing antibodies, the high rate of mutation within these regions and their resulting extreme sequence variability preclude the possibility of a single antibody specificity that will neutralize a diversity of HIV-1 isolates.

In spite of the aforementioned limitations in forming an effective neutralizing antibody response to HIV-1, there is a limited amount of data suggesting that antibodies play a role in HIV-1 containment. Considerable attention has been focused on characterizing neutralizing HIV-1–specific antibody responses since these may be of central importance in the creation of an HIV-1 vaccine. Much of

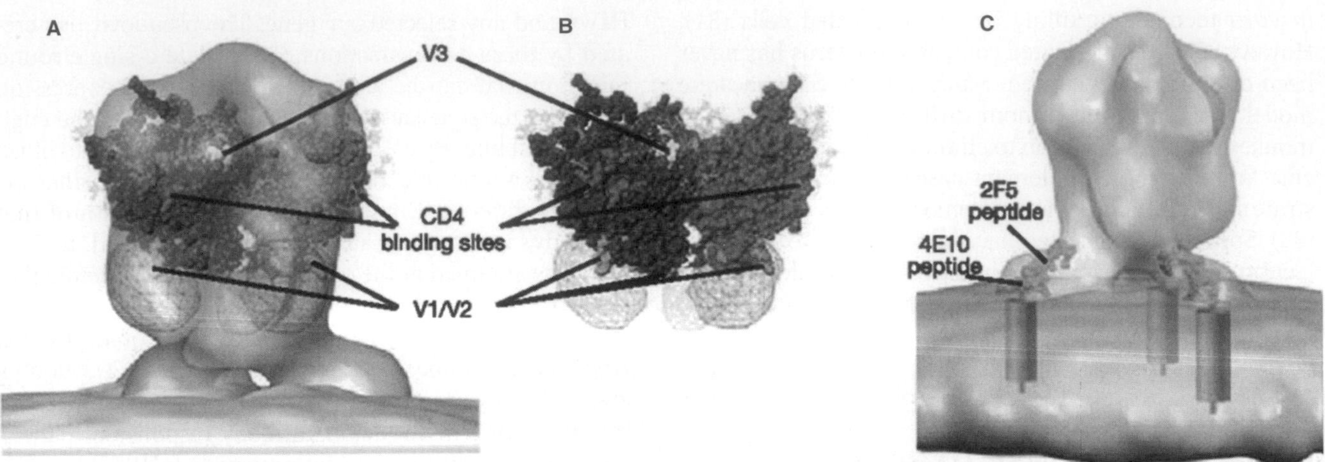

FIGURE 39.8 Tomographic reconstruction of an HIV-1 envelope glycoprotein trimer. A side view **(A, C)** and top view **(B)** of an envelope spike are shown. Structure modeling indicates the positions of the V1/V2 loops, the CD4 binding sites, and the V3 loop. The membrane proximal envelope region is shown **(C)** with the positions of two highly conserved neutralizing epitopes (the 4E10 and 2F5 epitopes). Adapted from (194).

the work in this area has been driven by a limited number of characterized monoclonal antibodies that are able to neutralize a diversity of HIV-1 isolates. Antibodies against three different neutralizing determinants of HIV-1 envelope have been studied in some depth: the third hypervariable loop of the envelope glycoproteins, the CD4-binding site of envelope, and the transmembrane envelope gp41 protein (Figure 39.8).

The third hypervariable domains of the HIV-1 envelope glycoproteins create a loop structure as a result of the formation of disulfide bonds (93). This so-called *V3 loop* has been implicated in the interactions of HIV-1 envelope glycoproteins with chemokine receptors (94). It is, therefore, reasonable that an antibody binding to this loop may interfere with the ability of the virus to bind to and enter a cell. In fact, the earliest antibodies that arise after an infection capable of neutralizing HIV-1 appear to recognize this V3 loop sequence (95,96). Considerable experimental work was done early in the AIDS epidemic in an attempt to develop the V3 loop as an immunogen for eliciting protective immune responses against HIV-1. However, a number of observations dampened enthusiasm for this approach. Extreme sequence variability exists among diverse HIV-1 isolates (97). Therefore, V3 loop–specific antibodies for the most part mediate type-specific neutralization. Moreover, it has become clear that in primary HIV-1 isolates, the V3 loop on the intact virion is not exposed to neutralizing antibodies (98). Thus, while antibodies do arise to the V3 loop, the antibodies are ultimately unable to access it and neutralize virions. At the time, these observations convinced investigators interested in vaccine development to shift their attention to the evaluation of more highly conserved sequences of the virus that might serve as targets for neutralization.

However, recently generated data has renewed interest in the V3 loop as a target for neutralizing antibodies. A limited number of monoclonal anti-V3 loop antibodies have been described that bind and neutralize a diversity of primary HIV-1 isolates (99). One such antibody, 447–52D, recognizes the GPGR motif at the tip of the V3 loop and neutralizes 47% of clade B HIV-1 isolates. Another antibody, 58.2, recognizes an epitope overlapping the tip of the loop and neutralizes a third of clade B isolates. Further, a homology between the V3 loop and the 40s loop of the CC chemokines has been described, suggesting that the V3 loop structure may have evolved to mimic a chemokine when the virus interacts with the cell-surface chemokine receptors CCR5 or CXCR4 (100). These findings have motivated continuing work to determine the ramifications of antibody–V3 loop interactions.

The CD4 binding sites of envelope represent another potential neutralizing determinant of HIV-1. Because the CD4 molecule is nonpolymorphic, the domains of HIV-1 that bind to CD4 must be relatively conserved among diverse isolates to maintain the viability of the virus. In fact, selected monoclonal antibodies specific for the CD4 binding domains of gp120 can be broadly neutralizing, recognizing and blocking a diversity of HIV-1 isolates from infecting cell populations *in vitro* (101,102). The best studied of these CD4 binding domain-specific neutralizing monoclonal antibodies is b12, an antibody that has been shown to occlude the CD4 binding site on gp120. The crystal structure of this monoclonal antibody has demonstrated a unique, long protruding CDR3 loop that may facilitate its ability to gain access to the deeply recessed CD4 binding pocket of the virus envelope (103). Importantly, however, the CD4 binding site–specific antibodies that have been assessed *in vivo* for their ability to protect chimpanzees from

HIV-1 challenge have not been protective. This observation has led to the suggestion that the CD4 binding site–specific antibodies, as a group, may not ultimately prove to be particularly potent as neutralizing antibodies.

The extraordinary degree of sequence conservation in the transmembrane gp41 protein of the envelope between various HIV-1 isolates makes it an attractive target for eliciting broadly neutralizing antibodies through vaccination. In fact, monoclonal antibodies have been developed that bind to the gp41 of a diversity of HIV-1 isolates and neutralize the virus *in vitro* (104). The most intensively studied of these monoclonal antibodies, 2F5 and 4E10, recognize distinct domains of the membrane proximal region of the ectodomain of gp41. Since these antibodies do not block receptor attachment, they are thought to inhibit the fusion process. While 2F5 binding is readily demonstrated to a linear peptide derived from this region of gp41, vaccination with this linear peptide cannot induce a neutralizing 2F5-like antibody. 4E10 has been shown to recognize an ordered helical peptide structure of gp41. No success has yet been achieved in attempts to elicit 2F5- or 4E10-like antibodies through subunit vaccination.

Several domains of HIV-1 only become exposed after CD4 binding of the envelope trimer. Coreceptor binding by gp120 triggers a change in the conformation of gp41 that exposes its hydrophobic fusion domain, facilitating the insertion of the N-terminal peptide of gp41 into the cytoplasmic membrane of the target cell. A peptide mimetic of a domain of gp41 has been shown to intercalate into the fusion apparatus and block the conformational changes required for viral fusion. This finding argues that it may be possible to generate antibodies that can similarly interfere with gp41-mediated fusion events. In fact, the well-defined series of molecular events leading to HIV-1 entry suggest that highly conserved amino acid sequences of both the C and N terminal regions of gp41 may prove useful targets for vaccine-induced neutralizing antibody responses (105,106).

Recent studies have shown convincing evidence that the envelope glycoproteins of HIV-1 undergo a continuous process of mutation that allow the virus to escape from neutralization by antibody (90,91). Pseudovirions created with envelopes of the HIV-1 isolated from chronically infected individuals cannot be neutralized by the antibody in the serum of those individuals at the time the envelopes were obtained. Since a selection process must be driving this viral evolution, this observation makes a strong argument for transient viral control by neutralizing antibodies in the setting of chronic infection.

Evidence in mouse models and in man suggests that neutralizing antibodies in individuals with established HIV-1 infections have little effect on ongoing viral replication. Immunodeficient mice reconstituted with human lymphoid tissue have been infected with HIV-1 and then infused with neutralizing anti–HIV-1 antibodies. These antibody treatments have little effect on HIV-1 replication (107). Intravenous administration of hyperimmune globulin with high titers of anti–HIV-1 antibodies in HIV-1–infected humans, similarly, has little effect on viral load or disease progression.

Thus, while antibodies may contribute to shaping the course of early viral infection, they ultimately do not appear to play a role in controlling viremia. Neutralizing monoclonal antibodies have been defined, yet they are difficult to elicit, and their antiviral activity can be readily circumvented as HIV-1 mutates to evade their binding. Importantly, however, preexisting circulating antibodies specific for HIV-1 envelope will likely be able to alter the clinical consequences of *de novo* HIV-1 infections. This is most convincingly demonstrated in nonhuman primate studies. The infusion of IgG derived from serum of an SIV-infected monkey into a naïve rhesus monkey caused a damping of viral replication and an attenuation of the pathogenicity of subsequent SIV infection (108). Moreover, the infusion of HIV-1–neutralizing monoclonal antibodies in macaques prior to their exposure to a highly pathogenic SHIV dramatically altered the consequences of both intravenous and mucosally initiated infections (109,110). In monkeys in which very high serum concentrations of neutralizing monoclonal antibodies are achieved, SHIV infections can be blocked or the pathogenic consequences of the infections can be significantly attenuated. These observations suggest that neutralizing antibodies specific for HIV-1 may have utility in the setting of vaccination to prevent HIV-1 infection.

CD8$^+$ T LYMPHOCYTE RESPONSE TO HIV-1

While little data have been generated to suggest that anti–HIV-1 antibodies play a role in containing replication of the virus in infected individuals, a number of studies have implicated HIV-1–specific CD8$^+$ CTL in controlling HIV-1 replication. This evidence comes from both *in vitro* and *in vivo* studies. HIV-1–specific CTLs have been found in large numbers in a variety of anatomic compartments in both HIV-1–infected humans and SIV-infected macaques: in peripheral blood lymphocytes, bronchoalveolar lavage lymphocytes, lymph nodes, spleen, skin, cerebrospinal fluid, and vaginal mucosal tissue (111). CD8$^+$ T lymphocytes have been shown to inhibit HIV-1 replication *in vitro* (112,113). A number of mechanisms have been implicated for this inhibition. Direct CTL lysis of HIV-1–infected cells *in vitro* can block the propagation of an *in vitro* infection. Soluble factors produced by CD8$^+$ T lymphocytes are also able to mediate this inhibition of virus replication. The beta chemokines MIP-1α, MIP-1β, and RANTES have been shown to inhibit HIV-1 replication *in vitro* (114). Other soluble factors most likely also play a role in this CD8$^+$ T lymphocyte–mediated inhibition of HIV-1 spread.

Further evidence demonstrates that clearance of the intense viral replication occurring during early days following infection correlates with the emergence of the HIV-1–specific CD8+ CTL response (115). A correlation also has been described between this early viral clearance and the appearance of an *in vivo* expansion of a clonal or oligoclonal population of CD8+ T lymphocytes as measured by their use of the same TCR V beta or V alpha gene family. Oligoclonal populations of T lymphocytes expressing TCR genes of the same family have been shown to emerge coincident with HIV-1 clearance during primary infection (116), suggesting that an HIV-specific CD8+ T lymphocyte population may be responsible for viral clearance. Temporal correlations between the emergence of oligoclonal populations of CD8+ CTL and viral clearance are particularly well delineated in the SIV/macaque model of AIDS. Using chromium release-type assays, Vß repertoire analyses, and tetramer assays, a tight correlation has been demonstrated between early viral clearance and the emergence of SIV-specific CTL responses (117–119) (Figure 39.9). The clinical status of HIV-1–infected individuals has also been shown to correlate with the strength of their virus-specific CTL responses. In chronically infected individuals, the HIV-1–specific CTL response, as measured with both precursor frequency CTL assays and tetramer binding assays, has been shown to be associated with clinical status and clinical prognosis (120,121).

Perhaps the most compelling evidence for the importance of CD8+ T cells in containing HIV-1 replication comes from studies in SIV-infected rhesus monkeys. In these studies, *in vivo* depletion of CD8+ cells in the monkeys, achieved by infusion of monoclonal anti-CD8 antibody, had profound effects on the replication of SIV (122) (Figure 39.10). When CD8 depletion lasted fewer than 21 days, the clearance of virus during primary infection was delayed by a full week as compared to control antibody treated monkeys. When the duration of depletion was greater than 28 days, primary viremia was never cleared following infection. The infected monkeys depleted of CD8+ T lymphocytes for more than 28 days during the period of primary infection died with a rapidly progressive AIDS-like syndrome. Moreover, the transient CD8+ T lymphocyte depletion of chronically SIV-infected rhesus monkeys was associated with a substantial rise in viral replication that returned to baseline levels with the reemergence of the CD8+ T cell population. These observations illustrate the central role played by CD8+ T lymphocytes in the control of HIV-1 replication.

CTL responses to HIV-1, like responses to many other pathogens, are specific for only a limited number of dominant epitopes. This extreme focusing of the immune response places extreme selection pressure on HIV-1 to mutate at these few dominant epitopes. Because of the high mutation rate of HIV-1, it was reasonable to postulate that HIV-1 would be particularly adept at this mechanism of immune evasion. In fact, studies in HIV-1–infected humans as well as SIV- and SHIV-infected rhesus monkeys have shown that viral mutational escape from CTL pressure does occur (123). This viral mutational escape was dramatically illustrated when a clonal population of Nef-specific CTL was infused into a chronically HIV-1–infected patient to evaluate the utility of adoptive immunotherapy

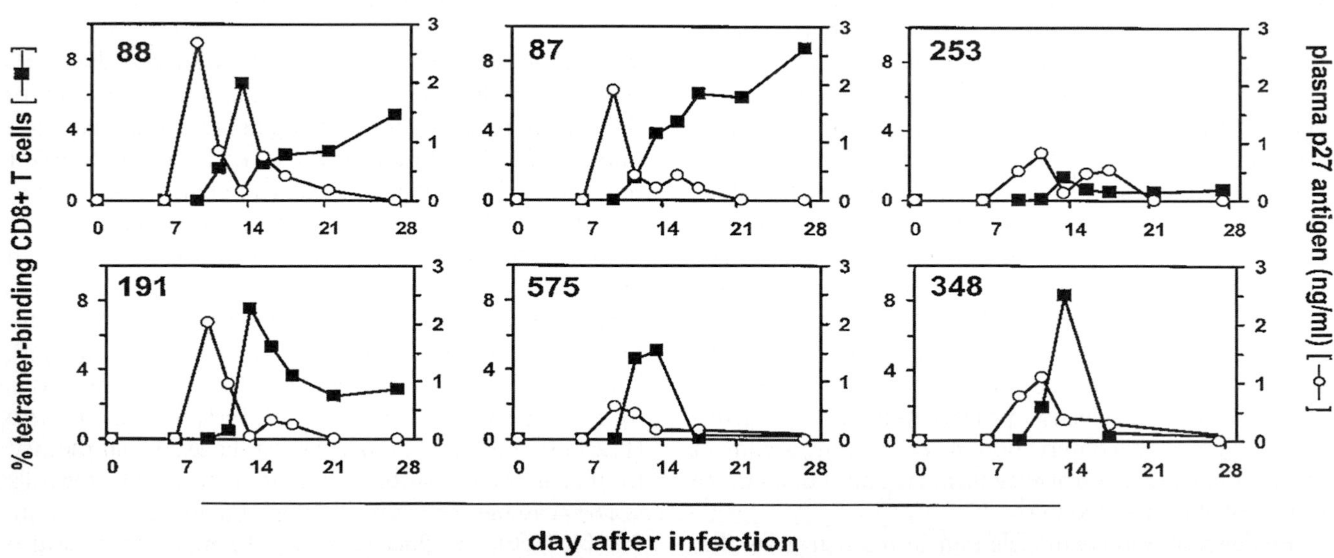

FIGURE 39.9 Temporal coincidence of early primate immunodeficiency virus control and the emergence of a virus-specific CD8+ T lymphocyte response. SIV replication, as measured by plasma viral antigen level, is partially controlled as the SIV-specific CD8+ T lymphocyte response emerges during the period of primary infection in six previously naïve rhesus monkeys. Adapted from (118).

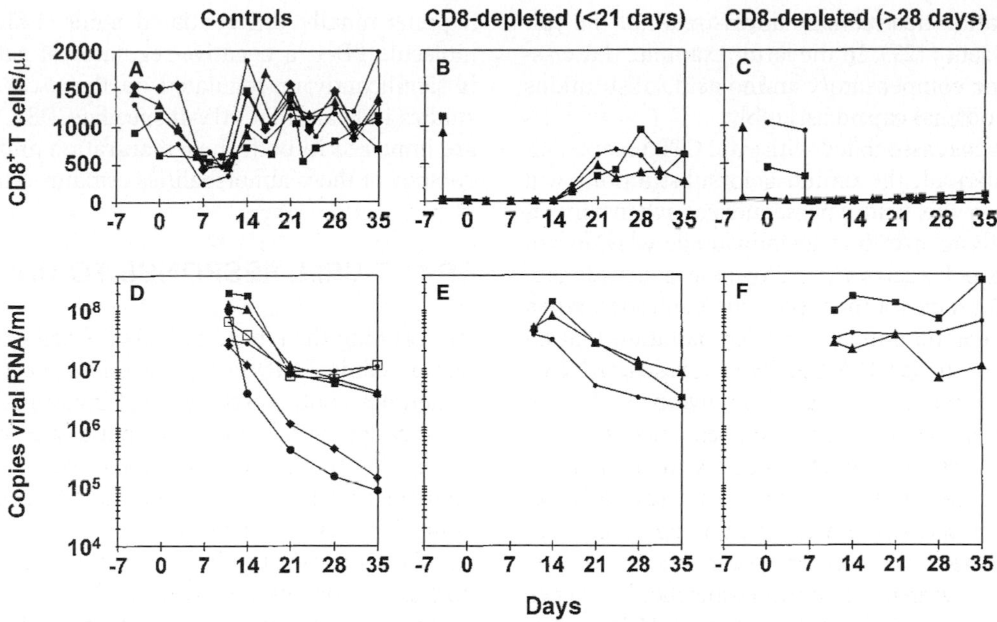

FIGURE 39.10 $CD8^+$ lymphocyte depletion is associated with loss of immune control of primate immunodeficiency virus replication in rhesus monkeys. Rhesus monkey $CD8^+$ lymphocytes were eliminated by monoclonal anti-CD8 antibody infusion for less than 21 days (B) or longer than 28 days (C). SIV containment to setpoint levels was delayed from 1 week in monkeys depleted of $CD8^+$ lymphocytes for less than 21 days (E), and SIV replication was never contained in monkeys depleted of $CD8^+$ lymphocytes for greater than 28 days (F). Adapted from (122).

for AIDS (124). An amino acid substitution in the patient's HIV-1 quasispecies in the epitope recognized by the Nef-specific CTL clone rapidly appeared, allowing the virus to escape from CTL recognition. As the phenomenon of viral escape from CTL pressure has been studied in greater depth, it has become clear that the virus quasispecies is shaped, on one hand, by viral avoidance of cellular immune pressure, and, on the other hand, by viral maintenance of optimal replication competency. This pressure to mutate away from CTL recognition underscores the importance of CTL in the control of HIV-1 infection.

The virus can employ a variety of mutational strategies to escape from CTL pressure (124). Most commonly, amino acid substitutions are selected for in the CTL epitopes of the virus that interfere with the binding of those CTL epitope peptides to MHC class I molecules. However, it has also been shown that extra-epitopic amino acid substitutions can be generated that interfere with the intracellular processing of the viral proteins, blocking the ability of epitope peptides to enter the MHC class I processing pathway. It has also been suggested that epitope mutations can occur that result in loss of TCR recognition of the epitope peptide/MHC class I complex without interfering with epitope peptide binding to MHC class I.

While a change in amino acid sequence may allow for viral escape from CTL, it is often associated with a conformational change in the protein containing the dominant epitope. CTL escape mutations that occur soon after infection are often those that do not exact a fitness cost on the virus. Some mutations in HIV-1, SIV, and SHIV have been reported to emerge in the viral quasispecies within a few weeks of infection, and viruses with these mutations can rapidly predominate in a population of replicating viruses (125). Such mutations appear to occur in regions of viral proteins that can tolerate the structural changes that are associated with those particular amino acid substitutions without impacting the function of those proteins. When these variant viruses are transmitted to MHC class I disparate individuals, individuals in whom there should be no CTL pressure on that particular region of the virus, the virus may not revert to its wild-type sequence, demonstrating that there is little fitness cost associated with the change.

Other mutations that facilitate viral escape from CTL recognition occur only after the virus has been replicating in an individual for a prolonged period of time. There is evidence that some of these epitope mutations can exact such a profound fitness cost on the virus that they are only tolerated if additional amino acid substitutions are incorporated into the virus as well. Thus, an HLA-B27–restricted CTL epitope mutation in HIV-1 has been described in which a position 2 epitope substitution that eliminates the anchor residue of the epitope can only be tolerated by the virus if an associated residue 6 epitope mutation is also present (126). Moreover, a dominant Gag epitope mutation is only tolerated by SIV/SHIV if a particular mutation upstream or downstream of the epitope is also present (127). In the latter example, these associated flanking compensatory amino acid substitutions are needed for normal capsid assembly.

If the fitness cost associated with viral CTL escape mutations is substantial, the amino acid substitutions will usually revert to the wild-type sequences when viruses are subsequently transmitted to individuals who do not carry MHC class I alleles that allow the generation of CTL responses specific for those particular epitopes. When an HIV-1 isolate containing an epitope mutation that allowed for escape from HLA-B57/58*01$^+$ restricted CTL was transmitted to HLA-B57/58*01$^-$ individuals, the epitope mutation reverted to the wild-type sequence (128). Interestingly, a study in SIV-infected monkeys demonstrated that episodic reversion to wild-type virus regularly occurred in monkeys in which viral mutational escape had previously occurred, but this reversion was rapidly reversed by the reemergence of epitope-specific CTL (129). This finding suggests that the maintenance of a CTL escape variant is a dynamic process in which there can be continuous change in the virus, reflecting the conflicting pressures of immune pressure and replication fitness. Moreover, the phenomenon of transmission-associated viral sequence reversion likely contributes to the relatively consistent pathogenicity of HIV-1 over extended periods of time in human populations.

The importance of CTL in containing viral replication in HIV-1–infected humans and SIV- and SHIV-infected monkeys is underscored by reports of dramatic clinical deterioration associated with single amino acid substitutions in dominant viral CTL epitopes that allow the infecting virus to escape from CTL recognition. The aforementioned chronically HIV-1–infected patient, who received infusions of a clonal population of Nef-specific CTL and developed a Nef escape viral variant that could not be recognized by CTL, demonstrated an abrupt rise in HIV-1 replication and a consequent loss of viral control associated with those CTL infusions (124). Similarly, a chronically SHIV-infected monkey that was successfully controlling viral replication to a very low level developed a CTL-escape virus and thereafter evidenced a rapid and profound clinical deterioration (130). These types of findings illustrate the role of CTL in controlling HIV-1 replication, the importance of CTL escape in AIDS immunopathogenesis, and finally the extent to which immune control of HIV-1 can depend on CTL recognition of a single dominant viral epitope.

Finally, studies have suggested that HIV-1–specific CD8$^+$ T lymphocytes do not function normally in infected individuals. When compared with cytomegalovirus-specific CD8$^+$ T lymphocytes, HIV-1–specific CD8$^+$ T lymphocytes in infected individuals express lower levels of perforin and higher levels of surface CD27 (131). There is also a skewing of these CD8$^+$ T lymphocytes toward a CD45RA$^-$CCR7$^-$ phenotype, consistent with a preterminally differentiated state (132). Further, the molecule PD-1, a negative regulator of activated T cells, is significantly up-regulated on these cells (133). These studies indicate that HIV-1–specific CD8$^+$ T lymphocytes are impaired in both their maturation and function. The etiology of these abnormalities remains unknown.

CD4$^+$ T CELL RESPONSE TO HIV-1

Determining the effects of helper T cell cytokine production on clinical AIDS progression has been an active and sometimes controversial area of investigation. A number of years ago, it was proposed that a bias of immune cells toward the production of specific networks of cytokines might either improve or impede immune control of HIV-1 (134). Work in murine models of the immune control of parasitic infections indicated that a bias toward production of TH1 cytokines interfered with parasite control, while a bias toward the production of TH2 cytokines improved containment of those pathogens. Since CD8$^+$ T lymphocytes have been shown to be of central importance in containing HIV-1 spread, and TH1 cytokines are known to support effector T lymphocyte responses *in vivo*, it was suggested that a bias toward production of TH1 cytokines may be beneficial for controlling HIV-1 replication. Moreover, it was proposed that a bias toward production of TH2 cytokines may interfere with immune containment of HIV-1 replication. Some even suggested that a vaccine-elicited immune response that was TH2 biased may accelerate disease progression in vaccinated individuals who subsequently become infected with HIV-1. While this hypothesis generated a substantial amount of investigative work, the general consensus of those working in the field has been that there is no evidence to support this paradigm of AIDS pathogenesis (135).

Since virus-specific CD4$^+$ T lymphocytes generated following infection with some viruses can have effector cytotoxic function, effort has gone into evaluating HIV-1–specific CD4$^+$ T lymphocytes for cytolytic capacity. However, no CD4$^+$ T lymphocyte-mediated killing activity has been observed. Therefore, the consensus in the field now is that CD4$^+$ T lymphocytes contribute to HIV-1 containment through providing help for the generation of virus-specific antibody and CD8$^+$ T lymphocyte responses.

Considerable attention has been focused on characterizing the functional capacity of CD4$^+$ T cells in HIV-1–infected individuals. T lymphocytes are functionally abnormal in those infected with the virus. In studies of peripheral blood lymphocytes of subjects with variable degrees of CD4$^+$ T lymphocyte loss, it was demonstrated that T lymphocyte responsiveness to soluble protein antigen is lost remarkably early after infection, earlier than responsiveness to alloantigen or mitogen (136). In fact, an inverse correlation exists in chronically infected individuals between virus load and HIV-1–specific $CD4^+$ T cell function as measured by viral protein driven proliferative responses (137). Moreover, early institution of highly active antiretroviral therapy during the period of primary infection can result in the preservation of considerable HIV-1–specific $CD4^+$ T cell function. These observations have led to the suggestion that the preservation of memory HIV-1–specific $CD4^+$ T cells as well as the cytokine production capacity of these cells may be crucial for the containment of HIV-1 in those individuals infected with the virus.

CHALLENGES IN THE CREATION OF AN HIV-1 VACCINE

Creation of an HIV-1 vaccine represents an unprecedented scientific challenge. The traditional approaches for creating effective antiviral vaccines have proven inadequate for making one against HIV-1. For example, vaccines based on live attenuated HIV-1 might mutate and regain their pathogenicity following inoculation into humans. Inactivated virus and protein-based vaccines have not generated antibodies that neutralize the genetically diverse viruses that are currently infecting human populations throughout the world. Moreover, these types of vaccines would not induce the cell-mediated immune responses that are needed to control the spread of HIV-1 in exposed individuals. A totally novel vaccine approach will therefore ultimately be required to stop the spread of this virus.

Despite the considerable efforts that have gone into developing an HIV-1 vaccine, few prototype immunogens have been evaluated for protective efficacy in human clinical trials. One of these vaccines, a recombinant form of the envelope glycoprotein gp120 administered with the adjuvant alum, was shown to confer protection against challenge by a highly attenuated HIV-1 isolate in chimpanzees (138). However, the vaccine had no protective efficacy in humans (139). In fact, most investigators involved in HIV-1 vaccine development were not surprised by the outcome of this trial. The vaccine elicited a gp120-specific antibody response, but the antibody did not neutralize HIV-1 isolates that were recently obtained from the blood of infected individuals (140–142). Moreover, because a vaccine antigen of this type does not enter the MHC class I pathway following administration, it cannot efficiently induce a CTL response. Since this subunit immunogen did not elicit neutralizing antibodies or CTL, there was little reason to suppose that it would confer protective immunity.

Another HIV-1 vaccine efficacy trial is currently underway to evaluate this same subunit immunogen in combination with a live recombinant viral vector using a prime-boost regimen. The vector being assessed in this clinical trial is a canary pox virus expressing HIV-1 genes. Although the canary pox virus has been shown to express genes *in vitro* in human cells, it does not replicate efficiently in these cells. It is hoped that this vector will express HIV-1 transgenes at a high enough level *in vivo* in humans to elicit a CTL response but will have no associated toxicity because it does not replicate. There is, however, also little optimism associated with this trial because of the low level of immunogenicity of the vector in humans observed in earlier clinical studies (143).

Although these advanced-phase human clinical trials for candidate vaccines have aroused little optimism, studies in nonhuman primates suggest that it should be possible to create an effective HIV-1 vaccine. Pretreatment of rhesus monkeys with SIV-specific immunoglobulin results in a reduction of viral replication following challenge with SIV (108). Infusion into rhesus monkeys of monoclonal antibodies that neutralize HIV-1 isolates *in vitro* has blocked the subsequent acquisition of primate immunodeficiency virus infection that is initiated by either intravenous or mucosal exposure to virus (109,110). Confidence that these findings might be translated into an effective antibody-based vaccine for HIV-1 is tempered by the observation that protection against infection in this experimental model has required levels of circulating antibody that are too high to be induced by routine vaccination strategies (144,145). Moreover, investigators remain unable to create a subunit immunogen that elicits broadly neutralizing antibodies. It is possible, however, that the rapid mobilization of a memory B cell population soon after exposure to HIV-1 might result in an early, robust antibody response that could eliminate or partially contain the replicating virus.

Studies in nonhuman primates have also shown that vaccine-elicited cellular immune responses, even in the absence of neutralizing antibodies, can confer significant protection against the clinical consequences of an immunodeficiency virus infection. Monkeys immunized with plasmid DNA, a live recombinant viral vector, or a combination of these vaccine modalities develop cellular immune responses that do not protect against the acquisition of infection, but do slow the rate of clinical disease progression that occurs following infection (146–148) (Figure 39.11). In comparison with control vaccinated animals, such vaccinated monkeys show a more rapid expansion of memory CTLs, a consequent reduction in peak and chronic levels of viral replication, a delay in the loss of $CD4^+$ T cells, and a delay in time to death.

Recent studies have begun to delineate the mechanisms underlying this prolonged survival of vaccinated, challenged monkeys. Because memory $CD4^+$ T cells express CCR5, the coreceptor for transmitted HIV-1 and SIV isolates, there is a rapid and dramatic loss of this lymphocyte subpopulation during the first days following infection as the virus targets these cells for destruction (25,58,149). By contributing to the control of early replication, vaccine-induced $CD8^+$ and $CD4^+$ T cell responses in rhesus monkeys provide some degree of protection against the

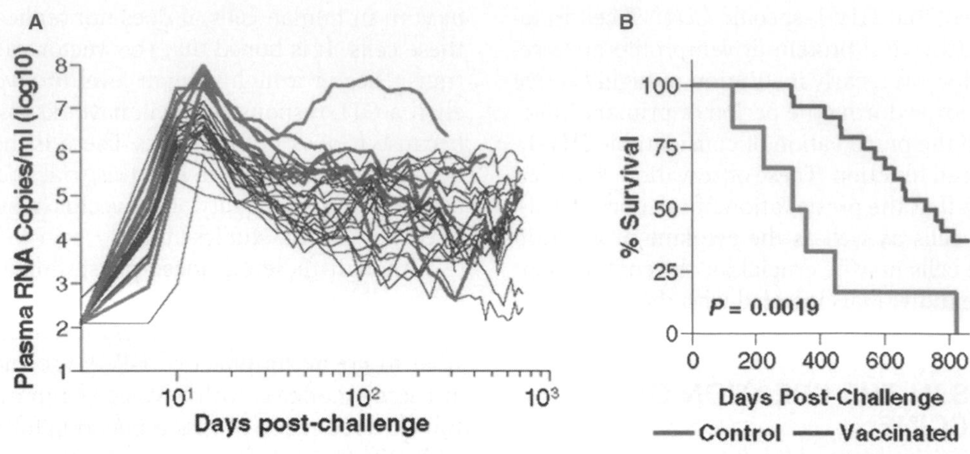

FIGURE 39.11 Vaccine-elicited cellular immunity confers partial protection against early primate immunodeficiency virus replication and an associated prolongation of survival in rhesus monkeys. Monkeys were vaccinated to induce a cell-mediated immune response and then infected with a highly pathogenic SIV. As shown in panel A, the vaccinated monkeys had lower levels of viral replication (blue lines) than did the control monkeys (red lines) through the first 120 days following infection. As shown in panel B, this blunting of viral replication in the vaccinated monkeys (blue line) was associated with a prolongation of survival. Adapted from (150).

destruction of these memory CD4$^+$ T cells (150,151). The protection of these cells confers a survival advantage, as the immune systems of the monkeys are better able to deal with potential opportunistic infections and malignancies.

Although the level of protection afforded by a CTL-based vaccine is certainly not ideal, the use of such a vaccine in human populations could have several important benefits. The prolonged survival of vaccinated individuals who subsequently become infected with HIV-1 would be an enormous advantage, particularly in resource-poor areas of the world where access to antiretroviral drugs remains limited. Further, if vaccinated individuals who become infected with HIV-1 maintain low levels of viral replication, the rapidity of viral spread from infected to uninfected people may slow (152). This is because low levels of HIV-1 replication in an individual should be associated with low levels of virus in their secretions, which in turn should be associated with the inefficient transmission of virus. In fact, levels of HIV-1 viremia in an infected individual have been shown to predict the likelihood of that individual transmitting virus (153). Therefore, a vaccine of this type could have benefits both for the individual and the population as a whole.

Nevertheless, accumulating evidence from nonhuman primate studies indicates that the duration of protection afforded by a CTL-based vaccine may ultimately be limited. Vaccine-related containment of primate immunodeficiency virus replication can be abruptly lost in monkeys following viral challenge, with a consequent dramatic clinical deterioration (130,154). In these monkeys, the change in clinical status was associated with viral acquisition of a mutation in a dominant CTL epitope that allowed the virus to escape from control by CTLs. The mutant viruses rapidly became the predominant viral quasispecies in the infected monkeys. These findings suggest that vaccine-elicited dominant-epitope–specific CTLs contain primate immunodeficiency virus replication, and that the immune pressure on the virus that is mediated by these CTLs selects for mutations that allow the virus to escape from recognition by this cellular immune response.

However, although it is reasonable to assume that virus will eventually escape from CTL control in this setting, protection may last for a relatively long period of time following infection. If viral replication is initially contained at a very low level, it may take a long time for escape variant viruses to be generated, as mutations will emerge in a population of viruses at a rate proportional to the rate of ongoing viral replication. Moreover, if CTLs are generated to multiple virus epitopes, escape of the virus at all of those epitopes may be required for the virus to evade T cell recognition and effective immune control. A CTL-based vaccine strategy may therefore be a viable approach to vaccine control of HIV-1 despite the phenomenon of viral escape from CTL recognition (155).

Bolstered by these rationales, two major CTL-based vaccines recently entered advanced-phase clinical testing: a recombinant adenovirus-based vaccine, and a plasmid DNA prime and recombinant adenovirus boost-based vaccine. However, the efficacy trials of the recombinant adenovirus-based vaccine as a sole immunogen were stopped early when an enterim analysis of the emerging results demonstrated on evidence of efficacy. Moreover, this analysis also raised the possibility that vaccinated men who were uncircumsized or vaccinees with serologic evidence of prior exposure to the vector may have had an increased rate of acquisition of HIV-1 infection. The impact of circumcision in this vaccine setting is consistent with the emerging evidence for the contribution of the foreskin in male acquisition of HIV-1. One theory that has been proposed to explain the impact of prior exposure to adenovirus is that exposure of adenovirus primed individuals to repeated administrations of an adenovirus vector may expand and activate adenovirus-specific $CD4^+$ T cells, increasing the number of activated $CD4^+CCR5^+$ T cells that can be infected by HIV-1. While these findings are discouraging, they do not indicate that an effective HIV-1 vaccine cannot be created. Rather, they suggest that other strategies are needed for generating protective immunity.

Although neutralizing antibodies do not play a pivotal role in early HIV-1 clearance, a vaccine-elicited neutralizing antibody response may confer substantial protection. For a vaccine to prevent infection by a diverse range of HIV-1 isolates, it must induce antibodies that neutralize genetically disparate HIV-1 isolates. However, the creation of a subunit immunogen that can elicit such an immune response has proven elusive. Some of the subunit envelope immunogens evaluated to date generate antibodies that block infection of HIV-1 isolates that have envelope proteins similar in sequence to those used in the vaccine. They also induce antibodies that have activity against a small subset of HIV-1 isolates that are particularly sensitive to neutralization. However, these vaccine-elicited antibodies do not neutralize most circulating HIV-1 strains (156–158). Nevertheless, it should be possible to configure an immunogen that will elicit a broadly neutralizing antibody response. This possibility is illustrated by the demonstration that monoclonal antibodies can be generated that neutralize diverse HIV-1 isolates (159,160).

Several strategies are currently being explored to create an effective subunit envelope immunogen. One of these approaches involves generating novel envelope-specific monoclonal antibodies that can neutralize a diverse range of HIV-1 isolates (161). By mapping the recognition specificities of these antibodies, domains of the virus will be identified that can serve as targets for broadly neutralizing antibodies. The underlying assumption in this strategy is that if a monoclonal antibody can be generated that neutralizes the virus, an immunogen can be configured to elicit an antibody with the same specificity and activity. However, it was recently reported that at least some of the monoclonal antibodies with broad neutralizing activity have polyspecific reactivity with autoantigens, and the production of these antibodies may be regulated by tolerance mechanisms (162). In fact, two of the most broadly reactive HIV-1 envelope-specific monoclonal antibodies are polyspecific autoantibodies that are reactive with the host phospholipid cardiolipin. It should be noted, however, that some investigators feel that this apparent cross-reactivity may reflect the hydrophobicity of the combining sites of these antibodies (163). This observation raises questions concerning the feasibility of generating antibodies in healthy individuals with these envelope specificities.

Another approach being explored to solve the difficult problem of inducing broadly neutralizing HIV-1–specific antibodies is to develop a more in-depth understanding of the structure of the HIV-1 envelope. It is hoped that this will suggest approaches for creating immunogens that approximate the native envelope glycoprotein in its biologically relevant three-dimensional conformations. Progress in this area has been slow because of the technical difficulties associated with determining the structure of the flexible, heavily glycosylated envelope protein. To date, structures of monomeric HIV-1 gp120 bound to CD4 and unbound monomeric SIV gp120 have been determined (164,165). However, the envelope glycoprotein of HIV-1 is comprised of two components, gp120 and the transmembrane part gp41. Moreover, it exists on the virus as a trimeric molecule and undergoes conformational changes as the virus fuses to the outer membrane of a cell during the process of infection. The structures of biologically relevant HIV-1 envelopes remain to be elucidated.

Although considerable effort is being expended to define conserved neutralizing epitopes of the HIV-1 envelope and to determine the structure of the prefusion envelope trimer, novel envelope immunogens continue to be created and evaluated as potential vaccine immunogens. These include baculovirus-expressed particles that express the envelope glycoprotein on their surface, chemically stabilized envelope trimers, and domains of the membrane-proximal region of the envelope expressed in membrane fragments.

Since much of the HIV-1 epidemic is fueled by sexual transmission of the virus, most investigators assume that an effective vaccine must elicit a mucosal immune response that will block the transmission of the virus at a mucosal surface. It is important to recognize that there are caveats associated with this assumption. First, it is still not proven that HIV-1 crosses an intact mucosal surface to initiate an infection. Epidemiological studies have clearly shown that the likelihood of HIV-1 acquisition is increased in individuals with genital ulcers, suggesting that sexual transmission of the virus may occur by hematogenous seeding (166–168). Moreover, it remains possible that many HIV-1 transmission events occur through microvascular tears in mucosal tissue rather across intact mucosa. It is, therefore, not proven beyond a doubt that sexual transmission of HIV-1 occurs across an intact mucosal surface.

Second, it is well-established that vaccine-induced systemic immune responses can confer effective protection against mucosally transmitted viruses. A clear example of this phenomenon is seen with the protection provided by the Salk polio vaccine (169). This inactivated-virus vaccine induces a systemic antibody response that does not block the transmission of the virus. Rather, it diminishes poliovirus replication systemically after mucosal transmission has occurred, blocking seeding of the CNS with the virus. This highly effective vaccine, therefore, aborts the natural course of a mucosally transmitted poliovirus infection without acting at the site of transmission.

Accepting these possible caveats, considerable effort is being focused on inducing both cellular and antibody responses that might contribute to containing the virus at a mucosal surface. At least some parenterally administered live recombinant vectors have been shown to elicit cellular immune responses at mucosal surfaces in nonhuman primates (170). Studies are being pursued to determine whether mucosal delivery of vectors, such as the gene-deleted adenoviruses, can actually enhance the mucosal cellular and humoral immune responses elicited by those vaccines. Novel live vector systems are also being explored that are specifically designed to induce mucosal immunity. Foremost among these strategies is the use of live recombinant Mycobacteria spp. and enteric bacteria such as Salmonella spp. These are nonpathogenic recombinant microorganisms that can be administered at a mucosal surface and should specifically elicit local cellular and humoral immune responses. Whether strategies specifically designed to generate potent mucosal immune responses can confer protection against sexually transmitted HIV-1 remains an open question.

Mutations rapidly accumulate in HIV-1 as it replicates, such that circulating strains of the virus can differ from one another by 20% in the more conserved proteins and by as much as 35% in the highly variable envelope proteins (171,172). Moreover, primary HIV-1 isolates have no principal neutralizing determinants, and each of these isolates can have a distinct target for the neutralizing antibody response. The implications of the sequence diversity of HIV-1 are also problematic for virus-specific $CD8^+$ T cell responses. Certainly there can be some antigenic cross-reactivity between isolates of HIV-1 in the cellular immune response, but single amino-acid substitutions can sometimes abrogate $CD8^+$ T cell recognition of a dominant epitope of the virus (173–175). HIV-1 vaccines that are based on a single sequence of the virus may therefore elicit immune responses that are too focused and type-specific to provide effective protection against the quasispecies of genetically diverse HIV-1 isolates that exist in a human population. A vaccine strategy for HIV-1 must therefore take into account the extreme sequence diversity of this virus.

One vaccine strategy being developed to deal with HIV-1 genetic variation involves the use of immunogens that incorporate a combination of variant genes or proteins from representative viruses. The rationale behind this approach is that immune responses to a particular portion of the virus may diversify following exposure to many related variant proteins, leading to the generation of memory T and B cells that can recognize sequences related to but distinct from those used to elicit the memory cell populations. In fact, a vaccine that includes three distinct envelope genes, encoding proteins from representative clade A, B, and C viruses, is moving forward into advanced-phase human clinical testing (176). Preliminary immunological evaluation of immune responses induced by this vaccination regimen suggests that the cellular and humoral immune responses to these distinct envelope proteins do not interfere with one another (177). However, although these vaccine-elicited immune responses have greater breadth than those elicited by envelope immunogens that employ a single gene sequence, the breadth of these responses has not proven to be greater than would be expected based on the additive properties of the immunogens.

Other approaches to dealing with the immunological problems created by the genetic diversity of HIV-1 isolates are also being evaluated. Several of these approaches make use of hypothetical viral gene sequences that are generated by phylogenetic reconstruction. These reconstructions are based on the data that have been accumulated to document the diversity of HIV-1 gene sequences that exist worldwide. Consensus sequences for each HIV-1 gene have been designed that encode the most common amino acid at each position of each viral protein. Ancestral sequences have also been constructed to approximate progenitor viral gene sequences (178). In both of these approaches, the sequences of these hypothetical genes are closer to the sequences of currently circulating viruses than most currently circulating viruses are to each other. Importantly, envelope proteins that have been constructed based on these types of hypothetical sequence have proven functional in several *in vitro* assay systems (172). These envelopes have been shown to bind to both CD4 and chemokine receptors and to bind several of the monoclonal antibodies that recognize conserved neutralizing determinants of HIV-1. It remains to be determined whether vaccines that are based on these hypothetical genes elicit immune responses with greater breadth than vaccines that incorporate single, naturally occurring viral genes.

Should it prove possible to create immunogens that induce both broadly neutralizing antibodies and broadly reactive CTLs, the magnitude, durability, and quality of the immune responses that can be generated with currently available technologies may still not be adequate for providing effective protection against HIV-1. In fact, studies have suggested that the level of circulating neutralizing antibody needed to prevent infection of macaques with a primate immunodeficiency virus are much higher than can be induced with traditional vaccine modalities (109,110). Moreover, the magnitude of the CTL responses that have been generated in human volunteers so far is not nearly as great as the vaccine-elicited responses in macaques that have controlled primate immunodeficiency virus spread (179,180).

Although live recombinant virus vectors continue to show promise as a viable approach for eliciting cellular immune responses to HIV-1, the magnitude of the responses in human volunteers immunized with such vaccines has been substantially lower than that seen in nonhuman primates. This reduced immunogenicity may be a consequence of preexisting vector-specific immunity. For example, adenovirus serotype 5 (Ad5)–specific immunity induced by naturally occurring adenovirus infections may reduce the immunogenicity of immunogens based on gene-deleted Ad5 vectors (181). Ad5-directed immunity does not, however, interfere with the immunogenicity of the Ad5-based vectors in macaques because nonhuman primates are infected with distinct families of adenoviruses with serological profiles that differ from human adenoviruses. To circumvent the problem of preexisting Ad5-specific immunity, novel adenovirus vectors are being developed for which there should be no preexisting immunity in human vaccine recipients. These novel vectors include selected human adenoviruses, such as adenovirus serotype 35, that rarely cause natural infections in humans (182). Adenoviruses that infect nonhuman primate species, including selected chimpanzee adenovirus isolates, are also being developed as potential vaccine vectors (183). Finally, chimeric adenovirus vectors are also being constructed that circumvent susceptibility to preexisting neutralizing antibodies against the vector but maintain high levels of immunogenicity (184).

In light of the concern that the durability of vaccine-elicited cellular immune responses will be important for an HIV-1 vaccine, several vectors are being explored that should persist in vaccinees. The assumption underlying this approach is that microorganisms that are never fully cleared in infected individuals should continue to make protein and therefore perpetuate an immune response. The most promising of the persisting vectors are those constructed with mycobacteria, including Mycobacterium bovis bacillus Calmette–Guérin (BCG). It should be noted, however, that emerging data indicate that the maximal generation of memory T cells might occur when antigen does not persist.

Plasmid DNA constructs have proven to be effective immunogens in mice for eliciting cellular immune responses and for priming antibody responses. It is now clear, however, that DNA vaccines are less immunogenic in nonhuman primates than they are in mice, and even less immunogenic in humans than in nonhuman primates. Therefore, strategies are being aggressively pursued to improve the immunogenicity of plasmid DNA vaccines. These strategies include formulating the plasmid DNAs with liposomes or polymers to increase their *in vivo* expression as well as protect them from rapid degradation (185). Novel delivery technologies are also being explored, including the use of *in vivo* electroporation to increase the efficiency of cellular transfection with DNA (186). In addition, studies have been done showing that coadministration of plasmid DNA immunogens with plasmids encoding cytokines has the potential to increase vaccine-elicited cellular immune responses (187). The best-studied of these approaches includes the use of cytokines that increase the clonal expansion of antigen-specific T cells, such as interleukin (IL)-2 and IL-15, and cytokines that attract and induce the maturation of antigen presenting cells, including granulocyte/macrophage colony-stimulating factor and β chemokines.

It remains unclear whether qualitative aspects of vaccine-elicited cellular immune responses or particular viral protein specificities of those cellular responses will prove important in protecting against viral replication and disease progression. The increasingly sophisticated use of polychromatic flow cytometry will allow the assessment of the functional capabilities of vaccine-induced T cell populations. It will be important to determine whether the production of certain cytokines or cytotoxic mediators by vaccine-elicited T cells is associated with particularly effective control of virus replication. Further, although there is a general consensus that it will be desirable to generate immune responses to several viral structural gene products, it is not yet clear whether cellular immune responses to some of the early viral regulatory proteins such as Tat and Nef will confer a substantial additional benefit to vaccinees.

Finally, effort is being focused on developing technologies that will augment humoral immune responses to subunit HIV-1 envelope immunogens. This is a particularly daunting challenge, as it will be important to deliver such immunogens in a manner that will not alter their natural structural conformations. The technologies receiving the most attention at the present time include oil and water emulsions and CpG motif-containing adjuvants that signal through Toll-like receptor 9.

Data from nonhuman primate studies indicate that existing technologies should allow for the creation of HIV-1 vaccines that preserve memory $CD4^+$ T cell populations and, as a result, attenuate the clinical course of infection. Importantly, several recent advances promise to improve the protection conferred by immunization. The magnitude and durability of vaccine-elicited immune responses should be dramatically improved by increasing the immunogenicity of plasmid DNA immunogens as well as the development of new generations of viral vectors that can escape recognition by preexisting vector-specific immunity. A greater breadth of immune recognition should be achieved using consensus gene sequences in these novel vectors. Moreover, investigations into the strategies for eliciting broadly neutralizing antibodies and mucosal immune responses should create strategies for further improving the effectiveness of HIV-1 vaccines. While the creation of an effective HIV-1 vaccine remains an enormous challenge, continuing progress in all of these areas provides reason for optimism about ultimately controlling the spread of AIDS.

NOTE: Portions of the text of this chapter were adapted from references (188) and (189).

REFERENCES

1. UNAIDS. *AIDS Epidemic Update* [online], http://www.searo.who.int/LinkFiles/Fact_and_FiguresPDFepi-update2005.pdf (2005).
2. Freed EO. HIV-1 and the host cell: an intimate association. *Trends Microbiol.* 2004;12:170–177.
3. Dalgleish AG, Beverley PC, Clapham PR, et al. The CD4 (T4) antigen is an essential component of the receptor for the AIDS retrovirus. *Nature.* 1984;312:763–767.
4. Alkhatib G, Combadiere C, Broder CC, et al. CC CKR5: a RANTES, MIP-1alpha, MIP-1beta receptor as a fusion cofactor for macrophage-trophic HIV-1. *Science.* 1996;272:1955–1958.
5. Feng Y, Broder CC, Kennedy PE, et al. HIV-1 entry cofactor functional cDNA cloning of a seven-transmembrane, G protein-coupled receptor. *Sciecne.* 1996;272:872–877.
6. Littman DR. Chemokine receptors: keys to AIDS pathogenesis? *Cell.* 1998;93:677–680.
7. Edinger AL, Mankowski JL, Doranz BJ, et al. CD4-independent, CCR5-dependent infection of brain capillary endothelial cells by a neurovirulent simian immunodeficiency virus strain. *Pro Natl Acad U S A.* 1997;94:14742–14747.
8. Cocchi F, DeVico AL, Garzino-Demo A, et al. Identification of RANTES, MIP-1 alpha, and MIP-1 beta as the major HIV-suppressive factors produced by CD8+ T cells. Science. 1995;270:1811–1815.
9. Connor RI, Ho DD. Transmission and pathogenesis of human immunodeficiency virus type 1. *AIDS Res Hum Retroviruses.* 1994;10:321–323.
10. Malim MH, Emerman M. HIV-1 sequence variation: drift, shift, and attenuation. *Cell.* 2001;104:469–472.
11. Sheehy AM, Gaddis NC, Choi JD, et al. Isolation of a human gene that inhibits HIV-1 infection and is suppressed by the viral Vif protein. *Nature.* 2002; 418:646–650.
12. Stremlau M, Owens CM, Perron MJ, et al. The cytoplasmic body component TRIM5alpha restricts HIV-1 infection in Old World monkeys. *Nature.* 2004;427:848–853.
13. Ganesh L, Burstein E, Guha-Niyogi A, et al. The gene product Murr1 restricts HIV-1 replication in resting CD4+ lymphocytes. *Nature.* 2003;426:853–857.
14. Hirsch VM, Olmsted RA, Murphey-Corb M, et al. An African primate lentivirus (SIVsm) closely related to HIV-2. *Nature.* 1989;339:389–392.
15. Keele BF, Van Heuverswyn F, Li Y, et al. Chimpanzee reservoirs of pandemic and nonpandemic HIV-1. *Science.* 2006;313:523–526.
16. Letvin NL, King NW. Immunologic and pathologic manifestations of the infection of rhesus monkeys with simian immunodeficiency virus of macaques. *J Acquir Immune Defic Syndr.* 1990;3:1023–1040.
17. Reimann KA, Li JT, Veazey R, et al. A chimeric simian/human immunodeficiency virus expressing a primary patient human immunodeficiency virus type 1 isolate env causes an AIDS-like disease after *in vivo* passage in rhesus monkeys. *J Virol.* 1996;70:6922–6928.
18. Watts DH. Management of human immunodeficiency virus infection in pregnancy. *N Engl J Med.* 2002;346:1879–1891.
19. Chiasson MA, Stoneburner RL, Lifson AR, et al. Risk factors for human immunodeficiency virus type 1 (HIV-1) infection in patients at a sexually transmitted disease clinic in New York City. *Am J Epidemiol.* 1990;131:208–220.
20. Spira AI, Marx PA, Patterson BK, et al. Cellular targets of infection and route of viral dissemination after an intravaginal inoculation of simian immunodeficiency virus into rhesus macaques. *J Exp Med.* 1996;183:215–225.
21. Haase AT. Perils at mucosal front lines for HIV and SIV and their hosts. *Nat Rev Immunol.* 2005;5:783–792.
22. Stahl-Hennig C, Steinman RM, Tenner-Racz K, et al. Rapid infection of oral mucosal-associated lymphoid tissue with simian immunodeficiency virus. *Science.* 1999;285:1261–1265.
23. Zhang Z, Schuler T, Zupancic M, et al. Sexual transmission and propagation of SIV and HIV in resting and activated CD4+ T cells. *Science.* 1999;286:1353–1357.
24. Mellors JW, Rinaldo CR Jr, Gupta P, et al. Prognosis in HIV-1 infection predicted by the quantity of virus in plasma. *Science.* 1996; 272:1167–1170.
25. Veazey RS, Mansfield KG, Tham IC, et al. Dynamics of CCR5 expression by CD4(+) T cells in lymphoid tissues during simian immunodeficiency virus infection. *J Virol.* 2000;74:11001–11007.
26. Fauci AS. Multifactorial nature of human immunodeficiency virus disease: implications for therapy. *Science.* 1993;262:1011–1018.
27. Dybul M, Fauci AS, Bartlett JG, et al. Panel on Clinical Practices for Treatment of HIV. Guidelines for using antiretroviral agents among HIV-infected adults and adolescents. *Ann Intern Med.* 2002;137:381–433.
28. Palella FJ Jr, Delaney KM, Moorman AC, et al. Declining morbidity and mortality among patients with advanced human immunodeficiency virus infection. HIV Outpatient Study Investigators. *N Engl J Med.* 1998;338(13):853–860.
29. Furtado MR, Callaway DS, Phair JP, et al. Persistence of HIV-1 transcription in peripheral-blood mononuclear cells in patients receiving potent antiretroviral therapy. *N Engl J Med.* 1999;340:1614–1622.
30. Ho DD, Neumann AU, Perelson AS, et al. Rapid turnover of plasma virions and CD4 lymphocytes in HIV-1 infection. *Nature.* 1995;373:123–126.
31. Siliciano JD, Kajdas J, Finzi D, et al. Long-term follow-up studies confirm the stability of the latent reservoir for HIV-1 in resting CD4+ T cells. *Nat Med.* 2003;9:727–728.
32. Pantaleo G, Menzo S, Vaccarezza M, et al. Studies in subjects with long-term nonprogressive human immunodeficiency virus infection. *N Engl J Med.* 1995;332:209–216.
33. Cao Y, Qin L, Zhang L, et al. Virologic and immunologic characterization of long-term survivors of human immunodeficiency virus type 1 infection. *N Engl J Med.* 1995;332:201–208.
34. Rodes B, Toro C, Paxinos E, et al. Differences in disease progression in a cohort of long-term non-progressors after more than 16 years of HIV-1 infection. *AIDS.* 2004;18:1109–1116.
35. Martinez V, Costagliola D, Bonduelle O, et al. Asymptomatiques a Long Terme Study Group. Combination of HIV-1-specific CD4 Th1 cell responses and IgG2 antibodies is the best predictor for persistence of long-term nonprogression. *J Infect Dis.* 2005;191:2053–2063.
36. Deacon NJ, Tsykin A, Solomon A, et al. Genomic structure of an attenuated quasi species of HIV-1 from a blood transfusion donor and recipients. *Science.* 1995;270:988–991.
37. Learmont JC, Geczy AF, Mills J, et al. Immunologic and virologic status after 14 to 18 years of infection with an attenuated strain of HIV-1. A report from the Sydney Blood Bank Cohort. *N Engl J Med.* 1999; 340:1715–1722.
38. Dean M, Carrington M, O'Brien SJ. *Annual Review of Genomics and Human Genetics.* 2002;3:263–292.
39. Keet IP, Tang J, Klein MR, et al. Consistent associations of HLA class I and II and transporter gene products with progression of human immunodeficiency virus type 1 infection in homosexual men. *J Infect Dis.* 1999;180:299–309.
40. Kaslow RA, Carrington M, Apple R, et al. Influence of combinations of human major histocompatibility complex genes on the course of HIV-1 infection. *Nat Med.* 1996;2:405–411.
41. Martin MP, Gao X, Lee JH, et al. Epistatic interaction between KIR3DS1 and HLA-B delays the progression to AIDS. *Nat Genet.* 2002;31:429–434.
42. Dean M, Carrington M, Winkler C, et al. Genetic restriction of HIV-1 infection and progression to AIDS by a deletion allele of the CKR5 structural gene. Hemophilia Growth and Development Study, Multicenter AIDS Cohort Study, Multicenter Hemophilia Cohort Study, San Francisco City Cohort, ALIVE Study. *Science.* 1996 27;273:1856–1862.
43. Huang Y, Paxton WA, Wolinsky SM, et al. The role of a mutant CCR5 allele in HIV-1 transmission and disease progression. *Nat Med.* 1996;2:1240–1243.
44. Smith MW, Dean M, Carrington M, et al. Contrasting genetic influence of CCR2 and CCR5 variants on HIV-1 infection and disease progression. Hemophilia Growth and Development Study (HGDS), Multicenter AIDS Cohort Study (MACS), Multicenter Hemophilia Cohort Study (MHCS), San Francisco City Cohort (SFCC), ALIVE Study. *Science.* 1997;277:959–965.
45. Anastassopoulou CG, Kostrikis LG. The impact of human allelic variation on HIV-1 disease. *Curr HIV Res.* 2003;1:185–203.

46. Rowland-Jones SL, McMichael A. Immune responses in HIV-exposed seronegatives: have they repelled the virus? *Curr Opin Immunol.* 1995;7:448–455.
47. Letvin NL, Walker BD. HIV versus the immune system: another apparent victory for the virus. *J Clin Invest.* 2001;107:273–275.
48. Zhu T, Corey L, Hwangbo Y, et al. Persistence of extraordinarily low levels of genetically homogeneous human immunodeficiency virus type 1 in exposed seronegative individuals. *J Virol.* 2003;77:6108–6116.
49. Casella CR, Finkel TH. Mechanisms of lymphocyte killing by HIV. *Curr Opin Hematol.* 1997;4:24–31.
50. Ho DD. Perspectives series: host/pathogen interactions. Dynamics of HIV-1 replication *in vivo*. *J Clin Invest.* 1997;99:2565–2567.
51. Ho DD, Neumann AU, Perelson AS, et al. Rapid turnover of plasma virions and CD4 lymphocytes in HIV-1 infection. *Nature.* 1995;373:123–126.
52. Perelson AS, Neumann AU, Markowitz M, et al. HIV-1 dynamics *in vivo*: virion clearance rate, infected cell life-span, and viral generation time. *Science.* 1996;271:1582–1586.
53. Wei X, Ghosh SK, Taylor ME, et al. Viral dynamics in human immunodeficiency virus type 1 infection. *Nature.* 1995;373:117–122.
54. Wolthers KC, Bea G, Wisman A, et al. T cell telomere length in HIV-1 infection: no evidence for increased CD4+ T cell turnover. *Science.* 1996;274:1543–1547.
55. Mohri H, Bonhoeffer S, Monard S, et al. Rapid turnover of T lymphocytes in SIV-infected rhesus macaques. *Science.* 1998;279:1223–1227.
56. Rosenzweig M, DeMaria MA, Harper DM, et al. Increased rates of CD4(+) and CD8(+) T lymphocyte turnover in simian immunodeficiency virus-infected macaques. *Proc Natl Acad Sci U S A.* 1998; 95:6388–93.
57. Hellerstein M, Hanley MB, Cesar D, et al. Directly measured kinetics of circulating T lymphocytes in normal and HIV-1 infected humans. *Nat Med.* 1999; 5:83–89.
58. Mattapallil JJ, Douek DC, Hill B, et al. Massive infection and loss of memory CD4+ T cells in multiple tissues during acute SIV infection. *Nature.* 2005;434:1093–1097.
59. Picker LJ. Immunopathogenesis of acute AIDS virus infection. *Curr Opin Immunol.* 2006;18:399–405.
60. Autran B, Carcelain G, Li TS, et al. Positive effects of combined antiretroviral therapy on CD4+ T cell homeostasis and function in advanced HIV disease. *Science.* 1997;277:112–116.
61. Pantaleo G, Graziosi C, Demarest JF, et al. Role of lymphoid organs in the pathogenesis of human immunodeficiency virus (HIV) infection. *Immunol Rev.* 1994;140:105–130.
62. Tenner-Racz K, Racz P. Follicular dendritic cells initiate and maintain infection of the germinal centers by human immunodeficiency virus. *Curr Top Microbiol Immunol.* 1995;201:141–159.
63. Harbol AW, Liesveld JL, Simpson-Haidaris PJ, et al. Mechanisms of cytopenia in human immunodeficiency virus infection. *Blood Rev.* 1994;8:241–251.
64. Schmitz JE, Kuroda MJ, Santra S, et al. Control of viremia in simian immunodeficiency virus infection by CD8+ lymphocytes. *Science.* 1999;283:857–860.
65. Douek DC, McFarland RD, Keiser PH, et al. Changes in thymic function with age and during the treatment of HIV infection. *Nature.* 1998;396:690–695.
66. Harbol AW, Liesveld JL, Simpson-Haidaris PJ, et al. Mechanisms of cytopenia in human immunodeficiency virus infection. *Blood Rev.* 1994;8:241–251.
67. Moses A, Nelson J, Bagby GC Jr. The influence of human immunodeficiency virus-1 on hematopoiesis. *Blood.* 1998;91:1479–1495.
68. Watanabe M, Ringler DJ, Nakamura M, et al. Simian immunodeficiency virus inhibits bone marrow hematopoietic progenitor cell growth. *J Virol.* 1990;64:656–663.
69. Biswas P, Poli G, Kinter AL, et al. Interferon gamma induces the expression of human immunodeficiency virus in persistently infected promonocytic cells (U1) and redirects the production of virions to intracytoplasmic vacuoles in phorbol myristate acetate-differentiated U1 cells. *J Exp Med.* 1992;176:739–750.
70. Poli G, Fauci AS. The effect of cytokines and pharmacologic agents on chronic HIV infection. *AIDS Res Hum Retroviruses.* 1992;8:191–197.
71. Tsunetsugu-Yokota Y, Honda M. Effect of cytokines on HIV release and IL-2 receptor alpha expression in monocytic cell lines. *J Acquir Immune Defic Syndr.* 1990; 3:511–516.
72. Posner MR, Hideshima T, Cannon T, et al. An IgG human monoclonal antibody that reacts with HIV-1/GP120, inhibits virus binding to cells, and neutralizes infection. *J Immunol.* 1991;146:4325–4332.
73. Boue F, Wallon C, Goujard C, et al. HIV induces IL-6 production by human B lymphocytes. Role of IL-4. *J Immunol.* 1992;148:3761–3767.
74. Rieckmann P, Poli G, Kehrl JH, et al. Activated B lymphocytes from human immunodeficiency virus-infected individuals induce virus expression in infected T cells and a promonocytic cell line, U1. *J Exp Med.* 1991;173:1–5.
75. Jacobson DL, McCutchan JA, Spechko PL, et al. The evolution of lymphadenopathy and hypergammaglobulinemia are evidence for early and sustained polyclonal B lymphocyte activation during human immunodeficiency virus infection. *J Infect Dis.* 1991; 163:240–246.
76. Pope M. Mucosal dendritic cells and immunodeficiency viruses. *J Infect Dis.* 1999;179 Suppl 3:S427–430.
77. Geijtenbeek TB, Kwon DS, Torensma R, et al. DC-SIGN, a dendritic cell-specific HIV-1-binding protein that enhances trans-infection of T cells. *Cell.* 2000; 100:587–597.
78. Muller F, Rollag H, Froland SS. Reduced oxidative burst responses in monocytes and monocyte-derived macrophages from HIV-infected subjects. *Clin Exp Immunol.* 1990;82:10–15.
79. Baldwin GC, Fleischmann J, Chung Y, et al. Human immunodeficiency virus causes mononuclear phagocyte dysfunction. *Proc Natl Acad Sci U S A.* 1990; 87:3933–3937.
80. Gendelman HE, Persidsky Y, Ghorpade A, et al. The neuropathogenesis of the AIDS dementia complex. *AIDS.* 1997; 11 Suppl A: S35–45.
81. Alter G, Altfeld M. NK cell function in HIV-1 infection. *Curr Mol Med.* 2006; 6:621–639.
82. Schmitz JE, Lifton MA, Reimann KA, et al. Effect of complement consumption by cobra venom factor on the the course of primary infection with simian immunodeficiency virus in rhesus monkeys. *AIDS Res Hum Retroviruses.* 1999;15:195–202.
83. Wyatt R, Kwong PD, Desjardins E, et al. The antigenic structure of the HIV gp120 envelope glycoprotein. *Nature.* 1998;393:705–711.
84. Li M, Gao F, Mascola JR, et al. Human immunodeficiency virus type 1 env clones from acute and early subtype B infections for standardized assessments of vaccine-elicited neutralizing antibodies. *J Virol.* 2005; 79:10108–10125.
85. Montefiori DC, Pantaleo G, Fink LM, et al. Neutralizing and infection-enhancing antibody responses to human immunodeficiency virus type 1 in long-term nonprogressors. *J Infect Dis.* 1996; 173:60–67.
86. Moog C, Fleury HJ, Pellegrin I, et al. Autologous and heterologous neutralizing antibody responses following initial seroconversion in human immunodeficiency virus type 1-infected individuals. *J Virol.* 1997;71:3734–3741.
87. Koup RA, Safrit JT, Cao Y, et al. Temporal association of cellular immune responses with the initial control of viremia in primary human immunodeficiency virus type 1 syndrome. *J Virol.* 1994;68:4650–4655.
88. Pellegrin I, Legrand E, Neau D, et al. Kinetics of appearance of neutralizing antibodies in 12 patients with primary or recent HIV-1 infection and relationship with plasma and cellular viral loads. *J Acquir Immune Defic Syndr Hum Retrovirol.* 1996;11:438–447.
89. Pilgrim AK, Pantaleo G, Cohen OJ, et al. Neutralizing antibody responses to human immunodeficiency virus type 1 in primary infection and long-term-nonprogressive infection. *J Infect Dis.* 1997;176: 924–932.
90. Wei X, Decker JM, Wang S, et al. Antibody neutralization and escape by HIV-1. *Nature.* 2003; 422:307–312.
91. Frost SD, Wrin T, Smith DM, et al. Neutralizing antibody responses drive the evolution of human immunodeficiency virus type 1 envelope during recent HIV infection. *Proc Natl Acad Sci U S A.* 2005;102: 18514–18519.
92. Kwong PD, Doyle ML, Casper DJ, et al. HIV-1 evades antibody-mediated neutralization through conformational masking of receptor-binding sites. *Nature.* 2002;420:678–682.

93. Leonard CK, Spellman MW, Riddle L, et al. Assignment of intrachain disulfide bonds and characterization of potential glycosylation sites of the type 1 recombinant human immunodeficiency virus envelope glycoprotein (gp120) expressed in Chinese hamster ovary cells. *J Biol Chem.* 1990;265:10373–10382.
94. Choe H, Farzan M, Sun Y, et al. The beta-chemokine receptors CCR3 and CCR5 facilitate infection by primary HIV-1 isolates. *Cell.* 1996;85:1135–1148.
95. Goudsmit J, Debouck C, Meloen RH, et al. Human immunodeficiency virus type 1 neutralization epitope with conserved architecture elicits early type-specific antibodies in experimentally infected chimpanzees. *Proc Natl Acad Sci U S A.* 1988; 85:4478–4482.
96. Javaherian K, Langlois AJ, McDanal C, et al. Principal neutralizing domain of the human immunodeficiency virus type 1 envelope protein. *Proc Natl Acad Sci U S A.* 1989;86:6768–6772.
97. LaRosa GJ, Davide JP, Weinhold K, et al. Conserved sequence and structural elements in the HIV-1 principal neutralizing determinant. *Science.* 1990; 249:932–935.
98. Burton DR, Montefiori DC. The antibody response in HIV-1 infection. AIDS. 1997;11 Suppl A:S87–98.
99. Gorny MK, Williams C, Volsky B, et al. Cross-clade neutralizing activity of human anti-V3 monoclonal antibodies derived from the cells of individuals infected with non-B clades of human immunodeficiency virus type 1. *J Virol.* 2006;80:6865–6872.
100. de Parseval A, Bobardt MD, Chatterji A, et al. A highly conserved arginine in gp120 governs HIV-1 binding to both syndecans and CCR5 via sulfated motifs. *J Biol Chem.* 2005;280:39493–39504.
101. Kang CY, Nara P, Chamat S, et al. Evidence for non-V3-specific neutralizing antibodies that interfere with gp120/CD4 binding in human immunodeficiency virus 1-infected humans. *Proc Natl Acad Sci U S A.* 1991;88:6171–6175.
102. Posner MR, Hideshima T, Cannon T, et al. An IgG human monoclonal antibody that reacts with HIV-1/GP120, inhibits virus binding to cells, and neutralizes infection. *J Immunol.* 1991;146:4325–4332.
103. Saphire EO, Parren PW, Pantophlet R, et al. Crystal structure of a neutralizing human IGG against HIV-1: a template for vaccine design. *Science.* 2001; 293:1155–1159.
104. Trkola A, Pomales AB, Yuan H, et al. Cross-clade neutralization of primary isolates of human immunodeficiency virus type 1 by human monoclonal antibodies and tetrameric CD4-IgG. *J Virol.* 1995;69:6609–6617.
105. Chan DC, Fass D, Berger JM, et al. Core structure of gp41 from the HIV envelope glycoprotein. *Cell.* 1997;89:263–273.
106. Chan DC, Kim PS. HIV entry and its inhibition. *Cell.* 1998;93:681–4.
107. Poignard P, Sabbe R, Picchio GR, et al. Neutralizing antibodies have limited effects on the control of established HIV-1 infection *in vivo*. *Immunity.* 1999;10:431–438.
108. Haigwood NL, Montefiori DC, Sutton WF, et al. Passive immunotherapy in simian immunodeficiency virus-infected macaques accelerates the development of neutralizing antibodies. *J Virol.* 2004;78: 5983–5995.
109. Mascola JR, Lewis MG, Stiegler G, et al. Protection of Macaques against pathogenic simian/human immunodeficiency virus 89.6PD by passive transfer of neutralizing antibodies. *J Virol.* 1999;73:4009–4018.
110. Mascola JR, Stiegler G, VanCott TC, et al. Protection of macaques against vaginal transmission of a pathogenic HIV-1/SIV chimeric virus by passive infusion of neutralizing antibodies. *Nat Med.* 2000;6:207–10.
111. Emini, E. Biology, Immunology and Therapy. *The Human Immunodeficiency Virus.* 2002;464.
112. Walker CM, Moody DJ, Stites DP, et al. CD8+ lymphocytes can control HIV infection *in vitro* by suppressing virus replication. *Science.* 1986;234:1563–1566.
113. Kannagi M, Chalifoux LV, Lord CI, et al. Suppression of simian immunodeficiency virus replication *in vitro* by CD8+ lymphocytes. *J Immunol.* 1988;140:2237–2242.
114. Cocchi F, DeVico AL, Garzino-Demo A, et al. Identification of RANTES, MIP-1 alpha, and MIP-1 beta as the major HIV-suppressive factors produced by CD8+ T cells. *Science.* 1995;270:1811–1815.
115. Koup RA, Safrit JT, Cao Y, et al. Temporal association of cellular immune responses with the initial control of viremia in primary human immunodeficiency virus type 1 syndrome. *J Virol.* 1994; 68:4650–4655.
116. Pantaleo G, Demarest JF, Soudeyns H, et al. Major expansion of CD8+ T cells with a predominant V beta usage during the primary immune response to HIV. *Nature.* 1994;370:463–467.
117. Chen ZW, Kou ZC, Lekutis C, et al. T cell receptor V beta repertoire in an acute infection of rhesus monkeys with simian immunodeficiency viruses and a chimeric simian-human immunodeficiency virus. *J Exp Med.* 1995;182:21–31.
118. Kuroda MJ, Schmitz JE, Charini WA, et al. Emergence of CTL coincides with clearance of virus during primary simian immunodeficiency virus infection in rhesus monkeys. *J Immunol.* 1999; 162:5127–5133.
119. Yasutomi Y, Reimann KA, Lord CI, et al. Simian immunodeficiency virus-specific CD8+ lymphocyte response in acutely infected rhesus monkeys. *J Virol.* 1993;67:1707–1711.
120. Musey L, Hughes J, Schacker T, et al. Cytotoxic-T-cell responses, viral load, and disease progression in early human immunodeficiency virus type 1 infection. *N Engl J Med.* 1997;337:1267–1274.
121. Ogg GS, Jin X, Bonhoeffer S, et al. Quantitation of HIV-1-specific cytotoxic T lymphocytes and plasma load of viral RNA. *Science.* 1998; 279:2103–2106.
122. Schmitz JE, Kuroda MJ, Santra S, et al. Control of viremia in simian immunodeficiency virus infection by CD8+ lymphocytes. *Science.* 1999;283:857–860.
123. Goulder PJ, Watkins DI. HIV and SIV CTL escape: implications for vaccine design. *Nat Rev Immunol.* 2004;4:630–640.
124. Koenig S, Conley AJ, Brewah YA, et al. Transfer of HIV-1-specific cytotoxic T lymphocytes to an AIDS patient leads to selection for mutant HIV variants and subsequent disease progression. *Nat Med.* 1995;1:330–336.
125. Allen TM, O'Connor DH, Jing P, et al. Tat-specific cytotoxic T lymphocytes select for SIV escape variants during resolution of primary viraemia. *Nature.* 2000;407:386–390.
126. Kelleher AD, Long C, Holmes EC, et al. Clustered mutations in HIV-1 gag are consistently required for escape from HLA-B27-restricted cytotoxic T lymphocyte responses. *J Exp Med.* 2001;193:375–386.
127. Peyerl FW, Barouch DH, Yeh WW, et al. Simian-human immunodeficiency virus escape from cytotoxic T-lymphocyte recognition at a structurally constrained epitope. *J Virol.* 2003; 77:12572–12578.
128. Leslie AJ, Pfafferott KJ, Chetty P, et al. HIV evolution: CTL escape mutation and reversion after transmission. *Nat Med.* 2004;10:282–289.
129. Barouch DH, Powers J, Truitt DM, et al. Dynamic immune responses maintain cytotoxic T lymphocyte epitope mutations in transmitted simian immunodeficiency virus variants. *Nat Immunol.* 2005;6:247–252.
130. Barouch DH, Kunstman J, Kuroda MJ, et al. Eventual AIDS vaccine failure in a rhesus monkey by viral escape from cytotoxic T lymphocytes. *Nature.* 2002;415:335–339.
131. Appay V, Nixon DF, Donahoe SM, et al. HIV-specific CD8(+) T cells produce antiviral cytokines but are impaired in cytolytic function. *J Exp Med.* 2000;192:63–75.
132. Champagne P, Ogg GS, King AS, et al. Skewed maturation of memory HIV-specific CD8 T lymphocytes. *Nature.* 2001;410:106–111.
133. Day CL, Kaufmann DE, Kiepiela P, et al. PD-1 expression on HIV-specific T cells is associated with T-cell exhaustion and disease progression. *Nature.* 2006;443:350–354.
134. Clerici M, Shearer GM. A TH1->TH2 switch is a critical step in the etiology of HIV infection. *Immunol Today.* 1993;14:107–111.
135. Graziosi C, Pantaleo G, Gantt KR, et al. Lack of evidence for the dichotomy of TH1 and TH2 predominance in HIV-infected individuals. *Science.* 1994;265:248–252.
136. Rosenberg ES, Billingsley JM, Caliendo AM, et al. Vigorous HIV-1-specific CD4+ T cell responses associated with control of viremia. Science. 1997; 278:1447–50.
137. Clerici M, Stocks NI, Zajac RA, et al. Detection of three distinct patterns of T helper cell dysfunction in asymptomatic, human immunodeficiency virus-seropositive patients. Independence of CD4+ cell numbers and clinical staging. *J Clin Invest.* 1989;84:1892–1899.
138. Berman PW, Gregory TJ, Riddle L, et al. Protection of chimpanzees from infection by HIV-1 after vaccination with recombinant glycoprotein gp120 but not gp160. *Nature.* 1990;345:622–625.

139. Cohen J. Public health. AIDS vaccine trial produces disappointment and confusion. Science. 2003; 299:1290–1.
140. Flynn NM, Forthal DN, Harro CD, et al. The rgp120 HIV Vaccine Study Group. Placebo-controlled phase 3 trial of a recombinant glycoprotein 120 vaccine to prevent HIV-1 infection. *J Infect Dis.* 2005;191:654–665.
141. Gilbert PB, Peterson ML, Follmann D, et al. Correlation between immunologic responses to a recombinant glycoprotein 120 vaccine and incidence of HIV-1 infection in a phase 3 HIV-1 preventive vaccine trial. *J Infect Dis.* 2005;191:666–677.
142. Graham BS, Mascola JR. Lessons from failure–preparing for future HIV-1 vaccine efficacy trials. *J Infect Dis.* 2005;191:647–649.
143. Goepfert PA, Horton H, McElrath MJ, et al. NIAID HIV Vaccine Trials Network. High-dose recombinant Canarypox vaccine expressing HIV-1 protein, in seronegative human subjects. *J Infect Dis.* 2005;192:1249–1259.
144. Parren PW, Marx PA, Hessell AJ, et al. Antibody protects macaques against vaginal challenge with a pathogenic R5 simian/human immunodeficiency virus at serum levels giving complete neutralization *in vitro*. *J Virol.* 2001;75:8340–8347.
145. Shibata R, Igarashi T, Haigwood N, et al. Neutralizing antibody directed against the HIV-1 envelope glycoprotein can completely block HIV-1/SIV chimeric virus infections of macaque monkeys. *Nat Med.* 1999;5:204–210.
146. Seth A, Ourmanov I, Schmitz JE, et al. Immunization with a modified vaccinia virus expressing simian immunodeficiency virus (SIV) Gag-Pol primes for an anamnestic Gag-specific cytotoxic T-lymphocyte response and is associated with reduction of viremia after SIV challenge. *J Virol.* 2000;74:2502–2509.
147. Barouch DH, Santra S, Schmitz JE, et al. Control of viremia and prevention of clinical AIDS in rhesus monkeys by cytokine-augmented DNA vaccination. *Science.* 2000;290:486–492.
148. Amara RR, Villinger F, Altman JD, et al. Control of a mucosal challenge and prevention of AIDS by a multiprotein DNA/MVA vaccine. *Science.* 2001;292:69–74.
149. Picker LJ, Hagen SI, Lum R, et al. Insufficient production and tissue delivery of CD4+ memory T cells in rapidly progressive simian immunodeficiency virus infection. *J Exp Med.* 2004; 200:1299–1314.
150. Letvin NL, Mascola JR, Sun Y, et al. Preserved CD4+ central memory T cells and survival in vaccinated SIV-challenged monkeys. *Science.* 2006;312:1530–1533.
151. Mattapallil JJ, Douek DC, Buckler-White A, et al. Vaccination preserves CD4 memory T cells during acute simian immunodeficiency virus challenge. *J Exp Med.* 2006;203:1533–1541.
152. Quinn TC, Wawer MJ, Sewankambo N, et al. Viral load and heterosexual transmission of human immunodeficiency virus type 1. Rakai Project Study Group. *N Engl J Med.* 2000;342:921–929.
153. Gray RH, Wawer MJ, Brookmeyer R, et al; Rakai Project Team. Probability of HIV-1 transmission per coital act in monogamous, heterosexual, HIV-1-discordant couples in Rakai, Uganda. *Lancet.* 2001;357:1149–1153.
154. Barouch DH, Kunstman J, Glowczwskie J, et al. Viral escape from dominant simian immunodeficiency virus epitope-specific cytotoxic T lymphocytes in DNA-vaccinated rhesus monkeys. *J Virol.* 2003;77:7367–7375.
155. Letvin NL. Progress toward an HIV vaccine. *Annu Rev Med.* 2005;56:213–223.
156. Mascola JR, Snyder SW, Weislow OS, et al. Immunization with envelope subunit vaccine products elicits neutralizing antibodies against laboratory-adapted but not primary isolates of human immunodeficiency virus type 1. The National Institute of Allergy and Infectious Diseases AIDS Vaccine Evaluation Group. *J Infect Dis.* 1996;173:340–348.
157. Bures R, Gaitan A, Zhu T, et al. Immunization with recombinant canarypox vectors expressing membrane-anchored glycoprotein 120 followed by glycoprotein 160 boosting fails to generate antibodies that neutralize R5 primary isolates of human immunodeficiency virus type 1. *AIDS Res Hum Retroviruses.* 2000;16:2019–2035.
158. Li M, Gao F, Mascola JR, et al. Human immunodeficiency virus type 1 env clones from acute and early subtype B infections for standardized assessments of vaccine-elicited neutralizing antibodies. *J Virol.* 2005;79:10108–10125.
159. D'Souza MP, Livnat D, Bradac JA, et al. Evaluation of monoclonal antibodies to human immunodeficiency virus type 1 primary isolates by neutralization assays: performance criteria for selecting candidate antibodies for clinical trials. AIDS Clinical Trials Group Antibody Selection Working Group. *J Infect Dis.* 1997;175:1056–1062.
160. Parren PW, Burton DR. The antiviral activity of antibodies *in vitro* and *in vivo*. *Adv Immunol.* 2001;77:195–262.
161. Burton DR, Desrosiers RC, Doms RW, et al. HIV vaccine design and the neutralizing antibody problem. *Nat Immunol.* 2004;5:233–236.
162. Haynes BF, Fleming J, St Clair EW, et al. Cardiolipin polyspecific autoreactivity in two broadly neutralizing HIV-1 antibodies. *Science.* 2005; 308:1906–1908.
163. Burton DR, Stanfield RL, Wilson IA. Antibody vs. HIV in a clash of evolutionary titans. *Proc Natl Acad Sci U S A.* 2005;102:14943–14948.
164. Kwong PD, Wyatt R, Robinson J, et al. Structure of an HIV gp120 envelope glycoprotein in complex with the CD4 receptor and a neutralizing human antibody. *Nature.* 1998;393:648–659.
165. Chen B, Vogan EM, Gong H, et al. Structure of an unliganded simian immunodeficiency virus gp120 core. *Nature.* 2005; 433:834–841.
166. Quinn TC, Glasser D, Cannon RO, et al. Human immunodeficiency virus infection among patients attending clinics for sexually transmitted diseases. *N Engl J Med.* 1988;318:197–203.
167. Stamm WE, Handsfield HH, Rompalo AM, et al. The association between genital ulcer disease and acquisition of HIV infection in homosexual men. *JAMA.* 1988;260:1429–1433.
168. Keet IP, Lee FK, van Griensven GJ, et al. Herpes simplex virus type 2 and other genital ulcerative infections as a risk factor for HIV-1 acquisition. *Genitourin Med.* 1990;66:330–333.
169. Henry JL, Jaikaran ES, Davies JR, et al. A study of poliovaccination in infancy: excretion following challenge with live virus by children given killed or living poliovaccine. *J Hyg (Lond).* 1966;64:105–120.
170. Baig J, Levy DB, McKay PF, et al. Elicitation of simian immunodeficiency virus-specific cytotoxic T lymphocytes in mucosal compartments of rhesus monkeys by systemic vaccination. *J Virol.* 2002;76:11484–11490.
171. Gaschen B, Taylor J, Yusim K, et al. Diversity considerations in HIV-1 vaccine selection. *Science.* 2002;296:2354–2360.
172. Gao F, Weaver EA, Lu Z, et al. Antigenicity and immunogenicity of a synthetic human immunodeficiency virus type 1 group m consensus envelope glycoprotein. *J Virol.* 2005;79:1154–63.
173. Yu XG, Lichterfeld M, Perkins B, et al. High degree of inter-clade cross-reactivity of HIV-1-specific T cell responses at the single peptide level. *AIDS.* 2005;19:1449–1456.
174. Geels MJ, Dubey SA, Anderson K, et al. Broad cross-clade T-cell responses to gag in individuals infected with human immunodeficiency virus type 1 non-B clades (A to G): importance of HLA anchor residue conservation. *J Virol.* 2005;79:11247–11258.
175. Coplan PM, Gupta SB, Dubey SA, et al. Cross-reactivity of anti-HIV-1 T cell immune responses among the major HIV-1 clades in HIV-1-positive individuals from 4 continents. *J Infect Dis.* 2005;191:1427–1434.
176. Chakrabarti BK, Ling X, Yang ZY, et al. Expanded breadth of virus neutralization after immunization with a multiclade envelope HIV vaccine candidate. *Vaccine.* 2005;23:3434–3445.
177. Seaman MS, Xu L, Beaudry K, et al. Multiclade human immunodeficiency virus type 1 envelope immunogens elicit broad cellular and humoral immunity in rhesus monkeys. *J Virol.* 2005;79:2956–2963.
178. Doria-Rose NA, Learn GH, Rodrigo AG, et al. Human immunodeficiency virus type 1 subtype B ancestral envelope protein is functional and elicits neutralizing antibodies in rabbits similar to those elicited by a circulating subtype B envelope. *J Virol.* 2005;79:11214–11224.
179. Catanzaro AT, Koup RA, Roederer M, et al; Vaccine Research Center 006 Study Team. Phase 1 Safety and Immunogenicity Evaluation of a Multiclade HIV-1 Candidate Vaccine Delivered by a Replication-Defective Recombinant Adenovirus Vector. *J Infect Dis.* 2006; 194:1638–1649.
180. Graham BS, Koup RA, Roederer M, et al; Vaccine Research Center 004 Study Team. Phase 1 Safety and Immunogenicity Evaluation of a Multiclade HIV-1 DNA Candidate Vaccine. *J Infect Dis.* 2006;194:1650–1660.
181. Sumida SM, Truitt DM, Kishko MG, et al. Neutralizing antibodies and CD8+ T lymphocytes both contribute to immunity to adenovirus serotype 5 vaccine vectors. *J Virol.* 2004;78:2666–2673.
182. Lemckert AA, Sumida SM, Holterman L, et al. Immunogenicity of heterologous prime-boost regimens involving recombinant

adenovirus serotype 11 (Ad11) and Ad35 vaccine vectors in the presence of anti-ad5 immunity. *J Virol.* 2005;79:9694–9701.

183. Tatsis N, Tesema L, Robinson ER, et al. Chimpanzee-origin adenovirus vectors as vaccine carriers. *Gene Ther.* 2006; 13:421–429.
184. Roberts DM, Nanda A, Havenga MJ, et al. Hexon-chimaeric adenovirus serotype 5 vectors circumvent pre-existing anti-vector immunity. *Nature.* 2006; 441:239–243.
185. Greenland JR, Liu H, Berry D, et al. Beta-amino ester polymers facilitate *in vivo* DNA transfection and adjuvant plasmid DNA immunization. *Mol Ther.* 2005;12:164–170.
186. Otten GR, Schaefer M, Doe B, et al. Potent immunogenicity of an HIV-1 gag-pol fusion DNA vaccine delivered by *in vivo* electroporation. *Vaccine.* 2006;24:4503–4509.
187. Sumida SM, McKay PF, Truitt DM, et al. Recruitment and expansion of dendritic cells *in vivo* potentiate the immunogenicity of plasmid DNA vaccines. *J Clin Invest.* 2004; 114:1334–1342.
188. Letvin NL, Walker BD. Immunopathogenesis and immunotherapy in AIDS virus infections. *Nat Med.* 2003;9:861–866.
189. Letvin NL. Progress and obstacles in the development of an AIDS vaccine. *Nat Rev Immunol.* 2006;6:931–939.
190. Freed EO. HIV-1 Gag Proteins: Divers Functions in the Virus Life Cycle. *J Virol.* 1998;251:1–15.
191. Moore JP, Doms RW. The entry of inhibitors: A fusion of science and medicine. *PNAS.* 2003;100:10598–10602.
192. Fauci AS, Pantaleo G, Stanley S, et al. Immunopathogenic Mechanisms of HIV Infection. *Ann Intern Med.* 1996; 124:654–663.
193. Sempowski GD, Hicks CB, Eron JJ, et al. Naive T cells are maintained in the periphery during the first 3 months of acute HIV-1 infection: implications for analysis of thymus function. *J Clin Immunol.* 2005;25:462–472.
194. Zhu P, Liu J, Bess J Jr, et al. Distribution and three-dimensional structure of AIDS virus envelope spikes. *Nature.* 2006;441:847–852.

Chapter 40

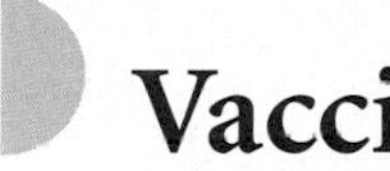

Vaccines

G.J.V. Nossal

INTRODUCTION

> *"Among the many pursuits of mankind, none can be more rewarding than that of preventing diseases by procedures which derive from the practice of vaccinology. Vaccines, together with sanitation and nutrition, have served as principal tools employed in public health to increase the health and life span of human beings. Vaccinology is a field in which dreams may be turned into realities."*

Thus wrote one of the pioneering giants of 20th century vaccine development, Maurice Hilleman, in 2003 (1). Vaccine research is once again very much in the public eye. Fields as diverse as HIV-AIDS, pandemic bird influenza, severe acute respiratory syndrome, and defense against bioterrorism attacks ensure that possible new vaccines remain in the spotlight. Vaccinology is poised at the interface of medical microbiology and immunology on the one hand, and of health policy and sociology on the other, and it has become a robust discipline in its own right. However, not every aspect of the scene is rosy. In the industrialized countries, the reduced prevalence of many infections has engendered a dangerous complacency. In the developing countries, resource constraints continue to loom large. In both situations, the activities of passionate but misguided antivaccine activists exert an influence disproportionate to their small numbers. Given the importance of the field, it is essential that all immunologists gain a good working knowledge of vaccinology.

This chapter describes how greatly knowledge of immune regulation in general, and of the relationship between innate and adaptive immunity in particular, contributes to vaccine research and design. Much technical material needs to be covered concerning adjuvants, choice of antigens, new routes of administration, and experimental vaccine design principles. At the same time, this chapter also addresses practical issues such as how to avoid a plethora of injections for our infants; how to reach those global citizens who most need vaccines, namely those in the poorer countries; and how to determine priorities to ensure that scarce health resources are deployed in the most efficient way.

The chief focus of the chapter naturally is on prevention of infection, although the possibility of vaccines playing a role in the control of established chronic infections such as HIV/AIDS or hepatitis C must also be explored. Beyond communicable diseases, there is a vast potential terrain, including vaccines to fight cancer, immunization approaches to autoimmunity or allergy, vaccination to prevent hemolytic disease of the newborn, or contraceptive vaccines. The cancer vaccine question is covered in Chapter 46, and the other issues are touched in Chapters 42 to 44. Here we can only cover the key concepts involved.

The world is waiting so eagerly for effective vaccines against the "big three" diseases—AIDS, tuberculosis and malaria—that it would be easy to lose sight of the devastating impact of diarrheal diseases, acute respiratory diseases, and largely nonfatal diseases such as schistosomiasis or hookworm, which cause extensive morbidity and loss of productivity. This chapter is not meant as a compendium of all new generation vaccines (2), which would require a work almost as long as the present book, but rather as an outline of the principles of vaccinology illustrated by specific examples of established or experimental vaccines. Many diseases are covered because of the protean nature and rich promise of the field.

HISTORICAL PERSPECTIVES

People who yearn for a simpler, Arcadian life less dominated by science and technology tend to forget that before the Industrial Revolution, life really was nasty, brutish, and short. Not only the great figures of music and literature, but also ordinary men, women, and children frequently died of infections easily prevented or cured today. It would be tempting to ascribe the improved situation only to medical science, particularly vaccines and antibiotics, but in fact the progressive lengthening of the average human lifespan much antedated these developments. Less grinding poverty, better sanitation, reduced overcrowding, and

TABLE 40.1 Chief Landmarks in the History of Vaccinology

1796	Edward Jenner introduces vaccination against smallpox
1880	Louis Pasteur develops attenuated fowl cholera vaccine, and soon after vaccines against anthrax and rabies.
1896	Robert Koch discovers the cholera vibrio. Killed, whole-cell bacterial vaccines against cholera, typhoid, plague, and other bacteria follow. They are very reactogenic.
1924	Bacille Calmette-Guerin (BCG) is introduced as a live attenuated tuberculosis vaccine.
Late 1920s, early 1930s	Progressively better diphtheria and tetanus vaccines are introduced based on toxins and then toxoids.
1935	17D strain of live attenuated yellow fever vaccine is introduced.
1945	Chick embryo allantoic fluid-derived killed influenza vaccine is developed.
1949	John Enders cultivates the poliomyelitis virus in tissue culture.
1955	Jonas Salk introduces the killed injectable poliomyelitis vaccine (IPV).
1961	Albert Sabin develops the live oral poliomyelitis vaccine (IPV).
1960–1969	Progressively improved live attenuated measles, mumps, and rubella vaccines are developed.
1974–1984	Polysaccharide vaccines against encapsulated gram-positive bacteria are introduced and progressively improved—Meningococcus, Pneumococcus, Hemophilus.
1981	Hepatitis B vaccine is licensed using surface antigen from human carrier plasma.
1983	*Hemophilus influenzae* carbohydrate-protein conjugate is developed as an effective vaccine for infants.
1986	Yeast-derived recombinant hepatitis B vaccine is licensed. This first vaccine derived thorough genetic engineering effectively begins a new paradigm that will dominate the next 20 years.

improved nutrition all played their part. But vaccines do have a proud place and count among the most cost-effective of all health interventions. Yet, the history of vaccines is not without its false starts and misadventures. The emergence of vaccines into the medical mainstream was in fact quite slow (Table 40.1).

Early civilizations that left written records, such as those of Egypt, India, Greece, and China, make reference to infectious diseases, but the accuracy of diagnosis is frequently questionable. It has been argued that the "leprosy" referred to in the Bible may well have represented a dermatological condition, such as psoriasis. Nevertheless, the fact that immunity was specific—that is, that one rarely contracted a given disease twice—was known to the ancient Greeks. The word *immunity* was first used in the 14th century for the example of plague. One disease that was particularly feared was smallpox, clearly described for the first time in China in the 4th century A.D. This was first because of its great prevalence, second because of the high case fatality rate (usually 20% to 30%), and third because when the pustules heal, they leave deep scars, therefore, recovering patients are disfigured for life. The history of vaccines begins with smallpox (3).

The Jennerian Era and Its Aftermath

Given that the microbial origin of infectious diseases was not discovered until the 19th century, it is hard to know what working hypothesis lay behind the first attempts to prevent smallpox. As early as the 10th century AD, the pustular fluid from smallpox lesions or the dried scabs from healing sores were given to susceptible individuals in an attempt to make them immune. This practice, known as *variolation,* involved inoculation into the skin in India, but into the nose in China. Surprisingly, variolation usually resulted in a much less severe disease than natural infection. There was a nasty lesion at the inoculation site, some satellite blisters, frequently a mild rash, and some constitutional symptoms of fever, myalgia, and lethargy, but mortality appeared to have been only 1% to 2%, and generalized scarring was also rare. One wonders what society thought about the fact that contacts of variolated individuals not infrequently developed the full, natural infection. Despite this, fear of smallpox epidemics was so great that even the august Royal Society of London debated the merits of variolation in the early 18th century. Clearly variolation worked, but the disadvantages were such that the medical profession as a whole remained skeptical.

Lady Mary Montague was the wife of the British ambassador in Constantinople and had her own 6-year-old son variolated in 1718. Returning to London, she interested several prominent members of the Royal College of Physicians in the practice as they struggled with the terrible smallpox epidemic of 1721. The president of the college, Sir Hans Sloane, became a convert following some experiments on convicted felons (no institutional ethics committees then!) and arranged the variolation of two royal princesses. Despite this, and perhaps fortunately, variolation did not become widespread in Britain or Europe.

Edward Jenner and the Rapid Spread of Smallpox Vaccination

Cows develop a smallpoxlike disease, cowpox, and lesions can appear on the udder and teats. Milkmaids can catch a mild version of cowpox, involving sores on the fingers and hand. In the 1760s and 1770s, several physicians drew attention to the fact that milkmaids were rarely pock-marked and that many could not be variolated. Several people—for example, farmer Benjamin Justy—claimed to have inoculated cowpox material into their children based on these observations. Be that as it may, it was the Gloucestershire general practitioner Edward Jenner who not only published first (4), but who was also actually intrepid enough to test the putative immunity by a challenge variolation. On May 17, 1796, milkmaid Sarah Nelmes donated a little fluid from her cowpox-affected hands, and Jenner forthwith inoculated James Phipps who promptly developed a lesion at the inoculation site. Jenner recorded (4):

> *"Notwithstanding the resemblance which the pustule thus excited on the boy's arm bore to variolous inoculation, yet as the indisposition attending to it was barely perceptible, I could scarcely persuade myself the patient was secure from the smallpox. However, on his being inoculated some months afterwards, it proved that he was secure."*

A further variolation five years later confirmed the maintenance of immunity.

Jenner's paper was rejected by the *Transactions of The Royal Society,* so he published his "Inquiry" privately. He must have derived great satisfaction from the speed with which vaccination, as the practice was termed, spread. In Europe, it became compulsory in several European countries early in the 19th century, and with stunning results. For example in Sweden, there were 5,126 smallpox deaths per 1 million population in 1800, but only 50 in 1821. Soon vaccination became popular in the United States and only slightly later throughout the world. In the second half of the 19th century, calf-derived fluid replaced the human source, and periodic revaccination was introduced. Jenner became famous in his own lifetime, but not nearly as revered as later. For example, in 1896 Britain extensively celebrated the centenary of the James Phipps experiment, secure in the knowledge that vaccination had proven brilliantly successful. Jenner has been recognized in memorials in many places, the statue in Kensington Gardens, London, among them, which represented the focal point for the great bicentenary events of 1996. Its plaque refers simply to "the country doctor who benefited mankind."

Who would have guessed that 181 years had to elapse between James Phipps' vaccination and the last case of naturally occurring smallpox? This is a reflection on the kind of world we inhabit. That said, smallpox eradication represented a signal public health achievement, which we shall now briefly summarize.

Global Eradication of Smallpox

Edward Jenner had speculated on the possibility that his vaccine could wipe out smallpox. It eventually became apparent that there was no animal reservoir of the smallpox virus and that it could live for only short periods outside the human body, so logically eradication was a possibility. North and Central America beat the scourge by 1951, Europe by 1953, and many countries in Asia by 1960, but at that time smallpox was still an enormous problem in Sub-Saharan Africa and most of the Indian sub-continent.

The World Health Assembly, the governing body of the World Health Organization (WHO), took a heady decision during its twelfth meeting in May 1959. As 977 million people still lived in smallpox endemic areas, global eradication was set as a new WHO goal. The preamble to the 1959 resolution mentioned a wildly optimistic timetable of 4 to 5 years for eradication. Given the huge scope of its mission, WHO has always been seriously under-resourced, and in fact little happened until 1966 when at last a significant budgetary allocation was made. Dr. Donald A. Henderson was appointed as head of the Smallpox Eradication Unit and Dr. Isao Arita as his medical officer. The 1967 plan called for 220 million people to be vaccinated that year. While Henderson set himself a 10-year target, he soon realized that immunizing all susceptible citizens was simply not feasible. He also recognized the challenge of quality control for the large number of vaccine doses required, as some suppliers proved thoroughly unreliable. Among the many other practical problems were data collection and handling, training of vaccinators and their supervisors, and certification of reference laboratories. The decision was taken to concentrate immunization efforts on known or possible contacts of actual cases. This put an enormous premium on a good surveillance strategy. The invention of a simple bifurcated needle to at once draw up and dispense vaccine fluid minimized wastage and improved vaccine take.

By 1971, such sufficient progress had been made toward global eradication that both the United States and the United Kingdom ceased their routine vaccination programs. In the early to mid 1970s, intense effort went into India and the Horn of Africa, but war between Ethiopia and Somalia certainly did not help. However, a large-scale emergency effort got on top of the disease, and the last case of naturally occurring smallpox was recorded in Merca, Somalia, on October 26, 1977.

Tragically, the story does not quite end there. A few laboratories continued their research on smallpox, and in 1978 a medical photographer at the University of Birmingham died from the disease, which she somehow caught from the smallpox laboratory one floor below her in the medical school. The small outbreak was soon controlled, but the 49-year-old head of the smallpox laboratory, Professor HS Bedson, felt so responsible that he committed suicide. The event highlights the dangers of variola virus stocks in laboratories, but both the United States and the former USSR refused to agree to the WHO's suggestion that all such stocks be destroyed. It well may be that further stocks are being held for biological warfare or bioterrorism purposes, although Iraq's "weapons of mass destruction" could never be found. The current major efforts that have gone into stockpiling smallpox vaccine, including improved vaccinia variants, just in case evil forces unleash secret sources of virulent variola virus is somewhat ironic.

On December 9, 1979—more than 4,000 years after the disease's first appearance and 183 years after young Master Phipps' adventure—the Global Commission on Smallpox Eradication certified that global eradication had been achieved. The campaign has rightly been hailed as the world's greatest public health triumph (Figure 40.1). Dr. Henderson is a revered figure and still a senior U.S. government advisor on control of epidemics and related matters. His self-imposed deadline slipped by only one year. The total cost of the WHO's program was $300 million, compared with an estimated cost burden of the disease of $1,350 million per annum prior to control.

The Dawn of Immunological Science (1875 to 1910): Pasteur, Koch, von Behring, Ehrlich

Jenner had no overarching theory for how vaccination provided immunity to smallpox. Two great giants, Louis Pasteur (1822 to 1895) and Robert Koch (1843 to 1910), established the true etiologic cause of infectious diseases and thus set the scene for a better understanding of the specificity of immunity. Pasteur (5) destroyed the spontaneous generation theory of bacteria, and Koch, his archrival and debating opponent, enunciated his famous postulates that, if fulfilled, established an agent as the cause of a disease. Pasteur made the critically important observation that bacteria grown for substantial periods in artificial

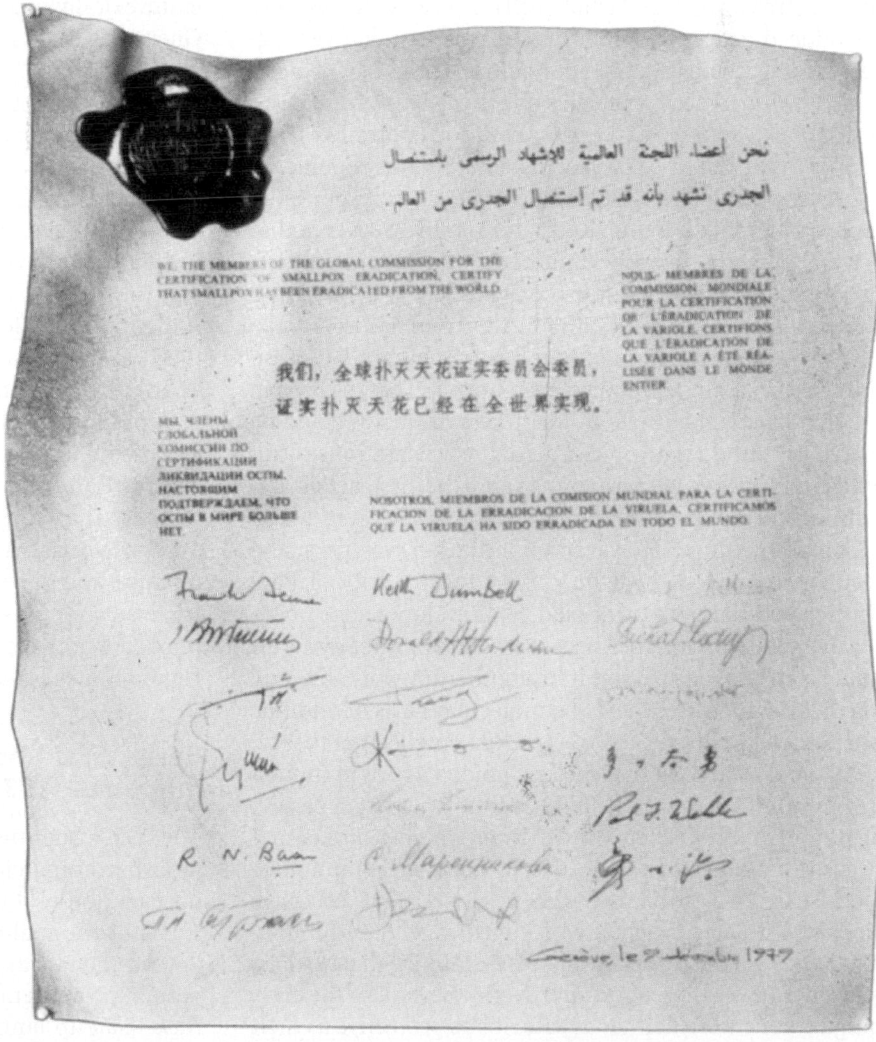

نحن أعضاء اللجنة العالمية للإشهاد الرسمي باستئصال
الجدري نشهد بأنه قد تم إستئصال الجدري من العالم.

WE, THE MEMBERS OF THE GLOBAL COMMISSION FOR THE CERTIFICATION OF SMALLPOX ERADICATION, CERTIFY THAT SMALLPOX HAS BEEN ERADICATED FROM THE WORLD.

NOUS, MEMBRES DE LA COMMISSION MONDIALE POUR LA CERTIFICATION DE L'ÉRADICATION DE LA VARIOLE, CERTIFIONS QUE L'ÉRADICATION DE LA VARIOLE A ÉTÉ RÉALISÉE DANS LE MONDE ENTIER.

我们，全球扑灭天花证实委员会委员，
证实扑灭天花已经在全世界实现。

МЫ, ЧЛЕНЫ ГЛОБАЛЬНОЙ КОМИССИИ ПО СЕРТИФИКАЦИИ ЛИКВИДАЦИИ ОСПЫ, НАСТОЯЩИМ ПОДТВЕРЖДАЕМ, ЧТО ОСПЫ В МИРЕ БОЛЬШЕ НЕТ.

NOSOTROS, MIEMBROS DE LA COMISION MUNDIAL PARA LA CERTIFICACION DE LA ERRADICACION DE LA VIRUELA, CERTIFICAMOS QUE LA VIRUELA HA SIDO ERRADICADA EN TODO EL MUNDO.

FIGURE 40.1 The parchment certifying global eradication of smallpox, 1979.

media lost their virulence. For example, *Pasteurella septica,* the cause of fowl cholera, when attenuated *in vitro* no longer caused disease. Rather, injection of such attenuated bacteria protected chickens from the effects of fresh, virulent cultures (6). With surprising speed, this idea was tested in a real-life setting. In 1881, the first tests of an attenuated anthrax vaccine were run, and in 1882, 85,000 sheep were immunized. Pasteur coined the word *vaccine* as a general term for immunizing preparations in homage to Edward Jenner and his use of vaccinia virus. Even though Pasteur did not know that rabies was caused by a virus rather than a bacterium and had to attenuate it in rabbit spinal cord rather than through culture, his introduction of rabies immunization on little Jacob Meister had a galvanic effect and was soon widely practiced. Crowned heads from all over the world came to pay honor to Pasteur, and he was able to build the Pasteur Institute in Paris entirely from benefactions. Founded in 1888, this Institute is of huge historic significance, as it was the first human institution entirely devoted to biomedical research.

Pasteur originally believed that microbes had to be alive to engender immunity, but following Koch's discovery of the cholera vibrio, killed whole-cell bacterial vaccines were introduced as early as 1896. Essentially similar, very reactogenic vaccines against typhoid fever and plague were shown to be at least partially effective. It is amazing to think that it took a further 60 years for controlled trials to show that this type of vaccine could confer significant short-term protection. But immunity research soon took quite a different direction. Roux and Yersin discovered that certain bacteria, notably diphtheria and tetanus bacilli, produced powerful soluble exotoxins, and von Behring and Kitasato discovered antibodies in 1890 and had some success in the passive immunotherapy of diphtheria, with antidiphtheria toxin antibodies from horses. This resulted in the first ever Nobel Prize in Medicine. Antitoxin could be mixed with the relatively crude toxin preparations available from culture supernatants, and the first active immunization against diphtheria or tetanus involved toxin-antitoxin mixtures. However, quantitation was poor and results variable. It took the genius and tenacity of Paul Ehrlich to bring rigor to the field. His development of quantitative methods for the measurement of antibody levels made von Behring's passive immunotherapy workable, and his theories on the cellular and molecular basis of immune phenomena gave the field tremendous intellectual thrust.

It could be argued that the first golden age of immunology (around 1880 to 1910) was accompanied by a certain degree of hubris. There was a time when it almost appeared that all that was needed to conquer communicable diseases was to isolate the causative agent, establish Koch's postulates, attenuate or kill the agent, and immunize. Yet from the earliest trials—for example, those of Pasteur on rabies—there was controversy. Several of the early preparations were neither as safe nor as protective as their protagonists claimed. Remember that neither production facilities nor regulatory agencies were well developed at this time, and the design of many of the clinical trials left much to be desired. Particular triumphs notwithstanding, broadly, the early promise of vaccines was not fully realized in the first golden age. There were significant professional reservations about vaccines and, in certain quarters, a distinctly antagonistic community reaction. The author was born in 1931, and it is quite clear that at that time, educated parents were by no means convinced about the advantages of immunization as a whole. Thus, the author had a good struggle with both diphtheria and whooping cough.

Early Bacterial Vaccines, Toxins, and Toxoids (1910 to 1930)

The flame of the live attenuated vaccine never died in the Pasteur Institute, and following Koch's isolation of the tubercle bacillus, the search for a tuberculosis (TB) vaccine began. Calmette and Guerin (7) started with an isolate of TB from a cow. After an amazing series of 213 subcultures over a period of 13 years, they intrepidly tried the culture orally in a newborn infant. Thus, Bacille Calmette-Guerin (BCG) was born. It was soon given intradermally rather than orally and was clearly effective in infants for the prevention of miliary TB and tuberculous meningitis, although its capacity to prevent adult pulmonary TB, the real killer in TB, is much more controversial.

World War I gave increased opportunity for the whole cell–killed bacterial vaccines to make their mark, especially in the case of typhoid, where systematic use seemed to control the disease despite the absence of a formal clinical trial. Another killed bacterial vaccine used fairly widely in the 1920s was that against *Bordetella pertussis*.

In 1923, Glenny discovered that formalin treatment of diphtheria toxin could render it harmless while preserving its immunogenic potential (8). At the Pasteur Institute, Ramon conducted similar studies. It was soon realized that these so-called toxoids were much more satisfactory as vaccines than the chancy toxin-antitoxin mixture, and their progressive introduction into the industrialized countries from about 1930 markedly lowered the impact of both diphtheria and tetanus. The decrease in the United States is over 99%.

Early Viral Vaccines: Yellow Fever and Influenza (1930 to 1950)

The 1920s saw the differences between viruses and bacteria becoming clear, and the 1930s was a heady period for isolation of disease-causing viruses, but tissue culture was still the realm of a few practitioners. An important development was Goodpasture's discovery of, and Burnet's improvement of, techniques for growing viruses and *Rickettsiae* in embryonated hen's eggs. Theiler's safe and effective live attenuated yellow fever vaccine, 17D, hails from this period, as do first-generation killed whole virus influenza vaccines and vaccines against typhus that were important for troops in World War II. Formalin-killed mouse brain–derived Japanese B encephalitis vaccine was also effective.

The Tissue Culture Revolution: Poliomyelitis, Measles, Mumps, Rubella (1950 to 1970)

The revolution in antiviral vaccines really began with the development of tissue culture as a way of growing viruses. The paper by Enders' group on the cultivation of the Lansing strain of the poliomyelitis virus in 1949 really was a watershed (9). It is difficult now to reconstruct the fear that surrounded poliomyelitis before 1955. Although the disease was epidemic in nature, waxing and waning with the summer seasons of maximum spread, it never went away. During a high incidence year, parents feared to send their children to the cinema or the swimming pool. Polio was a dreaded enemy. In the United States, for example, there were typically 20,000 or more cases of paralytic poliomyelitis per year. On April 12, 1955, the 10th anniversary of the death of Franklin D. Roosevelt, perhaps the most famous polio victim, a press conference at the University of Michigan revealed to the world that Dr. Jonas Salk's formalin-treated whole virus vaccine provided protection. Between 1955 and 1961, 300 million doses of the vaccine were administered, and polio declined dramatically. A major setback was the infamous Cutter Incident in which faulty production techniques allowed two lots of vaccine to slip through with inadequate formalin inactivation, resulting in 149 cases of polio, a disaster that lent impetus to the development of the live attenuated oral poliomyelitis vaccine of Sabin, first introduced in 1961. By 1965, this latter vaccine had essentially replaced the Salk vaccine in the United States, and soon after in most countries, although not in the Netherlands, Iceland, and Sweden. Being orally active, it was more convenient to use, and containing far fewer virions it was also much cheaper (Figure 40.2). Very rare reversions to neurovirulence, particularly in poliomyelitis virus type 3, (estimated at one case of acute flaccid paralysis per 2.7 million doses of oral poliomyelitis vaccine administered) have occasioned a rethink in the industrialized countries. Most now recommend injectable poliomyelitis vaccine again to obviate this very rare but extremely serious problem. The late Jonas Salk campaigned tirelessly for this reversion, the rivalry between him and Albert Sabin being legendary.

The great adventure of polio eradication is not quite finished, but there is no doubt that the dramatic success of polio immunization paved the way for a number of other live attenuated virus vaccines, again dependant on the principle of attenuation in tissue culture. Enders' original Edmondston strain of measles vaccine, first introduced in 1963, was a little bit "hot." When the author's younger son was born in 1964, the recommendation was to use this vaccine but to coadminister gamma globulin containing antimeasles antibodies! The problem was solved through the introduction of the more attenuated Moraten and Schwartz derivatives of the original Enders strain. This excellent measles vaccine was followed by a mumps vaccine first introduced in 1967 and a live attenuated rubella vaccine in 1968. Hilleman (10) records that a combined measles-mumps-rubella vaccine was the realization of a long-term dream achieved in 1969 and licensed in 1971. Now some firms have introduced a tetravalent measles-mumps-rubella-varicella vaccine. The potential to eliminate all four diseases from the industrialized countries is real. In several European countries, measles, mumps, and rubella transmission appears to have ceased, with the exception of imported cases.

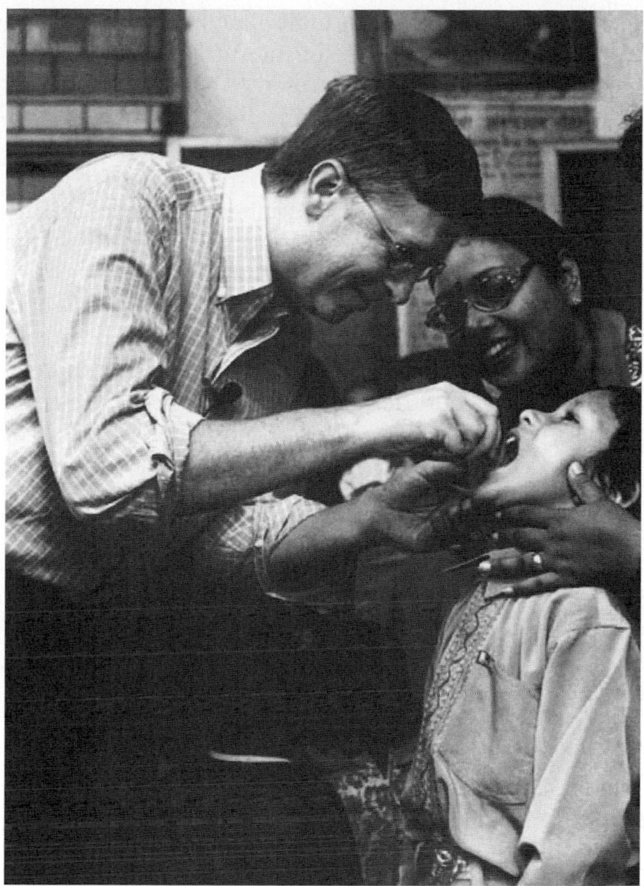

FIGURE 40.2 William H. Gates administering the Sabin oral poliomyelitis vaccine to an Indian child.

Dawn of the Molecular Era: Hepatitis B, Pneumococcus, *Hemophilus Influenzae B* (1970 to 1990)

Hepatitis B vaccine represented a watershed from several points of view. Although the toxoids and polysaccharide meningococcal vaccines are molecular or subunit vaccines from one point of view, use of the surface antigen of the hepatitis B virus (HBsAg) represented a new degree of purity of a single protein as a vaccine. It was also the first vaccine manufactured through recombinant DNA technology. It was the first example of a protein the tendency of which for self-assembly into 22nM virion-like particles greatly aided immunogenicity. Less obviously, it was the first time that a vaccine was introduced to the market as an expensive "boutique" vaccine for special risk groups such as doctors, nurses, and blood-bank workers, later to become a much cheaper public health tool of immense significance for developing countries. Given that there are 350 million carriers of hepatitis B worldwide and that 20% to 25% of carriers develop chronic liver disease, and a substantial proportion of these go on to primary hepatocellular carcinoma, the hepatitis B vaccine is the first anticancer vaccine in history. It is also unique in that the relevant antigen was originally thought to represent a protein polymorphism (Australia antigen) (11) and only later recognized as a viral component (12).

The great success of the hepatitis B vaccine has stilled many of society's fears about the use of recombinant DNA products and has certainly helped usher in the new era in which genetic engineering approaches have become the norm in vaccine research and development. It is to be hoped that the 18-year gap between Blumberg's discovery of Australia antigen and the development of the first generation blood-derived vaccine will not be repeated. Indeed, the time gap between cloning HBsAg and the yeast-derived vaccine was much shorter (13), and expression systems have improved enormously since that time.

Molecular vaccines of a different character were the subunit capsular polysaccharide vaccines against *Streptococcus pneumoniae, Neisseria meningitidis,* and *Hemophilus influenzae B* (Hib). These were licensed in the 1970s and early 1980s. Unfortunately, these vaccines do not work well in young infants, so another major molecular breakthrough was the conjugation of the carbohydrate antigens to a protein carrier, usually diphtheria or tetanus toxoid. This allowed effective T cell help and immunologic memory to develop. Various Hib conjugates were licensed in the late 1980s, effectively bringing us to the modern era. This progress will be summarized in the section on bacterial, viral, and parasitic vaccines.

KEY PRINCIPLES OF VACCINOLOGY

In the search for new vaccines, much effort is directed at identifying, isolating, and eventually manufacturing antigens from pathogens that are key to the pathogen's survival and multiplication within the host. These may be surface molecules, the neutralization of which may prevent infection; toxins that the invader uses for tissue destruction to provide a nidus for growth; or internal antigens, which can be processed and presented on infected cells provoking T cell–based destruction. It is important to realize that such pure antigens, when introduced into the body, do not necessarily induce an immune response. Indeed, pure, deaggregated proteins are more likely to induce immunologic tolerance. The first key principle in vaccinology, therefore, is to ensure immunogenicity of the material used.

Immunogenicity

To be immunogenic, a candidate vaccine generally has to reach an antigen presenting cell (APC), usually a dendritic cell. Furthermore, the APC, in its resting state, is not ready to initiate the immunoproliferative cascade; it must first be activated. In the past several years, our knowledge of these first important steps in the adoptive immune response has been greatly enhanced by analysis of innate immune responses used by invertebrate species against infection. The innate immune system is evolutionarily as old as multicellular life itself, namely around 2 billion years, but details of its molecular basis have only recently become apparent.

Janeway (14) first suggested the importance of "receptors that recognize patterns of microbial structure" and claimed a dual type of self/nonself discrimination, one among lymphocytes but the other based on APCs. It gradually became clear (15) that the innate immune system recognizes microorganisms via a limited number of germline-encoded pattern-recognition receptors (PRRs), whereas microbes possess pathogen-associated molecular patterns (PAMPs) that are integral to their structure and function. Different PRRs recognize different PAMPs, and although this limited germline-encoded and constitutively expressed repertoire of PRRs contrasts with the huge repertoire of rearranged T and B cell receptors, it nevertheless represents a valid and effective defense system. Amazingly, Janeway (14) foresaw in 1989 that the PRR–PAMP union would generate a stimulatory signal. The matter developed a new impetus with the strange saga of the Toll-like receptors (TLRs).

The Toll-like Receptors

Interleukin 1 (IL-1) is a key cytokine, and when it unites with the IL-1 receptor, a cascade of cellular signals is initiated that leads to activation of the NFκB transcription factor pathway and of MAP kinases. This in turn regulates the expression of genes involved in inflammation, immunity, and tissue repair. When it was found that a gene known as Toll, involved in dorsal-ventral polarization of the *Drosophila* embryo, was homologous to the cytoplasmic domain of the IL-1 receptor (16), insect scientists began to look for possible defense functions of the Toll gene. It was found that Toll was essential for protection against fungal infections (17). Toll was behaving like a PRR.

The search for mammalian homologues of Toll has been fruitful. To date, 12 members of the TLR family have been defined (15). All the TLRs are type 1 integral membrane glycoproteins with an extracellular domain containing leucine-rich repeats and an intracellular domain containing the IL-1-R homology. A given TLR can recognize two or more PAMPs that may not even be structurally related. Taken as an ensemble, the TLRs can recognize PAMPs of bacteria, viruses, parasites, fungi, and even some components of dead or dying cells. A partial list of TLR-PAMP interactions is given in Table 40.2 (modified from [15]). Note that TLRs can function as homodimers or heterodimers.

TLRs are expressed on dendritic cells (DCs) and macrophages, as well as on B and T cells, and nonimmunologic cells such as fibroblasts. Moreover, expression can be strongly upregulated—for example, by pathogens or cytokines. Some TLRs are expressed on the cell surface while others are found intracellularly—for example, in endosomes, in which case their ligands have to be internalized before TLR signaling can occur.

The complex signaling cascades that follow PAMP binding are gradually being unraveled. After ligand binding, TLRs dimerize and recruit adaptor molecules. Five have so far been identified (18), and it is likely that the differential responses mediated by different TLRs involve selective use of these adaptors. For example, the adaptor MyD88 (which is also used by the IL-1 receptor) initiates a cascade finally leading to the production of pro-inflammatory cytokines, whereas the adaptor TRIF sends the cascade in a direction ending with manufacture of type 1 interferons. In general terms, TLR stimulation leads to Th1 rather than Th2

TABLE 40.2 TLR Recognition of PAMPs

TLR	*PAMP*	*Bacterial Species*
TLR4	Lipopolysaccharide	Gram-negative bacteria
TLR2/TLR6	Diacyl lipopeptides	Mycoplasma
TLR1/TLR2	Triacyl lipopeptides	Mycobacteria and others
TLR2/TLR6	Lipoteichoic acid	Group B Streptococcus
TLR2	Peptidoglycan	Gram-positive bacteria
TLR2	Lipoarabinomannan	Mycobacteria
TLR5	Flagellin	Flagellated bacteria
TLR9	Unmethylated CpG motifs in DNA	Bacteria including mycobacteria
TLR11	Structure not determined	Uropathogenic bacteria
TLR	***PAMP***	***Viral Species***
TLR9	Unmethylated CpG motifs in DNA	DNA viruses (e.g., HSV-1 and 2
TLR3	Double-stranded RNA	RNA viruses-dsRNA as a replication intermediate
TLR7 and TLR8	Uridine or uridine/guaranosine rich single-stranded RNA	RNA viruses
TLR2 and TLR4	Various viral envelope glycoproteins	Various viruses such as measles, CMV and respiratory syncitial virus
TLR	***PAMP***	***Parasite Species***
TLR9	Hemozoin	*Plasmodium falciparum*
TLR2	Glycosylphosphatidyl isosital mucin	Trypanosomes
TLR4	Glycosylinositoll phospholipids	Trypanosomes
TLR11	Profilins	Toxoplasma
TLR	***PAMP***	***Fungal Species***
TLR6/TLR2	Zymosan	*Saccharomyces cerevisiae*
TLR2	Phospholipomannan	*Candida albicans*
TLR4	Mannan	*Candida albicans*
TLR2 and TLR4	Glucuronoxylomannan	*Cryptococcus neoformans*
TLR	***PAMPs That Are Host Components***	
TLR4	Heat shock proteins 60 and 70	
TLR4	Fibrinogen	
TLR12	So far an "orphan" TLR with PAMP not identified	

differentiation. However, some TLR-2 ligands can induce a Th2-bias (19), probably through the phosphorylation of ERK MAP kinase and induction of c-FOS, whereas other TLR-2 ligands such as zymosan can suppress T cell responses via a mechanism dependent on the anti-inflammatory cytokines IL-10 and TGF-β (20).

There are multiple subsets of DCs in both humans and mice. This raises the question of whether TLRs are differentially expressed within them and thus whether different DC subsets modulate immune responses (e.g., via Th1/Th2 balance) (21). For example, plasmacytoid DC in humans preferentially express TLR7 and TLR9 and also preferentially produce interferon-γ (22). At the same time activation of a given DC subset via distinct PRRs can differentially stimulate distinct types of T cell responses (23), illustrating the functional plasticity of DC. There is clearly a large amount of work that needs to be done before we can harness all this new knowledge for vaccine design. Nevertheless, in the section about adjuvants, we shall encounter examples of strategies critically involving TLRs.

Other PRRs in Innate Immunity

The avalanche of research on TLRs should not obscure the fact that there are other families of PRRs. Many pathogens activate complement via either the classical or alternative pathway, and complement fixation can be destructive. Pentraxins are a complex superfamily of multimeric (usually pentameric) proteins of which the best known are C-reactive protein, serum amyloid P component, and pentraxin 3 (PTX3). PTX3 is a key element of the humoral arm of innate immunity (24), and PTX3-deficient mice are highly susceptible to various bacterial and fungal infections. PTX3 activates complement and is an opsonin. It is evolutionarily conserved and has other functions in assembly of extracellular matrix and in fertility.

The mannose-binding lectin (MBL) is an evolutionarily conserved, circulating host defense protein with broad spectrum recognition capability against a wide variety of pathogens (25). It recognizes carbohydrate moieties such as D-mannose, L-fucose, and N-acetylglucosamine. MBL is synthesized predominantly in the liver and circulates as a multimer of homotrimers with the carbohydrate recognition domain attached via an α-helical coil to a collagen helix. MBL belongs to the collectin family of which four other members are known. There are endogenous as well as infectious ligands of MBL, including components of dying or of transformed cells. MBL is able to activate complement and act as an opsonin, and low levels of MBL can worsen susceptibility to infections in immunocompromised individuals. Interestingly, low levels of MBL render humans more susceptible to the SARS corona virus (26).

A second category of carbohydrate-binding lectins is the family of type II transmembrane proteins DC-SIGN, L-SIGN, SIGN-R1, and langerin (27). These molecules also have carbohydrate recognition domains, but this time associated with the surface of specific cells. As the name implies, DC-SIGN is specific for DCs and can recognize glycoproteins from several viruses and bacteria. Its homologues L-SIGN and (murine) SIGN-R1 show subtly different carbohydrate recognition profiles. Langerin is specific for Langerhans cells and plays an interesting role in presenting a nonpeptide (lipid) mycobacterial antigen to T cells (28). DC-SIGN can cluster into domains of 100 nm to 200 nm to help binding and internalization of virus particles (29) to increase the affinity for specific ligands. Finally, there is likely to be significant cross-talk between signaling through C-type lectins and through TLRs (27), indicating that the innate immune system is quite complex and sophisticated.

In the plant kingdom, there is a family of proteins, the plant R proteins, which are involved in resistance to pathogens (30). These exist both on the surface of plant cells and in the cytoplasm. The R proteins contain multiple leucine-rich repeats, a motif also found in the TLRs. It can be argued that all the surface R proteins resemble TLRs. What, then, might be the animal equivalent of the cytoplasmic R proteins? The best candidates are two closely related proteins, NOD1 and NOD2, which are capable of sensing bacterial lipopolysaccharide and bacterial muramyl dipeptide respectively (31). There is some evidence of synergy between NOD and TLR activation. An intriguing observation is that some familial cases of Crohn's disease have a partial loss of function mutation in the gene encoding NOD2. This raises the possibility that incorrect sensing of gut bacteria contributes to the intestinal inflammation, although NOD-"knockout" mice show no intestinal pathology. A number of other cytoplasmic pathogen recognition systems have recently been reviewed (15).

A further set of recognition phenomena relates to signals that warn an animal of "danger." Matzinger's original danger hypothesis suggested that the key signal came from stressed or damaged tissue (32), and this received support when necrotic, but not apoptotic, cells were shown to be capable of stimulating APC via TLR-2 (33). However, the notion can also be broadened to include danger signaled by pathogens. Both tissue injury and micro-organismal invasion provoke the rapid release of diverse host proteins that are potent immunostimulants and for which the novel term *alarmins* has been proposed (34). These mediators include defensins, cathelicidin, eosinophil-derived neurotoxin, and high-mobility group box protein 1. Members of the cationic host defense (antimicrobial) peptide family are found in every complex species (35). These amphipathic molecules are 12 to 50 amino acids long, are rich in arginine and lysine, and have up to 50% hydrophobic residues. Defensins and cathelicidins have direct antimicrobial activity against bacteria, viruses, parasites, and fungi, but also act as immune system modulators (36), stimulating immune activation but also defending the host against excessive inflammation. Therapeutic potential is being explored (e.g., for prevention of catheter-associated infections [37] or as adjuvants). Oppenhein and Yang believe many more alarmins remain to be identified (34). They cite recent evidence showing the DC-activating potential of several chemokines and granulysin and express the hope that further research on alarmins will lead to less toxic adjuvants.

Intensive though the work of the past decade has been on the interface between innate and adaptive immunity, the impression remains that we are really only at the beginning of this field. When we understand it more completely, we shall have powerful means of ensuring greater and safer immunogenicity of our vaccines.

REACTOGENICITY

Long before we knew about all the danger signals discussed in this chapter thus far, it was realized that effective vaccines often produced mild side-reactions. We shall consider serious adverse effects of vaccines in a later section, but the mild reactions fall under two headings. Live attenuated vaccines, such as those against smallpox or measles, involve the replication of the altered microorganism in the host, and in a proportion of cases a very minor version of the disease to be prevented can occur (e.g., with vaccinia, a nasty sore at the scarification site and local lymphadenopathy; with measles, a very mild rash and transient fever). Vaccines consisting of killed microbes or materials from them can cause local redness, swelling, and pain at the injection site and some mild systemic reactions such as transient fever, irritability, anorexia, headache, and general malaise. It must be stressed that in the vast majority of cases these reactions are mild, of short duration, and easily controlled by an antipyretic such as paracetamol.

These symptoms arise because immunogenic vaccines cause some inflammation and cytokine induction. Together they reflect the *reactogenicity* of a vaccine. Given that there is a great deal of individual variation, it is nevertheless the case that some vaccines are more reactogenic than others. Remembering that vaccines are given to healthy rather than sick individuals, and frequently to infants, a balance needs to be struck between acceptable reactogenicity and the seriousness of the disease to be prevented. A medical officer sent to control an outbreak of bubonic plague will accept greater reactogenicity than the mother of an infant needing protection against whooping cough. For the established vaccines, experience and progressive modification of formulations have provided the requisite balance. For vaccines still in the research phase, such as an anti-malaria vaccine, the equation is still being worked out. Paradoxically but fortunately, reactogenicity tends to be less in very young infants. On the other hand, it can be a real problem in immunocompromised individuals where the risk:benefit equation needs to be evaluated on a case-by-case basis.

Age at Immunization

A further key principle is that particular vaccines have to be given at the appropriate age. For example, hepatitis B can be acquired during the birth process, and immunization within the first 12 hours of life is recommended, followed by two later doses. However, the live attenuated measles vaccine is strongly inhibited by the presence of antibodies coming from the mother, so it is only given at 12 months of age in industrialized countries and at 9 months in developing countries. The standard "platform" of diphtheria-pertussis-tetanus vaccination consists of injections at 2, 4, and 6 months of age, with a booster at 15 to 18 months. In recent years, other vaccines have been added to this platform, as we shall see later in this chapter, while still others are not recommended before 12 months. Certain vaccines (e.g., against the pneumococcus or the influenza virus) are particularly relevant to saving lives among the aged, although progressively being recommended at younger ages. Some vaccines have their maximum value when given around the time of puberty (e.g., the human papilloma virus ([HPV] vaccine to prevent cervical cancer or the rubella vaccine for the prevention of intrauterine rubella, though the latter is now given earlier as part of a combination vaccine).

Vaccines for travelers represent a special case, particularly as some, such as those against cholera and typhoid fever, tend to protect for relatively short periods.

An area as yet insufficiently studied is that of booster-immunization in adolescence or adult life. We are all familiar with the tetanus "shots" given when we are injured to boost our childhood immunity. Recent epidemics of diphtheria have suggested that adults lose their immunity rather easily, so boosters every 10 years are recommended, but this is more honored in the breach than the observance. It is also likely that pertussis is a more common cause of severe respiratory disease in adults than is generally realized, so pertussis boosters could be useful.

Disease Burden and Cost-benefit Considerations

In the United States, there are new vaccines licensed against about 30 diseases, and the research pipeline shows that about 75 more diseases are being targeted for future prevention (38). In many cases, several different approaches are being taken to a particular disease. This illustrates the scope of the priority-setting exercise facing the world. In the industrialized countries, the key question is how many injections will the mothers of our infants tolerate, thus there is a big premium on the preparation of combinations of vaccines, where the large pharmaceutical firms are doing well, and on oral and other mucosal or transdermal delivery methods, where progress is slower. In the developing countries, cost is a major consideration, and a great deal of effort is going into the analysis of disease burden and cost-benefit considerations. This is no easy task as in many developing countries microbial diagnostic facilities are limited, so exact causation of pneumonia, meningitis or diarrhea is hard to establish. Furthermore, a surprising degree of variation in disease incidence between neighboring countries or different regions within a single country has been noted. This suggests that disease burden may have to be established in many places where the case for universal immunization is not self-evident. Of course there are diseases of such huge importance, such as HIV/AIDS, malaria, tuberculosis, or invasive pneumococcal disease, where a vaccine would clearly be a breakthrough product, but there are other examples, such as *Hemophilus influenzae B* in Asia, where some doubt remains. Dr. John Clemens, the director of the International Vaccine Institute in Seoul, Korea, believes there are examples where only an intervention trial involving vaccination and examining mortality statistics will provide reliable answers.

Societal Acceptance and Cultural Considerations

Vaccinology must also accommodate variations in societal acceptance of vaccines. There are some paradoxes here. In industrialized nations, the very success of immunization has made epidemics (e.g., of diphtheria, poliomyelitis, or measles) essentially things of the past. This gives anti-vaccine activists an advantage, but it is still the case that when immunization coverage rates fall below a threshold, typically around 80% of the population, a disease may become resurgent. As a further paradox, in developing countries where overall educational standards are low, an anti-vaccine rumor can gain extraordinarily wide acceptance. A recent case in point involved Nigeria, where the belief that the poliomyelitis vaccine represented a plot to render female Muslim babies sterile gained such currency that in mid-2003 immunization was essentially suspended. As a result, the resurgent virus caused disease not only in Nigeria but also through importation in many other countries.

The key to societal acceptance of vaccines is education. Well-planned and executed educational campaigns, especially involving the mass media, can have a major effect. Paradoxes remain, however. In the United Kingdom, a cleverly targeted campaign preceded the introduction of universal vaccination against *Neisseria meningitidis* serogroup C, including alerting people to the fact that only *some* forms of meningitis could be prevented. Immunization proved hugely successful. Yet a community of such sophistication was sufficiently scared by claims that the measles-mumps-rubella vaccine caused autism and Crohn's disease that a measles eradication campaign that had been going well was effectively derailed. It took some years for common sense to return.

A final reflection is that the proportion of people who strongly and consistently harbor anti-vaccine sentiments is actually quite small, perhaps 2%. The last paradox is that their refusal to have infants immunized does not matter as much as it might, because herd immunity will look after their children.

ADJUVANTS

The term *adjuvant* is a wide one and refers to the broad spectrum of substances or stratagems that are able to increase the immunogenicity of antigens incorporated into or coadministered with the adjuvant in question. O'Hagan and Valiente (39) have recently proposed a classification of adjuvants into immune potentiators on the one hand (e.g., TLR agonists), or antigen delivery systems on the other (e.g., emulsions or microparticles attractive to APC). The trouble with this otherwise useful suggestion is that many adjuvants represent a combination of these two principles. Pearse and Drane (40) have proposed the term *integrated adjuvants* for such cases.

One reflection of the difficulty of this field is that, despite the enormous amount of work that has been done, particularly in recent years, there are only two licensed adjuvant approaches. Overwhelmingly, the more common is alum, comprising aluminium phosphate and aluminium hydroxide, which we shall describe. Also, an emulsion adjuvant known as MF59 is licensed in Italy (41). Of course, some vaccines have their own "built in" adjuvanticity, such as BCG, a live attenuated tubercle bacillus, or the vaccinia virus for smallpox prevention. The difficulty in finding an ideal adjuvant rests in retaining adjuvant properties but avoiding worrying reactogenicity. We know from experimental animal work that different adjuvants bias the immune response toward antibody formation or cell-mediated immunity, and further toward particular antibody isotypes or certain T cell subsets. Now that pathogen genome mining as well as conventional vaccine research have yielded such a wealth of candidate antigens, the search for the right adjuvant for each vaccine has become somewhat of a "Holy Grail" in vaccinology.

To set the stage for a description of the more promising modern candidate adjuvants, we begin with a brief historical survey of the field.

Empirical Approaches to the Design of Adjuvants

Long before the TLRs were recognized, a great deal of empirical research had resulted in a variety of adjuvants that are now understood a little better. For example, it was realized that particulate antigens, readily scavenged by APCs, were much more immunogenic than soluble antigens. As early as 1926, Glenny et al. (42) noted that alum precipitation of diphtheria toxoid, creating a microparticulate antigen, considerably increased immunogenicity. It was found that killed bacteria could nonspecifically raise immune responsiveness, and *Mycobacterium tuberculosis* was very effective. Jules Freund combined killed tubercle bacteria with the absorption-delaying effects of mineral oil, creating the strong and widely used Freund's adjuvant (43). This caused far too serious local and systemic reactions for human use, and in many countries, is now no longer deemed appropriate for experimental animals either, prompting a search for less toxic bacteria-derived products retaining adjuvant properties. It was realized even in Freund's day, however, that the adjuvant could guide the direction of the immune response. Freund's adjuvant promotes both antibody formation and delayed-type hypersensitivity reactions, but when the mycobacteria are omitted, as in Freund's incomplete adjuvant, only antibody formation results.

In experimental immunology, various bacteria other than killed *M. tuberculosis* are used as adjuvants. It appears that if a killed bacterial preparation is itself highly antigenic, the adjuvant power spills over to the response to an antigen coadministered with it. Some guidance may also be given to the response. Killed *Bordetella pertussis* organisms are a strong Th2/antibody formation adjuvant for pure protein antigens. *Corynebacterium parvum* is more of a Th1 adjuvant. Turning to a parasite, *Nippostrongylus brasiliensis,* has long been used if one wishes to elicit powerful immunoglobulin E (IgE) responses.

Aluminum Compounds as Adjuvants

Aluminum hydroxide and aluminum phosphate are the two most commonly used adjuvants. Two chief methods underlie alum adjuvants: either *in situ* precipitation of aluminum compounds in the presence of antigen, or adsorption of antigen onto preformed aluminum gel. The latter is now more commonly used, as alum precipitation is quite demanding and batch-to-batch variation is a significant problem. The insoluble particles that result are less than 10 μM in diameter and may be as small as 0.1 μM. Alum adjuvants promote good antibody formation but little or no DTH or CD8$^+$ T cell–mediated cytotoxicity. They can lead to significant IgE responses, which on the one hand may be advantageous for anti-parasite vaccines, but on the other hand, can lead to hypersensitivity to the antigen in question. Overall, the safety record of alum is good, but occasionally local reactions can be troublesome. Properly formulated alum adjuvants are thus very satisfactory for diseases that can be prevented by serum IgG antibodies.

Emulsions as Adjuvants

Emulsions and emulsifying reagents have been central to adjuvant research. Incomplete Freund's adjuvant was used in the 1950s for the human influenza vaccine but never passed the regulatory hurdles. Companies have continued to improve their formulations, which may also contain one or more chemical promoters of immunogenicity. Both water-in-oil and oil-in-water emulsions can be used, and the oil can be of mineral, vegetable, animal, or synthetic origin. Stabilization by a surfactant is important, as is the nature of the emulsifying agent.

The firm SEPPIC has been promoting water-in-oil emulsions for human use, namely Montanide ISA51 and Montanide ISA720, which have been used in numerous phase I and II trials. Montanide ISA720 is of special interest because it has been used in HIV, malaria, and cytomegalovirus (CMV) vaccine trials. The adjuvant contains a natural, metabolizable oil and a highly refined mannide oleate emulsifier. Seventy parts of adjuvant are mixed with 30 parts of the aqueous, antigen-containing medium and homogenized, yielding watery droplets 0.3 to 3 μM in diameter, the emulsion being stable at 4°C for at least 2 years. The adjuvant promotes antibody formation and significant cytotoxic T cell activity.

The firm Chiron (now Novartis) has clinical experience going back 15 years with an oil-in-water emulsion known as MF59. This is now registered in Italy for use with an influenza vaccine (Fluad) and has been used in millions of doses. It has been found to be very safe and effective. The droplets of the metabolizable oil squalene are about 0.15 μM in diameter, and the other components are polysorbate 80, sorbitan trioleate, trisodium citrate dihydrate, and citric acid monohydrate. The preparation is surprisingly nonviscous, and thus easy to use and minimally reactogenic. The emulsion is stable at 2°C to 8°C for at least 3 years. MF59 is a good promoter of antibody formation and of Th2 type CD4$^+$ T cell responses but not of cytotoxic T cells in subhuman primates or human subjects.

The Syntex adjuvant formulation (SAF) is another oil-in-water emulsion, but it is noteworthy for also containing the immunostimulatory compound threonyl-muramyl dipeptide (threonyl-MDP) (44). This agent has an interesting history, going back to the early days of the search for the immunopotentiating chemicals in bacteria. Ellouz et al. (45), searching for the minimal structural requirements needed for the adjuvant properties of bacterial peptidoglycans, found that *N*-actetyl-muramyl- *L*-analyl- *D*-isoglutamine, or MDP, powerfully promoted both antibody formation and cell-mediated immunity. There have been variations on the theme; Allison and Byars (44) claimed that the threonyl derivative is less toxic and more powerful. The SAF emulsion vehicle also contains the nonionic block polymer surfactant poloxamer 401, which has adjuvant properties in its own right. The metabolizable oil is squalene, and the emulsifier is polysorbate 80. The adjuvant has elicited both cell-mediated and humoral immune responses with a variety of antigens. However, it does not appear to be progressing rapidly to clinical use, perhaps because the MDP component is, after all, too reactogenic.

Modern "Designer" Adjuvants

The major pharmaceutical companies involved in vaccine research have rapidly applied modern principles to rational adjuvant design. Up till now, each company has gone more or less its own way, and "head to head" comparisons of adjuvants are rare. This may soon change, as the Bill & Melinda Gates Foundation's Global HIV/AIDS Enterprise is funding research with precisely this aim. Some prominent examples of modern adjuvants follow.

AS02, GlaxoSmithKline Biologicals

AS02 is an integrated adjuvant comprising an oil-in-water emulsion to which two separate chemical immunostimulants have been added. These are 3D-MPL and QS21. Monophosphoryl lipid A (MPL) is the best product remaining from an important line of work. This sought to take the LPS endotoxins of gram-negative bacteria such as *Escherichia, Pseudomonas,* or *Salmonella* (now known to be strong TLR agonists) and to extract from them less toxic adjuvants. MPL is modified from lipid A and is much less toxic (46) but powerfully immunostimulatory; 3D-MPL is a further derivative. QS21 is an adjuvant derived from the bark of the South American tree *Quillaja saponaria.* Crude extracts consisting of a mixture of tannins, polyphenolics, and triterpene glycoside saponins were found to be immunostimulatory. A saponin mixture known as Quill A was a somewhat purer preparation, and when it was fractionated by high-performance liquid chromatography into at least 23 components, QS21 emerged as the saponin with the most power and least toxicity (47). QS21 strongly stimulates both T cell–dependent and T cell–independent antibody formation as well as cell-mediated immunity, including CD8$^+$ T cell cytotoxicity.

Not surprisingly, therefore, AS02 proved to be a powerful adjuvant in rodents, subhuman primates, and humans. In human malaria vaccine trials (see later discussion), it caused rapid and strong antibody formation, Th1 T cell proliferation with IFN-γ production, and CD8$^+$ cytotoxic T lymphocytes (CTL) responses (48). In HIV vaccine studies in Rhesus monkeys, the same results were obtained, and T cell immunity was impressive with two *M. tuberculosis* antigens in the same species. Given that antibody and T cell responses were both strong, GlaxoSmithKline saw this adjuvant as holding promise for HIV/AIDS, malaria, tuberculosis and cancer, obviously all in the long term.

Iscomatrix^{TM}, CSL Limited

Early immunologists were quick to realize that poorly immunogenic proteins could become more stimulatory as microparticles or microaggregates, such as through mild heat aggregation of serum proteins. Similarly, the property of physiological self-assembly can increase immunogenicity, as when the soluble hepatitis B protein self-assembles into virus-like particles. ISCOMs, or immunostimulating complexes, are a variation on this theme. Initially (49) these were microparticles consisting of lipids, saponins, and antigens (typically membrane proteins from enveloped viruses) that form spontaneously under the correct conditions. They are hollow, spherical particles of approximately 40nM diameter with a characteristic cage-like morphology when examined electron microscopically using negative staining techniques. The immunostimulatory properties of saponin derived from the bark of the *Quillaja saponaria* tree have long been known, but associated toxicity is considerable. Early ISCOM preparations used the purer forms Quil A and QS21, but reactogenicity was still observed, probably due to the hemolytic nature of the free saponin. ISCOMATRIX^{TM} is a further development of the technology (40) that appears to be suitable for human use. The saponin used is known as ISCOPREP and is a well-defined, extensively characterized fraction. The lipids used are Di-palmytoil phosphatidyl choline and cholesterol. These are chemically defined and synthetic. Saponin and lipid in the nonionic detergent Decanoyl-N-methylglucamide are incubated with a buffer and the ISCOMATRIX preparation forms. The incorporation of the saponin into the nanostructures removes the hemolytic activity and severe reactogenicity. At this stage, unlike the original ISCOMs, ISCOMATRIX has no antigen within it, which must now be added. If the protein is positively charged, electrostatic interactions with the negatively charged adjuvant will ensure tight association. Procedures for modifying either the protein or the adjuvant to maximize association have been developed, and a range of more specific coupling procedures has also been developed (50). Correctly formulated, these vaccines induce antibodies of all IgG isotypes, even in the presence of preexisting or passively acquired antibody. As well, strong CD8$^+$ T cell responses ensue.

Clinical experience with this adjuvant is now substantial. Two studies with an *E. coli* expressed, purified HPV16 E6E7 fusion protein in 60 women and men showed the vaccine to be safe and well tolerated, inducing humoral immune responses at all doses and cellular immune responses at the highest dose (51). Effective responses were also obtained in 55 people receiving intramuscular and 24 people receiving intranasal trivalent split virion influenza vaccine. A promising study has been conducted with the hepatitis C virus (HCV) core protein. Thirty male subjects received three immunizations of vaccine or placebo on days 0, 28, and 56. Antibody responses resulted in all but one of the HCV-immunized subjects, and specific T cell responses in subjects given the highest dose. A phase II study is underway in the hope that a therapeutic vaccine for chronic HCV infection might emerge.

Oligodeoxyribonucleotides Containing CpG motifs (CpG ODN)

There is a long history of attempting to use nucleic acids as adjuvants. In the 1960s, there was quite a vogue for using the polynucleotides polyI:C and polyA:U, known stimulators of interferon production, as experimental immunostimulators. The field took on an altogether different and more promising dynamic as a result of the work of Tokunaga et al. (52). These investigators were interested in the antitumor potential of BCG, noted that much of it was in the DNA fraction, and drew attention to particular sequences of oligodeoxyribonucleotides (ODN). Subsequently, using shorter ODN, they discovered that palindromic hexamers, each of which contains nonmethylated CpG dinucleotides, are responsible for immune activation, measured in their case by induction of interferon production by natural killer (NK) cells. Krieg et al. (53) established that the minimal immunostimulatory sequence was unmethylated 5′-Pur-Pur-CpG Pyr-Pyr-3′. Methylation of the cytosine was found to reduce activity. Because mammalian DNA contains fourfold fewer CpG dinucleotides than mammalian genomic DNA, and because 70% of these are methylated whereas bacterial cytosines rarely are, there arose the speculation that the mammalian innate immune system evolved to recognize the bacteria-specific pattern (54). This was well before the recognition of the TLR-9 receptor as the relevant PRR for CpG motifs as PAMPs.

Krieg and Davis of Coley Pharmaceuticals (55) have argued that CpG ODN is the strongest Th1-inducing adjuvant yet discovered. In humans, its PRR, TLR-9 is found only on B cells and plasmcytoid DC. Through its action on these cells, CpG ODN causes improved antigen presentation and the production of high levels of Th1 cytokines. Three main families of CpG ODN, termed *A, B,* and *C,* have been identified (56). The A class is a powerful activator of NK cells and DC but a poor stimulator of B lymphocytes. The B class, most frequently used in studies published to date, is a strong stimulator of B cells and DC but weaker for induction of NK cells or IFN-γ. The most recently discovered C class combines both sets of properties and also induces strong $CD8^+$ CTL responses. Species differences in effectiveness have been most extensively studies for the B class. The CpG that works best for mice is the hexamer GACGTT, but for humans GTCGTT is preferred. Two to three hexamers are optimal, best separated by at least two intervening bases, preferably Ts. The presence of poly-G flanking sequences is helpful as is a phosphorothioate backbone. The immune stimulatory effects are enhanced by a TpC dinucleotide on the 5′ end and by being pyrimidine rich on the 3′ side.

CpG ODN has been validated as a strong adjuvant in many studies (55). Model pure protein antigens, important pathogen-derived antigens such as hepatitis B surface antigen, hepatitis C envelope protein, influenza virus, and HIV gp160 have all been used, as well as many others. Further, CpG ODN can synergize with other adjuvants, such as alum, QS21, or MPL. Human studies have included trials with a commercial hepatitis B vaccine where, remarkably, a single dose induced sero-protection in 75% of subjects. In another trial involving 60 healthy volunteers, the B class ODN CPG7909, a 24-mer, was given with the influenza vaccine Fluarix^R and although the results were not dramatic, the suggestion was that lower vaccine doses could be used if the adjuvant was present (57).

Another company, Dynavax Technologies, terms its products *immunostimulatory sequences,* or ISS. Apart from infectious diseases, where targets include hepatitis B, hepatitis C, and HIV, Dynavax is especially interested in allergy, with ISS covalently linked to allergens being seen as a possible treatment. The motif AACGTTCG is considered superior to the hexamer AACGTT, and Dynavax has published extensively on the compound 1018, which is 5′-TGACTGTGAACGTTCGAGATGA-3′, but has also used other oligonucleotides. When 1018 was covalently coupled to the ragweed pollen antigen Amb a 1, the conjugate included a strong Th1-type response in mice, in contrast to Amb a 1 alone, which led to a Th2 response (58). Moreover, when peripheral blood mononuclear cell cultures from ragweed-allergic subjects were stimulated *in vitro* with the conjugate, the resulting cytokine profile was IFNγ dominated, and even when the cells had been pre-stimulated with Amb a 1 (leading to a Th2 response), the conjugate induced IFNγ production and partially inhibited IL-4 and IL-5 production.

Given these promising results, Dynavax went on to a phase II clinical trial in 27 hay fever sufferers, achieving good allergen-specific IgG levels. Randomized, placebo-controlled phase III trials have started. A phase I/II clinical trial of HBsAg linked to the ISS molecule has also begun.

It therefore appears that the CpG oligonucleotides have a promising future in both immunoprophylaxis and immunotherapy of various kinds. Further aspects of interest are that they can be used as mucosal adjuvants; that, in mice, they stimulate immune responses at a very young age; and that they allow immunogenicity even in the presence of preexisting antibody. Given this information, it is perhaps a matter of some concern that the clinical development of these adjuvants does not appear to have moved much further since the last edition of this textbook.

A further elaboration of the CpG ODN story comes from the work of Adamsson et al. (59). The ODN, in this case CpG ODN 2006, a 24-mer containing four CpGs, was chemically conjugated to the nontoxic B subunit of cholera toxin (CTB). Simple admixture of CTB (a well-known mucosal adjuvant) and ODN had no enhancing effect, but chemical linkage resulted in marked potentiation of cytokine and chemokine responses in human peripheral blood mononuclear cells or murine splenocytes. Mice immunized with tetanus toxoid and the conjugate showed much greater antibody responses and a tilting toward Th1 isotypes and IFNγ production. The effects were mediated through the expected TLR9/MyD88 and NFκB–dependant pathway.

Lipidated, T Cell-Helped, TLR2-Targeted Peptide Vaccines

Jackson's group (60) has come up with an interesting simple generic peptide-based vaccine structure that they term *self-adjuvating* and that promotes both antibody and cytotoxic T cell responses. The vaccines are totally synthetic and essentially consist of three components, namely a single helper T cell epitope, a target epitope of interest (which may concern either antibody or T cell receptors), and a TLR2-targeting lipid moiety with strong adjuvant properties. The T helper epitope is generic for different vaccines. The target epitope is specific for each particular vaccine and can be either a class I major histocompatibility complex (MHC)–restricted epitope for cytotoxic T cell responses or an epitope recognized by antibody where a humoral response is desired. The T helper epitope is contiguous with and N-terminal to the target epitope. In most cases the Th epitope was KLIPNASLIENCTKAEL from the canine distemper virus, but in some cases GALNNRFQIKGVELKS from influenza virus hemagglutinin. The Th epitope and the target epitope were separated by a single lysine residue. The lipid was Pam2Cys, a TLR2-targeting ligand closely related to the well-known Pam3Cys (N-palmytoil-S-[2,3bis (palmytoyloxy) propy]-cysteine), which has long been known as a strong adjuvant. Pam2Cys (Dipalmytoil-S-glycerylcysteine) is the lipid component of the macrophage-activating lipopeptide-2 isolated from mycoplasma and can readily be synthesized. It was attached to the lysine separating the two peptides through two serine residues. The use of a branched geometry in the construction of these vaccines is based on Jackson's previous work showing that a branched structure is significantly more immunogenic than the same epitopes in a tandem linear array, as well as more soluble.

In the mouse, the lipopeptides were effective experimental vaccines in diverse disease models requiring CD8^{+} T cell immunity including two tumor models, live *Listeria monocytogenes* challenge, or influenza virus recovery. Antibody responses to peptides from model hormone antigens were also markedly enhanced, the efficacy equaling that of complete Freund's adjuvant. The lipopeptides also work in dogs, and early clinical trials are being planned.

Inulin-derived Adjuvants

Inulin is a simple inert plant-derived polysaccharide consisting of a family of linear β-D-(2$\rightarrow$1) polyfructofuranosyl α-D-glucoses. A particulate form, known as gamma inulin (γ-IN) is a powerful complement activator and is an effective adjuvant capable of boosting both cell-mediated and humoral immunity (61). It appears to be remarkably nontoxic and has proven to be superior to alum in many animal models, on occasion outperforming Freund's complete adjuvant. A very small human study showed it to be effective in stimulating T cell responses to the ET protein of HPV16 in cervical cancer cases. More extensive human trials are now planned.

Liposomes, Virosomes, and Virus-like Particles

Liposomes have some but not all of the features of ISCOMs. Alving's group has obtained a good adjuvant effect using liposomes with cholera and malaria antigens. They have also obtained quite promising results using envelope protein peptides in a simian immunodeficiency virus (SIV) trial with macaque monkeys (62). The liposomes contain dimyristoyl phosphatidyl choline, dimyristoyl phosphatidyl glycerol, cholesterol, and monophosphoryl lipid A. In some experiments liposomes were alum adsorbed. Liposomes have also acted as adjuvants for diphtheria toxoid, tetanus toxoid, and a variety of hepatitis antigens. There is a great capacity to vary the particle size of liposomes, from approximately c.20 nM up to more than 10 μm in diameter. In general, liposomes are best used together with some other adjuvant.

Virosomes are multimeric aggregates of virus-derived transmembrane proteins (e.g., influenza hemagglutinin), and proteosomes are similar multimers of bacterial transmembrane proteins. They consist of 60 nM to 100 nM vesicles or membrane vesicle fragments. Amphipathic immunogens can be incorporated into these structures. These agents do not induce cell-mediated immunity unless an appropriate further adjuvant is added. Glück, of the Swiss Serum and Vaccine Institute, has been a strong proponent of the virosome approach. He has used influenza virus virosomes as a delivery system for, for example, hepatitis A and B or diphtheria and tetanus antigens (63), or as a mucosal vaccination strategy against influenza itself (64). In the latter case, hemagglutinin and neuraminidase were extracted from influenza virus, and phosphatidylcholine liposomes also containing the mucosal adjuvant *E. coli* heat-labile toxin at 1μg per dose were prepared. Two nasal spray immunizations induced good humoral responses in adult human volunteers, with significant salivary IgA. Elderly subjects also tolerated the vaccine well.

Virus-like particles (VLPs) are the results of self-assembly of virus capsid proteins. The considerable success of the hepatitis B vaccine owes much to the strong immunogenicity of the HBsAg particles. Similarly, the major capsid protein of the HPV is strongly immunogenic as a VLP. It has also been possible to incorporate other proteins into HBsAg VLPs and thus to enhance their immunogenicity.

Other Methods of Rendering Antigens Particulate

There are other ways of effecting a polymerization of antigens such as association with polymers. Nonionic block copolymers, usually used as additives to adjuvants employing an emulsion, are polymers of polyoxypropylene and polyoxyethylene, with which antigen can be associated. They have been used as components of complex adjuvant formulations by both Syntex and Ribi Chemical Co. These formulations induce a good Th1 response.

Carbohydrate polymers of mannose (e.g., mannan) or of β1-3 glucose (e.g., glucan) have been used in a similar manner. It is possible to conjugate peptides to mannan via an aminocaproic spacer and thereby produce a good antibody response. Mannan can also enhance the adjuvant properties of LPS. Part of the action may result from the stimulation of macrophages, which have a mannan-binding receptor.

Other surface active agents include dimethyl dioctadecyl ammonium bromide, avridine, and polyphosphazenes. Carbohydrate polymers with adjuvant properties include mannans as noted earlier, glucans, and dextrans. An interesting parasite-derived adjuvant is the *Leishmania* protein LeIF. This list is by no means exhaustive.

Microencapsulation of Antigens

This idea combines several desirable principles for adjuvants. Biodegradable microcapsules are particulate. They can enclose immunostimulatory molecules as well as antigen. They delay absorption of antigen and act as long-term depots. Best of all, they offer the hope that different chemical compositions will create particles that release their antigen as a pulse at various defined times after injection. Variables that affect the timing of release include particle size and the composition of the polymer. An ideal preparation would be a mixture of particles dissolving at intervals to mimic a primary dose and two booster doses.

Several laboratories share the credit for the development of controlled-release vaccine through encapsulation. The idea of biodegradable microcapsules containing antigens was promoted by Chang (65) and put into practice by Langer (66). The currently most popular material, the polymer poly(lactide-co-glycolide) (PLG), was first used by O'Hagan et al. (67) and by Eldridge et al. (68). This material was a happy choice because PLG has been used for many years as a biodegradable suture material. In that context, it has shown itself to be safe and nonreactogenic. PLG degrades by hydrolysis. How long this takes is determined both by chain length and by the ratio of lactide to glycolide in the polymer. The WHO has sponsored a considerable amount of work on PLG in the hope of coming up with a "one shot" formulation, which in the first instance could be applied to the problem of neonatal tetanus in developing countries. As infant immunization rates were low for women now of childbearing age, the WHO programs aim to immunize pregnant women with tetanus toxoid so that the newborn infants would be protected by antibodies crossing the placenta. However, it is difficult to persuade these women to make three trips to their local health center, which may require hours of walking. Once the controlled-release strategy has been perfected for this purpose, it could be adapted to other vaccines, such as hepatitis B or Hib.

Many frustrating problems have been encountered in this endeavor, but they are gradually being overcome one by one. The most important problem relates to stability of antigens in microparticles, both during the manufacturing process and *in vivo*. Further, although the lactide-to-glycolide ratio in PLG affects degradation rate, it was found in practice that a mixture of two different sets of microcapsules resulted not in sharp peaks of antigen release but rather in continuous release over a period. This seems to produce satisfactory antibody responses. It is now clear that, in preclinical studies, one injection of antigen in microcapsules can lead to higher and more sustained antibody formation than can two injections of antigen adsorbed onto alum.

Cyanoacrylates are another form of biodegradable polymer. For example, poly(butyl-2-cyanoacrylate) has been used as an adjuvant for oral immunization. Poly(methylmethacrylate) nanoparticles constitute another biodegradable adjuvant. The antigen can be either incorporated into the nanoparticles or adsorbed onto previously formed particles.

The use of PLG and other microparticles is under extensive investigation for the mucosal administration of vaccines. Particles of very small size (nanoparticles) may be even more suitable. Digestion in the stomach needs to be combated, perhaps by enteric-coated polymers, and coating with substances that increase intestinal absorption may be necessary. Delivery via the respiratory tract—for example, via intranasal immunization or aerosol administration—is a good possibility for respiratory pathogens. Rectal and vaginal delivery is also possible. Because there is a great deal of "cross-talk" between the various components of the mucosal immune system, and because oral delivery is by far the most practical, this deserves full experimental exploration in the first instance.

Biodegradable microparticles can induce T cell immunity, including CD8+ CTLs, as well as just antibody formation. For example, HIV envelope proteins contained in PLG particles induced HIV-specific CD4+ and CD8+ T cell responses in mice. Similarly, microparticles outperformed incomplete Freund's adjuvant in promoting Th1 CD4+ T cell responses with a subunit antigen from *M. tuberculosis* (69). The addition of cytokines or chemical adjuvants to further enhance these T cell effects remains to be explored.

Cytokines as Adjuvants

Cytokines have profound regulatory effects on all three cell types involved in immune responses (APCs, T cells, and B cells), so it is natural to ask whether they might find a use in adjuvant preparations, particularly inasmuch as some cytokines are noteworthy for guiding the immune response down particular pathways. This being so, it is interesting to note that the field of cytokines as adjuvants has not yet made much progress. Of course, cytokines are quite expensive and can exhibit marked, albeit dose-dependent, toxic effects. A variation on the theme explored in a later discussion is cytokine gene constructs as components of vectored or DNA vaccines, an approach that would have the advantage that the cytokine is delivered to the same milieu as the antigen, as opposed to systemically administered cytokines.

Several cytokines act on APCs. IFN-γ and TNF-α recruit and activate macrophages and help T cells develop antiviral effector functions, and IL-1α and IL-1β are also strongly pro-inflammatory. These cytokines have been assessed for their capacity to improve the response of mice to an inactivated rabies vaccine. All of them increased virus-specific IgG responses, IFN-γ raised resistance to challenge infection, and IFN-γ and IL-2 acted synergistically. Limited clinical trials have shown IFN-γ to accelerate the response of humans to hepatitis B vaccines. Granulocyte-macrophage colony-stimulating factor (GM-CSF) and FLT-3 ligand are strong stimulators of DCs; each has been claimed to have adjuvant properties in soluble form, and each has been used to stimulate DCs in various approaches to cell-based anticancer vaccines (70). The FLT-3 ligand stimulates both CD8α^+ (lymphoid type) and CD8α^- (myeloid type) DCs in the mouse and both CD11c$^+$ (monocytoid) and CD11c$^-$ (plasmacytoid) DCs in the human, whereas GM-CSF stimulates only the latter in each case. The former DC type tends to produce Th1-stimulating cytokines and the latter a Th2 bias. The differential mobilization of distinct DC subsets may have some potential in guiding immune responses. An early trial of FLT-3 ligand as an adjuvant in combination with alum failed to show an increase in the already strong immune response.

IL-2 has been explored most extensively (71). It can be highly effective in restoring immune responsiveness in mice with a deficient T cell system or in overcoming immune response gene-mediated low titers. Its effects in healthy animals are less impressive, although some enhanced protection in a variety of infectious disease models has been noted. IL-2 can improve survival in a variety of cancer immunotherapeutic models. One noteworthy clinical effect is its capacity to convert lepromatous leprosy into tuberculoid leprosy when injected directly into the lesions of patients. IL-4 and IL-10 have received some attention through their capacity to send the immune response veering into a Th2 direction, but currently the focus is on IL-10 as a possible therapy in autoimmunity rather than as an adjuvant. IL-12 can promote Th1 development, an effect that has been beneficial in a trial *Leishmania* vaccine. IL-23 has also been proposed for this purpose. One does not detect a great thirst within pharmaceutical industry to use soluble cytokines as adjuvants. In the longer term, it is conceivable that one or more could find a place in either vectored or DNA vaccines, as a gene construct rather than a finished product.

Molecular Targeting of Antigens

Antigens have to be brought to APCs, which in turn have to be activated to begin the adaptive immune response. Getting antigens to APC by linking them to ligands for which the APC have a counter-structure is a good first step. For example, fusing a protein antigen with C3d can increase murine anti–hen egg lysozyme responses by up to 10,000-fold (72), yielding responses much higher than with Freund's complete adjuvant. In mucosal immunity, coupling antigens covalently to a mucosal adjuvant can have profound effects, as discussed earlier. Now that the TLRs are being rapidly unraveled, one can anticipate more experimentation on antigens coupled to their various ligands. One novel development is the chemical conjugation of CpG ODN with the nontoxic CTB to create a highly immunostimulatory adjuvant (59). The rationale was to utilize the TLR-9 ligating properties of CpG ODN as well as the efficient ability of CTB to bind to immune cells, especially APC, and to transport the linked agent into endosomes and further to the trans-Golgi network and the endoplasmic reticulum. Using tetanus toxoid as an antigen, the conjugated molecule markedly enhanced IgG antibody formation and tilted the isotype pattern toward a Th1 response. Further, there was powerful *in vitro* stimulation of pro-inflammatory cytokines and chemokines by human peripheral blood mononuclear cells.

The reader by now has gathered that the field of adjuvants is not too rich in simplifying or overarching paradigms. It seems likely that empirical research will continue to dominate for some time. It may be well to end on a positive note. Combinations of the principles discussed here seem to be the way of the future. There have been any number of disappointing clinical trials of a malaria vaccine based on the *Plasmodium falciparum* circumsporozoite protein (CSP). Recently, when and only when three separate principles of adjuvanticity were combined did a vaccine capable of moderate protection against malaria result (73). The principles were incorporation of the malarial antigen into a virus-like particle, use of an oil-in-water emulsion, and addition of the chemical immunostimulants monophosphoryl lipid A and QS21. The Bill & Melinda Gates Foundation has recently supported head-to-head comparisons of various adjuvants for experimental HIV/AIDS vaccines, and this should promote progress in what is clearly a difficult area.

Viruses Can Activate Multiple TLRs

It may be that certain viruses have built in adjuvanticity through their capacity to engage multiple TLRs. Querec et al. (74) found that the live attenuated yellow fever vaccine 17D can activate multiple subsets of human and mouse DCs *in vitro*. It did so via no fewer than four TLRs, namely TLRs 2, 7, 8, and 9. As a result, the immune response is a mixed one of Th1 and Th2 helper cell induction as well as antigen-specific $CD8^+$ cytotoxic T cells. The Th1 responses are mediated by the adaptor protein MyD88, which is present downstream of most TLRs, but the Th2 responses require TLR-2 signaling, mediated by the adaptor protein TIRAP. Thus distinct TLRs might differentially regulate the Th1/Th2 balance. Incorporating different combinations of TLR ligands into vaccine candidates could therefore lead to immune responses appropriate to the disease in question. Yellow fever vaccine 17D is currently being manipulated to act as a carrier for a number of other antigens.

Yellow fever is not the only virus to activate TLRs. Measles and HCV appear to signal through TLR2 and Newcastle disease virus activates DCs through both TLR7 and TLR9, while Cocksackie virus B triggers TLR8.

Viruses and other pathogens can also signal via other PRRs, such as C-type lectins and mannose receptors (23). An intriguing possibility is that some of these interactions—for example, via DC-specific, ICAM-3 grabbing nonintegrin (DC-SIGN)—could actually induce regulatory T cells, thus suppressing the immune response and DC function (75). In this case the pathogen may in fact be manipulating the immune response to favor its own persistence, and, if so, learning more about the various PRRs and their functions could lead to novel strategies to treat chronic infections.

Mucosal Adjuvants

While conventional adjuvants can be considered for mucosally delivered vaccine preparations, there is a special class of lectin-like molecules endowed with immunostimulatory properties that are uniquely involved in enhancing mucosal responses. Cholera toxin (CT) is the most powerful mucosal adjuvant yet developed. The CTB retains much of the adjuvant property but not the toxicity. *E. coli* heat-stable enterotoxin (LT) is active, and fragment C of tetanus toxin has similar effects.

Obviously, the toxicity of CT and LT limits their usefulness as adjuvants. Pizza et al. (76) developed a clever strategy involving genetic modification of CT and LT resulting in derivatives that are still able to assemble into a holotoxin but have greatly diminished toxicity. These mutants act not only as mucosal immunogens, but also as adjuvants for coadministered bystander antigens. Recently, two equivalent derivatives of CT and LT, known as CTK63 and LTK63, have been prepared by substitution of a single, identical amino acid. The substitution is near the nicotinamide adenine dinucleotide (NAD) binding cleft. Interestingly, LTK63 worked much better than CTK63 both for the facilitation of serum antibody and as a coinducer of IgA in nasal or lung lavages of mice, being only slightly inferior to CT itself (77). The reasons for this difference are currently entirely obscure. Indeed, the mechanisms whereby the toxins mediate immunity are poorly understood.

Interestingly, when CT-B is covalently coupled to an antigen and is then given by a mucosal route, CT-B induces a strong mucosal IgA response to itself and, frequently, the conjugated antigen, but it actually causes systemic or peripheral immunological tolerance (78). Moreover, far less antigen is required than for normal mucosal immunity or tolerance induction. Further, the strategy works even in the presence of an already established state of systemic immunity. Impressive results have been obtained in animal models of autoimmune disease, including autoimmune encephalomyelitis, collagen-induced arthritis, and insulin-dependent diabetes mellitus. One possible mechanism may be the induction of T cells producing immunosuppressive cytokines such as transforming growth factor (TGF-β) and IL-10. Interestingly, even trace amounts of coadministered CT prevent tolerance induction.

Table 40.3 enunciates some of the principles underlying the design of adjuvants. Hopefully, some of these will lead to clinically successful new adjuvants after a disappointingly long waiting period.

CLASSIFICATION OF ESTABLISHED VACCINES

Dealing as it does with the administration of powerful biologicals to normal individuals, the vaccine community, including industry, is understandably conservative. Vaccines take time to establish themselves in the public consciousness, and then to change these vaccines for improved versions again takes time and effort. The world is facing some awkward decisions in the years immediately ahead as a

TABLE 40.3 Some Principles Underlying the Design of Adjuvants

- Uptake of antigens by APC is vital, hence rendering antigens polymeric or particulate helps.
- Activation of APC is essential; hence agents that engage TLR work well.
- Depot effects and delayed absorption can enhance immunity; hence emulsions and biodegradable microparticles underlie many adjuvant approaches.
- Bacteria and bacterial products were found early to stimulate immunity; many pure derivatives have resulted.
- A heterogeneous collection of natural or synthetic chemicals has been found empirically to enhance immunity.
- Many cytokines increase immune responses.
- Molecular targeting of antigens to APC through conjugation of ligands can enhance immune responses.
- Viruses and other pathogens may stimulate multiple TLRs and therefore possess built-in immunogenicity.
- Adjuvants are essential for good mucosal vaccine results, but much remains to be done in this field.

number of new vaccines have emerged from the research and development pipeline.

The purpose of a vaccine is to stimulate the immune response without subjecting an individual to the risk of actual infection. An ideal vaccine would confer the same degree of immunity as natural infection for diseases against which immunity is solid, or it would do better than nature for diseases in which immunity is not solid. Because most vaccines fall short of this ideal, it is frequently necessary to give vaccines more than once, making use of the phenomenon of immunological memory—namely, the capacity to respond more strongly to an antigen on re-exposure to it. Vaccines can elicit every kind of immune response, including antibody formation, Th1 and Th2–type $CD4^+$ T cell responses and $CD8^+$ T-cell responses, but most vaccine development programs for currently licensed vaccines have relied on the vaccine's capacity to evoke antibody formation. This will change as more ambitious targets are set and as capacity to guide immune responses down particular pathways improves. In particular, much more interest is being taken in whether a vaccine can lead to Th1-type and cytotoxic $CD8^+$ T cell responses.

Vaccines are designed primarily to prevent infection, although one of the first vaccines, the vaccine against rabies, was given after infection had been initiated. There is now increasing research on therapeutic vaccines—that is, vaccines administered after infection has been established. Such vaccines are designed to strengthen an immune response that is inadequate, particularly in cases of chronic or recurrent disease.

Obviously, microorganisms possess thousands of molecules that are foreign to a host animal or person and that are thus antigenic. Immune responses against the majority of these are entirely irrelevant to the prevention of infection. Therefore, increasing attention is being given to the identification, purification, and, frequently, molecular cloning of the antigens that evoke host-protective responses. With more complex pathogens such as parasites, it is not immediately apparent which antigens these are, and detective work needs to be done to establish correlates of immunity. The full genome sequence of many pathogens has been determined, and a new strategy is to search for likely transmembrane proteins or molecules involved in virulence, and then to conduct trials of these in mice for possible vaccine efficacy. This process is termed *genome mining*. Identification of the correct antigens is not the end of the story, however, because many pure, soluble proteins are poorly immunogenic. In fact, there is the need to balance the greater immunogenicity of whole microorganisms against the lower reactogenicity and greater conceptual elegance of molecular vaccines. This situation needs to be dissected on a case-by-case basis, although with more recent vaccines, such as Hib and acellular pertussis, the balance appears to be swinging in the latter direction.

Vaccines have potential usefulness beyond communicable diseases, such as anticancer vaccines, birth control vaccines, and vaccines aimed at lowering immune responses, such as in autoimmunity or allergy. These uses fall outside the scope of this chapter.

A classification of established vaccines is presented in Table 40.4.

Live Attenuated Vaccines

Ever since Jenner's smallpox vaccine, live attenuated vaccines have occupied a special place in the pantheon of vaccinology. Many viral vaccines of this type have an efficacy of >90%, and protection frequently lasts for many years. This is perhaps not surprising, because the multiplication of the pathogen in the host creates an antigenic stimulus not unlike that of a natural infection in terms of antigen amount, character, and location. This key advantage is also the source of potential disadvantage, as the "miniversion" of the relevant disease can assume dangerous proportions—for example, generalized vaccinia or BCG spread in immunodeficient or immunosuppressed children. In some vaccines, the mutations causing loss of virulence are not known. Further, mutations can restore virulence, as in the case of poliomyelitis. Much recent research has centered on more rationally planned attenuation based on an understanding of the molecular determinants of virulence. Relevant genetic engineering can result in improved vaccines in which reversion to virulence is impossible.

It must be recognized that the success of live attenuated vaccines poses some problems as to correct maintenance of immune status. For example, in many countries, measles vaccine is given only once, and nowhere is it mandated more than twice. Will this confer the same

TABLE 40.4 Classification of Licensed Vaccines

Types of Vaccine	Examples
Live attenuated viral	Poliomyelitis (OPV Sabin), measles, mumps, rubella, rabies, varicella, vaccinia, yellow fever, rotavirus, influenza (intranasal)
Live attenuated bacterial	BCG for tuberculosis or leprosy, Ty21a for typhoid fever
Killed whole virus	Poliomyelitis (IPV-Salk), influenza, hepatitis A, rabies
Killed whole-cell bacterial	Pertussis, cholera, anthrax, plague
Toxoids	Diphtheria, tetanus
Molecular vaccines—proteins	Acellular pertussis, subunit influenza, hepatitis B
Molecular vaccines—carbohydrate	Hib, Vi typhoid, meningococci, pneumococci
Molecular vaccines—carbohydrate-protein conjugate	Hib, meningococci, pneumococci
Combination vaccines	DPT, MMRV, DPT-Hib, DPT-Hib-IPV-hep B.

life-long immunity as an attack of measles? We cannot be sure and thus must maintain a level of alertness about booster doses in adult life. This has not been a priority area for live attenuated or any other kind of vaccine but is currently the subject of much debate. There are instances in which public health regulations mandate regular boosters—for example, the yellow fever vaccine for travelers to affected countries. Another vexing question is whether repeated environmental exposure to a common microbe provides a kind of natural booster. If so, problems may arise as a disease becomes uncommon in a community.

Surprisingly, giving a number of live attenuated vaccines together appears to cause no problems.

Vaccines Consisting of Killed Microorganisms

Because vaccines consisting of killed microorganisms are nonreplicating antigens, booster doses are essential. Some are excellent vaccines with high efficacy and safety, such as the Salk injectable poliomyelitis vaccine (IPV) or the hepatitis A vaccine. Others are of poor efficacy and short duration, such as the whole cell–killed injectable cholera vaccine, which has been all but abandoned. Others are partially effective but require improvement in terms of percentage of protection or duration of immunity. These include the older killed influenza and typhoid vaccines. Many of these vaccines have already been overtaken by new and improved versions, including subunit vaccines and orally active preparations.

Toxoids

When disease pathological processes are caused predominantly by a powerful exotoxin or enterotoxin, vaccines provoking antitoxin antibodies make good sense. In some cases, an exotoxin is a bacterium's device for creating sufficient tissue destruction to permit a rich growth medium to develop. That is the case in tetanus, diphtheria, and gas gangrene. For these cases, the relevant toxoids make good vaccines. Toxoids from enterotoxins have, in general, been less successful. However, a genetically detoxified derivative of the heat-labile enterotoxin (LT) of enterotoxigenic *Escherichia coli* is showing promise as a possible vaccine against traveler's diarrhea. This has been achieved through site-directed mutagenesis to inactivate the adenosine diphosphate–ribosyltransferase activity of the A subunit of LT. Equivalent mutants of CT may eventually prove important.

The current conventional diphtheria and tetanus vaccines contain many impurities; further, the formaldehyde treatment needed to turn the toxins into toxoids also causes cross-linkage of beef peptides present in the culture medium, resulting in the presence of unnecessary antigens in the final preparation. Scientifically, one could mount an argument for a mutant, nontoxic pure molecule, such as CRM197, as a new vaccine. CRM197 is a material cross-reacting to diphtheria toxin and containing a single glycine to glutamic acid substitution at position 52 rendering the toxin inactive. Despite scientific attractiveness, there is not much commercial pressure for changing vaccines that are working well. Doubtless, if the acellular pertussis component of diphtheria toxoid, whole-cell pertussis, and tetanus toxoid (DPT) vaccine continues to impress with their lack of reactogenicity, more pressure may build for the diphtheria and tetanus components to be free of side effects, and so ongoing research should be encouraged.

Molecular Vaccines: Protein

The recombinant DNA era has yielded a plethora of antigenic molecules that are pure and have been chosen in animal models through their capacity to provoke an immune response that is host protective. Some subunit vaccines, such as Hib and acellular pertussis, result from extremely elegant research that warrants description in its own right. Whereas some subunit vaccines, such as HBsAg, are highly immunogenic at low doses, others have been of disappointing strength and require adjuvants more powerful than the aluminum salts currently used to adsorb pure proteins onto small particles. As a group, subunit vaccines have been more expensive than older vaccines. This major barrier to developing country use can be partially countered by programs such as the Global Alliance for Vaccines and Immunization (discussed later) that create a large demand, whereby high volumes drive down costs of production.

Molecular Vaccines: Carbohydrate and Conjugate

The capsular polysaccharides of encapsulated bacteria are powerfully immunogenic and can make good vaccines. However, they suffer from three drawbacks. The carbohydrates are serotype specific—that is, they cover one variant of the pathogen only. Therefore, an effective vaccine may have to be a "cocktail" of many different carbohydrate molecules. Thus, the Merck pneumococcal vaccine has 23 separate components. Second, these vaccines work poorly or not at all in young infants. For a disease such as meningitis, in which the greatest rate of mortality is among children younger than 1 year, this represents a serious limitation. Third, being T-independent antigens, the vaccines engender suboptimal immunological memory. Therefore, the conjugation of these carbohydrates to protein carriers that engender T cell help represented a major step forward, which is described in detail in a later section.

Combination Vaccines

As more effective vaccines are developed, the question of the number of needle pricks to which young infants are subjected becomes an urgent one. Among the traditional vaccines, the DPT combination was standard for a long time, and whole-cell pertussis has been replaced by the subunit acellular pertussis in industrialized countries. As already mentioned, MMR is an extremely successful combination, and recently varicella has been successfully added to this, thus MMR-V. Considering DPT as a "platform," one can see logical additions to this, such as the addition of one or more of Hib, injectable killed polio (Salk) vaccine, and hepatitis B. In fact, such pentavalent and hexavalent formulations are now available. Antigenic competition has not yet become manifest, although the addition of Hib to DPT has caused problems for some manufacturers in the levels of antibodies reached. As successful vaccines for other types of meningitis become more popular (e.g., against *N. meningitidis* type C), the question of whether to add these or whether to create a second "meningitis/pneumonia" package will have to be faced. At least two companies are considering the possibility of heptavalent combinations, such as DPT–HiB–hepatitis B–meningitis A/C. Of course, the pneumococcal vaccine currently licensed (Prevnar from Wyeth) is already a 7-valent mixture, and more serotypes will soon be added. Consideration is also being given to a multiserotype meningococcus "cocktail," discussed in more detail later.

NEW APPROACHES TO VACCINE DESIGN

Table 40.5 outlines the main new approaches to vaccine design. In thinking about these approaches, it is important to remember that established public health practice is not easy to change, and it appears likely that the newer approaches will find more favor with regard to diseases for which no vaccine currently exists, such as HIV/AIDS or malaria, than in situations in which current vaccines are reasonably satisfactory.

Vectored Vaccines

Bernard Moss and Enzo Paoletti independently opened up a major chapter in vaccinology when they demonstrated that genes for important antigens could be introduced into the vaccinia virus without perturbing its replication and could be expressed in host cells in which the virus was

TABLE 40.5 Newer Approaches to Vaccine Design

Approach	*Purpose*
Vectored vaccines	To employ an attenuated virus or bacterium with limited replication potential to carry a gene or genes for antigens from a pathogen into the body
Nucleic acid vaccines	To use a plasmid containing genes coding for one or more antigens from a pathogen so the body itself becomes a factory for the antigen(s) in question; there are variations on the theme
Peptide vaccines	To construct a polymer out of a number of peptides, frequently T cell epitopes, creating an immunogen
Mucosal vaccines	To administer an antigen not by injection but via a mucosal surface (e.g., orally or intranasally) so as to engage the mucosal immune system in protection
Transdermal vaccines	To administer the antigen via the skin
Edible vaccines	To genetically engineer a plant such that it comes to contain antigen(s) in a form that is immunogenic when eaten
Prime-boost strategies	To administer two separate versions of a vaccine sequentially, typically a DNA vaccine followed by a vectored vaccine or either of these followed by a protein vaccine

dividing (79,80). This "Trojan Horse" concept, whereby harmless microorganisms act as vectors for antigen genes, has been extended in innumerable directions. Among other important vectors in use experimentally are vaccinia variants; avipoxviruses; adenoviruses; polioviruses; herpesviruses; crippled HIV, *Salmonella, Shigella,* and BCG bacterial species; and many more. The power of the concept is that it combines the best of two worlds: the force of a live attenuated vaccine, and the scientific precision of the rational subunit vaccine approach. Further, given the large size of the vaccinia genome or the genomes of some of the other vectors, it is feasible to consider the insertion of quite a few antigen genes, thus covering several diseases at once. It is also straightforward to incorporate one or more cytokine genes in the construct, should this be desirable for either the strength of the immune response or the direction it should take.

Although the concept was first introduced in the early 1980s, no relevant vaccine has yet come on the market. Clinical investigation has been somewhat limited so far, but, as discussed later, it has accelerated in the context of the so-called "prime-boost" strategy. There are understandable reservations about the use of unmodified vaccinia, particularly at a time when HIV is rife, because it can be dangerous in people with an ineffective T cell system, a reservation that could be partially countered by the inclusion of the IL-2 gene in the construct, which prevents athymic nude mice from succumbing to vaccinia (81). A number of vaccinia strains lacking genes that contribute to virulence have been prepared and are in clinical trial—for example, modified vaccinia Ankara (MVA). Also, nonreplicating viral vectors, such as canarypox or fowlpox in humans, can be considered. The field has doubtless been slowed somewhat by poor responses in early clinical trials of experimental HIV and malaria vaccines. Nevertheless, the overwhelming weight of preclinical data, with disease protection against at least 20 pathogens in at least 15 species, suggests that further research must eventually be crowned with success. It should be noted that the approach is designed to induce excellent T cell, including cytotoxic T cell, immunity.

Experimentation with bacterial vectors is not yet as far advanced, but examples are taken up when enteric and intracellular pathogens are discussed.

Nucleic Acid Vaccines

Few areas of experimental vaccinology have emerged as surprisingly and developed as explosively as that of nucleic acid vaccines. Two preludes to the actual discovery warrant mention. Wolff et al. (82), using plasmid DNA coding for a reporter gene, found that DNA injected as a saline solution and without the adjunct agents normally used for transfection could cause synthesis of the reporter protein in the recipient animal. This surprising finding came from a control group in which the real hope for the experimental group was uptake of liposomes containing DNA. Of various injection sites tested, intramuscular injection worked best. The total number of myotubes transfected within the injection region is 1% to 5%. The second prelude relates to a DNA delivery system, originally developed by an agricultural firm, Agrecetus, and first used as a means of transfecting plant cells. This Accell gene delivery system, also termed the *gene gun,* consists of a helium gas pressure–driven device capable of delivering into very superficial layers of tissue tiny gold particles coated with plasmid DNA. These DNA-coated microprojectiles could, for example, be delivered to the skin of mice, resulting in the synthesis of the relevant protein (83). It was not long before each of these two approaches was used to elicit immune responses in the mouse. The gene gun approach induced antibody formation against human growth hormone and human α-1 antitrypsin in the first demonstration that DNA immunization could work (84). Further, the prolonged persistence of encoded protein in the serum signaled the probability of continued antigenic stimulation. The first demonstration of a host-protective immune response came from the intramuscular injection approach (85). Mice were injected with plasmids encoding the nucleoprotein of influenza A virus. They developed both antibodies and class I MHC)-restricted CTLs. Upon challenge with a virulent influenza A strain, PR/8, 100% of treated mice survived, whereas 100% of controls were dead by day 9. Almost simultaneously, Fynan et al. (86) also protected mice against PR/8 by using the gene gun and DNA encoding the relevant hemagglutinin as the antigen. After these two striking results, the field really took off. A scant 4 years later, Donnelly et al. (87) were able to review an extraordinary range of preclinical studies showing humoral and T cell responses protective against a wide range of viruses, bacteria, and parasites, as well as various tumor models.

What are the essential features of nucleic acid vaccines? The key difference from the live vector approach is that the DNA encoding the antigen of interest cannot replicate in the human or animal body. The plasmids concerned are usually grown in *E. coli.* Their origin of replication is not suitable for mammalian cells. It is important to include a strong promoter element suitable for high-level gene expression in mammalian cells; for example, the immediate/early promoter of the human CMV works well. The construct should also have an appropriate messenger ribonucleic acid (RNA) transcript termination/polyadenylation sequence. After intramuscular injection, the DNA enters the cytoplasm and then the nucleus of the myocyte, but it is not integrated into the genome. Neither muscle cells nor the DCs, which are the targets of the gene gun approach, have a high rate of division, nor do they show extensive homology with the plasmid, and so homologous recombination is highly unlikely. Random integration remains a formal possibility, but, so far, no adverse effects have been noted. Gene expression is not at a high level. Antigen leaks out of myocytes for a considerable period, and, in the case of the gene gun, the gold particles deposited in the epidermis soon find their way into Langerhans cells, which then make their way to local lymph nodes. In the case of intramuscular injection, it is clear that the myocyte itself is not the inducer of immune responses. This was approached by Fu et al. (88) in an ingenious experiment. Parental into F1 bone marrow chimeric mice were prepared in such a way that the myocytes carried both parental MHC haplocytes but the professional APCs such as DCs, being (after an appropriate period) bone marrow derived, carried only the bone marrow donor parental haplotype. After reconstitution, the chimeric mice were given plasmid DNA coding for influenza virus nucleoprotein to generate CTLs. According to the rules of MHC restriction, because the mice possessed the thymic epithelial framework of the F1, their peripheral T cells, although of parental genotype, should be capable of recognizing antigen in the context of *both* parental haplotypes. However, when the CTLs were tested *in vitro,* they were clearly restricted only by the MHC alleles of the bone marrow donor. Had myocytes been the APCs creating the CTLs *in vivo,* this would not have been the case. In further chimeras, transplantation studies were done with an NP gene–transfected myoblast cell line. With appropriate choice of strains, it could be shown that H2-incompatible myoblasts could induce CTL responses, but these, when analyzed, were restricted to the MHC haplocyte not of the myoblast donor but of the bone marrow donor. This clearly showed that the myoblasts acted as a source of antigen that was somehow transferred to APCs in a way that allowed processing for the class I MHC pathway. This apparent exception to the dual pathway rules is an example of "cross-priming," which has also been noted in other systems. The efficacy of DNA vaccines in generating CTLs has been a common feature of most examples so far studied in mice.

The potential advantages of nucleic acid vaccines are numerous. The subunit approach to pure molecular vaccines can be seriously hampered by incorrect folding or glycosylation of antigens, which can present formidable problems and add to the cost of such vaccines. This should be largely obviated in DNA vaccines. Once an appropriate DNA vaccine has been engineered, it should be stable and batch variation should be minimal, facilitating quality control procedures. In terms of actual manufacturing procedure, nucleic acid vaccines should be relatively cheap. Multivalency could be achieved either by coinjection of a mixture of plasmids or by constructing complex plasmids.

A variation on the theme is the use of positive-strand RNA viruses such as alpha viruses that self-replicate within nondividing host cells and can be engineered to deliver inserted RNA coding for the antigen in question. It is also possible to engineer replicons in which the antigen-encoding RNA is substituted for viral structural genes and replicons can be packaged into infectious particles with helper viruses or split-genome packaging cell lines. DNA/RNA replicons can also be engineered and in some circumstances are more immunogenic than plasmid-based DNA vaccines.

Despite the justifiable excitement about nucleic acid vaccines, it has become clear that the responses achieved in subhuman primates and in humans are much lower than those in mice. In part, this may be a dosage question, because a human weighs 3,000 times more than a mouse, and it has not been practical to increase dosage commensurately. Considerable effort has therefore gone into enhancing the efficacy of DNA vaccines. Uptake of DNA has been enhanced by *in vivo* electroporation. DNA has been incorporated into microparticles or liposomes or has been given with an oil-in-water emulsion. Coinjection of cytokines or engineering the DNA to encode for a cytokine represents another approach. Of particular interest is the concept of encoding together with the DNA for the antigen DNA for a ligand that can target the fusion protein to an appropriate site. Boyle et al. (89) used L-selectin to target the antigen to high endothelial venule receptors, thus enhancing the amount going to lymphoid tissue, or CTL-associated antigen 4 to target the antigen to the counterstructures CD80 and CD86 on the surface of APCs. This strategy greatly increased antibody responses and improved protective efficacy in an influenza virus model. Moreover, the approach worked in a large animal—the sheep. Pig skin is believed to be a reasonable model for human skin, and when CTL-associated antigen 4–antigen fusion constructs were delivered into pig skin by the gene gun, the targeting strategy markedly enhanced the speed and magnitude of the antibody response.

Further aspects of nucleic acid vaccines are discussed later in the section on prime-boost strategies and in the specific context of HIV/AIDS and malaria vaccines.

It is clear that something as novel as nucleic vaccines will present substantial problems for the regulatory agencies. In addition to the carcinogenicity/insertional mutagenesis possibility, the conjectural hazards include autoimmunity to DNA or as a result of immune-mediated destruction of antigen-expressing cells. The latter could lead to direct damage or could occasion the release of intracellular antigens that would then provoke autoimmunity. In practice, however, induction of autoimmunity to autologous constituents is quite difficult and proceeds only with the use of strong adjuvants such as Freund's complete adjuvant. Another objection that has been raised is the possibility that a constant leak of small quantities of antigen over a prolonged period of time could lead to immunological tolerance, thus making the recipient incapable of responding to the antigen in question. This has not been encountered in any situation so far.

Peptide Vaccines

Peptide vaccines can be either synthetically prepared or encoded by DNA. Frequently, the plan is to include a multiplicity of epitopes, particularly T cell epitopes—for example, from several different antigens of a pathogen. The approach can also deal with serotype variation of antigens, epitopes being chosen from multiple strains. Peptide vaccines suffer from the constraint that many antibodies are directed to conformational determinants. The most interesting peptide vaccine research is in HIV, malaria, and tumor immunology.

An interesting variant involving highly polymerized peptides linked to a built-in adjuvant has already been considered earlier in this chapter.

Mucosal Vaccines

It has been estimated that the combined surface area of the mucosae of the gastrointestinal, respiratory, and urogenital tracts is 400 m^2. The total lymphocyte complement of the mucosal immune system is greater than that of the lymph nodes and spleen. In fact, the mucosa-associated lymphoid tissues (MALT) contribute three quarters of all immunocytes. The mucosal immune system includes organized collections of lymphoid tissue, such as the tonsils, adenoids, Peyer's patches, and appendix, and also single lymphoid follicles. These collections contain macrophages and DCs, sample antigens, and generate both T and B cell responses, including germinal center formation. There is a high proportion of immunoglobulin A (IgA) in the antibody formed. There is also extensive infiltration of epithelia and the lamina propria with lymphocytes and plasma cells. It is believed that these represent effector cells and that there is no immune induction within these latter sites. There are also large numbers of lymphoid cells in the parenchyma of exocrine glands.

Two types of antigen-capturing cells are of importance in mucosal immunity: the intraepithelial DCs and M cells. In stratified or pseudostratified epithelia, the DCs serve much the same function as skin Langerhans cells and extend right to the surface. In tracheal epithelium, for example, there are up to 700 such cells per mm^2 forming an almost contiguous network (90). As in the case of Langerhans cells, these DCs take antigens to draining lymph nodes for immune induction. The M cells are unique features of the mucosal immune system. They exist in the epithelium overlying organized collections such as Peyer's patches. Their job is to take up antigens from the mucosa and deliver them to the mucosal lymphoid tissue via a specialized pocket in the epithelium. M cells are active in taking up both macromolecular antigens and particulate antigens such as bacteria and essentially serve to channel them to professional APCs in the lymphoid collections beneath. M cell membranes contain the glycolipid GM1, to which CT can bind, and a variety of other carbohydrate structures with selective binding activity. Bacteria and viruses can also exploit this capacity of M cells to take them up efficiently to infect mucosae. This exploitation probably includes sexual transmission of HIV.

The lymphocyte traffic pattern differs for the mucosal immune system and the conventional immune system (91). There is a distinct tendency for mucosa-associated cells to home back to mucosal tissue but not necessarily to the same mucosa. The possibility therefore exists that immunization could occur via one mucosal surface, but an unrelated one could be protected. Nevertheless, the common mucosal immune system is more restricted than previously thought. In humans, studies with CTB administered by various mucosal routes have shown that the strongest response occurs at the directly exposed mucosa and the second strongest at adjacent mucosae (92). An exception is intranasal immunization that, apart from stimulating the respiratory tract, also induces a strong vaginal-genital tract immune response. As well as activating T and B cells, antigens delivered mucosally can also induce $CD4^+$ $CD25^+$ regulatory cells and therefore have strong suppressor activity.

Stimulation of immune responses via mucosal surfaces, leading to local IgA production and a variety of systemic B and T cell effects, suffers from two difficulties: Most nonreplicating antigens lead to immune responses only after large and multiple antigen doses, and these responses are of short duration. Even natural infection of mucus membranes leads to shorter-lived immunity than in the case of a systemic infection. This is why the field of mucosal adjuvants is particularly important.

Mucosal adjuvants include any substance or process that enhances uptake of antigen by mucosal lymphoid tissue. For example, bacteria are capable of recruiting large numbers of DCs into tracheal epithelium, and these DCs are critical to the induction of an immune response (93). Similarly, viruses can bring DCs into epithelia and can stimulate subsequent migration to draining lymph nodes. It has been argued that the increased susceptibility of neonates to respiratory infections results from the hyporesponsiveness of their immature DCs to such signals. In more mature individuals, the inherent immunogenicity of microorganisms suggests that the use of live vectors, be they bacterial or viral, engineered to express the antigen of interest, may in itself provide sufficient adjuvanticity, albeit perhaps with a limited duration of immunity.

Apart from specifically mucosal adjuvants, many adjuvant processes applicable to injectable vaccines have been used in experimental mucosal vaccines (reviewed in [92]). These include CpG ODN, VLPs, ISCOMs, liposomes, biodegradable particles, and bacterial spores.

Enteric and acute respiratory infections represent major public health problems, and HIV infection is frequently acquired through mucosal routes; therefore, vaccines protecting mucosal surfaces are highly desirable. With regard to their construction, it must be noted that mucosal surfaces are normally colonized by a rich flora of commensal bacteria. Remarkably little is known about what permits these commensals to remain but not to overgrow. There may well be some degree of immunological tolerance at work, and oral tolerance is a well-established phenomenon. At the same time, overgrowth and invasion would appear likely were there not some level of immune response. For the intelligent design of mucosal vaccines, better understanding of this balanced situation is required. Tolerance-including strategies may be valuable as well—for example, in autoimmune situations.

Cell-mediated immune responses within mucosal tissue must also be considered. These doubtless contribute to clearance of both bacteria and viruses from mucosal areas after infection: Holmgren makes the point that with some infections, such as *V. cholerae* or enterotoxigenic *E. coli*, the infection is so superficial that neither the bacteria nor their toxins penetrate into the epithelial cells, and in that case, antibodies alone (ideally mucosal IgA) are required for protection, whereas other pathogens, such as *Salmonella* and *Shigella* infections, penetrate deeper, where IgA but also systemic immunoglobulins M and G (IgM and IgG) antibodies may be important, as may the T cell component (94). Ideally, a mucosal vaccine should protect both against toxins produced by pathogens and against antigens involved in adhesion to epithelial cells (e.g., fimbriae) or invasion of tissue. In the case of viruses, $CD8^+$ $\alpha\beta$ TCR^+ cytotoxic T cells that are present intraepithelially clearly contribute to protection.

Vaccines that can be considered mucosal vaccines against five diseases have been licensed (although not in all countries). These are the oral Sabin-type polio vaccine; cholera vaccine, including killed bacteria, given with CTB or live attenuated bacteria; oral live attenuated typhoid vaccine; two different oral live attenuated rotavirus vaccines; and an intranasal influenza vaccine. In view of the power of the approach, it is hoped that more mucosal vaccines will follow. Much effort is going into the use of live recombinant microorganisms as mucosal delivery systems, such as live attenuated *Salmonella* bacteria given orally or adenoviruses given intranasally, but none of these have progressed very far.

Further aspects of the mucosal approach will be raised in the section on HIV/AIDS vaccines.

Transdermal Vaccines

It has been known for decades that antigens applied directly to the skin can cause an immune response, for that is exactly what contact sensitization represents. However, the realization that direct topical application of vaccines to the skin can cause systemic T and B cell responses is relatively novel (95). It is noteworthy that the Langerhans type of DC is really quite superficial in the epidermis, and once antigen has reached the cells, the question of their activation and consequent migration to the draining lymph node depends very much on the type of stimulus. For example, if the vaccine in question is administered together with an adjuvant such as CT, the immune cascade is initiated. Simple admixture with, for example, influenza virus hemagglutinin, suffices to initiate a boostable immune response involving both the systemic and mucosal compartments. Other exotoxins, including detoxified mutants, also work well. Simple skin manipulation, such as cleansing with alcohol or hydration of the skin, may enhance responses, and patches, gels, creams, and ointments are also under investigation.

Another concept being explored for transdermal administration of vaccines is a patch consisting essentially of extremely fine needles which would minimally abrade the skin but still target antigens within the patch to superficial Langerhans cells.

Edible Vaccines

Mason et al. (96) were stimulated by the call at the 1990 World Summit for Children for a radical new approach to vaccines for developing nations, so they set about creating transgenic plants that expressed putative vaccine antigens. The long-range idea was the possibility that a readily available food, such as bananas, might come to constitute a cheap source of edible vaccines. Apart from the considerable technical hurdles involved in expression of genes for antigens in edible portions of plants, a series of immunological questions needed to be addressed. These included the avoidance of oral tolerance, ensuring sufficient oral immunogenicity, ensuring some degree of protection against enzymic degradation of vaccines, and determining adequate dosage. Despite these constraints, progress has actually been remarkably rapid. A start was made with hepatitis B surface antigen in tobacco plants. Successful engineering resulted in the accumulation of VLPs in the tobacco leaf. Similar success was achieved with VLPs of Norwalk virus capsid protein. Next, potato plants were engineered to express the B subunit of heat-labile *E. coli* enterotoxin (LT-B), in the hope that a cheap source of a mucosal adjuvant would eventually result. Mice fed 5-g samples of raw potatoes on four occasions developed serum IgG and mucosal IgA specific for LT-B. The author had the pleasure of being a visiting professor in Dr. Myron Levine's laboratory in the University of Maryland on the very day that the first clinical trial of feeding raw, engineered potatoes to human volunteers was initiated. Both mucosal and systemic antitoxin immune responses were induced. Of course, it is not anticipated that potatoes will be used in the long run, because they need to be cooked. Rather, the aim is to engineer fruit that can be fed raw to infants and small children. To that end, a transformation system for bananas has been developed. Active research is being pursued on edible vaccines against hepatitis B, cholera, measles, and HPV.

It is envisaged that edible vaccines either will contain a mucosal adjuvant or will consist of VLPs. Either of these strategies should militate against oral tolerance. Coexpression of cytokine genes could also be envisaged. It is hoped that the plant cell wall, consisting of cellulose, pectins, and proteins, will be a partial barrier to enzymatic degradation of the enclosed antigen, allowing some to reach the small intestine, a major inductive site of mucosal immunity. Clearly, dosage for infants of various ages will have to be the subject of extensive research.

There is another and perhaps more practical dimension to the field of edible vaccines. This is to regard the transgenic plant itself not as the vaccine but rather as a factory for pharmaceutical proteins that are then extracted and processed much as they would have been from transformed bacteria or yeasts. It has been estimated that protein production costs from plants might be up to 1,000-fold cheaper than present fermentation methods (97). Three major strategies for antigens from pathogens have been developed: stable transformation of the nuclear genome, stable transformation of the chloroplast genome, and transient expression in plants using viral vectors (98). There is considerable interest in using such approaches for monoclonal antibody production as well. Of course, costs of the raw material represent only a fraction of the final vaccine cost. Field production costs have been computed for large batches of hepatitis B virus (HBV) grown in potato, tomato, corn, or tobacco leaf, and they varied from 1.36 U.S. cents to 7.11 U.S. cents per dose. Greenhouse production costs are somewhat higher. Contemplating plants as factories for pharmaceuticals obviously raises regulatory and environmental issues of an entirely new order. Yet one senses considerable excitement about the long-range possibilities.

Prime-boost Strategies

Most vaccines have to be administered on more than one occasion to achieve a satisfactory level of disease prophylaxis. Normally, booster vaccines are identical to the priming vaccines except that one or more components of a combination may be dropped. The initial impetus for a different approach came because of early disappointments with HIV envelope protein–based vaccines, which failed to produce antibodies capable of neutralizing primary isolates of HIV and failed to induce significant levels of HIV-specific $CD8^+$ CTLs. This prompted a search for alternative approaches. First, recombinant vaccinia virus engineered to express *env* was given as a primary dose to mice, followed by a booster dose of recombinant glycoprotein (gp) 160 (99). This endeavor was soon broadened to include priming with other vectored vaccines and boosting with either pure protein or VLPs. Viral vectors have included various modified vaccinia variants of diminished virulence and poxviruses of birds such as canarypox and fowlpox (which do not complete their replication cycle in mammalian hosts and yet express inserted genes) as well as various adenoviruses. Less commonly, alphaviruses, polio viruses, and crippled HIV have been suggested.

Prime-boost strategies can markedly enhance antibody formation but, more important, can engender strong $CD8^+$ and $CD4^+$ T lymphocyte responses. Just why the mixed-modality approach works so well is not entirely clear. "Focused priming" of T cells by naked DNA has been invoked, a $CD8^+$ T-cell response to one or a few immunodominant epitopes then being strongly amplified by, for example, a poxvirus boost. Certainly if the only antigen shared between the priming entity and the boosting entity is the antigen of interest, it seems logical that the immune system would react in a secondary manner to only that antigen. With DNA priming and protein boosting, it has been postulated that the low doses of protein associated with priming engender a high-affinity antibody response. Different mechanisms probably underlie the different regimens. There is, however, no doubt that the prime-boost approach has conferred excellent protection in animal models of various diseases, though early clinical trials have been less impressive. The matter is examined in more detail in the sections dealing with HIV/AIDS and malaria. A useful review of prime-boost strategies was published by Ramshaw and Ramsay (81).

BACTERIAL VACCINES

Diphtheria, Acellular Pertussis, and Tetanus

Historically, the diphtheria-pertussis-tetanus combination has come to be well accepted; only about 2% of the population harbor serious reservations. In view of its importance in a developing nation and the fact that health systems are geared to it, DPT has been regarded as a "platform" on which further vaccines, such as hepatitis B, Hib, and injectable poliomyelitis vaccines (IPV), and others, such as conjugate meningococcal or pneumococcal vaccines, could be placed. Different countries follow different schedules for a primary course of DPT, such as at 2, 3, or 4 months of age; 2, 4, and 6 months of age; or, in the setting of a developing country, 6, 10, and 14 weeks of age. It is generally agreed that three doses should be administered by 6 months of age. There is also variability between countries on the timing of a booster dose, such as DPT at 18 months or diphtheria toxoid only at 3 to 5 years. Tetanus toxoid plus a low dose of diphtheria toxoid is advised again at school-leaving age, and, ideally, a further booster should be given if a person suffers a penetrating wound (for tetanus) or travels to an epidemic or endemic area (for diphtheria). For tetanus, five doses are regarded as conferring life-long immunity, but this may not be correct. For diphtheria, a major epidemic in the countries of the former USSR, including many cases among adults, has shown that initial immunization had been inadequate, that immunity does wane with time, or both. In the United Kingdom, 25% of blood donors aged 20 to 29, but 53% of those aged 50 to 59, were found to have inadequate antibodies to diphtheria toxin. Relatively little attention has been given to adult reimmunization, but a movement for more aggressive immunization of older persons has begun. Boosters of diphtheria and tetanus every 10 years would be a very good idea.

It has already been mentioned that genetic detoxification of diphtheria and tetanus toxins is possible but that there has been little pressure to modify the traditional toxoid vaccines. Nevertheless, the mutant diphtheria protein CRM197 has been popular as the protein component of conjugate vaccines. Pertussis, however, has a reputation for being reactogenic and perhaps for causing rare more serious side effects.

For these reasons, there has been wide acceptance of a subunit (acellular pertussis, or aP) vaccine containing not killed bacteria but pure antigens derived from the bacteria. In fact, acellular pertussis vaccines have been in routine use in Japan since 1981. Renewed interest in the United States and in Europe has resulted in the testing of no fewer than 13 acellular pertussis vaccines. The key antigen is pertussis toxoid (PT), and other important antigens for protection are filamentous hemagglutinin and pertactin. Typical of the extensive clinical research that has been done on acellular pertussis vaccines is a trial in Italy, where immunization rates are relatively low and in which two acellular vaccines from SmithKlineBeecham and Chiron Biocine (renamed Chiron Vaccines in 1996) were compared with a whole-cell vaccine from Connaught Laboratories. The double-blind, randomized controlled trial involved 14,751 infants enrolled over a 1-year period in 1992 to 1993 (100). It involved 62 public health clinics and follow-up for an average of 17 months. Pertussis infection was confirmed by culture and quantitative serological tests. Unfortunately, the Connaught vaccine behaved quite atypically, giving only 36% protection. The two acellular vaccines behaved equivalently, giving 84% protection. Local and systemic adverse events were significantly less frequent with the two acellular vaccines, and their incidences were similar to those of a diphtheria toxoid vaccine without the pertussis component.

The chief difference between these two vaccines was that in the SmithKlineBeecham vaccine, the PT was detoxified by chemical treatment, whereas the Chiron Biocine vaccine contained a mutated, nontoxic form of PT that had been genetically detoxified. Site-directed mutagenesis introduced two point mutations (Arg 9→Lys and Glu 129→Gly) in the enzymic site of the PT. This vaccine caused a higher anti-PT response than that containing chemically inactivated PT, and continued blinded observation for a further year revealed significantly fewer pertussis cases in the Chiron Biocine group. A brief review by Rappuoli (101) gives a sobering insight into what is involved in bringing a new vaccine to the market. The project started in 1984. The cloning and sequencing of the PT gene was achieved in 1985; the amino acids that needed to be changed to remove toxicity were identified in 1987; the filamentous hemagglutinin was cloned in 1988 and the *B. pertussis* strain producing the nontoxic PT was constructed in 1989. Phased clinical trials were started as follows: phase I, 1989; phase II, 1990; phase III, 1992; end of phase III, 1995; filing of worldwide product license application worldwide, 1996. Introduction of new and improved vaccines is not for the faint-hearted!

An analysis of six acellular pertussis vaccines from nine trials was presented by Klein (102). In three of the trials, the acellular vaccine was about 10% less protective (84% versus 93%, 89% versus 98%, 85% versus 96%), but the differences did not reach statistical significance. The author is not aware of any meta-analysis of these data. However, an interesting review of all available clinical trial data was presented by Miller (103), reaching the tentative conclusion that a five-component vaccine—including not only pertussis toxin, filamentous hemagglutinin, and pertactin, but also fimbrial antigens 2 and 3—gave the greatest protection. These last two proteins are not the primary adhesins for the target cell surface but rather may serve to sustain attachment. Among other questions, it remains to be determined how long protection lasts with these newer vaccines. At the moment, there is no major push to switch over to these more expensive vaccines in developing countries, but the trend to the less reactogenic preparations is marked in the industrialized world and probably will prove irresistible globally.

Pertussis affects all ages, although morbidity and mortality rates are highest among children younger than 1 year. Because antibiotics appear to be of little use when symptoms are fully established, the intravenous administration of high-titered anti-pertussis immune globulin must be considered.

There are some doubts about the duration of immunity to pertussis, even with regard to the natural disease itself, and there is increasing evidence of this organism as a cause of prolonged cough illnesses in adolescents and adults. This raises the issues of regular booster immunization, not currently practiced, and of the highest possible infant coverage to achieve eventual herd immunity. There have been recent calls for tetanus-diphtheria-acellular pertussis (Tdap) boosters to replace Td boosters, especially for nurses and other healthcare workers.

Diarrheal Disease Vaccines: Typhoid, Cholera, Enterotoxigenic *E. coli,* and Shigellosis

Vaccines consisting of killed whole typhoid or cholera bacilli were among the earliest developed. However, efficacy was distinctly suboptimal, and local reactions at the injection site and within draining lymph nodes were marked. This approach has been virtually abandoned, and much progress has been made toward newer vaccines.

Typhoid Vaccines

Typhoid fever, which is far more than a diarrheal disease because *Salmonella typhi* is an invasive organism that causes severe parenteral toxicity, remains a serious public health problem. The disease is both waterborne and foodborne in countries with poor sanitation, but it is now quite rare in industrialized countries. There are an estimated 16 million to 33 million cases annually, with 500,000 to 700,000 deaths. In endemic countries, the majority of patients are between ages 5 and 19, which makes school-based immunization an attractive possibility. Unfortunately, routine immunization is not yet occurring, and the effective present-day vaccines are almost entirely confined to use by travelers and armed services personnel. This is a pity, as a study in Egypt concluded there were 59 cases per 100,000 population per year, of which 20% were multidrug resistant.

The live attenuated orally administered *S. typhi* strain Ty21a has been licensed in the United States since 1991. This was derived from the wild-type strain Ty2, which has been maintained in the laboratory since 1918, and the vaccine strain was developed in the early 1970s by chemical mutagenesis. The vaccine can be given orally as enteric-coated capsules. Tests on 200,000 children in Chile showed a protective efficacy of 62% for up to 7 years. Alternatively, a liquid formulation is now available that seems to be more effective, yielding 79% efficacy among 36,000 children aged 5 to 19 (104).

The second typhoid vaccine is an injectable form consisting of the Vi antigen. This is a linear homopolymer of galacturonic acid and forms a part of the capsular polysaccharide of the organism. A single dose of carbohydrate only is 55% effective, protecting for two but not three years. At the International Vaccine Institute in Korea, Clemens' group is coordinating a program known as DOMI (diseases of the most impoverished) funded by the Bill & Melinda Gates Foundation. They have tested a Chinese Vi antigen produced locally. A study of 118,588 persons aged 5 to 60 undertaken in southeast China (105) achieved vaccination coverage of 78% and showed mass immunization to be feasible and safe. The same vaccine had proven 71% effective during a 1999 outbreak. A Vi conjugate vaccine has been prepared in the hope that, like other conjugate vaccines, it might prove more effective and work at younger ages. A landmark study by Lin et al. (106) used the Vi polysaccharide conjugated to recombinant *Pseudomonas aeruginosa* exoprotein A in a double-blind, randomized, placebo-controlled trial on 11,091 Vietnamese children aged 2 to 5. Two doses were given, 6 weeks apart, and a 27-month follow-up study (including blood culture) showed a remarkable 91% to 95% efficacy (4 cases among 5,525 vaccinees and 47 among 5,566 controls). Even one injection caused good protection. This vaccine is clearly the best currently available.

Robbins' group at the National Institutes of Health have come up with an original idea that might materially cut costs. They have initiated a trial (not fully recruited in 2006) of a di-O-acetyl derivative of fruit pectin as a mimic resembling the Vi antigen. This carbohydrate is abundant, cheap, and contains no LPS, and the chemical conversion is straightforward (107). O-acetyl pectin has also been conjugated to *P. aeruginosa* exoprotein A.

Cholera Vaccines

Cholera is a much-feared disease caused by the waterborne and highly infectious bacterium *V. cholerae,* which has caused devastating epidemics in many parts of the world. Although oral rehydration represented a real breakthrough, case-fatality rates can still reach 20%; the very young and the very old are most susceptible. Through the decades, there has been much strain variation. Since 1961, the biotype El Tor of serogroup 01 has been dominant, and since 1992, the new and more virulent variant 0139 has been a threat (see later discussion). Cholera accounts for an estimated 120,000 deaths each year.

Humans are the only known natural host for *V. cholerae,* although it is also known to be able to survive in water for very long periods. Transmission is due to fecal contamination of water or food, and direct transmission from person to person is thought to be rare. Invasion does not occur, and pathological processes are caused by the toxin and the profuse watery diarrhea that it induces. Protection is through mucosal antibodies.

In a troubled world, a cholera vaccine would take on new significance. Refugee camps represent populations at special risk. In this situation, vaccination should be undertaken preemptively. Once an epidemic is under way, it is probably too late.

More than 100 years after Koch's discovery of the cholera bacterium, we still do not have wide use of a vaccine, although good candidates have been licensed. This is a pity, as a natural infection can produce fairly solid immunity of substantial duration. However, progress has been heartening, including some third-world production.

Extensive work has been done on a Swedish oral vaccine (108) consisting of a mixture of the CTB and killed whole bacteria. The rationale for recombinant CTB is that it, a nontoxic component of cholera toxin, can give rise to toxin-neutralizing antibodies that can fully protect animals not only after toxin administration, but also after challenge with virulent *Vibrio cholerae*. Further, CTB is stable in the intestinal milieu and binds with high affinity to M cells, thus initiating the immune cascade. This anti-toxic immunity synergizes with antibacterial intestinal immunity conferred by the killed whole-cell vibrios. As currently formulated, each dose of the vaccine Dukoral contains 1 mg of recombinant CTB and 10^{11} vibrios including inactivated Inaba, El Tor, and Ogawa strains.

A large clinical trial in Bangladesh conducted among 62,285 children and women showed good but transient vaccine efficacy (109). For the first 5 to 6 months, protection was 85% (100% in children aged 2 to 5), but this had fallen to 64% by 1 year, 52% at 2 years, and only 19% at 3 years. Adults showed 78% and 63% protection for the first or second year. It appeared important to establish the safety and efficacy of the vaccine in a region with high HIV/AIDS prevalence. Accordingly, the vaccine was used in a mass oral immunization program in Beira, Mozambique, where seropositivity to HIV is 20% to 30% in adults (110). The vaccine in two doses yielded 78% protection and was equally effective in young children and adults. Of the estimated 19,550 persons in the target population, 72% received the first dose and 57% both doses. Although cholera victims were not tested for HIV, the absence of serious side effects suggests that the vaccine is safe to use in seropositive individuals. The trial represents a significant step in validating oral cholera immunization where it is needed most.

A further variant of cholera has emerged in Madras, India. This variant, *V. cholerae* serogroup 0139, has spread rapidly in India, Bangladesh, and adjacent countries and has reached as far as Malaysia, Thailand, and China. Accordingly, formalin-killed 0139 *Vibrio* organisms were added to the existing 01 vaccine, and intestinal and systemic immune responses against both strains were elicited in a majority of human volunteers. This suggests that the development of a bivalent vaccine will be relatively straightforward.

Beautiful work has been done under difficult circumstances in Vietnam. Trach et al. (111) recently reported on an oral killed whole-cell *V. cholerae* vaccine without CTB, consisting of two doses of a mixture of Inaba and Ogawa strains, that was subjected to trials in 134,453 people in Vietnam. This vaccine was locally produced in Hanoi and was inexpensive at about U.S. 10 cents per dose. During an epidemic about 8 months after immunization, it proved 66% protective. Despite some admitted limitations in the trial protocol, the results are promising. Recently a bivalent vaccine containing also serogroup 0139 has been prepared and is undergoing trial.

Several live attenuated strains of *V. cholerae* have reached clinical trial. All these have been constructed to possess known genetic deletions to reduce virulence. The most advanced strain is CVD103-HgR, a live oral cholera vaccine strain constructed by recombinant DNA methods from a classical Inaba strain in which the A subunit of CT has been deleted. This was safe and immunogenic in North American volunteers, provides significant protection against experimental challenge (112), and in 1993 a large-scale, randomized, placebo-controlled field trial was initiated in North Jakarta involving a single oral dose of vaccine. About 67,000 subjects aged 2 to 42 were involved. Unfortunately, in a 4-year follow-up, the vaccine could not be shown to be efficacious. The results were somewhat confounded by an unexpectedly low incidence of cholera during the first year of the trial. Although the results showed 60% protection over the first 6 months and 24% protection during the first year, the low numbers make these results uncertain. Some good results did come out of this trial, however. The vaccine was well tolerated, even in infants as young as 3 months, and it did not interfere with the oral typhoid vaccine Ty21a. Further work on CVD103-HgR is in progress. It is reasonable to conclude that it is a good vaccine for travelers, because protection is evident already 7 days after a single dose and the product (Orochol) is licensed in several countries. Convincing protection in field situations remains to be demonstrated. An attenuated 0139 live oral vaccine, known as CD112, has also been prepared and confers good protection against challenge with wild-type 0139.

Pearson et al. (113) constructed a new series of live attenuated oral cholera vaccines that are based on the deletion of a whole "virulence cassette." Instead of deleting just the CT gene, additional associated virulence factors are deleted. These include the genes for zona occludens toxin, auxiliary cholera enterotoxin, and core-encoded pilus. Certain sequences encouraging recombination were also deleted to prevent the strain from regaining CT genes. Further, mobility-deficient variants were found to be less reactogenic. Volunteer studies with two of these, Peru-15 for *V. cholerae* 01 and Bengal-15 for *V. cholerae* 0139, look promising for a one-dose oral vaccine.

Vaccines Against Enterotoxigenic Escheria coli *(ETEC)*

Enterotoxigenic *E. coli* is a major cause of traveler's diarrhea and also causes illness ranging from mild to very severe in young children in developing countries. The pathogenesis of the disease is either heat-labile enterotoxin (LT), heat-stable enterotoxin (ST), or both. LT cross-reacts with CTB and so the oral CTB-whole cholera vaccine is partially protective against it. A specific ETEC vaccine should contain both an LT toxoid (as the ST toxin appears to be poorly immunogenic) and antigens from the fimbrial proteins, which help to attach the *E. coli* to the small intestinal mucosa. These attachment proteins or colonization factors (CFs) are strain specific, and the most prevalent ones would have to be included. In the meantime, an ETEC vaccine consisting of recombinant CTB and formalin-inactivated whole-cell ETEC bacteria expressing five CFs has been in clinical trial (114). In travelers, it has 77% to 82% protective efficacy against severe diarrhea, but protection against mild diarrhea was less impressive. In children in rural Egypt the vaccine failed to protect except in a subset with high immune responses. This argues that CFs plus LT toxoid should be tried.

Another strategy of some promise is to use attenuated *Shigella* bacteria as a vector in which both CFs and detoxified LT are expressed. In guinea pigs, this approach engenders good mucosal immunity (115). However, this is no guarantee that the approach would work in the real-life setting of the intestinal tract of third-world infants. The latest developments concerning this Shigella-ETEC approach are considered in the next section.

Shigella Vaccines

The author was probably among the majority of medical graduates to express surprise when he learned that shigellosis or bacillary dysentery was a bigger public health problem than either typhoid or cholera. It is one of the most serious diarrheal diseases in the world, with an estimated 175 million episodes per annum and 800,000 deaths (116). Both case numbers and estimates of mortality need to be reestimated, because diarrheal disease mortality as a whole is clearly falling. The most important organisms are *Shigella flexneri, Shigella sonnei, Shigella boydii,* and *Shigella dysenteriae. S. flexneri* predominates in developing countries, and *S. sonnei* in industrialized countries, the latter type of country accounting for fewer than 1% of episodes. Each species has multiple serotypes; there are about 30 serotypes altogether, a frustrating fact for the vaccine developer. Usually, a given serotype predominates in a given area at a given time.

Clinical findings of shigellosis include diarrhea, which can vary from mild to extremely severe with ulcerative lesions of the colon and significant blood in the motions. Fever, dehydration, and metabolic disturbances are common, and hemolytic uremic syndrome is a serious complication.

Shigella is, in fact, a facultative intracellular parasite that invades the colonic and rectal mucosa. Invasion of M cells and other APCs occurs, and lymphoid collections can be rapidly destroyed. Systemic and mucosal humoral immune responses are elicited by an infection, and the LPS of the organism is of great importance, because antibodies to it can protect against bacterial challenge. In fact, the two most advanced lines of research into a vaccine involve parenteral O-specific polysaccharide-protein conjugates and live attenuated mutant shigella organisms given orally. Further approaches include an intranasal proteosome vaccine, a ribosomal vaccine, and vectored vaccines.

Among the live attenuated orally active vaccines, much work has been done by Sansonetti and Phalipon (117) on a deletion mutant of *S. flexneri* serotype 2a strain SC602. This carries both an auxotrophic mutation (deletion of *ivcA*) and one diminishing virulence (deletion of *icsA*, also known as *virG*). An attractive feature of this vaccine is that oral administration of as few as 10^3 to 10^4 live organisms elicits a good local IgA response. In a series of clinical trials, a total of 58 North American volunteers experienced significant reactogenicity in 30% of cases, but interestingly this was not the case in an adult phase I trial in Bangladesh (120) in either adults or children. Unfortunately, these volunteers did not mount an antibody response, so for them at least SC602 appears to have been over-attenuated. Nevertheless, trials of higher doses are planned. This group has also developed a live attenuated *Shigella dysenteriae 1* vaccine strain SC599. The Pasteur Institute is currently (October 2006) recruiting for a phase II immunogenicity and safety clinical trial of two oral doses of this candidate.

Kotloff et al. (118) have developed the CVD series of attenuated vaccine candidates. CVD 1203 is an attenuated *S. flexneri 2a* with deletions in *aroA* and *icsA*, escalating doses showing increasing immunogenicity but also increasing reactogenitity. CVD 1207, with deletions that prevent enterotoxin formation, was less reactogenic but also less immunogenic. CVD 1208, with deletions in *guaBA, set,* and *sen,* was satisfactorily immunogenic with little reactogenicity. The University of Maryland group believes (119) that a multivalent *Shigella* vaccine providing broad coverage against disease will have to include *S. flexneri 2a, S. flexneri 3a, S. flexneri 6, S. sonnei,* and *S. dynenteriae 1.* Attenuated forms of *S. sonnei* (CVD1233) and *S. dysenteriae* (CVD1252) have been prepared. These strains are also being evaluated for use as live vectors for ETEC antigens including fimbrial and LT components. In a similar effort, SC608, a derivative of SC602, engineered to express ETEC fimbrial and enterotoxin antigens, performed well when given intranasally to guinea pigs as a combined Shigella-ETEC vaccine (120).

A further attenuated vaccine is the *S. sonnei* strain WRSS1 that contains an *icsA* deletion. Tested in Israeli army volunteers, it proved to be reasonably immunogenic and well tolerated.

As a final live attenuated approach, the typhoid vaccine strain Ty21a was engineered to carry *Shigella* LPS antigens. Early results look promising in both mice and a small number of human volunteers.

Parenteral vaccination represents a complete alternative and has been pioneered by Robbins and Schneerson (121), rightly honored for their role in the invention of the *Hemophilus influenzae B* conjugate vaccine. As the O-specific polysaccharide domain of the LPS of *Shigella* is essential for its virulence, this antigen conjugated to protein should make a good, T cell–dependent vaccine. In a small-scale efficacy trial, such a conjugate from *S. sonnei* conferred 74% protection to Israeli military recruits who suffered from a high rate of shigellosis during their basic training. Synthetic tetrasaccharides of increasing length corresponding to the O antigen of *S. dysenteriae* have also been prepared and conjugated, the optimal synthetic configuration proving to be significantly more immunogenic than the natural product. Altogether, this approach looks very promising.

Other inactivated vaccines under investigation include 3 to 5 oral doses of whole killed bacteria; an intranasal proteosome vaccine consisting of 1 mg of LPS noncovalently complexed with outer membrane proteins from *Neisseria meningitidis*, which proved reasonably protective in volunteers; purified ribosomes from *Shigella* bacteria, which have O antigen covalently bound and can be given parenterally; and 34kDa outer membrane protein from *Shigella flexneri* 2a, which, when injected, elicits a good protective response in animals (122).

So the research scene bristles with promising candidate *Shigella* vaccines, but clinical trials in developing country settings are now urgently required.

Helicobacter pylori Vaccines

In 1983, one of those rare true breakthroughs in medicine occurred. Peptic ulcer, a classical and common disease, had been thought to be caused by stress and hyperacidity. Instead, Marshall and Warren (123) attributed it to a spiral bacterium, soon identified as *Helicobacter pylori*. This discovery from Australia was greeted with great skepticism but was supported by Marshall's brave attempt to fulfill Koch's postulates through infecting himself, which resulted in gastritis and re-isolation of the organism, after which he cured himself with antibiotics. It is now generally accepted that *H. pylori* accounts not only for the majority of gastric and duodenal ulcers, but also for acute gastritis, chronic active gastritis, a significant proportion of gastric adenocarcinomas, and essentially 100% of B cell lymphomas of gastric MALT. Marshall and Warren's 2005 Nobel Prize was thoroughly well deserved.

Although the WHO had classified *H. pylori* as a class I carcinogen in 1994, it was only in 2001 that Uemura et al. (124) put the issue beyond doubt with a long-term prospective study of 1,526 Japanese patients with dyspepsia who were monitored for a mean period of 7.8 years. Of these, 1,246 had *H. pylori* infection and 280 did not. Within the study period, 36 gastric cancers developed, of which 23 were intestinal-type cancers and 13 were diffuse-type cancers. Every single cancer occurred among the infected patients ($p < 0.001$). Kaplan-Meier analysis showed the gastric cancer risk to be 5% in the infected group at 10 years.

Infection is acquired mostly during childhood and persists chronically if not treated, but it is reasonably easily cured by so-called "triple therapy" consisting of a proton-pump inhibitor and two antibiotics (e.g., metronidazole and ampicillin).

Many aspects of the epidemiology of *H. pylori* remain mysterious. Transmission is believed to be oral, through vomitus or diarrheal feces. Infection may result in a brief period of acute gastritis, after which the carrier has few or no symptoms for years or even decades. Infection is incredibly common, typically 40% in industrialized countries and up to 90% in some developing countries. However, of these infected people, only 15% to 20% eventually develop severe gastric or duodenal disease. The degree to which these bacteria represent a public health problem is still not generally appreciated. In the United States, it has been estimated that up to 25 million persons are ill with this infection at some stage of their lives. In these cases, re-infection after cure is rare, perhaps 1% per year, but in developing countries, it could be expected to be much higher. In such settings, a prophylactic vaccine would be especially desirable.

H. pylori is a gram-negative spiral, microaerophilic, flagellated bacterium that produces an amazing amount of the enzyme urease, which can make up 5% to 10% of the bacterium's protein. This converts gastric fluid urea to ammonia and carbon dioxide, a very efficient buffering system against stomach acid. Urease-negative *H. pylori* strains appear unable to colonize the stomach. We know much too little about why only some infected people develop chronic gastric disease. The best hint (125) comes from strain variation in the bacteria. Specifically, strains of type I possess a 40-kb fragment of DNA that comprises 31 genes and constitutes a pathogenicity island. Important within this area are the antigen CagA and genes that encode a secretion machinery that allows the active transfer of molecules from the bacterium to the gastric epithelial cell on which the bacteria reside. So-called type I strains express CagA (and appear to be more virulent), whereas type II strains do not. Further, type II strains are sometimes low expressers of another gene, that for the vacuolating cytotoxin VacA, which is thought to be important in pathogenesis. More work needs to be done on strain subtyping.

Neutrophil infiltration is a prominent feature in biopsy specimens from *H. pylori*–infected stomachs. An *H. pylori* 15-kDa protein that is chemotactic for neutrophils and monocytes and is a strong inducer of the production of reactive oxygen intermediates in neutrophils has been identified. This has been termed *neutrophil-activating protein* (NAP). Other possible candidate vaccine antigens of *H. pylori* include flagellin, various adhesins, heat-shock proteins, and LPS.

Animal models have provided proof of principle that both prophylactic and therapeutic *H. pylori* vaccines are feasible. Lee et al. (126) isolated a gastric spiral bacterium from cats, and this organism, *Helicobacter felis*, can colonize the mouse stomach and cause gastritis and even lymphoma. With this model in place, it was soon shown that a sonicate of *H. felis* was a protective vaccine in mice, providing 96% protection against oral challenge. A further important development was that of adapting fresh clinical isolates of *H. pylori* to grow in the mouse stomach by biweekly serial passage through specific pathogen-free mice. This resulted in the development of (a) one strain, derived from a type I clinical isolate, that caused gastric pathological processes mimicking those in the human, and (b) of another strain, derived from a type II clinical isolate, that caused only a mild inflammatory infiltrate without erosive lesions.

These considerations naturally led to the possibility of subunit vaccines. *H. pylori* urease was the first antigen in clinical trial, because it confers protection in animal models. The results of the first studies were not too impressive, although there was some reduction in the bacterial load. Both CagA and VacA are being assessed as possible oral immunogens in the *H. pylori* mouse model, with the addition of the genetically detoxified *E. coli* heat-labile enterotoxin, LTK63, as a mucosal adjuvant. Early results appear encouraging, as do those with CagA, VacA, and NAP in combination.

What about therapeutic intervention? Doidge et al. (127) achieved eradication of *H. felis* in infected mice with an oral administration of *H. felis* sonicate and CT as a mucosal adjuvant. Similarly, Corthesy-Theulaz et al. (128) successfully used the *H. pylori* urease B subunit as an oral treatment in mice. These results give encouragement for clinical therapeutic vaccine trials. It is probable that Th1 T cells are responsible for much of the inflammatory damage in the stomach, and a change in the balance toward a greater proportion of Th2 cells may be helpful. This accentuates the importance of a safe and effective adjuvant suitable for human use.

A beagle dog model of *H. pylori* infection has been developed, enabling serial gastric biopsies and thus dynamic evaluation of progressive pathological processes (129). In this model, encouraging results have been obtained with systemic immunization with a variety of recombinant proteins, including VacA, CagA, and NAP, simply adsorbed onto alum. A phase I human study validated the safety and immunogenicity of this combination. In view of the relatively low rate of acquisition of infection in industrialized countries, it is likely that any subunit combination vaccine arising from this research will have to be tested in areas with high transmission rates, such as in less developed countries or high-susceptibility ethnic minorities. However, this has not occurred, and one senses a degree of frustration from Doidge at the slow rate of progress (130). He considers the current generation of vaccines as insufficiently successful and pleads for new targets and adjuvants. The Chinese University of Military Medical Science is recruiting a phase III clinical trial of an oral *H. pylori* vaccine involving 10,000 volunteers, but no details of this vaccine are available.

If a safe, effective vaccine conferring a substantial period of protection can be developed, the approximately 1% lifetime risk of gastric cancer would, by itself, justify universal use; in view of the additional severe morbidity arising from chronic gastritis, gastric dysplasia, and peptic ulcer disease, the case becomes very strong indeed.

Vaccines Against Encapsulated Organisms

Haemophilus Influenzae B

Vaccines traditionally available for encapsulated organisms such as those just described have been prepared from purified capsular polysaccharide antigen. These vaccines suffer from two major disadvantages. First, being polysaccharide in nature, they do not engage the T cell limb of the immune response. This means that the antibodies are chiefly IgM, affinity maturation does not occur, and, most important, young infants do not respond well. Because the incidence of Hib meningitis peaks at around 10 to 11 months of age, a vaccine that is not really effective before the ages of 18 to 24 months is far from ideal.

The first-generation Hib vaccine, based on the polyribosylribitol phosphate (PRP) capsule, was developed almost simultaneously by Anderson et al. (131) and Rodrigues et al. (132). An extensive clinical trial involving 130,178 Finnish children was performed by Peltala et al. (133). No protection was noted in children younger than 18 months, even in those given a booster dose, but just a single dose in children aged 18 months to 5 years of age gave good protection against invasive Hib disease.

The second problem for these vaccines is that, in each case, there are multiple serotypes. With Hib, six capsular serotypes, a to f, are capable of causing disease in humans; fortunately, 99% of typeable strains causing invasive disease are type b. As we shall see, the problem is much worse for meningococci and pneumococci.

The same groups that pioneered the carbohydrate vaccine were involved in the breakthrough that yielded the extremely effective Hib conjugate vaccine (134,135). These researchers made use of the principle of conjugating antigenic Hib PRP saccharides to protein carriers to induce a T cell–dependent response, which matures much earlier in the human than does the T cell–independent response to saccharides alone. Different-length saccharides and different carriers were used by different companies; small, medium, and large polysaccharides were attached, with or without linkers, to diphtheria toxoid, the diphtheria toxin variant CRM_{197}, tetanus toxoid, or the group B meningococcal outer membrane complex. Eskola et al. (136) led the way with a clinical trial in Finland in 1986 to 1987 in which the vaccine was 83% effective and also eliminated oropharyngeal carriage. A further trial with an improved vaccine in 1988 to 1990 showed higher, more persistent antibody levels and better efficacy. From about 1990 on, there has been an increasing number of countries with national vaccination programs, and the result has been a dramatic decline in invasive Hib disease because of immunity, herd immunity, and lowered pathogen carriage rates. Already by 1991, meningitis incidence had decreased by 82% in the United States. In many countries, Hib meningitis is simply not seen anymore. It may not be too early to hope for the eventual control and near-eradication of this pathogen. Particularly encouraging is the fact that the conjugate vaccine works well in the setting of a developing country. Mulholland et al. (137) performed a double-blind randomized trial in The Gambia involving 42,848 infants who were given either DPT alone at 2, 3, and 4 months or DPT mixed with Hib polysaccharide-tetanus protein (PRP-T). Hib meningitis, Hib pneumonia, and five other forms of invasive Hib disease were evaluated over a 3-year period. Among the children (83%) who received all three doses, the efficacy of the vaccine for the prevention of all invasive Hib disease was 95%; for the prevention of Hib pneumonia, 100%; and of meningitis, 92%. Further, there was a 21.1% reduction of *all* cases of radiologically defined pneumonia.

Given the importance of acute respiratory disease as a killer of infants in developing countries, the Hib vaccine is progressively being added to routine infant immunization programs. Manufacturers are making vaccine available to poor countries at reasonable prices and combinations (e.g., DPT-hepatitis B-Hib) are helpful in reducing the number of injections required. There is evidence that Hib may be somewhat less of a problem in Asia than in Africa, and this is patiently being explored country by country. The conjugate vaccine is being widely used in Latin America.

Neisseria meningitidis

Neisseria meningitidis or the meningococcus causes a frightening disease with sudden onset and severe complications. Further, survivors may suffer lasting damage such as epilepsy, mental retardation or hearing loss. In contrast to Hib, which mainly strikes infants, meningococcal disease can occur at any age, with peak incidences in young children and adolescents and young adults. There are 13 identified serogroups based on the chemical structures of their capsular polysaccharide coats, of which the most important are A, B, C, Y, and W135. Most outbreaks in the industrialized world are serogroup B or C, whereas the commonest epidemic strain in Africa is A. There are also rare nontypeable strains, some of which have been proven to be serogroup B with poor expression of the capsular polysaccharide.

Two recent meningococcal public health measures are of particular interest. The first concerns control of African meningitis epidemics. These occur from December to June in the dry season in the countries of the so-called "meningitis belt" of Sub-Saharan Africa stretching from The Gambia and Senegal in the west to Ethiopia and Somalia in the east. The population at risk numbers 430 million people. A bad epidemic may result in 200,000 cases, with a 10% case fatality and 10% to 15% serious sequelae. Outbreak control previously depended on deployment of the meningococcal polysaccharide vaccine. In 2001, the Bill & Melinda Gates Foundation provided $70 million for the Meningitis Vaccine Project, a partnership between WHO and the Program for Appropriate Technology in Health (PATH). This called for expressions of interest in the development of a conjugate vaccine for *N. meningitidis* serogroup A, and eventually the Serum Institute of India in Pune was chosen as the commercial partner, with a view to providing 25 million doses annually at a cost of 40 U.S. cents per dose. The strategy called for industrialized country producers to supply both the serogroup A polysaccharide and the carrier tetanus toxoid, and for an experienced contract research organization to transfer the conjugation technology to India. In the event, all these steps were successfully completed and in March 2006 a successful phase I clinical study on 74 subjects found the vaccine to be safe and immunogenic. Phase II studies in The Gambia and Mali are commenced in late 2006. If all goes well, the vaccine will be through all testing and widely deployed in 1 to 29 year olds in 2009. Eventually infants will be immunized as well. As an epidemic of W135 meningitis has occurred in Burkina Faso, careful sero-surveillance will be required and a bi- or multivalent vaccine may eventually be needed.

The second series of programs relate to industrialized countries and the control of meningococcus C. A major campaign in the United Kingdom beginning in November 1999 introduced the conjugate vaccine into their routine 2, 3, and 4 months-of-age program. In addition, vaccine was offered to all persons under 18 in a catch-up campaign. The program was highly successful in virtually eliminating this form of meningitis (138), and follow-up studies have shown vaccine effectiveness to remain high 4 years later in those immunized from 5 months to 18 years of age, but less so in those immunized earlier (139). This suggests a booster in the second year of life might be wise. Herd immunity certainly played its part in the success. Successful programs have also been reported from Spain and Scotland, whereas in the Netherlands a single dose of vaccine at 14 months appears to be satisfactory.

A serious problem remains with meningococcus B, which causes 32% of meningococcal disease in the United States and more than 45% in Europe. The group B polysaccharide is composed of a homolinear polymer of (α2.3-8) N-acetyl neuraminic acid. Not only is this poorly immunogenic even when conjugated to protein, probably for reasons of immunologic tolerance, but also long-chain polysialated glycoproteins are abundant in immature brains, raising the specter of neurological damage if ways were found to break the tolerance. Attempts have been made to replace the native N-acetyl groups with N-propionyl groups, with some success. Alternatively and preferably, protein-based vaccines are being developed. Outer membrane vesicles can be prepared by detergent extraction from bacterial cells. These contain the major porin proteins as well as lipopolysaccharide and have had some success in outbreak control, but not in infants or young children (140). Further, the porins are subtype specific. A much more modern approach involves the technique of "genome mining" (141). In this project, the whole genome of the group B meningococcus MC58 was sequenced and 2,158 open reading frames were identified. Algorithms were used to identify proteins that might be exposed on the surface. Further, emphasis was placed on sequences homologous to group A meningococci and a *N. gonorrhea* strain. A total of 344 probably surface-exposed and conserved sequences were cloned, expressed in *E. coli* and injected into mice. Among these, 28 novel proteins that elicited antibodies that bound to the bacterial surface and had bactericidal activity were identified. A few elicited bactericidal titers comparable to those obtained by the outer membrane vesicle vaccine. From this group, five antigens were selected as inferred by high bactericidal activity or passive protection of mice or rats (142). These were combined into a multicomponent vaccine that was found to produce broad-based immunity. With alum as an adjuvant, mice made antibodies capable of killing 70% of a panel of 85 meningococcal strains from recent clinical isolates representative of global population diversity. When either CpG-ODN or MF59 was used as an adjuvant, this figure increased to 90%. Clinical trials are now planned. The genome mining "reverse vaccinology" approach involving isolation of new antigens and testing of resultant antisera against large collections of pathogen isolates holds promise for other protein-based vaccines.

In the meantime, a combined A, C, Y, W135 conjugate has been successfully trialed, and it remains to be seen where this will fit into the marketplace given that B and C are the dominant strains in the industrialized world. For the author, who feared missing the diagnosis of a meningitis case more than almost anything else during his hospital resident days, the thought of a "meningitis package" vaccine, including Hib and perhaps nontypable *Hemophilus*, would be like a dream come true.

Streptococcus pneumoniae

Streptococcus pneumoniae, the pneumococcus, is the leading cause of severe pneumonia in children and can also cause meningitis and septicemia, as well as less severe respiratory infections and otitis media. It also affects adults, particularly the elderly. It causes 800,000 to 1 million child deaths each year and an additional 800,000 deaths in adults. More than 90% of pneumococcal pneumonia deaths in children occur in developing countries, and children with HIV/AIDS are 20 to 40 times more likely to get invasive pneumococcal disease than other children. An effective vaccine is thus a tool of immense public health importance. There are more than 80 pneumococcus serotypes based on the polysaccharide capsule, but Merck's 23-valent carbohydrate vaccine, which has been available since 1983, covers most of the pathogenic isolates. This vaccine works well in children over 2 years and in adults, but for infants, a carbohydrate-protein conjugate is required. Several large firms have prepared and tested conjugate vaccines of 7 to 11 serotypes, but only one vaccine has been licensed, Wyeth's 7-valent Prevnar. A phase III clinical trial involving 37,000 Californian infants resulted in 22 observed cases of invasive pneumococcal disease caused by organisms of one of the 7 serotypes in the control group but zero cases in the immunized group ($p < 0.0001$). This 100% efficacy raises the question of whether any further controlled trials would be ethical. However, conditions in developing countries are different, so results of a large trial in The Gambia were greeted with great interest (143). A 9-valent conjugate vaccine containing 8 serotype-specific polysaccharides and one oligosaccharide conjugated to the diphtheria toxoid CRM-17 was used. The randomized, placebo-controlled, double-blind trial involved 8,718 vaccinees aged 6 to 51 weeks and 8,719 controls. Three doses were given at least 25 days apart, and over 95% of the children actually got all 3. The primary endpoint was radiologically proven pneumonia, and the vaccine efficacy was 37% against all causes of pneumonia. Secondary endpoints included invasive pneumococcal disease caused by vaccine serotypes, with 77% efficacy, and mortality from any cause at all, with a heartening 16% reduction. These results demonstrate that a pneumococcal conjugate vaccine would be a real boon in a developing country setting.

GlaxoSmithKline is developing an 11-valent pneumococcal vccine where the polysaccharides are conjugated to *Hemophilus influenzae* protein D as a carrier protein. An interesting large study conducted in the Czech Republic and Slovakia looked at the effects of this vaccine on otitis media, a very common childhood infection accounting for more than 20 million visits to a pediatrician each year in the United States (144). The two leading bacterial pathogens are *S. pneumoniae* and nontypable *H. influenzae*. The vaccine design was such as to kill two birds with one stone. In the randomized trial involving 4,968 infants, subjects received either this conjugate vaccine or hepatitis A vaccine as a control, and four doses were given at 3, 4, 5, and 12 to 15 months of age. Children were followed until the end of the second year of life. The vaccine was 34% effective against all otitis media, 58% effective against otitis media caused by pneumococcal serotypes included in the vaccine, and 35% effective against otitis caused by nontypable *H. influenzae*. The vaccine also reduced nasopharyngeal carriage of both pathogens. The efficacy against serotype-caused otitis was similar to that in prior Finnish studies. While pneumonia as such was not studied in this case, the combined vaccine must be considered quite promising. It is now being studied in a global clinical program but will not be available for several years.

Obviously, the more serotypes need to be included, the more expensive the conjugate vaccine will be. Therefore, it is a pleasure to record that in 2006 the Bill & Melinda Gates Foundation initiated a large granting program to speed the search for a common protein-based pneumococcal vaccine.

Intracellular Pathogens, Especially Tuberculosis and Leprosy

Bacteria that exploit the scavenger cell system and successfully learn to live inside cells present special challenges to the vaccine developer. Organisms of this sort include *Mycobacterium tuberculosis, Mycobacterium leprae,* and *Listeria monocytogenes.* Robust T-cell responses are the key to immune protection in these cases, involving Th1-type $CD4^+$ cells and $CD8^+$ CTLs, as well as γ/δ T cells and NK cells, each of which has been shown to be of importance. Induction of γ-interferon positive T cells is a central theme in the search for new vaccines (145). Because of its great public health importance, we shall consider mainly TB.

TB is one of the greatest communicable disease killers in the world. An astonishing 2 billion people harbor the bacterium in latent form; of these people, fewer than 10% develop active disease. However, there are about 9 million new active cases each year and about 2 million annual deaths. Unless something is done, between 2000 and 2020 there will be 1 billion people newly infected with TB, 200 million active cases, and 35 million deaths. Two huge threats are (a) combined infection with HIV and TB, in which death can occur within weeks of infection, and (b) the increased prevalence of strains of *M. tuberculosis* that are resistant to one or more antimicrobial agents. For example, in the United States, 13% of new TB cases are resistant to at least one first-line drug, and 3% are resistant to both isoniazid and rifampycin, the two most important drugs.

BCG was developed by serial passage of *Mycobacterium bovis* on media for an incredible 13 years, and it was introduced in 1921. It is the most widely used vaccine in the world, total usage having been over 3 billion doses. It is clearly effective in preventing severe childhood forms of TB, such as TB meningitis and military TB, estimates of efficacy varying from 50% to 80%, and in a developing country setting its broad immunostimulatory action may lower overall infant mortality in the first 6 months, although these studies are controversial. However, BCG is unreliable against adult TB. Early controlled trials suggested good efficacy, but half a dozen later trials, including one very large one in India, proved equivocal or negative. A general consensus today would be that the efficacy of BCG wanes after 10 to 15 years, and, curiously, booster doses do not seem to help, although they may (through cross-reaction) be partially effective for leprosy. The need for a more effective vaccine with a longer-lasting effect is clear. One possible reason for poor apparent efficacy in developing country trials is that prior exposure to environmental mycobacteria may either reduce or mask the protective effect of BCG. A hopeful vista for the longer-term future is that anti-microbial therapy and immunization will interact beneficially. Where it is assiduously pursued, "DOTS"—directly observed therapy, short course—is already having an effect, and DOTS is becoming more widely available through the WHO's Stop TB Partnership and the Global Fund to Fight AIDS, TB, and Malaria.

Attempts to develop a better TB vaccine fall under three broad headings (146), namely new and more planned attenuation of *M. tuberculosis,* restoring to BCG genes for important antigens that had been lost, and a subunit approach using antigens plus an adjuvant shown to be effective through animal models. Of course, such antigens could be coded for by DNA, either "naked" or via a vector, and "prime-boost" strategies could also be entertained.

All three approaches have been helped by the fact that the genome of *M. tuberculosis* has been sequenced (147), as have those of *M. bovis* and of BCG. This has helped the identification of genes deleted during the attenuation process and, through "reverse genetics," in the search for proteins that might represent credible vaccine candidates. Even before this analysis, more empirical research had thrown up at least 20 molecules capable of conferring protection.

Britton and Palendira (146) have summarized the single and double auxotrophic mutants of *M. tuberculosis* capable of protecting mice or guinea pigs. Some of these provide greater immunity than BCG—for example, a mutant unable to export the complex lipid phthiocerol dimycocerosate (148). Studies in immunodeficient mice have shown some of these mutants to be more virulent than BCG, and with the great prevalence of HIV in many countries with high TB incidence, this could constitute a grave problem. Risk of reversion to virulence is ever present, although less in doubly mutated strains. Finally, regulatory bodies may find it difficult to approve any *M. tuberculosis* derived strain.

Improving the current BCG essentially means adding genes that had been deleted and that code for credible candidate antigens. BCG has 14 regions of deletion and is missing 129 genes. Two recombinant BCG strains have entered phase I clinical trials, one over-expressing an antigen known as 85B and the other a urease-deficient strain expressing listeriolysin from *Listeria monocytogenes* (summarized in [145]).

With respect to the subunit approach, literally hundreds of proteins have been screened in experimental animal models (149), including systematic functional genomic antigen discovery and prioritization (150). Prominent targets include antigens secreted into bacterial culture filtrates such as the antigen 85 complex, a family of three closely related mycolyl transferases with homologues in all mycobacterial species, and ESAT-6, a protein restricted to *M. tuberculosis*. Ag85A, Ag85B, and ESAT-6 together represent a powerful combination (summarized in [151]). Mtb72f is a fusion protein derived from two cytoplasmic proteins mtb32 and mtb39 and has passed a phase I clinical trial promoted by GlaxoSmithKline and Corixa (150). The functional genomic approach including the use of human sera to identify proteins immunogenic for humans produced this promising candidate, which with the use of the ASO2A adjuvant induces a strong Th1 response. The final subunit vaccine already in clinical trial is a fusion protein of Ag85B and ESAT-6 given with an adjuvant IC31 from Intercell that contains CpG oligodeoxy-nucleotides and polycationic amino acids (Table 40.6).

Various alternative strategies are using these antigens as well. McShane et al. (152), trialing BCG vaccination followed by a boost with MVA containing Ag85A, are obtaining strong IFN-γ responses in trials both in the United Kingdom and The Gambia. Phase II human studies have commenced with this candidate. Preclinical studies have shown that combinations of multiple antigens as a DNA construct work well—for example, Ag85B plus ESAT-6 plus Ag64; further, the use of plasmid cytokines IL-12 or IL-23 increases T cell responses and vaccine efficacy using subunit DNA vaccines (153). A fuller list of the 20 or so DNA constructs that have shown efficacy in mice can be found in reference (148). Priming with Ag85B DNA and boosting with BCG gave good $CD4^+$ and $CD8^+$ T cell responses and better protection than BCG alone. Boosting with Ag85B as protein or priming with BCG and boosting with Ag85B DNA did not do as well. Recombinant adenovirus vectors represent an attractive alternative to MVA.

Any TB vaccine could be used in one of three ways: pre-exposure to prevent infection, post-exposure to prevent disease, or therapeutically to help to control established disease. Obviously in the third case the vaccine would be adjunct to a drug treatment program. Given the widespread use of BCG in developing countries, it is likely that any new vaccine would, in the first instance, be given to individuals who had already received BCG. Modeling the possible effects of a vaccine highlights that it would act synergistically with chemotherapy. A scenario that many favor is periodic mass vaccination and very intense search for active cases then promptly treated with chemotherapy.

Obviously clinical trials in a disease with such a long latent period will be lengthy, arduous, and expensive. Fortunately, the Bill & Melinda Gates Foundation, the European Commission, and the U.S. National Institutes of Health are all aware of this, and global collaboration toward a licensed vaccine by 2015 is impressive (151).

Leprosy

M. leprae has many similarities to *M. tuberculosis*. Some of the urgency has gone out of the search for a leprosy vaccine because of the remarkable success of multidrug therapy. There is good evidence that BCG itself is a moderately protective vaccine against leprosy, and Convit's vaccine, consisting of killed, armadillo-derived *M. leprae* plus live BCG, appears to be better. Other mycobacteria such as killed *Mycobacterium w* appear to be modestly effective. The subunit vaccine approach is not being actively pursued. One candidate is a 35-kDa protein that is a major target of the human T cell response to *M. leprae*. Sequencing of the *M. leprae* genome is now complete and may in time provide further candidate molecules.

Vaccines Against Group A Streptococci

Somewhat amazingly, since the development of penicillin during World War II, rheumatic fever and rheumatic heart disease nevertheless remain common in many developing countries, the prevalence being up to 20 per 1,000. *Streptococcus pyogenes* infections can also be followed by acute and chronic glomerulonephritis and otitis media. A good vaccine candidate would be the M protein, a coiled-coil alpha helical surface protein of the bacterium. However, the vaccine developer faces two major hurdles. First, there are more than 100 serotypes of group A streptococci, and

TABLE 40.6 Most Advanced Tuberculosis Vaccine Candidates (From 147,148,152,153)

Category	*Candidate*	*Key Investigator*	*Trial Phase*
Genetically engineered BCG	BCG overexpressing Ag85B	Horowitz, UCLA	I
	Urease-deficient BCG expressing listeriolysin	Kaufmann, Berlin	I
Subunit vaccines	Fusion protein of Ag85B and ESAT-6 with IC31 adjuvant	Anderson, Copenhagen	I
	Fusion protein of two secreted proteins, Mtb32 and Mtb39	Reed, Seattle	I
Vectored vaccine	MVA, a replication-deficient vaccinia virus, epxressing Ag85A boosts BCG-primed or naturally acquired TB immunity	McShane and Hill, Oxford	II

much of the variation is in the immunity-inducing but highly variable N-terminal portion of the M protein. Second, the major complications are almost certainly autoimmune in nature, and it would be a disaster if immunization triggered the very events that the vaccine is supposed to prevent. Brandt et al. (154) first identified a conserved, non–host cross-reactive peptide from the C-terminal half of the M protein and then linked this (in a manner that maintained the peptide's helical conformation) with a multiepitopic peptide consisting of seven N-terminal portions from seven different, relatively common serotypes, targeting northern Australian aboriginal isolates. The polymer technology, already described in the section on adjuvants, ensured full immunogenicity of all components. The vaccine was strongly immunogenic and protective in mice against a wide variety of strains and was not cross-reactive with any of many host self-proteins. The nature of the polymer backbone would allow peptides from other, non–M protein–derived vaccine candidates to be added as well. Such candidates include C5a peptidase, cysteine protease, and other streptococcal pyrogenic exotoxins. Some of these toxins can be rendered harmless through mutagenesis of the relevant genes. Another candidate is the major streptococcal adhesin, a protein known as sfbl.

Various formulations of these candidates, including parenteral injection, intranasal inoculation, and expression on the surface of *Streptococcus gordonii,* a commensal organism of the oral cavity, are in preclinical research. As antibiotic resistance becomes more of a problem, the pressure will build to take some of these candidates to the clinic.

VIRAL VACCINES

Viral vaccine research has produced both triumphs and tribulations. The triumphs include success against poliomyelitis, measles, mumps, rubella, varicella, hepatitis B, and, to a lesser extent, hepatitis A. The tribulations include struggles with HIV/AIDS, dengue, Epstein-Barr virus, and hepatitis C. Influenza and rotavirus are poised in between. It is not possible to run through the whole gamut of viral vaccines. Rather, the author wishes to highlight some of the complexities and remaining challenges and draw some lessons from them.

Hepatitis A, B, and C

These three viruses show an interesting spectrum of solved and unsolved problems that confront the vaccinologist. Hilleman (155) cited literature suggesting that contagious jaundice has been known to occur since the 5th century B.C. It became clear in the 1950s that "infectious hepatitis" and "homologous serum jaundice" had differing features, and this difference was cemented in the 1960s. Since the isolation of hepatitis A and B viruses and good serological tests for their recent presence, other forms of fecal-oral and of blood transmission of hepatitis have been discovered, of which the most important enterically transmitted agent is hepatitis E, and the most important parenterally transmitted is hepatitis C.

Hepatitis A is one of a group of diseases that also includes infectious mononucleosis, which is mild or entirely asymptomatic if contracted by young children but more severe if contracted in adolescents and adults. In rare cases, it causes fulminant hepatitis but is usually less severe, although it causes illness for up to several months. It is now only moderately common in industrialized countries, but very common in many developing countries. Immunization is a good idea for travelers, and both active immunization, giving long protection, and passive immunization with immune serum globulin, giving 3 months' protection, work well.

The virus initially proved very difficult to grow, and early studies depended on its identification by electron microscopy in fecal extracts. It was eventually grown in marmoset liver cells and a human hepatoma cell line, after which many types of cells were successfully infected. Growth of the virus in LLC-MK2 cells and availability of a marmoset model for vaccine testing led to a formalin-inactivated killed whole-virus vaccine, which, however, was not acceptable at that time because malignant cells were involved in growing the virus. Two groups eventually succeeded in obtaining growth in human diploid lung fibroblasts, and the resultant vaccines from (then) Smith KlineBeecham and Merck Sharp & Dohme work well. However, because virus yields are not enormous, hepatitis A is an expensive vaccine, and a live attenuated vaccine would be most beneficial in a developing nation. Several candidate vaccines exist; one has been extensively tested in China and found to be highly effective, but none has yet made it through to full registration.

Hepatitis B carrier rates vary from less than 0.1% to 15% of the population in different countries. Altogether, 2 billion people have serological evidence of past infection, and 350 million people are chronically infected. One million people die each year of cirrhosis or hepatocellular carcinoma. The acute attack is mild or insignificant. Hepatitis B virus does not grow in tissue culture, and there are two sources of vaccine: HBsAg isolated from chronic carriers of the virus, and the same material molecularly cloned in yeast or Chinese hamster ovary cells. The carrier-derived vaccine was, for a long time, far cheaper and has been widely used in developing countries. Now the recombinant vaccine has become much cheaper. Some recent tenders for the public sector in developing countries have come in at around 30 U.S. cents per dose, so recombinant vaccine has essentially replaced the human-derived material. Both vaccines are about equally effective; response rates to protective levels of antibody vary from 85% to 95%

in different studies. Protection may be achieved with lower levels of antibody than those generally believed to be protective, perhaps because of $CD8^+$ T cell effects. One worry is that some vaccinated people become carriers of what have been called "escape mutants," which persist despite the presence of good antibody levels to the native virus. The most common change is an arginine-for-glycine substitution in the *a* loop, against which antibodies are usually directed. Although it is not yet certain that the mutation changes the virus to one of lower infectivity, M. H. Kane (personal communication) pointed out that there is no evidence yet of escape mutants having spread from one person to another. There is therefore no need yet to worry about the univalency of the current vaccine. Presumably, if escape mutants become a problem but if the number of different serotypes is limited, the variants could be included in a recombinant vaccine. It is encouraging to note that universal infant immunization is now being widely adopted. Further, the vaccine is frequently given in combination with others.

The hepatitis C virus was the first of the non-A, non-B viruses identified. Hepatitis C is transmitted in the same way as hepatitis B but is an even nastier disease, inasmuch as about 80% of people who contract the infection become chronic carriers, and many of these go on to develop chronic liver disease. Further, a significant proportion develop hepatocellular carcinoma; in Japan, where about 2% of people are carriers, hepatitis C is a more common cause of liver cancer than is hepatitis B.

Research on hepatitis C has been severely hampered by the fact that attempts to culture the virus in standard tissue culture have failed. In view of this, the cloning of the virus by Choo et al. (156) was considered a major triumph, particularly because it soon led to the development of an assay for antibodies useful in screening blood donations. However, development of a vaccine against hepatitis C faces difficulties. The virus is a rapidly mutating RNA virus with a single open reading frame encoding a polyprotein of about 3,000 amino acids. There are two envelope proteins, E1 and E2, identified by analogy with other flaviviruses, which are produced by proteolytic cleavage. Study of these by genomic analysis of hepatitis C cloned from patients in different parts of the world shows a great degree of structural (and therefore antigenic) diversity. Further, experimentation on vaccine candidates is rendered difficult by the fact that the only animal model is the chimpanzee. This makes it hard to characterize and quantitate neutralizing antibodies, although it is known that plasma from a chronic carrier can protect chimpanzees from infection.

Recently, the cloned viral genome has been used to produce infectious hepatitis C virus in tissue culture (157), and a number of different replicon systems have been developed (reviewed in [158]). Further, the functional hepatitis C virus replication complex has been directly visualized by green fluorescent protein insertion or by immunogold staining. This has revealed many of the details of the infectious process.

The primary event in the virus entering a liver cell is high-affinity binding of HCV E2 protein to a large external loop of the cell surface molecule CD81, a tetraspannin molecule present on several cell types. However, cofactors are certainly required, and both high- and low-density lipoproteins have been implicated. Binding of E2 to CD81 can be inhibited by neutralizing antibodies, and there was a surprising degree of cross-neutralization between greatly disparate virus isolates. This raises the hope that binding may be at least partly independent of E2 sequence variation. Clinical trials of an E1/E2 vaccine are in progress.

Another approach to immunization involves raising $CD8^+$ T lymphocytes to nonenvelope glycoproteins. A variety of these have been tested, particularly the core antigen. A collaboration between Chiron (now Novartis) and CSL Ltd has shown that the use of ISCOMs promotes good $CD8^+$ CTL development in both monkeys and human volunteers. The hope, in the first instance, is for a therapeutic vaccine in chronic carriers, used in combination with antiviral chemotherapy.

Rotavirus Vaccines

In 1973, Bishop and Holmes in Australia discovered 70-nM virus particles possessing a distinctive double-shelled outer capsid in duodenal epithelium and stool filtrates from children with acute gastroenteritis. These so-called *rotaviruses* turned out to be an extremely important cause of diarrheal illness. In industrialized countries, rotavirus accounts for about one third of the hospitalizations of infants and young children for diarrhea. Although the mortality rate is quite low because of intravenous rehydration, both the cost and distress are high. It has been estimated that 2 million to 7 million children in the United States suffer rotavirus diarrhea each year, which results in 500,000 physician visits, 50,000 hospitalizations, and $274 million in direct medical costs. In developing countries, rotavirus is devastating, causing over 600,000 deaths per year. In a developing country like Bangladesh, it has been estimated that up to 1% of all children die of rotavirus diarrhea. The disease is widespread around the world, infection being via the fecal-oral route. By the age of 5 years, 95% of children have encountered the virus. Natural immunity develops (159). Severe diarrhea is rare on second infection. This is interesting, because there are four commonly encountered strains, so some degree of cross-protection is likely. The virus has 11 segments of double-stranded RNA, each of which encodes a protein. The outer capsid (against which protection is required) consists of G and P proteins, both of which induce neutralizing antibodies. The 10 known G proteins and the 8 known P proteins of the human virus could theoretically reassort into 80 different serotypes, but only four strains—P8G1, P8G3, P8G4, and

P4G2—are globally important. For the future, two nonstructural proteins could emerge as vaccine candidates: a putative enterotoxin NSP4, and the inner capsid protein VP6. Rarer serotypes are not to be entirely neglected and crop up in some surveys.

Early vaccine trials were with a live attenuated bovine rotavirus and were predicated on the view that animal and human rotaviruses shared a common group antigen. Next, a Rhesus rotavirus was tested. These early vaccines gave variable results. Then a Rhesus–human reassortant vaccine was generated by coinfecting cell cultures with a Rhesus rotavirus possessing G serotype 3 and three different human rotaviruses of G serotypes 1, 2, and 4. The three reassortants possessing a Rhesus genetic background but the human capsid protein 1, 2, or 4 were combined with the G3 Rhesus strain to create a tetravalent vaccine. Each of the four viruses was tested at 10^4 and later 10^5 plaque forming units (PFU), vaccine being administered in three oral doses, and the final vaccine submitted for licensure contained 10^5 PFU of each virus, thus 4×10^5 PFU per dose, all told. In clinical trials involving about 10,000 infants, no major adverse events were noted, except one to be discussed. Vaccine efficacy was 48% to 60% in terms of all disease but 61% to 100% against severe disease. In the United States, 80% of very severe episodes and 100% of dehydrating rotavirus illnesses were prevented. The vaccine, produced by Wyeth-Lederle, was duly licensed in August 1998. It was recommended for all children in the United States, to be given orally at 2, 4, and 6 months. By July 1999, 1.5 million doses had been given to 800,000 children.

In the 27 prelicensing trials of candidate rotavirus vaccines, five cases of a rare form of bowel obstruction were noted. In this syndrome, known as intussusception, a portion of bowel prolapses into a more distal portion, and peristalsis propels it further, causing a painful and potentially fatal blockage. The incidence was 0.05%, in comparison with a 0.02% incidence in the placebo control group; this difference did not reach statistical significance but was sufficient to warrant listing in the manufacturer's product insert. In any event, 15 cases of intussusception were reported between September 1998 and July 1999. As a result, this vaccine (RotaShield) was voluntarily withdrawn from the market in October 1999, a distressing and expensive event.

Notwithstanding this setback, Merck Inc. continued with the development of an oral, live, pentavalent human-bovine reassortant rotavirus vaccine, Rotateq, with activity against G1, G2, G3, G4, and P[8] serotypes. A phase III trial in 68,000 healthy infants aged 6 to 12 weeks involved vaccine or placebo, with two further doses at 4 to 10 week intervals (160). Intussusception occurred in 12 recipients of the vaccine and 15 recipients of placebo within 1 year after the first dose, including 6 and 5 respectively within the first 6 weeks. Full vaccination reduced gastroenteritis severe enough for an emergency department visit of hospitalization by 94.5%, clinic visits by 86% and any rotavirus gastroenteritis by 74%. This vaccine was licensed in 2006.

A different approach was taken by GlaxoSmithKline. Its vaccine Rotarix is a live attenuated monovalent G1P[8] human rotavirus strain, relying on cross-reactivity to give broad protection. A phase III study was conducted on 63,225 healthy infants from 11 Latin American countries and Finland who received two oral doses at approximately 2 and 4 months of age. Only 13 children developed intussusception during a 31-day window after each dose, 6 vaccine recipients and 7 in the placebo group. The vaccine was 85% effective against severe rotavirus gastroenteritis and actually reduced hospitalization from *all* causes of diarrhea by 42% (161).

Yet another strategy exploits the fact that some strains of rotavirus, so-called *nursery strains,* seem to cause asymptomatic infection in neonates but protect against later rotavirus infection. One of these, RV3, is a G3P[6] virus, which has been in a phase II trial (162) and is now being further developed in association with BioFarma in Indonesia. Another nursery strain is being progressed in India and is in phase II trial. One obvious advantage of having a vaccine of just one strain is lower cost.

Further ideas being explored are parenteral injection of baculovirus-expressed VLPs containing structural rotavirus proteins from multiple serotypes; DNA vaccines; or incorporating rotavirus into microspheres for use as an oral mucosal vaccine. Rotavirus genes have also been inserted into Sabin poliovirus or vaccinia.

The intussusception saga illustrates some of the very real problems in vaccine development. Rare complications can be quite significant when a whole population is the object of study. The more clinical prelicensure work needs to be done, the greater the research and development costs for the manufacturer and the more the pressure to charge a high price. The higher the price, the lower is the likelihood of extensive use in developing nations. Clearly, risk–benefit and cost–benefit analyses will need to form a prominent part of the landscape for the vaccines of the future.

Influenza Vaccines

Influenza is by no means a trivial disease. In industrialized countries, the regular winter attacks provoke a usually self-limited febrile illness that causes many lost hours of work. Further, flu can be the prelude to fatal pneumonia in the elderly. Annual vaccination is widely recommended for this age group, and in many countries is becoming common for children and younger adults as well. About three times per century, much more serious pandemics of influenza have occurred, which we shall consider in detail.

The influenza virus is an RNA virus; the genome consists of eight segments of single-strand RNA. The most important antigen for neutralization is the hemagglutinin (HA), one of two dominant surface proteins; antibodies to the other, the neuraminidase, can also be neutralizing. The big problem in influenza immunization is the virus' capacity to change its antigenic type. This happens in two ways. Point mutations in the HA occur with a frequency of $10^{-5.5}$ per generation. These lead to subtle but important changes in HA epitopes. This tendency to mutate away from antibody attack is referred to as *drift.* It means that the antibodies made one winter may not be as effective against the next winter's flu. Accordingly, an elaborate system of monitoring and nomenclature has arisen around the world; several WHO Collaborating Centers are responsible for providing seed lots of vaccine twice a year that reflect the most recent and dominant antigenic types. Influenza viruses also infect animals, such as pigs and horses; birds, such as geese, ducks, and chickens; and marine mammals. There are 15 distinct HA types in influenza A, and only some are infectious for humans. There are nine distinct neuraminidase types, only some of which occur in humans. Thus, influenza A viruses are frequently referred to by their serotype (e.g., H3N1). Influenza B virus is also highly adapted to humans. This virus has no subtypes, and the infections on the whole tend to be less severe.

The segmented nature of the viral genome and the existence of a variety of animal hosts makes for the possibility of coinfection of cells with human-adapted and animal-adapted strains, a reassortment of genes and the emergence of novel strains with the sudden appearance of a new antigenic subtype. Such a major change is referred to as *antigenic shift.* There may be little or no cross-reactivity with antibody provoked by previously circulating strains. The stage is then set for a major pandemic. In the 20th century, there were three such pandemics: the so-called swine flu of 1918 to 1919, the "Asian" flu of 1957, and the "Hong Kong" flu of 1969. The swine flu (which was in fact a bird flu) killed 20 million to 40 million people, while the latter two pandemics killed an estimated 1 million people each, older adults accounting for the great majority of deaths. It would appear that the risk for such reassortants is greatest in areas where humans and animals such as chickens or pigs live in close contact.

In 1997, a virus highly virulent in birds was isolated in Hong Kong. This H5N1 strain had been carried to chickens by infected migratory waterfowl and is nearly 100% fatal in chickens. Since then, this virus has spread rapidly throughout Southeast Asia and onward to Central Asia, Europe, the Middle East, Northern and Western Africa, and even West Papua. About 200 million birds have died from the virus or have been killed to prevent its spread. Humans in close contact with chickens are at risk of catching the virus. So far (September 2006) 246 people in 10 countries have fallen ill, with 144 deaths, a far greater case fatality rate than any influenza virus previously reported. Fortunately, human to human transmission rarely occurs. In May 2006, there were two instances in Indonesia where very close contact (e.g., nursing a patient for 6 days) might have caused infection. However, mutation or reassortment with a human strain for easier transmissibility is an ever-present risk. There is already evidence of more than one clade showing the virus is mutating. Accordingly, most industrialized countries have emergency plans that include stockpiling of antiviral drugs, development of point-of-care diagnostic tests, quarantine plans, public health measures, and development of suitable vaccines. A second bird flu, H9N2, has also been encountered and appears to be less virulent.

The standard influenza vaccine consists of formalin-inactivated whole virus, still grown in fertile hen's eggs and frequently rendered less reactogenic by "splitting" through ether or detergent treatment. Tissue cultured variants are in development. In Italy, a vaccine incorporating MF59 adjuvant is registered. The standard vaccine is reasonably effective, but protection is of short duration. Typically, the killed vaccine is 60% to 70% effective. Helpful though such a vaccine is, the search for better vaccines is lively.

Obvious areas to explore are live attenuated vaccines and mucosal administration. These are combined in the efforts of Aviron (now MedImmune) with their preparation FluMist. Cold-adapted viruses, initially developed at the University of Michigan, are produced in specific pathogen-free eggs, and a trivalent preparation consisting of two A and one B strains is given via a nasal spray–syringe delivery system. A single dose is safe and effective. The largest trial achieved 93% efficacy in the first year and in the second, 100% efficacy against strains included in the vaccine, and 86% against the emergent mismatched strain A/Sydney/05/97 (H3N2). This new vaccine was licensed in 2003 for administration to 5 to 49 year-old subjects. Prelicensure studies showed results to be significantly superior to those of the inactivated injectable vaccine. Glück's intranasal virosome-based vaccine, already mentioned, appeared to significantly increase the risk of Bell's palsy, so is not being further marketed. By 2006, FulMist had been administered to more than 4 million individuals with a total of only 5 Bell's palsy cases reported, a causal association not being established, and thus represents a safe, effective and probably superior addition to the armamentarium.

Bird Flu Vaccines

As there is no preexisting immunity, conventional influenza vaccines containing the H5N1 virus do not perform particularly well in humans. For example, Treanor et al. (163) found that 2 doses of 90 mg of influenza virus (3 to 6 times the normal dose) raised a neutralizing antibody titer of 1:40 (the theoretically protective level) in only 54% of adult subjects, with lower doses giving lower responses. This can certainly be improved with either alum or MF59 adjuvant. As quantity of vaccine would be a real issue early in a pandemic, other approaches must be explored. An adenovirus vector genetically engineered to express H5 hemagglutinin on its surface was 100% effective in protecting mice and also very potent in chickens against authentic H5N1 virus (164). Curiously, subcutaneous injection worked much better than intranasal vaccine in the latter case. This vaccine causes both B and T cell immunity. Other possibilities include live attenuated cold-adapted intranasal vaccine—MedImmune has been given a large contract to develop such a variant—and a platform or backbone vaccine against all 15 variations of the H antigen, with the hope of one generic influenza vaccine stockpile. DNA vaccines, of course, would avoid the need for eggs. There is also rapid development of mammalian cell culture methods for the virus. Plant-made vaccines are another possibility. If and when a shift variant with global pandemic potential emerges, it will be important to ramp up production as rapidly as possible, as well as to prioritize those recipients (e.g., doctors, nurses, quarantine officers) needing the vaccine first.

Antibody-based Vaccines Against Human Immunodeficiency Virus

The human immunodeficiency virus 1 (HIV-1) has developed some devilishly clever strategies to foil the human immune response. It exhibits an astonishing rate of mutation, particularly in the portion of its envelope protein that is involved in infectivity, allowing the virus to escape the antibody response. It finds several levels of "safe haven" refuges unreachable by antibodies—for example, persistence within macrophages and DCs, or penetration into the brain. Further, integration of provirus DNA into the host cell genome, with no external evidence of the virus's presence, represents an escape resistant to CTL attack. It targets the first lymphocyte in the immune cascade, the $CD4^+$ T cell, which may delay an effective immune response and will certainly facilitate the disastrous upsurge in viral load late in the disease, because T cell levels fall so low that resistance essentially disappears. It has an extraordinarily high rate of replication. We now know that the immune system is a pitched battleground from the first entry of the virus.

The most common mode of transmission of HIV is sexual intercourse. The virus infects $CD4^+$ T cells and spreads within this population and also in DCs. By about 1 week, virus can be detected in local lymph nodes and soon in the blood. Seeding to gut-associated lymphoid tissue is particularly extensive. Viremia reaches a peak around 3 weeks with $\sim 10^7$ virus particles per ml of blood, or more. But then $CD8^+$ cytotoxic T cells help to control the early infection (165), HIV-specific cells comprising 10% of the circulating $CD8^+$ pool. The virus load falls up to a 100-fold to reach a relatively stable level (the "set point") by 2 to 6 months after infection. The set point has prognostic significance: The lower it is, the slower the rate of progression to AIDS. But sooner or later the $CD4^+$ T cell count falls, and when it reaches 200/ml to 400/ml, virus levels rise and AIDS supervenes.

Two to three months after primary infection, neutralizing antibodies appear, but escape mutant viruses immediately become manifest, so the natural antibody response (166) is always faced with persisting, fast-changing virus. The question then is: Could a vaccine elicit an antibody response that prevents the virus from gaining a foothold in the first place?

Early attempts to develop an AIDS vaccine followed the classical path of seeking to induce antibodies to the most prominent antigens on the viral surface: namely, the envelope (*env*) glycoproteins gp160 or the products it yields, the exterior viral protein gp120, and the transmembrane glycoprotein gp41. Two unfortunate findings from phase II trials of recombinant *env* antigens caused early disappointment. First, the data showed a small number of "breakthrough" infections despite immunization; second, antibodies engendered by immunization, although capable of neutralizing HIV grown in transformed T cell lines, were much less effective against freshly isolated virus grown in peripheral blood mononuclear cells. Since those early days, we have learned much about how HIV infects its target cells (reviewed in [166]). Gp120 and noncovalently associated gp41 exist as homodimers on the viral surface. So from the beginning much of gp120 is hidden, while its exposed surface is heavily glycosylated, handicapping a putative neutralizing antibody seeking access. The CD4-binding site is deeply recessed and "guarded" by the V1/V2 loops so the virus can vary extensively. When gp120 binds to CD4, the envelope protein undergoes a conformational change that exposes a high-affinity binding site for one of two coreceptors, CCR5 and CXCR-4, members of the chemokine receptor family. After this second binding event, gp41 in turn changes shape, leading to the insertion of a hydrophobic amino-terminal fusion peptide into the target cell membrane to mediate membrane fusion and viral entry. Much of the current effort in HIV vaccine research seeks to "freeze" these various highly transitory structures. The well-hidden binding sites are relatively conserved compared with the rest of the envelope protein. Be that as it may, the use of recombinant envelope proteins as vaccines has not been successful so far. The firm VaxGen took its recombinant gp120 vaccine AIDSVAX^{TM} to two sizable phase III trials without obtaining significant protection.

Before looking at other antibody-evoking vaccine strategies, we must recall the great heterogeneity of this virus. There are three main types of HIV-1, which probably represent three separate infections of humans from chimpanzees, namely M, N, and O. Both N and O strains are quite rare and are very close to simian immunodeficiency virus. The main M type can be broken in to subtypes or clades of which the most important are A, B, C, D (which may be part of B), E, and G. All clades are present in central Africa. The most important clade in the Americas,

Europe, and Australia is B; in South and East Asia it is C; and in Southeast Asia it is E. Vaccines will probably have to be clade specific. To complicate matters further, inter-subtype recombination is frequent, and the recombinant forms AD, AE, AG, and BC are readily recognized. Clade classification is on the basis of genotype, and the correlation between genotype and immunotype is by no means clear-cut. There is a complex matrix of cross-reactivities in both humoral and cellular responses that will have to be sorted out antigen by antigen when particular antigens are chosen for an eventual vaccine.

There are two reasons why it is too early to give up on antibody production as a key to HIV prophylaxis: First, passively administered antibody can prevent infection of macaque monkeys with SIV–HIV hybrid virus (SHIV), a widely used model for HIV (167). Second, there are five monoclonal antibodies that have the capacity to neutralize a broad variety of freshly isolated HIV subtypes (reviewed in [166]). One is against conserved elements of the CD4 binding site; one sees the coreceptor binding site; one is directed against mannans linked to *env*; and two bind to the membrane-proximal region of gp41. These last two resemble certain auto-antibodies in that they are broadly cross-reactive and bind with high affinity to cardiolipin (168). It has been suggested that these antibodies are rare because of self tolerance, and if a way could be found to evoke plentiful anti-*env* antibodies of this character, a vaccine against HIV might ensue.

There is no shortage of good ideas for novel antibody-inducing vaccines. Conformationally altered gp120 to which CD4 has been bound represents one possibility, and the most promising variant of this idea is a single-chain gp120-CD4 fusion protein (169) that fortunately does not appear to elicit anti-CD4 antibodies. There are also attempts to create synthetic mimotopes of the suddenly exposed binding structure, utilizing the extensive three-dimensional information that has become available, as well as epitopes exposed during HIV-mediated cell fusion. One proposal seeks to use computational methods to identify those pieces of HIV that are targets for neutralization and to synthesize hundreds of these to create antigens, antibodies against which could be broadly neutralizing. In another endeavor, it is proposed to screen very large numbers of human or experimental animal antibodies for broad neutralization potential and then work backward from the antibodies to the appropriate HIV epitopes. A somewhat similar concept is that of the firm Maxygen, where chimaeric or "shuffled" *env* genes from several different HIV isolates are expressed and tested for reactivity with powerfully neutralizing antibodies, positive proteins then being used to immunize mice to determine whether they generate the requisite antibodies (170). These newer ideas have not yet reached the clinical trial stage. Some of them, as well as projects discussed in the next section, will be supported by a $287 million initiative from the Bill & Melinda Gates Foundation announced in July 2006 as part of the Global HIV/AIDS Vaccine Enterprise, which gave 16 grants to 165 researchers from 19 countries to support collaborative research. By October, 2006, Gates Foundation grants for AIDS vaccine research had totaled $528 million.

T Cell–Based Vaccines Against HIV

All over the world, great effort is being put into attempts to create an AIDS vaccine based on the induction of powerful T cell immunity, particularly the induction of cytotoxic $CD8^+$ T cells active against virus-infected cells. There are good reasons to believe that $CD8^+$ T cells play a critical role in the control of HIV. Relevant findings include a close correlation between CTL appearance and a fall in virus levels in SHIV-1–infected Rhesus macaque monkeys and the detection of significant numbers of HIV-specific CTLs in a variety of seronegative individuals at high risk, such as babies born to HIV-positive mothers, a small proportion of female African professional sex workers, and a proportion of subjects with needlestick injuries. Among seropositive individuals, those who do not progress or progress slowly to AIDS have robust CTL responses. In view of this evidence, it is important to include in a vaccine virally encoded proteins produced in the cytosol of the infected cell, so that peptide fragments of such proteins could be presented at the surface of the infected cell in association with class I MHC molecules. Further, it would be advantageous to use adjuvants or other techniques known to favor $CD8^+$ T cell production. Use of a multiplicity of antigens might counteract mutations occurring in any single component within the virus-infected cells that should be eliminated. Finally, a procedure evoking mucosal as well as lymph node and splenic CTLs would be ideal.

In a resurgent and now well-financed AIDS vaccine effort, a large number of antigens or genes for antigens have been the subject of intensive research. These include *env, gag, pol, nef, rev, tat,* and HIV protease. Further, an incredible variety of vector systems has been included in preclinical research. Among these are vaccinia; vaccinia modified to be less aggressive (e.g., modified vaccinia Ankara); adenoviruses; avipox viruses, including canarypox and fowlpox; and (although less frequently) other viruses, including recombinant avirulent poliovirus, mengovirus, herpesvirus, Venezuelan equine encephalitis virus, vesicular stomatitis virus, Semliki Forest virus and influenza virus. Possible bacterial vectors include *Salmonella,* BCG, *Shigella, Listeria,* and *Lactobacillus.* Many of these have been through a variety of animal models of protection with a measure of success.

Among the 100 or so vaccine candidates, there is no doubt that the prime-boost strategies described earlier hold pride of place (171–173). Increasing use is being made of the SHIV virus (HIV envelope and SIV core) model in macaques.

There is by now substantial literature on virtually every conceivable variation on this prime-boost scheme, with many preclinical successes. A constant undercurrent in the literature is strong $CD8^+$ CTLs as a signpost of promise. Among the many additions to prime-boost strategies, a recurring theme is either strong adjuvants accompanying particularly a protein boost or coadministration of cytokine gene expression cassettes with DNA immunogens.

A mucosal approach is also being pursued in a variety of ways. Mucosal surfaces are a major natural route of HIV entry, and protection through the mucosal immune system would therefore be valuable. Berzofsky et al. (174) have long been championing the idea of a multideterminant peptide vaccine comprising epitopes for both T helper cells and CTLs. The mucosal study (175) focused on the antigens *env, pol,* and *gag,* using *env* from HIV and *pol* and *gag* from SIV. The study design involved macaque monkeys and a challenge with virulent SHIV intrarectally. The investigators compared two vaccine approaches: a subcutaneous injection with Montanide ISA51 as an adjuvant, versus intrarectal inoculation of the vaccine with a mutant heat-labile *E. coli* toxin as a mucosal adjuvant. The latter provided significantly better protection, because (at least in part) of a strong intestinal mucosal CTL response. This group is also exploring the concept of epitope enhancement—that is, slightly modifying T helper cell epitope sequences to increase epitope affinity for class II MHC. This results in more effective helper T cells and also more CTLs (176). It must be remembered, however, that appropriate systemic immunization can also raise enough CTLs to protect against rectal challenge. For example, a prime-boost regimen consisting of priming with a cytokine-augmented DNA vaccine and boosting with a recombinant MVA construct, each vaccine containing multiple viral antigens, completely protected against intrarectal SHIV challenge in the same macaque model. But what is the situation in the human?

There have been at least 40 clinical trials of HIV vaccines, most of them phase I but about a quarter of them having progressed to phase II. The harvest has been disappointing. $CD8^+$ T cell responses have usually fallen below those in macaques to SHIV models, and responses in mice have been of poor predictive value. DNA vaccines have been poor performers, and while DNA priming with an MVA-HIV boost is more immunogenic, it is mainly a $CD4^+$ T cell response (177). Prime-boost works better than two injections of MVA. Recombinant replication-defective adenovirus-5 gives one of the best $CD8^+$ responses to *gag* peptides, but preexistent antibodies reduce immunogencity. However, MVA-HIV markedly amplified both $CD4^+$ and $CD8^+$ vaccine-specific T cell responses in HIV-infected individuals undergoing highly active antiretroviral therapy for chronic HIV infection (178). One prime-boost protocol has reached phase III trial, namely recombinant canarypox priming with *env, gag, pol, nef,* and protease, followed by a gp120 protein boost. Results are not yet available.

The reader wishing to learn more about the many clinical trials should consult www.iavireport.org/trialsdb.

One very positive development in this rather gloomy scene is that recent efforts, particularly by the Bill & Melida Gates Foundation, the National Institutes of Health, and the European Union, have prompted a great deal more coordination and collaboration among the global AIDS vaccine research community. No one expects a licensed AIDS vaccine within the next 10 years, but the author confidently predicts that by the 7th edition of this book a number of credible candidates will have reached "proof of principle" stage. The distance then left to travel should not be underestimated. Perhaps the greatest practical problem in HIV vaccine research is where to go after encouraging phase I and II studies. Large prophylactic studies are horrendously expensive. Results would be most rapidly obtained in developing countries because of the high rate of carriage, but such trials are beset with practical and ethical problems. Practically, will it be possible to conduct trials whose results will meet U.S. Food and Drug Administration standards? Ethically, will it be possible to give trial participants sufficient safe sex education? Will it be possible to guarantee to developing country governments that, if the trial in which their citizens have taken part is successful, the relevant vaccine will be made available to the population at an affordable price? Clearly, the eventual development of a successful vaccine remains an immense scientific and humanitarian challenge.

Dengue Vaccines

Dengue is a mosquitoborne flavivirus infection caused by four dengue virus (DEN) serotypes, DEN-1, 2, 3, and 4. It is found in tropical and subtropical regions around the world, being endemic in more than 100 countries. The problem is worst in Southeast Asia, but recent spread to the Middle East and even to the U.S. states of Texas and Hawaii has caused great concern. Classical dengue fever is a serious but self-limited infection with fever, headache, myalgia, arthralgia, and rashes. The worst problem is a curious and potentially lethal complication, the dengue hemorrhagic fever-dengue shock syndrome (DHF/DSS). This still incompletely understood syndrome usually arises when a person who has been infected with one DEN serotype contracts another. Similarly, an infant possessing maternal antibodies against one strain is susceptible when infected with another. There is some kind of antibody-dependent enhancement of pathology. This increased susceptibility of the partially immune certainly introduced a note of caution into the development of a vaccine.

Much effort has gone into conventional serially tissue-culture passaged tetravalent live attenuated vaccines (reviewed in [179]). GlaxoSmithKline is working with the Walter Reed Army Institute of Research and started a phase II trial in March 2006. This research involves 132 adults aged 18 to 45 years and 51 infants aged 12 to 15 months. Follow-up will be for at least 4 years. Unfortunately, some "interference" between the serotypes has been encountered, and two injections do not elicit neutralizing levels of antibodies in all vaccinees. Sanofi-Aventis has the license to develop a tetravalent vaccine originating from Mahidol University in Thailand. Again, two doses appeared to be followed by breakthrough infections and three doses were needed for consistent neutralizing antibody responses.

Sanofi-Aventis has a second string to its bow because it has licensed a product from Acambis that is a chimaeric yellow fever-dengue virus tetravalent formulation in which pre-membrane and envelope genes from DEN serotypes 1 to 4 were substituted for the same genes of yellow fever (180). This worked well in monkeys, and human studies are in train involving two injections 5 to 9 months apart. No significant adverse reactions have been reported.

Blaney et al. (181) are developing a live attenuated tetravalent dengue vaccine using reverse genetics. The strategy involves attenuating deletions and chimaerization of C, M, and e genes to create a virus with tetravalent specificity. Preliminary clinical studies indicate that the vaccine was well tolerated and immunogenic. Maxygen, in collaboration with the U.S. Naval Medical Research Center, is thrusting in the same direction, but via a DNA vaccine created by DNA shuffling of envelope genes to create a tetravalent construct (182). This vaccine is still at the preclinical stage.

We can anticipate with some confidence that one or more of these approaches will have led to a licensed vaccine by the time of the next edition of this book or soon thereafter.

VACCINES AGAINST PARASITIC DISEASES

If viruses and bacteria have evolved elaborate strategies to defeat the vertebrate immune system, parasites, with their much larger complement of DNA, possess an even wider and more diverse range. Although no vaccine against any human parasitic disease has been licensed, the feasibility of such vaccines has been demonstrated in the veterinary field, where several successful vaccines are in use to deal with both protozoan and metazoan infestations. The difficulty of overcoming all the necessary hurdles for human vaccines is evidenced by the fact that over the past 30 years, some of the best minds in vaccinology have applied themselves to the problem, but only in malaria have vaccines moved to the stage of phase IIb trials, with moderate success. Nevertheless, parasitism is so important from a public health viewpoint and the progress in understanding of parasite molecular biology and genetics so significant that the research effort must continue. Moreover, the progressive resistance of some parasites to chemotherapy and of vectors to insecticides highlights the importance of vaccines for disease control.

Malaria Vaccines

Malaria is the most prevalent vectorborne disease in the world. It is caused by protozoa of four species of *Plasmodium.* It threatens 2 billion people in 90 countries and causes approximately 500 million to 600 million clinical cases and 1 million to 2 million deaths per year. Overwhelmingly, the worst continent for malaria is Africa, where 90% of the deaths occur, chiefly in children younger than 5 years. *P. falciparum* is by far the most dangerous of the four species that affect humans, and cerebral malaria, in which parasitized erythrocytes develop cytoadherence antigens and block up cerebral arterioles, is the most prominent cause of death. It is known that antibodies can be therapeutic, and the hope that a vaccine will eventually be developed is sustained by the observation that inhabitants of endemic areas eventually become relatively immune to attacks, although this immunity is not sterilizing, as small quantities of parasites are left in the host.

The next most important species is *P. vivax,* famous for attacks that can recur long after exposure. From a practical point of view, a vaccine that could protect against both *P. falciparum* and *P. vivax* would have much to commend it. Industry could then charge high prices for a traveler's vaccine in industrialized countries. However, the preclinical research is being pursued separately for the two species with a heavy concentration on the bigger killer.

In view of the considerable amount of research that has been done, it is legitimate to ask why no effective malaria vaccine yet exists. This involves both theoretical and practical considerations. The best vaccines are for diseases in which nature provides solid immunity if an individual survives a first attack. This is not the case in malaria, in which immunity in endemic areas is tenuous at best and easily lost if the individual leaves to live in a malaria-free country. Clearly, the parasite has evolved powerful strategies to evade the host immune response. From a practical viewpoint, the parasite is difficult to grow; *P. falciparum* requires human blood, and *P. vivax* does not even replicate *in vitro* in red blood cells. Investigators are thus driven to recombinant DNA technology with all of the difficulties of choice of antigen among hundreds of candidates and correct refolding of every candidate. Add to this the fact that no animal model is a good imitation of the human disease, and the difficulties for the investigator mount.

Among the evolutionary strategies of the parasite, two stand out. The first is high mutability in most of the antigens that have been studied, resulting in extensive allelic polymorphism, so that multiple forms of the antigen exist in the parasite population as a whole, which presumably reflects selection of mutants because parental forms are eliminated by antibody. Second, a very key antigen of *P. falciparum*, the so-called *P. falciparum* erythrocyte membrane protein 1 (PfEMP1), which is prominent on the surface of infected red blood cells, is represented in the genome by approximately 50 variant copies (183). As a clone of parasites emerges and reaches a sufficient size to strongly signal the immune system, eliminating most parasites, a variant expressing a different PfEMP1 arises, grows, reaches a critical size, and in turn is eliminated by antibody, and so the cycle repeats itself until, eventually, immunity to all the forms of PfEMP1 is achieved.

Life Cycle of Plasmodium falciparum

With these preliminary considerations out of the way, we should now look at the parasite's life cycle (with *P. falciparum* as the model) to determine where the different points of attack might be. Figure 40.3 shows this schematically. Invasion of the human is initiated when the female anopheline mosquito bites the human subject, thereby injecting a mobile form known as a sporozoite into the skin. The dominant surface antigen of the sporozoite is the circumsporozoite antigen or CSP, first identified by the Nussenzweigs (184) in the early 1980s and cloned soon thereafter. This candidate vaccine antigen has been the subject of intensive research. The sporozoite rapidly and efficiently invades hepatocytes. Two to 10 sporozoites can initiate infection within 5 to 30 minutes, probably involving an interaction between CSP and the glycosaminoglycan chains of heparin sulfate proteoglycans. A second sporozoite surface protein, the thrombospondin-related adhesion protein (TRAP), has a region highly homologous to a part of CSP and is probably also involved in binding to hepatocyte heparin sulfate proteoglycans. TRAP is required for sporozoite mobility and infectivity.

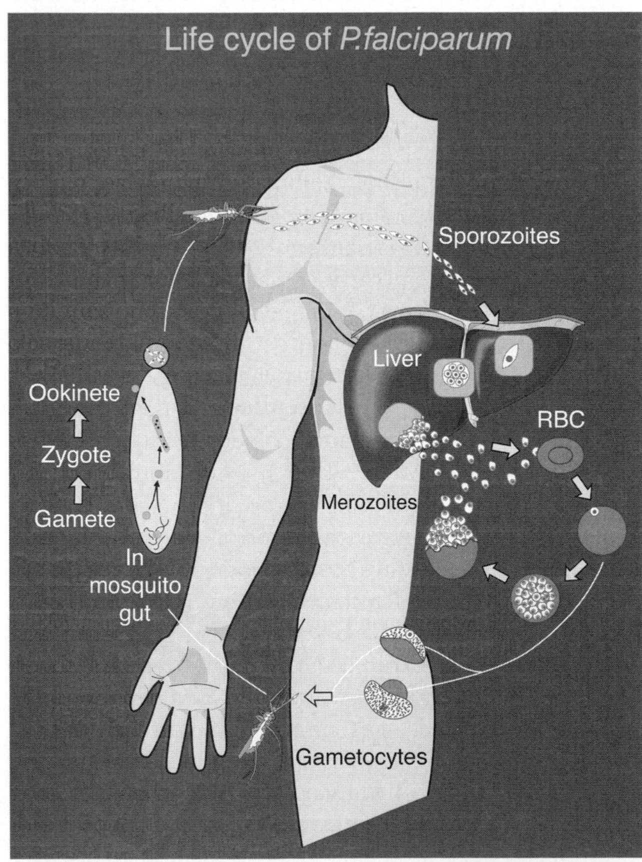

FIGURE 40.3 Life cycle of *Plasmodium falciparum*. Note particularly four life-cycle stages that could be vaccine targets: the sporozoites, the infected liver cell, the merozoites, and the gametocytes.

Within the hepatocyte, each sporozoite develops into a schizont containing 10,000 to 30,000 merozoites. Over this period, the hepatocyte presents on its surface peptides from a number of preerythrocytic stage proteins. A $CD8^+$ cytotoxic T cell attack on infected liver cells could materially lower the number of merozoites formed and thus lessen the attack on erythrocytes. As long as the parasite is confined to the liver, there are no clinical symptoms of malaria. Within 10 days or less, the liver schizont ruptures, and the merozoites are released and begin to invade erythrocytes, there to undergo another asexual amplification. The erythrocytic cycle is responsible for disease manifestation, inasmuch as development, rupture, and reinvasion initiate a vicious cycle.

Merozoite invasion of erythrocytes is a complex process involving multiple steps. The merozoite attaches to the erythrocyte, reorients itself so that its apical end faces the red blood cell, after which a tight junction develops, and parasite organelles known as rhoptries discharge their contents onto the red blood cell membrane. A progressively deeper vacuole forms and eventually closes to surround the engulfed parasite. The best-studied erythrocyte surface receptor for a parasite ligand is the Duffy blood group antigen for *P. vivax*. In contrast, *P. falciparum* seems capable of using multiple pathways for invasion, including sialic acids on glycophorins A, B, and C, as well as peptide sequences on glycophorins. As for the parasite ligands, a Duffy binding-like (DBL) superfamily has been defined. For *P. vivax*, the most important member is a 140-kDa Duffy-binding protein (PvDBP) (185), and for *P. falciparum*, EBA-175 appears to be the prototype. But additional merozoite proteins play a role in invasion, inasmuch as quite a number of monoclonal antibodies against them can block invasion *in vitro*. These include various merozoite surface proteins (MSPs) and proteins translocated from the apical organelles, the rhoptries and the micronemes, to the surface before invasion.

An important event in clinical malaria is the adherence of infected erythrocytes to vascular endothelium. When this occurs in small vessels in the brain, blockage can follow, resulting in cerebral malaria and death. The chief molecular mediator of cytoadherence is the variant surface antigen PfEMP1, as already mentioned (183). The receptors for adherence are various and include CD36, intracellular adhesion molecule 1, vascular cell adhesion molecule 1, E-selectin, and chondroitin sulfate A.

In addition to producing merozoites, the erythrocytic cycle is also responsible for the production of the sexual forms known as gametocytes. These are taken up by the mosquito and mature into gametes. A vaccine capable of producing antigametocyte antibodies could destroy them in the blood of the vaccinee or could interfere with their maturation in the mosquito, or both. The life cycle of the parasite is, of course, completed in the mosquito, in which sexual union occurs, sporozoites emerge from mature oocysts 10 to 14 days after an infective blood meal, and invasion of salivary glands occurs soon thereafter.

Possible Vaccine Approaches

Given the complexity of this life cycle, many observers believe that a final malaria vaccine will contain key molecules from various and perhaps all stages. However, it is necessary to consider the best candidates from each stage in turn. Much knowledge has accumulated over the past 25 years (reviewed in [186,187]).

The sporozoite stage is an attractive target, inasmuch as a 100% effective vaccine would prevent infection completely and a partially effective one would lower the eventual invasive merozoite burden. Like most malarial antigens, the CSP presents as a dominant antigen multiple tandem repeats, in this case of the sequence NANP, which can absorb a large proportion of the anti-CSP antibodies both of the serum of patients and of CSP (or irradiated sporozoite) immunized persons. Promising results have been obtained with GlaxoSmithKline's vaccine known as RTS,S, given with the adjuvant AS02. RTS,S is a fusion protein of the carboxy-terminal half of CSP (which includes both part of the tandem repeat, thus R, and also important T cell epitopes, thus T) fused to the HBsAg. This is coexpressed in yeast with (nonfused) HBsAg (thus, S), which self-assembles into virion-like structures, aiding immunogenicity. The adjuvant AS02, already described, has strong T and B cell–stimulatory properties. In a human challenge model, this significantly protected malaria-naïve volunteers, although immunity was of short duration. In a field study in a rural area of The Gambia involving 306 men aged 18 to 45 years, the vaccine was safe and well-tolerated although fairly reactogenic, evoked strong anti-CSP antibody and T cell responses, and clearly gave partial protection in that it significantly delayed *P. falciparum* infection and reduced symptomatic malaria (188). Again, immunity waned rather quickly, but some immunological memory resulted, inasmuch as a booster dose given the following year reduced the incidences of infection and of symptomatic malaria. A phase IIb study in 1- to 4-year-old children in Mozambique also gave some protection (73), which appeared to be maintained for 18 months (189). There is also considerable research interest in vaccines consisting of whole irradiated sporozoites or live attenuated sporozoites (reviewed in [187]).

Anti–Liver-stage Vaccine

T cell immunity clearly plays a role in malaria and the most clear-cut example is in relation to parasite T cell epitopes on the surface of the infected liver cell. The most extensively investigated antigen is TRAP (thrombospondin-related adhesion protein), and it has been used alone or combined with a string of up to 15 epitopes from various parasite life stages. There have been multiple small clinical trials of the "prime-boost" approach, using the vectors naked DNA, MVA, an attenuated strain of fowlpox virus, FP9, or other vectors. Some of these have clearly reduced the liver-stage parasite load (reviewed in [187]). Priming with FP9 followed by boosting with MVA presently appears the best combination. An argument can be mounted for combined immunization with RTS,S and TRAP.

Blood-stage Antigens and Vaccines

There is a plethora of blood stage antigens at various stages of testing. The subject of the largest amount of work has been the protein MSP-1, a 195-kDa major merozoite protein, and various fragments of it. Considerable protective efficacy has been shown in murine and simian vaccine trials, although in the human, the highly polymorphic nature of this antigen may prove problematic. Efforts are being directed toward defining conserved protective epitopes of MSP-1. Other significant merozoite surface candidates are MSP-2, MSP-3, MSP-4, and MSP-5. The combination 4/5 looks attractive because it is relatively less polymorphic.

As noted, rhoptry-associated proteins (RAPs) perform as yet ill-defined tasks in merozoite invasion of erythrocytes. The antigens RAP-1 and RAP-2 show less polymorphism and have been partially successful in a Saimiri monkey model. The apical merozoite antigen 1 (AMA-1) is strongly protective in murine and simian trials, has been in phase I human trials, and is in continuing clinical development (190). Because this antigen has 16 conserved cysteine residues and exhibits a three-domain structure, correct refolding after expression is essential and presents a challenge.

In view of the importance of the initial docking events involving PvDBP for *P. vivax* and EBA-175 for *P. falciparum,* these represent further interesting candidates. For PvDBP, the cysteine-rich amino-terminal region II is conserved and constitutes the receptor-binding domain. This fragment, PvRII, when correctly refolded, represents an interesting *P. vivax* candidate. The same may be true for a homologous region of EBA-175.

Although the highly variant surface antigen family PfEMP1, which mediates cytoadherence, also exhibits DBL domains, it remains to be determined whether there is enough conservation in the RII domain for a polypeptide vaccine to hold promise.

Transmission Blocking Vaccines

Vaccines directed against the sexual stages of the parasite would not protect the vaccinee but could have profound effects at the community level if widely deployed. Antibodies made by the vaccinee would be taken up by the biting mosquito in its blood meal and could hamper the complex parasite life cycle within the vector. To date, studies have focused on the gametocyte-specific surface antigens Pfs48/45 and pfs230, the ookinete-specific surface molecules P25 and P28, and a variety of secreted ookinete proteins (reviewed in [186]). Phase I human trials have begun.

Antidisease Vaccines: Glycophosphatidylinositol Toxin of Malaria as a New Candidate Vaccine Molecule

An imaginative new approach to malaria immunization is being investigated by Schofield (reviewed in [191]). This is predicated on the idea that much of the pathological processes in malaria result from an inflammatory cascade initiated by a malarial toxin. GPI of parasite origin is the candidate and an oligosaccharide of the *P. falciparum* GPI glycan was synthesized, conjugated to a protein carrier, and injected into mice. Following challenge with *P. berghei*, the vaccine substantially reduced severe pathology, cerebral malaria, and mortality, but with no effect on parasite growth rate. There was also protection against blood acidosis, pulmonary edema, and vascular occlusion. It is hoped to take this approach into the clinic in the near future.

The Gates Malaria Vaccine Initiative

The analysis just described, which is by no means exhaustive, shows that the malaria vaccine field fairly bristles with promise. A critical block has been the capacity to take candidate molecules that look interesting on the basis of preclinical research to phase I and phase II clinical trials. Therefore, the Malaria Vaccine Initiative funded by the Bill & Melinda Gates Foundation is highly welcome. It will fund the preparation of vaccine pilot lots in accordance with Good Manufacturing Practice criteria, improve facilities for clinical and field trials, and provide coordination and cooperation between various major groups, thus optimizing their potential. However, this is not to deny the many hurdles that must still be overcome before this badly needed vaccine emerges.

Regretfully, vaccines against other human parasitic diseases have not progressed as far. There is considerable preclinical research in schistosomiasis, leishmaniasis, toxoplasmosis, amoebiasis, hookworm, hydatid disease, trypanosomiasis, and many other parasites. Let us hope that future editions of this book may see at least some of these progress to phase III trials in humans.

ADVERSE EFFECTS OF VACCINES

Three considerations dictate that adverse effects of vaccines must be taken very seriously. First, vaccines are normally given to healthy individuals, as opposed to most other biopharmaceuticals, which are given to the sick. Second, most vaccines are given to infants and young children, deemed to be both very precious and very vulnerable. Third, in the industrialized countries, the very success of immunization programs, combined with good personal hygiene, environmental sanitation, and improved living conditions, has made epidemic disease seem like something unfamiliar and perhaps something with which antibiotics and other medical treatments can cope. In other words, opponents of immunization can be excused for not understanding the risk-benefit equation of vaccines because of a lack of personal experience. This has to be countered by good education.

Fortunately, serious adverse events are very rare with currently used vaccines. This creates what at first seems a curious problem. Because nearly all children get quite a few vaccine injections in the first year of life, a reasonable proportion of all infants coming down with some rare complaint, such as encephalitis, will have had an immunization within, for example, a week of that illness. The assumption of a causative rather than coincidental relationship is quite human and can be contested only by statistical arguments, which are unfamiliar to most people. The more serious claimed side effects are considered first.

The most controversial vaccine from the viewpoint of side effects has been DPT, containing whole killed pertussis bacteria. Reactions such as fever, irritability, local redness, swelling and pain, anorexia, and drowsiness are quite common, although of short duration and easily ameliorated by a drug such as paracetamol. Febrile convulsions occur in about 1 case in 2,000 to 3,000 and cause no long-term harm. Follow-up study has shown no evidence of neurological damage or intellectual impairment. The question of serious acute neurological illness, such as encephalopathy, has caused the most concern. The incidence was put at 1 case per 330,000 vaccine doses in the United Kingdom in 1981, but reanalysis of the data, coupled with a large study in the United States by the Institute of Medicine, challenged this conclusion. The American Academy of Pediatrics found that, although "the data accumulated to date may not prove that pertussis vaccine can never cause brain damage, they indicate that if it does so, such occurrences must be exceedingly rare" (192). The Institute of Medicine concluded that the risk of serious neurological complications was somewhere between 0 and 1 per 200,000. Because the number of cases of whooping cough has fallen by a factor of 50 in the United States since the introduction of the vaccine, and because the disease is accompanied by permanent brain damage in about 1% of cases and by death in 0.1% to 4% of cases, depending on the study, the risk-benefit equation is still enormously on the side of vaccination, even with the worst assumptions about brain damage from vaccination. The acellular pertussis vaccine has effectively terminated this debt.

The next important area of concern is poliomyelitis. Adverse reactions to this vaccine are of particular importance because there have been no cases of wild poliomyelitis in the industrialized countries for many years. In fact, poliomyelitis transmission ceased in the western hemisphere in 1991. Thus, even a single case of vaccine-associated poliomyelitis is a real tragedy. Unfortunately, a reversion to neurovirulence of the Sabin poliovirus, although excessively rare, is not absolutely unknown. It appears that for approximately 2.7 million doses of the oral poliovirus vaccine, there is one case of paralytic polio, most commonly of Sabin type 3. On average, there have been about five such cases in the United States per year. Some have been in vaccinees and some in their contacts.

A major survey of paralytic poliomyelitis in England and Wales between 1985 and 1991 was reported by Joce et al. (193). In total, 21 confirmed cases were found. Thirteen were vaccine-associated, nine being in vaccinees and four in contacts. Five were imported cases, and three were cases whose source of infection was unknown. The estimated risk of vaccine-associated paralysis was 1.46 per million for the first dose but 0.49 per 10^6 for the second and 0 for the third and fourth. In all, nine cases of paralysis arose from 18.4 million doses of vaccine administered over 7 years, with a risk of paralysis of 0.49% per 10^6 immunizations, which is remarkably similar to the U.S. figure of 1 per 2.7 million. Two vaccine-associated cases occurred in immunodeficient children, for whom inactivated poliomyelitis vaccine should have been offered.

Whereas the risks of oral polio vaccine are truly minuscule, the industrialized world has largely gone back to the injectable, Salk-type vaccine (IPV).

One can draw up a panoply of other "accusations" against vaccines. Live attenuated virus vaccines can certainly cause damage in immunodeficient or immunosuppressed children; generalized vaccinia was probably the worst example. Now that smallpox has been eradicated, this risk has disappeared. If a vaccinia variant is rescued as a vaccine vector, it will be one of lessened virulence.

One can examine the existing vaccines one by one and identify claims for side reactions. Mild measles rash can follow the measles vaccine. Certainly, measles is a nasty disease for the unimmunized, with a case-fatality rate in developing nations of about 2% to 3% in unimmunized infants. In the industrialized world, the measles case-fatality rate is vastly lower, at 0.01% to 0.02%. However, nonfatal complications are common, including otitis media, pneumonia, and subacute sclerosing pan-encephalitis. As far as the live attenuated vaccine is concerned, encephalitis and similar problems are very occasionally reported, but their origins have been hard to pin down, and the feasibility of reducing these rare, conjectural complications, as well as the acknowledged commoner ones (e.g., febrile convulsions), remains problematic at this stage.

Both the measles vaccine and its companions (mumps, rubella, and soon, perhaps, varicella) have good track records in *not* causing serious complications. Suffice it to say that these are live attenuated vaccines, which can cause problems in particular patients. Reactions are mild and include malaise, fever, mild rash, and (rarely) febrile convulsions. One report (194) surveyed the incidence of thrombocytopenic purpura after MMR vaccination. The incidence was 1 per 500,000 for measles or rubella alone, 1 per 120,000 for measles and rubella, and 1 per 105,000 for the combined MMR vaccine. The syndrome resembled the purpura that can occur after natural measles or rubella infections. Complete recovery occurred in 89.5% of cases; normalization followed by relapse was noted in 7%. No deaths have been reported. This French study accords with conclusions reached in several other countries. Although a plausible causal relationship can be argued, the usually favorable outcome ensures that this rare complication does not modify the risk-benefit equation significantly. The mumps vaccine occasionally causes aseptic meningitis.

From time to time, somewhat exotic claims of adverse events are made. For example, measles vaccination was claimed to cause autism and Crohn's disease. Nine studies have now refuted this. The hepatitis B vaccine was supposed to cause multiple sclerosis; exhaustive analysis has failed to support the association. No matter how bizarre, each claim must be examined carefully.

Excipients in the vaccine or adjuvant substances can occasion side reactions varying from inflammation to abscess formation. More seriously, vaccines can occasionally cause anaphylaxis, thrombocytopenia, or acute arthritis. These serious complications occur in fewer than 1 case in 100,000.

In summary, vaccines that have been through the current stringent regulatory process are incredibly safe. This fact deserves to be widely promulgated, and the media in particular need to be educated through a consistent and nonconfrontational effort.

RECOMMENDED IMMUNIZATION SCHEDULE

In the United States, routine immunization is recommended against 14 diseases, and this is likely to rise quite soon with the recent development of rotavirus and HPV vaccines. The schedule has become quite complex, and pharmaceutical companies are working hard to develop new combinations. Table 40.7 gives the current recommendations for children and adolescents in the

TABLE 40.7

DEPARTMENT OF HEALTH AND HUMAN SERVICES • CENTERS FOR DISEASE CONTROL AND PREVENTION

Recommended Immunization Schedule for Persons Aged 0–6 Years—UNITED STATES • 2007

Vaccine ▼ Age ►	Birth	1 month	2 months	4 months	6 months	12 months	15 months	18 months	19–23 months	2–3 years	4–6 years
Hepatitis B[1]	HepB	HepB		see footnote 1			HepB			HepB Series	
Rotavirus[2]			Rota	Rota	Rota						
Diphtheria, Tetanus, Pertussis[3]			DTaP	DTaP	DTaP		DTaP				DTaP
Haemophilus influenzae type b[4]			Hib	Hib	*Hib*[4]	Hib			Hib		
Pneumococcal[5]			PCV	PCV	PCV	PCV				PCV PPV	
Inactivated Poliovirus			IPV	IPV		IPV					IPV
Influenza[6]								Influenza (Yearly)			
Measles, Mumps, Rubella[7]						MMR					MMR
Varicella[8]						Varicella					Varicella
Hepatitis A[9]								HepA (2 doses)		HepA Series	
Meningococcal[10]										MPSV4	

Range of recommended ages

Catch-up immunization

Certain high-risk groups

This schedule indicates the recommended ages for routine administration of currently licensed childhood vaccines, as of December 1, 2006, for children aged 0–6 years. Additional information is available at http://www.cdc.gov/nip/recs/child-schedule.htm. Any dose not administered at the recommended age should be administered at any subsequent visit, when indicated and feasible. Additional vaccines may be licensed and recommended during the year. Licensed combination vaccines may be used whenever any components of the combination are indicated and other components of the vaccine are not contraindicated and if approved by the Food and Drug Administration for that dose of the series. Providers should consult the respective Advisory Committee on Immunization Practices statement for detailed recommendations. Clinically significant adverse events that follow immunization should be reported to the Vaccine Adverse Event Reporting System (VAERS). Guidance about how to obtain and complete a VAERS form is available at **http://www.vaers, hhs.gov** or by telephone, **800-822-7967**.

1. **Hepatitis B vaccine (HepB).** *(Minimum age: birth)*
   At birth:
   - Administer monovalent HepB to all newborns before hospital discharge.
   - If mother is hepatitis surface antigen (HBsAg)-positive, administer HepB and 0.5 mL of hepatitis B immune globulin (HBIG) within 12 hours of birth.
   - If mother's HBsAg status is unknown, administer HepB within 12 hours of birth. Determine the HBsAg status as soon as possible and if HBsAg-positive, administer HBIG (no later than age 1 week).
   - If mother is HBsAg-negative, the birth dose can only be delayed with physician's order and mother's negative HBsAg laboratory report documented in the infant's medical record.

   After the birth dose:
   - The HepB series should be completed with either monovalent HepB or a combination vaccine containing HepB. The second dose should be administered at age 1–2 months. The final dose should be administered at age ≥24 weeks. Infants born to HBsAg-positive mothers should be tested for HBsAg and antibody to HBsAg after completion of ≥3 doses of a licensed HepB series, at age 9–18 months (generally at the next well-child visit).

   4-month dose:
   - It is permissible to administer 4 doses of HepB when combination vaccines are administered after the birth dose. If monovalent HepB is used for doses after the birth dose, a dose at age 4 months is not needed.
2. **Rotavirus vaccine (Rota).** *(Minimum age: 6 weeks)*
   - Administer the first dose at age 6–12 weeks. Do not start the series later than age 12 weeks.
   - Administer the final dose in the series by age 32 weeks. Do not administer a dose later than age 32 weeks.
   - Data on safety and efficacy outside of these age ranges are insufficient.
3. **Diphtheria and tetanus toxoids and acellular pertussis vaccine (DTaP).** *(Minimum age: 6 weeks)*
   - The fourth dose of DTaP may be administered as early as age 12 months, provided 6 months have elapsed since the third dose.
   - Administer the final dose in the series at age 4–6 years.
4. ***Haemophilus influenzae* type b conjugate vaccine (Hib).** *(Minimum age: 6 weeks)*
   - If PRP-OMP (PedvaxHIB® or ComVax® [Merck]) is administered at ages 2 and 4 months, a dose at age 6 months is not required.
   - TriHiBit® (DTaP/Hib) combination products should not be used for primary immunization but can be used as boosters following any Hib vaccine in children aged ≥12 months.
5. **Pneumococcal vaccine.** *(Minimum age: 6 weeks for pneumococcal conjugate vaccine [PCV]; 2 years for pneumococcal polysaccharide vaccine [PPV])*
   - Administer PCV at ages 24–59 months in certain high-risk groups. Administer PPV to children aged ≥2 years in certain high-risk groups. See *MMWR* 2000;49(No. RR-9):1–35.
6. **Influenza vaccine.** *(Minimum age: 6 months for trivalent inactivated influenza vaccine [TIV]; 5 years for live, attenuated influenza vaccine [LAIV])*
   - All children aged 6–59 months and close contacts of all children aged 0–59 months are recommended to receive influenza vaccine.
   - Influenza vaccine is recommended annually for children aged ≥59 months with certain risk factors, health-care workers, and other persons (including household members) in close contact with persons in groups at high risk. See *MMWR* 2006;55(No. RR-10):1–41.
   - For healthy persons aged 5–49 years, LAIV may be used as an alternative to TIV.
   - Children receiving TIV should receive 0.25 mL if aged 6–35 months or 0.5 mL if aged ≥3 years.
   - Children aged <9 years who are receiving influenza vaccine for the first time should receive 2 doses (separated by ≥4 weeks for TIV and ≥6 weeks for LAIV).
7. **Measles, mumps, and rubella vaccine (MMR).** *(Minimum age: 12 months)*
   - Administer the second dose of MMR at age 4–6 years. MMR may be administered before age 4–6 years, provided ≥4 weeks have elapsed since the first dose and both doses are administered at age ≥12 months.
8. **Varicella vaccine.** *(Minimum age: 12 months)*
   - Administer the second dose of varicella vaccine at age 4–6 years. Varicella vaccine may be administered before age 4–6 years, provided that ≥3 months have elapsed since the first dose and both doses are administered at age ≥12 months. If second dose was administered ≥28 days following the first dose, the second dose does not need to be repeated.
9. **Hepatitis A vaccine (HepA).** *(Minimum age: 12 months)*
   - HepA is recommended for all children aged 1 year (i.e., aged 12–23 months). The 2 doses in the series should be administered at least 6 months apart.
   - Children not fully vaccinated by age 2 years can be vaccinated at subsequent visits.
   - HepA is recommended for certain other groups of children, including in areas where vaccination programs target older children. See *MMWR* 2006;55(No. RR-7):1–23.
10. **Meningococcal polysaccharide vaccine (MPSV4).** *(Minimum age: 2 years)*
    - Administer MPSV4 to children aged 2–10 years with terminal complement deficiencies or anatomic or functional asplenia and certain other high-risk groups. See *MMWR* 2005;54(No. RR-7):1–21.

The Recommended Immunization Schedules for Persons Aged 0–18 Years are approved by the Advisory Committee on Immunization Practices (http://www.cdc.gov/nip/acip), the American Academy of Pediatrics (http://www.aap.org), and the American Academy of Family Physicians (http://www.aafp.org).

SAFER • HEALTHIER • PEOPLE™

(Continued)

DEPARTMENT OF HEALTH AND HUMAN SERVICES • CENTERS FOR DISEASE CONTROL AND PREVENTION

Recommended Immunization Schedule for Persons Aged 7–18 Years—UNITED STATES • 2007

Vaccine ▼ / Age ▶	7–10 years	11–12 YEARS	13–14 years	15 years	16–18 years
Tetanus, Diphtheria, Pertussis[1]	see footnote 1	Tdap	Tdap		
Human Papillomavirus[2]	see footnote 2	HPV (3 doses)	HPV Series		
Meningococcal[3]	MPSV4	MCV4	MCV4	MCV4[3] MCV4	MCV4
Pneumococcal[4]	PPV	PPV	PPV	PPV	PPV
Influenza[5]	Influenza (Yearly)	Influenza (Yearly)	Influenza (Yearly)	Influenza (Yearly)	Influenza (Yearly)
Hepatitis A[6]	HepA Series	HepA Series	HepA Series	HepA Series	HepA Series
Hepatitis B[7]	HepB Series	HepB Series	HepB Series	HepB Series	HepB Series
Inactivated Poliovirus[8]	IPV Series	IPV Series	IPV Series	IPV Series	IPV Series
Measles, Mumps, Rubella[9]	MMR Series	MMR Series	MMR Series	MMR Series	MMR Series
Varicella[10]	Varicella Series	Varicella Series	Varicella Series	Varicella Series	Varicella Series

Legend: Range of recommended ages; Catch-up immunization; Certain high-risk groups

This schedule indicates the recommended ages for routine administration of currently licensed childhood vaccines, as of December 1, 2006, for children aged 7–18 years. Additional information is available at **http://www.cdc.gov/nip/recs/child-schedule.htm.** Any dose not administered at the recommended age should be administered at any subsequent visit, when indicated and feasible. Additional vaccines may be licensed and recommended during the year. Licensed combination vaccines may be used whenever any components of the combination are indicated and other components of the vaccine are not contraindicated and if approved by the Food and Drug Administration for that dose of the series. Providers should consult the respective Advisory Committee on Immunization Practices statement for detailed recommendations. Clinically significant adverse events that follow immunization should be reported to the Vaccine Adverse Event Reporting System (VAERS). Guidance about how to obtain and complete a VAERS form is available at **http://www.vaers.hhs.gov** or by telephone, **800-822-7967.**

1. **Tetanus and diphtheria toxoids and acellular pertussis vaccine (Tdap).** *(Minimum age: 10 years for BOOSTRIX® and 11 years for ADACEL™)*
   - Administer at age 11–12 years for those who have completed the recommended childhood DTP/DTaP vaccination series and have not received a tetanus and diphtheria toxoids vaccine (Td) booster dose.
   - Adolescents aged 13–18 years who missed the 11–12 year Td/Tdap booster dose should also receive a single dose of Tdap if they have completed the recommended childhood DTP/DTaP vaccination series.
2. **Human papillomavirus vaccine (HPV).** *(Minimum age: 9 years)*
   - Administer the first dose of the HPV vaccine series to females at age 11–12 years.
   - Administer the second dose 2 months after the first dose and the third dose 6 months after the first dose.
   - Administer the HPV vaccine series to females at age 13–18 years if not previously vaccinated.
3. **Meningococcal vaccine.** *(Minimum age: 11 years for meningococcal conjugate vaccine [MCV4]; 2 years for meningococcal polysaccharide vaccine [MPSV4])*
   - Administer MCV4 at age 11–12 years and to previously unvaccinated adolescents at high school entry (at approximately age 15 years).
   - Administer MCV4 to previously unvaccinated college freshmen living in dormitories; MPSV4 is an acceptable alternative.
   - Vaccination against invasive meningococcal disease is recommended for children and adolescents aged ≥2 years with terminal complement deficiencies or anatomic or functional asplenia and certain other high-risk groups. See *MMWR* 2005;54(No. RR-7):1–21. Use MPSV4 for children aged 2–10 years and MCV4 or MPSV4 for older children.
4. **Pneumococcal polysaccharide vaccine (PPV).** *(Minimum age: 2 years)*
   - Administer for certain high-risk groups. See *MMWR* 1997;46(No. RR-8):1–24, and *MMWR* 2000;49(No. RR-9):1–35.
5. **Influenza vaccine.** *(Minimum age: 6 months for trivalent inactivated influenza vaccine [TIV]; 5 years for live, attenuated influenza vaccine [LAIV])*
   - Influenza vaccine is recommended annually for persons with certain risk factors, health care workers, and other persons (including household members) in close contact with persons in groups at high risk. See *MMWR* 2006;55 (No. RR-10):1–41.
   - For healthy persons aged 5–49 years, LAIV may be used as an alternative to TIV.
   - Children aged <9 years who are receiving influenza vaccine for the first time should receive 2 doses (separated by ≥4 weeks for TIV and ≥6 weeks for LAIV).
6. **Hepatitis A vaccine (HepA).** *(Minimum age: 12 months)*
   - The 2 doses in the series should be administered at least 6 months apart.
   - HepA is recommended for certain other groups of children, including in areas where vaccination programs target older children. See *MMWR* 2006;55 (No. RR-7):1–23.
7. **Hepatitis B vaccine (HepB).** *(Minimum age: birth)*
   - Administer the 3-dose series to those who were not previously vaccinated.
   - A 2-dose series of Recombivax HB® is licensed for children aged 11–15 years.
8. **Inactivated poliovirus vaccine (IPV).** *(Minimum age: 6 weeks)*
   - For children who received an all-IPV or all-oral poliovirus (OPV) series, a fourth dose is not necessary if the third dose was administered at age ≥4 years.
   - If both OPV and IPV were administered as part of a series, a total of 4 doses should be administered, regardless of the child's current age.
9. **Measles, mumps, and rubella vaccine (MMR).** *(Minimum age: 12 months)*
   - If not previously vaccinated, administer 2 doses of MMR during any visit, with ≥4 weeks between the doses.
10. **Varicella vaccine.** *(Minimum age: 12 months)*
    - Administer 2 doses of varicella vaccine to persons without evidence of immunity.
    - Administer 2 doses of varicella vaccine to persons aged <13 years at least 3 months apart. Do not repeat the second dose, if administered ≥28 days after the first dose.
    - Administer 2 doses of varicella vaccine to persons aged ≥13 years at least 4 weeks apart.

The Recommended Immunization Schedules for Persons Aged 0–18 Years are approved by the Advisory Committee on Immunization Practices (http://www.cdc.gov/nip/acip), the American Academy of Pediatrics (http://www.aap.org), and the American Academy of Family Physicians (http://www.aafp.org).

SAFER • HEALTHIER • PEOPLE™

(Continued)

Catch-up Immunization Schedule

UNITED STATES • 2007

for Persons Aged 4 Months–18 Years Who Start Late or Who Are More Than 1 Month Behind

The table below provides catch-up schedules and minimum intervals between doses for children whose vaccinations have been delayed. A vaccine series does not need to be restarted, regardless of the time that has elapsed between doses. Use the section appropriate for the child's age.

Vaccine	Minimum Age for Dose 1	Minimum Interval Between Doses			
		Dose 1 to Dose 2	Dose 2 to Dose 3	Dose 3 to Dose 4	Dose 4 to Dose 5
CATCH-UP SCHEDULE FOR PERSONS AGED 4 MONTHS–6 YEARS					
Hepatitis B[1]	Birth	4 weeks	8 weeks (and 16 weeks after first dose)		
Rotavirus[2]	6 wks	4 weeks	4 weeks		
Diphtheria, Tetanus, Pertussis[3]	6 wks	4 weeks	4 weeks	6 months	6 months[3]
Haemophilus influenzae type b[4]	6 wks	**4 weeks** if first dose administered at age <12 months **8 weeks (as final dose)** if first dose administered at age 12-14 months **No further doses needed** if first dose administered at age ≥15 months	**4 weeks[4]** if current age <12 months **8 weeks (as final dose)[4]** if current age ≥12 months and second dose administered at age <15 months **No further doses needed** if previous dose administered at age ≥15 months	**8 weeks (as final dose)** This dose only necessary for children aged 12 months–5 years who received 3 doses before age 12 months	
Pneumococcal[5]	6 wks	**4 weeks** if first dose administered at age <12 months and current age <24 months **8 weeks (as final dose)** if first dose administered at age ≥12 months or current age 24–59 months **No further doses needed** for healthy children if first dose administered at age ≥24 months	**4 weeks** if current age <12 months **8 weeks (as final dose)** if current age ≥12 months **No further doses needed** for healthy children if previous dose administered at age ≥24 months	**8 weeks (as final dose)** This dose only necessary for children aged 12 months–5 years who received 3 doses before age 12 months	
Inactivated Poliovirus[6]	6 wks	4 weeks	4 weeks	4 weeks[6]	
Measles, Mumps, Rubella[7]	12 mos	4 weeks			
Varicella[8]	12 mos	3 months			
Hepatitis A[9]	12 mos	6 months			
CATCH-UP SCHEDULE FOR PERSONS AGED 7–18 YEARS					
Tetanus, Diphtheria/ Tetanus, Diphtheria, Pertussis[10]	7 yrs[10]	4 weeks	**8 weeks** if first dose administered at age <12 months **6 months** if first dose administered at age ≥12 months	**6 months** if first dose administered at age <12 months	
Human Papillomavirus[11]	9 yrs	4 weeks	12 weeks		
Hepatitis A[9]	12 mos	6 months			
Hepatitis B[1]	Birth	4 weeks	8 weeks (and 16 weeks after first dose)		
Inactivated Poliovirus[6]	6 wks	4 weeks	4 weeks	4 weeks[6]	
Measles, Mumps, Rubella[7]	12 mos	4 weeks			
Varicella[8]	12 mos	**4 weeks** if first dose administered at age ≥13 years **3 months** if first dose administered at age <13 years			

1. **Hepatitis B vaccine (HepB).** *(Minimum age: birth)*
   - Administer the 3-dose series to those who were not previously vaccinated.
   - A 2-dose series of Recombivax HB® is licensed for children aged 11–15 years.
2. **Rotavirus vaccine (Rota).** *(Minimum age: 6 weeks)*
   - Do not start the series later than age 12 weeks.
   - Administer the final dose in the series by age 32 weeks. Do not administer a dose later than age 32 weeks.
   - Data on safety and efficacy outside of these age ranges are insufficient.
3. **Diphtheria and tetanus toxoids and acellular pertussis vaccine (DTaP).** *(Minimum age: 6 weeks)*
   - The fifth dose is not necessary if the fourth dose was administered at age ≥4 years.
   - DTaP is not indicated for persons aged ≥7 years.
4. ***Haemophilus influenzae* type b conjugate vaccine (Hib).** *(Minimum age: 6 weeks)*
   - Vaccine is not generally recommended for children aged ≥5 years.
   - If current age <12 months and the first 2 doses were PRP-OMP (PedvaxHIB® or ComVax® [Merck]), the third (and final) dose should be administered at age 12– 15 months and at least 8 weeks after the second dose.
   - If first dose was administered at age 7–11 months, administer 2 doses separated by 4 weeks plus a booster at age 12–15 months.
5. **Pneumococcal conjugate vaccine (PCV).** *(Minimum age: 6 weeks)*
   - Vaccine is not generally recommended for children aged ≥5 years.
6. **Inactivated poliovirus vaccine (IPV).** *(Minimum age: 6 weeks)*
   - For children who received an all-IPV or all-oral poliovirus (OPV) series, a fourth dose is not necessary if third dose was administered at age ≥4 years.
   - If both OPV and IPV were administered as part of a series, a total of 4 doses should be administered, regardless of the child's current age.
7. **Measles, mumps, and rubella vaccine (MMR).** *(Minimum age: 12 months)*
   - The second dose of MMR is recommended routinely at age 4–6 years but may be administered earlier if desired.
   - If not previously vaccinated, administer 2 doses of MMR during any visit with ≥4 weeks between the doses.
8. **Varicella vaccine.** *(Minimum age: 12 months)*
   - The second dose of varicella vaccine is recommended routinely at age 4–6 years but may be administered earlier if desired.
   - Do not repeat the second dose in persons aged <13 years if administered ≥28 days after the first dose.
9. **Hepatitis A vaccine (HepA).** *(Minimum age: 12 months)*
   - HepA is recommended for certain groups of children, including in areas where vaccination programs target older children. See *MMWR* 2006;55(No. RR-7):1–23.
10. **Tetanus and diphtheria toxoids vaccine (Td) and tetanus and diphtheria toxoids and acellular pertussis vaccine (Tdap).** *(Minimum ages: 7 years for Td, 10 years for BOOSTRIX®, and 11 years for ADACEL™)*
    - Tdap should be substituted for a single dose of Td in the primary catch-up series or as a booster if age appropriate; use Td for other doses.
    - A 5-year interval from the last Td dose is encouraged when Tdap is used as a booster dose. A booster (fourth) dose is needed if any of the previous doses were administered at age <12 months. Refer to ACIP recommendations for further information. See *MMWR* 2006;55(No. RR-3).
11. **Human papillomavirus vaccine (HPV).** *(Minimum age: 9 years)*
    - Administer the HPV vaccine series to females at age 13–18 years if not previously vaccinated.

Information about reporting reactions after immunization is available online at **http://www.vaers.hhs.gov** or by telephone via the 24-hour national toll-free information line 800-822-7967. Suspected cases of vaccine-preventable diseases should be reported to the state or local health department. Additional information, including precautions and contraindications for immunization, is available from the National Center for Immunization and Respiratory Diseases at **http://www.cdc.gov/nip/default.htm** or telephone, **800-CDC-INFO (800-232-4636)**.

DEPARTMENT OF HEALTH AND HUMAN SERVICES • CENTERS FOR DISEASE CONTROL AND PREVENTION • SAFER • HEALTHIER • PEOPLE

(Continued)

United States. Schedules will vary somewhat from country to country.

ACCELERATED EFFORTS IN GLOBAL IMMUNIZATION

In recent years, markedly greater effort is going into the attempt to bring the benefits of vaccines to all the world's children. The Global Alliance for Vaccines and Immunization (GAVI), generously funded by the Bill & Melinda Gates Foundation, Norway, and several other donors, is making a big impact (195). Its focus is on a country-driven approach and high accountability, with concrete rewards for good results. In 2005, the G8 group of countries pledged to double aid to Africa, and planning is at an advanced stage for a new and innovative method of financing known as the International Finance Facility for Immunization (IFFIm). The idea is to raise $4 billion through the issue of bonds to be redeemed via unbreakable pledges by the donor countries. Spent over 10 years, it is estimated that this extra money for GAVI would prevent an additional 5 million child deaths by 2015 and more than 5 million future adult deaths from liver cirrhosis and cancer due to hepatitis B (196). In due time, when vaccines become available, the various sizeable bodies devoted to HIV/AIDS, malaria, and TB, such as the Global Fund to Fight AIDS, Tuberculosis, and Malaria, will ensure wide distribution. On the research side, most major donors are getting behind the Global HIV/AIDS Vaccine Enterprise (GHAVE), which seeks to harmonize and coordinate HIV vaccine research around the world.

It is to be hoped that the large polio eradication effort is crowned with success in the next several years. If so, the question will have to be asked whether there should be further eradication attempts. Measles would be a real possibility, but it must be admitted that total eradication is quite an expensive effort. The polio example has shown us that cessation of infant immunization while there is still polio in another country is dangerous. Some argue that control as a public health threat is a more sensible goal to set than elimination of the last virus from the planet. Still, what a magnificent argument to be able to have! Over time, the argument will recur for every organism for which we have an excellent vaccine and no animal or environmental reservoir.

VACCINATION OF THE VERY YOUNG AND THE OLD

Both extremes of age offer special challenges for the designer of new and improved vaccines. Some vaccines should be delivered very early in life, such as at birth, to be maximally useful. These include vaccines for diseases carried by the mother, such as hepatitis B, hepatitis C, HIV, or CMV. Early infant immunization is also good for encapsulated bacteria and rotavirus. Traditionally, BCG has also been given within a few days of birth in developing countries. Other vaccines are recommended for the elderly, including (in many countries) influenza and pneumococcal vaccines. There has been an up-surge of interest in protecting the elderly.

Although much more mature than that of the newborn mouse, the newborn infant's immune system is not yet hugely responsive, and neonatal immunization does not generally lead to extensive antibody formation. However, neonatal immunization can lead to useful priming of both B and T cell memory responses and thus serves a useful purpose (197). Preclinical studies suggest that the immaturity is not so much in $CD4^+$ or $CD8^+$ T cells themselves but rather in APCs and the APC–T cell interaction. This suggests that suitable adjuvant formulations could overcome the problem. Another feature of neonates is that they appear deficient in the capacity to form long-lived, bone marrow–seeking, antibody-forming plasma cells.

Maternally acquired antibodies can interfere with primary active immune responses. This is a serious point for many infant vaccines, including live and nonlive preparations, although it appears not to be an issue for hepatitis B. Inhibition is highly epitope specific and is much more important for B cell than for T cell responses. From a practical viewpoint, each case must be investigated specifically. For the most important vaccines of the future, maternal antibodies should not be a problem for HIV or TB, but for malaria, in which antibodies are of at least equal importance to T cells, the matter may be more germane. In the important example of measles, an aerosolized vaccine may overcome the problem.

At the other end of life, several factors militate against robust immune responses. The thymic cortex is largely replaced by fat, and few or no new T cells are exported from there. Thus, T cell immunity to new antigens must depend on cross-reactions with previously encountered ones. Similarly, the number of progenitors of B cells in the bone marrow is also reduced, although not as markedly. Interestingly, DCs from the peripheral blood of individuals older than 65 years are present in somewhat *increased* numbers, normal in appearance and surface markers, and unimpaired in antigen-presenting function. This may partly militate against the reduced proliferative capacity of aged T cells. While the capacity to mount a serum antibody response may be reduced, some vaccine boosters work well (e.g., tetanus and influenza).

A curious phenomenon in old age is the progressive accumulation of a differentiated $CD8^+$ T cell population specific for CMV, which may leave the rest of the repertoire depleted (198). Yet the elderly do not have too much trouble mounting a CD4^{+} T cell response to vaccines such as rabies or tickborne encephalitis (199). Overall, the elderly may require higher antigen doses or more frequent boosters than young adults. An interesting example is Merck's recently introduced vaccine for the prevention of herpes zoster and post–herpetic neuralgia in the ageing. It works well but requires 14 times the dose of live attenuated varicella virus than the formulation for infant immunization.

As more vaccines become available, and as the lowered impact of epidemic diseases prompts complacency in the minds of many, health authorities will have to give much more thought to the whole question of booster immunizations in adult life. In terms of policy, this area is currently a bit of a mess. It should not be left to the vagaries of choices by travelers.

CONCLUSION

There is no doubting the current renaissance in vaccinology. The field veritably bristles with new and exciting possibilities, and although the commercial potential is not as great as for prescription drugs, the healthy percentage sales growth of the sector has not gone unnoticed in the boardrooms of the big pharmaceutical companies. Of the new vaccination approaches discussed, mucosal delivery systems, new adjuvant formulations, and extensive combinations are the most promising. DNA vaccines, viral vectors, and prime-boost approaches are intellectually exciting but some distance away. Transdermal delivery systems, methods to circumvent the need for a cold chain, plant production systems for antigens, and microencapsulation technologies are fertile research areas. Despite his enthusiasm for such novel developments, the author is also aware of the fact that changes to national immunization programs can be made only after extensive clinical research, particularly in cases in which an effective vaccine already exists. The future, therefore, represents a judicious balance between conservatism in a measure already regarded skeptically by a minority and cautious activism as thorough research documents the value of each new and improved vaccine. Nor should a healthy pluralism be opposed. Some countries will move faster on some vaccines because of their particular perspectives and problems. All of this means that the widespread introduction of the rich panoply of vaccines coming from the research sector will probably be slower than the scientific community would like. In the long run, however, the approach to many communicable diseases will be revolutionized by the new vaccinology. Further, the thrusting programs bringing vaccines to the developing countries need to be strongly applauded. The legacy of Jenner and Pasteur is in good hands.

ACKNOWLEDGMENTS

The author thanks Ms. Jill Van Es for her careful typing of the manuscript; Ms. Josephine Marshall and Ms. Wendy Hertan for help with references; and many kind colleagues around the world for supplying up-to-date information.

REFERENCES

1. Hilleman MR. Overview of vaccinology in historic and future perspective. In: Hildegrund CJ, ed. *DNA Vaccines*. Kluwer Academic/Plenum Publishers; 2003. p. 1–37.
2. Levine MM, Woodrow GC, Kaper JB, Cobon GS. *New generation vaccines*. New York: Marcel Dekker, Inc; 2004.
3. Fenner F, Henderson DA, Arita I, Jezek Z, Ladnyi ID. *Smallpox and its eradication*. Geneva: World Health Organization; 1988.
4. Jenner E. *An inquiry into the causes and effects of the variolae vaccinae, a disease discovered in some of the Western Counties of England, particularly Gloucestershire, and known by the name of cow pox*. London: Published privately; 1778.
5. Pasteur L, Joubert J, Chamberland C. The germ theory of disease. *C R Hebd Seances Acad Sci*. 1878;86:1037–1052.
6. Pasteur L. De l'attenuation du virus du cholera des poules. *C R Acad Sci Paris*. 1880;91:673–680.
7. Calmette LCA, Guérin C, Weill-Hallé B. Essai d'immunisation contre l'infection tuberculeuse. *Bull Acad Med (Paris)*. 1924;91:787–796.
8. Glenny AT, Hopkins BE. Diphtheria toxoid as an immunising agent. *Brit J Exp Path*. 1923;4:283–288.
9. Enders JF, Weller TH, Robbins RC. Cultivation of the Lansing strain of poliomyelitis virus in cultures of various human embryonic tissues. *Science*. 1949;109:85–87.
10. Hilleman MR. The development of live attenuated mumps virus vaccine in historic perspective and its role in the evolution of combined measles-mumps-rubella. In: Plotkin S. FB, editor. *Vaccinia, vaccination and vaccinology: Jenner, Pasteur and their successors*. Paris: Elsevier; 1996. p. 283–292.
11. Blumberg BS, Alter HJ, Visnich S. A "new" antigen in leukemia sera. *J Am Med Assoc*. 1965;191:541–546.
12. Blumberg BS. Australia antigen, hepatitis, and leukemia. *Tokyo J Med Sci*. 1968;76:1.
13. Valenzuela P, Medina A, Rutter WJ, et al. Synthesis and assembly of hepatitis B virus surface antigen particles in yeast. *Nature*. 1982;298:347–350.
14. Janeway CA, Jr. Approaching the asymptote? Evolution and revolution in immunology. In: Cold Spring Harbor Symposia on Quantitative Biology; 1989. p. 1–14.
15. Akira S, Uematsu S, Takeuchi O. Pathogen recognition and innate immunity. *Cell*. 2006;124:783–801.
16. Gay NJ, Keith FJ. Drosophila Toll and IL-1 receptor. *Nature*. 1991;351(6325):355–356.
17. Lemaitre B, Nicolas E, Michaut L, et al. The dorsoventral regulatory gene cassette spatzle/Toll/cactus controls the potent antifungal response in Drosophila adults. *Cell*. 1996;86:973–983.
18. O'Neill AJ. How Toll-like receptors signal: what we know and what we don't know. *Curr Opin Immunol*. 2006;18:3–9.
19. Dillon S, Agrawal A, Van Dyke T, et al. A TLR2 ligand stimulates Th2 responses *in vivo*, via induction of ERK MAP kinase and c-Fos in dendritic cells. *J Immunol*. 2004;172:4733–4743.
20. Dillon S, Agrawal A, Banerjee K, et al. Yeast zymosan, a ligand for TLR-2 and dectin-1, induces reglatory antigen-presenting cells and immunological tolerance. *J Clin Invest*. 2006;116:916–928.
21. Pulendran B, Ahmed R. Translating innate immnity into immunological memory: implications for vaccine development. *Cell*. 2006;124:849–863.
22. Liu YJ. IPC: professional type 1 interferon-producing cells and plasmacytoid dendritic cell precursors. *Annu Rev Immunol*. 2005;23:275–306.

23. Pulendran B. Variegation of the immune response with dendritic cells and pathogen recognition receptors. *J Immunol.* 2005;1:2457–2465.
24. Bottazi B, Garlanda C, Salvatori G, et al. Pentraxins as a key component of innate immunity. *Cur Opin Immunol.* 2006;18.
25. Takahashi K, Ip WK, Michelow IC, et al. The mannose-binding lectin: a prototypic pattern recognition molecule. *Curr Opin Immunol.* 2006;18:16–23.
26. Ip WK, Chan KH, Law HK, et al. Mannose-binding lectin in severe acute respiratory syndrome coronavirus infection. *J Infect Dis.* 2005;191:1697–1704.
27. Cambi A, Figdor CG. Levels of complexity in pathogen recognition by C-type lectins. *Curr Opin Immunol.* 2005;17:345–351.
28. Hunger RE, Sieling PA, Ochoa MT, et al. Langerhans cells utilize CD1a and langerin to efficiently present nonpeptide antigens to T cells. *J Clin Invest.* 2004;113:658–660.
29. Cambi A, F dL, van Maarseveen NM, et al. Microdomains of the C-type lectin DC-SIGN are portals for virus entry into dendritic cells. *J Cell Biol.* 2004;164:145–155.
30. Jones DA, Takemoto D. Plant innate immunity—direct and indirect recognition of general and specific pathogen-associated molecules. *Curr Opin Immunol.* 2004;16:48–62.
31. Murray PJ. NOD proteins: an intracellular pathogen-recognition system or signal transduction modifiers? *Curr Opin Immunol.* 2005;17:352–358.
32. Matzinger P. The danger model: a renewed sense of self. *Science.* 2002(296):301–305.
33. Li M, Carpio DF, Zheng Y, et al. An essential role of the NF-kappa B/Toll-like receptor pathway in induction of inflammatory and tissue-repair gene expression by necrotic cells. *J Immunol.* 2001;166(12):7128–7135.
34. Oppenheim JJ, Yang D. Alarmins: chemotactic activators of immune responses. *Curr Opin Immunol.* 2005;17:359–365.
35. Hancock REW, Diamond G. The role of cationic antimicrobial peptides in innate host defences. *Trends Microbiol.* 2000;8:402–410.
36. Brown KL, Hancock REW. Cationic host defense (antimicrobial) peptides. *Curr Opin Immunol.* 2006;18:24–30.
37. Zhang L, Falla TJ. Cationic antimicrobial peptides—an update. *Expert Opin Investig Drugs.* 2004;13:97–106.
38. Heilman C. Accelerated development of vaccines 2002. In: *The Jordan Report: Division of Microbiology and Infectious Diseases.* Bethesda, Maryland: NIAID, NIH; 2002.
39. O'Hagan DT, Valiante NM. Recent advances in the discovery and delivery of vaccine adjuvants. *Nature Rev Drug Discov.* 2003;2:727–735.
40. Pearse MJ, Drane D. ISCOMATRIX adjuvant for antigen delivery. *Adv Drug Deliv Rev.* 2005;57:465–474.
41. Ott G, Barchfeld GL, Chernoff R, et al. MF59: Design and evaluation of a safe and potent adjuvant for human vaccines. In: Powell MF, Newman MJ, eds. *Vaccine Design: The Subunit and Adjuvant Approach.* New York: Plenum Press; 1995. p. 277–296.
42. Glenny AT, Pope CG, Waddington H, Wallace V. The antigenic value of toxoid precipitated by potassium alum. *J Pathol Bacteriol.* 1926;29:38–45.
43. Freund J, McDermott K. Sensitization to horse serum by means of adjuvants. *Proc Soc Exp Biol Med.* 1942;49:548–553.
44. Allison AC, Byars NE. An adjuvant formulation that selectively elicits the formation of antibodies of protective isotypes and of cell-mediated immunity. *J Immunol Methods.* 1986;95(2):157–168.
45. Ellouz F, Adam A, Ciorbaru R, et al. Minimal structural requirements for adjuvant activity of bacterial peptidoglycans. *Biochem Biophys Res Commun.* 1974;59:1317–1325.
46. Johnson AG, Tomai M, Solem L, et al. Characterization of a non-toxic monophosphoryl lipid A. *Rev Infect Dis.* 1987;9 Suppl 5:S512–S516.
47. Kensil CR, Patel U, Lennick M, et al. Separation and characterization of saponins with adjuvant activity from Quillaja saponaria Molina cortex. *J Immunol.* 1991;146(2):431–437.
48. Stoute JA, Slaoui M, Heppner DG, et al. A preliminary evaluation of a recombinant circumsporozoite protein vaccine against Plasmodium falciparum malaria. RTS,S Malaria Vaccine Evaluation Group. *N Engl J Med.* 1997;336(2):86–91.
49. Morein B, Sundquist B, Höglund S, et al. Iscom, a novel structure for antigenic presentation of membrane proteins from enveloped viruses. *Nature.* 1984;308:457–460.
50. Drane D, Pearse MJ. The ISCOMATRIX^{TM} adjuvant. In: Schijns VE, O'Hagan DT, editors. *Immunopotentiators in Modern Vaccines.* Boston: Elsevier Academic Press; 2006. p. 191–215.
51. Frazer IH, Quinn M, Nicklin JL, et al. Phase 1 study of HPV16-specific immunotherapy with E6E7 fusion protein and ISCOMATRIX adjuvant in women with cervical intraepithelial neoplasia. *Vaccine.* 2004;23:172–181.
52. Tokunaga T, Yamamoto H, Shimada S, et al. Antitumor activity of deoxyribonucleic acid fraction from Mycobacterium bovis BCG. I. Isolation, physicochemical characterization, and antitumor activity. *J Natl Cancer Inst.* 1984;72(4):955–962.
53. Krieg AM, Yi AK, Matson S, et al. CpG motifs in bacterial DNA trigger direct B-cell activation. *Nature.* 1995;374(6522):546–549.
54. Medzhitov R, Janeway CA, Jr. Innate immunity: the virtues of a nonclonal system of recognition. *Cell.* 1997;91(3):295–298.
55. Kreig AM, Davis HL. CpG ODN as a Th1 immune enhancer for prophylactic and therapeutic vaccines. In: *Vaccine Adjuvants. Immunological and Clinical Principles.* 2005. p. 87–110.
56. Vollmer J, Weeratna R, Payette PJ, et al. Characterization of three CpG oligodeoxynucleotide classes with distinct immunostimulatory activities. *Eur J Immunol.* 2004;34:251–262.
57. Cooper CL, Davis HL, Morris ML, et al. Safety and immunogenicity of CPG 7909 injection as an adjuvant to Fluarix influenza vaccine. *Vaccine.* 2004;22:3136–3143.
58. Tighe H, Takabayashi K, Schwartz D, et al. Conjugation of immunostimulatory DNA to the short ragweed allergen Amb a 1 enhances its immunogenicity and reduces its allergenicity. *J Allergy Clin Immunol.* 2000;106(1 Pt 1):124–134.
59. Adamsson J, Lindblad M, Lundqvist A, et al. Novel immunostimulatory agent based on CpG oligodeoxynucleotide linked to the non-toxic B subunit of cholera toxin. *J Immunol.* 2006;176:4902–4913.
60. Jackson DC, Lau YF, Le T, et al. A totally synthetic vaccine of generic structure that targets Toll-like receptor 2 on dendritic cells and promotes antibody or cytotoxic T cell responses. *Proc Natl Acad Sci U S A.* 2004;101:15440–15445.
61. Silva DG, Cooper PD, Petrovsky N. Inulin-derived adjuvants efficiently promote both Th1 and Th2 immune reponses. *Immunol Cell Biol.* 2004;82:611–616.
62. Alving CR, Detrick B, Richards RL, et al. Novel adjuvant strategies for experimental malaria and AIDS vaccines. *Ann NY Acad Sci.* 1993;690:265–275.
63. Mengiardi B, Berger R, Just M, et al. Virosomes as carriers for combined vaccines. *Vaccine.* 1995;13(14):1306–1315.
64. Gluck U, Gebbers JO, Gluck R. Phase 1 evaluation of intranasal virosomal influenza vaccine with and without Escherichia coli heat-labile toxin in adult volunteers. *J Virol.* 1999;73(9):7780–7786.
65. Chang TMS. Biodegradable, semi-permeable microcapsules containing enzymes hormones, vaccines and other biologicals. *J Bioeng.* 1976;1:25–32.
66. Langer R. Polymers for the sustained release of macromolecules: their use in a single step method of immunization. *Meth Enzymol.* 1981;73:57–75.
67. O'Hagan DT, Rahman D, McGee JP, et al. Biodegradable microparticles as controlled release antigen delivery systems. *Immunology.* 1991;73(2):239–242.
68. Eldridge JH, Staas JK, Meulbroek JA, et al. Biodegradable and biocompatible poly(DL-lactide-co-glycolide) microspheres as an adjuvant for staphylococcal enterotoxin B toxoid which enhances the level of toxin-neutralizing antibodies. *Infect Immun.* 1991;59(9):2978–2986.
69. Vordermeier HM, Coombes AG, Jenkins P, et al. Synthetic delivery system for tuberculosis vaccines: immunological evaluation of the M. tuberculosis 38 kDa protein entrapped in biodegradable PLG microparticles. *Vaccine.* 1995;13(16):1576–1582.
70. Pulendran B, Palucka K, Banchereau J. Sensing pathogens and tuning immune responses. *Science.* 2001;293:253–256.
71. Giedlin MA. Cytokines as vaccine adjuvants: the use of interleukin-2. In: O'Hagan DT, editor. *Vaccine Adjuvants. Preparation Methods and Research Protocols.* Totowa, NJ: Humana Press; 2000. p. 283–297.

72. Dempsey PW, Allison ME, Akkaraju S, et al. C3d of complement as a molecular adjuvant: bridging innate and acquired immunity. *Science.* 1996;271(5247):348–350.
73. Alonso PL, Sacarlal J, Aponte JJ, et al. Efficacy of the RTS,S/AS02A vaccine against Plasmodium falciparum infection and disease in young African children: randomised controlled trial. *Lancet.* 2004;364:1411–1420.
74. Querec T, Bennouna S, Alkan S, et al. Yellow fever vaccine YF-17D activates multiple dendritic cell subsets via TLR2, 7, 8, and 9 to stimulate polyvalent immunity. *J Exp Med.* 2006;203:413–424.
75. Geijtenbeek TB, Van Vliet SJ, Koppel EA, et al. Mycobacteria target DC-SIGN to suppress dendritic cell function. *J Exp Med.* 2003;197: 7–17.
76. Pizza M, Fontana MR, Giuliani MM, et al. A genetically detoxified derivative of heat-labile Escherichia coli enterotoxin induces neutralizing antibodies against the A subunit. *J Exp Med.* 1994;180(6):2147–2153.
77. Douce G, Fontana M, Pizza M, et al. Intranasal immunogenicity and adjuvanticity of site-directed mutant derivatives of cholera toxin. *Infect Immun.* 1997;65(7):2821–2828.
78. Sun J-B, Holmgren J, Czerkinsky C. Cholera toxin B subunit: an efficient transmucosal carrier-delivery system for induction of peripheral immunological tolerance. *Proc Natl Acad Sci U S A.* 1994;91:10795–10799.
79. Mackett M, Smith GL, Moss B. Vaccinia virus: a selectable eukaryotic cloning and expression vector. *Proc Natl Acad Sci U S A.* 1982;79:7415–7419.
80. Panicali D, Paoletti E. Construction of pox viruses as cloning vectors: insertion of the thymidine kinase gene from herpes simplex virus into the DNA of infectious vaccinia virus. *Proc Natl Acad Sci U S A.* 1982;79:4927–4931.
81. Ramshaw IA, Ramsay AJ. The prime-boost strategy: exciting prospects for improved vaccination. *Immunol Today.* 2000; 21(4):163–165.
82. Wolff JA, Malone RW, Williams P, et al. Direct gene transfer into mouse muscle in vivo. *Science.* 1990;247(4949 Pt 1):1465–1468.
83. Williams RS, Johnstone SA, Reidy M, et al. Introduction of foreign genes into tissues of living mice by DNA-coated microprojectiles. *Proc Natl Acad Sci U S A.* 1991;88:2726–2730.
84. Tang DC, Devit M, Johnston SA. Genetic immunization is a simple method for eliciting an immune response. *Nature.* 1992;356:152–154.
85. Ulmer JB, Donnelly JJ, Parker SE, et al. Heterologous protection against influenza by injection of DNA encoding a viral protein. *Science.* 1993;259:1745–1749.
86. Fynan EF, Webster RG, Fuller DH, et al. DNA vaccines - protective immunizations by parenteral, mucosal and gene-gun inoculations. *Proc Natl Acad. Sci U S A.* 1993;90:11478–11482.
87. Donnelly JJ, Ulmer JB, Shiver JW, et al. DNA vaccines. *Annu Rev Immunol.* 1997;15:617–648.
88. Fu TM, Ulmer JB, Caulfield MJ, et al. Priming of cytotoxic T lymphocytes by DNA vaccines: requirement for professional antigen presenting cells and evidence for antigen transfer from myocytes. *Mol Med.* 1997;3(6):362–371.
89. Boyle JS, Brady JL, Lew AM. Enhanced responses to a DNA vaccine encoding a fusion antigen that is directed to sites of immune induction. *Nature.* 1998;392(6674):408–411.
90. Holt PG, Schon-Hegrad MA, McMenamin PG. Dendritic cells in the respiratory tract. *Int Rev Immunol.* 1990;6(2–3):139–149.
91. Picker LJ, Butcher EC. Physiological and molecular mechanisms of lymphocyte homing. *Annu Rev Immunol.* 1994;62:561–569.
92. Holmgren J, Czerkinsky C. Mucosal immunity and vaccines. *Nature Medicine Suppl.* 2005;11:S45–S53.
93. McWilliam AS, Nelson D, Thomas JA, et al. Rapid dendritic cell recruitment is a hallmark of the acute inflammatory response at mucosal surfaces. *J Exp Med.* 1994;179:1331–1336.
94. Holmgren J, Rudin A. Mucosal immunity and bacteria. In: Ogra P, Mestecky J, Lamm M, et al, eds. *Mucosal Immunology.* San Diego: Academic Press; 1999. p. 685–693.
95. Glenn GM, Scharton-Kersten T, Vassell R, et al. Transcutaneous immunization with bacterial ADP-ribosylating exotoxins as antigens and adjuvants. *Infect Immun.* 1999;67(3):1100–1106.
96. Mason HS, Lam DM, Arntzen CJ. Expression of hepatitis B surface antigen in transgenic plants. *Proc Natl Acad Sci U S A.* 1992;89(24):11745–11749.
97. Peterson RK, Arntzen CJ. On risk and plant-based biopharmaceuticals. *Trends Biochem.* 2004;22:64–66.
98. Amtzen C, Plotkin S, Dodet B. Plant-derived vaccines and antibodies: potential and limitations. *Vaccine.* 2005;23:1753–1756.
99. Hu SL, Klaniecki J, Dykers T, et al. Neutralizing antibodies against HIV-1 BRU and SF2 isolates generated in mice immunized with recombinant vaccinia virus expressing HIV-1 (BRU) envelope glycoproteins and boosted with homologous gp160. *AIDS Res Hum Retroviruses.* 1991;7(7):615–620.
100. Greco D, Salmaso S, Mastrantonio P, et al. A controlled trial of two acellular vaccines and one whole-cell vaccine against pertussis. Progetto Pertosse Working Group. *N Engl J Med.* 1996;334(6):341–348.
101. Rappuoli R. Rational design of vaccines. *Nat Med.* 1997;3(4):374–376.
102. Klein D. Pertussis vaccines: a continuing saga. In: Baker PJ, ed. *The Jordan Report. Accelerated Development of Vaccines.* Bethesda: Division of Microbiology and Infectious Diseases, NIAID, NIH; 1996 p. 29–32.
103. Miller E. Overview of recent clinical trials of acellular pertussis vaccines. *Biologicals.* 1999;27:79–86.
104. Ivanoff B, Levine MM, Lambert PH. Vaccination against typhoid fever: present status. *Bull WHO.* 1994;72:957–971.
105. Yang J, Acosta CJ, Si GA, et al. A mass vaccination campaign targeting adults and children to prevent typhoid fever in Hechi; expanding the use of Vi polysaccharide vaccine in southeast China: a cluster-randomized trial. *BMC Public Health.* 2005;5:49–58.
106. Lin FY, Ho VA, Khiem HB, et al. The efficacy of a Salmonella typhi Vi conjugate vaccine in two-to-five-year-old children. *N Engl J Med.* 2001;344:1263–1269.
107. Szu SC, Bystricky S, Hinojosa-Ahumada M, et al. Synthesis and some immunologic properties of an O-acetyl pectin [poly(1–4)-alpha-D-GalpA]-protein conjugate as a vaccine for typhoid fever. *Infect Immun.* 1994;62:5545–5549.
108. Sanchez JL, Vasquez B, Begue RE, et al. Protective efficacy of oral whole-cell/recombinant-B-subunit cholera vaccine in Peruvian military recruits. *Lancet.* 1994;344:1273–1276.
109. van Loon FPL, Clemens JD, Chakraborty J, et al. Field trial of inactivated oral cholera vaccines in Bangladesh: results from 5 years of follow-up. *Vaccine.* 1996;14:162–166.
110. Lucas ME, Deen JL, von Seidlein L, et al. Effectiveness of mass oral cholera vaccination in Beira, Mozambique. *N Engl J Med.* 2005;352:757–767.
111. Trach DD, Clemens JD, Ke NT, et al. Field trial of a locally produced, killed, oral cholera vaccine in Vietnam. *Lancet.* 1997;349(9047):231–235.
112. Tacket CO, Losonsky G, Nataro JP, et al. Onset and duration of protective immunity in challenged volunteers after vaccination with live oral cholera vaccine CVD 103-HgR. *J Infect Dis.* 1992;166(4):837–841.
113. Pearson GD, Woods A, Chiang SL, et al. CTX genetic element encodes a site-specific recombination system and an intestinal colonization factor. *Proc Natl Acad Sci U S A.* 1993;90(8):3750–3754.
114. Svennerholm AM, Savarino SJ. Oral inactivated whole cell B subunit combination vaccine against enterotoxigenic *Escherichia coli.* In: Levine MM, Kaper JB, Rappouli R, et al, eds. *New Generation Vaccines.* 3rd ed. New York: Marcel Dekker; 2004. p. 737–750.
115. Barry E, Altboum Z, Losonsky G, et al. Immune responses elicited against multiple enterotoxigenic *Escherichia coli* fimbriae and mutant LT expressed in attenuate *Shigella* vaccine strains. *Vaccine.* 2003;21:333–340.
116. Kotloff KL, Winickoff JP, Ivanoff B, et al. Global burden of *Shigella* infections: implicatons for vaccine development and implementation of control strategies. *Bull WHO.* 1999;77(8):651–666.
117. Sansonetti P, Phalipon A. Shigellosis: from molecular pathogenesis of infection to protective immunity and vaccine development. *Res Immunol.* 1996;147(8–9):595–602.
118. Kotloff KL, Noriega FR, Samandari T, et al. Shigella *flexneri* 2a strain CVD 1207, with specific deletions in *vir*G, *sen*, *set*, and *gua*BA, is highly attenuated in humans. *Infect Immun.* 2000;68(3): 1034–1039.

119. Weekly epidemiological record. World Health Organization 2006; 81:49–60.
120. Ranallo RT, Fonseka CP, Cassels F, et al. Construction and characterization of bivalent *Shigella flexneri* 2a vaccine strains SC608(pCFAI) and SC608(pCFAI/LTB) that express antigens from enterotoxigenic *Escherichia coli*. *Infect Immun.* 2005;73:258–267.
121. Robbins JB, Schneerson R. Future vaccine development at NICHD. *Ann NY Acad Sci.* 2004;1038:49–59.
122. Mukhopadhaya A, Mahalanabis D, Chakrabarti MK. Role of Shigella flexneri 2a 34 kDa outer membrane protein in induction of protective immune response. *Vaccine.* 2006;24:6028–6036.
123. Marshall BJ, Warren JR. Unidentified curved bacilli in the stomach of patients with gastritis and peptic ulceration. *Lancet.* 1983;1:1311–1315.
124. Uemura N, Okamoto S, Yamamoto S, et al. Helicobacter pylori infection and the develoment of gastric cancer. *N Engl J Med.* 2001;345(11):784–789.
125. Del Giudice G, Covacci A, Telford JL, et al. The design of vaccines against Helicobacter pylori and their development. *Annu Rev Immunol.* 2001;19:523–563.
126. Lee A, Hazell SL, O'Rourke J, Kouprach S. Isolation of a spiral-shaped bacterium from the cat stomach. *Infect Immun.* 1988;56(11):2843–2850.
127. Doidge C, Crust I, Lee A, et al. Therapeutic immunization against *Helicobacter* infection. *Lancet.* 1994;343(8902):914–915.
128. Corthesy-Theulaz I, Porta N, Glauser M, et al. Oral immunization with *Helicobacter pylori* urease B subunit as a treatment against *Helicobacter* infection in mice. *Gastroenterology.* 1995;109(1):115–121.
129. Rossi G, Fortuna D, Pancotto L, et al. Immunohistochemical study of lymphocyte populations infiltrating the gastric mucosa of beagle dogs experimentally infected with *Helicobacter pylori*. *Infect Immun.* 2000;68(8):4769–4772.
130. Sutton P, Doidge C. Helicobacter vaccines spiral into the new millennium. *Digestive & Liver Disease.* 2003;35:675–687.
131. Anderson P, Peter G, Johnston RB, Jr., et al. Immunization of humans with polyribophosphate, the capsular antigen of *Hemophilus influenzae*, type b. *J Clin Invest.* 1972;51(1):39–44.
132. Rodrigues LP, Schneerson R, Robbins JB. Immunity to *Hemophilus influenzae* type b. I. The isolation, and some physicochemical, serologic and biologic properties of the capsular polysaccharide of *Hemophilus influenzae* type b. *J Immunol.* 1971;107(4):1071–1080.
133. Peltala H, Käyhty H, Sivonen A, et al. *Haemophilus influenzae* type b capsular polysaccharide vaccine in children: a double-blind field study of 100,000 vaccines 3 months to 5 years of age in Finland. *Pediatrics.* 1977;60:730–737.
134. Anderson P. Antibody responses to *Haemophilus influenzae* type b and diphtheria toxin induced by conjugates of oligosaccharides of the type b capsule with the non-toxic protein CRM197. *Infect Immun.* 1983;39:233–238.
135. Schneerson R, Robbins JB, Chu C, et al. Semi-synthetic vaccines composed of capsular polysaccharides of pathogenic bacteria covalently bound to proteins for the prevention of invasive diseases. *Prog Allergy.* 1983;33:144–158.
136. Eskola J, Kayhty H, Takala AK, et al. A randomized, prospective field trial of a conjugate vaccine in the protection of infants and young children against invasive Haemophilus influenzae type b disease. *N Engl J Med.* 1990;323(20):1381–1387.
137. Mulholland K, Hilton S, Adegbola R, et al. Randomised trial of *Haemophilus influenzae* type-b tetanus protein conjugate vaccine [corrected] for prevention of pneumonia and meningitis in Gambian infants. *Lancet.* 1997;349(9060):1191–1197.
138. Miller E, Salisbury D, Ramsay M. Planning, registration and implementation of an immunisation campaign against meningococcal serogroup C disease in the UK: a success story. *Vaccine.* 2002;20:S58–S67.
139. Trotter CL, Andrews NJ, Kaczmarski EB, et al. Effectiveness of meningococcal serogroup C conjugate vaccine 4 years after introduction. *Lancet.* 2004;364:365–367.
140. Jodar L, Feavers IM, Salisbury D, et al. Development of vaccines against meningococcal disease. *Lancet.* 2002;359:1499–1508.
141. Pizza M, Scarlato V, Masagnani V, et al. Identification of vaccine candidates against serogroup B meningococcus by whole-genome sequencing. *Science.* 2000;287:1816–1895.
142. Giuliani MM, Adu-Bobie J, Comanducci M, et al. A universal vaccine for serogroup B meningococcus. *Proc Natl Acad Sci U S A.* 2006;103:10834–10839.
143. Cutts FT, Zaman SM, Enwere G, et al. Efficacy of nine-valent pneumococcal conjugate vaccine against pneumonia and invasive pneumococcal disease in The Gambia: randomised, double-blind, placebo-controlled trial. *Lancet.* 2005;365:1139–1146.
144. Prymula R, Peeters P, Chrobok V, et al. Pneumococcal capsular polysaccharides conjugated to protein D for prevention of acute otitis media caused by both Streptococcus pneumoniae and non-typable Haemophilus influenzae: a randomised double-blind efficacy study. *Lancet.* 2006;367:740–748.
145. Kaufmann SH. Recent findings in immunology give tuberculosis vaccines a new boost. *Trends Immunol* 2006;in press.
146. Britton WJ, Palendira U. Improving vaccines against tuberculosis. *Immunol Cell Biol.* 2003;81:34–45.
147. Cole ST, Brosch R, Parkhill J, et al. Deciphering the biology of *Mycobacterium tuberculosis* from the complete genome sequence. *Nature.* 1998;393:537–544.
148. Pinto R, Saunders BM, Camacho LR, et al. Mycobacterium tuberculosis defective in phthiocerol dimycocerosate translocation provides greater protective immunity against tuberculosis than the existing bacille Calmette-Guerin vaccine. *J Infect Dis.* 2004;189:105–112.
149. Orme IM. Preclinical testing of new vaccines for tuberculosis: a comprehensive review. *Vaccine.* 2006;24:2–19.
150. Reed S, Lobet Y. Tuberculosis vaccine development; from mouse to man. *Microbes & Infection.* 2005;7:922–931.
151. Young D, Dye C. The development and impact of tuberculosis vaccines. *Cell.* 2006;124:683–687.
152. McShane H, Pathan AA, Sander CR, et al. Recombinant modified vaccinia virus Ankara expressing antigen 85A boosts BCG-primed and naturally acquired antimycobacterial immunity in humans. *Nat Med.* 2004;10:1240–1244.
153. Wozniak TM, Ryan AA, Triccas JA, et al. Plasmid interleukin-23 (IL-23), but not plasmid IL-27, enhances the protective efficacy of a DNA vaccine against Mycobacterium tuberculosis infection. *Infect Immun.* 2006;74:557–565.
154. Brandt ER, Sriprakash KS, Hobb RI, et al. New multi-determinant strategy for a group A streptococcal vaccine designed for the Australian Aboriginal population. *Nat Med.* 2000;6(4):455–459.
155. Hilleman MR. Hepatitis and hepatitis A vaccine: a glimpse of history. *J Hepatol.* 1993;18(Suppl 2):S5–S10.
156. Choo QL, Richman KH, Han JH, et al. Genetic organization and diversity of the hepatitis C virus. *Proc Natl Acad Sci U S A.* 1991; 88(6):2451–2455.
157. Wakita T, Pietschmann T, Kato T, et al. Production of infectious hepatitis C virus in tissue culture from a cloned viral genome. *Nat Med.* 2005;11:791–796.
158. Brass V, Moradpour D, Blum HE. Molecular virology of hepatitis C virus (HCV): 2006 update. *Int J Med Sci.* 2006;3:29–34.
159. Bishop RF, Barnes GL, Cipriani E, et al. Clinical immunity after neonatal rotavirus infection. A prospective longitudinal study in young children. *N Engl J Med.* 1983;309(2):72–76.
160. Vesikari T, Matson DO, Dennehy P, et al. Safety and efficacy of a pentavalent human-bovine (WC3) reassortant rotavirus vaccine. *N Engl J Med.* 2006;354:23–33.
161. Ruiz-Palacios GM, Perez-Schael I, Velazquez FR, et al. Safety and efficacy of an attenuated vaccine against severe rotavirus gastroenteritis. *N Engl J Med.* 2006;354:11–22.
162. Barnes GL, Lund JS, Mitchell SV, et al. Early phase II trial of human rotavirus vaccine candidate RV3. *Vaccine.* 2002;20:2950–2956.
163. Treanor JJ, Campbell JD, Zangwill KM, et al. Safety and immunogenicity of an inactivated subvirion influenza A (H5N1) vaccine. *N Engl J Med.* 2006;354:1343–1351.
164. Gao W, Soloff AC, Lu X, et al. Protection of mice and poultry from lethal H5N1 avian influenza virus through adenovirus-based immunization. *J Virol.* 2006;80:1959–1964.
165. Ho DD, Neumann AU, Perelson AS, et al. Rapid turnover of plasma virions and CD4 lymphocytes in HIV-1 infection. *Nature.* 1995;373(6510):123–126.

166. McMichael AJ. HIV vaccines. *Annu Rev Immunol.* 2006;24:227–255.
167. Parren PW, Marx PA, Hessell AJ, et al. Antibody protects macaques against vaginal challenge with a pathogenic R5 simian/human immunodeficiency virus at serum levels giving complete neutralization in vitro. *J Virol.* 2001;75:8340–8347.
168. Haynes BF, Fleming J, St Clair EW, et al. Cardiolipin polyspecific autoreactivity in two broadly neutralizing HIV-1 antibodies. *Science.* 2005;308:1906–1908.
169. Fouts T, Godfrey K, Bobb K, et al. Crosslinked HIV-1 envelope-CD4 receptor complexes elicit broadly cross-reactive neutralizing antibodies in rhesus macaques. *Proc Natl Acad Sci U S A.* 2002;99:11842–11847.
170. News. "Breeding" antigens for new vaccines. *Science.* 2001;19(13 July):236–238.
171. Letvin NL, Montefiori DC, Yasutomi Y, et al. Potent, protective anti-HIV immune responses generated by bimodal HIV envelope DNA plus protein vaccination. *Proc Natl Acad Sci U S A.* 1997;94(17):9378–9383.
172. Amara RR, Villinger F, Altman JD, et al. Control of a mucosal challenge and prevention of AIDS by a multiprotein DNA/MVA vaccine. *Science.* 2001;292(5514):69–74.
173. Barouch DH, Santra S, Schmitz JE, et al. Control of viremia and prevention of clinical AIDS in rhesus monkeys by cytokine-augmented DNA vaccination. *Science.* 2000;290(5491):486–492.
174. Berzofsky JA, Ahlers JD, Derby MA, et al. Approaches to improve engineered vaccines for human immunodeficiency virus and other viruses that cause chronic infections. *Immunol Rev.* 1999;170:151–172.
175. Belyakov IM, Hel Z, Kelsall B, et al. Mucosal AIDS vaccine reduces disease and viral load in gut reservoir and blood after mucosal infection of macaques. *Nat Med.* 2001;7(12):1320–1326.
176. Ahlers JD, Belyakov IM, Thomas EK, et al. High-affinity T helper epitope induces complementary helper and APC polarization, increased CTL, and protection against viral infection. *J Clin Invest.* 2001;108(11):1677–1685.
177. Goonetilleke N, Moore S, Dally L, et al. Induction of multifunctional human immunodeficiency virus type 1 (HIV-1)-specific T cells capable of proliferation in healthy subjects by using a prime-boost regimen of DNA- and modified vaccinia virus Ankara-vectored vaccines expressing HIV-1 Gag coupled to CD8+ T-cell epitopes. *J Virol.* 2006;80:4717–4728.
178. Dorrell L, Yang H, Ondondo B, et al. Expansion and diversification of virus-specific T cells following immunization of human immunodeficiency virus type 1 (HIV-1)-infected individuals with a recombinant modified vaccinia virus Ankara/HIV-1 Gag vaccine. *J Virol.* 2006;80:4705–4716.
179. Almond J, Clemens J, Engers H, et al. Accelerating the development and introduction of a dengue vaccine for poor children, 5–8 December 2001, Ho Chi Minh City, VietNam. *Vaccine.* 2002;20:3043–3046.
180. Guirakhoo F, Pugachev K, Zhang Z, et al. Safety and efficacy of chimeric yellow Fever-dengue virus tetravalent vaccine formulations in nonhuman primates. *J Virol.* 2004;78:4761–4775.
181. Blaney JE, Burbin AP, Murphy BR, Whitehead SS. Development of a live attenuated dengue virus vaccine using reverse genetics. *Viral Immunol.* 2006;19:10–32.
182. Apt D, Raviprakash K, Brinkman A, et al. Tetravalent neutralizing antibody response against four dengue serotypes by a single chimeric dengue envelope antigen. *Vaccine.* 2006;24:335–344.
183. Biggs BA, Anders RF, Dillon HE, et al. Adherence of infected erythrocytes to venular endothelium selects for antigenic variants of Plasmodium falciparum. *J Immunol.* 1992;149(6):2047–2054.
184. Nussenzweig V, Nussenzweig RS. Circumsporozoite proteins of malaria parasites. *Cell.* 1985;42(2):401–403.
185. Singh S, Pandey K, Chattopadhayay R, et al. Biochemical, biophysical and functional characterization of bacterially expressed and refolded receptor binding domain of *Plasmodium vivax* duffy-binding protein. *J Biol Chem.* 2001;276(20):17111–17116.
186. Matuschewski K. Vaccine development against malaria. *Curr Opin Immunol.* 2006(18):449–457.
187. Hill AVS. Pre-erythrocytic malaria vaccines: toward greater efficacy. *Nature Rev.* 2006;6:21–32.
188. Bojang KA, Milligan PJM, Pinder M, et al. Efficacy of RTS,S/ASO2 malaria vaccine against *Plasmodium falciparum* infection in semi-immune adult men in The Gambia: a randomised trial. *Lancet.* 2001;358:1927–1934.
189. Alonso PL, Sacarlal J, Aponte JJ, et al. Duration of protection with RTS,S/AS02A malaria vaccine in prevention of Plasmodium falciparum disease in Mozambican children: single-blind extended follow-up of a randomised controlled trial. *Lancet.* 2005;366:2012–2018.
190. Saul A, Lawrence G, Allworth A, et al. A human phase 1 vaccine clinical trial of the Plasmodium falciparum malaria vaccine candidate apical membrane antigen 1 in Montanide ISA720 adjuvant. *Vaccine.* 2005;23:3076–3083.
191. Schofield L, Mueller I. Clinical immunity to malaria. *Curr Mol Med.* 2006;2006:205–221.
192. American Academy of Pediatrics Committee on Infectious Diseases. The relationship between pertussis vaccine and brain damage: reassessment. *Pediatrics.* 1991;88:397–400.
193. Joce R, Wood D, Brown D, et al. Paralytic poliomyelitis in England and Wales 1985–1991. *Brit Med J.* 1992;305:79–82.
194. Jonville-Béra AP, Autret E, Galy-Eyraud C, et al. Thrombocytopenic purpura after measles, mumps and rubella vaccination: a retrospective survey by the French Regional Pharmacovigilance Centres and Pasteur-Mérieux Sérums et Vaccins. *Pediatr Infect Dis J.* 1996;15:44–48.
195. Nossal GJV. Gates, GAVI, the glorious global funds and more: all you ever wanted to know. *Immunol Cell Biol.* 2003;81:20–22.
196. Lob-Levyt J, Affolder R. Innovative financing for human development. *Lancet.* 2006;367.
197. 197. Lambert P-H, Liu MA, Siegrist C-A. Can successful vaccines teach us how to induce efficient protective immune responses? *Nature Med Supp.* 2005;11:S54–S62.
198. Pawelec G, Akbar A, Caruso C, et al. Is immunosenescence infectious? *Trends Immunol.* 2004;25:406–410.
199. Gomez I, Marx F, Gould EA, et al. T cells from elderly persons respond to neoantigenic stimulation with an unimpaired IL-2 production and an enhanced differentiation into effector cells. *Exp Gerontol.* 2004;39x:597–605.

SECTION VIII

Immunologic Mechanisms in Disease

Chapter 41

Systemic Autoimmunity

Betty Diamond

INTRODUCTION

Our understanding of basic immunology has grown immensely over the last decades, leading to a new appreciation of autoimmunity and autoimmune disease. This chapter will provide a re-evaluation of systemic autoimmune disease focusing on general principles that will then be reviewed in the context of some selected diseases, systemic lupus erythematosus (SLE), inflammatory arthritis, scleroderma, vasculitis, and autoimmune muscle disease.

Conceptual Framework

There are several major concepts to be presented:

1. Autoreactivity can be beneficial as well as harmful.
2. Clinical disease depends on an infelicitous interplay of genes and environment.
3. Antigen is important in the maintenance of autoreactivity.
4. Pathologic autoreactivity or autoimmune disease is often accompanied by reduced immunocompetence, with an increased susceptibility to both infection and malignancy.
5. Different cellular and molecular processes characterize the inductive phase of autoimmune disease, the early effector phase of target organ inflammation, and the late phase of irreversible tissue damage.
6. Tissue injury in autoimmune disease involves the recruitment of resident cells within the target organ into the inflammatory process, as well as the infiltration of blood-borne inflammatory cells.
7. Optimal treatment strategies for these diseases should restore immune homeostasis rather than solely diminish immune activation.

These concepts arise from studies of murine models of disease and studies of patients. Increasingly, studies demonstrate the multiple potential pathoetiologies of each autoimmune disease and suggest an as-yet-unclassified heterogeneity of disease. As clearer phenotypic analyses of patient subsets develop, it will be possible to design better therapies for these diseases, and even prevention strategies.

GENERAL PRINCIPLES

Defining Autoimmune Disease

It is important to note that the list of systemic autoimmune diseases is not fixed. There is no definition of autoimmune disease that meets with universal approval. There are a number of inflammatory diseases mediated by cells and effector mechanisms of the innate immune system, without evidence of activation of the adaptive immune response and without evidence of an inciting exposure to foreign antigen. These diseases, familial Mediterranean fever and other autoinflammatory diseases caused by mutations in molecules of the innate immune system such as pyrin, cryopyrin, and NOD2 (1), Behcet disease, perhaps even atherosclerosis, are not classified as systemic autoimmune diseases, despite immune activation and multiple organ involvement. Rather, in the clinical setting, an operational definition of a systemic autoimmune disease is a disease in which tissue damage is mediated by T cells and antibodies, most often displaying autoreactivity (2). Despite defining autoimmune diseases as the consequence of a dysregulated adaptive immune system, it is clear that the innate and the adaptive immune responses are both involved in systemic autoimmune diseases. The innate immune system may contribute to the initial induction of antigen-specific autoreactivity and may also participate in the effector mechanisms responsible for tissue damage, but activated T cells, antibodies, or both, must be present in lesional tissue.

The immune activation present in patients with systemic autoimmune diseases must occur in the absence of any detectable ongoing infection (2). This definition allows for the possibility that many autoimmune diseases may be the late sequelae of infection by either a particular microbial pathogen or a range of different microbial pathogens. It also means that some diseases currently referred to as autoimmune may in the future be diagnosed as an immune response to an ongoing infection or an ongoing exposure to an environmental toxin. Thus, the immunosuppressive or immunomodulatory therapies currently in use or under investigation for autoimmune disease may give way, in some clinical contexts, to antibiotic therapy or to behavioral modification to avoid toxic exposures.

In animal models, the operative definition of an autoimmune disease is more straightforward; whether or not defects in the innate immune system and dendritic cell function are involved, an autoimmune disease can be replicated in a syngeneic host by adoptive transfer of T cells or B cells, or both, and does not occur in the absence of T cells or B cells, or both. Because these diseases, whether in humans or mice, require, by definition, the activation of T cells and B cells, there is a presumption of antigenic specificity in the immune response, although the full range of the targeted autoantigens is not known for most autoimmune diseases. It is also important to be aware that the autospecificities of either disease-associated T cells or antibodies that have been recognized thus far may not be the autospecificities important in eliciting the pathogenic response or the autospecificities leading to target organ injury. New autoantigens and new cross-reactivities continue to be identified; some of these provide novel and important insights into pathogenesis.

Prevalence of Disease

When autoimmune diseases were first described, it was apparent that each disease was relatively uncommon. Increasingly, a relationship among apparently distinct autoimmune diseases is being recognized. This re-evaluation began with epidemiologic studies showing that multiple autoimmune diseases can cluster within a single family and has progressed to the identification of genes that function as susceptibility factors for a number of different autoimmune diseases (3). The close relationship among these diseases is further supported by clinical trials showing that the same therapeutic intervention can provide clinical benefit in multiple distinct diseases. When autoimmune diseases are considered together, they are present in 5% to 7% of the population and constitute a major cause of morbidity and early mortality. There is also some evidence that the incidence of some diseases may be increasing. A recent report suggested a rise, for unknown reasons, in the incidence of systemic lupus (4). As most autoimmune diseases are multigenic in origin and require some environmental trigger, it is possible that genetic admixture, changes in diet, and environmental exposures, as well as changes in microbial exposures, may affect both the incidence and phenotypic characteristics of autoimmune disease.

Normal Self-tolerance

Immune tolerance is discussed in detail in Chapter 29, and is reviewed here only briefly to highlight aspects of immune regulation that may be disturbed in systemic autoimmune diseases. Immune homeostasis depends on the appropriate function of multiple intercellular and intracellular pathways. The innate immune system requires an appropriate threshold for activation and balanced effector functions. The B- and T-cell repertoires must display sufficient autoreactivity for self-regulation but lack pathogenic autoreactivity. Thresholds for activation, survival, and downregulation of the adaptive immune response must permit memory formation, but preclude a chronic inflammatory state. Finally, self-antigens must be effectively sequestered from immune recognition or presented through a tolerogenic pathway. Exactly where normal tolerance mechanisms fail in individuals with systemic autoimmune diseases is a matter of some debate, but increasingly, studies in mice suggest that intrinsic abnormalities in the innate immune system and dendritic cell function, a failure of central and peripheral tolerance checkpoints for T and B cells, and abnormal exposure to self-antigen can all predispose to systemic autoimmunity, and usually more than one defect in homeostatic regulation is present.

T-Cell Tolerance

It is clear that the random V (D) J and VJ gene rearrangements necessary to generate the diversity of T-cell receptors (TCRs) and B-cell receptors (BCRs) that characterize the normal T- and B-cell repertoire give rise to a high percentage of autoreactive antigen receptors. The elimination or regulation of self-reactive T cells begins in the thymus with the deletion of T cells that have high affinity for self-peptide/self-MHC complexes and with the generation of self-reactive regulatory T cells (5). Studies of T-cell selection have focused on transgene-encoded TCRs present in mice with organ-specific autoimmunity or on artificial model systems. With few exceptions, the actual antigens recognized by T cells in systemic autoimmune diseases are unknown. Histone-reactive T cells can be identified in both murine (6) and human lupus (7), and T-cell reactivity to collagen can be identified in mice with collagen-induced arthritis (8) and in rheumatoid arthritis (RA) in humans (9). However, T-cell specificities in myositis, scleroderma, Sjogren syndrome, and vasculitis are unknown, and it can be presumed that the antigenic specificities of most disease-enhancing T cells in lupus and rheumatoid arthritis are also unknown. Studies in mice suggest that even nonautoreactive activated T cells can sustain autoantibody production and autoimmune disease.

Although deficiency of the transcriptional regulator, AIRE, causes a failure to delete autoreactive T cells in the thymus and leads to generalized autoreactivity in mice, especially in endocrine organs (10), there are surprisingly few models of systemic autoimmune disease with an identified defect in thymic selection. The MRL mouse strain displays reduced stringency in central tolerance, but autoimmune disease occurs only late in life in MRL mice, unless there is an impairment in Fas or Fas ligand expression (11). There is, however, evidence that negative selection of autoreactive T cells is critical to the prevention of systemic autoimmune disease. Mice that lack class II expression on bone marrow–derived cells display thymic maturation of autoreactive T cells. When T cells from these mice are transferred into syngeneic hosts that exhibit normal peripheral expression of class II molecules, systemic autoimmunity ensues (12). Thus, the thymus plays a role in the elimination of T cells reactive with nuclear antigens.

Peripheral T-cell tolerance is maintained, in part, by tolerogenic dendritic cells, and dysregulation of these cells can lead to autoimmunity (13). This may be genetically determined; alternatively, dendritic cell dysfunction may be a consequence of environment, such as vitamin D deficiency (14) or continuous exposure to Toll-like receptor (TLR) agonists (15). Once an inflammatory milieu has been established, dendritic cell activation can lead to the activation of autoreactive T cells that rely on peripheral tolerance mechanisms for their control.

Regulatory T cells are among the enforcers of peripheral tolerance. In organ-specific autoimmunity in mice, these regulatory cells have been clearly demonstrated to be important in containing autoreactivity. In systemic autoimmunity, there is increasing evidence for a decreased number of some regulatory T-cell subsets, but restoration of self-tolerance through the administration of additional regulatory T cells has not yet been achieved.

B-Cell Tolerance

The failure of B-cell tolerance is a major feature of most systemic autoimmune diseases. B-cell tolerance begins in the bone marrow, where antigen engagement of the BCR triggers deletion, anergy, or receptor editing (16). Evidence continues to accumulate that receptor editing or the replacement of a light chain that associates with the heavy chain to form an autoantibody with a novel light chain that does not produce autoreactivity is the first line of defense against autoimmunity; impaired tolerance has been seen both with a deficiency of receptor editing and with indiscriminate receptor editing that leads to novel light chains conferring autoreactivity. Thus far, defects in receptor editing have not been identified in individuals with autoimmune disease. There is some evidence that receptor editing can occur in the rheumatoid synovium, but this appears to be a pathogenic rather than a protective process (17).

BCR signaling thresholds are critical to the maintenance of B-cell tolerance, as all mechanisms of B-cell tolerance depend, at least in part, on BCR engagement. Overexpression of CD19, mutations of CD45, and deletion of CD22 or SHP-1 all enhance BCR signaling and lead to systemic autoimmunity (18), yet inhibition of BCR signaling through enhanced activity of CD22 or Ly108 also leads to autoreactivity because the attenuated signal fails to activate early tolerance mechanisms (19). Because inhibitors of molecules in the BCR signaling pathway are available, understanding the critical balance between overexuberant B-cell activation (strong BCR signaling) and deficient B-cell tolerance induction (weak BCR signaling) is crucial for proper therapeutic targeting of the BCR signaling pathways.

The study of mice with transgene-encoded BCRs has provided much information about normal tolerance mechanisms and has identified a role for all the above-mentioned tolerance mechanisms as well as developmental arrest and active tolerance that occurs when B cells are chronically exposed to self-antigen and IL-6 (20). There are also data showing that regulatory checkpoints exist for B cells not just during the maturation to immunocompetence but even after exposure to antigen, in the germinal center and in the late stages of B-cell differentiation to memory or long-lived plasma cells (21,22). For example, anti-Sm B cells fail to become plasma cells upon exposure to antigen in a nonautoimmune host, but will mature to a plasma cell phenotype in MRL/lpr autoimmune mice (23). Similarly, a deficiency of the inhibitory Fc receptor, FcRIIb, permits plasma-cell differentiation of autoreactive B cells (24). Finally, B-cell tolerance depends on normal cell death pathways; there is abundant evidence that autoreactive B cells fail to die when there is an excess of antiapoptotic or a deficit in proapoptotic molecules within the cell (25). B-cell tolerance can be broken both by intrinsic defects in B-cell function as mentioned in this section and by the extrinsic provision of excess growth and survival factors such as CD40, BAFF, and cytokines within the B-cell microenvironment (26).

Healthy Autoreactivity

Early immunologists recognized that a major challenge to the immune system is to distinguish self- from foreign antigen. Because they recognized that pathogenic autoreactivity is usually avoided, they inferred a global prohibition on the survival of autoreactive lymphocytes. Since the early days of the "horror autotoxicus" of Ehrlich and the clonal selection theory of Burnet, awareness has grown that autoreactivity is an intrinsic and necessary feature of the healthy immune system, and that the selection against autoreactive cells is not absolute. Most important, there is now an understanding that the immune system responds to antigen, whether it is self- or foreign, only when certain conditions are met. Exquisite regulation of immune activation at multiple levels prevents pathogenic autoreactivity and also ensures an appropriate response to non–self-antigens.

It is now abundantly clear that the repertoire of naïve, immunocompetent T and B cells is shaped by self-antigen. Selection of the T-cell repertoire occurs within the thymus as T cells mature to immunocompetence and continues in the periphery as T cells recognize self-peptide/self-MHC complexes on tolerogenic dendritic cells. Mature immunocompetent T cells are positively selected on the basis of displaying some degree of reactivity with self-peptide/self-MHC complexes on epithelial cells in the thymic cortex and are negatively selected when the interaction with peptide/MHC complexes on thymic medullary epithelial cells or dendritic cells is overly strong (5). Thus, all T cells that mature to immunocompetence display autoreactivity. The autoantigenic epitopes will vary depending on MHC haplotype and on the degree of TCR engagement required to mediate negative selection. Because the genes encoding the molecules that transduce the TCR signal and control MHC expression display functional polymorphisms that affect either their activity or their level of expression, a different degree of receptor engagement may be required to transduce a survival or a death signal in different individuals (27). Similarly, polymorphisms exist in genes encoding molecules that govern apoptotic pathways, also leading to differences in stringency of negative selection (28,29). Finally, polymorphisms in self-antigens may affect their ability to mediate either positive or negative selection (30). Thus, each individual has a unique spectrum of autoreactive T cells that exit the thymus. Further negative selection occurs in the periphery when these cells either encounter self-antigens presented in a non-inflammatory setting in the absence of costimulatory signals or are suppressed by regulatory T cells. The presence of multiple subsets of regulatory cells in the periphery attests to the importance of these cells in maintaining immune homeostasis (31). Autoreactive T cells, or T cells that were not appropriately subjected to tolerance mechanisms, are present in all systemic autoimmune diseases, yet little is known of the nature of the tolerance defect. In animal models of these diseases, a small amount of evidence exists suggesting a defect in thymic selection, but the major problem(s) is believed to be in peripheral tolerance.

It is not yet clear whether there is a requirement that B cells display some degree of autoreactivity for maturation to immunocompetence, but there is a growing body of data to suggest that positive selection of B cells also occurs. Recent studies show that in healthy individuals a very high percentage of the unselected immature B-cell repertoire in the bone marrow is reactive with nuclear antigens. These studies further show that autoreactive cells are routinely eliminated in both the bone marrow and the spleen but that significant autoreactivity remains in the naïve repertoire, with approximately 10% of naïve B cells displaying reactivity with a small panel of autoantigens (32). This observation perhaps provides a clue to the high percentage of nonautoimmune individuals who have antibody reactivity to nuclear antigens and the frequency of this autospecificity in individuals with systemic autoimmune diseases.

Two populations of B lymphocytes straddle the innate and the adaptive immune system, marginal-zone B cells and B1 cells. Both these populations display limited antigen-receptor heterogeneity, both are skewed to autoreactivity, and both perform protective functions in the immune system (33). B1 cells, in particular, have been studied in some detail. They arise in the fetal liver and are a self-regenerating population thereafter. They express a limited repertoire of immunoglobulin-variable (V) region genes; because they do not express terminal deoxynucleoside transferase, they display limited junctional diversity as well. It is now well appreciated that these cells make antibodies with specificity for phosphatidylserine that bind to apoptotic cells and apoptotic debris (34). Opsonization by antibody enhances macrophage phagocytosis and degradation of apoptotic debris. In the absence of the "natural autoantibodies" made by B1 cells, apoptotic material can be ingested by dendritic cells (35). The ingested DNA and RNA bind to TLRs, activate the dendritic cells, and create an immunogenic environment for the presentation of self-antigen (36). These antibodies are but one of a host of substances, including SAP, C1q, mannose-binding lectin, and C-reactive protein, that coat apoptotic cells to direct them to degradative pathways (37). Apoptotic cells activate lipases that convert phosphatidylcholine to lysophosphatidylcholine (LPC) (35). Natural autoantibodies also bind LPC; interestingly, antibodies to phosphatidylserine and lysophosphatidylcholine are present even in mice raised in a germ-free environment, suggesting that self-antigen may be responsible for triggering antibody secretion (38). These antibodies also cross-react with oxidized low-density lipoproteins (LDLs) and may be protective against atherosclerosis.

Consistent with the hypothesis that natural IgM autoantibodies protect against the development of pathogenic autoimmunity is a study showing that nonspontaneously autoimmune mice will develop anti DNA antibodies and a consequent lupu-like renal disease when they have no circulating IgM (39). Furthermore, when mice with a genetic deficiency of secreted IgM were challenged with lupospolysaccharide (LPS), they developed increased titers of IgG anti-DNA antibodies. Another study suggesting the beneficial effect of IgM autoantibodies demonstrates that NZB/W lupus-prone mice develop less disease when given IgM anti-DNA antibody. In this study, however, the effect of the IgM autoantibody appeared to relate more to renal protection than to a decrease in activation of IgG-producing DNA-reactive B cells (40). Thus, natural autoantibodies may both impede activation of pathogenic autoreactive B cells and prevent pathogenic antibodies from binding their target autoantigens.

It has been suggested that rheumatoid factor (RF), antibody to the constant region of the IgG heavy chain, also exerts a protective effect. RF is among the natural autoantibodies that are present in nonautoimmune individuals. Titers of RF increase in individuals with chronic infections. Nonpathogenic RF is exclusively IgM, whereas pathogenic, rheumatoid arthritis-related RF may be IgG as well (41). In healthy individuals, RF is thought to serve two important functions. By binding preferentially to antigen-aggregated

IgG, it assists in the removal of immune complexes, thus hastening the degradation of antigens that may be toxins. RF is also thought to assist in the presentation of microbial antigen to the immune system, because immune complexes are more immunogenic than soluble antigen (42). In normal individuals, once the antigen has been cleared and immune complexes are no longer present, the RF B cells are tolerized by soluble IgG and do not enter the memory or plasma cell compartments (43).

Relationship between Healthy and Pathogenic Autoreactivity

A major unsolved question is the relationship between natural autoantibodies and the autoantibodies of autoimmune disease. To date, there is little evidence in humans that natural autoantibodies contribute to autoimmune disease or that B1 cells are the sources of pathogenic autoreactivity, although there are murine models of systemic lupus in which B1 cells or marginal-zone B cells are the source of pathogenic autoantibodies. It is clear from studies of mice expressing transgene-encoded natural autoantibodies that B cells expressing these antibodies are not routinely subject to tolerance induction, even in nonspontaneously autoimmune strains; however, they rarely become memory cells or long-lived plasma cells (33). Thus, these B cells do not inevitably lead to autoimmune disease. Studies of B cells producing transgene-encoded RF have shown that these cells can be activated by immune complexes and T-cell help to secrete low-affinity RF, but that B cells producing high-affinity antibody are deleted (44). Furthermore, in human disease and many mouse models of disease, pathogenic autoantibodies are not derived from B cells making natural autoantibodies but are produced by B2 cells that have undergone extensive somatic mutation (45). Some studies of murine B-cell genealogies demonstrate low-affinity autoreactivity in the precursor B cell, but similar studies of human autoantibodies are scarce and fail to reveal this phenomenon.

It is important to note that autoreactive B cells are routinely activated following exposure to microbial antigen, but the response resolves after the microbial antigen is eradicated. Yet the induction of autoreactivity or failure to control the autoreactivity that routinely arises during the response to microbial antigen is usually not sufficient to cause autoimmune disease. Whether the transition to frank disease requires an increased array of autospecificities, particular pathogenic subsets of autoantibodies, concomitant defects of innate immunity or T-cell tolerance, or vulnerable target organs is not known. Whether systemic autoimmune disease begins with a failure to downregulate the autoreactivity that is activated by infection remains uncertain, but the autoantibodies that characterize autoimmune disease differ significantly from those that are part of a healthy immune response (21,41).

Unifying Features of Systemic Autoimmune Diseases

The general theories or observations regarding autoimmunity that are discussed in this chapter will not apply to all systemic autoimmune diseases. Although it is reasonable to think of these diseases together, it is important to recognize that each disease has unique features. It is also important to note that although it has been a convention to define autoimmune diseases as systemic or organ-specific, this dichotomy is somewhat artificial. Organ-specific and systemic diseases may share susceptibility genes and can coexist within a family and, indeed, within an individual. Organ-specific autoimmune disease as well as systemic autoimmune disease may target autoantigens that are ubiquitously expressed.

Antinuclear Antibodies

A unifying feature of most systemic autoimmune diseases is the presence of autoantibodies to nuclear antigens. It is interesting to note that autoantibodies are made to these same autoantigens in approximately 5% to 10% of a healthy population, with a greater incidence in women and older individuals (46). Antinuclear antibodies are also present in 20% of individuals receiving IFN therapy or TNFα blockade. Only a small percent of these individuals will progress from autoimmunity to autoimmune disease (47). The frequency of elevated titers of antinuclear antibodies (ANAs) in systemic autoimmunity may reflect the autoreactivity present in the unselected B-cell repertoire. Studies documenting an early dysregulation of B-cell selection in systemic lupus and RA support the notion that B-cell dysfunction is a key component of these diseases (48). A study of factors that predispose to ANA reactivity may reveal aspects of the genetic basis for autoreactivity and may illuminate pathways that are dysregulated in systemic autoimmune disease.

Female Predisposition

Another feature of many autoimmune diseases is an increased incidence in women. Overall, there is a threefold greater incidence of autoimmune disease in women, but for some diseases the female predominance is much stronger. This occurs in both systemic and organ-specific diseases. Interestingly, autoantibodies to nuclear antigens are more common in women than in men. These antibodies are present in many autoimmune diseases and, as stated earlier, appear to represent a substrate on which clinical autoimmune disease develops. It is not yet established how much this reflects a sex-determined difference and how much it reflects hormonal influences. Most systemic autoimmune diseases have an age of onset after puberty. For example, in systemic lupus, the female:male incidence is 3:1 for disease onset prior to puberty, 9:1 after puberty, and reverts to 2:1 after menopause (49). However, several studies now show that autoantibodies can be present years before onset of clinical disease; thus, preclinical disease may precede puberty more frequently than previously recognized (50). It is important to note, however, that not all autoimmune diseases appear to be exacerbated by female hormones. Rheumatoid arthritis, for example, is less frequent in women on oral contraceptive therapy and often improves during pregnancy (51).

Hormones can affect the function of all cells in the immune system. Estradiol can promote the survival of high-affinity autoreactive B cells at both the immature and the transitional stages of development, in part by decreasing the strength of BCR signaling (49). Some studies suggest that there are polymorphisms of estrogen receptor α (ERα) that predispose to autoimmunity and some studies suggest a preferential metabolism of estradiol in autoimmune individuals to its more estrogenic metabolites, but the role of estrogen in systemic autoimmunity remains controversial (52). Prolactin also has been shown to rescue autoreactive B cells from negative selection, but prolactin appears to operate through enhancing the T-cell–mediated rescue of B cells destined for apoptosis.

Recent data suggest that sex-determined differences may also contribute to the female predisposition to disease. The Yaa gene, which accelerates autoimmune disease in men, is present in a region of the Y chromosome that represents a translocation of a portion of the X chromosome; this locus contains the gene encoding TLR 7, for which the natural ligand is RNA (53). Although it is not yet known whether one TLR7 allele is routinely silenced in women, a possible implication is that women routinely express more TLR7, thereby permitting more immune activation by microbial or self-RNA. Finally, it is worth remembering that the effect of sex hormones may not be on immune activation, but may in fact be on target-organ display of autoantigen or target-organ response to the production of inflammatory mediators. Thus, the effects of sex hormones on kidney, joint, muscle, and other targeted organs need to be more fully investigated.

Flares and Remissions

A characteristic of autoimmune diseases is their waxing and waning activity. Most individuals with autoimmune disease experience a succession of exacerbations and remissions; however, some individuals can experience a chronic, smoldering course of disease, whereas others can experience a self-limited disease. In systemic lupus and scleroderma, flares can be accompanied by inflammation and damage in previously unaffected organs. In RA and myositis, flares can involve previously unaffected joints or muscles, respectively. Novel autoreactivities may account for novel organ involvement in some diseases, but this explanation is inadequate to explain the changes in affected joints in RA, muscles in myositis, or skin regions in scleroderma that occur during disease flares. However, the remission of RA in the joints of a limb that is immobilized, while disease is sustained in a mobile limb, suggests that activation or injury of resident cells as a result of joint motion may be required to sustain target-organ inflammation (54).

Although flares and remissions are typical in autoimmune disease, it is still not established whether flares are secondary to the activation of memory cells or result from a new wave of activation of naïve cells. It is also not clear whether the defects in central and peripheral tolerance that are permissive for disease are always present, or whether normal or near-normal immune homeostasis may characterize periods of remission. Recent studies of systemic lupus suggest the presence of a defect in early B-cell selection and in memory-cell repertoire even in a time of drug-free clinical remission (32). Finally, the mechanisms responsible for naturally occurring remissions have not been identified in systemic autoimmune diseases. Whether regulatory T cells play a role in these remissions is a question of intense current interest.

There are several reasons that such seemingly obvious and critical questions remain unanswered. First, most spontaneous animal models of systemic autoimmunity are characterized by a persistent progression of immune activation and tissue injury. Some induced models exhibit remissions, but rarely do they exhibit subsequent flares. Thus, the animal models for these diseases have not been extremely informative regarding fluctuations in disease activity. Second, the only routinely available tissue to sample from patients is blood, and the cells present in blood may not fully reflect those involved in disease pathogenesis. Furthermore, especially, in the case of B cells and dendritic cells, the number of cells that can be analyzed may be limiting. Currently, it is also difficult to study disease in individuals who are not receiving some form of immunomodulatory therapy. Thus, there are few spontaneous remissions available for study in most patient cohorts.

Genetic Susceptibility

Clinically, it has been known for decades that autoimmune diseases have a genetic component. Children and siblings of individuals with an autoimmune disease have an increased risk of developing that disease. Concordance rates for autoimmune diseases are approximately 5% in dizygotic twins and approximately 30% in monozygotic twins (55). It is also clear that different autoimmune diseases may be present within a single family and that an individual may exhibit more than one autoimmune disease. These observations led to the recognition that these diseases share susceptibility genes even before those genes were identified. Now it is clear from genetic studies that several genes, CTLA-4, PTPN22, and CARD15 (NOD-2), for example, predispose to more than one autoimmune disease (3).

Monogenic Diseases

Although there is a genetic component to essentially every autoimmune disease, only a few diseases appear to be monogenic. The human disease, APECED, a disease of inflammation in multiple endocrine organs, results from a deletion of the AIRE gene (56). The AIRE gene encodes a molecule that causes tissue-specific proteins to be expressed in medullary epithelial cells in the thymus. The consequence of this ectopic protein expression is the deletion of many developing thymocytes with specificity for peptides from tissue-specific proteins (57). In hosts with a deletion of the AIRE gene, autoreactive thymocytes develop to immunocompetence and initiate an immune attack primarily on endocrine organs. It is clear from both murine and human studies that even in this disease, phenotypic features of disease are determined by genetic background (58). It is also clear that regulatory T cells develop normally in AIRE-deficient mice (59), thus suggesting that regulatory T-cell function is insufficient for the prevention of autoimmune disease when there is a significant failure of central T-cell tolerance.

IPEX, immune dysregulation, polyendocrinopathy, enteropathy, X-linked, is caused by a mutation in the gene encoding Foxp3, a forkhead transcription factor that is critical for function of regulatory T cells. Infants with this disease develop diarrhea, diabetes, hypothyroidism, cytopenias, and an eczema that is apparently related to high IgE levels, although predisposing allergens have not been identified (60). The antigenic specificities of the overexuberant T-effector cells have not yet been determined. Just as the antigenic specificities of autoreactive T cells in patients with APECED will identify autoantigens for which there is central tolerance, the identification of the antigenic specificities of autoreactive T cells in IPEX may provide insight into autospecificities that are routinely regulated in the periphery by regulatory cells.

Deficiency of the gene encoding either Fas or Fas ligand also leads to a systemic autoimmune disease. The Fas protein interacts with Fas ligand to mediate activation-induced cell death in a number of cell lineages within the immune system. In mice, Fas or Fas ligand deficiency confers features of systemic lupus, with production of antinuclear antibodies and glomerulonephritis. In contrast, Fas deficiency in humans causes a disease called autoimmune lymphoproliferative syndrome (ALPS), characterized by generalized lymphadenopathy and hypergammaglobulinemia. In general, these patients produce antibodies to red blood cells or platelets, resulting in anemia or thrombocytopenia, respectively (61). Interestingly, there is an increased incidence of malignancy in these patients, suggesting that a common mechanism of immune dysregulation may be responsible for both autoimmunity and malignancy. However, not all individuals with deficient Fas expression have a disease phenotype; thus, other genes modulate the phenotypic expression of Fas deficiency (62).

Recently, it has been appreciated that mutations in the gene encoding TACI, a receptor for BAFF and APRIL, can lead to both immunodeficiency and the subsequent development of autoantibodies (63). Mice deficient in TACI similarly develop antinuclear antibodies and a lupos-like glomerulonephritis that appears to reflect a release from TACI-mediated B-cell apoptosis and inhibition of B-cell activation, and perhaps a loss of protective IgM autoantibodies (63).

Polygenic Diseases

Most autoimmune diseases are multigenic, with three or more genetic loci involved in disease expression. Each locus represents a chromosomal region that has been mapped by linkage analysis with a particular disease phenotype. It is now becoming clear that a susceptibility locus may identify not merely a susceptibility gene but rather a susceptibility haplotype, as each locus often includes more than one susceptibility gene. This is perhaps best exemplified in the genetic dissection of the NZM 2410 lupus-prone mouse, in which three susceptibility loci were initially described. Subsequent analysis has shown that there are multiple genes within each locus that contribute to disease susceptibility. For example, within the SLE 1 locus on chromosome 1, genes encoding Fc receptors, the complement receptor CR2, and Ly108, the SLAM family member, have all been implicated in disease pathogenesis (64). The analysis of this mouse strain also exemplifies another general principle: There are resistance loci that prevent autoimmunity as well as susceptibility loci that facilitate autoimmunity (64). Thus, an individual's genetic risk is the summation of susceptibility and resistance loci. Yet another principle is embedded within this observation. In general, each susceptibility gene or locus is compatible with normal immune homeostasis. Only when a number of susceptibility loci coexist is normal self-tolerance abrogated. Thus, it may be possible to develop the same disease phenotype from entirely distinct combinations of susceptibility loci. Indeed, it is increasingly clear that the critical susceptibility loci may differ in ethnically or racially different populations. This is perhaps most apparent in RA. In Caucasians and Asians, homozygosity of a DR4 allele with a sequence termed the "shared epitope" (Q/R/D R/K RAA at positions 70 to 74 of HLADRβ1) increases the risk of developing disease from 1 in 100 to 1 in 7 (65); however, in individuals of African descent with RA, the shared epitope is rarely present (66).

Multiple Immune Pathways Contribute to the Genetic Risk for Systemic Autoimmunity

Most genes associated with systemic autoimmunity have been identified in studies of patients with lupus or rheumatoid arthritis. Much less is understood of genetic risk for other systemic autoimmune diseases. It may be helpful to identify four areas of immune cell function that have been genetically implicated in the induction of autoimmunity (a) lymphocyte selection and antigen-receptor signaling, (b) lymphocyte activation and costimulatory molecules, (c) lymphocyte survival and pro- and antiapoptotic pathways, and (d) antigen accessibility.

Lymphocyte Selection

HLA haplotype represents a susceptibility factor in almost all autoimmune diseases. As stated earlier, in rheumatoid arthritis, particular alleles of DR4 represent a strong susceptibility factor only in some populations, yet patients of all ethnic and racial backgrounds respond equally well to current treatment modalities, suggesting a similar pathogenetic mechanism to this disease even in individuals who differ in MHC haplotype

In SLE, class II alleles do not determine disease predisposition so much as autoantibody specificity, with anti-Ro antibodies occurring in DR3 individuals and anti-DNA antibodies in DR2 individuals (67). Interestingly, and in contrast to the response to therapy in rheumatoid arthritis, there are some recent data suggesting that patients who differ with respect to these antigenic specificities also differ with respect to response to B-cell ablation therapy (68). While most autoimmune diseases are associated with particular class II alleles, some are associated with class I alleles. Ankylosing spondylitis and reactive arthritis are associated with HLA B27, and to a lesser degree, B7 (67).

It has long been assumed that the HLA association reflects the importance of HLA molecules in determining T-cell repertoire, but this has not been proven for any autoimmune disease. Many genes besides those encoding class I and class II molecules reside within the MHC locus and may contribute to or be responsible for disease susceptibility. For example, genes encoding TNFα and complement components reside within the MHC locus, and polymorphisms or deletions of these genes can predispose to particular autoimmune diseases (69).

Genes that modulate antigen receptor (TCR or BCR) signaling are associated with lupus and RA in murine models and in the human population (48,64). Some of these genes may alter the threshold for negative selection and tolerance induction early in lymphocyte development, whereas others may alter thresholds for the activation of immunocompetent lymphocytes. Both decreased and increased BCR signaling can predispose to autoimmunity. Although this might seem paradoxical, there is accumulating evidence that signaling pathways and the signaling thresholds that govern cell-fate decisions may differ in immature and mature lymphocytes. Thus, a diminished signal during B-cell development will increase the survival and maturation of autoreactive cells, whereas an enhanced signal after the achievement of immunocompetence may increase B-cell activation. Most disease-susceptibility genes that alter BCR signaling affect the naïve B-cell repertoire. However, some modulators of BCR signaling, such as FcRIIB, a downregulator of BCR signaling, appear to affect antigen-activated cells.

Modulators of TCR signaling can also lead to autoreactivity. In mice, deletion of the gene encoding IBP (IRF4-binding protein), an activator of Rho GTPases, leads to altered TCR signaling and antinuclear antibody production (18). Similarly, deletion of Rasgrp1 leads to a lupus-like disease in mice (18). Whether these signaling defects alter T-cell repertoire or thresholds for activation by cross-reactive antigen or self-antigen is not yet known.

Lymphocyte Activation and Costimulation

Cytokines and costimulatory molecules, including classic costimulatory pathways and those mediated through engagement of toll-like receptors and cytokines, can alter lymphocyte selection, resulting in the rescue of immature autoreactive B cells from negative selection or modulating thresholds for peripheral activation of lymphocytes. Several alterations in costimulatory pathways may be most important after antigen activation. For example, deletion of the roquin gene leads to increased inducible costimulator (ICOS) expression on T cells within the germinal center reaction and enhanced autoantibody production (70). CTLA-4 is a molecule involved in downregulation of activated T cells and in the initial activation of regulatory T cells. Deletion of CTLA-4 in mice is associated with a fulminant inflammatory disease (71). A polymorphism of CTLA-4 in humans that leads to a decrease in soluble CTLA-4 is associated with several autoimmune diseases (72). Soluble CTLA-4 may act as an endogenous inhibitor of CD28-B7 interactions or may induce indoleamine 2,3-deoxygenase (IDO), an enzyme involved in tryptophan metabolism, resulting in local immunosuppression (73). Similarly, PD-1 is an inhibitory receptor on both T and B cells; polymorphisms or deletion of PD-1 may function both in the selection of the naïve repertoire or after the initial encounter with antigen (74).

Inappropriate cytokine production may also predispose to autoimmunity. For example, a polymorphism of osteopontin is associated with autoimmunity in humans (75). Increased osteopontin protects murine T cells from activation-induced death and may assist in the inappropriate survival of antigen-activated autoreactive T cells. In mice, deficiency of TNFα can predispose to the development of SLE (76). Similarly, TNFα blockade in humans has been associated with the development of SLE in a small percentage of treated patients (77).

Lymphocyte Survival

It is now clear that many genes involved in cell survival constitute susceptibility factors for autoimmune disease, most notably, members of the Bcl-2 family. Increased expression or functional polymorphisms of Bcl-2 can induce a lupos-like disease (78). Recent data suggest cross-talk between apoptotic and antigen-receptor pathways. Interestingly, the combined presence of a lupus-susceptibility allele of Bcl-2 and a lupus-susceptibility allele of IL-10 leads to a 40-fold increased risk of disease (79). Whether the IL-10 allele cooperates with Bcl-2 to decrease stringency of negative selection in the immature B-cell compartment or functions independently of Bcl-2 to alter lymphocyte function later in disease, or both, is not known.

Antigen

Antigen accessibility or antigen load may influence autoimmunity. Murine models clearly demonstrate that an increase in apoptotic debris or defective clearance of apoptotic debris results in a lupos-like phenotype (18). Individuals who are deficient in C1q or DNase demonstrate impaired clearance of apoptotic material and a predisposition to lupus (80). Whether deficiencies in C2 and C4 contribute to lupus because they also lead to reduced clearance of apoptotic cells or whether they lead to reduced BCR signaling and a reduced stringency of negative selection is not known.

Induction of potentially pathogenic autoreactivity is insufficient for autoimmune disease. It is clear that inflammatory effector mechanisms must be activated in target organs, because damage to these organs is usually the result of infiltration by inflammatory cells and release of soluble inflammatory mediators. Thus, genes that govern cell trafficking help modulate the inflammatory response in target organs. In addition, target organs must be vulnerable to autoimmune attack. This vulnerability may be genetically determined, as in rodent models of rheumatic carditis, tubular nephritis, and lupos-like glomerulonephritis, but it can also be altered by nongenetic or environmental factors.

Other Genes of Clinical Significance

There are some genes that are known to be involved in predisposition to autoimmune disease, with an as-yet-undetermined effect on either immune activation or target-organ vulnerability. Estrogen-receptor α alleles associate with both lupus and RA (81). Paradoxically, the effect of estrogen on these two diseases, while still a matter of some uncertainty, seems to be contradictory. Exogenous estrogen appears to increase risk and exacerbate lupus in at least some individuals, while it protects against RA (82). Polymorphisms of the vitamin D receptor and the hydroxylase gene involved in vitamin D metabolism have been implicated as risk factors in several autoimmune diseases. Vitamin D helps maintain dendritic cells in a tolerogenic state, facilitating peripheral tolerance mechanisms. Thus, adequate vitamin D levels may be important in the proper presentation of self-antigen and immune homeostasis, and several studies now suggest that vitamin D deficiency may predispose to both organ-specific and systemic autoimmunity (83).

Antigens in Systemic Autoimmune Disease

B-Cell Antigens

The major evidence for a role for antigen in spontaneous autoimmunity is the observation that increasing antigen exposure in animal models leads to increased B-cell autoreactivity.

Self-antigen

The frequent observation that autoimmune disease may be triggered or exacerbated by exposure to UV light suggests that self-antigen can drive autoimmunity, because UV light clearly induces cell death and alters vascular permeability, thus exposing cells of the immune system to an array of tissue antigens (84). This observation is entirely consistent with the fact that a lupos-like phenotype develops in many murine models characterized by an increase in apoptotic debris, most commonly consequent to impaired clearance. Furthermore, administration of apoptotic cells to certain mouse strains results in the production of antinuclear antibodies (85). Interestingly, many autoantibodies bind to neoantigenic determinants that are exposed on molecules following cleavage by granzyme B, a protease present in cytolytic T cells (86). The implication is that the immune system is tolerant to the peptides derived from self-proteins that are generated by caspase cleavage but not to the peptides generated by granzyme cleavage. A further implication is a potential viral etiology to autoimmune disease, as cytolytic T cells are activated in response to viral infection. Both autoantibodies and autoreactive B cells may then lead to epitope spreading and drive pathogenic inflammation independent of the initial viral insult. Thus, viral infection may initiate autoimmunity but may not be required to perpetuate disease. This suggestion is consistent with the clinical observation that new autoantibody specificities arise over time in individuals with an existing autoimmune disease or progressing toward autoimmune disease (50). As autoreactive B cells become activated, they may present novel (cryptic) peptides of autoantigen to T cells (87). Because these peptides are not routinely presented on thymic dendritic cells, thymic epithelial cells, or peripheral dendritic cells, there may have been no deletions of T cells specific for these self-peptides.

Although genetic differences can modulate antigen load, environmental influences can also affect exposure to autoantigen. UV light induces cellular apoptosis. Smoking increases the citrullination of proteins in the respiratory epithelium; smoking is a known risk factor for RA, a disease in which antibodies to citrullinated peptides are both diagnostic and pathogenic. The recent recognition of the pathogenicity of antibodies to citrullinated proteins in RA has led to studies showing that mice unable to reverse the citrullination of proteins develop autoimmunity (88). Studies in a murine model for induction of RF have shown that activation of autoreactive B cells requires an adequate exposure to autoantigen. Similarly, administering the Sm antigen, a targeted autoantigen in lupus, to autoimmune mice increases titers of anti-Sm antibody (89). Furthermore, certain immune complexes, such as those containing DNA, RNA, phospholipids, or other ligands for pattern recognition and Toll-like receptors, once formed, can activate dendritic cells and can create a proinflammatory milieu that promotes and perpetuates autoreactivity by converting tolerogenic into immunogenic dendritic cells (90).

Just as apoptotic cells can provide a source of targeted autoantigen in systemic autoimmune diseases, so can the regenerating cells in damaged tissues, which have been shown in some diseases, most notably myositis, to express high levels of targeted autoantigens (91). Thus, the very process of repair of tissue injury may fuel established autoimmunity. In organ-specific autoimmune disease, the removal of the autoantigen can lead to the diminution in number and activation of autoreactive lymphocytes (92); in systemic autoimmune diseases, the targeted autoantigens tend to be ubiquitous, precluding their removal.

Idiotype Networks

Several models suggest that idiotype–anti-idiotype networks can drive B-cell autoreactivity. This phenomenon has been demonstrated in murine models for the induction of anti-DNA and anti-cardiolipin antibodies (93). Although anti-idiotypes to autoantibodies have been found in patients with autoimmune disease, their role in either the induction or the regulation of autoreactivity remains speculative.

Microbial Antigen

Molecular mimicry may operate to permit foreign antigen to initiate autoimmune responses. Autoantibodies have frequently been shown to cross-react with microbial antigen. Some of the more intriguing instances of molecular mimicry are the cross-reactivity of anti-DNA antibodies with bacterial antigens and with the EBNA protein of Epstein–Barr virus (EBV) (94). In lupus, there are reports of high titers of antibody to EBV, consistent with, but not proof of, the hypothesis that EBV may be a causative agent (95). It is also possible that microbial antigens trigger T-cell dependent B-cell responses, with the consequent somatic hypermutation of immunoglobulin-variable region genes leading to the acquisition of autoreactivity. Clearly, somatic mutation in B cells responding to non–self-antigens can generate autoreactivity. Interestingly, the experimental back-mutation of a very few anti-DNA antibodies derived from lupus patients to their germline configuration has demonstrated an apparent lack of autoreactivity in the precursor B cells (96). This observation is consistent with the argument that pathogenic autoantibodies may be generated in response to microbial antigen. Furthermore, this hypothesis is consistent with the observation that the somatically mutated V-region genes that encode pathogenic autoantibodies are distinct from those that encode natural autoantibodies.

It is interesting to speculate that the mild immunodeficiency that accompanies many systemic autoimmune diseases permits more prolonged microbial infections, fueling the production of autoantibodies. Because autoantibodies induced perhaps by molecular mimicry, perhaps by exposure of usually sequestered self-antigen to B or T cells, or perhaps as a result of bystander B-cell activation, are normally generated in the course of a response to any microbial antigen, it is important to determine when such a response is aberrant and may lead to autoimmune disease. Persistence of autoantibody production is clearly abnormal. Usually, autoantibody titers in nonautoimmune individuals decrease as microbial antigen is eradicated. Epitope spreading is a critical phenomenon in protective immunity, but epitope spreading to autoantigens is not present in the routine autoreactivity seen in response to infectious agents. In autoimmune disease, epitope spreading to an increased number of autoantigenic epitopes occurs, leading ultimately to an expansion in the number of targeted autoantigens (97). Both retrospective and prospective studies now show that there is a slow but steady increase in the number of self-antigens bound by autoantibodies in individuals with clinical disease (50). Indeed, the progression from autoreactivity to autoimmune disease may take several years. Whether this progressive increase is necessary because a particular pathogenic autoantibody must arise, or because multiple autospecificities are necessary for adequate recruitment of inflammatory cells by immune complexes, or because multiple autoreactive B cells are needed to present cryptic peptides of self-antigens to T cells and provide a diverse autoreactive T-cell response is not known.

T-Cell Antigens

T-cell autoreactivity in systemic autoimmune disease is harder to identify than B-cell autoreactivity. In systemic lupus, T cells to histone epitopes have been identified in both mice and humans (98). T cells infiltrate muscle tissue in polymyositis and dermatomyositis, joints in RA, and salivary glands in Sjogren syndrome, but their target antigens have not been determined. Often the T cells in systemic autoimmune disease appear to recognize posttranslational modulations of self-proteins (88,99). For example, T cells in rodent models of RA induced by collagen immunization recognize glycosylated collagen (100). T cells in murine models of SLE recognize iso-aspartyl–modified peptides; mice deficient in the protein L-isoaspartate O-methyl transferase, which cannot repair isoaspartyl modifications, develop antinuclear antibodies and glomerulonephritis (101). Whatever the important antigenic specificities, T cells are critical effectors in these diseases, because preventing their function ameliorates disease. Furthermore, the antibodies present in these diseases have features characteristic of T-cell–dependent responses, including heavy-chain class switching and somatic mutation. In RA and Sjogren syndrome, ectopic germinal centers can sometimes be seen in target organs (102). It is highly probable that multiple autoantigens are targeted, as the T-cell-receptor repertoire of organ-infiltrating T cells is polyclonal (102), and in murine models, a diverse T-cell repertoire is needed for the development of lupus nephritis (103).

Environmental Antigens

In additional to microbial antigens, drugs or antigens in the environment are potential triggers of disease. Drug-induced lupus can occur following exposure to hydralazine, procainamide, chlorpromazine, diphenylhydantoin, and other agents (104). It is not clear if any of these drugs binds to self-antigen to generate a neoantigen. Some clearly cause hypomethylation of DNA, leading to increased expression of adhesion molecules on T cells and a lower threshold for T-cell activation. When this occurs, even non-autoreactive T cells can activate autoreactive B cells. Although procainamide has been demonstrated to alter T-cell selection in the thymus in mice (105), it is unlikely that this is a major mechanism for disease induction in humans, as thymic maturation of new T cells is minimal in most individuals receiving these drugs and developing lupuslike autoreactivity.

Mercuric chloride induces a lupuslike phenotype with antinuclear antibodies and nephritis (106). Scleroderma, in particular, has been linked to toxin exposure (107). Polyvinylchloride, L-tryptophan, rapeseed oil, gadolinium, and bleomycin have all been associated with the development of a progressive fibrosis; all but gadolinium- and bleomycin-induced disease are characterized by the presence of many eosinophils in lesional tissue. The presence of eosinophils may be a unique feature of exposure to an external agent, as these cells are not routinely present in primary scleroderma.

Much controversy surrounds the potential role of silica as a trigger for autoimmune disease. It has been linked to both systemic lupus and scleroderma. Recent epidemiologic studies have suggested that silica exposure may be a surrogate marker for exposure to bacterial lipopolysaccharide (LPS), as both these exposures occur primarily in individuals who work in proximity to the soil (108). In animal models, repeated exposure to LPS can induce lupuslike autoreactivity but has not been shown to induce a sclerodermalike phenotype (109). At one time there was a concern that silicon breast implants might precipitate autoimmune disease in women, but a number of impartial reviews of the epidemiologic, clinical, and animal data failed to confirm an association.

Mechanisms of Tissue Damage

It is important to consider mechanisms of tissue damage in autoimmune diseases, as these can differ significantly from mechanisms of immune activation. The clear implication of this observation is that whereas some therapeutic interventions may lessen both the inductive and effector phases of autoimmunity, others may be therapeutic with respect to one phase, but not both. The concept that the profile of cytokines and soluble mediators produced by cells in lymphoid organs may differ from those of cells involved in tissue inflammation is now well established. This observation further suggests that it is no longer useful to consider certain mediators to be strictly proinflammatory or anti-inflammatory. For example, TNFα protects against the development of autoantibodies, but contributes to tissue destruction (110). Similarly, TGFβ may limit the inductive phase of autoimmunity, but it causes fibrosis in tissues, leading to irreversible damage. IL-10 may also play a dual role in disease, inhibiting antigen presentation initially but driving T-cell proliferation, antibody class switching, and autoantibody production as disease progresses (111). IFNγ also has been suggested to have dualistic properties, as an enhanced level of IFNγ following treatment of MRL/Ipr mice with an agonistic antibody to CD137 is associated with disease prevention, but is later associated with augmenting the production of pathogenic autoantibodies and exacerbating tissue injury (112). Recently, it has become apparent that a newly described subset of effector T cells, T_H17 cells, induced by IL6, IL23, and TGFβ and producing large amounts of IL-17, is crucial in the collagen-induced model of RA. TGFβ, paradoxically, is responsible for induction of both T_H17 cells and regulatory T cells; these T-cell subsets are likely to establish an important counterpoint in systemic autoimmune disease. Thus, it is clear that disease stages include initiation, progression, and tissue destruction, that the critical pathways for disease exacerbation or remission can differ in each stage, and that particular signaling pathways may be operative in both the activation and the regulation of pathogenic autoimmunity. In murine models, the disease is largely synchronized, but in human disease, all three stages may exist simultaneously. Studies of therapeutic interventions in animal models and human disease have shown that it is possible to prevent tissue damage while immune activation continues uninterrupted (113), and conversely, one can perform immunoablation in animals and humans and tissue damage may continue unabated (114).

Therapeutic Considerations

For many decades, the therapy for systemic autoimmune disease was based on a strategy of global immunosuppression. Corticosteroids are cytotoxic to plasma cells (they are a major component of the therapy for multiple myeloma), suppress many of the effector mechanisms of inflammation, and are used in many autoimmune diseases. Interestingly, they may, in fact, exacerbate scleroderma, perhaps because the disease is characterized more by fibrosis and less by inflammation. In addition, a number of cytotoxic agents have been used in all systemic autoimmune diseases. These include cyclophosphamide, azathioprine, and, more recently, methotrexate and mycophenolate mofetil. These therapies are designed for use during major flares, and are generally continued in lower dose for maintenance of remission. Recently, a large number of new therapies have been attempted or are under design. The reason for the extraordinary increase in interest in designing therapeutics for autoimmune disease reflects, at least in part, the recognition that these diseases may share common pathogenetic mechanisms.

A major triumph of rational drug design and immunomodulatory therapy has been the success of TNFα blockade in the treatment of RA. This approach targets the effector phase of pathogenesis. Both soluble TNFα receptor and anti-TNFα antibody display equivalent efficacy in the treatment of RA, even though only anti TNFα antibody blocks membrane-bound as well as soluble TNFα (115) and appears to carry a greater risk of activating latent tuberculosis and other opportunistic infections (116).

The experience with TNFα blockade is also a cautionary tale. Effector pathways and inductive pathways differ in autoimmune diseases, and interfering with one may exacerbate the other. TNFα blockade with either soluble receptor or with anti-TNFα antibody leads to a 20% frequency of ANA positivity. Of these ANA-positive individuals, 10% display anti-DNA antibodies and approximately 1% develop frank lupus (115). The data suggest that withdrawal of TNFα blockade leads to a loss of anti-DNA antibodies and a return to ANA negativity in almost all cases. This observation is consistent with the demonstration of reduced TNFα expression in lupus-prone NZB/W mice and the demonstration of a therapeutic effect of administration of exogenous TNFα in this strain (117). The tolerance checkpoint(s) that is compromised is not known, and whether the primary effect is on the T- or B-cell repertoire remains uncertain.

Two other therapies have recently received U.S. Food and Drug Administration (FDA) approval for the treatment of RA and have potential efficacy in other autoimmune diseases as well. These are both designed to target the inductive phase of autoimmunity. CTLA-4Ig blocks T-cell activation by interfering with the interaction of B7 molecules on antigen-presenting cells with CD28 on naïve T cells. In addition, the binding of CTLA-4Ig to B7 induces expression of IDO in antigen-presenting cells, which degrades tryptophan, thereby limiting T-cell proliferation (73). This therapy appears as effective as TNFα blockade in reducing joint pain and inflammation. There are, as yet, no data on the incidence of bone erosions or cardiovascular disease in patients receiving CTLA-4Ig. Inhibition of both the inductive and the effector of the immune system may lead to unacceptable immunosuppression; the combination of TNFα blockade and CTLA-4Ig was more immunosuppressive than either agent alone, as evidenced by a higher rate of infection (118).

Antibody to CD20, rituximab, is a B-cell–depleting agent that has also recently received FDA approval for the treatment of RA. The success of this therapeutic agent suggests the importance of B cells as antigen-presenting cells in RA. It is important to state, however, that B-cell depletion may also work by reducing the titer of pathogenic antibodies. The clinical studies of rituximab therapy show a nonimmediate reduction in titer of IgG RF and antibodies to citrulinated cyclic peptides (anti-CCP antibodies, another antibody specific to patients with RA), but no change in titer of IgM RF (119). Different antibody specificities respond differently to B-cell depletion, almost certainly depending on the B-cell subset responsible for antibody production. In general, a decrease in IgG autoantibodies in the systemic autoimmune diseases is more likely to be beneficial than a decrease in IgM autoantibody titers, as IgG antibodies are more closely linked to disease pathogenesis. Based on a strategy of targeting the B cell in autoimmune disease, antibody to BAFF, a B-cell survival factor, is also being tested in RA and in lupus.

Thus far, no therapeutic agent has been able to induce a long-term drug-free remission, suggesting either a strong genetic component to disease or the persistence of pathogenic cells after cessation of therapy. It is highly likely that different therapeutic agents will be needed to block the inductive and the effector phases of disease, and that it will be necessary to treat patients indefinitely with agents that maintain a clinical remission once the disease phenotype has become manifest. Most important, effective therapy may well require targeting more than one pathway in disease pathogenesis; agents that alone exert a small effect on disease, may, in combination, demonstrate a very significant effect.

SYSTEMIC AUTOIMMUNE DISEASES

The remainder of this chapter will address specific diseases, focusing on human disease, relationships to the proposed concepts of autoimmunity, and supporting evidence from animal models. Critical aspects of each disease that are shared or are distinct will be identified.

SYSTEMIC LUPUS ERYTHEMATOSUS

SLE in humans is characterized by antinuclear antibody production and pathologic findings of inflammation, vasculitis, vasculopathy, and immune-complex deposition in multiple target organs. Susceptibility to SLE is clearly modulated by ethnicity and gender. Although it affects both males and females of all age groups, it most commonly presents in women during their child-bearing years, with a striking female-to-male ratio of 9:1. This ratio is approximately 3:1 in younger and older populations, supporting a role for hormonal factors in the induction of disease. Incidence rates reported during the last 25 years in North America vary from 2 to 7 per 100,000, with rates in African-American, Afro-Caribbean, Hispanic, and Asian populations approximately three times greater than in Caucasian populations. The worldwide prevalence of lupus ranges from 17 to 48 per 100,000, but has been reported as high as 207/100,000 in an Afro-Caribbean population in the United Kingdom. While a precise etiology of SLE is not known, serendipitous combinations of genetic, hormonal, and environmental factors are thought to contribute to the loss of self-tolerance.

Clinical Manifestations

The diversity of disease manifestations and severity in SLE is quite striking and includes constitutional complaints as well as the involvement of every organ system. Given the protean manifestations of disease, the American College of Rheumatology (ACR) criteria for diagnosis of SLE were developed for the purpose of allowing comparisons across studies (Table 41.1) (120). Meeting four of the 11 criteria establishes disease with approximately 95% certainty. There are, however, many patients with SLE who display only two or three criteria; this syndrome is termed incomplete lupus.

The production of autoantibodies is a unifying feature for all SLE patients. Antinuclear antibodies (ANAs) are present in 98% of SLE patients; a positive ANA test is very sensitive for SLE, although not specific, as ANA positivity is a feature of 5% to 30% of a healthy population, most of whom will never develop an autoimmune disease (121). Individual autoantibody specificities to nuclear and intracellular components, such as double-stranded (ds) DNA and Sm, are more specific but occur with lower frequency (Table 41.2). Most autoantibody levels do not correlate with disease activity; antibodies to dsDNA, in contrast, often rise in flare and subside in remission. Individual autoantibodies have been shown to associate with specific disease manifestations. These associations include anti-dsDNA antibodies with lupus nephritis, anti-Ro antibodies

TABLE 41.1 Classification Based on the Criteria of the American College of Rheumatology (ACR) for the Diagnosis of Systemic Lupus Erythematosus[a]

ACR criteria 1982 (updated 1997) description	
Malar rash	Fixed erythema, flat or raised, over the malar eminences, sparing the nasolabial folds
Discoid rash	Erythematous raised patches with adherent keratotic scaling and follicular plugging
Photosensitivity	Reaction to sunlight, resulting in the development of or increase in skin rash
Oral ulcers	Oral or nasopharyngial ulceration, usually painless
Arthritis	Nonerosive arthritis involving two or more peripheral joints
Serositis	Pleuritis or pericarditis
Renal disorder	Proteinuria >0.5 g/day and/or cellular casts
Neurologic disorder	Seizures and/or psychosis in the absence of drug toxicity or metabolic disturbances
Hematologic disorder	Hemolytic anemia, leukopenia, lymphopenia, or thrombocytopenia
ANA	Positive test for antinuclear antibodies in the absence of drugs known to induce it
Immunologic disorder	Elevated serum antibody titers to dsDNA, Sm, phospholipids, or false positive VDRL

[a]These criteria were developed for the purpose of allowing comparison of patients from different centers enrolled in clinical studies. Patients meeting at least four of the 11 criteria may be diagnosed with 95% certainty, but individual patients with systemic lupus erythematosus may exhit fewer than four criteria.

TABLE 41.2 Autoantibodies in Systemic Lupus Erythematosus (SLE)

Autoantibody	*Frequency (% positive at any time)*	*Clinical Association*
Anti-dsDNA	50–70	Nephritis
Anti-Sm	5–30	Pathognomonic for SLE
Anti-SSA/Ro	40–50	Dry eyes and mouth, SCLE, neonatal lupus, cytopenias, photosensitivity
Anti-SSB/La	10–15	
Anti-RNP	40–60	MCTD, myositis, Raynauds
Anti-NMDAR	40–50	Cognitive dysfunction, depression
Antiphospholipid	15–50	Thrombosis, pregnancy loss, cutaneous ulcers
Anti-ribosomal P	10–20	Psychosis, depression

SCLE, subacute cutaneous lupus; MCTD, mixed connective tissue disease with SICCA syndrome (dry eyes and dry mouth) as well as subacute cutaneous lupus and neonatal lupus, anti-RNP antibodies with Raynaud phenomenon, arthritis, myositis, and lung disease (122), and anti-NMDA receptor antibodies with depression and possibly cognitive impairment in SLE (123,124). The recent finding that autoantibodies may precede the clinical diagnosis of SLE by many years suggests that progression to pathologic autoimmunity in SLE need not be an acute process (50). Increases in autoantibody titer and antigenic diversity up to the time of diagnosis suggest that pathologic autoimmunity evolves over time and that the inductive phase may precede the effector phase of disease by many years. Whether a tissue-specific trigger is needed to initiate target-organ inflammation is not known but is highly probable.

Pathogenesis and Genetic Susceptibility

Familial disease clustering and a higher disease concordance in monozygotic than dizygotic twins support an underlying genetic susceptibility. Increasingly, it is recognized that multiple genetic polymorphisms and specific HLA haplotypes contribute to disease susceptibility. Most SLE-associated alleles are present in healthy individuals in the population. The presence of a single SLE-associated allele is insufficient to cause disease; generation of a lupuslike phenotype requires the presence of combinations of several SLE-associated alleles. Many SLE-associated alleles have also been implicated in other autoimmune diseases (e.g., CTLA-4 polymorphisms associated with Graves disease and type 1 diabetes, PTPN22 polymorphisms associated with RA and type 1 diabetes), suggesting that specific patterns of autoimmunity are determined by particular combinations of autoimmune-associated alleles, some of which govern target vulnerability, and environmental stimuli (3). The evidence for a common set of susceptibility genes in multiple autoimmune diseases also helps to explain familial clustering of diverse autoimmune diseases.

At least eight genetic loci with significant linkage to SLE have been identified (Table 41.3) (125). Associations between HLA alleles and specific autoantibodies appear to be modulated by ethnicity (Table 41.4). Presumed susceptibility genes from human studies in SLE include those affecting selection and survival of B cells, T-lymphocyte activation and survival, cytokine production, antigen presentation, and clearance of apoptotic debris (126).

Failure of B-Cell Tolerance

Recent analyses of antibodies cloned from circulating B cells in SLE patients demonstrate a failure to establish self-tolerance during B-cell development and are consistent with an intrinsic B-cell defect at this stage of differentiation (127). Repertoire analyses of antibodies cloned from B cells derived from bone marrow and peripheral blood of healthy donors provide evidence for both a central tolerance checkpoint in the bone marrow and a second peripheral checkpoint, as evidenced by a decrease in the frequency of autoreactive antibodies from 75% in the bone marrow to 20% in the circulating naïve compartment (128). The low-affinity, self-reactive, polyclonal IgM antibodies produced by circulating mature naïve B cells in healthy individuals are thought to facilitate clearance of apoptotic cells, thereby decreasing the development of a potentially pathogenic T- and B-cell response to self-antigen (129). Virtually none of these antibodies binds dsDNA. Although the checkpoint between immature B cells in the bone marrow and newly emigrated cells in blood appears to be intact in the small number of SLE patients studied, the mature naïve B-cell compartment in

TABLE 41.3 Chromosomal Regions with Confirmed Linkage to Systemic Lupus Erythematosus

Chromosome	Cytogenic Location	Locus Name	Candidate Genes
1	1q23		*CRP* FcγRIIa FcγRIIb FcγRIIIa
1	1q25-31		
1	1q41-42	*SLEB1*	*PARP* *TLR5*
2	2q35-37	*SLEB2*	*PDCD1*
4	4p16-15.2	*SLEB3*	
6	6p11-21		MHC II : DRB1 *TNFα* *C2, C4*
12	12q24	*SLEB4*	
16	16q12		NOD2 OAZ

CRP, C-reactive protein; FcγR, IgG Fc gamma receptor; *PARP*, poly(ADP-ribose) polymerase; TLR5, Toll-like receptor 5; *PDCD1*, programmed cell death 1; MHC, major histocompatibility complex; *TNF*, tumor necrosis factor; *NOD2*, nucleotide oligomerization domain 2; *OAZ*, OLF1/EBF-associated zinc finger protein.

TABLE 41.4 MHC Class II Autoantibody Associations in Systemic Lupus Erythematosus

Autoantibody	HLA-DRB1	HLA-DQA1	HLA-DQB1	Ethnic Association
Anti-Sm			*0602	Caucasian,
			*0601	African-American
Anti-Ro	*0301	*0501	*0201	Caucasian
	*0803	*0103	*0601	Japanese
Anti-RNP	*04		*0302	Caucasian
		*0101	*0501	African-American

SLE is enriched for autoreactive clones (40% to 50% in SLE, 20% in controls). Mechanisms responsible for this implied failure of the peripheral checkpoint have not been clearly elucidated.

Because signaling through the BCR is a primary mechanism for triggering deletion, anergy, or receptor editing, abnormal BCR signaling is likely to play a role in the breakdown of tolerance (130). As discussed previously, both decreased and increased signaling through the BCR may predispose to an increased risk of autoantibody production. Mouse models support a paradigm of decreased BCR signaling leading to laxity in B-cell negative selection, increased autoreactivity in the naïve B-cell population, and increased risk of autoantibody production. Although the enhanced autoreactivity of the naïve repertoire appears to be a permissive substrate for the development of SLE, back-mutation of two mutated anti-DNA antibodies to their germline-encoded precursors demonstrates a lack of autospecificity in the original antibody.

Circulating mature B cells from SLE patients demonstrate a heightened response to BCR crosslinking, demonstrated by increased levels of intracellular calcium and increased tyrosine phosphorylation. Several mechanisms for enhanced BCR signaling in mature B cells have been identified. Lyn is an intracellular protein tyrosine kinase that can diminish BCR signaling through phosphorylation of CD22, FcRIIb, and other ITIM-containing inhibitory receptors (131). Studies of SLE patients show that Lyn expression may be decreased by 50% or more in resting and activated B cells, with a positive correlation between reduced levels of Lyn and the production of anti-DNA antibodies (132). FcRIIb is an inhibitory receptor that downregulates the BCR when both receptors are co-ligated. Increased intracellular Ca^{2+} flux noted in SLE B cells may be due to defective upregulation of FcRIIb on memory B cells (133), decreased availability of the intracellular SHIP protein that is part of the FcRIIb signaling cascade (134), or an FcRIIb polymorphism (Ile 232 Thr) that prevents partitioning of the receptor into lipid rafts (135), where it must reside to associate with the BCR.

In addition, costimulatory molecules and cytokines whose expression is dysregulated in SLE can rescue autoreactive B cells from BCR-mediated deletion. Expression of some of these molecules, for example, BAFF, CD40, CD40L, IL-10, correlates with disease activity and increased anti-DNA antibody titers (136). BAFF, in particular, is implicated in the pathogenesis of SLE, because mice that overexpress BAFF have a lupuslike disease, NZB/NZW and MRL-*lpr* mice have elevated levels of BAFF, and treatment with anti-BLyS antibody ameliorates progression of disease in these lupus-prone mice (137). The elevated serum levels of BAFF reported in SLE patients may be secondary to the lymphopenia often seen in SLE or may result from exposure of plasmacytoid dendritic cells to DNA or RNA containing immune complexes (138). Marginal-zone B cells in mice (IgM memory cells in humans) are easily stimulated by BAFF to exhibit enhanced function as antigen-presenting cells, potentially activating autoreactive T cells (139).

The presence of extensive somatic mutation seen in autoantibodies derived from SLE patients strongly supports germinal-center maturation of pathogenic, autoreactive B cells. Somatic hypermutation with random point mutations gives rise to self-reactive clones at high frequency, but in nonautoimmune individuals these rarely exit from the germinal center. In SLE, checkpoints at the germinal-center response have been studied through an analysis of antibodies expressing the 9G4 idiotype, which is encoded by the VH 4.34 heavy-chain variable-region gene (129). These antibodies bind N-acetyl-lactosamine (NAL) determinants on blood-group antigens, gangliosides, gastrointestinal mucins, glycolipids, and CD45 on B lymphocytes. Though virtually undetectable in normal sera, 9G4 IgM antibody titers are greatly increased in response to mycoplasma, Epstein–Barr virus, and cytomegalovirus infections. 9G4 B cells constitute 5% to 10% of the naïve and IgM memory B-cell populations in healthy donors; they are, however, excluded from IgG memory B-cell and plasma-cell compartments and are not seen within normal tonsillar germinal centers, suggesting the presence of a tolerance checkpoint at germinal-center entry. Evaluation of lymphoid tissue from tonsillar biopsies and spleens of SLE patients reveals that the frequency of germinal-center 9G4 B cells is 15% to 20%, thereby identifying another failed tolerance checkpoint in SLE (21). The suggestion that transition to the IgM^+ memory B-cell compartment is another checkpoint for selection against autoreactive cells is supported by data showing a decrease in frequency of autoreactive IgM^+ memory B cells to 2% from 20% in the mature naïve B-cell population in healthy individuals; whether this checkpoint is abrogated in SLE is not yet determined (140).

These data are consistent with data from murine studies identifying multiple tolerance checkpoints during B-cell development and activation. B-cell autonomous properties can alter these checkpoints, as can interactions with other cell types or soluble mediators. The loss of B-cell tolerance in SLE is critical to the initiation of target-organ injury but also has implications beyond autoantibody formation. B cells are essential for antigen presentation and cytokine production (141). B cells with self-reactive specificity are likely to present self-peptides to autoreactive T cells (141); this pathway provides a rationale for B-cell depletion therapy even in autoimmune diseases in which T cells are the critical effectors (142).

Lymphocyte Activation

The presence of class-switched, high-affinity, somatically mutated autoantibodies in SLE patients suggests that cognate B-cell/T-cell interactions and antigen-specific T-cell activation have occurred. Specific HLA DR haplotypes (DR2, DR3) have been associated with a two- to threefold increased susceptibility for SLE and with particular autoantibody specificities, consistent with the model of an antigen-driven process involving antigen-specific T-cell activation.

By providing help to autoreactive B cells, T cells in lupus contribute to the abrogation of self-tolerance. Lupus T cells display increased expression of activation markers. Some studies show that stimulation of the TCR on SLE T cells leads to an abnormally high increase in intracellular Ca^{tt}. This appears to be a consequence of a decreased association of the ζ chain and an increased association of the γ chain of the Fc receptor with the TCR (143). Although there is a heightened Ca^{tt} influx after TCR stimulation, IL 2 production is decreased. Lupus T cells display increased expression of Crem α, which is perhaps responsible for the reduced IL-2 production, and for their decreased susceptibility to activation-induced cell death (AICD) (144).

Several polymorphisms of genes involved in T-cell regulation have been reported in SLE. The protein tyrosine phosphatase N22 (PTPN22) contributes to the downregulation of T-cell–receptor activation. Polymorphisms in PTPN22 associated with overexuberant T-cell activation have been reported in Caucasian and Spanish SLE populations (145). A polymorphism of the gene encoding PD-1, a receptor in the TNF superfamily that has an ITIM motif in its cytoplasmic tail and is involved in downregulation of activated T and B cells, has been associated with SLE susceptibility in Mexican and European populations (146).

Self-tolerance is maintained, in part, by the suppressive actions of regulatory T cells (Treg). $CD4^+CD25^+$ Treg suppress proliferation and effector functions of $CD4^+CD25^-$ T cells. Studies of Treg in patients with SLE have demonstrated reduced numbers of peripheral $CD4^+CD25^+$ cells in patients with active disease (147). The basis for this has not yet been ascertained, but IL 2 is critically important for maintenance and survival of Treg cells; decreased expression may contribute to the abnormalities in Treg function noted in SLE (147).

The Innate Immune Response

It has become increasingly apparent that upregulation of the type I interferon pathways plays an important role in the pathogenesis of SLE (148). Elevated levels of IFNα, correlating with disease activity, severity, and titers of anti-DNA antibodies, were originally reported three decades ago. Causality was demonstrated in the 1990s with the use of recombinant IFNα for treatment of hepatitis C and the subsequent reports of IFNα-induced autoantibody production and the development of a lupuslike syndrome. Several studies have demonstrated the upregulation of a set of IFN-inducible genes in the peripheral blood mononuclear cells of SLE patients (148). The expression of this "interferon signature" has been shown to correlate with disease activity and with the presence of antibodies to RNA containing antigens.

Plasmacytoid dendritic cells have been identified as the major producers of IFNα. These cells are identified by surface expression of blood dendritic cell antigens (BDCA) 2 and 4 and CD123 and intracellular expression of both TLR7 and TLR9. SLE serum has been shown to induce IFNα production in normal peripheral blood mononuclear cells in culture; the IFN-inducing factor in SLE serum is DNA- or RNA-containing immune complexes (148). Chromatin-containing immune complexes are internalized by plasmacytoid dendritic cells through binding of nucleic acid–containing immune complexes to an activating Fc receptor. After internalization, chromatin is delivered to TLR9 or TLR7 located in an intracellular lysosomal compartment. Ligation of TLR9 by DNA or TLR7 by RNA triggers a signaling cascade resulting in transcription of several proinflammatory molecules including IFNα, IL-6, -8, -18, MIP-1α and MIP-1β, RANTES, and BAFF (149). FcR engagement alone by immune complexes is insufficient to promote dendritic cell activation and blockade of TLR7 and 9 with hydroxychloroquine and of TLR9 with inhibitory oligonucleotides will abrogate IFNα production. The proinflammatory effects of IFNα include dendritic cell activation and promotion of B-cell differentiation and Ig isotype switching. By promoting dendritic cell maturation, IFNα also increases the potential for activation of autoreactive T cells. Polymorphisms in the tyrosine kinase 2 (tyk2) gene have been associated with increased expression of type I interferon in SLE (150). Recently, a polymorphism of IRF-5, a transcription factor involved in TLR signaling pathways that regulates the expression of inflammatory cytokines including type 1 IFN and IL-6, IL-12, and TNFα, has been associated with SLE in several patient cohorts (3). It is important to note, however, that in some of the lupus-prone mouse models, decreases in type 1 interferon unexpectedly lead to a worsening of disease, suggesting that the effect of IFNα on autoimmunity is more complex than is currently appreciated (151). Whether there are patients whose disease might also be exacerbated by a reduction in type 1 interferon is unknown.

The anti-inflammatory effects of IL-10 include diminished antigen presentation by dendritic cells and decreased macrophage activation, leading to decreased T-cell activation overall and a reduced Th1 response. In NZB/W lupus-prone mice, IL-10 paradoxically increases disease severity. Correspondingly, treatment of a small number of lupus patients with anti-IL-10 antibody resulted in clinical improvement (152), and promoter polymorphisms in the IL-10 gene leading to enhanced production have been reported to associate with SLE (126).

Tissue Injury

Although the presence of autoantibodies is essential for a diagnosis of SLE, it is recognized that antibodies are not responsible for all of the tissue damage and organ destruction seen in clinical disease. Although specific autoantibodies have been identified in affected organs in SLE patients (anti-dsDNA antibodies in the kidney, anti-Ro antibodies in skin and fetal heart conducting systems, anti-NMDA receptor antibodies in brain), autoantibodies have also been found in nonlesional tissue, demonstrating that antibody deposition alone is insufficient for inflammation and tissue damage. It has become increasingly apparent that much of the tissue destruction appears to be cytokine-mediated. IFNγ, IL-Iβ, TNFα, TGFβ, IL-18, and IL-6 are all expressed at high levels in kidney biopsy tissue from SLE patients with active glomerulonephritis (153), and skin biopsies from SLE patients have shown increased expression of IFNα and IL-6 in lesional sites (154).

TNFα is a pleiotropic cytokine with well-known proinflammatory effects, including T-cell and macrophage activation and release of other proinflammatory cytokines such as IL-1, -6, -18 and IFNγ (153). Although TNFα blockade has proved to be enormously successful in RA and Crohn's disease, the role of TNFα in SLE is more complex. Low TNFα levels in mice are associated with autoantibody production, and TNFα blockade leads to antinuclear antibody production in 20% of treated individuals. TNFα blockade may be used successfully in active SLE to modulate effector mechanisms of renal injury, but it leads to increased titers of anti-DNA and anticardiolipin autoantibodies. Several polymorphisms for genes encoding TNFα and TNFβ (lymphotoxin-α) have been associated with SLE; their functional effects are not fully determined.

Monocyte chemoattractant protein (MCP-1) is a potent chemoattractant for monocytes, memory T cells, and natural-killer T cells. Expression of this protein is increased in renal tubular cells and glomeruli in lupus nephritis, and urinary levels of MCP-1 are increased in patients with active nephritis (155). A functional MCP-1 polymorphism resulting in increased production of MCP-1 has been associated with SLE nephritis (126), providing evidence that there are genetic determinants of target-organ susceptibility to immune attack.

Antigen Exposure

Reduced uptake of apoptotic cells leads to initiation of disease in murine models of SLE and has been identified histopathologically in lymph nodes of lupus patients (156). Complement components, mannose-binding lectin (MBL), and C-reactive protein (CRP) are all acute-phase reactant proteins that contribute to the opsonization of apoptotic debris, thereby facilitating clearance and reducing the likelihood that apoptotic debris will become immunogenic. Homozygous deficiencies of early complement components C2, C4, and C1q are rare but confer substantial risk for SLE (126). Polymorphisms of both MBL and CRP genes have also been associated with SLE susceptibility; MBL-susceptibility alleles appear to be more important in Chinese and Spanish populations than in Northern European populations (126).

Efficient uptake of immune complexes and opsonized debris is mediated by Fc receptors expressed predominantly on hematopoietic cells (B cells, neutrophils, macrophages, and dendritic cells). FcRI, IIa, IIIa, and IIIb all contain immunoreceptor tyrosine-based activation motifs (ITAMs) in their cytoplasmic tails. Crosslinking of these receptors by IgG immune complexes results in mast-cell and neutrophil degranulation, phagocytosis, antibody-dependent cellular cytotoxicity, upregulation of cytokine gene transcription, and release of inflammatory mediators (157). These activating receptors also enhance dendritic cell maturation (157). Single-nucleotide substitutions in the activating FcR genes result in molecules with altered binding to IgG immune complexes. Associations between the FcRIIA R131H low-affinity allele and disease susceptibility or nephritis have been reported in Brazilian, Thai, Korean, German, and African-American populations (158). FcRIIIA F158V and FcγRIIIB NA2/NA2 polymorphisms are reported to associate with disease susceptibility in Dutch, Korean, Thai, and Caucasian populations (158). The recent finding that FcRIIa R131 is a significant predictor of the efficacy of B-cell depletion in SLE patients treated with anti-CD20 antibody suggests that identification of FcR polymorphisms may also be useful in predicting response to some therapeutic agents.

DNase I is an endonuclease that creates single-stranded nicks in DNA (159). DNase I–deficient mice develop a lupuslike illness characterized by autoantibodies, nephritis, and early death, and in NZB/W lupus-prone mice, low serum DNase 1 activity is detectable before the onset of renal disease. A small number of patients with SLE have a mutation in DNase 1 leading to low serum DNase activity and markedly elevated IgG titers against nucleosomal antigens, including dsDNA. Several studies of lupus patients have demonstrated low serum DNase 1 activity; low DNase I activity is not associated with coding-region polymorphisms, but could potentially be associated with polymorphisms in noncoding regions that regulate gene expression. It was initially speculated that reduced DNase 1 activity might reflect a loss of serum DNase through damaged kidneys, but low DNase 1 activity has been detected even in patients without kidney disease.

Cell Survival

Polymorphisms in Bcl-2, an antiapoptotic molecule that defines the threshold for cell death and survival, have been implicated in susceptibility to SLE in Chinese and Mexican populations (160). Importantly, the combination of a Bcl-2–susceptibility allele and an IL-10–susceptibility allele has been reported to confer a 40-fold increased risk of

SLE, buttressing the theory that combinations of susceptibility alleles markedly increase risk. Although SLE patients do not have mutations leading to Fas or FasL deficiency, elevated serum levels of soluble Fas have been reported in SLE, and lymphopenia in SLE has been associated with increased Fas expression on circulating lymphocytes.

Hormonal Influences

The greater frequency of lupus in women has fueled the hypothesis that sex hormones play a role in disease pathogenesis (49). Recently, three randomized, placebo-controlled trials of the use of estrogen in SLE patients determined the existence of a subset of patients whose disease is exacerbated by hormone. All three studies concluded that exogenous estrogens were well tolerated in patients with stable disease and lacking in antiphospholipid antibodies, but mild to moderate flare rates were significantly increased in postmenopausal women treated with hormone replacement (161–163). The response to estrogen is mediated by two intracellular receptors, ERα and ERβ, and polymorphisms of the ERα gene have been associated with age of disease onset and disease severity in some human SLE populations.

Twenty percent of SLE patients are reported to have elevated prolactin levels; nonetheless, treatment with bromocriptine, a blocker of prolactin secretion, has displayed equivocal benefit. Prolactin receptors are found on a variety of cells including T and B, and ligation of these transmembrane receptors results in upregulation of CD40, CD40L, and Bcl-2, all of which might facilitate the survival of autoreactive B cells.

New Therapeutic Approaches

For many years, there were few clinical trials on systemic lupus and no new therapeutic options. Therapy consisted of corticosteroids to decrease immune activation and inflammation. Azathioprine was recommended as a steroid-sparing agent, and cyclophosphamide was given to patients with aggressive disease. Hydroxychloroquine was also recommended for most patients and was thought to decrease antigen presentation by interfering with phagolysomal fusion; it is now believed to function by preventing the activation of TLR7 and TLR9 that reside in a lysosomal compartment, thereby blocking DC activation by DNA-containing immune complexes.

Recently, many new therapeutic options have been proposed, and many are currently in clinical trial. First, mycophenolate mofetil was shown to be as efficacious as cyclophosphamide in the treatment of acute lupus nephritis. Trials to determine if mycophenolate is as effective as cyclophosphamide in maintenance of renal remission are underway. Mycophenolate may have a better toxicity profile, as it does not cause ovarian failure and infertility.

High-dose cyclophosphamide treatment followed by autologous stem-cell reconstitution has been performed in lupus patients; a randomized study is now in process. With increasing interest in the potential role of the B cell as the antigen-presenting cell for self-antigen, B-cell–depletion strategies are being explored with antibodies to CD20 and to CD22. A related approach targets BAFF and its three receptors (BAFF-R, TACI, and BCMA). An initial study of anti-BAFF antibody failed to show clinical efficacy, although it did lead to a modest reduction in anti-DNA antibodies.

Costimulatory blockade using an antibody to CD40 ligand (CD40L) to prevent the CD40L interaction with CD40 on B cells and antigen-presenting cells was attempted in lupus patients. The suggestion of clinical efficacy in a few patients, however, was tempered by an unanticipated increase in the incidence of thrombotic events. Subsequent studies have now shown that human platelets, unlike murine platelets, also express CD40L. Antagonistic antibodies to CD40 are now under development to attempt again to target this pathway.

A clinical study of CTLA-4Ig in lupus is currently underway. Interestingly, a therapeutic effect of CTLA-4Ig on established kidney disease in NZB/W mice is seen even though autoantibody titers do not decrease; thus, CTLA-4Ig may have a direct effect on renal pathology. Engagement of CD28 may be required for expression of chemokine and chemokine receptors that allow extravasation of activated cells into tissue. CTLA-4Ig may block this phase of disease pathogenesis or may work directly on renal cells expressing B7 molecules. Studies of ICOS blockade are in development, as are studies of agents that block type I interferon. The murine models show that the efficacy of these interventions are strain-specific and depend on the mechanism for autoantibody production. It is highly likely, therefore, that each of these interventions will be effective in only a subset of patients; identifying each subset in advance of treatment initiation remains a challenge.

Most therapies focus on the inductive phase of autoimmune disease, however, the therapeutic benefits of uncoupling links in the inflammatory cascade and targeting molecules that mediate end-organ damage are increasingly recognized. A small number of patients with refractory lupus nephritis have been treated with TNFα blockade with marked decreases in proteinuria despite an increase in autoantibody production. TNFα-receptor expression on renal epithelial cells appears to be crucial for induction of antibody-mediated glomerulonephritis, although it remains uncertain whether TNFR1 or TNFR2 or both must be present. Thus, the effect of TNFα blockade on renal nephritis is likely to be an effect on resident renal cells.

Studies of antigen-specific therapies are in their infancy. LJP 394 is a multimeric DNA compound that has been demonstrated to reduce anti-DNA antibody titer and to reduce numbers of DNA-reactive B cells in the BXSB murine lupus model. In clinical trials in lupus patients, it has been shown to reduce titers of high-affinity anti-DNA antibodies, but it has a modest effect, if any, on reduction of renal flares. It may be that LJP394 fails to induce tolerance in the proinflammatory milieu of lupus patients, it may not have been used at an adequate dose, or there may be too many nephritogenic antibodies in lupus patients that are not bound by LJP394.

Mouse Models of SLE

Systemic lupus is a disease that has attracted much attention from immunologists, in part because a very large number of genetic manipulations in mice give rise to a lupus-like disease. Indeed, susceptibility loci have been identified on every murine chromosome, and >30 susceptibility loci have been reported (18). Initial studies of lupus focused on spontaneously arising strains that displayed serum titers of anti-DNA antibodies and glomerulonephritis.

NZB/W Mouse

The NZB/W mouse develops high-affinity anti-DNA antibodies and a proliferative glomerulonephritis. Of interest, female mice develop earlier and more aggressive disease. The disease is hormonally responsive; estrogen exacerbates disease and androgen protects against disease, and studies demonstrate a defect in central tolerance, with high-affinity autoreactive immature B cells maturing to immunocompetence. The mice are characterized by hyperreactivity of naïve B cells with an early spontaneous increase in IgG-producing B cells. The pathogenic anti-DNA antibodies in this strain are IgG, predominantly IgG2a and IgG2b, and many display extensive somatic mutation with some evidence for affinity maturation to DNA, suggesting a requirement for T-cell help and a defect in selection of germinal-center B cells. A B-cell autonomous defect has been shown in adoptive transfer studies, but full disease expression requires the presence of NZB/W T cells as well.

The genetic analysis of the NZB/W strain has revealed a locus on chromosome 1 to be critical in autoreactivity. This same region is a susceptibility locus in the related NZM2410 strain, and an orthologous region of chromosome 1 in humans is also a lupus-susceptibility locus. The locus includes the genes encoding Fc receptors. The NZB/W mouse has been demonstrated to have low-level expression of the inhibitory FcRIIB and, similar to human patients, a failure to upregulate expression of this receptor on memory B cells. Interestingly, a forced increase in expression of FcRIIB in B cells in this strain markedly reduces autoantibody production and renal disease (164). There are, however, many candidate genes in this locus besides FcγRIIB. The IFNγ-inducible gene Ifi202 has also been implicated in disease susceptibility; the susceptibility allele is linked to increased resistance to p53-mediated apoptosis of B cells (165). Consistent with the hypothesis that an IFNγ-inducible gene is involved in disease pathogenesis, IFNγ itself contributes to disease severity (166).

IFNγ blockade reduces IgG anti-DNA antibody production and glomerular immunoglobulin deposition, in part by preventing class switching to IgG2b and IgG2a; the recent identification of FcR IV with high-affinity binding to IgG2a has led to the speculation that the absence of activation of this receptor may be responsible for reduced renal inflammation when IgG2a antibodies are reduced (167). It has, in fact, been demonstrated in this strain that the deletion of the γ chain of activating Fc receptors leads to a marked reduction in renal inflammation, although it causes no diminution in autoantibody production (168). Several other loci have also been suggested to play a role in autoimmune disease in this strain (18). Of note, the putative susceptibility loci derive from both the NZB and the NZW parental strains. A promoter polymorphism in the gene encoding TNFα leading to decreased expression of TNFα associates with disease; administration of exogenous TNFα reduces autoantibody production in this strain (117). Paradoxically, TNFα contributes to kidney inflammation. The potentially conflicting role of cytokines in the inductive and pathogenic phases of diseased complicates the design of therapeutic strategies. Because TLR signaling and consequent production of IFNα has been implicated in murine and human lupus, NZB/W mice lacking the IFNα receptor have been generated; these mice lack a disease phenotype; conversely, administration of IFNα to NZB/W mice markedly accelerates disease (169,170).

The NZB/W strain has been of substantial utility in preclinical studies of lupus therapeutics. Early studies demonstrated the efficacy of either continuous or intermittent cyclophosphamide in NZB/W lupus; cyclophosphamide remains a major agent in the therapeutic armamentarium in SLE. Anti-CD3 and anti-CD4 therapy was also shown to be effective therapy in this model, leading to a therapeutic focus on the T cell. Anti-CD40 ligand antibody diminishes autoantibody production in NZB/W mice and leads to improved renal function. T cells from the NZB/W mouse have been shown to respond to an immunoglobulin heavy-chain variable-region peptide. A tolerogenic exposure to this peptide leads to a markedly less severe disease. Because T cells of lupus patients also recognize this peptide, a protocol to induce tolerance with peptide is currently in early trials in patients.

CTLA-4Ig was also tested as a therapeutic agent in this strain and demonstrated good efficacy. When CTLA-4Ig is used together with even a single dose of cyclophosphamide, there is not only a cessation of progression of renal disease, but also a reversal of ongoing renal disease. This has led to speculation that some critical effects of CTLA-4Ig are on effector mechanisms of renal injury, both extravasation of inflammatory cells into renal tissue and recruitment of resident renal cells to the inflammatory cascade (113). BAFF blockade also diminishes renal disease. Only a modest decrease in IgG autoantibodies is observed following either BAFF-R-Ig or TACl-Ig; their mechanism of action may be a reduction in B-cell number with a consequent decrease in T-cell activation (171). Agonistic antibody to CD137 (4-1BB), a T-cell costimulatory molecule belonging to the TNFR family, leads to near-normal life span in NZB/W mice, and a short treatment given after disease onset reduces ongoing disease severity (112). The mechanisms for this effect have not fully been elucidated, but current hypotheses include induction of anergy, deletion of autoreactive CD4 T cells, generation of regulatory T cells, or IFNγ-dependent regulation of T-cell function. This treatment is interesting because it shows that long-lasting restoration of tolerance can be achieved in mice with spontaneous SLE in which B and T cells are continuously being activated. This approach has not yet been applied to human disease.

NZM Mice

The NZM mouse strains are closely related to the NZB/W mice; they derive from extensive intercrossing of NZB/W mice. The NZM 2410 strain, in particular, has been studied in detail. Three large regions (SLE 1, 2, and 3) on chromosomes 1, 4, and 7 have been identified as susceptibility loci. The chromosome 1 locus includes the region identified as a susceptibility locus in NZB/W mice, and it contributes to ANA reactivity. The chromosome 4 locus also contributes to ANA reactivity, but also to T-cell activation. The chromosome 9 locus contributes both a dendritic cell activation phenotype and renal vulnerability. Together these susceptibility loci, derived from both parental strains, are sufficient to confer full lupus susceptibility on nonautoimmune C57Bl/6 mice. Extensive subsequent analyses have demonstrated that multiple susceptibility genes are present within each locus. Within the chromosome 1 locus are genes encoding Fc receptors, complement receptors, and Ly108. The Ly108 allele present in the NZM2410 mouse has been demonstrated to attenuate BCR signaling, leading to diminished negative selection in the naïve B-cell repertoire. Thus, despite the hyperreactivity of mature B cells in this strain, there may be hyporesponsiveness of immature B cells. This model is consistent with some new data discussed earlier from human patients demonstrating a persistent lack of stringency in central B-cell tolerance that could be attributable to decreased BCR signaling (reviewed in 64).

The renal pathology in the NZM2410 strain is characterized by more glomerulosclerosis and less proliferative disease than the renal disease in the NZB/W mice. Studies in the NZM strains have linked glomerular disease to stat 6 activation, as stat 6–deficient mice have high titers of autoantibodies but little renal disease. Surprisingly, stat 4–deficient NZM mice fail to develop strong T_H1 responses and fail to produce high titers of IgG2b and IgG2a anti-DNA antibodies, yet they develop accelerated renal disease. These studies support the model that the genetic basis for induction of autoreactivity differs from the genetic basis for target-organ damage (172).

SNF1 Mouse

The F1 progeny of SWR × NZB (SNF1) also develop a lupuslike disease. T-cell reactivity to histone peptides was first identified in this strain and, subsequently, in other lupus-prone strains and in humans with SLE. In particular, a conserved peptide in H4 is recognized in the context of multiple mouse and human class II molecules, and administration of soluble peptide has been demonstrated in mice to prevent disease when presented in the appropriate fashion; trials are planned in lupus patients (173).

MRL/lpr Mouse

The MRL/lpr mouse has also been a subject of intense investigation. This mouse has a defect in Fas expression. On other genetic backgrounds, the Fas mutation can lead to no phenotype or to lymphoproliferation without autoantibody production. On the MRL background, the fas mutation leads to lymphoproliferation, autoantibody production and inflammation in the kidney and salivary glands. The most obvious phenotypic abnormality is an expansion of B220$^+$, CD4$^-$, CD8$^-$ T cells, which contribute to autoantibody production. Anti-DNA antibodies are a dominant specificity, but anti-Sm antibodies, RF, and anti-Ro and La antibodies are also present (174). MRL/lpr mice, like NZB/W mice, display low-level expression of FcRIIB on B cells. Increased FcRIIB expression leads to a marked attenuation of autoantibody production, even though the expansion of abnormal T cells persists (164).

Not all aspects of disease pathogenesis are similar between MRL/lpr and NZB/W mice. Paradoxically, TLR9 deficiency in the MRL/lpr background leads to enhanced disease, whereas TLR7 deficiency leads to attenuated disease (175). Furthermore, MRL/lpr mice deficient in Fc receptor γ-chain expression still develop renal disease (176). Finally, type I IFN attenuates disease in this strain (151). The reasons for the differences between the strains are not understood, but they raise the specter that similar heterogeneity in etiopathogenesis and response to therapy will exist in the human population and complicate the design of clinical trials.

Motheaten Mouse

The motheaten mouse (me/me) has a defective SHP-1 gene. It also develops anti-DNA antibodies and glomerulonephritis (177). Although the anti-DNA antibodies in

NZB/W, NZM, and MRL/lpr mice display extensive somatic mutation, the anti-DNA antibodies in motheaten mice appear to derive from B1 cells. B cells in this strain display marked hyperreactivity. Because SHP-1 is the phosphatase that is activated by engagement of CD22, it is not surprising that the same phenotype is observed as in CD22-deficient mice. Whether B1 cells in humans can produce pathogenic anti-DNA antibodies is not known.

BXSB Mouse

The BXSB mouse is unique in that male mice are preferentially affected. They possess a chromosomal translocation of a region of the X chromosome inserted into the Y chromosome. Because the X chromosome region includes the gene encoding TLR7, there is increased TLR7 expression in these mice, perhaps leading to increased dendritic cell and B-cell activation in the presence of RNA-containing immune complexes (178).

Other Lupus-prone Strains

The past decades have seen an enormous proliferation of genetically altered mice that develop a lupuslike serology. One feature of these models is that the disease phenotype is only apparent on particular genetic backgrounds. Appearance of clinical disease is determined by the presence of cooperating susceptibility loci, whereas absence of clinical disease in a particular strain may reflect a lack of cooperating susceptibility loci or the presence of suppressor loci that interfere with disease expression. Similar to studies of lupus genetics in the human population, susceptibility genes include those that govern antigen exposure, lymphocyte survival, activation pathways, antigen-receptor signaling, and target-organ vulnerability (reviewed in 64). Several gene deletions that affect the removal of apoptotic cells and apoptotic debris result in a lupuslike syndrome. For example, deletion of DNase 1, C1q, or SAP leads to the production of anti-DNA antibodies. Similarly, deletion of c mer, a membrane tyrosine kinase critical to the process of phagocytosis by macrophages, also leads to autoantibody production and glomerulonephritis. Overexpression of genes that prevent B-cell apoptosis, such as Bcl-2 and BAFF, are also associated with a lupuslike syndrome. A third category of genes implicated in lupus pathogenesis is those encoding inflammatory cytokines or costimulatory molecules. Deletions or overexpression of genes regulating the TCR or BCR signaling pathway may also lead to a lupuslike syndrome. The genetic manipulations that increase the strength of BCR signaling appear to lead to anti-DNA antibody production by marginal-zone or B1 cells. Recently, a few models of lupus have been developed in which the critical defect in B-cell selection appears to be within the germinal center or in the differentiation to a plasma cell. Deletion of the roquin gene leads to increased expression of ICOS on follicular T-helper cells, enlarged germinal centers, anti-DNA production, and nephritis (70). Mice with a deletion of IBP (IRF4-binding protein) also display enlarged germinal centers and anti-DNA–antibody production (179). Although the enlarged germinal centers in this model suggest that they are the site of dysregulation of B-cell selection, this has not yet been proven. The FcRIIB deletion appears to interfere with a tolerance checkpoint before plasma cell differentiation in both T-independent and T-dependent responses (180). These genetically engineered mice very clearly demonstrate that a multiplicity of pathways of immune selection and activation and a multiplicity of tolerance checkpoints can be implicated in lupus; which of these are most frequently involved in the human disease has not yet been established.

One feature of many mouse models is activation of dendritic cells, sometimes a primary feature of disease and sometimes secondary to ingestion of nucleic acid–containing immune complexes. The proinflammatory milieu created by the presence of stimulatory immune complexes is thought to lead to a continuing expansion in the number of targeted autoantigens. Consistent with this pathophysiology, most murine models display elevated expression of BAFF, probably secondary to TLR signaling in dendritic cells, and BAFF blockade is therapeutic in some murine models of disease (181). Despite this general feature of murine models of lupus, there is as yet no predictable response to deletion of TLRs or to type I IFN blockade, as some models are exacerbated by deletion of a TLR or improved by administration of IFN (182).

Induced Models of Lupus

There are also several induced models of lupus. One model that has been studied extensively is graft-versus-host disease. Injection of some strains with immunocompetent cells of another strain leads to the production of anti-DNA antibodies by host B cells activated by donor T cells. These anti-DNA antibodies cause glomerulonephritis (183). More recently, there has been much interest in pristane-induced lupus. In this model, there appears to be activation of the innate immune response, leading to anti-DNA antibody production (184). There are also antigen-induced models. BALB/c mice immunized with a peptide mimetope of DNA develop antipeptide, anti-DNA cross-reactive antibodies. This response is T-cell–dependent, with antigen-specific T cells displaying a T_H1 pattern of cytokine production (185). Immunization with DNA-binding proteins can also induce anti-DNA antibodies, presumably because a DNA–protein complex forms in vivo and functions in a hapten-carrier fashion (186).

Finally, estradiol and prolactin have been shown to induce autoantibody production in a nonautoimmune BALB/c mouse transgenic for the heavy chain of an anti-DNA antibody. Estradiol alters B-cell selection, permitting high-affinity DNA-reactive B cells that normally undergo deletion to mature to immunocompetence. The altered selection reflects an estrogen-induced decrease in BCR signaling. Prolactin, likewise, leads to the survival of high-affinity DNA-reactive B cells that are normally subject to negative selection, but the effects of prolactin are T-cell–dependent and appear to reflect a prolactin-induced rescue of autoreactive B cells through simultaneous upregulation of CD40 on B cells and CD40L on T cells (52).

Drug-induced lupus in humans can be caused by exposure to a number of drugs, including, most notably, hydralazine and procainamide. One important consequence of hydralazine exposure in mice is decreased DNA methylation, thereby increasing transcription of multiple genes, some of which contribute to B-cell activation. In particular, increased transcription of LFA-1 augments T-cell help to autoreactive B cells; nonautoreactive T cells that overexpress LFA-1 can induce autoantibody production in non-spontaneously autoimmune mice (187).

INFLAMMATORY ARTHRITIS

The inflammatory arthritides share a strong association with MHC haplotype and are manifested clinically by differing patterns of joint involvement and constitutional symptoms that are modulated by age, gender, and ethnicity.

RHEUMATOID ARTHRITIS

RA is a chronic inflammatory disease that targets synovial joints and can be accompanied by significant systemic symptoms and extra-articular manifestations. Disease severity, ranging from mild, nondeforming arthritis to extremely aggressive, destructive, and crippling arthritis, is influenced by an array of genetic, hormonal, and environmental factors. RA has an overall prevalence of 1% in most populations. Several epidemiologic studies using the revised American College of Rheumatology (ACR) criteria for diagnosis have concluded that the most significant risk factors include increasing age, female gender, family history, and smoking. The reported female-to-male ratio in RA ranges from 2:1 to 3:1, with the gender discrepancy being most marked in premenopausal women. Whether this female preponderance is the result of hormonal differences or other sex-associated genetic determinants is not clear; however, in contrast to systemic lupus, use of exogenous estrogen has been reported to decrease the risk of developing RA.

Clinical Manifestations

The diagnosis of RA remains a clinical determination based on the presence of symmetric polyarticular inflammatory arthritis involving the small joints of the hands and feet (excluding the distal interphalangeal joints), continuing over a minimum period of 6 weeks. The presence of morning stiffness lasting for 30 minutes or more associated with the arthritis is quite specific for RA. Joint erosions on plain radiographs are the most specific radiographic feature of RA, heralding an aggressive disease course; however, the sensitivity of radiographs for detecting articular erosions within the first 2 years of disease activity is low. Magnetic resonance imaging (MRI) and joint ultrasound are more sensitive for detecting erosive disease. The most frequent radiographic findings in early disease are soft-tissue swelling and periarticular osteopenia. Joint damage is directly attributable to the presence of destructive proteases and osteoclast-activating cytokines within the synovial tissue. Upregulation of transcription of synovial tissue proteases has been demonstrated within 2 weeks of clinical symptoms. Similarly, MRI studies demonstrate that joint erosions may be present within weeks of the onset of symptoms (188). These observations are consistent with the finding that autoantibodies and elevation of acute-phase reactants can precede onset of symptoms by years, and confirm the presence of checkpoints between autoreactivity and tissue destruction.

Many patients have constitutional complaints of fatigue, myalgias, and occasionally weight loss and fever, consistent with the elevated serum levels of IL-1, IL-6, and TNFα. Extra-articular manifestations such as rheumatoid nodules, interstitial lung disease, and leukocytoclastic vasculitis are associated almost exclusively with the presence of high titers of IgG RF and tend to occur late in the disease.

Patients with RA have increased mortality rates, with life expectancies 10 to 15 years shorter than predicted. This has been attributed to increased susceptibility to infection secondary to the disease itself and to immunosuppressive therapy, gastrointestinal bleeding secondary to therapy, accelerated atherosclerotic heart disease secondary to chronic inflammation, and lymphoproliferative disorders secondary to both the disease itself and to immunosuppressive therapy. Factors that have been associated with poor outcome include the presence of an HLA allele with the shared epitope (HLA-DRB1 haplotype), rheumatoid factor, and rheumatoid nodules (189). Both lupus and RA are associated with an increased incidence of Sjogren syndrome, which, in turn, is associated with an increased incidence of lymphoid malignancy.

Pathogenesis and Genetic Susceptibility

HLA-DRB1 alleles encoding a common amino acid sequence (the shared epitope) in the third variable region of the DRB1 molecule have been identified as the strongest genetic risk factor for RA in patients of Caucasian descent. Apart from this strong association of the MHC-encoded shared epitope with disease susceptibility, several other disease-associated loci have been confirmed using the large North American Rheumatoid Arthritis Cohort (NARAC) (190). These include the PTPN22 polymorphism also found in SLE, the CTLA4 CT60 allele also found in type 1 diabetes, and peptidylarginine deiminase 4 (see below). CTLA-4 is upregulated on the surface of $CD4^+$ T cells following T-cell activation and outcompetes CD28 for B7 binding. CTLA4 engagement on T cells leads to inhibition of effector function. The CT60 CTLA-4 autoimmune disease–associated polymorphism has been reported to result in decreased production of soluble CTLA-4, which may act as an endogenous inhibitor of T-cell activation (3).

Synovial Architecture

Pathogenesis involves the activation of resident cells within the joint in addition to the influx of inflammatory cells in response to chemoattractants. The normal synovial membrane consists of a continuous surface of connective tissue. The intimal or lining layer is populated by two cell types; a bone marrow–derived synoviocyte with macrophagelike properties (type A) and a mesenchymal fibroblastlike synoviocyte (type B). The subintimal layer is composed of numerous blood vessels and connective tissue fibroblasts. Synovial tissue extracellular matrix is composed of a loose structure of large amounts of hyaluronan along with collagen (types III, IV, V, VI), laminin, fibronectin, and proteoglycan.

The hallmarks of synovial abnormalities in RA include microvasculature damage, synovial-lining hyperplasia, neoangiogenesis, and an inflammatory cell infiltrate of lymphocytes, macrophages, and neutrophils (191). Although the relative importance of each of these cell types is controversial, it is likely that all contribute to the synovial lesion in RA. Three patterns of lymphoid organization in rheumatoid synovial tissue have been described: (a) ectopic germinal-center arrangement with T and B cells surrounding a network of dendritic cells; (b) aggregates of T and B cells without dendritic cells and without germinal centers; and (c) T and B cells diffusely infiltrating the stroma. A very few patients will have a form of granulomatous synovitis that histologically resembles rheumatoid nodules. The organization of synovial tissue into ectopic lymphoid structures may provide advantageous conditions for antigen presentation and subsequent cellular activation.

Synovial tissues containing germinal centers produce the highest amount of IgG (192). Lymphotoxin β (LT-β) and CXCL13 (BLC) production also correlates with germinal-center structures. Interestingly, the mantle zones of these germinal centers also contain IFNγ-producing $CD8^+$ T cells, and depletion of these cells causes disintegration of the germinal centers, decreased production of lymphotoxin β, and cessation of immunoglobulin secretion. SCID mice engrafted with germinal center–containing synovial tissue and exposed to BAFF and APRIL blockade mediated by TACI-Ig showed a marked decrease in T-cell and dendritic cell activation and IgG production, supporting the hypothesis that B cells also sustain the activation of T cells and dendritic cells. Conversely, BAFF and APRIL blockade in SCID mice engrafted with the aggregate and diffuse forms of synovitis result in enhanced IFNγ production and T-cell activation. These data suggest the potential influence of synovial architecture in response to immunobiologic therapies.

Fibroblastlike synoviocyte proliferation occurs early in the disease process (193). Proliferation and activation of synoviocytes are early features of the rheumatoid synovial membrane, known as pannus, that extends to the cartilage and erodes periarticular bone at the margin between synovium and bone. Upregulation of the adhesion molecules VCAM-1 and integrin $\alpha(v)\beta(3)$ on activated fibroblastlike synoviocytes allows these cells to adhere to the extracellular matrix of articular cartilage and triggers intracellular signaling cascades that lead to proliferation and escape from contact inhibition. Activation of synoviocytes leads to increased production of matrix metalloproteinases (MMPS), whose potent catalytic activity is normally kept under control by endogenous inhibitors of MMPs (TIMPS). TNFα and IL-1 induce MMPs, but TNFα-independent pathways of synoviocyte activation also exist, perhaps providing an explanation for the 30% to 40% of RA patients who fail to respond to TNF blockade. Other destructive enzymes released by activated fibroblastlike synoviocytes include cathepsins B, L, and K.

Synovial fibroblasts stimulated with IL-1 and TLR-2 ligand demonstrate increased production of IL-5, MMPs, and chemokines, and several studies have now documented increased expression of TLR-2, -3, -4, and -7 and their ligands in fibroblasts and macrophages in the synovial lining of rheumatoid joints (194). Stimulation of rheumatoid dendritic cells with HSPB8, a heat-shock protein that is an endogenous ligand for TLR4, results in activation and secretion of IL-6, TNFα, and several chemokines (194). The recent finding that a functional polymorphism of TLR 2 significantly associates with susceptibility to RA in a Korean population adds to the growing appreciation of the importance of TLR signaling in this disease (195).

Autoantibodies

Although immunization with type II collagen, the cartilage protein gp39, and proteoglycans induce arthritis in animal models, and patients with RA may have antibodies that are reactive with these proteins, evidence that these molecules are inciting antigens in human disease is not strong. Several groups have demonstrated oligoclonal B-cell populations in the rheumatoid synovium with a more restricted B-cell repertoire in the synovium than in the blood (196). The identification of persistent B-cell clones in synovial fluid from patients obtained at different times is also consistent with the theory of clonal B-cell expansion. However, most autoantibodies commonly seen in RA, in particular RF and antibodies to citrullinated proteins, are directed against ubiquitous antigens and are not joint-specific.

RF, an antibody directed against the Fc portion of IgG, remains the major laboratory finding in RA and is present in approximately 70% of patients (197). RFs are polyclonal antibodies of predominantly IgM isotype; IgG and IgA RF correlate more with aggressive disease. The "natural" low-affinity RF produced by $CD5^+$ B cells found in healthy individuals and a variety of chronic infections, inflammatory conditions, malignancies, organ transplants, and pregnancy are germline-encoded polyreactive IgM antibodies (198). In RA, the RF is high-affinity, monoreactive, and somatically mutated, and may be produced by B cells within the synovium. Furthermore, RF displays higher-affinity binding to agalactosyl IgG, which is enhanced in active disease. Deposition of immune complexes containing RF in cartilage and vasculitic lesions appears to contribute to local inflammatory changes through activation of the complement cascade and NK-cell activation. RF-positive patients have a worse prognosis, but joint histology in patients lacking RF is not obviously different than in patients who have RF.

Antibodies directed against cyclic citrullinated proteins (anti-CCP) display equal sensitivity and higher specificity for RA. Citrullinated peptides are have been identified in synovium from patients with RA, osteoarthritis, and psoriatic arthritis, but the presence of anti-CCP antibodies either in the serum or synovial fluid appears to be restricted to RA. Citrullination of proteins including fibrin, vimentin, and histones is mediated by peptidylarginine deaminases. PAD14, a peptidylarginine deiminase, has been identified as an RA-susceptibility gene (190), and citrullinated peptides have been shown to bind with high affinity to the HLA-DRB1 0401 shared epitope allele that is associated with disease (199). It has recently been demonstrated in an animal model of collagen-induced arthritis that anti-CCP antibodies bind to inflamed synovial tissue, thereby enhancing joint inflammation and damage (200). Furthermore, citrullination of proteins is enhanced in inflamed joints and is a hallmark of stressed and proapoptotic cells; therefore, both RF and anti-CCP autoantibodies appear to contribute to the synovial lesions in RA, and both are predictive of aggressive disease. Interestingly, smoking, a risk factor for disease, increases the density of citrullinated proteins in lung epithelial cells.

Both RF and anti-CCP antibodies have been shown to appear in the serum years before onset of clinical disease. Patients show significantly higher percentages of autoreactive B cells in both the new emigrant and mature naïve B-cell compartments compared to healthy controls, and 10% to 20% of these express RF or anti-CCP antibodies (198).

An excess of V*k*J*k*1 light-chain rearrangements in new emigrant B cells in some patients suggests premature termination of secondary recombination and impaired receptor editing, whereas other new emigrant B cells show evidence of a failure to downregulate recombination events. Patients who do not show evidence of defective secondary recombination may display unusually long *k* chains containing 11 or more amino acids in CDR3, suggesting aberrant regulation of deoxynucleotidyl transferase (TdT) (198).

Because of the therapeutic focus on macrophage activation and secretion of TNF and IL-1β and the absence of identified autoantibodies in approximately 30% of patients, B cells were considered for a long time to be peripheral players in pathogenesis. However, recent studies have highlighted a potential role of B cells in rheumatoid synovium other than autoantibody production (192). One of the most clinically compelling arguments for B-cell involvement in RA is the surprising efficacy of rituximab, an anti-CD20 chimeric B-cell–depleting antibody (201). Interestingly, rituximab often displays clinical efficacy before altering serum titers of RF, implying a potential role for B cells in antigen presentation and cytokine production.

T Cells

The strong association between specific HLA haplotypes and disease susceptibility has led to a T-cell–centric model of disease. However, numerous studies attempting to define the antigenic specificity of infiltrating oligoclonal T cells in rheumatoid synovium failed to demonstrate consistent results. Despite the failure to isolate oligoclonal T-cell populations in joints, the HLA-DRB1 shared epitope association remains a powerful susceptibility determinant.

The T cell has recently become the focus of studies linking RA to premature immune senescence (102). Aging T cells lose surface expression of CD28 and are no longer able to upregulate CD40L on their surface; without the obligate costimulatory molecules, they function poorly in MHC class II–restricted interactions. With age, T cells also acquire surface expression of the stimulatory killer immunoglobulinlike receptors (KIRs) and NKG2D that normally regulate activation of NK cells. The finding that RA patients have increased numbers of circulating $CD4^+CD28^-$ T cells with shortened telomeres suggests a senescent $CD4^+CD28^-$ profile. T cells expressing KIR receptors have also been identified in rheumatoid synovium, and an allele of KIR2DS2, one of the stimulatory KIR receptors on $CD28^-$ T cells, has been identified as a risk factor for disease (202). Furthermore, the number of $CD4^+CD28^-$ cells in patients correlates with the presence of extra-articular manifestations, erosive disease, and the risk of atherosclerotic complications of disease (102), and reversal of the T-cell phenotype has been observed in individuals treated with TNFα blockade. Synoviocytes express fractaline, which binds to CX3CR1 present on senescent T cells. Engagement of CX3CR1 by fractalkine results in IFNγ and TNFα secretion, thereby promoting ongoing T-cell activation and inflammation. Thus, it is possible that senescent T cells are particularly responsive to stimuli from the synovium, although they are less responsive to antigen-specific stimuli.

Antigen Exposure

The role of HLA class II molecules has been intensively studied in RA because of the compelling data showing that the shared epitope constitutes a major risk factor for disease susceptibility (203). Interestingly, homozygosity for the shared epitope confers greater risk than heterozygosity, arguing against the hypothesis that disease-related class II molecules are critical in presenting certain self-peptides to CD4$^+$ T cells. Rather, it has been speculated that the shared epitope itself may be immunogenic and homologous sequences have been identified in both bacterial and viral proteins. The exact role of the predisposing class II molecules remains unclear, because no dominant self peptides have been recovered from class II molecules in rheumatoid synovial tissue and no search for virus or bacteria has demonstrated an infectious etiology.

Cytokines

TNFα and IL-1 are potent proinflammatory cytokines secreted by macrophages, and both stimulate fibroblastlike synoviocytes to proliferate and secrete IL-6, IL-8, GM-CSF, FGF, and MMPs (204). They also act to induce adhesion molecules such as VCAM-1 and E-selection on endothelial cells, thereby contributing to endothelial-cell activation and diapedesis of additional leukocytes to sites of inflammation. TNFα, IL-8, and VEGF also promote angiogenesis, a feature of rheumatoid synovium.

Osteoclast differentiation and activation result from the binding of RANK (receptor activator of nuclear-receptor factor NFκB) to its ligand, RANKL. The relative expressions of RANK, RANKL, and osteoprotegerin (OPG), a molecule that competitively binds RANKL and thus prevents osteoclast activation, determines the amount of bone resorption at a given site. Rheumatoid joint tissue has been shown to contain increased amounts of RANKL and decreased amounts of OPG. TNFα, IL-1, and M-CSF are capable of acting directly on osteoclast precursors to promote osteoclast differentiation or indirectly by modulating RANKL and OPG expression (205).

New Therapeutic Approaches

Better understanding of the cytokines and effector molecules in rheumatoid synovium has led to the development of a number of biologic agents that selectively target pathways of disease. Clinical responses to these therapies continue to inform us about the complex interactions in the immune system. Early biologic therapies targeting CD4 cells depleted CD4 cells in the peripheral blood but had less effect on activated and synovial T-cell populations and disappointingly little effect on disease course. In contrast, the revolutionary success of TNFα blockade for RA, and more recently, blockade of IL-6, is testimony to the fact that control of inflammatory mediators, regardless of the inciting triggers in disease pathogenesis, can provide effective treatment for this disease. Recently, the role of the adaptive immune system has been re-established with the demonstrated efficacy of CTLA-4Ig and B-cell depletion (rituximab) as treatment modalities, and additional B-cell–targeted therapies are under investigation. Blockade of RANK and RANKL has been shown to prevent bone loss in inflammatory arthritis in rodents but has not yet been used in rheumatoid arthritis.

Mouse Models of RA

Although multiple strains of mice display the spontaneous production of anti-DNA antibodies and a lupuslike disease, there are fewer spontaneous rodent models of RA (206). The MRL/lpr mouse strain, which spontaneously develops lupus, also develops an inflammatory arthritis with pannus formation and synovial proliferation. This strain may develop serologic features of RA, with both IgM and IgG RF and antibody to citrullinated peptides; it also displays an increase in a galactosyl IgG that appears to be independent of the development of arthritis (184). This coexistence of both diseases in a genetically susceptible host is of interest because lupus patients may also develop an erosive arthritis with the antibody specificities and histologic features that are present in classical RA, and some genes predisposing to RA also predispose to lupus.

More recently, inbred recombinant strains derived from C57Bl/6 and DBA/2 mice have been demonstrated to develop a rheumatoidlike arthritis. The genetic basis for this susceptibility is currently under investigation. Interestingly, female mice are predominantly affected, consistent with the 2:1 female:male incidence observed in the human disease.

In addition, genetically manipulated mice develop a rheumatoidlike disease. Mice deficient in the inhibitory receptor for IL-1, IL1Ra, will spontaneously develop inflammatory arthritis, demonstrating the critical role of IL-1 in disease pathogenesis and providing a rational for the therapeutic targeting of IL-1. As is the case in essentially all autoimmune diseases, this genetic manipulation leads to disease only in certain strains.

Similarly, mice that overexpress TNFα will develop an inflammatory arthritis with bone erosions, reinforcing the importance of TNFα in joint destruction in RA. Mice that are deficient in Zap 70 also spontaneously develop an inflammatory arthritis. The pathogenesis in this model appears to reflect a failure in thymic tolerance mechanisms and the maturation to immunocompetence of autoreactive T cells (207).

Susceptible strains of both rat and mouse will develop an inflammatory arthritis after systemic administration of pristane or incomplete Freund adjuvant (206). This observation raises the possibility that activation of the innate immune system can lead to a non–antigen-specific inflammation localized to joints, and suggests that inhibition of TLR signaling may be of clinical benefit. In fact, hydroxychloroquine, which impedes signaling by intracellular TLRs, is an effective treatment modality. Furthermore, speculation continues regarding a relationship between RA and microbial exposure. An inciting role for microbial exposure in RA is exemplified by the streptococcal cell-wall model of disease. The bacterial peptidoglycan activates the innate immune system, triggering an inflammatory cascade that subsequently requires T-cell activation for transformation from a self-limited arthritis into a chronic inflammatory disease (208).

Injection of mycobacterium into skin or footpads causes arthritis in rats. The rat model of adjuvant-induced arthritis has been exploited extensively in studies of effector mechanisms in joint destruction, and the model has been critical in suggesting a role for heat-shock proteins (HSP) in RA pathogenesis. T cells reactive with a heat-shock protein, HSP65, can transfer disease to a syngeneic host, and prior immunization with HSP65 will prevent development of arthritis, apparently through the activation of regulatory T cells (209). Despite this, neonatal thymectomy does not offer disease protection, although it abrogates T-cell responses to protein antigens

Certain strains of rat and mouse immunized with type II collagen also develop an inflammatory joint disease (210). This model is dependent on both T- and B-cell activation and has excited significant interest because of the presence of collagen-reactive T and B cells in some patients with RA. In this model, T_H1 cells producing IFNγ are not critical to disease; rather, T_H17 cells are central to joint destruction (211). Moreover, a deficiency of IFNγ leads to enhanced disease in this model, perhaps reflecting the IFNγ-mediated inhibition of T_H17 cells. The role of the DR4 shared epitope has also been addressed in the collagen-induced model of disease. Mice transgenic for either a DR4 or DQ8 susceptibility allele develop accelerated and aggressive disease in response to collagen immunization (212); yet, as discussed previously, the role of collagen as an inciting antigen in human disease remains unproven.

Interestingly, immunization with a joint-specific antigen is not always necessary for the induction of inflammatory arthritis. Mouse strains that develop an inflammatory arthritis after immunization with type II collagen develop a similar histopathology after immunization with ovalbumin or bovine serum albumin. In mice expressing human DR-susceptibility alleles, antibody to the inciting antigen is critical for the development of arthritis.

The role of antibody in disease initiation has been elegantly studied in the KRN model of RA. Mice with a transgene-encoded T-cell receptor specific for glucose 6-phosphate isomerase (GPl) develop a RA-like disease (213). Passive transfer of anti-GPI antibody leads to joint edema and inflammation. The antibody, directed to a ubiquitous antigen, forms immune complexes that lead to mast-cell and neutrophil degranulation, and vascular permeability within the joint. The immune complexes initiate an inflammatory response through activation of the alternate pathway of complement and engagement of activating Fc receptors. It has been speculated that the inflammatory process occurs unabated in the joint because of the absence of inhibitors of the complement cascade on the surface of cartilage. Progression to chronic inflammation requires T-cell activation, but an acute inflammatory response occurs with immune complexes alone. Indeed, it appears that a similar mechanism of acute joint inflammation is responsible for the arthritis that can accompany many infectious processes and serum sickness.

Once an inflammatory reaction is initiated in the joint, there is increased citrullination of proteins locally, providing the host with a novel antigen presented in a proinflammatory milieu and providing a substrate for binding of anti-CCP antibody and the initiation or persistence of an inflammatory response (200). The contribution of T cells to histopathology is, in part, a result of their production of RANKL, which is critical in the conversion of blood-borne monocytes to bone-resorbing osteoclasts. Furthermore, all these models identify a critical role for TNFα in activating the RANK/RANKL pathway (214). These observations suggest that a rheumatoidlike histopathology in the joint may be a common final pathway that can be initiated by both antigen-specific and antigen-nonspecific exposures. These models also suggest an important role for antibody in the inductive phase of joint inflammation, consistent with the known existence of anti-CCP antibodies and RF before disease onset and a requirement for T-cell activation for progression to chronic inflammation. The actual diversity of triggers for RA in the human population is not known. So far, effective immunomodulatory therapies in RA have focused on the innate immune system and effector mechanisms, although the success of both B-cell depletion (anti-CD20) and T-cell blockade (CTLA-4Ig) suggests that blockade of the adaptive immune system will also provide benefit.

REACTIVE ARTHRITIS

The seronegative inflammatory spondyloarthropathies include reactive arthritis, ankylosing spondylitis, psoriatic arthritis, and arthritis associated with inflammatory bowel disease. All of these arthropathies are characterized clinically by spinal and peripheral joint oligoarthritis, enthesitis (inflammation of the attachment of tendons to bone), and occasional involvement of ocular, mucocutaneous, and cardiac tissues. Reactive arthritis (ReA), also referred to as Reiter syndrome, has been selected for review in this chapter as an inflammatory arthritis with a clear genetic association and known bacterial triggers.

Clinical Manifestations

ReA was originally described as a sterile arthritis and enthesitis initiated by an infection distant from the involved joints. However, subsequent findings of viable persistent organisms and bacterial fragments in synovial tissue many years after the clinical initial infection have made this definition obsolete. The term ReA is currently used for a spectrum of clinical manifestations (arthritis, urethritis, conjunctivitis) following an infectious episode. In developed countries, ReA most frequently follows urogenital infections with *Chlamydia trachomatis;* in underdeveloped countries, ReA follows intestinal infections. *Salmonella (typhimurium* and *enteritidis)*, *Shigella*, *Campylobacter jejuni*, and *Yersinia enterocolitica* are the most common triggers for postdysenteric ReA. All of these pathogenic strains are obligate intracellular organisms, and all contain LPS in their outer membrane. The prevalence of ReA is modulated by frequency of the HLA-B27 haplotype in a given population as well as by bacterial exposure. Overall prevalence is reported as 1/1,000. A distinct male predilection with a male-to-female ratio of 9:1 in ReA following genitourinary infection may be represent an ascertainment bias, as there is no gender difference in prevalence of ReA secondary to enteric infections.

Clinical manifestations usually begin 2 to 4 weeks after the triggering infection. Classic musculoskeletal symptoms are an acute, asymmetric oligoarthritis with a predilection for the sacroiliac joints, knees, ankles, and feet. Joint fluid findings are consistent with an inflammatory process, and bacterial organisms cannot be grown using routine cultures. Constitutional signs and symptoms are not common features of this disease, and extra-articular manifestations are rare. Although most patients with ReA recover completely within 6 to 12 months, some (15%) will have a relapsing, progressive course. The majority of patients who develop a chronic course and have extra-articular manifestations are HLA-B27–positive, highlighting the importance of this genotype for disease severity as well as susceptibility.

Pathogenesis and Genetic Susceptibility

Initial hypotheses regarding pathogenesis focused on the role of HLA-B27 as an antigen-presenting molecule and molecular mimicry between bacterial and self-peptides. The finding of HLA-B27–restricted T-cell responses to bacterial antigens from *Chlamydia* and *Klebsiella* and B27-restricted epitopes derived from human aggrecanase support this theory (215). A recent comparative analysis of T-cell receptor (TCR) CDR3 sequences from synovial fluid $CD8^+$ T cells found a conserved motif in 12 patients infected with four types of enteric bacteria, suggesting the presence of a ubiquitous immunodominant antigen (216). However, the lack of $CD8^+$ T-cell involvement in rodent models transgenic for B27 does not support this model.

An alternative theory that has recently been proposed suggests that the unusually slow folding rate of the B27 polypeptide promotes the generation of misfolded molecules that accumulate in the endoplasmic reticulum leading to a proinflammatory "unfolded protein response" (217). Another consequence of the unique structure of B27 may be the formation of surface homodimers leading to increased immunogenicity. A recent study found significantly higher levels of homodimer expression in ReA patients compared to HLA-B27–positive controls and increased expression of homodimers on cells of B27–positive patients following LPS stimulation (218).

It is important to note that HLA-B27 constitutes only part of overall risk for development of ReA. Less than 5% of HLA-B27–positive individuals develop one of the B27-associated diseases. Functional polymorphisms in genes for IL-10 and TNFα have been linked to susceptibility for ReA in some populations, and longitudinal analysis of ReA patients has shown that low secretion of TNFα by circulating T lymphocytes at onset of arthritis is predictive of a chronic course. Furthermore, IL-10 is upregulated in synovial tissue from patients with chronic ReA, whereas levels of TNFα and IFNγ mRNA are decreased (219). Two pilot studies of TNFα inhibition with in ReA failed to show benefit, consistent with these data.

Role of Infection

Intact antigens from *Chlamydia, Yersinia,* and *Salmonella* have been demonstrated in synovial tissue and fluid years after initial infection in patients with ReA. Furthermore, detection of bacterial RNA by polymerase chain-reaction assays have established the presence of viable, albeit noncultivable, *Chlamydia* organisms in synovial tissue in several studies (220). These findings, together with T-cell proliferation in response to the infectious agents, suggest that there is impaired ability to eliminate triggering bacteria in patients with ReA. In vitro studies indicate that HLA-B27–expressing monocytes have an impaired ability to control intracellular replication of *Salmonella*. Interestingly, intracellular, viable, nonreplicating *Chlamydia* within monocytes isolated from synovial fluid and tissue of ReA patients show an aberrant phenotype characterized by downregulation of outer membrane protein (omp-1) genes and upregulation of HSP 60 genes, which encode a highly immunogenic protein that may account for the inflammatory response to persistent *Chlamydia* (221).

Mouse Models of Spondylarthritis and ReA

Because of the salience of B27 as a susceptibility factor for spondylarthritis and ReA, rodents transgenic for B27 and human $\beta 2$ microglobulin have been generated (222). Rats expressing these transgenes develop arthritis, spondylitis, skin lesions, and colitis. Unfortunately, the model has not resolved whether the disease is characterized by an unfolded protein response or by an antigen-specific response. On the one hand, microarray data demonstrate an unfolded protein signature in lesional tissue (223); on the other hand, disease can be transferred by T cells (224). One hypothesis that allows for the coexistence of both pathogenetic mechanisms involves the presentation of enterobacteria-derived peptides by B27 molecules to T cells that cross-react with a peptide from a joint-specific protein. This model is consistent with the attenuated disease that occurs when B27 transgenic animals are bred in germ-free conditions.

VASCULITIS

The primary systemic vasculitides are a heterogenous group of frequently devastating diseases, renowned for their diversity of clinical manifestations that make classification schemes based on clinical and histologic data extremely difficult. Other than the well-known association between some of the medium- to small-vessel vasculitides and antineutrophilic cytoplasmic autoantibodies (ANCA), there are no known specific serologic markers for these diseases. The currently accepted classification scheme is based on vessel size.

Large-vessel Vasculitis

The large-vessel vasculitides include giant-cell arteritis (GCA) (also known as temporal arteritis) and Takayasu Arteritis (TA).

Clinical Manifestations

GCA is a disease of the elderly with few, if any, well-documented cases in individuals under the age of 50 years. The incidence of GCA is reported as 7 to 33/100,000, with highest rates seen in Northern Europe; the disease is rare in black and Hispanic populations. GCA is frequently dominated by constitutional symptoms such as malaise, fever, weight loss, stiffness of the shoulder and pelvic girdle muscles, and depression. Laboratory testing generally reveals a normochromic, normocytic anemia and markedly elevated levels of acute-phase reactants including CRP and IL-6. Localized symptoms suggestive of tissue ischemia include loss of vision, jaw claudication, and temporal artery tenderness.

GCA targets certain vascular beds while sparing others with remarkable regularity. The most likely sites of vascular involvement are the second to fifth branches of the aorta and the thoracic aorta. Diagnosis is made on the basis of a temporal artery biopsy that reveals panarteritis with mononuclear cells arranged in granulomatous infiltrates throughout the vessel wall.

In contrast, TA is a disease of young women, with a female-to-male ratio of 8 to 9:1 and an estimated incidence of 2.6 per million. The disease appears to be more common in Asian women. The vascular lesions in TA target the subclavian and carotid arteries most commonly, although there is some evidence that vascular distribution is modulated by ethnicity (225).

Pathogenesis

GCA and TA may be histologically indistinguishable. Importantly, both diseases involve only large elastic arteries that have well-developed layers, including the intima, internal elastic lamina, tunica media, external elastic lamina, and adventitia. Arterial damage occurs in response to granulomatous inflammation and takes the form of neointimal proliferation and vessel occlusion rather that arterial wall destruction, aneurism formation, and hemorrhage. Mechanistic studies of large-vessel vasculitis have focused on GCA because temporal artery biopsies are easily obtainable.

The role of adaptive immune response in GCA is supported by its association with HLA-DR4 and the presence of $CD4^+$ T cells in the inflammatory infiltrates (226). Clonally expanded, activated $CD4^+$ T cells are centered in the adventitial layer and produce abundant amounts of IFNγ. Removal of T cells from temporal artery biopsies engrafted into SCID mice results in resolution of the vasculitic lesions, and adoptive transfer of tissue-derived T cells accelerates the inflammatory response (227).

The finding of large numbers of activated dendritic cells (DCs) in the media and adventitia in temporal artery biopsies from GCA patients has led to the speculation that these DCs are responsible for T-cell recruitment and initiation of the granulomatous inflammatory response. Phenotypically, these are myeloid dendritic cells; their depletion abrogates arteritis in SCID mice transplanted with GCA arteries (228). Activated macrophages reside mostly in the tunica media of the GCA lesion, where they form granulomatous infiltrates along the media–intima border, releasing matrix metalloproteinases (MMPs) and reactive oxygen intermediates that promote tissue destruction and disruption of the elastic lamina.

Medium- and Small-sized-vessel Vasculitis

Unlike the chronic granulomatous infiltrates seen in large-vessel vasculitis, the small- and medium-sized-vessel vasculitides are characterized by a necrotizing infiltrate in the vessel wall. In contrast to the model proposed for the large-vessel vasculitides, in which the immunologic injury is thought to occur in the adventitia, the inflammatory process is initiated on the luminal side of the vessel. This chapter will focus on ANCA-associated vasculitis.

ANCA-Associated Vasculitis

Three forms of ANCA-associated vasculitis have been identified: Wegeners granulomatosis (WG), Churg-Strauss syndrome (CSS), and microscopic polyangiitis (MPA). These are rare entities; a population-based study in England reported incidences of 8.5, 3.6, and 2.4 per million for WG, MPA, and CSS, respectively (229). Disease onset typically occurs in the fifth decade and there is a slight gender difference, with a male-to-female ratio of 2:1. Clinical features overlap substantially. Classically, WG patients demonstrate involvement of the upper airway and ears, lungs, and kidneys. MPA classically presents as a pulmonary-renal syndrome with pulmonary capillaritis and glomerulonephritis. Of the three, CSS is perhaps the easiest to distinguish because of the characteristic eosinophilia and obligatory history of allergic rhinitis and progressive asthma. Coronary arteritis and myocarditis secondary to eosinophilic infiltrates are a leading cause of morbidity and mortality in CSS, but are rarely seen in WG or MPA.

Role of ANCA in Disease Pathogenesis

The major antigenic specificities for ANCA are proteinase 3 (PR3), also known as cANCA because of the diffuse cytoplasmic staining pattern on immunofluorescence studies, and myeloperoxidase (MPO), also known as pANCA because of its perinuclear immunofluorescence pattern (230). PR3 is a serine proteinase located in azurophilic granules of neutrophils and lysosomes of monocytes, but also found on the surface of resting neutrophils. The amount of surface PR3 appears to be genetically determined, and increased expression is associated with an increased risk of disease. MPO localizes to the same intracellular compartments as PR3 but does not appear to be displayed on the surface of resting neutrophils (231). Generally, anti-PR3 antibodies associate with WG, and anti-MPO antibodies associate with MPA and CSS.

Currently, clinical, in vitro, in vivo, and animal model data support, but do not prove, a pathogenic role for ANCA (230). Multiple studies demonstrate that both PR3 and MPO ANCA are capable of activating neutrophils primed with TNFα, GM-CSF, or microbial products in vitro to degranulate, release IL-1β, IL-8, and reactive-oxygen free radicals. ANCA IgG has also been shown to stabilize adhesion of neutrophils to cultured endothelial cells, by inducing a conformational change in β2 integrins on the neutrophil surface.

Passive transfer of anti-MPO IgG derived from MPO knockout mice immunized with mouse MPO to both immune-competent and Rag2$^{-/-}$ mice results in glomerulonephritis and small-vessel vasculitis that is histologically similar to human ANCA-mediated disease, indicating that antigen-specific T cells are not required to induce the acute injury (232). However, neutrophil depletion in recipient mice completely abrogated the induction of vasculitis and glomerulonephritis (233). Although these data support a pathogenic, contributory role for ANCA, there is still no explanation for the development of ANCA. In addition, the clinical utility of ANCA titers in predicting disease flares is limited.

Treatment

Corticosteroids and cytotoxic agents constitute the current treatment strategies for the systemic vasculitides. Antibiotic therapy helps maintain remission in WG, probably through anti-inflammatory rather than microbial effects. TNF blockade has failed to show benefit in WG and in fact resulted in an increased risk of solid-tumor development (234).

SCLERODERMA

Scleroderma (systemic sclerosis; SSc) is an autoimmune disease characterized by microvascular injury, autoantibody production, and excessive collagen deposition leading to progressive cutaneous and visceral fibrosis.

Clinical Manifestations

Reports on the incidence and prevalence of SSc vary widely and appear to be heavily influenced by ethnicity and geography. The highest overall prevalence rates of 276 cases per million adults are reported in the United States, with African-Americans affected more commonly and more severely than Caucasians. An apparent increase in prevalence since 1950 may reflect a true increase, ascertainment differences, or improved survival and earlier diagnosis. Women are at higher risk of developing disease than men, with reported femal-to-male ratios of 3 to 8:1. The mean age at diagnosis tends to be in the fourth to fifth decade for Caucasian women and in the third or fourth decade for African-American women.

The two major disease subsets, diffuse cutaneous SSc (dcSSc) and limited cutaneous SSc (lcSSC), are distinguished by the extent of skin involvement. dcSSc is defined by the presence of skin thickening proximal to the elbows and knees and/or involving the torso, whereas lc SSc is characterized by skin thickening distal to the elbows and knees. Facial involvement does not distinguish between the two major disease subtypes. Defining and assigning

TABLE 41.5 Scleroderma-Specific Autoantibodies

Disease Subset	Autoantibody	HLA Association	Frequency (%)
dcSSc	Antitopoisomerase 1 (Scl-70)	DRB1*1101, *1104 DPB1*1301	10–20
	Anti-RNA-polymerase I, III		20
dcSSc and lcSSc	Anti-U-3 RNP (antifibrillarin)		5–20
	Anti-PM/Scl		3
lcSSc	Anticentromere	DRB1*01, *04 DQB1*05	20–30
	Anti-Th/To	DRB1*11	2–5
	Anti-U-1 RNP		

dcSSc, diffuse cutaneous scleroderma; lcSSc, limited cutaneous scleroderma.

individual patients to disease subsets is clinically extremely useful; dcSSC is more aggressive and is commonly associated with internal-organ involvement, whereas limited disease is more indolent but more often associated with pulmonary hypertension.

Pathogenesis and Genetic Susceptibility

Strong evidence for a genetic basis for susceptibility comes from the increased familial clustering of disease. As seen in SLE, while several studies have yielded only a very modest disease association with HLA haplotypes, the associations are much more pronounced and significant between HLA subsets and autoantibodies (Table 41.5) (235). Similarly, although the concordance for the clinical phenotype between monozygotic and dizygotic twins is the same (approximately 5%), the concordance rate for antinuclear antibodies is much higher in monozygotic (95%) compared to dizygotic twins (60%) (236). It is generally felt that SSc is triggered by an environmental insult to the susceptible host, and many infectious and chemical agents have been implicated in disease development. Geographic clusters of SSc provide strong evidence for environmental triggers (237).

Autoantibodies and Immune Dysregulation

ANA are found in more than 95% of SSc patients, and a number of scleroderma-specific autoantibodies that associate strongly with disease subsets have been identified (238). Although these autoantibodies are highly specific for SSc, biopsies of involved tissue are remarkable for the paucity of antibody or immune-complex deposition, and there is currently little data to support a causal role of these autoantibodies in disease pathogenesis.

The activated $CD4^+$ T cells in SSc skin are skewed toward a Th2 phenotype with increased production of profibrotic cytokines, IL-4, -5, -6, -8, -10, and -13 (239). Although the cutaneous $CD4^+$ T-cell infiltrate has been shown to be oligoclonal, suggestive of an antigen-driven response, no inciting antigen has been elucidated.

Collagen Synthesis

SSc fibroblasts explanted from involved tissue demonstrate unique abilities to continue producing extracellular matrix components after serial passages in vitro. TGFβ, one of the most potent inducers of collagen and proteoglycan production, appears to be essential to the sclerosing process in SSc for the following reasons: (a) SSc fibroblasts have an increased expression of TGFβ receptors and therefore may be more sensitive to stimulatory effects of TGFβ; (b) there are increased plasma levels of TGFβ; and (c) TGFβ is present in early skin lesions, before collagen deposition (240,241).

Recent evidence suggests an antibody-mediated mechanism for fibroblast proliferation and collagen gene expression. Serum from SSc patients contains antibodies directed against the platelet-derived growth receptor (PDGFR) (242). Ligation of PDGFRs trigger an intracellular signaling pathway that leads to increased collagen gene expression. These studies are the first to directly imply a causal role of autoantibodies in tissue fibrosis in SSc.

New Therapeutic Approaches

The treatment of scleroderma remains difficult, and there are few effective options for the skin disease or the inflammatory lung disease. A recent blinded study of cyclophosphamide for the treatment of alveolitis yielded marginal results, consistent with previous data suggesting that anti-inflammatory and immunosuppressive agents are of limited use in SSc, perhaps reflecting the fibrotic rather than inflammatory pathology. Disappointingly, a recent Phase II clinical trial of an anti-TGFβ reagent in early scleroderma showed no efficacy and more adverse events in the treatment group (243), indicating that TGFβ blockade alone is insufficient to halt the fibrotic process. Recently, imatinib mesylate, an inhibitor of PDGF, has been shown to reverse pulmonary hypertension in animal models (244), and a few case reports have suggested efficacy in humans.

Mouse Models of Scleroderma

There are several interesting rodent models of scleroderma, all of which suggest the centrality of TGFβ in this disease. The tight skin mouse (tsk) displays intradermal collagen deposition, autoimmunity, and vascular abnormalities. The genetic defect is a duplication of the fibrillin gene (245). Homozygosity of this duplication is an embryonic lethal mutation. Although the tsk mouse makes several of the autoantibodies that are present in patients with scleroderma, these antibodies are not crucial to disease pathogenesis. B cells, however, are critical, as CD19-deficient tsk mice display a marked attenuation of collagen deposition (246). Further genetic analyses of this strain have shown that tsk mice deficient in one or both copies of the IL-4 gene also have a markedly reduced disease phenotype, reflecting the impact of IL-4 on TGFβ transcription (247).

The bleomycin-induced model of scleroderma displays primarily an interstitial lung disease when bleomycin is administered by an intratracheal route and dermal fibrosis when bleomycin is administered subcutaneously. The disease phenotype is exaggerated in TNF-receptor–deficient mice, presumably because a TNFα-mediated pathway is responsible for collagen degradation and restoration of more normal extracellular matrix composition following the initial inflammatory response (248,249).

The skin changes of scleroderma are similar to those seen in graft-versus-host disease; not surprisingly, therefore, transfer of spleen cells to irradiated or RAG-deficient hosts has also been exploited as a model of scleroderma. The transfer of B10D2 splenocytes to RAG-deficient mice results not only in dermal and visceral fibrosis but also in the production of antibodies to Scl-70 (250).

MYOSITIS

Inflammatory myositis is a rare condition that may occur alone or in association with other autoimmune diseases such as SLE or scleroderma. Although the major clinical feature of both inflammatory myopathies, dermatomyositis (DM) and polymyositis (PM), is symmetric proximal muscle weakness, the two diseases are quite different in terms of their epidemiology, associated clinical manifestations, pathologic findings, and suspected immunopathogenesis. Both are considered autoimmune diseases on the basis of autoantibody associations, the presence of T-cell infiltrates in affected tissue, and response to immunosuppressive medications.

Clinical Manifestations

Both PM and DM are characterized by the insidious onset of symmetric proximal muscle weakness involving the neck extensor muscles, shoulder girdle, and hip girdle, with sparing of the facial and extraocular muscles. DM has additional dermatologic findings and is often associated with malignancy (251). An accurate assessment of disease prevalence is very difficult becaue of discrepancies in classification criteria; however, estimates of incidence range from 0.5 to 8.4 cases per million. DM has a bimodal age distribution, with peak incidences in the teenage years and between the fifth and sixth decades, whereas PM is extremely unusual in children and even in adults is the less common of the two. The female-to-male ratio is approximately 3:1. There is evidence that ethnicity plays a role in disease susceptibility; African-Americans are three to four times more likely to develop disease than Caucasians (252).

Biopsy is the gold standard for diagnosis of myositis (253). Histologic findings in DM characteristically include an inflammatory infiltrate invading the perivascular space and the interfascicular septae. The intramuscular vessels reveal endothelial hyperplasia with fibrin thrombi, and complement membrane attack complex (C5b-9) deposition in vessel walls. A similar type of perivascular infiltrate with CD4^{+} cells is seen on skin biopsy in DM.

The findings in PM are strikingly different, with infiltrating CD8^{+} T cells in an endomysial pattern. Together with activated macrophages, they flank healthy-appearing muscle fibers expressing class I MHC antigens. When class 1 antigens are seen in DM biopsies, they are expressed by damaged muscle fibers only. The diagnosis of PM relies on the finding of MHC-I/CD8^{+} complexes in healthy muscle fibers.

Pathogenesis

Current understanding of the immunopathogenesis of the inflammatory myopathies proposes quite distinct entities; DM is traditionally regarded as a humorally mediated microangiopathy, whereas PM is felt to be an HLA-restricted, T-cell–mediated myotoxic immune response (251). Despite these differences, some inflammatory responses are common to both disease subsets.

The increased expression of CXCR3 and its IFNγ-inducible ligand CXCL10 in infiltrating inflammatory cells in both PM and DM, together with increased expression of MCP-1, suggests a Th1 skewing of the immune response in these diseases (254). These data are further substantiated by increased serum levels of IL-18 that parallel equally elevated levels of IFNγ in both PM and DM (255). The recent finding of large numbers of perivascular and perimysial plasmacytoid dendritic cells associated with upregulation of IFNα-inducible genes strongly suggests a role for the innate immune system in pathogenesis of DM (256). In contrast, myeloid dendritic cells are present in PM lesions. The presence of dendritic cells in PM muscle suggests that phaocytosis and antigen presentation followed by T-cell recruitment are occurring at the involved sites or in local lymph nodes.

$CD8^+$ T cells obtained from PM biopsies are cytotoxic to autologous myotubes in vitro. Several studies have demonstrated clonally expanded circulating and invasive $CD8^+$ T cells. These data suggest an antigen-driven response; however, the nature of the antigenic target on myocytes remains unknown.

A role for MHC class I in muscle fiber damage unrelated to antigen presentation and lymphocyte response is suggested by the observations that class I expression precedes the inflammatory infiltrate in PM and persists in the absence of infiltrating cells. Similarly, class I transgenic mice develop weakness before an inflammatory infiltrate appears, and gene transfer of class I plasmids in vitro and in vivo diminishes muscle regeneration and differentiation (257). Inappropriate overexpression of class I may lead to a stress response in the endoplasmic reticulum, as has been proposed for B27-related disease. The inciting triggers for upregulation of class I, however, remain speculative and include viral infections, trauma, or denervation and hypoxia.

Autoantibodies

Autoantibodies are found in 50% of patients with inflammatory myositis; some are specific for inflammatory myositis (MSAs) and some are associated with other connective tissue diseases as well (MAAs) (Table 41.6). The antigenic targets of most MSAs are cytoplasmic proteins or ribonucleoprotein complexes involved in protein synthesis and translocation. Of the six reported antibodies to aminoacyl-transfer RNA synthetases (anti-tRNA synthetases), the most common is the anti-Jo-1 antibody to histidyl-tRNA synthetase. Apoptotic muscle cells release the NH_2-terminal fragment of Jo-1 that acts as a chemoattractant for activated lymphocytes to the damaged tissue. Other MSAs are directed against nuclear helicase (anti–Mi-2) and signal-recognition particle (anti-SRP) (258).

Seasonal patterns of disease onset—increased incidence of Jo-1–associated disease in the spring and increased incidence of SRP-associated disease in the winter and spring months—suggest an infectious trigger for myositis, but none has been successfully identified (251).

It has recently been reported that regenerating myositis muscle provides a rich source of autoantigen (Mi-2, Jo-1, U-1 RNP, and DNA PKS). These data implicate regenerating muscle cells as a source of ongoing antigen drive, accounting for the observed self-sustaining nature of the disease (91). This paradigm does not address the nature of the initial inciting event leading to immune activation in myositis, but it is theorized that muscle damage leading to regeneration may initiate disease in a predisposed patient.

Treatment

The treatment of inflammatory muscle disease is generally confined to the use of corticosteroids or immunosuppressive agents. Dermatomyositis associated with malignancy is most responsive to reduction in tumor mass. As therapies become more focused, it is likely that each disease will respond to different agents, as polymyositis is characterized by the activation of cytotoxic $CD8^+$ cells and dermatomyositis by antibody production and activation of $CD4^+$ cells.

TABLE 41.6 Autoantibodies in Inflammatory Myositis

Autoantibody	*Antigenic Target*	*Frequency*
Myositis-specific antibodies		
Anti-tRNA-synthetases	Aminoacyl-tRNA-synthetase	
Anti-Jo-1	Histidyl-tRNA-sythetase	20% PM/DM
Anti-PL-7	Threonyl-tRNA-synthetase	<5% PM/DM
Anti-PL-12	Alanyl-tRNA-synthetase	<5% PM/DM
Anti-EJ	Glycyl-tRNA-synthetase	<5% PM/DM
Anti-OJ	Isoleucyl-tRNA-synthetase	<5% PM/DM
Anti-KS	Asparaginyl-tRNA-synthetase	<5% PM/DM
Anti-SRP (signal-recognition particle)	325-kDa ribonucleoprotein translocation regulation factor	<5% PM
Anti-Mi-2	Nuclear helicase	5–10% DM
Myositis-associated antibodies		
Anti-PM-ScL	Nucleolar exosome	5–25% DM/SSc
Anti-Ro, La		3–27%
Anti-U1 snRNP	Ribonuclearprotein	5–60%

Mouse Models of Myositis

Models of myositis support the hypothesis that muscle damage followed by muscle regeneration may trigger inflammation and autoreactivity. Synaptotagmin VII is a lysosomal protein involved in lysosomal exocytosis, a process that contributes to the repair of wounds in the plasma membrane. Mice deficient in this protein develop inflammation in muscle, muscle weakness, and antinuclear antibodies, suggesting that the failure to repair damaged cells can potentially trigger an autoimmune attack on muscle (259). Similarly, ectopic expression of MHC class I molecules in skeletal muscle leads to autoantibody production and muscle inflammation. Once enhanced class I expression is present on muscle, an inflammatory response develops that may reflect the antigen-presenting capacity of myocytes but more likely represents a misfolded protein response (260).

The peptide-binding motif of H-2 K^d is similar to that of HLA A2402, an MHC allele associated with polymyositis. Because polymyositis is characterized by an infiltration of $CD8^+$ cells, peptides associating with H-$2K^d$ and A2404 were sought. Pyruvate kinase M1/M2 is abundantly expressed in skeletal muscle and contains a peptide that can be anchored in the H-2 K^d abd A2404 peptide-binding grooves. Administration of dendritic cells pulsed with this peptide to BALB/c (H-2^d) mice leads to muscle inflammation with infiltration of predominantly $CD8^+$ T cells (261).

CONCLUSION

The systemic autoimmune diseases have in common the targeting of the musculoskeletal system, although other organ systems can also be affected. A major shared feature is the presence of ANA. Reactivity to nuclear antigens may be more than a fortuitous communality and may signal a shared abnormality in B-cell development and tolerance. Alternatively, nuclear antigens may contribute little to either the elicitation or the pathogenicity of ANA; as new cross-reactivities continue to be identified, they may provide greater insight into pathogenic processes.

SLE and RA clearly share some susceptibility genes with each other and with organ-specific autoimmune diseases; however, there is as yet no evidence for a shared genetic predisposition between these diseases and vasculitides, scleroderma, or inflammatory myopathies. Indeed, pathogenetic mechanisms appear to differ among these diseases, with different effector T-cell subsets.

Nonpathogenic autoreactivity, in particular the presence of the autoantibodies of systemic autoimmune diseases, is far more widespread than pathogenic autoreactivity. Major, and poorly understood, checkpoints exist between normal serology and ANA and then between enhanced autoreactivity and tissue damage. Finally, in persistent disease, an additional progression from cellular infiltration and inflammation to fibrosis occurs; the molecular switch for this change in tissue response is not well characterized. Nevertheless, this complicates the treatment of these diseases, as stage of disease may be a determinant in response to therapy.

The major advances in our understanding of these diseases in the past decade have been a function of the improved methodologies for the study of human cells and tissue. Although animal models continue to be critical to our understanding, it is now possible and necessary to test the validity of animal models against the human disease and to choose those models most similar to patient subsets for the design of therapeutic interventions.

REFERENCES

1. Stojanov S, Kastner DL. Familial autoinflammatory diseases: genetics, pathogenesis and treatment. *Curr Opin Rheumatol.* 2005;17(5):586–599.
2. Davidson A, Diamond B. Autoimmune diseases. *N Engl J Med.* 2001;345(5):340–350.
3. Gregersen PK, Behrens TW. Genetics of autoimmune diseases—disorders of immune homeostasis. *Nat Rev Genet.* 2006;7(12):917–928.
4. Trends in deaths from systemic lupus erythematosus—United States, 1979–1998. *MMWR.* 2002;51(17):371–374.
5. Gallegos AM, Bevan MJ. Central tolerance: good but imperfect. *Immunol Rev.* 2006;209:290–296.
6. Kaliyaperumal A, Michaels MA, Datta SK. Naturally processed chromatin peptides reveal a major autoepitope that primes pathogenic T and B cells of lupus. *J Immunol.* 2002;168(5):2530–2537.
7. Datta SK. Major peptide autoepitopes for nucleosome-centered T and B cell interaction in human and murine lupus. *Ann NY Acad Sci.* 2003;987:79–90.
8. Fournier C. Where do T cells stand in rheumatoid arthritis? *Joint Bone Spine.* 2005;72(6):527–532.
9. Snowden N, Reynolds I, Morgan K, Holt L. T cell responses to human type II collagen in patients with rheumatoid arthritis and healthy controls. *Arthritis Rheum.* 1997;40(7):1210–1218.
10. Notarangelo LD, Gambineri E, Badolato R. Immunodeficiencies with autoimmune consequences. *Adv Immunol.* 2006;89:321–370.
11. Nose M, Nishihara M, Kamogawa J, et al. Genetic basis of autoimmune disease in MRL/lpr mice: dissection of the complex pathological manifestations and their susceptibility loci. *Rev Immunogenet.* 2000;2(1):154–164.
12. Bhandoola A, Tai X, Eckhaus M, et al. Peripheral expression of self-MHC-II influences the reactivity and self-tolerance of mature CD4(+) T cells: evidence from a lymphopenic T cell model. *Immunity.* 2002;17(4):425–436.
13. Steinman RM, Hawiger D, Nussenzweig MC. Tolerogenic dendritic cells. *Annu Rev Immunol.* 2003;21:685–711.
14. Adorini L, Penna G, Giarratana N, et al. Dendritic cells as key targets for immunomodulation by vitamin D receptor ligands. *J Steroid Biochem Mol Biol.* 2004;89–90(1–5):437–441.
15. Anders HJ, Zecher D, Pawar RD, et al. Molecular mechanisms of autoimmunity triggered by microbial infection. *Arthritis Res Ther.* 2005;7(5):215–224.
16. Melchers F, Rolink AR. B cell tolerance—how to make it and how to break it. *Curr Top Microbiol Immunol.* 2006;305:1–23.
17. Meffre E, Schaefer A, Wardemann H, et al. Surrogate light chain expressing human peripheral B cells produce self-reactive antibodies. *J Exp Med.* 2004;199(1):145–150.
18. Kono DH, Theofilopoulos AN. Genetics of SLE in mice. *Springer Semin Immunopathol.* 2006;28(2):83–96.

19. Kumar KR, Li L, Yan M, et al. Regulation of B cell tolerance by the lupus susceptibility gene Ly108. *Science*. 2006;312(5780):1665–1669.
20. Kilmon MA, Rutan JA, Clarke SH, et al. Low-affinity, Smith antigen-specific B cells are tolerized by dendritic cells and macrophages. *J Immunol.* 2005;175(1):37–41.
21. Cappione A 3rd, Anolik JH, Pugh-Bernard A, et al. Germinal center exclusion of autoreactive B cells is defective in human systemic lupus erythematosus. *J Clin Invest.* 2005;115(11):3205–3216.
22. William J, Euler C, Primarolo N, et al. B cell tolerance checkpoints that restrict pathways of antigen-driven differentiation. *J Immunol.* 2006;176(4):2142–2151.
23. Culton DA, O'Conner BP, Conway KL, et al. Early preplasma cells define a tolerance checkpoint for autoreactive B cells. *J Immunol.* 2006;176(2):790–802.
24. Ravetch JV, Bolland S. IgG Fc receptors. *Annu Rev Immunol.* 2001; 19:275–290.
25. Deming PB, Rathmell JC. Mitochondria, cell death, and B cell tolerance. *Curr Dir Autoimmun.* 2006;9:95–119.
26. Noelle RJ, Erickson LD. Determinations of B cell fate in immunity and autoimmunity. *Curr Dir Autoimmun.* 2005;8:1–24.
27. Muller-Hilke B, Mitchison NA. The role of HLA promoters in autoimmunity. *Curr Pharm Des.* 2006;12(29):3743–3752.
28. Chiocchetti A, Indelicato M, Bensi T, et al. High levels of osteopontin associated with polymorphisms in its gene are a risk factor for development of autoimmunity/lymphoproliferation. *Blood.* 2004;103(4): 1376–1382.
29. Nolsoe RL, Kelly JA, Pociot F, et al. Functional promoter haplotypes of the human FAS gene are associated with the phenotype of SLE characterized by thrombocytopenia. *Genes Immun.* 2005;6(8):699–706.
30. Haller K, Kisand K, Pisarev H, et al. Insulin gene VNTR, CTLA-4 +49A/G and HLA-DQB1 alleles distinguish latent autoimmune diabetes in adults from type 1 diabetes and from type 2 diabetes group. *Tissue antigens.* 2007;69(2):121–127.
31. Scalzo K, Plebanski M, Apostolopoulos V. Regulatory T-cells: immunomodulators in health and disease. *Curr Top Med Chem.* 2006; 6(16):1759–1768.
32. Yurasov S, Tiller T, Tsuiji M, et al. Persistent expression of autoantibodies in SLE patients in remission. *J Exp Med.* 2006;203(10):2255–2261.
33. Martin F, Kearney JF. B-cell subsets and the mature preimmune repertoire. Marginal zone and B1 B cells as part of a "natural immune memory." *Immunol Rev.* 2000;175:70–79.
34. Arnold LW, Spencer DH, Clarke SH, et al. Mechanisms that limit the diversity of antibody: three sequentially acting mechanisms that favor the spontaneous production of germline encoded antiphosphatidyl choline. *Int Immunol.* 1993;5(11):1365–1373.
35. Peng Y, Kowalewski R, Kim S, et al. The role of IgM antibodies in the recognition and clearance of apoptotic cells. *Mol Immunol.* 2005;42(7):781–787.
36. Marshak-Rothstein A. Toll-like receptors in systemic autoimmune disease. *Nat Rev Immunol.* 2006;6(11):823–835.
37. Grimsley C, Ravichandran KS. Cues for apoptotic cell engulfment: eat-me, don't eat-me and come-get-me signals. *Trends Cell Biol.* 2003;13(12):648–656.
38. Kim SJ, Gershov D, Ma X, et al. I-PLA(2) activation during apoptosis promotes the exposure of membrane lysophosphatidylcholine leading to binding by natural immunoglobulin M antibodies and complement activation. *J Exp Med.* 2002;196(5):655–665.
39. Ehrenstein MR, Cook HT, Neuberger MS. Deficiency in serum immunoglobulin (Ig)M predisposes to development of IgG autoantibodies. *J Exp Med.* 2000;191(7):1253–1258.
40. Werwitzke S, Trick D, Kamino K, et al. Inhibition of lupus disease by anti-double-stranded DNA antibodies of the IgM isotype in the (NZB × NZW)F1 mouse. *Arthritis Rheum.* 2005;52(11):3629–3638.
41. Davidson A, Bridges SL. Autoimmunity in rheumatoid arthritis. In: St. Clair W, Pisetsky D, Haynes B, eds. *Textbook of Rheumatoid Arthritis*. Philadelphia: Lippincott Williams & Wilkins; 2004:197–212.
42. Roosnek E, Lanzavecchia A. Efficient and selective presentation of antigen-antibody complexes by rheumatoid factor B cells. *J Exp Med.* 1991;173(2):487–489.
43. Tighe H, Heaphy P, Baird S, et al. Human immunoglobulin (IgG) induced deletion of IgM rheumatoid factor B cells in transgenic mice. *J Exp Med.* 1995;181(2):599–606.
44. Wang H, Shlomchik MJ. High affinity rheumatoid factor transgenic B cells are eliminated in normal mice. *J Immunol.* 1997;159(3): 1125–1134.
45. Diamond B, Katz JB, Paul E, et al. The role of somatic mutation in the pathogenic anti-DNA response. *Annu Rev Immunol.* 1992;10: 731–757.
46. Egner W. The use of laboratory tests in the diagnosis of SLE. *J Clin Pathol.* 2000;53(6):424–432.
47. Eriksson C, Engstrand S, Sundqvist KG, et al. Autoantibody formation in patients with rheumatoid arthritis treated with anti-TNF alpha. *Ann Rheum Dis.* 2005;64(3):403–407.
48. Dorner T, Lipsky PE. Signalling pathways in B cells: implications for autoimmunity. *Curr Top Microbiol Immunol.* 2006;305: 213–240.
49. Grimaldi CM. Sex and systemic lupus erythematosus: the role of the sex hormones estrogen and prolactin on the regulation of autoreactive B cells. *Curr Opin Rheumatol.* 2006;18(5):456–461.
50. Arbuckle MR, McClain MT, Rubertone MV, et al. Development of autoantibodies before the clinical onset of systemic lupus erythematosus. *N Engl J Med.* 2003;349(16):1526–1533.
51. Brennan P, Bankhead C, Silman A, et al. Oral contraceptives and rheumatoid arthritis: results from a primary care-based incident case-control study. *Semin Arthritis Rheum.* 1997;26(6):817–823.
52. Cohen-Solal JF, Jeganathan V, Grimaldi CM, et al. Sex hormones and SLE: influencing the fate of autoreactive B cells. *Curr Top Microbiol Immunol.* 2006;305:67–88.
53. Subramanian S, Tus K, Li QZ, et al. A Tlr7 translocation accelerates systemic autoimmunity in murine lupus. *Proc Natl Acad Sci U S A.* 2006;103(26):9970–9975.
54. Keyszer G, Langer T, Kornhuber M, et al. Neurovascular mechanisms as a possible cause of remission of rheumatoid arthritis in hemiparetic limbs. *Ann Rheum Dis.* 2004;63(10):1349–1351.
55. Worthington J, Silman AJ. Genetic control of autoimmunity, lessons from twin studies. *Clin Exp Immunol.* 1995;101(3):390–392.
56. Villasenor J, Benoist C, Mathis D. AIRE and APECED: molecular insights into an autoimmune disease. *Immunol Rev.* 2005;204:156–164.
57. Anderson MS, Venanzi ES, Chen Z, et al. The cellular mechanism of Aire control of T cell tolerance. *Immunity.* 2005;23(2):227–239.
58. Jiang W, Anderson MS, Bronson R, et al. Modifier loci condition autoimmunity provoked by Aire deficiency. *J Exp Med.* 2005;202(6): 805–815.
59. Kekalainen E, Tuovinen H, Joensuu J, et al. A defect of regulatory T cells in patients with autoimmune polyendocrinopathy-candidiasis-ectodermal dystrophy. *J Immunol.* 2007;178(2):1208–1215.
60. Wan YY, Flavell RA. Regulatory T-cell functions are subverted and converted owing to attenuated Foxp3 expression. *Nature.* 2007;445:766–770.
61. Worth A, Thrasher AJ, Gaspar HB. Autoimmune lymphoproliferative syndrome: molecular basis of disease and clinical phenotype. *Br J Haematol.* 2006;133(2):124–140.
62. Clementi R, Chiocchetti A, Cappellano G, et al. Variations of the perforin gene in patients with autoimmunity/lymphoproliferation and defective Fas function. *Blood.* 2006;108(9):3079–3084.
63. Seshasayee D, Valdez P, Yan M, et al. Loss of TACI causes fatal lymphoproliferation and autoimmunity, establishing TACI as an inhibitory BLyS receptor. *Immunity.* 2003;18(2):279–288.
64. Fairhurst AM, Wandstrat AE, Wakeland EK. Systemic lupus erythematosus: multiple immunological phenotypes in a complex genetic disease. *Adv Immunol.* 2006;92:1–69.
65. Deighton C, Criswell LA. Recent advances in the genetics of rheumatoid arthritis. *Curr Rheumatol Rep.* 2006;8(5):394–400.
66. McDaniel DO, Alarcon GS, Pratt PW, et al. Most African-American patients with rheumatoid arthritis do not have the rheumatoid antigenic determinant (epitope). *Ann Intern Med.* 1995; 123(3):181–187.
67. Reveille JD. The genetic basis of autoantibody production. *Autoimmun Rev.* 2006;5(6):389–398.
68. Anolik JH, Campbell D, Felgar RE, et al. The relationship of FcgammaRIIIa genotype to degree of B cell depletion by rituximab in

the treatment of systemic lupus erythematosus. *Arthritis Rheum.* 2003;48(2):455–459.
69. Prahalad S. Genetics of juvenile idiopathic arthritis: an update. *Curr Opin Rheumatol.* 2004;16(5):588–594.
70. Vinuesa CG, Cook MC, Angelucci C, et al. A RING-type ubiquitin ligase family member required to repress follicular helper T cells and autoimmunity. *Nature.* 2005;435(7041):452–458.
71. Tivol EA, Borriello F, Schweitzer AN, et al. Loss of CTLA-4 leads to massive lymphoproliferation and fatal multiorgan tissue destruction, revealing a critical negative regulatory role of CTLA-4. *Immunity.* 1995;3(5):541–547.
72. Ueda H, Howson JM, Esposito L, et al. Association of the T-cell regulatory gene CTLA4 with susceptibility to autoimmune disease. *Nature.* 2003;423(6939):506–511.
73. Mellor AL, Chandler P, Baban B, et al. Specific subsets of murine dendritic cells acquire potent T cell regulatory functions following CTLA4-mediated induction of indoleamine 2,3 dioxygenase. *Int Immunol.* 2004;16(10):1391–1401.
74. James ES, Harney S, Wordsworth BP, et al. PDCD1: a tissue-specific susceptibility locus for inherited inflammatory disorders. *Genes Immun.* 2005;6(5):430–437.
75. D'Alfonso S, Barizzone N, Giordano M, et al. Two single-nucleotide polymorphisms in the 5′ and 3′ ends of the osteopontin gene contribute to susceptibility to systemic lupus erythematosus. *Arthritis Rheum.* 2005;52(2):539–547.
76. Jacob CO, Hwang F, Lewis GD, et al. Tumor necrosis factor alpha in murine systemic lupus erythematosus disease models: implications for genetic predisposition and immune regulation. *Cytokine.* 1991;3(6):551–561.
77. Atzeni F, Turiel M, Capsoni F, et al. Autoimmunity and anti-TNF-alpha agents. *Ann NY Acad Sci.* 2005;1051:559–569.
78. Lopez-Hoyos M, Carrio R, Merino R, et al. Constitutive expression of bcl-2 in B cells causes a lethal form of lupuslike autoimmune disease after induction of neonatal tolerance to H-2b alloantigens. *J Exp Med.* 1996;183(6):2523–2531.
79. Mehrian R, Quismorio FP Jr., Strassmann G, et al. Synergistic effect between IL-10 and bcl-2 genotypes in determining susceptibility to systemic lupus erythematosus. *Arthritis Rheum.* 1998;41(4):596–602.
80. Gaipl US, Sheriff A, Franz S, et al. Inefficient clearance of dying cells and autoreactivity. *Curr Top Microbiol Immunol.* 2006;305:161–176.
81. Deroo BJ, Korach KS. Estrogen receptors and human disease. *J Clin Invest.* 2006;116(3):561–570.
82. Cutolo M, Lahita RG. Estrogens and arthritis. *Rheum Dis Clin N Am.* 2005;31(1):19–27, vii.
83. Valdivielso JM, Fernandez E. Vitamin D receptor polymorphisms and diseases. *Clin Chim Acta; Int J Clin Chem.* 2006;371(1–2):1–12.
84. Caricchio R, McPhie L, Cohen PL. Ultraviolet B radiation-induced cell death: critical role of ultraviolet dose in inflammation and lupus autoantigen redistribution. *J Immunol.* 2003;171(11):5778–5786.
85. Georgiev M, Agle LM, Chu JL, et al. Mature dendritic cells readily break tolerance in normal mice but do not lead to disease expression. *Arthritis Rheum.* 2005;52(1):225–238.
86. Schachna L, Wigley FM, Morris S, et al. Recognition of Granzyme B-generated autoantigen fragments in scleroderma patients with ischemic digital loss. *Arthritis Rheum.* 2002;46(7):1873–1884.
87. Mamula MJ. Epitope spreading: the role of self peptides and autoantigen processing by B lymphocytes. *Immunol Rev.* 1998;164: 231–239.
88. Yang ML, Doyle HA, Gee RJ, et al. Intracellular protein modification associated with altered T cell functions in autoimmunity. *J Immunol.* 2006;177(7):4541–4549.
89. Shores EW, Pisetsky DS, Grudier J, et al. Immunization with the Sm nuclear antigen induces anti-Sm antibodies in normal and MRL mice. *Immunology.* 1988;65(3):473–478.
90. Deane JA, Bolland S. Nucleic acid-sensing TLRs as modifiers of autoimmunity. *J Immunol.* 2006;177(10):6573–6578.
91. Casciola-Rosen L, Nagaraju K, Plotz P, et al. Enhanced autoantigen expression in regenerating muscle cells in idiopathic inflammatory myopathy. *J Exp Med.* 2005;201(4):591–601.
92. Chiovato L, Latrofa F, Braverman LE, et al. Disappearance of humoral thyroid autoimmunity after complete removal of thyroid antigens. *Ann Intern Med.* 2003;139(5 Pt 1):346–351.
93. Shoenfeld Y. Anti-DNA idiotypes: from induction of disease to novel therapeutical approaches. *Immunol Lett.* 2005;100(1):73–77.
94. Poole BD, Scofield RH, Harley JB, et al. Epstein-Barr virus and molecular mimicry in systemic lupus erythematosus. *Autoimmunity.* 2006;39(1):63–70.
95. Harley JB, Harley IT, Guthridge JM, et al. The curiously suspicious: a role for Epstein-Barr virus in lupus. *Lupus.* 2006;15(11): 768–777.
96. Wellmann U, Letz M, Herrmann M, et al. The evolution of human anti-double-stranded DNA autoantibodies. *Proc Natl Acad Sci U S A.* 2005;102(26):9258–9263.
97. Deshmukh US, Gaskin F, Lewis JE, et al. Mechanisms of autoantibody diversification to SLE-related autoantigens. *Ann NY Acad Sci.* 2003;987:91–98.
98. Suen JL, Chuang YH, Tsai BY, et al. Treatment of murine lupus using nucleosomal T cell epitopes identified by bone marrow-derived dendritic cells. *Arthritis Rheum.* 2004;50(10):3250–3259.
99. Anderton SM. Post-translational modifications of self-antigens: implications for autoimmunity. *Curr Opin Immunol.* 2004;16(6):753–758.
100. Backlund J, Carlsen S, Hoger T, et al. Predominant selection of T cells specific for the glycosylated collagen type II epitope (263–270) in humanized transgenic mice and in rheumatoid arthritis. *Proc Natl Acad Sci U S A.* 2002;99(15):9960–9965.
101. Doyle HA, Gee RJ, Mamula MJ. A failure to repair self-proteins leads to T cell hyperproliferation and autoantibody production. *J Immunol.* 2003;171(6):2840–2847.
102. Goronzy JJ, Henel G, Sawai H, et al. Costimulatory pathways in rheumatoid synovitis and T-cell senescence. *Ann NY Acad Sci.* 2005; 1062:182–194.
103. Busser BW, Adair BS, Erikson J, Laufer TM. Activation of diverse repertoires of autoreactive T cells enhances the loss of anti-dsDNA B cell tolerance. *J Clin Invest.* 2003;112(9):1361–1371.
104. Vasoo S. Drug-induced lupus: an update. *Lupus.* 2006;15(11):757–761.
105. Rubin RL, Kretz-Rommel A. A nondeletional mechanism for central T-cell tolerance. *Crit Rev Immunol.* 2001;21(1–3):29–40.
106. Mayes MD. Epidemiologic studies of environmental agents and systemic autoimmune diseases. *Environ Health Perspect.* 1999;107 (suppl 5):743–748.
107. D'Cruz D. Autoimmune diseases associated with drugs, chemicals and environmental factors. *Toxicol Lett.* 2000;112–113:421–432.
108. Parks CG, Cooper GS. Occupational exposures and risk of systemic lupus erythematosus: a review of the evidence and exposure assessment methods in population- and clinic-based studies. *Lupus.* 2006;15(11):728–736.
109. Liu B, Yang Y, Dai J, et al. TLR4 up-regulation at protein or gene level is pathogenic for lupuslike autoimmune disease. *J Immunol.* 2006;177(10):6880–6888.
110. Kollias G. TNF pathophysiology in murine models of chronic inflammation and autoimmunity. *Semin Arthritis Rheum.* 2005;34 (5 suppl 1):3–6.
111. Groux H, Cottrez F. The complex role of interleukin-10 in autoimmunity. *J Autoimmun.* 2003;20(4):281–285.
112. Sun Y, Chen HM, Subudhi SK, et al. Costimulatory molecule-targeted antibody therapy of a spontaneous autoimmune disease. *Nat Med.* 2002;8(12):1405–1413.
113. Schiffer L, Sinha J, Wang X, et al. Short term administration of costimulatory blockade and cyclophosphamide induces remission of systemic lupus erythematosus nephritis in NZB/W F1 mice by a mechanism downstream of renal immune complex deposition. *J Immunol.* 2003;171(1):489–497.
114. Jayne D, Tyndall A. Autologous stem cell transplantation for systemic lupus erythematosus. *Lupus.* 2004;13(5):359–365.
115. Desai SB, Furst DE. Problems encountered during anti-tumour necrosis factor therapy. *Best Pract Res Clin Rheumatol.* 2006;20(4): 757–790.
116. Winthrop KL. Risk and prevention of tuberculosis and other serious opportunistic infections associated with the inhibition of tumor necrosis factor. *Nat Clin Pract Rheumatol.* 2006;2(11):602–610.
117. Jacob CO, McDevitt HO. Tumour necrosis factor-alpha in murine autoimmune "lupus" nephritis. *Nature.* 1988;331(6154):356–358.

118. Weinblatt M, Combe B, Covucci A, et al. Safety of the selective co-stimulation modulator abatacept in rheumatoid arthritis patients receiving background biologic and nonbiologic disease-modifying antirheumatic drugs: a one-year randomized, placebo-controlled study. *Arthritis Rheum.* 2006;54(9):2807–2816.
119. Cambridge G, Leandro MJ, Edwards JC, et al. Serologic changes following B lymphocyte depletion therapy for rheumatoid arthritis. *Arthritis Rheum.* 2003;48(8):2146–2154.
120. Tan EM, Cohen AS, Fries JF, et al. The 1982 revised criteria for the classification of systemic lupus erythematosus. *Arthritis Rheum.* 1982;25(11):1271–1277.
121. Tan EM, Feltkamp TE, Smolen JS, et al. Range of antinuclear antibodies in "healthy" individuals. *Arthritis Rheum.* 1997;40(9):1601–1611.
122. Hoffman IE, Peene I, Meheus L, et al. Specific antinuclear antibodies are associated with clinical features in systemic lupus erythematosus. *Ann Rheum Dis.* 2004;63(9):1155–1158.
123. Kowal C, DeGiorgio LA, Nakaoka T, et al. Cognition and immunity; antibody impairs memory. *Immunity.* 2004;21(2):179–188.
124. Omdal R, Brokstad K, Waterloo K, et al. Neuropsychiatric disturbances in SLE are associated with antibodies against NMDA receptors. *Eur J Neurol.* 2005;12(5):392–398.
125. Tsao BP. Update on human systemic lupus erythematosus genetics. *Curr Opin Rheumatol.* 2004;16(5):513–521.
126. Krishnan S, Chowdhury B, Tsokos GC. Autoimmunity in systemic lupus erythematosus: integrating genes and biology. *Semin Immunol.* 2006;18(4):230–243.
127. Yurasov S, Wardemann H, Hammersen J, et al. Defective B cell tolerance checkpoints in systemic lupus erythematosus. *J Exp Med.* 2005;201(5):703–711.
128. Yurasov S, Hammersen J, Tiller T, et al. B-cell tolerance checkpoints in healthy humans and patients with systemic lupus erythematosus. *Ann N Y Acad Sci.* 2005;1062:165–174.
129. Milner EC, Anolik J, Cappione A, Sanz I. Human innate B cells: a link between host defense and autoimmunity? *Springer Semin Immunopathol.* 2005;26(4):433–452.
130. Kamradt T, Mitchison NA. Tolerance and autoimmunity. *N Engl J Med.* 2001;344(9):655–664.
131. Pugh-Bernard AE, Cambier JC. B cell receptor signaling in human systemic lupus erythematosus. *Curr Opin Rheumatol.* 2006;18(5): 451–455.
132. Flores-Borja F, Kabouridis PS, Jury EC, et al. Decreased Lyn expression and translocation to lipid raft signaling domains in B lymphocytes from patients with systemic lupus erythematosus. *Arthritis Rheum.* 2005;52(12):3955–3965.
133. Mackay M, Stanevsky A, Wang T, et al. Selective dysregulation of the Fc{gamma}IIB receptor on memory B cells in SLE. *J Exp Med.* 2006;203:2157–2164.
134. Enyedy EJ, Mitchell JP, Nambiar MP, et al. Defective FcgammaRIIb1 signaling contributes to enhanced calcium response in B cells from patients with systemic lupus erythematosus. *Clin Immunol.* 2001;101(2):130–135.
135. Floto RA, Clatworthy MR, Heilbronn KR, et al. Loss of function of a lupus-associated FcgammaRIIb polymorphism through exclusion from lipid rafts. *Nat Med.* 2005;11(10):1056–1058.
136. Bijl M, Horst G, Limburg PC, et al. Expression of costimulatory molecules on peripheral blood lymphocytes of patients with systemic lupus erythematosus. *Ann Rheum Dis.* 2001;60(5):523–526.
137. Kayagaki N, Yan M, Seshasayee D, et al. BAFF/BLyS receptor 3 binds the B cell survival factor BAFF ligand through a discrete surface loop and promotes processing of NF-kappaB2. *Immunity.* 2002;17(4):515–524.
138. Cheema GS, Roschke V, Hilbert DM, et al. Elevated serum B lymphocyte stimulator levels in patients with systemic immune-based rheumatic diseases. *Arthritis Rheum.* 2001;44(6):1313–1319.
139. Attanavanich K, Kearney JF. Marginal zone, but not follicular B cells, are potent activators of naive CD4 T cells. *J Immunol.* 2004; 172(2):803–811.
140. Tsuiji M, Yurasov S, Velinzon K, et al. A checkpoint for autoreactivity in human IgM+ memory B cell development. *J Exp Med.* 2006;203(2):393–400.
141. Chan OT, Hannum LG, Haberman AM, et al. A novel mouse with B cells but lacking serum antibody reveals an antibody-independent role for B cells in murine lupus. *J Exp Med.* 1999;189(10):1639–1648.
142. Yan J, Harvey BP, Gee RJ, et al. B cells drive early T cell autoimmunity in vivo prior to dendritic cell-mediated autoantigen presentation. *J Immunol.* 2006;177(7):4481–4487.
143. Enyedy EJ, Nambiar MP, Liossis SN, et al. Fc epsilon receptor type I gamma chain replaces the deficient T cell receptor zeta chain in T cells of patients with systemic lupus erythematosus. *Arthritis Rheum.* 2001;44(5):1114–1121.
144. Budagyan VM, Bulanova EG, Sharova NI, et al. The resistance of activated T-cells from SLE patients to apoptosis induced by human thymic stromal cells. *Immunol Lett.* 1998;60(1):1–5.
145. Kyogoku C, Langefeld CD, Ortmann WA, et al. Genetic association of the R620W polymorphism of protein tyrosine phosphatase PTPN22 with human SLE. *Am J Hum Genet.* 2004;75(3):504–507.
146. Prokunina L, Castillejo-Lopez C, Oberg F, et al. A regulatory polymorphism in PDCD1 is associated with susceptibility to systemic lupus erythematosus in humans. *Nat Genet.* 2002;32(4):666–669.
147. Mudd PA, Teague BN, Farris AD. Regulatory T cells and systemic lupus erythematosus. *Scand J Immunol.* 2006;64(3):211–218.
148. Ronnblom L, Eloranta ML, Alm GV. The type I interferon system in systemic lupus erythematosus. *Arthritis Rheum.* 2006;54(2):408–420.
149. Means TK, Luster AD. Toll-like receptor activation in the pathogenesis of systemic lupus erythematosus. *Ann NY Acad Sci.* 2005;1062: 242–251.
150. Sigurdsson S, Nordmark G, Goring HH, et al. Polymorphisms in the tyrosine kinase 2 and interferon regulatory factor 5 genes are associated with systemic lupus erythematosus. *Am J Hum Genet.* 2005;76(3):528–537.
151. Hron JD, Peng SL. Type I IFN protects against murine lupus. *J Immunol.* 2004;173(3):2134–2142.
152. Llorente L, Richaud-Patin Y, Garcia-Padilla C, et al. Clinical and biologic effects of anti-interleukin 10 monoclonal antibody administration in systemic lupus erythematosus. *Arthritis Rheum.* 2000;43(8):1790–1800.
153. Aringer M, Smolen JS. Tumour necrosis factor and other proinflammatory cytokines in systemic lupus erythematosus: a rationale for therapeutic intervention. *Lupus.* 2004;13(5):344–347.
154. Blomberg S, Eloranta ML, Cederblad B, et al. Presence of cutaneous interferon-alpha producing cells in patients with systemic lupus erythematosus. *Lupus.* 2001;10(7):484–490.
155. Wada T, Furuichi K, Segawa-Takaeda C, et al. MIP-1alpha and MCP-1 contribute to crescents and interstitial lesions in human crescentic glomerulonephritis. *Kidney Int.* 1999;56(3):995–1003.
156. Baumann I, Kolowos W, Voll RE, et al. Impaired uptake of apoptotic cells into tingible body macrophages in germinal centers of patients with systemic lupus erythematosus. *Arthritis Rheum.* 2002;46(1): 191–201.
157. Nimmerjahn F, Ravetch JV. Fcgamma receptors: old friends and new family members. *Immunity.* 2006;24(1):19–28.
158. Reefman E, Dijstelbloem HM, Limburg PC. Fcgamma receptors in the initiation and progression of systemic lupus erythematosus. *Immunol Cell Biol.* 2003;81(5):382–389.
159. Tsukumo S, Yasutomo K. DNaseI in pathogenesis of systemic lupus erythematosus. *Clin Immunol.* 2004;113(1):14–8.
160. Mevorach D. Systemic lupus erythematosus and apoptosis: a question of balance. *Clin Rev Allergy Immunol.* 2003;25(1):49–60.
161. Buyon JP, Petri MA, Kim MY, et al. The effect of combined estrogen and progesterone hormone replacement therapy on disease activity in systemic lupus erythematosus: a randomized trial. *Ann Intern Med.* 2005;142(12 Pt 1):953–962.
162. Petri M, Kim MY, Kalunian KC, et al. Combined oral contraceptives in women with systemic lupus erythematosus. *N Engl J Med.* 2005;353(24):2550–2558.
163. Sanchez-Guerrero J, Uribe AG, Jimenez-Santana L, et al. A trial of contraceptive methods in women with systemic lupus erythematosus. *N Engl J Med.* 2005;353(24):2539–2549.
164. McGaha TL, Sorrentino B, Ravetch JV. Restoration of tolerance in lupus by targeted inhibitory receptor expression. *Science.* 2005;307(5709):590–593.
165. Xin H, D'Souza S, Jorgensen TN, et al. Increased expression of Ifi202, an IFN-activatable gene, in B6.Nba2 lupus susceptible mice

inhibits p53-mediated apoptosis. *J Immunol.* 2006;176(10):5863–5870.

166. Lawson BR, Prud'homme GJ, Chang Y, et al. Treatment of murine lupus with cDNA encoding IFN-gammaR/Fc. *J Clin Invest.* 2000; 106(2):207–215.
167. Nimmerjahn F, Bruhns P, Horiuchi K, et al. FcgammaRIV: a novel FcR with distinct IgG subclass specificity. *Immunity.* 2005; 23(1):41–51.
168. Clynes R, Dumitru C, Ravetch JV. Uncoupling of immune complex formation and kidney damage in autoimmune glomerulonephritis. *Science.* 1998;279(5353):1052–1054.
169. Kono DH, Baccala R, Theofilopoulos AN. Inhibition of lupus by genetic alteration of the interferon-alpha/beta receptor. *Autoimmunity.* 2003;36(8):503–510.
170. Mathian A, Weinberg A, Gallegos M, et al. IFN-alpha induces early lethal lupus in preautoimmune (New Zealand Black × New Zealand White) F1 but not in BALB/c mice. *J Immunol.* 2005;174(5):2499–2506.
171. Ramanujam M, Wang X, Huang W, et al. Similarities and differences between selective and nonselective BAFF blockade in murine SLE. *J Clin Invest.* 2006;116(3):724–734.
172. Singh RR, Saxena V, Zang S, et al. Differential contribution of IL-4 and STAT6 vs STAT4 to the development of lupus nephritis. *J Immunol.* 2003;170(9):4818–4825.
173. Kang HK, Michaels MA, Berner BR, et al. Very low-dose tolerance with nucleosomal peptides controls lupus and induces potent regulatory T cell subsets. *J Immunol.* 2005;174(6):3247–3255.
174. Theofilopoulos AN, Dixon FJ. Murine models of systemic lupus erythematosus. *Adv Immunol.* 1985;37:269–390.
175. Christensen SR, Shupe J, Nickerson K, et al. Toll-like receptor 7 and TLR9 dictate autoantibody specificity and have opposing inflammatory and regulatory roles in a murine model of lupus. *Immunity.* 2006;25(3):417–428.
176. Matsumoto K, Watanabe N, Akikusa B, et al. Fc receptor-independent development of autoimmune glomerulonephritis in lupus-prone MRL/lpr mice. *Arthritis Rheum.* 2003;48(2):486–494.
177. Shultz LD, Rajan TV, Greiner DL. Severe defects in immunity and hematopoiesis caused by SHP-1 protein-tyrosine-phosphatase deficiency. *Trends Biotechnol.* 1997;15(8):302–307.
178. Pisitkun P, Deane JA, Difilippantonio MJ, et al. Autoreactive B cell responses to RNA-related antigens due to TLR7 gene duplication. *Science.* 2006;312(5780):1669–1672.
179. Fanzo JC, Yang W, Jang SY, et al. Loss of IRF-4-binding protein leads to the spontaneous development of systemic autoimmunity. *J Clin Invest.* 2006;116(3):703–714.
180. Fukuyama H, Nimmerjahn F, Ravetch JV. The inhibitory Fcgamma receptor modulates autoimmunity by limiting the accumulation of immunoglobulin G+ anti-DNA plasma cells. *Nat Immunol.* 2005;6(1):99–106.
181. Boule MW, Broughton C, Mackay F, et al. Toll-like receptor 9-dependent and -independent dendritic cell activation by chromatin-immunoglobulin G complexes. *J Exp Med.* 2004;199(12):1631–1640.
182. Davidson A, Aranow C. Pathogenesis and treatment of systemic lupus erythematosus nephritis. *Curr Opin Rheumatol.* 2006;18(5): 468–475.
183. Eisenberg R. The chronic graft-versus-host model of systemic autoimmunity. *Curr Dir Autoimmun.* 2003;6:228–244.
184. Kuroda Y, Ono N, Akaogi J, et al. Induction of lupus-related specific autoantibodies by non-specific inflammation caused by an intraperitoneal injection of *n*-hexadecane in BALB/c mice. *Toxicology.* 2006;218(2–3):186–196.
185. Khalil M, Inaba K, Steinman R, et al. T cell studies in a peptide-induced model of systemic lupus erythematosus. *J Immunol.* 2001; 166(3):1667–1674.
186. Desai DD, Marion TN. Induction of anti-DNA antibody with DNA-peptide complexes. *Int Immunol.* 2000;12(11):1569–1578.
187. Yung RL, Quddus J, Chrisp CE, et al. Mechanism of drug-induced lupus. I. Cloned Th2 cells modified with DNA methylation inhibitors in vitro cause autoimmunity in vivo. *J Immunol.* 1995;154(6):3025–3035.
188. Cunnane G, Fitzgerald O, Beeton C, et al. Early joint erosions and serum levels of matrix metalloproteinase 1, matrix metalloproteinase 3, and tissue inhibitor of metalloproteinases 1 in rheumatoid arthritis. *Arthritis Rheum.* 2001;44(10):2263–2274.
189. Alamanos Y, Drosos AA. Epidemiology of adult rheumatoid arthritis. *Autoimmun Rev.* 2005;4(3):130–136.
190. Plenge RM, Padyukov L, Remmers EF, et al. Replication of putative candidate-gene associations with rheumatoid arthritis in >4,000 samples from North America and Sweden: association of susceptibility with PTPN22, CTLA4, and PADI4. *Am J Hum Genet.* 2005; 77(6):1044–1060.
191. Goronzy JJ, Weyand CM. Rheumatoid arthritis. *Immunol Rev.* 2005;204:55–73.
192. Weyand CM, Seyler TM, Goronzy JJ. B cells in rheumatoid synovitis. *Arthritis Res Ther.* 2005;7(suppl 3):S9–S12.
193. Huber LC, Distler O, Tarner I, et al. Synovial fibroblasts: key players in rheumatoid arthritis. *Rheumatology (Oxf).* 2006;45(6):669–675.
194. Roelofs MF, Boelens WC, Joosten LA, et al. Identification of small heat shock protein B8 (HSP22) as a novel TLR4 ligand and potential involvement in the pathogenesis of rheumatoid arthritis. *J Immunol.* 2006;176(11):7021–7027.
195. Lee EY, Yim JJ, Lee HS, et al. Dinucleotide repeat polymorphism in intron II of human Toll-like receptor 2 gene and susceptibility to rheumatoid arthritis. *Int J Immunogenet.* 2006;33(3):211–215.
196. Itoh K, Patki V, Furie RA, et al. Clonal expansion is a characteristic feature of the B-cell repetoire of patients with rheumatoid arthritis. *Arthritis Res.* 2000;2(1):50–58.
197. Westwood OM, Nelson PN, Hay FC. Rheumatoid factors: what's new? *Rheumatology (Oxf).* 2006;45(4):379–385.
198. Samuels J, Ng YS, Coupillaud C, et al. Human B cell tolerance and its failure in rheumatoid arthritis. *Ann NY Acad Sci.* 2005;1062:116–126.
199. Hill JA, Southwood S, Sette A, et al. Cutting edge: the conversion of arginine to citrulline allows for a high-affinity peptide interaction with the rheumatoid arthritis-associated HLA-DRB1*0401 MHC class II molecule. *J Immunol.* 2003;171(2):538–541.
200. Kuhn KA, Kulik L, Tomooka B, et al. Antibodies against citrullinated proteins enhance tissue injury in experimental autoimmune arthritis. *J Clin Invest.* 2006;116(4):961–973.
201. Emery P, Fleischmann R, Filipowicz-Sosnowska A, et al. The efficacy and safety of rituximab in patients with active rheumatoid arthritis despite methotrexate treatment: results of a phase IIB randomized, double-blind, placebo-controlled, dose-ranging trial. *Arthritis Rheum.* 2006;54(5):1390–1400.
202. Yen JH, Moore BE, Nakajima T, et al. Major histocompatibility complex class I-recognizing receptors are disease risk genes in rheumatoid arthritis. *J Exp Med.* 2001;193(10):1159–1167.
203. Dieude P, Cornelis F. Genetic basis of rheumatoid arthritis. *Joint Bone Spine.* 2005;72(6):520–526.
204. Firestein GS. Evolving concepts of rheumatoid arthritis. *Nature.* 2003;423(6937):356–361.
205. Walsh NC, Crotti TN, Goldring SR, et al. Rheumatic diseases: the effects of inflammation on bone. *Immunol Rev.* 2005;208: 228–251.
206. Kannan K, Ortmann RA, Kimpel D. Animal models of rheumatoid arthritis and their relevance to human disease. *Pathophysiology.* 2005;12(3):167–181.
207. Sakaguchi S, Sakaguchi N. Animal models of arthritis caused by systemic alteration of the immune system. *Curr Opin Immunol.* 2005;17(6):589–594.
208. Joosten LA, Heuvelmans-Jacobs M, Lubberts E, et al. Local interleukin-12 gene transfer promotes conversion of an acute arthritis to a chronic destructive arthritis. *Arthritis Rheum.* 2002;46(5): 1379–1389.
209. van Eden W, Hauet-Broere F, Berlo S, et al. Stress proteins as inducers and targets of regulatory T cells in arthritis. *Int Rev Immunol.* 2005;24(3–4):181–197.
210. van den Berg WB. Animal models of arthritis. What have we learned? *J Rheumatol Suppl.* 2005;72:7–9.
211. Lubberts E, van den Bersselaar L, Oppers-Walgreen B, et al. IL-17 promotes bone erosion in murine collagen-induced arthritis through loss of the receptor activator of NF-kappa B ligand/ osteoprotegerin balance. *J Immunol.* 2003;170(5):2655–2662.

212. Szanto S, Bardos T, Szabo Z, et al. Induction of arthritis in HLA-DR4-humanized and HLA-DQ8-humanized mice by human cartilage proteoglycan aggrecan but only in the presence of an appropriate (non-MHC) genetic background. *Arthritis Rheum.* 2004; 50(6):1984–1995.
213. Mandik-Nayak L, Allen PM. Initiation of an autoimmune response: insights from a transgenic model of rheumatoid arthritis. *Immunol Res.* 2005;32(1–3):5–13.
214. Neumann E, Gay S, Muller-Ladner U. The RANK/RANKL/osteoprotegerin system in rheumatoid arthritis: new insights from animal models. *Arthritis Rheum.* 2005;52(10):2960–2967.
215. Kuon W, Kuhne M, Busch DH, et al. Identification of novel human aggrecan T cell epitopes in HLA-B27 transgenic mice associated with spondyloarthropathy. *J Immunol.* 2004;173(8):4859–4866.
216. May E, Dulphy N, Frauendorf E, et al. Conserved TCR beta chain usage in reactive arthritis; evidence for selection by a putative HLA-B27-associated autoantigen. *Tissue Antigens*. 2002;60(4):299–308.
217. Vahamiko S, Penttinen MA, Granfors K. Aetiology and pathogenesis of reactive arthritis: role of non-antigen-presenting effects of HLA-B27. *Arthritis Res Ther*. 2005;7(4):136–141.
218. Raine T, Brown D, Bowness P, et al. Consistent patterns of expression of HLA class I free heavy chains in healthy individuals and raised expression in spondyloarthropathy patients point to physiological and pathological roles. *Rheumatology (Oxf)*. 2006;45(11): 1338–1344.
219. Gerard HC, Wang Z, Whittum-Hudson JA, et al. Cytokine and chemokine mRNA produced in synovial tissue chronically infected with *Chlamydia trachomatis* and *C. pneumoniae*. *J Rheumatol.* 2002;29(9):1827–1835.
220. Gerard HC, Schumacher HR, El-Gabalawy H, et al. Chlamydia pneumoniae present in the human synovium are viable and metabolically active. *Microbial Pathogenesis*. 2000;29(1):17–24.
221. Rihl M, Kohler L, Klos A, Zeidler H. Persistent infection of *Chlamydia* in reactive arthritis. *Ann Rheum Dis*. 2006;65(3):281–284.
222. Lories RJ. Animal models of spondyloarthritis. *Curr Opin Rheumatol.* 2006;18(4):342–346.
223. Turner MJ, Sowders DP, DeLay ML, et al. HLA-B27 misfolding in transgenic rats is associated with activation of the unfolded protein response. *J Immunol.* 2005;175(4):2438–2448.
224. Hacquard-Bouder C, Ittah M, Breban M. Animal models of HLA-B27-associated diseases: new outcomes. *Joint Bone Spine*. 2006;73(2):132–138.
225. Moriwaki R, Noda M, Yajima M, et al. Clinical manifestations of Takayasu arteritis in India and Japan—new classification of angiographic findings. *Angiology*. 1997;48(5):369–379.
226. Weyand CM, Hicok KC, Hunder GG, et al. The HLA-DRB1 locus as a genetic component in giant cell arteritis. Mapping of a disease-linked sequence motif to the antigen binding site of the HLA-DR molecule. *J Clin Invest*. 1992;90(6):2355–2361.
227. Weyand CM, Ma-Krupa W, Goronzy JJ. Immunopathways in giant cell arteritis and polymyalgia rheumatica. *Autoimmun Rev.* 2004;3(1):46–53.
228. Weyand CM, Ma-Krupa W, Pryshchep O, et al. Vascular dendritic cells in giant cell arteritis. *Ann NY Acad Sci.* 2005;1062:195–208.
229. Lane SE, Watts RA, Shepstone L, et al. Primary systemic vasculitis: clinical features and mortality. *QJM*. 2005;98(2):97–111.
230. Bosch X, Guilabert A, Font J. Antineutrophil cytoplasmic antibodies. *Lancet*. 2006;368(9533):404–418.
231. von Vietinghoff S, Schreiber A, Otto B, et al. Membrane proteinase 3 and Wegener's granulomatosis. *Clin Nephrol*. 2005;64(6):453–459.
232. Xiao H, Heeringa P, Hu P, et al. Antineutrophil cytoplasmic autoantibodies specific for myeloperoxidase cause glomerulonephritis and vasculitis in mice. *J Clin Invest*. 2002;110(7):955–963.
233. Xiao H, Heeringa P, Liu Z, et al. The role of neutrophils in the induction of glomerulonephritis by anti-myeloperoxidase antibodies. *Am J Pathol*. 2005;167(1):39–45.
234. Stone JH, Holbrook JT, Marriott MA, et al. Solid malignancies among patients in the Wegener's Granulomatosis Etanercept Trial. *Arthritis Rheum*. 2006;54(5):1608–1618.
235. Gilchrist FC, Bunn C, Foley PJ, et al. Class II HLA associations with autoantibodies in scleroderma: a highly significant role for HLA-DP. *Genes Immun*. 2001;2(2):76–81.
236. Feghali-Bostwick C, Medsger TA Jr, et al. Analysis of systemic sclerosis in twins reveals low concordance for disease and high concordance for the presence of antinuclear antibodies. *Arthritis Rheum.* 2003;48(7):1956–1963.
237. Arnett FC, Howard RF, Tan F, et al. Increased prevalence of systemic sclerosis in a Native American tribe in Oklahoma. Association with an Amerindian HLA haplotype. *Arthritis Rheum.* 1996;39(8):1362–1370.
238. Steen VD. Autoantibodies in systemic sclerosis. *Semin Arthritis Rheum.* 2005;35(1):35–42.
239. Abraham DJ, Varga J. Scleroderma: from cell and molecular mechanisms to disease models. *Trends Immunol.* 2005;26(11):587–595.
240. Higley H, Persichitte K, Chu S, et al. Immunocytochemical localization and serologic detection of transforming growth factor beta 1. Association with type I procollagen and inflammatory cell markers in diffuse and limited systemic sclerosis, morphea, and Raynaud's phenomenon. *Arthritis Rheum.* 1994;37(2):278–288.
241. Rudnicka L, Varga J, Christiano AM, et al. Elevated expression of type VII collagen in the skin of patients with systemic sclerosis. Regulation by transforming growth factor-beta. *J Clin Invest*. 1994; 93(4):1709–1715.
242. Baroni SS, Santillo M, Bevilacqua F, et al. Stimulatory autoantibodies to the PDGF receptor in systemic sclerosis. *N Engl J Med.* 2006;354(25):2667–2676.
243. Denton CP, Merkel PA, Furst DE, et al. Recombinant human anti-transforming growth factor beta1 antibody therapy in systemic sclerosis: a multicenter, randomized, placebo-controlled Phase I/II trial of CAT-192. *Arthritis Rheum.* 2006;56(1):323–333.
244. Schermuly RT, Dony E, Ghofrani HA, et al. Reversal of experimental pulmonary hypertension by PDGF inhibition. *J Clin Invest.* 2005;115(10):2811–2821.
245. Lemaire R, Bayle J, Lafyatis R. Fibrillin in Marfan syndrome and tight skin mice provides new insights into transforming growth factor-beta regulation and systemic sclerosis. *Curr Opin Rheumatol.* 2006;18(6):582–587.
246. Hasegawa M, Hamaguchi Y, Yanaba K, et al. B-lymphocyte depletion reduces skin fibrosis and autoimmunity in the tight-skin mouse model for systemic sclerosis. *Am J Pathol.* 2006;169(3):954–966.
247. Kodera T, McGaha TL, Phelps R, et al. Disrupting the IL-4 gene rescues mice homozygous for the tight-skin mutation from embryonic death and diminishes TGF-beta production by fibroblasts. *Proc Natl Acad Sci U S A.* 2002;99(6):3800–3805.
248. Murota H, Hamasaki Y, Nakashima T, et al. Disruption of tumor necrosis factor receptor p55 impairs collagen turnover in experimentally induced sclerodermic skin fibroblasts. *Arthritis Rheum.* 2003;48(4):1117–1125.
249. Yamamoto T. The bleomycin-induced scleroderma model: what have we learned for scleroderma pathogenesis? *Arch Dermatol Res.* 2006;297(8):333–344.
250. Christner PJ, Jimenez SA. Animal models of systemic sclerosis: insights into systemic sclerosis pathogenesis and potential therapeutic approaches. *Curr Opin Rheumatol.* 2004;16(6):746–752.
251. Dalakas MC, Hohlfeld R. Polymyositis and dermatomyositis. *Lancet*. 2003;362(9388):971–982.
252. Oddis CV, Conte CG, Steen VD, et al. Incidence of polymyositis-dermatomyositis: a 20-year study of hospital diagnosed cases in Allegheny County, PA 1963–1982. *J Rheumatol.* 1990;17(10): 1329–1334.
253. Dalakas MC. Muscle biopsy findings in inflammatory myopathies. *Rheum Dis Clin N Am*. 2002;28(4):779–798, vi.
254. De Paepe B, De Keyzer K, Martin JJ, et al. Alpha-chemokine receptors CXCR1–3 and their ligands in idiopathic inflammatory myopathies. *Acta Neuropathol.* 2005;109(6):576–582.
255. Tucci M, Quatraro C, Dammacco F, et al. Interleukin-18 overexpression as a hallmark of the activity of autoimmune inflammatory myopathies. *Clin Exp Immunol.* 2006;146(1):21–31.
256. Greenberg SA, Pinkus JL, Pinkus GS, et al. Interferon-alpha/beta-mediated innate immune mechanisms in dermatomyositis. *Ann Neurol.* 2005;57(5):664–678.
257. Nagaraju K. Role of major histocompatibility complex class I molecules in autoimmune myositis. *Curr Opin Rheumatol.* 2005;17(6): 725–730.

258. Sordet C, Goetz J, Sibilia J. Contribution of autoantibodies to the diagnosis and nosology of inflammatory muscle disease. *Joint Bone Spine*. 2006;73(6):646–654.
259. Chakrabarti S, Kobayashi KS, Flavell RA, et al. Impaired membrane resealing and autoimmune myositis in synaptotagmin VII-deficient mice. *J Cell Biol*. 2003;162(4):543–549.
260. Nagaraju K, Casciola-Rosen L, Lundberg I, et al. Activation of the endoplasmic reticulum stress response in autoimmune myositis: potential role in muscle fiber damage and dysfunction. *Arthritis Rheum*. 2005;52(6):1824–1835.
261. Kawachi I, Tanaka K, Tanaka M, et al. Dendritic cells presenting pyruvate kinase M1/M2 isozyme peptide can induce experimental allergic myositis in BALB/c mice. *J Neuroimmunol*. 2001;117 (1–2):108–115.

Chapter 42

Organ-Specific Autoimmunity

Matthias G. von Herrath and Dirk Homann

Misdirection and improper control of immune responses can lead to organ-specific destruction, which is classified as autoimmunity, if cells reactive to self antigens can be identified. Although a certain genetic predisposition is associated with most organ-specific autoimmune disorders, other contributing etiologic factors remain to be identified. It is not clear whether some of the diseases that selectively affect one or few organs are due to a yet-unidentified viral infection and autoimmune responses arise secondary to such a primary attack. Once a destructive process has taken root, the outcome depends on a multitude of internal and external factors and can be influenced therapeutically. For example, alteration of the systemic or local, organ-specific cytokine milieu has proven to be of benefit. In addition to the immunopathology and etiology, novel treatments that are based on redirecting the immune system into a state of benign autoreactivity are discussed in this chapter.

GENERAL CONCEPTS IN ORGAN-SPECIFIC AUTOIMMUNITY

Immunity and Autoimmunity

Autoimmunity is the "Other" (1) of immunity, and in true dialectical fashion, immunity's inception as a scientific discipline encapsulated the conceptual problem that was to shape the immunologic debates in the first 15 and last 50 years of the 20th century. As much as the prefix *auto* assigns a specific place apart from immunity proper, the idea of immunity is not conceivable (for better or worse), without the notion of the self (2). Immunity's distinct association with the individual self stretches from its etymologic roots in the Roman legal concept of an *individual's* exemption from duty, service, or tax to its official induction into the canon of medical terminology [defined as "*idio*syncratic condition" in the 1878 edition of Littré's *Dictionnaire de Médecine* (3)] and beyond. However, with the dawn of the 20th century, in the wake of the seminal discoveries of immune protection by active immunization with attenuated pathogens (4) or passive transfer of convalescent serum (5) and the seemingly unstoppable success of the "New Immunology," the notion of the immunologic self underwent a dramatic reconfiguration. The price for immunity, it appeared, was autoimmunity, a concept so problematic that its existence had to be relegated to the realm of the almost unspeakable (that is, the Greco-Latin neologism of a "horror autotoxicus") (6). Paradoxically, the very time that saw the concept of "horror autotoxicus" acquire a quasi-dogmatic status as the "law of immunity research" (7) was also the time that A. Silverstein termed the "classical period" of autoimmunity research (8). Although declared anathema, autoimmune phenomena were reported in a quick succession of widely publicized observations. In 1902, Portier and Richet reported the phenomenon of anaphylaxis (as opposed to *pro*phylaxis) (9); Maurice Arthus characterized the local inflammatory response that was to bear his name in 1903 (10); Donath and Landsteiner described the first human autoimmune disease (paroxysmal cold hemoglobinuria) in 1904 (11); and the term allergy ("altered reactivity") was coined by von Pirquet and Schick in their analysis of serum sickness in 1905 (12). The idea that tissue destruction may lead to expanded immunopathology (nowadays referred to as determinant spreading) was proposed by Weil and Braun in 1909: In the course of an infectious disease, "tissue alterations lead to the generation of complement-binding factors that, ... based on their affinity to bodily cells, themselves attack and damage the cells of the organism" (13). Even the concepts of organ specificity (14), immunoprivilege, and the breakdown of regulatory mechanisms as a cause for autoimmunity (7) were developed in the early days of autoimmunity research.

This period of extraordinary productivity was followed by an almost 40-year hiatus (the "dark ages of autoimmunity research") (8). The reasons for a generalized disinterest in autoimmune phenomena are manifold and included political reconfigurations after World War I, the death of both Ehrlich (1915) and Metchnikoff (1916), a misconception of "horror autotoxicus" as the immune system's *inability* to generate responses against self, and a paradigm shift in the field of immunology in favor of immunochemical approaches (8). The renaissance of autoimmunity research had to await observations about immunologic tolerance of mice congenitally infected with lymphocytic choriomeningitis virus (LCMV) (15), description of tolerance in chimeric cattle twins (16), and Peter Medawar's work on skin transplant rejection (17–20), as well as the integration of these findings into a conceptual framework of self and non-self as determinants for immunologic reactivity (21). Burnet subsequently developed and extended these ideas into the "clonal selection theory of antibody formation" (22) thereby establishing the conceptual centrality of self, non-self, and immunologic tolerance. Although the dogmatic reading of "horror autotoxicus" was still prevalent [Ernest Witebsky delayed his publication about thyroid antibodies (23) for several years, assuming an experimental error (8)], Ehrlich's original conception as "regulatory contrivances" that prevent autoimmunity was now validated within the context of the clonal selection theory.

Again, however, the usefulness of self and non-self as distinguishing parameters was challenged at the very time they began their rise to prominence. Ludwik Fleck, in his *Genesis and Development of a Scientific Fact*, questioned the capacity of an immune system that only interacts with structures that are strictly non-self: "it is very doubtful whether an invasion in the old sense is possible, involving as it does an inference by completely foreign organisms in natural conditions. A completely foreign organism could find no receptors capable of reaction and thus could not generate a biological process" (24). This view was echoed and elaborated on in the work of Jerne (25) and Coutinho (26), and even the possibility of a beneficial role for autoimmune processes was postulated by concepts such as "physiologic autoimmunity" (27), "positive autoimmunity" (28), and "protective autoimmunity" (29). The importance of autoreactivity as an integral aspect of immunity is furthermore demonstrated by the processes of "positive selection," T cell development in the thymus, and the T cell–mediated destruction of transformed or infected tissues, which are based on the recognition of foreign (e.g., viral peptides, or even self, as in the case of some tumor-derived antigens) in the context of "self" (major histocompatibility complexes). In fact, events associated with danger or the preservation of tissue integrity rather than the discrimination between self/non-self have been postulated as a primary driving force that engages the immune system (30,31). More recently, the notion that immune reactivity is generated by the introduction of strong antigenic discontinuities ("criterion of continuity") has been proposed and may offer an elegant solution to some of the conceptual problems outlined earlier (32,33). Still, the idea of recognition (2,34,35) remains a central element common to all of these models because the immune system's principal task is cast as a differentiation between organismal states (self vs. non-self, safety vs. danger, integrity vs. damage, continuity vs. discontinuity, etc.). Such operational distinctions are indeed powerful tools for conceptualizing the functions of the immune system—with impressive success, as well as some obvious shortcomings. Yet they may also insinuate a proximity of logical and functional categories that can culminate in the postulate of a principal objective, a veritable *raison d'être* for the immune system. However, rather than rejecting the need for a comprehensive conceptual framework in favor of pure experimental work (36), we endorse continuing efforts to develop a theoretical basis for the phenomenon of "auto/immunity" and favor an evolutionary perspective that conceives of the immune system, devoid of a particular purpose (37), as "the cause of its own necessity" (38).

The notion of autoimmunity as an aberrant phenomenon has informed much of our current understanding about the immune system and its functions, and there appears to be a growing awareness that immunity and autoimmunity are both historically and conceptually intertwined. An emerging consensus indicates that the anthropomorphisms of self and non-self should be overcome [e.g., as suggested in the respective forewords to two major autoimmunity textbooks (39,40)] and that autoimmunity is likely a universal phenomenon in the evolution of the vertebrate immune system. As part of the evolving organism, the immune system processes antigen stimuli in a deterministic fashion restricted by genetics, previous antigenic experience of the host, nature of the antigen, and the conditions of its presentation (39). However, any effort to imbue the immune system's function with an overriding purpose, no matter how important for our conceptualization and experimentation, has to recognize that evolution is ignorant of teleology. In this respect, the remark by the Darwinist Paul Ehrlich that production of autoantibodies is "dysteleological in the extreme" (6) may be extended to the functionality of the immune system as a whole; there is no teleology in autoimmunity or immunity, just the workings of a complex system under evolutionary constraints. The rules that inform immunity are the same ones that govern autoimmunity.

The Burden of Autoimmune Diseases

The existence of autoimmune diseases in humans has been known for 100 years. By now, autoimmune pathogenesis has been attributed to more than 40 human diseases (41), yet it is still far from clear which features can conclusively be proven to have an underlying autoimmune pathogenesis. It has been suggested, somewhat provocatively, that with knowledge about an infectious origin, diseases are called immunopathologically mediated, whereas lack of such knowledge results in reference to such diseases as autoimmune (42). Although this argument is akin to the medical taxonomy in which diseases of unknown origin are assigned to the domain of the "endogenous," "idiotypic," "essential," or "primary," a "positive" definition for autoimmune disease is very much needed to provide a specific diagnostic framework that allows for unequivocal identification of distinct autoimmune disorders yet remains flexible enough to accommodate new insights in etiologic and symptomatologic processes. A first attempt to provide such a basis for the establishment of the autoimmune origin of human diseases was formulated by Witebsky et al., who modeled their postulates on those of Koch: "recognition of an autoimmune response; autoantibody or cell-mediated, identification of a corresponding autoantigen, as well as induction of an analogous autoimmune response and disease in experimental animals" (43). A timely update for these criteria was proposed by Rose and Bona, who suggested a combination of direct evidence (transfer of pathogenic antibodies or T cells), indirect evidence (reproduction of disease in experimental animals), and circumstantial evidence (clinical clues) to determine an underlying autoimmune etiology for human diseases (41). However, it is important to note that any specific guidelines have to be tailored to individual autoimmune disorders. For instance, an exemplary catalogue of diagnostic criteria has been developed by the International Autoimmune Hepatitis Group to facilitate and improve the diagnosis of autoimmune hepatitis (44). This report also illustrates the importance of distinguishing between an autoimmune and infectious origin for hepatitis (44): Immunosuppressive therapy has a beneficial effect on the course of autoimmune hepatitis (AIH), and although responsiveness to such therapy is one of the diagnostic criteria for AIH, this therapy may be detrimental when used for treatment of virus-induced hepatitis.

As a first of its kind, a metastudy published in 1997 provided a comprehensive evaluation of prevalence and incidence studies conducted for 24 autoimmune diseases since 1965 (45). Overall, 1 in 31 Americans, or approximately 8.5 million people, were estimated to be afflicted by an autoimmune disease. The most prevalent disorders, divided into organ-specific and systemic conditions (and ranked in order of prevalence), are listed in Table 42.1. The study by Jacobson and colleagues also documents some striking, if not entirely unexpected, findings. Many autoimmune conditions are clearly understudied, and some of the most frequently studied diseases exhibit comparatively low prevalence rates. The cause for this imbalance between the public health burden posed by some autoimmune disorders and their attraction as objects for scientific study remains to be elucidated but will likely include the presence or absence of effective therapy. Pernicious anemia, the sixth-most-common autoimmune disease in the United States, can be effectively managed and therefore elicits only limited epidemiologic interest. In contrast, some rare conditions may pose a pronounced burden to afflicted individuals and thus warrant continued efforts to develop more effective prophylactic and therapeutic interventions. Furthermore, the availability of certain models for autoimmune diseases (again not necessarily a reflection of the epidemiologic importance of the corresponding human autoimmune disease) has an impact on choices made by researchers charting their field of study. Finally, as in other areas of research or clinical medicine, the funds and resources available are the result of multiple factors that may or may not include the public health burden exerted by a particular autoimmune disease. Balancing these aspects appropriately to appreciate and address the burden of autoimmune diseases based on both the afflicted individual and society at large is a challenge that will require continued efforts to identify, investigate, inform, and, it is hoped, improve the therapies for many autoimmune diseases.

Differentiating Organ-specific and Systemic Autoimmune Diseases

A perennial approach in the quest to make sense of complex phenomena is the establishment of dichotomies, however fraught with shortcomings, inconsistencies, and exceptions to the rule. Steeped in clinical traditions and immediately intelligible, the distinction between systemic and organ-specific autoimmune diseases is as useful as it is inadequate. Given that the evolving understanding of autoimmune diseases requires a constant reevaluation of concepts pertaining to etiopathogenesis and effective

TABLE 42.1 Prevalence of Autoimmune Diseases

Autoimmune Disease	*Organ*	*Weighted Mean Prevalence Rate/100,000*	*Weighted Mean Incidence Rate/100,000*
Thyroiditis/hypothyroidism	**Thyroid**	**1,323.8**	**21.8**
Grave's disease/hyperthyroidism	**Thyroid**	**1,151.5**	**13.9**
Rheumatoid arthritis	Joints, lung, heart, other	860.0	23.7
Vitiligo	**Skin**	**400.2**	
Type 1 diabetes	**Pancreatic β cells**	**192.0**	**12.2**
Pernicious anemia	**Stomach**	**150.9**	[a]
Multiple sclerosis	**Brain/spinal cord**	**58.3**	**3.2**
Glomerulonephritis (primary)	**Kidney**	**40.0**	**3.6**
Systemic lupus erythematosus	Skin, joints, kidney, brain, lung, heart, other	23.8	7.3
Glomerulonephritis (IgA)	**Kidney**	**23.2**	**2.4**
Sjögren's syndrome	—	14.4	[a]
Addison's disease	**Adrenal**	**5.0**	[a]
Myasthenia gravis	**Muscle**	**5.1**	**0.4**
Polymyositis/dermatomyositis	Muscle, lung, heart, joints, other	5.1	1.8
Scleroderma	Skin	4.4	0.8
Primary billiary cirrhosis	**Liver bile ducts**	**3.5**	**0.9**
Uveitis	**Eye**	**1.7**	**18.9**
Chronic active hepatitis	**Liver**	**0.4**	**0.7**

Data taken from Jacobson et al. (45), which should be consulted for details.
Organ-specific autoimmune diseases in bold, systemic autoimmune diseases in regular type face.
The prevalence/incidence rate from each study within a disease category contributed proportionately based on the population size of that study. The proportion or weight was calculated by dividing the study population denominator by the total of all the study population denominators for each disease.
[a] No studies on disease incidence are available.

treatment modalities, it would be premature to abandon such a simple and still useful classification. Instead, that porous juncture between systemic and organ-specific disorders may reveal hitherto unappreciated aspects of pathogenesis. On the surface, the patterns of pathology result from the distribution of anatomic niches that provide a suitable environment to interface antigens and immune effectors. Leaving aside the difficulties pertaining to the identification of initiating autoantigens in many human autoimmune diseases (and the challenging task of correlating markers of immunologic activity, such as autoantibodies, with cause or consequence of tissue destruction), a particularly puzzling phenomenon is the apparent organ specificity of some disorders in the face of autoimmune responses that target ubiquitous antigens. For instance, the ribonucleoprotein antigens implicated in Sjögren's syndrome or the transfer RNA synthetases targeted in polymyositis are widely expressed intracellular antigens, yet the pathology of these diseases is relatively circumscribed. Another intriguing example is the K/BxN arthritis model in which pathogenic antibodies recognize the ubiquitous cytoplasmic enzyme glucose-6-phosphate isomerase (GPI). Here, the preferential involvement of the joints apparently results from unique properties of the regional vasculature that allow for an antibody-mediated increase of vasopermeability and amplification of pathology by extracellular GPI deposition in the articular cavities (46,47). The observation that autoimmune damage is critically dependent on aspects of the local microanatomy emphasizes the importance of considering autoimmune processes in the larger context of interdependent organ systems.

Finally, an examination of some animal models used for the study of particular organ-specific autoimmune disorders further challenges the simple notion of restricted pathology and may provide clues about etiologic commonalities of ostensibly disparate clinical autoimmune syndromes. The nonobese diabetic (NOD) mouse is the most widely used animal model for the study of type 1 diabetes (T1D), a severe condition caused by autoimmune destruction of the insulin-producing β cells in the pancreas (48,49). However, NOD mice also exhibit aspects of type 2 diabetes (T2D) (50) and are prone to autoimmune sialitis, thyroiditis, peripheral neuropathy, and prostatitis (a lupus erythematosus–like syndrome that develops after exposure to killed mycobacteria), as well as, under certain circumstances, exocrine pancreatitis (49). Similar to the etiology of T1D, specific T cells are involved in the pathogenesis of all of these disorders, although antigenic targets and requirements for costimulatory interactions are distinct. Thus, as in human T1D, the NOD mouse combines a generalized genetic susceptibility to multiorgan autoimmunity that is focused on pancreatic β cells but not limited to endocrine organs.

Central and Peripheral Tolerance: Implementing an Operational Concept

A detailed historical discussion of the concept of tolerance is beyond the scope of this chapter, but some aspects of the use of the term tolerance require clarification at the outset. Tolerance in adaptive immunity, *strictu sensu*, is the absence of specific lymphocyte activity, the consequence of physical deletion or functional silencing of specific T and B cells. Some researchers refer to these tolerance mechanisms as "passive" or "recessive" tolerance to distinguish them explicitly from "active" or "dominant" tolerance. Although the latter constitutes bona fide immune responses (and therefore other researchers do not categorize them as a mode of tolerance), their particular nature results in a phenotype that is comparable to that achieved by means of passive/recessive tolerance. Distinct effector mechanisms (e.g., immunosuppressive cytokines) and possibly dedicated classes of immune cells (e.g., T regulatory cells [Tregs]) ensure that local or systemic autoimmunity is avoided. The concept of T cell suppressors, first proposed in the early 1970s by Gershon (51), has recently been resurrected in the form of professional $CD25^+FoxP3^+CD4^+$ and adaptive Tregs and has attracted considerable attention. However, although there is indeed a population of $CD25^+$ T cells committed to regulatory activity in naive, nonimmunized mice, we underscore that regulatory functions, including those that limit autoimmunity, are a feature of the immune system as a whole and can be exercised by other classes of immune cells as well (e.g., $CD8^+$ T cells, $\gamma\delta$T cell receptor [TcR], T cells, NKT cells). Thus, although $CD25^+CD4^+$ regulatory T cells occupy a distinct and important niche in the complex dynamic network of immune functions, not all Tregs are $CD25^+CD4^+$, nor do all $CD25^+CD4^+$ T cells function as suppressors. Indeed, novel markers might characterize regulatory function better; among these is the expression of the forkhead/winged helix transcription "FoxP3" (52–58) and secretion of cytokines with regulatory function such as interleukin (IL)-10 (59,60) or transforming growth factor-β (TGFβ) (61). The many efforts to understand the nature of $CD25^+CD4^+$ Tregs have been expertly reviewed elsewhere (62,63).

T Cell Tolerance

Autoreactivity, by definition, designates a specific immune response to self-antigens. Antigen-nonspecific responses such as inflammation and innate immune processes should not be considered autoimmune in the strict sense, although they may accompany, enhance, or even trigger adaptive autoimmune responses. Thus, antigen-specific T or B cell immunity would have to underlie a genuine autoimmune disorder. Furthermore, for organ-specific autoimmune diseases, antigen specificity of primary effector lymphocytes must be largely restricted to autoantigens derived from defined organs or tissues. Once initiated, organ-specific responses that precipitate or drive the localized autoimmune reaction may diversify to comprise additional specificities (determinant spreading) and pathogenic mechanisms.

How does the adaptive immune system restrict generation and activation of autoreactive lymphocytes? The central process by which the generation of T cell receptor diversity is limited is called thymic selection. Thymic selection is a developmental process that selects T cells with a biased repertoire for export into the periphery (64–68). T cells that interact at least weakly with self-peptides presented in the context of major histocompatibility class (MHC) molecules are chosen in the course of positive selection (69,70), whereas those that do not effectively interact with MHC:peptide complexes die by neglect. However, interactions above a certain avidity threshold result in elimination by negative selection and constitutes the basis for central tolerance (64,68). Thus, central tolerance prevents widespread autoimmunity as a function of lymphocyte/antigen-complex avidity and preferentially selects T cells with specificities for antigens not expressed in thymic epithelium for export into the periphery. However, central tolerance is not a complete mechanism, and a sizeable pool of T cells with intermediate avidity can escape negative selection and is exported to the periphery. The presence of these autoreactive T cells can be considered physiologic and they are not noxious for two reasons: Either they are usually not activated and exhibit a naive phenotype, or they exhibit regulatory effector functions and act as adaptive Tregs following activation. Thus, not all self-reactive lymphocytes necessarily need to exhibit an aggressive phenotype. Depending on their specific effector function, autoreactive T cells could exhibit regulatory functions and critically modulate or even abort local autoimmune processes. Such autoreactive regulators might occur physiologically and constitute the majority of autoimmune responses present in healthy individuals. Only an encounter under appropriate stimulatory conditions (i.e., presentation of autoantigen-derived peptides presented in the context of MHC class I or II molecules accompanied by antigen-nonspecific costimulatory interactions and strong inflammatory signals) can lead to their full activation and detrimental effector functions in the periphery. As "armed effectors," autoreactive T cells are potentially very dangerous and may initiate organ-specific autoimmunity if they recognize the autoantigens or closely related proteins in a defined tissue. It is thought that a few autoaggressive "driver clones" with highly detrimental effector function can sustain a localized autoimmune process.

The presence of autoreactive T cells in the periphery might suggest that detrimental autoimmunity should occur quite frequently if organ-specific autoantigens are not expressed in the thymus. Alternatively, such physiologically occurring autoimmunity is not of a regulatory nature. Yet there are several additional mechanisms that maintain tolerance in the periphery. "Peripheral tolerance" involves a set of mechanisms that ensures that autoreactive T lymphocytes are not activated in the periphery. These mechanisms pertain to both autoreactive and heteroreactive T cells and involve the following pathways. First, it has been observed that naive T cells triggered by a strong signal through the TcR alone may lose the ability to proliferate, and some but not all effector functions become anergic (74–76). Presence of certain cytokines or costimulatory interactions can avoid the induction of anergy or may reverse an anergic state. Second, highly activated T cells will eventually undergo activation-induced cell death (AICD) (77). AICD is thought to be essential for the downmodulation of immune responses and the reestablishment of immune homeostasis. Impairment of AICD may lead to continued immune activation and generalized autoreactivity. For CD4 lymphocytes, AICD is FAS/FAS-L dependent (78,79); it is not clear which interactions precisely control AICD in CD8 cells. Third, molecules that can deliver specific negative signals, such as the B7-binding CTLA-4, are involved in "turning off" the antigen-specific T cells (80,81). Finally, other factors such as regulatory lymphocytes and regulatory antigen-presenting cells (APCs) might play important roles in maintaining peripheral tolerance (51,62,82).

B Cell Tolerance

Although they are not selected in the thymus, developing B cells are subject to similar selection processes that comprise central and peripheral tolerance mechanisms. After B cells mature in the bone marrow, clonal selection occurs after recognizing antigens in the periphery, is avidity dependent, and allows the B cells to undergo further receptor editing. Because T helper (TH) lymphocytes are needed to optimize B cell responses to most protein antigens, the T cell–dependent antibody production is referred to as "thymus dependent." TH cell–independent B cell responses occur mostly to bacterial and lipid antigens, for example, to lipopolysaccharide (LPS), and are therefore rarely autoaggressive. Thus, T cell tolerance controls directly B cell reactivity to autoantigens. In general, systemic autoimmune disorders such as systemic lupus erythematosus (SLE) are B cell dependent, and organ-specific diseases such as multiple sclerosis (MS) and T1D are less dependent on autoantibodies, although B cells could play important roles because APCs and antibodies could enhance disease pathogenesis. In both T1D and MS, autoantibodies correlate with disease progression. In thyroiditis, autoantibodies are instrumental in causing disease, and in autoimmune hepatitis their role is thought to be crucial (see later organ-specific sections).

In conclusion, central and peripheral tolerance mechanisms effectively control the vast majority of autoreactive lymphocytes, which ensures that autoaggressive immune responses are relatively rare (less than 5% overall population). Some of the considerations described in this subsection are illustrated in Figure 42.1.

Organ-specific Tuning: Regulatory and Destructive Autoimmunity

As indicated in the section The Burden of Autoimmune Diseases, although autoimmune disorders must conform to a set of general criteria, organ-specific autoimmunity must be considered in addition to the specific context of the target organ affected. Certain effector functions exerted by autoreactive lymphocytes will be detrimental only to particular cells or tissues. For example, the pancreatic β cells are more sensitive to the damaging effect of inflammatory cytokines than neighboring β cells (both cell types are part of the islets of Langerhans) and other cells in their vicinity (e.g., fibroblasts or acinar tissue of the pancreas) (83). On the other hand, some organs provide a microenvironment that suppresses inflammatory responses. For example, both the gut and the central nervous system contain relatively large amounts of TGFβ, which can have direct antiinflammatory effector functions on T cells and APCs and activate Tregs, unless IL-6 is present (61,84–87). In addition, certain large organs such as the liver may better tolerize lymphocyte responses directed toward them because they contain a high number of cells that are incapable of costimulation (e.g., hepatocytes) and consequently would shut down naive autoreactive lymphocytes that recognize them (30). Finally, the precise activation state, phenotype, and effector function of an autoreactive cell are critical in determining their impact on tissues expressing their cognate antigen. Some molecules will exert beneficial functions, for example, IL-4 and probably IL-10 and TGFβ in T1D (88–90). Antigen-specific adaptive and professional regulatory cells are likely participants of every local autoimmune process and could be essential in delaying or preventing clinical disease altogether. Although their induction is a clear therapeutic goal, phenotype and mechanistic aspects essential for regulatory function are not understood in detail. One hypothesis is that professional and adaptive Tregs exert their function by targeting and altering APC function. They may act as true bystander processors if their suppressive action via APC modulation is extended to aggressive immune responses regardless of specificity located in the microenvironment of the affected organ (Figure 42.2). Indeed, such cells have been identified in several animal models (89,91–93), but their existence and function in humans are not well defined. Alternatively, regulatory lymphocytes

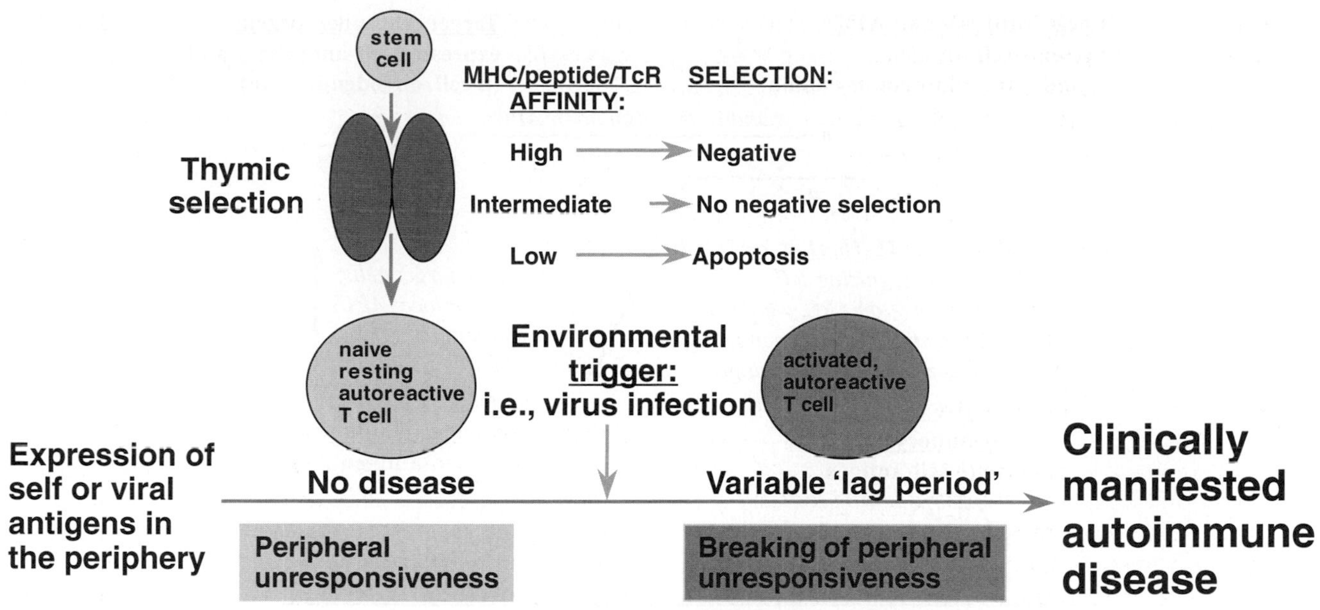

FIGURE 42.1 Events important for the pathogenesis of autoimmunity. Autoreactive lymphocytes can escape thymic negative selection if they are of lower avidity. Such initially naive cells can become activated to turn into autoreactive aggressive as well as regulatory (Treg) cells. Mechanisms that play a role in addition to the genetic predisposition are probably viral infections, other inflammatory processes, and release of cytokines and chemokines. It is noteworthy that not all inflammatory processes need to foster autoimmunity because it is known that many viral infections can protect from the development of autoimmune disease. APCs, antigen-presenting cells; MHC, major histocompatibility complex.

may directly affect activated or naive aggressive lymphocytes and induce anergy or apoptosis. Furthermore, by changing the overall cytokine milieu of a given inflammatory process, the number and function of aggressive cells and cytokines/chemokines may be dampened in a localized area (94). Probably the best-understood balancing circuits used by autoreactive adaptive Tregs are the TH1/TH2 paradigm (95–97) and signaling by IL-10 (60) and/or TGFβ (61). In light of these observations, autoreactivity is not necessarily detrimental or even essential as regards Tregs.

Finally, it might be difficult or even impossible to define a general phenotype of autoaggressive lymphocytes that will cause damage at any site or organ. Instead, autoaggression has to be defined in relation to the target organ or cell that is under attack. Lymphocytes detrimental in one organ/disease might not necessarily be detrimental to other organs, with ubiquitous autoimmunity rarely occurring.

Initiating Autoimmunity: Antigens, Genes, and Environment

Antigens

A central challenge in most human autoimmune disorders is the identification of an initiating autoantigen or autoantigens. For example, several candidate autoantigens have been identified in T1D; however, it is unclear and controversial whether any are actually involved in initiation of the disease. A similar situation exists for MS and rheumatoid arthritis (RA). Because it is unclear which antigens initiate destructive autoimmunity in the majority of human autoimmune diseases, it is important to better define the requisite properties of such antigens. A more detailed understanding of the earliest events during the development of autoimmune pathogenesis should be of direct benefit to the development of therapeutic interventions that forestall development of clinical disease.

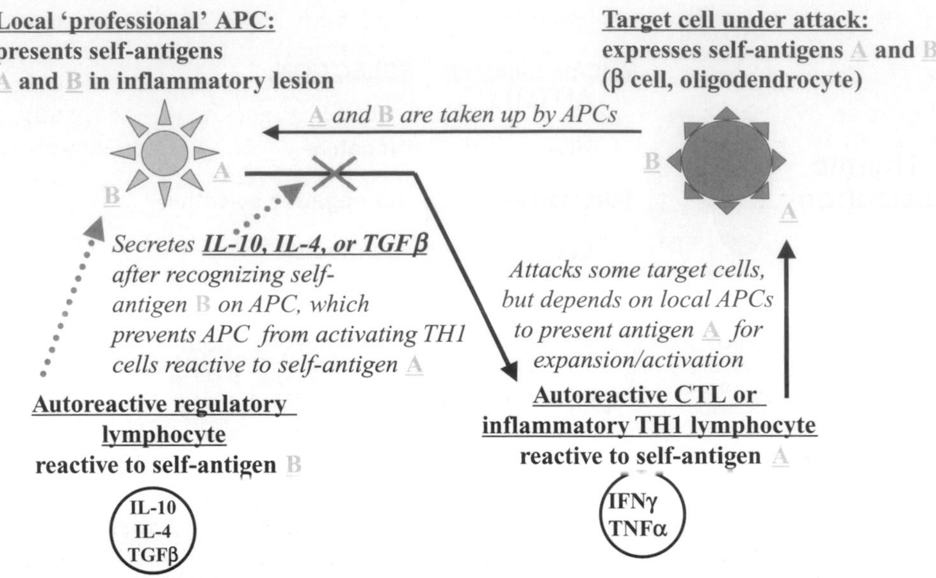
Local 'professional' APC:
presents self-antigens
A and B in inflammatory lesion
Target cell under attack:
expresses self-antigens A and B
(β cell, oligodendrocyte)
A and B are taken up by APCs
Secretes IL-10, IL-4, or TGFβ
after recognizing self-antigen B on APC, which prevents APC from activating TH1 cells reactive to self-antigen A
Attacks some target cells, but depends on local APCs to present antigen A for expansion/activation
Autoreactive regulatory lymphocyte
reactive to self-antigen B
Autoreactive CTL or inflammatory TH1 lymphocyte
reactive to self-antigen A
IL-10
IL-4
TGFβ
IFNγ
TNFα

FIGURE 42.2 The concepts of bystander suppression and infectious tolerance. Organ (cell)-specific autoantigens are taken up and presented by professional antigen-presenting cells (APCs) locally in the organ or draining lymph node. Such autoantigens can then activate autoreactive lymphocytes with diverse effector functions (aggressive vs. Treg). As a consequence, aggressive T cells directed toward antigen A could be regulated by Tregs specific for a different autoantigen B, a process termed bystander suppression by Howard Weiner. In theory, one Treg could suppress aggressive cells with multiple specificities and also foster induction of more heterologous Tregs to the same or other antigens by conditioning APCs, a process termed infectious tolerance by Hermann Waldman. Regulatory cytokines that can dampen or modulate APCs are interleukin (IL)-10, IL-4, and transforming growth factor-β (TGFβ). CTL, cytotoxic T lymphocyte; IFNγ, interferon-γ; TFNα, tissue necrosis factor-α.

The concept of processing antigens to determine self was introduced by Sercarz (98,99). Autoantigens that are not expressed in the thymus or are of cryptic nature (98,100,101) may encounter a more extensive T cell repertoire of higher avidity. Such antigens appear to be better targets. Low levels of thymic antigen expression or limited numbers of thymic medullary cells may lead to partial tolerance (102,103). In addition, the precise timing of antigen expression during embryonic development may play a major role in the establishment of tolerance. Antigens that are cryptic or not expressed during early embryonic development might become better targets later because more autoreactive T cells will be present in the periphery. It should be considered that certain embryonic antigens are involved in initiating autoimmune diseases (104).

Other parameters of importance are the constraints with which particular antigens can be presented to the immune system in a given target organ. Exogenous uptake of soluble antigens usually results in processing via the MHC class II presentation pathway. Such antigens may also be processed through the MHC class I pathway by dendritic cells (DCs), a mechanism termed cross-presentation. Cross-presentation appears to be less efficient than direct endogenous presentation of antigens through the MHC class I pathway. At this point it is not clear which properties will make an antigen a more efficient candidate for cross-presentation. The class I pathway may be very important in the effector phase for many autoimmune disorders because cytotoxic CD8$^+$ T lymphocytes (CTLs) can be induced in this fashion and CTLs have profound detrimental effector functions (interferon-γ [IFNγ] and tumor necrosis factor-α [TNFα] secretion and lysis of target cells) (107). Clearly, recent observations have shown that cross-presentation can lead to immunity, as well as tolerance, and in this way propagate or, alternatively, halt autoimmune disease (105,108). It is less likely that autoantigens that are not presented by professional APCs or within lymphoid organs after their release from target cells/organs can initiate autoimmunity. Only under special circumstances (i.e., extremely high-density presentation of an antigen on a target cell or highly inflammatory conditions including chemotaxis) would this appear to be possible. This could possibly occur during localized or systemic viral infections and could also be an important event in lymphocyte entry into target organs, especially if chemotaxis is involved and endothelial cells present autoantigens (109). In addition, experienced or primed autoaggressive lymphocytes would be capable of becoming activated after seeing antigen in the absence of costimulation, and thus accumulating a memory pool of autoaggressive T cells might be inherently dangerous to an organism.

Thus, the type of autoantigen will define its own potential "candidacy" in an autoimmune process. Autoantigens that are not expressed during development or were cryptic for an extended period of time, as well as antigens secreted and cross-presented in lymphoid organs by APCs, appear to be better suited for assuming the role as primary culprits.

Genes

An abundance of empirical evidence indicates the association of many organ-specific autoimmune diseases with certain human leukocyte antigen (HLA) haplotypes, as well as other susceptibility or protective genes. The principal specific genetic linkages will be discussed later separately for each condition. In general, MHC I (such as HLA-B27) (110,111) or class II (such as DR4) genes might predispose to a certain disease by enhanced presentation of pathogenic peptides in the periphery or inefficacious presentation of autoantigen-derived peptides in the thymus. For example, the human HLA-DQ8 molecule has a striking structural similarity to the mouse I-A^{g7} class II that predisposes NOD mice to spontaneous autoimmune diabetes (112,113). However, the link to disease appears not to be as simple as reasoned earlier in the chapter, and more complex mechanisms might be in place. Presentation of the pathogenic peptide in gluten-induced celiac disease involves acidic modification of the protein to generate the peptide ultimately presented by MHC class II (114), and other chemical modifications can be expected to alter peptide binding to MHC and the resulting conformation.

Other genes that encode immunoregulatory or inflammatory proteins may be involved in the disease process. Genes that support tissue or wound repair (e.g., islet cell regeneration in T1D) may be of help in preventing disease development (115). For most organ-specific autoimmune disorders the genetic links are complex and not absolute. Many susceptibility and resistance genes act in concert to modulate the clinical phenotype. Noteworthy newly emerging themes in the genetics of autoimmunity are the fact that small nucleotide polymorphisms might result in alternate forms of the same gene and the fact that the overall MHC region genes are becoming unraveled (116). A striking example for the former is the existence of an alternate splice form of the inhibitor of cellular function (CTLA-4). Vijayakrishnan et al. discovered that the presence of a secondary splice variant of the CTLA-4 gene lacking the B7.1/B7.2 binding motif could be instrumental in defining the genetic penetration of diabetes pathogenesis (117). An important area that is still largely unexplored relates to genes responsible for transcriptional control of other proteins. Experimental models indicate that transcription factors can have profound effects on the development of autoimmune disease, and variations in expression and activity levels may be observed between susceptible and protected individuals. In summary, a complex interplay of many genes will predispose for a certain autoimmune disease, but the concordance of clinical manifestation is frequently not higher than 30% to 40% in monozygotic twins (118–124). For this reason, other factors are to be considered in studying the triggering or propagation of the organ-specific disease process.

Environment

Viral Infections

For many years viral infections have been discussed as potential candidates for triggering autoimmunity in susceptible individuals because of their capacity directly to infect target tissues and induce strong inflammatory responses. Although the association between viral infections and organ-specific autoimmune disorders is a very intriguing possibility, it has been exceedingly difficult to demonstrate a causative role for specific viruses in human autoimmune diseases. In addition to the many obstacles are the possibilities that (a) all individuals undergo a multitude of viral infections during their lifetime, (b) one has to assume that viruses are frequently cleared at the time of diagnosis, and viral footprints can be difficult to find in individuals affected by an autoimmune disease (hit and run event), (c) the precise viral strain, infection kinetics, number of T cells, and type of effector functions induced may play an instrumental role in determining its effect in an individual genetically at risk, necessitating a very detailed immunologic profiling (125), (d) due to MHC polymorphism, there is a significant variation in specificity of the antiviral response, (e) viral infections might not trigger autoimmunity per se but affect an ongoing autoimmune process in a detrimental way, and (f) there is increasing evidence that viral and other (126) infections rather prevent than enhance ongoing autoimmune responses, either by apoptosing aggressive T cells or by augmenting the Treg pool (127) (C. F. Filippi and M. G. von Herrath, unpublished). Thus, a successful approach should first explore the underlying mechanisms in virally induced autoimmunity and then apply the precise insight and paradigms developed specifically to the human situation.

The most important mechanisms to be considered are summarized in Figure 42.3:

1. Molecular mimicry implies that the cross-reactivity between viral and self determinants is a principle cause or mechanism of enhancing autoimmunity (128,129).
2. Bystander activation postulates that APCs and autoreactive lymphocytes will become activated indirectly as a consequence of the cytokine/chemokine by virus infection of a particular organ (130).

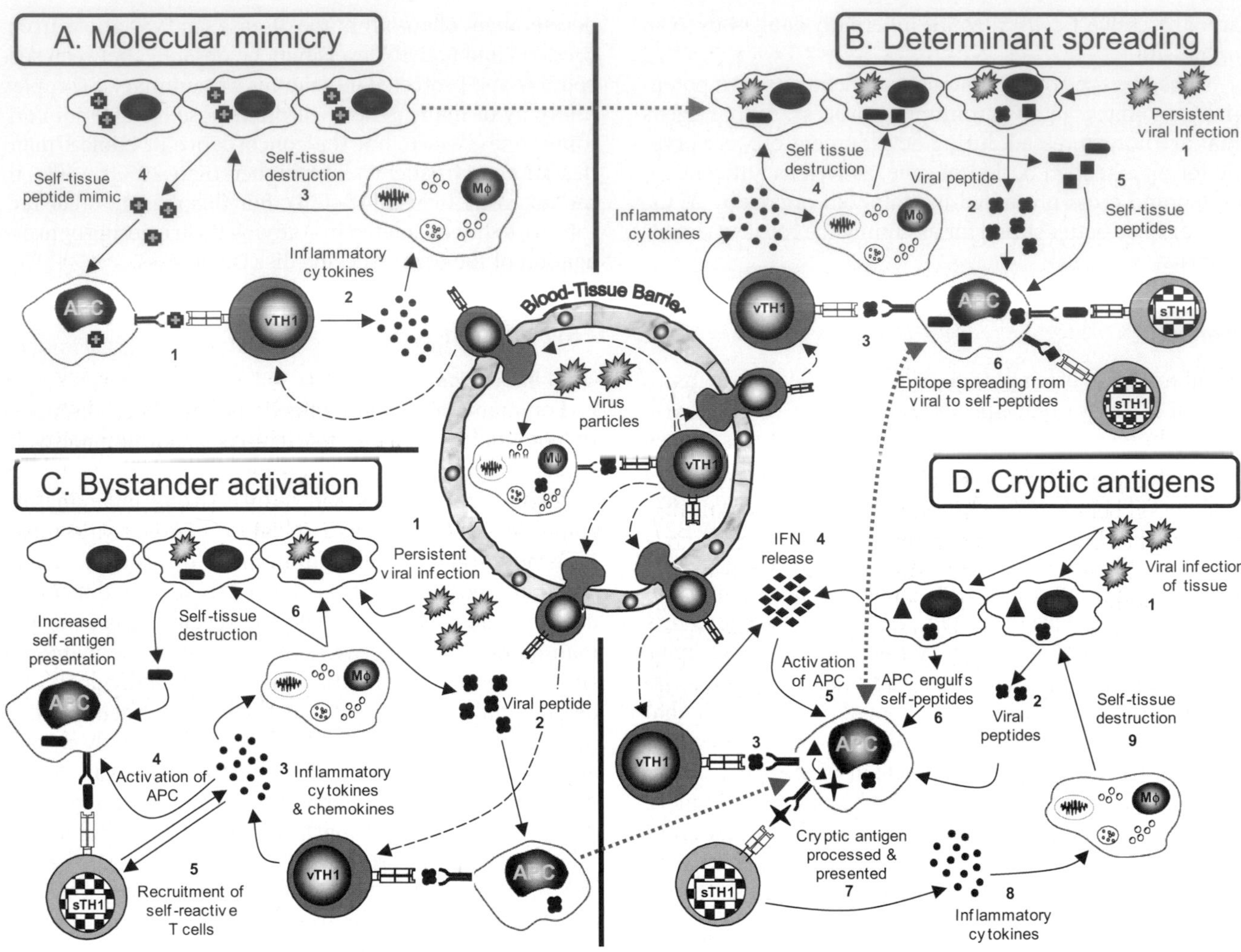

FIGURE 42.3 Potential mechanisms of autoimmune disease induction. After a viral infection, activated virus-specific T helper cells (vTH1) and CD8 cytotoxic T lymphocytes (CTLs) will migrate more readily through blood–tissue barriers to infected and noninfected organs. **(A)** Molecular mimicry describes the activation of cross-reactive lymphocytes that recognize the original viral epitope and a self-epitope (1), which leads to the release of cytokines and chemokines (2), which enhance local inflammation, activate antigen-presenting cells (APCs), and indirectly or directly cause tissue destruction (3) and spreading of the autoimmune process (4). **(B)** In the epitope spread model, persistent viral infections (1) could result in the activation of virus-specific T cells (2, 3), which cause tissue damage by killing virally infected cells (4), leading to the release (5) and (cross-) presentation of more autoantigens (6). **(C)** The bystander activation model describes the non–antigen-specific activation of autoreactive T cells. Infiltration by virus-specific T cells (1, 2) leads to inflammation and upregulation of immunity throughout the tissue (3, 4), involving the activation of APCs, which now differentially process autoantigens (also *de novo* or previously cryptic antigens). This can lead to activation of lymphocytes by TcR-specific or TcR-independent mechanisms (5), which can then cause tissue damage (6). **(D)** The cryptic antigen model describes the initiation of autoimmunity by differential processing of self-antigen/peptides, which can occur under inflammatory conditions. After viral infections, interferons (IFN) (1) are secreted by antiviral T cells and infected cells (2–4). APCs are activated in this way (5), which enables them to engulf self-peptides (6, *triangle*), or to differentially process endogenous autoantigens. Cytokines can activate proteases more strongly, which might result in the presentation and processing of previously cryptic autoantigens (7–9). The displayed pathways are not mutually exclusive and are probably operational at different levels in many autoimmune responses. Currently of high interest is the presentation of neoantigens and strategies to define them. Mϕ, macrophage. (Courtesy of Steve Miller and Ludovich Croxford, Northwestern University, Chicago, Illinois.)

3. Virally induced determinant spreading involves the presentation of autoantigens (possibly previously cryptic) by virus-activated APCs (131–133).

The experimental evidence for all of these three scenarios obtained in different mouse models *in vivo* is well documented. However, none of these has been proven for any human autoimmune disorder due to the large size of human trials and the invasive nature of *in vivo* diagnostics required at the present stage. Thus, in the near future we will continue to depend on animal models until noninvasive human *in vivo* diagnostic strategies have advanced to allow for imaging of trafficking of antigen-specific lymphocytes. In addition, the prospect of directly visualizing immune processes in target organs of afflicted patients may offer improved diagnostics as well as custom-tailored therapeutic interventions. A final remark pertains to the negative association between viral infections and autoimmune disease that has been observed in several experimental models (134). These observations support the so-called "hygiene hypothesis," that is, the epidemiologic finding that the incidence of many autoimmune disorders is decreased in equatorial countries that exhibit a higher prevalence of various infectious diseases. However, no firm associations have been established.

Other Environmental Causes

Similar to viral infections, other inflammatory stimuli may trigger or enhance autoimmunity. The gut deserves particular attention in this respect. At this site each individual harbors thousands of different bacterial strains, and viral infections are common. Furthermore, the mucosal lining is permeable for nutrients and constitutes a very large interactive surface with the environment. Again, the complete absence of all bacteria results in severe immune dysfunction and possibly autoimmunity. However, it would be incorrect to conclude that infections are therefore always protective. Indeed, the commensal flora appears to be crucial in maintaining proper immune activation and function, with certain pathogens definitely eliciting strong gut immune responses that could lead to autoimmune disease (135,136).

Regulatory Circuits in Autoimmune Processes

Cytokines

Cytokines and chemokines are essential regulators of cellular and humoral immune responses and lymphocyte trafficking (137–139). They play a central role in orchestrating immune processes and constitute a multitude of positive, as well as negative, feedback loops (140). Certain cytokines can negatively or positively influence the production of other cytokines [e.g., the TH1/TH2 paradigm and the recently discovered TGFβ-mediated differentiation of IL-17–producing T cells in the presence of IL-6–secreting cells or Tregs in the absence of IL-6 (84,95)] and therefore determine the balance between pro- and antiinflammatory factors in the local environment. Furthermore, autocrine production feedback can augment or shut down production of a given cytokine by one cell. Cytokine networks operate with a fair amount of redundancy, and cytokines and chemokines share common receptors. They are the most likely mediators of "bystander activation" and "suppression" processes and also offer an effective and versatile therapeutic target via the temporarily restricted use of cytokine- or chemokine-blocking antibodies. Their precise function can vary quite dramatically with respect to the autoimmune disease under investigation and will be discussed in the various disease-oriented sections. Furthermore, their level and timing of expression during an ongoing disease process will determine whether they have a positive or negative effect (or any at all; see later discussion).

Apoptosis

It appears to be a general paradigm of great functional consequence that activation of the immune system is followed by a process that reverses the activation and reestablishes homeostatic baseline levels of immunity (77,79). In the absence of such regulatory mechanisms, immune responses will overshoot their goals and excessive immunopathology will occur. Thus, activation-induced cell death is believed to play an important role in regulating autoimmunity. Apoptotic lymphocytes, for example, are easily detected in islet infiltrates in T1D (141), and targeted induction of limited apoptosis may even prevent onset of autoimmune disease (142). Although increased apoptosis of aggressive lymphocytes that exceeds the supply of newly activated cells may directly limit an ongoing autoimmune process, limited apoptosis of target tissues may indirectly facilitate induction of protective regulatory responses. On the other hand, whereas apoptosis of target cells should be limited, decreased apoptosis of autoreactive aggressive lymphocytes will propagate autoimmunity. It is important to consider precisely which cells undergo apoptosis to predict the possible outcome.

- If too many target cells die by apoptosis, organ destruction occurs more rapidly; however, at the same time, antigens released from apoptotic cells appear to propagate tolerance rather than immunity (142,143).
- If Tregs die by apoptosis, autoimmunity will be enhanced (144).
- If aggressive lymphocytes die by apoptosis, this should in general ameliorate disease. However, because they have to first be activated, they might induce organ damage during their activation phase.

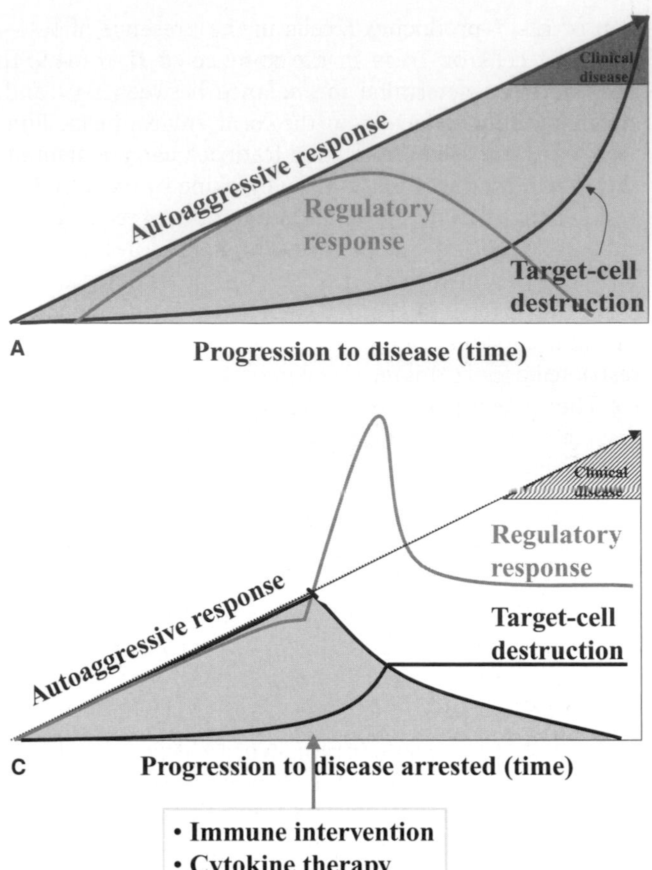

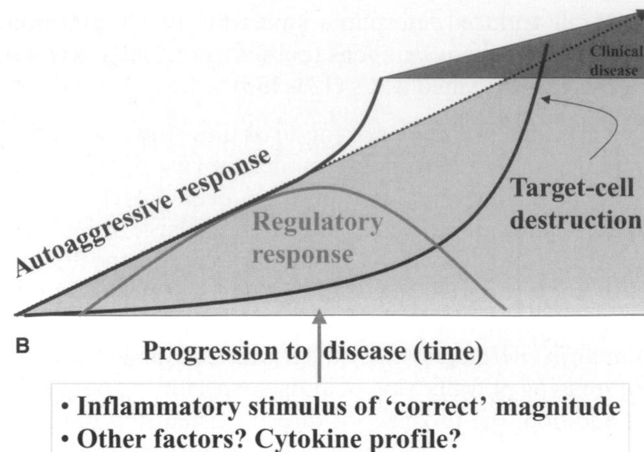

FIGURE 42.4 Kinetic issues in autoimmune diseases. Clinical manifestation of autoimmunity is the consequence of a disequilibrium between protective (regulatory) and aggressive (effector) responses **(A).** An important consideration is that the destruction of the target cell or organ will usually lag somewhat behind the peak of the aggressive responses because organ regeneration is common. **(B)** Inflammatory stimuli will augment the effector arm of the autoreactive response, resulting in more rapid disease development. In contrast, induction of Tregs and increased regulation can delay or dampen organ destruction **(C).**

Thus, an ongoing autoimmune process can be viewed as a rather fine-tuned and fragile equilibrium of aggressive and regulatory components, and the precise activation kinetics and survival times of all lymphocyte types implicated in the process will determine the outcome. We are unable to delineate the precise *in vivo* cellular kinetics, and a more thorough understanding will require improved noninvasive diagnostic techniques.

Kinetic

One of the most important emerging areas for an improved understanding of the pathogenesis of autoimmunity is concerned with the kinetics of immune responses. The pathophysiologic or therapeutic effect of a given lymphocyte population depends not only on specificity, activation state, and effector functions, but also on the timing of each phase of the disease. Indeed, inflammatory cytokines such as IFNγ or TNFα exhibit opposing effects in T1D, depending on the precise time point of generation (145). Early expression enhances islet destruction and disease development, whereas late expression ameliorates disease by inducing apoptosis of autoaggressive cells. These kinetic issues constitute a major obstacle for successful immune intervention because they preclude the use of specific blocking agents or administration of cytokines without precise knowledge of their kinetically differential role in the disease process. Figure 42.4 illustrates these kinetic considerations in relation to target cell destruction. A better understanding of the underlying "autoimmune kinetics" is essential, and treatments will likely have to be individualized, in particular, for antigen-specific immune-based therapies.

Therapeutic Considerations

Efficacy, Specificity, and Undesired Effects

Treatment of autoimmune disorders is not that different conceptually from cancer therapy. A fine balance must be found between efficacy of the intervention and acceptable undesired effects. The main goal of autoimmune disorder therapy is suppression of the pathologic autoimmune response. Therapeutic options range in principle from continuous immunosuppression of the entire immune system to specific, targeted, temporarily limited and local immunosuppression. Systemic immune modulation or antiinflammatory therapy will affect the entire immune system and may compromise the immune status of the individual. One of the more recent examples for effective systemic treatment is the blockade of TNFα to ameliorate RA (146,147). Although undesired effects are relatively low, SLE-like symptoms have been observed in a few patients, as has the enhanced susceptibility to tuberculosis. This is especially encouraging because blockade of TNFα affects inflammatory pathways distinct from the targets of conventional antiinflammatory therapy with corticosteroids or nonsteroidal antiinflammatory drugs.

Autoantigen-specific immune interventions, in contrast, bear the promise of lower systemic side effects because they can be targeted to antigens that are exclusively expressed in the diseased organ (148,149). However, the efficacy might be lower, and suitable target antigens have to be chosen carefully because enhancement of autoimmunity is an important concern. The goal is either deletion of aggressive autoreactive T cells or induction of regulatory cells (150). To achieve the latter, response modifiers are probably required at the time of immunization to skew the resulting immune response to exert regulatory effector functions. Deletion of autoaggressive lymphocytes or anergy induction is even more risky because only suboptimal immunization (i.e., in the absence of costimulators) will result in this outcome. To control this *in vivo* is rather difficult. Ultimately, antigen-specific therapy will likely have to be individualized due to MHC polymorphism and distinct T cell repertoires among individual patients and should be combined with other systemically acting agents, for example, antibodies against CD3 or CD4 or costimulation blockade. Indeed, there is intriguing recent evidence along these lines in animal models; combination of a non–Fc-binding anti-CD3 antibody with mucosal immunization of insulin or insulin-derived peptides exhibited clear synergy and enhanced efficacy in reversing recent-onset diabetes in the NOD mouse (151). In this case, induction of insulin-specific adaptive Tregs and their effector function were enhanced, and protection by these Tregs was transferable and highly effective in that it prevented recent-onset T1D.

Promising Targets

For antiinflammatory interventions, the factor to be targeted should be as disease specific as possible. Therefore, blockade of TNF works well for RA but not for T1D or MS (152). Experimental evidence supports this observation because TNFα is a crucial mediator discovered to be elevated in affected joints (147) but has clearly positive, as well as negative, effector function in murine models for MS and T1D (153,154). Targeting ubiquitously present chemokines or cytokines will likely not bear much success because of the resulting generalized immune modulation or suppression.

For antigen-specific interventions, antigens that are already targeted by regulatory autoreactivity are likely to constitute good targets to augment such a preexisting response (155). These antigens should not be selected to delete autoreactive cells, which may precipitate a loss of regulation. Instead, the induction of apoptosis or anergy should be reserved for specific lymphocytes involved in destructive autoimmune responses. However, the fact that autoimmune responses demonstrate changes in preferentially targeted antigens over time ("determinant spreading") makes such interventions difficult to design, and individualization would be necessary.

Reestablishment of Tissue-specific Immune Regulation

One of the factors that pose a challenge to understanding the pathogenesis of distinct autoimmune diseases may also hold a clue to developing effective and specific treatment strategies. Each target cell, tissue, or organ exhibits specific features that distinguish it from other sites in the body. These site-specific features of autoimmunity will likely offer unique target sites for interventions and lower systemic side effects. However, one concern is that reestablishing proper immune homeostasis and regulation in one organ may still affect homeostasis systemically or at another site. Therefore, thorough preclinical evaluation and careful monitoring of undesired effects is urgently needed. Ideally, treatments have to be administered before complete organ destruction has occurred in patients identified by genetic screening to be at risk of developing full blown clinical disease. During the preclinical state, frequently regulatory autoreactive responses are still strong, and their augmentation can result in protection (Figure 42.5). During advanced stages of autoimmunity, Treg

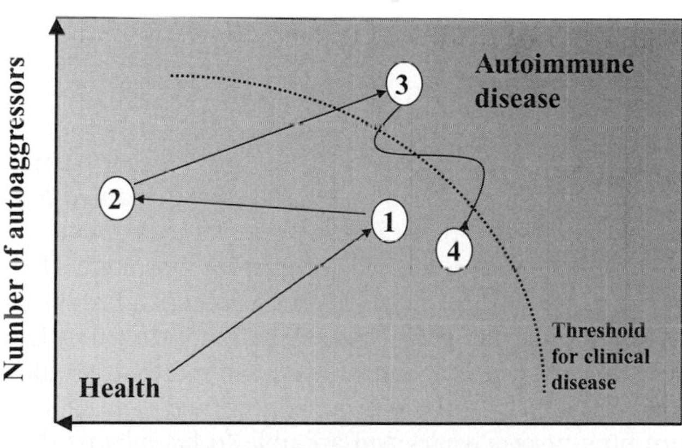

FIGURE 42.5 Development of autoimmune disease as a function of aggression versus regulation. After induction of disease (1), distinct numbers of autoaggressive and autoreactive Tregs will be generated and activated. Oscillations between protective states and diseases states follow (2, 3), that is, the so-called "honeymoon phase" in type 1 diabetes, which can eventually lead to an irreversible state of clinical manifestation of disease (4). An additional important factor the ability of the target organ to regenerate.

function or susceptibility of effector T cells to regulation might decrease (156). The goal to reestablish homeostasis and proper regulation after initial organ-specific inflammation appears to be a natural countermeasure to which a specific immune response could be harnessed. An intriguing example is the recently emerging concept of organ repair, which could potentially be enhanced by drug therapy. In T1D, regeneration and replication of β cells could occur after giving exenatide, a glucagon-like peptide-1 agonist. This is an established intervention in T2D and in T1D is under investigation in combination with other drugs, for example, anti-CD3.

ORGAN-SPECIFIC AUTOIMMUNE DISORDERS

A comprehensive and balanced discussion of organ-specific autoimmune diseases at large is well beyond the scope of this chapter. Our choice of individual diseases for this part of the chapter was guided by their relevance to human health, that is, disease prevalence and severity, as well as recent insights into pathogenetic mechanisms that may contribute to the development of novel treatment modalities. Given these limitations, we extend our apologies to all those scientists and clinicians whose work on organ-specific autoimmune disease is not mentioned in this discussion.

Endocrine Autoimmune Diseases

Thyroid: Grave's Disease and Hashimototo's Thyroiditis

Introduction and Disease Description

The year 1956 was seminal for the field of human autoimmunity, given the discoveries of Hashimoto's thyroiditis as an autoimmune disease and of Grave's disease as caused by an autoantibody. These discoveries prompted some straightforward and relatively uncomplicated treatments *(157,158)*. In Grave's disease, autoantibodies directed against the thyroid-stimulating hormone (TSH) receptor on thyroid cells stimulate excessive production of thyroid hormone, which is normally controlled by feedback regulation. In contrast, in Hashimoto's thyroiditis, autoantibodies to thyroid peroxidase and thyroglobulin are present over years and are able to fix sublytic doses of complement to cells of the thyroid. The result is an inflammatory reaction, which is also associated with T cell–mediated cytotoxicity. Thyroid damage due to painful Hashimoto's thyroiditis may be associated with the development of Grave's disease, indicating that there is a tendency for spreading of the autoimmune reaction in humans. Treatment of thyroiditis is relatively straightforward with antithyroid drugs (methimazole) and radioactive iodine.

Autoimmune Features

Autoantigens targeted in thyroiditis are thyroid peroxidase, a cell surface protein (Hashimoto's thyroiditis), and the TSH receptor (Grave's disease). Autoimmune responses to thyroglobulin are also seen in animal models. The B cell epitopes to these autoantigens have been mapped relatively well; however, as in the case of other human autoimmune disorders, T cell responses, their tracking and specificity, and their eliciting antigens in humans have remained largely elusive *(157)*. Aberrant T cell immunity has been linked to the CTLA-4 locus, which is supported by studies of thyroiditis in NOD mice. The usual suspects, that is, APC dysfunction, autoaggressive lymphocytes, and links to viral infections, have been examined, but no conclusive etiologic or mechanistic evidence has been obtained. It is noteworthy that a role for Tregs has been established in Mason's animal model for thyroiditis *(159)*.

Genetic Features and Environmental Factors

Of interest, numerous viruses have been implicated in the pathogenesis of different thyroid diseases, but firm evidence for a direct involvement of viruses or virus-induced immune responses leading to clinically manifest disease is scarce. Subacute thyroiditis is a clinical and pathologic form of thyroid involvement that appears after infection with viruses such as measles, influenza, adenovirus, Epstein-Barr virus, and coxsackie virus *(160)*. Again, however, a causative role *in vivo* has not been shown for any single infectious agent *(161)*. Presence of viral material in the thyroid and elevated virus-specific antibody titers were found to correlate with subacute thyroiditis. In other instances direct virally induced thyroiditis has been documented epidemiologically with thyroid or parathyroid disease.

Retroviruses, in particular human immunodeficiency virus (HIV) infections, have generated much interest. Although HIV infection and acquired immunodeficiency syndrome (AIDS) may affect multiple endocrine organ systems *(162–165)*, thyroid dysfunction usually reflects weight loss, anorexia, and cachexia of advanced HIV disease rather than a direct viral effect on the thyroid *(166,167)*. Thus, direct involvement of the thyroid by HIV or by opportunistic infections is uncommon and may include subclinical hypothyroidism and "euthyroid sick syndrome." The clinical relevance is probably limited because overt hyper- or hypothyroidism does not occur with greater frequency in HIV-infected and AIDS patients as compared to patients with other nonthyroidal illnesses [HIV and the thyroid gland are reviewed elsewhere *(166)*]. Involvement of the parathyroid in patients with AIDS could be shown by reduced basal and maximal parathyroid hormone levels, but the mechanisms underlying these findings have not been elucidated *(168)*. To account for a possible role of HIV in thyroid autoimmunity, a 66% homology between the HIV-1 Nef protein and the human TSH receptor has been noted. However, reactivity of sera from Grave's patients against a Nef peptide showed no significant difference as compared to normal controls *(169)*. This does not rule out the presence of conformationally shared T or B cell epitopes with HIV proteins. In analyzing mechanisms of molecular mimicry, studies of potential antigenic surfaces have emerged as an important supplement to analysis of sequence similarity *(170)*.

In addition, antibodies from a Grave's patient showed reactivity to the Gag proteins of another retrovirus, human foamy virus (HFV) *(170)*. The association of HFV with Grave's disease or subacute thyroiditis is controversial. Whereas one study demonstrated HFV-related sequences in the DNA of peripheral blood in two thirds of the Grave's patients but none in normal controls *(171)*, another study could not confirm these findings *(172)*.

In other studies, an association between human T cell leukemia lymphoma virus (HTLV) I and II and the occurrence of autoimmune thyroiditis or Grave's disease was reported *(172–175)*. Furthermore, as in the case of HIV, hepatitis C virus was shown to lead to a wide variety of autoimmune disorders including involvement of the thyroid gland *(176–180)*. Moreover, treatment of chronic hepatitis B and C with IFNα leads to induction or enhancement of autoimmune disease *(181–183)*. For congenital rubella infection, which has been associated with T1D, Addison's disease, growth hormone deficiencies, and thyroid disorders *(184)*, it is not clear whether thyroid involvement is the result of a direct viral effect or a more generalized dysfunction of the immune system *(161)*.

Animal Models

Animal models in mice and chicken have been used to study virus-induced thyroiditis [reviewed elsewhere *(161)*]. Mice persistently infected with LCMV showed reductions of thyroglobulin mRNA and circulating thyroid hormones in the absence of thyroid cell destruction *(185)*. Thyroiditis characterized by focal destruction of the follicular structures, inflammatory infiltration, and generation of antibodies against thyroglobulin and thyroid peroxidase was observed in a reovirus type 1 mouse model of thyroiditis *(186)*. The reovirus gene responsible for autoantibody induction was identified, and the encoded polypeptide as shown to bind to tissue-specific surface receptors *(187)*. Spontaneous lymphocytic infiltration of the thyroid is observed in the obese strain of chickens. Such chickens express an endogenous retrovirus, avian leukosis virus (ev22), not detected in healthy normal inbred strains *(188)*. Although ev22 appears to be a genetic marker rather than a cause for thyroiditis, infection of normal chicken embryos with avian leukosis virus can cause hypothyroidism *(189)*. Moreover, aberrant MHC class II expression is demonstrated in obese strain chickens, and elevated levels of 2.5-oligoadenylate synthetase and 2,5-oligoadenylate polymer levels in the cytosol of thyroid epithelial cells occur, suggesting viral involvement *(190)*. Again, not all cross-reactivities with self ligands need to increase autoimmunity *(191)*, and regulatory cells also play a major role in modulating autoimmune thyroiditis *(159)*.

Endocrine Pancreas: T1D

Introduction and Disease Description

Although the distinct symptoms of diabetes mellitus have been known since antiquity, the underlying pathophysiologic processes were only identified in the late 19th and early 20th centuries. The proof of the involvement of the pancreas in diabetes etiology was conducted by von Mering and Minkowski, who demonstrated in 1890 that extirpation of the canine pancreas resulted in the classic symptomatology of hyperglycemia, abnormal hunger, increased thirst, polyuria, and glycosuria *(192)*. Subsequently, inflammatory changes in the endocrine pancreas, that is, the islets of Langerhans, were correlated with diabetes by Schmidt in 1902 *(193)*, and two decades later, Banting and Best identified insulin as a pancreatic hormone *(194)*. This provided the basis for insulin substitution therapy, which remains the cornerstone for T1D management. In a classic 1965 paper, Gepts noted the histopathologic similarity between thyroiditis and insulitis and suggested an immune basis for the disease *(195)*. By 1974, the concept of T1D as an autoimmune syndrome was firmly established by the discovery of islet cell antibodies and an association between T1D and certain HLA genes *(196–198)*.

Autoimmune Features

More than three decades later, the possible autoimmune origin of T1D is understood in much greater detail. However, the lymphocytic infiltration of the islets of Langerhans (Figure 42.6) and the presence of antibodies specific for β cell antigens associated with the progressive destruction of insulin-producing β cells *(199,200)* still constitute the cardinal evidence for an autoimmune etiology. Although there is a reasonably strong genetic linkage to certain HLA molecules, the disease has to be considered polygenic in nature (118), and a significant discordance of disease among monozygotic twins suggests that environmental factors contribute to trigger and/or exacerbate the disease. Furthermore, it is unclear which islet antigens are the primary targets. The earliest islet cell–specific antibodies in human individuals at risk are directed to insulin *(201,202)*, and evidence from relevant animal models and recent human studies points toward insulin as a primary antigenic target *(203)*, IGRP (islet-specific glucose-6-phosphatase catalytic subunit–related protein) *(204,205)*, and possibly glutamic acid decarboxylase (GAD) *(206)*, but definitive proof for a pathogenic role has only be ascertained in the NOD mouse model and not yet in humans *(207)*. The cellular infiltrates found in the islets contain

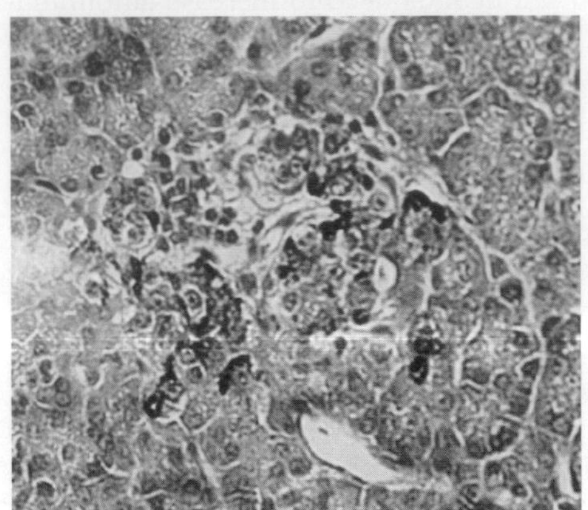

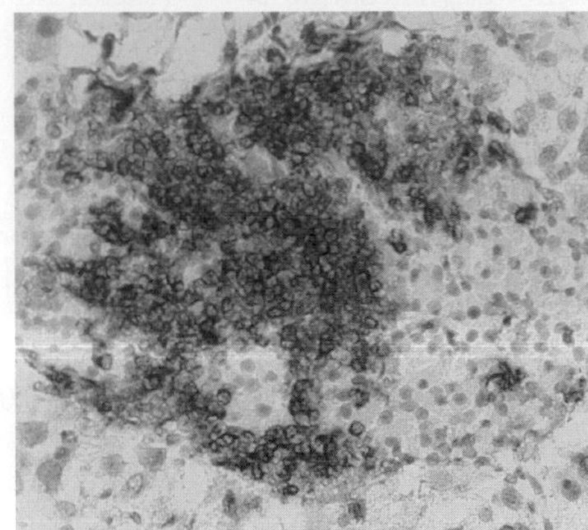

FIGURE 42.6 Human and mouse insulitic lesions. Comparison of human insulitis **(left)** and insulitis from a rat insulin promoter-lymphocytic choriomeningitis virus (LCMV) mouse 14 days postinfection with LCMV **(right)**. (Left panel courtesy of Francesco Dotta, University La Sapienzia, Rome, Italy; right panel courtesy of von Herrath laboratory, La Jolla Institute for Allergy and Immunology, La Jolla, California.) (See Color insert.)

both $CD4^+$ and $CD8^+$ T lymphocytes, and their irreducible role in β cell destruction has been documented in several animal models *(208–210)*. $CD8^+$ T cells can exert direct cytotoxic effects toward MHC class I–expressing β cells, whereas $CD4^+$ T cells secrete inflammatory cytokines and can provide help to $CD8^+$ T cells as well as B cells. Ultimately, it is important to consider that β cells constitute about 60% of the islets, which in turn contribute only approximately 2% to the pancreas mass and demonstrate, unlike many other tissues targeted in autoimmune disorders, an exquisite sensitivity to cytokines such as IL-1, TNF, and IFNs that will result in their apoptotic cell death after prolonged exposure (83).

The detection of islet-antigen specific antibodies remains an essential tool in identifying prediabetic subjects and monitoring the progression of subclinical and clinical disease. Procedures for autoantibody determination have been substantially refined and standardized worldwide. Emerging data from clinical studies support the notion that with progression of the prediabetic phase, generation of islet antibodies also is increased *(211–213)*. Usually, antibodies to insulin become discernible first, then GAD, and then insulinoma antigen 2 (IA-2). Individuals with islet antibodies to three or more distinct antigens have a greater than 90% risk of developing T1D (124). Thus, islet antibodies are an excellent marker for disease risk. However, they appear not to play a role pathogenetically, because transfer of antibodies from mothers to children does not increase the risk for T1D, and B cells are not needed for human diabetes *(214–216)*. In this crucial respect the NOD mouse appears to provide a paradigm that might not be applicable to human diabetes because maternal antibodies are an essential factor for diabetes development in offspring of NOD mice *(217)*.

Human T cell responses to islet antigens are not yet standardized and can vary considerably among different laboratories. One reason for this may be the source of T cells that are generally subjected to specificity analysis: Blood-borne $CD4^+$ or $CD8^+$ T cells may not reflect the specificity distribution and frequencies of islet-specific T cells observed in the target organ, that is, pancreas and its draining lymph nodes. Even the study of spleen-derived islet-specific T cells readily obtained from NOD mice and analyzed in standardized proliferation assays has shown variations among different NOD mouse colonies *(218)*. Therefore, measurement of multiple effector functions (i.e., cytokine production) in highly standardized assays are likely required to assess T cell autoreactivity on a routine basis *(219)*. Even under those circumstances, T cell responses are expected to vary among individuals and depend on the HLA haplotype and individual trigger(s) that precipitate T1D. A recent remarkable paper *(220)* showed that tracking of immune responses to naturally processed peptide epitopes (NPPEs) can discern differences between healthy individuals and those afflicted with T1D; whereas the number of overall T cells reacting with the NPPEs was similar, individuals with T1D produced more IFNγ relative to IL-10, and the ratio was the opposite in healthy individuals.

Genetic Features and Environmental Factors

Because the discordance of T1D is significant in monozygotic twins (concordance rate approximately 35%), environmental factors have to act in concert with diabetes-susceptibility genes to orchestrate the autoimmune destruction of β cells. The initial hope that only a few genes would contribute to disease pathogenesis and that genetic links would help to directly understand the mechanistic aspects of T1D pathogenesis has been progressively eroded. Instead, a complex network of susceptibility and resistance genes in both humans and animals (e.g., the NOD mouse) has slowly taken shape. Human T1D-associated loci "insulin-dependent type I diabetes" (IDDM1-15) comprise MHC class II genes (IDDM1), insulin (IDDM2), insulin-like growth factor 1 (IDDM3), immune-related proteins (IDDM4, intercellular adhesion molecule [ICAM]; CD3, IDDM7; HOXD8 (homeo box D8); and IDDM12, CTLA-4), as well as other candidate genes that do not have an apparent link to immune functions and/or β cells. In addition, certain maintenance, developmental, or growth factors may be involved (120). Many of these genes exhibit direct parallels to NOD mouse diabetes-susceptibility genes *(221)*.

The association between particular HLA/MHC class II haplotypes and the occurrence of human diabetes has been of particular interest. DRB1/04-DQA1/0301/B1 and DRB1/03-DQA1/0501/0201 strongly predispose to T1D, and more than 80% of patients carry either one or both alleles *(222)*. In contrast, other MHC class II haplotypes can protect from disease, as evidenced by the sixfold-reduced risk to T1D in DRB1/15-DQA1/B1/0602–expressing individuals. Recent evidence indicates that other genes in the MHC region would likely contribute significantly to T1D risk (116).

An intriguing mechanistic hypothesis was put forth in relation to McDevitt's observation that predisposing HLA class II alleles appear to express small neutral amino acids at position 57 of the DQ allele of white populations, whereas an aspartic acid is located in resistant alleles at the same position. Because position 57 is part of the peptide-anchoring pocket, amino acid substitutions in this area would affect peptide binding. Indeed, the susceptibility alleles prefer different peptides, but the contribution to T1D development is not yet clear, and a mechanistic link has to be established. Both central and peripheral tolerance mechanisms have been implicated, but no direct proof has been obtained. It is important to realize that the human susceptibility MHC class II alleles share amino acids at position 57 with the I-A^{g7} alleles expressed in the NOD mouse and are required for NOD T1D predisposition. However, as previously mentioned, polymorphisms in the MHC class II coding region alone cannot explain diabetes pathogenesis. The amount of complexity involved in the immunogenetics of T1D has been well described by Serreze and Leiter *(223,224)*:

> Many genes contributing to T1D may contribute to dysregulate different biochemical steps in a common developmental or metabolic pathway. For example, sequential expression of hundreds, if not thousands of genes would be expected in the developmental and functional maturation of a macrophage or dendritic cell from stem cell precursors. This process does not occur in a vacuum, but is contingent upon cues provided by the physical environment. In the case for APC development, the microfloral and dietary environments are crucial.

Thus, diabetes susceptibility and resistance genes contribute to disease in a polygenetic/multifactorial fashion that appears to gain in complexity as it is being unraveled. The link to environmental factors will be defined to shape gene expression and disease development. Major contributors in this respect appear to be associated with gut and viral infections.

With more than 400 m^2 of mucosal epithelium, the gut constitutes the largest interactive surface area of the human body connecting us with the environment and its pathogens (135). Therefore, exposure to antigens or pathogens through the gut, mediated by the largest outpost of the immune system, the gut-associated lymphoid tissue (GALT), will strongly affect specific and general immune functions. It is intriguing that immune tolerance to the numerous foreign protein antigens found in food, as well as bacterial antigens derived from the commensal flora, is generally well maintained *(225)*. This may be attributable to the high levels of immunoglobulin A (IgA) and TGFβ in the gut and to the phenomenon of "oral tolerance" (OT) *(226)*. OT has been observed in animal models and humans and is defined as tolerance induction to protein antigens present in the gut. It occurs via two principal mechanisms: Low amounts of antigen will induce a nonaggressive immune-regulatory response, whereas high amounts of antigen can lead to lymphocyte anergy or deletion *(227–229)*. This is likely achieved via APC modulation. In addition, the profound immune dysregulation found in the absence of a bacterial flora in both animals and humans points to an important physiologic role that foreign antigens play in immune homeostasis in the gut *(230)*. Furthermore, NOD mice only exhibit high levels of autoimmunity when kept in a clean, specific pathogen-free environment and do not develop T1D when housed under "dirty" conditions *(200)*. It is unclear whether a baseline level of immune stimulation is needed for proper development and tuning of the immune system, and which types and quantities of gut-derived or gut-induced regulatory cells are involved in the maintenance of immune tolerance. Nevertheless, $CD4^+$ TH2–like regulators, as well as $\gamma\delta$ intraepithelial lymphocytes (30% in mice, 15% in humans) *(231)*, have been associated through various lines of evidence with active mucosal tolerance. Thus, changes in mucosal functions and infections of the gut or certain dietary components may play a role in T1D pathogenesis.

Several reports and studies have attempted to establish a link between the introduction of cow's milk and development of T1D in young infants. This link was not observed in the German, Australian, and American infant diabetes studies, but it was described in a Finnish epidemiologic study *(232,233)*. The Finnish study differed from most of the others by an extended observation time involving infant as well as childhood consumption of cow's milk. Therefore, a dietary link between milk feeding and T1D can be considered unlikely but not excluded after long-term exposure to cow albumin or other milk proteins. Similarly, wheat-derived gluten and milk-derived insulin have been implicated as a cause for childhood diabetes. The evidence, however, is not convincing at this point, and no firm links have been established. Some intriguing observations were published more recently supporting the concept of a viral etiology for T1D. The mechanistic links between viral infections and autoimmunity can be manifold and have been discussed in detail in the introductory section of this chapter. A significant association between rotavirus infection in young infants and the first occurrence of islet autoantibodies was established by Harrison's group in Australia *(234)* but not in Finnish populations *(235)*. Rotavirus is a double-stranded RNA virus, infects the intestinal mucosa, and is a common cause of seasonal childhood diarrhea. It can polyclonally activate T and B lymphocytes and might possibly harbor antigens that could immunologically mimic islet cell-derived self proteins. However, it is not clear whether it infects the pancreas or islets directly. Another case can be made for enteroviruses. Coxsackie (Cox) B4 virus has been isolated from islets of a child with acute-onset T1D *(236–238)*, and CoxB3 and 4 strains commonly infect the gut, pancreas, and heart *(239)*. They lead to profound pancreatitis if they replicate at high enough titers and might harbor a mimicry antigen (P2C protein) *(200)* cross-reactive on the T cell level with a human GAD epitope. However, this evidence could not be replicated by other laboratories and is controversial. Recently, it has become apparent, however, that CoxB3 viral strains can effectively prevent T1D in the NOD mouse *(240)*, which might be a more common scenario than enhancement of T1D. Overall, findings such as this might support the "hygiene hypothesis," which implies that infections protect from rather than enhance autoimmunity.

Similar to coxsackie, other enteroviruses such as polio or echoviruses have been detected in the pancreas and might therefore at least have enhancing effects on ongoing islet destruction in prediabetic individuals at risk *(236)*. The establishment of a firm association between viral infections and T1D is difficult because the underlying mechanistic links established in several animal models allow for the virus to be cleared before autoimmunity develops (e.g., in the rat insulin promoter, RIP-LCMV); viruses need not necessarily directly induce islet reactive T cell responses but can act as bystander activators, and, in many cases, viral infections have been found capable of preventing autoimmunity.

Animal Models

Because the pancreas and its draining lymphoid organs are notoriously difficult to access, many important insights about diabetes immunology have been gained from suitable animal models that continue to refine our understanding of the pathogenesis and the development of potential prophylactic and therapeutic strategies. There is a multiplicity of animal models for T1D. The most commonly used models take advantage of natural mutations that give rise to spontaneous diabetes onset or antigen-specific induction of disease using transgenic technology. Other models use β cell damage initiated by treatment with specific chemicals (e.g., streptozodozin) or virus infection. Encephalomyocarditis virus is diabetogeneic in mice, and the incidence of disease depends on both virus and mouse strains used (129,*237,238,241–246*). Similarly, coxsackie virus, associated with diabetes development in humans, causes extensive pancreatic tissue damage and release of sequestered autoantigens that lead to rapid diabetes development in some mouse strains *(247)*.

Models of Spontaneous Diabetes Onset. There are several animal models of spontaneous T1D *(248)*. The two most extensively used are the Bio Breeding (BB) rat, introduced in 1974 at the Bio Breeding Laboratories in Canada, and the NOD mouse strain established in 1974 in Osaka, Japan *(248)*. Because the BB rat is associated with leukopenia and other abnormalities *(248)*, the NOD mouse has been the model of choice due to its genetic linkages, which are reminiscent of human T1D *(248)*. In both models, adoptive transfer of T cells can induce disease *(249)*. Of interest, administration of viral infections, first shown with LCMV, can prevent IDDM in both BB rats and NOD mice *(250,251)*. This occurs in the absence of a general immune suppression. Although the mechanism involved is unclear, the generation of suppresser T cells has been suggested *(251,252)*.

Models of Antigen-Specific Diabetes Induction. Expression of influenza virus hemagglutinin (HA) under the control of the RIP resulted in a low incidence (10% to 20%) of spontaneous T1D, with no significant enhancement of disease occurring after infection of such RIP-HA mice with influenza virus. However, in RIP-HA mice expressing a transgenic TcR specific for a determinant of the influenza virus HA, the incidence of spontaneous T1D increased to 100% *(253)*. These studies clearly demonstrate the importance of autoreactive T cells present at sufficient numbers for induction of autoimmune disease. Thus, the inability of influenza strain PR8 to cause T1D in RIP-HA mice likely reflects the low precursor frequency of self-reactive $CD8^+$ T cells. Of interest, recent studies from the Sherman laboratory have demonstrated that spontaneous disease in this model is associated with cross-presentation of HA. It has been postulated that cross-presentation constitutes an important mechanism for unmasking of islet-specific antigens to autoaggressive $CD8^+$ T cells. When the model antigen ovalbumin (OVA) was expressed as a self-antigen in β cells using the RIP, similar observations were made, underscoring the likely importance of cross-presentation in autoimmune diabetes. These studies also demonstrated that the clinical outcome correlated with the number of autoreactive CD4$^+$ and CD8$^+$ cells generated and determined a cutoff level below which the autoimmune reaction would not take hold in the pancreas *(254–256)*.

Similar to RIP-HA and RIP-OVA mice, the RIP was also used to express the nucleoprotein (NP) or glycoprotein (GP) of LCMV in the insulin-producing β cells *(208,257,258)*. Diabetes develops 2 to 4 weeks after infection with LCMV due to a strong CD8$^+$ or combined CD8$^+$/CD4$^+$ T cell response directed to the viral/self GP or NP in the β cells. Insulitis is initiated only when the systemic antiviral response reaches its peak and continues well after the LCMV infection has been eliminated (118,259). Therefore, the localized, islet-specific autoimmune process, although initiated by a response to the viral/self transgene, can be regarded as an autoimmune process that follows kinetics distinctly, in contrast to from systemic antiviral immunity. Indeed, antigenic spreading to insulin and GAD is observed during the prediabetic phase *(211)*. Destruction of β cells requires activation of APCs *(260)* in the islets and is mediated by both perforin and inflammatory cytokines, predominantly IFNγ *(261)*. Thus, the RIP-LCMV model reproduces many features found in human diabetes as well as other mouse models. A distinct advantage of RIP-LCMV mice is that the time point for induction of the autoaggressive, LCMV-NP specific response can be chosen experimentally and that virus-specific, destructive CD4$^+$ and CD8$^+$ T cells can be enumerated, functionally evaluated, and localized using limiting dilution analysis, MHC tetramers, or intracellular cytokine stains *(262,263)*. These aspects constituted an advantage in a recently published study, in which we could demonstrate that feeding of insulin during the prediabetic period induces insulin β chain–specific CD4$^+$ regulatory lymphocytes that act as bystander suppressors and can locally downregulate the autoaggressive diabetogenic response in the pancreatic draining lymph node and the islets *(263)*. Other studies in the RIP-LCMV model have underlined the role of thymic selection in allowing sufficient numbers of low-avidity autoaggressive T cells to emerge in the periphery *(264)*, the role of non-MHC–linked genes in influencing the kinetics and severity of T1D even in the presence of high numbers of autoaggressive T cells *(263)*, and the importance of APCs in breaking tolerance and sustaining autoaggressive T cell responses *(265–267)*.

Under some conditions, CD4$^+$ or CD8$^+$ T cells can induce T1D by adoptive immunization *(249,268)*. In general, T1D develops more slowly or not at all in the absence of CD8$^+$ CTL, MHC I, or perforin (83,*269*). Similar considerations are true for MHC class II and costimulatory molecules, unless their elimination affects the generation of regulatory lymphocytes *(270,271)*. Cytokines, however, frequently play dual roles in T1D pathogenesis in animal models. IFNγ, in general known as a proinflammatory mediator that upregulates MHC molecules, can "unmask" β cells for immune recognition by induction of MHC class I expression, but also can exert direct antiviral effects and might be beneficial by increasing apoptosis of aggressive T lymphocytes later in the disease (83). A similar dual role is true for TNFα, which appears to enhance early disease (possibly by directly causing β cell death in conjunction with other cytokines) but ameliorates advanced autoimmunity just prior to onset of clinical disease (145,*272*). For these reasons, blockade of such inflammatory mediators might be problematic in T1D. Dual roles were also described for IFNα *(273–275)*, IL-2 *(276)*, and IL-10 *(277,278)*. In some of these studies the level of the cytokine might play as important a role as the precise timing of expression. The only cytokine with largely beneficial effects has been IL-4, which ameliorates the disease and therefore might be a good candidate for treating or preventing T1D *(279)*. In general, those chemokines that attract lymphocytes to the islets and activate macrophages worsen the course of autoimmune diabetes. Figure 42.7 illustrates the pathogenetic hypotheses generated through research in multiple animal models.

Treatment and Prevention

Despite intensive research, no effective prophylaxis, therapy, or cure of T1D is available. However, even under optimal disease management with insulin substitution therapy, T1D significantly shortens life expectancy due to eventual vascular complications in multiple organs. All of the strategies that look promising have either been evaluated in animal models or are in early clinical trials in humans (see next paragraphs). Part of the problem in devising such prophylactic or interventive immune-based approaches is that the only endpoints in human trials are disease prevention and insulin requirements, as well as remaining insulin production (C-peptide levels). No precise interim staging is yet possible, which makes efficient clinical evaluation very difficult compared to MS or RA, in which access to the target organ either visually by magnetic resonance imaging (MRI) or directly by sampling fluids is much easier to achieve. Animal models have provided interesting ideas and evidence for a variety of antigen-specific and systemic interventions that bear promise for human diabetes.

Antigen-specific Immunoregulation. Immunization with DNA plasmids that express islet self-antigens, with or without cytokines, that act as response modifiers can induce autoreactive regulatory CD4$^+$ T cells. These cells are able to suppress autoaggressive CD4 and CD8 cells locally in the pancreatic draining lymph node, where they act as bystander suppressors. Phenotypically they behave very similar to the TH2-like regulators (155,*280–283*) induced after oral antigen administration. In treated mice (using

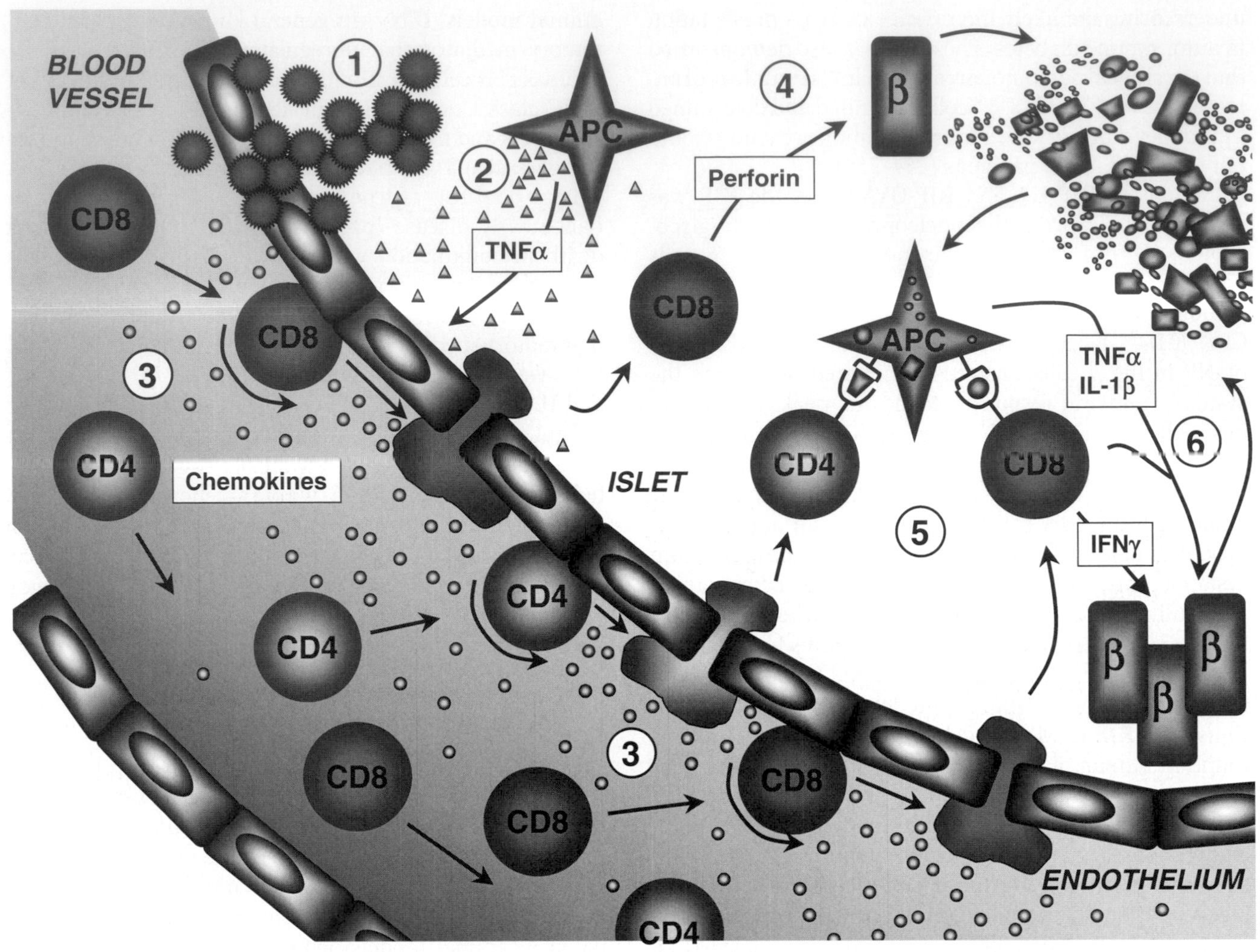

FIGURE 42.7 Immunopathogenesis of type 1 diabetes. Viral infections and other inflammatory stimuli (1) can activate antigen-presenting cells (APCs) (2), which secrete chemotactic mediators that entice lymphocytes in blood vessels to "roll" and enter into the pancreatic islet tissue (3). Entering lymphocytes might directly destroy β cells (4) or activate APCs locally (5) and also propagate inflammation by secreting proinflammatory cytokines (6). It is unknown how long effector cells remain in a given islet and how many β cells they can eliminate in a given time frame. IFNγ, interferon-γ; IL-1β interferon-1β; TFNα, tissue necrosis factor-α. (Courtesy of Urs Christen, University of Frankfurt, Frankfurt, Germany.)

several distinct diabetes models), insulitis is permanently reduced, and progression to clinical diabetes can be prevented in 50% to 80% of the animals (149,155,*280,281*). To bring this approach to the clinic as a preventive therapy, a suitable marker would be needed that can predict early outcome, for example, levels and isotypes of autoantibodies. Like other antigen-specific interventions, this strategy will not likely be effective in late stages of the prediabetic phase and should therefore be thought of and tested as an early preventive therapy. The important advantage of this and other antigen-specific approaches is that the risk for systemic side effects is low because the effector cells will act antigen specifically only in the area, where autoimmune destruction is ongoing and their cognate antigen (e.g., GAD, insulin, or heat shock protein) is presented. Cytokine response modifiers will be needed to avoid deleterious augmentation of aggressive responses.

Altered Peptide Ligands. Modified insulin peptides that favor a TH2-like deviation of responder cells have been developed by Neurocrine (San Diego, CA) and showed great promise in the NOD mouse model. These are being tested in preclinical safety studies, and clinical trials have not yet shown efficacy *(284–286)*.

Anergy-inducing Compounds. This strategy is based on the observation that immunization with antigen in the absence of (professional) costimulation by B7 molecules will lead to incomplete T cell activation and may result in anergy. *In vitro* and animal studies show much promise, in that antigen-specific cells can be selectively deleted.

Modulatory DCs. A few recent studies have shown that DCs can be modulated in such a way that they can induce tolerance in an antigen-specific fashion. This is an emerging area, and it is unclear how these modulations occur and what the precise *in vivo* effector mechanisms are (59).

Combination Therapies. Safe induction of autoantigen-specific long-term tolerance is the Holy Grail for the treatment of autoimmune diseases. In animal models of T1D, oral or intranasal immunization with islet antigens induces Tregs that are capable of bystander suppression; however, such interventions are only effective early in the prediabetic phase. We demonstrated that a novel combination treatment with anti–CD3ϵ-specific antibody and intranasal proinsulin peptide can reverse recent-onset diabetes in two murine diabetes models with much higher efficacy than monotherapy with anti-CD3 or antigen alone. *In vivo*, expansion of $CD25^{+}FoxP3^{+}$ and insulin-specific Tregs producing IL-10, TGFβ, and IL-4 was strongly enhanced. These cells could transfer dominant tolerance to immune-competent, recent-onset diabetic recipients and suppressed heterologous autoaggressive CD8 responses. Thus, combining a systemic immune modulator with antigen-specific Treg induction is more efficacious in reverting diabetes. Because Tregs act site specifically, this strategy should also be expected to reduce the potential for systemic side effects (151).

Therapeutic Concepts Under Clinical Evaluation. These include the following:

1. Anti-CD3 treatment. One of the more recent promising ongoing trials evaluates systemic administration of non–complement binding anti-CD3/Fab_2' *(287)* in human diabetes and recipients of transplants. The effector mechanism is systemic and likely relies on the induction of antigen-nonspecific regulators *(270)* that are $CD62L^{high}$ and $CD25^{high}$, as well as anergy or deletion of activated aggressive lymphocytes. From data in animal models and initial data in humans, systemic immune suppression is not too profound, indicating good feasibility for this strategy. The recent completion of a randomized, controlled trial confirms the effectiveness of this approach for treatment of individuals recently diagnosed with T1D *(288)*.

2. Oral tolerance. As for MS and RA, oral antigen trials have failed so far for T1D, except in a distinct subgroup of patients *(289)*, necessitating repeat investigations. The reasons for these failures after initially very promising animal data have become increasingly clear from follow-up animal experimentation. It is likely that the dose of antigen was significantly too low (presumably by a factor of 10 to 100). This problem may be overcome by coupling the orally administered proteins to gut response modifiers such as the cholera toxin B subunit. Second, the choice of antigen is very important, and even minor amino acid changes can modify the dose–response curves. Without a reliable preclinical marker it will be very difficult to tune this treatment to the human situation *(230)*.

3. Heat shock proteins. The first very promising diabetes prevention trial has recently been published and indicates a very good reduction of insulin requirements in patients treated with a heat shock protein peptide derived from an islet heat shock protein putative autoantigen. The precise mechanism needs to be evaluated, and long-term beneficial effects are uncertain *(290)*.

4. Immunization with insulin B peptides and incomplete Freund's adjuvant. This intervention, again evaluated and developed in the NOD mouse, is in clinical phase 1 trial. The mechanism might involve immune deviation or deletion of insulin-specific effector cells; the use of incomplete Freund's adjuvant has been proven to be uncomplicated in this trial so far.

5. Islet transplants. A promising therapeutic advance was made by developing a specific protocol for gentle isolation and purification of human islets (Edmonton protocol) that appear to be less prone to rejection after intraportal implantation into diabetic subjects *(291)*. However, continued immune suppressive treatment is still necessary in recipients of such transplants to prevent renewed autoimmune destruction of islet transplants, emphasizing the need for effective immune-based strategies of T1D prevention.

Perspective and Conclusions

No single animal model accurately reflects all aspects of human T1D. Consequently, translating the successful T1D prevention and reversion strategies developed in a variety of animal models into clinical applications faces significant obstacles, as is evident from failures in recent clinical trials. For example, more than 140 therapeutic options have been developed to prevent T1D in the NOD mouse *(199)*, but not a single one is as effective in humans. To improve this situation there is a dire need for preclinical markers that accurately predict the potential success of an intervention being evaluated by a clinical trial. Better tracking reagents for blood autoreactive T cells such as tetramers, noninvasive, high-resolution *in vivo* imaging systems, and perhaps isotype profiles of islet antigen autoantibodies and their change after a given preclinical intervention are good candidates *(292)*. Similar considerations apply to the maintenance of long-term tolerance after islet transplantation, where prolonged systemic immunosuppression might not be feasible *(293–296)*. Lastly, treatment modalities will likely have to be tailored to the specific needs of individual patients.

Central Nervous System and Ocular Autoimmune Diseases

Multiple Sclerosis

Introduction and Disease Description

MS is the most predominant human demyelinating disease of the central nervous system (CNS). An autoimmune etiology is suggested by elevated frequencies of myelin basic protein (MBP)–specific T cells documented in several independent studies of individuals diagnosed with MS *(297–300)*. Furthermore, demonstrations that adoptive transfer of T cells specific for myelin or other CNS antigens can cause a CNS autoimmune syndrome in experimental animals resembling human MS support the concept of a direct T cell–mediated pathogenesis. In addition, myelin-specific and lipid-specific antibodies have been found in MS cerebrospinal fluid *(301)*. These antibodies are able to fix complement and induce antibody-dependent cellular cytotoxicity (ADCC) and may be involved in the demyelinating process. In spite of these clues, the etiology of MS is unclear, and a complex interplay of genetic and environmental factors (similar to T1D etiology) has to be postulated.

MS is a rather heterogeneous disease. However, we are only beginning to understand how clinical and pathologic differences may point toward distinct etiologies and, potentially, treatment strategies of differential applicability and efficacy. Different subtypes of MS are somewhat better histologically defined (e.g., the distinction between T cell–rich and macrophage-rich lesions, as well as the balance between demyelination and remyelination, which can vary dramatically) than those of T1D because many tissues from patients with clinically active disease are available post mortem, whereas pancreatic islets are mostly destroyed in T1D and no immunologic correlates can be established at the end stage *(302,303)*. MS predominantly affects younger women, and its frequency, dependent on geographic location, may approach up to 3 in 1,000 *(304)*. Clinically, the disease can take a mild or very debilitating course, and, intriguingly, neuritis of the optical nerve is frequently the first sign of MS. Diagnosis is usually obtained by electroencephalography and direct imaging that allows for identification of individual lesions, their development over time, and the success of therapeutic interventions. Immune-based approaches such as the use of IFNβ or Copaxone combined with systemic immune-modulatory agents has brought some limited success for certain forms of MS. Thus, a cure for MS appears possibly a little closer than for T1D.

Autoimmune Features

Although MBP- and proteolipoprotein (PLP)-specific T cells have been documented in patients with MS, some follow-up studies have reported similar frequencies in normal individuals *(305)*. More recent studies have documented increased numbers of MBP-specific T cells in MS patients reactive to six different MBP epitopes, supporting the concept of determinant spreading as a potential pathogenetic factor. Furthermore, their activation appears to be increased selectively in MS patients, and they are less dependent on costimulation *(306)*. Thus, it appears plausible that resting T cells specific for CNS antigens are present in both healthy and affected individuals, but their activation is selectively increased under conditions of disease and their epitope/antigen recognition repertoire has expanded. In addition to cellular infiltrations, MS is usually marked by edema and inflammatory signs such as MHC upregulation, cytokine, and chemokine induction. A breakdown of the blood–brain barrier facilitates antibody access to the CNS. Antibodies specific for myelin structures and lipid components *(307)* are commonly found in MS patients, and some studies indicate fluctuations, similar to T cell responses of antibody titers in parallel to exacerbations and remissions of disease. These findings await confirmation in larger patient cohorts. It is important to note that such antibodies can be directed to MBP, myelin oligodendrocyte associated protein (MOG), and other myelin constituents *(308)*. The fact that they can fix complement and enhance complement-mediated cytotoxicity implicates them as possible agents of demyelination.

Genetic Features and Environmental Factors

There is a definite genetic link between both progressive (HLA-DR3) and remitting relapsing MS (DR2) and human MHC class II alleles. However, similar to T1D, there is a significant discordance among monozygotic twins (greater than 55%). A pronounced geographic gradient (higher incidence in northern as compared to southern regions) argues for additional environmental triggers or modulators *(304)*. Many viruses have been implicated in the pathogenesis of MS, but a causal link has not been established. For example, human herpes virus 6 was discovered around MS lesions, but follow-up studies did not discover any differences comparing healthy, Alzheimer's, or Parkinson's tissues with MS lesions *(309)*. Furthermore, antibodies to corona virus have been detected in serum of MS patients, which indicates that demyelination might occur similar to the mouse hepatitis virus model. Mechanistically, the same paradigms as for diabetes might apply (described in the introductory section), but a persistent viral infection might more likely be the culprit, based on similar observations in some mouse models (e.g., the Theiler murine encephalitis virus [TMEV] model). The difficulty in establishing conclusive proof is the multiplicity of infections during the course of a lifetime and the manifold viral traces that can usually be detected in both healthy and diseased individuals. Even if the same levels of viral antigen, RNA, or DNA are observed when comparing healthy patients with MS patients, this still does not rule out the possibility that a certain virus will only induce CNS disease in conjunction with a distinct MHC haplotype. Indeed, animal models indicate that this is in fact the case. With the introduction of improved vaccination and antiviral treatment protocols for multiple infectious agents we may be able to infer a causal relationship if the incidence of MS should recede after introduction of such an intervention.

Animal Models

Experimental allergic encephalitis (EAE) is one of the oldest and most widely studied animal models for a human autoimmune disease (99,*310,311*). EAE, a primarily CD4$^+$ T cell–mediated disease, can be induced in susceptible mouse strains (SJL, PL/J) by immunization with MBP, PLP, MOG proteins, or their respective MHC class II–restricted epitopes together with complete Freund's adjuvant and pertussis toxin. More recently, a role for CD8$^+$ T cells has also been documented. The clinical picture resembles that of a relapsing remitting disease with profound neurologic symptoms. CNS histologic findings include T cell infiltration (mainly CD4$^+$ T cell lymphocytes; Figure 42.8), APC and microglia activation, and disruption of the blood–brain barrier. Some demyelination occurs, and histologic changes can undergo periods of remission that are accompanied by remyelination. The predominant cytokine profile is TH1-like, and TH2 cytokines have protective function *(312)*. Epitope spreading occurs, and activated APCs take a central role as "drivers" of the autoimmune process (133). A shortcoming of this model is the major extent of external manipulation required to break tolerance (adjuvant, pertussis). These might be necessary to affect the blood–brain barrier, skew the systemic cytokine profile to TH1 phenotype, and support prolonged inflammation.

A lesser degree of additional nonspecific inflammatory condition is required for some virus-induced animal models for MS. Infection with TMEV, which replicates predominantly in neurons (particularly motor neurons during initial stages of infection), results in a poliomyelitis-like syndrome, including flaccid paralysis. Certain strains of mice that survive the primary infection become persistently infected and develop a chronic progressive inflammatory demyelinating disease (133). Demyelination is the consequence of the CD4$^+$ T cell response to persisting TMEV and involves determinant spreading as a consequence of infection and local inflammation (133). Studies from S. Miller's laboratory have recently shown that APCs in the CNS are crucial for diversification/epitope-spreading of the initiating anti-TMEV response to other brain self-antigens such as MBP and PLP. Furthermore, when recombinant TMEV expressing PLP epitopes or modified mimic epitopes were employed, infection resulted in enhanced disease. These experiments provided *in vivo* evidence for a possible role of molecular mimicry in CNS autoimmune disease *(313)*.

Somewhat similar to TMEV, infection with neurotropic strains of mouse hepatitis virus (MHV) induces neurologic disease accompanied by demyelination *(314)*. An interesting difference is that MHV will not persist and therefore allows for easier differentiation between the antiviral and the autoimmune responses. CD4$^+$ and CD8$^+$ lymphocytes accompanied by inflammatory cytokines are needed for destruction. These virus-induced models of demyelination suggest that a transient or persisting presence of virus in the CNS may be needed in conjunction with a nontolerized antiviral response for disease induction and/or propagation *(314)*. Indeed, another animal model of virally induced CNS disease, the transgenic MBP-LCMV model developed in analogy to the RIP-LCMV model for T1D, only exhibits mild motor dysfunction, despite good lymphocytic infiltration *(315)*. It is possible that activation of APCs is insufficient in this model to locally propagate systemically induced autoaggressive lymphocytes once they have entered the parenchyma of the CNS. These considerations are depicted in Figure 42.9.

Treatment and Prevention

Similar to observations in the diabetes models *(282)*, DNA vaccines that aim to skew the autoreactive response to MBP or PLP from a TH1 to a TH2 phenotype have shown some success in the EAE model. However, it

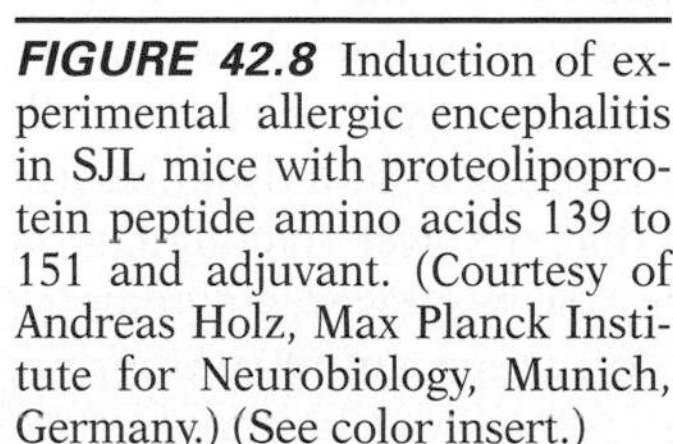

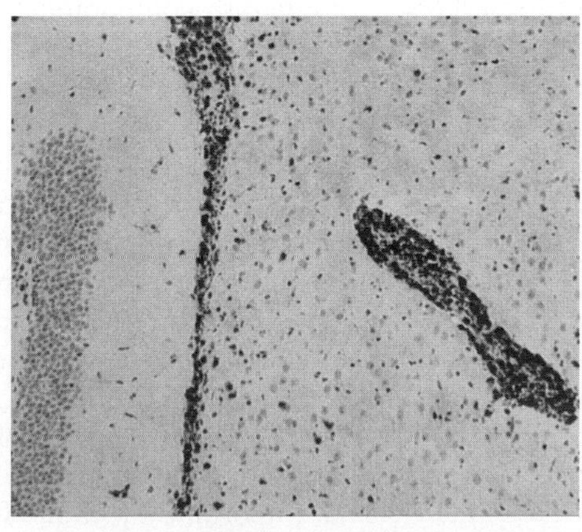

CD4 infiltrate, hippocampus

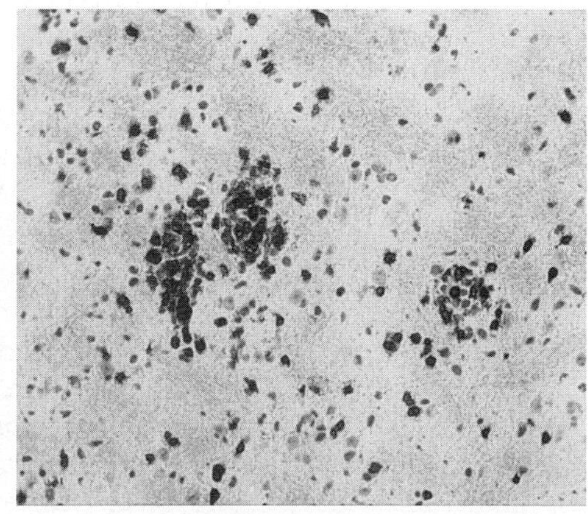

CD4 infiltrate, brain stem

FIGURE 42.8 Induction of experimental allergic encephalitis in SJL mice with proteolipoprotein peptide amino acids 139 to 151 and adjuvant. (Courtesy of Andreas Holz, Max Planck Institute for Neurobiology, Munich, Germany.) (See color insert.)

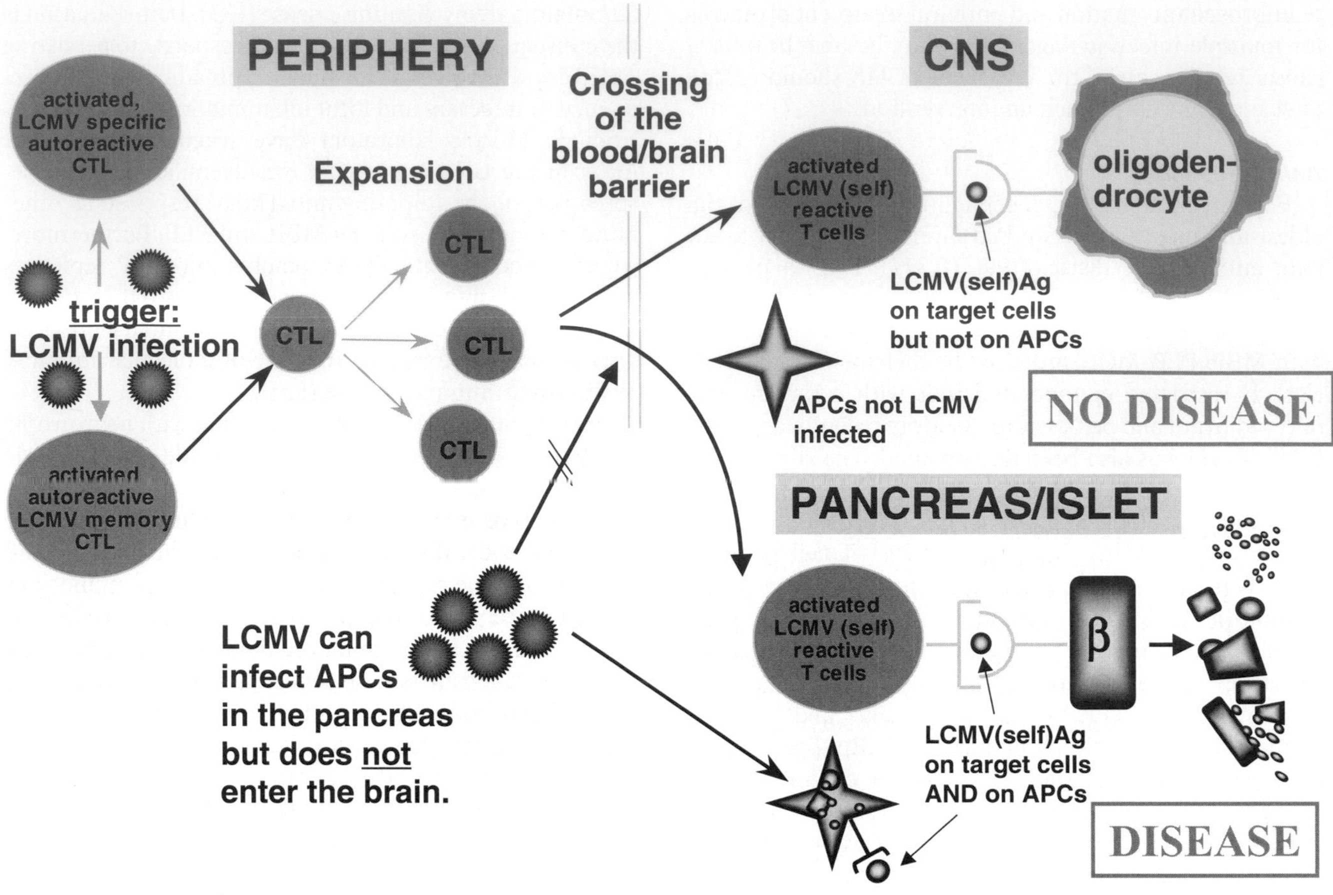

FIGURE 42.9 Induction of profound autoimmune disease of the islets but only mild autoimmune infiltration in the central nervous system (CNS) in rat insulin promoter– versus myelin basic protein–lymphocytic choriomeningitis virus (LCMV) transgenic mice. Activated antigen-presenting cells (APCs) might be a crucial local driver once an autoimmune process has been initiated. This issue is illustrated well when one compares the LCMV transgenic brain and self (transgene)-directed organ-specific autoimmunity; LCMV only infects the pancreas but not the brain. Of interest, clinical disease only evolves in islets (type 1 diabetes), whereas infiltration of the brain tissue is transient, causing little damage. Ag, antigen; CTL, cytotoxic T lymphocyte.

remains to be seen whether these findings can be directly translated to humans, and clinical phase 1-2 trials are being conducted by BayHill Therapeutics (Palo Alto, CA). At least for MS there are preclinical markers that can noninvasively and continuously track the size and appearance of current lesions and in this way indicate success or failure of a given therapy in a more immediate way as compared to T1D *(316,317)*. Oral tolerance induction had shown much promise in EAE models but recently failed in a human trial *(318)*. Strong placebo effects were observed after feeding irrelevant protein versus MBP, and the outcome was therefore not conclusive, leaving a smaller read-out window. Blockade of TNFα has shown promise in animal models but not in humans (152). The antidepressive agent Rolipram is under clinical evaluation after it exhibited anti-TNF effects in animal models for MS.

From the immunologic point of view, treatment of MS is further advanced than treatment of T1D. It should be noted that life expectancy in MS is more reduced because no therapy comparable to insulin substitution is possible. Of the current regimens, IFNβ has shown very promising results in phase 3 clinical trials *(319)*. Of interest, IFNγ, in contrast, has aggravated MS *(320)*. Furthermore, Copaxone might act as a mixture of altered peptide ligands (as a polymer MBP analog), and in this way it may skew the immune responses systemically to a less aggressive phenotype and has shown promise for certain forms of early MS *(321)*. In addition, phosphodiesterase inhibitors might induce TH2 skewing, as recently demonstrated in a small-scale trial *(322)*. Finally, generalized immunosuppressive therapy with corticosteroids that are given in conjunction with relapses and thereafter slowly phased out remains an important backbone for MS treatment. Azathioprine, cyclophosphamide, and plasmapheresis are not effective. Cyclosporin A is helpful but has profound side effects. Altered peptide ligands (APLs) to human MBP epitopes have shown strong allergic side effects and have worsened disease in one study indicating that APLs might activate both *in vivo* aggressive and regulatory lymphocytes *(323,324)*. It appears that the success of APLs can therefore vary from individual to individual. Some setbacks have been encountered with monoclonal antibodies. It is noteworthy that anti-CD40L exhibited some efficacy but led to coagulation disturbances in humans *(325)* and is on hold. In addition, integrin blockers have shown promise and have returned to clinical trials after they were on hold because combination with IFNβ had lead to reemergence of CNS viral infection in three patients.

Perspective and Conclusions

Therapeutic interventions in MS are becoming more effective but will likely have to be individualized and fine tuned with respect to the subtype of MS in a given patient. Antigen-specific therapy is in development, but better understanding of the role of T cells in MS will be needed to translate experimental findings into clinical applications. Combination of systemically acting antibodies shows good promise and will have to be further developed.

Ocular Autoimmune Diseases

Various inflammatory diseases of the eye accompany other systemic or organ-specific autoimmune disorders and are shown in Figure 42.12. Some of these diseases will be discussed very briefly because they are described in a separate chapter in this book.

Bechterew's Disease/Spondylarthoropathies

Iridocyclitis is frequently associated with Bechterew's disease (ankylosing spondylitis), which is characterized by a chronic spondylarthrosis of the ileosacral joints resulting in profound kyphosis and is associated in 30% to 50% of cases with the HLA-B27 allele *(326–328)*. Of interest, mucosal inflammation, ulcers, and vasculitis are frequently associated with this disease group. The immunologic pathogenesis is not clearly defined, but cross-reactive antibodies to bacterial proteins are frequently observed in the sera of patients with spondarthopathies such as Bechterew's disease, Reiter's syndrome, psoriasis, Crohn's disease, or ulcerative colitis. Therefore, molecular mimicry has been hypothesized as a cause for these disorders, but proof has been difficult to obtain. Several animal models have been developed, the most intriguing of which is probably a HLA-B27 transgenic rat that develops joint diseases, genital ulceration, and eye disease. Systemic immunosuppressive interventions are not effective, and the treatment of choice is nonsteroidal antiinflammatory drugs. Local steroids are frequently administered for symptoms affecting the eye.

Rheumatoid Arthritis

RA is an autoimmune joint disease (see later discussion) that is frequently associated with scleritis and episcleritis. Inflammatory infiltrates are found in the peripheral cornea leading to ulcerations. Local treatments are usually without effect, and symptoms are ameliorated in conjunction with systemic immunosuppressive therapy. In contrast, juvenile arthritis is accompanied in about 20% of patients with cataracts and iridocyclitis, and ocular symptoms are often sensitive to local and systemic immunosuppression.

Sarcoidosis

Sarcoidosis is a chronic, systemic granulomatous inflammatory disease that involves the eye (uveitis in 20% of cases) and constitutes the cause for uveitis in about 10% of patients. Multiple organs are affected, in particular the lungs. The etiology is unclear, and an autoimmune pathogenesis is suspected, with multiple inflammatory changes occurring in the eye (see Figure 42.10). Local therapy with steroids is usually helpful, and systemic immunosuppression could be considered.

Idiopathic Uveitis

About half of the cases of uveitis are not associated with a known primary syndrome, and in young adults the association (50%) with HLA-B27 is striking. Only a few of these patients will ultimately develop Bechterew's disease. Again, the etiology is quite unclear, but some evidence suggests that molecular mimicry between ocular and viral antigens, for example, herpes virus, could play a role. Peptide therapy is being evaluated; otherwise steroids are the only effective choice.

Figure 42.10 gives a summary of the eye structures and some of the systemic diseases that are associated with possible autoimmune disorders of the eye.

Animal Models

Small rodent models for autoimmune uveitis and herpes virus keratitis have been very useful for understanding the underlying immunopathology of inflammatory eye disorders.

Experimental Autoimmune Uveoretinitis (EAU). EAU is induced, similar to EAE, by immunizing susceptible rodent strains with retinal proteins such as the receptor retinoid binding protein (IRBP) *(329)*. Extensive studies by R. Caspi and colleagues have revealed that EAU follows very similar autoimmune paradigms as other experimental autoimmune diseases, including EAE and induced forms of diabetes. For example, a TH1-like response drives the aggressive EAU process *(330)*, whereas IL-10 in synergy with IL-4 has a pronounced protective function *(331,332)*.

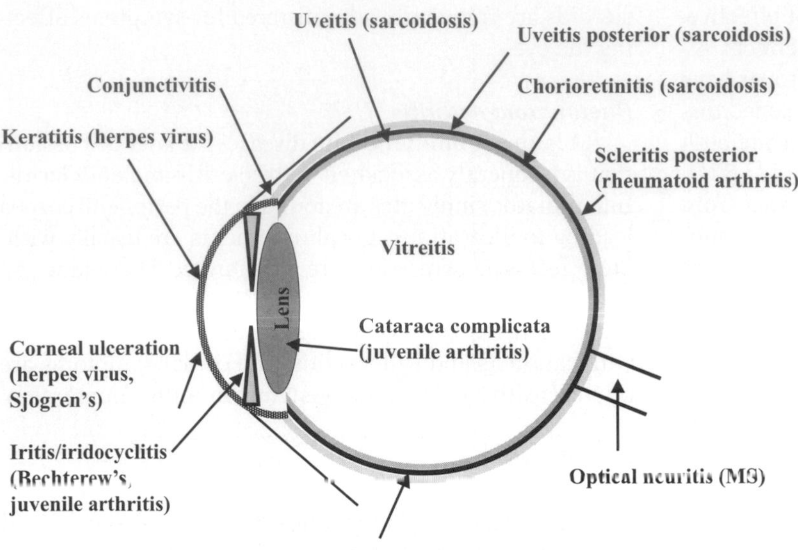

FIGURE 42.10 Overview of the structure of the eye and some of its inflammatory diseases and their association with other systemic disorders. MS, multiple sclerosis.

Similarly, disease-resistant mice exhibit a predominantly TH2-like response to IRBP. Experimental evidence indicates that sequestration and local immune privilege of IRBP and possibly other retinal antigens leads to a lack of systemic tolerance to these proteins, and, consequently, destructive autoimmune responses can be readily induced. Conversely, tolerance can be reestablished by therapeutic application of tolerizing retinal-Ag/Ig fusion proteins, an approach that is supported by experimental induction of peripheral tolerance using transgenic antigen expression under an MHC class II promoter. Of interest, peptide therapy using an HLA-B27–restricted peptide appears to be effective in humans. The immunopathology of this EAU model in comparison to human uveitis, as found in sarcoidosis, is displayed in Figure 42.11.

Herpes Virus-induced Keratitis. Herpes virus–induced keratitis has been explored in several animal models. The most intriguing studies have come from the laboratory of H. Cantor. Inoculation of a genetically susceptible mouse strain with herpes simplex virus (HSV)-1 results in a viral infection of the eye and cornea that is accompanied by an immune response to HSV-1 (128). Of interest, damage to the eye is only initiated by the virus and strongly depends on $CD4^+$ T cells that can cross-react with a self-protein. This animal model is one of the few that strongly indicate a direct immunopathologic role for molecular mimicry in an *in vivo* model for autoimmune disease. Studies by Rouse and colleagues have focused on the role of inflammatory bystander effects in the HSV-keratitis model *(333,334)*. In these studies, inflammatory cytokines were shown to play a major role in mediating local damage, and administration of DNA vaccine constructs expressing certain beneficial cytokines such as IL-10 ameliorated disease *(335)*. It is important to point out that these studies were performed using a different HSV strain, and that the precise immunopathogenic process (mimicry vs. bystander effects) indeed depends on the strain of HSV used *(336)*. Additional observations have underscored the importance of regulatory cells in downmodulating a virally induced autoimmune disease. It is worthwhile mentioning that Streilein and colleagues previously demonstrated regulatory cells in ocular autoimmune disease and discovered an important role for tolerizing antigen-presenting cells *(337,338)*.

Treatment and Prevention

Due to the associated side effects, it is desirable to avoid systemic immunosuppressive interventions, as well as the local application of corticosteroids. Recently, a Munich group identified a HLA-B27–derived peptide that could function as a mimic to the retinal S antigen and induce EAU in Lewis rats *(339)*. This mimic peptide was used as an orally administered antigen and produced very promising results in two human pilot trials in Germany. Thus, antigen-specific immune modulation using retinal self-antigens or their peptide mimics may be developed as an effective therapeutic choice. It remains to be seen whether combination of such a treatment with cytokine-DNA vaccines, as demonstrated by Rouse's group for HSV keratitis or by Caspi's group for EAU, both in mouse models, might enhance efficacy. In addition, systemic immune modulation bears promise. Recently, a trial using anti-CD25 monoclonal antibody (dacluzimab) was conducted at the National Institutes for Health with promising results. It is noteworthy that in this case the dampening of effector cells rather than any effects on $CD25^+$ Tregs appears to explain the efficacy.

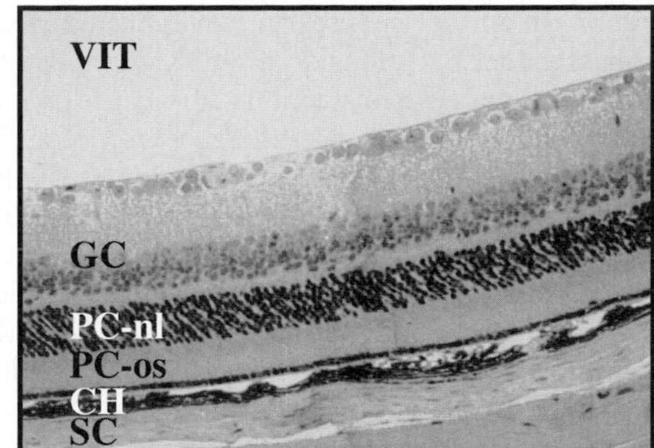

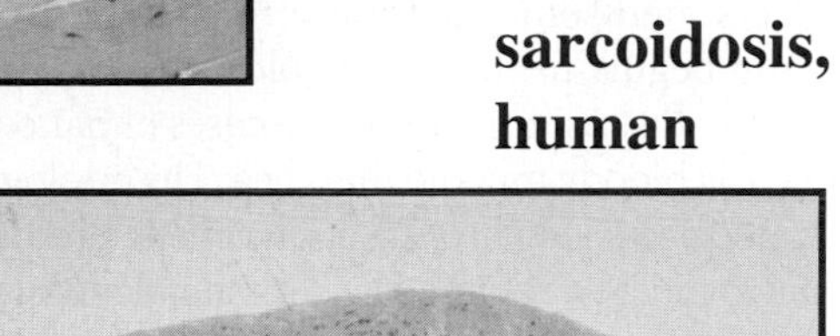

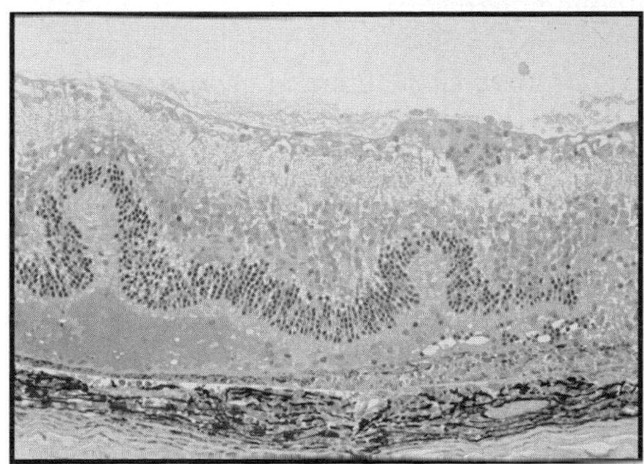

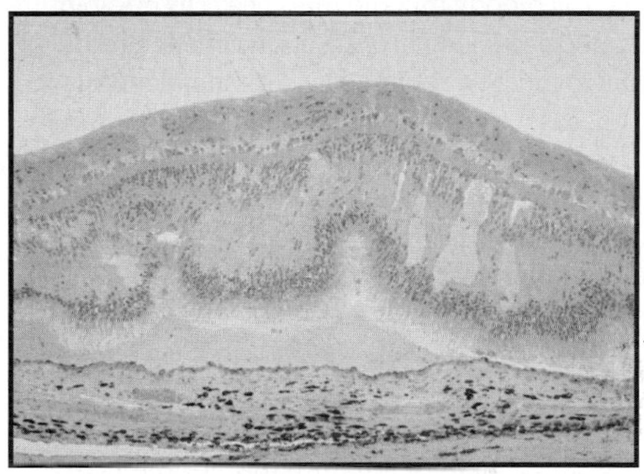

FIGURE 42.11 Histopathologic comparison of human and mouse uveitis. (Courtesy of Rachel Caspi, National Eye Institute, Bethesda, Maryland.) EAU, experimental autoimmune uveoretinitis. (See color insert.)

Gastrointestinal Autoimmune Diseases

The gut constitutes a unique immunologic environment, given its large interactive mucosal surface area and the need to maintain tolerance toward food antigens and bacteria normally present within the gut flora. The gut-associated immune system has an important regulatory and barrier function. Immune responses are usually initiated within the Peyer's patches, which obtain a significant amount of antigen via the M cells located within the mucosa and specialized in antigen uptake and transport (136,*340,341*). Lymphocytes will circulate through the Peyer's patches, where B or T cell responses can be initiated. Of interest, the B cell responses are characteristically IgA high. After antigen encounter, these cells will circulate to the mesenteric lymph nodes and enter the systemic circulation. Specifically for the gut there are other extralymphoid locations where immune cells are located and where immune responses (aggressive or regulatory) can be initiated. One is the intestinal lamina propria, where MHC class II is expressed and bacterial products can be presented. Predominantly CD4 T and B cells may assume regulatory functions, and IgA is secreted with the mucus into the gut lumen. The second are intraepithelial lymphocytes (IELs). A significant proportion of IELs expresses the ©™ T cell receptor and have cytotoxic as well as immune-regulatory functions *(342,343)*. Certain studies after oral or intranasal feeding of autoantigens have attributed regulatory function to $\gamma\delta$ lymphocytes. Overall, the hypothesis that the gut environment is ideally suited to induce a tolerizing or regulatory immune response to antigens present in the gut lumen is of high interest and well supported by evidence from animal models (e.g., "oral tolerance") *(344)*. The rationale is that the immune system must have evolved unique mechanisms to deal with the multitude of foreign antigens present in the gut and needed as nutrients and for digestive purposes. Indeed, mice housed within a sterile environment have a shorter life span and multiple immune defects, indicating that the gut's immune system is vital for regular immune development and functions.

Pernicious Anemia and Autoimmune Gastritis

Pernicious anemia is the end stage of autoimmune gastritis observed in about 10% to 20% of patients *(345)* and represents the most common cause of vitamin B_{12} deficiency *(346)*. Autoimmune gastritis is associated with autoantibody production to parietal cells and to its secreted product, intrinsic factor. In addition, a role for CD8 and $CD4^+$ T cells has been demonstrated *(347)*. Animal models have been developed *(348)*. Standard therapy is paternal B_{12} administration. Of interest, this disease also develops in mice after thymectomy and is characterized by a relative lack of $CD25^+$ regulatory $CD4^+$ T cells (150,*349,350*).

Ulcerative Colitis

Ulcerative colitis is a chronic inflammatory disease of the gut that affects men somewhat more frequently than women. It usually begins in the distal colon and rectum and spreads proximally, resulting in severe cases of pancolitis. The hallmark is bloody mucoid diarrhea. The etiology is unclear; evidence points toward a certain genetic predisposition that has to meet triggering environmental factors. Unlike Crohn's disease, the inflammatory foci are not granulomatous and not discontinuous. Overall, inflammatory mediators are increased, but systemic symptoms are rare. Treatment is usually achieved by corticosteroids. In severe cases ulcerative colitis may require removal of the colon.

Crohn's Disease

As opposed to ulcerative colitis, Crohn's disease begins as a discontinuous, granulomatous inflammation of the proximal ileum. Ulcerations are frequent, and the disease is more severe than ulcerative colitis. The permeability of the mucosal epithelium is enhanced, which leads to a local breakdown of barrier functions and upregulation of TNF, IL-1, IL-6, and other cytokines. The immune reaction involves the whole mucosa and regional lymph nodes. In addition to standard immunosuppressive treatments, blockade of TNF appears to be promising in recent clinical trials, similar to the situation in RA *(351)*.

Hepatic Autoimmune Diseases

As an anatomic site for the induction and perpetuation of immune responses, the liver exhibits distinctive immunologic features that appear to favor an overall "tolerogenic" microenvironment. This perspective is supported by the apparent absence of liver pathology in spite of the continuous exposure to nutritional antigens and components of commensal gut flora *(352)*, the ability of viral (hepatitis B and C) and parasitic (malaria falciparum) pathogens to establish persistence, and chronic hepatitis *(353,354)*, as well as the ready acceptance of liver allografts without immunosuppression in experimental models *(355)*. Moreover, successful liver transplants in humans require comparatively less immunosuppressive therapy *(356)*, and in some cases, complete weaning of immunosuppressive drugs has been achieved without compromising the functionality of the transplant *(357)*. The prevailing notion that the liver preferentially promotes abortive immune responses and tolerance was recently challenged in a meticulous study by Klein and Crispe. Having optimized the considerable surgical feat of orthotopic liver transplants in mice, the authors conclusively demonstrated that the liver effectively initiates the bona fide activation and differentiation of specific T cell responses *(358)*. Thus, the mechanisms operative in "liver tolerance" are not the consequence of altered antigen presentation, maturation failure, or premature T cell death but instead appear to rely on the activation of poorly defined regulatory circuits by persisting antigens.

Conversely, a breakdown of such tolerance mechanisms, presciently postulated almost 100 years ago as a cause for autoimmune diseases at large (7), may contribute to pathogenesis of hepatic autoimmune disorders. Here, we discuss the three major autoimmune diseases of the liver: autoimmune hepatitis (AIH) *(359–361)*, which primarily targets hepatocytes; primary biliary cirrhosis (PBC) *(362–364)*, in which small bile ducts are destroyed; and primary sclerosing cholangitis (PSC) *(365,366)*, in which the damage is mainly focused on medium to large bile ducts. In addition, we include "halothane hepatitis" as a paradigm for an immune-mediated adverse drug reaction *(367)*.

Autoimmune Hepatitis

Introduction and Disease Description

Autoimmunity was invoked as a cause for hepatitis in the early 1950s *(368–370)*, and based on the association of AIH and antinuclear antibodies (ANAs) the term lupoid hepatitis was proposed *(371)*. AIH preferentially affects women but is observed worldwide in children and adults of both sexes in diverse ethnic groups; it represents an estimated 10% to 20% of all cases of chronic hepatitis (which for the most part is due to infections with hepatitis viruses B, C, and D) *(359,360)*. Clinical symptoms range from inapparent to fulminant disease courses, and differential diagnosis is guided by an exemplary scoring system developed by the International Autoimmune Hepatitis Group (44,*372*). The presence of autoantibodies targeting different subcellular components is commonly used to differentiate two types of AIH. The etiology of AIH is undefined, but a contribution of environmental/microbial factors and genetic predisposition, as in so many other autoimmune diseases, is invoked as a trigger for T cell–mediated, destructive autoimmunity. Finally, it is also possible that as-yet-unidentified hepatitis viruses or other chronic viral infections contribute to some AIH cases *(180,373)*.

Autoimmune Features

The presence of specific autoantibodies in AIH is a key feature in the diagnostic scoring system and the foundation for the clinical distinction of type 1 and type 2 AIH (see Table 42.2). Type 1 AIH is characterized by ANAs, a class of antibodies also observed in PBC, PSC, and other forms of chronic hepatitis. Although smooth muscle and antiactin antibodies, atypical perinuclear antineutrophilic antibodies, and antibodies directed against soluble liver antigen and liver-pancreas antigen are specific for type 1 AIH, their combined measurements allow for a reasonable distinction from type 2 AIH and, to a certain extent, other chronic liver diseases. Ant–liver-kidney microsomal (LKM) antibodies are a serologic marker for type 2 AIH, with the majority binding the LKM1 antigen identified as cytochrome monooxygenase P450 IID6 (CYP2D6). In addition, less than 20% of type 2 AIH patients also carry autoantibodies specific for uridine diphosphate glucoronosyltransferase, designated LKM3, and 30% to 50% of patients generate antibody responses against formiminotransferase cyclodeaminase (FTCD). Of all of these targets in AIH, only one, the hepatocyte-specific asialoglycoprotein receptor (ASGPR), is cell surface expressed and may thus function as a direct immunogen for antibody-mediated hepatocyte damage. ASGPR-reactive antibodies, also not disease specific, are observed in 50% to 75% of AIH patients *(359,360,374)*. Because the generation of these autoantibodies is T helper cell dependent, it is not surprising that loss of tolerance also occurs on the T cell level, and lymphocytes isolated from the livers of patients with AIH type 2 can react *in vitro* and expand after exposure to P4502D6 antigen. This finding supports the concept of a lymphocyte-driven autoaggression and might underlie pathogenesis. Furthermore, mononuclear infiltration of the periportal areas and liver parenchyma is usually present when the disease progresses and causes the AIH-typical "piecemeal" appearance of the liver. Although evidence from animal models and human studies gives some indication that cytotoxic killing of hepatocytes could play a role, further analysis is hampered by the fact that intrahepatic lymphocytes are difficult to access in humans. The notion that defective suppressor T cell activity contributes to AIH pathogenesis, proposed more than two decades ago, was supported by recent work documenting reduced frequencies of peripheral $CD4^+CD25^+$ Treg in AIH patients as compared to healthy controls *(375)*. Cytokines also appear to play an important role in human AIH. Administration of type 1 IFN led to strong exacerbation of AIH, showing that it may play a central role in liver destruction *(376)*. IFNs upregulate MHC I and II molecules, enhance inflammation, and have strong antiviral effects. The outcome of these studies therefore argues against a role for an ongoing chronic (or acute) viral infection in patients with AIH who test negative for hepatitis virus antigen or antibodies. A negative regulatory role could possibly be attributed to IL-6 and TNFα. These two cytokines are reduced in the livers of AIH patients and have a negative effect on cytochrome P450 regulation *(377)*. As a consequence, the lower levels of IL-6 and TNF might enhance CYP2D6 expression and in this way support autoimmunity directed against CYP2D6 in patients with type 2 AIH. Finally, AIH pathogenesis is not necessarily controlled by the TH1/TH2 paradigm: $CD4^+$ T cells expressing TH1 cytokines are elevated in type 1 AIH, whereas TH2 cytokines are augmented in type 2 AIH in agreement with the high levels of CYP2D6-specific antibodies present in these patients.

Is production of autoantibodies important for AIH pathogenesis, or is it just an epiphenomenon signifying the breaking of tolerance to self-antigens? Evidence suggests that autoantibodies in AIH play a role that can be situated somewhere between T1D, in which autoantibodies and B lymphocytes likely play no pathogenetically important role in humans, and SLE, in which autoantibodies are complement fixing and enhance organ destruction. LKM antibodies found in AIH, for example, can inhibit cytochrome P450 function *in vitro* but not *in vivo* and may participate in hepatocyte dysfunction or destruction. Epitope mapping of the CYP2D6 antigen in type 2 AIH revealed two immunodominant regions spanning amino acids 256 to 269 and 181 to 245 that are recognized by most of the AIH type 2 patients' sera. Because there is a significant genetic polymorphism in humans for the CYP2D6 antigen, it is possible that patients with AIH target CYP2D6 protein selectively (LKM-1 antibodies), whereas cytochrome P4502D9 (LKM-2) is targeted in patients with drug-induced hepatitis, disulfide isomerase in halothane induced hepatitis, or UDP-glycosyltransferases in hepatitis D virus–associated autoimmunity. As so often, identification of the major target antigens, clearly a decisive step toward a better understanding of the underlying disease process, has not yielded compelling hypotheses as to the precise pathogenetic mechanisms.

Genetic Features and Environmental Factors

No single genetic locus capable of explaining AIH etiology has been identified. HLA-DR3 and HLA-DR4 are associated with type 1 AIH, and the HLA-A1-B8-DR3 haplotype exhibits a particularly strong association with early disease onset, relapse, and the eventual necessity for liver transplantation. In contrast, type 2 AIH is associated with carriage of HLA-DR7. Genes outside the HLA loci potentially conferring disease susceptibility include complement component C4, CTLA-4, vitamin D receptor, Fas receptor, and others *(359,360,374)*.

The association with hepatitis C, D, and E virus–induced hepatitis and autoimmunity is very intriguing. However, at this point, the prevalence of hepatitis C virus (HCV) for example, exhibits drastic variations among studies performed in different countries, and autoantibody titers appear much higher in patients with HCV-negative AIH. In a more recent study it was observed that sera of 38% of chronic hepatitis C patients reacted specifically with CYP2D6, whereas none of the sera obtained from patients with chronic hepatitis B showed CYP2D6 reactivity *(376)*. Furthermore, it was discovered that HCV has the potential to induce autoreactive $CD8^+$ T cells that cross-reactively recognize the cytochrome P450 isoforms 2A6 and 2A7, which contain sequence homology to HCV amino acids 178 to 187. In this context it may be important to emphasize that molecular mimicry also seems to be an important factor in other immune-mediated diseases of the liver. Hence, trifluoroacetyl (TFA)–protein adducts, as generated during the metabolism of halothane by CYP2E1, confer molecular mimicry to the lipoic acid prosthetic group of the pyruvate dehydrogenase complex (PDC) and other members of the 2-oxoacid dehydrogenase family (71,*208,258,378*), which in turn are major autoantigens in PBC (103). Consequently, halothane hepatitis and PBC may be linked on the level of cross-reactive autoantibodies that recognize similar target antigens. It remains to be seen whether novel subtypes of hepatitis viruses can be observed in AIH patients and whether further studies will corroborate such an association. It is likely, however, that viruses play a multifactorial role in AIH pathogenesis (similar to T1D) and that no single virus will be identified as a specific cause for liver autoimmunity.

Animal Models

Over the last 30 years, many attempts have been made to develop animal models for AIH; however, no reliable model is available that reproduces the spontaneous relapsing chronic disease course of type 1 AIH *(379,380)*.

1. In the hepatitis B virus surface antigen (HbsAg) transgenic mouse, the HBsAg is expressed in hepatocytes under control of the mouse albumin promoter. Induction of transient hepatitis is possible after adoptive transfer of activated T cells from HBsAg-primed donor mice *(381,382)*. Although not designed to reproduce features of AIH, this model has been extraordinarily helpful in understanding the role of IFNs in inducing liver damage, as well as clearing hepatitis B virus (HBV) from the liver. Results have shown that IFNs, in the absence of cytotoxicity, can purge virus from infected hepatocytes. Furthermore, induction of HBV-specific $CD4^+$ and $CD8^+$ T cell responses can be evaluated in this model. The transgenic mice exhibited profound liver damage and infiltration after transfer of HBV-specific T lymphocytes.

2. In another model system, the MHC class I molecule H-$2K^b$ is transgenically expressed in the liver of mice that also carry transgenic T cells specific for H-$2K^b$. Hepatitis induction was only successful when such mice were infected with a liver-specific pathogen, indicating that bystander activation within the liver microenvironment can be very potent in causing autoimmune damage *(383)*. A similar approach was chosen in yet another model that combines liver-specific expression of a transgene [here, the immunodominant LCMV glycoprotein epitope (GP_{33})] and transgenic T cells specific for the transgene *(384)*. These mice remain tolerant to the transgene even in the presence of transferred GP_{33}-specific T cells. However, under conditions of LCMV infection and TcR-transgenic T cell transfer, these mice develop a transient form of hepatitis as indicated by elevated alanine amino transferase (ALT) levels *(384)*. Together, the foregoing findings emphasize the importance of both autoreactive T cells and generalized inflammatory alterations in the wake of microbial infection.

3. The potential pathogenic contribution of autoantibodies was recently demonstrated in a new mouse model. Injection of a monoclonal antibody derived from a patient with type 1 AIH and specific for an undefined 190-kDa cell surface protein promoted predominantly perivenular hepatocellular necrosis in mice *(385)*. However, the validity of this model remains to be critically evaluated because the pathology does not appear to closely resemble that of type 1 AIH.

4. Arguably, more compelling models have been developed for the study of type 2 AIH. DNA immunization of mice with human CYPD6 and FTCD antigens leads to the generation of LMK1 and anti-liver–cytosol type 1 autoantibodies (targeting CYPD6 and FTCD, respectively) and specific CTLs, pronounced lymphocytic infiltration of the liver, and an elevation of ALT levels indicative of liver damage *(386)*. Of interest, recent work with this model has reproduced some aspects of the genetic predisposition exerted on disease development because C57BL/6 mice demonstrated more pronounced disease than 129/Sv mice and no inflammation was observed in Balb/c mice *(387)*. Lastly, infection with a recombinant adenovirus expressing the 2D6 antigen (U. Christen and M. von Herrath, unpublished) can lead to focal and confluent liver necrosis in mice resembling that of autoimmune hepatitis (Figure 42.12). In summary, the success of most mouse models has only been partial because hepatitis was transient and induction of chronic disease appeared to be difficult to achieve. Figure 42.13 illustrates the possible pathogenetic mechanisms implicated in autoimmune hepatitis.

Treatment and Prevention

Immunosuppression is the therapy of choice for AIH. Since their introduction in 1968 *(388)*, predinisolone and azathioprine have become standard treatment regimens *(360,389)*. To a certain extent, the impressive success rate of this therapeutic approach (greater than 85% of AIH patients) may have removed the urgency to pursue basic AIH research *(380)*. Immunosuppressive therapy also improves survival of patients with severe AIH *(390)*, but no guidelines are available for individuals with minimal symptoms. End-stage AIH is an important indication for liver transplantation *(391)*. Recurrence of AIH has been reported after liver transplantation *(392)*, but was not as frequent as observed for islet transplants in T1D patients. Therapeutic

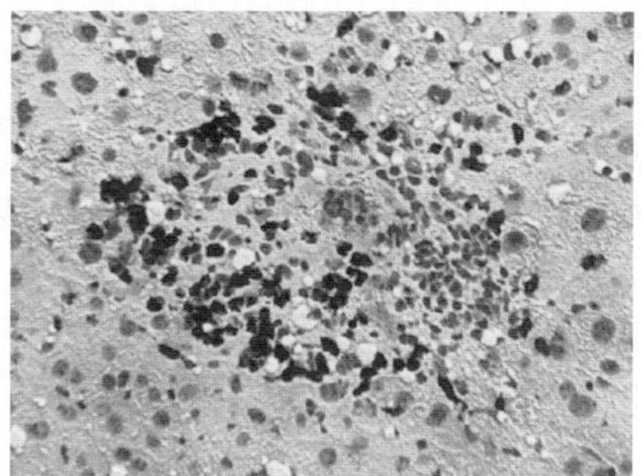

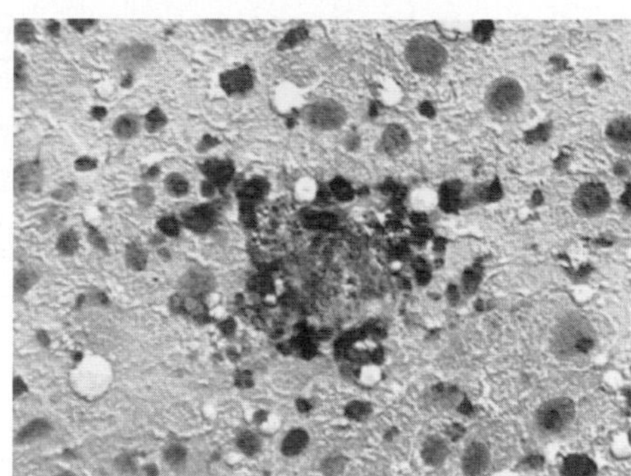

FIGURE 42.12 Liver necrosis in 2D6 transgenic mice infected with an adenoviral recombinant expressing 2D6. (Courtesy of Urs Christen and Matthias von Herrath, University of Frankfurt, Germany, and La Jolla Institute for Allergy and Immunology, La Jolla, California.)

use of IFNs, effective for treatment of viral hepatitis, can worsen autoimmune liver disease *(376)* and challenges the assumption that unknown chronic viral infections of the liver, although possible initiators, maintain the active disease process.

Primary Biliary Cirrhosis

Introduction and Disease Description

PBC is a slowly progressive hepatic autoimmune disorder that primarily affects women. The disease is typically associated with high titers of antimitochondrial autoantibodies (AMAs) that presage onset of clinical disease by 5 to 10 years. Histopathologic changes include portal inflammation and destruction of intrahepatic bile ducts, which occur at various rates and degrees in different patients. The resulting decrease of bile secretion and retention of toxic substances within the liver leads to further hepatic damage, fibrosis, cirrhosis, and eventual liver failure *(362–364)*.

Autoimmune Features

Although speculation about the autoimmune pathogenesis of PBC centers around the usual suspects of genetic and environmental/microbial factors, PBC may serve as an example of how advanced knowledge about the targeted autoantigens can give rise to novel and intriguing hypotheses. The presence of AMAs in PBC were first described in the 1950s, the autoantigens cloned in the 1980s and 1990s, and B cell, $CD4^+$, and $CD8^+$ T cell epitopes of the major autoantigen PDC-E2 mapped in the 1990s and 2000s. More than 90% of PBC patients have high titers of autoantibodies directed against the 2-oxo-acid dehydrogenase complex (2-OADC) E2 subunit, in particular the

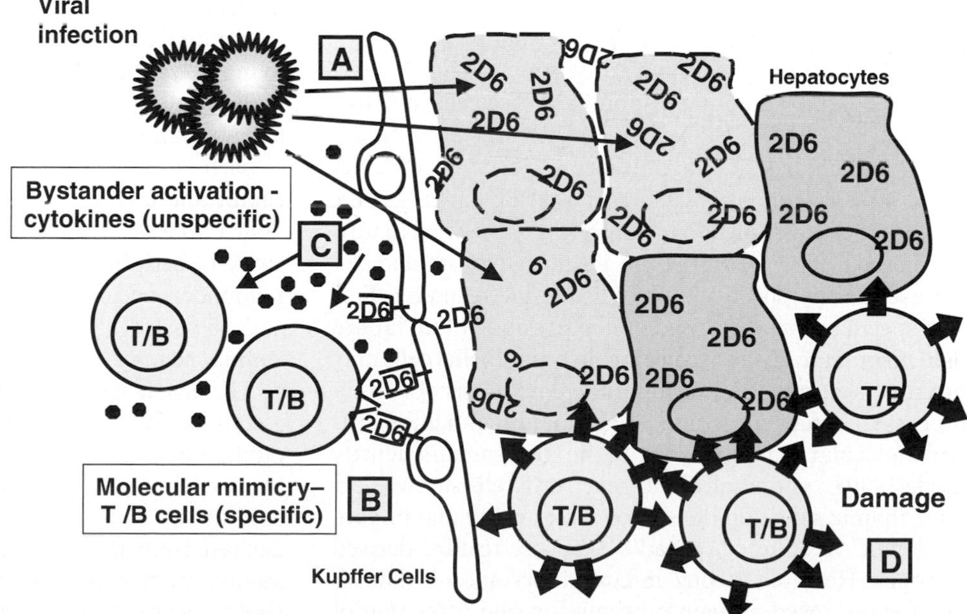

FIGURE 42.13 Pathogenesis of liver autoimmunity after viral infection in the 2D6 animal model. Viral infection leads to expression of high cytokine levels in the liver **(A).** The infection will probably also activate resident macrophages (Kupffer cells) **(B).** Antiviral T cells react against virally infected cells and destroy them. This leads to release of autoantigens from hepatocytes, which can be (cross-) presented, leading to pathogenic responses against autoantigens such as cytochrome P450 2D6. Chemokine and cytokine release **(C)** leads to enhanced inflammation and antigen presentation **(D).**

TABLE 42.2 Autoantibodies and Autoantigens in Autoimmune Liver Disease

	Type I AIH	*Type II AIH*	*PBC*	*PSC*
Autoantibodies	**ANA:** centromere, ribonucleoprotein, cyclin A, histone **SMA:** F actin, anti-ASGPR anti-SLA/LP **pANCA:** myeloid-specific nuclear envelope protein	**Anti-LKM-1:** CYP450, 2D6 **Anti-LC-1:** formiminotrans-ferase cyclodeaminase	**AMA:** PDC-E2, BCOADC-E2, OGDC-E2, PDC-ERBP, PDC-E1α **ANA:** nuclear pore complex, anti-gp210, anti-p62, nuclear dot pattern, anti-Sp 100, anti-PML, anti-SUMOs	**pANCA:** myeloid-specific nuclear envelope protein **ANA:** anticardiolipin, thyroperoxidase, rheumatic factor, *Helicobacter pylori* immunoglobulin G
B cell infiltrate in liver	+ with plasma cells	+ with plasma cells	+ with plasma cells	+/−

AIH, autoimmune hepatitis; AMA, antimitochondrial autoantibodies; ANA, antinuclear antibodies; LKM-1, liver-kidney microsomal-1; LP-1, lipocortin-1; pANCA, perinuclear anti-neutrophil cytoplasmic antibody; PBC, primary biliary cirrhosis; PSC, primary sclerosing cholangitis; SMA, smooth muscle antibodies.
From Moritoki Y, Lian ZX, Ohsugi Y, et al. B cells and autoimmune liver diseases. *Autoimmun Rev.* 2006;5:449, with permission.

E2 component of the pyruvate dehydrogenase complex (PDC-E2) (Table 42.2). Mapping studies have identified determinants within the PDC-E2 lipoyl domains as primary targets for antibody and T cell reactivity, motifs that are also located in the E2 subunit of other 2-OADC members (OGDC-E2, BCKD-E2; the same motif is also found in E3-BP) *(363)*. Antibody reactivity to nuclear envelope proteins gp210 and p62 was observed in 10% to 30% of patients and is apparently associated with more active disease. The obvious question emerging from the identification of these autoantigens pertains to the fact that they are (a) found in every cell type and (b) located on the inner surface of the inner mitochondrial membrane, and are thus separated from immune effectors by three membranes. In addition, the existence of a clinical entity known as AMA-negative PBC, a disease very similar to PBC but without detectable AMA, appears to further argue against a pathogenic role for these autoantibodies *(364)*. Yet, certain particularities of bile duct epithelial cells may predispose them to be targets for humoral immune responses. These cells, just like salivary epithelial cells, express receptors involved in the transcytosis of IgA, and high titers of PDC-E2–specific IgA are observed in bile, saliva, and urine of PBC patients. AMA IgA was recently shown to induce apoptosis, which in turn may lead to PDC accumulation in the cytoplasm and cell surface and amplification of the immune response. Further speculation has focused on the possibility that failure of PDC glutathionylation specifically in epithelial cells may promote accumulation of immunogenic forms of PDC, a process that may be initiated by xenobiotic-modified PDC and molecular mimicry *(363)*. In the "determinant density model" *(393)*, potentially PDC-reactive T cells survive negative thymic selection due to low TcR avidity and remain "dormant" in spite of sporadic exposure to PDC-derived epitopes. However, strong inflammatory stimuli that allow for improved antigen presentation and activation of Toll-like receptors (TLRs; monocytes from PBC patients exhibit enhanced sensitivity to TLR signals), for example, through microbial molecular mimicry, may induce the breakdown of tolerance that precipitates the disease. It should be noted that the general validity of this hypothesis, including a key role for low-avidity T cells and TLRs, is fully supported by elegant studies in models for induction of autoimmune diabetes (102,*394*). Finally, a model has been proposed in which a primary dysfunction of endothelial cells results in overproduction of endothelins, inflammatory alterations, and ischemic damage due to vasoconstriction and the generation of PDC-specific humoral and cellular responses as a secondary event *(364)*. These hypotheses are not mutually exclusive and may be critically evaluated in two recently introduced animal models.

Genetic Features and Environmental Factors

Familial clustering of PBC and a high concordance rate in monozygotic twins (63%) indicate a genetic component to PBC pathogenesis. However, no consistent associations have been found between PBC susceptibility and carriage of particular HLA genes. Polymorphisms in vitamin D receptor and CTLA-4 genes have been suggested to be conducive to PBC development, and X chromosome monosomy in peripheral white blood cells may explain female preponderance of the disease *(363,374)*.

Animal Models

The absence of a suitable animal model has long been a serious obstacle to PBC research. However, two recent publications document important progress on this front by describing the spontaneous onset of a PBC-like disease in two mouse strains. NOD.c3c4 mice congenically derived from the NOD strain generate PDC-E2–specific autoantibodies and exhibit biliary pathology characterized by destructive cholangitis, granuloma formation, and eosinophilic infiltration. It is significant that T cells were observed in affected areas of the biliary epithelium and that transfer of splenocytes or CD4$^+$ T cells induces disease in NOD.c3c4-SCID recipients, suggesting a central role for T cells in pathogenesis *(395)*. In the second model, abolition of TGFβ signaling in T cells (achieved by T cell–specific expression of a dominant-negative TGFβRII) resulted in the production of AMAs directed against PDC-E2, BCOADC-E2, and OGDC-E2, as well as lymphocytic liver infiltration with periportal inflammation analogous to the histologic profile in human PBC. These observations implicated the TGFβ pathway in PBC pathogenesis and suggested that the activation of intrinsically self-reactive T cells was a consequence of impaired regulatory T cell function rather than molecular mimicry *(396)*.

Treatment and Prevention

It is noteworthy that despite its presumed autoimmune etiology, PBC is not ameliorated by immunosuppressive therapy. In the absence of optimized therapeutic protocols, treatment is tailored according to individual responsiveness of PBC patients and includes management of disease symptoms (pruritus, osteoporosis, hyperlipidemia, and portal hypertension) and therapy of the underlying disease by stepwise addition of ursodeoxycholic acid (UDCA), colchicin, and methotrexate. Nevertheless, the use of colchicin and low-dose methotrexate, presumably acting as an immunomodulatory rather than antimetabolic agent, is controversial. In cases of liver failure, orthotopic liver transplantation is the only effective treatment *(362)*.

Primary Sclerosing Cholangitis

Introduction and Disease Description

PSC is a chronic cholestatic liver disease (cholestasis: suppression of biliary flow) frequently associated with inflammatory bowel disease (greater than 75% of PSC patients). It is characterized by fibrotic inflammation and destruction of the large intra- and extrahepatic bile ducts and may lead to the development of cholangiocarcinoma (in 10% to 30% of PSC patients) and ultimately death by liver failure.

Autoimmune Features

Although the etiology of PSC is undefined, a complex multistep process has been delineated and involves cholangiocyte activation through bacterial pathogen-associated molecular patterns (PAMP), production of proinflammatory cytokines in conjunction with aberrant chemokine expression and endothelial cell adhesion molecules, and the recruitment of T cells presumably specific for enterocyte antigens and primed in GALT *(366)*. The generation of autoantibodies is a common feature (Table 42.2), but most antibodies are not specific for PSC and their contribution to disease pathogenesis is unclear *(374)*.

Genetic Features and Environmental Factors

As in AIH, susceptibility to PSC is conferred by HLA-B8 and DR3. Whether a CTLA-4 polymorphism is associated with disease susceptibility is controversial *(366)*. The relative risk of PSC among first-degree relatives of PSC patients is almost 100-fold increased compared to the general population *(365)*.

Animal Models

None of the animal models developed reproduce all pertinent aspects of human PSC *(397)*. Rat models of small bowel bacterial overgrowth and administration of bacterial cell wall components have provided some support for an ethiopathogenetic role of PAMPs. Other models include injury of biliary epithelial or vascular endothelial cells (rodents, dog, monkey) and toxic, infectious, or intraluminal biliary injury (rodents) permitting the study of cytokines, chemokines, and inflammation in the development of diffuse bile duct sclerosis *(397)*.

Treatment and Prevention

There is no effective medical therapy for PSC *(398)*. Treatment with the hydrophilic bile acid UDCA improves liver enzymes, but its effect on liver histology and prognosis is inconclusive. Orthotopic liver transplant constitutes the only established long-term treatment for PSC, with cumulative 5-year survival in approximately 70% of patients.

Halothane Hepatitis

Halothane hepatitis is a severe, life-threatening form of hepatic damage that affects a small subset of individuals exposed to the anesthetic agent halothane *(399)*; it is believed to have an immunologic basis. Sera of afflicted individuals contain autoantibodies directed against the native and the TFA form of hepatic proteins. TFA proteins are generated during the oxidative metabolism of halothane (2-bromo-2-chloro-1,1,1-trifluoroethane) and include cytochrome P450, protein disulfide isomerase, microsomal carboxlesterase, calreticulin, Erp72, GRP78 (BiP), and GRP94. Evidence suggests that such TFA proteins arise in all individuals exposed to halothane. However, the vast majority of individuals appear to tolerate this covalent protein modification. The lack of immunologic responsiveness was suggested to occur due to tolerance induced through the presence of structures in the repertoire of self-determinants, which immunochemically and structurally mimic TFA proteins very closely. In fact, lipoic acid, the prosthetic group of the constitutively expressed E2 subunits of members of the 2-oxoacid dehydrogenase complex family, was demonstrated by immunochemical and molecular modeling analysis to perfectly mimic

N^6-trifluoroacteyl-L-lysine, the major haptenic group of TFA proteins. Of interest, a fraction of patients with halothane hepatitis exhibited irregularities in the hepatic expression levels of these cross-reactive proteins. Thus, molecular mimicry of TFA-lysine by lipoic acid or the impairment thereof could be considered a susceptibility factor for individuals developing halothane hepatitis *(400)*. A small-animal model for chemically induced liver diseases has been described *(401)*.

Perspective and Conclusions

The presence of autoantibodies in AIH, PBC, and PSC is indicative of autoimmune processes, but none of the antibodies described is liver specific, and their contribution to pathogenesis is unclear. Although the complex role of T cells is subject to investigations, the same caveats regarding specificity and pathogenicity discussed earlier apply for autoimmune liver diseases *(402)*. Although the success of immunosuppressive therapy—in fact a criterion for the diagnostic scoring system for AIH (44,372)—further supports autoimmune etiology for AIH, it is conceivable that a viral infection might initiate disease as a "hit-and-run" event. Following elimination of viral antigens, disease may be perpetuated by immune-mediated processes and preclude the identification of a particular virus as a causative agent at the time of liver disease diagnosis. Again, the role of "foreign" and "self"-antigens becomes blurred, and their interactions with the immune system in terms of immunity or autoimmunity are conceptually problematic. Future investigations should seek to improve animal models and focus on human autoantigens and the application of contemporary tools for identification and isolation of specific lymphocytes. On the basis of such developments, future *in vivo* tracking of autoaggressive lymphocytes with noninvasive methods should substantially improve our insight into disease pathogenesis.

Renal Autoimmune Diseases

Glomerolunephritis (GN) is the major cause of chronic renal disease and kidney failure and exhibits a wide spectrum of histopathologic alterations, disease severity, and clinical outcomes. In most cases, evidence for an immune-mediated pathogenesis, including humoral and cellular responses, has been obtained *(403–406)*. The precise incidence of defined renal autoimmune disease is difficult to establish because definite diagnosis requires histologic evaluation of the kidneys. In this respect, the Italian registry of renal biopsies provides a unique repository, and information about selected glomerular disease obtained from this resource is displayed in Table 42.3 *(407,408)*. The identity of nephritogenic antigens targeted in most renal autoimmune diseases is poorly defined, with the notable exception of Goodpasture's syndrome, a form of anti–glomerular basement membrane (GBM) disease in which autoantibodies bind to α3(IV) collagen in the GBM and are associated with rapidly progressive GN and pulmonary hemorrhage. Conformational epitopes have been mapped to two regions within the noncollagenous (NC1) domain of the α3(IV) chain *(409)*. A role for T cells, both in providing help for autoantibody production and exerting direct effector functions, has also emerged in recent years. Cast within the reigning concept of balanced TH1 and TH2 immunity, it appears that TH1 responses are associated with proliferative and crescentic forms of GN that cause severe injury, whereas TH2 responses are associated with membranous patterns of injury *(403)*. These distinctions have also given rise to speculations that have harnessed the "hygiene hypothesis" as a potential explanation for the observation that proliferative GNs have a relatively high incidence in developing countries, whereas minimal-change disease and IgA nephropathy predominate in developed countries. Therapeutically, immunosuppression with corticosteroids, in combination with cyclophosphamide and plasma exchange (to remove damaging antibodies), is employed to manage diseases. Based on the TH1/TH2 paradigm and its role in developing therapies for other autoimmune diseases that aim to target the TH1-TH2 balance, therapeutic approaches such as oral tolerance, cytokine-based immune modulation (anti-TNFα and IL-12p40 antibodies, recombinant IL-10), antiadhesion molecules, and chemokine receptor blockade are being evaluated for use in the treatment of autoimmune renal diseases *(403)*.

TABLE 42.3 Incidence of Glomerular Diseases in 1993

Disease	*Incidence per Million Population*
Immunoglobulin A nepthropathy	8.4
Membranous glomerulonephritis	4.9
Focal segmental glomerulonephritis	2.3
Minimal change disease	1.6
Mesangiocapillary glomerulonephritis	1.4
Poststreptococcal glomerulonephritis	0.7

From Schena FP. Survey of the Italian Registry of Renal Biopsies. Frequency of the renal diseases for 7 consecutive years. The Italian Group of Renal Immunopathology. *Nephrol Dial Transplant.* 1997;12:418, with permission.

Cutaneous Autoimmune Diseases

Cutaneous autoimmune disorders are commonly divided into non–organ-specific and organ-specific diseases. The former group contains skin manifestations of systemic autoimmune disorders such as SLE, Crohn's disease, and ulcerative colitis, and this group is detailed in Chapter 41. The organ-specific autoimmune skin disorders discussed

TABLE 42.4 Autoimmune Bullous Dermatoses

Disorder	Acantholysis	Autoantigen	Autoantibody Class	T Cell Subset
Pemphigus vulgaris (PV)	Suprabasilar	Desmoglein-3 > desmoglein-1	IgG4, IgG1, IgA (occasionally)	TH1, TH2, Tr1, CD8$^+$ CD28$^-$ Treg
Pemphigus folicaeus (PF)	Subcorneal	Desmoglein-1	IgG4, IgG1	TH1, TH2
Bullous pemphigoid (BP)	Subepidermal	BP180, BP230	IgG1, IgG4, IgA (occasionally)	TH1, TH2
Cicatricial pemphigoid (CP)	Subepidermal	BP180 > BP230, laminin 5	IgG1, IgG4, IgA (occasionally)	TH1
Pemphigus gestationis (PG)	Subepidermal	BP180, BP230	IgG1, IgG3	TH1, TH2
Dermatitis herpetiformis (DH) (associated with gluten-sensitive enteropathy)	Subepidermal	Epidermal transglutaminase	IgA	TH2
Linear IgA disease	Subepidermal	BP180, BP230	IgA	TH1, TH2
Epidermolysis bullosa acquisita (EBA)	Subepidermal	Collagen VII	IgG, IgA, IgM (occasionally)	TH1, TH2, no Treg contribution

Ig, immunoglobulin.

here include several autoimmune bullous dermatoses, as well as pigmentation disorder vitiligo. Despite a relative paucity of animal models for human autoimmune skin disorders, the skin is one of the few organs that offer direct access to target antigens and effector cells; consequently, advanced insights into mechanisms of disease induction and perpetuation have been obtained in recent years.

Autoimmune Bullous Dermatoses

Autoimmune bullous dermatoses comprise a group of severe, possibly fatal skin disorders characterized by erosions and blisters of skin and/or mucous membranes (Table 42.4, Figure 42.14). The term "pemphigus" (from the Greek and Latin for "pustule") that is featured in the name of several of these diseases dates to "pemphigoid fever" described by Hippocrates nearly 2,400 years ago and has been used to describe chronic blistering skin conditions since the mid-18th century. All forms of pemphigus have distinctive characteristics, but they exhibit the common feature of epidermal cell-to-cell detachment known as acantholysis. On occasion, pemphigus syndromes are associated with other autoimmune diseases such as SLE, RA, myasthenia gravis, pernicious anemia, and Hashimoto's thyroiditis.

Pemphigus Vulgaris

Pemphigus vulgaris (PV) is the most common and severe form of pemphigus in the United States, constituting more than 80% of reported cases *(410,411)*. With a worldwide incidence of 1 to 5 cases per million per year in the general population, PV remains a rare disease and preferentially affects individuals in the fourth to sixth decade of life. Clinical features include flaccid, fragile, and noninflammatory bullae (from the Latin for "bubble") that arise on normal-appearing skin. These lesions tend to coalesce and rupture, leaving larger areas of denuded skin

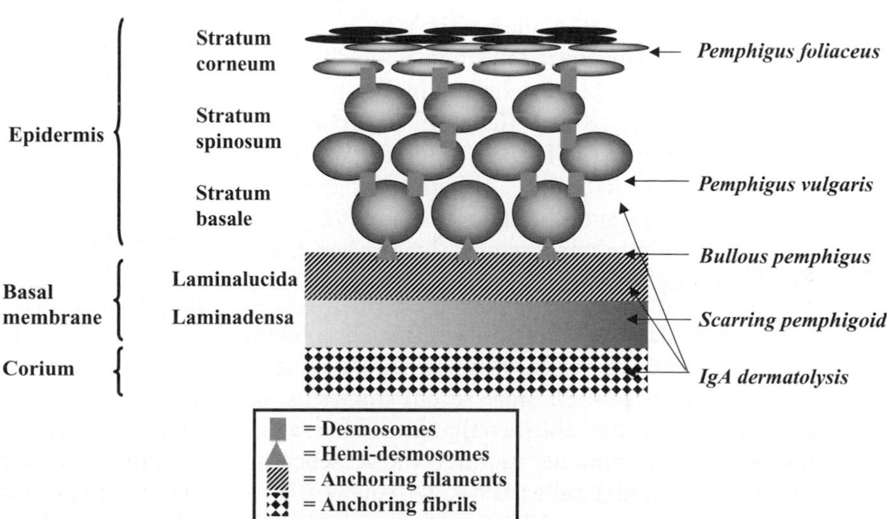

FIGURE 42.14 Different layers of the skin and their involvement in autoimmune skin syndromes. IgA, immunoglobulin A.

that often heal poorly *(410–412)*. About half of the patients initially present with lesions confined to the oral mucosa, although any surface with squamous epithelial tissue may be affected. Blister formation begins with edema of epidermal intracellular spaces and progresses to complete loss of cohesion between epidermal cells. In PV, blisters occur in the suprabasilar region of the epidermis while leaving attachment of basal cells to the dermis largely intact *(410–414)*.

Autoimmune Features. The hallmark of PV is the presence of autoantibodies generated against the desmosomal glycoprotein desmoglein-3 (Dsg3) (Table 42.4). In fact, the unequivocal identification of this antigen makes PV one of a few human autoimmune diseases for which the relevant autoantigen has been defined. Although the pathogenic contribution of Dsg3 antibodies has been demonstrated in passive transfer experiments, recent work has emphasized the importance of specific T cells *(415)*. Peripheral $CD4^+$ and occasional $CD8^+$ T cell responses targeting Dsg3 with varying functional profiles (TH1 and TH2) have been described. These autoreactive $CD4^+$ T cells may be involved in the coordination of specific B cell responses as evidenced by TH1-regulated IgG1 and TH2-regulated Dsg3 antibodies in patient sera. Of interest, IL-10–producing, Dsg3-reactive T cells have also been identified in the majority of healthy individuals carrying PV-associated HLA alleles (see later discussion) but were described in less than 20% of PV patients *(416)*. Given these functional attributes reminiscent of the Tr1 regulatory T cell subset as well as the documentation of $CD8^+CD28^-$ T cells with potential regulatory function in remittent PV patients (cited in ref. *415*), it has been proposed that clinical disease may emerge as a consequence of an imbalance between autoreactive pathogenic and Tregs *(415)*.

Genetic Features and Environmental Factors. Although PV can affect anyone, an enhanced prevalence is observed in people of Mediterranean or Jewish ancestry. Associations with certain HLA alleles (HLA-26, HLA-B38, SC21, HLA-DR4) in Ashkenazi Jews and non-Ashkenazi Jews (HLA-Drw6) have been detected in PV patients, and it has been suggested that the third hypervariable region of the $\beta 1$ chain of the DRB1 allele may constitute a susceptibility locus *(410–412)*. Although PV may be associated with other autoimmune diseases *(414)*, its occurrence with certain malignant diseases has been defined as a separate entity *(417)*.

Animal Models. The pathogenic role of autoantibodies has been demonstrated by passive transfer of PV patient sera into neonatal mice *(418)*. More recent studies using Dsg3-deficient mice have established that loss of tolerance and induction of autoimmunity required the presence of both autoreactive B and T cells *(419–421)*. Finally, $CD4^+$ T cells from Dsg3-immunized, HLA transgenic mice target Dsg3 epitopes identical to those identified in humans and thus constitute a promising model with which to further analyze the regulation of Dsg3-specific T cells and autoantibody production *in vivo (415)*.

Treatment and Prevention. Corticosteroids are the treatment of choice, and supplementary immunosuppressive agents (cyclophosphamide, azathioprine, and methotrexate) are commonly used to reduce the side effects of steroids. In severe cases, plasmapheresis may be of short-term benefit.

Other Autoimmune Bullous Disorders

These include pemphigus foliaceus (PF), bullous pemphigoid (BP), cicatricial (scarring) pemphigoid, epidermolysis bullosa acquisita, dermatitis herpitiformis, and linear immunoglobulin A disease (Table 42.4). Two forms of PF are recognized, one affecting individuals irrespective of ethnic background or geography and the other, PF fogo selvagem (Portuguese for “savage fire”), endemic to certain regions of Brazil. Antibodies found in the circulation of PF patients preferentially target desmoglein-1, are of the IgG4 subclass, and, similar to PV, can induce aspects of the disease in a neonatal mouse transfer model *(410)*; TH1 and TH2 T cells specific for the same antigen have also been described *(415)*. Information about genetic association is incomplete due to the rarity of PF. However, PF fogo selvagem demonstrates associations with HLA-DR1 and HLA-DR4. Prior to the introduction of corticosteroids, fewer than 10% of patients underwent spontaneous remission, and fatalities reached up to 40% within the first 2 years of disease. Compared to PV, PF patients respond more rapidly and to smaller doses of corticosteroids *(410)*.

Together with PV, BP belongs to the best-characterized bullous disorders with regard to pathogenesis. In BP, IgG autoantibodies are directed against components of the dermoepidermal basement membrane such as BP antigens BP180 and BP230. Again, these antigens are also recognized by $CD4^+$ T cells and comprise both TH1- and TH2-type subsets *(415)*. Systemic corticosteroids with facultative addition of other immunosuppressive agents are used as treatment. The principal autoimmune targets and basic pathologic features of the remaining bullous dermatoses are listed in Table 42.4.

Perspective and Conclusions

The identification of relevant autoantigens, a task that is far from complete in the majority of human autoimmune diseases, is usually considered to be a critical step in understanding pathogenetic mechanisms and an important step toward the development of targeting immunomodulatory therapies. However, the case of PV and BP is a telling reminder that even with established knowledge about such primary autoantigens, the development of specific immunotherapies faces continuing challenges.

Vitiligo

Introduction and Disease Description

Vitiligo is an acquired, noncontagious disorder of pigmentation resulting from melanocyte loss *(422,423)*. The disease is characterized by defined areas of depigmentation that range from limited numbers of macules (focal vitiligo) to bilateral, symmetric distribution of the lesions (generalized vitiligo, the most common type) to involvement of the complete body surface area (universal vitiligo). Vitiligo is arguably the most common pigmentary disorder, affecting 0.5% to 2% of the population worldwide, and it demonstrates no predilection for gender or ethnicity. Although commonly regarded as a pathophysiologic entity with distinct clinical manifestations, recent work suggests the existence of a spectrum of vitiligo disorders with different etiologies. The potential autoimmune etiology of vitiligo has been discussed for some time and has gained traction through recent studies on genetic epidemiology. A combination of environmental, genetic, and immunologic factors is thought to contribute to autoimmune melanocyte destruction. This hypothesis is further strengthened by the reported association of vitiligo with other autoimmune diseases such as autoimmune thyroid disease, SLE, Addison's disease, and pernicious anemia *(424)*. Nevertheless, the specific causes of vitiligo are obscure, and progress is limited due to a lack of a clear definition of the disorder as well as a dearth of experimental animal models *(423)*.

Autoimmune Features

T cell infiltrates were reported in generalized vitiligo and exhibited molecular signatures indicative of CTL and TH1 responses (TNFα and IFNγ) *(425)*. CD8$^+$ T cells tend to predominate in vitiligo lesions, and high frequencies of MelanA-specific CD8$^+$ T cell subsets apparently correlate with disease severity *(426,427)*. Additional infiltrating cells include macrophages, monocytes, and DCs that produce proinflammatory cytokines. The role of DCs in local immune responses is unclear, but the DC-mediated killing of melanocytes has been suggested as a mechanism for depigmentation *(428)*. Finally, circulating autoantibodies, including those specific for the melanocyte antigen tyrosinase-related protein-1 (TRP1), have been identified in the sera of vitiligo patients, and TRP1-specific antibodies can induce melanocyte loss in mice *(429)*. Nevertheless, there appears to be an emerging consensus that alterations of humoral immunity are secondary to T cell–mediated autoimmune destruction.

Genetic Features and Environmental Factors

Evidence for genetic factors contributing to onset of generalized vitiligo has been obtained in studies of vitiligo patients' close relatives *(424,430)*. The largest vitiligo twin study demonstrated concordance for generalized vitiligo in monozygotic twins of 23%, far greater than the risk for nonidentical siblings (6.3%) and the general population risk *(424)*. At the same time, these data highlight the critical importance of environmental factors. Genetic association and linkage studies have revealed an association between vitiligo and HLA-DRB1, DLRB4, and DQB1 alleles as well as other genes, many of which await confirmation *(422,423)*. It is worth noting that the first vitiligo linkage data excluded a single candidate gene, the microophthalmia-associated transcription factor (MITF). MITF appeared to be a relevant candidate due to numerous mutations at the mouse microphthalmia (*mi*) locus associated with reduced or absent pigmentation and with the *mivit/vit* mutation presenting postnatal depigmentation that resembles human vitiligo *(431)*.

Animal Models

The lack of a tractable experimental animal model has clearly hampered progress in vitiligo research. Nevertheless, the mutant Smyth line of chickens exhibited several relevant clinical features, including melanocyte loss as a consequence of T cell infiltration *(432)*. Furthermore, the potential contribution of herpes virus infection to vitiligo induction in Smyth-line chickens *(433)* emphasizes the role of environmental factors and warrants further investigation into this model.

Treatment and Prevention

Routine nonsurgical repigmentation strategies include phototherapy, topical steroids, and inhibitors of the calcineurin pathway. These treatment modalities, although interfering with a multitude of complex pathophysiologic pathways, modulate in particular the activity of local T cell responses.

Perspective and Conclusions

In addition to genes involved in aberrant immune regulation, more than 120 genes are known to participate in the coordination of mammalian pigmentation. However, the recent identification of several candidate genes and genetic linkages associated with vitiligo will facilitate the elucidation of biological pathways involved in vitiligo pathogenesis and allow for a better differentiation of the spectrum of vitiligo disorders. As a result, novel therapeutic and prophylactic approaches will likely be developed in the near future.

Cardiac Autoimmune Diseases

The etiology for primary myocarditis is unclear, and an autoimmune cause has to be taken into account. The heart muscle is infiltrated mainly by CD4$^+$ T cells and macrophages, and the infiltrates are usually diffuse and nonfocal. The infiltrating cells produce considerable amounts of IFNγ and TNFα. As a consequence of the inflammation, heart muscle cells can swell, the heart can dilate, and severe disturbances of the electrical conduction can occur. It is noteworthy that myocarditis can also occur in conjunction with certain systemic autoimmune diseases such as SLE, scleroderma, RA, polymyositis, and polyarteritis nodosa. Two specific scenarios are noteworthy.

The first is myocarditis occurring after Chagas' disease. In this case, cross-reactivity between antigens presented by the parasite causing Chagas' disease (*Trypanosoma cruzi*), and cardiac myosin has been observed in patients with myocarditis *(434)*. The scarcity of parasites in the chronic phase of the disease contrasts with the severe cardiac pathology observed in approximately 30% of persistently infected patients and suggests a role for autoimmunity as the origin of the pathology. In these cases, various *T. cruzi* antigens, such as B13, cruzipain, and Cha, cross-react with host antigens at the B or T cell level, and their role in pathogenesis has been widely studied. Immunization with those antigens and/or passive transfer of autoreactive T lymphocytes in mice leads to clinical disturbances similar to those observed in Chagas' disease patients. On the other hand, the parasite is becoming increasingly detected in chronically infected hosts and may also be the cause of pathology either directly or through parasite-specific mediated inflammatory responses. Thus, the issue of autoimmunity versus parasite persistence as the cause of Chagas' disease pathology is being hotly debated.

The second scenario is coxsackie B virus–associated myocarditis. Also in this situation, immunopathology outlasts the direct presence of the virus in heart muscle. This disease has been extensively studied in experimental models by Rose and colleagues *(435)*. They developed two murine models of myocarditis—one elicited by cardiotropic CoxB3 virus infection and the other by cardiac myosin immunization—to better analyze the pathogenetic mechanisms responsible for immune-mediated heart muscle disease. Both virus infection and myosin immunization produce myocardial inflammation and elicit heart-reactive antibodies that bind to the myocardium *in vivo* and recognize the cardiac myosin heavy chain. Each model offers unique advantages. The virus-induced disease more closely resembles human myocarditis; myosin immunization isolates the autoimmune components of the disease because no virus infection is involved. They also distinguished strains of mice resistant to autoimmune myocarditis (such as B10.A) from those susceptible to the autoimmune phase of disease (such as A.CA and A/J). Mice from a resistant strain to virus- or myosin-induced autoimmune heart disease develop myocardial inflammation and myosin antibodies if cotreated with TNFα or IL-1 when infected or immunized. Thus, cytokines can modulate the outcome of cardiotropic virus infection and enhance its autoimmune sequela. They also found that blocking IL-1 receptor inhibits autoimmune myocarditis in genetically susceptible mice. Of interest, there is no regulatory function of TH2 cytokines such as IL-4, illustrating that immune regulation is an organ-specific concept rather than a global paradigm applicable to all autoimmune disease equally.

Rheumatoid Arthritis

Although RA is commonly classified as a systemic autoimmune disease, we believe that it can offer insights and paradigms that are important for understanding organ-specific diseases such as T1D and MS. A particularly interesting aspect is that diagnostic or therapeutic access to the target organ is comparatively easy achieved, and this has facilitated the development of rational and highly effective immunotherapies. In this case high levels of TNFα were detected in affected joints, and TNF blockade has proven to be a highly effective intervention in RA (see more detailed description later).

Introduction and Disease Description

RA is a severe debilitating disease with unknown etiology. Epidemiologically, the prevalence is about 1% in the overall population; women are affected three times more frequently than men, and the peak of incidence is within the fourth to sixth decades of life (147,*436*). Diagnostic criteria include typical morning stiffness, joint swelling with fluid accumulation, defined radiologic changes, subcutaneous rheumatic nodes, and positive rheumatoid factor (autoantibodies). The prognosis is worse in HLA-DR4–positive patients, and, similar to diabetes and MS, there is genetic linkage with certain MHC haplotypes (Figure 42.15). Without systemic immunosuppressive or antiinflammatory therapy, the disease eventually

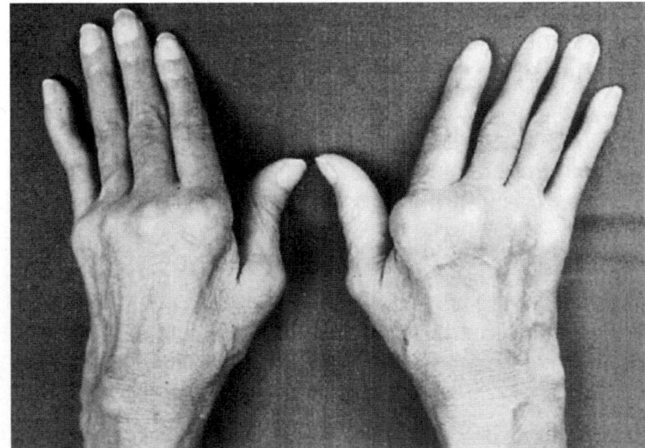

Typical ulnar deviation and swan's neck deformation of the hands in rheumatoid arthritis

FIGURE 42.15 Rheumatoid arthritis.

results in destruction of many major joints and immobilizes the patient. The major cause of death is infections that easily take a more severe course in immobile individuals (147).

The etiology of RA is ill defined. Because there is a possible overlap with infection-associated arthropathies (e.g., Reiter's syndrome), bacteria have always been good candidates as a cause for arthritis, and molecular mimicry has been implicated because cross-reactivity of autoantibodies between self and bacterial proteins have been detected (111). However, although it is quite possible to demonstrate cross-reactive antibodies and T cells in human blood, proof of their pathogenetic involvement is exceedingly difficult to obtain. The immune system is likely to have developed to tolerate a low-level cross-reactivity, which might even be necessary for its proper function, and it is very difficult to prove a mechanistic link between autoreactive cells and pathologic autoimmunity in humans.

Autoimmune Features

The evidence that RA is an autoimmune disease stems, as in the case of MS and T1D, from the observation that T lymphocytes in a patient's blood can react with joint-derived autoantigens, and IgM autoantibodies, as well as ANAs, are readily found in humans *(437)*. Inflammatory signs in the serum include complement activation and increased erythrocyte sedimentation rate, which indicates that the antibodies could possibly play a role in the disease process. Similarly, immunization with collagen can induce arthritis in susceptible mouse strains. Figure 42.16 summarizes the major pathogenetic pathways leading to progressive joint destruction. As in many other autoimmune disease animal

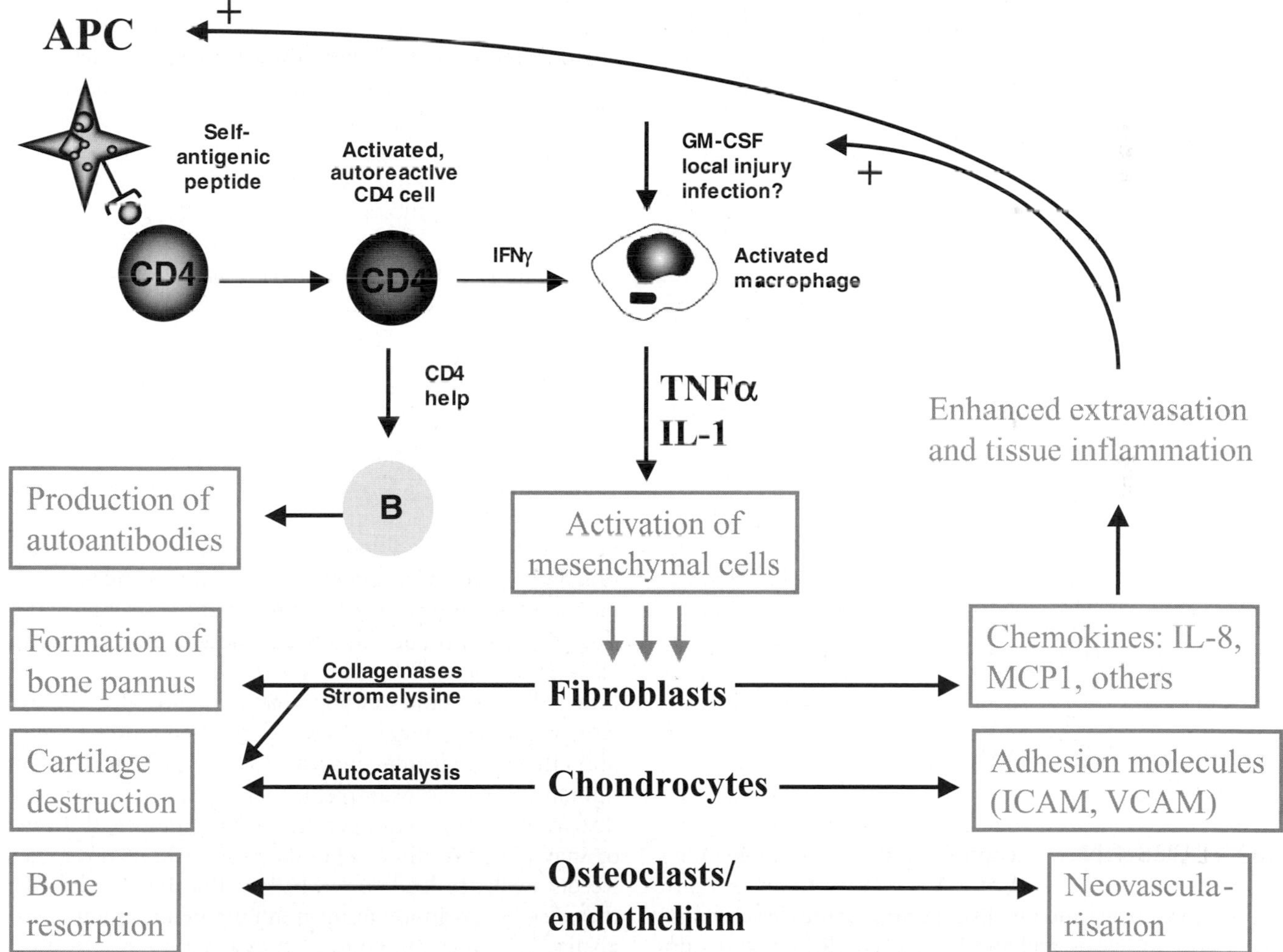

FIGURE 42.16 Pathogenic pathways leading to joint destruction in rheumatoid arthritis (RA). Note the central role of tissue necrosis factor-α (TNFα), which is strongly supported by the fact that TNF blockade ameliorates RA in humans. APC, antigen-presenting cell; GM-CSF, granulocyte-monocyte colony-stimulating factor; ICAM, intercellular adhesion molecule; IFNγ, interferon-γ; IL, interleukin; MCP1, monocyte chemotactic protein-1; VCAM, vascular cell adhesion molecule.

models, collagen-induced arthritis models require strong immunization with autoantigens and adjuvant, supporting the concept that breaking of self-tolerance, even on a genetically susceptible background, requires a rather pronounced inflammatory stimulus. In contrast, how disease is initiated in humans is unclear.

Treatment and Prevention

Treatment of RA is a difficult task because the medications that adequately suppress joint inflammation also have strong systemic side effects. Therefore, a delicate balance between different therapeutic approaches that target different stages of the inflammatory process needs to be established. Corticosteroids and nonsteroidal antiinflammatory drugs can provide some baseline relief but are not able to halt progressive joint destruction. Gold compounds, methotrexate, and cyclophosphamide are more effective but also have profound systemic side effects. For this reason, progress with novel immunomodulatory interventions is of important benefit for RA patients.

Application of cyclosporin A was shown to be effective by suppressing proliferation and activation of T lymphocytes. More recently, a more selective intervention has been established based on research by M. Feldman's group (146). TNFα was found to play a key role in an *in vitro* model of synovial destruction using human cells, and TNFα-blocking agents to be applied *in vivo* were subsequently developed. After promising preclinical results in animal models, this intervention was tested in clinical trials and is now licensed for treatment of RA. Although side effects do occur, as expected, they appear tolerable, and clinical improvement of disease is pronounced. In some patients, SLE-like symptoms were observed, indicating that blocking a cytokine beneficial for one autoimmune disorder might be detrimental for another. Indeed, TNF blockade is not helpful in MS and T1D because this cytokine exhibits complex dual functions, depending on the disease stage. Based on encouraging results with TNF blockade in RA, it may be possible to find similar key cytokines for T1D or MS treatment. It should be stressed that the successful intervention was developed based on human cell cultures and not animal models, underlining the need for direct research on human materials, if and when possible.

CONCLUSION

A common trait among diverse animal models for autoimmune diseases and the human conditions they aim to model appears to be the difficulty with which experimental autoimmunity is achieved. Breaking of tolerance to self-antigens requires in most cases strong inflammatory (e.g., pertussis toxin and adjuvant in EAE or collagen-induced arthritis) or infectious (e.g., RIP-LCMV model for T1D, and TMEV/MHV models for MS) stimuli. In addition, many animal models require a genetically susceptible background or have to rely on artificial autoantigen expression by means of transgenic technology. In contrast to the relatively easy detection of autoreactive lymphocytes in antigen-induced animal models, it has been a daunting endeavor in humans (as well as spontaneous disease models such as the NOD mouse), and data obtained often vary considerably among different patients as well as laboratories. What are the implications for our understanding of autoimmune diseases in humans, given these challenges? First, it is unlikely that strong inflammatory stimuli could be provided under natural conditions in the absence of infectious disease. Thus, viral and bacterial infections remain prime candidates for causing secondary autoimmunity (see Miller's TMEV model of APC-mediated determinant spreading to autoantigens). Infectious pathogens could provide the "danger signals" (P. Matzinger) needed for propagation of extended inflammation leading to clinical disease. Nevertheless, proof of a causal relationship is exquisitely difficult (if not impossible) because traces of pathogens detected may have no relation to the underlying disease process or may be cleared from the system by the time of secondary clinical disease. In addition, disease is likely to depend on individual pathogen strains, making a very detailed immunologic profiling in prospective clinical trials necessary. It is possible that the introduction of new antiviral treatments might unmask such an association in the future. Second, a genetically susceptible background could be required to provide a fertile field for initiating a chronic inflammation involving autoantigens. This probably occurs via a multifaceted network of multiple susceptibility and protective genes, and it will be impossible to treat a respective disease just by analyzing the background genes involved. Lastly, autoreactive lymphocytes might predominantly be present in the affected organ or site and not in the peripheral blood, which makes their identification and characterization in humans rather difficult.

A note of caution should be devoted to our interpretation of specific findings obtained in individual animal models. Animal models should serve to teach us paradigms of how a disease could develop kinetically *in vivo*. The precise parameters, targeted antigens, susceptibility genes, and effector molecules may be considerably different in humans. Thus, for example, if there is an indication that insulin is a primary antigen in the NOD mouse, this may or may not have direct relevance to the human disease. Recent evidence leads us to believe that insulin, indeed, may also be a primary antigen in human autoimmune diabetes, but other antigens such as GAD might also play a role. The opportunities as well as limits of each animal model have to be delineated. Again, the NOD mouse appears to be prone to multiorgan autoimmunity [induction of EAE *(438)*, neuritis *(439)*, arthritis, and hepatitis have all been observed in NOD or NOD-congenic mouse strains] and exhibits, in addition to diabetes, thyroiditis, sialitis, and orchitis. Thus, diabetes in the NOD mouse is clearly different from typical human T1D. Therefore, treatments capable of correcting the systemic immune dysregulation that predominates in the NOD model may not directly apply to human T1D, where no such pronounced systemic dysregulation is present. Based on these considerations, it is not surprising that of the more than 140 therapeutic strategies that prevent diabetes in the NOD mouse, only a handful have made it to phase 1 human trials. Experiments with human cells or materials should be undertaken to solidify the choice of molecules or target antigens. The successful story with respect to blockade of TNFα to treat RA underlines the importance of this step. Employment of a multiplicity of models thus becomes imperative to evaluate potential candidate interventions, as does a careful proceeding, objective evaluation, and avoidance of premature conclusions. In addition to the researchers and clinicians, publishers as well as news media will have to share this responsibility. Continued research will undoubtedly provide us eventually with sufficient insight into the complexities of organ-specific autoimmunity, but patience and perseverance coupled with experimental objectivity will be required.

Recent therapeutic progress has been very good using monoclonal antibodies to dampen autoimmune processes in humans. One example is a non–Fc-binding anti-CD3 antibody, which has now delayed β cell destruction in two independent trials in recent-onset T1D *(288,440)*. Combination of this antibody with antigen-specific induction of regulatory cells might be a future important strategy based on its initial success in various mouse models (151). Other antibody-based therapies have been effective in psoriasis, Crohn's disease, RA, MS, and uveitis. Thus, the road map to ultimate therapeutic success might lie in a well-tuned combination of such therapeutics, likely in conjunction with autoantigen-specific approaches that involve the transfer or induction of regulatory cells (Tregs). Augmentation of adaptive as well as intrinsic Tregs might be, in the end, the key for achieving site-specific tolerance (involving bystander suppression of effector responses and "infectious" induction of more Tregs) and is being explored with much success in many preclinical models.

REFERENCES

1. Lacan J. The field of the other and back to the transference. In: Miller JA, ed. *The four fundamental concepts of psycho-analysis*. New York: WW Norton, 1981:203–260.
2. Tauber AI. The biological notion of self and non-self. In: Zalta EN, ed. *Stanford Encyclopedia of Philosophy*. Stanford, CA: The Metaphysics Research Lab, 2006. Available at http://plato.stanford.edu/entries/bilogy-self/#Rel.
3. Littré E, Robin CH. *Dictionnaire de médecine, de chirugie, de pharmacie et de l'art vétérinaire*, 1878.
4. Pasteur L. De l'attenuation du virus cholera des poules. *C R Acad Sci*. 1880;91:673–680.
5. von Behring E, Kitasato S. Über das Zustandekommen der Diphtherie-Immunität und der Tetanus-Immunität bei Thieren. *Dtsch Med Wochenschr*. 1890;16:1113–1114.
6. Ehrlich P, Morgenroth J. Zytotoxine als Antikorper. *Berl Klin Wochenschr*. 1901;38:251–260.
7. Römer P, Gebb H. Beiträge zur Frage der Anaphylaxie durch Linseneiweiss und Eiweiss aus andern Geweben des Auges. *Graefes Arch Ophtalmol*. 1912;81:367–402.
8. Silverstein A. *A History of Immunology*. San Diego, CA: Academic Press, 1989.
9. Portier P, Richet C. De l'action anaphylactique de certain venins. *C R Soc Biol* (Paris). 1902;54:170–172.
10. Arthus, M. Injections repetées de serum du cheval chez le lapin. *C R Soc Biol* (Paris). 1903;55:817–820.
11. Donath J, Landsteiner K. Uber paroxysmale Hamoglobinurie. *Munch Med Wochenschr*. 1904;51:1590–1601.
12. von Pirquet C, Schick B. *Die Serumkrankeit*. Leipzig: Deuticke, 1905.
13. Weil E, Braun H. Über das Wesen der luetischen Erkrankung auf Grund der neueren Forschungen. *Wien Klin Wochenschr*. 1909; 22:372.
14. Uhlenhuth P. *Festschrift zum 60. Geburtstag von Robert Koch*. Jena: Fisher, 1903.
15. Traub E. Persistence of lymphocytic choriomeningitis vieus in immune animals and its relation to immunity. *J Exp Med*. 1936;63:847–861.
16. Owen RD. Immunogenetic consequences of vascular anastomoses between bovine cattle twins. *Science*. 1945;102:400–401.
17. Medawar PB. The behaviour and fate of skin autografts and skin homografts in rabbits. *J Anat*. 1944;78:176–199.
18. Medawar PB. A second study of the behaviour and fate of skin homografts in rabbits. *J Anat*. 1945;79:157–176.
19. Medawar PB. Immunity to homologous grafted skin. I. The suppression of cell division in grafts transplanted to immunized animals. *Br J Exp Pathol*. 1946;27:9–14.
20. Medawar PB. Immunity to homologous grafted skin. II. The immunity relationship between the antigens of blood and skin. *Br J Exp Pathol*. 1946;27:15–24.
21. Burnet FM, Fenner F. *The production of antibodies*. New York: Macmillan, 1949.
22. Burnet FM. *The clonal selection theory of acquired immunity*. Cambridge: Cambridge University Press, 1957.
23. Witebsky E, Rose NR. Studies on organ specificity. V. Changes in the thyroid glands of rabbits following active immunization with rabbit thyroid extracts. *J Immunol*. 1956;76:417–427.
24. Fleck L. *Entstehung und Entwicklung einer wissenschaftlichen tatsache. Einfurung in die Lehre vom Dekstil und Denkkollektiv*. Basel: B. Schwabe, 1935.
25. Jerne NK. Towards a network theory of the immune system. *Ann Immunol*. 1974:373–389.
26. Coutinho A, Forni L, Holmberg D, et al. From an antigen-centered, clonal perspective of immune responses to an organism-centered, network perspective of autonomous activity in a self-referential immune system. *Immunol Rev*. 1984;79:151–168.
27. Grabar P. Hypothesis. Auto-antibodies and immunological theories: an analytical review. *Clin Immunol Immunopathol*. 1975;4:453–466.
28. Wigzell H. Positive autoimmunity. In: Talal N, ed. *Autoimmunity: genetic, immunologic, virologic and clinical aspects*. New York: Academic Press, 1997:693–707.
29. Schwartz M, Cohen IR. Autoimmunity can benefit self-maintenance. *Immunol Today*. 2000;21:265–268.
30. Matzinger P. Tolerance, danger, and the extended family. *Annu Rev Immunol*. 1994;12:991–1045.
31. Dembic Z. Immune system protects integrity of tissues. *Mol Immunol*. 2000;37:563–569.
32. Pradeu T, Carosella ED. Analyse critique du modèle immunologique du soi et du non-soi et de ses fondements métaphysiques implicites. *C R Biol*. 2004;327:481–492.
33. Pradeu T, Carosella ED. On the definition of a criterion of immunogenicity. *Proc Natl Acad Sci U S A*. 2006;103:17858–17861.
34. Cohn, M. A commentary on the Zinkernagel-Hengartner 'Credo 2004'. *Scand J Immunol*. 2005;62:187–194.
35. Sercarz EE, Maverakis E. Recognition and function in a degenerate immune system. *Mol Immunol*. 2004;40:1003–1008.

36. Vance RE. Cutting edge: cutting edge commentary: a Copernican revolution? Doubts about the danger theory. *J Immunol.* 2000;165:1725–1728.
37. Tada T. The immune system as a supersystem. *Annu Rev Immunol.* 1997;15:1–13.
38. Hedrick SM. The acquired immune system: a vantage from beneath. *Immunity*. 2004;21:607–615.
39. Rose NR, Mackay IR. Prelude. In: Rose NR, Mackay IR, eds. *The autoimmune diseases*. San Diego, CA: Academic Press, 1998: 1–4.
40. Schwartz R. Foreword. In: Lahita RG, Chiorazzi N, Reeves WH, eds. *Textbook of the autoimmune diseases*. Philadelphia: Lippincott Williams & Wilkins, 2000.
41. Rose NR, Bona C. Defining criteria for autoimmune disease (Witebsky's postulates revisited). *Immunol Today*. 1993;114:426–430.
42. Zinkernagel RM. Anti-infection immunity and autoimmunity. *Ann NY Acad Sci*. 2002;958:3–6.
43. Witebsky E, Rose NR, Terplan K, et al. Chronic thyroiditis and autoimmunization. *J Am Med Assoc*. 1957;164:1439–1447.
44. Alvarez F, Berg PA, Bianchi FB, et al. International Autoimmune Hepatitis Group Report: review of criteria for diagnosis of autoimmune hepatitis. *J Hepatol*. 1999;31:929–938.
45. Jacobson DL, Gange SJ, Rose NR, et al. Epidemiology and estimated population burden of selected autoimmune diseases in the United States. *Clin Immunol Immunopathol*. 1997;84:223–243.
46. Matsumoto I, Maccioni M, Lee DM, et al. How antibodies to a ubiquitous cytoplasmic enzyme may provoke joint-specific autoimmune disease. *Nat Immunol*. 2002;3:360–365.
47. Binstadt BA, Patel PR, Alencar H, et al. Particularities of the vasculature can promote the organ specificity of autoimmune attack. *Nat Immunol*. 2006;7:284–292.
48. Shoda LK, Young DL, Ramanujan S, et al. A comprehensive review of interventions in the NOD mouse and implications for translation. *Immunity*. 2005;23:115–126.
49. Anderson MS, Bluestone JA. The NOD mouse: a model of immune dysregulation. *Annu Rev Immunol*. 2005;23:447–485.
50. Chaparro RJ, Konigshofer Y, Beilhack GF, et al. Nonobese diabetic mice express aspects of both type 1 and type 2 diabetes. *Proc Natl Acad Sci U S A*. 2006;103:12475–12480.
51. Gershon RK, Kondo K. Infectious immunological tolerance. *Immunology*. 1971;21:903–914.
52. Schubert LA, Jeffery E, Zhang Y, et al. Scurfin (FOXP3) acts as a repressor of transcription and regulates T cell activation. *J Biol Chem*. 2001;276:37672–37679.
53. Ziegler SF. FOXP3: of mice and men. *Annu Rev Immunol*. 2006;24: 209–226.
54. Hori S, Nomura T, Sakaguchi S. Control of regulatory T cell development by the transcription factor Foxp3. *Science*. 2003;299:1057–1061.
55. Khattri R, Cox T, Yasayko SA, et al. An essential role for Scurfin in $CD4^+CD25^+$ T regulatory cells. *Nat Immunol*. 2003;4:337–342.
56. Fontenot JD, Gavin MA, Rudensky AY. Foxp3 programs the development and function of $CD4^+CD25^+$ regulatory T cells. *Nat Immunol*. 2003;4:330–336.
57. Fontenot JD, Rasmussen JP, Williams LM, et al. Regulatory T cell lineage specification by the forkhead transcription factor foxp3. *Immunity*. 2005;22:329–341.
58. Wan YY, Flavell RA. Identifying Foxp3-expressing suppressor T cells with a bicistronic reporter. *Proc Natl Acad Sci U S A*. 2005;102:5126–5131.
59. Haase C, Ejrnaes M Juedes, et al. Immunomodulatory dendritic cells require autologous serum to circumvent nonspecific immunosuppressive activity *in vivo*. *Blood*. 2005;106:4225–4233.
60. Roncarolo MG, Gregori S, Battaglia M, et al. Interleukin-10-secreting type 1 regulatory T cells in rodents and humans. *Immunol Rev*. 2006;212:28–50.
61. Li MO, Wan YY, Sanjabi S, et al. Transforming growth factor-beta regulation of immune responses. *Annu Rev Immunol*. 2006;24:99–146.
62. Shevach EM. Regulatory T cells in autoimmmunity. *Annu Rev Immunol*. 2000;18:423–449.
63. Shevach EM. $CD4^+$ $CD25^+$ suppressor T cells: more questions than answers. *Nat Rev Immunol*. 2002;2:389–400.
64. Ashton-Rickardt PG, Bandeira A, Delaney J, et al. Evidence for a differential avidity model of T-cell selection in the thymus. *Cell*. 1994;76:651–663.
65. Hoffmann MW, Heath WR, Ruschmeyer D, et al. Deletion of high-avidity T cells by thymic epithelium. *Proc Natl Acad Sci U S A*. 1995; 92:9851–9855.
66. Jameson SC, Bevan MJ. T-cell selection. *Curr Opin Immunol*. 1998; 10:214–219.
67. Sebzda E, Mariathasan S, Ohteki T, et al. Selection of the T cell repertoire. *Annu Rev Immunol*. 1999;17:829–874.
68. Kishimoto H, Sprent J. The thymus and negative selection. *Immunol Res*. 2000;21:315–323.
69. Nikolic-Zugic J, Bevan MJ. Role of self-peptides in positively selecting the T-cell repertoire. *Nature*. 1990;344:65–67.
70. Surh CD, Lee DS, Fung-Leung WP, et al. Thymic selection by a single MHC/peptide ligand produces a semidiverse repertoire of $CD4^+$ T cells. *Immunity*. 1997;7:209–219.
71. Steinman L. A few autoreactive cells in an autoimmune infiltrate control a vast population of nonspecific cells: A tale of smart bombs and the infantry. *Proc Natl Acad Sci U S A*. 1996;93:2253–2256.
72. van den Elzen P, Menezes JS, Ametani A, et al. Limited clonality in autoimmunity: drivers and regulators. *Autoimmun Rev*. 2004;3:524–529.
73. Han B, Serra P, Amrani,A, et al. Prevention of diabetes by manipulation of anti-IGRP autoimmunity: high efficiency of a low-affinity peptide. *Nat Med*. 2005;11:645–652.
74. Allison JP. CD28-B7 interactions in T-cell activation. *Curr Opin Immunol*. 1994;6:414–419.
75. Harding FA, Allison JP. CD28-B7 interactions allow the induction of $CD8^+$ cytotoxic T-lymphocytes in the absence of exogenous help. *J Exp Med*. 1993;177:1791–1796.
76. Schwartz RH. A cell culture model for T lymphocyte clonal anergy. *Science*. 1990;248:1349–1356.
77. Lenardo M, Chan KM, Hornung F, et al. Mature T lymphocyte apoptosis—immune regulation in a dynamic and unpredictable antigenic environment. *Annu Rev Immunol*. 1999;17:221–253.
78. Abbas AK. Die and let live: eliminating dangerous lymphocytes. *Cell*. 1996;84:655–657.
79. Van Parijs L, Abbas AK. Homeostasis and self-tolerance in the immune system: turning lymphocytes off. *Science*. 1998;280:243–248.
80. Chambers CA, Kuhns MS, Egen JG, et al. CTLA-4-mediated inhibition in regulation of T cell responses: mechanisms and manipulation in tumor immunotherapy. *Annu Rev Immunol*. 2001;19:565–594.
81. Salomon B, Bluestone JA. Complexities of CD28/B7: CTLA-4 costimulatory pathways in autoimmunity and transplantation. *Annu Rev Immunol*. 2001;19:225–252.
82. Weiner HL, Friedman A, Miller A, et al. Oral tolerance: immunologic mechanisms and treatment of animal and human organ-specific autoimmune diseases by oral administration of autoantigens. *Annu Rev Immunol*. 1994;12:809–837.
83. Seewaldt S, Thomas HE, Ejrnaes M, et al. Virus-induced autoimmune diabetes: most beta-cells die through inflammatory cytokines and not perforin from autoreactive (anti-viral) cytotoxic T-lymphocytes. *Diabetes*. 2000;49:1801–1809.
84. Bettelli E, Carrier Y, Gao W, et al. Reciprocal developmental pathways for the generation of pathogenic effector TH17 and regulatory T cells. *Nature*. 2006;441:235–238.
85. Marth T, Strober W, Seder RA, et al. Regulation of transforming growth factor-beta production by interleukin-12. *Eur J Immunol*. 1997;27:1213–1220.
86. Seder RA, Marth T, Sieve MC, et al. Factors involved in the differentiation of TGF-β-producing cells from naive $CD4^+$ T cells: IL-4 and IFN-γ have opposing effects, while TGF-β positively regulates its own production. *J Immunol*. 1998;160:5719–5728.
87. King C, Davies J, Mueller R, et al. TGF-b1 alters APC preference, polarizing islet antigen responses toward a Th2 phenotype. *Immunity*. 1998;8:601–613.
88. Rizzo LV, Morawetz RA, Miller-Rivero NE, et al. IL-4 and IL-10 are both required for the induction of oral tolerance. *J Immunol*. 1999;162:2613–2622.

89. Homann D, Holz A, Bot A, et al. Autoreactive CD4+ lymphocytes protect from autoimmune diabetes via bystander suppression using the IL-4/STAT6 pathway. *Immunity*. 1999;11:463–472.
90. King C, Hoenger RM, Cleary MM, et al. Interleukin-4 acts at the locus of the antigen-presenting dendritic cell to counter-regulate cytotoxic CD8+ T-cell responses. *Nat Med.* 2001;7:206–214.
91. Zhang ZY, Lee CS, Lider O, et al. Suppression of adjuvant arthritis in Lewis rats by oral administration of type II collagen. *J Immunol.* 1990;145:2489–2493.
92. Maron R, Blogg NS, Polanski M, et al. Oral tolerance to insulin and the insulin B-chain: cell lines and cytokine patterns. *Ann NY Acad Sci*. 1996;778:357.
93. Hancock WW, Polanski M, Zhang J, et al. Suppression of insulitis in non-obese diabetic (NOD) mice by oral insulin administration is associated with selective expression of interleukin-4 and -10, transforming growth factor-beta, and prostaglandin-E. *Am J Pathol.* 1995;147:1193–1199.
94. Bergerot I, Arreaza GA, Cameron MJ, et al. Insulin B-chain reactive CD4+ regulatory T-cells induced by oral insulin treatment protect from type 1 diabetes by blocking the cytokine secretion and pancreatic infiltration of diabetogenic effector T-cells. *Diabetes*. 1999;48:1720–1729.
95. Charlton B, Lafferty KJ. The Th1/Th2 balance in autoimmunity. *Curr Opin Immunol.* 1995;7:793–798.
96. Paul WE. Interleukin-4: a prototypic immunoregulatory lymphokine. *Blood.* 1991;77:1859–1870.
97. Lepault F, Gagnerault MC. Characterization of peripheral regulatory CD4+ T cells that prevent diabetes onset in nonobese diabetic mice. *J Immunol.* 2000;164:240–247.
98. Sercarz EE. Processing creates the self. *Nat Immunol.* 2002;3:110–112.
99. Anderton SM, Viner NJ, Matharu P, et al. Influence of a dominant cryptic epitope on autoimmune T cell tolerance. *Nat Immunol.* 2002;3:175–181.
100. Moudgil KD, Sekiguchi D, Kim SY, et al. Immunodominance is independent of structural constraints: each region within hen eggwhite lysozyme is potentially available upon processing of native antigen. *J Immunol.* 1997;159:2574–2579.
101. Bhardwaj V, Kumar V, Geysen HM, et al. Degenerate recognition of a dissimilar antigenic peptide by myelin basic protein-reactive T cells. *J Immunol.* 1993;151:5000–5010.
102. Zehn D, Bevan MJ. T cells with low avidity for a tissue-restricted antigen routinely evade central and peripheral tolerance and cause autoimmunity. *Immunity*. 2006;25:261–270.
103. Ashton-Rickardt PG, Bandeira A, Delaney JR, et al. Evidence for a differential avidity model of T cell selection in the thymus. *Cell.* 1994;76:651–663.
104. Moudgil KD, Sercarz EE. Understanding crypticity is the key to revealing the pathogenesis of autoimmunity. *Trends Immunol.* 2005;26:355–359.
105. Carbone FR, Kurts C, Bennett SRM, et al. Cross-presentation: a general mechanism for CTL immunity and tolerance. *Immunol Today*. 1998;19:368–373.
106. van Stipdonk MJ, Lemmens EE, Schoenberger SP. Naive CTLs require a single brief period of antigenic stimulation for clonal expansion and differentiation. *Nat Immunol.* 2001;2:423–429.
107. Blattman JN, Sourdive DJ, Murali-Krishna K, et al. Evolution of the T cell repertoire during primary, memory, and recall responses to viral infection. *J Immunol.* 2000;165:6081–6090.
108. Heath WR, Kurts C, Miller JFAP, et al. Cross-tolerance: a pathway for inducing tolerance to peripheral tissue antigens. *J Exp Med.* 1998;187:1549–1553.
109. Savinov AY, Wong FS, Stonebraker AC, et al. Presentation of antigen by endothelial cells and chemoattraction are required for homing of insulin-specific CD8+ T cells. *J Exp Med.* 2003;197:643–656.
110. Taurog JD, Maika SD, Satumtira N, et al.. 1999. Inflammatory disease in HLA-B27 transgenic rats. *Immunol Rev.* 169:209–223.
111. Schwimmbeck P, Yu DT, Oldstone MBA. Autoantibodies to HLA-B27 in sera of patients with ankylosing spondylitis and Reiter's syndrome. *J Exp Med.* 1987;166:173–181.
112. McDevitt HO. The role of MHC class II molecules in susceptibility and resistance to autoimmunity. *Curr Opin Immunol.* 1998;10:677–681.
113. Sonderstrup G, McDevitt HO. DR, DQ, and you: MHC alleles and autoimmunity. *J Clin Invest*. 2001;107:795–796.
114. Molberg O, Kett K, Scott H, et al. Gliadin specific, HLA DQ2-restricted T cells are commonly found in small intestine biopsies from coeliac disease patients, but not from controls. *Scand J Immunol*. 1997;46:103–108.
115. von Herrath MG, Wolfe T, Möhrle U, et al. Protection from type 1 diabetes in the face of high levels of activated autoaggressive lymphocytes in a viral transgenic mouse model crossed to the SV129 strain. *Diabetes.* 2001;50(12):2700–2708.
116. de Bakker PI, McVean G, Sabeti PC, et al. A high-resolution HLA and SNP haplotype map for disease association studies in the extended human MHC. *Nat Genet*. 2006;38:1166–1172.
117. Vijayakrishnan L, Slavik JM, Illes Z, et al. An autoimmune disease-associated CTLA-4 splice variant lacking the B7 binding domain signals negatively in T cells. *Immunity*. 2004;20:563–575.
118. Bach J-F. Organ-specific autoimmunity. *Immunol Today*. 1995; 16:353–355.
119. Bach J-F. Insulin dependent diabetes mellitus as an autoimmune disease. *Endocrine Rev*. 1994;15:516–542.
120. Bach J-F. Predictive medicine in autoimmune diseases: from the identification of genetic predisposition and environmental influence to precocious immunotherapy. *Clin Immunol Immunopathol.* 1994;72:156–161.
121. Todd JA. The role of MHC class II genes in susceptibility to insulin-dependent diabetes mellitus. *Curr Top Microbiol Immunol.* 1990;164:17–40.
122. Vyse TJ, Todd JA. Genetic analysis of autoimmune disease. *Cell.* 1996;85:311–318.
123. Redondo MJ, Rewers M, Yu L, et al. Genetic determination of islet cell autoimmunity in monozygotic twin, dizygotic twin, and non-twin siblings of patients with type 1 diabetes: prospective twin study. *BMJ*. 1999;318:698–702.
124. Aly TA, Ide A, Jahromi MM, et al. Extreme genetic risk for type 1A diabetes. *Proc Natl Acad Sci U S A*. 2006103:14074–14079.
125. Sevilla N, Homann D, von Herrath MG, et al. Virus-induced diabetes in a transgenic model: role of cross-reacting viruses and quantitation of effector T cells needed to cause disease. *J Virol.* 2000;74:3284–3292.
126. Raine T, Zaccone P, Mastroeni P, et al. *Salmonella typhimurium* infection in nonobese diabetic mice generates immunomodulatory dendritic cells able to prevent type 1 diabetes. *J Immunol.* 2006;177:2224–2233.
127. Christen U, Benke D, Wolfe T, et al. Cure of prediabetic mice by viral infections involves lymphocyte recruitment along an IP-10 gradient. *J Clin Invest*. 2004;113:74–84.
128. Zhao ZS, Granucci F, Yeh L, et al. Molecular mimicry by herpes simplex virus-type 1: autoimmune disease after viral infection. *Science*. 1998;279:1344–1347.
129. Oldstone MBA. Molecular mimicry and autoimmune disease. *Cell.* 1987;50:819–820.
130. Horwitz MS, Bradley LM, Harbertson J, et al. Diabetes induced by coxsackie virus: Initiation by bystander damage and not molecular mimicry. *Nat Med*. 1998;4:781–785.
131. Olson JK, Girvin AM, Miller SD. Direct activation of innate and antigen-presenting functions of microglia following infection with Theiler's virus. *J Virol*. 2001;75:9780–9789.
132. Miller SD, Vanderlugt CL, Begolka WS, et al. Persistent infection with Theiler's virus leads to CNS autoimmunity via epitope spreading. *Nat Med*. 1997;3:1133–1136.
133. Katz-Levy Y, Neville KL, Girvin AM, et al. Endogenous presentation of self myelin epitopes by CNS-resident APCs in Theiler's virus-infected mice. *J Clin Invest*. 1999;104:599–610.
134. Oldstone MB. Prevention of type I diabetes in nonobese diabetic mice by virus infection. *Science*. 1988;239:500–502.
135. Blumberg RS, Saubermann LJ, Strober W. Animal models of mucosal inflammation and their relation to human inflammatory bowel disease. *Curr Opin Immunol.* 1999;11:648–656.
136. Kelsall BL, Strober W. Dendritic cells of the gastrointestinal tract. *Springer Semin Immunopathol*. 1997;18:409–420.
137. La Cava A, Sarvetnick N. The role of cytokines in autoimmunity. *Curr Dir Autoimmun*. 1999;1:56–71.

138. von Andrian UH, Mackay CR. T-cell function and migration. Two sides of the same coin. *N Engl J Med*. 2000;343:1020–1034.
139. Godessart N, Kunkel SL. Chemokines in autoimmune disease. *Curr Opin Immunol*. 2001;13:670–675.
140. O'Shea JJ, Ma A, Lipsky P. Cytokines and autoimmunity. *Nat Rev Immunol*. 2002;2:37–45.
141. Kim S, Kim KA, Hwang DY, et al. Inhibition of autoimmune diabetes by Fas ligand: the paradox is solved. *J Immunol*. 2000;164:2931–2936.
142. Hugues S, Mougneau E, Ferlin W, et al. Tolerance to islet antigens and prevention from diabetes induced by limited apoptosis of pancreatic beta cells. *Immunity*. 2002;16:169–181.
143. Gallucci S, Lolkema M, Matzinger P. Natural adjuvants: endogenous activators of dendritic cells. *Nat Med*. 1999;5:1249–1255.
144. Delovitch TL, Singh B. The nonobese diabetic mouse as a model of autoimmune diabetes: immune dysregulation gets the NOD. *Immunity*. 1997;7:727–738.
145. Christen U, Wolfe T, Mohrle,U, et al. A dual role for TNF-alpha in type 1 diabetes: islet-specific expression abrogates the ongoing autoimmune process when induced late but not early during pathogenesis. *J Immunol*. 2001;166:7023–7032.
146. Maini RN, Elliott M, Brennan FM, et al. TNF blockade in rheumatoid arthritis: implications for therapy and pathogenesis. *APMIS*. 1997;105:257–263.
147. Feldmann M, Brennan FM, Maini RN. Rheumatoid arthritis. *Cell*. 1996;85:307–310.
148. Tisch R, McDevitt H. Antigen specific immunotherapy: Is it a real possibility to combat T-cell medicated autoimmunity? *Proc Natl Acad Sci U S A*. 1994;91:437–438.
149. Tisch R, Wang B, Weaver DJ, et al. Antigen-specific mediated suppression of beta cell autoimmunity by plasmid DNA vaccination. *J Immunol*. 2001;166:2122–2132.
150. Shevach EM, McHugh RS, Piccirillo CA, et al. Control of T-cell activation by CD4$^+$ CD25$^+$ suppressor T cells. *Immunol Rev*. 2001;182:58–67.
151. Bresson D, Togher L, Rodrigo E, et al. Anti-CD3 and nasal proinsulin combination therapy enhances remission from recent-onset autoimmune diabetes by inducing Tregs. *J Clin Invest*. 2006;116:1371–1381.
152. Sicotte NL, Voskuhl RR. Onset of multiple sclerosis associated with anti-TNF therapy. *Neurology*. 2001;57:1885–1888.
153. Riminton DS, Korner H, Strickland DH, et al. Challenging cytokine redundance: Inflammatory cell movement and clinical course of experimental autoimmune encephalomyelitis are normal in lymphotoxin-deficient, but not tumor necrosis factor-deficient, mice. *J Exp Med*. 1998;187:1517–1528.
154. Sedgwick JD, Riminton DS, Cyster JG, et al. Tumor necrosis factor: a master-regulator of leukocyte movement. *Immunol Today*. 2000;21:110–113.
155. Coon B, An L-L, Whitton JL, et al. DNA immunization to prevent autoimmune diabetes. *J Clin Invest*. 1999;104:189–194.
156. Tang Q, Henriksen KJ, Bi M, et al. *In vitro*-expanded antigen-specific regulatory T cells suppress autoimmune diabetes. *J Exp Med*. 2004;199:1455–1465.

Chapter 43

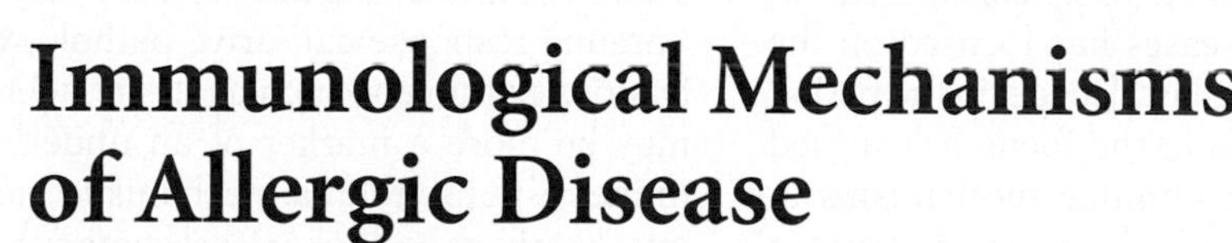

Immunological Mechanisms of Allergic Disease

Marsha Wills-Karp

INTRODUCTION

This chapter will provide an overview of our current understanding of diseases gathered under the rubric of "allergy." These diverse diseases (anaphylaxis, asthma, allergic rhinitis, atopic dermatitis, food allergy) are united at least superficially by the facts that: (a) these conditions all result from the expression of harmful immune responses; (b) the implicated immune responses are all associated with the generation of immunoglobin E (IgE) (whether or not IgE is integral to pathogenesis); and (c) the antigens that driveg such immune responses are not derived from infectious pathogens. The basic cellular and molecular mechanisms that underlie the pathogenesis of allergic disorders, as well as the environmental and genetic substrates for their generation, will be closely considered. Although the study of allergic diseases has focused on the adaptive immune response in the last decade, in the period since the last edition of this book, the focus has shifted to dissecting the role of innate immune mechanisms in regulating susceptibility to the development of aberrant immune responses in allergic diseases. Thus this edition will reflect this change in perspective when possible. Although much of our current understanding of mechanism in allergic disease has derived from the study of animal models, mechanistic data on human disease will be discussed wherever possible. The chapter finishes with a brief survey of the clinical and therapeutic characteristics of the major human allergic disorders. Readers are referred to clinically oriented texts for a fuller discussion of such issues.

Historical Perspective

The term *allergy* was coined in 1906 by the astute pediatrician Clemens von Pirquet, who argued that antigenic stimuli led to two distinct categories or patterns of response: immunity and allergy *(1)*. The former, an old concept, referred to those responses that lead to protection from infectious challenge. The latter, a novel theoretical construct, referred to "altered reactivity" that itself led to host damage. This idea of allergy, that is, the notion that the immune response can itself be a cause of disease, was a powerful conceptual advance that led to novel insights into the pathogenesis of a variety of diseases. Quite naturally, this concept of allergy initially included autoimmune diseases in addition to those conditions that are classified as allergic diseases today. As has been noted, current usage largely restricts allergy to diseases caused by the subset of harmful immune responses (to pathogen-unrelated antigens) that is associated with the generation of IgE. There is some artificiality to this. Very similar patterns of immune response can drive pathology in response to infectious pathogens such as tissue helminths. Further, IgE may be more a marker of an underlying pattern of immune response than a mechanistic participant in the immunopathogenesis of at least some subtypes of allergic disease. As long as these caveats are kept in mind, however, this concept of allergic disease, long enshrined by clinical subspecialists, has considerable theoretical and practical utility.

The trail leading to the specific identification of IgE began with demonstration by Prausnitz and Kuster in 1921 that hypersensitivity to an antigen could be passively transferred in serum from one individual to another *(2)*. The instigating antigens (allergens, in contemporary parlance) were known as atopens, and the mysterious plasma factor that conferred sensitivity was called atopic reagin. It was not until 1966 that Teruko and Kimishige Ishizaka demonstrated that reaginic activity was carried by a novel class of immunglobulin, IgE (3,4,5). The word *atopy* has since come to denote the propensity for developing allergic reactions to common environmental antigens (allergens), a propensity defined operationally by elevations in serum levels of IgE reactive with, or by skin test reactivity to, such antigens. Definitions of other key terms are given in Table 43.1.

Before proceeding to a direct focus on allergic diseases, it is useful to consider the classification scheme for harmful immune responses, or hypersensitivity reactions, initially outlined by Coombs and Gell *(6)*. This widely used formulation, modified by Janeway and Travers *(7)*

TABLE 43.1 Definitions of Key Terms

Allergen	An environmental antigen that typically elicits allergic responses in susceptible individuals. These antigens ordinarily have little or no intrinsic toxicity.
Allergy	Clinically adverse reactions to environmental antigens reflecting acquired immune responses that are marked phenotypically by the presence of allergen-specific IgE, along with mast-cell and eosinophil recruitment and/or activation. $CD4^+$ T cells that produce a Th2 profile of cytokines (IL-4, IL-5, and IL-13) are thought to be central to the development of allergic responses.
Atopy	The propensity for developing immediate hypersensitivity reactions to common environmental allergens, defined operationally by elevations in serum levels of IgE reactive with allergens or by skin-test reactivity to allergens.
Allergic diseases	The group of clinical disorders (such as allergic asthma, allergic rhinitis [hay fever], and atopic dermatitis) in which IgE-associated immune responses, typically directed against otherwise innocuous environmental allergens, are thought to have a pathogenic role.

and Kay *(8)*, systematizes the major mechanisms initiating injurious processes that are mediated by the adaptive (as opposed to the innate) immune system (Table 43.2). The scheme delineates four classes of hypersensitivity: (a) type I, or immediate hypersensitivity, in which allergens interact with specific IgE (and/or IgG1 in the mouse) on the surface of mast cells or basophils, leading to the release of a variety of pharmacoactive inflammatory mediators; (b) type II hypersensitivity, or cytotoxic reactions, in which antibodies react with cell surface–associated antigens or receptors, leading to tissue injury and/or altered receptor function; (c) type III hypersensitivity, or immune complex reactions, in which damage is mediated by immune complexes generated by antibody in the presence of antigen excess; and (d) type IV, or delayed-type hypersensitivity, in which harmful T-cell–driven inflammatory processes proceed without any necessary role for antibodies.

In light of this classification scheme, beloved of generations of immunologists and medical students alike, allergic reactions seem to fall squarely into the category of type I hypersensitivity responses. Enhanced mechanistic understanding of allergic processes has inevitably complicated matters, however. Most allergic responses are multiphasic, combining elements of diverse hypersensitivity types into one "allergic cascade." For example, the initial phase of the clinical asthmatic response to an aeroallergen is often due to immediate (type I) hypersensitivity. However, this is frequently followed by late-phase responses that are more characteristic of delayed-type (type IV) hypersensitivity reactions.

General Features of Atopic Disorders

Allergic disorders are categorized by the anatomic site where disease is manifested: atopic dermatitis (skin), atopic rhinitis (nasal passages), atopic asthma (lung), food allergy (gut), and anaphylaxis (systemic) (Table 43.3). These clinical entities all involve a similar allergic effector cascade, at least superficially, with differences in presentation likely reflecting variation in the physiochemical characteristics of the allergen, the site of initial sensitization to the allergen, the route and dose of allergen exposure, and the programmed response of resident cells (e.g., epithelial cells), to injury and inflammation. Anaphylaxis aside, there is often a stereotypical sequence in the development of allergic manifestations of disease in patients with atopy, with early expression of food sensitivities or atopic dermatitis and the subsequent development of either atopic rhinitis or asthma. Many individuals will have all three of the latter clinical entities, which form the "atopic triad."

Atopic disorders represent a major health problem worldwide, affecting 5% to 30% of the population. The incidence of atopic diseases, including asthma, atopic rhinitis, and atopic dermatitis, has increased dramatically in recent years in Westernized countries *(9–11)*. In such countries, 30% of the population manifests some form of atopic disease at some time in their lives. Interestingly, the low baseline level of atopic diseases in developing countries has not changed over the same time period, suggesting that factors associated with the Westernized lifestyle predispose to atopic disease. The widespread prevalence and morbidity of atopic diseases imposes a heavy burden on society.

The defining feature of atopy is the production of IgE in response to exposure (via muocosa or the skin) to a variety of ubiquitous, and otherwise innocuous, antigens. Such IgE production is a tightly regulated process, part of a complex network of cellular and molecular events necessary for the development of the allergic response. Initiation of this response appears to occur when allergen is taken up in the mucosae by antigen presenting cells which then traffick to the draining lymph nodes where they present allergens to $CD4^+$ T cells (a process referred to as sensitization). In atopic individuals, responding allergen-specific T cells polarize to a Th2 pattern of production, with the elaboration of cytokines such as IL-4, IL-13, IL-5, and IL-9 (vide infra). Although T cells from nonatopic individuals clearly recognize these same environmental antigens, the expansion and differentiation of such T cells does not involve Th2 deviation. Instead, it is thought that nonatopic individuals develop "tolerance" to these innocuous environmental antigens. The mechanisms controlling allergen-associated Th2 polarization in atopic individuals or tolerance in non-affected individuals are not completely understood. It appears likely that genetic and environmental factors affecting the antigen-presenting process play a key role.

The elaboration of Th2 cytokines sets into motion a complex series of events leading to IgE production; the development, recruitment, and activation of effector cells such as mast cells, basophils, eosinophils, and effector T cells; and a variety of downstream effector cascades. Once an atopic individual is sensitized, the manifestations of allergy are readily induced upon re-exposure to the allergen (the elicitation phase). Although the effector phases of IgE-associated atopic disorders generally appear as a continuum, it is useful to define three temporal patterns: (a) acute reactions (developing within seconds to minutes of allergen exposure); (b) delayed or late reactions (developing hours after allergen exposure); and (c) chronic reactions (developing over days to years). Acute reactions result from crosslinking of high-affinity FcεR (FcεRI) on the surface of mast cells/basophils, induced by the interaction of allergen with cell-bound IgE. Such crosslinking results in the release of vasoactive mediators, chemotactic factors, and cytokines that initiate the so-called allergic cascade. This early reaction may resolve within minutes,

TABLE 43.2 Modified Coombs/Gell Classification of the Four Major Types of Initiating Mechanisms of Immunologically-Mediated Adverse (i.e., "Hypersensitivity") Reactions

Immunologic Specificity	*Type 1: IgE Antibody (+ IgG_1 in Mouse)*	*Type II: IgG Antibody*		*Type III: IgG Antibody*	*Type IV: T Cells*		
		a	*b*		*a1* *Th1 Cel.*	*a2* *Th2 Cell*	B Cytolytic *T Cells*
Antigen	Soluble antigen "allergen"	Cell- or matrix-associated antigen	Cell surface receptors	Soluble antigen	Soluble antigen	Soluble antigen	Cell-associated antigen
Effector mechanism	$Fc\epsilon RI$ or $Fc\gamma RIII$-dependent mast cell/basophil activation, with release of mediators/cytokines	Complement, $Fc\gamma R^+$ professional phagocytes, NK cells	Antibody alters signaling	$Fc\gamma R^+$ cells, complement	Th1-associated effectors (e.g., macrophages)	Th2-associated effectors (e.g., eosinophils, basophils)	Direct cytotoxicity
Initial consequences	Rapidly developing (seconds to minutes) effects of mediators on target cells (usually not involving direct cytotoxicity)	Cell death and/or tissue injury	Pathology due to increased or diminished receptor-dependent cell function	Inflammation associated with recruitment and activation of neutrophils and other leukocytes	Chronic inflammation Reactions develop slowly (hours to days) and can persist for long periods	Chronic inflammation	Death of target cells
Examples and notes	IgE- (or, in mouse, IgG_1-) dependent anaphylaxis (potentially fatal systemic reaction) or passive cutaneous anaphylaxis (a local reaction)	Certain drug reactions and reactions to incompatible blood transfusions	Graves disease (thyroid-stimulating agonist antibody); myasthenia gravis (antagonist antibody to acetylcholine receptor)	(Including mast cells in the mouse); Arthus reaction and other "immune complex-" mediated reactions	Contact dermatitis, tuberculin reaction	Chronic allergic inflammation (type I reactions may also contribute to chronic allergic inflammation)	Reactions to certain viral infected cells, certain forms of graft rejection

Source: Reprinted from Galli and Lantz, IN: W. Paul, ed. *Fundamental Immunology.* 4th ed. Philadelphia: Lippincott-Raven Press; 1999.

TABLE 43.3 Major Features of Allergic Immune Responses

1. Responses are elicited by certain groups of environmental allergens such as foods, drugs, and proteins derived from pollens, insects (house dust mite), and animal dander.
2. In susceptible individuals, allergens are presented to naïve T cells by dendritic cells residing in the mucosa of the skin, gastrointestinal tract, or respiratory tract. For reasons that are not well understood, T cells of atopic individuals undergo differentiation to a Th2 cytokine-producing pattern.
3. Elaboration of Th2 cytokines (IL-4, IL-5, IL-3, IL-9) initiates the allergic cascade via their combined ability to regulate IgE production, FcεRI expression, mast-cell phenotype, and development, recruitment, and activation of eosinophils.
4. Under the control of Th2 cell–derived signals (IL-4, IL-13, and CD40L), B cells undergo class switching to production of the IgE subclass.
5. Upon re-exposure to the offending allergen, acute responses occurring within minutes of allergen exposure, resulting from release of preformed mediators (histamine, tryptase) from FcεRI-bearing cells via the crosslinking of allergen and IgE on their surface. Cells activated during the acute phase also release cytokines and mediators that perpetuate the Th2-driven response.
6. Late-phase responses are due to the combined effects of inflammatory cells (eosinophils and T cells) recruited to the tissues within 6 to 24 hours after the initial allergen exposure
7. Repeated allergen exposures in the context of an already-inflamed tissue results in structural changes (remodeling) such as smooth muscle thickening, tissue fibrosis, and mucus cell hyperplasia.

but it is often followed by late-phase responses that begin 3 to 6 hours after antigen challenge and may persist for days in the absence of therapy. The pathophysiologic consequences of chronic reactions are associated with the migration of eosinophils and lymphocytes from the blood into affected tissues.

ALLERGENS

Definition and General Characteristics of Allergens

Allergens are, by definition, antigens that can elicit specific IgE responses in genetically susceptible individuals. The list of structures that have been identified as allergens represents a tiny subset of the antigenic universe to which humans are routinely exposed to. Allergens are generally subdivided by route of exposure and source. Such allergens include aeroallergens (pollens, mold spores, animal dander, fecal material excreted by mites and cockroaches), food allergens, stinging insects, pharmaceuticals, and latex.

Allergen Classification

Purified allergens are named in accordance with guidelines published in 1994 by the World Health Organization International Union of Immunologic Societies Allergen Nomenclature Sub-Committee, based on their source and the order in which they were discovered *(12)*. The names incorporate the first three letters of the genus and the first letter of the species from which the allergen is derived, plus an Arabic numeral that is used to denote structurally homologous allergens from the same species. For example, the two major species of dust mite (*Dermatophagoides pteronyssinus* and *Dermatophagoides farinae*) are designated as *Der p* (*Der p 1*, *Der p 2*), and *Der f* (*Der f 1*, *Der f 2*). Other major allergens include *Fel d 1* from the cat, *Bet v 1* from birch pollen, *Amb a 1* from ragweed pollen, *Phl p 1* from the pollen of timothy grass, and *Bla g 2* from cockroach.

Biologic Properties of Allergens

The major allergens are a diverse group of proteins in which no one biologic property appears to be dominant. However, recent studies suggest that allergens may be proteins that activate the innate immune response, either through their intrinsic enzymatic activity or through activation of pattern-recognition receptors (PRRs) on mucosal epithelial cells or antigen-presenting cells (APCs) directly. Allergens from diverse sources have enzymatic activity that may bias the immune response toward a Th2 phenotype. For example, the cysteine protease of dust mite, *Der p 1*, the aspartic protease of cockroach, *Bla g 2*, the serine protease of *Aspergillus fumigatus*, and the bacterial subtilisins are all major allergenic molecules associated with the development of atopy and asthma. It is thought that these proteases induce Th2-driven inflammatory responses in the airways by disrupting the epithelial cell junctions so that these, and other molecules, gain access to, and alter the function of, underlying cells of the innate immune system (dendritic cells, mast cells, basophils, and macrophages) and B and T cells. In support of this hypothesis, *Der p 1* has been shown to activate the innate immune response via cleavage of complement components into their active components at the mucosal surface *(13)*. Moreover, through its ability to disrupt epithelial architecture, *Der p 1* may also facilitate its own passage across the (mucosal surface) epithelium, thus enhancing its own access to immune cells. Yet another potential mechanism by which proteolytic allergens such as *Der p 1* may alter the immune response is by cleaving CD25, the 55-kDa α subunit of IL-2R *(14*,15). As a result of cleavage of CD25, peripheral blood T cells show markedly diminished proliferation and IFN-γ secretion in response to potent stimulation by anti-CD3 mAb. These findings suggest that *Der p 1* decreases the growth and expansion of antigen-specific Th1 cells, augmenting expansion of the antigen-specific Th2 cells that favor a proallergic response. *Der p 1* may also contribute to the allergic phenotype by cleaving CD23 on murine B cells that would normally serve to inhibit IgE synthesis, thereby disrupting an important negative regulator of IgE production *(16)*. Along these lines, a recent comparison of various allergenic astigmatid mite extracts showed that all mites contain some type of enzymatic activity (phosphatase, esterase, aminopeptidase, glycosidase activity) (17). Cockroach allergens have been shown to contain serine proteases that lead to metalloproteinase (MMP) induction and proinflammatory cytokine production in the airway epithelium (18). Moreover, the potent peanut allergen *Ara h 2* is homologous to and functions as a trypsin inhibitor *(19)*. Other allergens, such as ragweed pollen, have been shown to contain intrinsic NADPH oxidases. Recently, birch pollen has been shown to contain phytoprostanes that are similar in structure to PGE_2 (20). Pollen-derived NADPH oxidases have been shown to rapidly increase the levels of reactive oxygen species (ROS) in lung epithelium as well as the amount of oxidized glutathione (GSSG) and 4-hydroxynonenal (4-HNE) in airway-lining fluid. These oxidases, as well as products of oxidative stress (such as GSSG and 4-HNE) generated by these enzymes, are thought to play a pivotal role in the development of lung inflammation (21).

Alternatively, it has recently been recognized, with the discovery of PRRs, that allergens and their soluble components may contain pathogen-associated molecular patterns (PAMPs) that actively interact with innate recognition systems present in the mucosal layer of various tissues. Specifically, it has long been appreciated that allergens contain substances such as endotoxin, chitin, or β-glycans, which are recognized by pattern-recognition receptors (TLR4, TLR2, dectin-1, mannose receptor) on cells lining mucosal surfaces such as the epithelium or on underlying dendritic cells. Activation of these PRRs both directly and indirectly provides signals required for productive interactions between dendritic cells (DCs) and T cells at mucosal surfaces. The ability to provide these danger signals to DCs likely underlies the unique ability of allergens to initiate allergic responses. Nonetheless, although many of these allergens can potentially create a microenvironment conducive to Th2 cell differentiation and expansion, normal individuals do not mount Th2 responses when exposed to these allergens, which suggests that despite the nature of these antigens, other factors are necessary for the development of allergic outcomes in susceptible individuals.

Specific Allergens

Aeroallergens

Aeroallergens are airborne proteins or glycoproteins derived from a variety of different sources, including pollinating trees and grasses, mold spores, animal dander (cat, dog, and rodent), and particulates secreted by dust mites and cockroaches. Factors that affect the growth or accumulation of these latter organisms (high humidity, well-insulated homes, fitted carpets) increase the levels of these allergens in the indoor environment. Exposure to such indoor allergens is also dependent on a variety of geographic, climatic, and socioeconomic factors. Interestingly, whereas indoor allergens are more closely associated with development of asthma, outdoor allergens (e.g., ragweed pollen) appear to be more important to the development of allergic rhinitis. The mechanisms underlying such associations remain obscure. Speculation has focused on the physiochemical nature (size, chemical structure) and pattern of exposure (acute versus chronic).

Food Allergens

Although hundreds of different foods are ingested, only a small number account for the vast majority of food allergy. The most common foods responsible for childhood food allergy are milk, egg, peanut, soy, and wheat. Responses to food allergens are relatively common in children <2 years old, but usually disappear as the child matures. In contrast, in adult food allergy, the most common offending foods are peanuts, tree nuts, fish, and shellfish. Most food allergens have been found to be water-soluble glycoproteins ranging in size from 10 to 40 kDa that are heat- and acid-stable and and resistant to proteolytic degradation. Exceptions to this are fruit and vegetable allergens. Reactions to food allergens can be fatal, with one of the most severe food reactions occurring in response to peanut allergens.

Latex Allergens

A new class of antigens associated with immediate hypersensitivity reactions to latex rubber has been identified in the last few years. Latex allergy is frequently seen in health care workers, rubber industry workers, and subjects undergoing multiple surgical procedures in early infancy *(22,23)*. Symptoms manifest as contact urticaria, rhinoconjunctivitis, asthma, and mucosal swelling. However, severe reactions and death have occurred upon exposure of patients to latex balloons on the rectal mucosa, especially in children with spina bifida. Multiple individual latex allergens have been identified, eight of which have received an international nomenclature designation. These include *Hev b 1*, rubber elongation factor; *Hev b 2*, B-1,3-glucanase; *Hev b 3*, homologous to *Hev b 1*; *Hev b 4*, a microhelix component; *Hev b 6*, prohevein/hevein; and *Hev b 7*, a patatinlike protein *(24)*. It has recently been appreciated that individuals with allergies to certain fruits such as banana, avocado, kiwi, and chestnut develop clinical symptoms upon initial contact with latex *(25)*. This phenomenon has been coined "the latex–fruit syndrome." It is thought to occur as a result of the presence of IgE reactive to enzymes such as β-glucanase and chitinases that are present in both fruits and rubber. Interestingly, mammalian chitinases have been identified as being inducible by Th2 cytokines such as IL-13.

Pharmaceuticals

Adverse drug reactions are relatively common clinical problems. Most conventional pharmaceutical agents are relatively low-molecular-weight compounds that become allergens only after their haptenization to endogenous proteins. The penicillins are classic instigators of allergic reactions. Penicillin is associated with a relatively high incidence of allergic reactions because of the chemical reactivity of penicillin and its metabolites. Although penicillin itself is the major allergen, its metabolic products, penicilloate and penilloate, are minor allergens but are responsible for a disproportionate share of severe, life-threatening reactions. Moreover, the drug is often administered parenterally, which greatly increases the probability that an adverse IgE-associated response will be fatal. Cephalosporin drugs are structurally similar to penicillin, and penicillin-allergic individuals may have IgE antibodies that cross-react with cephalosporin. Other agents, such as quaternary ammonium compounds (neuromuscular blocking agents) and sulfonamides (antibiotics) are relatively common stimuli of allergic reactions.

Insect Venom Allergens

Stinging-insect hypersensitivity develops in both nonatopic and atopic individuals. Individuals are sensitized when relatively high levels of proteins (approximately 50 μg) in venom are injected subcutaneously during a sting. The venom-associated allergens of several vespids (yellow jacket, wasp, fire ants, and white-faced hornet) are cross-reactive and include antigen 5, phospholipase, and hyaluronidase. The honeybee venom contains distinct allergens, including two major ones, phospholipase A_2 and hyaluronidase, and a less important one, melittin. Many of these allergens have proteolytic activity.

CD4+ TH2 POLARIZED IMMUNE RESPONSES IN ATOPY

As the primary orchestrators of specific immune responses to foreign antigens, the T lymphocyte has been implicated in the pathogenesis of allergic diseases. Several lines of evidence support a causal role for T lymphocytes in allergic disorders. Increased numbers of T lymphocytes are found in the bronchial mucosa, nasal mucosa, and skin of patients with allergic asthma, rhinitis, and dermatitis, respectively, when compared with nonatopic controls (26–28). In asthma and allergic rhinitis, $CD4^+$ T cells predominate. In atopic dermatitis, however, excess $CD4^+$ and $CD8^+$ T populations are both present in skin lesions (18). Further, there is a generalized increase in T-cell activation in allergic individuals, both at the site of disease and systemically. Increased cell surface expression of T-cell activation markers such as the interleukin-2 receptor (IL-2R), class II histocompatibility antigens (HLA-DR), and very-late-activation antigen-1 (VLA-1) have been observed in all disorders in the atopic triad (27,28).

As has been covered in detail in other chapters, functional subsets of $CD4^+$ T cells have been distinguished at both clonal and population levels by the unique profiles of cytokines that they produce (29,30). The differential presence of these cytokine phenotypes in a variety of allergic and infectious diseases both in mice and in humans has provided descriptive power and theoretical insight into disease pathogenesis (30,31,*32*). Th1 cells producing TNF-β, and interferon-gamma (IFN-γ), are critical in the development of cell-mediated immunity, macrophage activation, and the production of complement-fixing antibody isotypes (29,30). Th2 cells producing IL-4, IL-13, IL-5, IL-9, and IL-6 are important in the stimulation of IgE production, mucosal mastocytosis, eosinophilia, and macrophage deactivation (29,30). Another subpopulation of T cells, referred to as regulatory T cells (Treg), have immunosuppressive functions and cytokine profiles distinct from either Th1 or Th2 cells. These cells are thought to play an important role in limiting immune responses to self- or exogenous antigens by preventing the activation and function of nonregulatory effector T cells through through cell-to-cell interactions or through elaboration of IL-10 and/or TGF-β.

Until recently, the development of allergies had been thought to be due solely to an imbalance between allergen-specific Th1 and Th2 cells, with a skew toward Th2 immune responses. However, several lines of evidence suggest that allergic diseases may arise as a result of an imbalance between allergen-specific Treg and Th2 cells resulting in a loss of tolerance mediated via Treg cells. Whether this imbalance occurs due to overzealous Th2 immune responses, to impaired Treg responses, or a combination of both, is an open question. Evidence for each will be discussed below.

Th2 Polarized Immune Responses in Atopy Disorders

Several lines of evidence support the involvement of Th2 cytokines in the pathogenesis of allergic disorders. First, T cells at the site of disease (bronchoalveolar lavage, bronchial biopsies, nasal biopsies) in allergic individuals (allergic asthma, atopic rhinitis) express elevated levels of mRNA for IL-4, IL-13, GM-CSF, and IL-5 (28–31). In atopic dermatitis patients, elevated Th2 cytokines (IL-4, IL-13, IL-5) and their receptors (IL-4R, IL-5R) are found in skin lesions in acute disease *(33)*, whereas cytokine patterns in chronic lesions are mixed, with both Th2 cytokines (IL-5 and IL-13) and Th1 cytokines (IFN-γ) being expressed (*34*,35). Second, it has been shown that successful therapeutic treatment of these disorders is associated with a reduction in the Th2 cytokine pattern. For example, both steroid treatment and immunotherapeutic regimes result in reductions in Th2 cytokine levels in the nasal mucosa (36) and allergen-stimulated PBMCs (37) of patients with allergic rhinitis and in bronchoalveolar lavage (BAL) of asthmatic patients (35).

Although considerable descriptive evidence suggests that CD4$^+$ T lymphocytes and Th2 cytokines are important in the pathogenesis of atopic disorders in humans, definitive proof is of course difficult to obtain. As a result, experimental animal models have been extremely useful in mechanistic delineation of the role of CD4$^+$ T cells and T-cell–derived cytokines in the pathogenesis of allergic disorders. Murine models of antigen-driven asthma have consistently revealed a causal role for CD4$^+$ T cells in the development of the signs of allergic airway disease (38,39). In these models, sensitization with various allergens (ovalbumin, house dust mite, ragweed, aspergillius) by either intraperitoneal injections or airway challenge, followed by direct airway challenge, induces a phenotype closely resembling that observed in human asthmatics (38,39). Specifically, allergen sensitization and challenge results in airway hyperresponsiveness, eosinophilic inflammation, elevations in allergen-specific IgE levels, and mucus hypersecretion. Regardless of mouse strains or exposure protocols, an absolute requirement for CD4$^+$ T cells for the development of allergic responses is clear in such models (38). A lack of CD4$^+$ T cells, achieved either by antibody depletion (38) or gene targeting (40), is associated with prevention of the development of allergen-induced airway responses. Conversely, depletion of CD8$^+$ T cells does not affect airway responses to allergen challenge in mice (41). Furthermore, adoptive transfer of Th2 clones into the mouse lung is sufficient for the development of allergic airway symptoms (48). On the other hand, transfer of Th1 clones *(42)*, or administration of agents such as IL-12 and IFN-γ that inhibit Th2 cytokine production and stimulate Th1 pathways, prevent the development of allergen-induced airway hyperresponsiveness and eosinophilic inflammation in murine models (43,44,*45*). Conversely, mice that are deficient in T-bet, a transcription factor important in IFN-γ secretion, spontaneously develop Th2-mediated allergic airway responses *(46)*. Several studies have shown evidence of association between polymorphisms in the T-bet gene and asthma phenotypes in humans *(47)*.

The involvement of each of the specific Th2 cytokines in atopic airway responses has been demonstrated in studies in which IL-4, IL-5, IL-13, and IL-9 have been manipulated through either antibody blockade (48,49), or gene targeting (50,51,*52*,53). Similar roles for CD4$^+$ T cells and Th2 cytokines have been demonstrated in experimental mouse models of each of the atopic disorders, including atopic rhinitis *(54,55)*, food allergy *(56)*, and atopic dermatitis (53). Collectively, the Th2 cytokines orchestrate the elicitation of the allergic response via their ability to regulate IgE production and recruitment and activation of various effector cells (e.g., mast cells, eosinophils). In particular, IL-4, through its critical role in Th2 differentiation, has been shown to be essential in the initiation of allergic airway responses (*57*,58). IL-5 clearly plays a role in eosinophil development, recruitment, and activation at the site of Th2-inflammatory responses (59), whereas IL-9 appears to be an important regulator of mast-cell activation *(60)*. IL-13 has been shown to have a singular role in the effector phase of the allergic response (39,61). Specifically, it is sufficient to induce many of the manifestations of allergic disease, including airway inflammation, airway hyperresponsiveness, and mucus cell hypersecretion in allergic airway diseases (39,61). Recently, another Th2-specific cytokine, IL-21, which is a member of the common γ-chain family of cytokines, has been shown to be important in the development of Th2 immune responses (62) IL-21R–deficient mice have impaired development of airway hyperresponsiveness (AHR), and eosoinophilic inflammation concomitant with a reduction in IL-13 levels in BAL fluids. Although the mechanisms by which IL-21 regulates allergic inflammation are unknown, IL-21 is not thought to be required for Th2 differentiation, but may be important for migration and/or survival of Th2 cells.

Role of NK T Cells in Allergic Disease

Although allergic diseases have clearly been associated with polarized Th2 cytokine production in tissues, the source of these Th2 cytokines has been recently debated. Specifically, recent studies have implicated invariant TCR$^+$ CD1d-restricted CD4$^+$ natural killer T cells (NKT cells) as one of the major sources of Th2 cytokines (63–65). Akbari et al. demonstrated that NKT-deficient mice do not develop airway hyperresponsiveness in response to systemtic ovalbumin priming in the presence of adjuvants and subsequent allergen aerosol challenge. The resistance of these mice to the development of allergen-specific airway hyperrepsonsiveness can be overcome by adoptive transfer of tetramer-purified NKT cells producing IL-4 and IL-13 or by rIL-13 treatment. In support of a role for NKT cells, Morishima et al. have shown that priming of mice with ovalbumin plus the NKT cell ligand, α-GalCer, overcomes the tolerance that is normally seen with airway exposure to OVA alone *(66)*. In this model, the development of Th2-mediated AHR is CD1d$^+$-dependent; however, it does not occur in mice that are deficient in MHC class II, suggesting that NKT cells are necessary but not sufficient to induce Th2-mediated responses. Interestingly, a single administration of α-GalCer to the mouse airway induces AHR, suggesting that NKT cells may serve as effector cells in the absence of conventional Th2 responses through their ability to produce Th2 cytokines such as IL-13. The effect of NKT cell activation appears to depend on the timing and context of activation, as other studies have shown that activation of NKT cells with α-GalCer + OVA in OVA-primed mice actually inhibits AHR, and Th2 cytokine production, in a NKT cell– and IFN-γ–dependent manner *(66,67)*. In support of a role for NKT cells in human asthma, Akbari et al. demonstrated that a large fraction of $CD4^+CD3^+$ cells in the lungs of allergic asthmatic individuals are not MHC class II–restricted, but rather natural killer T cells (68). Similarly, Sen et al. (69) found that $V\alpha24^+$-invariant natural killer T cells (iNKT cells) in the blood of patients with asthma selectively expressed CCR9, and that large numbers of $CCR9^+$ and $V\alpha24^+$ cells were present in bronchial biopsy samples from patients with asthma, but not from control subjects. They also showed that conventional $CD3^+$ α/β T cells could be polarized to a Th2 phenotype by cell-to-cell contact with $V\alpha24^+$-invariant natural killer T cells, with enhanced expression of CCR9, from patients with asthma. The induction of Th2 cytokine production requires CCL25 and CCR9 to activate adjacent membrane signaling by CD226, a leukocyte-adhesion molecule, that is expressed on monocytes. CD226 appears to be critical for activating $V\alpha24^+$-invariant natural killer T cells for the induction of a Th2 bias in conventional T cells. Dendritic cells and epithelial cells are major sources of CCL25. They also showed that the numbers of $CCR9^+$ $V\alpha24^+$ NKT cells in the peripheral blood of symptomatic patients with asthma decreased after steroid treatment and when asthma was clinically silent. Interestingly, iNKT cells do not appear to be required for the development of another allergic disorder, namely, atopic dermatitis (70). Taken together, these studies suggest that NKT cells play a prominent role in the development of some Th2 immune allergic responses; however, the exact nature of their role depends on both the timing and dose of the activating ligand. Thus, NKT cells can function as an adjuvant when iNKT cells are activated during adminstration of a protein antigen, can direct induction of AHR when they are activated in the absence of other signals, or can function to prevent the development of AHR when they are activated by strong NKT cell–activating agents once inflammation is established. The most likely scenario is one in which NKT cells and conventional $CD4^+$ T cells responding to their respective glycolipid and peptide antigens work in concert to mediate the development of allergic responses. Although the exact mechanisms by which NKT cells are activated during Th2 immune responses are currently unknown, there are several possibilities: (a) allergens such as pollens may contain glycolipids that are recognized by the invariant TCR of NKT cells (71,72); (b) self-glycolipid antigens may be released and/or recognized during the course of inflammatory responses; or (c) conventional T cells may augment the numbers of NKT cells at mucosal surfaces through cytokine production, costimulatory molecules, or through other mechanisms in the absence of NKT cell ligands. Further studies will be required to determine the extent of the contribution of NKT cells in various allergic disorders and to determine the specific endogenous or exogenous glycoplipid antigens that are activating NKT cells in allergic patients.

Impaired Treg Cell Function in Atopic Individuals

It has recently been hypothesized that under noninflammatory conditions the outcome of immune responses to innocuous environmental allergens is the development of immunologic tolerance. Moreover, it is thought that a loss of tolerance results in Th2-biased immune responses at mucosal surfaces. Although the specific immunologic events that mediate tolerance in this setting are not well understood, recent studies have suggested that regulatory T cells protect against the development of allergic disease and that their function is impaired in genetically susceptible individuals. As is described in depth in other chapters, T-regulatory cells (Treg) are cells that inhibit the development and function of other nonregulatory T cells. To date, two major categories of Treg cells have been described. The first is the naturally occurring, thymically derived $CD4^+CD25^+$ Treg cells that express high levels of the transcription factor Foxp3, which is essential for their development and function. The other major category is the antigen-specific Treg, which can be induced in vitro and in vivo under particular conditions of antigen stimulation. These antigen-specific Treg secrete anti-inflammatory cytokines such as IL-10 and TGF-β, and regulate immune responses and inflammatory pathologies. Antigen-induced Treg that secrete IL-10 are oftern referred to as IL-10 Treg cells, or Tr1 cells, whereas those that secrete TGF-β have been referred to as Th3 cells.

Several lines of evidence from both human and animal studies have suggested that alterations in Treg populations and function may contribute to susceptibility to allergic disease. In animal models, several studies show that adoptive transfer of $CD4^+CD25^+$ Treg can reverse established airway inflammation through an IL-10–dependent process. Conversely, reduced expression of membrane-bound TGF-β exacerbates airway pathology in an asthma model (73). Furthermore, environmental exposures to agents that induce Treg cell expansion have been shown to ameliorate the development of asthma. In particular, exposure of mice early in life to lipopolysaccharide (LPS) resulted in the expansion of T cells expressing CD25 and IL-10 concomitant with reduced allergic manifestations upon sensitization and challenge compared to those mice without exposure to LPS *(74)*. Treatment of mice with mycobacterium-induced allergen-specific Treg cells producing IL-10 and TGF-β protected against airway inflammation (75). Similarly, heat-killed *Listeria monocytogenes* treatment induced allergen-specific Treg producing IFN-γ and IL-10, which protected against food allergy in dogs *(76)*.

Although fewer conclusive studies have been conducted in humans, several studies support the hypothesis that impaired Treg function may contribute to development of Th2-dependent pathologies in humans. For example, the frequency of allergen-specific IL-10–secreting cells was significantly decreased in allergic patients compared to nonatopic individuals (77). Whether the IL-10 is derived from Treg or activated effector T cells is unknown. In addition to a relative lack of Treg in atopic individuals, Ling et al. (78) have shown that CD4$^+$CD25$^+$ cells from atopic individuals have impaired ability to suppress effector T-cell cytokine production. Another interesting observation regarding the role of Treg in susceptibility to atopy is the finding that children who outgrew milk allergy had higher numbers of CD4$^+$CD25$^+$ cells in their blood (79). Furthermore, therapies shown to be beneficial in the treatment of allergy and asthma, such as allergen immunotherapy or glucocorticoid therapy, have been shown to increase the induction of allergen-specific IL-10–secreting Treg cells, concomitant with a reduction in allergen-specific Th2 responses (80).

Although the mechanisms by which Treg regulate the development of allergic inflammation are not completely understood, they are thought to prevent allergic symptoms by suppression of Th2-cell effector function through the elaboration of the suppressive cytokines, IL-10 and TGF-β. However, recent studies now support the concept that Treg may alter sensitization and ongoing Th2 immune responses by regulating airway DC function. Mice lacking the transcription factor RunX3, which is involved in downstream TGF-β signaling, spontaneously develop symptoms of asthma concomitant with increased numbers of lung DCs, displaying a mature phenotype with increased expression of MHC II, OX40 ligand, and CCR7 (81). Moreover, dendritic cells from RunX3-deficient mice induce inflammatory responses to otherwise harmless inhaled antigens, possibly through their lack of responsiveness to locally secreted TGF-β. In further support of a role for T regulation of DCs, it has been shown that in mice (C3H/HeJ) that are resistant to HDM-induced asthma and airway hyperresponsiveness, Treg depletion with the CD25-depleting antibody similarly led to increased numbers of pulmonary myeloid DCs with increased expression of MHC II, CD80, and CD86 and an increased capacity to stimulate T-cell proliferation and Th2 cytokine production (82). In contrast, Treg from normally susceptible A/J mice do not suppress inflammation and AHR. These data suggest that resistance to allergen-driven AHR is mediated in part by CD4$^+$CD25$^+$ Treg suppression of DC activation and that the absence of this regulatory pathway contributes to susceptibility.

The lack of allergen-specific tolerance in allergic individuals has been hypothesized to be related to improved hygiene in industrialized countries, possibly due to reduced infections, alterations in commensal microflora in the intestinal tract, and/or reduced Toll-like receptor (TLR) signaling. This will be discussed in more detail in the following sections. Taken together, these studies suggest that Treg may induce tolerance to or provide protection from inhaled allergens in healthy individuals and that an imbalance between allergen-specific Treg and Th2 cytokine–producing cells may underlie susceptibility to the development of atopic diseases.

Determinants of Susceptibility to Th2 Immune Responses in Atopic Individuals

Overview

Very little is known conclusively about the underlying causes of the aberrant expansion of Th2 cytokine-producing cells in atopic humans. However, the skewed Th2 immune responses in atopic disorders may be due to either overzealous Th2 immune responses, impaired ability to generate either Th1 or T regulatory responses, a lack of exposure to Th1- and Treg-promoting agents, or a combination of these. This balance is influenced by a number of genetic and environmental factors that control both the innate and adapative immune responses to allergens at mucosal surfaces. There is supportive data for each of these determinants in atopic diseases (Figure 43.1).

Genetic Influences on Allergen Sensitization

There is substantial evidence suggesting that the development of atopic diseases is genetically controlled *(83,84)*. Familial aggregation and twins studies have confirmed a fundamental contribution of genetic factors to the development of atopy and specific clinical atopic phenotypes (85). Specifically, individuals with a first-degree relative with atopic phenotypes are at a significantly greater risk of developing atopy. Moreover, individuals with two "atopic" parents are at a greater risk of developing an allergic disease than those with only one atopic parent. However, inheritance of atopic disorders appears to be preferentially associated with the atopic status of the mother *(86)*. Further support for a genetic basis of asthma is the fact that there is a greater concordance for atopic disease between monozygotic twins compared to dizygotic twins (*87,88,*89). The concordance is not 100%, suggesting that asthma is a polygenic disorder with strong environmental influences. Despite the complex genetic nature of atopic disorders, multiple studies have reported evidence of linkage of atopic-related traits with six primary chromosomal regions, including (a) the Th2 cytokine gene cluster on 5q31-q33, including the IL-4, IL-13, CD14, SPINK5, LTC4S, and CYFIP2 genes; (b) the HLA region on 6p21, including both classical (HLA-DRB1, HLA-DQB1, HLA-G)

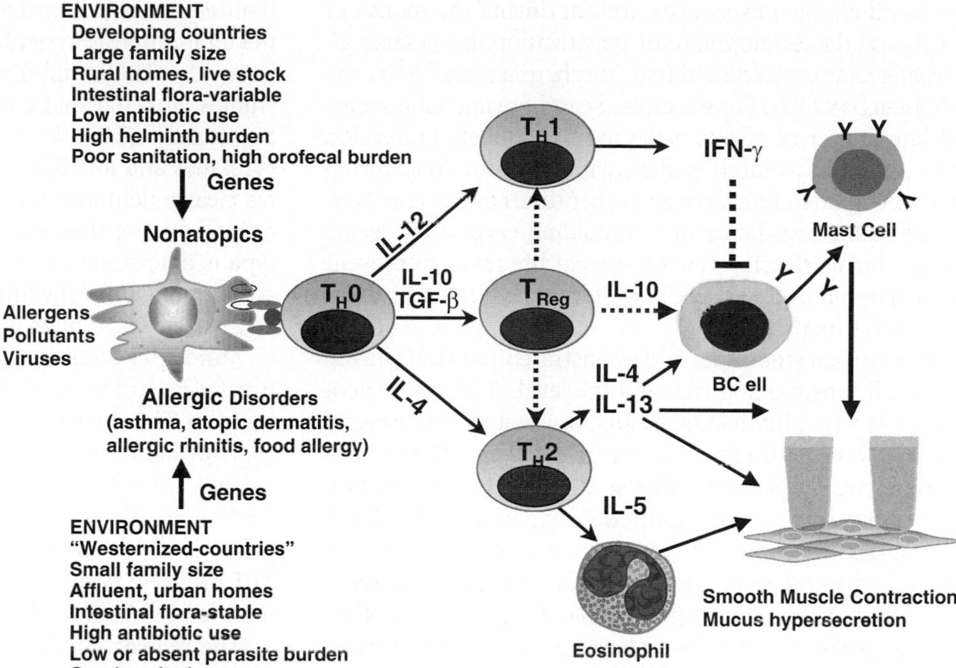

FIGURE 43.1 Allergic diseases are associated with aberrant adaptive immune responses to innocuous environmental antigens. The development of allergic responses to harmless antigens is influenced both by environmental factors and by the genetic background of the individual. Under conditions in which microbial exposure is minimal, such as in Westernized countries, T cells differentiate along a Th2 pattern with elaboration of IL-4, IL-13, IL-5, IL-9, and IL-21. In contrast, microbial exposure in early life protects against the development of harmful Th2 immune responses via the induction of regulatory T cells.

and nonclassical HLA genes (TNF, LTA); (c) the region that contains the high-affinity IgE receptor gene (FcεRIb) on 11q13; (d) a large region on chromosome 12q14 that spans several candidate genes (Stat6, interferon-γ, stem cell factor, nitric oxide synthase 1); (e) a region of 16q containing the IL4RA; and (f) a region of 20p containing the first positionally cloned asthma gene, ADAM33. In addition, >100 genes have been associated with atopic disorders through candidate gene and positional cloning efforts (see reviews in 90,91) (Table 43.4). The involvement of specific candidate genes in atopic disease pathogenesis will be addressed in relevant sections throughout the text.

Environmental Influences on Development of Atopic Disease

Despite the clear heritable component of asthma, the incomplete concordance of disease in twins studies and the rapid shift in the rate at which the incidence of atopic disorders is rising suggest a recent change in environmental influences on this process. Changes in exposures to allergens, infectious agents or their by-products, and/or pollutants have all been suspected. It is likely that multiple environmental factors influence the development of allergic diseases, and that there may be complex interactions between these individual factors.

Timing and Dose of Allergen Exposure

The spectrum of antigens an asthmatic individual is sensitized to is dependent on their environment in early life. This tenet is based on the positive correlations observed

TABLE 43.4 Genes Associated with Atopic and Asthmatic Phenotypes in at Least Two or More Published Studies

2–5 Studies		*6–10 Studies*	*>10 Studies*
KCNS33	NAT2	GSTM1	IL-4
ACP1	DEFB1	L10	IL13
IL-1A	TLR4	CTLA4	CD14
IL-1B	C5	SPINKS	ADRB2
DPP10	GATA3	LTC4S	HLA-DRB1
CCR5	ALOX5	LTA	HLA-DQB1
IL5RA	CRTH2	GRPA	TNF
TLR6	IL18	NOD1	FCER1B
TLR10	AICDA	CC16	IL4RA
TLR2	VDR	GSTP1	ADAM33
CSF2	IFNG	STAT6	
IL5	PHF11	NOS1	
IL12B	CYSLTR2	CCL5	
TIM1	TCRA/D	TBXA2R	
TM3	CMA1	TGFB1	
HLA-G	PTGDR		
HLA-DQA1	CARD15		
HLA-DPB1	NOS2A		
TAP1	CRHR1		
PAFAH	CCL11		
EDN1	TBX21		
IFNGR1	STAT3		
CCL24	ITGB3		
CCL26	ACE		
CFTR	C3		
NOS3	GSTT1		
IL1RN	MIF		

Source: Adapted from Ober and Hoffjan, *Genes and Immunity.* 2006;7:95–100

between allergen exposures present during the month of birth and the development of sensitization to the same allergens later in childhood (e.g., birch, grass, and dust mite allergens) *(92,93)*. For example, Scandinavian babies born in late winter or early spring are more likely to develop IgE antibody to birch pollen, which is prevalent during the spring, than those born at other times of the year *(92)*. In addition, avoidance or withholding certain allergenic foods during the first few months of life tends to prevent sensitization and subsequent allergic responses to these particular foods.

Numerous studies have demonstrated the relationship between sensitization risk and the level of allergen exposure *(94,95)*. This has been best studied in relationship to dust mite and cat antigens in early life. When both parents are atopic, dust mite sensitization occurred with <1% prevalence when infants were exposed to <0.1 μg of house dust mite allergen per gram of dust, but this value increased to 6% with allergen levels >10 μg per gram of dust *(94)*. Although antigen dose is positively correlated with sensitization, recent studies suggest that the relationship may be more complex. Specifically, high exposure to animal dander early in life has been shown to be protective against manifestations of asthma *(96)*. Whether this represents immune tolerance as a result of high antigen dose or concomitant exposure to other factors such as endotoxin as a result of living in close proximity to a pet is unknown.

More important than the actual dose of allergen is the age at which exposure occurs. It has recently been hypothesized that exposure to environmental antigens occurs both prenatally and postnatally. In this regard, several independent studies have provided support for the postulate that prenatal events may influence susceptibility to allergic diseases (84,97). For example, it has been shown that cord-blood mononuclear cells respond to inhalant and food allergens, suggesting that initial priming of allergen-specific T-cell responses may occur before birth (84,97). It has been demonstrated that the responding cord-blood T cells were indeed of fetal origin, as they did not respond to common vaccine antigens such as tetanus toxoid, against which the majority of adults in the study population expressed active immunity (84). These findings suggest that transfer of substances from mother to child (e.g., allergens, antibodies, toxins, hormones, or other immune mediators via the placenta) may occur during gestation, which might prime or sensitize the developing infant to environmental antigens. In addition, factors present in the *in utero* environment may serve to influence the nature of the immune response of the fetus to allergens that cross the placenta. Indeed, mediators such as PGE2 and high levels of progesterone, which has been shown to alter the Th1/Th2 balance by either suppressing Th1 cytokine production or inducing a Th2 pattern, are present during pregnancy. Th2 skewing is thought to take place to suppress IFN-γ production, which is toxic to the fetus. Accordingly, exogenous antigens that leak across the placenta are likely to be presented to the fetal immune system within a milieu conducive to selection for Th2 immunity. This contention is supported by studies showing that cord-blood cells from both allergic and nonallergic infants both produce high levels of Th2 cytokines and low IFN-γ levels *(98)*. Although these studies clearly demonstrate that initial allergen priming may occur *in utero*, they also suggest that the Th2 cell phenotype is determined to a substantial degree after birth, as only a minority of the infants who exhibit allergen-specific Th2 responses at birth go on to develop disease.

Although immune responses in neonates are skewed toward a Th2 phenotype, studies of human infants indicate that this Th2 skew gradually diminishes during the first 2 years of life in nonallergic individuals (84,99). In allergic infants, the reverse occurs, with the strength of neonatal Th2 responses increasing over a similar period (84,99). The persistence of this neonatal bias and the failure to produce Th1 or T-regulatory type responses may be an important feature of the atopic disease state *(100)*.

The redirection of Th2 responses is thought to occur simultaneously with childhood bacterial or viral infections in early life. This relationship has been capsulated in the "hygiene hypothesis," which argues that early childhood infections inhibit the tendency to develop allergic disease (101). Several epidemiologic studies have provided support for this hypothesis. For example, Von Mutius (102) compared allergic sensitization and atopy in children from West Germany and East Germany. She noted that the frequency of atopy was considerably higher in West German children (36.7%) than in their peers in East Germany (18.2%). The authors attributed the increase in allergy to the "Western lifestyle," with decreased family size, improved housing, and prevention of infectious diseases in early childhood. Further epidemiologic support for this hypothesis comes from studies demonstrating an inverse relationship between farm living, pet ownership, daycare attendance in early life, and atopy. Although the general implication of these studies is that protection from allergy seems to be associated with an increase in microbial exposure, the link has remained fairly indirect. One study that has addressed the relationship between asthma and a specific pathogen is a cross-sectional study of Italian military recruits (103). The authors found a significant inverse association between the presence of antibodies to hepatitis A and various measures of atopy. In all likelihood, such evidence of previous infection with hepatitis A merely provides evidence of a risk of exposure to fecal–oral pathogens. However, recent studies suggested that perhaps exposure to hepatitis A is protective against the development of atopy, as polymorphisms in the receptor for hepatitis A, TIM-1 (T-cell immunoglobulin– and mucin domain–containing molecule-1), are associated with protection from atopy (104). Interestingly, the association of TIM-1 mutations with protection is only observed in patients who show serologic evidence of HepA infection. At a population level, Shirakawa et al. *(105)* found that among Japanese schoolchildren there was a strong inverse association between delayed-type hypersensitivity (Th1-mediated immune response) to Bacillus Calmette-Guerin (BCG) and atopy. Positive tuberculin responses predicted a lower incidence of asthma, lower serum IgE levels, and cytokine profile biases toward a type 1 profile. These results suggest that exposure and response to bacteria may, by modification of immune cytokines profiles, inhibit atopic disorders. In a study of defined infectious exposures, Aaby et al. documented that vaccination with *Mycobacterium bovis* BCG was associated with a reduction in the prevalence of allergy in Guinea-Bissau *(106)*. However, such protection was not observed in a similar retrospective study of BCG vaccination in Swedish children with a family history of allergy.

The complex interface with the microbial world provided by the gastrointestinal tract might well be important to the interrelationship between infection and allergy. The endogenous flora of the gut provide a wealth of stimuli for the developing immune system at birth. There seem to be both quantitative and qualitative differences in early-childhood patterns of bacterial colonization between the developed and developing world. For example, a study of Swedish and Pakistani infants indicates that intestinal colonization with aerobic gram-negative bacteria tends to occur later in Westernized than in developing countries (107). Once they are colonized, infants in developed countries tend to carry the same enterobacterial strains, whereas infants in developing countries are often colonized serially with different strains. Differences in intestinal flora have also been found between allergic and nonallergic children in Europe *(108,109)*. Allergic children seem to be colonized less often with lactobacilli in Sweden and Estonia than nonallergic controls (110). This idea is consistent with the observation that oral tolerance cannot be induced in germ-free mice *(111)*. Furthermore, elimination of commensal intestinal microflora and toll like receptor (TLR) signaling with broad-spectrum antibiotics also prevented oral tolerance from developing, enhanced allergic sensitization, and resulted in susceptibility to intestinal inflammation. These observations suggest that TLR signaling by commensal bacteria under normal steady-state conditions is required for maintenance of intestinal epithelial homeostatsis, and possibly for the induction of some forms of Treg. The intestine has been shown to affect immune response at other mucosal surfaces, including the respiratory tract, lacrimal, salivary and mammary glands, through secretory IgA antibodies *(112,113)*.

Further support for this hypothesis is the striking association between polymorphisms in genes in the Toll pathways and atopic phenotypes. Specifically, an association has been consistently reported between a polymorphism in the CD14 gene, increased levels of sCD14, and decreased levels of IgE, reflecting the importance of bacterial LPS in downregulating Th2 responses (114). Moreover, a polymorphism in the coding region of the TLR4 gene (A/G 896) resulting in reduced cell surface expression of TLR4 and subsequent disruption of LPS-mediated signaling has been associated with atopy in children (115). However, the data in asthma are conflicting, with some studies showing an association between asthma and TLR4 polymorphisms (115), whereas others do not (116). Interestingly, inheritance of both the TLR4 SNP (A/G+896) and the IL-4 SNP (−590) confers greater risk of asthma pathogenesis in females *(117)*. Clearly, these innate immune pathways play a critical role in determining the inflammatory reactions of the airways and the outcome of T-cell respones to inhaled allergens.

Although the hygiene hypothesis is likely oversimplified, it is theoretically possible that DCs at mucosal surfaces in atopic individuals receive less innate immune stimulation in the form of microbial stimuli (LPS, peptidoglycans, mycobacterial antigens) and therefore fail to redirect weak Th2 responses into protective Th1 responses or T-regulatory responses. This hypothesis may provide a plausible explanation for the rising prevalence of these disorders in Westernized countries.

Exposure to other environmental agents such as diesel particles, ozone, second-hand tobacco smoke, and viruses (respiratory synctial virus (RSV), rhinoviruses) can also enhance sensitization to allergens in young children (110). Numerous epidemiologic studies illustrate clear associations between exposure to these agents and enhanced antigenic sensitization and worsening of disease. Nasal challenge with diesel particles alone increased IgE production in both atopic and nonatopic individuals, suggesting that diesel particles indeed may be a sensitizer *(118)*. When evaluated together with allergen, diesel exposure of ragweed-sensitive subjects resulted in a significant increase in allergen-specific IgE, with an increase in Th2 cytokine production. Ozone can alter both immediate and late-phase responses of asthmatics and allergic rhinitics to inhaled allergen *(119)*. Epidemiologic studies have shown that exposure to environmental tobacco smoke (ETS) in childhood is associated with increased skin-test reactivity, serum IgE, and prevalence of eosinophilia *(120–122)*. Recently, it has been shown that controlled chamber exposures of ragweed-sensitive subjects to ETS resulted in enhanced production of allergen-specific IgE, Th2 cytokines, and decreased IFN-γ levels in nasal lavage fluids (123). Although there is controversy regarding whether RSV is an inducer of allergic asthma or rather a predictor of aberrant immune responses, severe RSV infections are strongly associated with asthma *(124)*. Similarly, rhinoviral infections are strongly associated with exacerbations in atopic airway disease *(125)*. In summary, the complex interplay between genetic and environmental factors likely governs susceptibility to the development of atopic disorders.

FACTORS REGULATING TH2 IMMUNE RESPONSES IN ALLERGIC INDIVIDUALS

Antigen Presentation in Atopic Individuals

The nature of the T-cell response to antigens encountered at the mucosal surface depends on three signals provided by professional APCs (Figure 43.2). Although a number of professional APCs, such as dendritic cells, Langerhans cells (LCs), B cells, and macrophages, are present at mucosal surfaces and have the cellular specialization to capture and process antigen for presentation to T cells, it has become increasingly clear over the last decade that DCs and Langerhan cells are the most important professional APCs at mucosal surfaces. DCs migrate as precursor cells to sites of the body where antigen entry

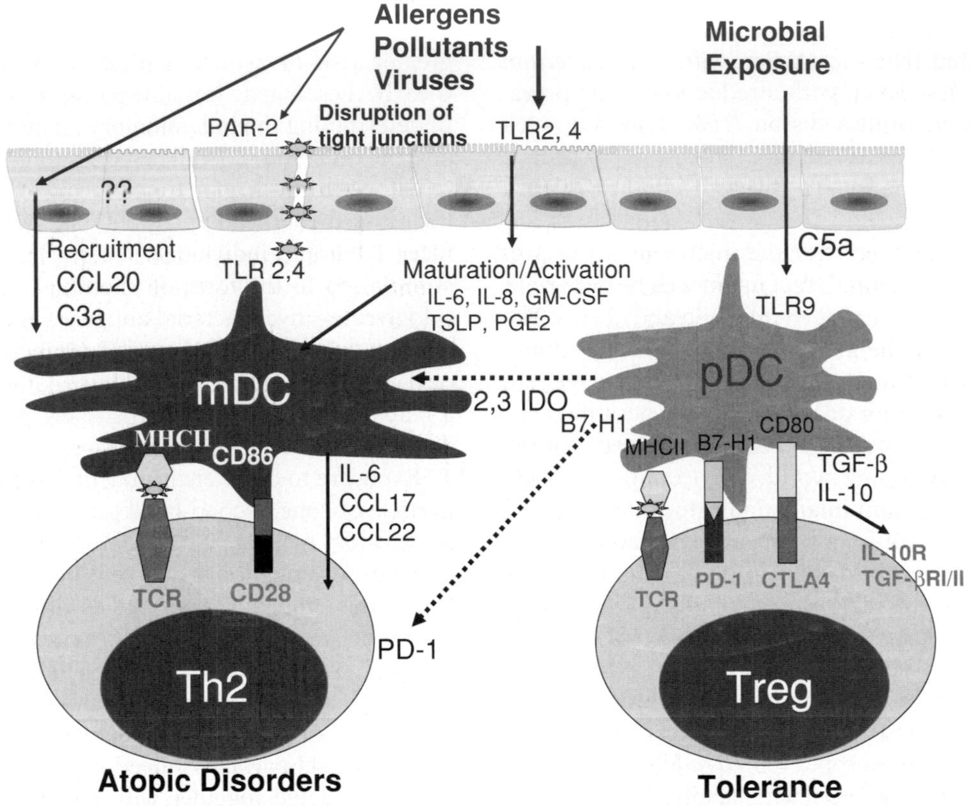

FIGURE 43.2 Postulated factors regulating dendritic cell instruction of T-cell differentiation in atopic disorders. Dendritic cell recruitment, activation, and maturation are controlled both by direct stimulation by PAMPs contained in allergens themselves and through indirect signals derived from surrounding resident cells such as epithelial cells. Immature DCs are recruited to mucosal surfaces following the release of chemokines (i.e., CCL20) and inflammatory mediators (IL-8, IL-6) by epithelial cells in response to inflammatory stimuli such as allergens, pollutants, irritants, and/or viral infections. Although the mechanisms by which these stimuli elicit chemokine release are unknown, certain allergens contain protease activity that has been shown to activate epithelial cells via stimulation of PAR-2 receptors on the epithelium. In addition to activating epithelial cells to release chemokines and cytokines, allergen-derived proteases can also cause disruption of epithelial tight junctions and allow antigens to gain access to DCs located beneath their surface. Allergens are taken up, processed, and presented to T cells in the context of MHC class II molecules. DCs mature and express costimulatory molecules (i.e., CD86, OX40) under the influence of cytokines (GM-CSF, IL-6) and mediators (TSLP, PGE2) derived from surrounding tissues or through direct stimulation of PRRs (likely TLR4, 2) expressed on their surface. In atopic individuals, it has been postulated that myeloid DCs appear to be the predominant population of DCs taking up antigen and driving the differentiation of naïve T cells toward a Th2 profile. In contrast, in nonatopics, allergen is taken up in the context of microbial signals, which preferentially stimulate plasmacytoid DCs through TLR9 expression. Activation of pDCs results in the stimulation of naïve T cells to differentiate into T-regulatory cells expressing an array of inhibitory molecules such as CTLA4, PD-1, IL-10R, and TGF-βRI and II. Activation of the production of IL-10 and TGF-β as well as 2,3-IDO results in the inhibition of Th2 effector cell function as well as inhibition of myeloid DC activation, leading to the development of immunological tolerance to environmental antigen exposure.

occurs (i.e., lung, skin, GI tract). At these sites they form an extensive network of cells, extending cell projections in between resident cell types that ensure accessibility to allergens. DCs that reside in the periphery have an immature phenotype, specialized for uptake and recognition of antigens, but are not yet capable of stimulating naïve T cells, because they lack costimulatory molecules on their surface (CD80, CD86). Normally, DCs present antigens quite inefficiently; however, when antigen is encountered in an inflammatory context (e.g., in the presence of antigen-derived danger signals) or through indirect sensing of "danger" from surrounding cells via the release of inflammatory cytokines (IL-1β, TNF-α, IL-6, PGE_2, GM-CSF), DCs undergo a developmental program referred to as maturation. During maturation, they lose their ability to take up antigen and acquire a phenotype of professional APCs expressing all the costimulatory molecules and chemokines required to attract and stimulate naïve T cells. Once DCs have acquired antigens at the mucosal surface, they migrate to T-cell areas of draining lymph nodes and present their antigen cargo to naïve T cells. During this interaction with naïve T cells in the lymph nodes, DCs have an opportunity to influence T-cell differentiation along a Th1, Th2, or regulatory T-cell pattern, by secretion of a specific cytokine pattern, depending on their lineage, their maturation status, and the consequent costimulatory molecule pattern. Thus, alterations in the signals provided by DCs to T cells may underlie the development of polarized Th2-cell responses in the context of allergic disease. Considerable evidence is accumulating to support this tenet.

Indeed, several lines of evidence in murine models of allergic disease as well as in atopic humans support a pivotal role for DCs in the development of allergic responses. For example, Lambrecht et al. (126) have demonstrated that infusion of antigen-pulsed bone marrow–derived DCs into the respiratory tract of mice primed them for development of Th2-mediated immune responses upon subsequent antigen challenge. Conversely, using a suicide-gene approach to specifically deplete DCs, it was demonstrated that antigen exposure did not induce allergic responses in the absence of DCs (126). In humans, a critical role for DC in generation of allergic responses is the demonstration that regular use of budesonide and fluticasone, which is associated with improvement in lung function, is associated with a reduction in the number of $CD1a^+$ $HLA\text{-}DR^+$ DCs in the airways of asthmatic patients (127).

Altered DC Phenotype and Function in Allergic Diseases

DCs play a major role in the surveillance of peripheral tissue sites for incoming antigens, a function that is dependent on their capacity for tightly controlled migration between different compartments. Under steady-state conditions, there is a continuous turnover of DC at mucosal surfaces, with the recruitment of immature DC from circulating precursors balanced by the exit of mature, antigen-loaded cells to regional lymph nodes. In both humans and mice, DCs are not constitutively present in the tracheal-bronchial mucosa in the first year of life; their occurrence appears to be dependent on exposure to inflammatory stimuli from the local environment (128,129). Indeed, the numbers of HLA-DR expressing dendritic cell numbers are increased in the mucosal tissues of asthmatic, allergic rhinitic, and atopic dermatitis patients when compared to the low level of DCs found in specimens from normal controls (127,*130–133)*. Although the exact signals that regulate the rapid recruitment of immature DCs from the blood into the mucosal tissues are not fully understood, exposure to a number of environmental triggers (allergens, particulate matter, smoke, RSV, ozone) have been shown to dramatically increase the recruitment of DCs in both animal models of atopic disease and atopic humans (134–136). These triggers likely attract DCs to mucosal surfaces through their ability to induce a set of chemokines that bind to receptors expressed exclusively on immature DCs. Indeed, it has been shown that epithelial cells synthesize and secrete the CCR6 ligand, MIP-3α/CCL20, in response to allergens and particulate matter (137,*138*). Interestingly, though *Der p 1* stimulation of bronchial epithelial cells from patients with asthma results in CCL20 production and migration of LC precursors, this effect is not observed in cells from healthy individuals (139). The ability of these triggers to induce DC chemokines may explain the adjuvant effect of each of these irritants in induction of allergic responses. Taken together, these studies suggest that responsiveness of mucosal epithelial cells to certain pathogens and/or environmental stimuli early in childhood may enhance or inhibit sensitization to allergens by affecting DC recruitment.

The maturational state of DCs is thought to be an important determinant of the development of tolerance or immunity. It has been suggested that DC immaturity may contribute to the development of tolerance *(140)*. Indeed, studies from both animal models and atopic humans suggest that the magnitude and pattern of costimulatory molecule expression on DCs is strongly associated with susceptibility to atopic disease. In this regard, DCs influence the nature of the immune response to antigen stimulation through the balance of positive signals provided by CD28 engagement of B7-1, B7-2, B7-H3, and B7-H4 on resting T cells and negative signals provided through ligation of CTLA4 and PD-1 on resting T cells. Indeed, differences in the relative expression of these positive and negative signals have been shown to be important in various murine models of allergic disease. Specifically, it has been reported in numerous studies that Th2-mediated immune responses are predominantly dependent on DC expression of CD86, not CD80 *(141)*. In contrast, stimulation of CTLA4,

TIM-3, and BTLA have all been shown to decrease allergic responses *(142)*. CTLA4 in particular is predominantly expressed on Treg and is thought to mediate its inhibitory effects through Treg suppressive functions. More recently, it has been shown that the PD-1 ligand B7-H1 may also be an important regulator of tolerance through its ability to induce Treg (143). Several studies have shown that B7RP–ICOS interactions mediate tolerance through the induction of IL-10–secreting Tr1 cells (144,*145*), but other studies report that ICOS positively regulates allergic responses (146).

Several studies have suggested that DCs from atopic individuals have a different phenotype from those of nonatopic individuals (147,148,*149*). First, the functional capacity of DCs from atopic individuals has been elegantly studied in a humanized severe combined immune deficiency mouse model (150). In this model, it has been demonstrated that adoptive transfer of DC from atopic individuals reconstitutes Th2 polarized immunity associated with allergic inflammation in the lungs of mice. In contrast, transfer of DC from nonatopics resulted in combined Th1/Th2 responses. In another study, it has shown that *Der p 1* stimulation of monocyte-derived DC from *Der p 1*–sensitive patients resulted in preferential upregulation of CD86 expression and proinflammatory cytokine production (IL-1β, TNF-α, IL-6) when compared to cells from nonallergic patients or pollen-sensitive subjects (148). Purified T cells from house dust mite (HDM)-sensitive patients stimulated by autologous *Der p 1*–pulsed DC preferentially produced IL-4. Interestingly, DCs from nonatopic individuals stimulated with *Der p 1* expressed CD80, produced IL-12, and stimulated IFN-γ production in T cells. Another intriguing finding of this study was that the effects of *Der p 1* on costimulatory molecule expression in DC from allergic patients was dependent on the enzymatic activity of *Der p 1*, as a cysteine protease inhibitor prevented these effects. It has also been shown that differences in inhibitory molecule expression may play a role in susceptibility to allergic disease. Specifically, Akdis et al. showed that allergen-specific (*Der p 1*) T cells from nonatopics produced high levels of IL-10 that were associated with elevated T-cell surface expression of IL-10R, CTLA4, TGF-βR1 and II, CD25, and PD-1 compared to those of atopic individuals. Neutralization of these suppressor pathways led to increased production of Th2 cytokines, suggesting that ligation of these inhibitory receptors on T cells by their DC ligands is critical in maintaining the balance between Th2 and tolerogenic T-cell responses (151). Taken together, these studies suggest that DCs from atopic individuals display altered costimulatory molecule patterns compared to normal individuals in response to direct stimulation with allergens and the PAMPs they may contain. Although the pattern and level of expression of costimulatory molecules on DCs and their ligands on T cells may be controlled by exogenous signals, polymorphisms in several costimulatory molecules have been shown to be associated with increased risk of development of Th2-mediated immune responses and atopic diseases such as asthma and atopic dermatitis. Specifically, polymorphisms in ICOS (1413G/A) are associated with allergic sensitization and Th2 cytokine production (152), and polymorphisms in the CTLA4 gene are associated with early-onset infant atopic dermatitis (153) and asthma (154).

Innate Immune Responses to Environmental Antigens

Allergens interact with innate recognition systems present in the mucosal layer and with various receptors present on a diversity of cells at the mucosal surface of the respiratory tract, skin, and GI tract, including epithelial cells, and phagocytic cells (dendritic cells, macrophages). As the primary interface with the environment, the epithelial cell layer represents the front-line defense against injury by pathogens or environmental irritants. Emerging evidence suggests that epithelial cells play a critical role in both antigen recognition and danger recognition. Although it is not entirely clear whether they present antigens, they actively interact with environmental antigens/allergens, both in healthy individuals and patients with allergic diseases. Allergenic particles and their associated soluble components interact directly with epithelial cells through a variety of diverse mechanisms, including (a) binding of pattern-recognition receptors, including various members of the Toll-like receptor family; and (b) activation of protease receptors (PARs). Activation of epithelial cells through these diverse pathways can induce the release of cytokines, chemokines, and growth factors that both facilitate entry of antigens into mucosa and interation with APCs, providing instructive signals to dendritic cells in the mucosa. There is mounting evidence that alterations in innate immune responses occurring at the epithelial–environmental interface may be important determinants of susceptibility or resistance to the development of allergic diseases.

Although allergens are not infectious in nature, they contain bio-organic substances (pollens, excreta of insects and mites, degraded plant products) that are actively recognized by PRRs such as TLRs. Indeed, epithelial cells cultured with various triggers of asthma have been shown to produce a number of inflammatory chemokines and cytokines in a TLR-dependent manner (155). Whether this is due to recognition of PAMPs within the allergens themselves or to endotoxin contamination is currently unknown. However, there is emerging evidence that allergens do indeed contain PAMPs that interact with various PRRs, including TLR4, TLR2, and TLR9. A requirement for PAMP recognition to induce sensitization to inhaled antigens has been shown for LPS in a murine model of OVA-induced asthma. In this model, wild-type mice were sensitized to inhaled OVA, whereas TLR4-deficient mice were not (151).

However, the relationship is complex, depending on the timing and dose of LPS exposure. LPS exposure during sensitization inhibits Th2-driven immune responses and drives a tolerogenic response *(156)*. In contrast, delivery of LPS to sensitized mice exacerbates Th2 responses (157). Moreover, the dose of LPS has been shown to be critical, as high dose exposure induces Th1 responses, whereas low-dose LPS drives Th2 immune responses (158). The exact explanation for this complexity is unknown, but it may reflect differences in the types of cells activated at different times during an immune response or to the differential expression of TLRs on different populations of DCs, as will be discussed later. The role of TLR2in Th2-mediated immune responses is complex as well. For example, delivery of the TLR2 agonist Pam3Cys along with allergen at the time of sensitization enhanced the prominent Th2-biased immune response and the symptoms of asthma in mice (159). Activation of APCs by Pam3Cys resulted in the induction of Th2-associated effector molecules such as IL-13, IL-1β, and GM-CSF and upregulation of B7RP-1 expression. In contrast, if TLR2 agonists are administered to mice previously sensitized and challenged with OVA, they markedly reduced Th2 cytokine production, airway inflammation, and IgE production *(160)*. Although Pam3CSK4 (a synthetic bacterial lipopeptide) therapy increased IFN-γ, IL-12, and IL 10 production, the anti-inflammatory effect of Pam3CSK4 was independent of IL-10 or TGF-β, but was critically dependent on IL-12. In contrast, stimulation of TLR9 by allergens as well as bacterial antigens has been shown to provide protection from the development of allergic responses (161). Despite our rudimentary understanding of the role of PAMPs in allergic responses, one may speculate that either differences in exposures to microbial products or polymorphisms in genes of the TLR pathway may both be important determinants of the risk of developing allergic disease through altering the phenotype and function of DCs. Along these lines, genetic studies show that polymorphisms of different components of innate recognition pathways may partly explain susceptibility to atopy. For instance, polymorphisms in CD14 have been shown to be associated with sCD14 levels, total IgE levels, and positive skin tests (162,163). Similarly, a polymorphism in the TLR2 gene (TLR2–16934) was shown to be a major susceptibility gene for children living on farms (164). Polymorphisms of the intracellular NOD1 protein, which binds cell wall peptidoglycans of gram-negative bacteria, were shown to be especially associated with atopic eczema and asthma (165).

Several of the common allergens (*Der p 3*, *Der p 9*, cockroach extracts, pollens) have been shown to have protease activity. Allergens containing protease activity, such as *Der p 1*, a cysteine protease, have been demonstrated to produce functional changes in the barrier function of the epithelium, probably by disrupting the epithelial tight junctions by degrading the tight junction proteins ZO-1 and desmoplakin (166). Disruption of the tight junctions may facilitate access of allergens to the underlying cells including DCs but may also directly initiate inflammatory cascades (modulate the function or immune and structural cells) in DCs and/or airway epithelium. Although the cellular mechanisms by which protease activity induces cytokine release remain unclear, members of a recently identified G-protein–coupled family of cell surface receptors, designated protease-activated receptors (PARs), have been implicated. Indeed, allergens such as the house dust mite serine proteases, *Der p 3*, *Der p 9*, cockroach extracts, and pollens activate PARs. Asokananthan et al. (167) showed that endogenous peptidases caused the release of cytokines through the activation of PAR receptors on the respiratory epithelium, and that all four members of the PAR family were expressed on respiratory epithelial cells. PAR-2 receptor activation leads to two main functional responses: production of prostaglandin E2 and production of proinflammatory cytokines (IL-8, MCP-1, IL-6). In vivo experiments in experimental allergen models support the contention that activation of PAR receptor pathways is associated with enhanced allergic responses. Specifically, PAR-2 overexpression enhanced ovalbumin-induced eosinophilia and bronchial hyperresponsiveness, whereas PAR-2 deficiency was associated with reduced allergen-driven eosinophilia and IgE production (168). As alluded to earlier, differences in DC responsiveness to allergen-derived proteases may be an important determinant of DC activation and atopic sensitization. Indeed, there is evidence that alterations in the expression of the protease receptor PAR-2 on epithelial cells may lead to greater *Der p 1* induction of DC chemokines and mediators from these cells obtained from asthmatics compared to nonatopic individuals. Taken together, these studies suggest that altered recognition and/or responsiveness to activators of the innate immune response at the epithelial–DC interface may contribute to sensitization to environmental antigens.

Altered DC Subset Distribution and Activation in Atopic Disorders

Recent evidence suggests that the development of tolerance may also be a function of specialized DC subsets (169,*170*,*171*). Although classification of DC subsets is an evolving field, in humans and in mice, multiple DC subsets have been identified based on their origin, phenotype, and function (169,*170–172*,173). Briefly, in humans, two major DC subsets have been identified that include CD11c^{high} myeloid cells (mDC) and CD11c^{low} plasmacytoid cells (pDC). mDCs are monocyte-derived cells and were originally referred to as DC1, as they were thought to produce predominantly IL-12 and drive Th1 immune responses. Plasmacytoid DCs were originally referred to as DC2, as they could promote Th2 immune responses. However, they also have the unique potential of promoting Th1 responses by releasing large amounts of type 1 IFN in the presence of viruses (174) and dampening immune responses by inducing IL-10–producing CD4$^+$ regulatory T cells *(175)*. Recent studies suggest that the function of these two subsets is variable, depending on their location and the inflammatory context. Interestingly, these two subsets have unique expression profiles of immune molecules such as TLRs and chemokine receptors, suggesting distinctive compartmentalization and specific functions of these DC subsets (176). mDCs express TLR2, TLR4, TLR5, and/or TLR3, whereas pDCs express a more restricted profile of TLRs, including TLR9 and TLR7. Thus differences in recruitment, antigen uptake, or activation of DC subsets may play a role in altered immune responses in atopic individuals.

Several lines of evidence suggest that alterations in the relative proportion of specific DC subsets taking up antigen at mucosal surfaces may play an important role in the development of immunity or tolerance. For example, adoptive transfer of myeloid DCs to the murine airway prior to antigen exposure has been shown to induce Th2-mediated immune responses to a tolerogenic antigen (177). On the other hand, Lambrecht and colleagues (178) have shown that depletion of pDCs in mice during inhalation of the normally inert antigen OVA via the airways without systemic priming led to a Th2 response and all the features of asthma, whereas adoptive transfer of pDCs before sensitization prevented disease. These results strongly suggested that pDCs may provide intrinsic protection against inflammatory responses to harmless antigens. Although the precise mechanisms by which pDCs promote tolerance are unknown, several possibilities exist. First, pDCs may deliver a negative signal to T cells or mDCs directly, through their high-level of expression of programmed death ligand 1 (179). Additionally, pDCs can produce the tryptophan-metabolizing enzyme indoleamine 2,3-dioxygenase, which has a strong inhibitory activity on T-cell proliferation (180). Another explanation for the tolerogenic properties of pDCs is related to their immature phenotype, because it has been demonstrated that immature DCs can induce Treg ex vivo (181). Moreover, human pDCs activated by CpG oligonucleotides induce the generation of Treg (175). In contrast, it is speculated that mDCs may drive the development of Th2 responses by producing IL-6, which counteracts the suppression by naturally occurring CD4$^+$CD25$^+$ Treg. Further support for the importance of DC subsets to Th2 immune responses was provided by Lewkowich et al. (82), who reported that differential susceptibility of certain murine strains to allergen-induced asthma is associated with differences in the ratio of pDCs to mDCs recruited to the lung following allergen exposure. Although the exact factors regulating the recruitment and/or activation of different DC subsets is unknown, Kohl et al. (182) have shown that complement activation at the airway surface is an important regulator of DC subset recruitment and activation. Specifically, they demonstrate that C5a preferentially results in the recrutment of pDCs to the lung, which is associated with protection against the development of Th2-mediated allergic airway responses. Taken together, these studies suggest that the balance between mDCs and pDCs may play a pivotal role in T-cell responses to antigen encounter at mucosal surfaces, with myeloid cells driving immunity while pDCs mediate tolerance to mucosal antigens. Dysregulation of the balance of mDCs and pDCs present in tissues in early life might predispose to atopic sensitization.

Because of the difficulty in sampling DC populations in tissues from atopic individuals, the role of mDC and pDCs in atopic individuals remains controversial. For example, Hagendorens et al. *(183)* compared DC populations in cord blood from children at low versus high risk of atopy and did not detect any differences. In contrast, a moderate reduction in pDC numbers in the blood was reported in atopic asthmatic children compared with healthy controls, which the authors suggested might be due to increased migration of pDCs to the target organ. In contrast, Matsuda et al. *(184)* showed that adult patients with asthma have increased numbers of pDCs in the blood compared to healthy controls. However, Upham showed that mDC numbers were reduced in the blood of patients after allergen challenge, suggesting that circulating mDCs are being recruited to the airway mucosa (136). In atopic dermatitis patients, Hashizume et al. reported an overall increase in the numbers of DCs in the blood, with a relative increase in pDCs over mDCs *(185)*. However, when DCs were evaluated in the nasal epithelium of atopic rhinitis patients, the number of pDCs was reduced. Although there is controversy as to the relative proportion of individual DC subsests present in the blood and tissues of atopic individuals, there is evidence that DC subsets may be functionally different between atopic and healthy individuals. Specifically, *Der p 1*–pulsed mDCs from healthy donors produced IL-10, whereas mDCs from allergic patients did not *(186)*. Although the study of DC subsets in human disease is in its infancy, taken together, these studies suggest that differences in the balance of DC subsets and their activation state may play an important role in determining the development of tolerance or immunity to environmental antigens. However, additional studies of DC subsets in relevant tissues are needed.

DC Cytokine Regulation of Th2 Differentiation in Allergic Disease

One of the most important variables in instruction of T-cell differentiation comes from the local cytokine milieu at the time of antigen presentation. Although much is still to be learned about these factors, well-documented examples are Th1 cell polarizing factors such as IL-12, and IL-27. Th2 cell polarizing factors include IL-6, TSLP,

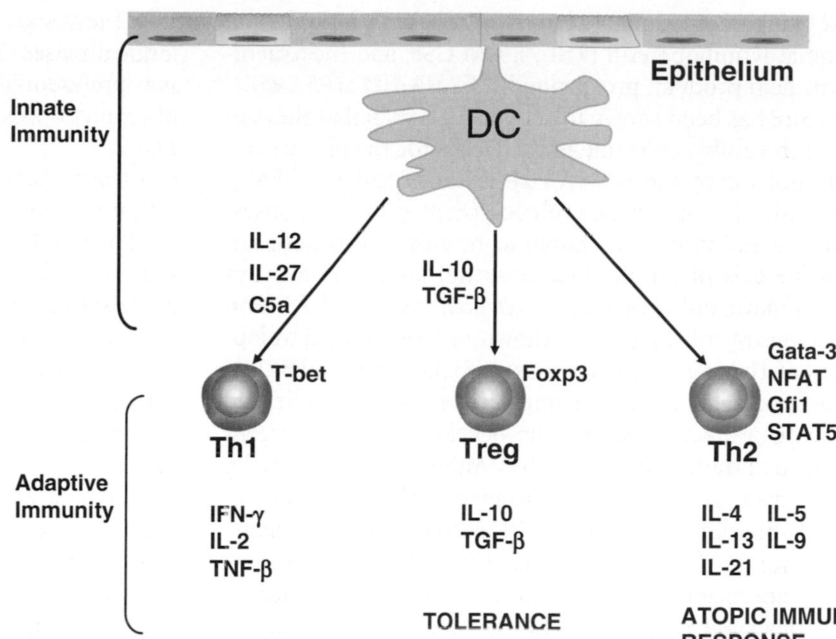

FIGURE 43.3 Cytokines and downstream transcription factors are important in instructing T-cell differentiation to Th1-cells (IL-12, IL-27), Th2-cells (IL-6, TSLP, GM-CSF, PGE_2, IL-4), or T-regulatory cells (IL-10, TGF-β).

GM-CSF, PGE_2, and IL-4. Treg cell polarizing factors include IL-10 and TGF-β (Figure 43.3). Alterations in either the production of, or responsiveness to, these signals could lead to the development of aberrant Th2 immune responses in atopic individuals. Indeed, there is evidence to support each of these possibilities.

Potential Dysregulation of Th2 Differentiation Factors in Atopy

The exact mechanisms regulating differentiation of uncommitted T-cell responses into Th2 cells remain obscure. However, factors released by DC themselves (IL-6) or factors produced by the surrounding tissues (TSLP, PGE_2, GM-CSF) may play an important role in regulating DC cytokine production and subsequent T-cell responses. In addition, T cells in atopic individuals may respond more strongly to Th2-differentiating stimuli as a result of primary alterations in transcription factors regulating Th2 differentiation.

IL-6 has been shown to be an important determinant of Th2 cell differentiation, as it is secreted by cells of the innate immune system and induces the expansion of Th2 effector cells *(187)*. The mechanism by which IL-6 drives Th2 differentiation is controversial, as some studies suggest that IL-6 is able to polarize naïve $CD4^+$ T cells to effector Th2 cells by inducing the initial production of IL-4 in $CD4^+$ T cells (188), whereas other studies suggest that IL-6 produced by mucosal DCs impedes Th1 immune responses via suppression of DC IL-12 rather than through induction of IL-4 *(189)*. Additionally, IL-6 released by DCs has been shown to inhibit the suppressive function of $CD4^+CD25^+$ Treg cells, thus inhibiting the development of tolerance (190). More recent studies suggest that IL-6 plays a complex role in Th2 differentiation through distinct actions mediated via its binding of the membrane and soluble forms of its receptor *(191)*. Specifically, IL-6 can bind to the soluble IL-6R, and through a mechanism called trans signaling, induces proliferation of cells expressing the cognate receptor gp130. This mechanism appears to be used for proliferation by developed Th2 cells in the airways, as blockade of the soluble IL-6R with the fusion protein gp130Fc reduces Th2 cells in the lung. In contrast, through the membrane-bound IL-6R, IL-6 controls $CD4^+CD25^+$ survival, as well as the initial stages of Th2 cell development in the lung. In support of a role for IL-6 in allergic disorders, serum levels of sIL-6R are increased in patients with asthma and are further increased during a spontaneous attack or following experimental allergen challenge (192). Although the mechanisms of altered IL-6 production are unknown, several triggers of allergic asthma (i.e., allergens, pollutants, ozone) induce IL-6 production in the epithelial cells lining mucosal tissues. Furthermore, variants in the IL-6 gene have been associated with hayfever and atopy *(193)*. Through the ability of IL-6 both to suppress Treg function and to inhibit Th1 differentiation, IL-6 signaling may drive Th2 cell differentiation in atopic disorders.

Epithelial cells lining mucosal tissues release a number of mediators in response to triggers of allergic disease such as allergens (i.e., *Der p 1*, *Pen ch 13* [aspergillus], cockroach antigens (194), viral infections (RSV), and pollutants (cigarette smoke, ozone, particulate matter) that may contribute to the instruction of T cells by DCs to polarize to a

Th2 cytokine–producing phenotype. These include thymic stromal lymphopoietin (TSLP), GM-CSF, and the arachidonic acid product, prostaglandin E2 (PGE2) *(195,196)*.

TSLP has been shown to activate DCs such that they acquire the ability to prime naïve T cells for the production of pr-inflammatory cytokines while downregulating IFN-γ and IL-10. In support of a role for TSLP in Th2 responses, TSLP levels have been shown to be elevated in both animal models of atopic disease as well as in the airways of asthmatic individuals *(197)*. Overexpression of TSLP in the lungs of mice has been shown to lead to the development of Th2 immune responses (198). In contrast, TSLPR-knockout mice develop strong Th1 responses to allergen and are protected against the development of allergen-driven asthmatic responses (199). Although the underlying mechanism of TSLP's ability to prime DCs is not known, TSLP-stimulated dendritic cells have been shown to prime human CD4$^+$ T cells into Th2 cytokine–producing cells in the absence of exogenous IL-4 and APCs. Interestingly, IL-4 blockade inhibited TSLP-mediated Th2 differentiation, demonstrating that IL-4 is involved in this process. Further analysis has shown that TSLP-induced Th2 differentiation is dependent on Stat6 and independent of IL-2. Moreover TSLP treatment leads to immediate, direct IL-4 gene transcription *(200)*. Although the mechanisms by which TSLP induces Th2 cytokine production are unknown, one mechanism that has been postulated is that TSLP induces DCs to express OX40 ligand (OX40L) but not IL-12. In support of this contention, TSLP-induced OX40L on DCs was required for triggering naïve CD4$^+$ T cells to produce IL-4, -5, and -13 (201). Taken together, these studies suggest that TSLP production at the mucosal surface may be an important determinant of polarized Th2 immune responses to environmental stimuli. The mechanisms regulating TSLP production remain to be elucidated.

GM-CSF is produced by airway epithelial cells in response to several triggers of allergic disease. It is thought to contribute to the recruitment, priming, and survival of DCs in the airways. Interestingly, overexpression of GM-CSF in the murine lung has been shown to be sufficient to prime Th2-mediated immune responses (202). Indeed, GM-CSF–dependent priming of Th2 responses occurred following challenge with ragweed *(203)*, but not when the innocuous antigen ovalbumin was delivered to the airways in the absence of added adjuvants. Although the mechanism(s) by which it preferentially leads to Th2 responses are unknown, it has been shown to be a preferential growth factor for myloid DCs.

The arachidonic acid product prostaglandin E2 (PGE2) has been shown to influence the local polarization of T cells by impairing the ability of maturing DCs to produce bioactive IL-12 p70. It has also been shown to cause early development of immature DC1 into Th2-promoting cells. In support of a role for PGE2 in Th2 immune responses, PGE2 levels are consistently elevated in patients with allergic diseases (204,*205*). As described earlier, birch pollen may preferentially induce Th2 immune responses by virtue of its phytoprostanecontent, which is a plant homolog of PGE2.

Clearly, the presence of IL-4 at the site of antigen presentation is a dominant factor in determining the likelihood for Th2 polarization of the naïve Th cell in both mice and humans. It has been noted that intranodal Th2 cells deviate bystander Th1 responses within the same lymph node toward the Th2 phenotype via secretion of IL-4, thus providing a potential mechanism for progressive spreading of sensitization to encompass additional allergen specificities in chronic atopic asthma. In support of a central role for IL-4 in Th2 polarization in atopic disorders, the results of several studies suggest that genes regulating IL-4 production may be altered in atopic diseases and in particular in asthma. First, a specific polymorphism in the IL-4 gene itself has been shown to correlate with high serum IgE levels and enhanced IL-4 gene expression *(206)*. A similar association has been reported between the T allele of the −590C/T polymorphism of the IL-4 gene promoter region and atopic dermatitis *(207)*. Moreover, several groups have shown that expression of a mutant form of the IL-4 receptor α chain in allergic patients is associated with increased IL-4 signaling (110). Furthermore support for the role of IL-4 signaling in Th2 polarization in atopic disorders is the demonstration of the importance of the signal transducer and activator of transcription protein 6 (STAT6) in development of Th2 differentiation and development of allergic responses in mice *(208)*. Indeed, elevations in STAT6 expression in asthmatic tissues have been reported *(209)*. Moreover, a GT repeat polymorphism in the first exon of the STAT6 gene has recently been associated with increased prevalence of several atopic disorders (bronchial asthma, atopic dermatitis, food allergies) *(210)*.

Another factor expressed in Th2 cells that appears to function as a potent coactivator of IL-4 gene transcription is NFAT (nuclear factor of activated T cells). Several studies in mice have shown that alterations in a number of the family members of the NFAT protein family may result in altered IL-4 gene expression and polarization of T-cell responses toward the type 2 pattern. NFAT proteins are expressed on T cells, B cells, and mast cells, and control the transcription of a number of genes relevant to allergic disorders, including IL-4. Several studies have now shown that loss of NFATC1 activity results in impaired T-lymphocyte activity and secretion of IL-4 in mice (211,212). These experiments suggest that deficiencies in this transcription factor may lead to the development of the allergic phenotype.

A transcription factor that may be more widely involved in the induction and maintenance of the Th2 pattern of cytokine secretion is GATA-3. GATA-3 belongs to a subfamily of zinc-finger transcription factors that interact with specific DNA-binding sequences in the regulatory regions of genes encoding T-helper 2–like cytokines. GATA-3, has been shown to be differentially expressed in Th2 and Th1 cells, and expression of this gene is sufficient to drive Th2 differentiation *(213)*. Altered regulation of GATA-3 expression may be important in atopy, as GATA-3 expression has been shown to be elevated in bronchoalveolar lavage fluids and bronchial biopsies of asthmatics when compared to normals *(209,214)*. Furthermore, blockade of this gene with a dominant negative mutant of GATA-3 inhibits allergic inflammation in mice (215). Recent evidence suggests that STAT5A can induce IL-4 production in naïve T cells by rendering the IL-4 gene accessible (216). However, overexpression of both STAT5A and GATA-3 provides maximal IL-4 production. Interestingly, a role for the transcriptional repressor gene growth factor independent 1 (Gfi1) in Th2 expansion has also been recently shown *(217)*.

Several other genes or chromosomal regions have been shown to be important in susceptibility to mounting Th2-driven immune responses in murine models; these include CNS-1 and TIM (T-cell immunoglobulin– and mucin domain–containing molecule). It has been shown that deletion of a noncoding segment, CNS-1 on murine chromosome 11 (human 5q), which is in the intergenic region between the IL-4 and IL-13 genes, results in the diminution of Th2 cytokine production in T cells (218). Similarly, a member of the TIM family of genes, also located on murine chromosome 11, has been shown to confer susceptibility to asthma in mice. Recent studies confirm an association of variants in TIM-1 and susceptibility to asthma (219). Although it is not currently known whether inheritance of a single gene variant or a combination of genetic variants is required to drive Th2 cell commitment in atopic individuals, considerable evidence is mounting to suggest that genetic differences in factors important in Th2 cell commitment may underlie susceptibility to development of atopic disorders.

Altered Th1-Promoting Cytokines in Atopic Disorders

Although Th2 cell polarization in atopic disorders can clearly arise as a result of aberrant expression of the genes important in Th2 differentiation, alterations in factors controlling expansion of the opposing Th1 pathways may also play an important role. In this regard, IL-12, a product of monocytes and DCs, is a primary determinant of T-cell differentiation to a Th1 pattern (220). Impaired IL-12 production has been reported in each of the atopic disorders *(221,222)*. Furthermore, successful steroid treatment was characterized by a significant increase in the numbers of cells expressing IL-12 mRNA, whereas steroid therapy in steroid-resistant patients did not result in an increase in IL-12–expressing cells. Further support for the importance of IL-12 in prevention of antigen-induced allergic airway responses has been provided by the observation that blockade of endogenous production of IL-12 in naturally resistant murine strains (C3H/HeJ) renders them susceptible to the development of allergen-induced AHR and eosinophilic inflammation *(223)*. Taken together, these studies suggest that dysregulation of endogenous IL-12 levels may be an important mechanism governing the pathogenesis of allergic disorders.

The mechanisms that give rise to alterations in IL-12 production are unclear at the present time; however, several possibilities exist, such as altered expression of the genes encoding either one or both of the individual subunits of the functional cytokine, or alternations in pathways regulating IL-12 production in DCs. To date, several studies have shown an association between IL-12B (IL-12p40) promoter polymorphisms and allergic phenotypes *(224,225)*, whereas others do not *(226)*. Alternatively, the deficient production of IL-12 in atopic disorders may occur as a result of altered regulation of DC IL-12 production by mediators and cytokines, which either positively (IFN-γ, C5a), or negatively (IL-4, PGE_2, IL-10, C3a), regulate its production. Recent studies suggest that perhaps complement components produced by cells in the mucosa, such as epithelial cells, may regulate IL-12 production *(227)*. It is postulated that C5a and C3a play a reciprocal role in regulating IL-12 production, with C5a inducing IL-12 and C3a inhibiting its production *(227)*. Interestingly, allergens such as house dust mite contain proteases that cleave both C5 and C3 into their active fragments, suggesting that allergens may directly activate complement and thereby regulate the type of immune response elicited at the mucosal surface *(13)*. Consistent with a potential role for complement, several studies have now demonstrated that animals deficient in either C3 or C3a do not develop allergic airway responses and have reduced Th2 cytokine production compared to wild-type mice (228,229). Conversely, lack of a functional C5 gene renders mice susceptible to development of allergen-driven Th2 immune responses (230). Support for a role for complement in human atopic diseases is provided by recent studies demonstrating enhanced expression of complement components in airway tissues from asthmatics (228) and the association of polymorphisms in complement genes, C5 *(140,141)*, and C3 *(231,232)*, with asthma phenotypes.

Another member of the IL-12 family, IL-27, has been shown to play an important role in the initiation of Th1 differentiation. In addition, IL-27 has been shown to regulate the Th2 differentiation factor, GATA-3. IL-27 consists of two subunits, the Epstein–Barr virus–induced gene 3 (EBI3) and p28. The actions of IL-27 are mediated by the WSX-1 receptor chain, which is highly expressed on $CD4^+$ T lymphocytes and NK cells. IL-27/WSX-1 signaling has been shown to inhibit allergen-driven airway hyperreactivity and lung inflammation in mice (233). Moreover, a recent study suggests that a polymorphism in the IL-27p28 gene (G964A) is associated with susceptibility to asthma *(234)*. Taken together, these studies support the possibility that alterations in Th1-promoting pathways may contribute to the aberrant Th2 polarization observed in atopic disorders.

Altered Treg Cell–Promoting Cytokines in Atopic Disorders

Several lines of evidence suggest that the production of cytokines by DCs leading to Treg generation is altered in atopic individuals. The DC cytokines that are known to regulate Treg differentiation are IL-10 and TGF-β. Although altered levels of IL-10 have been observed in atopic disorders, the relationship is not straightforward. For example, there are conflicting reports about the levels of IL-10 in atopic patients, with some studies demonstrating elevations in IL-10 levels in bronchial biopsies *(235)*, PBMCs *(236)*, bronchoalveolar lavage fluids *(237)*, and in the gut mucosa of asthmatic patients *(238)*, while others report diminished IL-10 production in sputum from asthmatic patients *(239)* and isolated T cells from children with asthma or atopic dermatitis *(240)*. Results from animal studies show similar disparities. IL-10–knockout mice have been shown to have both reduced allergic responses *(241)* as well as enhanced responses to allergen challenge (242). Investigators have suggested that the discrepancies in the results of studies with IL-10–deficient mice may be dependent on the genetic background of the strain (242). In contrast, studies in which animals have been treated with recombinant IL-10 *(243)* or overexpress the IL-10 gene (244) uniformly demonstrate that IL-10 suppresses inflammation and decreases development of Th2-mediated immune responses. Moreover, adoptive transfer of IL-10–expressing DC cells induced tolerance to allergen exposure (245). The variability in the results may reflect the pleiotrophic actions of IL-10 during the course of allergic reactions. IL-10 can clearly influence T-cell differentiation through its inhibitory actions on IL-12 as well as its ability to reduce antigen presentation to T cells by limiting class II, CD80 and CD86 expression on APCs. IL-10 not only generates tolerance in T cells, it is a potent anti-inflammatory cytokine, which can serve to dampen inflammation once initiated *(246)*. In this regard, it has been shown to reduce total and specific IgE production while increasing protective IgG4 levels *(247)*. The fact that steroids *(248)*, lactobacillus *(249)*, and standard immunotherapy regimes *(250)*, all of which successfully resolve symptoms in atopic diseases, induce IL-10 production suggests that perhaps IL-10 is protective and that IL-10 production may be impaired in atopic individuals. Diminished IL-10 production may lead both to loss of tolerance to environmental antigens as well as an inability to control inflammation once initiated. The elevations in IL-10 tissue levels observed during challenge with allergens may reflect compensatory mechanisms designed to suppress harmful inflammatory responses. In this regard, genetic polymorphisms in the promoter of the IL-10 gene (C to A change at position 571) have been associated with asthma and elevated serum IgE levels (251).

Another DC-derived factor that regulates Treg differentiation is TGF-β. Although TGF-β is a pleiotrophic cytokine, it has been shown to play an important role in Treg differentiation and function. Specifically, it plays a role in the conversion of naïve CD4 T cells into the regulatory phenotype and has been reported to mediate the cell contact–dependent suppressive activity of Treg (252). Elemental to this conversion process is induction of expression of the forkhead transcription factor, Foxp3, in $CD4^+CD25^-$ T cells by TGF-β. Importantly, in a murine asthma model, administration of these TGF-β–induced suppressor T cells prevented house dust mite–induced allergic responses *(253)*. More recent studies show that the induction of Treg suppressor function and FoxP3 expression by TGF-β is dependent on TGF-β's ability to enhance CD80:CTLA-4 interactions on T cells. Consistent with an important role for TGF-β in regulation of T-cell differentiation, several studies (253), but not all *(254)*, suggest that SNPs in the TGF-β1 gene may be associated with atopic and asthma phenotypes *(255)*.

Several other mediators commonly present in inflamed tissues regulate Treg function as well. These include the arachidonic acid product prostaglandin D2 (PGD2) and heme-oxygenase (HO-1). The mast-cell mediator, PGD2, through stimulation of the DP1 receptor, has been shown to enhance Treg function through inhibiting DC IL-12p70 and p40 expression (256,257) and increasing $Foxp3^+$ $CD4^+$ regulatory T cells that suppress inflammation in an IL-10–dependent pathway (258). HO-1 enhances the secretion of IL-10 and increases the percentage of Treg *(259)*. Collectively, these studies suggest that dysregulation of factors controlling Treg cell differentiation and/or function may predispose to the development of deleterious Th2-mediated allergic responses to environmental antigens.

Role of DCs in Secondary Immune Responses

In addition to their contribution to the primary immune response leading to sensitization, DCs are likely to contribute to secondary immune responses in atopic individuals. Several lines of evidence support the absolute requirement of these cells in the secondary response, despite the previously held view that memory/effector T cells are less dependent on costimulation and, in theory, respond to any APC such as B cells, macrophages, and even eosinophils. First, during secondary immune responses, both human and rodent DC are rapidly recruited to mucosal surfaces (134). Second, depletion of DC in allergen-primed mice completely prevented the development of Th2-mediated allergic inflammation *(260)*. Lastly, Hammad et al. (148) showed that adoptive transfer of myeloid DCs into PBMC-reconstituted hu-SCID mice boosted the production of house dust mite–specific IgE, illustrating that DCs stimulate memory Th2 cells to enhance secondary immune responses. These results provide strong evidence that DCs play a pivotal role in the primary as well as secondary response to allergens, although the mechanisms remain obscure.

Dendritic cells may play a role in secondary immune responses via their surface expression of the high-affinity IgE receptor. Indeed, CD1a$^+$ airway DCs express the α chain of the high-affinity IgE receptor. When allergen is recognized via the FcεRI on DCs, it is very efficiently targeted to the MHC class II–rich endocytic compartment, the site of peptide loading onto MHC class II. It has been suggested that the presence of IgE on DCs lowers the threshold for allergen recognition, boosting the secondary immune response by efficiently stimulating memory T cells. In support of this concept, Coyle et al. (261) showed that when allergen-specific IgE was captured by a nonanaphylactogenic anti-IgE antibody in sensitized mice, the mice failed to produce Th2 cytokines upon re-exposure to the sensitizing allergen. This perpetuation of the allergic response may indeed occur in atopic patients, in that the proportion of DCs expressing the α subunit of the high-affinity IgE receptor is significantly increased in asthmatic and atopic dermatitis patients compared to nonatopic controls *(262)*. This increase in FcεRI on DCs may also be the result of higher endogenous levels of IL-4, a known modulator of immunoglobulin Fc receptors.

Collectively, these studies suggest that altered DC function may underlie the propensity of atopic individuals to mount Th2-biased immune responses to environmental allergens. More detailed information regarding the exact mechanisms awaits further study of DC biology.

TH2 CYTOKINE REGULATION OF ALLERGIC INFLAMMATION

The dependence of the immunopathogenic consequences of allergic immune responses on Th2 cells likely stems from their pivotal role in regulating the primary effectors of both the acute and late-phase reactions, namely, IgE and eosinophils. In addition, as will be discussed in a later section, Th2 cell-derived cytokines, themselves, also serve as effector cells of the allergic response.

One of the major roles of IL-4 in allergic inflammation is as the primary inducer of immunoglobulin-class switching in B cells that leads to the synthesis and secretion of IgE (263). The importance of IL-4 to IgE synthesis has been demonstrated by the fact that neither IL-4– nor STAT6–deficient mice produce IgE *(208)*. The exact mechanisms by which IL-4 regulates IgE class switching will be discussed later. IL-13 is also able to regulate IgE synthesis in humans, but its role in IgE synthesis in mice is controversial. The combination of IL-4's effects on IgE synthesis and mast-cell growth suggests a primary role for IL-4 in the development of the early-phase response. As will be discussed in greater detail in a later section, IgE activation of mast cells leads to the synthesis and release of a number of inflammatory mediators that may contribute to the vascular, smooth muscle, and mucus changes observed in the early-phase response to allergen challenge.

Through their unique and overlapping actions IL-4, IL-13, and IL-5 coordinately regulate the development, recruitment, and activation of eosinophils. IL-4 and IL-13 have both been shown to contribute to the recruitment of eosinophils into sites of inflammation, as evidenced by the fact that inhibition of either IL-4 or IL-13 by antibody blockade, or gene deletion eliminates allergen-driven increases in tissue eosinophils (58,61). Conversely, overexpression of these cytokine genes in mice results in tissue eosinophilia (51,264). Because IL-5 has been shown to be the primary determinant of eosinophil differentiation, activation, and survival, it plays a critical role in eosinophil regulation in allergic responses. The importance of IL-5 in antigen-induced eosinophilia has been examined in numerous animal studies *(265)*. For example, blockade of endogenous IL-5 levels in antigen-sensitized guinea pigs *(265)* and in mice (49) has resulted in significant suppression of both BAL and tissue eosinophilia. More definitively, mice in which the IL-5 gene has been disrupted do not develop eosinophilic inflammation (50). Reconstitution of these mice with IL-5 completely restored aeroallergen-induced eosinophilia. Thus, through the coordinate regulation of IgE and eosinophilia, Th2 cytokines orchestrate the elicitation phase of allergic immune responses. In the next section we will discuss in more detail the steps involved in IgE regulation.

REGULATION OF IGE SYNTHESIS

Ishizaka and colleagues purified immunoglobulin E in 1966 (4,266). IgE has the shortest half-life (2.5 days) of all classes of immunoglobulins. In addition, it is present in serum at levels considerably lower than those of other immunoglobulin classes such as IgG. There is considerable heterogeneity in the levels of IgE among individuals. For example, levels of <100 ng/mL are observed in most normals, whereas IgE levels can reach as high as 1,000 ng/mL in parasitized or atopic individuals. The high variability in serum levels contrasts strikingly to other immunoglobulin isotypes and suggests that tight control of IgE may therefore be important to prevent the potentially lethal consequences of IgE-mediated inflammation. Indeed, synthesis of IgE and its receptor expression appear to be regulated by a series of steps involving both cell–cell contact with CD4+ Th2 cells and activation by cytokines secreted by these cells. In this section we will discuss our current knowledge of the complex steps involved in regulation of IgE synthesis, and expression of its receptors.

Isotype Class Switching to IgE Production

The production of IgE antibodies by B cells is triggered by a complex series of secreted signals and cell surface interactions, followed by molecular genetic rearrangements at the immunoglobulin heavy-chain locus, IgH (Figure 43.4). The first step in IgE production is the binding of allergen to allergen-specific B cells via their membrane-bound immunoglobulin receptor (BCR). The B cells then internalize and process the allergen, and present the processed allergen to T cells as peptide fragments in association with MHC class II molecules. The peptide–MHC II complex is then recognized by the TCR on Th2 cells. Initially, all B cells produce IgM antibodies. At this point, a $V_H(D)J_H$ cassette of sequences encoding the variable domain is immediately adjacent to the Cμ exons, which encode the IgM-constant regions at the 5′ end of the IgH locus. Farther downstream in IgH are several widely spaced clusters of exons. C regions encode the constant-region domains of the IgG, IgE, and IgA heavy-chain isotypes. Upon stimulation by cytokines, along with critical cell–cell interactions with CD4+ T-cell surface accessory molecules, B cells can change the isotype of the antibodies (or effector functions) they produce while retaining their original antigenic specificity. This process requires that genomic DNA be spliced and rejoined to move the VDJ elements from their location proximal to Cμ to a position many kilobases downstream, next to the C-region exons encoding the heavy chains of other isotypes. A large amount of intervening DNA is excised and discarded in this irreversible process, and therefore the mechanism is referred to as deletional switch recombination.

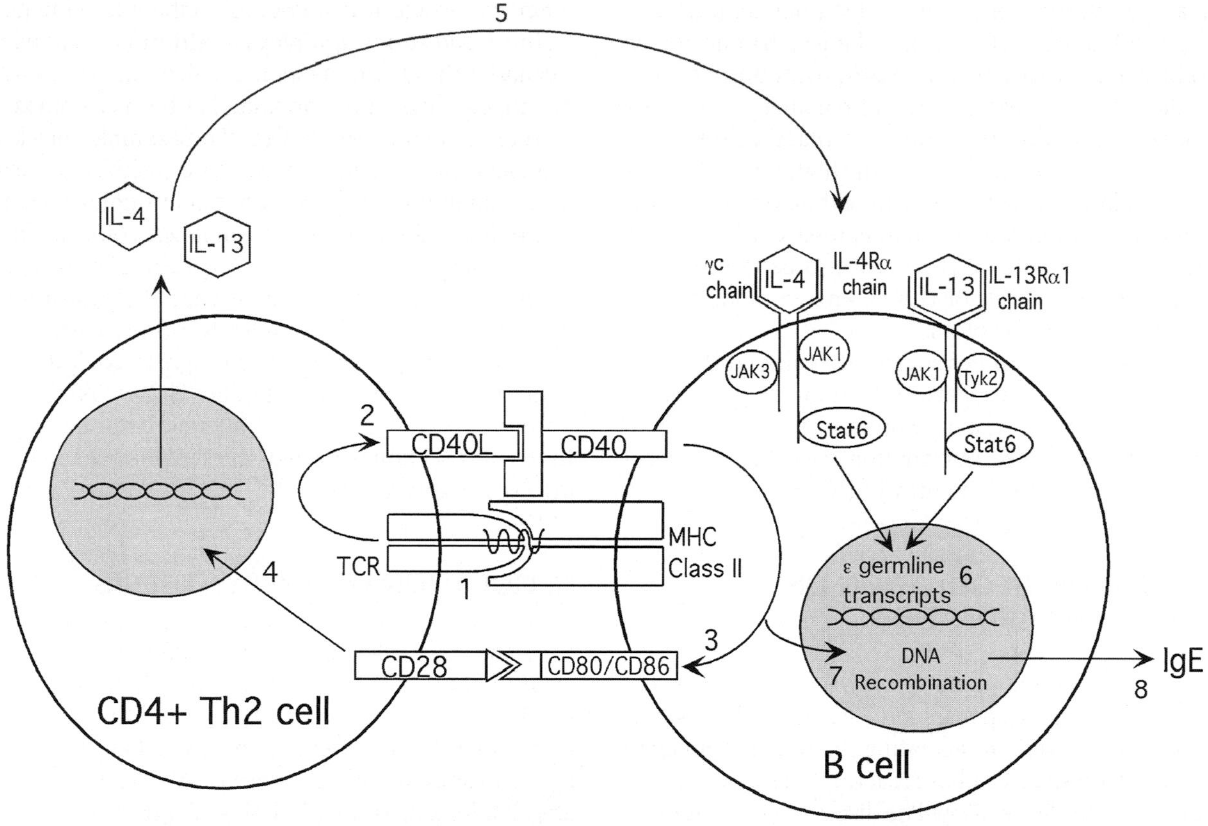

FIGURE 43.4 The regulation of IgE synthesis involves many sequential steps: *(1)* recognition of antigen/MHC class II by the T-cell receptor; *(2)* TCR activation leads to the induction of CD40 ligand on the T cell, which is then recognized by CD40 on the B cell; *(3)* CD40/CD40L cognate interaction leads to induction of CD80/CD86 on the B cell, which can then interact with CD28; *(4)* the Th2 cell secretes IL-4 and IL-13; *(5)* IL-4 and IL-13 bind their cognate receptors on B cells and result in activation of Stat6; *(6)* IL-4 and IL-13 signaling events result in initiation of transcription at the Iε promotor and the production of immature germline ε transcripts; *(7)* the CD40/CD40L interaction provides the necessary second signal required for recombination of the germline locus; *(8)* transcription of mature ε transcripts from the rearranged locus followed by translation and secretion of IgE.

Isotype switching to IgE production requires two signals (267). The first signal is provided by the Th2 cytokines IL-4 and IL-13 and is IgE isotype–specific. IL-4 and IL-13 stimulate transcription at the Cε gene locus, which contains the exons encoding the constant-region domains of the IgE ε heavy chain. This transcription is initiated at a site upstream the ε switch region designated Iε. The second signal is a B-cell–activating signal provided through CD40/CD40L interactions. Together these interactions result in induction of the necessary deletional switch recombination that brings into proximity all of the elements of a functional ε heavy chain.

The first signal for IgE class switching is provided by the T-cell–derived cytokines IL-4/IL-13. IL-4 induces RNA transcription at the Cε locus via stimulation of STAT6 through binding the type I IL-4 receptor composed of the IL-4Rα chain and the γ c chain. IL-13 has also been shown to regulate IgE class switching in humans through binding the type II IL-4 receptor composed of the IL-4Rα and IL-13Rα1 chains. However, there is considerable controversy about the role of IL-13 in IgE class switching in mice. Following either IL-4 or IL-13 binding to its respective receptor complex, JAK kinases phosphorylate tyrosine residues in the intracellular domains of the receptor chains, providing docking sites for STAT6. These STAT6 molecules become phosphorylated and then form homodimers that translocate to the nucleus. In the nucleus they bind to specific sequences (TTCN(N)GAA) in the promoter of IL-4/IL-13–responsive genes, including Iε. The importance of STAT6 in IL-4–induced isotype switching is supported by the fact that germline transcription and IgE class switching are markedly impaired in STAT6-deficient mice (268). Other transcription factors are also important in induction of germline transcription of the Cε locus. The importance of NF-κB for the induction of germline transcripts has been recently confirmed by the finding that expression of germline transcripts for Cε are severely diminished in NF-κB p50 knockout mice *(269)*.

IL-4– and/or IL-13–induced transcription factor binding to the Cε locus results in germline transcription of the Cε locus (Figure 43.5). Germline transcripts originate from a 5′ promoter of the Iε exon, which is located just upstream of the 4 Cε exons. IL-4 induces the appearance of 1.7- to 1.9-kb germline Cε transcripts that contain an Iε exon, located 2 kb upstream of Sε, spliced to the Cε1 to Cε4 exons. After processing, the mature germline mRNA's include the 140-bp Iε exon and exons Cε1 to Cε4. These transcripts have been referred to as sterile, because of the presence of stop codons in each of the three reading frames of Iε . However, it is the process of transcription itself that appears to facilitate the deletional switch recombination event. For example, Harriman et al. (270) analyzed IgA switching using mice retaining a normal Iα promoter in which the Iα exon was replaced by an HPRT minigene, and found that switching can occur to the locus despite the absence of complete Iα-containing transcripts. This has been

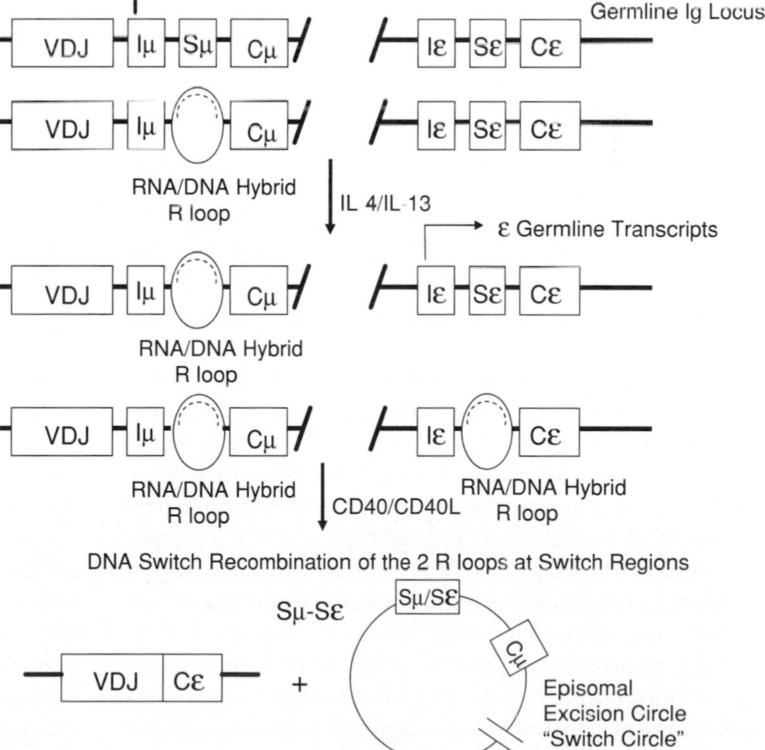

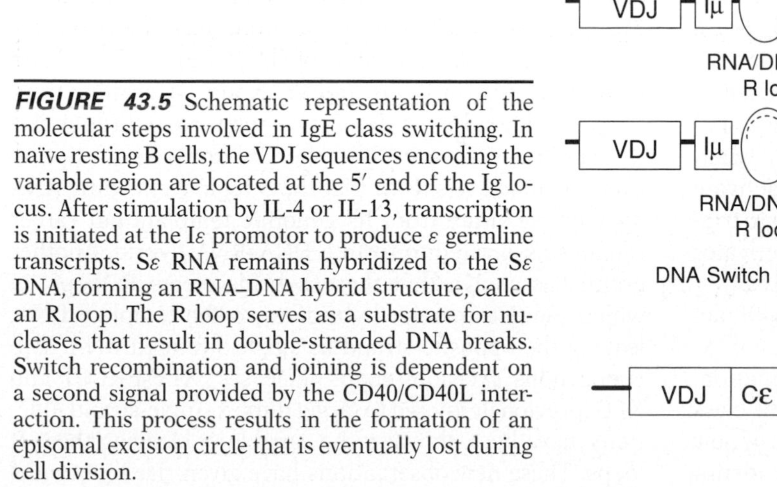

FIGURE 43.5 Schematic representation of the molecular steps involved in IgE class switching. In naïve resting B cells, the VDJ sequences encoding the variable region are located at the 5′ end of the Ig locus. After stimulation by IL-4 or IL-13, transcription is initiated at the Iε promotor to produce ε germline transcripts. Sε RNA remains hybridized to the Sε DNA, forming an RNA–DNA hybrid structure, called an R loop. The R loop serves as a substrate for nucleases that result in double-stranded DNA breaks. Switch recombination and joining is dependent on a second signal provided by the CD40/CD40L interaction. This process results in the formation of an episomal excision circle that is eventually lost during cell division.

demonstrated at the Cε locus in that switch recombination occurred at the Cε locus when the Iε exon and promoter were intact but Cε exons were absent (271).

The second signal for IgE class switching is dependent on cell-to-cell contact between T and B cells. Specifically, the interaction between CD40 on the surface of B cells with CD40L on the T-cell surface is critical to drive the IgE switch to completion and lead to IgE production. CD40 is a 50-kDa surface glycoprotein that is constitutively expressed on all human B lymphocytes. CD40L is transiently induced on T cells after stimulation of the T-cell receptor by antigen/MHC complexes. Binding of newly expressed CD40L with CD40 on B cells provides the second signal for induction of deletional switch recombination to IgE.

Several lines of evidence support a critical role for CD40/CD40L interactions in isotype switching. First, it had been shown by numerous groups that isotype switching requires the presence of and contact with T cells. After an extensive search for the T-cell contact signal, it was discovered that CD40/CD40L interactions were responsible for the T-cell dependency of this process. Proof of this was provided by the observation that activation of CD40L could completely substitute for T-cell help (272). Furthermore, a soluble form of CD40 inhibits its interactions with CD40L, blocking IL-4–driven IgE synthesis in human B cells (273). Lastly, genetic deficiencies in CD40L or CD40 in humans and mice, respectively, disrupt IgE synthesis. In humans, CD40L is encoded on the X chromosome, and individuals with the X-linked hyper-IgM syndrome are deficient in CD40L. Their B cells are unable to produce IgG, IgA, or IgE *(274)*. Similarly, mice that are deficient in either the CD40L or CD40 genes have the same defect in antibody production (275,276).

CD40/CD40L interactions are thought to provide a second signal via stimulation of a number of signaling pathways that likely synergize with those initiated by IL-4 and IL-13 to achieve e-germline transcription. Specifically, after interaction with CD40L on the B-cell surface, CD40 aggregation triggers signal tranduction through four intracellular proteins, which belong to the family of TNF receptor–associated factors (TRAFs). TRAFs 2, 5, 6 are known to associate with the intracytoplasmic domain of CD40 after its multimerization by interaction with CD40L. TRAF-2, TRAF-5, and TRAF-6 promote the dissociation of NF-κB from its inhibitor, IκB. In turn, NF-κB can synergize with STAT6 induced by IL-4/IL-13 signaling to activate the Iε promoter, as described previously. In addition to triggering TRAF associations, engagement of CD40 activates protein tyrosine kinases (PTKs), such as JAK kinases.

Another mechanism by which cytokine and CD40L activation may induce class switching is via induction of expression of proteins required in deletional recombination. Specifically, both cytokine and CD40L induction of class switching have been shown to require the synthesis of new proteins. One of these proteins has been recently identified as activation-induced cytidine deaminase (AID) *(277)*. AID is expressed in activated B cells and in germinal centers of lymph nodes. Mice that are deficient in AID have a dramatic impairment in isotype switching, with elevated IgM levels and low or absent IgE, IgG, and IgA isotypes (278). Interestingly, a rare autosomal form of hyper-IgM syndrome has now been attributed to mutations in this gene *(279)*. Although these studies suggest that this protein is critical to isotype switching, the mechanisms by which it participates in switch recombination remain obscure at present. AID has homology to the RNA editing enzyme APOBEC, which modifies specific sites in ApoB precursor RNA to give rise to a transcript encoding the functional apoB48 protein. AID might execute a similar RNA-editing function in B cells, processing pre-RNA–encoding proteins involved in the mechanisms of switch recombination and hypermutation. Alternatively, AID might mediate the construction of ribozymes, complex RNA structures with nuclease activity, or it could act directly on DNA substrates in the heavy-chain locus. Currently, the weight of evidence favors the action of AID as a DNA-editing enzyme.

Deletional Switch Recombination

Following the delivery of both IL-4 and CD40/CD40L signals, deletional switch recombination occurs through a series of molecular events that are not yet fully understood (271,280). However, the current data are consistent with a model in which IL-4/IL-13–driven transcription originating at the Iε promoter alters the ε heavy-chain locus in a way that permits isotype switch recombination. However, because the ε-germline transcripts do not encode a functional protein, their precise role in isotype switching has long eluded investigators. Recently a number of reports have begun to shed light on this subject. It appears that germline transcripts participate in the assembly of complex DNA–RNA hybrid structures, which then target nucleases to the ε locus for the initial DNA cleavage in the cut-and-paste reaction of deletional switch recombination. In deletional switch recombination at the ε locus, DNA cleavage and ligation are carried out within the switch (Sε) cassette, which contains repeats of GAGCT and GGGGT and is located between the Iε and Cε exons. ε-Germline transcripts, originating at the Iε promoter, pass through the Sε region and then on into the Cε exons. Transcription experiments have shown that the S region–encoding RNA does not separate from its genomic template but rather remains associated to form a DNA–RNA hybrid. Another group has shown that these hybrids create R loops, in which the S transcript hybridizes to the template DNA, leaving the opposite strand as single-stranded DNA. Two endogenous excision-repair nucleases, XPF-ERCC1 and XPG, previously known to target duplex single-strand junctions, have been shown to be capable of cleaving these R loops. These new observations have given rise to a model in which R loops formed by the association of Sε RNA with its Sε genomic template serve as substrates for nucleases that generate double-strand DNA breaks in the first step of deletional switching. In later steps, these breaks can be annealed by DNA end joining to analogous breaks in Sμ, located between $V_H(D)J_H$ and the Cμ exons. This rearrangement brings the $V_H(D)J_H$ segments encoding the antigen-binding site into the immediate proximity of the Cε exons encoding the constant domains. The product of this recombination is the de novo generation of a complete multiexon gene that can be transcribed as a single message encoding the full ε heavy chain. Although these new reports establish the existence of R loops and demonstrate that these two nucleases can cleave these structures, it has not been definitively shown that these enzymes are the nucleases relevant to the deletional isotype switch mechanism. The specific nucleases used by B cells still need to be identified. These proteins may be constitutively expressed in B cells, but, as discussed previously, proteins such as AID may be induced as a result of either IL-4/IL-13 or CD40/CD40L interactions.

Negative Regulation of IgE Synthesis

Several cytokines, including TGF-β, IFN-α, and IFN-γ, can inhibit IL-4-dependent IgE synthesis in both mice *(281)* and humans *(282)*. IFN-γ suppresses the expression of ε-germline transcripts in murine B cells stimulated with IL-4 and LPS. IFN-γ may affect recombination events without affecting the expression of ε-germline transcripts. Other agents, including IL-12 *(283)* and IL-10 (247), have been reported to inhibit IgE while enhancing IgG4 *(283)*. Interestingly, the Th2 cytokine IL-21 has recently been shown to inhibit IgE isotype class switching and IgE^+ cell clonal expansion (284). Although the exact mechanism by which IL-21 regulates IgE production is not entirely understood, it is thought that IL-21 directly antagonizes IL-4 and LPS-induced Iε switch recombination (285). Because IL-21 does not alter proliferation or STAT6 phosphorylation of murine B cells in response to IL-4, the mechanism is unknown. Another mechanism of regulation of IgE is through the competition with IL-4–driven IgG4-blocking antibodies. IgE-mediated hypersensitivity reactions are rare in patients with chronic helminth infections, even though FcεRI-bearing cells are sensitized with antiparasite IgE. The inhibition of allergic reactivity is due mainly to IgG4-blocking antibodies, as evidenced by the fact that the depletion of IgG4 specifically removes the blocking activity from the sera of microfilaremic patients. IgG4-blocking activity has also been detected in patients receiving immunotherapy for insect venom *(286)* and house dust mite hypersensitivity *(287)*. Blocking IgG4 competes with cell-bound IgE for allergen binding. Because the IgG4 molecule is functionally monovalent, does not fix complement, and binds weakly to Fcγ receptors, antigen binding to IgG4 has no harmful consequences. However, competition between IgG4 and IgE can occur only if the two antibody isotypes have at least in part the same antigen specificity. A molecular mechanism for this overlap in specificity was provided by the demonstration that isotype switching can occur sequentially from IgM to IgE through IgG4. This has been formally demonstrated, in that IgG antibody in mice can completely suppress IgE-mediated anaphylaxis (288).

IgE Receptors

The two major Fc receptors for IgE are called FcεRI and FcεRII (CD23) *(289)*. They are distinguished by their structure and their relative affinities for IgE. The high-affinity IgE receptor FcεRI binds monomeric IgE with an affinity constant of 1010 M^{-1}, whereas CD23 binds with a much lower affinity (10^8 M^{-1}). The high-affinity receptors are constitutively expressed at high levels on mast cells and basophils. They are also found, albeit at lower levels, on peripheral blood dendritic cells, monocytes, and human Langerhans cells. The low-affinity receptor is also expressed on a wide variety of cells, including B cells, T cells, Langerhans cells, monocytes, macrophages, platelets, and eosinophils.

FcεRI-Mediated Signal Transduction

The FcεRI is a member of the multisubunit immune response receptor (MIRR) family of cell surface receptors that lack intrinsic enzymatic activity but transduce intracellular signals through association with cytoplasmic tyrosine kinases *(289)*. In rodents, FcεRI is expressed on mast cells and basophils as a heterotetramer consisting of a single IgE-binding α subunit, a β subunit, and two disulfide-linked γ subunits. The α chain consists of two extracellular Ig-like loops, a single transmembrane region containing an aspartic acid residue, and a short cytoplasmic domain that lacks signal transduction motifs. The charged amino acid within the transmembrane domain mediates the association of the α subunit with the signaling component of the γ subunit. The β subunit consists of four membrane-spanning domains and a cytoplasmic tail capable of transducing intracellular signals that amplify γ-mediated signaling events. In rodents, all three subunits are required for the cell surface expression of FcεRI *(289,290)*. In contrast, in humans the receptor can be expressed as two different isoforms, a tetramer ($\alpha,\beta,\gamma 2$) or a trimer ($\alpha\gamma 2$). The tetrameric complex ($\alpha\beta\gamma 2$) is expressed on mast cells and basophils, whereas the trimer is expressed on Langerhans cells, dendritic cells, monocytes and macrophages, and eosinophils.

FcεRI signaling occurs upon IgE binding to the receptor. This requires two sequential events: (a) binding of IgE antibody to the FcεRI and (b) crosslinking of IgE antibody by bivalent or multivalent antigen. Crosslinking of the receptor initiates a coordinated sequence of biochemical and morphologic events that result in: (a) exocytosis of secretory granules containing histamine and other performed mediators; (b) synthesis and secretion of newly formed lipid mediators, such as prostaglandins and leukotrienes; and (c) synthesis and secretion of cytokines. Although the exact signaling pathways governing each of these functions are not known, the following model has been proposed. The β and γ subunits each contain a conserved immunoreceptor tyrosine-based activation motif (ITAM) within their cytoplasmic tails that is rapidly phosphorylated on tyrosine after FcεRI aggregation (*290*,291). Tyrosine phosphorylation of the β and γ ITAMs is mediated by Lyn, which is constitutively associated with the β subunit and activated after antigen-mediated FcεRI aggregation. FcεRI crosslinking leads to recruitment and activation of the tyrosine kinase Syk, which binds to the tyrosine-phosphorylated γ ITAMS through its tandem SH2 domains *(289)*. Recruitment of Syk occurs upstream of several signal transduction pathways. The importance of Syk is demonstrated by using Syk-deficient mast cells, which fail to degranulate, synthesize leukotrienes, and secrete cytokines after FcεRI stimulation *(292)*. Ultimately, this pathway leads to the activation of MAP kinases, and activation of PKC pathways. PKC pathways are thought to be important in exocytosis and granule-content release and gene expression. Activation of MAP kinases also regulates the enzymatic activity of PLA_2, leading to generation of a variety of lipid mediators (PAF, PGD_2, and LTC_4). Antigen-mediated aggregation of FcεRI also stimulates the recruitment and activation of p21ras, which has been implicated in FcεRI-induced cytokine transcription and secretion *(289)*.

Regulation of FcεRI Surface Expression

Although the expression of FcεRI on the surface of mast cells appears to occur early in their differentiation and/or maturation in vivo, the levels are known to be regulated by several factors postmaturation. Studies in both mice and humans have revealed that the levels of FcεRI on mast cells can be regulated by IgE itself as well as by Th2 cytokines. Indeed, atopic individuals with high serum IgE levels show markedly upregulated mast cell and basophil FcεRI levels (293,*294*). Moreover, anti-IgE treatment of atopic individuals results in downregulation of FcεRI expression on human basophils *(295)*. Further evidence is provided by murine studies in which IgE-deficient mice exhibit dramatically reduced levels of receptors on mast cells and basophils. Because IgE-deficient mice still express receptors, albeit at lower levels, other mechanisms of regulation are thought to exist. In fact, cytokines such as IL-4 and IL-13 have been shown to upregulate FcεRIα expression on mast cells, basophils, and monocytes. Glucocorticoids have been shown to inhibit IL-4– and IL-13–induced upregulation of the FcεRIα chain on monocytes *(296)*. Together these results suggest that, through a multistep positive feedback process, Th2 cytokines enhance both the production of IgE and the expression of its receptor, which lead to further mast-cell activation and release of Th2 cytokines in the local microenvironment, serving to perpetuate the allergic response.

Mast-cell activation is subject to negative regulation by a growing family of structurally and functionally related inhibitory receptors. These include FcγRIIB, CTLA4, killer cell inhibitory receptors (KIRs), and gp^{49b1} on mast cells. Indeed, gp^{45b1}-deficient mice exhibit more severe anaphylactic reactions than their normal counterparts (297). Each of these receptors possesses an immunoreceptor tyrosine-based inhibitory motif (ITIM). Coaggregation of FcεRI and these inhibitory receptors on the surface of mast cells results in inhibition of FcεRI-induced mast-cell activation *(298,299)*. In general, inhibitory receptors are thought to inhibit the actions of activation receptors containing ITAM motifs by recruiting phosphatases through an immunoreceptor tyrosine-based inhibition motif (ITIM) (300).

FcεRII (CD23)

In humans, CD23 (FcεRII, B-cell differentiation antigen) is a Ca^{2+}-dependent C-type lectin of 45 kDa. It has wide distribution among hematopoietic and structural cells and exists in two forms, CD23a, and CD23b, resulting from alternative splicing at the N terminus and differing by five amino acids in the cytoplasmic domain. The isoforms of CD23 are found on B cells; one is constitutively expressed (CD23a), whereas the other form, CD23b, is induced by factors such as IL-4 (301) and CD40L in conjunction with IL-4. CD23b is also found on non-B cells such as T cells, Langerhans cells, monocytes, macrophages, platelets, and eosinophils *(302,303)* and mediates different biologic functions. The b form has been shown to be associated with phagocytosis of soluble IgE complexes, while the a form is associated with endocytosis of IgE-coated particules *(304)*.

Structurally, CD23 presents a single membrane-spanning domain followed by an extracellular domain that consists of three regions: the α-helical coiled-coil stalk region, which mediates the formation of trimers, followed by the lectin head, which binds IgE, and at the C terminus a short tail containing an inverse RGD sequence, a common recognition site of integrins *(305,306)*. CD23 is cleaved at the membrane to yield a series of soluble fragments. sCD23s of varying molecular weights arise by an autocatalytic process involving matrix metalloproteinase cleavage of membrane-bound CD23. The endogenous proteases that participate in CD23 shedding have not been identified. However, interestingly, *Der p 1*, the major house dust mite antigen, has been shown to selectively cleave CD23 and to promote IgE synthesis (16). CD23 expression is upregulated by several factors, including by its ligand, IgE *(307)*, and by IL-4 (301). On the other hand, IFN-γ counteracts the inducing effect of IL-4 on CD23 expression.

CD23 is thought to mediate a number of effects, including regulation of IgE synthesis, antigen presentation, proliferation and differentiation of B cells, and activation of monocytes, effects that can be ascribed to the membrane and soluble forms of CD23 *(306,308)*. Binding of IgE to the membrane-bound form of the receptor transduces an inhibitory signal that prevents further IgE synthesis *(309)*. In contrast, the soluble forms described previously upregulate IgE production, and their release has been found to be inhibited by IgE binding *(310)*. Soluble CD23 also ligates CD11b/CD11c to promote release of proinflammatory mediators such as IL-1β, IL-6, and TNF-α (311).

CD23 expression on B cells and monocytes and sCD23 production is markedly increased in allergic disorders *(33,312,313)*. Moreover, reduction of allergen-induced CD23 expression on B cells has been observed after successful desensitization therapy *(314)*. Dysregulation of the CD23 pathway in atopic patients might be part of their propensity to develop IgE antibodies and of an enhancement of the inflammatory reaction, through the action of sCD23 as well as through IgE-dependent triggering of CD23 on non–B cells.

EFFECTOR CELLS OF THE ALLERGIC RESPONSE

Overview

Once a genetically susceptible individual is sensitized to a given allergen and IgE antibody has been formed, subsequent exposure to allergens readily induces the manifestations of atopic disease. Although these responses are generally a continium, they have been categorized into three types based on their temporal sequence: (a) acute or immediate responses, (b) late-phase reactions, and (c) chronic allergic inflammation.

Exposure of a sensitized individual to allergens results in immediate reactions, the characteristics of which depend on the site of entry of the allergen. In the nasal mucosa, allergen provocation of sensitized individuals results in sneezing, itching, and nasal discharge. Acute allergic reactions, elicited in the skin at the sites of allergen injection, are characterized by intense itching, redness, and edema. In asthmatic patients subjected to allergen inhalation, these mediators rapidly elicit bronchial mucosa edema, mucus production, and smooth muscle constriction. Acute or immediate responses are thought to be due to the release of preformed mediators released by antigen interaction with Fc receptors and IgE on IgE-bearing cells (mast cells and basophils). The release of mast-cell products produces multiple local effects, including enhanced local vascular permeability (leading to leakage of plasma proteins, including fibrogen, resulting in local deposition of cross-linked fibrin and tissue swelling), increased cutaneous blood flow, with intravascular fluid from postcapillary venules, producing erythema), and other effects, such as itching, due to the stimulation of cutaneous sensory nerves by histamine. Typically, these reactions are detectable within a few minutes of allergen challenge, reach a maximum in 30 to 60 minutes, then rapidly wane.

In many individuals the acute phase is followed by what has been termed a late-phase reaction (LPR) that occurs within 6 to 48 hours after allergen exposure and can persist for several days in the absence of therapy. The characteristic signs and symptoms of late-phase reactions are reddening and swelling of the skin, sneezing and nasal discharge, and wheezing and cough upon lower-airway challenge. Late-phase reactions are thought to occur as a result of recruitment of circulating leukocytes to the site of allergen exposure following antigen presentation to T cells. Both eosinophils and T cells are assumed to mediate the late-phase response. However, mast cells may also contribute to the late-phase response. The importance of leukocyte recruitment is supported by the fact that a variety of treatments, which are associated with a reduction in leukocyte recruitment that is elicited at sites of LPRs, can also reduce the signs and symptoms of these responses.

In naturally occurring allergic diseases, patients typically experience repeated exposure to the offending allergens over a period of weeks to years. Although the specific features of pathology of each of these diseases vary according to the anatomic site affected, it has been generally recognized that the structural changes that occur in each tissue are due to the persistence of inflammation. These tissue changes range from thickened skin and fibrotic papules to extensive remodeling of the airway wall with smooth muscle hypertrophy, subepithelial fibrosis, and mucus cell hypertrophy. In each case, these structural changes are associated with significant alterations in their function.

Development of Mast Cells and Basophils

History and Overview

Mast cells and basophils were discovered by Paul Ehrlich in the late 1800s, based on staining of their cytoplasmic granules with aniline and basophilic dyes, respectively *(315)*. It was once thought that basophils might be circulating precursors of mast cells or that mast cells were "tissue basophils," but current evidence suggest that they are indeed distinct cell types. Although these cell types have unique functions and release a unique profile of mediators, they also produce an overlapping array of mediators that are known to contribute to the allergic diathesis. It is hypothesized that IgE produced by allergen-reactive

B cells binds to FcεR receptors present on the surface of mast cells and basophils, and that when challenged with allergen, these cells release vasoactive mediators as well as chemotactic factors and cytokines that promote leukocyte infiltration and exacerbate the inflammatory response. Through the production and release of these proinflammatory molecules, mast cells and basophils set into motion a series of events that result in immediate responses to allergens in the skin, lungs, and nose of atopic individuals and may also contribute to the late-phase response.

Basophils

Basophils are a small population of peripheral blood leukocytes containing cytoplasmic granules that stain with basophilic dyes. They typically exhibit a segmented nucleus with marked condensation of nuclear chromatin and contain round or oval cytoplasmic granules. Basophils are thought to arise from pluripotent $CD34^+$ progenitors found in cord blood, peripheral blood, and bone marrow. They have been suggested to evolve from $CD34^+$/IL-$3R\alpha^+$/IL-5^+ eosinophil/basophil progenitors, as supported by the occurrence of granulocytes with a hybrid eosinophil/basophil phenotype in patients with chronic or acute myelogenous leukemia or in cell culture *(316–318)*. Unlike mast cells, basophils differentiate and mature in the bone marrow and then circulate in the blood, where they constitute <1% of circulating leukocytes. IL-3 appears to be an important developmental factor for basophils *(319)*, although many other growth factors, such as IL-5, GM-CSF, TGF-α, and nerve growth factor, likely influence their development *(320–322)*. Like mast cells, basophils possess high-affinity IgE receptors (FcεR1) that are cross-linked upon engagement of receptor-bound IgE with corresponding antigens, resulting in release of a number of mediators that are in part common for both cell types.

The study of basophil biology has been severely hampered by the lack of specific markers for detection of basophils in tissues and the inability to isolate significant numbers of these cells from peripheral blood. Participation of basophils in allergic reactions has traditionally been documented by indirect means, such as by determining the pattern of mast-cell– or basophil–specific mediators such as histamine (derived from both), PGD_2 (mast cells only), and LTC_4 (primarily from basophils). Despite the difficulties in studying basophils, recent studies suggest that they rapidly produce large amounts of the immunoregulatory cytokines IL-4 and IL-13 and constitutively express CD40L and CCR3 on their surface. These findings, taken together with the demonstration that they are rapidly recruited to the skin (323), lung *(324)*, and nose *(325)* after allergen challenge, suggests that these cells likely play an important role in allergic diseases. However, because much more is known about the role of mast cells in the immune response, we will confine our discussion to mast cells except where specific information about basophils is available.

Mast Cells

Mast cells typically appear as round or elongated cells with a nonsegmented or occasionally bi- or multinucleated nucleus. Their intracellular granules stain purple when stained with aniline blue dyes. This change in color represents the interaction of the dyes with the highly acidic heparin contained in the mast-cell granules. Mast cells, like other granulocytes, are derived from $CD34^+$ hematopoietic progenitor cells; however, they are distinct from other granulocytes in that they mature in the periphery. Several lines of evidence suggest that interactions between the tyrosine kinase receptor c-kit, which is expressed on the surface of mast cells, and the c-kit ligand, stem cell factor (SCF), are essential for normal mast-cell development and survival. For example, mice with mutations that result in either markedly impaired c-kit function or a reduction in c-kit virtually lack mast cells. Reconstitution with rSCF can induce mast-cell hyperplasia in vivo in mice, rats, primates, and humans *(326)*.

Mast cells are distributed throughout normal connective tissues, where they often lie adjacent to blood and lymphatic vessels, near or within nerves, beneath epithelial surfaces that are exposed to the external environment, such as those of the respiratory tract, GI tract, and skin (Figure 43.6). At these locations they are ideally situated to encounter foreign antigens and to release their products in close proximity to their respective target cells (i.e., epithelial cells, vascular endothelium, smooth muscle, and fibroblasts). In humans and mice, the number of mast cells in a tissue varies markedly, depending on the anatomic site and the immunologic status of the host.

The mast-cell population is composed of a heterogeneous group of cells with respect to their structure and function *(327)*. On the basis of their content of neutral serine proteases, they had previously been divided into two phenotypes. One subset, designated MC_{TC}, contains tryptase, chymase, cathespsin G, and carboxypeptidase, whereas the other phenotype, designated MC_T, contains only tryptase. MC_{TC} is found predominantly in skin and at subepithelial locations in the bronchial, nasal, and GI mucosa, whereas the MC_T is located predominantly in alveolar walls, intestinal epithelium, and in airway epithelium in patients with allergic disease. However, more recent studies in both humans and animal models suggest that mast cells in different anatomic sites and even within a single site can vary in several aspects of their phenotype, including morphology, responsiveness to various stimuli, and activation and mediator content.

The tissue levels of mast cells and their specific phenotypes are likely controlled by a complex interplay between SCF, other growth factors, and cytokines. SCF is

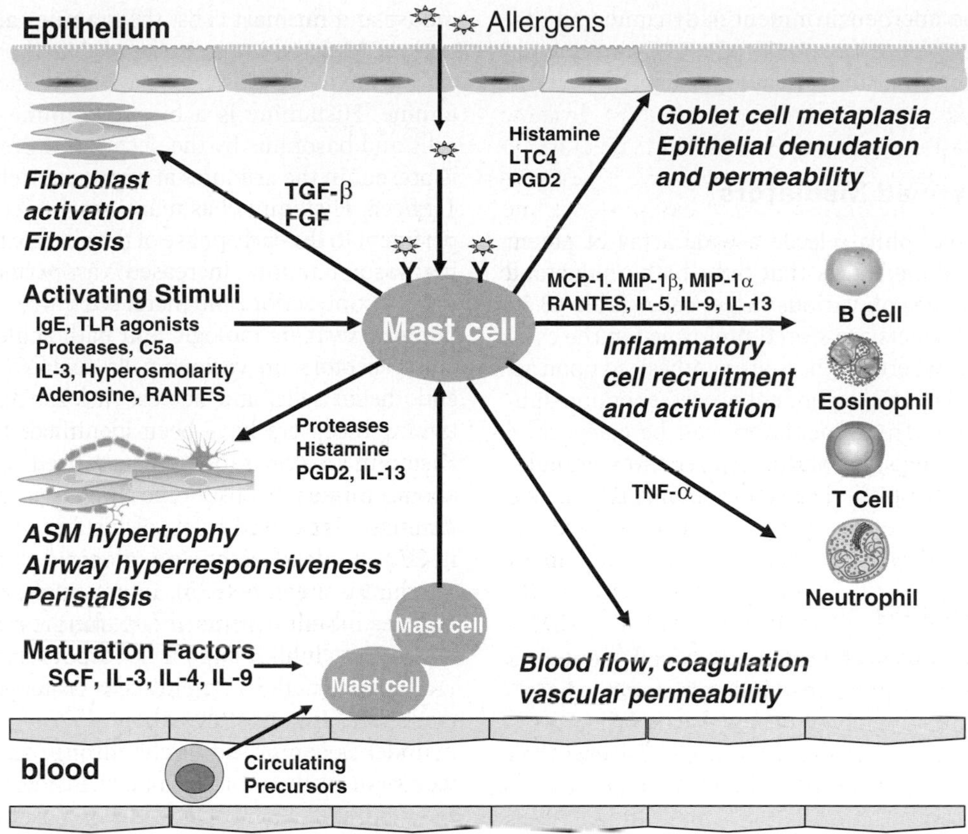

FIGURE 43.6 Mast cells are produced in the bone marrow and released into the circulation as immature precursors. They mature in tissues under the influence of stem cell factor, SCF, IL-3, IL-4, and IL-9. Once activated by either antigen crosslinking of surface IgE or via a variety of other factors (TLR ligands, proteases, C5a, IL-3, hyperosmolarity, adenosine, RANTES), mast cells degranulate and release a variety of mediators, including vasoactive and bronchoactive mediators (histamine, LTC4, PGD_2, proteases), chemokines (MCP-1, MIP-1α, MIP-1β, RANTES), cytokines (IL-9, IL-13, IL-5, TNF-α), and growth factors (TGF-β and FGF). Through the release of this vast array of mediators, mast cells induce many features of the early-phase allergic response, including enhanced vascular and epithelial permeability, mucus secretion, and airway hyperresponsiveness. They also contribute to the late-phase allergic response via the recruitment and activation of a number of inflammatory cells, including neutrophils, eosinophils, T cells, and B cells. Through the activation of inflammatory cells as well as direct effects on mucosal cells, mast cells also contribute to the remodeling (goblet cell metaplasia, tissue fibrosis, and smooth muscle hypertrophy) of mucosal tissues observed in chronic statges of the allergic response.

necessary to elicit the c-kit–mediated signaling that ensures the expansion of cells of the mast-cell lineage, whereas the development of different phenotypes appears to be determined by their responsiveness to signals from T cells. Specifically MC_T-cell expansion appears to be T-cell–dependent, whereas expansion of the MC_{TC} population is T-cell–independent. This contention is supported by the fact that humans with T-cell deficiencies have a lack of intraepithelial intestinal mast cells, while maintaining submucosal mast-cell populations *(328)*. Similarly, athymic mice lack intraepithelial cells and are unable to expand this population in the GI tract in response to helminthic infections (329). IL-3, IL-4, and IL-9, in particular, are among the T-cell–derived cytokines known to influence mast-cell development and phenotypic characteristics. A role for IL-3 in mast-cell hyperplasia has been demonstrated in intestinal helminthic infections in which IL-3 depletion inhibits the intraepithelial mast cell hyperplasia normally observed in the jejunum of infected mice (330). A similar case can be made for IL-9, because IL-9 transgenic mice spontaneously develop intraepithelial mast-cell hyperplasia in the jejunum *(331)*. The action of IL-9 can be blocked by depletion of SCF. Moreover, IL-9 and IL-10 reversibly induce MMCP-1 and MMCP-2 expression in mast cells through transcript stabilization, suggesting that T-cell–derived cytokines can influence the spectrum of mediators produced by a given mast cell. Taken together, these studies suggest that the regulation of mast-cell phenotype in the microenvironment is dynamic and that T-cell–derived cytokines are major determinants of the numbers, distribution, and phenotype of mast cells in tissues.

Mast-Cell–Derived Mediators

Mast cells and basophils release a wide array of potent biologically active mediators that have both unique and overlapping activities on various target cells (Table 43.5). Some of these products are stored preformed in the cytoplasmic granules, whereas others are synthesized upon activation of the cell by IgE-dependent processes or non–IgE-dependent stimuli. These mediators can be categorized into three main groups: (a) preformed secretory granule–associated mediators, (b) lipid-derived mediators, and (c) cytokines.

Preformed Mediators

The secretory granules of human mast cells contain a crystalline complex of preformed inflammatory mediators bound ionically to a matrix of proteoglycan. When mast-cell activation occurs, the granules swell and lose their crystalline nature and the individual mediators are released by exocytosis. The mediators stored in mast cells include histamine, proteoglycans, serine proteases, carboxypeptidase A, and small amounts of sulphatases. In mouse and rat mast cells, the granules also contain serotonin *(332–334)*.

The mediator most associated with the mast cell is histamine. Histamine is a biogenic amine formed in mast cells and basophils by the decarboxylation of histidine. It is present in the granules at approximately 100 mmol/L or 1 pg/cell. Histamine has many potent activities which are pertinent to the early phase of the allergic response, including vasodilatation, increased vasopermeability, smooth muscle contraction, and increased mucus production. Histamine exerts its biologic and pathologic effects via specific receptors on various cells such as smooth muscle, endothelial cells, and nerves. At least three types of histamine receptors have been identified: H1, H2, and H3. Histamine is very rapidly metabolized, with a half-life of about 1 minute, by histamine N-methyltransferase and histaminase. Increased levels of histamine have been found in BAL fluids of asthmatic, atopic dermatitis, and allergic rhinitis patients (335). Interestingly, although antihistamines inhibit the immediate allergic responses, they do not seem to inhibit late-phase responses.

Heparin is the predominant proteoglycan in human mast cells. It constitutes about 75% of the total. The remainder is comprised of chondroitin sulfhates. The proteoglycan is the storage matrix inside the granule, and the acid sulfate groups of the glycosaminoglycans provide binding sites for the other preformed mediators. Proteoglycans also have anticoagulant, anticomplement, and

TABLE 43.5 Products of Mast Cells and Basophils

Mediators	*Actions*
Preformed mediators	
Histamine	Increase vascular permeability, smooth muscle contraction
Neutral proteases	
Tryptase, chymase	Physiologic function uncertain (different mast-cell populations express diffrent combinations of proteases)
Cathepsin G	
Carboxypeptidase	
Lipid mediators	
PGD_2	Smooth muscle contraction
LTC_4	Increase vascular Permeability, smooth muscle constration, increase mucus production
LTB_4	Neutrophil chemotaxis
TXA_2	Vasoconstrictor, platelet aggregation, smooth muscle constraction
PAF	Vasoconstrictor, platelet aggregation, smooth muscle constraction, chemotactic for neutrophils and eosinophils
Cytokines	
TNF-α,IL-6,IL-8,IL-1α	Numerous proinflammatory action
IL-4,IL-13	Switch factor for Ige, VCAM-1 expression
IL-5	Regulation of eosinophils
Chemokines	
MIP-1α,MCP-1, MIP-1B, RANTES	Chemotactic for monocyte/macrophages
Growth factors	
FGP, VEGF	Include growth of fibroblasts and endothelial cells, respectively

PGD2, prostaglandin D2; LTC4, leukotrene C4; PAF, plalelet-activating factor; FGP, fibroblast growth factor; VEGF, vascular endothelial growth factor.

antikallikrein effects. In addition to regulating the kinetics of release of mediators from the granule matrices, proteoglycans can also regulate the activity of some of the associated mediators.

The major mast-cell protease, which is present in all types of mast cells, is tryptase. Tryptase is a serine protease, and it is stored fully active in the granule. There are two distinct forms of tryptase with 90% amino acid sequence homology: α-tryptase and β-tryptase *(336,337)*. The β-tryptase form is a useful clinical biomarker for anaphylaxis. Tryptase levels measured within 4 hours of a presumed anaphylactic reaction are more sensitive than serum or urine histamine in implicating mast-cell activation and degranulation *(338,*339,*340)*. By weight, tryptase is the major enzyme stored in the cytoplasmic granules of human mast cells, and it occurs in all human mast-cell populations. It has many activities, including cleavage of peptides such as vasoactive intestinal peptide, bronchodilator peptides, and calcitonin gene-related peptide, but not substance P; sensitization of smooth muscle; cleavage of type IV collagen, fibronectin, and type VI collagen; upregulation of ICAM-1 on epithelial cells; and mitogenic activity for fibroblasts and epithelial cells *(334)*. Some of these activities have led to speculation that mast cells may be involved in chronic inflammation and tissue remodeling *(341)*.

The other major neutral protease in mast cells is chymase. It is also a serine protease that is stored in the active form in the granules of some human mast cells. Unlike tryptase, chymase is only present in a subset of mast cells. Chymase can cleave angiotensin I and neurotensin, but it has no activities on VIP or substance P. Importantly, it can degrade IL-4. Some subsets of mast cells also contain other proteinases, such as carboxypeptidase and cathepsin G.

Newly Synthesized Mediators

Lipid Mediators

Activation of mast cells not only results in release of preformed granule-associated mediators, it can also initiate the de novo synthesis of certain lipid-derived substances. Of particular importance are the cycloxygenase and lipoxygenase metabolites of arachidonic acid, because these products possess potent inflammatory activity. Lipoxygenases generate leukotrienes (LTs), hydroperoxyeicosatetraenoic acids (HPETEs), and the reduced products of HPETES, hydroxyeicosatetrenoic acids (HETEs), whereas cycloxygenase products include prostaglandins and thromboxanes.

Leukotrienes are produced by the activity of 5-lipoxygenase on arachidonic acid (AA). Arachidonic acid is converted to 5-HPETE, which can then be converted to LTB_4 through the action of the LTA_4 hydrolase or to LTC_4 via LTC_4 synthase. LTC_4 can then be converted to LTD_4 and LTE_4. Human mast cells generally produce more LTC_4 than LTB_4. The leukotrienes were originally discovered in 1938 and referred to as the slow-reacting substance of anaphylaxis until their structural elucidation in 1979 *(342,343)*. In 1983, Samuelson identified the slow-reacting substance of anaphylaxis (SRS-A) as the cysteinyl leukotrienes, LTC_4, D_4, and E_4.

Leukotrienes induce a prolonged cutaneous wheal-and-flare response, stimulate prolonged bronchoconstriction (10 to 1,000 times more potently than histamine), enhance vascular permeability, promote bronchial mucus secretion *(344)*, and induce constriction of arterial and intestinal smooth muscle (345,*346–348*). Cysteinyl leukotrienes have been detected in the BAL fluid of asthmatic patients and in the urine of patients following inhaled allergen challenge or aspirin challenge in sensitive individuals. Cysteinyl leukotriene receptor antagonists and leukotriene synthesis blockers have been introduced into clinical practice as novel therapies for asthma. In asthmatic patients, clinical trials have demonstrated that approximately 80% of the early bronchoconstrictor response can be eliminated with cysteinyl leukotriene antagonists *(349–351)*. These blockers also block 50% of the late-phase response to inhaled allergen, supporting the importance of cysteinyl leukotrienes in the late phase of the allergic response *(349–351)*. However, the fact that PGD_2 and tryptase are not found in BAL fluid during the late-phase reaction suggests that the cysteinyl leukotrienes noted in the late phase are the product of basophils or eosinophils and not mast cells.

In contrast to the cysteinyl leukotrienes, mast cells produce very little LTB_4. LTB_4 is a potent chemotactic factor for neutrophils and to a lesser extent for eosinophils *(352)*. Certain mast-cell types, including bone-marrow–derived murine mast cells and human lung mast cells, may also secrete platelet-activating factor (PAF) *(353,354)*. PAF has several actions that suggest that it is an important mediator of anaphylaxis, including (a) its ability to induce aggregation and degranulation of platelets; (b) its induction of wheal-and-flare reactions in human skin, (c) its ability to increase lung resistance, and (d) induction of systemic hypotension.

The major cyclo-oxygenase–derived product in mast cells is PGD_2, which is a potent bronchoconstrictor. PGD_2 is rapidly degraded to $9\alpha,11\beta$-PGF_2, producing another potent bronchoconstrictor. Maximal activation of mast cells yields 50 to 100 ng PGD_2 per 10^6 mast cells *(355)*. Although PGD_2 is 100-fold less potent than cysteinyl leukotrienes, it is released in larger molar amounts and thus is important in the early bronchoconstrictor response to airway allergen challenge (356). PGD_2 exerts its effects by interacting with the thromboxane receptor on airway smooth muscle *(357)*. PGD_2 is also chemotactic for neutrophils and is an inhibitor of platelet aggregation. There is considerable evidence that prostanoids are generated during allergic reactions in vivo. PGD_2 is elevated in the BAL of asthmatic subjects following inhaled allergen challenge *(358)*. Furthermore, the metabolite of PGD_2, 9α,11β-PGF_2, increases markedly in the urine after allergen or aspirin challenge of sensitive asthmatics *(359)*. Significantly raised PGF2α and PGE_2 levels are reported in the serum of asthmatics *(360,361)*. These findings are confused by the fact that there is no therapeutic benefit from cyclo-oxygenase (COX) inhibitors and, in fact, COX inhibitors often exacerbate underlying asthma *(362,363)*.

Mast-Cell–Derived Cytokines

Mast cells may be important initiators of both the early- and late-phase allergic reaction by their ability to synthesize and secrete cytokines. Mast cells express message for a number of cytokines, including proinflammatory cytokines, immunoregulatory cytokines, and chemokines.

Mast cells contain preformed stores of several proinflammatory cytokines, including TNF-α, IL-8, IL-6, and IL-1α. Release of these cytokines early in the immune response likely contributes to the recruitment of leukocytes during the late-phase response via their ability to increase expression of adhesion molecules such as P- and E-selectin, vascular cell adhesion molecule (VCAM-1),and intercellular adhesion molecule-1 (ICAM-1) on vascular endothelial cells. Mast cells appear to be an important initial source of TNF-α during allergic responses. Mast cells produce a number of immunoregulatory cytokines, such as IL-3, IL-4, IL-5, GM-CSF, IL-13, and IL-16. In the human bronchial mucosa, IL-4 immunoreactivity is seen in approximately 80% of mast cells (364,*365*). Indeed, it has been suggested that mast cells are the primary source of IL-4 protein in inflamed airways. Although cytokine production by basophils has not been as extensively studied as that in mast cells, they have been shown to produce large quantities of IL-4 and IL-13. The rapid and perhaps sustained production of cytokines by these cells at sites of allergic inflammation may intensify or perpetuate IgE production and Th2 cell differentiation. Mast cells have also been shown to produce a number of chemokines such as MCP-1, MIP-1β, MIP-1α, and RANTES. Elaboration of these chemokines may contribute to the cellular component of the late-phase response.

Mast-Cell Activation

Mast-cell activation may be initiated upon interaction of a multivalent antigen with its specific IgE antibody attached to the cell membrane via its high-affinity receptor, FcεR1. Cross-linking of IgE by the interaction of allergen with specific determinants on the Fab portion of the molecule brings the receptors into juxtaposition and initiates mast-cell activation and mediator generation and release. Mast cells may also be activated by non-IgE–mediated stimuli such as neuropeptides, complement components, and drugs such as opiates. In addition to IgE-dependent stimuli, several non–IgE-dependent stimuli activate mast cells and basophils. C5a, IL-3, fMLP, and certain chemokines (RANTES) are known to induce histamine and mediator release in mast cells and basophils. Hyperosmolarity itself also stimulates mediator secretion from these cells. Degranulation produced by both IgE-dependent and non–IgE dependent stimuli appear similar. However, the biochemical processes that lead to mediator release may differ.

Role of Mast Cells in Acute-Phase Responses

Several lines of evidence suggest that mast cells and basophils play a pivotal role in the generation of acute-phase responses. First, allergen provocation of atopic individuals is associated with extensive activation of mast cells, as judged by the detection of the release of mast-cell–associated mediators (histamine, tryptase) at the site of allergen challenge. Second, therapeutics that inhibit the release of these mediators (mast-cell stabilizers) or their actions (antihistamines) effectively attenuate acute allergic responses. Despite this evidence in humans, the data in animal models is conflicting. The preponderance of studies in mice suggests that acute responses are mast-cell– and IgE–dependent, but others suggest that these responses are IgE–independent. For example, it has been shown that responses induced in mice by passive transfer of allergen-specific IgE antibodies and subsequent intravenous allergen challenge are inhibited in genetically mast-cell–deficient Kit^{w}/Kit^{W-v} mice. When these mice were reconstituted with mast cells by adoptive transfer, their acute-phase responses were restored *(366)*. In contrast, some investigators have reported that anaphylactic responses develop normally in IgE-deficient mice (367). Although these conflicting results may reflect inherent differences in mast-cell biology between humans and mice, they imply that both mast-cell– and IgE–dependent and –independent processes are likely involved in the expression of the physiologic features of the acute-phase reaction.

Role of Mast Cells in Late-Phase Responses

Although it has long been thought that mast cells contribute only to the early acute response, recent evidence demonstrates their potential contribution to the late-phase response. First, through the elaboration of proinflammatory cytokines, chemokines, and immunoregulatory cytokines as discussed previously, mast cells may contribute to the cellular component of the late-phase response as well as favor the acquisition of the Th2 phenotype by providing a continuously high concentration of IL-4. Second, mast-cell–derived mediators may also contribute to the chronic remodeling of mucosal tissues, because many of the mediators they release influence turnover of connective tissue. Specifically, histamine and tryptase have been shown to stimulate fibroblast growth and collagen synthesis in vitro and in vivo. Lastly, studies in humans have shown that stabilization of mast cells with sodium nedocromil effectively inhibits both the early- and late-phase responses to allergen exposure *(368)*. Furthermore, recent clinical trials utilizing a monoclonal antibody against IgE resulted in reductions in symptoms and improvement in lung function in asthmatics (369). Although together these reports support a role for mast cells in the late-phase response, studies of animal models of atopic dermatitis and asthma suggest that late-phase reactions are similar in wild-type and IgE-deficient mice (53,*370*) suggesting that although mast cells are capable of inducing late-phase responses, additional mast-cell–independent processes also contribute to the development of late-phase responses.

EOSINOPHIL BIOLOGY

Eosinophil blood and tissue levels are generally quite low in the absence of parasitic infection or atopy. One of the hallmarks of allergic disorders is heightened production of eosinophils in the bone marrow and the accumulation of eosinophils in tissues and blood. Eosinophil differentiation, recruitment, and activation are under the regulation of a series of molecular events orchestrated by Th2 cytokines. Although the exact role of eosinophils in the pathology of allergic responses is not known, eosinophils are known to release a myriad of mediators and cytokines that have the potential to induce the symptoms of allergy as well as amplify the allergic response through the release of immunoregulatory and proinflammatory cytokines.

Eosinophils are bone marrow–derived granulocytes that are characterized by their bilobed nuclei and their distinctive cytoplasmic granules (Figure 43.7) (371,372). They contain three distinct types of cytoplasmic granules: (a) eosinophil-specific granules, which contain electron-dense crystalloid cores; (b) primary granules, which lack a crystalloid core and develop early in eosinophil maturation; and (c) smaller granules, which contain arylsulfatase and other enzymes. Eosinophils also contain varying numbers of lipid bodies. Lipid bodies are non–membrane-bound, lipid-rich inclusions that are also found in macrophages and mast cells, and are thought to contribute to the formation of eicosanoid mediators. Eosinophils are generally identified in blood and tissues by the affinity of their cytoplasmic granules for acid aniline dyes such as eosin and in tissues by immunostaining for eosinophil-specific proteins (in particular, major basic protein [MBP]).

Eosinophil-Derived Mediators

Eosinophil-Specific Cationic Proteins

Eosinophils store four highly basic, low-molecular-weight proteins in their cytoplasmic granules: MBP, eosinophil-derived neurotoxin (EDN), eosinophil peroxidase (EPO), and eosinophil cationic protein (ECP). MBP, EPO, and ECP are potent toxins for helminths and bacteria, and they are strongly implicated as mediators of allergic diseases such as asthma, atopic dermatitis, and allergic rhinitis (Figure 43.7). MBP is potently toxic for mammalian cells in vitro, and high levels of MBP are found in the body fluids of patients with asthma and other allergic disorders (373). Both MBP and ECP exert their toxicity by damaging target-cell membranes through charge-mediated interactions. In addition to its toxic properties, MBP activates platelets, mast cells, and basophils, which in turn release histamine. Furthermore, MBP administration to primates induces airway hyperresponsiveness. MBP may induce AHR through its demonstrated ability to competitively inhibit binding to cholinergic muscarinic M2 receptors on parasympathetic nerves *(374)*. These receptors normally function as autoreceptors that inhibit the release of acetylcholine from the nerve ending. Thus, inhibition of these receptors by MBP would enhance the release of acetylcholine in the airway wall, resulting in heightened contractile responses. Both ECP and EDN have partial sequence identity with pancreatic ribonucleases; however, EDN is more potent as a ribonuclease than is ECP.

Eosinophil peroxidase (EPO), which is distinct from the myeloperoxidase of neutrophils and monocytes, consists of two polypeptides of about 15 and 55 kDa. It catalyzes the formation of hypobromous acid from hydrogen peroxidase and halide ions (preferentially bromide). HOBr reacts with primary amines to form bromamines, and it converts tyrosine to 3-bromotyrosine. Increases in the levels of 3-bromotyrosine in BAL proteins have been observed in asthmatics following allergen provocation (375). Thus, the oxidative pathways induced in activated eosinophils may damage biomolecules in vivo (375).

Another prominent component of eosinophil primary granules is Charcot Leyden crystals (CLC). This protein comprises up to 10% of the total cellular protein in human eosinophils. Although the CLC protein possesses lysophospholipase activity, structural analysis suggest that the CLC protein is similar to that of galectins 1 and 2, members of the "S-type" lectin superfamily *(376)*. Recent studies in the mouse lung suggest that CLC may contain a protein called YM-1 (T-lymphocyte–derived eosinophil chemotactic factor), which has sequence homology to chitinase *(377)*. Chitinase activity of these proteins may explain the strong association between eosinophilia and parasite infestations. These crystals are often found in sputum, feces, and tissues in patients with allergic asthma and

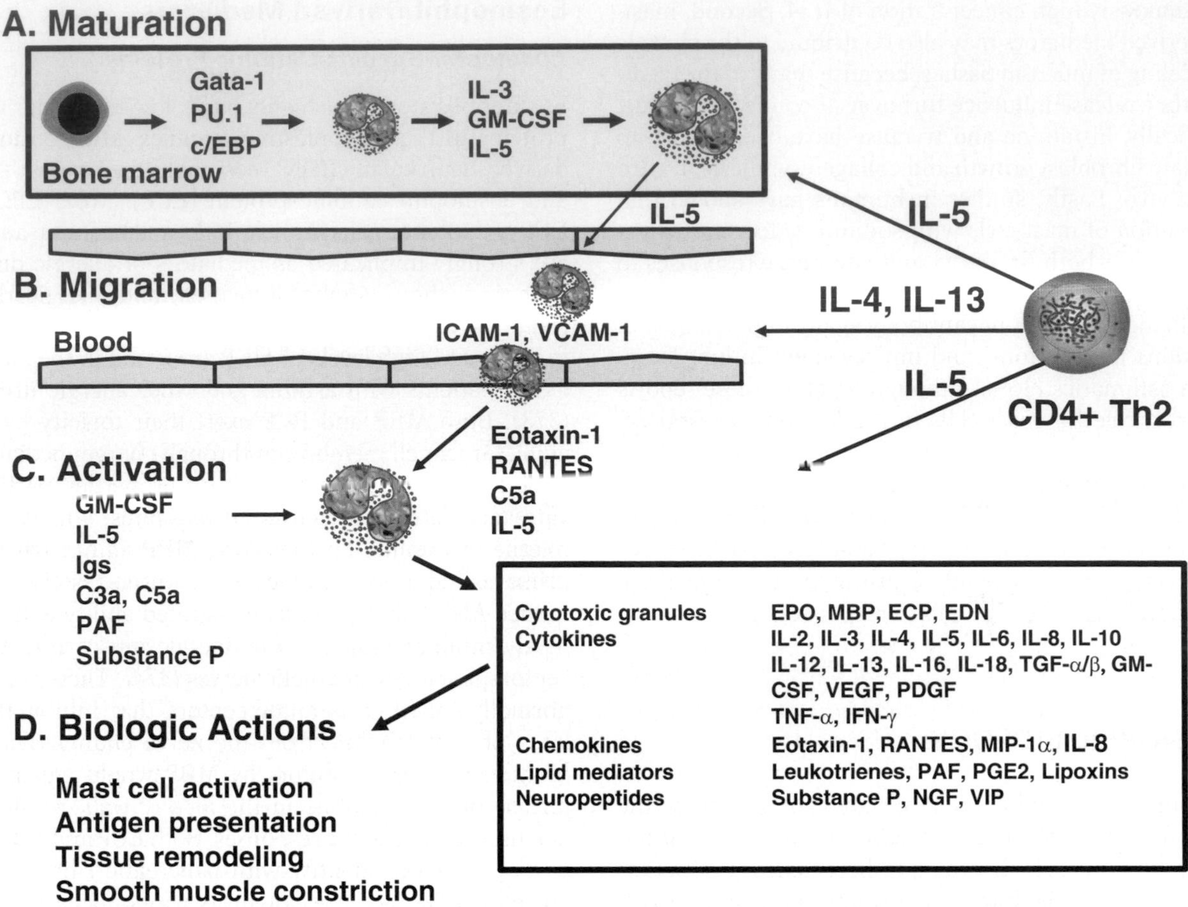

FIGURE 43.7 Schematic representation of eosinophil: **(A)** maturation, **(B)** migration, **(C)** activation, and (D) pleiotrophic actions during allergic immune responses. Eosinophils develop in the bone marrow, where they differentiate from hematopoietic progenitor cells into mature eosinophils under the control of several transcription factors, including GATA-1, PU.1, and c/EBP. Th2 cytokines coordinately regulate eosinophil recruitment, activation, and accumulation at the site of antigen exposure. Following allergen-specific induction of Th2 cytokine production (IL-5, IL-4, IL-13, IL-3, GM-CSF), IL-5 rapidly induces differentiation of eosinophils from myeloid precursors in the bone marrow to stimulate their release into the bloodstream. IL-4 and/or IL-13 promote eosinophil egress from the vascular compartment by upregulating VCAM-1 expression on vascular endothelial cells. Subsequently, IL-4 and IL-13 guide eosinophils to the site of allergen exposure by regulating the production of various chemokines (e.g., RANTES, eotaxin) by local cells such as macrophages and epithelial cells. Once these cells accumulate in tissues, locally produced IL-5, along with other cytokines, such as GM-CSF, and IL-3 promote their actions by prolonging their survival in tissues. Eosinophils store and release a number of proteins in their specific granules. Specifically, MBP is stored in the core of the granule, whereas ECP, EDN, EPO are found in the matrix of the granules. Eosinophils also contain lipid bodies in which products of lipoxygenase and cycloxygenase are formed. Eosinophils also release a number of cytokines, chemokines, and neuropeptides that are important in the allergic diathesis.

other eosinophil-related diseases characterized by significant eosinophilia.

Lipid Mediators

Upon stimulation, eosinophils elaborate several bioactive lipids, including products of the 5- and 15-lipooxygenase pathway; products of the cyclooxygenase pathway, and platelet-activating factor (PAF). Lipid bodies, or intracellular lipid-rich domains, are induced to develop in many activated eosinophils in vivo and are sites for enhanced synthesis of both lipoxygenase- and cyclo-oxygenase–derived eicosanoids. The activities of eosinophil-derived lipids, which are generally proinflammatory, are multiple and include potent smooth muscle contraction, vasoactivity, and mucus secretion activities.

Cytokines

In recent years it has been recognized that eosinophils are a major source of cytokines and appear to store some if not all of these cytokines in cytoplasmic specific granules. Triggering of eosinophils by engagement of receptors for cytokines Ig and C3 can lead to secretion of an array of proinflammatory and immunoregulatory cytokines, chemokines, and growth factors, including IL-2, IL-3, IL-4, IL-5, IL-6, IL-8, IL-10, IL-12, IFN-γ, TNF-α, GM-CSF, TGF-β, TGF-α, RANTES, MIP-1α, eotaxin, VEGF, PDGF-β, and heparin-binding epidermal growth factor (see 59). Through the quick release of this diverse array of cytokines at the inflammatory loci, the eosinophil is poised to perpetuate and/or intensify the eosinophil-mediated inflammatory response, both by enhancing its own activation and through the release of Th2 cytokines.

Recruitment of Eosinophils to Sites of Inflammation

Preferential accumulation of eosinophils at sites of allergic inflammation involves multiple molecular events that are integrated and controlled by Th2 cytokines *(378)*. These include (a) differentiation and release of mature eosinophils from the bone marrow into the bloodstream; (b) upregulation of specific adhesion molecules on eosinophils and endothelium; (c) stimulation of C-C chemokine production and egress of eosinophils from the blood into the tissues; and (d) production of eosinophil-active cytokines that increase eosinophil survival in tissues.

Eosinophils are terminally differentiated granulocytes that develop from CD34$^+$ hematopoietic progenitor cells in the bone marrow. Under the influence of GM-CSF, IL-3, and IL-5, they differentiate into mature eosinophils. These cytokines likely promote eosinophilopoiesis via induction of GATA-1, PU.1, or C/EPS through their shared common β-chain (379,380). Of these, IL-5 has the most specific effects on eosinophil differentiation and production. In addition to its effects on eosinophil differentiation, IL-5 can rapidly induce the release of developed eosinophils from the bone marrow into the peripheral circulation. The importance of IL-5 to blood and tissue eosinophilia has been repeatedly shown in in vitro and in vivo studies of gene-targeted and overexpressing mouse lines (50,381).

Circulating eosinophils are recruited to sites of inflammation by the combined actions of inflammatory mediators, adhesion molecules, and chemoattractants (Figure 43.7). Several cell adhesion molecules have been implicated in eosinophil adherence to cytokine-stimulated vascular endothelium, including ICAM-1, E-selectin, L-selectin, and the very late antigen-4/VCAM-1. The importance of VCAM-1 to eosinophil recruitment has been shown in primate and mouse studies in which blockade of VCAM-1/VLA-4 interactions inhibits eosinophil infiltration of tissues *(382)*. IL-4 and IL-13 induce VCAM-1 expression on the surface of vascular endothelial cells, leading to preferential recruitment of eosinophils into sites of allergic inflammation.

Eosinophil migration to the sites of inflammatory loci is mediated by a number of chemoattractants. Until the last decade, mediators such as PAF, C5a, and LTB_4 were considered to be the most important eosinophil chemoattractants. Although they are potent chemoattractants, they do not show any specificity for eosinophils. However, there are a number of C-C chemokines that are eosinophil chemoattractants (RANTES [regulation on activated, normal T-cell expression and secretion, CCL5], eotaxin [CCL11], monocyte chemoattractant proteins MCP-4 [CCL13], MCP-3 [CCL7], and MIP-α [CCL3]). The levels of most of these chemokines have been shown to be upregulated in the mucosal tissues of asthmatics, atopic rhinitics, and atopic dermatitis patients. Although each of these chemokines is implicated in eosinophil chemotaxis, it was originally hypothesized that eotaxin would play a pivotal role in eosinophilic inflammation in that it binds specifically to the chemokine receptor 3 (CCR3), whereas the other C-C chemokines bind multiple receptors. The fact that CCR3 is highly expressed on eosinophils, basophils, and Th2 cells, but not on neutrophils, suggested that it plays an important role in Th2-mediated inflammatory responses (383,384). Surprisingly, though, eotaxin-deficient mice have shown only minor defects in eosinophil accumulation (385,386), indicating that eotaxin is not uniquely required for eosinophil accumulation. Along these lines, complete abrogation of eosinophil migration has not been observed by inhibition of any one chemokine (41,385,387,388,*389*), suggesting that multiple chemokines working in concert are required to direct leukocytes to specific sites of inflammation. Thus it has been postulated that a panopy of chemokines may be required to establish the multiple chemical gradients required for eosinophils to migrate through several local compartments from the vascular spaces to the mucosal surfaces in the nose, airway, and skin.

Lastly, eosinophils rapidly undergo apoptosis unless provided with signals from eosinophil growth factors such as IL-5, GM-CSF, and IL-3. Prolonged survival of eosinophils under the influence of locally generated growth factors is thought to be an important mechanism for selective eosinophil accumulation in atopic diseases. Direct evidence for prolonged survival of eosinophils in atopic disease comes from the fact that glucocorticoid treatment of atopic individuals results in a rapid loss of tissue eosinophils.

Based on the independent and overlapping roles of IL-4, IL-13, and IL-5, discussed previously, we can envision the following paradigm for regulation of allergen-induced tissues eosinophilia. Following allergen-specific induction of Th2 cytokine production, IL-5 would rapidly induce differentiation of eosinophils from myeloid precursors in the bone marrow and stimulate their release into the bloodstream. IL-4 and/or IL-13 would promote eosinophil egress from the vascular compartment by upregulating VCAM-1 expression on vascular endothelial cells. Once the cells accumulate in tissues, locally produced IL-5 along with other mediators such as eotaxin would promote their actions by prolonging their survival in tissues. Within this paradigm, allergen-driven eosinophil recruitment into tissues is coordinately regulated by the Th2 cytokines, IL-4, IL-13, and IL-5.

Mechanisms of Eosinophil Activation

The effector functions of eosinophils are mediated by stimuli that induce degranulation. Eosinophil degranulation can be regulated by multiple components, including those that primarily stimulate the cells (e.g., immunoglobulins and lipid mediators), priming agents (e.g., cytokines), and chemokines. However, the precise mechanisms by which eosinophil degranulation occurs in vivo are still poorly understood.

Eosinophils express receptors for several immunoglobulins, including IgG, IgA, and IgE. Surfaces coated with IgG, IgA, and secretory IgA stimulate eosinophil degranulation in vitro. Of these immunoglobulins, sIgA is best for inducing eosinophil degranulation and does not stimulate neutrophil degranulation. Because IgA is the most abundant immunoglobulin isotype in mucosal secretions of the respiratory and gastrointestinal tracts, it may be an important regulator of eosinophil activation at these sites. IgE may also be important for eosinophil activation, because eosinophils can bind IgE via three distinct structures: the S-type lectin galectin-3, FcεRII/CD23, and FcεRI. It was initially shown that eosinophils, isolated from patients with parasite-induced eosinophilia, degranulate in response to IgE antibody or IgE-coated parasites (390,*391*). Subsequent studies showed that local allergen provocation induces expression of FcεRI by eosinophils infiltrating into the airways *(392)* and skin of patients with allergic diseases *(393,394)*. In studies using sera from ragweed-allergic patients with hay fever, ragweed-specific IgG, but not IgE, induced allergen-dependent eosinophil degranulation in vitro *(395,396)*. Thus it remains to be determined whether IgE is an important regulator of eosinophil degranulation in atopy.

Eosinophil degranulation may also be induced by soluble stimuli alone. Cytokines, especially those with eosinophilopoietic activity, such as GM-CSF and IL-5, are potent inducers of eosinophil granule protein release. Interestingly, eosinophil granule proteins themselves, including MBP and EPO, stimulate eosinophils and cause degranulation, suggesting an autocrine mechanism of eosinophil degranulation *(397)*. Other physiologic stimuli for eosinophil degranulation include PAF, the complement fragments C5a and C3a, and the neuropeptide, substance P *(398)*. As discussed briefly previously, chemokines may also activate eosinophils by binding CCR3. In this regard, eotaxin induces eosinophil degranulation and leukotriene C_4 (LTC_4) release.

Eosinophils as Effector Cells in Allergic Responses

Eosinophils, through the elaboration of a plethora of preformed mediators and lipid mediators described previously, are postulated to play a role in several aspects of the allergic response, including antigen presentation, T-cell proliferation and differentiation, as well as mast-cell activation and airway remodeling. Although it remains controversal, it has recently been shown that eosinophils may function in antigen presentation *(399)*. Specifically, eosinophils have been shown to effectively present soluble parasitic antigens to $CD4^+$ T cells, thereby promoting T-cell proliferation and polarization. They may also regulate T-cell proliferation, activation, and polarization via the array of cytokines they produce, as well as through their ability to synthesize indoleamine 2,3-dioxygenase (IDO) *(400)*.

Circumstantial evidence for a causative role of eosinophils in allergic inflammation as well as the clinical symptoms of atopic disorders comes from a variety of studies (401). First, elevated levels of activated eosinophils and their protein products (MBP, ECP, EPO, EDN) have been consistently demonstrated in BAL fluids and airway biopsy tissues from patients with asthma (401), in nasal biopsy specimens from allergic rhinitic patients (nasal fluids and nasal biopsies) (402), and in skin lesions from patients with atopic dermatitis (403). Second, in each of these diseases, increased levels of eosinophils and their proteins correlate with disease severity. Lastly, successful steroid treatment is associated with a marked reduction in both blood and tissue eosinophil levels in asthma and atopic rhinitis *(404–406)*.

Despite the substantial body of circumstantial evidence that supports a causative role for eosinophils in the pathophysiology of atopic disorders, the results of studies designed to define a pathogenic role for eosinophils in atopic disorders are conflicting. Studies in IL-5 gene knockout (50) and transgenic mice (381) show that both eosinophilia and AHR are IL-5–dependent. In addition, anti-IL-5 treatment of cynomolgus monkeys inhibits allergen-induced airway reactivity and BAL eosinophilia *(407)*. In contrast, other investigators have demonstrated that blockade of eosinophils by IL-5 ablation did not affect AHR (50,408). This dissociation between eosinophils and the late-phase response has recently been confirmed in a multiple-center study in human asthmatics that demonstrated that whereas anti-IL-5 treatment suppressed pulmonary eosinophils, it did not inhibit either early or late responses to inhaled allergens or improve lung function (409). There may be multiple explanations for a lack of effect in this study, including the small study size, dosing schedule, and/or acute nature of treatment, but these studies suggest that blockade of eosinophils and IL-5 alone are not sufficient to inhibit clinical symptoms of atopic disease. Arguably, the study was underpowered and the dosing regime did not result in complete ablation of eosinophils in lung tissues, leaving the question open as to whether complete ablation is necessary to achieve therapeutic benefit. In a follow-up study using a multiple dosing regime, it was shown that anti-IL-5 attenuated several indices of airway remodeling, including enhanced matrix protein deposition (procollagen, tenascin, laminin), profibrotic molecule expression (TGF–β), and airway smooth muscle hypertrophy, without effects on airway physiology. The failure of anti–IL-5 treatment to ameliorate allergic symptoms in humans has brought into question the importance of eosinophils in human asthma. However, as long as existing therapies do not completely eliminate tissue eosinophils, the issue will not be resolved.

In order to address this issue, several groups have undertaken the task of developing eosinophil-deficient mice (410,*411*). One group generated an eosinophil-deficient mouse via insertion of a cytocidal protein (diphtheria toxin A) in the promoter of the eosinophil peroxidase (EPO) gene. These mice were reported to be completely devoid of eosinophils in all tissues (410). Moreover, all features of the allergic phenotype were absent (AHR, mucus, eosinophilia, Th2 cytokine production) in these mice following allergen challenge. The other eosinophil-deficient mouse line harbors a deletion of a high-affinity GATA-binding site in the GATA-1 promoter, leading to the specific ablation of the eosinophil lineage *(411)*. In this line, eosinophil depletion had no effect on AHR, mucus production, or Th2 cytokine production, but did reduce airway remodeling assessed by collagen deposition. Interestingly, the results of this study mirror that observed in the human anti–IL-5 trials. However, the exact reasons for the discrepancies in the mouse models are unknown. However, they may be due to the presence of residual eosinophils in the dbl-GATA mice or to unappreciated hematologic abnormalities, or toxic effects of diptheria toxin on noneosinophils in the EPO-diphtheria toxin A mice.

Th2 Cells as Effector Cells

Our recent understanding of the role of Th2 cells in the allergic diathesis suggest that they are important effector cells in the allergic response in addition to their well-accepted role as orchestrators of the inflammatory process. Specifically, the Th2 cytokine IL-13 has been implicated as an effector molecule in allergic disease. Evidence for this contention comes from studies in which blockade of endogenous levels of IL-13 in antigen-sensitized mice by administration of a soluble form of the IL-13RA2 chain, which binds only IL-13, completely reversed AHR and pulmonary mucus cell hyperplasia (39,61). Furthermore, it was shown that recombinant IL-13 was able to re-create the symptoms of asthma (airway hyperresponsiveness, mucus hypersecretion, eosinophilia) in the absence of functional T cells or B cells (39). These effects were shown to be independent of eosinophils as well *(412)*. These results suggested that IL-13's effects were not due to its known role in regulating IgE or eosinophil recruitment. Interestingly, despite the similarities in function between IL-13 and IL-4, IL-4 blockade at the time of antigen challenge does not ablate airway hyperresponsiveness *(413)*. This was further supported by the finding that transfer of Th2 cells derived from IL-4–deficient mice was still able to confer airway hyperresponsiveness *(42)*. Moreover chronic expression of IL-13 in the mouse lung results in development of these features, as well as subepithelial fibrosis and the formation of Charcot-Leyden crystals (264). In contrast, overexpression of the IL-4 gene in the murine lung does not result in AHR or subepithelial fibrosis *(414)*. Taken together, these studies suggest that IL-4 is essential for the initiation of Th2 polarized immune responses to allergenic peptides, whereas IL-13 alone may mediate the main physiologic consequences of allergic airway disease, namely, airway hyperresponsiveness, mucus hypersecretion, and subepithelial fibrosis.

As IL-4 and IL-13 share a functional receptor, one of the questions puzzling immunologists is how IL-13 may play a preferential role in the effector arm of the allergic response. Several explanations have been postulated, including the possibility that IL-4 production at the site of inflammation is short-lived and that IL-13 may persist, giving the allusion that IL-13 is the more important mediator of the effector phase of the response. This hypothesis is not without merit, as IL-4 is difficult to measure at the site of inflammation and kinetic studies have shown sustained IL-13 production in the lungs of asthmatic patients *(415)*. However, several in vitro studies have also claimed to observe unique functions of these cytokines in systems in which the level of cytokines is controlled. It can always be debated that any differences observed in these systems may be due to differences in degradation of these two proteins in culture or that the recombinant forms of these proteins do not have equivalent potency. Another potential hypothesis is that IL-13 may act through an as-yet-unidentified receptor complex. In support of this hypothesis, a recent study demonstrated that although AHR and eosinophilia induced by adoptive transfer of IL-13–sufficient T cells are STAT6-dependent, these effects appear to occur independently of the IL-4Rα chain *(416)*. These studies suggest that an as-yet-unidentified IL-13–binding chain may exist or that different configurations of the existing chains may mediate distinct effects of

IL-13 stimulation. As will be discussed later, the IL-13Rα2 chain may play a role in mediating processes unique to IL-13 under some circumstances. Alternatively, it has recently been shown that IL-4 may induce inhibitory pathways through the type I receptor that limit its proallergic effects mediated through the type II receptor *(417)*. On the other hand, it has been shown that IL-13 induces a small set of epithelial-specific genes that are not upegulated by IL-4 in vivo but are, however, STAT6-dependent. This apparent IL-13 selectivity occurs either via IL-13 stimulation of a unique receptor complex or as a result of IL-4 inhibition of these putative pathways. Although the mystery underlying the unique functions of IL-4 and IL-13 is far from solved, multiple explanations for their apparently unique functions are emerging.

IL-13 has several actions that implicate it as an effector in the allergic diathesis, such as its role in mucus production, fibrotic processes, and perhaps bronchoconstriction (Figure 43.8). First, it has been shown to play an important role in mucus hypersecretion. Mucus hypersecretion is a consistent feature of the allergic phenotype in both the upper and lower respiratory tracts. In fact, extensive plugging of the airway lumen has been associated with fatal episodes of asthma. This response is a Th2 cell-dependent process, as adoptive transfer of Th2 cells into the murine lung reconstitutes the effect of antigen challenge *(42)*. Several lines of evidence suggest that mucus cell metaplasia is an IL-13–, not IL-4–, dependent process. For example, transfer of Th2 cells devoid of IL-4 or IL-5 genes still induce extensive goblet cell metaplasia in the murine lung. However, blockade of the IL-4Rα chain or deficiency in STAT6 prevents the development of mucus cell metaplasia following allergen challenge, suggesting that IL-13 may be the ligand for the IL-4/STAT6 pathway in mucus cell changes *(208)*. Indeed, administration of soluble IL-13RA2 reversed the metaplastic response of goblet cells induced by allergen sensitization and challenge. Administration of rIL-13 in vivo or overexpression of the IL-13 gene

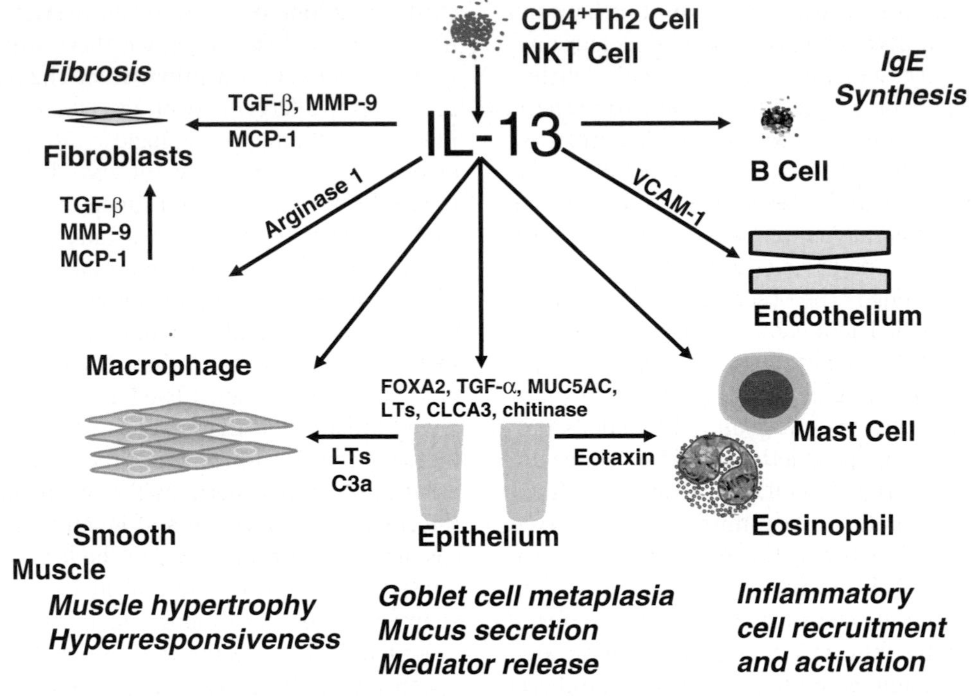

FIGURE 43.8 Schematic representation of the role of interleukin-13 (IL-13) in the effector phase of the allergic response. IL-13 is produced in the airway by a variety of cells, including T cells ($CD4^+$, NK T cells), eosinophils, and mast cells. IL-13 binds its receptor on multiple cell types and induces the expression of a variety of genes in target cells. The consequencecs of IL-13 receptor activation include IgE synthesis, adhesion molecule expression on endothelial cells (VCAM-1) and egress of inflammatory cells into mucosal tissues, inflammatory cell activation (eosinophils and mast cells), epithelial cell activation leading to mucus hypersecretion (FOXA2, CLCA1/3, TGF-α, MUC5AC) and mediator release (LTs, C3, eotaxin), smooth muscle activation and hypertrophy, airway hyperresponsiveness, activation of macrophages and fibroblasts leading to the production of various enzymes involved in collagen synthesis (arginase I, MMP-9, TGF-β, PDGF-AA), and deposition leading to tissue fibrosis. C3a, complement factor 3; VCAM-1, vascular cell adhesion molecule 1; CLCA1/2, Ca^{2+}, activating chloride channel gene 1/3; MMP9, metalloproteinase 9; TGF-α, transforming growth factor-α; FOXA2, forkhead box a2 transcription factor; MUC5AC, mucin gene 5AC.

recapitulates antigen effects on mucus production. Conversely, allergen-induced goblet cell metaplasia is significantly reduced in IL-13–deficient mice *(418)*. This was not further reduced when IL-4 was blocked with neutralizing antibodies, suggesting that indeed IL-13 is the primary regulator in vivo of mucus cell hyperplasia. The mechanisms by which IL-13 regulates mucus production are not entirely clear, but it has been shown to coordinately regulate a number of processes in the airway epithelium, which may contribute to mucus hypersecretion such as the induction of mucin gene expression, and ion-channel gene expression and activity *(419)*.

Another feature of the chronic inflammatory response in both the skin and the airways is the presence of a fibrotic process. Recent data suggest that IL-13 is an important regulator of fibrotic processes. For example, overexpression of IL-13 in the murine lung induces a dramatic fibrotic response in the airway wall (264). Furthermore, IL-13 transgenic mice express matrix proteases such as MMP and cathepsins that are thought to be important in the fibrotic response (420). A clear demarcation of function for IL-4 and IL-13 in fibrosis has been demonstrated in Th2-mediated pathology of *Schistosome mansoni* infection in mice. Schistosome-induced collagen deposition is reduced in the lungs of STAT-6–deficient animals, but not in IL-4–deficient mice (421). Furthermore, sIL-13RA2-Ig delivery completely prevented the fibrotic response in parasite-infected mice. Thus in several models of Th2-mediated fibrosis, blockade of IL-13 selectively inhibited fibrotic remodeling processes, suggesting that this cytokine may be an important mediator of inflammation-induced tissue fibrosis.

Although the mechanisms by which IL-13 induces tissue fibrosis are far from understood, several recent studies have begun to shed light on the sequence of events leading to IL-13–induced fibrosis. IL-13 likely regulates tissue fibrosis through a series of coordinated actions on a number of cells types within the lung. First, IL-13 has been shown by several investigators to upregulate the synthesis of arginase I (422,423). Arginase I is an enzyme that hydrolyzes L-arginine to urea and L-ornithine, which is a necessary metabolite for the production of polyamines and prolines required for collagen synthesis by fibroblasts. Evidence of an in vivo role for this pathway in tissues fibrosis was provided by Hesse et al. (422). Specifically, they showed that blockade of ornithine-aminodecarboxylase, which ultimately results in the generation of proline, markedly enhanced parasite-driven tissue fibrosis. Consistent with a role for arginase I in asthma, Rothenberg et al. (423) demonstrated that the enzyme is upregulated in an ovalbumin model of asthma and in animals exposed to recombinant IL-13 as well as in lung tissues of asthmatics, compared to normal individuals.

Second, IL-13–dependent lung fibrosis is mediated via its ability to induce and activate the profibrotic mediator TGF-β *(424)*. In this regard, IL-13 induces the production of TGF-β both directly in epithelial cells *(425)*, and indirectly in monocytes/macrophages via its ability to recruit and activate these cells *(424)*. This is thought to occur via the interaction of MCP-1 with its receptor CCR2 on monocyte/macrophages, as both lung fibrosis and TGF-β production in IL-13 transgenic mice are diminished in mice devoid of CCR2 *(426)*. Further support for this argument is the fact that MCP-1 has been shown to stimulate TGF-β1 production in lung fibroblasts *(427)*. In addition to stimulation of TGF-β synthesis, IL-13 also activates latent TGF-β through the induction of MPP9 *(424)*.

Lastly, IL-13 may also have a direct effect on fibrotic processes by stimulating the proliferation of myofibroblasts via a STAT6-dependent process involving platelet-derived growth factor AA (PDGF-AA) *(428)*. Lung fibrosis may also arise as a result of IL-13's ability to stimulate the accumulation of the nucleoside, adenosine (429). Specifically, it has been shown that IL-13–overexpressing mice have increased adenosine levels and reduced adenosine deaminase (ADA) gene expression and enzyme activity, while exhibiting marked increases in lung collagen. Furthermore, blockade of adenosine levels in the lung by ADA enzyme therapy diminished IL-13–induced fibrosis concomitant with a reduction in elaboration of a selective set of chemokines (MCP-1, -2, -3, -5 and eotaxin). Collectively these studies suggest that a number of IL-13–driven processes culminate in the generation of fibrogenic processes in the lung.

Airway hyperresponsiveness (AHR) or an exaggerated response to specific and nonspecific stimuli is a hallmark of asthma. The exact mechanisms by which IL-13 induces airway hyperresponsiveness are currently unknown. Several lines of evidence suggest that IL-13 can induce airway hyperresponsiveness in the absence of inflammatory cells. The initial IL-13Rα2Ig studies showed that IL-13 blockade inhibited AHR without affecting inflammatory cell recruitment or IgE synthesis (61). Moreover, Grunig et al. (39) demonstrated that T and B cells were not essential for IL-13's effects on AHR. Support for this contention is provided by Vargaftig et al. (430), who demonstrated that pretreatment of mice with vinblastine, a granulocyte inhibitor, failed to inhibit IL-13–induced AHR. In support of this theory, IL-13 has been shown to induce hyperresponsiveness as early as 6 hours after administration, long before significant inflammation has occurred *(431)*. In addition, Kibe et al. *(432)* reported that glucocorticoid treatment that inhibits lung eosinophilia did not attenuate AHR induced by IL-13. More definitely, studies in mast-cell–deficient *(433)* and eotaxin/IL-5 double-knockout mice *(412)* confirm the contention that the traditional effector cells, B cells, mast cells, and eosinophils, are not required for IL-13 to induce AHR. Collectively, these results suggest that although IL-13 is able to direct the recruitment of inflammatory cells into the airways, they are likely not necessary for induction of

AHR. Alternatively, IL-13 may induce AHR via direct effects on resident airway cells.

Whether airway hyperresponsiveness is mediated by direct effects on airway smooth muscle (ASM) or indirectly via effects on resident airway cells such as the epithelium is currently a matter of debate. IL-13 could potentially induce direct effects on ASM, as these cells do indeed express the IL-13 receptor chains including the IL-4Rα, the IL-13Rα1, and the IL-13Rα2 chain, but not the common γ chain. In this regard, several investigators have shown in both murine *(434)* and rabbit tracheal strips *(435)* that IL-13 treatment enhanced maximal carbachol- and KCL-induced force generation, while IL-4 had no effect. One group has provided strong evidence that this effect is likely mediated via resident airway cells, as IL-13 overexpression in mice with STAT6 expressed only in the airway epithelium are hyperresponsive (208). Nonetheless, IL-13 has been shown to enhance bradykinin-, histamine-, and acetylcholine-induced intracellular calcium fluxes in isolated smooth muscle cells *(436)*. Consistent with these findings, Shore et al. have shown that IL-13 increases LTD4-stimulated changes in isolated smooth muscle cell stiffness—a surrogate of contraction. It is speculated that these changes may be mediated via the ability of IL-13 to increase cysteinyl leukotriene receptor (CysLT1) expression on smooth muscle cells *(437)*. This is particularly interesting, as IL-4 does not upregulate CysLT1 expression. However, this would likely not explain the effects of IL-13 on responses to other contractile agonists. A more general mechanism by which IL-13 may alter contractile function of ASM has been recently been postulated by Panettieri et al. (438). Specifically, they showed that IL-13 induces calcium fluxes in ASM via increasing CD38 expression and cADP-ribosyl cyclase (cADPR) activity, as evidenced by the ability of an cADPR inhibitor to block these responses. Taken together, these results suggest that although no one to date has shown direct contraction of ASM in response to IL-13, it is likely that through its ability to induce calcium activation pathways and/or LTD4-receptor expression, it enhances responses to other endogenous contractile agonists. Alternatively, IL-13 may also affect contractile properties of smooth muscle by altering the ability of smooth muscle to relax once contracted. For example, several groups have reported that IL-13 significantly reduces B-adrenoceptor–induced relaxation of airway smooth muscle *(435,439)*. The effects of IL-13 on smooth muscle function may also be a result of significant increases in the area of airway smooth muscle in the airway wall. Although IL-13 likely does not directly mediate smooth muscle proliferation, it may influence muscle proliferation indirectly via stimulation of CysLTs *(437)*. Specifically, although IL-13 treatment of ASM cells in culture alone did not induce smooth muscle proliferation, pretreatment of cells with IL-13 enhanced proliferation induced by LTD4. Similar effects were also observed with TGF-β treatment of cells. The enhanced proliferation was prevented by pretreatment of the cytokine-primed cells with a selective Cys-LT receptor antagonist. The authors speculate that muscle thickening may be due to positive feedback interactions between leukotrienes, IL-13 and TGF-β. Alternatively, IL-13 may induce smooth muscle proliferation through its ability to increase vascular endothelial growth factor (VEGF) from human airway smooth muscle that in turn induces fibronectin expression in these cells *(440)*. Fibronectin also promotes ASM mitogenesis in vitro *(441)*. Although the exact mechanism(s) through which IL-13 regulates smooth muscle function are only beginning to be understood, the collective data support the ability of IL-13 to alter airway smooth muscle function both indirectly and perhaps directly via binding its receptors on smooth muscle.

Another potential mechanism by which IL-13 may regulate airway tone is via the induction of the AMCase chitinase gene (442). In an elegant paper, Zhu et al. have recently shown that IL-13 induces the expression of an acidic mammalian chitinase (AMCase) in airway epithelium and macrophages and that either inhibition of chitinase enzyme activity or treatment of mice with antiserum directed against the chitinase abolished IL-13–induced AHR. Although the exact mechanisms by which IL-13 induction of chitinase results in the development of airway hyperresponsiveness are currently unknown, expression of the chitinase gene in mouse airway epithelial cells resulted in elaboration of several chemokines, namely, eotaxin and MCP-1. As discussed previously, both of these chemokines have been shown to be important in allergic inflammation and airway reactivity.

Chitin is a common carbohydrate polymer found in nematodes, insects, and fungi. In this regard, it is also found in organisms that provide a rich source of allergens, such as house dust mite and cockroaches. As such, it is interesting to speculate that these chitins may serve as environmental triggers for Th2 immune responses in general. Thus, one may envision a scenario in which the Th2 immune response likely arose as a defense against chitin-containing parasitic organisms, but for some unknown reason, in susceptible individuals, this response has been co-opted to defend against chitin-containing organisms (HDM, cockroaches) that are neither infectious nor inherently harmful. Clearly, defining the role of chitinases in allergic asthma and more broadly in Th2-mediated immune responses is an area ripe for study.

Whether IL-13 mediates AHR via sequential activation of the above-mentioned pathways, through a combination of these pathways, or by yet-unidentified pathways, the stimulation of IL-13 receptors on the epithelium clearly plays an important role in IL-13–mediated airway hyperresponsiveness. Nonetheless, as the studies referenced previously suggest that IL-13 also has direct effects on airway smooth muscle, airway hyperresponsiveness likely arises via the combined actions of IL-13 on the epithelium and airway smooth muscle.

Although IL-13 does not appear to have direct effects on T-cell differentiation, several lines of evidence suggest that it may affect or perpetuate the Th2 response via several pathways. First, it induces the expression of several chemokines that are thought to selectively recruit Th2 cells, namely, TARC and MDC (443). Second, it can recruit additional dendritic cells to the site of allergen exposure via the induction of MMP9 and TARC *(444)*. Further, it appears to promote its own production via regulation of the production of several mediators such as adenosine and histamine, which, in turn, stimulate cells such as eosinophils, mast cells, basophils, and smooth muscle cells to produce more IL-13. Through stimulation of these pathways, IL-13 may be an important contributor to the chronicity of allergic disease. Thus, blockade of IL-13 may have the added benefit of breaking this vicious Th2-promoting positive feedback loop.

The importance of IL-13 in allergic disorders in humans is supported by numerous reports of exaggerated IL-13 production in asthma, atopic rhinitis, and allergic dermatitis (445). In asthma in particular, both message and protein levels of IL-13 are elevated in bronchial biopsy specimens and BAL cells from allergic individuals when compared with those of control subjects *(222)*. Conversely, IL-13 levels are reduced in asthmatic and rhinitis patients undergoing allergen desensitization treatment regimes or steroid treatment *(222)*. Moreover, a recent cohort study of neonates demonstrates that high IL-13 productive capacity of cord-blood $CD4^+$ T cells is a significant predictor of risk for subsequent development of atopic diseases *(446)*. In support of the notion that IL-13 is a central effector of allergic immune responses, several groups have reported strong associations of polymorphisms in the IL-13 promoter and coding region with various features of the asthmatic phenotype (447,448). Of particular interest is the Arg130/Gln substitution in the coding region of IL-13 noted by multiple groups and detected across multiple ethnic groups. Moreover, Arima et al. have recently provided evidence that the Arg110Gln may be a functional variant *(449)*. Utilizing a mutant recombinant IL-13, they show that recombinant IL-13 containing the Gln110 variant bound the IL-13 receptor α2 chain with lower affinity than the wild-type IL-13, resulting in a lower clearance rate of the cytokine. Interestingly, they demonstrated that although the IL-13 variant did not alter any biologic properties of IL-13, asthmatic patients homozygous for the Gln110 variant have higher serum levels of IL-13 than those without the variant. They postulated that impaired binding of IL-13 by the soluble IL-13Rα2 chain leads to higher serum levels and prolonged activity of IL-13 in vivo. Vercelli et al. (450) have also shown that the -1112T variant of the IL-13 promoter is functional, as expression of it in human and murine $CD4^+$ Th2 lymphocytes enhanced IL13 promoter activity. Interestingly, increased expression of IL13-1112T in Th2 cells was associated with the creation of a Yin-Yang 1 binding site that overlapped a STAT motif involved in negative regulation of IL-13 expression and attenuated STAT6-mediated transcriptional repression. The enhanced IL-13 secretion in IL13-1112TT homozygotes suggests that expression of this allele may underlie its association with susceptibility to allergic inflammation.

Unifying Hypothesis

The elicitation of allergic airway responses in a sensitized individual upon re-exposure to offending allergens is likely the culmination of a complex network of cellular and molecular events (Figure 43.). Following antigen challenge, cross-linking of antigen and IgE on IgE-bearing cells leads to the immediate release of substances such as histamine, leukotrienes, PGD_2, and tryptase. The actions of these mediators account for the immediate symptoms, such as smooth muscle constriction, vasodilation, and increased vascular permeability. It is possible that the release of IL-13 by either mast cells or basophils can also induce many of these same symptoms. Secretion of chemokines (eotaxin) and cytokines (IL-4, IL-5) by basophils and mast cells also serve to attract more T cells, antigen-presenting cells, and effector cells such as eosinophils to the site of insult. Simultaneously, dendritic cells within the mucosa are presenting allergen to T cells and, within 6 to 48 hours, additional T cells are recruited to the area. The expression of FcεRI on the surface of dendritic cells greatly facilitates their uptake, processing, and presentation of allergens to T cells during the elicitation phase of the response. Furthermore, the cytokine milieu created as a result of mast-cell and basophil activation, namely, a Th2 cytokine environment, most likely drives a polarized Th2 response. Further production of Th2 cytokines at the local site augments the recruitment and activation of additional eosinophils and T cells. During the late phase, release of mediators from mast cells, basophils, eosinophils, and T cells act in concert to induce the vascular changes, bronchoconstrictor, and mucus changes observed during the late-phase response. Many repetitions of this sequence lead to persistent inflammation, resulting in alterations in the structure and function of resident mucosal cells such as smooth muscle, fibroblasts, and epithelial cells. As many of the actions of these effector cells are redundant, it is not surprising that neither depletion of mast cells nor depletion of eosinophils has been sufficient to significantly ablate the physiologic consequences of allergen exposure. One point of convergence is the production of IL-13 by all of the likely suspects (e.g., basophils, mast cells, eosinophils, and T cells). Given its ability to induce effector functions, elevations in IL-13 levels may not only provide a unifying explanation for the

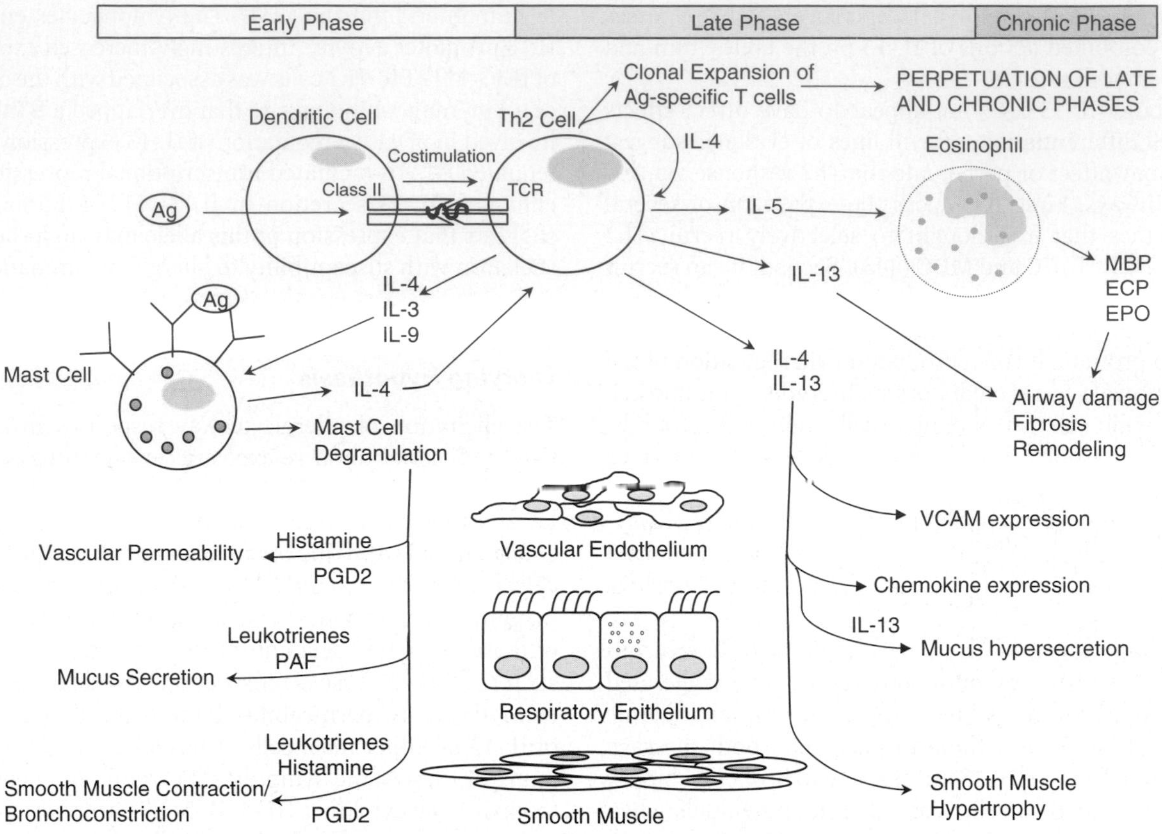

FIGURE 43.9 Overview of the acute, late, and chronic phases of the allergic response. Crosslinking of surface IgE on sensitized mast cells by antigen results in mast-cell degranulation and release of numerous mediators, including histamine, tryptase, PDG_2, and cytokines. These mediators are largely responsible for the early phase of the allergic response. Antigen presentation by dendritic cells to Th2 cells results in activation and clonal expansion of antigen-specific T cells and the subsequent release of Th2 cytokines, IL-4, IL-5, and IL-13. These cytokines result in recruitment of eosinophils, chemokine expression, smooth muscle hypertrophy, and mucus hypersecretion. Ultimately, long-term exposure to IL-13 and eosinophilic effector molecules leads to the structural changes observed in tissues of individuals with chronic disease.

importance of multiple effector cells in allergic responses, it may also provide an ideal target for therapy.

CHARACTERISTICS OF SPECIFIC ATOPIC DISORDERS

In this section, we will briefly discuss the clinical manifestations, pathogenesis, and therapeutic strategies for the treatment of the classical atopic syndromes, including anaphylaxis, allergic rhinitis, atopic dermatitis, and asthma. Readers should consult clinical allergy textbooks for further details on these disorders.

Anaphylaxis

Anaphylaxis refers to a systemic, immediate hypersensitivity reaction that results from IgE-mediated release of vasoactive and inflammatory mediators from mast cells and basophils. Death from anaphylaxis is most often due to respiratory obstruction and/or cardiovascular collapse. The initial experimental description of the phenomenon dates to a paper published in 1902, in which Portier and Richet *(451)* described the sensitization of dogs to sea anemone venom, a process with fatal sequelae upon subsequent exposure to nonlethal doses of the venom. In opposition to prophylaxis, this was termed *anaphylaxis,* meaning against or without protection. Common causes of anaphylaxis in humans include exposure to antibiotics and other drugs, radiocontrast media, latex, venom, and foods. The cause of anaphylaxis remains unidentified in up to two thirds of patients. Whereas anaphylactic reactions involve IgE-mediated mast cell and basophil degranulation by definition, anaphylactoid reactions result from mast-cell and basophil degranulation by IgE-independent means. Underlying etiologies, where known, include drugs, biologic agents, and physical factors (e.g., pressure, cold, sunlight); a substantial proportion of cases are idiopathic.

Allergic Rhinitis

In 1819, John Bostock first described catarrus aestivus or hay fever *(452)*. In 1873, Charles Blackley recognized that pollen grains were the causative agents of hay fever. In the 1800s, hay fever was considererd a rare disorder, restricted to the privileged class. This is certainly no longer the case. According to recent estimates, up to 40% of children in the United States are affected by allergic rhinitis *(453)*, making it the most common atopic disorder in the industrial North. Allergic rhinitis is an IgE-mediated disease characterized by sneezing, rhinorrhea, nasal congestion, and nasal pruritis *(454,455)*. The seasonal form is caused by allergens released during tree, grass, or weed pollination; the perennial form is associated with allergies to animal dander, dust mites, and/or mold spores. Skin testing—the experimental interrogation of the ability of a panel of antigen extracts to induce cutaneous immediate-type hypersensitivity responses—is often employed for diagnostic confirmation of atopy, and to determine the allergens to which an individual is sensitized.

Treatment strategies include allergen avoidance, antihistamines, α-adrenergic agonists, intranasal steroids, topical ipratropium bromide, and immunotherapy regimes. Immunotherapy, introduced by Noon and Freeman in 1911 as a method for protecting patients against the effects of "pollen toxin" *(456)*, has been used since as a treatment for patients with allergic rhinitis and allergic asthma. Conventional allergen immunotherapy involves the subcutaneous injection of graded quantities of allergen. Although such immunotherapy has been associated with therapeutic benefit, the relevant immunologic mechanisms remain obscure. In patients with venom anaphylaxis, allergen immunotherapy is the prophylactic treatment of choice.

Food Allergy

Food allergy needs careful distinction from the more common adverse reactions to ingested substances (e.g., food intolerance, dose-related toxic reactions) that are not immune-mediated. True food allergy afflicts approximately 8% of children under the age of 3 years, and 2% of the adult population. Such food hypersensitivity comprises several disorders that vary in time of onset, severity, and persistence. The most common type of food allergy is immediate gastrointestinal hypersensitivity. Symptoms, consisting of nausea, abdominal pain, colic, vomiting, and/or diarrhea, develop within minutes to 2 hours of antigen exposure. Infants with this syndrome may present with intermittent vomiting and poor weight gain. The predominant response to orally ingested antigens is the induction of tolerance. Food allergy represents an aberration of this process. Only a small number of foodstuffs account for the vast majority of offending allergens. In childhood, the most common allergens derive from milk, egg, peanut, soy, and wheat. In adults, the most common foods implicated are peanuts, tree nuts, fish, and shellfish. Most food allergens are relatively small, water-soluble, heat- and acid-stable glycoproteins that are resistant to proteolytic degradation. The higher incidence of disease in childhood is presumably related to factors regulating the ontogeny of the gut and immune system development *(457,458)*. Therapy revolves around avoidance of the offending allergen. Interestingly, patients with atopic dermatitis commonly have subclinical food hypersensitivity, with ingestion of the relevant allergen leading to worsening of their dermatitis.

Oral allergy syndrome represents a second type of food hypersensitivity. This is an immediate-type contact allergy that leads to pruritus, tingling, and swelling of the lips, palate, and throat following ingestion of the offending allergen, usually in fruits or vegetables. Oral allergy syndrome affects up to 40% of adults with defined pollen allergy, due to cross-reacting allergens. Therapy involves allergen avoidance.

The eosinophilic gastroenteritides (eosinophilic esophagitis, gastritis, gastroenteritis), though not thought in general to be due to food allergy, deserve brief mention here. These syndromes are characterized pathologically by eosinophil infiltration, and clinically by a variety of nonspecific symptoms, including abdominal pain, nausea, vomiting, and diarrhea, although the etiology and pathogenesis remain unclear in most cases. Some cases are due to hypersensitivity reactions to antigens derived from *Anycylostoma caninum*, a common dog hookworm that is poorly adapted to, and causes nonpatent infection of, humans *(459)*. Some cases may indeed be due to food allergy.

Atopic Dermatitis

Atopic dermatitis is a common, chronic, relapsing, inflammatory skin disease characterized by dry skin, severe pruritis, secondary excoriation which can lead to lichenification, and a heightened susceptibility to cutaneous infections. Atopic dermatitis can lead to significant suffering, both physical and psychologic. The prevalence of atopic dermatitis has increased in the last few decades; currently, 10% are affected at some point during childhood in the United States. Both environmental and genetic factors seem to play a role in susceptibility. Given the fact that the hereditability of atopy appears to be largely disease type–independent, it is notable that parental atopic dermatitis confers a higher risk for the development of atopic dermatitis than for either allergic asthma or allergic rhinitis in offspring, suggesting the likelihood of atopic dermatitis–specific genes *(460)*. Disease generally presents early in childhood and is associated with sensitivity to food and/or inhalant allergens. In adults, disease is primarily associated with sensitivity to inhalant allergens. Apart from exposure to specific food and inhalant allergens, environmental triggers such as irritating substances, emotional stress, climactic factors, hormones, and local infections are all known to be important in the expression of atopic dermatitis. Skin lesions generally display evidence of mast-cell, eosinophil, and T-cell infiltration and activation. In contrast to other atopic disorders, a biphasic pattern of T-cell polarization or reactivity is present in atopic dermatitis: Th2 cytokines predominate in acute lesions, whereas chronic lesions express a mix of Th1 and Th2 cytokines.

Current treatment of atopic dermatitis is directed at symptomatic relief, skin hydration, the reduction of cutaneous inflammation, and avoidance of inciting antigens. Therapies include antihistamines, topical immunosuppressive agents (glucocorticoids, FK506), moisturizers, environmental control measures for inhalant allergens, and food-elimination diets for food allergens. Recent Phase I and II studies have supported the efficacy of short-term IFN-γ therapy in the treatment of severe atopic dermatitis *(461)*, although the mechanism of action remains unclear.

Asthma

The term *asthma* was coined by Hippocrates to refer to attacks of breathlessness and wheezing. Asthma is a complex inflammatory disease of the lung in which the prevalence, morbidity, and mortality have been increasing markedly over the last few decades. Asthma is a heterogeneous disorder with variations in the age of onset, severity of disease, and underlying pathogenesis. Although asthma is multifactorial in origin, with both environmental and genetic influences, atopy is the strongest identifiable predisposing factor for the development of asthma. Most childhood asthma is allergic in nature and is referred to as extrinsic or atopic asthma; however, asthma that develops in adulthood and some forms of childhood asthma are not associated with elevated IgE, and this form is referred to as intrinsic or nonatopic asthma. In the most common form of the disease, extrinsic asthma, the inflammatory process is thought to arise as a result of inappropriate immune responses to commonly inhaled antigens. The inflammatory response in the asthmatic lung is characterized by infiltration of the airway wall with lymphocytes, predominantly $CD4^+$ T cells, eosinophils, and degranulated mast cells. Structurally, the airways of asthmatics are characterized by mucus cell hyperplasia, subepithelial membrane thickening, and loss of epithelial cell integrity. These cellular findings have consistently been associated with the main physiologic abnormalities of the disease, including variable airflow obstruction and airway hyperresponsiveness. As discussed extensively in this chapter, the pathologic consequences of this disease are thought to arise as a result of skewed T-cell responses to inhaled antigens, which in turn lead to activation and recruitment of the primary effector cells, mast cells, eosinophils, and T cells. Activation of these cells results in the release of a plethora of mediators that individually or in concert induce changes in airway geometry and produce the symptoms of the disease.

Current guidelines for asthma management emphasize environmental control measures, objective monitoring, and pharmacotherapy for comprehensive asthma management. The exact combination of pharmacotherapy is dependent on the severity of disease, with short-acting bronchodilators (β-adrenergic agonists) being recommended for mild intermittent asthma, with the addition of anti-inflammatory medication including inhaled or oral corticosteroids, cromolyn or nedocromil, or a leukotriene antagonists being indicated for more severe disease. Several new therapies have been introduced over the last few years, including the anti-IgE monoclonal antibody omalizumab (Xolair), which is a recombinant humanized monoclonal anti-IgE antibody that has demonstrated efficacy in allergic asthma and other IgE-related allergic illnesses (seasonal and perennial allergic rhinitis). In three pivotal, placebo-controlled trials in patients with moderate-to-severe allergic asthma, omalizumab provided effective disease control, significantly reducing exacerbations and the need for unscheduled outpatient visits, emergency room visits, and hospitalizations (see review, 462). Trials in humans have shown that Amb a 1, a ragweed-pollen antigen, conjugated to a phosphorothioate oligodeoxyribonucleotide immunostimulatory sequence of DNA, greatly reduced allergenicity, and may offer long-term clinical efficacy in the treatment of allergic rhinitis (463). Clinical trials aimed at blocking IL-13 and/or IL-4 pathways are underway, and early reports suggest that this approach may be promising: however, as clinical testing of these new therapies is in early stages, determination of their efficacy in asthma therapy awaits further study.

ACKNOWLEDGMENTS

The authors would like to thank Christopher Karp for editorial assistance. The author acknowledges the support of National Institute of Health grants, HL076383, PO1 ES009606, and HL67736 to MWK.

REFERENCES

4. Ishizaka K, Ishizaka T, Hornbrook MM. Physico chemical properties of human reaginic antibody. IV. Presence of a unique immunoglobulin as a carrier of reaginic activity. *J Immunol.* 1966;97:75–85.
5. Ishizaka K, Ishizaka T, Hornbrook MM. Physicochemical properties of reaginic antibody. V. Correlation of reaginic activity wth gamma-E-globulin antibody. *J Immunol.* 1966;97:840–853.
15. Schulz O, Sewell HF, Shakib F. Proteolytic cleavage of CD25, the alpha subunit of the human T cell interleukin 2 receptor, by

Der p 1, a major mite allergen with cysteine protease activity. *J Exp Med*. 1998;187:271–275.
17. Morgan MS, Arlian LG. Enzymatic activity in extracts of allergy-causing astigmatid mites. *J Med Entomol*. 2006;43:1200–1207.
18. Page K, Hughes VS, Bennett GW, et al. German cockroach proteases regulate matrix metalloproteinase-9 in human bronchial epithelial cells. *Allergy*. 2006;61:988–995.
20. Traidl-Hoffmann C, Mariani V, Hochrein H, et al. Pollen-associated phytoprostanes inhibit dendritic cell interleukin-12 production and augment T helper type 2 cell polarization. *J Exp Med*. 2005;201:627–636.
21. Boldogh I, Bacsi A, Choudhury BK, et al. ROS generated by pollen NADPH oxidase provide a signal that augments antigen-induced allergic airway inflammation. *J Clin Invest*. 2005;115:2169–179.
26. Karlsson MG, Davidsson A, Hellquist HB. Increase in CD4$^+$ and CD45RO$^+$ memory T cells in the nasal mucosa of allergic patients. *APMIS*. 1994;102:753–758.
27. Azzawi M, Bradley B, Jeffery PK, et al. Identification of activated T lymphocytes and eosinophils in bronchial biopsies in stable atopic asthma. *Am Rev Respir Dis*. 1990;142:1407–1413.
28. Corrigan CJ, Kay AB. CD4 T-lymphocyte activation in acute severe asthma. Relationship to disease severity and atopic status. *Am Rev Respir Dis*. 1990;141:970–977.
29. Mosmann TR, Cherwinski H, Bond MW, et al. Two types of murine helper T cell clone. I. Definition according to profiles of lymphokine activities and secreted proteins. *J Immunol*. 1986;136:2348–2357.
30. Street NE, Mosmann TR. Functional diversity of T lymphocytes due to secretion of different cytokine patterns. *FASEB J*. 1991;5:171–177.
31. Kapsenberg ML, Wierenga EA, Bos JD, et al. Functional subsets of allergen-reactive human CD4$^+$ T cells. *Immunol Today*. 1991;12:392–395.
35. Werfel T, Morita A, Grewe M, et al. Allergen specificity of skin-infiltrating T cells is not restricted to a type-2 cytokine pattern in chronic skin lesions of atopic dermatitis. *J Invest Dermatol*. 1996;107:871–876.
36. Fokkens WJ, Godthelp T, Holm AF, et al. Allergic rhinitis and inflammation: the effect of nasal corticosteroid therapy. *Allergy*. 1997;52:29–32.
37. Secrist H, Chelen CJ, Wen Y, et al. Allergen immunotherapy decreases interleukin 4 production in CD4$^+$ T cells from allergic individuals. *J Exp Med*. 1993;178:2123–2130.
38. Gavett SH, Chen X, Finkelman F, et al. Depletion of murine CD4$^+$ T lymphocytes prevents antigen-induced airway hyperreactivity and pulmonary eosinophilia. *Am J Respir Cell Mol Biol*. 1994;10:587–593.
39. Grunig G, Warnock M, Wakil AE, et al. Requirement for IL-13 independently of IL-4 in experimental asthma. *Science*. 1998;282:2261–2263.
40. Corry DB, Grunig G, Hadeiba H, et al. Requirements for allergen-induced airway hyperreactivity in T and B cell-deficient mice. *Mol Med*. 1998;4:344–355.
41. Gonzalo JA, Lloyd CM, Kremer L, et al. Eosinophil recruitment to the lung in a murine model of allergic inflammation. The role of T cells, chemokines, and adhesion receptors. *J Clin Invest*. 1996;98:2332–2345.
43. Gavett SH, O'Hearn DJ, Li X, et al. Interleukin 12 inhibits antigen-induced airway hyperresponsiveness, inflammation, and Th2 cytokine expression in mice. *J Exp Med*. 1995;182:1527–1536.
48. Gavett SH, O'Hearn DJ, Karp CL, et al. Interleukin-4 receptor blockade prevents airway responses induced by antigen challenge in mice. *Am J Physiol*. 1997;272:L253–L261.
49. Kung TT, Stelts DM, Zurcher JA, et al. Involvement of IL-5 in a murine model of allergic pulmonary inflammation: prophylactic and therapeutic effect of an anti-IL-5 antibody. *Am J Respir Cell Mol Biol*. 1995;13:360–365.
50. Foster PS, Hogan SP, Ramsay AJ, et al. Interleukin 5 deficiency abolishes eosinophilia, airways hyperreactivity, and lung damage in a mouse asthma model. *J Exp Med*. 1996;183:195–201.
51. Brusselle G, Kips J, Joos G, et al. Allergen-induced airway inflammation and bronchial responsiveness in wild-type and interleukin-4-deficient mice. *Am J Respir Cell Mol Biol*. 1995;12:254–259.
53. Spergel JM, Mizoguchi E, Oettgen H, et al. Roles of TH1 and TH2 cytokines in a murine model of allergic dermatitis. *J Clin Invest*. 1999;103:1103–1111.
58. Coyle AJ, Le G Gros, Bertrand C, et al. Interleukin-4 is required for the induction of lung Th2 mucosal immunity. *Am J Respir Cell Mol Biol*. 1995;13:54–59.
59. Rothenberg ME, Hogan SP. The eosinophil. *Annu Rev Immunol*. 2006;24:147–174.
61. Wills-Karp M, Luyimbazi J, Xu X, et al. Interleukin-13: central mediator of allergic asthma. *Science*. 1998;282:2258–2261.
62. Frohlich A, Marsland BJ, Sonderegger I, et al. IL-21 receptor signaling is integral to the development of Th2 effector responses in vivo. *Blood*. 2007;109:2023–2031.
63. Akbari O, Stock P, Meyer E, et al. Essential role of NKT cells producing IL-4 and IL-13 in the development of allergen-induced airway hyperreactivity. *Nat Med*. 2003;9:582–588.
64. Lisbonne M, Diem S, de Castro Keller A, et al. Cutting edge: invariant V alpha 14 NKT cells are required for allergen-induced airway inflammation and hyperreactivity in an experimental asthma model. *J Immunol*. 2003;171:1637–1641.
65. Meyer EH, Goya S, Akbari O, et al. Glycolipid activation of invariant T cell receptor$^+$ NK T cells is sufficient to induce airway hyperreactivity independent of conventional CD4$^+$ T cells. *Proc Natl Acad Sci U S A*. 2006;103:2782–2787.
68. Akbari O, Faul JL, Hoyte EG, et al. CD4$^+$ invariant T-cell-receptor$^+$ natural killer T cells in bronchial asthma. *N Engl J Med*. 2006;354:1117–1129.
69. Sen Y, Yongyi B, Yuling H, et al. V alpha 24-invariant NKT cells from patients with allergic asthma express CCR9 at high frequency and induce Th2 bias of CD3$^+$ T cells upon CD226 engagement. *J Immunol*. 2005;175:4914–4926.
70. Elkhal A, Pichavant M, He R, et al. CD1d restricted natural killer T cells are not required for allergic skin inflammation. *J Allergy Clin Immunol*. 2006;118:1363–1368.
71. Agea E, Russano A, Bistoni O, et al. Human CD1-restricted T cell recognition of lipids from pollens. *J Exp Med*. 2005;202:295–308.
72. Zhou D, Mattner J, Cantu C 3rd, et al. Lysosomal glycosphingolipid recognition by NKT cells. *Science*. 2004;306:1786–1789.
73. Scherf W, Burdach S, Hansen G. Reduced expression of transforming growth factor beta 1 exacerbates pathology in an experimental asthma model. *Eur J Immunol*. 2005;35:198–206.
75. Zuany-Amorim C, Sawicka E, Manlius C, et al. Suppression of airway eosinophilia by killed *Mycobacterium vaccae*-induced allergen-specific regulatory T-cells. *Nat Med*. 2002;8:625–629.
77. Matsumoto K, Inoue H, Fukuyama S, et al. Decrease of interleukin-10-producing T cells in the peripheral blood of severe unstable atopic asthmatics. *Int Arch Allergy Immunol*. 2004;134:295–302.
78. Ling EM, Smith T, Nguyen XD, et al. Relation of CD4$^+$CD25$^+$ regulatory T-cell suppression of allergen-driven T-cell activation to atopic status and expression of allergic disease. *Lancet*. 2004;363:608–615.
79. Karlsson MR, Rugtveit J, Brandtzaeg P. Allergen-responsive CD4$^+$CD25$^+$ regulatory T cells in children who have outgrown cow's milk allergy. *J Exp Med*. 2004, 199:1679–1688.
80. Karagiannidis C, Akdis M, Holopainen P, et al. Glucocorticoids upregulate FOXP3 expression and regulatory T cells in asthma. *J Allergy Clin Immunol*. 2004;114:1425–1433.
81. Fainaru O, Woolf E, Lotem J, et al. Runx3 regulates mouse TGF-beta-mediated dendritic cell function and its absence results in airway inflammation. *EMBO J*. 2004;23:969–979.
82. Lewkowich IP, Herman NS, Schleifer KW, et al. CD4$^+$CD25$^+$ T cells protect against experimentally induced asthma and alter pulmonary dendritic cell phenotype and function. *J Exp Med*. 2005;202:1549–1561.
84. Prescott SL, Macaubas C, Holt BJ, et al. Transplacental priming of the human immune system to environmental allergens: universal skewing of initial T cell responses toward the Th2 cytokine profile. *J Immunol*. 1998;160:4730–4737.
85. Ober C. Susceptibility genes in asthma and allergy. *Curr Allergy Asthma Rep*. 2001;1:174–179.
89. Marsh DG, Neely JD, Breazeale DR, et al. Linkage analysis of IL4 and other chromosome 5q31.1 markers and total serum immunoglobulin E concentrations. *Science*. 1994;264:1152–1156.
90. Ober C, Hoffjan S. Asthma genetics. 2006: the long and winding road to gene discovery. *Genes Immun*. 2006;7:95–100.
91. Wills-Karp M, Ewart SL. Time to draw breath: asthma-susceptibility genes are identified. *Nat Rev Genet*. 2004;5:376–387.

97. Warner JA, Miles EA, Jones AC, et al. Is deficiency of interferon gamma production by allergen triggered cord blood cells a predictor of atopic eczema? *Clin Exp Allergy*. 1994;24:423–430.
99. Prescott SL, Macaubas C, Smallacombe T, et al. Reciprocal age-related patterns of allergen-specific T-cell immunity in normal vs. atopic infants. *Clin Exp Allergy*. 1998;28(suppl 5):39–44; discussion 50–51.
101. Strachan DP. Hay fever, hygiene, and household size. *Br Med J*. 1989;299:1259–1260.
102. von Mutius E, Martinez FD, Fritzsch C, et al. Prevalence of asthma and atopy in two areas of West and East Germany. *Am J Respir Crit Care Med*. 1994;149:358–364.
103. Matricardi PM, Rosmini F, Ferrigno L, et al. Cross sectional retrospective study of prevalence of atopy among Italian military students with antibodies against hepatitis A virus. *Br Med J*. 1997;314:999–1003.
104. McIntire JJ, Umetsu SE, Macaubas C, et al. Immunology: hepatitis A virus link to atopic disease. *Nature*. 2003;425:576.
107. Adlerberth I, Carlsson B, de Man P, et al. Intestinal colonization with Enterobacteriaceae in Pakistani and Swedish hospital-delivered infants. *Acta Paediatr Scand*. 1991;80:602–610.
110. Bjorksten B. The environmental influence on childhood asthma. *Allergy*. 1999;54:17–23.
114. Gao PS, Mao XQ, Baldini M, et al. Serum total IgE levels and CD14 on chromosome 5q31 (letter). *Clin Genet*. 1999;56:164–165.
115. Fageras Bottcher M, Hmani-Aifa M, Lindstrom A, et al. A TLR4 polymorphism is associated with asthma and reduced lipopolysaccharide-induced interleukin-12(p70) responses in Swedish children. *J Allergy Clin Immunol*. 2004;114:561–567.
116. Raby BA, Klimecki WT, Laprise C, et al. Polymorphisms in toll-like receptor 4 are not associated with asthma or atopy-related phenotypes. *Am J Respir Crit Care Med*. 2002;166:1449–1456.
123. Diaz-Sanchez D, Rumold R, Gong H, Jr. Challenge with environmental tobacco smoke exacerbates allergic airway disease in human beings. *J Allergy Clin Immunol*. 2006;118:441–446.
126. Lambrecht BN. The dendritic cell in allergic airway diseases: a new player to the game. *Clin Exp Allergy*. 2001;31:206–218.
127. Moller GM, Overbeek SE, Van Helden-Meeuwsen CG, et al. Increased numbers of dendritic cells in the bronchial mucosa of atopic asthmatic patients: downregulation by inhaled corticosteroids. *Clin Exp Allergy*. 1996;26:517–524.
128. Tschernig T, Debertin AS, Paulsen F, et al. Dendritic cells in the mucosa of the human trachea are not regularly found in the first year of life. *Thorax*. 2001;56:427–431.
129. Hamada K, Goldsmith CA, Goldman A, et al. Resistance of very young mice to inhaled allergen sensitization is overcome by coexposure to an air-pollutant aerosol. *Am J Respir Crit Care Med*. 2000;161:1285–1293.
134. Jahnsen FL, Moloney ED, Hogan T, et al. Rapid dendritic cell recruitment to the bronchial mucosa of patients with atopic asthma in response to local allergen challenge. *Thorax*. 2001;56:823–826.
135. McWilliam AS, Napoli S, Marsh AM, et al. Dendritic cells are recruited into the airway epithelium during the inflammatory response to a broad spectrum of stimuli. *J Exp Med*. 1996;184:2429–432.
136. Upham JW, Denburg JA, O'Byrne PM. Rapid response of circulating myeloid dendritic cells to inhaled allergen in asthmatic subjects. *Clin Exp Allergy*. 2002;32:818–823.
137. Reibman J, Hsu Y, Chen LC, et al. Airway epithelial cells release MIP-3alpha/CCL20 in response to cytokines and ambient particulate matter. *Am J Respir Cell Mol Biol*. 2003;28:648–654.
139. Pichavant M, Charbonnier AS, Taront S, et al. Asthmatic bronchial epithelium activated by the proteolytic allergen Der p 1 increases selective dendritic cell recruitment. *J Allergy Clin Immunol*. 2005;115:771–778.
143. Krupnick AS, Gelman AE, Barchet W, et al. Murine vascular endothelium activates and induces the generation of allogeneic $CD4^{+}25^{+}Foxp3^{+}$ regulatory T cells. *J Immunol*. 2005;175:6265–6270.
144. Akbari O, Freeman GJ, Meyer EH, et al. Antigen-specific regulatory T cells develop via the ICOS-ICOS-ligand pathway and inhibit allergen-induced airway hyperreactivity. *Nat Med*. 2002;8:1024–1032.
146. Tesciuba AG, Subudhi S, Rother RP, et al. Inducible costimulator regulates Th2-mediated inflammation, but not Th2 differentiation, in a model of allergic airway disease. *J Immunol*. 2001;167:1996–2003.
147. Bellinghausen I, Brand U, Knop J, et al. Comparison of allergen-stimulated dendritic cells from atopic and nonatopic donors dissecting their effect on autologous naïve and memory T helper cells of such donors. *J Allergy Clin Immunol*. 2000;105:988–996.
148. Hammad H, Charbonnier AS, Duez C, et al. Th2 polarization by Der p 1-pulsed monocyte-derived dendritic cells is due to the allergic status of the donors. *Blood*. 2001;98:1135–1141.
150. Hammad H, Lambrecht BN, Pochard P, et al. Monocyte-derived dendritic cells induce a house dust mite-specific Th2 allergic inflammation in the lung of humanized SCID mice: involvement of CCR7. *J Immunol*. 2002;169:1524–1534.
151. Akdis M, Verhagen J, Taylor A, et al. Immune responses in healthy and allergic individuals are characterized by a fine balance between allergen-specific T regulatory 1 and T helper 2 cells. *J Exp Med*. 2004;199:1567–1575.
152. Shilling RA, Pinto JM, Decker DC, et al. Cutting edge: polymorphisms in the ICOS promoter region are associated with allergic sensitization and Th2 cytokine production. *J Immunol*. 2005;175:2061–2065.
153. Jones G, Wu S, Jang N, et al. Polymorphisms within the CTLA4 gene are associated with infant atopic dermatitis. *Br J Dermatol*. 2006;154:467–471.
154. Howard TD, Postma DS, Hawkins GA, et al. Fine mapping of an IgE-controlling gene on chromosome 2q: Analysis of CTLA4 and CD28. *J Allergy Clin Immunol*. 2002;110:743–751.
155. Becker S, Fenton MJ, Soukup JM. Involvement of microbial components and toll–like receptors 2 and 4 in cytokine responses to air pollution particles. *Am J Respir Cell Mol Biol*. 2002;27:611–618.
157. Strohmeier GR, Walsh JH, Klings ES, et al. Lipopolysaccharide binding protein potentiates airway reactivity in a murine model of allergic asthma. *J Immunol*. 2001;166:2063–2070.
158. Eisenbarth SC, Piggott DA, Huleatt JW, et al. Lipopolysaccharide-enhanced, toll-like receptor 4-dependent T helper cell type 2 responses to inhaled antigen. *J Exp Med*. 2002;196:1645–1651.
159. Redecke V, Hacker H, Datta SK, et al. Cutting edge: activation of Toll-like receptor 2 induces a Th2 immune response and promotes experimental asthma. *J Immunol*. 2004;172:2739–2743.
161. Hessel EM, Chu M, Lizcano JO, et al. Immunostimulatory oligonucleotides block allergic airway inflammation by inhibiting Th2 cell activation and IgE-mediated cytokine induction. *J Exp Med*. 2005;202:1563–1573.
162. Choudhry S, Avila PC, Nazario S, et al. CD14 tobacco gene-environment interaction modifies asthma severity and immunoglobulin E levels in Latinos with asthma. *Am J Respir Crit Care Med*. 2005;172:173–182.
163. Vercelli D, Baldini M, Stern D, et al. CD14: a bridge between innate immunity and adaptive IgE responses. *J Endotoxin Res*. 2001;7:45–48.
164. Eder W, Klimecki W, Yu L, et al. Toll-like receptor 2 as a major gene for asthma in children of European farmers. *J Allergy Clin Immunol*. 2004;113:482–488.
165. Weidinger S, Klopp N, Rummler L, et al. Association of NOD1 polymorphisms with atopic eczema and related phenotypes. *J Allergy Clin Immunol*. 2005;116:177–184.
166. Wan H, Winton HL, Soeller C, et al. Der p 1 facilitates transepithelial allergen delivery by disruption of tight junctions (see comments). *J Clin Invest*. 1999;104:123–133.
167. Asokananthan N, Graham PT, Stewart DJ, et al. House dust mite allergens induce proinflammatory cytokines from respiratory epithelial cells: the cysteine protease allergen, Der p 1, activates protease-activated receptor (PAR)-2 and inactivates PAR-1. *J Immunol*. 2002;169:4572–4578.
168. Schmidlin F, Amadesi S, Dabbagh K, et al. Protease-activated receptor 2 mediates eosinophil infiltration and hyperreactivity in allergic inflammation of the airway. *J Immunol*. 2002;169:5315–5321.
169. Guermonprez P, Valladeau J, Zitvogel L, et al. Antigen presentation and T cell stimulation by dendritic cells. *Annu Rev Immunol*. 2002;20:621–667.

173. Rissoan MC, Soumelis V, Kadowaki N, et al. Reciprocal control of T helper cell and dendritic cell differentiation. *Science*. 1999;283:1183–1186.
174. Cella M, Jarrossay D, Facchetti F, et al. Plasmacytoid monocytes migrate to inflamed lymph nodes and produce large amounts of type I interferon. *Nat Med*. 1999;5:919–923.
176. Iwasaki A, Medzhitov R. Toll-like receptor control of the adaptive immune responses. *Nat Immunol*. 2004;5:987–995.
177. Chen L. Co-inhibitory molecules of the B7-CD28 family in the control of T-cell immunity. *Nat Rev Immunol*. 2004;4:336–347.
178. Lambrecht BN, De Veerman M, Coyle AJ, et al. Myeloid dendritic cells induce Th2 responses to inhaled antigen, leading to eosinophilic airway inflammation. *J Clin Invest*. 2000;106:551–559.
179. Fallarino F, Asselin-Paturel C, Vacca C, et al. Murine plasmacytoid dendritic cells initiate the immunosuppressive pathway of tryptophan catabolism in response to CD200 receptor engagement. *J Immunol*. 2004;173:3748–3754.
180. Hayashi T, Beck L, Rossetto C, et al. Inhibition of experimental asthma by indoleamine 2,3-dioxygenase. *J Clin Invest*. 2004;114:270–279.
181. de Heer HJ, Hammad H, Soullie T, et al. Essential role of lung plasmacytoid dendritic cells in preventing asthmatic reactions to harmless inhaled antigen. *J Exp Med*. 2004;200:89–98.
182. Kohl J, Baelder R, Lewkowich IP, et al. A regulatory role for the C5a anaphylatoxin in type 2 immunity in asthma. *J Clin Invest*. 2006;116:783–796.
188. Rincon M, Anguita J, Nakamura T, et al. Interleukin (IL)-6 directs the differentiation of IL-4-producing CD4+ T cells. *J Exp Med*. 1997;185:461–469.
190. Doganci A, Eigenbrod T, Krug N, et al. The IL-6R alpha chain controls lung CD4+CD25+ Treg development and function during allergic airway inflammation in vivo. *J Clin Invest*. 2005;115:313–325.
192. Yokoyama A, Kohno N, Sakai K, et al. Circulating levels of soluble interleukin-6 receptor in patients with bronchial asthma. *Am J Respir Crit Care Med*. 1997;156:1688–1691.
194. Page K, Hughes VS, Odoms KK, et al. German cockroach proteases regulate interleukin-8 expression via nuclear factor for interleukin-6 in human bronchial epithelial cells. *Am J Respir Cell Mol Biol*. 2005;32:225–231.
198. Zhou B, Comeau MR, De Smedt T, et al. Thymic stromal lymphopoietin as a key initiator of allergic airway inflammation in mice. *Nat Immunol*. 2005;6:1047–1053.
199. Al-Shami A, Spolski R, Kelly J, et al. A role for TSLP in the development of inflammation in an asthma model. *J Exp Med*. 2005;202:829–839.
201. Ito T, Wang YH, Duramad O, et al. TSLP-activated dendritic cells induce an inflammatory T helper type 2 cell response through OX40 ligand. *J Exp Med*. 2005;202:1213–1223.
202. Xing Z, Ohkawara Y, Jordana M, et al. Transfer of granulocyte-macrophage colony-stimulating factor gene to rat lung induces eosinophilia, monocytosis, and fibrotic reactions. *J Clin Invest*. 1996;97:1102–1110.
204. van der Pouw Kraan TC, Boeije LC, Smeenk RJ, et al. Prostaglandin-E2 is a potent inhibitor of human interleukin 12 production. *J Exp Med*. 1995;181:775–779.
211. Yoshida H, Nishina H, Takimoto H, et al. The transcription factor NF-ATc1 regulates lymphocyte proliferation and Th2 cytokine production. *Immunity*. 1998;8:115–124.
212. Ranger AM, Hodge MR, Gravallese EM, et al. Delayed lymphoid repopulation with defects in IL-4-driven responses produced by inactivation of NF-ATc. *Immunity*. 1998;8:125–134.
215. Zhang DH, Yang L, Cohn L, et al. Inhibition of allergic inflammation in a murine model of asthma by expression of a dominant-negative mutant of GATA-3. *Immunity*. 1999;11:473–482.
216. Zhu J, Cote-Sierra J, Guo L, et al. Stat5 activation plays a critical role in Th2 differentiation. *Immunity*. 2003;19:739–748.
218. Mohrs M, Blankespoor CM, Wang ZE, et al. Deletion of a coordinate regulator of type 2 cytokine expression in mice. *Nat Immunol*. 2001;2:842–847.
219. McIntire JJ, Umetsu SE, Akbari O, et al. Identification of Tapr (an airway hyperreactivity regulatory locus) and the linked Tim gene family. *Nat Immunol*. 2001;2:1109–1116.
220. Hsieh CS, Macatonia SE, Tripp CS, et al. Development of TH1 CD4+ T cells through IL-12 produced by Listeria- induced macrophages. *Science*. 1993;260:547–549.
228. Humbles AA, Lu B, Nilsson CA, et al. A role for the C3a anaphylatoxin receptor in the effector phase of asthma. *Nature*. 2000;406:998–1001.
230. Karp CL, Grupe A, Schadt E, et al. Identification of complement factor 5 as a susceptibility locus for experimental allergic asthma. *Nat Immunol*. 2000;1:221–226.
233. Miyazaki Y, Inoue H, Matsumura M, et al. Exacerbation of experimental allergic asthma by augmented Th2 responses in WSX-1-deficient mice. *J Immunol*. 2005;175:2401–2407.
242. Grunig G, Corry DB, Leach MW, et al. Interleukin-10 is a natural suppressor of cytokine production and inflammation in a murine model of allergic bronchopulmonary aspergillosis. *J Exp Med*. 1997;185:1089–1099.
244. Stampfli MR, Cwiartka M, Gajewska BU, et al. Interleukin-10 gene transfer to the airway regulates allergic mucosal sensitization in mice. *Am J Respir Cell Mol Biol*. 1999;21:586–596.
245. Akbari O, DeKruyff RH, Umetsu DT. Pulmonary dendritic cells producing IL-10 mediate tolerance induced by respiratory exposure to antigen. *Nat Immunol*. 2001;2:725–731.
251. Hobbs K, Negri J, Klinnert M, et al. Interleukin-10 and transforming growth factor-beta promoter polymorphisms in allergies and asthma. *Am J Respir Crit Care Med*. 1998;158:1958–1962.
252. Zheng SG, Wang JH, Stohl W, et al. TGF-beta requires CTLA-4 early after T cell activation to induce FoxP3 and generate adaptive CD4+CD25+ regulatory cells. *J Immunol*. 2006;176:3321–3329.
256. Faveeuw C, Gosset P, Bureau F, et al. Prostaglandin D2 inhibits the production of interleukin-12 in murine dendritic cells through multiple signaling pathways. *Eur J Immunol*. 2003;33:889–898.
257. Theiner G, Gessner A, Lutz MB. The mast cell mediator PGD2 suppresses IL-12 release by dendritic cells leading to Th2 polarized immune responses in vivo. *Immunobiology*. 2006;211:463–472.
258. Hammad H, Kool M, Soullie T, et al. Activation of the D prostanoid 1 receptor suppresses asthma by modulation of lung dendritic cell function and induction of regulatory T cells. *J Exp Med*. 2007;204:357–367.
261. Coyle AJ, Wagner K, Bertrand C, et al. Central role of immunoglobulin (Ig) E in the induction of lung eosinophil infiltration and T helper 2 cell cytokine production: inhibition by a non-anaphylactogenic anti-IgE antibody. *J Exp Med*. 1996;183:1303–1310.
263. Finkelman FD, Katona IM, Urban JF Jr, et al. IL-4 is required to generate and sustain in vivo IgE responses. *J Immunol*. 1988;141:2335–2341.
264. Zhu Z, Homer RJ, Wang Z, et al. Pulmonary expression of interleukin-13 causes inflammation, mucus hypersecretion, subepithelial fibrosis, physiologic abnormalities, and eotaxin production. *J Clin Invest*. 1999;103:779–788.
266. Ishizaka K, Ishizaka T. Identification of g E-antibodies as a carrier of reaginic activity. *J Immunol*. 1967;99:1187.
267. Vercelli D. The functional genomics of CD14 and its role in IgE responses: an integrated view. *J Allergy Clin Immunol*. 2002;109: 14–21.
268. Linehan LA, Warren WD, Thompson PA, et al. STAT6 is required for IL-4-induced germline Ig gene transcription and switch recombination. *J Immunol*. 1998;161:302–310.
270. Harriman GR, Bradley A, Das S, et al. IgA class switch in I alpha exon-deficient mice. Role of germline transcription in class switch recombination. *J Clin Invest*. 1996;97:477–485.
271. Oettgen HC, Geha RS. IgE in asthma and atopy: cellular and molecular connections. *J Clin Invest*. 1999;104:829–835.
272. Jabara HH, Fu SM, Geha RS, et al. CD40 and IgE: synergism between anti-CD40 monoclonal antibody and interleukin 4 in the induction of IgE synthesis by highly purified human B cells. *J Exp Med*. 1990;172:1861–1864.
273. Armitage RJ, Fanslow WC, Strockbine L, et al. Molecular and biological characterization of a murine ligand for CD40. *Nature*. 1992;357:80–82.
275. Kawabe T, Naka T, Yoshida K, et al. The immune responses in CD40-deficient mice: impaired immunoglobulin class switching and germinal center formation. *Immunity*. 1994;1:167–178.

276. Renshaw BR, Fanslow WC 3rd, Armitage RJ, et al. Humoral immune responses in CD40 ligand-deficient mice. *J Exp Med*. 1994;180:1889–1900.
278. Muramatsu M, Kinoshita K, Fagarasan S, et al. Class switch recombination and hypermutation require activation-induced cytidine deaminase (AID), a potential RNA editing enzyme. *Cell*. 2000;102:553–563.
280. Shapira SK, Vercelli D, Jabara HH, et al. Molecular analysis of the induction of immunoglobulin E synthesis in human B cells by interleukin 4 and engagement of CD40 antigen. *J Exp Med*. 1992;175:289–292.
284. Ozaki K, Spolski R, Feng CG, et al. A critical role for IL-21 in regulating immunoglobulin production. *Science*. 2002;298:1630–1634.
285. Suto A, Nakajima H, Hirose K, et al. Interleukin 21 prevents antigen-induced IgE production by inhibiting germ line C(epsilon) transcription of IL-4-stimulated B cells. *Blood*. 2002;100:4565–4573.
288. Strait RT, Morris SC, Finkelman FD. IgG-blocking antibodies inhibit IgE-mediated anaphylaxis in vivo through both antigen interception and Fc gamma RIIb cross-linking. *J Clin Invest*. 2006;116;833–841
291. Turner H, Kinet JP. Signalling through the high-affinity IgE receptor Fc epsilonRI. *Nature*. 1999;402:B24–B30.
293. Malveaux FJ, Conroy MC, Adkinson NF Jr, et al. IgE receptors on human basophils. Relationship to serum IgE concentration. *J Clin Invest*. 1978;62:176–181.
297. Daheshia M, Friend DS, Grusby MJ, et al. Increased severity of local and systemic anaphylactic reactions in gp49B1-deficient mice. *J Exp Med*. 2001;194:227–234.
300. Long EO. Regulation of immune responses through inhibitory receptors. *Annu Rev Immunol*. 1999;17:875–904.
301. Yokota A, Kikutani H, Tanaka T, et al. Two species of human Fc epsilon receptor II (Fc epsilon RII/CD23): tissue-specific and IL-4-specific regulation of gene expression. *Cell*. 1988;55:611–68.
311. Lecoanet-Henchoz S, Gauchat JF, Aubry JP, et al. CD23 regulates monocyte activation through a novel interaction with the adhesion molecules CD11b-CD18 and CD11c-CD18. *Immunity*. 1995;3:119–125.
323. Charlesworth EN, Hood AF, Soter NA, et al. Cutaneous late-phase response to allergen. Mediator release and inflammatory cell infiltration. *J Clin Invest*. 1989;83:1519–1526.
329. Ruitenberg EJ, Elgersma A. Absence of intestinal mast cell response in congenitally athymic mice during Trichinella spiralis infection. *Nature*. 1976;264:258–260.
330. Lantz CS, Boesiger J, Song CH, et al. Role for interleukin-3 in mast-cell and basophil development and in immunity to parasites. *Nature*. 1998;392:90–93.
335. Casale TB, Wood D, Richerson HB, et al. Elevated bronchoalveolar lavage fluid histamine levels in allergic asthmatics are associated with methacholine bronchial hyperresponsiveness. *J Clin Invest*. 1987;79:1197–1203.
339. Schwartz LB, Bradford TR, Rouse C, et al. Development of a new, more sensitive immunoassay for human tryptase: use in systemic anaphylaxis. *J Clin Immunol*. 1994;14:190–194.
345. Weiss JW, Drazen JM, McFadden ERJ, et al. Airway constriction in normal humans produced by inhalation of leukotriene D. Potency, time course, and effect of aspirin therapy. *JAMA*. 1983;249:2814–2817.
356. Hardy CC, Robinson C, Tattersfield AE, et al. The bronchoconstrictor effect of inhaled prostaglandin D2 in normal and asthmatic men. *N Engl J Med*. 1984;311:209–213.
364. Bradding P, Feather IH, Howarth PH, et al. Interleukin 4 is localized to and released by human mast cells. *J Exp Med*. 1992;176:1381–1386.
367. Oettgen HC, Martin TR, Wynshaw-Boris A, et al. Active anaphylaxis in IgE-deficient mice. *Nature*. 1994;370:367–370.
369. Fahy JV, Fleming HE, Wong HH, et al. The effect of an anti-IgE monoclonal antibody on the early- and late-phase responses to allergen inhalation in asthmatic subjects. *Am J Respir Crit Care Med*. 1997;155:1828–1834.
371. Weller PF. Eosinophils: structure and functions. *Curr Opin Immunol*. 1994;6:85–90.
372. Gleich GJ. Mechanisms of eosinophil-associated inflammation. *J Allergy Clin Immunol*. 2000;105:651–663.
373. Weller PF, Lim K, Wan HC, et al. Role of the eosinophil in allergic reactions. *Eur Respir J Suppl*. 1996;22:109s–115s.
375. Wu W, Samoszuk MK, Comhair SA, et al. Eosinophils generate brominating oxidants in allergen-induced asthma. *J Clin Invest*. 2000;105:1455–1463.
379. Nerlov C, Graf T. PU.1 induces myeloid lineage commitment in multipotent hematopoietic progenitors. *Genes Dev*. 1998;12:2403–2412.
380. Nerlov C, McNagny KM, Doderlein G, et al. Distinct C/EBP functions are required for eosinophil lineage commitment and maturation. *Genes Dev*. 1998;12:2413–2423.
381. Lee JJ, McGarry MP, Farmer SC, et al. Interleukin-5 expression in the lung epithelium of transgenic mice leads to pulmonary changes pathognomonic of asthma. *J Exp Med*. 1997;185:2143–2156.
383. Ponath PD, Qin S, Post TW, et al. Molecular cloning and characterization of a human eotaxin receptor expressed selectively on eosinophils. *J Exp Med*. 1996;183:2437–2448.
384. Uguccioni M, Mackay CR, Ochensberger B, et al. High expression of the chemokine receptor CCR3 in human blood basophils. Role in activation by eotaxin, MCP-4, and other chemokines. *J Clin Invest*. 1997;100:1137–1143.
385. Rothenberg ME, MacLean JA, Pearlman E, et al. Targeted disruption of the chemokine eotaxin partially reduces antigen- induced tissue eosinophilia. *J Exp Med*. 1997;185:785–790.
387. Collins PD, Marleau S, Griffiths-Johnson DA, et al. Cooperation between interleukin-5 and the chemokine eotaxin to induce eosinophil accumulation in vivo. *J Exp Med*. 1995;182:1169–1174.
388. Gonzalo JA, Lloyd CM, Wen D, et al. The coordinated action of CC chemokines in the lung orchestrates allergic inflammation and airway hyperresponsiveness. *J Exp Med*. 1998;188:157–167.
390. Gounni AS, Lamkhioued B, Ochiai K, et al. High-affinity IgE receptor on eosinophils is involved in defence against parasites. *Nature*. 1994;367:183–16.
401. Seminario MC, Gleich GJ. The role of eosinophils in the pathogenesis of asthma. *Curr Opin Immunol*. 1994;6:860–864.
402. Terada N, Konno A, Fukuda S, et al. Interleukin-5 gene expression in nasal mucosa and changes in amount of interleukin-5 in nasal lavage fluid after antigen challenge. *Acta Otolaryngol*. 1994;114:203–208.
403. Kiehl P, Falkenberg K, Vogelbruch M, et al. Tissue eosinophilia in acute and chronic atopic dermatitis: a morphometric approach using quantitative image analysis of immunostaining. *Br J Dermatol*. 2001;145:720–729.
408. Corry DB, Folkesson HG, Warnock ML, et al. Interleukin 4, but not interleukin 5 or eosinophils, is required in a murine model of acute airway hyperreactivity (published erratum appears in *J. Exp. Med.* 185(9):1715). *J Exp Med*. 1996;183:109–117.
409. Leckie MJ, ten Brinke A, Khan J, et al. Effects of an interleukin-5 blocking monoclonal antibody on eosinophils, airway hyper-responsiveness, and the late asthmatic response. *Lancet*. 2000;356:2144–2148.
410. Lee JJ, Dimina D, Macias MP, et al. Defining a link with asthma in mice congenitally deficient in eosinophils. *Science*. 2004;305:1773–1776.
420. Zheng T, Zhu Z, Wang Z, et al. Inducible targeting of IL-13 to the adult lung causes matrix metalloproteinase- and cathepsin-dependent emphysema. *J Clin Invest*. 2000;106:1081–1093.
421. Chiaramonte MG, Donaldson DD, Cheever AW, et al. An IL-13 inhibitor blocks the development of hepatic fibrosis during a T-helper type 2-dominated inflammatory response. *J Clin Invest*. 1999;104:777–785.
422. Hesse M, Modolell M, La Flamme AC, et al. Differential regulation of nitric oxide synthase-2 and arginase-1 by type 1/type 2 cytokines in vivo: granulomatous pathology is shaped by the pattern of L-arginine metabolism. *J Immunol*. 2001;167:6533–6544.
423. Zimmermann N, King NE, Laporte J, et al. Dissection of experimental asthma with DNA microarray analysis identifies arginase in asthma pathogenesis. *J Clin Invest*. 2003;111:1863–1874.
429. Blackburn MR, Lee CG, Young HW, et al. Adenosine mediates IL-13-induced inflammation and remodeling in the lung and interacts in an IL-13-adenosine amplification pathway. *J Clin Invest*. 2003;112:332–344.
430. Vargaftig BB, Singer M. Leukotrienes mediate murine bronchopulmonary hyperreactivity, inflammation, and part of mucosal

metaplasia and tissue injury induced by recombinant murine interleukin-13. *Am J Respir Cell Mol Biol*. 2003;28:410–419.

438. Deshpande DA, Dogan S, Walseth TF, et al. Modulation of calcium signaling by interleukin-13 in human airway smooth muscle: role of CD38/cyclic adenosine diphosphate ribose pathway. *Am J Respir Cell Mol Biol*. 2004;31:36–42.
442. Zhu Z, Zheng T, Homer RJ, et al. Acidic mammalian chitinase in asthmatic Th2 inflammation and IL-13 pathway activation. *Science*. 2004;304:1678–1682.
443. Zhu Z, Ma B, Zheng T, et al. IL-13-induced chemokine responses in the lung: role of CCR2 in the pathogenesis of IL-13-induced inflammation and remodeling. *J Immunol*. 2002;168:2953–2962.
445. Humbert M, Durham SR, Kimmitt P, et al. Elevated expression of messenger ribonucleic acid encoding IL-13 in the bronchial mucosa of atopic and nonatopic subjects with asthma. *J Allergy Clin Immunol*. 1997;99:657–665.
447. Graves PE, Kabesch M, Halonen M, et al. A cluster of seven tightly linked polymorphisms in the IL-13 gene is associated with total serum IgE levels in three populations of white children. *J Allergy Clin Immunol*. 2000;105:506–513.
448. Heinzmann A, Mao XQ, Akaiwa M, et al. Genetic variants of IL-13 signalling and human asthma and atopy. *Hum Mol Genet*. 2000;9:549–559.
450. Cameron L, Webster RB, Strempel JM, et al. Th2 cell-selective enhancement of human IL13 transcription by IL13–1112CT, a polymorphism associated with allergic inflammation. *J Immunol*. 2006;177:8633–8642.
462. Spector S. Omalizumab: efficacy in allergic disease. *Panminerva Med*. 2004;46:141–148.
463. Creticos PS, Schroeder JT, Hamilton RG, et al. Immunotherapy with a ragweed-toll-like receptor 9 agonist vaccine for allergic rhinitis. *N Engl J Med*. 2006;355:1445–1455.

Chapter 44

Transplantation Immunology

Megan Sykes, Kathryn Wood, and David H. Sachs

The transplantation of organs and cells between individuals saves or prolongs thousands of lives each year. The growing list of organs transplanted includes corneas, kidneys, livers, hearts, lungs, small intestines, pancreata, and even hands and faces. Currently, clinical cellular transplantation includes islets of Langerhans and hematopoietic cells, but the list is likely to expand in the future to include other cell types, such as hepatocytes and myoblasts, which are currently under investigation in experimental models. Success of all types of transplants depends on the ability to avoid rejection due to a host-versus-graft immune response. Hematopoietic cell transplantation is, in addition, associated with some special considerations because the administration of a donor graft that contains mature T cells to a conditioned, and consequently immunoincompetent, recipient is associated with the risk of rejection in the graft-versus host direction, that is, graft-versus-host disease (GVHD). Because all of these transplants are performed between different humans, that is, members of the same species, they are referred to as *allotransplants*. However, improvements in immunosuppressive therapies have increased the success of allotransplantation to the point that a new limitation has been encountered, namely, the insufficient supply of human organs.

Although this insufficiency can be partly overcome by the increasing use of living donors as sources of kidneys, liver, and lungs, such procedures are associated with significant risks to the donor, and some organs (e.g., the heart) can obviously be obtained only from cadaveric donors. This organ shortage has led to considerable interest in alternatives, such as artificial organs, tissue grafts engineered *in vitro* from stem cells, and organs from other species. Transplants from other species, referred to as *xenografts*, are a promising solution to the organ shortage, but present even greater immunologic challenges than allografts, as well as potentially novel infectious risks, and these problems must be addressed before xenotransplantation can be effectively used in the clinic. This chapter presents an overview of the immunology of organ and cellular allotransplantation, as well as xenotransplantation. Allogeneic and xenogeneic responses differ from other immunologic responses in at least two fundamental ways. First, they exhibit extraordinary strength and, probably for that reason, include unusual types of responses that cannot be detected in other areas of immunology. Second, they can be stimulated by two different sets of antigen-presenting cells, those of the donor and those of the recipient. In this chapter, we will emphasize these differences from classical immunology as we describe our current understanding of the immune responses that cause graft rejection.

ORIGINS OF TRANSPLANTATION IMMUNOLOGY

Early History

Although there were sporadic reports of tissue transplants in ancient times *(1)*, skin grafting did not become an accepted practice until the late 1800s. However, even then many workers did not distinguish between autografts (donor and recipient the same individual) and allografts (donor and recipient of the same species) or even, sometimes, xenografts (donor and recipient of different species). The last of these formed the basis for an extensive practice known as zoografting in which patients were subjected to grafts from animals ranging from pigs to frogs *(2)*. Billingham *(3)* points out that no one apparently cared whether the grafted skin "took" or merely promoted healing of the wound. The results of these efforts led to a period of confusion in transplantation. Without any clear understanding of the processes involved, surgeons embarked on all sorts of transplants, and a series of operations were reported that we know, from our present understanding of the laws of transplantation, could not possibly have been successful. The transplantation of internal organs awaited the development of techniques for vascular anastomosis. In 1908, Carrel *(4)*, one of the pioneers of vascular surgery, reported the results of *en bloc* allotransplantation of both kidneys in a series of nine cats. He was able to obtain up to 25 days of urine output in some cats, but ultimately all of them died. Although other investigators repeated and modified Carrel's experiments, no major advances in prolonging the function of allografts or in understanding the cause for their failure were made for the following 3 decades.

During this same period, the closely related field of tumor transplantation gained momentum *(3)*. Although many of the experiments with tumor transplants provided information essential to an understanding of transplantation immunology, this was not clear at the time. Many workers were committed to the idea that they were studying an effect peculiar to tumor tissues. In his Harvey Lecture, Medawar summed up the confusion neatly by the statement, "Nearly everyone who supposed that he was using transplantation to study tumors was in fact using tumors to study transplantation" (5).

In 1936, Voronoy, a Russian surgeon, reported the first clinical renal allograft *(1)*. There was apparently a mismatch of blood types and the patient died having demonstrated only minimal renal function. The early postwar years saw reports of attempts at clinical renal homotransplantation from various locales around the world. In 1952, the first successful renal transplant was performed in Boston using the kidney of an identical twin (6).

One of the important contributions to the understanding of transplantation in this era was the work of Medawar. In 1943, Gibson and Medawar reported their experience with autologous and allogeneic skin grafts on a woman who had suffered extensive third-degree burns. The allografts in this case were taken from the patient's sibling, and for clinical reasons were transplanted in two different stages separated by about a week. The authors observed accelerated rejection of the second grafts. Appreciating the possible significance of these observations, Medawar *(5)* followed them with a series of grafting experiments in rabbits and mice. By 1945, he was able to conclude that "resistance to homologous grafted skin therefore belongs to the general category of actively acquired immune reactions" *(5)*, thereby establishing the relationship of clinical transplantation to the field of immunology.

History, Principles, and Discoveries of Immunogenetics

Inbred Strains

Rodents have provided an invaluable model for the study of the genetic basis for graft rejection. One of the main features that has made them so valuable is the availability of a large number of inbred strains. Such strains consist of animals that have been produced by sequential pedigreed brother-sister matings for at least 20 generations and which are, therefore, essentially genetically identical. With the exception of the sex chromosomes, chromosomes in such strains are homozygous and therefore produce identical homozygous progeny.

The reason that sequential inbreeding leads to homozygosity is illustrated in Figure 44.1. For the sake of simplicity, the first generation illustrated in this figure is indicated as a brother-sister mating in which, for any given autosomal locus, the alleles being bred will be of the form AB × AB. The more general case of AB × CD can also be analyzed statistically by a similar, although slightly more complicated, mathematical treatment. The ratio of genotypes of the offspring from this breeding is given by the binomial formula (AA:AB:BB = 1:2:1). Thus, as illustrated at the second generation, when a single brother-sister pair is chosen, the chance that both animals will have the genotype AA at the locus in question is 1/16. Similarly, the probability that the second-generation mating will take the form BB × BB is also 1/16. In either of these eventualities, all future generations will be fixed as homozygotes (either AA or BB) and therefore we speak of the locus as being fixed. Thus, the probability of fixation of a given autosomal locus at this generation is 1/8.

For segregation of a large number of independent loci, it is mathematically equivalent to state that the probability of fixing a given locus is 1/8, or that on the average 1/8 of the segregating loci will be fixed. If the locus in question is not fixed during this random breeding, then the chances that it will be fixed at the next breeding are still approximately 1/8 (actually a little higher). In other words, 1/8 of the loci would be expected to fix at the second inbreeding generation, 1/8 of the remaining unfixed loci would be expected to fix at the next generation, and so on. As indicated in Figure 44.1, the probability of fixation (Pfix) is given by the formula:

$$P_{fix} = 1 - \left(\frac{7}{8}\right)^{n-1}$$

This equation describes a curve that rises asymptotically toward a probability of 100% fixation (Figure 44.2). Because genes travel at meiosis in groups rather than individually, there is a finite number of units of genetic

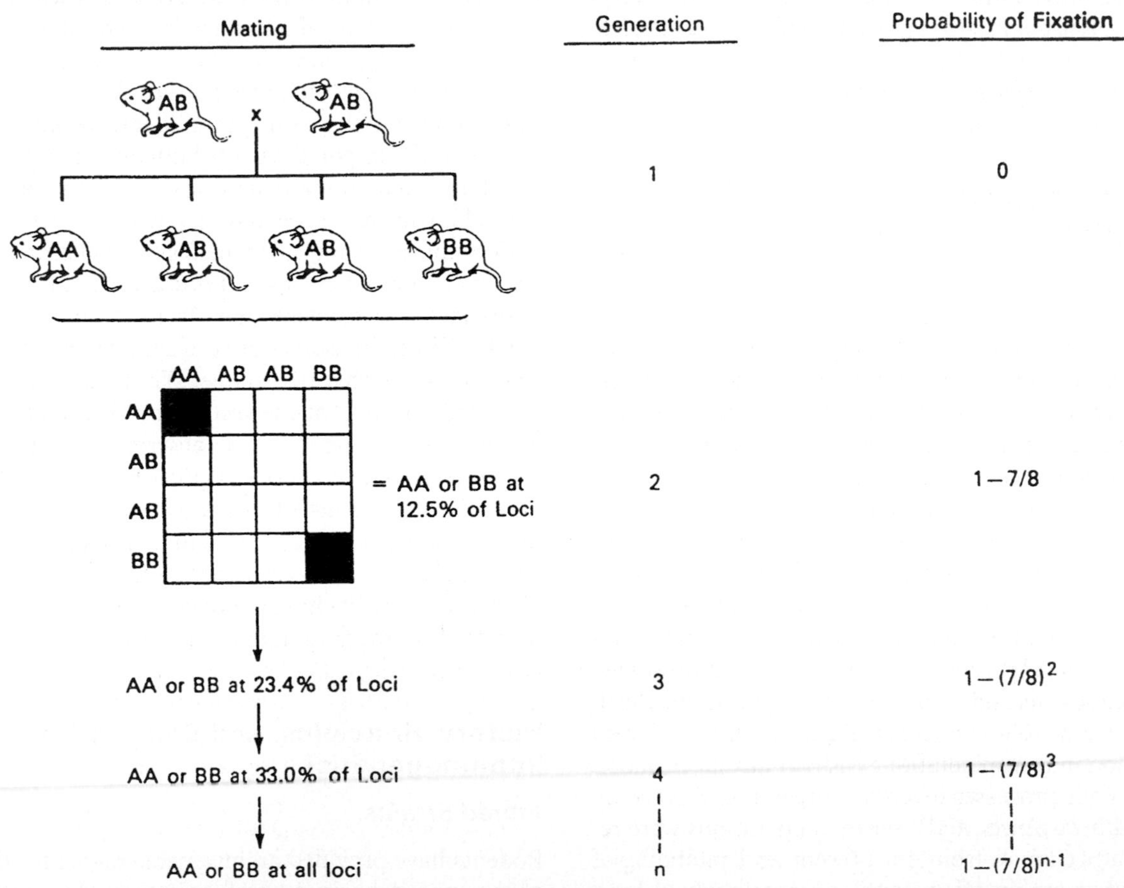

FIGURE 44.1 Breeding scheme for inbred strains.

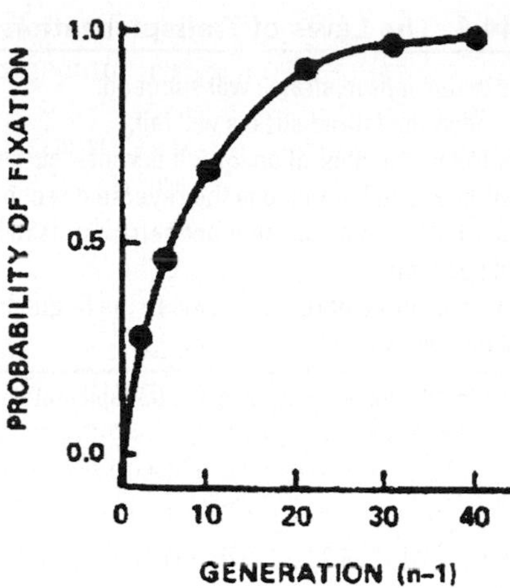

FIGURE 44.2 Probablity of fixation curve.

information that segregate. Therefore, for practical purposes, one can consider a strain inbred after 20 such brother-sister matings because at this point there is a very small chance that any locus will not have reached homozygosity. All loci will be of the genotype either AA or BB, and there will no longer be any loci of the heterozygous form AB. The strain so derived is defined as an inbred strain. Hundreds of such well-characterized inbred strains are now available.

Inbred strains have also been produced in several other species including rats, guinea pigs, and rabbits. However, both space requirements and other genetic features, such as gestation times, age of sexual maturity, and litter size, make production of inbred strains in larger species much more difficult. Indeed, until recently, there were no inbred large-animal species available. However, during the past 35 years, studies in one of our laboratories (D. H. Sachs, Boston, MA, USA) have produced highly inbred miniature swine (7,8). Swine were chosen for this purpose because they represent one of the few large-animal species in which breeding characteristics make genetic experiments possible. Swine have a relatively large litter size (three to ten offspring) and a short gestation time (3 months). They reach sexual maturity at approximately 6 months of age, and sows have an estrous cycle every 3 weeks. These breeding characteristics made it possible to develop major histocompatibility complex (MHC) homozygous lines of miniature swine in a relatively short time *(7)*, to isolate new MHC recombinants and breed them to homozygosity, and to carry out short-term backcross experiments in order to identify and study the segregation of genetic characteristics. These miniature swine now represent the only large-animal model in which MHC genetics can be reproducibly controlled. As such, these animals have been particularly useful in assessing the effects of MHC matching on rejection and/or tolerance induction *(9)*.

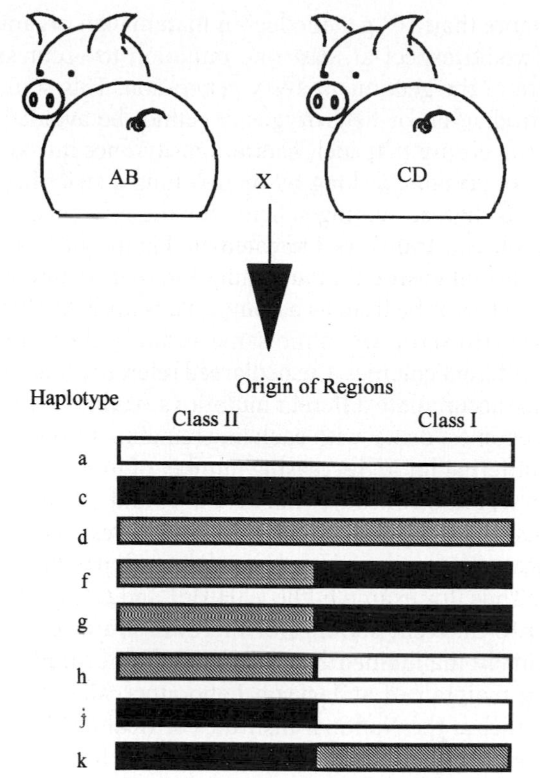

FIGURE 44.3 Origin of miniature swine haplotypes.

At present, swine of three homozygous SLA haplotypes, SLA^a, SLA^c, SLA^d, and five lines bearing intra-SLA recombinant haplotypes are maintained, as illustrated in Figure 44.3. All of these lines differ by minor histocompatibility loci, thus providing a model in which most of the transplantation combinations relevant to human transplantation can be mimicked. Thus, for example, transplants within an MHC homozygous herd simulate transplants between HLA identical siblings, while transplants between herds resemble cadaveric or nonmatched sibling transplants. Likewise, transplants between pairs of heterozygotes can be chosen to resemble parent into offspring or one-haplotype mismatched sibling transplants. In addition, one subline of SLA^{dd} animals was selected for further inbreeding in order to produce a fully inbred line of miniature swine. This subline has now reached a coefficient of inbreeding of more than 94%, and is now sufficiently inbred for histocompatibility, that is, reciprocal skin grafts among the offspring have not been rejected (8). These animals should be particularly useful in permitting adoptive transfer studies for the first time in a large-animal model.

One problem in maintaining true homozygosity of inbred strains is that of mutation. The average mutation frequency for mammalian genes has been estimated to be approximately 10^{-6} per base pair per meiosis. Because there are more than 10^6 genetic loci in mammalian organisms, one would expect at least one mutation to occur somewhere in the genome at every generation. This source of reintroduction of heterozygosity cannot be avoided, but one can ensure that such heterozygosity, once introduced, will not remain for long by maintaining a strict brother-sister pedigreed mating scheme for the reference line of any inbred strain. As indicated in Figure 44.1, such a scheme will ensure that any mutation that occurs will either be lost or be fixed as a homozygous allele by this procedure. However, when the same strain is maintained in two different colonies, the pedigreed reference lines will of course accumulate different mutations, leading to the phenomenon of "drift," with each line remaining truly inbred, but differing for an increasing number of fixed mutations. Such separated lines are called *sublines* and are designated by a series of letters following the strain designation that indicate the origin and location of the pedigreed reference line. Thus, for example, the C3H/HeJ and C3H/HeN lines are two different sublines of the C3H strain. Both were originally maintained by Heston (He), one subline then being maintained at Jackson Laboratory (C3H/HeJ) and the other at the National Institutes of Health (C3H/HeN). Although these strains are still quite similar for many properties, there are already several known differences between them, such as the responsiveness of their lymphocytes to lipopolysaccharide. Often differences between sublines are first detected when results from one laboratory are found difficult to reproduce in another.

Genetic Principles Governing Tissue Transplantation: The "Laws of Transplantation"

In the early 1900s it was noted by tumor biologists that tumors arising in inbred animals could frequently be transplanted successfully to other animals of the same line, while this was usually impossible in outbred animals. Little *(10)* then studied this phenomenon systematically, and in the process produced and characterized a large number of inbred strains of mice. In summarizing the results of these studies of tumor grafting in mice, Little described what have since been called the "five laws of transplantation" (Table 44.1). Little's remarkable insight was to reconcile these observations with the classical Mendelian principles by proposing that recipients would reject grafts if the donor expressed a product of any histocompatibility (tissue compatibility) locus that was not expressed by the recipient. His explanation for the unusual inheritance pattern in Table 44.1 was to suggest, first, that there must be codominant expression of the histocompatibility genes, and second, that there must be a relatively large number of histocompatibility loci. Under these conditions, members of the F1 generation would express both parental alleles at all histocompatibility loci (and thus would fail to reject grafts from parental, F2, or subsequent generations) and members of the F2 generation would be unlikely to express all of the products of histocompatibility genes that are expressed by either parental generation (and thus would usually reject parental allografts).

TABLE 44.1 The Laws of Transplantation

1. Transplants within inbred strains will succeed.
2. Transplants between inbred strains will fail.
3. Transplants from a member of an inbred parental strain to an F_1 offspring will succeed but those in the reverse direction will fail.
4. Transplants from F_2 and all subsequent generations to F_1 animals will succeed.
5. Transplants from inbred parental strains to the F_2 generation will usually, but not always, fail.

Adapted from Little CC. The genetics of tissue transplantation in mammals. *Cancer Res.* 1924;8:75–95.

Estimating the Number of Histocompatibility Genes

One can experimentally determine the number of histocompatibility loci by which any two inbred strains differ by breeding a large F2 population between these strains and then transplanting tissues from one of the parental strains to all of the F2 offspring, measuring the fraction of grafts that survive. As illustrated in Figure 44.4, if the two strains were to differ at only one histocompatibility locus, one would predict that 3/4 of the grafts would survive. If, however, if the two strains differed by two independently segregating histocompatibility loci, then one would predict that $(3/4)^2$ or 9/16 of the grafts would survive. Similarly, if there were n loci by which these two strains differed, one would expect $(3/4)^n$ to be the fraction of surviving grafts. When this equation has been solved for "n" experimentally, using skin grafts as the challenging transplant, numbers as high

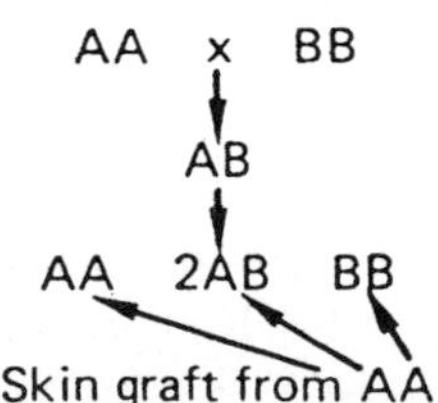

No. Loci	Expected Survivals
1	3/4
2	$(3/4)^2$
.	.
.	.
n	$(3/4)^n$

FIGURE 44.4 Estimating the number of histocompatibility loci.

as 30 to 50 have been reported (11). Because there are only 20 chromosome pairs in the mouse genome, these larger numbers imply that many chromosomes carry more than one histocompatibility locus.

Producing Congenic Strains: Identifying the Major Histocompatibility Complex

A process to generate strains differing from one another genetically at only a single one of these numerous histocompatibility loci was pursued by Snell *(12)* at Jackson Laboratory, and involved the production of congenic strains (inbred strains that differ from one another at only one independently segregating genetic locus) using the rejection of parental skin grafts as the trait used to select successive matings. It became apparent during this process that one histocompatibility locus could be distinguished from all the others by the speed with which it caused skin graft rejection. This is now called the *major histocompatibility complex* (MHC). All of the other 30 to 50 histocompatibility loci have since been called minor histocompatibility loci. There are now a very large number of H-2 congenic strains of mice available (Table 44.2), as well as some that isolate minor histocompatibility loci and some rat congenic strains.

TABLE 44.2 List of H-2 Congenic Resistant Strains

Strain	*H-2 Haplotype*	*Origin of Background*	*MHC*
A	a	A	—
A./BY	b	A	Brackyury
A./CA	f	A	Caracal
A./SW	s	A	Swiss
BALB/c	d	BALB/c	BALB/c
BALB.B	b	BALB/c	C57BL/10
BALB.K	k	BALB/c	C3H
B6.AKR-H-2^k	k	C57BL/6	AKR
B6.SJl	s	C57BL/6	SJL
B10	b	C57BL/10	C57BL/10
B10.A	a	C57BL/10	A
B10.D2	d	C57BL/10	DBA/2
B10.M	f	C57BL/10	Outbred
B10.BR	k	C57BL/10	C57BR
B10.SM	v	C57BL/10	SM
B10.RIII	r	C57BL/10	RIII
B10.PL	u	C57BL/10	PL/J
C3H	k	C3H	C3H
C3H.SW	b	C3H	Swiss
C3H.JK	j	C3H	JK
C3H.NB	p	C3H	NB
D1.C	d	DBA/1	BALB/c
D1.LP	b	DBA/1	LP
LP.RIII	r	LP	RIII

MHC, major histocompatibility complex.

One of the most useful breeding schemes to produce CR lines is illustrated in Figure 44.5. Starting with two inbred strains, labeled for simplicity strain A and strain B, the objective is to obtain a strain that will share its entire genome with strain A except for the major histocompatibility locus H-2, which will be derived from strain B. The end product will be designated strain A.B. Using the cross-intercross scheme illustrated in Figure 44.4, a skin graft or tumor graft from strain A is placed onto all F2 offspring. Animals that reject the graft must be of genotype bb in at least one histocompatibility locus. Obviously, because there are many histocompatibility loci, most animals at this generation will reject the graft. However, if only animals rejecting vigorously are chosen, and if numerous such animals are selected, then one can be reasonably certain to have selected bb homozygotes at the H-2 locus by this procedure. The process is then repeated sequentially, mating rejectors back to strain A animals at each F2 generation. At each sequential F2 generation, the fraction of animals rejecting grafts vigorously will be smaller than it was at the previous generation. By selecting only vigorous rejectors one will ensure the selection of the bb homozygote at the H-2 locus. By the time nine cycles have been completed, one would expect only one histocompatibility locus to be segregating, so that only 25% of the intercross offspring should be capable of rejecting the graft. Assuming that vigorous rejection has been demanded throughout, one can be relatively certain that the selected locus will be H-2. In addition, the chances that any other nonselected locus will still be heterozygous rather than having reverted to the homozygous aa genotype will have fallen to less than 0.2%. Stated another way, more than 99.8% of nonselected loci will be expected to be identical to their counterparts in strain A. A male and a female homozygote from the final intercross are selected and used to establish a pedigreed inbred congenic line A.B.

Because mammalian genes are transferred as linked units in chromosomes, this process will always lead to the retention of a variable amount of bb genetic information at genes closely linked to the locus being selected. However, as described later, the occurrence of recombination during intercrossing generations leads also to fixation of the aa genotype at loci on the same chromosome as the MHC (chromosome 17 in mice) but at a variable distance from H-2. For practical purposes, animals that have been through at least nine cycles of such selected breeding are considered to be congenic.

As indicated in Table 44.2, there are now a large number of H-2 congenic mouse strains available on a variety of backgrounds. In general, the names of each of these strains follow the rule A.B, with strain A being the background strain used in the production of the congenic, and strain B being the other parental strain from which the alternate allele at H-2 was selected. All of the early inbred mouse strains were assigned a small-letter designation to

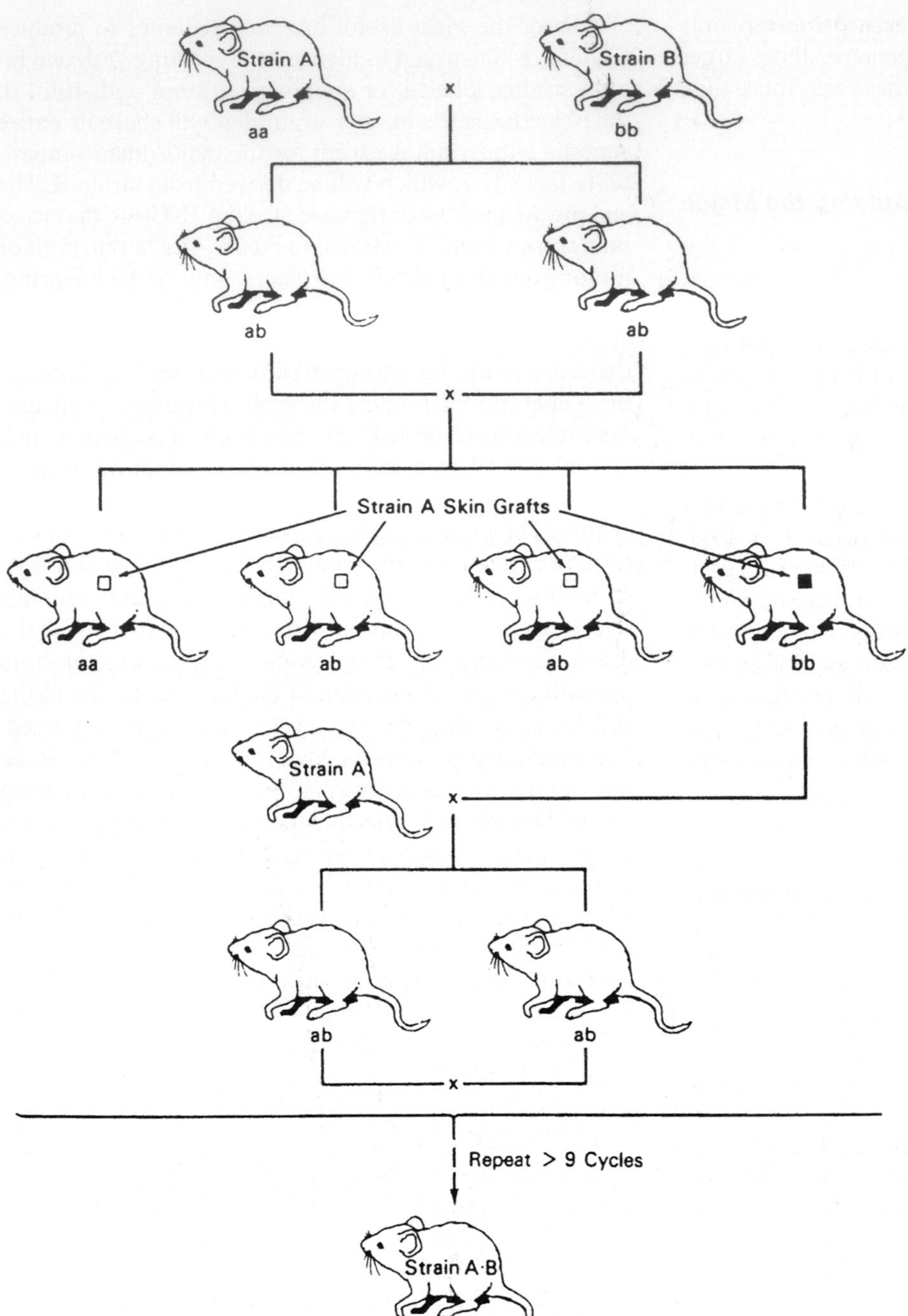

FIGURE 44.5 Schematic representation for production of a congenic line.

represent the particular constellation of alleles that they possessed at genes in the MHC. This small-letter designation is often called the *haplotype designation*, as indicated in Table 44.2. Thus, for example, strain C57BL/10 (or B10) is assigned the haplotype designation H-2b, and strain DBA/2 the haplotype designation H-2d. Thus, the congenic strain B10.D2 represents a line in which the background is derived from the C57BL/10 and the MHC from the DBA/2. It thus resembles in almost every way the C57BL/10 congenic partner, except that it differs from this partner for all properties controlled by MHC-linked genes.

Intra-MHC Recombinant Strains: Class I and II Antigens

As can be seen in Figure 44.5, every alternate generation in this mating scheme involves the crossing of animals heterozygous at H-2. Whenever heterozygotes are bred, there is always a possibility of recombination between autosomal chromosomes at meiosis. During the production of congenic lines, such recombination will tend to decrease the amount of linked genetic information carried into the congenic from the H-2 source. Therefore, the more backcrosses a particular congenic line has been subjected to, the closer will be the boundaries on either side of H-2 at

TABLE 44.3 List of H-2 Recombinant Strains

Recombinant Interval Haplotypes	*Parental Haplotypes*	*Haplotypes Designation*	*KAESD*	*Presence of Additional Recombinant Site*	*Strain Bearing Recombinant*
K-A	b/m	bq1	b/k k k q	Yes	B10.MBR
	s/a1	t1	slk k k d	Yes	A.TL
A-E	a/b	h4	k klb b b	No	B10.A(4R)
	b/a	i5	b blk d d	Yes	B10.A(5R)
	b/a	i3	b blk d d	Yes	B10.A(3R)
E-S	k/d	a	k k kld d	No	A, B10.A
S-D	d/b	g	d d d dlb	No	HTG, B10.HTG
	d/k	o2	d d d dlk	No	C3H.OH
	a/b	h1,h2	k k k dlb	Yes	B10.A(2R)
	k/q	m	k k k klq	No	AKR.M, B10.AKM
	q/a	y2	q q q qld	No	B10.T(6R)
	s/A	t2	s s s sld	No	A.TH

Notes: Congenic recombinant haplotypes available from The Jackson Laboratory.
Note that many of the recombinants involve at least one haplotype already containing a point of recombination. These are indicated by "Yes" and are listed only under the recombinant interval representing the most recent recombination in the haplotype's history.

which the chromosome reverts to the background strain. Because it soon became apparent that the MHC was in fact made up of multiple loci, there was also the possibility for recombination within H-2 to occur during such crosses. Fortunately, mouse geneticists were aware of this possibility and saved numerous recombinants during the production of H-2 congenic lines. Indeed, it was through the detection and characterization of such recombinants that the linkage map of H-2 was constructed. Thus, for example, there are now a series of recombinants between strain C57BL/10(H-2b) and A/WySn(H-2a) that were isolated by Stimpfling during production of the B10.A CR line and which have provided a great deal of information on the genetic fine structure of the H-2 complex. Strains B10.A(2R) and B10.A(4R), for example, have been used to map a variety of immune response genes within the MHC. Table 44.3 presents a listing of many of the most useful congenic recombinant strains now available and their known or presumed points of recombination. Among the most important contributions that came from the study of intra-MHC recombinant strains was the progressive understanding that the loci within the MHC encoded two general types of MHC antigens, now referred to as class I and class II MHC antigens.

DONOR ANTIGENS RESPONSIBLE FOR GRAFT REJECTION

Major Histocompatibility Antigens

MHC antigens are called *histocompatibility* antigens because of their powerful role in causing graft rejection; yet they did not evolve in nature to prevent tissue grafting. Although the name serves to emphasize the historical importance of transplantation in the discovery of the MHC, the essential role of MHC antigens is now understood to involve the presentation of peptides of foreign antigens to responding T cells (see Chapter 19). Table 44.4 summarizes important aspects of the MHC antigens that are worth emphasizing in this chapter on transplantation, while a much more detailed description of their structure and function can be found in Chapter 19.

Basic Features of MHC Antigens

Class I and Class II Antigens

Different loci within the complex encode two general types of MHC antigens, termed *class I and class II antigens*. Originally, the class I antigens were identified most easily by serologic techniques, while class II antigens were defined by their ability to induce proliferative responses

TABLE 44.4 Summary of Features of MHC

Class I antigens	Single polymorphic chain Three domains: alpha 1, 2, and 3 MW: 45,000 Associated with beta 2 microglobulin A, B, and C loci in humans Expressed on all tissues and cells
Class II antigens	Two polymorphic chains: alpha and beta Each with two domains: alpha 1 and 2, beta 1 and 2 MW: 33,000 and 28,000 DP, DQ, and DR loci in humans Expressed on macrophages, dendritic cells and B cells; vascular endothelium; activated human T cells

MHC, major histocompatibility complex.

of allogeneic lymphocytes *(13)*. Class I and class II MHC antigens evoke allogeneic responses that differ in magnitude, as will be discussed later.

Polymorphism

The MHC antigens exhibit extraordinary polymorphism. This polymorphism presumably provides an advantage to members of the species by ensuring a broad capacity to present the peptides of, and thus respond to, a large number of foreign antigens. In the human HLA complex, for example, there are currently at least 300 known alleles at each of the HLA-B (class I) and DRB1 (class II) loci (14). The high degree of polymorphism has important consequences for transplantation. Given that there are three class I loci (A, B, and C) and three to four class II loci (DQ, DP, DRB1, ± an expressed DRB 3,4 or 5 locus present in some haplotypes) on each haplotype, the likelihood of achieving identity for MHC antigens in two unrelated humans is extremely small.

Tissue Distribution

The tissue distribution of the two types of MHC antigens differs. Class I antigens are present on all nucleated cells of the body, but may be sparsely represented on some types of cells *(15)*. Class II MHC antigens are more selective in their distribution *(16)*. They are especially frequent on macrophages, dendritic cells (DCs), and B lymphocytes. They are present on other lymphoid cells under some circumstances, and on vascular endothelium. Their expression on some tissues of the body is regulated according to various stimuli *(17)* and differs between species. One of the important distinctions between rodents and many larger species is the lack of constitutive expression of class II antigens on the vascular endothelium and other cell populations in rodents. In contrast, pigs, monkeys and humans express class II antigens on these tissues *(18)*.

The Importance of MHC Antigens in Alloreactivity. Alloreactivity is the immune response to foreign antigens of other members of the same species. MHC antigens are exceptionally important in stimulating alloresponses, both *in vivo* and *in vitro*.

VIGOROUS GRAFT REJECTION. Early experiments showed that mouse skin grafts differing only in their MHC antigens were typically rejected in 8 to 10 days, whereas grafts differing by only a few minor histocompatibility antigens were typically rejected in 3 or more weeks. Subsequent experiments have confirmed the importance of MHC antigens for other types of grafts. In pigs, primarily-vascularized organs, such as the kidney, may survive indefinitely in some cases, even without immunosuppression, if all of their MHC antigens are matched, whereas MHC-mismatched kidneys are always rejected within 2 weeks *(18)*. However, the importance of MHC antigen matching becomes harder to detect, especially for highly immunogenic skin graft survival, when comparing MHC-mismatched grafts with grafts differing for multiple minor histocompatibility antigens.

STRONG *in vitro* ALLORESPONSES. Allogeneic MHC antigens also stimulate an extraordinarily strong T-cell response *in vitro*. This strength is manifested partly by the ability to readily achieve primary *in vitro* cell-mediated responses to allogeneic MHC antigens, whereas *in vitro* responses to non-MHC antigens generally require *in vivo* priming. The standard *in vitro* assay of helper function in cellular immunity is the mixed lymphocyte response. This assay uses uptake of radiolabeled thymidine or loss of a fluorescent intracellular dye on successive cell divisions *(19)* to measure proliferation of T cells after allogeneic stimulation. Such analyses have led to frequency estimates of approximately 1% to 7% of T cells proliferating in a particular alloresponse *(19–22)*, while naïve T cells reactive with an exogenous peptide generally represent only approximately one in tens to hundreds of thousands of the same T-cell pool (*23*,*24*,*25*). Much higher precursor frequencies of alloreactive T cells compared with those for a particular peptide presented by a self-MHC molecule are measurable in limiting dilution assays. The helper response can also be quantified and characterized by measuring the production of particular cytokines such as interleukin 2 (IL-2) using biologic assays, enzyme-linked immunosorbent assay (ELISA), and enzyme-linked immunosorbent spot (ELISPOT) assay (*26*,*27*), intracellular cytokine staining with flow cytometry *(28)*, and polymerase chain reaction (PCR).

Likewise, strong primary direct alloresponses of $CD8^+$ T cells can be measured *in vitro*, either in standard cell-mediated lympholysis (CML) assays, in limiting dilution assays measuring cytotoxic T lymphocyte (CTL) precursor frequencies or in cytokine production assays similar to those previously described for CD4 cells. The CML assay measures T-cell–mediated cytotoxicity against allogeneic targets. Alloreactive CTLs can easily be generated from naïve T cells after about 5 to 7 days of *in vitro* stimulation with MHC-disparate cells. Generation of CTLs to peptides of minor antigens presented by self MHC molecules, however, requires that the T cells first be primed *in vivo*. The amount of cytotoxicity measured *in vitro* is a function of both the helper activation and the number of precursor CTLs available at the start of the *in vitro* culture. Therefore, to focus on just the cytotoxic effector function the assay is often performed with the addition of exogenous helper factors, such as IL-2, in order to provide an excess of help.

The presence of T cells that can kill donor targets without a period of *in vitro* sensitization (direct cytolytic activity) *(29)*, an increased precursor frequency of alloreactive T cells, and development of CTL under modified conditions *(30)* has been used to demonstrate *in vivo* activation

TABLE 44.5 ***In vitro* Pathways of Alloreactivity**

	Helper Pathways				Cytotoxic Pathways	
	Direct		Indirect			
	I	II	I	II	I	II
$CD4^+$	–	++++	–	+++	–	++
$CD8^+$	++	–	+/–	–	++++	++

by alloantigens. More recently developed techniques, including ELISPOT and intracellular cytokine staining, have enhanced the ability to detect nonproliferating or noncytolytic CD8 T cells that have been sensitized *in vivo (28)*.

In general, the rule that CD4 cells recognize class II antigens and CD8 cells recognize class I antigens has been borne up by extensive investigation of the pathways of alloreactivity. However, this strong bias for recognition of each class of MHC antigen is more stringent for CD4 cells than for CD8 cells. The summary shown in Table 44.5 indicates the relative magnitude of the response for each T-cell subpopulation in response to each type of antigenic challenge. It should be noted that in some cases where the response is shown in Table 44.5 to be absent (based on bulk culture experiments), there have been T-cell clones derived (presumably exceptional cases) that demonstrate this specificity.

Direct Recognition of Allogeneic MHC Antigens. As indicated in Table 44.5, the extraordinary strength of alloreactivity largely reflects the ability of T cells to recognize allogeneic MHC antigens presented on donor APC, which is referred to as "direct" allorecognition. "Indirect" allorecognition, on the other hand, denotes presentation of donor-derived peptides on MHC antigens of recipient APC. Although these responses are much weaker than direct alloresponses, they are nevertheless important (see later discussion). Three different, but not mutually exclusive, hypotheses have been proposed to explain the high frequency of directly alloreactive T cells: (i) a genetic bias favoring T-cell receptor genes that bind to MHC antigens, (ii) a high density of individual allogeneic MHC determinants on the surface of allogeneic APCs, and (iii) a large number of different allogeneic MHC/peptide determinants expressed on the donor APCs.

GENETIC BIAS. Because the thymus only positively selects T cells with some degree of MHC reactivity, a T-cell receptor (TCR) gene pool that encodes a broad range of specificities (as is the case for B cells) would produce many useless precursors. A narrower pool of T-cell receptor genes, however, would allow for more efficient thymic selection. Considerable evidence supports the hypothesis that TCRs have intrinsic affinity for MHC molecules before positive and negative selection (*31–37*,38,*39*). Although thymocytes must survive positive selection in order to mature and enter the peripheral T-cell pool, the TCR affinity for self-MHC/peptide complexes required for positive selection is much lower than that involved in negative selection (38). Positive selection results in enrichment for TCRs capable of seeing modified self-MHC antigens. Those receptors with strong affinity for the same MHC antigens plus self-peptides are deleted through negative selection. Because TCRs are not normally negatively selected in the presence of allogeneic MHC molecules, intrinsic allogeneic MHC reactivity persists within a T-cell repertoire that has been negatively selected only by "self" MHC-peptide complexes. Alloreactivity can occur despite the influence of positive selection because negative selection never occurs for the vast majority of T cells recognizing allogeneic MHC antigens.

THE "DETERMINANT DENSITY" HYPOTHESIS. As illustrated in Figure 44.6A, the density of a given specific peptide determinant expressed by a self-APC would be quite low (as most MHC antigens present other peptides), whereas the density of a peptide-independent allogeneic MHC determinant on allogeneic APCs would be very high (as every MHC antigen would include the foreign determinant). According to this hypothesis, a high frequency

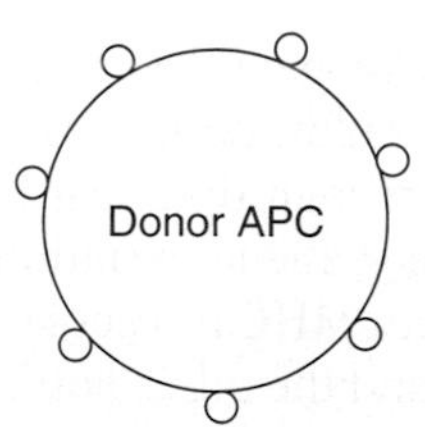

Donor APC with donor MHC antigens (O), all of which are foreign.

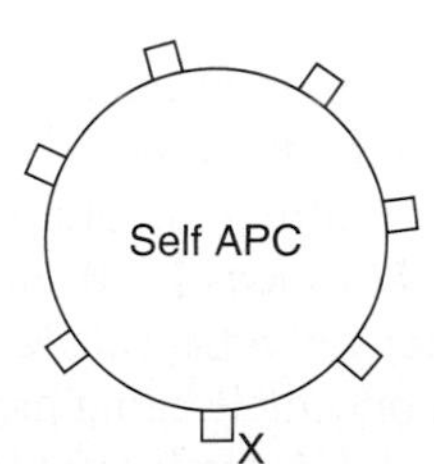

Self APC with self MHC molecules (□). The rare self MHC molecule presents a peptide (X) of an environmental pathogen.

A

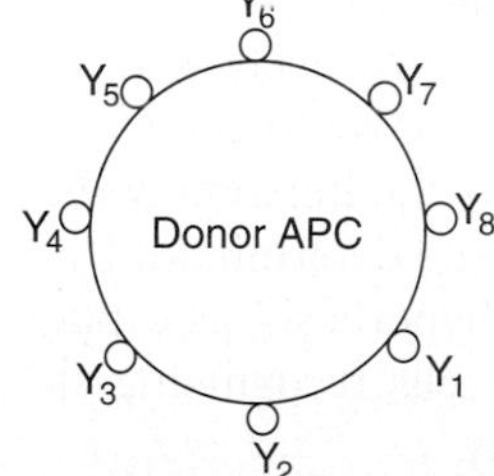

Donor MHC antigens (O). Each presents different "self peptides," generating different foreign determinants.

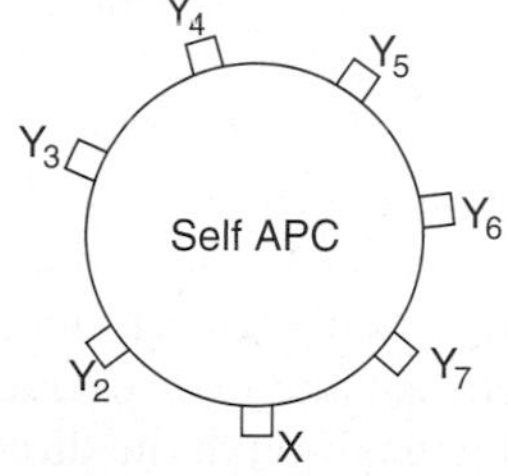

Self MHC molecules (□) also present self peptides ($Y_{1...N}$), but these are all self determinants.

B

FIGURE 44.6 **A:** Determinant density hypothesis. **B:** Determinant frequency hypothesis. APC, antigen-pressenting cell; MHC, major histocompatibility complex.

of alloreactive T cells might be apparent because abundant allogeneic MHC determinants would activate many cross-reactive T cells with relatively low affinities. This hypothesis implies that allogeneic MHC molecules can be recognized at least partly independently of the peptides they present, and T-cell clones recognizing MHC antigens in a completely or partially peptide-independent manner have indeed been demonstrated in the alloreactive TCR repertoire (40,*41–46*).

THE "DETERMINANT FREQUENCY" HYPOTHESIS. T cells specific for allogeneic MHC antigens are influenced by the peptides presented by these MHC molecules *(47)*. Whereas MHC molecules on self-APCs present peptides of self proteins (say $X_{1,2,\ldots n}$), allogeneic MHC antigens may present peptides of polymorphic allogeneic "self" proteins (e.g., "Allo + X_1, Allo + X_2, . . . Allo + X_n") (Fig. 44.6B). Alternatively, the self-peptides presented by self or allogeneic MHC molecules might be identical, but these complexes would stimulate different TCRs because crystal structure data indicate that both peptide and MHC alpha helix residues contribute to the surface that is recognized by a TCR *(48–51)*. In both cases, the set of determinants represented by "Self + $X_{1\ldots n}$" would differ from that represented by "Allo + $X_{1\ldots n}$". T cells responsive to self-peptides on self-APCs (Self + X_1, Self + $X_{2,\ldots}$ etc.) are eliminated by the induction of self-tolerance, leaving only self-MHC molecules presenting peptides of foreign antigens to stimulate an immune response. On the other hand, self-tolerance would not affect the response to the many self-peptides on allogeneic APCs (Allo + X_1, Allo + $X_{2,\ldots}$ etc.). Thus, alloreactive T cells are more frequent because each allogeneic MHC antigen generates a large number of different foreign determinants. Consistent with this hypothesis, many alloreactive T cells have been shown to be peptide-specific or at least partially peptide-selective *(41,42,52–59)*. Cardiac allografting studies using $DM^{-/-}$ mice, which lack the capacity to replace invariant chain-derived CLIP peptide with a more diverse array of peptides, provide strong *in vivo* evidence for the importance of peptides in direct allorecognition (60).

Clearly, both peptide-dependent and -independent alloreactive TCRs exist, and both types are likely to contribute to the high frequency of alloreactive TCRs. Overall, the available information supports the inherent MHC binding capacity of TCRs, as well as the determinant frequency and the determinant density hypothesis, as explanations for the high frequency of T cells recognizing alloantigens through the direct pathway.

Minor Histocompatibility Antigens

Although initially defined by their ability to cause rapid graft rejection, major histocompatibility antigens are currently defined in part by the location of the genes encoding them and in part by the well-characterized structure of both class I and class II antigens (see Chapter 19). For example, Qa and Tla antigens are generally considered class I-like products because of their structure and location in the genome, even though they are weak transplantation antigens in terms of rejection. Minor histocompatibility antigens, on the other hand, are those capable of eliciting a T-cell immune response, but which lack the structural characteristics of MHC products *(61)*. Rather than being allelic cell surface proteins, minor histocompatibility antigens, like other antigens recognized by T cells, are peptides of donor proteins that are presented by MHC molecules (*62–66*,67,*68*,*69*). In mice, antigens derived from enzymes encoded by mitochondrial DNA are presented by nonclassical class I molecules and may function as maternally inherited minor histocompatibility antigens (70). Because individuals are tolerant to the peptides derived from their own proteins, they only respond to the peptides of another individual's proteins that have allelic variation, that is, polymorphism. Antigens that can cause rejection through B-cell responses without a T-cell response are not considered to be minor histocompatibility antigens.

It has been estimated that there may be as many as 720 minor histocompatibility loci in mice (71), and at least 50 have been mapped to autosomes in the murine genome. Minor histocompatibility antigens can be expressed ubiquitously or in a tissue-selective or tissue-specific manner *(72)*. Some of the peptides representing minor histocompatibility antigens have been isolated in mice and humans, and the proteins from which they are derived have been identified (67,*68*,*69*,71,73,*74*,75,76,77,78,*79–83*,84). These proteins are often intracellular proteins such as nuclear transcription factors and myosin. However, CD31 is a polymorphic cell-surface glycoprotein that functions as a minor histocompatibility antigen with controversial significance for GVHD risk in bone marrow transplant (BMT) recipients *(85,86)*. Presumably any cellular protein with allelic variation could function as a minor histocompatibility antigen as long as a peptide expressing that allelic variation can be processed and presented by an MHC antigen.

Some minor antigens are diallelic peptides, both of which can be represented by a particular MHC molecule (73,75), resulting in bidirectional recognition (e.g., the murine *H13* locus [75]). Alternatively, allelic variation in the capacity of a peptide to bind to an MHC molecule can result in one allele being presented and the other not (e.g., the human HA-1 minor antigen, in which only one of two allelic peptides binds effectively to HLA-A2 [73]). Minor antigenic determinants can also result from the failure of one allele to be processed to a peptide, as has been observed for the HLA-A2–restricted minor determinant HA-8. Although both alleles, when provided as peptides, can be recognized by HA-8–specific CTL, only one allele is naturally produced, apparently because the other is transported poorly by the TAP (transporter associated with antigen presentation) complex (76).

It is very difficult to detect humoral responses to minor antigens, presumably because individual peptide/MHC complexes are too low in abundance on the cell surface to either stimulate an antibody response or be detected on the cell surface with antibodies. An exception is the recent discovery of antibodies against H-Y (Y chromosome-encoded) antigens in association with chronic GVHD *(87)*. Additionally, antibody responses to tumor-associated antigens, which, similar to minor antigens, are presented as peptides in the context of MHC molecules, have been detected in humans with various malignancies *(88)*.

When multiple minor antigenic disparities exist, the immune response to one of these antigens often predominates in a phenomenon known as *immunodominance (89–94)*. Removal of the immunodominant recognition sometimes produces strong responses to antigens that previously evoked weak or no responses. This phenomenon may be due to competition between peptides of different minor antigens for presentation by MHC molecules (71). The duration of antigen presentation and TCR avidities may also determine immunodominance *(95)*. An exceptionally immunodominant peptide, H60, which is derived from an NKG2D-binding protein, produces responses that are comparable in potency to those elicited by MHC alloantigens, apparently because of the existence of a very high frequency of TCR in the naïve repertoire with specificity for this peptide (96). However, immunodominance of CTL responses measured *in vitro* does not necessarily reflect the immunodominance of the same antigens *in vivo*, as has been revealed by studies of GVHD in mice (71,97). This discrepancy may reflect the importance of tissue distribution of minor antigen expression or of helper T-cell responses to minor antigens in inducing GVHD *(80)*.

The H-Y antigens are encoded by several genes on the Y chromosome, and are therefore expressed only by males of a given species (71,78,*98–101*). Some mouse strains are capable of rejecting H-Y-disparate (otherwise histocompatible) grafts while others are not. Such rejection requires that the antigen generate both helper determinants, recognized by $CD4^+$ cells in association with class II MHC antigens, and cytotoxic determinants, recognized by $CD8^+$ cells in association with class I antigens, suggesting that to be identifiable as minor histocompatibility antigen, proteins must generate at least two different peptide fragments with allelic variation (102). Exceptions are observed in TCR transgenic mice with an unphysiologically high frequency of a single clone recognizing an H-Y peptide *(103)*.

Because of the relative ease with which CTL assays can be used to measure peptide-specific responses, minor histocompatibility antigens have been identified as determinants recognized by CTL. In humans, these have been identified mainly in the setting of HLA-identical sibling donor bone marrow transplantation, in association with GVHD and marrow graft rejection (*74*,76,*80,81,104,105*). Immunodominance of CTL responses to particular H-Y and HA determinants as well as expansion of minor antigen-specific CTL detected with tetrameric complexes of HLA molecules and minor antigenic peptides (*81,105*,106) have been associated with GVHD and marrow graft rejection (107), and certain incompatibilities (e.g., HA-1) may predispose to GVHD *(74,108)*. The use of DCs as APC has permitted the recent molecular identification of minor antigenic peptide epitopes recognized by $CD4^+$ Th *(109)*.

Other Antigens of Potential Importance in Transplantation

Superantigens

Like MHC antigens, superantigens can stimulate primary *in vitro* T-cell proliferative responses and activate a high proportion of the T-cell repertoire. However, these antigens are not presented as peptides in the binding groove of MHC molecules, but instead bind to distinct regions of class II MHC molecules, and engage nonvariable portions of $V\beta$ components of the TCR, rather than the hypervariable regions that recognize peptides. Endogenous superantigens are not classical transplantation antigens, perhaps because of their restricted tissue expression patterns *(110–114)*. However, they may contribute to GVHD in mice (115).

Tissue-Specific Antigens

Some peptides presented by MHC molecules may be derived from proteins with limited tissue distribution *(116–119)*. Responses to such peptides will not be detected by *in vitro* assays to measure T-cell responsiveness to donor antigens when lymphohematopoietic cells are used as the stimulating cell population. The existence of tissue-specific antigens suggests that transplantation tolerance induced by one set of donor cells might not always induce complete tolerance to donor cells of a different sort. For example, the existence of skin-specific antigens may result in skin graft rejection despite the presence of stable hematopoietic chimerism induced by hematopoietic cell transplantation (HCT) (120). Tissue-specific proteins do not necessarily need to show allelic variation to be regarded as alloantigens in bone marrow chimeras as the determinant formed by a given peptide with an allogeneic MHC molecule would be different from that formed by the same peptide with a recipient MHC molecule.

Several human minor histocompatibility antigens may be expressed only on hematopoietic cells (*72*,121). GVH-alloreactive donor T cells that recognize such antigens could potentially achieve graft-versus-leukemia (GVL) effects without GVHD. However, disparities for some of these minor antigens (e.g., HA-1) have in fact been associated with an increased incidence of GVHD *(74,108)*. It is of interest that effector and regulatory CD8 T cells recognizing the donor HA-1 peptide have been detected, in association with microchimerism, in HLA-identical kidney graft recipients (122).

Endothelial Glycoproteins

Blood Group Antigens

Blood group antigens are important in relation to blood transfusion but also in the context of transplantation. The blood group antigens do not evoke cell-mediated immune responses and hence are not classified as minor histocompatibility antigens. They are expressed on erythrocytes and other cells and, importantly, on vascular endothelium, where they may serve as the targets for antibody-mediated attack on blood vessels of organ grafts. Blood group antigens are the products of glycosylation enzymes that are not the same in all individuals. Blood group A and B individuals each express their respective antigen but O individuals have neither. The natural antibodies against blood group antigens an individual lacks probably arise because of cross-reactions with common carbohydrate determinants of environmental microorganisms. Thus, type O individuals have antibodies to the antigens of A and B donors, while A and B individuals only have antibodies reactive with antigens from each other, and AB individuals have antibodies to neither. Therefore, O recipients can only receive transfusions from O donors; A and B recipients can receive transfusions from O donors or from individuals sharing their blood type; and AB recipients can receive blood from donors of any blood type. The same rules apply to the transplantation of most primarily vascularized organs in man *(123)*. Recently, advances have been made in the ability to successfully transplant kidneys across ABO barriers by adsorbing antibody from the plasma and depleting B cells (124). Blood group antigens are of lesser importance, but nevertheless significant, in hematopoietic cell transplantation. ABO incompatibility in the host-versus-graft direction can lead to prolonged red cell aplasia following HCT; incompatibility in the GVH direction can result in initial hemolytic anemia, but this complication can be avoided by washing the donor HCT preparation to rid it of plasma *(125)*. In addition to the ABO locus, there are other loci determining blood group antigens on erythrocytes, but these are irrelevant to organ transplantation because they are not expressed on vascular endothelium.

Other Allogeneic Endothelial Glycoproteins

Other glycoproteins expressed on the vascular endothelium may serve as targets for humoral responses. Very rarely, preformed antibodies to these antigens may give rise to hyperacute rejection of primarily-vascularized organs *(126)*. Although antibody responses to non-HLA, non-ABO endothelial antigens have been associated with chronic rejection *(127–129)*, the specificity and pathogenic role of these antibodies is unknown.

Species-specific Carbohydrate Determinants

Closely analogous to the blood group antigens are the carbohydrate determinants expressed on vascular endothelium that show species specificity. For example, pigs, which are of interest as a potential xenograft source animal (see later discussion), as well as most other species, express an α-1,3-galactosyltransferase (αGal transferase) enzyme that is not expressed by humans. This enzyme glycosylates β-galactosyl N-acetyl glucosamine to form a Galα1-3Galβ1-4GlcNAc (αGal) determinant. During evolution, at the level of Old World primates, the gene for this transferase lost its function because of mutation. Because the Gal antigen is found on bacteria and other environmental antigens, humans and Old World primates make a large amount of antibody against Gal. Thus, "natural" antibodies are present in human serum, which reacts to the non–self-pig determinant αGal (130,*131*), and these can cause hyperacute rejection of primarily vascularized xenogeneic transplants. αGal may also be recognized by other components of the innate immune system, such as macrophages (132).

"Missing Self" and Natural Killer Cell Recognition

In apparent violation of the laws of transplantation previously described, (AxB) F1 mice are capable of rejecting bone marrow from parental donors, a phenomenon termed *hybrid resistance*. This phenomenon, as well as rapid rejection of fully allogeneic marrow, is mediated by natural killer (NK) cells *(133)*. NK cells are large granular lymphocytes that lack TCRs, and that have the ability to mediate cytolysis against certain tumor targets and hematopoietic cells. NK cells also produce a number of proinflammatory, hematopoietic, and even anti-inflammatory cytokines, and may be divided into subsets on the basis of their cytokine production pattern *(134)*.

The originally puzzling specificity of NK cell-mediated marrow rejection is due to the expression by NK cells of inhibitory receptors that recognize specific groups of class I MHC alleles on target cells and prevent cytolysis by the NK cell. These class I receptors are type II C lectins (Ly49 family) or dimers of CD94 with NKG2 lectins in the mouse, and are either immunoglobulin family members (KIR) or CD94/NKG2 in humans. Recognition by an inhibitory receptor of a class I ligand results in intracellular transmission of an inhibitory signal via an immune receptor tyrosine-based inhibitory motif that interacts with a tyrosine phosphatase and counteracts activating signals transmitted from other cell-surface molecules. Recognition of "self" class I inhibitory ligands is believed to be important in preventing the NK cell from killing normal autologous cells *(135,136)*. Additional inhibitory NK cell receptors recognize ligands other than class I MHC (137). Molecules of the KIR, Ly-49, and NKG2 families lacking an intracellular immune receptor tyrosine-based inhibitory motif are

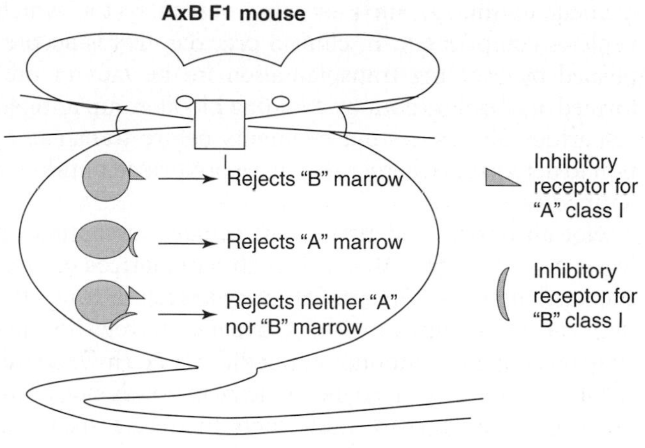

FIGURE 44.7 An explanation for hybrid resistance. Each *filled circle* represents a subset of natural killer cells.

capable of associating with molecules that contain tyrosine-based activating motifs (DAP-10 and DAP-12) *(138–140)* that activate cytolytic activity by NK cells (see Chapter 16). There are several other types of NK cell-activating receptors as well, including Fc receptors and natural cytotoxicity receptors (141). The effects of at least some activating receptors can be overridden by inhibitory signals *(142)*. Thus, the ability of an NK cell to kill an allogeneic target will depend on the interplay of inhibitory and activating receptors on the NK cell and the respective ligands expressed by the potential target cells.

Inhibitory receptors are clonally distributed on NK cells, each of which may express one or more different inhibitory receptor. For NK cells to be functional yet tolerant of "self" they must express at least one inhibitory receptor for a self-class I MHC molecule (*143*,144). Thus, as is illustrated in Figure 44.7, an AxB F1 recipient will have subsets of NK cells with inhibitory receptors that recognize MHC of either the A parent, the B parent, or both. The absence of "B" class I molecules on, for example, AA parental hematopoietic cells, permits subsets of (AxB)F1 NK cells that have inhibitory receptors only for class I molecules from the B parent, to destroy AA cells. Thus, hybrid resistance and NK cell-mediated resistance to fully allogeneic marrow grafts can be explained on the basis of "missing self" *(136)*. The possible role of NK cells in mediating graft rejection is discussed in a later section.

MECHANISMS OF GRAFT REJECTION

At least four distinct mechanisms that can cause graft rejection have been defined according to the time frame in which they tend to occur in clinical practice. Although their names (hyperacute rejection, accelerated rejection, acute rejection, and chronic rejection) have a clear temporal distinction, it is increasingly possible to characterize these mechanisms according to the cell types and processes involved and, in some cases, they may occur at uncharacteristic times.

Rejection Caused by Preformed Antibodies (Hyperacute Rejection)

Hyperacute rejection occurs within minutes to hours after blood flow is established to a transplanted vascularized organ (145,*146*,*147*). The phenomenon is visible and dramatic: the organ turns blue and its function ceases. Microscopically, there is extensive evidence of vascular thrombosis and hemorrhage.

There are several important components involved in the mechanism of hyperacute rejection. First, there are donor endothelial MHC antigens or carbohydrate determinants (see previous discussion). Second, there are preformed antibodies that can bind these antigens. Third, the complement and coagulation cascades are activated by the binding of preformed antibodies to the donor antigens on the vascular endothelium. The interaction of these components leading to hyperacute rejection is diagrammed in Figure 44.8.

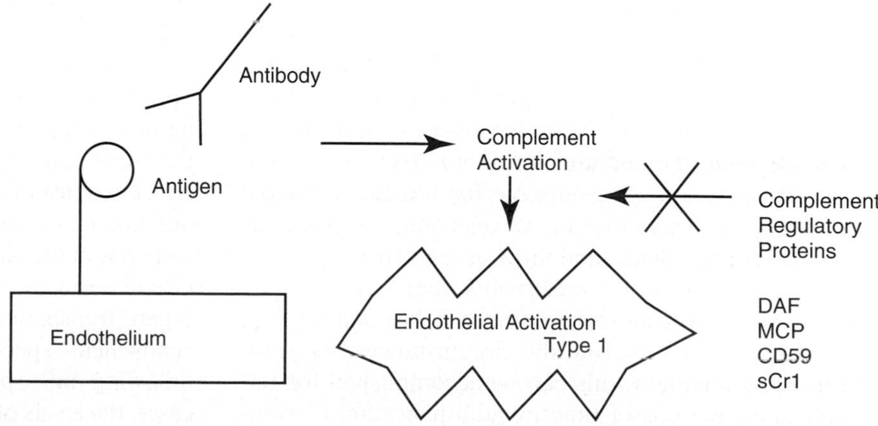

FIGURE 44.8 Schematic representation of hyperacute rejection.

The role of complement in hyperacute rejection is inferred both from the accumulation of various complement components in the grafts and from the fact that complement depletion leads to prolonged survival of xenografts *(148)*. Complement activation leads to production of active protein fragments and complexes of complement components, which cause tissue injury either directly or by recruiting effector cells that mediate destruction of the graft. In allogeneic combinations, this is initiated by antibody-mediated activation of complement through the classical pathway, while in xenogeneic combinations, the alternative pathway may also be involved (149). In both cases the membrane attack complex, produced by the ordered interaction of several complement components, initiates the destructive pathway.

Complement activation is controlled by several regulatory molecules, including complement receptor 1, decay accelerating factor (DAF, CD55), membrane cofactor protein (MCP, CD46), and CD59, which act at different stages along the cascade (see Chapter 33). Many of these molecules are produced by the vascular endothelial cells. Because these regulatory proteins prevent unwanted complement activation in the face of low levels of perturbation to the system, the titer and avidity of the preformed antibodies must be high enough to activate despite these down-regulating molecules. Thus, preformed antibodies directed at MHC antigens almost always accomplish this activation, whereas the lower-affinity blood group antibodies lead to hyperacute rejection in only about 25% of kidneys. One of the reasons that hyperacute rejection is such an important feature in xenogeneic transplantation is that the complement regulatory proteins produced by the donor vascular endothelium of one species do not always function effectively with complement molecules derived from a different species. Because of this homologous restriction, lower levels of an initial triggering signal lead to explosive complement activation.

Although the membrane attack complex is often thought of as a lytic molecule, its effect on the donor vascular endothelium, even before cell lysis, is to cause endothelial activation. This occurs rapidly, before there is time for new gene transcription or protein synthesis, and has been referred to as *type I endothelial activation*. The two principal manifestations of this activation are cell retraction, leading to gaps between endothelial cells, and initiation of coagulation pathways due to the loss of antithrombotic molecules from the endothelium *(150)*. Thus, type I endothelial activation is responsible for the two principal pathologic findings in hyperacute rejection: extravascular hemorrhage and edema, and intravascular thrombosis.

There are no known treatments that can stop the process of hyperacute rejection once it has started and, thus, it is essential to avoid the circumstances that initiate it. Experimentally, this can be accomplished for relatively short periods of time by administration of complement inhibitors, such as cobra venom factor, which depletes complement. In clinical practice, this is accomplished by avoiding transplantation in the face of preformed antibodies, both by avoiding blood group antigen disparities and by testing recipients before transplantation to determine whether they have preformed antidonor antibodies.

Not all organs and tissues are equally susceptible to hyperacute rejection. Most primarily vascularized organs, such as kidneys and hearts, are very susceptible, but the liver can often survive without hyperacute rejection despite pre-existing antidonor antibodies *(151)*. However, resistance of the liver to hyperacute rejection is not absolute. The other types of transplants that are resistant to hyperacute rejection are those that do not immediately expose donor vascular endothelium to the recipient's circulation, such as skin grafts, whose blood vessels are not in communication with those of the recipient until about a week after transplantation. After this, large doses of exogenously administered antidonor antibodies can destroy skin grafts through a complement-dependent mechanism *(152)*. Free cellular transplants, such as bone marrow cells or hepatocytes, as well as islet grafts *(153)* are not fed by their own blood vessels and thus are not susceptible to the mechanisms of hyperacute rejection. However, in many cases these cell transplants do express some of the antigens recognized by preformed antibodies, and antibodies can impair engraftment *(154)*. In the case of HCT, this resistance can be overcome by transplanting larger numbers of cells *(154–156)*. Additionally, antibody-independent complement activation has been shown to be a significant factor diminishing the engraftment of xenogeneic bone marrow (157).

Acute Humoral Rejection (Accelerated Rejection)

A second mechanism of rejection, also caused by antibodies, occurs as a result of antibodies that are induced very rapidly after a transplant is performed. This type of rejection has been called *acute humoral* or *accelerated* rejection because it typically occurs within the first 5 days posttransplant. The process is characterized by fibrinoid necrosis of donor arterioles with intravascular thrombosis (158).

Accelerated rejection is rare in allogeneic combinations because it requires that an antibody response occur before the T-cell response that is typically responsible for acute rejection episodes (see later discussion). Indeed, it is very difficult experimentally to induce an allogeneic B-cell response in the absence of T-cell immunity. The best examples of accelerated rejection are observed in vascularized organ transplants between closely related concordant xenogeneic species and between discordant species following adsorption of anti-Gal antibodies. In these cases, the levels of preformed antibodies are not sufficient to cause hyperacute rejection, but antidonor antibodies appear rapidly (within 3 to 4 days), causing rejection. The pathology of acute humoral rejection reveals a paucity of lymphocytes infiltrating the donor graft, antibody binding to donor vascular endothelium, and fibrinoid necrosis of the donor vessels. Vigorous anti–T-cell immunosuppression has little effect on acute humoral rejection, whereas immunosuppression with reagents that affect B-cell responses, such as cyclophosphamide, delays its onset until more typical T-cell–mediated rejection occurs *(159)*.

Like hyperacute rejection, acute humoral rejection is usually initiated by antibody binding to antigens on the donor vascular endothelium. In this case, however, the subsequent endothelial changes occur more slowly, allowing time for gene transcription and new protein synthesis. This later form of activation has been called *type II endothelial activation* (149,160). Many of its features appear to be mediated by the transcription factor NFκB, which generates many of the responses associated with inflammation, including the secretion of inflammatory cytokines such as IL-1 and IL-8 and the expression of adhesion molecules such as E-selectin and intercellular adhesion molecule (ICAM)-1 *(161)*. In addition, type II endothelial activation causes the loss of thrombomodulin and other prothrombotic changes *(162)*. Thus, the events following type II endothelial activation are associated with the pathologic changes that occur with "accelerated" rejection, including the tendency toward intravascular thrombosis and the inflammatory destruction of donor vessels that occurs in the absence of infiltrating lymphocytes.

Just as there are regulatory processes for complement activation, there are regulatory molecules that counter the tendency toward intravascular coagulation and the process of type II endothelial activation, for example, tissue factor protein inhibitor (expressed by vascular endothelium, which inhibits factor Xa of the clotting cascade) and a number of other protective molecules, including Bcl-x_L, Bcl-2, and A20 (149,163). Although these are often thought of as antiapoptotic molecules, they also tend to inhibit activation mediated by NFκB. Like the regulatory molecules of complement, some of these regulators may not function across species differences, leading to disordered regulation of the coagulation system *(164)*.

Although vigorous early antibody responses generate type II endothelial activation and accelerated rejection, later antibody responses usually fail to do so. The process that enables transplanted organs to survive in the face of circulating antibodies that can bind endothelial antigens has been called *accommodation* (149,*165*). In xenogeneic combinations, and some allogeneic combinations with preformed blood group antibodies, accommodation has been achieved by the removal of preformed antibodies for a period of 1 to 2 weeks and the allowance of their slow return after this time. Similarly, resistance to type II endothelial activation has been achieved *in vitro* by pretreatment with low levels of antiendothelial antibodies that are insufficient to trigger activation *(166)*. The achievement of accommodation is associated with increased expression of the antiapoptotic genes previously described and with changes in the isotype of the recipient's antibody responses (160,*167*). However, accommodation has not yet been convincingly demonstrated in a pig-to-primate xenograft model.

An important difference between hyperacute and acute humoral rejection is that there is no known therapy to stop graft destruction by hyperacute rejection, whereas acute humoral rejection can sometimes be reversed by plasmapheresis to remove antidonor antibodies and treatment with anti–B-cell reagents *(159,168)*.

Acute Cellular Rejection and Acute Graft-versus-Host Disease

"Acute cellular rejection," which is characterized by a mononuclear cell infiltrate in the graft, is the most common type of organ allograft rejection treated by clinicians. Acute rejection occurs with decreasing frequency after the first 3 months, but rejection by apparently similar mechanisms may occur much later, especially if immunosuppressive medication is withdrawn. Acute rejection is T-cell–dependent, as demonstrated in humans by the efficacy of reagents that specifically block T-cell responses in preventing and treating rejection. Treatment of acute rejection usually includes increased doses of standard immunosuppressive drugs or antilymphocyte antibodies. These strategies are so likely to be successful that the diagnosis of acute rejection is doubtful if they are not.

Whereas 30 years ago the majority of transplant recipients suffered one or more rejection episode, and only about half of the recipients were able to keep their transplanted organ for a full year, the use of newer immunosuppressive drugs and anti–T-cell antibodies has changed these numbers considerably. Currently, as many as 80% of kidney transplant recipients never experience an episode of acute rejection *(169)*, and it is now quite rare to lose a transplanted organ to cell-mediated rejection during the first year after transplantation. However, the use of these highly effective immunosuppressive treatments is associated with significant morbidity.

The study of cell-mediated rejection *in vivo* has used four types of experiments. First, there have been the studies of clinical transplants, which are obviously highly relevant, but which are always performed in the presence of immunosuppression and without the capacity to control and manipulate important variables. Second, there have been studies of skin grafts, heart graft fragments, artificial "sponge" allografts or islet transplants in rodents, which provide large amounts of controlled data on highly immunogenic grafts, but which may not accurately reflect the processes of rejection for primarily vascularized organs. Third, there have been studies of heart and other types of primarily vascularized organ transplants in rodents, but these types of transplants are more tolerogenic and hence more easily accepted than similar transplants in large animals and humans. Finally, there have been studies of primarily vascularized organ transplants in large animals, such as monkeys or pigs, which have obvious clinical relevance. Unfortunately, these studies are expensive, difficult to perform in large numbers, and are limited by the lack of monitoring and support at the same level that is possible in humans. The conclusions suggested by these different approaches have not always been the same, and thus, the description of the general mechanisms of T-cell–mediated rejection is complicated by the need to identify exceptions and features that occur only in special cases.

Acute GVHD is the counterpart of cellular rejection that involves graft-versus-host alloreactivity in the context of HCT and certain organ transplants in which significant amounts of donor lymphoid tissue are implanted (e.g., liver and small bowel transplantation). Like acute rejection, acute GVHD is T-cell–dependent, as illustrated by its effective prevention by T-cell–depletion of the graft, and by the ability of T-cell–suppressive or depleting agents to prevent and treat acute GVHD. T-cell depletion of the donor graft prevents GVHD, but it is associated with increased rates of graft rejection and relapse of malignant diseases.

Extensive study has suggested a major role for interactions between alloreactive CD4 helper cells producing cytokines of the "Th1" type and alloreactive cytotoxic $CD8^+$ effector cells in mediating rejection (reviewed in ref. *170*) and GVHD. Nevertheless, a number of additional pathways contribute to acute rejection and GVHD, involving both the innate and the adaptive immune systems (reviewed in ref. 171). There is extraordinary redundancy in the many different pathways that can cause rejection and GVHD, making it impossible to suppress rejection without strong immunosuppression or tolerance induction.

The concepts of "direct" and "indirect" allorecognition previously introduced must be considered at both the sensitization and effector phases of an immune response. As shown in Figure 44.9, there are three major T-cell pathways to consider in relation to graft rejection. These include: (i) direct recognition of donor alloantigens by $CD4^+$ T cells, which generate effector CD4 cells and provide help for the generation of effector CD8 cells; (ii) direct activation of CD8 T cells by donor APC; and (iii) $CD4^+$ T-cell activation by recipient APCs presenting reprocessed donor antigens (the indirect pathway of sensitization). This pathway is important in providing help for immunoglobulin (Ig) production by B cells. *Cross-priming* is a term specifically denoting sensitization of CD8 T cells through the indirect pathway. A role in rejection for cross-primed $CD8^+$ T cells is not included in Figure 44.9 because this pathway has not been shown to play a role in solid organ allograft rejection. However, such a pathway may play a role under certain circumstances, as described later. The multiplicity of T-cell sensitization and effector pathways involved in graft rejection and GVHD is demonstrated by the frequent failure of elimination of either $CD4^+$ or $CD8^+$ T cells from the recipient to prevent graft rejection or GVHD *(172–174)*. As a result of the high precursor frequency of T cells that respond to allogeneic MHC antigens directly, populations of T cells that ordinarily have minimal significance become functionally important.

Table 44.5 summarizes the pathways and specificities that have been identified *in vitro* for recognition by helper and cytotoxic CD4 and CD8 T cells. These *in vitro* studies provide a framework from which to understand the role of the various cell populations in allograft rejection.

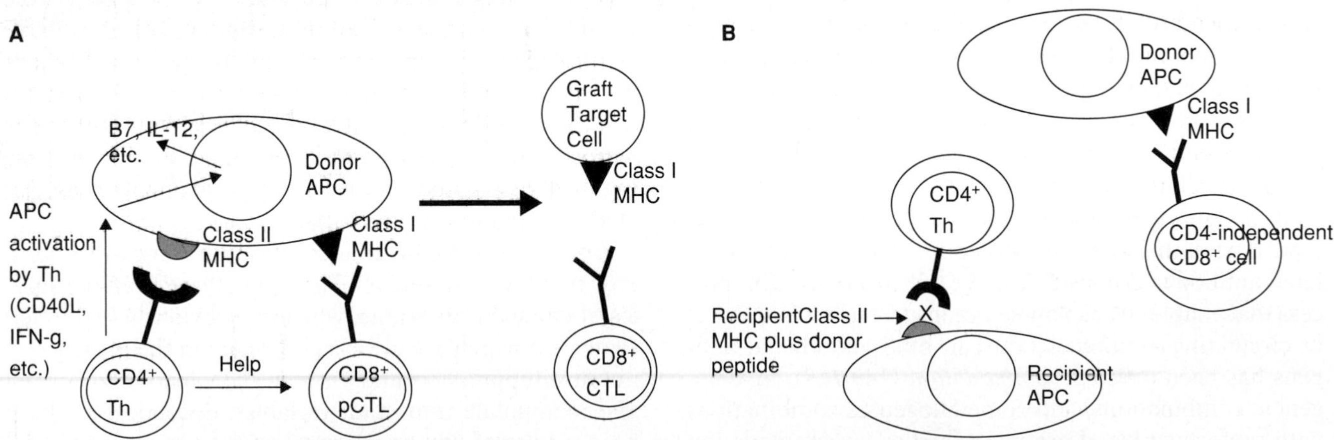

FIGURE 44.9 Model of T-cell–mediated rejection. **A:** Interactions between $CD4^+$ Th, donor antigen-presenting complex (APC), and $CD8^+$ cytotoxic T lymphocyte (CTL). **B:** Additional pathways of T-cell sensitization that can lead to rejection. MHC, major histocompatibility complex.

Sensitization and Cell Trafficking During Rejection and GVHD

Transplanted tissue contains passenger leukocytes of donor origin that have the characteristics of immature DCs *(175)*. In response to the inflammatory signals that are triggered by retrieval and transplantation, both within the tissue itself as well as in the recipient, the donor-derived passenger leukocytes rapidly leave the graft and migrate to the secondary lymphoid tissues of the recipient (176). Secondary lymphoid tissues comprise the spleen, lymph nodes, and gut or mucosal-associated lymphoid tissue and depending on the location of the graft, the passenger leukocytes will migrate to the tissue that drains the graft site where they encounter naïve T cells. After transplantation, *in situ* within the tissue and during migration, the passenger leukocytes acquire the phenotypic and functional characteristics of mature DCs, expressing high levels of MHC class I and II molecules as well as other cell-surface costimulatory molecules necessary to fully activate naïve $CD4^+$ and $CD8^+$ T cells *(177)*. Once in the secondary lymphoid tissues they act as professional APCs, presenting antigens expressed in the transplanted tissue to recipient T cells via the direct pathway of allorecognition.

Naïve T cells recirculate around the body and are constantly moving through the secondary lymphoid tissues sampling the APC, both host- and (after transplantation) donor-derived, for antigen (178). If a naïve T cell with a TCR that can recognize a donor MHC molecule encounters the donor-derived passenger leukocyte in the draining lymphoid tissue as it recirculates, it will stop, interact, and differentiate into an antigen-experienced, effector T cell. In support of the secondary lymphoid tissue being the primary site for sensitization of naïve T cells and initiation of rejection after solid organ transplantation, Lakkis and colleagues (179) showed that cardiac allografts were not rejected in splenectomized aly/aly mice that lack secondary lymphoid tissue as a result of a recessive mutation in the gene encoding Nf-kb–inducing kinase *(180)*, and suggested that in this situation permanent graft acceptance was not due to tolerance but rather immunologic ignorance. Other studies indicating that secondary lymphoid tissues draining the graft are the key site for initiation of the immune response have followed the fate of T cells of a known specificity for donor antigen as they respond *(181)*. It should be noted after transplantation of a primarily vascularized graft, it takes time for the lymphatic drainage to be reestablished; thus in the early posttransplant period, the spleen and the graft itself may be important (176). Similarly, after bone marrow transplantation, the initiation of GVHD takes place in the secondary lymphoid tissue, with evidence for the initial proliferation of donor $CD4^+$ T cells followed by $CD8^+$ T cells in secondary lymphoid organs with subsequent homing to the intestines, liver, and skin (*182*,183). Another study had suggested that Peyer's patches played a critical role in the initiation of GVHD (184). Visualizing the T cells as they respond during the initiation of GVHD showed that while Peyer's patches are involved, they are not the only secondary lymphoid tissue to contribute to the activation of T cells that can home to the gut; mesenteric lymph nodes and spleen are also sites where gut homing T cells were activated (183).

However, in solid-organ transplantation, exclusive initiation of rejection in the secondary lymphoid tissues conflicts with the earlier hypothesis that rejection was initiated within the graft itself by donor endothelial cells lining the vessels of vascularized organ and tissue grafts that could activate T cells directly as they passed through the graft (*185*,186). Since publication of these early articles, there have been a number of studies that support this hypothesis. For example, human endothelial cells have been shown to activate naïve T cells *in vitro (187)* and in the mouse, APCs that are not of hematopoietic origin have been shown to activate $CD8^+$ T cells *in vitro* and *in vivo (188)*, thus supporting the concept that T cells may be activated in the graft rather than in the secondary lymphoid tissue. Moreover, splenectomized lymphotoxin α and lymphotoxin β knockout mice that also lack secondary lymphoid tissues were found to reject cardiac allografts, albeit at a slower tempo (189). Each of these models is subtly different immunologically, and therefore different components of the immune response to an allograft may be differentially affected by the presence or absence of secondary lymphoid tissue. Clearly in the absence of secondary lymphoid tissue, the initiation of the rejection response by naïve T cells is less aggressive.

Although antigen presentation via the direct pathway plays a dominant role in initiating the response to a transplant, there are a finite number of donor-derived passenger leukocytes transferred within a transplanted organ. Thus, the role of the direct pathway in allograft rejection diminishes with time as eventually only "nonprofessional" APCs such as endothelial cells remain to stimulate direct pathway T cells. Endothelial cells within the graft may assume a greater significance with time after transplantation both for the initiation and as a target for direct pathway effector cells. Activation of naïve T cells may occur predominantly in the secondary lymphoid tissue after transplantation, activation of memory T cells in presensitized recipients is quite different. Unlike naïve T cells, memory T cells can migrate to nonlymphoid tissues in the periphery *(190)* and can trigger rejection through pathways that are independent of secondary lymphoid tissues (191). Thus, in humans where there are likely to be both naïve and memory T cells that can recognize or cross-react with donor MHC molecules, rejection may be initiated both within the secondary lymphoid tissue and within the allograft by naïve and memory T cells, respectively.

At the same time that donor-derived passenger leukocytes are leaving the graft, recipient leukocytes, including

APCs, are attracted to the graft by the inflammatory mediators and chemokines released in the vicinity of the transplanted tissue. As these cells traffic through the graft they phagocytose debris arising from tissue damage at the time of transplantation before migrating to the draining lymphoid tissue. The ingested antigens are processed and presented on recipient MHC molecules to T cells in the recipient lymphoid tissue *(192)*. In addition, soluble antigens released from the graft will also be transported in the blood to the draining lymphoid tissue, where they will be taken up and presented by resident APCs. Common antigenic peptides presented by the indirect pathway are the hypervariable peptide binding regions of MHC molecules (193). Indirect pathway responses undoubtedly contribute to acute rejection, although the tempo of rejection may be slower because of the lower frequency of T cells that can respond. However, unlike direct pathway allorecognition, the indirect pathway is available for antigen presentation for as long as the graft remains *in situ*, and therefore becomes the dominant mode of allorecognition long term.

Traffic of naïve lymphocytes is usually restricted to recirculation between the blood and lymphatic systems. However, once they have been primed in the secondary lymphoid tissues, activated lymphocytes as well as other activated leukocytes must be able to migrate into the graft in order to destroy the transplanted tissue, a process known as *leukocyte recruitment*.

The inflammatory processes at the site of transplantation generate chemotactic cytokines called chemokines, and up-regulation of chemokine receptor expression by activated leukocytes enables them to migrate along the chemoattractant gradient to reach the graft *(194)*.

Inflammatory signals also affect blood vessels in the vicinity of the transplant, causing vasodilation and endothelial activation. Activated endothelial cells rapidly externalize preformed granules called Weibel-Palade bodies that contain the adhesion molecule P-selectin *(195)* and rapidly up-regulate expression of VCAM and CD62E (E-selectin). At the same time, chemokines released from the graft become tethered to the endothelium, and these alterations in endothelial surface markers advertise to passing leukocytes that an inflammatory process is occurring in the neighboring tissue.

Leukocytes are usually conveyed within the fast laminar flow at the center of blood vessels, but once activated leukocytes reach postcapillary venules in proximity to the graft, they are able to leave this rapid flow and move toward the edge of the vessel. This occurs in response to the local chemokine gradient and is assisted by the slower blood flow in the vasodilated blood vessels near the graft. Leukocyte extravasation is a multistep process (see Chapters 13,26). Initially, low affinity interactions develop between endothelial P-selectin and sialyl-Lewis^X moieties that are present on the surface of activated leukocytes. These interactions continually form and break down and the leukocyte "rolls" along the endothelial surface. If chemokines are present on the endothelial surface, conformational changes in leukocyte integrin molecules occur that allow them to bind other endothelial adhesion molecules such as ICAM-1. These higher-affinity interactions cause arrest of the leukocyte on the endothelial surface, allowing it to commence extravasation. Having entered the tissues, the activated leukocytes continue to migrate along chemokine gradients in order to invade the graft.

Antigen Recognition and T-Cell Help in Graft Rejection and GVHD

Role of Direct CD4 Allorecognition

Figure 44.9A depicts a model whereby direct CD4 T-cell sensitization by donor class II MHC antigens may both generate CD4$^+$ effector cells and provide help for the activation, differentiation, and proliferation of cytotoxic CD8$^+$ cells. These recipient CD8$^+$ cells directly recognize donor class I MHC antigens. In the classical Th1 CD4/CD8 pathway of rejection, CD4 cells provide help for the differentiation of cytotoxic CD8 effector cells that destroy the graft. Priming of naïve, directly alloreactive T cells requires professional APC that leave the graft and enter the recipient's lymphoid tissues. The CD4 help for CD8 cells consists of both cytokine (e.g., IL-2) production and "conditioning" of the APC, for example, by production of interferon (IFN)-γ and by interactions of CD40 on the APC with CD40L on the activated CD4 cell. These interactions induce APC expression of CD80, CD86, and other costimulatory molecules, cytokines such as IL-12, and MHC, making it more effective at activating both CD4 and CD8 cells. Virus-specific CD8 cells primed to antigen in the absence of CD4 help are defective in the ability to clear viral infections and lack full effector function *(196)*, and "helpless" CD8 cells seem to die via a TRAIL-mediated pathway on secondary antigen encounter *(197)*. IL-2 during the priming phase can be critical for the ability of CD8 memory cells to expand on later encounter with the antigen *(198)*. A third pathway of CD4 help may involve direct interactions with CD40 induced on the surface of activated CD8 cells *(199)*.

Studies involving very limited (not clinically relevant) antigenic disparities between donors and recipients suggested that a "three-cell cluster" model involving interactions between helper T cells, effector T cells, and APCs was essential for rejection (200,*201–203*). For example, tail skin grafts from class I mutant mice (bm7) placed on B6 recipients are not rejected, apparently because of a lack of helper stimulation. On the other hand, grafts from (bm12 × bm7)F1 mice, which express an additional class II antigen disparity, are rejected. A bm12 graft on one side of a B6 mouse, although itself rejected, does not induce the rejection of a bm7 graft on the other side of the same animal, whereas a (bm12 × bm7)F1 graft on one side of a recipient does induce rejection of a bm7 graft on the other side. These results suggest that the CD4 help elicited during rejection of a bm12 graft cannot function elsewhere in the body to assist potential effector cells specific for the bm7 graft. On the other hand, when both the bm12 and bm7 antigens are expressed on the same graft, and therefore on the same APCs, effector cells are generated that can function elsewhere in the body. However, these observations may not be applicable to more clinically relevant histoincompatibilities, and other experimental evidence *(204,205)* suggests that CD4 helper cells sensitized by antigen presented on recipient APCs can provide help for CD8$^+$ effector cells recognizing antigen presented by donor APCs. One possible explanation for such results is that a three-cell cluster is still essential for CD4 cells to provide help to CD8 cells mediating rejection, and that, for example, donor class I MHC/peptide complexes might be transferred and picked up by recipient MHC so recipient directly alloreactive CD8 T cells encounter their ligands on the same recipient APC that an indirectly alloreactive CD4 cell recognizes. Transfer of class I/peptide antigens from dead cells, leading to such "cross-dressing" of APC, has recently been described (206).

Depletion of donor APCs can markedly prolong graft survival *(207–211)*, illustrating the importance of direct allorecognition in inducing rejection. Direct allorecognition by recipient CD4 T cells is necessary to induce cardiac allograft rejection in mice (212).

CD4$^+$ T cells alone can cause rejection of many types of grafts in the absence of CD8 cells, indicating that CD4 T cells can mediate effector functions in addition to functioning as helper cells. Directly alloreactive CD4 cells alone can reject grafts with full MHC disparities (212,*213*), class II antigen disparities alone, and multiple minor antigen disparities alone (*173*,214,*215*). In BMT recipients, they can induce GVHD in the absence of CD8 cells in the setting of class II, full MHC, or multiple minor histoincompatibilities (*216,217*,218,*219*). CD4$^+$ cells have been shown to reject class II and minor antigen-mismatched bone marrow grafts (220,*221*).

Role of Indirect CD4 Cell-Mediated Allorecognition

There is considerable evidence for a role for the indirect pathway of CD4 cell-mediated allorecognition in skin and solid-organ graft rejection (*222–226*,*227*,*228–229*). One major role of the indirect pathway is to induce class-switched alloantibody responses *(230)* through cognate interactions between recipient class II-restricted indirectly alloreactive CD4 cells and host B cells that recognize donor MHC molecules through their Ig receptors, process them, and present donor MHC peptides with their class II molecules. CD4 cells contribute to rejection of bone marrow grafts differing only at class I MHC loci, suggesting a role for indirect allorecognition (220,*221*).

Rejection by CD4 cells of skin grafts lacking class II antigen expression shows that the indirect pathway of rejection can be powerful *(204,222)*. Rejection of islet xenografts from highly disparate species in mice is very dependent on CD4$^+$ T cells, even though CD4$^+$ direct activation measured *in vitro* is very weak *(231)*, suggesting a dominant role for the indirect pathway in this setting. Clinically, sensitization of indirect CD4 responses to donor MHC-derived peptides has been demonstrated in patients undergoing graft rejection, and some studies have suggested that an increase in the precursor frequency of T cells responding through the indirect pathway provides the best correlation with clinical events *(232–239)*. A major role for indirect allorecognition has been suggested in the setting of chronic rejection (193,240,*241*), in part because this pathway is critical for the induction of antibody responses, which have been implicated in the pathogenesis of chronic rejection (*242,243*,244,245,*246–248*). Moreover, the eventual replacement of donor APC by recipient APC suggests that the latter may be responsible for fueling the immune response on a long-term basis. Experimental *(210,249)* and clinical *(238,246)* evidence has supported this hypothesis. Indeed, direct alloresponses tend to subside over time in patients with heart or kidney allografts (250,*251,252*).

In view of the apparent importance of the indirect pathway of allorecognition in graft rejection, it is not obvious why donor APC depletion or the lack of donor class II MHC expression should be effective in preventing rejection in some situations (*207–211*,212). An essential role for indirect allorecognition has been difficult to demonstrate in acute rejection, and this pathway alone may simply be too weak to induce it. CD4$^+$ cells alone are incapable of rejecting some skin grafts with minimal class I or minor histoincompatibilities (200,*253,254*) or of inducing GVHD when class I and minor histocompatibility barriers alone are present *(216,217)*. In the case of renal and cardiac allografts, donor APC depletion may allow the inherent tolerogenicity of the parenchymal tissue to prevail and spread to the indirect pathway. Initial sensitization through the direct pathway may be essential in producing the inflammatory conditions necessary to promote indirect pathway sensitization, so that the latter does not occur or is tolerogenic in the absence of the former. An alternative explanation might be that donor APCs are essential for the sensitization of the effector cells responsible for graft rejection, while indirect presentation is important for the sensitization of helper cells. In the absence of donor APCs, potential effector cells might become anergic as a result of encountering donor antigens directly only on parenchymal cells of a graft.

Role of Helper-Independent CD8$^+$ T Cells

CD8 T cells can readily reject allografts in the absence of CD4 cells, suggesting that CD4 help is not critical in the presence of the high frequency of alloreactive CD8 cells existing in the naïve repertoire. Indeed, CD8$^+$ T cells alone can reject skin and bone marrow grafts with isolated MHC class I antigen disparity (*172*,200,220,*221*,*255*,*256*) and alloreactive CD8 T-cell memory can be generated and maintained in the absence of CD4 cells (*181*).

CD8 cells can induce GVHD without CD4 T cells in the setting of full MHC, class I only, and minor antigen histoincompatibility (*257,258*). Direct recognition of recipient minor histocompatibility antigens on recipient APCs has shown to be essential for the induction of CD8-dependent, CD4-independent GVHD in an MHC-identical, lethally irradiated mouse model (*259*), but indirect CD8 recognition of recipient antigens presented by donor APC amplifies the process (*260*).

Grafts expressing only class I antigen disparities are usually rejected more slowly than class II disparate grafts, and responses dependent on CD8$^+$ helper responses are more easily suppressed by cyclosporine (*261–263*). Many primarily vascularized grafts that express only a class I antigen disparity still require CD4$^+$ cells to initiate rejection, probably because of the defects in function, survival, and secondary expansion described previously for "helpless" CD8 cells. Probably as a result of these limitations, CD4-independent rejection by CD8$^+$ cells is influenced by several factors that do not seem to be as important for CD4$^+$ T cells. First, CD8$^+$ direct activation is very dependent on the number of donor APCs in a graft (*172,222*). Second, CD8$^+$ direct activation fails to initiate rejection of grafts with only a small number of minor antigen disparities and provides only a weak helper response even when there are a large number of foreign minor antigens. CD8$^+$ helper cells also differ from CD4$^+$ helper cells in being unable to provide help for other cell populations (264). Apparently the IL-2 produced by these cells is used by the cells themselves as they develop effector function. CD8$^+$ helper cells cannot provide help for CD8$^+$ cells with a different specificity and cannot provide help for B-cell antibody responses.

Although Table 44.5 includes CD8$^+$ CTL with specificity for class II antigens because these have been detected *in vitro*, CD8$^+$ cells alone cannot reject skin grafts with only limited class II antigen disparities (200,218,*253*,*265*).

Cross-Primed CD8 Cells

Peptides of exogenous antigens were originally thought to be presented by MHC class II antigens while those of endogenous antigens are presented by MHC class I molecules (*266,267*). However, it has more recently become clear that class I presentation of exogenous peptides is essential for many immune responses (*169,268–270*), and several pathways have now been delineated for the processing and presentation of exogenous antigens by class I molecules (271). The phenomenon, termed *cross-priming*, was originally demonstrated in a transplantation model by Bevan (*66*), who showed that when minor antigen-disparate grafts with MHC antigens of type A were placed on MHC (AxB) F1 recipients, the CD8$^+$ cells of these recipients became sensitized to the minor antigens presented by both A and B types of class I MHC molecules. Activation of cross-primed CD8 cells has been shown to be strongly dependent on CD4 help and IL-2 (*272*). Cross-primed CD8 cells seem most likely to play a significant role in rejection because of donor minor histocompatibility antigens and MHC-derived peptides when there is sharing of class I alleles between the donor and recipient. In the absence of class I MHC sharing between donor and recipient (273), the self-class I/allogeneic peptide epitope cannot be presented by the parenchymal or endothelial cells of the graft. However, even without class I sharing, indirect CD8$^+$ cell sensitization can lead to the rejection of skin allografts, perhaps because of recognition of donor peptides presented by recipient endothelial cells on host-derived vessels that revascularize the graft (274,*275*). Cross-primed CD8 cells might also contribute to graft rejection via indirect effector mechanisms on antigen recognition on host APC in the graft or by producing cytokines that contribute to the overall regulation of the immune response (*275,276*). Thus, the question of how CD8$^+$ indirect sensitization might affect graft rejection remains one of the open issues in transplantation immunology.

Effector Mechanisms of Acute Rejection and GVHD

Although CD4$^+$ and CD8$^+$ cytotoxic T cells are important effectors of graft rejection and GVHD and can account for the precise selectivity of graft destruction that is sometimes observed, the role of additional tissue-destructive mechanisms, and particularly of "indirect" effector mechanisms initiated by T cells specific for modified self-MHC antigens, is being increasingly appreciated. Some of these mechanisms involve effector cells of the innate immune system and cytokines as final mediators of tissue destruction. The net result of this multiplicity of pathways is that there is considerable redundancy between the mechanisms of graft rejection. A brief review of the available data on these issues ensues.

Cytotoxic Mechanisms of Acute Cellular Graft Rejection and GVHD

Solid-organ graft rejection can be correlated with the presence in the graft of proteins and mRNA encoding perforin, granzymes, and proteases associated with cell-mediated cytotoxicity (*277–284*). The presence in urine of cell-derived RNA encoding perforin and granzyme B has been associated with renal allograft rejection in humans (285). A functional analysis of the role of various cytotoxic pathways in graft rejection and GVHD has been facilitated by the use of mice deficient in one or more effector proteins involved in CTL activity, particularly perforin, granzyme, and Fas/Fas ligand (*286,287*). Although the perforin/granzyme pathway is the major cytolytic pathway for CD8 T cells and CD4 cells tend to use the Fas/FasL pathway (288), both subsets are capable of both types of cytolytic activity (*289*,290), and the perforin pathway is available to both T-cell subsets mediating GVHD *(286)*. All of these cytotoxic proteins play contributory roles and no single protein has been found to be critical for the induction of solid-organ graft rejection *(287,291–293)*, GVHD *(294–297)*, or bone marrow graft rejection *(298)* in the presence of clinically relevant mismatches. Critical cytotoxic interactions have been identified in a few special situations. For example, GVHD directed at isolated class II MHC disparities is markedly reduced in the absence of Fas/FasL interactions *(297)*, and the survival of K^b mutant class I-only mismatched heart allografts is markedly prolonged in perforin-deficient recipients *(287)*. Fas ligand may be critical role for induction of lymphoid hypoplasia (299) and skin and liver GVHD (299). Although the perforin-granzyme pathway contributes to GVHD (297,299), the Fas-mediated cytotoxic pathway appears to be of greater overall importance in causing GVHD. In contrast, the perforin/granzyme pathway and TRAIL pathways may play a predominant role in antileukemic effects, especially of CD8 cells, and selective blockade of the Fas/FasL pathway may ameliorate CD8-mediated GVHD without eliminating GVL effects *(296,300–303)*.

Evidence for a Role for Non-CTL Mechanisms in Graft Rejection and GVHD

Strong evidence supports the ability of T cells to effect rejection of grafts whose parenchymal cells do not express the ligand of the TCR, that is, the existence of indirect effector mechanisms. When syngeneic skin from bone marrow chimeras in which the APCs of the skin had been replaced by cells derived from an allogeneic donor bone marrow was transplanted, the entire graft was rejected (304). Thus, entire skin grafts can be rejected when only the APCs are foreign, indicating that nonselective destruction of grafted tissue can occur, especially if the inflammatory response is sufficiently vigorous. Several studies have clearly shown a role for indirect CD4 cell-mediated rejection of skin *(305,306)* and cardiac (307) allografts lacking the determinant recognized by the CD4 T-cell population. In the case of cardiac allografts, replacement of graft endothelium by the host was shown to be a key element in the induction of acute and chronic rejection through this indirect effector mechanism (307). Moreover, GVHD, mediated in part by cytokines but associated with significant liver and intestinal injury, can be induced by donor T cells in MHC-deficient hosts receiving wild type host DCs, suggesting that indirect effector mechanisms may mediate GVHD *(308,309)*. However, the capacity of CD4 T cells to mediate GVHD across minor histocompatibility barriers is markedly attenuated when the target antigens are expressed only on hematopoietic cells (310). Together, these results suggest that indirect effector mechanisms can destroy transplanted tissue (or recipient tissue, in the case of HCT) under some circumstances, but less efficiently than direct mechanisms.

The lack of correlation between rejection and the ability to detect CTL *in vitro* in some situations also suggests the existence of noncytotoxic rejection mechanisms. CD4 effector cells can reject class I-only disparate grafts in recipients depleted of CD8 T cells (200,218,*253,265,311,312*,313), even though *in vitro* assays have generally failed to reveal cytotoxic CD4 cells specific for class I alloantigens. Some studies suggest that mice depleted of CD8 T cells by antibody treatment still have a population of cytotoxic precursors (apparently of the CD8 lineage despite the absence of the CD8 antigen) *(314,315)*, and others suggest that there is an effector mechanism mediated by CD4 cells specific for class I peptides presented by class II molecules *(316)*. These results do not distinguish a direct from an indirect effector mechanism because the donor and recipient class II molecules were identical in these experiments, but they do suggest that noncytotoxic cells may be effectors of rejection, as $CD4^+$ cytotoxic T cells were not detectable.

Because CTL activity to minor histocompatibility antigens can only be measured *in vitro* after *in vivo* priming, minor disparate graft rejection provides an opportunity to test whether every case of rejection is associated with the development of CTL activity. Skin grafts that differ by only the H-Y antigens are rejected by some, but not other strains of mice, and rejection does not correlate with the generation of *in vitro* cytotoxicity. In some cases, CTLs are detectable *in vitro* despite the absence of graft rejection, and vice versa *(317–319)*, again suggesting the existence of noncytotoxic mechanisms.

Graft-Infiltrating Cells

Many types of cells infiltrate rejecting grafts, including CD4 and CD8 T cells, NK cells, and macrophages (313,*320,321*,322,323.*324–327*). There are, however, relatively few B cells *(328)*. Repertoire analysis of alloresponses revealed marked polyclonality (*21*,329), and propagation of graft-infiltrating cells reveals polyclonal cytotoxic and IL-2–producing lymphocytes of both CD4 and CD8 lineages *(330,331)*. Many T cells seem to be recruited nonspecifically into rejecting grafts, as only a fraction of them recognize donor antigens, but only the donor-reactive CTL show evidence of having been activated *in vivo*, as indicated by their ability to respond to donor antigens without further antigen-specific stimulation *(332)*. Early reports suggesting that an oligoclonal T-cell response occurs during allograft rejection *(333)* might have been subject to *in vitro* culturing artefacts and sampling error *(328)*. A polyclonal TCR repertoire was detected in rejecting rodent heart allografts, whereas evidence of oligoclonal dominance was detected in heart grafts of animals that were rendered tolerant to their grafts *(334)*. However, graft-infiltrating

T cells of long-term rejected human kidneys *(335)* and of acutely rejecting rat heart allografts *(336)* have been reported to show skewed CDR3 length distributions within some Vβ families, suggesting some degree of oligoclonal dominance. T cells infiltrating xenografts did not show such skewing, suggesting an even broader use of the TCR repertoire in xenograft rejection *(336–338)*. Analyses of T cells mediating GVHD in the setting of multiple minor histoincompatibilities have revealed a markedly skewed repertoire, but still with the involvement of several different Vβ families, each exhibiting an oligoclonal response *(339,340)*. Clinical studies suggest that the antiminor histocompatibility antigen TCR repertoire is most often polyclonal (341).

The number of invading T cells in a graft is not necessarily correlated with the speed of rejection. Whole MHC and class II disparate grafts generally elicit dense cellular infiltrates, while class I-disparate grafts are generally sparsely infiltrated, and only to a similar extent as syngeneic grafts *(328)*. The number of cells within minor antigen disparate grafts is generally far greater than the number invading grafts with class I-only differences, even when the rejection of the class I grafts is faster *(328)*.This finding has suggested that certain critical elements of the graft, such as its blood vessels, are the actual site of graft destruction and, indeed, endothelialitis is an important hallmark of clinically significant rejection activity (342).

Role of Natural Killer Cells

Although the role of NK cells in mediating hybrid resistance and allogeneic marrow rejection is well established in mice, the amount of resistance mediated by NK cells to allogeneic pluripotent hematopoietic stem cells (PHSC) is limited, and can be readily overcome by increasing the dose of donor stem cells administered *(343,344)*. Furthermore, a role for NK cells in resisting human allogeneic marrow engraftment has not been clearly demonstrated. However, their role may become more significant if mismatched transplants are attempted with less toxic, nonmyeloablative regimens instead of more traditional myeloablative conditioning. Consistent with this possibility, patients with severe combined (T and B cell) immunodeficiency (SCID) who have functional NK cells require cytotoxic conditioning to permit engraftment of haploidentical marrow. In contrast, those lacking NK cells have a low incidence of rejection in the absence of any such treatment *(345)*.

A strategy for exploiting the ability of NK cells to be triggered by "missing self" has recently been reported in patients receiving HLA-mismatched related donor HCT and in mice (346). Donor-derived NK cells with graft-versus-host reactivity due to the lack of donor class I MHC inhibitory ligands in the recipient can apparently kill residual host leukemia cells and alloreactive cells that resist the marrow graft without causing GVHD. The alloreactive donor NK cells may actually reduce susceptibility to GVHD by killing recipient APCs needed to activate donor T cells (346). Although striking antileukemia effects of such killer cell immunoglobulin-like receptor (KIR) mismatching were detected in heavily conditioned patients receiving high doses of haploidentical CD34 stem cells (346), the effect of KIR incompatibility has been more variable in other clinical studies *(347–349)*.

The possible role of NK cells in rejecting solid-organ grafts is somewhat controversial. NK cells are prominent among cells infiltrating rejecting organ allografts, and may be the earliest producers of inflammatory cytokines and chemokines and inducers of DC maturation (*350,351*,352,*353*). If NK cells make an important contribution to solid-organ allograft rejection under normal circumstances they must be dependent on T cells, as mice lacking T cells are unable to reject nonhematopoietic allografts. Furthermore, whereas bone marrow allografts from class I-deficient donors ($\beta 2m^{-/-}$) are subject to potent NK-mediated rejection (because these cells cannot trigger inhibitory receptors on host NK cells *[354]*), $\beta 2m^{-/-}$ skin grafts are not rejected by $\beta 2m^{+}$ recipients *(355)*. However, NK cells have recently been reported to play a critical role in cardiac allograft rejection in CD28 knockout mice *(356,357)*. Interactions between NK cells and T cells have also been implicated in chronic allograft vasculopathy in a murine cardiac allograft model (352).

Inhibitory receptors on NK cells are quite broad in their class I specificity (358), and recognition of even fully allogeneic class I molecules can confer some protection from NK-mediated marrow destruction compared with that observed for cells deficient in class I expression (*354–357*,358,*359*). Because of the increased disparity of xenogeneic compared with allogeneic MHC molecules, NK cells may receive fewer inhibitory signals from xenogeneic than allogeneic cells. Indeed, transduction of human HLA molecules into porcine endothelial cells has proven to be an effective means of reducing NK cell-mediated xenogeneic cell adhesion and cytotoxicity (*360*,361,362). However, some inhibitory receptors, such as killer cell lectin-like receptor G1 (KLRG1), do recognize xenogeneic ligands such as E-cadherin *(363)*. In addition to failing to receive inhibitory signals from xenogeneic MHC molecules, NK cells may also be activated by interactions of activating receptors with ligands on xenogeneic cells *(364–366)*. Examples include the effective activation achieved by interactions of human NKG2D and NKp44 with their ligands on porcine endothelial cells *(366)*. There is some evidence that activating human NK cell receptors may bind to carbohydrate epitopes expressed by pigs and not humans *(367)*.

On balance, many xenogeneic NK cell-target interactions appear to show a predominance of functional activating interactions over inhibitory ones, resulting in high levels of reactivity. Indeed, NK cells resist xenogeneic marrow engraftment to a greater extent than allogeneic marrow (*343,368,369*,370). NK cells have also been implicated in the acute vascular rejection (371) that can destroy solid-organ xenografts that have escaped hyperacute rejection (see later discussion) and in xenogeneic skin graft rejection (372). Because one mechanism by which NK cells mediate cytolysis is antibody-dependent cell-mediated cytotoxicity, it is possible that IgG natural antibodies play a significant role in initiating NK cell-mediated rejection. NK cells also release cytokines, such as IFN-γ and tumor necrosis factor-α (TNF-α), which activate macrophages and endothelial cells and induce inflammation (371).

Role of NKT Cells

A subset of murine and human T cells expresses NK cell-associated phenotypic surface markers. Many of these recognize glycolipid antigens presented by CD-1 nonclassical class I molecules, and major subsets express an "invariant" TCR α chain and restricted β chains *(373)*. They produce a variety of cytokines, the most prominent of which are IFN-γ and IL-4 *(374)*, have cytolytic activity, and may provide an important link between innate and adaptive immunity *(375,376)*. Most NKT cells are either $CD4^+CD8^-$ or $CD4^-CD8^-$. Although these cells have apparent inhibitory effects on graft rejection (377,*378–380*), GVHD (381,*382*), and other immune responses, NKT cells also promote antimicrobial and antitumor immunity and have been reported to participate in islet allograft *(383)* and isograft (384) rejection in mice.

Role of Monocytes/Macrophages and Eosinophils as Effectors of Rejection

Classical delayed-type hypersensitivity responses are thought to depend on the activation of macrophages by helper T cells through production of IFN-γ. It is likely that proinflammatory cytokines and chemokines produced by activated monocytes and macrophages play a role in endothelial cell activation and lymphocyte recruitment. Additionally, activated macrophages may damage tissue through the production of toxic molecules such as nitric oxide (385).

Macrophages play an especially important role in the rejection of cellular xenografts such as islets *(386,387)*, whose rejection they can effect after activation in the presence of T cells *(388)*. Macrophages cause almost immediate rejection of xenogeneic bone marrow, even in the absence of adaptive immunity *(389–391)*. Human macrophages can phagocytose porcine cells in an antibody- and complement-independent manner (392). Additional studies have implicated macrophages in solid-organ and skin xenograft rejection *(393–398)*. These powerful effects of xenogeneic macrophages may be accounted for by the combined ability of certain xenogeneic receptors to activate macrophages *(399)* while important inhibitory interactions, such as that between CD47 and its macrophage ligand SIRPα, are not effective (400).

Eosinophils recruited to allografts by Th2 T-cell responses have been reported to be effectors of graft rejection in some experimental models, and eosinophils are often found clinically in rejecting allografts (reviewed in ref. 171). Th2-derived IL-4 and IL-5 recruit and activate eosinophils, which release highly cytotoxic substances from granules into the tissue. Th2-mediated rejection is apparently down-modulated by alloreactive CD8 CTL, which kill donor DCs in the T-cell areas of lymph nodes, thereby limiting direct alloantigen presentation to CD4 cells *(401)*. These results emphasize the fact that Th2 responses are not necessarily benign and conducive to graft acceptance.

Cytokines as Mediators of Graft Rejection and GVHD

Cytokines have complex roles as both regulators and effectors of immune reactivity, and studies of their role in transplantation have consequently yielded many paradoxical findings. Many studies have correlated the onset of graft rejection with the presence of cytokines or mRNA encoding them in the graft and, with renal transplantation, in the urine (285). Although the "classical" rejection pathway involves the Th1 cytokines IFN-γ and IL-2 and cytotoxic T cells, a great redundancy of rejection pathways is suggested by studies detecting both Th1 (IL-2, IFN-γ) and Th2 (IL-4, IL-5, IL-10) cytokines in rejecting allografts *(283,402–409)*. Although the concept that Th2 cytokines are anti-inflammatory and may suppress rejection and GVHD has attracted considerable interest *(410–413*,414–417,*418)*, Th2 responses have been clearly shown to contribute to both graft rejection *(410,419–421)* and GVHD *(422–425)*. With a few special exceptions *(426–428)*, studies using various cytokine knockout mice as recipients have failed to reveal any single molecule that is essential for rejection (*429–434*,435) or GVHD (*422*,436,*437*). In a model involving adoptive transfer of T cells to immunodeficient mice, allogeneic heart allografts required IFN-γ receptor expression in order to be rejected by $CD4^+$ cells, and additional data suggested that IFN-γ may itself be a critical effector molecule of graft destruction in this system (438).

In GVHD, cytokines such as TNF-α and IFN-γ play a role in the inflammatory cascade involving macrophage activation by lipopolysaccharide from the damaged gut epithelium and by IFN-γ to release TNF-α, nitric oxide, and other mediators of tissue injury (385,*439–442*). In certain models, TNF-α had been shown to play a critical role in wasting disease and intestinal GVHD *(443,444)*. Although the relative contribution of cytokine-dependent mechanisms versus direct cell-mediated cytotoxicity to GVHD is still a matter of debate, the capacity to induce GVHD with T cells lacking both the perforin-mediated and the Fas-mediated pathways of cytotoxicity, even in mice also lacking TNF receptor1 (TNFR1)-mediated signaling pathways *(297,445,446)*, demonstrates the redundancy of GVHD effector mechanisms.

The generation of a newly discovered class of cytokine-producing CD4 T cell, the "Th-17" cell, is antagonized by Th-1 cells and promoted by IL-23, transforming growth factor (TGF)-β, and IL-6. Th-17 cells produce IL-17, a proinflammatory cytokine that has been implicated in various models of immune injury, including allergic, autoimmune, and infectious diseases (447). A role for Th-17 has been suggested in animal models of heart and aortic allograft rejection and in clinical lung transplantation (447). A more complete understanding of the role of Th-17 in transplantation is likely to emerge in the near future.

Chronic Rejection and Chronic GVHD

Most experimental studies of rejection are performed without immunosuppression and, therefore, graft destruction usually occurs within the first several days or weeks by one of the mechanisms previously described. In clinical practice, however, the use of immunosuppression usually allows graft survival for much longer periods of time. Nonetheless, clinical survival statistics reveal that even when 1-year graft survival has been achieved, the loss of transplanted organs continues to occur at a rate of about 3% to 5% per year and a significant proportion of this delayed or late graft failure appears to be due to immunologic mechanisms.

The term *chronic rejection* has been used to describe this later process of delayed graft destruction. As immunosuppressive reagents have become more effective at controlling acute rejection, chronic rejection has emerged as one of the most important problems in clinical practice. There has been ongoing improvement during the past 30 years in the 1-year graft survival rates for kidney transplants, but the half-life for organs that have survived for 1 year has not changed significantly during that entire period of time and, as a result of this ongoing loss, only about 50% of transplants are still functioning 10 years later.

Although almost every type of organ transplant suffers from chronic rejection, the pathologic manifestations are different in each case. Kidney biopsies tend to show interstitial fibrosis along with arterial narrowing from hyalinization of the vessels. In the heart, the process is manifested principally as a diffuse myointimal hyperplasia proceeding to fibrosis of the coronary arteries that has often been referred to as *accelerated atherosclerosis* or *transplant arteriosclerosis*. Chronic rejection in lung transplants primarily affects the bronchioles with progressive narrowing of these structures, and is referred to as *bronchiolitis obliterans*. The liver may be the one type of organ transplant that is relatively resistant to chronic rejection, but the progressive destruction of bile ducts referred to as the *vanishing bile duct syndrome* may be another manifestation of this process.

Some of the causes of chronic graft destruction may not be immunologic in origin *(448,449)*. Analysis of sequential kidney transplant biopsies suggests that chronic rejection represents cumulative and incremental damage to the graft from time-dependent nonimmunologic and immunologic causes (450). Potential nonimmunologic factors that have been considered to contribute to the development of chronic rejection include the initial ischemic insult, the reduced mass of transplanted tissue (especially in the case of kidney transplants leading to hyperfiltration injury), the denervation of the transplanted organ, the hyperlipidemia and hypertension associated with immunosuppressive drugs, the immunosuppressive drugs themselves, and chronic viral injury, among others. Nonetheless, although these factors undoubtedly contribute to the process, there is a marked difference in survival between syngeneic and allogeneic transplants in experimental models. Thus, there is almost certainly an important immunologic component in most cases of chronic rejection.

Several important observations regarding the pathogenesis of chronic rejection have emerged from clinical practice, particularly the analysis of biopsy samples. In kidney transplants, two distinctive phases of injury as chronic allograft nephropathy evolved have been described (450). Previous studies have suggested that there is a high correlation between the onset of chronic rejection and a history of early acute and subclinical rejection episodes *(451,452)*. Analysis of protocol biopsies has revealed that the onset of mild chronic rejection by 1 year after kidney transplantation is associated with an initial phase of early tubulointerstitial damage from ischemic injury that occurs before severe rejection is detected. Beyond 1 year, a later phase of chronic allograft nephropathy was characterized by microvascular and glomerular injury (450). Importantly for long-term outcomes, the clinical data show that the process of chronic rejection is usually refractory to increases in immunosuppressive therapy, in contrast to acute rejection episodes that almost always respond to treatment. The development of chronic rejection has also frequently been associated with the presence of antidonor antibodies *(453,454)* and the deposition of complement component C4d in the allograft.

Taken together, these clinical observations have suggested to some that chronic rejection is the result of chronic B-cell alloantibody production, while others believe that chronic rejection requires the early sensitization of the immune system to donor antigens. Moreover, there are also now data emerging to suggest that components of the innate immune system such as NK cells can also contribute *(455)*. Alloantibody production might equally well be a marker for other rejection mechanisms as opposed to a cause of chronic rejection. Moreover, the presence of alloantibody and C4d may be transient and there are clear examples of chronic changes in the graft in their absence *(456)*. In addition, early rejection episodes probably reflect primarily the degree of antidonor immunoreactivity, and may not be required for chronic rejection themselves. Therefore, even if sufficient immunosuppression were given to prevent acute rejection, chronic rejection might still occur when the suppression was reduced to levels tolerable to the recipient over the long term, even if acute rejection had never occurred. Finally, experimental studies have suggested that the mechanisms of chronic rejection are not absolutely dependent on either antibody formation or on the occurrence of acute rejection episodes.

The uncertainties that arise from the interpretation of the clinical data make it important to develop experimental models for studying the mechanisms of chronic rejection. It is difficult in the laboratory, however, to mimic a process that may take 5 or 10 years to develop in patients treated with immunosuppressive drugs. Thus, the effort to study chronic rejection experimentally has depended on surrogate short-term pathologic markers that are thought to predict the long-term changes of chronic rejection. In particular, these studies have concentrated on the development of the myointimal proliferation that is thought to be the precursor of the chronic vascular changes typically observed in patients. In rodents, pigs, and primates this has often been done with grafts after an initial period of immunosuppression that prevents acute rejection *(457–459)*. All of these experimental studies are subject to the caveat that the surrogate pathologic lesion occurs much earlier than the typical changes of chronic rejection in patients. Thus, the process being studied experimentally may not be the same as the clinical process.

Pathologic Manifestations of Experimental Chronic Rejection

The typical pathologic features of the experimental lesion associated with chronic rejection are shown in Figure 44.10 *(460)*. The marked narrowing of the vascular lumen is caused by the substantial proliferation of endothelial and then smooth muscle cells that can be host-derived *(461)*. Associated with this proliferation is progressive destruction of the media. In time, the cellular proliferation becomes less pronounced and is replaced by concentric fibrosis that narrows the vascular lumen. Immunohistologic staining indicates that there is increased expression of several adhesion molecules *(460)*, intracellular proteins such as vimentin *(462,463)*, and easily detectable levels of several molecules, including nitric oxide synthase *(464)*, acidic fibroblast growth factor, insulinlike growth factor, IFN-γ *(465)*, and endothelin, each *(466)* of which may play a role. Ultimately, the ischemia resulting from vascular occlusion results in fibrosis in the parenchyma of the organ, and consequent organ dysfunction (467). In the case of the lung or the liver, chronic injury may cause changes most prominently in the bronchioles or the bile ducts, but this is also associated with arterial lumen loss, which may be the primary lesion causing bronchiolitis obliterans or bile duct fibrosis, respectively (467).

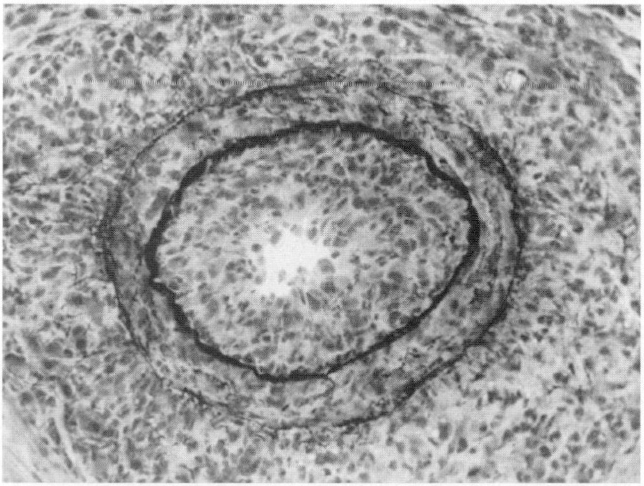

FIGURE 44.10 Histology of chronic rejection.

Immunologic Mechanisms of Chronic Rejection

Rejection requires a dialogue between the innate and adaptive immune system. Innate immunity is most likely involved at the outset of the process that leads to the development of chronic rejection and there is evidence to suggest that NK cells *(455,468)* and complement activation can be involved (469). At the level of the adaptive response, because it is assumed that stimulation of direct pathway T cells is likely to diminish over time as donor APCs are replaced by recipient APC (see previous discussion), it is commonly assumed that the predominant immune response that causes chronic rejection occurs through the indirect pathway.

Studies in pigs have suggested that the vascular changes of chronic rejection are more apt to develop when there are class I antigenic disparities than when there are only class II disparities and have suggested that the development of the lesion depend especially on CD8 T cells. In mouse models, in contrast, there is evidence that either CD4 or CD8 T cells can produce the lesion and that either class I or class II antigenic disparities are sufficient to stimulate chronic rejection *(470)*. The finding that class II antigenic disparities are themselves sufficient to induce this pathology is consistent with the observation of class II MHC expression on the vascular endothelium and medial smooth muscle cells of mouse cardiac allografts with these vascular lesions *(471)*. Because class II MHC is not constitutively expressed by mouse vascular endothelial cells, indirect recognition of donor class II transferred from passenger leukocytes may be responsible for inducing an inflammatory response that leads to subsequent up-regulation of class II on the donor vascular endothelium. In keeping with the prediction of many clinical studies, adoptive transfer experiments into SCID mice have shown that alloantibodies in the absence of T cells can induce the typical pathologic vascular changes, and lesions can develop in T-cell–deficient mice (245). However, T cells without B cells have also been shown to cause the lesion, although there may be somewhat less tendency to progress to end-stage fibrosis (244).

Several studies have indicated that the induction of donor-specific tolerance can prevent the development of the vascular changes of chronic rejection, although not all of the short-term manipulations that have been effective in preventing acute rejection have necessarily prevented the later onset of chronic rejection. Remarkably, mice rendered tolerant by neonatal injection of donor splenocytes, or by the induction of high levels of lasting, multilineage mixed chimerism with demonstrated central deletion of donor-reactive T cells and permanent acceptance of donor-specific skin grafts, demonstrate graft vasculopathy in donor cardiac allografts *(468)*. Thus, in the complete absence of antidonor T-cell reactivity, other cell types such as NK cells may induce these types of lesions in cardiac allografts. In addition, T-cell recognition of cardiac-specific antigens presented by donor MHC and not shared by donor hematopoietic cells could play a possible role in the development of these lesions in immunocompetent, tolerant mice *(455)*.

From these data, it seems likely that multiple immunologic mechanisms may be capable of creating the graft arteriosclerotic lesions that are characteristic of chronic rejection, and that T-cell alloreactivity is not essential for their induction. Whether there is a critical final common mediator involved in all of these pathways is not currently known. However, IFN-γ has been shown to play an important role in the development of lesions in several models *(465,472)*, and STAT4-deficient mice, which do not respond to IL-12 and therefore cannot generate Th1 responses, show markedly reduced severity of graft vasculopathy compared with wild type mice *(473)*. TGF-β has been shown to attenuate the lesions, but has also been detected within the lesions and implicated in the development of fibrosis *(474)*.

Chronic Graft-versus-Host Disease

Chronic graft-versus-host disease (cGVHD) is the most common and severe complication among patients surviving for more than 100 days after allogeneic bone marrow transplantation. Clinically, acute and cGVHD can be distinguished on the basis of the time of onset, clinical manifestations, and distinct pathobiologic mechanisms. Acute GVHD usually occurs within 2 to 6 weeks following allogeneic BMT and primarily affects the skin, liver, and the gastrointestinal tract with T-cell infiltration of the epithelia of the skin, mucous membranes, bile ducts, and gut. However, acute GVHD has been noted to occur later in recent protocols involving nonmyeloablative conditioning for HCT. In contrast, cGVHD involves a wider range of organs and clinical manifestations include scleroderma, liver failure, immune complex disease, glomerulonephritis, and autoantibody formation.

The pathogenesis of cGVHD, like chronic rejection, is poorly understood. The disease involves T-cell responses to alloantigens or autoantigens. Because most BMT is performed between HLA-identical or closely HLA-matched pairs, alloreactivity may be directed against minor histocompatibility antigens (miHA) presented by shared MHC molecules, or against MHC alloantigens when present. T cells developing *de novo* in a recipient thymus that is damaged by GVHD may result in the emergence of autoreactive T cells into the peripheral repertoire (475). The injury to target organs is poorly understood, but may involve TGF-β, which promotes fibrosis and other cytokines, as well as B-cell activation and production of autoantibodies.

The main risk factors for the onset of cGVHD are donor and patient age and sex, source of progenitor cells, graft composition, and previous acute GVHD. cGVHD can be treated, but infections resulting from immunosuppression due to the disease itself and its treatment are a major source of morbidity. Extensive skin involvement, thrombocytopenia, and progression are poor prognostic factors.

PHYSIOLOGIC INTERACTIONS THAT MODULATE GRAFT REJECTION AND GVHD

All immune responses are modulated by down-regulatory components that help to limit or terminate the response. Although graft rejection and GVHD often involve exceptionally strong immune responses, these responses are still accompanied by down-regulatory components that can be manipulated to promote graft survival. Many of these manipulations are described in the section on tolerance, but some of the regulatory components of the rejection response are briefly described here.

Down-modulating Signals Following T-Cell Activation

Interactions between Fas and Fas Ligand (FasL), which is up-regulated during rejection responses, may help to mitigate GVHD and graft rejection by mediating destruction of activated T cells and APCs *(293)*. Consistent with this concept, FasL-deficient recipients are more susceptible than normal mice to the development of GVHD *(476)* and high levels of FasL in the microenvironment may help to explain the resistance to rejection of tissues transplanted to some "privileged sites," such as the testis or the anterior chamber of the eye *(477)*. Although investigators have attempted to exploit this pathway to achieve graft survival, the overexpression of FasL causes a nonspecific inflammatory syndrome associated with prominent neutrophil infiltration *(478)*, and overexpression of Fas ligand in pancreatic islets has made them more susceptible to destruction (479). Forced FasL overexpression on donor DCs also induces this neutrophil response, which augments graft rejection *(480)*.

CTLA4 is clearly important in the maintenance of self-tolerance, as evidenced by the T-cell lymphoproliferative autoimmune syndrome that develops in CTLA4 knockout mice *(481,482)*. Blockade of CTLA4 accelerates cardiac allograft rejection *(483)* and increases GVHD *(484)*, and CTLA4 has been shown to play a role in T-cell tolerance in many systems (435,485,*486–497*). CD28 knockout mice can reject allografts, despite unopposed signaling through CTLA-4 *(498)*, but their capacity to induce GVHD is diminished *(484)*. PD1, an additional down-regulatory molecule expressed by activated T cells that recognizes the B7 family members PDL-1 and PDL-2, also mitigates graft rejection (499) and GVHD *(500)*. Studies of cardiac allograft rejection suggest that PD1 plays an important modulatory role in the presence of extensive antigenic disparities between the donor and recipient, but that the BTLA-HVEM inhibitory pathway plays a predominant role in the presence of more restricted antigenic disparities *(501)*.

Regulatory Cytokines

The inflammatory condition that develops in IL-2 knockout mice is clear evidence of the important immunomodulatory role of this cytokine, and studies in several graft rejection *(502)* and GVHD *(503)* models have confirmed such a role in transplantation. Much of this effect is the result of the important role of IL-2 in activating and expanding regulatory cells (504,*505*), as is discussed elsewhere in this chapter, and IL-2 can also promote activation-induced cell death of alloreactive CD8 cells (504,*506*). Although IFN-γ can also promote graft rejection, rejection occurs rapidly in IFN-γ knockout mice *(434,507)* and is even accelerated in certain models *(508)*. Moreover, IFN-γ has been shown to play a down regulatory role in GVHD (*422*,436) and solid-organ graft survival *(509,510)*. Although the mechanism by which IFN-γ inhibits graft rejection is not fully understood, this cytokine has antiproliferative effects on CD4 and CD8 cells *(437,512)*, increases T-cell apoptosis via the Fas/FasL pathway *(511,512)*, up-regulates the production of nitric oxide *(513–516)*, which has immunomodulatory properties (385), and promotes regulatory T-cell function (517). IFN-γ inhibits both CD4- and CD8-mediated GVHD, and mitigates the expansion of both T-cell subsets (436,*518*). Moreover, the major cytokines that induce IFN-γ, IL-12, and IL-18, can down-modulate graft rejection (*433*,435,*519*) and GVHD (436,*520,521*). This down-modulatory role of IL-12 and IL-18 is dependent on IFN-γ and the Fas-FasL pathway (436,*521,522*).

Despite interest in the concept that Th2 cytokines are anti-inflammatory and may suppress rejection and GVHD (*410–413*,414,415,*416*,417,*418*), IL-4 deficiency does not accelerate graft rejection *(508,523)* and can actually down-modulate GVHD (422). However, there clearly are situations in which the balance of cytokines allows an immunomodulatory effect to be achieved by Th2 cytokines. For example, the use of total lymphoid irradiation can alter the balance between NKT cells and conventional T cells in BMT recipients, and IL-4 production by enriched recipient NKT cells down-modulates GVHD *(524)*. This approach has recently been extended to a clinical trial of HLA-identical HCT, and impressively low rates of acute GVHD were reported (525).

Anti-inflammatory cytokines such as IL-10 or TGF-β, given either exogenously or via gene transfer, may down-modulate the process of graft destruction *(526–529)*. Cardiac allograft rejection was accelerated in transiently immunosuppressed IL-10–deficient mice *(508)* and GVHD was accelerated when donors were IL-10–deficient *(423)*, suggesting a physiologically relevant role for this cytokine in modulating these responses *in vivo*. The important role of these cells in regulatory T-cell function is discussed elsewhere in this chapter. On the other hand, IL-10 can enhance cytolytic mechanisms of islet graft rejection *(530)* and high doses can accelerate GVHD *(423)*.

The Presence of the Transplanted Organ

Although early rejection episodes occur with most types of organ transplants, there are some exceptions to this rule. Kidney and liver transplants in mice can survive for long periods without immunosuppression, even with MHC disparities (*531,532*,533), and there have been cases of prolonged liver transplant survival in pigs without immunosuppression *(534)*. In addition, many types of rodent transplants, such as heart grafts, require only a short course of immunosuppression to achieve prolonged survival *(535,536)*. In these experimental systems, the long survival of these transplanted organs often diminishes, or even prevents, the subsequent rejection of antigenically identical donor skin grafts *(531,537)*. In the porcine model, the presence of a tolerogenic class I-mismatched renal allograft can promote the survival of a donor-matched cardiac allograft with a short course of immunosuppression *(538)*. Even in clinical transplantation, it appears that the long survival of a transplanted organ may diminish the rejection response because much less immunosuppression is required late after transplantation than in the early period. Thus, the mere survival of a transplanted organ can markedly down-modulate the specific antidonor immune response. Extensive data implicate regulatory cells induced by tolerogenic organs as a major mechanism of this type of immune modulation (see later discussion).

There are two important features to emphasize regarding the capacity of transplanted organs to regulate their own survival. First, their capacity to do so often confuses the results of experimental studies designed to test tolerance-inducing strategies. For example, it is frequently reported that a particular form of immunosuppression induces tolerance when provided at the time of murine cardiac transplantation. However, the conclusion that the form of immunosuppression employed leads to tolerance is not justified. The heart, which is initially protected from rejection by the immunosuppression, may be largely responsible for the tolerant condition. Second, the processes that down-regulate graft rejection may be inhibited by the standard forms of immunosuppression that are used clinically to achieve excellent graft survival *(539)* because these drugs inhibit T cell signaling and therefore may inhibit active processes of tolerance induction.

Role of Graft and Tissue Injury

Graft injury, such as that associated with ischemia-reperfusion, and host tissue injury induced by conditioning therapy in the case of HCT, play an important role in promoting graft rejection and GVHD, respectively, probably because of the effects of tissue injury on both T-cell activation and recruitment. As discussed in the section "Sensitization and Cell Trafficking during Rejection and GVHD," APC migration from tissues to lymph nodes, where T-cell priming occurs, is promoted by inflammatory signals in the tissues. For example, the inflammatory cytokines TNF-α and IL-1α promote migration of Langerhans cells from the skin to the lymphoid tissues *(540–544)*.

The impact of tissue inflammation on trafficking of activated T cells to tissues is illustrated dramatically in murine allogeneic HCT models. Administration of large numbers of nontolerant donor lymphocytes to established mixed bone marrow chimeras (i.e., animals not recently treated with conditioning therapy) leads to a GVH response that attacks only lymphohematopoietic tissues and does not cause GVHD, a disease of epithelial tissues such as skin, intestines, and liver *(545,546)*. In contrast, similar numbers of T cells cause rapidly lethal, severe GVHD in freshly irradiated hosts (*545*,547). Both ablative and nonmyeloablative conditioning with syngeneic hematopoietic reconstitution *(548)* are associated with very early production of chemokines in the GVHD target tissues. The conditioning-induced chemokine up-regulation is followed by immigration of T cells that then elicit a further cascade of chemokines that amplifies the response *(548)*. A similar scenario likely applies to adhesion molecules that promote leukocyte infiltration through the microvasculature of these tissues. Lethal TBI and cyclophosphamide, for example, up-regulate the proinflammatory cytokines IL-1, IL-6 and TNF-α *(549–551)*, which can up- regulate endothelial cell E-selectin, P-selectin, ICAM-1, and VCAM-1 *(552,553)*. In the absence of such host target tissue inflammation, mature, activated GVH-reactive effector T cells are unable to traffic into skin and induce injury (547). Provision of a local toll-like receptor (TLR) stimulus promotes the entry of such cells into the skin and induces localized GVHD (547), indicating that tissue inflammation provides a critical checkpoint for T-cell recruitment to GVHD target tissues. Nevertheless, GVHD can occur when very large numbers of nontolerant parental T cells are administered to genetically tolerant F1 hosts *(554)*, indicating that, in the presence of sufficiently powerful GVH responses, the need for tissue inflammation to induce GVHD can be bypassed.

All forms of organ and tissue transplantation involve ischemic and traumatic injury to the donor tissue, which may be one of the reasons that rejection episodes occur most frequently early after transplantation. The surgical trauma associated with even a syngeneic skin or heart graft *(350,555)* is associated with very early production of chemokines in the graft. Allogeneic but not syngeneic skin grafts are then infiltrated by NK cells that induce further chemokine production (350). Chemokines produced in response to ischemia-reperfusion injury promote the early infiltration of neutrophils *(556)*, which in turn perpetuate inflammation that promotes subsequent T-cell infiltration *(557)*. These observations collectively support the concept that a "danger" signal helps regulate graft rejection (558). These danger signals likely include products of cell death such as nucleic acids that function as endogenous ligands for TLRs (see later discussion) and other receptors for products of stressed cells. In addition, later inflammation may trigger late rejection episodes. Nevertheless, skin and cardiac allografts that are allowed to heal in before being exposed to alloreactive T cells developing *de novo* posttransplant or following adoptive transfer, are rapidly rejected if there is sufficient antigenic disparity between donor and host (*559*,560). Skin grafts bearing only minimal antigenic disparities from the host may have a more absolute requirement for innate immune stimuli or other sources of inflammation to induce rejection *(561)*. Similarly, even achieving organ transplant survival for many years in clinical practice is rarely sufficient to allow the cessation of immunosuppression without rejection. Therefore, nonspecific danger signals are not a critical requirement for graft rejection and it is better to picture the antigenic disparity and the recipient's immune responsiveness as the dominant features controlling graft rejection, while danger signals may influence the timing, intensity, or character of the rejection response.

Role of the Innate Immune System

The innate immune system comprises a group of cells and molecules that provide a first line of defence against pathogens, and which also play an important role in allograft rejection. Primary adaptive immune system responses that rely on the activation and expansion of antigen-specific T and B cells take several days to reach maturity. In contrast, the innate immune system can be considered as a "preformed" defense mechanism that is immediately available to defend the host until either the dangerous stimulus is cleared or the adaptive immune system is able to mount an antigen-specific response *(562)*. Clearly, this is a somewhat simplistic view; while many components of the innate immune system can be recruited very quickly after transplantation, their activity can be amplified after activation.

As previously discussed, the physical process of graft retrieval and implantation generates signals within the graft and the recipient that trigger rejection *(562)*. Pattern recognition receptors exist to detect the unwanted presence of bacterial or viral pathogen-associated molecular patterns, but after transplantation the TLRs that form part of the pattern recognition receptor family can also be used to detect the molecules produced as a result of implantation of the graft. These signals include heat shock proteins, reactive oxygen species, nucleic acids, complement breakdown products, and molecules associated with tissue fibrosis that activate cells of the innate immune system via TLR ligation (see Chapter 14).

Dying cells are an inevitable consequence of the ischemia and reperfusion injury that is caused by organ and tissue retrieval. Macrophages and other phagocytic cells ingest necrotic tissue and, when activated, release cytokines such as TNF-α, IL-1, and IL-6 that all contribute to the local inflammatory environment. IFN-γ, whose early production may require CD8 T-cell activation, also activates macrophages to become effective APCs and release chemokines *(563–565)*. The early infiltration of macrophages into a graft at the onset of rejection has been suggested to be a poor prognostic sign for transplant survival. Macrophage colony-stimulating factor (M-CSF) produced by tubular and mesangial cells promotes macrophage infiltration and proliferation and may play a pathogenic role in acute rejection.

Damaged tissue can also trigger complement activation in the absence as well as the presence of antibody, and complement has been demonstrated to contribute to ischemia reperfusion injury (566). Activated complement components constitute a proteolytic cascade that generates a range of effector molecules. The anaphylatoxins C5a and C3a are chemoattractant molecules that assist leukocytes to home to the graft while other soluble mediators are able to opsonize cells, targeting them for destruction by phagocytes. Recognition of C3b, C4b, or their fragments covalently bound to target cells by complement receptors on the surface of leucocytes facilitates antigen presentation and T- and B-cell activation *(567,568)*. Generation of the terminal components of the complement cascade (C5b-9) results in formation of the membrane attack complex within the target cell membrane and initiation of target cell lysis. This has been demonstrated to play an important role in ischemia-reperfusion injury (566). In addition to the potential of the damaged tissue itself to activate complement, there is also evidence that natural IgM antibody can trigger the complement activation via both the classical and mannose binding lectin pathway *(569)*. Studies in muscle reperfusion models initially identified natural IgM as a major initiator of pathology through the activation of the complement system and recruitment of inflammatory cells. When the repertoire of natural IgM antibodies was altered, significant protection of the myocardial tissue was observed with only limited apoptosis of cardiomyocytes and decreased neutrophil infiltration compared with when natural antibody was present (570). As previously mentioned, there is also increasing evidence that complement can influence graft outcomes, contributing to the development of acute and/or chronic rejection, either directly or through antibody-dependent mechanisms *(469,571)*.

The potential role of NK cells in graft rejection has been discussed earlier. Polymorphism of NK cell-receptor targets should theoretically generate alloreactive NK cells that could contribute to tissue damage following transplantation. However, to date there has been no direct demonstration that they play an essential role in acute allograft rejection *(572)*, although as previously mentioned, there is evidence that they may contribute to the development to chronic rejection *(455)*. Interestingly, NK cells have recently been shown to promote tolerance induction (see later discussion) by killing donor APCs *(573)*.

Increasing evidence demonstrates the important role that components of the innate immune system play in activating the adaptive immune system. In particular, ligation of TLRs on DCs induces maturation, as defined by up-regulation of costimulatory molecules and MHC class II, enhancing their ability to act as a bridge between the innate and adaptive immune system *(574)*. TLRs are critical sentinels of the innate immune system and contribute to the early response after transplantation. Using HY grafts, Goldstein and colleagues *(575)* showed that rejection was not triggered in the absence of MyD88 TLR signaling pathway because of the migration of a reduced number of mature DCs to the draining lymph nodes that resulted in the impaired generation of antigraft-reactive T cells and Th1 immunity. Further studies using fully allogeneic grafts have shown that multiple TLR signaling pathways contribute to the initiation of rejection (*575,576,577*). As well as stimulating rejection, TLR signaling and activation of the innate immune system may also prevent or increase the difficulty of inducing tolerance to alloantigens *(578)* (see later discussion).

MANIPULATIONS TO PREVENT GRAFT REJECTION

The importance of transplantation immunology lies ultimately in the application of its principles to clinical transplantation. Thus, the critical issue is to determine how the components and regulatory interactions involved in graft rejection might be manipulated to allow graft acceptance. One level of immunosuppression involves nonspecific approaches, reducing the overall immunocompetence of the recipient to all foreign antigens, and the second level seeks to prevent responses only to the antigens of a particular donor. Ultimately, the goal is to achieve tolerance, which is lasting donor-specific nonresponsiveness.

Nonspecific Techniques

Standard Drugs

Reviewing the pharmacology of the nonspecific immunosuppressive drugs commonly used in clinical transplantation is beyond the scope of this chapter. It is important to note, however, that most of the major advances in clinical transplantation that have occurred over the past 4 decades have been made possible largely because of these agents. Most recipients of allogeneic organs today receive exogenous immunosuppression in the form of combination therapy with several drugs (Table 44.6), including steroids, a calcineurin inhibitor (cyclosporine or tacrolimus), and an antimetabolite (e.g., azathioprine or mycophenolate mofetil). Newer drugs, including sirolimus and several other agents, are tested as substitutes for the calcineurin inhibitors in some regimens, and both steroid-free and single-drug regimens are being tested *(579–582)*, as are strategies incorporating immunosuppressive antibodies (583). In general terms, both standard and experimental immunosuppressive drugs suppress immune responses either by depleting immune cells, by blocking costimulation, or by inhibiting lymphocyte gene transcription (e.g., cyclosporine, tacrolimus), cytokine signal transduction (e.g., rapamycin), or nucleotide synthesis (e.g., azathioprine, mycophenolate mofetil).

Experimental Drugs

The list of standard drugs will almost certainly be modified in the near future by the addition of drugs that are now considered experimental (Table 44.6). 15-Deoxyspergualin is a distinctly different agent that has no effect on IL-2 production or utilization. It appears to prevent activated T and B cells from differentiating into mature effector cells. It is currently under clinical evaluation for rejection crises and for prophylaxis in highly sensitized patients. Leflunomide is an orally bioavailable prodrug that is converted to the active metabolite A77 1726, which has shown promise in treating acute and chronic rejection in animal models. It prevents lymphocyte proliferation both by inhibiting *de novo* pyrimidine synthesis and by inhibiting the activity of tyrosine kinases associated with cytokine receptors. Leflunomide can also prevent smooth muscle proliferation, and hence may be beneficial in preventing graft vasculopathy. Leflunomide has not only prolonged allo- and xenograft survival, but has also prevented the production of antidonor antibodies in animal models. Clinical trials are also in progress using a new immunosuppressive agent called FTY720. This drug has the unusual effect of altering T-cell trafficking, apparently in ways that prevent entry of the cells into donor grafts *(584)*.

Anti–T-Cell Antibodies

Another form of nonspecific immunosuppressive therapy used both clinically and experimentally is that achieved with antibodies specific for T cells of the recipient. Originally, anti–T-cell antibodies were obtained from heterologous antisera prepared against lymphocytes (ALG) or thymocytes (ATG) of the recipient species. These powerful immunosuppressants are still used in some induction regimens and for the treatment of rejection episodes. Their

TABLE 44.6 Immunosuppressive Medications

Type of Drug	*Examples*	*Mode of Action*
Antirejection medication		
1st Generation	Prednisone	Anti-inflammatory; inhibition of cytokines
	Azathioprine	Anti-metabolite (purine analog)
2nd Generation	Cyclosporin	Calcineurin inhibition (down-regulates IL-2)
	FK-506	Calcineurin inhibition (down-regulates IL-2)
	MMF	Inhibitor of nucleotide synthesis
	Rapamycin	Inhibitor of signal transduction
Polyclonal Abs	ATG	T-cell depletion
	Thymoglobulin	T-cell depletion
Monoclonal Abs	Anti-CD3	T-cell sequestration
	Anti-CD25	Activated T cells
	Anti-CD2	T-cell depletion and costimulation blockade
	Anti-CD154	Costimulation blockade
	CTLA4-Ig	Costimulation blockade
	Anti-CD40	Costimulation blockade

IL, interleukin.

major side effects include serum sickness and infectious complications. A variety of monoclonal antibodies (mAb) are also being used actively in clinical transplantation or are being tested in clinical trials (Table 44.6). These include OKT3, the first mouse anti-CD3 mAb to be used in this way, Campath-1, an anti-CD52 mAb that depletes T and B cells, and numerous other, newer mAbs. In general, these antibodies are now either "humanized" from the mouse versions by genetic engineering or prepared in mice carrying human immunoglobulin genes *(585)* to avoid immunization of the recipients.

Monoclonal antibodies to the α chain of the IL-2 receptor (CD25) have been used in an effort to achieve greater antigen specificity with anti–T-cell antibodies, based on the hypothesis that these mAbs might selectively eliminate only those T cells activated by the transplant. Clinical results using humanized anti-CD25 mAbs have so far demonstrated immunosuppression, but not tolerance induction *(586)* perhaps because CD25^{+} regulatory T cells are also depleted. Some mAbs have also been used in attempts to block the effector mechanism of graft rejection, including anti-ICAM antibodies and anti-TNF antibodies. Costimulatory blockers have shown promise, and will be discussed later.

Donor-specific Tolerance Induction

The Need for Tolerance-inducing Regimens

Immune tolerance denotes a state in which donor-specific nonresponsiveness is maintained without immunosuppressive agents. This definition might include allograft acceptance without immunosuppression, regardless of whether or not the immune system will accept other organs and tissues from the same donor (i.e., whether or not tolerance is "systemic" throughout the immune system); others define tolerance as a systemic state of immune nonresponsiveness to the donor. In both definitions, the recipient can reject organs from a third-party donor. For the purpose of this discussion, we will define tolerance as specific acceptance of a donor organ, and will qualify the term as "systemic" when it applies to the entire immune system. Systemic tolerance seems less likely to be perturbed and permit graft rejection when environmental conditions change in the recipient; for example, when a viral infection involves the donor organ.

Transplantation tolerance is a desirable goal for three major reasons. First, although improvements in immunosuppressive therapy have dramatically increased the success of clinical organ transplantation, these drugs are associated with life–long increased risks of infection and malignancy. Second, despite improved immunosuppression, chronic rejection still contributes to constantly downsloping long-term survival curves for organ allografts. Chronic rejection is less likely to occur in tolerant recipients. Third, a critical shortage of allogeneic organs has increased interest in the use of other species as organ and tissue sources. However, immune barriers to xenografts are greater than those to allografts, and the induction of both B-cell and T-cell tolerance may be essential to the ultimate success of xenotransplantation.

Central and Peripheral Tolerance

Other chapters in this book describe the mechanisms by which tolerance to self-antigens is achieved (see Chapter 29). For most developing T cells, these processes take place in the thymus, which is the central organ for T-cell development. Induction of deletional tolerance or anergy among developing thymocytes is referred to as *central*, as distinguished from the *peripheral* tolerance that may develop among already-mature T cells when they encounter antigen in the peripheral tissues. Peripheral tolerance may result from the action of regulatory T cells or other cell types, or by deletion or anergy. Peripheral tolerance mechanisms play an important role in tolerizing T cells that recognize tissue-specific self-antigens that may not be encountered in the thymus during T-cell development. However, a remarkable number of antigens previously thought to be "tissue-specific" and present only on peripheral tissues have recently been found to be expressed in the thymus and to induce central tolerance *(587,588)*. Expression of many of these genes in the thymus is controlled by the *AIRE* transcription factor, and humans and mice with a defect in *AIRE* develop multiorgan autoimmune syndromes *(589,590)*. B cells are also susceptible to tolerance induction by several mechanisms during development in the marrow or on encounter with antigens in the periphery, as is discussed later.

Mechanisms of Transplantation Tolerance

The known mechanisms for inducing T- and B-cell tolerance can be grouped into the categories deletion, anergy, and suppression. In addition, a graft may simply be ignored by recipient lymphocytes but in most transplant settings this is unlikely to be a reliable mechanism for sustaining tolerance. Each of these mechanisms will be described briefly, and our current understanding of the role of each mechanism is then discussed in relation to particular strategies to induce transplantation tolerance.

Clonal Deletion

B cells: Studies using Ig receptor transgenic mice suggest that B cells are susceptible to deletion at particular stages of development on recognition of membrane-bound antigen *(591)*. Antigen expression on either radioresistant host cells or on a small population of hematopoietic cells appears to be sufficient to delete immature B cells specific for that antigen *(592)*. When a developing B cell with autoreactivity encounters self-antigen, it undergoes developmental arrest. *RAG* gene-dependent light chain receptor editing then takes place; if this results in the formation of a nonautoreactive Ig receptor, the B cell survives; if not, the B cell undergoes apoptosis. The mechanisms of these processes have recently been reviewed (593). Cells of the B-1 subset, which produce natural antibodies responsible for xenograft hyperacute rejection *(594)*, can be deleted by an apoptotic process in mice when their surface Ig is cross-linked by cell-bound antigen *(595)*. Deletion and/or receptor editing is responsible for the long-term tolerance of natural antibody-producing B-1 cells in mice rendered mixed chimeric with bone marrow expressing an antigen for which natural antibody-producing cells pre-exist in the recipient *(156,596,597)*.

T cells. Most central T-cell tolerance occurs via a deletional mechanism due to recognition of self-antigens presented by hematopoietic cells and thymic epithelial cells (reviewed in refs. *598* and 599). In addition, T cells recognizing self-antigens presented only by nonhematopoietic thymic stromal cells may be rendered anergic to such antigens *(600)*. Antigens presented by thymic epithelium may also lead to the development of regulatory cells that recognize them and tolerize other T cells in the periphery *(601–603)*. Deletion of self-reactive T cells is believed to occur when the avidity of an interaction between an immature thymocyte and an APC in the thymus is sufficiently high to induce apoptotic cell death *(604,605)*. This high avidity includes a relatively high-affinity interaction between a rearranged TCR and a self-peptide/MHC complex presented in the thymus. TCR with lower affinity for such complexes are more likely to survive this process, and other mechanisms are required to prevent their activation in the periphery under conditions of, for example, inflammation and antigen up-regulation on normal tissues. Several hematopoietic cell types, including DCs *(606)*, B cells *(607)*, and thymocytes *(608,609)*, as well as nonhematopoietic cells of the thymic stroma *(610,611)* (reviewed in refs. 558 and *612*), have the capacity to induce intrathymic tolerance by deletional and nondeletional mechanisms. Transplantation tolerance induced by intrathymic deletion should be very reliable, as the absence of lymphocytes with reactivity to the donor would ensure that a specific response to donor antigens could not be induced under any circumstances.

Peripheral deletion has also been described for mature T cells on exposure to antigen *in vivo (613–615)*. Deletion seems to be the natural consequence, under noninflammatory conditions, of cross-presentation by lymph node DCs of self-antigen expressed in parenchymal tissues to CD8 CTL *(616–618)*. Peripheral CD8 cells may undergo clonal deletion in a process termed *exhaustion* in the presence of a large antigen load that persists *(619,620)*. A possibly related phenomenon has been observed for host-reactive CTL in the context of GVHD *(621,622)*. Peripheral deletion of donor-reactive T cells has been demonstrated in several transplantation tolerance models involving costimulatory blockade with donor lymphocyte or bone marrow infusion (485,*623,624*) and was suggested in recipients of allografts with anti-CD154 and rapamycin (625). In addition, veto cells (see later discussion) can delete alloreactive CTL precursors. Recently, a non-veto mechanism mediated by $CD4^-CD8^-$ cytotoxic regulatory cells has been reported to lead to the deletion of alloreactive CD8 T cells with the same specificity as the regulatory cells *(626)*.

Anergy

Anergy is a state that may result when T cells recognize peptide/MHC complexes, but without receiving adequate accessory or costimulatory signals (*600*,*627,628,629*). A lymphocyte is considered to be "anergic" if it cannot proliferate in response to the antigen for which it is specific. T-cell anergy has been associated with altered signaling and tyrosine phosphorylation patterns *(630–633)* and with a lack of IL-2 production. T-cell anergy can often *(634)*, but not always *(635)*, be overcome by providing exogenous IL-2. In some cases anergy has been associated with TCR down-modulation *(615,636–638)*.

T cells may become anergic if they encounter antigen without costimulation (639), or if they encounter peptide ligands for which they have low affinity *(604,605)*. In addition to mature peripheral T cells, thymocytes are also susceptible to anergy induction by antigens presented on hematopoietic *(607)* or nonhematopoietic stromal *(640–642)* cells. Anergy is generally reversible *in vivo* and can be overcome by infection *(643)* or by removal of antigen *(644–647)*, and therefore may not be as robust a form of tolerance as deletion. Although deletion has been reported to follow the induction of anergy of T cells in the continued presence of antigen *(648,649)*, this is not a universal outcome, and anergic T cells may persist for long periods of time *(650,651)*. In a transplantation model involving BMT under cover of costimulatory blockade, peripheral donor-reactive CD4 T cells have been shown to be rendered anergic prior to their deletion over a period of weeks (652). Anergic T cells may also down-regulate the activity of other T cells, so that they function as "suppressor" or "regulatory" T cells *(653,654)*. This regulation may occur via conditioning of an APC by an anergic T cell so that naïve T cells recognizing the same or different antigens on the same APC are also tolerized *(655)*.

Anergy is an important tolerance mechanism for the many self-reactive B cells that escape deletion in the bone marrow *(656,657)*. Most of these B cells die within the peripheral lymphoid tissues or are anergic, particularly if they recognize abundant but low-avidity antigens (*591*, reviewed in ref. 593). Anergy requires persistent antigen and is characterized by Ig receptor down-regulation *(591)*, altered signaling patterns, and increased apoptosis on antigen encounter *(592)*. The failure of anergic B cells to up-regulate BAFF receptors plays an important role in their inability to compete for survival in germinal centers. T-cell tolerance and the resulting absence of help is important for the maintenance of B-cell anergy, as anergic B cells can be activated in the presence of high-avidity antigen and T-cell help (593). Anergy is responsible for the early tolerance of natural antibody-producing B-1 cells in mice rendered mixed chimeric with bone marrow cells expressing an antigen recognized by natural antibody-producing cells in the recipient *(155,596,597)*.

Suppression

Regulatory T Cells. The concept of antigen-specific suppression and the existence of a specialized population of T cells, known initially as suppressor cells and more recently as regulatory T cells (Treg), that could control immune responsiveness originated in the 1970s from the studies of Gershon and Kondo *(658)* among others, who demonstrated the existence of complex regulatory networks involving several levels of T-cell–mediated suppression. In the specific setting of transplantation, a role for suppressor cells in transplantation tolerance was also identified *(659)*. However, despite the efforts of many groups through the. 1980s, the cellular and molecular characteristics of these suppressor cells were never defined with any precision, even though the phenomenon of suppression was highly reproducible *in vivo*, particularly in transplant models.

In 1990, Hall and colleagues *(660)* re-examined the function of T-cell subpopulations present in rats with long-term surviving cardiac allografts after cyclosporine treatment and, interestingly, reported that tolerance could be adoptively transferred by $CD25^+CD4^+$ cells. However, interest in characterizing suppressor/regulatory T cells was not fully revived until Sakaguchi and colleagues *(661)* followed up on data showing that susceptible strains of neonatally thymectomized mice developed multiorgan autoimmune disease. These workers found that neonatal thymectomy resulted in a loss of T cells with suppressor or regulatory properties that could be enriched among T cells expressing CD25, the alpha chain of the IL-2 receptor.

Naturally occurring $CD25^+CD4^+$ T cells with regulatory properties are generated in the thymus through interaction between the developing thymocytes with an intermediate affinity ligand, too low for negative selection, expressed on nonhematopoietic cells of the thymus for their positive selection (*662*,663). Cortical thymic epithelium has been found to be the site of the MHC class II expression required for the development of functional Treg *(601)*. In addition to the naturally occurring populations of $CD25^+CD4^+$ T cells with regulatory activity, populations of T cells with regulatory properties that also express CD25 can be induced in the periphery following exposure to antigen under certain conditions (664). It is likely that following transplantation or exposure to alloantigen, Treg that can control the immune response and prevent rejection will be derived from both the naturally occurring and induced populations (see later discussion). In addition to the wealth of data in mice, $CD4^+$ T cells expressing high levels of CD25 in the peripheral blood and thymus have also been shown to have suppressive activity in humans *(665–670)* and are present in transplant recipients with long-term surviving allografts *(671)*.

CD25 is by no means an exclusive marker for T cells with regulatory activity. Although the kinetics of expression are different, CD25 is also expressed by activated T cells. Indeed in transplantation, monoclonal antibodies targeting CD25 are licensed for use as antirejection therapies. Thus, there is a need to define other markers for Treg. The list of potential cell surface markers has been growing steadily, and includes CD152 (CTLA4), CD103, and glucocorticoid-induced TNFR-related protein, among many others. However, as yet, the "perfect marker" has not been identified. As well as cell surface and intracellular proteins, transcription factors can also potentially provide a tool for identifying committed cell lineages. In both humans and mice, *foxp3*, a forkhead/winged-helix transcription factor designated Scurfin in mice has been shown to be a potential master regulator for the development and function of Treg as mutations in the *Fox p3* gene lead to uncontrolled activation/expansion of $CD4^+$ T cells *(672,673)*. A direct link between *Foxp3* expression and regulatory activity came from retroviral gene transfer studies where transduction of naïve mouse T cells with *foxp3* resulted in acquisition of regulatory function *(674)*. This correlation between *Foxp3* and regulation has been strengthened by the generation of *Foxp3* transgenic mice where cells expressing *Foxp3* protein express either green *(675)* or red fluorescent protein *(676)*, allowing such cells to be identified and their function explored. Although in mice the relationship between *Foxp3* expression and regulation may be tightly linked, the situation may not be so straightforward in humans, as Foxp3 protein has also been found in activated T cells in some situations *(677)*.

Recipient-derived $CD25^+CD4^+$ T cells were shown to have potent regulatory properties in both the induction and maintenance phases of tolerance to alloantigens *in vivo* in mice (e.g., *678*,679,*680*,*681*). In BMT, donor $CD25^+CD4^+$ T cells present in the bone marrow inoculum were found to protect from GVHD (*682*,*683*,684). In humans, $CD25^{high}CD4^+$ T cells have been found in the peripheral blood of immunosuppression-free allograft recipients *(671)* and their presence may contribute to long-term graft survival. As mentioned previously, Treg with capacity to control immune responses to a transplant most likely comprise naturally occurring and induced Treg populations. Naturally occurring Treg present in naïve, unmanipulated adult mice have been shown to be capable of preventing rejection of allografts mismatched for a single minor histocompatibility antigen, for example, H-Y. However, they appear to be much less potent than Treg induced following exposure to alloantigen, as studies comparing the activity of naturally occurring and induced Treg directly suggest that 10 times fewer induced Treg are needed to prevent allograft rejection. These findings may explain why in situations where grafts are mismatched for multiple major and minor histocompatibility antigens, it has sometimes been difficult to demonstrate that naturally occurring Treg can control the rejection response.

After transplantation, the ability to generate Tregs *in vivo* may be influenced by the microenvironment. It has been shown that the balance between the presence of IL-6 and TGF-β *in vivo* can have a dramatic impact on which T-cell population develops. Importantly, Treg generation can be prevented by inflammation *(685,686)*, a situation that occurs commonly *in vivo* after cell or organ transplantation, leading instead to the generation of cells capable of mediating tissue damage, including T_H17 cells *(685–687)*.

The mechanisms of regulation effected by Treg to prevent allograft rejection involve a variety of different pathways. When Tregs are reactivated by their cognate antigen through TCR they can rapidly and transiently produce IFN-γ that is needed to mediate their regulatory activity and prevent rejection (517). Interestingly, IFN-γ has been shown previously to be an essential mediator for the induction of tolerance in mouse models in which costimulation blockade was used to prevent graft rejection *(688)*. The transient production of IFN-γ by Tregs can have multiple effects on cells with which they interact (689), including other T cells, mediated either directly or indirectly through effects on APCs *(690)*. Treg activity can result in inhibition of cytokine production and secretion, down-regulation of costimulatory and/or adhesion molecule expression, inhibition of proliferation, induction of anergy, elimination of the effector population by promoting cell death, or even conversion of naïve and/or effector T cells to a regulatory phenotype, a process known as *infectious tolerance (691–694)*. IL-2, IL-10 and TGF-β may have roles in this phenomenon *(695)*. If this process is effective, any new T cells entering the repertoire after transplantation where immunoregulation is the dominant mechanism of tolerance will be converted to Treg, thereby propagating and reinforcing the tolerant state throughout the posttransplant course.

Indoleamine 2,3 dioxygenase (IDO), an enzyme that catalyses the initial and rate limiting step of the kynurenine pathway of tryptophan catabolism, is known to be subject to transcriptional regulation by IFN-γ *(696 699)*, dependent on STAT-1 signalling *(698)*. IFN-γ released by Treg can lead to the development of IDO-competent DCs that may acquire the capacity to control T cells locally through tryptophan depletion; overexpression of IDO inhibits alloimmune responses (e.g., *[699–701]*). The molecular mechanism responsible for the conversion of DCs to become IDO competent requires further investigation, but roles for TGF-β and IL-10 have been suggested *(692,693)*.

In addition, the activity of Treg *in vivo* in transplant models has been shown to be dependent on IL-10 *(680)*, TGF-β *(702)*, and CTLA-4 (e.g., refs. *492,679,703–706*). CTLA-4 (CD152) is constitutively expressed by Treg and engagement of CD80/86 on DC can also induce IDO (707). In addition, CTLA-4 has been found to modulate T-cell motility by activating LFA-1 clustering and adhesion *(708)*, thereby altering the threshold for T-cell activation *(709)*. Although the mechanistic links between each of these mediators still requires clarification, it is important to note that many of the same molecules have also been found to be required for Treg activity in other settings, including autoimmune diseases, suggesting that Treg capable of controlling disease states *in vivo* have many properties in common.

One property of Tregs that can potentially be exploited in the context of transplantation is their ability to mediate bystander regulation in a defined microenvironment *in vivo*. To elaborate their functional activity, Treg need to be activated through their TCR. Data obtained by Thornton and Shevach *(709) in vitro* showed that reactivation of Treg with a defined antigen specificity through their TCR-enabled the cells to suppress the response of other cells present in the same *in vitro* cultures. Karim and colleagues (710) have shown that it is possible to exploit this observation *in vivo* to enable Tregs that are generated and respond to an unrelated protein antigen, such as human gamma globulin, to control rejection when the cells are restimulated through TCR immediately before they are asked to function *in vivo*.

Despite the current interest in the role of $CD25^+CD4$ Treg, it is important to remember that regulatory activity is not exclusive to CD4 T cells, and CD8 *(711–713)*, $CD8CD28^-$ *(714)*, $TCR^+CD4^-CD8^-$ ("double negative") *(626)*, and NKT cells (377,715) have also been shown to have regulatory activities in different situations after transplantation. In fact, regulatory mechanisms in both the innate and adaptive immune systems will most likely contribute to the overall outcome after transplantation. This is highlighted by the finding that both NKT cells and $CD25^+CD4$ Treg play a role in preventing acute GVHD after allogeneic BMT *(682,683*,684,*715)* and a recent study showing that inhibitory NK cell receptors can play a regulatory role in T-cell homeostasis *(716)*.

It may be possible to exploit Treg to control the immune response after transplantation either by developing strategies using immunosuppressive agents that promote Treg generation and/or do not inhibit their function or by generating Treg *ex vivo* and using them as a cellular therapy at different stages in the posttransplant course to prevent rejection and re-establish control. Understanding the impact of immunosuppressive drugs on Treg generation and

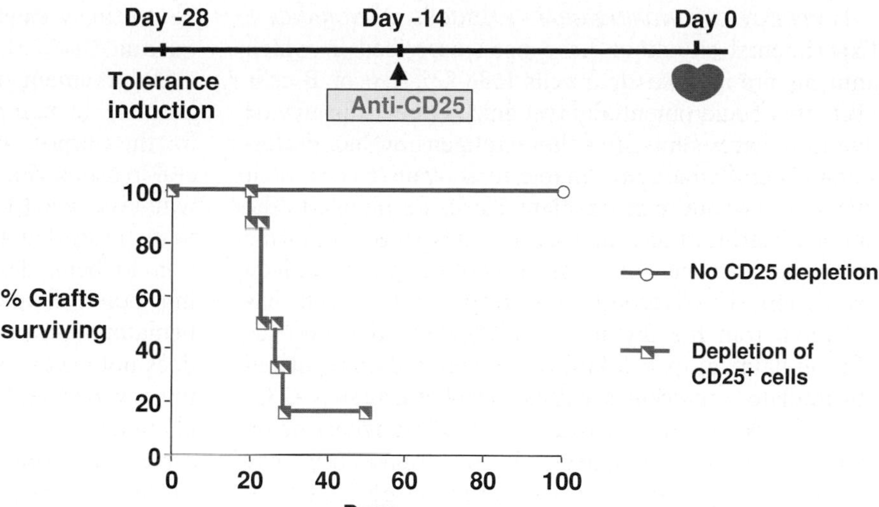

FIGURE 44.11 Administration of anti-CD25 monocloncal antibodies after the induction of Treg (regulatory T cells) can prevent long-term graft survival.

function is an important part of using the potential of Treg *in vivo*. Data from mouse models suggest that the calcineurin inhibitors have the capacity to inhibit T-cell apoptosis after activation, thereby preventing a reduction in the frequency of effector T cells that would allow Tregs to assume a more dominant functional role (625,*717*; Bushell and Wood, personal communication). Similarly, administration of anti-CD25 monoclonal antibodies after the induction of Treg can prevent long-term graft survival (Figure 44.11). On the other hand, other classes of immunosuppressive drug, such as the mTOR inhibitors sirolimus and everolimus, may enhance the generation of Tregs. Strategies to generate and/or expand Tregs *ex vivo* for therapeutic purposes are being developed with potential application in cell and organ transplantation. A variety of different approaches have been shown to be successful for generating and/or expanding T cells with regulatory capacity in both mice and humans including exposure to TGF-β, IFN-γ, and stimulation with anti-CD3/CD28 in the presence of IL-2, to name just some (e.g., refs. *718* and *719*). The development, maintenance, and expansion of Treg is critically dependent on IL-2 *(720,721)*. In each case at the end of the culture period, T cells that emerge have been shown either *in vitro,* and in some studies *in vivo*, to have regulatory activity that can prevent allograft rejection or GVHD *(722)*.

Antibody-mediated Suppression. Idiotypes are unique antigenic determinants that characterize the binding sites of antibody or T-cell receptors. These determinants can be antigenic and induce the production of anti-idiotypic antibodies *(723)*. Antibody-mediated suppression could theoretically occur through the recognition of idiotypes of antidonor Ig receptors. Anti-idiotypic antibodies can suppress antibody reactivity by directly binding to the antigen-binding site of the antibody, and the development of such antibodies has been suggested as one of the possible benefits of pre–kidney transplant blood transfusions. Such antibodies have also been suggested to contribute to the apparent hyporesponsiveness to noninherited maternal antigens in renal allograft recipients. In the past, it was also considered possible that anti-idiotypic antibodies might inhibit T-cell recognition of antigen, but this now seems unlikely, given that T cells recognize peptide/MHC complexes, whereas antibodies recognize epitopes of intact molecules. It continues to be an intriguing question whether normal regulatory mechanisms for B-cell responses might include anti-idiotypes, as suggested by Jerne. However, efforts to control transplantation using exogenous anti-idiotypic antibodies to either T- or B-cell receptors have been disappointing *(724)*.

Antibodies can also induce tolerance through a process known as *enhancement*. Enhancement is defined as prolongation of graft survival achieved by the presence of antigraft antibodies *(725)*. This phenomenon was first described in experiments involving allogeneic tumor growth. Subsequently, enhancing regimens using anti-MHC antibodies and/or soluble antigen were shown to produce long-term tolerance for rodent allogeneic kidney transplants *(726)*. The simple interpretation was that anti-MHC antibodies bind to the antigen and thereby block the immune response, but this explanation has not turned out to be sufficient. For example, tolerance following enhancement can be transferred by cells and not serum from enhanced recipients. Apparently, the administered antibody sets up a host reaction that leads to specific immunosuppression. An idiotype/anti-idiotype network would be an attractive explanation for this phenomenon. Unfortunately, the spectacular success obtained using enhancement for kidney graft survival in rats has not been observed for grafts in other species and this approach has largely been abandoned, at least for the present.

LYMPHOCYTES IGNORING GRAFT ANTIGENS ("IGNORANCE"). Experimental situations have been described in which antigens are ignored by T cells *(638,727,728)* or B cells *(591)* that could potentially recognize them. This may be due to the presentation of these antigens by "nonprofessional APCs," which are unable to activate T cells, or it may reflect a failure of recipient T cells to migrate to the antigen-bearing tissue, as has been described in murine solid-tumor models *(729)*. The level of peripheral antigen expression, how recently the responding T cell has emerged from the thymus *(638,730)*, and the presence of proinflammatory cytokines *(731,732)* and up-regulated costimulatory molecules within peripheral tissues *(733)* may all influence the decision of a T cell to ignore or respond to peripheral antigens. However, "ignorance" may be a precarious state that can be upset by additional immunologic stimuli provoked by inflammation that may be induced, for example, by infection *(728)* or by presentation of antigen on professional APCs, as has been described for endocrine allografts that are depleted of APCs prior to transplantation *(734)*.

Strategies for Inducing Transplantation Tolerance

Strategies to Achieve Central Tolerance

Mixed Chimerism. It has been known for 60 years that hematopoietic chimerism induced *in utero* is associated with transplantation tolerance (reviewed in ref. 735). The capacity of hematopoietic cells to induce tolerance results largely from their ability to induce intrathymic clonal deletion of thymocytes that recognize them. Thus, bone marrow engraftment can reliably induce tolerance to the most immunogenic allografts, such as fully MHC-mismatched skin and small bowel grafts *(368,736,737)*. Despite this powerful tolerance-inducing capacity, HCT has not yet been routinely applied to the induction of tolerance in man. HCT for tolerance induction in rodents originally involved recipient treatment with lethal whole-body irradiation. Removal of mature donor T cells before transplantation was shown to prevent GVHD *(738–741)*, which allowed the development of a new immune system that is tolerant to both donor and recipient antigens. For wide application for organ allograft tolerance, HCT must be successful and safe across MHC barriers. However, MHC-mismatched allogeneic HCT in larger animals, including humans, has proved to be less successful and more dangerous than in rodents because of the toxicity associated with myeloablative conditioning, and the inordinately high risks of GVHD and engraftment failure (reviewed in ref. 742). Marrow rejection is increased when donor marrow is T-cell–depleted to prevent GVHD. Therefore, it will be essential to develop more specific and effective methods of overcoming the barriers to marrow engraftment with minimal GVHD risk before this highly effective approach to tolerance induction can be routinely used in patients to achieve organ allograft tolerance.

Achievement of a state of mixed rather than full allogeneic hematopoietic chimerism would be desirable for the purpose of allograft tolerance induction for several reasons. First, mixed chimerism can be achieved with less toxic (nonmyeloablative) conditioning regimens than those that lead to full donor chimerism. In addition to being less toxic than myeloablative conditioning, nonmyeloablative regimens allow recovery of host hematopoiesis, so that life-threatening marrow failure does not occur, even in the event that rejection of donor marrow occurs. Secondly, compared with fully allogeneic chimeras, improved immunocompetence has been observed in mixed chimeras, which contain host-type APC in the periphery, allowing optimal antigen presentation to T cells that have developed in the host thymus, and which therefore preferentially recognize peptide antigens presented by host-type MHC molecules (120,*743*). Although the premise that hematopoietic cells do not participate in positive selection is controversial and has recently been challenged *(744)*, studies of antiviral CTL responses in mixed chimeras showed exquisite specificity for recipient-derived MHC-restricting elements *(745)*. Third, mixed chimeras contain hematopoietic cells from both the recipient and the donor in the thymus and hence delete both host-reactive and donor-reactive T cells, resulting in a peripheral T-cell repertoire that is deleted of cells that recognize the donor or the host *(746,747)*. Although nonhematopoietic thymic stromal cells have some capacity to induce deletional tolerance, the capacity of hematopoietic cells, especially DCs, to do so, is particularly powerful. Thus, intrathymic deletion of host-reactive cells in addition to donor-reactive cells occurs in mixed chimeras to a greater extent than in full chimeras *(746,748)*. As might be expected, tolerance induced by intrathymic deletional mechanisms is systemic, as shown by both *in vivo* and *in vitro* studies (reviewed in ref. 599).

Several nonmyeloablative approaches have been recently developed to permit the use of BMT to achieve mixed chimerism and specific tolerance, bringing the approach toward clinical application. In mixed chimeras prepared with a nonmyeloablative regimen consisting of low-dose (3-Gy) TBI, T-cell depleting mAbs and thymic irradiation *(368)*, intrathymic deletion was shown to be the major mechanism maintaining donor-specific tolerance *(746)*. Although anergy may play a role in tolerizing the few peripheral T cells that escape depletion with mAbs in this model, long-term tolerance appears to be maintained purely by a deletional mechanism. Administration of donor MHC-specific antibody to eliminate donor chimerism from established mixed chimeras results in loss of tolerance, and in the *de novo* appearance in the periphery of T cells with receptors that recognize donor antigens. However, if the recipient thymus is removed prior to elimination of chimerism with antidonor antibody, specific tolerance to the donor is preserved, and donor-reactive TCRs do not appear in the periphery (749). Thus, chimerism is needed *only* in the thymus and not in the periphery in order to ensure persistent tolerance. This is consistent with a purely central deletional mechanism, as peripheral anergy and suppression generally require the relevant antigen to maintain the tolerance. Because thymic APCs are continually turning over, this observation emphasizes the need for hematopoietic stem cell engraftment at sufficient levels in order to ensure an uninterrupted supply of donor APCs in the recipient thymus for the life of the mixed chimera. The absence of suppressive tolerance mechanisms makes these animals particularly vulnerable to breaking of tolerance when nontolerant T cells emerge from the thymus after intentional depletion of donor antigen, or after exogenous administration of nontolerant host-type T cells (652,749).

These and other studies have led to an evolving understanding of the minimal requirements for achievement of lasting chimerism. These requirements are summarized in Figure 44.12. T-cell alloreactivity in both the thymus and periphery must be overcome in order to permit allogeneic stem cell engraftment and early seeding of the thymus with allogeneic APC. Intrathymic alloreactivity can be overcome with thymic irradiation *(368)*, high doses of T-cell–depleting antibodies *(750)*, or costimulatory blockers such as anti-CD154 or CTLA4Ig (751,*752*). Peripheral T-cell–mediated alloreactivity can be overcome with T-cell–depleting mAbs *(368,753)*, or with costimulatory blockers (751). Low-dose TBI or busulfan is often used in nonmyeloablative regimens to achieve mixed chimerism, creating an environment that facilitates the engraftment of donor hematopoietic stem cells in the host *(750,754)*. Although such myelosuppressive treatments can be omitted by administering very high marrow doses *(753)*, and all preconditioning can be eliminated by giving a high dose of fully MHC-mismatched donor marrow followed by a single injection of each of two costimulatory blockers *(755)* or repeated injections of anti-CD154 *(756)*, methods of obtaining sufficient donor stem cells to permit engraftment without some minimal host myelosuppression do not yet exist clinically. The mechanisms of peripheral tolerance achieved with the combination of costimulatory blockade and allogeneic BMT are discussed later in the section on peripheral tolerance (see "Costimulatory Blockade with Infusion of Donor Hematopoietic Cells.").

Mixed chimerism induced with costimulatory blockade or T-cell–depleting antibodies is associated with a systemic state of tolerance, as evidenced by specific unresponsiveness to the donor in mixed lymphocyte response and CML assays and the acceptance of donor skin grafted at any time post-BMT *(368,752,755,757)*. In contrast, tolerance approaches that do not lead to mixed chimerism generally do not induce systemic tolerance, suggesting that tolerance might be less robust.

Additional approaches to achieving mixed chimerism for tolerance induction include the use of total lymphoid irradiation plus BMT, which has been more successful in rodents *(758,759)* than in humans *(760,761)*. Other regimens involving various combinations of anti–T-cell antibodies, irradiation, and immunosuppressive drugs have also permitted the achievement of mixed chimerism in both large (762,*763–765*) and small *(766–769)* animals. The successful induction of tolerance in a primate model using a nonmyeloablative approach to inducing mixed chimerism (762), combined with murine studies demonstrating the utility of mixed chimerism followed by delayed donor lymphocyte infusions (DLI) as an approach to achieving

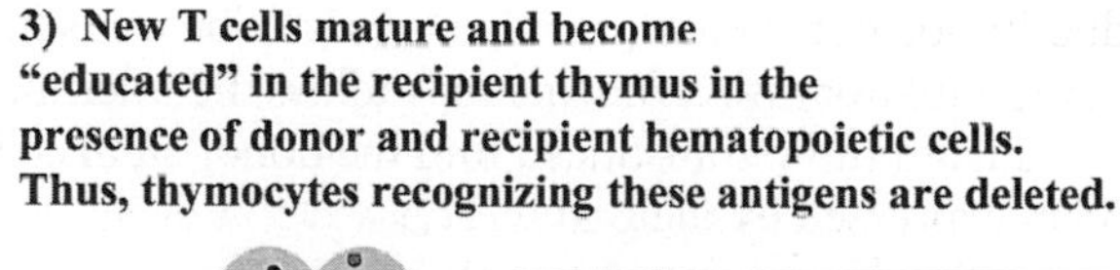

3) New T cells mature and become "educated" in the recipient thymus in the presence of donor and recipient hematopoietic cells. Thus, thymocytes recognizing these antigens are deleted.

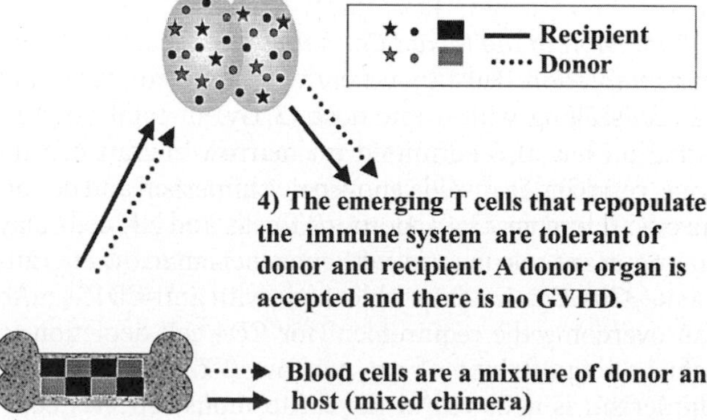

FIGURE 44.12 Requirements for induction of long-term mixed hematopoietic chimerism. GVHD, graft-versus-host disease.

GVL effects without GVHD *(545,546)*, has been used as the basis for a clinical trial of mixed chimerism induction followed by DLI for the treatment of patients with hematologic malignancies *(770,771)*. Success with this approach led to a pilot evaluation of combined HLA-identical kidney and bone marrow transplantation with this nonmyeloablative regimen in patients with renal failure due to multiple myeloma, which provided the first demonstration that transplantation tolerance could be intentionally induced in humans (772).

The ability to replace recipient T-cell depletion with costimulatory blockade in the murine models is encouraging for several reasons. First, it has been difficult to achieve T-cell depletion with antibodies in large animals and humans that is as exhaustive as that achieved in the previously mentioned rodent models, perhaps because of the use of inadequate doses or suboptimal reagents. A second concern is that, if sufficiently exhaustive T-cell depletion could be achieved in humans, T-cell recovery from the thymus might be dangerously slow, especially in older individuals (reviewed in ref. 773). The ability to replace some *(757)* or all (751,*755,756*) T-cell depleting antibodies with costimulatory blockade is therefore of considerable interest.

GVHD does not occur in the rodent models previously discussed, despite the use of unseparated donor bone marrow cells. This is most readily explained by the continued presence of the T-cell–depleting or costimulatory blocking antibodies in the serum of the hosts at the time of BMT *(774)*. These levels are sufficient to prevent alloreactivity by the relatively small number of mature T cells in the donor marrow.

An alternative to using allogeneic hematopoietic engraftment to achieve tolerance is to reconstitute recipients with autologous bone marrow cells that have been transduced with genes encoding foreign transplantation antigens *(775)*. Although this approach is limited because the full spectrum of donor antigens cannot be transduced, active regulatory mechanisms may allow the tolerance to spread from those transduced into the donor stem cells to others expressed by the graft *(776)*.

Extension of the Mixed Chimerism Approach to Xenotransplantation. Host treatment with mAbs to T cells and NK cells along with a low dose (3 Gy) of total body irradiation has also permitted rat marrow engraftment in mice, resulting in mixed xenogeneic chimerism and donor-specific tolerance *(369)*. Both $\gamma\delta$ T cells and NK cells play an important role in resisting xenogeneic marrow engraftment (370). Costimulatory blockade with anti-CD154 mAb can overcome the requirement for CD4 cell depletion to achieve engraftment of rat marrow *(777)*. Once mixed chimerism is achieved in the rat to mouse species combination, donor-specific tolerance is observed at the level of both T cells and B cells *(59,369,778–780)*. Pigs are widely believed to be the most suitable xenogeneic donor species for transplantation to humans, but transplantation from this species is impeded by the presence in human sera of "natural" antibody (Nab) that cause hyperacute rejection of porcine vascularized xenografts. The major specificity recognized by human natural antibody on porcine tissues is a ubiquitous carbohydrate epitope, Galα1–3Galß1–4GlcNAc-R (αGal). Humans lack a functional α1–3Gal transferase (GalT) enzyme, as do GalT knockout mice, which also make anti-αGal Nab. Both pre-existing and newly developing B cells producing anti-αGal antibodies are tolerized by the induction of mixed chimerism in GalT knockout mice receiving αGal-expressing allogeneic or xenogeneic marrow *(156,596,781)*. The induction of mixed xenogeneic chimerism prevents hyperacute rejection, acute vascular rejection, and cell-mediated rejection of primarily vascularized cardiac xenografts *(779)*. Long-term mixed xenogeneic chimeras produced in GalT knockout mice lack anti-Gal surface Ig-bearing cells in the spleen, and show tolerance in ELISPOT assays *(596,779)*. The major IgM Nab-producing cell population in mice is a B-1b cell population in the spleen *(594)*, and these are tolerized rapidly by an anergy mechanism, which is followed later by clonal deletion and/or receptor editing of Gal-specific B cells *(597)*. Splenic B cells, possibly of a similar subset, are also, along with immature plasma cells, the major anti-Gal IgM-producing population in nonhuman primates and baboons *(782)*.

Studies in mixed allogeneic chimeras show that recipient NK cells are tolerized to the donor *(783)* and studies in the rat to mouse combination also indicate a state of tolerance *(784)*. Despite this T, B, and NK cell tolerance, the levels of donor chimerism decline gradually over time, the result of a competitive advantage of recipient mouse marrow over xenogeneic rat marrow as the host recovers from low-dose TBI *(785)*. Species specificity or selectivity of cytokines, adhesion molecules, and other interactions that regulate hematopoiesis *(786)* probably account for this advantage. Achievement of xenogeneic hematopoietic repopulation has proved to be an even more formidable challenge in highly disparate (discordant) species combinations. Administration of exogenous donor species-specific cytokines can partially overcome this barrier *(787,788)*, and high levels of porcine hematopoietic stem cell engraftment have been achieved in immunodeficient mice transgenically expressing the porcine hematopoietic cytokines IL-3, stem cell factor, and GM-CSF *(789)*. The use of these mice has permitted demonstration that mouse T cells *(790)* and, importantly, using a humanized mouse model, that human T cells *(791)* can be centrally tolerized to porcine xenoantigens via induction of mixed xenogeneic chimerism.

Macrophages also play a significant role in resisting engraftment of xenogeneic marrow from highly disparate species *(389,390)*. It seems likely that macrophages and other cellular components of the innate system recognize foreign lipids and carbohydrates on highly disparate xenogeneic cells via specific activating receptors and that the failure of inhibitory interactions may increase susceptibility to destruction by such cells, as suggested by recent studies (400).

Xenogeneic Thymic Transplantation

An alternative approach to achieving xenogeneic T-cell tolerance involves replacement of the recipient thymus with a xenogeneic donor thymus after host T-cell depletion and thymectomy. Immunocompetent mice treated in this way reconstitute $CD4^+$ T cells in xenogeneic porcine thymic grafts *(792)*. These cells repopulate the periphery, are competent to resist infection *(793)*, and are tolerant of porcine donor antigens *(792,794)*. Tolerance to both donor and host develops, at least in part, by intrathymic deletional mechanisms in these animals, reflecting the presence of class IIhigh APCs from both species within the thymic graft *(794,795)*. T cells that differentiate in a xenogeneic thymus respond to peptide antigens presented by host MHC *(793)*. Studies using TCR transgenic mouse recipients showed that positive selection in such grafts is mediated only by porcine thymic MHC, with no influence of mouse MHC (796,797). However, the excellent immune function achieved in these mice *(793)* and in humans receiving HLA-mismatched allogeneic thymic transplantation for the treatment of congenital thymic aplasia (DiGeorge syndrome) *(798,799)*, suggests that "restriction incompatibility" due to MHC disparity between the positive selecting cells in the thymus and the APCs in the periphery may not be a major obstacle to the achievement of adequate immune function, perhaps reflecting the fact that MHC reactivity is inherent in unselected TCR sequences (*33*,38). Importantly, human T cells can also be rendered specifically tolerant of the porcine donor by developing in xenogeneic porcine thymus grafts (800). This approach has been applied and has demonstrated promise in pig-to-primate xenograft models (*801*,802).

Transplantation of allogeneic *(803)* and concordant xenogeneic *(804)* thymic epithelial tissue obtained from fetuses before seeding with hematopoietic cells can also induce tolerance. The mechanism of tolerance in such animals seems to predominantly involve generation of donor-specific regulatory cells (*805*,806). Transplantation of xenogeneic thymic tissue into congenitally athymic recipients has frequently resulted in the development of a multiorgan autoimmune syndrome, possibly resulting from the lack of recipient-type thymic epithelium needed for the development of regulatory cells with specificity for certain recipient antigens (*601,602,807,808,809*,810). This complication occurs much less frequently in thymectomized, T-cell–depleted mice than in congenitally athymic mice receiving porcine thymic transplants *(811)*, probably because of the persistence of regulatory cells derived from the host thymus prior to thymectomy and T-cell depletion.

Development of Chimerism Without Host Conditioning

Developmentally Immunoincompetent Recipients. One of the first demonstrations of acquired tolerance was obtained in Freemartin cattle, which are fraternal twins that share a placental circulation and develop mixed chimerism spontaneously *in utero* (812,813). Because prenatal diagnosis of a number of congenital diseases has become possible, injection of allogeneic PHSC to preimmune human fetuses has been explored and used successfully to correct immunodeficiency diseases diagnosed *in utero* (*814,815*,816). Chimerism was detected in the T-cell compartment afflicted by the congenital deficiency, and not in other hematopoietic lineages. Low levels of chimerism have also been achieved in preimmune normal mouse fetuses and sheep receiving *in utero* transplants *(817)*. In a large-animal model, successful engraftment of enriched human PHSC populations has been successfully achieved without GVHD (*818,819*,820). Although the ability of *in utero* HCT to induce transplantation tolerance has been somewhat unpredictable *(821,822)*, durable chimerism and renal allograft tolerance have recently been achieved in a porcine model involving *in utero* transplantation of T-cell–depleted adult bone marrow *(823)*.

Acquired immune tolerance was first demonstrated by Billingham and colleagues *(824)*, who injected allogeneic cells and tissue lysates into untreated neonatal mice, which then demonstrated unresponsiveness to donor skin grafts. Lasting microchimerism and even sufficient levels of chimerism for flow cytometric detection (macrochimerism) have been observed in some neonatally tolerized mice (825,*826,827*). Both intrathymic and extrathymic deletional mechanisms of tolerance have been implicated in some strain combinations (825,*826*). The presence of microchimerism does not predict skin graft tolerance in perinatally injected mice, and nontolerant animals can maintain microchimerism following donor graft rejection *(828,829)*. Regulatory cells probably play a role in rodents in which neonatal tolerance has been induced, as tolerance cannot be easily broken by the infusion of nontolerant host–type lymphocytes (825,*830,831*). In contrast, when deletional tolerance is induced in animals in which the pre-existing peripheral T-cell response has been fully ablated (e.g., mixed chimeras prepared with the myeloablative or nonmyeloablative regimens previously described), the absence of suppressive cell populations makes it easy to abolish tolerance by the infusion of nontolerant host-type lymphocytes (749,*832*). Neonatal mice tend to produce Th2 responses, which may promote donor-specific skin graft acceptance (*413*,414). However, neonatal mice are capable of mounting CTL and Th1 responses under certain conditions *(833,834)*. The ability of allogeneic spleen cell infusions to induce tolerance may also reflect the high ratio of non-costimulatory APCs (T and B cells) in donor inocula to recipient T cells in the neonate, rather than to any unique susceptibility to tolerance induction *(835)*.

Adult Recipients. Based on the recent observation that microchimerism can exist for many years in the tissues of human recipients of solid-organ allograft recipients who did not receive hematopoietic cell transplants *(836)*, it has been hypothesized that microchimerism, resulting from emigration of passenger leukocytes from the graft to recipient tissues, leads to donor-specific tolerance *(837)*. "Microchimerism," which requires highly sensitive techniques for its detection, should be distinguished from the mixed chimerism previously discussed, in which multilineage chimerism is readily measurable by flow cytometry. Mechanisms by which microchimerism might conceivably promote peripheral T cell tolerance include nonprofessional APC function of donor-derived B or T cells *(838–840)* and veto activity of T cells, NK cells, and other cell types, eliminating CTL reactive against antigens expressed on the veto cells *(841)*. If low numbers of donor hematopoietic stem cells engraft, donor leukocytes migrating to recipient thymi might induce central tolerance among T cells that develop subsequently. Adult rodent liver grafts contain self-renewing hematopoietic stem cells *(842,843)*, and DC progenitors have been detected in the marrow of mice that spontaneously accept mouse liver allografts *(844)*.

However, the hypothesis that microchimerism leads to tolerance is controversial (845), and it is currently unclear whether microchimerism is even associated with tolerance. Lasting microchimerism does not appear to play a role in several animal models of tolerance in which the issue has been carefully examined *(846–848)*, and tolerance is by no means assured in the presence of microchimerism *(849)*. It is also clear in humans that microchimerism neither denotes a state of tolerance nor is required to maintain an allograft under all circumstances (845,*849–851*).

Recently, several groups have evaluated the ability of donor bone marrow cell infusions given without recipient myelosuppression or T-cell depletion to enhance graft survival in recipients of standard chronic immunosuppressive therapy *(852,853)*. Such transplants can be associated with significant risks from possible immunosuppressive effects of the transplant and from GVHD *(854,855)*. Although no significant impact on acute rejection episodes or immunosuppressive medication doses were observed *(854)*, the incidence of chronic renal allograft rejection was significantly reduced on longer follow-up in one of these series (856). Studies with living donor renal transplantation *(857)* or cadaveric liver transplantation (858) did not reveal significant improvements in outcomes or reductions in immunosuppression in recipients of donor bone marrow, despite the persistence of and gradual increase in low levels of chimerism *(857)*.

These studies did not include intentional peripheral T-cell depletion of the hosts. In a nonhuman primate model that includes recipient pretreatment with antilymphocyte serum for T-cell depletion, and, for optimal results, total lymphoid irradiation (TLI), veto cells in donor bone marrow that inactivate recipient CTLp may promote graft acceptance *(859)*. However, only a fraction of recipients show long-term graft acceptance, with the best results obtained when the donor and recipient share a DR class II MHC allele (860). The combination of anti-lymphocyte globulin and TLI with donor BMT has begun to be evaluated in pilot clinical studies (see "From Animal Models to Clinical Transplantation Tolerance").

In contrast to the model using anti-lymphocyte serum without irradiation, macroscopically detectable, though transient, chimerism has been observed in an otherwise similar primate model that includes a sublethal dose of host irradiation (762). The mechanism by which myelosuppressive conditioning promotes marrow engraftment may include both the creation of physical niches due to the destruction of host hematopoietic cells, and the up-regulation of cytokines that promote hematopoiesis. Recent studies have implicated up-regulation of chemokine SDF-1, which binds to stem cell CXCR4, and complement (C3) cleavage fragments in radiation-induced marrow injury and promotion of stem cell homing to that microenvironment *(861)*. In mice, myelosuppression is required to promote engraftment of syngeneic marrow cells given in numbers similar to those that could be obtained from marrow of living human allogeneic marrow donors *(750)*. However, this requirement can be overcome by the administration of very high doses of syngeneic marrow *(862,863)*. Furthermore, engraftment of high doses of allogeneic marrow can be achieved without myelosuppressive treatment in mice that receive T-cell–depleting mAbs *(753)* or costimulatory blockade *(755,756)*. This approach has been successfully extended to a full haplotype-mismatched porcine model *(764)*. These studies demonstrate that multilineage mixed chimerism and lasting, systemic deletional tolerance can be achieved without requiring recipient T-cell depletion or myelosuppression. However, practical approaches to obtaining such numbers of allogeneic PHSC in humans have not yet been developed.

Strategies to Achieve Peripheral Tolerance

Donor Specific Transfusion/Gene Therapy with Autologous Cells

In rodents, donor-specific transfusions (DSTs) have the ability to prolong allograft survival *(864)*, and in certain donor/recipient combinations have been shown to induce operational tolerance *(865)*. In most other species, DST alone has a less dramatic impact on graft outcome, but there is no doubt that it can influence graft survival in a positive manner and even in humans has been shown to be beneficial to graft outcome *(866,867)*. However, alongside these potential positive effects, infusion of cells expressing alloantigens from the organ donor can also have negative effects, including sensitizing the recipient to donor alloantigens, thereby increasing the risk of hyperacute rejection. Moreover, with the introduction of erythropoietin into clinical practice there was no longer a medical need to use transfusions to treat dialysis patients on transplant waiting this; thus, the practice has largely stopped.

Investigations into the mechanisms by which alloantigen infusion or donor antigens released from the graft at the time of transplantation can manipulate the immune response to a subsequent transplant have provided important insights into how the adult immune system can be manipulated *in vivo*. Studies in rodents have shown that the level of unresponsiveness induced varies considerably depending on the quantity and source of alloantigen infused as well as the immune status of the recipient *(868)*. Interestingly, it was not found necessary to pretreat recipients with every donor major and minor histocompatibility antigen they would subsequently encounter on the allograft. Exposure to a single-donor alloantigen was sufficient to induce some graft prolongation as long as the allograft also expressed the same alloantigen (*869*,870). This phenomenon was demonstrated in a number of experimental systems both in models of transplantation and autoimmune disease and is referred to as *linked unresponsiveness* or *suppression* (871,*872,873*). The mechanisms underpinning this effect have subsequently been elucidated and involve regulatory or suppressor T cells *(874)* that once activated can mediate so-called bystander suppression, a mechanism identified initially *in vitro (709)* that also operates *in vivo*, thereby influencing the functional activity of other leukocytes present in the same microenvironment *in vivo* (710).

An alternative strategy to using allogeneic cells for inducing specific unresponsiveness is to manipulate recipient cells to express defined MHC molecules that are subsequently expressed by the graft. The first proof of concept study using this approach transfected a fibroblast cell line of recipient origin with a mouse MHC class I gene, *H2K*^{b} (870). When the transfectants were used to pretreat recipient mice before transplantation, graft survival was prolonged. Obviously, cell lines are not applicable to the clinical situation and therefore recipient or autologous bone marrow cells and hematopoietic stem cells were investigated as alternatives. This approach, using either replication defective retroviral or adenovirus constructs, has permitted markedly prolonged survival of class I–disparate skin grafts bearing the class I gene that was introduced into the autologous marrow *(775)* and fully allogeneic heart allografts *(875)*. In some settings, tolerance to the transduced antigens can be induced either by infusing the transduced cells alone *(876)*, or by combining the transduced cells with other immune modulating agents (*776*,877,*878*).

As with other approaches to tolerance induction, the persistence of the antigen, either in the form of the transduced cells, or after transplantation, from the graft is critical to the maintenance of the unresponsive state *in vivo (879)*.

Tolerogenic APCs

DCs are central to the activation/priming of an immune response, but paradoxically they can also promote the development of tolerance (*880*,881). The key to both functions center on the state of maturation of the DC when it functions *in vivo* and/or its lineage. Initially, immature myeloid DCs that express low levels of MHC class II and costimulatory molecules at the cell surface were identified as the dominant form of DC that had the capacity to induce T-cell tolerance. In contrast, mature myeloid DCs that express much higher levels of both MHC and costimulatory molecules were required for priming T-cell responses. However, mature DCs have subsequently also been shown to have the capacity induce tolerance; therefore, the relationship between the state of maturity of a DC and its tolerogenic potential is now less clear. In addition, plasmacytoid DCs (pDCs) have also been found to have a role in tolerance induction. pDCs were originally defined by their capacity to secrete large amounts of type I interferons in response to viruses and to play an essential role in protecting individuals against inflammatory responses to harmless antigens but they have now also been shown to be able to induce human regulatory T cells *in vitro* that produce significant amounts of IL-10, low IFN-γ, and no IL-4, IL-5, or TGF-β *(712)*. pDCs, unlike myeloid DCs, can rapidly express ICOS-L (ligand of inducible costimulatory protein) on maturation, which has been found to play a key role in the generation of IL-10–producing regulatory T cells *(882)*. In mice, preplasmacytoid DCs appear to be capable of facilitating hematopoietic stem cell engraftment, thereby promoting donor-specific skin graft tolerance in allogeneic recipients *(883)*. However, the exact role and practicality of using preplasmacytoid DCs in this setting requires clarification, as T cells are more abundant and hence more powerful in promoting engraftment. Significantly, donor-derived preplasmacytoid DCs infused 7 days before transplant were found to prolong subsequent heart allograft survival (from 9 to 22 days) in the absence of immunosuppressive therapy *(884)*, but this effect was markedly enhanced by anti-CD154 mAb administration *(885)*.

Immature DCs have been shown to promote tolerance to solid-organ allografts and bone marrow grafts. For example, a single injection of immature donor-derived DCs 7 days before transplantation of an MHC-mismatched heart allograft extends *(886)* or prolongs survival indefinitely *(887)* in a donor-specific manner. The potential tolerogenic effects of immature DCs can be potentiated by the coadministration of immune modulating agents such as costimulation blockade *(888)*. Among several distinct approaches to generate stably immature DCs, pharmacologic manipulation may offer a promising and clinically applicable option. For example, sirolimus has been found to inhibit DC maturation and effector function *(889)*. "Alternatively activated" or "regulatory" DCs, which have low costimulatory ability, were also found to protect MHC-mismatched skin grafts from rejection *(890)* and to protect mice from lethal acute GVHD when administered 7 days before transplantation *(891)*.

Reports showing that mature DCs can induce tolerance despite expressing high levels of MHC and costimulatory molecules include *in vitro* data with human cells demonstrating that maturation of human monocyte-derived DC with TNF-α and prostaglandin E2 triggered cross-priming and proliferation of $CD8^+$ T cells with tolerogenic properties *(892)* and that mature but not immature DCs can prime $CD4^+$ T cells that inhibit allogeneic mixed leukocyte reactions *(893)*. *In vivo*, bone marrow-derived DC matured with TNF-γ, but not lipopolysaccharide or antibody to CD40, protected mice from $CD4^+$ T cell-mediated experimental autoimmune encephalomyelitis, despite the expression of high levels of MHC class II and costimulatory molecules *(894)*.

Taking the data using different populations of DC together, it seems that both myeloid and pDCs can promote tolerance, and that maturation by itself is not the distinguishing feature that separates their immunogenic from their tolerogenic function. Indeed, maturation is more of a continuum than an "on-off" switch, and a "semimature" state, in which DCs are phenotypically mature but remain poor producers or proinflammatory cytokines, appears to be linked to tolerogenic function (895). The combination of DCs administered with costimulatory blockade may be the most promising approach identified thus far.

T-cell Depleting Antibodies

Many tolerance induction strategies that have been investigated in small- and large-animal studies have used depletion of leukocytes (antithymocyte globulin, anti-CD52) or T cells (anti-CD3 with or without immunotoxin, CD2, CD4, and CD8) to create an environment *in vivo* that allows "reprogramming of the immune system" (896). In small animals, the short-term depletion of T cells, in combination with an allograft, appears to be sufficient in some situations for tolerance to develop and be maintained in the long term. The success rate can be enhanced by removing the thymus before transplantation to prevent repopulation of the periphery with T cells after transplantation *(897)*. Initial data from primates using immunotoxin conjugated anti-CD3 alone before transplantation or in combination with deoxyspergualin, a drug which inhibits NF-κB and therefore monocytes and macrophages, at the time of transplantation suggested that T-cell depletion can be used to induce tolerance to donor alloantigens *(898–900)*. However, follow-up trials in humans undergoing renal transplantation and T-cell depletion with the anti-CD52 monoclonal antibody alemtuzumab with or without deoxyspergualin revealed that neither profound T-cell depletion alone or in combination with deoxyspergualin induced tolerance in humans *(901,902)*. However, clinical results, across organ systems, reveal that steroid-free regimens with reduced maintenance doses of immunosuppression may be used after alemtuzumab therapy (*903*,904,*905*).

Depletion of leukocytes at the time of transplantation creates a transient immunodeficiency in the recipient, compromising the recipient's ability to reject the transplant. The degree and duration of leukocyte depletion achieved determine how effective and for how long the graft is protected from immune attack *(906,907)*. The downstream events that occur once leukocytes begin to reappear in the recipient's circulation are not understood clearly. Studies using TCR transgenic recipients have shown that when leukocytes are depleted, the maintenance of tolerance depends on transplantation of the graft within a time window of depletion of donor-reactive cells in the thymus and periphery *(908)*. If the organ graft is transplanted at the appropriate time, donor-reactive cells fail to repopulate from the thymus in an antigen-selective manner. Although donor-reactive cells do not reappear in the periphery, cells with reactivity to other antigens repopulated the periphery of recipients with long-term surviving organ grafts. These data can be used to suggest a mechanism for the long-term survival observed in primates treated with anti-CD3 immunotoxin complex. In this case one can argue that the $CD3^+$ T cells are depleted by the immunotoxin before transplantation. A window of opportunity is created such that when a renal allograft is transplanted, no donor-reactive cells are present in the periphery. As cells repopulate the periphery with time after the transplantation, donor-reactive cells are deleted or eliminated as a result of the presence of the surviving graft.

Costimulatory Blockade and Other Biological Proteins

With Solid Organs. T-cell activation, and hence rejection, depends on multiple signals. Cell-surface costimulatory molecules provide "signal 2." which, when combined with "signal 1" through TCR, triggers the activation of naïve T cells *(909,910)*. When signal 1 is forced to act on its own, T cells have been shown to undergo anergy or apoptosis (627). The original concept of a single costimulatory pathway has long been superseded and it is now clear that there are multiple levels at which costimulation can participate both in initiating and determining the direction that an immune response takes (911). Nevertheless, targeting costimulatory pathways with either monoclonal antibodies or recombinant fusion proteins specific for the costimulatory molecule itself or the ligand with which it interacts can be very effective at suppressing immune responses and in some cases may have the capacity to induce tolerance to donor antigens *in vivo*.

Members of the immunoglobulin and TNF/TNFR superfamilies make up many of the costimulatory molecules that are integral to positive costimulation in the pathway of T-cell activation. Two pairs of ligand-receptor interactions that seem to play key roles in positive costimulation are CD40/CD40-ligand (CD154), which are members of the TNF/TNFR superfamily and CD80/CD86 and CD28, which belong to the Ig superfamily (911). Although the precise role that each of these costimulatory pathways plays during rejection and tolerance is still not completely understood, the complete abrogation or attenuation of either of these pathways can modulate the immune response to an allograft *in vivo*. Recent development of CD28 blockade by CTLA-4Ig (Abatacept) for rheumatoid arthritis and clinical trials with modified CTLA-4 Ig (Belatacept) for transplantation shows promise for the utilization of costimulation blockade in suppressing effector responses (912,913).

The B7:CD28/CTLA-4 Pathway. CD80(B7-1) and CD86(B7-2) are expressed as cell surface molecules by APCs and are responsible for delivering additional signals to T cells when they interact with CD28. CD86 and CD80 can also interact with a second molecule, CD152 (CTLA4), which is expressed by T cells later in the activation process and is expressed constitutively by regulatory T cells. CD86 and CD80 can exhibit preferential binding to CD28 and CD152, respectively *(914)*. In contrast to CD28, CTLA4 negatively regulates T-cell activation when it engages its ligand on the APC and, as described previously, is implicated in normal homeostasis in the immune system *(915)*. However, the precise role that CTLA4 plays during T-cell activation and regulation requires further clarification *(916)*. CTLA4 is pivotal in regulating the threshold of signals during T-cell activation and recent findings suggest that up-regulation of CTLA-4 expression increases T-cell motility and overrides the TCR-induced stop signal required for stable conjugate formation between T cells and APCs. This results in reduced contact periods between T cells and APCs, leading to decreased cytokine production and proliferation *(916)*.

Using the B7:CD28/CTLA-4 Pathway for Therapeutics. When CTLA4Ig, an immunoglobulin fusion protein of CTLA4, was produced, it was shown to inhibit graft rejection in xenogeneic and allogeneic systems *(917,918)*. In rodent models, CTLA4Ig therapy has been shown to have the capacity to induce tolerance to some types of grafts (*917*,919), an effect that was enhanced when infused donor antigen was included in the treatment protocol (919,*920,921*). This effect has not been found in every experimental model examined, however. For example, the use of CTLA4Ig monotherapy in primates has not been reported to be capable of inducing long-term graft survival *(922)*.

The mechanism by which CTLA4Ig promotes graft survival has been investigated in a mouse model. Blockade of CD80 and CD86 at the time of alloantigen recognition has been suggested to trigger T-cell apoptosis in the early phase after transplantation (625); however, it should be noted that no specific markers for alloantigen-specific T cells were incorporated into this analysis and therefore more detailed studies to confirm this property would add value. When an antiapoptotic gene, *bcl-*x_L, was expressed in the responding lymphocytes, deletion did not occur, and graft prolongation was prevented. This finding suggests that CTLA4Ig facilitates the development of long-term graft function by reducing the number of donor-reactive cells that have to be controlled downstream in the posttransplant course.

Although primate models using CTLA4Ig to induce tolerance proved to be largely unsuccessful, the theoretical foundation of blocking this pathway to promote graft survival continued to intrigue researchers. Additionally, it was known that the binding properties of CTLA4 could be manipulated to optimize the ligation of both CD80 and CD86, a crucial component to experimental efforts at tolerance induction (912).

Belatacept. Experiments using CTLA4Ig laid the groundwork for further development of therapeutic agents targeting the B7:CD28/CTLA4 pathway. Belatacept, LEA29Y, was originally derived from the fusion protein CTLA4Ig, or Abatacept (913,*923*). It differs from CTLA4Ig by two amino acids, conferring an approximately twofold increased binding capacity to CD80 and CD86. This increase in avidity allows for a tenfold increase in the *in vitro* suppression of T-cell activation when compared with CTLA4Ig and in nonhuman primate studies, Belatacept was found to prolong renal allograft survival and inhibit donor-specific alloantibody production both alone and in combination with other traditionally used immunosuppressive regimens *(923)*. These and other findings allowed for the translation of LEA29Y to renal transplant patients in the clinics. To date, results of phase 2 trials comparing Belatacept with cyclosporine in partially randomized studies across 22 centers in North America and Europe of more than 200 patients suggest that Belatacept is not inferior to cyclosporine. In fact, results of this trial revealed that patients with Belatacept-based therapy had improved renal function, reduction in chronic allograft nephropathy, and decreased calcineurin-related toxicity *(924)*. Additionally, recent experiments in nonhuman primates using neonatal porcine islet grafts have revealed long-term xenograft survival under the cover of CD28-CD154 blockade with maintenance immunosuppression of sirolimus and Belatacept (925). Although promising, further trials and vigilant follow-ups are necessary to accurately assess the efficacy of these new therapeutic regimens.

CD40-CD154 Pathway. The CD40-CD154 pathway has been targeted to inhibit graft rejection using monoclonal antibody therapy either alone (*926,927,928*) or in combination with alloantigen infusion (*929*). CD154, or CD40-ligand, is a type 2 membrane protein of the TNF family and is expressed predominantly by activated CD4$^+$ T cells and by a small proportion of CD8$^+$ T cells, NK cells and eosinophils (*930*), and, significantly, on platelets as well (*931*). Structural models predict that CD154 forms a homotrimer that binds to CD40 on the surface of APCs. CD40 is expressed by B cells, macrophages, DCs, thymic epithelium, and is inducible on the surface of endothelial cells and fibroblasts.

The CD40-CD154 pathway interaction is pivotal for the induction of humoral and cellular responses to nominal antigens as well as alloantigens. A CD40-Ig fusion protein and a blocking monoclonal antibody to CD154 were shown to inhibit B-cell cycling, proliferation, and differentiation into plasma cells in response to T-cell–dependent antigens (*932*). *In vivo* studies using CD154 monoclonal antibody or CD40 or CD154 knockout mice (*933,934*) demonstrated a crucial role for this interaction in the generation of primary and secondary humoral responses to T-cell–dependent antigens, class switching, and development of germinal centers. The lack of a humoral response in the absence of CD40-CD40L interaction is caused not only by a lack of signalling through CD40 on the B-cell surface, but also the inhibition of priming of CD4$^+$ T cells through CD40L (*935*).

CD40 triggering on the APC primes the APC for stimulation. Signals through CD40 have been shown to upregulate expression of CD80 and CD86, as well as induce IL-12 (*936*). Activation of DCs through CD40 promotes their ability to present antigen to T cells; this may explain why targeting CD154 and blocking its ability to interact with CD40 has a profound effect on T-cell–dependent immune responses *in vivo*. If modification of APC function is also a route to the development of tolerance *in vivo*, as previously outlined, blocking CD154-CD40 interactions may also influence tolerance induction by altering both the interaction and signals between APC and immunoregulatory and suppressor T cells (*937*).

Using the CD40-CD154 Pathway for Therapeutic Intervention in Cell and Organ Transplantation. Long-term acceptance of cardiac, renal, and islet allografts in several mouse and nonhuman primate models has been achieved with CD40 blockade using anti-CD154 monoclonal antibody as monotherapy or in conjunction with CTLA4Ig (*926,929,938,939*). With the exception of BMT, in which durable chimerism and tolerance can be achieved with anti-CD154 mAb (see later discussion), so-called tolerant states generated by anti-CD154 therapy alone have been shown to disappear when therapy is withdrawn, leading to rejection. Even with CD28 blockade, anti-CD154 therapy must be sustained to promote permanent engraftment of cardiac or islet grafts (*938,940,941*).

Although promising results were reported in experimental models, anti-CD154 therapy was found to have the unexpected complication of thrombogenesis. It was then that CD154 was found to play key roles in coagulation and clotting, with some reports suggesting that CD154 acts to stabilize thrombi while others implicate CD154 in platelet activation (*933*). Whatever the role that CD154 may play in transplantation tolerance, it is clear that this molecule acts via independent pathways in a variety of cascades unrelated to tolerance induction.

Interest in this approach was also reflected in reports that a humanized monoclonal antibody specific for CD154 (hu5c8) was capable of prolonging the survival of renal and islet allografts in rhesus monkeys (*922,927,942*). The initial data from these primate studies appeared encouraging, with rejection-free survival of the kidney grafts, provided that antibody therapy at a relatively high dose (25 mg/kg) was continued in the first 6 months posttransplant. When anti-CD154 therapy was discontinued after the first month posttransplant, rejection episodes did occur. Analysis of the status of recipients with long-term surviving grafts showed that peripheral lymphocytes from the monkeys failed to respond *in vitro* to donor antigens, but the recipients developed antidonor antibodies, and biopsy samples from some of the long-term surviving grafts revealed T-cell infiltrates. Together, these observations were sufficiently encouraging to initiate a pilot clinical study using hu5c8 in renal transplantation. In this study, hu5c8 was administered to seven patients with low-dose steroid alone and five patients experienced episodes of rejection (943).

Other variants of costimulatory blockade that target different epitopes of CD154 have been developed with hopes of improved tolerance induction and without promotion of thrombogenesis. Recent experimental results in cardiac allografts of cynomolgus monkeys treated with an inhibitor of CD154, IDEC-131, either alone or in combination with leukocyte depletion in the form of antithymocyte globulin prolonged allograft survival; however, tolerance was not induced, as alloantibody production and transplant vasculopathy, while delayed, still occurred (944). Recently, the utilization of triple therapy with an abbreviated course of mTOR inhibition (sirolimus), a donor-specific transfusion, and IDEC-131 prevented allograft rejection and induced operational tolerance in rhesus monkeys undergoing MHC-mismatched renal transplantation (945). Still other anti-CD154 antibodies, such as ABI793, have been developed, but have also been plagued with continued thromboembolic complications (946).

To understand why CD154 blockade was effective in some but not other settings, an analysis in the mouse revealed that that only when rejection depended on CD4$^+$ T cells was CD154 blockade on its own effective at prolonging graft survival. In fact, in donor-recipient combinations in which CD8 T cells also play a role in rejection, many studies have shown that the CD8 T cell subset is unaffected by CD154 monoclonal antibody therapy *(947,948)* such that CD8 T cells become activated, proliferate, and home to the graft in the presence of high-dose continued anti-CD154 monoclonal antibody therapy *in vivo (948)*.

Further studies have been undertaken to evaluate antibodies to CD40 in order to bypass the potential ramifications of CD154 blockade. Initial animal knockout models revealed a propensity of CD154 knockout mice to develop unstable thrombi, a phenomenon not seen in CD40 knockout mice *(949)*. Preliminary studies in the rhesus monkey renal allograft model reveal somewhat promising results with a short course of low-dose calcineurin inhibitor administered concomitantly with anti-CD40/anti-CD86 costimulation blockade (950). In this study, two of four animals developed 3-year drug-free graft survival, and none of the animals developed alloantibodies to the donor, suggestive of tolerance induction (950).

Targeting CD3 and Accessory Molecules. Initially, administration of depleting anti-CD4 and anti-CD8 monoclonal antibodies was shown to result in prolonged graft survival *(951–953)*. That this treatment strategy resulted in antigen-specific tolerance was first shown most clearly when a protein antigen was administered in conjunction with a depleting anti-CD4 monoclonal antibody *(954–956)*. Refinements of these types of protocols have resulted in the ability to achieve long-term T-cell unresponsiveness to protein and alloantigens in the absence of T-cell depletion in experimental models *(957–959)*. In fact, many other accessory molecules, other than anti-CD4 and anti-CD8, have been targeted in an attempt to induce tolerance in models of bone marrow *(960,961)*, islet *(962–964)*, renal *(965)*, and cardiac allografts *(961,966,967)*, to name a few.

OKT3, a murine antihuman CD3 monoclonal antibody, received approval for human use in 1986 in kidney transplant patients undergoing rejection and eventually for liver and cardiac transplant recipients as well (968). Although widely used, OKT3 brings with it the undesired complications of the human antimouse antibody response as well as a first-dose reaction characterized by fevers, chills, gastrointestinal, respiratory, and cardiac complications *(969,970)*. These ramifications are thought to be the result of T-cell activation and subsequent cytokine release (968). Therefore, many investigators have attempted to construct pharmacotherapeutics that mimic the efficacy of OKT3 with less immunogenicity. A few of these OKT3-derived molecules in preliminary studies such as hu12F6, hOKT3gamma1 (Ala-Ala), and ChAglyCD3 have proven to be more effective in T-cell suppression and less immunogenic when compared with OKT3 (968,*971,972*).

Along with anti-CD3, antibodies to CD11a (leukocyte function associated antigen-1, LFA-1) and its ligands, ICAM-1, -2, and -3, have been investigated and have led to prolonged graft survival in many of the aforementioned models. LFA-1 has been implicated as an essential molecule for cellular trafficking and motility as well as T-cell activation *(973,974)*. Additionally, reports also suggest that the interaction of LFA-1 and the ICAM molecules serve as a costimulatory pairing for T-cell activation *(975)*.

Operational tolerance induced by these strategies has been shown to develop over several weeks after the initial antigen encounter *(976,977)*. When a combination of donor antigen and monoclonal antibody therapy targeting accessory molecules is used, the precise mechanism of tolerance induction in part depends on the amount of antigen infused *(959)*. Deletion also may be used as one of the mechanisms of tolerance initially *(868,978)*, but in the absence of complete deletion of donor-reactive cells, immunoregulation develops. When antibodies targeting accessory molecules are used as therapeutic agents at the time of transplantation, immunoregulation is the dominant mechanism that comes into play to maintain tolerance in the longer term *(979)*.

In these systems, tolerance to donor antigens is induced and/or maintained as a result of the development of a population of regulatory and suppressor T cells that can mediate unresponsiveness to the initiating donor antigen as well as other antigens present on the graft, the phenomenon of linked unresponsiveness *(980)*. In mice and rats, this type of tolerance has been shown to be infectious *(691)*; it can be transferred from one generation of cells to another, provided there is sufficient period of contact between the two populations.

The maintenance of tolerance in these systems requires the persistent presence of antigen in the form of the organ when the thymus is still functional *(981)*. In the absence of donor antigen, tolerance is eventually lost, presumably as a result of the export of naïve cells T cells from the thymus into the periphery. Quantitatively, if these cells fail to encounter antigen, they eventually outnumber the unresponsive T cells induced by the monoclonal antibody therapy.

Costimulatory Blockade with Infusion of Donor Hematopoietic Cells

Although long-term tolerance is maintained by intrathymic deletion in mixed chimeras prepared with costimulatory blockade (751,*755,757*), initial tolerance of peripheral T cells involves specific deletion of donor-reactive CD4 (652,751,*982,983*) and CD8 (485) T cells. The deletion of CD4 cells achieved following BMT with anti-CD154 is not due to binding of anti-CD154 mAb to activated T cells, and only requires failure of the CD154-CD40 interaction *(984)*. This CD4 cell deletion is Fas-independent and is not blocked by cyclosporine, arguing against a role for "activation-induced cell death" *(983)*, which, in contrast, is thought to be involved in tolerance induction with anti-CD154 mAb plus rapamycin *(717)*. Peripheral deletion of donor-reactive CD8 cells has been observed both in mice receiving donor-specific transfusions and/or BMT with costimulatory blockade (485,*623,624*). CD8 deletion occurs within 1 to 2 weeks and requires the presence of CD25-negative CD4 cells (485). CD4 regulatory cells are not required for maintenance of tolerance after this initial 2-week period (485). Deletion of donor-reactive CD4 cells occurs more slowly, over 4 to 5 weeks, and is preceded by a state of specific anergy toward the donor (652,*984*). Regulatory cells do not appear to play a major role in maintaining the long-term tolerance induced by costimulatory blockade with BMT because tolerance and chimerism are obliterated by the infusion of relatively small numbers of nontolerant recipient-type spleen cells in this model and linked suppression is not observed (652). Because hematopoietic stem cell engraftment ensures complete central deletional tolerance in these long-term chimeras (751,*755,757,982*), and specific peripheral deletion is quite complete, there may be insufficient donor-reactive T cells present to induce the expansion and maintenance of specific regulatory cells.

Administration of DST under cover of blocking anti-CD40L mAb prevents islet allograft rejection *(938)*. Like BMT, the use of DST involves administration of hematopoietic cells, but only BMT with mixed chimerism induction leads to engraftment of hematopoietic stem cells and intrathymic deletion as the mechanism maintaining long-term tolerance *(752,755)*. In thymectomized mice, the combination of DST and anti-CD40L leads to long-term skin graft survival in fully MHC-mismatched recipients *(491)*. In euthymic mice, only a small fraction of animals achieve long-term skin graft survival with this treatment *(929)* indicating the failure to establish central tolerance without hematopoietic stem cell chimerism *(623)*. In addition, the inability to resist breaking of tolerance by new thymic emigrants in this model argues that powerful peripheral regulatory mechanisms (suppression) are not operative in these animals. However, regulatory mechanisms may play a role in the initial suppression of alloresponses, as depletion of CD4 cells abrogated skin graft acceptance *(491)*. Both CTLA4 and IFN-γ have been shown to play an important role in the induction of tolerance in this model *(491,496,985)*. CTLA4 appears to also be critical for the achievement of mixed chimerism and tolerance with BMT and anti-CD154 mAb (J. Kurtz and M. Sykes, unpublished data, 1998), but IFN-γ and IL-2 do not play a requisite role (485), consistent with the lack of requirement for "natural" regulatory cells. DST in this model promotes peripheral deletion of donor-reactive CD8 T cells *(623)*, and can be replaced by CD8 depletion with mAb *(985)*. The combination of anti-CD154, BMT and DST seems to be particularly effective in achieving mixed chimerism, largely because of the capacity of DST to overcome residual CD8 T cell-mediated alloresistance *(624,986)*.

Costimulatory blockers have been explored for the induction of graft-versus-host tolerance in order to prevent GVHD in BMT recipients. GVHD has been inhibited by B7/CD28 blockade or anti-CD154 mAb *(987–989)*. Pre-BMT exposure of donor T cells to recipient alloantigens in the presence of anti-CD40L inhibits GVHD via a mechanism involving CD25$^+$ regulatory CD4 cells (682). Clinically, a reduced incidence of acute GVHD has been observed in leukemic patients receiving HLA-mismatched bone marrow transplants that had been exposed to recipient alloantigens in the presence of CD28 blockade with CTLA4Ig *(990)*. Blockade of 4–1BB/4–1BBL costimulatory interaction can also suppress GVHD and GVL *(991)*.

A Large animal Tolerance Model

MHC-defined, inbred miniature swine have provided an instructive model for delineation of the role of various histoincompatibilities in tolerance and rejection in large animals. Studies of pig renal transplantation have demonstrated that spontaneous tolerance can be induced by organ grafts when MHC antigens are matched. The ability to achieve such tolerance depends on one or possibly two non–MHC-linked genetic loci in the recipient animals. The presence of the "acceptor" phenotype also permits the spontaneous acceptance of single haplotype class I–mismatched kidney grafts *(9)*. Graft acceptance is associated with donor-specific CTL unresponsiveness, apparently because of a deficiency in help for these CTL, and not because of a deletional mechanism. Thus, in class II–matched, class I–mismatched porcine donor-recipient pairs, a 12-day course of high-dose (10 mg/kg/day) CsA permits long-term renal allograft acceptance in 100% of cases *(9)*.

The requirement that class II antigens be matched between donor and recipient in order for this tolerance to be achieved may reflect the influence of a major difference in class II antigen expression that exists between large and small animals. Unlike large animals and man, in which class II antigens are expressed constitutively on vascular endothelial cells, the corresponding endothelial cells of rodent species do not express MHC class II molecules *(992,993)*. Consistent with this interpretation, the use of a short course of CsA can facilitate the ability of renal allografts to induce tolerance in rodents across fully MHC-mismatched barriers, but tolerance induction in swine requires class II matching between donor and recipient for uniform success.

Animals accepting class II matched allografts are systemically tolerant to the donor's class I and minor antigens, as indicated by the fact that the accepted graft can be removed and replaced by a second donor-matched graft, which is accepted without immunosuppressive therapy. This ability of CsA to facilitate tolerance induction, and the ability of exogenous IL-2 to prevent the induction of tolerance in this model *(9)*, are consistent with the interpretation that induction of tolerance of donor class I–reactive CTL is due, at least in part, to the absence of adequate T-cell "help" during the time of initial exposure to antigen. A selective decrease of expression of the Th1-associated cytokine IFN-γ relative to the Th2-associated cytokine IL-10 has been observed in these accepted grafts *(994)*. The thymus appears to play a role in the induction of tolerance among pre-existing peripheral T cells in this model, as removal of the host thymus prior to kidney allotransplantation leads to rejection *(995)*. The possible mechanisms responsible for this role of the thymus in inducing peripheral tolerance phenomena are discussed elsewhere in this chapter. The kidney allograft itself clearly plays an important role in the tolerance induced in this model. Class II–matched cardiac allografts are not accepted after a similar short course of CsA, but they are accepted if grafted to animals that are tolerized in this manner to kidney allografts bearing the same mismatched class I alleles as the donor heart *(538)*. The mechanisms of this tolerance have been demonstrated to involve regulatory T cells that can specifically suppress antidonor CTL responses (*996,997,998,999*).

The Relationship Between Peripheral T-Cell Tolerance and Central Tolerance

In the pig model previously described, the thymus plays a role in the induction of tolerance among pre-existing peripheral T cells *(995)*. It is possible that T cells that are activated in the periphery by the organ allograft recirculate to the thymus *(1000)*, and may be tolerized there, with or without encounter with donor antigen. Alternatively, the migration of donor antigens or cells to the thymus may induce the development of regulatory T cells that specifically recognize the donor antigens and down-regulate alloreactive T cells when they enter the periphery *(1001,1002)*. The role of the thymus in the development of Treg has already been discussed previously. Finally, it is possible that recent thymic emigrants are required for the peripheral development of regulatory cells.

A second model involving the thymus in peripheral tolerance involves injection of donor antigens intrathymically. The initial idea underlying this approach was to use antibody treatment to deplete peripheral T cells and to induce central tolerance among recovering T cells by direct introduction of antigen into the thymus. However, more recent studies have shown that tolerance can be induced by intrathymic injection of soluble alloantigens without peripheral T-cell depletion *(1003)*. Because removal of the thymus before or within the first few days of allografting results in rejection of the allograft *(1004)*, the thymus must play an active role in tolerizing pre-existing peripheral T cells, possibly by one of the mechanisms proposed in the preceding paragraph. Evidence has been obtained for recirculation of activated donor-reactive T cells to the recipient thymus in this model *(1005,1006)*, and active regulatory cell populations have been described *(1007)*. Transferable tolerance is not induced by intrathymic marrow injection alone without an organ allograft in rats *(1008)*, suggesting that the graft itself helps to tolerize the pre-existing T-cell repertoire. The intrathymic injection approach has not been successful in "high-responder" rat strain combinations *(1008,1009)*, and has not successfully allowed xenotolerance induction. Furthermore, chronic rejection of cardiac allografts was not prevented by intrathymic injection of donor spleen cells in antilymphocyte serum-treated rats *(1010)*. While one attempt to use this approach in nonhuman primates was discouraging *(1011)*, donor-specific skin graft prolongation was reported in three animals receiving allogeneic or xenogeneic (human) CD34^{+} cells intrathymically *(1012)*.

From Animal Models to Clinical Transplantation Tolerance

Almost every transplant clinician has treated patients who have chosen to withdraw immunosuppressive therapy for a variety of reasons. The majority of such patients reject their allograft, but rare cases achieve "spontaneous" tolerance in this manner, demonstrating that tolerance can be achieved in humans. Extensive efforts are underway to identify markers that would distinguish such tolerant patients prospectively before withdrawal of immunosuppression, but so far none have been proven to be reliable. Although clinical trials have already begun in which tolerance inducing strategies are combined with conventional pharmacologic immunosuppression, none of the strategies for achieving transplantation tolerance have been used to replace such chronic therapy in a large clinical series. In general, short-term results of most organ allograft transplants are excellent, making it essential to have extremely reliable methods of inducing tolerance in order to ethically justify their use in place of conventional chronic immunosuppressive therapies. Because the risk of rejection due to immunosuppression withdrawal is difficult to accept in patients, it is our opinion that extension of results from animal models to humans should only be attempted after: (i) rodent studies have demonstrated robust tolerance in multiple strain combinations using extensively histoincompatible, highly immunogenic grafts such as skin; (ii) efficacy has been demonstrated in large animal models; and (iii) acceptable toxicity has been demonstrated in large-animal models. When complete removal of immunosuppression can be achieved, the level of toxicity accepted in the short term may be somewhat higher than that which could be accepted on a long-term basis.

Although induction of central deletional tolerance with hematopoietic cell grafts is a reliable and durable approach to achieving permanent graft survival, earlier techniques for achieving central tolerance have involved more vigorous ablation of the lymphohematopoietic system than can be safely achieved in larger animals. Thus, the major challenge in bringing the mixed chimerism/central tolerance approach to clinical application is to develop highly specific, nontoxic methods of conditioning the host for acceptance of a hematopoietic allograft or xenograft. The extensive animal data that have been accumulated on the ability of mixed chimerism induced with reduced intensity conditioning to achieve robust transplantation tolerance, including its demonstration in large-animal models (762,*1013*), combined with clinical data obtained in patients with a more conventional indication for HCT, have allowed clinical evaluation of this approach for tolerance induction. Mixed chimerism can be achieved with reduced toxicity using nonmyeloablative conditioning in patients with hematologic malignancies *(770)*, and lymphohematopoietic GVH reactions induced by DLI can be used to achieve graft-versus-tumor effects *(771)*. These observations provided an opportunity to evaluate the potential of this approach to induce transplantation tolerance in patients with a hematologic malignancy, multiple myeloma, and consequent renal failure. Six patients have received a simultaneous nonmyeloablative bone marrow transplant and renal allograft from HLA-identical siblings, and have accepted their kidney grafts without any immunosuppression for periods as long as 9 years, with very good tumor responses. Similar to the primate model previously described, in which BMT has been shown to be essential for tolerance induction *(1014)*, chimerism in several of these patients was only transient (772), suggesting that the kidney graft itself may participate in tolerance induction and/or maintenance after chimerism has played its initial role. Mechanistic studies performed in these patients suggest that tolerance may be specific for donor antigens expressed by the kidney, while responses to antigens expressed on hematopoietic cells but not the kidney may even be sensitized (772). Additional data suggest a possible role for regulatory cells in maintaining tolerance in such patients, but the precise nature of these cells is unclear (772). The promising results obtained in these patients have provided an important proof of principle, and another trial has now been initiated at the Massachusetts General Hospital in patients without malignancy who receive HLA-mismatched haploidentical bone marrow and kidney grafts with a regimen that leads to transient mixed chimerism without GVHD. Four of five patients receiving combined kidney and bone marrow transplantation with this protocol have achieved graft survival of immunosuppression for periods of one to >4 years. These patients show *in vitro* evidence of systemic donor-specific underesponsivness (1015). Thus, proof of principle has been obtained that organ allograft tolerance can be achieved across HLA barriers in humans using non-myeloablative bone marrow transplantation. Efforts to achieve HLA-mismatched kidney allograft tolerance with donor BMT using the TLI/anti-thymocyte globulin conditioning regimen were unsuccessful *(761)*, but this approach did succeed in one patient receiving an HLA-identical donor transplant (1016).

Most techniques to achieve peripheral tolerance in larger animals have not been as effective as in rodent models. Furthermore, peripheral mechanisms alone have not been sufficient to reliably overcome the most stringent transplantation barrier imposed by fully MHC-mismatched primary skin allografts in rodents. The "infectious" nature of suppressive mechanisms of tolerance makes them potentially attractive as a means of inducing robust and durable tolerance. However, it will be difficult to control the development of such mechanisms until they are better understood. It seems likely that the optimal approach to achieving clinical transplantation tolerance might require combinations of both central and peripheral strategies.

TRANSPLANTATION OF SPECIFIC ORGANS AND TISSUES

Kidney Transplantation

Kidneys are the most frequently transplanted human organs, with approximately 10,000 kidney transplants being performed annually in the United States. Renal allograft survival has increased steadily since its inception, and at present there is more than 95% patient survival and more than 91% organ survival at 1 year *(1017)* However, even well-matched recipients of renal transplants must continue to take immunosuppressive medications for the rest of their lives, with complications including an increased risk of infection, cancer, hypertension, and metabolic bone disease. In addition, even when immunosuppression is well managed, there is an inexorable loss of kidneys to chronic rejection at a rate of approximately 5% to 7% per year. Both of these problems might be eliminated by the induction of tolerance. However, the success of clinical transplantation using immunosuppressive drugs has made it difficult to justify the risk of new approaches to tolerance. Only recently have clinical trials of tolerance induction for renal transplantation begun in earnest ([772,1015,1016] and see previous section).

As for other organs, a major obstacle in kidney transplantation is the shortage of organs, which has been a paradoxical consequence of the success of this field. Unlike hearts and livers, where the inadequate supply of cadaveric organs spells death for many potential recipients, candidates for renal transplants are instead faced with long periods on dialysis while they wait for a kidney. This waiting time can be 4 or more years even for unsensitized candidates, and even greater for those with high levels of sensitization. To avoid this delay, many patients are now being offered kidneys from living donors, and in many transplant centers the number of living donor renal transplants performed per year now exceeds the number of transplants from cadaveric donors.

Sensitization of renal transplant candidates usually results from prior antigen exposure, either by blood transfusions or previous transplants. Such highly sensitized patients are said to have "high panel reactivity"; they may wait many years to obtain a kidney that is crossmatch–negative, and some never receive a transplant at all. Indeed, as discussed later, these patients may be among the first to benefit if and when xenotransplantation becomes a clinical reality (1018).

Finally, as previously discussed, "chronic rejection" of kidney transplants is a continuing problem to the field and probably involves both immunologic reactivity and other factors, including the effects of the early ischemic injury and the ongoing effects of drugs and metabolic abnormalities in the recipient *(452)*. This process leads to an inexorable loss of organs at the rate of approximately 5% to 7% per year. Thus, although the 1-year survival rate for kidney transplants has improved from approximately 40% to more than 90% during the past 40 years, at 5 years there is only 71% graft survival and the half-life for kidney transplants has barely increased, remaining less than 10 years.

Liver Transplantation

Transplantation of the liver represents a major technical challenge. For this reason the organ and patient survival rates have not been as high as those for renal transplantation, but have nevertheless increased yearly, with a current 1-year organ survival rate of about 80% and patient survival rate of about 86% *(1017)*. There are currently about 6,000 liver transplants carried out in the United States per year. The severe shortage of available organs has recently led to use of living donors, although the number is still small, accounting for only about 5% of liver transplants, or about 300 cases per year in the United States. Living donation constitutes a higher proportion of liver transplants in countries such as Japan, where cadaveric donation is less widely accepted.

Immunologically, the liver is relatively resistant to early antibody-mediated rejection, allowing successful transplantation even across blood group barriers and in the face of a positive crossmatch, although a negative crossmatch is generally considered preferable *(1019–1021)*. In addition, long-term survival of liver transplants does not appear to be improved by HLA matching between donor and recipient *(1021)*. Both of these immunologic features may be responsible for the fact that the long-term results of liver transplantation are almost as good as those for kidney, with 65% graft survival and 71% patient survival at 5 years. Finally, transplantation of the liver carries with it large numbers of donor lymphoid cells, thus creating the potential for inducing GVHD *(1023)*. The symptoms can range from antibody-dependent hemolysis of recipient red blood cells across a blood group incompatibility to severe or even fatal, full-blown GVHD.

Heart and Lung Transplantation

There are approximately 2,000 heart transplants performed annually in the United States. As might be expected for this vital organ, the 1-year statistics for heart transplantation are approximately the same for patient (87%) and graft (86%) survival *(1017)*. One of the immunologic issues of particular importance in heart transplantation is the high rate of atherosclerotic disease in the coronary arteries of the donor organ, due at least partly to chronic rejection, as previously discussed. Nevertheless, patient and graft survivals are about 70% for heart transplants at 5 years.

The number of lung transplants performed annually in the United States is approximately 1,200, while only about 30 combined heart and lung transplants are performed. The statistics for lung transplant survival are about the same as for liver (82% graft survival and 83% patient survival) over the first year, but then decrease much faster, with 5-year survivals of only about 45% for grafts and 46% for patients *(1017)*. A major cause of graft loss is a process called *bronchiolitis obliterans*, thought to be the pulmonary manifestation of chronic rejection *(1024)*. However, these patients are also highly susceptible to pulmonary infections, which undoubtedly contributes to the poor long-term statistics.

Pancreas and Islet Transplantation

Transplantation of the whole pancreas was almost without success until about. 1980, largely for technical reasons. More recently, successful pancreas transplantation to treat diabetes mellitus has been achieved using new technical approaches, and with success rates of about 92% at 1 year, approaching those for kidney transplantation, as long as the two organs are transplanted together. There are approximately 850 simultaneous kidney/pancreas transplants per year in the United States. The lower survival rates (77% graft survival at 1 year) achieved when pancreas transplantation is performed alone (about 500 cases annually) probably reflect the difficulty in diagnosing rejection episodes involving this organ. By the time blood sugar levels begin to rise, destruction of the pancreas is generally so far advanced that it cannot be reversed by immunosuppressive therapy. Measurement of the serum creatinine, reflecting early dysfunction of a simultaneous kidney transplant, allows much earlier detection of rejection activity and, thus, better outcomes.

Simultaneous transplantation of both a kidney and a pancreas from a single donor has demonstrated, surprisingly, that rejection activity in one organ is not always associated with rejection activity in the other. It is not known whether this occasional dichotomy reflects tissue-specific antigens or localized inflammatory events in one, but not the other organ.

Most pancreas transplantation is carried out as a curative treatment for diabetes mellitus. For this purpose, the potential also exists of transplanting only the insulin-producing islet cells rather than the whole pancreas. In rodent models, both allogeneic and xenogeneic islet transplants have successfully achieved normoglycemia in diabetic animals *(1025,1026)*. Attempts to extend these results to patients, however, have met with limited success *(1027,1028)*, and until recently, the results of whole-organ pancreas transplantation in correcting the hyperglycemia of diabetes have been far superior to those of islet transplantation *(1029–1031)*. In 2000, the "Edmonton Protocol" (1032) showed much improved survival of islet transplants at 1 year in 4 of 12 patients, using a new combination of immunosuppressive drugs that appeared to cause less damage to transplanted islets. However, this protocol required use of two or sometimes three pancreases for a single recipient, and by 5 years, in a much larger series of patients, only 10% of patients have remained insulin-independent *(1033–1035)*. Thus, these results, while representing an improvement, remain much inferior to the results of whole-organ pancreas transplantation.

Hematopoietic Cell Transplantation

Bone marrow transplants, and more recently, transplants of hematopoietic stem cells and progenitors mobilized from the marrow into peripheral blood by treatment with G-CSF, are used most commonly for the treatment of otherwise incurable leukemias and lymphomas, aplastic anemia, and congenital immunodeficiency states. Additional applications include hemoglobinopathies and inborn errors of metabolism. Autologous HCT is used for hematologic rescue following high-dose chemotherapy/radiotherapy for the treatment of malignancies and is currently being explored as a treatment for autoimmune diseases. However, autologous HCT will not be considered further here as it does not involve the broaching of any immunologic barriers.

One fundamental difference between HCT and the transplantation of all other organs is that the recipient's treatment for his or her malignancy usually results in ablation of the immune and hematopoietic systems prior to transplantation, that is, the "conditioning" for transplantation is myeloablative. Originally, hematopoietic cell allografts were administered only as a means of replacing ablated host hematopoiesis. However, clinical experience revealed that one of the main therapeutic benefits of allogeneic HCT is due to the GVL effect of donor lymphocytes (reviewed in ref. 1036). With the recognition of this immunotherapeutic benefit of allogeneic HCT, clinicians began to evaluate less toxic, nonmyeloablative conditioning as a means of allowing allogeneic marrow to engraft so that donor lymphocytes can mediate GVL effects *(770,771,1037,1038)*. In contrast to HCT for malignancies and other indications in immunocompetent recipients, transplantation for immunodeficiency states does not require myeloablation or immunoablation in order to achieve alloengraftment, which is often associated with reconstitution only of the deficient immune system and not other hematopoietic lineages.

Another major distinguishing feature of HCT is that the recovering immune system in bone marrow transplant recipients is tolerant to the donor alloantigens, so there is no requirement for immunosuppressive therapy to prevent allograft rejection once the initial immune resistance to the allograft has been overcome.

A third unique feature of HCT (as well as transplants of other organs that are rich in lymphoid tissue, such as small intestinal grafts and, to a lesser extent, liver grafts) is the ability of T cells in the allograft to mount an immunologic attack on the recipient's tissues, resulting in GVHD. GVHD rates and severity are reduced using prophylaxis with nonspecific immunosuppressive drugs, but still afflicts about 50% of recipients of HLA-matched sibling HCT. The frequency and severity of the GVHD that develops when extensive HLA barriers are traversed has essentially precluded the routine performance of such transplants, making HCT unavailable to many for whom no other curative treatment exists. The establishment of large marrow donor registries has permitted the performance of closely matched transplants from unrelated donors, but these transplants are also associated with a high incidence of severe GVHD, resulting from the existence of HLA mismatches that are undetected by conventional serologic HLA typing techniques (1039), which are now being replaced by more specific molecular typing techniques (see "HLA and Hematopoietic Cell Transplantation"). Additionally, greater minor histoincompatibilities can be expected in unrelated compared with related donor transplants.

The GVL effect of allogeneic lymphocytes, especially T cells, transferred with the donor graft, is due largely to recognition by donor T cells of host alloantigens, which are also expressed on malignant cells. Therefore, while T-cell depletion of the donor graft decreases the incidence of GVHD, this benefit is offset by increased relapse rates (1040) and increased risk of engraftment failure due to rejection *(1041)*. Graft rejection can be offset by more intensive host conditioning and high doses of donor hematopoietic stem cells, even with extensively (one haplotype) HLA-mismatched stem cell grafts *(1042)*, but at the expense of delayed immune reconstitution *(1043)*. While T-cell–mediated GVL effects due to GVH reactivity are greatly diminished with such an approach, this may be compensated for by the ability of NK cells to mediate GVL when the host lacks inhibitory MHC ligands recognized by the donor, at least for patients with acute myelogenous leukemia (346). Such alloreactive NK cells may also help to promote donor engraftment by eliminating alloresistant host T cells (346).

A major and elusive goal in the HCT field has been to separate the GVL effect of donor T cells from their potential to cause GVHD. Recently, several new approaches for inhibiting GVHD have been attempted. The use of costimulatory blockade has already been discussed. Because these approaches might be expected to block donor-antihost responses, including those that eliminate residual leukemia in the host, it seems quite likely that they would also impair GVL responses and might have their greatest utility in the treatment of nonmalignant diseases. Alternative approaches involve immunostimulatory cytokines such as IL-2, IFN-γ, IL-12, IL-11, and IL-18, all of which, paradoxically, inhibit GVHD in mouse models *(503,520,1044,1045)*. These cytokines have been shown to preserve or enhance GVL effects while GVHD is inhibited *(518,1046–1048)*. The inhibitory effect of IL-12 on GVHD is mediated by IFN-γ, which also promotes the GVL effect of CD8 T cells (436,1050). Keratinocyte growth factor also appears to inhibit GVHD while preserving GVL and promoting alloengraftment, through mechanisms that are not fully understood (*1051*,1052). Blockade of Fas/FasL, perforin, TNF-α, and IL-1 pathways have shown some efficacy in animal models and the latter have entered clinical trials (reviewed in ref. 437). Many other strategies, such as immune deviation and the use of NKT cells have been discussed elsewhere in the chapter.

Another approach to separating GVL from the GVHD-inducing capacity of MHC-directed alloreactivity is to separate the hematopoietic cell transplant and the administration of donor T cells in time, so that the T cells are given after some host recovery from the initial conditioning regimen has occurred. Mixed chimeras are immunologically tolerant of their original marrow donor's antigens and a GVH reaction occurs after administration of nontolerant DLIs, resulting in conversion of mixed hematopoietic chimerism to full donor chimerism. Remarkably, this powerful GVH alloreaction against lymphohematopoietic cells is not associated with GVHD in mice, even though donor T cells are given in numbers that would cause rapidly lethal GVHD in freshly conditioned recipients *(545,546)*. Although antihost MHC alloreactivity mediates the most potent GVL effects (1053,*1054*) and GVH-reactive donor T cells can clearly be shown to be activated and proliferating in mixed chimeric recipients of DLI *(547, 1054)*, these cells do not migrate to epithelial GVHD target tissues in the absence of inflammatory signals in those tissues *(547)*, as is discussed in the section "Role of Graft and Tissue Injury." The observation that GVH reactions can be confined to the lymphohematopoietic system suggests an approach to separating GVHD from GVL reactions, as hematologic malignancies reside largely in the lymphohematopoietic system. Proof of principle has been obtained that similar results can be achieved in patients receiving nonmyeloablative BMT with *in vivo* T-cell depletion of the donor and recipient, followed by delayed DLI for the treatment of lymphomas (772,1055), but the desired outcome is not always achieved, and further understanding should lead to refinements in this approach. In addition to recovery of epithelial GVHD target tissues from conditioning-induced injury, increasing resistance to GVHD with time may be conferred by recovering T-cell populations that down-regulate GVH reactions (1056,*1057*) while permitting GVL effects to be achieved (1058). Eradication of relapsed leukemia following delayed DLI is somewhat variably associated with GVHD in patients, but generally to a lesser degree than would be expected in freshly conditioned recipients of similar cell numbers (1036,*1059*).

Additional strategies for separating GVHD from allogeneic graft-versus-tumor effects include the transduction of donor T cells with suicide genes so that the alloresponse can be turned off at will, hopefully after residual tumor has been eradicated (*1060*,1061). Another approach is to avoid the GVH alloresponse, and try to target the donor immune response to tumor-specific antigens (1062). Idiotypic determinants associated with unique Ig receptors and TCRs on the surface of B- and T-cell malignancies, respectively, may trigger an immune response when presented by professional APCs such as DCs *(1063,1064)*. However, limitations to this approach include the low frequency of tumor antigen-specific T cells pre-existing in a given T-cell repertoire. These frequencies are even lower than those against minor histocompatibility antigens, and the generation of meaningful tumor-specific responses is likely to necessitate donor presensitization along with *in vitro* expansion of tumor-specific effector cells, a process that can limit the homing capacity of injected cells. Such prolonged cultures may be impractical for use in the setting of HCT, in which leukemia-reactive cells must eliminate exponentially expanding leukemic cells. Immunization of HCT donors with tumor antigens could potentially overcome these limitations. Minor histocompatibility alloantigens expressed by lymphohematopoietic cells (including leukemias and lymphomas) but not by the epithelial GVHD target tissues may also be targeted using *in vitro* expanded CTL. Such antigens have recently been identified *(72)*. Recently, it was shown that administration of primed T cells specific for a single immunodominant class I-restricted minor histocompatibility antigen could mediate GVL without GVHD. Avoidance of GVHD was dependent on the absence of GVH-reactive T cells with additional specificities in the donor inoculum *(1065)*. In theory, the less-risky strategy of generating tumor-specific responses from autologous T cells could achieve similar outcomes. However, T-cell immunity may be markedly impaired in the tumor-bearing host *(1066)*, and the use of immunologically unimpaired allogeneic donors is therefore appealing. Another approach to overcoming such immune suppression, which may be mediated in part by regulatory T cells, is to use chemotherapy to deplete regulatory cells and create space for lymphopenia-driven expansion of autologous lymphocytes, which may then mediate significant antitumor effects (1067).

Xenogeneic Transplantation

During the past decade, the increasing shortage of allogeneic donor organs has evoked a worldwide resurgence of interest in xenotransplantation, that is, the replacement of human organs or tissues with those from a donor of a different species. Routine clinical application of this therapeutic modality is still in the future. However, recent progress, which is reviewed briefly here, offers cause for optimism.

Concordant versus Discordant Xenotransplantation

Xenotransplants have been classified into two groups—"concordant" and "discordant"—on the basis of phylogenetic distance between the species combination, speed of the rejection, and levels of detectable preformed antibodies *(1068)*. Animals that are evolutionarily closely related and that have minimal or no preformed natural antibodies specific for each other are called *concordant,* while animals that belong to evolutionarily distant species and reject organs in a hyperacute manner are termed *discordant*. There are, of course, many gradations between these extremes, and there are also a variety of known exceptions to the rule, making this nomenclature less than ideal.

Choice of Donor Species for Clinical Xenotransplantation

From a phylogenetic viewpoint, nonhuman primates would undoubtedly be the most similar to allotransplants immunologically. However, because of considerations of size, availability, and likelihood of transmission of infectious disease, most investigators have decided against the use of primates as a future source of xenogeneic organs. Instead, the discordant species, swine, has been chosen by many as the most suitable xenograft donor. The pig has essentially unlimited availability, as well as favorable breeding characteristics, and many of its organ systems are similar to those of humans. Partially inbred miniature swine are a particularly attractive choice because of their size (adult weights of approximately 120 kg), their physiology (also similar to humans for many organ systems), and their breeding characteristics, which have permitted inbreeding and genetic manipulation (1069).

Mechanisms of Xenograft Rejection

Xenografts are subject to all four of the rejection mechanisms described earlier in this chapter and give rise to more powerful immune responses than allografts, probably for each type of rejection. There are two fundamental reasons for this finding. First, xenografts offer more foreign antigens as targets for an immune response. Second, there are frequently molecular incompatibilities between members of different species that prevent the normal function of receptor–ligand interactions. Because in many cases the occurrence of "homologous restriction" for receptor–ligand pairs has been found to impair the regulatory processes that normally control immune and inflammatory responses, the result is that rejection mechanisms that may be relatively weak in allogeneic combinations become explosive following xenogeneic transplantation.

The well-recognized susceptibility of xenografts to hyperacute rejection illustrates both of these fundamental problems. As is discussed in the section on transplantation antigen, (see "Species-specific Carbohydrate Determinats") primates have large amounts of anti-αGal natural antibodies that then react with pig tissues after xenotransplantation, causing vigorous rejection.

As already discussed, the hyperacute rejection that occurs with pig-to-primate transplantation is more vigorous than in the case of allogeneic blood group disparities, at least in part because the complement regulatory proteins expressed by pig endothelium are less efficient in controlling human complement activation than are the human regulatory proteins expressed by human organs. Thus, these molecular incompatibilities also contribute to the increased intensity of the hyperacute rejection mechanism.

Similarly, the factors responsible for accelerated graft rejection are more prominent in xenogeneic than in allogeneic transplantation, probably also because the process is magnified considerably by the failure of regulatory molecules to function effectively with human coagulation factors, thus increasing the tendency toward intravascular thrombosis (163). The biological reasons for the likely participation of NK cells in this form of xenograft rejection *(1070)* have been discussed previously.

The available evidence also suggests that cell-mediated immune responses to xenografts are more powerful than those directed to allografts *(1071)*. Initially, there was some uncertainty about this point because cell-mediated immune responses to xenogeneic stimulating cells were first studied using mouse T cells, for which molecular incompatibilities with human cells lead to weaker direct recognition of xenogeneic than allogeneic stimulators *in vitro*. In this case, the incompatibilities turned out to involve the accessory molecules that are required for T-cell activation rather than a lack of antigens that stimulate TCRs. Thus, it seemed that cell-mediated rejection *in vivo* might also be weak. However, cell-mediated xenograft rejection, even by mice, has consistently been found to be extremely powerful *in vivo,* apparently initiated by $CD4^+$ T cells responding to the many additional antigenic peptides through the indirect pathway.

For reasons of potential clinical applicability, greatest attention has been directed at investigation of the human-antipig cellular response. In contrast to the murine studies, direct responses by human CD4 and CD8 T cells to pig stimulators can be readily measured *in vitro (1072)*. In addition, the cell-mediated reaction *in vitro* has been found to include a significant contribution by NK cells that can lyse pig targets. Most of the other molecular interactions involved in cellular immunity that have been examined appear to be at least partially functional in primate antipig responses. Therefore, human-antipig T-cell responses are likely to be as great as or greater than those in allogeneic combinations.

Therapeutic Strategies for Xenotransplantation

There are three main strategies that have been pursued to achieve long-term survival of xenogeneic transplants. The first has been to seek nonspecific immunosuppressive drugs that might prove especially effective for xenotransplantation. Unfortunately, none of the new drugs that have contributed to improved outcomes for allografts have proven sufficient to make xenografting possible, and considering the immunologic barriers to xenotransplantation discussed earlier, it is unlikely that any such drug exists. Furthermore, the heightened immune response to xenografts compared with allografts suggests that larger amounts of exogenous immunosuppression will be required to achieve xenograft survival comparable to that of allografts. Given the narrow therapeutic window that already exists in allogeneic transplantation, most investigators believe that more than just immunosuppressive drugs will be needed to accomplish widespread clinical application of xenogeneic transplantation. Data so far for long term survival of functioning pig-to-primate transplants of organs (802) and of islets (925,*1073*) support this impression.

The second therapeutic approach has been to use genetic engineering of donor animals to lessen the immunologic barriers to xenografts. Because the two features that distinguish xenografts from allografts are the larger number of antigens and the molecular incompatibilities between species, these genetic modifications have been aimed primarily at correcting these two disadvantages of xenografts (Figure 44.13). The first transgenic pigs produced by genetic engineering for xenotransplantation attempted to make use of the species specificity of complement regulatory proteins. Transgenic pigs were produced that expressed human genes for several of these proteins. Organs from animals expressing one of these molecules (hDAF) have been studied extensively, and appear to be more resistant to hyperacute rejection than are those from wild type pigs *(1074)*, but nevertheless susceptible to acute humoral rejection *(1075)*. Numerous other transgenes (Figure 44.13) have been tested in attempts to further alter the primate host's humoral response to pig xenografts, but none to date has prolonged the survival of organ transplants beyond the survivals achieved with hDAF organs (163).

The alternative genetic engineering strategy to the addition of transgenes is the removal or inactivation of genes through knockout technology *(1076)*. In mice, the availability of embryonic stem cells has made it possible to use homologous recombination to generate numerous knockouts *(1076,1077)*, including mice that do not express the α-1,3-galactosyltransferase that is responsible for generating the Gal determinant. Until recently, this technology was not available in larger animals because embryonic stem cells have only been derived in certain strains of mice. However, the advent of cloning through nuclear transfer technology, first demonstrated in the famous sheep

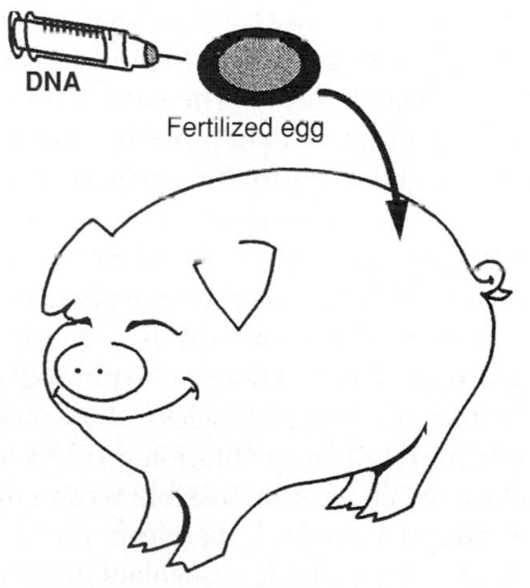

DNA

Fertilized egg

Transgenics

- Complement inhibition
  - DAF
  - CD46
  - CD59
- Growth factors
  - pIL-3, pSCF
  - Human GF receptors
- MHC genes
  - Class I (NK inhibition)
- Macrophage inhibition
  - CD47
- Inhibition of coagulation and thrombosis
  - CD39
  - Thrombomodulin
  - Hirudin
  - Tissue Factor Pathway Inhibitor

Knockouts

- α 1,3 Gal Transferase
- PERV (via knockout or RNAi)

FIGURE 44.13 Genetically modified pigs as xenograft source animals. GF, growth factors; NK, natural killer; PERV, pig endogenous retroviruses.

"Dolly" *(1078)*, has made knockout technology possible in several large-animal species, including pigs. Because, as described earlier, the major stumbling block in pig-to-primate xenotransplantation has been the large amount of natural antibody directed toward the Gal determinant, investigators have used this technology to eliminate the Gal-producing enzyme from pigs (1079,*1080–1082*). These new knockout pigs (called *GalT-KO*), like humans and Old World primates, do not put Gal onto the surface of their cells. As a result, xenotransplants can now be performed without the powerful rejection previously caused by natural anti-Gal antibodies. The results have been remarkable, with increased survivals of both heart and kidney transplants from pigs to baboons (802,*1083*). Using immunosuppressive drugs, organ survivals were prolonged using these new Gal knockout (GalT-KO) pigs, but new antibodies soon appeared, causing rejection (802,*1083*). However, using a regimen directed toward induction of tolerance (see later discussion), organ survivals were prolonged markedly, and no rejection was seen (802). There are still problems to be resolved before such transplants will be attempted in patients, but survivals are now being measured in months rather than in days, as they were only a few years ago.

The third strategy to achieve successful xenotransplantation is the induction of tolerance to donor antigens. Potential applications of this strategy have been described earlier in this chapter, with reference mainly to transplantation in rodent models (see previous discussion). There have been attempts to use either mixed chimerism or thymic transplantation to induce tolerance across xenogeneic barriers in primates. So far, long-term success by the mixed chimerism approach has been attained only for concordant cynomolgus monkey-to-baboon renal transplants *(1084)*. Both mixed chimerism and thymic transplantation approaches had been attempted for the discordant pig-to-baboon combination before the availability of GalT-KO swine, but with limited success *(1085–1087)*. However, combining the thymic transplantation approach with the use of the GalT-KO as a source of pig kidneys has extended survivals to more than 3 months (802). Thus, it seems possible that elimination of the natural antibody problem along with tolerance induction could make discordant xenotransplantation as successful as allogeneic transplantation in providing a long-term solution for patients waiting for transplants. Of course, it is possible that when these barriers are overcome, other obstacles, not yet apparent, will still limit the survival of xenogeneic transplants, and additional measures will be required to achieve success.

Nonimmunologic Barriers to Xenotransplantation

In addition to the immunologic mechanisms that prevent successful xenografting, there are two other potentially important obstacles to clinical application. First, molecular incompatibilities between species may cause physiologic dysfunction of xenogeneic organs. This kind of incompatibility is least likely for the heart, for which the function, albeit vital, is relatively simple. It could certainly become an obstacle, however, for the liver, as the liver is known to produce so many different products, including serum proteins and enzymes, that it is likely that at least some of these products may not function properly in a primate host. On the other hand, if the number of incompatibilities leading to physiologic dysfunction is limited, they could be correctable through knockout and transgenic technology. Thus, the physiologic dysfunction of xenogeneic organs is unlikely to be an insurmountable barrier to xenotransplantation.

The other nonimmunologic barrier to xenotransplantation is the risk of cross-species transfer of infectious agents, potentially creating a health hazard, not only for the recipient, but also for society as a whole. This possibility has gained significant attention, both in the scientific literature and in the lay press, and the issue has become confused by enormous uncertainties about the true risks that are involved. *Zoonosis* is a term that has been used for some time to describe the general process of cross-species infection, and the term *xenozoonosis* has been developed to describe infection transmission that might occur as a result of xenotransplantation (1088). It is important to realize that from the point of view of the individual recipient, the risk of transmitting infection by xenotransplantation is likely to be less than by current clinical allotransplantation, both because of the natural resistance to cross-species transmission of infectious diseases and because it should be possible to screen for and eliminate the presence of known pathogens from the herd of donor pigs.

The major infectious concern, therefore, is that endogenous retroviral sequences from donor cells might infect the recipient's cells, giving rise to previously unrecognized pathogenic viruses *(1089)*. The concern has been raised that such new viruses might prove hazardous to other human beings in addition to the xenograft recipient *(1090)*. However, to date there is no evidence that such cross-species transfer after a pig-to-human transplant would generate a virus that would be infectious or pathogenic. Indeed, studies of humans exposed to pig tissues have not revealed any cases of detectable pig endogenous retroviruses *(1091,1092)*. Nevertheless, the concern about infections from xenotransplantation involves fear of the unknown, for which it is impossible to assign an accurate level of risk. At this time, therefore, public health agencies and members of the transplant community are attempting to design rational approaches for identifying the true risks of xenotransplantation and detecting untoward events rapidly, while at the same time allowing further progress in this potentially enormously important field of transplantation *(1093)*.

Clinical Progress in Xenotransplantation

Early clinical efforts in xenotransplantation took place in the 1960s, and involved organ transplants from nonhuman primates (163). One of the patients survived for 9 months with normal renal function provided by the kidney of a chimpanzee *(1094)*. Additional clinical trials thereafter, using baboon hearts and livers, were considerably less successful. More recent clinical trials have involved fetal pig cells transplanted into the brains of patients with Parkinson or Huntington diseases. Survival of pig tissue 8 months after the transplant was documented in a patient taking only moderate doses of immunosuppression *(1095)*. These studies suggest that cellular xenotransplantation may be achieved more easily, and thus may be performed sooner, than solid-organ transplants, especially because free cellular transplants lack the vascular endothelium that is the target for both hyperacute and accelerated rejection. For organ xenotransplantation, most investigators believe that further clinical trials should await a reasonable expectation of success on the basis of pig-to-nonhuman primate experimental studies, a goal that is becoming closer but has not yet been realized.

SOME IMMUNOLOGIC ISSUES IN CLINICAL TRANSPLANTATION

The Effect of Antigen Matching on Organ Graft Survival

Clinical Data

In the absence of transplantation-antigen disparities, graft rejection does not occur. However, the importance of antigen matching is one of the controversial issues in clinical transplantation. The debate is frequently confused by failure to focus on the quantitative issue of whether improved, but incomplete, antigen matching influences the outcome of organ transplantation sufficiently to warrant its logistical difficulties.

The evidence from transplantation of kidneys using living related donors provides a clinical demonstration of the importance of antigen matching in subsequent graft survival. Two siblings may share all of their HLA antigens (25% likelihood), half of their HLA antigens (50% likelihood), or none of their HLA antigens (25% likelihood). Identical twins share all of their transplantation antigens, but siblings are generally matched for only about half of the minor antigens that distinguish their parents, even if they are HLA-identical. Data from a large international database on kidney allograft survival from 1985 to 1999 showed a survival half-life of HLA-identical sibling allografts of 23.4 years, as compared with 12.8 years for haploidentical-related allografts (14). These data support the basic concept that antigen matching matters, and for related donors, MHC antigen matching is widely agreed to be advantageous.

In the absence of a living related donor, transplantation is performed with organs from unrelated donors, usually from cadaveric sources. Because of the extensive polymorphism of MHC antigens, unrelated donors selected in a random fashion would not be expected to share many HLA antigens with the recipient. Similarly, there would only be sporadic matching of the minor histocompatibility antigens. Correspondingly, the survival of organs from cadaveric donors (half-life of 11.1 years in the large registry referred to previously [14]) has generally been shorter than that of HLA-identical or one-haplotype–mismatched-related transplants. Although longer ischemic time of cadaveric compared with living donor kidney transplants could account for some of this difference, a significant inverse correlation between graft survival and number of (serologically determined) HLA mismatches was evident among cadaveric donor recipients, and was still evident among the subgroup with short ischemic times. A similar effect could also be seen in recipients of living unrelated donor transplants with various mismatches (14). A long-term benefit for increased HLA matching could also be seen in recipients of cardiac, but not liver, allografts (14). Because all of these analyses are retrospective, an unanswered question is whether the potential added ischemic time required for nonrandom distribution of cadaveric organs to achieve a larger number of matched antigens would lead to better results.

A second question for all unrelated transplants is whether the more specific information provided by molecular typing confers a graft survival advantage over serologic typing. It appears that the typing for loci that cannot be typed serologically, such as HLA-DP, as well as DNA typing within a serotype, can benefit the survival of cadaveric transplants in heavily presensitized recipients, but probably not in unsensitized recipients (14). Thus, for the majority of recipients, it remains unclear that the distribution of organs to achieve better matching would be worth the effort, expense, and increased ischemic time, which might negatively affect outcome.

Experimental Data

As previously discussed, miniature swine provide a particularly useful large-animal model for testing experimentally the importance of antigen matching. Over the past 30 years, three herds of these animals have been developed for studies of transplantation biology, with each herd bred to homozygosity for a different allele at the MHC (termed *SLA* in swine) (Figure 44.3). Subsequent breeding was intentionally randomized within herds in order to maintain a variety of segregating minor histocompatibility loci, so that transplants among these

TABLE 44.7 Graft survival and antigen matching in minipigs

	Mismatch			
Graft	*Minors only*	*Major and minors*	*Class I*[a]	*Class II*[a]
Skin	11.8 ± 0.9	7.0 ± 0.4	10.8 ± 2.3	7.8 ± 1.0
Kidney	30.0 ± 15.0 (2/3) >120 (1/3)	12 ± 1.9	19.5 ± 6.8 (2/3) >120 (1/3)	21.8 ± 10.4

[a]Single haplotype mismatch.

animals resemble the situation within human families, that is, HLA-identical versus nonidentical siblings.

Studies of skin and renal allografts between these animals produced the results shown in Table 44.7. The difference observed for skin graft survival between SLA-matched and SLA-mismatched animals was modest, but matching had a much more profound effect on kidney graft survival. One third of the grafts between SLA-matched animals survived indefinitely without immunosuppression, despite the existence of multiple minor histoincompatibilities. The ability to reject renal allografts across minor differences was found to depend on an autosomal dominant gene, not linked to the MHC *(9)*.

Using intra-MHC recombinants between miniature swine haplotypes, the relative importance of class I versus class II matching on renal allograft survival was examined in these large animals *(9)*. The survival of renal allografts with class I–only differences and with class II–only differences is shown in Table 44.7. As in the mouse, both class I and class II differences appeared sufficient to cause prompt skin graft rejection. However, for kidney allografts, class II matching was of particular importance in determining the outcome. In fact, the results for minor plus class I differences were indistinguishable from those for minor histocompatibility antigen differences alone.

These experimental data were obtained without the exogenous immunosuppression always administered in clinical studies. They demonstrate the biological principle that antigen matching is important to graft survival and further indicate that class II antigen matching is likely to be particularly important. No experimental system is likely to settle the empirical issue in clinical medicine, however, of how much benefit will be obtained under the conditions of current practice.

HLA and Hematopoietic Cell Transplantation

In contrast to the results described previously for solid-organ transplants, the importance of HLA matching for unrelated HCT is unquestioned. Until quite recently, HCT was performed almost exclusively in HLA-identical (or single HLA-antigen mismatched) sibling pairs. Although this restriction has severely limited the use of HCT (only 25% of individuals have an HLA-identical sibling; another 5% has a single antigen-mismatched–related donor), the complications of HLA-mismatched transplantation have prohibited its widespread use. Among these complications, GVHD is the most prevalent and severe, with a severe form of the disease occurring in 75% to 80% of recipients of related donor transplants differing at one to three HLA A, B, or DR loci *(1096)*. Additionally, the incidence of marrow graft rejection increases in the presence of HLA disparity: while only 2% of HLA-identical related donor grafts are rejected, the figure increases to approximately 12% in recipients of unmodified haploidentical-related donor grafts (1039,*1097*).

Similar to solid-organ graft rejection, GVHD appears to be a particularly severe problem in the setting of class II MHC mismatching (1039,*1098*), but class I mismatching can also confer GVHD risk *(1099)* and synergizes with class II disparity (1039).

With respect to marrow graft rejection, class I (including HLA-A,B, and C) disparities have been most strongly associated with increased risk, which increases in proportion to the number of such disparities (14,1039,*1097*). Although the importance of class I mismatching, and particularly that of HLA-C, might suggest a role for NK cell-mediated rejection, antidonor NK reactivity was not demonstrable during the time of rejection in a patient receiving marrow from a donor whose HLA class I alleles would be incapable of triggering recipient KIRs recognizing recipient class I alleles *(1100)*. Thus far, a role for NK cells in mediating marrow allograft rejection has not been demonstrated in heavily conditioned hosts, but their role may become more significant if mismatched transplants are attempted with less toxic, nonmyeloablative regimens. In contrast, a role for classical CTL is well established in the rejection of even HLA-identical donor marrow following myeloablative conditioning *(1011)*. Rejection of HLA-identical HCT is rare unless the donor product is T-cell depleted *(1038,1102,1103)*, but occurs quite frequently in the setting of HLA-mismatched transplants, even without T-cell depletion *(1097)*, and increases even further with T-cell depletion *(1104,1105)*. Antidonor CTL specific for the mismatched donor class I allele have been associated with marrow rejection following unrelated donor transplantation *(1105)*. Class II disparities may also play a role in unrelated donor stem cell graft rejection (1039), and such rejection may be mediated by $CD4^+$ CTL *(29)*.

High resolution, PCR-based HLA typing methods have increased the capacity to avoid HLA disparities that would have previously (when only serologic HLA typing was available) gone unrecognized. However, higher-resolution HLA typing will obviously reduce the chance of finding a fully matched unrelated donor, even with the availability of large registries such as the National Marrow Donor Program in the United States, which currently contains more than 5 million volunteer registrants. Already, many patients do not succeed in finding an unrelated donor, and thus the identification of "acceptable" mismatches in the unrelated donor setting is of the utmost importance.

Crossmatch

There are several tests designed to detect pre-existing antibodies with specificity for donor antigens in the serum of potential recipients. First, recipients and donors must be matched for ABO blood type because, with the exception of organs from donors of the A_2 blood group, transplantation across blood group barriers may cause hyperacute rejection (see previous discussion). Second, immediate pretransplant sera from prospective recipients are tested for reactivity against lymphocytes of potential donors. This "crossmatch" is generally performed by a two-step, antibody-mediated, complement-dependent cytotoxicity assay, although methods using flow cytometry are now becoming more popular in many centers.

"Sensitized" Candidate for Organ Transplantation

Because kidneys and many other vascularized organs cannot be transplanted safely into recipients with pre-existing antibodies, the clinical goal is to avoid the formation of antibodies reactive with donor antigens or to find organs that do not express the particular HLA antigens against which the recipient has been sensitized. Except for blood group antibodies, recipient sensitization to transplantation antigens generally occurs by prior exposure to allogeneic tissue. This may occur as a result of blood transfusion, as a result of previous organ transplantation, or, in women, by exposure to paternal antigens on fetal cells during parturition. The degree of sensitization of a potential kidney recipient is measured regularly by testing sera on a panel of lymphocytes selected from individuals who collectively express a broad representation of the HLA antigens, resulting in assessment of high panel reactivity, as defined earlier. Highly sensitized candidates may wait many years to receive a kidney transplant.

The level of sensitization manifested by transplantation candidates fluctuates over time. As a result, it is possible for recipients to have a negative crossmatch with a donor's cells using recently obtained serum, but a positive crossmatch using previously collected sera. Transplantation in the face of this "historical positive crossmatch" has been performed successfully. Obtaining crossmatch-negative donors by locating well-matched organs or waiting for a decline in the level of sensitization represent the primary solutions currently available for sensitized patients. Recently, however, there have been successful reports of renal transplants in the face of antidonor antibodies as a means of using otherwise available kidneys, through plasmapheresis and treatment with anti-CD20 mAb and/or IVIG, followed by immunosuppression geared toward preventing antibody responses *(1107,1108)*.

The Diagnosis of Rejection

In clinical organ transplantation, the most obvious manifestation of the rejection process is usually diminished function of the transplanted organ, but it is important to confirm the immunologic origin of the event before increasing immunosuppression. Unfortunately, no clinical sign is by itself sufficient to diagnose rejection and *in vitro* assays have been disappointing. Recent reports suggest that measurement of urinary perforin and granzyme B levels may be useful in this diagnosis (285,*1109,1110*). Nevertheless, the gold standard remains histologic examination of the biopsy of the transplanted organ itself. Pathologists have been able to identify the abnormal lymphocytic infiltrate within grafts, to grade the intensity of the infiltrate, and, for some organs, to describe histologic findings characterizing the effects of immunologic injury *(1111)*. Some pathologic changes, including a lymphocytic infiltrate of the vascular wall, seem to be well correlated with rejection activity *(1011,1012)*. In addition, pathologic changes suggesting nonimmunologic causes of renal dysfunction may be helpful in patient management. Recently, the immunohistologic finding of deposition of the complement component C4d in the peritubular capillaries has been reported to be indicative of rejection, especially in the kidney (*1113*), although controversy remains as to whether this finding can also be indicative of accommodation *(1113,1114)*, the phenomenon of organ graft prolongation in the presence of antidonor antibodies (see previous discussion).

Despite the widespread reliance on the biopsy to define episodes of rejection, however, diagnosis of rejection is often difficult even by this means because of problems differentiating this diagnosis from drug toxicity and/or viral infection. Furthermore, when routine "protocol" biopsies of transplanted organs have been performed instead of biopsies for suspected rejection, they have revealed a poor correlation between histologic findings and clinical evidence of rejection. These results are consistent with several experimental models of tolerance induction that have shown intense lymphocytic infiltrates in organs that go on to survive indefinitely and/or in recipients who develop tolerance to the donor antigens *(117,1114)*. These studies suggest that the amount of lymphocytic infiltrate detected pathologically may not be helpful in diagnosing rejection episodes and determining the need for treatment.

How Much Immunosuppression Is Enough?

Although the majority of transplant recipients respond immunologically to their new organ despite immunosuppression, some patients seem never to generate any rejection activity and maintain their transplanted organ with very small doses of immunosuppressive drugs. Indeed, a few patients have been known to stop all of their medications but have kept their transplant for years without rejection. On the other hand, some patients seem to require and tolerate very high doses of exogenous immunosuppression, while others seem to be severely immunocompromised by low doses of these drugs. These observations make it clear that the amount of immunosuppression that is required or that is safe is not the same for every individual or for all grafts. Unfortunately there is no well-established assay to determine the amount of immunosuppression an individual requires and can safely tolerate for their particular transplant.

CONCLUSION

The great danger in any textbook chapter is that the need to summarize what we think is known will obscure the much greater amount still left to be learned. In recent years, enormous progress has been made in the study of the major histocompatibility antigens, yet we still know too little about the products of the numerous other histocompatibility loci that encode the minor histocompatibility antigens. Recently we have gained important insight into the role of antigen-presenting cells in T-cell sensitization, but we still have not explored adequately the role that indirect presentation of alloantigens plays in graft rejection. During the past 2 decades we have learned much about the generation and function of cytotoxic T lymphocytes and about their likely role in some mechanisms of graft rejection and GVHD; however, our understanding of noncytolytic mechanisms of rejection and GVHD, which clearly exist, is much more limited.

Finally, this chapter has outlined several techniques for the generation of immunologic tolerance to alloantigens in experimental systems; however, as is described earlier, the first human beings have only recently been transplanted with a tolerance-inducing regimen (nonmyeloablative allogeneic BMT with simultaneous donor kidney transplantation) that allows the early discontinuation of nonspecific immunosuppression. The encouraging initial results achieved with this approach raise hopes that routine tolerance induction may soon become a clinical reality. It is, of course, the great fascination of transplantation immunology that new insights into basic immunologic issues will likely have important consequences for clinical transplantation in the future.

REFERENCES

6. Groth CG. Landmarks in clinical renal transplantation. *Surg Gynecol Obstet*. 1972;134:327–328.
8. Mezrich JD, Haller GW, Arn JS, et al. Histocompatible miniature swine: an inbred large-animal model. *Transplantation*. 2003;75:904–907.
11. Bailey DW, Mobraaten LE. Estimates of the number of loci contributing to the histoincompatibility between C57BL-6 and BALB-c strains of mice. *Transplantation*. 1969;7:394–400.
14. Erlich HA, Opelz G, Hansen J. HLA DNA typing and transplatation. *Immunity*. 2001;14:347–356.
24. The HS, Harley E, Phillips RA, et al. Quantitative studies on the precursors of cytotoxic lymphocytes I. Characterization of a clonal assay and determination of the size of clones derived from single precursors. *J Immunol*. 1977;118:1049–1056.
27. Benichou G, Valujskikh A, Heeger PS. Contributions of direct and indirect T cell alloreactivity during allograft rejection in mice. *J Immunol*. 1999;162:358.
38. Huseby ES, White J, Crawford F, et al. How the T cell repertoire becomes peptide and MHC specific. *Cell*. 2005;122:247–260.
40. Bevan MJ. High determinant density may explain the phenomenon of alloreactivity. *Immuno Today*. 1984;5:128–130.
60. Felix NJ, Brinckey WJ, Griffiths R, et al. H2-DM alpha(−/−)mice show the importance of major histocompatibility complex-bound peptide in cardiac allograft rejection. *J Exp Med*. 2000;192: 31–40.
67. Wallny HJ, Rammensee HG. Identification of classical minor histocompatibility antigen as cell-derived peptide. *Nature*. 1990;343 (6255):275–278.
70. Lindahl KF, Vyers DE, Dabhi VM, et al. H2-H3, a full-service class Ib histocompatibility antigen. *Ann Rev Immunol*. 1997;15:851–879.
71. Perreault C, Roy DC, Fortin C. Immunodominant minor histocompatibility antigens: the major ones. *Immunol Today*. 1998;19: 69–74.
73. den Haan JMM, Meadows LM, Wang W, et al. The minor histocompatibility antigen HA-1: A diallelic gene with a single amino acid polymorphism. *Science*. 1998;279:1054–1057.
75. Mendoza LM, Paz P, Zuberi A, et al. Minors held by major: The H13 minor histocompatibility locus defied as a peptide/MHC class I complex. *Immunity*. 1997;7:461–472.
76. Brickner AG, Warren EH, Caldwell JA, et al. The immunogenicity of a new human minor histocompatibility antigen results from differential antigen processing. *J Exp Med*. 2001;193:195–206.
78. Simpson E, Roopenian D, Goulmy E. Much ado about minor histocompatibility antigens. *Immunol Today*. 1998;19:108–111.
84. Malarkannan S, Horng T, Eden P, et al. Differences that matter: major cytotoxic T cell-stimulating minor histocompatibility antigens. *Immunity*. 2000;13:333–344.
96. Choi EY, Christianson GJ, Yoshimura Y, et al. Immunodominance of H60 is caused by an abnormally high precursor T cell pool directed against its unique minor histocompatibility antigen peptide. *Immunity*. 2002;17:593–603.
97. Korngold R, Wettstein PJ. Immunodominance in the graft-vs-host disease T cell response to minor histocompatibility antigens. *J Immunol*. 1990;145:4079–4088.
102. Roopenian DC, David AP, Christianson GJ, et al. The functional basis of minor histocompatibility loci. *J Immunol*. 1993;151:4595–4605.
106. Mutis T, Gillespie G, Schrama E, et al. Tetrameric HLA class I-minor histocompatibility antigen peptide complexes demonstrate minor histocompatibility antigen-specific cytotoxic T lymphocytes in patients with graft-versus-host disesae. *Nature Med*. 1999;5:839–842.
107. Rufer N, Wolpert E, Helg C, et al. HA-1 and the SMCY-derived peptide FIDSYICQV (H-Y) are immunodominant minor histocompatibility antigens after bone marrow transplantation. *Transplantation*. 1998;66:910–916.
115. Jones MS, Riley R, Hamilton BL, et al. Endogenous superantigens in allogeneic bone marrow transplant recipients rapidly and selectively expand donor T cells which can produce IFN-gamma. *Bone Marrow Transplant*. 1994;14:725–735.
120. Ildstad ST, Wren SM, Bluestone JA, et al. Characterization of mixed allogeneic chimeras. Immunocompetence, in vitro reactivity, and genetic specificity of tolerance. *J Exp Med*. 1985;162: 231–244.
121. Warren EH, Greenberg PD, Riddell SR. Cytotoxic T-lymphocyte-defined human minor histocompatibility antigens with a restricted tissue distribution. *Blood*. 1998;91:2197–2207.

122. Cai J, Lee J, Jankowska-Gan E, et al. Minor H Antigen HA-1-specific Regulator and Effector CD8+ T Cells, and HA-1 Microchimerism, in Allograft Tolerance. *J Exp Med.* 2004;199: 1017–1023.
124. Gloor JM, Lager DJ, Fidler ME, et al. A Comparison of splenectomy versus intensive posttransplant antidonor blood group antibody monitoring without splenectomy in ABO-incompatible kidney transplantation. *Transplantation.* 2005;80:1572–1577.
130. Platt JL, Bach FH. The barrier to xenotransplantation. *Transplantation.* 1991;52:937–947.
132. Jin R, Greenwald A, Peterson MD, et al. Human monocytes recognize porcine endothelium via the interaction of galectin 3 and alpha-GAL. *J Immunol.* 2006;177:1289–1295.
137. Kumar V, McNerney ME. A new self: MHC-class-I-independent natural-killer-cell self-tolerance. *Nat Rev Immunol.* 2005;5:363–374.
141. Moretta A, Bottino C, Vitale M, et al. Activating receptors and coreceptors involved in human natural killer cell-mediated cytolysis. *Annu Rev Immunol.* 2001;19:197 223.
144. Raulet DH, Vance RE. Self-tolerance of natural killer cells. *Nat Rev Immunol.* 2006;6:520–531.
145. Alwayn IP, Basker M, Buhler L, et al. The problem of anti-pig antibodies in pig-to-primate xenografting: current and novel methods of depletion and/or suppression of production of anti-pig antibodies. *Xenotransplantation.* 1999;6:157–168.
149. Robson SC, Schulte AE, Bach FH. Factors in xenograft rejection. *Ann N Y Acad Sci.* 1999;875:261–276.
157. Yang Y-G, Chen AM, Sergio JJ, et al. Role of antibody-independent complement activation in rejection of porcine bone marrow cells in mice. *Transplantation.* 1999;69:163–190.
158. Trpkov K, Campbell P, Pazderka F, et al. Pathologic features of acute renal allograft rejection associated with donor-specific antibody. Analysis using the Banff grading schema. *Transplantation.* 1996;61:1586–1592.
160. Bach FH, Ferran C, Hechenleitner P, et al. Accomodation of vascularized xenografts: expression of "protective genes" by donor endothelial cells in a host Th2 cytokine environment. *Nat Med.* 1997;3:196–204.
163. Sachs DH, Sykes M, Robson SC, et al. Xenotransplantation. *Adv Immunol.* 2001;79:129–223.
171. Le Moine A, Goldman M. Non-classical pathways of cell-mediated allograft rejection: new challenges for tolerance induction? *Am J Transplant.* 2003;3:101–106.
176. Larsen C, Morris P, Austyn J. Migration of dendritic leukocytes form cardiac allografts into host spleens: a novel pathway for initiation of rejection. *J Exp Med.* 1990;171:307–314.
179. Lakkis F, Arakelov A, Konienczny B. et al. Immunologic "ignorance" of vascularised organ transplants in the absence of secondary lymphoid tissue. *Nature Medicine.* 2000;6:686–688.
183. Beilhack A, Schulz S, Baker J, et al. In vivo analyses of early events in acute graft-versus-host disease reveal sequential infiltration of T-cell subsets. *Blood.* 2005;106:1113–1122.
184. Murai M, Yoneyama H, Ezaki T, et al. Peyer's patch is the essential site in initiating murine acute and lethal graft-versus-host reaction. *Nature Immunology.* 2003;4:154–160.
186. Barker C, Bilingham R. The role of afferent lymphatics in the rejection of skin homografts. *J Exp Med.* 1968;128:197–221.
189. Zhou P, Hwang K, Palucki D, et al. Secondary lymphoid organs are important but not absolutely required for allograft responses. *American Journal of Transplantation.* 2003;3:259–266.
191. Chalasani G, Dai Z, Konieczny BT, et al. Recall and propagation of allospecific memory T cells independent of secondary lymphoid organs. *PNAS.* 2002;99:6175–6180.
193. Benichou G, Takizawa PA, Olson CA, et al. Donor major histocompatibility complex (MHC) peptides are presented by recipient MHC molecules during graft rejection. *J Exp Med.* 1992;175: 305–308.
200. Rosenberg AS, Mizuochi T, Sharrow SO, et al. Phenotype, specificity, and function of T cell subsets and T cell interactions involved in skin allograft rejection. *J Exp Med.* 1987;165:1296 1315.
206. Dolan BP, Gibbs KD, Jr., Ostrand-Rosenberg S. Dendritic cells cross-dressed with peptide MHC class I complexes prime CD8+ T cells. *J Immunol.* 2006;177:6018–6024.
212. Pietra BA, Wiseman A, Bolwerk A, et al. CD4 T cell-mediated cardiac allograft rejection requires donor but not host MHC class II. *J Clin Invest.* 2000;106:1003–1010.
214. Rosenberg AS, Singer A. Cellular basis of skin allograft rejection: an in vivo model of immune-mediated tissue destruction. *Ann Rev Immunol.* 1992;10:333–358.
218. Sprent J, Schaefer M, Lo D, et al. Properties of purified T cell subsets. II. In vivo responses to class I vs. class II H-2 differences. *J Exp Med.* 1986;163:998–1011.
220. Sharabi Y, Sachs DH, Sykes M. T cell subsets resisting induction of mixed chimerism across various histocompatibility barriers. In: Gergely J, Benczur M, Falus A, et al., eds. *Progress in Immunology VIII.* Proceedings of the Eighth International Congress of Immunology, Budapest, Springer-Verlag, Heidelberg. 1992: 801–805.
227. Rogers NJ, Lechler RI. Allorecognition. *Am J Transplant.* 2001;1: 97–102.
240. Bradley JA, Mowat AM, Bolton EM. Processed MHC class I alloantigen as the stimulus for CD4+ T-cell dependent antibody-mediated graft rejection. *Immunol Today.* 1992;13:434 437.
244. Russell PS, Chase CM, Colvin RB. Alloantibody- and T cell-mediated immunity in the pathogenesis of transplant arteriosclerosis: lack of progression to sclerotic lesions in B cell-deficient mice. *Transplantation.* 1997;64:1531–1536.
245. Shi C, Lee WS, He Q, et al. Immunologic basis of transplant-associated arteriosclerosis. *Proc Natl Acad Sci U S A.* 1996;93:4051–4056.
250. Mason PD, Robinson CM, Lechler RI. Detection of donor-specific hyporesponsiveness following late failure of human renal allografts. *Kidney Int.* 1996;50:1019–1025.
264. Rosenberg AS, Mizuochi T, Singer A. Evidence for involvement of dual-function T cells in rejection of MHC class I disparate skin grafts. Assessment of MHC class I alloantigens as in vivo helper determinants. *J Exp Med.* 1988;168:33–45.
271. den Haan JM, Bevan MJ. Antigen presentation to CD8(+) T cells: cross-priming in infectious diseases. *Curr Opin Immunol.* 2001; 13:437–441.
273. Valujskikh A, Zhang Q, Heeger PS. CD8 T cells specific for a donor-derived, self-restricted transplant antigen are nonpathogenic bystanders after vascularized heart transplantation in mice. *J Immunol.* 2006;176:2190 2196.
274. Valujskikh A, Lantz O, Celli S, et al. Cross-primed CD8(+) T cells mediate graft rejection via a distinct effector pathway. *Nat Immunol.* 2002;3:844–851.
285. Li B, Hartono C, Ding R, et al. Noninvasive diagnosis of renal-allograft rejection by measurement of messenger RNA for perforin and granzyme B in urine. *New Engl J Med.* 2001;344:947–954.
288. Graubert TA, Russell JH, Ley TJ. The role of Granzyme B in murine models of acute graft-versus-host disease and graft rejection. *Blood.* 1996;87:1232–1237.
290. Hahn S, Gehri R, Erb P. Mechanism and biological significance of CD4-mediated cytotoxicity. *Immunol Rev.* 1995;146:57–79.
299. Baker MB, Altman NH, Podack ER, et al. The role of cell-mediated cytotxicity in acute GVHD after MHC-matched allogeneic bone marrow transplantation in mice. *J Exp Med.* 1996;183. 2645–2656.
304. Doody DP, Stenger KS, Winn HJ. Immunologically nonspecific mechanisms of tissue destruction in the rejection of skin grafts. *J Exp Med.* 1994;179:1645–1652.
307. Kapessidou Y, Habran C, Buonocore S, et al. The replacement of graft endothelium by recipient-type cells conditions allograft rejection mediated by indirect pathway CD4(+) T cells. *Transplantation.* 2006;81:726–735.
310. Jones SC, Murphy GF, Friedman TM, et al. Importance of minor histocompatibility antigen expression by nonhematopoietic tissues in a CD4+ T cell-mediated graft-versus-host disease model. *J Clin Invest.* 2003;112:1880–1886.
313. Bradley AJ, Bolton EM. The T-cell requirements for allograft rejection. *Transplant.* 1992;6:115–129.
322. Hall B, Dorsch S. Cells mediating allograft rejection. *Immunologic Reviews.* 1984;77:570.
323. Ascher NL, Hoffman RA, Hanto DW, et al. Cellular basis of allograft rejection. *Immunol Rev.* 1984;77:216–230.

329. Douillard P, Cuturi M-C, Brouard S, et al. T cell receptor repertoire usage in allotransplantation: An overview. *Transplantation*. 1999;68:913–921.
341. Scheinberg P, Price DA, Ambrozak DR, et al. Alloreactive T cell clonotype recruitment in a mixed lymphocyte reaction: implications for graft engineering. *Exp Hematol*. 2006;34:788–795.
342. Colvin RB. The renal allograft biopsy. *Kidney Int*. 1996;50:1069–1082.
346. Ruggeri L, Capanni M, Urbani E, et al. Effectiveness of donor natural killer cell alloreactivity in mismatched hematopoietic transplants. *Science*. 2002;295:2097–2100.
352. Kitchens WH, Uehara S, Chase CM, et al. The changing role of natural killer cells in solid organ rejection and tolerance. *Transplantation*. 2006;81:811–817.
358. Renard V, Cambiaggi A, Vely F, et al. Transduction of cytotoxic signals in natural killer cells: a general model of fine tuning between activatory and inhibitory pathways in lymphocytes. *Immunol Rev*. 1997;155:205–221.
361. Forte P, Pazmany L, Matter-Reissmann UB, et al. HLA-G Inhibits Rolling Adhesion of Activated Human NK Cells on Porcine Endothelial Cells. *J Immunol*. 2001;167:6002–6008.
362. Forte P, Baumann BC, Weiss EH, et al. HLA-E expression on porcine cells: protection from human NK cytotoxicity depends on peptide loading. *Am J Transplant*. 2005;5:2085–2093.
370. Nikolic B, Cooke DT, Zhao G, et al. Both T cells and NK cells inhibit the engraftment of xenogeneic rat bone marrow cells in mice. *J Immunol*. 2001;166:1398–1404.
371. Goodman DJ, Millan MT, Ferran C, et al. Mechanisms of delayed xenograft rejection. In: Cooper DKC, Kemp E, Platt JL, et al., eds. *Xenotransplantation: The transplantation of organs and tissues between species*. Heidelberg: Springer, 1997:77–94.
372. Gourlay WA, Chambers WH, Monaco A, et al. Importance of natural killer cells in the rejection of hamster skin xenografts. *Transplantation*. 1998;65:727–734.
377. Seino KK, Fukao K, Muramoto K, et al. Requirement for natural killer T (NKT) cells in the induction of allograft tolerance. *Proc Natl Acad Sci U S A*. 2001;98:2577–2581.
381. Zeng D, Lewis D, Dejbakhsh-Jones S, et al. Bone marrow NK1.1– and NK1.1+ T cells reciprocally regulate acute graft versus host disease. *J Exp Med*. 1999;189:1073–1081.
384. Yasunami Y, Kojo S, Kitamura H, et al. Valpha14 NK T cell-triggered IFN-gamma production by Gr-1$^+$CD11b$^+$ cells mediates early graft loss of syngeneic transplanted islets. *J Exp Med*. 2005;202:913–918.
385. Bogdan C. Nitric oxide and the immune response. *Nat Immunol*. 2001;2:907–916.
392. Ide K, Ohdan H, Kobayashi T, et al. Antibody- and complement-independent phagocytotic and cytolytic activities of human macrophages toward porcine cells. *Xenotransplant*. 2005;12:181–188.
400. Wang H, Verhalen J, Madariaga ML, et al. Attenuation of phagocytosis of xenogeneic cells by manipulating CD47. *Blood*. 2007;109:836–842.
414. Donckier V, Wissing M, Bruyns C, et al. Critical role of interleukin 4 in the induction of neonatal transplantation tolerance. *Transplantation*. 1995;59:1571–1576.
415. Inoue Y, Konieczny BT, Wagener ME, et al. Failure to induce neonatal tolerance in mice that lack both IL-4 and IL- 13 but not in those that lack IL-4 alone. *J Immunol*. 2001;167:1125–1128.
417. Antin JH, Ferrara JLM. Cytokine dysregulation in acute graft-versus-host disease. *Blood*. 1992;80:2964–2968.
435. Lakkis FG, Dai Z. The role of cytokines, CTLA-4 and costimulation in transplant tolerance and rejection. *Curr Opin Immunol*. 1999;11:504–508.
436. Yang Y-G, Dey B, Sergio JJ, et al. Donor-derived Interferon g is required for inhibition of acute GVHD by interleukin 12. *J Clin Invest*. 1998;102:2126–2135.
438. Wiseman AC, Pietra BA, Kelly BP, et al. Donor IFN-gamma receptors are critical for acute CD4(+) T cell-mediated cardiac allograft rejection. *J Immunol*. 2001;167:5457–5463.
447. Steinman L. A brief history of T(H)17, the first major revision in the T(H)1/T(H)2 hypothesis of T cell-mediated tissue damage. *Nat Med*. 2007;13:139–145.
450. Nankivell BJ, Borrows RJ, Fung CLS, et al. The Natural History of Chronic Allograft Nephropathy. *N Engl J Med*. 2003;349:2326–2333.
467. Libby P, Pober J. Chronic rejection. *Immunity*. 2001;14:387–397.
469. Pratt J, Basheer A, Sacks S. Local synthesis of complement component C3 regulates acute renal transplant rejection. *Nature Medicine*. 2002;8:582–587.
475. Sakoda Y, Hashimoto D, Asakura S, et al. Donor-derived thymic-dependent T cells cause chronic graft-versus-host disease. *Blood*. 2007;109(4):1756–1764.
479. Kang S-M, Schneider DB, Lin Z, et al. Fas ligand expression in islets of Langerhans does not confer immune privilege and instead targets them for rapid destruction. *Nature Med*. 1997;3:738–743.
485. Fehr T, Takeuchi Y, Kurtz J, et al. Rapid peripheral deletion of donor- reactive CD8 T cells permits mixed allogeneic chimerism and tolerance induction in recipients of anti-CD40L and allogeneic BMT: Short-term regulation by CD4 cells. *Eur J Immunol*. 2005;35:2679–2690.
499. Sandner SE, Clarkson MR, Salama AD, et al. Role of the programmed death-1 pathway in regulation of alloimmune responses in vivo. *J Immunol*. 2005;174:3408–3415.
504. Malek TR, Bayer AL. Tolerance, not immunity, crucially depends on IL-2. *Nat Rev Immunol*. 2004;4:665–674.
517. Sawitzki B, Kingsley CI, Oliveira V, et al. IFN-gamma production by alloantigen-reactive regulatory T cells is important for their regulatory function in vivo. *J Exp Med*. 2005;201:1925–1935.
525. Lowsky R, Takahashi T, Liu YP, et al. Protective conditioning for acute graft-versus-host disease. *N Engl J Med*. 2005;353:1321–1331.
533. Qian S, Thai NL, Lu L, et al. Liver transplant tolerance: mechanistic insights from animal models, with particular reference to the mouse. *Transplant Rev*. 1997;11:151–164.
547. Chakraverty R, Cote D, Buchli J, et al. An inflammatory checkpoint regulates recruitment of graft-versus-host-reactive T cells to peripheral tissues. *J Exp Med*. 2006;203:2021–2031.
558. Matzinger P. Tolerance, danger, and the extended family. *Ann Rev Immunol*. 1994;12:991–1045.
560. Anderson CC, Carroll JM, Gallucci S, et al. Testing time-, ignorance-, and danger-based models of tolerance. *J Immunol*. 2001;166:3663–3671.
566. Sacks S, Chowdhury P, Zhou W. Role of the complement system in rejection. *Current Opinion in Immunology*. 2003;15:487–492.
570. Zhang M, Michael L, Grosjean S, et al. The role of natural IgM in myocardial ischemia-reperfusion injury. *J Mol Cell Cardiol*. 2006;41:62–67.
576. Obhrai JS, Goldstein DR. The role of toll-like receptors in solid organ transplantation. *Transplantation*. 2006;81:497–502.
583. Krieger NR Knechtle SJ. Novel immunosuppressive agents in tolerance induction. *Curr Drug Targets Cardiovasc Haematol Disord*. 2002;2:97–103.
593. Ferry H, Leung JC, Lewis G, et al. B-cell tolerance. *Transplantation*. 2006;81:308–315.
599. Sykes M. Mixed Chimerism and transplant tolerance. *Immunity*. 2001, 14:417–424.
625. Wells AD, Li XC, Li Y, et al. Requirement for T cell apoptosis in the induction of peripheral transplantation tolerance. *Nature Med*. 1999;5:1303–1312.
627. Schwartz RH. A cell culture model for T lymphocyte clonal anergy. *Science*. 1990;248:1349–1356.
639. Appleman LJ, Boussiotis VA. T cell anergy and costimulation. *Immunol Rev*. 2003;192:161–180.
652. Kurtz J, Shaffer J, Anosova N, et al. Mechanisms of early peripheral CD4 T cell tolerance induction by anti-CD154 monoclonal antibody and allogeneic bone marrow transplantation: Evidence for anergy and deletion, but not regulatory cells. *Blood*. 2004;103:4336–4343.
663. Seddon B, Mason D. The third function of the thymus. *Immunol Today*. 2000;21:95–99.
664. Wood KJ, Sakaguchi S. Regulatory T cells in transplantation tolerance. *Nature Immunology Reviews*. 2003;3:199–210.
679. Kingsley CI, Karim M, Bushell AR, et al. CD25$^+$CD4$^+$ Regulatory T Cells Prevent Graft Rejection: CTLA-4- and IL-10-Dependent Immunoregulation of Alloresponses. *J Immunol*. 2002;168:1080–1086.

684. Cohen JL, Trenado A, Vasey D, et al. $CD4^+CD25^+$ Immunoregulatory T Cells: New Therapeutics for Graft-Versus-Host Disease. *J Exp Med*. 2002;196:401–406.
689. Wood KJ, Sawitzki B. Interferon gamma: a crucial role in the function of induced regulatory T cells *in vivo*. *Trends in Immunology*. 2006;27:183–187.
707. Fallarino F, Grohmann U, Hwang K, et al. Modulation of tryptophan catabolism by regulatory T cells. *Naure Immunology*. 2003;4:1206–12012.
710. Karim M, Feng G, Wood KJ, et al. $CD25^+CD4^+$ regulatory T cells generated by exposure to a model protein antigen prevent allograft rejection: antigen specific reactivation in vivo is critical for bystander regulation. *Blood*. 2005;105:4871–4877.
742. Martin P. Overview of marrow transplantation immunology. In: Forman SJ, Blume KG, Thomas ED, eds. *Hematopoietic Cell Transplantation*. Cambridge: Blackwell Scientific Publications, 1999: 19–27.
749. Khan A, Tomita Y, Sykes M. Thymic dependence of loss of tolerance in mixed allogeneic bone marrow chimeras after depletion of donor antigen. Peripheral mechanisms do not contribute to maintenance of tolerance. *Transplantation*. 1996;62:380–387.
751. Wekerle T, Sayegh MH, Hill J, et al. Extrathymic T cell deletion and allogeneic stem cell engraftment induced with costimulatory blockade is followed by central T cell tolerance. *J Exp Med*. 1998;187:2037–2044.
762. Kawai T, Cosimi AB, Colvin RB, et al. Mixed allogeneic chimerism and renal allograft tolerance in cynomologous monkeys. *Transplantation*. 1995;59:256–262.
772. Fudaba Y, Spitzer TR, Shaffer J, et al. Myeloma Responses and Tolerance Following Combined Kidney and Nonmyeloablative Marrow Transplantation: In Vivo and In Vitro Analyses. *Am J Transplant*. 2006;6:2121–2133.
773. Haynes BF, Markert ML, Sempowski GD, et al. The role of the thymus in immune reconstitution in aging, bone marrow transplantion, and HIV-1 infection. *Ann Rev Immunol*. 2000;18: 529–560.
796. Zhao Y, Swenson K, Sergio JJ, et al. Pig MHC mediates positive selection of mouse $CD4^+$ T cells with a mouse MHC-restricted TCR in pig thymus grafts. *J Immunol*. 1998;161:1320–1326.
800. Nikolic B, Gardner JP, Scadden DT, et al. Normal development in porcine thymus grafts and specific tolerance of human T cells to porcine donor MHC. *J Immunol*. 1999;162:3402–3407.
802. Yamada K, Yazawa K, Shimizu A, et al. Marked prolongation of porcine renal xenograft survival in baboons through the use of alpha1,3-galactosyltransferase gene-knockout donors and the cotransplantation of vascularized thymic tissue. *Nat Med*. 2005;11:32–34.
806. Modigliani Y, Pereira P, Thomas-Vaslin V, et al. Regulatory T cells in thymic epithelium-induced tolerance. I. Suppression of mature peripheral non-tolerant T cells. *Eur J Immunol*. 1995;25:2563–2571.
810. Yan Y, Devos T, Yu L, et al. Pathogenesis of autoimmunity after xenogenic thymus transplantation. *J Immunol*. 2003;170:5936–5946.
812. Owen RD. Immunogenetic consequences of vascular anastomoses between bovine twins. *Science*. 1945;102:400–401.
813. Anderson D, Billingham RE, Lampkin GH, et al. The use of skin grafting to distinguish between monozygotic and dizygotic twins in cattle. *Heredity*. 1951;5:379–397.
816. Flake AW, Roncarolo M-G, Puck JM, et al. Treatment of X-linked severe combined immunodeficiency by in utero transplantation of paternal bone marrow. *New Engl J Med*. 1996;335:1806–1810.
820. Flake AW, Zanjani ED. In utero hematopoietic stem cell transplantation: Ontogenic opportunities and biologic barriers. *Blood*. 1999;94:2179–2191.
825. Streilein JW. Neonatal tolerance of H-2 alloantigens. *Transplantation*. 1991;52:1–10.
845. Wood K, Sachs DH. Chimerism and transplantation tolerance: cause and effect. *Immunol Today*. 1996;17:584–588.
856. Ciancio G, Miller J, Garcia-Morales RO, et al. Six-year clinical effect of donor bone marrow infusions in renal transplant patients. *Transplantation*. 2001;71:827–835.
858. Tryphonopoulos P, Tzakis AG, Weppler D, et al. The role of donor bone marrow infusions in withdrawal of immunosuppression in adult liver allotransplantation. *Am J Transplant*. 2005;5: 608–613.
860. Thomas JM, Verbanac KM, Smith JP, et al. The facilitating effect of one-DR antigen sharing in renal allograft tolerance induced by donor bone marrow in rhesus monkeys. *Transplantation*. 1995;59:245–255.
870. Madsen JC, Superina RA, Wood KJ, et al. Immunological unresponsiveness induced by recipient cells transfected with donor MHC genes. *Nature*. 1988;332:161–164.
871. Davies JD, Leong LY, Mellor A, et al. T cell suppression in transplantation tolerance through linked recognition. *J Immunol*. 1996;156:3602–3607.
877. Bagley J, Tian C, Sachs DH, et al. Induction of T-cell tolerance to an MHC class I alloantigen by gene therapy. *Blood*. 2002;99:4394–4399.
881. Barratt-Boyes, SM, Thomson AW. Dendritic Cells: Tools and Targets for Transplant Tolerance. *Am J Transplant*. 2005;5: 2807–2813.
895. Lutz MB, Schuler G. Immature, semi-mature and fully mature dendritic cells: which signals induce tolerance or immunity? *Trends in Immunology*. 2002;23:445–449.
896. Waldmann H. Reprogramming the immune system. *Immunological Review*. 2002;185:227–235.
904. Watson C, Bradley J, Friend P, et al. Alemtuzumab (CAMPATH 1H) induction therapy in cadaveric kidney transplantation—efficacy and safety after five years. *American Journal of Transplantation*. 2005;5:1347–1353.
911. Greenwald RJ, Freeman GJ, Sharpe AH. The B7 Family Revisited *Annu Rev Immunol*. 2005;23:515–548.
912. Larsen CP, Knechtle SJ, Adams A, et al. A new look at blockade of T-cell costimulation: A therapeutic strategy for long-term maintenance immunosuppression. *Am J Transplant*. 2006:876–883.
913. Bluestone JA, St. Clair EW, Turka LA. CTLA4Ig: Bridging the Basic Immunology with Clinical Application. *Immunity*. 2006;24: 233–238.
919. Pearson T, Alexander D, Hendrix R, et al. CTLA4-Ig plus bone marrow induces long-term allograft survival and donor-specific unresponsiveness in the murine model. *Transplantation*. 1996;1996;61:997–1004.
925. Cardona K, Korbutt GS, Milas Z, et al. Long-term survival of neonatal porcine islets in nonhuman primates by targeting costimulation pathways. *Nat Med*. 2006;12:304–306.
927. Kirk A, Burkly L, Batty D, et al. Treatment with humanised monolconal antibody against CD154 prevents acute renal allograft rejection in nonhuman primates. *Nature Medicine*. 1999;5:686–693.
943. Kirk AD, Knechtle SJ, Sollinger HW, et al. Preliminary results of the use of humanized anti CD154 in human renal allotransplantation *American Journal of Transplantation*. 2001;1:S191.
944. Azimzadeh AM, Pfeiffer S, Wu G, et al. Alloimmunity in primate heart recipients with CD154 blockade: evidence for alternative costimulation mechanisms. *Transplantation*. 2006;81:255–264.
945. Preston EH, Xu H, Dhanireddy KK, et al. IDEC-131 (anti-CD154), sirolimus and donor-specific transfusion facilitate operational tolerance in non-human primates. *Am J Transplant*. 2005;2005;5:1032–1041.
946. Kanmaz T, Fechner JH, Jr., Torrealba J, et al. Monotherapy with the novel human anti-CD154 monoclonal antibody ABI793 in rhesus monkey renal transplantation model 1. *Transplantation*. 2004;77:914–920.
950. Haanstra KG, Sick EA, Ringers J, et al. Costimulation blockade followed by a 12-week period of cyclosporine A facilitates prolonged drug-free survival of rhesus monkey kidney allografts. *Transplantation*. 2005;79:1623–1626.
968. Li B, Wang H, Dai J, et al. Construction and characterization of a humanized anti-human CD3 monoclonal antibody 12F6 with effective immunoregulation functions. *Immunology*. 2005;116:487–498.
997. Mezrich JD, Kesselheim JA, Johnston DR, et al. The role of regulatory cells in miniature swine rendered tolerant to cardiac allografts by donor kidney cotransplantation. *Am J Transplant*. 2003;3:1107–1115.

1015. Kawai T, Cosimi AB, Spitzer TR, et al. HLA-mismatched renal transplantation without maintenance immunosuppression. *N Engl J Med.* 1008;358:353–361.
1016. Scandling JD, Basque S, Dejbakhsh-Jones S, et al. Tolerance and chimerism after renal and hematopoietic-cell transplantation. *N Engl J Med.* 2008;358:362–368.
1017. Wong BS, Yamada K, Okumi M, et al. Allosensitization does not increase the risk of xenoreactivity to alpha1,3-galactosyltransferase gene-knockout miniature swine in patients on transplantation waiting lists. *Transplantation.* 2006;82:314–319.
1032. Shapiro AM, Lakey JR, Ryan EA, et al. Islet transplantation in seven patients with type 1 diabetes mellitus using a glucocorticoid-free immunosuppressive regimen. *N Engl J Med.* 2000;343:230–238.
1036. Antin JH. Graft-versus-leukemia: No longer an epiphenomenon. *Blood.* 1993;82:2273–2277.
1039. Petersdorf E, Anasetti C, Martin PJ, et al. Genomics of unrelated-donor hematopoietic cell transplantation. *Curr Opin Immunol.* 2001;13:582–589.
1040. Fefer A. Graft-versus-tumor responses. In: Thomas ED, Blume KG, Forman SJ, eds. *Hematopoietic Cell Transplantation.* Malden, MA: Blackwell Science, 1999;316–326.
1050. Yang Y-G, Qi J, Wang M-G, et al. Donor-derived interferon separates graft-versus-leukemia effects and graft-versus-host disease induced by donor CD8 T cells. *Blood.* 2002;99:4207–4215.
1052. Panoskaltsis-Mortari A, Taylor PA, Rubin JS, et al. Keratinocyte growth factor facilitates alloengraftment and ameliorates graft-versus-host disease in mice by a mechanism independent of repair of conditioning-induced tissue injury. *Blood.* 2000;96: 4350–4356.
1053. Mapara MY, Kim Y-M, Wang S-P, et al. Donor lymphocyte infusions mediate superior graft-versus-leukemia effects in mixed compared to fully allogeneic chimeras: a critical role for host antigen-presenting cells. *Blood.* 2002;100:1903–1909.
1055. Spitzer TR, MCafee S, Dey BR, et al. Non-myeloablative haploidentical stem cell transplantation using anti-CD2 monoclonal antibody (MEDI-507)-based conditioning for refractory hematologic malignancies. *Transplantation.* 2003;75:1748–1751.
1056. Johnson BD, Becker EE, LaBelle JL, et al. Role of immunoregulatory donor T cells in suppression of graft-versus-host disease following donor leukocyte infusion therapy. *J Immunol.* 1999;163:6479–6487.
1058. Johnson BD, Becker EE, Truitt RL. Graft-vs.-host and graft-vs.-leukemia reactions after delayed infusions of donor T-subsets. *Biol Blood Marrow Transplant.* 1999;5:123–132.
1061. Contassot E, Ferrand C, Angonin R, et al. Ganciclovir-sensitive acute graft-versus-host disease in mice receiving herpes simplex virus-thymidine kinase-expressing donor T cells in a bone marrow transplantation setting. *Transplantation.* 2000;69:503–508.
1062. Falkenburg JHF, Wafelman ARJP, Smit WM, et al. Complete remission of accelerated phase chronic myeloid leukemia by tratment with leukemia-reactive cytotoxic T lymphocytes. *Blood.* 1999;94:1201–1208.
1067. Dudley ME, Wunderlich JR, Robbins PF, et al. Cancer regression and autoimmunity in patients after clonal repopulation with antitumor lymphocytes. *Science.* 2002;298:850–854.
1069. Sachs DH. The pig as a potential xenograft donor. *Vet Immunol Immunopathol.* 1994;43:185–191.
1079. Lai L, Kolber-Simonds D, Park KW, et al. Production of alpha-1,3-galactosyltransferase knockout pigs by nuclear transfer cloning. *Science.* 2002;295:1089–1092.
1088. Fishman JA, Patience C. Xenotransplantation: infectious risk revisited. *Am J Transplant.* 2004;4:1383–1390.

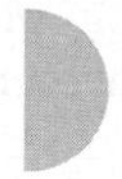

Tumor Immunology

Nicholas P. Restifo, Paul F. Robbins, and Steven A. Rosenberg

INTRODUCTION

In recent years, the field of tumor immunology has grown explosively, and the boundaries of the field, never particularly clear, have become less distinct. If one were to consider tumor immunology as comprising all of the possible interactions of immune cells with tumors, it seems that the topic of tumor immunology is enormous and would include components of fields as diverse as angiogenesis and carcinogenensis. Although our focus in the present chapter is on harnessing the immune system to control tumor growth, it has become clear that tumor growth can be promoted by inflammatory immune responses. Immune cells have been shown to express a variety of factors that promote angiogenesis as well as metastasis (1). Anti-inflammatory medications reduce the rate of intestinal neoplasia, and ulcerative colitis is associated with an increase in the incidence of human colorectal cancers (2). Studies in murine model systems indicate that pro-inflammatory cytokines such as tumor necrosis factor (TNF)-α play a role in enhancing cell growth and development through activation of NF-κB, which enhances the expression of a variety of anti-apoptotic genes *(3–5)*. The complexity of these regulatory pathways was revealed by a recent report demonstrating enhanced tumorogeneis in hepatocytes that fail to up-regulate NF-kB, an effect that results from sustained activation of c-Jun N-terminal kinase in response to TNF-α treatment (6). In a recent report, production of interleukin (IL)-23 appeared to play role in up-regulating expression of pro-angiogenic factors in the tumor environment *(7)*. Although transforming growth factor (TGF)-β has been shown to suppress tumor growth, in some circumstances it can actually promote the growth of tumor cells that have developed resistance to the pro-apoptotic actions of TGF-β (reviewed in [8]). In a murine model system, catecholamines produced in response to stress were found to promote tumor growth by stimulating angiogenesis *(9)*. Overall, these results indicate that the immune system can act through a variety of mechanisms to promote rather than suppress tumor growth. Nevertheless, results of a variety of animal model studies as well human clinical trials have demonstrated that cells of the immune system can be effective at controlling and eliminating even large tumor deposits, which is a primary focus of our review.

Studies first carried out in the 1940s using transplantable murine tumors indicated that T cells could recognize antigens expressed on tumor cells and that these cells were capable of mediating tumor regression. These findings lead to the identification in the 1980s of genes that encoded tumor rejection antigens expressed on murine tumors as well as the subsequent identification of antigens recognized by human tumor reactive T cells. The observation that many of the human tumor antigens represented widely expressed, nonmutated gene products lead to the expectation that effective vaccine therapies could be developed for the treatment of cancer patients. The results of vaccination therapies that boost the immune response of individuals with cancer have, however, to this point been disappointing. Vaccination with virus like particles expressing human papilloma virus (HPV) proteins appear to be successful in preventing the establishment of cervical cancer, which should lead to a significant reduction in the mortality resulting from this form of cancer. However, the HPV vaccine prevents viral infection, interfering with events that lead to cellular proliferation and transformation. Thus the HPV vaccine represents and extension of the success of vaccines against infectious disease and should not be viewed as a therapeutic cancer vaccine *per se*: In spite of the presence of highly immunogenic HPV epitopes, vaccination appears to be ineffective at treating patients with existing diseases that appear to result from infection with this virus. Therapies have been developed, however, that are capable of resulting in the regression of large established tumor metastases. In a current clinical protocol involving the adoptive transfer of melanoma reactive T cells, objective clinical responses have been observed in approximately 50% of treated patients, and in between 10% and 15% of treated, long-term tumor regression has been seen. A better understanding of the basic mechanisms that regulate immune responses will hopefully lead to the development of even more effective adoptive immunotherapies and may also lead to the development of effective cancer vaccines.

INITIAL DEMONSTRATIONS OF TUMOR RECOGNITION BY CELLS OF THE IMMUNE SYSTEM

Studies first carried out in the 1980s demonstrated that normal spleen cells cultured in IL-2, termed lymphokine activated killer cells (*LAK* cells), had the ability to lyse fresh as well as cultured tumor cells. Uncultured cells derived from normal tissues were not lysed by LAK cells. Lysis of autologous as well as allogeneic tumor cells was observed, demonstrating that recognition of target cells was not MHC restricted.

Evidence for specific tumor recognition by cells of the immune system was obtained in experiments first conducted over 5 decades ago using murine tumors generated through the use of the mutagen methylcholanthrene (MCA). Mice that received a surgical resection of previously inoculated tumors could be protected against a subsequent tumor challenge *(10)*; however, while these mice were protected against challenge with the immunizing tumor, either no or limited protection was observed against challenge with other MCA tumors (11,*12*). Subsequent observations indicated that $CD8^+$ cytotoxic T cells were the cells that were primarily responsible for mediating the rejection of MCA induced tumors as well as other tumors (13,*14,15*).

The nature of antigens recognized by T cells was first revealed by studies carried out using the mouse mastocytoma P815. Variants of P815 generated by mutagenesis resulted in the generation of variants, termed *tum-*, that were rejected by syngeneic mice (16). The *in vitro* stimulation of T cells derived from the mice that had rejected the tum- cell lines resulted in the generation of several cytotoxic T lymphocyte (CTL) clones that appeared to recognize tumor antigens, some of which were also expressed on the parental P815 cell line. Tumors that arose following the injection of relatively low numbers of P815 cells would partially regress in the majority of injected mice, followed by regrowth of the tumor, leading to the eventual death of injected mice *(17)*. The recurrent tumors had lost the expression of antigens detected with P815-specific T cell clones, indicating that *in vivo* immunoselection had occurred and providing evidence that these antigens represented tumor rejection antigens.

The genes encoding tumor antigens expressed on mutagenized P815 cells that were initially cloned by screening with tumor reactive CTL clones were found to contain point mutations (18). These mutations resulted in the generation of the specific peptide epitopes that were the target of the CTL clones that appeared to be responsible for tumor rejection. Subsequent studies, however, indicated that tumor rejection antigens could be derived from normal cellular genes. The P1A antigen, which was isolated from P815, represented a nonmutated product (19). This gene product was also expressed on a mastocytoma cell line and was found to represent a differentiation antigen with a limited tissue distribution. Immunization of mice with a transfectant of L1210 leukemia cells that coexpressed P1A as well as the costimulatory molecule B7–1 resulted in the protection against lethal challenge with wild-type P815 tumor cells (20). These observations, as well as subsequent studies carried out in human clinical trials, described below, provide evidence that nonmutated self-antigens represent potent targets for tumor rejection.

Approaches to the Identification of Tumor Antigens

Three major approaches have been used to identify the molecular nature of antigens that are naturally processed and presented on tumor cells, which to date comprise more than 100 antigenic proteins and/or epitopes (Table 45.1). Most antigens have been identified using T cells with the ability to recognize intact cancer cells, as assessed by either specific cytokine release or lysis when T cells and cancer cells are co-cultured. These T cells can be derived by repeated *in vitro* sensitization with tumor cells or by the culture of tumor infiltrating lymphocytes (TIL). These anti-tumor T cells can be used to screen tumor cDNA libraries transfected into target cells containing the appropriate restriction element. Alternatively, peptides can be eluted from cancer cells and used to pulse HLA-matched target cells that are then tested for recognition by the anti-tumor T cells. To identify HLA class II–restricted tumor antigens, cellular proteins can be fractionated and fed to antigen presenting cells (APC) until a single protein species is identified.

A second approach to identify cancer antigens uses a "reverse immunology" method in which putative antigens are used to generate tumor reactive T cells by repeated *in vitro* sensitization with candidate peptides from proteins that were primarily identified through the use of previously described peptide–MHC binding motifs. For example, the HLA-binding motif for the HLA-A2 class I molecule, which is expressed by approximately 50% of Caucasians, consists of an optimal methionine, leucine, or isoleucine anchor residue at position two and a valine at the carboxy-terminal anchor residue position, generally position nine or ten (21). The peptide reactive T cells are then tested for the ability to recognize intact cancer cells to determine whether the identified peptides are naturally processed and presented on the surface of cancer cells. Alternatively, mice transgenic for human major histocompatibility complex (MHC) molecules have been immunized with candidate antigens and the murine T cells used to test for cancer cell recognition. Observations indicate that only a small percentage of the potential epitopes are naturally presented on the cell surface at sufficient levels to allow detection by T cells, which results at least in part from the fact that the majority of peptides that are presented on the cell surface in association with class I molecules appear to be processed in the proteasome, a multi-subunit catalytic complex that is responsible for generating the carboxy-terminus of processed peptides (22). Thus, although it has been surprisingly easy to use these techniques to generate T cells against individual peptides, only a limited number of these peptides are naturally presented on the surface of tumor cells.

A third approach to the identification of tumor antigens is a method that has been termed *SEREX* (serological

TABLE 45.1 Representative Human Leukocyte Antigen (HLA) Class I and Class II Restricted T-cell Epitopes

	Tumor Expression				
Category	*Pattern*	*Epitope*	*Amino Acid*	*HLA Restriction Element*	*Reference*
Cancer testis					
MAGE-A1	Many	EADPTGHSY	161–169	A1	319
MAGE-A3	Many	EVDPIGHLY	168–176	A1	*25*
NY-ESO-1	Many	SLLMWITQC	157–165	A2	30
NY-ESO-1	Many	SLLMWITQCFLPVF	157–170	DPβ1*0401/2	35
Melanocyte differentiation antigen					
MART-1	Melanoma	AAGIGILTV	27–35	A2	40
gp100	Melanoma	ITDQVPSFV	209–217	A2	47
gp100	Melanoma	YLEPGPVTA	280–288	A2	48
Tyrosinase	Melanoma	YMDGTMSQV	369–377	A2	*136*
Tyrosinase	Melanoma	QNILLSNAPLGPQFP	56–70	DRβ1*0401	57
Tyrosinase	Melanoma	SYLQDSDPDSFQD	450–462	DRβ1*0401	57
gp100	Melanoma	TTEWVETTARELPIPEPE	420–437	DRβ1*0701	*61*
Overexpressed gene product					
PRAME	Melanoma	LYVDSLFFL	301–309	A24	63
FGF-5	Renal carcinoma	NTYASPRFK	172–176 and 204–207	A3	137
Mutated antigen					
CDK4	Melanoma	ACDPHSGHFV	23–32	HLA-A2	*83*
p14ARF:125–133,	Many	AVCPWTWLR	125–133	HLA-A*1101	87
p16INK4a:111–119	Many	AVCPWTWLR	111–119	HLA-A*1101	87
HLA-A*1101	Melanoma	—	—	HLA-A*1101	87

analysis of recombinant cDNA expression libraries) (23). This method, which utilizes antisera from cancer patients to screen cDNA libraries constructed from tumor cells, has resulted in the identification of thousands of target molecules (online list available at http://www2.licr.org/CancerImmunomeDB, registration is required). Although some of the proteins identified using this technique are expressed in a tumor-specific manner, many of the proteins identified using this technique are expressed in normal tissues but appear to be overexpressed in tumor cells. Normal proteins released from large masses of necrotic and apoptotic tumor cells may also be processed by dendritic cells (DC) and may also lead to the generation of antibodies against intracellular products that are normally sequestered from the immune system.

CATEGORIES OF TUMOR ANTIGENS CAN BE DEFINED BY EXPRESSION PATTERNS

Nonmutated Self-antigens Recognized by CD8$^+$ and CD4$^+$ T Cells

Cancer/Testis Antigens

The genes that encode a wide variety of antigens expressed in both murine and human tumors have now been identified either using T cells that have been deliberately sensitized against tumor cells or by culturing TIL cells *in vitro* with IL-2. The first antigen shown to be recognized by human tumor reactive T cells, termed *MAGE-1,* was isolated by screening a melanoma genomic DNA library derived from the MZ2-MEL cell line with a CTL clone that recognized MZ2-MEL cells (24). MAGE-1 was found to be a nonmutated gene that was a member of a large, previously unidentified gene family. The T cell epitope identified using the MAGE-1 reactive CTL clone was recognized in the context of the HLA-A1 restriction element. Several additional members of the MAGE gene family have now been shown to encode T cell epitopes recognized by tumor reactive T cells *(25,26)*. These genes are expressed exclusively either in the testes alone or in testes and placenta, but not in other normal tissues, and have been termed *cancer/testis antigens.* These tissues fail to express HLA molecules and thus are not recognized by T cells reactive with members of this gene family. Members of the MAGE gene family are expressed in a variety of tumor types, including melanoma, breast, prostate and esophageal cancer. Although variable levels of expression were observed in these tumor types, DNA methylation was found to play a predominant role in regulating expression of MAGE family genes. Cells in which the MAGE-1 gene was highly methylated failed to express this gene product, and treatment of cultured cells with the demethylating agent 5-aza-2′-deoxycytidine upregulated gene expression in tumor cells as well as normal cultured fibroblasts (27,*28*).

The NY-ESO-1 antigen, which was initially identified using the SEREX technique (29), represents a cancer/testis antigen that is unrelated to the MAGE family of genes. The peripheral blood of a melanoma patient with a high serum titer of anti-NY-ESO-1 antibodies was found to contain HLA class I–restricted T cells directed against this antigen, and further studies resulted in the identification of the NY-ESO-1:157-165 peptide as a dominant epitope recognized by HLA-A2–restricted, NY-ESO-1–reactive T cells (30,*31*). The NY-ESO-1 molecule is expressed in approximately 30% of breast, prostate, as well as melanoma tumors. In contrast to other antigens such as tyrosinase and MAGE-1, for which infrequent antibody responses have been observed, 10 out of 12 patients with NY-ESO-1–positive tumors possessed serum antibodies directed against this antigen *(32)*. In addition, tumor burden was positively associated with the titer of anti-NY-ESO-1 antibodies *(31)*, and the presence of NY-ESO-1 antibodies was associated with the presence of T cells directed against the NY-ESO-1:157-165 HLA-A2–restricted epitope (33).

The presence of relatively high-affinity anti-NY-ESO-1 IgG antibodies is indicative of the presence of cognate help resulting either from the recognition of NY-ESO-1 class II–restricted epitopes that are presented on the tumor cell surface or epitopes that are processed and presented by APC that have taken up NY-ESO-1 protein released from tumor cells. Multiple NY-ESO-1 epitopes that are recognized by CD4$^+$ T cells have been identified by *in vitro* stimulation with candidate epitopes (*34*,35,36). It is not clear that these epitopes are naturally processed and presented *in vivo*, however, as evidence that T cells generated *in vitro* using these peptides recognized tumor cells or APCs that have been pulsed with tumor cell lysates was not presented in many of these studies.

Melanocyte Differentiation Antigens

The gene encoding the melanoma antigen designated MART-1 (37) or Melan-A (38) was isolated following the screening of melanoma cDNA libraries with an HLA-A2–restricted tumor reactive TIL and a CTL clone derived by *in vitro* sensitization, respectively. The MART-1 gene encoded a 118 amino acid protein that is expressed in between 80% and 90% of fresh melanomas and cultured melanoma cell lines *(39)*. The majority of melanoma-reactive, HLA-A2–restricted TIL were shown to recognize MART-1, indicating that this is a highly immunodominant antigen (40,*41*).

The MART-1 antigen is representative of a set of gene products, termed *melanocyte differentiation antigens* (MDAs), that are expressed in melanoma as well as in normal melanocytes present in the skin as well as in the retina. Tumors arising from glial cells have also been shown to express MDAs, and low levels of expression of these products have been detected in normal brain tissue *(42–44)*. Expression of these genes products results from the activity of tissue-specific promoters *(45)*, an observation that is consistent with the fact that that normal melanocytes as well as glial cells are derived from neuroectrodermal tissue.

In an attempt to identify the dominant T cell epitope recognized by MART-1–reactive, HLA-A2–restricted T cells, a set of 23 candidate peptides from MART-1 were synthesized and tested for their ability to be recognized by MART-1–reactive T cells. The peptides that were synthesized conformed to the optimal HLA-A2–binding motif, which consists of a leucine, isoleucine, or methionine at the primary anchor position 2 and a valine at the carboxy-terminal primary anchor position (21). In addition, MART-1 peptides that contained an optimal residue at one of the primary anchor positions but a conservative substitution at the second primary anchor position were synthesized. The results of peptide screening assays demonstrated that HLA-A2–restricted, MART-1–reactive T cells recognized a single nonamer peptide AAGIGILTV(MART-1:27-35) as well as two overlapping decamers EAAGIGILTV and AAGIGILTVI (40). Nine out of 10 HLA-A2–restricted TIL cultures recognized the MART-1 gene product, and each of these cultures recognized that MART-1:27-35 epitope. Subsequent studies carried out by mass spectrometric analysis of peptides eluted from HLA-A2 molecules isolated from the surface of melanoma cells indicated that the AAGIGILTV(MART-1:27-35) nonamer represented the predominant MART-1 epitope that was naturally processed and presented on the surface of melanomas, as neither of the overlapping decamer peptides were isolated using this technique *(46)*. The MART-1:27-35 peptide did not conform to the optimal HLA-A2 binding motif, as it contained an alanine residue at the second position and was found to bind HLA-A2 with a relatively low affinity (47). These results have lead to further studies to explore the factors that may be involved with the expansion of T cells reactive with this epitope, as well as attempts to sensitize T cells using peptide variants that bind HLA-A2 with a higher affinity, which are discussed later in this chapter.

Several proteins were initially shown to be involved in the synthesis of melanin but were subsequently found to represent MDAs, including the gp100, tyrosinase, tyrosine-related protein (TRP-1), and TRP-2 gene products. In one study, pools of peptides eluted from the surface of melanoma cells were separated on HPLC columns and tested for their ability to sensitize target cells for T cell recognition (48). Candidate peptides present in positive subpools were then sequenced using a triple quadrupole mass spectrometer. They were then synthesized and tested for T cell recognition, resulting in the identification of the gp100 peptide YLEPGPVTA (gp100:280-288) as an epitope that was recognized by 5 out of 5 *in vitro* cultured CTL lines. Further studies resulted in the identification of multiple immunodominant HLA-A2–restricted epitopes from the 661 amino acid gp100 glycoprotein. Following the screening of four gp100-reactive TIL lines with 169 peptides from the gp100 protein identified as potential candidates based on the use of the HLA-A2 binding motif, three additional gp100 epitopes, ITDQVPFSA(gp100:209-217), KTWGQYWQV (gp100:154-162), and VLYRYGSFSV (gp100:476- 485) were identified (47). As noted earlier for the MART-1 epitope, the ITDQVPFSA(gp100:209-217) and KTWGQYWQV (gp100:154–162) peptides do not conform to the consensus HLA-A2 binding motif, which lead to further studies described later in this chapter examining the antigenicity and immunogenicity of variants of these epitopes that conformed to this binding motif.

Epitopes from many of the MDAs have been found to be recognized in the context of restriction elements other than HLA-A2, and in addition, epitopes on these molecules recognized by murine tumor reactive T cells have been identified. Tyrosinase *(49,50)*, TRP-1- and TRP-2-reactive T cells (*51,52*,53) have been shown to these gene products in the context of a variety of HLA class I alleles. A peptide epitope recognized by HLA-A2–restricted, TRP-2–reactive T cells, SVYDFFVWL (TRP-2:180-188), also represented a dominant epitope recognized by H-2K^b restricted T cells (54). Adoptive immunotherapy studies carried out using the B16 murine melanoma also demonstrated that this represented a tumor rejection antigen.

One of the epitopes of tyrosinase found initially to be recognized by CD8$^+$ T cells in the context of HLA-A2 was also found to be recognized by CD4$^+$ T cells (55), an observation that, while unusual, has been reported for another melanoma-reactive CD4$^+$ T cell (56). The lack of dependence on CD8 for target cell recognition indicates that these cells may express particularly high-affinity T cell receptors (TCR).

Several of the MDAs initially identified as the targets of class I–restricted T cells have also been shown to be recognized by class II–restricted CD4$^+$ T cells. Two epitopes of tyrosinase were found to be recognized in the context of HLA-DRβ1*0401 (57). Additional shared class II–restricted epitopes that have been described include an epitope that is shared between TRP-1 and TRP-2 *(58)* as well as multiples epitopes derived from the gp100 glycoprotein *(59–61)*.

Overexpressed Gene Products

Gene products that are expressed at low levels in normal tissues but that are overexpressed in a variety of tumor types have also been shown to be recognized by T cells. Screening of an autologous renal carcinoma cDNA library with a tumor reactive, HLA-A3–restricted T cell clone resulted in the isolation of FGF5 (62), a protein that was expressed only at low levels in normal tissues but upregulated in multiple renal carcinomas as well as prostate and breast carcinomas. Use of a similar approach with an HLA-A24–restricted melanoma-reactive T cell clone resulted in the isolation of a previously undescribed gene that was termed *PRAME* (63). This gene product appeared to be expressed are relatively high levels in melanomas as well as additional tumor types, but was also detected in a variety of normal tissues that included testis, endometrium, ovary, and adrenals. The HLA-A24–restricted PRAME-reactive T cell clone, however, expressed the natural killer (NK) inhibitory receptor p58.2, and tumor cell recognition was dependent upon loss of expression of the HLA Cw-7 allele that represented the ligand for the inhibitory receptor, which may explain the lack of recognition of normal tissues that express relatively high levels of this HLA gene product. Products derived from endogenous retroviral sequences that are overexpressed specifically in tumor cells have been shown to be recognized by murine *(64)* as well as human T cells *(65)*.

Generation of T Cells Using Candidate Epitopes ("Reverse Immunology")

Candidate epitope approaches have been utilized to generate T cells reactive with peptides derived from overexpressed gene products, as well as to generate T cells reactive with additional epitopes of previously identified tumor antigens. In many cases, HLA binding motifs have been used to identify a panel of peptides that are then synthesized and tested for their ability to bind to a particular MHC allele, followed by *in vitro* sensitization or *in vivo* immunization with candidate peptides. Using this approach, immunogenic peptides have been identified in the human carcinoembryonic antigen (CEA) (66), a protein that is overexpressed in colon and breast carcinomas. Similar approaches have been used to identify epitopes in proteins that are overexpressed in prostate carcinomas such as prostate-specific antigen (PSA) *(67)* and prostate specific membrane antigen (PSMA) *(68)*.

Attempts to generate T cells reactive with Her-2/neu, a protein that is frequently overexpressed in a variety of tumor type including breast carcinomas, have primarily focused on the Her-2/neu:369-377 peptide, a peptide that binds with high affinity to HLA-A2. Initial studies indicated that T cells generated with this peptide recognized the appropriate tumor targets (69). Subsequently, immunization of patients with the same peptide in Freund's incomplete adjuvant was found to result in the generation of peptide-reactive T cells following two *in vitro* stimulations of postvaccination peripheral blood mononuclear cell (PBMC) from three out of the four patients who were tested (70). Although these T cells recognized targets cells that were pulsed with relatively low concentrations of the Her-2/neu:369-377 peptide, they failed to recognize HLA-A2$^+$/Her-2/neu$^+$ tumor cells, and objective clinical responses were not observed in this trial.

A peptide corresponding to amino acids 540-548 of the human telomerase catalytic subunit (hTERT) was initially reported to generate tumor reactive T cells (71). The results reported by additional investigators, however, have failed to provide evidence that T cells generated using this peptide recognized tumor targets (72,73). Inefficient processing may be responsible for these findings, as the incubation of a long peptide corresponding to amino acids 534-554 of the telomerase protein with purified proteasomes resulted in the production of multiple cleavage products but did not result in the generation of peptides containing the appropriate carboxy terminus (72), in contrast to results observed with naturally processed T cell epitopes.

It is not clear why there is disagreement with regard to the ability of T cells generated using candidate antigens to recognize unmanipulated tumor cells. Factors such as patient-to-patient variation, as well as the use of different treatments, such as incubation of *in vitro* cultured cell lines with interferon (INF)-γ, may play a role in these findings. Inadequate specificity controls as well as the use of bulk, uncloned T cell lines, however, may also at least in part be responsible for these discrepancies.

Another factor that appears to contribute to the difficulty in identifying naturally processed T cell epitopes is the fact that only a small percentage of the potential epitopes that are capable of binding to a particular MHC molecule are naturally processed and presented on the cell surface at sufficient levels to activate a T cell. The carboxy-terminus of the majority of processed peptides is generated within the proteasome, a multi-subunit complex of proteolytic enzymes that possess preferential polypeptide cleavage sites. Based on these findings, additional techniques have been used to identify naturally processed peptides. In one study, 27-mer polypeptides that encompassed 19 potential HLA-A2 binding peptides from the PRAME antigen were incubated with proteasomes, followed by the analysis of the peptides that resulted from proteasomal degradation (75). Four peptides were identified as potential candidates on the basis of the production of peptides containing the correct carboxy-terminus as well as the lack of internal cleavage of the peptides following proteasomal digestion, and T cells generated using these peptides were shown to recognize endogenously processed antigen. Using a similar approach, an immunogenic epitope was identified from the widely expressed antigen SSX-2 *(76)*.

Another method that has been used to identify naturally processed epitopes is the use of mass spectrometry to sequence peptides that have been eluted from MHC molecules isolated from the surface of human tumor cells. Use of this technique, coupled with microarray gene expression profiling, resulted in the identification of peptides that were derived from proteins that were overexpressed in tumor cells (77). Peptides identified using this approach may in many cases not be immunogenic, as the expression of these proteins at some level in normal tissues may lead to self-tolerance; however, one of the peptides that was identified in this study also appeared to be recognized by human tumor reactive T cells.

Epitopes Identified through the Use of HLA Transgenic Mice

Transgenic mice that express human HLA molecules have also been immunized in an attempt to identify T cell epitopes that are naturally processed and presented on tumor cells. Mis-sense mutations have been shown to result in overexpression of p53 in a wide variety of tumor types; however, self-tolerance due to the wide expression of p53 in normal cells appears to be responsible for the difficulty in generating T cells capable of recognizing nonmutated p53 epitopes (*78,79,*80). High-affinity, p53 reactive T cells, however, were generated by immunization of HLA transgenic mice with the human p53:264-272 peptide that contained only a single substitution of asparagine for aspartic acid at the fifth position (81). Human T cells that were transduced with the murine p53 TCR were capable of recognizing a variety of human tumor cells that overexpressed p53 (82). Both CD8$^+$ and CD4$^+$ T cells that were transduced with the murine p53 TCR recognized p53 overexpressing tumors, as expected on the basis of previous observation of a high affinity.

Transgenic mice expressing human MHC molecules have also been used to identify HLA class II restricted T cell epitopes. Mice expressing the human HLA-DRβ1*0401 class II restriction element were immunized with the NY-ESO-1 protein and screened for their ability to recognize peptides derived from the native protein. One of the epitopes that was identified using this approach, NY-ESO-1:160-180, was then used to sensitize human T cells. The T cells that were generated using this approach were found to recognize an epitope of NY-ESO-1 in the context of the HLA-DPβ1*0401 and 0402 alleles, which are expressed by more than 80% of patients (35). This epitope overlapped with a previously described immunodominant HLA-A2–restricted epitope NY-EOS-1:157-165. Subsequent studies, however, have failed to confirm the association between expression of the HLA-DP4 allele and NY-ESO-1 immunity *(83)*, and peripheral CD4$^+$ T cells from 11 out of 13 melanoma patients were found to recognize additional NY-ESO-1 epitopes in the context of multiple HLA class II alleles (36). Immunization of HLA-DRβ1*0401 mice has also resulted in the identification of T cells that recognize epitopes of gp100 *(60)*.

T Cell Epitopes Identified Using Full Length Recombinant Tumor Antigens

Recombinant proteins, as well as viruses that encode full-length tumor antigens, have also been used to carry out *in vitro* sensitization of human T cells to identify T cell epitopes. Pulsing of PBMC with recombinant gp100 protein followed by *in vitro* sensitization resulted in the identification of an HLA class II–restricted epitope of gp100 (61). The use of T cell–depleted PBMC infected with recombinant adenovirus, vaccinia virus, or fowl pox virus encoding NY-ESO-1 to stimulate autologous T cells resulted in the identification of NY-ESO-1 epitopes that were recognized in a variety of MHC class II gene products (36).

Mutated Antigens

Mutated Gene Products Recognized by CD8$^+$ and CD4$^+$ T cells

A variety of mutated antigens have also been identified as targets of tumor reactive T cells. While these studies have not providing generally useful targets for therapy, they have in some cases provided insights into mechanisms involved with tumor development. The CDK4 gene product that was cloned using a CTL clone contained a point mutation that enhanced the binding to the HLA-A2 restriction element (84). This mutation, which was identified in one out of an additional 28 melanomas that were analyzed, lead to inhibition of binding to the cell cycle inhibitory protein p16^{INK4a} and may have played a role in the loss of growth control in this tumor cell. A point-mutated product of the β-catenin gene containing a substitution of phenylalanine for serine at position 37 was isolated by screening a cDNA library with an HLA-24–restricted, melanoma reactive TIL line (85). The peptide epitope corresponded to amino acids 27 to 35 of the mutated β-catenin gene product, and the phenylalanine substitution appeared to have generated an optimal peptide for binding to HLA-A24. This mutation was found to stabilize the β-catenin gene product by altering a critical serine phosphorylation site, and two out of 24 additional melanoma cell lines were found to express transcripts with identical mutations (86). Previous studies demonstrating that β-catenin functions as a transcriptional activator are consistent with the hypothesis that the mutated gene products may have played a role in the development of these tumors. A mutated caspase-8 transcript was identified using T cells reactive with head and neck cancer (87), and overlapping frameshifted transcripts of the p14ARF and p16INK4 genes were found to encode an epitope recognized by melanoma reactive T cells (88). These observations provide support for the notion that mutated gene products that play a role in promoting tumorlogenesis may frequently serve as the targets of tumor reactive T cells, as there may have been selective pressure to maintain expression of these products (89–91).

The observations made in murine studies indicating that immunization against an individual tumor does not generally result in cross-protection against multiple tumors has lead to the suggestion that mutant T cell epitopes represent the dominant antigens responsible for tumor rejection *(92)*. The identification of mutated antigens is also more difficult due to the problems with identifying the appropriate class I or class II restriction element and may have lead to their being underrepresented in studies attempting to identify human cancer antigens. In addition, the nature of mutated antigens may make them more potent targets, as T cells reactive with these epitopes may not have undergone the same degree of negative selection as those that are reactive with normal, nonmutated self-antigens. Nevertheless, the studies described in this chapter suggest that normal self-proteins can represent tumor rejection antigens, as the adoptive transfer of cells whose predominant reactivity is directed against MDAs such as MART-1 and gp100 can lead to the regression of even bulky tumor deposits.

Common Mutations Can Provide Candidate Epitopes for T Cell Generation

Attempts have been made to generate tumor reactive T cells using epitopes that result from mutational hot spots that are present in some oncogenes. This approach has been used to generate responses against p21ras, which is frequently mutated at position 12 and 61, as well as peptides that result from junctional sequences present in bcr-abl fusion products that are frequently expressed in cancers such as acute lymphoblastic leukemia (reviewed in [93]). While caution is needed in evaluating the reactivity of T cells generated using candidate epitope approaches, antigen presentation of class II–restricted epitopes may not result from direct recognition of tumor cells. Constitutive expression of HLA class II has been observed in some tumor types, in particular melanoma, but is not generally observed in other tumor histologies. APCs such as DCs and monocytes, however, can process and present exogenous proteins derived from tumor cells to class II–restricted T cells *(94)*. Cross-priming of HLA class I–restricted tumor reactive T cells has been observed *(94,95)*, and thus it is also theoretically possible that these epitopes could be presented by DC. These observations have been made in experimental systems and may not contribute significantly to normal *in vivo* immune responses to human tumors, however, as tumors generally appear to be capable of directly presenting HLA class I–restricted epitopes to appropriately activated T cells.

Cancers with Viral Etiologies May Provide Potent Targets for Immune Responses

Although the expression of viral oncogenes has been shown in experimental systems to lead to the development of a wide variety of cancers, viruses have not been shown to play a role in the development of the majority of human cancers. Nevertheless, it is now clear that viruses play an important role in the etiology of cancers such as genital and hepatic carcinomas. Infection with papilloma viruses, a group of double-stranded DNA viruses that infect squamous epithelium, is highly associated with the development of a variety of genital lesions that range from warts to carcinoma. Cancer of the cervix is now the second most common cancer in women worldwide and poses a particular threat to women in third-world countries where routine pap smears are not carried out. Nearly 100 HPV genotypes have been identified, and infection with HPV 16 and 18 as well as several additional genotypes is highly associated with the development of genital cancers (reviewed in [96]). The viral proteins E6 and E7 have been shown to lead to cellular transformation *in vitro (97)* and appear to be responsible for the induction of tumorogeneis following *in vivo* infection with HPV. The role of the immune system in controlling HPV infection and development of malignancy was demonstrated by the observation that neutralizing antibodies directed against the major viral capsid protein L1 are highly protective, as demonstrated in passive transfer studies carried out in animals (98). Cell-mediated immunity may also play a protective role, however, as spontaneously regressing genital warts have been found to contain dense infiltrates of lymphocytes and macrophages *(99)*. Recombinant vaccines have been produced by the generation of virus-like particles (VLP), self-assembling particles that form following the expression of the HPV L1 protein in recombinant viral and yeast systems, were initially found to be protective in animal models (98,*100*). The results of a phase II trial in which 2,392 women between 16 and 23 years of age were immunized with HPV16 VLPs indicated that 100% of the vacinees protected against infection with HPV 16 (101). The results of another hase II trail carried out with an HPV 6,11,16,18 quadrivalent vaccine demonstrated a reduction of infection with HPV 6,11,16 and 18 by 90% compared with placebo (102). Although vaccination with VLP does not lead to the regression of established disease, a variety of therapeutic vaccination strategies are also being tested.

A role for both hepatitis B virus (HBV) and hepatitis C virus (HCV) infection in the development of cirrhosis as well as hepatocellular carcinoma has been clearly demonstrated. Hepatitis is a noncytopathic virus, and infection of normal healthy individuals generally lead to spontaneous regression as a result of immune responses directed against HBV; however, in about 3% of individuals, chronic infection leads to cirrhosis and hepatocellular carcinoma (103). Damage to the liver appears to result in the most part from immune responses directed against HBV-infected cells and nonspecific inflammatory responses (reviewed in [104]). In contrast to HPV, studies have failed to provide evidence that oncogenic proteins derived from HBV or HCV result in transformation. The increased cell turnover resulting from chronic hepatitis infection may lead to carcinoma development by increasing the number of somatic mutations generated in normal hepatocytes *(105)*. Vaccination with HBV has been found to be effective at reducing the rate of development of hepatic carcinoma; however, immunization is only partially effective in some populations, particularly children born to HBV positive women *(106)*. The challenge for the future is to develop effective preventive vaccines for HCV as well as effective therapeutic vaccines for HBV and HCV.

Functional TCR Avidity/Affinity and Diversity

Observations made in several studies suggest that there are wide variations in functional avidity of T cells reactive with a particular peptide epitope. Vaccination with the MART-1:26-35 native peptide was reported to increase the avidity of T cells present in peripheral blood reactive with this epitope, as defined by the ability of those cells to recognize target cells pulsed with titrated doses of the cognate peptide (107). Analysis of the T cell repertoire in this study indicated that the increase in avidity resulted from an oligoclonal T cell expansion.

The identification and isolation of T cells with high affinity has also been carried out through the use of specific peptide–MHC tetramers, complexes that can be generated by incubating biotinylated MHC molecules that have been refolded in the presence of a specific MHC-binding peptide with streptavidin *(108)*. The levels of binding of HLA-A2 MART-1:27-35 tetramers was found to correlate with functional T cell avidity (109), and similar findings were reported for additional T cell epitopes *(110)*. A lack of correlation between tetramer binding and avidity, however, has been noted in some studies (111,*112*), which may reflect the fact that many variables can affect tetramer binding. These findings have lead to attempts to devise methods to more reliably evaluate TCR affinity. Measurement of the off-rate of tetramer binding has been shown to be more directly correlated with affinity than direct binding *(113)*. Tetramers prepared with mutated MHC molecules that fail to interact with CD8 have also been used to identify high-affinity TCRs. While the wild-type HLA-A2 molecule was found to bind to CD8 with an estimated affinity of 137 μM, binding of an HLA-A2 mutant containing both a substitution of aspartic acid for lysine at position 227 and of threonine for alanine at position 228, termed D227K/T228A, to CD8 was essentially undetectable (>10,000 μM) (114). A comparison of the levels of binding of native and A2 227/228 KA tetramers has provided the means to distinguish high affinity from low affinity TCR *(115)*. Further studies carried out using the D227K/228A mutant have demonstrated that antibodies to CD8 can enhance or inhibit T cell activation, and this activity appears to be independent of the binding of CD8 to MHC molecules *(116)*. Observations indicating that the CD8 molecule present on the cell surface plays an important role in organizing the TCR on the cell surface *(117)* and may in fact directly interact with the TCR *(118,119)* are consistent with these findings.

In a recent study, a panel of MART-1 reactive T cell clones were examined for their ability to recognize tumor and peptide pulsed target cells, as well as for their ability to bind to the wild-type or mutant D227K/T228A HLA-A2 tetramers (120). The T cell clones that produced high levels of cytokines in response to tumors as well as peptide pulsed targets bound to both the wild-type and mutant tetramers, whereas clones that produced relatively low levels of cytokines bound to the wild type-but not the mutant tetramer, results that were confirmed by studies carried out using the TCRs that were isolated from these cells.

Additional studies have provided evidence for a restriction in the repertoire of MART-1 reactive T cells. While a variety of TCR beta chain variable (TR-BV) sequences have been associated with recognition of MART-1 *(121)*, the majority of receptors directed against this epitope were found in multiple studies to express TR-AV 12 (120,122). The dominant usage of particular TCR α chains observed in responses against both tumor and viral antigens suggests that structural features of germline encoded α chain residues may play an important role in dictating TCR specificity, while α chain junctional diversity along with β chain usage may influence TCR affinity *(123)*.

Multiple Mechanisms Involved with Generating T Cell Epitopes Revealed by Tumor Antigen Studies

A variety of previously unconventional mechanisms have been shown to be involved with generating epitopes that have been identified using T cells derived either by *in vitro* or *in vivo* tumor stimulation. While introns are normally spliced from RNA transcripts prior to being exported to the cytoplasm, multiple T cell epitopes have been found to encoded by intronic sequences *(124–127)*. Although unspliced transcripts may occur at relatively low frequencies in both normal and malignant cells, a transcript containing an intronic sequence of the N-acetylglucosaminyltransferase V gene that encoded a T cell epitope recognized by tumor reactive T cells was found to be expressed in approximately 50% of melanomas (128). Normal cells did not express transcripts containing intronic sequences, indicating that splicing was altered in tumor cells. Alternative open reading frames have also been found to antigens recognized by tumor reactive T cells *(129–132)*. An influenza epitope translated from an alternative open reading frame appears to result from read-through of the normal initiation codon at a low frequency that is dependent on the context of that codon and the number of additional start codons that precede the alternative open reading frame (133), and the open reading frame encoding an antigen expressed in renal cancer cells was initiated from a non-AUG codon (134). A T cell epitope was found be encoded by frame-shifted transcripts of p16^{INK4a}, and p14^{ARF} was identified using melanoma reactive T cells (88). Alternative splicing of transcripts derived from the CDKN2A tumor suppressor gene locus gives rise to both p16^{INK4a} and p14^{ARF}, and small exonic deletions that result in frame-shifted transcripts of this locus have been frequently observed in tumor types such as acute myeloid leukemia (AML) and melanoma *(135,136)*.

Unconventional mechanisms of protein processing are also involved with generating tumor antigen epitopes. An HLA-A2–restricted epitope from tyrosinase was found to contain an aspartic acid residue that resulted from deglycosylation of an asparagine residue that represented a glycosylation site in the native protein (137). In addition, an epitope derived from the FGF-5 molecule that was recognized by renal cancer reactive T cells was generated as a result of protein splicing (138,*139*), a mechanism of protein processing that had not previously been shown to occur in eukaryotes, having only been demonstrated in unicellular organisms (140) and plants *(141)*.

Additional results have demonstrated altered antigen processing in cells expressing the immunoproteasome, which is expressed in professional APCs as well as interferon gamma (IFN-γ)–treated cells and differs in substrate specificity from the proteasome as a result of the replacement of the $\beta 1$, $\beta 2$, and $\beta 5$ subunits with the INF-γ inducible subunits LMP2, MECL1, and LMP7 (74). The results of *in vitro* studies suggested that the MART-1:26–35 and gp100:209-217 epitopes were inefficiently processed in melanomas that had been treated for several daya with IFN-γ to induce expression of the immunoproteasome (142). Expression of the immunoproteasome is needed, however, for the efficient processing of many additional T cell epitopes (143,*144*).

Enhanced Antigenicity and Immunogenicity of High-affinity Altered Peptide Ligands

Peptide binding studies have revealed that the native MART-1:27-35 peptide as well as the gp100:209-217 and 280-288 peptides possessed relatively low binding affinities to HLA-A2. The observation that the sequence of these peptides does not conform to the consensus HLA-A2 binding motif lead to studies aimed at generating a higher affinity peptide that is more immunogenic than the native peptide. The substitution of methionine for the threonine at position two in the native gp100:209-217 peptide lead to a peptide with a nine-fold higher affinity for HLA-A2 than the native peptide, and the substitution of an optimal valine for the alanine present at position nine in the gp100:280-288 peptide lead to a 10-fold higher affinity than the native peptide (145). Variants containing additional modifications at these positions as well as at positions one and three were generated and found in some cases to bind with higher affinity to HLA-A2 than these variants; however, gp100 reactive TIL recognized the gp100:209-217 2M and gp100:280-288 9V peptides as well as the wild-type peptides, in contrast to many of the other variants tested. Tumor reactive T cells were also more efficiently induced when the modified gp100:209-217 2M and 280-288 9V peptides were used to carry out *in vitro* sensitizations of PBMC from HLA A2^{+} individuals.

Recent results have demonstrated that the off rate of the gp100:209-217 2M peptide for binding to HLA-A2 is enhanced by seven-fold over the native peptide, while crystallographic studies have demonstrated that the structure of the complex of HLA-A2 with both the native and modified peptides is essentially identical *(146)*. The analysis of peripheral blood samples from 95 melanoma patients also indicated that the frequencies of T cells that recognize either the native or the modified peptides were essentially identical, further supporting the use of the gp100:209-217 2M peptide in vaccination strategies.

In murine studies, immunization of mice with a vaccinia virus construct encoding the human gp100 protein resulted in the induction of T cells that cross-reacted with murine gp100 (147). A dominant T cell epitope that was recognized in the context of H-2D^{b}, gp100:25-33, contained three differences in the amino terminus of the peptide that were responsible for enhancing the binding of the peptide to H-2D^{b} by a factor of between 100 and 1,000-fold.

Modified variants of the MART-1 peptide that have enhanced binding to HLA-A2 have also been identified and utilized for *in vitro* sensitization of T cells. The peptides ALGIGILTV (MART-1:27-35[28L]) and AMGIGILTV (MART-1:27-35[28M]) that contained substitutions of optimal position-two anchor residues, leucine or methionine, for the alanine in the MART-1:27-35 nonamer AAGIGILTV, bound with high affinity to HLA-A2 (148). Multiple T cell clones that reacted with the wild-type peptide, however, failed to recognize the modified nonamers peptides containing substitutions at the second position. The peptide decamer ELAGIGILTV containing a substitution of a leucine for the alanine at position two in the MART-1:26-35 decamer (MART-1:26-35[2L]) bound to HLA-A2 with a nine-fold higher affinity than the native nonamer. The majority of T cell clones reactive with the native MART-1 peptide recognized targets pulsed with the MART-1:26-35(2L) peptide, and the five CTL clones that were tested in this study recognized targets pulsed with between 30-fold and 20,000-fold lower concentrations of the MART-1:26-35(2L) peptide than the native peptide. The MART-1:26-35(2L) peptide exhibited a significantly slower dissociation rate from HLA-A2 than the native peptide, which may be the primary factor responsible for the significant enhancement of the antigenicity of the modified peptide. In addition, *in vitro* sensitization with the MART-1:26-35(2L) peptide was more efficient at inducing peptide and tumor reactive T cells than sensitization with the native peptide. Modification of the native nonamer by substitution of a leucine for the alanine at position one, MART-1:27-35(1L), also resulted in a peptide that appeared to possess increased immunogenicity, although this did not result in enhanced binding to HLA-A2 (148). Stimulation with the

MART-1:27-35(1L) peptide was also reported to enhance the secretion of IL-2 by MART-1 reactive T cells *(149)*.

Additional studies have further extended the observation that high frequencies of T cells reactive with the MART-1:27-35 epitope are present in HLA-A2 individuals. Limiting dilution analysis demonstrated the presence of high frequencies of MART-1 reactive T cells in the peripheral blood of melanoma patients, as the frequency of MART-1 reactive T cells was found to be >1 in 2,000 peripheral blood cells in four out of nine melanoma patients who were analyzed, while in the remaining patients frequencies on the order of 1 in 40,000 cells were detected (150). Using HLA-A2 tetramers that were prepared with the MART-1:26-35(2L) peptide because of the instability of the native MART-1 peptide complexes with HLA-A2, it was demonstrated that detectable levels of MART-1 reactive T cells were found in the peripheral blood of 10 out of 13 melanoma patients and 6 out of 10 healthy HLA-A2 individuals (151). Further investigations have revealed that MART-1 reactive T cells can recognize peptides derived from self-proteins as well as foreign pathogens (152,*153*), indicating that the relatively high frequencies of T cells reactive with the MART-1 epitope in normal individuals as well as melanoma patients may at least in part result from the presence of subsets of cross-reactive T cells.

The immunogenicity of the dominant NY-ESO-1:157-165 HLA-A2 epitope was also enhanced by the substitution of an optimal valine for the carboxyl-terminal cysteine residue (154). Crystallographic data indicated that complementarity between the peptide and MHC binding groove, as well as between the TCR and the peptide–MHC complex was enhanced by the valine substitution. The immunogenicity of the native cysteine containing peptide was also enhanced by inclusion of reducing agents in *in vitro* assays to reduce cysteinylation as well as dimerization of the native peptide *(155)*.

Multiple Factors Influence *in vivo* T Cell Function

Phenotype of Tumor Reactive T Cells in vivo

Relatively high percentages of tumor reactive T cells have been detected in both the peripheral blood and tumor tissues of patients with growing melanomas, but far less so if at all in patients with other types of solid cancers. These observations in melanoma patients have lead to the analysis of the state of differentiation and activation of cells present in these sites. The majority of MART-1:27-35 tetramer reactive T cells in the peripheral blood of healthy donors expressed a naïve phenotype, whereas those present in the peripheral blood of melanoma patients contained a mixture of T cells with a naïve and effector phenotype (151,156,*157*).

The tumor reactive T cells present in melanoma patients were found in many reports to respond normally to *in vitro* peptide stimulation; however, peripheral T cells isolated from a melanoma patient that were reactive with the MART-1:27-35 and tyrosinase:369-377 epitopes were shown in one study to be deficient in their ability to release cytokines in response to mitogens, as well as their ability to lyse melanoma target cells (158). Peripheral T cell responses to recall antigens such as tetanus toxoid, as well as responses to polyclonal activators, have been reported to be depressed in patients with breast cancer *(159)* as well as additional tumor types *(160)*, and specific effects on the responsiveness of CD4$^+$ T cells has been noted *(161)*. Diminished immune responses may, however, also result from chemotherapy or other treatments administered to patients, rather than reflecting systemic immune suppression resulting from tumor cell growth. Peripheral T cells isolated from the majority of cancer patients do not, however, appear to exhibit a state of either generalized immunosuppression or suppression of specific tumor antigen responses, as demonstrated by the ability of patients with progressive disease to respond to vaccination with tumor antigen peptides (162–164). In addition, many of the tumor antigen epitopes that have been studied represent self-antigens that bind MHC molecules with relatively low affinities and may not efficiently activate peripheral T cells, which are generally in a resting state.

Immunosuppression in the Tumor Micro-environment

Considerable evidence exists, however, for the functional impairment of T cells present within the tumor micro-environment. The analysis of T cells present within melanomas as well as tumor-invaded lymph nodes has provided evidence for the functional impairment of T cells present at these sites, whereas T cells present in the peripheral blood analyzed simultaneously did not show evidence for impairment (165). Myeloid cells present in the tumor micro-environment have also been shown to express arginase, resulting in down-regulation of TCR zeta chain expression and impaired T cell function in a mouse tumor model *(166)*, and have been observed in human renal cancer patients *(167)*. Expression of arginase as well as nitric oxide synthase, which also plays a role in arginine metabolism, has also been observed in human prostate carcinomas (168). Expression of the inhibitory molecule indoleamine 2,3 dioxygenase, which is involved with degradation of tryptophan, was also observed in plasmacytoid DCs within tumor-draining lymph nodes *(169)*. Mouse studies have provided evidence that a subpopulation of monocytes that express the Gr-1 molecule can down-regulate T cell responses *(170,171)*. The ability of tumors to secrete granulocyte macrophage colony stimulating factor (GM-CSF) has been associated with the accumulation of a population of CD34$^+$ suppressor cells that may correspond in humans to a recent described population of cells termed *myeloid suppressor cells* (172).

The identification of T regulatory (Treg) cells as potent modulators of immune responses has lead to an examination of their potential role in modulating anti-tumor responses. In a murine tumor model system, Gr-1^+ monocytes have been reported to induce T regulatory cells (173). Recent analyses carried out using antibodies directed against the Forkhead box P3 (FoxP3) protein indicate that relatively high numbers of regulatory T cells may be present in the tumor micro-environment (164,174,*175,176*), which may act to limit anti-cancer immune responses. The expansion of Treg cells may result from expression of TGF-β in the tumor environment *(177)*.

Additional data have suggested that the levels of T cell subsets detected within tumors can be associated with enhanced or decreased survival of patients with a variety of tumor types, including ovarian cancer *(178)*, melanoma *(179)*, and colon cancer (180). Conflicting data concerning the exact phenotypic properties associated with prognosis has led to considerable confusion in this area. These findings may reflect the presence of an ongoing anti-tumor immune response that may act to limit the growth of malignant cells. The cross-presentation of tumor antigens by DC, which can be influenced by many factors *(181)*, may also be important for priming effective immune responses. Thus, the balance between factors that act to promote effective anti-tumor immune responses and suppressive factors that act to limit those responses may thus be responsible for determining progression of tumor growth.

CANCER THERAPIES

A wide variety of therapies have been evaluated in model systems and are now being developed for treatment of patients with cancer, which include those that involve direct immunization of patients with a variety of immunogens, as well as the adoptive transfer of activated effector cells. The identification of multiple antigens recognized by T cells has provided targets that can be utilized in a variety of contexts. Vaccination has been carried out using peptides either in saline or in adjuvants such as incomplete Freund's adjuvant, DCs that have been pulsed with peptides, with naked DNA encoding T cell epitopes, preparations of heat shock proteins prepared from tumor cells, as well as whole tumor cells and tumor lysates that have been pulsed on APCs. In addition, recombinant immunogens have been incorporated into viruses such as vaccinia, bird poxviruses, and adenoviruses that have been used successfully to protect against infectious diseases (182). The use of standard oncologic criteria is, however, needed to properly evaluate and compare the results of therapy trials. One commonly used definition of clinical response developed by the World Health Organization is a decrease in the sum of the products of the perpendicular diameters of all lesions by greater than 50% with less than a 25% increase in any lesion, a criterion that has been used to evaluate all of the studies carried out in the Surgery Branch, National Cancer Institute (NCI). Another set of criteria that has recently been proposed is the Response Evaluation Criteria in Solid Tumors (RECIST), which defines a response as a 30% reduction in the sum of the maximum diameters of all lesions and no new or progressive lesions. Another important issue is the application of results obtained from animal model systems to human clinical trials. Although these have provided important clues that may lead to improved therapies, it is important to note that model systems that employ tumor protection do not appear to be relevant to the treatment of patients with bulky metastases. Short-term lung metastasis models involve the treatment of relatively small, nonvascularized tumors, and again may not be directly relevant to the majority of tumors that are the targets of current clinical trials.

Nonantigen-specific Therapies

IL-2 Therapy

The best available evidence that immunologic reactions can mediate the regression of large, vascularized metastatic cancers comes from humans who have received the administration of recombinant IL-2. Initial murine tumor treatment model studies demonstrated that the administration of high-dose IL-2 could result in substantial tumor regression (183). In subsequent clinical trials employing treatment with high-dose IL-2, objective tumor regression was observed in between 10% and 20% of treated melanoma and renal cancer patients (184). Almost half of the responses are complete, and more than 80% of these are ongoing beyond 10 years. Thus, although the frequency of response is relatively low, response durations can be substantial, and in many cases curative. These results led to the approval of IL-2 by the FDA for the treatment of patients with metastatic melanoma and renal cancer. The factors that influence clinical responses to IL-2 therapy are not clear; however, recent findings demonstrate that IL-2 administration can lead to the expansion of peripheral Treg cells (185,*186*). Many tumors have also been shown to contain relatively high frequencies of Treg cells, and thus the relative balance between Treg and effector T cells within the tumor environment may at least in part influence the degree of responsiveness to this therapy.

Anti-CTLA-4 Antibody Therapy

CTL-associated antigen 4 (CTLA-4) is an immunomodulatory molecule expressed on both $CD8^+$ and $CD4^+$ T cells that maintains peripheral tolerance by suppressing T cell activation and proliferation. Triggering through CTLA-4 results in a decrease in T cell responsiveness and raises the threshold for T cell activation (reviewed in [187]). Mice genetically deficient in the expression of CTLA-4 develop profound autoimmunity and die of a lymphoproliferative disease at 4 weeks of age. Similarly, in humans, CTLA-4 gene polymorphisms have been linked to the development of various autoimmune diseases, including autoimmune hypothyroidism and type 1 diabetes.

Blockade of CTLA-4 function provides a compelling means of enhancing anti-tumor immunity since tumors primarily express nonmutated, self-antigens. Administration of an anti-CTLA-4 blocking antibody has been shown to result in enhanced regression in murine tumor model systems when administered in combination with an anti-CD25 antibody and tumor vaccination *(188)* or with antibodies directed against activating molecules such as 4-1BB (189). More significantly, recent translation of these findings in clinical trials demonstrated that the administration of an anti–CTLA-4 blocking antibody mediates objective responses in approximately 15% to 20% of patients with metastatic melanoma (190). Objective responses correlated with grade III/IV autoimmune manifestations, including dermatitis, enterocolitis, hepatitis, and hypophysitis. Recent evidence using a knock-in humanized CTLA-4 transgenic mouse model indicates that cancer immunity can occur also in the absence of autoimmune disease (191).

While these results clearly demonstrate the importance of signaling through CTLA-4 in regulating T cell activation, the cellular mechanisms underlying the blockade of CTLA-4 negative regulation remain poorly defined. Some groups have shown that CTLA-4 blockade directly enhances $CD8^+$ T cell activation, proliferation, and cytotoxic activity even in the absence of $CD4^+$ T cell help (192). Blockade of CTLA-4 together with GM-CSF–producing vaccines was ineffective in treating large, vascularized subcutaneous murine tumors, however, and results obtained by other investigators indicate that the lack of CTLA-4 expression on $CD8^+$ T cells alone was insufficient to break peripheral tolerance and enhance effector functions of self-/tumor reactive T cells (193). In tumor treatment as well as prevention studies carried out with pmel-1 transgenic T cells expressing a TCR directed against an unmutated murine gp100 epitope, deletion of the CTLA-4 locus through a genetic knockout failed to enhanced the efficacy of $CD8^+$ pmel-1 T cells. Unlike previous reports indicating that the absence of CTLA-4 had a greater impact on activated rather than on naïve T cells *(194)*, CTLA-4 blockade did not appear to enhance the function of activated pmel-1 T cells.

These findings do not appear to be restricted to self-antigen systems, because similar results have been observed with T cells that recognize foreign epitopes. The lack of CTLA-4 did not affect the ability of adoptively transferred $CD8^+$ transgenic T cells expressing the alloreactive 2C TCR on a Rag-2 knockout background to control B16 SIY growth (195). Moreover, in the lymphocytic choriomeningitis viral model, the absence of CTLA-4 on p33-specific transgenic TCR $CD8^+$ T cells did not affect antiviral T cell responses (196). Removal of $CD4^+$ T cells by crossing the pmel-1 CLTA-$4^{-/-}$ mouse onto a Rag-$1^{-/-}$ background resulted in the complete abrogation of $CD8^+$ T cell activation and autoimmune manifestations; nevertheless, the effects of $CD4^+$ CLTA-$4^{-/-}$ T cells were dependent on the absence of CTLA-4 on $CD8^+$ T cells. These results indicated that dysregulation of $CD4^+$ T cell function through inactivation of CTLA-4 promoted the autoimmunity as well as tumor immunity that was mediated by $CD8^+$ CLTA-$4^{-/-}$ T cells.

Active Immunization Approaches to Cancer Therapy

Cancer vaccines aim to stimulate the adaptive arm of the immune system directly *in vivo*. Despite a wealth of knowledge relevant to basic aspects of tumor immunology, however, the clinical realization of effective therapeutic vaccines for solid tumors have not yet been convincingly achieved. There is a telling paucity of murine tumor models that suggest that active vaccine approaches can mediate the regression of established vascularized tumors, so it is not surprising that these approaches have shown little efficacy in humans. Enthusiasm about the effectiveness of cancer vaccines has often been grounded in surrogate and subjective endpoints, rather than reliable objective cancer regressions using standard oncologic criteria. In a recent review of 1,306 vaccine treatments, including those conducted in the Surgery Branch at the NCI, a 3.3% overall objective response rate was observed (197). In addition to the relatively low response rates observed in these studies, however, in many cases relatively soft criteria such as stable disease or the regression of individual metastases in the presence of progressive disease at other sites have been reported. The presence of numerous and redundant negative influences of the host immune system and tumor microenvironment also may act to limit the effectiveness of "active immunotherapy" with therapeutic vaccines. These observations underscore the need to improve current cancer vaccines and to develop alternative immunotherapeutic strategies for the treatment of metastatic cancer.

Peptide Vaccines

Multiple trials have also been carried out by administering peptides to patients either in saline or oil-in-water emulsions such as Montanide. Immunization resulted in the expansion of T cells reactive with peptides such as the dominant gp100:280–288 (198) and tyrosinase:369-377 (199) peptides; however, the levels of T cells reactive with these epitopes was generally less than 0.01% of peripheral $CD8^+$ T cells. Similar levels have been observed using recombinant viral vaccines directed against epitopes derived from carcinoembryonic antigen *(200)* and prostate-specific antigen (201). Prime-boost regimens employing immunization with recombinant viral constructs followed by boosting with peptide immunization is a strategy that has been found to result in enhanced frequencies of T cells reactive with viral epitopes. In one study, immunization with a canarypox (Alvac) recombinant virus containing a minigene construct encoding the HLA-A1–restricted MAGE-1:161-169 and MAGE-3:168-176 epitopes followed by peptide immunization did appear to enhance the frequencies of tumor reactive T cells. In this trial, a partial response was observed in 1 out of the 40 treated patients, but again the frequency of reactive cell was less than 0.001% of peripheral blood CD8$^+$ T cells. Further studies revealed that the frequency of T cells reactive with additional antigens such as the gp100:209-217 and MAGE-C2:336-344 epitopes was increased after vaccination to approximately 0.01% of peripheral blood CD8$^+$ T cells (202). The analysis of individual T cell clonotypes that recognize these antigens that were identified on the basis of specific TCR beta chain variable region (TCR-BV) sequences revealed that the high frequencies of T cells approached 10% of the CD8$^+$ T cells in regressing cutaneous metastasis and an invaded lymph node, while prior to vaccination frequencies of less than 0.1% of CD8$^+$ T cells were observed. The expansion of cells that recognize epitopes that are not included in the vaccine may have occurred through a bystander effect; however, it is difficult to interpret observations made with a single tumor metastasis that may have regressed due to unrelated mechanisms. The results of *in vitro* sensitization with the NY-ESO-1:157-165 peptide demonstrated that peptide reactive T cells could be induced from PBMC of 2 out of 10 HLA-A2$^+$ melanoma patients who were evaluated *(31)*. In addition, a low frequency of tetramer+ T cells, corresponding to 0.04% of peripheral blood CD8$^+$ T cells, was detected in 1 out of the 10 HLA-A2$^+$ patients who were examined. In an additional trial, immunization with the modified gp100:209-217 2M peptide in combination with IL-2 appeared to result in significantly higher response rates than treatment with IL-2 alone (203); however, the majority of responses that were observed in this trial were found to be transient, and most of the responding patients succumbed to recurrent tumors.

A variety of studies have demonstrated that T cells directed against the MART-1:27-35 epitope can be more readily detected than those directed against additional tumor epitopes, which are compatible with studies suggesting that responses against this epitope are highly dominant in HLA-A2$^+$ melanoma patients. In one study, *in vitro* sensitization with the MART-1:27-35 peptide resulted in the induction of tumor reactive T cells from 13 out of 13 HLA-A2$^+$ melanoma patients, as well as 5 out of 9 HLA-A2$^+$ healthy donors (204). In addition, vaccination appeared to enhance the generation of tumor reactive T cells resulting from *in vitro* peptide sensitization *(205)*. Subsequent studies carried out with MART-1 tetramers demonstrated that significant levels of T cells reactive with the MART-1:27-35 epitope could be detected in the peripheral blood of a significant percentage of unimmunized HLA-A2$^+$ melanoma patients as normal individuals. Significant percentages of T cells reactive with the MART-1 tetramer could be detected in the peripheral blood of 7 out of 10 HLA-A2$^+$ melanoma patients and 6 out of 10 healthy donors at levels between 0.04% and approximately 0.2% of peripheral CD8$^+$ T cells (151).

Patients have also been immunized with multiple peptides in attempts to circumvent the escape of antigen loss variants. Evidence has been presented indicating that it is possible to generate T cell responses directed against multiple melanoma antigen (206), and increases in the frequency of T cells reactive with multiple peptides used for immunization were observed in peripheral blood as well as in sentinel lymph nodes that drain the immunization site (207). In one report, however, immunization with multiple peptides mixed together in incomplete Freund's adjuvant altered peptide immunogenicity (208).

Synthetic oligodeoxynucleotides containing CpG motifs that are potent stimulators of the Toll-like receptor (TLR) TLR9 have been identified and have been used as adjuvants in peptide vaccination trials *(209)*. In a recent study, immunization with the MART-1:26-35 peptide in combination with CpG oligodeoxynucleotide Vaccimmune/CPG 7909 was found to generate an enhanced frequency of peptide reactive T cells in the blood of melanoma patients (164). Immunization was not associated with enhanced frequencies of peptide reactive tumor infiltrating T cells, however, but appeared to be associated with high frequencies of FoxP3$^+$ T regulatory cells within the tumor.

Several clinical trials have been carried out involving immunization with serologically defined antigens such as GM2 ganglioside, which represents one of the most immunogenic gangliosides expressed on melanoma cells. Early studies demonstrated that administration of GM2 with combination with *Bacillus* Calmette-Guérin (BCG) induced immunoglobulin (Ig)M anti-GM2 antibodies in the majority of immunized patients, and a correlation between antibody responses with improved recurrence free survival and overall survival in stage 3 melanoma patients was noted (210). Studies comparing different vaccine formulations resulted in selection of a commercial formulation consisting of GM2 coupled to keyhole limpet hemocyanin (GMK) in combination with the QS-21 adjuvant, which, in contrast to earlier trials, induced high titers of IgM antibodies in more than 80% of patients as well as IgG antibodies, which had not been previously observed with GM2 plus BCG. The results of a large randomized study comparing GMK to high-dose interferon alpha (IFN-α-2b), however, indicated that the GMK vaccine was inferior to IFN-α-2b (211).

Although the expansion of T cells directed against the immunizing peptide was generally observed in these trials, generally less than 5% of the treated patients demonstrated clinical responses, and strict oncologic criteria have not always been utilized in reporting these results. One possible explanation for the lack of clinical responses is the fact that these immunizations generally have been shown to result in the stimulation of frequencies of peptide reactive T cells that are less than 0.1% of peripheral T cells. It has been estimated that frequencies on the order of 1% or more of peripheral blood T cells, however, may be required to mount an effective anti-tumor response (212,*213*), though little reliable data is available to support this statement. Additional findings demonstrate, however, that tumor progression can occur even in the presence of relatively high frequencies of tumor antigen reactive T cells. In an adjuvant trial of patients with no evidence of disease at the start of the course of vaccination, multiple course of peptide immunization carried out over a course of approximately 1 year with the modified gp100:209-217 2M peptide was shown to result in the induction of high levels of peptide and tumor reactive T cells (163). Analysis of reactivity of PBMC obtained following multiple ELISPOT assays indicated that in 44% of the immunized patients between 1% and 10% of all peripheral $CD8^+$ T cells recognized the immunogen, and in 17% of patients >10% of peripheral $CD8^+$ T cells recognized this peptide. Although immunoselection for loss of antigen or HLA-A2 expression could have been partially responsible for some of the recurrences, recurrences of tumors that clearly expressed both antigen and HLA-A2 were observed in this trial.

Whole Cell Vaccines

Clinical trials employing whole tumor cells as vaccines represents can theoretically activate cells reactive against multiple antigenic targets, and early model studies have demonstrated the ability of autologous tumor cell vaccination to protect mice from subsequent tumor inoculation (11,*12*). In a trial comparing treatment with a combination of an allogeneic melanoma vaccine with the adjuvant DETOX, there was no significant increase in relapse free survival when compared to patients randomized to observation without further therapy (214). Treatment with a combination of three irradiated allogeneic melanoma cells with BCG (Canvaxin trial) resulted in an overall survival rate of 49%, as opposed to a rate of 37% in patients who did not receive the vaccine (215). Further evaluation of this approach in phase III trials, however, showed no significant difference in survival of patients with stage III or IV melanoma receiving this treatment compared to controls receiving BCG alone (216).

Gene modified cells have been evaluated for their effectiveness in cancer therapy protocols. In a murine model system, mice that were immunized with B16 melanoma cells transduced with genes encoding 10 cytokines were examined for their resistance to a subsequent inoculation of the wild-type B16 tumor (217). The results indicated that tumors transduced with the GM-CSF gene provided significant protection against B16 tumor challenge, and a lower level of protection was observed in mice immunized with IL-4 and IL-6 transduced tumors. In a clinical trial involving immunization of patients with autologous renal carcinoma cells that had been transduced with the GM-CSF gene, immune responses against the parental renal carcinomas were observed, as measured by delayed type hypersensitivity (DTH) responses, and an objective clinical response was observed in 1 out of the 16 fully evaluable patients (218). Melanoma patients have also been immunized with allogeneic irradiated melanomas transduced with GM-CSF. Analysis of DTH responses provided evidence for priming of reactivity against autologous tumor cells in 17 out of 25 patients, and one complete and one partial response was observed (219), but again it is difficult to evaluate the effectiveness of this approach in this relatively small trial.

DC Vaccines

Other approaches have utilized immunization with professional APCs such as autologous DC. In one trial, patients were vaccinated with autologous DC that were pulsed either with peptide or melanoma lysates. Objective clinical responses were observed in 5 out of 16 treated patients (220); however, follow-up studies involving treatment of larger numbers of patients using this approach have not been reported by this group. Another approach has employed immunization of patients with DCs that have been transfected either with mRNA encoding individual tumor antigens or bulk mRNA isolated from tumor cells (221,*222*). Although expansion of tumor reactive T cells following these treatments has been reported, only sporadic cases of tumor regression were observed in these trials. In one study carried out by the Dendreon Corporation (Seattle, WA), an APC vaccine loaded with an antigen called prostatic acid phosphatase linked to GM-CSF was used to treat men with hormone-refractory prostate cancer (223), and in a retrospective subset analysis, limited clinical efficacy was claimed. Additional trials are also being carried out using DCs pulsed with either tumor lysates or using hybrids of DCs and cancer cells (224).

Recombinant Vaccines

Multiple trials have been carried out using either recombinant viral constructs or naked DNA encoding particular tumor antigens. In these trials, recombinants containing either full-length gene products or mini-genes containing individual or multiple T cell epitopes were evaluated. The failure in general to detect enhanced precursor frequencies directed against the tumor antigens may have resulted from the dominance of viral epitopes.

Attempts have also been made to enhance the potency of vaccination protocols through the provisions of costimulatory signals. In studies carried out in a mouse model system, evidence for enhanced immunity was obtained following immunization with a recombinant virus that contained the genes encoding the candidate tumor antigen CEA along with genes encoding LFA-3, ICAM-1, and B7–1, termed *TRICOM* (225). In an ongoing clinical trial, injection of a vaccinia virus TRICOM construct directly into melanoma lesion resulted in one partial response and one complete response out of the 12 treated patients (226). One objective response was also observed in 58 patients with advanced CEA-expressing cancers that were treated with TRICOM-CEA (227), but larger randomized patient studies will be needed to establish the efficacy of this approach.

Heat Shock Proteins (HSP)

The first autologous HSP vaccine introduced in clinical trials was Oncophage or, HSPPC-96 (heat shock protein-peptide complex 96; Antigenics Inc., Woburn, MA) produced from surgically resected cancer tissue and formulated for intradermal or subcutaneous injection. Numerous HSP vaccine trials have been carried out in a variety of patients including those with resected pancreatic adenocarcinoma, renal cell carcinoma, melanoma, colorectal cancer, non-Hodgkin's lymphoma, and gastric cancer. The results of these trials, however, have failed to demonstrate the effectiveness of HSP-based vaccines (reviewed in [228]).

Idiotypic Determinants as Therapeutic Targets

The presence of idiotypic determinants on the Ig molecules expressed by B cell lymphomas has presented investigators with unique targets for vaccine trials of patients with hematopoietic malignancies. Immunization with idiotypic proteins that have been coupled to carrier proteins has been shown to result in long-term tumor regression in significant numbers of treated patients (229). These responses were associated with serological anti-idiotypic responses as well as FcγRIIIa polymorphisms, suggesting that humoral immunity may play a significant role in these responses. Immunization with DCs that have been pulsed with idiotype protein was also shown to result in tumor regression in 4 out of 10 vaccinated patients (230).

In summary, although some success has been achieved in clinical vaccination studies carried out with leukemias and lymphomas, possibly as a result of the unique nature of the antigenic targets expressed on these tumors, the results of active immunization trials carried out in patients with other malignancies have been disappointing. These have included trials involving treatment of patients with melanoma, a patient population demonstrating significant response rates to cellular therapies, as described later in this chapter. Many of the murine model systems that have been studied employed either prevention protocols in which the vaccination may have prevented implantation of the tumor or relied on the treatment of relatively small, nonvascularized tumors. Another problem encountered in these early trials is the observation that antigenically complex vaccines such as those employing recombinant viral constructs contain immunodominant determinants that overshadow responses to relatively weak tumor antigens present in these constructs.

Passive Immunological Treatments

Adoptive Cell Transfer

The transfer of in vitro cultured LAK cells to syngeneic mice along with IL-2 was found to lead to the regression of relatively small established pulmonary metastases as well as prolonged survival *(231)*. Subsequent studies in human adoptive immunotherapy trials resulted in durable complete tumor responses (232); however, there was no significant differences in long-term survival between patients treated with LAK cells plus IL-2 compared to IL-2 alone.

Further studies carried out using TILs demonstrated that cultured TIL contained potent effector cells that, in mouse models, were between 50- and 100-fold more active than LAK cells (233) and lead to TIL adoptive immunotherapy trials. The identification of CD8$^+$ T cells as potent effectors of the adaptive anti-tumor immune response has lead to the extensive use of these cells in both experimental model systems and clinical trials. Tumor-specific CD4$^+$ T cells have been also identified, but their functionality can be manifold because CD4$^+$ T cells can help or hinder anti-tumor immune responses. The target antigens recognized by tumor reactive T cells have been described earlier. A number of advances in basic immunology have made a substantial impact on therapies based on the adoptive transfer of T cells. The molecular signals that modulate T cell activation, function, and memory are being elucidated. Both positive and negative signals from costimulatory molecules have been shown to shape the anti-tumor response. Cytokines, including those with receptors that contain the common cytokine-receptor γ-chain, have been shown to alter the programming of T cells.

Adoptive cell transfer (ACT) therapies accomplish T cell stimulation *ex vivo* by activating and expanding autologous self-/tumor reactive T cells to large numbers that are then transferred back to the patient. Early attempts of ACT therapies using TILs in immuno-replete patients met with some success (234), although the lack of persistence of the transferred cells appeared to limit their clinical effectiveness. Previous preclinical studies, however, had indicated that immune ablation is an effective preconditioning regimen that can enhance T cell responses after adoptive transfer (235). The adoptive transfer of TILs after

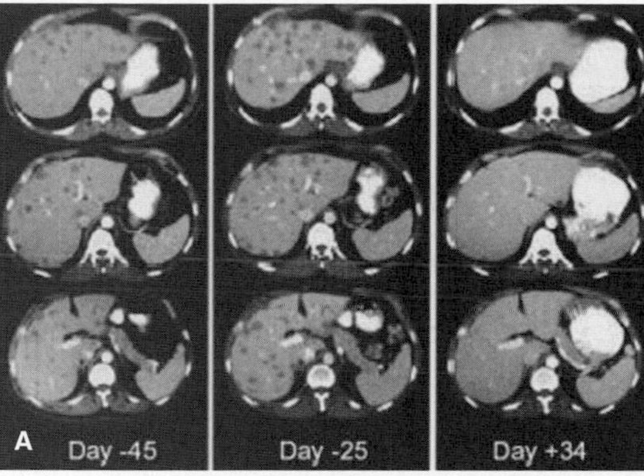

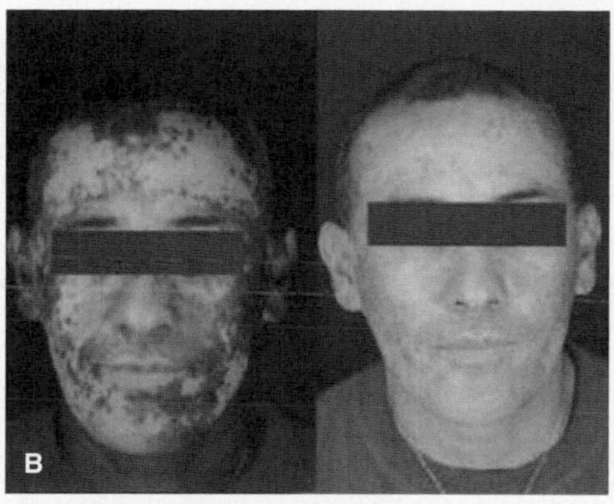

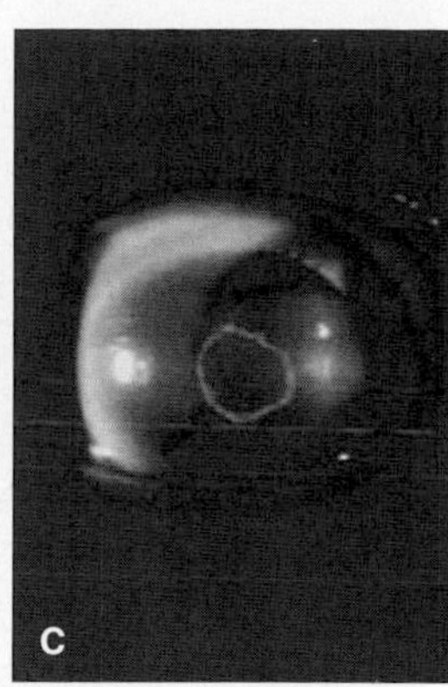

FIGURE 45.1 Tumor destruction and autoimmunity following the adoptive cell transfer of TILs, in the setting of chemotherapy-mediated lymphoablation. **A:** Computed tomography (CT) scan of liver metastases in a melanoma patient. Metastatic lesions progressed rapidly before the treatment (from day −45 to day −25), then regressed dramatically after adoptive T cell transfer (day +34). **B:** Extensive destruction of normal melanocytes (vitiligo) in a patient who experienced a remarkable clinical response. **C:** Anterior uveitis (inflammation of the eye) in a patient who exhibited >99% tumor reduction (*320*).

nonmyeloablative but lymphodepleting systemic chemotherapy can induce objective anti-cancer responses in approximately 50% of patients with metastatic, multivisceral, bulky melanoma that is refractory to standard treatments including chemotherapy, radiation therapy, and IL-2 administration (236) (Figure 45.1).

These clinical studies that combine a lymphodepleting preparative regimen followed by the administration of activated anti-tumor T cells and IL-2 provide the clearest evidence that antigen-specific immunotherapies can result in cancer regression when appropriate treatment and host factors are combined. Studies carried out in both animal model systems as well as in patients have now provided clues as to the factors that influence tumor regression following the transfer of self-/tumor-reactive T cells into lymphopenic recipients. Further studies have begun to elucidate the phenotypic and functional characteristics of tumor-specific T cells that mediate anti-tumor responses *in vivo*. Many of these factors, which are described in the following section, provide the bases for rational design of new ACT-based immunotherapies that incorporate vaccines, increased intensity preconditioning regimens with hematopoietic stem cell (HSC) transplantation, and alternative methods for the generation and selection of T cells for transfer.

Lymphodepletion Increases the Efficacy of ACT through a Variety of Mechanisms

It has long been observed in mice that depletion of immune cells prior to ACT can dramatically improve the anti-tumor efficacy of transferred $CD8^+$ T cells, but the specific mechanisms that contribute to this increased immunity have only recently begun to be elucidated. Although it seems counterintuitive that the efficacy of ACT-based tumor immunotherapy can be improved by the removal of the host immune system, several mechanisms might underlie the augmented efficacy of tumor reactive T cells in the lymphopenic environment. These factors include the elimination of immunosuppressive cells such as $CD4^+CD25^+$ Treg cells, the depletion of endogenous cells that compete for activating cytokines, and the increased function and availability of APCs (Figure 45.2).

Elimination of Immunosuppressive Cells

Extensive studies have now demonstrated that Treg cells are critically involved in the maintenance of peripheral self-tolerance; however, more recent studies have provided evidence that Treg cells may also down-regulate anti-tumor immune responses. These cells constitutively express high levels of the transcription factor FoxP3 as well as several cell-surface molecules associated with T cell activation. These include IL-2Rα (CD25), which together with the IL2-Rβ and γ chains forms the high-affinity IL-2 receptor, glucocorticoid-induced TNF receptor–related protein (GITR) and CTL-associated antigen-4 (CTLA4). An exclusive molecular signature for human Treg cells does not currently exist, however, because activation of $CD4^+$ T cells can also result in up-regulation of FoxP3 expression. Experiments using mice lacking Treg cells owing to specific gene defects, as well as the "add-back" of these cells, have convincingly shown that they are capable of suppressing the anti-tumor activities of adoptively transferred self-/tumor reactive T cells. Augmented anti-tumor responses were observed after ACT of self-/tumor reactive effector $CD8^+$ T cells to tumor-bearing $CD4^{-/-}$, but not $CD8^{-/-}$, mice, indicating that the immunoregulatory cells are contained in the $CD4^+$ T cell population. The suppressive activity was restricted to the $CD25^+$ T cell subset because

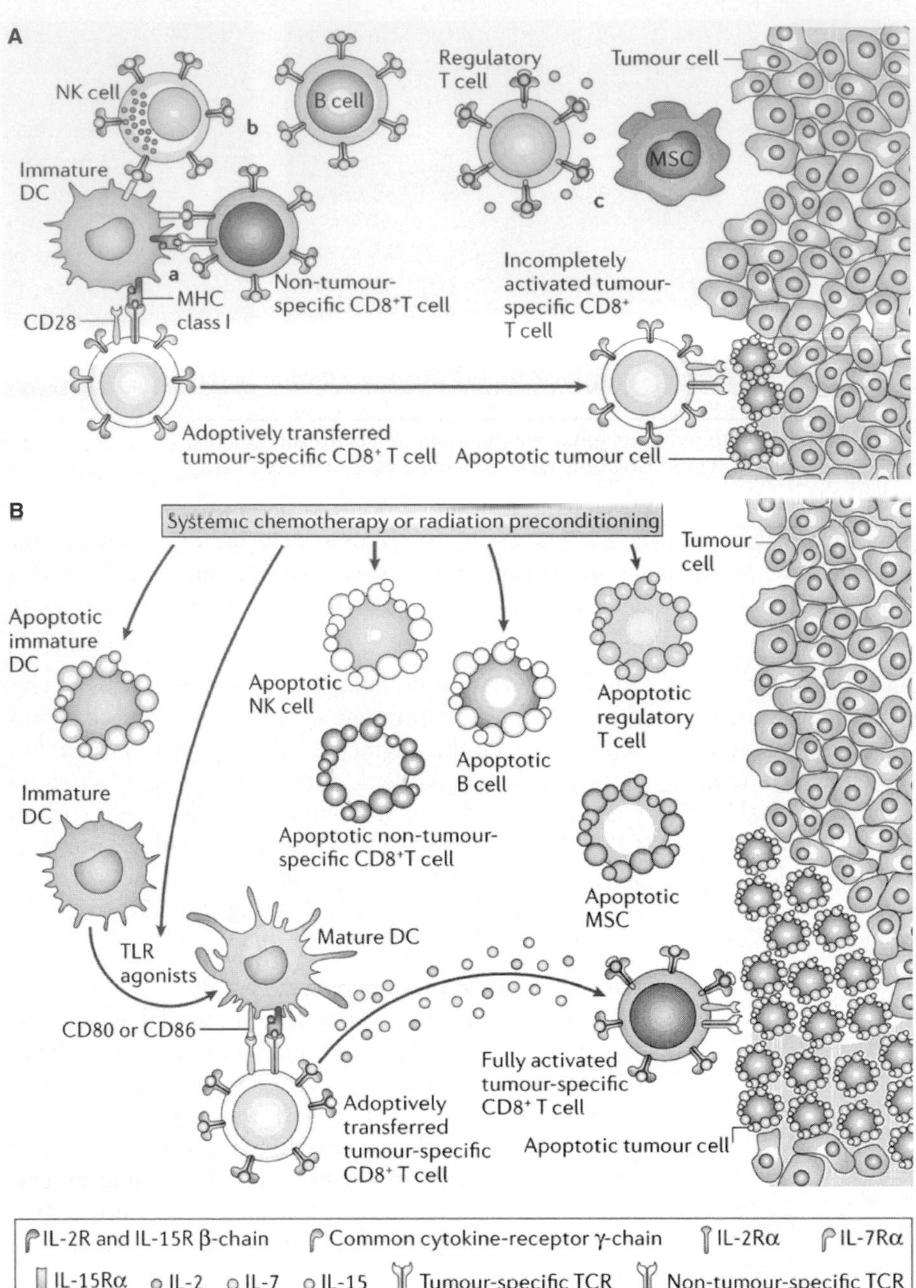

FIGURE 45.2 The rationale for lymphodepletion. **A:** In immunoreplete hosts, competition for homeostatic and activating cytokines such as IL-2, IL-7, and IL-15 can inhibit the functions of adoptively transferred T cells. Treg, NK cells, and other immune cell populations (e.g., macrophages) can display suppressive activity either by direct cell-to-cell contact or release of suppressive cytokines, and the tumor itself might act as a negative regulator of T cell activation. **B:** Lymphodepleting preconditioning using systemic chemotherapy or radiation can augment the functions of adoptively transferred T cells by reducing competing "cytokine sinks" and regulatory elements. In addition, the pro-inflammatory environment can activate immature DCs as well as enhancing MHC expression on tumor cells. Abbreviations: DC, dendritic cell; IL, interleukin; NK cells, natural killer cells (271).

transfer of $CD4^+CD25^+$ Treg cells alone, or in combination with $CD4^+CD25^-$ T helper (T_H) cells, to mice receiving $CD8^+$ anti-tumor cells inhibited effective immunotherapy in lymphopenic mice. By contrast, transfer of T_H cells alone in this setting resulted in profound autoimmunity and eradication of established tumors. The maintenance and function of effector $CD8^+$ T cells required the presence of T_H cells able to produce IL-2.

The immunosuppressive role of Treg cells in patients with cancer has only recently begun to be explored. Treg cells have been reported to be overrepresented in tumor lesions from patients with ovarian and lung cancer (237). Cells that possess characteristics of Treg cells have been isolated following the *in vitro* culture of melanoma TIL (238,239), although the *in vivo* significance of these observation has not been established. Reduced survival was reportedly associated with increased tumor infiltration by Treg cells in patients with ovarian cancer (240), although these findings have been recently contradicted (241). Therefore, at present, no conclusive data link the *in vivo* function of Treg cells and the progression of cancer. Nevertheless, the suppressive effects of Treg cells might contribute to the poor clinical response rates reported in patients with cancer who receive immunotherapy in nonlymphodepleting settings. Selective elimination of Treg cells from patient TILs might further improve the efficacy of ACT approaches in the lymphodepleting setting, because the proliferation of Treg cells can be enhanced by the lymphopenic environment and the presence of exogenous IL-2. Further, removal of Treg cells from PBMC might enrich for a T_H-cell population able to bolster the response of self-/tumor-specific $CD8^+$ T cells *in vivo*.

Other immune cells including NKT cells, NK cells, and $CD11b^+Gr1^+$ myeloid suppressor cells (MSCs) have been shown to dampen T cell function. Some studies have suggested that NKT cells mediate suppression through the production of cytokines such as IL-13 (242). Although the precise lineage of MSCs has not been clearly defined, these cells appear to comprise a heterogeneous population of cells that comprises myeloid cells at various stages of differentiation, including monocytes, granulocytes, and a subset of immature myelo-monocytic cells (170). Increased frequencies of MSCs are found in conditions characterized by impaired T cell function, including tumors and chronic infections (243), and MSCs may play an important role in the induction of Treg cells in the tumor environment (173). The expression of arginase and inducible nitric oxide synthase (iNOS) by MSCs leads to the release highly reactive peroxynitrates may play an important role in mediating T cell suppression (168), but MSCs may also mediate suppression through direct contact with T cells. Depletion of MSCs using a Gr1-specific antibody has also been shown to result in protection from tumor challenge (244). Therefore, removal of MSCs, and thereby their suppressive activity, might contribute to the increased anti-tumor T cell responses observed after ACT in patients who have been lymphodepleted.

Minimizing Cellular Cytokine Sinks

Transfer of small numbers of antigen-specific T cells into a lymphopenic host results in T cell clonal expansion and activation, a process known as *homeostatic proliferation*. In the lymphopenic environment, antigen-experienced T cells proliferate independently of self-peptide–MHC complexes. However, either cotransferring an "irrelevant" population of T cells or increasing the number of transferred cells can reduce the level of homeostatic proliferation in a dose-dependent manner showing that other elements exist that limit homeostatic proliferation. Although host-mediated inhibition of the proliferation of adoptively transferred T cells might involve direct cellular contact, competition might also exist between transferred and host T cells for a limited amount of the cytokines that are required to support $CD8^+$ T cell homeostasis, and such competition is known as the "cytokine sink" effect.

The importance of the availability of these cytokines has been shown in experiments in which mice deficient for IL-7 or IL-15 showed impaired homeostatic maintenance and proliferation of memory $CD8^+$ T cells (245). Conversely, transgenic mice overexpressing IL-7 or IL-15 have increased numbers of T cells owing to the preferential expansion of the memory $CD8^+CD44^{high}$ T cell population (246). In the pmel-1 mouse model of ACT therapy, lymphodepletion before cell transfer increased the persistence of self-/tumor-specific T cells, as well as their effector function and tumor regression, compared to immunoreplete hosts (247). Conversely, increased anti-tumor responses were seen when these cytokines were exogenously administered or when the endogenous competition (that is host lymphocytes) for these cytokines was removed by using mice lacking both recombination-activating gene 2 (RAG2) and γ_C (247). These findings show that a key mechanism underlying the improved efficacy of ACT therapies after lymphodepletion is the transient eradication of endogenous lymphocytes, which serve as cellular cytokine sinks. The use of cytokines such as IL-7, which is capable of supporting the survival of $CD4^+$ and $CD8^+$ T effector and memory T cells but does not promote the survival of Treg cells, might also be advantageous for adoptive cell transfer therapy. Depletion of cells expressing NK1.1 (using an NK1.1-specific antibody) improves the efficacy of ACT therapy in tumor-bearing *Rag1*$^{-/-}$ mice and implicates NK cells as key players in the cytokine sink effect, a process that might be mediated by consumption of IL-15, a critical cytokine for the survival and proliferation of both T and NK cells *in vivo*.

Another cytokine whose receptor contains the γ_C signaling chain IL 2 is a T cell growth factor commonly used to promote the expansion and function of self-/tumor-specific T cell populations *in vitro* and *in vivo*. Perhaps more importantly, however, IL-2 is essential for the maintenance of peripheral self-tolerance. Mice deficient in either IL-2 or components of the IL-2 receptor spontaneously develop lymphoproliferative and autoimmune disorders (248). These observations have been linked to impaired Treg cell homeostasis and "metabolic fitness" *in vivo,* rather than suppressive function, because Treg cells from either IL-2– or IL-2Rα (CD25)–deficient mice are competent when tested in *in vitro* assays of suppressive function. More recent findings, however, have shown that *in vivo* IL-2 signaling is important not only for maintaining Treg-cell "fitness" but also for their suppressive function. The anti-tumor activity of adoptively transferred self-/tumor-specific $CD8^+$ T cells was inhibited in wild-type but not IL-2Rα–deficient mice, despite both animals having comparable numbers of $FoxP3^+$ Treg cells (249). Further, blockade of IL-2Rα with specific antibody has been shown to induce profound autoimmunity resulting from impaired Treg cell function, rather than depletion of these cells (250). These results indicate that *in vivo* immunoregulation by Treg cells might, in part, be a product of their constitutive expression of the component of the IL-2 receptor with highest affinity for IL-2, IL-2Rα (CD25), and their increased capacity to consume IL-2. Therefore, removal of Treg cells by lymphodepletion might result in increased anti-tumor reactivity of adoptively transferred CD8$^+$ T cells not only by the elimination of direct cellular inhibition, but also by increasing the availability of IL-2.

Improved APC Function and Availability

Systemic chemotherapy and total body irradiation have both been used before ACT to deplete the lymphoid compartment of the host and create a niche for the transferred cells. Investigators have long hypothesized that these treatments might also cause necrosis or apoptosis of tumor cells, resulting in APC uptake of tumor antigens and the subsequent cross-presentation of these antigens to the adoptively transferred self-/tumor reactive CD8$^+$ T cells. Although lymphodepletion can reduce the absolute number of APCs *in vivo*, it can also promote their transition to an activated state. In mice, the expression of the activation markers CD86 and I-A (MHC class II) has been reported to be up-regulated on the surface of splenic DCs after irradiation (251). Further, DCs isolated after irradiation released substantially more IL-12 in comparison with DCs isolated from nonirradiated mice (252). Activation of DCs after chemotherapy or irradiation might be triggered by translocation of bacterial products, such as lipopolysaccharide (LPS) and other TLR agonists, into the bloodstream following damage to the integrity of mucosal barriers. The production of pro-inflammatory cytokines such as TNF, IL-1, and IL-4 by host cells might be also involved in mediating DC maturation. In addition, the lymphopenic environment might facilitate the activation of transferred self-/tumor reactive T cells through decreased competition at the surface of antigen-bearing APCs. Although the net effect of lymphodepletion on APC function is less clear than its impact on Treg cells and cellular cytokine sinks, ablation might ultimately increase the anti-tumor reactivity of transferred T cells by increasing the activation and availability of APCs.

T Cell Differentiation State and ACT-Based Immunotherapies

Lymphodepletion can have a marked impact on ACT-based immunotherapies, but it is not the only factor that has been shown to impact clinical responses. Emerging findings from both mouse studies and clinical trials indicate that intrinsic properties related to the differentiation state of the adoptively transferred T cell populations are critical to the success of ACT-based approaches.

In both mice and humans, CD8$^+$ T cell subsets have been categorized into distinct differentiation states using a variety of phenotypic and functional attributes. A progressive pathway of CD8$^+$ T cell differentiation has gained acceptance based on the findings of *ex vivo* phenotypic analyses of virus-specific T cells, measurement of telomere length, gene-expression profiling, and *in vitro* differentiation studies. Within this paradigm, activation of naïve CD8$^+$ T cells results in proliferation and progressive differentiation through early, intermediate, and late effector stages depending on signal strength. Memory CD8$^+$ T cells might reflect T cells arrested at intermediate stages of the differentiation pathway, but there remains some debate regarding the pathways by which effector and memory T cells develop.

The phenotypic and functional characteristics of self-/tumor-specific CD8$^+$ T cells that are associated with optimal *in vivo* tumor responses in the pmel-1 mouse model of ACT therapy have recently been elucidated. Self-/tumor-specific CD8$^+$ T cells at progressive stages of differentiation were generated using multiple *in vitro* stimulations with antigen. Surprisingly, CD8$^+$ T cells that acquired terminal effector properties and had increased anti-tumor activity *in vitro* were found to be less effective at triggering tumor regression *in vivo* (253). Terminally differentiated CD8$^+$ T cells were nearly 100-fold less effective *in vivo* on a per cell basis than T cells at an early stage of differentiation. Similar findings have been reported by other groups employing different mouse tumor and allogeneic HSC transplantation models. The *in vitro* expansion of T cells for ACT—as it is currently performed for clinical use—induces progressive CD8$^+$ T cell differentiation toward a late effector state resulting in phenotypic and functional changes that may render T cells less "fit" to mediate anti-tumor responses *in vivo* and less able to benefit from the activating cues present in the lymphopenic host (Figure 45.3). For example, less differentiated, central memory–like T cells have a high proliferative potential, are less prone to apoptosis than more differentiated cells, and have a higher ability to respond to homeostatic cytokines, because they express receptors such as IL-7Rα. Therefore, less differentiated central memory–like T cells might proliferate and become fully activated in the lymphopenic environment, which is rife with homeostatic cytokines such as IL-7.

The Importance of Trafficking to Lymph Nodes

Tumor immunologists have long sought to cause T cells to specifically traffic to their tumor targets. The loss of expression of the lymphoid homing molecule CD62L and the acquisition of CD44 expression were reported to be associated with increased anti-tumor effects of adoptively transferred T cells (254). It is now clear in both tumor and viral models, however, that T cells able to home to secondary lymph nodes, where they can be effectively stimulated by DCs, are more effective in adoptive immunotherapy (253,255). Anti-tumor responses have also been found to be abrogated in hosts devoid of peripheral lymphoid tissues and with a disrupted splenic structure (256), which is consistent with additional studies that indicate that that tumors alone are inefficient at triggering effective immune responses. Similarly, CD62L$^-$ T cells were less effective at mediating allo-responses in an allogeneic HSC

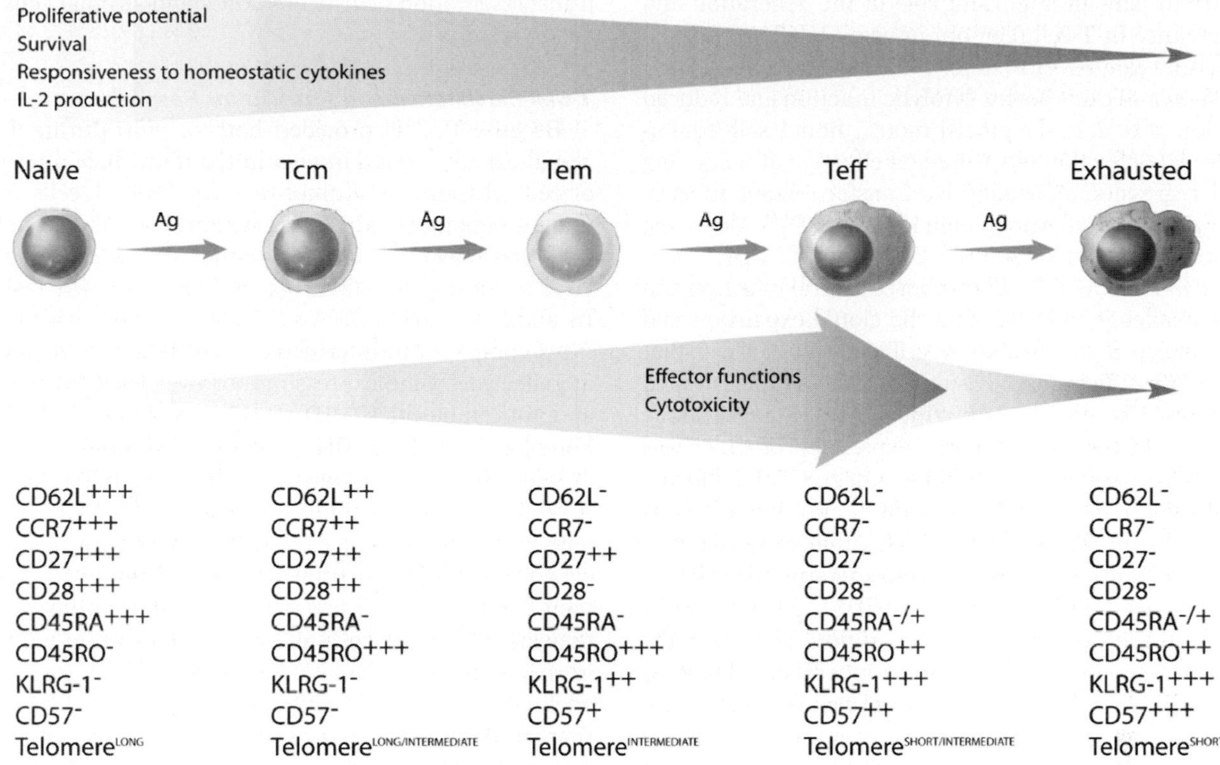

FIGURE 45.3 Inverse relationship of *in vitro* and *in vivo* antitumor functions of adoptively transferred naive and effector T cell subsets. As time and the strength of stimulation increases, naïve CD8$^+$ T cells proliferate and progressively differentiate through early, intermediate, and late effector stages. The phenotypic and functional changes that characterize this process are illustrated as no expression (–), intermediate expression (+), and high expression (hi) of the various markers. The progressive acquisition of full effector functions (dashed burgundy line) is associated with a decreased ability of T cells to cause tumor regression after adoptive transfer (black line). This may result from progressive telomere shortening, loss of proliferative potential, decreased expression by T cells of lymph-node homing and costimulatory molecules and the inability of terminally differentiated T cells to produce IL-2, as well as a reduction in the levels of receptors required to receive activating signals from homeostatic cytokines. KLRG1, killer-cell lectin-like receptor G1 (*321*).

transplantation model (257). Therefore, down-regulation of expression of lymph node homing molecules at the intermediate and late stages of effector CD8$^+$ T cell differentiation can result in impairment of their anti-tumor capacity. The principle that T cells must home to lymph nodes to be effective has not been established in humans, as CD62L$^-$ and CCR7$^-$ TILs were able to engraft, proliferate, and ultimately lead to objective responses in approximately 50% of treated patients. Nevertheless, it is possible that the expression of additional T cell homing molecules may play an important role in these therapies.

Costimulatory Molecules and T Cell Persistence

Transition from an early to an intermediate effector stage is marked by down-regulation of CD28 expression. The interaction of CD28 with CD80 or CD86 on APCs amplifies TCR-mediated T cell activation and proliferation. Enhanced IL-2 secretion, the induction of anti-apoptotic molecules, as well as increases in cell-cycle progression have been associated with T cell expression of CD28. The role of CD28 expression in ACT-based clinical trials has been recently investigated in detail. Self-/tumor-specific TILs express low but detectable levels of CD28. After cell infusion, immediate and high expression of CD28 was detected on circulating self-/tumor reactive T cells, indicating that either rapid up-regulation of CD28 expression or early selective expansion and survival of the CD28$^+$ T cell population had occurred (258). Analysis of clonotypes derived from TIL that either did or did not persist after adoptive transfer provided some evidence for the preferential survival of clones that expressed the highest levels of CD28 (259), indicating that there may be a survival advantage for transferred T cells that possess an early effector phenotype.

Engagement of the costimulatory molecule CD27 can also augment TCR-induced T cell proliferation and appears to play an important role in the generation and maintenance of T cell memory *in vivo* (260,261). Consistent with a late effector state, T cells lacking CD27 have been shown to exert potent cytolytic function and reduced secretion of IL-2. In the pmel-1 mouse model, self-/tumor-specific late effector cells were less effective at mediating tumor regression after adoptive transfer relative to early effector T cells that express high levels of CD27. Moreover, the administration of soluble CD27 ligand, CD70, augmented *in vivo* $CD8^+$ T cell responses to viral infection and tumor challenge by increasing the clonal expansion and maintenance of antigen-specific T cells, indicating that CD27 expression is not only a marker of less differentiated T cells but also functionally critical for optimal immune responses. In the clinical arena, expression of CD27 was found to be up-regulated to varying degrees by culturing TIL in the absence of IL-2 for 2 days, and based on this analysis, the numbers of $CD27^+$ TILs that were administered to patients who responded to therapy were significantly higher than the numbers of $CD27^+$ cells administered to nonresponders (262). In addition, after ACT, the percentage of persistent T cells in peripheral blood that expressed CD27 gradually increased and was associated with the long-term maintenance of stable tumor reactive T cells in treated patients (258,*263*). These results, taken together with results obtained in studies carried out with viral epitopes, indicate that T cells expressing CD27 may selectively persist *in vivo* and give rise to a stable memory $CD8^+$ T cell population.

Homeostatic Cytokine Signals and T Cell Persistence

Increased access to homeostatic cytokines has been shown to be critical for the increased anti-tumor responses following ACT to lymphodepleted hosts. Homeostatic signals can be regulated by both the availability of cytokines in the host and the level of expression of the cytokine receptors on the surface of transferred $CD8^+$ T cells. Expression of IL-7Rα by a subset of effector $CD8^+$ T cells might identify precursors destined to become long-lived memory cells. IL-7Rα^{low} self-/tumor-specific late effector $CD8^+$ T cells transferred to tumor-bearing mice persisted at decreased numbers and were less effective at inducing anti-tumor responses than IL-7Rα^{high} early effector $CD8^+$ T cells. In patients, IL-7Rα was expressed at low levels on all TIL populations at the time of ACT but was up-regulated immediately after infusion on the surface of robustly proliferating self-/tumor-specific T cells that persisted (258). Therefore, IL-7 signaling seems to be important for the immediate and long-term survival of self-/tumor-specific T cells after ACT. Only low levels of IL-15Rα were detected on the majority of cells present in TILs used for ACT and, unlike IL-7Rα, IL-15Rα was not up-regulated on persisting self-/tumor-specific T cells after ACT (258). Nevertheless, IL-15 signaling might play an important role in the *in vivo* persistence of adoptively transferred T cells because transpresentation of IL-15 by APCs and stromal cells can occur.

T Cell Persistence and Anti-Tumor Responses

Because IL-2 is provided both *in vitro* during T cell clonal expansion and *in vivo* in the immediate aftermath of cell infusion, self-/tumor-reactive $CD8^+$ T cells might undergo apoptosis after IL-2 withdrawal. As early effector T cells have the capacity to release IL-2, selective survival of these cells might occur in an autocrine fashion. In addition, early effector T cells have survival advantages compared to intermediate and late effector T cells, as reflected by the expression of lower levels of the pro-apoptotic molecules, BID (B-cell lymphoma 2 [BCL-2]–homology domain 3 [BH3]–interacting-domain death agonist), BAD (BCL-2-antagonist of cell death), and CD95L (CD95 ligand; also known as FASL), and higher levels of anti-apoptotic molecules (253). The intrinsic proliferative capacity of adoptively transferred T cells might also affect their ability to engraft and persist. Greater proliferation of the early effector T cell subset has been seen *in vitro* and *in vivo* following stimulation with cognate antigen. In parallel with T cell proliferation and progressive differentiation, gradual telomere erosion occurs until a critical degree of shortening results in chromosomal abnormalities and cell death or senescence. This process might be partially compensated for by telomerase activity, and therefore telomere length and telomerase activity can critically influence T cell replicative capacity. Interestingly, recent analyses of human TILs have shown a correlation between the telomere length of transferred cells and persistence of T cells *in vivo* following ACT, indicating that in addition to self-/tumor-antigen recognition, the intrinsic proliferative capacity of adoptively transferred T cells might also be a factor affecting persistence and successful tumor treatment (259).

Optimizing Tumor-Reactive T cells for ACT

The finding that less differentiated, central memory–like T cells might be the optimal population for ACT-based immunotherapies raises a relevant clinical problem. Data from animal studies indicate a direct correlation between the number of adoptively transferred T cells and anti-tumor responses *in vivo,* fostering the notion that high numbers of self-/tumor reactive T cells must be administered to patients to obtain therapeutically effective anti-tumor responses. Therefore, in clinical trials, tumor reactive $CD8^+$ T cells are expanded to large numbers *in vitro* with CD3-specific antibody and IL-2 or specific antigen stimulation and IL-2, which drives differentiation of T cells to intermediate and late effector stages of differentiation. New findings in mice emphasize that the quantity of transferred T cells is a critical factor when T cells with the same quality and fitness are being used for ACT (253). To this end, increased anti-tumor responses were observed in mice after adoptive transfer of lower numbers of early effector T cells compared to higher numbers of late effector T cells. Therefore, one of the greatest challenges in the field is currently the generation of large numbers of "fit" T cells for ACT.

Modifications of Current* in vitro *Expansion Protocols

Using a standard rapid expansion protocol, TILs for transfer are selected and populations are expanded for about 2 weeks with CD3-specific antibody, high doses of IL-2, and irradiated allogeneic feeder cells (Figure 45.4). This procedure results in the differentiation of self-/tumor-specific $CD8^+$ T cells to an intermediate and late effector state. Limiting the *in vitro* expansion phase to a short duration might markedly improve the "fitness" of the transferred T cells because a greater percentage of self-/tumor reactive T cells express CCR7, costimulatory molecules, and IL-7Rα and are actively dividing in the first week of growth. The question remains whether this improvement in fitness can compensate for the reduced number of cells generated soon after activation.

Cytokines, acting in concert with signals through the TCR and costimulatory molecules, can function as accelerators or brakes for T cell proliferation and differentiation. IL-2 has been shown to be an effective T cell growth factor but has undesirable effects, including

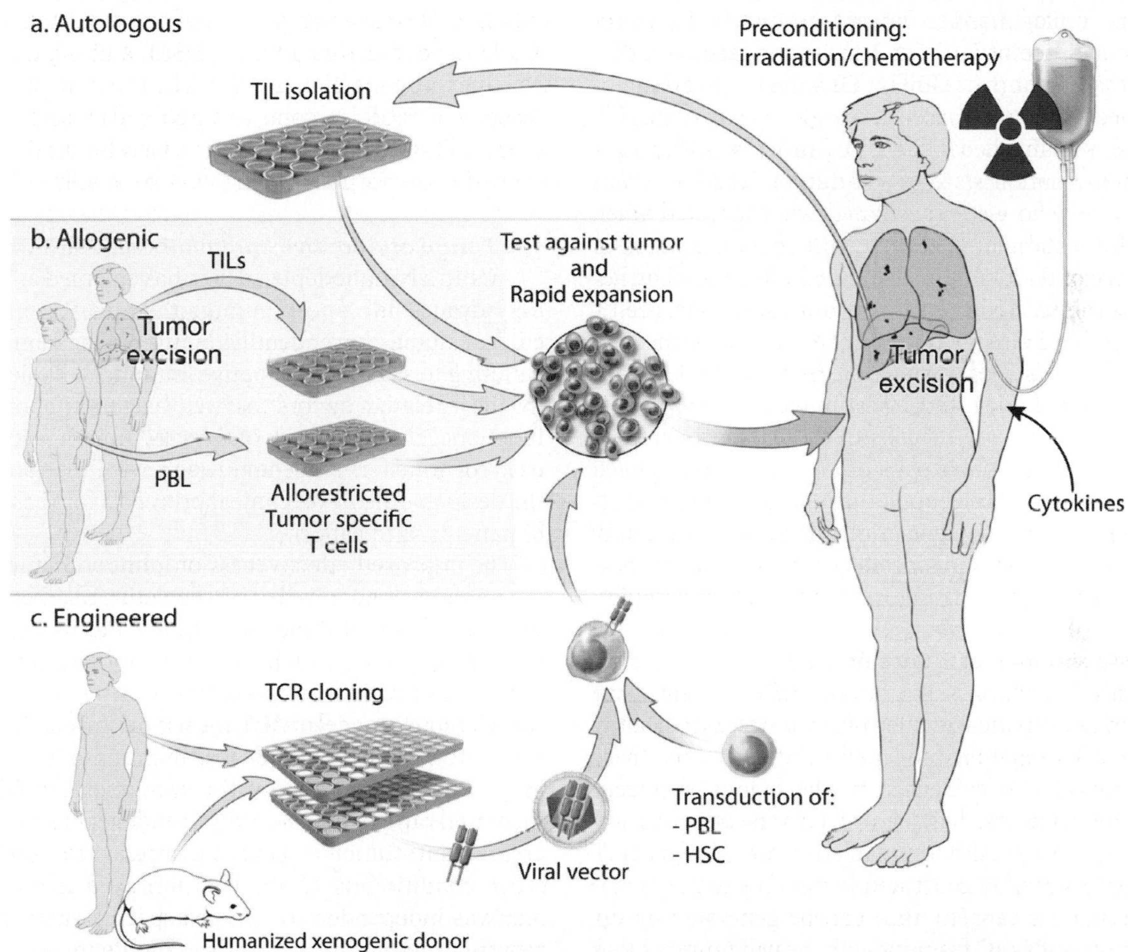

FIGURE 45.4 Three general approaches to adoptive cell transfer using a preconditioning lymphodepleting regimen consisting of chemoradiotherapy in conjunction with administration of exogenous cytokines. **A:** Autologous TILs isolated from patient tumor samples are tested, expanded, and reinfused. **B:** Allogeneic cells derived from TILs that are harvested from another patient or generated *in vitro* from peripheral blood lymphocytes of an allogeneic healthy donor are selected for their ability to recognize patient tumor cells. **C:** Effector T cells are generated by the transduction of recombinant lentiviral or retroviral vectors that encode TCRs, directed against tumor antigens. Tumor-reactive T cells generated using any of these approaches can be further manipulated cells before transfer by the transduction of genes that encode cytokines, adhesion molecules, or anti-apoptotic molecules. Abbreviations: HSC, hematopoietic stem cells; PBL, peripheral blood lymphocytes; TCR, T-cell receptor; TIL, tumor-infiltrating lymphocyte (*322*).

the ability to decrease the expression of lymphoid-organ homing molecules and promote the terminal differentiation of T cells, predisposing them to activation-induced cell death. Other cytokines with a receptor that contains γc such as IL-15 can analogously induce the *in vitro* expansion of self-/tumor reactive $CD8^+$ T cell populations for ACT. Studies carried out in a mouse model indicate that IL-15 may be superior to IL-2 in promoting the development of long-lasting viral immunity, perhaps through the generation of cells with more of a central memory than an effector memory phenotype (264). The ability of murine transgenic gp100 reactive pmel T cells stimulated *in vitro* with IL-15 to more effectively treat B16 tumors than cells generated with IL-2 is consistent with this model (256). Additional γc receptor chain cytokines, including IL-7 and IL-21, evaluated in a similar manner did not promote robust proliferation or differentiation of self-/tumor reactive $CD8^+$ T cells *in vitro*, but the resultant cells had a greater antitumor efficacy *in vivo* than cells expanded *in vitro* with IL-2 (N. Restifo, unpublished data). By contrast, no differences in the differentiation state of self-/tumor reactive T cells from patients who were vaccinated were detected when the cells were stimulated *ex vivo* with cognate antigen in the presence of IL-2, IL-7, or IL-15 (265). Results using human cells probably reflect the use of antigen-experienced T cells, which have already differentiated into intermediate and late effector stages, instead of the naïve populations used in mouse studies. Indeed, stimulation of naïve human self-/tumor reactive T cells in the presence of IL-21 induced the preferential expansion of a less differentiated $CD28^{high}CD45RO^+$ T cell population able to release IL-2 after stimulation with cognate antigen. Therefore, the ability to obtain naïve self-/tumor-specific $CD8^+$ T cells may provide the means to improving current ACT-based therapies.

Genetic Modification of T Cells for ACT

Naturally occurring self-/tumor-specific T cells have been described in patients with cancer, as well as in healthy individuals. The inability to appropriately trigger these endogenous cells, as evidenced by the failure of current vaccination strategies, has lead to current adoptive immunotherapy trials. Although effective tumor reactive T cells cannot be readily generated in patients with the majority of common cancers, they can be generated by the transduction of PBMC from patients bearing tumors that express widely shared antigens with TCR that recognize those epitopes. In a recent study, PBMCs that were transduced with a TCR recognizing the MART-1/HLA-A2 epitope, in addition to efficiently recognizing appropriate tumor cell targets *in vitro*, mediated tumor regression in 2 out of the 17 treated melanoma patients (266). The affinity of the TCR selected for transduction, the level of transduced TCR expressed on the cell surface, and the differentiation state of the transduced T cells used for ACT might critically contribute to the success of trials following TCR transduction. Additional screening has identified TCR that appear to possess a higher functional avidity than the MART-1 TCR used in the initial clinical trial cited earlier (120). Natural variations between the sequences of particular peptide epitopes between species has also facilitated the generation of high-affinity TCRs, such as the murine TCR identified for a nonmutated, HLA-A2–restricted human p53 epitope (81). In addition, random mutagenesis of TCR complementary-determining regions generated in an *in vitro* phage display system resulted in the isolation of TCRs with up to a million-fold higher affinity than the nonmutated receptor with no apparent loss of binding specificity (267). Additional studies have demonstrated that T cells that were genetically engineered to express mutated TCRs with enhanced affinities displayed a higher degree of cross-reactivity with variants of the native epitope than cells expressing a wild-type TCR (268), and further, T cells expressing high-affinity variants of the murine alloreactive 2C TCR, in contrast to cells expressing the wild-type 2C TCR, recognized endogenously processed antigens expressed on normal autologous spleen cells (269).

The Future of Adoptive Immunotherapy

ACT to a lymphodepleted host has emerged as a promising advance in cancer immunotherapy. Preclinical and clinical studies have identified multiple mechanisms contributing to successful adoptive immunotherapies, including host-related factors, as well as the phenotypic and functional characteristics of the self-/tumor reactive T cells used for transfer. These findings provide the rationale for the design of the novel clinical protocols for the treatment of patients with cancer.

The improved effectiveness of immunotherapy following a nonmyeloablative lymphodepleting regimen provides the rational basis for the evaluation of more intensive conditioning regimens, such as a myeloablative treatment in conjunction with autologous HSC transplantation. In the pmel-1 mouse model of ACT, the use of a myeloablative regimen profoundly depleted host immunosuppressive cells and cellular sinks for activating cytokines, resulting in an increased ratio of effector cells to endogenous cells and increased anti-tumor responses compared to nonmyeloablative conditioning (270). The improved therapeutic effect was independent of antigen-specific vaccination but required the transfer of HSCs, which enhanced the proliferation and survival of coadministered self-/tumor reactive T cells possibly through the release of cytokines, growth factors, and anti-apoptotic factors. The finding that myeloablative conditioning with a HSC transplant obviated the need for specific vaccination has important implications for ACT-based immunotherapies in humans, which employ polyclonal TILs with often-unknown specificity for which effective vaccines are not available. The use of a myeloablative preconditioning regimen involving chemotherapy and total body irradiation together with

HSC transplantation in humans is currently under evaluation.

Increased immunity might be achieved with the use of more selective approaches to lymphodepletion to eliminate the toxicities associated with the use of nonspecific preconditioning regimens based on chemotherapy and radiation. For example, Treg cells and other immunosuppressive cells might be selectively depleted with directed immunotoxins. To overcome the sink effect of competing endogenous cells, saturating levels of activating cytokines might be provided exogenously. Alternatively, T_H cells able to produce manifold cytokines might be cotransferred with self-/tumor reactive T cells. Selective engagement of activation-associated molecules such as TLRs can also be utilized to activate APCs. Further, the use of combinatorial approaches might be of greater clinical benefit compared to single modality strategies.

Murine models have now shown that early effector T cells mediate superior *in vivo* anti-tumor responses compared to intermediate and late effector T cells on the basis of their increased proliferative and survival potential, receptiveness to homeostatic and costimulatory signals, homing to secondary lymphoid tissues, and ability to secrete IL-2 (reviewed in [271]). In humans, suggestive data supports the preclinical finding that less differentiated T cells may represent the ideal cells for ACT. These findings indicate that the measurement of IFN-γ release or cytolytic ability represents inadequate criteria for selection of T cells for ACT and suggest that additional factors such as T cell phenotype, telomere length, TCR affinity, as well as the ability of cells to secrete cytokines such as IL-2 should be considered in selecting cells for therapy. The next generation of ACT-based immunotherapies might rely upon the ability to endow "fit" cells with elevated cell-surface expression of high-affinity, self-/tumor-specific TCRs by gene transfer technology that can be used in conjunction with specific vaccines. Ultimately, the TCR gene therapy approach might hold the key to the widespread application of ACT-based therapy to the treatment of cancers of multiple histologies.

Stem Cell Transplantation and the Potential Role of NK Cells in Cancer Therapies

Several clinical trials have evaluated the use of allogeneic HSC transplantation (HCT) for the treatment of patients with leukemia, and results suggest that a subset of T cells that mediate graft versus host responses may be directed against antigens that are expressed specifically on leukemia cells, or what has been termed *graft versus leukemia* (reviewed in [272]). Minor histocompatibility antigens that are limited in their expression to hematopoietic cells and that are recognized by T cells have been identified (273). The transfer of donor lymphocytes is also associated with enhanced survival of patients who relapsed following transplantation of T cell–depleted bone marrow (274). The significant improvement in survival noted in many of these study of donor lymphocyte infusions provides further evidence that a graft versus leukemia effect mediated by T cells that recognize target antigens on tumor cells are responsible for tumor regression. These products have also been shown to be recognized by specific T cells and may play an important role in mediating graft versus leukemia effects. Additional results, however, indicate that NK cells may play an important role in mediating the anti-tumor effects of bone marrow transplantation. The presence of killer inhibitory receptors (KIRs) that recognize HLA gene products on target cells is responsible for blunting the response of NK cells to targets that express those molecules, and in patients with leukemia who are receiving cells from HLA nonidentical donors, responses were associated with a lack of expression of the appropriate KIRs on recipient cells (275). In addition, an improved outcome was noted in patients who received transplants from HLA-identical siblings if the recipient cells lacked the presence of KIR recognized by donor NK cells (276). Although these results indicate that these approaches may provide a treatment option for patients with tumors arising from hematopoietic cells, it is not clear that these treatments will be effective for patients with solid tumors.

Antibody-based Therapies

Cell surface proteins that are overexpressed on tumors have been targeted with either unmodified antibodies or antibodies that have been linked to toxins or radionuclides. The glycoprotein CEA is overexpressed on colon and breast cancer, although significant expression of this protein is observed in normal tissues, particularly in intestinal crypts. Antibodies that bind to monocytes or DCs through Fc receptors have been shown to mediate the lysis of target cells *in vitro* through antibody dependent cellular cytotoxicity (ADCC), and the *in vitro* effectiveness of immunotoxins has been clearly demonstrated. There has, however, been a lack of success in the treatment of solid tumors with these reagents, which appears to arise from the lack of effective penetration of tumor tissues *in vivo* by these reagents.

There have been examples of successful treatments using antibody-based therapies. Substantial clinical responses have been observed in breast cancer patients who have been treated with antibodies directed against Her-2/neu (277). The Her-2/neu protein is involved with signaling through a growth factor receptor, and thus the function of the protein may play an important role in the therapy mediated by this antibody *(278)*. The antibody rituximab, which is directed against the B cell surface protein CD20, has also been shown to mediate effective anti-cancer effects against B cell leukemias (reviewed in [279]). It is not clear how the effects of the unconjugated antibody are mediated but may involve the induction of apoptosis, complement mediated lysis of tumor cells, as well as through ADCC mechanisms. Additional trials have tested the use of rituximab that has been conjugated with radionuclides for cancer treatment *(280)*. The treatment of a blood-borne tumor by an antibody, however, may represent a special case, as antibodies administered intravenously may be particularly effective against these tumors, as they would have a direct access to tumor cells which are present in the blood.

Chimeric T Cell Receptors

Cell surface antigens that are overexpressed on tumor cells such as ERB-b2 also provide potential targets for cellular therapies, as antibodies linked to intracellular signaling domains have been shown to deliver activation signals to gene-modified T cells. In an initial demonstration of the function of these receptors, constructs generated by linking antibody heavy and light chain variable regions to TCR α and β constant regions were shown to function in a murine T cell hybridoma (281). Subsequent studies have primarily been carried out using single chain antibody constructs in which an amino terminal antibody heavy chain variable region is followed by an appropriate light chain variable region. This single chain Fv fragment has been linked through a flexible spacer to the transmembrane and cytoplasmic domains derived either from the Fc receptor γ chain (282) or the TCR ζ signaling chain (283). Additional studies have revealed that the proliferation and survival of T cells that have been engineered to express recombinant "T-bodies" appears to be enhanced by the linkage of intracellular signaling domains from costimulatory molecules such as CD28 *(284)* and OX40 *(285)*.

Initial studies carried out in model systems have provided evidence for the ability of T cells that have been redirected using T-bodies to mediate tumor regression. Intratumoral injection of human T cells transduced with a T-body directed against a protein that is overexpressed in a variety of tumors, erbB2, was found to cause regression of established prostatic adenocarcinomas in a mouse xenograft model (286). Similarly, murine T cells transduced with a chimeric construct that encoded a single chain antibody directed against prostate-specific membrane antigen eradicated human prostate tumors in a xenogeneic murine model system *(287)*. Clinical trials have now been carried out using single chain antibodies directed against the human folate binding protein, a molecule that is overexpressed on ovarian carcinomas (288), as well as carbonic anhydrase IX, an antigen that is overexpressed in renal carcinomas (289). Objective responses were not observed in either trial, and there was evidence of liver toxicity in the renal cancer trial that limited the cell doses that could be administered to patients. Nevertheless, these reagents may provide tools for the development of widely applicable cancer therapies, as the recognition of target cells is not restricted by the MHC molecules expressed on the tumor cell surface.

Single chain constructs containing a flexible linker between conventional TCR α and β chains as well as intracellular signaling domains similar to those present in T-bodies have also been found to confer on T cells the ability to recognize cognate peptide antigen–MHC complexes *(290)*. Single chain TCRs possess potential advantages over dual chain TCRs, which can interact with endogenous α and β chains, leading to a significant reduction in the number of appropriately paired receptors on the T cell surface. In one study comparing a single chain TCR with the corresponding dual chain TCR, the dual chain TCR conferred more potent effector functions on the gene modified T cells than the single chain receptor (291); however, additional modifications such as those employed in T-bodies may enhance single chain TCR signaling.

INFLUENCE OF IMMUNE SYSTEM ON TUMOR DEVELOPMENT

Immunosurveillance

Although appropriate T cell activation can lead in some cases to tumor regression, the normal role of the immune system in controlling tumor development is unclear. Burnet and Thomas theorized in the 1950s that the immune system played an important role in preventing the outgrowth of tumors, a concept that was termed *immunosurveillance* (292). Further studies demonstrated that immunodeficient mice that lacked T cells did not generally develop high rates of tumors; however, additional cells such as NK cells that were present in T cell–deficient mice may have been responsible for controlling tumor growth (293). Immunodeficient patients exhibit only a slightly higher rate of solid malignancies, with the exception of relatively rare diseases such as Kaposi's sarcoma, which develop in HIV patients. More recent studies in mice have provided some evidence that the immune system may prevent the outgrowth of tumors bearing highly immunogenic antigens, while tumors that possess mechanisms that prevent the immune system from responding appropriately can grow progressively, a mechanism that has been termed "immunoediting" (reviewed in [294]). Factors that influence tumor cell growth include the immunogenicity of antigens expressed by that cell as well as the sensitivity to host factors that regulate immune responses. Tumors isolated from immunodeficient mice in many cases are rejected following injection into normal mice *(295)*, and enhanced rates of tumor development in response to carcinogen treatment have been observed in mice that lack responsiveness to IFN-γ *(296)*. Expression of proinflammatory cytokines such as IFN-γ may be necessary to overcome the effects of soluble inhibitory factors such as TGF-β and IL-10, as well as products expressed in T cells such as CTLA-4 and PD-1 that act to limit normal anti-tumor responses *(297,298)*.

Examination of the association between lymphocyte infiltration of tumor sites and patient survival has provided some support for the role of immunosurveillance in controlling tumor growth. The presence of brisk infiltrates of TIL in a variety of tumor types has been associated with improved survival multiple studies (*178,179*,180,*299*). As the presence of a higher ratio of T regulatory cells to $CD8^+$ T cells within tumors has been associated with poor prognosis (240,*300*), further analysis of tumor as well as other sites may be needed to evaluate this issue.

Immune Escape

One of the correlates of immunoediting models is that selective pressure exerted by the immune system can then lead to the outgrowth of tumor variants containing mutations that lead to the loss of recognition by cells of the immune system. Relatively small groups of malignant or premalignant cells that avoid detection by the immune system initially develop random mutations, and pressure exerted by immune cells can then lead to the selective outgrowth of variants that have lost expression of gene products such as HLA class I molecules. Recent studies have demonstrated a complex interplay of positive and negative factors that regulate responses to tumors, however, and thus it is difficult to evaluate the role of any individual factors in tumor progression. The laws of natural selection may also be at work when cancer cells that possess genetic and epigenetic traits that are beneficial to their survival or proliferation are conferred growth advantage over others, and the outcome of this passive process is determined by multiple factors in the tumor environment such as growth factors, nutrient supply, and immune pressure. Nevertheless, it is reasonable to assume that the immune system can play some role in sculpting the phenotypic characteristics of spontaneously arising tumors. In addition, anti-tumor immunotherapies that lead to partial tumor cell elimination represents an additional scenario where selective pressure can lead to the outgrowth of preexisting tumor escape variants.

Loss or Down-regulation of HLA Class I Antigens

Tumor antigens are processed largely by the proteasome to generate peptides, which are transported by transporter associated with antigen processing (TAP) to the endoplasmic reticulum, where they bind to HLA class I heavy chain in association with β_2-microglobulin. The HLA–peptide complexes are then transported through the Golgi to cell surface. Several mechanisms have been shown to result in the loss or down-regulation of HLA class I expression. β_2-microglobulin mutation/deletion results in HLA class I total loss. Defects in components of the antigen-processing machinery that lead to decreased HLA class I expression on the cell surface of human tumors have been described (301). Selective loss of an HLA class I haplotype, locus, or allele has also been observed in human tumor cells *(302)*, as well as the loss of β_2-microglobulin *(303)*, although a causal relationship between these changes and tumor growth in such clinical scenarios is difficult to demonstrate unequivocally.

While partial or complete losses of HLA class I could theoretically lead to immune escape, those cells should then be more susceptibility to lysis by NK cells. Recent studies have shown, however, that NK cells express activating receptors such as NKG2D, which bind to stressed-induced ligands (MICA and MICB) that can be up-regulated in a variety of tumors (reviewed in [304]). Activation of NK cells through this signaling pathway can overcome the inhibitory effect of HLA class I binding receptors (KIRs). From these data, it is clear that HLA class I–negative tumors should be susceptible to NK killing. Loss or down-regulation of MICA/B expression by actively growing tumors has been suggested as an escape strategy, but there is no experimental evidence for this, and actively proliferating tumor cells have been found to express MICA/B independently of cellular stress.

An alternative explanation for why tumor cells that have lost HLA class I are not destroyed by NK cells may be derived from the activation-inhibition model. NK cells are rapidly activated in the presence of stimulatory factors such as IL-12, IL-2, or type 1 INFs that are released in response to inflammatory conditions associated with microbial infections. In "sterile" environments, as seen with tumors or transplantation, such stimulatory factors may not be readily available and the cross-talk between DCs and resting NK cells that normally leads to NK cell activation may not occur. In addition, the production of immunomodulatory cytokines such as TGF-β or macrophage migration inhibitory factor (MIF) by tumor cells may directly inhibit NK cell activation and function. Loss of expression of surface antigens can occur independently of the dysregulation of HLA class I expression. It is possible that increases in the potency of T cell–based tumor immunotherapy may increase the prominence of escape mechanisms such as antigen loss.

Defective Death Receptor Signaling

Defective death receptor signaling is another mechanism that may contribute to the survival and proliferation of tumor cells. Recent studies have shown the expression of the caspase-8 inhibitor cFLIP (cellular FLICE inhibitory protein) in various tumors. In these cases, cFLIP may render tumor cells resistant to death receptor–mediated apoptosis and may contribute to immunoresistance to T cells *in vivo* (305,*306*). Down-regulation or loss of Fas expression in tumors may also contribute to their resistance to apoptosis. Missense mutations and loss of the Fas gene have been identified in hematological cancers such as multiple myeloma *(307)* as well as in melanomas (308).

Lack of Costimulation

As discussed earlier, most tumors seem to grow in a noninflammatory microenvironment that is not conducive to immune activation. Histologically, tumors generally coexist innocuously with normal tissues, apparently without giving or inducing immune activating signals, especially during the early stage of growth. Recognition of tumor antigens by DCs in this condition will not lead to DC activation and maturation. In addition, like most normal tissues, tumor cells usually do not express costimulatory molecules such as B7-1 (CD80), B7-2 (CD86), and CD40. Recognition of tumor antigens by $CD4^+$ and $CD8^+$ T lymphocytes without adequate costimulation will lead to T cell anergy. Insertion of the genes encoding B7-1, B7-2, or both into tumor in the experimental setting will generally increase the immunogencity of a tumor but does not *necessarily* lead to regression.

Immunosuppressive Cytokines

Activation or inhibition of T cells also depends on the presence or absence of cytokines in their immediate microenvironment. Tumor cells have been known to elaborate a variety of cytokines and chemokines that can negatively effect maturation and function of immune cells. Vascular endothelial growth factor (VEGF), which is a cytokine that is produced by most tumors, has been shown in several *in vitro* studies to inhibit DC differentiation and maturation through suppression of the transcription factor NF-κB in HSCs (309). In patients with lung, head and neck, and breast cancers, there was a decrease in function and number of mature DCs, which was associated with increased plasma level of VEGF (310). Elevated levels of IL-10, a molecule that has been shown to inhibit DC maturation, has also frequently been detected in serum of patients with cancer (*311*,312). Additionally, IL-10 may protect tumor cells from CTL by down-regulation of HLA class I, class II, and ICAM-1. Further, the loss of HLA class I expression may be due to IL-10–mediated down-regulation of TAP1 and TAP2 proteins in tumor cells. Prostaglandin E2 (PGE-2) represents an immunosuppressive factor that is expressed by tumors owing to enhanced expression of the enzyme cyclooxygenase 2 (COX2), which is the rate-limiting enzyme for PGE-2 synthesis. Relatively high levels of PGE-2 have been found in the serum of renal cancer patients *(313)*. Increased expression of PGE-2 in the blood of cancer patients has also been associated increased production of IL-10 from monocytes (314); however, the results of another study suggest that IL10 may inhibit PGE-2 production (315).

High levels of transforming growth factor (TGF)-β are frequently found in cancer patients and are associated with progression of disease and poor response to immunotherapy, an observation that may reflect the ability of this cytokine to inhibit the activation and proliferation of lymphocytes. Tumors may not necessarily produce these cytokines as escape mechanisms, however, as the hypothesized immunosuppressive functions may be mere side effects of the angiogenic and growth factor functions of these cytokines.

The Controversy Involving Apoptosis of Activated T Cells

One of the more controversial mechanisms of tumor escape is the expression of death receptor ligands by tumor cells. A variety of cancer cells have been reported to express functional FasL that induces apoptosis of Fas+ susceptible target cells (316). These include lung carcinoma, melanoma, colon carcinoma, and hepatocellular carcinoma. The most recent study on this controversial topic asserted that FasL was coexpressed with melanosomal and lysosomal markers in multivesicular bodies (MVB) in human melanoma cells (317). These data have been questioned, however, due to a lack of appropriate negative controls, technical concerns such as the use of nonspecific antibodies, nonintron spanning polymerase chain reaction (PCR) primers without proper controls, and in functional assays that employ the Jurkat cell line, which itself can be induced to express FasL. Additional studies have failed to provide evidence of FasL expression in melanoma either at mRNA or protein levels, however, and Fas susceptible targets were not lysed by melanoma cells in controlled functional assays (318). In fact, all well-controlled *in vivo* experiments using FasL-transfected tumor cells have shown accelerated rejection accompanied by neutrophil infiltration (319). The activity of FasL may be modulated by the presence or absence of certain cytokines within the tumor microenvironment, and TGF-β has been shown to regulate the pro-inflammatory effects of FasL. It is now apparent that upon activation by tumor antigen recognition, T cells express high levels of FasL, which induces apoptosis in themselves ("suicide") and each other ("fratricide").

Tumor Escape and Immunotherapy

Despite recent progress in tumor immunobiology and technical advances in the field of tumor immunotherapy, current antigen-specific immunotherapeutic strategies have only been successful in patients with melanoma and not other cancer types. It is not clear whether tumor escape accounts for these failures, or whether lack of observed tumor regression is due to inadequacies of the immunotherapies themselves.

The balance of immune activation and immune inhibition must be in favor of the former if tumors are to come under immune pressure. However, even in some instances where effective anti-tumor responses can be achieved with immunotherapy, tumors often recur. It seems likely that as the tumor immunologist's armamentarium becomes more powerful and immunotherapies become more effective, the selection of tumor variants with immunoresistant phenotypes will be observed with greater frequency. Tumor escape may ultimately thwart some dramatic responses to immunotherapy. Indeed, some tumors that recur after successful immunotherapy often possess immunoresistant phenotypes.

CONCLUSION

The identification of antigens that are either specifically expressed or are overexpressed on tumor cells has provided an opportunity to explore therapies for the treatment of patients with a wide variety of tumor types. The results of an extensive series of clinical trials employing a wide variety of treatments, however, have in general failed to provide evidence that vaccination can lead to tumor regression. With the exception of trials employing treatments against tumor of hematopoietic origin such as lymphomas and leukemias, responses have generally been observed in 5% or less of treated patients, which may in some cases reflect a low background of spontaneous tumor regression. The development of preventive vaccination protocols against cancers such as HPV has demonstrated the ability of the immune system to control the development of virally induced cancers but unfortunately may not be relevant to the control of naturally arising tumors of nonviral origin. Adoptive immunotherapy approaches have demonstrated that expanded populations of tumor reactive T cells can lead to the destruction of bulky metastatic lesions; however, long-term tumor regressions are observed in only a minority of treated patients.

These clinical trial results clearly point to the need to develop a better understanding of the basic mechanisms that regulate anti-cancer immune responses. The presence of regulatory T cells, inhibitory factors expressed by tumor cells and by infiltrating monocytes or other cell types, represent some of the factors that may limit these responses. In addition, the failure to generate appropriately activated APCs within the tumor microenvironment may contribute to the lack of responses observed in patients undergoing therapy. Nevertheless, these and other studies provide opportunities to explore the role of factors such as host conditioning on response to therapy and will hopefully facilitate the development of treatments that result in long-term tumor regression in the majority of treated patients.

REFERENCES

1. Coussens LM, Werb Z. Inflammation and cancer. *Nature*. 2002;420:860–867.
2. Clevers H. At the crossroads of inflammation and cancer. *Cell*. 2004;118:671–674.
6. Sakurai T, Maeda S, Chang L, et al. Loss of hepatic NF-kappa B activity enhances chemical hepatocarcinogenesis through sustained c-Jun N-terminal kinase 1 activation. *Proc Natl Acad Sci U S A*. 2006;103:10544–10551.
8. Wakefield LM, Roberts AB. TGF-beta signaling: positive and negative effects on tumorigenesis. *Curr Opin Genet Dev*. 2002;12:22–29.
11. Prehn RT, Main JM. Immunity to methylcholanthrene-induced sarcomas. *J Natl Cancer Inst*. 1957;18:769–778.
13. Old LJ, Boyse EA. Immunology of experimental tumors. *Annu Rev Med*. 1964;15:167–186.
16. Boon T. Antigenic tumor cell variants obtained with mutagens. *Adv Cancer Res*. 1983;39:121–151.
18. Lurquin C, Van Pel A, Mariamë B, et al. Structure of the gene of tum-transplantation antigen P91A: the mutated exon encodes a peptide recognized with Ld by cytolytic T cells. *Cell*. 1989;58:293–303.
19. Van den Eynde B, Lethe B, Van Pel A, et al. The gene coding for a major tumor rejection antigen of tumor P815 is identical to the normal gene of syngeneic DBA/2 mice. *J Exp Med*. 1991;173:1373–1384.
20. Brandle D, Bilsborough J, Rulicke T, et al. The shared tumor-specific antigen encoded by mouse gene P1A is a target not only for cytolytic T lymphocytes but also for tumor rejection. *Eur J Immunol*. 1998;28:4010–4019.
21. Parker KC, Bednarek MA, Coligan JE. Scheme for ranking potential HLA-A2 binding peptides based on independent binding of individual peptide side-chains. *J Immunol*. 1994;152:163–175.
22. Princiotta MF, Finzi D, Qian SB, et al. Quantitating protein synthesis, degradation, and endogenous antigen processing. *Immunity*. 2003;18:343–354.
23. Preuss KD, Zwick C, Bormann C, et al. Analysis of the B-cell repertoire against antigens expressed by human neoplasms. *Immunol Rev*. 2002;188:43–50.
24. van der Bruggen P, Traversari C, Chomez P, et al. A gene encoding an antigen recognized by cytolytic T lymphocytes on a human melanoma. *Science*. 1991;254:1643–1647.
27. Weber J, Salgaller M, Samid D, et al. Rosenberg. Expression of the MAGE-1 tumor antigen is up regulated by the demethylating agent 5-aza-2'-deoxycytidine. *Cancer Res*. 1994;54:1766–1771.
29. Chen YT, Scanlan MJ, Sahin U, et al. A testicular antigen aberrantly expressed in human cancers detected by autologous antibody screening. *Proc Natl Acad Sci U S A*. 1997;94:1914–1918.
30. Jager E, Chen YT, Drijfhout JW, et al. Simultaneous humoral and cellular immune response against cancer-testis antigen NY-ESO-1: definition of human histocompatibility leukocyte antigen (HLA)-A2-binding peptide epitopes. *J Exp Med*. 1998;187:265–270.
33. Jager E, Nagata Y, Gnjatic S, et al. Monitoring CD8 T cell responses to NY-ESO-1: correlation of humoral and cellular immune responses. *Proc Natl Acad Sci U S A*. 2000;97:4760–4765.
35. Zeng G, Wang X, Robbins PF, et al. CD4(+) T cell recognition of MHC class II-restricted epitopes from NY- ESO-1 presented by a prevalent HLA DP4 allele: association with NY-ESO- 1 antibody production. *Proc Natl Acad Sci U S A*. 2001;98:3964–3969.
36. Gnjatic S, Atanackovic D, Jager E, et al. Survey of naturally occurring $CD4^+$ T cell responses against NY-ESO-1 in cancer patients: correlation with antibody responses. *Proc Natl Acad Sci U S A*. 2003;100:8862–8867.
37. Kawakami Y, Eliyahu S, Delgado CH, et al. Cloning of the gene coding for a shared human melanoma antigen recognized by autologous T cells infiltrating into tumor. *Proc Natl Acad Sci U S A*. 1994;91:3515–3519.
38. Coulie PG, Brichard V, Van Pel A, et al. A new gene coding for a differentiation antigen recognized by autologous cytolytic T lymphocytes on HLA-A2 melanomas. *J Exp Med*. 1994;180:35–42.
40. Kawakami Y, Eliyahu S, Sakaguchi K, et al. Identification of the immunodominant peptides of the MART-1 human melanoma antigen recognized by the majority of HLA-A2-restricted tumor infiltrating lymphocytes. *J Exp Med*. 1994;180:347–352.
47. Kawakami Y, Eliyahu S, Jennings C, et al. Recognition of multiple epitopes in the human melanoma antigen gp100 by tumor-infiltrating T lymphocytes associated with in vivo tumor regression. *J Immunol*. 1995;154:3961–3968.

48. Cox AL, Skipper J, Chen Y, et al. Identification of a peptide recognized by five melanoma-specific human cytotoxic T cell lines. *Science*. 1994;264:716–719.
53. Parkhurst MR, Fitzgerald EB, Southwood S, et al. Identification of a shared HLA-A*0201-restricted T-cell epitope from the melanoma antigen tyrosinase-related protein 2 (TRP2). *Cancer Res*. 1998;58:4895–4901.
54. Bloom MB, Perry-Lalley D, Robbins PF, et al. Identification of tyrosinase-related protein 2 as a tumor rejection antigen for the B16 melanoma. *J Exp Med*. 1997;185:453–459.
55. Nishimura MI, Avichezer D, Custer MC, et al. MHC class I-restricted recognition of a melanoma antigen by a human CD4+ tumor infiltrating lymphocyte [In Process Citation]. *Cancer Res*. 1999;59:6230–6238.
56. Somasundaram R, Robbins P, Moonka D, et al. CD4(+), HLA class I-restricted, cytolytic T-lymphocyte clone against primary malignant melanoma cells. *Int J Cancer*. 2000;85:253–259.
57. Topalian SL, Gonzales MI, Parkhurst M, et al. Melanoma-specific CD4+ T cells recognize nonmutated HLA-DR-restricted tyrosinase epitopes. *J Exp Med*. 1996;183:1965–1971.
62. Hanada K, Perry-Lalley DM, Ohnmacht GA, et al. Identification of fibroblast growth factor-5 as an overexpressed antigen in multiple human adenocarcinomas. *Cancer Res*. 2001;61:5511–5516.
63. Ikeda H, Lethe B, Lehmann F, et al. Characterization of an antigen that is recognized on a melanoma showing partial HLA loss by CTL expressing an NK inhibitory receptor. *Immunity*. 1997;6:199–208.
66. Tsang KY, Zaremba S, Nieroda CA, et al. Generation of human cytotoxic T cells specific for human carcinoembryonic antigen epitopes from patients immunized with recombinant vaccinia-CEA vaccine. *J Natl Cancer Inst*. 1995;87:982–990.
69. Fisk B, Blevins TL, Wharton JT, et al. Identification of an immunodominant peptide of HER-2/neu protooncogene recognized by ovarian tumor-specific cytotoxic T lymphocyte lines. *J Exp Med*. 1995;181:2109–2117.
70. Zaks TZ, Rosenberg SA. Immunization with a peptide epitope (p369–377) from HER-2/neu leads to peptide-specific cytotoxic T lymphocytes that fail to recognize HER-2/neu+ tumors. *Cancer Res*. 1998;58:4902–4908.
71. Vonderheide RH, Hahn WC, Schultze JL, et al. The telomerase catalytic subunit is a widely expressed tumor-associated antigen recognized by cytotoxic T lymphocytes. *Immunity*. 1999;10:673–679.
72. Ayyoub M, Migliaccio M, Guillaume P, et al. Lack of tumor recognition by hTERT peptide 540–548-specific CD8(+) T cells from melanoma patients reveals inefficient antigen processing. *Eur J Immunol*. 2001;31:2642–2651.
74. Rock KL, Goldberg AL. Degradation of cell proteins and the generation of MHC class I-presented peptides. *Annu Rev Immunol*. 1999;17:739–779.
75. Kessler JH, Beekman NJ, Bres-Vloemans SA, et al. Efficient identification of novel HLA-A(*)0201-presented cytotoxic T lymphocyte epitopes in the widely expressed tumor antigen PRAME by proteasome-mediated digestion analysis. *J Exp Med*. 2001;193:73–88.
77. Weinschenk T, Gouttefangeas C, Schirle M, et al. Integrated functional genomics approach for the design of patient-individual antitumor vaccines. *Cancer Res*. 2002;62:5818–5827.
80. Kuball J, Schuler M, Antunes Ferreira E, et al. Generating p53-specific cytotoxic T lymphocytes by recombinant adenoviral vector-based vaccination in mice, but not man. *Gene Ther*. 2002;9:833–843.
81. Theobald M, Biggs J, Dittmer D, et al. Targeting p53 as a general tumor antigen. *Proc Natl Acad Sci U S A*. 1995;92:11993–11997.
82. Cohen CJ, Zheng Z, Bray R, et al. Recognition of fresh human tumor by human peripheral blood lymphocytes transduced with a bicistronic retroviral vector encoding a murine anti-p53 TCR. *J Immunol*. 2005;175:5799–5808.
84. Wolfel T, Hauer M, Schneider J, et al. A p16INK4a-insensitive CDK4 mutant targeted by cytolytic T lymphocytes in a human melanoma. *Science*. 1995;269:1281–1284.
85. Robbins PF, El-Gamil M, Li YF, et al. A mutated ?-catenin gene encodes a melanoma-specific antigen recognized by tumor infiltrating lymphocytes. *J Exp Med*. 1996;183:1185–1192.
86. Rubinfeld B, Robbins P, El-Gamil M, et al. Stabilization of beta-catenin by genetic defects in melanoma cell lines [see comments]. *Science*. 1997;275:1790–1792.
87. Mandruzzato S, Brasseur F, Andry G, et al. A CASP-8 mutation recognized by cytolytic T lymphocytes on a human head and neck carcinoma. *J Exp Med*. 1997;186:785–793.
88. Huang J, El-Gamil M, Dudley ME, et al. T cells associated with tumor regression recognize frameshifted products of the CDKN2A tumor suppressor gene locus and a mutated HLA class I gene product. *J Immunol*. 2004;172:6057–6064.
93. Cheever MA, Chen W, Disis ML, et al. T-cell immunity to oncogenic proteins including mutated ras and chimeric bcr-abl. *Ann NY Acad Sci*. 1993;690:101–112.
96. Stanley MA. Human papillomavirus vaccines. *Rev Med Virol*. 2006;16:139–149.
98. Suzich JA, Ghim SJ, Palmer-Hill FJ, et al. Systemic immunization with papillomavirus L1 protein completely prevents the development of viral mucosal papillomas. *Proc Natl Acad Sci U S A*. 1995;92:11553–11557.
101. Koutsky LA, Ault KA, Wheeler CM, et al. A controlled trial of a human papillomavirus type 16 vaccine. *N Engl J Med*. 2002;347:1645–1651.
102. Villa LL, Costa RL, Petta CA, et al. Prophylactic quadrivalent human papillomavirus (types 6, 11, 16, and 18) L1 virus-like particle vaccine in young women: a randomised double-blind placebo-controlled multicentre phase II efficacy trial. *Lancet Oncol*. 2005;6:271–278.
103. Lee WM. Hepatitis B virus infection. *N Engl J Med*. 1997;337:1733–1745.
104. Rehermann B, Nascimbeni M. Immunology of hepatitis B virus and hepatitis C virus infection. *Nat Rev Immunol*. 2005;5:215–229.
107. Valmori D, Dutoit V, Schnuriger V, et al. Vaccination with a Melan-A peptide selects an oligoclonal T cell population with increased functional avidity and tumor reactivity. *J Immunol*. 2002;168:4231–4240.
109. Yee C, Savage PA, Lee PP, et al. Isolation of high avidity melanoma-reactive CTL from heterogeneous populations using peptide-MHC tetramers. *J Immunol*. 1999;162:2227–2234.
111. al-Ramadi BK, Jelonek MT, Boyd LF, et al. Lack of strict correlation of functional sensitization with the apparent affinity of MHC/peptide complexes for the TCR. *J Immunol*. 1995;155:662–673.
114. Hutchinson SL, Wooldridge L, Tafuro S, et al. The CD8 T cell coreceptor exhibits disproportionate biological activity at extremely low binding affinities. *J Biol Chem*. 2003;278:24285–24293.
120. Johnson LA, Heemskerk B, Powell DJ, Jr., et al. Gene transfer of tumor-reactive TCR confers both high avidity and tumor reactivity to nonreactive peripheral blood mononuclear cells and tumor-infiltrating lymphocytes. *J Immunol*. 2006;177:6548–6559.
122. Sensi M, Traversari C, Radrizzani M, et al. Cytotoxic T-lymphocyte clones from different patients display limited T-cell-receptor variable-region gene usage in HLA-A2-restricted recognition of the melanoma antigen Melan-A/MART-1. *Proc Natl Acad Sci U S A*. 1995;92:5674–5678.
128. Guilloux Y, Lucas S, Brichard VG, et al. A peptide recognized by human cytolytic T lymphocytes on HLA-A2 melanomas is encoded by an intron sequence of the N- acetylglucosaminyltransferase V gene. *J Exp Med*. 1996;183:1173–1183.
133. Bullock TN, Patterson AE, Franlin LL, et al. Initiation codon scanthrough versus termination codon readthrough demonstrates strong potential for major histocompatibility complex class I-restricted cryptic epitope expression. *J Exp Med*. 1997;186:1051–1058.
134. Ronsin C, Chung-Scott V, Poullion I, et al. A non-AUG-defined alternative open reading frame of the intestinal carboxyl esterase mRNA generates an epitope recognized by renal cell carcinoma-reactive tumor-infiltrating lymphocytes in situ. *J Immunol*. 1999;163:483–490.
137. Skipper JC, Hendrickson RC, Gulden PH, et al. An HLA-A2-restricted tyrosinase antigen on melanoma cells results from post-translational modification and suggests a novel pathway for processing of membrane proteins. *J Exp Med*. 1996;183:527–534.
138. Hanada K, Yewdell JW, Yang JC. Immune recognition of a human renal cancer antigen through post-translational protein splicing. *Nature*. 2004;427:252–256.

140. Paulus H. Protein splicing and related forms of protein autoprocessing. *Ann Rev Biochem*. 2000;69:447–496.
142. Morel S, Levy F, Burlet-Schiltz O, et al. Processing of some antigens by the standard proteasome but not by the immunoproteasome results in poor presentation by dendritic cells. *Immunity*. 2000;12:107–117.
143. Van den Eynde BJ, Morel S. Differential processing of class-I-restricted epitopes by the standard proteasome and the immunoproteasome. *Curr Opin Immunol*. 2001;13:147–153.
145. Parkhurst MR, Salgaller ML, Southwood S, et al. Improved induction of melanoma-reactive CTL with peptides from the melanoma antigen gp100 modified at HLA-A*0201-binding residues. *J Immunol*. 1996;157:2539–2548.
147. Overwijk WW, Tsung A, Irvine KR, et al. gp100/pmel 17 is a murine tumor rejection antigen: induction of "self"-reactive, tumoricidal T cells using high-affinity, altered peptide ligand. *J Exp Med*. 1998;188:277–286.
148. Valmori D, Fonteneau JF, Lizana CM, et al. Enhanced generation of specific tumor-reactive CTL in vitro by selected Melan-A/MART-1 immunodominant peptide analogues. *J Immunol*. 1998;160:1750–1758.
150. Anichini A, Molla A, Mortarini R, et al. An expanded peripheral T cell population to a cytotoxic T lymphocyte (CTL)-defined, melanocyte-specific antigen in metastatic melanoma patients impacts on generation of peptide-specific CTLs but does not overcome tumor escape from immune surveillance in metastatic lesions. *J Exp Med*. 1999;190:651–668.
151. Pittet MJ, Valmori D, Dunbar PR, et al. High frequencies of naive Melan-A/MART-1-specific CD8(+) T cells in a large proportion of human histocompatibility leukocyte antigen (HLA)-A2 individuals. *J Exp Med*. 1999;190:705–715.
152. Loftus DJ, Castelli C, Clay TM, et al. Identification of epitope mimics recognized by CTL reactive to the melanoma/melanocyte-derived peptide MART-1(27–35). *J Exp Med*. 1996;184:647–657.
154. Chen JL, Stewart-Jones G, Bossi G, et al. Structural and kinetic basis for heightened immunogenicity of T cell vaccines. *J Exp Med*. 2005;201:1243–1255.
156. D'Souza S, Rimoldi D, Lienard D, et al. Circulating Melan-A/Mart-1 specific cytolytic T lymphocyte precursors in HLA-A2+ melanoma patients have a memory phenotype. *Int J Cancer*. 1998;78:699–706.
158. Lee PP, Yee C, Savage PA, et al. Characterization of circulating T cells specific for tumor-associated antigens in melanoma patients. *Nat Med*. 1999;5:677–685.
162. Rosenberg SA, Yang JC, Schwartzentruber DJ, et al. Immunologic and therapeutic evaluation of a synthetic peptide vaccine for the treatment of patients with metastatic melanoma. *Nat Med*. 1998;4:321–327.
163. Rosenberg SA, Sherry RM, Morton KE, et al. Tumor progression can occur despite the induction of very high levels of self/tumor antigen-specific $CD8^+$ T cells in patients with melanoma. *J Immunol*. 2005;175:6169–6176.
164. Appay V, Jandus C, Voelter V, et al. New generation vaccine induces effective melanoma-specific $CD8^+$ T cells in the circulation but not in the tumor site. *J Immunol*. 2006;177:1670–1678.
165. Zippelius A, Batard P, Rubio-Godoy V, et al. Effector function of human tumor-specific CD8 T cells in melanoma lesions: a state of local functional tolerance. *Cancer Res*. 2004;64:2865–2873.
168. Bronte V, Kasic T, Gri G, et al. Boosting antitumor responses of T lymphocytes infiltrating human prostate cancers. *J Exp Med*. 2005;201:1257–1268.
172. Serafini P, Borrello I, Bronte V. Myeloid suppressor cells in cancer: recruitment, phenotype, properties, and mechanisms of immune suppression. *Semin Cancer Biol*. 2006;16:53–65.
173. Huang B, Pan PY, Li Q, et al. Gr-1+$CD115^+$ immature myeloid suppressor cells mediate the development of tumor-induced T regulatory cells and T-cell anergy in tumor-bearing host. *Cancer Res*. 2006;66:1123–1131.
174. Beyer M, Kochanek M, Giese T, et al. In vivo peripheral expansion of naive CD4+CD25high $FoxP3^+$ regulatory T cells in patients with multiple myeloma. *Blood*. 2006;107:3940–3949.
180. Galon J, Costes A, Sanchez-Cabo F, et al. Type, density, and location of immune cells within human colorectal tumors predict clinical outcome. *Science*. 2006;313:1960–1964.
182. Restifo NP, Rosenberg SA. Developing recombinant and synthetic vaccines for the treatment of melanoma. *Curr Opin Oncol*. 1999;11:50–57.
183. Rosenberg SA, Mule JJ, Spiess PJ, et al. Regression of established pulmonary metastases and subcutaneous tumor mediated by the systemic administration of high dose recombinant IL-2. *J Exp Med*. 1985;161:1169–1188.
184. Rosenberg SA, Yang JC, Topalian SL, et al. Treatment of 283 consecutive patients with metastatic melanoma or renal cell cancer using high-dose bolus interleukin-2. *JAMA*. 1994;271:907–913.
185. Ahmadzadeh M, Rosenberg SA. IL-2 administration increases CD4+ CD25(hi) Foxp3+ regulatory T cells in cancer patients. *Blood*. 2006;107:2409–2414.
187. Sansom DM, Walker LS. The role of CD28 and cytotoxic T-lymphocyte antigen-4 (CTLA-4) in regulatory T-cell biology. *Immunol Rev*. 2006;212:131–148.
189. Kocak E, Lute K, Chang X, et al. Combination therapy with anti-CTL antigen-4 and anti-4–1BB antibodies enhances cancer immunity and reduces autoimmunity. *Cancer Res*. 2006;66:7276–7284.
190. Attia P, Phan GQ, Maker AV, et al. Autoimmunity correlates with tumor regression in patients with metastatic melanoma treated with anti-cytotoxic T-lymphocyte antigen-4. *J Clin Oncol*. 2005;23:6043–6053.
191. Lute KD, May Jr. KF, Lu P, et al. Human CTLA4 knock-in mice unravel the quantitative link between tumor immunity and autoimmunity induced by anti-CTLA-4 antibodies. *Blood*. 2005;106:3127–3133.
192. McCoy KD, Hermans IF, Fraser JH, et al. Cytotoxic T lymphocyte-associated antigen 4 (CTLA-4) can regulate dendritic cell-induced activation and cytotoxicity of CD8(+) T cells independently of CD4(+) T cell help. *J Exp Med*. 1999;189:1157–1162.
193. Gattinoni L, Ranganathan A, Surman DR, et al. CTLA-4 dysregulation of self/tumor-reactive CD8+ T cell function is CD4+ T cell-dependent. *Blood*. 2006.
195. Blank C, Brown I, Peterson AC, et al. PD-L1/B7H-1 inhibits the effector phase of tumor rejection by T cell receptor (TCR) transgenic CD8+ T cells. *Cancer Res*. 2004;64:1140–1145.
196. Bachmann MF, Waterhouse P, Speiser DE, et al. Normal responsiveness of CTLA-4-deficient anti-viral cytotoxic T cells. *J Immunol*. 1998;160:95–100.
197. Rosenberg SA, Yang JC, Restifo NP. Cancer immunotherapy: moving beyond current vaccines. *Nat Med*. 2004;10:909–915.
198. Slingluff Jr, CL, Yamshchikov G, Neese P, et al. Phase I trial of a melanoma vaccine with gp100(280–288) peptide and tetanus helper peptide in adjuvant: immunologic and clinical outcomes. *Clin Cancer Res*. 2001;7:3012–3024.
199. Schaed SG, Klimek VM, Panageas KS, et al. T-cell responses against tyrosinase 368–376(370D) peptide in HLA*A0201+ melanoma patients: randomized trial comparing incomplete Freund's adjuvant, granulocyte macrophage colony-stimulating factor, and QS-21 as immunological adjuvants. *Clin Cancer Res*. 2002;8:967–972.
201. Eder JP, Kantoff PW, Roper K, et al. A phase I trial of a recombinant vaccinia virus expressing prostate-specific antigen in advanced prostate cancer. *Clin Cancer Res*. 2000;6:1632–1638.
202. Lurquin C, Lethe B, De Plaen E, et al. Contrasting frequencies of antitumor and anti-vaccine T cells in metastases of a melanoma patient vaccinated with a MAGE tumor antigen. *J Exp Med*. 2005;201:249–257.
203. Rosenberg SA, Yang JC, Schwartzentruber DJ, et al. Immunologic and therapeutic evaluation of a synthetic peptide vaccine for the treatment of patients with metastatic melanoma. *Nat Med*. 1998;4:321–327.
204. Marincola FM, Rivoltini L, Salgaller ML, et al. Differential anti-MART-1/MelanA CTL activity in peripheral blood of HLA- A2 melanoma patients in comparison to healthy donors: evidence of in vivo priming by tumor cells. *J Immunother Emphasis Tumor Immunol*. 1996;19:266–277.
206. Valmori D, Dutoit V, Ayyoub M, et al. Simultaneous CD8+ T cell responses to multiple tumor antigen epitopes in a multipeptide melanoma vaccine. *Cancer Immun*. 2003;3:15.
207. Chianese-Bullock KA, Pressley J, Garbee C, et al. MAGE-A1-, MAGE-A10-, and gp100-derived peptides are immunogenic when combined with granulocyte-macrophage colony-stimulating factor and

montanide ISA-51 adjuvant and administered as part of a multipeptide vaccine for melanoma. *J Immunol*. 2005;174:3080–3086.
208. Rosenberg SA, Sherry RM, Morton KE, et al. Altered CD8(+) T-cell responses when immunizing with multiepitope peptide vaccines. *J Immunother*. 2006;29:224–231.
210. Livingston PO, Wong GY, Adluri S, et al. Improved survival in stage III melanoma patients with GM2 antibodies: a randomized trial of adjuvant vaccination with GM2 ganglioside. *J Clin Oncol*. 1994;12:1036–1044.
211. Atkins LS, Flaherty L, Sosman JA, et al. A prospective randomized phase III trial of concurrent biochemotherapy (BCT) with cisplatin, vinblastin, dacarbazine (CVD), IL-2 and interferon alpha-2b (IFN) versus CVD alone in patients with metastatic melanoma (E3695): An ECOG-coordinated intergoup trial. *Proc Am Soc Clin Oncol*. 2003;22:708.
212. Clay TM, Hobeika AC, Mosca PJ, et al. Assays for monitoring cellular immune responses to active immunotherapy of cancer. *Clin Cancer Res*. 2001;7:1127–1135.
214. Sondak VK, Liu PY, Tuthill RJ, et al. Adjuvant immunotherapy of resected, intermediate-thickness, node-negative melanoma with an allogeneic tumor vaccine: overall results of a randomized trial of the Southwest Oncology Group. *J Clin Oncol*. 2002;20:2058–2066.
215. Hsueh EC, Essner R, Foshag LJ, et al. Prolonged survival after complete resection of disseminated melanoma and active immunotherapy with a therapeutic cancer vaccine. *J Clin Oncol*. 2002;20:4549–4554.
216. Faries MB, Morton DL. Therapeutic vaccines for melanoma: current status. *Bio Drugs*. 2005;19:247–260.
217. Dranoff G, Jaffee E, Lazenby A, et al. Vaccination with irradiated tumor cells engineered to secrete murine granulocyte-macrophage colony-stimulating factor stimulates potent, specific, and long-lasting anti-tumor immunity. *Proc Natl Acad Sci U S A*. 1993;90:3539–3543.
218. Simons JW, Jaffee EM, Weber CE, et al. Bioactivity of autologous irradiated renal cell carcinoma vaccines generated by ex vivo granulocyte-macrophage colony-stimulating factor gene transfer. *Cancer Res*. 1997;57:1537–1546.
219. Soiffer R, Hodi FS, Haluska F, et al. Vaccination with irradiated, autologous melanoma cells engineered to secrete granulocyte-macrophage colony-stimulating factor by adenoviral-mediated gene transfer augments antitumor immunity in patients with metastatic melanoma. *J Clin Oncol*. 2003;21:3343–3350.
220. Nestle FO, Alijagic S, Gilliet M, et al. Vaccination of melanoma patients with peptide- or tumor lysate-pulsed dendritic cells. *Nat Med*. 1998;4:328–332.
221. Heiser A, Coleman D, Dannull J, et al. Autologous dendritic cells transfected with prostate-specific antigen RNA stimulate CTL responses against metastatic prostate tumors. *J Clin Invest*. 2002;109:409–417.
223. Rini BI. Technology evaluation: APC-8015, Dendreon. *Curr Opin Mol Ther*. 2002;4:76–79.
224. Ribas A, Butterfield LH, Glaspy JA, et al. Current developments in cancer vaccines and cellular immunotherapy. *J Clin Oncol*. 2003;21:2415–2432.
225. Hodge JW, Sabzevari H, Yafal AG, et al. A triad of costimulatory molecules synergize to amplify T-cell activation. *Cancer Res*. 1999;59:5800–5807.
226. Kaufman HL, Cohen S, Cheung K, et al. Local delivery of vaccinia virus expressing multiple costimulatory molecules for the treatment of established tumors. *Hum Gene Ther*. 2006;17:239–244.
227. Marshall JL, Gulley JL, Arlen PM, et al. Phase I study of sequential vaccinations with fowlpox-CEA(6D)-TRICOM alone and sequentially with vaccinia-CEA(6D)-TRICOM, with and without granulocyte-macrophage colony-stimulating factor, in patients with carcinoembryonic antigen-expressing carcinomas. *J Clin Oncol*. 2005;23:720–731.
228. Wang HH, Mao CY, Teng LS, et al. Recent advances in heat shock protein-based cancer vaccines. *Hepatobiliary Pancreat Dis Int*. 2006;5:22–27.
229. Weng WK, Czerwinski D, Timmerman J, et al. Clinical outcome of lymphoma patients after idiotype vaccination is correlated with humoral immune response and immunoglobulin G Fc receptor genotype. *J Clin Oncol*. 2004;22:4717–4724.
230. Timmerman JM, Czerwinski DK, Davis TA, et al. Idiotype-pulsed dendritic cell vaccination for B-cell lymphoma: clinical and immune responses in 35 patients. *Blood*. 2002;99:1517–1526.
232. Rosenberg SA, Lotze MT, Yang JC, et al. Prospective randomized trial of high-dose interleukin-2 alone or in conjunction with lymphokine-activated killer cells for the treatment of patients with advanced cancer. *J Natl Cancer Inst*. 1993;85:622–632.
233. Rosenberg SA, Spiess P, Lafreniere R. A new approach to the adoptive immunotherapy of cancer with tumor-infiltrating lymphocytes. *Science*. 1986;233:1318–1321.
234. Rosenberg SA, Yannelli JR, Yang JC, et al. Treatment of patients with metastatic melanoma with autologous tumor-infiltrating lymphocytes and interleukin 2. *J Natl Cancer Inst*. 1994;86:1159–1166.
235. Rosenberg SA, Spiess P, Lafreniere R. A new approach to the adoptive immunotherapy of cancer with tumor-infiltrating lymphocytes. *Science*.. 1986;233:1318–1321.
236. Dudley ME, Wunderlich JR, Yang JC, et al. Adoptive cell transfer therapy following non-myeloablative but lymphodepleting chemotherapy for the treatment of patients with refractory metastatic melanoma. *J Clin Oncol*. 2005;23:2346–2357.
237. Woo EY, Chu CS, Goletz TJ, et al. Regulatory CD4(+)CD25(+) T cells in tumors from patients with early- stage non-small cell lung cancer and late-stage ovarian cancer. *Cancer Res*. 2001;61:4766–4772.
238. Wang HY, Lee DA, Peng G, et al. Tumor-Specific Human CD4(+) Regulatory T Cells and Their Ligands. Implications for Immunotherapy. *Immunity*. 2004;20:107–118.
239. Wang HY, Peng G, Guo Z, et al. Recognition of a new ARTC1 peptide ligand uniquely expressed in tumor cells by antigen-specific CD4+ regulatory T cells. *J Immunol*. 2005;174:2661–2670.
240. Curiel TJ, Coukos G, Zou L, et al. Specific recruitment of regulatory T cells in ovarian carcinoma fosters immune privilege and predicts reduced survival. *Nat Med*. 2004;10:942–949.
241. Loddenkemper C, Schernus M, Noutsias M, et al. In situ analysis of FOXP3+ regulatory T cells in human colorectal cancer. *J Transl Med*. 2006;4:52.
242. Terabe M, Matsui S, Noben-Trauth N, et al. NKT cell-mediated repression of tumor immunosurveillance by IL-13 and the IL-4R-STAT6 pathway. *Nat Immunol*. 2000;1:515–520.
243. Makarenkova VP, Bansal V, Matta BM, et al. CD11b+/Gr-1+ myeloid suppressor cells cause T cell dysfunction after traumatic stress. *J Immunol*. 2006;176:2085–2094.
244. Seung LP, Rowley DA, Dubey P, et al. Synergy between T-cell immunity and inhibition of paracrine stimulation causes tumor rejection. *Proc Natl Acad Sci U S A*. 1995;92:6254–6258.
245. Tan JT, Ernst B, Kieper WC, et al. Interleukin (IL)-15 and IL-7 jointly regulate homeostatic proliferation of memory phenotype CD8+ cells but are not required for memory phenotype CD4+ cells. *J Exp Med*. 2002;195:1523–1532.
246. Kieper WC, Tan JT, Bondi-Boyd B, et al. Overexpression of interleukin (IL)-7 leads to IL-15-independent generation of memory phenotype CD8+ T cells. *J Exp Med*. 2002;195:1533–1539.
247. Gattinoni L, Finkelstein SE, Klebanoff CA, et al. Removal of homeostatic cytokine sinks by lymphodepletion enhances the efficacy of adoptively transferred tumor-specific CD8+ T cells. *J Exp Med*. 2005;202:907–912.
248. Malek TR. The main function of IL-2 is to promote the development of T regulatory cells. *J Leukoc Biol*. 2003.
249. Antony PA, Paulos CM, Ahmadzadeh M, et al. Interleukin-2-dependent mechanisms of tolerance and immunity in vivo. *J Immunol*. 2006;176:5255–5266.
250. Kohm AP, McMahon JS, Podojil JR, et al. Cutting Edge: Anti-CD25 monoclonal antibody injection results in the functional inactivation, not depletion, of CD4+CD25+ T regulatory cells. *J Immunol*. 2006;176:3301–3305.
251. Torihata H, Ishikawa F, Okada Y, et al. Irradiation up-regulates CD80 expression through two different mechanisms in spleen B cells, B lymphoma cells, and dendritic cells. *Immunology*. 2004;112:219–227.
252. Shigematsu A, Adachi Y, Koike-Kiriyama N, et al. Effects of low-dose irradiation on enhancement of immunity by dendritic cells. *J Radiat Res (Tokyo)*. 2007;48:51–55.

253. Gattinoni L, Klebanoff CA, Palmer DC, et al. Acquisition of full effector function in vitro paradoxically impairs the in vivo antitumor efficacy of adoptively transferred CD8+ T cells. *J Clin Invest.* 2005;115:1616–1626.
254. Kagamu H, Touhalisky JE, Plautz GE, et al. Isolation based on L-selectin expression of immune effector T cells derived from tumor-draining lymph nodes. *Cancer Res.* 1996;56:4338–4342.
255. Wherry EJ, Teichgraber V, Becker TC, et al. Lineage relationship and protective immunity of memory CD8 T cell subsets. *Nat Immunol.* 2003;4:225–234.
256. Klebanoff CA, Gattinoni L, Torabi-Parizi P, et al. Central memory self/tumor-reactive $CD8^{+}$ T cells confer superior antitumor immunity compared with effector memory T cells. *Proc Natl Acad Sci U S A.* 2005;102:9571–9576.
257. Chen BJ, Cui X, Sempowski GD, et al. Transfer of allogeneic CD62L- memory T cells without graft-versus-host disease. *Blood.* 2004;103:1534–1541.
258. Powell Jr, DJ, Dudley ME, Robbins PF, et al. Transition of late stage effector T cells to CD27+ CD28+ tumor-reactive effector memory T cells in humans after adoptive cell transfer therapy. *Blood.* 2005;105:241–250.
259. Zhou J, Shen X, Huang J, et al. Telomere length of transferred lymphocytes correlates with in vivo persistence and tumor regression in melanoma patients receiving cell transfer therapy. *J Immunol.* 2005;175:7046–7052.
260. Hendriks J, Xiao Y, Borst J. CD27 promotes survival of activated T cells and complements CD28 in generation and establishment of the effector T cell pool. *J Exp Med.* 2003;198:1369–1380.
261. Ochsenbein AF, Riddell SR, Brown M, et al. CD27 expression promotes long-term survival of functional effector-memory $CD8^{+}$ cytotoxic T lymphocytes in HIV-infected patients. *J Exp Med.* 2004;200:1407–1417.
262. Huang J, Kerstann KW, Ahmadzadeh M, et al. Modulation by IL-2 of CD70 and CD27 expression on CD8+ T cells: importance for the therapeutic effectiveness of cell transfer immunotherapy. *J Immunol.* 2006;176:7726–7735.
264. Oh S, Berzofsky JA, Burke DS, et al. Coadministration of HIV vaccine vectors with vaccinia viruses expressing IL-15 but not IL-2 induces long-lasting cellular immunity. *Proc Natl Acad Sci U S A.* 2003;100:3392–3397.
265. Liu S, Riley J, Rosenberg S, et al. Comparison of common gamma-chain cytokines, interleukin-2, interleukin-7, and interleukin-15 for the in vitro generation of human tumor-reactive T lymphocytes for adoptive cell transfer therapy. *J Immunother.* 2006;29:284–293.
266. Morgan RA, Dudley ME, Wunderlich JR, et al. Cancer regression in patients after transfer of genetically engineered lymphocytes. *Science.* 2006;314:126–129.
267. Li Y, Moysey R, Molloy PE, et al. Directed evolution of human T-cell receptors with picomolar affinities by phage display. *Nat Biotechnol.* 2005;23:349–354.
268. Donermeyer DL, Weber KS, Kranz DM, et al. The study of high-affinity TCRs reveals duality in T cell recognition of antigen: specificity and degeneracy. *J Immunol.* 2006;177:6911–6919.
270. Wrzesinski C, Paulos CM, Gattinoni L, et al. Hematopoietic stem cells promote the expansion and function of adoptively transferred antitumor CD8 T cells. *J Clin Invest.* 2007;117:492–501.
271. Gattinoni L, Powell, Jr. DJ, Rosenberg SA, et al. Adoptive immunotherapy for cancer: building on success. *Nat Rev Immunol.* 2006;6:383–393.
272. Riddell SR, Bleakley M, Nishida T, et al. Adoptive transfer of allogeneic antigen-specific T cells. *Biol Blood Marrow Transplant.* 2006;12:9–12.
273. Brickner AG, Evans AM, Mito JK, et al. The PANE1 gene encodes a novel human minor histocompatibility antigen that is selectively expressed in B-lymphoid cells and B-CLL. *Blood.* 2006;107:3779–3786.
274. van Rhee F, Lin F, Cullis JO, et al. Relapse of chronic myeloid leukemia after allogeneic bone marrow transplant: the case for giving donor leukocyte transfusions before the onset of hematologic relapse. *Blood.* 1994;83:3377–3383.
275. Ruggeri L, Capanni M, Urbani E, et al. Effectiveness of donor natural killer cell alloreactivity in mismatched hematopoietic transplants. *Science.* 2002;295:2097–2100.
276. Hsu KC, Keever-Taylor CA, Wilton A, et al. Improved outcome in HLA-identical sibling hematopoietic stem-cell transplantation for acute myelogenous leukemia predicted by KIR and HLA genotypes. *Blood.* 2005;105:4878–4884.
277. Slamon DJ, Leyland-Jones B, Shak S, et al. Use of chemotherapy plus a monoclonal antibody against HER2 for metastatic breast cancer that overexpresses HER2. *N Engl J Med.* 2001;344:783–792.
279. Held G, Poschel V, Pfreundschuh M. Rituximab for the treatment of diffuse large B-cell lymphomas. *Expert Rev Anticancer Ther.* 2006;6:1175–1186.
281. Gross G, Gorochov G, Waks T, et al. Generation of effector T cells expressing chimeric T cell receptor with antibody type-specificity. *Transplantation Proceedings.* 1989;21:127–130.
282. Hwu P, Shafer GE, Treisman J, et al. Lysis of ovarian cancer cells by human lymphocytes redirected with a chimeric gene composed of an antibody variable region and the Fc receptor gamma chain. *J Exp Med.* 1993;178:361–366.
283. Eshhar Z, Waks T, Gross G, et al. Specific activation and targeting of cytotoxic lymphocytes through chimeric single chains consisting of antibody-binding domains and the gamma or zeta subunits of the immunoglobulin and T-cell receptors. *Proc Natl Acad Sci U S A.* 1993;90:720–724.
286. Pinthus JH, Waks T, Kaufman-Francis K, et al. Immuno-gene therapy of established prostate tumors using chimeric receptor-redirected human lymphocytes. *Cancer Res.* 2003;63:2470–2476.
288. Kershaw MH, Westwood JA, Parker LL, et al. A phase I study on adoptive immunotherapy using gene-modified T cells for ovarian cancer. *Clin Cancer Res.* 2006;12:6106–6115.
289. Lamers CH, van Elzakker P, Langeveld SC, et al. Process validation and clinical evaluation of a protocol to generate gene-modified T lymphocytes for imunogene therapy for metastatic renal cell carcinoma: GMP-controlled transduction and expansion of patient's T lymphocytes using a carboxy anhydrase IX-specific scFv transgene. *Cytotherapy.* 2006;8:542–553.
291. Willemsen RA, Weijtens ME, Ronteltap C, et al. Grafting primary human T lymphocytes with cancer-specific chimeric single chain and two chain TCR. *Gene Ther.* 2000;7:1369–1377.
292. Burnet FM. The concept of immunological surveillance. *Prog Exp Tumor Res.* 1970;13:1–27.
293. Stutman O. Tumor development after 3-methylcholanthrene in immunologically deficient athymic-nude mice. *Science.* 1974;183:534–536.
294. Dunn GP, Old LJ, Schreiber RD. The immunobiology of cancer immunosurveillance and immunoediting. *Immunity.* 2004;21:137–148.
301. Restifo NP, Esquivel F, Kawakami Y, et al. Identification of human cancers deficient in antigen processing. *J Exp Med.* 1993;177:265–272.
304. Gonzalez S, Groh V, Spies T. Immunobiology of human NKG2D and its ligands. *Curr Top Microbiol Immunol.* 2006;298:121–138.
305. Rippo MR, Moretti S, Vescovi S, et al. FLIP overexpression inhibits death receptor-induced apoptosis in malignant mesothelial cells. *Oncogene.* 2004;23:7753–7760.
308. Shin MS, Park WS, Kim SY, et al. Alterations of Fas (Apo-1/CD95) gene in cutaneous malignant melanoma. *Am J Pathol.* 1999;154:1785–1791.
309. Gabrilovich D, Ishida T, Oyama T, et al. Vascular endothelial growth factor inhibits the development of dendritic cells and dramatically affects the differentiation of multiple hematopoietic lineages in vivo. *Blood.* 1998;92:4150–4166.
310. Almand B, Resser JR, Lindman B, et al. Clinical significance of defective dendritic cell differentiation in cancer. *Clin Cancer Res.* 2000;6:1755–1766.
312. Knauf WU, Ehlers B, Bisson S, et al. Serum levels of interleukin-10 in B-cell chronic lymphocytic leukemia. *Blood.* 1995;86:4382–4383.
314. Hidalgo GE, Zhong L, Doherty DE, et al. Plasma PGE-2 levels and altered cytokine profiles in adherent peripheral blood mononuclear cells in non-small cell lung cancer (NSCLC). *Mol Cancer.* 2002; 1:5.
315. Berg DJ, Zhang J, Lauricella DM, et al. Il-10 is a central regulator of cyclooxygenase-2 expression and prostaglandin production. *J Immunol.* 2001;166:2674–2680.

316. Griffith TS, Brunner T, Fletcher SM, et al. Fas ligand-induced apoptosis as a mechanism of immune privilege. *Science* 1995;270:1189–1192.
317. Hahne M, Rimoldi D, Schroter M, et al. Melanoma cell expression of Fas(Apo-1/CD95) ligand: implications for tumor immune escape [see comments]. *Science*. 1996;274:1363–1366.
318. Chappell DB, Zaks TZ, Rosenberg SA, et al. Human melanoma cells do not express Fas (Apo-1/CD95) ligand. *Cancer Res*. 1999;59:59–62.
319. Allison J, Georgiou HM, Strasser A, et al. Transgenic expression of CD95 ligand on islet beta cells induces a granulocytic infiltration but does not confer immune privilege upon islet allografts. *Proc Natl Acad Sci U S A*. 1997;94:3943–3947.

Chapter 46

Primary Immunodeficiency Diseases

Rebecca H. Buckley

INTRODUCTION

Recognition of the first human primary immunodeficiency diseases more than a half century ago (1,2) set the stage for an exponential increase in information about the functions of the various components of the immune system. Since then, more than 200 human primary immunodeficiency disorders have been recognized (3,4). These discoveries, together with several naturally occurring immune defects in animal species and the ability to create "knockout mice," have seemingly opened the door to the ultimate dissection of the immune system.

Primary, or genetically determined, immunodeficiency disorders may affect one or more components of the immune system, including T, B, and NK lymphocytes, phagocytic cells, and complement proteins. This chapter focuses on the genetic bases of and/or faulty immunologic mechanisms underlying some of the most important human immunodeficiency diseases involving lymphocytes (Table 46.1).

Immunodeficiency diseases are characterized by undue susceptibility to infection. Paradoxically, many immunodeficiency syndromes are also characterized by autoimmune diseases and/or excessive production of

TABLE 46.1 Abnormal Genes Known to Cause Primary Immunodeficiency

Chromosome	Disease
1q21	MCH class II antigen deficiency caused by RFX5 mutation[a]
1q22-q25	SCID due to CD3 ζ chain deficiency[a]
1q23	ALPS type 1b caused by deficiency of Fas ligand (CD178)[a]
1q25	Chronic granulomatous disease (CGD) caused by gp67^{phox} deficiency[a]
1q31-q32	SCID due to CD45 deficiency[a]
1q42-q43	Chediak-Higashi syndrome[a]
2p11	Kappa-chain deficiency[a]
2p12	CD8 deficiency due to CD8 antigen α polypeptide deficiency[a]
2q12	CD8 lymphocytopenia caused by ZAP70 deficiency[a]
2q33	Autosomal recessive CVID due to ICOS deficiency[a]
2q33-q34	ALPS types IIa and IIb caused by deficiencies of caspase 10 or 8[a]
2q35	CID with microcephaly due to Cernunnos deficiency[a]
5p13	SCID or Omenn's syndrome due to IL-7 receptor α-chain deficiency[a]
5q31.1-q33.1	IL-12 p40 deficiency[a]
6p21.3	MHC class I antigen defects caused by TAP1, TAP2, or tapasin deficiency[a]
6p21.3	(?) CVID and selective IgA deficiency
6q23-q24	IFNγ receptor 1 deficiency due to α chain deficiency[a]
7q11.23	CGD caused by gp47^{phox} deficiency[a]
8q21	Nijmegen breakage syndrome due to mutations in *Nibrin*[a]
9p13	Cartilage hair hypoplasia due to deficiency of RNA component of mitochondrial RNA-processing endoribonuclease[a]
10p13	SCID (Athabascan, radiation sensitive) due to mutations in the *Artemis gene*[a]
10p13	DiGeorge's syndrome/velocardiofacial syndrome
10q23.2-q23.33	Agammaglobulinemia due to BLNK deficiency[a]
10q23-q24	ALPS type 1a due to CD95 (Fas) deficiency[a]
11p13	IL-2 receptor α chain deficiency[a]
11p13	SCID or Omenn's syndrome caused by RAG-1 or RAG-2 deficiency[a]
11q14.3-q21	LAD2 due to deficiency of sialyl-Lewis^{X}
11q22.3	AT, attributable to AT mutation, causing deficiency of DNA-dependent kinase[a]
11q23	SCID or non-SCID due to CD3 γ, δ, or ε chain deficiency[a]
12	Hyper IgM syndrome cause by deficiency of uracil-DNA glycosylase[a]
12p13	Hyper IgM caused by deficiency of activation-induced cytidine deaminase[a]
12q12	Interleukin-1 receptor-associated kinase-4 deficiency[a]
13q	MHC class II antigen deficiency caused by RFXAP deficiency[a]
13q33-q34	Ligase 4 deficiency
14q13.1	Purine nucleoside phosphorylase deficiency[a]
14q32.3	Immunoglobulin heavy-chain deletion[a]
15q21	Griscelli's syndrome due to myosin VA or Rab27a deficiency[a]
16p11.2	CVID due to CD19 deficiency[a]
16p13	MHC class II antigen deficiency caused by CIITA deficiency[a]
17p11.2	CVID or IgA deficiency due to TACI deficiency[a]
16q24	CGD caused by gp22^{phox} deficiency[a]
17q11-q12	Human nude defect due to *FOXN1* deficiency[a]
19p12	MHC class II antigen deficiency caused by RFXANK deficiency[a]
19p13.1	IL-12R β chain deficiency[a]
19p13.1	SCID caused by Janus kinase 3 deficiency[a]
19p13.2	Agammaglobulinemia caused by mutations in *Ig*α gene[a]
20q12-q13.2	Hyper IgM syndrome due to CD40 deficiency
20q13.2-q13.11	SCID caused by adenosine deaminase deficiency[a]
21q22.1-q22.2	IFNγ receptor 2 deficiency due to β chain deficiency[a]
21q22.3	APCED due to AIRE deficiency[a]
21q22.3	Leukocyte adhesion deficiency type 1, caused by CD18 deficiency[a]
22q11.2	Agammaglobulinemia caused by mutations in λ5 surrogate light chain gene[a]
22q11.2	DiGeorge's/velocardiofacial syndrome
22q13.1-q13.3	CVID due to BAFF-R deficiency
Xp21.1	CGD caused by gp91^{phox} deficiency[a]

(continued)

TABLE 46.1 Abnormal Genes Known to Cause Primary Immunodeficiency (Continued)

Chromosome	*Disease*
Xp11.22	WAS caused by WAS protein deficiency[a]
Xp11.23	IPEX due to FOXP3 deficiency[a]
Xp11.3-p21.1	Properdin deficiency[a]
Xq13.1-q13.3	X-linked SCID caused by common γ-chain deficiency[a]
Xq22	X-linked agammaglobulinemia caused by Bruton tyrosine kinase deficiency[a]
Xq25-26	X-linked lymphoproliferative syndrome caused by mutations in the *SH2D1A* gene[a]
Xq26	Immunodeficiency with hyper IgM caused by CD154 (CD40 ligand) deficiency[a]
Xq28	Anhidrotic ectodermal dysplasia with immunodeficiency caused by mutations in the nuclear factor κB essential modulator[a]

AIRE, autoimmune regulator; ALPS, autoimmune lymphoproliferative syndrome; APECED, autoimmune polyendocrinopathy-candidiasis ectodermal dysplasia; AT, ataxia-telangiectasia; BAFF-R, B cell–activating factor of the tumor necrosis factor family receptor; BLNK, B cell linker; CGD, chronic granulomatous disease; CID, combined immunodeficiency; CIITA, MHC class II transactivator; CVID, common variable immunodeficiency; FOXP3, forkhead box P3; ICOS, inducible costimulator; IFN, interferon; Ig, immunoglobulin; IL, interleukin; IPEX, immune dysregulation, polyendocrinopathy, enteropathy, X-linked syndrome; LAD, leukocyte adhesion deficiency; MCH, major histocompatibility complex; RAG, recombination activating gene; RFXAP, RFX-associated protein; SCID, severe combined immunodeficiency; TACI, transmembrane activator, calcium-modulator and cyclophilin ligand interactor; WAS, Wiskott-Aldrich syndrome; ZAP70, ζ-chain–associated protein-70.

[a]Gene cloned and sequenced; gene product known.

immunoglobulin E (IgE) antibodies. Due to the ability of antibiotics to control many types of infections, diagnosis of these diseases is often delayed, and autoimmunity or allergy may be the presenting manifestation. Finally, there is an increased incidence of malignancy in patients with immunodeficiency diseases (5). Whether this is due to increased susceptibility to infection with agents predisposing to malignancy or to defective tumor immunosurveillance is unknown.

With the exception of selective IgA deficiency, genetically determined immunodeficiency is considered to be rare (3). However, the true incidence and prevalence of these diseases are unknown because there is no screening for any of these disorders at birth or during infancy, childhood, or adulthood anywhere in the world. B cell defects appear to far outnumber those affecting T cells, phagocytic cells, or complement proteins. It has been estimated that agammaglobulinemia occurs with a frequency of 1:50,000 and severe combined immunodeficiency with a frequency of 1:40,000 to 1:100,000 live births. Selective absence of serum and secretory IgA is the most common defect, with reported incidences ranging from 1:333 to 1:700 (6,7). Primary immunodeficiency is seen more often in infants and children than in adults.

MOLECULAR GENETICS OF PRIMARY IMMUNODEFICIENCY

Until 1993, there was little insight into the fundamental problems underlying a majority of human primary immunodeficiency disorders. It is impressive that the underlying genetic defects have now been identified in more than 150 of these diseases (Table 46.1) (4). Within the last decade and a half the molecular bases of seven X-linked immunodeficiency disorders have been discovered (Figure 46.1, Table 46.1): X-linked agammaglobulinemia (8,9),

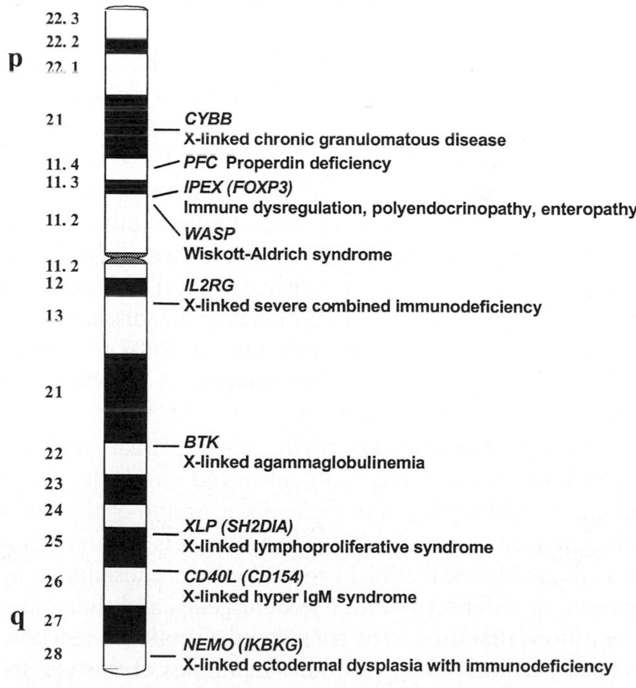

FIGURE 46.1 Locations of the X-linked immunodeficiency disease loci. Correspondence with the cytogenetic map of the X chromosome is indicated on the left. Most of these defects have been discovered over the last decade.

TABLE 46.2 Mutated Immune System Genes with Variable Phenotypic Expression

Mutated Gene	*Normal Gene Product*	*Classic Syndrome*	*Variant Syndrome*
RAG1	Recombinase activating gene 1	SCID	1. Omenn's syndrome 2. Oligoclonal γ/δ T cells, autoimmune disease, and CMV infection
BTK	Bruton tyrosine kinase	Agammaglobulinemia	Polysaccharide antibody deficiency
WASP	Wiskott-Aldrich syndrome protein	Wiskott-Aldrich syndrome	X-linked thrombocytopenia
SH2D1A	Slam-associated protein (SAP)	Fatal infectious mononucleosis	1. Common variable immunodeficiency 2. Hemophagocytic lymphohistiocytosis
CD3ε	CD3 ε chain	SCID	Moderate susceptibility to infection
IL2RG	Interleukin-2 receptor γ [common gamma chain (γc)]	SCID	Moderate combined immunodeficiency
ADA	Adenosine deaminase	SCID	Moderate combined immunodeficiency
JAK3	Jak3	SCID	Moderate combined immunodeficiency

CMV, cytomegalovirus; SCID, severe combined immunodeficiency. From Buckley RH. Variable phenotypic expression of mutations in genes of the immune system. *J Clin Invest.* 2005;115(11):2974, with permission.

X-linked immunodeficiency with hyper IgM (10,11), the Wiskott-Aldrich syndrome (12,13), X-linked severe combined immunodeficiency (14,15), X-linked lymphoproliferative disease (16,17), immune dysregulation, polyendocrinopathy, enteropathy, X-linked (IPEX) syndrome (18), and nuclear factor of κB essential modulator (NEMO) deficiency (19,20) (Table 46.1). The abnormal gene in X-linked chronic granulomatous disease (CGD) had been identified several years earlier (21), and the gene encoding properdin (mutated in properdin deficiency) has also been cloned (22).

In addition to these X-linked defects, the underlying bases for numerous autosomal recessive immunodeficiencies have also been identified (Table 46.1) (4). The rapidity of these advances suggests that there will soon be many more. The discovery and cloning of the genes for these diseases have obvious implications for the potential of gene therapy (23). A committee of the World Health Organization has published several versions of a classification of primary immunodeficiency diseases over the last three decades, most recently in 2007 (3). Table 46.1 lists some of the numerous conditions for which the molecular bases are known (4).

Discovery of mutated genes that cause primary immunodeficiencies has significantly advanced our understanding of the pathogenesis of these diseases and of the functions of normal gene products. However, it is apparent that seemingly identical clinical conditions are caused by mutations in different immune system genes and that some conditions that used to be considered a single disease now must be defined as a syndrome. Examples of this are severe combined immunodeficiency, which is now known to be caused by mutations in 12 different genes; hyper IgM syndrome, which can result from mutations in any one of at least 6 different genes; Omenn's syndrome, which can be caused by mutations in at least 4 different genes; and common variable immunodeficiency (CVID), which can be caused by mutations in any one of at least 10 different genes, although the molecular basis for most common form of CVID is unknown. To make matters even more complicated, it is becoming abundantly clear that the phenotypic presentation of mutations in a single gene can be quite different even within the same family, depending on the location and type of mutation but also probably on other genetic factors and environmental influences (Table 46.2) (24).

DEFECTS CHARACTERIZED BY ANTIBODY DEFICIENCY

X-Linked Agammaglobulinemia

Most boys afflicted with X-linked agammaglobulinemia (XLA), also known as Bruton's agammaglobulinemia (2), remain well during the first 6 to 9 months of life by virtue of maternally transmitted IgG antibodies (25). Thereafter, they repeatedly acquire infections with extracellular pyogenic organisms such as pneumococci, streptococci, and *Haemophilus* unless given prophylactic antibiotics or γ-globulin therapy. Chronic fungal infections are not usually present, and *Pneumocystis jiroveci* pneumonia rarely occurs unless there is an associated neutropenia (26). Viral infections are also usually handled normally, with the notable exceptions of the hepatitis viruses and the enteroviruses (27). In addition to septic arthritis, patients with this condition may have joint inflammation similar to that seen in rheumatoid arthritis (25). Infections with *Ureaplasma urealyticum* and viral agents such as echoviruses, coxsackie viruses, and adenovirus have been identified from joint fluid cultures of patients even on intravenous immune globulin (IVIG) replacement therapy. These observations suggest a primary role for antibody, particularly secretory IgA, in host defense against this group of viruses, because normal T cell numbers and function are present in X-linked agammaglobulinemia. Concentrations of immunoglobulins of all isotypes are very low, and circulating B cells are usually absent. Pre-B cells are present in reduced numbers in the bone marrow. Tonsils are usually very small, and lymph nodes are rarely palpable due to absence of germinal centers from these lymphoid tissues. Thymus architecture, including Hassall's corpuscles, is normal, as are the thymus-dependent areas of spleen and lymph nodes.

In 1993, two groups of investigators independently and almost simultaneously discovered the mutated gene in XLA (8,9). Because XLA had been precisely mapped to position Xq22 (Figure 46.1), one group successfully used the technique of positional cloning to identify an abnormal gene in patients with this defect (Table 46.1) (9). For other reasons, the second group sought and found a B cell–specific tyrosine kinase important in murine B lymphocyte signaling (8); the kinase was found to be encoded by a gene on the mouse X chromosome. When the human gene counterpart was cloned, it was found to reside at Xq22, and the gene product was identical to that found by the first group. This intracellular signaling tyrosine kinase has been named Bruton tyrosine kinase (or Btk) in honor of O. C. Bruton. Btk is a member of the Tec family of cytoplasmic protein tyrosine kinases (28). It is expressed at high levels in all B-lineage cells, including pre-B cells. This kinase appears to be necessary for pre-B cell expansion and maturation into surface Ig-expressing B cells, but it probably has a role at all stages of B cell development (8,9). It has not been detected in any cells of T lineage, but it has been found in cells of the myeloid series (8). Thus far, all males with known XLA (by family history) have had low or undetectable Btk mRNA and kinase activity.

Female carriers of XLA can be identified by the finding of nonrandom X chromosome inactivation in their B cells or by the detection of the mutated gene (if known in the family) (29). Prenatal diagnosis of affected or nonaffected male fetuses has also been accomplished by detection of the mutated gene in chorionic villous or amniocentesis samples. Studies of Btk protein enzymatic activity or mRNA have also permitted identification of X-linked inheritance in some agammaglobulinemic boys with no family history. The fact that Btk is also expressed in cells of myeloid lineage is of interest in light of the occurrence of intermittent neutropenia in boys with XLA, particularly at the onset of an acute infection (26). It is conceivable that Btk is only one of several signaling molecules participating in myeloid maturation and that neutropenia would be observed in XLA only when rapid production of such cells is needed. XLA has also been reported in association with growth hormone deficiency in nine cases (30) and with sensorineural hearing loss in three cases (31).

A mutation at position 28 of the murine *btk* gene has been shown to be the basis for the B cell defect in CBA/N mice (32). Because such mice have a much milder antibody deficiency than boys with XLA have, speculation had been that humans with mutations in the non–kinase-encoding part of the *Btk* gene might have a less severe immunodeficiency. However, many different mutations of the human *Btk* gene (more than 550) have been described (33), encompassing most parts of the coding portions of the gene, and there has not been any clear correlation between the location of the mutation and the clinical phenotype.

Autosomal Recessive Agammaglobulinemia

Autosomal recessive conditions that resemble XLA phenotypically are caused by mutations in the genes that encode immunoglobulin heavy or light chains or their associated signaling molecules, leading to a- or hypogammaglobulinemia (Table 46.1). In μ chain (34), λ5/14.1 (surrogate light chain) (35), Igα (B cell antigen receptor signaling molecule) (36), and B cell linker (*BLNK*) gene mutations (37), circulating B cells are absent. In the case of other heavy-chain gene mutations, deficiencies of individual immunoglobulin classes or subclasses are seen, and circulating B cells are present (38). Mutations in the κ-chain gene result in molecules with only λ light chains.

Immunodeficiency with Elevated IgM

The hyper IgM syndrome is characterized by defective class switch recombination (39) resulting in very low serum IgG, IgA, and IgE levels but either a normal or a markedly elevated concentration of polyclonal IgM. Patients with this syndrome resemble agammaglobulinemics in their susceptibility to encapsulated bacterial infections (40). The hyper IgM syndrome may be caused by mutations in at least six different genes (41). Thus far, two X-linked and four autosomal recessive defects have been found to cause this syndrome, and there are likely to be more. Distinctive clinical features permit presumptive recognition of the type of mutation in these patients, thereby aiding proper choice of therapy (Table 46.3). However, all such patients should undergo molecular analysis to ascertain the affected gene for purposes of genetic counseling, carrier detection, and definitive therapy.

X-Linked Hyper IgM Due to CD154 (CD40 Ligand) Deficiency (HIGM1)

Like boys with XLA, those with X-linked hyper IgM (HIGM1) may become symptomatic during the first or second year of life with recurrent pyogenic infections. However, they also are highly prone to have *Pneumocystis*

TABLE 46.3 Hyper Immunoglobulin M (HIGM) Syndrome: Clinical Features of the Different Molecular Types

HIGM Type	PJ Pneumonia	Neutropenia	Lymphadenopathy	Early Death
HIGM1 (CD40L Def)	Yes	Yes	No	Yes
NEMO	No	No	No	Unknown
HIGM2 (AICDA Def), HIGM5 (UNG Def)	No	No	Yes	No
HIGM3 (CD40 Def)	Yes	Yes	No	Unknown
HIGM4 (molecular defect unknown)	No	No	Yes	No

AICDA, activation-dependent cytidine deaminase; Def, defect; NEMO, nuclear factor of κB essential modulator; PJ, *Pneumocystis jiroveci*; UNG, uracil-DNA glycosylase.

jiroveci pneumonia and to have profound neutropenia (40,42). Normal numbers of B lymphocytes are usually present in the circulation of these patients.

Until 1993 this condition was classified as a B cell defect because only IgM is produced. However, B cells from HIGM1 patients were shown more than two decades ago to have the capacity to synthesize IgM, IgA, and IgG normally when cocultured with a "switch" T cell line, suggesting that in those patients the defect lay in T lineage cells (43). This was puzzling because routine tests of T cell function were usually normal in such patients. In 1993, the abnormal gene in HIGM1 was localized to Xq26 (Figure 46.1) and identified by five groups almost simultaneously (10,44–46). The gene product is a surface molecule known as CD154 (or CD40 ligand) on the surfaces of activated helper T cells (47), which interacts with CD40 molecules on B cells (Figure 46.2) (10). Cross-linking of CD40 on either normal or HIGM1 B cells with a monoclonal antibody to CD40 or with soluble CD154 in the presence of cytokines (interleukin [IL]-2, IL-4, or IL-10) causes the B cells (which are intrinsically normal in HIGM1) to undergo proliferation and isotype switching and to secrete various types of immunoglobulins. CD154 is a type II integral membrane glycoprotein with significant sequence homology to tumor necrosis factor (TNF); it is found only on activated T cells, primarily of the CD4 phenotype (Figure 46.2) (47). Mutations in the gene encoding CD154 on HIGM1 patients' T cells result in a lack of signaling of their normal B cells when their T cells are activated. Therefore, HIGM1 B cells fail to undergo isotype switching and produce only IgM, and there is an absence of $CD27^+$ memory B cells (48). Lymph node histology shows only abortive germinal center formation and a severe depletion and phenotypic abnormalities of follicular dendritic cells. Of further importance to effective immune responses, the lack of stimulation of CD40 also results in these patients' B cells not upregulating CD80 and CD86. The latter are important costimulatory molecules that interact with CD28/CTLA4 on T cells (49). The failure of interaction of the molecules of those pathways results in a propensity for tolerogenic T cell signaling and defective recognition of tumor cells.

Many distinct point mutations or deletions in the gene encoding CD154 have been identified, giving rise to frame shifts, premature stop codons, and single amino acid substitutions, most of which were clustered in the TNF homology domain located in the carboxy-terminal region (39).

In a retrospective study of 56 European patients with HIGM1, 13 (23.3%) had died, and the mean age at death was 11.7 years (42). In addition to opportunistic infections such as *Pneumocystis jiroveci* pneumonia, there is an increased incidence of cryptosporidial enteritis and

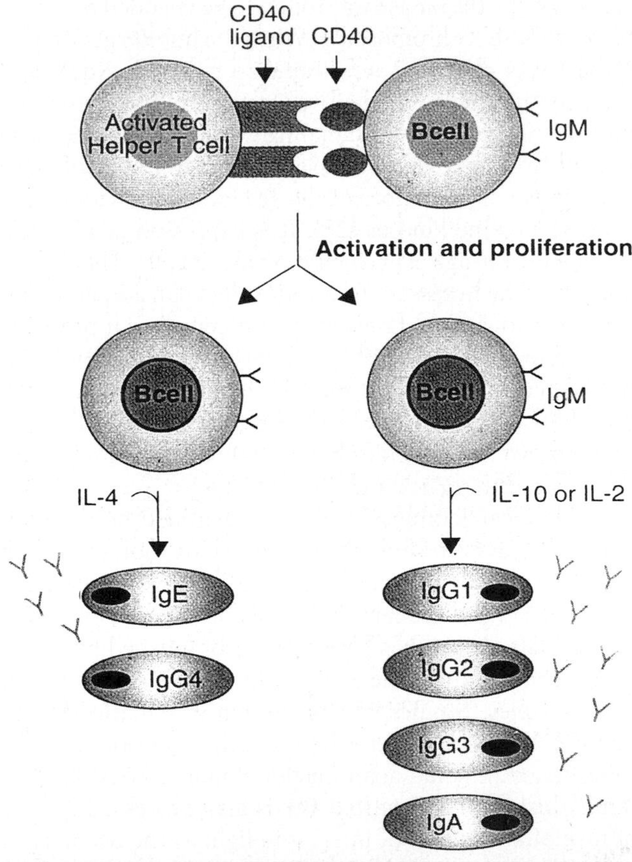

FIGURE 46.2 The role of the CD40 ligand (CD154) in B cell class switching. The *CD154* gene is mutated in X-linked hyper immunoglobulin M (IgM) syndrome. Thus, this is a T cell, not a B cell, defect. IL, interleukin. (From Allen RC, Armitage RJ, Conley ME, et al. CD40 ligand gene defects responsible for X-linked hyper IgM syndrome. *Science*. 1993;259:990, with permission.)

subsequent liver disease in this syndrome. There is also an increased risk of malignancy. Because of the poor prognosis, the treatment of choice is an HLA-identical sibling bone marrow transplant at an early age (50). Treatment for this condition also includes monthly IVIG infusions (51). In patients with severe neutropenia, the use of granulocyte colony-stimulating factor has been beneficial.

X-Linked Hyper IgM Due to Nuclear Factor κB Essential Modulator (NEMO or Iκκγ) Deficiency

This condition is characterized most often clinically as anhidrotic ectodermal dysplasia with associated immunodeficiency (EDA-ID) in males and incontinentia pigmenti in females (19,20). It results from mutations in the *IKBKG* gene at position 28q on the X chromosome (Figure 46.1), which encodes nuclear factor of κB (NFκB) essential modulator (NEMO). NEMO is a regulatory protein that serves as a scaffold for two kinases necessary for activation of the transcription factor NFκB. Activation of NFκB by proinflammatory stimuli normally leads to increased expression of genes involved in inflammation, such as TNFα and IL-12. B cells from patients with NEMO deficiency fail to undergo class switch recombination, and their antigen-presenting cells fail to produce TNFα and IL-12 (20). Germline loss-of-function mutations cause the X-linked dominant condition incontinentia pigmenti and are lethal in male fetuses. Mutations in the coding region of *IKBKG* are associated with EDA-ID.

The immunodeficiency has been variable, with most EDA-ID patients showing impaired antibody responses to polysaccharide antigens (19). However, two patients with EDA-ID presented with hyper IgM (20). Pharmacologic inhibitors of NFκB activation have been shown to downregulate CD154 mRNA and protein levels, suggesting the mechanism of hyper IgM in this condition (52). Stop codon mutations in *IKBKG* are associated with osteopetrosis, lymphedema, EDA, and immunodeficiency (OL-EDA-ID). Neither type of mutation abolishes NFκB signaling entirely. OL-EDA-ID patients' immune cells respond poorly to lipopolysaccharide, IL-1, IL-18, TFNα, and CD154, accounting for the seriousness of their infections. Although most hyper IgM patients with this defect should be easily recognizable because of the presence of ectodermal dysplasia, some have presented with immunodeficiency but no ectodermal dysplasia (53).

Autosomal Recessive Hyper IgM

Autosomal Recessive Hyper IgM Due to Activation-induced Cytidine Deaminase Deficiency (HIGM2)

It has been known for some time that not all males with hyper IgM have a mutation in the gene encoding CD154, and there are many examples in females (54), indicating that this condition has more than one genetic cause. As in HIGM1, concentrations of serum IgG, IgA, and IgE are very low in this autosomal recessive form of hyper IgM. However, in contrast to X-linked CD40L deficiency, where the IgM level is normal or only slightly elevated, the serum IgM concentration in patients with autosomal recessive hyper IgM is often markedly elevated and polyclonal (55). Patients with autosomal recessive hyper IgM are generally older at age of onset of infections, do not have susceptibility to *Pneumocystis jiroveci* pneumonia, often do have isohemagglutinins, and are less likely to have anemia, neutropenia, or thrombocytopenia (Table 46.3) (55). Normal numbers of B lymphocytes are usually present in the circulation of these patients. However, in further contrast to HIGM1 patients, B cells from patients with autosomal hyper IgM are not able to switch from IgM-secreting to IgG-, IgA-, or IgE-secreting cells, even when cocultured with monoclonal antibodies to CD40 and a variety of cytokines (39). Thus, in these patients, the condition truly is a B cell defect.

The defect in many patients with autosomal recessive hyper IgM has been identified as mutations in a gene on chromosome 12p13 that encodes an activation-dependent cytidine deaminase (AICDA), an RNA- and DNA-editing enzyme specifically expressed in germinal center B cells (55,56). A deficiency of AICDA results in impaired terminal differentiation of B cells and a failure of isotype switching, and there is a lack of immunoglobulin gene somatic hypermutation (Figure 46.3). Unlike HIGM1 patients, who have minimal lymphoid tissue, patients with this defect have lymphoid hyperplasia because they have enhanced although defective germinal center formation. Nearly all such patients have markedly elevated polyclonal serum IgM levels, and, when their B cells are cultured *in vitro*, they spontaneously secrete large amounts of IgM. This IgM secretion is not further augmented by the addition of IL-4 or anti-CD40 with IL-4 or other cytokines. Their B cells are positive for CD27 (56).

With early diagnosis and treatment with IVIG (51), as well as good management of infections with antibiotics, patients with AICDA mutations generally have a more benign course than do those with HIGM1 (Table 46.3).

Autosomal Recessive Hyper IgM Due to Uracil-DNA Glycosylase Deficiency (HIGM5)

AICDA deaminates cytosine into uracil in targeted DNA, followed by uracil removal by uracil-DNA glycosylase (UNG). Three patients with hyper IgM were found to have mutations in the gene encoding UNG (57). Their B cells had profoundly impaired class switch recombination and a partial defect in somatic hypermutation. They had clinical characteristics similar to those of patients with AICDA deficiency, that is, susceptibility to bacterial infections, lymphoid hyperplasia, and elevated serum concentrations of

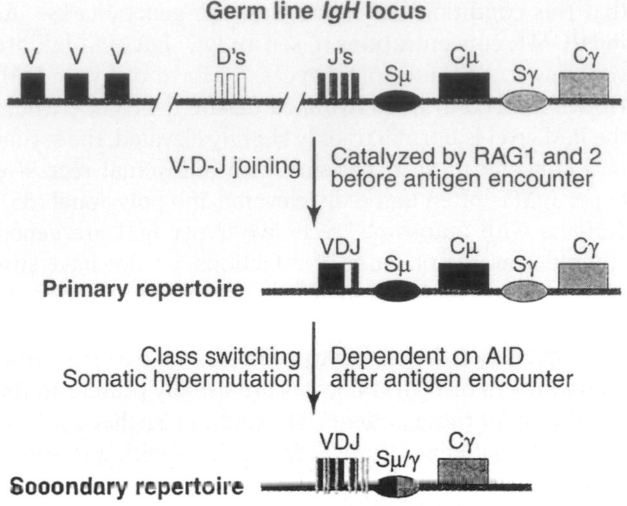

FIGURE 46.3 Schematic representation of the generation of antibody repertoires. Rearrangement of antigen receptor genes from their germline configuration occurs through the actions of the products of recombinase activating genes (RAGs) 1 and 2 without antigen encounter to generate a primary antibody repertoire composed of immunoglobulin M (IgM) antibodies. However, class switch recombination and somatic hypermutation requires the action of activation-induced cytidine deaminase (AID) following antigen encounter. The *AID* gene is mutated in one autosomal recessive form of hyper IgM. Thus, this is truly a B cell defect because the B cells are unable to generate a secondary repertoire. (From Neuberger MS, Scott J. RNA editing AIDS antibody diversification? *Science*. 2000;289:1705, with permission.)

IgM with profoundly decreased serum IgG and IgA concentrations (Table 46.3).

Autosomal Recessive Hyper IgM Due to Mutations in CD40 (HIGM3)

CD40 is a type I integral membrane glycoprotein encoded by a gene on chromosome 20 and belonging to the TNF and nerve growth factor receptor superfamily. It is expressed on B cells, macrophages, dendritic cells, and a few other types of cells (Figure 46.2). Three patients with autosomal recessive hyper IgM were identified who failed to express CD40 on their B cell surfaces (58). Their clinical presentations were similar to those with XHIM due to CD40L deficiency (Table 46.3). Sequence analysis of their CD40 genomic DNA showed that one patient carried a homozygous silent mutation at the fifth base pair position of exon 5, involving an exonic splicing enhancer and leading to exon skipping and premature termination; the other two patients showed a homozygous point mutation in exon 3, resulting in a cysteine-to-arginine substitution. These findings show that mutations of the CD40 gene can also cause an autosomal recessive form of hyper IgM that is clinically indistinguishable from HIGM1 due to CD40L deficiency (58).

X-Linked Lymphoproliferative Disease

X-linked lymphoproliferative disease (XLP), also referred to as Duncan's disease (after the original kindred in which it was described), is a recessive trait characterized by an inadequate immune response to infection with Epstein-Barr virus (EBV), resulting in (usually) fatal malignant or nonmalignant immune cell proliferation or in immunodeficiency syndromes (59,60). Affected boys are apparently healthy until they experience infectious mononucleosis (59). There are three major clinical phenotypes: (a) fulminant, often fatal, infectious mononucleosis (FIM) (50% of cases), (b) lymphomas, predominantly involving B lineage cells (25%), and (c) acquired hypogammaglobulinemia (25%) (59). The mononucleosis is fatal primarily because of extensive liver necrosis caused by polyclonally activated CD8$^+$ cytotoxic T cells that recognize EBV-infected autologous B cells. The mean age at presentation is less than 5 years. Most patients surviving the primary infection develop lymphomas or hypogammaglobulinemia. Natural killer (NK) function is also markedly depressed (61).

The defective gene in XLP was localized to the Xq26-q27 region and cloned; it is now known officially as *SH2D1A* (Figure 46.1, Table 46.1) (16,17,62). The gene encodes a novel T cell–specific adaptor protein composed of a single SH2 domain. It functions as an inhibitory adaptor protein for a high-affinity self-ligand called signaling lymphocyte activation molecule (SLAM) present on the surfaces of T and B cells. The adaptor protein, called SAP (for SLAM-associated protein) or SH2D1A, normally serves to inhibit signal transduction by SLAM so that T cell proliferation does not continue unchecked in response to EBV and possibly other types of infections. Boys who have mutations in SH2D1A fail to inhibit this signaling. The SH2D1A protein also associates with 2B4 on NK cells (61). Ligation of 2B4 on NK cells from a SAP- deficient XLP patient failed to initiate cytotoxicity. Despite this, CD2- or CD16-induced cytotoxicity of SAP-deficient NK cells was similar to that of normal NK cells. Thus, selective impairment of 2B4-mediated NK cell activation may contribute to the immunopathology of XLP (61).

Two pedigrees have been reported in which boys in one arm of each pedigree had been diagnosed with common variable immunodeficiency (CVID), whereas those in the other arms had FIM (Figure 46.4) (63). The family members with CVID never gave a history of infectious mononucleosis. However, all of affected members of each pedigree had the same distinct *SH2D1A* mutation, despite the different clinical phenotypes. Because the *SH2D1A* mutation was the same but the phenotype varied in these families, XLP should be considered in all males with a diagnosis of CVID, particularly if there is more than one male family member with this phenotype. A patient with an *SH2D1A* mutation was recently reported who developed systemic

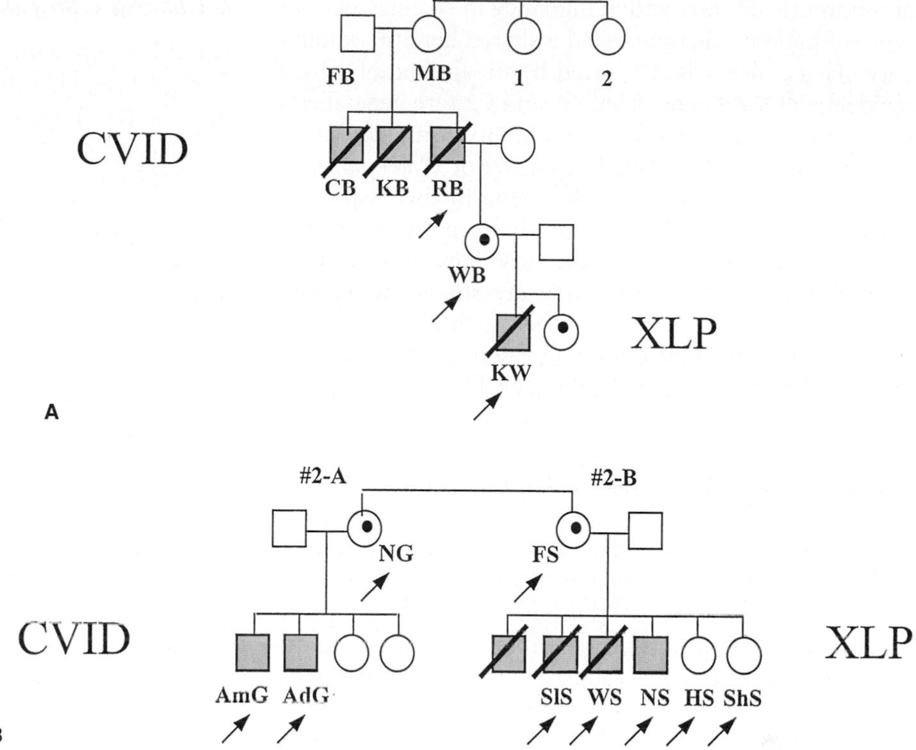

FIGURE 46.4 **A, B:** Two pedigrees in which boys in one arm of each had the clinical phenotype of common variable immunodeficiency (CVID) and in the other fulminating infectious mononucleosis, leading to a diagnosis of X-linked lymphoproliferative disease (XLP). The pedigree-unique mutations in *SH2DIA* were the same in those with CVID as in those with XLP. Thus, boys with CVID should be screened for this mutation. (From Morra M, Silander O, Calpe-Flores S, et al. Alterations of the X-linked lymphoproliferative disease gene *SH2DIA* in common variable immunodeficiency syndrome. *Blood*. 2001;98(5):1321–1325, with permission.)

vasculitis, hypogammaglobulinemia, and hemophagocytic lymphohistiocytosis (64).

XLP overall has an unfavorable prognosis: 70% of affected boys die by age 10 years. Only two XLP patients are known to have survived beyond 40 years. Approximately half of the limited number of patients with XLP given HLA-identical related or unrelated unfractionated bone marrow transplants are surviving without sign of the disease (50).

Common Variable Immunodeficiency

CVID is a syndrome characterized by hypogammaglobulinemia with B cells. Most patients have no known molecular diagnosis, but it is highly likely that this syndrome consists of many different genetic defects. Also known as "acquired" hypogammaglobulinemia because of a generally later age of onset of infections, the patients may appear similar clinically to those with XLA in the kinds of infections experienced and bacterial etiologic agents involved (3,65). In comparing the two defects, it is noted that in CVID there is an almost equal sex distribution, a tendency to autoantibody formation, normal-sized or enlarged tonsils and lymph nodes, and splenomegaly in approximately 25% of those affected. Lymphoid interstitial pneumonia, pseudolymphoma, amyloidosis, and noncaseating granulomata of the lungs, spleen, skin, and liver have also been seen. There is a 438-fold increase in lymphomas in affected women in the fifth and sixth decades (66).

The serum immunoglobulin and antibody deficiencies in CVID may be as profound as in XLA. Despite normal numbers of circulating immunoglobulin-bearing B lymphocytes and the presence of lymphoid cortical follicles, blood B lymphocytes from CVID patients do not differentiate into immunoglobulin-producing cells when stimulated with PWM *in vitro*, even when cocultured with normal T cells. From these observations, it was believed that the defect(s) in this syndrome are intrinsic to the B cell. However, B cells from some CVID patients can be stimulated to both isotype-switch and synthesize and secrete immunoglobulin when stimulated with anti-CD40 plus IL-4 or IL-10 (67). T cells and T cell subsets are usually present in normal percentages, but a dominance of T cells has been observed in some patients, and depressed T cell function has been reported in others. Tonsils and lymph nodes are either normal sized or enlarged, and splenomegaly occurs in approximately 25% of patients with CVID. In addition, there is a tendency to autoantibody formation, and there are now several cases of lupus erythematosus converting to CVID (68). Rarely, CVID has been reported to resolve transiently or permanently when some such patients acquired HIV infection (69).

Because this disorder occurs in first-degree relatives of patients with selective IgA deficiency (A Def) and some patients with A Def become panhypogammaglobulinemic, it has long been suspected that these diseases have a common genetic basis (70). The high incidences of abnormal immunoglobulin concentrations, autoantibodies, autoimmune disease, and malignancy in families of both types of patients also suggested a shared hereditary influence. This concept is supported by the finding of a high incidence of C4-A gene deletions and C2 rare gene alleles in the class III major histocompatibility complex (MHC) region in individuals with either A Def or CVID, suggesting that there is a susceptibility gene in this region on chromosome 6 (71). However, the abnormal gene has not yet been identified. These studies also have shown that a small number of HLA haplotypes are shared by individuals affected with CVID and A Def, with at least one of two particular haplotypes being present in 77% of those affected (71). In one large family with 13 members, 2 had A Def and 3 had CVID (70). All of the immunodeficient patients in the family had at least one copy of an MHC haplotype shown to be abnormally frequent in A Def and CVID: HLA-DQB1*0201, HLA-DR3, C4B-Sf, C4A-deleted, G11-15, Bf-0.4, C2a, HSP70-7.5,TNF-5, HLA-B8 and HLA-A1. However, four immunologically normal members of the pedigree also possessed this haplotype, indicating that its presence alone is not sufficient for expression of the defects (70). Environmental factors, particularly drugs such as phenytoin, have been suspected as providing the triggers for disease expression in individuals with the permissive genetic background.

The foregoing notwithstanding, it is clear that CVID is still best thought of as a syndrome that includes many different genetic defects. Most cases of CVID are sporadic or follow an autosomal dominant pattern of inheritance for which the underlying genetic defect(s) have not been discovered. As noted, however, two pedigrees have been reported in which boys in one arm of each pedigree had CVID, whereas those in the other had FIM (Figure 46.4) (63). Thus, the *SH2D1A*, *Btk*, and *CD154* genes should be studied in male CVID patients because patients with these mutations may present clinically with CVID. In addition, both males and females should be evaluated for mutations in the *AID*, *UNG*, and *CD40* genes for the same reason. Four other known causes of this syndrome are discussed below.

Inducible Costimulator Deficiency in Autosomal Recessive CVID

In the Black Forest of Germany, patients with CVID have been found who have an autosomal recessive pattern of inheritance and who lack the "inducible costimulator" (ICOS), a surface protein on activated T cells (72). Binding of ICOS to its ligand induces a significant increase in T cell proliferation and cytokine production, especially of IL-10, which has been implicated in the differentiation of B cells to plasma cells. Nine such patients from six families have been found to have identical homozygous large genomic deletions of the *ICOS* gene, suggesting a founder effect. Thus far, no examples of ICOS deficiency have been found in the United States.

B Cell Signaling Defects in CVID

Other patients with a clinical presentation of CVID have recently been identified with mutations involving intermediates in B cell signaling and developmental pathways (65). Specifically, mutations in CD19, B cell–activating factor of the TNF family receptor (BAFF-R), and transmembrane activator, calcium-modulator, and cyclophilin ligand interactor (TACI) genes have been identified in such patients (73–75). BAFF and APRIL serve as ligands for BAFF-R, TACI, and B cell maturation antigen (BCMA). It is postulated that the patients with mutations in BAFF-R or TACI most likely lack the necessary B cell signaling provided through interaction with BAFF and APRIL to promote proper maturation and generation of a diverse antibody repertoire. These findings further emphasize the known heterogeneity of CVID. As the molecular bases of more and more primary immunodeficiency syndromes are being identified, it will be important to consider a variety of genetic mutations that can lead to the hypogammaglobulinemia seen in CVID.

The treatment of patients with CVID is essentially the same as that for XLA (51). Anaphylactic reactions caused by IgE antibodies to IgA are always a possibility in patients with CVID; thus, caution should be used when therapy is initiated with IVIG preparations containing IgA (76). Nonanaphylactic adverse reactions to IVIG infusions in patients with CVID (usually those with chronic lung or sinus disease) have been associated with elevated plasma TNFα levels. The prognosis for patients with CVID is reasonably good unless severe autoimmune disease or malignancy develops.

Selective IgA Deficiency

An isolated absence or near-absence (i.e., less than 10 mg/dL) of serum and secretory IgA is believed to be the most common well-defined immunodeficiency disorder, with a frequency of 1:333 being reported among some blood donors (6). Although this disorder has been observed in apparently healthy individuals (6), it is commonly associated with ill health. As would be expected when there is a deficiency of the major immunoglobulin of external secretions, infections occur predominantly in the respiratory, gastrointestinal, and urogenital tracts (65). Bacterial agents responsible are essentially the same as in other types of antibody deficiency syndromes. There is no clear evidence that patients with this disorder have an undue susceptibility to viral agents. Similar to CVID, there is a frequent association of A Def with collagen-vascular and autoimmune diseases. In further similarity to patients with CVID, there is an increased incidence of malignancy.

Serum concentrations of other immunoglobulins are usually normal in patients with A Def, although IgG2 subclass deficiency has been reported, and IgM (usually elevated) may be monomeric. Children with A Def vaccinated with killed poliovirus intranasally produced local IgM and

IgG antibodies. Of possible etiologic and great clinical significance is the presence of antibodies to IgA in the sera of as high as 44% of patients with A Def (6). A number of A Def patients have had severe or fatal anaphylactic reactions after intravenous administration of blood products containing IgA, and anti-IgA antibodies [particularly IgE anti-IgA antibodies (76)] have been implicated. For this reason, only five-times washed (in 200-mL volumes) normal donor erythrocytes or blood products from other IgA-absent individuals should be administered to these patients. Patients with A Def also frequently have IgG antibodies against cow milk and ruminant serum proteins (77). These antiruminant antibodies often falsely detect "IgA" in immunoassays that employ goat (but not rabbit) antisera (7). A high incidence of autoantibodies has also been noted.

The basic defect leading to A Def is unknown. *In vitro* cultures of B cells from some IgA-deficient patients could be stimulated to produce IgA by the combination of anti-CD40 and IL-10. Treatment with Dilantin, sulfasalazine (78), *d*-penicillamine, or gold has been suspected as being the cause of A Def; the condition has also been known to remit following discontinuation of Dilantin therapy or spontaneously. Usually when this happens the remission is permanent. The occurrence of A Def in both males and females and in families is consistent with autosomal inheritance; in most families this appears to be dominant with variable expressivity (70). As noted, this defect occurs in pedigrees with CVID patients, some patients with IgA deficiency have gone on to develop CVID, and recent studies suggest that the susceptibility genes for these two defects may reside in the MHC class III region as an allelic condition on chromosome 6 (Table 46.1) (70,71).

Immunodeficiency with Thymoma

Patients with immunodeficiency with thymoma are adults who almost simultaneously develop recurrent infections, panhypogammaglobulinemia, deficits in cell-mediated immunity, and benign thymoma (3). They may also have eosinophilia or eosinopenia, aregenerative or hemolytic anemia, agranulocytosis, thrombocytopenia, or pancytopenia. Antibody formation is poor, and progressive lymphopenia develops, although percentages of Ig-bearing B lymphocytes are usually normal. The thymomas are predominantly of the spindle cell variety, but other types of benign and malignant thymic tumors have been seen.

IgG Subclass Deficiencies

A number of patients have been reported to have deficiencies of one or more subclasses of IgG, despite normal or elevated total IgG serum concentrations (79). IgG_2 deficiency would be suspected if patients had repeated problems with encapsulated bacterial pathogens, because a majority of the antipolysaccharide antibody molecules are of the IgG_2 isotype. Most of those with absent or very low concentrations of IgG_2 have been patients with A Def. However, not all A Def patients who have recurrent infections have IgG_2 deficiency, and some A Def patients have defective antipolysaccharide antibody responses despite normal levels of IgG_2. Similarly, patients with the Wiskott-Aldrich syndrome, who have a profound antipolysaccharide antibody deficiency, have normal levels of IgG_2. Marked deficiencies of antipolysaccharide antibodies have also been noted in other non–Wiskott-Aldrich children and adults with recurrent infections who had normal concentrations of IgG_2, as well as normal concentrations of all of the other immunoglobulin isotypes (80). Conversely, a number of healthy children have been described who had low levels of IgG_2 but normal responses to polysaccharide antigens when immunized. In other patients with IgG_2 deficiency, continued follow-up revealed an evolving pattern of immunodeficiency (such as into CVID), suggesting that the presence of IgG subclass deficiency may be a marker for more general immune dysfunction (81). Thus, the more relevant question to ask is "What is the capacity of the patient to make specific antibodies to protein and polysaccharide antigens?" It is, therefore, difficult to know the biological significance of the multiple moderate deficiencies of IgG subclasses that have been reported, particularly when completely asymptomatic individuals have been described who totally lacked IgG_1, IgG_2, IgG_4, and IgG_1 due to gene deletion (Table 46.1) (38).

CELLULAR IMMUNODEFICIENCY

In general, patients with partial or absolute defects in T cell function have infections or other clinical problems for which there is no effective treatment or which are of a more severe nature than those with antibody deficiency disorders. It is also rare that such individuals survive beyond infancy or childhood.

Thymic Hypoplasia (DiGeorge's Syndrome)

Thymic hypoplasia results from dysmorphogenesis of the third and fourth pharyngeal pouches during early embryogenesis, leading to hypoplasia or aplasia of the thymus and parathyroid glands (82). Other structures forming at the same age are also frequently affected, resulting in anomalies of the great vessels (right-sided aortic arch), esophageal atresia, bifid uvula, upper limb malformations, congenital heart disease (conotruncal, atrial and ventricular septal defects), a short philtrum of the upper lip, hypertelorism, an antimongoloid slant to the eyes, mandibular hypoplasia, and low-set, often notched ears (82). A variable degree of hypoplasia of the thymus and parathyroid glands (partial DiGeorge's syndrome) is more frequent than total aplasia (83). Those with complete DiGeorge's syndrome are susceptible to infections with opportunistic pathogens and to graft-versus-host disease (GVHD) from nonirradiated blood transfusions. There are many clinical similarities among DiGeorge's syndrome, the velocardiofacial syndrome, the fetal alcohol syndrome, and retinoic acid toxicity.

Patients with DiGeorge's syndrome are usually only mildly lymphopenic (83). However, the percentage of $CD3^+$ T cells is variably decreased. Immunoglobulin concentrations are usually normal, although sometimes IgE is elevated and IgA may be low (83). Responses of blood lymphocytes after mitogen stimulation have been absent, reduced, or normal, depending on the degree of thymic deficiency (83). Thymic tissue, when found, does contain Hassall's corpuscles and a normal density of thymocytes; corticomedullary distinction is present. Lymphoid follicles are usually present, but lymph node paracortical areas and thymus dependent regions of the spleen show variable degrees of depletion.

DiGeorge's syndrome has occurred in both males and females. It is rarely familial, but three cases of apparent autosomal dominant inheritance have been reported. Microdeletions of specific DNA sequences from chromosome 22q11.2 (the DiGeorge chromosomal region) have been shown in a majority of patients, and several candidate genes have been identified in this region (82). There appears to be an excess of 22q11.2 deletions of maternal origin (84). Another deletion associated with DiGeorge's and velocardiofacial syndromes has been identified on chromosome 10p13 (85).

No immunologic treatment is needed for the partial form. If patients with the partial DiGeorge syndrome do not have a severe cardiac lesion, they have few clinical problems, except that some experience seizures and developmental delay. Transplantation of cultured, mature thymic epithelial explants has successfully reconstituted the immune function of several infants with the complete DiGeorge syndrome (86).

COMBINED IMMUNODEFICIENCY DISORDERS

Severe Combined Immunodeficiency

Severe combined immunodeficiency (SCID) is a fatal syndrome of diverse genetic cause characterized by profound deficiencies of T and B cell (and sometimes NK cell) function (87–90). Affected infants present in the first few months of life with frequent episodes of diarrhea, pneumonia, otitis, sepsis, and cutaneous infections. Persistent infections with opportunistic organisms such as *Candida albicans, Pneumocystis jiroveci*, varicella-zoster virus, parainfluenza 3 virus, respiratory syncytial virus, adenovirus, cytomegalovirus, Epstein-Barr virus, and bacillus Calmette-Guérin lead to death. These infants also lack the ability to reject foreign tissue and are, therefore, at risk for GVHD from maternal T cells that cross into the fetal circulation while the SCID infant is *in utero* or from T lymphocytes in nonirradiated blood products or allogeneic bone marrow (50).

Infants with SCID are lymphopenic (87,88,91). They have an absence of lymphocyte proliferative responses to mitogens, antigens, and allogeneic cells *in vitro*, even on samples collected *in utero* or from the cord blood (92). Therefore, physicians caring for newborns need to be aware of what the normal range for the cord blood absolute lymphocyte count is (2,000 to 11,000/mm^3) and arrange for T cell phenotypic and functional studies to be performed on blood from neonates with values below this range (87,91–93). Even though all forms of SCID could be diagnosed at birth by detecting lymphopenia or an absence of T cells, there is currently no newborn screening for this syndrome anywhere in the world. The normal absolute lymphocyte count is much higher at 6 to 7 months of age, when most SCIDs are diagnosed, so that any count below 4,000/mm^3 at that age is lymphopenic (94). Serum immunoglobulin concentrations are diminished to absent, and no antibody formation occurs after immunization. Typically, all SCID patients have very small thymuses (usually less than 1 g), which fail to descend from the neck, contain no thymocytes, and lack corticomedullary distinction and Hassall's corpuscles. However, the thymic epithelium is normal, and results of bone marrow stem cell transplantation have shown that these tiny thymuses are capable of supporting normal T cell development (95). Thymus-dependent areas of the spleen are depleted of lymphocytes in SCID patients, and lymph nodes, tonsils, adenoids, and Peyer's patches are absent or extremely underdeveloped.

In the more than 50 years since the initial description of SCID (1), it has become evident that the genetic origins of this condition are quite diverse (Table 46.4) (88,96). X-linked SCID (SCID-X1) is the most common form, accounting for approximately 46% of U.S. cases

TABLE 46.4 Twelve Abnormal Genes in Severe Combined Immunodeficiency

Cytokine receptor genes
IL2RG
JAK3
IL7Rα
Antigen receptor genes
RAG1
RAG2
Artemis
Ligase 4
CD3δ
CD3ε
CD3ζ
Other genes
ADA
CD45

TABLE 46.5 Severe Combined Immunodeficiency Lymphocyte Phenotypes

$T^-B^+NK^-$	γ chain deficient Jak3 deficient
$T^-B^+NK^+$	IL-7Rα deficient CD3δ deficient CD3ε deficient CD3ζ deficient CD45 deficient
$T^-B^-NK^-$	ADA deficient
$T^-B^-NK^+$	RAG1/RAG2 deficient *Artemis* deficient *Ligase 4* deficient

ADA, adenosine deaminase; IL-7Rα, interleukin-7 receptor α chain; Jak3, Janus kinase-3; RAG, recombination activating gene.

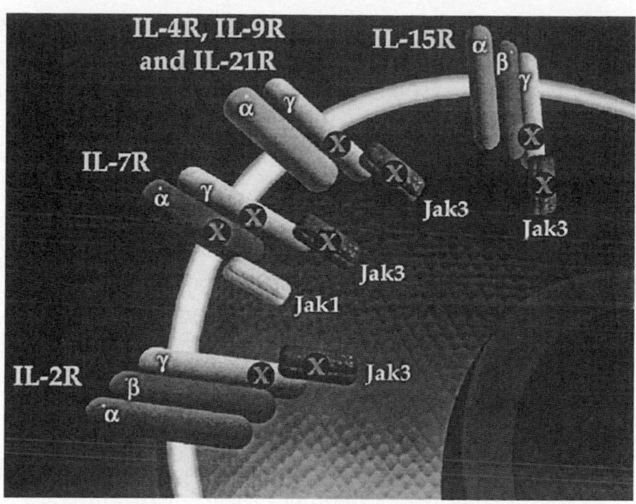

FIGURE 46.5 Diagram showing that Janus kinase 3 (Jak3) is the major signal transducer for the common γ chain shared by multiple cytokine receptors. Mutations in the *IL2RG* gene cause X-linked severe combined immunodeficiency (X-SCID), whereas mutations in the *JAK3* gene result in a form of autosomal recessive SCID that mimics X-SCID in lymphocyte phenotype (i.e., $T^-B^+NK^-$). Mutations in the alpha chain of the IL-7 receptor also cause SCID, but unlike X-linked and Jak3-deficient SCID, IL-7Rα chain–deficient SCID infants have both B and NK cells (i.e., are $T^-B^+NK^+$). (From Buckley RH. Primary cellular immunodeficiencies. *J Allergy Clin Immunol.* 2002;109(5):747, with permission.)

(Figure 46.7) (88,96). Mutated genes on autosomal chromosomes have been identified in 11 genetic types of SCID: adenosine deaminase (ADA) deficiency, Janus kinase 3 (Jak3) deficiency, IL-7 receptor α-chain deficiency (IL-7Rα), recombination-activating gene (*RAG-1* or *RAG-2*) deficiencies, *Artemis* deficiency, CD3 α-, ε-, and ζ-chain deficiencies, and CD45 deficiency; and there are likely other causes yet to be discovered (Table 46.1) (88,96).

X-Linked Recessive Severe Combined Immunodeficiency Disease (SCID-X1)

Despite the uniformly profound lack of T or B cell function, patients with SCID-X1 usually have few or no T or NK cells but a normal or elevated number of B cells (Table 46.5) (87,91,93). However, SCID-X1 B cells do not produce immunoglobulin normally, even after T cell reconstitution by bone marrow transplantation (91). The abnormal gene in SCID-X1 was mapped to the Xq13 region and identified as the gene encoding a common gamma chain (γc) shared by several cytokine receptors, including those for IL-2, IL-4, IL-7, IL-9, IL-15, and IL-21 (Figures 46.1, 46.5) (14,15,97). Of the first 136 patients studied, 95 distinct mutations spanning all eight *IL2RG* exons were identified, most of them consisting of small changes at the level of one to a few nucleotides (Figure 46.6) (98). These mutations resulted in abnormal γc's in two thirds of the cases and absent γc protein in the remainder. The finding that the mutated gene results in faulty signaling through several cytokine receptors explains how multiple cell types can be affected by a mutation in a single gene (97,99,100).

Autosomal Recessive Severe Combined Immunodeficiency Disease Caused by Adenosine Deaminase Deficiency

An absence of the enzyme adenosine deaminase (ADA) has been observed in approximately 16% of patients with SCID (Figure 46.7) (87,88,91). The gene encoding ADA is on chromosome 20q13-ter and was cloned and sequenced more than a decade ago (101). There are certain distinguishing features of ADA deficiency, including the presence of multiple skeletal abnormalities of chondroosseous dysplasia on radiographic examination; these occur predominantly at the costochondral junctions, at the apophyses of the iliac bones, and in the vertebral bodies (causing a "bone-in-bone" effect) (101). ADA deficiency results in pronounced accumulations of adenosine, 2′-deoxyadenosine, and 2′-*O*-methyladenosine (101). The latter metabolites directly or indirectly lead to apoptosis of thymocytes and circulating lymphocytes, which causes the immunodeficiency. As a consequence, ADA-deficient infants usually have a much more profound lymphopenia than those with other types of SCID, with mean absolute lymphocyte counts of less than 500/mm^3 and deficiencies of all types of lymphocytes (Table 46.5) (88,91). As with other types of SCID, ADA deficiency can be cured by HLA-identical or haploidentical T cell–depleted bone marrow transplantation, which is the treatment of choice (50,88,91). Enzyme replacement therapy with polyethylene glycol–modified bovine ADA (PEG-ADA) administered subcutaneously once weekly has resulted in both clinical and immunologic improvement in more than 100 ADA-deficient patients (102). However, the immunocompetence achieved is not nearly so great as with bone marrow

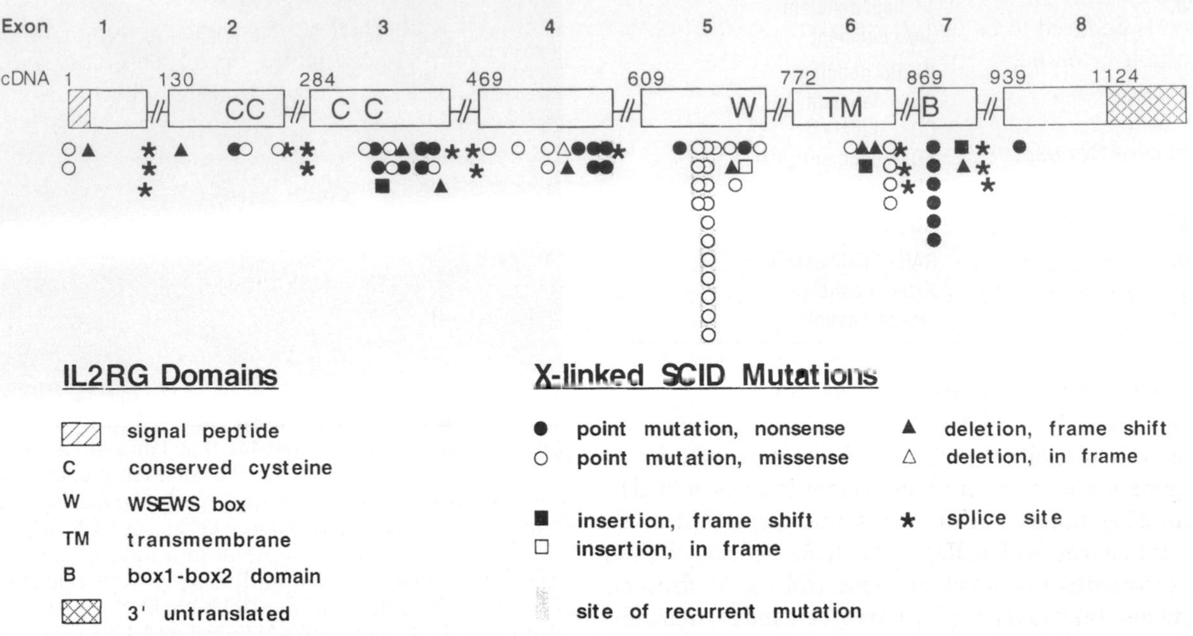

FIGURE 46.6 *IL2RG* cDNA map showing exons, cDNA numbers corresponding to the first coding nucleotide of each exon, protein domains, and sites of mutations found in 87 unrelated families with X-linked severe combined immunodeficiency (X-SCID). Identical mutations found in unrelated patients are surrounded by shaded boxes. (From Puck JM, Pepper AE, Henthorn PS, et al. Mutation analysis of IL2RG in human X-linked severe combined immunodeficiency. *Blood.* 1997;89:1968, with permission.)

transplantation (103). In view of this, PEG-ADA therapy should not be initiated if bone marrow transplantation is contemplated because it will confer graft-rejection capability on the infant. After T cell function is effected by bone marrow transplantation (without pretransplantation chemotherapy), infants with ADA deficiency generally have B cell function.

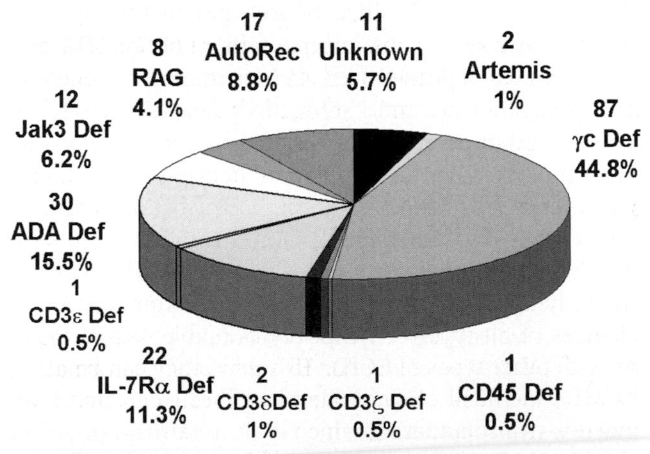

FIGURE 46.7 Relative frequencies of the different genetic types of severe combined immunodeficiency among 194 patients seen consecutively by the author over three and a half decades. ADA, adenosine deaminase; Def, defect; γc, γ chain; IL-7Rα, IL-7 receptor α chain; RAG, recombinase activating gene.

Autosomal Recessive Severe Combined Immunodeficiency Disease Caused by Janus Kinase 3 Deficiency

SCID patients with autosomal recessive SCID caused by Janus kinase 3 (Jak3) deficiency resemble all other types in their susceptibility to infection and to graft-versus-host disease from allogeneic T cells. However, they have lymphocyte characteristics most closely resembling those of patients with X-linked SCID, including an elevated percentage of B cells and very low percentages of T and NK cells (Table 46.5) (88,104). Because Jak3 is the only signaling molecule known to be associated with γc, it's gene was a candidate for mutations leading to autosomal recessive SCID of unknown molecular type (Table 46.4, Figure 46.6) (105). Thus far, more than 30 patients who lack Jak3 have been identified (Figure 46.6) (88,104,106). Like SCID-X1 patients, they have very low or no NK cells (88). Even after successful immune reconstitution by bone marrow transplantation, they fail to develop NK cells (50). Moreover, as with SCID-X1 patients, they often fail to develop normal B cell function after transplantation despite their high numbers of B cells. Their failure to develop NK cells or B cell function is believed to be due to the defective function of the multiple cytokine receptors that share γc.

Autosomal Recessive Severe Combined Immunodeficiency Caused by Interleukin 7 Receptor α-Chain Deficiency

Because mice whose genes for either the α chain of the IL-7 receptor or of IL-7 itself have been mutated are profoundly deficient in T and B cell function but have normal natural killer cell function, naturally occurring mutations in these genes were sought in some of the author's patients who had $T^-B^+NK^+$ SCID and who had previously been shown not to have either γc or Jak3 deficiency. Mutations in the gene for IL-7Rα on chromosome 5p13 have been found in 22 of the author's patients, making it the third-most-common cause of SCID (Figure 46.7) (88,107). These findings imply that the T cell but not the NK cell defect in SCID-X1 and Jak3-deficient SCID results from an inability to signal through the IL-7 receptor (Figure 46.6). The fact that these patients developed normal B cell function after nonablative haploidentical bone marrow stem cell transplantation despite lacking donor B cells also suggests that the B cell defect in SCID-X1 is not due to failure of IL-7 signaling.

Autosomal Recessive Severe Combined Immunodeficiency Caused by Recombination-Activating Gene (RAG-1 or RAG-2) Deficiencies

Infants with autosomal recessive SCID caused by mutations in recombination activating genes *RAG-1* and *RAG-2* resemble all others in their infection susceptibility and complete absence of T or B cell function. However, their lymphocyte phenotype differs from those of patients with SCID caused by γc, Jak3, IL-7Rα, or ADA deficiencies in that they lack both B and T lymphocytes and have primarily NK cells in their circulation ($T^-B^-NK^+$ SCID, Table 46.5) (88). This particular phenotype suggested a possible problem with their antigen receptor genes, leading to the discovery of mutations in *RAG-1* and *RAG-2* in some (but not all) such SCID infants (108–110). These genes, on chromosome 11p13, encode proteins necessary for somatic rearrangement of antigen receptor genes on T and B cells. The proteins recognize recombination signal sequences (RSSs) and introduce a DNA double-stranded break, permitting V, D, and J gene rearrangements. *RAG-1* or *RAG-2* mutation results in a functional inability to form antigen receptors through genetic recombination.

Patients with Omenn's syndrome also have mutations in *RAG1* or *RAG2* genes, resulting in partial and impaired V(D)J recombinational activity (109,110). Omenn's syndrome is characterized by the development soon after birth of a generalized erythroderma and desquamation, diarrhea, hepatosplenomegaly, hypereosinophilia, and markedly elevated serum IgE levels. The latter are caused by circulating activated, oligoclonal T lymphocytes that do not respond normally to mitogens or antigens *in vitro* (111). Circulating B cells are not found, and lymph node architecture is abnormal due to a lack of germinal centers. The condition is fatal unless corrected by bone marrow transplantation (50).

Autosomal Recessive Severe Combined Immunodeficiency Caused by Deficiencies of the Artemis *Gene*

SCID may also be caused by a deficiency of a novel V(D)J recombination/DNA repair factor that belongs to the metallo-β-lactamase superfamily. It is encoded by a gene on chromosome 10p called *Artemis* (110,112). A deficiency of this factor results in an inability to repair DNA after double-stranded cuts have been made by *RAG1* or *RAG2* gene products in rearranging antigen receptor genes from their germline configuration. Similar to *RAG1*- and *RAG2*-deficient SCID, this defect results in another form of $T^-B^-NK^+$ SCID, also called Athabascan SCID (Table 46.5). In addition, there is increased radiation sensitivity of both skin fibroblasts and bone marrow cells of those affected with this type of SCID (110,112).

Autosomal Recessive Severe Combined Immunodeficiency Caused by Deficiencies of the Ligase 4 *Gene Product*

Another recently described cause of radiation-sensitive $T^-B^-NK^+$ SCID (Tables 46.4, 46.5) is mutation in the *Ligase 4* gene (113). The gene product is necessary for catalyzing the ligation step in the nonhomologous end-joining (NHEJ) pathway of DNA double-strand break (DSB) repair. Sequencing analysis of the *LIG4* gene in a female Turkish infant with $T^-B^-NK^+$ SCID (Table 46.5) who was not microcephalic and who had normal development revealed the presence of a homozygous deletion of three nucleotides CAA at nucleotide positions 5333 to 5335 (National Center for Biotechnology Information [NCBI] AF479264). Deletion of these three nucleotides resulted in deletion of glutamine Q433 in the protein (NCBI NP_996820). *LIG4* transcripts were present, but the absence of detectable LIG4 protein suggested that this mutation affects protein stability. The mutations in *LIG4* that had been previously reported were hypomorphic and resulted in radiosensitivity and leukemia in two patients or in pancytopenia, micro-cephaly, and developmental and growth delay—collec-tively called the LIG4 syndrome—in eight other patients (114,115).

Autosomal Recessive Severe Combined Immunodeficiency Caused by CD45 Deficiency

Another molecular defect causing SCID is a mutation in the gene encoding the common leukocyte surface protein CD45 (116,117). This hematopoietic cell–specific transmembrane protein tyrosine phosphatase functions to regulate Src kinases required for T and B cell antigen receptor signal transduction. A 2-month-old male infant presented with a clinical picture of SCID and was found to have a very low number of T cells but a normal number of B cells. The T cells failed to respond to mitogens, and serum immunoglobulins diminished with time. He was found to have a large deletion at one *CD45* allele and a point mutation causing an alteration of the intervening sequence 13 donor splice site at the other (116). A second case of SCID due to CD45 deficiency has been reported (117), and the author and her associates have recently evaluated yet a third case (unpublished observations) confirming that the lymphocyte phenotype is $T^-B^+NK^+$ SCID (Table 46.5). Figure 46.7 shows the frequency of the various genetic forms of SCID that I have evaluated over the last three and a half decades.

Autosomal Recessive Severe Combined Immunodeficiency Caused by Mutations in Genes Encoding Chains of the CD3 Complex

Dadi et al. (118) discovered in 2003 that mutations in the gene encoding the δ chain of the CD3 complex caused SCID. Later, de Saint Basile et al. (119) studied three families with fetuses/infants who had SCID of unknown molecular type. All of the fetuses/infants had the $T^-B^+NK^+$ lymphocyte phenotype (Table 46.5), that is, they had no T cells but did have phenotypically normal B cells and natural killer (NK) cells, the same phenotype as in the SCID infants reported by Dadi et al. (118). Mutations in the gene encoding the CD3δ chain were found in only two of the families. In the third family, the investigators found a homozygous mutation in the CD3ε gene that created a premature stop codon near the start of the extracellular domain, resulting in the absence of CD3 expression in those individuals affected. The author has evaluated a similar patient. More recently, mutations in the CD3 ζ-chain gene were found by the author and her associates to also result in $T^-B^+NK^+$ SCID (Table 46.5) (120). In the latter case, the infant had $CD16^+$ NK cells but no $CD56^+$ NK cells.

Hypomorphic mutations in the CD3ε gene had been previously reported in a 4-year-old boy who had had recurrent *Haemophilus influenzae* pneumonia early in life but was later healthy (121). His T cells had low expression of the CD3 complex but did respond to antigens. Defective expression of the T cell receptor CD3 complex was also reported in two male siblings in a Spanish family who were found to have mutations in the CD3γ gene (122). One of the siblings died at age 31 months with autoimmune hemolytic anemia and viral pneumonia, but the other was healthy. Both had very low expression of CD3 on their T cells, but they were capable of making antigen-specific responses and had IgG_2 subclass deficiency.

Treatment and Prognosis

SCID is a pediatric emergency (87,88,91,92). Replacement therapy with IVIG fails to halt the progressively downhill course (51). Unless bone marrow transplantation from HLA-identical or haploidentical donors can be performed, death usually occurs before the patient's first birthday and almost invariably before the second. On the other hand, transplantation in the first 3.5 months of life offers a greater than 96% chance of survival (88,91,92). Therefore, early diagnosis is essential. Recent studies have shown that the immune reconstitution effected by stem cell transplants is due to thymic education of the transplanted allogeneic stem cells (95). The thymic output appears to occur sooner and to a greater degree in those infants transplanted in the neonatal period than in those transplanted after that time (92). There are more than 500 SCID patients surviving worldwide as a result of successful bone marrow transplantation (50).

ADA deficiency was the first genetic defect in which gene therapy was attempted; these early efforts were unsuccessful (23). However, within the last decade, normal γc cDNA was successfully transduced into autologous marrow cells of nine infants with SCID-X1 in France by retroviral gene transfer, with subsequent full correction of their T and NK cell defects (123). Thus the efficacy of gene therapy in conferring immune function in those infants with SCID-X1 seemed to be superior to that of allogeneic hematopoietic stem-cell transplantation. Tragically, however, serious adverse events occurred in four of them, who developed leukemia-like processes, with expanded clonal populations of T cells (124). The leukemias are considered to have been induced by the retroviral gene therapy by a process called insertional mutagenesis. More recently, this complication also occurred in a SCID-X1 patient treated in England, but it has not occurred in eight ADA-deficient patients successfully treated with gene therapy in Italy (125). In view of the early successes with gene therapy in SCID-X1 and ADA deficiency (23), the hope is that in the future those and other primary immunodeficiencies for which the molecular defects have been identified will be correctable by gene therapy.

Reticular Dysgenesis

This condition was first described in 1959 in identical twin male infants who exhibited a total lack of both lymphocytes and granulocytes in their peripheral blood and bone marrow. Seven of the eight infants thus far reported with this defect died between 3 and 119 days of age from overwhelming infections; the eighth underwent complete immunologic reconstitution from a bone marrow transplant. Recombinant granulocyte colony-stimulating factor was not successful in the treatment of an infant with this condition. The thymuses have all weighed less than 1 g, no Hassall's corpuscles have been present, and few or no thymocytes have been seen. The molecular basis of this autosomal recessive disorder is unknown (3).

Combined Immunodeficiency

The term combined immunodeficiency (CID) is used to distinguish patients with low but not absent T cell function from those with SCID. Several examples will be given.

Purine Nucleoside Phosphorylase Deficiency

More than 40 patients with CID have been found to have purine nucleoside phosphorylase (PNP) deficiency (101,126). Deaths have occurred from generalized vaccinia, varicella, lymphosarcoma, and graft-versus-host disease mediated by T cells from nonirradiated allogeneic blood or bone marrow. Two thirds of patients have had neurologic abnormalities ranging from spasticity to mental retardation. One third of patients developed autoimmune diseases, the most common of which is autoimmune hemolytic anemia. Most patients have normal or elevated concentrations of all serum immunoglobulins. PNP-deficient patients are as profoundly lymphopenic as those with ADA deficiency, with absolute lymphocyte counts usually less than 500/mm^3. T cell function is low but not absent and is variable with time. The gene encoding PNP is on chromosome 14q13.1, and it has been cloned and sequenced. A variety of mutations have been found in the PNP gene in patients with PNP deficiency (101). Unlike ADA deficiency, serum and urinary uric acid are deficient because PNP is needed to form the urate precursors hypoxanthine and xanthine. Prenatal diagnosis is possible. PNP deficiency is invariably fatal in childhood unless immunologic reconstitution can be achieved. Bone marrow transplantation is the treatment of choice but has been successful in only six such patients (50,127,128).

Ataxia-Telangiectasia

Ataxia-telangiectasia (AT) is a complex combined immunodeficiency syndrome with associated neurologic, endocrinologic, hepatic, and cutaneous abnormalities (129,130). The most prominent features are progressive cerebellar ataxia, oculocutaneous telangiectasias, chronic sinopulmonary disease, a high incidence of malignancy, and variable humoral and cellular immunodeficiency (131). The ataxia typically becomes evident soon after the child begins to walk and progresses until he or she is confined to a wheelchair, usually by 10 to 12 years of age. The telangiectasias develop at between 3 and 6 years of age. Recurrent, usually bacterial, sinopulmonary infections occur in roughly 80% of these patients. Fatal varicella occurred in one patient, and transfusion- associated graft-versus-host disease has also been reported. Selective IgA deficiency is found in from 50% to 80% of those affected (131). IgE concentrations are usually low, and IgG2 or total IgG may be decreased. Specific antibody titers may be decreased or normal. The percentages of CD3$^+$ and CD4$^+$ T cells are only modestly low, and *in vitro* tests of lymphocyte function have generally shown moderately depressed proliferative responses to T and B cell mitogens. The thymus is hypoplastic, exhibits poor organization, and is lacking in Hassall's corpuscles. Cells from patients, as well as those of heterozygous carriers, have increased sensitivity to ionizing radiation, defective DNA repair, and frequent chromosomal abnormalities (131). The malignancies reported in this condition usually have been of the lymphoreticular type, but adenocarcinoma and other forms also have been seen; there is also an increased incidence of malignancy in unaffected relatives.

Inheritance of AT follows an autosomal recessive pattern. The mutated gene (*ATM*) responsible for this defect was mapped by restriction fragment length polymorphism analysis to the long arm of chromosome 11 (11q22–23) and was cloned (130,132). The gene product is a DNA-dependent protein kinase localized predominantly to the nucleus and believed to be involved in mitogenic signal transduction, meiotic recombination, and cell cycle control (130). Of the mutations identified, a majority were expected to completely inactivate the ATM protein by truncating it, by abolishing correct initiation or termination of translation, or by deleting large segments (130). No satisfactory definitive treatment has been found (131). The prognosis is exceedingly poor for patients with this condition, although a number have reached adulthood. The most common causes of death are lymphoreticular malignancy and progressive neurologic disease.

Immunodeficiency with Thrombocytopenia and Eczema (Wiskott-Aldrich Syndrome)

The Wiskott-Aldrich syndrome (WAS) is an X-linked recessive syndrome characterized by eczema, thrombocytopenic purpura with normal-appearing megakaryocytes but small defective platelets, and undue susceptibility to infection (13,89,133). Patients usually present during infancy with prolonged bleeding from the circumcision site, bloody diarrhea, or excessive bruising. Atopic dermatitis and recurrent infections usually also develop during the first year of life. Infections are usually those produced by pneumococci and other encapsulated bacteria, resulting in otitis media, pneumonia, meningitis, or sepsis. Later, infections with opportunistic agents such as *Pneumocystis jiroveci* and the herpesviruses become more problematic. Autoimmune cytopenias and vasculitis are common in those who live beyond infancy. Survival beyond the teens is rare; infections and bleeding may cause death, and there is also a 12% incidence of fatal malignancy in this condition (13,133).

Patients with WAS have an impaired humoral immune response to polysaccharide antigens, as evidenced by absent or greatly diminished isohemagglutinins and poor or absent antibody responses to polysaccharide antigens (13). In addition, antibody titers to protein antigens fall with time. Most often there is a low serum IgM, elevated IgA and IgE, and a normal or slightly low IgG concentration. Flow cytometry of blood lymphocytes has shown a moderately reduced percentage of T cells, and lymphocyte responses to mitogens are moderately depressed (13).

The mutated gene responsible for this defect was mapped to Xp11.22–11.23 and isolated in 1994 by Derry et al. (12). It was found to be limited in expression to lymphocytic and megakaryocytic lineages (12). The gene product, a 501–amino acid, proline-rich protein that lacks a hydrophobic transmembrane domain, was designated WAS protein (WASP). It has been shown to bind CDC42H2 and rac, members of the Rho family of GTPases, which are important in actin polymerization (13,134). A large and varied number of mutations in the *WASP* gene have been identified in WAS patients, with some correlation of the site of the mutation with severity of infection susceptibility or other problems in one series (135) but not in others. Mutations in the *WASP* gene have been shown to affect not only platelet (136) and T cell function but also dendritic cell and B cell adhesion, homing, and function (137,138) and NK cell cytotoxicity (139). Isolated X-linked thrombocytopenia is also caused by mutations in the *WASP* gene, as are some cases of severe congenital neutropenia (140). Carriers can be detected by the finding of nonrandom X chromosome inactivation in several hematopoietic cell lineages or by detection of the mutated gene (if known in the family). Prenatal diagnosis of WAS can also be made by chorionic villous sampling or amniocentesis if the mutation is known in that family. Two families with apparent autosomal inheritance of a clinical phenotype similar to WAS have been reported (141,142), and in one case a girl was shown to have this as an X-linked defect (143).

Numerous patients with WAS have had complete corrections of both the platelet and the immunologic abnormalities by HLA-identical sibling bone marrow transplants after being conditioned with irradiation or busulfan and cyclophosphamide (50). Success has been minimal with T cell–depleted haploidentical stem cell transplants in WAS, primarily because of the requirement for pretransplant immunosuppression to permit engraftment, the long time course to immunoreconstitution when T cells are depleted, resistance to engraftment, and a high mortality from preexisting opportunistic infections in that setting (50). However, success has been achieved in the treatment of WAS with matched unrelated donor transplants when done in children younger than 5 years of age (144). It is likely that matched related or unrelated cord blood transplants will be similarly successful because in both cases T cells can be left in the donor cell suspension. Several patients who required splenectomy for uncontrollable bleeding had impressive rises in their platelet counts and did well clinically while being administered prophylactic antibiotics and IVIG (145). Based on success in *in vitro* transfection studies (146), the first gene therapy trials for this condition are underway (147). The most common cause of death in WAS patients is EBV-induced lymphoreticular malignancy (133).

Cartilage-hair Hypoplasia

In 1965, an unusual form of short-limbed dwarfism with frequent and severe infections was reported among the Pennsylvania Amish; non-Amish cases have since been described (148). These patients have short and pudgy hands with redundant skin, metaphyseal chondrodysplasia, hyperextensible joints of hands and feet but an inability to extend the elbows completely, and fine, sparse light hair and eyebrows. These features led to the name cartilage-hair hypoplasia (CHH). Radiographically the bones show scalloping and sclerotic or cystic changes in the metaphyses. In contrast to ADA deficiency, in which the predominant changes are in the apophyses of the iliac bones, the ribs, and vertebral bodies, the chondrodysplasia in CHH principally affects the limbs. Severe and often fatal varicella infections, progressive vaccinia, and vaccine-associated poliomyelitis have been observed. Associated conditions include deficient erythrogenesis, Hirschsprung's disease, and an increased risk of malignancies.

Three patterns of immune dysfunction have emerged: defective antibody-mediated immunity, defective cellular immunity (most common form), and severe combined immunodeficiency. NK cells, however, are increased in number and function.

CHH is an autosomal recessive condition, and the defective gene was mapped to chromosome 9p21-p13 in Amish and Finnish families. Numerous mutations have been found in the untranslated *RMRP* gene that cosegregates with the CHH phenotype (149).The gene product, endoribonuclease RNase MRP (mitochondrial RNA processing), consists of an RNase molecule bound to several proteins. It has at least two functions: cleavage of RNA in mitochondrial DNA synthesis and nucleolar cleaving of pre-RNA. Mutations in *RMRP* cause CHH by disrupting a function of RNase MRP RNA that affects multiple organ systems (149). Bone marrow transplantation has resulted in immunologic reconstitution in some cartilage-hair hypoplasia patients with the SCID phenotype (91). Those with milder types of immune deficiency have lived to adulthood, some even to old age.

Nijmegen Breakage Syndrome

This is a rare autosomal recessive condition in which the immunologic, cytogenetic, and radiation-sensitivity findings are almost identical to those in ataxia-telangiectasia (150,151). However, the patients are quite distinct from those with ataxia-telangiectasia clinically in that they have short stature, a "birdlike" facies, and microcephaly from birth. They lack the classic clinical features of ataxia-telangiectasia, including ataxia and telangiectasia, and they have normal serum α-fetoprotein levels. Intelligence can vary from normal to moderate mental retardation. The immunodeficiency appears to be more severe than in ataxia-telangiectasia. Most patients have recurrent respiratory infections. The tendency to express rearrangements of chromosomes 7 and 14 and to develop a malignancy is much higher than in ataxia-telangiectasia. More than 40 patients from approximately 30 families have been reported, and most are of eastern European origin (150,151). Complementation studies have indicated that patients with this syndrome are genetically distinct from those with ataxia-telangiectasia. The abnormal gene in this condition has been mapped to chromosome 8q21 (Table 46.1) (152).

Defective Expression of Major Histocompatibility Complex Antigens

There are two main forms: (a) class I MHC antigen deficiency (bare lymphocyte syndrome) and (b) class II MHC antigen deficiency.

MHC Class I Antigen Deficiency

An isolated deficiency of MHC class I antigens is rare, and the resulting immunodeficiency is milder than that in SCID, contributing to a later age of presentation (153). Sera from affected individuals contain normal quantities of class I MHC antigens and β_2-microglobulin, but class I MHC antigens are not detected on any cells in the body. There is a deficiency of $CD8^+$ but not of $CD4^+$ T cells. Mutations have been found in two genes within the MHC locus on chromosome 6 that encode the peptide transporter proteins TAP1 and TAP2 (Table 46.1) (153–155). TAP proteins function to transport peptide antigens from the cytoplasm across the Golgi apparatus membrane to join the α chain of MHC class 1 molecules and β_2-microglobulin. The complex can then move to the cell surface; if the assembly of the complex cannot be completed because there is no peptide antigen, the MHC class I complex is destroyed in the cytoplasm.

MHC Class II Antigen Deficiency

Many individuals affected with this autosomal recessive syndrome are of North African descent.. More than 70 patients have been identified. They present in infancy with persistent diarrhea, often associated with cryptosporidiosis; bacterial pneumonia; pneumocystis; septicemia; and viral or monilial infections. Nevertheless, their immunodeficiency is not as severe as in SCID, as evidenced by their failure to develop BCGosis or GVHD from nonirradiated blood transfusions (156). MHC class II–deficient patients have a very low number of $CD4^+$ T cells but normal or elevated numbers of $CD8^+$ T cells. Lymphopenia is only moderate. The MHC class II antigens HLA-DP, -DQ, and -DR are undetectable on blood B cells and monocytes. The patients have impaired antigen-specific responses caused by the absence of these antigen-presenting molecules. In addition, MHC antigen–deficient B cells fail to stimulate allogeneic cells in mixed leukocyte culture. Lymphocytes respond normally to mitogens but not to antigens. The thymus and other lymphoid organs are severely hypoplastic. The lack of class II molecules results in abnormal thymic selection because recognition of HLA molecules by thymocytes is central to both positive and negative selection. The latter results in circulating $CD4^+$ T cells that have altered CDR3 profiles. The associated defects of both B and T cell immunity and of HLA expression emphasize the important biological role for HLA determinants in effective immune cell cooperation.

Four different molecular defects resulting in impaired expression of MHC class II antigens have been identified (Table 46.1) (156). In one, there is a mutation in the gene on chromosome 1q that encodes a protein called RFX5, a subunit of RFX, a multiprotein complex that binds the X box motif of MHC II promoters (157). A second form is caused by mutations in a gene on chromosome 13q that encodes a second, 36-kDa subunit of the RFX complex called RFX-associated protein (RFXAP) (158). The most recently discovered and most common cause of MHC class II defects are mutations in RFXANK, the gene encoding a third subunit of RFX (159). In a fourth type, there is a mutation in the gene on chromosome 16p13 that encodes a novel MHC class II transactivator (CIITA), a non–DNA-binding coactivator that controls the cell-type specificity and inducibility of MHC II expression (160). All of these defects cause impairment in the coordinate expression of MHC class II molecules on the surface of B cells and macrophages (156).

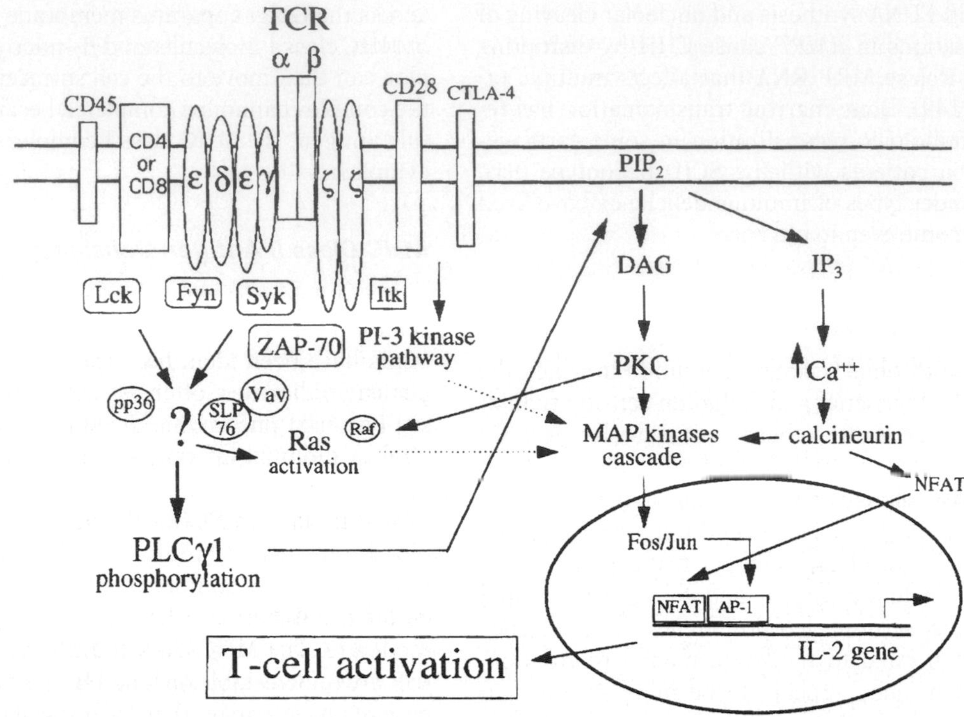

FIGURE 46.8 T cell signal transduction pathway. The T cell receptor (TCR) spans the plasma membrane in association with CD3 and ζ, CD4 or CD8, CD28, and CD45. Cytoplasmic protein tyrosine kinases (PTKs) associated with the TCR are activated on antigen binding to the TCR. These PTKs include Lck, Fyn, ζ-chain–associated protein-70 (ZAP-70), and Syk. PTK activation results in the phosphorylation of phospholipase Cγ1 (PLCγ1) and the activation of other signaling molecules. Distal signaling events, including PKC activation and Ca^{2+} mobilization, result in the transcription of genes encoding interleukin-2 (IL-2) and other proteins, culminating in T cell activation, differentiation, and proliferation. Ionomycin and phorbol myristate acetate (PMA) can be used to mimic distal signaling events. Mutations in the gene encoding ZAP-70 result in markedly impaired T cell activation, in addition to abnormal thymic selection resulting in CD8 deficiency. AP-1, activated protein; DAG, diacylglycerol; IP_3, inositol phosphate 3; MAP, mitogene-activated protein kinase; NFAT, nuclear factor of activated T cells; PIP_2, phosphatidyl inositol 2; PL-3, phospholipase 3. (Modified from Elder ME. Severe combined immunodeficiency due to a defect in the tyrosine kinase ZAP-70. *Pediatr Res*. 1996;39:743, with permission.)

CD8 Deficiency Due to a Mutation in the CD8α Gene

Another cause for CD8 deficiency (in addition to ζ-chain–associated protein-70 deficiency and MHC class I antigen deficiency) was discovered in a 25-year-old Spanish man with a history of recurrent respiratory infections since childhood. Immunoglobulins and antibodies were normal, as were T cell proliferation studies and NK cell function. However, he was found to have a complete absence of $CD8^+$ T cells. Molecular studies revealed a missense mutation in both alleles of the immunoglobulin domain of the CD8α gene in the patient and in two of his sisters (161,162).

T CELL ACTIVATION DEFECTS

These conditions are characterized by the presence of normal or elevated numbers of blood T cells that appear phenotypically normal but fail to proliferate or produce cytokines in response to stimulation with mitogens, antigens, or other signals delivered to the T cell antigen receptor (TCR) due to defective signal transduction from the TCR to intracellular metabolic pathways (Figure 46.8) (163). This condition can be caused mutations in genes for a variety of cell surface molecules or signal transduction molecules. These patients have problems similar to those of other T cell–deficient individuals, and some with severe T cell activation defects may resemble SCID patients clinically. Two examples are described.

Defective Ca^{2+} Release–Activated Ca^{2+} Channels

Two male infants born to consanguineous parents had SCID-like infection susceptibility despite phenotypically normal blood lymphocytes. However, their T cells were unable to produce IL-2, IFNγ, IL-4, and TNFα. Electrophoretic mobility shift assays were used to examine the DNA binding of AP-1, Oct, CREB, SP1, NFκB, and NF-AT, and the binding of all but NF-AT was normal (164). This problem was subsequently shown to be secondary to defective store-operated Ca^{2+} entry and calcium release–activated calcium (CRAC) channel function. The molecular defect responsible for this was recently discovered (165). It was found that the infants are homozygous for a single missense mutation in the gene that encodes a novel protein called Orai1. The protein contains four putative transmembrane segments. Expression of wild-type Orai1 in SCID T cells restored store-operated Ca^{2+} influx and the CRAC current. The authors propose that Orai1 is an essential component or regulator of the CRAC channel complex.

CD8 Lymphocytopenia Due to ζ-Chain–Associated Protein-70 Deficiency

Patients with CD8 lymphocytopenia caused by ζ-chain–associated protein-70 (ZAP-70) deficiency present during infancy with severe, recurrent, sometimes fatal infections similar to those in SCID patients; however, they often live longer and present later than SCID patients (163). More than eight cases have been reported, and a majority were Mennonites (163,166,167). They have normal, low, or elevated serum immunoglobulin concentrations and normal or elevated numbers of circulating $CD4^+$ T lymphocytes but essentially no $CD8^+$ cells. These $CD4^+$ T cells fail to respond to mitogens or to allogeneic cells *in vitro* or to generate cytotoxic T lymphocytes. By contrast, NK activity is normal. The thymus of one patient exhibited normal architecture; there were normal numbers of CD4:CD8 double-positive thymocytes but an absence of CD8 single-positive thymocytes. This condition has been attributed to mutations in the gene encoding ZAP-70, a non–src family protein tyrosine kinase important in T cell signaling (Figure 46.8) (163). The gene is on chromosome 2 at position q12. ZAP-70 has been shown to have an essential role in both positive and negative selection in the thymus (Table 46.1) (166). The hypothesis as to why there are normal numbers of $CD4^+$ T cells is that thymocytes can use the other member of the same tyrosine kinase family, Syk, to facilitate positive selection of $CD4^+$ cells. In addition, there is a stronger association of Lck with $CD4^+$ than with $CD8^+$ cells. Syk is present at fourfold-higher levels in thymocytes than in peripheral T cells, possibly accounting for the lack of normal responses by the $CD4^+$ blood T cells.

AUTOIMMUNE AND LYMPHOPROLIFERATIVE SYNDROMES

Immune Dysregulation, Polyendocrinopathy, Enteropathy, X-Linked Syndrome (IPEX)

IPEX syndrome is a fatal, X-linked recessive immunologic disorder characterized by multisystem autoimmunity, most commonly in the form of early-onset type 1 diabetes mellitus, severe enteropathy with watery, often bloody diarrhea associated with eosinophilic inflammation and an eczematous dermatitis, and moderate to severe recurrent infections caused by *Enterococcus and Staphylococcus* species. The condition is due to mutations in the forkhead box P3 (*FOXP3*) gene on Xp11.23 (Figure 46.1), which encodes a forkhead domain–containing protein, FOXP3 (168). *FOXP3* is predominantly expressed in the $CD4^+CD25^{high}$ subset of regulatory T cells (Tregs), and studies in mutant mice indicate that FOXP3 is essential for the development of Tregs. The number and phenotype of $CD4^+CD25^{high}$ T cells appears to be normal in IPEX patients, but there is either no FOXP3 protein in these cells or mutant protein with abnormal regulatory function (169). The findings demonstrate a key role for FOXP3 in the maintenance of self-tolerance and in the prevention of autoimmune and allergic diseases.

Autoimmune Polyendocrinopathy-Candidiasis Ectodermal Dysplasia (APCEP)

Patients with this syndrome present with chronic mucocutaneous candidiasis and polyendocrinopathy, usually affecting the parathyroid or adrenal glands and less frequently the thyroid, liver, and skin. Autoimmune polyendocrinopathy-candidiasis ectodermal dysplasia, or autoimmune polyendocrinopathy syndrome type I (APS1), is due to a mutation in the autoimmune regulator (*AIRE*) gene (170,171). The gene product, AIRE, is expressed at high levels in purified human thymic medullary stromal cells and is believed to regulate the cell surface expression of tissue-specific proteins such as insulin and thyroglobulin. Expression of these self-proteins allows for the negative selection of autoreactive T cells during their development. Failure of negative selection results in organ-specific autoimmune destruction. The overall significance of AIRE in the establishment and maintenance of T cell self-tolerance is not well understood.

Autoimmune Lymphoproliferative Syndrome (ALPS)

Autoimmune lymphoproliferative syndrome (ALPS) is a disorder of apoptosis in which the inability of lymphocytes to die leads to nonmalignant massive lymphadenopathy, hypersplenism, and autoimmune cytopenias of childhood onset (172). Consistent immunologic findings include polyclonal hypergammaglobulinemia and an expansion of T cells lacking either CD4 or CD8 on their surfaces (double-negative T cells). The most frequent genetic cause of ALPS is germline dominant, heterozygous mutations in the tumor necrosis factor receptor superfamily member 6 (*TNFRSF6*) gene (ALPS type Ia), which encodes CD95 (also known as Fas), a mediator of apoptosis. Somatic mutations in the gene have also been found. Other causes are mutations in genes encoding either the CD95 ligand (ALPS type Ib), caspase 10 (ALPS type IIa), or caspase 8 (ALPS type IIb). Major determinants of morbidity and mortality in ALPS are the severity of the autoimmune disease, hypersplenism, and the risk of Hodgkin's or non-Hodgkin's lymphoma (173). Penetrance and range of disease manifestations in ALPS are highly variable, even among family members who share the same dominant *TNFRSF6* mutation (172). Although most episodes of cytopenias respond to courses of conventional immunomodulatory agents, some ALPS patients with massive splenomegaly may require splenectomy and/or ongoing immunosuppressive treatment. This disorder underscores the critical role played by cell surface receptor–mediated apoptosis in eliminating redundant proliferating lymphocytes with autoreactive and oncogenic potential.

Interleukin 2 Receptor α Chain (IL-2Rα, CD25) Mutation

A male infant born of a consanguineous union presented at 6 months of age with cytomegalovirus pneumonia, persistent oral and esophageal candidiasis, adenoviral gastroenteritis, and failure to thrive. He developed lymphadenopathy, hepatosplenomegaly, and chronic inflammation of his lungs and mandible. Biopsies revealed extensive lymphocytic infiltration of his lung, liver, gut, and bone. Serum IgG and IgM were elevated, but IgA was low. He had a T cell lymphocytopenia, with an even CD4:CD8 ratio. The T cells responded poorly to anti-CD3, phytohemagglutinin and other mitogens, and IL-2. He was found to have a truncated mutation of the IL-2R α chain (CD25) (Table 46.1) (174). He could not reject an allogeneic skin graft. He was given a successful allogeneic bone marrow transplant following cytoreduction.

Young mutant mice lacking the IL-2R α chain have phenotypically normal T and B cell development (175). However, as adults, they develop massive lymphoid organ enlargement and polyclonal T and B cell expansion attributed to defective apoptosis. They also develop autoimmune disorders, including hemolytic anemia and inflammatory bowel disease. Similarly, gene targeted mice lacking the IL-2R β chain develop exhaustive differentiation of B cells into plasma cells, elevated IgG1 and IgE, and autoantibodies that cause hemolytic anemia (176). Their T cells did not respond to polyclonal or antigen-specific activators. It is known that IL-2 programs murine $\alpha\beta$ T lymphocytes for apoptosis (177). From these observations, it is deduced that both IL-2R α and β chains play an important role in influencing the activation programs of T cells, the balance between clonal expansion and cell death following lymphocyte activation, and the prevention of autoimmunity.

DEFECTS IN INNATE IMMUNITY

Leukocyte Adhesion Deficiencies 1 and 2

Leukocyte Adhesion Deficiency-1 (LAD-1)

This condition is attributable to mutations in the gene on chromosome 21 at position q22.3 encoding CD18, a 95-kDa β subunit shared by three adhesive heterodimers: LFA-1 on B, T, and NK lymphocytes; complement receptor type 3 (CR3) on neutrophils, monocytes, macrophages, eosinophils, and NK cells; and p150,95 (another complement receptor) (Table 46.1) (178). The α chains of these three molecules (encoded by genes on chromosome 16) are not expressed because of the abnormal β chain. Those so affected have histories of delayed separation of the umbilical cord, omphalitis, gingivitis, recurrent skin infections, repeated otitis media, pneumonia, septicemia, ileocolitis, peritonitis, perianal abscesses, and impaired wound healing (178). Life-threatening bacterial and fungal infections account for the high mortality. Affected people do not have increased susceptibility to viral infections or malignancy. Blood neutrophil counts are usually significantly elevated even when no infection is present because of an inability of the cells to adhere to vascular endothelium and migrate out of the intravascular compartment. All cytotoxic lymphocyte functions are considerably impaired because of a lack of the adhesion protein LFA-1; deficiency of LFA-1 also interferes with immune cell interaction and immune recognition. CR3 binds fixed iC3b fragments of C3 and β-glucans; its absence causes abnormal phagocytic cell adherence and chemotaxis and a reduced respiratory burst with phagocytosis. Deficiencies of these glycoproteins can be screened for by flow cytometry with monoclonal antibodies to CD18 or to CD11a, b, or c. Because the CD18 gene has been cloned and sequenced, this disorder is another potential candidate for gene therapy (23).

Leukocyte Adhesion Deficiency-2 (LAD-2)

LAD-2 is attributable to the absence of neutrophil sialyl-Lewis^X, a ligand of E-selectin on vascular endothelium (178). This disorder was discovered in two unrelated Israeli boys 3 and 5 years of age, each the offspring of consanguineous parents. Both had severe mental retardation, short stature, a distinctive facial appearance, and the Bombay (hh) blood phenotype, and both were secretor- and Lewis-negative. They both had had recurrent severe bacterial infections similar to those seen in patients with LAD-1, including pneumonia, peridontitis, otitis media, and localized cellulitis. Similar to that in patients with LAD-1, their infections were accompanied by pronounced leukocytosis (30,000 to 150,000/mm^3) but an absence of pus formation at sites of recurrent cellulitis. *In vitro* studies revealed a pronounced defect in neutrophil motility. Because the genes for the red blood cell H antigen and for the secretor status encode for distinct $\alpha_{1,2}$-fucosyltransferases and the synthesis of Sialyl-Lewis^X requires an $\alpha_{1,3}$-fucosyltransferase, it was postulated that a general defect in fucose metabolism is the basis for this disorder. It was subsequently found that GDP-L-fucose transport into Golgi vesicles was specifically impaired (179), and then missense mutations in the GDP-fucose transporter cDNA of three patients with LAD II were discovered. Thus, GDP-fucose transporter deficiency is a cause of LAD-2 (180).

Interferon-γ Receptor-1 and 2 Mutations

Disseminated BCG infections occur in infants with SCID or with other severe T cell defects. However, in approximately half of the cases no specific host defect has been found. One possible explanation for this predilection was found in a 2.5-month-old Tunisian female infant who had fatal idiopathic disseminated BCG infection (181) and in four children from Malta who had disseminated atypical mycobacterial infection in the absence of a recognized immunodeficiency (182). In the case of all five children, there was consanguinity in their pedigrees. All affected were found to have a functional defect in the upregulation of TNFα production by their blood macrophages in response to stimulation with IFNγ. Furthermore, all lacked expression of IFNγR's on their blood monocytes or lymphocytes, and each was found to have a mutation in the gene on chromosome 6q22-q23 that encodes IFNγR1. Of interest, these children did not appear to be susceptible to infection with agents other than mycobacteria. Th1 responses appeared to be normal in these patients. The susceptibility of these children to mycobacterial infections thus apparently results from an intrinsic impairment of the IFNγ pathway response to these particular intracellular pathogens, showing that IFNγ is obligatory for efficient macrophage antimycobacterial activity. Since the initial discoveries of IFNγR1-deficient humans, many more examples have been found, and IFNγR2-deficient individuals have been found as well (183,184).

IL-12 and IL-12 Receptor β1 Mutations

IL-12 is produced by activated antigen-presenting cells (dendritic cells, macrophages) (183). It promotes the development of Th1 responses and is a powerful inducer of IFNγ production by T and NK cells (184). A child with BCG and *Salmonella enteritidis* infection was found to have a large homozygous deletion within the IL-12 p40 subunit gene, precluding expression of functional IL-12 p70 cytokine by activated dendritic cells and phagocytes. As a result, IFNγ production by the child's lymphocytes was markedly impaired (185). This suggested that IL-12 is essential for protective immunity to intracellular bacteria such as mycobacteria and *Salmonella*. In further support of this, T and NK cells from seven unrelated patients who had severe idiopathic mycobacterial and *Salmonella* infections failed to produce IFNγ when stimulated with IL-12 (186,187). The patients were otherwise healthy. They were found to have mutations in the IL-12 receptor β1 chain, resulting in premature stop codons in the extracellular domain, resulting in unresponsiveness to this cytokine, again demonstrating IL-12's crucial role in host defense (186,187).

Germline STAT 1 Mutation

Interferons induce the formation of two transcriptional activators: gamma-activating factor (GAF) and interferon-stimulated gamma factor 3 (ISGF3). A natural heterozygous germline STAT1 mutation associated with susceptibility to mycobacterial but not viral disease was found in two unrelated patients with unexplained mycobacterial disease (188). This mutation caused a loss of GAF and ISGF3 activation but was dominant for one cellular phenotype and recessive for the other. It impaired the nuclear accumulation of GAF but not of ISGF3 in cells stimulated by interferons, implying that the antimycobacterial but not the antiviral effects of human interferons are mediated by GAF. More recently, two patients have been identified with homozygous *STAT-1* mutations who developed both post–BCG vaccination disseminated disease and lethal viral infections. The mutations in these patients caused a complete lack of STAT 1 and resulted in a lack of formation of both GAF and ISGF3 (189).

Il-1R–Associated Kinase 4 Deficiency

Members of interleukin-1 receptor and the Toll-like receptor superfamily share an intracytoplasmic Toll-IL-1 receptor (TIR) domain, which mediates recruitment of the interleukin-1 receptor–associated kinase (IRAK) complex via TIR-containing adapter molecules (190). Three unrelated, otherwise healthy children with recurrent pyogenic infections due to pneumococci and staphylococci had normal immunocompetence by standard immune studies. They had normal titers of antipneumococcal antibodies. However, their blood and fibroblast cells did not activate nuclear factor κB and mitogen-activated protein kinase and failed to induce downstream cytokines in response to any of the known ligands of TIR-bearing receptors. Each was found to have an inherited deficiency of IRAK-4. Thus, the TIR-IRAK signaling pathway appears to be crucial for protective immunity against specific bacteria but is redundant against most other microorganisms (190).

Chediak-Higashi Syndrome

This rare disease is characterized by oculocutaneous albinism and susceptibility to recurrent respiratory tract and other types of infections (191). The hallmark of the disease is giant lyosomal granules, not only in neutrophils, but also in most of the other cells of the body, including melanocytes, neural Schwann cells, renal tubular cells, gastric mucosa, pneumatocytes, hepatocytes, Langerhans cells of the skin, and adrenal cells (191). The granules in neutrophils are positive for peroxidase, acid phosphatase, and esterase. The abnormal lysosomes are unable to fuse with phagosomes, so that ingested bacteria cannot be lysed normally. In addition, there is nearly complete absence of cytotoxic T lymphocyte and NK cell activity as a result of abnormal lysosomal granule function (191). Abnormal chemotaxis has also been reported, and there is evidence of a profound alteration of the cytoskeleton of the neutrophils. There are reports of a decreased number of centriole-associated microtubules and abnormalities in tubulin tyrosinolation.

The fundamental defect in this autosomal recessive disorder was recently found to be caused by mutations in a gene on human chromosome 1 at position q42-43 (Table 46.1) (192,193). This gene is similar to the one mutated in the murine beige defect (192). The gene product is postulated to function with other proteins as components of a vesicle membrane–associated signal transduction complex that regulates intracellular protein trafficking (192).

Approximately 85% of the patients develop an "accelerated phase" of the disease, with fever, jaundice, hepatosplenomegaly, lymphadenopathy, pancytopenia, bleeding diathesis, and neurologic changes (194). Once the accelerated phase occurs, the disease is usually fatal within 30 months unless successful treatment with an unfractionated HLA-identical bone marrow transplant following cytoreductive conditioning can be accomplished (50,195).

HYPERIMMUNOGLOBULINEMIA E SYNDROME

The hyperimmunoglobulinemia E (hyper IgE) syndrome is a relatively rare primary immunodeficiency syndrome characterized by recurrent severe staphylococcal abscesses of the skin, lungs, and viscera and greatly elevated levels of serum IgE (196,197). I first reported the disorder in two young boys in 1972 (196). Since then I have evaluated more than 40 patients with the condition, and many other examples have been reported (197). These patients all have histories of staphylococcal abscesses involving the skin, lungs, joints, and other sites from infancy; persistent pneumatoceles develop as a result of their recurrent pneumonias. The pruritic dermatitis that occurs is not typical atopic eczema, and it does not always persist; respiratory allergic symptoms are usually absent. I noted coarse facial features in the first two patients (196), and this has been a consistent feature of all of the patients I have evaluated with this syndrome. Hyper IgE syndrome patients look very different from their nonaffected family members. Distinctive facial characteristics were again pointed out recently by Grimbacher et al. (198). Among the findings reported were a prominent forehead, deep-set eyes, a broad nasal bridge, a wide, fleshy nasal tip, mild prognathism, facial asymmetry, and hemihypertrophy. They also found that the mean nasal interalar distance in these patients was above the 98th percentile ($p < 0.001$). These findings were present in all patients in that study by age 16 years (198). High incidences of scoliosis and hyperextensible joints were also noted. An interesting observation in that group of patients that had not been previously reported was a 72% incidence of failure or delayed shedding of the primary teeth, owing to lack of root resorption (198). Unexplained osteopenia is also present in most patients with the hyper IgE syndrome, many of whom have problems with recurrent fractures from even minor trauma (198,199).

Laboratory features include exceptionally high serum IgE; elevated serum IgD; usually normal concentrations of IgG, IgA, and IgM; pronounced blood and sputum eosinophilia; abnormally low anamnestic antibody responses to booster immunizations; and poor antibody-mediated and cell-mediated responses to neoantigens. *In vitro* studies have shown normal percentages of all lymphocytes. Most patients have normal lymphocyte-proliferative responses to mitogens but very low or absent responses to antigens or allogeneic cells from family members. Blood, sputum, and histologic sections of lymph nodes, spleen, and lung cysts show striking eosinophilia. Hassall's corpuscles and normal thymic architecture were observed at postmortem examination of one patient. Phagocytic cell ingestion, metabolism, killing, and total hemolytic complement activity have been normal in all patients. Variable defects of mononuclear or polymorphonuclear chemotaxis have been present in some but not all patients and hence are not the basic problem in these patients (197).

The fundamental problem in this condition was recently discovered and found to be due to mutations in the STAT 3 gene. I have observed a decreased percentage of T cells of the memory (CD45RO) phenotype in the blood of these patients, and such a decrease possibly is related to these patients' impaired anamnestic antibody responses, impaired antigen-specific T cell responses, and abnormal mixed leukocyte responses (201,202). Paradoxically, B cells from these patients do not produce as much IgE as normal or atopic B cells do when they are cultured with IL-4 and anti-CD40 *in vitro* (200). The latter indicates that the B cells may have already been exposed to IL-4 *in vivo* and were no longer sensitive to it because they had already isotype-switched *in vivo*. Because of the very short half-life of IL-4, serum levels cannot be detected; therefore it has been difficult to prove that the condition is caused by excessive IL-4 production. The presence of increased numbers of eosinophils in blood, sputum, and tissues suggests that some of the pathology seen may be eosinophil mediated. The fact that both men and women have been affected, just as members of succeeding generations have, is consistent with an autosomal dominant form of inheritance with incomplete penetrance.

The most effective management for this condition is long-term therapy with a penicillinase-resistant penicillin or cephalosporin, with the addition of other antibiotics or antifungal agents as required for specific infections, and appropriate thoracic surgery for superinfected pneumatoceles or those persisting beyond 6 months. Interferon-γ therapy has been tried but had no clinical benefit, and neither did bone marrow transplantation. If the diagnosis is made early and antistaphylococcal antibiotic therapy is rendered in treatment doses continuously, the prognosis is good. Three patients are known to have died of lymphoreticular malignancy, and three experienced cryptococcal meningitis.

CONCLUSION

Since the discovery of X-linked agammaglobulinemia more than five decades ago, more than 200 genetically determined immunodeficiencies have been identified, and the list is rapidly growing. Recent research has led to major breakthroughs in the definition of the molecular bases of a large number of these disorders, and, undoubtedly, this will soon be the case for many others. This information will obviously be of great value in clarifying variant forms of these diseases, in carrier detection, in prenatal diagnosis, and, it is hoped, eventually in permitting gene therapy for many of these conditions.

In addition to the knowledge gained about the immune system from studying the clinical and immunologic features of these rare patients, even greater information about the functioning of the immune system should come from the integrated and comparative study of immune abnormalities in patients and those in gene-targeted mutant mice deficient. Moreover, these studies should lead to the design of more specific and effective therapies.

Although treatment of these rare defects has not advanced quite as rapidly as the discovery of new primary immunodeficiency diseases and the fundamental causes of a large number of them, major therapeutic advances have been made over the last three decades. These include (a) the development of safe intravenous forms of human immunoglobulin that make it possible to deliver high quantities of missing antibodies to antibody-deficient patients, (b) the development of T cell depletion techniques that permit the use of half-matched parents as donors of corrective stem cells for human infants with SCID, and (c) the recent success in achieving successful gene therapy in both X-linked and ADA-deficient SCID. The creation of human chimeras by nonablative allogeneic bone marrow stem cell transplantation has also made it possible to study early human T, B, and NK cell ontogeny, tolerance induction, and MHC restriction mechanisms (i.e., "thymic education") in a manner heretofore not possible. In the next few years, humans with genetically determined immunodeficiency diseases, as well as artificially created immunodeficient animals, will undoubtedly provide many more insights into the normal workings of the immune system.

REFERENCES

1. Glanzmann E, Riniker P. Essentielle lymphocytophtose. Ein neues krankeitsbild aus der Sauglingspathologie. *Ann Paediat*. 1950;174:1–5.
2. Bruton OC. Agammaglobulinemia. *Pediatrics*. 1952;9:722–728.
3. Geha RS, Notarangelo LD, Casanova JL, et al. Primary immunodeficiency diseases: an update from the International Union of Immunological Societies Primary Immunodeficiency Diseases Classification Committee. *J Allergy Clin Immunol.* 2007;120:776–794.
4. Ochs HD, Smith CIE, Puck JM. *Primary immunodeficiency diseases: a molecular and genetic approach*, 2nd ed. Oxford: Oxford University Press, 2007.
5. Elenitoba-Johnson KSJ, Jaffe ES. Lymphoproliferative disorders associated with congenital immunodeficiencies. *Semin Diag Pathol.* 1997;14:35–47.
6. Clark JA, Callicoat PA, Brenner NA. Selective IgA deficiency in blood donors. *Am J Clin Pathol.* 1983;80:210–213.
7. Buckley RH. Clinical and immunologic features of selective IgA deficiency. In: Bergsma D, Good RA, Finstad J, et al., eds. *Immunodeficiency in man and animals*. Stamford, CT: Sinauer Associates, 1975:134–142.
8. Tsukada S, Saffran DC, Rawlings DJ, et al. Deficient expression of a B cell cytoplasmic tyrosine kinase in human X-linked agammaglobulinemia. *Cell*. 1993;72:279–290.
9. Vetrie D, Vorechovsky I, Sideras P, et al. The gene involved in X-linked agammaglobulinaemia is a member of the src family of protein-tyrosine kinases. *Nature*. 1993;361:226–233.
10. Allen RC, Armitage RJ, Conley ME, et al. CD40 ligand gene defects responsible for X-linked hyper IgM syndrome. *Science*. 1993;259: 990–993.
11. Disanto JP, Bonnefoy JY, Gauchat JF, et al. CD40 ligand mutations in X-linked immunodeficiency with hyper-IgM. *Nature*. 1993; 361(6412):541–543.
12. Derry JMJ, Ochs HD, Francke U. Isolation of a novel gene mutated in Wiskott-Aldrich syndrome. *Cell*. 1994;78:635; Erratum, *Cell*. 1994;79:922a].
13. Ochs HD, Thrasher AJ. The Wiskott-Aldrich syndrome. *J Allergy Clin Immunol*. 2006;117(4):725–738.
14. Noguchi M, Yi H, Rosenblatt HM, et al. Interleukin-2 receptor gamma chain mutation results in X-linked severe combined immunodeficiency in humans. *Cell*. 1993;73:147–157.
15. Puck JM, Deschenes SM, Porter JC, et al. The interleukin-2 receptor gamma chain maps to Xq13.1 and is mutated in X-linked severe combined immunodeficiency, SCIDX1. *Hum Mol Genet*. 1993;2:1099–1104.
16. Sayos J, Wu C, Morra M, et al. The X-linked lymphoproliferative-disease gene product SAP regulates signals induced through the co-receptor SLAM. *Nature*. 1998;395(6701):462–469.
17. Nichols KE, Harkin DP, Levitz S, et al. Inactivating mutations in an SH2 domain-encoding gene in X-linked lymphoproliferative syndrome. *Proc Natl Acad Sci U S A*. 1998;95(23):13765–13770.
18. Bennett CL, Christie J, Ramsdell F, et al. The immune dysregulation, polyendocrinopathy, enteropathy, X-linked syndrome (IPEX) is caused by mutations of FOXP3. *Nat Genet*. 2001;27(1):20–21.
19. Doffinger R, Smahi A, Bessia C, et al. X-linked anhidrotic ectodermal dysplasia with immunodeficiency is caused by impaired NF-kappaB signaling. *Nat Genet*. 2001;27(3):277–285.

20. Jain A, Ma CA, Liu S, et al. Specific missense mutations in NEMO result in hyper-IgM syndrome with hypohydrotic ectodermal dysplasia. *Nat Immunol*. 2001;2(3):223–228.
21. Dinauer MC, Orkin SH, Brown R. The glycoprotein encoded by the X-linked chronic granulomatous disease locus is a component of the neutrophil cytochrome b complex. *Nature*. 1987;327:717.
22. Westberg J, Fredrikson GN, Truedsson L, et al. Sequence-based analysis of properdin deficiency: identification of point mutations in two phenotypic forms of an X-linked immunodeficiency. *Genomics*. 1995;29:1–8.
23. Candotti F, Fischer A. Gene therapy. In: Ochs HD, Smith CIE, Puck JM, eds. *Primary immunodeficiency diseases: a molecular and genetic approach*. Oxford: Oxford University Press, 2007:688–705.
24. Buckley RH. Variable phenotypic expression of mutations in genes of the immune system. *J Clin Invest*. 2005;115(11):2974–2976.
25. Winkelstein JA, Marino MC, Lederman HM, et al. X-linked agammaglobulinemia: report on a United States registry of 201 patients. *Medicine* (Baltimore). 2006;85(4):193.
26. Buckley RH, Rowlands DR. Allergy rounds: agammaglobulinemia, neutropenia, fever and abdominal pain. *J Allergy Clin Immunol*. 1973;51:308–318.
27. Wilfert CM, Buckley RH, Mohanakumar T, et al. Persistent and fatal central nervous system echovirus infections in patients with agammaglobulinemia. *N Engl J Med*. 1977;296:1485–1489.
28. Kitanaka A, Mano H, Conley ME, et al. Expression and activation of the nonreceptor tyrosine kinase Tec in human B cells. *Blood*. 1998;91(3):940–948.
29. Smith CIE, Satterthwaite AB, Witte ON. X-linked agammaglobulinemia: a disease of Btk tyrosine kinase. In: Ochs HD, Smith CIE, Puck JM, eds. *Primary immunodeficiency diseases: a molecular and genetic approach*. Oxford: Oxford University Press, 2007:279–303.
30. Conley ME, Burks AW, Herrod HG, et al. Molecular analysis of X-linked agammaglobulinemia with growth hormone deficiency. *J Pediatr*. 1991;119:392–397.
31. Richter D, Conley ME, Rohrer J, et al. A contiguous deletion syndrome of X-linked agammaglobulinemia and sensorineural deafness. *Pediatr Allergy Immunol*. 2001;12(2):107–111.
32. Scher I. The CBA/N mouse strain: an experimental model illustrating the influence of X-chromosome on immunity. *Adv Immunol*. 1982;33:1.
33. Lindvall JM, Blomberg KE, Valiaho J, et al. Bruton's tyrosine kinase: cell biology, sequence conservation, mutation spectrum, siRNA modifications, and expression profiling. *Immunol Rev*. 2005;203:200–215.
34. Yel L, Minegishi Y, Coustan-Smith E, et al. Mutations in the mu heavy chain gene in patients with agammaglobulinemia. *N Engl J Med*. 1996;335:1486–1493.
35. Minegishi Y, Coustan-Smith E, Wang YH, et al. Mutations in the human lambda 5/14.1 gene result in B cell deficiency and agammaglobulinemia. *J Exp Med*. 1998;187:71–77.
36. Minegishi Y, Coustan-Smith E, Rapalus L, et al. Mutations in Igalpha (CD79a) result in a complete block in B-cell development. *J Clin Invest*. 1999;104(8):1115–1121.
37. Minegishi Y, Rohrer J, Coustan-Smith E, et al. An essential role for BLNK in human B cell development. *Science*. 1999;286(5446):1954–1957.
38. Lefranc MP, Hammarstrom L, Smith CIE, et al. Gene deletions in the human immunoglobulin heavy chain constant region locus: molecular and immunological analysis. *Immunol Rev*. 1991;2:265–281.
39. Notarangelo LD, Lanzi G, Peron S, et al. Defects of class-switch recombination. *J Allergy Clin Immunol*. 2006;117(4):855–864.
40. Winkelstein JA, Marino MC, Ochs H, et al. The X-linked hyper-IgM syndrome: clinical and immunologic features of 79 patients. *Medicine* (Baltimore) 2003;82(6):373–384.
41. Durandy A, Revy P, Fischer A. Autosomal hyper-IgM syndromes caused by an intrinsic B cell defect. In: Ochs HD, Smith CIE, Puck JM, eds. *Primary immunodeficiency diseases: a molecular and genetic approach*. Oxford: Oxford University Press, 2007:269–278.
42. Levy J, Espanol-Boren T, Thomas C, et al. Clinical spectrum of X-linked hyper IgM syndrome. *J Pediatr*. 1997;131:47–54.
43. Mayer L, Swan SP, Thompson C. Evidence for a defect in "switch" T cells in patients with immunodeficiency and hyperimmunoglobulinemia M. *N Engl J Med*. 1986;314:409–413.
44. Korthauer U, Graf D, Mages HW. Defective expression of T cell CD40 ligand causes X-linked immunodeficiency with hyper IgM. *Nature*. 1993;361:539–541.
45. Di Santo JP, Bonnefoy JY, Gauchat JF, et al. CD40 ligand mutations in X-linked immunodeficiency with hyper IgM. *Nature*. 1993;361:541–543.
46. Aruffo A, Farrington M, Hollenbaugh D, et al. The CD40 ligand, gp39, is defective in activated T cells from patients with X-linked hyper IgM syndrome. *Cell*. 1993;72:291–300.
47. Noelle RJ, Roy M, Shepherd DM, et al. A 39-kDa protein on activated helper T cells binds CD40 and transduces the signal for cognate activation of B cells. *Proc Natl Acad Sci U S A*. 1992;89:6550–6554.
48. Agematsu K, Nagumo H, Shinozaki K, et al. Absence of IgD-CD27(+) memory B cell population in X-linked hyper-IgM syndrome. *J Clin Invest*. 1998;102(4):853–860.
49. Yang Y, Wilson JM. CD40 ligand-dependent T cell activation: requirement of B7-CD28 signaling through CD40. *Science*. 1996;273:1862–1864.
50. Buckley RH, Fischer A. Bone marrow transplantation for primary immunodeficiency diseases. In: Ochs HD, Smith CIE, Puck JM, eds. *Primary immunodeficiency diseases: a molecular and genetic approach*. Oxford: Oxford University Press, 2007:669–687.
51. Orange JS, Hossny EM, Weiler CR, et al. Use of intravenous immunoglobulin in human disease: a review of evidence by members of the Primary Immunodeficiency Committee of the American Academy of Allergy, Asthma and Immunology. *J Allergy Clin Immunol*. 2006;117(4 Suppl):S525–S553.
52. Srahna M, Remacle JE, Annamalai K, et al. NF-kappaB is involved in the regulation of CD154 (CD40 ligand) expression in primary human T cells. *Clin Exp Immunol*. 2001;125(2):229–236.
53. Puel A, Reichenbach J, Bustamante J, et al. The NEMO mutation creating the most-upstream premature stop codon is hypomorphic because of a reinitiation of translation. *Am J Hum Genet*. 2006;78(4):691–701.
54. Oliva A, Quinti I, Scala E, et al. Immunodeficiency with hyperimmunoglobulinemia M in two female patients is not associated with abnormalities of CD40 or CD40 ligand expression. *J Allergy Clin Immunol*. 1995;96:403–410.
55. Minegishi Y, Lavoie A, Cunningham-Rundles C, et al. Mutations in activation-induced cytidine deaminase in patients with hyper IgM syndrome. *Clin Immunol*. 2000;97(3):203–210.
56. Revy P, Muto T, Levy Y, et al. Activation-induced cytidine deaminase (AID) deficiency causes the autosomal recessive form of the Hyper-IgM syndrome (HIGM2). *Cell*. 2000;102:565–575.
57. Imai K, Catalan N, Plebani A, et al. Hyper-IgM syndrome type 4 with a B lymphocyte-intrinsic selective deficiency in Ig class-switch recombination. *J Clin Invest*. 2003;112(1):136–142.
58. Ferrari S, Giliani S, Insalaco A, et al. Mutations of CD40 gene cause an autosomal recessive form of immunodeficiency with hyper IgM. *Proc Natl Acad Sci U S A*. 2001;98(22):12614–12619.
59. Morra M, Howie D, Grande MS, et al. X-linked lymphoproliferative disease: a progressive immunodeficiency. *Annu Rev Immunol*. 2001;19:657–682.
60. Schuster V, Terhorst C. X-linked lymphoproliferative disease due to defects of *SH2D1A*. In: Ochs HD, Smith CIE, Puck JM, eds. *Primary immunodeficiency diseases: a molecular and genetic approach*. Oxford: Oxford University Press, 2007:470–484.
61. Tangye SG, Phillips JH, Lanier LL, et al. Functional requirement for SAP in 2B4-mediated activation of human natural killer cells as revealed by the X-linked lymphoproliferative syndrome. *J Immunol*. 2000;165(6):2932–2936.
62. Coffey AJ, Brooksbank RA, Brandau O, et al. Host response to EBV infection in X-linked lymphoproliferative disease results from mutations in an SH2-domain encoding gene. *Nat Genet*. 1998;20(2):129–135.
63. Morra M, Silander O, Calpe-Flores S, et al. Alterations of the X-linked lymphoproliferative disease gene *SH2DIA* in common variable immunodeficiency syndrome. *Blood*. 2001;98(5):1321–1325.
64. Kanegane H, Ito Y, Ohshima K, et al. X-linked lymphoproliferative syndrome presenting with systemic lymphocytic vasculitis. *Am J Hematol*. 2005;78(2):130–133.

65. Hammarstrom L, Smith CIE. Genetic approach to common variable immunodeficiency and IgA deficiency. In: Ochs HD, Smith CIE, Puck JM, eds. *Primary immunodeficiency diseases: a molecular and genetic approach*. Oxford: Oxford University Press, 2007:313–325.
66. Cunningham-Rundles C, Cooper DL, Duffy TP, et al. Lymphomas of mucosal-associated lymphoid tissue in common variable immunodeficiency. *Am J Hematol*. 2002;69(3):171–178.
67. Punnonen J, Kainulainen L, Ruuskanen O, et al. IL-4 synergizes with IL-10 and anti-CD40 MoAbs to induce B cell differentiation in patients with common variable immunodeficiency. *Scand J Immunol*. 1997;45:203–212.
68. Baum CG, Chiorazzi N, Frankel S, et al. Conversion of systemic lupus erythematosus to common variable hypogammaglobulinemia. *Am J Med*. 1989;87:449–456.
69. Wright JJ, Birx DL, Wagner DK, et al. Normalization of antibody responsiveness in a patient with common variable hypogammaglobulinemia and HIV infection. *N Engl J Med*. 1987;317:1516–1519.
70. Ashman RF, Schaffer FM, Kemp JD, et al. Genetic and immunologic analysis of a family containing five patients with common variable immune deficiency or selective IgA deficiency. *J Clin Immunol*. 1992;12:406–414.
71. Schroeder HW, Zhu Z, March RE, et al. Susceptibility locus for IgA deficiency and common variable immunodeficiency in the HLA-DR3, -B8, -A1 haplotypes. *Mol Med*. 1998;4:72–86.
72. Grimbacher B, Hutloff A, Schlesier M, et al. Homozygous loss of ICOS is associated with adult-onset common variable immunodeficiency. *Nat Immunol*. 2003;4(3):261–268.
73. van Zelm MC, Reisli I, van der BM, et al. An antibody-deficiency syndrome due to mutations in the CD19 gene. *N Engl J Med*. 2006;354(18):1901–1912.
74. Salzer U, Chapel HM, Webster AD, et al. Mutations in TNFRSF13B encoding TACI are associated with common variable immunodeficiency in humans. *Nat Genet*. 2005;37(8):820–828.
75. Castigli E, Wilson SA, Garibyan L, et al. TACI is mutant in common variable immunodeficiency and IgA deficiency. *Nat Genet*. 2005;37(8):829–834.
76. Burks AW, Sampson HA, Buckley RH. Anaphylactic reactions after gamma globulin administration in patients with hypogammaglobulinemia. *N Engl J Med*. 1986;314:560–564.
77. Buckley RH, Dees SC. The correlation of milk precipitins with IgA deficiency. *N Engl J Med*. 1969;281:465–469.
78. Leickly FE, Buckley RH. Development of IgA and IgG2 subclass deficiency after sulfasalazine therapy. *J Pediatr*. 1986;108: 481–482.
79. Sandler SG, Trimble J, Mallory DM. Coexistent IgG2 and IgA deficiencies in blood donors. *Transfusion*. 1996;36:256–258.
80. Ambrosino DM, Umetsu DT, Siber GR, et al. Selective defect in the antibody response to *Haemophilus influenzae* type b in children with recurrent infections and normal IgG subclass levels. *J Allergy Clin Immunol*. 1988;81:1175–1179.
81. Shackelford PG, Granoff DM, Polmar SH, et al. Subnormal serum concentrations of IgG2 in children with frequent infections associated with varied patters of immunologic dysfunction. *J Pediatr*. 1990;116:529–538.
82. Driscoll DA, Sullivan KE. DiGeorge syndrome: a chromosome 22q11.2 deletion syndrome. In: Ochs HD, Smith CIE, Puck JM, eds. *Primary immunodeficiency diseases: a molecular and genetic approach*. Oxford: Oxford University Press, 2007:485–495.
83. Junker AK, Driscoll DA. Humoral immunity in DiGeorge syndrome. *J Pediatr*. 1995;127:231–237.
84. Demczuk S, Levy A, Aubry M, et al. Excess of deletions of maternal origin in the DiGeorge/velo-cardio-facial syndromes. A study of 22 new patients and review of the literature. *Hum Genet*. 1995;96(1): 9–13.
85. Daw SC, Taylor C, Kraman M, et al. A common region of 10p deleted in DiGeorge and velocardiofacial syndromes. *Nat Genet*. 1996;13:458–460.
86. Markert ML, Sarzotti M, Ozaki DA, et al. Thymus transplantation in complete DiGeorge syndrome: immunologic and safety evaluations in 12 patients. *Blood*. 2003;102(3):1121–1130.
87. Buckley RH, Schiff RI, Schiff SE, et al. Human severe combined immunodeficiency (SCID): Genetic, phenotypic and functional diversity in 108 infants. *J Pediatr*. 1997;130:378–387.
88. Buckley RH. Molecular defects in human severe combined immunodeficiency and approaches to immune reconstitution. *Annu Rev Immunol*. 2004;22:625–655.
89. Buckley RH. Primary immunodeficiency diseases due to defects in lymphocytes. *N Engl J Med*. 2000;343:1313–1324.
90. Buckley RH. Primary cellular immunodeficiencies. *J Allergy Clin Immunol*. 2002;109(5):747–757.
91. Buckley RH, Schiff SE, Schiff RI, et al. Hematopoietic stem cell transplantation for the treatment of severe combined immunodeficiency. *N Engl J Med*. 1999;340:508–516.
92. Myers LA, Patel DD, Puck JM, et al. Hematopoietic stem cell transplantation for severe combined immunodeficiency in the neonatal period leads to superior thymic output and improved survival. *Blood*. 2002;99(3):872–878.
93. Buckley RH. Molecular defects in human severe combined immunodeficiency and approaches to immune reconstitution. *Ann Rev Immunol*. 2004;55:625–656.
94. Altman PL. Blood leukocyte values: man. In: Dittmer DS, ed. *Blood and other body fluids*. Washington, DC: Federation of American Societies for Experimental Biology, 1961:125–126.
95. Patel DD, Gooding ME, Parrott RE, et al. Thymic function after hematopoietic stem-cell transplantation for the treatment of severe combined immunodeficiency. *N Engl J Med*. 2000;342(18):1325–1332.
96. Buckley RH. The multiple causes of human SCID. *J Clin Invest*. 2004;114(10):1409–1411.
97. Vosshenrich CA, Di Santo JP. Cytokines: IL-21 joins the gamma(c)-dependent network? *Curr Biol*. 2001;11(5):R175–R177.
98. Puck JM, Pepper AE, Henthorn PS, et al. Mutation analysis of IL2RG in human X-linked severe combined immunodeficiency. *Blood*. 1997;89:1968–1977.
99. Russell SM, Keegan AD, Harada N, et al. Interleukin-2 receptor gamma chain: a functional component of the interleukin-4 receptor. *Science*. 1993;262:1880–1883.
100. Noguchi M, Nakamura Y, Russell SM, et al. Interleukin-2 receptor gamma chain: a functional component of the interleukin-7 receptor. *Science*. 1993;262:1977–1880.
101. Hirschhorn R, Candotti F. Immunodeficiency due to defects of purine metabolism. In: Ochs HD, Smith CIE, Puck JM, eds. *Primary immunodeficiency diseases: a molecular and genetic approach*. Oxford: Oxford University Press, 2007:169–196.
102. Hershfield MS, Buckley RH, Greenberg ML, et al. Treatment of adenosine deaminase deficiency with polyethylene glycol-modified adenosine deaminase (PEG-ADA). *N Engl J Med*. 1987;316:589–596.
103. Chan B, Wara D, Bastian J, et al. Long-term efficacy of enzyme replacement therapy for adenosine deaminase (ADA)-deficient severe combined immunodeficiency (SCID). *Clin Immunol*. 2005;117(2):133–143.
104. Roberts JL, Lengi A, Brown SM, et al. Janus Kinase 3 (JAK3) deficiency: clinical, immunologic and molecular analyses of 10 patients and outcomes of stem cell transplantation. *Blood*. 2004;103:209–218.
105. Candotti F, Notarangelo LD. Autosomal recessive severe combined immunodeficiency due to defects in cytokine signalling pathways. In: Ochs HD, Smith CIE, Puck JM, eds. *Primary immunodeficiency diseases: a molecular and genetic approach*. Oxford: Oxford University Press, 2007:137–152.
106. Russell SM, Tayebi N, Nakajima H, et al. Mutation of Jak3 in a patient with SCID: essential role of Jak3 in lymphoid development. *Science*. 1995;270:797–800.
107. Puel A, Ziegler SF, Buckley RH, et al. Defective IL7R expression in T(−)B(+)NK(+) severe combined immunodeficiency. *Nat Genet*. 1998;20(4):394–397.
108. Schwarz K, Gauss GH, Ludwig L, et al. RAG mutations in human B cell-negative SCID. *Science*. 1996;274:97–99.
109. Corneo B, Moshous D, Gungor T, et al. Identical mutations in RAG1 or RAG2 genes leading to defective V(D)J recombinase activity can cause either T-B-severe combined immune deficiency or Omenn syndrome. *Blood*. 2001;97(9):2772–2776.
110. de Villartay J-P, Schwarz K, Villa A. V(D)J recombination defects. In: Ochs HD, Smith CIE, Puck JM, eds. *Primary immunodeficiency diseases: a molecular and genetic approach*. Oxford: Oxford University Press, 2007:153–168.

111. Rieux-Laucat F, Bahadoran P, Brousse N, et al. Highly restricted human T cell repertoire in peripheral blood and tissue-infiltrating lymphocytes in Omenn's syndrome. *J Clin Invest*. 1998;102(2):312–321.
112. Moshous D, Callebaut I, de Chasseval R, et al. Artemis, a novel DNA double-strand break repair/V(D)J recombination protein, is mutated in human severe combined immune deficiency. *Cell*. 2001;105(2):177–186.
113. van der Burg M, van Veelen LR, Verkaik NS, et al. A new type of radiosensitive T-B-NK$^+$ severe combined immunodeficiency caused by a LIG4 mutation. *J Clin Invest*. 2006;116(1):137–145.
114. Enders A, Fisch P, Schwarz K, et al. A severe form of human combined immunodeficiency due to mutations in DNA ligase IV. *J Immunol*. 2006;176(8):5060–5068.
115. Buck D, Moshous D, de Chasseval R, et al. Severe combined immunodeficiency and microcephaly in siblings with hypomorphic mutations in DNA ligase IV. *Eur J Immunol*. 2006;36(1):224–235.
116. Kung C, Pingel JT, Heikinheimo M, et al. Mutations in the tyrosine phosphatase CD45 gene in a child with severe combined immunodeficiency disease. *Nat Med*. 2000;6(3):343–345.
117. Tchilian EZ, Wallace DL, Wells RS, et al. A deletion in the gene encoding the CD45 antigen in a patient with SCID. *J Immunol*. 2001;166(2):1308–1313.
118. Dadi HK, Simon AJ, Roifman CM. Effect of CD3delta deficiency on maturation of alpha/beta and gamma/delta T-cell lineages in severe combined immunodeficiency. *N Engl J Med*. 2003;349(19):1821–1828.
119. de Saint Basile G, Geissmann F, Flori E, et al. Severe combined immunodeficiency caused by deficiency in either the delta or the epsilon subunit of CD3. *J Clin Invest*. 2004;114(10):1512–1517.
120. Roberts JL, Lauritsen JHP, Cooney M, et al. T$^-$B$^+$NK$^+$ severe combined immunodeficiency caused by complete deficiency of the CD3 zeta subunit of the T cell antigen receptor complex. *Blood*. 2007;109(8):3198.
121. Soudais C, De Villartay JP, Le Deist F, et al. Independent mutations of the human CD3-epsilon gene resulting in a T cell receptor/CD3 complex immunodeficiency. *Nat Genet*. 1993;3(1):77–81.
122. Arnaiz-Villena A, Timon M, Rodriguez-Gallego C, et al. T lymphocyte signalling defects and immunodeficiency due to the lack of CD3 gamma. *Immunodeficiency*. 1993;4(1–4):121–129.
123. Hacein-Bey-Abina S, Le Deist F, Carlier F, et al. Sustained correction of X-linked severe combined immunodeficiency by ex vivo gene therapy. *N Engl J Med*. 2002;346(16):1185–1193.
124. Hacein-Bey-Abina S, Von Kalle C, Schmidt M, et al. A serious adverse event after successful gene therapy for X-linked severe combined immunodeficiency. *N Engl J Med*. 2003;348(3):255–256.
125. Aiuti A, Slavin S, Aker M, et al. Correction of ADA-SCID by stem cell gene therapy combined with nonmyeloablative conditioning. *Science*. 2002;296(5577):2410–2413.
126. Markert ML. Purine nucleoside phosphorylase deficiency. *Immunodef Rev*. 1991;3:45–81.
127. Broome CB, Graham ML, Saulsbury FT, et al. Correction of purine nucleoside phosphorylase deficiency by transplantation of allogeneic bone marrow from a sibling. *J Pediatr*. 1996;128(3):373–376.
128. Myers LA, Hershfield MS, Neale WT, et al. Purine nucleoside phosphorylase deficiency (PNP-def) presenting with lymphopenia and developmental delay: successful correction with umbilical cord blood transplantation. *J Pediatr*. 2004;145(5):710–712.
129. Chun HH, Gatti RA. Ataxia-telangiectasia, an evolving phenotype. *DNA Repair* (Amsterdam). 2004;3(8–9):1187–1196.
130. Lavin MF, Shiloh Y. Ataxia-telangiectasia. In: Ochs HD, Smith CIE, Puck JM, eds. *Primary immunodeficiency diseases: a molecular and genetic approach*. Oxford: Oxford University Press, 2007:402–426.
131. Nowak-Wegrzyn A, Crawford TO, Winkelstein JA, et al. Immunodeficiency and infections in ataxia-telangiectasia. *J Pediatr*. 2004;144(4):505–511.
132. Savitsky K, Bar-Shira A, Gilad S, et al. A single ataxia telangiectasia gene with a product similar to PI-3 kinase. *Science*. 1995;268:1749–1753.
133. Ochs HD, Rosen FS. Wiskott-Aldrich syndrome. In: Ochs HD, Smith CIE, Puck JM, eds. *Primary immunodeficiency diseases: a molecular and genetic approach*. Oxford: Oxford University Press, 2007:454–469.
134. Haddad E, Zugaza JL, Louache F, et al. The interaction between Cdc42 and WASP is required for SDF-1-induced T- lymphocyte chemotaxis. *Blood*. 2001;97(1):33–38.
135. Jin Y, Mazza C, Christie JR, et al. Mutations of the Wiskott-Aldrich syndrome protein (WASP): hotspots, effect on transcription, and translation and phenotype/genotype correlation. *Blood*. 2004;104(13):4010–4019.
136. Sabri S, Foudi A, Boukour S, et al. Deficiency in the Wiskott-Aldrich protein induces premature proplatelet formation and platelet production in the bone marrow compartment. *Blood*. 2006;108(1):134–140.
137. Westerberg L, Larsson M, Hardy SJ, et al. Wiskott-Aldrich syndrome protein deficiency leads to reduced B-cell adhesion, migration, and homing, and a delayed humoral immune response. *Blood*. 2005;105(3):1144–1152.
138. Olivier A, Jeanson-Leh L, Bouma G, et al. A partial down-regulation of WASP is sufficient to inhibit podosome formation in dendritic cells. *Mol Ther*. 2006;13(4):729–737.
139. Orange JS, Ramesh N, Remold-O'Donnell E, et al. Wiskott-Aldrich syndrome protein is required for NK cell cytotoxicity and colocalizes with actin to NK cell-activating immunologic synapses. *Proc Natl Acad Sci U S A*. 2002;99(17):11351–11356.
140. Ancliff PJ, Blundell MP, Cory GO, et al. Two novel activating mutations in the Wiskott-Aldrich syndrome protein result in congenital neutropenia. *Blood*. 2006;108(7):2182–2189.
141. Kondoh T, Hayashi K, Matsumoto T, et al. Two sisters with clinical diagnosis of Wiskott-Aldrich syndrome: is the condition in the family autosomal recessive? *Am J Med Genet*. 1995;60:364–369.
142. Rocca B, Bellacosa A, de Cristofaro R, et al. Wiskott-Aldrich syndrome: report of an autosomal dominant variant. *Blood*. 1996;87:4538–4543.
143. Parolini O, Ressmann G, Haas OA, et al. X-linked Wiskott-Aldrich syndrome in a girl. *N Engl J Med*. 1998;338(5):291–295.
144. Filipovich AH, Stone JV, Tomany SC, et al. Impact of donor type on outcome of bone marrow transplantation for Wiskott-Aldrich syndrome: collaborative study of the International Bone Marrow Transplant Registry and the National Marrow Donor Program. *Blood*. 2001;97(6):1598–1603.
145. Mullen CA, Anderson KD, Blaese RM. Splenectomy and/or bone marrow transplantation in the management of the Wiskott-Aldrich syndrome: long-term follow-up of 62 cases. *Blood*. 1993;82:2961–2966.
146. Dewey RA, Avedillo DI, Ballmaier M, et al. Retroviral WASP gene transfer into human hematopoietic stem cells reconstitutes the actin cytoskeleton in myeloid progeny cells differentiated *in vitro*. *Exp Hematol*. 2006;34(9):1161–1169.
147. Boztug K, Dewey RA, Klein C. Development of hematopoietic stem cell gene therapy for Wiskott-Aldrich syndrome. *Curr Opin Mol Ther*. 2006;8(5):390–395.
148. Abinun M, Kaitila I, Casanova J-L. Immunodeficiencies with associated manifestations of skin, hair, teeth and skeleton. In: Ochs HD, Smith CIE, Puck JM, eds. *Primary immunodeficiency diseases: a molecular and genetic approach*. Oxford: Oxford University Press, 2007:513–524.
149. Ridanpaa M, Sistonen P, Rockas S, et al. Worldwide mutation spectrum in cartilage-hair hypoplasia: ancient founder origin of the major70A$\rightarrow$G mutation of the untranslated RMRP. *Eur J Hum Genet*. 2002;10(7):439–447.
150. Weemaes CMR, Smeets DFCM, van der Burgt CJAM. Nijmegen breakage syndrome: a progress report. *Int J Radiat Biol*. 1994;66:S185–S188.
151. Chrzanowska KH, Kleijer WJ, Krajewska-Walasek M, et al. Eleven Polish patients with microcephaly, immunodeficiency, and chromosomal instability: the Nijmegen breakage syndrome. *Am J Med Genet*. 1995;57:462–471.
152. Saar K, Chrzanowska KH, Stumm M, et al. The gene for the ataxia-telangiectasia variant, Nijmegen breakage syndrome, maps to a 1-cM interval on chromosome 8q21. *Am J Hum Genet*. 1997;60:605–610.
153. de la Salle H, Donato L, Hanau D. Peptide transporter defects in human leukocyte antigen class I deficiency. In: Ochs HD, Smith CIE, Puck JM, eds. *Primary immunodeficiency diseases: a molecular and genetic approach*. Oxford: Oxford University Press, 2007:242–250.

154. de la Salle H, Zimmer J, Fricker D, et al. HLA class I deficiencies due to mutations in subunit 1 of the peptide transporter TAP1. *J Clin Invest*. 1999;103(5):R9.
155. Donato L, de la Salle H, Hanau D, et al. Association of HLA class I antigen deficiency related to a TAP2 gene mutation with familial bronchiectasis. *J Pediatr*. 1995;127(6):895–900.
156. Reith W, Lisowska-Grospierre B, Fischer A. Molecular basis of major histocompatibility complex class II deficiency. In: Ochs HD, Smith CIE, Puck JM, eds. *Primary immunodeficiency diseases: a molecular and genetic approach*. Oxford: Oxford University Press, 2007:227–241.
157. Steimle V, Durand B, Barras E, et al. A novel DNA-binding regulatory factor is mutated in primary MHC class II deficiency (bare lymphocyte syndrome). *Genes Dev*. 1995;9(9):1021–1032.
158. Durand B, Sperisen P, Emery P, et al. RFXAP, a novel subunit of the RFX DNA binding complex is mutated in MHC class II deficiency. *EMBO J*. 1997;16(5):1045–1055.
159. Masternak K, Barras E, Zufferey M, et al. A gene encoding a novel RFX-associated transactivator is mutated in the majority of MHC class II deficiency patients. *Nat Genet*. 1998;20(3):273–277.
160. Zhou H, Glimcher LH. Human MHC class II gene transcription directed by the carboxyl terminus of CIITA, one of the defective genes in type II MHC combined immune deficiency. *Immunity*. 1995;2:545–553.
161. Calle-Martin O, Hernandez M, Ordi J, et al. Familial CD8 deficiency due to a mutation in the CD8 alpha gene. *J Clin Invest*. 2001;108(1):117–123.
162. Regueiro JR, Espanol T. CD3 and CD8 deficiencies. In: Ochs HD, Smith CIE, Puck JM, eds. *Primary immunodeficiency diseases: a molecular and genetic approach*. Oxford: Oxford University Press, 2007:216–226.
163. Elder ME. Severe combined immunodeficiency due to defects in T cell receptor-associated protein tyrosine kinases. In: Ochs HD, Smith CIE, Puck JM, eds. *Primary immunodeficiency diseases: a molecular and genetic approach*. Oxford: Oxford University Press, 2007:203–211.
164. Feske S, Muller JM, Graf D, et al. Severe combined immunodeficiency due to defective binding of the nuclear factor of activated T cells in T lymphocytes of two male siblings. *Eur J Immunol*. 1996;26:2119–2126.
165. Feske S, Gwack Y, Prakriya M, et al. A mutation in Orai1 causes immune deficiency by abrogating CRAC channel function. *Nature*. 2006;441(7090):179–185.
166. Negishi I, Motoyama N, Nakayama K, et al. Essential role for ZAP-70 in both positive and negative selection of thymocytes. *Nature*. 1995;376:435–438.
167. Elder ME. Severe combined immunodeficiency due to a defect in the tyrosine kinase ZAP-70. *Pediatr Res*. 1996;39:743–748.
168. Bennett CL, Ochs HD. IPEX is a unique X-linked syndrome characterized by immune dysfunction, polyendocrinopathy, enteropathy, and a variety of autoimmune phenomena. *Curr Opin Pediatr*. 2001;13(6):533–538.
169. Bacchetta R, Passerini L, Gambineri E, et al. Defective regulatory and effector T cell functions in patients with FOXP3 mutations. *J Clin Invest*. 2006;116(6):1713–1722.
170. Aaltonen J, Bjorses P, Prheentupa J, et al. An autoimmune disease, APECED, caused by mutations in a novel gene featuring two PHD-type zinc-finger domains. The Finnish-German APECED Consortium. Autoimmune Polyendocrinopathy-Candidiasis-Ectodermal Dystrophy. *Nat Genet*. 1997;17(4):399–403.
171. Peltonen-Palotie L, Halonen M, Perheentupa J. Autoimmune polyendocrinopathy, candidiasis, ectodermal dystrophy. In: Ochs HD, Smith CIE, Puck JM, eds. *Primary immunodeficiency diseases: a molecular and genetic approach*. Oxford: Oxford University Press, 2007:342–353.
172. Puck JM, Rieux-Laucat F, LeDiest F, et al. Autoimmune lymphoproliferative syndrome. In: Ochs HD, Smith CIE, Puck JM, eds. *Primary immunodeficiency diseases: a molecular and genetic approach*. Oxford: Oxford University Press, 2007:326–341.
173. Worth A, Thrasher AJ, Gaspar HB. Autoimmune lymphoproliferative syndrome: molecular basis of disease and clinical phenotype. *Br J Haematol*. 2006;133(2):124–140.
174. Sharfe N, Dadi HK, Shahar M, et al. Human immune disorder arising from mutation of the alpha chain of the interleukin-2 receptor. *Proc Natl Acad Sci U S A*. 1997;94:3168–3171.
175. Willerford DM, Chem J, Ferry JA, et al. Interleukin-2 receptor α chain regulates the size and content of the peripheral lymphoid compartment. *Immunity*. 1995;3:521–530.
176. Suzuki H, Kundig TM, Furlonger C, et al. Deregulated T cell activation and autoimmunity in mice lacking interleukin-2 receptor β. *Science*. 1995;268:1472–1476.
177. Lenardo MJ. Interleukin-2 programs mouse $\alpha\beta$ T lymphocytes for apoptosis. *Nature*. 1991;353:858–861.
178. Etzioni A, Harlan JM. Cell adhesion and leukocyte adhesion defects. In: Ochs HD, Smith CIE, Puck JM, eds. *Primary immunodeficiency diseases: a molecular and genetic approach*. Oxford: Oxford University Press, 2007:550–564.
179. Sturla L, Puglielli L, Tonetti M, et al. Impairment of the Golgi GDP-L-fucose transport and unresponsiveness to fucose replacement therapy in LAD II patients. *Pediatr Res*. 2001;49(4): 537–542.
180. Lubke T, Marquardt T, Etzioni A, et al. Complementation cloning identifies CDG-IIc, a new type of congenital disorders of glycosylation, as a GDP-fucose transporter deficiency. *Nat Genet*. 2001;28(1):73–76.
181. Jouanguy E, Altare F, Lamhamedi S, et al. Interferon-gamma-receptor deficiency in an infant with fatal bacille Calmette-Guerin infection. *N Engl J Med*. 1996;335:1956–1961.
182. Newport MJ, Huxley CM, Huston S, et al. A mutation in the interferon-gamma-receptor gene and susceptibility to mycobacterial infection. *N Engl J Med*. 1996;335:1941–1949.
183. Dorman SE, Holland SM. Interferon-gamma and interleukin-12 pathway defects and human disease. *Cytokine Growth Factor Rev*. 2000;11(4):321–333.
184. Newport MJ, Holland SM, Levin M, et al. Inherited disorders of the interleukin-12/23-interferon gamma axis. In: Ochs HD, Smith CIE, Puck JM, e eds. *Primary immunodeficiency diseases: a molecular and genetic approach*. Oxford: Oxford University Press, 2007: 390–401.
185. Altare F, Lammas D, Revy P, et al. Inherited interleukin 12 deficiency in a child with bacille Calmette-Guerin and *Salmonella enteritidis* disseminated infection. *J Clin Invest*. 1998;102(12):2035–2040.
186. Altare F, Durandy A, Lammas D, et al. Impairment of mycobacterial immunity in human interleukin-12 receptor deficiency. *Science*. 1998;280:1432–1435.
187. de Jong R, Altare F, Haagen I, et al. Severe mycobacterial and *Salmonella* infections in interleukin-12 receptor-deficient patients. *Science*. 1998;280:1435–1438.
188. Dupuis S, Dargemont C, Fieschi C, et al. Impairment of mycobacterial but not viral immunity by a germline human STAT1 mutation. *Science*. 2001;293(5528):300–303.
189. Dupuis S, Jouanguy E, Al Hajjar S, et al. Impaired response to interferon-alpha/beta and lethal viral disease in human STAT1 deficiency. *Nat Genet*. 2003;33(3):388–391.
190. Ku CL, Yang K, Bustamante J, et al. Inherited disorders of human Toll-like receptor signaling: immunological implications. *Immunol Rev*. 2005;203:10–20.
191. Spritz RA. Chediak-Higashi syndrome. In: Ochs HD, Smith CIE, Puck JM, eds. *Primary immunodeficiency diseases: a molecular and genetic approach*. Oxford: Oxford University Press, 2007:570–588.
192. Nagle DL, Karim MA, Woolf EA, et al. Identification and mutation analysis of the complete gene for Chediak-Higashi syndrome. *Nat Genet*. 1996;14:307–311.
193. Certain S, Barrat F, Pastural E, et al. Protein truncation test of LYST reveals heterogenous mutations in patients with Chediak-Higashi syndrome. *Blood*. 2000;95(3):979–983.
194. Aslan Y, Erduran E, Gedik Y, et al. The role of high dose methylprednisolone and splenectomy in the accelerated phase of Chediak-Higashi syndrome. *Acta Haematol*. 1996;96:105–107.
195. Haddad E, Le Deist F, Blanche S, et al. Treatment of Chediak-Higashi syndrome by allogenic bone marrow transplantation: report of 10 cases. *Blood*. 1995;85:3328–3333.
196. Buckley RH, Wray BB, Belmaker EZ. Extreme hyperimmunoglobulinemia E and undue susceptibility to infection. *Pediatrics*. 1972;49:59–70.

197. Buckley RH. The hyper-IgE syndrome. *Clin Rev Allergy Immunol.* 2001;20(1):139–154.
198. Grimbacher B, Holland SM, Gallin JI, et al. Hyper-IgE syndrome with recurrent infections–an autosomal dominant multisystem disorder. *N Engl J Med.* 1999;340(9):692–702.
199. Buckley RH. The hyper-IgE syndrome. *Clin Rev Allergy Immunol.* 2001;20(1):139–154.
200. Minegishi Y, Saito M, Tsuchiya S, et al. Dominant-negative mutations in the DNA-binding domain of STAT3 cause hyper-IgE syndrome. *Nature.* 2007;448(7157):1058–62.
201. Holland SM, Deleo FR, Elloumi HZ, et al. STAT3 mutations in the hyper-IgE syndrome. *N Engl J Med.* 2007;357:1608–19.
202. Claassen JL, Levine AD, Schiff SE, et al. Mononuclear cells from patients with the hyper IgE syndrome produce little IgE when stimulated with recombinant interleukin 4 *in vitro*. *J Allergy Clin Immunol*. 1991;88:713–721.

INDEX

Note: Page numbers followed by *f* indicate figures; page numbers followed by *t* indicate tables.

E

H

J

K

M

O

Q

R

S